FERRI'S
CLINICAL
ADVISOR

FERRI'S

CLINICAL ADVISOR

Instant Diagnosis and Treatment

FRED F. FERRI, M.D., F.A.C.P.

Clinical Professor
Department of Community Health
Brown University School of Medicine
Chief, Division of Internal Medicine
St. Joseph's Health Services and Fatima Hospital
Providence, Rhode Island

2003 EDITION

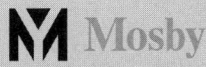 Mosby

An Imprint of Elsevier Science
St. Louis London Philadelphia Sydney Toronto

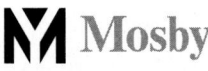

Mosby

An Imprint of Elsevier Science

11830 Westline Industrial Drive
St. Louis, Missouri 63146

NOTICE

Pharmacology is an ever-changing field. Standard safety precautions must be followed, but as
new research and clinical experience broaden our knowledge, changes in treatment and drug
therapy may become necessary or appropriate. Readers are advised to check the most current
product information provided by the manufacturer of each drug to be administered to verify
the recommended dose, the method and duration of administration, and contraindications.
It is the responsibility of the licensed prescriber, relying on experience and knowledge of the
patient, to determine dosages and the best treatment for each individual patient. Neither the
publisher nor the editor assumes any liability for any injury and/or damage to persons or
property arising from this publication.

Previous editions copyrighted 1999, 2000, 2001, 2002.

International Standard Book Number 0-323-01303-1
International Standard Book Number 0-323-01304-X (Package)

Acquisitions Editors: Steven Merahn, Quincy McDonald
Developmental Editor: Kristen Mandava
Publishing Services Manager: Patricia Tannian
Senior Project Manager: Suzanne C. Fannin
Book Design Manager: Gail Morey Hudson
Cover Design: Teresa Breckwoldt

GW/MVB

Printed in the United States of America

Last digit is the print number: 9   8   7   6   5   4   3   2   1

Section Editors

GEORGE T. DANAKAS, M.D., F.A.C.O.G.
Clinical Assistant Professor
Department of Obstetrics and Gynecology
State University of New York at Buffalo
Buffalo, New York
Section I

MARK J. FAGAN, M.D.
Director, Medical Primary Care Unit
Rhode Island Hospital
Associate Professor of Medicine
Brown University School of Medicine
Providence, Rhode Island
Section I

FRED F. FERRI, M.D., F.A.C.P.
Clinical Professor
Department of Community Health
Brown University School of Medicine
Chief, Division of Internal Medicine
St. Joseph's Health Services and Fatima Hospital
Providence, Rhode Island
Sections I-V

JOSEPH R. MASCI, M.D.
Chief of Infectious Diseases
Associate Director of Medicine
Elmhurst Hospital Center Associate Professor of Medicine
Mount Sinai School of Medicine
Elmhurst, New York
Section I

LONNIE R. MERCIER, M.D.
Clinical Instructor
Department of Orthopedic Surgery
Creighton University School of Medicine
Omaha, Nebraska
Section I

WILLIAM H. OLSON, M.D.
Professor, Department of Neurology
University of Louisville School of Medicine
Louisville, Kentucky
Section I

PETER PETROPOULOS, M.D., F.A.C.C.
Clinical Assistant Professor
Brown University School of Medicine
Department of Veterans Affairs
Providence, Rhode Island
Section I

TOM J. WACHTEL, M.D.
Physician-in-Charge, Division of Geriatrics
Rhode Island Hospital
Professor of Community Health and Medicine
Brown University School of Medicine
Providence, Rhode Island
Section I

Contributors

PHILLIP J. ALIOTTA, M.D., M.S.H.A., F.A.C.S.
Clinical Instructor
Department of Urology
School of Medicine and Biomedical Sciences
State University of New York at Buffalo
Buffalo, New York
Medical Director
Center for Urologic Research of Western New York
Williamsville, New York

GEORGE O. ALONSO, M.D.
Attending Physician, Division of Infectious Diseases
Elmhurst Hospital Center
Elmhurst, New York
Instructor in Medicine, Mount Sinai School of Medicine
New York, New York

VASANTHI ARUMUGAM, M.D.
Instructor, Department of Medicine
Mount Sinai School of Medicine
New York, New York
Attending, Division of Infectious Diseases/Department of
Medicine
Elmhurst Hospital Center
Elmhurst, New York

SUDEEP KAUR AULAKH, M.D., C.M., F.R.C.P.C.
Fellow, General Internal Medicine
Rhode Island Hospital
Clinical Instructor of Medicine
Brown University School of Medicine
Providence, Rhode Island

WILLIAM F. BOYD, M.D., M.P.H.
Staff Physician
Academic Medical Center
Internal Medicine Inpatient Service
Rhode Island Hospital/The Miriam Hospital
Providence, Rhode Island

MANDEEP K. BRAR, M.D.
Clinical Assistant Professor
Department of Obstetrics and Gynecology
State University of New York at Buffalo
Buffalo, New York

REBECCA S. BRIENZA, M.D., M.P.H.
Assistant Professor
Department of Internal Medicine
Yale University School of Medicine
New Haven, Connecticut

JENNIFER CLARKE, M.D.
Staff Physician, Division of General Internal Medicine
Rhode Island Hospital
Clinical Instructor of Medicine
Brown University School of Medicine
Providence, Rhode Island

MARIA A. CORIGLIANO, M.D., F.A.C.O.G.
Clinical Assistant Professor
Department of Obstetrics and Gynecology
State University of New York at Buffalo
Buffalo, New York

KAROLL CORTEZ, M.D.
Fellow in Infectious Disease
Division of Infectious Disease
Rhode Island Hospital
Providence, Rhode Island

CLAUDIA L. DADE, M.D.
Attending Physician, Division of Infectious Diseases
Elmhurst Hospital Center
Elmhurst, New York
Instructor in Medicine, Mount Sinai School of Medicine
New York, New York

GEORGE T. DANAKAS, M.D., F.A.C.O.G.
Clinical Assistant Professor
Department of Obstetrics and Gynecology
State University of New York at Buffalo
Buffalo, New York

JANE V. EASON, M.D.
Attending Physician, Division of Infectious Diseases
Elmhurst Hospital Center
Elmhurst, New York
Instructor in Medicine, Mount Sinai School of Medicine
New York, New York

PEGGY L. EL-MALLAKH, B.S.N., M.S.N.
College of Nursing
University of Kentucky
Lexington, Kentucky

RIF S. EL-MALLAKH, M.D.
Associate Professor
Department of Psychiatry and Behavioral Sciences
University of Louisville School of Medicine
Louisville, Kentucky

MARILYN FABBRI, M.D.
Instructor, Department of Medicine
Mount Sinai School of Medicine
New York, New York
Attending, Division of Infectious Diseases/Department of
Medicine
Elmhurst Hospital Center
Elmhurst, New York

MARK J. FAGAN, M.D.
Director, Medical Primary Care Unit
Rhode Island Hospital
Assistant Professor of Medicine
Brown University School of Medicine
Providence, Rhode Island

GIL FARKASH, M.D.
Assistant Clinical Professor
State University of New York at Buffalo
School of Medicine
Buffalo, New York

FRED F. FERRI, M.D., F.A.C.P.
Clinical Professor
Department of Community Health
Brown University School of Medicine
Chief, Division of Internal Medicine
St. Joseph's Health Services and Fatima Hospital
Providence, Rhode Island

TIFFANY B. GENEWICK, M.D.
Clinical Instructor
Department of Obstetrics and Gynecology
State University of New York at Buffalo
Buffalo, New York

DAVID R. GIFFORD, M.D., M.P.H.
Assistant Physician, Division of Geriatrics
Rhode Island Hospital
Assistant Professor of Community Health and Medicine
Brown University School of Medicine
Providence, Rhode Island

REBECCA A. GRIFFITH, M.D.
Fellow, General Internal Medicine
Rhode Island Hospital
Assistant Instructor of Medicine
Brown University School of Medicine
Providence, Rhode Island

MICHAEL GRUENTHAL, M.D., PH.D.
Assistant Professor, Department of Neurology
University of Louisville School of Medicine
Louisville, Kentucky

MICHELE HALPERN, M.D.
Attending Physician, Division of Infectious Diseases
New Rochelle Hospital
New Rochelle, New York
Clinical Assistant Professor of Medicine
New York Medical College
Valhalla, New York

SAJEEV HANDA, M.D.
Medical Director, Academic Medical Center
Internal Medicine Inpatient Service
Rhode Island Hospital/The Miriam Hospital
Clinical Instructor of Medicine
Brown University School of Medicine
Providence, Rhode Island

MICHAEL P. JOHNSON, M.D.
Staff Physician, Division of General Internal Medicine
Rhode Island Hospital
Associate Professor of Medicine
Brown University School of Medicine
Providence, Rhode Island

WAN J. KIM, M.D.
Clinical Instructor
Department of Obstetrics and Gynecology
State University of New York at Buffalo
Buffalo, New York

MELVYN KOBY, M.D.
Assistant Clinical Professor of Medicine
Department of Ophthalmology
University of Louisville School of Medicine
Louisville, Kentucky

JOSEPH J. LIEBER, M.D.
Chief, Medical Consultation Service
Elmhurst Hospital Center
Elmhurst, New York
Clinical Associate Professor of Medicine
Mount Sinai School of Medicine
New York, New York

ZEENA LOBO, M.D.
Attending Physician
Division of Infectious Diseases
Elmhurst Medical Center
Elmhurst, New York

EUGENE J. LOUIE-NG, M.D.
Clinical Instructor
Department of Obstetrics and Gynecology
State University of New York at Buffalo
Buffalo, New York

JOSEPH R. MASCI, M.D.
Associate Director of Medicine
Elmhurst Hospital Center
Elmhurst, New York
Associate Professor of Medicine
Mount Sinai School of Medicine
New York, New York

KELLY MCGARRY, M.D.
Associate Director
General Internal Medicine Residency Program
Rhode Island Hospital
Assistant Professor
Brown University School of Medicine
Providence, Rhode Island

LONNIE R. MERCIER, M.D.
Clinical Instructor
Department of Orthopedic Surgery
Creighton University School of Medicine
Omaha, Nebraska

DENNIS J. MIKOLICH, M.D.
Chief, Division of Infectious Diseases
VA Medical Center
Clinical Associate Professor of Medicine
Brown University School of Medicine
Providence, Rhode Island

ANNE W. MOULTON, M.D.
Director, General Internal Medicine Fellowship
Rhode Island Hospital
Associate Professor of Medicine
Brown University School of Medicine
Providence, Rhode Island

TAKUMA NEMOTO, M.D.
Research Associate Professor of Surgery
State University of New York at Buffalo
Buffalo, New York

JAMES J. NG, M.D.
Fellow, General Internal Medicine
Rhode Island Hospital
Assistant Clinical Instructor of Medicine
Brown University School of Medicine
Providence, Rhode Island

†PETER NICHOLAS, M.D.
Chief, Division of Infectious Diseases
Elmhurst Hospital Center
Elmhurst, New York
Associate Professor of Medicine
Mount Sinai School of Medicine
New York, New York

GAIL M. O'BRIEN, M.D.
Associate Director of Clinical Operations
Medical Primary Care Unit
Rhode Island Hospital
Clinical Assistant Professor of Medicine
Brown University School of Medicine
Providence, Rhode Island

JEANNE M. OLIVA, M.D.
Staff Physician
Division of General Internal Medicine
Rhode Island Hospital
Providence, Rhode Island

WIILIAM H. OLSON, M.D.
Professor, Department of Neurology
University of Louisville School of Medicine
Louisville, Kentucky

PETER PETROPOULOS, M.D., F.A.C.C.
Clinical Assistant Professor
Brown University School of Medicine
Department of Veterans Affairs
Providence, Rhode Island

MICHAEL PICCHIONI, M.D.
Attending Physician
Baystate Medical Center
Assistant Professor of Medicine
Tufts University School of Medicine
Springfield, Massachusetts

MAURICE POLICAR, M.D.
Attending Physician, Division of Infectious Diseases
Elmhurst Hospital Center
Elmhurst, New York
Assistant Professor of Medicine
Mount Sinai School of Medicine
New York, New York

LUTHER K. ROBINSON, M.D.
Associate Professor of Pediatrics
Director, Dysmorphology and Clinical Genetics
State University of New York at Buffalo
Buffalo, New York

CARLOS SALAMA, M.D.
Attending Physician
Division of Infectious Diseases
Elmhurst Medical Center
Elmhurst, New York
Assistant Professor of Medicine
Mount Sinai School of Medicine
New York, New York

HARVEY M. SHANIES, M.D., PH.D.
Associate Director of Medicine for Clinical & Academic
    Pulmonary & Critical Care Medicine
Elmhurst Hospital Center
Elmhurst, New York
Clinical Associate Professor of Medicine
Mount Sinai School of Medicine
New York, New York

DEBORAH L. SHAPIRO, M.D.
Chief, Division of Rheumatology
Elmhurst Hospital Center
Elmhurst, New York
Clinical Assistant Professor of Medicine
Mount Sinai School of Medicine
New York, New York

MARIA ELENA SOLER, M.D.
Clinical Instructor
Department of Obstetrics and Gynecology
State University of New York at Buffalo
Buffalo, New York

ANNE SPAULDING, M.D.
Staff Physician
Divisions of General Internal Medicine and Infectious
    Diseases
Rhode Island Hospital
Clinical Assistant Professor of Medicine
Brown University School of Medicine
Providence, Rhode Island

JULIE ANNE SZUMIGALA, M.D.
Clinical Instructor
Department of Obstetrics and Gynecology
State University of New York at Buffalo
Buffalo, New York

DOMINICK TAMMARO, M.D.
Associate Director, Categorical Internal Medicine
    Residency
Co-Director, Medicine-Pediatrics Residency
Division of General Internal Medicine
Rhode Island Hospital
Assistant Professor of Medicine
Brown University School of Medicine
Providence, Rhode Island

PETER E. TANGUAY, M.D.
Ackerly Professor of Child & Adolescent Psychiatry
Department of Psychiatry and Behavioral Sciences
University of Louisville School of Medicine
Louisville, Kentucky

†Deceased.

TOM J. WACHTEL, M.D.
Physician-in-Charge, Division of Geriatrics
Rhode Island Hospital
Professor of Community Health and Medicine
Brown University School of Medicine
Providence, Rhode Island

DENNIS M. WEPPNER, M.D., F.A.C.O.G.
Associate Professor of Clinical Gynecology/Obstetrics
State University of New York at Buffalo
Clinical Chief
Department of Gynecology/Obstetrics
Millard Fillmore Hospital
Buffalo, New York

LAUREL M. WHITE, M.D.
Clinical Assistant Professor
Department of Obstetrics and Gynecology
Division of Maternal Fetal Medicine
State University of New York at Buffalo
Buffalo, New York

JOHN M. WIECKOWSKI, M.D., PH.D., F.A.C.O.G.
Director
Reproductive Medicine and In Vitro Fertilization
Williamsville, New York

MATTHEW L. WITHIAM-LEITCH, M.D.
Clinical Instructor
Department of Obstetrics and Gynecology
State University of New York at Buffalo
Buffalo, New York

BETH J. WUTZ, M.D.
Clinical Assistant Professor of Medicine
Division of Internal Medicine/Pediatrics
Kajeida Health–Buffalo General Hospital
State University of New York at Buffalo
Buffalo, New York

MADHAVI YERNENI, M.D.
Staff Physician, Academic Medical Center
Internal Medicine Inpatient Service
Rhode Island Hospital/The Miriam Hospital
Providence, Rhode Island

SCOTT J. ZUCCALA, D.O., F.A.C.O.G.
Staff Physician
Mercy Hospital of Buffalo
Buffalo, New York

To

OUR FAMILIES

Their constant support and encouragement
made this book a reality

Preface

This book is intended to be a clear and concise reference for the primary care physician. It is available in clinical text and CD-ROM format. Its user-friendly format was designed to provide a fast and efficient way to identify important clinical information and to offer practical guidance in patient management. The book is divided into five sections and an appendix, each with emphasis and clinical information useful to primary care physicians.

The tremendous success of the previous editions and the enthusiastic comments from numerous colleagues have brought about several positive changes. Each section has been significantly expanded from the first edition, bringing the total number of medical topics covered in this book to more than 1000. Illustrations have been added to several topics to enhance recollection of clinically important facts. A detailed table of contents facilitates identification and retrieval of topics. The addition of ICD-9-CM codes will expedite claims submission and reimbursement.

Section I contains 615 medical disorders of clinical importance to primary care physicians. Medical topics in this section are arranged alphabetically, and the material in each topic is presented in outline format for ease of retrieval. Key, quick-access information is consistently highlighted, and clinical photographs are used to further illustrate selected medical conditions. ICD-9-CM codes are included to expedite claims submission and reimbursement. Most references focus on current peer-reviewed journal articles rather than outdated textbooks and old review articles. Topics in this section use the following structured approach:

1. Basic Information (Definition, Synonyms, ICD-9-CM Codes, Epidemiology and Demographics, Physical Findings and Clinical Presentation, Etiology)
2. Diagnosis (Differential Diagnosis, Workup, Laboratory Tests, Imaging Studies)

3. Treatment (Nonpharmacologic Therapy, Acute General Rx, Chronic Rx, Disposition, Referral)
4. Pearls and Considerations (Comments, References)

Section II has been expanded to include the differential diagnosis, etiology, and classification of 472 signs and symptoms. This is a practical section that allows the user investigating a physical complaint or abnormal laboratory value to follow a "workup" leading to a diagnosis. The physician then can easily look up the presumptive diagnosis in Section I for the information specific to that illness.

Section III now includes 179 clinical algorithms to guide and expedite the patient's workup and therapy. This section is particularly valuable in today's managed care environment.

Section IV includes normal laboratory values and interpretation of results of 183 commonly ordered laboratory tests. By providing interpretation of abnormal results, this section facilitates the diagnosis of medical disorders and further adds to the comprehensive, "one stop" nature of our text. The cost of each laboratory test has also been added to this section for this edition.

Section V focuses on preventive medicine and offers essential guidelines from the U.S. Preventive Services Task Force. Information in this section on clinical preventive services includes recommendations for the periodic health examination, screening for major diseases and disorders, patient counseling, and immunization and chemoprophylaxis recommendations.

The **Appendix** contains common definitions used in Complementary and Alternative Medicine (CAM), a listing of frequently used herbals with documented or suspected risks, and selected resources for complementary/alternative medicine. CAM has gained tremendous popularity; however, the gap between allopathy and CAM remains substantive. With the material in this appendix we hope to lessen the current scarcity of exposure of allopathic physicians to the diversity of CAM therapies.

As practicing physicians, we all realize the importance of patient education and the need for clear communication with our patients. Toward that end, we have included on a companion CD-ROM easy-to-use, practical patient instruction sheets, organized alphabetically and covering the majority of the topics in this book. Several new patient teaching guides have been added to the 2003 edition. These patient teaching guides (PTGs) are available in English and Spanish. They are a valuable addition to patient care and useful to improve physician-patient communication, patient satisfaction, and quality of care. For ease of identification, each clinical topic in Section I of the book with a

corresponding patient teaching guide on the CD is marked with *"(PTG)"* after the topic name, at the top of the page in the book. In addition, the cross-references to the CD are included in the table of contents.

I strongly believe that we have produced a state of the art information system with significant differences from existing texts. I hope that its user-friendly approach, its numerous unique features, and yearly updates will make our book and CD-ROM valuable medical references not only to primary care physicians, but also to physicians in other specialties, medical students, and allied health professionals.

Fred F. Ferri, M.D.

Contents

Detailed Contents

SECTION I DISEASES AND DISORDERS

PTG indicates that a patient teaching guide is available on the companion CD-ROM.

SECTION II DIFFERENTIAL DIAGNOSIS, ETIOLOGY, AND CLASSIFICATION OF COMMON SIGNS AND SYMPTOMS

SECTION III   CLINICAL ALGORITHMS

SECTION IV LABORATORY TESTS AND INTERPRETATION OF RESULTS

SECTION V CLINICAL PREVENTIVE SERVICES

APPENDIX   COMPLEMENTARY AND ALTERNATIVE MEDICINE

Diseases and Disorders

BASIC INFORMATION

DEFINITION
Abruptio placentae is the separation of placenta from the uterine wall before delivery of the fetus. There are three classes of abruption based on maternal and fetal status, including an assessment of uterine contractions, quantity of bleeding, fetal heart rate monitoring, and abnormal coagulation studies (fibrinogen, PT, PTT).
- Grade I: mild vaginal bleeding, uterine irritability, stable vital signs, reassuring fetal heart rate, normal coagulation profile (fibrinogen 450 mg %)
- Grade II: Moderate vaginal bleeding, hypertonic uterine contractions, orthostatic blood pressure measurements, unfavorable fetal status, fibrinogen 150 mg % to 250 mg %
- Grade III: severe bleeding (may be concealed), hypertonic uterine contractions, overt signs of hypovolemic shock, fetal death, thrombocytopenia, fibrinogen <150 mg %

ICD-9CM CODES
641.2 Premature separation of placenta

EPIDEMIOLOGY & DEMOGRAPHICS
INCIDENCE (IN U.S.): 1/86-206 births; incidence by grade: I = 40%, II = 45%, III = 15%; 80% occur before the onset of labor
RISK FACTORS: Hypertension (greatest association), trauma, polyhydramnios, multifetal gestation, smoking, use of crack cocaine, chorioamnionitis, preterm premature rupture of membranes
RECURRENCE RATE: 5% to 17%; with two prior episodes, 25%

PHYSICAL FINDINGS & CLINICAL PRESENTATION
- Triad of uterine bleeding (concealed or per vagina), hypertonic uterine contractions or signs of preterm labor, and evidence of fetal compromise exists.
- More than 80% of cases have external bleeding; 20% of cases have no bleeding but have indirect evidence of abruption, such as failed tocolysis for preterm labor.
- Tetanic uterine contractions are found in only 17% of cases, unless grade II or III abruption.

ETIOLOGY
- Primary etiology: unknown
- Hypertension: found in 40% to 50% of grade III abruptions

- Rapid decompression of uterine cavity, such as is found with polyhydramnios or multifetal gestation
- Blunt external trauma (motor vehicle accident, spousal abuse)

 DIAGNOSIS

DIFFERENTIAL DIAGNOSIS
Placenta previa, cervical or vaginal trauma, labor, cervical cancer, rupture of membranes. The differential diagnosis of vaginal bleeding in pregnancy is described in Box 2-252.

WORKUP
- Initial assessment should evaluate for the source of bleeding, ruling out placenta previa and associated conditions that contraindicate any type of vaginal examination, e.g., pelvic speculum examination.
- Continuous fetal heart monitoring is indicated for all viable gestations (60% incidence of fetal distress in labor); may show early signs of maternal hypovolemia (late decelerations or fetal tachycardia) before overt maternal vital sign changes.
- Actual amount of blood loss is often greater than initially perceived because of the possibility of concealed retroplacental bleeding and the apparent "normal" vital signs. The relative hypervolemia of pregnancy initially protects the gravida until late in the course of bleeding, when abrupt and sudden cardiovascular collapse can occur without warning.

LABORATORY TESTS
- Baseline Hgb and Hct help quantify blood loss and, even more important, with every four to six determinations can demonstrate significant trends during expectant management.
- Coagulation profile: platelets, fibrinogen, prothrombin, and partial thromboplastin time. DIC can develop with severe abruption. If fibrinogen is <150 mg %, estimated blood loss equals 2000 ml, and if fibrinogen is <100 mg %, consider FFP to prevent further bleeding.
- Type and antibody screen is important to identify Rh-negative patients who may need Rh immune globulin.

IMAGING STUDIES
Ultrasound should include fetal presentation and status, amniotic fluid volume, placental location, as well as any evidence of hematoma (retroplacental, subchorionic, or preplacental).

 TREATMENT

Treatment is dependent on gestational age of the fetus, severity of the abruption, and maternal status. Stabilization of the mother is the first priority.

ACUTE GENERAL Rx
- Initial assessment for signs of maternal hemodynamic compromise or hemorrhagic shock; large-bore intravenous access, with crystalloid fluid resuscitation using a replacement of 3 ml LR solution for every 1 ml estimated blood loss.
- Indwelling Foley catheter to monitor urine output and maternal volume status, with a goal of 30 ml/hr urine output.
- Assess fetal status and gestational age, using sonogram and continuous fetal heart rate monitoring.
- Because of the unpredictable nature of abruptions, cross-matched blood should be made available during the initial resuscitation period.

CHRONIC Rx
- In the term fetus or where lung maturity has been documented, delivery is indicated.
- In the preterm fetus or with an immature lung profile, consideration should be given for betamethasone 12.5 mg IM q24h for two doses and then delivery, depending on the severity of the abruption and the likelihood of fetal complications from preterm birth.
- C-section should be reserved for cases of fetal distress or for standard obstetric indications.
- In select cases, such as severe prematurity with a stable mother and mild contractions, magnesium sulfate can be used for tocolysis, 6 g IV loading dose then 3 g/hr maintenance, to allow for course of steroids.

DISPOSITION
Because of the unpredictable nature of abruptions, expectant management should occur only under controlled circumstances.

REFERRAL
Abruptio placentae places mother and fetus in a high-risk situation and should be managed by a qualified obstetrician in a facility with capability for neonatal and maternal resuscitation and ability to perform emergency C-sections.
Author: **Scott J. Zuccala, D.O.**

BASIC INFORMATION

■ DEFINITION
A brain abscess is a focal, intracerebral infection that begins as a localized area of cerebritis and develops into a collection of pus surrounded by a well-vascularized capsule.

ICD-9CM CODES
324.0 Brain abscess

■ EPIDEMIOLOGY & DEMOGRAPHICS
- Quite uncommon (occur about 2% as commonly as brain tumors)
- Occur at any age
- Peak incidences in preadolescence and middle age
- Most common source of underlying infection: contiguous spread from the paranasal sinuses, middle ear, or teeth

■ PHYSICAL FINDINGS & CLINICAL PRESENTATION
- Classic triad: fever, headache, and focal neurologic deficit are present in <50% of cases.
- A dull, aching, poorly localized headache is the most common presenting symptom (70%).
- Fever is present in only 50% of patients.
- Focal neurologic findings (e.g., hemiparesis, aphasia, ataxia) depend on the location of the abscess and are seen in 30% to 50% of cases.
- Papilledema is present in 25% of cases.
- Presence of adjacent infections (dental abscess, otitis media, and sinusitis) may be a clue to the underlying diagnosis and should be sought in any suspected case.
- Time course from symptom onset to presentation ranges from hours in fulminant cases to more than 1 month; 75% present in the first 2 weeks.

- The nonspecific presentation of a brain abscess warrants that clinicians maintain a high index of suspicion.

■ ETIOLOGY
- Brain abscesses arise from:
  Contiguous infection
  Hematogenous spread from a remote site
- They are classified based on the likely portal of entry.
Likely source of abscess:
A. Contiguous focus or primary infection (55% of all brain abscesses):
  1. Paranasal sinus: occur in frontal lobe; streptococci, *Bacteroides, Haemophilus,* and *Fusobacterium* species
  2. Otitis media/mastoiditis: occur in temporal lobe and cerebellum; streptococci, Enterobacteriaceae, *Bacteroides,* and *Pseudomonas* species
  3. Dental sepsis: occur in frontal lobe; mixed *Fusobacterium, Bacteroides,* and *Streptococcus* species
  4. Penetrating head injury: site of abscess depends on site of wound; *Staphylococcus aureus, Clostridium* species, Enterobacteriaceae species
  5. Postoperative: *Staphylococcus epidermidis* and *S. aureus,* Enterobacteriaceae, and Pseudomonadaceae
B. Hematogenous spread/distant site of infection (25% of all brain abscesses): abscesses most commonly multiple, especially in middle cerebral artery distribution; infecting organisms depend on source.
  1. Congenital heart disease: streptococci, *Haemophilus* species
  2. Endocarditis: *S. aureus,* viridans streptococci
  3. Urinary tract: Enterobacteriaceae, Pseudomonadaceae
  4. Intraabdominal: streptococci, Enterobacteriaceae, anaerobes
  5. Lung: streptococci, *Actinomyces* species, *Fusobacterium* species

  6. Immunocompromised host: *Toxoplasma* species, fungi, Enterobacteriaceae, *Nocardia* species
C. Cryptogenic (unknown source): 20% of all brain abscesses

DIAGNOSIS

■ DIFFERENTIAL DIAGNOSIS
- Other parameningeal infections: subdural empyema, epidural abscess, thrombophlebitis of the major dural venous sinuses and cortical veins
- Embolic strokes in patients with bacterial endocarditis
- Mycotic aneurysms with leakage
- Viral encephalitis (usually resulting from herpes simplex)
- Acute hemorrhagic leukoencephalitis
- Parasitic infections: toxoplasmosis, echinococcosis, cysticercosis
- Neoplasm
- Cerebral infarction
- CNS vasculitis
- Chronic subdural hematoma

■ WORKUP
Physical examination, laboratory tests, and imaging studies

■ LABORATORY TESTS
- WBC counts are often normal.
- ESR is usually elevated, but may be normal.
- Blood cultures are most often negative (10% positive).
- Lumbar puncture is contraindicated in patients with suspected abscess (20% die or suffer neurologic decline).
- The yield of Gram stain and culture of material aspirated at time of surgical drainage approaches 100%.

■ IMAGING STUDIES

- MRI is the diagnostic procedure of choice; provides superior detail compared to CT scan (higher sensitivity and specificity than CT scan, but not always immediately available).
- CT scan (Fig. 1-1) with intravenous contrast is still an excellent test (sensitivity 95% to 99%).
- Serial CT or MRI scanning is recommended to follow the response to therapy.

℞ TREATMENT

Effective treatment involves a combination of empiric antibiotic therapy and timely excision or aspiration of the abscess.

■ ACUTE GENERAL Rx

- If evidence of edema or mass effect, treatment of elevated intracranial pressure is paramount (includes hyperventilation of the mechanically ventilated patient, dexamethasone, mannitol).
- Medical therapy is never a substitute for surgical intervention to relieve increased intracranial pressure.
- Steroids should be limited to patients with severe cerebral edema or midline shift.

■ MEDICAL Rx

Empiric antibiotic therapy guided by:
- Abscess location
- Suspicion of primary source
- Presence of single or multiple abscesses
- Patient's underlying medical conditions (i.e., HIV, immunocompromised)

Selection of empiric antibiotic therapy:
- Primary infection or contiguous source:
  1. Otitis media/mastoiditis, sinusitis, dental infection: third-generation cephalosporin (cefotaxime 2 g q4h IV or ceftriaxone 2 g q12h IV) plus metronidazole 7.5 mg/kg q6h IV or 15 mg/kg q12h IV
  2. Postsurgical: nafcillin or oxacillin 2 g q4h IV plus third-generation cephalosporin or vancomycin 1 g q12h IV plus third-generation cephalosporin
  3. Penetrating trauma: nafcillin or oxacillin 2 g q4h IV plus third-generation cephalosporin
- Hematogenous spread (congenital heart disease, endocarditis, urinary tract, lung, intraabdominal): nafcillin plus metronidazole plus third-generation cephalosporin

Duration of antibiotic therapy is unclear. Most recommend parenteral treatment for 2 to 6 wk, followed by 2 to 4 mo of oral therapy until response evident by neuroimaging (CT/MRI).

■ SURGICAL Rx

- Stereotactic biopsy or aspirate of the abscess if surgically feasible
- Essential to selection of targeted antimicrobial coverage
- Timing and choice of surgery depends on:
  Primary infection source
  Number and location of the abscesses
  Whether the procedure is diagnostic or therapeutic
  Neurologic status of the patient

■ DISPOSITION

- Prompt diagnostic consideration, early institution of appropriate antimicrobial therapy, and advanced neuroradiologic imaging have reduced the mortality resulting from brain abscesses from 40% to 80% in the preantibiotic era to 0% to 30% at present.
- Morbidity is usually manifest as persistent neurologic sequelae (seizures, intellectual or behavioral impairment, motor deficits) seen in 30% to 55% of patients.

■ REFERRAL

Consultation with a neurosurgeon is mandatory.
Author: **Kelly McGarry, M.D.**

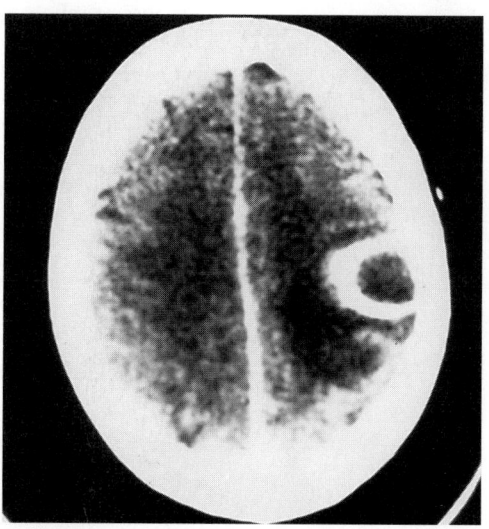

Fig. 1-1 Computed tomography (CT) scan showing a brain abscess. A woman presented to physicians after a focal seizure followed by headache and weakness of the arm. Dental work had been performed several weeks before. CT scan revealed a contrast-enhanced, ringlike mass surrounded by edema. It is not possible on this scan to differentiate tumor from abscess. At surgery a well-encapsulated abscess was encountered. (From Andreoli TE [ed]: *Cecil essentials of medicine,* ed 4, Philadelphia, 1997, WB Saunders.)

BASIC INFORMATION

■ DEFINITION
Breast abscess is an acute inflammatory process resulting in the formation of a collection of pus. Typically there is painful erythematous mass formation in the breast, occasionally with draining through the overlying skin or nipple duct opening.

■ SYNONYMS
Subareolar abscess
Lactational or puerperal abscess

ICD-9CM CODES
6.110 Abscess of the breast
675.0 Abscess of the nipple related to childbirth
675.1 Abscess of the breast related to childbirth

■ EPIDEMIOLOGY & DEMOGRAPHICS
- 10% to 30% of all breast abscesses are lactational.
- Acute mastitis occurs in 2.5% of nursing mothers, with 1 in 15 of these women developing abscess.

■ PHYSICAL FINDINGS & CLINICAL PRESENTATION
Painful erythematous induration involving the part of the breast leading to fluctuant abscess

■ ETIOLOGY
- Lactational abscess: milk stasis and bacterial infection leading to mastitis, then to abscess, with *Staphylococ-cus aureus* the most common causative agent
- Subareolar abscess:
  1. Central ducts involved, with obstructive nipple duct changes leading to bacterial infection
  2. Cultured organisms mixed, including anerobes, staphylococci, streptococci, and others

DIAGNOSIS

■ DIFFERENTIAL DIAGNOSIS
- Inflammatory carcinoma
- Advanced carcinoma with erythema, edema, and/or ulceration
- Rarely, tuberculous abscess
- Hydradenitis of breast skin
- Sebaceous cyst with infection

■ WORKUP
- Clinical examination sufficient
- If abscess suspected, referral to surgeon for incision, drainage, and biopsy
- If possible abscess or advanced carcinoma, referral for workup required

■ LABORATORY TESTS
- Perform C&S test of abscess contents.
- If mammogram or ultrasound prevented by discomfort, perform after resolution of abscess if required.

TREATMENT

■ NONPHARMACOLOGIC THERAPY
- Established abscess: incision and drainage, preferably with general anesthesia
- Biopsy of abscess cavity wall to exclude carcinoma

■ ACUTE GENERAL Rx
- Antibiotics: the pathogen is generally staphylococci in lactational abscess. Recommended initial antibiotic therapy is with nafcillin or oxacillin 2g q4h IV or cefazolin 1g q8h IV.
- If acute mastitis is treated early, resolution without drainage is possible.
- Subareolar abscess: broad-spectrum antibiotic treatment and drainage are needed to control acute phase.

■ CHRONIC Rx
Further surgical treatment for recurrences or fistula

■ DISPOSITION
- Lactational abscess: possible to continue breast-feeding without apparent risk of infection to the infant
- Subareolar abscess:
  1. Notorious for recurrence or complication of fistula formation
  2. Patient informed and referred for subsequent care

■ REFERRAL
- If abscess drainage required
- For surgical consultation if subareolar abscess involved

Author: **Takuma Nemoto, M.D.**

BASIC INFORMATION

DEFINITION
Liver abscess is a necrotic infection of the liver usually classified as pyogenic or amebic.

SYNONYMS
Pyogenic hepatic abscess
Amebic hepatic abscess

ICD-9CM CODES
572.0 Abscess of liver

EPIDEMIOLOGY & DEMOGRAPHICS
- Worldwide, amebic liver abscess is more common than pyogenic liver abscess.
- In the U.S., pyogenic liver abscess is more common than amebic liver abscess.
- Incidence of pyogenic liver abscess is 6 to 10 cases per 100,000.
- Amebic liver abscesses complicate amebic colitis in nearly 10% of cases.
- Most abscesses occur on the right lobe of the liver.
- More common in men than women.

PHYSICAL FINDINGS & CLINICAL PRESENTATION
- Fever, chills, and sweats
- Anorexia with weight loss
- Nausea, vomiting, and diarrhea
- Cough with pleuritic chest pain
- Right upper quadrant abdominal pain
- Hepatomegaly
- Splenomegaly
- Jaundice
- Pleural effusions, rales, and friction rubs may be present.

ETIOLOGY
- Pyogenic liver abscess is usually polymicrobial (*E. coli*, *K. pneumoniae*, *P. aeruginosa*, *Proteus*, *Bacteroides*, *Fusobacterium*, *Actinomyces*, gram-positive anaerobes and *S. aureus*).
- Amebic hepatic abscess is caused by the parasite *Entamoeba histolytica*.
- Pyogenic liver abscess occurs from:
  1. Biliary disease with cholangitis
  2. Gallbladder disease with contiguous spread to the liver
  3. Diverticulitis or appendicitis with spread via the portal circulation
  4. Hematogenous spread via the hepatic artery
  5. Penetrating wounds
  6. Cryptogenic
- Amebiasis is usually due to fecal-oral contamination and invades the intestinal mucosa gaining entry into the portal system to reach the liver.

DIAGNOSIS

The diagnosis of liver abscess requires a high index of suspicion after a detailed history and physical examination. Imaging studies confirm the presence of a liver abscess.

DIFFERENTIAL DIAGNOSIS
- Cholangitis
- Cholecystitis
- Diverticulitis
- Appendicitis
- Perforated viscus
- Mesentery ischemia
- Pulmonary embolism
- Pancreatitis

WORKUP
- The workup of a liver abscess should focus on differentiating between amebic and pyogenic causes.
- Features suggesting an amebic cause are: travel to an endemic area, single abscess rather than multiple abscesses, subacute onset of symptoms, and absence of conditions predisposing to pyogenic liver abscess as highlighted under "Etiology."
- Laboratory studies are not specific but useful as adjunctive tests.
- Imaging studies cannot differentiate between the two and bacteriologic cultures may be sterile in 50% of the cases.

LABORATORY TESTS
- CBC showing leukocytosis
- Liver function tests: Alkaline phosphatase is most commonly elevated (95%); AST and ALT elevated in 50% of cases
- PT (INR) prolonged (70%)
- Blood cultures positive in 50% of cases
- Aspiration (50% sterile)
- Stool samples for *E. histolytica* trophozoites (positive in 10% to 15% of amebic liver abscess cases)
- Serologic testing for *E. histolytica* does not differentiate acute from old infections

IMAGING STUDIES
- CXR abnormal in 50% of the cases showing elevated right hemidiaphragm, pleural effusions, and consolidating infiltrates
- Ultrasound (80% to 100% sensitivity in detecting abscesses)
- CT scans more sensitive in detecting hepatic abscesses and contiguous organ extension (Fig. 1-2)
- Most liver abscesses are single; however, multiple liver abscesses are seen with systemic bacteremia

TREATMENT

NONPHARMACOLOGIC THERAPY
- The management of pyogenic liver abscess differs from that of amebic liver abscess.
- Medical management is the cornerstone of therapy in amebic liver abscess, whereas early intervention in the form of surgical therapy or catheter drainage and parenteral antibiotics is the rule in pyogenic liver abscess.

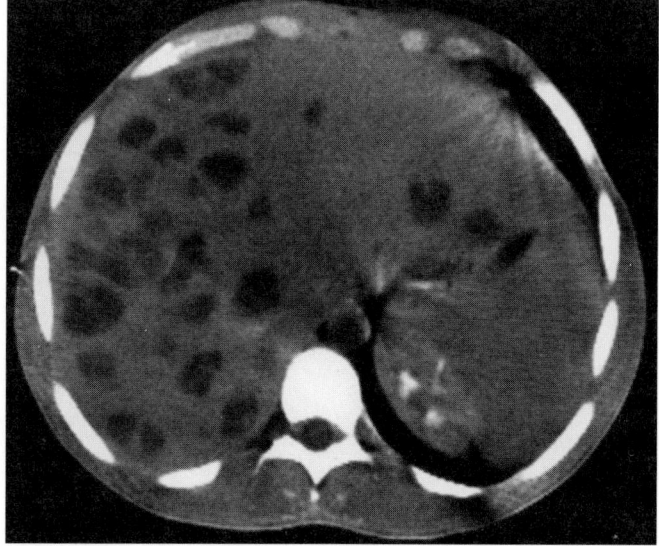

Fig. 1-2 CT scan demonstrating multiple pyogenic liver abscesses in a 25-year-old man. (From Goldman L, Bennett JC [ed]: *Cecil textbook of medicine*, ed 21, Philadelphia, 2000, WB Saunders.)

■ **ACUTE GENERAL Rx**

- Percutaneous drainage under CT or ultrasound guidance is essential in the treatment of pyogenic liver abscesses.
- Aspiration of hepatic amebic abscesses is not required unless there is no response to treatment or a pyogenic cause is being considered.
- Antibiotic treatment for pyogenic liver abscess initially is empirical triple therapy with penicillin, aminoglycoside, and metronidazole.
  1. Parenteral antibiotics are continued for 2 wk and followed by 4 to 6 wk PO therapy.
  2. Clindamycin with an aminoglycoside or imipenem alone are alternative choices.
- Antibiotic coverage for amebic liver abscesses include:
  1. Metronidazole 750 mg PO tid for 10 days
  2. Dehydroemetine 1 mg/kg/day IM for 5 days followed by chloroquine 1 g/day for 2 days; then 500 mg/day for 2 to 3 wk can be used as an alternative to metronidazole

■ **CHRONIC Rx**

If fever persists for 2 wk despite percutaneous drainage and antibiotic therapy as outlined under "Acute General Rx," surgery is indicated.

■ **DISPOSITION**

- Most patients with pyogenic liver abscesses defervesce within 2 wk of treatment with antibiotics and drainage.
- Pyogenic liver abscess cure rates using percutaneous drainage and antibiotics have been reported to have cure rates between 88% and 100%.
- Mortality of untreated pyogenic liver abscess is nearly 100%.
- Most patients with amebic liver abscesses defervesce within 4 to 5 days of treatment.
- Amebic liver abscess mortality rate is <1% unless complications occur (see under Comments).

■ **REFERRAL**

Infectious disease, interventional radiology, and general surgical consultations are recommended in any patient with a single hepatic abscess or multiple abscesses.

☼ PEARLS & CONSIDERATIONS

■ **COMMENTS**

- Complications of pyogenic and amebic liver abscesses include:
  1. Pleuropulmonary extension resulting in empyema, abscess, and fistula formation
  2. Peritonitis
  3. Purulent pericarditis
  3. Sepsis

REFERENCES

Kar P, Kapoor S, Jain A: Pyogenic liver abscess: aetiology, clinical manifestations and management, *Trop Gastroenterol* 19(4):136, 1998.

Sharma MP, Ahuja V: Management of amebic and pyogenic liver abscess, *Indian J Gastroenterol Suppl* 1:C33, 2001.

Williams CN: Hepatic abscess, *Can J Gastroenterol* 12(4):249, 1998.

Author: **Peter Petropoulos, M.D.**

BASIC INFORMATION

■ **DEFINITION**

A lung abscess is an infection of the lung parenchyma resulting in a necrotic cavity containing pus.

■ **SYNONYMS**

Pulmonary abscess

ICD-9CM CODES

513.0 Abscess of lung

■ **EPIDEMIOLOGY & DEMOGRAPHICS**

- Incidence has decreased over the last 30 years as a result of antibiotic therapy.
- Lung abscess in patients age 50 and over is associated with primary lung neoplasia in 30% of the cases.
- Lung abscesses commonly coexist with empyemas.
- Risk factor population includes patients with:
  1. Alcohol-related problems
  2. Seizure disorders
  3. Cerebrovascular disorders with dysphagia
  4. Drug abuse
  5. Esophageal disorders (e.g., scleroderma, esophageal carcinoma, etc.)
  6. Poor oral hygiene
  7. Obstructive malignant lung disease
  8. Bronchiectasis

■ **PHYSICAL FINDINGS & CLINICAL PRESENTATION**

- Symptoms are generally insidious and prolonged, occurring for weeks to months
- Fever, chills, and sweats
- Cough
- Sputum production (purulent with foul odor)
- Pleuritic chest pain
- Hemoptysis
- Dyspnea
- Malaise, fatigue, and weakness
- Tachycardia and tachypnea
- Dullness to percussion, whispered pectoriloquy, and bronchophony

■ **ETIOLOGY**

- The most important factor predisposing to lung abscess is aspiration.
- Following aspiration as a major predisposing factor is periodontal disease.
- Lung abscess is rare in an edentulous person.
- Approximately 90% of lung abscesses are caused by anaerobic microorganisms (*Bacteroides fragilis, Fusobacterium nucleatum, Peptostreptococcus*, microaerophilic *Streptococcus*).

- In most cases anaerobic infection is mixed with aerobic or facultative anaerobic organisms (*S. aureus, E. coli, K. pneumoniae, P. aeruginosa*).

 DIAGNOSIS

Lung abscess may be primary or secondary.

- Primary lung abscess refers to infection from normal host organisms within the lung (e.g., aspiration, pneumonia).
- Secondary lung abscess results from other preexisting conditions (e.g., endocarditis, underlying lung cancer, pulmonary emboli).

Lung abscess may be acute or chronic.

- Acute lung abscess is present if symptoms are of less than 4 to 6 wk.
- Chronic lung abscess is present if symptoms are greater than 6 wk.

■ **DIFFERENTIAL DIAGNOSIS**

The differential diagnosis is similar to cavitary lung lesions:

- Bacterial (anaerobic, aerobic, infected bulla, empyema, actinomycosis, tuberculosis)
- Fungal (histoplasmosis, coccidioidomycosis, blastomycosis, aspergillosis, cyptococcosis)
- Parasitic (amebiasis, echinococcosis)
- Malignancy (primary lung carcinoma, metastatic lung disease, lymphoma, Hodgkin's disease)
- Wegener's granulomatosis, sarcoidosis, endocarditis, and septic pulmonary emboli

■ **WORKUP**

- The workup of a patient with lung abscess attempts to elicit a primary or a secondary cause.
- Blood tests are not specific in diagnosing lung abscesses.
- Most diagnoses are made from imaging studies; however, to diagnose a specific cause bacteriologic studies are needed.

■ **LABORATORY TESTS**

- CBC with leukocytosis
- Bacteriologic studies
  1. Sputum Gram stain and culture (commonly contaminated by oral flora)
  2. Percutaneous transtracheal aspiration
  3. Percutaneous transthoracic aspiration
  4. Fiberoptic bronchoscopy using bronchial brushings or bronchoalveolar lavage are the most widely used intervention when

trying to obtain diagnostic bacteriologic cultures
- Blood cultures on some occasions may be positive
- If an empyema is present, obtaining empyema fluid via thoracentesis may isolate the organism

■ **IMAGING STUDIES**

- CXR makes the diagnosis of lung abscess showing the cavitary lesion with an air fluid level.
- Lung abscesses are most commonly found in the posterior segment of the right upper lobe.
- Chest CT scan can localize and size the lesion and assist in differentiating lung abscesses from other pathologic processes (e.g., tumor, empyema, infected bulla, etc.) (Fig. 1-3).

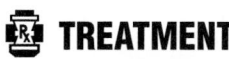 **TREATMENT**

■ **NONPHARMACOLOGIC THERAPY**

- Oxygen therapy
- Postural drainage
- Respiratory therapy maneuvers

■ **ACUTE GENERAL Rx**

- Penicillin 1 to 2 million units IV q4h until improvement (e.g., afebrile, decrease in sputum production, etc.) followed by penicillin VK 500 mg PO qid for the next 2 to 3 wk but usually requiring longer 6- to 8-wk courses.
- Metronidazole is given with penicillin at doses of 7.5 mg/kg IV q6h followed by PO 500 mg bid to qid dosing.
- Clindamycin is an alternative choice if concerned about penicillin-resistant organisms. The dose is 600 mg IV q8h until improvement, followed by 300 mg PO q6h.

■ **CHRONIC Rx**

- Brochoscopy to assist with drainage and/or diagnosis is indicated in patients who fail to respond to antibiotics or if there is suspected underlying malignancy.
- Surgery is indicated on rare occasions (<10%) in patients with complications of lung abscess mentioned below.

■ **DISPOSITION**

- Over 95% of patients are cured with the use of antibiotics alone.
- Complications of lung abscesses include:
  1. Empyema
  2. Massive hemoptysis
  3. Pneumothorax
  4. Bronchopleural fistula

- Mortality is low in community-acquired lung abscess (2.5%)
- Hospital-acquired lung abscess carry a high mortality rate (65%)

▪ REFERRAL
If lung abscess is present, consultation with pulmonary and infectious disease specialist is recommended.

☼ PEARLS & CONSIDERATIONS

▪ COMMENTS
- Complications of lung abscesses include:
  1. Empyema
  2. Bronchopleural fistula
  3. Hepatobronchial fistula
  4. Brain abscess
  5. Bronchiectasis

- Refractory cases are usually the result of:
  1. Large cavity size (>6 cm)
  2. Recurrent aspiration
  3. Thick-walled cavities
  4. Underlying lung carcinoma
  5. Empyema formation
- Necrotizing pneumonia is similar to a lung abscess but differs in size (<2 cm in diameter) and number (usually multiple suppurative cavitory lesions)

REFERENCES
Finegold SM: Lung abscess. In *Mandell, Douglas, and Bennett's principles and practice of infectious diseases,* ed 5, New York, 2000, Churchill Livingstone.

Mwandumba HC, Beeching NJ: Pyogenic lung infections: factors for predicting clinical outcome of lung abscess and thoracic empyema, *Curr Opin Pulm Med* 6(3):234, 2000.

Cassiere HA, Niederman MS: Aspiration pneumonia, lipoid pneumonia, and lung abscess. In Baum GL et al: *Textbook of pulmonary diseases,* ed 6, New York, 1998, Lippincott-Raven.

Wiedemann HP, Rice TW: Lung abscess and empyema, *Semin Thorac Cardiovasc Surg* 7:119, 1995.

Author: **Peter Petropoulos, M.D.**

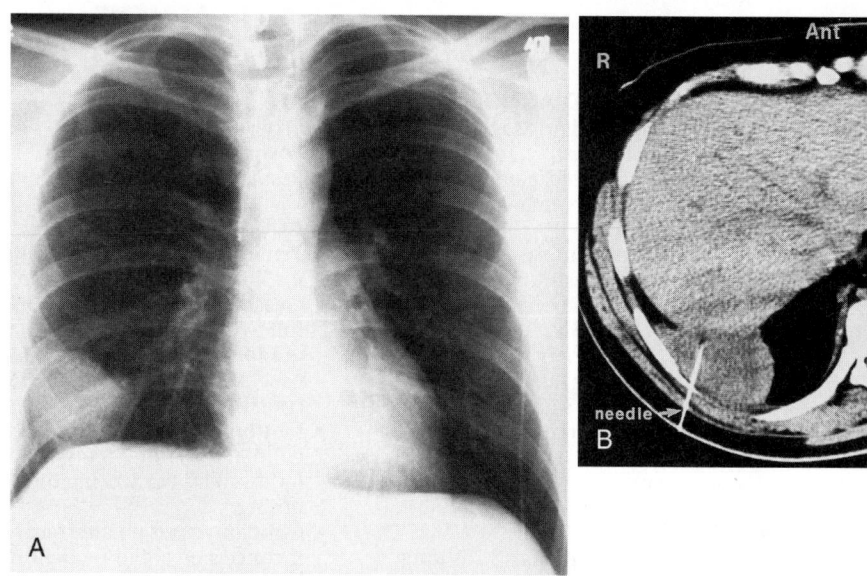

Fig. 1-3 Lung abscess. On a chest radiograph, a lung abscess may look to be a solid rounded lesion **(A),** or, if it has a connection with the bronchus, there may be an air-fluid level in a thick-walled cavitary lesion. CT scanning **(B)** can be used to localize the lesion and to place a needle for drainage and aspiration of contents for culture. (From Mettler FA [ed]: *Primary care radiology,* Philadelphia, 2000, WB Saunders.)

BASIC INFORMATION

■ **DEFINITION**

Pelvic abscess is an acute or chronic infection, most commonly involving the pelvic viscera, initially localized and thus creating its own unique environment, so that treatment and possible cure require specific therapy. There are four categories based on etiologic factors:

- Ascending infection, spreading from cervix through endometrial cavity to adnexa, forming a tuboovarian complex
- Infection occurring in the puerperium, which spreads to the adnexa from the endometrium or myometrium via hematogenous or lymphatic route
- Abscess complicating pelvic surgery
- Involvement of the pelvic viscera secondary to spread from contiguous organs, such as appendicitis or diverticulitis

■ **SYNONYMS**

Tuboovarian abscess (TOA)
Vaginal cuff abscess

ICD-9CM CODES

614.2 Salpingitis and oophoritis not specified as acute, subacute, or chronic

■ **EPIDEMIOLOGY & DEMOGRAPHICS**

INCIDENCE:

- 34% of hospitalized patients with PID
- 1% to 2% of patients undergoing hysterectomy, most with vaginal approach
- Peak incidence third to fourth decade
- 25% to 50% are nulliparous

RISK FACTORS: Same risk factors as for PID, although in 30% to 50% of patients there is no prior history of salpingitis before abscess forms.

■ **PHYSICAL FINDINGS & CLINICAL PRESENTATION**

- Abdominal or pelvic pain (90%)
- Fever or chills (50%)
- Abnormal bleeding (21%)
- Vaginal discharge (28%)
- Nausea (26%)
- Up to 60% to 80% present in the absence of fever or leukocytosis; lack of these findings should not rule out diagnosis

■ **ETIOLOGY**

- Mixed flora of anaerobes, aerobes, and facultative anaerobes, such as *E. coli, B. fragilis, Prevotella* species, aerobic streptococci, *Peptococcus,* and *Peptostreptococcus*

- *N. gonorrhoeae* and *Chlamydia* are the major etiologic factors in cervicitis and salpingitis but are rarely found in abscess cavity cultures.

 DIAGNOSIS

■ **DIFFERENTIAL DIAGNOSIS**

- Pelvic neoplasms, such as ovarian tumors and leiomyomas
- Inflammatory masses involving adjacent bowel or omentum, such as ruptured appendicitis or diverticulitis
- Pelvic hematomas, as may occur after C-section or hysterectomy
- Fig. 3-128 describes the diagnostic approach to patients with a pelvic mass; the differential diagnosis of pelvic mass is described in Box 2-195
- The differential diagnosis of pelvic pain is described in Box 2-196
- Physical examination
- Sonogram or CT scan: commonly employed because, owing to associated pain and guarding, a suboptimal abdominal or pelvic examination is the rule rather than the exception
- Most common cause of preventable death: physician delay in diagnosis

■ **LABORATORY TESTS**

- CBC including WBC with differential, Hgb, and Hct
- Aerobic as well as anaerobic cultures of cervix, blood, urine, sputum, peritoneal cavity (if entered), and abscess cavity before starting antibiotics
- Pregnancy test in patients of reproductive age if the possibility of pregnancy exists

■ **IMAGING STUDIES**

- Sonogram: noninvasive, inexpensive study to confirm diagnosis, estimate size of abscess, and monitor response to therapy; sensitivity >90%
- CT scan: used for both diagnosis and therapy (CT-guided drainage)
  1. Primary focus where sonogram provided insufficient information, as with intraabdominal vs. pelvic abscesses
  2. Success rate with CT-guided abscess drainage: unilocular, 90%; multilocular, 40%

 TREATMENT

Major concerns:
1. Desire for future fertility
2. Likelihood of rupture of abscess, with resulting peritonitis, septic shock, and morbid sequelae

■ **ACUTE GENERAL Rx**

- Decision as to whether patient requires immediate surgery (uncertain diagnosis or suspicion of rupture) or management with IV antibiotics, reserving surgery for those with inadequate clinical response (e.g., 48 to 72 hr of therapy, with persistent fever or leukocytosis, increasing size of mass, or suspicion of rupture)
- Poor response to medical therapy in those with adnexal masses >8 cm, bilateral disease, or immunocompromise
- Antibiotic combinations:
  1. Clindamycin 900 mg IV q8h or metronidazole 500 mg IV q6-8h plus gentamicin either 5 to 7 mg/kg q24h or 1.5 mg/kg q8h
  2. Alternatives: ampicillin sulbactam 3 g IV q6h or cefoxitin 2 g IV q6h or cefotetan 2 g IV q12h plus doxycyline 100 mg IV q12h
- During medical management, high index of suspicion for acute rupture, such as acute worsening of abdominal pain or new-onset tachycardia and hypotension, mandating immediate surgical intervention after patient stabilization
- Surgical options:
  1. Laparoscopy with drainage and irrigation
  2. Transvaginal colpotomy (abscess must be midline, dissect rectovaginal septum, and be adherent to vaginal fornix)
  3. Laparotomy, including total abdominal hysterectomy with bilateral salpingo-oophorectomy or unilateral salpingo-oophorectomy

■ **DISPOSITION**

- Of patients treated with medical therapy, response in 75%, with a 50% pregnancy rate
- No response in 30% to 40%; can be treated with either CT-guided drainage or surgical intervention, keeping in mind that unilateral adnexectomy may give equal chance of cure vs. hysterectomy, yet preserve reproductive potential

■ **REFERRAL**

If patient has a TOA, refer to gynecologist.

 PEARLS & CONSIDERATIONS

■ **COMMENTS**

If *Actinomyces* species is isolated from culture, treatment with penicillin is required for an extended period of time (6 wk to 3 mo).

Author: Scott J. Zuccala, D.O.

BASIC INFORMATION

■ DEFINITION

A perirectal abscess is a localized inflammatory process that can be associated with infections of soft tissue and anal glands based on anatomic location. Perianal and perirectal abscesses may be simple or complex, causing suppuration. Infections in these spaces may be classified as superficial perianal or perirectal with involvement in the following anatomic spaces: ischiorectal, intersphincteric, pestianal, and supraelevator (Fig. 1-4).

■ SYNONYMS

Rectal abscess
Perianal abscess
Anorectal abscess

ICD-9CM CODES

566 Perirectal abscess

■ EPIDEMIOLOGY & DEMOGRAPHICS

INCIDENCE (IN U.S.): Commonly encountered
PREDOMINANT SEX: Male > female
PREDOMINANT AGE: All ages
PEAK INCIDENCE: Not seasonal; common
GENETICS: None known

■ PHYSICAL FINDINGS & CLINICAL PRESENTATION

- Localized perirectal or anal pain—often worsened with movement or straining
- Perirectal erythema or cellulitis
- Perirectal mass by inspection or palpation
- Fever and signs of sepsis with deep abscess
- Urinary retention

■ ETIOLOGY

Polymicrobial aerobic and anaerobic bacteria involving one of the above anatomic spaces, often associated with localized trauma.
Microbiology: most bacteria are polymicrobial, mixed enteric and skin flora
Predominant anaerobic bacteria:
- *Bacteroides fragilis*
- *Peptostreptococcus* spp.
- *Prevotella* spp.
- *Fusobacterium* spp.
- *Porphyromonas* spp.
- *Clostridium* spp.
Predominant aerobic bacteria:
- *Staphylococcus aureus*
- *Streptococcus* spp.
- *Escherichia coli*

DIAGNOSIS

Many patients will have predisposing underlying conditions including:
- Malignancy or leukemia
- Immune deficiency
- Diabetes mellitus
- Recent surgery
- Steroid therapy

■ DIFFERENTIAL DIAGNOSIS

- Neutropenic enterocolitis
- Crohn's disease (inflammatory bowel disease)
- Pilonidal disease
- Hidradenitis suppurativa
- Tuberculosis or actinomycosis; Chagas' disease
- Cancerous lesions
- Chronic anal fistula
- Rectovaginal fistula
- Proctitis—often STD-associated, including:
  Syphilis
  Gonococcal
  Chlamydia
  Chancroid
  Condylomata acuminata
- AIDS-associated:
  Kaposi's sarcoma
  Lymphoma
  CMV

■ WORKUP

- Examination of rectal, perirectal/perineal areas
- Rule out necrotic process and crepitance suggesting deep tissue involvement
- Local aerobic and anaerobic culture

- Blood cultures if toxic, febrile, or compromised
- Possible sigmoidoscopy

■ IMAGING STUDIES

Usually not indicated unless extensive disease abscess

TREATMENT

- Incision and drainage of abscess
- Debridement if necrotic tissue
- Rule out need for fistulectomy
- Local wound care—packing
- Sitz baths

Antibiotic treatment: Directed toward coverage for mixed skins and enteric flora

Outpatient—oral:	Amoxacillin clavulanic acid (Augmentin) Ciprofloxacin plus metronidazole or clindamycin
Inpatient—intravenous:	Ampicillin/ sulbactam (Unasyn) Cefotetan Piperacillin/ tazobactam Imipenem

REFERENCE

Nelson RL et al: Prevalence of benign anorectal disease in a randomly selected population, *Dis Colon Rectum* 88:341, 1994.
Author: **Dennis J. Mikolich, M.D.**

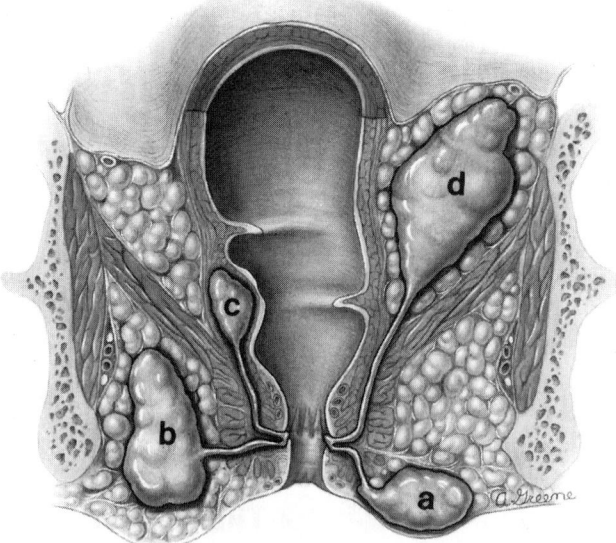

Fig. 1-4 Common sites of anorectal abscesses: perianal *(a)*, ischiorectal *(b)*, intersphincteric *(c)*, and supralevator *(d)*. (From Noble J [ed]: *Textbook of primary care medicine,* ed 2, St Louis, 1996, Mosby.)

BASIC INFORMATION

■ DEFINITION

Child abuse refers to the intentional maltreatment by a caregiver of any child under the age of 18 yr. Four categories generally defined:
1. Neglect: failure to provide basic needs such as food, shelter, supervision
2. Physical abuse: infliction of bodily injury or harm
3. Sexual abuse: passive or active use or exposure of children to sexual acts
4. Emotional abuse: humiliating, coercive behavior that retards a child's psychologic development

■ SYNONYMS

Child maltreatment
Child neglect
Sexual abuse
"Shaken baby syndrome"
"Battered child syndrome"

ICD-9CM CODES
995.5 Child maltreatment syndrome

■ EPIDEMIOLOGY & DEMOGRAPHICS
INCIDENCE (IN U.S.):
- 1.2 cases/100,000 persons/yr (70% physical abuse, 25% sexual abuse, 5% neglect)
- Death rate: 1000 to 4000 children/yr
- 10% of emergency injuries for children <5 yr of age
PREVALENCE (IN U.S.): More than 5% of children <18 yr of age

PREDOMINANT SEX: Females may be at a slightly greater risk.
PREDOMINANT AGE:
- Incidence of all forms of abuse increases with age; teenagers are at twice the risk of infants.
- Risk of death is much higher in children <5 yr.
- Of the 1000 to 4000 annual deaths attributable to abuse, 80% are in children <5 yr, and 40% are in children <1 yr of age. For children <6 mo of age, abuse is the second cause of death (sudden infant death is first).
PEAK INCIDENCE:
- Approximately one third before the age of 1 yr, one third between 1 yr and 6 yr, and one third above age 6 yr
- Handicapped children at a much greater risk throughout childhood
GENETICS:
- No genetic factors are known.
- Sexual abuse is equally distributed throughout all socioeconomic groups, but physical abuse and neglect are more prevalent in lower socioeconomic groups, because abuse increases with severe stress, family violence, and substance abuse.
- Approximately 30% of abused children will abuse their children.

■ PHYSICAL FINDINGS & CLINICAL PRESENTATION
- Presence of multiple injuries of various ages, particularly in the setting of a discrepancy in the history and severity of injury

- Injuries of childhood usually on bony prominences; soft tissue injuries more commonly inflicted by others (Fig. 1-5)
- Burns occur in 10% of abused children; usually result from cigarettes or immersion of buttocks or extremities in scalding hot water
- Retinal hemorrhage diagnostic for "shaken baby syndrome," because it occurs with head injury or sudden compression of the chest (Purtscher's retinopathy)
- Subdural bleeding exceedingly rare in children unless child has suffered shaking or significant head trauma
- Presence of sperm or acid phosphatase in the vaginal vault diagnostic of intercourse within 72 hr and indicates sexual abuse of female child
- Sexually transmitted diseases in a child highly suggestive of sexual abuse
- Disruption of normal genital anatomy often associated with recurrent sexual abuse (e.g., a lax anal sphincter, thickening or darkening of labial skin, significantly enlarged hymen opening)

■ ETIOLOGY
- Sexual abuse of girls: passive mother and domineering father (or stepfather)
- Physical abuse: severe psychosocial stressors such as poverty, unemployment, drug abuse, or marital discord
- History of abuse in the parent or the presence of violence in the family of origin: may predispose to child abuse

MARKS from INSTRUMENTS

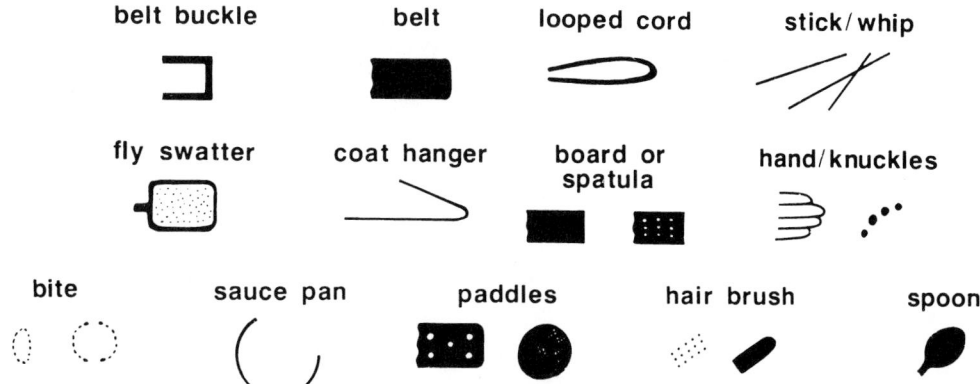

belt buckle   belt   looped cord   stick/whip

fly swatter   coat hanger   board or spatula   hand/knuckles

bite   sauce pan   paddles   hair brush   spoon

Fig. 1-5 A variety of instruments may be used to inflict injury on a child. Often the choice of an instrument is a matter of convenience. Marks tend to silhouette or outline the shape of the instrument. The possibility of intentional trauma should prompt a high degree of suspicion when injuries to a child are geometric, paired, mirrored, of various ages or types, or on relatively protected parts of the body. Early recognition of intentional trauma is important to provide therapy and prevent escalation to more serious injury. (From Behrman RE: *Nelson textbook of pediatrics,* Philadelphia, 1996, WB Saunders.)

- Neglect associated with similar factors, particularly if child's birth was unplanned

DIAGNOSIS

■ DIFFERENTIAL DIAGNOSIS
Distinction from accidental injuries is crucial.

■ WORKUP
- History from the child, caregivers, and other individuals living in the home to reconstruct events and determine any inconsistency or implausibility in the story (Caution is required not to taint the history with the way in which it is obtained or the interviewer's own bias.)
- Physical examination to determine developmental parameters (height, weight) and to document extent and age of bruises
- Examinations for sexual abuse performed within the first 72 hr to be conducted by a rape-crisis team
- Fig. 1-6 describes the management of suspected child abuse

■ LABORATORY TESTS
- Examine fluids in the vaginal vault for sperm and acid phosphatase if intercourse was believed to have occurred within 72 hr.
- Culture oral, vaginal, and anal orifices for sexually transmitted diseases.
- Do bleeding studies if bruising is thought to be secondary to clotting abnormality.
- Examine nutritional, hematopoietic, and endocrine parameters for patients with neglect or failure to thrive.

■ IMAGING STUDIES
- For children ages 2 to 5 yr: obtain a bone survey (skull, thorax, pelvis, spine, arms, and legs).

- In children older than 5 yr: obtain more focused x-rays.
- Do brain imaging if head trauma or shaking is suspected.
- Take color photographs of skin lesions if legal action is anticipated. (NOTE: Parental consent is not required for photos documenting suspected child abuse.)

TREATMENT

■ NONPHARMACOLOGIC THERAPY
- Gear initial interventions toward stabilizing the injuries and preventing further abuse.
- Contact Child Protective Services. (NOTE: Physicians are mandated to report suspected abuse.)
- Where hospitalization is not required, arrange for emergency foster care if possible.
- If a child is returned to abusive environment, 5% mortality rate and 35% severe injury rate is to be expected.

■ ACUTE GENERAL Rx
Pharmacologic intervention is limited to that required to stabilize the injuries.

■ CHRONIC Rx
- Treatment in abusive families is generally poor. A review of several studies including some 3000 families found that a third of abusive parents will continue abuse while in treatment and half may revert to abuse at end of treatment.
- Separation of child via foster care may be traumatic to the child.
- Preventive programs for young single mothers at high risk are thought more effective than other interventions.
- Treatment of sexual abusers is marred by a high recurrence rate.

- In <5% of cases the abuse is related to a psychotic illness that can be treated directly.

■ DISPOSITION
- Victims of abuse and neglect may die or suffer lifelong emotional or physical disability.
- Abused children are more aggressive and have greater interpersonal difficulties. As adults they suffer from depression, anxiety, and substance abuse at twice the rate of the general population, and 30% are likely to abuse their children.
- Victims of sexual abuse will experience problems with sexual identity and function. Of women with borderline personality disorder, 60% have suffered physical or sexual abuse.

■ REFERRAL
- The physician is mandated to report suspected abuse to Child Protective Services.
- Rape-crisis teams exist in most urban areas and are usually better prepared to deal with issues of sexual abuse.
- People at high risk may benefit from prophylactic counseling.
- Most abused children need some therapy to cope with abuse and resulting separation from the family of origin.

REFERENCES
Bethea L: Primary prevention of child abuse, *Am Fam Physician* 59:1577, 1999.
Coury DL: Recognition of child abuse: notes from the field, *Arch Pediatr Adolesc Med* 154:9, 2000.
Lahoh SL et al: Evaluating the child for sexual abuse, *Am Fam Physician* 63:883, 2001.
Taylor SE: The lifelong legacy of childhood abuse, *Am J Med* 107:399, 1999.
Author: **Rif S. El-Mallakh, M.D.**

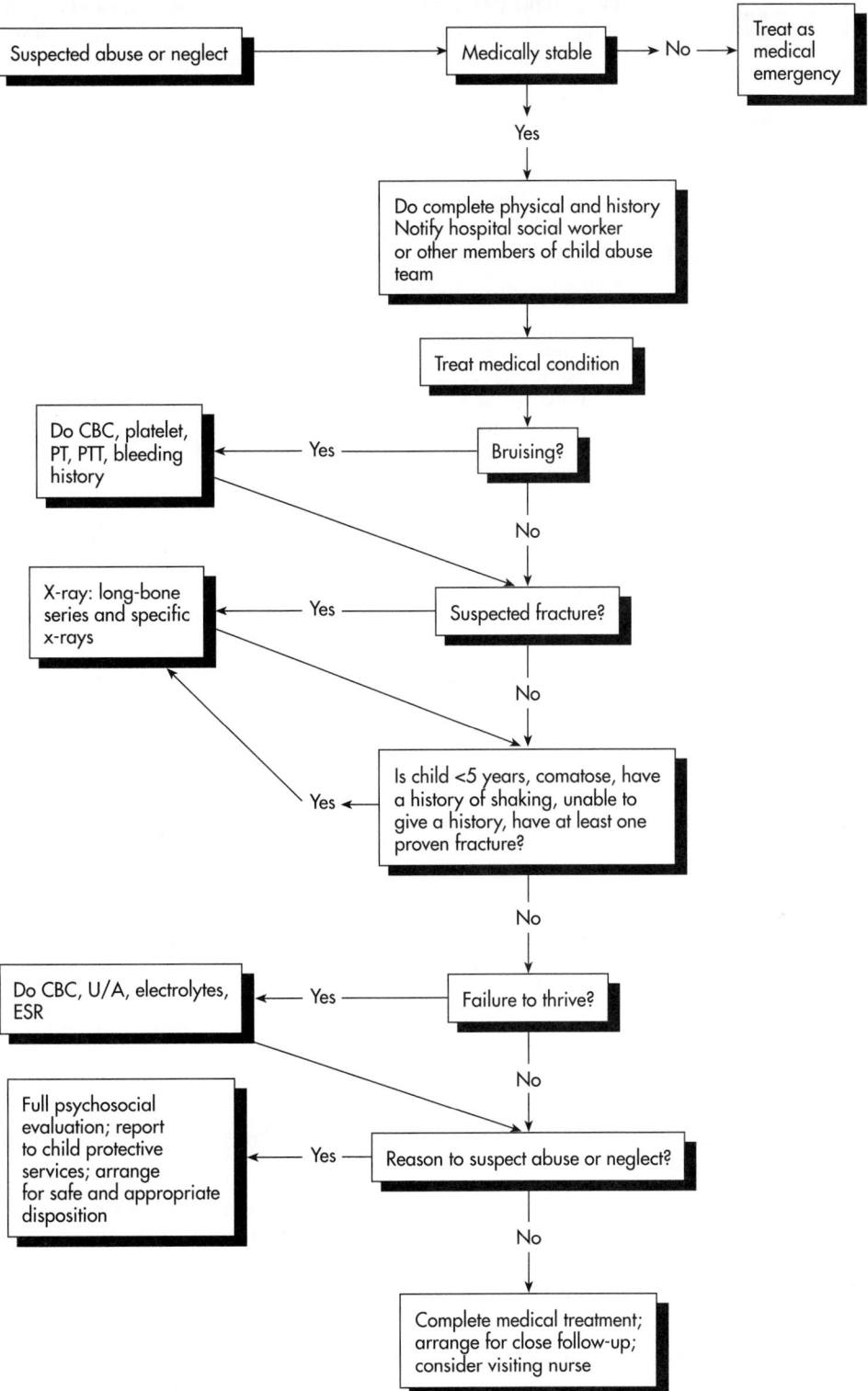

Fig. 1-6   Management of suspected child abuse. *CBC,* Complete blood count; *ESR,* erythrocyte sedimentation rate; *PT,* prothrombin time; *PTT,* partial thromboplastin time; *U/A,* urinalysis. (From Rosen P [ed]: *Emergency medicine,* ed 4, St Louis, 1998, Mosby.)

BASIC INFORMATION

■ DEFINITION
Drug abuse is a recurring pattern of harmful use of a substance despite adverse consequences of the substance in work, school, relationships, the legal system, or personal health. This may occur concurrently with or independently from *substance dependence*, in which there is the presence of physiologic tolerance, discontinuation-induced withdrawal, or inability to willfully control rate or discontinue substance.

■ SYNONYMS
Substance abuse
Addiction

ICD-9CM CODES
Defined by specific substance F10-F19 (DSM-IV code is also defined by specific substance 291-292, 303-305).

■ EPIDEMIOLOGY & DEMOGRAPHICS
INCIDENCE (IN U.S.): For alcohol the incidence is 7%/yr.
PREVALENCE (IN U.S.):
- For alcohol: lifetime
- For cocaine abuse: lifetime prevalence is 0.2%
- For marijuana abuse: lifetime prevalence is 4%
- For amphetamine abuse: lifetime prevalence is 2%
- For hallucinogens: rate is 0.3%
- For opiates: rate is 0.7%
- For nicotine: lifetime prevalence of dependence is 20%

PREDOMINANT SEX:
- Males abuse substances more frequently than females.
- The rates of male:female substance abusers are as follows:
  Alcohol 5:1
  Opiates 3-4:1
  Amphetamines 3-4:1
  Hallucinogens 2:1
  Marijuana 1-2:1
  Cocaine 1:1
PREDOMINANT AGE:
- Problematic use of substances may begin in early life (8 to 10 yr).
- The mean age of onset of problem drinking is about 25 yr for men and 30 yr for women.
PEAK INCIDENCE:
- For most substances: 18 to 30 yr of age
- Men: average >20 yr of heavy drinking
- Women: average 15 yr of heavy drinking
GENETICS
- There is evidence of a nonspecific genetic factor.
- Vulnerability to alcohol abuse is increased in Asians with the alcohol dehydrogenase type 2 isozyme and the aldehyde dehydrogenase type 2 isozyme.

■ PHYSICAL FINDINGS & CLINICAL PRESENTATION
- Abuse of several substances generally occurs together; e.g., alcohol abuse is often found in association with abuse of or dependence on nicotine.
- Symptoms of anxiety, depression, insomnia, cognitive and memory dysfunction, and emotional/behavioral dyscontrol are frequent.

- Alcohol and cocaine abuse are specifically associated with violence and accidents; e.g., more than half of all murderers *and* their victims are intoxicated at the time of the crime.

■ ETIOLOGY
Two models of addiction: (1) Conditioning—substance use paired with enforcing and triggering stimuli, and (2) Homeostatic—either preexisting abnormalities or drug-induced abnormalities lead to initial or continued use of the drug.

🔬 **DIAGNOSIS**

■ DIFFERENTIAL DIAGNOSIS
- Psychiatric disorders such as depression, mania, social phobia, or other anxiety disorders that coexist or occur as a consequence of substance abuse
- Cannot diagnose these disorders accurately in the setting of active substance abuse (Table 1-1)

■ WORKUP
- The history is crucial for diagnosis of any substance abuse disorder; because of frequent denial and poor insight into problem substance abuse, collateral information from family, friends, and co-workers is often helpful.
- Observation of problematic behavior during intoxication or withdrawal is diagnostic.
- Physical examination findings are limited and not diagnostic (e.g., needle scars from repeated intravenous injections, rhinorrhea secondary to intranasal cocaine).

TABLE 1-1 Diagnostic Criteria for Dependence and Drug Abuse

DEPENDENCE (>3 NEEDED)	ABUSE (>1 FOR 12 MO)
1. Tolerance	1. Recurrent substance use resulting in failure to fulfill major role obligations at work, school, or home
2. Withdrawal	
3. The substance is often taken in larger amounts over a longer period than intended	2. Recurrent substance use in situations in which it is physically hazardous
4. Any unsuccessful effort or a persistent desire to cut down or control substance use	3. Recurrent substance-related legal problems
5. A great deal of time is spent in activities necessary to obtain the substance or recover from its effects	4. Continued substance use despite having persistent or recurrent social or interpersonal problems caused or exacerbated by the effects of the substance
6. Important social, occupational, or recreational activities given up or reduced because of substance use	Never met criteria for dependence
7. Continued substance use despite knowledge of having had persistent or recurrent physical or psychological problems that are likely to be caused or exacerbated by the substance	

From Goldman L, Bennett JC (eds): *Cecil textbook of medicine*, ed 21, Philadelphia, 2000, WB Saunders.

■ LABORATORY TESTS
Most helpful tests: toxicology screen or blood alcohol level

■ IMAGING STUDIES
- Not helpful in routine diagnosis and management of substance abuse, but possibly useful in the management of sequelae of substance abuse; e.g., head CT scan to evaluate the alcohol abuse–associated increased risk of subdural hematomas or increased evidence of cerebral atrophy
- Liver ultrasound to evaluate for alcohol-related fatty changes
- Two-dimensional echo for intravenous drug use–associated valvular lesions

℞ TREATMENT

■ NONPHARMACOLOGIC THERAPY
- Relapse prevention by avoidance of trigger stimuli or by uncoupling trigger stimuli from substance ingestion
- Self-help groups such as Alcoholics Anonymous, Narcotics Anonymous, and Al-Anon

■ ACUTE GENERAL Rx
- Acute interventions are usually confined to safe withdrawal in the setting of dependence.
- Benzodiazepines are safe and effective in acute alcohol withdrawal.
- Anticonvulsants, particularly carbamazepine, are used effectively in Europe.
- β-Blockers and clonidine should be avoided in alcohol withdrawal, because they mask markers of the severity of the withdrawal (blood pressure and pulse rate).
- Clonidine alleviates the discomfort of opiate and nicotine withdrawal.
- Nicotine patches and gum reduce withdrawal symptoms.

■ CHRONIC Rx
- Few agents are useful in prevention of substance abuse relapse.
- Disulfiram (Antabuse) workup and metronidazole (Flagyl): possible interaction with alcohol causes physical discomfort.
- Naltrexone helps reduce craving for alcohol.
- Adjunctive use of antidepressants or lithium is helpful when substance use is associated with anxiety and mood symptoms.

- Methadone replacement is used in opiate abuse/dependence (controversial).

■ DISPOSITION
- Substance abuse is a chronic relapsing illness.
- The goal of treatment is always abstinence, but success of treatment is measured by return of function and increasing duration between relapses.
- When substance abuse is complicated by another psychiatric illness, prognosis for both conditions is quite poor.

■ REFERRAL
- Always refer to self-help groups (AA, NA) for patient, Al-Anon for significant others.
- Intensive substance abuse treatment is nearly always indicated in substance-dependent individuals.
- Individuals with coexisting primary psychiatric illness and substance abuse nearly always require the care of a psychiatrist.

Author: **Rif S. El-Mallakh, M.D.**

BASIC INFORMATION

■ **DEFINITION**
Geriatric abuse is the willful infliction of physical pain or injury; emotional pain, injury, humiliation, or intimidation; exploitation or misappropriation of money or property; or neglect by the designated caregiver of nutritional hygiene or medical needs (Box 1-1).

■ **SYNONYMS**
Elder abuse
Battered elder syndrome

■ **ICD-9CM CODES**
995.81 Adult maltreatment syndrome

■ **EPIDEMIOLOGY & DEMOGRAPHICS**
INCIDENCE (IN U.S.): Unknown
PREVALENCE (IN U.S.):
• 3.2% in a large study in Boston.
• Estimated up to 10% of individuals >65 yr of age.
• Only 15% of elder abuse comes to the attention of authorities.
• Most (>60%) abuse is committed by one spouse against another.
• Approximately 25% of abuse is committed by an adult child of the victim who is living in the same home and is usually financially dependent on the victim.

PREDOMINANT SEX:
• No data available
• Women thought to be at greater risk
PREDOMINANT AGE: Risk increases as level of disability, not age, increases
PEAK INCIDENCE: >80 yr old

■ **PHYSICAL FINDINGS & CLINICAL PRESENTATION**
• Physical abuse with multiple injuries at various stages with implausible or inconsistent descriptions of their origins
• Extreme fear, hypervigilance, or withdrawal
• Torn or blood-stained underwear or new onset of a sexually transmitted disease signaling sexual abuse
• Toxicologic evidence of unprescribed medications

■ **ETIOLOGY**
• Relatives with mental illness or substance abuse
• Excessive dependence on the elderly individual for financial, housing, and other necessities
• A history of violence, particularly within the family

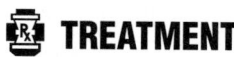 **DIAGNOSIS**

■ **DIFFERENTIAL DIAGNOSIS**
Risk increases as the elder's level of disability increases. Consequently, poor hygiene, poor nutrition, confusion,

psychosis in the setting of dementia, and poor compliance with prescribed treatments may all occur without ongoing abuse.

■ **WORKUP**
• Interview patient separately from the suspected abuser.
• Build trust; patients may be reticent.
• Ask direct questions.
• Be aware that physical findings are usually unexplained injuries or burns.
• An algorithm for the management of suspected domestic violence is described in Fig. 3-55.

■ **LABORATORY TESTS**
• Toxicology screens or therapeutic drug monitoring
• If sexual abuse suspected, screening for sexually transmitted diseases

■ **IMAGING STUDIES**
X-rays as indicated

TREATMENT

■ **NONPHARMACOLOGIC THERAPY**
• Reporting abuse to Adult Protective Services is mandatory in most states. This also provides the physician access to specialized personnel who can aid in evaluation and disposition.
• Separate patient and abuser.
• If the burden of care underlies the abuse, refer to respite services.

■ **ACUTE GENERAL Rx**
As indicated for injury or pain relief

■ **CHRONIC Rx**
If the patient's level of disability does not allow for independent living, institutionalization may be required.

■ **REFERRAL**
Referral to Adult Protective Services is mandatory in 42 states.

REFERENCES
Gerbert B et al: A qualitative analysis of how physicians with expertise in domestic violence approach the identification of victims, *Ann Intern Med* 131:578, 1999.
Hirsh CH et al: The primary care of elder mistreatment, *West J Med* 170:353, 1999.
Kyriacou D et al: Risk factors for injury to women from domestic violence, *N Engl J Med* 341:1892, 1999.
Author: **Rif S. El-Mallakh, M.D.**

BOX 1-1   Types of Geriatric Abuse

Physical abuse
    Assault
    Rough handling
    Burns
    Sexual abuse
    Unreasonable physical confinement
Physical neglect
    Dehydration
    Malnutrition
    Poor hygiene
    Inappropriate or soiled clothing
    Medications given improperly
    Lack of medical care
Psychological abuse
    Verbal or emotional abuse
    Threats
    Isolation/confinement
Material abuse
    Withholding finances
    Misuse of funds
    Theft
    Withholding means for daily living

From Bosker G et al: *Geriatric emergency medicine*, St Louis, 1990, Mosby.

BASIC INFORMATION

■ **DEFINITION**
Acetaminophen poisoning is a disorder manifested by hepatic necrosis, jaundice, somnolence, and potential death if not treated appropriately. Pathologically there is hepatic necrosis.

■ **SYNONYMS**
Paracetamol poisoning

■ **ICD-9CM CODES**
965.4 Acetaminophen poisoning

■ **EPIDEMIOLOGY & DEMOGRAPHICS**
• Potentially toxic ingestions of acetaminophen-containing medications exceed 100,000 cases annually.
• Death rate is approximately 1/1000 persons. Nearly 50% of exposures occur in children <6 yr.
• Hepatic necrosis is most likely to occur in people who are chronically malnourished, who regularly abuse alcohol, and who are using other potentially hepatotoxic medications.

■ **PHYSICAL FINDINGS & CLINICAL PRESENTATION**
• The physical examination may vary depending on the number of hours lapsed from the ingestion of acetaminophen (see Table 1-2).
• Initially, symptoms may be mild or absent and may consist of diaphoresis, malaise, nausea, and vomiting.
• After the initial 12 to 24 hr, patient may complain of RUQ pain with associated vomiting, diaphoresis, and subsequent somnolence.
• In massive overdoses, jaundice may occur within the initial 72 hr.
• Subsequent coma, somnolence, and confusion follow and can ultimately lead to death if not treated appropriately.

■ **ETIOLOGY**
The amount of acetaminophen necessary for hepatic toxicity varies with the patient's body size and hepatic function. Using standardized nomograms,[1] calculating the acetaminophen plasma level and the number of hours after ingestion, the clinician can determine potential hepatic toxicity (see Fig. 1-7).

■ **DIAGNOSIS**

■ **DIFFERENTIAL DIAGNOSIS**
• Liver disease from alcohol abuse or hepatitis
• Ingestion of other hepatotoxic substances

■ **WORKUP**
Initial workup is aimed at confirming acetaminophen overdose with plasma acetaminophen level and assessment of hepatic damage and potential damage to other organ systems, such as kidneys, pancreas, and heart (see "Laboratory Tests"). An acetaminophen overdose algorithm is described in Fig. 1-8.

■ **LABORATORY TESTS**
• Initial laboratory evaluation consists of plasma acetaminophen level with a second level drawn approximately 4 to 6 hr after the initial level. Subsequent levels can be obtained q2-4h until the levels stabilize or decline. These levels can be plotted using the Rumack-Matthew nomogram to calculate potential hepatic toxicity.
• Transaminases (AST, ALT), bilirubin level, prothrombin time, BUN, and creatinine should be initially obtained on all patients.
• Serum and urine toxicology screen for other potential toxic substances is also recommended on admission.

■ **TREATMENT**

■ **NONPHARMACOLOGIC THERAPY**
Consultation with Poison Control Center for management recommendations is recommended in patients with large ingestions of acetaminophen and/or ingestion of other toxic substances. A toxic dose of acetaminophen usually exceeds 7.5 g in the adult or 140 mg/kg.

■ **ACUTE GENERAL Rx**
• Perform gastric lavage and administer activated charcoal if the patient is seen within 1 hr of ingestion or the clinician suspects polydrug ingestion.
• Determine blood levels 4 hr after ingestion; if in the toxic range, start *N*-acetylcysteine (Mucomyst), 140 mg/kg PO as a loading dose, followed by 70 mg/kg PO q4h for 48 hr. (*N*-Acetylcysteine therapy should be started within 24 hr of acetaminophen overdose.) If charcoal therapy was initially instituted, lavage the stomach and recover as much charcoal as possible; then instill *N*-acetylcysteine, increasing the loading dose by 40%.
• Monitor acetaminophen level; use graph to plot possible hepatic toxicity.
• Provide adequate IV hydration (e.g., $D_5\frac{1}{2}NS$ at 150 ml/hr).
• If acetaminophen level is nontoxic, acetylcysteine therapy may be discontinued.

■ **DISPOSITION**
Most patients will recover fully without persisting hepatic abnormalities. Hepatic failure is particularly unusual in children <6 yr.

■ **REFERRAL**
Psychiatric referral is recommended following intentional ingestions.
Author: **Fred F. Ferri, M.D.**

TABLE 1-2   Stages in the Clinical Course of Acetaminophen Toxicity

STAGE	TIME FOLLOWING INGESTION	CHARACTERISTICS
I	½-24 hr	Anorexia, nausea, vomiting, malaise, pallor, diaphoresis
II	24-48 hr	Resolution of above; right upper quadrant abdominal pain and tenderness; elevated bilirubin, prothrombin time, hepatic enzymes; oliguria
III	72-96 hr	Peak liver function abnormalities; anorexia, nausea, vomiting, malaise may reappear
IV	4 days-2 wk	Resolution of hepatic dysfunction or complete liver failure

From Behrman RE: *Nelson textbook of pediatrics,* ed 16, Philadelphia, 2000, WB Saunders.

[1]Rumack BH, Matthew H: *Pediatrics* 55:871, 1975.

Fig. 1-7 Rumack-Matthew nomogram for acetaminophen poisoning. (From Rumack BH, Matthew H: *Pediatrics* 55:871, 1975. In Rosen P [ed]: *Emergency medicine,* ed 4, St Louis, 1998, Mosby.)

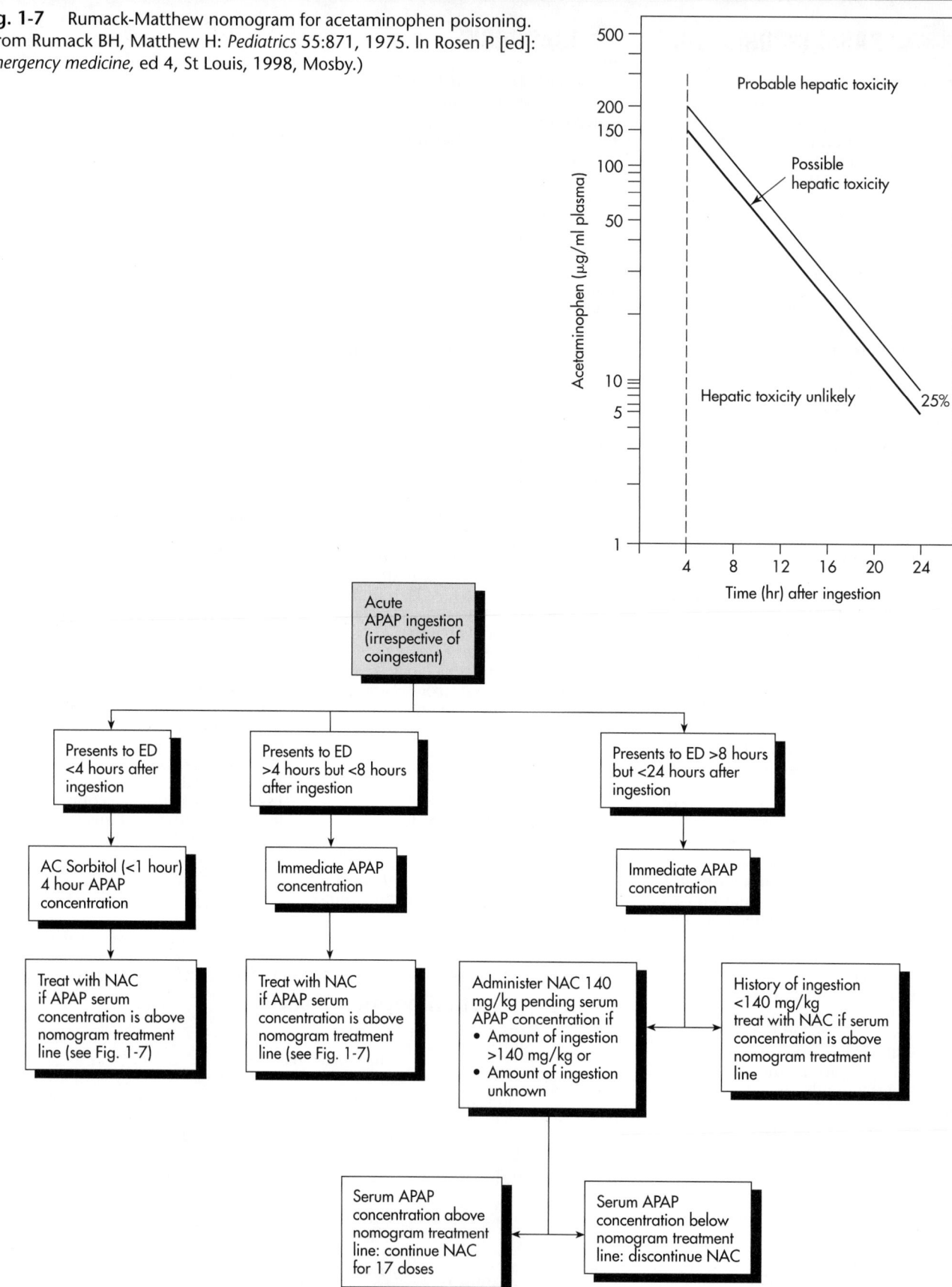

Fig. 1-8 **Treatment of acetaminophen ingestion.** *APAP,* Acetaminophen; *ED,* emergency department; *NAC, N*-acetylcysteine. (From Rosen P [ed]: *Emergency medicine,* ed 4, St Louis, 1998, Mosby.)

BASIC INFORMATION

■ DEFINITION
Achalasia is a motility disorder of the esophagus characterized by inadequate relaxation of the lower esophageal sphincter (LES) and ineffective peristalsis of esophageal smooth muscle. The result is functional obstruction of the esophagus.

■ SYNONYMS
Esophageal achalasia
Esophageal cardiospasm

ICD-9CM CODES
530.0 Achalasia

■ EPIDEMIOLOGY & DEMOGRAPHICS
• Annual incidence is about 1 in 100,000 persons.
• Although the onset of symptoms may occur at any age, it is more common in persons 30 to 50 yr old.
• Men and women are affected equally.

■ PHYSICAL FINDINGS & CLINICAL PRESENTATION
Symptoms:
• Dysphagia to both solid and liquid
• Chest pain and vomiting of undigested food
• Symptoms of aspiration such as nocturnal cough; possible dyspnea and pneumonia
Physical findings:
• If severe and prolonged, then possible weight loss
• Focal lung examination abnormalities and wheezing also possible

■ ETIOLOGY
• Etiology is incompletely understood.
• This motility disorder is likely due to viral or autoimmune degeneration of the esophageal myenteric plexus.
• Herpes zoster and measles virus have been implicated.
• Association with the HLA class II antigen, DQw1, has been noted.

DIAGNOSIS

■ DIFFERENTIAL DIAGNOSIS
• Angina
• Bulimia
• Anorexia nervosa
• Gastric bezoar
• Gastritis
• Peptic ulcer disease
• Esophageal disease:
  GERD
  Sarcoidosis
  Amyloidosis
  Esophageal stricture
  Esophageal webs and rings
  Scleroderma
  Barrett's esophagus
  Lymphoma
  Chagas' disease
  Esophagitis
  Diffuse esophageal spasm
  Infiltrating gastric cancer
  Postvagotomy dysmotility

■ WORKUP
• Physical examination and laboratory analyses to rule out other causes and assess complications
• Imaging studies and manometry for diagnosis

■ LABORATORY TESTS
• Assessment of nutritional status with albumin and prealbumin if indicated
• CBC, ECG, stress test, stool and emesis for occult blood if diagnosis is in doubt

■ IMAGING STUDIES
Barium swallow with fluoroscopy may demonstrate the following findings:
• Uncoordinated or absent esophageal contractions
• An acutely tapered contrast column ("bird's beak," Fig. 1-9)
• Dilation of the distal (smooth muscle portion) esophagus
• Esophageal air fluid level
Manometry may be indicated if barium swallow is inconclusive. Characteristic abnormalities are as follows:
• Low-amplitude disorganized contractions
• High intraesophageal resting pressure
• High LES pressure
• Inadequate LES relaxation after swallow
Direct visualization by endoscopy can rule out other causes of dysphagia.

TREATMENT

Three modalities of treatment:
• Medical:
  Smooth muscle relaxants including nitrates and calcium channel blockers are effective in up to 70% of patients.
  Botulinum toxin injection will benefit up to 90% of patients but will require repeat injections.
• Mechanical dilation:
  Fixed or pneumatic dilators may benefit up to 90%. Esophageal rupture or perforation is a rare complication that can be managed conservatively in some stable patients.
• Surgical
  Open and thoracoscopic esophagomyotomy are available and effective (90%). This approach currently offers the most durable symptom relief. About 10% of patients undergoing surgery will have symptomatic reflux disease.

■ DISPOSITION
Prognosis is excellent in patients who respond to therapy. In long-standing disease or inadequately treated disease, there is an increased risk of squamous cell carcinoma. Chronic GERD, as a result of treatment, may be complicated by Barrett's esophagus and malignant transformation.

■ REFERRAL
Choice of and response to therapy will determine referral. Some surgeons may not be facile with thoracoscopic procedures.

REFERENCES
Spiess AE, Kahrilas PJ: Treating achalasia, *JAMA* 280:638, 1998.
Vaezi MF, Richter JE: Practice guidelines: diagnosis and management of achalasia, *Am J Gastroenterol* 94(12):3406, 1999.
Vaezi MF et al: Botulinum toxin versus pneumatic dilatation in the treatment of achalasia: a randomized trial, *Gut* 44:231, 1999.
Author: **James J. Ng, M.D.**

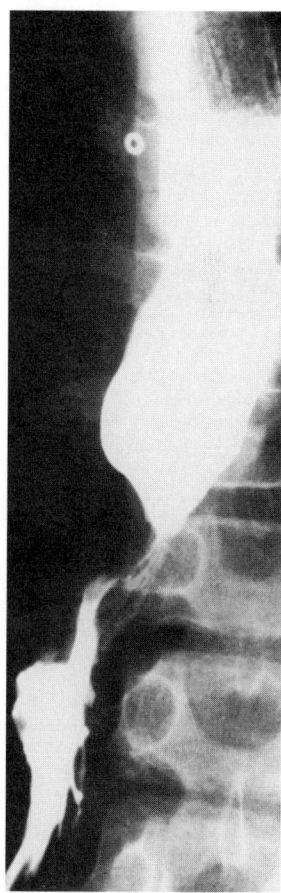

Fig. 1-9 Classic appearance of achalasia of the esophagus. The dilated esophagus ends in a narrow segment. (From Hoekelman R [ed]: *Primary pediatric care,* ed 3, St Louis, 1997, Mosby.)

BASIC INFORMATION

■ **DEFINITION**
Achilles tendon rupture refers to the loss of continuity of the tendo Achillis, usually from attrition.

ICD-9CM CODES
845.09 Achilles tendon rupture

■ **EPIDEMIOLOGY & DEMOGRAPHICS**
PREDOMINANT AGE: 30 to 55 yr

■ **PHYSICAL FINDINGS & CLINICAL PRESENTATION**
Injury often occurs during an activity that puts great stress on the tendon. Sudden "pop" is often felt followed by weakness and swelling.
• Patient walks flat-footed and is unable to stand on the ball of the foot.
• Tenderness and hemorrhage are present at the site of injury, and a sulcus is usually palpable but may be obscured by an organizing clot if the examination is delayed.
• Although active plantar flexion is usually lost, some plantar flexion occasionally remains because of the activity of the other posterior compartment muscles.
• Thompson's test is usually positive. Test measures plantar flexion of the foot when the calf is squeezed with the patient kneeling on a chair; normal foot plantarflexes with calf compression, but movement is absent when tendo Achillis is ruptured.
• Excessive passive dorsiflexion of the foot is also present on the injured side (Fig. 1-10).

■ **ETIOLOGY**
• Relative hypovascularity predisposing to tendon rupture in several tendons (Achilles, biceps, and supraspinatus)
• With advancing age, vascular supply to the tendon further compromised
• Repetitive trauma leading to degeneration of this critical area and weakness
• Rupture of tendo Achillis usually 2.5 to 5 cm from the insertion of the tendon into the os calcis
• Most common causative event leading to rupture: sudden dorsiflexion of the plantar flexed foot (landing from a height) or sudden pushing off with the weight on the forefoot

 DIAGNOSIS

■ **DIFFERENTIAL DIAGNOSIS**
• Incomplete (partial) tendo Achillis rupture
• Partial rupture of gastrocnemius muscle, often medial head (previously thought to be "plantaris tendon rupture")

■ **WORKUP**
• Clinical diagnosis of tendo Achillis rupture is usually obvious.
• If bony injury is suspected, plain roentgenograms are indicated.
• Other studies are usually unnecessary.

 TREATMENT

• Early referral is necessary for surgical repair.
• If surgery is contraindicated, a short leg cast applied with the foot in equinus may allow healing.
• In cases of neglected rupture, reconstruction is usually indicated.

■ **DISPOSITION**
• Prognosis for recovery after surgical repair of the acute rupture is good, but recurrence is not uncommon regardless of treatment.
• Tendo Achillis must be protected from excessive activity for up to 1 yr.
• Results of reconstruction for neglected cases are worse than with primary repair.

REFERENCE
Moller M et al: Acute rupture of the tendo achilles, *J Bone Joint Surg* 83(B):843, 2001.
Author: **Lonnie R. Mercier, M.D.**

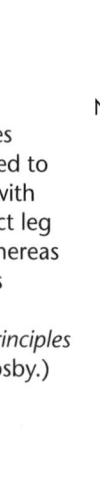
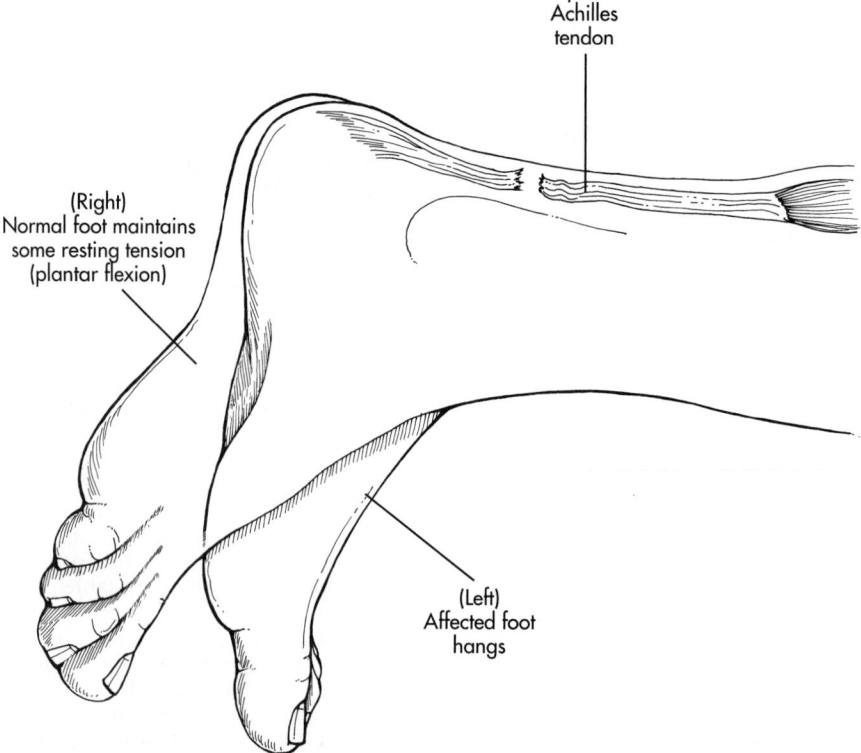

Fig. 1-10 Observation of Achilles tendon rupture. The patient is asked to lie prone on the examining table with feet hanging off the end. The intact leg retains inherent plantar flexion, whereas on the injured side, the foot hangs straight down with gravity. (From Scudieri G [ed]: *Sports medicine: principles of primary care,* St Louis, 1997, Mosby.)

BASIC INFORMATION

■ **DEFINITION**
Acne vulgaris is a chronic disorder of the pilosebaceous apparatus caused by abnormal desquamation of follicular epithelium leading to obstruction of the pilosebaceous canal, resulting in inflammation and subsequent formation of papules, pustules, nodules, comedones, and scarring.

■ **SYNONYMS**
Acne

ICD-9CM CODES
706.1 Acne vulgaris

■ **EPIDEMIOLOGY & DEMOGRAPHICS**
• Acne is the most common skin disease in the U.S.
• It is most common in teenagers (highest incidence between ages of 16 and 18 yr).

■ **PHYSICAL FINDINGS & CLINICAL PRESENTATION**
• Open comedones (blackheads), closed comedones (whiteheads)
• Greasiness (oily skin)
• Presence of scars from prior acne cysts
• Various stages of development and severity may be present concomitantly
• Common distribution of acne: face, back, and upper chest
• Inflammatory papules, pustules, and ectatic pores

■ **ETIOLOGY**
• Overactivity of the sebaceous glands and blockage in the ducts. The obstruction leads to the formation of comedomes, which can become inflamed because of overgrowth of *Propionibacterium acnes*.
• Exacerbated by environmental factors (hot, humid, tropical climate), medications (e.g., iodine in cough mixtures, hair greases), industrial exposure to halogenated hydrocarbons.

DIAGNOSIS

■ **DIFFERENTIAL DIAGNOSIS**
• Gram-negative folliculitis
• Staphylococcal pyoderma
• Acne rosacea
• Drug eruption
• Sebaceous hyperplasia
• Angiofibromas, basal cell carcinomas, osteoma cutis
• Occupational exposures to oils or grease
• Steroid acne

■ **WORKUP**
History and physical examination:
• Inquire about previous treatment
• Careful drug history
• Family history, history of cyclic menstrual flares
• History of use of cosmetics and cleansers
• Oral contraceptive use

■ **LABORATORY TESTS**
• Laboratory evaluation is generally not helpful.
• Patients who are candidates for therapy with isotretinoin (Accutane) should have baseline liver enzymes, cholesterol, and triglycerides checked, because this medication may result in elevation of lipids and liver enzymes.
• A negative serum pregnancy test should also be obtained in females 1 wk before initiation of isotretinoin; it is also imperative to maintain effective contraception during and 1 mo after therapy with isotretinoin ends because of its teratogenic effects.

TREATMENT

■ **NONPHARMACOLOGIC THERAPY**
• Contrary to popular belief, diet has little or no bearing on acne. Greasy foods do not cause acne. If the patient, however, feels that a particular food is exacerbating the acne, it should be avoided.
• Acne is not caused by dirt; therefore, excessive washing is unnecessary.
• Long-term exposure to coal tar, machine oil, lubricating oils, and greases should be avoided; use of hair pomades containing oils should also be avoided; topical exposure to cocoa butter can also exacerbate acne and should be avoided.

■ **ACUTE GENERAL Rx**
Treatment generally varies with the type of lesions (comedomes, papules, pustules, cystic lesions) and the severity of acne.
• Comedones can be treated with tretinoin (Retin-A); it is applied generally once qhs; large open comedones (blackheads) should be expressed.
• Patients should be reevaluated after 4 to 6 wk. Benzoyl peroxide gel (2.5% or 5%) may be added if the comedones become inflamed or form pustules. Topical antibiotics (erythromycin, clindamycin lotions or pads) can also be used in patients with significant inflammation. The combination of 5% benzoyl peroxide and 3% erythromycin (Benzamycin) is highly effective in patients who

have a mixture of comedonal and inflammatory acne lesions.
• Pustular acne can be treated with tretinoin and benzoyl peroxide gel applied on alternate evenings; drying agents (sulfacetamide-sulfa lotions [Novacet, Sulfacet]) are also effective when used in combination with benzoyl peroxide; oral antibiotics (doxycycline 100 mg qd or erythromycin 1 g qd given in two to three divided doses) are effective in patients with moderate to severe pustular acne; patients not responding well to these antibiotics can be switched over to minocycline 50 to 100 mg bid; however, this medication is more expensive.
• Patients with nodular cystic acne can be treated with systemic agents: antibiotics (erythromycin, tetracycline, doxycycline, minocycline), isotretinoin (Accutane), or oral contraceptives. Periodic intralesional triamcinolone (Kenalog) injections by a dermatologist are also effective. The possibility of endocrinopathy should be considered in patients responding poorly to therapy.
• Isotretinoin is indicated for acne resistant to antibiotic therapy and severe acne; dosage is 0.5 to 1 mg/kg/day in two divided doses (maximum of 2 mg/kg/day); duration of therapy is generally 20 wk for a cumulative dose ≥120 mg/kg for severe cystic acne; before using this medication patients should undergo baseline laboratory evaluation (see above). This drug is absolutely contraindicated during pregnancy because of its teratogenicity.
• Oral contraceptives reduce androgen levels and therefore sebum production. They represent a useful adjunctive therapy for all types of acne in women and adolescent girls.

■ **REFERRAL**
Referral for intralesional injection and dermabrasion should be considered in patients with severe acne unresponsive to conventional therapy.

PEARLS & CONSIDERATIONS

■ **COMMENTS**
Indications for systemic therapy of acne are:
• Painful deep papules or nodules
• Extensive lesions
• Active acne with severe scarring or hyperpigmentation
• Patient's morale
Patients should be educated that in most cases acne can be controlled but not cured and that at least 4 to 6 wk of initial therapy should be required before significant improvement is noted.
Author: **Fred F. Ferri, M.D.**

BASIC INFORMATION

■ **DEFINITION**

Acoustic neuroma is a benign proliferation of the Schwann cells that cover the vestibular branch of the eighth cranial nerve (CN VIII). Symptoms are commonly a result of compression of the acoustic branch of CN VIII, the facial nerve (CN VII), and the trigeminal nerve (CN V). The glossopharyngeal nerve (CN IX) and vagus nerve (CN X) are less commonly involved. In extreme cases, compression of the brainstem may lead to obstruction of CSF outflow and elevated intracranial pressure (ICP).

■ **SYNONYMS**

Vestibular schwannoma

ICD-9CM CODES

225.1 Acoustic neuroma

■ **EPIDEMIOLOGY &**
   DEMOGRAPHICS

Annual incidence is about 1 in 100,000 patients per year. There may be a slight female predominance. The tumor most commonly presents in the fifth and sixth decades.

■ **PHYSICAL FINDINGS & CLINICAL**
   PRESENTATION

• Hearing loss, unilateral tinnitus, balance problems, vertigo, facial pain (trigeminal neuralgia) and weakness, difficulty swallowing, fullness or pain of the involved ear, and headache may occur.
• With elevated ICP, patients may also suffer from vomiting, fever, and visual changes.
• Hearing loss is the most common presenting complaint and is usually high frequency.

■ **ETIOLOGY**

The etiology is incompletely understood. Bilateral acoustic neuromas may be inherited in an autosomal dominant manner as part of neurofibromatosis type 2. This disease is associated with a defect on chromosome 22q1.

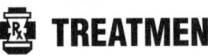 **DIAGNOSIS**

■ **DIFFERENTIAL DIAGNOSIS**

Benign positional vertigo, Meniere's disease, trigeminal neuralgia, cerebellar disease, normal-pressure hydrocephalus, presbycusis, glomus tumors, vertebrobasilar insufficiency, ototoxicity from medications, and other tumors: meningioma, glioma, facial nerve schwannoma, cavernous hemangioma, metastatic tumors

■ **WORKUP**

Physical examination, laboratory analysis, and imaging studies

■ **PHYSICAL EXAMINATION**

• A detailed neurologic examination with special attention to the cranial nerves is crucial.
• Otoscopic evaluation may help to rule out other causes of hearing loss.

■ **LABORATORY TESTS**

CSF protein may be elevated.

■ **IMAGING STUDIES**

• CT scan with contrast can detect tumors 1 cm in diameter or larger (Fig. 1-11).
• MRI with gadolinium is the most sensitive noninvasive test and can detect tumors as small as 2 mm in diameter.

℞ TREATMENT

Treatment decisions should be based on the size of the tumor, rate of growth (older patients tend to have slower-growing tumors), degree of neurologic deficit, life expectancy, age of the patient, and surgical risk.

• Surgery is the definitive treatment. Choice of approach (middle cranial fossa, translabyrinthine or posterior cranial fossa) may vary depending on the size of the tumor, amount of residual hearing, and degree of surgical risk that can be tolerated. Partial resection is sometimes undertaken to minimize the risk of injury to nearby structures. Intraoperative facial nerve monitoring is recommended.
• Radiotherapy has been used to treat tumors that are less than 3 cm in diameter. Radiotherapy following partial resection has also been used to minimize complications.
• Observation may be appropriate for older or frail patients with small tumors, but serial scanning may not be able to detect neurologically significant growth and risk may be higher if surgery is delayed.

■ **DISPOSITION**

Hearing can be preserved at near preoperative levels in more than two thirds of patients with small- to medium-sized tumors.

■ **REFERRAL**

Prompt referral to an ENT specialist who is facile with all three surgical approaches is recommended.

REFERENCES

Kondziolka D et al: Long-term outcomes after radiosurgery for acoustic neuromas, *N Engl J Med* 339:1426, 1999.
Pitts LH, Jackler RK: Treatment of acoustic neuromas, *N Engl J Med* 339:1471, 1998.
Poen JC et al: Fractionated stereotactic radiosurgery and preservation of hearing in patients with vestibular schwannoma: a preliminary report, *Neurosurgery* 45(6):1299, 1999.
Author: **James J. Ng, M.D.**

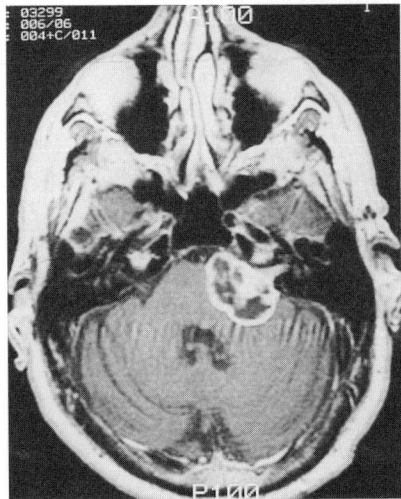

Fig. 1-11 Acoustic schwannoma. Axial, postcontrast-enhanced T1-weighted image demonstrates an inhomogeneously contrast-enhancing mass in the left cerebellopontine angle with extension into the left internal auditory canal. There is associated displacement of the brainstem. (From Specht N [ed]: *Practical guide to diagnostic imaging,* St Louis, 1998, Mosby.)

BASIC INFORMATION

■ DEFINITION
Acquired immunodeficiency syndrome (AIDS) is a disorder caused by infection with the human immunodeficiency virus, type 1 (HIV-1) and marked by progressive deterioration of the cellular immune system, leading to secondary infections or malignancies.

■ SYNONYMS
AIDS

ICD-9CM CODES
042.9 AIDS, unspecified

■ EPIDEMIOLOGY & DEMOGRAPHICS
INCIDENCE (IN U.S.):
- 27.1 cases/100,000 persons
- Varies widely by location
- 85% of cases in large cities

PREVALENCE (IN U.S.): 62 cases/100,000 persons

PREDOMINANT SEX: Males 84%, females 16% (through 1998) 40% of newly reported U.S. cases in 1999 were in women.

PREDOMINANT AGE: 80% between ages 20 and 40 yr

PEAK INCIDENCE: See above

GENETICS:
- Familial disposition: no clear genetic predisposition
- Congenital infection:
  1. Transmittable from an infected mother to the fetus in utero in as many as 30% of pregnancies.
  2. No specific congenital malformations associated with infection; low birth weight and spontaneous abortion are possible.
- Neonatal infection: transmission possible to the neonate intrapartum or postpartum through breast-feeding

■ PHYSICAL FINDINGS & CLINICAL PRESENTATION
- Nonspecific findings: fever, weight loss, anorexia
- Specific syndromes:
  1. Seen in association with opportunistic infection and malignancies, so-called indicator diseases
  2. Most common:
     Respiratory infections (*Pneumocystis carinii* pneumonia, TB, bacterial pneumonia, fungal infection)
     CNS infections (toxoplasmosis, cryptococcal meningitis, TB)
     GI (cryptosporidiosis, isosporiasis, cytomegalovirus); Table 2-98 and Table 3-5 describe organisms associated with diarrhea in patients with AIDS
     Eye infections (cytomegalovirus, toxoplasmosis)
     Kaposi's sarcoma (cutaneous or visceral) or lymphoma (nodal or extranodal)
- Possibly asymptomatic

- Diagnosis of AIDS if T-lymphocyte subset analysis demonstrating CD4 cell count <200 or <14% of total lymphocyte in the presence of proven HIV infection even in the absence of other infections
- The various manifestations of HIV infection are described in Boxes 2-127 to 2-131 and Tables 2-95 to 2-102

■ ETIOLOGY
- Caused by infection with human immunodeficiency virus, type 1 (HIV-1)
- Transmitted by heterosexual or male homosexual contact, needle-sharing (during IV drug use), transfusion of contaminated blood or blood products, and from infected mother to fetus or neonate as described above

DIAGNOSIS

■ DIFFERENTIAL DIAGNOSIS
- Other wasting illnesses mimicking the nonspecific features of AIDS:
  1. TB
  2. Neoplasms
  3. Disseminated fungal infection
  4. Malabsorption syndromes
  5. Depression
- Other disorders associated with dementia or demyelination producing encephalopathy, myelopathy, or neuropathy

■ WORKUP
Prompt evaluation of respiratory, CNS, GI complaints

■ LABORATORY TESTS
- HIV antibody testing
- T-lymphocyte subset analysis: performed to determine the degree of immunodeficiency
- Viral load assay: to plan long-term antiviral therapy consider genotype or phenotype sensitivity testing for patients failing therapy
- CSF examination: for meningitis
- Serologic tests for syphilis, hepatitis B, hepatitis C, and toxoplasmosis

■ IMAGING STUDIES
- Cerebral CT for encephalopathy or focal CNS complications (e.g., toxoplasmosis, lymphoma)
- Pulmonary gallium scanning to aid in the diagnosis of a *Pneumocystis carinii* pneumonia

TREATMENT

■ NONPHARMACOLOGIC THERAPY
- Maintain adequate caloric intake
- Encourage good oral hygiene, regular dental care

■ ACUTE GENERAL Rx
Acute management of opportunistic infections and malignancies is reviewed elsewhere in this text under specific AIDS-related disorders.

■ CHRONIC Rx
For all HIV-infected patients, particularly those meeting the case definition of AIDS:
- Preventive therapy for *Pneumocystis carinii* pneumonia and TB (see specific chapters elsewhere in this text).
- Antiretroviral therapy employing combinations of nucleoside derivative agents: zidovudine (AZT), didanosine (DDI), zalcitabine (DDC), lamivudine (3TC), stavudine (D4T), abacavir in addition to protease inhibitors (saquinavir, ritonavir, indinavir, nelfinavir, agenerase, ritonavir/lopinavir) nonnucleoside reverse transcriptase inhibitors (nevirapine, delavirdine, efavirenz) or the nucleotide agent tenofovir according to current recommendations based on clinical stage and viral load studies.
- An approach to evaluating chronic diarrhea in patients with HIV infection is described in Fig. 3-53. Fig. 3-80 describes the approach to the acutely ill HIV-infected patient. Evaluation of respiratory complaints is described in Fig. 3-81. Approach to a patient with a suspected CNS lesion is described in Fig. 3-103.
- Genotypic resistance testing should be strongly considered for any patient failing antiretroviral therapy.

■ REFERRAL
All patients with AIDS: to a physician knowledgeable and experienced in the management of the disease and its complications

REFERENCES
Carpenter C et al: Antiretroviral therapy in adults, updated recommendations of the International AIDS Society-USA Panel, *JAMA* 283:381, 2000.

Henry K: The case for more cautious, patient-focused antiretroviral therapy, *Ann Intern Med* 132(4):307, 2000.

Isada CM: New developments in long-term treatment of HIV: the honeymoon is over, *Cleve Clin J Med* 68(9):804, 2001.

Kaplan JE et al: Epidemiology of human immunodeficiency virus–associated opportunistic infections in the United States in the era of highly active antiretroviral therapy, *Clin Infect Dis* 30(suppl 1):S5, 2000.

Palmer S et al: Tenofovir, adefovir and zidovudine susceptibilities of primary human immunodeficiency virus type 1 isolates with non-B subtypes or nucleoside resistance, *AIDS Res Hum Retroviruses* 17(12):1167, 2001.

Piot P et al: The global impact of HIV/AIDS, *Nature* 410:968, 2001.

Richman DD: HIV chemotherapy, *Nature* 410:995, 2001.
Author: **Joseph R. Masci, M.D.**

BOX 1-2   Conditions Included in the 1993 AIDS Surveillance I Case Definition

Bacterial infections, multiple or recurrent*
Candidiasis of bronchi, trachea, or lungs
Candidiasis, esophageal
Cervical cancer, invasive†
Coccidioidomycosis, disseminated or extrapulmonary
Cryptococcosis, extrapulmonary
Cryptosporidiosis, chronic intestinal (>1-mo duration)
Cytomegalovirus disease (other than liver, spleen, or nodes)
Cytomegalovirus retinitis (with loss of vision)
Encephalopathy, HIV related
Herpes simplex, chronic ulcer(s) (>1-mo duration); or bronchitis, pneumonitis, or esophagitis
Histoplasmosis, disseminated or extrapulmonary
Isoporiasis, chronic intestinal (>1-mo duration)
Kaposi's sarcoma

Lymphoid interstitial pneumonia and/or pulmonary lymphoid hyperplasia*
Lymphoma, Burkitt's (or equivalent term)
Lymphoma, primary, of brain
Mycobacterium avium-intracellulare complex or *Myobacterium kansasii,* disseminated or extrapulmonary
Mycobacterium tuberculosis, any site (pulmonary† or extrapulmonary)
Mycobactrium, other species or unidentified species, disseminated or extrapulmonary
Pneumocystis carinii pneumonia
Pneumonia, recurrent†
Progressive multifocal leukoencephalopathy
Salmonella septicemia, recurrent
Toxoplasmosis of brain
Wasting syndrome of HIV infection

*Children younger than 13 years.
†Added in the 1993 expansion of the AIDS surveillance case definition for adolescents and adults.

TABLE 1-3   Approved Nucleoside Reverse Transcriptase Inhibitors

AGENT	TRADE NAME	ORAL BIOAVAIL-ABILITY (%)	SERUM HALF-LIFE (H)	INTRACELLULAR HALF-LIFE OF TRIPHOSPHATE (H)	ELIMINATION	DOSE*	AVAILABIILITY	MAJOR ADVERSE EFFECTS‡
Zidovudine	Retrovir	63	1.1	3-4	Hepatic glucuronidation Renal excretion	Adults: 200 mg PO q8h or 300 mg PO q12h Pediatric: 90-180 mg/m² PO q6-12h, up to adult dose	300-mg tablets 100-mg capsules 10-mg/ml syrup 10-mg/ml solution for IV infusion	Headache Insomnia Gastrointestinal intolerance Fatigue Anemia Neutropenia Myositis
Didanosine	Videx	40	1.5	8-24	Cellular metabolism Renal excretion	Adult ≥60 kg: powder 250 mg PO q12h; tablets 200 mg PO q12h Adult <60 kg: powder 167 mg PO q12h; tablets 125 mg PO q12h Pediatric: 90-150 mg/m² PO q12h of solution up to adult dose	25-mg, 50-mg, 100-mg, 150-mg chewable tablets 100-mg, 167-mg, 250-mg powder packets 10-mg/ml solution	Diarrhea Abdominal discomfort Nausea Peripheral neuropathy Pancreatitis
Zalcitabine	Hivid	87	1.2	2.6	Renal excretion	Adult: 0.75 mg PO q8h	0.375-mg, 0.75-mg tablets	Peripheral neuropathy Pancreatitis Oral ulcers
Stavudine	Zerit	86	1.1	3	Renal excretion	Adult ≥60 kg: 40 mg PO q12h Adult <60 kg: 30 mg PO q12h Pediatric: 1 mg/kg q12h, up to adult dose	15-mg, 20-mg, 30-mg, 40-mg capsules 1-mg/ml solution	Peripheral neuropathy
Lamivudine	Epivir	86	2.5	11-14	Renal excretion	Adult: 150 mg PO q12h Pediatric: 4 mg/kg PO q12h, up to adult dose	150-mg tablets 10-mg/ml solution	Headache Fatigue
Abacavir	Ziagen	83	1.5	3.3	Hepatic glucuronidation and carboxylation	Adult: 300 mg PO q12h Pediatric: 8 mg/kg PO q12h, up to adult dose	300-mg tablets 20-mg/ml solution	Hypersensitivity reaction
Zidovudine + Lamivudine	Combivir†					Adult: One tablet PO q12h	300-mg zidovudine/150-mg lamivudine tablet	

From Mandell GL: *Mandell, Douglas, and Bennett's principles and practice of infectious diseases,* ed 5, New York, 2000, Churchill Livingstone.
*Neonatal dose may differ significantly from pediatric dose described here.
†Pharmacokinetic properties, adverse effects, and drug interactions are similar to those of lamivudine and zidovudine used separately.
‡All nucleoside reverse transcriptase inhibitors may also be associated with rare occurrence of potentially fatal lactic acidosis and hepatomegaly with steatosis.

TABLE 1-3   Approved Nonnucleoside Reverse Transcriptase Inhibitors—cont'd

AGENT	TRADE NAME	ORAL BIOAVAIL-ABILITY (%)	SERUM HALF-LIFE (H)	ELIMINATION	DOSE*	AVAILABIILITY	MAJOR ADVERSE EFFECTS
Nevirapine	Viramune	>90	>24	Hepatic cytochrome P450	Adult: 200 mg PO qd for 14 d, then 200 mg PO q12h if no rash develops Pediatric: 120 mg/m² PO qd for 14 d then increase to 120-200 mg/m² PO q12h if no rash develops, up to adult dose	200-mg tablets	Rash Elevated hepatic transaminases
Delavirdine	Rescriptor	85	5.8	Hepatic cytochrome P450	Adult: 400 mg PO q8h	100-mg tablets	Rash Dizziness
Efavirenz	Sustiva		>24	Hepatic cytochrome P450	Adult: 600 mg PO qd	50 mg-, 100 mg-, 200 mg-capsules	Headache Rash

*Neonatal dose may differ significantly from pediatric dose described here.

TABLE 1-4   Approved Protease Inhibitors

AGENT	TRADE NAME	ORAL BIOAVAIL-ABILITY (%)	SERUM HALF-LIFE (H)	ELIMINATION	DOSE*	AVAILABIILITY	MAJOR ADVERSE EFFECTS†
Saquinavir (soft gel capsule)	Fortovase		1-2	Hepatic cytochrome P450	Adult: 1200 mg PO q8h	200-mg soft gel capsules	Nausea Diarrhea Abdominal discomfort
Saquinavir (hard capsule)	Invirase	4	1-2	Hepatic cytochrome P450	Adult: When used in combination with ritonavir, 400-600 mg PO q12h	200-mg hard capsules	Nausea Diarrhea Abdominal discomfort
Ritonavir	Norvir	70	3.2	Hepatic cytochrome P450	Adult: 300 mg PO q12h with escalation over 1-2 wk to 600 mg PO q12h When used in combination with saquinavir, dose often decreased to 400 mg PO q12h Pediatric: 250 mg/m² of solution PO q12h with escalation over 1-2 wk to 400 mg/m² PO q12h, up to adult dose	100-mg capsules 80-mg/ml solution	Nausea, vomiting Diarrhea Abdominal discomfort Circumoral or peripheral paresthesias Fatigue Altered taste Hypercholesterolemia Hypertriglyceridemia Elevated hepatic transaminases
Indinavir	Crixivan	60-65	1.8	Hepatic cytochrome P450	Adults: 800 mg PO q8h	200-mg, 400-mg capsules	Nausea Abdominal discomfort Nephrolithiasis Hyperbilirubinemia
Nelfinavir	Viracept	20-80	3.5-5	Hepatic cytochrome P450	Adult: 750 mg PO q8h Pediatric: 20-30 mg/kg q8h, up to adult dose	250-mg tablets 50-mg/g powder	Diarrhea
Amprenavir	Agenerase		9	Hepatic cytochrome P450	Adult: Capsule 1200 mg PO q12h Pediatric: Capsule 20 mg/kg PO q12h or 15 mg/kg PO q8h, up to adult dose; solution 22.5 mg/kg PO q12h or 17 mg/kg PO q8h, up to 2800	50-mg, 150-mg capsules 15 mg/ml solution	Nausea, vomiting Rash
Lopinavir/ ritonavir	Kaletra	Not yet established	5-6	Hepatic cytochrome P450	3 capsules 2×/day	Soft-gel capsules 133.3 mg lopinavir 33.3 mg ritonavir	Diarrhea, pancreatitis

From Mandell GL: *Mandell, Douglas, and Bennett's principles and practice of infectious diseases*, ed 5, New York, 2000, Churchill Livingstone.
*Neonatal dose may differ significantly from pediatric dose described here.
†All protease inhibitors may be associated with hyperglycemia and changes in body fat distribution. They may also be associated with rare episodes of hemorrhage in persons with hemophilia.

TABLE 1-4A   Approved Nucleotide Reverse Transcriptase Inhibitor

AGENT	TRADE NAME	ORAL BIO-AVAILABILITY (%)	SERUM HALF-LIFE (H)	ELIMINATION	DOSE	AVAILABILITY	MAJOR ADVERSE EFFECTS
Tenofovir	Viread	25	—	Renal	300-mg/d	300-mg tablet	Nausea, vomiting, diarrhea

TABLE 1-5   Therapy for Opportunistic Infections in Patients with HIV Infection

CLINICAL DISEASE	DRUG	DOSE	ROUTE	INTERVAL	DURATION
Pneumocystis pneumonia	Trimethoprim with sulfamethoxazole	5 mg/kg with 25 mg/kg	PO, IV	q8h	21 d
	or				
	Trimethoprim plus dapsone	300 mg	PO	18h	21 d
	or	100 mg	PO	qd	
	Pentamidine	3-4 mg/kg	IV (IM)	qd	21 d
	or				
	Atovaquone	750 mg	PO	q12h	21 d
	or				
	Clindamycin plus primaquine	300-450 mg	PO, IV	q6h	21 d
	or	15 mg	PO	qd	
	Trimetrexate plus leucovorin	45 mg/m^2	IV	q24h	21 d
		20 mg/m^2	PO, IV	q6h	
	Prednisone (adjuctive tehrapy for severe episode)	40 mg	PO	q12h*	21 d
Pneumocystis pneumonia (maintenance)	Trimethoprim plus sulfamethoxazole	1 single- or double-strength tablet	PO	q24h	Lifelong¶
	or				
	Dapsone	100 mg	PO	q24h	Lifelong
Toxoplasmosis	Sulfadiazine plus pyrimethamine plus leucovorin	1-2 g	PO	q6h	Lifelong
		100 mg†	PO	qd	Lifelong
	or	10-25 mg	PO, IV	qd	Lifelong
	Clindamycin plus pyrimethamine	450-600 mg	PO	q6h	Lifelong
		50-100 mg†	PO	qd	Lifelong
Cryptosporidiosis	Paromomycin	1.0 g	PO	bid	Lifelong
Microsporidiosis	Albendazole	400 mg	PO	bid	Lifelong
Isosporiasis	Trimethoprim wih sulfamethoxazole	160 mg	PO, IV	q6h	10 d
	followed by	800 mg			
	Trimethoprim plus sulfamethaxazole	160 mg	PO	bid	14 d
Candidiasis		800 mg			
Oral	Fluconazole	100-200 mg	PO, IV	q24h	5-10 d
Esophageal	Fluconazole	100-400 mg	PO, IV	q24h	14-21 d
Vaginal	Fluconazole	150 mg	PO	—	One dose
Coccidioidomycosis (Pulmonary)	Amphotericin B	0.5-1.0 mg/kg	IV	q24h	≥56 d
	followed by				
	Itraconazole	300 mg	PO	bid	3 d
	followed by	200 mg	PO	bid	Lifelong
	Fluconazole	400-800 mg	PO	q24h	Lifelong
Cryptococcal infection	Amphotericin B with flucytosine	0.7 mg/kg with	IV	q24h	≥14 d
	followed by	25 mg/kg	PO	q6h	≥14 d
	Fluconazole	400 mg	PO	q24h	8 wk
	followed by				
	Fluconazole	200 mg	PO	q24h	Lifelong
Histoplasmosis	Amphotericin B	0.5-1.0 mg/kg	IV	q24h	≥28-56 d
	followed by				
	Itraconazole	200 mg	PO	q24h	Lifelong
Herpes simplex	Acyclovir	200 mg	PO	5/d	10-14 d
	or				
	Famciclovir	125-250 mg	PO	q12h	10-14 d
	or				
	Valacyclovir	500 mg	PO	q12h	10-14 d
Varicella-zoster virus					
Dermatomal	Acyclovir	800 mg	PO	5/d	7-10 d
	or				
	Famciclovr	500 mg	PO	q8h	7-10 d
	or				
	Valacyclovir	1000 mg	PO	q8h	7-10 d
Disseminated	Acyclovir	10-12 mg/kg	IV	q8h	7-14 d

From Mandell GL: *Mandell, Douglas, and Bennett's principles and practice of infecitous diseases,* ed 5, New York, 2000, Churchill Livingstone.
*Prednisone, 40 mg q12h × 5 d, followed by 20 mg bid × 5 d, followed by 20 mg qd × 11 d.
†Following a single loading dose of pyrimethamine, 200 mg.
‡With probenecid as described in package insert.
§With pyridoxine 50 mg PO qd.
¶For patients who have sustained response to HAART (see text for criteria for discontinuation of maintenance therapy).

TABLE 1-5   Therapy for Opportunistic Infections in Patients with HIV Infection—cont'd

CLINICAL DISEASE	DRUG	DOSE	ROUTE	INTERVAL	DURATION
Cytomegalovirus	Ganciclovir *followed by*	5 mg/kg	IV	q12h	14-21 d
	Ganciclovir *or*	5 mg/kg	IV	q24h	Lifelong¶
	Foscarnet *followed by*	60 mg/kg	IV	q8h	14-21 d
	Foscarnet *or*	90-120 mg/kg	IV	q24h	Lifelong¶
	Ganciclovir implant *or*	—	—	q6-9m	Lifelong¶
	Cidofovir‡ *followed by*	5 mg/kg 5 mg/kg	IV IV	qwk q2wk	2 wk Lifelong¶
Mycobacterium tuberculosis	Isoniazid§ *and*	300 mg	PO, IM	q24h	At least 6 mo
	Rifampin *and*	600 mg	PO, IV	q24h	At least 6 mo
	Ethambutol *and*	15-25 mg/kg	PO	q24h	Depends on sensitivity
	Pyrazinamide	15-25 mg/kg	PO	q24h	2 mo
Mycobacterium avium complex	Clarithromycin Ethambutol	500 mg 15 mg/kg	PO PO	q12h q24h	Lifelong¶ Lifelong
Bartonella (Rochalimaea) spp.	Erythromycin *or*	500 mg	PO	q6h	≥12 wk
	Doxycycline	100 mg	PO	q12h	≥12 wk

From Mandell GL: *Mandell, Douglas, and Bennett's principles and practice of infecitous diseases,* ed 5, New York, 2000, Churchill Livingstone.
*Prednisone, 40 mg q12h × 5 d, followed by 20 mg bid × 5 d, followed by 20 mg qd ×11 d.
†Following a single loading dose of pyrimethamine, 200 mg.
‡With probenecid as described in package insert.
§With pyridoxine 50 mg PO qd.
¶For patients who have sustained response to HAART (see text for criteria for discontinuation of maintenance therapy).

TABLE 1-6   Prophylaxis for Human Immunodeficiency Virus–Related Opportunistic Infections

PATHOGEN	INDICATION FOR PROPHYLAXIS	FIRST CHOICE	ALTERNATIVES	COMMENTS
Pneumocystis	CD4$^+$ <200/mm^3 Persistent unexplained fever Chronic oropharyngeal candidiasis	Trimethoprim-sulfamethoxazole, 1 DS qd or SS	Dapsone, 50 mg qd, + pyrimethamine, 50 mg/wk Dapsone alone (100 mg qd) Aerosolized pentamidine	SS tablets are effective and may be less toxic than DS. Aerosol pentamidine should be delivered by Respirgard nebulizer.
Mycobacterium avium complex	CD4$^+$ <100/mm^3	Clarithromycin, 500 mg bid	Azithromycin (1200 mg qwk) Rifabutin, 300 mg qd	Rifabutin increases hepatic metabolism of other drugs.
Toxoplasma	No consensus	Trimethoprim-sulfamethoxazole, 1 DS qd	—	Pyrimethamine alone is not effective.
Mycobacterium tuberculosis	PPD >5 mm "High risk"	Sensitive: Isoniazid, 300 mg × 9 mo Resistant: ?	Rifampin* 600 mg, or Rifabutin* 300 mg, and pyrizinamide (15-25 mg/kg	For resistant strains, two-drug regimens using combinations of rifampin, pyrazinamide, or a quinolone can be considered.
Candida	Multiple recurrences	Fluconazole, 200 mg daily	qd × 2 mo)	Include pyridoxine, 500 mg qd for isoniazid-containing regimens. Recommended only if recurrences are severe or frequent.
Herpes simplex	Multiple recurrences	Acyclovir, 200 mg qd 3-4 ×/day Famciclovir, 125 mg PO bid Valacyclovir, 500 mg PD bid	Itraconazole, 100 mg qd —	
Cytomegalovirus	None	—	—	Oral ganciclovir is not recommended currently.
Pneumococcus	All patients	Pneumovax	—	Trimethoprim-sulfamethoxazole, clarithromycin, and azithromycin appear to prevent some disease.
Influenza	All patients	Influenza vaccine	—	—

From Mandell GL: *Mandell, Douglas, and Bennett's principles and practice of infectious diseases,* ed 5, New York, 2000, Churchill Livingstone.
DS, Double strength; *PPD,* purified protein derivative; *SS,* single strength.
*For patients receiving HAART, dose adjustments may be necessary.

BASIC INFORMATION

■ DEFINITION
Acromegaly is a chronic debilitating disease with an insidious onset, resulting from the effects of either hypersecretion of growth hormone (GH) or increased amounts of an insulin-like growth factor I (IGF-I).

■ SYNONYMS
Marie's disease

ICD-9CM CODES
253.0 Acromegaly

■ EPIDEMIOLOGY & DEMOGRAPHICS
INCIDENCE: 3 to 4 new cases/1,000,000 persons
PREVALENCE: 50 to 60 cases/1 million persons, with some estimates as high as 90 cases/1 million persons
PREDOMINANT SEX: No sexual predominance
MEAN AGE AT DIAGNOSIS: Males: 40 yr; females: 45 yr
RISK FACTORS
• Increased mortality, primarily from cardiovascular and respiratory causes
• Death in 50% of untreated patients by age 50 yr (twice the rate of the general population)
• Increased prevalence of colon carcinoma and other malignancies

■ PHYSICAL FINDINGS & CLINICAL PRESENTATION
• Coarse features resulting from growth of soft tissue
• Coarse, oily skin
• Hands and feet that are spade-like, fleshy, and moist
• Prognathism, which can give an underbite
• Carpal tunnel syndrome
• Excessive sweating
• Arthralgias and severe osteoarthritis
• History of increased hat, glove, and/or shoe size
• Hypertension
• Skin tags
• Muscle weakness and decreased exercise capacity
• Headache, often severe
• Diabetes mellitus
• Visual field defects

■ ETIOLOGY
Cause is usually a pituitary adenoma, affecting the anterior lobe.

DIAGNOSIS

■ DIFFERENTIAL DIAGNOSIS
Ectopic production of growth hormone–releasing hormone (GHRH) from a carcinoid or other neuroendocrine tumor

■ WORKUP
1. First screening test: measure serum IGF-I level.
   a. Direct measurement of the GH level is not as useful, because it is secreted in a pulsatile fashion and a random level may be falsely normal.
   b. Upper limits of a normal IGF-I level, depending on the assay: >380 ng/ml or 2.5 U/ml.
2. Failure to suppress serum GH to less than 2 ng/ml after 100 g oral glucose is considered conclusive.
   a. Patients may show suppression of GH or a paradoxical response.
   b. Patients will not suppress GH to 2 ng/ml or less (the normal response).
   c. GHRH level >300 ng/ml is indicative of an ectopic source of GH.

■ LABORATORY TESTS
• Elevated serum phosphate
• Elevated urine calcium

■ IMAGING STUDIES
• Imaging studies of choice: MRI of the pituitary and hypothalamus
• CT of the pituitary and hypothalamus used initially

TREATMENT

■ SURGERY
Treatment of choice: transsphenoidal microsurgical adenomectomy
• Surgical failure rate: about 13.3% for microadenomas (tumors <10 mm) and 11.1% for macroadenomas (tumors >10 mm confined to the sella)
• Preoperative IGF-I level: indicator of surgical outcome with higher levels in the surgical failure group

■ RADIOTHERAPY
• Irradiation to reduce further growth of the tumor in most patients
• Major complication: hypopituitarism, which may occur in up to 50% of patients; this complication is more likely in patients who had surgery irradiation

■ MEDICAL Rx
• Indicated when patients have failed surgical therapy, when surgery is contraindicated, and in patients waiting for the effects of radiotherapy to begin
• Octreotide
  1. A somatostatin analog given tid at a dose of 100 μg subcutaneously
  2. Important side effects: biliary sludge and gallstones; nausea, cramps, and steatorrhea; suppression of GH levels to about 5 μg/L in 52% of patients; IGF-I levels normalized to about 53%
  3. Important in the preoperative shrinkage of pituitary tumors and softening of adenomatous tissue
• Bromocriptine
  1. A dopamine analog given at a dosage of 10 to 60 mg PO tid to qid
  2. Less effective than octreotide
  3. Important advantages: less expensive than octreotide and taken orally
  4. Important side effects: orthostatic hypotension, lightheadedness, nausea, constipation, and nasal stuffiness
  5. Suppresses GH levels to <5 μg/L in about 20% of patients; normalizes GH levels in approximately 10%, and shrinks pituitary adenomas in 10% to 20%; IGF-I levels normalized to about 10%
• Pegvisomant is a growth hormone receptor antagonist that has shown promising results in the treatment of acromegaly.

■ CHRONIC Rx
Combination of bromocriptine and octreotide may be synergistic, allowing a lower combination dosage than alone.

■ DISPOSITION
• Patients receiving radiotherapy need long-term follow-up to monitor the potential development of hypopituitarism.
• Continuation of medical therapy should be based on the normalization of IGF-I levels.

REFERENCE
Trainer et al: Treatment of acromegaly with the growth hormone-receptor antagonist pegvisomant, *N Engl J Med* 342:1172, 2000.
Author: **Beth J. Wutz, M.D.**

BASIC INFORMATION

■ DEFINITION
Actinomycosis is a chronic bacterial infection characterized by the formation of painful abscesses, soft tissue infiltration, and draining sinuses.

■ SYNONYMS
Actinomyces infection

ICD-9CM CODES
039.9 Actinomycosis

■ EPIDEMIOLOGY & DEMOGRAPHICS
- Actinomycosis is worldwide in distribution.
- Commonly found as normal flora of the oral cavity, pharynx, tracheobronchial tree, gastrointestinal tract, and female urogenital tract.
- Incidence 1:300,000.
- Males infected more often than females 3:1.
- Can occur at any age but commonly seen in midlife.
- Incidence has decreased since the 1950s and is attributed to better oral hygiene and antibiotics.

■ PHYSICAL FINDINGS & CLINICAL PRESENTATION
Actinomycosis can affect any organ and characteristically manifests as:
- Cervicofacial disease (most common site):
  1. Occurs in the setting of poor dental hygiene, recent dental surgery, or minor oral trauma
  2. Painful soft tissue swelling commonly seen at the angle of the mandible
  3. Fever, chills, and weight loss
  4. Trismus
  5. Soft tissue facial infection with sinus tract or fistula formation
- Thoracic disease:
  1. Can involve the lungs, pleura, mediastinum, or chest wall.
  2. Presumed secondary to aspiration of *Actinomyces* organisms in patients with poor oral hygiene.
  3. Fever, cough, weight loss, and pleuritic chest pains are common symptoms.
  4. Signs of pneumonia or pleural effusion may be present.
  5. With extension beyond the lungs to mediastinal structures and the chest wall, signs and symptoms of pericarditis, empyema, chest wall sinus drainage, and tracheoesophageal fistula can all occur (Fig. 1-12).
- Abdominal disease:
  1. Occurs most commonly after appendectomy, perforated bowel, diverticulitis, or surgery to the gastrointestinal tract.
  2. Lesions develop most commonly in the ileocecal valve, causing abdominal pain, fever, weight loss, and a palpable mass.
  3. Extension may occur to the liver, causing jaundice and abscess formation.
  4. Sinus tracts to the abdominal wall can occur.
- Pelvic disease:
  1. Commonly occurs by extension from abdominal disease of the ileocecal valve to the right adnexa (80% of cases).
  2. Endometritis.

■ ETIOLOGY
- Actinomycosis is most commonly caused by *Actinomyces israelii*. Other causes are *A. naeslundii, A. odontolyticus, A. viscosus, A. meyeri,* and *A. gerencseriae.*
- *Actinomyces* are gram-positive, non-spore-forming, anaerobic or microaerophilic rods.
- Actinomycosis infections are polymicrobial, usually associated with *Streptococcous, Bacteroides, Eikenella corrodens, Enterococcus,* and *Fusobacterium.*
- Infects individuals only after entry into disrupted mucosa or tissue injury.

DIAGNOSIS

Isolating the bacteria in the proper clinical setting makes the diagnosis of actinomycosis.

■ DIFFERENTIAL DIAGNOSIS
Nocardiosis, botryomycosis, chromomycosis, intestinal tuberculosis, ameboma, Crohn's disease, colon cancer, and other causes of acute, subacute, or chronic infections of the lung, abdomen, hepatic, GI, GU, musculoskeletal, and CNS system.

■ WORKUP
The workup includes obtaining specimens either by aspirating abscesses, excising sinus tracts, or tissue biopsies.

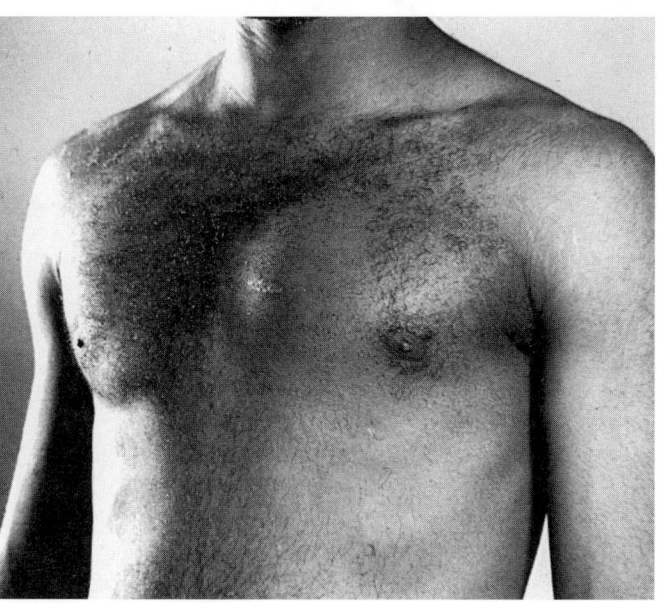

A

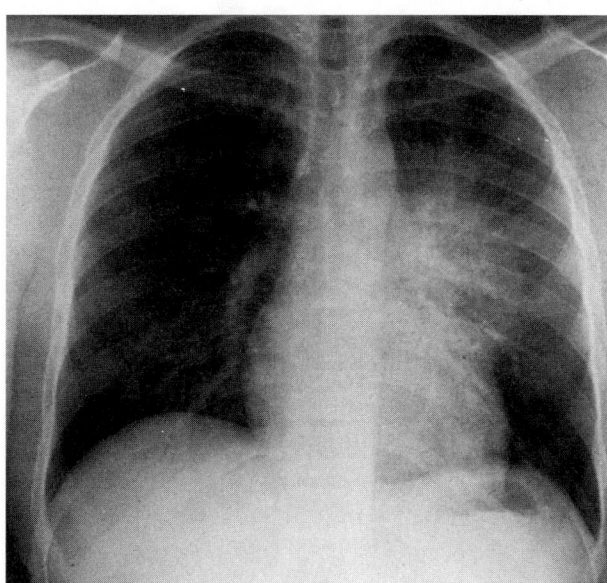

B

Fig. 1-12 Thoracic actinomycosis. **A,** Initial presentation with a bulging mass lesion in the left chest wall with a central sinus tract. **B,** The chest radiograph with the associated pulmonary infiltrate. (From Gorbach SL: *Infectious diseases,* ed 2, Philadelphia, 1998, WB Saunders.)

■ LABORATORY TESTS
- Isolating "sulfur granules" from tissue specimens or draining sinuses confirm the diagnosis of actinomycosis.
  1. Sulfur granules are nests of *Actinomyces* species. Sulfur granules may be macroscopic or microscopic (Fig. 1-13).
  2. Sulfur granules are crushed and stained for identification of *Actinomcyes* organisms and may take up to 3 wk to grow in culture media.

■ IMAGING STUDIES
- Imaging studies are useful adjunctive tests in localizing the site and spread of infection.
  1. CXR
  2. CT scan of the head, chest, abdomen, and pelvic areas is useful

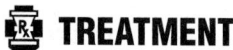

℞ TREATMENT

■ NONPHARMACOLOGIC THERAPY
- Incision and drainage of abscesses
- Excision of sinus tract

■ ACUTE GENERAL Rx
- Penicillin 10 to 20 million units per day in 4 divided doses for 4 to 6 wk.
- In penicillin-allergic patients, erythromycin, tetracycline, clindamycin, or cephalosporins (depending on the type of penicillin allergy) are reasonable alternatives.
- Chloramphenicol 50 to 60 mg/kg/day has been used for CNS actinomycosis.

■ CHRONIC Rx
- Following 4 to 6 wk IV penicillin, oral penicillin V 500 mg PO qid for 6 to 12 mo.
- Treatment of associated microorganisms is not needed.

■ DISPOSITION
- Clinical actinomycosis, if not treated, spreads to contiguous tissues and structures ignoring tissue planes. Hematogenous spread, although possible, is rare.
- Actinomycosis is very sensitive to antibiotics but requires chronic long-term treatment to prevent relapse.

■ REFERRAL
If the diagnosis of actinomycosis is suspected, consultation with an infectious disease specialist is suggested. General surgical consultation for excision of sinus tracts and abscess incision and drainage is recommended.

☼ PEARLS & CONSIDERATIONS

■ COMMENTS
- There is no person-to-person transmission of *Actinomyces*.
- Isolation of the organism in an asymptomatic individual does not mean the person has actinomycosis. Active symptoms must be present to make the diagnosis.
- Pelvic actinomycosis has been associated with use of an intrauterine device (IUD).
- Actinomycosis can also involve the CNS, causing multiple brain abscesses.

REFERENCES
Russo TA: Agents of actinomycosis. In *Mandell, Douglas, and Bennett's principles and practice of infectious diseases,* ed 5, New York, 2000, Churchill Livingstone.
Smego RA, Foglia G: Actinomycosis, *Clin Infect Dis* 26:1255, 1998.
Author: **Peter Petropoulos, M.D.**

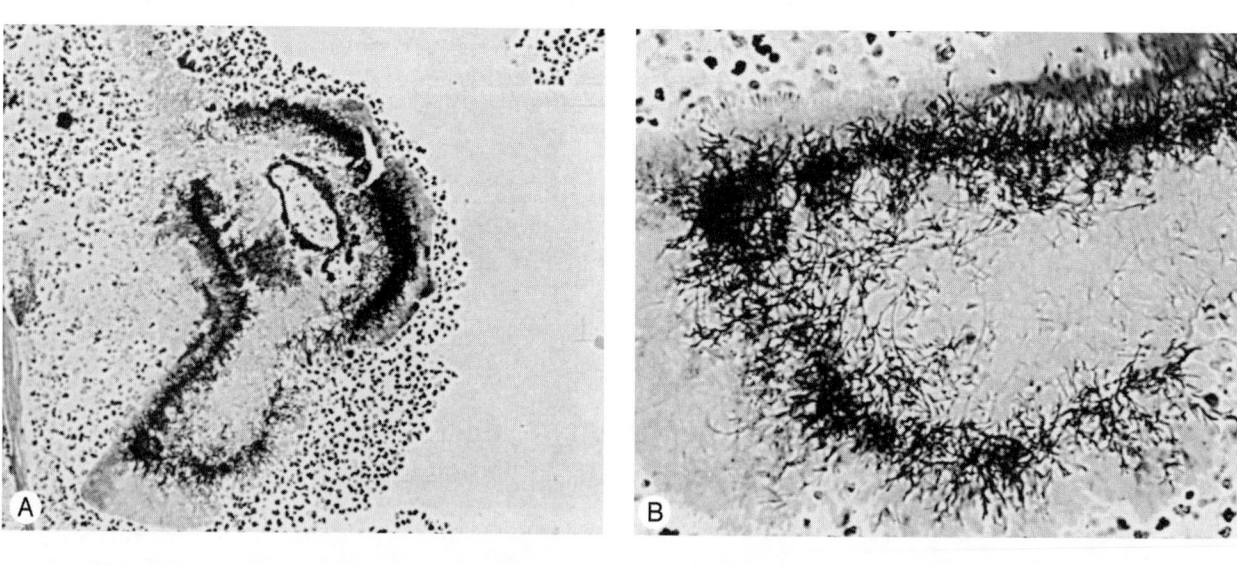

Fig. 1-13 A, Actinomycotic sulfur granule surrounded by inflammatory cells (Brown-Brenn stain, ×250). **B,** Increased magnification (×1000) demonstrates the delicate, branched filaments of *Actinomyces.* (From Mandell GL [ed]: *Mandell, Douglas, and Bennett's principles and practice of infectious diseases,* ed 5, New York, 2000, Churchill LIvingstone.)

BASIC INFORMATION

■ DEFINITION

Addison's disease is characterized by inadequate secretion of corticosteroids resulting from partial or complete destruction of the adrenal glands.

■ SYNONYMS

Primary adrenocortical insufficiency

ICD-9CM CODES

255.4 Addison's disease

■ EPIDEMIOLOGY & DEMOGRAPHICS

PREVALENCE: 5 cases/100,000 persons
PREDOMINANT SEX: Female:male ratio of 2:1

■ PHYSICAL FINDINGS & CLINICAL PRESENTATION

- Hyperpigmentation: more prominent in palmar creases, buccal mucosa, pressure points (elbows, knees, knuckles), perianal mucosa, and around areolas of nipples
- Hypotension
- Generalized weakness
- Amenorrhea and loss of axillary hair in females

■ ETIOLOGY

- Autoimmune destruction of the adrenal glands (80% of cases)
- Tuberculosis (15% of cases)
- Carcinomatous destruction of the adrenal glands
- Adrenal hemorrhage (anticoagulants, trauma, coagulopathies, pregnancy, sepsis)
- Adrenal infarction (arteritis, thrombosis)
- Other: sarcoidosis, amyloidosis, postoperative, fungal infections, AIDS

DIAGNOSIS

■ DIFFERENTIAL DIAGNOSIS

Sepsis, hypovolemic shock, acute abdomen, apathetic hyperthyroidism in the elderly, myopathies, GI malignancy, major depression, anorexia nervosa, hemochromatosis, salt-losing nephritis, chronic infection

■ WORKUP

- If the clinical picture is highly suggestive of adrenocortical insufficiency, the diagnosis can be made with the rapid ACTH (Cortrosyn) test:
  1. Give 250 μg ACTH by IV push and measure cortisol levels at 0 and 30 min.
  2. Cortisol level <18 μg/dl at 30 or 60 min is suggestive of adrenal insufficiency.
  3. Measure plasma ACTH. A high ACTH level confirms primary adrenal insufficiency.
- Secondary adrenocortical insufficiency (caused by pituitary dysfunction) can be distinguished from primary adrenal insufficiency by the following:
  1. Normal or low plasma ACTH level following rapid ACTH (Cortrosyn test)
  2. Absence of hyperpigmentation
  3. No significant impairment of aldosterone secretion (because aldosterone secretion is under control of the renin-angiotensin system)
  4. Additional evidence of hypopituitarism (e.g., hypogonadism, hypothyroidism)
- Fig. 1-14 describes a diagnostic algorithm for adrenal insufficiency.

■ LABORATORY TESTS

- Increased potassium, decreased sodium and chloride
- Decreased glucose
- Increased BUN/creatinine ratio (prerenal azotemia)
- Mild normocytic, normochromic anemia, neutropenia, lymphocytosis, eosinophilia (significant dehydration may mask hyponatremia and anemia)
- PPD and antiadrenal antibodies

■ IMAGING STUDIES

- Chest x-ray examination may reveal a small heart.
- Abdominal x-ray film: adrenal calcifications may be noted if the adrenocortical insufficiency is secondary to TB or fungus.
- Abdominal CT scan: small adrenal glands generally indicate either idiopathic atrophy or long-standing TB, whereas enlarged glands are suggestive of early TB or potentially treatable diseases.

TREATMENT

■ NONPHARMACOLOGIC THERAPY

- Perform periodic monitoring of serum electrolytes, vital signs, and body weight; liberal sodium intake is suggested.
- Periodic measurement of bone density may be helpful in identifying patients at risk for the development of osteoporosis.

Patients should carry a Medic Alert bracelet and an emergency pack containing hydrocortisone 100 mg ampule, syringe, and needle. Patients and partners should be educated on how to give IM injection in case of vomiting or coma.

■ ACUTE GENERAL Rx

Addisonian crisis is an acute complication of adrenal insufficiency characterized by circulatory collapse, dehydration, nausea, vomiting, hypoglycemia, and hyperkalemia.

1. Draw plasma cortisol level; do not delay therapy while waiting for confirming laboratory results.
2. Administer dexamethasone sodium phosphate 4 mg q12h or hydrocortisone 100 mg IV q6h for 24 hr; if patient shows good clinical response, gradually taper dosage and change to oral maintenance dose (usually prednisone 7.5 mg/day).
3. Provide adequate volume replacement with D_5NS solution until hypotension, dehydration, and hypoglycemia are completely corrected. Large volumes (2 to 3 L) may be necessary in the first 2 to 3 hr to correct the volume deficit and hypoglycemia and to avoid further hyponatremia.

Identify and correct any precipitating factor (e.g., sepsis, hemorrhage).

■ CHRONIC Rx

- Give hydrocortisone 15 to 20 mg PO every morning and 5 to 10 mg in late afternoon or prednisone 5 mg in morning and 2.5 mg hs.
- Give fludroxycortisone acetate 0.1 mg/day: this mineralocorticoid is necessary if the patient has primary adrenocortical insufficiency.
- Instruct patients to increase glucocorticoid replacement in times of stress and to receive parenteral glucocorticoids if diarrhea or vomiting occurs.
- The administration of dehydroepiandrosterone 50 mg PO qd improves well-being and sexuality in women with adrenal insufficiency.

■ DISPOSITION

- Lifelong medical supervision is necessary to monitor adequacy of therapy and prevent complications.
- Adrenal function is rarely recovered.
- Life expectancy is in the normal range if adequately treated.

PEARLS & CONSIDERATIONS

■ COMMENTS

Patient education material may be obtained from the National Addison's Disease Foundation, 505 Northern Blvd., Suite 200, Great Neck, NY 11021, phone: (516) 487-4992.
Author: **Fred F. Ferri, M.D.**

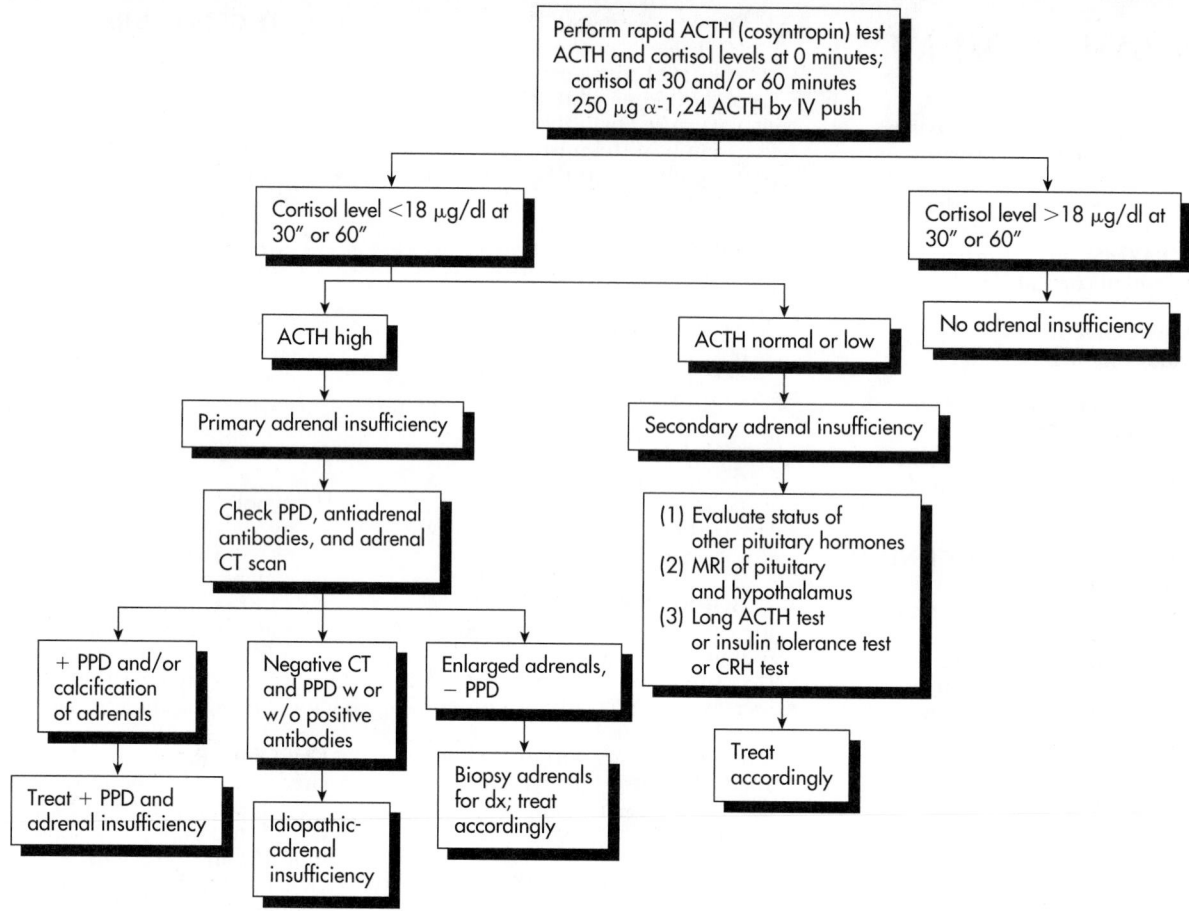

Fig. 1-14 **Evaluation of adrenal insufficiency.** *ACTH,* Adrenocorticotropic hormone;
CRH, corticotropin-releasing hormone; *CT,* computed tomography; *MRI,* magnetic resonance imaging;
PPD, purified protein derivative. (From Noble J: *Primary care medicine,* ed 3, St Louis, 2001, Mosby.)

BASIC INFORMATION

■ DEFINITION
In the U.S., agoraphobia is considered part of the continuum of panic attacks and panic disorder. In Europe, agoraphobia is conceptualized as a phobic condition independent of panic. A *panic attack* is a relatively brief, sudden episode of intense fear or apprehension, often associated with a sense of impending doom and various uncomfortable and disquieting physical symptoms. *Panic disorder* is diagnosed if at least one panic attack is followed by a significant degree of concern about future attacks or a major change in behavior related to these attacks. Agoraphobia is anxiety about, or avoidance of, places or situations in which the ability to leave suddenly is limited or impossible in the event of having a panic attack.

■ SYNONYMS
Anxiety attacks
Fear attacks

ICD-9CM CODES
F 41.0 Panic disorder without agoraphobia (DSM-IV: 300.01)
F 40.01 Panic disorder with agoraphobia (DSM-IV: 300.01)

■ EPIDEMIOLOGY & DEMOGRAPHICS
INCIDENCE (IN U.S.): 1% 1-mo incidence of panic attacks
PREVALENCE (IN U.S.):
- 15% lifetime prevalence of panic attacks
- Panic disorder much more uncommon, with a lifetime prevalence of 1.5% to 3.5%; chronicity of condition reflected by a similar 1-yr prevalence rate of 1% to 2%
- Agoraphobia relatively rare; 0.3% to 1% lifetime prevalence

PREDOMINANT SEX:
- Women more commonly affected (>85% of clinical population)
- Panic disorder twice as common in women
- Panic disorder with agoraphobia three times as common in women

PREDOMINANT AGE:
- Age of onset earlier in males (24 yr) than females (28 yr)
- Onset after age 45 yr rare

PEAK INCIDENCE:
- Chronic condition with a waxing and waning course
- Bimodal incidence peaks noted, with the first peak between ages 15 and 24 yr and second peak between 35 and 44 yr

GENETICS:
- Risk of developing panic disorder in first-degree relatives of individuals with panic disorder four to seven times that of general population
- Findings in twin studies: about 60% of contributing factors to panic are genetic

■ PHYSICAL FINDINGS & CLINICAL PRESENTATION
- Panic disorder
  1. Present either with a panic attack or with fear and anxiety related to anticipation of a future panic attack
  2. Typical presentation: unexpected, untriggered periods of intense anxiety and fear with associated physiologic changes (e.g., palpitations, sweating, tremulousness, shortness of breath, chest pain, GI distress, faintness, derealization, paresthesia)
  3. Emergency or physician visits often occasioned by physical symptoms
- Agoraphobia
  1. Rare complaints to physician
  2. Activities usually self-limited by avoiding public situations where the patient might experience a panic attack and would be unable to exit readily, such as the following:
     Crowded public areas (stores, public transportation, church)
     Individual interactions (hair dresser, neighborhood meetings)
  3. On exposure to or anticipation of exposure to such situations, significant anxiety occurs

■ ETIOLOGY
Hypotheses (NOTE: There are sufficient data to support each model.)
  1. Central dyscontrol of autonomic arousal (typically localized to the locus ceruleus)
  2. Cognitive overreaction to relatively mild physiologic cues
  3. Dysfunction of a central suffocation alarm mechanism

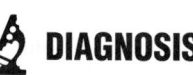

DIAGNOSIS

■ DIFFERENTIAL DIAGNOSIS
- Medical conditions
  1. Arrhythmias
  2. Hyperthyroidism
  3. Hyperparathyroidism
  4. Seizure disorders
  5. Respiratory diseases
  6. Pheochromocytoma
- Therapeutic (theophylline, steroids) and recreational (cocaine, amphetamine, caffeine) drugs and drug withdrawal (alcohol, barbiturates, benzodiazepines)
- Phobias (e.g., specific phobia or social phobia)

- Obsessive-compulsive disorder (cued by exposure to the object of the obsession)
- Posttraumatic stress disorder (cued by recall of a stressor)

■ WORKUP
- Emergency presentation: cardiac, respiratory, or neurologic symptoms
- History and physical examination to rule out a concomitant medical condition

NOTE: Panic disorder and agoraphobia are not diagnoses of exclusion, but exclusion of other conditions is usually required.

■ LABORATORY TESTS
- Thyroid profile
- Electrolyte measures, including calcium
- Toxicology screen
- ECG
- Acute cases: possible monitoring and cardiac enzymes to rule out arrhythmia or ischemia

■ IMAGING STUDIES
- For temporal lobe dysfunction (e.g., temporal lesions or as ictal or interictal manifestation of temporal lobe seizures): brain CT scan or MRI and/or an EEG in some patients
- Holter monitor to rule out occult or episodic arrhythmias
- Chest x-ray examination, ABG, or pulmonary function tests if respiratory compromise suspected

TREATMENT

■ NONPHARMACOLOGIC THERAPY
- Psychotherapy: generally very effective; long-term follow-up studies of panic patients suggest that therapy is possibly superior to pharmacologic interventions
- Interpersonal and cognitive-behavioral therapy modalities: most extensively studied

■ ACUTE GENERAL Rx
- Benzodiazepines, particularly alprazolam: very effective in acute setting
- Low-dose alprazolam for patients with rare panic attacks and asymptomatic interattack periods (0.25 to 0.5 mg PO or sublingually prn)

■ CHRONIC Rx
- Because disorder patients, as a group, have a low likelihood of abusing benzodiazepines, uncomplicated cases managed with low-dose benzodiazepines on a schedule or prn
- Preferred pharmacologic agents: antidepressants with a significant serotonin reuptake inhibitory action
- Imipramine quite effective in both panic disorder and agoraphobia

- Newer antidepressants (paroxetine, sertraline, and fluoxetine) quite effective in preventing panic attacks and ameliorating agoraphobia

■ DISPOSITION
- Typical course chronic but with significant waxing and waning (common to have long periods of remission)
- Presence of agoraphobia associated with a more chronic course
- Findings with long-term follow-up studies: 6 to 10 yr after treatment some 30% in remission, 40% to 50% improved with residual symptoms, and the remainder either unchanged or worse

■ REFERRAL
Referral needed if:
- Patients do not respond to a serotonin reuptake inhibitor
- Therapy is the preferred treatment

REFERENCE
Pohl RB et al: Sertraline in the treatment of panic disorder: a double-blind multicenter trial, *Am J Psychiatry* 155:1188, 1998.
Author: **Rif S. El-Mallakh, M.D.**

BASIC INFORMATION

■ DEFINITION

Although it is impossible to define alcoholism precisely, among the commonly used screening instruments for this disorder are the CAGE questionnaire, short Michigan Alcoholism Screening Test (SMAST), National Council on Alcoholism criteria, and DSM-III-A criteria.

Although not generally included under the topic alcoholism, hazardous or at-risk drinking should also be considered. For men, at-risk drinking is defined as greater than 14 drinks/week or more than 4 drinks/occasion. For women, at-risk drinking is defined as about half that given for men.

■ SYNONYMS

Alcohol abuse
Substance abuse

ICD-9CM CODES

303.9 Alcoholism

■ EPIDEMIOLOGY & DEMOGRAPHICS

INCIDENCE (IN U.S.):
• See "Prevalence."
• 20% achieve abstinence without help, 70% achieve sobriety for 1 yr.
PREVALENCE (IN U.S.): 7% of population 18 yr or older
PREDOMINANT SEX:
• Lifetime risk for males 8% to 10%
• Lifetime risk for females 3% to 5%
PEAK INCIDENCE: 20 to 40 yr
GENETICS: More common with a family history of alcoholism and in patients of Irish, Scandinavian, and Native American descent

■ PHYSICAL FINDINGS & CLINICAL PRESENTATION

• Recurring minor trauma
• GI bleeding
• Pancreatitis

• Liver disease
• Odor of alcohol on breath
• Tremulousness
• Tachycardia
• Peripheral neuropathy
• Recent memory loss
• Table 1-7 describes some alcohol-related medical disorders.

■ ETIOLOGY

• Social and genetic factors important
• Risk factors:
  1. Broken homes
  2. Unemployment
  3. Divorce
  4. Recurrent depression
  5. Addiction to another substance, including tobacco

DIAGNOSIS

■ WORKUP

• Screening tests (CAGE or SMAST)
• Blood studies
• Stool for occult blood
• Fig. 1-15 describes an algorithm for evaluation of alcohol abuse

■ LABORATORY TESTS

• γ-Glutamyltransferase (GGT)
• Aspartate aminotransferase (SGOT, AST)
• Mean corpuscular volume (MCV)

■ IMAGING STUDIES

Indicated only if there is a history of trauma

TREATMENT

■ NONPHARMACOLOGIC THERAPY

• Abstinence.
• Depression, if present, should be treated at same time ETOH is withdrawn.

■ ACUTE GENERAL Rx

• Observe for delirium tremens (DTs): if tachycardia or visual hallucinations occur, administer lorazepam or other benzodiazepines (Box 1-3).
• IM thiamine is mandatory in DTs and in acute extraocular disorders.

■ CHRONIC Rx

• See "Referral."
• Pharmacotherapies for alcoholism include the opiate antagonists (naltrexone 50 mg PO qd or nalmefene 10 to 40 mg qd), disulfiram, acamprosate, lithium, and SSRIs.

■ DISPOSITION

See "Referral"

■ REFERRAL

• To Alcoholics Anonymous or Adult Children of Alcoholics
• Family members to Al-Anon or Al-A-Teen
• Many cities have Salvation Army Adult Rehabilitation centers; all patients accepted, regardless of ability to pay

✿ PEARLS & CONSIDERATIONS

■ COMMENTS

The cure rate for alcoholism is very disappointing, regardless of the modality. Only those who want to be helped will be helped. An effective strategy for the primary care physician is a prominently displayed sign in the office that states, "If you think you consume too much alcoholic beverage, please discuss it with me." Those who do open up the discussion can be given the facts in a nonjudgemental way and often can be helped. All too often, problem drinkers lie on the questionnaire until they face a life-threatening health issue—and even then denial often reigns supreme.

BOX 1-3   Management of Alcohol Withdrawal

Observe and normalize vital signs
Administer thiamine, 100 mg, then replace fluid and electrolytes
Sedate with chlordiazepoxide, 25 mg PO qid
Administer chlordiazepoxide, 25-50 mg IM prn for signs of withdrawal
Use haloperidol (1-2 mg PO q4h prn) or thorazine cautiously for hallucinations or agitation
Replace folic acid (1 mg/day PO) and thiamine (100 mg IM and then 100 mg/day PO)
Give multivitamin daily
Begin β-blocker (atenolol, 50 mg) or clonidine (0.2 mg PO bid) to reduce adrenergic signs

From Andreoli TE (ed): *Cecil essentials of medicine,* ed 5, Philadelphia, 2001, WB Saunders.

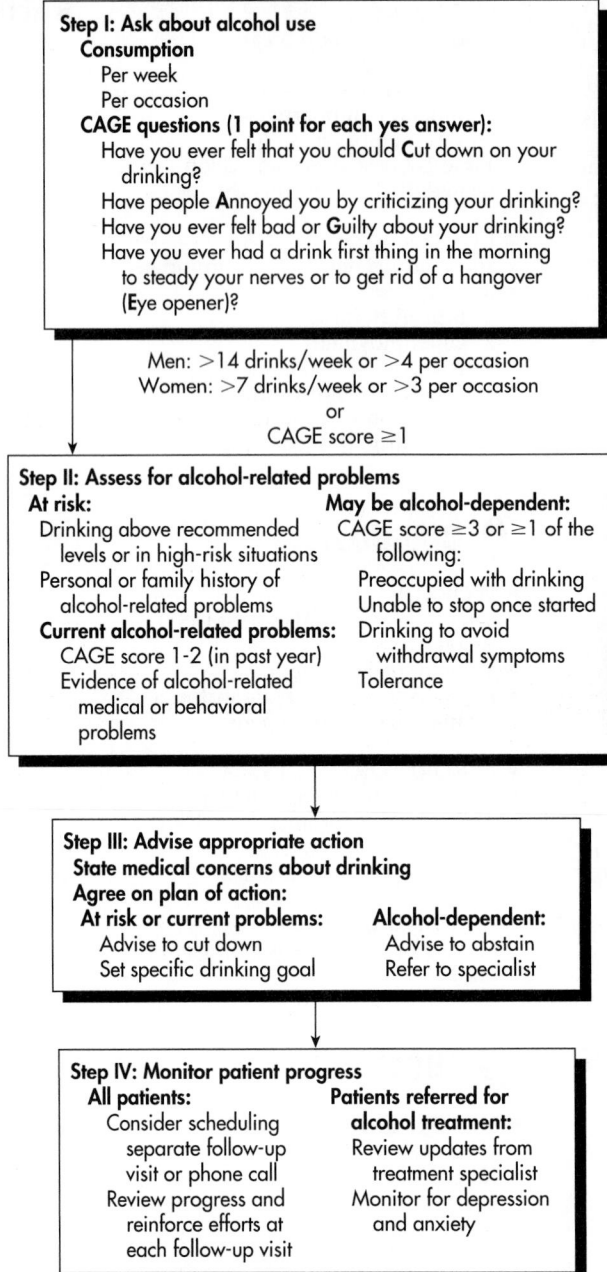

Step I: Ask about alcohol use
 Consumption
  Per week
  Per occasion
 CAGE questions (1 point for each yes answer):
  Have you ever felt that you should **C**ut down on your
   drinking?
  Have people **A**nnoyed you by criticizing your drinking?
  Have you ever felt bad or **G**uilty about your drinking?
  Have you ever had a drink first thing in the morning
   to steady your nerves or to get rid of a hangover
   (**E**ye opener)?

Men: >14 drinks/week or >4 per occasion
Women: >7 drinks/week or >3 per occasion
or
CAGE score ≥1

Step II: Assess for alcohol-related problems
 At risk: **May be alcohol-dependent:**
  Drinking above recommended   CAGE score ≥3 or ≥1 of the
   levels or in high-risk situations   following:
  Personal or family history of   Preoccupied with drinking
   alcohol-related problems   Unable to stop once started
 Current alcohol-related problems: Drinking to avoid
  CAGE score 1-2 (in past year)   withdrawal symptoms
  Evidence of alcohol-related   Tolerance
   medical or behavioral
   problems

Step III: Advise appropriate action
 State medical concerns about drinking
 Agree on plan of action:
  At risk or current problems: **Alcohol-dependent:**
   Advise to cut down   Advise to abstain
   Set specific drinking goal   Refer to specialist

Step IV: Monitor patient progress
 All patients: **Patients referred for**
  Consider scheduling   **alcohol treatment:**
   separate follow-up   Review updates from
   visit or phone call   treatment specialist
  Review progress and   Monitor for depression
   reinforce efforts at   and anxiety
   each follow-up visit

Fig. 1-15   Screening and brief intervention for alcohol problems in clinical practice. (From Goldman L, Bennett JC [eds]: *Cecil textbook of medicine,* ed 21, Philadelphia, 2000, WB Saunders.)

TABLE 1-7   Alcohol-Related Medical Disorders

AFFECTED ORGAN OR SYSTEM	DISORDERS

Nutrition	Deficiencies of primarily thiamine but also the following:
	    Vitamins: Folate, thiamine, pyridoxine, niacin, riboflavin
	    Minerals: Magnesium, zinc, calcium
	    Protein

Metabolites and electrolytes	Hypoglycemia, ketoacidosis, hyperlipidemia, hyperuricemia, hypomagnesemia, hypophosphatemia
GI tract	Liver: Fatty liver, hepatitis, cirrhosis Gut: Esophagitis, gastritis Pancreatitis
Nervous system	Brain: Hepatic encephalopathy, Wernicke-Korsakoff syndrome, cerebellar degeneration, central pontine myelinolysis, Marchiafava-Bignami disease, cerebral atrophy with dementia Neuromuscular: Neuropathy, myopathy Amblyopia
Cardiovascular	Heart: Arrhythmia, cardiomyopathy Hypertension
Bone marrow	Macrocytosis, anemia, thrombocytopenia, leukopenia
Endocrine	Pseudo-Cushing's syndrome, testicular atrophy, amenorrhea
Other	Traumatic injury Osteopenia Fetal alcohol syndrome

From Goldman L, Bennett JC (eds): *Cecil textbook of medicine,* ed 21, Philadelphia, 2000, WB Saunders.

REFERENCES

Fiellin DA et al: Outpatient management of patients with alcohol problems, *Ann Intern Med* 133:816, 2000.

Garbutt JC et al: Pharmacological treatment of alcohol dependence: a review of the evidence, *JAMA* 281:1318, 1999.

Jaeger TM et al: Symptom triggered therapy for alcohol withdrawal syndrome in medical in patients, *Mayo Clin Proc* 76:695, 2001.

O'Connor PG, Schotrenfeld RS: Patients with alcohol problems, *N Engl J Med* 9:592, 1998.

Reid MC et al: Hazardous and harmful alcohol consumption in primary care, *Arch Intern Med* 159:1681, 1999.

Schneekloth TD et al: Point prevalence of alcoholism in hospitalized patients: continuing challenges of detection, assessment, and diagnosis, *Mayo Clin Proc* 76:460, 2001.

Author: **William H. Olson, M.D.**

BASIC INFORMATION

■ DEFINITION
Primary aldosteronism is a clinical syndrome characterized by hypokalemia, hypertension, low plasma renin activity (PRA), and excessive aldosterone secretion.

■ SYNONYMS
Hyperaldosteronism
Conn's syndrome

■ ICD-9CM CODES
255.1 Primary aldosteronism

■ EPIDEMIOLOGY & DEMOGRAPHICS
INCIDENCE/PREVALENCE: 1% to 2% of patients with hypertension; more common in females

■ PHYSICAL FINDINGS & CLINICAL PRESENTATION
- Generally asymptomatic
- If significant hypokalemia is present, possible muscle cramping, weakness, paresthesias
- Hypertension
- Polyuria, polydipsia

■ ETIOLOGY
- Aldosterone-producing adenoma (>60%)
- Idiopathic hyperaldosteronism (>30%)
- Glucocorticoid-suppressible hyperaldosteronism (<1%)
- Aldosterone-producing carcinoma (<1%)

DIAGNOSIS

■ DIFFERENTIAL DIAGNOSIS
- Diuretic use
- Hypokalemia from vomiting, diarrhea
- Renovascular hypertension
- Other endocrine neoplasm (pheochromocytoma, deoxycorticosterone-producing tumor, renin-secreting tumor)

■ WORKUP
In patients with hypokalemia and a low PRA, confirming tests for primary hyperaldosteronism include the following:
- 24-hr urine test for aldosterone and potassium levels (potassium >40 mEq and aldosterone >15 μg).
- Captopril test: administer 25 to 50 mg of captopril (ACE inhibitor) and measure plasma renin and aldosterone levels 1 to 2 hr later. A plasma aldosterone level >15 ng/dl confirms the diagnosis of primary aldosteronism. This test is more expensive and is best reserved for situations in which the 24-hr urine for aldosterone is ambiguous.
- 24-hr urinary tetrahydroaldosterone (<65 μg/24 hr) and saline infusion test (plasma aldosterone >10 ng/dl) can also be used in ambiguous cases.
- The renin-aldosterone stimulation test (posture test) is helpful in differentiating IHA from aldosterone-producing adenoma (APA). Patients with APA have a decrease in aldosterone levels at 4 hr, whereas patients with IHA have an increase in their aldosterone levels.
- As a screening test for primary aldosteronism, an elevated plasma aldosterone-renin ratio (ARR), drawn randomly from patients on hypertensive drugs, is predictive of primary aldosteronism (positive predictive value 100% in a recent study). ARR is calculated by dividing plasma aldosterone (mg/dl) by plasma renin activity (mg/ml/hour). ARR >100 is considered elevated.
- Bilateral adrenal venous sampling may be done to localize APA when adrenal CT scan is equivocal. In APA, ipsilateral/contralateral aldosterone level is >10:1, and ipsilateral venous aldosterone concentration is very high (>1000 ng/dl).
- A diagnostic evaluation of hypertensive patients with suspected aldosteronism is described in Fig. 1-16.

■ LABORATORY TESTS
Routine laboratory tests can be suggestive but are not diagnostic of primary aldosteronism. Common abnormalities are:
- Spontaneous hypokalemia or moderately severe hypokalemia while receiving conventional doses of diuretics
- Possible alkalosis and hypernatremia

■ IMAGING STUDIES
- Adrenal CT scans (with 3-mm cuts) may be used to localize neoplasm.
- Adrenal scanning with iodocholesterol (NP-59) or 6-beta-iodomethyl-19-norcholesterol after dexamethasone suppression. The uptake of tracer is increased in those with aldosteronoma and absent in those with idiopathic aldosteronism and adrenal carcinoma.

TREATMENT

■ NONPHARMACOLOGIC THERAPY
- Regular monitoring and control of blood pressure
- Low-sodium diet, tobacco avoidance, maintenance of ideal body weight, and regular exercise program

■ ACUTE GENERAL Rx
- Control of blood pressure and hypokalemia with spironolactone, amiloride, or ACE inhibitors
- Surgery (unilateral adrenalectomy) for APA

■ CHRONIC Rx
Chronic medical therapy with spironolactone, amiloride, or ACE inhibitors to control blood pressure and hypokalemia is necessary in all patients with bilateral idiopathic hyperaldosteronism.

■ DISPOSITION
Unilateral adrenalectomy normalizes hypertension and hypokalemia in 70% of patients with APA after 1 yr. After 5 yr, 50% of patients remain normotensive.

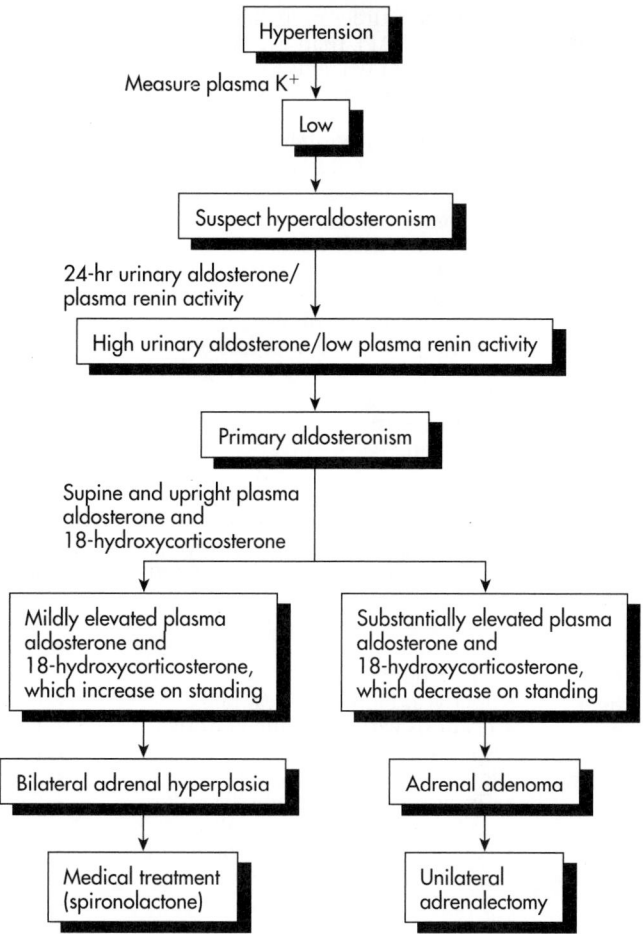

Fig. 1-16   **Flow chart for evaluating a patient with suspected primary hyperaldosteronism.**
(From Andreoli TE [ed]: *Cecil essentials of medicine,* ed 5, Philadelphia, 2001, WB Saunders.)

■ REFERRAL
Surgical referral for unilateral adrenal-ectomy following confirmation of uni-lateral APA or carcinoma

☼ PEARLS & CONSIDERATIONS

■ COMMENTS
• Frequent monitoring of blood pres-sure and electrolytes postoperatively is necessary, because normotension after unilateral adrenalectomy may take up to 4 mo.
• Fig. 1-16 describes a diagnostic ap-proach to patients with adrenal mass.

REFERENCES
Gallay BJ et al: Screening for primary al-dosteronism without discontinuing hy-pertensive medications: plasma aldosterone-renin ratio, *Am J Kidney Dis* 37:699, 2001.

Montori VM et al: Validity of the aldosterone-renin ratio used to screen for primary aldosteronism, *Mayo Clin Proc* 76:877, 2001.
Sawka A et al: Primary aldosteronism: factors associated with normalization of blood pressure after surgery, *Ann Intern Med* 135:258, 2001.
Author: **Fred F. Ferri, M.D.**

BASIC INFORMATION

■ DEFINITION

Altitude sickness refers to a spectrum of illnesses related to hypoxia occurring in people rapidly ascending to high altitudes. The three types of altitude sickness are acute mountain sickness, high-altitude pulmonary edema, and high-altitude cerebral edema (see Table 1-8).

■ SYNONYMS

Acute mountain sickness (AMS)
High-altitude pulmonary edema (HAPE)
High-altitude cerebral edema (HACE)

ICD-9CM CODES

289 Mountain sickness, acute
993.2 High altitude, effects

■ EPIDEMIOLOGY & DEMOGRAPHICS

- Over 30 million people are at risk of developing altitude sickness.
- In Summit County, Colorado, the incidence of acute mountain sickness was 22% at altitudes of 1850 to 2750 m (7000 to 9000 ft) and 42% at altitudes of 3000 m (10,000 ft).
- Approximately 0.01% of tourists to Colorado ski resorts experience HAPE or HACE.

- Men are 5 times more likely to develop HAPE than women.
- AMS and HACE affect men and women equally.

■ PHYSICAL FINDINGS & CLINICAL PRESENTATION

Acute mountain sickness
- Occurs within hours to a few days after rapid ascent over 8000 feet (2500 m)
- Headache
- Dizziness and lightheadedness
- Nausea, vomiting, and loss of appetite
- Fatigue
- Sleep disturbance
- AMS can evolve into HAPE and HACE

High-altitude pulmonary edema (Figs. 1-17 and 1-18)
- Occurs usually during the second night after rapid ascent over 8000 feet (2500 m)
- Dyspnea at rest
- Dry cough
- Chest tightness
- Tachycardia, tachypnea, rales, cyanosis with pink-tinged frothy sputum

High-altitude cerebral edema
- Usually presents several days after AMS
- Confusion, irritability, drowsiness, stupor, hallucinations
- Headache, nausea, vomiting
- Ataxia, paralysis, and seizures

- Coma and death may develop within hours of the first symptoms

■ ETIOLOGY

- As one ascends to altitudes above sea level, the atmospheric pressure decreases. Although the percentage of oxygen in the air remains the same, the partial pressure of oxygen decreases with altitude.
- Thus the cause of altitude sickness is primarily hypoxia resulting from low partial pressures of oxygen.
- The body responds to low oxygen partial pressures through a process of acclimitization (see "Comments").

DIAGNOSIS

The diagnosis of altitude sickness is made by clinical presentation and physical findings described above.

■ DIFFERENTIAL DIAGNOSIS

- Dehydration
- Carbon monoxide poisoning
- Hypothermia
- Infection
- Substance abuse
- Congestive heart failure
- Pulmonary embolism
- Cerebrovascular accident

■ WORKUP

Typically the diagnosis is self-evident after history and physical examination. Laboratory tests and imaging studies help monitor cardiopulmonary and CNS status in patients admitted to the intensive care unit for pulmonary and/or cerebral edema.

■ LABORATORY TESTS

Laboratory tests are not very useful in diagnosing altitude sickness.

■ IMAGING STUDIES

CXR showing Kerley B-lines and patchy edema (see Fig. 1-17)
CT scan of the head showing diffuse or patchy edema

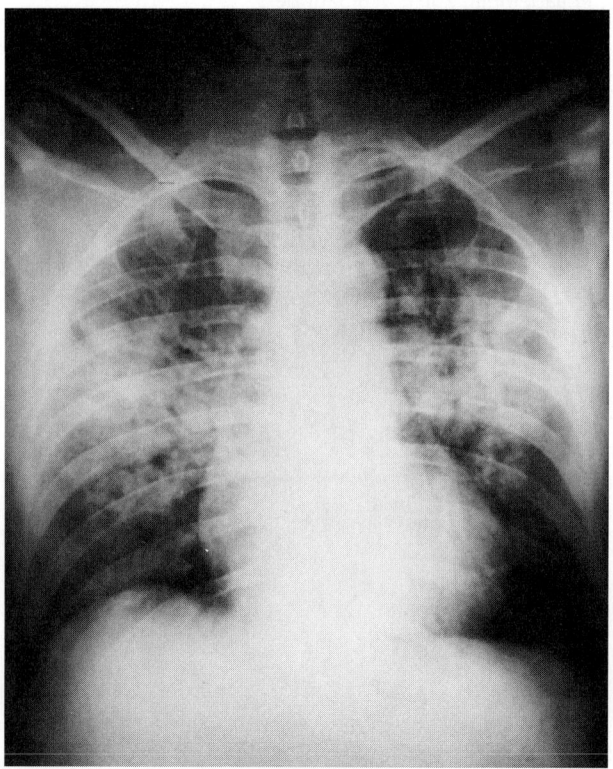

Fig. 1-17   Chest radiograph showing high-altitude pulmonary edema. (From Strauss RH [ed]: *Sports medicine,* ed 2, Philadelphia, 1991, WB Saunders.)

TABLE 1-8   High-Altitude Sickness

	ACUTE MOUNTAIN SICKNESS	HIGH-ALTITUDE PULMONARY EDEMA	HIGH-ALTITUDE CEREBRAL EDEMA
Diagnostic findings	Nausea, vomiting, headache, lethargy, sleep disturbance, tinnitus, vertigo	Shortness of breath, tachypnea, tachycardia, cough, variable cyanosis	Headache, mental confusion, delirium, ataxia, hallucination, seizure, focal neurologic signs, coma
Onset	4-6 hr after reaching high altitude	24-96 hr	48-72 hr
Altitude	>8000 ft	8000-14,000 ft	Usually >12,000 ft
Ancillary data (in addition to those indicated for diagnostic evaluation)	ABG Chest x-ray study Electrolytes	ABG Chest x-ray study ECG Bleeding screen	ABG Electrolytes CT head
Differential considerations			
Trauma	Concussion Gastroenteritis	Pulmonary contusion	Head Meningitis
Infection	Respiratory or CNS infection	Pneumonia	Encephalitis
Metabolic		Uremia	Diabetic ketoacidosis Uremia Encephalopathy $\downarrow\uparrow$ Na$^+$, $\uparrow$ Ca^{++}
Intoxication	Salicylates	Multiple	Narcotics
Vascular		CHF	Subarachnoid hemorrhage
Management (all respond to descent)			
Admit	Variable	Yes	Yes
Oxygen	Yes	Yes	Yes
Acetazolamide	Prophylactic	Prophylactic	Prophylactic
Bronchodilator	No	Yes	No
Steroids	Controversial	Yes	Yes
Ventilation with PEEP	No	Yes, if severe	Hyperventilation

From Barkin RM, Rosen P: *Emergency pediatrics*, St Louis, 1999, Mosby.
ABG, Arterial blood gas; *CHF,* congestive heart failure; *CNS,* central nervous system; *CT,* computed tomography; *ECG,* electrocardiogram; *PEEP,* peak end-expiratory pressure.

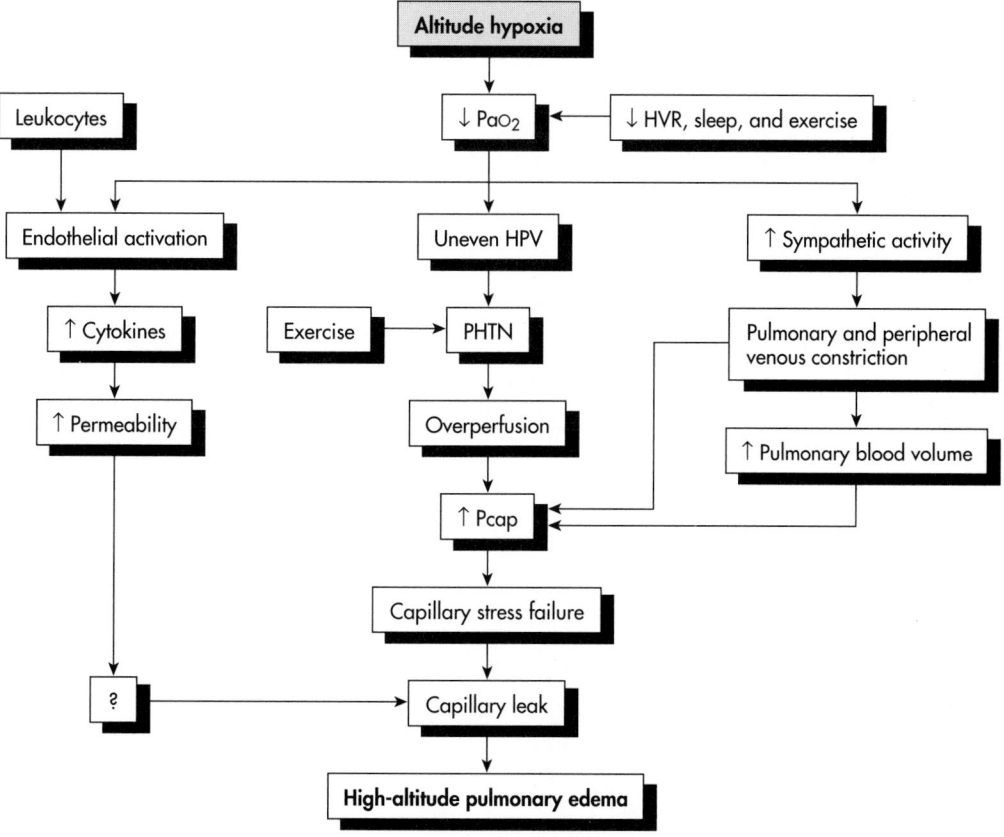

Fig. 1-18   Proposed pathophysiology of high-altitude pulmonary edema. *HPV,* Hypoxic pulmonary vasoconstriction; *HVR,* hypoxic ventilatory response; *Pcap,* capillary pressure; *PHTN,* pulmonary hypertension. (From Auerbach PS: *Wilderness medicine,* ed 4, St Louis, 2001, Mosby.)

℞ TREATMENT

■ NONPHARMACOLOGIC THERAPY

- Stop the ascent to allow acclimatization or start to descend until symptoms have resolved.
- Oxygen 4 to 6 L/min is used for severe AMS, HAPE, and HACE.
- Portable hyperbaric bags are useful if available at the site.
- Avoid dehydration.

■ ACUTE GENERAL Rx

- Aspirin 325 mg PO q6h can be used for headaches in AMS.
- Acetazolamide 125 mg to 250 mg PO bid is used in patients with AMS and HAPE.
- Nifedipine 10 mg sublingual followed by long-acting nifedipine 30 mg bid is used for patients with HAPE who cannot descend immediately.
- Dexamethasone 4 mg PO is used in patients with severe AMS, HAPE, and HACE.

■ CHRONIC Rx

- Prevention therapy is the most prudent therapy.

1. Slow staged ascent to avoid altitude sickness.
2. Start the ascent below 8000 feet.
3. Ascend 1000 ft/day and rest.
4. Spend two nights at the same altitude every 3 days.
5. Sleep at lower heights than the altitude climbed ("climb high, sleep low").

■ DISPOSITION

- AMS improves over a period of 2 to 3 days.
- HAPE is the most common cause of death among the altitude illnesses.
- More than 60% of patients with HAPE will have recurrence of symptoms on subsequent climbs.
- Neurologic deficits may persist for weeks but eventually resolve. If coma occurs, prognosis is poor.

■ REFERRAL

Cardiology and neurology referrals are made in patients with pulmonary edema and CNS findings respectively.

☼ PEARLS & CONSIDERATIONS

■ COMMENTS

- Acclimatization is the process whereby the body adapts to hypoxia by optimizing oxygen delivery to cells. Adaptive mechanism includes:
  1. Hyperventilation to increase O_2 in the setting of hypoxia
  2. Tachycardia secondary to hypoxemia
  3. Pulmonary hypertension developed to improve ventilation perfusion mismatch
  4. Cerebral vasodilatation to increase blood flow to the brain
  5. Rise in hemoglobin and hematocrit
- Risk factors for the development of altitude sicknesses are:
  1. Rapid ascent
  2. Strenuous exertion on arrival
  3. Obesity
  4. Previous history of altitude sickness
  5. Male gender
- Physical fitness is not protective against high-altitude illness.

REFERENCES

Hachett PH, Roach RC: High-altitude illness, *N Engl J Med* 345:107, 2001.
Harris MD et al: High-altitude medicine, *Am Fam Physician* 57(8):1907, 1998.
Klocke DL, Decker WW, Stepanek J: Altitude-related illnesses, *Mayo Clin Proc* 73:988, 1998.
Author: **Peter Petropoulos, M.D.**

BASIC INFORMATION

■ DEFINITION

DSM-IV defines Alzheimer's as follows:

A. The development of multiple cognitive deficits manifested by both:

1. Memory impairment (impaired ability to learn new information and to recall previously learned information)
2. One (or more) of the following cognitive disturbances:
   a. Aphasia (language disturbance)
   b. Apraxia (impaired ability to carry out motor activities despite intact motor function)
   c. Agnosia (failure to recognize or identify objects despite intact sensory function)
   d. Disturbance in executive functioning (i.e., planning, organizing, sequencing, abstracting)

B. The cognitive deficits in criteria A1 and A2 each cause significant impairment in social or occupational functioning and represent a significant decline from a previous level of functioning.

C. The course is characterized by gradual onset and continuing cognitive decline.

D. The cognitive deficits in criteria A1 and A2 are not a result of any of the following:

1. Other central nervous system conditions that cause progressive deficits in memory and cognition (e.g., cerebrovascular disease, Parkinson's disease, Huntington's disease, subdural hematoma, normal-pressure hydrocephalus, brain tumor)
2. Systemic conditions that are known to cause dementia (e.g., hypothyroidism, vitamin B_{12} or folic acid deficiency, niacin deficiency, hypercalcemia, neurosyphilis, HIV infection)
3. Substance-induced conditions

E. The deficits do not occur exclusively during the course of a delirium.

F. The disturbance is not better accounted for by another Axis I disorder (e.g., major depressive disorder, schizophrenia).

ICD-9CM CODES
331.0 Alzheimer's disease

■ EPIDEMIOLOGY & DEMOGRAPHICS
INCIDENCE (IN U.S.): 3.5% of Americans ages 65 to 74 yr
PREDOMINANT SEX: Female
PREDOMINANT AGE: 85+ yr
PEAK INCIDENCE: 65 to 74 yr
GENETICS: Patients with trisomy 21 (Down syndrome) develop Alzheimer's in middle age.
There is a gene on chromosome 109 that appears to be linked to increased levels of amyloid B_{42}, a neurotoxic molecule associated with both early-onset and late-onset Alzheimer's disease.

■ PHYSICAL FINDINGS & CLINICAL PRESENTATION
Families often bring patient to medical attention because of memory problems (e.g., repetitive questions, misplacement of items, missed appointments, getting lost away from home), hallucinations, disruptive behavior, insomnia, and anxiety/depression disorders.
Initial screen of cognitive function: diagnosis requires a documentation of a decline in cognition from a previous level. Perform Folstein Mini-Mental Status Examination.

- Orientation to time and space: based on intact registration and recall (short-term memory); orientation to space is preserved longer than orientation to time.
- Registration: depends on hearing and paying attention; if patient unable to complete task, consider the diagnosis of delirium (see above).
- Attention and calculation: to avoid educational bias, use simple tasks such as saying the days of the week forward and backward or counting backward from 20 to 0; because this function is preserved very late in Alzheimer's disease, if patient unable to complete task, consider a frontal lobe dementia such as Pick's disease or delirium.
- Recall: patients with early stages of dementia will make first errors in this function, often with no other errors in the examination. Errors in orientation follow next.
- Language: patients with early stages of Alzheimer's disease will have specific difficulty drawing a clock showing a given time. This is a measure of the characteristic visual-spatial impairment.
- Consider comprehensive neuropsychologic testing by a qualified neuropsychologist to confirm screening mental status testing. This testing can help differentiate parietal-temporal dementias (AD or PD) from frontal-temporal dementias, such as Pick's, or focal dementias, such as vascular dementias.

DIAGNOSIS

■ WORKUP
Lumbar puncture if chronic CNS infection is suspected

■ LABORATORY TESTS
- CBC
- Serum electrolytes
- Glucose
- BUN/creatinine
- Liver and thyroid function tests
- Serum vitamin B_{12} and methylmalonic acid
- Syphilis serology
- HIV, sedimentation rate, urinalysis

■ IMAGING STUDIES
CT scan or MRI to rule out hydrocephalus and mass lesions and to document cerebral atropy

TREATMENT

■ NONPHARMACOLOGIC THERAPY
Patients must have a caregiver; enrollment in adult day care centers is helpful.

■ ACUTE GENERAL Rx
None

■ CHRONIC Rx
- Above all, make sure the patient does not have a treatable cause of dementia.
- Estrogen replacement may reduce incidence in women.
- Donepezil (Aricept) 5 mg PO at hs initially, subsequently increased to 10 mg qd may improve both cognition and global function in mild to moderate Alzheimer's dementia. This drug is very expensive and may not be cost effective. Not indicated in severe Alzheimer's.
- Rivastigmine (Exelon) is a reversible cholinesterase inhibitor recently approved for the treatment of mild to moderate dementia of Alzheimer's type. Starting dose is 1.5 mg bid, gradually increasing to 3 mg bid if well tolerated after a minimum of 2 weeks. Not indicated in severe Alzheimer's.
- Galantamine (Reminyl) is a newer agent for the treatment of mild to moderate dementia of the Alzheimer's type. Its precise mechanism of action is unknown but is thought to include acetylcholinesterase inhibition. Initial starting dose is 4 mg PO bid. This medication is contraindicated in patients with severe hepatic or renal impairment.

PEARLS & CONSIDERATIONS

■ COMMENTS
The physician must make a thorough search for the treatable causes of dementia.

REFERENCES

Bertram L et al: Guidance for genetic linkage of Alzheimer's disease to chromosome 109, *Science* 290:2302, 2000.

DSM-IV: Diagnostic and statistical manual of mental disorders, ed 4, Washington, DC, 1994, American Psychiatric Association.

Richards S, Hendric HC: Diagnosis, management, and treatment of Alzheimer's disease, *Arch Intern Med* 159:789, 1999.

Author: **William H. Olson, M.D.**

BASIC INFORMATION

■ DEFINITION
Amaurosis fugax is a temporary loss of vision in one eye caused by transient interference with its blood supply.

ICD-9CM CODES
362.34 Amaurosis fugax

■ EPIDEMIOLOGY & DEMOGRAPHICS
INCIDENCE (IN U.S.): An uncommon presentation of carotid artery disease
PEAK INCIDENCE: 55 yr and older

■ PHYSICAL FINDINGS & CLINICAL PRESENTATION
- There are usually no physical findings.
- Acute stage: cholesterol emboli may be seen in retinal artery (Hollenhorst plaque): carotid bruits or other evidence of generalized atherosclerosis.
- If embolus is cardiac in origin, atrial fibrillation is often present.

■ ETIOLOGY
Usually embolic

DIAGNOSIS

■ DIFFERENTIAL DIAGNOSIS
- Embolic from carotid artery, aorta and great vessels, heart
- Ocular causes: glaucoma, central retinal vein or artery occlusion
- Neurologic causes: optic neuritis, multiple sclerosis, optic nerve compression
- Systemic disorders: migraine, giant cell arteritis, blood dyscrasia

■ WORKUP
- Careful examination of retina; embolus may be visible and confirm the diagnosis (Fig. 1-19)
- Auscultation of arteries for bruits
- Examination of all pulses

■ LABORATORY TESTS
- CBC with sedimentation rate.
- PT and PTT.
- Serum chemistries, including lipid profile.
- Anticardiolipin antibody, protein C, and protein S should be considered in younger patients with a personal or family history of coagulopathy or strokes at a young age.
- VDRL and toxicology screen are discretionary tests based on patient's age and history.

■ IMAGING STUDIES
- Carotid Dopplers followed by MRA or four-vessel angiography as indicated.
- Transthoracic echocardiography (TTE) is indicated to screen for embolization in patients with evidence of heart disease and in patients without an evident source for their transient neurologic deficit. Transesophageal echocardiography (TEE) is more sensitive for detecting cardiac sources of embolization (ventricular mural thrombus, patent foramen ovale, aortic arch, mitral valve disorders); however, it is more uncomfortable and expensive and is best reserved for patients with an unknown source of TIA or when cardiac embolization cannot be completely ruled out on TTE.

TREATMENT

■ NONPHARMACOLOGIC THERAPY
- Diet (decrease saturated fatty acids and high-cholesterol foods)
- Exercise
- Cessation of tobacco use if thought to be atherosclerotic in origin

■ ACUTE GENERAL Rx
- Treat as an emergency.
- Give aspirin, heparin if there is no intracranial hemorrhage.

■ CHRONIC Rx
Reduce risks by carotid endarterectomy if stenosis >80%. Control hypertension and manage risk factors for increased cholesterol levels.

■ DISPOSITION
If significant stenosis not found and emboli are from carotid, consider other causes in differential diagnosis.

■ REFERRAL
Vascular surgeon or neurosurgeon if significant stenosis found
- Carotid endarterectomy is indicated in the following settings:
  1. High-grade (≥80%) isolateral stenosis and surgery can be done early and at low risk
  2. Greater than 50% stenosis associated with a large carotid artery ulcer
  3. Multiple TIAs despite medical therapy, in the setting of high-grade or ulcerative ipsilateral disease, and surgery can be done at low to medium risk
  4. Crescendo attacks in the setting of high-grade or ulcerative ipsilateral disease and surgery can be done at low to medium risk
- Patient preference and the experience of the surgical team should be considered whenever surgery is contemplated.

PEARLS & CONSIDERATIONS

■ COMMENTS
Although amaurosis fugax is relatively rare, this classic presentation of carotid artery disease is often accompanied by a transient contralateral hemiparesis.

REFERENCES
Benauente D et al: Prognosis after transient monocular blindness associated with carotid-artery stenosis, *N Engl J Med* 345:1084, 2001.
Ryan MR, Combs G, Penix L: Preventing stroke in patients with transient ischemic attacks, *Am Fam Physician* 60:2329, 1999.
Author: **William H. Olson, M.D.**

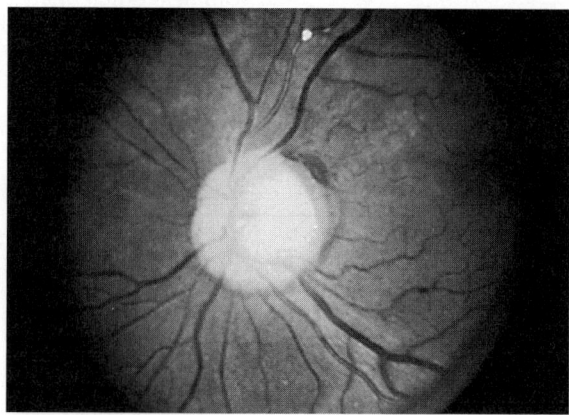

Fig. 1-19 A cholesterol crystal embolus lodged at an arterial bifurcation. (From Stein JH [ed]: *Internal medicine,* ed 5, St Louis, 1998, Mosby.)

BASIC INFORMATION

■ **DEFINITION**
Amblyopia refers to a decrease in vision in one or both eyes in the presence of an otherwise normal ophthalmologic examination.

■ **SYNONYMS**
Deprivation amblyopia
Occlusion amblyopia
Strabismus amblyopia
Refractive amblyopia
Organic or toxic amblyopias
Lazy eye

■ **ICD-9CM CODES**
368.00 Amblyopia

■ **EPIDEMIOLOGY & DEMOGRAPHICS**
INCIDENCE (IN U.S.): 1% to 4% of the general population
PREVALENCE (IN U.S.): High incidence in premature infants with drug-dependent mothers and in neurologically impaired children

PREDOMINANT SEX: None
PREDOMINANT AGE: Childhood
PEAK INCIDENCE: Childhood

■ **PHYSICAL FINDINGS & CLINICAL PRESENTATION**
Decreased vision using best refraction in the presence of normal corneal, lens, retinal, and optic nerve appearance (Fig. 1-20)

■ **ETIOLOGY**
• Visual deprivation
• Strabismus
• Occlusion with patching
• Refractive error organic lesions in the nervous system
• Toxins

🔬 **DIAGNOSIS**

■ **DIFFERENTIAL DIAGNOSIS**
• Central nervous system (CNS) disease (brainstem)
• Optic nerve disorders
• Corneal or other eye diseases

■ **WORKUP**
• Complete eye examination
• Motility evaluation

■ **LABORATORY TESTS**
Usually none

■ **IMAGING STUDIES**
Usually not necessary unless CNS lesion suspected

℞ **TREATMENT**

■ **NONPHARMACOLOGIC THERAPY**
• Glasses
• Patches
• Removal of the cause of the amblyopia if possible
• Surgery to align the eyes

■ **CHRONIC Rx**
Patching or optics, including prisms

■ **DISPOSITION**
Immediate patching, alternating eyes daily

■ **REFERRAL**
To ophthalmologist if vision is compromised

💡 **PEARLS & CONSIDERATIONS**

■ **COMMENTS**
The earlier the referral, the better the outcome.
Author: **Melvyn Koby, M.D.**

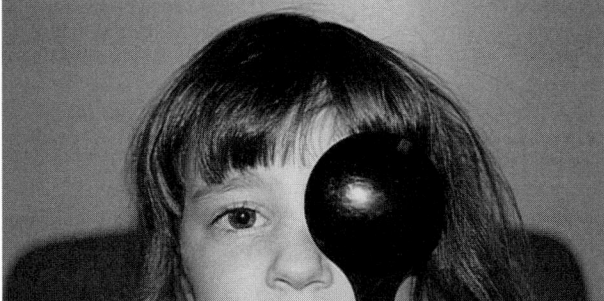

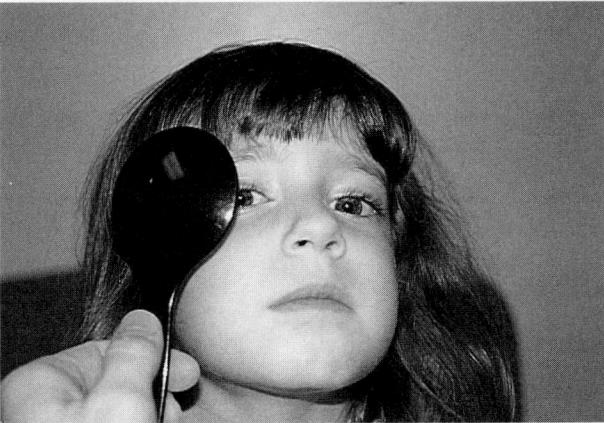

Fig. 1-20   A, This child happily fixes with her right eye and does not object if the left eye is covered. **B,** When the right eye is covered she moves her head away and tries to remove the cover, demonstrating a fixation preference for the right eye and amblyopia of the left eye. (From Hoekelman R [ed]: *Primary pediatric care,* ed 3, St Louis, 1997, Mosby.)

BASIC INFORMATION

■ DEFINITION
Amebiasis is an infection caused by the protozoal parasite *Entamoeba histolytica*. Although primarily an infection of the colon, amebiasis may cause extraintestinal disease, particularly liver abscess.

■ SYNONYMS
Amebic dysentery (when severe intestinal infection)

ICD-9CM CODES
006.9 Amebiasis

■ EPIDEMIOLOGY & DEMOGRAPHICS
INCIDENCE (IN U.S.): Highest in institutionalized patients, sexually active homosexual men
PREVALENCE (IN U.S.): 4% (80% of infections asymptomatic)
PREDOMINANT SEX:
- Equal sex distribution in general
- Striking male predominance of liver abscess
PREDOMINANT AGE: Second through sixth decades
PEAK INCIDENCE: Peaks at age 2 to 3 yr and >40 yr
GENETICS: Infection more likely to be fulminant in young infants

■ PHYSICAL FINDINGS & CLINICAL PRESENTATION
- Often nonspecific
- Approximately 20% of cases symptomatic
  1. Diarrhea, which may be bloody
  2. Abdominal and back pain
- Abdominal tenderness in 83% of severe cases
- Fever in 38% of severe cases
- Hepatomegaly, RUQ tenderness, and fever in almost all patients with liver abscess (may be absent in fulminant cases)

■ ETIOLOGY
- Caused by the protozoal parasite *E. histolytica* (Fig. 1-21)
- Transmission by the fecal-oral route
- Infection usually localized to the large bowel, particularly the cecum where a localized mass lesion (ameboma) may form
- Extraintestinal infection in which the organism invades the bowel mucosa and gains access to the portal circulation

DIAGNOSIS

■ DIFFERENTIAL DIAGNOSIS
- Severe intestinal infection possibly confused with ulcerative colitis or other infectious enterocolitis syndromes, such as those caused by

Shigella, Salmonella, Campylobacter, or invasive *Escherichia coli*
- In elderly patients: ischemic bowel possibly producing a similar picture

■ WORKUP
- Three stool specimens over a period of 7 to 10 days to exclude the diagnosis (sensitivity 50% to 80%)
- Concentration and staining the specimen with Lugol's iodine or methylene blue to increase the diagnostic yield
- Available culture (rarely necessary in routine cases)

■ LABORATORY TESTS
- Stool examination is generally reliable.
- Mucosal biopsy is occasionally necessary.
- Serum antibody may be detected and is particularly sensitive and specific for extraintestinal infection or severe intestinal disease.
- Aspiration of abscess fluid is used to distinguish amebic from bacterial abscesses.

■ IMAGING STUDIES
Abdominal imaging studies (sonography or CT scan) to diagnose liver abscess

TREATMENT

■ ACUTE GENERAL Rx
- Metronidazole (750 mg PO tid for 10 days) is used in the treatment of mild to severe intestinal infection and amebic liver abscess; it may be administered intravenously when necessary.
- Follow with iodoquinol (650 mg PO tid for 20 days) to eradicate persistent cysts.

- For asymptomatic patients with amebic cysts on stool examination, use iodoquinol or paromomycin (500 mg PO tid for 7 days).
- Avoid antiperistaltic agents in severe intestinal infections to avoid risk of toxic megacolon.
- Liver abscess is generally responsive to medical management but surgical intervention indicated for extension of liver abscess into pericardium or, occasionally, for toxic megacolon.

■ DISPOSITION
Host immunity incomplete and reinfection rate high for patients remaining at risk

■ REFERRAL
- For consultation with infectious diseases specialist for extraintestinal infection or persistent or relapsing intestinal infection
- For surgical consultation:
  1. For toxic megacolon
  2. For impending rupture of or extension of liver abscess into adjacent structures

PEARLS & CONSIDERATIONS

■ COMMENTS
- Infection with other intestinal parasites, particularly *Giardia lamblia,* may coexist with amebiasis.
- Clinical algorithms for evaluation of patients with diarrhea are described in Figs. 3-51 and 3-52.

REFERENCE
Stanley SL: Protective immunity to amebiasis: new insights and new challenges, *J Infect Dis* 184(4):504, 2001.
Author: **Joseph R. Masci, M.D.**

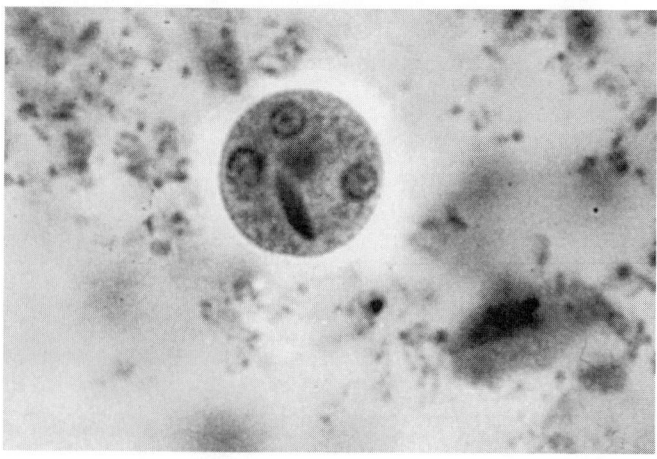

Fig. 1-21 Mature cyst of *Entamoeba histolytica.* Three of the four nuclei are seen in the plane of focus of this photomicrograph. (From Mandell GL [ed]: *Mandell, Douglas, and Bennett's principles and practice of infectious diseases,* ed 5, New York, 2000, Churchill Livingstone.)

BASIC INFORMATION

■ DEFINITION
Amyloidosis is a generic term describing the deposition of amyloid fibrils in body tissues. *Amyloid* is an amorphous, eosinophilic material; it is birefringent and usually extracellular. Electron microscopy reveals nonbranching fibrils that are soluble and relatively resistant to proteolytic digestion.

ICD-9CM CODES
277.3 Amyloidosis

■ EPIDEMIOLOGY & DEMOGRAPHICS
- Amyloidosis affects primarily males between the ages of 60 and 70 yr.
- There are between 1500 and 3500 new cases annually in the U.S.
- The most common type in the U.S. is immunoglobulin light chain related (AL).

■ PHYSICAL FINDINGS & CLINICAL PRESENTATION
- Findings are variable with organ system involvement. Symmetric polyarthritis, peripheral neuropathy, and carpal tunnel syndrome may be present with joint involvement.
- Signs and symptoms of nephrotic syndrome may be present with renal involvement.
- Fatigue and dyspnea may occur with pulmonary involvement.
- Diarrhea, macroglossia (20% of patients), malabsorption, hepatomegaly, and weight loss may occur with GI involvement.
- Cardiac involvement is common and can lead to predominantly right-sided CHF, JVD, peripheral edema, and hepatomegaly.
- Vascular involvement can result in easy bleeding and periorbital purpura ("racoon-eyes").

■ ETIOLOGY
The source of amyloid protein is a population of monoclonal plasma cells in the bone marrow. There are several chemically documented amyloidoses that can be principally subdivided into:
1. Acquired systemic amyloidosis (immunoglobulin light chain, multiple myeloma, hemodialysis amyloidosis)
2. Heredofamilial systemic (polyneuropathy, familial Mediterranean fever)
3. Organ-limited (Alzheimer's disease)
4. Localized endocrine (pancreatic islet, medullary thyroid carcinoma)

■ DIAGNOSIS

■ DIFFERENTIAL DIAGNOSIS
Variable, depending on the organ involvement:
- Renal involvement (toxin- or drug-induced necrosis, glomerulonephritis, renal vein thrombosis)
- Interstitial lung disease (sarcoidosis, connective tissue disease, infectious etiologies)
- Restrictive cardiac (endomyocardial fibrosis, viral myocarditis)
- Carpal tunnel (rheumatoid arthritis, hypothyroidism, overuse)
- Mental status changes (multiinfarct dementia)
- Peripheral neuropathy (alcohol abuse, vitamin deficiencies, diabetes mellitus)

■ WORKUP
Diagnostic approach is aimed at demonstration of amyloid deposits in tissues. This may be accomplished with rectal biopsy (positive in >60% of cases). Renal, myocardial, and bone marrow biopsy are other options. Abdominal fat pad biopsy can also be diagnostic.

■ LABORATORY TESTS
- Initial laboratory evaluation should include CBC, TSH, renal functions studies, ALT, AST, alkaline phosphatase, bilirubin, urinalysis, and serum and urine protein immunoelectrophoresis.
- Various laboratory abnormalities include proteinuria (found in >70% of cases), anemia, renal insufficiency, liver function abnormalities, hypothyroidism (10% to 20% of patients), and elevated monoclonal proteins. The finding of a monoclonal light chain in the serum or urine is very useful for diagnosis.

■ IMAGING STUDIES
- Chest x-ray may reveal hilar adenopathy and mediastinal adenopathy.
- Two-dimensional Doppler echocardiography to study diagnostic filling is useful to evaluate for cardiac involvement.
- Nuclear imaging with technetium-labeled aprotinin may detect cardiac amyloidosis.

■ TREATMENT

■ NONPHARMACOLOGIC THERAPY
Lifestyle changes with low-salt diet in patients with CHF; protein and sodium restrictions in patients with renal failure

■ ACUTE GENERAL Rx
Therapy is variable, depending on the type of amyloidosis. Amyloidosis associated with plasma cell disorders may be treated with melphalan and prednisone, along with colchicine. Colchicine may also be effective in renal amyloidosis.

■ CHRONIC Rx
Renal transplantation is needed in patients with renal amyloidosis. Peritoneal dialysis in place of hemodialysis in patients with renal failure may improve hemodialysis amyloidosis by clearing β-2 microglobulin.

■ DISPOSITION
Prognosis is determined primarily by the presence or absence of cardiac involvement and with the form of amyloidosis:
- In reactive amyloidosis, eradication of the predisposing disease slows and can occasionally reverse the progression of amyloid disease. Survival of 5 to 10 yr after diagnosis is not uncommon.
- Patients with familial amyloidotic polyneuropathy generally have a prolonged course lasting 10 to 15 yr.
- Amyloidosis associated with immunocytic processes carries the worst prognosis (life expectancy <1 yr).
- The progression of amyloidosis associated with renal hemodialysis can be improved with newer dialysis membranes that can pass β-2 microglobulin.
- Median survival in patients with overt CHF is approximately 6 mo, 30 mo without CHF.

■ REFERRAL
Surgical referral for biopsy of subcutaneous abdominal fat, skin, gingival, or rectal tissue

✦ PEARLS & CONSIDERATIONS

■ COMMENTS
Amyloidosis should be considered in any patient older than 40 yr presenting with nonischemic CHF, nephrotic syndrome, unexplained hepatomegaly, and idiopathic peripheral neuropathy.

REFERENCES
Dember LM et al: Effect of dose-intensive intravenous melphalan and autologous blood stem-cell transplantation on a1 amyloidosis-associated renal disease, *Ann Intern Med* 134:746, 2001.
Gertz MA et al: Amyloidosis, confirmation, prognosis, and therapy, *Mayo Clin Proc* 74:490, 1999.
Author: **Fred F. Ferri, M.D.**

BASIC INFORMATION

■ DEFINITION
Amyotrophic lateral sclerosis (ALS) is a progressive neuromuscular condition affecting upper and lower motor neurons, characterized pathologically by degeneration of motor neurons in the brainstem and spinal cord and by degeneration of neurons in the motor cortex and corticospinal tracts.

■ SYNONYMS
ALS
Lou Gehrig's disease

ICD-9CM CODES
335.20 Amyotrophic lateral sclerosis

■ EPIDEMIOLOGY & DEMOGRAPHICS
INCIDENCE: 0.5 to 2 cases/100,000 persons. Onset is usually between the ages of 50 and 70 years. The male:female ratio is 2:1.
PREVALENCE: 5 in 100,000 persons
GENETICS: 5% of cases are familial in an autosomal dominant pattern; some but not all families map to the gene for superoxide dismutase on chromosome 21.

■ PHYSICAL FINDINGS & CLINICAL PRESENTATION
- Lower motor neuron signs (asymmetric muscle weakness, wasting, fasciculations)
- Upper motor neuron signs (Babinski's sign, clonus)
- Unexplained weight loss, slurring of speech
- Difficulty walking and swallowing
- Hyperreflexia

■ ETIOLOGY
- The cause of ALS is unknown. Mutations in a single gene can initiate a process that leads to the selective degeneration of motor neurons.
- A familial form is transmitted in an autosomal dominant pattern.
- Ingestion of the cycad nut may be associated with ALS-Parkinson-dementia complex of Guam.

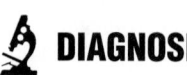

DIAGNOSIS

■ DIFFERENTIAL DIAGNOSIS
- Cervical spondylotic myelopathy
- Spinal stenosis with compression of lumbosacral nerve roots

- Lead axonal neuropathy
- Multifocal motor neuropathy with conduction block
- Syphilitic myelitis with amyotrophy
- Delayed effects of electrical injury to spinal cord
- Late-onset hexosaminidase deficiency
- Polyglucosan body disease
- Syringomyelia
- Spinal AV malformations

■ WORKUP
- EMG and nerve conduction studies
- Lumbar puncture and CSF analysis
- Bone marrow examination to exclude myeloma, Waldenstrom disease, or other lymphoproliferative disease if CSF protein content exceeds 75 mg/dl

■ LABORATORY TESTS
- Serum protein immunofixation electrophoresis on warm blood (allowed to clot at 37° C to avoid loss of the monoclonal proteins as a cryoglobulin)
- Quantitative immunoglobulin analysis
- Antibodies to GM1 and myelin-associated glycoprotein
- Heavy metal testing: generally not indicated

■ IMAGING STUDIES
- Chest x-ray examination
- MRI in selected cases to exclude disorders listed in differential diagnosis
- Modified barium swallow to evaluate risk of choking

TREATMENT

■ NONPHARMACOLOGIC THERAPY
- Family planning for chronic illness (discussion of living will, financial matters, and DNR orders)
- Emotional support for patient and family members
- Prosthetic devices (e.g., wheelchair)
- Discussion regarding preparation for tracheostomy
- Noninvasive positive-pressure ventilation for patients with ALS and respiratory insufficiency
- Physical therapy, speech therapy

■ ACUTE GENERAL Rx
Riluzole (Rilutek) is the only medication approved to extend survival in patients with ALS. Dosage is 50 mg q12h,

at least 1 hr before or 2 hr after meals. Benefits are marginal (prolonged survival by 3-6 months) and the medication is very expensive.

■ CHRONIC Rx
- Supportive care to prevent complications (aspiration, decubitus ulcerations, malnutrition)
- Relief of spasticity with baclofen, dantrolene, or diazepam
- Treatment of depression

■ DISPOSITION
- Mean duration of symptoms is 2 to 4 yr.
- About 20% of patients survive >5 yr.
- There have been reports of spontaneous arrest of the disease.

■ REFERRAL
- Referral to a neurologist is recommended to confirm diagnosis.
- Surgical referral for tracheostomy may be needed to prevent aspiration as the disease progresses.
- Psychiatric referral for counseling on associated anxiety and depression may be necessary in selected cases.
- Nursing home placement and/or hospice may be necessary in advanced stages of the disease.
- GI referral for PEG placement may be needed.

☼ PEARLS & CONSIDERATIONS

■ COMMENTS
- Patient education material may be obtained through the ALS Association, 21021 Ventura Boulevard, Suite 321, Woodland Hills, CA 91364, phone: (800) 782-4727; or the Muscular Dystrophy Association, 3561 East Sunrise Drive, Tucson, AZ 85718-3204; phone: (602) 529-2000.
- Variants of ALS include progressive spinal atrophy (lower motor neuron signs alone are evident) and primary lateral sclerosis (only upper motor neuron signs are seen).

REFERENCES
Ganzini L et al: Attitudes of patients with amyotrophic lateral sclerosis and their care givers toward assisted suicide, *N Engl J Med* 339:957, 1998.
Rowland LP, Shneider NA: Amyotrophic lateral sclerosis, *N Engl J Med* 344:1688, 2001.
Author: **Fred F. Ferri, M.D.**

BASIC INFORMATION

■ DEFINITION

An anaerobic infection is caused by one of a group of bacteria that require a reduced oxygen tension for growth.

ICD-9CM CODES
See specific condition.

■ EPIDEMIOLOGY & DEMOGRAPHICS

INCIDENCE (IN U.S.): Statistics incomplete for various reasons: unavailable specimens, fastidious organisms, inadequate culture techniques

■ PHYSICAL FINDINGS & CLINICAL PRESENTATION

- May occur at any site, but most are anatomically related to mucosal surfaces
- Should be suspected when there is foul-smelling tissue, soft-tissue gas, necrotic tissue, or abscesses
- Head and neck
  1. Odontogenic infections from dental or soft tissue possibly progressing to periapical abscesses, at times extending to bone
  2. Both anaerobic and aerobic pathogens in chronic sinusitis, chronic mastoiditis, and chronic otitis media
  3. Peritonsillar abscess possible
  4. Complications: deep neck space infections, brain abscesses, mediastinitis
- Pleuropulmonary
  1. May involve anaerobes present in the oropharynx
  2. Aspiration more common in persons with altered mental status or seizures
  3. Anaerobic bacteria more likely in those with gingivitis or periodontitis
  4. Manifestations: necrotizing pneumonia, empyema, lung abscess
- Intraabdominal
  1. Disruption of intestinal integrity leading to infection involving anaerobic bacteria
  2. Bacteria from colonic neoplasm, perforated appendicitis, diverticulitis, or bowel surgery, causing bacteremia, peritonitis, at times intraabdominal abscesses
  3. Resulting infections usually mixed, containing both anaerobes and aerobes
- Female genital tract
  1. Anaerobes in bacterial vaginosis, salpingitis, endometritis, pelvic abscesses, septic abortion; infections tend to be mixed
  2. Possible pelvic thrombophlebitis when resolving pelvic infection is accompanied by new or persistent fever
- Other anaerobic infections
  1. Skin and soft-tissue infection at any site
  2. More commonly associated infections: synergistic gangrene, bite wound infections, infected decubitus ulcers
  3. Clinical significance of anaerobes in diabetic foot infections unclear
  4. Anaerobic bacteremia uncommon with source usually intraabdominal, followed by female genital tract, pleuropulmonary, and head and neck infections
  5. Osteomyelitis especially when associated with decubitus ulcers or vascular insufficiency
  6. Facial bone osteomyelitis from adjacent infections of the teeth or sinuses

■ ETIOLOGY

- Most commonly endogenous, arising from bacteria that normally line mucosal surfaces
- Disruption of mucosal barriers resulting from various conditions (trauma, ischemia, surgery, perforation), with infection occurring when organisms gain access to normally sterile sites, causing tissue destruction and abscess formation
- Synergy between different anaerobes or between anaerobes and aerobes important

- Most commonly involved: gram-negative anaerobic bacilli
  1. *Bacteroides*
     a. Many organisms, including those in the *B. fragilis* group, which can be found in most intraabdominal infections
     b. May also play a part in infections of the female genital tract, only occasionally causing infections above the diaphragm
  2. *Prevotella:* may be involved in oral and pleuropulmonary infections, as well as infections of the female genital tract
  3. *Porphyromonas:* important in dental infections
  4. *Fusobacterium:* may be involved in infections related to oral flora (pleuropulmonary, otitis, sinusitis, brain abscess)
- Gram-positive anaerobic cocci
  1. *Peptostreptococcus* and anaerobic *Streptococcus*
  2. More commonly associated with head and neck infections, female genital tract infections, and, at times, skin and soft-tissue infections
- Anaerobic gram-positive bacilli
  1. Less common
  2. Include *Clostridium difficile*–associated diarrhea and *C. perfringens* wound infections
  3. Bacteremia with *C. septicum, C. perfringens,* or *C. tertium* possibly associated with colonic malignancy
  4. Potent toxins produced by *C. botulinum* and *C. tetani* potential cause of severe disease
  5. *Propionibacterium:* can occasionally cause serious disease, but a frequent contaminant of blood cultures
  6. *Actinomyces,* most commonly *A. israelii,* causes infections that cross tissue planes and result in draining sinuses

Oral-cervicofacial, pleuropulmonary, and abdominal disease most common. Pelvic disease usually related to use of intrauterine contraceptive device. Sulfur granules may be found in clinical specimens.

DIAGNOSIS

■ **DIFFERENTIAL DIAGNOSIS**
- Clinically similar to focal infections caused by other organisms, but have an increased propensity toward tissue destruction and abscess formation
- Aerobic gram-negative organisms involved in gas formation, although more commonly associated with anaerobes
- Abscesses differentiated from other space-occupying lesions
- Diarrhea associated with *C. difficile* a mimic of other causes of infectious diarrhea

■ **WORKUP**
- Specimens submitted for culture processed within 30 min
- Large volume of material more likely to have significant growth; swabs less efficient for transporting infected material
- Blood cultures—preferably before antibiotic administration

■ **LABORATORY TESTS**
- Elevated WBC count, with extremely high WBC counts sometimes seen with pseudomembranous colitis
- Positive stool *C. difficile* toxin assay
- Increased lactate levels in ischemia or perforation
- Possible positive blood or wound cultures, but failure to grow anaerobes in culture may be common, attributed to inadequate culturing techniques and/or fastidious organisms

■ **IMAGING STUDIES**
- Plain film of an affected area to show gas in tissues, free air resulting from a perforated viscus, or an air/fluid level inside an abscess
- Ultrasound, CT scan, or MRI to reveal abscesses or tissue destruction

■ **TREATMENT**

■ **NONPHARMACOLOGIC THERAPY**
- Removal of necrotic tissue
- Drainage of abscesses (accomplished by CT scan–guided percutaneous drainage)

■ **ACUTE GENERAL Rx**
Oral antibiotics with anaerobic activity: clindamycin, metronidazole, and chloramphenicol
- Broader spectrum of activity with amoxicillin/clavulanate
- Penicillin VK in odontogenic infections
- Oral metronidazole for *C. difficile*–associated diarrhea, with oral vancomycin reserved for recurrent or recalcitrant infections
Parenteral antibiotics for more serious illness
- IV clindamycin, metronidazole, and chloramphenicol
- Cephalosporins (anaerobic or mixed infections): cefoxitin and cefotetan
- Extended-spectrum penicillins (i.e., piperacillin) and combination β-lactamase plus β-lactamase inhibitor drugs
  1. Significant anaerobic activity, plus various degrees of broad-spectrum coverage
  2. Include ampicillin/sulbactam, ticarcillin/clavulanate, and piperacillin/tazobactam

- Imipenem: a broad-spectrum agent with extensive anaerobic activity
- Actinomycosis treated with penicillin for 6 to 12 mo
- SMX/TMP and fluoroquinolones: ineffective
- Table 1-9 describes antimicrobial susceptibility patterns for anaerobic bacteria.

■ **CHRONIC Rx**
Some infections (lung abscess, osteomyelitis, and empyema) require weeks to months of therapy.

■ **DISPOSITION**
- Most infections are curable if adequate surgical and medical therapy is provided.
- Those involving sites with compromised vasculature are more likely to require surgical manipulation, including amputation.

■ **REFERRAL**
If other than mild disease

☼ **PEARLS & CONSIDERATIONS**

■ **COMMENTS**
- Chloramphenicol is associated with aplastic anemia, although this is an extremely rare complication.
- Imipenem is a possible cause of thrombocytopenia and may lower the seizure threshold, especially in elderly patients with renal insufficiency.

REFERENCE
Ortiz E, Sande MA: Routine use of anaerobic blood cultures: are they still indicated? *Am J Med* 108:445, 2000.
Author: **Maurice Policar, M.D.**

TABLE 1-9 Antimicrobial Susceptibility Patterns for Anaerobic Bacteria*

BACTERIA	PENICILLIN	β-LACTAMASE†	CEFOXITIN	CEFOTETAN	IMIPENEM/ MEROPENEM	TROVA- FLOXACIN	CLINDAMYCIN	METRON- IDAZOLE
B. fragilis	−	+	+	+	+	+	v	+
B. thetaiotaomicron	−	+	v	v	+	v	v	+
B. fragilis group, other	−	+	v	v	+	+	v	+
Prevotella species	v	+	+	+	+	+	+	+
Fusobacterium nucleatum	v	+	+	+	+	v	+	+
Fusobacterium necrophorum	+	+	+	+	+	v	+	+
Porphyromonas species	+	+	+	+	+	+	+	+
Peptostreptococci	+	+	+	+	+	+	+	+
Propionibacterium acnes	+	+	+	+	+	+	+	+
Veillonella	+	+	+	+	+	+	+	+
Actinomyces	+	+	+	+	+	+	+	+

From Goldman L, Bennett JC (eds): *Cecil textbook of medicine*, ed 21, Philadelphia, 2000, WB Saunders.
−, Resistant; +, susceptible; *v*, variable.
*Based on a variety of in vitro susceptibility studies from different laboratories and using different techniques.
†β-Lactamase inhibitor, β-lactam combination (e.g., ticarcillin/clavulanate, amipicillin/sulbactam, pipericillin/tazobactam).

BASIC INFORMATION

■ DEFINITION
A fissure is a tear in the epithelial lining of the anal canal (i.e., from the dentate line to the anal verge).

■ SYNONYMS
Anorectal fissure
Anal ulcer

■ ICD-9CM CODES
565.0 Anal fissure

■ EPIDEMIOLOGY & DEMOGRAPHICS
- Can occur at any age
- Most common in young and middle-aged adults
- Occurs in men > women
- Women more likely to have anterior fissure than men (10% vs. 1%, respectively)
- Most common cause of rectal bleeding in infants
- Common in women before and after childbirth

■ PHYSICAL FINDINGS & CLINICAL PRESENTATION
With separation of the buttocks will see a tear in the posterior midline or, less frequently, in the anterior midline (Fig. 1-22)
- Acute anal fissure:
  1. Sharp burning or tearing pain exacerbated by bowel movements
  2. Bright-red blood on toilet paper, a streak of blood on the stool or in the water
- Chronic anal fissure:
  1. Pruritus ani
  2. Pain seldom present
  3. Intermittent bleeding
  4. Sentinel tag at the caudal aspect of the fissure, hypertrophied anal papilla at the proximal end
- Underlying disease possible if the fissure:
  1. Is ectopically located
  2. Extends proximal to the dentate line
  3. Is broad-based or deep
  4. Is especially purulent

■ ETIOLOGY
- Most initiated after passage of a large, hard stool
- May result from frequent defecation and diarrhea
- Bacterial infections: TB, syphilis, gonorrhea, chancroid, lymphogranuloma venereum
- Viral infections: herpes simplex virus, cytomegalovirus, human immunodeficiency virus
- Inflammatory bowel disease (IBD): Crohn's disease, ulcerative colitis
- Trauma: surgery (hemorrhoidectomy), foreign bodies, anal intercourse
- Malignancy: carcinoma, lymphoma, Kaposi's sarcoma

DIAGNOSIS

■ DIFFERENTIAL DIAGNOSIS
- Proctalgia fugax
- Thrombosed hemorrhoid

■ WORKUP
- Digital rectal examination after lubricating the entire anus with anesthetic jelly (i.e., 2% lidocaine) and waiting 5 to 10 min
- Anoscopy
- Proctosigmoidoscopy to exclude inflammatory or neoplastic disease
- Biopsy if doubt exists about the etiology of the condition
- All studies done under adequate anesthesia

■ IMAGING STUDIES
- Colonoscopy or barium enema: if diagnosis of IBD or malignancy is suspected
- Small bowel series: occasionally obtained for similar reasons
- Biopsy to reveal caseating granuloma if TB is suspected
- Wet prep with darkfield examination to demonstrate treponemes if syphilis is suspected

TREATMENT

■ NONPHARMACOLOGIC THERAPY
- Sitz baths
- High-fiber diet
- Increased oral fluid intake

■ ACUTE GENERAL Rx
- Bulk-producing agent (i.e., Metamucil)/stool softener
- Local anesthetic jelly (may exacerbate pruritus ani)
- Nitroglycerin ointment
- Suppositories *not* recommended
- Surgery

■ CHRONIC Rx
- Surgery: lateral internal anal sphincterotomy
- Injection of botulinum toxin (an injection into each side of the internal anal sphincter) is effective in healing chronic anal fissures in over 90% of patients.

■ DISPOSITION
Outpatient surgery

■ REFERRAL
- If fissure does not resolve with conservative therapy in 4 to 6 wk
- If patient prefers surgery for acute fissure
- If patient has chronic fissure

PEARLS & CONSIDERATIONS

■ COMMENTS
HIV-positive patients should be referred to clinicians who are well versed in the myriad infectious and neoplastic conditions that masquerade as anal ulcers in these patients.

REFERENCES
Brisinda G et al: A comparison of injection of botulinum toxin and topical nitroglycerin ointment for the treatment of chronic anal fissure, *N Engl J Med* 341:65, 1999.
Pfenninger JL, Zainea GG: Common anorectal conditions, *Am Fam Physician* 64:77, 2001.
Author: **Maria Elena Soler, M.D.**

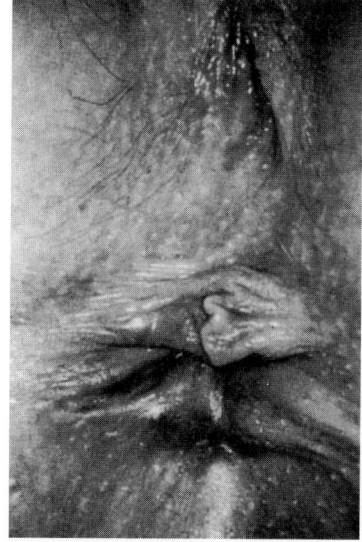

Fig. 1-22 Lateral anal fissure. (Courtesy of Gershon Efron, MD, Sinai Hospital of Baltimore. In Seidel HM et al: *Mosby's guide to physical examination,* ed 3, St Louis, 1995, Mosby.)

BASIC INFORMATION

■ DEFINITION
Anaphylaxis is a sudden-onset, life-threatening event characterized by bronchial contractions in conjunction with hemodynamic changes. Its clinical presentation may include respiratory, cardiovascular, cutaneous, or gastrointestinal manifestations.

■ SYNONYMS
Anaphylactoid reaction is closely related to anaphylaxis. It is caused by release of mast cells and basophil mediatros triggered by non–IgE-mediated events.

ICD-9CM CODES
995.0 Anaphylactic shock
995.60 Anaphylaxis due to food
999.4 Anaphylaxis due to immunization
977.9 Anaphylaxis due to drugs
989.5 Anaphylaxis following stings

■ EPIDEMIOLOGY & DEMOGRAPHICS
INCIDENCE: 20,000 to 50,000 persons/yr in the U.S. Anaphylaxis rates are 0.0004% for food, 0.7% to 10% for penicillin, 0.22% to 1% for radiocontrast media, and 0.5% to 5% after insect stings. It is estimated that 1 in every 3000 inpatients in U.S. hospitals develops an anaphylactic reaction.

■ PHYSICAL FINDINGS & CLINICAL PRESENTATION
- Urticaria, pruritus, skin flushing, angioedema, weakness, dizziness
- Dyspnea, cough, malaise, difficulty swallowing
- Wheezing, tachycardia, diarrhea
- Hypotension, vascular collapse

■ ETIOLOGY
Virtually any substance may induce anaphylaxis in a given individual.
- Commonly implicated medications are antibiotics, insulin, allergen extracts, opiates, vaccines, NSAIDs, contrast media, streptokinase
- Foods and food additives, nuts, egg whites, shellfish, fish, milk, fruits, and berries
- Blood products, plasma, immunoglobulin, cryoprecipitate, whole blood
- Venoms such as snake venom, fire ant venom, bee sting (*Hymenoptera* stings)
- Latex

DIAGNOSIS

■ DIFFERENTIAL DIAGNOSIS
- Endocrine disorders (carcinoid, pheochromocytoma)
- Globus hystericus, anxiety disorder
- Systemic mastocytosis
- Pulmonary embolism, serum sickness, vasovagal reactions

■ WORKUP
Workup is aimed mainly at eliminating other conditions that may mimic anaphylaxis (e.g., vasovagal syncope may be differentiated by the presence of bradycardia as opposed to the tachycardia seen in anaphylaxis; the absence of hypoxemia in ABG analysis may be useful to exclude pulmonary embolism or foreign body aspiration).

■ LABORATORY TESTS
- Laboratory evaluation is generally not helpful, because the diagnosis of anaphylaxis is a clinical one.
- ABG analysis may be useful to exclude pulmonary embolism, status asthmaticus, and foreign body aspiration.
- Elevated serum and urine histamine levels can be useful for diagnosis of anaphylaxis, but these tests are not commonly available.

■ IMAGING STUDIES
Generally not helpful.
- Chest x-ray is indicated in patients presenting with acute respiratory compromise.
- Radiologic evaluation for epiglottitis is useful in patients with acute respiratory compromise.
- ECG should be considered in all patients with sudden loss of consciousness or complaints of chest pains or dyspnea and in any elderly patient.

TREATMENT

■ NONPHARMACOLOGIC THERAPY
- IV access should be rapidly established, and intravenous fluids (i.e., saline) should be administered.
- Supplemental oxygen and cardiac monitoring are also recommended.

■ ACUTE GENERAL Rx
- Epinephrine should be rapidly administered as an SC or IM injection at a dose of 0.01 ml/kg of aqueous epinephrine 1:1000 (maximum adult dose 0.3 to 0.5 ml). The dose may be repeated approximately q5-10 min if there is persistence or recurrence of symptoms. Endotracheal epinephrine should be considered if IV access is not possible during life-threatening reactions.
- Administration of H_1- and H_2-receptor antagonists is also recommended in the initial treatment of anaphylaxis.

1. Administer diphenhydramine 25 to 50 mg IV or IM.
2. Cimetidine 300 mg IV over 3 to 5 min, or ranitidine 50 mg IV, should be given initially; subsequent doses of H_1- and H_2-blockers can be given orally q6h for 48 hr.

- Corticosteroids are not useful in the acute episode because of their slow onset of action; however, they should be administered in most cases to prevent prolonged or recurrent anaphylaxis. Commonly used agents are hydrocortisone sodium succinate 250 to 500 mg IV q4-6h in adults (4 to 8 mg/kg for children) or methylprednisolone 60 to 125 mg IV in adults (1 to 2 mg/kg in children).
- Aerosolized β-agonists (i.e., albuterol, 2.5 mg, repeat PRN 20 min) are useful to control bronchospasm.
- Additional useful agents in specific circumstances: atropine for refractory bradycardia, dopamine for refractory hypotension (despite volume expansion), and glucagon in patients on β-blocking drugs.

■ DISPOSITION
Prognosis is generally good if treated immediately.

PEARLS & CONSIDERATIONS

■ COMMENTS
- Patient education regarding the nature of the illness and preventive measures is recommended. A documented history of previous anaphylactic episodes or known anaphylaxis triggers is the most reliable method of identifying individuals at risk.
- Prescription for prefilled epinephrine syringe (EpiPen) should be given, and the patient should be instructed on the use of this emergency epinephrine kit in case of recurrent anaphylactic episodes.
- Patients should also be advised to carry or wear Medic Alert ID describing substances that have caused anaphylaxis.
- Avoidance of radiologic contrast is also recommended.
- Venom immunotherapy immediately after a sting is effective and recommended for up to 5 years after the anaphylactic incident.

REFERENCE
Neugut AI et al: Anaphylaxis in the United States, *Arch Intern Med* 161:15, 2001.
Author: **Fred F. Ferri, M.D.**

BASIC INFORMATION

■ DEFINITION
Aplastic anemia is a bone marrow failure resulting from a variety of causes and characterized by stem cell destruction or suppression leading to pancytopenia.

■ SYNONYMS
Refractory anemia
Hypoplastic anemia

ICD-9CM CODES
284.9 Aplastic anemia
284.8 Acquired aplastic anemia
284.0 Congenital aplastic anemia

■ EPIDEMIOLOGY & DEMOGRAPHICS
• There is no predominant age or sex for the acquired form.
• The annual incidence of aplastic anemia in the U.S. is 3 to 9 cases/1 million persons.

■ PHYSICAL FINDINGS & CLINICAL PRESENTATION
• Skin pallor, ecchymosis, petechiae, retinal hemorrhage
• Possible fever, mouth and tongue ulceration, pharyngitis
• Possible short stature or skeletal and nail anomalies in the congenital form
• Possible audible systolic ejection murmur with profound anemia

■ ETIOLOGY
• In most patients with acquired aplastic anemia, bone marrow failure results from immunologically mediated, tissue-specific organ destruction.
• Common etiologic factors in aplastic anemia:
  Toxins (e.g., benzene, insecticides)
  Drugs (e.g., Felbatol, cimetidine, busulfan and other myelosuppressive drugs, gold salts, chloramphenicol, sulfonamides, trimethadione, quinacrine, phenylbutazone)
  Ionizing irradiation
  Infections (e.g., hepatitis C, HIV)
  Idiopathic
  Inherited (Fanconi's anemia)
  Other: immunologic, pregnancy

DIAGNOSIS

■ DIFFERENTIAL DIAGNOSIS
• Bone marrow infiltration from lymphoma, carcinoma, myelofibrosis
• Severe infection
• Hypoplastic acute lymphoblastic leukemia in children

• Hypoplastic myelodysplastic syndrome or hypoplastic acute myeloid leukemia in adults
• Hypersplenism
• Hairy cell leukemia

■ WORKUP
• Diagnostic workup consists primarily of bone marrow aspiration and biopsy and laboratory evaluation (CBC and examination of blood film).
• Bone marrow examination generally reveals paucity or absence of erythropoietic and myelopoietic precursor cells; patients with pure red cell aplasia demonstrate only absence of RBC precursors in the marrow.
• A clinical algorithm for the diagnosis of anemia is described in Fig. 3-10.

■ LABORATORY TESTS
• CBC reveals pancytopenia. Macrocytosis and toxic granulation of neutrophils may also be present. Isolated cytopenias may occur in the early stages.
• Reticulocyte count reveals reticulocytopenia.
• Additional initial laboratory evaluation should include Ham test to exclude paroxysmal nocturnal hemoglobinuria (PNH) and testing for hepatitis C.

■ IMAGING STUDIES
• Chest x-ray examination
• Abdominal sonogram or CT scan to evaluate for splenomegaly
• Radiography of hand and forearm in patients with constitutional anemia
• CT scan of thymus region if thymoma-associated RBC aplasia is suspected

TREATMENT

■ NONPHARMACOLOGIC THERAPY
• Discontinuation of any offending drugs or agents
• Evaluation for bone marrow transplantation

■ ACUTE GENERAL Rx
• Aggressive treatment of neutropenic fevers with parenteral broad-spectrum antibiotics
• Platelet and RBC transfusions PRN; however, avoidance of transfusions in patients who are candidates for bone marrow transplantation
• Immunosuppressive therapy with antithymocyte globulin (ATG) and/or cyclosporine (CSP); ATG in combination with prednisone (1 to 2 mg/kg/day initially) to avoid complications of serum sickness
• Transplantation of allogeneic marrow or peripheral blood stem cell

transplantation from a histocompatible sibling usually cures the underlying bone marrow failure
• In patients with severe aplastic anemia who are not candidates for allogenic bone marrow, use of high-dose cyclophosphamide therapy without bone marrow transplantation represents a third option for initial treatment of aplastic anemia. Survival at 2 yr has been reported at 84%; however, the study was small and uncontrolled.

■ CHRONIC Rx
Long-term patient monitoring with physical examination and routine laboratory evaluation to screen for relapse

■ DISPOSITION
• Patients with severe aplastic anemia who have marrow transplants before the onset of transfusion-induced sensitization have an excellent probability of long-term survival and normal life; age is a significant factor; the incidence of graft vs. host disease increases with age and is >90% in patients >30 yr of age.
• Following bone marrow transplantation from an HLA-identical sibling, >70% of patients are long-term survivors and can be considered cured.
• Response to immunosuppression in aplastic anemia is independent of age, but treatment is associated with increased mortality in older patients.
• Overall 5-yr survival rate for aplastic anemia is now 70% to 90%.

■ REFERRAL
Hematology referral is indicated in all patients with aplastic anemia.

PEARLS & CONSIDERATIONS

■ COMMENTS
Additional patient information on aplastic anemia can be obtained from Aplastic Anemia Foundation of America, PO Box 22689, Baltimore, MD 21203; phone number: (410) 955-2803.

REFERENCES
Brodsuy RA et al: Durable treatment-free remission after high-dose cyclophosphamide therapy for previously untreated severe aplastic anemia, *Ann Intern Med* 135:477, 2001.
Tichelli A et al: Effectiveness of immunosuppression therapy in older patients with aplastic anemia, *Ann Intern Med* 130:193, 1999.
Young NS: Acquired aplastic anemia, *JAMA* 282:271, 1999.
Author: **Fred F. Ferri, M.D.**

BASIC INFORMATION

■ **DEFINITION**
Autoimmune hemolytic anemia is anemia secondary to premature destruction of red blood cells caused by the binding of autoantibodies and/or complement to red blood cells.

ICD-9CM CODES
283.0 Autoimmune hemolytic anemia

■ **EPIDEMIOLOGY & DEMOGRAPHICS**
Autoimmune hemolytic anemia is most common in women <50 yr.

■ **PHYSICAL FINDINGS & CLINICAL PRESENTATION**
• Pallor
• Tachycardia
• Hepatomegaly, splenomegaly

■ **ETIOLOGY**
• Warm antibody mediated: IgG (often idiopathic or associated with leukemia, lymphoma, thymoma, myeloma, viral infections, and collagen-vascular disease)
• Cold antibody mediated: IgM and complement in majority of cases (often idiopathic, at times associated with infections, lymphoma, or cold agglutinin disease)
• Drug induced: three major mechanisms:
   1. Antibody directed against Rh complex (e.g., methyldopa)
   2. Antibody directed against RBC-drug complex (hapten-induced, e.g., penicillin)
   3. Antibody directed against complex formed by drug and plasma proteins; the drug-plasma protein-antibody complex causes destruction of RBCs (innocent bystander, e.g., quinidine).

■ **DIAGNOSIS**

■ **DIFFERENTIAL DIAGNOSIS**
• Hemolytic anemia caused by membrane defects (paroxysmal nocturnal

hemoglobinuria, spur-cell anemia, Wilson's disease)
• Non–immune mediated (microangiopathic hemolytic anemia, hypersplenism, cardiac valve prosthesis, giant cavernous hemangiomas, march hemoglobinuria, physical agents, infections, heavy metals, certain drugs [nitrofurantoin, sulfonamides])

■ **WORKUP**
• Evaluation consists primarily of laboratory evaluation to confirm hemolysis and to exclude other causes of the anemia.
• A clinical algorithm for evaluation of anemia is described in Fig. 3-10.
• Box 2-23 describes the differential diagnosis of megaloblastic anemia. Box 2-21 describes drug-induced anemia.

■ **LABORATORY TESTS**
• Initial laboratory tests: CBC (anemia), reticulocyte count (elevated), liver function studies (elevated indirect bilirubin, LDH), evaluation of peripheral smear, Coombs' test (positive direct Coombs' test indicates presence of antibodies or complement on the surface of RBC, positive indirect Coombs' test implies presence of anti-RBC antibodies freely circulating in the patient's serum), haptoglobin level (decreased)
• IgG antibody and IgM antibody
• Hepatitis serology, ANA

■ **IMAGING STUDIES**
• Chest x-ray
• CT scan of chest and abdomen to rule out lymphoma should also be considered

■ **TREATMENT**

■ **NONPHARMACOLOGIC THERAPY**
• Discontinuation of any potentially offensive drugs

• Plasmapheresis-exchange transfusion for severe life-threatening cases only
• Avoid cold exposure in patients with cold antibody

■ **ACUTE GENERAL Rx**
• Prednisone 1 to 2 mg/kg/day in divided doses initially
• Splenectomy in patients responding inadequately to corticosteroids when RBC sequestration studies indicate splenic sequestration
• Immunosuppressive drugs and/or immunoglobulins only after both corticosteroids and splenectomy (unless surgery is contraindicated) have failed to produce an adequate remission
• Danazol, usually used in conjunction with corticosteroids (may be useful in warm antibody autoimmune hemolytic anemia)

■ **DISPOSITION**
Prognosis is generally good unless anemia is associated with underlying disorder with a poor prognosis (e.g., leukemia, myeloma).

■ **REFERRAL**
Surgical referral for splenectomy in refractory cases

■ **PEARLS & CONSIDERATIONS**

■ **COMMENTS**
Monitor for potential complications such as thromboembolism or severe anemia with shock.
Author: **Fred F. Ferri, M.D.**

BASIC INFORMATION

■ **DEFINITION**
Iron deficiency anemia is anemia secondary to inadequate iron supplementation or excessive blood loss.

ICD-9CM CODES
280.9 Iron deficiency anemia
648.2 Iron deficiency anemia complicating pregnancy

■ **EPIDEMIOLOGY & DEMOGRAPHICS**
Dietary iron deficiency occurs often in infants as a result of unsupplemented milk diets. It is also commonly seen in women during their reproductive years, as a result of heavy menstrual periods, and during pregnancy (increased demand).

■ **PHYSICAL FINDINGS & CLINICAL PRESENTATION**
• Most patients have a normal examination.
• Skin pallor and conjunctival pallor may be present.

■ **ETIOLOGY**
• Blood loss from GI or menstrual bleeding (GU blood loss less often the cause)
• Dietary iron deficiency (rare in adults)
• Poor iron absorption in patients with gastric or small bowel surgery
• Repeated phlebotomy

• Increased requirements (e.g., during pregnancy)
• Other: traumatic hemolysis (abnormally functioning cardiac valves), idiopathic pulmonary hemosiderosis (iron sequestration in pulmonary macrophages), paroxysmal nocturnal hemoglobinuria (intravascular hemolysis)

 DIAGNOSIS

■ **DIFFERENTIAL DIAGNOSIS**
• Anemia of chronic disease
• Sideroblastic anemia
• Thalassemia trait
• The differential diagnosis of iron deficiency is described in Table 1-10.

■ **WORKUP**
Diagnostic workup consists primarily of laboratory evaluation. Most patients with iron deficiency anemia are asymptomatic in the early stages. With progressive anemia, the major complaints are fatigue, dizziness, exertional dyspnea, pagophagia (ice eating), pica. Patient's history may also suggest GI blood loss (melena, hematochezia, hemoptysis).
• A clinical algorithm for the evaluation of anemia is described in Fig. 3-10.

■ **LABORATORY TESTS**
• Laboratory results vary with the stage of deficiency (see Box 1-4).

• Absent iron marrow stores and decreased serum ferritin are the initial abnormalities.
• Decreased serum iron and increased TIBC are the next abnormalities.
• Hypochromic microcytic anemia is present with significant iron deficiency.
• Peripheral smear in patients with iron deficiency generally reveals microcytic hypochromic RBCs with a wide area of central pallor, anisocytosis, and poikilocytosis when severe.
• Laboratory abnormalities consistent with iron deficiency are low serum ferritin level, elevated RBC distribution width (RDW) with values generally >15, low MCV, elevated TIBC, and low serum iron.
• The reticulocyte hemoglobin content (CHr) may be a good screening test for iron deficiency. It can be measured on an automated hematology analyzer and represents a relatively inexpensive and fast way to detect iron deficiency.

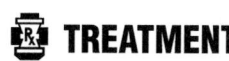 **TREATMENT**

■ **NONPHARMACOLOGIC THERAPY**
Patients should be instructed to consume foods containing large amounts of iron, such as liver, red meat, and legumes.

TABLE 1-10 Differential Diagnosis of Iron Deficiency: Clinical and Laboratory Features

HISTORY/PHYSICAL EXAMINATION	IRON	TOTAL IRON-BINDING CAPACITY	FERRITIN	SMEAR	RED CELL DISTRIBUTION WIDTH	MARROW IRON
Iron Deficiency						
Bleeding	↓	↑	↓	Microcytosis	↑	Absent
Pica				Hypochromia		
Angular cheilosis				Pencil shapes		
Koilonychia						
Dysphagia						
Anemia of Chronic Disease						
Chronic infection or inflammation	↓	↓	↑	RBC normal (¼ microcytosis)	Normal	↑ (In reticuloendothelial system, not RBC precursors)
Thalassemia Trait						
Family history	Normal/↑	Normal	↑	Microcytosis		
Splenomegaly (±)				Targets Hypochromia	Normal	↑

From Carlson KJ et al: *Primary care of women*, St Louis, 1995, Mosby.
RBC, Red blood cells.

BOX 1-4   Development of Iron Deficiency Anemia

STAGE I: IRON DEPLETION	STAGE II: IRON-DEFICIENT ERYTHROPOIESIS	STAGE III: IRON DEFICIENCY ANEMIA
Serum ferritin ↓	Serum ferritin ↓	Serum ferritin ↓
Bone marrow iron ↓	Bone marrow iron ↓	Bone marrow iron ↓
	Serum iron ↓	Serum iron ↓
	TIBC ↑	TIBC ↑
		Hemoglobin ↓
		Hematocrit ↓
		MCV ↓
		RDW ↑

From Roper D et al: Anemias caused by impaired production of erythrocytes. In Rodak BF (ed): *Diagnostic hematology,* Philadelphia, 1995, WB Saunders.
↑, increased; ↓, decreased, *MCV,* Mean corpuscular volume; *RDW,* red blood cell distribution width; *TIBC,* total iron-binding capacity.

■ ACUTE GENERAL Rx

- Treatment consists of ferrous sulfate 325 mg PO qd-tid for at least 6 mo. Calcium supplements can decrease iron absorption; therefore, these two medications should be staggered.
- Parenteral iron therapy is reserved for patients with poor tolerance, noncompliance with oral preparations, or malabsorption.
- Transfusion of packed RBCs is indicated in patients with severe symptomatic anemia (e.g., angina) or life-threatening anemia.

■ CHRONIC Rx

Patients should be instructed to continue their iron supplements for at least 6 mo or longer to correct depleted body iron stores.

■ DISPOSITION

Most patients respond rapidly to iron supplementation with improvement in CBC and general well-being. GI side effects from oral iron therapy are common and may require decreased dose to once daily.

■ REFERRAL

GI referral for evaluation of GI malignancy is recommended in all patients with iron deficiency and suspected GI blood loss.

☼ PEARLS & CONSIDERATIONS

■ COMMENTS

If the diagnosis of iron deficiency anemia is made, it is mandatory to try to locate the suspected site of iron loss.

REFERENCES

Brugnara C et al: Reticulocyte hemoglobin content to diagnose iron deficiency in children, *JAMA* 281:2225, 1999.

US Dept of Health & Human Services: Recommendations to prevent and control iron deficiency in the US, *MMWR* 47:RR-3, 1998.

Author: **Fred F. Ferri, M.D.**

BASIC INFORMATION

DEFINITION
Pernicious anemia is an autoimmune disease resulting from antibodies against intrinsic factor and gastric parietal cells.

SYNONYMS
Megaloblastic anemia resulting from vitamin B_{12} deficiency

ICD-9CM CODES
281.0 Pernicious anemia

EPIDEMIOLOGY & DEMOGRAPHICS
- Increased incidence in females and older adults (diagnosis is unusual before age 35 yr)
- The overall prevalence of undiagnosed PA over age 60 yr is 1.9%
- Prevalence is highest in women (2.7%), particularly in black women (4.3%)
- Increased incidence of autoimmune disease (e.g., type 1 DM, Graves' disease, Addison's disease), *Helicobacter pylori* infection

PHYSICAL FINDINGS & CLINICAL PRESENTATION
- Mucosal pallor, glossitis
- Peripheral sensory neuropathy with paresthesias initially and absent reflexes in advanced cases
- Loss of joint position sense, pyramidal or long track signs
- Possible splenomegaly and mild hepatomegaly
- Generalized weakness and delirium/dementia

ETIOLOGY
- Antigastric parietal cell antibodies in >70% of patients, antiintrinsic factor antibodies in >50% of patients
- Atrophic gastric mucosa

DIAGNOSIS

DIFFERENTIAL DIAGNOSIS
- Nutritional vitamin B_{12} deficiency
- Malabsorption
- Chronic alcoholism (multifactorial)
- Chronic gastritis related to *H. pylori* infection
- Folic acid deficiency
- Myelodysplasia
- The differential diagnosis of megaloblastic anemia is described in Box 2-23. A clinical algorithm for evaluation of anemia is described in Fig. 3-10.

WORKUP
- The clinical presentation of pernicious anemia varies with the stage. Initially, patient may be asymptomatic. In advanced stages, patients may present with impaired memory, depression, gait disturbances, paresthesias, and complaints of generalized weakness.
- Investigation consists primarily of laboratory evaluation.
- Endoscopy and biopsy for atrophic gastritis may be performed in selected cases.
- Diagnosis is crucial because failure to treat may result in irreversible neurologic deficits.

LABORATORY TESTS
- CBC generally reveals macrocytic anemia and leukopenia with hypersegmented neutrophils.
- MCV is generally significantly elevated in the advanced stages.
- Reticulocyte count is low/normal.
- Falsely low serum cobalamin levels can occur in patients with severe folate deficiency, in patients using high doses of ascorbic acid, and when cobalamin levels are measured following nuclear medicine studies (radioactivity interferes with cobalamin RIA measurement).
- Falsely high normal levels in patients with cobalamin deficiency can occur in severe liver disease or chronic granulocytic leukemia.
- The absence of anemia or macrocytosis does not exclude the diagnosis of cobalamin deficiency. Anemia is absent in 20% of patients with cobalamin deficiency, and macrocytosis is absent in >30% of patients at the time of diagnosis. It can be blocked by concurrent iron deficiency or anemia of chronic disease and may be masked by thalassemia trait.
- Schilling test is abnormal in part I; part II corrects to normal after administration of intrinsic factor.
- Laboratory tests used for detecting cobalamin deficiency in patients with normal vitamin B_{12} levels include serum and urinary methylmalonic acid level (elevated), total homocysteine level (elevated), intrinsic factor antibody (positive).
- An increased concentration of plasma methylmalonic acid (P-MMA) does not predict clinical manifestations of vitamin B_{12} deficiency and should not be used as the only marker for diagnosis of B_{12} deficiency.
- Additional laboratory abnormalities can include elevated LDH, direct hyperbilirubinemia, and decreased haptoglobin.

TREATMENT

NONPHARMACOLOGIC THERAPY
Avoid folic acid supplementation without proper vitamin B_{12} supplementation.

ACUTE GENERAL Rx
Traditional therapy of a cobalamin deficiency consists of IM injections of vitamin B_{12} 1000 µg/wk for the initial 4 to 6 wk followed by 1000 µg/mo IM indefinitely. When hematologic parameters have returned to normal range, intranasal cyanocobalamin may be used in place of IM cyanocobalamin. The initial dose of intranasal cyanocobalamin (Nascobal) is one spray (500 µg) in one nostril once per week. Monitor response and increase dose if serum B_{12} levels decline. Consider return to intramuscular vitamin B_{12} supplementation if decline persists.

CHRONIC Rx
Parenteral vitamin B_{12} 1000 µg/mo or intranasal cyanocobalamin 500 µg/wk (see above) for the remainder of life

DISPOSITION
Anemia generally resolves with appropriate treatment. Neurologic deficits, if present at diagnosis, may be permanent.

REFERRAL
GI referral for endoscopy upon diagnosis of pernicious anemia and surveillance endoscopy every 5 yr to rule out gastric carcinoma

PEARLS & CONSIDERATIONS

COMMENTS
- Patients must understand that therapy is lifelong.
- Self-injection of vitamin B_{12} may be taught in selected patients.

REFERENCES
Avas A et al: Increased plasma methylmalonic acid level does not predict clinical manifestations of vitamin B_{12} deficiency, *Arch Intern Med* 161:1534, 2001.

Snow CF: Laboratory diagnosis of vitamin B_{12} and folate deficiency, *Arch Intern Med* 159:1289, 1999.

Author: **Fred F. Ferri, M.D.**

BASIC INFORMATION

■ DEFINITION
Sickle cell anemia is a hemoglobinopathy characterized by the production of hemoglobin S caused by substitution of the amino acid valine for glutamic acid in the sixth position of the γ-globin chain. When exposed to lower oxygen tension, RBCs assume a sickle shape resulting in stasis of RBCs in capillaries. Painful crises are caused by ischemic tissue injury resulting from obstruction of blood flow produced by sickled erythrocytes.

■ SYNONYMS
Sickle cell disease
Hemoglobin S disease

ICD-9CM CODES
286.60 Sickle cell anemia

■ EPIDEMIOLOGY & DEMOGRAPHICS
- Sickle cell hemoglobin S is transmitted by an autosomal recessive gene. It is found mostly in blacks (1 in 400 black Americans).
- Sickle cell trait occurs in nearly 10% of black Americans.
- There is no predominant sex.

■ PHYSICAL FINDINGS & CLINICAL PRESENTATION
- Physical examination is variable depending on the degree of anemia and presence of acute vasoocclusive syndromes or neurologic, cardiovascular, GU, and musculoskeletal complications.
- There is no clinical laboratory finding that is pathognomonic of painful crisis of sickle cell disease. The diagnosis of a painful episode is made solely on the basis of the medical therapy and physical examination.
- Bones are the most common site of pain. Dactylitis, or hand-foot syndrome (acute, painful swelling of the hands and feet), is the first manifestation of sickle cell disease in many infants. Irritability and refusal to walk are other common symptoms. After infancy, musculoskeletal pain can be symmetric, asymmetric, or migratory, and it may or may not be associated with swelling, low-grade fever, redness, or warmth.
- In both children and adults, sickle vasoocclusive episodes are difficult to distinguish from osteomyelitis, septic arthritis, synovitis, rheumatic fever, or gout.
- When abdominal or visceral pain is present, care should be taken to exclude sequestration syndromes (spleen, liver) or the possibility of an acute condition such as appendicitis,

pancreatitis, cholecystitis, urinary tract infection, PID, or malignancy.
- Pneumonia develops during the course of 20% of painful events and can present as chest and abdominal pain. In adults chest pain may be a result of vasoocclusion in the ribs and often precedes a pulmonary event. The lower back is also a frequent site of painful crisis in adults.
- The "acute chest syndrome" manifests with chest pain, fever, wheezing, tachypnea, and cough. Chest x-ray reveals pulmonary infiltrates. Common causes include infection (mycoplasma, chlamydia, viruses), infarction, and fat embolism.
- Musculoskeletal and skin abnormalities seen in sickle cell anemia include leg ulcers (particularly on the malleoli) and limb-girdle deformities caused by avascular necrosis of the femoral and humeral heads.
- Endocrine abnormalities include delayed sexual maturation and late physical maturation, especially evident in boys.
- Neurologic abnormalities on examination may include seizures and altered mental status.
- Infections, particularly involving *Salmonella, Mycoplasma,* and *Streptococcus,* are relatively common.
- Severe splenomegaly secondary to sequestration often occurs in children before splenic atrophy.

DIAGNOSIS

■ DIFFERENTIAL DIAGNOSIS
- Thalassemia
- Iron deficiency anemia, leukemia
- The differential diagnosis of patients presenting with a painful crisis is discussed in "Physical Findings" (see above)

■ WORKUP
- Screening of all newborns regardless of racial background is recommended. Screening can be performed with sodium metabisulfite reduction test (Sickledex test).
- Hemoglobin electrophoresis will also confirm the diagnosis and is useful to identify hemoglobin variants such as fetal hemoglobin and hemoglobin A2.

■ LABORATORY TESTS
- Anemia (resulting from chronic hemolysis), reticulocytosis, leukocytosis, and thrombocytosis are common.
- Elevations of bilirubin and LDH are also common.
- Peripheral blood smear may reveal sickle cells, target cells, poikilocytosis, and hypochromia (Fig. 1-23).

- Elevated BUN and creatinine may be present in patients with progressive renal insufficiency.
- Urinalysis may reveal hematuria and proteinuria.

■ IMAGING STUDIES
- Chest x-ray examination is useful in patients presenting with "chest syndrome." Cardiomegaly may be present on chest x-ray examination.
- Bone scan is useful to rule out osteomyelitis (usually secondary to salmonella). MRI scan is also effective in diagnosing osteomyelitis.
- CT scan or MRI of brain is often needed in patients presenting with neurologic complications such as TIA, CVA, seizures, or altered mental status.
- Transcranial Doppler is a useful commodity to identify children with sickle cell anemia who are at risk for stroke.

TREATMENT

■ NONPHARMACOLOGIC THERAPY
- Patients should be instructed to avoid conditions that may precipitate sickling crisis, such as hypoxia, infections, acidosis, and dehydration.
- Maintain adequate hydration (PO or IV).
- Correct hypoxia.

■ ACUTE GENERAL Rx
- Aggressively diagnose and treat suspected infections (*Salmonella* osteomyelitis and pneumococcal infections occur more often in patients with sickle cell anemia because of splenic infarcts and atrophy). Combination therapy with a cephalosporin and erythromycin plus incentive spirometry and bronchodilators are useful in patients with acute chest syndrome.
- Provide pain relief during the vasoocclusive crisis. Medications should be administered on a fixed time schedule with a dosing interval that does not extend beyond the duration of the desired pharmacologic effect.
  1. Meperidine is contraindicated in patients with renal dysfunction or CNS disease because its metabolite, normeperidine (which is excreted by the kidneys) can cause seizures.
  2. Narcotics should be given on a fixed schedule (not prn for pain), with rescue dosing for breakthrough pain as needed.
  3. Except when contraindications exist, concomitant use of NSAIDs should be standard treatment.

4. Nurses should be instructed not to give narcotics if the patient is heavily sedated or respirations are depressed.

5. When the patient shows signs of improvement, narcotic drugs should be tapered gradually to prevent withdrawal syndrome. It is advisable to observe the patient on oral pain relief medications for 12 to 24 hr before discharge from the hospital.

- Aggressively diagnose and treat any potential complications (e.g., septic necrosis of the femoral head, priapism, bony infarcts, and acute "chest syndrome").
- Avoid "routine" transfusions but consider early transfusions for patients at high risk for complications. Indications for transfusion: aplastic crises, severe hemolytic crises (particularly during third trimester of pregnancy), acute chest syndrome, and high risk of stroke.
- Hydroxyurea (500 to 750 mg/day) increases hemoglobin F levels and reduces the frequency of painful crises.

■ CHRONIC Rx

- Guidelines for prompt management of fever, infections, pain, and specific complications should be reviewed.
- Genetic counseling is recommended in all cases.
- Avoid unnecessary transfusions. Exchange transfusions may be necessary for patients with acute neurologic signs, in aplastic crisis, or undergoing surgery.
- Allogeneic stem cell transplantation can be curative in young patients with symptomatic sickle cell disease; however, the death rate from the procedure is nearly 10%, the marrow recipients are likely to be infertile, and there is an undefined risk of chemotherapy-induced malignancy.

- Penicillin V 125 mg PO bid should be administered by age 2 months and increased to 250 mg bid by age 3. Penicillin prophylaxis can be discontinued after age 5 except in children who have had splenectomy.

■ REFERRAL

- Hospitalization is generally recommended for most crises and complications.
- Psychosocial counseling and support structures should be developed.

☼ PEARLS & CONSIDERATIONS

■ COMMENTS

- Patients and their families should receive genetic counseling and should be made aware of the difference between sickle cell trait and sickle cell disease.
- Regular immunizations and pneumococcal vaccination are recommended. The prophylactic administration of penicillin soon after birth and the timely administration of pneumococcal and *H. influenzae* type b vaccines have resulted in a significant decline in the incidence of these infections. The heptavalent conjugated pneumococcal vaccine (Prevan) should be administered from 2 months of age. The 23-valent unconjugated pneumococcal vaccine is given from age 2 and can be boosted once 3 years later. Influenza vaccination can be given after 6 months of age.
- Patients should be instructed on a well-balanced diet and appropriate folic acid supplementation.
- Sickle cell variants are described in Table 2-183.
- The presence of dactylitis, Hb <7, or leukocytosis in the absence of infection during the first 2 yr of life, indi-

cates a higher risk of severe sickle cell disease later in life.
- Among patients with sickle cell disease, the acute chest syndrome is commonly precipitated by fat embolism and infection, especially community-acquired pneumonia. Among older patients and those with neurologic symptoms, the syndrome often progresses to respiratory failure.
- Poloxamer 188, a nonionic surfactant with hemorheological and antithrombotic properties, has been reported to produce a significant but relatively small decrease in the duration of painful episodes and an increase in the proportion of patients who achieved resolution of the symptoms. A more significant effect was observed in patients who received concomitant hydroxyurea.

REFERENCES

Adams RJ et al: Prevention of a first stroke by transfusions in children with sickle cell anemia and abnormal results on transcranial Doppler ultrasonography, *N Engl J Med* 339:5, 1998.

Miller ST et al: Prediction of disease outcomes in children with sickle cell disease, *N Engl J Med* 342:83, 2000.

Orringer E et al: Purified poloxamer 188 for treatment of acute vaso-occlusive crisis of sickle cell disease, *JAMA* 286:2099, 2001.

Vichinski EP et al: Causes and outcomes of the acute chest syndrome in sickle cell disease, *N Engl J Med* 342:1855, 2000.

Wethers DL: Sickle cell disease in childhood, *Am Fam Physician* 62:1013, 2000.

Author: **Fred F. Ferri, M.D.**

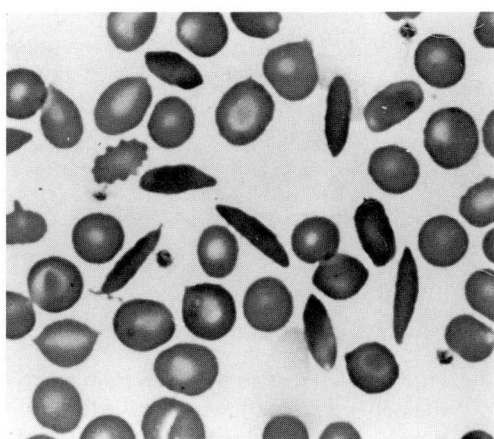

Fig. 1-23 Photomicrograph of peripheral blood smear, sickle cells, typical of sickle cell anemia. (From Andreoli TE [ed]: *Cecil essentials of medicine,* ed 4, Philadelphia, 1997, WB Saunders.)

BASIC INFORMATION

■ DEFINITION
Sideroblastic anemia is a group of disorders characterized by hypochromic anemia associated with tissue iron overload and the presence of ringed sideroblasts in the bone marrow. The disorder can be hereditary or acquired.

■ SYNONYMS
- Primary hereditary sideroblastic anemia
- Primary acquired refractory anemia with ringed sideroblasts (RARS)
- Secondary toxin associated

ICD-9CM CODES
285.0 Sideroblastic anemia

■ EPIDEMIOLOGY & DEMOGRAPHICS
- Hereditary sideroblastic anemia, being sex-linked, primarily affects males.
- Primary acquired sideroblastic anemia is usually a disease of the elderly.

■ PHYSICAL FINDINGS & CLINICAL PRESENTATION
The symptoms for sideroblastic anemia are the same for any anemia:
- Symptoms include fatigue, weakness, palpitations, shortness of breath, headaches, irritability, and chest pain.
- Physical findings may include pallor, tachycardia, hepatosplenomegaly, S_3, JVD, and rales.

■ ETIOLOGY
- Primary hereditary sideroblastic anemia is usually inherited as a sex-linked recessive disease.
- Primary acquired sideroblastic anemia is idiopathic.
- Secondary acquired sideroblastic anemia can be caused by alcohol, isoniazid, pyrazinamide, cycloserine, chloramphenical, and copper deficiency.

DIAGNOSIS

■ DIFFERENTIAL DIAGNOSIS
- Sideroblastic anemia must be differentiated from other causes of microcytic hypochromic anemia: iron deficiency anemia, thalassemia, anemia of chronic disease, lead poisoning, and blood loss.
- Tissue iron overload from sideroblastic anemia may act similar to hereditary hemochromatosis with liver cirrhosis, diabetes, congestive heart failure, and cardiac arrhythmias.

■ WORKUP
The diagnostic workup of suspected sideroblastic anemia includes laboratory evaluation and bone marrow aspiration and biopsy.

■ LABORATORY TESTS
- CBC (low Hgb, low Hct, low MCV, high RDW)
- Peripheral smear: dimorphic large and small cells revealing "Pappenheimer bodies" or siderocytes when stained for iron.
- Bone marrow shows the classic ringed sideroblasts not seen in normal bone marrow tissue (Fig. 1-24). The ringed sideroblasts represent iron storage in the mitochondria of normoblasts.

TREATMENT

■ NONPHARMACOLOGIC THERAPY
- Avoid alcohol.
- Secondary sideroblastic anemia due to isoniazid, pyrazinamide, and cycloserine can expect a full recovery by withdrawing the medication and by the use of vitamin B_6 (50 to 200 mg/day).

■ ACUTE GENERAL Rx
- Hereditary sideroblastic anemia:
  1. Nearly 35% of patients receiving vitamin B_6 (50 to 200 mg/day) will improve their red blood cell to near normal values.
  2. The remainder of patients will require blood transfusions to treat symptoms of anemia.
- Primary acquired sideroblastic anemia:
  1. Most patients do not respond to vitamin B_6.
  2. Erythropoietin has shown some success in improving the anemia.
  3. Blood transfusions are indicated for patients with symptomatic anemia.

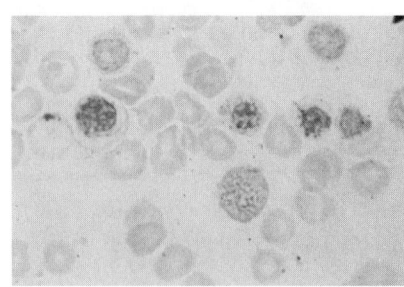

Fig. 1-24 Prussian blue iron stain of the bone marrow shows ringed sideroblasts. (From Goldman L, Bennett JC [eds]: *Cecil textbook of medicine,* ed 21, Philadelphia, 2000, WB Saunders.)

■ CHRONIC Rx
- Hereditary sideroblastic anemia:
  1. Organ dysfunction resulting from iron overload will require periodic phlebotomies.
  2. In advanced cases, desferoxamine 40 mg/kg/day IV is given.
- Primary acquired sideroblastic anemia:
  1. As in the hereditary form, periodic phlebotomies are indicated when serum iron levels increase to >500 µg/L and desferoxamine is used in patients requiring frequent blood transfusions.

■ DISPOSITION
- Hereditary sideroblastic anemia:
  1. With above mentioned treatment, prognosis is good for a normal life expectancy.
- Primary acquired sideroblastic anemia:
  1. In patients with anemia alone, life expectancy is normal. In patients dependent on blood transfusions one can expect morbidity from organ dysfunction.
  2. Some patients with acquired sideroblastic anemia can go on to develop leukemia.

■ REFERRAL
- Hematology

PEARLS & CONSIDERATIONS

■ COMMENTS
- Sideroblastic anemia can be thought of as an iron-loading anemia secondary to defective heme synthesis. Protein enzymes necessary for heme synthesis are located in the mitochondria of erythroid cells. A decrease in the activity of these enzymes (d-aminolevulinic acid synthetase, ferrochelatase) impedes protoporphyrin formation and the incorporation of iron into protoporphyrin preventing heme synthesis. Iron continues to be absorbed from the GI tract accumulating in the mitochondria surrounding the nucleus of the normoblast and forming the "ringed sideroblast."
- Vitamin B_6, pyridoxal phosphate, is a required cofactor in heme synthesis and drugs such as isoniazid, cycloserine, and pyrazinamide can inhibit its function.

REFERENCES
Bridges KR: Sideroblastic anemia: a mitochondrial disorder, *J Pediatr Hematol Oncol* 19(4):274, 1997.
Massey AC: Microcytic anemia: differential diagnosis and management of iron deficiency anemia, *Med Clin North Am* 76(3):549, 1992.
Author: **Peter Petropoulos, M.D.**

BASIC INFORMATION

■ DEFINITION
An abdominal aortic aneurysm is a permanent localized dilatation of the abdominal aortic artery to at least 50% when compared with the normal diameter. The normal diameter in men is 2.3 cm, and in women it is 1.9 cm.

■ SYNONYMS
AAA

ICD-9CM CODES
441.4 Aneurysm, abdominal (aorta)
441.3 Ruptured abdominal aortic aneurysm

■ EPIDEMIOLOGY & DEMOGRAPHICS
- The incidence of abdominal aortic aneurysms has been rising from 12.2 cases/100,000 persons to 36.2 cases/100,000 persons from 1951 to 1980.
- The prevalence ranges from 2% to 5% in men >60 yr.
- AAA is predominantly a disease of the elderly, affecting men > women (4:1).
- Rupture of an abdominal aortic aneurysm is the tenth leading cause of death in men >55 yr (15,000 deaths/yr in the U.S.).
- The risk of rupture is 0% per year in aneurysms <4 cm, 1% per year in aneurysms 4.0 to 4.9 cm, 11% per year in aneurysms 5.0 to 5.9 cm, and 25% per year in aneurysms >6 cm.
- Mortality after rupture is >90%. Of those patients who reach the hospital, it is estimated 50% will survive.

■ PHYSICAL FINDINGS & CLINICAL PRESENTATION
- Pulsatile epigastric mass that may or may not be tender.
- Discoloration and pain of the feet if the thrombus within the aneurysm embolizes.
- Shock, hypoperfusion, abdominal distention if rupture occurs.
- Rare presentations include hematemesis or melena with abdominal and back pain in patients with aorto-enteric fistulas. Aortocaval fistula produces loud abdominal bruits.

■ ETIOLOGY
Multifactorial
- Atherosclerotic (degenerative or nonspecific)
- Genetic, e.g., Ehlers-Danlos syndrome
- Trauma
- Cystic medial necrosis (Marfan's syndrome)
- Arteritis, inflammatory
- Mycotic, infected (syphilis)

DIAGNOSIS

■ DIFFERENTIAL DIAGNOSIS
Almost 75% of abdominal aneurysms are asymptomatic and are discovered on routine examination or serendipitously when ordering studies for other complaints. This must be considered in the differential of anyone presenting with abdominal pain or back pain.

■ IMAGING STUDIES
- Abdominal ultrasound is nearly 100% accurate in identifying an aneurysm and estimating the size to within 0.3 to 0.4 cm. It is not very good in estimating the proximal extension to the renal arteries or involvement of the iliac arteries.
- CT scan is recommended for preoperative aneurysm imaging and estimating the size to within 0.3 mm. There are no false-negatives, and the CT scan can localize the proximal extent, detect the integrity of the wall, and rule out rupture.
- Angiography gives detailed arterial anatomy, localizing the aneurysm relative to the renal and visceral arteries. This is the definitive preoperative study for surgeons.
- MRI can also be used, but it is more expensive and not as readily available.

TREATMENT

■ NONPHARMACOLOGIC THERAPY
- Treat atherosclerotic risk factors (diet and exercise for blood pressure, cholesterol, and diabetes, and abstinence from tobacco).
- Definitive treatment depends on the size of the aneurysm (see "Chronic Rx").

■ ACUTE GENERAL Rx
- Abdominal aortic rupture is an emergency. Surgery is the only chance for survival.
- Surgical mortality rates for ruptured aneurysms average 50% compared with 4% for elective repair of the nonruptured aorta.

■ CHRONIC Rx
Diagnosing, sizing, and repairing the aneurysm in an asymptomatic patient is crucial.

- For aneurysms 5 cm or greater, prosthetic graft replacement is recommended, providing there is no contraindication (e.g., MI within 6 mo, refractory CHF, life expectancy <2 yr, severe residual from CVA).
- For aneurysms between 4 and 5 cm, there is still controversy. Some recommend follow-up every 6 mo with ultrasound to look for expansion. If there is >0.5 cm expansion in this group, most would proceed with surgery.
- For aneurysms <4 cm, most would follow up with ultrasounds every 6 mo. For the high-risk patient deemed inoperable for such major surgery, endovascular stent-anchored grafts under local anesthesia have provided an alternative approach.

■ DISPOSITION
For aneurysms <5 cm, the course is variable but estimates of expansion rates average 0.4 cm/yr, with larger aneurysms expanding more rapidly.

■ REFERRAL
Vascular surgical referral should be made in asymptomatic patients with aneurysms 4 cm or greater or in rapidly expanding aneurysms of 0.5 cm/yr, especially if symptoms are present.

PEARLS & CONSIDERATIONS

■ COMMENTS
- Most abdominal aortic aneurysms are infrarenal. Surgical risk is increased in patients with coexisting coronary artery disease, pulmonary disease (Pao$_2$ <50 mm Hg, FEV$_1$ <11), liver cirrhosis, and chronic renal failure (Cr >3 mg/dl). Detailed cardiac workup with radionuclide perfusion studies for ischemia and aggressive perioperative hemodynamic monitoring help identify high-risk patients and decrease postoperative complications.

REFERENCES
Gorski Y, Ricotta JJ: Weighing risks in abdominal aortic aneurysm: best repaired in an elective, not an emergency procedure, *Postgrad Med* 106:2, 75, 1999.
Hallett JW: Management of abdominal aortic aneurysms, *Mayo Clin Proc* 75:395, 2000.
Santilli JD, Santilli DM: Diagnosis and treatment of abdominal aortic aneurysm, *Am Fam Physician* 56(4):1081, 1997.
Author: **Peter Petropoulos, M.D.**

BASIC INFORMATION

■ DEFINITION

Angina pectoris is characterized by discomfort that occurs when myocardial oxygen demand exceeds the supply. Myocardial ischemia can be asymptomatic (silent ischemia), particularly in diabetics. Angina is classified as follows:

1. CHRONIC (STABLE):
- Usually follows a precipitating event, e.g., climbing stairs, sexual intercourse, a heavy meal, emotional stress, cold weather
- Generally same severity as previous attacks; relieved by the customary dose of nitroglycerin
- Caused by a fixed coronary artery obstruction secondary to atherosclerosis

2. UNSTABLE (REST OR CRESCENDO):
- Recent onset
- Increasing severity, duration, or frequency of chronic angina
- Occurs at rest or with minimal exertion

3. PRINZMETAL'S VARIANT:
- Occurs at rest
- Manifests electrocardiographically as episodic ST-segment elevations
- Caused by coronary artery spasms with or without superimposed coronary artery disease
- Patients also more likely to develop ventricular arrhythmias

4. MICROVASCULAR ANGINA (SYNDROME X):
- Refers to patients with normal coronary angiograms and no coronary spasm but chest pain resembling angina and positive exercise test

- Defective endothelium-dependent dilation in the coronary microcirculation contributing to the altered regulation of myocardial perfusion and the ischemic manifestations in these patients
- Excellent prognosis

5. OTHER:
Angina due to aortic stenosis and idiopathic hypertrophic subaortic stenosis, cocaine-induced coronary vasoconstriction.

■ FUNCTIONAL CLASSIFICATION

- New York Heart Association Functional Classification of Angina:
  Class I—Angina only with unusually strenuous activity.
  Class II—Angina with slightly more prolonged or rigorous activity than usual.

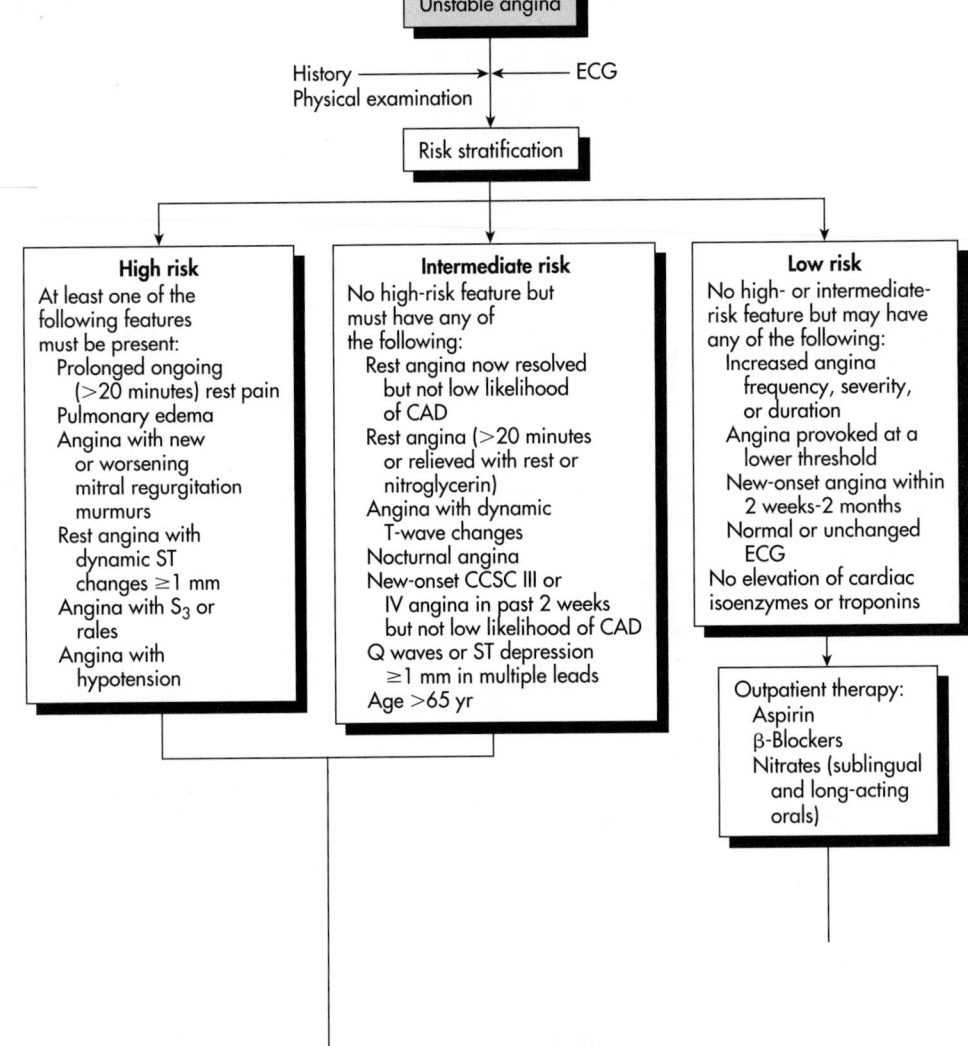

Fig. 1-25   Approach to the patient with unstable angina. *CAD,* Coronary artery disease; *CCSC,* Canadian Cardiovascular Society Classification; *ECG,* electrocardiogram. (Modified from Greene HL, Johnson WP, Lemcke DL: *Decision making in medicine,* ed 2, St Louis, 1998, Mosby.)

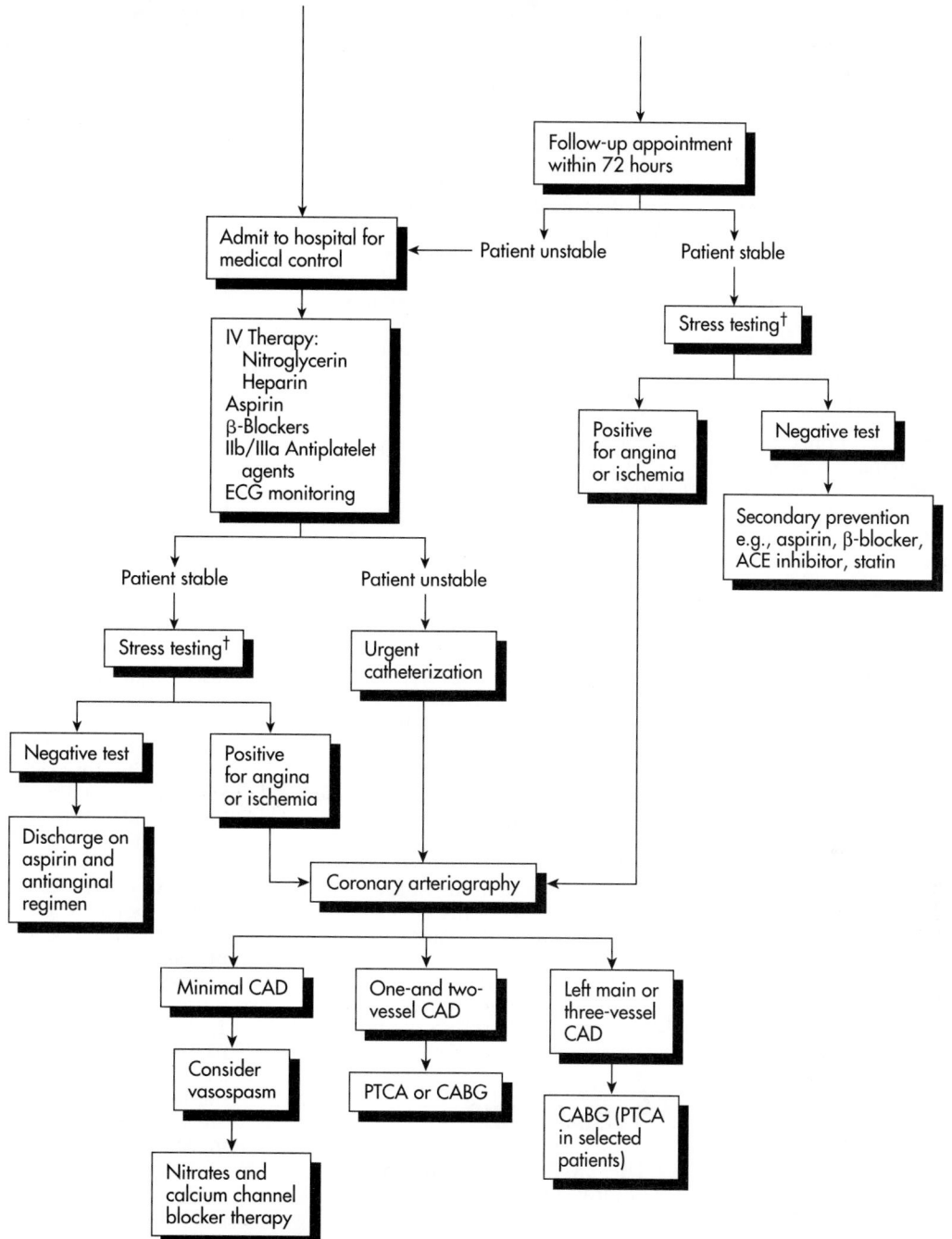

Fig. 1-25, cont'd   Approach to the patient with unstable angina. *CABG,* Coronary artery bypass graft surgery; *CAD,* coronary artery disease; *CCSC,* Canadian Cardiovascular Society Classification; *ECG,* electrocardiogram; *PTCA,* percutaneous transluminal coronary angioplasty. (Modified from Greene HL, Johnson WP, Lemcke DL: *Decision making in medicine,* ed 2, St Louis, 1998, Mosby.)
*May consider use of low-molecular-weight heparin (LMWH) SC instead of IV heparin.
†Exercise myocardial perfusion imaging, pharmacologic stress with vasodilator, dobotamine stress echocardiography.

Class III—Angina with usual daily activity.

Class IV—Angina at rest.

- Grading of Angina by the Canadian Cardiovascular Society Classification System:

  Class I—Ordinary physical activity does not cause angina, such as walking, climbing stairs. Angina (occurs) with strenuous, rapid, or prolonged exertion at work or recreation.

  Class II—Slight limitation of ordinary activity. Angina occurs on walking or climbing stairs rapidly; walking uphill; walking or stair climbing after meals, in cold, in wind, or under emotional stress; or only during the few hours after awakening. Angina occurs on walking more than two blocks on the level and climbing more than one flight of ordinary stairs at a normal pace and in normal condition.

  Class III—Marked limitations of ordinary physical activity. Angina occurs on walking one to two blocks on the level and climbing one flight of stairs in normal conditions and at a normal pace.

  Class IV—Inability to carry on any physical activity without discomfort—anginal symptoms may be present at rest.

ICD-9CM CODES
411.1 Angina, stable
413 Angina pectoris
413.1 Prinzmetal's angina
413.9 Angina, unspecified

■ EPIDEMIOLOGY & DEMOGRAPHICS

- Angina is most common in middle-aged and elderly males.
- Females are usually affected after menopause.
- Prevalence of angina pectoris in people older than 30 yr is >3%.
- Within 12 mo of initial diagnosis, 10% to 20% of patients with diagnosis of stable angina progress to MI or unstable angina.

■ PHYSICAL FINDINGS & CLINICAL PRESENTATION

- Although there is significant individual variation, most patients complain of substernal chest pain (pressure, tightness, heaviness, sharp pain, sensation similar to intestinal gas or dysphagia).
- The pain is of short duration (30 sec to 30 min), nonpleuritic, and often accompanied by shortness of breath, nausea, diaphoresis, and numbness or pain in the left arm, jaw, or shoulder.

■ ETIOLOGY
The various causes of myocardial ischemia are described in Box 2-173.

UNCONTROLLABLE RISK FACTORS FOR ANGINA:
- Advanced age
- Male sex
- Genetic predisposition

MODIFIABLE RISK FACTORS FOR ANGINA:
- Smoking (risk is almost double)
- Hypertension (risk is double if systolic blood pressure is >180 mm Hg)
- Hyperlipidemia
- Impaired glucose tolerance or diabetes mellitus
- Obesity (weight >30% over ideal)
- Hypothyroidism
- Left ventricular hypertrophy (LVH)
- Sedentary lifestyle
- Oral contraceptive use
- Cocaine use (Cocaine is used by >5,000,000 Americans regularly and is responsible for >64,000 ER evaluations yearly to rule out myocardial ischemia.)
- Low serum folate levels. (Folate is required for conversion of homocysteine to methionine.) Hyperhomocystinemia has a toxic effect on vascular endothelium and interferes with proliferation of arterial wall smooth muscle cells. Folate deficiencies are associated with an increased risk of fatal coronary heart disease.)
- Elevated homocysteine levels
- Elevated levels of highly sensitive C-reactive protein (hs-CRP, cardio CRP)
- Elevated levels of lipoprotein-associated phospholipase A2
- Elevated fibrinogen levels
- Depression in men
- Vasculitis

🔬 DIAGNOSIS

■ DIFFERENTIAL DIAGNOSIS
Noncardiac pain mimicking angina may be caused by:
- Pulmonary diseases (pulmonary hypertension, pulmonary embolism, pleurisy, pneumothorax, pneumonia)
- GI disorders (peptic ulcer disease, pancreatitis, esophageal spasm or spontaneous esophageal muscle contraction, esophageal reflux, cholecystitis, cholelithiasis)
- Musculoskeletal conditions (costochondritis, chest wall trauma, cervical arthritis with radiculopathy, muscle strain, myositis)
- Acute aortic dissection
- Herpes zoster

■ WORKUP
- The most important diagnostic factor is the history.
- The physical examination is of little diagnostic help and may be totally normal in many patients, although the presence of an S_4 gallop is suggestive of ischemic chest pain.
- An ECG taken during the acute episode may show transient T-wave inversion or ST-segment depression or elevation, but some patients may have a normal tracing. (Table 2-189 and Fig. 2-7 describe the differential diagnosis of ST-segment elevation.)
- Treadmill exercise tolerance test is useful to identify patients with coronary artery disease who would benefit from cardiac catheterization. Stress echocardiogram of radionuclide testing (e.g., thallium, persantine, dobutamine) are useful and sensitive in the detection of myocardial ischemia.
- Although invasive x-ray coronary angiography remains the gold standard for the identification of clinically significant coronary artery disease, coronary magnetic resonance angiography can accurately detect coronary artery disease of the proximal and middle segments. This noninvasive approach, where available, can be used to reliably identify (or rule out) left main coronary artery or three-vessel disease.

■ LABORATORY TESTS
- Initial laboratory tests in patients with chronic stable angina should include hemoglobin, fasting glucose, and fasting lipid panel.
- Cardiac isoenzymes (CK-MB q8h × 2) should be obtained to rule out MI in patients with unstable angina.
- Cardiac troponin I and T are specific markers of myocardial necrosis and are useful in evaluating patients with unstable angina. Elevation of either of these proteins in the setting of an acute coronary syndrome identifies patients with a several-fold increased risk of death in subsequent weeks. Patients with negative troponin assays on arrival in the ER and repeated 4 hours later are at a low level of risk for cardiac events within the following 30 days, and most of these patients can be safely discharged from the ER. Troponin T tests can be false-positive in patients with renal failure, sepsis, rhabdomyolysis, fibrin clots, and heterophile antibodies. The presence of jaundice or the concurrent use of heparin can result in underestimation of troponin.
- Circulating interleukin-6 (IL-6), a cytokine with both proinflammatory

and antiinflammatory effects, is a strong independent marker of increased mortality in unstable coronary artery disease and identifies patients who benefit most from a strategy of early intervention.

- New markers for risk stratification in acute coronary syndromes based on neurohormonal activation and inflammation have recently been identified. A single measurement of B-type natriuretic peptide, a natriuretic and vasodilative peptide regulated by ventricular wall tension and stored mainly in the ventricular myocardium, obtained in the first few days after the onset of ischemic symptoms, provides predictive information for risk stratification in acute coronary syndromes. Pregnancy-associated plasma protein A (PAPP-A), which is found in both men and women, is an activator of insulin-like growth factor I (IGF-I), or a mediator of atherosclerosis may be a marker for unstable plaques. Elevated plasma levels of PAPP-A can identify patients with unstable angina in the absence of elevations of either troponin I or C-reactive protein.

■ IMAGING STUDIES
- Echocardiography is indicated only in patients with suspected valvular abnormalities; it is also useful to evaluate LV function.
- Coronary angiography is performed to define the location and extent of coronary disease; this is indicated in selected patients who are candidates for CABG surgery or angioplasty. Noninvasive methods for assessing myocardial viability to predict which patients will have increased LVEF and improved survival after revascularization include positron-emission tomography, dobutamine echocardiography, and contrast-enhanced MRI. Additional studies are needed to determine the cost effectiveness of these studies in patients with ischemic cardiomyopathy

■ TREATMENT

■ NONPHARMACOLOGIC THERAPY
- Aggressive modification of preventable risk factors (weight reduction in obese patients, regular aerobic exercise program, correction of folate deficiency, estrogen replacement in postmenopausal women, low-cholesterol and low-sodium diet, cessation of cigarette smoking)

- Correction of possible aggravating factors (e.g., anemia, thyrotoxicosis, hypertension, diabetes mellitus, hypercholesterolemia)

■ ACUTE GENERAL Rx
The major classes of antiischemic agents are nitrates, β-adrenergic blockers, calcium channel blockers, aspirin, and heparin; they can be used alone or in combination.

- Nitrates cause venodilation and relaxation of vascular smooth muscle; the decreased venous return from venodilation decreases diastolic ventricular wall tension (preload) and thereby reduces mechanical activity (and myocardial oxygen consumption) during systole. Relaxation of vascular smooth muscle increases coronary blood flow and reduces systemic pressure. Tolerance to nitrates can be minimized by avoiding sustained blood levels with a daily nitrate-free period (e.g., omission of bedtime dose of oral isosorbide dinitrate or 12 hr on/12 hr off transdermal nitroglycerin therapy). Nitrates are relatively contraindicated in patients with hypertrophic obstructive cardiomyopathy, and should also be avoided in patients with severe aortic stenosis.

- β-Adrenergic blockers achieve their major antianginal effect by reducing heart rate and systolic blood pressure. Absent contraindications, they should be regarded as initial therapy for stable angina for all patients. Their dose should generally be adjusted to reduce the resting heart rate to 50-60 beats/min.

- Calcium channel blockers play a major role in preventing and terminating myocardial ischemia induced by coronary artery spasm. They are particularly effective in treating microvascular angina. Short-acting calcium channel blockers should be avoided. Calcium channel blockers should generally also be avoided after complicated MI (CHF) and in patients with CHF secondary to systolic dysfunction (unless necessary to control heart rate).

- Aspirin: give initial dose of at least 160 mg/day followed by 81 to 325 mg/day. Aspirin inhibits cyclooxygenics and synthesis of thromboxane A_2 and reduces the risk of adverse cardiovascular events by 33% in patients with unstable angina. Patients intolerant to aspirin can be treated with the antiplatelet agent clopidogrel.

- Heparin is useful in patients with unstable angina and reduces the frequency of MI and refractory angina. Patients with unstable angina treated with aspirin plus heparin have a 32% reduction in the risk of MI and death compared with those treated with aspirin alone; therefore, unless heparin is contraindicated, most hospitalized patients with unstable angina should be treated with both aspirin and heparin. Enoxaparin (low–molecular weight heparin) 1 mg bid SC is as effective as continuous unfractionated heparin in reducing the incidence of unstable angina. It is usually given for 3-8 days, or until coronary revascularization is performed. Longer administration does not provide additional cardiac benefits and may increase risk of hemorrhage.

- Early administration of platelet glycoprotein IIb/IIIa receptor antagonists tirofiban and eptifibatide is useful in unstable angina, in high-risk patients with positive troponin tests, or those undergoing percutaneous revascularization. Abciximab, the first GP IIb/IIa inhibitor, is an important component of percutaneous revascularization. Started in the catheterization lab, it reduces the incidence of ischemic events. Contraindications to the use of GP IIb/IIa inhibitors are: severe hypertension (>180/110), internal bleeding within 30 days, history of intracranial hemorrhage, neoplasm, NVM, aneurysm, CVA within 30 days or history of hemorrhagic CVA, thrombocytopenin (<100 k), acute pericarditis, history or symptoms suggestive of aortic dissection, and major surgical procedures or severe physical trauma within previous month.

■ CHRONIC Rx
Use of lipid-lowering drugs (e.g., statins) is recommended in patients with coronary heart disease and in patients with hyperlipidemia refractory to diet and exercise. Statins (e.g., pravastatin) also decrease the level of the inflammatory marker hs-CRP independently of the magnitude of change in lipid parameters.

■ REFERRAL
SURGICAL THERAPY: *CABG surgery* is recommended for patients with left main coronary disease, for those with symptomatic three-vessel disease, and for those with left ventricular EF <40% and critical (>70% stenosis) in all three major coronary arteries. Surgical therapy improves prognosis, particularly in diabetic patients with multivessel disease.

Minimally invasive direct coronary artery bypass (MIDCAB) is a variation of CABG for patients in whom sternotomy and cardiopulmonary bypass is either contraindicated or unnecessary. In this procedure the left internal mammary is anastomosed to the LAD through a thoracic incision without cardiopulmonary bypass. This operation is generally preformed for patients with only single-vessel CAD.

The Port-Access Procedure is another type of minimally invasive technique; however, it is performed on an arrested heart and with the use of cardiopulmonary bypass.

ANGIOPLASTY AND CORONARY STENTS: *Percutaneous transluminal coronary angioplasty (PTCA)* should be considered for patients with one- or two-vessel disease that does not involve the main left coronary artery and in whom ventricular function is normal or near normal. Patients selected for PTCA must also be candidates for CABG. The types of lesions best suited for angioplasty are proximal lesions, noncalcified, concentric, and preferably shorter than 5 mm (should not exceed 10 mm). Approximately 80% of patients show immediate benefit after PTCA. Restenosis with recurrence of angina occurs in approximately 30% of patients, usually within the first 3 months after PTCA. In these patients PTCA can be repeated. The frequency of abrupt closure postangioplasty can be reduced by pretreatment with IV glycoprotein IIb/IIIa receptor inhibitors, which block the final common pathway of platelet aggregation. In patients with clinically documented acute coronary syndrome who are treated with GP IIb/IIa inhibitors, even small elevations in cTmI and cTmT identify high-risk patients who derive a large clinical benefit from an early invasive strategy. Abciximab (Reopro) and eptifibatide (Integrilin) are approved for use before and during percutaneous coronary interventions. They are expensive (>$1400 per dose of abciximab) and can cause thrombocytopenia in 0.5% to 1% of patients.

Platelet counts should be monitored for 24 hours after starting glycoprotein IIb/IIIa inhibitors. Reversal of thrombocytopenia (e.g., patients undergoing emergency CABG) can be achieved with platelet transfusions.

The development of *coronary stents* has broadened the number of patients who can be treated in the cardiac laboratory. Stents are currently used in nearly 70% of all percutaneous interventional lesions. The rate of restenosis may be reduced by placing a stent electively in primary atheromatous lesions. Common stent types include coil, slotted tube, mesh, and ring. They provide a safety net during PTCA and reduce restenosis rates afterward in about 30% of patients. In patients with symptomatic isolated stenosis of the proximal left anterior descending artery, stenting has advantages over standard coronary angioplasty in that it is associated with both a lower rate of restenosis and a better clinical outcome. The major limitations of stenting are subacute thrombosis, restenosis within the stent, bleeding complications when anticoagulants are used poststenting, and higher cost ($1500 average unit price). The combination of aspirin and clopidogel is effective in preventing coronary stent thrombosis. The recent development of coated stents may eventually eliminate the risk of agstenosis. Although trials have failed to show that stents favorably influence mortality, they have fulfilled their goal of decreasing the morbidity associated wtih angina and the need for repeated revascularization after PTCA. In patients with elevated total homocysteine levels, treatment with a combination of folic acid, vitamin B_{12} and pyridoxine significantly reduces homocysteine levels and decreases the rate of restenosis and the need for revascularization of the target lesion after coronary angioplasty.

CARBON DIOXIDE LASER: Transmyocardial revascularization with carbon dioxide laser significantly improves outcome in patients with angina refractory to medical treatment and who are not candidates for CABG or PTCA. This procedure is available only in selected centers.

REFERENCES

Ambrose JA, Dangas G: Unstable angina, *Arch Intern Med* 160:25, 2000.

Bayes-Genis A et al: Pregnancy associated plasma protein A as a marker of acute coronary syndromes, *N Engl J Med* 345:1022, 2001.

De Lemos J et al: The prognostic value of B-type natriurectic peptide in patients with acute coronary syndromes, *N Engl J Med* 345:1014, 2001.

Fihn SD et al: Guidelines for the management of patients with chronic stable angina: treatment, *Ann Intern Med* 135:616, 2001.

Kim RJ et al: The use of contrast-enhanced MRI to identify reversible myocardial dysfunction, *N Engl J Med* 343:1445, 2000.

Kim WY et al: Coronary magnetic resonnance angiography for the detection of coronary stenosis, *N Engl J Med* 345:1863, 2001.

Lindmarm E et al: Relationship between interleukin-6 and mortality in patients with unstable coronary disease, *JAMA* 286:2107, 2001.

Mehran R et al: One-year clinical outcome after minimally invasive direct coronary bypass circulation, *Circulation* 102:2799, 2000.

Morrow D et al: Ability of minor elevations of troponins I and T to predict benefit from an early invasive strategy in patients with unstable angina and non-ST elevation MI, *JAMA* 286:2405, 2001.

Schnyder G et al: Decreased rate of coronary restenosis after lowering of plasma homocysteine levels, *N Engl J Med* 345:1543, 2001.

Yeghiazarians Y et al: Unstable angina pectoris, *N Engl J Med* 342:101, 2000.

Author: **Fred F. Ferri, M.D.**

BASIC INFORMATION

■ DEFINITION

- The cutaneous swelling caused by the release of vasoactive mediators is called urticaria and angioedema.
- Urticaria causes edema of the superficial dermis.
- Angioedema involves the deep layers of the dermis and the subcutaneous tissue.

■ SYNONYMS

Angioneurotic edema

ICD-9CM CODES
995.1 Angioedema (allergic)
277.6 Angioedema (hereditary)

■ EPIDEMIOLOGY & DEMOGRAPHICS

- Approximately 20% of the population experiences urticaria and/or angioedema at some time during life.
- Race: No predilection.
- Sex: More occurrences in women than men.
- Angioedema can occur together with urticaria (50%) or alone (10%).
- Angioedema commonly occurs after adolescence in the third decade of life.
- Incidence of hereditary angioedema is 1/150,000 persons.

■ PHYSICAL FINDINGS & CLINICAL PRESENTATION

- Angioedema may be acute or chronic.
  1. Acute angioedema is defined as symptoms lasting <6 wk.
  2. Chronic angioedema is defined as symptoms lasting >6 wk.
- Urticaria is commonly known as "hives" and is characterized by:
  1. Pruritus
  2. Palpable
  3. Erythematous
  4. Millimeters to centimeters in size
  5. Multiple in number
  6. Fades within 12 to 24 hr
  7. Reappears at other sites
- Angioedema is characterized by the following:
  1. Nonpruritic
  2. Burning
  3. Not well demarcated
  4. Involves eyelids (Fig. 1-26), lips, tongue and extremities
  5. Can involve the larynx causing respiratory distress
  6. Resolves slowly

■ ETIOLOGY

- Angioedema, with or without urticaria, is classified as allergic, heredity, or idiopathic.
- Angioedema is primarily due to mast cell activation and degranulation

with release of vasoactive mediators (e.g., histamine, serotonin, bradykinins) resulting in postcapillary venule inflammation, vascular leakage, and edema in the deep layers of the dermis and subcutaneous tissue.

- Pathologically angioedema has both immunological and nonimmunological mediated mechanisms
  1. Immunoglobulin E (Ig E)-mediated angioedema may result from antigen exposure (e.g., foods [milk, eggs, peanuts, shell fish, tomatoes, chocolate, sulfites] or drugs [penicillin, aspirin, NSAIDs, phenytoin, sulfonamides]).
  2. Complement-mediated angioedema involving immune complex mechanisms can also lead to mast cell activation that manifests as serum sickness.
  3. Hereditary angioedema is an autosomal dominant disease due to a deficiency of C1 esterase inhibitor (C1-INH). C1-INH is a protease inhibitor that is normally present in high concentrations in the plasma. C1-INH serves many functions, one of which is to inhibit plasma kallikrein, a protease that cleaves kininogen and releases bradykinin. A deficiency in C1-INH results in excess concentration of kininogen and the subsequent release of kinin mediators.
  4. Acquired angioedema is usually associated with other diseases, most commonly B-cell lymphoproliferative disorders, but may also result from the formation of auto-antibodies directed against C1 inhibitor protein.
  5. Other causes of angioedema include infection (e.g., herpes simplex, hepatitis B, cox sackie A and B, streptococcus, candida,

ascoris, and strongyloides), insect bites and stings, stress, physical factors (e.g., cold, exercise, pressure, and vibration), collagen vascular diseases (e.g., SLE, Henoich-Schönlein purpura), and idiopathic causes.

DIAGNOSIS

A detailed history and physical examination usually makes the diagnosis of angioedema. Extensive lab testing is of limited value.

■ DIFFERENTIAL DIAGNOSIS

The differential diagnosis of angioedema includes:
1. Cellulitis
2. Hypothyroidism
3. Contact dermatitis
4. Atopic dermatitis
5. Mastocytosis
6. Granulomatous cheilitis
7. Bullous pemphigoid
8. Urticaria pigmentosa
9. Anaphylaxis
10. Erythema multiforme
11. Epiglottitis
12. Peritonsillar abscess

■ WORKUP

- An extensive workup searching for the cause of angioedema is often unrevealing (90%).
- Workup including diagnostic blood tests and allergy testing is performed based on the history and physical examination.

■ LABORATORY TESTS

- CBC, ESR, and urinalysis are sometimes helpful as part of the initial evaluation.
- Stools for ova and parasites

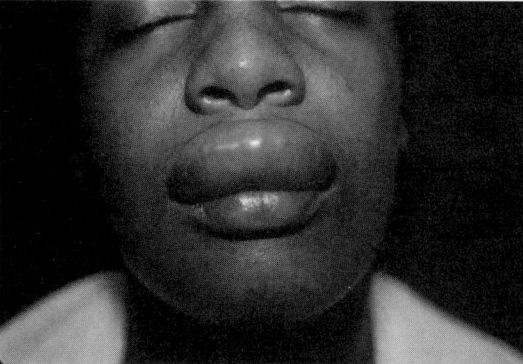

Fig. 1-26 Angioedema of the upper lip, with severe swelling of deeper tissues. (From Goldstein BG, Goldstein AO: *Practical dermatology*, ed 2, St Louis, 1997, Mosby.)

Gwendolyn R. Lee, M.D.
Internal Medicine

- Serology testing
- C1 esterase inhibitor concentration in suspected hereditary angioedema
- Complement C4 measurements is decreased in C1-INH deficiency.
- Skin and radioallergosorbent (RAST) testing may be done if food allergies are suspected.
- Skin biopsy is usually done in patients with chronic angioedema refractory to corticosteroid treatment.

℞ TREATMENT

■ NONPHARMACOLOGIC THERAPY
- Eliminate the offending agent
- Avoid triggering factors (e.g., cold, stress)
- Cold compresses to affected areas

■ ACUTE GENERAL Rx
- Acute life-threatening angioedema involving the larynx is treated with:
  1. Epinephrine 0.3 mg in a solution of 1:1000 given subcutaneously
  2. Diphenhydramine 25 to 50 mg IV or IM
  3. Cimetidine 300 mg IV or ranitidine 50 mg IV
  4. Methylprednisolone 125 mg IV
- Mainstay therapy in angioedema is H1 antihistamines.
  1. Diphenhydramine 25 to 50 mg q6h

2. Chlorpheniramine 4 mg q6h
3. Hydroxyzine 10 to 25 mg q6h
4. Cetirizine 5 to 10 mg qd
5. Loratidine 10 mg qd
6. Fexofenadine 60 mg qd
- H2 antihistamines can be added to H1 antihistamines.
  1. Ranitidine 150 mg bid
  2. Cimetidine 400 mg bid
  3. Famotidine 20 mg bid
- Tricyclic antidepressants
  1. Doxepin 25 to 50 mg qd can be tried.
- Corticosteroids are rarely required for symptomatic relief of acute angioedema.

■ CHRONIC Rx
- Chronic angioedema is treated as described under "Acute General Rx."
- Corticosteroids are used more often in chronic angioedema.
- Prednisone 1 mg/kg/day for 5 days and then tapered over a period of weeks.
- Androgens are used for the treatment of hereditary angioedema.

■ DISPOSITION
- Antihistamines achieve symptomatic relief in over 80% of patients with angioedema.
- In chronic angioedema, corticosteroid is given in addition to antihistamines.

- A small percentage of people will have recurrence of symptoms after steroid treatment.
- Chronic angioedema can last for months and even years.

■ REFERRAL
Dermatology consultation is recommended in patients with chronic angioedema, hereditary angioedema, and recurring angioedema.

☼ PEARLS & CONSIDERATIONS

■ COMMENTS
- Identifying a cause for angioedema in patients is often difficult and met with frustration.
- Chronic angioedema, unlike acute angioedema, is rarely caused by an allergic reaction.

REFERENCES
Beltrani VS: Urticaria and angioedema, *Dermatol Clin* 14:171, 1996.

Kwong KY, Mallouf N, Jones CA: Urticaria and angioedema: pathophysiology, diagnosis, and treatment, *Pediatr Ann* 27:719, 1998.

Wagner WO: Angioedema: frightening and frustrating, *Cleve Clin J Med* 66(4):203, 1999.

Author: **Peter Petropoulos, M.D.**

BASIC INFORMATION

■ DEFINITION

Ankle fractures involve the lateral, medial, or posterior malleolus of the ankle and may occur either alone or in some combination. Associated ligamentous injuries are included.

ICD-9CM CODES
824.8 Ankle fracture (malleolus) (closed)
824.2 Lateral malleolus fracture (fibular)
824.0 Medial malleolus fracture (tibial)

■ PHYSICAL FINDINGS & CLINICAL PRESENTATION
- Deformity usually dependent on extent of displacement
- Pain, tenderness, and hemorrhage at the site of injury
- Gentle palpation of ligamentous structures (especially deltoid ligament) to determine the extent of soft tissue injury
- Evaluation of distal neurovascular status; results recorded

■ ETIOLOGY
- The ankle depends on its ligamentous and bony support for stability. The joint, or *mortise,* is an inverted U with the dome of the talus fitting into the medial and lateral malleoli. The posterior margin of the tibia is often called the *third* or *posterior malleolus.*
- Most common ankle fractures are the result of eversion or lateral rotation forces on the talus (in contrast to common sprains, which are caused usually by inversion).

DIAGNOSIS

■ IMAGING STUDIES
Standard AP and lateral views accompanied by an AP taken 15° internally rotated. The last view is taken to properly visualize the mortise.

TREATMENT

All fractures: elevation and ice to control swelling for 48 to 72 hr.

■ ACUTE GENERAL Rx
- Clinical and roentgenographic assessment of the status of the ankle mortise and stability of the injury is mandatory to determine treatment.

- There is potential for displacement if both sides of the joint are significantly injured (e.g., fracture of the lateral malleolus with deltoid ligament injury).
- Deviation of the position of the talus in the mortise could lead to traumatic arthritis.
- If there is no widening of the ankle mortise, many injuries can be safely treated with simple casting without reduction:
1. Undisplaced or avulsion fractures of either malleolus below the ankle joint line:
   a. Stability of the joint is not compromised and a short leg walking cast or ankle support is sufficient.
   b. Weight bearing is allowed as tolerated.
   c. In 4 to 6 wk, protection may be discontinued.
2. Isolated undisplaced fractures of the medial, lateral, or posterior malleolus:
   a. Usually stable and require only the application of a short leg walking cast with the ankle in the neutral position or fracture cast boot.
   b. Immobilization should be continued for 8 wk.
   c. Fracture line of lateral malleolus may persist roentgenographically for several months, but immobilization beyond 8 wk is usually unnecessary.
   d. Undisplaced bimalleolar fractures are treated with a long leg cast flexed 30° at the knee to prevent motion and displacement of the fracture fragments. In 4 wk, a short leg walking cast may be applied for an additional 4 wk.
3. Isolated fractures of the lateral malleolus that are slightly displaced:
   a. May be treated with casting if no medial injury is present.
   b. A below-knee walking cast is applied with ankle in the neutral position and weight bearing is allowed as tolerated.
   c. Six weeks of immobilization is sufficient.
   d. If medial tenderness is present, suggesting deltoid ligament rupture, a carefully molded cast may suffice if weight bearing is not allowed and the patient is followed closely for signs of instability, especially after swelling recedes. If significant widening of the medial ankle mortise (increase in the "medial clear space") develops as a result of lateral displacement of the talus,

referral for possible reduction is indicated.
   e. If signs of instability are already present at initial examination (widening of the medial clear space with medial tenderness), referral is indicated.
4. Undisplaced fracture of the distal fibular epiphysis:
   a. Diagnosed clinically.
   b. There is tenderness over the epiphyseal plate.
   c. Roentgenographic findings are often negative.
   d. A short leg walking cast is applied for 4 wk.
   e. Growth disturbance is rare.
5. Isolated posterior malleolar fractures involving less than 25% of the joint surface on the lateral roentgenogram:
   Safely treated by applying a short leg walking cast or fracture brace. (Fractures involving >25% of the weight-bearing surface should be referred because of the potential for instability and subsequent traumatic arthritis)

■ CHRONIC Rx
- Early motion is encouraged through a home exercise program.
- Protection from reinjury is appropriate for 4 to 6 wk following cast or brace removal.
- Temporary increase in lower extremity swelling that frequently occurs after short leg cast removal may benefit from the use of support hose.

■ DISPOSITION
Significant factors involved in the development of traumatic arthritis:
- Amount of joint trauma at the time of injury
- Eventual position of the talus in the mortise
Fracture nonunion is uncommon unless displacement is significant.

■ REFERRAL
Orthopedic consultation for:
- Unstable ankle joint
- Widened ankle mortise
- Posterior malleolar fracture over 25% of joint with incongruity
- Marked displacement of fracture fragment

REFERENCES
Kay RM, Matthys GA: Pediatric ankle fractures: evaluation and treatment, *J Am Acad Orthop Surg* 9:268, 2001.
Makwana NK et al: Conservative versus operative treatment for displaced ankle fractures in patients over 55 years of age, *J Bone Joint Surg* 83(B):525, 2001.

Author: **Lonnie R. Mercier, M.D.**

BASIC INFORMATION

■ DEFINITION
An ankle sprain is an injury to the ligamentous support of the ankle. Most (85%) involve the lateral ligament complex (Fig. 1-27). The anterior inferior tibiofibular (AITF) ligament, deltoid ligament, and interosseous membrane may also be injured. Damage to the tibiofibular syndesmosis is sometimes called a *high sprain* because of pain above the ankle.

ICD-9CM CODES
845.00 Sprain, ankle or foot

■ EPIDEMIOLOGY & DEMOGRAPHICS
PREVALENCE: 1 case/10,000 people each day
PREDOMINANT SEX: Varies according to age and level of physical activity

■ PHYSICAL FINDINGS & CLINICAL PRESENTATION
• Often a history of a "pop"
• Variable amounts of tenderness and hemorrhage
• Possible abnormal anterior drawer test (pulling the plantar flexed foot forward to determine if there is any abnormal increase in forward movement of the talus in the ankle mortise) (Fig. 1-28)
• Inversion sprains: tender laterally; syndesmotic injuries: area of tenderness is more anterior and proximal
• Evaluation of motor function (Fig. 1-29)

■ ETIOLOGY
• Lateral injuries usually result from inversion and plantar flexion injuries.
• Eversion and rotational forces may injure the deltoid or AITF ligament or the interosseous membrane.

DIAGNOSIS

■ DIFFERENTIAL DIAGNOSIS
• Fracture of the ankle or foot, particularly involving the distal fibular growth plate in the immature patient
• Avulsion fracture of the fifth metatarsal base

■ WORKUP
• History and clinical examination are usually sufficient to establish the diagnosis.
• Plain radiographs are always needed.

■ IMAGING STUDIES
Roentgenographic evaluation
1. Usually normal but always performed
2. Should include the fifth metatarsal base
3. All minor avulsion fractures noted
Varying opinions on the usefulness of arthrograms, tenograms, and stress films

TREATMENT

■ ACUTE GENERAL Rx
Ankle sprains are often graded I, II, or III, according to severity, with Grade III injury implying complete rupture. The first line of treatment is described by the mnemonic device, *RICE:*
• Rest
• Ice
• Compression
• Elevation
• Varying opinions regarding the initial use of NSAIDs
• In 48 to 72 hr, active range of motion and weight bearing as tolerated
• In 4 to 5 days, exercise against resistance added
• Possible cast immobilization for some patients who require early independent walking; short leg orthoses also available for the same purpose
• Surgery is rarely recommended, even for Grade III sprains; reports of equally satisfactory outcomes with nonsurgical treatment

■ CHRONIC Rx
• Lateral heel and sole wedge to prevent inversion
• Protective taping or bracing during vigorous activities (Fig. 1-30)
• Strengthening exercises

■ DISPOSITION
• Lateral sprains of any severity may cause lingering symptoms for weeks and months.
  1. Some syndesmotic sprains take even longer to heal.
  2. Heterotopic ossification may even develop in the interosseous membrane, but long-term results do not seem to be affected by such ossification.
• Continuing lateral symptoms may require surgical reconstruction, although late traumatic arthritis or chronic instability is rare regardless of treatment.

■ REFERRAL
For orthopedic consultation for cases that fail to respond to conservative treatment

PEARLS & CONSIDERATIONS

■ COMMENTS
If healing seems delayed (over 6 wk), the following conditions should be considered:
1. Talar dome fracture
2. Reflex sympathetic dystrophy
3. Chronic tendinitis
4. Peroneal tendon subluxation
5. Other occult fracture
6. Peroneal weakness (poor rehabilitation)
Repeat plain roentgenograms, bone scan, or MRI may be indicated.

REFERENCE
Wolfe M et al: Management of ankle sprains, *Am Fam Physician* 63:83, 2001.
Author: **Lonnie R. Mercier, M.D.**

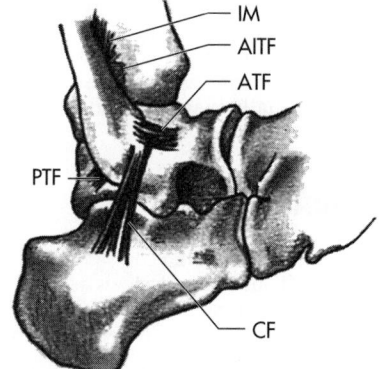

Fig. 1-27 The lateral ankle ligaments, anterior and posterior talofibular *(ATF, PTF)* and calcaneofibular *(CF)*. Also shown are the anterior inferior tibiofibular ligament *(AITF)* and the beginning of the interosseous membrane *(IM)*. (From Mercier LR [ed]: *Practical orthopaedics,* ed 4, St Louis, 1995, Mosby.)

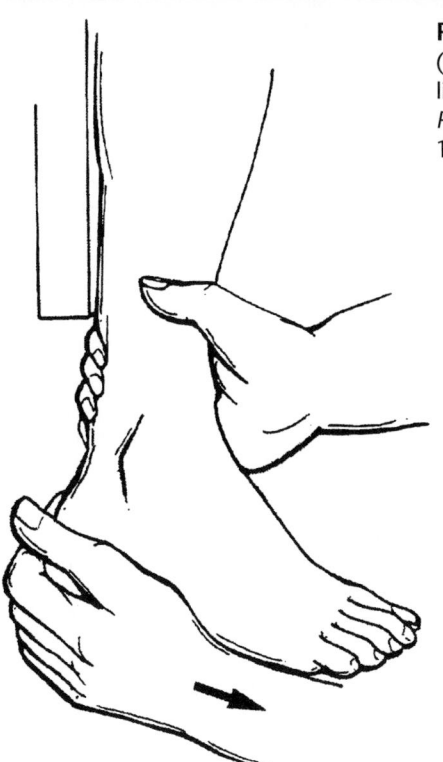

Fig. 1-28   Anterior drawer test of the ankle (tests the integrity of the anterior talofibular ligament). (From Brinker MR, Miller MD: *Fundamentals of orthopaedics,* Philadelphia, 1999, WB Saunders.)

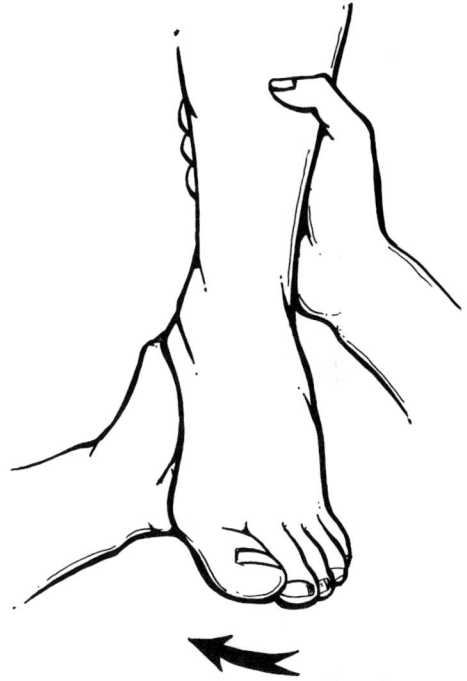

Fig. 1-29   Talar tilt test (inversion stress) of the ankle (tests the integrity of the anterior talofibular ligament and the calcaneofibular ligament). (From Brinker MR, Miller MD: *Fundamentals of orthopaedics,* Philadelphia, 1999, WB Saunders.)

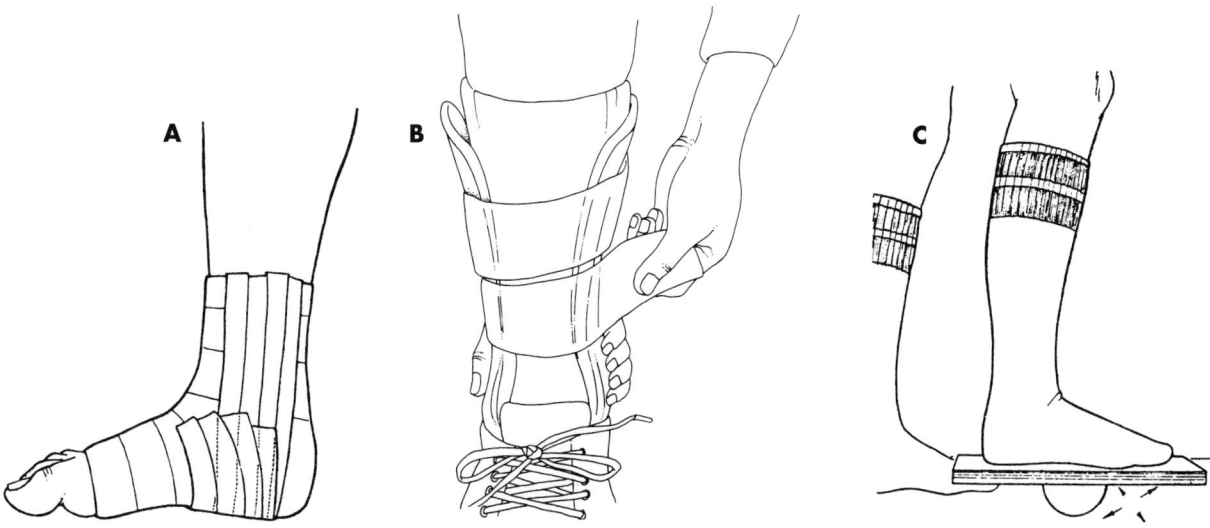

Fig. 1-30   A, The most effective method of supporting most acute ankle sprains is by using an Ace wrap reinforced with 1-in medial and lateral tape strips. The anterior and posterior aspects of the ankle are left free to allow the patient to flex and extend the ankle. The patient is encouraged to bear weight with crutches. **B,** Diagram of an air splint. Straps are adjusted to heel size, the lower straps are wrapped about the ankle, and the side extensions are centered. The splint is then pressurized and straps adjusted until comfortable support and pressure are attained. **C,** As the ankle pain subsides, about the third to fifth day, balancing exercises can begin to allow the patient to regain ankle proprioception and avoid recurrent instability problems. (From Jardon OM, Mathews MS: Orthopedics. In Rakel RE [ed]: *Textbook of family practice,* ed 5, Philadelphia, 1995, WB Saunders.)

BASIC INFORMATION

■ DEFINITION
Ankylosing spondylitis is a chronic inflammatory condition involving the sacroiliac joints and axial skeleton. It is one of a group of several overlapping syndromes, including spondylitis associated with Reiter's syndrome, psoriasis, and IBD. Patients are typically seronegative for the rheumatoid factor, and these disorders are now commonly called *rheumatoid variants* or *seronegative spondyloarthropathies.*

■ SYNONYMS
Marie-Strumpell disease

ICD-9CM CODES
720.0 Ankylosing spondylitis

■ EPIDEMIOLOGY & DEMOGRAPHICS
PREVALENCE: 0.15% of male population (rare in blacks)
PREDOMINANT AGE AT ONSET: 15 to 35 yr
PREDOMINANT SEX: Male:female ratio of 10:1

■ PHYSICAL FINDINGS & CLINICAL PRESENTATION
- Morning stiffness
- Fatigue, weight loss, anorexia, and other systemic complaints in more severe forms
- Bilateral sacroiliac tenderness (sacroiliitis)
- Limited lumbar spine motion (Fig. 1-31)
- Loss of chest expansion measured at the nipple line <2.5 cm, reflecting rib cage involvement
- Occasionally, peripheral joint involvement (large joints are more commonly affected)
- Possible extraskeletal manifestations affecting the cardiovascular system (aortic insufficiency, heart block, cardiomegaly), lungs (pulmonary fibrosis), and eye (uveitis)

■ ETIOLOGY
Unknown

DIAGNOSIS

■ DIFFERENTIAL DIAGNOSIS
- Other spondyloarthropathies (see Table 2-188 and Box 2-199)
- A clinical algorithm for the evaluation of back pain is described in Fig. 3-28.

■ WORKUP
The modified New York criteria are often used for diagnosis:
- Low back pain of at least 3 mo duration improved by exercise and not relieved by rest

- Limitation of lumbar spine movement in sagittal and frontal planes
- Decreased chest expansion below normal values for age and sex
- Bilateral sacroiliitis of minimal grade or greater
- Unilateral sacroiliitis of moderate grade or greater

■ LABORATORY TESTS
- Elevated sedimentation rate
- Absence of rheumatoid factor and ANA
- Possible mild hyperchromic anemia
- Presence of HLA/B27 antigen in >90% of patients

■ IMAGING STUDIES
- Early roentgenographic features are those of bilateral sacroiliitis on plain films.
- Vertebral bodies may become demineralized and a typical "squaring off" occurs.
- With progression, calcification of the annulus fibrosus and paravertebral ligaments develop, giving rise to the so-called bamboo spine appearance.
- End result may be a forward protruding cervical spine and fixed dorsal kyphosis.

TREATMENT

■ NONPHARMACOLOGIC THERAPY
- Exercises primarily to maintain flexibility; general aerobic activity also important
- Postural training
  1. Patients must be instructed to sit in the erect position and to avoid stooping; otherwise, a flexion contracture of the spine may develop, which can become so severe that the patient cannot see forward.
  2. Sleeping should be in the supine position on a firm mattress;

pillows should not be placed under the head or knees.

■ CHRONIC Rx
NSAIDs: indomethacin is often successful in relieving symptoms; newer nonsteroidal agents may be tried as well.
- New research into the use of DMARDs such as tumor necrosis factor antagonists appears promising.

■ DISPOSITION
- Most patients have a normal life span.
- The usual course of the disease is not life-threatening, but death may occur as a result of aortic insufficiency or secondary amyloidosis with renal disease.

■ REFERRAL
- Orthopedic consultation for pain or deformity
- Ophthalmologic consultation for ocular complications
- Rheumatology consultation for uncontrolled symptoms

PEARLS & CONSIDERATIONS

■ COMMENTS
Years may pass between the onset of symptoms and the ultimate diagnosis because of the frequency of nonspecific low back pain from other disorders.

REFERENCES
Braun J, De Keyser F et al: New treatment options in spondyloarthropathies: increasing evidence for significant efficacy of anti-tumor necrosis therapy, *Curr Opin Rheumatol* 13:245, 2001.
Olivieri I et al: Ankylosing spondylitis and undifferentiated spondyloarthropathies: a clinical review and description of a disease subset with older age at onset, *Curr Opin Rheumatol* 13:280, 2001.
Author: **Lonnie R. Mercier, M.D.**

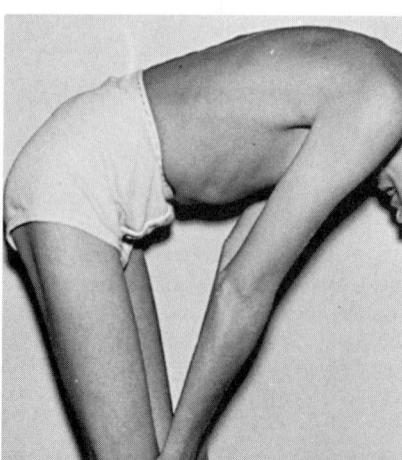

Fig. 1-31   Loss of lumbodorsal spine mobility in a boy with ankylosing spondylitis: the lower spine remains straight when the patient bends forward. (From Behrman RE: *Nelson textbook of pediatrics,* Philadelphia, 1996, WB Saunders.)

BASIC INFORMATION

■ **DEFINITION**
A fistula is an inflammatory tract with a secondary (external) opening in the perianal skin and a primary (internal) opening in the anal canal at the dentate line. It originates in an abscess in the intersphincteric space of the anal canal. Fistulas can be classified as follows:
1. Intersphincteric: fistula track passes within the intersphincteric plane to the perianal skin; most common
2. Transsphincteric: fistula track passes from the internal opening, through the internal and external sphincter, and into the ischiorectal fossa to the perianal skin; frequent
3. Suprasphincteric: after passing through the internal sphincter, fistula tract passes above the puborectalis and then tracts downward, lateral to the external sphincter, into the ischiorectal space to the perianal skin; uncommon; if abscess cavity extends cephalad, a supralevator abscess possibly palpable on rectal examination
4. Extrasphincteric: fistula tract passes from the rectum, above the levators, through the levator muscles to the ischiorectal space and perianal skin; rare
With a horseshoe fistula, the tract passes from one ischiorectal fossa to the other behind the rectum.

■ **SYNONYMS**
Fistula-in-ano

ICD-9CM CODES
565.1 Anal fistula

■ **EPIDEMIOLOGY & DEMOGRAPHICS**
• Common in all ages
• Occurs equally in men and women
• Associated with constipation
• Pediatric age group: more common in infants; boys > girls

■ **PHYSICAL FINDINGS & CLINICAL PRESENTATION**
• Acute stage: perianal swelling, pain, and fever
• Chronic stage: history of rectal drainage or bleeding; previous abscess with drainage
• Tender external fistulous opening, with 2 to 3 cm of the anal verge, with purulent or serosanguineous drainage on compression; the greater the distance from the anal margin, the greater the probability of a complicated upward extension
• Goodsall's rule:
1. Location of the internal opening related to the location of the external opening.

2. With external opening anterior to an imaginary line drawn horizontally across the midpoint of the anus: fistulous tract runs radially into the anal canal.
3. With opening posterior to the transanal line: tract is usually curvilinear, entering the anal canal in the posterior midline.
4. Exception to this rule: an external, anterior opening that is >3 cm from the anus. In this case the tract may curve posteriorly and end in the posterior midline.
• If perianal abscess recurs, presence of a fistula is suggested.

■ **ETIOLOGY**
• Most common: nonspecific cryptoglandular infection (skin or intestinal flora)
• Fistulas more common when intestinal microorganisms are cultured from the anorectal abscess
• Tuberculosis
• Lymphogranuloma venereum
• Actinomycosis
• Inflammatory bowel disease (IBD): Crohn's disease, ulcerative colitis
• Trauma: surgery (episiotomy, prostatectomy), foreign bodies, anal intercourse
• Malignancy: carcinoma, leukemia, lymphoma
• Treatment of malignancy: surgery, radiation

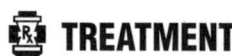 **DIAGNOSIS**

■ **DIFFERENTIAL DIAGNOSIS**
• Hidradenitis suppurativa
• Pilonidal sinus
• Bartholin's gland abscess or sinus
• Infected perianal sebaceous cysts

■ **WORKUP**
• Digital rectal examination:
1. Assess sphincter tone and voluntary squeeze pressure
2. Determine the presence of an extraluminal mass
3. Identify an indurated track
4. Palpate an internal opening or pit
• Gentle probing of external orifice to avoid creating a false tract; 50% do not have clinically detectable opening
• Anoscopy
• Proctosigmoidoscopy to exclude inflammatory or neoplastic disease
• All studies done under adequate anesthesia

■ **LABORATORY TESTS**
• CBC
• Rectal biopsy if diagnosis of IBD or malignancy suspected; biopsy of external orifice is useless

■ **IMAGING STUDIES**
• Colonoscopy or barium enema if:
1. Diagnosis of IBD or malignancy is suspected
2. History of recurrent or multiple fistulas
3. Patient <25 yr old
• Small bowel series: occasionally obtained for reasons similar to above
• Fistulography: unreliable; but may be helpful in complicated fistulas

Rx **TREATMENT**

■ **NONPHARMACOLOGIC THERAPY**
Sitz baths

■ **ACUTE GENERAL Rx**
• Treatment of choice: surgery
• Broad-spectrum antibiotic given if:
1. Cellulitis present
2. Patient is immunocompromised
3. Valvular heart disease present
4. Prosthetic devices present
• Stool softener/laxative

■ **CHRONIC Rx**
• Surgery
• Surgical goals are as follows:
1. Cure the fistula
2. Prevent recurrence
3. Preserve sphincter function
4. Minimize healing time
• Methods for the management of anal fistulas: fistulotomy, setons, rectal advancement flaps, colostomy

■ **DISPOSITION**
Outpatient surgery

■ **REFERRAL**
Refer to a surgeon with expertise in this area.

PEARLS & CONSIDERATIONS

■ **COMMENTS**
• HIV-positive and diabetic patients with perirectal abscesses/fistulas are true surgical emergencies.
• Risk of septicemia, Fournier's gangrene, and other septic complications make immediate drainage imperative.

REFERENCE
Pfenninger JL, Zainea GG: Common anorectal condition, *Am Fam Physician*, 64:22, 2001.
Author: **Maria Elena Soler, M.D.**

BASIC INFORMATION

■ DEFINITION
Anorexia nervosa is a psychiatric disorder characterized by abnormal eating behavior, severe self-induced weight loss, and a specific psychopathology (see "Workup").

ICD-9CM CODES
307.1 Anorexia nervosa

■ EPIDEMIOLOGY & DEMOGRAPHICS
INCIDENCE/PREVALENCE (IN U.S.):
- Anorexia nervosa occurs in 0.2% to 1.3% of the general population, with an annual incidence of 5 to 10 cases/100,000 persons.
- Participation in activities that promote thinness (athletics, modeling) are associated with a higher incidence of anorexia nervosa.

PREDOMINANT SEX: Female:male ratio is 9:1. Approximately 0.5% to 1% of women between the ages of 15 and 30 yr have anorexia nervosa.
PREDOMINANT AGE: Adolescence to young adulthood is the predominant age. Mean age of onset is 17 yr.

■ PHYSICAL FINDINGS & CLINICAL PRESENTATION
- Primary care physicians must be skilled at recognizing this disorder because patients with mild cases usually present with nonspecific symptoms such as asthenia, lack of energy, or dizziness. The physical examination may be normal in the early stages or in mild cases. Patients with moderate to severe anorexia have the physical characteristics described below.
- Patient is emaciated and bundled in clothing.
- Skin is dry and has excessive growth of lanugo. Skin may also be yellow-tinged from carotenodermia.
- Brittle nails, thinning scalp hair are present.
- Bradycardia, hypotension, hypothermia, and bradypnea are common.
- Female fat distribution pattern is no longer evident.
- Axillary and pubic hair is preserved.
- Peripheral edema may be present.

■ ETIOLOGY
- Etiology is unknown, but probably multifactorial (sociocultural, psychologic, familial, and genetic factors).
- A history of sexual abuse has been reported in as many as 50% of patients with anorexia nervosa.
- Psychologic factors: anorexics often have an incompletely developed personal identity. They struggle to maintain a sense of control over their environment, they usually have a low self-esteem, and they lack the sense that they are valued and loved for themselves.

DIAGNOSIS

■ DIFFERENTIAL DIAGNOSIS
- Depression with loss of appetite
- Schizophrenia
- Conversion disorder
- Occult carcinoma, lymphoma
- Endocrine disorders: Addison's disease, diabetes mellitus, hypothyroidism or hyperthyroidism, panhypopituitarism
- GI disorders: celiac disease, Crohn's disease, intestinal parasitosis
- Infectious disorders: AIDS, TB
- A clinical algorithm for the evaluation of anorexia is described in Fig. 3-16.

■ WORKUP
- A diagnosis can be made using the following DSM-IV diagnostic criteria for anorexia nervosa:
  1. Refusal to maintain body weight (BW) at or above a minimally normal weight for age and height (e.g., weight loss leading to maintenance of BW <85% of that expected or failure to make expected weight gain during a period of growth, leading to BW <85% of that expected)
  2. Intense fear of gaining weight or becoming fat, even though underweight
  3. Disturbance in the way in which BW or shape is experienced, undue influence of BW or shape on self-evaluation, or denial of the seriousness of the current low BW

  4. In postmenarchal females, amenorrhea, i.e., the absence of at least three consecutive menstrual cycles (A woman is considered to have amenorrhea if her periods occur only following hormone, e.g., estrogen, administration.)
  Specify type:
  Restricting type: During the current episode of anorexia nervosa, the person has not regularly engaged in binge-eating or purging behavior (i.e., self-induced vomiting or the misuse of laxatives, diuretics, or enemas).
  Binge-eating/purging type: During the current episode of anorexia nervosa, the person has regularly engaged in binge-eating or purging behavior (i.e., self-induced vomiting or the misuse of laxatives, diuretics, or enemas).
- The SCOFF questionnaire is a useful screening tool used in England for eating disorders. It consists of the following five questions:
  1. Do you make yourself *S*ick because you feel full?
  2. Have you lost *C*ontrol over how much you eat?
  3. Have you lost more than *O*ne stone (about 6 kg) recently?
  4. Do you believe yourself to be *F*at when others say you are thin?
  5. Does *F*ood dominate your life?
- A positive response to two or more questions has a reported sensitivity of 100% for anorexia and bulimia, and an overall specificity of 87.5%.
- Baseline ECG should be performed on all patients with anorexia nervosa. Routine monitoring of patients with prolonged QT interval is necessary; sudden death in these patients is often caused by ventricular arrhythmias related to QT interval prolongation.

■ LABORATORY TESTS
- Endocrine abnormalities:
  1. Decreased FSH, LH, T_4, T_3, estrogens, urinary 17-OH steroids, estrone, and estradiol
  2. Normal free T_4, TSH
  3. Increased cortisol, GH, rT_3, T_3RU
  4. Absence of cyclic surge of LH

- Leukopenia, thrombocytopenia, anemia, reduced ESR, reduced complement levels, reduced CD4 and CD8 cells may be present.
- Metabolic alkalosis, hypocalcemia, hypokalemia, hypomagnesemia, hypercholesterolemia, and hypophosphatemia may be present.
- Increased plasma β-carotene levels are useful to distinguish these patients from others on starvation diets.

℞ TREATMENT

■ NONPHARMACOLOGIC THERAPY

- A multidisciplinary approach with psychologic, medical, and nutritional support is necessary.
- A goal weight should be set and the patient should be initially monitored at least once a week in the office setting (Box 1-5). The target weight is 100% of ideal BW for teenagers and 90% to 100% for older patients.
- Weight gain should be gradual (1 to 3 lb/wk) to prevent gastric dilation.
- Electrolyte levels should be strictly monitored.
- Mealtime should be a time for social interaction, not confrontation.
- Postprandially, sedentary activities are recommended. The patient's access to a bathroom should be monitored to prevent purging.

■ ACUTE GENERAL Rx

- Criteria to decide on the appropriate initial course of treatment for patients with anorexia nervosa are usually based on the presence of complications, percentage of ideal body weight, and severity of body image distortion.
- Outpatient treatment is adequate for most patients.
- Indications for hospitalization are described in the "Referral" section.
- Medically stable patients who are within 85% of ideal body weight can be followed up by the primary care physician at 3- or 4-wk intervals, which can be lengthened as the patient improves.
- Pharmacologic treatment generally has no role in anorexia nervosa unless major depression or another psychiatric disorder is present. SSRIs can be used to alleviate the depressed mood and moderate obsessive-compulsive behavior in some individuals.

■ CHRONIC Rx

- Psychotherapy continued for years and focused specifically on self-image, family and peer interactions, and relapse prevention is an integral part of a successful recovery.
- Family therapy is also recommended, especially in younger patients.

■ DISPOSITION

- The long-term prognosis is generally poor and marked by recurrent exacerbations. The percentage of patients with anorexia nervosa who fully recover is modest. Most patients continue to suffer from a distorted body image, disordered eating habits, and psychic difficulties.
- Most patients with anorexia nervosa will recover menses within 6 months of reaching 90% of their ideal body weight. It is important to note that patients with anorexia nervosa can become pregnant despite amenorrhea.
- Mortality rates vary from 5% to 20%. Frequent causes of death are electrolyte abnormalities, starvation, or suicide.
- A prolonged QT interval is a marker for risk of sudden death.

■ REFERRAL

Hospitalization should be considered in the following situations:
1. Severe dehydration or electrolyte imbalance
2. ECG abnormalities (prolonged QT interval, arrhythmias)
3. Significant physiologic instability (hypotension, orthostatic changes)
4. Intractable vomiting, purging, or bingeing
5. Patient having suicidal thoughts
6. Weight loss exceeds 30% of ideal BW and is unresponsive to outpatient treatment
7. Rapidly progressing weight loss (>2 lbs in a week)
8. Failure to progress in nutritional rehabilitation in outpatient treatment

REFERENCES

American Psychiatric Association: Practice guideline for the treatment of patients with eating disorders, *Am J Psychiatry* 157(suppl):4, 2000 (revision).

Becker AE et al: Eating disorders, *N Engl J Med* 340:1092, 1999.

Mehler PS: Diagnosis and care of patients with anorexia nervosa in primary care setting, *Ann Intern Med* 134:1048, 2001.

Morgan JF et al: The SCOFF questionnaire: assessment of a new screening tool for eating disorders, *BMJ* 319:1467, 1999.

Author: **Fred F. Ferri, M.D.**

> **BOX 1-5   Example of Refeeding Protocol**
>
> 1. Contract with patient for a weight goal. Goal should not exceed 1 to 2 pounds in the first week and 3 to 5 pounds afterwards.
> 2. Begin 800 to 1200 kcal in frequent small meals (to avoid bloating sensation).
> 3. Increase calories to 1500 to 3000 depending on height and age (consult with nutrition service).
> 4. Add, as necessary, vitamin and mineral supplements.
> 5. In severe cases, total parenteral nutrition must be used (starting at 800 to 1200 kcal/day).

From Goldberg RJ (ed): *Practical guide to the care of the psychiatric patient,* ed 2, St Louis, 1998, Mosby.

BASIC INFORMATION

■ DEFINITION
Anthrax is an acute infectious disease caused by the spore-forming bacterium *Bacillis anthracis*.

ICD-9CM CODES
0.22.0 Cutaneous anthrax
0.22.1 Inhalation anthrax
0.22.2 Gastrointestinal anthrax
022.3 Sepsis from anthrax

■ EPIDEMIOLOGY & DEMOGRAPHICS
- Anthrax most commonly occurs in hoofed animals and can only incidentally infect humans who come in contact with infected animals or animal products. Between 20,000 and 100,000 cases of cutaneous anthrax occur worldwide annually. In the U.S. the annual incidence was about 130 cases before 2001.
- Until the recent bioterrorism attack in 2001, most cases of anthrax occurred in industrial environments (contaminated raw materials used in manufacturing process) or in agriculture.
- In 2001 there were more than 20 confirmed cases of anthrax resulting from bioterrorism, most of which

were associated with handling of contaminated mail. Inhalation anthrax is the most lethal form of anthrax and results from inspiration of 8000-50,000 spores of *Bacillus anthracis*. Before 2001 there had not been a case of inhalation anthrax in the U.S. for 20 years.
- Direct person-to-person spread of anthrax is extremely unlikely, if it occurs at all; therefore, there is no need to immunize or treat contacts of persons ill with anthrax, such as household contacts, friends, or co-workers, unless they also were exposed to the same source of infection.

■ PHYSICAL FINDINGS & CLINICAL PRESENTATION
Symptoms of disease vary depending on how the disease was contracted, but usually occur within 7 days after exposure. The serious forms of human anthrax are inhalation anthrax, cutaneous anthrax, and intestinal anthrax.
- **Inhalation anthrax** begins with a brief prodrome resembling a viral respiratory illness followed by development of hypoxia and dyspnea, with radiographic evidence of mediastinal widening. Host factors, dose of exposure, and chemoprophylaxis may affect the duration of the incubation period. Initial symptoms include mild fever, muscle aches,

and malaise and may progress to respiratory failure and shock; meningitis often develops.
- **Cutaneous anthrax** is characterized by a skin lesion evolving from a papule, through a vesicular stage, to a depressed black eschar (Fig. 1-32, *A*). The incubation period ranges from 1-12 days. The lesion is usually painless, but patients also may have fever, malaise, headache, and regional lymphadenopathy. The eschar dries and falls off in 1-2 wk with little scarring.
- **Gastrointestinal anthrax** is characterized by severe abdominal pain followed by fever and signs of septicemia. Bloody diarrhea and signs of acute abdomen may occur. This form of anthrax usually follows after eating raw or undercooked contaminated meat and can have an incubation period of 1-7 days. Gastric ulcers may occur and may be associated with hematemesis. An oropharyngeal and an abdominal form of the disease have been described. Involvement of the pharynx is usually characterized by lesions at the base of the tongue, dysphagia, fever, and regional lymphadenopathy. Lower bowel inflammation typically causes nausea, loss of appetite, and fever followed by abdominal pain, hematemesis, and bloody diarrhea.

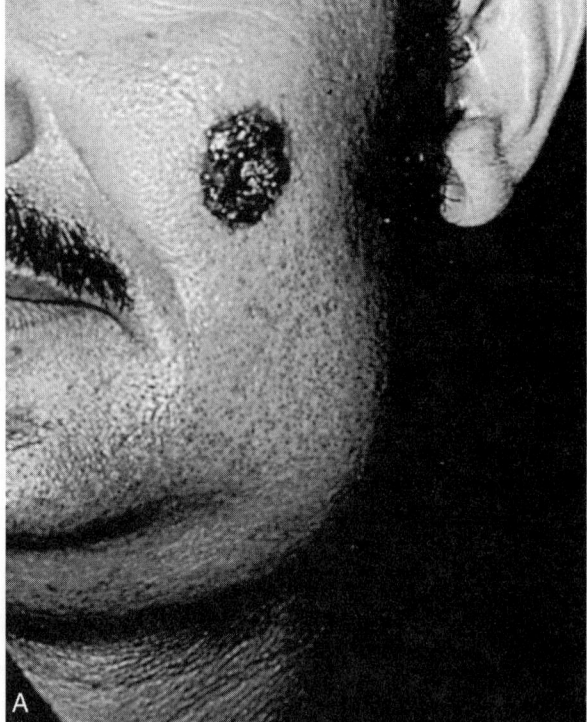
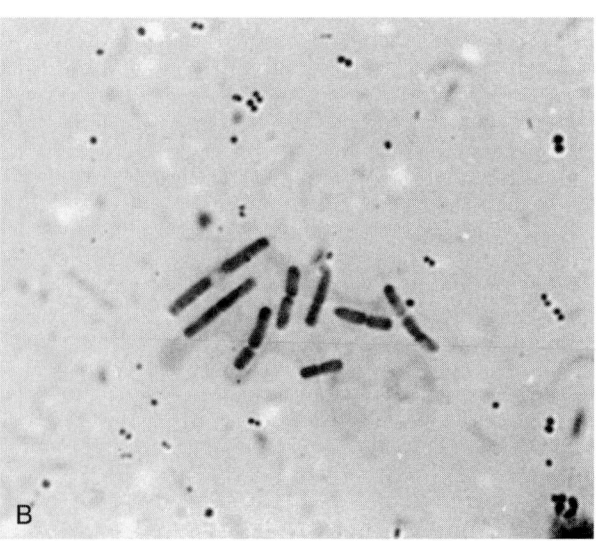

Fig. 1-32 **A,** A shepherd from Morocco was seen with a painless pruritic facial lesion associated with regional lymphadenopathy. **B,** Gram stain of the vesicular fluid revealed characteristic boxcar-shaped encapsulated bacilli. (**A** Courtesy of Professor Jean-Hilaire Saurat, Chief, Dermatology Clinic, Geneva University Hospital, Geneva, Switzerland. **B** From Mandell GL, Bennett JE, Dolin R: *Principles and practice of infectious diseases,* ed 5, New York, 2000, Churchill Livingstone.)

■ ETIOLOGY

The disease is caused by *Bacillus anthracis,* a gram-positive, spore-forming bacillus. It is aerobic, nonmotile, non-hemolytic on sheep's blood agar, and grows readily at temperature of 37° C, forming large colonies with irregularly tapered outgrowths (a Medusa's head appearance). In the host it appears as single organisms or chains of two or three bacilli (Fig. 1-32, *B*).

🔬 DIAGNOSIS

■ DIFFERENTIAL DIAGNOSIS

* Inhalation anthrax must be distinguished from influenza-like illness (ILI) and tularemia. Most cases of ILI are associated with nasal congestion and rhinorrhea, which are unusual in inhalation anthrax. Additional distinguishing factors are the usual absence of abnormal chest x-ray in ILI (see below).
* Cutaneous anthrax should be distinguished from staphylococcal disease, ecthyma, ecthyma gangrenosum, plague, brown recluse spider bite, and tularemia.
* The differential diagnosis of gastrointestinal anthrax includes viral gastroenteritis, shigellosis, and yersiniosis.

■ WORKUP

* The clinical evaluation of persons with possible inhalation anthrax is described in Fig. 1-33.
* Fig. 1-34 describes the clinical evaluation of persons with possible cutaneous anthrax.

■ LABORATORY TESTS

* Presumptive identification is based on Gram stain of material from skin lesion, CSF, or blood showing encapsulated gram-positive bacilli.
* Confirmatory tests are performed at specialized labs. Virulent strains grow on nutrient agar in the presence of 5% CO_2. Susceptibility to lysis by gamma phage or DFA staining of cell-wall polysaccharide antigen are also useful confirmatory tests.

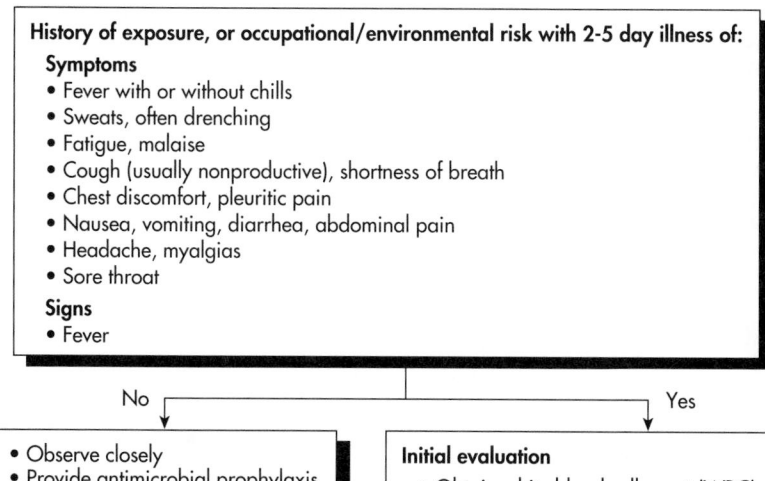

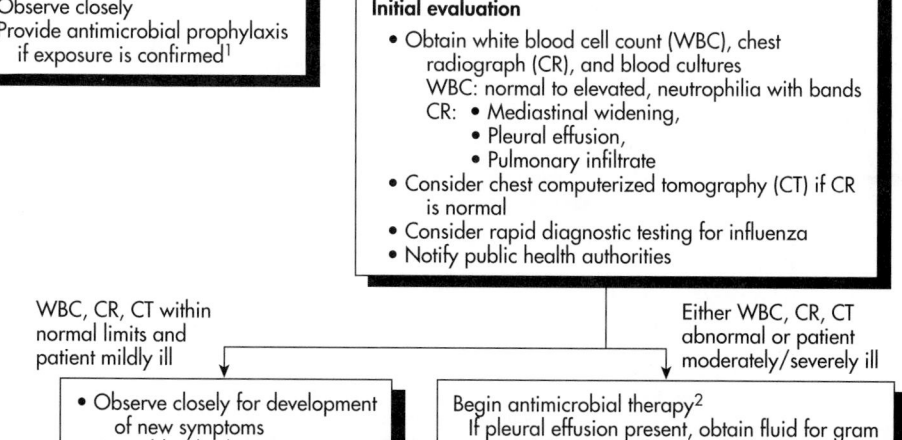

*Available through CDC or LRN. Cell block obtained by centrifugation of pleural fluid.
†Serologic testing available at CDC may be an additional diagnostic technique.

References
1. CDC: Update: investigation of anthrax associated with intentional exposure and interim public health guidelines, *MMWR* 50:889, 2001.
2. CDC: Update: investigation of bioterrorism-related anthrax and interim guidelines for exposure management and antimicrobial therapy, *MMWR* 50:909, 2001.

Fig. 1-33 Clinical evaluation of persons with possible inhalational anthrax.

- Nasal swab culture to determine inhalation exposure are of limited diagnostic value. A negative result does not exclude the possibility of exposure. It may be used by public health officials to assist in epidemiologic investigations of exposed persons to evaluate the dispersion of spores.
- Serologic testing by enzyme-linked immunosorbent assay (ELISA) can confirm the diagnosis.
- A skin test (Anthracin Test) that detects anthrax cell-mediated immunity is also available in specialized labs.

■ IMAGING STUDIES
Chest x-ray usually reveals mediastinal widening. Additional findings include infiltrates and pleural effusion.

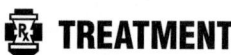 **TREATMENT**

■ NONPHARMACOLOGIC THERAPY
IV hydration and ventilator support may be necessary in inhalation anthrax

■ ACUTE GENERAL THERAPY
- Table 1-11 describes a treatment protocol for inhalation anthrax.
- The treatment protocol for cutaneous anthrax is described in Table 1-12.
- Initial postexposure prophylaxis therapy in adults is with ciprofloxacin, 500 mg PO bid or doxycycline 100 mg bid. The total duration of treatment is 60 days.

■ CHRONIC Rx
None

■ DISPOSITION
- Case fatality estimates for inhalation anthrax are extremely high (>90%).
- The case fatality rate for cutaneous anthrax is 20% without and <1% with antibiotic treatment.
- The case fatality rate for gastrointestinal anthrax is estimated to be 25% to 60%.

■ REFERRAL
Consultation with an infectious disease specialist is recommended in all cases of anthrax. Local state authorities should also be notified of suspected cases of anthrax.

☼ PEARLS & CONSIDERATIONS

■ COMMENTS
Postexposure prophylaxis: If the exposure to *Bacillus anthracis* is confirmed and anthrax vaccine is available, 3 doses of the vaccine should be given at 0, 2, and 4 wk, and antibiotics should be continued throughout the 4-wk period. If vaccine is not available, antibiotics should be continued for 60 days.

REFERENCES
Interim guidelines for investigation of and response to *Bacillus anthracis* exposures, *MMWR* 50:987, 2001.
Post-exposure anthrax prophylaxis, *Med Lett Drugs Ther* 43:91, 2001.
Swartz MN: Recognition and management of anthrax: an update, *N Engl J Med* 345:1621, 2001.
Author: **Fred F. Ferri, M.D.**

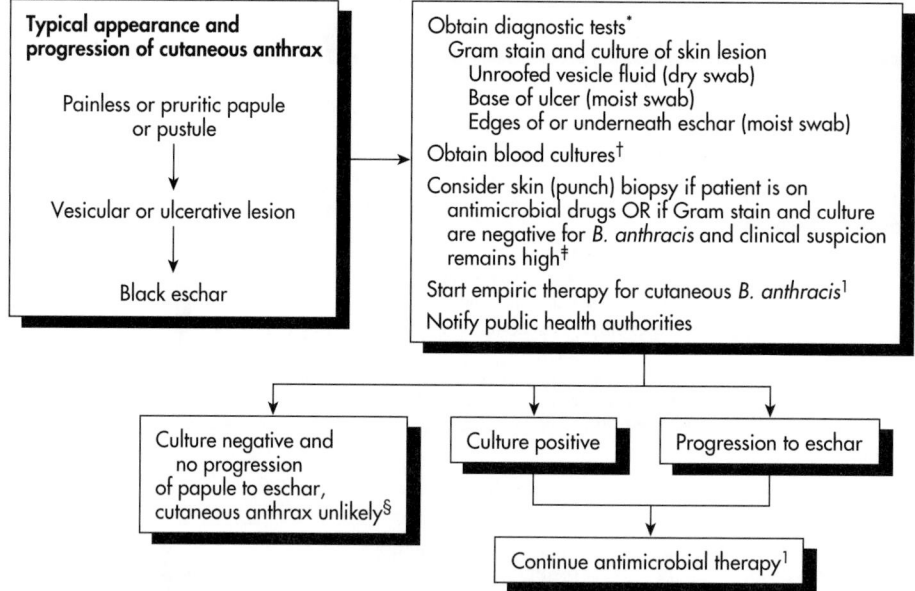

References
1. CDC: Update: investigation of bioterrorism-related anthrax and interim guidelines for exposure management and antimicrobial therapy, *MMWR* 50:909, 2001.
2. CDC: Update: investigation of anthrax associated with intentional exposure and interim public health guidelines, *MMWR*, 50:899, 2001.

*Serologic testing available at CDC may be an additional diagnostic technique for confirmation of cases of cutaneous anthrax.
†If blood cultures are positive for *B. anthracis*, treat with antimicrobials as for inhalational anthrax.[1]
‡Punch biopsy should be submitted in formalin to CDC. Polymerase chain reaction can also be done on formalin-fixed specimen. Gram stain and culture are often negative for *B. anthracis* after initiation of antimicrobials.
§Continued antimicrobial prophylaxis for inhalational anthrax for 60 days if aerosol exposure to *B. anthracis* is known or suspected.[2]

Fig. 1-34 Clinical evaluation of persons with possible cutaneous anthrax.

TABLE 1-11 Inhalational Anthrax Treatment Protocol[a,b]

CATEGORY	INITIAL THERAPY (INTRAVENOUS)[c,d]	DURATION
Adults	Ciprofloxacin 400 mg every 12 hr[a] **or** Doxycycline 100 mg every 12 hr[f] **and** One or two additional antimicrobials[d]	IV treatment initially.[e] Switch to oral antimicrobial therapy when clinically appropriate: Ciprofloxacin 500 mg PO bid **or** Doxycycline 100 mg PO bid Continue for 60 days (IV and PO combined)[g]
Children	Ciprofloxacin 10-15 mg/kg every 12 hr[h,i] **or** Doxycycline[f,j]: >8 yr and >45 kg: 100 mg every 12 hr >8 yr and ≤45 kg: 2.2 mg/kg every 12 hr ≤8 yr: 2.2 mg/kg every 12 hr **and** One or two additional antimicrobials[d]	IV treatment initially.[e] Switch to oral antimicrobial therapy when clinically appropriate: Ciprofloxacin 10-15 mg/kg PO every 12 hr[i] **or** Doxycycline[j]: >8 yr and >45 kg: 100 mg PO bid >8 yr and ≤45 kg: 2.2 mg/kg PO bid ≤8 yr: 2.2 mg/kg PO bid Continue for 60 days (IV and PO combined)[g]
Pregnant women[k]	Same for nonpregnant adults (the high death rate from the infection outweighs the risk posed by the antimicrobial agent)	IV treatment initially. Switch to oral antimicrobial therapy when clinically appropriate.[b] Oral therapy regimens same for nonpregnant adults
Immunocompromised persons	Same for nonimmunocompromised persons and children	Same for nonimmunocompromised persons and children

MMRW 5:987, 2001.

[a]For gastrointestinal and oropharyngeal anthrax, use regimens recommended for inhalational anthrax.
[b]Ciprofloxacin or doxycycline should be considered an essential part of first-line therapy for inhalational anthrax.
[c]Steroids may be considered as an adjunct therapy for patients with severe edema and for meningitis based on experience with bacterial meningitis of other etiologies.
[d]Other agents with in vitro activity include rifampin, vancomycin, penicillin, ampicillin, chloramphenicol, imipenem, clindamycin, and clarithromycin. Because of concerns of constitutive and inducible beta-lactamases in *Bacillus anthracis,* penicillin and ampicillin should not be used alone. Consultation with an infectious disease specialist is advised.
[e]Initial therapy may be altered based on clinical course of the patient; one or two antimicrobial agents (e.g., ciprofloxacin or doxycycline) may be adequate as the patient improves.
[f]If meningitis is suspected, doxycycline may be less optimal because of poor central nervous system penetration.
[g]Because of the potential persistence of spores after an aerosol exposure, antimicrobial therapy should be continued for 60 days.
[h]If intravenous ciprofloxacin is not available, oral ciprofloxacin may be acceptable because it is rapidly and well absorbed from the gastrointestinal tract with no substantial loss by first-pass metabolism. Maximum serum concentrations are attained 1-2 hours after oral dosing but may not be achieved if vomiting or ileus are present.
[i]In children, ciprofloxacin dosage should not exceed 1 g/day.
[j]The American Academy of Pediatrics recommends treatment of young children with tetracyclines for serious infections (e.g., Rocky Mountain spotted fever).
[k]Although tetracyclines are not recommended during pregnancy, their use may be indicated for life-threatening illness. Adverse effects on developing teeth and bones are dose related; therefore, doxycycline might be used for a short time (7-14 days) before 6 months of gestation.

TABLE 1-12 Cutaneous Anthrax Treatment Protocol*

CATEGORY	INITIAL THERAPY (ORAL)†	DURATION
Adults*	Ciprofloxacin 500 mg bid **or** Doxycycline 100 mg bid	60 days‡
Children*	Ciprofloxacin 10–15 mg/kg every 12 hr (not to exceed 1 g/day)† **or** Doxycycline§: >8 yr and >45 kg: 100 mg every 12 hr >8 yr and ≤45 kg: 2.2 mg/kg every 12 hr ≤8 yr: 2.2 mg/kg every 12 hr	60 days‡
Pregnant women*¶	Ciprofloxacin 500 mg bid **or** Doxycycline 100 mg bid	60 days‡
Immunocompromised persons*	Same for nonimmunocompromised persons and children	60 days‡

MMRW 5:987, 2001.

*Cutaneous anthrax with signs of systemic involvement, extensive edema, or lesions on the head or neck require intravenous therapy, and a multidrug approach is recommended.
†Ciprofloxacin or doxycycline should be considered first-line therapy. Amoxicillin 500 mg PO tid for adults or 80 mg/kg/day divided every 8 hours for children is an option for completion of therapy after clinical improvement. Oral amoxicillin dose is based on the need to achieve appropriate minimum inhibitory concentration levels.
‡Previous guidelines have suggested treating cutaneous anthrax for 7-10 days, but 60 days is recommended in the setting of this attack, given the likelihood of exposure to aerosolized *B. anthracis.*
§The American Academy of Pediatrics recommends treatment of young children with tetracyclines for serious infections (e.g., Rocky Mountain spotted fever).
¶Although tetracyclines or ciprofloxacin are not recommended during pregnancy, their use may be indicated for life-threatening illness. Adverse effects on developing teeth and bones are dose related; therefore, doxycycline might be used for a short time (7-14 days) before 6 months of gestation.

BASIC INFORMATION

■ DEFINITION
The antiphospholipid antibody syndrome (APS) is characterized by antibodies directed against either phospholipids or proteins bound to anionic phospholipids. The syndrome is referred to as primary APS when it occurs alone and as secondary APS when in association with SLE and other rheumatic disorders (Fig. 1-35). APS can affect all organ systems and includes venous and arterial thrombosis, recurrent fetal losses, and thrombocytopenia.
Four types of antiphospholipid antibodies have been characterized:
- False-positive serologic tests for syphilis
- Lupus anticoagulants
- Anticardiolipin antibodies
- Anti-β2 glycoprotein-1 antibodies

■ ICD-9CM CODES
795.79 Antiphospholipid antibody syndrome

■ EPIDEMIOLOGY & DEMOGRAPHICS
- Some APS-positive families exist, and HLA studies have suggested associations with HLA DR7, DR4, and Dqw7 plus Drw53.
- Other risk factors: underlying SLE and collagen-vascular diseases; other autoimmune disorders including rheumatoid arthritis, Sjögren's syndrome, Behçet's syndrome, and ITP; drug-induced; and AIDS.
- Most individuals are otherwise healthy and have no underlying medical condition.
- Several studies assessing presence of aPL in patients with cardiovascular and cerebrovascular disease have found a higher than expected prevalence of antibody.

■ PHYSICAL FINDINGS & CLINICAL PRESENTATION (BOX 1-6)
Associated conditions and effects on various systems of APS include:
- **Neurology:** stroke, TIA, migraine, multiinfarct dementia, epilepsy, chorea, movement disorders, transverse myelopathy, dysarthria
- **Rheumatology:** SLE, DLE, subacute cutaneous (Ro-positive) LE, Sjögren's syndrome; rare in RA and inflammatory vasculitides
- **Cardiology:** pulmonary hypertension, valvular disease (especially mitral valve involvement), intracardiac thrombosis (can mimic culture negative bacterial endocarditis), CAD, MI
- **Nephrology:** renal vein thrombosis, glomerulosclerosis secondary to glomerular thrombosis, ARF, hypertension (malignant and nonmalignant), intrarenal vascular lesions, thrombotic microangiopathy

---

BOX 1-6   Clinical Manifestations of the Antiphospholipid Antibody Syndrome

Common
Venous thrombosis
Arterial thrombosis
Stroke
Extremity gangrene
Visceral infarction
Recurrent fetal loss
Thrombocytopenia
Livedo reticularis

Uncommon
Coombs'-positive hemolysis
Valvular heart disease
Chorea
Nonstroke ischemia syndrome
Transverse myelopathy

From Andreoli TE (ed): *Cecil essentials of medicine,* ed 4, Philadelphia, 1997, WB Saunders.

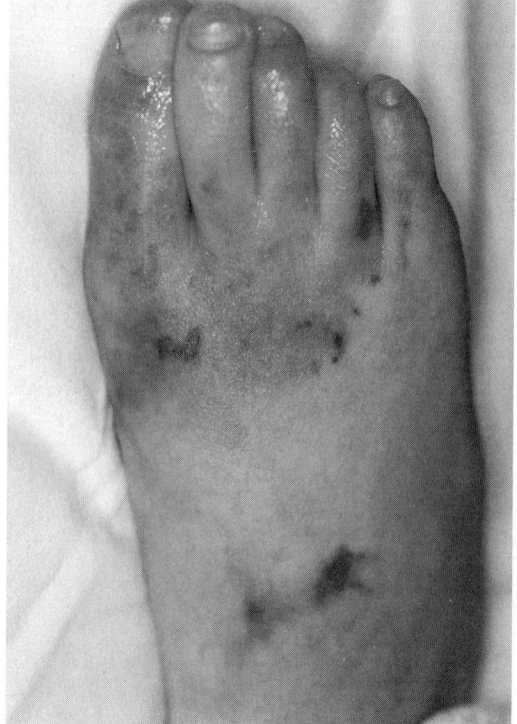

Fig. 1-35 A 12-year-old girl with systemic lupus erythematosus and antiphospholipid antibodies with painful cutaneous vasculitis of the right foot. Arterial thrombosis documented by angiography resulted in cyanosis of the large toe. Symptoms resolved with treatment with heparin and corticosteroids. (From Behrman RE [ed]: *Nelson textbook of pediatrics,* ed 16, Philadelphia, 2000, WB Saunders.)

- **Endocrinology:** Addison's disease secondary to adrenal thrombosis, "autoimmune Addison's" may be secondary to thrombosis
- **Gastroenterology:** gut ischemia, hepatic vein thrombosis, Budd-Chiari syndrome (second most common cause of BCS)
- **Dermatology:** livedo reticularis, recurrent skin ulcers, skin nodules
- **Hematology:** thrombocytopenia, autoimmune hemolytic anemia
- **Obstetrics:** recurrent spontaneous abortion (secondary to placental vessel thrombosis and ischemia)
- **Critical care:** acute multisystem organ failure: thrombocytopenia, ARDS, jaundice, death; "catastrophic antiphospholipid syndrome" with widespread multiorgan thrombosis
- **Surgical:** no large studies on risk of postoperative thrombosis in aPL-positive individuals; some evidence that orthopedic patients may have increased risk of avascular necrosis of femoral head

■ ETIOLOGY

- Antibodies to phospholipids reacting with negatively charged phospholipids
- Range of possible mechanisms of thrombosis includes: effects of aPL on platelet membranes, endothelial cells, and clotting components such as prothrombin, protein C or S
- Recently shown that prephospholipids are not immunogenic and that a binding protein (β_2-glycoprotein I) may be the key immunogen in the APS

🔬 DIAGNOSIS

■ DIFFERENTIAL DIAGNOSIS

- Other hypercoagulable states (inherited or acquired)
- Inherited: ATIII/protein C, S deficiencies
- Acquired: heparin-induced thrombopathy, myeloproliferative syndromes, cancer

■ WORKUP

History: hypercoagulability patient and family
- Criteria from an international consensus conference are at least one of the following clinical criteria **and** at least one of the following laboratory criteria:
  Clinical: Either one or more episodes of venous, arterial, or small vessel thrombosis, and/or morbidity with pregnancy.
  Laboratory: The presence of IgG and/or IgM anticardiolipin antibody and/or lupus anticoagulant activity (no standardized assay; must use Russell viper venom test), found on two or more occasions, at least 6 wk apart.

■ LABORATORY TESTS

Laboratory testing indicated in:
- Patient with underlying SLE or collagen-vascular disease with thrombosis
- Patient with recurrent, familial, or juvenile DVT or thrombosis in an unusual location (mesenteric or cerebral)
- Possibly in patients with lupus or lupuslike disorders in high-risk situations, e.g., surgery, prolonged immobilization, pregnancy
Abnormal tests include:
- Positive test for syphilis (RPR/VDRL), "false-positive"
- Positive lupus anticoagulant will cause prolongation of apTT and Russell viper venom time
- IgG anticardiolipin (ELISA for anticardiolipin is most sensitive and specific test [>80%])
- Presence of anti β_2-glycoprotein I antibody

■ PROGNOSIS

Limited data on natural history in untreated patients.

💊 TREATMENT

■ ACUTE GENERAL Rx

- Anticoagulant agents: heparin, warfarin

Prophylaxis:
- Positive aPL and major thrombotic events or recurrent thrombotic events: lifelong warfarin treatment, INR 3-4: Aspirin alone appears to be of no benefit for the thrombotic manifestations of APS. The addition of aspirin or dipyridamole to warfarin may help prevent recurrent arterial thrombosis.
Asymptomatic with abnormal laboratory results, no previous thrombosis:
- Questionable whether ASA (81 mg) is effective
- No routine prophylaxis
- Antithrombotic prophylaxis for major surgery, prolonged immobilization, and pregnancy
Pregnant women:
- Positive aPL antibodies, no history of nonplacental thrombotic event (e.g., DVT) or positive aPL antibodies and history of ≥2 spontaneous abortions: ASA, 81 mg at conception and SQ heparin, 10,000 IU q12h to midinterval PTT.
- Positive aPL antibodies, diagnosis of APS and history of nonplacental thrombotic event (e.g., DVT): ASA, 81 mg and heparin to PTT of 1.5 to 2 × control value
- In pregnancy warfarin should not be used; low-dose subcutaneous heparin and aspirin are effective and safe; IVIG and prednisone have also been used with success if aspirin and heparin fail.

■ CHRONIC Rx

Cerebral features of lupus may be more related to thrombosis than inflammation, may respond better to anticoagulants than immunosuppression.

REFERENCES

Bick RL: Syndromes of thrombosis and hypercoagulability: congenital and acquired causes of thrombosis, *Med Clin North Am* 82(3):409, 1998.

McCrae KR: Antiphospholipid antibody associated thrombosis: a consensus for treatment? *Lupus* 5:560, 1996.

Petri M: Pathogenesis and treatment of the antiphospholipid antibody syndrome, *Med Clin North Am* 81:151, 1997.

Wilson WA et al: International consensus statement on preliminary classification criteria for definite antiphospholipid syndrome: report of an international workshop, *Arthritis Rheum* 42:1309, 1999.

Author: **Rebecca S. Brienza, M.D., M.P.H.**

BASIC INFORMATION

■ DEFINITION
Anxiety may present as a symptom in a wide range of psychiatric and medical conditions. Generalized anxiety disorder (GAD) is a condition in which the individual experiences excessive anxiety, fear, and worry for most of the time, continuously for at least 6 mo. The subjective anxiety must be accompanied by at least three somatic symptoms (e.g., restlessness, irritability, sleep disturbance, muscle tension, difficulty concentrating, or fatigability).

■ SYNONYMS
Anxiety neurosis
Chronic anxiety
GAD

ICD-9CM CODES
F41.1 (DSM-IV Code 300.02)

■ EPIDEMIOLOGY & DEMOGRAPHICS
INCIDENCE (IN U.S.): 31% in 1 yr
PREVALENCE (IN U.S.):
- In general population: 4.1% to 6.6% lifetime
- In primary care setting: 2.9% (It is the most common anxiety disorder in this setting.)
PREDOMINANT SEX: Females are more frequently affected (2:1 ratio), but they present for treatment less frequently (3:2 female:male).
PREDOMINANT AGE:
- 30% of patients report onset of symptoms before age 11 yr.
- 50% of patients have onset before age 18 yr.
PEAK INCIDENCE: Chronic condition with onset in early life
GENETICS: Concordance rates in dizygotic twins and monozygotic twins are not different (0% to 5%), but detailed analysis of 1033 female twin pairs finds that heredity contributes about 30% of the factors that may cause GAD.

■ PHYSICAL FINDINGS & CLINICAL PRESENTATION
- Report of being "anxious" all of their lives
- Excessive worry, usually regarding family, finances, work, or health
- Sleep disturbance, particularly early insomnia
- Muscle tension (typically in the muscles of neck and shoulders)
- Headaches (muscle tension)
- Difficulty concentrating
- Day form of fatigue
- Gastrointestinal symptoms compatible with IBD (one third of patients)
- Physical consequences of anxiety are the driving force for patients seeking medical attention
- Comorbid psychiatric illness (e.g., dysthymia or major depression) and substance abuse (e.g., alcohol abuse) are frequent

■ ETIOLOGY
- There is no clear etiology.
- Several hypotheses centering on neurotransmitter (catecholamines, indolamines) and developmental psychology are used as framework for treatment recommendations.

DIAGNOSIS

■ DIFFERENTIAL DIAGNOSIS
- Wide range of psychiatric and medical conditions; however, for a diagnosis of GAD to be made a person must experience anxiety with coexisting physical symptoms the majority of the time continuously for at least 6 mo
- Cardiovascular and pulmonary disease
- Hyperthyroidism
- Parkinson's disease
- Myasthenia gravis
- Consequence of recreational drug use (e.g., cocaine, amphetamine, and PCP) or withdrawal (e.g., alcohol or benzodiazepines)

■ WORKUP
- History: required for diagnosis
- Physical examination: confirm the patient's physical complaints
- Exclusion of organic basis for the complaints possibly requiring additional workup

TREATMENT

■ NONPHARMACOLOGIC THERAPY
- Cognitive-behavioral therapy
- Relaxation training
- Biofeedback
- Psychodynamic psychotherapy
NOTE: Studies directly comparing medications with psychotherapy are not available, but the general clinical impression is that the psychotherapies are probably superior to pharmacotherapies.

■ ACUTE GENERAL Rx
- Acute treatment is rarely indicated because GAD is a chronic condition.
- Occasionally, patients are in acute distress, requiring physician to respond quickly; benzodiazepines are given under these conditions as drug of choice for both daytime anxiety and initial insomnia.

■ CHRONIC Rx
- Benzodiazepines provide long-term symptom control with only occasional problems with tolerance or abuse; however, rate of relapse after discontinuation of benzodiazepines may be twice the rate after discontinuation of the available nonbenzodiazepine anxiolytic buspirone.
- SSRIs and venlafaxine are also effective in generalized anxiety disorders.
- Buspirone is effective without any potential for tolerance or abuse.
- Tricyclic antidepressants are useful if an element of comorbid depression exists.
- Sedating antidepressants are also useful in ameliorating initial insomnia.
- Trazodone and nefazodone possibly have unique benefits for these patients.

■ DISPOSITION
- This condition is chronic with periodic exacerbations.
- Treatment is given to provide a significant degree of improvement, but symptoms and dysfunction may persist.

■ REFERRAL
- If the symptoms are refractory to treatment
- If the case is complicated with a comorbid psychiatric condition
- If treatment response is suboptimal with residual dysfunction

Author: **Rif S. El-Mallakh, M.D.**

BASIC INFORMATION

■ DEFINITION
Aortic dissection occurs when an intimal tear allows blood to dissect between medial layers of the aorta.

ICD-9CM CODES
441.00 Aortic dissection
444.01 Aortic dissection, thoracic

■ SYNONYMS
Dissecting aortic aneurysm, unspecified site

■ EPIDEMIOLOGY & DEMOGRAPHICS
PREDOMINANT SEX: Males > females
PEAK INCIDENCE: Sixth and seventh decades
RISK FACTORS: Hypertension

■ CLASSIFICATION
- Stanford type A (includes DeBakey types I and II) involves ascending aorta (Fig. 1-36)
- Stanford type B (DeBakey type III) limited to descending aorta

■ PHYSICAL FINDINGS & CLINICAL PRESENTATION
- Abrupt onset of severe chest pain
- May present with back and/or abdominal pain
- 12% of patients present with syncope
- Hypertension or hypotension
- Unequal or absent pulses
- Murmur of aortic insufficiency possible
- Neurologic abnormalities caused by carotid obstruction (hemiplegia) or spinal cord ischemia (paraplegia)
- Mass effect can cause Horner's syndrome, superior vena cava syndrome, hoarseness, dysphagia, airway compromise
- Cardiac tamponade caused by dissection into pericardial sac

■ ETIOLOGY
- Hypertension
- Cystic medial necrosis
- Marfan's syndrome
- Congenital aortic valve abnormalities
- Previous cardiac surgery

DIAGNOSIS

■ DIFFERENTIAL DIAGNOSIS
- Acute MI
- Aortic insufficiency
- Nondissecting aortic aneurysm
- Musculoskeletal pain
- Pericarditis
- Angina
- Cholecystitis

■ WORKUP
Physical examination and imaging

■ LABORATORY TESTS
ECG may suggest LVH or pericardial effusion.

■ IMAGING STUDIES
- Chest x-ray may show widened mediastinum (62%), displacement of aortic intimal calcium
- Transesophageal echocardiography, sensitivity 97% to 100%, can detect aortic insufficiency and pericardial effusion; study of choice in many centers
- MRI, sensitivity 90% to 100%, difficult for unstable intubated patients
- CT, sensitivity 83% to 100%, involves IV contrast, cannot detect aortic insufficiency (Fig. 1-37)
- Aortography, sensitivity 81% to 91%, involves IV contrast, allows visualization of coronary arteries

TREATMENT

■ ACUTE GENERAL Rx
- Admit to ICU for hemodynamic monitoring.
- Decrease contractility and BP using β-blocker IV; labetalol 20 mg initially, then 40 to 80 mg q10min, titrate to systolic BP 120 mm Hg and pulse 60.
- Decrease BP using sodium nitroprusside by IV infusion pump 0.3 to 10 mg/kg/min, titrate to systolic BP 120 mm Hg.
- Type A (proximal) dissections usually require emergent or urgent surgery.
- Percutaneous fenestration and/or stent placement for selected patients

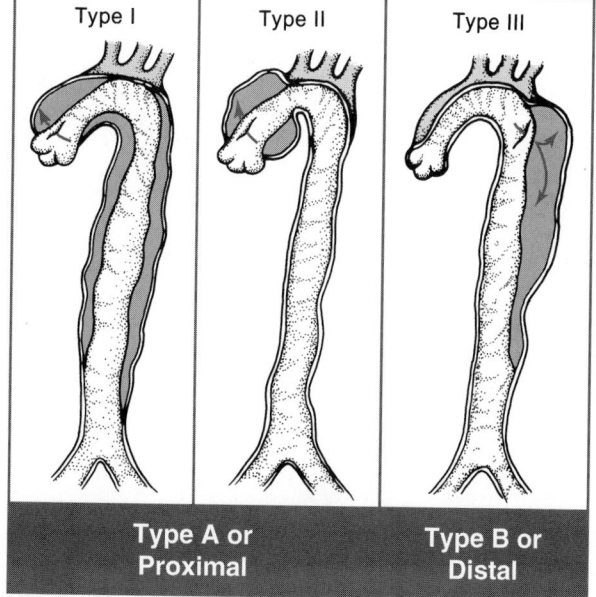

Fig. 1-36   Classification systems for aortic dissection. (From Isselbacher EM, Eagle KA, DeSanctis RW: Diseases of the aorta. In Braunwald E [ed]: *Heart disease: a textbook of cardiovascular medicine,* ed 5, Philadelphia, 1997, WB Saunders.)

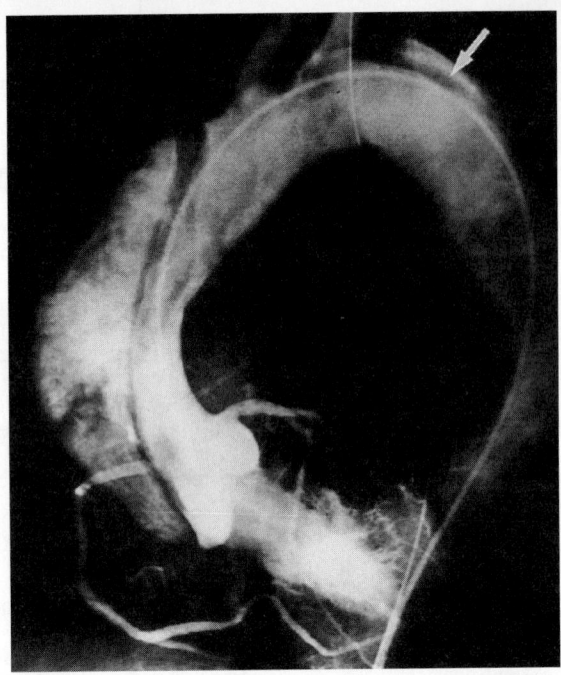

Fig. 1-37   Aortic dissection. An angiogram demonstrates a type A dissection beginning in the aortic root and causing severe aortic regurgitation. Both coronary arteries fill from the true channel. A separate retrograde dissection entry is noted distal to the origin of the left subclavian artery, causing partial occlusion of this vessel. (From Miller SW: *Cardiac radiology: the requisites,* St Louis, 1996, Mosby.)

- Type B (distal) dissection, if stable, can be treated medically and monitored for signs of propagation, branch compromise, continued pain, or impending rupture.

■ DISPOSITION
- Untreated, mortality is 85% within 2 wk.
- Type A dissections surgically treated, mortality is 15% to 20%.
- Type B dissections treated medically, mortality is 15% to 20%.

■ REFERRAL
For ICU management and surgery

REFERENCE
Hagan PG et al: The international registry of acute aortic dissection: new insights into an old disease, *JAMA* 283:897, 2000.
Author: **Mark J. Fagan, M.D.**

BASIC INFORMATION

■ DEFINITION

Aortic regurgitation is retrograde blood flow into the left ventricle from the aorta secondary to incompetent aortic valve.

■ SYNONYMS

Aortic insufficiency
AI
AR

■ ICD-9CM CODES

424.1 Aortic valve disorders

■ EPIDEMIOLOGY & DEMOGRAPHICS

- The most common cause of isolated severe aortic regurgitation is aortic root dilation.
- Infectious endocarditis is the most frequent cause of acute aortic regurgitation.

■ PHYSICAL FINDINGS & CLINICAL PRESENTATION

- Widened pulse pressure (markedly increased systolic blood pressure, decreased diastolic blood pressure) is present.
- Bounding pulses, head "bobbing" with each systole (de Musset's sign) are present; "water hammer" or collapsing pulse (Corrigan's pulse) can be palpated at the wrist or on the femoral arteries ("pistol shot" femorals) and is caused by rapid rise and sudden collapse of the arterial pressure during late systole; capillary pulsations (Quincke's pulse) may occur at the base of the nail beds.
- A to-and-fro "double Duroziez" murmur may be heard over femoral arteries with slight compression.
- Popliteal systolic pressure is increased over brachial systolic pressure ≥40 mm Hg (Hill's sign).
- Cardiac auscultation reveals:
  1. Displacement of cardiac impulse downward and to the patient's left
  2. S_3 heard over the apex
  3. Decrescendo, blowing diastolic murmur heard along left sternal border
  4. Low-pitched apical diastolic rumble (Austin-Flint murmur) caused by contrast of the aortic regurgitant jet with the left ventricular wall
  5. Early systolic apical ejection murmur

■ ETIOLOGY

- Infective endocarditis
- Rheumatic fibrosis
- Trauma with valvular rupture
- Congenital bicuspid aortic valve

- Myxomatous degeneration
- Syphilitic aortitis
- Rheumatic spondylitis
- SLE
- Aortic dissection
- Fenfluramine, dexfenfluramine
- Takayasu's arteritis, granulomatous arteritis

DIAGNOSIS

■ DIFFERENTIAL DIAGNOSIS

- Patent ductus arteriosus, pulmonary regurgitation, and other valvular abnormalities
- The differential diagnosis of cardiac murmurs is described in Table 2-35

■ WORKUP

- Echocardiogram, chest x-ray, ECG, and cardiac catheterization (selected patients)
- Medical history and physical examination focused on the following clinical manifestations:
  1. Dyspnea on exertion
  2. Syncope
  3. Chest pain
  4. CHF

■ IMAGING STUDIES

- Chest x-ray study
  1. Left ventricular hypertrophy (chronic aortic regurgitation)
  2. Aortic dilation
  3. Normal cardiac silhouette with pulmonary edema: possible in patients with acute aortic regurgitation
- ECG: left ventricular hypertrophy
- Echocardiography: coarse diastolic fluttering of the anterior mitral leaflet; LVH in patients with chronic aortic regurgitation
- Cardiac catheterization: assesses degree of left ventricular dysfunction, confirms the presence of a wide pulse pressure, assesses surgical risk, and determines if there is coexistent coronary artery disease

TREATMENT

■ NONPHARMACOLOGIC THERAPY

- Avoidance of competitive sports and strenuous activity
- Salt restriction

■ ACUTE GENERAL Rx

MEDICAL:

- Digitalis, diuretics, ACE inhibitors, and sodium restriction for CHF; nitroprusside in patients with acute aortic regurgitation

- Long-term vasodilator therapy with ACE inhibitors or nifedipine for reducing or delaying the need for aortic valve replacement in asymptomatic patients with severe aortic regurgitation and normal left ventricular function
- Bacterial endocarditis prophylaxis for surgical and dental procedures (see Boxes 5-1 to 5-3 and Tables 5-25 and 5-26)

SURGICAL: Reserved for:

- Symptomatic patients with chronic aortic regurgitation despite optimal medical therapy
- Patients with acute aortic regurgitation (i.e., infective endocarditis) producing left ventricular failure
- Evidence of systolic failure:
  1. Echocardiographic fractional shortening <25%
  2. Echocardiographic and diastolic dimension >55 mm
  3. Angiographic ejection fraction <50% or end-systolic volume index (ESVI) >60 ml/m^2
- Evidence of diastolic failure:
  1. Pulmonary pressure >45 mm Hg systolic
  2. Left ventricular end-diastolic pressure (LVEDP) >15 mm Hg at catheterization
  3. Pulmonary hypertension detected on examination
- In general, the "55 rule" has been used to determine the timing of surgery: surgery should be performed before EF <55% or end-systolic dimension >55 mm.

■ DISPOSITION

Variable depending on underlying condition and left ventricular function; aortic regurgitation (except when secondary to infective endocarditis) is generally well tolerated, and patients remain asymptomatic for years.

■ REFERRAL

Surgical referral (see "Acute General Rx" for indications)

PEARLS & CONSIDERATIONS

■ COMMENTS

The operative mortality rate for aortic regurgitation is 3% to 5%.

REFERENCE

Bonow RO et al: Guidelines for the management of patients with valvular heart disease: executive summary. A report of the American College of Cardiology/AHA Task Force on practice guidelines, *Circulation* 98:1949, 1998.

Author: **Fred F. Ferri, M.D.**

BASIC INFORMATION

■ DEFINITION

Aortic stenosis is obstruction to systolic left ventricular outflow across the aortic valve. Symptoms appear when the valve orifice decreases to <1 cm^2 (normal orifice is 3 cm^2). The stenosis is considered severe when the orifice is <0.5 cm^2/m^2 or the pressure gradient is 50 mm Hg or higher.

■ SYNONYMS

Aortic valvular stenosis
AS

■ ICD-9CM CODES

424.1 Aortic valvular stenosis

■ EPIDEMIOLOGY & DEMOGRAPHICS

- Aortic stenosis is the most common valve lesion in adults in Western countries.
- Calcific stenosis (most common cause in patients >60 yr old) occurs in 75% of patients.

■ PHYSICAL FINDINGS & CLINICAL PRESENTATION

- Rough, loud systolic diamond-shaped murmur, best heard at base of heart and transmitted into neck vessels; often associated with a thrill or ejection click; may also be heard well at the apex
- Absence or diminished intensity of sound of aortic valve closure (in severe aortic stenosis)
- Late, slow-rising carotid upstroke with decreased amplitude
- Strong apical pulse
- Narrowing of pulse pressure in later stages of aortic stenosis

■ ETIOLOGY

- Rheumatic inflammation of aortic valve
- Progressive stenosis of congenital bicuspid valve
- Idiopathic calcification of the aortic valve
- Congenital (major cause of aortic stenosis in patients <30 yr)

DIAGNOSIS

■ DIFFERENTIAL DIAGNOSIS

- Hypertrophic cardiomyopathy
- Mitral regurgitation
- Ventricular septal defect
- Aortic sclerosis
- The differential diagnosis of cardiac murmurs is described in Table 2-35.

■ WORKUP

- Echocardiography
- Chest x-ray examination, ECG

- Cardiac catheterization in selected patients (see below)
- Medical history focusing on symptoms and potential complications:
  1. Angina
  2. Syncope (particularly with exertion)
  3. CHF
  4. GI bleeding: in patients with associated hemorrhagic telangiectasia (AVM)

■ IMAGING STUDIES

- Chest x-ray examination
  1. Poststenotic dilation of the ascending aorta
  2. Calcification of aortic cusps
  3. Pulmonary congestion (in advanced stages of aortic stenosis)
- ECG:
  1. Left ventricular hypertrophy (found in >80% of patients)
  2. ST-T wave changes
  3. Atrial fibrillation: frequent
- Echocardiography: thickening of the left ventricular wall; if the patient has valvular calcifications, multiple echos may be seen from within the aortic root and there is poor separation of the aortic cusps during systole. Gradient across the valve can be estimated but is less precise than with cardiac catheterization.
- Cardiac catheterization: indicated in symptomatic patients; it confirms the diagnosis and estimates the severity of the disease by measuring the gradient across the valve, allowing calculation of the valve area. It also detects coexisting coronary artery stenosis that may need bypass at the same time as aortic valve replacement.

TREATMENT

■ NONPHARMACOLOGIC THERAPY

- Strenuous activity should be avoided.
- Sodium restriction is needed if CHF is present.

■ ACUTE GENERAL Rx

MEDICAL:
- Diuretics and sodium restriction are needed if CHF is present; digoxin is used only to control rate of atrial fibrillation.
- ACE inhibitors are relatively contraindicated.
- Calcium channel blocker verapamil may be useful only to control rate of atrial fibrillation.
- Antibiotic prophylaxis is necessary for surgical and dental procedures (see Boxes 5-1 to 5-3 and Tables 5-25 and 5-26)

SURGICAL:
- Valve replacement is the treatment of choice in symptomatic patients because the 5-yr mortality rate after onset of symptoms is extremely high, even with optimal medical therapy; valve replacement is indicated if cardiac catheterization establishes a pressure gradient >50 mm Hg and valve area <1 cm^2.
- Balloon aortic valvotomy for adult acquired aortic stenosis is useful only for palliation.

■ DISPOSITION

- 15% to 20% of patients with severe aortic stenosis die before age 20 yr.
- The 5-yr survival rate in adults is 40%.
- The average duration of symptoms before death is as follows: angina, 60 mo; syncope, 36 mo; CHF, 24 mo.
- About 75% of patients with symptomatic aortic stenosis will be dead 3 yr after onset of symptoms unless the aortic valve is replaced.

■ REFERRAL

- Surgical referral for valve replacement in symptomatic patients. However, the presence of moderate or severe valvular calcification, together with a rapid increase in aortic-jet velocity, identifies patients with a very poor prognosis who should be considered for early valve replacement rather than have surgery delayed until symptoms develop.
- Surgical mortality rate for valve replacement is 3% to 5%; however, it varies with patient's age (>8% in patients >75 yr old).

PEARLS & CONSIDERATIONS

■ COMMENTS

- Balloon valvuloplasty is useful in infants and children or poor surgical candidates who do not have calcified valve apparatus; it can be done as an intermediate procedure to stabilize high-risk patients before surgery.
- When performed in adults who have calcified valves, balloon valvuloplasty is useful only for short-term reduction in severity of aortic stenosis when surgery is contraindicated, since restenosis occurs rapidly.

REFERENCES

Bonow RO et al: Guidelines for the management of patients with valvular heart disease: executive summary. A report of the American College of Cardiology/AHA Task Force on practice guidelines, *Circulation* 98:1949, 1998.
Rosenhek R et al: Predictors of outcome in severe, asymptomatic aortic stenosis, *N Engl J Med* 343:611, 2000.
Author: **Fred F. Ferri, M.D.**

BASIC INFORMATION

■ DEFINITION
Appendicitis is the acute inflammation of the appendix.

ICD-9CM CODES
540.9 Appendicitis
540.0 Appendicitis with generalized peritonitis

■ EPIDEMIOLOGY & DEMOGRAPHICS
- Appendicitis occurs in 10% of the population, most commonly between the ages of 10 and 30 yr.
- It is the most common abdominal surgical emergency.
- Incidence of appendicitis has declined over the past 30 yr.
- Male:female ratio is 3:2 until mid-20s; it equalizes after age 30 yr.

■ PHYSICAL FINDINGS & CLINICAL PRESENTATION
- Abdominal pain: initially the pain may be epigastric or periumbilical in nearly 50% of patients; it subsequently localizes to the RLQ within 12 to 18 hr. Pain can be found in back or right flank if appendix is retrocecal or in other abdominal locations if there is malrotation of the appendix.
- Pain with right thigh extension (psoas sign), low-grade fever: temperature may be >38° C if there is appendiceal perforation.
- Pain with internal rotation of the flexed right thigh (obturator sign) is present.
- RLQ pain on palpation of the LLQ (Rovsing's sign): physical examination may reveal right-sided tenderness in patients with pelvic appendix.
- Point of maximum tenderness is in the RLQ (McBurney's point).
- Nausea, vomiting, tachycardia, cutaneous hyperesthesias at the level of T12 can be present.

■ ETIOLOGY
Obstruction of the appendiceal lumen with subsequent vascular congestion, inflammation, and edema; common causes of obstruction are:
- Fecaliths: 30% to 35% of cases (most common in adults)
- Foreign body: 4% (fruit seeds, pinworms, tapeworms, roundworms, calculi)
- Inflammation: 50% to 60% of cases (submucosal lymphoid hyperplasia

[most common etiology in children, teens])
- Neoplasms: 1% (carcinoids, metastatic disease, carcinoma)

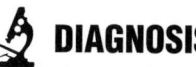

DIAGNOSIS

■ DIFFERENTIAL DIAGNOSIS
- Intestinal: regional cecal enteritis, incarcerated hernia, cecal diverticulitis, intestinal obstruction, perforated ulcer, perforated cecum, Meckel's diverticulitis
- Reproductive: ectopic pregnancy, ovarian cyst, torsion of ovarian cyst, salpingitis, tuboovarian abscess, Mittelschmerz endometriosis, seminal vesiculitis
- Renal: renal and ureteral calculi, neoplasms, pyelonephritis
- Vascular: leaking aortic aneurysm
- Psoas abscess
- Trauma
- Cholecystitis
- Mesenteric adenitis

■ WORKUP
- Patients presenting with RLQ pain, nausea, vomiting, anorexia, and RLQ rebound tenderness should undergo prompt clinical and laboratory evaluation. Imaging studies are generally not necessary in typical appendicitis. They are useful when the diagnosis is uncertain.
- A clinical algorithm for the evaluation of abdominal pain is described in Fig. 3-1.

■ LABORATORY TESTS
- CBC with differential reveals leukocytosis with a left shift in 90% of patients with appendicitis. Total WBC count is generally lower than 20,000/mm^3. Higher counts may be indicative of perforation. Less than 4% have a normal WBC and differential. A low Hgb and Hct in an older patient should raise suspicion for carcinoma of the cecum.
- Microscopic hematuria and pyuria may occur in <20% of patients.

■ IMAGING STUDIES
- Appendiceal CT scan as a noninvasive diagnostic aid has an accuracy of more than 90%. It improves patient care and reduces the use of hospital resources.
- Ultrasound is useful, especially in younger women when diagnosis is unclear. Normal ultrasonographic

findings should not deter surgery if the history and physical examination are indicative of appendicitis. Ultrasound followed by CT with rectal contrast is more than 90% accurate in detecting acute appendicitis in children.
- Laparoscopy may be useful as both a diagnostic and a therapeutic modality.

TREATMENT

■ NONPHARMACOLOGIC THERAPY
- NPO
- Do not administer analgesics or antibiotics until the diagnosis is made (may mask signs of peritonitis).

■ ACUTE GENERAL Rx
- Urgent appendectomy (laparoscopic or open), correction of fluid and electrolyte imbalance with vigorous IV hydration and electrolyte replacement
- IV antibiotic prophylaxis to cover gram-negative bacilli and anaerobes (cefotetan, clindamycin and gentamicin, or metronidazole with gentamicin)

■ DISPOSITION
In general, prognosis is excellent. Mortality is <1% in young adults without complications; however, it exceeds 10% in elderly patients with ruptured appendix.

■ REFERRAL
Surgical referral as soon as diagnosis is suspected

PEARLS & CONSIDERATIONS

■ COMMENTS
Perforation is common (20% in adult patients). Indicators of perforation are pain lasting >24 hr, leukocytosis >20,000/mm^3, temperature >102° F, palpable abdominal mass, and peritoneal findings.

REFERENCE
Garcia Pena BM et al: Cost and effectiveness of ultrasonography and limited CT for diagnosing appendicitis in children, *Pediatrics* 106:672, 2000.
Author: **Fred F. Ferri, M.D.**

BASIC INFORMATION

■ DEFINITION

The prototype of granulomatous arthritis is tuberculous arthritis. Atypical mycobacteria, sarcoidosis, and sporotrichosis can cause granulomatous involvement of the synovium, but these entities are much less common.

■ SYNONYMS

Tuberculous arthritis
Pott's disease

■ ICD-9CM CODES

711.40 Arthropathy associated with other bacterial disease
730.88 Other infection involving bone

■ EPIDEMIOLOGY & DEMOGRAPHICS

INCIDENCE (IN U.S.): Unknown
PREVALENCE (IN U.S.): Unknown
PREDOMINANT SEX: Male = female
PREDOMINANT AGE: Rare in childhood
PEAK INCIDENCE: No seasonal predilection

■ PHYSICAL FINDINGS

- Often no constitutional symptoms (fever and weight loss)
- Possibly no clinical or radiographic evidence of pulmonary TB
- Spinal infection most often in the thoracic or upper lumbar area, with back pain as the most common symptom
- Considerable local muscle spasm possible
- Kyphosis and neurologic symptoms resulting from spinal cord compression in advanced disease
- Chronic monoarticular arthritis in the peripheral joints
- Single joint involved in 85% of patients
- Pain, swelling, limitation of motion, and joint stiffness less dramatic than in acute bacterial arthritis; possibly present for months to years
- Seen more often in persons from developing countries, elderly patients, and hemodialysis patients

■ ETIOLOGY

- Hematogenous spread of organisms from a distant site of infection or by direct spread from bone
- Most commonly affected area: 50% of cases in the spine; next most commonly affected area: large joints (knee and hip)
- Primary infection beginning in the lungs and spreading to the highly vascular synovium
- Tuberculous osteomyelitis commonly involving an adjacent joint

- In peripheral joints, a granulomatous reaction in the synovium causing joint effusion and eventual destruction of underlying bone
- In the spine, infection of the intervertebral disk spreading to adjacent vertebrae
- Osteomyelitis of vertebrae causing collapse, kyphosis, or gibbous deformity, and possibly paraspinal "cold" abscess

 DIAGNOSIS

■ DIFFERENTIAL DIAGNOSIS

- Sarcoidosis
- Fungal arthritis
- Metastatic cancer
- Primary or metastatic synovial tumors

■ WORKUP

- High index of suspicion needed
- Gold standard: synovial biopsy
- Joint aspiration and culture of the synovial fluid performed while awaiting biopsy
- Positive synovial fluid smear for acid-fast bacilli in 20% of cases; positive culture in 80%
- Elevated synovial fluid protein, low glucose
- Considerable variation in synovial fluid WBC count, but values of 10,000 to 20,000 cells/mm³ typical; may be predominantly polymorphonuclear leukocytes
- Usually positive tuberculin skin test
- Anergy in elderly patients or in advanced disease
- In spinal infections, percutaneous or open biopsy to obtain accurate C&S data

■ LABORATORY TESTS

Peripheral WBC count and ESR are elevated but nonspecific.

■ IMAGING STUDIES

- Plain radiographs of the affected joint
  1. Typically demonstrate bony destruction with little new bone formation
  2. Osteopenia and soft tissue swelling in early infections
  3. Later, erosions at the joint margins
  4. In the spine, disk space narrowing with vertebral collapse (wedging) causing characteristic kyphosis
- CT scan: useful in early diagnosis of infections of the spine and to detect paraspinal abscess
- Technetium and gallium scintigraphic scans: may be positive, but do not permit differentiation from inflammation or osteoarthritis

 TREATMENT

■ NONPHARMACOLOGIC THERAPY

Encourage range-of-motion exercises of the affected joint to prevent contractures.

■ ACUTE GENERAL Rx

- Combination chemotherapy
  1. If sensitive TB suspected, give isoniazid 5 mg/kg/day (maximum 300 mg/day) plus rifampin 10 mg/kg/day (maximum 600 mg/day) for at least 6 mo and pyrazinamide 15 to 30 mg/kg/day (maximum 2 g/day) for at least the first 2 mo plus ethambutol 15 to 25 mg/kg/day until sensitivity results are available.
  2. Most patients are treated successfully with chemotherapy alone.
  3. Urgent surgical intervention is necessary if spinal cord compression causes neurologic changes.
- Surgical debridement in cases of extensive bone involvement

■ CHRONIC Rx

In long-standing extensive disease, arthrodesis of weight-bearing joints

■ DISPOSITION

Loss of cartilage and destruction of underlying bone if treatment is not initiated promptly

■ REFERRAL

- To a physician experienced in the management of TB
- For consultation with an infectious diseases specialist if drug resistance is suspected or documented
- For neurosurgical and/or orthopedic consultation if neurologic impairment suspected

PEARLS & CONSIDERATIONS

■ COMMENTS

- As TB has become more prevalent in the U.S. in the last 10 to 20 yr, TB arthritis and osteomyelitis have also become more common.

REFERENCES

Emery P et al: Detection of *Mycobacterium tuberculosis* group organisms in human and mouse joint tissue by reverse transcriptase PCR: prevalence in diseased synovial tissue suggests lack of specific association with rheumatoid arthritis, *Infect Immun* 69(30):1821, 2001.

Miyata K, Kanzaki T: Early onset sarcoidosis masquerading as juvenile rheumatoid arthritis, *J Am Acad Dermatol* 43:969, 2001.

Shanahan EM, Hanley SD: Tuberculosis of the wrist, *Arth Rheum* 42(12):2724, 1999.
Author: **Deborah L. Shapiro, M.D.**

BASIC INFORMATION

■ **DEFINITION**
Bacterial arthritis is a highly destructive form of joint disease most often caused by hematogenous spread of organisms from a distant site of infection. Direct penetration of the joint as a result of trauma or surgery and spread from adjacent osteomyelitis may also cause bacterial arthritis. Any joint in the body may be affected. Gonococcal arthritis causes a distinct clinical syndrome and is often considered separately.

■ **SYNONYMS**
Septic arthritis
Pyogenic arthritis

ICD-9CM CODES
711 Pyogenic arthritis, site unspecified

■ **EPIDEMIOLOGY & DEMOGRAPHICS**
INCIDENCE (IN U.S.): Unknown
PREVALENCE (IN U.S.): Unknown
PREDOMINANT SEX: Gonococcal arthritis in males
PREDOMINANT AGE: Gonococcal arthritis in sexually active adults
PEAK INCIDENCE:
• Gonococcal arthritis: young adults
• Other bacterial causes: all ages

■ **PHYSICAL FINDINGS & CLINICAL PRESENTATION**
• Hallmark: acute onset of a swollen, painful joint
• Limited range of motion of the joint
• Effusion, with varying degrees of erythema and increased warmth around the joint
• Single joint affected in 80% to 90% of cases of nongonococcal arthritis
• Gonococcal dermatitis-arthritis syndrome
  1. Typical pattern is a migratory polyarthritis or tenosynovitis
  2. Small pustules on the trunk or extremities
• Febrile patient at presentation
• Most commonly affected joints in adult: knee and hip, but any joint may be involved; in children: hip

■ **ETIOLOGY**
• Bacteria spread from another locus of infection
  1. Highly vascular synovium is invaded by hematogenously spread bacteria.
  2. WBC enzymes cause necrosis of synovium, cartilage, and bone.
  3. Extensive joint destruction is rapid if infection is not treated with appropriate IV antibiotics and drainage of necrotic material.
• Predisposing factors: rheumatoid arthritis, prosthetic joints, advanced age, immunodeficiency
• The most common nongonococcal organisms are *Staphylococcus aureus,*

β-hemolytic streptococci, and gram-negative bacilli.

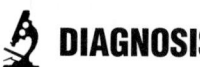 **DIAGNOSIS**

■ **DIFFERENTIAL DIAGNOSIS**
• Gout
• Pseudogout
• Trauma
• Hemarthrosis
• Rheumatic fever
• Adult or juvenile rheumatoid arthritis
• Spondyloarthropathies such as Reiter's syndrome
• Osteomyelitis
• Viral arthritides
• Septic bursitis

■ **WORKUP**
• Joint aspiration, Gram stain, and culture of the synovial fluid
• Immediate arthrocentesis before other studies are undertaken or antibiotics instituted

■ **LABORATORY TESTS**
• Joint fluid analysis
  1. Synovial fluid leukocyte count is usually elevated >50,000 cells/mm^3 with a differential count of 80% or more polymorphonuclear cells.
  2. Counts are highly variable, with similar findings in gout, pseudogout, or rheumatoid arthritis.
  3. The differential diagnosis of synovial fluid abnormalities is described in Table 2-192.
• Blood cultures
• Culture of possible extraarticular sources of infection
• Elevated peripheral WBC count and ESR (nonspecific)

■ **IMAGING STUDIES**
• X-ray examination of the affected joint to rule out osteomyelitis
• CT scan for early diagnosis of infections of the spine, hips, and sternoclavicular and sacroiliac joints
• Technetium and gallium scintigraphic scans (positive, but do not permit differentiation of infection from inflammation)
• Indium-labeled WBC scans (less sensitive, but more specific)

■ **TREATMENT**

■ **NONPHARMACOLOGIC THERAPY**
• Affected joints aspirated daily to remove necrotic material and to follow serial WBC counts and cultures
• If no resolution with IV antibiotics and closed drainage: open debridement and lavage, particularly in nongonococcal infections
• Prevention of contractures:

1. After acute stage of inflammation, range-of-motion exercises of the affected joint
2. Physical therapy helpful

■ **ACUTE GENERAL Rx**
• IV antibiotics immediately after joint aspiration and Gram stain of the synovial fluid
• For infections caused by gram-positive cocci: penicillinase-resistant penicillin, such as nafcillin (2 g IV q4h), unless there is clinical suspicion of methicillin-resistant *Staphylococcus aureus,* in which case vancomycin (1 g IV q12h)
• Infections caused by gram-negative bacilli: treated with a third-generation cephalosporin or an antipseudomonal penicillin plus an aminoglycoside, pending C&S results
• For suspected gonococcal infection, including young adults when the synovial fluid Gram stain is nondiagnostic: ceftriaxone 1 g IV q24h

■ **CHRONIC Rx**
See indications for surgical drainage.

■ **DISPOSITION**
• With prompt treatment, complete resolution is expected.
• Delay in treatment may result in permanent destruction of cartilage and loss of function of the affected joint.

■ **REFERRAL**
To an orthopedist for open drainage if the infected joint fails to improve on appropriate antibiotics and closed aspiration

PEARLS & CONSIDERATIONS

■ **COMMENTS**
• Any patient with an acute monoarticular arthritis should undergo an urgent joint aspiration to rule out septic arthritis, even if there is a history of gout.

REFERENCES
Ike RW: Bacterial arthritis, *Curr Opin Rheumatol* 10(4):330, 1998.
Kothari NA, Pelchovitz DJ, Meyer JS: Imaging of musculoskeletal infections, *Radiol Clin North Am* 39(40):653, 2001.
Turpin S, Lambert R: Role of scintigraphy in musculoskeletal and spinal infections, *Radiol Clin North Am* 39(2):169, 2001.
Van der Heijden IM, Wilbrink B: Detection of bacterial DNA in serial synovial samples obtained during antibiotic treatment from patients with septic arthritis, *Arth Rheum* 42(10):2198, 1999.
Author: **Deborah L. Shapiro, M.D.**

BASIC INFORMATION

■ DEFINITION
Juvenile rheumatoid arthritis is arthritis beginning before the age of 16 yr.

■ SYNONYMS
Still's disease
Juvenile chronic arthritis
Juvenile polyarthritis

■ ICD-9CM CODES
714.3 Juvenile chronic polyarthritis

■ EPIDEMIOLOGY & DEMOGRAPHICS
PREVALENCE (IN U.S.): 250,000 to 300,000 cases
PREVALENT SEX: Female:male ratio of 2:1
PREVALENT AGE: Two peak incidences, between ages of 1 and 3 yr and ages 8 and 12 yr.

■ PHYSICAL FINDINGS & CLINICAL PRESENTATION
Usually one of three types:

SYSTEMIC OR ACUTE FEBRILE JUVENILE RHEUMATOID ARTHRITIS (20% OF CASES):
- Characterized by extraarticular manifestations, especially spiking fevers and a typical rash that frequently appears in the evening and may be elicited by gently scratching the skin in susceptible areas (Koebner's phenomenon)
- Possible splenomegaly, generalized lymphadenopathy, pericarditis, and myocarditis
- Often, minimal articular findings overshadowed by systemic symptoms

PAUCIARTICULAR OR OLIGOARTICULAR FORM (50% OF CASES):
- Involves fewer than 5 joints
- Usually involves the larger joints, such as the knees, elbows, and ankles
- Systemic features often minimal, and only one to three joints usually involved
- Rarely causes impairment but chronic iridocyclitis develops in approximately 30% of cases with this form, and permanent loss of vision will develop in a high percentage of these patients (Fig. 1-38)
- Accelerated growth of the affected limb from chronic hyperemia possibly resulting in a temporary leg length discrepancy that is eventually equalized in most cases on control of the inflammation

POLYARTICULAR JUVENILE RHEUMATOID ARTHRITIS (30% OF CASES):
- Involves five or more joints
- Resembles the adult disease in its symmetric involvement of the small joints of the hands and feet (Fig. 1-39)
- Cervical spine involvement common and may produce marked loss of motion

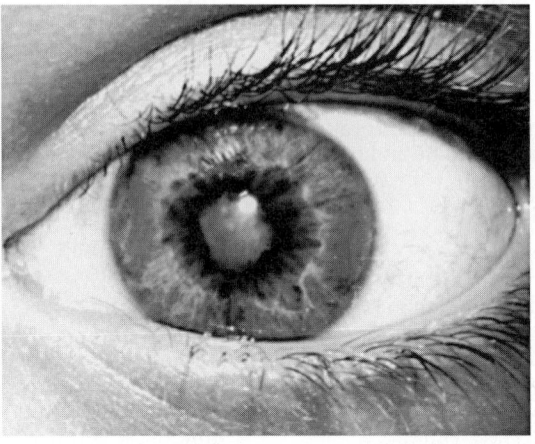

Fig. 1-38 Chronic iridocyclitis of juvenile rheumatoid arthritis. Extensive posterior synechiae have resulted in a small, irregular pupil. There is a well-developed cataract and early band keratopathy at the medial and lateral margins of the cornea. (From Behrman RE [ed]: *Nelson textbook of pediatrics,* ed 16, Philadelphia, 2000, WB Saunders.)

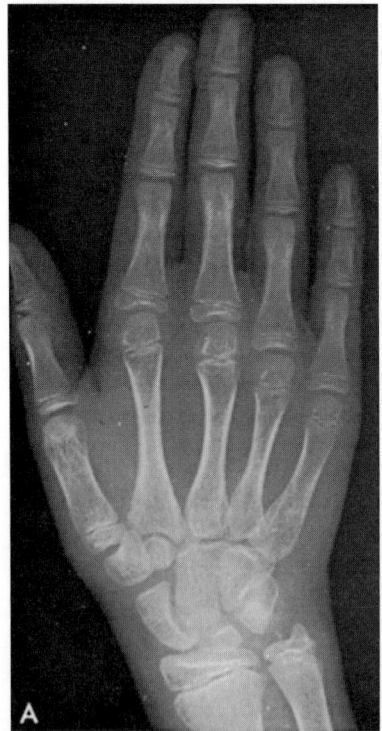
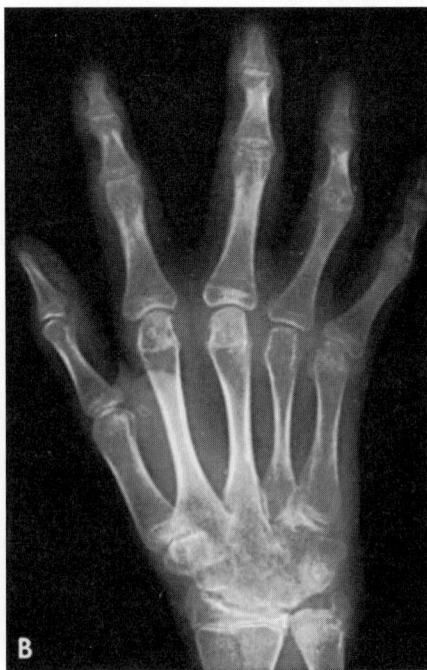

Fig. 1-39 Progression of joint destruction in a girl with rheumatoid factor–positive juvenile rheumatoid arthritis despite doses of corticosteroids sufficient to suppress symptoms in the interval between *A* and *B.* **A,** Roentgenogram of the hand at onset. **B,** Roentgenogram 4 years later, showing a loss of articular cartilage and destruction changes in the distal and proximal interphalangeal and metacarpophalangeal joints and destruction and fusion of wrist bones. (From Behrman RE [ed]: *Nelson textbook of pediatrics,* ed 16, Philadelphia, 2000, WB Saunders.)

- Early closure of the ossification centers of the mandible, often producing a markedly receding chin, a characteristic of this form
- Systemic manifestations similar to the febrile variety but not as dramatic

ETIOLOGY

Unknown. There is increasing evidence that the inflammation and destruction of bone and cartilage that occurs in many rheumatic diseases are the result of the activation, by some unknown mechanism, of proinflammatory cells that infiltrate the synovium. These cells, in turn, release various substances, such as cytokines and tumor necrosis factor (TNF) alpha, which subsequently cause the pathologic changes typical of this group of diseases. Many of the newer therapeutic agents are directed at the suppression of these final mediators of inflammation.

DIAGNOSIS

DIFFERENTIAL DIAGNOSIS
- Infectious causes of fever
- SLE
- Rheumatic fever
- Drug reaction
- Serum sickness
- "Viral arthritis"
- Lyme arthritis

WORKUP
Initial laboratory and imaging studies are often nonspecific in children with rheumatoid arthritis.

LABORATORY TESTS
- Increased ESR
- Low-grade anemia

- Very high peripheral WBC count
- Rheumatoid factor: rarely demonstrable in the serum of children
- Antinuclear antibodies: often found in children with ocular complications

IMAGING STUDIES
- Roentgenographic findings are similar to those in adult, with soft tissue swelling and osteoporosis early in the disease.
- Joint destruction is less frequent.
- Bony erosion and cyst formation may be present as a result of synovial hypertrophy.

TREATMENT

NONPHARMACOLOGIC THERAPY
Proper management requires close cooperation among primary physician, therapist, rheumatologist, and orthopedist.
- Rest
- Physical and occupational therapy
- Patient and family education
- Proper diet and weight maintenance

ACUTE GENERAL Rx
- Aspirin (stopped during childhood viral illnesses to avoid Reye's syndrome)
- Other NSAIDs
- DMARDs and biologic response modifiers (BMRs)
- Intraarticular steroids
- Systemic corticosteroids

DISPOSITION
- Complete remission occurs in the majority of patients and may occur at any age.
- 70% to 85% of children regain normal function.

- Mortality rate is 2%.
- Children with a protracted systemic phase of the disease are most at risk for developing serious intercurrent infection and potentially fatal amyloidosis.
- Myocarditis may develop in the systemic form.
- Blindness is the most serious complication of the pauciarticular form; joint deformity is the most serious problem of polyarticular disease.

REFERRAL
- For ophthalmology consultation when ocular involvement is suspected (frequent eye examinations, especially in oligoarticular form)
- For orthopedic consultation for corrective surgery

PEARLS & CONSIDERATIONS

COMMENTS
Patient information on juvenile rheumatoid arthritis can be obtained from the National Arthritis Foundation, 1330 West Peachtree Street, Atlanta, GA 30309; phone: 1-800-283-7800.

REFERENCES
Choy EHS, Panayi G: Cytokine pathways and joint inflammation in rheumatoid arthritis, *N Engl J Med* 344:907, 2001.
Uremer JM: Rational use of new and existing disease-modifying agents in rheumatoid arthritis, *Ann Intern Med* 134:695, 2001.
Wulffaact NM, Kuis W: Treatment of refractory juvenile kliopathic arthritis, *J Rheumatol* 28:929, 2001.
Author: **Lonnie R. Mercier, M.D.**

BASIC INFORMATION

■ DEFINITION
Psoriatic arthritis is an inflammatory spondyloarthritis occurring in patients with psoriasis who are usually seronegative for rheumatoid factor. It is often included in a class of disorders called *rheumatoid variants* or *seronegative spondyloarthropathies.*

■ ICD-9CM CODES
696.0 Psoriatic arthritis

■ EPIDEMIOLOGY & DEMOGRAPHICS
PREVALENCE: 5% to 10% of patients with psoriasis (psoriasis affects 1% to 1.5% of general population)
PREVALENT SEX: Males = females
PREVALENT AGE: 30 to 55 yr

■ PHYSICAL FINDINGS & CLINICAL PRESENTATION
- Usually gradual clinical onset
- Asymmetric involvement of scattered joints
- Selective involvement of the DIP joints (described in "classic" cases but present in only 5% of patients; Fig. 1-40)
- Symmetric arthritis similar to RA in 15% of patients
- Possible development of predominant sarcoiliitis in a small number of cases
- Advanced form of hand involvement (arthritis mutilans) in some patients
- Dystrophic changes in the nails (pitting, ridging) in many patients with DIP involvement

■ ETIOLOGY
Unknown

DIAGNOSIS

■ DIFFERENTIAL DIAGNOSIS
- Rheumatoid arthritis
- Erosive osteoarthritis
- Gouty arthritis
- Ankylosing spondylitis
- The differential diagnosis of spondyloarthropathies is described in Table 2-189 and Box 2-232.

■ WORKUP
- Early diagnosis may be difficult to establish because the arthritis may develop before skin lesions appear.
- Laboratory studies show no specific abnormalities in most cases.

■ LABORATORY TESTS
- Slight elevation of ESR
- Possible mild anemia
- Possible HLA-B27 antigen (especially in patients with sarcoiliitis)

■ IMAGING STUDIES
- Peripheral joint findings similar to those in rheumatoid arthritis but erosive changes in the distal phalangeal tufts characteristic of psoriatic arthritis
- Bony osteolysis; periosteal new bony formation
- Changes in axial skeleton: sacroiliitis, development of vertebral syndesmophytes (osteophytes) that often bridge adjacent vertebral bodies
- Paravertebral ossification
- Spinal changes: do not have same appearance as ankylosing spondylitis; however, spine abnormalities are less common than sacroiliitis

TREATMENT

■ NONPHARMACOLOGIC THERAPY
- Rest
- Splinting
- Joint protection
- PT

■ ACUTE GENERAL Rx
- NSAIDs
- Occasional intraarticular steroid injections
- DMARDs: rarely are required

■ DISPOSITION
- Different from rheumatoid arthritis in both prognosis and response to treatment
- Generally, mild joint symptoms in psoriatic arthritis
- Disease-free intervals lasting for several years in many patients

■ REFERRAL
Orthopedic consultation for painful joint deformity

REFERENCES
Crotty JG et al: Interventions for psoriatic arthritis, Cochrane Database System Rev 3: CD 000212, 2000.
Hohkr T, Marker-Hermann E: Psoriatic arthritis: clinical aspects genetics, and the role of T-cells, *Curr Opin Rheumatol* 13:245, 2001.
Patel S et al: Psoriatic arthritis-emerging concepts, *Rheumatology* (Oxford) 40:243, 2001.
Author: **Lonnie R. Mercier, M.D.**

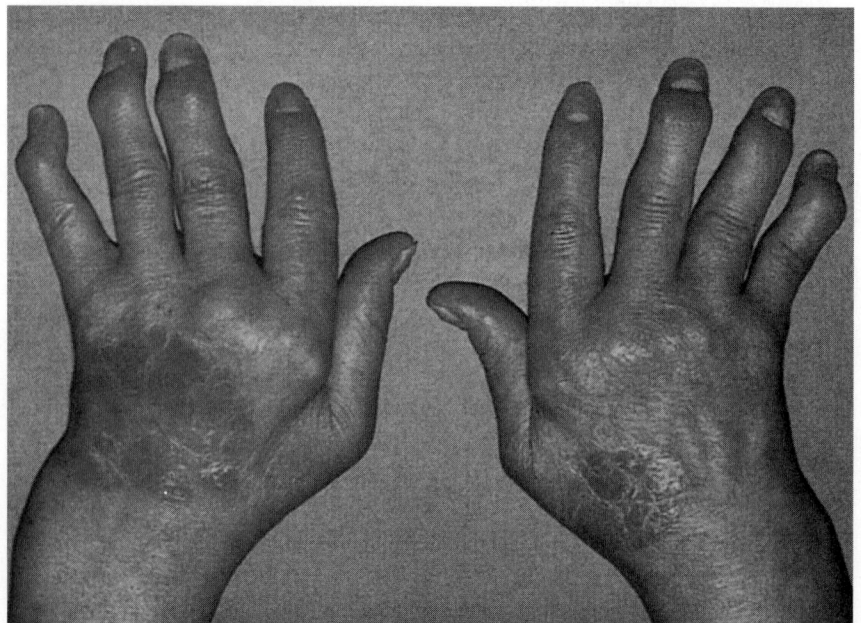

Fig. 1-40 The hands of a woman with symmetric polyarthritis. Initially, this was indistinguishable from rheumatoid disease, but note the distal interphalangeal joint involvement, which is uncommon in rheumatoid arthritis, as well as the skin psoriasis. (From Klippel J, Dieppe P, Ferri F [eds]: *Primary care rheumatology,* London, 1999, Mosby.)

BASIC INFORMATION

■ DEFINITION
Rheumatoid arthritis (RA) is a systemic disorder characterized by chronic joint inflammation that most commonly affects peripheral joints.

ICD-9CM CODES
714.0 Rheumatoid arthritis

■ EPIDEMIOLOGY & DEMOGRAPHICS
PREVALENCE: 5 cases/1000 adults
PREVALENT AGE: 35 to 45 yr
PREDOMINANT SEX:
- Female:male ratio of 3:1
- After age 50 yr, sex difference less marked

■ PHYSICAL FINDINGS & CLINICAL PRESENTATION
- Usually gradual onset; common prodromal symptoms of weakness, fatigue, and anorexia
- Initial presentation: multiple symmetric joint involvement, most often in the hands and feet, usually MCP, MTP, and PIP joints (Fig. 1-41)
- Joint effusions, tenderness, and restricted motion usually present early in the disease
- Eventual characteristic deformities: subluxations, dislocations, and joint contractures
- Extraarticular findings:
  1. Tendon sheaths and bursae frequently affected by chronic inflammation
  2. Possible tendon rupture
  3. Rheumatoid nodules over bony prominences such as the elbow and shaft of the ulna
  4. Splenomegaly, pericarditis, and vasculitis
  5. Findings of carpal tunnel syndrome resulting from flexor tenosynovitis

■ ETIOLOGY
Unknown. There is increasing evidence that the inflammation and destruction of bone and cartilage that occurs in many rheumatic diseases are the result of the activation by some unknown mechanism of proinflammatory cells that infiltrate the synorium. These cells, in turn, release various substances, such as cytokines and tumor necrosis factor (TNF) alpha, which subsequently cause the pathologic changes typical of this group of diseases. Many of the newer therapeutic agents are directed at the suppression of these final mediators of inflammation.

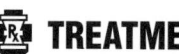

DIAGNOSIS

■ DIFFERENTIAL DIAGNOSIS
- SLE
- Seronegative spondyloarthropathies
- Polymyalgia rheumatica
- Acute rheumatic fever
- Scleroderma

According to the American College of Rheumatology, RA exists when four of seven criteria are present, with criteria 1 to 4 being present for at least 6 wk.
1. Morning stiffness over 1 hr
2. Arthritis in three or more joints with swelling
3. Arthritis of hand joints with swelling
4. Symmetric arthritis
5. Rheumatoid nodules
6. Roentgenographic changes typical of RA
7. Positive serum rheumatoid factor

■ LABORATORY TESTS
- Increase in rheumatoid factor in 80% of cases (rheumatoid factor also present in the normal population)
- Possible mild anemia
- Usually, elevated acute phase reactants (ESR, C-reactive protein)
- Possible mild leukocytosis
- Usually, turbid joint fluid, which forms a poor mucin clot; elevated cell count, with an increase in polymorphonuclear leukocytes

■ IMAGING STUDIES
Plain radiography
- Usually reveals soft-tissue swelling and osteoporosis early (Fig. 1-42)
- Eventually, joint space narrowing, erosion, and deformity visible as a result of continued inflammation and cartilage destruction

TREATMENT

■ NONPHARMACOLOGIC THERAPY
Proper management requires close cooperation among primary physician, therapist, rheumatologist, and orthopedist.
- Patient education is important.
- Rest with proper exercise and splinting can prevent or correct joint deformities.
- Maintain proper diet and control obesity.

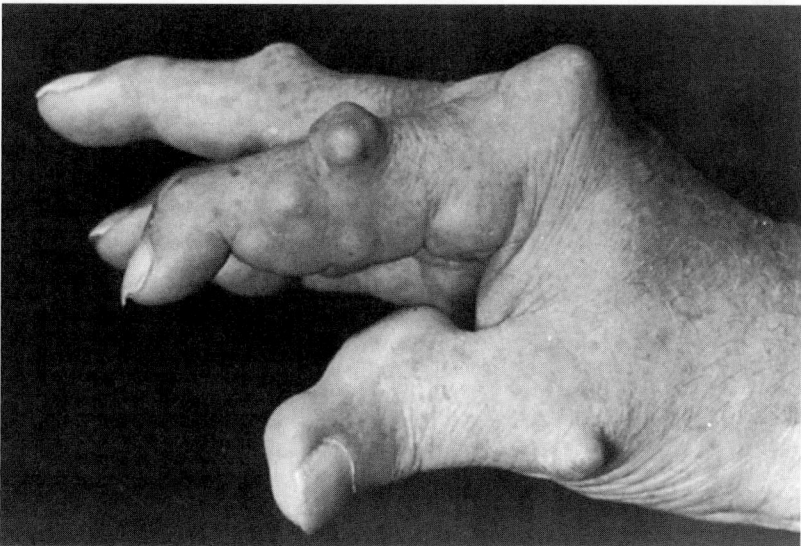

Fig. 1-41 Rheumatoid arthritis. Hand of a 60-year-old man with seropositive rheumatoid arthritis. There are fixed deformities and gross rheumatoid nodules. (From Canoso JJ: *Rheumatology in primary care,* Philadelphia, 1997, WB Saunders.)

■ CHRONIC Rx

- NSAIDs: commonly used as the initial treatment to relieve inflammation (drug of choice for most patients: aspirin, but other NSAIDs also effective)
- Disease-modifying drugs (DMARDs): are traditionally begun when NSAIDs are not effective; current recommendations favor early aggressive treatment with DMARDs, seeking to minimize long-term joint damage. Commonly used agents are methotrexate, cyclosporine, hydroxychloroquine, sulfasalazine, leflunomide, and infliximab. Most of these are associated with potential toxicity and require close monitoring. They are also usually slow-acting drugs that require more than 8 wk to become effective (see Table 1-13)
- Oral prednisone
- Intrasynovial steroid injections
- Etanercept (Enbrel), a tumor necrosis factor alpha blocker is indicated in moderately to severely active RA in patients who respond inadequately to DMARDs. The combination of etanercept and methotrexate has been reported to be effective and promising in the treatment of RA.

■ DISPOSITION

- Remissions and exacerbations are common, but condition is chronically progressive in the majority of cases.
- Joint degeneration and deformity often lead to disability.
- Early diagnosis and treatment are important and can improve quality of life.

■ REFERRAL

Orthopedic consultation for corrective surgery

REFERENCES

Choy EHS, Panayi GS: Cytokine pathways and joint inflammation in rheumatoid arthritis, *N Engl J Med* 344:907, 2001.

Kremer JM: Rational use of new and existing disease-modifying agents in rheumatoid arthritis, *Ann Intern Med* 134:695, 2001.

Lipsky PE et al: Infliximab and methotrexate in the treatment of rheumatoid arthritis, *N Engl J Med* 343:1594, 2000.

Matteson FL: Current treatment strategies for rheumatoid arthritis, *Mayo Clin Proc* 75:69, 2000.

Pincus T et al: Combination therapy with multiple disease-modifying antirheumatic drugs in rheumatoid arthritis: a preventive strategy, *Ann Intern Med* 131:768, 1999.

Weinblatt ME et al: A trial of etanercept, a recombinant tumor necrosis factor receptor: Fe fusion protein, in patients with rheumatoid arthritis receiving methotrexate, *N Engl J Med* 340:253, 1999.

Author: **Lonnie R. Mercier, M.D.**

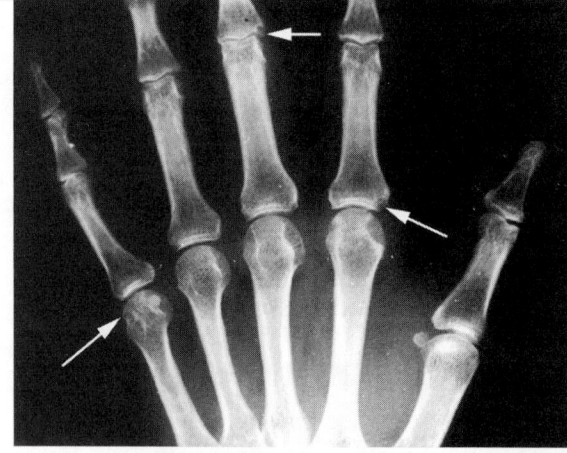 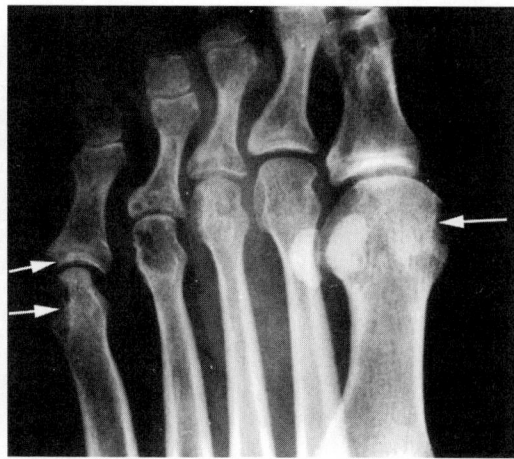

Fig. 1-42   Rheumatoid arthritis. **A,** Periarticular osteopenia and marginal erosions in MCPs and a PIP *(arrows).* **B,** In the same patient, marginal erosions at metatarsal heads. (From Canoso JJ [ed]: *Rheumatology in primary care,* Philadelphia, 1997, WB Saunders.)

TABLE 1-13   Selected Disease-Modifying Antirheumatic Drugs

TYPE/GENERIC (TRADE) NAME	RECOMMENDED DOSAGES	TOXIC EFFECTS	RECOMMENDED MONITORING
Gold compounds (Myochrysine)	IM: 10 mg followed by 25 mg 1 wk later, then 25-50 mg wkly until there is toxicity, major clinical improvement, or cumulative dose = 1 g. If effective, interval between doses is increased.	Pruritus, dermatitis (frequent—$\frac{1}{3}$ of pts), stomatitis, nephrotoxicity, blood dyscrasias, "nitritoid" reaction: flushing, weakness, nausea, dizziness 30 min after injection.	CBC, platelet count before every other injection. Urinalysis before each dose.
Aurothioglucose (Solganal)	IM: 10 mg; 2nd and 3rd doses 25 mg, 4th and subsequent 50 mg. Interval between doses: 1 wk. If improvement, no toxicity→decrease dose to 25 mg or increase interval between doses.	Dermatitis, stomatitis, nephrotoxicity, blood dyscrasias.	CBC, platelet count every 2 wk. Urinalysis before each dose.
Auranofin (Ridaura)	Oral: 3 mg bid or 6 mg qd. May increase to 3 mg tid after 6 months.	Loose stools, diarrhea (up to 50%), dermatitis.	Baseline CBC, platelet count, U/A, renal, liver function, at onset then CBC with platelet count, U/A 9 months.
Antimalarial Hydroxychloroquine (Plaquenil)	Oral: 400-600 mg qd with meals then 200-400 mg qd.	Retinopathy, dermatitis, muscle weakness, hypoactive DTRs, CNS.	Ophthalmologic examination every 3 months (visual acuity, slitlamp, funduscopic, visual field tests), neuromuscular examination.
Penicillamine (Cuprimine, Depen)	Oral: 125-250 mg qd, then increasing at monthly intervals doses to max 750-1000 mg by 125-250 mg.	Pruritus, rash/mouth ulcers, bone marrow depression, proteinuria, hematuria, hypogeusia, myesthenia, myositis, GI distress, pulmonary toxicity, teratogenic.	CBC every 2 weeks until dose stable, then every month. U/A weekly until dose stable, then every month. HCG as needed.
Methotrexate (Rheumatrex)	Oral: 7.5-15 mg weekly.	Pulmonary toxicity, ulcerative stomatitis, leukopenia, thrombocytopenia, GI distress, malaise, fatigue, chills, fever, CNS, elevated LFTs/liver disease, lymphoma, infection.	CBC with platelet count, LFTs weekly × 6 wk then monthly LFTs, U/A periodically, HCG as needed.
Azathioprine (Imuran)	Oral: 50-100 mg qd, increase at 4-wk intervals by 0.5 mg/kg/d up to 2.5 mg/kg/d.	Leukopenia, thrombocytopenia, GI, neoplastic if previous Rx with alkylating agents.	CBC with platelet count, wkly × 1 mo, 2×/mo. × 2 mo, then monthly, HCG as needed.
Sulfasalazine (Azulfidine)	Oral: 500 mg daily then increase up to 3 g daily.	GI, skin rash, pruritus, blood dyscrasias, oligospermia.	CBC, U/A q 2 wk × 3 mo, then monthly × 9 mo, then every 6 mo.
Alkylating agents Cyclophosphamide (Cytoxan)	Oral: 50-100 mg daily up to 2.5 mg/kg/d.	Leukopenia, thrombocytopenia, hematuria, GI, alopecia, rash, bladder cancer, non-Hodgkin's lymphoma, infection.	CBC with platelet count, regularly. HCG as needed.
Chlorambucil (Leukeran)	Oral: 0.1-0.2 mg/kg/d.	Bone marrow suppression, GI, CNS, infection.	CBC with platelet count every wk. WBCs 3-4 days after each CBC during 1st 3-6 wk at therapy. HCG as needed.
Cyclosporine (Sandimmune)	Oral 2.5-5 mg/kg/d.	Nephrotoxicity, tremor, hirsutism, hypertension, gum hyperplasia.	Renal function, liver function.
Pyrimidine, synthesis inhibitors Leflunomide (Arava)	Loading dose: 100 mg/d for 3 days. Maintenance therapy: 20 mg/d; if not tolerated, 10 mg/d.	Hepatotoxicity, carcinogenesis. Immunosuppression, long half-life.	LFTs every month, drug levels after discontinuation (after 1 month therapy, remains in blood for 2 years without use of cholestyramine).

From Rakel RE (ed): *Principles of family practice*, ed 6, Philadelphia, 2002, WB Saunders.
Bid, Twice a day; *CBC*, complete blood count; *CNS*, central nervous system; *DTR*, deep tendon reflex; *GI*, gastrointestinal; *HCG*, human chorionic gonadotropin; *IM*, intramuscular; *LFT*, liver function test; *qd*, every day; *tid*, three times a day; *U/A*, urinalysis; *WBC*, white blood cell count.

BASIC INFORMATION

■ DEFINITION
Asbestosis is a slowly progressive diffuse interstitial fibrosis resulting from dose-related inhalation exposure to fibers of asbestos.

ICD-9CM CODES
501 Asbestosis

■ EPIDEMIOLOGY & DEMOGRAPHICS
- In U.S.: 5 to 10 new cases/100,000 persons/yr
- Prolonged interval (20 to 30 yr) between exposures to inhaled fibers and clinical manifestations of disease
- Most common in workers involved in the primary extraction of asbestos from rock deposits and in those involved in the fabrication and installation of products containing asbestos (e.g., naval shipyards in World War II, installation of floor tiles, ceiling tiles, acoustic ceiling coverings, wall insulation, and pipe coverings in public buildings)

■ PHYSICAL FINDINGS & CLINICAL PRESENTATION
- Insidious onset of shortness of breath with exertion is usually the first sign of asbestosis.
- Dyspnea becomes more severe as the disease advances; with time, progressively less exertion is tolerated.
- Cough is frequent and usually paroxysmal, dry, and nonproductive.
- Scant mucoid sputum may accompany the cough in the later stages of the disease.
- Fine end respiratory crackles (rales, crepitations) are heard more predominantly in the lung bases.
- Digital clubbing, edema, jugular venous distention are present.

■ ETIOLOGY
Inhalation of asbestos fibers

DIAGNOSIS

■ DIFFERENTIAL DIAGNOSIS
- Silicosis
- Siderosis, other pneumonoconioses
- Lung cancer
- Atelectasis

■ WORKUP
Documentation of exposure history, diagnostic imaging, pulmonary function testing

■ LABORATORY TESTS
- Generally not helpful
- Possible mild elevation of ESR, positive ANA and RF (These tests are nonspecific and do not correlate with disease severity or activity.)
- Pulmonary function testing: decreased vital capacity, decreased total lung capacity, decreased carbon monoxide gas transfer
- ABGs: hypoxemia, hypercarbia in advanced stages

■ IMAGING STUDIES
Chest x-ray examination (Fig. 1-43):
- Small, irregular shadows in lower lung zones
- Thickened pleural, calcified plaques (present under diaphragms and lateral chest wall)
CT scan of chest confirms the diagnosis.

TREATMENT

■ NONPHARMACOLOGIC THERAPY
- Smoking cessation, proper nutrition, exercise program to maximize available lung function

- Home oxygen therapy PRN
- Removal of patient from further asbestos fiber exposure

■ ACUTE GENERAL Rx
- Prompt identification and treatment of respiratory infections
- Supplemental oxygen on a PRN basis
- Annual influenza vaccination, pneumococcal vaccination

■ CHRONIC Rx
See "Acute General Rx."

■ DISPOSITION
- There is no specific treatment for asbestosis.
- Death is usually secondary to respiratory failure from cor pulmonale.
- Patients with asbestosis have increased risk for mesotheliomas, lung cancer, and TB. Recent reports indicate that the risk of asbestos-induced lung cancer may be overestimated.
- Survival in patients following development of mesothelioma is 4 to 6 yr.

■ REFERRAL
To pulmonologist initially

PEARLS & CONSIDERATIONS

■ COMMENTS
Patient information on asbestosis can be obtained from the American Lung Association, 1740 Broadway, New York, NY 10019.

REFERENCES
Camus M et al: Nonoccupational exposure to chrysotile asbestos and the risk of lung cancer, *N Engl J Med* 338:1565, 1998.
Author: **Fred F. Ferri, M.D.**

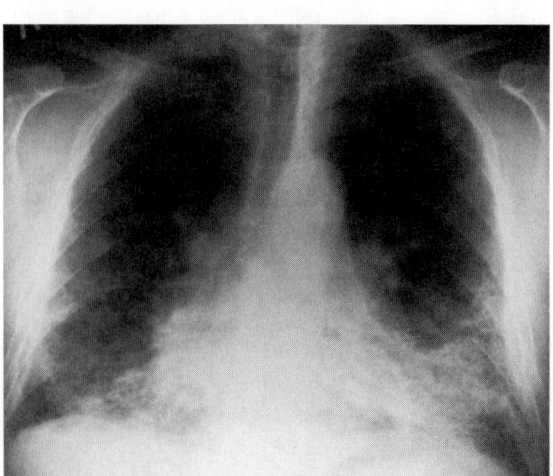

Fig. 1-43 Asbestosis. PA radiograph shows coarse linear opacities at both lung bases obscuring the cardiac borders. (From McLoud TC: *Thoracic radiology: the requisites,* St Louis, 1998, Mosby.)

BASIC INFORMATION

■ DEFINITION

Ascariasis is a parasitic infection caused by the nematode *Ascaris lumbricoides*. The majority of those infected are asymptomatic; however, clinical disease may arise from pulmonary hypersensitivity, intestinal obstruction, and secondary complications.

ICD-9CM CODES

127.0 Ascariasis

■ EPIDEMIOLOGY & DEMOGRAPHICS

INCIDENCE (IN U.S.):
- Unknown
- Three times the infection rates found in blacks as in whites

PREVALENCE (IN U.S.): Estimated at 4,000,000, the majority of which live in the rural southeastern part of the country

PREDOMINANT SEX: Both sexes probably equally affected, with a possible slight female preponderance

PREDOMINANT AGE: Most common in children, with estimated mean age of approximately 5 yr based on surveys in highly endemic areas

PEAK INCIDENCE: Unknown

NEONATAL INFECTION: Probable transmission, though not specifically studied

■ PHYSICAL FINDINGS & CLINICAL PRESENTATION

- Occurs approximately 9 to 12 days after ingestion of eggs (corresponding to the larva migration through the lungs)
- Nonproductive cough
- Substernal chest discomfort
- Fever
- In patients with large worm burdens, especially children, intestinal obstruction associated with perforation, volvulus, and intussusception
- Migration of worms into the biliary tree giving clinical appearance of biliary colic and pancreatitis as well as acute appendicitis with movement into that appendage
- Rarely, infection with *A. lumbricoides* producing interstitial nephritis and acute renal failure
- In endemic areas in Asia and Africa, malabsorption of dietary proteins and vitamins as a consequence of chronic worm intestinal carriage

■ ETIOLOGY

- Transmission is usually hand to mouth, but eggs may be ingested via transported vegetables grown in contaminated soil.
- Eggs are hatched in the small intestine, with larvae penetrating intestinal mucosa and migrating via the circulation to the lungs.
- Larval forms proceed through the alveoli, ascend the bronchial tree, and return to the intestines after swallowing, where they mature into adult worms.
- Estimated time until the female adult worm to begin producing eggs is 2 to 3 mo.
- Eggs are passed out of the intestines with feces.
- Within human host, adult worm lifespan is 1 to 2 yr.

DIAGNOSIS

■ DIFFERENTIAL DIAGNOSIS

- Radiologic manifestations and eosinophilia to be distinguished from drug hypersensitivity and Löffler's syndrome
- The differential diagnosis of intestinal helminths is described in Table 2-93.

■ LABORATORY TESTS

- Examination of the stool for *Ascaris* ova
- Expectoration or fecal passage of adult worm
- Eosinophilia: most prominent early in the infection and subsides as the adult worm infestation established in the intestines
- Anti-ascaris IgG4 blood levels by ELISA is a sensitive and specific marker of infection and may be useful in the evaluation of treatment

■ IMAGING STUDIES

- Chest x-ray examination to reveal bilateral oval or round infiltrates of varying size (Löffler's syndrome); NOTE: infiltrates are transient and eventually resolve.
- Plain films of the abdomen and contrast studies to reveal worm masses in loops of bowel
- Ultrasonography and endoscopic retrograde cholangiopancreatography (ERCP) to identify worms in the pancreaticobiliary tract

TREATMENT

■ NONPHARMACOLOGIC THERAPY

Aggressive IV hydration, especially in children with fever, severe vomiting, and resultant dehydration

■ ACUTE GENERAL Rx

- Mebendazole (Vermox)
  1. Drug of choice for intestinal infection with *A. lumbricoides*
  2. 100 mg PO tid given for 3 days
- Albendazole, given as a single 400-mg dose PO
- Both mebendazole and albendazole are contraindicated in pregnancy.
- Pyrantel pamoate (Antiminth)
  1. Given at a dose of 11 mg/kg PO (maximum dose of 1 g/day)
  2. Considered safe for use in pregnant women
- Piperazine citrate
  1. Recommended in cases of intestinal or biliary obstruction
  2. Administered as a syrup, given via nasogastric tube, a 150 mg/kg loading dose, followed by six doses of 65 mg/kg q12h
  3. Considered safe in pregnancy, but cannot be given concurrently with chlorpromazine
- Complete obstruction should be managed surgically.

■ DISPOSITION

Overall prognosis is good.

■ REFERRAL

To gastroenterologist in cases of visualized pancreaticobiliary tract or appendiceal obstruction

To surgeon in cases of complete obstruction or suspected secondary complication (e.g., perforation or volvulus)

PEARLS & CONSIDERATIONS

■ COMMENTS

- Hepatic abscess, containing both viable and dead worms, complicating *Ascaris*-induced biliary duct disease has been documented.
- Given the known transmission of the parasite, routine hand washing and proper disposal of human waste would significantly decrease the prevalence of this disease.

REFERENCES

Amjad N et al: An unusual presentation of acute cholecystitis: biliary ascariasis *Hosp Med* 62(6):370, 2001.

Bude RO et al: Case 20 Biliary ascariasis, *Radiology* 214(3):844, 2000.

Hui JY et al: A woman with ascites and abdominal masses, *Lancet* 355(9203): 546, 2000.

Santra A et al: Serodiagnosis of ascariasis with specific IgG4 antibody and its use in an epidemiological study, *Trans R Soc Trop Med Hyg* 95(3):289, 2001.

Yamamoto R et al: Effect of intestinal helminthiasis on nutritional status of school children, *Southeast Asian J Trop Med Public Health* 31(4):755, 2000.

Author: **George O. Alonso, M.D.**

BASIC INFORMATION

DEFINITION
Aspergillosis refers to several forms of a broad range of illnesses caused by infection with *Aspergillus* species.

ICD-9CM CODES
117.3 Aspergillosis
117.3 Aspergillosis with pneumonia
117.3 *Aspergillus (flavus) (fumigatus)* (infection) *(terreus)*

EPIDEMIOLOGY & DEMOGRAPHICS
- *Aspergillus* species are ubiquitous in the environment internationally
- Cause a variety of illness from hypersensitivity pneumonitis to disseminated overwhelming infection in immunosuppressed patients
- Frequently cultured from samples obtained in hospital wards from unfiltered outside air circulating through open windows
- Reaches the patient by airborne conidia (spores) that are small enough (2.5 to 3 µm) to reach the alveoli on inhalation
- Can also invade the nose and paranasal sinuses, external ear, or traumatized skin
- The clinical syndrome and pathologic spectrum of *Aspergillus* lung disease is dependent on the underlying lung architecture, the host's immune response, and the degree of inoculum.

ETIOLOGY
- *Aspergillus fumigatus* is the usual cause.
- *A. flavus* is the second most important species, particularly in invasive disease of immunosuppressed patients and in lesions beginning in the nose and paranasal sinuses.

ALLERGIC ASPERGILLOSIS:
- Represents a hypersensitivity pneumonitis
- Presents as cough, dyspnea, fever, chills, and malaise typically 4 to 8 hr after exposure
- Repeated attacks can lead to granulomatous disease and pulmonary fibrosis

ALLERGIC BRONCHOPULMONARY ASPERGILLOSIS (ABPA):
- Hypersensitivity reaction of the airways to *Aspergillus* fungal antigens present in the bronchial tree
- Results from an initial type I (immediate hypersensitivity) and a type III reaction (immune complexes), which is most likely responsible for the roentgenographic features and more destructive changes of the bronchi

ASPERGILLOMAS ("FUNGUS BALLS"):
- In the absence of invasion or significant immune response, *Aspergillus* can colonize a preexisting cavity, causing pulmonary aspergilloma
- Forms masses of tangled hyphal elements, fibrin, and mucus
- Patients typically have a history of chronic lung disease, tuberculosis, sarcoidosis, or emphysema
- Manifests commonly as hemoptysis: blood-streaked sputum to active bleeding necessitating surgical reaction
- Many are asymptomatic

INVASIVE ASPERGILLOSIS:
- Patients with prolonged and profound granulocytopenia are predisposed to rapidly progressive *Aspergillus* pneumonia
- Lungs typically manifest a necrotizing bronchopneumonia, ranging from small areas of infiltrate to intensive bilateral hemorrhagic infarction
- Most common presentation is that of unremitting fever and a new pulmonary infiltrate despite broad-spectrum antibiotic therapy in an immunosuppressed patient
- Dyspnea and nonproductive cough are common; sudden pleuritic pain and tachycardia, sometimes with a pleural rub, may mimic pulmonary embolism; hemoptysis is uncommon
- Roentgenograms may reveal patchy bronchopneumonic, nodular densities, consolidation, or cavitation
- Immunocompromised patients: invasive pulmonary *Aspergillus* (IPA) generally is acute and evolves over days to weeks; less commonly, patients with normal or only mild abnormalities of their immune systems may develop a more chronic, slowly progressive form of IPA

EXTRAPULMONARY DISSEMINATION:
- Cerebral infarction from hematogenous dissemination may occur in immunosuppressed individuals
- Abscess formation may occur from direct extension of invasive disease in the sinuses
- Esophageal or gastrointestinal ulcerations caused by *Aspergillus* may occur in the immunosuppressed host
- Fatal perforation of the viscus or bowel infarction may occur
- Necrotizing skin ulcers involving the extremities (Fig. 1-44)
- Osteomyelitis
- Endocarditis

Patients with AIDS and a CD4 count of below 50 mm³ have increased susceptibility to invasive aspergillosis.

DIAGNOSIS

DIFFERENTIAL DIAGNOSIS
- Tuberculosis
- Cystic fibrosis
- Carcinoma of the lung
- Eosinophilic pneumonia
- Bronchiectasis
- Sarcoidosis
- Lung abscess

WORKUP
Physical examination and laboratory evaluation

LABORATORY TESTS
ALLERGIC BRONCHOPULMONARY ASPERGILLOSIS:
1. Peripheral blood eosinophilia
2. Skin test with *Aspergillus* antigenic extract usually is positive but is nonspecific
3. *Aspergillus* serum precipitating antibody is present in 70% to 100% of cases
4. Sputum cultures may be positive for *Aspergillus* spp. but are nonspecific

ASPERGILLOMAS:
1. Sputum culture
2. Serum precipitating antibody

INVASIVE ASPERGILLOSIS:
Definitive diagnosis requires the demonstration of tissue invasion as seen on a biopsy specimen (i.e., septate, acute branching hyphae) or a positive culture from the tissue obtained by an invasive procedure such as transbronchial biopsy.
1. Sputum and nasal cultures: in high-risk patients a positive culture is strongly suggestive of invasive aspergillosis.
2. Serologic studies not helpful, rarely elevated in patients with invasive disease
3. Blood cultures: usually negative
4. Lung biopsy is necessary for definitive diagnosis
5. Biopsy and culture of extrapulmonary lesions

IMAGING STUDIES
ALLERGIC BRONCHOPULMONARY ASPERGILLOSIS:
- Chest roentgenograms show a variety of abnormalities from small, patchy, fleeting infiltrates (commonly in the upper lobes) to lobar consolidation and/or cavitation
- A majority of patients eventually develop central bronchiectasis

ASPERGILLOMAS:
Chest roentgenograms or CT scans usually show the characteristic intracavity mass partially surrounded by a crescent of air (Fig. 1-45).

INVASIVE ASPERGILLOSIS:
Chest roentgenograms and CT scanning may reveal cavity formation.

TREATMENT

ACUTE GENERAL Rx
ALLERGIC BRONCHOPULMONARY ASPERGILLOSIS:
- Prednisone (0.5 to 1 mg/kg PO) until the chest roentgenogram has

cleared, followed by alternate-day therapy at 0.5 mg/kg PO (3 to 6 mo)
- Bronchodilators and physiotherapy
- Serial chest roentgenograms and serum IgE useful in guiding treatment
- Antifungals are not recommended

ASPERGILLOMAS:
- Controversial and problematic
- Up to 10% of aspergillomas may resolve clinically without overt pharmacologic or surgical intervention
- Observation for asymptomatic patients
- Surgical resection/arterial embolization for those patients with severe hemoptysis or life-threatening hemorrhage
- For those patients at risk for marked hemoptysis with inadequate pulmonary reserve, consider itraconazole 200 to 400 mg/day PO

INVASIVE ASPERGILLOSIS:
- Amphotericin B 0.8 to 1.2 mg/kg IV qd to a total dose of 2 to 2.5 g; itraconazole 200 to 400 mg/d PO for 1 yr
- Amphotericin B lipid complex (ABLC) 5 mg/kg IV qd in those intolerant of or refractory to amphotericin B
- Amphotericin B colloidal dispersion (ABCD) 3 to 6 mg/kg IV qd; stepwise approach in those who have failed amphotericin B
- Liposomal amphotericin B (L-AMB) 3 to 5 mg/kg IV q day; stepwise approach is indicated as empiric therapy for presumed fungal infection in febrile neutropenic patients who are refractory to or intolerant of amphotericin B
- Itraconazole 200 mg IV bid × 4 doses followed by 200 mg IV qd or

200 mg tid for 4 days, then 200 mg bid PO—first-line therapy if not taking p450 inducers.
- Voriconazole 6 mg/kg IV bid followed by 6 mg/kg IV for up to 27 days, then 400 mg/day PO for up to 24 weeks. Note that the optimal dose regimens have yet to be defined.

■ REFERRAL
Consultation with an infectious diseases specialist is highly recommended.

REFERENCE
Ferry TG, Yates RR: Aspergillomas: should we treat them all? *Infect Dis Clin Pract* 7:122, 1998.
Author: **Sajeev Handa, M.D.**

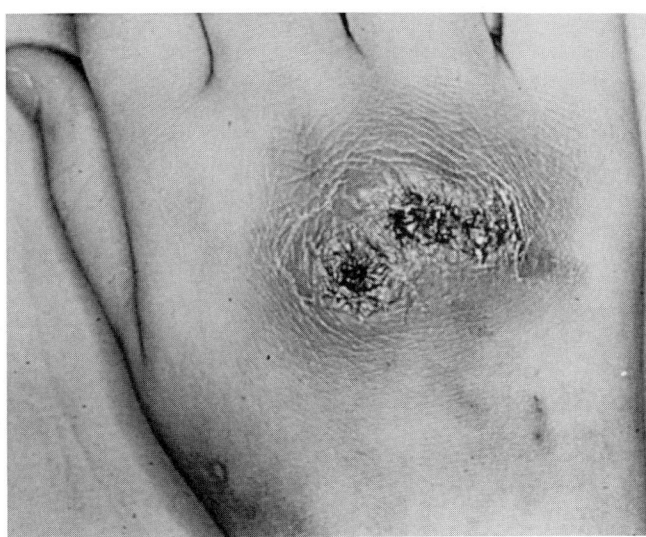

Fig. 1-44 Cutaneous aspergillosis in a patient with acute leukemia and marked neutropenia. The lesion developed at the site where a steel needle had been left for several days of intravenous infusion. (From Mandell GL [ed]: *Mandell, Douglas, and Bennett's principles and practice of infectious diseases,* ed 5, New York, 2000, Churchill Livingstone.)

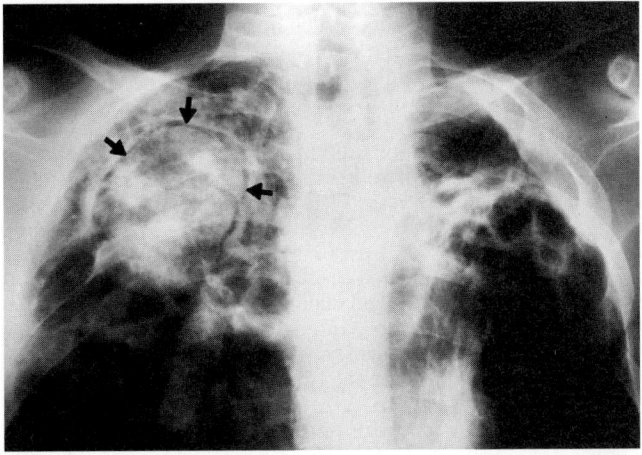

Fig. 1-45 Fungus ball or mycetoma caused by *Aspergillus.* Coned-down PA view of the chest of a patient with biapical fibrocavitary tuberculosis accompanied by volume loss. There is a mass in a large right upper-lobe cavity with air dissecting into the cavity producing "air crescents" *(arrows).* (From McLoud TC: *Thoracic radiology: the requisites,* St Louis, 1998, Mosby.)

BASIC INFORMATION

■ DEFINITION

The American Thoracic Society defines asthma as a "disease characterized by an increased responsiveness of the trachea and bronchi to various stimuli and manifested by a widespread narrowing of the airways that changes in severity either spontaneously or as a result of treatment." *Status asthmaticus* can be defined as a severe continuous bronchospasm.

■ SYNONYMS

Bronchospasm
Reactive airway disease
Bronchial asthma

ICD-9CM CODES
493.9 Asthma, unspecified
493.1 Intrinsic asthma
493.0 Extrinsic asthma

■ EPIDEMIOLOGY & DEMOGRAPHICS
- Asthma affects 5% of the population.
- It is more common in children (10% of children, 5% of adults).
- 50% to 80% of children with asthma develop symptoms before 5 yr of age.
- Overall asthma mortality in the U.S. is 20 per 1 million persons.

■ PHYSICAL FINDINGS & CLINICAL PRESENTATION
Physical examination varies with the stage and severity of asthma and may reveal only increased inspiratory and expiratory phases of respiration. Physical examination during status asthmaticus may reveal:
- Tachycardia and tachypnea
- Use of accessory respiratory muscles
- Pulsus paradoxus (inspiratory decline in systolic blood pressure >10 mm Hg)
- Wheezing: absence of wheezing (silent chest) or decreased wheezing can indicate worsening obstruction
- Mental status changes: generally secondary to hypoxia and hypercapnia and constitute an indication for urgent intubation
- Paradoxic abdominal and diaphragmatic movement on inspiration (detected by palpation over the upper part of the abdomen in a semirecumbent position): important sign of impending respiratory crisis, indicates diaphragmatic fatigue
- The following abnormalities in vital signs are indicative of severe asthma:
  1. Pulsus paradoxus >18 mm Hg
  2. Respiratory rate >30 breaths/min
  3. Tachycardia with heart rate >120 beats/min

■ ETIOLOGY
- Intrinsic asthma: occurs in patients who have no history of allergies; may be triggered by upper respiratory infections or psychologic stress
- Extrinsic asthma (allergic asthma): brought on by exposure to allergens (e.g., dust mites, cat allergen, industrial chemicals)
- Exercise-induced asthma: seen most frequently in adolescents; manifests with bronchospasm following initiation of exercise and improves with discontinuation of exercise
- Drug-induced asthma: often associated with use of NSAIDs, β-blockers, sulfites, certain foods and beverages

DIAGNOSIS

■ DIFFERENTIAL DIAGNOSIS
- CHF
- COPD
- Pulmonary embolism (in adult and elderly patients)
- Foreign body aspiration (most frequent in younger patients)
- Pneumonia and other upper respiratory infections
- Rhinitis with postnasal drip
- TB
- Hypersensitivity pneumonitis
- Anxiety disorder
- Wegener's granulomatosis
- Diffuse interstitial lung disease
- The differential diagnosis of childhood asthma is described in Table 2-16.

■ WORKUP
Medical history, physical examination, pulmonary function studies and peak flow meter determination, blood gas analysis and oximetry (during acute bronchospasm), chest radiography if infection is suspected

■ LABORATORY TESTS
Laboratory tests can be normal if obtained during a stable period. The following laboratory abnormalities may be present during an acute bronchospasm:
- ABGs can be used in staging the severity of an asthmatic attack:
  Mild: decreased PaO_2 and $PaCO_2$, increased pH
  Moderate: decreased PaO_2, normal $PaCO_2$, normal pH
  Severe: marked decreased PaO_2, increased $PaCO_2$, and decreased pH
- CBC, leukocytosis with "left shift" may indicate the existence of bacterial infection.
- Sputum: eosinophils, Charcot-Leyden crystals; PMNs, and bacteria may be found on Gram stain in patients with pneumonia.

- Useful diagnostic tests for asthma:
  1. Pulmonary function studies: during acute severe bronchospasm, FEV_1 is <1 L and peak expiratory flow rate (PEFR) <80 L/min
  2. Methacholine challenge test
  3. Skin test: to assess the role of atopy (when suspected)

■ IMAGING STUDIES
- Chest x-ray film: usually normal, may show evidence of thoracic hyperinflation (e.g., flattening of the diaphragm, increased volume over the retrosternal air space)
- ECG: tachycardia, nonspecific ST-T wave changes; may also show cor pulmonale, right bundle-branch block, right axial deviation, counterclockwise rotation

TREATMENT

■ NONPHARMACOLOGIC THERAPY
- Avoidance of triggering factors (e.g., salicylates, sulfites)
- Encouragement of regular exercise (e.g., swimming)
- Patient education regarding warning signs of an attack and proper use of medications (e.g., correct use of inhalers)

■ ACUTE GENERAL Rx
The Expert Panel of the National Asthma Education and Prevention Program (NAEPP) based on the classification of asthma severity (Table 1-14) recommends the following stepwise approach in the pharmacologic management of asthma in adults and children older than 5 yr:

STEP 1 (MILD INTERMITTENT ASTHMA): No daily medications are needed.
- Short-acting inhaled β₂-agonists as needed (e.g., albuterol [Ventolin, Proventil], terbutaline [Brethaire], bitolterol [Tornalate], pirbuterol [Maxair])

STEP 2 (MILD PERSISTENT ASTHMA): Daily treatment may be needed.
- Low-dose inhaled corticosteroid (e.g., beclomethasone [Beclovent, Vanceril], flunisolide [AeroBid], triamcinolone [Azmacort]) can be used.
- Cromolyn (Intal) or nedocromil (Tilade) can also be used.
- Additional considerations for long-term control are the use of leukotriene receptor antagonists—montelukast (Singulair) or safirlukast (Accolade).
- Quick relief of asthma can be achieved with short-acting inhaled β₂-agonists (see above).

STEP 3 (MODERATE PERSISTENT ASTHMA): Daily medication is recommended.

- Low-dose or medium-dose inhaled corticosteroids (See above) plus long-acting inhaled β_2-agonist (salmeterol [Serevent]), or long-acting oral β_2-agonists (e.g., albuterol, sustained-release tablets). Salmeterol is also available as a dry powder inhaler (Discus) that does not require a spacer device; the dosage is one puff bid. A salmeterol-fluticasone combination for the Disnus inhaler (Advair) is now available and simplifies therapy for patients with asthma. It generally should be reserved for patients with at least moderately severe asthma not controlled by an inhaled corticosteroid alone.
- Use short-acting inhaled β-agonists on a PRN basis for quick relief.

STEP 4 (SEVERE PERSISTENT ASTHMA):

- Daily treatment with high-dose inhaled corticosteroids plus long-acting inhaled β-agonists (e.g., long-acting oral β_2-agonist plus long-term systemic corticosteroids (e.g., methylprednisolone, prednisolone, prednisone) can be used.

- Short-acting β_2-agonists can be used on a PRN basis for quick relief.

Treatment of *status asthmaticus* is as follows:

- Oxygen generally started at 2 to 4 L/min via nasal cannula or Venti-Mask at 40% Fio_2; further adjustments are made according to the ABGs.
- Sympathomimetics: various agents and modalities are available.
  1. Epinephrine (1:1000 dilution)
     a. Dosage range is 0.3 to 0.5 ml SC; may repeat after 15 to 20 min.
     b. Onset of action is within 15 min.
     c. Duration is 1 to 4 hr.
     d. Use with caution in patients >40 yr or anyone with heart disease.
  2. Terbutaline (Brethine)
     a. May be given SC, 0.25 mg q6-8h.
     b. Clinically significant increase in FEV_1 occurs within 15 min and persists 90 min to 4 hr.
     c. Generally, has fewer cardiac stimulating effects than epinephrine; however, systemic vasodilation with compensatory tachycardia can occur.

3. Metaproterenol (Alupent)
   a. May be administered via aerosol nebulizer, bulb nebulizer, or IPPB (e.g., 0.3 ml of metaproterenol in 3 ml of saline solution, given via nebulizer).
   b. Onset of action is within 5 min; duration is 3 to 4 hr.
4. Isotharine (Bronkosol): 0.25 to 0.5 ml in 3 ml of saline solution via nebulizer q4h is also effective; however, its duration is less than that of metaproterenol.
5. Albuterol (Proventil, Ventolin): 0.5 to 1 ml (2.5 to 5 mg) in 3 ml of saline solution tid or qid via nebulizer.

- Corticosteroids
  1. Early administration is advised, particularly in patients using steroids at home.
  2. Patients may be started on hydrocortisone (Solu-Cortef) 2.5 to 4 mg/kg or methylprednisolone (Solu-Medrol) 0.5 to 1 mg/kg IV loading dose, then q6h PRN; higher doses may be necessary in selected patients (particularly those receiving steroids at home); steroids given by inhalation (e.g., beclomethasone 2 inhalations qid,

TABLE 1-14   Classification of Asthma Severity

CLINICAL FEATURES BEFORE TREATMENT*	SYMPTOMS†	NIGHTTIME SYMPTOMS	LUNG FUNCTION
Step 4			
Severe Persistent	Continual symptoms Limited physical activity Frequent exacerbations	Frequent	■ FEV_1 or PEFR ≤60% predicted ■ PEFR variability >30%
Step 3			
Moderate Persistent	Daily symptoms Daily use of inhaled short-acting β_2-agonist Exacerbations affect activity Exacerbations ≥2 times a week; may last days	>1 time a week	■ FEV_1 or PEFR >60%-<80% predicted ■ PEFR variability >30%
Step 2			
Mild Persistent	Symptoms >2 times a week but <1 time a day Exacerbations may affect activity	>2 times a month	■ FEV_1 or PEFR ≥80% predicted ■ PEFR variability 20%-30%
Step 1			
Mild Intermittent	Symptoms ≤2 times a week Asymptomatic and normal PEFR between exacerbations Exacerbations brief (from a few hours to a few days); intensity may vary	≤2 times a month	■ FEV_1 or PEFR ≥80% predicted ■ PEFR variability <20%

Modified from National Asthma Education and Prevention Program, National Heart, Lung, and Blood Institute, Expert Panel Report 2: *Guidelines for the diagnosis and management of asthma.* Washington, DC, NIH Pub No 97-4051, July 1997.

*The presence of one of the features of severity is sufficient to place a patient in that category. An individual should be assigned to the most severe grade in which any feature occurs. The characteristics noted in this figure are general and may overlap because asthma is highly variable. Furthermore, an individual's classification may change over time.

†Patients at any level of severity can have mild, moderate, or severe exacerbations. Some patients with intermittent asthma experience severe and life-threatening exacerbations separated by long periods of normal lung function and no symptoms.

PEFR, Peak expiratory flow rate.

maximum 20 inhalations/day) are also useful for controlling bronchospasm and tapering oral steroids and should be used in all patients with severe asthma.

3. Rapid but judicious tapering of corticosteroids will eliminate serious steroid toxicity; long-term low-dose methotrexate may be an effective means of reducing the systemic corticosteroid requirement in some patients with severe refractory asthma.

4. The most common errors regarding steroid therapy in acute bronchospasms are the use of "too little, too late" and too rapid tapering with return of bronchospasm.

• Atropine analog (e.g., ipratropium bromide [Atrovent] 2 inhalations qid, maximum 12 inhalations in 24 hr) is useful in patients not responding well to β-agonists and whose bronchospasm is secondary to bronchitis; when ipratropium is used with a β₂-agonist there is additive effect.

• Theophylline or aminophylline
1. Its role in acute exacerbation of asthma has been questioned; IV theophylline or aminophylline has been used in patients with asthma because of its primary bronchodilating effect and its antiinflammatory actions. However, most studies indicate that in patients with acute asthma, the addition of IV aminophylline to β₂-agonists does not lead to additional bronchodilation and may result in significant adverse effects.

2. Most authorities now believe that aminophylline should not be used routinely in the treatment of acute exacerbations of asthma. The addition of aminophylline may be justified only for those few patients who do not respond to β-agonists, corticosteroids, and anticholinergic medications. Aminophylline has potential toxic effects (e.g., cardiac arrhythmias, seizures).

3. When used, frequent monitoring of blood levels is indicated to prevent toxicity, particularly in elderly patients.

• IV hydration: judicious use is necessary to avoid CHF in elderly patients.

• IV antibiotics are indicated when there is suspicion of bacterial infection (e.g., infiltrate on chest x-ray, fever, or leukocytosis).

• Intubation and mechanical ventilation are indicated when above measures fail to produce significant improvement.

• General anesthesia: halothane may reverse bronchospasm in a severe asthmatic who cannot be ventilated adequately by mechanical means.

• IV magnesium sulfate supplementation in children with low or borderline-low magnesium levels may improve acute bronchospasm.

Several reports in recent literature point to the beneficial effect on bronchospasm with a 20-min infusion of 40 mg/kg, up to a maximum of 2 g of magnesium sulfate in patients with acute asthma attack.

• Fig. 1-46 describes management of asthma exacerbations in the emergency department and for inpatients.

• Fig. 1-47 describes home management of acute asthma.

■ REFFERRAL
Box 1-7 describes indications for referral to an asthma specialist.

☼ PEARLS & CONSIDERATIONS

■ COMMENTS
Additional patient information on asthma can be obtained from the Asthma and Allergy Foundation of America, Suite 305, Washington, DC 20036.

REFERENCES
Ciarallo L et al: Higher dose IV magnesium therapy for children with moderate to severe acute asthma, *Arch Pediatr Adol Med* 154:979, 2000.

Holgate ST: Therapeutic options for persistent asthma, *JAMA* 285:2637, 2001.

National Asthma Education and Prevention Program: *Expert panel report 2: guidelines for diagnosis and management of asthma*, Bethesda, Md, 1997, National Institutes of Health.

Naureckas ET, Solway J: Mild asthma, *N Engl J Med* 345:1257, 2001.

Parameswaran K et al: Ashilition of IV aminophylline to beta-2 agonists in adults with acute asthma, *Cochrane Database Syst Rev* 200.

Author: **Fred F. Ferri, M.D.**

BOX 1-7 Possible Indications for Referral to an Asthma Specialist

Severe, acute asthma that has caused loss of consciousness, hypoxia, respiratory failure, convulsions, or near death

Poorly controlled asthma as indicated by admission to a hospital, frequent need for emergency care, need for oral corticosteroids, absence from school or work, disruption of sleep, interference with quality of life

Severe, persistent asthma requiring step 4 care (consider for patients who require step 3 care)

Patient less than 3 years old who requires step 3 or 4 care (consider for patient less than 3 years old who requires step 2 care)

Requirement for continuous oral corticosteroids or high-dose inhaled corticosteroids or more than two short courses of oral corticosteroids within 1 year

Need for additional diagnostic testing such as allergy skin testing, rhinoscopy, provocative challenge, complete pulmonary function testing, bronchoscopy

Consideration for immunotherapy

Need for additional education regarding asthma, complications of asthma and treatment of asthma, problems with adherence to management recommendations, or allergen avoidance

Uncertainty of diagnosis

Complications of asthma, including sinusitis, nasal polyposis, aspergillosis, severe rhinitis, vocal cord dysfunction, gastroesophageal reflux

Modified from National Asthma Education and Prevention Program, National Heart, Lung, and Blood Institute, Expert Panel Report 2: *Guidelines for the diagnosis and management of asthma.* Washington, DC, NIH Pub No 97-4051, July 1997.

TABLE 1-15   Classification of Severity of Acute Asthma Exacerbations

	MILD	MODERATE	SEVERE	RESPIRATORY ARREST IMMINENT
Symptoms				
Breathlessness	While walking	While talking (infant—softer, shorter cry; difficulty feeding)	While at rest (infant—stops feeding)	
	Can lie down	Prefers sitting	Sits upright	
Talks in	Sentences	Phrases	Words	
Alertness	May be agitated	Usually agitated	Usually agitated	Drowsy or confused
Signs				
Respiratory rate	Increased	Increased	Often >30/min	
Use of accessory muscles; suprasternal retractions	Usually not	Commonly	Usually	Paradoxical thoracoabdominal movement
Wheeze	Moderate, often only end expiratory	Loud; throughout exhalation	Usually loud; throughout inhalation and exhalation	Absence of wheeze
Pulse/minute	<100	100-120	>120	Bradycardia
Pulsus paradoxus	Absent <10 mg Hg	May be present 10-25 mm Hg	Often present >25 mm Hg (adult) 20-40 mm Hg (child)	Absence suggests respiratory muscle fatigue

Guide on rates of breathing in awake children:

Age	Normal Rate
<2 mo	<60/min
2-12 mo	<50/min
1-5 yr	<40/min
6-8 yr	<30/min

Guide to normal pulse rates in children:

Age	Normal Rate
2-12 mo	<160/min
1-2 yr	<120/min
2-8 yr	<110/min

Functional Assessment				
PEF % predicted or % personal best	80%	Approx. 50%-80%	<50% predicted or personal best or response lasts <2 hr	
Pao_2 (on air)	Normal (test not usually necessary)	>60 mm Hg (test not usually necessary)	<60 mm Hg: possible cyanosis	
and/or				
Pco_2	<42 mm Hg (test not usually necessary)	<42 mm Hg (test not usually necessary)	≥42 mm Hg: possible respiratory failure	
Sao_2 % (on air) at sea level	>95% (test not usually necessary)	91%-95%	<91%	

Hypercapnia (hypoventilation) develops more readily in young children than in adults and adolescents.

NOTE:
- The presence of several parameters, but not necessarily all, indicates the general classification of the exacerbation.
- Many of these parameters have not been systematically studied, so they serve only as general guides.

From National Asthma Education and Prevention Program, National Heart, Lung, and Blood Institute, Expert Panel Report 2: *Guidelines for the diagnosis and management of asthma.* NIH Pub No 97, July 1997.

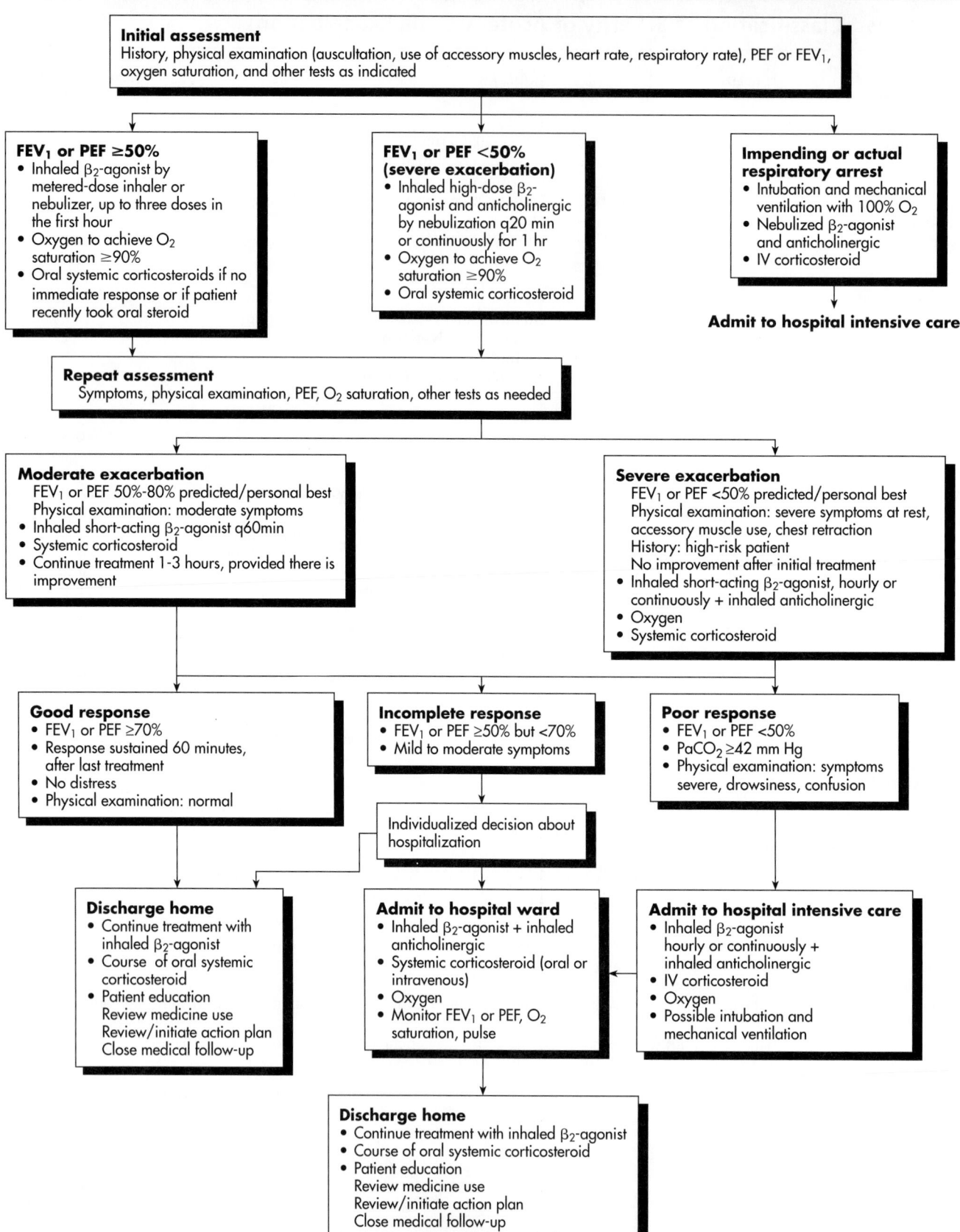

Initial assessment
History, physical examination (auscultation, use of accessory muscles, heart rate, respiratory rate), PEF or FEV₁, oxygen saturation, and other tests as indicated

FEV₁ or PEF ≥50%
- Inhaled β₂-agonist by metered-dose inhaler or nebulizer, up to three doses in the first hour
- Oxygen to achieve O₂ saturation ≥90%
- Oral systemic corticosteroids if no immediate response or if patient recently took oral steroid

FEV₁ or PEF <50% (severe exacerbation)
- Inhaled high-dose β₂-agonist and anticholinergic by nebulization q20 min or continuously for 1 hr
- Oxygen to achieve O₂ saturation ≥90%
- Oral systemic corticosteroid

Impending or actual respiratory arrest
- Intubation and mechanical ventilation with 100% O₂
- Nebulized β₂-agonist and anticholinergic
- IV corticosteroid

Admit to hospital intensive care

Repeat assessment
Symptoms, physical examination, PEF, O₂ saturation, other tests as needed

Moderate exacerbation
FEV₁ or PEF 50%-80% predicted/personal best
Physical examination: moderate symptoms
- Inhaled short-acting β₂-agonist q60min
- Systemic corticosteroid
- Continue treatment 1-3 hours, provided there is improvement

Severe exacerbation
FEV₁ or PEF <50% predicted/personal best
Physical examination: severe symptoms at rest, accessory muscle use, chest retraction
History: high-risk patient
No improvement after initial treatment
- Inhaled short-acting β₂-agonist, hourly or continuously + inhaled anticholinergic
- Oxygen
- Systemic corticosteroid

Good response
- FEV₁ or PEF ≥70%
- Response sustained 60 minutes, after last treatment
- No distress
- Physical examination: normal

Incomplete response
- FEV₁ or PEF ≥50% but <70%
- Mild to moderate symptoms

Poor response
- FEV₁ or PEF <50%
- PaCO₂ ≥42 mm Hg
- Physical examination: symptoms severe, drowsiness, confusion

Individualized decision about hospitalization

Discharge home
- Continue treatment with inhaled β₂-agonist
- Course of oral systemic corticosteroid
- Patient education
  Review medicine use
  Review/initiate action plan
  Close medical follow-up

Admit to hospital ward
- Inhaled β₂-agonist + inhaled anticholinergic
- Systemic corticosteroid (oral or intravenous)
- Oxygen
- Monitor FEV₁ or PEF, O₂ saturation, pulse

Admit to hospital intensive care
- Inhaled β₂-agonist hourly or continuously + inhaled anticholinergic
- IV corticosteroid
- Oxygen
- Possible intubation and mechanical ventilation

Discharge home
- Continue treatment with inhaled β₂-agonist
- Course of oral systemic corticosteroid
- Patient education
  Review medicine use
  Review/initiate action plan
  Close medical follow-up

Fig. 1-46   Management of asthma exacerbations: emergency department and hospital-based care. *FEV₁,* Forced expiratory volume in 1 second; *PEF,* peak expiratory flow. (From National Asthma Education and Prevention Program: *Guidelines for the diagnosis and management of asthma,* NIH Pub No 97-4051A, Bethesda, Md, 1997, National Institutes of Health, National Heart, Lung, and Blood Institute.)

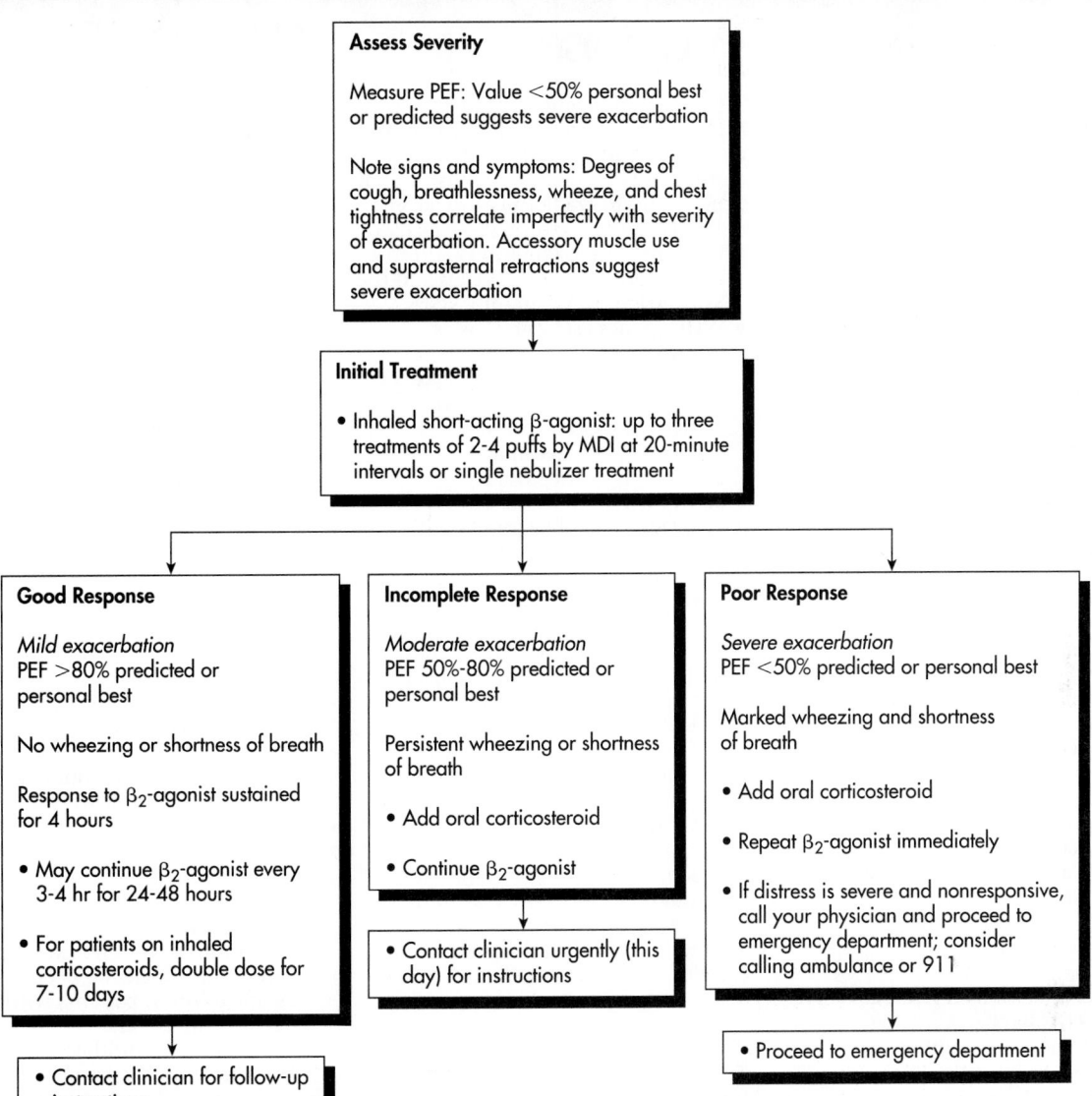

Assess Severity

Measure PEF: Value <50% personal best or predicted suggests severe exacerbation

Note signs and symptoms: Degrees of cough, breathlessness, wheeze, and chest tightness correlate imperfectly with severity of exacerbation. Accessory muscle use and suprasternal retractions suggest severe exacerbation

Initial Treatment

• Inhaled short-acting β-agonist: up to three treatments of 2-4 puffs by MDI at 20-minute intervals or single nebulizer treatment

Good Response

Mild exacerbation
PEF >80% predicted or personal best

No wheezing or shortness of breath

Response to β$_2$-agonist sustained for 4 hours

• May continue β$_2$-agonist every 3-4 hr for 24-48 hours

• For patients on inhaled corticosteroids, double dose for 7-10 days

Incomplete Response

Moderate exacerbation
PEF 50%-80% predicted or personal best

Persistent wheezing or shortness of breath

• Add oral corticosteroid

• Continue β$_2$-agonist

Poor Response

Severe exacerbation
PEF <50% predicted or personal best

Marked wheezing and shortness of breath

• Add oral corticosteroid

• Repeat β$_2$-agonist immediately

• If distress is severe and nonresponsive, call your physician and proceed to emergency department; consider calling ambulance or 911

• Contact clinician urgently (this day) for instructions

• Proceed to emergency department

• Contact clinician for follow-up instructions

Fig. 1-47   Home management of acute asthma. *MDI,* Metered dose inhaler; *PEF,* peak expiratory flow rate. (Modified from National Asthma Education and Prevention Program, National Heart, Lung, and Blood Institute, Expert Panel Report 2: *Guidelines for the diagnosis and management of asthma,* NIH Pub No 97-4051, July 1997.)

BASIC INFORMATION

■ DEFINITION
Astrocytoma refers to a brain neoplasia arising from glial precursor cells (astrocytes).

■ SYNONYMS
Astroglial neoplasms

ICD-9CM CODES
191.9 Astrocytoma, unspecified site

■ EPIDEMIOLOGY & DEMOGRAPHICS
- Incidence of primary brain tumors is 6/100,000 persons.
- Approximately 18,000 primary brain tumors are diagnosed each year in the United States.
- In adults, glioblastoma is the most common brain tumor, followed by meningioma and astrocytoma. In children, astrocytomas are second only to medulloblastoma.
- Astrocytomas can be found at all ages, with an early peak between 0 to 4 years of age followed by a trough between the ages of 15 to 24 and then a steady rise in incidence occurs.
- Peak age incidence of low-grade astrocytoma is 34 yr.
- Peak age incidence of anaplastic astrocytoma is 41 yr.
- Peak age incidence of glioblastoma is 53 yr.

■ PHYSICAL FINDINGS & CLINICAL PRESENTATION
- Astrocytomas classically present with any one or more of the following features:
  1. Headache
  2. New-onset seizure
  3. Nausea and vomiting
  4. Focal neurologic deficit
  5. Change in mental status
  6. Papilledema

■ ETIOLOGY
- The specific etiology of astrocytoma is unknown.
- Genetic abnormalities leading to defective tumor suppressing genes or activation of protooncogenes has been proposed.

DIAGNOSIS

A provisional diagnosis of astrocytoma is made on clinical grounds and radiographic imaging studies. Tissue pathology is needed to establish the diagnosis and to grade the astrocytoma.
- Two common grading systems used for astrocytomas are the World Health Organization (WHO) and the Saint Anne–Mayo grading system.
- WHO grades astrocytomas as follows:
  1. Grade I juvenile pilocytic astrocytoma, subependymal giant cell astrocytoma, and peliomorphic xanthroastrocytoma.
  2. Grade II astrocytoma
  3. Grade III anaplastic astrocytoma
  4. Grade IV glioblastoma multiforme
- The Saint Anne–Mayo system grades astrocytomas according to the presence or absence of four histologic features: nuclear atypia, mitoses, endothelial proliferation, and necrosis.
  1. Grade I tumors have none of the features.
  2. Grade II tumors have one feature.
  3. Grade III tumors have two features.
  4. Grade IV tumors have three or more features.
- Grades I and II astrocytomas are commonly called low-grade astrocytomas.
- Grades III and IV astrocytomas are called high-grade malignant astrocytomas.

■ DIFFERENTIAL DIAGNOSIS
The differential diagnosis is vast and includes any cause of headache, seizures, change in mental status, and focal neurologic deficits.

■ WORKUP
A CT scan or MRI of the head essentially makes the diagnosis of an intracranial brain tumor. However, tissue is needed to establish a diagnosis of astrocytoma.

■ LABORATORY TESTS
Blood tests are not very specific in the diagnosis of astrocytoma.

■ IMAGING STUDIES
MRI is the diagnostic imaging study of choice (Fig. 1-48). MRI and MRA are used to locate the margins of the tumor, distinguish vascular masses from tumors, detect low-grade astrocytomas not seen by CT scan, and provide clear views of the posterior fossa.

■ ACUTE GENERAL Rx
- Surgery is the initial treatment of almost all astrocytomas. Surgery helps in:
  1. Establishing a pathologic diagnosis
  2. Debulking the tumor
  3. Alleviating intracranial pressure
  4. Offering complete excision with hope for a cure
- Before surgery, dexamethasone 10 mg IV is given followed by 4 to 6 mg IV q6h.
- Phenytoin 300 mg qd is used for seizure control.

■ CHRONIC Rx
- Radiation therapy is used postoperatively in patients with low-grade astrocytoma (controversial) and in high-grade astrocytoma. Some authorities recommend waiting for symptoms to occur following surgery in patients with low-grade astrocytoma before using XRT.
- Chemotherapy has not been recommended in low-grade astrocytoma.
- Chemotherapeutic drugs carmustine and lomustine have been used with some effect in patients with high-grade astrocytoma.
- High-dose chemotherapy followed by autologous bone marrow transplantation is a consideration.

■ DISPOSITION
- Approximately 10% to 35% of astrocytomas (usually grade I pilocytic astrocytomas) are amenable to complete surgical excision and cure.
- The management of low-grade astrocytomas depends in part on the location of the tumor.
- In low-grade astrocytomas, the tumor is more infiltrative and therefore not amenable to complete excision. Nevertheless, most studies recommend surgery to remove as much of the tumor burden as possible.

- The prognosis of patients with low-grade astrocytoma is highly variable. A median of 7 yr is cited.
- Malignant astrocytomas, grades III and IV, usually require surgery for debulking. It is not known from prospective studies if surgery improves survival; however, retrospective studies suggest a survival benefit in the surgical treated group.
- Median survival for patients with high-grade astrocytomas is 2 yr for anaplastic type and 1 yr for glioblastoma multiforme.

■ REFERRAL
A team of specialty consultations is indicated in patients diagnosed with astrocytoma. A neurosurgeon, radiation oncologist, and neurooncologist are all needed to assist in establishing the diagnosis and to provide immediate and follow-up treatment.

☼ PEARLS & CONSIDERATIONS

■ COMMENTS
- Anaplastic astrocytomas and glioblastomas constitute more than 60% of all primary brain tumors.

- Other treatment modalities including stereotaxic radiosurgery using a gamma knife and interstitial brachytherapy are available.

REFERENCES
Black PM: Brain tumors. Part 1. *N Engl J Med* 324(21):1471, 1991.
Black PM: Brain tumors. Part 2. *N Engl J Med* 324(22):1555, 1991.
Wen PY et al: High-grade astrocytomas, *Neurol Clin* 13(4):875, 1995.
Author: **Peter Petropoulos, M.D.**

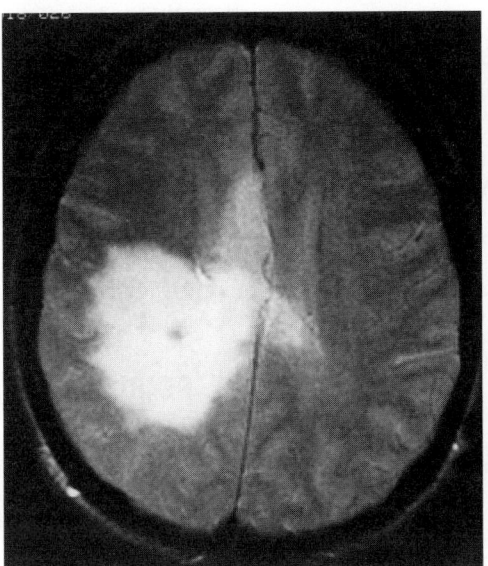
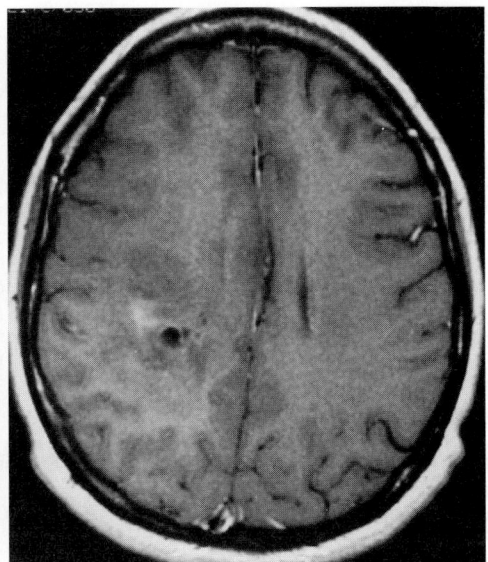

Fig. 1-48   Low-grade astrocytoma as imaged by MRI. On the left, T2-weighted image; on the right, T1-weighted image, gadolinium contrast with minimum enhancement. The images are typical of this tumor, which is being detected with increasing frequency in seizure patients by MRI. Many are invisible on CT scans. (From Goldman L, Bennett JC [eds]: *Cecil textbook of medicine,* ed 21, Philadelphia, 2000, WB Saunders.)

BASIC INFORMATION

■ DEFINITION
Atelectasis is the collapse of lung volume.

ICD-9CM CODES
518.0 Atelectasis

■ EPIDEMIOLOGY & DEMOGRAPHICS
- Occurs frequently in patients receiving mechanical ventilation with higher Fio_2
- Dependent regions of the lung are more prone to atelectasis: they are partially compressed, they are not as well ventilated, and there is no spontaneous drainage of secretions with gravity

■ PHYSICAL FINDINGS & CLINICAL PRESENTATION
- Decreased or absent breath sounds
- Abnormal chest percussion
- Cough, dyspnea, decreased vocal fremitus and vocal resonance
- Diminished chest expansion, tachypnea, tachycardia

■ ETIOLOGY
- Mechanical ventilation with higher Fio_2
- Chronic bronchitis
- Cystic fibrosis
- Endobronchial neoplasms
- Foreign bodies
- Infections (e.g., TB, histoplasmosis)
- Extrinsic bronchial compression from neoplasms, aneurysms of ascending aorta, enlarged left atrium
- Sarcoidosis
- Silicosis
- Anterior chest wall injury, pneumothorax
- Alveolar injury (e.g., toxic fumes, aspiration of gastric contents)
- Pleural effusion, expanding bullae
- Chest wall deformity (e.g., scoliosis)
- Muscular weaknesses or abnormalities (e.g., neuromuscular disease)
- Mucus plugs from asthma, allergic bronchopulmonary aspergillosis, postoperative state

DIAGNOSIS

■ DIFFERENTIAL DIAGNOSIS
- Neoplasm
- Pneumonia
- Encapsulated pleural effusion
- Abnormalities of brachiocephalic vein and of the left pulmonary ligament

■ WORKUP
- Chest x-ray (Fig. 1-49)
- CT scan and fiberoptic bronchoscopy (selected patients)

■ IMAGING STUDIES
- Chest x-ray will confirm diagnosis.
- CT scan is useful in patients with suspected endobronchial neoplasm or extrinsic bronchial compression.
- Fiberoptic bronchoscopy (selected patients) is useful for removal of foreign body or evaluation of endobronchial and peribronchial lesions.

TREATMENT

■ NONPHARMACOLOGIC THERAPY
- Deep breathing, mobilization of the patient
- Incentive spirometry
- Tracheal suctioning
- Humidification
- Chest physiotherapy with percussion and postural drainage

■ ACUTE GENERAL Rx
- Positive-pressure breathing (CPAP by face mask, positive end-expiratory pressure [PEEP] for patients on mechanical ventilation)
- Use of mucolytic agents (e.g., acetylcysteine [Mucomyst])
- Recombinant human DNase (dornase alpha) in patients with cystic fibrosis
- Bronchodilator therapy in selected patients

■ CHRONIC Rx
Chest physiotherapy, humidification of inspired air, frequent nasotracheal suctioning

■ DISPOSITION
Prognosis varies with the underlying etiology.

■ REFERRAL
- Bronchoscopy for removal of foreign body or plugs unresponsive to conservative treatment
- Surgical referral for removal of obstructing neoplasms

PEARLS & CONSIDERATIONS

■ COMMENTS
Patients should be educated that frequent changes of position are helpful in clearing secretions. Sitting the patient upright in a chair is recommended to increase both volume and vital capacity relative to the supine position.

Author: **Fred F. Ferri, M.D.**

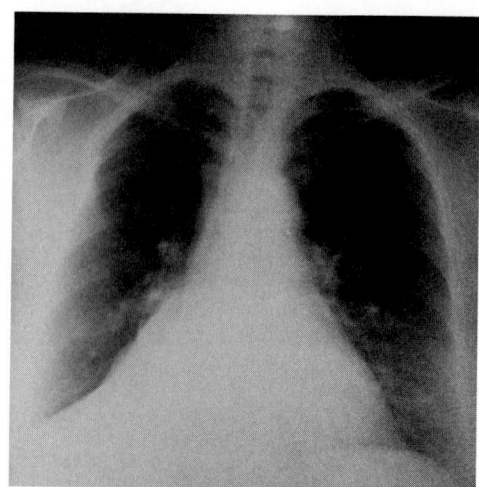

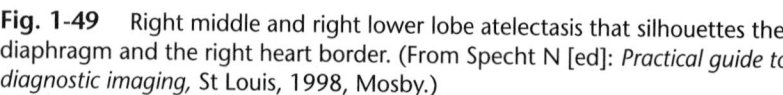

Fig. 1-49 Right middle and right lower lobe atelectasis that silhouettes the diaphragm and the right heart border. (From Specht N [ed]: *Practical guide to diagnostic imaging,* St Louis, 1998, Mosby.)

BASIC INFORMATION

■ DEFINITION
Atrial fibrillation is totally chaotic atrial activity caused by simultaneous discharge of multiple atrial foci.

■ SYNONYMS
AF
A-fib

■ ICD-9CM CODES
427.31 Atrial fibrillation

■ EPIDEMIOLOGY & DEMOGRAPHICS
The prevalence of atrial fibrillation increases with age, from 2% in the general population to 5% in patients older than 60 yr.

■ PHYSICAL FINDINGS & CLINICAL PRESENTATION
Clinical presentation is variable:
- Most common complaint: palpitations
- Fatigue, dizziness, light-headedness in some patients
- A few completely asymptomatic patients
- Cardiac auscultation revealing irregularly irregular rhythm

■ ETIOLOGY
- Coronary artery disease
- MS, MR, AS, AR
- Thyrotoxicosis
- Pulmonary embolism, COPD
- Pericarditis
- Myocarditis, cardiomyopathy
- Tachycardia-bradycardia syndrome
- Alcohol abuse
- MI
- WPW syndrome
- Other causes: left atrial myxoma, atrial septal defect, carbon monoxide poisoning, pheochromocytoma, idiopathic

DIAGNOSIS

■ DIFFERENTIAL DIAGNOSIS
- Multifocal atrial tachycardia
- Atrial flutter
- Frequent atrial premature beats

■ WORKUP
New-onset atrial fibrillation: ECG, echocardiogram, Holter monitor, and laboratory evaluation

■ LABORATORY TESTS
- TSH, free T_4
- Electrolytes

■ IMAGING STUDIES
- ECG (see Fig. 1-51 for "Atrial flutter and atrial fibrillation")
  1. Irregular, nonperiodic wave forms (best seen in V1) reflecting continuous atrial reentry
  2. Absence of P waves
  3. Conducted QRS complexes showing no periodicity
- Echocardiography to evaluate left atrial size and detect valvular disorders
- Holter monitor: useful to evaluate paroxysmal atrial fibrillation

TREATMENT

■ NONPHARMACOLOGIC THERAPY
- Avoidance of alcohol in patients with suspected excessive alcohol use
- Avoidance of caffeine and nicotine

■ ACUTE GENERAL Rx
- Fig. 1-50 describes an approach to the management of newly diagnosed atrial fibrillation or atrial fibrillation of recent onset.
- If the patient is hemodynamically stable, treatment options include IV diltiazem, verapamil, digoxin, or propranolol (Table 1-16).
- IV heparin or SC low-molecular-weight heparin
- Cardioversion is indicated if the ventricular rate is >140 bpm and the patient is symptomatic (particularly in acute MI, chest pain, dyspnea, CHF) or when there is no conversion to normal sinus rhythm after 3 days of pharmacologic therapy. The likelihood of cardioversion-related clinical thromboembolism is low in patients with atrial fibrillation lasting <48 hr. Patients with atrial fibrillation lasting >2 days have a 5% to 7% risk of clinical thromboembolism if cardioversion is not preceded by several weeks of warfarin therapy. However, if transesophageal echocardiography reveals no atrial thrombus, cardioversion may be performed safely after only a short period of anticoagulant therapy. Anticoagulant therapy should be continued for at least 1 mo after cardioversion to minimize the incidence of adverse thromboembolic events following conversion from atrial fibrillation to sinus rhythm.
- Anticoagulate with warfarin (unless patient has specific contraindications).

- Long-term anticoagulation with warfarin (adjusted to maintain an INR of 2 to 3) is indicated in all patients with atrial fibrillation and associated cardiovascular disease, including the following:
  1. Rheumatic valvular disease (MS, MR, AI)
  2. Aortic stenosis
  3. Prostatic mitral valve
  4. History of previous embolism
  5. Known cardiac thrombus
  6. CHF
  7. Cardiomyopathy with poor left ventricular function
  8. Nonrheumatic heart disease (e.g., hypertensive cardiovascular disease, coronary artery disease, ASD)
  9. Anticoagulation is generally not recommended in young patients with lone atrial fibrillation.

■ CHRONIC Rx
- Anticoagulation with warfarin (see "Acute General Rx")
- Rate control with digoxin

■ DISPOSITION
Factors associated with maintenance of sinus rhythm following cardioversion:
- Left atrium diameter <60 mm
- Absence of mitral valve disease
- Short duration of atrial fibrillation

■ REFERRAL
Surgical treatment of atrial fibrillation:
- The maze procedure with its recent modifications creating electrical barriers to the macroreentrant circuits that are thought to underlie atrial fibrillation is being performed with good results in several medical centers (preservation of sinus rhythm in >95% of patients without the use of long-term antiarrhythmic medication). Clear indications for its use remain undefined. Generally surgery is reserved for patients with rapid heart rate refractory to pharmacologic therapy or who cannot tolerate pharmacologic therapy.
- Catheter-based radiofrequency ablation procedures designed to eliminate atrial fibrillation are being performed; studies on long-term survival of these patients are pending.
- Implantable atrial defibrillators combine the option of atrial defibrillation with the capacity for ventricular defibrillation. Clinical experience for these devices remains limited. Their main indication is patients with highly symptomatic paroxysmal atrial fibrillation resistant to other therapies or patients with paroxysmal atrial fibrillation and coexisting ventricular arrhythmias.

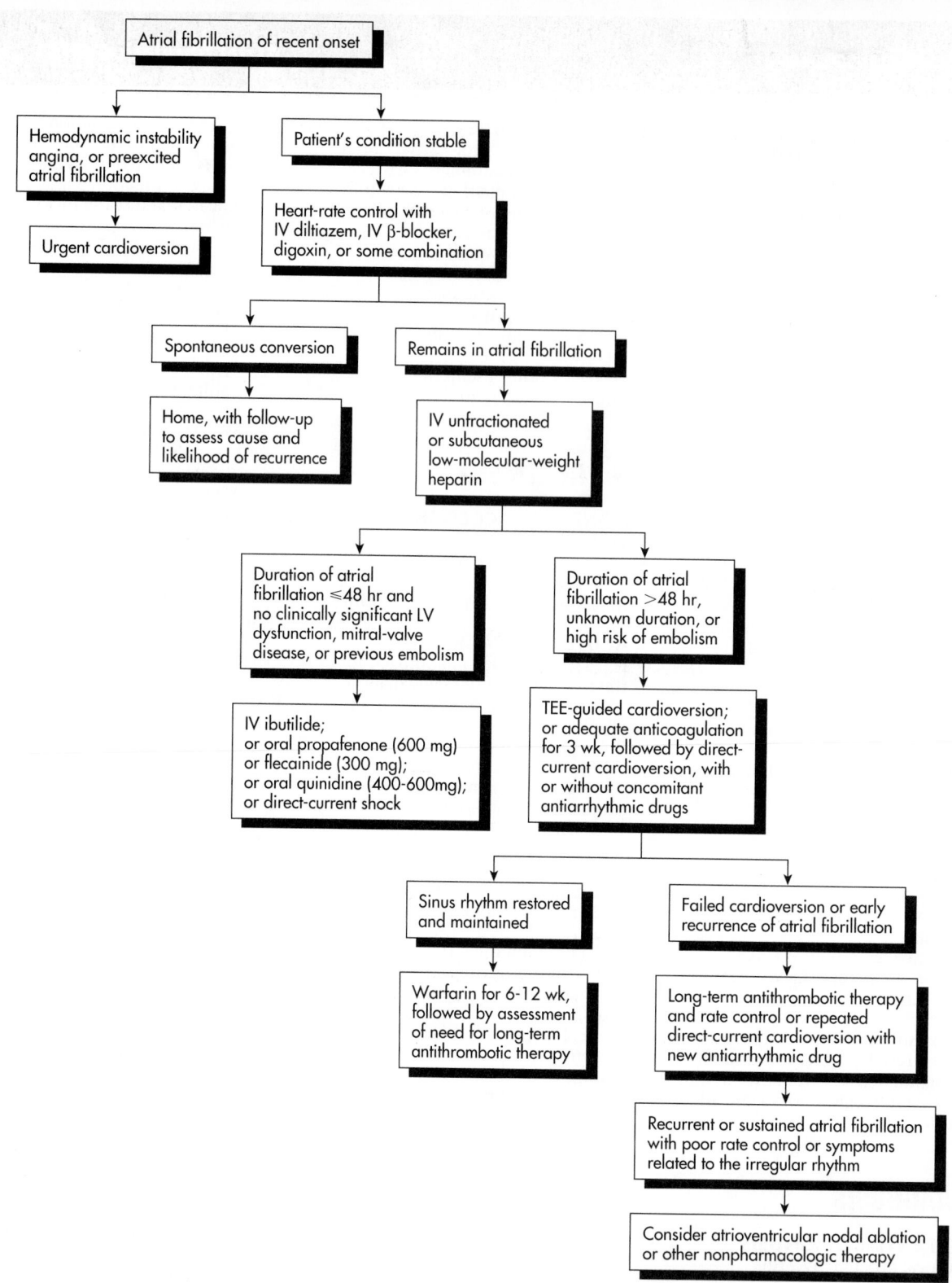

Fig. 1-50 **An approach to the management of newly diagnosed atrial fibrillation or atrial fibrillation of recent onset.** The pharmacologic therapies suggested for the termination of atrial fibrillation of less than 48 hours' duration are not presented in order of preference; to avoid drug interactions, no more than one should be used. Direct-current cardioversion can be attempted as the initial strategy or used if drug therapy fails. This figure does not detail the investigation into the cause of atrial fibrillation. Strong consideration should be given to the performance of echocardiography and thyroid-function tests, at minimum, for the evaluation of the cause and evaluation of ventricular function. Although low-molecular-weight heparin has not been compared in a clinical trial with unfractionated heparin in patients with atrial fibrillation of recent onset, it has been found at least as effective as unfractionated heparin in other situations when used for the prevention of arterial thromboembolism. It should also be noted that intravenous unfractionated heparin has never been formally evaluated as a therapy for atrial fibrillation of recent onset. Although the Food and Drug Administration has not approved low-molecular-weight heparin for use in atrial fibrillation, it is a logical alternative to intravenous unfractionated heparin. Both intravenous ibutilide and oral quinidine may provoke torsade de pointes. Although oral quinidine is quite effective for the termination of an episode of acute atrial fibrillation, long-term oral quinidine is not recommended for the maintenance of sinus rhythm. *IV,* Intravenous; *LV,* left ventricular; *TEE,* transesophageal echocardiography. (From Falk RH: *N Engl J Med,* 344[14]:1069, 2001.)

TABLE 1-16   Pharmacologic Heart-Rate Control in Atrial Fibrillation

DRUG	CONTROL OF ACUTE EPISODE	CONTROL OF SUSTAINED ATRIAL FIBRILLATION	COMMENTS
Calcium-channel blockers			
Diltiazem	20-mg bolus followed, if necessary, by 25 mg given 15 min later. Maintenance infusion of 5-15 mg/hr.	Oral controlled-release formulation, 180-300 mg daily.	Long-term control may be better with the addition of digoxin.
Verapamil	5-10 mg IV over 2-3 min, repeated once, 30 min later. Maintenance infusion rate is not reliably documented.	Slow-release formulation, 120-240 mg once or twice daily.	Causes elevation in digoxin level. May be more negatively inotropic than diltiazem.
Beta-blockers*			
Esmolol	0.5 mg/kg of body weight IV, repeated if necessary. Follow with infusion at 0.05 mg/kg/min, increasing as needed to 0.2 mg/kg/min.	Not available in oral forms.	Hypotension may be troublesome but responds to drug discontinuation.
Metoprolol	5-mg bolus IV, repeated twice at intervals of 2 min. No data on maintenance infusion.	50-400 mg daily in divided doses.	Useful if there is concomitant coronary disease.
Propranolol	1-5 mg IV, given over 10 min.	30-360 mg in divided doses or in long-acting form.	Noncardioselective: use cautiously in patients with a history of bronchospasm.
Digoxin	1.0-1.5 mg IV or orally over 24 hr in doses of 0.25 to 0.5 mg.	0.125-0.5 mg daily.	Renally excreted. Slow onset even if given IV, with less effective control than other agents, although may be synergistic with them. Poor efficacy for exertional heart-rate control.

From Falk RH: *N Engl J Med* 344(14):1070, 2001.
IV, Intravenously.
*The beta-blockers listed are representative of agents in this category. Other intravenous or oral beta-blockers may be equally acceptable.

☼ PEARLS & CONSIDERATIONS

■ COMMENTS

Aspirin may be a suitable alternative to warfarin in men >70 yr with increased risk of bleeding and in low risk patients (no recent history of CHF, previous thromboembolism, or systolic BP >160 mm Hg) between 65 and 75 yr of age.

- Amiodarone or sotalol can be used to maintain sinus rhythm in selected patients with recurrent, symptomatic atrial fibrillation. Both drugs are very expensive and associated with common side effects (pulmonary, GI, thyroid abnormalities).

REFERENCES
Falk RH: Atrial fibrillation, *N Engl J Med* 344:1067, 2001.
Klein AL et al: Use of transesophageal echocardiography to guide cardioversions in patients with atrial fibrillation, *N Engl J Med* 344:1411, 2001.
Roy D et al: Amiodarone to prevent recurrence of atrial fibrillation, *N Engl J Med* 342:13, 2000.
Author: **Fred F. Ferri, M.D.**

BASIC INFORMATION

■ DEFINITION
Atrial flutter is a rapid atrial rate of 280 to 340 bpm with varying degrees of intraventricular block.

■ ICD-9CM CODES
427.32 Atrial flutter

■ EPIDEMIOLOGY & DEMOGRAPHICS
Atrial flutter is common during the first week after open heart surgery.

■ PHYSICAL FINDINGS & CLINICAL PRESENTATION
- Fast pulse rate (approximately 150 bpm)
- Symptoms of cardiac failure, light-headedness, and angina pectoris

■ ETIOLOGY
- Atherosclerotic heart disease
- MI
- Thyrotoxicosis
- Pulmonary embolism
- Mitral valve disease
- Cardiac surgery
- COPD

DIAGNOSIS

■ DIFFERENTIAL DIAGNOSIS
- Atrial fibrillation
- Paroxysmal atrial tachycardia

■ WORKUP
- ECG
- Laboratory evaluation

■ LABORATORY TESTS
- Thyroid function studies
- Serum electrolytes

■ IMAGING STUDIES
ECG (Fig. 1-51)
- Regular, "sawtooth," or "F" wave pattern, best seen in II, III, and AVF and secondary to atrial depolarization
- AV conduction block (2:1, 3:1, or varying)

TREATMENT

■ NONPHARMACOLOGIC THERAPY
- Valsalva maneuver or carotid sinus massage usually slows the ventricular rate (increases grade of AV block) and may make flutter waves more evident.
- Electrical cardioversion is given at low energy levels (20 to 25 J).

■ ACUTE GENERAL Rx
- In absence of cardioversion, IV diltiazem or digitalization may be tried to slow the ventricular rate and convert flutter to fibrillation. Esmolol, verapamil, and adenosine may also be effective.
- Atrial pacing may also terminate atrial flutter.
- Atrial flutter is frequently associated with intermittent atrial fibrillation. It may be prudent to anticoagulate patients with atrial flutter and coexisting medical disorders (e.g., dia-

betes mellitus, hypertension, cardiac disease) before cardioversion.

■ CHRONIC Rx
- Chronic atrial flutter may respond to amiodarone.
- Radiofrequency ablation to interrupt the atrial flutter is also effective for patients with chronic or recurring atrial flutter.

■ DISPOSITION
Over 85% of patients convert to regular sinus rhythm following cardioversion with as little as 25 to 50 J.

■ REFERRAL
For radiofrequency ablation in patients with chronic or recurring atrial flutter

PEARLS & CONSIDERATIONS

■ COMMENTS
Patient education material can be obtained from American Heart Association, 7320 Greenville Avenue, Dallas, TX 75231.
Author: **Fred F. Ferri, M.D.**

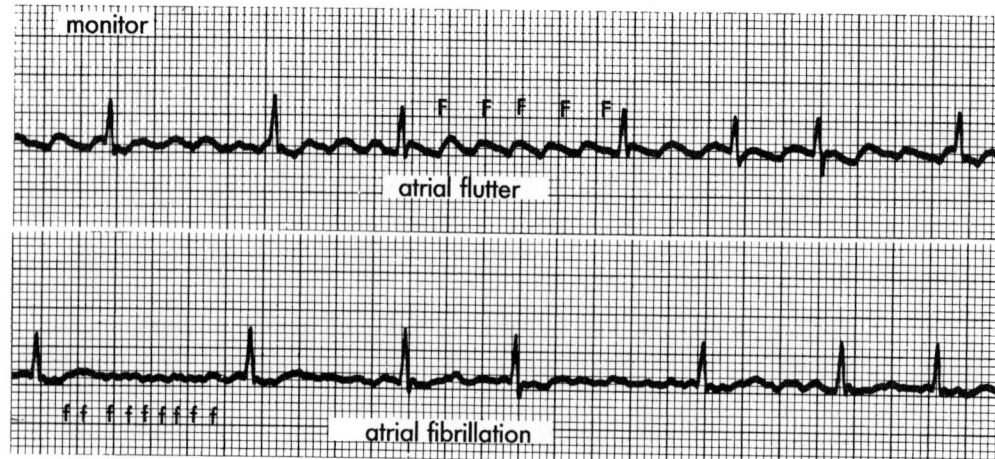

Fig. 1-51 Atrial flutter and fibrillation. Notice the sawtooth waves with atrial flutter *(F)* and the irregular fibrillatory waves with atrial fibrillation *(f)*. (From Goldberger AL [ed]: *Clinical electrocardiography,* ed 5, St Louis, 1994, Mosby.)

BASIC INFORMATION

■ DEFINITION

Atrial septal defect (ASD) is an abnormal opening in the atrial septum that allows for blood flow between the atria. There are several forms (Fig. 1-52)
- Ostium primum: defect low in the septum
- Ostium secundum: occurs mainly in the region of the fossa ovalis
- Sinus venous defect: less common form, involves the upper part of the septum

■ SYNONYMS

ASD

ICD-9CM CODES

429.71 Atrial septal defect

■ EPIDEMIOLOGY & DEMOGRAPHICS

- 80% of cases of ASD involve persistence of ostium secundum.
- Incidence is higher in females.
- ASD accounts for 8% to 10% of congenital heart abnormalities.

■ PHYSICAL FINDINGS & CLINICAL PRESENTATION

- Pansystolic murmur best heard at apex secondary to mitral regurgitation (ostium primum defect)
- Widely split S_2
- Visible and palpable pulmonary artery pulsations
- Ejection systolic flow murmur
- Prominent right ventricular impulse
- Cyanosis and clubbing (severe cases)
- Exertional dyspnea
- Patients with small defects: generally asymptomatic

■ ETIOLOGY

Unknown

DIAGNOSIS

■ DIFFERENTIAL DIAGNOSIS

- Primary pulmonary hypertension
- Pulmonary stenosis
- Rheumatic heart disease
- Mitral valve prolapse
- Cor pulmonale

■ WORKUP

- ECG
- Chest x-ray examination
- Echocardiography
- Cardiac catheterization

■ IMAGING STUDIES

- ECG
  1. Ostium primum defect: left axis deviation, RBBB, prolongation of PR interval
  2. Sinus venous defect: leftward deviation of P axis
  3. Ostium secundum defect: right axis deviation, right bundle-branch block
- Chest x-ray: cardiomegaly, enlargement of right atrium and ventricle, increased pulmonary vascularity, small aortic knob
- Echocardiography with saline bubble contrast and Doppler flow studies: may demonstrate the defect and the presence of shunting. Transesophageal echocardiography is much more sensitive than transthoracic echocardiography in identifying sinus venous defects and is preferred by some for the initial diagnostic evaluation.
- Cardiac catheterization: confirms the diagnosis in patients who are candidates for surgery. It is useful if the patient has some anatomic finding on echocardiography that is not completely clear or has significant elevation of pulmonary artery pressures.

TREATMENT

■ NONPHARMACOLOGIC THERAPY

Avoidance of strenuous activity in symptomatic patients

■ ACUTE GENERAL Rx

- Children and infants: closure of ASD before age 10 yr is indicated if pulmonary:systemic flow ratio is >1.5:1.
- Adults: closure is indicated in symptomatic patients with shunts >2:1.
- Surgery should be avoided in patients with pulmonary hypertension with reversed shunting (Eisenmenger's syndrome) because of increased risk of right heart failure.
- Transcatheter closure is advocated in children when feasible.
- Prophylactic β-blocker therapy to prevent atrial arrhythmias should be considered in adults with ASD.
- Surgical closure is indicated in all patients with ostium primum defect and significant shunting unless patient has significant pulmonary vascular disease.

■ CHRONIC Rx

See "Acute General Rx."

■ DISPOSITION

- Mortality is high in patients with significant ostium primum defect.
- Patients with small shunts have a normal life expectancy.
- Surgical mortality varies with the age of the patient and the presence of cardiac failure and systolic pulmonary artery hypertension; mortality ranges from <1% in young patients (<45 yr old) to >10% in elderly patients with presence of heart failure and systolic pulmonary hypertension.
- Preoperative atrial fibrillation is a risk factor for immediate postoperative and long-term atrial fibrillation.
- Thromboembolism after surgical repair of an ASD in an adult can occur in the early postoperative period. Giving early postoperative anticoagulation in patients >35 yr of age at the time of ASD repair and continuing it for at least 6 months will decrease the risk.

REFERENCE

Moodie DS, Sterba R: Long-term outcomes excellent for ASD repair in adults, *Cleve Clin J Med* 67:591, 2000.
Author: **Fred F. Ferri, M.D.**

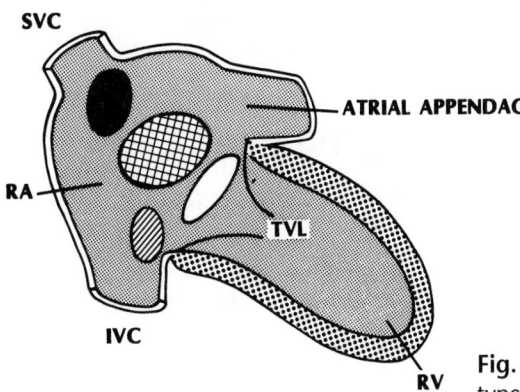

Fig. 1-52 Location of the four types of atrial septal defect. *SVC,* Superior vena cava; *RA,* right atrium; *IVC,* inferior vena cava; *RV,* right ventricle; *TVL,* tricuspid valve leaflet. (From Noble J [ed]: *Primary care medicine,* ed 2, St Louis, 1996, Mosby.)

BASIC INFORMATION

■ DEFINITION

Attention deficit hyperactivity disorder (ADHD) follows a persistent pattern (lasting at least 6 mo) of inattention *or* hyperactivity/impulsivity that is greater than expected for age and that begins before age 7 yr. The disorder is further defined by dysfunction in at least two settings (e.g., home, school, day care).

■ SYNONYMS

Hyperactivity
Attention deficit disorder (ADD)

ICD-9CM CODES
F90.X (DMS-IV 314.XX)

■ EPIDEMIOLOGY & DEMOGRAPHICS

PREVALENCE (IN U.S.): 35% of school-age children
PREDOMINANT SEX: Males > females, with rates ranging from 4:1 to 9:1
PREDOMINANT AGE:
- Onset must occur before age 7 yr.
- At least 20% experience spontaneous remissions by adolescence; however, the disorder may persist into adulthood.

PEAK INCIDENCE: Diagnosis is usually made after child begins school (ages 6 to 9 yr).
GENETICS:
- Familial pattern in many patients with ADHD
- Specific thyroid hormone abnormality in a very small fraction of familial ADHD

■ PHYSICAL FINDINGS & CLINICAL PRESENTATION

- Usually diagnosed in elementary school, where achievement is compromised and behavioral dyscontrol is less tolerated
- Wide array of symptoms, including difficulty sustaining attention, frequent careless mistakes, failure to follow instructions, difficulty organizing activities, distractability, forgetfulness, fidgeting, inability to sit still or play quietly, excessive activity or speech, inability to await turn, or intrusiveness
- May exhibit bossiness, stubbornness, demoralization, mood lability, and poor self-esteem
- IQ scores slightly lower than the general population

■ ETIOLOGY

- Probability of multiple etiologies
- Associated and possibly etiologic factors: comorbid Tourette's, a history of abuse or neglect, lead poisoning, previous encephalitis, drug exposure in utero, low birth weight, and mental retardation. If possible, a specific diagnosis should be made.
- Thyroid hormone metabolism abnormalities identified in a pedigree of familial ADHD

🔬 DIAGNOSIS

■ DIFFERENTIAL DIAGNOSIS

- In early childhood, may be difficult to distinguish from normal active children.
- ADHD may overlap symptoms in children with disruptive behavior such as conduct disorder or oppositional defiant disorders.
- School and behavioral problems are associated with a learning disability (these disorders often coexist).
- Bipolar disorder may be confused with ADHD, but it can be distinguished by the episodic nature of bipolar illness and the pervasive presence of ADHD.

■ WORKUP

- History with collateral information from parents and teachers is central to the diagnosis.
- Neurologic examination including imaging studies is used to uncover nonspecific, nonvocal, soft neurologic signs that frequently can be found in ADHD children.
- Questionnaires for parents and adolescents aid in the diagnosis.
- Psychologic testing is useful to diagnose a learning disability.

🏥 TREATMENT

■ NONPHARMACOLOGIC THERAPY

Children generally do better in special education settings with behavioral management of the disruptive behavior.

■ ACUTE GENERAL Rx

- Stimulants: mainstay of treating ADHD; include methylphenidate (Ritalin), dextroamphetamine (Dexedrine), and pemoline (Cylert)
- The amphetamine-dextroamphetamine combination Adderall is also useful in children with ADHD. Once-daily Adderall is as effective as twice-daily methylphenidate and both are superior to once-daily methylphenidate.
- Adjuncts: antidepressants (rare cardiac deaths in children and adolescents warrant caution); serotonin reuptake–inhibiting antidepressants (safer but efficacy not as well documented), clonidine, and neuroleptics

■ DISPOSITION

- Severity generally decreases with age.
- In late adolescence, the symptom severity is quite mild in many individuals.
- Full or partial aspects of the disorder are possibly persistent into mid-adulthood and require ongoing pharmacotherapy.

■ REFERRAL

- If diagnosis is complicated by coexisting conditions
- If treatment with stimulants is not adequately effective

REFERENCES

Pecham WG et al: Once-a-day concerta methylphenidate versus three-times daily methylphenidate in laboratory and natural settings, *Pediatrics* 107:105, 2001.

Pelham WE et al: A comparison of morning only and morning/late afternoon Adderall to morning-only, twice-daily, and three times daily methylphenidate in children with ADHD, *Pediatrics* 104:1300, 1999.

Smucker WD et al: Evaluation and treatment of ADHD, *Am Fam Physician* 64:817, 2001.

Szymanski ML, Zolotor A: Attention-deficit/hyperactivity disorder: management, *Am Fam Physician* 64:1355, 2001.

Zametrin AJ et al: Problems in the management of attention deficit hyperactivity disorder, *N Engl J Med* 340:40, 1999.

Author: **Rif S. El-Mallakh, M.D.**

BASIC INFORMATION

■ **DEFINITION**
The term *autistic disorder* refers to impairment in the development of language, communication, and reciprocal social interaction along with a restricted behavioral repertoire, with onset before age 3 yr.

■ **SYNONYMS**
Autism
Early infantile autism
Childhood autism
Kanner's autism

■ **ICD-9CM CODES**
F84.0 Autistic disorder
(DSM-IV coded 299.0 Autistic disorder)

■ **EPIDEMIOLOGY & DEMOGRAPHICS**
PREVALENCE (IN U.S.): 2 to 5 cases/10,000 persons (10 to 15 cases/10,000 persons when broader definitions are used)
PREDOMINANT SEX: Male:female ratio of 3-4:1
PREDOMINANT AGE: Lifelong illness
PEAK INCIDENCE: Before age 3 yr
GENETICS: Unknown genetic component; risk for sibling of affected individual: increases to 3%

■ **PHYSICAL FINDINGS & CLINICAL PRESENTATION**
• Marked impairment in the understanding and use of both verbal and nonverbal communication (probably underlies the profound impairment in social interaction)
• Stereotypic behavior or language

■ **ETIOLOGY**
• Majority of cases of autism are not associated with a medical condition.
• There is a significant increase in comorbid seizure disorder (25%) and mental retardation.
• Autism is sometimes associated with other neurologic conditions (e.g., encephalitis, phenylketonuria, fragile X, and others), suggesting that it may result from nonspecific neuronal injury.
• Specific abnormality that produces autistic symptoms has not been identified.

 DIAGNOSIS

■ **DIFFERENTIAL DIAGNOSIS**
• Other pervasive developmental disorders
• Rett's syndrome: occurs in females, exhibits head growth deceleration, loss of previously acquired motor skills, and incoordination
• Childhood disintegration disorder: development normal until age 2 yr, followed by regression
• Childhood-onset schizophrenia: follows period of normal development
• Asperger's syndrome: lacks the language developmental abnormalities of autism
• Isolated symptoms of autism: when occurring in isolation, defined as disorders, e.g., selective mutism, expressive language disorder, mixed receptive-expressive language disorder, or stereotypic movement disorder

■ **WORKUP**
A two-part process:
1. Establish the diagnosis.
2. Determine if there are any associated medical conditions.

■ **LABORATORY TESTS**
• PKU screen (usually done at birth in the U.S.)
• Chromosome analysis to rule out fragile X in both boys and girls (carrier girls may exhibit mild symptoms.)

■ **IMAGING STUDIES**
• EEG to diagnose coexisting seizure disorder (a normal EEG does not rule out a seizure disorder.)
• Head CT scan or MRI to rule out tuberous sclerosis
• Possible BAER to rule out hearing deficit
• IQ testing to help determine functional level of the child

TREATMENT

■ **NONPHARMACOLOGIC THERAPY**
• A behavioral training program that is consistent in both the home and school environments is important.

• Educational needs should focus on language and social development.
• Most children need a highly structured environment.
• Educating the parents and teachers is of great value.

■ **ACUTE GENERAL Rx**
• Haloperidol or other high-potency neuroleptics are helpful in reducing aggression and stereotypy.
• Serotonin reuptake inhibitor antidepressants (fluoxetine, clomipramine, sertraline, paroxetine) are possibly useful in children with coexisting depression or with marked obsessive or ritualistic behaviors.
• Naltrexone is useful for children with self-injurious behaviors.
• Valproic acid and carbamazepine are preferred to phenytoin or phenobarbital for seizure control.

■ **CHRONIC Rx**
• Extended use of all medications used for acute management
• Potential for tardive dyskinesia with chronic use of neuroleptics
• Large doses of vitamin B_6 and magnesium supplementation (mild ameliorating effect)

■ **DISPOSITION**
• Most children (70%) will require some degree of assistance as adults, will not be able to work, and will not achieve proper social adjustment.
• Some 10% (particularly if IQ is in the normal range and speech is achieved by age 5 yr) may have a reasonable outcome.
• Children with Asperger's syndrome may have a very good outcome despite ongoing symptoms.

■ **REFERRAL**
Assistance may be needed in diagnosis, management, parental teaching, or intervention with the school system.
Authors: **Rif S. El-Mallakh, M.D., and Peter E. Tanguay, M.D.**

BASIC INFORMATION

■ DEFINITION

Babesiosis is a tick-transmitted protozoan disease of animals, caused by intraerythrocytic parasites of the genus *Babesia.* Humans are incidentally infected, resulting in a nonspecific febrile illness.

ICD-9CM CODES
088.82 Babesiosis

■ EPIDEMIOLOGY & DEMOGRAPHICS
INCIDENCE (IN U.S.): Unknown
PREVALENCE (IN U.S.):
- In areas of high endemicity, seropositivity ranging from 9% (Rhode Island) to 21% (Connecticut)
- Highest number of reported cases in New York

PREDOMINANT SEX: Males (most likely through increased exposure to vectors during recreational or occupational activities)
PREDOMINANT AGE: Severity apparently increasing with age >40 yr
PEAK INCIDENCE: Spring and summer months, May through September
GENETICS: None known
CONGENITAL INFECTION: At least one case of probable vertical transmission
NEONATAL INFECTION: At least two cases of perinatal transmission

■ PHYSICAL FINDINGS & CLINICAL PRESENTATION
- Incubation period 1 to 4 wk, or 6 to 9 wk in transfusion-associated disease
- Gradual onset of irregular fever, chills, diaphoresis, headache, myalgia, arthralgia, fatigue, and dark urine
- On physical examination: petechiae, frank or mild hepatosplenomegaly, and jaundice
- Infection with *B. divergens* producing a more severe illness with a rapid onset of symptoms and increasing parasitemia progressing to massive intravascular hemolysis and renal failure

■ ETIOLOGY
- Vector: Deer tick, *Ixodes scapularis* (also known as *I. dammini*)
  1. Feeds on rodents during the spring and summer while in its larval and nymphal stages and on deer as an adult
  2. During the warmer months in endemic areas, humans are readily infected while engaging in outdoor activities
- *Babesia microti,* along with *B. divergens* and *B. bovis,* account for most human infections.
- In the U.S., cases caused by *B. microti* are acquired on offshore islands of the northeastern coast, including Nantucket Island, Cape Cod, and Martha's Vineyard in Massachusetts; Block Island in Rhode Island; and Long Island, Fire Island, and Shelter Island in New York; as well as the nearby mainland including Connecticut.
- Sporadic cases reported from California, Georgia, Maryland, Minnesota, Virginia, Wisconsin, and most recently the WA-1 strain from Washington State and the MO-1 strain from Missouri.
- *B. divergens* and *B. bovis* are implicated in human disease in Europe, where the disease remains rare and predominantly associated with asplenia.
- Majority of cases are symptomatic.
- May be transmissible by transfusion, through platelets and erythrocytes.
- Mixed infections (*B. microti* and *Borrelia burgdorferi*) are estimated to occur in 10% (Rhode Island and Connecticut) to 60% (New York) of cases.

DIAGNOSIS

■ DIFFERENTIAL DIAGNOSIS
- Ambeiasis
- Ehrlichiosis
- Hepatic abscess
- Leptospirosis
- Malaria

- Salmonellosis, including typhoid fever
- Acute viral hepatitis
- Hemorrhagic fevers

■ WORKUP
Should be suspected in any febrile patient living or traveling in an endemic area, irrespective of exposure history to ticks or tick bites, especially if asplenic

■ LABORATORY TESTS
- CBC to reveal mild to moderate pancytopenia
- Abnormally elevated serum chemistries, including creatinine, liver function profile, lactate dehydrogenase, and direct and total bilirubin levels
- Urinalysis to reveal proteinuria and hemoglobinuria
- Examination of Giemsa- or Wright-stained thick and thin blood films for intraerythrocytic parasites
  1. In its classic, though infrequently seen, form a "tetrad" or "Maltese Cross" composed of four daughter cells attached by cytoplasmic strands is observed (Fig. 1-53).
  2. More commonly, smaller forms composed of a single chromatin dot are eccentrically located within bluish cytoplasm.
  3. Parasitized erythrocytes may be multiply infected but not enlarged, or they may show evidence of pigment deposition, seen with *Plasmodium* species.
- Diagnosis achieved serologically by indirect immunofluorescence assay (IFA) is specific for *B. microti.*
  1. Titer of ≥1:64 is indicative of seropositivity, whereas one ≥1:256 is considered diagnostic of acute infection.
  2. Assay is hampered by the inability to distinguish between exposed patients and those who are actively infected.
  3. Immunoglobulin M indirect immunofluorescent-antibody test may be highly sensitive and specific for diagnosis.

TREATMENT

■ NONPHARMACOLOGIC THERAPY
Supportive care with adequate hydration

■ ACUTE GENERAL Rx
- In patients with intact spleens: predominantly asymptomatic or if symptomatic, generally self-limited
- Therapy reserved for the severely ill patient, especially if asplenic or immunosuppressed
- Combination of quinine sulfate 650 mg PO tid plus clindamycin 600 mg PO tid (1.2 g parenterally bid) taken for 7 to 10 days: effective but may not eliminate parasites
- Exchange transfusions in addition to therapy with quinine and clindamycin: successful treatment for severe infections in asplenic patients associated with high levels of *B. microti* or *B. divergens* parasitemia

■ DISPOSITION
Prognosis is usually good and fatal outcomes are rare.

■ REFERRAL
- For prompt consultation with an infectious disease specialist if the diagnosis is acutely suspected, especially in the asplenic, elderly, or immunocompromised patient
- For hospitalization for the severely ill patient who may require exchange transfusions in addition to antibiotic therapy

PEARLS & CONSIDERATIONS

■ COMMENTS
- Prevention of babesiosis in asplenic or immunocompromised hosts is best achieved by avoidance of areas where the vector is endemic, especially during the months of May through September.
- If residence or travel in endemic areas is unavoidable, advise patients to perform daily cutaneous self-examination, wear light-colored clothing (to facilitate removal of ticks), and apply tick repellent (diethyltoluamide and dimethylphthalate) to skin or clothing.
- Advise a daily inspection for ticks in family pets (e.g., cats and dogs).
- Infection with *B. divergens*, especially in the asplenic patient, is often fatal.
- At least one case of concurrent babeosis and Lyme disease has been documented.

REFERENCES

Dacey MJ et al: Septic shock due to babesiosis, *Clin Infect Dis* 33(5):E37, 2001.

Dorman et al: Fulminant babesiosis treated with clindamycin, quinine and whole-blood exchange transfusion, *Transfusion* 40(3):375, 2000.

Hatcher JC et al: Severe babesiosis in Long Island: review of 34 cases and their complications, *Clin Infect Dis* 32(8):1117, 2001.

Javed MJ et al: Concurrent babesiosis and ehrlichiosis in an elderly host, *Mayo Clin Proc* 76(5):563, 2001.

Mylonakis E: When to suspect and how to monitor babesiosis, *Am Fam Physician* 63(10):1969, 2001.

Weinberg GA: Laboratory diagnosis of ehrlichosis and babesiosis, *Pediatr Infect Dis J* 20(4):435, 2001.

Author: **George O. Alonso, M.D.**

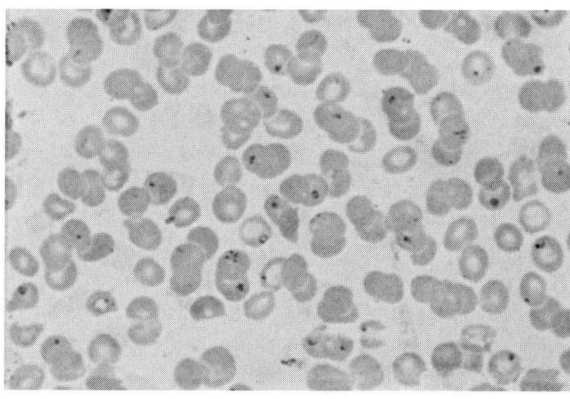

Fig. 1-53 *Babesia microti*–infected erythrocytes from a case of transfusion-induced babesiosis. Note ring and one tetrad form. (From Gorbach SL: *Infectious diseases,* ed 2, Philadelphia, 1998, WB Saunders.)

BASIC INFORMATION

■ **DEFINITIONS**
Baker's cyst refers to a fluid-filled popliteal bursa located along the medial border of the popliteal fossa.

■ **SYNONYMS**
Popliteal cyst

ICD-9CM CODES
727.51 Baker's cyst (knee)

■ **EPIDEMIOLOGY & DEMOGRAPHICS**
- Popliteal cysts occur at all ages.
- Incidence of Baker's cysts is unknown.
- Between 2% to 6 % of all patients thought to have clinical DVT turn out to have symptomatic Baker's cysts.
- Approximately 5% of MRIs of the knees reveal popliteal cysts.

■ **PHYSICAL FINDINGS & CLINICAL PRESENTATION**
- Pain in the popliteal space
- Knee swelling
- Leg edema
- Prominence of the popliteal fossa
- Decreased range of motion of the knee
- Locking of the knee
- Foucher's sign: The cyst becomes hard with knee extension and soft with knee flexion.
- Neuropathic lancinating pains radiating from the knee down the back of the leg.
- Deep vein thrombosis (DVT)

■ **ETIOLOGY**
- Baker's cysts are believed to represent fluid distention of the bursal sac separating the semimembranous tendon from the medial head of the gastrocnemius.
- In children, Baker's cysts are thought to be secondary to trauma and irritation of the knee.

- In adults, Baker's cysts are usually associated with pathologic changes of the knee joint:
  1. Rheumatoid arthritis
  2. Osteoarthritis of the knee
  3. Meniscal tears
  4. Patellofemoral chondromalacia
  5. Fracture
  6. Gout
  7. Pseudogout
  8. Infection (tuberculosis)

 DIAGNOSIS

Baker's cysts, like deep vein thrombosis, are very difficult to diagnose on clinical grounds alone. In fact, Baker's cyst frequently mimics a DVT and is sometimes called *pseudothrombophlebitis syndrome.*

■ **DIFFERENTIAL DIAGNOSIS**
- DVT
- Popliteal aneurysms
- Abscess
- Tumors
- Lymphadenopathy
- Varicosities
- Ganglion

■ **WORKUP**
Anyone suspected of having a popliteal cyst should undergo imaging studies to exclude other causes.

■ **LABORATORY TESTS**
Blood tests are not very specific in the diagnosis of Baker's cysts.

■ **IMAGING STUDIES**
- Plain x-ray (AP and lateral views) may show calcification in a solid tumor or in the posterior meniscal area.
- Ultrasound is easy, cost effective, and excludes other causes of popliteal fossa pathology.
- MRI of the knee identifies coexisting joint pathology (e.g., osteoarthritis, torn meniscus).
- Noninvasive venous studies to rule out DVT.

 TREATMENT

Treatment is directed at the underlying pathology leading to the formation of the popliteal cyst.

■ **NONPHARMACOLOGIC THERAPY**
- Rest
- Strenuous activity avoidance
- Knee immobilization possibly necessary in some cases

■ **ACUTE GENERAL Rx**
- NSAIDs, ibuprofen 400 to 800 mg PO tid, or naproxen 250 to 500 mg PO bid can be used to treat Baker's cyst caused by RA, gout, and pseudogout.
- Intraarticular injection or injection of the cyst with corticosteroids, triamcinolone acetonide 40 mg is sometimes tried.

■ **CHRONIC Rx**
- Surgical procedures addressing the underlying cause or aimed at the cyst include:
  1. Arthroscopic surgery to remove loose cartilaginous fragment
  2. Partial or total meniscectomy
  3. Open excision of the cyst (Fig. 1-54)

■ **DISPOSITION**
- Baker's cyst may spontaneously resolve without treatment.
- Complications of Baker's cysts are:
  1. Rupture
  2. DVT
  3. Nerve impingement

■ **REFERRAL**
Because Baker's cysts are commonly the result of underlying rheumatologic causes, a consultation with rheumatology is often recommended.

☼ PEARLS & CONSIDERATIONS

■ COMMENTS

- Popliteal cysts was first described in 1877 by Baker in connection with disease of the knee joint.

- Baker's cyst and DVT can coexist. It is imperative to exclude the diagnosis of DVT before discharging the patient from the emergency room, hospital, or office.
- In the setting of meniscus injury, Baker's cysts commonly originate from the posterior horn of the medial meniscus with or without a tear.

REFERENCES

Drescher MJ, Smally AJ: Thrombophlebitis and pseudothrombophlebitis in the ED, *Am J Emerg Med* 15(7):683, 1997.
Stone KR et al: The frequency of Baker's cysts associated with meniscal tears, *Am Sports Med* 24(5):670, 1996.
Author: **Peter Petropoulos, M.D.**

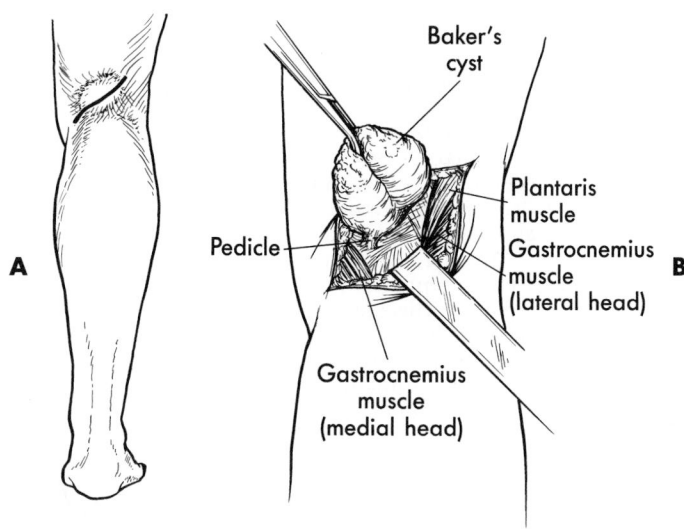

Fig. 1-54 Removal of midline Baker's cyst. **A,** Skin incision. **B,** After being exposed, pedicle is clamped, ligated, divided, and inverted. (Redrawn and modified from Meyerding HW, Van Demark GE: *JAMA* 122:858, 1943.)

BASIC INFORMATION

■ DEFINITIONS
Balanitis is an inflammation of the superficial tissues of the penile head (Fig. 1-55).

■ ICD-9CM CODES
112.2 Balanitis

■ EPIDEMIOLOGY & DEMOGRAPHICS
INCIDENCE (IN U.S.): Unknown
PREVALENCE (IN U.S.): Unknown
PREDOMINANT SEX: Exclusive to males
PEAK INCIDENCE: All ages, especially in sexually active men

■ PHYSICAL FINDINGS & CLINICAL PRESENTATION
- Itching and tenderness
- Pain, dysuria, and local edema
- Rarely, ulceration and lymph node enlargement
- Severe ulcerations leading to superimposed bacterial infections
- Inability to void: unusual, but a more distressing and serious complication

■ ETIOLOGY
- Poor hygiene, causing erosion of tissue with erythema and promoting growth of *Candida albicans*
- Sexual contact, urinary catheters, and trauma
- Allergic reactions to condoms or medications

 DIAGNOSIS

■ DIFFERENTIAL DIAGNOSIS
- Leukoplakia
- Reiter's syndrome
- Lichen planus
- Balanitis xerotica obliterans
- Psoriasis
- Carcinoma of the penis
- Erythroplasia of Queyrat

■ WORKUP
- Sexually active males: assessment for evidence of other sexually transmitted diseases
- Biopsy if lesions do not heal

■ LABORATORY TESTS
- VDRL
- Serum glucose
- Wet mount
- KOH prep
- Microculture

■ TREATMENT

■ NONPHARMACOLOGIC THERAPY
- Maintenance of meticulous hygiene
- Retraction and bathing of prepuce several times a day
- Warm sitz baths to ease edema and erythema
- Consideration of circumcision, especially when symptoms are severe or recurrent
- With Foley catheters, strict catheter care strongly advised

■ MEDICATIONS
- Analgesics, such as acetaminophen and/or codeine
- Clotrimazole 1% cream applied topically twice daily to affected areas
- Bacitracin or Neosporin ointment applied topically four times daily
- With more severe bacterial superinfection: cephalexin 500 mg PO qid
- Topical corticosteroids added four times daily if dermatitis severe
- Patients with suspected urinary tract infections: trimethoprim-sulfa DS twice daily or ciprofloxacin 500 mg PO bid after obtaining appropriate cultures

■ REFERRAL
- For surgical evaluation for circumcision if symptoms are recurrent, especially if phimosis or meatitis occurs (NOTE: Severe phimosis with an inability to void may require prompt slit drainage.)
- For biopsy to rule out other diagnosis such as premalignant or malignant lesions if lesions are not healing

REFERENCE
Fungus infections of the skin. In Rakel RE (ed): *Saunders manual of medical practice,* Philadelphia, 1996, WB Saunders.
Author: **Joseph J. Lieber, M.D.**

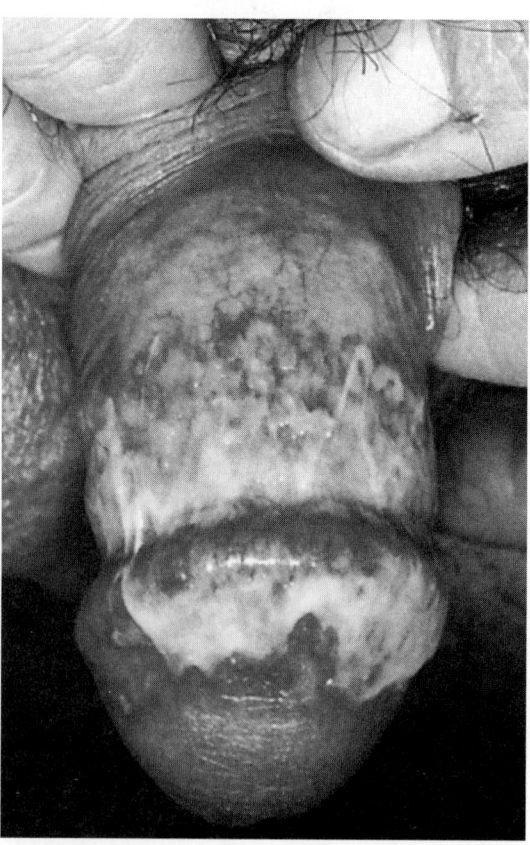

Fig. 1-55 *Candida* balanitis. The moist space between the skin surfaces of the uncircumcised penis is an ideal environment for *Candida* infection. This thick white exudate is typical of a severe acute infection. (From Habif TP: *Clinical dermatology: a color guide to diagnosis and therapy,* ed 3, St Louis, 1996, Mosby.)

BASIC INFORMATION

■ DEFINITION
Barrett's esophagus occurs when the squamous lining of the lower esophagus is replaced by columnar epithelium. The condition is associated with an increased risk of esophageal cancer.

■ SYNONYMS
Intestinal metaplasia of the lower esophagus

ICD-9CM CODES
530.2 Barrett's syndrome or ulcer

■ EPIDEMIOLOGY & DEMOGRAPHICS
- Male predominance with a 4:1 ratio of men to women
- Mean age of onset is 40 yr with a mean age of diagnosis of 55 to 60 yr
- Occurs more frequently in Caucasians and Hispanics than in African-Americans with a ratio of 10-20:1
- Mean prevalence of 9.6% in patients undergoing endoscopy for symptoms of GERD

■ PHYSICAL FINDINGS & CLINICAL PRESENTATION
Symptoms:
- Heartburn
- Asymptomatic, incidental finding
- Dysphagia for solid food
- Less frequent: chest pain, hematemesis, or melena
Physical findings:
- Nonspecific
- Ranges from epigastric tenderness on palpation to completely normal

■ ETIOLOGY
- Metaplasia is thought to be secondary to irritation of esophageal lining secondary to chronic gastroesophageal reflux (Fig. 1-56).
- Because not all individuals with GERD develop Barrett's esophagus, there is probably also a genetic propensity for the disease.

DIAGNOSIS

■ DIFFERENTIAL DIAGNOSIS
- GERD, uncomplicated
- Erosive esophagitis
- Gastritis
- Hiatal hernia
- Peptic ulcer disease
- Angina
- Malignancy
- Stricture

■ DIAGNOSTIC CRITERIA: CONTROVERSIAL
- Long segment
- Short segment
- Junctional intestinal metaplasia

■ DIAGNOSTIC TESTS
- Endoscopy with biopsy necessary for diagnosis
- Histologic hallmark is intestinal metaplasia in esophagus (see Fig. 1-57)
- Upper GI with barium may reveal ulcer crater in esophagus (Fig. 1-58); however, UGI is nonspecific and insensitive for the diagnosis

TREATMENT

■ NONPHARMACOLOGIC THERAPY
Same as treatment for GERD alone for symptoms of acid reflux (life-style modifications and pharmacologic therapy)

■ ACUTE GENERAL Rx
- Proton pump inhibitors (PPIs) are most effective
- Adequate system control of GERD in patients with Barrett's esophagus may control symptoms and adequate acid suppression may impede the progression to dysplasia.
- If asymptomatic and incidentally found to have Barrett's esophagus, medication is unnecessary

■ CHRONIC Rx
- Laser ablation, photodynamic therapy, endoscopic mucosal resection.
- Surgery for: (1) management of GERD and associated sequelae or (2) cancer or precursor lesions

■ SCREENING
- GERD highly prevalent in general population
- Only 4% to 10% of patients with reflux symptoms develop Barrett's esophagus

- ACG recommends that patients with Barrett's undergo surveillance endoscopy and biopsy at intervals determined by the presence and grade of dysplasia, with a range of every 6 months to 3 years
- Patients should be treated aggressively for GERD before surveillance

■ DISPOSITION
- Overall, 30 to 50 times increased risk of adenocarcinoma of the esophagus in patients with Barrett's esophagus than in general population
- This risk corresponds to 500 cancers per year per 100,000 persons with Barrett's esophagus
- Specifics of frequency of monitoring is controversial, no prospective controlled studies to prove that surveillance increases life expectancy
- Usual recommendation is periodic surveillance by endoscopy and biopsy for detection of carcinoma or high-grade dysplasia
- Current generally accepted follow-up recommendations for patients with Barrett's esophagus (no dysplasia) include endoscopy every 2 to 3 yr and q6mo (×2), then once/yr for those with low-grade dysplasia

■ REFERRAL
- For endoscopy with biopsy in patients with chronic GERD symptomatology who have not had previous endoscopy
- For surveillance in those with a previous biopsy-proven diagnosis of Barrett's esophagus
- For those with high-grade dysplasia, biopsies should be confirmed by an expert pathologist, then esophageal resection or intensive surveillance should be offered.

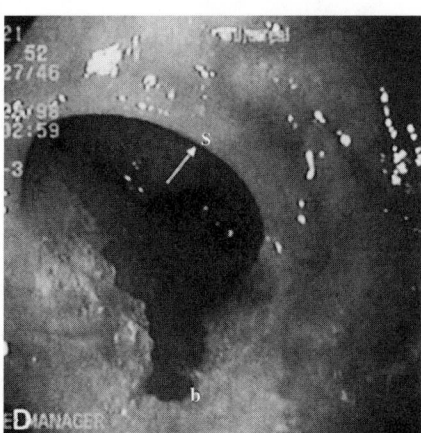

Fig. 1-56 Endoscopic view of the distal esophagus from a patient with gastroesophageal reflux disease showing a tongue of Barrett's mucosa *(b)* and a Schatzki's ring *(s) (arrow).* (From Goldman L, Bennett JC [eds]: *Cecil textbook of medicine,* ed 21, Philadelphia, 2000, WB Saunders.)

REFERENCES

Bammer T et al: Rationale for surgical therapy of Barrett esophagus, *Mayo Clin Proc* 76:335, 2001.

Cameron A: Management of Barrett's esophagus, *Mayo Clin Proc* 73:5, 1998.

Falk GW: Current challenges in Barrett's esophagus, *Cleve Clin J Med* 68:415, 2001.

Morales TG, Sampliner RE: Barrett's esophagus, *Arch Intern Med* 159:1411, 1999.

Oatu-Lasear R, Fitzgerald RC, Triadafilopoulas G: Differentiation and proliferation in Barrett's esophagus and the effects of acid suppression, *Gastroenterology* 117:327, 1999.

Provenzale D, Schmitt C, Wong JB: Barrett's esophagus: a new look at surveillance based on emerging estimates of cancer risk, *Am J Gastroenterol* 94:2043, 1999.

Rajan E, Burgart LJ, Gostout CJ: Endoscopic and histologic diagnosis of Barrett esophagus, *Mayo Clin Proc* 76:217, 2001.

Samplinear RE: Practice guidelines on the diagnosis, surveillance, and therapy of Barrett's esophagus: the Practice Parameters Committee of the American College of Gastroenterology, *Am J Gastroenterol* 93:1028, 1998.

Sharma P: Short segment Barrett esophagus and specialized columnar mucosa at the gastroesophageal junction, *Mayo Clin Proc* 76:331, 2001.

Wang KK, Samplinear RE: Mucosal ablation therapy of Barrett esophagus, *Mayo Clin Proc* 76:433, 2001.

Author: **Rebecca S. Brienza, M.D., M.P.H.**

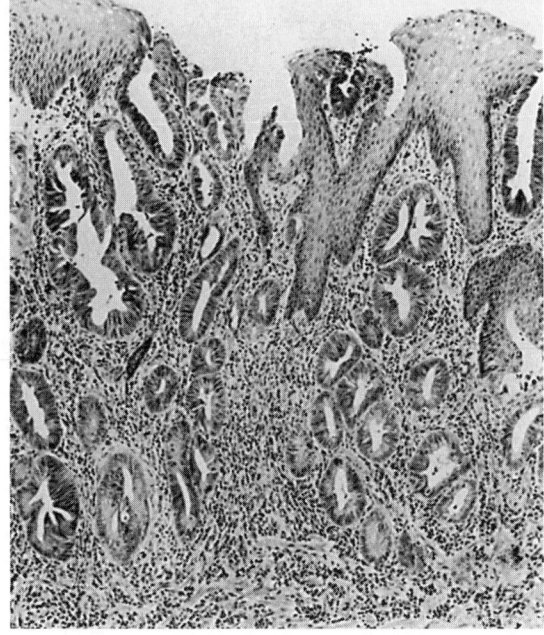

Fig. 1-57 Epithelial metaplasia (original magnification, ×16). The esophageal mucosa consists of columnar epithelium (Barrett's esophagus) intermixed with squamous epithelium. (Photomicrograph courtesy Frank Mitros, MD, Department of Pathology, University of Iowa. (From Stein JH [ed]: *Internal medicine,* ed 5, St Louis, 1998, Mosby.)

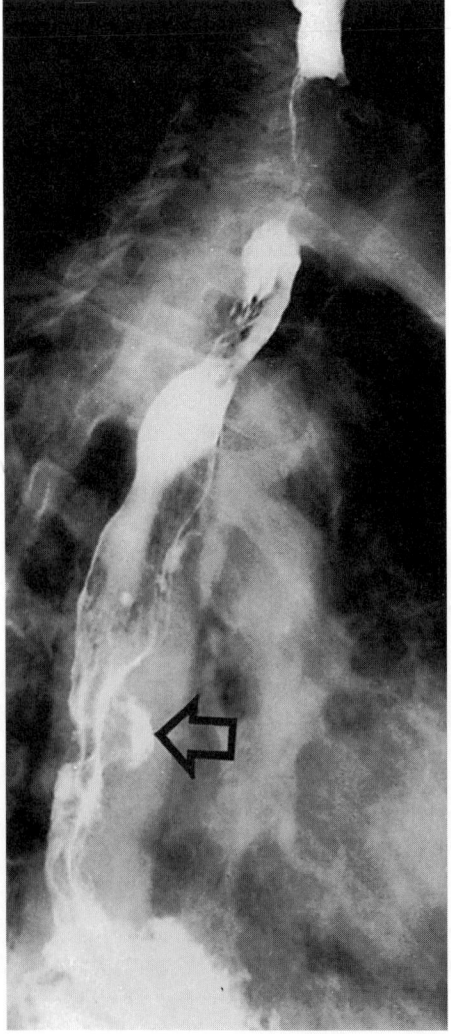

Fig. 1-58 Peptic esophageal ulcer. The occurrence of an ulcer crater *(arrow)* in the esophagus is indicative of Barrett's esophageal mucosal metaplasia. (Radiograph courtesy Charles C. Lu, MD, Department of Radiology, University of Iowa. From Stein JH [ed]: *Internal medicine,* ed 5, St Louis, 1998, Mosby.)

BASIC INFORMATION

■ DEFINITION
Basal cell carcinoma is a malignant tumor of the skin arising from basal cells of the lower epidermis and adnexal structures. It may be classified as one of six types (nodular, superficial, pigmented, cystic, sclerosing or morpheaform, and nevoid). The most common type is nodular (21%); the least common is morpheaform (1%); a mixed pattern is present in approximately 40% of cases. Basal cell carcinoma advances by direct expansion and destroys normal tissue.

■ SYNONYMS
BCC

ICD-9CM CODES
179.9 Basal cell carcinoma, site unspecified
173.3 Basal cell carcinoma, face
173.4 Basal cell carcinoma, neck, scalp
173.5 Basal cell carcinoma, trunk
173.6 Basal cell carcinoma of the limb
173.7 Basal cell carcinoma, lower limb

■ EPIDEMIOLOGY & DEMOGRAPHICS
- Most common cutaneous neoplasm in humans (>400,000 cases/yr)
- 85% appear on the head and neck region
- Most common site: nose (30%)
- Increased incidence with age >40 yr
- Increased incidence in men
- Risk factors: fair skin, increased sun exposure, use of tanning salons with ultraviolet A or B radiation, history of irradiation (e.g., Hodgkin's disease), personal or family history of skin cancer, impaired immune system

■ PHYSICAL FINDINGS & CLINICAL PRESENTATION
Variable with the histologic type:
- Nodular: dome-shaped, painless lesion that may become multilobular

and frequently ulcerates (rodent ulcer); prominent telangiectatic vessels are noted on the surface; border is translucent, elevated, pearly white (Fig. 1-59); some nodular basal cell carcinomas may contain pigmentation giving an appearance similar to a melanoma.
- Superficial: circumscribed scaling black appearance with a thin raised pearly white border; a crust and erosions may be present; occurs most frequently on the trunk and extremities.
- Morpheaform: flat or slightly raised yellowish or white appearance (similar to localized scleroderma); appearance similar to scars, surface has a waxy consistency.

■ ETIOLOGY
Sun exposure and use of tanning salons with equipment that emits ultraviolet A or B radiation

DIAGNOSIS

■ DIFFERENTIAL DIAGNOSIS
- Keratoacanthoma
- Melanoma (pigmented basal cell carcinoma)
- Xeroderma pigmentosa
- Basal cell nevus syndrome
- Molluscum contagiosum
- Sebaceous hyperplasia
- Psoriasis

■ WORKUP
Biopsy to confirm diagnosis

TREATMENT

■ NONPHARMACOLOGIC THERAPY
Avoidance of excessive tanning, use of sun screens to prevent damage from excessive sun exposure

■ ACUTE GENERAL Rx
Variable with tumor size, location, and cell type:

- Excision surgery: preferred method for large tumors with well-defined borders on the legs, cheeks, forehead, and trunk
- Mohs' micrographic surgery: preferred for lesions in high-risk areas (e.g., nose, eyelid), very large primary tumors, recurrent basal cell carcinomas, and tumors with poorly defined clinical margins
- Electrodesiccation and curettage: useful for small (<6 mm) nodular basal cell carcinomas
- Cryosurgery with liquid nitrogen: useful in basal cell carcinomas of the superficial and nodular types with clearly definable margins; no clear advantages over the other forms of therapy; generally reserved for uncomplicated tumors
- Radiation therapy: generally used for basal cell carcinomas in areas requiring preservation of normal surround tissues for cosmetic reasons (e.g., around lips); also useful in patients who cannot tolerate surgical procedures or for large lesions and surgical failures

■ CHRONIC Rx
Periodic evaluation for at least 5 yr because of increased risk of recurrence of another basal cell carcinoma (>40% risk within 5 yr of treatment)

■ DISPOSITION
- More than 90% of patients are cured.
- A lesion is considered low risk if it is <1.5 cm in diameter, is nodular or cystic, is not in a difficult-to-treat area (H zone of face), and has not been previously treated.
- Nodular and superficial basal cell carcinomas are the least aggressive.
- Morpheaform lesions have the highest incidence of positive tumor margins (>30%) and the greatest recurrence rate.

REFERENCE
Jerant AF et al: Early detection and treatment of skin cancer, *Am Fam Physician* 62:357, 2000.
Author: **Fred F. Ferri, M.D.**

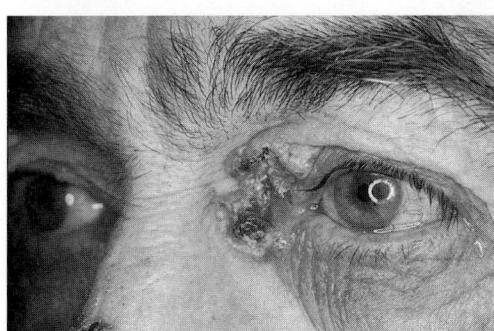

Fig. 1-59   Basal cell carcinoma. Note rolled translucent border and central ulceration in typical facial location. (From Noble J et al: *Textbook of primary care medicine,* ed 2, St Louis, 1995, Mosby.)

BASIC INFORMATION

■ DEFINITION
Behçet's disease is an inflammatory disorder characterized by the presence of oral aphthous ulcers, genital ulcers, uveitis, and skin lesions (Figs. 1-60 and 1-61).

ICD-9CM CODES
136.1 Behçet's syndrome

■ EPIDEMIOLOGY & DEMOGRAPHICS
Behçet's disease is observed in two different geographic locations.
- One is observed in individuals living in Japan, Korea, Turkey, and the Mediterranean basin.
  1. Prevalence ranges from 1:7000 to 1:10,000.
  2. Turley has the highest prevalence at 80 to 370 cases per 100,000.
- The other is observed in individuals living in North America and Northern Europe.
  1. Prevalence ranges from 1:20,000 to 1:100,000.
  2. Prevalence of Behçet's disease in the U.S. is 0.12 to 0.33 cases per 100,000.
- In those areas the prevalence of HLA-B51 is higher in patients with Behçet's disease.
- Incidence in men and women 1:1.

■ PHYSICAL FINDINGS & CLINICAL PRESENTATION
- Behçet's disease typically affects individuals in the third to fourth decade of life and primarily presents with painful aphthous oral ulcers. The ulcers occurs in crops measuring 2 to 10 mm in size and found on the mucous membrane of the cheek, gingiva, tongue, pharynx, and soft palate.
- Genital ulcers are similar to the oral ulcers.
- Decreased vision secondary to either uveitis, keratitis, vitreous hemorrhage, or occlusion of the retinal artery or vein may occur.
- Skin findings including papules, vesicles, folliculitis, and acneiform and erythema nodosum–like lesions can be found on the proximal extremities and trunk.
- Arthritis and arthralgias.
- CNS meningeal findings including headache, fever, and stiff neck can occur. Cerebellar ataxia and pseudobulbar palsy occur with involvement of the brainstem.
- Vasculitis leading to both arterial and venous inflammation or occlusion can result in signs and symptoms of a myocardial infarction, intermittent claudication, deep vein thrombosis, hemoptysis, and aneurysm formation.

■ ETIOLOGY
The etiology of Behçet's disease is unknown. An immune-related vasculitis is thought to lead to many of the manifestations of Behçet's disease. What triggers the immune response and activation is not yet known.

DIAGNOSIS

According to the International Study Group for Behçet's disease, the diagnosis of Behçet's disease is established when recurrent oral ulceration is present along with at least two of the following:
- Recurrent genital ulceration
- Eye lesions
- Skin lesions
- Positive pathergy test

■ DIFFERENTIAL DIAGNOSIS
- Ulcerative colitis
- Crohn's disease
- Lichen planus
- Pemphigoid
- Herpes simplex infection
- Reiter's syndrome
- Ankylosing spondylitis
- AIDS
- Hypereosinophilic syndrome.
- Sweet's syndrome

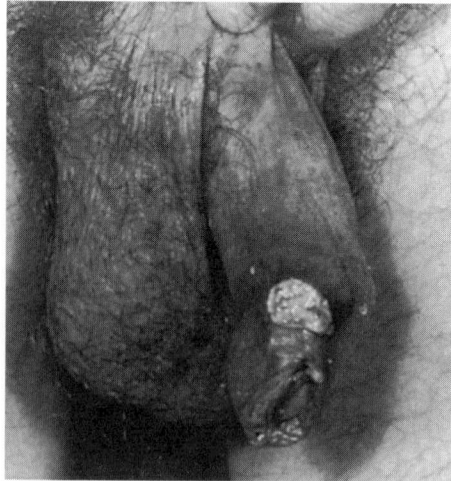
Fig. 1-60 Behçet's syndrome. Painful prepuceal ulcer in a male with superficial thrombophlebitis, oral ulcers, and bowel vasculitis. (From Canoso J: *Rheumatology in primary care,* Philadelphia, 1997, WB Saunders.)

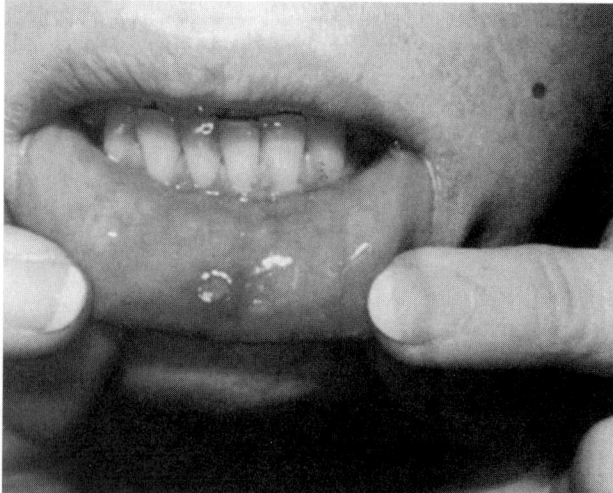
Fig. 1-61 Behçet's syndrome. Painful aphthous inner lower lip ulcer in a 30-year-old Chinese woman with relapsing oral and genital ulcers and uveitis. She did well on low-dose prednisone plus colchicine. (From Canoso J: *Rheumatology in primary care,* Philadelphia, 1997, WB Saunders.)

■ WORKUP

The diagnosis of Behçet's disease is a clinical diagnosis. Laboratory tests and x-ray imaging may be helpful in working up the complications of Behçet's disease or excluding other diseases in the differential.

■ LABORATORY TESTS

There are no diagnostic laboratory tests for Behçet's disease.

■ IMAGING STUDIES

CT scan, MRI, and angiography are useful for detecting CNS and vascular lesions

 TREATMENT

Treatment is directed at the patient's clinical presentation (e.g., mucocutaneous lesions, ocular lesions, arthritis, GI, CNS, or vascular lesions).

■ NONPHARMACOLOGIC THERAPY

Supportive care

■ ACUTE GENERAL Rx

- Oral and genital ulcers are treated with:
  1. Topical corticosteroids (e.g., triamcinolone acetonide ointment applied tid).
  2. Tetracycline tablets 250 mg dissolved in 5 cc water and applied to the ulcer for 2 to 3 min.
  3. Colchicine 0.5 to 1.5 mg/kg/day PO.
  4. Thalidomide 100 to 300 mg PO daily.
  5. Dapsone 100 mg PO daily.
  6. Pentoxifyline 300 mg/day PO.

- Ocular lesions
  1. Anterior uveitis is treated by an ophthalmologist with topical corticosteroids (e.g., betamethasone drops 1 to 2 drops tid). Topical injection with dexamethasone 1 to 1.5 mg has also been tried.
- CNS disease
  1. Chlorambucil 0.1 mg/kg/day is used in the treatment of posterior uveitis, retinal vasculitis, or CNS disease. Patients not responding to chlorambucil can be tried on cyclosporine 5 to 7 mg/kg/day.
  2. In CNS vasculitis, cyclophosphamide 2 to 3 mg/kg/day is used. Prednisone can be used as an alternative.
- Arthritis
  1. NSAIDs, e.g., ibuprofen 400 to 800 mg tid orally or indomethacin 50 to 75 mg/day PO.
  2. Sulfasalzine 1 to 3 g/day PO is an alternative treatment.
- GI lesions
  1. Sulfasalzine 1 to 3 g/day PO.
  2. Prednisone 40 to 60 mg/day PO.
- Vascular lesions
  1. Prednisone 40 to 60 mg/day PO.
  2. Cytotoxic agents as mentioned above.
  3. Heparin 5000 to 20,000 U/day followed by oral warfarin.

■ CHRONIC Rx

- Chronic therapy is usually continued for approximately 1 yr after remission.
- Surgery may be indicated in patients with complications of bowel perforation, vascular occlusive disease, and aneurysm formation.

■ DISPOSITION

- The aphthous oral ulcers last 1 to 2 wk recurring more frequently than genital ulcers.
- Approximately 25% of patients with ocular lesions become blind.
- The disease course is unpredictable.
- Complications include:
  1. Meningitis
  2. Cerebrovascular accident (stroke)
  3. Aneurysm rupture
  4. Peripheral lower-extremity ischemia
  5. Mesenteric ischemia
  6. Myocardial infarction

■ REFERRAL

If the diagnosis of Behçet's disease is suspected, a referral to both rheumatology and ophthalmology is indicated because the disease is so rare.

☼ PEARLS & CONSIDERATIONS

■ COMMENTS

The pathergy test refers to the formation of a nodule or pustule at the site of a sterile puncture with a 20- or 22-gauge needle.

REFERENCES

Ehrlich GE: Behcet's disease: an update, *Compr Ther* 25(4):216, 1999.
International Study Group for Behçet's Disease: Criteria for diagnosis of Behçet's disease, *Lancet* 335:1078, 1990.
Sakane T et al: Behcet's disease, *N Engl J Med* 341(17):1284, 1999.
Yazici H, Yurdakul S, Hamuryudan V: Behçet's syndrome, *Curr Opin Rheumatol* 11:53, 1999.
Author: **Peter Petropoulos, M.D.**

BASIC INFORMATION

■ DEFINITION
Bell's palsy is facial weakness affecting the muscles supplied by the seventh cranial nerve (facial nerve, Fig. 1-62).

■ SYNONYMS
Idiopathic facial paralysis

ICD-9CM CODES
351.0 Bell's palsy

■ EPIDEMIOLOGY & DEMOGRAPHICS
INCIDENCE: 25 cases/100,000 persons
GENETICS: A predisposition to cranial neuropathies, especially seventh and third nerve palsies, has been reported.
RISK FACTORS: Diabetes, pregnancy, age >30 yr

■ PHYSICAL FINDINGS & CLINICAL PRESENTATION
- Unilateral paralysis of the facial muscles (<1% of the facial palsies are bilateral)
- Ipsilateral loss of taste
- Possible ipsilateral ear pain
- Increased or decreased unilateral eye tearing

■ ETIOLOGY
- Most cases are idiopathic
- The cause is often viral (herpes simplex).
- Herpes zoster can cause Bell's palsy in association with herpetic blisters affecting the outer ear canal or the area behind the ear.
- Bell's palsy can also be one of the manifestations of Lyme disease.

DIAGNOSIS

■ DIFFERENTIAL DIAGNOSIS
- Neoplasms affecting the base of the skull or the parotid gland
- Bacterial infectious process (meningitis, otitis media, osteomyelitis of the base of the skull)
- Brainstem stroke
- Multiple sclerosis
- Sarcoidosis
- Head trauma with fracture of temporal bone
- Other: Guillain-Barré, carcinomatous or leukemic meningitis, leprosy, Melkersson-Rosenthal syndrome
- Box 2-95 describes the differential diagnosis of facial palsy.

■ WORKUP
Bell's palsy is a clinical diagnosis. A focused history and neurologic examination will confirm the diagnosis.

■ LABORATORY TESTS
- FBS to evaluate for diabetes
- VDRL in selected patients
- Lyme titer in endemic areas

■ IMAGING STUDIES
- Contrast-enhanced MRI to exclude neoplasms is indicated only in patients with atypical features or course.
- Chest x-ray examination may be useful to exclude sarcoidosis or to rule out TB in selected patients before treating with steroids.

TREATMENT

■ NONPHARMACOLOGIC THERAPY
- Reassure patient that the disease is most likely a result of a virus attacking the nerve, not a stroke. It is also important to inform the patient that the prognosis is good.
- Avoid corneal drying by applying skin tape to the upper lid to keep the palpebral fissure narrowed. Lacri-Lube ophthalmic ointment at night and artificial tears during the day are also useful to prevent excessive drying.
- The patient should use dark glasses when going outside to minimize sun exposure.

■ ACUTE GENERAL Rx
- Although the benefits of corticosteroid therapy remain unproven, most practitioners use a brief course of prednisone therapy.
- If used, prednisone therapy should be started within 4 days of onset of Bell's palsy.
- Optimal steroid dose is unknown. Prednisone can be given as one 50-mg tablet qd for 7 days without tapering or can be started at 80 mg and tapered by 5 mg/day until finished.
- Combination therapy with acyclovir and prednisone has been reported to result in a modest improvement in clinical outcome.

■ CHRONIC Rx
Patients should be monitored for evidence of corneal abrasion and ulceration or hemifacial spasm.

■ DISPOSITION

- Of affected individuals, 95% recover satisfactorily within few months.
- Recurrence is experienced in 5% of Bell's palsy cases.

■ REFERRAL

- Persistent redness or irritation of the eye requires referral to an ophthalmologist.
- Neurology referral is recommended if diagnosis is unclear or if the clinical course is atypical.

☼ PEARLS & CONSIDERATIONS

■ COMMENTS

A patient brochure discussing facial nerve problems can be obtained from the American Academy of Otolaryngology—Head and Neck Surgery (AAO-HNS), phone: (703) 519-1528.
Author: **Fred F. Ferri, M.D.**

I

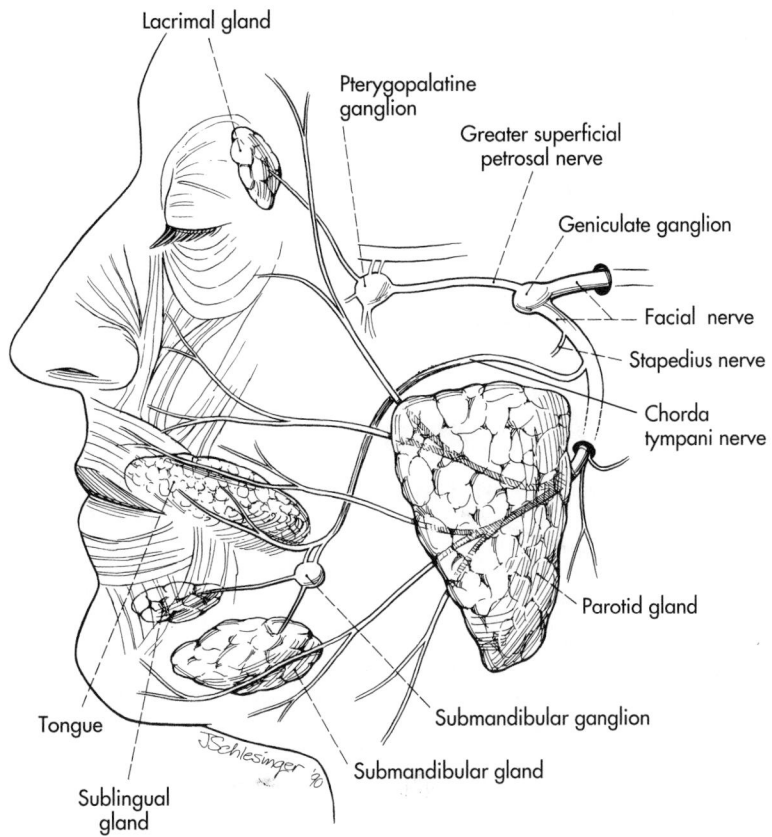

Fig. 1-62 Course of the facial nerve demonstrating motor branches to the mimetic musculature; parasympathetic innervation to the submandibular, sublingual, lacrimal, and minor salivary glands; and taste fibers emanating from the anterior two thirds of the tongue. (From Woodson GE: *Ear, nose and throat disorders in primary care,* Philadelphia, 2001, WB Saunders.)

BASIC INFORMATION

■ DEFINITION

Bipolar disorder is an episodic, recurrent, and frequently progressive condition in which the afflicted individual suffers periods of mania and, possibly, depression. Depressive episodes are not essential for the diagnosis. However, the individual must experience at least one manic episode in which he/she experiences at least 1 wk of continuous symptoms of elevated, expansive, or irritable mood in association with three or four of the following:

- Decreased need for sleep
- Grandiosity
- Pressured speech
- Subjective or objective flight of ideas
- Distractibility
- Increased level of goal-directed activity
- Problematic behavior

■ SYNONYMS

Manic-depression
Cycloid psychosis

ICD-9CM CODES

296.4-6 Circular manic, circular depressed, circular type mixed

■ EPIDEMIOLOGY & DEMOGRAPHICS

INCIDENCE (IN U.S.): Approximately 1% of the population
PREVALENCE (IN U.S.): 0.4% to 1.6%
PREDOMINANT SEX: Equal distribution among male and female
PREDOMINANT AGE: Lifelong condition with age of onset 14 to 30 yr
PEAK INCIDENCE: Onset in 20s
GENETICS:

- Concordance rates for monozygotic twins: 0.7 to 0.9, for dizygotic twins: 0.2 to 0.4
- Risk of offspring with one affected parent: 0.2 to 0.4, with two affected parents: 0.4 to 0.7
- Displays the phenomenon of genetic anticipation (earlier onset with successive generations), which is a hallmark phenomenon of trinucleotide repeat diseases
- CAG trinucleotide repeats increased by approximately 30 repeats but location unknown
- Displays a parent of origin effect in which there is a higher frequency of the disease in maternal relatives
- Susceptibility locus mapped to chromosome 18p

■ PHYSICAL FINDINGS & CLINICAL PRESENTATION

- Mania associated with psychomotor activation that is usually goal-directed but not necessarily productive
- Elevated and frequently labile mood
- Flight of ideas with rapid, loud, pressured speech
- Psychosis with delusions, hallucinations, and formal thought disorder possible
- Depressive episodes resembling major depression (see "Major Depression"); however, retardation usually extreme
- Catatonia possible in severe cases

■ ETIOLOGY

- Unknown
- Hypotheses:
  1. Abnormalities of membrane function
  2. Second messenger abnormalities
  3. Noradrenergic excess

DIAGNOSIS

■ DIFFERENTIAL DIAGNOSIS

- Secondary manias caused by medical disorder (e.g., renal disease, AIDS, stroke, digoxin toxicity) are frequent.
- Onset of mania after age 40 yr is suggestive of secondary mania.
- Less severe, and probably distinct, conditions of bipolar type II and cyclothymia are possible.
- Cross-sectional examination of acutely manic patient can be confused with schizophreniform or a paranoid psychosis.

■ WORKUP

- History
- Physical examination
- Mental status examination

■ LABORATORY TESTS

- Because of high rate of secondary manias, initial presentation to confirm health of all major organ systems (routine chemistries, complete blood count, urinalysis, sedimentation rate)
- Low threshold for examination of CSF

■ IMAGING STUDIES

Imaging of anatomy (CT scan or MRI) as well as function (EEG) should be part of initial workup.

TREATMENT

■ NONPHARMACOLOGIC THERAPY

- Psychotherapy to help patients cope with consequences of the disease and improve compliance with medications
- Bright light therapy in the northern latitudes in individuals exhibiting a seasonal pattern of winter depression

■ ACUTE GENERAL Rx

- First-line agents for acute mania: lithium, valproate, and carbamazepine
- Useful adjuncts to acute treatment: antipsychotics and benzodiazepines
- Problematic because antidepressants can induce manic episodes

■ CHRONIC Rx

- Goal of long-term treatment: prevention
- Best agents for prophylaxis: lithium, valproate, and carbamazepine
- Useful second-line agents: antipsychotics (particularly the atypical agents such as clozapine)
- Long-term use of antidepressants: frequently destabilizes patient and leads to more frequent relapses

■ DISPOSITION

- Course is variable.
- Over 90% of patients having a single manic episode are likely to experience others.
- Uncontrolled manic or depressive episodes can lead to additional episodes ("illness begets illness").
- Untreated suicide rate approaches 20%; drops to only 8% to 10% with treatment.
- Psychosocioeconomic consequences of both mania and depression can be severe and disabling.
- Cost of condition is about $48 billion annually (in 1991 dollars).

■ REFERRAL

- If use of antidepressant contemplated
- If patient is severely manic or suicidal

REFERENCE

El-Mallakh RS: *Lithium: actions and mechanisms,* Washington, DC, 1996, American Psychiatric Press.
Author: **Rif S. El-Mallakh, M.D.**

BASIC INFORMATION

■ DEFINITION
A bite wound can be animal or human, accidental or intentional.

ICD-9CM CODES
879.8 Bite wound, unspecified site

■ EPIDEMIOLOGY & DEMOGRAPHICS
- Bite wounds account for 1% of emergency department visits.
- More than 1 million bites occur in humans annually in the U.S.
- Dog bites account for 85% to 90% of all bites and result in 10 to 20 fatalities yearly in the U.S.; cat bites, 10% to 20%. Typically the animal is owned by the victim.
- Infection rates are highest for cat bites (30% to 50%), followed by human bites (15% to 30%) and dog bites (5%).
- The extremities are involved in 75% of bites.

■ PHYSICAL FINDINGS & CLINICAL PRESENTATION
- The appearance of the bite wound is variable (e.g., puncture wound, tear, avulsion).
- Cellulitis, lymphangitis, and focal adenopathy may be present in infected bite wounds.
- Patient may experience fever and chills.

■ ETIOLOGY
- Increased risk of infection: human and cat bites, closed fist injuries, wounds involving joints, puncture wounds, face and lip bites, bites with skull penetration, bites in immunocompromised hosts
- Most frequent infecting organisms:
  1. *Pasteurella* spp.: responsible for majority of infections within 24 hr of dog (*Pasteurella canis*) and cat (*Pasteurella multocida, Pasteurella septica*) bites
  2. *Capnocytophaga canimorsus* (formerly DF-2 bacillus): a gram-negative organism responsible for late infection, usually following dog bites
  3. Gram-negative organisms *(Pseudomonas, Haemophilus):* often found in human bites
  4. *Streptococcus* spp., *Staphylococcus aureus*
  5. *Eikenella corrodens* in human bites

🔬 DIAGNOSIS

■ DIFFERENTIAL DIAGNOSIS
- Bite from a rabid animal (often the attack is unprovoked)
- Factitious injury

■ WORKUP
- Determination of the time elapsed since the patient was bitten, status of rabies immunization of the animal, and underlying medical conditions that might predispose the patient to infection (e.g., DM, immunodeficiency)
- Documentation of bite site, notification of appropriate authorities (e.g., police department, animal officer)

■ LABORATORY TESTS
- Generally not necessary
- Hct if there has been significant blood loss
- Wound cultures (aerobic and anaerobic) if there is evidence of sepsis or victim is immunocompromised patient; cultures should be obtained before irrigation of the wound but after superficial cleaning

■ IMAGING STUDIES
X-rays are indicated when bony penetration is suspected or if there is suspicion of fracture or significant trauma; x-rays are also useful for detecting presence of foreign bodies (when suspected).

💊 TREATMENT

■ NONPHARMACOLOGIC THERAPY
- Local care with debridement, vigorous cleansing, and saline irrigation of the wound; debridement of devitalized tissue
- High-pressure irrigation to clean bite wound and ensure removal of contaminants (e.g., use saline solution with a 30- to 35-ml syringe equipped with a 20-gauge needle or catheter with tip of syringe placed 2 to 3 cm above the wound)

- Avoid blunt probing of wounds (increased risk of infection)

■ ACUTE GENERAL Rx
- Avoid suturing of hand wounds and any wounds that appear infected.
- Puncture wounds should be left open
- Give antirabies therapy and tetanus immune globulin and toxoid as needed (Table 1-17).
- Use empiric antibiotic therapy in high-risk wounds (e.g., cat bite, hand bites, face bites, genital area bites, bites with joint or bone penetration, human bites, immunocompromised host): amoxicillin-clavulanate (Augmentin) 500 to 875 mg bid for 7 days or cefuroxime (Ceftin) 250 to 50 mg bid for 7 days.
- In hospitalized patients, IV antibiotics of choice are cefoxitin 1 to 2 g q6h, ampicillin-sulbactam 1.5 to 3 g q6h, ticarcillin-clavulanate 3 g q6h, or ceftriaxone 1 to 2 g q24h.
- Prophylactic therapy for persons bitten by others with HIV (see Table 5-30) and hepatitis B (see Table 5-28)

■ DISPOSITION
Prognosis is favorable with proper treatment.

■ REFERRAL
- Hospitalization and IV antibiotic therapy for infected human bites; bites with injury to joints, nerves, or tendons; or any animal bites unresponsive to oral therapy.
- In the outpatient setting, bite wounds should be reevaluated within 48 hours to assess for signs of infection.

■ COMMENTS
Box 1-8 describes risk factors for infection from animal bite.

REFERENCES
Presutti RJ: Prevention and treatment of dog bites, *Am Fam Physician* 63:1567, 2001.

Talan DA et al: Bacteriologic analysis of infected dog and cat bites, *N Engl J Med* 340:85, 1999.

Weiss HB et al: Incidence of dog bite injuries treated in emergency departments, *JAMA* 279:51, 1998.
Author: **Fred F. Ferri, M.D.**

BOX 1-8   Risk Factors For Infection From Animal Bite

High Risk
Location

Hand, wrist, or foot
Scalp or face in patients with high risk of cranial perforation; CT or skull radiograph examination is mandatory
Over a major joint (possibility of perforation)
Through-and-through bite of cheek

Type of wound

Punctures that are difficult or impossible to irrigate adequately
Tissue crushing that cannot be debrided (typical of herbivores)
Carnivore bite over vital structure (artery, nerve, joint)

Patient

Older than 50 years
Asplenic
Chronic alcoholic
Altered immune status (chemotherapy, acquired immunodeficiency syndrome [AIDS], immune defect)
Diabetic
Peripheral vascular insufficiency
Chronic corticosteroid therapy
Prosthetic or diseased cardiac valve (consider systemic prophylaxis)
Prosthetic or seriously diseased joint (consider systemic prophylaxis)

Species

Large cat (canine teeth produce deep punctures that can penetrate joints, cranium)
Primates
Pigs (anecdotal evidence only)
Alligators, crocodiles

Low Risk
Location

Face, scalp, ears, and mouth (all facial wounds should be sutured)
Self-bite of buccal mucosa that does not go through to skin

Type of wound

Large, clean lacerations that can be thoroughly cleansed (the larger the laceration, the lower the infection rate)
Partial-thickness lacerations and abrasions

Species

Rodents
Quokkas
Bats (although high risk for rabies)

From Auerbach PS: *Wilderness medicine,* ed 4, St Louis, 2001, Mosby.
CT, Computed tomography.

TABLE 1-17   Tetanus Prophylaxis

HISTORY OF IMMUNIZATION (DOSES)	CLEAN MINOR WOUNDS		MAJOR DIRTY WOUNDS	
	TOXOID*	TIG†	TOXOID	TIG
Unknown	Yes	No	Yes	Yes
None to one	Yes	No	Yes	Yes
Two	Yes	No	Yes	No (unless wound older than 24 hr)
Three or more				
Last booster within 5 years	No	No	No	No
Last booster within 10 years	No	No	Yes	Yes
Last booster more than 10 years ago	Yes	No	Yes	Yes

From Auerbach PS: *Wilderness medicine,* ed 4, St Louis, 2001, Mosby.
*Toxoid: Adult: 0.5 ml DT intramuscularly (IM). Child less than 5 years old: 0.5 ml DPT IM. Child older than 5 years: 0.5 ml DT IM.
†Tetanus immune globulin (TIG): 250 to 500 units IM in limb contralateral to toxoid.

BASIC INFORMATION

■ DEFINITION
- Bees, wasps, and ants that sting
- Flies, mosquitoes, fleas, and lice that bite
- Two major classes of arthropods: insects, arachnida

ICD-9CM CODES
989.5 Anaphylactic shock or reaction
910-915 For bites/injury, superficial by site (0.4 if not infected, 0.5 if infected)

■ EPIDEMIOLOGY & DEMOGRAPHICS
- Occur during warm weather, near nests
- Bees attracted to bright clothing and perfumes
- Mosquitoes near standing water
- Flies near horses
- Fleas from pets
- Lice and scabies from person to person or clothing
- 0.4% to 4% of population allergic to venom of one or more stinging insects

■ PHYSICAL FINDINGS & CLINICAL PRESENTATION
BEE, WASP, AND ANT STINGS:
Local Reaction:
- Erythema
- Edema surrounding site; can be life threatening if involves mouth or throat and causes airway obstruction
- Stings around eye can lead to iris or lens damage
Toxic Reaction:
- Usually with more than 10 stings
- Vomiting, diarrhea, syncope or urticaria, or bronchospasm
Systemic or Anaphylactic Reaction:
- Rapid onset, symptoms intensify rapidly
- Urticaria, dry cough, progresses to chest constriction, wheezing, vertigo, vomiting, shock, within 30 min or less
Delayed Reaction:
- Serum sickness–like symptoms 10 to 14 days after sting
FLEA, LICE, AND SCABIES BITES:
- Similar lesions, small red spots or lines become erythematous
- Highly pruritic, thus usually see linear scratch marks
- Scabies concentrates on hands and feet, leaves zig-zag red burrows
SPIDER AND SCORPION BITES:
- The class *Arachnida* contains the largest number of venomous species known and includes black widow spiders and brown recluse spiders (see Fig. 1-63)
- The classic symptomatology of the black widow spider is initially a pin-prick sensation followed by swelling and redness; two small fang marks may be noticed

■ ETIOLOGY
- Various insects
- Systemic reaction thought to be IgE-mediated, causing release of histamine and other anaphylactic mediators
- Venoms contain histamine and various antigens

DIAGNOSIS

■ DIFFERENTIAL DIAGNOSIS
History is crucial in attempting to correctly identify bees or hornets, which may be important if immunotherapy is a future consideration. Patients can usually identify fleas, flies, and mosquitoes. Body lice concentrate about waist, shoulder, neck, axillae. Head lice look like dandruff but can't be brushed out. Pubic lice appear as bluish spots on abdomen and thighs. Scabies causes burrows on hands and feet.

■ WORKUP
Physical examination: look for stingers and remove if possible. Scabies burrows can have mites that can be scraped with a blade and identified under a microscope.

TREATMENT

Stings:
- Remove stinger by scraping; do not use tweezers because this can squeeze venom into wound
- Local reactions: ice pack, oral antihistamines, analgesics, prednisone; elevate involved limbs
- Systemic reaction: epinephrine 1:1000, 0.3 to 0.5 ml SC; massage injection site to hasten absorption; second injection every 15 min as necessary; antihistamines IV
- Bronchospasm: β_2-agonist as necessary; intubate, if necessary, for airway obstruction
- Hypotension supportive care with isotonic fluids
- IV steroids: limit urticaria and edema
Fly, mosquito, and flea bites:
- Symptomatic treatment similar to stings, clean to prevent secondary infection
- Head lice: permethrin 5% (Elimite), repeat in 7 to 10 days; comb with fine comb to remove nits; safe in children over 2 mo
- Body lice: sterilization of clothing, disposal if possible
- Scabies: permethrin 5% cream, chin to toes; leave on 8 to 10 hr, repeat in 7 days

- Second-line agent for scabies is lindane 1%: not safe in children or pregnancy
Spider bite (black widow):
- Apply ice pack to bite area, immediate transport to ER
- Tetanus immunization should be instituted
- Symptomatic treatment (e.g., controlling muscle cramps with calcium gluconate, dantrolene sodium, diazepam)
- Cardiac monitoring, antivenin

■ DISPOSITION
- For patients with systemic reactions, send home with emergency epinephrine kit
- If severe or anaphylactic reaction, admit and observe for 48 hr for cardiac, renal, or neurologic problems

■ REFERRAL
For patients with systemic reactions, refer to allergist for immunotherapy; 95% to 98% effective in preventing anaphylaxis
Author: **Gail M. O'Brien, M.D.**

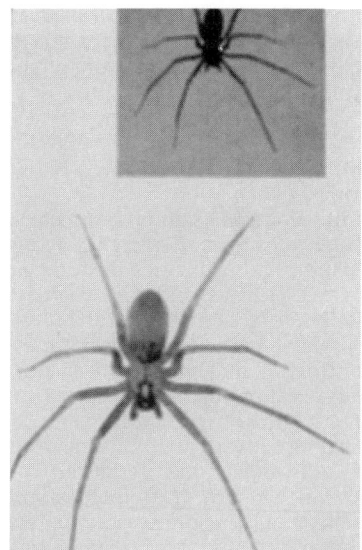

Fig. 1-63 Brown recluse and black widow spiders may produce extensive tissue necrosis and ulceration. (From Noble J [ed]: *Primary care medicine,* ed 2, St Louis, 1996, Mosby.)

BASIC INFORMATION

■ DEFINITION
The normal effect of a bee, wasp, brown recluse spider, or fire ant bite or sting is to cause intense local pain, some immediate erythema, and often a small area of edema by injecting venom. Allergic reactions can be either local or generalized.

■ SYNONYMS
Venom allergy

ICD-9CM CODES
989.5 Stings (bees, wasps)
989.5 Bites (fire ant, brown recluse spider)

■ EPIDEMIOLOGY & DEMOGRAPHICS
PREVALENCE (OF BEE STINGS AND INSECT BITES):
- Unknown
- Between 0.4% and 4% of the population is allergic to the venom of one or more stinging insects
- Bites by fire ants and brown recluse spiders are less likely to cause systemic disease

INCIDENCE (IN U.S.): 50 to 150 people die each year from insect sting anaphylaxis; anaphylaxis occurs more often within 10 to 30 min of a sting

■ PHYSICAL FINDINGS & CLINICAL PRESENTATION
Stings:
- Cutaneous: the skin is the most common site of an allergic reaction. Manifestations include flushing, urticaria, pruritus, and angioedema.
- Respiratory: hoarseness, difficulty speaking, choking, throat tightness or tingling may progress to stridor, laryngeal edema, laryngospasm, and bronchoconstriction. This is the leading cause of anaphylactic death.
- Cardiovascular: manifestations include tachycardia, hypotension, arrhythmia, in some cases progressing to profound hypovolemic shock. Myocardial infarction is rare. Cardiac manifestations are the second leading cause of death from anaphylaxis.
- Other symptoms: abdominal pain, nausea, vomiting, and diarrhea.

Bites:
Brown recluse spider:
- Erythematous, violaceous, or hemorrhagic discoloration at site within 8 hr
- Central necrosis: lesions <1 cm heal within weeks; lesions >1 cm take months to heal
- Mild hemolysis, mild coagulopathy
- Fevers, chills, vomiting, joint pain

Fire ant:
- Circularly arrayed pustules

■ ETIOLOGY
Stings:
- Most systemic reactions to insect stings are classic IgA-mediated allergic reactions.
- Reactions occur in previously sensitized patients who have produced high titers of IgE antibody to insect venom antigens
- Sensitization to wasp venom requires only a few stings and can occur after a single sting.
- Sensitization to bee venom occurs mainly in people who have been stung frequently by bees.

Bites:
- Brown recluse spider venom contains enzymes that can cause tissue necrosis.
- Fire ant venom contains proteins toxic to the skin.

DIAGNOSIS

■ DIFFERENTIAL DIAGNOSIS
- Stings: cellulitis, bites
- Bites: stings, cellulitis

■ WORKUP
History is essential for accurate diagnosis including timing of sting or bite and type of insect (bee, wasp, spider, or ant) if known.

■ LABORATORY TESTS
- Skin test: either skin prick test or intradermal with bee and wasp venom.
- Measurement of serum bee-specific or wasp-specific IgE measured by radioallergosorbent tests (RAST) or other assays.

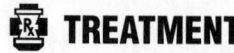

TREATMENT

■ ACUTE GENERAL Rx
Sting:
- Treatment with oral antihistamines if limited reaction
- Treatment for larger swellings and associated systemic symptoms is IM antihistamines, intravenous corticosteroids, adrenaline, IM epinephrine, and IV fluids

Bite:
- Supportive
- Application of ice

Brown recluse spider:
- Excision of lesion
- Dapsone
- IV corticosteroids

■ DISPOSITION
Sting:
Prognosis for a limited reaction is excellent. Anywhere from 20% to 80% of patients who have had generalized reaction to a sting will have no such reaction on subsequent sting and there is no evidence that the next sting will necessarily cause a more severe reaction. The reasons for the variable outcome include patient's immune status at the time of sting, dose of venom injected, and site of sting.

Bite:
- Prognosis for fire ant bite is excellent. Large lesions from brown recluse spider bites may take months to heal.

■ FURTHER MANAGEMENT
Patients with a history of sting allergies should carry syringes preloaded with epinephrine (EpiPen) and oral antihistamines to take if they are stung again. Consider a referral to an allergist for immunotherapy.

REFERENCES
Ewan PW: ABC of allergies: venom allergy, *BMJ* 316(7141):1365, 1998.
Kemp ED: Bites and stings of the arthropod kind, *Postgrad Med* 103(6):88, 1998.
Koh WL: When to worry about spider bites: inaccurate diagnosis can have serious, even fatal, consequences, *Postgrad Med* 103(4):235, 1998.
Author: **Anne W. Moulton, M.D.**

BASIC INFORMATION

■ **DEFINITION**
Injury resulting from snake biting a human.

ICD-9CM CODES
989.5 Venomous poisoning

■ **EPIDEMIOLOGY & DEMOGRAPHICS**
• There are 45,000 snake bites in the United States each year, 8000 of which are caused by poisonous snakes. This results in approximately 9 to 15 fatalities, most among children, the elderly, and those in whom treatment has been delayed.
• In the United States at least one species of poisonous snake has been identified in every state except Alaska, Hawaii, and Maine. The majority of venomous snakes are members of the family *Crotalidae,* which includes rattlesnakes, copperheads, and cottonmouths. The *Elapidae* family, which includes the coral snake, accounts for the remainder.

■ **PHYSICAL FINDINGS & CLINICAL PRESENTATION**
The initial signs and symptoms vary with species, but a general description is provided below.
CROTALIDAE (PIT VIPERS): Signs and symptoms:
• Fang puncture(s)
• Pain within 5 min
• Edema within 30 min
• Erythema of site and adjacent tissues
If no edema or erythema is manifested within 4 to 8 hr after the snakebite, it is safe to assume envenomation did not occur. Other manifestations include:
• Perioral paresthesias, metallic taste, and tingling of fingers or toes (especially with rattlesnake bites)
• Fasciculations, may be generalized
• Systemic reactions: chills, fever, nausea, vomiting, headache, lymphangitis, hypotension, weakness
ELAPIDAE (CORAL SNAKES): Signs and symptoms:
• Little or no pain or swelling immediately after the bite
Systemic symptoms most common but there may be a delay of 1 to 5 hr before onset:
• Ptosis
• Dysphagia
• Dysarthria
• Intense salivation
• Later: loss of DTRs and respiratory depression

■ **DIAGNOSIS**

■ **DIFFERENTIAL DIAGNOSIS**
• Harmless snake bite
• Scorpion bite
• Insect bite
• Cellulitis
• Laceration or puncture wound
Harmless snakebites are usually characterized by four rows of small scratches (teeth in upper jaw) separated from two rows of scratches (teeth in lower jaw) (Fig. 1-64). This is in distinction to venomous snake bites, which should have puncture wounds produced by the snake's fangs. There may also be teeth marks other than fang marks present. Not all bites from venomous snakes result in envenomation, but observation in suspected cases is critical.

■ **WORKUP**
• Physical examination and laboratory evaluation with emphasis on assessing the severity of the envenomation
• No standardized classification system for grading envenomations; the following classification was first described by Russell in 1964:
    Minimal: confined to the site of the bite, no significant systemic symptoms or signs, no laboratory abnormalities
    Moderate: manifestations extend beyond the site of the bite but no life-threatening systemic symptoms
    Severe: symptoms involve entire limb or part and include severe systemic symptoms and signs, may have laboratory abnormalities including abnormal coagulation studies

■ **LABORATORY TESTS**
• For all envenomations, draw blood for CBC, platelet count, coagulation profile (PT, PTT, fibrinogen); send urinalysis and perform ECG
• More severe bites may require further tests including sedimentation rate, serum electrolytes, BUN, serum creatinine, creatine kinase, liver functions, and type and crossmatch
It is important to remember that the severity of envenomation should be continually assessed and based on the most severe symptom, sign, or laboratory result at that time. Grading may change.

■ **TREATMENT**

■ **ACUTE GENERAL Rx**
IN THE FIELD: For a suspected snakebite
• Immobilize affected part below level of the heart
• Remove any constricting items
• Keep victim warm but avoid alcohol, stimulants (caffeine)
• DO NOT use ice
• Tourniquet and incision and suction use by those not skilled in snake bite management are discouraged
• Transport immediately to nearest medical facility
IN THE HOSPITAL:
• Obtain time of bite, description of snake if possible, medical history, including previous snake bites and treatment
• Ask about allergies, specifically to horse serum
• Record vital signs: BP, HR, T, RR
• Inspect site of bite for fang marks, local symptoms
• Measure circumference of bitten part at two or more proximal sites and compare with unaffected limb; repeat every 15 to 20 min
• Neurologic examination
• Gauge the severity of the bite and decide whether administration of antivenin is necessary
• For minimal envenomation without progressive manifestations
  1. Clean and immobilize affected part
  2. Immunize against tetanus
  3. Observe patient for at least 6 hr
• Patients who have progressive symptoms (local or systemic) and/or moderate to severe envenomation should be considered for antivenin
• The same antivenin works for all bites in this country except those of the coral snake (which has its own antivenin)
• Zoos with exotic snakes are required to maintain a supply of snake-specific antivenin on their premises
• Antivenin is most effective when given within 4 hr of the bite and less so after 12 hr
Once the decision is made to use antivenin
• Skin test for sensitivity to horse serum should be done (instructions in antivenin brochure)
• If positive, risks and benefits need to be considered, antivenin given if life or limb is threatened and in a critical care setting; contact regional poison control center for desensitization

- If negative, initially dilute antivenin and be ready to treat anaphylaxis
- Administer antivenin in accordance with information provided in the antivenin brochure

Guidelines to dosage:
- For *pit viper* bites
  - Mild   5 vials
  - Moderate   10 vials
  - Severe   15 vials
  - Shock   20 vials
- For *coral snake* bites
  - 3 vials, if symptoms evolve, repeat with 5 vials

Other considerations:
- Initial dose of antivenin should be repeated until progression of symptoms has abated, but observation of bitten part should be continued for another 48 hr
- Children require more antivenin; increase dose by 50%
- Pregnancy is not a contraindication to antivenin
- Immunize against tetanus if no booster within past 5 yr; if never immunized, give immunoglobulin as well as toxoid

- Manage pain as needed (acetaminophen, codeine, meperidine)
- Avoid sedation in Mojave rattlesnake, eastern diamondback rattlesnake, and coral snake bites
- Antibiotics reserved for moderate to severe cases; use those with broad-spectrum coverage (which includes gram negatives, i.e., quinolone derivatives)

■ DISPOSITION
Prognosis is good with prompt evaluation and treatment.

■ REFERRAL
To medical facility with ICU for administration of antivenin

☼ PEARLS & CONSIDERATIONS

■ COMPLICATIONS
Most frequent complication of treated envenomations is serum sickness; occurs 7 to 14 days after antivenin administration and is characterized by fever, rash, arthralgias, and lymphadenopathy. It can be treated with PO prednisone 60 mg/d, tapered over 7 to 10 days

Acutely, there is the risk of anaphylaxis to antivenin as mentioned previously. This occurs within 30 min and is treated with
- IV epinephrine
- IV diphenhydramine
- IV hydrocortisone

Injuries also result from
- Tourniquet placement
- Cryotherapy

Author: **Rebecca A. Griffith, M.D.**

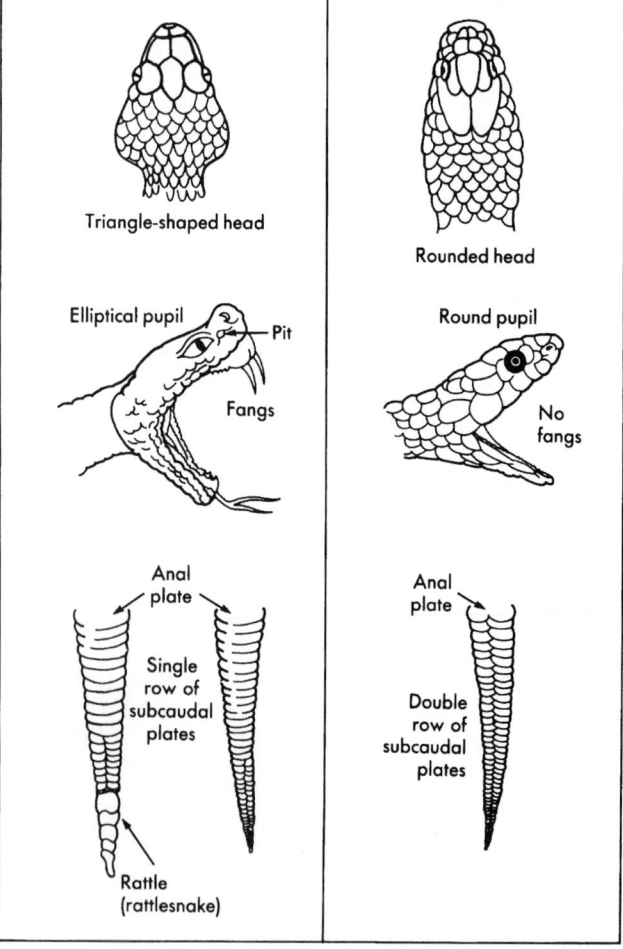

Fig. 1-64 Identification of venomous snakes. (From Rosen P [ed]: *Emergency medicine,* ed 4, St Louis, 1998, Mosby.)

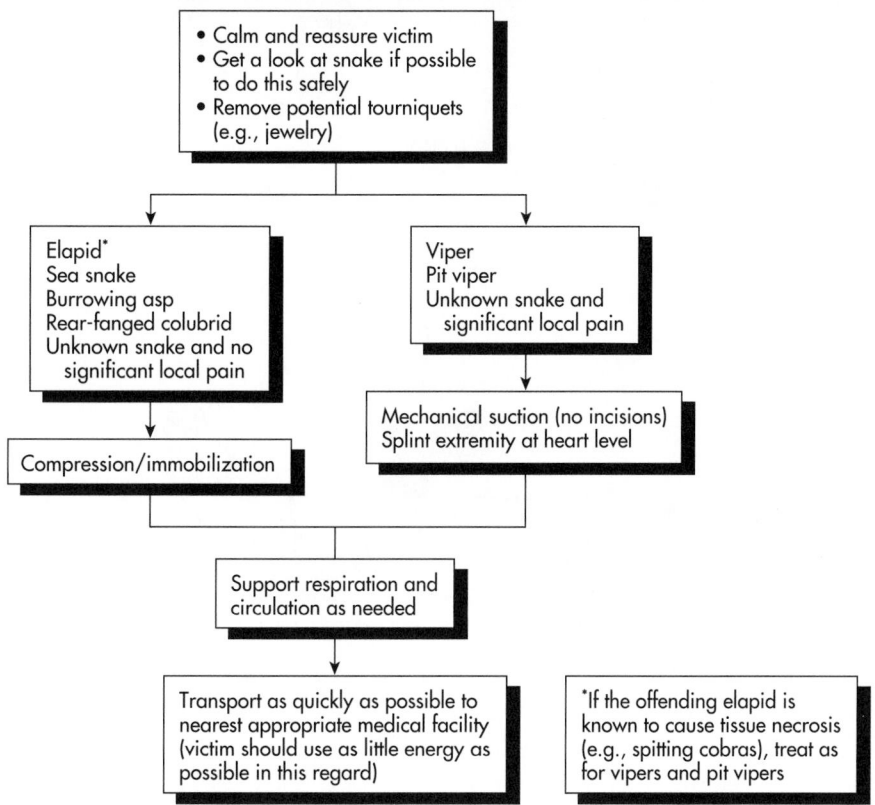

Fig. 1-65 First-aid measures for venomous snakebites. (From Auerbach PS: *Wilderness medicine,* ed 4, St Louis, 2001, Mosby.)

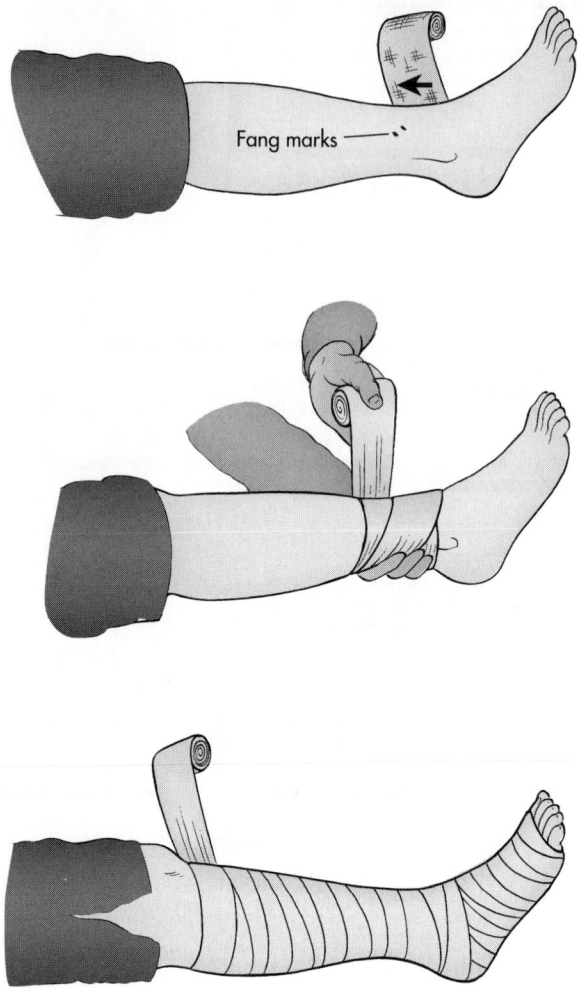

Fang marks

Fig. 1-66   Australian compression and immobilization technique has proved effective in the management of elapid and sea snake envenomations. Its efficacy in viper bites has yet to be evaluated clinically. (From Auerbach PS: *Wilderness medicine,* ed 4, St Louis, 2001, Mosby.)

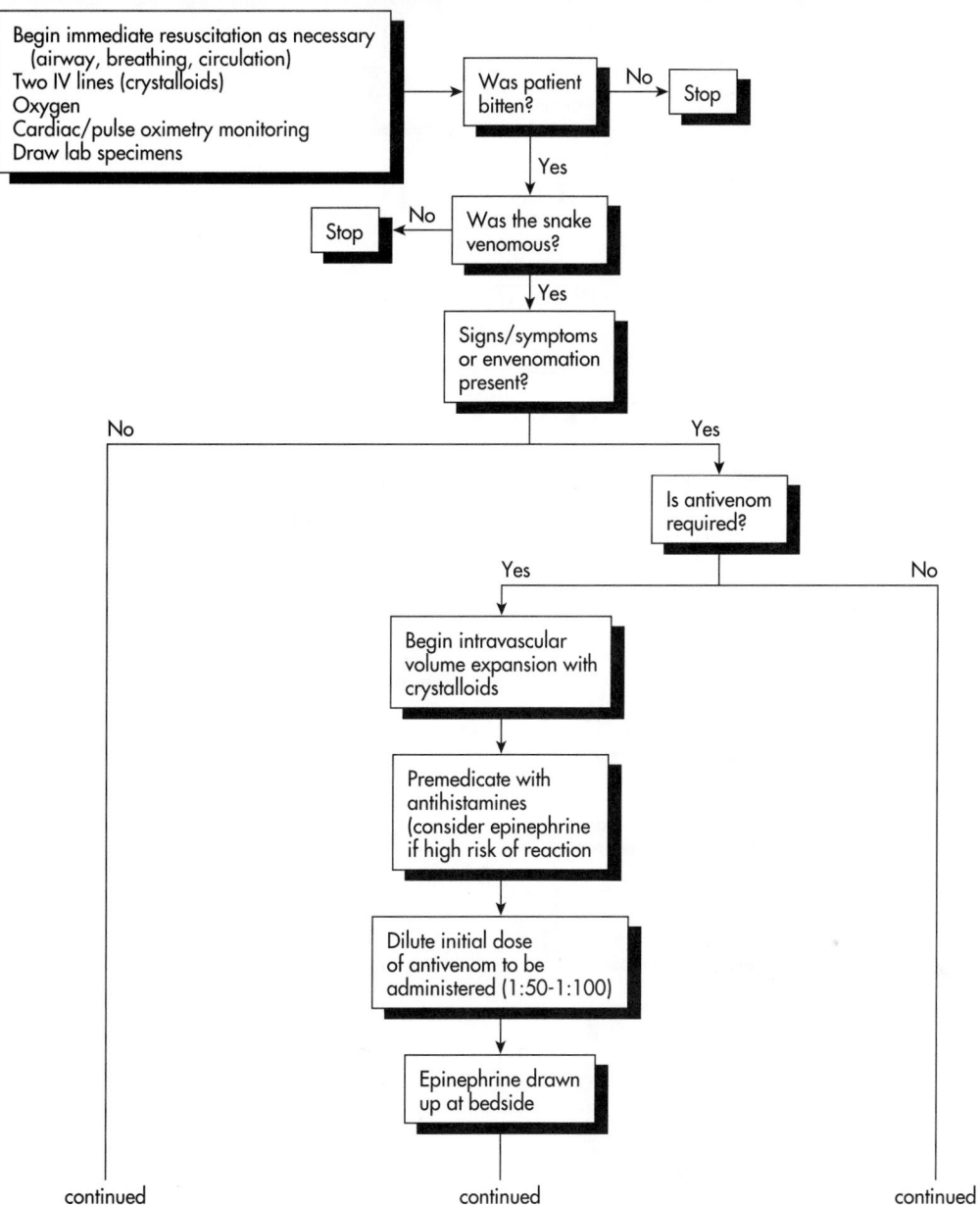

Fig. 1-67 Guidelines for the hospital management of venomous snakebite. *IV,* Intravenous. (From Auerbach PS: *Wilderness medicine,* ed 4, St Louis, 2001, Mosby.)

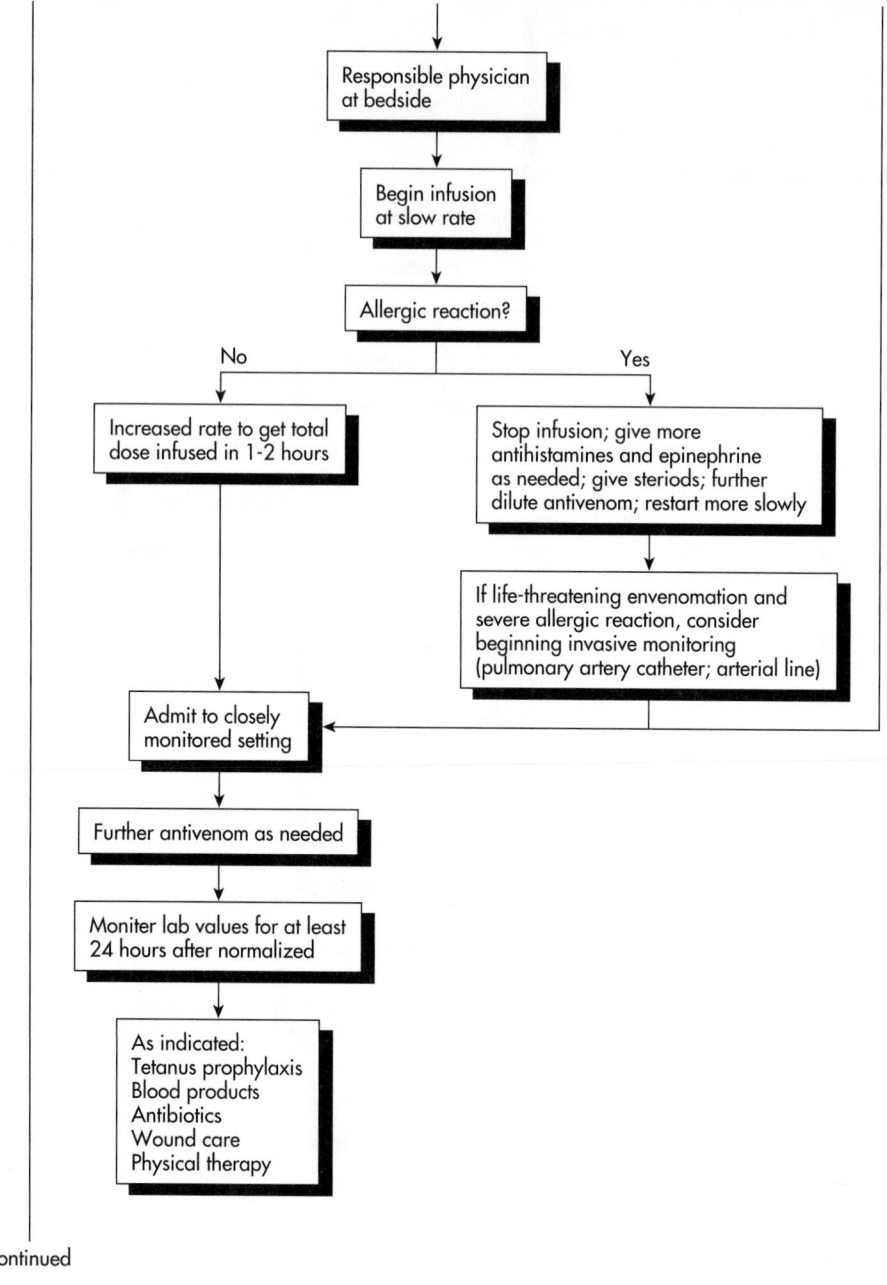

Responsible physician
at bedside

Begin infusion
at slow rate

Allergic reaction?

No   Yes

Increased rate to get total   Stop infusion; give more
dose infused in 1-2 hours   antihistamines and epinephrine
                                     as needed; give steriods; further
                                     dilute antivenom; restart more slowly

                                     If life-threatening envenomation and
                                     severe allergic reaction, consider
                                     beginning invasive monitoring
                                     (pulmonary artery catheter; arterial line)

Admit to closely
monitored setting

Further antivenom as needed

Moniter lab values for at least
24 hours after normalized

As indicated:
Tetanus prophylaxis
Blood products
Antibiotics
Wound care
Physical therapy

continued

Fig. 1-67, cont'd   (From Auerbach PS: *Wilderness medicine,* ed 4, St Louis, 2001, Mosby.)

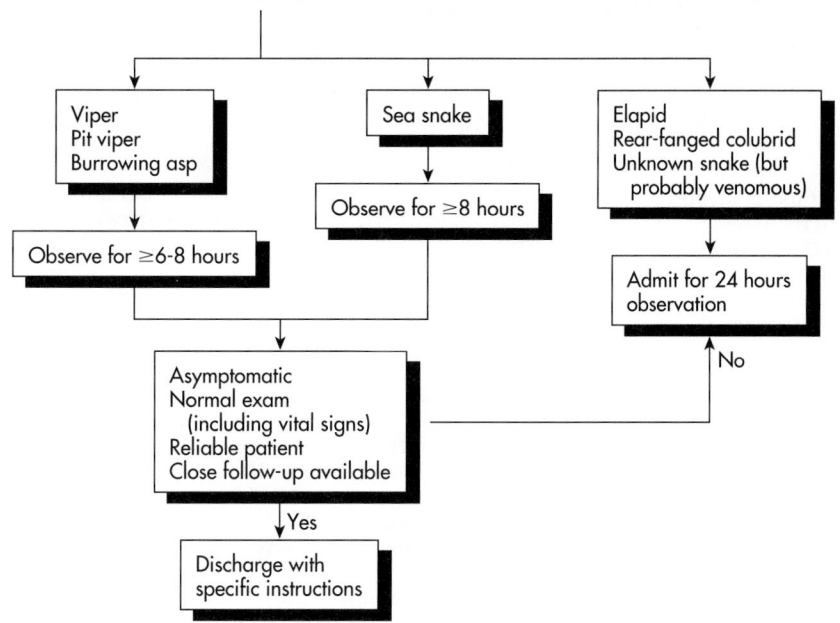

Fig. 1-67, cont'd (From Auerbach PS: *Wilderness medicine,* ed 4, St Louis, 2001, Mosby.)

BOX 1-9   Diagnostic Studies in Evaluation of Venomous Snakebite Victims

Blood and Serum

Type and cross-match
Complete blood cell count
Peripheral smear
Coagulation studies (fibrinogen, fibrin degradation products, D-dimer, partial thromboplastin time, prothrombin time)
Electrolytes, glucose, creatinine, blood urea nitrogen, liver enzymes, bilirubin
Arterial blood gases
Myoglobin, creatine kinase

Urine

Bedside tests (glucose, blood, myoglobin [on each voided specimen])
Urinalysis

Stool

Test for blood

Radiographs

Chest (if over 40 yr old, history of underlying cardiopulmonary disease, or severe envenomation)
Bite site soft tissue films (if retained fangs possible; poor sensitivity)
Computed tomography of the brain (if presentation suggests intracranial hemorrhage)

Electrocardiogram

If patient is over 40 yr old, has a history of underlying cardiopulmonary disease, or has a severe envenomation

From Auerbach PS: *Wilderness medicine,* ed 4, St Louis, 2001, Mosby.

BASIC INFORMATION

■ DEFINITION

Bladder cancer is a heterogeneous spectrum of neoplasms ranging from non–life-threatening, low-grade, superficial papillary lesions to high-grade invasive tumors, which often have metastasized at the time of presentation. It is a field change disease in which the entire urothelium from the renal pelvis to the urethra may be susceptible to malignant transformation. *Types:* Transitional cell carcinoma (TCCa), squamous cell carcinoma, and adenocarcinoma.

ICD-9CM CODES
Primary: 188.9
Secondary: 198.1
CIS: 233.7
Benign: 223.3
Uncertain behavior: 236.7
Unspecified: 239.4

■ EPIDEMIOLOGY & DEMOGRAPHICS

Each year approximately 54,000 new cases are diagnosed and over 12,000 deaths are attributed to bladder cancer. Until 1990, the incidence of bladder cancer in the U.S. was rising. Since 1990, the incidence of bladder cancer is decreasing at a rate of 0.8% per year (1.2% among men and 0.4% among women).

PREDOMINANT SEX: In males, it is the fourth most common cancer; it accounts for 10% of all cancers. In females, it is the eighth most common cancer; it accounts for 4% of all cancers.

RISK: The lifetime risk of developing bladder cancer is 2.8% in white males, 0.9% in black males, 1% in white females, and 0.6% in black females.
Smoking:
• Users of "black" tobacco in place of "blond" tobacco have a twofold to threefold increase in developing bladder cancer.
• Smoking risk is based on consumption:
  With a twofold to threefold increase for subjects smoking at least 10 cigarettes per day
  The risk increases again when the daily consumption rises above 40-60 cigarettes per day
• Smokers of low tar and nicotine cigarettes have a lower risk when compared with higher tar and nicotine cigarettes.
• Unfiltered cigarettes have a 50% increased risk of bladder cancer compared with those who smoke filtered cigarettes.
• Pipe smokers have a lower risk of bladder cancer compared with cigarette smokers.
• Cigar smoking, snuff, and chewing tobacco, although implicated in nonurologic cancers, is not believed to influence bladder cancer risk.

Diet:
• Diets rich in beef, pork, and animal fat consumption increases risk of bladder cancer.
• There is no indication that consumption of nonbeer alcoholic drinks contributes to bladder cancer development.
• Beer consumption has been linked to bladder cancer development as a result of the presence of nitrosamines in the beer. Similarly, these nitrosamines have been implicated in the development of rectal cancer.
• Drinking coffee is not believed to contribute to bladder cancer risk. There is additional evidence that coffee consumption is protective for colorectal cancers, possibly by diminishing fecal transit time.

PEAK INCIDENCE: Incidence increases with age, high >60 yr, uncommon <40 yr.

GENETICS: It is thought to be multifactorial in etiology, involving both genetic and environmental interactions. Overall, it is estimated that approximately 20% to 25% of the male population in the U.S. with bladder cancer has the disease as a result of occupational exposure.

DISTRIBUTION: In North America, transitional cell carcinomas comprise 93%, squamous cell carcinomas comprise 6%, and adenocarcinomas account for 1% of bladder cancers.

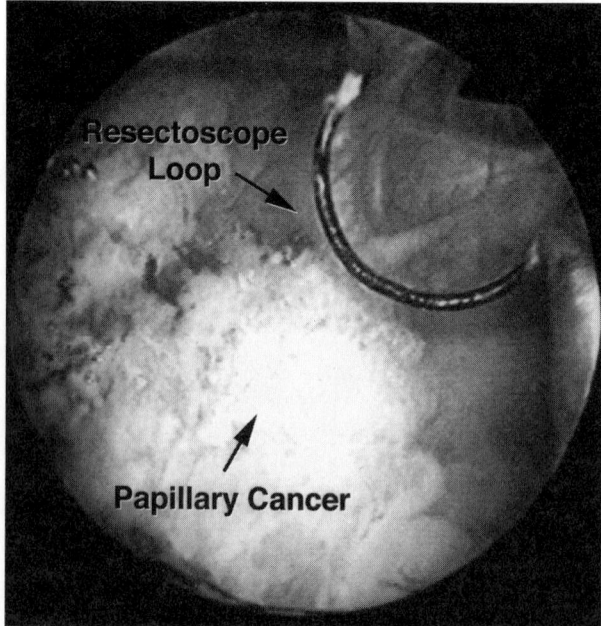
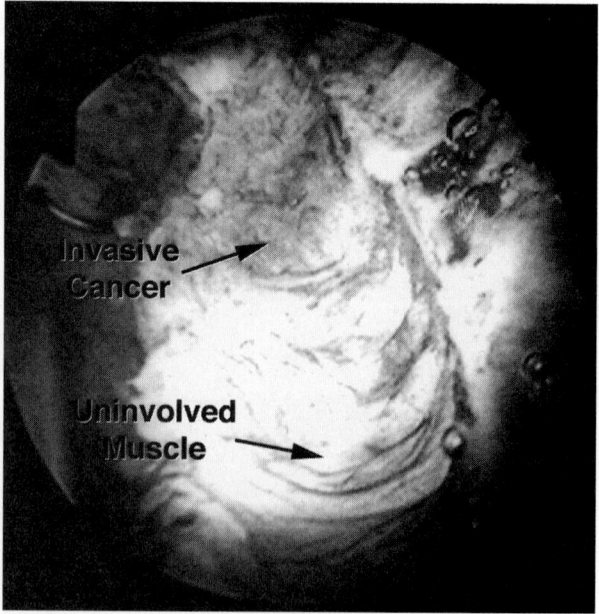

Fig. 1-68   A, Papillary bladder cancer in right lower aspect of photograph, with resection loop poised to begin transurethral resection. **B,** Demonstration of grossly uninvolved muscularis propria *(bottom)* and cancer grossly invading the bladder wall *(top).* (From Abeloff MD [ed]: *Clinical oncology,* ed 2, New York, 2000, Churchill Livingstone.)

PATHOGENESIS: Two pathways exist for bladder cancer (TCCa):

1. Papillary superficial disease occasionally leading to invasive cancer (75%)
2. Carcinoma-in-situ (CIS) and solid invasive cancer with high risk of disease progression (25%)

Two distinct forms of "Superficial Cancer" exist:

T_a	Papillary low-grade tumor High rate of recurrence Disease progression occurs <5%
T_1	Higher-grade papillary tumors that infiltrate the lamina propria Often associated with flat CIS that may involve the urothelium diffusely Disease progression occurs between 30% to 50% Subdivided into:
T_{1a}	Penetration of tumor up to the muscularis mucosae Disease progression 5.3%
T_{1b}	Penetration of tumor through the muscularis mucosae Disease progression 53%

Flat CIS:

Entirely different and separate pathway of cancer development whose mechanism is manifested by dysplasia, which leads to the occurrence of poorly differentiated malignant cells that replace or undermine the normal urothelium and extend along the plane of the bladder wall. It penetrates the basement membrane and lamina propria in 20% to 30% of the cases and is associated with the development of solid tumor growth. A defect in chromosome 17p53 occurs in 50% of the cases.

At presentation, 72% of cancers are localized to the bladder, 20% of the cancers extend to the regional lymph nodes, and 3% present with distant metastases. 80% of superficial TCCa recur with up to 30% progressing to a higher stage or grade. Younger patients most commonly develop low-grade papillary noninvasive TCCa and are less likely to have recurrences when compared with older patients with similar lesions. Involvement of the upper tracts with tumor occurs in 25% to 50% of the cases.

STAGING (BASED ON THE TNM SYSTEM):

T_0	No tumor in specimen
T_{is}	CIS
T_a	Papillary TCCa noninvasive
T_1	Papillary TCCa into lamina propria
T_2	TCCa invasive of superficial ms
T_{3a}	Invasive of deep ms
T_{3b}	Invasive of perivesical fat
T_{4a}	Invasive of adjacent pelvic organ
T_{4b}	Invasive of pelvic wall with fixation

Invasive of nodal status:

N_0	No nodal involvement
N_{1-3}	Pelvic nodes
N_4	Nodes above bifurcation
N_x	Unknown

Invasive of metastatic status:

M_0	No distant metastases
M_1	Distant metastases
M_x	Unknown

MOLECULAR EPIDEMIOLOGY: TCCa is usually a field change disease with tumors arising at different times and sites in the urothelium suggesting a polyclonal etiology of bladder cancer. Bladder cancers have been associated with abnormalities on chromosomes 1, 4, 11, 5, 7, 3, 9, 21, 18, 13, 8; with alterations in suppressor genes P53, retinoblastoma gene, and P16; and with alterations in oncogenes H-ras and epidermal growth factor receptor.

■ PHYSICAL FINDINGS

- Gross painless hematuria
- Microhematuria
- Frequency, urgency, occasional dysuria

With locally invasive to distant metastatic disease, the presentation can include:

- Abdominal pain
- Flank pain
- Lymphedema
- Renal failure
- Anorexia
- Bone pain

■ ETIOLOGY

Bladder cancer is a potentially preventable disease associated with specific etiologic factors:

- Cigarette smoking is associated with 25% to 65% of the cases. The risk of developing a TCCa is 2 to 4 times higher in smokers than in nonsmokers, and that risk persists for many years, being equal to nonsmokers only after 12 to 15 yr of smoking abstinence. Smoking tomacco is associated with tumors that are characterized by higher histologic grade, increased tumor stage, increase in the numbers of tumor present, and increased tumor size.
- Occupational exposures: dye workers, textile workers, tire and rubber workers, petroleum workers
- Chemical exposure: O-toluidine, 2-naphthylamine, benzidine, 4-amino-biphenyl, and nitrosamines
- Exposure to HPV type 16

Squamous carcinomas are associated with:

- Schistosomiasis
- Urinary calculi
- Indwelling catheters
- Bladder diverticula

Miscellaneous causes:

- Phenacetin abuse
- Cyclophosphamide
- Pelvic irradiation
- Tuberculosis

Adenocarcinomas are associated with:

- Exstrophy
- Endometriosis

BOX 1-10 American Urological Association Guideline Recommendations

1. Undiagnosed bladder tumor: obtain a histologic diagnosis of the tumor: Transurethral resection of the tumor is the most common method.
2. Stage Ta or T1 cancer: Complete surgical eradication of all visible tumors. The lesion can be treated with electrocautery resection, fulguration, or laser ablation. Adjuvant intravesical therapy is recommended for patients with carcinoma-in-situ, T1, or high-grade Ta tumors. The agent recommended is BCG or mitomycin C. Cystectomy is an option for this set of tumors because of risk of progression to muscle-invasive disease even after intravesical chemotherapy.

An increased risk of disease progression is associated with large tumor, high-grade tumor, location of the tumor in a site that is poorly accessible to complete resection, diffuse disease, infiltration of lymphatic or vascular spaces, and prostatic urethral involvement.

3. Carcinoma-in-situ or high-grade T1 cancer and prior intravesical chemotherapy: Cystectomy is the recommendation based on the panel's expert opinion rather than evidence from outcomes data. The data show a substantial risk of progression to muscle-invasive cancer in patients with diffuse carcinoma-in-situ and high-grade T1 tumors. The response to intravesical chemotherapy in terms of altering this disease progression is unknown, and as a result of this, cystectomy is an option for the afflicted patient.

American Urological Association, Guideline Division, 1120 North Charles Street, Baltimore, MD 21201.

- Neurogenic bladder
- Urachal abnormalities
- As a secondary site for distant metastases from other organs (i.e., colon cancer)

 DIAGNOSIS

- History and physical examination
- Urinalysis
- Cystoscopy with bladder barbotage and biopsy
- Transurethral resection of bladder tumor(s) (Fig. 1-68)
- There is insufficient evidence to determine whether a decrease in mortality from bladder cancer occurs with hematuria testing, urinary cytology, or a variety of other tests on exfoliated urinary cells or other substances.
- In addition to urinary cytologies and bladder barbotage, BTA, NMP22, and Fibrin Degradation Products (FDP) have been approved by the FDA as bladder cancer tumor markers. No marker has general, widespread acceptance because the results are affected by the presence of stents, recent urologic manipulation, stones, infection, bowel interposition, and prostatitis creating false-positive results.

■ **DIFFERENTIAL DIAGNOSIS**
- Urinary tract infection
- Frequency-urgency syndrome
- Interstitial cystitis
- Stone disease
- Endometriosis
- Neurogenic bladder

■ **LABORATORY TESTS**
RADIOLOGIC TESTS:
- IVP, renal ultrasound, retrograde pyelography, CT scan, and MRI.
- One or a combination of studies can be used. In the absence of skeletal symptoms, bone scan is not recommended.

 TREATMENT

■ **NONPHARMACOLOGIC THERAPY**
- Initially, transurethral resection of bladder tumor (TURBT)
- Loop biopsy of the prostatic urethra if high-grade TCCa is suspected
- If superficial disease, follow-up pro-

tocol with repeat TURBT and/or the use of intravesical agents is recommended
- For advanced bladder cancer, radical cystectomy with urethrectomy (unless orthotopic diversion is planned) and either ileal loop conduit or orthotopic diversion

BLADDER PRESERVATION APPROACHES: Following cystectomy for muscle invasive disease, 50% or more of the patients will develop metastases. Most patients develop metastases at distant sites, a third relapse locally. Bladder preservation management is offered in those individuals who refuse surgery or who might not be suitable radical cystectomy patients. Bladder-sparing protocols include extensive TURBT or partial cystectomy with external beam or interstitial radiotherapy and systemic chemotherapy. Radiotherapy as a single treatment modality is not effective. The best predictor of successful bladder preservation is a complete response following the combination of initial TURBT and two cycles of CMV (cisplatin, methotrexate, vinblastine) chemotherapy seen with stages T2-T3a.

INDICATIONS FOR PARTIAL CYSTECTOMY:
- Tumor within a bladder diverticulum
- Solitary, primary, and muscle-invasive or high-grade lesion of a region of the bladder that allows complete excision with adequate surgical margins
- Inability to adequately resect tumor by TURBT alone because of size or location
- Tumor overlying a ureteral orifice requiring ureteral reimplantation
- Biopsy of a radiation-induced ulceration
- Palliation of severe local symptoms
- Patient refusal or urinary diversion
- Poor-risk patient who is not a diversion candidate

Contraindications:
- Multiple tumors
- CIS
- Cellular atypia on biopsy
- Prostatic invasion
- Invasion of the trigone
- Inability to achieve adequate surgical margins
- Prior radiotherapy
- Inability to maintain adequate bladder volume after resection
- Evidence of extravesical tumor extension
- Poor surgical risk

■ **ACUTE GENERAL Rx**
INDICATIONS FOR INTRAVESICAL CHEMOTHERAPY:
- High-grade tumor
- Tumor size >5 cm
- Tumor multiplicity
- Presence of CIS
- Positive urinary cytologies following a resection
- Incomplete tumor resection
Intravesical agents: thiotepa, Adriamycin, mitomycin C, AD-32, BCG, interferon, bropirimine, Epodyl, interleukin-2, and keyhole-limpet hemocyanin. Photodynamic therapy with hematoporphyrin derivatives has also been used.

INDICATIONS FOR CYSTECTOMY:
- Large tumors not amenable to complete TURBT
- High-grade tumor
- Multiple tumors with frequent recurrences
- Diffuse CIS not responsive to intravesical chemotherapy
- Prostatic urethra involvement
- Irritative bladder symptoms with upper tract deterioration
- Muscle-invasive disease
- Disease outside of the bladder

SYSTEMIC CHEMOTHERAPY: Used as neoadjuvant and adjuvant therapy for systemic disease. The most effective agents are cisplatin, methotrexate, vinblastine, Adriamycin (MVAC). Other agents include: mitoxantrone, vincristine, etoposide (VP16), 5FU, ifosfamide, Taxol, gemcitabine, Piritrexim, and gallium nitrate. Chemotherapy in combination can provide palliation and modest survival benefit.

RADIOTHERAPY: Conflicting reports suggest that superficial bladder cancer is more sensitive to radiotherapy. Squamous changes within the tumor and secretion of human chorionic gonadotropin by the lesion are associated with poor response to radiotherapy. Only 20% to 30% of patients with invasive bladder cancer can be cured by external beam radiation therapy alone. It is used in combination with surgery or with systemic agents to treat bladder cancer primarily in those patients who are not surgical candidates or who refuse surgery.

■ **CHRONIC Rx**
FOLLOW-UP RECOMMENDATIONS FOR SUPERFICIAL BLADDER CANCER:
- Cystoscopy, bladder barbotage, and bimanual examination every 3 mo for 2 yr, then every 6 mo for 2 yr, and annually thereafter.

- Upper tract studies are based on the risk of upper tract tumor development, generally every 2 to 5 yr.

FOLLOW-UP RECOMMENDATIONS FOR ADVANCED DISEASE:

Bladder Preservation:

- Cystoscopy, barbotage, bimanual examination, biopsy (when indicated), every 3 mo for 2 yr, then every 6 mo for 2 yr, yearly thereafter.
- CT scan of abdomen and pelvis every 6 mo for 2 yr in addition to chest x-ray examination, liver function testing, and serum creatinine.

Cystectomy with Ileal Loop/Orthotopic Bladder:

- Neobladder endoscopy and IVP yearly.
- CT scan of abdomen and pelvis every 6 mo for 2 yr in addition to chest x-ray examination, liver function tests, and serum creatinine.
- Loopogram every 6 mo for 2 yr, then yearly.

PEARLS & CONSIDERATIONS

COMMENTS

- The most useful prognostic parameters for bladder tumor recurrence and subsequent cancer progression are tumor grade, depth of tumor penetration, multifocal tumors, frequency of recurrence, tumor size, CIS, lymphatic invasion, papillary or solid tumor configuration.
- Box 1-7 describes the American Urological Association Guideline Recommendations for bladder cancer.

Author: **Philip J. Aliotta, M.D., M.S.H.A.**

BASIC INFORMATION

■ DEFINITION

Blastomycosis is a systemic pyogranulomatous disease caused by a dimorphic fungus, *Blastomyces dermatitidis.*

ICD-9CM CODES
116.0 Blastomycosis
116.0 Primary pulmonary
116.1 Brazilian
116.1 South American
116.2 Keloidal
117.5 European

■ EPIDEMIOLOGY & DEMOGRAPHICS

Most patients reside in the southeastern and south central states, especially those bordering the Mississippi and Ohio River valleys, the Midwestern states, and Canadian provinces bordering the Great Lakes. Rare cases have been reported outside the United States. Widely disseminated disease is most common in immunocompromised hosts, especially those with acquired immunodeficiency syndrome (AIDS).

■ PHYSICAL FINDINGS & CLINICAL PRESENTATION

- Acute infection: 50% symptomatic, median incubation 30 to 45 days, symptoms are nonspecific: mimic influenza or bacterial infection with abrupt onset of myalgias, arthralgias, chills and fever; transient pleuritic pain, cough that is initially nonproductive; resolution within 4 wk is usual
- Chronic or recurrent infection: indolent and progressive; manifestations are diverse including pulmonary or extrapulmonary disease

Pulmonary manifestations: Symptoms and signs of chronic pneumonia: productive cough, hemoptysis, pleuritic chest pain, weight loss, low-grade pyrexia

Extrapulmonary manifestations:
1. Cutaneous: most common; may occur with or without pulmonary disease. Two different lesions:
   Verrucous: beginning as a small papulopustular lesion on exposed body areas that may develop into an eschar with peripheral microabscesses
   Ulcerative
Subcutaneous nodules (cold abscesses) may also occur.
2. Bone and joint: 10% to 50% of patients have osteolytic lesions; affects long bones, vertebrae, and ribs; lesions may present with a contiguous soft-tissue abscess or draining sinus that may spread to a joint resulting in a pyarthrosis
3. Genitourinary: 10% to 30% of patients; prostatic involvement is

most common and may manifest as obstruction; epididymis and testes may also be affected
4. Central nervous system: 5% normal host; 40% AIDS patients; meningitis and abscess formation

■ ETIOLOGY

B. dermatitidis exists in warm, moist soil that is rich in organic material. When these microfoci are disturbed, the aerosolized spores or conidia are inhaled into the lungs. Disease at other sites is a result of dissemination from the initial pulmonary infection; the latter may be acute or chronic.

DIAGNOSIS

■ DIFFERENTIAL DIAGNOSIS
PULMONARY INFECTION:
- Tuberculosis
- Bronchogenic carcinoma
- Histoplasmosis
- Bacterial pneumonia
CUTANEOUS INFECTION:
- Bromoderma
- Pyoderma gangrenosum
- *Mycobacterium marinum* infection
- Squamous cell carcinoma
- Giant keratoacanthoma

■ WORKUP
- Physical examination and laboratory evaluation
- Definitive diagnosis established by culture

■ LABORATORY TESTS
- Presumptive diagnosis can be made by visualizing the distinctive yeast forms in clinical specimens.
- Culture: on Sabouraud's or more enriched media
  1. Aspirated material from abscesses
  2. Skin scrapings
  3. Prostatic secretions (urine culture with prostatic massage)
- Direct examination of clinical specimens
  1. Wet preparation with 10% KOH
  2. Histopathology: typically demonstrates pyogranulomas; yeast identification requires special stains
- Serologic tests: currently, a negative serologic test cannot be used to exclude blastomycosis, nor should a positive titer be an indication to start treatment.

■ IMAGING STUDIES
In chronic disease, chest radiographic findings are nonspecific but lobar or segmental alveolar infiltrates, especially of the upper lobes, are most common and may progress to cavitation.

TREATMENT

■ ACUTE BLASTOMYCOSIS
- Indication for chemotherapy remains controversial in patients with acute pulmonary blastomycosis.
- Since the acute form may be benign and self-limited, patients may be closely observed.
- Some patients progress to chronic infection with attendant significant morbidity and therefore may require treatment.
- Patients who are immunocompromised, or have extrapulmonary disease or progressive pulmonary disease should be treated.

■ CHRONIC BLASTOMYCOSIS
- Itraconazole 200 mg IV bid × 4 doses followed by 200 mg IV qd or itraconazole 200 to 400 mg/day for 6 mo remains the drug of choice except for those patients with CNS disease or with fulminant illness who require amphotericin B.
- Ketoconazole 400 mg/day PO for 6 mo is an alternative in mild-moderate disease.
- Amphotericin B: total dose of 1.5 to 2.5 g IV is recommended in immunocompromised patients, those with life-threatening disease or CNS disease, or those for whom azole treatment has failed. In addition, amphotericin B is the only drug approved for treating blastomycosis in pregnant women.
- Amphotericin B lipid complex (ABLC) 5 mg/kg/day IV may be considered in patients who are intolerant of or refractory to amphotericin.
- Fluconazole 400 mg/day to 800 mg/day PO for 6 mo in those who cannot take itraconazole or who are unable to tolerate a full course of amphotericin B.
- Surgery may be indicated with antifungal therapy for drainage of large abscesses.

■ PROGNOSIS
- Before the development of antifungal chemotherapy the disease had a progressive course with eventual extrapulmonary disease and a mortality exceeding 60%.
- Relapse rate for patients treated with amphotericin B is 5%; relapse is more common in AIDS patients.

■ REFERRAL
Consultation with an infectious diseases specialist is highly recommended, especially in chronic blastomycosis.
Author: **Sajeev Handa, M.D.**

BASIC INFORMATION

■ DEFINITION

Blepharitis is an acute or, most often, chronic inflammation of the eyelid margins that is often refractory to treatment.

ICD-9CM CODES

373.0 Blepharitis

■ PHYSICAL FINDINGS & CLINICAL PRESENTATION

- Chronically infected lids are usually diffusely erythematous, with collarettes (fibrin exudate) at the base of the lashes (Fig. 1-69)
- Lid margins thicken over time, with associated loss of eyelashes (madarosis), misdirected growth of lashes (trichiasis), and overflow or inspissation of the meibomian glands
- Associated conjunctivitis with erythema and edema is common, but it is usually without discharge
- Chalazia may develop
- Superficial punctate erosions of the inferior corneal epithelium are common
- More severe findings, such as corneal pannus, ulcerative keratitis, or lid ectropion, are less common

■ ETIOLOGY

Multiple: bacterial and nonbacterial causes
- Staphylococcal infection
- Seborrheic dermatitis
- Rosacea
- Dry eye (keratoconjunctivitis sicca): includes a decrease in tear volume and/or increased rate of evaporation
- Meibomian gland dysfunction: normally there is keratinization of the meibomian gland duct; hyperkeratinization can plug up the duct
- Two categories of blepharitis:
  1. Anterior blepharitis, most often associated with staphylococcal infection or seborrheic dermatitis
  2. Posterior blepharitis, associated with meibomian gland dysfunction

Note: Most often bacteria isolated from blepharitis patients are normal skin microflora, but in greater amounts (mostly *S. epidermidis* and *P. acnes*). (*S. aureus* and coagulase-negative staphylococci can be cultured from the eyelid margins of 10% to 35% and 90% to 95% of healthy persons, respectively.)

DIAGNOSIS

■ DIFFERENTIAL DIAGNOSIS

- Keratoconjunctivitis sicca
- Eyelid malignancies
- Herpes simplex blepharitis
- Molluscum contagiosum
- Phthiriasis palpebrarum
- Phthirus pubis (pubic lice)
- Demodex folliculorum (transparent mites)
- Allergic blepharitis

■ WORKUP

- Scrapings of the eyelids to show polymorphonuclear leukocytes and gram-positive cocci

■ LABORATORY TESTS

Eyelid cultures and antibiotic sensitivity testing (usually not done unless patient fails to respond to initial treatment regimen)

TREATMENT

■ NONPHARMACOLOGIC THERAPY

- Lid scrubs are the oldest and most effective treatment.
- Alkaline soaps may be beneficial; alcohol and some detergents may be effective in removing surface lipids and microflora.
- Hot compresses applied to closed lids for 5 to 10 min: heat loosens debris from lid margins and increases meibomian gland fluidity.
- Firm massage of the lid margins to enhance the flow of secretions from glands, followed by cleansing of the lids with cotton-tipped applicators dipped in a 50:50 mixture of baby shampoo and water.
- Lashes and lid margins scrubbed vigorously while the eyelids are closed, followed by thorough rinsing.
- Following local massage and cleansing, the mainstay of treatment is application of topical antibiotic ointment to the eyelid margins.
- Antibiotics must be in ointment form for lids and drops or ointment for the ocular surface.
  1. Most effective topical antibiotics available are bacitracin and erythromycin ophthalmic ointments; also effective are many aminoglycosides and fluoroquinolones.
  2. Ointment is applied one to four times daily, depending on the severity of inflammation, for 1 to 2 wk.
  3. Treatment is continued once daily, at bedtime, for another 4 to 8 wk.
  4. Treatment is continued for 1 mo after all signs of inflammation have disappeared.

For patients with rosacea:
1. Tetracycline 250 mg orally qid or doxycycline 100 mg orally bid along with local treatment
2. Dosing reduced to once daily for several mo, depending on the clinical situation

Recalcitrant cases with antibiotic resistance:
1. Vancomycin eyedrops 1%
2. Ciprofloxacin or ofloxacin eyedrops

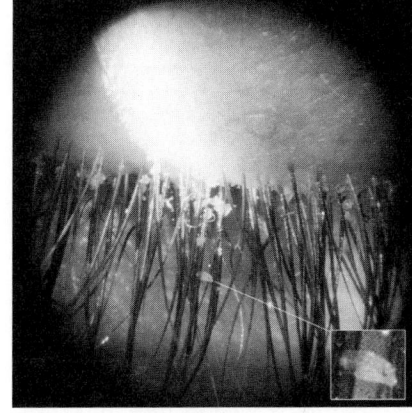
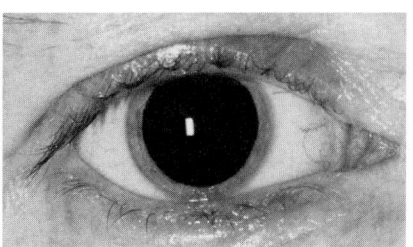

Fig. 1-69 A, Seborrheic blepharitis. The typical scales (scurf) are translucent and easily removed. **B,** Staphylococcal blepharitis showing the typical lid margin erythema and discharge. (From Palay D [ed]: *Ophthalmology for the primary care physician,* St Louis, 1997, Mosby.)

■ **CHRONIC Rx**

By definition, this is a chronic condition for which there is often no cure. This is complicated by the fact that long-term use of antibiotics results in development of resistance and cross-resistance.

Some newer agents being evaluated are flavonoid-type compounds (resveratrol, silymarin) that have antioxidant properties (may have a role in reducing the inflammatory response), and azelaic acid and glycolic acid (used to treat acne and have antikeratinizing effects).

Adapalene gel is also useful in treating acne; it has antiinflammatory properties and an antiproliferative effect on keratinocytes.

■ **DISPOSITION**

This condition is often refractory to treatment, and often requires prolonged courses of treatment. It is important that patients receive adequate education about treatment and compliance.

■ **REFERRAL**

To an ophthalmologist if patient fails to respond to local therapy.

REFERENCE

McCulley JP, Shine WE: Changing concepts in the diagnosis and management of blepharitis, *Cornea* 19(5):650, 2000.

Author: **Jane V. Eason, M.D.**

BASIC INFORMATION

■ DEFINITION
Primary malignant bone tumors are invasive, anaplastic, and have the ability to metastasize. Most arise from the marrow (myeloma), but tumors may develop from bone, cartilage, fat, and fibrous tissues. Leukemia and lymphoma are excluded from this discussion.
FIBROSARCOMA AND LIPOSARCOMA:
Extremely rare. They are similar to those tumors arising in soft tissue.
OSTEOSARCOMA: A rare primary malignant tumor of bone characterized by malignant tumor cells that produce osteoid or bone. Several variants have been described: parosteal sarcoma, periosteal sarcoma, multicentric, and telangiectatic forms.
CHONDROSARCOMA: A malignant cartilage tumor that may develop primarily or secondarily from transformation of a benign osteocartilaginous exostosis or enchondroma.
EWING'S SARCOMA: A malignant tumor of unknown histogenesis.
MULTIPLE MYELOMA: A neoplastic proliferation of plasma cells.

■ SYNONYMS
Multiple myeloma:
1. Plasma cell myeloma
2. Plasmacytoma

ICD-9CM CODES
203.0 Multiple myeloma
170.9 Neoplasma, bone (periosteum), primary malignant
M9180/3 Osteosarcoma
N9220/3 Chondrosarcoma
M9260/3 Ewing's sarcoma

■ EPIDEMIOLOGY & DEMOGRAPHICS
MULTIPLE MYELOMA:
- The most common tumor in bone
- Age at onset: usually >40 yr
- Male:female ratio of 2:1
OSTEOGENIC SARCOMA:
- Average age at onset: 10 to 20 yr
- Males > females
- Parosteal sarcoma in older patients
CHONDROSARCOMA:
- Age at onset: 40 to 60 yr
- Male:female ratio of 2:1
EWING'S SARCOMA:
- Age at onset: 10 to 15 yr

■ PHYSICAL FINDINGS
MULTIPLE MYELOMA:
- May present as a systemic process or, less commonly, as a "solitary" lesion
- Early manifestations: anorexia, weight loss, and bone pain; majority of cases present initially with back pain that often leads to the detection of a destructive skeletal lesion
- Other organ systems eventually become involved, resulting in more bone pain, anemia, renal insufficiency, and/or bacterial infections, usually as a result of the dysproteinemia typical of this disorder
- Possible secondary amyloidosis, leading to cardiac failure or nephrotic syndrome
OSTEOSARCOMA:
- Most originating in the metaphysis
- 50% to 60% around the knee
- Possible pain and swelling, but otherwise healthy patient
- Osteosarcoma in conjunction with Paget's disease, manifested primarily as a sudden increase in bone pain
CHONDROSARCOMA:
- Tumor most commonly involving the pelvis, upper femur, and shoulder girdle
- Painful swelling
EWING'S SARCOMA:
- Painful soft tissue mass often present
- Possibly increased local heat
- Midshaft of a long bone usually affected (in contrast to other tumors)
- Weight loss, fever, and lethargy

DIAGNOSIS

■ DIFFERENTIAL DIAGNOSIS
- Osteomyelitis
- Metastatic bone disease
The age of the patient and the initial radiographic features often determine the next appropriate diagnostic steps.

■ LABORATORY TESTS
- Slightly elevated alkaline phosphatase in osteosarcoma
- In Ewing's sarcoma: reflective of systemic reaction; include anemia, an increase in WBC count, and an elevated sedimentation rate
- In multiple myeloma:
  1. Bence Jones protein in the urine
  2. Anemia and elevated sedimentation rate
  3. Characteristic dysproteinemia on serum protein electrophoresis
  4. Diagnostic feature: peak in the electrophoretic pattern suggestive of a monoclonal gammopathy
  5. Rouleaux formation in the peripheral blood smear
  6. Often, presence of hypercalcemia, but alkaline phosphatase levels usually normal

■ IMAGING STUDIES
- Classic osteogenic sarcoma penetrates the cortex early in many cases.
  1. A blastic (dense), lytic (lucent), or mixed response may be seen in the affected bone.
  2. An aggressive perpendicular sunburst pattern may be present as a result of periosteal reaction, and peripheral Codman's triangles are often noted.
  3. Margins of the tumor are poorly defined.
- Speckled calcifications in a destructive radiolucent lesion are usually suggestive of chondrosarcoma.
- Ewing's sarcoma is characterized radiographically by mottled, irregular destructive changes with periosteal new bone formation. The latter may be multilayered, producing the typical "onion skin" appearance.
- Typical roentgenographic finding in multiple myeloma is the "punched out" lesion with sharply demarcated edges.
  1. Multiple lesions are usual.
  2. Diffuse osteoporosis may be the only finding in many cases.
  3. Pathologic fractures are common.

TREATMENT

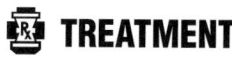

The evaluation and treatment of malignant bone tumors are complicated. Diagnostic studies and treatment should be supervised by an orthopedic cancer specialist and oncologist.

■ DISPOSITION
- In the past 20 yr, dramatic improvements have been made in the treatment protocols for osteosarcoma with the use of adjuvant multidrug regimens and limb-sparing surgery.
- 70% 5-yr survival rates have been obtained in some series.
- Prognosis of multiple myeloma remains poor despite new therapies.
  1. Complete remissions are uncommon.
  2. Survival with a solitary lesion may be long, but most patients succumb after a median of 3 yr.
- Prognosis for Ewing's sarcoma has improved with a combination of chemotherapy, local resection, and radiation therapy.
- Chondrosarcomas are not sensitive to chemotherapy or radiation, and prognosis will depend on the grade of the tumor and the ability to obtain an adequate resection.

REFERENCES
Abe S et al: Long-term local intensive preoperative chemotherapy and joint-preserving conservative surgery for osteosarcoma around the knee, *Orthopedics* 24:671, 2001.
Papagelopoulos PJ et al: Current concepts in the evaluation and treatment of osteosarcoma, *Orthopedics* 23:858, 2000.
Author: **Lonnie R. Mercier, M.D.**

BASIC INFORMATION

■ **DEFINITION**
Botulism is an illness caused by a neurotoxin produced by *Clostridium botulinum*. Three types of disease can occur: foodborne botulism, wound botulism, and infant intestinal botulism. Recent concern has increased about a possible fourth type of disease: inhalational botulism. Does not occur naturally, but may occur as a result of bioterrorism.

ICD-9CM CODE
005.1 Botulism

■ **EPIDEMIOLOGY & DEMOGRAPHICS**
INCIDENCE (IN U.S.): Approximately 24 cases/yr of foodborne illness, 3 cases/yr of wound botulism, and 71 cases/yr of infant botulism

■ **PHYSICAL FINDINGS & CLINICAL PRESENTATION**
• Symptoms usually begin 12 to 36 hr following ingestion.
• Severity of illness is related to the quantity of toxin ingested.
• Significant findings:
  1. Cranial nerve palsies, with ocular and bulbar manifestations being most frequent (diplopia, ophthalmoplegia, ptosis, dysphagia, dysarthria, and dry mouth)
  2. Usually bilateral nerve involvement that may progress to a descending flaccid paralysis
  3. Typically, absence of sensory findings; sensorium intact
  4. GI symptoms (nausea, vomiting, diarrhea, or cramps)
  5. Usually no fever
• Wound botulism
  1. Occurs mostly in injecting drug users (subcutaneous heroin injection—"skin popping") or with traumatic injury.
  2. Presentation is similar to that of foodborne disease, except for a longer incubation period and the absence of GI symptoms.
  3. Wound infection is not always apparent, but injection sites frequently reveal cellulitis, draining pus, or abscess formation.

■ **ETIOLOGY**
• Cause is one of several types of neurotoxins (usually A, B, or E) produced by *C. botulinum,* an anaerobic, gram-positive bacillus. Spore production guarantees survival of the organism in extreme conditions. Botulinum toxin is the most powerful neurotoxin known.
• Disease results from absorption of toxin into the circulation from a

mucosal surface or wound. Botulinum toxin does not penetrate intact skin.
• In foodborne variety, disease is caused by ingestion of preformed toxin. Although rapidly inactivated by heat, the toxin can survive the proteolytic environment of the stomach.
• In wound botulism, toxin is elaborated by organisms that contaminate a wound. Most cases reported are from California.
• In infant botulism, toxin is produced by organisms in the GI tract.
• Inhalational botulism has been demonstrated experimentally in primates. This manufactured form results from aerosolized toxin, and has been attempted by bioterrorists.

■ **DIAGNOSIS**

■ **DIFFERENTIAL DIAGNOSIS**
• Myasthenia gravis
• Guillain-Barré syndrome
• Tick paralysis
• CVA

■ **WORKUP**
Search made for toxin and the organism (see "Laboratory Tests")
• Electrophysiologic studies (EMG) may aid in the diagnosis.

■ **LABORATORY TESTS**
• Samples of food and stool are cultured for the organism.
• Food, serum, and stool are sent for toxin assay.

■ **TREATMENT**

■ **NONPHARMACOLOGIC THERAPY**
• Supportive care with intubation if respiratory failure occurs
• Debridement of the wound in wound botulism

■ **ACUTE GENERAL Rx**
• Give trivalent equine botulinum antitoxin as early as possible. Once a clinical diagnosis is made, antitoxin should be administered before laboratory confirmation.
  1. Give one vial by IM injection and one vial IV.
  2. The antitoxin is available from the Centers for Disease Control and Prevention [(404) 639-2206 or (404) 639-2888]; it is derived from horse serum, so there is a significant incidence of serum sickness.

  3. Skin testing, and possible desensitization, is recommended before treatment.
• Give wound botulism patients penicillin, 2 million U IV q4h.

■ **CHRONIC Rx**
• Supportive
• Rehabilitation/physical therapy

■ **DISPOSITION**
• Highest mortality in the first case in an outbreak, with subsequent cases receiving rapid treatment
• Complete recovery for most individuals

■ **REFERRAL**
Immediate for all cases to an ER and an infectious disease consultant

PEARLS & CONSIDERATIONS

■ **COMMENTS**
• Routine cooking inactivates the toxin, but spores are resistant to environmental factors. At room temperature, spores can germinate and produce toxin.
• Most outbreaks are associated with home-canned foods, especially vegetables.
• Patients must be closely monitored for progression to respiratory paralysis.
• There is increasing concern over the potential use of botulinum toxin as a biologic weapon, either by the enteric route or by aerosolization.
• Notify public health authorities.

REFERENCES
Amon SS et al: Botulinum toxin as a biological weapon, *JAMA* 285(8):1059, 2001.
Bleck TP: *Clostridium botulinim (botulism).* In Mandell GL, Bennett JE, Dolin R (eds): *Principles and practice of infectious diseases,* ed 5, New York, 2000, Churchill Livingstone.
Maselli RA: Pathogenesis of human botulism, *Ann N Y Acad Sci* 841:122, 1998.
Shapiro RL et al: Botulism in the United States: a clinical and epidemiologic review, *Ann Intern Med* 129:221, 1998.
Werner SB et al: Wound botulism in California, 1951-1998: recent epidemic in heroin injectors, *Clin Infect Dis* 31:1018, 2000.
Author: **Maurice Policar, M.D.**

BASIC INFORMATION

■ DEFINITION
Brain neoplasms are primary (non-metastatic) tumors arising from one of many intracranial cellular substrates. Specific tumors and prognosis are listed under other headings.

■ SYNONYMS
Brain tumors
Primary tumors of the central nervous system

ICD-9CM CODES
225.0 Brain neoplasm (benign)
239.2 Brain neoplasm (unspecified)

■ EPIDEMIOLOGY & DEMOGRAPHICS
INCIDENCE (IN U.S.): Male: 9.2 cases/100,000 persons/yr; female: 8.1 cases/100,000 persons/yr
PREVALENCE (IN U.S.): Not reported
PREDOMINANT SEX: Male > female
PREDOMINANT AGE: Male: 75+ yr; female: 65 to 74 yr
PEAK INCIDENCE: Over age 64 yr
GENETICS:
- Some tumor types are associated with specific chromosomal abnormalities.
- Incidence is increased in certain inherited diseases (e.g., neurofibromatosis, tuberous sclerosis).

■ PHYSICAL FINDINGS & CLINICAL PRESENTATION
- Varies with tumor location, size, and rate of growth

- Generally: progressive signs and symptoms
- Headache as presenting symptom is seen in 20% of patients and develops later in 60%
- Seizures in 33% of patients

■ ETIOLOGY
- Most cases are idiopathic.
- Specific chromosomal abnormalities and prior cranial irradiation are sometimes implicated.

DIAGNOSIS

■ DIFFERENTIAL DIAGNOSIS
- Stroke
- Abscess
- Metastatic tumors

■ WORKUP
- Thorough history and physical examination to help resolve differential diagnosis
- MRI of brain, histologic confirmation if needed

■ LABORATORY TESTS
CSF cytology may yield histologic diagnosis.

■ IMAGING STUDIES (Fig. 1-70)
A neuroradiologist is able to diagnose tumor type with greater than 80% accuracy, but all tumors should be biopsied for 100% accuracy. The biopsy should be subjected to histochemical analysis.
- Use of chronic steroids will prevent edema for a limited time.
- MRI with contrast is highly sensitive.
- CT scan is useful if calcification or hemorrhage suspected.

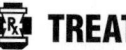

TREATMENT

■ NONPHARMACOLOGIC THERAPY
- Surgical removal or debulking possibly required, especially if the tumor is of a benign nature (e.g., meningioma, acoustic neuroma, oligodendroglioma, low-grade astrocytoma). No further therapy is usually required.
- Radiation is useful for certain types of tumors.

■ ACUTE GENERAL Rx
Steroids (e.g., dexamethasone 4 mg PO q6h) may be used as a temporizing measure to reduce edema.

■ CHRONIC Rx
- If the diagnosis is glioblastoma multiforme, results of radiation and chemotherapy are very disappointing, and how the therapy affects the quality of life measured in months must be carefully considered.
- Most neurosurgeons prescribe dilantin prophylactically for seizures; others wait until a seizure actually occurs.

■ DISPOSITION
- Varies as a function of histologic type and age

■ REFERRAL
All cases warrant evaluation by an oncologist.

REFERENCE
Meyer FB et al: Awake craniotomy for aggressive resection of primary gliomas located in gloanent brain, *Mayo Clin Proc* 76:677, 2001.
Author: **Michael Gruenthal, M.D., Ph.D.**

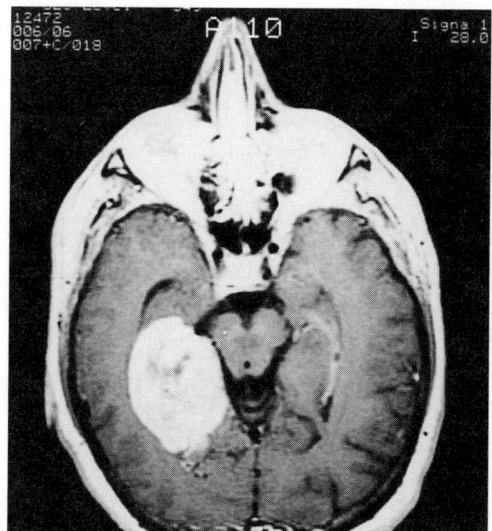

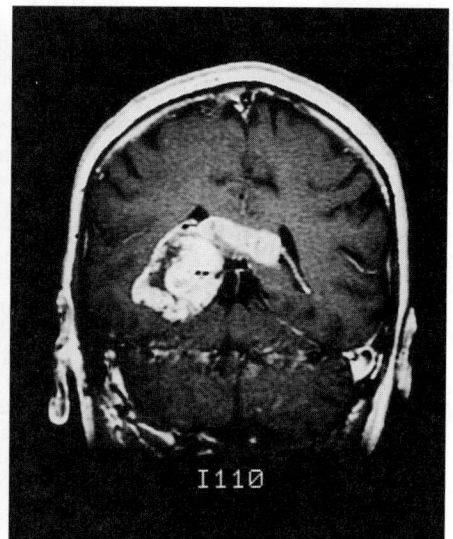

Fig. 1-70 Glioblastoma multiforme. Axial, **A**, and coronal, **B**, postcontrast enhanced T1-weighted image showing a large homogeneously contrast-enhancing mass in the right medial temporal lobe with extension across the midline. (From Specht N [ed]: *Practical guide to diagnostic imaging,* St Louis, 1998, Mosby.)

BASIC INFORMATION

DEFINITION
The term *breast cancer* refers to invasive carcinoma of the breast, whether ductal or lobular.

SYNONYMS
Carcinoma of the breast

ICD-9CM CODES
174.9 Malignant neoplasm female breast

EPIDEMIOLOGY & DEMOGRAPHICS
- Nearly exclusively the disease of women, with only 1% of breast cancers in males
- Steady increase in its incidence in the U.S., with 180,000 new patients annually
- Annual mortality of 44,000
- Risk steadily increases with age
- Genetically defined group of women with BRCA-1 or BRCA-2 identified to carry lifetime risk as high as 85%

PHYSICAL FINDINGS
- Increasing number of small breast cancers found by mammograms
- Patients usually completely free of physical findings
- Palpable tumors possibly as small as 1 cm or even smaller
- Size of the mass and its location measured and documented
- Skin and/or nipple retraction and skin edema/erythema/ulcer/satellite nodule
- Nodal enlargement in axilla and supraclavicular areas
- Advanced disease: clinical signs of pleural effusion and/or hepatomegaly
- Rare instances: clear, serous, or bloody discharge only symptom
- Nipple evaluation (see "Paget's disease of the breast")

ETIOLOGY
- Precise mechanism of carcinogenesis not understood
- Possibly interaction of ovarian estrogen, nonovarian estrogen, estrogens of exogenous origin with breast tissue of varied carcinogenic susceptibility to develop cancer
- Other known or suspected variables: childbearing, breast-feeding practice, diet, physical activities, body mass, alcoholic intake
- Have identified families with known high risk
- Women with BRCA-1 and BRCA-2 associated with high risk

 DIAGNOSIS

DIFFERENTIAL DIAGNOSIS
The following nonmalignant breast lesions can simulate breast cancer on both physical and mammogram examinations:
1. Fibrocystic changes
2. Fibroadenoma
3. Hamartoma

IMAGING STUDIES
Mammograms: 30% to 50% of breast cancers detected by screening mammograms only as a spiculated mass, a mass with or without microcalcifications, or a cluster of microcalcifications (Fig. 1-71)

WORKUP
- Physical examination:
  1. Mass detected by patient or medical professional: workup required
  2. Negative mammogram: breast cancer not ruled out
  3. Sonogram: to demonstrate mass to be cyst, usually eliminating need for further workup
- To establish diagnosis:
  1. Positive aspiration cytology on a clinically and mammographically malignant mass—highly accurate but still requires open biopsy confirmation
  2. Stereotactic core needle biopsy diagnosis: reliable with invasive carcinoma identified, but negative or equivocal results require careful evaluation
  3. Atypical hyperplasia or in situ carcinoma found by core needle biopsy: open surgical biopsy confirmation still required
  4. Excisional or incisional biopsy: establishes diagnosis
- NOTE: Do not rely on negative mammogram or negative aspiration cytology to exclude malignancy. Make appropriate referral. Obtain imaging studies such as bone scan, chest x-ray examination, CT scan of abdomen, or CT scan of liver.
- Breast radiologic evaluation is described in Fig. 3-33. An algorithm for breast cancer screening and evaluation is described in Fig. 3-34. Table 2-31 describes the differential diagnosis of breast lumps.

TREATMENT

NONPHARMACOLOGIC THERAPY
- Early breast cancer: primarily surgical or surgical and radiotherapeutic
- Choice in 60% to 70% of women between modified mastectomy and breast-conserving treatment, which consists of lumpectomy, axillary staging with sentinel node biopsy or axillary dissection, and breast irradiation

ACUTE GENERAL Rx
- May require adjuvant chemotherapy or endocrine therapy
- Evaluation and treatment by medical oncologist

CHRONIC Rx
Follow-up required after proper treatment of primary breast cancer includes:
1. Periodic clinical evaluations
2. Annual mammograms
3. Other tests as indicated
4. Patient instruction in monthly breast self-examination technique

DISPOSITION
- Prognosis after curative therapy: depends on size of tumor, extent of nodal metastasis, and pathologic grade of tumor
  1. Patient with 1-cm tumor with no axillary node metastasis: 10-yr disease-free survival rate of 90%
  2. Patient with 3-cm tumor with metastasis in four nodes: 10-yr disease-free survival rate of 15% if no systemic adjuvant therapy given
  3. Outlook for most patients is between these extremes
- Systemic adjuvant therapy: improves prognosis significantly

REFERRAL
Referral is necessary as soon as breast cancer is even remotely suspected.

PEARLS & CONSIDERATIONS

Breast cancer in pregnancy and lactation:
1. Frequency in women 40 yr old or younger reported to be 15%
2. May carry worse prognosis because disease discovery delayed by engorged and nodular breast changes and/or because disease progression more rapid in pregnancy

3. Survival rates similar to those for nonpregnant early-stage breast cancer patients in same age group
4. Mass usually found by patient or obstetrician
5. Expedient workup recommended, including mammography and sonography
6. Diagnosis to be made without delay
7. Choice of mastectomy or lumpectomy with axillary dissection for treatment
8. Adjuvant chemotherapy delayed until third trimester or after delivery
9. Irradiation to breast after lumpectomy delayed until after delivery

Duct carcinoma in situ (DCIS, intraductal carcinoma):
1. "New" disease mostly found by mammogram as cluster of microcalcification and/or density
2. Less often, presents as palpable mass or nipple discharge
3. Before mammogram screening, DCIS accounted for 1% of all breast cancers
4. Now, 15% to 20% or even higher proportion present with DCIS

5. Formerly treated with mastectomy, now lumpectomy
6. Cure rates 98% to 99%
7. No axillary dissection required
8. With radiation, breast recurrences reduced
9. Mastectomy possibly required with extensive and/or high-grade DCIS
10. Systemic adjuvant treatment is not indicated

Inflammatory carcinoma:
1. Rare but rapidly progressive and often lethal form of breast cancer
2. Presents as erythematous and edematous breast resembling mastitis
3. Biopsy required, including skin
4. Treatment with combination chemotherapy followed by surgery and radiation therapy
5. Prognosis once dismal, now 5-yr disease-free survival in 50% of patients

■ COMMENTS
• Patient education material can be obtained from the following:
1. SHARE: Self-Help for Women with Breast Cancer, 19 W 44th Street, No 415, New York, NY 10036-5902.

2. Y-ME National Organization of Breast Cancer Information and Support, 18220 Harwood Avenue, Homewood, IL 80430.
• Breast radiologic evaluation is described in Fig. 3-33; evaluation of nipple discharge is noted in Fig. 3-32, and evaluation of palpable mass is described in Fig. 3-34.

REFERENCES
Barton MB, Harris R, Fletcher SW: Does this patient have breast cancer? *JAMA* 282:1270, 1999.

Hellekson KL: NIH statement on adjuvant therapy for breast cancer, *Am Fam Physician* 63:1857, 2001.

Hortobagyi GN: Treatment of breast cancer, *N Engl J Med* 339:974, 1998.

Slamon DJ et al: Use of chemotherapy plus a monoclonal antibody against HER2 for metastatic breast cancer that overexpresses HER2, *N Engl J Med* 344(11):783, 2001.

Author: **Takuma Nemoto, M.D.**

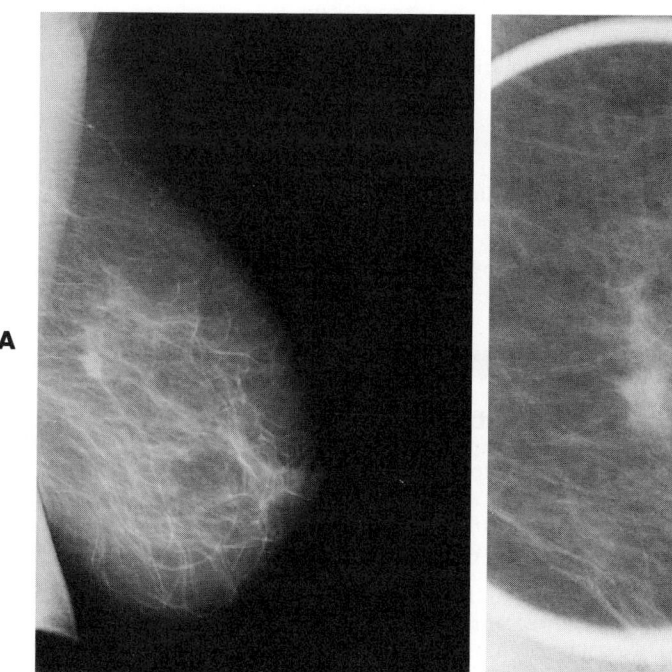
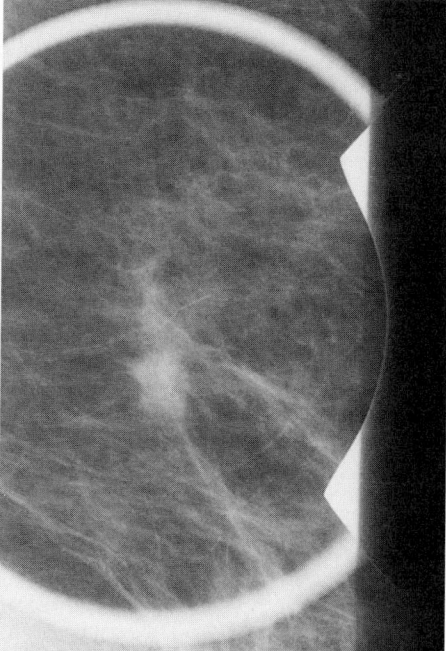

Fig. 1-71 **A,** Right mediolateral and, **B,** spot magnification view from routine screening mammography demonstrates a small, ill-defined mass with minimal spiculation. This was nonpalpable, and biopsy demonstrated infiltrating ductal carcinoma. (From Specht N [ed]: *Practical guide to diagnostic imaging,* St Louis, 1998, Mosby.)

BASIC INFORMATION

■ DEFINITION
Breech presentation exists when the fetal longitudinal axis is such that the cephalic pole occupies the uterine fundus. Three types exist, with respective percentages at term, frank (48% to 73%, flexed hips, extended thighs), complete (4.6% to 11.5%, flexed hips and knees), and footling (12% to 38%, hips extended).

ICD-9CM CODES
652.2 Breech presentation without mention of version

■ EPIDEMIOLOGY & DEMOGRAPHICS
INCIDENCE: Gestational age dependent: 3% to 4% overall, 14% at 29 to 32 wk, 33% at 21 to 24 wk
PERINATAL MORTALITY: 9% to 25%, or three to five times increase over vertex presentation at term. If one corrects for the associated increase in congenital anomalies and complications of prematurity, the morbidity and mortality approach that of the vertex presentation at term regardless of route of delivery.

■ PHYSICAL FINDINGS & CLINICAL PRESENTATION
- Maintain a high index of suspicion
- Lack of presenting part on vaginal examination
- Fetal heart tones heard above the umbilicus
- Leopold maneuvers revealing mobile fetal part in the uterine fundus

■ ETIOLOGY
- Abnormal placentation (fundal), uterine anomalies (fibroids, septa), pelvic or adnexal masses, alterations in fetal muscular tone, or fetal malformations
- Associated conditions: trisomy 13, 18, 21, Potter syndrome, myotonic dystrophy, prematurity

DIAGNOSIS

■ DIFFERENTIAL DIAGNOSIS
Vertex, oblique, or transverse lie

■ WORKUP
- If possible, determine reason for breech presentation, history of uterine anomalies, gestational age, or associated fetal congenital anomalies.

- Assess fetal status, by either continuous fetal heart rate monitoring or ultrasound.
- Assess pelvis to determine feasibility of vaginal delivery.
- Assess risk for safety of vaginal vs. abdominal delivery.

■ IMAGING STUDIES
Ultrasound to evaluate for:
- Fetal anomalies, such as hydrocephalus
- Placental location
- Position of fetal head relative to spine (check for hyperextension)
- Estimated fetal weight (2500 to 3800 g)
- Type of breech (frank, complete, footling)

■ CRITERIA FOR TRIAL OF LABOR
- Estimated fetal weight 2000 to 3800 g
- Frank breech
- Adequate pelvis
- Flexed fetal head
- Continuous fetal monitoring
- Normal progress of labor
- Bedside availability of anesthesia and capability for immediate C-section
- Informed consent
- Obstetrician trained in vaginal breech delivery

■ CRITERIA FOR C-SECTION
- Estimated fetal weight <1500 g or >4000 g
- Footling presentation (20% risk of cord prolapse, usually late in course of labor)
- Inadequate pelvis
- Hyperextended fetal head (21% risk of spinal cord injury)
- Nonreassuring fetal status
- Abnormal progress of labor
- Lack of trained obstetrician

TREATMENT

■ ACUTE GENERAL Rx
- Vaginal delivery in selected patient: allow maternal expulsive forces to deliver fetus until scapula visible (avoiding traction); with flexion and/or Piper forceps, deliver fetal head.
- Perform C-section for the above-mentioned reasons.
- External cephalic version, success 60% to 75%, after 37 wk, contraindicated with placental abruption, low-lying placenta, maternal hypertension, previous

uterine incision, multiple gestation, nonreassuring fetal status.

■ COMPLICATIONS
- Head entrapment: leading cause of death (with the exception of anomalous fetuses), 88 cases/1000 deliveries, avoid by maintaining flexion of fetal head, use of Piper forceps or Dührssen's incisions. Before 36 wk, HC > AC, thus fetal predisposition. Tentorial tears secondary to hyperextended head. Association with trisomy 21 in 3% to 5% of cases. Avoid hyperextension of head during delivery.
- Cord prolapse: usually occurs late in the course of labor. Incidence depends on type of breech—frank (0.5%), complete (4% to 5%), footling (10%).
- Nuchal arm: arm extended above fetal head, occurs when there is undue traction before delivery of fetal scapulas. Treatment depends on bringing trapped arm across infant's face.

■ DISPOSITION
If confounding variables are corrected for, such as prematurity and associated congenital anomalies (6.3% of breeches vs. 2.4% in general population), route of delivery plays a less important role in fetal outcome than previously thought.

■ REFERRAL
An obstetrician trained in delivery of the vaginal breech is a prerequisite for attempting vaginal route, although it must be explained to the patient that with C-section certain risks (such as hyperextension of the fetal head with resultant spinal cord injury) may be minimized but not eliminated.

PEARLS & CONSIDERATIONS

■ COMMENTS
For breech presentation, in general, mortality is increased thirteenfold and morbidity sevenfold. The main reasons are an increase in congenital anomalies, perinatal hypoxia, birth injury, and prematurity.
There is no contraindication to induction of labor in the breech presentation, nor is labor prohibited in a primigravida.
Author: **Scott J. Zuccala, D.O.**

BASIC INFORMATION

■ DEFINITION
Bronchiectasis is the abnormal dilation and destruction of bronchial walls, which may be congenital or acquired.

ICD-9CM-CODES
494.0 Bronchiectasis

■ EPIDEMIOLOGY & DEMOGRAPHICS
- Cystic fibrosis is responsible for nearly 50% of all cases of bronchiectasis.
- Acquired primary bronchiectasis is uncommon because of rapid diagnosis of pulmonary infections and frequent use of antibiotics.

■ PHYSICAL FINDINGS & CLINICAL PRESENTATION
- Moist crackles at lung bases
- Cough with expectoration of large amount of purulent sputum
- Fever, night sweats, generalized malaise, weight loss
- Hemoptysis
- Halitosis, skin pallor
- Clubbing (infrequent)

■ ETIOLOGY
- Cystic fibrosis
- Lung infections (pneumonia, lung abscess, TB, fungal infections, viral infections)
- Abnormal host defense (panhypogammaglobulinemia, Kartagener's syndrome, AIDS, chemotherapy)
- Localized airway obstruction (congenital structural defects, foreign bodies, neoplasms)
- Inflammation (inflammatory pneumonitis, granulomatous lung disease, allergic aspergillosis)

DIAGNOSIS

■ DIFFERENTIAL DIAGNOSIS
- TB
- Asthma
- Chronic bronchitis or chronic sinusitis
- Interstitial fibrosis
- Chronic lung abscess
- Foreign body aspiration
- Cystic fibrosis
- Lung carcinoma

■ WORKUP
Sputum for Gram stain and C&S, chest x-ray examination, bronchoscopy, spirometry

■ LABORATORY TESTS
- Sputum for Gram stain, C&S, and acid-fast bacteria (AFB)
- CBC with differential (leukocytosis with left shift, anemia)
- Serum protein electrophoresis to evaluate for hypogammaglobulinemia
- Antibody test for aspergillosis
- Sweat test in patients with suspected cystic fibrosis

■ IMAGING STUDIES
- Chest x-ray examination: hyperinflation, crowded lung markings, small cystic spaces at the base of the lungs (Fig. 1-72)
- High-resolution CT scan of the chest: to detect cystic lesions and exclude underlying obstruction from neoplasm
- Bronchography only when surgery is contemplated
- Pulmonary function tests: generally reveal obstructive or mixed ventilatory defect
- Bronchoscopy: helpful to evaluate hemoptysis, rule out obstructive lesions, and remove mucus plugs

TREATMENT

■ NONPHARMACOLOGIC THERAPY
- Postural drainage and chest percussion
- Adequate hydration
- Supplemental oxygen for hypoxemia

■ ACUTE GENERAL Rx
- Antibiotic therapy is based on the results of sputum, Gram stain, and C&S; in patients with inadequate or inconclusive results, empiric therapy with amoxicillin/clavulanate 500 mg to 875 mg q12h, TMP-SMX q12h, doxycycline 100 mg bid, or cefuroxime 250 mg bid for 10 to 14 days is recommended.
- Bronchodilators are useful in patients with demonstrable air flow obstruction.

■ CHRONIC Rx
- Avoidance of tobacco
- Maintenance of proper nutrition and hydration
- Prompt identification and treatment of infections
- Pneumococcal vaccination and annual influenza vaccination

■ DISPOSITION
Prognosis is variable with severity of the disease and underlying etiology of bronchiectasis.

■ REFERRAL
Surgical referral for partial lung resection in patients with localized severe disease unresponsive to medical therapy or in patients with massive hemoptysis

PEARLS & CONSIDERATIONS

■ COMMENTS
Patient education material on bronchiectasis can be obtained from the American Lung Association, 1740 Broadway, New York, NY 10019.
Author: **Fred F. Ferri, M.D.**

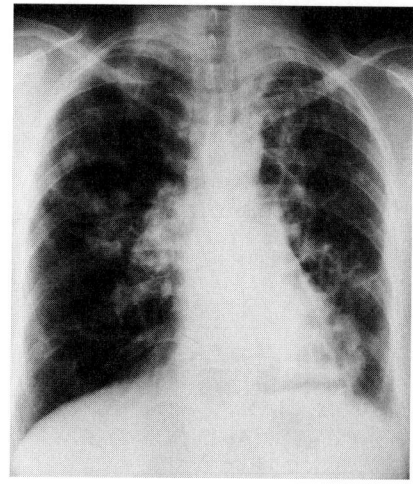

Fig. 1-72 Cystic changes are demonstrated in both lung fields and are most pronounced at the left lung base secondary to cystic bronchiectasis. (From Specht N [ed]: *Practical guide to diagnostic imaging,* St Louis, 1998, Mosby.)

BASIC INFORMATION

■ **DEFINITION**
Acute bronchitis is the inflammation of trachea and bronchi.

ICD-9CM CODES
466.0 Acute bronchitis

■ **EPIDEMIOLOGY & DEMOGRAPHICS**
- Highest incidence in smokers, older adults, young children, and in winter months
- In the U.S. there are nearly 30 million ambulatory visits annually for cough, leading to more than 12 million diagnoses of "bronchitis."

■ **PHYSICAL FINDINGS & CLINICAL PRESENTATION**
- Cough, usually worse in the morning, often productive. It is mainly caused by transient bronchial hyperresponsiveness.
- Low-grade fever
- Substernal discomfort worsened by coughing
- Postnasal drip, pharyngeal injection
- Rhonchi that may clear after cough, occasional wheezing

■ **ETIOLOGY**
- Viral infections are the leading cause of bronchitis (rhinovirus, influenza virus, adenovirus, respiratory syncytial virus)
- Atypical organisms (*Mycoplasma, Chlamydia pneumoniae*)
- Bacterial infections (*Haemophilus influenzae, Moraxella, Streptococcus pneumoniae*)
- Table 1-18 describes common infectious agents

DIAGNOSIS

■ **DIFFERENTIAL DIAGNOSIS**
- Pneumonia
- Asthma
- Sinusitis
- Bronchiolitis
- Aspiration
- Cystic fibrosis
- Pharyngitis
- Cough secondary to medications
- Neoplasm (elderly patients)
- Influenza
- Allergic aspergillosis
- GERD
- CHF (in elderly patients)
- Bronchogenic neoplasm

■ **WORKUP**
Seldom necessary (e.g., to rule out pneumonia, neoplasm)

■ **LABORATORY TESTS**
- Tests are generally not necessary.
- CBC may reveal mild leukocytosis.

- Sputum culture, Gram stain, and blood cultures are generally not indicated.

■ **IMAGING STUDIES**
Chest x-ray examination is usually reserved for patients with suspected pneumonia, influenza, or underlying COPD and no improvement with therapy.

TREATMENT

■ **NONPHARMACOLOGIC THERAPY**
- Avoidance of tobacco and other pulmonary irritants
- Increased fluid intake
- Use of vaporizer to increase room humidity

■ **ACUTE GENERAL Rx**
- Inhaled bronchodilators (e.g., albuterol, metaproterenol) PRN for 1 to 2 weeks in patients with wheezing or troublesome cough. Inhaled albuterol has been proven effective in reducing the duration of cough in adults with uncomplicated acute bronchitis.
- Cough suppression with guaifenesin; addition of codeine for cough suppression (e.g., Robitussin-AC) if cough is severe and is significantly interrupting patient's sleep pattern
- Use of antibiotics (TMP-SMX, amoxicillin, doxycycline, cefuroxime) for acute bronchitis is generally not indicated; should be considered only in patients with concomitant COPD and purulent sputum or in patients unresponsive to prolonged conservative treatment

- Antibiotics are overused in patients with acute bronchitis (70% to 90% of office visits for acute bronchitis result in treatment with antibiotics); this practice pattern is contributing to increases in resistant organisms

■ **CHRONIC Rx**
Avoidance of tobacco and other pulmonary irritants

■ **DISPOSITION**
Complete recovery within 7 to 10 days in most patients

■ **REFERRAL**
For pulmonary function testing only in patients with recurrent bronchitis and suspected underlying asthma

PEARLS & CONSIDERATIONS

■ **COMMENTS**
- Patient education material may be obtained from the American Lung Association, 1740 Broadway, New York, NY 10019.
- Intervention studies reveal that patient and physician education are effective in reducing the use of antibiotic therapy

REFERENCES
Heston WJ, Mainous AG: Acute bronchitis, *Am Fam Physician* 6:1270, 1998.
Snow V et al: Principles of appropriate antibiotic use for treatment of acute bronchitis in adults, *Ann Intern Med* 136:518, 2001.
Author: **Fred F. Ferri, M.D.**

TABLE 1-18   Acute Bronchitis: Infectious Agents and Treatment

AGENT	TREATMENT
Viral	
Influenza A virus	Amantadine or rimantadine
Influenza B virus	—
Parainfluenza virus	—
Coronavirus	—
Respiratory syncytial virus	—
Rhinovirus	—
Adenovirus	—
Bacterial and Bacteria-Like	
Mycoplasma pneumoniae	Doxycycline or macrolide*
Chlamydia pneumoniae	Doxycycline or macrolide*
Bordetella pertussis	Erythromycin

From Gorbach SL: *Infectious diseases,* ed 2, Philadelphia, 1998, WB Saunders.
*Macrolides are erythromycin, azithromycin, and clarithromycin.

BASIC INFORMATION

■ DEFINITION

Brucellosis is a zoonotic infection caused by one of four species of *Brucella*. It commonly presents as a nondescript febrile illness.

■ SYNONYMS

Malta fever
Bang's disease

ICD-9CM CODES

023.9 Brucellosis

■ EPIDEMIOLOGY & DEMOGRAPHICS

INCIDENCE (IN U.S.): About 100 cases/yr (may be underreported)
PREDOMINANT SEX: Male
PREDOMINANT AGE: Adult
CONGENITAL INFECTION: Recent evidence suggests a high rate of spontaneous abortions in untreated pregnant women during the first and second trimesters.
NEONATAL INFECTION: Can occur if mother is infected during pregnancy.

■ PHYSICAL FINDINGS

- Incubation period is 1 wk to 3 mo.
- Patients may be asymptomatic or have nonspecific symptoms such as fever, sweats, malaise, weight loss, and depression.
- Bacteremic patients may have arthralgias or arthritis. Patients may rarely present with abdominal pain.
- Fever is the most common finding.
- Hepatomegaly, splenomegaly, or lymphadenopathy is possible.
- Localized disease:
  1. Related to a single organ
  2. Includes endocarditis, meningitis, and osteomyelitis (especially vertebral)
  Chronic hepatosplenic suppurative brucellosis (CHSB) presents with hepatic or splenic abscesses. This form is thought to be a reactivation, and can occur years after the acute infection.

■ ETIOLOGY

- Caused by infection with *Brucella* species:
  1. Most commonly *melitensis,* but also *suis, abortus,* or *canis*
  2. A small, gram-negative coccobacillus
- Acquired through breaks in the skin or by inhalation or ingestion of organisms.

- Most cases occur after exposure to animals (sheep, goats, swine, cattle, or dogs), or animal products (i.e., milk, hides, tissue).
- Most cases (in U.S.) occur in men with occupational exposure to animals (farmers, ranchers, veterinarians, abattoir workers).
- Laboratory acquisition is possible.
- May occur in tourists to other countries who ingest goat milk or cheese.

⚗ DIAGNOSIS

■ DIFFERENTIAL DIAGNOSIS

Many febrile conditions without localizing manifestations (i.e., TB, endocarditis, typhoid fever, malaria, autoimmune diseases)

■ WORKUP

- Cultures of blood, bone marrow, or other tissue (lymph node, liver) should be sent and held for 4 wk, since *Brucella* grows slowly in vitro.
- Granulomas on biopsy are suggestive of diagnosis.

■ LABORATORY TESTS

- WBC count: normal or low
- Serology:
  1. Serum agglutination test (SAT) to detect antibodies to *B. abortus, melitensis,* and *suis*
  2. Specific antibody test to identify antibodies to *B. canis*
  3. False-negative SAT possibly resulting from a prozone effect
  Serologic studies may be nondiagnostic in CHSB

■ IMAGING STUDIES

- Radiographs to show splenic calcifications in chronic disease
- Bone scan and radiographs of the spine to suggest osteomyelitis
- Ultrasound or CT scan of the abdomen to show an enlarged liver or spleen
- Echocardiogram to reveal vegetations in endocarditis
In CHSB, abscesses and calcifications may be seen in the liver and spleen

℞ TREATMENT

■ NONPHARMACOLOGIC THERAPY

- Drainage of abscesses
- Valve replacement for endocarditis

■ ACUTE GENERAL Rx

Combination antibiotics required:
- Doxycycline 100 mg PO bid plus streptomycin 15 mg/kg IM qd for 6 wk
- Less effective: doxycycline 100 mg PO bid plus rifampin 600 mg PO qd or sulfamethoxazole 800 mg/trimethoprim 160 mg one DS tablet PO qid
Courses <6 wk are associated with higher relapse rates; longer courses are recommended for complicated disease.

■ CHRONIC Rx

See "Acute General Rx."

■ DISPOSITION

Relapse is possible weeks to months after the completion of therapy, usually because of noncompliance with a prolonged medical regimen or a persistent focus of infection that requires surgical drainage.
Reactivation with CHSB has been reported up to 35 yr after initial illness.

■ REFERRAL

For all cases to an infectious disease specialist

☼ PEARLS & CONSIDERATIONS

■ COMMENTS

- Alert the microbiology laboratory to the possibility of *Brucella.*
- Do not use doxycycline in children or pregnant women.
- Avoid aminoglycosides in pregnant women.

REFERENCES

Ariza J et al: Current understanding and management of chronic hepatosplenic suppurative brucellosis, *Clin Infect Dis* 32(7):995, 2001.
Fernandez MD et al: *Brucella* acute abdomen mimicking appendicitis, *Am J Med* 108:599, 2000.
Khan MY et al: Brucellosis in pregnant women, *Clin Infect Dis* 32(8):1172, 2001.
Memish Z et al: *Brucella* bacteremia: clinical and laboratory observations in 160 patients, *J Infect Dis* 40:59, 2000.
Author: **Maurice Policar, M.D.**

BASIC INFORMATION

■ DEFINITION

Budd-Chiari syndrome (BCS) is the obstruction of hepatic venous blood flow. The site of obstruction may be anywhere from the small central lobar veins of the liver to the proximal inferior vena cava (IVC). Although BCS is frequently caused by thrombosis, extrinsic compression and venous malformations may also cause obstruction. BCS may result in portal hypertension, cirrhosis, and liver failure.

■ SYNONYMS

Hepatic vein thrombosis
Postsinusoidal obstruction
Hepatic venous outflow obstruction

ICD-9CM CODES

453.0 Budd-Chiari syndrome

■ EPIDEMIOLOGY & DEMOGRAPHICS

BCS is a rare disorder. Etiology varies with geography. In the U.S., BCS is more commonly associated with myeloproliferative disease, hypercoagulable states, IVC membranes, and tumors.

■ PHYSICAL FINDINGS & CLINICAL PRESENTATION

Variable according to the degree, location, and acuity of the obstruction.
- Fulminant: Severe abdominal pain, jaundice, hepatomegaly, ascites, acute liver failure, and encephalopathy. Early recognition and treatment are essential to survival. This presentation is more commonly seen in pregnant women.
- Acute: Abdominal pain, hepatomegaly, and progressive liver dysfunction. Without treatment this presentation of BCS may evolve into the chronic form.
- Chronic: This presentation is the result of chronic portal hypertension with or without cirrhosis; ascites, esophageal varices, splenomegaly, coagulopathy, and encephalopathy.

■ ETIOLOGY

Hypercoagulable states:
- Myeloproliferative disease:
    Polycythemia vera
    Essential thrombocytosis
- Protein C deficiency
- Antithrombin III deficiency
- Protein S deficiency
- Activated protein C resistance
- Antiphospholipid antibody
- Pregnancy
- Oral contraceptive pills
- Sickle cell anemia
- Metastatic cancer

Infection:
- Liver abscess
- Filariasis
- Schistosomiasis
- Hydatid cyst
- Syphilis
- Tuberculosis
Malignancy:
- Adrenal
- Ovarian
- Bronchogenic
- Renal
- Hepatocellular
- Leiomyosarcoma
Other:
- Sarcoid
- IVC membrane
- Trauma

DIAGNOSIS

■ DIFFERENTIAL DIAGNOSIS

- Shock liver
- Viral hepatitis
- Toxic hepatitis
- Alcoholic hepatitis
- Pancreatitis
- Cholecystitis
- Perforated viscus
- Peptic ulcer disease
- Cardiac cirrhosis
- Alcoholic cirrhosis
- Cirrhosis of other etiologies:
    Wilson's
    Hemochromatosis
    α-1-Antitrypsin deficiency
    Autoimmune

■ WORKUP

Physical examination, laboratory analysis, and imaging studies

■ LABORATORY TESTS

Assessment of liver function:
- Transaminases, prothrombin time, albumin, bilirubin, and platelet count
Diagnostic tests:
- Viral hepatitis panel, α-1-antitrypsin, serum iron, transferrin saturation, alkaline phosphatase, ceruloplasmin, toxicology screen, antismooth muscle antibody, antimitochondrial antibody, and double-stranded DNA antibody

■ IMAGING STUDIES

Doppler ultrasound is usually sufficient. If this study is technically limited, MRI and CT scan may demonstrate collateral circulation and poor visualization of the hepatic veins (Fig. 1-73). MRI and CT scan may also be able to localize any masses. Venography may be indicated if the diagnosis is still in doubt.

TREATMENT

■ ACUTE GENERAL Rx

- Supportive measures
- Liver transplant may be indicated for fulminant BCS
- Shunting, stenting, or angioplasty to decompress the portal circulation may be indicated for acute BCS in patients in stable condition
- Thrombolytic therapy can also be used to decompress the portal circulation

■ CHRONIC Rx

- Chronic anticoagulation may be needed to maintain shunt patency or in patients with thrombotic BCS
- Liver transplantation
- Shunt thrombosis is a common complication

■ DISPOSITION

Prognosis is dependent on time to recognition and treatment, etiology, acuity, and the type of intervention.

■ REFERRAL

Prompt referral to a surgeon specializing in hepatobiliary disease is recommended.

REFERENCE

Granger DR et al: Transjugular intrahepatic portosystemic shunt (TIPS) for Budd Chiari syndrome or portal vein thrombosis, *Am J Gastroenterol* 94(3):559, 1999.
Author: **James J. Ng, M.D.**

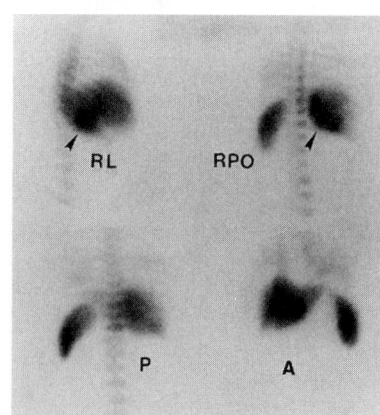

Fig. 1-73 Budd-Chiari syndrome. Good Tc-99m SC uptake in the region of the caudate lobe *(arrowheads)* in a patient with hepatic vein thrombosis. Images were acquired in the right lateral *(RL)*, right posterior oblique *(RPO)*, posterior *(P)*, and anterior *(A)* projections. Note increased marrow uptake. (From Thrall JH, Ziessman HA [eds]: *Nuclear medicine: the requisites*, St Louis, 1995, Mosby.)

BASIC INFORMATION

■ DEFINITION
Bulimia nervosa is a prolonged illness characterized by a specific psychopathology (see below).

ICD-9CM CODES
783.6 Bulimia

■ EPIDEMIOLOGY & DEMOGRAPHICS
INCIDENCE/PREVALENCE: Affects 1% to 3% of female adolescents and young adults
PREDOMINANT SEX: Female:male ratio of 10:1
PREDOMINANT AGE: Adolescence to young adulthood; mean age of onset: 17 yr

■ PHYSICAL FINDINGS & CLINICAL PRESENTATION
- Parotid and salivary gland swelling
- Scars on the back of the hand and knuckles (Russell's sign) from rubbing against the upper incisors when inducing vomiting
- Eroded enamel, particularly on the lingual surface of the upper teeth; pyorrhea and other gum disorders possible
- Petechial hemorrhages of the cornea, soft palate, or face possibly noted after vomiting
- Loss of gag reflex, well-developed abdominal musculature
- Usually no emaciation; normal physical examination possible

■ ETIOLOGY
Etiology is unknown but likely multifactorial (sociocultural, psychologic, familial factors). Bulimia is much more common in Western societies where there is a strong cultural pressure to be slender. According to the American Psychiatric Association, patients with eating disorders display a broad range of symptoms that occur along a continuum between those of anorexia nervosa and bulimia.

DIAGNOSIS

■ DIFFERENTIAL DIAGNOSIS
- Schizophrenia
- GI disorders
- Neurologic disorders (seizures, Kleine-Levin syndrome, Klüver-Bucy syndrome)
- Brain neoplasms
- Psychogenic vomiting

■ WORKUP
- The following questions are useful to screen patients for bulimia:
  1. "Are you satisfied with your eating habits?"
  2. "Do you ever eat in secret?"
- Answering "no" to the first question and/or "yes" to the second question has 100% sensitivity and 90% specificity for bulimia. The SCOFF questionnaire can also be used as a screening tool for eating disorders (see "Anorexia Nervosa" topic).
- A diagnosis can also be made using the following DSM-IV diagnostic criteria for bulimia nervosa:
  1. Recurrent episodes of binge eating (rapid consumption of a large amount of food in a discrete period of time)
  2. A feeling of lack of control over eating behavior during the eating binges
  3. Self-induced vomiting, use of laxatives or diuretics, strict dieting or fasting, or rigorous exercise to prevent weight gain
  4. A minimum of two binge-eating episodes a week for at least 3 mo
  5. Persistent overconcern with body shape and weight

■ LABORATORY TESTS
- Electrolyte abnormalities secondary to vomiting (hypokalemia and metabolic alkalosis) or to diarrhea from laxative abuse (hypokalemia and hyperchloremic metabolic acidosis)
- Hyponatremia, hypocalcemia, hypomagnesemia (caused by laxative abuse)
- Elevated cortisol, decreased LH, decreased FSH

TREATMENT

■ NONPHARMACOLOGIC THERAPY
- Cognitive behavioral therapy to control abnormal behaviors
- Use of food diaries, nutritional counseling, and planning meals at least a day in advance is useful to counter abnormal eating behaviors
- Correction of electrolyte abnormalities

■ ACUTE GENERAL Rx
- SSRIs are generally considered to be the safest medication option in these patients. They are useful in severely depressed patients and in those who fail to benefit from cognitive behavioral therapy.
- Prompt recognition and treatment of complications:
  1. Ipecac cardiotoxicity from laxative abuse
  2. Electrolyte abnormalities (see above)
  3. Esophagitis and Mallory-Weiss tears; esophageal rupture from repeated vomiting
  4. Aspiration pneumonia and pneumomediastinum
  5. Menstrual irregularities (including amenorrhea)
  6. GI abnormalities: acute gastric dilatation, pancreatitis, abdominal pain, constipation

■ CHRONIC Rx
- Psychotherapy continued for years and focused specifically on self-image and family and peer interactions is an integral part of successful recovery.
- Family therapy is also recommended, especially in younger patients.

■ DISPOSITION
Course is variable and marked by frequent recurrence of exacerbations.

■ REFERRAL
- In addition to the primary care physician, the multidisciplinary team should include a dietician, a psychiatrist, and a family therapist.
- Hospitalization should be considered for patients with severe electrolyte abnormalities or those with suicidal thoughts.

✷ PEARLS & CONSIDERATIONS

■ COMMENTS
Bulimia has a close association with depression, bipolar disorder, obsessive-compulsive disorder, alcoholism, and substance abuse.

REFERENCES
American Psychiatric Association: Practice guideline for the treatment of patients with eating disorders, *Am J Psychiatry* 157(suppl):4, 2000.
Becker AG: Eating disorders, *N Engl J Med* 340:1092, 1999.
Keel PK et al: Long-term outcome of bulimia nervosa, *Arch Gen Psychiatry* 56:63, 1999.
McGilley BM, Pryor TL: Assessment and treatment of bulimia nervosa, *Am Fam Physician* 57:2743, 1998.
Author: **Fred F. Ferri, M.D.**

BASIC INFORMATION

■ **DEFINITION**
Bullous pemphigoid refers to an autoimmune, subepidermal blistering disease seen in the elderly.

■ **SYNONYMS**
Subepidermal autoimmune bullous dermatoses

■ **ICD-9CM CODES**
694.5 Pemphigoid

■ **EPIDEMIOLOGY & DEMOGRAPHICS**
• Commonly seen in the elderly over 70 yr old
• Incidence 10/1 million
• Equal prevalence between males and females
• No racial predilection
• Most common of the autoimmune bullous dermatoses

■ **PHYSICAL FINDINGS & CLINICAL PRESENTATION**
History
• Bullous pemphigoid typically starts as an eczematous or urticarial rash on the extremities.
• Blisters form between 1 wk to several months.
Physical findings
• Anatomic distribution
  1. Flexor surfaces of the arms, legs, groin, axilla, and lower abdomen
  2. Spares the head and neck
  3. Rare involvement of mucous membranes
• Lesion configuration
  1. May be localized to the extremities or generalized
  2. Lesions irregularly grouped but sometimes can be serpiginous (Fig. 1-74)
• Lesion morphology
  1. Blistering bullae characteristic findings measuring anywhere from 5 mm to 2 cm in diameter
  2. Contains clear or bloody fluid
  3. Arises from normal skin or from an erythematous base
  4. Heals without scarring if denuded

■ **ETIOLOGY**
Bullous pemphigoid is an autoimmune disease with IgG and/or C3 complement component reacting with antigens located in the basement membrane zone.

 DIAGNOSIS

The diagnosis of bullous pemphigoid should be considered in any elderly individual with pruritic bullae.

■ **DIFFERENTIAL DIAGNOSIS**
• Cicatricial pemphigoid
• Herpes gestationis
• Epidermolysis bullosa acquisita
• Systemic lupus erythematosus
• Erythema multiforme
• Pemphigus
• Drug eruptions
• Pemphigoid nodularis

■ **WORKUP**
The clinical presentation and characteristic skin lesions assist in making the diagnosis of bullous pemphigoid. Specific laboratory tests, skin biopsy staining, and immunofluoroscence studies confirm the diagnosis (Fig. 1-75).

■ **LABORATORY TESTS**
• Antibodies to the basement membrane zone are detected in the serum in 70% of patients with bullous pemphigoid.
• Skin biopsy staining with hematoxylin-eosin reveals subepidermal blisters.

• Direct and indirect immunofluorescence studies using salt-split skin detect the presence of IgG and C3 immune complexes on the basement membrane zone and can differentiate bullous pemphigus from other autoimmune blistering diseases.
• Immunoelectron microscopy also reveals immune deposits on the basement membrane zone.

■ **IMAGING STUDIES**
X-ray imaging studies are not very useful in the workup of patients with bullous pemphigoid.

℞ **TREATMENT**

Treatment of bullous pemphigoid is based on the degree of involvement and rate of disease progression.

■ **NONPHARMACOLOGIC THERAPY**
• Avoid scratching.
• Use mild soaps and emollients after bathing to prevent dryness of the skin.

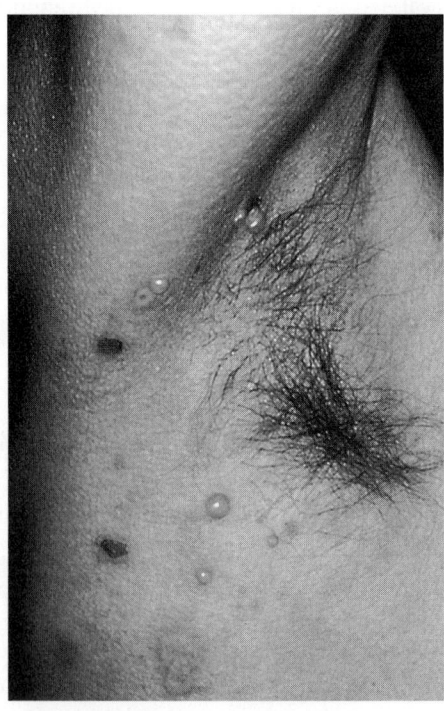

Fig. 1-74   Bullous pemphigoid. Note intact bullae with erosions in aflexural distribution. (From Goldstein BG, Goldstein AO: *Practical dermatology,* ed 2, St Louis, 1997, Mosby.)

■ ACUTE GENERAL Rx

- Topical steroids can be used in patients with localized disease.
- Systemic steroids is the usual treatment for more advanced bullous pemphigoid.
  1. Prednisone 60 to 100 mg PO qd is initiated and continued until new blister formation ceases. The dose is tapered to 20 to 40 mg. Thereafter, the dose is gradually tapered according to the clinical findings.
- If patients cannot take corticosteroids, dapsone, combination tetracycline and nicotinamide or azathioprine can be tried.

■ CHRONIC Rx

- Combination prednisone and azathioprine protocols are available in the treatment of bullous pemphigoid.
- Cyclophosphamide can be considered in attempt to reduce chronic long-term use of corticosteroids.

■ DISPOSITION

- Left untreated, patients with bullous pemphigoid run the risk of sepsis from infected bullae.
- Mortality rates are estimated at 19% at 1 year, 6% at 2 yr, and 28% to 30% at 3 yr.

■ REFERRAL

If bullous pemphigoid is suspected, a dermatology consultation is recommended to assist with decisions regarding diagnosis, monitoring, and therapy.

☼ PEARLS & CONSIDERATIONS

■ COMMENTS

- Bullous pemphigoid has been associated with diabetes, multiple sclerosis, pernicious anemia, rheumatoid arthritis, lichen planus, psoriasis, and vitiligo.
- Not known to transform into malignancies or represent a dermatologic manifestation of harboring malignancies.

REFERENCES

Korman NJ: Bullous pemphigoid: bullous diseases, *Dermatol Clin* 11:483, 1993.

Korman NJ: Bullous pemphigoid: the latest in diagnosis, prognosis and therapy, *Arch Dermatol* 134(9):1137, 1998.

Scott JE, Ahmed AR: The blistering diseases, *Med Clin North Am* 82(6):1239, 1998.

Vaillant L, et al: Evaluation of clinical criteria for diagnosis of bullous pemphigoid, *Arch Dermatol* 134(9):1075, 1998.

Author: **Peter Petropoulos, M.D.**

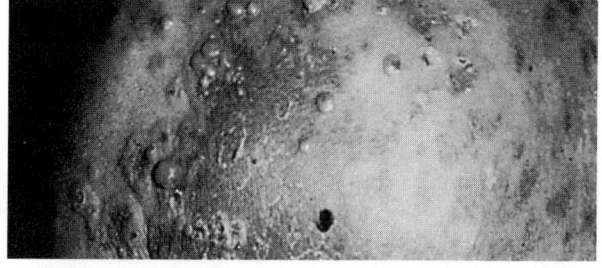

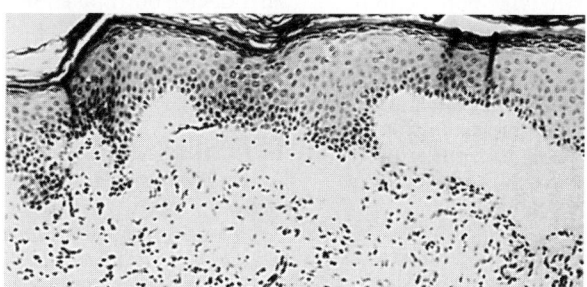

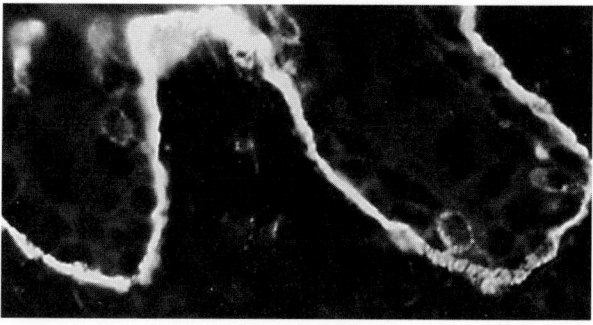

Fig. 1-75 Bullous pemphigoid. **A,** Clinical presentation with intact bullae and healing lesions. **B,** Hematoxylin and eosin stain of a blister reveals dermal-epidermal separation and a dermal inflammatory cell infiltrate. **C,** Indirect immunofluorescence performed on cryosections of rat tongue using serum from a patient with bullous pemphigoid, and fluorescein-labeled antihuman IgG. Note the binding of antibodies to the basement membrane zone in a linear and continuous pattern. (From Stein JH [ed]: *Internal medicine*, ed 5, St Louis, 1998, Mosby.)

BASIC INFORMATION

■ **DEFINITION**
Burn injuries consist of thermal injuries (flames, scalds, cigarettes), as well as chemical and electrical burns.

■ **SYNONYMS**
Thermal injury

ICD-9CM CODES
942-949 (by region, % burn)

■ **EPIDEMIOLOGY & DEMOGRAPHICS**
PREVALENCE (IN U.S.): 100,000 hospitalizations and 12,000 deaths annually
PREDOMINANT SEX: Male:female ratio of 2:1
PREVALENT AGE: 18 to 35 yr with high incidence of scalds in ages 1 to 5 yr

■ **PHYSICAL FINDINGS & CLINICAL PRESENTATION**
• Burns are defined by size and depth (Fig. 1-76).
• *First-degree burns* involve the epidermis only and appear painful and red.
• *Second-degree (partial-thickness) burns* involve the dermis and appear blistered or moist and red.
• *Third-degree (full-thickness) burns* extend through the dermis with associated destruction of hair follicles and sweat glands. The skin is charred, pale, *painless,* and leathery.
• The "rule of nines" is useful for rapidly assessing the extent of a burn (see Fig. 1-77). Second- and third-degree burns are used to calculate the total burn surface area (TBSA) (Fig. 1-78).

■ **DIAGNOSIS**

■ **CLASSIFICATION**
Major burns: Partial-thickness burns >25% TBSA; full-thickness burns >10% TBSA; burns crossing major joints or involving the hands, face, feet, or perineum; electrical or chemical burns; those complicated by inhalation injury, or involving poor-risk patients (extremes of age/intercurrent diseases)
Moderate burns: Partial-thickness burns >15% to 25% TBSA; full-thickness burns >2% to 10% TBSA and not involving the specific conditions above
Minor burns: Partial-thickness burns <15% TBSA or full-thickness burns <2% TBSA

■ **WORKUP**
Diagnosis is based on clinical findings

■ **LABORATORY STUDIES**
• CBC, electrolytes, BUN, creatinine, and glucose
• Serial ABG and carboxyhemoglobin if smoke inhalation suspected
• Urinalysis, urine myoglobin, and CPK levels if concern for rhabdomyolysis

■ **IMAGING STUDIES**
Chest x-ray and bronchoscopy if smoke inhalation suspected

■ **TREATMENT**

Minor burns are amenable to outpatient treatment, whereas moderate and major burns should be treated in specialized burn care facilities according to the principles described below.

■ **ACUTE GENERAL Rx**
• Establish airway: inspect for inhalation injury and intubate for suspected airway edema (often seen 12 to 24 hr later); supplemental O_2
• Remove jewelry and clothing and place one or two large-bore peripheral IVs (if TBSA > 20%)
• Fluid resuscitation with Ringer's lactate at 2 to 4 ml/kg per %TBSA per 24 hr with half the calculated fluid given in the first 8 hr; may titrate to urine output of 0.5 to 1 ml/kg/hr
• Foley catheter and NG tube (20% of patients develop an ileus)
• Td booster
• IV morphine in 2- to 6-mg doses
• Stress ulcer prophylaxis with H_2-blockers in high-risk patients
• Prophylactic antibiotics are not recommended

■ **BURN WOUND Rx**
• Wash burned skin with cool water or saline (1° to 5° C; immerse approximately 30 min if able) and cleanse with mild soap
• Sharp debridement of ruptured or tense blisters (except palms and soles)
• There are several approaches to burn dressings after cleansing and debriding:
1. Apply thin layer of antibiotic ointment (silver sulfadiazine can be used unless sulfa allergy or facial burn) and cover with a nonadherent dressing (e.g., Telfa or petroleum-soaked gauze) followed by a sterile gauze wrap. Wash wound and change dressing bid.
2. Apply saline-soaked gauze (Xeroform, Owen's), cover with 4×4 dressing and a bulky absorbent dressing such as Kerlex. Reevaluate in 5 to 7 days.
3. Apply occlusive dressing (Duoderm, Tegaderm, Biobrane), remove in 7 to 10 days.
• Excision and autografting are required for deep second-degree or third-degree burns and should be done as soon as 24 hr after burn injury.

■ **DISPOSITION**
• Respiratory injury, sepsis, and multi-organ failure may complicate severe burns.
• Scarring can be expected in many second-degree and all third-degree burns.

■ **REFERRAL**
For surgical debridement and grafting evaluation

PEARLS & CONSIDERATIONS

■ **COMMENTS**
First-degree burns (e.g., sunburns) can be treated with cool compresses, antihistamines, emollients, and at times, a rapidly tapering dose of steroids.

REFERENCES
Cohen R, Moelleken B: Disorders due to physical agents. In Tierney L, McPhee S, Papadakis M (eds): *Current medical diagnosis and treatment,* ed 37, Stamford, Conn, 1998, Appleton & Lange.
Edlich R, Moghtader J: Thermal burns. In Rosen P (ed): *Emergency medicine: concepts and clinical practice,* ed 4, vol 1, St Louis, 1998, Mosby.
Fulcher W: Thermal and environmental injuries. In Rakel R (ed): *Textbook of family practice,* ed 5, Philadelphia, 1995, WB Saunders.
Schwartz L: Thermal burns. In Tintinalli J (ed): *Emergency medicine: a comprehensive study guide,* New York, 1996, McGraw-Hill.
Author: **Michael P. Johnson, M.D.**

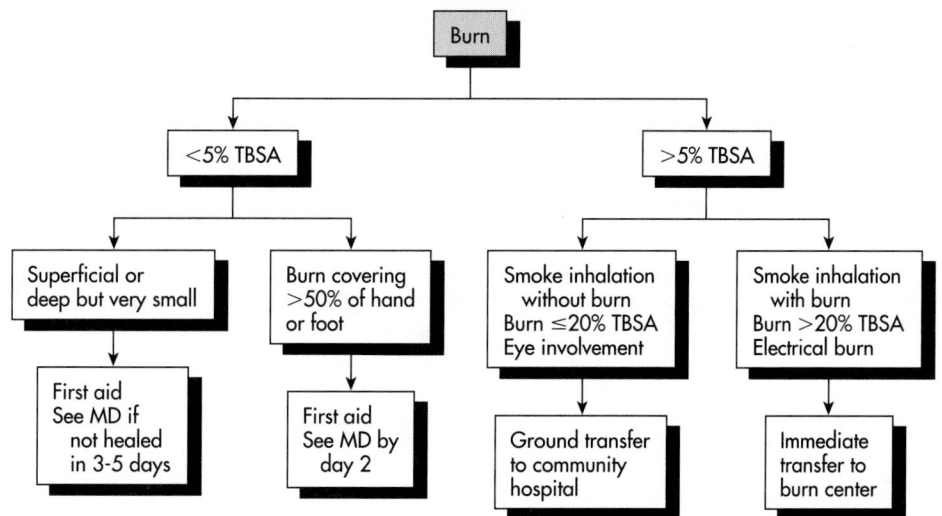

Fig. 1-76 **Algorithm for decision making at the scene.** *TBSA,* Total body surface area. (From Auerbach PS: *Wilderness medicine,* ed 4, St Louis, 2001, Mosby.)

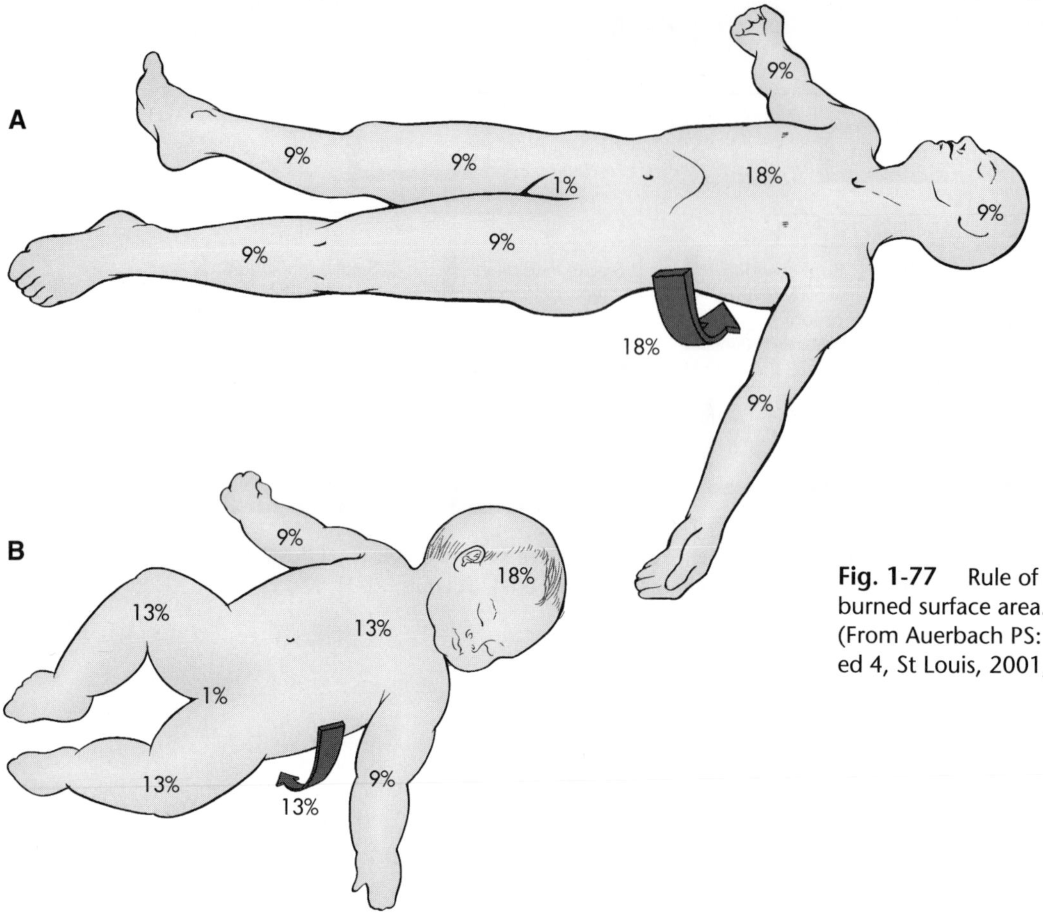

A

9%

9%   9%

1%

18%

9%

9%   9%

18%

9%

B

9%

18%

13%   13%

1%

13%   9%

13%

Fig. 1-77   Rule of nines used for estimating burned surface area. **A**, Adult. **B**, Infant. (From Auerbach PS: *Wilderness medicine*, ed 4, St Louis, 2001, Mosby.)

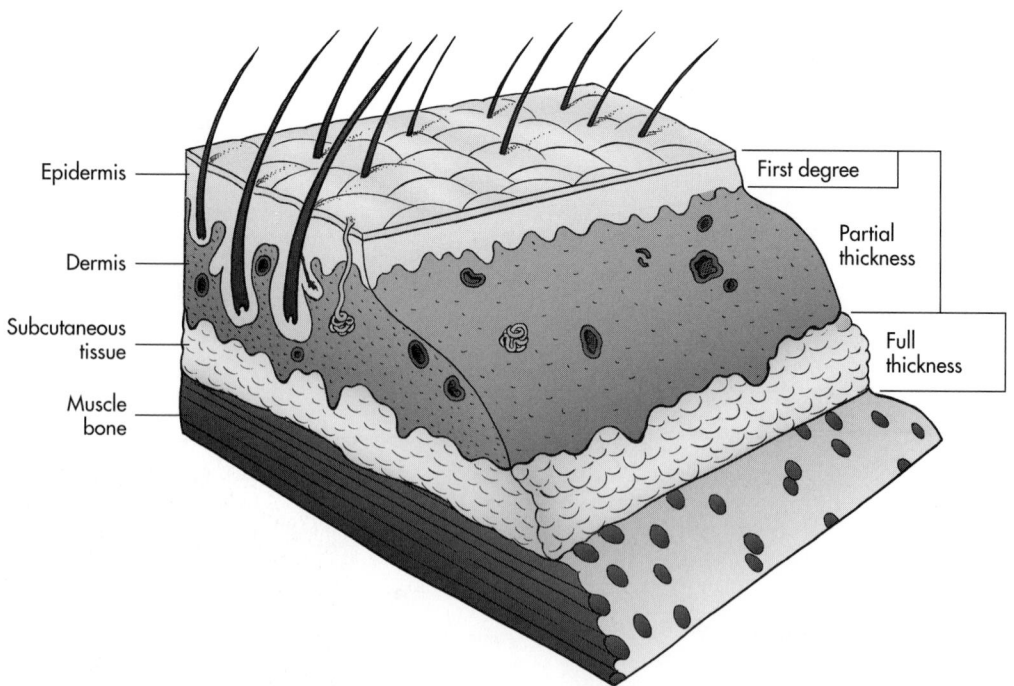

Epidermis

Dermis

Subcutaneous tissue

Muscle bone

First degree

Partial thickness

Full thickness

Fig. 1-78   Skin anatomy. (From Auerbach PS: *Wilderness medicine*, ed 4, St Louis, 2001, Mosby.)

BASIC INFORMATION

■ DEFINITION
Bursitis is an inflammation of a bursa and is usually aseptic. A *bursa* is a closed sac lined with a synovial-like membrane that sometimes contains fluid that is found or that develops in an area subject to pressure or friction.

■ SYNONYMS
Housemaid's knee (prepatellar bursitis)
Weaver's bottom (ischial gluteal bursitis)
Baker's cyst (gastrocnemius-semimembranosus bursa)

ICD-9CM CODES
726.19 Subacromial bursitis
726.33 Olecranon bursitis
726.5 Ischiogluteal bursitis (hip)
726.5 Iliopsoas bursitis (hip)
726.61 Anserine bursitis
726.5 Trochanteric bursitis
726.65 Prepatellar bursitis
727.51 Baker's cyst
726.79 Retrocalcaneal bursitis

■ PHYSICAL FINDINGS & CLINICAL PRESENTATION
- Swelling, especially if bursa is superficial (olecranon, prepatellar)
- Local tenderness with pain on pressure against bursa
- Pain with joint movement
- Referred pain
- Palpable occasional fibrocartilaginous bodies (most common in olecranon and prepatellar bursae)

■ ETIOLOGY
- Acute trauma
- Repetitive trauma
- Sepsis
- Crystalline deposit disease

DIAGNOSIS

■ DIFFERENTIAL DIAGNOSIS
- Degenerative joint disease
- Tendinitis (sometimes occurs in conjunction with bursitis)
- Cellulitis (if bursitis is septic)
- Infectious arthritis

■ WORKUP
Aspiration with Gram stain and C&S

■ IMAGING STUDIES
- Plain radiography to rule out other potential or coexisting bone or joint problems (Fig. 1-79)
- MRI

TREATMENT

■ NONPHARMACOLOGIC THERAPY
- If chronic, elimination of cause of pressure or irritation
- Use of relief pads, avoidance of direct pressure
- Rest
- Elevation
- Ice for acute trauma

■ ACUTE GENERAL Rx
- Septic:
  1. Appropriate antibiotic coverage and drainage
  2. Aspiration of purulent fluid with a large-bore needle (if there is no rapid clinical response, incision and drainage are indicated)
- Nonseptic:
  1. Aspiration of blood from acute trauma
  2. Application of compression dressing

■ CHRONIC Rx
- Aspiration if excessive fluid volume present, followed by application of compression dressing to prevent fluid reaccumulation (repeat aspiration may be required)
- Steroid injection into bursa (1 ml of triamcinolone, 40 mg, mixed with 1 to 3 cc of xylocaine depending on size of bursa.)
- NSAIDs

■ DISPOSITION
- Many bursal sacs "dry up" eventually.
- Nonsurgical treatment is effective in most cases.

■ REFERRAL
For orthopedic consultation to assist in treatment of sepsis or for excision of chronic enlarged bursa when indicated

PEARLS & CONSIDERATIONS

■ COMMENTS
- Injection of trochanteric bursa may require spinal needle in large patient.
- Sterile bursae should not be incised and drained because a chronic draining sinus tract may develop.
- Involvement of the iliopsoas bursa may cause groin pain, although the diagnosis is difficult to make because of the inaccessibility of the area to direct examination. (This also makes steroid injection impossible even if the diagnosis could be established.)

Author: **Lonnie R. Mercier, M.D.**

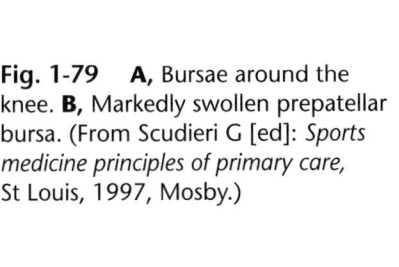

Fig. 1-79 A, Bursae around the knee. **B,** Markedly swollen prepatellar bursa. (From Scudieri G [ed]: *Sports medicine principles of primary care,* St Louis, 1997, Mosby.)

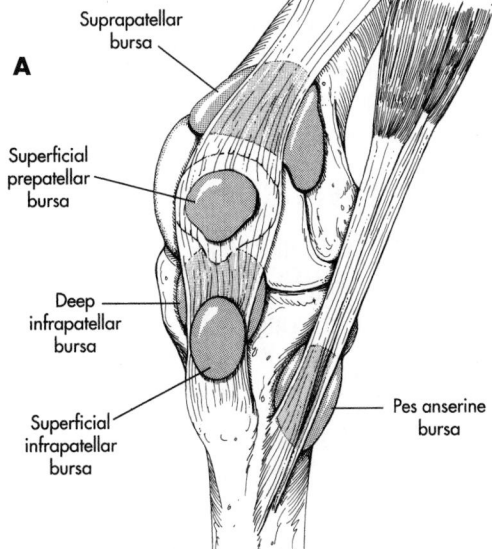

A

Suprapatellar bursa

Superficial prepatellar bursa

Deep infrapatellar bursa

Superficial infrapatellar bursa

Pes anserine bursa

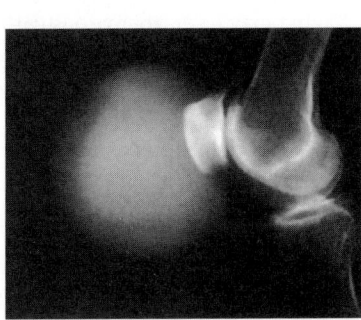

B

BASIC INFORMATION

■ DEFINITION
Candidiasis is an inflammatory process involving the vulva and/or the vagina and is caused by superficial invasion of epithelial cells by *Candida* species.

■ SYNONYMS
Moniliasis
Thrush
Candidosis

ICD-9CM CODES
112.1 Moniliasis
112.0 Thrush
112 Candidosis

■ EPIDEMIOLOGY & DEMOGRAPHICS
- This is the second most common form of vaginitis in the U.S. It is estimated that up to 75% of women will have at least one episode of vulvovaginal candidiasis (VVC) during their childbearing years and about 45% will have a second attack. A small subpopulation of probably <5% of adult women has recurrent, often intractable episodes. *Candida* may be isolated in up to 20% of asymptomatic women of childbearing age.
- Factors that predispose to development of symptomatic VVC include pregnancy, antibiotic use, and diabetes. Antibiotic use disturbs normal vaginal flora and allows overgrowth of fungi; pregnancy and diabetes are associated with decrease in cell-mediated immunity.
- Factors associated with increased rates of asymptomatic vaginal colonization: pregnancy, high-estrogen oral contraceptives, uncontrolled diabetes mellitus, attendance at STD clinics.

■ PHYSICAL FINDINGS & CLINICAL PRESENTATION
Symptoms of VVC consist of:
- Vulvar pruritus with vaginal discharge that typically resembles cottage cheese
- Erythema and edema of labia and vulvar skin; possible discrete pustulopapular peripheral lesions (satellite lesions)
- Vagina may be erythematous with an adherent, whitish discharge
- Cervix may appear normal.
- Symptoms characteristically exacerbated in the week preceding menses with some relief after onset of menstrual flow.

■ ETIOLOGY
- *Candida* are dimorphic fungi (spores and mycelial forms).
- *C. albicans* is responsible for 85% to 90% of vaginal yeast infections.
- *C. glabrata, C. tropicalis* (non-*albicans* species) also cause vaginitis and may be more resistant to conventional therapy.

DIAGNOSIS

■ DIFFERENTIAL DIAGNOSIS
- Bacterial vaginosis
- Trichomoniasis

■ WORKUP
- Discharge may vary from watery to homogeneously thick. May have complaints of vaginal soreness, dyspareunia, vulvar burning, and irritation. External dysuria may be present.
- Usually normal vaginal pH (<4.5).
- Budding yeast forms or mycelia will appear in as many as 80% of cases. Saline wet prep of vaginal secretions usually is normal; may be increased in inflammatory cells in severe cases.
- Whiff test negative (KOH).
- 10% KCl useful and more sensitive than wet mount for microscopic identification.
- Can make a presumptive diagnosis based on symptomatology in the absence of microscopy-proven fungal elements if the pH and wet prep are normal. Fungal culture is recommended to confirm diagnosis.
- In chronic/recurrent, burning replaces itching as prominent symptom. Confirm diagnosis with direct microscopy and culture. Many may actually have chronic or atrophic dermatitis.

■ LABORATORY TESTS
If sending cultures, send on Nickerson's media or semiquantitative slide-stix cultures. There is no reliable serologic technique for diagnosis.

TREATMENT

■ ACUTE GENERAL Rx
TOPICAL BUTOCONAZOLE: 2% vaginal cream 5 g intravaginally for 3 days
TOPICAL CLOTRIMAZOLE:
  1% cream 5 g intravaginally for 7 to 14 days

100-mg vaginal tablet for 7 days
100-mg vaginal tablets, two tablets for 3 days
500-mg vaginal tablet, single dose
TOPICAL MICONAZOLE:
  2% cream 5 g intravaginally for 7 days
  200-mg vaginal suppository for 3 days
  100-mg vaginal suppository for 7 days
TOPICAL TIOCONAZOLE: 6.5% ointment 5 g intravaginally, single dose
TOPICAL TERCONAZOLE:
  0.4% cream 5 g intravaginally for 7 days
  0.8% cream 5 g intravaginally for 3 days
  80-mg suppository for 3 days
ORAL FLUCONAZOLE: 150-mg single PO dose

■ CHRONIC Rx
Ketoconazole 400 mg PO qd or fluconazole 200 mg PO qd until symptoms resolve. Then maintenance on prophylactic doses of these agents for 6 mo (ketoconazole 100 mg/day, fluconazole 150 mg/wk).

■ DISPOSITION
Usually relatively limited in duration and occurrence. If chronic or recurrent, may consider screening for diabetes, HIV, or other immune deficiencies.

PEARLS & CONSIDERATIONS

■ COMMENTS
Azoles are more effective than nystatin. Symptoms usually take 2 to 3 days to resolve. Adjunctive treatment with weak topical steroid such as 1% hydrocortisone cream may help with relief of symptoms.

REFERENCE
CDC 1998 guidelines for treatment of sexually transmitted diseases, *MWWR* 47(RR-1)1, 1998.
Author: **Eugene J. Louie-Ng, M.D.**

BASIC INFORMATION

■ DEFINITION
Carbon monoxide is a colorless, odorless, tasteless, nonirritating gas. When inhaled it produces toxicity by causing cellular hypoxia.

ICD-9CM CODES
986 Carbon monoxide poisoning

■ EPIDEMIOLOGY & DEMOGRAPHICS
- Carbon monoxide poisoning is seen more frequently during the winter months.
- Most common cause of lethal poisoning in the U.S.

■ PHYSICAL FINDINGS & CLINICAL PRESENTATION
Symptoms of toxicity are seen most frequently in organs with highest oxygen consumption, especially the heart and brain.
- Severity of symptoms usually, but not always, correlates with measured carboxyhemoglobin levels (Table 1-19).
- Cherry-red skin color and bright red venous blood are infrequent and late findings of carbon monoxide poisoning.

■ ETIOLOGY
Carbon monoxide causes tissue hypoxia by a number of mechanisms.
- Carbon monoxide binds to hemoglobin with an affinity 250 times greater than oxygen, thus displacing oxygen from hemoglobin and decreasing the oxygen-carrying capacity of blood.
- Carbon monoxide shifts the oxyhemoglobin curve to the left, thus decreasing oxygen release to tissue.
- Cellular respiration is depressed by inhibition of the cytochrome oxidase system.
- Cardiac function is depressed by direct binding to cardiac myoglobin.
Carbon monoxide poisoning occurs when individuals are exposed to smoke from fires, automobile exhaust, faulty stoves, or heating systems in poorly ventilated areas.

DIAGNOSIS

■ DIFFERENTIAL DIAGNOSIS
- Cyanide
- Hydrogen sulfide
- Methemoglobinemia
- Amphetamines and derivatives
- Cocaine
- Cyclic antidepressants
- Phencyclidine (PCP)
- Phenothiazines
- Theophylline

■ WORKUP
History of exposure to carbon monoxide, physical examination, laboratory tests

■ LABORATORY TESTS
- Carboxyhemoglobin concentration
- Direct measurement of arterial oxygen saturation
NOTE: Pulse oximetry and arterial blood gas may be falsely normal because neither measures oxygen saturation directly. Pulse oximetry is inaccurate because of the similar absorption characteristics of oxyhemoglobin and carboxyhemoglobin. An arterial blood gas is inaccurate because it measures oxygen dissolved in plasma (which is not affected by carbon monoxide) and then calculates oxygen saturation.
- Electrolytes, glucose, BUN, creatinine (because lactic acidosis and rhabdomyolysis may develop)
- ECG (rule out ischemia)
- Pregnancy test (fetus at high risk)

TREATMENT

■ ACUTE GENERAL Rx
- Remove from site of carbon monoxide exposure
- Ensure adequate airway
- Continuous ECG monitor
- 100% oxygen by tight-fitting nonrebreather mask or endotreacheal tube (this decreases the half-life of carboxyhemoglobin from 4 to 6 hr to 60 to 90 min)
- Measure carboxyhemoglobin level every 2 to 4 hr
- Continue oxygen until carboxyhemoglobin level is less than 5%
Hyperbaric oxygen (3 ATM) decreases half-life of carbon monoxide to 20 to 30 min
- Controversial if there is any beneficial effect over regular 100% oxygen
- Consider for individuals with:
  1. Severe intoxication (carboxyhemoglobin >25%, neurologic signs, ischemic ECG changes, severe metabolic acidosis, rhabdomyolysis, pulmonary edema, shock)
  2. Those who do not respond rapidly to oxygen at room air
  3. Pregnant women with carboxyhemoglobin >15%
  4. Newborns
- Consult local poison control center
- Treat seizures and coma
- Consider concomitant poisoning with other toxic gases that may be present in smoke (i.e., cyanide, methemoglobinemia, other irritant gases) and/or thermal injury to the airway

■ DISPOSITION
- Depends on severity of exposure
- Survivors are at risk for neurologic sequelae ranging from parkinsonism to neuropychiatric symptoms (personality and memory disorders).
- Fetal demise is likely because fetal hemoglobin is more sensitive to carbon monoxide binding (fetal/neonatal carboxyhemoglobin levels may be twice as high as maternal levels).

■ REFERRAL
- Regional poison control center
- +/− Hyperbaric chamber

REFERENCE
Ernst A, Zibrak JD: Carbon monoxide poisoning, *N Engl J Med* 339:1603, 1998.
Author: **Sudeep K. Aulakh, M.D., F.R.C.P.C.**

TABLE 1-19 Carboxyhemoglobin Level and Signs and Symptoms

CARBOXYHEMOGLOBIN (%)	SYMPTOMS	PHYSICAL FINDINGS
<10	Mild headache, dyspnea on vigorous exertion	
20 to 40	Nausea, dizziness, irritability, fatigue, severe headache, confusion, decreased visual acuity, dyspnea on moderate excretion	Retinal hemorrhages
41 to 70	Tachycardia, tachypnea, lethargy, ataxia, syncope, seizures, myocardial ischemia, pulmonary edema, metabolic acidosis, coma	ECG: ST segment changes, conduction blocks, arrhythmia
>80	Rapidly fatal	

BASIC INFORMATION

■ DEFINITION
Carcinoid syndrome is a symptom complex characterized by paroxysmal vasomotor disturbances, diarrhea, and bronchospasm. It is caused by the action of amines and peptides (serotonin, bradykinin, histamine) produced by tumors arising from neuroendocrine cells.

■ SYNONYMS
Flush syndrome
Argentaffinoma syndrome

ICD-9CM CODES
259.2 Carcinoid syndrome

■ EPIDEMIOLOGY & DEMOGRAPHICS
INCIDENCE: Carcinoid tumors are found incidentally in 0.5% to 0.75% of autopsies.

■ PHYSICAL FINDINGS & CLINICAL PRESENTATION
- Cutaneous flushing (75% to 90%)
  1. The patient usually has red-purple flushes starting in the face, then spreading to the neck and upper trunk.
  2. The flushing episodes last from a few minutes to hours (longer-lasting flushes may be associated with bronchial carcinoids).
  3. Flushing may be triggered by emotion, alcohol, or foods, or it may occur spontaneously.
  4. Dizziness, tachycardia, and hypotension may be associated with the cutaneous flushing.
- Diarrhea (>70%): often associated with abdominal bloating and audible peristaltic rushes
- Intermittent bronchospasm (25%): characterized by severe dyspnea and wheezing
- Facial telangiectasia
- Tricuspid regurgitation from carcinoid heart lesions

■ ETIOLOGY
- The carcinoid syndrome is caused by neoplasms originating from neuroendocrine cells.
- Carcinoid tumors are principally found in the following organs: appendix (40%), small bowel (20%; 15% in the ileum), rectum (15%), bronchi (12%), esophagus, stomach, colon (10%), ovary, biliary tract, pancreas (3%).
- Carcinoid tumors do not usually produce the syndrome unless liver metastases are present or the primary tumor does not involve the GI tract.

DIAGNOSIS

■ DIFFERENTIAL DIAGNOSIS
- The carcinoid syndrome must be distinguished from idiopathic flushing (IF); patients with IF more often are females, younger, and with a longer duration of symptoms; palpitations, syncope, and hypotension occur primarily in patients with IF.
- An algorithm for the diagnosis and treatment of carcinoid tumors is described in Fig. 1-80.

■ LABORATORY TESTS
- The biochemical marker for carcinoid syndrome is increased 24-hr urinary 5-hydroxyindoleacetic acid (5-HIAA), a metabolite of serotonin (5-hydroxytryptamine).
- False elevations can be seen with ingestion of certain foods (bananas, pineapples, eggplant, avocados, walnuts) and certain medications (acetaminophen, caffeine, guaifenesin, reserpine); therefore patients should be on a restricted diet and should avoid these medications when the test is ordered.
- Liver function studies are an unreliable indicator of liver involvement.

■ IMAGING STUDIES
- Chest x-ray examination is useful to detect bronchial carcinoids.
- CT scans of abdomen or a liver and spleen radionuclide scan is useful to detect liver metastases (palpable in >50% of cases).
- Iodine-123 labeled somatostatin (123-ISS) can detect carcinoid endocrine tumors with somatostatin receptors.
- Scanning with radiolabeled octreotide can visualize previously undetected or metastatic lesions.

TREATMENT

■ NONPHARMACOLOGIC THERAPY
Avoidance of ethanol ingestion (may precipitate flushing)

■ ACUTE GENERAL Rx
- Surgical resection of the tumor can be curative if the tumor is localized or palliative and result in prolonged asymptomatic periods if metastases are present. Surgical manipulation of the tumor can, however, cause severe vasomotor abnormalities and bronchospasm (carcinoid crisis).
- Percutaneous embolization and ligation of the hepatic artery can decrease the bulk of the tumor in the liver and provide palliative treatment of tumors with hepatic metastases.
- Cytotoxic chemotherapy: combination chemotherapy with 5-fluorouracil and streptozotocin can be used in patients with unresectable or recurrent carcinoid tumors; however, it has only limited success.
- Control of clinical manifestations:
  1. Diarrhea usually responds to diphenoxylate with atropine (Lomotil).
  2. Flushing can be controlled by the combination of H_1- and H_2-receptor antagonists (e.g., diphenhydramine 25 to 50 mg PO q6h and ranitidine 150 mg bid).
  3. Somatostatin analog (SMS 201-995) is effective for both flushing and diarrhea in most patients.
  4. Bronchospasm can be treated with aminophylline and/or albuterol.
- Nutritional support: supplemental niacin therapy may be useful to prevent pellagra, because the tumor uses dietary tryptophan for serotonin synthesis, resulting in a nutritional deficiency in some patients.

■ CHRONIC Rx
- Subcutaneous somatostatin analogues (octreotide 150 μg SC tid) have been used successfully for long-term control of symptoms in patients with unresectable neoplasms.
- Echocardiography and monitoring for right-sided CHF are recommended for patients with unresectable disease because endocardial fibrosis, involving predominantly the endocardium, chordae, and valves of the right side of the heart, can occur and result in right-sided CHF.

■ DISPOSITION
- Prognosis varies with the stage and location of the tumor.
- Carcinoids of the appendix and rectum have a low malignancy potential and rarely produce the clinical syndrome; metastases are also uncommon if the size of the primary lesion is <2 cm in diameter.

REFERENCE
Kulke MH, Mayer RJ: Carcinoid tumors, *N Engl J Med* 340:898, 1999.
Author: **Fred F. Ferri, M.D.**

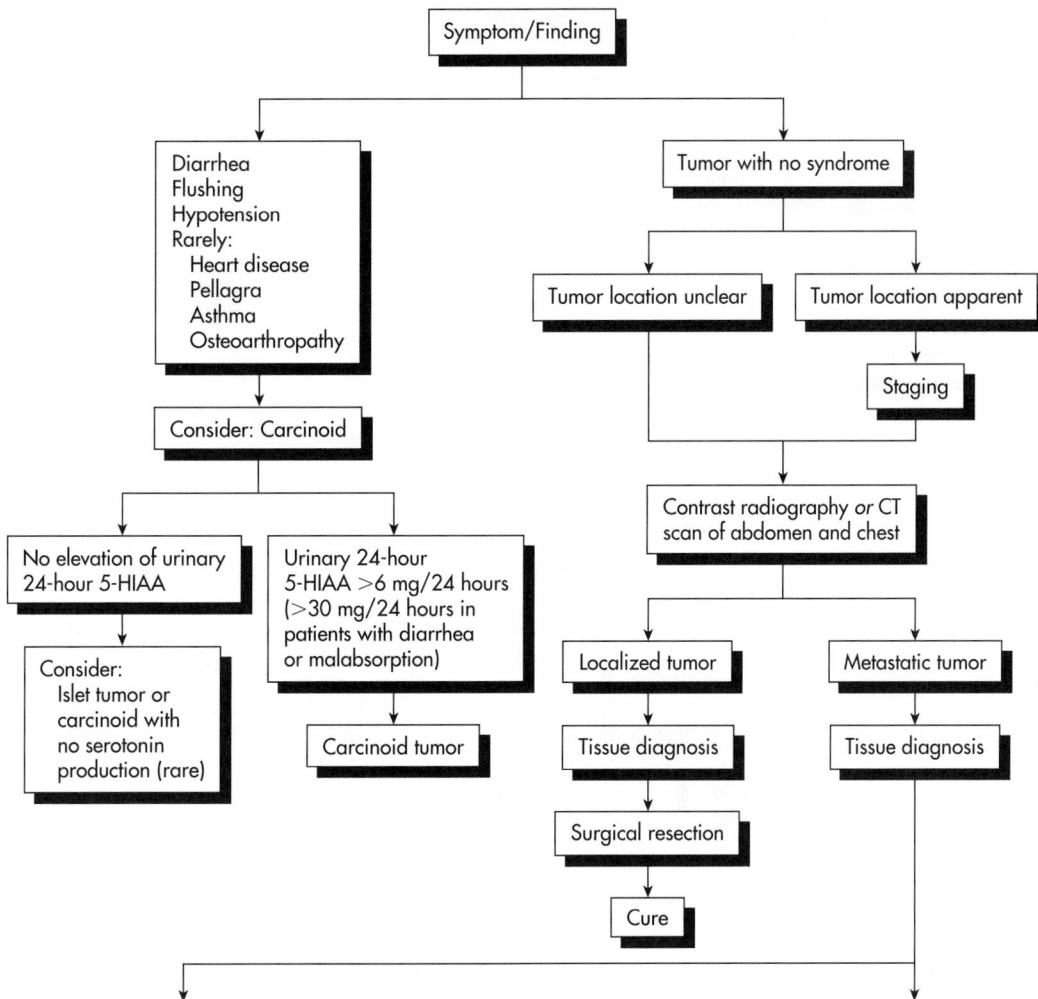

Fig. 1-80 **Diagnosis and treatment of carcinoid tumors.** *5-HIAA,* 5-Hydroxyindoleacetic acid. (From Abeloff MD: *Clinical oncology,* ed 2, New York, 2000, Churchill Livingstone.)

Gwendolyn R. Lee, M.D.
Internal Medicine

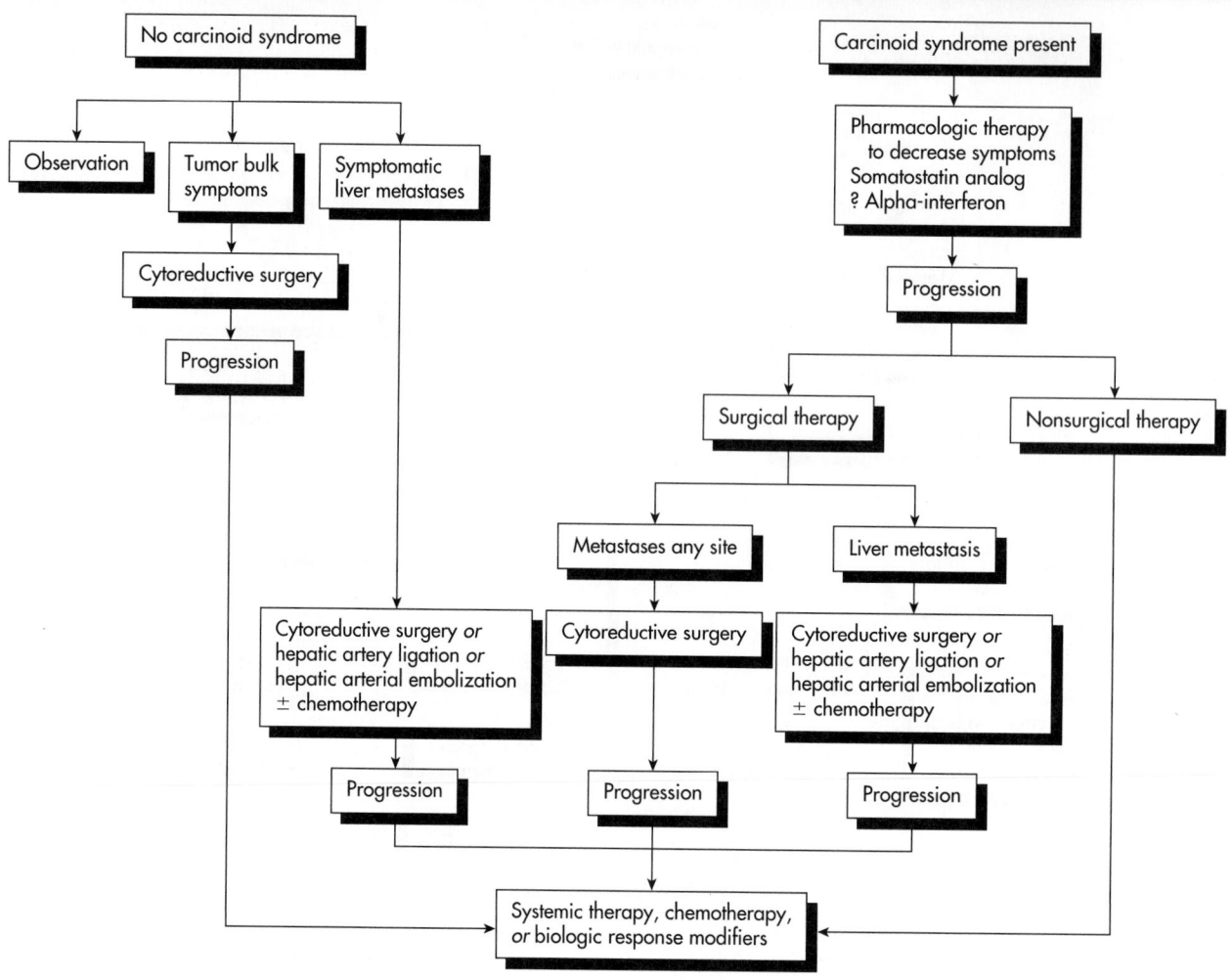

Fig. 1-80, cont'd Diagnosis and treatment of carcinoid tumors. *5-HIAA*, 5-Hydroxyindoleacetic acid. (From Abeloff MD: *Clinical oncology*, ed 2, New York, 2000, Churchill Livingstone.)

BASIC INFORMATION

■ DEFINITION

Cardiac tamponade is compression of the heart by fluid within the pericardial sac that impairs dilation and filling of the ventricles during diastole.

ICD-9CM CODES

423.9 Unspecified diseases of the pericardium

■ PHYSICAL FINDINGS & CLINICAL PRESENTATION

Acute cardiac tamponade (e.g., penetrating wounds, iatrogenic, aortic dissection)
1. Beck's triad
   a. Decrease in systemic arterial pressure
   b. Elevated central venous pressure
   c. Small, quiet heart

Chronic accumulating pericardial effusion leading to tamponade
1. Pericardial friction rub may be present
2. Tachypnea and tachycardia
3. Raised jugular venous distention (prominent *x* descent with absent *y* descent)
4. Pulsus paradoxus (>10 mm Hg fall in systolic blood pressure during inspiration)
5. Soft heart sounds

■ ETIOLOGY

Acute
1. Penetrating trauma
2. Aortic dissection
3. Myocardial rupture after treatment of MI with thrombolytics and/or heparin
4. Iatrogenic (central line and pacemaker insertions, postcoronary bypass surgery)

Chronic accumulating pericardial effusion leading to tamponade
1. Malignancy (e.g., lung, breast, lymphoma)
2. Viral pericarditis (e.g., coxsackie, HIV)
3. Uremia
4. Bacterial, fungal, and tuberculosis
5. Myxedema (rare)
6. Collagen-vascular disease (e.g., SLE, RA, scleroderma)
7. Radiation

DIAGNOSIS

■ DIFFERENTIAL DIAGNOSIS

COPD, constrictive pericardial disease, restrictive cardiomyopathy, right ventricular infarction, and pulmonary embolism can all lead to elevated jugular venous pressure, decreased systemic pressure, and pulsus paradoxus.

■ WORKUP

Cardiac tamponade is a clinical diagnosis made at the bedside by noting the above-mentioned physical findings. The echocardiogram will support the clinical diagnosis. Thereafter, one must pursue the etiology with specific laboratory work (see below).

■ LABORATORY TESTS

- Electrolytes, BUN, Cr, ESR, thyroid function tests, ANA, RF, PPD, blood cultures, viral titers, and pericardial fluid analysis and cultures will all help in identifying or excluding a possible etiology of the effusion leading to tamponade.
- 12-lead ECG findings are suggestive but not diagnostic.
  1. Low voltage (<5 mm QRS amplitude in the limb leads and <10 mm in the chest leads)
  2. PR depression
  3. Electrical alternans (alternating amplitude of the QRS complex in any or all leads)

■ IMAGING STUDIES

- The chest x-ray examination is not very specific. The heart size can be normal in acute tamponade or massive (water bottle configuration) in slow-forming effusions.
- The echocardiogram can detect effusions as small as 20 ml and can strongly suggest tamponade physiology (collapse of the right atrium and right ventricle during diastole).
- Right-sided cardiac catheterization and intrapericardial pressure measurements confirm the diagnosis.
- Typical findings are diastolic equalization of pressures (pulmonary artery pressure = right ventricular diastolic pressure = right atrial pressure = intrapericardial pressure).

TREATMENT

■ NONPHARMACOLOGIC THERAPY

Cardiac tamponade should be treated urgently. Avoid drugs that will reduce preload and exacerbate tamponade (e.g., nitrates, diuretics).

■ ACUTE GENERAL Rx

- The acute forms of tamponade as mentioned earlier (see "Etiology") usually require emergency cardiothoracic surgery.
- Provide hemodynamic support with volume expansion and vasopressors along with emergency subxiphoid pericardiocentesis in the suspected tamponade code situation (e.g., electromechanical dissociation, patient in shock).

■ CHRONIC Rx

- Depends on etiology
- Semiacute treatment includes:
  1. Right-side heart catheter with echocardiographic guided pericardiocentesis (can be done by cardiology). The catheter can be left in place for 48 hr to allow for continued drainage until a more definitive procedure is performed or the etiology is resolved (e.g., dialysis for uremia, levothyroxine for myxedema).
- Other surgical drainage procedures include:
  1. Subxiphoid pericardial drainage
  2. Limited pericardiectomy draining the pericardial fluid into the left hemithorax
  3. Complete pericardiectomy

■ DISPOSITION

The prognosis of cardiac tamponade depends on the underlying cause.

■ REFERRAL

- Cardiology consultation is made if the clinical suspicion of tamponade exists.
- Cardiothoracic surgeon consultation is made when tamponade is confirmed.

PEARLS & CONSIDERATIONS

■ COMMENTS

As little as 200 ml of fluid can lead to acute cardiac tamponade, whereas in the chronic formation, the pericardial sac can hold up to 5 L of fluid before tamponade occurs.

REFERENCE

Spodick DH: Pathophysiology of cardiac tamponade, *Chest* 113(5):1372, 1998.
Author: **Peter Petropoulos, M.D.**

BASIC INFORMATION

■ DEFINITION
Cardiomyopathies are a group of diseases primarily involving the myocardium and characterized by myocardial dysfunction that is not the result of hypertension, coronary atherosclerosis, valvular dysfunction, or pericardial abnormalities. In dilated cardiomyopathy, the heart is enlarged, and both ventricles are dilated.

■ SYNONYMS
Congestive cardiomyopathy

ICD-9CM CODES
425.4 Other primary cardiomyopathies

■ EPIDEMIOLOGY & DEMOGRAPHICS
- The prevalence of dilated cardiomyopathy in the general adult population is approximately 1%.
- Incidence increases with age and approaches 10% at age 80 yr.

■ PHYSICAL FINDINGS & CLINICAL PRESENTATION
- Increased jugular venous pressure
- Small pulse pressure
- Pulmonary rales, hepatomegaly, peripheral edema
- S_3, S_4
- Mitral regurgitation, tricuspid regurgitation (less common)

■ ETIOLOGY
- Idiopathic
- Alcoholism
- Collagen-vascular disease (SLE, RA, polyarteritis, dermatomyositis)
- Postmyocarditis
- Peripartum (last trimester of pregnancy or 6 mo postpartum)
- Heredofamilial neuromuscular disease
- Toxins (cobalt, lead, phosphorus, carbon monoxide, mercury, doxorubicin, daunorubicin)
- Nutritional (beri-beri, selenium deficiency, carnitine deficiency, thiamine deficiency)
- Cocaine, heroin, organic solvents ("glue sniffer's heart")
- Irradiation
- Acromegaly, osteogenesis imperfecta, myxedema, thyrotoxicosis, diabetes
- Hypocalcemia

- Antiretroviral agents (zidovudine, didanosine, zalcitabine)
- Phenothiazines
- Infections (viral [HIV], rickettsial, mycobacterial, toxoplasmosis, trichinosis, Chagas' disease)
- Hematologic (e.g., sickle cell anemia)
- Table 2-37 describes the classification of cardiomyopathies.

DIAGNOSIS

■ DIFFERENTIAL DIAGNOSIS
- Frank pulmonary disease
- Valvular dysfunction
- Pericardial abnormalities
- Coronary atherosclerosis
- Psychogenic dyspnea

■ WORKUP
- Chest x-ray examination, ECG, echocardiogram
- Medical history with emphasis on the following symptoms:
  1. Dyspnea on exertion, orthopnea, PND
  2. Palpitations
  3. Systemic and pulmonary embolism
- Cardiac troponin T levels: Persistently elevated troponin T levels are a marker of poor outcome in cardiomyopathy patients.

■ IMAGING STUDIES
CHEST X-RAY EXAMINATION:
- Massive cardiac enlargement
- Interstitial pulmonary edema
ECG:
- Left ventricular hypertrophy with ST-T wave changes
- RBBB or LBBB
- Arrhythmias (atrial fibrillation, PVC, PAC, ventricular tachycardia)
ECHOCARDIOGRAM:
- Low ejection fraction with global akinesia

TREATMENT

■ NONPHARMACOLOGIC THERAPY
- Bed rest when CHF is present
- Treatment of underlying disease (SLE, alcoholism)

■ ACUTE GENERAL Rx
- Treat CHF (cause of death in 70% of patients) with sodium restriction, diuretics, ACE inhibitors, and digitalis.

- Vasodilators (combined with nitrates and ACE inhibitors) are effective agents in dilated cardiomyopathy.
- Prevent thromboembolism with oral anticoagulants.
- Low-dose β-blockade with metoprolol may improve ventricular function by interrupting the cycle of reflex sympathetic activity and controlling tachycardia.
- Diltiazem has also been reported to have a long-term beneficial effect in idiopathic dilated cardiomyopathy.
- Preliminary studies have revealed that growth hormone administered for 3 mo to patients with idiopathic dilated cardiomyopathy increased myocardial mass and reduced the size of the left ventricular chamber, resulting in improvement in hemodynamics and clinical status.
- Use antiarrhythmic treatment as appropriate.

■ DISPOSITION
Annual mortality is 20% in patients with moderate heart failure, and it exceeds 50% in patients with severe heart failure.

■ REFERRAL
Consider heart transplant for young patients (<60 yr old) who are no longer responsive to medical therapy.

PEARLS & CONSIDERATIONS

■ COMMENTS
Patents should be encouraged to restrict alcohol and sodium intake.

REFERENCE
Sato Y et al: Persistently increased serum concentrations of cardiac troponin T in patients with idiopathic dilated cardiomyopathy are predictive of adverse outcomes, *Circulation* 103:368, 2001.
Author: **Fred F. Ferri, M.D.**

BASIC INFORMATION

■ DEFINITION
Cardiomyopathies are a group of diseases primarily involving the myocardium and characterized by myocardial dysfunction that is not the result of hypertension, coronary atherosclerosis, valvular dysfunction, or pericardial abnormalities. In hypertrophic cardiomyopathy there is marked hypertrophy of the myocardium and disproportionally greater thickening of the intraventricular septum than that of the free wall of the left ventricle (asymmetric septal hypertrophy [ASH]).

■ SYNONYMS
Idiopathic hypertrophic subaortic stenosis (IHSS)
Hypertrophic obstructive cardiomyopathy (HOCM)
ASH
HCM

■ ICD-9CM CODES
425.4 Cardiomyopathy, hypertrophic nonobstructive
425.1 Cardiomyopathy, hypertrophic obstructive
746.84 Cardiomyopathy, hypertrophic congenital

■ EPIDEMIOLOGY & DEMOGRAPHICS
The disease occurs in two major forms:
1. A familial form, usually diagnosed in young patients and gene mapped to chromosome 14q
2. A sporadic form, usually found in elderly patients

■ PHYSICAL FINDINGS & CLINICAL PRESENTATION
- Harsh, systolic, diamond-shaped murmur at the left sternal border or apex that increases with Valsalva maneuver and decreases with squatting
- Paradoxic splitting of S_2 (if left ventricular obstruction is present)
- S_4
- Double or triple apical impulse
- Increased obstruction
  1. Drugs: digitalis, β-adrenergic stimulators (isoproterenol, dopamine, epinephrine), nitroglycerin, vasodilators, diuretics, alcohol
  2. Hypovolemia
  3. Tachycardia
  4. Valsalva maneuver
  5. Standing position
- Decreased obstruction
  1. Drugs: β-adrenergic blockers, calcium channel blockers, disopyramide, α-adrenergic stimulators
  2. Volume expansion
  3. Bradycardia
  4. Hand grip exercise
  5. Squatting position

■ ETIOLOGY
- Autosomal dominant trait with variable penetrance
- Sporadic occurrence
- Table 2-37 describes the classification of cardiomyopathies.

DIAGNOSIS

■ DIFFERENTIAL DIAGNOSIS
- Coronary atherosclerosis
- Valvular dysfunction
- Pericardial abnormalities
- Chronic pulmonary disease
- Psychogenic dyspnea

■ WORKUP
- Chest x-ray examination, ECG, echocardiography
- Medical history with emphasis in the following manifestations:
  1. Dyspnea
  2. Syncope (usually seen with exercise)
  3. Angina (decreased angina in recumbent position)
  4. Palpitations
- 24-hr Holter monitor to screen for potential lethal arrhythmias (principal cause of syncope or sudden death in obstructive cardiomyopathy)

■ IMAGING STUDIES
- Chest x-ray examination: normal or cardiomegaly
- ECG: left ventricular hypertrophy, abnormal Q waves in anterolateral and inferior leads
- Echocardiography: ventricular hypertrophy, ratio of septum thickness to left ventricular wall thickness >1.3:1, increased ejection fraction

TREATMENT

■ NONPHARMACOLOGIC THERAPY
Advise avoidance of alcohol; alcohol use (even in small amounts) results in increased obstruction of the left ventricular outflow tract.

■ ACUTE GENERAL Rx
- Propranolol 160 to 240 mg/day. The beneficial effects of β-blockers on symptoms (principally dyspnea and chest pain) and exercise tolerance appear to be largely a result of a decrease in the heart rate with consequent prolongation of diastole and increased passive ventricular filling. By reducing the inotropic response, β-blockers may also lessen myocardial oxygen demand and decrease the outflow gradient during exercise, when sympathetic tone is increased.
- Verapamil also decreases left ventricular outflow obstruction by improving filling and probably reducing myocardial ischemia.
- IV saline infusion in addition to propranolol or verapamil is indicated in patients with CHF.
- Disopyramide is a useful antiarrhythmic.
- Use antibiotic prophylaxis for surgical procedures (see Boxes 5-1 to 5-3 and Tables 5-25 and 5-26).
- Avoid use of digitalis, diuretics, nitrates, and vasodilators.
- Encouraging results have been reported on the use of DDD pacing for hemodynamic and symptomatic benefit in patients with drug-resistant hypertrophic obstructive cardiomyopathy.
- Implantable defibrillators are a safe and effective therapy in HCM patients prone to ventricular arrhythmias.

■ DISPOSITION
Patients with hypertrophic cardiomyopathy are at increased risk of sudden death, especially if there is onset of symptoms during childhood. Adult patients can be considered low risk if they have no symptoms or mild symptoms and also if they have none of the following:
- A family history of premature death caused by hypertrophic cardiomyopathy
- Nonsustained ventricular tachycardia during Holter monitoring
- A marked outflow tract gradient
- Substantial hypertrophy (>20 mm)
- Marked left atrial enlargement
- Abnormal blood pressure response during exercise

■ REFERRAL
Surgical treatment (myotomy-myectomy) is reserved for patients who have both a large outflow gradient (≥50 mm Hg) and severe symptoms of heart failure that are unresponsive to medical therapy. The risk of sudden death from arrhythmias is not altered by surgery.

PEARLS & CONSIDERATIONS

■ COMMENTS
Screening of family members with echocardiography is indicated.

REFERENCES
Fananapazir L: Advances in molecular genetics and management of hypertrophic cardiomyopathy, *JAMA* 281:1746, 1999.
Maron BJ et al: Clinical course of hypertrophic cardiomyopathy in a regional United States cohort, *JAMA* 281:650, 1999.
Author: **Fred F. Ferri, M.D.**

BASIC INFORMATION

■ DEFINITION

Cardiomyopathies are a group of diseases primarily involving the myocardium and characterized by myocardial dysfunction that is not the result of hypertension, coronary atherosclerosis, valvular dysfunction, or pericardial abnormalities. Restrictive cardiomyopathies are characterized by decreased ventricular compliance, usually secondary to infiltration of the myocardium.

ICD-9CM CODES
425.4 Other primary cardiomyopathies

■ EPIDEMIOLOGY & DEMOGRAPHICS
Relatively uncommon cardiomyopathy that is most frequently caused by amyloidosis (Fig. 1-81), myocardial fibrosis (after open heart surgery), and radiation

■ PHYSICAL FINDINGS & CLINICAL PRESENTATION
- Edema, ascites, hepatomegaly, distended neck veins
- Fatigue, weakness (secondary to low output)
- Kussmaul's sign: may be present
- Regurgitant murmurs
- Possible prominent apical impulse

■ ETIOLOGY
- Infiltrative and storage disorders (glycogen storage disease, amyloidosis, sarcoidosis, hemochromatosis)
- Scleroderma
- Radiation
- Endocardial fibroelastosis
- Endomyocardial fibrosis
- Idiopathic
- Toxic effects of anthracycline
- Carcinoid heart disease, metastatic cancers
- Diabetic cardiomyopathy
- Eosinophilic cardiomyopathy (Löffler's endocarditis)

Table 2-37 describes the classification of cardiomyopathies.

DIAGNOSIS

■ DIFFERENTIAL DIAGNOSIS
- Coronary atherosclerosis
- Valvular dysfunction
- Pericardial abnormalities
- Chronic lung disease
- Psychogenic dyspnea

■ WORKUP
- Chest x-ray examination, ECG, echocardiogram
- Cardiac catheterization, MRI (selected cases)

■ IMAGING STUDIES
- Chest x-ray examination:
  1. Moderate cardiomegaly
  2. Possible evidence of CHF (pulmonary vascular congestion, pleural effusion)
- ECG:
  1. Low voltage with ST-T wave changes
  2. Possible frequent arrhythmias, left axis deviation, and atrial fibrillation
- Echocardiogram: increased wall thickness and thickened cardiac valves (especially in patients with amyloidosis)
- Cardiac catheterization to distinguish restrictive cardiomyopathy from constrictive pericarditis
  1. Constrictive pericarditis: usually involves both ventricles and produces a plateau of elevated filling pressures
  2. Restrictive cardiomyopathy: impairs the left ventricle more than the right (PCWP > RAP, PASP >50 mm Hg)
- MRI may also be useful to distinguish restrictive cardiomyopathy from constrictive pericarditis (thickness of the pericardium >5 mm in the latter)

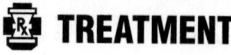

TREATMENT

■ NONPHARMACOLOGIC THERAPY
Control CHF by restricting salt.

■ ACUTE GENERAL Rx
- Cardiomyopathy caused by hemochromatosis may respond to repeated phlebotomies to decrease iron deposition in the heart.
- Sarcoidosis may respond to corticosteroid therapy.
- Corticosteroid and cytotoxic drugs may improve survival in patients with eosinophilic cardiomyopathy.
- There is no effective therapy for other causes of restrictive cardiomyopathy.

■ CHRONIC Rx
Death usually results from CHF or arrhythmias; therefore therapy should be aimed at controlling CHF by restricting salt, administering diuretics, and treating potentially fatal arrhythmias.

■ DISPOSITION
Prognosis varies with the etiology of the cardiomyopathy.

■ REFERRAL
Cardiac transplantation can be considered in patients with refractory symptoms and idiopathic or familial restrictive cardiomyopathies.

Author: **Fred F. Ferri, M.D.**

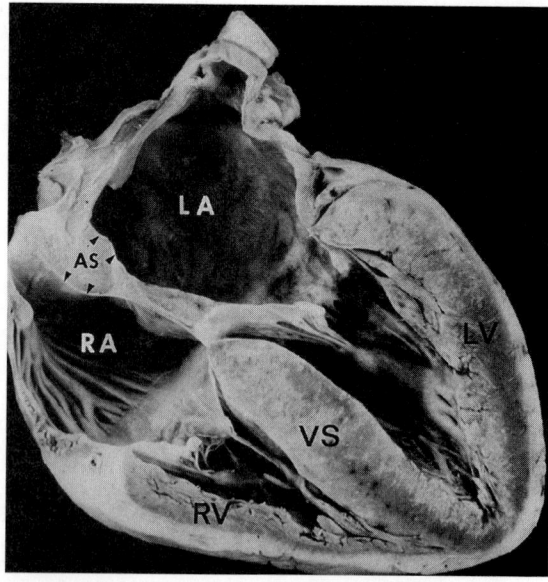

Fig. 1-81 A necropsy specimen of an amyloid heart demonstrating the thickened ventricular septum *(VS)*, atrial septum *(AS)*, and free wall of the left ventricle *(LV)* and right ventricle *(RV)*, and the dilated left atrium *(LA)*. *RA*, Right atrium. (Courtesy Dr. William Edwards, Mayo Clinic, Rochester, Minn. In Goldman L, Bennett JC [eds]: *Cecil textbook of medicine*, ed 21, Philadelphia, 2000, WB Saunders.)

BASIC INFORMATION

■ DEFINITION
Dizziness, presyncope, or syncope in a patient with carotid sinus hypersensitivity is defined as *carotid sinus syndrome.* Carotid sinus hypersensitivity is the exaggerated response to carotid stimulation resulting in bradycardia, hypotension, or both.

■ SYNONYMS
Carotid sinus syncope
CSS

■ ICD-9CM CODES
337.0 Idiopathic peripheral autonomic neuropathy
Carotid sinus syncope or syndrome

■ EPIDEMIOLOGY & DEMOGRAPHICS
• The incidence of carotid sinus hypersensitivity is 10% in the adult population.
• The incidence increases with age.
• Men are affected more often than women (2:1).
• Carotid sinus syndrome is rarely found before the age of 50 yr.

■ PHYSICAL FINDINGS & CLINICAL PRESENTATION
Properly performed carotid sinus massage at the bedside is diagnostic. This maneuver can elicit three types of responses in the appropriate patient (see "Diagnosis").
1. Carotid sinus massage (CSM) should be done in the supine position while monitoring the patient's blood pressure by cuff and heart rate by ECG.
2. CSM should not be performed on patients with carotid bruits or recent TIA/CVA.
3. CSM should be performed on only one artery at a time.
4. CSM should be applied for approximately 5 sec.

■ ETIOLOGY
• Idiopathic
• Head and neck tumors (e.g., thyroid)
• Significant lymphadenopathy
• Carotid body tumors
• Prior neck surgery

DIAGNOSIS

• The diagnosis of CSS is made when carotid sinus hypersensitivity is diagnosed by CSM and no other cause of syncope is identified.
• CSM can elicit three types of responses that are diagnostic of carotid sinus hypersensitivity:

1. Cardioinhibitory type: CSM producing asystole for at least 3 sec
2. Vasodepressor type: CSM producing a decrease in systolic blood pressure of 50 mm Hg or 30 mm Hg in the presence of neurologic symptoms
3. Mixed type: CSM producing both types of responses
• It is not absolutely necessary to produce symptoms with CSM to diagnose CSS.

■ DIFFERENTIAL DIAGNOSIS
All causes of syncope, e.g., cardiac tachyarrhythmias and bradyarrhythmias, cardiac valvular disease and obstructive cardiomyopathy, cerebrovascular events, seizures, drug-induced, autonomic dysfunction, orthostasis/hypovolemia, cough, micturition, hypoxemia, and hypoglycemia

■ WORKUP
The workup must exclude other causes of syncope as guided by the history and the physical examination. Blood tests, cardiac noninvasive studies (Holter, echocardiograms, ECG, tilt test, treadmill testing), cardiac invasive testing (electrophysiologic studies), EEG, and CT scan should be ordered in the appropriate clinical setting.

TREATMENT

■ NONPHARMACOLOGIC THERAPY
Avoidance of triggering factors such as straining or applying neck pressure from tight collars, shaving, or rapid head turning.

■ ACUTE GENERAL Rx
Treatment will vary according to the type of carotid hypersensitivity response (e.g., cardioinhibitory, vasodepressor, or mixed) and symptoms present (see "Chronic Rx"). Acute treatment is usually not needed, because most patients at presentation are hemodynamically stable but present with either a fall resulting in an injury (e.g., hip fracture, laceration) or a complaint of true syncope with no injury.

■ CHRONIC Rx
For asymptomatic carotid sinus hypersensitivity of either the cardioinhibitory or vasodepressor type, it is generally agreed that pacemaker implantation is not necessary.
For patients with CSS with a cardioinhibitory response to CSM:
• Dual-chamber permanent pacemaker is indicated.

• Controversy exists as to whether to implant the pacemaker after the first syncopal episode or after a recurrent episode.
For patients with CSS with a vasodepressor response to CSM:
• Measures to maintain systolic blood pressure are tried:
1. Sympathomimetics (ephedrine has been tried with success but has significant side effects, e.g., palpitations, tremors.)
2. Fludrocortisone with its mineralocorticoid effect also has been tried with limited success.
3. Dual-chamber pacemaker is *not* indicated in the patient with pure vasodepressor response.
4. Elastic knee-high or thigh-high stockings help to maintain systolic blood pressure.
5. Carotid sinus denervation is reserved for those patients refractory to the above mentioned treatment.
For patients with CSS with a mixed response to CSM:
• Dual-chamber permanent pacemaker and atropine can effectively treat the bradycardic response but have no major effect on the hypotensive response. The vasodepressor response should be treated as mentioned above.

■ DISPOSITION
CSS occurs in the elderly population and presents with falls or syncope often resulting in injury. Up to 50% of the patients who present with symptoms will have recurrent symptoms. This is reduced in the group of patients for whom a pacemaker is indicated. There is no difference in survival in this group of patients when compared with the general population.

■ REFERRAL
Cardiology referral is indicated if a pacemaker is considered.

PEARLS & CONSIDERATIONS

■ COMMENTS
The most common type of response to CSM in this population is cardioinhibitory response followed by mixed and vasodepressor responses.

REFERENCE
Fachinetti P et al: Carotid sinus syndrome: a review of the literature and our experience using carotid sinus denervation, *J Neurosurg Sci* 42(4):189, 1998.
Author: **Peter Petropoulos, M.D.**

BASIC INFORMATION

■ DEFINITION
Carpal tunnel syndrome is an entrapment neuropathy involving the median nerve at the wrist (Fig. 1-82). It is the most common entrapment neuropathy in the upper extremity.

ICD-9CM CODES
354.0 Carpal tunnel syndrome

■ EPIDEMIOLOGY & DEMOGRAPHICS
PREVALENT AGE: 30 to 60 yr (bilateral up to 50%)
PREVALENT SEX: Females are affected two to five times as often as males

■ PHYSICAL FINDINGS & CLINICAL PRESENTATION
- Nocturnal pain
- Occasional median nerve sensory impairment (often only index and long fingers)
- Positive Tinel's sign at wrist (tapping over the median nerve on the flexor surface of the wrist produces a tingling sensation radiating from the wrist to the hand)
- Positive Phalen's test (reproduction of symptoms after 1 min of gentle, unforced wrist flexion)
- Carpal compression test: Pressure with the examiner's thumb over the patient's carpal tunnel for 30 sec elicits symptoms
- Thenar atrophy in long-standing cases

■ ETIOLOGY
- Idiopathic in most cases
- Space-occupying lesions in carpal tunnel (tenosynovitis, ganglia, aberrant muscles)
- Often associated with hypothyroidism, hormonal changes of pregnancy
- Job-related mechanical overuse may be a risk factor
- Traumatic injuries to wrist

DIAGNOSIS

■ DIFFERENTIAL DIAGNOSIS
- Cervical radiculopathy
- Chronic tendinitis
- Vascular occlusion
- Reflex sympathetic dystrophy
- Osteoarthritis
- Other arthritides
- Other entrapment neuropathies

■ IMAGING STUDIES
Routine roentgenograms may be helpful in establishing cause or ruling out other conditions.

■ ELECTRODIAGNOSTIC STUDIES
Nerve conduction velocity tests and electromyography are useful in establishing the diagnosis and ruling out other syndromes.

TREATMENT

■ ACUTE GENERAL Rx
- Elimination of repetitive trauma
- Occupational splints or braces
- NSAIDs
- Injection of carpal canal (avoiding median nerve)
- Low-dose oral corticosteroids (e.g., prednisolone 20 mg qd for 2 wk, followed by 10 mg qd for 2 more wk) are also effective for symptom relief in selected patients.

■ DISPOSITION
Prognosis is variable. Some cases resolve spontaneously. Relief from local injection appears transient and symptoms recur in the majority of cases following injection.
Carpal tunnel syndrome is common in the third trimester of pregnancy, but symptoms subside after delivery in most cases, often dramatically. Symptoms may recur with subsequent pregnancies. Surgery is not recommended in pregnant patients because of the likelihood of spontaneous recovery.

■ REFERRAL
Surgical referral in cases of failed medical management

REFERENCES
Bagatur AE, Zorer G: The carpal tunnel syndrome is a bilateral disorder, *J Bone Joint Surg Br* 83(5):655, 2001.
Chang MH et al: Oral drug of choice in carpal tunnel syndrome, *Neurology* 51:390, 1998.
Dammers JW et al: Injection with methylprednisolone proximal to the carpal tunnel: randomized double blind trial, *BMJ* 319:884, 1999.
D'Arcy C, McGee S: Does this patient have carpal tunnel syndrome? *JAMA* 283:3110, 2000.
Gonzalez MH, Bylak J: Steroid injection and splinting in the treatment of carpal tunnel syndrome, *Orthopedics* 24:479, 2001.
Nagle DJ: Evaluation of chronic wrist pain, *J Am Acad Orthop Surg* 8:45, 2000.
Robinson LR: Role of neurophysiologic evaluation in diagnoses, *J Am Acad Orthop Surg* 8:190, 2000.
Wong SM et al: Local vs. systemic caricosteroids in the treatment of carpal tunnel syndrome, *Neurology* 56:1565, 2001.
Author: **Lonnie R. Mercier, M.D.**

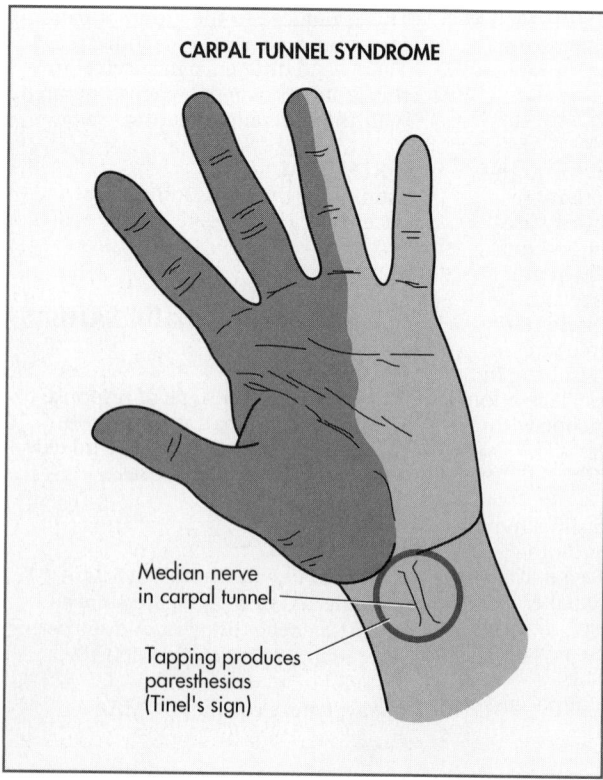

CARPAL TUNNEL SYNDROME

Median nerve in carpal tunnel

Tapping produces paresthesias (Tinel's sign)

Fig. 1-82 Distribution of pain and/or paresthesias *(dark-shaded area)* when the median nerve is compressed by swelling in the wrist (carpal tunnel). (From Arnett FC: Rheumatoid arthritis. In Andreoli TE [ed]: *Cecil essentials of medicine,* ed 4, Philadelphia, 1997, WB Saunders.)

BASIC INFORMATION

■ DEFINITION
Cataracts are the clouding and opacification of the crystalline lens of the eye. The opacity may occur in the cortex, the nucleus of the lens, or the posterior subcapsular region, but it is usually in a combination of areas.

■ SYNONYMS
Congenital cataracts (e.g., from rubella)
Metabolic cataracts (e.g., caused by diabetes)
Collagen-vascular disease cataracts (caused by lupus)
Hereditary cataracts
Age-related senile cataracts
Traumatic cataracts
Toxic or drug-induced cataracts (e.g., caused by steroids)

ICD-9CM CODES
366 Cataract

■ EPIDEMIOLOGY & DEMOGRAPHICS
INCIDENCE (IN U.S.): Highest cause of treatable blindness; cataract removal most frequent surgical procedure in patients >65 yr old (1.3 million operations/yr, with an annual cost of approximately $3 billion).
PREDOMINANT AGE: Elderly; some stage of cataract development is present in >50% of persons 65 to 74 yr old and 65% of those >75 yr old.
PEAK INCIDENCE:
• In early life: congenital and hereditary causes predominant
• In older age group: senile cataracts (after 40 yr of age)

GENETICS: Hereditary with such syndromes as galactosemia, homocystinuria, diabetes

■ PHYSICAL FINDINGS & CLINICAL PRESENTATION
Cloudiness and opacification of the crystalline lens of the eye (Fig. 1-83)

■ ETIOLOGY
• Heredity
• Trauma
• Toxins
• Age-related
• Drug-related
• Congenital
• Inflammatory

 # DIAGNOSIS

■ DIFFERENTIAL DIAGNOSIS
• Corneal lesions
• Retinal lesions

■ WORKUP
Complete eye examination, including slit lamp examination, funduscopic examination, and brightness acuity testing

■ LABORATORY TESTS
• Rarely, urinary amino acid screening and CNS imaging studies with congenital cataracts
• Fasting glucose in young adults with cataracts

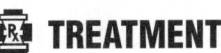 # TREATMENT

■ NONPHARMACOLOGIC THERAPY
• Wait until vision is compromised before doing surgery.
• Surgery is indicated when corrected visual acuity in the affected eye is >20/30 in the absence of other ocular disease; however, surgery may be justified when visual acuity is better in specific situations (especially disabling glare, monocular diplopia).

■ ACUTE GENERAL Rx
None necessary

■ CHRONIC Rx
• Change glasses as cataracts develop.
• Myopia is common, and glasses can be adjusted until surgery is contemplated.

■ DISPOSITION
Refer if sight compromised.

■ REFERRAL
Refer to ophthalmologist for extraction when vision is compromised (see "Nonpharmacologic Therapy").

☼ PEARLS & CONSIDERATIONS

■ COMMENTS
Success rate with surgery is 95% to 98%.
Author: **Melvyn Koby, M.D.**

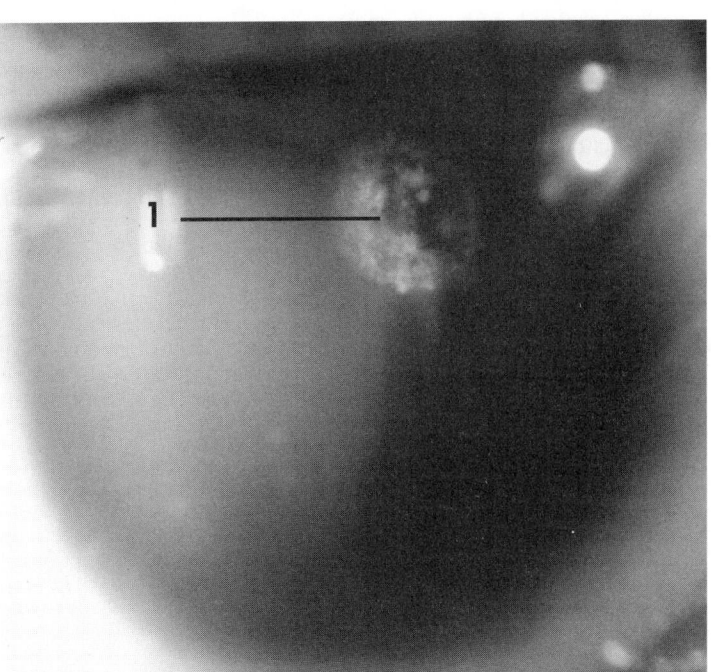

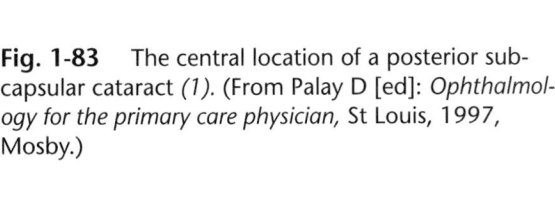
Fig. 1-83   The central location of a posterior subcapsular cataract *(1)*. (From Palay D [ed]: *Ophthalmology for the primary care physician,* St Louis, 1997, Mosby.)

BASIC INFORMATION

■ DEFINITION
Cat-scratch disease (CSD) is a syndrome consisting of gradually enlarging regional lymphadenopathy occurring after contact with a feline. Atypical presentations are characterized by a variety of neurologic manifestations as well as granulomatous involvement of the eye, liver, spleen, and bone. The disease is usually self-limiting, and recovery is complete; however, patients with atypical presentations, especially if immunocompromised, may suffer significant morbidity and mortality.

■ SYNONYMS
Cat-scratch fever
Benign inoculation lymphoreticulosis
Nonbacterial regional lymphadenitis

ICD-9CM CODES
078.3 Cat-scratch disease

■ EPIDEMIOLOGY & DEMOGRAPHICS
PREVALENCE: Unknown
INCIDENCE (IN U.S.):
- Unknown
- Majority of reported cases in children

PEAK INCIDENCE: August through January
GENETICS: Unknown

■ PHYSICAL FINDINGS & CLINICAL PRESENTATION
- Classic, most common finding: regional lymphadenopathy occurring within 2 wk of a scratch or contact with felines
- Tender, swollen lymph nodes most commonly found in the head and neck, followed by the axilla and the epitrochlear, inguinal, and femoral areas
- Erythematous overlying skin, showing signs of suppuration from involved lymph nodes
- On careful examination; evidence of cutaneous inoculation in the form of a nonpruritic, slightly tender pustule or papule (Fig. 1-84)
- Fever in most patients
- Malaise and headache in fewer than a third of patients

- Atypical presentations in fewer than 15% of cases
  1. Usually in association with lymphadenopathy and a low-grade or frank fever (>101° F, >38.3° C)
  2. Include granulomatous involvement of the conjunctiva (Parinaud's oculoglandular syndrome) and focal masses in the liver, spleen, and mesenteric nodes
- CNS involvement: neuroretinitis, encephalopathy, encephalitis, transverse myelitis, seizure activity, and coma
- Possible osteomyelitis in children

■ ETIOLOGY
- Major cause: *Bartonella (Rochalimaea) henselae*
- Mode of transmission: predominantly by direct inoculation through the scratch, bite, or lick of a cat, especially a kitten
- Limited evidence in support of an arthropod (flea) as an alternative vector of infection arising from bacteremic felines.
- Rarely, associated with dogs, monkeys, and inanimate objects with which a feline has been in recent contact
- Approximately 2 wk after introduction of the bacteria into the host, regional lymphatic tissues displaying granulomatous infiltration associated with gradual hypertrophy
- Possible dissemination to distant sites (e.g., liver, spleen, and bone), usually characterized by focal masses or discrete parenchymal lesions

🔬 DIAGNOSIS

■ DIFFERENTIAL DIAGNOSIS
Granulomas of this syndrome must be differentiated from those associated with tularemia, tuberculosis, sarcoidosis, sporotrichosis, toxoplasmosis, lymphogranuloma venerum, fungal diseases, and benign and malignant tumors.

■ WORKUP
Diagnosis should be considered in patients who present with a predominant complaint of gradually enlarging regional (focal) lymphadenopathy, often with fever and a recent history of having contact with a cat.

■ LABORATORY TESTS
- Three of four of the following criteria are required:
  1. History of animal contact in the presence of a scratch, dermal, or eye lesion
  2. Culture of lymphatic aspirate that is negative for other causes
  3. Positive CSD skin test
  4. Biopsied lymph node histology consistent with CSD
- Enhanced culture techniques and serologies will augment establishment of the diagnosis.
- Histopathologically, Warthin-Starry silver stain has been used to identify the bacillus.
- Routine laboratory findings:
  1. Mild leukocytosis or leukopenia
  2. Infrequent eosinophilia
  3. Elevated ESR
- Abnormalities of bilirubin excretion and elevated hepatic transaminases are usually secondary to hepatic obstruction by granuloma, mass, or lymph node
- In patients with neurologic manifestations, lumbar puncture usually reveals normal CSF, although there may be a mild pleocytosis and modest elevation in protein.

💊 TREATMENT

■ NONPHARMACOLOGIC THERAPY
- Warm compresses to the affected nodes
- In cases of encephalitis or coma: supportive care

■ ACUTE GENERAL Rx
- There is no consensus over therapy, especially as the disease is self-limited in a majority of cases.
- It would be prudent to treat severely ill patients, especially if immunocompromised, with antibiotic therapy, because these patients tend to suffer dissemination of infection and increased morbidity.
- *Bartonella* is usually sensitive to aminoglycosides, tetracycline, erythromycin, and the quinolones.
- When the isolate is proven by culture, the patient should receive antibiotic therapy as directed by the obtained sensitivities.

- Antipyretics and NSAIDs may also be used.

■ DISPOSITION
Overall prognosis is good.

■ REFERRAL
- To an appropriate subspecialist to evaluate specific lesions
- For diagnostic aspiration or excision in presence of regional lymph-adenopathy, bone lesions, and mesenteric lymph nodes and organs
- To ophthalmologist for ocular granulomas
  1. Usually diagnosed clinically
  2. Rarely require excision

✹ PEARLS & CONSIDERATIONS

■ COMMENTS
- A typical presentation of this syndrome may be as fever of unknown origin.

- Hepatic and splenic granulomas, coronary valve infections may offer few physical clues to diagnosis, emphasizing the need for a complete history.
- CSD should be considered in the differential diagnosis of school-aged children presenting with status epilepticus.
- Chronically immunocompromised patients considering the acquisition of a young feline should be made aware of the possible risk of infection.
- No signs of illness may be apparent in bacteremic kittens.

REFERENCES
De La Rosa GR: Native valve endocarditis due to *Bartonella henselae* in a middle-aged human immunodeficiency virus-negative woman, *J Clin Microbiol* 39(9):3417, 2001.

Eskow E et al: Concurrent infection of the central nervous system by *Borrelia burgdorferi* and *Bartonella henselae:* evidence for a novel tick-borne disease complex, *Arch Neurol* 58(9):1357, 2001.
Fournier PE: Epidemiologic and clinical characteristics of *Bartonella quintana* and *Bartonella henselae* endocarditis: a study of 48 patients, *Medicine* 80(4):245, 2001.
Goldstein DA et al: Acute endogenous endophthalmitis due to *Bartonella henselae, Clin Infect Dis* 33(5):718, 2001.
Labalette P et al: Cat-scratch disease neuroretinitis diagnosed by a polymerase chain reaction approach, *Am J Ophthalmol* 132(4):575, 2001.
Modi SP et al: Cat-scratch disease presenting as multifocal osteomyelitis with thoracic abscess, *Pediatr Infect Dis J* 20(10):1006, 2001.
Murano I et al: Giant hepatic granuloma caused by *Bartonella henselae, Pediatr Infect Dis J* 20(3):319, 2001.
Author: **George O. Alonso, M.D.**

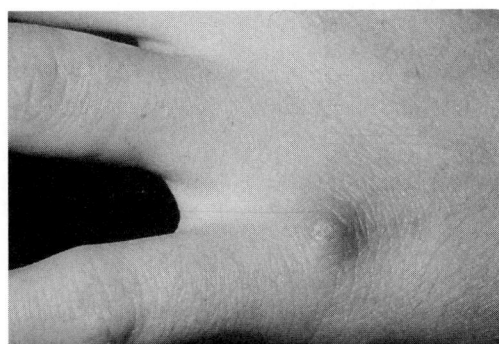

Fig. 1-84   Primary lesion of cat-scratch disease is a tender papule occurring 3 to 10 days after a scratch. (From Noble J [ed]: *Primary care medicine,* ed 2, St Louis, 1996, Mosby.)

BASIC INFORMATION

■ DEFINITION

Cavernous sinus thrombosis is an uncommon diagnosis usually stemming from infections of the face or paranasal sinuses resulting in thrombosis of the cavernous sinus and inflammation of its surrounding anatomic structures, including cranial nerves III, IV, V (ophthalmic and maxillary branch), and VI, and the internal carotid artery.

■ SYNONYMS

Intracranial venous sinus thrombosis or thrombophlebitis

ICD-9CM CODES

325 Phlebitis and thrombophlebitis of intracranial venous sinus

■ EPIDEMIOLOGY & DEMOGRAPHICS

- Cavernous sinus thrombosis is rare.
- Before antibiotics the mortality rate from cavernous sinus thrombosis was 80% to 100%.
- With antibiotics, the mortality rates range between 20% and 30%.
- Morbidity remains high (between 25% and 50%).

■ PHYSICAL FINDINGS & CLINICAL PRESENTATION

The classic findings include:
- Ptosis
- Proptosis
- Chemosis
- Cranial nerve palsies (III, IV, V, VI)
  1. Sixth nerve palsy is the most common.
  2. Sensory deficits of the ophthalmic and maxillary branch of the fifth nerve are common.

Other findings:
- Decreased visual acuity and blindness may occur.
- Venous engorgement and papilledema on funduscopic examination may be found.
- Fever, tachycardia, sepsis may be present.
- Headache with nuchal rigidity may occur.
- Pupil may be dilated and sluggishly reactive.

■ ETIOLOGY

- *Staphylococcus aureus* is the most common infectious microbe, found in 50% to 60% of the cases.
- *Streptococcus* is the second leading cause.
- Gram-negative rods and anaerobes may also lead to cavernous sinus thrombosis.

- The most common primary site of infection leading to cavernous sinus thrombosis is sphenoid sinusitis; however, other sites of infection, including the middle ear, orbit, eye, eyelid, and face, can result in the same sequelae.

DIAGNOSIS

- The diagnosis of cavernous sinus thrombosis is made clinically.
- Proptosis, ptosis, chemosis, and cranial nerve palsy beginning in one eye and progressing to the other eye establish the diagnosis.

■ DIFFERENTIAL DIAGNOSIS

- Orbital cellulitis
- Internal carotid artery aneurysm
- CVA
- Migraine headache
- Allergic blepharitis
- Thyroid exophthalmos
- Brain tumor
- Meningitis
- Mucormycosis
- Trauma

■ WORKUP

Cavernous sinus thrombosis is a clinical diagnosis with laboratory tests and imaging studies confirming the clinical impression.

■ LABORATORY TESTS

- CBC, ESR, blood cultures, and sinus cultures help establish and identify an infectious primary source.
- Lumbar puncture is necessary to rule out meningitis.

■ IMAGING STUDIES

- Sinus films are helpful in the diagnosis of sphenoid sinusitis. Opacification, sclerosis, and air-fluid levels are typical findings.
- CT scan is the best study to diagnose sphenoid sinusitis; however, CT scan is not very sensitive in diagnosing cavernous sinus thrombosis.
- MRI is the imaging study of choice to diagnose cavernous sinus thrombosis.
- Cerebral angiography can be performed, but it is invasive and not very sensitive.
- Orbital venography is difficult to perform, but it is excellent in diagnosing occlusion of the cavernous sinus.

TREATMENT

■ NONPHARMACOLOGIC THERAPY

Recognizing the primary source of infection (e.g., facial cellulitis, middle ear, and sinus infections) and treating the primary source expeditiously is the best way to prevent cavernous sinus thrombosis.

■ ACUTE GENERAL Rx

- Broad-spectrum intravenous antibiotics are used until a definite pathogen is found.
  1. Nafcillin 1.5 g IV q4h
  2. Cefotaxime 1.5 to 2 g IV q4h
  3. Metronidazole 15 mg/kg load followed by 7.5 mg/kg IV q6h
- Anticoagulation with heparin is controversial. Retrospective studies show conflicting data. This decision should be made with subspecialty consultation.
- Steroid therapy is also controversial.

■ CHRONIC Rx

Surgical drainage with sphenoidotomy is indicated if the primary site of infection is thought to be the sphenoid sinus.

■ DISPOSITION

Cavernous sinus thrombosis can be a life-threatening, rapidly progressive infectious disease with high morbidity and mortality rates despite antibiotic use.

■ REFERRAL

If the diagnosis is suspected, this should be considered a medical emergency. Depending on the primary site of infection, appropriate consultation should be made (e.g., ENT, ophthalmology, and infectious disease.)

PEARLS & CONSIDERATIONS

■ COMMENTS

Realizing the cavernous sinus lies just above and lateral to the sphenoid sinus and drains the middle portion of the face via the superior and inferior ophthalmic veins and knowing that cranial nerves III, IV, V, and VI pass alongside or through the cavernous sinus make the clinical findings and diagnosis easier to understand.

Author: **Peter Petropoulos, M.D.**

BASIC INFORMATION

DEFINITION
Celiac disease is a chronic disease characterized by malabsorption and diarrhea precipitated by ingestion of food products containing gluten.

SYNONYMS
Gluten enteropathy
Celiac sprue

ICD-9CM CODES
579.0 Celiac disease

EPIDEMIOLOGY & DEMOGRAPHICS
- Estimates of the incidence and prevalence of celiac sprue in the U.S. range from 50 to 500 cases/100,000 persons; it is highest in whites of northern European ancestry (1 in 300).
- Incidence is highest during infancy and the initial 36 mo (secondary to the introduction of foods containing gluten), in the third decade (frequently associated with pregnancy and severe anemia during pregnancy), and in the seventh decade.
- There is a slight female predominance.

PHYSICAL FINDINGS & CLINICAL PRESENTATION
- Physical examination may be entirely within normal limits.
- Weight loss, dyspepsia, short stature, and failure to thrive are noted in children and infants.
- Weight loss, fatigue, and diarrhea are common in adults.
- Abdominal pain, nausea, and vomiting are unusual.
- Pallor as a result of iron deficiency anemia is common.
- Manifestations of calcium deficiency, such as tetany and seizures, are rare and can be exacerbated by coexistent magnesium deficiency.
- Angular cheilitis, aphthous ulcers, atopic dermatitis, and dermatitis herpetiformis are frequently associated with celiac disease.

ETIOLOGY
Sensitivity to gliadin, a protein fraction of gluten found in wheat, rye, barley, and oats

 DIAGNOSIS

DIFFERENTIAL DIAGNOSIS
- IBD
- Laxative abuse
- Intestinal parasitic infestations
- Other: irritable bowel syndrome, tropical sprue, chronic pancreatitis, Zollinger-Ellison syndrome, cystic fibrosis (children), lymphoma, eosinophilic gastroenteritis, short bowel syndrome, Whipple's disease

WORKUP
Initial evaluation consists of laboratory tests followed by radiographic studies and upper GI endoscopy with biopsy of duodenum or proximal jejunum.

LABORATORY TESTS
- Iron deficiency anemia
- Folic acid deficiency
- Vitamin B_{12} deficiency, hypomagnesemia, hypocalcemia
- Antigliadin IgA and IgG antibodies are elevated in >90% of patients; however, they are nonspecific. IgA endomysial antibodies are more specific for celiac sprue and are the best screening test for celiac disease, except in the case of patients with IgA deficiency. Tissue transglutinase autoantibody by ELISA is a newer serologic test for celiac sprue.
- Biopsy of the small bowel reveals absence or shortening of villi, intraepithelial lymphocytes, and crypt lengthening and hyperplasia (Fig. 1-85). Several biopsy specimens should be obtained for proper diagnosis.
- Tests for malabsorption are abnormal: fecal fat estimation for 72 hr is elevated (>7 g/day), D-xylose testing reveals malabsorption of sugar.

IMAGING STUDIES
Small bowel follow-through reveals altered mucosal folds and luminal dilation.

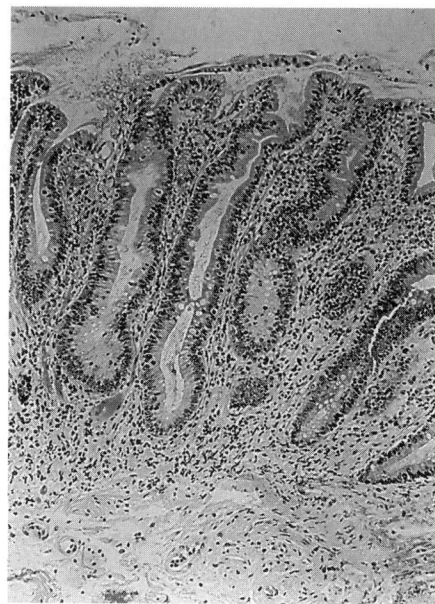

Fig. 1-85 Intestinal biopsy appearance of flattened villi and hyperplastic crypts. (Courtesy Heidron Rotterdam, MD. In Goldman L, Bennett JC [eds]: *Cecil textbook of medicine,* ed 21, Philadelphia, 2000, WB Saunders.)

TREATMENT

NONPHARMACOLOGIC THERAPY
Patients should be instructed on gluten-free diet (avoidance of wheat, rye, and barley). Recent studies show that oats do not damage the mucosa in celiac disease.

ACUTE GENERAL Rx
- Correct nutritional deficiencies with iron, folic acid, calcium, vitamin B_{12} as needed.
- Prednisone 20 to 60 mg qd gradually tapered is useful in refractory cases.

CHRONIC Rx
- Lifelong gluten-free diet is necessary.
- Repeat small bowel biopsy following treatment generally reveals significant improvement. It is also useful to evaluate for increased risk of small bowel T-cell lymphoma in these patients (10%), especially in untreated patients.

DISPOSITION
- Prognosis is good with adherence to gluten-free diet. Rapid improvement is usually seen within a few days of treatment.
- Serial antigliadin or antiendomysial antibody tests can be used to monitor the patient's adherence to a gluten-free diet.

REFERRAL
GI referral for small bowel biopsy.

PEARLS & CONSIDERATIONS

COMMENTS
- Patient education material can be obtained from the American Celiac Society, 45 Gifford Ave., Jersey City, NJ 07304.
- Celiac disease should be considered in patients with unexplained metabolic bone disease or hypocalcemia, especially because GI symptoms may be absent or mild.
- The prevalence of celiac disease in patients with dyspepsia is twice that of the general population. Screening for celiac disease should be considered in all patients with persistent dyspepsia.

REFERENCES
Bardella M et al: Increased prevalence of celiac disease in patients with dyspepsia, *Arch Intern Med* 160:1489, 2000.
Feighery C: Celiac disease, *BMJ* 319:236, 1999.
Author: **Fred F. Ferri, M.D.**

BASIC INFORMATION

■ DEFINITION
Cellulitis is a superficial inflammatory condition of the skin. It is characterized by erythema, warmth, and tenderness of the area involved.

■ SYNONYMS
Erysipelas (cellulitis generally secondary to group A β-hemolytic streptococci)

ICD-9CM CODES
682.9 Cellulitis

■ EPIDEMIOLOGY & DEMOGRAPHICS
Cellulitis occurs most frequently in diabetics, immunocompromised hosts, and patients with venous and lymphatic compromise.

■ PHYSICAL FINDINGS & CLINICAL PRESENTATION
Variable with the causative organism
- Erysipelas: superficial-spreading, warm, erythematous lesion distinguished by its indurated and elevated margin; lymphatic involvement and vesicle formation are common.
- Staphylococcal cellulitis: area involved is erythematous, hot, and swollen; differentiated from erysipelas by nonelevated, poorly demarcated margin; local tenderness and regional adenopathy are common; up to 85% of cases occur on the legs and feet.
- *H. influenzae* cellulitis: area involved is a blue-red/purple-red color; occurs mainly in children; generally involves the face in children and the neck or upper chest in adults.
- *Vibrio vulnificus:* larger hemorrhagic bullae, cellulitis, lymphadenitis, myositis; often found in critically ill patients in septic shock.

■ ETIOLOGY
- Group A β-hemolytic streptococci (may follow a streptococcal infection of the upper respiratory tract)
- Staphylococcal cellulitis
- *H. influenzae*
- *Vibrio vulnificus:* higher incidence in patients with liver disease (75%) and in immunocompromised hosts (corticosteroid use, diabetes mellitus, leukemia, renal failure)
- *Erysipelothrix rhusiopathiae:* common in people handling poultry, fish, or meat

- *Aeromonas hydrophila:* generally occurring in contaminated open wound in fresh water
- Fungi *(Cryptococcus neoformans):* immunocompromised granulopenic patients
- Gram-negative rods *(Serratia, Enterobacter, Proteus, Pseudomonas):* immunocompromised or granulopenic patients

DIAGNOSIS

■ DIFFERENTIAL DIAGNOSIS
- Necrotizing fasciitis
- DVT
- Peripheral vascular insufficiency
- Paget's disease of the breast
- Thrombophlebitis
- Acute gout
- Psoriasis
- Candida intertrigo
- Pseudogout
- Osteomyelitis

■ WORKUP
Physical examination and laboratory evaluation

■ LABORATORY TESTS
- Gram stain and culture (aerobic and anaerobic)
1. Aspirated material from:
   a. Advancing edge of cellulitis
   b. Any vesicles
2. Swab of any drainage material
3. Punch biopsy (in selected patients)
- Blood cultures
- ALOS titer (in suspected streptococcal disease)

Despite the above measures the cause of cellulitis remains unidentified in most patients.

■ IMAGING STUDIES
CT or MRI in patients with suspected necrotizing fasciitis (deep-seated infection of the subcutaneous tissue that results in the progressive destruction of fascia and fat): patients present with diffuse swelling of an arm or leg followed by the appearance of bullae filled with clear fluid or maroon, violaceous fluid.

TREATMENT

■ NONPHARMACOLOGIC THERAPY
Immobilization and elevation of the involved limb

■ ACUTE GENERAL Rx
Erysipelas
- PO: penicillin V 250 to 500 mg qid
- IM: penicillin G (procaine) 600,000 U bid
- IV: penicillin G (aqueous) 4 to 6 million U/day
NOTE: Use erythromycin, cephalosporins, clindamycin, or vancomycin in patients allergic to penicillin.
Staphylococcus cellulitis
- PO: dicloxacillin 250 to 500 mg qid
- IV: nafcillin, 1 to 2 g q4-6h
- Cephalosporins (cephalothin, cephalexin, cephradine) also provide adequate antistaphylococcal coverage except for MRSA.
- Use vancomycin in patients allergic to penicillin or cephalosporins and in patients with methicillin-resistant *S. aureus* (MRSA)
H. influenzae cellulitis
- PO: amoxicillin, cefaclor, cefixime, or cefuroxime
- IV: cefuroxime or ampicillin; TMP-SMX in patients allergic to penicillin
- Amoxicillin is ineffective in ampicillin-resistant strains (approximately 30%), IV cefuroxime is indicated in severely ill patients.
Vibrio vulnificus
- Aminoglycoside plus tetracycline or chloramphenicol
- IV support and admission into ICU (mortality rate >50% in septic shock)
Erysipelothrix
- Penicillin
Aeromonas hydrophila
- Aminoglycosides
- Chloramphenicol

■ DISPOSITION
Prognosis is good with prompt treatment.

■ REFERRAL
For surgical debridement in addition to antibiotics in patients with suspected necrotizing fasciitis
Author: **Fred F. Ferri, M.D.**

BASIC INFORMATION

■ DEFINITION
Cerebral palsy refers to a group of motor impairment syndromes secondary to lesions or anomalies of the brain that arise in the early stages of in utero development or at birth. The term *cerebral palsy* is archaic; congenital static encephalopathy is preferred and encompasses a wide range of nonprogressive brain abnormalities present at birth.

■ SYNONYMS
Little's disease
Congenital static encephalopathy
Congenital spastic paralysis

■ ICD-9CM CODES
343 Infantile cerebral palsy
343.9 Infantile cerebral palsy, unspecified

■ EPIDEMIOLOGY & DEMOGRAPHICS
INCIDENCE (IN U.S.): 1.5 to 2.5 cases/1000 live births
PREVALENCE (IN U.S.): Close to incidence (0 nonprogressive disease)
PREDOMINANT SEX: Male = female
PREDOMINANT AGE: 3 to 5 yr
PEAK INCIDENCE: At birth

■ PHYSICAL FINDINGS & CLINICAL PRESENTATION
- Mental retardation (30%)
- Seizures (30%)
- Hemiplegia
- Diplegia
- Extrapyramidal findings
- Delay in motor milestones
- Hypotonia

■ ETIOLOGY
Multifactorial: low birth weight, congenital malformations, thyroid or estrogen therapy during pregnancy, low Apgar scores, difficult delivery, prematurity, hyperbilirubinemia

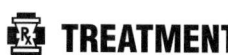

DIAGNOSIS

■ DIFFERENTIAL DIAGNOSIS
Spinal cord abnormalities

■ WORKUP
Follow motor milestones and primitive reflexes

■ LABORATORY TESTS
- Thyroid function
- Urine amino acid screen
- Chromosomal analysis

■ IMAGING STUDIES
CT scan, MRI, and ultrasonography may show periventricular leukomalacia and/or periventricular hemorrhage.

TREATMENT

■ NONPHARMACOLOGIC THERAPY
- Physical therapy
- Special education

■ ACUTE GENERAL Rx
Not applicable unless seizures are present.

■ CHRONIC Rx
- Physical therapy
- Special schooling
- Treatment of seizures, if present

■ DISPOSITION
Have child remain at home if at all possible.

■ REFERRAL
If the child is seriously handicapped, physical medicine and rehabilitation referrals are especially helpful.

PEARLS & CONSIDERATIONS

■ COMMENTS
- Prevention is the most rational approach and involves close monitoring of pregnancy, ultrasound, and the avoidance of all drugs and alcohol.
- Patient education information on cerebral palsy can be obtained from the United Cerebral Palsy Association, 7 Penn Plaza, Suite 804, New York, NY 10001; phone: 1-800-USA-1UCP.
- *Cerebral palsy* is an old-fashioned term; obviously children can have congenital brain damage without motor impairment.

Author: **William H. Olson, M.D.**

BASIC INFORMATION

■ **DEFINITION**
Cerebrovascular accident (CVA) describes acute brain injury caused by decreased blood supply or hemorrhage.

■ **SYNONYMS**
Stroke
CVA

■ **ICD-9CM CODES**
436 Acute stroke

■ **EPIDEMIOLOGY & DEMOGRAPHICS**
INCIDENCE (IN U.S.):
• Occurs in 5 to 10/100,000 persons <40 yr of age
• Occurs in 10 to 20/100,000 persons >65 yr of age
PREVALENCE (IN U.S.): Estimated at 2 million persons
PREDOMINANT SEX: Incidence is 30% higher in males
PREDOMINANT AGE: 60+ yr
PEAK INCIDENCE: 80 to 84 yr
GENETICS: Family history a risk factor, but no distinct genetic etiology has been identified.

■ **PHYSICAL FINDINGS & CLINICAL PRESENTATION**
Motor and/or sensory and/or cognitive deficits, depending on distribution and extent of involved vascular territory.

■ **ETIOLOGY**
• From 70% to 80% are caused by ischemic infarcts; 20% to 30% are hemorrhagic.
• 80% of ischemic infarcts are from occlusion of large vessels caused by atherosclerotic vascular disease, 15% are caused by cardiac embolism, 5% are from other causes, including hypercoagulable states and vasculitis.
• Small vessel occlusion is most often caused by lipohyalinosis along with chronic hypertension.

• Risk factors for ischemic stroke are described in Box 1-11.

 DIAGNOSIS

■ **DIFFERENTIAL DIAGNOSIS**
• TIA
• Migraine
• Seizure
• Mass lesion

■ **WORKUP**
• Thorough history and physical examination, including detailed neurologic and cardiovascular evaluation to identify vascular territory and likely etiology (Fig. 1-87 and Table 1-20)
• Mandatory ECG
• Echocardiography, Holter monitor, or carotid Doppler should be seriously considered

■ **LABORATORY TESTS**
• CBC
• Platelet count
• PT (INR)
• PTT
• BUN, creatinine
• Lipid panel
• Glucose
• Electrolytes
• Urinalysis
• Additional tests, depending on suspected etiology (in younger patients; e.g., coagulopathies)

■ **IMAGING STUDIES**
• CT scan without contrast to identify hemorrhage or infarct (Figs. 1-86 and 1-88).
• An MRI identifies abnormalities in the posterior fossa and, in particular, lacunar infarcts. A flair image sequeue is mandatory in acute stage (less than 6 hr).
• Possibly MRA or x-ray angiography to identify aneurysms or other vascular malformations.

■ **TREATMENT**

■ **NONPHARMACOLOGIC THERAPY**
• Above the knee elastic stockings to prevent venous stairs
• Carotid endarterectomy in suitable patients with carotid territory stroke associated with 70% to 99% ipsilateral carotid stenosis, performed by an experienced surgeon with low morbidity and mortality
• Modification of risk factors

■ **ACUTE GENERAL Rx**
• Box 1-12 describes initial considerations for patients with stroke.
• Judicious control of blood pressure; patients with chronic hypertension may extend the area of infarction if the blood pressure is lowered into the "normal" range.
• If patient presents <3 hr after onset of a nonhemorrhagic stroke, thrombolytic therapy in a specialized stroke center may be beneficial.

■ **ACUTE SPECIFIC Rx**
• If a lacunar infarct is demonstrated by MRI and this coincides with physical findings, no further therapy is necessary other than control of hypertension and rehabilitation. This is the most common scenario.

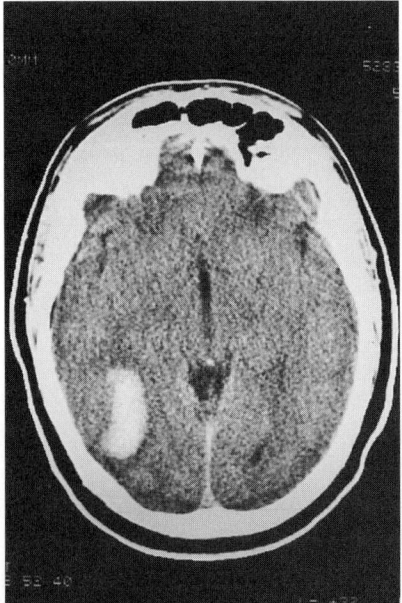

Fig. 1-86 Intracerebral hemorrhage. Noncontrast CT scan demonstrates an intracerebral hemorrhage in the right occipital lobe. (From Specht N [ed]: *Practical guide to diagnostic imaging,* St Louis, 1998, Mosby.)

BOX 1-11 Risk Factors for Ischemic Stroke

Diabetes
Hypertension
Smoking
Family history of premature vascular disease
Hyperlipidemia
Atrial fibrillation
History of transient ischemic attack (TIA)
History of recent myocardial infarction
History of congestive heart failure (left ventricular [LV] ejection fraction <25%)
Drugs (sympathomimetics, oral contraceptive pill, cocaine)

From Andreoli TE (ed): *Cecil essentials of medicine,* ed 5, Philadelphia, 2001, WB Saunders.

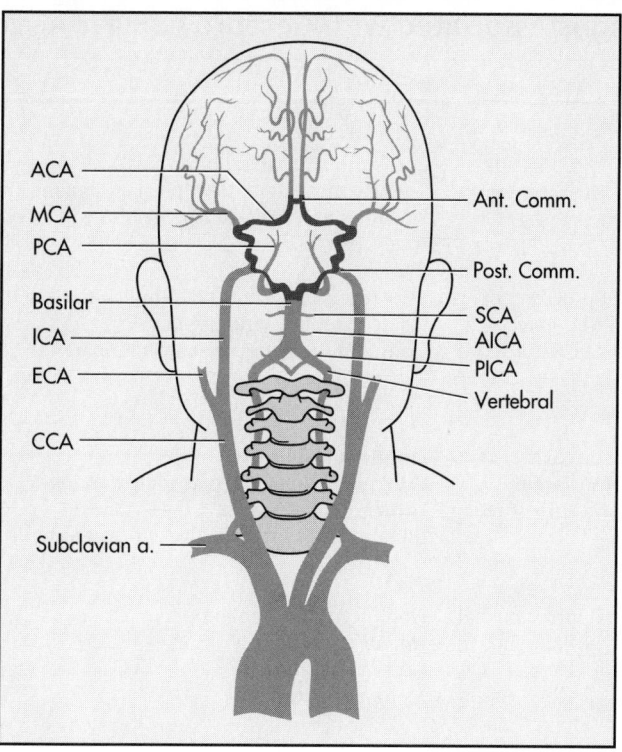

Fig. 1-87   Coronal view of the extracranial and intracranial arterial supply to brain. Vessels forming the circle of Willis are highlighted. *ACA,* Anterior cerebral artery; *AICA,* anterior inferior cerebellar artery; *Ant. Comm.,* anterior communicating artery; *CCA,* common carotid artery; *ECA,* external carotid artery; *ICA,* internal carotid artery; *MCA,* middle cerebral artery; *PCA,* posterior cerebral artery; *PICA,* posterior inferior cerebellar artery; *Post. Comm.,* posterior communicating artery; *SCA,* superior cerebellar artery. (From Andreoli TE [ed]: *Cecil essentials of medicine,* ed 5, Philadelphia, 2001, WB Saunders.)

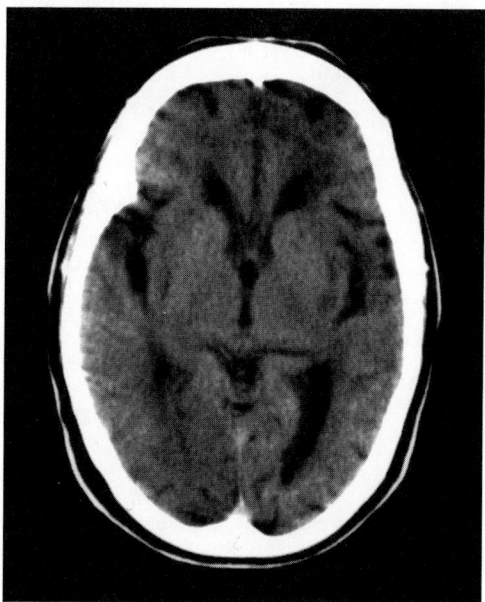

Fig. 1-88   Occipital lobe infarct (posterior cerebral artery territory). Note the large right occipital hypodensity with mass effect caused by infarction and subsequent edema. (From Cwinn AA, Grahovac SZ [eds]: *Emergency CT scans of the head: a practical atlas,* St Louis, 1998, Mosby.)

TABLE 1-20   Neurologic Signs Associated with Cerebrovascular Accident by Location

ARTERY AFFECTED	NEUROLOGIC SIGNS
Internal Carotid Artery	
(Supplies the cerebral hemispheres and diencephalon by the ophthalmic and ipsilateral hemisphere arteries)	Occasional unilateral blindness Severe contralateral hemiplegia, hemianesthesia, and hemianopia Profound aphasia if left hemisphere involved
Middle Cerebral Artery	
(Supplies structures of higher cerebral processes of communication; language interpretation; perception and interpretation of space, sensation, form, and voluntary movement)	Alterations in communication, cognition, mobility, and sensation Homonymous hemianopia Contralateral hemiplegia or hemiparesis
Anterior Cerebral Artery	
(Supplies medial surfaces and upper convexities of frontal and parietal lobes and medial surface of hemisphere, which includes motor and somesthetic cortex serving the legs)	Emotional lability Confusion, amnesia, personality changes Urinary incontinence Impaired mobility, with weakness greater in lower extremities than in upper
Posterior Cerebral Artery	
(Supplies medial and inferior temporal lobes, medial occipital lobe, thalamus, posterior hypothalamus, and visual receptive area)	Homonymous hemianopia Hemianesthesia Cortical blindness Memory deficits
Vertebral or Basilar Arteries	
(Supply the brainstem and cerebellum) Incomplete occlusion	Drop attacks Unilateral and bilateral weakness of extremities Diplopia, homonymous hemianopia Nausea, vertigo, tinnitus, and syncope Dysphagia Dysarthria Sometimes confusion and drowsiness
Anterior portion of pons	"Locked-in" syndrome—no movement except eyelids; sensation and consciousness preserved
Complete occlusion or hemorrhage	Coma Miotic pupils Decerebrate rigidity Respiratory and circulatory abnormalities Death
Posterior Inferior Cerebellar Artery	
(Supplies the lateral and posterior portion of the medulla)	Wallenberg syndrome Dysphagia, dysphonia Ipsilateral anesthesia of face and cornea for pain and temperature (touch preserved) Ipsilateral Horner syndrome Contralateral loss of pain and temperature sensation in trunk and extremities Ipsilateral decompensation of movement (cerebellar signs)
Anterior Inferior and Superior Cerebellar Arteries	
(Supply the cerebellum)	Difficulty in articulation, swallowing, gross movements of limbs; nystagmus (cerebellar signs)
Anterior Spinal Artery	
(Supplies the anterior spinal cord)	Flaccid paralysis, below level of lesion Loss of pain, touch, temperature sensation (proprioception preserved, sensory level)
Posterior Spinal Artery	
(Supplies the posterior spinal cord)	Sensory loss, particularly proprioception, vibration, touch, and pressure (movement preserved)

Adapted from Seidel HM (ed): *Mosby's guide to physical examination,* ed 4, St Louis, 1999, Mosby.

BOX 1-12   Initial Considerations for Patients with Strokes

Initial care
  Stabilize the patient, secure the airway, and provide adequate oxygenation
  Assess level of consciousness, language, visual fields, eye movements, and pupillary movements
  Obtain history and perform physical examination
  Perform CT of head without contrast
  Obtain CBC with platelets and differential, electrolytes, creatinine, BUN, glucose, PT/PTT, arterial blood gas, or oxygen
    saturation
  Consider a toxicology screen
  Consider special coagulation studies such as antiphospholipid antibodies, factor V Leiden assay, protein C and protein
    S, antithrombin III, ANA, fibrinogen, RPR, homocysteine, serum protein electrophoresis
Consider acute intervention with t-PA if symptoms for less than 3 hr
Consider the following with admission orders
  Transthoracic echocardiogram (consider transesophageal echocardiogram if transthoracic echocardiogram is equivocal
    or there is a high suspicion of cardiogenic thromboembolism)
  Carotid duplex ultrasonography
  Telemetry
  Supplemental oxygen and appropriate oxygen saturation monitoring
  Antiplatelet therapy
  Fluid restriction if infarct is large, to reduce cerebral edema
  Close monitoring of intake and output
  Regular determinations of blood glucose levels to avoid hyperglycemia
  NPO if there are concerns about the pharyngeal reflex pending swallowing evaluation
  Elevate the head of the bed 20-30 degrees to reduce cerebral edema
  Bed rest for the first 24 hr with fall precautions, then advance as appropriate
  Vital signs and neurologic checks every 2 hr times four until stable
  Prophylaxis for DVT if immobile (elastic stockings at a minimum)
  Speech therapy consultation to evaluate swallowing
  Neurology, physical therapy, occupational therapy, nutrition, and social services consultations

From Rakel RE (ed): *Principles of family practice,* ed 6, Philadelphia, 2002, WB Saunders.
ANA, Antinuclear antibodies; *BUN,* blood urea nitrogen; *CBC,* complete blood count; *CT,* computed tomography; *DVT,* deep vein thrombosis; *NPO,* nothing by mouth; *PT/PTT,* prothrombin time/partial thromboplastin time; *RPR,* rapid plasma reagin; *t-PA,* tissue plasminogen activator.

BOX 1-13   Criteria for Tissue Plasminogen Activator (alteplase [Activase]) Use in Patients with Thromboembolic Stroke

Criteria for considering t-PA as a treatment option
  Age ≥18 yr
  Noncontrast CT without evidence of hemorrhage
  Time since onset of symptoms clearly <3 hr before t-PA administration would begin
Criteria for excluding t-PA as a treatment option
Historical and clinical findings
  Clinical presentation suggests subarachnoid hemorrhage, even if CT is normal
    Sudden, severe headache, often with loss of consciousness at onset
    Vomiting common
  Active internal bleeding, increased risk of bleeding, or known bleeding diathesis, including:
    Recent use of warfarin with a prolonged international normalized ratio (INR)—some would add current use of war-
      farin regardless of INR
    Use of heparin within 48 hr with a prolonged aPTT
    Platelet count <100,000/mm^3
    History of intracranial hemorrhage
    Known arteriovenous malformation or aneurysm
    GI or GU bleeding within the past 21 days
    Arterial puncture within the past 7 days
  Recent lumbar puncture
  Stroke, intracranial surgery, or head trauma within the previous 3 mo
  Major surgery or serious trauma within the preceding 14 days
  Persistent systolic blood pressure >185 mm Hg or diastolic blood pressure >110 mm Hg
  Seizure at stroke onset
  Rapidly improving neurologic signs
  Isolated, mild neurologic deficits
  Acute myocardial infarction
  Post–myocardial infarction pericarditis
  Blood glucose <50 mg/dl or >400 mg/dl
  Patient pregnant or lactating
CT findings
  Evidence of intracranial hemorrhage
  Hypodensity or effacement of the sulci in $\frac{1}{3}$ of the territory of the middle cerebral artery

From Rakel RE (ed): *Principles of family practice,* ed 6, Philadelphia, 2002, WB Saunders.
aPTT, Activated partial thromboplastin time; *CT,* computed tomography; *GI,* gastrointestinal; *GU,* genitourinary; *t-PA,* tissue plasminogen activator.

- If on *diffusion weighted MRI* a fresh infarct is demonstrated and if onset of symptoms is less than 3 to 4 hrs, including evaluation, rt PA is indicated. This is a relatively rare situation, even in large centers with stroke teams. Box 1-13 describes criteria for thrombolytic therapy in patients with thromboembolic stroke.
- If patient is in atrial fibrillation and/or a cardiac mural thrombus is found on echocardiography, heparin followed by warfarin is indicated.
- If a subarachnoid or intracerebral hemorrhage is found on CT, cerebral angiography is indicated to identify aneurysm. If no aneurysm is found and clot is expanding, neurosurgical evaluation of clot may be attempted, but outcomes are generally poor.
- If an *interventional* neuroradiologist is available, and if onset of symptoms is less than 6 hr, direct injection of the clot with a clot-busting agent can have an excellent outcome.

■ **CHRONIC Rx**
- Antiplatelet therapy (aspirin, clopidogrel [Plavix], or ticlopidine) reduces the risk of subsequent stroke.
- Aspirin alone is used first, and another agent is added if TIAs continue. Coumadin is usually reserved for patients with cardioembolic stroke.

■ **DISPOSITION**
1-yr mortality: 28% to 40%

■ **REFERRAL**
- The primary care physician should seriously consider referring all nonlacunar stroke patients to a stroke center on an emergency basis.
- If uncertain about diagnosis, etiology, or management.
- For intracerebral hemorrhage (possible neurosurgical intervention).

REFERENCES
American Heart Association Scientific Statement: Primary prevention of ischemic stroke: a statement for health care professionals from the stroke council of the American Heart Association, *Circulation* 103:167, 2001.

Benevante D, Hart RG: Stroke: management of acute ischemic stroke, *Am Fam Physician* 59:2828, 1999.

Caplan LR: Stroke treatment: promising but still struggling, *JAMA* 279:1304, 1998.

Qureshi A et al: Spontaneous intracranial hemorrhage, *N Engl J Med* 344:1450, 2001.

Sacco RL et al: High-density lipoprotein cholesterol and ischemic stroke in the elderly, *JAMA* 285:2729, 2001.

Author: **Michael Gruenthal**, M.D., Ph.D.

BASIC INFORMATION

■ DEFINITION
Cervical cancer is penetration of the basement membrane and infiltration of the stroma of the uterine cervix by malignant cells.

ICD-9CM CODES
180 Malignant neoplasm of cervix uteri

■ EPIDEMIOLOGY & DEMOGRAPHICS
INCIDENCE: There are approximately 15,000 new cases annually, with 4000 to 5000 associated deaths. The U.S. has an age-adjusted mortality of 2.6 cases/100,000 persons for cervical cancer.
PREDOMINANCE: Higher incidence rates occur in developing countries. Among the U.S. population, Hispanics have a higher incidence than African-Americans, who likewise have a higher incidence than whites.
RISK FACTORS: Smoking, early age at first intercourse, multiple sexual partners, immunocompromised state, non-barrier methods of birth control, infection with high-risk HPV (types 16 and 18), multiparity.

■ PHYSICAL FINDINGS & CLINICAL PRESENTATION
• Unusual vaginal bleeding, particularly postcoital
• Vaginal discharge and/or odor
• Advanced cases may present with lower extremity edema or renal failure
• In early stages there may be little or no obvious cervical lesion, more advanced cases may present with large, bulky, friable lesions encompassing the majority of the vagina (Fig. 1-89)
• **ETIOLOGY**
• Dysplastic cells progress to invasive carcinoma.
• Thought to be linked to the presence of HPV types 16, 18, 45, and 56 via interaction of E6 oncoproteins on p53 gene product.
• There may be an association between past infection with *Chlamydia trachomatis.*

DIAGNOSIS

■ DIFFERENTIAL DIAGNOSIS
• Cervical polyp or prolapsed uterine fibroid
• Preinvasive cervical lesions
• Neoplasia metastatic from a separate primary

■ WORKUP
• Thorough history and physical examination
• Pelvic examination with careful rectovaginal examination
• Colposcopy with directed biopsy and endocervical curettage

■ LABORATORY TESTS
• CBC, chemistry profile
• Squamous cell carcinoma (SCC) antigen in research setting
• Carcinoembryonic antigen (CEA)

■ IMAGING STUDIES
• Chest x-ray examination
• IVP
• Depending on stage, may need cystoscopy, sigmoidoscopy or BE, CT scan or MRI, lymphangiography

TREATMENT

■ NONPHARMACOLOGIC THERAPY
• FIGO stage Ia: cone biopsy or simple hysterectomy
• FIGO stage Ib or IIa: type III radical hysterectomy and pelvic lymphadenectomy *or* pelvic radiation therapy
• Advanced or bulky disease: multimodality therapy (radiation, chemotherapy, and/or surgery)

■ ACUTE GENERAL Rx
Cervical cancer may present with massive and acute vaginal bleeding requiring volume and blood replacement, vaginal packing or other hemostatic modalities, and/or high-dose local radiotherapy.

■ CHRONIC Rx
• Physical examination with Pap smear every 3 mo for 2 yr, every 6 mo during the third to fifth year, and annually thereafter
• Chest x-ray examination annually

■ DISPOSITION
Five-year survival varies by stage:
• Stage I 60% to 90%
• Stage II 40% to 80%
• Stage III <60%
• Stage IV <15%
Early detection by Pap smear imperative to long-term improvements in survival.

■ REFERRAL
Gynecologic oncologist for all invasive disease

REFERENCES
Anttila T et al: Serotypes of *Chlamydia trachomatis* and risk for development of cervical squamous cell carcinoma, *JAMA* 285:47, 2001.
Morris M et al: Pelvic radiation with concurrent chemotherapy compared with pelvic and para-aortic radiation for high-risk cervical cancer, *N Engl J Med* 340:1137, 1999.
Nuono J et al: New tests for cervical cancer screening, *Am Fam Physician* 64:780, 2001.
Author: **Gil Farkash, M.D.**

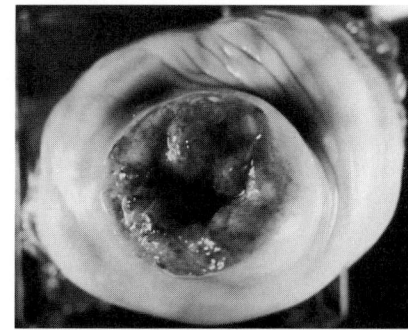

Fig. 1-89 Carcinoma of cervix (gross specimen). (From Mishell D [ed]: *Comprehensive gynecology,* ed 3, St Louis, 1997, Mosby.)

BASIC INFORMATION

■ DEFINITION
Cervical disk syndromes refer to diseases of the cervical spine resulting from disk disorder, either herniation or degenerative change (spondylosis) (Fig. 1-90). When posterior osteophytes compress the anterior spinal cord, lower extremity symptoms may result, a condition termed *cervical spondylotic myelopathy*.

ICD-9CM CODES
722.4 Degenerative intervertebral cervical disk
722.71 Degenerative cervical disk with myelopathy

■ EPIDEMIOLOGY & DEMOGRAPHICS
PREVALENCE: 10% of general adult population (symptoms in 50% of population at some time in their life)
PREDOMINANT SEX: Male = female
PREDOMINANT AGE: 30 to 60 yr

■ PHYSICAL FINDINGS & CLINICAL PRESENTATION
- Neck pain, radicular symptoms, or myelopathy, either alone or in combination
- Limited neck movement
- Pain with neck motion, especially extension (Fig. 1-91)
- Referred unilateral interscapular pain, resulting in a local trigger point
- Radicular arm pain (usually unilateral), numbness, and tingling possible, most commonly involving the C6 (C5-C6 disk) or C7 (C6-C7 disk) nerve root (Fig. 1-92)
- Weakness and reflex changes (C6—biceps, C7—triceps)
- Myelopathy possibly resulting in gait disturbance, weakness, and even spasticity
- Sensory examination usually not helpful

■ ETIOLOGY
Unknown

DIAGNOSIS

■ DIFFERENTIAL DIAGNOSIS
- Rotator cuff tendinitis
- Carpal tunnel syndrome
- Thoracic outlet syndrome
- Brachial neuritis
A clinical algorithm for evaluation of neck pain is described in Fig. 3-119.

■ WORKUP
In most cases, the diagnosis can be established on a clinical basis alone. Fig. 1-94 describes an algorithm for suspected cervical disc syndrome.

■ IMAGING STUDIES
- Plain roentgenograms within the first few weeks
  1. Usually normal in soft disk herniation
  2. With chronic degenerative disk disease, usually loss of height of the disk space, anterior and posterior osteophyte formation, and encroachment on the intervertebral foramen by osteophytes (see Fig. 1-90)
- Myelography, CT scanning, and MRI indicated in patients whose symptoms do not resolve or when other spinal pathology suspected
- Electrodiagnostic studies to confirm the diagnosis or rule out peripheral nerve disorders

TREATMENT

■ NONPHARMACOLOGIC THERAPY
- Rest and cervical collar if needed
- Local modalities such as heat
- Physical therapy (Fig. 1-93)

■ ACUTE GENERAL Rx
- NSAIDs
- "Muscle relaxants" for their sedative effect
- Analgesics as needed
- Epidural steroid injection for radicular pain

■ DISPOSITION
- Usually improve with time
- Surgical intervention in <5%

■ REFERRAL
Orthopedic or neurosurgical consultation for intractable pain or neurologic deficit

PEARLS & CONSIDERATIONS

■ COMMENTS
- Pain relief with physical therapy seems anecdotal and short-lived; any overall improvement usually parallels what would have probably occurred naturally.
- Sometimes carpal tunnel syndrome and cervical radiculopathy occur together; this is termed the *double-*

crush syndrome and results from nerve compression at two separate levels. Proximal compression may decrease the ability of the nerve to tolerate a second, more distal compression.
- Surgical intervention is indicated primarily for relief of radicular pain caused by nerve root compression or for the treatment of myelopathy; it is generally not helpful when chief complaint is neck pain alone.
- In many cases of cervical spondylosis with myelopathy, the lower-extremity symptoms are much more disabling than the neck symptoms, a situation that can cause some difficulty in determining their etiology.

REFERENCES
Albert TJ, Murrell SE: Surgical management of cervical radiculopathy, *J Am Acad Orthop Surg* 7:368, 1999.
Linton SJ: A review of psychological risk factors in back and neck pain, *Spine* 25:1148, 2000.
Robinson LR: Role of neurophysiologic evaluation in diagnosis, *J Am Acad Orthop Surg* 8:190, 2000.
Author: **Lonnie R. Mercier, M.D.**

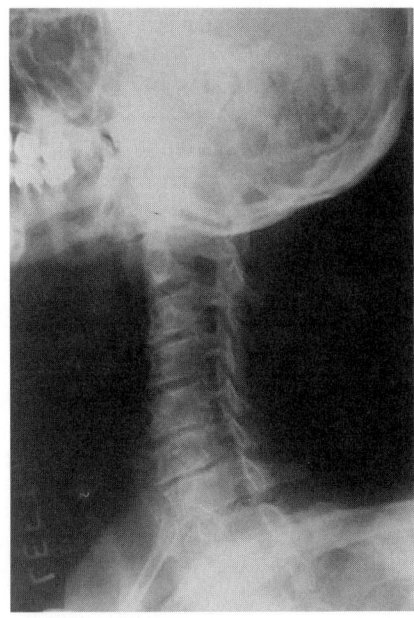

Fig. 1-90 Cervical spondylosis. Right anterior oblique x-ray of cervical spine demonstrates multilevel neural canal stenosis from C3-4 through C6-7 secondary to chronic degenerative spur formation arising from the uncinate processes. (From Goetz CG: *Textbook of clinical neurology,* Philadelphia, 1999, WB Saunders.)

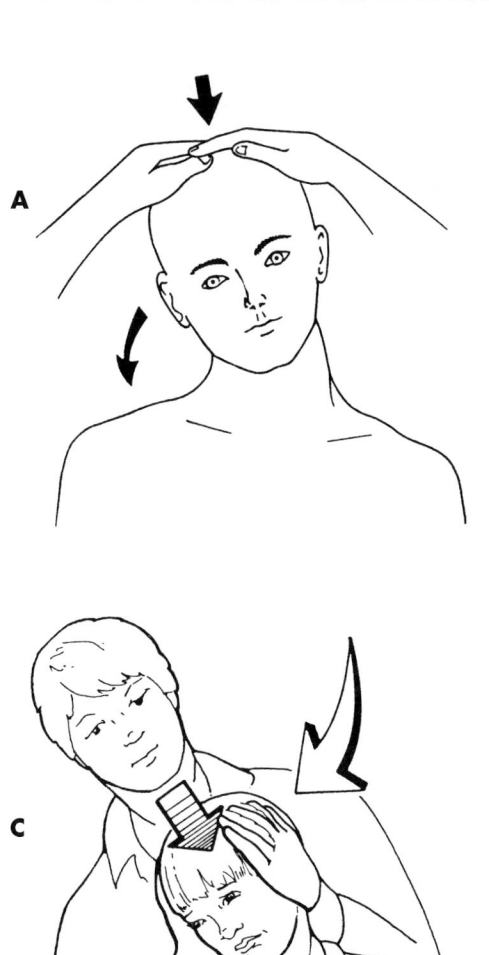

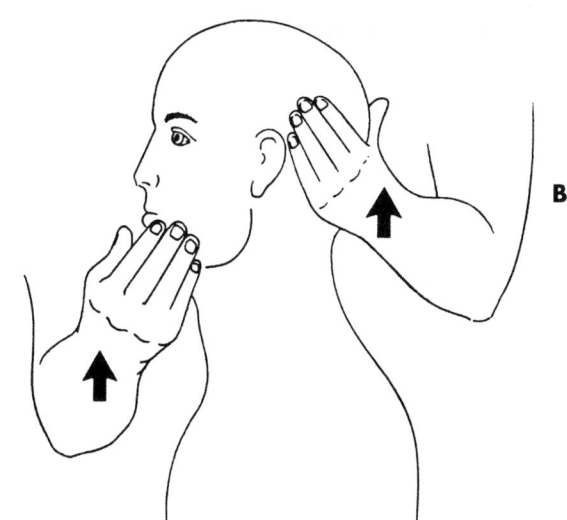

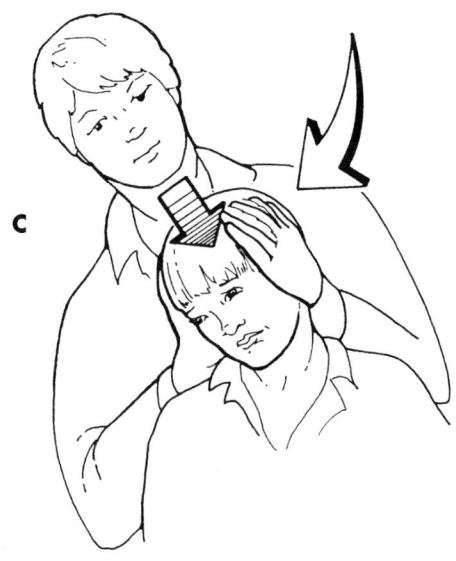

Fig. 1-91 Nerve root encroachment tests. **A,** A compression test can cause radicular symptoms on the affected side. **B,** Distraction can relieve these symptoms. **C,** Spurling's test. Lateral flexion and rotation with compression may cause nerve root encroachment and pain on the ipsilateral side in patients with cervical nerve root impingement. (From Brinker MR, Miller MD: *Fundamentals of orthopaedics,* Philadelphia, 1999, WB Saunders.)

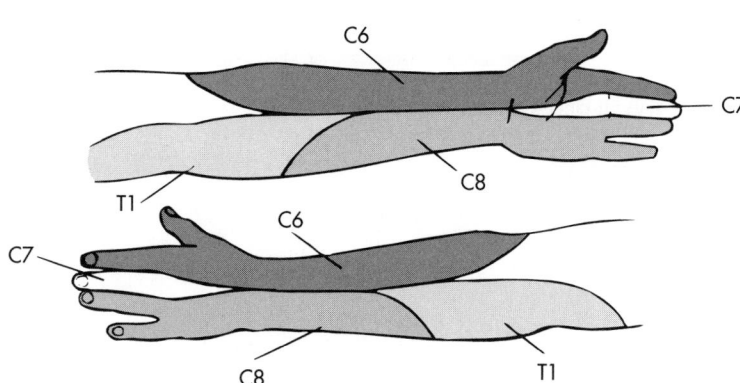

Fig. 1-92 Volar and dorsal dermatome pattern of the forearm and hand. Pain and paresthesias may radiate into these areas when the affected nerve root is compressed. *Note:* Extremity symptoms caused by disk disease are almost always unilateral. (From Mercier LR [ed]: *Practical orthopaedics,* ed 4, St Louis, 1995, Mosby.)

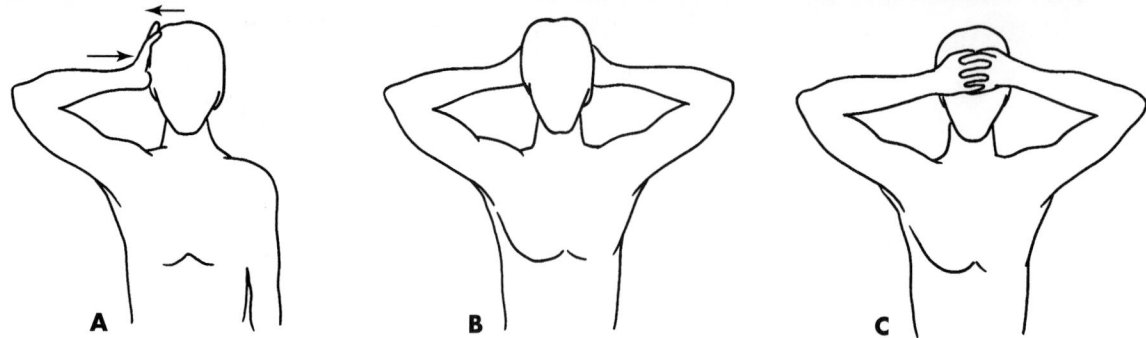

Fig. 1-93   Isometric neck exercises. **A,** The hand is placed against the side of the head slightly above the ear, and pressure is gradually increased while resisting with the neck muscles and keeping the head in the same position. The position is held 5 seconds, relaxed, and repeated five times. **B,** The exercise is performed on the other side and then from the back and front **(C).** The exercise should be performed three to four times daily. (From Mercier LR [ed]: *Practical orthopaedics,* ed 4, St Louis, 1995, Mosby.)

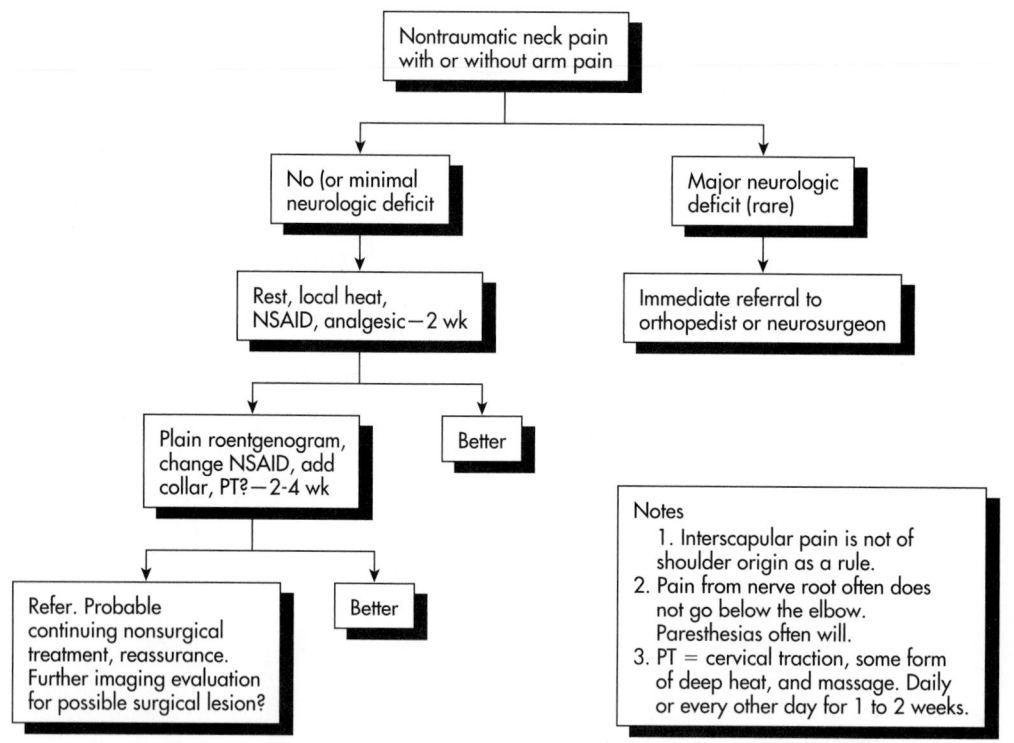

Fig. 1-94   Algorithm for suspected cervical disk syndrome. *NSAID,* Nonsteroidal antiinflammatory drug; *PT,* physical therapy. (From Mercier LR [ed]: *Practical orthopaedics,* ed 4, St Louis, 1995, Mosby.)

BASIC INFORMATION

■ **DEFINITION**

Cervical dysplasia refers to atypical development of immature squamous epithelium that does not penetrate the basement epithelial membrane. Characteristics include increased cellularity, nuclear abnormalities, and increased nuclear to cytoplasm ratio. A progressive polarized loss of squamous differentiation exists beginning adjacent to the basement membrane and progressing to the most advanced stage (severe dysplasia), which encompasses the complete squamous epithelial layer thickness (Fig. 1-95).

Classification systems:

Modified Papanicolaou: Class I, II, III, IV, and V

Dysplasia: Normal, atypia (mild, moderate, and severe), carcinoma in situ, and cancer

CIN: Normal, atypia (CIN I, II, or III), and cancer

Bethesda classification:

Normal/benign, AGCUS, ASCUS, LGSIL (including HPV), HGSIL, and cancer

■ **SYNONYMS**

Class III or class IV Pap smear

Cervical intraepithelial neoplasia (CIN)

Low-grade or high-grade squamous intraepithelial lesion (LGSIL or HGSIL)

ICD-9CM CODES

622.1 Dysplasia of cervix (uteri)

■ **EPIDEMIOLOGY & DEMOGRAPHICS**

PEAK INCIDENCE:

• Age 35 yr
• Abnormal Pap smear rate revealing dysplasia approximates 2% to 5%, depending on population risk factors and false-negative rate variance
• False-negative rate approaching 40%
• Average age-adjusted incidence of severe dysplasia 35 cases/100,000 persons

PREVALENCE:

• Dysplasia: peak age, 26 yr (3600 cases/100,000 persons)
• CIS: peak age, 32 yr (1100 cases/100,000 persons)
• Invasive cancer: peak age, 77 yr (800 cases/100,000 persons)

■ **PHYSICAL FINDINGS & CLINICAL PRESENTATION**

• Cervical lesions associated with dysplasia usually are not visible to the naked eye; therefore physical findings are best viewed by colposcopy of a 3% acetic acid–prepared cervix.
• Patients evaluated by colposcopy are identified by abnormal cervical cytology screening from Pap smear screening
• Colposcopic findings:
  1. Leukoplakia (white lesion seen by the unaided eye that may represent condyloma, dysplasia, or cancer)
  2. Acetowhite epithelium with or without associated punctation, mosaicism, abnormal vessels
  3. Abnormal transformation zone (abnormal iodine uptake, "cuffed" gland openings)

■ **ETIOLOGY**

• Not clearly elucidated
• May be caused by abnormal reserve cell hyperplasia resulting in atypical metaplasia and dysplastic epithelium
• Strongly associated and initiated by oncogenic HPV infection (high-risk HPV types 16, 18, 31, 33, 35, 45, 51, 52, 56, and 58; low-risk HPV types 6, 11, 42, 43, and 44)
• Risk factors:
  1. Any heterosexual coitus
  2. Coitus during puberty (T-zone metaplasia peak)
  3. DES exposure
  4. Multiple sexual partners
  5. Lack of prior Pap smear screening
  6. History of STD
  7. Other genital tract neoplasia
  8. HIV
  9. TB
  10. Substance abuse
  11. "High-risk" male partner (HPV)
  12. Low socioeconomic status
  13. Early first pregnancy
  14. Tobacco use
  15. HPV

🔬 **DIAGNOSIS**

■ **DIFFERENTIAL DIAGNOSIS**

• Metaplasia
• Hyperkeratosis
• Condyloma
• Microinvasive carcinoma
• Glandular epithelial abnormalities
• Adenocarcinoma in situ
• VIN
• VAIN
• Metastatic tumor involvement of the cervix

■ **WORKUP**

Periodic history and physical examination (including cytologic screening), depending on age, risk factors, and history of preinvasive cervical lesions

• Consider screening for sexually transmitted disease (Gc, *Chlamydia*, VDRL, HIV, HPV)
• Abnormal cytology (HGSIL/LGSIL, initial ASCUS in high-risk patients, recurrent ASCUS in low-risk/postmenopausal patients) and grossly evident suspicious lesions; refer for colposcopy and possible directed biopsy/ECC (examination should include cervix, vagina, vulva, and anus)
• For glandular cell abnormalities (AGCUS): refer for colposcopy and possible directed biopsy/ECC, and consider endometrial sampling
• In pregnancy: abnormal cytology followed by colposcopy in the first trimester and at 28 to 32 wk; only high-grade lesions suspect for cancer biopsied; ECC contraindicated
• Fig. 3-126 describes an approach to Pap smear abnormalities

■ **LABORATORY TESTS**

• Gc, *Chlamydia* to rule out STD
• Pap cytology screening (requires appropriate sampling, preparation, cytologist interpretation and reporting)
• Colposcopy and directed biopsy, ECC for indications (see "Workup")
• HPV-DNA typing considered

■ **IMAGING STUDIES**

• Cervicography
• Computer-enhanced Pap cytology screening (e.g., PAPNET)

💊 **TREATMENT**

■ **NONPHARMACOLOGIC THERAPY**

• Superficial ablative techniques (cryosurgery, CO_2 laser, and electrocoagulation diathermy) considered for colposcopy-identified dysplasia (moderate to severe dysplasia or CIS) and negative ECC; mild dysplasia followed conservatively in a compliant patient
• Cone biopsy (LEEP, CO_2 laser, "cold knife" cone biopsy) considered for colposcopy-identified dysplasia (moderate to severe dysplasia or CIS) and positive ECC or if there is a two-

grade or more discrepancy between the Pap smear, colposcopy, and biopsy or ECC findings
- Hysterectomy if patient has completed child bearing and has persistent or recurrent severe dysplasia or CIS
- In pregnancy: treatment for cervical dysplasia deferred until after delivery

■ ACUTE GENERAL Rx
Topical 5-fluorouracil (5-FU) is rarely used for recurrent cervicovaginal lesions.

■ CHRONIC Rx
- Because of the risk for persistent and recurrent dysplasia, long-term follow-up is individualized based on patient risk factors, Pap smear and colposcopy results, treatment history, and presence of high-risk HPV (e.g., Pap smear q3-4mo/yr, then q6mo/1 yr, then annually [if all normal], or repeat colposcopy examination and treat as indicated).
- Mild dysplasia with negative ECC should be followed conservatively in a compliant patient as a majority of these lesions persist or regress.

■ DISPOSITION
- Because of the large numbers of women in high-risk groups, the prevalence of HPV, and the high false-negative Pap smear rate,

routine Pap smear screening should be reinforced for all women, especially those with a history of cervical dysplasia.
- Success rates for treatment approach 80% to 90%.
- Detection of persistence of recurrence requires careful follow-up.
- Cervical treatment possibly results in infertility (cervical stenosis or incompetence), which requires careful consideration and discretion for use of LEEP and cone biopsy.
- Appropriate counseling and informed consent needed when considering any form of management of cervical dysplasia.
- There has been no case of cervical dysplasia progressing to invasive cancer with appropriate screening, diagnosis, treatment, and follow-up.

■ REFERRAL
- Patients with abnormal Pap cytology should not be followed by repeat Pap smear screening.
- Patients with identified abnormal cytology should be evaluated by a skilled colposcopist (defined as documented didactic and preceptorship training including 50 cases of identified pathology, ongoing colposcopy activity with a minimum of 2 cases/wk, Q.A. log, and periodic CME).

- If treatment is required, patient should be referred to a gynecologist or gynecologic oncologist skilled in the diagnosis and treatment of preinvasive cervical disease.

⚙ PEARLS & CONSIDERATIONS

■ COMMENTS
- Patient education material available from American College of Obstetricians and Gynecologists.
- A clinical algorithm for workup of Pap smear abnormalities is described in Fig. 3-126.

REFERENCES
Nuono J et al: New tests for cervical cancer screening, *Am Fam Physician* 64:780, 2001.
Solomon D et al: Comparison of three management strategies for patients with atypical squamous cells of undetermined significance: baseline results from a randomized trial, *J Natl Cancer Inst* 93:293, 2001.
Author: **Dennis M. Weppner, M.D.**

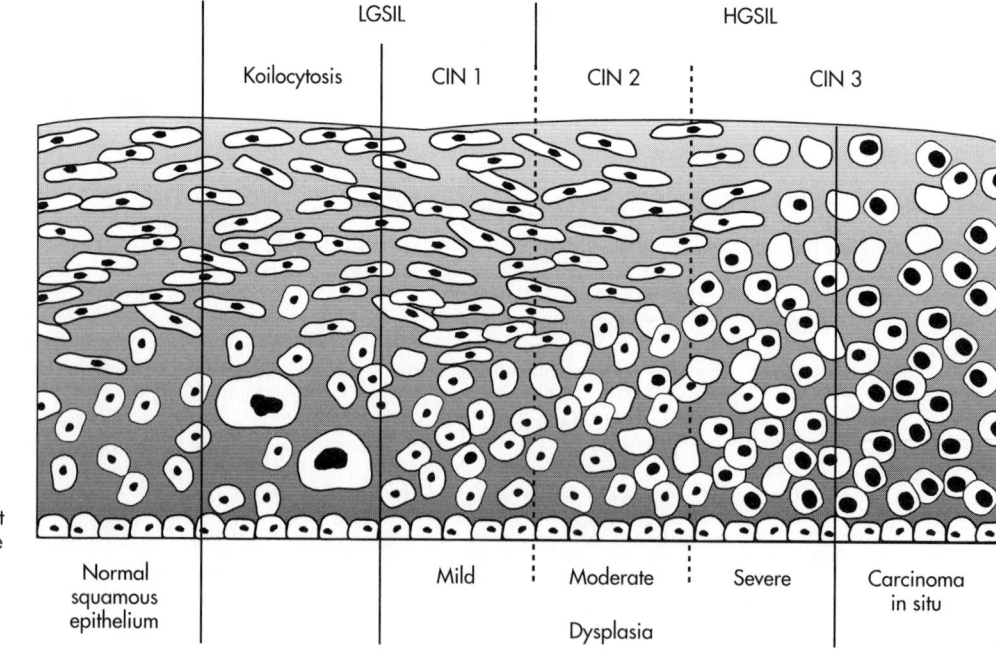

Fig. 1-95 Diagram of cervical epithelium showing various terminologies used to characterize progressive degrees of cervical neoplasia. (From Mishell D [ed]: *Comprehensive gynecology,* ed 3, St Louis, 1997, Mosby.)

BASIC INFORMATION

■ **DEFINITION**
A cervical polyp is a growth protruding from the cervix or endocervical canal. Polyps that arise from the endocervical canal are called *endocervical polyps*. If they arise from the ectocervix, they are called *cervical polyps*.

■ **ICD-9CM CODES**
622.7 Mucous polyp of cervix

■ **EPIDEMIOLOGY & DEMOGRAPHICS**
Cervical polyps are common. Found in approximately 4% of all gynecologic patients. Most commonly present in perimenopausal and multigravid women between the ages of 30 and 50 yr. Endocervical polyps are more common than cervical polyps and are almost always benign (Fig. 1-96). Malignant degeneration is extremely rare.

■ **PHYSICAL FINDINGS & CLINICAL PRESENTATION**
Polyps may be single or multiple and vary in size from being extremely small (a few mm) to large (4 cm). They are soft, smooth, reddish-purple to cherry-red in color. They bleed easily when touched. Very large polyps can cause some cervical dilation. There may be vaginal discharge associated with cervical polyps if the polyp has become infected.

■ **ETIOLOGY**
• Most unknown
• Inflammatory
• Traumatic
• Pregnancy

DIAGNOSIS

■ **DIFFERENTIAL DIAGNOSIS**
• Endometrial polyp
• Prolapsed myoma
• Retained products of conception
• Squamous papilloma
• Sarcoma
• Cervical malignancy

■ **WORKUP**
Polyps are most commonly asymptomatic and are usually found at the time of annual gynecologic pelvic examination. Polyps are also found in women who present for evaluation of intermenstrual or postcoital bleeding and for profuse vaginal discharge. Polyps are painless. Unless a patient has a bleeding abnormality that necessitates her being evaluated by a physician, polyps would go undiagnosed until her next Pap smear was obtained.

TREATMENT

■ **NONPHARMACOLOGIC THERAPY**
Simple surgical excision can be done in the office. The physician should be prepared for bleeding, which can easily be controlled with silver nitrate or Monsel's solution. Most commonly, a polyp is excised by grasping it at the stalk and twisting it off. Polyps can also be excised by electrocautery or, in the case of very large polyps, in an outpatient surgical suite. Sexual intercourse and tampon usage are to be avoided until the patient's follow-up visit. Also, douching is not to be performed.

■ **ACUTE GENERAL Rx**
Generally, no medication is needed.

■ **CHRONIC Rx**
Patient is followed up in 2 wk for recheck of the surgical excision site unless there is active bleeding, in which case she would be seen immediately. The cervix should be checked at the patient's routine gynecologic visits.

■ **DISPOSITION**
Since these are almost always benign, usually no further treatment is needed. Annual gynecologic examinations should be performed to check for any regrowths.

■ **REFERRAL**
To a gynecologist for removal of polyps

PEARLS & CONSIDERATIONS

■ **COMMENTS**
A Pap smear should be obtained before removing the polyp. If an abnormal Pap smear is obtained, more than likely the cause will be secondary to the polyp. If a colposcopic evaluation is needed, this should also be performed. During pregnancy, the cervix is highly vascularized. If the polyps are stable and benign-appearing, they should just be observed during the pregnancy and removed only if they are causing bleeding.

REFERENCE
Copeland L: *Textbook of gynecology,* ed 2, Baltimore, 1999, Saunders.
Author: **George T. Danakas, M.D.**

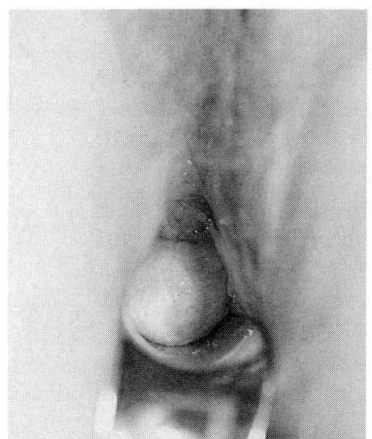 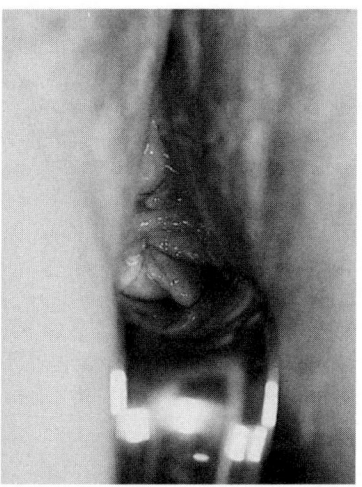

Fig. 1-96   A, Fibroid polyp protruding through the external cervical os. **B,** Small endocervical polyp. (From Symonds EM, Macpherson MBA: *Color atlas of obstetrics and gynecology,* St Louis, 1994, Mosby.)

BASIC INFORMATION

■ DEFINITION
Cervicitis is an infection of the cervix. It may result from direct infection of the cervix, or it may be secondary to uterine or vaginal infection.

■ SYNONYMS
Endocervicitis
Ectocervicitis
Mucopurulent cervicitis

■ ICD-9CM CODES
616.0 Cervicitis
098.15 Acute gonococcal cervicitis
079.8 Chlamydia infection

■ EPIDEMIOLOGY & DEMOGRAPHICS
Cervicitis accounts for 20% to 25% of patients presenting with abnormal vaginal discharge, and this affects women only. It is most common in adolescents, but it can be found in any sexually active woman. Practicing unsafe sex with multiple sexual partners increases the risk of developing cervicitis, as well as other sexually transmitted diseases.

■ PHYSICAL FINDINGS
Cervicitis is usually asymptomatic or associated with mild symptoms. Copious vaginal discharge (Fig. 1-97), pelvic pain, and dyspareunia may be present if cervicitis is severe. The cervix can be erythematous and tender on palpation during bimanual examination. The cervix may also bleed easily when obtaining cultures or a Pap smear.

■ ETIOLOGY
- *Chlamydia*
- *Trichomonas*
- *Neisseria gonorrhoeae*
- Herpes simplex
- *Trichomonas vaginalis*
- Human papillomavirus

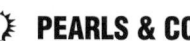 **DIAGNOSIS**

■ DIFFERENTIAL DIAGNOSIS
- Carcinoma of the cervix
- Cervical erosion
- Cervical metaplasia

■ WORKUP
The patient usually presents with a vaginal discharge or history of postcoital bleeding. Otherwise the patient is diagnosed asymptomatically during routine examination. On examination there is gross visualization of yellow, mucopurulent material on the cotton swab.

■ LABORATORY TESTS
On a smear there will be ten or more polymorphonuclear leukocytes per microscopic field. Positive Gram stain is found. Cultures should be obtained for *Chlamydia* and *N. gonorrhoeae.* Use a wet mount to look for trichomonads. Obtain a Pap smear.

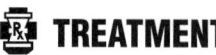 **TREATMENT**

■ NONPHARMACOLOGIC THERAPY
Cervicitis is treated in an outpatient setting. Cryosurgery is an option for treatment of cervicitis with negative cultures and negative biopsies. Safe sex should be practiced with the use of condoms. Partners should be treated in all cases of infection proven by culture.

■ ACUTE GENERAL Rx
Because *Chlamydia* and *N. gonorrhoeae* make up >50% of the cause of infectious cervicitis, if it is suspected, treat without waiting for culture results. Administer ceftriaxone 125-mg IM single dose followed by doxycycline 100 mg PO bid for 7 days. If the patient is pregnant, treat with azithromycin (Zithromax) 1-g single dose instead of using doxycycline, which is contraindicated in pregnant or nursing mothers. If *Trichomonas* is the etiologic agent, treat with metronidazole 2-g single dose. For herpes, treat with acyclovir 200 mg PO five times qd for 7 days.

■ DISPOSITION
Cervicitis responds well to antibiotics. Possible complications to watch for are a subsequent PID and infertility (found in 5% to 10% of patients). Repeat cultures should be performed after treatment. Sexual relations can be resumed after negative cultures.

■ REFERRAL
If subsequent PID develops, consider hospital admission for IV antibiotics.

PEARLS & CONSIDERATIONS

■ COMMENTS
Patient educational material can be obtained from local health clinics and clinics for sexually transmitted diseases.

REFERENCE
Centers for Disease Control: Sexually transmitted disease treatment guideline, *MMWR* 47(RR-1), 1998.
Author: **George T. Danakas, M.D.**

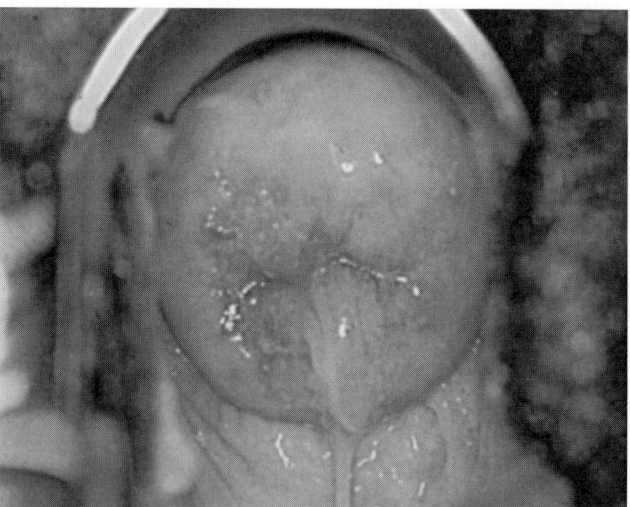

Fig. 1-97 Colposcopy of a woman with mucopurulent cervicitis and purulent discharge from endocervical os. (Courtesy Dr. David Soper, Richmond, Va. From Mandell GL [ed]: *Mandell, Douglas, and Bennett's principles and practice of infectious diseases,* ed 5, New York, 2000, Churchill Livingstone.)

BASIC INFORMATION

■ **DEFINITION**

Chagas' disease is a infection caused by the protozoan parasite *Trypanosoma cruzi*. The disease is characterized by an acute nonspecific febrile illness that may be followed, after a variable latency period, by chronic cardiac, GI, and neurologic sequelae.

■ **SYNONYMS**

American trypanosomiasis

ICD-9CM CODES
086.2 Chagas' disease

■ **EPIDEMIOLOGY & DEMOGRAPHICS**

INCIDENCE (IN U.S.):
- Four cases of autochthonous transmission in California and Texas
- In the last two decades, six cases of laboratory-acquired infection, three cases of transfusion-associated transmission, and nine cases of imported disease reported to the Centers for Disease Control and Prevention (none of the imported cases involving returning tourists)

PREVALENCE (IN U.S.): Based on regional seroprevalence studies in Hispanic blood donors, it is estimated that between 50,000 and 100,000 persons infected with *T. cruzi* are currently residing in the U.S.

PREDOMINANT SEX: Male = female

PREDOMINANT AGE:
- In highly endemic areas, mean age of acute infection: approximately 4 yr old
- Variable age distribution for both types of chronic disease, depending on geography
- Mean age of onset: usually between 35 and 45 yr

PEAK INCIDENCE: Unknown

GENETICS:

Congenital Infection: Congenital transmission has been documented with attendant high fetal mortality and morbidity in surviving infants.

Neonatal Infection: In rural areas, within substandard housing, transmission is likely to occur.

■ **PHYSICAL FINDINGS & CLINICAL PRESENTATION**

- Inflammatory lesion that develops about 1 wk after contamination of a break in the skin with infected insect feces (chagoma)
  1. Area of induration and erythema
  2. Usually accompanied by local lymphadenopathy

- Presence of Romaña's sign, which consists of unilateral painless palpebral and periocular edema, when conjunctiva is portal of entry
- Constitutional symptoms of fever, fatigue, and anorexia, along with edema of the face and lower extremities, generalized lymphadenopathy, and mild hepatosplenomegaly after the appearance of local signs of disease
- Myocarditis in a small portion of patients, sometimes with resultant CHF
- Uncommonly, CNS disease, such as meningoencephalitis, which carries a poor prognosis
- Symptoms and signs of disease persisting for weeks to months, followed by spontaneous resolution of the acute illness; patient then in the indeterminate phase of the disease (asymptomatic with attendant subpatent parasitemia and reactive antibodies to *T. cruzi* antigens)
- Chronic disease may become manifest years to decades after the initial infection:
  1. Most common organ involved: heart, followed by GI tract, and to a much lesser extent the CNS
     a. Cardiac involvement takes the form of arrhythmias or cardiomyopathy, but rarely both.
     b. Cardiomyopathy is bilateral but predominantly affects the right ventricle and is often accompanied by apical aneurysms and mural thrombi.
     c. Arrhythmias are a consequence of involvement of the bundle of His and have been implicated as the leading cause of sudden death in adults in highly endemic areas.
     d. Right-sided heart failure, thromboembolization, and rhythm disturbances associated with symptoms of dizziness and syncope are characteristic.
  2. Patients with megaesophagus: dysphasia, odynophagia, chronic cough, and regurgitation, frequently resulting in aspiration pneumonitis
  3. Megacolon: abdominal pain and chronic constipation, which, when severe, may lead to obstruction and perforation
  4. CNS symptoms: most often secondary to embolization from the heart or varying degrees of peripheral neuropathy

■ **ETIOLOGY**

- *T. cruzi*
  1. Found only in the Americas, ranging from the southern half of the U.S. to southern Argentina
  2. Transmitted to humans by various species of bloodsucking reduviid ("kissing") insects, primarily those of the genera *Triatoma, Panstrongylus,* and *Rhodnius*
  3. Usually found in burrows and trees where infected insects transmit the parasite to nonhuman mammals (e.g., opossums and armadillos), which constitute the natural reservoir
  4. Intrusion into enzootic areas for farmland, allowing insects to take up residence in rural dwellings, thus including humans and domestic animals in the cycle of transmission
  5. Initial infection of insects by ingesting blood from animals or humans that have circulating flagellated trypanosomes (trypomastigotes)
  6. Multiplication of ingested parasites in the insect midgut as epimastigotes, then differentiation into infective metacyclic trypomastigotes in the hindgut whereby the parasites are discharged with the feces during subsequent blood meals
  7. Transmission to the second mammalian host through contamination of mucous membranes, conjunctivae, or wounds with insect feces containing infected forms.
- In the vertebrate host
  1. Movement of parasites into various cell types, intracellular transformation and multiplication in the cytoplasm as amastigotes, and thereafter differentiation into trypomastigotes
  2. Following rupture of the cell membrane, parasitic invasion of local tissues or hematogenous spread to distant sites, maintaining a parasitemia infective for vectors
- In addition to insect vectors, *T. cruzi* is transmitted through blood transfusions, transplacentally, and, occasionally, secondary to laboratory accidents.

DIAGNOSIS

■ DIFFERENTIAL DIAGNOSIS
Acute disease
- Early African trypanosomiasis
- New World cutaneous and mucocutaneous leishmaniasis

Chronic disease
- Idiopathic cardiomyopathy
- Idiopathic achalasia
- Congenital or acquired megacolon

■ WORKUP
Principal considerations in diagnosis:
- A history of residence where transmission is known to occur
- Recent receipt of a blood product while in an endemic area
- Occupational exposure in a laboratory

■ LABORATORY TESTS
For acute diagnosis:
- Demonstration of *T. cruzi* in wet preparations of blood, buffy coat, or Giemsa-stained smears
- Xenodiagnosis, a technique involving laboratory-reared insect vectors fed on subjects with suspected infection thereafter examined for parasites, and culture of body fluids in liquid media to establish diagnosis
  1. Hampered by the length of time required for completion
  2. Of limited use in clinical decision making with regard to drug therapy
  3. Although xenodiagnosis and broth culture are considered to be more sensitive than microscopic examination of body fluids, sensitivities may not exceed 50%.
- Recent advances in serologic testing, including immunoblot assay, in situ indirect fluorescent antibody, and PCR-based techniques
  1. Show increased sensitivity and specificity for *T. cruzi* in acute and chronic infections
  2. Not widely available, limiting their usefulness in the diagnosis of acute disease

For chronic *T. cruzi* infection:
- Traditional serologic tests including: complement fixation (CF), indirect immunofluorescence (IIF), indirect hemagglutination, enzyme-linked immunosorbent assay (ELISA), and radioimmune precipitation assay
- Persistent problem with these tests: in addition to sensitivity and specificity, false-positive results

- Saliva ELISA may be useful as a screening diagnostic test in epidemiologic studies of chronic trypanosomiasis infection in endemic areas.

℞ TREATMENT

■ NONPHARMACOLOGIC THERAPY
- Chronic chagasic heart disease: mainly supportive
- Megaesophagus: symptoms usually amenable to dietary measures or pneumonic dilation of the esophagogastric junction
- Chagasic megacolon: in its early stages responsive to a high-fiber diet, laxatives, and enemas

■ ACUTE GENERAL Rx
Nifurtimox (Lampit, Bayer 2502):
- Only drug available in the U.S. for the treatment of acute, congenital, or laboratory-acquired infection
- Recommended oral dosage for adults: 8 to 10 mg/kg/day given in four divided daily doses and continued for 90 to 120 days
- Parasitologic cure in approximately 50% of those treated; should be begun as early as possible

Benznidazole, a nitroimidazole derivative:
- Has demonstrated similar efficacy as nifurtimox in limited trials
- Recommended oral dosage: 5 mg/kg/day for 60 days

■ CHRONIC Rx
- In patients with indeterminate phase or chronic disease: no evidence of benefit with pharmacologic therapy
- In patients exhibiting bradyarrhythmias: pacemakers
- In individuals with congestive heart failure:
  1. Treat with modalities appropriate for dilated, especially right-sided, cardiomyopathic disease.
  2. Cardiac transplant is a controversial alternative for end-stage cardiomyopathy; however, reactivation rate found to be low and amenable to therapy without subsequent infection of the allograft in one study.
  3. Myotomy or esophageal resection is reserved for patients with advanced disease.

- In advanced chagasic megacolon associated with chronic fecal impaction, perforation, or, less commonly, volvulus: surgical resection

■ DISPOSITION
Based on few prospective studies, most patients infected with *T. cruzi* will not develop symptomatic Chagas' disease.

■ REFERRAL
- For consultation with an infectious disease specialist or communication with the Centers for Disease Control and Prevention when the disease is acutely suspected
- To a cardiologist for pacemaker implantation for patients with bradyarrhythmias
- To a surgeon for symptomatic disease in individuals with chagasic megaesophagus or megacolon

☼ PEARLS & CONSIDERATIONS

■ COMMENTS
- In recipients of solid organ or bone marrow transplants, patients with AIDS, or those receiving chemotherapy, there may be reactivation of indeterminate phase disease.
- Prognosis in patients with chagasic cardiomyopathy who develop CHF is poor, with death often ensuing in a matter of months.
- Patients with chagasic esophageal disease have an increased incidence of esophageal malignancy.

REFERENCES
Lages-Silva E et al: Relationship between *Trypanosoma cruzi* and human chagasic megaesophagus: blood and tissue parasitism, *Am J Trop Med Hyg* 65(5):435, 2001.

Rassi A et al: Chagas' heart disease, *Clin Cardiol* 23(12):883, 2000.

Solari A et al: Identification of *Trypanosoma cruzi* genotypes circulating in Chilean chagasic patients, *Exp Parasitol* 97(4):226, 2001.

Teixeira AR et al: Emerging Chagas disease: trophic network and cycle of transmission of *Trypanosoma cruzi* from palm trees in the Amazon, *Emerg Infect Dis* 7(1):100, 2001.
Author: **George O. Alonso, M.D.**

BASIC INFORMATION

DEFINITION
Chancroid is a sexually transmitted disease characterized by painful genital ulceration and inflammatory inguinal adenopathy.

SYNONYMS
Soft chancre
Ulcus molle

ICD-9CM CODES
099.0 Chancroid

EPIDEMIOLOGY & DEMOGRAPHICS
- Exact incidence is unknown.
- Occurs more frequently in men (male:female ratio of 10:1).
- Clinical infection is rare in women.
- There is a higher incidence in uncircumcised men and in tropical and subtropical regions.
- Incubation period is 4 to 7 days but may take up to 3 wk.

PHYSICAL FINDINGS & CLINICAL PRESENTATION
- One to three extremely painful ulcers (Fig. 1-98), accompanied by tender inguinal lymphadenopathy (especially if fluctuant)
- May present with inguinal bubo and several ulcers
- In women: initial lesion in the fourchette, labia minora, urethra, cervix, or anus; inflammatory pustule or papule that ruptures leaving a shallow, nonindurated shallow ulceration, usually 1- to 2-cm diameter with ragged, undermined edges
- Unilateral lymphadenopathy develops 1 wk later in 50% of patients

ETIOLOGY
Haemophilus ducreyi, a bacillus

 DIAGNOSIS

DIFFERENTIAL DIAGNOSIS
- Other genitoulcerative diseases such as syphilis, herpes, LGV, granuloma inguinale.
- A clinical algorithm for the initial management of genital ulcer disease is described in Fig. 3-69.
- Table 2-84 describes the differential diagnosis of genital sores.

WORKUP
- Diagnosis based on history and physical examination is often inadequate. Must rule out syphilis in women because of the consequences of inappropriate therapy in pregnant women. Base initial diagnosis and treatment recommendations on clinical impression of appearance of ulcer and most likely diagnosis for population. Definitive diagnosis is made by isolation of organism from ulcers by culture or Gram stain.

LABORATORY TESTS
Darkfield microscopy, RPR, HSV cultures, *H. ducreyi* culture, HIV testing recommended

TREATMENT

NONPHARMACOLOGIC THERAPY
Fluctuant nodes should be aspirated through healthy adjacent skin to prevent formation of draining sinus. I&D not recommended, delays healing.

Use warm compresses to remove necrotic material.

ACUTE GENERAL Rx
- Azithromycin 1 g PO (single dose) *or*
- Ceftriaxone 250 mg IM (single dose) *or*
- Ciprofloxacin 500 mg PO bid for 3 days *or*
- Erythromycin 500 mg PO qid for 7 days

NOTE: Ciprofloxacin is contraindicated in patients who are pregnant, lactating, or less than 18 yr of age.

DISPOSITION
- All sexual partners should be treated with a 10-day course of one of the above regimens.
- Patients should be reexamined 3 to 7 days after initiation of therapy. Ulcers should improve symptomatically within 3 days and objectively within 7 days after initiation of successful therapy.

PEARLS & CONSIDERATIONS

COMMENTS
- In the U.S. HSV-1 and syphilis are the most common causes of genital ulcers, followed by chancroid, LGV, and granuloma inguinale.

REFERENCE
Center for Disease Control: Guidelines for treatment of sexually transmitted, *MMWR* 47(RR-1), 1998.
Author: **Eugene J. Louie-Ng, M.D.**

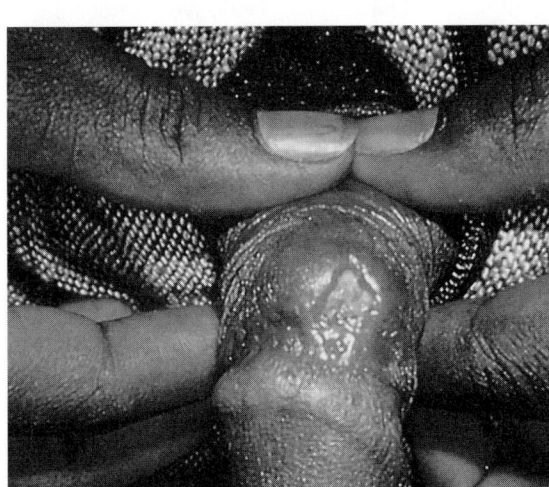

Fig. 1-98 Chancroid. Note shaggy, ragged-edged ulcer with edema and exudative base. (Courtesy Beverly Sanders, MD. From Goldstein B [ed]: *Practical dermatology,* ed 2, St Louis, 1997, Mosby.)

BASIC INFORMATION

■ DEFINITION
Charcot-Marie-Tooth disease is a heterogeneous group of noninflammatory inherited peripheral neuropathies.

■ SYNONYMS
Peroneal muscular atrophy
Hereditary motor and sensory neuropathy (HMSN)
Idiopathic dominantly inherited hypertrophic polyneuropathy

■ ICD-9CM CODES
356.1 Charcot-Marie-Tooth disease, paralysis, or syndrome

■ EPIDEMIOLOGY & DEMOGRAPHICS
PREDOMINANT AGE: Onset usually 10 to 20 yr but can be delayed to 50 to 60 yr
PREDOMINANT SEX: Male:female ratio of 3:1

■ PHYSICAL FINDINGS & CLINICAL PRESENTATION
- Variable presentation from family to family, but affected individuals in a family tend to have similar symptomatology
- Usually, gradual onset, with slowly progressive disorder
- Foot deformity producing a high arch (cavus) and hammer toes
- Atrophy of the lower legs producing a stork-like appearance (muscle wasting does not involve the upper legs) (Fig. 1-99)
- Nerve enlargement
- Sensory loss or other neurologic signs, although the sensory involvement is usually mild
- Scoliosis
- Decreased proprioception that often interferes with balance and gait
- Painful paresthesias
- In late cases, possible involvement of hands
- Absence of DTRs in many cases
- Poorly healing foot ulcers in some patients

■ ETIOLOGY
Chronic segmental demyelination of peripheral nerves with hypertrophic changes caused by remyelination

DIAGNOSIS

■ DIFFERENTIAL DIAGNOSIS
- Other inherited neuropathies
- Toxic, metabolic, and nutritional polyneuropathies

■ WORKUP
- The early onset, slow progression, and familial nature of the disorder are usually sufficient to establish diagnosis.
- Electrophysiologic studies are often diagnostic and may also be helpful in defining various subtypes of this group of neuropathies.
- Occasionally, muscle and nerve (sural) biopsy may be required.

TREATMENT

■ ACUTE GENERAL Rx
- Genetic counseling
- Supportive physical therapy and occupational therapy
- Prevention of injury to limbs with diminished sensibility
- Bracing

■ CHRONIC Rx
Occasionally, surgery to add stability and restore a plantigrade foot

■ DISPOSITION
- Disability is usually mild and compatible with a long life.
- 10% to 20% of patients are asymptomatic.
- A small number of cases are nonambulators by the sixth or seventh decade.

■ REFERRAL
- For orthopedic consultation for bracing and treatment of deformity
- For genetic counseling

PEARLS & CONSIDERATIONS

■ COMMENTS
Patient information on Charcot-Marie-Tooth disease is available from the Muscular Dystrophy Association, 3300 East Sunrise Drive, Tucson, Arizona 85718; phone: 1-800-572-1717.
Author: **Lonnie R. Mercier, M.D.**

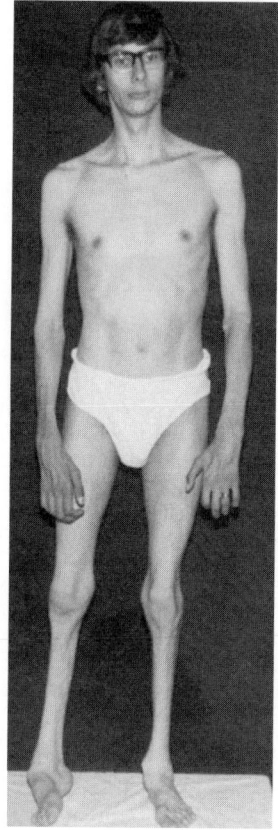

Fig. 1-99   Patient with Charcot-Marie-Tooth disease showing marked wasting of calf muscles and intrinsic foot muscles. (From Dubowitz V: *Muscle disorders in childhood,* London, 1995, WB Saunders. In Goetz CG: *Textbook of clinical neurology,* Philadelphia, 1999, WB Saunders.)

BASIC INFORMATION

■ DEFINITION
Charcot's joint is a chronic, progressive joint degeneration, often devastating, seen most commonly in peripheral weight-bearing joints and vertebrae, which develops as a result of the loss of normal sensory innervation of the joint. It was described by Charcot as a result of tabes dorsalis.

■ SYNONYMS
Neuropathic arthropathy

ICD-9CM CODES
094.0 Charcot's arthropathy

■ EPIDEMIOLOGY & DEMOGRAPHICS
PREVALENCE:
- 1 case/750 patients with diabetes mellitus; 5 cases/100 of those with peripheral neuropathy (foot is most commonly involved)
- 20% to 40% of patients with syringomyelia (shoulder most commonly involved)
- 5% to 10% of patients with tabes dorsalis; usually >60 yr (spine, hip, and knee most commonly involved)

■ PHYSICAL FINDINGS & CLINICAL PRESENTATION
Neuropathic joint disease is relatively painless, often in spite of considerable destruction
- Often, diffusely warm, swollen, and occasionally erythematous involved joint, the latter suggesting sepsis
- Possible progression of joint instability; palpable osseous debris; crepitus common
- Often, frank dislocation, leading to bony deformity, especially in more superficial joints

■ ETIOLOGY
The most widely accepted theory is the "neurotraumatic" theory:
- Impairment and loss of joint sensitivity decreases the protective mechanism about the joint.
- Rapid destruction occurs.
- Chronic inflammation and repetitive effusions develop, eventually contributing to joint instability and incongruity.

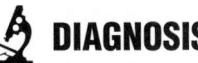

DIAGNOSIS

■ DIFFERENTIAL DIAGNOSIS
- Osteomyelitis, cellulitis, abscess
- Infectious arthritis
- Osteoarthritis
- Rheumatoid and other inflammatory arthritides

■ WORKUP
- An underlying neurologic disorder must always be present.
- Diabetes mellitus with peripheral neuropathy is the most common cause (Fig. 1-100).
- Syringomyelia, tabes dorsalis, Charcot-Marie-Tooth disease, congenital indifference to pain, alcoholism, and spinal dysraphism can all lead to the disorder.

■ LABORATORY TESTS
In questionable cases, aspiration, sometimes including biopsy, to rule out sepsis

■ IMAGING STUDIES
Plain roentgenography
- Sufficient to establish diagnosis in most cases, especially if etiology is known

- Findings: variable degrees of destruction and dislocation

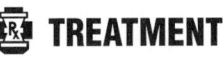

TREATMENT

■ ACUTE GENERAL Rx
- Protection of effusions, sprains, and fractures until all hyperemic response has resolved
- Braces, special shoes with molded inserts, and elevation of the extremity
- Patient education with avoidance of weight bearing when lower extremity joints are involved
- Surgery: only limited value

■ DISPOSITION
Once the full-blown neuropathic joint has developed, treatment is difficult.

REFERENCE
Pinzur MS et al: Current practice patterns in the treatment of Charcot foot, *Foot Ankle Int* 21:916, 2000.
Author: **Lonnie R. Mercier, M.D.**

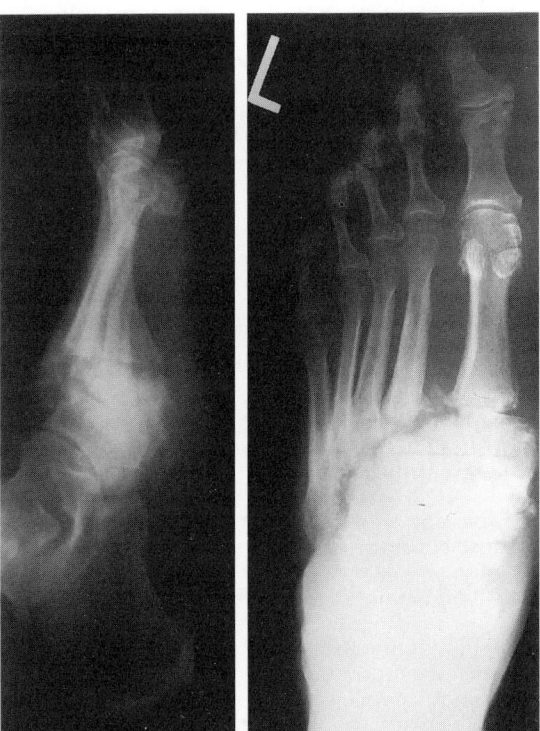

Fig. 1-100 Diabetes mellitus and neuropathic arthritis. Note lateral displacement of metatarsals *(left)* and fragmentation and osseous debris *(right)*. (From Goldman L, Bennett JC [eds]: *Cecil textbook of medicine,* ed 21, Philadelphia, 2000, WB Saunders.)

BASIC INFORMATION

■ DEFINITION
Chickenpox is a common viral illness characterized by acute onset of generalized vesicular rash and fever.

■ SYNONYMS
Varicella

■ ICD-9CM CODES
052.9 Varicella

■ EPIDEMIOLOGY & DEMOGRAPHICS
- The incubation period of chickenpox ranges from 9 to 21 days.
- Peak incidence is in the springtime.
- The predominant age is 5 to 10 yr.
- Infectious period begins 2 days before onset of clinical symptoms and lasts until all lesions have crusted.
- Most patients will have lifelong immunity following an attack of chickenpox; protection from chickenpox following varicella vaccine is approximately 6 yr.

■ PHYSICAL FINDINGS & CLINICAL PRESENTATION
- Findings vary with the clinical course. Initial symptoms consist of fever, chills, backache, generalized malaise, and headache.
- Symptoms are generally more severe in adults.
- Initial lesions generally occur on the trunk (centripetal distribution) and occasionally on the face; these lesions consist primarily of 3- to 4-mm red papules with an irregular outline and a clear vesicle on the surface (dew drops on a rose petal appearance).
- Intense pruritus generally accompanies this stage.
- New lesion development generally ceases by the fourth day with subsequent crusting by the sixth day.
- Lesions generally spread to the face and the extremities (centrifugal spread).
- Patients generally present with lesions at different stages at the same time.
- Crusts generally fall off within 5 to 14 days.
- Fever is usually highest during the eruption of the vesicles; temperature generally returns to normal following disappearance of vesicles.
- Signs of potential complications (e.g., bacterial skin infections, neurologic complications, pneumonia, hepatitis) may be present on physical examination.
- Mild constitutional symptoms (e.g., anorexia, myalgias, headaches, restlessness) may be present (most common in adults).
- Excoriations may be present if scratching is prominent.

■ ETIOLOGY
Varicella-zoster virus is a human herpesvirus III that can manifest with either varicella or herpes zoster (i.e., shingles, which is a reactivation of varicella).

DIAGNOSIS

■ DIFFERENTIAL DIAGNOSIS
- Other viral infection (see Tables 2-61 and 2-72 for differential diagnosis of exanthems and fever and rash)
- Impetigo
- Scabies
- Drug rash
- Urticaria
- Dermatitis herpetiformis

■ WORKUP
Diagnosis is usually made based on patient's history and clinical presentation.

■ LABORATORY TESTS
- Laboratory evaluation is generally not necessary.
- CBC may reveal leukopenia and thrombocytopenia.
- Serum varicella titers (significant rise in serum varicella IgG antibody level), skin biopsy, or Tzanck smear are used only when diagnosis is in question.

TREATMENT

■ NONPHARMACOLOGIC THERAPY
- Use antipruritic lotions for symptomatic relief.
- Avoid scratching to prevent excoriations and superficial skin infections.
- Use a mild soap for bathing; hands should be washed often.

■ ACUTE GENERAL Rx
- Use acetaminophen for fever and myalgias; aspirin should be avoided because of the increased risk of Reye's syndrome.
- Oral acyclovir (20 mg/kg qid for 5 days) initiated at the earliest sign (within 24 hr of illness) is useful in healthy, nonpregnant individuals 13 yr of age or older to decrease the duration and severity of signs and symptoms. Immunocompromised hosts should be treated with IV acyclovir 500 mg/m^2 or 10 mg/kg q8h IV for 7 to 10 days.
- Varicella-zoster immunoglobulin (VZIG) is effective in preventing chickenpox in susceptible individuals. Dose is 12.5 U/kg IM (up to a maximum of 625 U). May repeat dose 3 wk later if the exposure persists; VZIG must be administered as early as possible after presumed exposure.
- Varicella vaccine is available for children and adults; protection lasts at least 6 yr. Patients with HIV or other immunocompromised patients should not receive the live attenuated vaccine.
- Pruritus from chickenpox can be controlled with antihistamines (e.g., hydroxyzine 25 mg q6h) and oral antipruritic lotions (e.g., calamine).
- Oral antibiotics are not routinely indicated and should be used only in patients with secondary infection and infected lesions (most common infective organisms are *Streptococcus* sp. and *Staphylococcus* sp.).

■ DISPOSITION
- The course is generally benign in immunocompetent adults and children.
- Infants who develop chickenpox are incapable of controlling the infection and should be given varicella-zoster immunoglobulin or γ-globulin if VZIG is not available.

■ REFERRAL
Hospitalization and IV acyclovir are recommended for immunocompromised patients with chickenpox and for patients who develop neurologic complications or pneumonia.

PEARLS & CONSIDERATIONS

■ COMMENTS
- VZIG can be obtained from the nearest regional Red Cross Blood Center or the Centers for Disease Control and Prevention in Atlanta, Georgia.
- Varicella immunization (Varivax) is recommended for all who have not had chickenpox; dosage for adults and adolescents (≥13 yr old) is two 0.5-ml doses 4 to 8 wk apart.

REFERENCE
Cohen JI: Recent advances in varicella-zoster virus infection, *Ann Intern Med* 130:922, 1999.
Author: **Fred F. Ferri, M.D.**

BASIC INFORMATION

■ DEFINITION
Genital infection with *Chlamydia trachomatis* may result in urethritis, epididymitis, cervicitis, and acute salpingitis, but often it is asymptomatic in women (see "Pelvic Inflammatory Disease").

ICD-9CM CODES
597.80 Urethritis
604.0 Epididymitis
616.0 Cervicitis
381.51 Acute salpingitis

■ EPIDEMIOLOGY & DEMOGRAPHICS
- *Chlamydia trachomatis* is the most common cause of sexually transmitted disease in the U.S. More than 4 million infections occur annually, although the exact number is unknown because reporting is not required in all states. Occurrence is common worldwide, and recognition has been increasing steadily over the last two decades in the U.S., Canada, Australia, and Europe.
- Most women with endocervical or urethral infections are asymptomatic.
- Up to 45% of cases of gonococcal infection may have concomitant chlamydial infection.
- Infertility or ectopic pregnancy can result as a complication from symptomatic or asymptomatic chronic infections of the endometrium and fallopian tubes.
- Conjunctival and pneumonic infection of the newborn may result from infection in pregnancy.

■ PHYSICAL FINDINGS & CLINICAL PRESENTATION
Clinical manifestations may be similar to those of gonorrhea: mucopurulent endocervical discharge, with edema, erythema, and easily induced endocervical bleeding caused by inflammation of endocervical columnar epithelium. Less frequent manifestations may include bartholinitis, urethral syndrome with dysuria and pyuria, perihepatitis (Fitz-Hugh–Curtis syndrome).

■ ETIOLOGY
- *Chlamydia trachomatis*, serotypes D through K
- Obligate, intracellular bacteria

DIAGNOSIS

■ DIFFERENTIAL DIAGNOSIS
Gonorrhea, nongonococcal urethritis (nonchlamydial etiologies)

■ WORKUP
Diagnosis based on laboratory demonstration of evidence of infection in intraurethral or endocervical swab by various tests. The intracellular organism is less readily recovered from the discharge.

■ LABORATORY TESTS
- Cell culture is the reference method for diagnosis (single culture sensitivity 80% to 90%), but it is labor intensive and takes 48 to 96 hr; it is not suited for large screening programs
- Nonculture methods:
  Direct fluorescent antibody (DFA) tests
  Enzyme immunoassay (EIA)
  DNA probes
  Polymerase chain reaction (PCR)
- With the exception of PCR, the other tests are probably less specific than cell culture and may yield false-positive results.
- Because this is an intracellular organism, purulent discharge is not an appropriate specimen. An adequate sample of infected cells must be obtained.

TREATMENT

Urethritis, cervicitis, conjunctivitis (except for LGV):
- Azithromycin 1 g PO × 1 *or*
- Doxycycline 100 mg PO bid for 7 days

- Alternatives
  1. Erythromycin base 500 mg PO qid for 7 days *or*
  2. Erythromycin ethylsuccinate 800 mg PO qid for 7 days *or*
  3. Ofloxacin 300 mg PO bid for 7 days

Infection in pregnancy:
- Erythromycin base 500 mg PO qid for 7 days *or*
- Amoxicillin 500 mg PO tid for 7 days

Alternatives:
  1. Erythromycin base 250 mg PO qid for 7 days *or*
  2. Erythromycin ethylsuccinate 800 mg PO qid for 7 days *or*
  3. Erythromycin ethylsuccinate 400 mg PO qid for 14 days *or*
  4. Azithromycin 1 g PO (single dose)

NOTE: Doxycycline and ofloxacin are contraindicated in pregnancy. Safety and efficacy of azithromycin are not established in pregnancy and lactation, although preliminary data indicate that it may be safe and effective. Erythromycin estolate is contraindicated in pregnancy because of drug-related hepatotoxicity.

■ DISPOSITION
See "Gonorrhea." In all patients being treated for chlamydia, presumptive treatment for concomitant infection with gonorrhea should be done. Also see "Treatment" in "Pelvic Inflammatory Disease."

REFERENCE
Centers for Disease Control: Guidelines for treatment of sexually transmitted diseases, *MMWR* 47(RR-1):1, 1998.
Author: **Eugene J. Louie-Ng, M.D.**

BASIC INFORMATION

■ DEFINITION
Cholangitis refers to an inflammation and/or infection of the hepatic and common bile ducts associated with obstruction of the common bile duct.

■ SYNONYMS
Biliary sepsis
Ascending cholangitis
Suppurative cholangitis

ICD-9CM CODES
576.1 Cholangitis

■ EPIDEMIOLOGY & DEMOGRAPHICS
INCIDENCE (IN U.S.): Complicates approximately 1% of cases of cholelithiasis
PREVALENCE (IN U.S.): 2 cases/1000 hospital admissions
PREDOMINANT SEX:
- Females, for cholangitis secondary to gallstones
- Males, for cholangitis secondary to malignant obstruction and HIV infection

PREDOMINANT AGE: Seventh decade and older; unusual <50 yr of age
PEAK INCIDENCE: Seventh decade

■ PHYSICAL FINDINGS & CLINICAL PRESENTATION
- Usually acute onset of fever, chills, abdominal pain, tenderness over the RUQ of the abdomen, and jaundice (Charcot's triad)
- All signs and symptoms in only 50% to 85% of patients
- Often, dark coloration of the urine resulting from bilirubinuria
- Complications:
  1. Bacteremia (50%) and septic shock
  2. Hepatic abscess and pancreatitis

■ ETIOLOGY
Obstruction of the common bile duct causing rapid proliferation of bacteria in the biliary tree
- Most common cause of common bile duct obstruction: stones, usually migrated from the gallbladder
- Other causes: prior biliary tract surgery with secondary stenosis, tumor (usually arising from the pancreas or biliary tree), and parasitic infections from *Ascaris lumbricoides* or *Fasciola hepatica*
- Iatrogenic after contamination of an obstructed biliary tree by endoscopic retrograde cholangiopancreatoscopy (ERCP) or percutaneous transhepatic cholangiography (PTC)

- Primary sclerosing cholangitis (PSC)
- HIV-associated sclerosing cholangitis: associated with infection by CMV, *Cryptosporidium,* Microsporida, and *Mycobacterium avium* complex

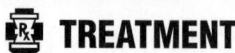

DIAGNOSIS

■ DIFFERENTIAL DIAGNOSIS
- Biliary colic
- Acute cholecystitis
- Liver abscess
- PUD
- Pancreatitis
- Intestinal obstruction
- Right kidney stone
- Hepatitis
- Pyelonephritis

■ WORKUP
- Blood cultures
- CBC
- Liver function tests

■ LABORATORY TESTS
- Usually, elevated WBC count with a predominance of polynuclear forms
- Elevated alkaline phosphatase and bilirubin in chronic obstruction
- Elevated transaminases in acute obstruction
- Positive blood cultures in 50% of cases, typically with enteric gram-negative aerobes (e.g., *E. coli, Klebsiella pneumoniae*), enterococci, or anaerobes

■ IMAGING STUDIES
- Ultrasound:
  1. Allows visualization of the gallbladder and bile ducts to differentiate extrahepatic obstruction from intrahepatic cholestasis
  2. Insensitive but specific for visualization of common duct stones
- CT scan:
  1. Less accurate for gallstones
  2. More sensitive than ultrasound for visualization of the distal part of the common bile duct
  3. Also allows better definition of neoplasm
- ERCP:
  1. Confirms obstruction and its level
  2. Allows collection of specimens for culture and cytology
  3. Indicated for diagnosis if ultrasound and CT scan are inconclusive
  4. May be indicated in therapy (see "Treatment")

TREATMENT

■ NONPHARMACOLOGIC THERAPY
Biliary decompression
- May be urgent in severely ill patients or those unresponsive to medical therapy within 12 to 24 hr
- May also be performed semielectively in patients who respond
- Options:
  1. ERCP with or without sphincterotomy or placement of a draining stent
  2. Percutaneous transhepatic biliary drainage for the acutely ill patient who is a poor surgical candidate
  3. Surgical exploration of the common bile duct

■ ACUTE GENERAL Rx
- Nothing by mouth
- Intravenous hydration
- Broad-spectrum antibiotics directed at gram-negative enteric organisms, anaerobes, and enterococcus: if infection is nosocomial, post-ERCP, or the patient is in shock, strong consideration of broader coverage to include hospital organisms such as *Pseudomonas aeruginosa,* resistant *Staphylococcus aureus,* and others.

■ CHRONIC Rx
Repeated decompression may be necessary, particularly when obstruction is related to neoplasm.

■ DISPOSITION
Excellent prognosis if obstruction is amenable to definitive surgical therapy; otherwise relapses are common.

■ REFERRAL
- To biliary endoscopist if obstruction is from stones or a stent needs to be placed
- To interventional radiologist if external drainage is necessary
- To a general surgeon in all other cases
- To an infectious disease specialist if blood cultures are positive or the patient is in shock or otherwise severely ill

REFERENCE
Hanau LH, Steibigel NH: Acute (ascending) cholangitis, *Infect Dis Clin North Am* 14(3):521, 2000.
Author: **Michele Halpern, M.D.**

BASIC INFORMATION

■ **DEFINITION**

Cholecystitis is an acute or chronic inflammation of the gallbladder generally secondary to gallstones (>95% of cases)

■ **SYNONYMS**

Gallbladder attack

ICD-9CM CODES

575.0 Acute cholecystitis
574.0 Calculus of the gallbladder with acute cholecystitis
575.1 Cholecystitis without mention of calculus

■ **EPIDEMIOLOGY & DEMOGRAPHICS**

• Acute cholecystitis occurs most commonly in females during the fifth and sixth decades.
• The incidence of gallstones is 0.6% in the general population and much higher in certain ethnic groups (>75% of Native Americans by age 60 yr).

■ **PHYSICAL FINDINGS & CLINICAL PRESENTATION**

• Pain and tenderness in the right hypochondrium or epigastrium; pain possibly radiating to the infrascapular region
• Palpation of the RUQ eliciting marked tenderness and stoppage of inspired breath (Murphy's sign)
• Guarding
• Fever (33%)
• Jaundice (25% to 50% of patients)
• Palpable gallbladder (20% of cases)
• Nausea and vomiting (>70% of patients)
• Fever and chills (>25% of patients)
• Medical history often revealing ingestion of large, fatty meals before onset of pain in the epigastrium and RUQ

■ **ETIOLOGY**

• Gallstones (>95% of cases)
• Ischemic damage to the gallbladder, critically ill patient (acalculous cholecystitis)
• Infectious agents, especially in patients with AIDS (CMV, *Cryptosporidium*)
• Strictures of the bile duct
• Neoplasms, primary or metastatic

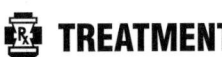 **DIAGNOSIS**

■ **DIFFERENTIAL DIAGNOSIS**

• Hepatic: hepatitis, abscess, hepatic congestion, neoplasm, trauma
• Biliary: neoplasm, stricture

• Gastric: PUD, neoplasm, alcoholic gastritis, hiatal hernia
• Pancreatic: pancreatitis, neoplasm, stone in the pancreatic duct or ampulla
• Renal: calculi, infection, inflammation, neoplasm, ruptured kidney
• Pulmonary: pneumonia, pulmonary infarction, right-sided pleurisy
• Intestinal: retrocecal appendicitis, intestinal obstruction, high fecal impaction
• Cardiac: myocardial ischemia (particularly involving the inferior wall), pericarditis
• Cutaneous: herpes zoster
• Trauma
• Fitz-Hugh–Curtis syndrome (perihepatitis)
• Subphrenic abscess
• Dissecting aneurysm
• Nerve root irritation caused by osteoarthritis of the spine

■ **WORKUP**

Laboratory evaluation and imaging studies

■ **LABORATORY TESTS**

• Leukocytosis (12,000 to 20,000) is present in >70% of patients.
• Elevated alkaline phosphatase, ALT, AST, bilirubin; bilirubin elevation >4 mg/dl is unusual and suggests presence of choledocholithiasis.
• Elevated amylase may be present (consider pancreatitis if serum amylase elevation exceeds 500 U).

■ **IMAGING STUDIES**

• Nuclear imaging (HIDA scan) is useful for diagnosis of acalculous cholecystitis: sensitivity and specificity exceed 90% for acute cholecystis. This test is only reliable when bilirubin is <5 mg/dl. A positive test will demonstrate obstruction of the cystic or common hepatic duct; the test will not demonstrate the presence of stones.
• Ultrasound of the gallbladder will demonstrate the presence of stones and also dilated gallbladder with thickened wall and surrounding edema in patients with acute cholecystitis.
• CT scan of abdomen is useful in cases of suspected abscess, neoplasm, or pancreatitis.
• Plain film of the abdomen generally is not useful, because <25% of stones are radiopaque.

TREATMENT

■ **NONPHARMACOLOGIC THERAPY**

Provide IV hydration; withhold oral feedings.

■ **ACUTE GENERAL Rx**

• Cholecystectomy (laparoscopic is preferred, open cholecystectomy is acceptable); conservative management with IV fluids and antibiotics may be justified in some high-risk patients in order to convert an emergency procedure into an elective one with a lower mortality.
• ERCP with sphincterectomy and stone extraction can be performed in conjunction with laparoscopic cholecystectomy for patients with choledochal lithiasis; approximately 7% to 15% of patients with cholelithiasis also have stones in the common bile duct.
• IV fluids, broad-spectrum antibiotics, pain management (meperidine PRN) should be used.

■ **DISPOSITION**

• Prognosis is good; elective laparoscopic cholecystectomy can be performed as outpatient procedure.
• Hospital stay (when necessary) varies from overnight with laparoscopic cholecystectomy to 4 to 7 days with open cholecystectomy.
• Complication rate is approximately 1% (hemorrhage and bile leak) for laparoscopic cholecystectomy and <0.5% (infection) with open cholecystectomy.

■ **REFERRAL**

Hospitalization and surgical referral in all patients with acute cholecystitis

☼ **PEARLS & CONSIDERATIONS**

■ **COMMENTS**

• Patients should be instructed that stones may recur in bile ducts.
• Gallbladder aspiration in which all fluid visualized by ultrasound is aspirated represents a nonsurgical treatment when patients who are at high operative risk develop acute cholecystitis. Salvage cholecystectomy is reserved for nonresponders.

REFERENCE

Chopra S et al: Treatment of acute patients at high surgical risk: comparison of clinical outcomes after gallbladder aspiration and after percutaneous cholecystoctomy, *AJR Am J Roentgenol* 176:1025, 2001.
Author: **Fred F. Ferri, M.D.**

BASIC INFORMATION

■ DEFINITION
Cholelithiasis is the presence of stones in the gallbladder.

■ SYNONYMS
Gallstones

ICD-9CM CODES
574.2 Calculus of the gallbladder without mention of cholecystitis
574.0 Calculus of the gallbladder with acute cholecystitis

■ EPIDEMIOLOGY & DEMOGRAPHICS
- Gallstone disease can be found in 20 million Americans. Of these, 2% to 3% (500,000 to 600,000) are treated with cholecystectomies each year.
- Annual medical expenditures for gallbladder surgeries in the U.S. exceed $5 billion.
- Incidence of gallbladder disease increases with age. Highest incidence is in the fifth and sixth decades. Predisposing factors for gallstones are female sex, pregnancy, age >40 yr, family history of gallstones, obesity, ileal disease, oral contraceptives, diabetes mellitus, rapid weight loss, estrogen replacement therapy.
- Patients with gallstones have a 20% chance of developing biliary colic or its complications at the end of a 20-yr period.

■ PHYSICAL FINDINGS & CLINICAL PRESENTATION
- Physical examination is entirely normal unless patient is having a biliary colic; 80% of gallstones are asymptomatic.
- Typical symptoms of obstruction of the cystic duct include intermittent, severe, cramping pain affecting the RUQ.
- Pain occurs mostly at night and may radiate to the back or right shoulder. It can last from a few minutes to several hours.

■ ETIOLOGY
- 75% of gallstones contain cholesterol and are usually associated with obesity, female sex, diabetes mellitus; mixed stones are most common (80%), pure cholesterol stones account for only 10% of stones.
- 25% of gallstones are pigment stones (bilirubin, calcium, and variable organic material) associated with hemolysis and cirrhosis. These tend to be black pigment stones that are refractory to medical therapy.
- 50% of mixed-type stones are radiopaque.

 DIAGNOSIS

■ DIFFERENTIAL DIAGNOSIS
- PUD
- GERD
- IBD
- Pancreatitis
- Neoplasms
- Nonnuclear dyspepsia

■ LABORATORY TESTS
Generally normal unless patient has biliary obstruction (elevated alkaline phosphatase, bilirubin).

■ IMAGING STUDIES
- Ultrasound of the gallbladder will detect small stones and biliary sludge (sensitivity, 95%; specificity, 90%); the presence of dilated gallbladder with thickened wall is suggestive of acute cholecystitis.
- Nuclear imaging (HIDA scan) can confirm acute cholecystitis (>90% accuracy) if gallbladder does not visualize within 4 hr of injection and the radioisotope is excreted in the common bile duct.

 TREATMENT

■ NONPHARMACOLOGIC THERAPY
Life-style changes (avoidance of diets high in polyunsaturated fats, weight loss in obese patients—however, avoid rapid weight loss)

■ ACUTE GENERAL Rx
- The management of gallstones is affected by the clinical presentation.
- Asymptomatic patients do not require therapeutic intervention.
- Surgical intervention is generally the ideal approach for symptomatic patients. Laparoscopic cholecystectomy is generally preferred over open cholecystectomy because of the shorter recovery period.
- Patients who are not appropriate candidates for surgery because of coexisting illness or patients who refuse surgery can be treated with oral bile salts: ursodiol (Actigall) 8 to 10 mg/kg/day in two to three divided doses for 16 to 20 mo, or chenodiol (Chenix) 250 mg bid initially, increasing gradually to a dose of 60 mg/kg/day. Candidates for oral bile salts are patients with cholesterol stones (radiolucent, noncalcified stones), with a diameter of ≤15 mm and having three or fewer stones.
- Direct solvent dissolution with methyl *tert*-butyl ether (MTBE) can be used in patients with multiple stones with diameter ≥3 cm; this method should be used only by physicians experienced with contact dissolution. Administration of the solvent is either through percutaneous transhepatic placement of a catheter into the gallbladder or endoscopic retrograde catheter placement with subsequent continuous infusion and aspiration of the solvent either manually or by automatic pump system. MTBE is a powerful cholesterol solvent and can dissolve stones in a few hours (>90% dissolution over a 2-hr infusion).
- Extracorporeal shock wave lithotripsy (ESWL) is another form of medical therapy. It can be used in patients with stone diameter of ≤3 cm and having three or fewer stones.
- Candidates for medical therapy must have a functioning gallbladder and must have absence of calcifications on CT scans.

■ DISPOSITION
- Recurrence rate after bile acid treatment is approximately 50% in 5 yr. Periodic ultrasound is necessary to assess the effectiveness of treatment.
- Gallstones recur after dissolution therapy with MTBE in >40% of patients within 5 yr.
- Following extracorporeal shock wave lithotripsy, stones recur in approximately 20% of patients after 4 yr.
- Patients with at least 1 gallstone <5 mm in diameter have a greater than fourfold increased risk of presenting with acute biliary pancreatitis. A policy of watchful waiting in such cases is generally unwarranted.
- A potential serious complication of gallstones is acute cholangitis. ERCP and endoscopic sphincterectomy (EC) followed by interval laparoscopic cholecystectomy is effective in acute cholangitis.

■ REFERRAL
Surgical referral for cholecystectomy in symptomatic patients who are surgical candidates

REFERENCES
Ahmed A et al: Management of gallstones and their complications, *Am Fam Physician* 61:1673, 2000.
Poon RT et al: Management of gallstone cholangitis in the era of laparoscopic cholecystectomy, *Arch Surg* 136:11, 2001.
Author: **Fred F. Ferri, M.D.**

BASIC INFORMATION

DEFINITION
Cholera is an acute diarrheal illness caused by *Vibrio cholerae*.

ICD-9CM CODES
001 Cholera

EPIDEMIOLOGY & DEMOGRAPHICS
INCIDENCE (IN U.S.): Approximately 50 cases/yr, most in travelers returning from endemic areas
PREDOMINANT AGE:
- In nonendemic areas, attack rates equal in all age groups
- In epidemic areas, children >2 yr old most commonly infected
PEAK INCIDENCE:
- None in the U.S.
- Summer and fall in endemic areas
GENETICS:
Neonatal Infection: Illness uncommon before age 2 yr, probably because of passive immunity

PHYSICAL FINDINGS & CLINICAL PRESENTATION
- Asymptomatic illness or a mild diarrhea
- Classic illness: abrupt onset of voluminous watery diarrhea, which may lead to severe dehydration, acidosis, shock, and death
- Vomiting early in the illness, but usually absence of fever and abdominal pain
- Typical "rice water" stools, pale with flecks of mucus and no blood
- Possibly prominent muscle cramps attributable to loss of fluid and electrolytes
- Untreated illness: results in hypovolemic shock and death in hours to days
- With adequate fluid and electrolyte repletion, a self-limited illness that resolves in a few days
- Antimicrobials shorten the course of illness

ETIOLOGY
Responsible organism is one of several strains of *V. cholerae,* with most infections from the O1 serotype, the *El Tor* biotype.
- In the U.S., one outbreak occurred from the ingestion of illegally imported crab, and sporadic infection has been associated with the consumption of contaminated shellfish in Gulf Coast states.
- Most cases occur in returning travelers.
- Transmission during epidemics results from ingestion of contaminated water and, in some instances, contaminated food.
- Achlorhydria or the use of gastric acid–suppressing agents can increase susceptibility to infection.
- Cholera toxin acts on intestinal epithelial cells to cause secretion of massive amounts of fluid and electrolytes.

DIAGNOSIS

DIFFERENTIAL DIAGNOSIS
- Mild illness mimicking gastroenteritis from a variety of etiologies
- Sudden, voluminous diarrhea causing marked dehydration uncommon in other illnesses
A differential diagnosis of infectious diseases in travelers is described in Table 2-110.

WORKUP
Send stool for culture and microscopy. NOTE: Treatment should not be delayed while awaiting culture results.

LABORATORY TESTS
- Possibly elevated WBC count; increased Hgb as a result of hemoconcentration
- Elevated BUN and creatinine suggesting prerenal azotemia
- Hypoglycemia
- Stool cultures on appropriate media to grow the organism
- Wet mount of stool under dark-field or phase contrast microscopy to show organisms with characteristic darting motility

TREATMENT

NONPHARMACOLOGIC THERAPY
Adequate fluid and electrolyte replacement:
- Usually achieved using oral rehydration solutions containing salts and glucose
- The addition of an orally administered nonabsorbed starch (e.g., 50 g of high amylose maize starch per liter of oral rehydration solution) reduces fecal fluid loss and shortens the duration of diarrhea in adolescents and adults with cholera.
- IV fluid and electrolyte replacement sometimes required

ACUTE GENERAL Rx
Antimicrobial therapy to decrease shedding of fluid and organisms and shorten the course of illness:
- Doxycycline 100 mg PO bid for 5 days *or*
- Septra one DS tablet PO bid for 5 days

CHRONIC Rx
It is likely that asymptomatic chronic carriers exist, but since they are difficult to identify and their role in transmission of disease appears limited, there is no recommendation for treatment of these individuals.

DISPOSITION
Mortality of adequately hydrated patients is <1%.

REFERRAL
If more than mild illness occurs

PEARLS & CONSIDERATIONS

COMMENTS
- Currently, there is no indication for vaccination of travelers to endemic areas: the risk of infection is small, protection from available vaccines is limited, and side effects are prominent and frequent.
- Doxycycline should not be used to treat children or pregnant women.

REFERENCES
Ramakrishna BS et al: Amylase-resistant starch plus oral rehydration solution for cholera, *N Engl J Med* 342:308, 2000.
Raufman JP: Cholera, *Am J Med* 104:386, 1998.
Author: **Maurice Policar, M.D.**

BASIC INFORMATION

■ DEFINITION
Chronic fatigue syndrome (CFS) is characterized by four or more of the following symptoms, present concurrently for at least 6 mo:
- Impaired memory or concentration
- Sore throat
- Tender cervical or axillary lymph nodes
- Muscle pain
- Multijoint pain
- New headaches
- Unrefreshing sleep
- Postexertion malaise

■ SYNONYMS
Yuppie flu
CFS
Chronic Epstein-Barr syndrome

ICD-9CM CODES
780.7 Chronic fatigue syndrome
300.8 Neurasthenia

■ EPIDEMIOLOGY & DEMOGRAPHICS
PREVALENCE IN U.S.: 100 to 300 cases/100,000 persons
PREDOMINANT AGE: Young adulthood and middle age
PREDOMINANT SEX: Female > male

■ PHYSICAL FINDINGS & CLINICAL PRESENTATION
- There are no physical findings specific for CFS.
- The physical examination may be useful to identify fibromyalgia and other rheumatologic conditions that may coexist with CFS.

■ ETIOLOGY
- The etiology of CFS is unknown.
- Many experts suspect that a viral illness may trigger certain immune responses leading to the various symptoms. Most patients often report the onset of their symptoms with a flulike illness.
- Initial reports indicated a possible role of Epstein-Barr virus, but subsequent studies disproved this theory.

DIAGNOSIS

■ DIFFERENTIAL DIAGNOSIS
- Psychosocial depression, dysthymia, anxiety-related disorders, and other psychiatric diseases
- Infectious diseases (SBE, Lyme disease, fungal diseases, mononucleosis, HIV, chronic hepatitis B or C, TB, chronic parasitic infections)
- Autoimmune diseases: SLE, myasthenia gravis, multiple sclerosis, thyroiditis, RA
- Endocrine abnormalities: hypothyroidism, hypopituitarism, adrenal insufficiency, Cushing's syndrome, diabetes mellitus, hyperparathyroidism, pregnancy, reactive hypoglycemia
- Occult malignant disease
- Substance abuse
- Systemic disorders: chronic renal failure, COPD, cardiovascular disease, anemia, electrolyte abnormalities, liver disease
- Other: inadequate rest, sleep apnea, narcolepsy, fibromyalgia, sarcoidosis, medications, toxic agent exposure, Wegener's granulomatosis
- Table 2-70 describes the differential diagnosis of fatigue.

■ WORKUP
Because CFS is a clinical diagnosis and the symptoms are generally subjective, the history and physical examination are essential for excluding other causes of fatigue. A detailed mental status examination is necessary. Abnormalities should be further evaluated with appropriate psychiatric, psychologic, or neurologic examination. Fig. 3-66 describes an algorithmic approach to the patient presenting with fatigue.

■ LABORATORY TESTS
- No specific laboratory tests exist for diagnosing CFS. Initial laboratory tests are useful to exclude other conditions that may mimic or may be associated with CFS.
  1. Screening laboratory tests: CBC, ESR, ALT, total protein, albumin, globulin, alkaline phosphatase, calcium, phosphorus, glucose, BUN, creatinine, electrolytes, TSH, and urinalysis are useful.
  2. Serologic tests for Epstein-Barr virus, *Candida albicans,* human herpesvirus 6, and other studies for immune cellular abnormalities are not useful; these tests are expensive and generally not recommended.
- Other tests may be indicated depending on the history and physical examination (e.g., ANA, RF in patients presenting with joint complaints or abnormalities on physical examination, Lyme titer in areas where Lyme disease is endemic).

■ IMAGING STUDIES
Generally not recommended unless history and physical examination indicate specific abnormalities (e.g., chest x-ray examination in any patient suspected of TB or sarcoidosis)

TREATMENT

■ NONPHARMACOLOGIC THERAPY
- Education and counseling help to develop realistic goals and expectations.
- Support groups (see below) are useful.
- Patients should be reassured that the illness is not fatal and that most patients improve over time.
- An initially supervised exercise program to preserve and increase strength is beneficial for most patients and can improve symptoms.

■ ACUTE GENERAL Rx
Therapy is generally palliative. The following medications may be helpful:
- Antidepressants: The choice of antidepressant varies with the desired side effects. Patients with difficulty sleeping or fibromyalgia-like symptoms may benefit from low-dose tricyclics (doxepin 10 mg hs or amitriptyline 25 mg qhs). When sedation is not desirable, low-dose SSRIs (paroxetine 20 mg qd) often help alleviate fatigue and associated symptoms.
- NSAIDs can be used to relieve muscle and joint pain and headaches.
- Fludrocortisone as monotherapy for neurally mediated hypotension is no more efficacious than placebo.
- Low-dose hydrocortisone therapy provides a few benefits in quality of life; however, it is associated with frequent side effects and is not recommended.
"Alternative" medications (herbs, multivitamins, nutritional supplements) are very popular with many CFS patients but are generally not very helpful.

■ CHRONIC Rx
Psychiatric referral and treatment are helpful in coping with the disease in the majority of patients.

■ DISPOSITION
Moderate to complete recovery at 1 yr occurs in 22% to 60% of patients with CFS.

PEARLS & CONSIDERATIONS

■ COMMENTS
In CFS the symptoms are serious enough to reduce daily activities by >50% and in absence of any other medically identifiable disorders.

REFERENCES
Rowe PC et al: Fludrocortisone acetate to treat neurally mediated hypotension in chronic fatigue syndrome, *JAMA* 285:52, 2001.

Whiting P et al: Interventions for the treatment and management of chronic fatigue syndrome, *JAMA* 286:1360, 2001.
Author: **Fred F. Ferri, M.D.**

BASIC INFORMATION

■ DEFINITION
Chronic obstructive pulmonary disease (COPD) is a disorder characterized by the presence of airflow limitation that is not fully reversible. COPD encompasses *emphysema*, characterized by loss of lung elasticity and destruction of lung parenchyma with enlargement of air spaces, and *chronic bronchitis*, characterized by obstruction of small airways and productive cough greater than 3 months' duration for more than 2 successive years. Patients with COPD are classically subdivided in two major groups based on their appearance:

1. "Blue bloaters" are patients with chronic bronchitis; the name is derived from the bluish tinge of the skin (secondary to chronic hypoxemia and hypercapnia) and from the frequent presence of peripheral edema (secondary to cor pulmonale); chronic cough with production of large amounts of sputum is characteristic.
2. "Pink puffers" are patients with emphysema; they have a cachectic appearance but pink skin color (adequate oxygen saturation); shortness of breath is manifested by pursed-lip breathing and use of accessory muscles of respiration.

■ SYNONYMS
COPD
Emphysema
Chronic bronchitis

ICD-9CM CODES
496 COPD
492.8 Emphysema

■ EPIDEMIOLOGY & DEMOGRAPHICS
- COPD affects 16 million Americans and is responsible for >80,000 deaths/yr.
- Highest incidence is in males >40 yr.
- 16 million office visits, 500,000 hospitalizations, and >$18 billion in direct health care costs annually can be attributed to COPD.

■ PHYSICAL FINDINGS & CLINICAL PRESENTATION
- Blue bloaters (chronic bronchitis): peripheral cyanosis, productive cough, tachypnea, tachycardia
- Pink puffers (emphysema): dyspnea, pursed-lip breathing with use of accessory muscles for respiration, decreased breath sounds
- Possible wheezing in both patients with chronic bronchitis and emphysema

- Features of both chronic bronchitis and emphysema in many patients with COPD
- Acute exacerbation of COPD is mainly a clinical diagnosis and generally manifests with worsening dyspnea, increase in sputum purulence, and increase in sputum volume

■ ETIOLOGY
- Tobacco exposure
- Occupational exposure to pulmonary toxins (e.g., cadmium)
- Atmospheric pollution
- α-1 antitrypsin deficiency (rare; <1% of COPD patients)

DIAGNOSIS

■ DIFFERENTIAL DIAGNOSIS
- CHF
- Asthma
- Respiratory infections
- Bronchiectasis
- Cystic fibrosis
- Neoplasm
- Pulmonary embolism
- Sleep apnea, obstructive
- Hypothyroidism

■ WORKUP
Chest x-ray examination, pulmonary function testing, blood gases (in patients with acute exacerbation)

■ LABORATORY TESTS
- CBC may reveal leukocytosis with "shift to the left" during acute exacerbation.
- Sputum may be purulent with bacterial respiratory tract infections.
- ABGs: normocapnia, mild to moderate hypoxemia may be present.
- α-1 antitrypsin level is low in patients with α-1 antitrypsin deficiency (do not order this test routinely).
- Pulmonary function testing: abnormal diffusing capacity, increased total lung capacity and/or residual volume, fixed reduction in FEV_1 are present with emphysema; normal diffusing capacity, reduced FEV_1 are present with chronic bronchitis. Generally, acute spirometry should not be used to diagnose an exacerbation or assess its severity.

■ IMAGING STUDIES
Chest x-ray examination:
- Hyperinflation with flattened diaphragm, tending of the diaphragm at the rib, and increased retrosternal chest space (Fig. 1-101)
- Decreased vascular markings and bullae in patients with emphysema
- Thickened bronchial markings and enlarged right side of the heart in patients with chronic bronchitis

TREATMENT

■ NONPHARMACOLOGIC THERAPY
- Weight loss in patients with chronic bronchitis.
- Avoidance of tobacco use and elimination of air pollutants.
- Oxygen therapy on a PRN basis.
- Pulmonary toilet: careful nasotracheal suction is indicated in patients with excessive secretions and inability to expectorate. Mechanical percussion of the chest as applied by a physical or respiratory therapist is ineffective with acute exacerbations of COPD.

■ ACUTE GENERAL Rx
- Acute exacerbation of COPD can be treated with:
  1. Inhaled anticholinergic bronchodilators such as ipratropium are very productive.
  2. Inhaled short-acting B_2 agonists or use of a nebulizer to provide alauterol or a similar agent with saline and oxygen enhances delivery of the medications to the airways.
  3. IV methylprednisolone 50- to 100-mg bolus, then q6-8h; taper as soon as possible. Inhaled corticosteroids are useful in patients with moderate to severe COPD and in patients with frequent exacerbations.
  4. Judicious oxygen administration (hypercapnia and further respiratory compromise may occur after high-flow oxygen therapy); use of a Venturi-type mask delivering an inspired oxygen fraction of 24% to 28% is preferred to nasal cannula.
  5. Noninvasive positive pressure ventilation delivered by a facial or nasal mask in the treatment of chronic restrictive thoracic disease may obviate the need for intratracheal intubation.
- Antibiotics are indicated in suspected respiratory infection.
  1. *Haemophilus influenzae, Streptococcus pneumoniae* are frequent causes of acute bronchitis.
  2. Oral antibiotics of choice are azithromycin, levofloxacin, or cefuroxime.
  3. The use of antibiotics is beneficial in exacerbations of COPD presenting with increased dyspnea and sputum purulence (especially if the patient is febrile).
- Guaifenesin may improve cough symptoms and mucus clearance; however, mucolytic medications are generally ineffective. Their benefits may be greatest in patients with more advanced disease.

- Intubation and mechanical ventilation may be necessary if above measures fail to provide improvement.
- An algorithm for the general management of COPD is described in Fig. 1-102.

■ DISPOSITION
- Following the initial episode of respiratory failure, 5-yr survival is approximately 25%.

- Development of cor pulmonale or hypercapnia and persistent tachycardia are poor prognostic indicators.

⚙ PEARLS & CONSIDERATIONS

■ COMMENTS
- All patients with COPD should receive pneumococcal vaccine and yearly influenza vaccine.

REFERENCES
Bach PB et al: Management of acute exacerbations of chronic obstructive pulmonary disease: a summary and appraisal of published evidence, *Ann Intern Med* 134:600, 2001.

Barnes PJ: Chronic obstructive lung disease, *N Engl J Med* 343:269, 2000.

Snow V et al: Evidence base for management of acute exacerbations of chronic obstructive pulmonary disease, *Ann Intern Med* 134:595, 2001.

Author: **Fred F. Ferri, M.D.**

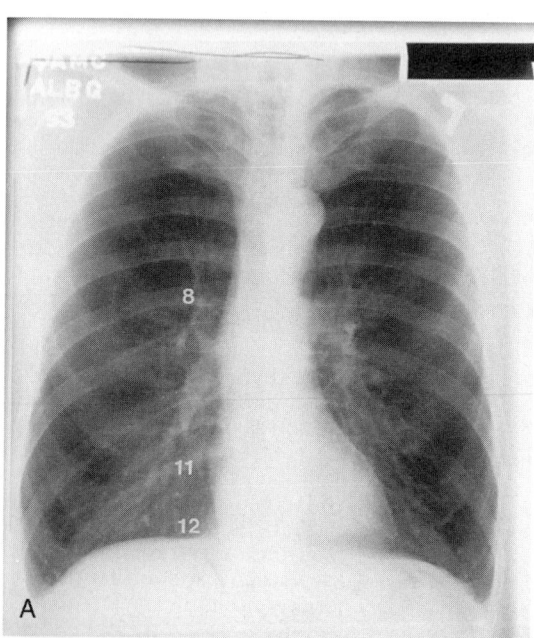

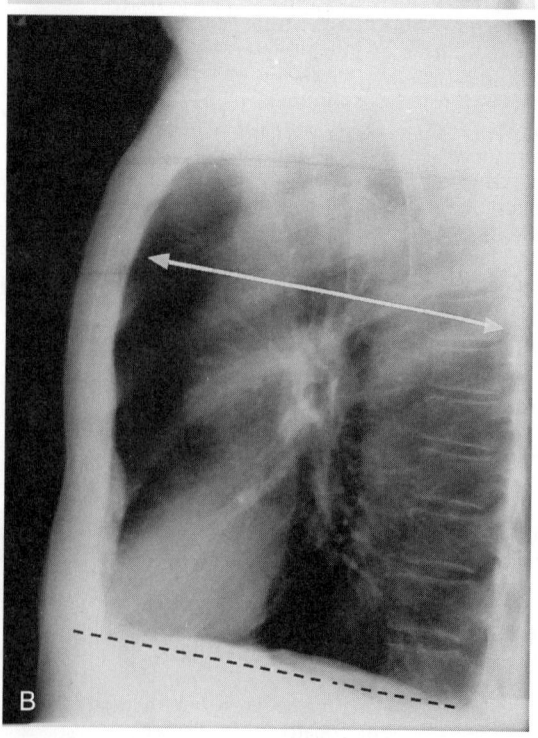

Fig. 1-101 Chronic obstructive pulmonary disease (COPD). The posteroanterior view **(A)** shows that the superior aspect of the hemidiaphragms is at the same level as the posterior aspect of the 12th ribs. Hyperinflation is also seen on the lateral view **(B)** as an increase in the anteroposterior diameter and flattening of the hemidiaphragms. (From Mettler FA [ed]: *Primary care radiology,* Philadelphia, 2000, WB Saunders.)

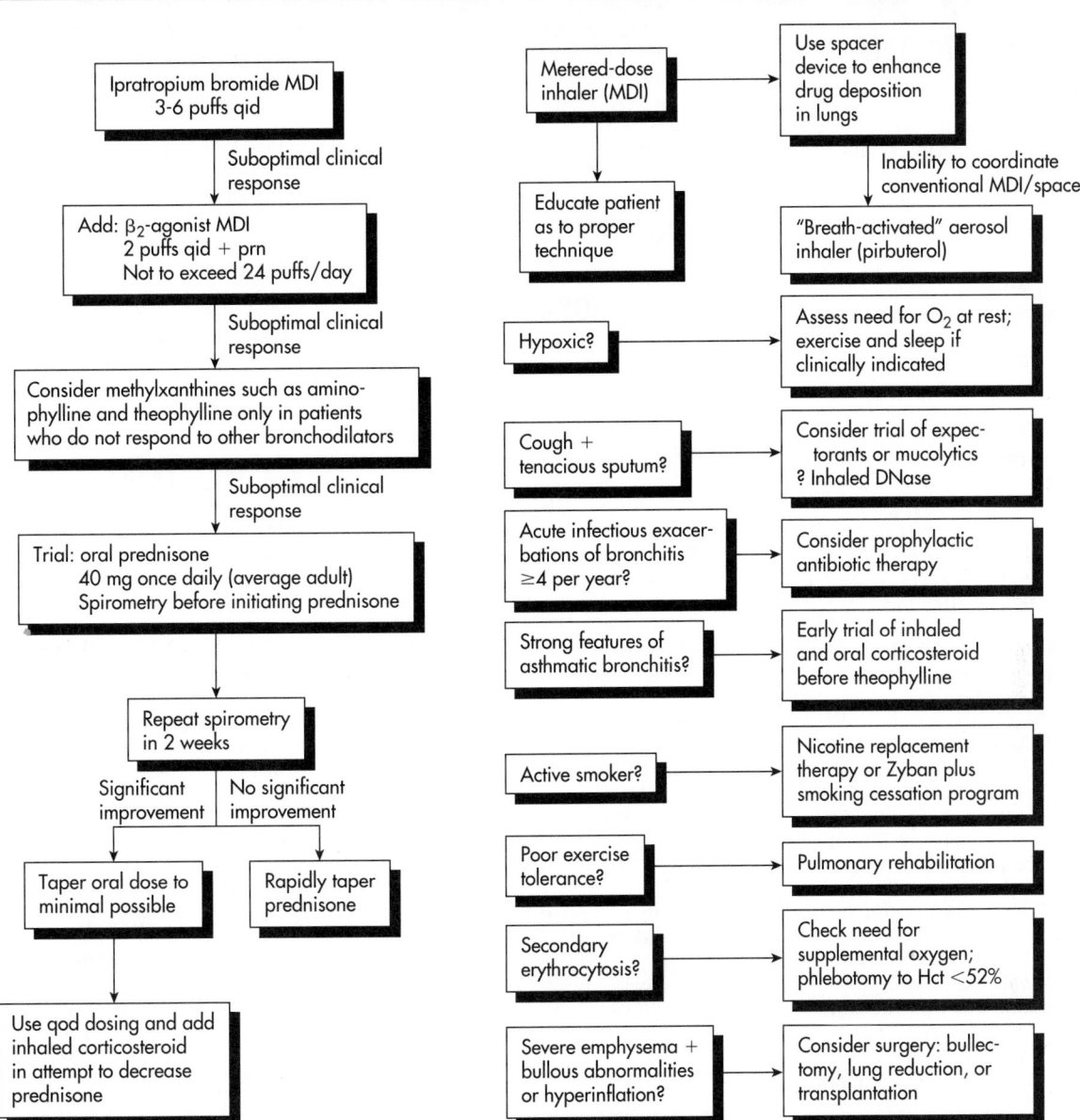

Fig. 1-102 Managed care guide: pharmacotherapy and general management approaches for chronic obstructive pulmonary disease (COPD). *DNase,* Deoxyribonuclease; *Hct,* hematocrit; *prn,* as needed; *qid,* four times a day; *qod,* every other day. (Modified from Noble J: *Primary care medicine,* ed 3, St Louis, 2001, Mosby.)

BASIC INFORMATION

■ DEFINITION

Churg-Strauss syndrome refers to a systemic vasculitis involving small-sized arteries characterized by asthma, hypereosinophilia, and necrotizing vasculitis with extravascular eosinophil granulomas.

■ SYNONYMS

Allergic angiitis and granulomatosis

ICD-9CM CODES

446.4 Angiitis, allergic granulomatous

■ EPIDEMIOLOGY & DEMOGRAPHICS

- Churg-Strauss syndrome is a rare disease
- At the Mayo Clinic, 90 cases were observed over a 19 year period from 1976-1995
- Affects males > females (2:1)
- Can occur at any age but usually affects young to middle-aged adults (~40 years of age)

■ PHYSICAL FINDINGS & CLINICAL PRESENTATION

Churg-Strauss syndrome can be described as occuring in three distinct phases:
1. The prodromal phase or allergic phase characterized by severe astina, either with or without allergic rhinitis, sinusites, headache, cough, and wheezing.
2. The eosinophilic phase characterized by peripheral eosinophilia and eosinophilic tissue infiltration producing signs and symptoms of cough, fever, anorexia, weight loss, sweats, malaise, abdominal pain, and diarrhea.
3. The vasculitic phase, which may involve any organ, including the heart (most frequent), lung, CNS, kidney, lymph nodes, muscle, and skin, and manifesting in chest pain, dyspnea, hemophysis, arthralgia, myalgias, peripheral neuropathy (mononeuritis multiplex), joint swelling, skin rash, and signs of CHF.

■ ETIOLOGY

- The cause of Churg-Strauss syndrome is unknown—a hypersensitivity immunological etiology has been proposed.
- Although similar and at times grouped with patients with polyarteritis nodosa (PAN), Churg-Strauss syndrome differs:
  1. Churg-Strauss syndrome vasculitis involves not only small-sized arteries but also veins and venules.
  2. Churg-Strauss syndrome, unlike PAN, predominantly involves the lung. Other organs affected include heart, GI, CNS, kidney, and skin.
  3. Churg-Strauss biopsy show necrotizing vasculitis along with a granulomatous extravascular reaction infiltrated by eosinophils.

DIAGNOSIS

The American College of Rheumatology has established criteria for the diagnosis of Churg-Strauss syndrome. For the diagnosis to be made at least 4 of the following 6 criteria must be met:
- Asthma
- Eosinophilia >10%
- Mononeuropathy or polyneuropathy
- Pulmonary infiltrates
- Paranasal sinus abnormalities
- Extravascular eosinophils

The presence of any 4 or more of the 6 criteria yields a sensitivity of 85% and a specificity of 99.7%.

■ DIFFERENTIAL DIAGNOSIS

- Polyarteritis nodosa
- Wegener's granulomatosis
- Sarcoidosis
- Loeffler syndrome
- Henoch-Schöenlein purpura
- Allergic bronchopulmonary aspergillosis
- Rheumatoid arthritis
- Leukocytoclastic vasculitis

■ WORKUP

If the clinical suspicion of Churg-Strauss is raised, further workup including blood tests, x-rays, and tissue biopsy help establish the diagnosis.

■ LABORATORY TESTS

- CBC with differential may reveal one diagnostic criterion: eosinophilia with counts ranging from 5000 to 10,000 eosinophils/mm³.
- ESR is usually elevated and a marker of inflammation.
- BUN/creatinine may be elevated, suggesting renal involvement.
- Urinalysis may show hematuria and proteinuria.
- 24-hour urine for protein if greater than 1 g/day is a poor prognostic factor.
- Antineutrophil cytoplasmic antibodies (ANCA), although not diagnostic of Churg-Strauss syndrome, are found in up to 70% of patients.
- AST, ALT, and CPK may indicate liver or muscle (skeletal or cardiac) involvement.

- RA and ANA may be positive.
- Biopsy substantiates the diagnosis if the characteristic findings as described above are seen.

■ IMAGING STUDIES

- Chest x-ray is abnormal in >50% of the cases and can show patchy migratory infiltrates, interstitial lung disease, or nodular infiltrates (Fig. 1-103).
- Paranasal sinus films may reveal sinus opacification.
- Angiography is sometimes done in patients with mesenteric ischemia or renal involvement.

TREATMENT

■ NONPHARMACOLOGIC THERAPY

Oxygen therapy in severe asthmatic exacerbations

■ ACUTE GENERAL Rx

- Corticosteroids are the treatment of choice. Prednisone 1 mg/kg/day is the starting dose and is continued for the first month. Thereafter, prednisone is tapered progressively to 10 mg/day at 1 yr.
- A drop in the eosinophil count and the ESR documents a response.

■ CHRONIC Rx

- Cyclophosphamide plus corticosteroids are used in patients with multiorgan involvement and poor prognostic factors.
- Many with persistent symptoms of asthma will require long-term corticosteroids even if vasculitis is no longer present.

■ DISPOSITION

- Clinical remissions are obtained in over 90% of patients.
- With treatment, long-term prognosis is good, with a 5-yr survival rate of 80%.
- The 5-year survival of untreated Churg-Strauss is 25%.
- Death usually occurs from progressive refractory vasculitis, myocardial involvement, or severe GI involvement (mesenteric ischemia, pancreatitis, etc.).

■ REFERRAL

If a patient is suspected of having Churg-Strauss syndrome, a pulmonary referral for diagnosis and management is appropriate.

PEARLS & CONSIDERATIONS

■ COMMENTS
• Poor prognostic factors include:
1. Renal insufficiency
2. Proteinuria >1g/day
3. GI involvement
4. Cardiac involvement
5. CNS involvement
• Churg-Strauss syndrome was first described by Churg and Strauss in 1951

after reviewing a number of autopsy cases previously classified as polyarteritis nodosa.

REFERENCES
Guillevin L et al: Prognostic factors in polyarteritis nodosa and Churg-Strauss syndrome: a prospective study of 342 patients, *Medicine* 75(1):17, 1996.
Guillevin L et al: Churg-Strauss syndrome: clinical study and long-term follow-up of 96 patients, *Medicine* 78(1):26, 1999.
Masi AT et al: American College of Rheumatology 1990 criteria for the classification of Churg-Strauss syndrome, *Arthritis Rheumatol* 33:1094, 1990.
Vogel P, Schissel D: Churg-Strauss syndrome (allergic granulonatosis), e *Medicine Journal* 2(10), 2001. (www.emedicine.com).
Author: **Peter Petropoulos, M.D.**

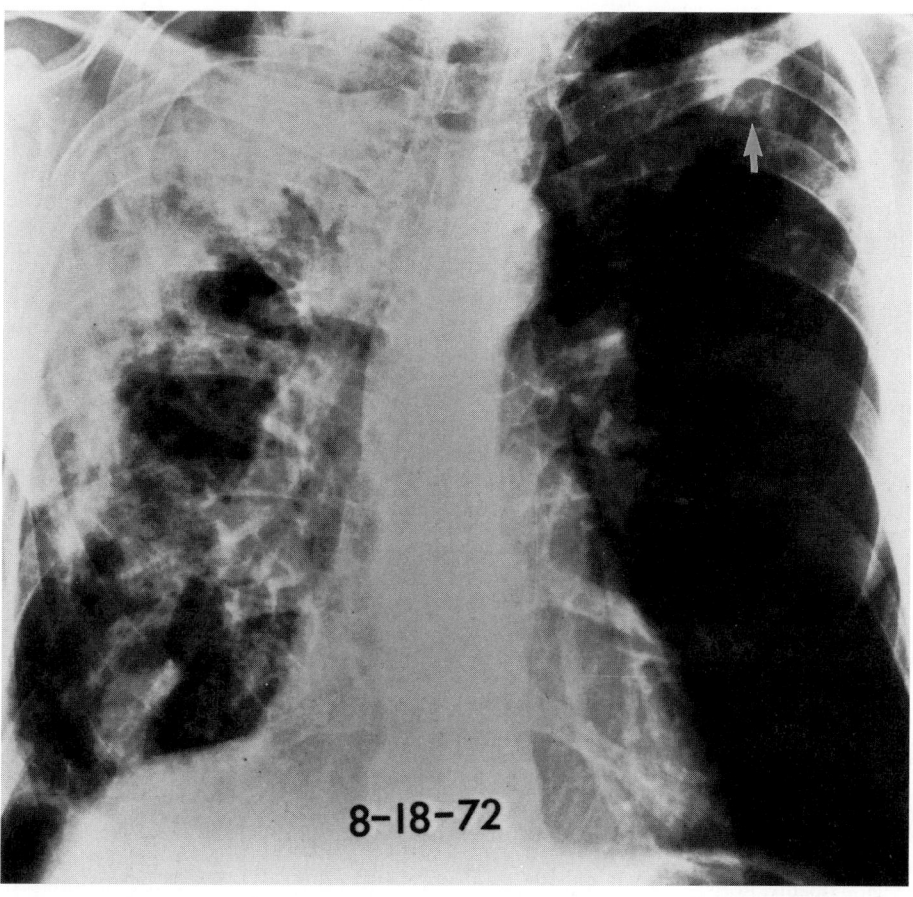

Fig. 1-103   Allergic angitis and granulomatosis. PA chest radiograph demonstrates peripheral air-space consolidation in the right lung and a nodule *(arrow)* in the left upper lobe in this asthmatic patient. (From McLoud TC [ed]: *Thoracic radiology, the requisites,* St Louis, 1998, Mosby.)

BASIC INFORMATION

■ DEFINITION

Cirrhosis is defined histologically as the presence of fibrosis and regenerative nodules in the liver. It can be classified as micronodular, macronodular, and mixed; however, each form may be seen in the same patient at different stages of the disease. Cirrhosis manifests clinically with portal hypertension, hepatic encephalopathy, and variceal bleeding.

ICD-9CM CODES
571.5 Cirrhosis of the liver
571.2 Cirrhosis of the liver secondary to alcohol

■ EPIDEMIOLOGY & DEMOGRAPHICS
- Cirrhosis is the eleventh leading cause of death in the U.S. (death rate 9 deaths/100,000 persons/yr).
- Alcohol abuse and viral hepatitis are the major causes of cirrhosis in the U.S.

■ PHYSICAL FINDINGS & CLINICAL PRESENTATION
SKIN: Jaundice, palmar erythema (alcohol abuse), spider angiomata, ecchymosis (thrombocytopenia or coagulation factor deficiency), dilated superficial periumbilical vein (caput medusae), increased pigmentation (hemochromatosis), xanthomas (primary biliary cirrhosis), needle tracks (viral hepatitis)
EYES: Kayser-Fleischer rings (corneal copper deposition seen in Wilson's disease; best diagnosed with slit lamp examination), scleral icterus
BREATH: Fetor hepaticus (musty odor of breath and urine found in cirrhosis with hepatic failure)
CHEST: Possible gynecomastia in men
ABDOMEN: Tender hepatomegaly (congestive hepatomegaly), small, nodular liver (cirrhosis), palpable, nontender gallbladder (neoplastic extrahepatic biliary obstruction), palpable spleen (portal hypertension), venous hum auscultated over periumbilical veins (portal hypertension), ascites (portal hypertension, hypoalbuminemia)
RECTAL EXAMINATION: Hemorrhoids (portal hypertension), guaiac-positive stools (alcoholic gastritis, bleeding esophageal varices, PUD, bleeding hemorrhoids)

GENITALIA: Testicular atrophy in males (chronic liver disease, hemochromatosis)
EXTREMITIES: Pedal edema (hypoalbuminemia, failure of right side of the heart), arthropathy (hemochromatosis)
NEUROLOGIC: Flapping tremor, asterixis (hepatic encephalopathy), choreoathetosis, dysarthria (Wilson's disease)

■ ETIOLOGY
- Alcohol abuse
- Secondary biliary cirrhosis, obstruction of the common bile duct (stone, stricture, pancreatitis, neoplasm, sclerosing cholangitis)
- Drugs (e.g., acetaminophen, isoniazid, methotrexate, methyldopa)
- Hepatic congestion (e.g., CHF, constrictive pericarditis, tricuspid insufficiency, thrombosis of the hepatic vein, obstruction of the vena cava)
- Primary biliary cirrhosis
- Hemochromatosis
- Chronic active hepatitis caused by hepatitis B or C
- Wilson's disease
- α-1 antitrypsin deficiency
- Infiltrative diseases (amyloidosis, glycogen storage diseases, hemochromatosis)
- Nutritional: jejunoileal bypass
- Others: parasitic infections (schistosomiasis), idiopathic portal hypertension, congenital hepatic fibrosis, systemic mastocytosis, autoimmune hepatitis, hepatic steatosis, IBD

DIAGNOSIS

■ DIFFERENTIAL DIAGNOSIS
Refer to "Etiology."

■ WORKUP
Diagnostic workup is aimed at identifying the most likely cause of cirrhosis. The history is extremely important:
- Alcohol abuse: alcoholic liver disease
- History of hepatitis B (chronic active hepatitis, primary hepatic neoplasm, or hepatitis C)
- History of IBD (primary sclerosing cholangitis)
- History of pruritus, hyperlipoproteinemia, and xanthomas in a middle-aged or elderly female (primary biliary cirrhosis)
- Impotence, diabetes mellitus, hyperpigmentation, arthritis (hemochromatosis)

- Neurologic disturbances (Wilson's disease, hepatolenticular degeneration)
- Family history of "liver disease" (hemochromatosis [positive family history in 25% of patients], α-1 antitrypsin deficiency)
- History of recurrent episodes of RUQ pain (biliary tract disease)
- History of blood transfusions, IV drug abuse (hepatitis C)
- History of hepatotoxic drug exposure
- Coexistence of other diseases with immune or autoimmune features (ITP, myasthenia gravis, thyroiditis, autoimmune hepatitis)

■ LABORATORY TESTS
- Decreased Hgb and Hct, elevated MCV, increased BUN and creatinine (the BUN may also be "normal" or low if the patient has severely diminished liver function), decreased sodium (dilutional hyponatremia), decreased potassium (as a result of secondary aldosteronism or urinary losses)
- Decreased glucose in a patient with liver disease indicating severe liver damage
- Other laboratory abnormalities:
  1. Alcoholic hepatitis and cirrhosis: there may be mild elevation of ALT and AST, usually <500 IU; AST > ALT (ratio >2:3).
  2. Extrahepatic obstruction: there may be moderate elevations of ALT and AST to levels <500 IU.
  3. Viral, toxic, or ischemic hepatitis: there are extreme elevations (>500 IU) of ALT and AST.
  4. Transaminases may be normal despite significant liver disease in patients with jejunoileal bypass operations or hemochromatosis or after methotrexate administration.
  5. Alkaline phosphatase elevation can occur with extrahepatic obstruction, primary biliary cirrhosis, and primary sclerosing cholangitis.
  6. Serum LDH is significantly elevated in metastatic disease of the liver; lesser elevations are seen with hepatitis, cirrhosis, extrahepatic obstruction, and congestive hepatomegaly.
  7. Serum γ-glutamyl transpeptidase (GGTP) is elevated in alcoholic liver disease and may also be elevated with cholestatic disease

(primary biliary cirrhosis, primary sclerosing cholangitis).

8. Serum bilirubin may be elevated; urinary bilirubin can be present in hepatitis, hepatocellular jaundice, and biliary obstruction.
9. Serum albumin: significant liver disease results in hypoalbuminemia.
10. Prothrombin time: an elevated PT in patients with liver disease indicates severe liver damage and poor prognosis.
11. Presence of hepatitis B surface antigen implies acute or chronic active hepatitis B.
12. Presence of antimitochondrial antibody suggests primary biliary cirrhosis, chronic active hepatitis.
13. Elevated serum copper, decreased serum ceruloplasmin, and elevated 24-hr urine may be diagnostic of Wilson's disease.
14. Protein immunoelectrophoresis may reveal decreased α-1 globulins (α-1 antitrypsin deficiency), increased IgA (alcoholic cirrhosis), increased IgM (primary biliary cirrhosis), increased IgG (chronic active hepatitis, cryptogenic cirrhosis).
15. An elevated serum ferritin and increased transferrin saturation are suggestive of hemochromatosis.
16. An elevated blood ammonia suggests hepatocellular dysfunction; serial values are not useful in following patients with hepatic encephalopathy because there is poor correlation between blood ammonia level and degree of hepatic encephalopathy.
17. Serum cholesterol is elevated in cholestatic disorders.
18. Antinuclear antibodies (ANA) may be found in autoimmune hepatitis.
19. Alpha fetoprotein: levels >1000 pg/ml are highly suggestive of primary liver cell carcinoma.
20. Anti–hepatitis C virus identifies patient with prior hepatitis C virus infection.
21. Elevated level of serum globulin (especially γ-globulins) may occur with autoimmune hepatitis.

■ IMAGING STUDIES
- Ultrasonography is the procedure of choice for detection of gallstones and dilation of common bile ducts.
- CT scan is useful for detecting mass lesions in liver and pancreas, assess-ing hepatic fat content, identifying idiopathic hemochromatosis, early diagnosing of Budd-Chiari syndrome, dilation of intrahepatic bile ducts, and detection of varices and splenomegaly.
- Technetium-99m sulfur colloid scanning is useful for diagnosing cirrhosis (there is a shift of colloid uptake to the spleen, bone marrow), identifying hepatic adenomas (cold defect is noted), diagnosing Budd-Chiari syndrome (there is increased uptake by the caudate lobe; see Fig. 1-73).
- ERCP is the procedure of choice for diagnosing periampullary carcinoma, common duct stones; it is also useful in diagnosing primary sclerosing cholangitis.
- Percutaneous transhepatic cholangiography (PTC) is useful when evaluating patients with cholestatic jaundice and dilated intrahepatic ducts by ultrasonography; presence of intrahepatic strictures and focal dilation is suggestive of PSC.
- Percutaneous liver biopsy is useful in evaluating hepatic filling defects, diagnosing hepatocellular disease or hepatomegaly, evaluating persistently abnormal liver function tests, and diagnosing hemachromatosis, primary biliary cirrhosis, Wilson's disease, glycogen storage diseases, chronic hepatitis, autoimmune hepatitis, infiltrative diseases, alcoholic liver disease, drug-induced liver disease, and primary or secondary carcinoma.

℞ TREATMENT

■ NONPHARMACOLOGIC THERAPY
Avoid any hepatotoxins (e.g., ethanol, acetaminophen); improve nutritional status.

■ ACUTE GENERAL Rx
- Correct any mechanical obstruction to bile flow (e.g., calculi, strictures).
- Provide therapy for underlying cardiovascular disorders in patients with cardiac cirrhosis.
- Remove excess body iron with phlebotomy and deferoxamine in patients with hemochromatosis.
- Remove copper deposits with D-penicillamine in patients with Wilson's disease.
- Long-term ursodiol therapy will slow the progression of primary biliary cirrhosis. It is, however, ineffective in primary sclerosing cholangitis.
- Glucocorticoids (prednisone 20 to 30 mg/day initially or combination therapy or prednisone and azathioprine) is useful in autoimmune hepatitis.
- Liver transplantation may be indicated in otherwise healthy patients (age <65 yr) with sclerosing cholangitis, chronic hepatitis cirrhosis, or primary biliary cirrhosis with prognostic information suggesting <20% chance of survival without transplantation; contraindications to liver transplantation are AIDS, most metastatic malignancies, active substance abuse, uncontrolled sepsis, uncontrolled cardiac or pulmonary disease.

■ CHRONIC Rx
- Treatment of complications of portal hypertension (ascites, esophagogastric varices [see Fig. 3-27], hepatic encephalopathy, and hepatorenal syndrome)
- Table 3-3 describes prognostic variables based on the Child-Pugh score.

■ DISPOSITION
- Prognosis varies with the etiology of the patient's cirrhosis and whether there is ongoing hepatic injury. Mortality rate exceeds 80% in patients with hepatorenal syndrome.
- Two markers of portal hypertension, thrombocytopenia and splenomegaly, moderately increase the likelihood of large esophageal varices.
- If advanced cirrhosis is present and transplantation is not feasible, survival is 1 to 2 yr.

■ REFERRAL
- Hospital admission for bleeding varices, hepatic encephalopathy, or onset of hepatorenal syndrome
- Liver transplantation in suitable candidates is the only effective long-term treatment of complications resulting from cirrhosis

☼ PEARLS & CONSIDERATIONS

■ COMMENTS
Thrombocytopenia and advanced Child-Pugh cases are associated with the presence of varices. These factors are useful to identify cirrhotic patients who benefit most from referral for endoscopic screening for varices.
Author: **Fred F. Ferri, M.D.**

BASIC INFORMATION

DEFINITION

Primary biliary cirrhosis (PBC) is a chronic progressive disease, most often affecting women, characterized by progressive destruction of the small intrahepatic bile ducts with portal inflammation leading to fibrosis, cirrhosis, liver failure, and the need for liver transplantation.

ICD-9CM CODES
571.6 Biliary cirrhosis

EPIDEMIOLOGY & DEMOGRAPHICS
- PBC affects all races and accounts for 0.6% to 2% of deaths from cirrhosis worldwide.
- Approximately 95% of patients are female.
- PBC is reported only rarely in Africa and the Indian subcontinent.
- Prevalence estimates range from 19 to 151 cases per million population whereas incidence estimates range from 3.9 to 15 cases per million population per year.
- Genetic factors are important in the development of PBC; however, there is no clear dominant or recessive pattern of inheritance. Prevalence in families with one affected member is estimated to be 100 times higher than the general population. There is a weak association between PBC and HLA-DR8.
- Onset typically occurs between the ages of 30 and 65 yr.
- Associated with Sjögren's syndrome, arthritis, Raynaud's phenomenon, and scleroderma.

PHYSICAL FINDINGS & CLINICAL PRESENTATION
SYMPTOMS:
- Variable dependent on stage of diagnosis. Fatigue and pruritus are the usual presenting symptoms. However, as many as 48% to 60% may be asymptomatic.
- Pruritus may first occur during pregnancy but is distinguished from pruritus of pregnancy because it persists into the postpartum period.
- Pruritus is worse at night, under constricting, coarse garments; in association with dry skin; and in hot, humid weather.
- Musculoskeletal complaints caused by inflammatory arthropathy in 40% to 70% of patients: 5% to 10% develop chronic RA; 10% develop "arthritis of PBC."
- Unexplained RUQ pain.

PHYSICAL:
- Variable: dependent on stage of disease at time of presentation. Early may be completely normal.
- 25% to 50% have hypopigmentation of skin
- Excoriations may be present.
- Hepatomegaly and splenomegaly may be present in more advanced disease.
- Xanthomas, jaundice, and features of chronic liver disease/cirrhosis are all features of advanced disease.

ETIOLOGY
- Cause remains unknown.
- Most data point to inherited abnormality of immunoregulation.

DIAGNOSIS

DIFFERENTIAL DIAGNOSIS
Other etiologies of chronic liver disease and cirrhosis:
- Alcoholic cirrhosis
- Viral hepatitis (chronic)
- Primary sclerosing cholangitis
- Autoimmune chronic active hepatitis
- Chemical/toxin-induced cirrhosis
- Other hereditary or familial disorders (e.g., CF, α1-antitrypsin deficiency)

WORKUP
History, physical examination, laboratory evaluation, and liver biopsy

LABORATORY TESTS
- Antimitochondrial antibodies (found in 95% of patients with PBC and are 98% specific)
- Elevated alkaline phosphatase (of hepatic origin)
- Elevated GGTP
- Normal or slightly elevated aminotransferases
- Bilirubin normal early; increases with disease progression (direct and indirect)
- Elevated serum lipids (total cholesterol, HDL, and LDL)
- Percutaneous liver biopsy
- Eosinophilia

IMAGING STUDIES
If history, physical examination, blood tests, and liver biopsy are all consistent with PBC, neither imaging nor cholangiography is necessary.

PROGNOSIS
- Progressive but variable
- Median survival asymptomatic: 10 to 16 yr; symptomatic: 7 yr
- Neither presence nor titer of antimitochondrial antibodies predicts survival
- Prognostic laboratory measures: serum bilirubin, albumin, prothrombin time
- At risk for both osteoporosis and osteomalacia
- Presence of cirrhosis, increased risk for hepatocellular carcinoma

TREATMENT

- Management decisions vary depending on clinical status of patient.
- No generally accepted treatment of underlying disease process.
- Treatment focuses on management of complications (pruritus, metabolic bone diseases, hyperlipidemia).

ACUTE GENERAL Rx
- Ursodiol, colchicine, and methotrexate have shown encouraging results.
- Ursodiol extends survival and lengthens the time before liver transplantation; normalizes bilirubin, may mask need for transplantation.
- Colchicine and methotrexate yield less impressive results but are still modestly effective.
- Prednisone, azathioprine, penicillamine, and cyclosporine have limited efficacy and predictable toxicity.

CHRONIC Rx
- Liver transplantation definitive.
- 85% to 90% survival at 1 yr; survival rates thereafter resemble age/sex-matched healthy persons.
- PBC does not recur if appropriate immunosuppression is used.
- Pruritus: use cholestyramine resin, antihistamines, colestipol, rifampin, ursodiol, or naloxone.
- Monitoring antimitochondrial antibody titer is *not* useful in assessing response to therapy.

DISPOSITION
Definitive treatment requires liver transplantation; survival is 7 to 16 yr, dependent on symptoms.

REFERRAL
Evaluation for liver transplantation or treatment of refractory variceal bleeding

Author: **Rebecca S. Brienza, M.D., M.P.H.**

BASIC INFORMATION

■ **DEFINITION**
Claudication refers to leg pain brought on by exertion and relieved with rest.

■ **SYNONYMS**
Intermittent claudication

ICD-9CM CODES
443.9 Peripheral vascular disease, unspecified
440.21 Intermittent claudication due to atherosclerosis

■ **EPIDEMIOLOGY & DEMOGRAPHICS**
INCIDENCE: 3 to 8 cases/1000 persons
PREVALENCE: 2% to 4% in the general population
RISK: Major risk factors of tobacco, hypertension, diabetes, and hypercholesterolemia increase the chance of developing claudication. Cigarette smoking is the major determinant of disease progression.

■ **PHYSICAL FINDINGS & CLINICAL PRESENTATION**
• Diminished pulses
• Bruits over the distal aorta, iliac or femoral arteries heard
• Pallor of the distal extremities on elevation
• Rubor with prolonged capillary refill on dependency
• Cool skin temperature
• Trophic changes of hair loss and muscle atrophy noted
• Nonhealing ulcers, necrotic tissue, and gangrene possible

■ **ETIOLOGY**
Primary cause of claudication is atherosclerosis with subsequent stenosis of peripheral vessels and inability to supply blood to working muscle.

 DIAGNOSIS

The history of buttock, thigh, or calf pain or fatigue brought on by exertion and relieved by rest along with the above-mentioned physical findings makes the diagnosis of claudication fairly certain. Noninvasive studies help confirm the diagnosis.

■ **DIFFERENTIAL DIAGNOSIS**
Spinal stenosis, muscle cramps, degenerative osteoarthritic joint disease particularly of the lumbar spine and hips, and compartment syndrome may all resemble claudication.

■ **WORKUP**
• Noninvasive vascular testing confirms the clinical impression of claudication and aids in locating the major occlusive site. Noninvasive testing uses continuous-wave Doppler to measure systolic arterial pressures and reports the ankle-brachial index (ABI) and segmental systolic pressures as well as Doppler waveforms.
• Ankle-brachial index (ABI): The ratio of ankle pressure to brachial pressure is usually about 1.
  1. In claudication the ABI ranges from 0.5 to 0.8.
  2. In patients with rest pain or impending limb loss, ABI $\leq$0.3.
• Segmental systolic pressures usually are measured from the high thigh, above the knee, below the knee, and the ankle. Normally there should not be >20 mm Hg difference in pressures between adjacent segments. If the gradient is >20 mm Hg, significant narrowing is suspected in the intervening segment.
• Both ABI and segmental pressures can be done before and after exercise.

■ **IMAGING STUDIES**
• Duplex ultrasound can be used to locate the occluded areas and assess the patency of the distal arterial system or prior vein grafts.
• MRA and spiral CT angiography are newer imaging techniques available.
• Angiography remains the gold standard for imaging peripheral arterial occlusions. Complications can occur, and the study should be done only if surgical reconstruction is being considered.

TREATMENT

■ **NONPHARMACOLOGIC THERAPY**
• Avoidance of tobacco is vital.
• Diet to control diabetes and blood pressure, as well as to reduce cholesterol, should be followed.
• Exercise must be emphasized. Exercise along with abstaining from tobacco is the best medical treatment available for the exertional claudication patient. Exercise will increase walking distances before symptoms occur and provides an overall better functioning status. Walking 30 to 60 min/day for 5 days at about 2 mi/hr is recommended.

■ **ACUTE GENERAL Rx**
Most patients with claudication respond to conservative management mentioned above. If this fails, medicines can be tried (see "Chronic Rx"). Surgical reconstruction has its specific indications reserved for patients with impending limb loss (see "Chronic Rx").

■ **CHRONIC Rx**
• Pentoxifylline (Trental) and cilostazol (Pletal) have been approved for use in patients with intermittent claudication who have not responded well to conservative measures. Pentoxifylline 400 mg tid or cilostazol 100 mg bid for 3 mo should be tried. If there is no improvement in symptoms, the medicine can be discontinued.
• Surgical reconstruction is indicated in patients with refractory rest pain, limb ischemia, nonhealing ulcers, or gangrene and in a select group of patients with functional disability. Common surgical procedures:
  1. Aortoiliofemoral reconstruction: perioperative mortality <3%.
  2. Infrainguinal bypass, e.g., femoropopliteal, femorotibial: perioperative mortality, 2% to 5%.
  3. Extraanatomic bypass, e.g., axillofemoral or femorofemoral bypass.
  4. Angioplasty is used on short, discrete stenotic lesions in the iliac or femoropopliteal artery.
  5. Atherectomy, stents, and lasers are newer techniques.

■ **DISPOSITION**
Intermittent claudication progressing to an ischemic leg or limb loss is an unusual course, especially if maintaining the conservative treatment of exercise and abstaining from tobacco.

■ **REFERRAL**
Consultation with the vascular surgeon is recommended in the patient with threatened limb loss, rest pain, nonhealing ulcers, functional disability from pain, and gangrene.

PEARLS & CONSIDERATIONS

■ **COMMENTS**
Claudication is a marker for generalized atherosclerosis. This group of patients has a higher risk of death from cardiovascular events than from limb loss. This should be kept in mind when deciding to proceed with surgical evaluation. Every effort should be made toward conservative measures.

REFERENCE
Dormandy JA, Rutherford RB: Management of peripheral arterial disease (PAD): TASC Working Group, *J Vasc Surg* 31(1Pt2):S1, 2000.
Author: **Peter Petropoulos, M.D.**

BASIC INFORMATION

DEFINITION
Cocaine is an alkaloid derived from the coca plant *Erythroxylon coca,* native to South America, which contains approximately 0.5% to 1% cocaine. The drug produces physiologic and behavioral effects when administered orally, intranasally, intravenously, or via inhalation following smoking. Cocaine has potent pharmacologic effects on dopamine, norepinephrine, and serotonin neurons in the central nervous system (CNS) involving alteration and blockade of cellular membrane transport and prevention of reputake.

SYNONYMS
Cocaine hydrochloride: topical solution (FDA approved as a topical anesthetic)
Free base: aqueous solution of cocaine hydrochloride converted to a more volatile base state by the addition of alkali, thereby extracting the cocaine base in a residue or precipitate
Crack: potent, purified smokable form; produces effects similar to those of intravenous administration
Street names include Bernice, Bernies, C, Cadillac or Champagne of drugs, Carrie, Cecil, Charlie, Coke, Dust, Dynamite, Flake, Gin, Girl, Gold dust, Green gold, Jet, Powder, Star dust, Paradise, Pimp's drug, Snowflake, Stardust, White girl
Liquid lady = alcohol + cocaine
Speedball = heroin + cocaine
Street measures: Hit (2-200 mg), snort, line, dose, spoon (approximately 1 g)

ICD-9CM CODES
304.2 Cocainism

EPIDEMIOLOGY & DEMOGRAPHICS
The 1993 National Household Survey on Drug Abuse estimated that 4.5 million Americans used cocaine in 1992, with 1.3 million reporting use at least monthly.
Between 1993 and 1994, intravenous cocaine and heroin abusers accounted for a major new group of persons with human immunodeficiency virus (HIV) in several metropolitan areas.
Although there has been an encouraging trend of decreased cocaine abuse by young persons, the National Institute on Drug Abuse 1995 report *Epidemiologic Trends in Drug Abuse* noted that "cocaine (including crack) remains the nation's most serious drug problem."

PHYSICAL FINDINGS & CLINICAL PRESENTATION
PHASE I:
- CNS: euphoria, agitation, headache, vertigo, twitching, bruxism, nonintentional tremor
- Nausea, vomiting, fever, hypertension, tachycardia
PHASE II:
- CNS: lethargy, hyperreactive deep tendon reflexes, seizures (status epilepticus)
- Sympathetic overdrive: tachycardia, hypertension, hyperthermia
- Incontinence
PHASE III:
- CNS: flaccid paralysis, coma, fixed dilated pupils, loss of reflexes
- Pulmonary edema
- Cardiopulmonary arrest
Psychologic dependence manifests with habituation, paranoia, hallucinations (cocaine "bugs").

Central nervous system: cerebral ischemia and infarction, cerebral arterial spasm, cerebral vasculitis, cerebral vascular thrombosis, subarachnoid hemorrhage, intraparenchymal hemorrhage, seizures, cerebral atrophy, movement disorders
Cardiac: acute myocardial ischemia and infarction, arrhythmias and sudden death, dilated cardiomyopathy and myocarditis, infective endocarditis, aortic rupture
Pulmonary: (secondary to smoking crack cocaine) inhalation injuries: cartilage and nasal septal perforation, oropharyngeal ulcers; immunologically mediated diseases: hypersensitivity pneumonitis, bronchiolitis obliterans; pulmonary vascular lesions and hemorrhage, pulmonary infarction, pulmonary edema secondary to left ventricular failure, pneumomediastinum, and pneumothorax
Gastrointestinal: gastroduodenal ulceration and perforation; intestinal infarction and/or perforation, colitis
Renal: acute renal failure secondary to rhabdomyolysis and myoglobinuria; renal infarction; focal segmental glomerulosclerosis
Obstetric: placental abruption, low infant weight, prematurity, and microcephaly
Psychiatric: anxiety, depression, paranoia, delirium, psychosis, and suicide

ETIOLOGY
Cocaine may be absorbed through different routes with varying degrees of speed
- Nasal insufflation/snorting: 2.5 min
- Smoking: <30 sec
- Oral: 2 to 5 min
- Mucosal: <20 min
- Intravenous injection: <30 sec

DIAGNOSIS

■ DIFFERENTIAL DIAGNOSIS
- Methamphetamine ("speed") abuse
- Methylenedioxyamphetamine ("ecstasy") abuse
- Cathione ("khat") abuse
- Lysergic acid diethylamide (LSD) abuse

■ WORKUP
Physical examination and laboratory evaluation

■ LABORATORY TESTS
- Toxicology screen (urine): Cocaine is metabolized within 2 hr by the liver to major metabolites, benzoylecogonine and ecgonine methylester, that are excreted in the urine. Metabolites can be identified in urine within 5 min of IV use and up to 48 hr after oral ingestion
- Blood: CBC, electrolytes, glucose, BUN, creatinine, calcium
- ABG analysis
- ECG

TREATMENT

There is no specific antidote and, at present, no drug therapy is uniquely effective in treating cocaine abuse and dependence. In addition, adulterants, contaminants, and other drugs may be admixed with street cocaine. Amantadine may provide effective treatment for cocaine-dependent patients with severe cocaine withdrawal symptoms, as well as the other dopamine agonist bromocriptine (1.5 mg PO tid), which may alleviate some of the symptoms of craving associated with acute cocaine withdrawal.

■ ACUTE GENERAL Rx
Acute cocaine toxicity requires following advanced poisoning treatment and life support. A suspected "body-packer" should have an abdominal radiograph to detect the continued presence of cocaine-containing condoms in the intestinal tract. If present, gentle catharsis with charcoal and mineral oil should be performed with ICU admission and monitoring. Management of cocaine-related toxicity is also outlined in Table 1-21.

■ SPECIFIC TREATMENT
For an outline of treatment, see Table 1-21
INHALATION: Wash nasal passages
ANXIETY: Diazepam 15 to 20 mg PO IV for severe agitation
SEIZURE MANAGEMENT (STATUS EPILEPTICUS):
- Diazepam 5 to 10 mg IV over 2 to 3 min, may be repeated every 10 to 15 min
- Lorazepam 2 to 3 mg IV over 2 to 3 min, may be repeated
- Phenytoin loading dose 15 to 18 mg/kg IV at a rate not to exceed 25 to 50 mg/min under cardiac monitoring

- Phenobarbital loading dose 10 to 15 mg/kg IV at a rate of 25 mg/min; an additional 5 mg/kg may be given in 30 to 45 min if seizures are not controlled.
- Refractory seizures, consider:
  Pancuronium 0.1 mg/kg IV
  Halothane general anesthesia
  Both require EEG monitoring to determine brain seizure activity.

HYPERTENSION:
- Nifedipine 10 mg SL
- Labetalol 10 to 80 mg IV
- Propranolol 1 mg IV/qmin, up to 6 mg
- Phentolamine may be required (unopposed adrenergic effects)
- If diastolic pressure >120 mm Hg: hydralazine hydrochloride 25 mg IM or IV; may repeat q1h
- If hypertension uncontrolled or hypertensive encephalopathy is present: sodium nitroprusside initially at 0.5 μg/kg/min not to exceed 10 μg/kg/min

VENTRICULAR ARRHYTHMIAS:
- Propranolol 1 mg/min IV for up to 6 mg
- Lidocaine 1.5 mg/kg IV bolus followed by IV infusion (controversial: may cause seizures)
- Termination of ventricular arrhythmias may be resistant to lidocaine and even cardioversion

■ REFERRAL
Consider psychotherapy and/or behavioral therapy once stable.
Author: **Sajeev Handa, M.D.**

TABLE 1-21 Management of Cocaine-Related Toxicity

CONDITION	DIAGNOSIS	MANAGEMENT
Rhabdomyolysis	CK <5-10 times normal Muscle tenderness Urine dip insensitive	Vigorous hydration, urine output at least 2 ml/kg Mannitol or bicarb for rhabdomyolysis resistant to hydration
Hyperthemia	Rectal temperature CK Electrolytes	Continuous rectal probe. Bring temperature down to 101° F within 30-45 min
Hyptertension	Continuous blood pressure monitoring; consider arterial line	Nitroprusside, phentolamine, labetalol
Chest pain	Chest x-ray film, ECG, cardiac enzymes for patients with abnormal ECGs or persistant cardiac-sounding chest pain	Benzodiazepines for agitation; aspirin and nitroglycerin drip for ischemic pain; see text for discussion of indications for admission; PCTA possibly better than thrombolysis for presumed cocaine-associated MI
Agitation	Clinical evaluation; stat glucose	Benzodiazepines

From Rosen P (ed): *Emergency medicine,* ed 4, St Louis, 1998, Mosby.

BASIC INFORMATION

■ **DEFINITION**

Coccidioidomycosis is an infectious disease caused by the fungus *Coccidioides immitis*. It is usually asymptomatic and characterized by a primary pulmonary focus with infrequent progression to chronic pulmonary disease and dissemination to other organs.

■ **SYNONYMS**

San Joaquin Valley fever

ICD-9CM CODES
114.0 Coccidioidax pneumonia
114.1 Cutaneous or extrapulmonary (primary) coccidioidomycosis
114.3 Disseminated or prostate coccidioidomycosis
114.5 Pulmonary coccidioidomycosis
114.2 Meninges coccidioidomycosis
114.4 Chronic coccidioidomycosis

■ **EPIDEMIOLOGY & DEMOGRAPHICS**

PREVALENCE: Unknown
INCIDENCE (IN U.S.): Estimated annual infection rate 100,000 persons, predominantly in southwest U.S.
PREDOMINANT SEX: Males, between the ages of 25 to 55 yr
PEAK INCIDENCE: Unknown
GENETICS:
Familial Disposition: Unknown
Congenital Infection: Documented, but considered to occur rarely
Neonatal Infection:
• Occurs equally between the sexes
• Clinical disease more severe than in older children and adults

■ **PHYSICAL FINDINGS & CLINICAL PRESENTATION**
• Asymptomatic infections or illness consistent with a nonspecific upper respiratory tract infection in at least 60%
• Symptoms of primary infection—cough, malaise, fever, chills, night sweats, anorexia, weakness, and arthralgias (desert rheumatism)—in remaining 40% within 3 wk of exposure
• Skin rashes, such as erythema nodosum and erythema multiforme, usually with a significant female preponderance
• Scattered rales and areas that are dull on percussion with auscultation
• Spontaneous improvement within 2 wk of illness, with complete recovery usual

• Subsequent pulmonary residua in the form of pulmonary nodules and cavities in <10% of those patients with primary infection; half of these patients asymptomatic
• In a small portion of these patients: a progressive pneumonitis, often with a fatal outcome
• Some, especially if immunocompromised and/or diabetic, progressing to chronic pulmonary disease
• Over many years, granulomas rupture, leading to new cavity formation and continued fibrosis, often accompanied by hemoptysis
• Possible bronchiectasis with acute or chronic disease
• Disseminated or extrapulmonary disease in approximately 0.5% of acutely infected patients
  1. Early signs of probable dissemination: fever, malaise, hilar adenopathy, and elevated ESR persisting in the setting of primary infection
  2. Most organs are susceptible to dissemination, with heart and GI tract generally spared
• Musculoskeletal involvement
  1. Occurs one third of the time in disseminated disease
  2. Usually presents with local pain, swelling of a joint, bone, or muscle
  3. Majority of bone lesions unifocal and usually involve the skull, metacarpals, metatarsals, and tibia
  4. Vertebral column possibly affected with usually multiple lesions involving the arch and contiguous ribs and sparing the intravertebral disk
  5. Joint lesions predominantly unifocal, most commonly involving the ankle and knee, and often accompanying adjacent sites of osteomyelitis
• Meningeal involvement
  1. Occurs approximately one third of the time with dissemination
  2. Usually presents within 6 mo of primary infection or may appear concurrently
  3. Mass lesions rare, with approximately 40 cases reported this century
  4. Usually, absence of classic signs of meningeal irritation, but possible focal deficits, seizure activity, and stiff neck
  5. Most common complaint: headache
  6. Presenting symptoms: fever, weakness, confusion, lethargy, vomiting

• Cutaneous involvement, excluding rash
  1. Variable in appearance, taking the form of pustules, papules, plaques, nodules, ulcers, abscesses, or proliferative lesions
  2. Lesions most characteristically verrucous
  3. Dissemination and fatal outcomes most common in men, pregnant women, neonates, immunocompromised hosts, and individuals of dark-skinned races, especially those of African, Filipino, Mexican, and Native American ancestry

■ **ETIOLOGY**
• *Coccidioides immitis* is endemic to the American continent, including northern, central, and southern parts.
• In the U.S., most cases are acquired in Arizona, California, New Mexico, and Texas.
• Endemic areas coincide with the Lower Sonoran Life Zone, with semi-arid climate, sparse flora, and alkaline soil.
• Fungus exists in the mycelial phase in soil, having barrel-shaped hyphae (arthroconidia).
• Windswept spores from easily fragmented arthroconidia are dispersed to infect other soil (saprophytic cycle) or are inhaled by animals, including rodents and humans.
• Arthrospore deposits in the alveoli, then fungus converts to thick-walled spherule.
• Internal spherical spores (endospores) are released through spherule rupture and mature into new spherules (parasitic cycle).
• Fungus incites a granulomatous reaction in host tissue, usually with caseation necrosis.

🔬 **DIAGNOSIS**

■ **DIFFERENTIAL DIAGNOSIS**
• Acute pulmonary coccidioidomycoses:
  1. Community-acquired pneumonias caused by *Mycoplasma* and *Chlamydia*
  2. Granulomatous diseases, e.g., *Mycobacterium tuberculosis* and sarcoidosis
  3. Other fungal diseases, such as *Blastomyces dermatitidis* and *Histoplasma capsulatum*
• Coccidioidomas: true neoplasms

■ WORKUP

- Suspected in patients with a history of residence or travel in an endemic area, especially during periods favorable to spore dispersion (e.g., dust storms and drought followed by heavy rains)
- Suspected with a patient history of handling fomites from endemic areas (e.g., fruit and cotton), as in textile workers or fruit handlers

■ LABORATORY TESTS

- CBC to reveal eosinophilia, especially with erythema nodosum
- Routine chemistries: usually normal but may reveal hyponatremia
- Elevated serum levels of IgE; associated with progressive disease
- CSF cell counts and chemistry: pleocytosis with mononuclear cell predominance associated with hypoglycorrhachia and elevated protein level
- Definitive diagnosis based on demonstration of the organism by culture from body fluids or tissues (Fig. 1-104)
  1. Greatest yield with pus, sputum, synovial fluid, and soft tissue aspirations, varying with the degree of dissemination
  2. Possible positive cultures of blood, gastric aspirate, pleural effusion, peritoneal fluid, and CSF, but less frequently obtained
  3. In patients with AIDS: failure of sputum cultures to grow the fungus, so pulmonary biopsy is needed
- Serologic evaluations
  1. Latex agglutination and complement fixation
  2. Elevated serum complement-fixing antibody (CFA) titers ≥1:32 (Smith and Saito) strongly correlated with disseminated disease, except with meningitis where lower titers seen
  3. Variable discriminating titers depending on method, so must be based on reference ranges provided
  4. In meningeal disease: CFA detected in CSF except with high serum CFA titers secondary to concurrent extraneural disease
  5. Enzyme-linked immunosorbent assay (ELISA) against a 33-kDa spherule antigen to detect and monitor CNS disease
- Coccidioidin, the mycelial phase antigen, and spherulin, the parasitic phase antigen
  1. Positive (>5 mm) 1 mo following onset of symptomatic primary infection

  2. Useful in assessing prior infection
  3. Negative skin test with primary infection: latent or future dissemination

■ IMAGING STUDIES

Chest x-ray examination:
- Reveals unilateral infiltrates, hilar adenopathy, or pleural effusion in primary infection
- Shows areas of fibrosis containing usually solitary, thin-walled cavities that persist as residua of primary infection
- Possible coccidioidoma, a coin-like lesion representing a healed area of previous pneumonitis

℞ TREATMENT

NONPHARMACOLOGIC THERAPY

- Supportive care in mild symptomatic disease
- In patients with extrapulmonary manifestations involving draining skin, joint, and soft tissue infection: local wound care to avoid possible bacterial superinfection

■ ACUTE GENERAL Rx

- In general, drug therapy is not required for patients with asymptomatic pulmonary disease and most patients with mild symptomatic primary infection.
- Chemotherapy is indicated under the following circumstances:
  1. Severe symptomatic primary infection
  2. High serum CFA titers
  3. Persistent symptoms >6 wk
  4. Prostration
  5. Progressive pulmonary involvement
  6. Pregnancy
  7. Infancy
  8. Debilitation
  9. Concurrent illness (e.g., diabetes, asthma, COPD, malignancy)
  10. Acquired or induced immunosuppression
  11. Racial group with known predisposition for disseminated disease
- Fluconazole
  1. Oral therapy with 200 to 400 mg/day appears to be the drug of choice for meningeal and deep-seated mycotic infections.
  2. In patients with AIDS, fluconazole may be considered the drug of choice for initial and maintenance therapy.
  3. All patients with coccidioidal meningitis should continue azole therapy indefinitely.

- Itraconazole
  1. 400 mg/day achieves 90% response in bone, joint, soft tissue, lymphatic, and genitourinary infections.
  2. Pulmonary infections have been less responsive.
  3. Insufficient data exist for treatment of meningeal disease.
- Amphotericin B is the classic therapy for disseminated extraneural disease, dose 1 to 1.5 mg/kg/day, qd for the first week and qid thereafter, for a total dose of 1 to 2.5 g or until clinical and serologic remission is accomplished.
  1. Local instillation into body cavities such as sinuses, fistulae, and abscesses has been adjunct to therapy.
  2. Liposomal amphotericin B is probably equally effective, but further studies are needed.
  3. Duration of therapy for extraneural disease is undefined but probably about 1 yr.
- With meningeal disease:
  1. Intrathecal amphotericin B remains the traditional treatment modality, given alone or preceding the use of oral agents.
  2. Begin in doses of 0.01 to 0.025 mg/day, gradually increasing the dose as tolerated, to 0.5 mg/day with the patient in Trendelenburg's position.
  3. If given via Ommaya reservoir, as in ventriculitis, dose may be increased to 1.5 mg/day if tolerated.
  4. Concomitant parenteral therapy with amphotericin B is used for simultaneous extraneural disease as standard doses and with purely meningeal disease in smaller doses, although not strictly indicated.
  5. Intrathecal therapy is usually given three times a week for at least 3 mo, then discontinued or gradually tapered until once every 6 wk through 1 yr of therapy.
  6. Patients need routine monitoring of CSF, CFA, cell count, and chemistries for at least 2 yr following cessation of therapy.
- For osteomyelitis, soft-tissue closed space infections, and pulmonary fibrocavitary disease: surgical debridement, drainage, or resection, respectively, in addition to oral azole therapy or parenteral administration of amphotericin B

■ CHRONIC Rx

For chronically immunocompromised patients, lifelong therapy with oral azoles or amphotericin B

■ DISPOSITION

- Prognosis for primary symptomatic infection is good.
- Immunocompromised patients are most likely to have disseminated disease and higher morbidity and mortality.

■ REFERRAL

- To surgeon for the evaluation of chronic hemoptysis, enlarging cavitary lesions despite chemotherapy and intrapleural rupture, osteomyelitis, and other synovial or soft tissue closed space infections
- For neurosurgical consultation in patients with meningeal disease to establish the delivery route of intrathecal drug therapy

☼ PEARLS & CONSIDERATIONS

■ COMMENTS

- Infected body fluids contained within a closed moist environment (e.g., sputum in a specimen cup)

provide the opportunity for the fungus to revert to its hyphal form whereby spores may be made airborne on opening of the container. Purulent drainage into a cast, allowing conversion of fungus to the saprophytic phase, has been responsible for acute disease when the cast was opened and the spores were unintentionally made airborne.

- Patients with a remote history of exposure, especially if immunosuppressed by medication or disease, may reactivate primary disease and suffer rapid dissemination.
- Although cardiac disease is rare, constrictive pericarditis in the setting of disseminated coccidioidomycosis has been documented and is potentially fatal.

REFERENCES

Galgiani JN et al: Practice guidelines for the treatment of coccidioidomycosis. Infectious Disease Society of America, *Clin Infect Dis* 30(4):658, 2000.

Rosen EJ: Reactivated laryngeal coccidioidomycosis, *Otolaryngol Head Neck Surg* 125(1):120, 2001.

Rosenstein NE et al: Risk factors for severe pulmonary and disseminated coccidioidomycosis: Kern County, California, 1995-1996, *Clin Infect Dis* 32(5):708, 2001.

Sydorak RM et al: Coccidioides immitis in the gallbladder and biliary tree, *J Pediatr Surg* 36(7):1054, 2001.

Woods CW et al: Coccidioidomycosis in human immunodeficiency virus-infected persons in Arizona, 1994-1997: incidence, risk factors and prevention, *J Infect Dis* 181(4):1428, 2000.

Wrobel CJ et al: Clinical presentation, radiological findings and treatment results of coccidioidomycosis involving the spine: report on 23 cases, *J Neurosurg* 95(1 Suppl):33, 2001.

Author: **George O. Alonso, M.D.**

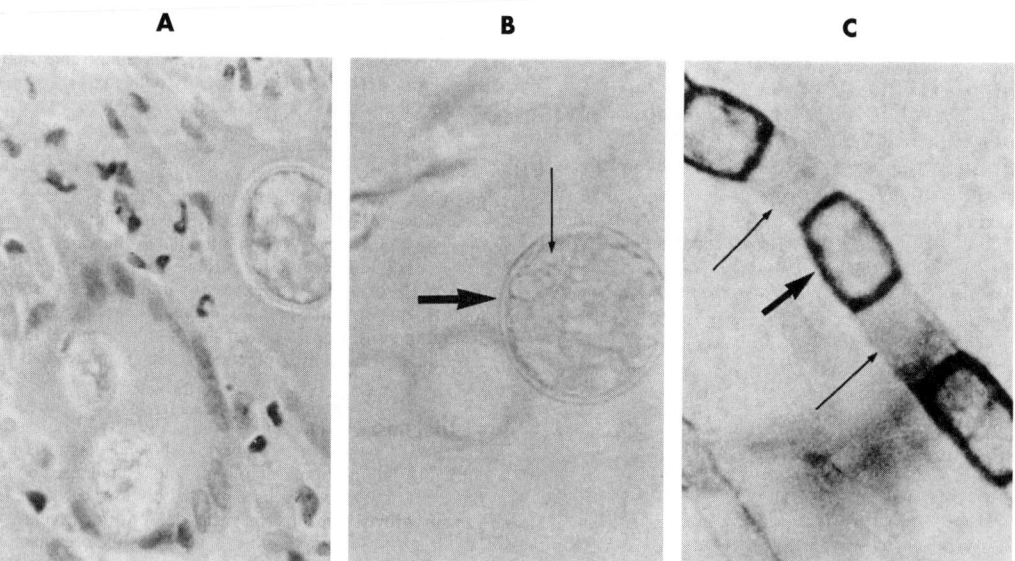

Fig. 1-104 Morphologic appearance of *Coccidioides immitis*. **A,** Spherules within Langerhans' giant cells, shown by hematoxylin and eosin stain. **B,** Spherule in unstained potassium hydroxide preparation. The endospores within spherule *(small arrow)* and the clearly defined double wall of spherule *(large arrow)* are evident. **C,** Mycelial form with barrel-shaped arthroconidia *(large arrow)* spaced between intercalating "ghost cells" *(small arrows)*. (From Stein JH [ed]: *Internal medicine,* ed 5, St Louis, 1998, Mosby.)

BASIC INFORMATION

■ DEFINITION

Colorectal cancer is a neoplasm arising from the luminal surface of the large bowel: descending colon (40% to 42%), rectosigmoid and rectum (30% to 33%), cecum and ascending colon (25% to 30%), transverse colon (10% to 13%).

ICD-9CM CODES
154.0 Colorectal cancer

■ EPIDEMIOLOGY & DEMOGRAPHICS

- Colorectal cancer is the second leading cause of cancer deaths in the U.S. (>135,000 new cases and >50,000 deaths/year).
- Peak incidence is in the seventh decade of life.
- 50% of rectal cancers are within reach of the examiner's finger, 50% of colon cancers are within reach of the flexible sigmoidoscope.
- Colorectal cancer accounts for 14% of all cases of cancer (excluding skin malignancies) and 14% of all yearly cancer deaths.
- Risk factors:
  1. Hereditary polyposis syndromes
     a. Familial polyposis (high risk)
     b. Gardner's syndrome (high risk)
     c. Turcot's syndrome (high risk)
     d. Peutz-Jeghers syndrome (low to moderate risk)
  2. IBD, both ulcerative colitis and Crohn's disease
  3. Family history of "cancer family syndrome"
  4. Heredofamilial breast cancer and colon carcinoma
  5. History of previous colorectal carcinoma
  6. Women undergoing irradiation for gynecologic cancer
  7. First-degree relatives with colorectal carcinoma
  8. Age >40 yr
  9. Possible dietary factors (diet high in fat or meat, beer drinking, reduced vegetable consumption)
  10. Hereditary nonpolyposis colon cancer (HNPCC): autosomal-dominant disorder characterized by early age on onset (mean age of 44 yr) and right-sided or proximal colon cancers, synchronous and metachronous colon cancers, mucinous and poorly differentiated colon cancers; it accounts for 1% to 5% of all cases of colorectal cancer
  11. Previous endometrial or ovarian cancer, particularly when diagnosed at an early age

■ PHYSICAL FINDINGS & CLINICAL PRESENTATION

- Physical examination may be completely unremarkable.
- Digital rectal examination can detect approximately 50% of rectal cancers.
- Palpable abdominal masses may indicate metastasis or complications of colorectal carcinoma (abscess, intussusception, volvulus).
- Abdominal distention and tenderness are suggestive of colonic obstruction.
- Hepatomegaly may be indicative of hepatic metastasis.

■ ETIOLOGY

Colorectal cancer can arise through two mutational pathways: microsatellite instability or chromosomal instability.

DIAGNOSIS

■ DIFFERENTIAL DIAGNOSIS
- Diverticular disease
- Strictures
- IBD
- Infectious or inflammatory lesions
- Adhesions
- Arteriovenous malformations
- Metastatic carcinoma (prostate, sarcoma)
- Extrinsic masses (cysts, abscesses)

■ WORKUP
- The clinical presentation of colorectal malignancies is initially vague and nonspecific (weight loss, anorexia, malaise). It is useful to divide colon cancer symptoms into those usually associated with right side of colon and those commonly associated with left side of colon, since the clinical presentation varies with the location of the carcinoma.
  1. Right side of colon
     a. Anemia (iron deficiency secondary to chronic blood loss).
     b. Dull, vague, and uncharacteristic abdominal pain may be present or patient may be completely asymptomatic.
     c. Rectal bleeding is often missed because blood is mixed with feces.
     d. Obstruction and constipation are unusual because of large lumen and more liquid stools.
  2. Left side of colon
     a. Change in bowel habits (constipation, diarrhea, tenesmus, pencil-thin stools).
     b. Rectal bleeding (bright red blood coating the surface of the stool).
     c. Intestinal obstruction is frequent because of small lumen.

- Early diagnosis of patients with surgically curable disease (Dukes' A, B) is necessary, because survival time is directly related to the stage of the carcinoma at the time of diagnosis. Appropriate screening recommendations are discussed in Section V.
- Dukes' and UICC classification for colorectal cancer:
  A Confined to the mucosa-submucosa (I)
  B Invasion of muscularis propria (II)
  C Local node involvement (III)
  D Distant metastasis (IV)

■ LABORATORY TESTS
- Positive fecal occult blood test
- Microcytic anemia
- Elevated plasma carcinoembryonic antigen (CEA)
- Liver function tests

■ IMAGING STUDIES
- Colonoscopy with biopsy (primary assessment tool)
- CT scan of abdomen to assist in pre-operative staging
- Chest x-ray examination to look for evidence of metastatic disease
- Air-contrast barium enema (Fig. 1-105) only in patients refusing colonoscopy or unable to tolerate colonoscopy

TREATMENT

■ NONPHARMACOLOGIC THERAPY
Decrease fat intake to 30% of total energy intake, increase fiber, fruit, and vegetable consumption. Recent literature reports do not support a protective effect from dietary fiber against colorectal cancer in women.

■ ACUTE GENERAL Rx
- Surgical resection: 70% of colorectal cancers are resectable for cure at presentation; 45% of patients are cured by primary resection.
- Radiation therapy is a useful adjunct to fluorouracil and levamisole therapy for stage II or III rectal cancers.
- Adjuvant chemotherapy with combination of 5-fluorouracil (5-FU) and levamisole substantially increases cure rates for patients with stage III colon cancer and should be considered standard treatment for all such patients and selected patients with high-risk stage II colon cancer.
- Weekly treatment with irinotecar plus fluorouracil and leucovorin is superior to a widely used regimen of fluorouracil and leucovorin for metastatic colorectal cancer in terms of progression-free survival and overall survival.

- In patients who undergo resection of liver metastases from colorectal cancer, postoperative treatment with a combination of hepatic arterial infusion of floxuridine and IV fluorouracil improves the outcome at 2 yr.
- Irinotecan (Camptosar), a potent inhibitor of topoisomerase I, a nuclear enzyme involved in the unwinding of DNA during replication, can be used to treat metastatic colorectal cancer refractory to other drugs, including 5-FU; it may offer a few months of palliation but is expensive and associated with significant toxicity.

■ CHRONIC Rx
Follow-up is indicated with:
- Fecal occult blood testing every 6 mo for 4 yr, then yearly
- Colonoscopy yearly for the initial 2 yr, then every 3 yr
- CEA level should be obtained baseline; if elevated, it can be used postoperatively as a measure of completeness of tumor resection or to monitor tumor recurrence; if used to monitor tumor recurrence, CEA should be obtained every 2 mo for 2 yr, then every 4 mo for 2 yr, and then yearly. The role of CEA for monitoring patients with resected colon cancer has been questioned because of the small number of cures attributed to CEA monitoring despite the substantial cost in dollars and physical and emotional stress associated with monitoring.

■ DISPOSITION
- The 5-yr survival varies with the stage of the carcinoma:
  1. Dukes' A 5-yr survival, >80%
  2. Dukes' B 5-yr survival, 60%
  3. Dukes' C 5-yr survival, 20%
  4. Dukes' D 5-yr survival, 3%
- Overall 5-yr disease-free survival is approximately 50% for colon cancer.
- High-frequency microsatellite instability in colorectal cancer is independently predictive of a relatively favorable outcome and, in addition, reduces the likelihood of metastases.
- In patients with Dukes' C (stage III) colorectal cancer there is improved 5-year survival among women treated with adjuvant chemotherapy (53% with chemotherapy vs. 33% without) and among patients with right-sided tumors treated with adjuvant chemotherapy.
- Retention of 18q alleles in microsatellite-stable cancers and mutation of the gene for the type I receptor for TGF-B1 in cancers with high levels of microsatellite instability point to a favorable outcome after adjuvant chemotherapy with fluorouracil-based regimens for stage II colon cancer.

■ REFERRAL
- Surgical referral for resection
- Oncology referral for adjuvant chemotherapy in selected patients
- Radiation oncology referral for patients with stage II or III rectal cancers

☼ PEARLS & CONSIDERATIONS

■ COMMENTS
- The National Cancer Institute has published consensus guidelines for universal screening for hereditary nonpolyposis colon cancer (HNPCC) in patients with newly diagnosed colorectal cancer. Tumors in mutation carriers of HNPCC typically exhibit microsatellite instability, a characteristic phenotype that is caused by expansions or contractions of short nucleotide repeat sequences. These guidelines (Bethesda Guidelines) are useful for selective patients for microsatellite instability testing. Screening patients with newly diagnosed colorectal cancer for HNPCC is cost effective, especially if the benefits to their immediate relatives are considered.
- Expression of guanylyl cyclase C mRNA in lymph nodes is associated with recurrence of colorectal cancer in patients with stage II disease. Analysis of guanylyl cyclase mRNA expression by RT-PCR may be useful for colorectal cancer staging.
- The use of either annual or biennial fecal occult-blood testing significantly reduces the incidence of colorectal cancer.

REFERENCES
Cagir B et al: Guanylyl cyclase C messenger RNA is a biomarker for recurrent stage II colorectal cancer, *Ann Intern Med* 131:805, 1999.

Elsaleh H et al: Association of tumor site and sex with survival benefit from adjuvant chemotherapy in colorectal cancer, *Lancet* 355:1745, 2000.

Gryfe R et al: Tumor microsatellite instability and clinical outcome in young patients with colorectal cancer, *N Engl J Med* 342:69, 2000.

Raedle J et al: Bethesda guidelines: relation to microsatellite instability and MLH1 promoter methylation in patients with colorectal cancer, *Ann Intern Med* 135:566, 2001.

Saltz LB et al: Irinotecan plus fluorouracil and leucovorin for metastatic colorectal cancer, *N Engl J Med* 343:905, 2000.

Watanabe T et al: Molecular predictors of survival after adjustment chemotherapy for colon cancer, *N Engl J Med* 344:1186, 2001.
Author: **Fred F. Ferri, M.D.**

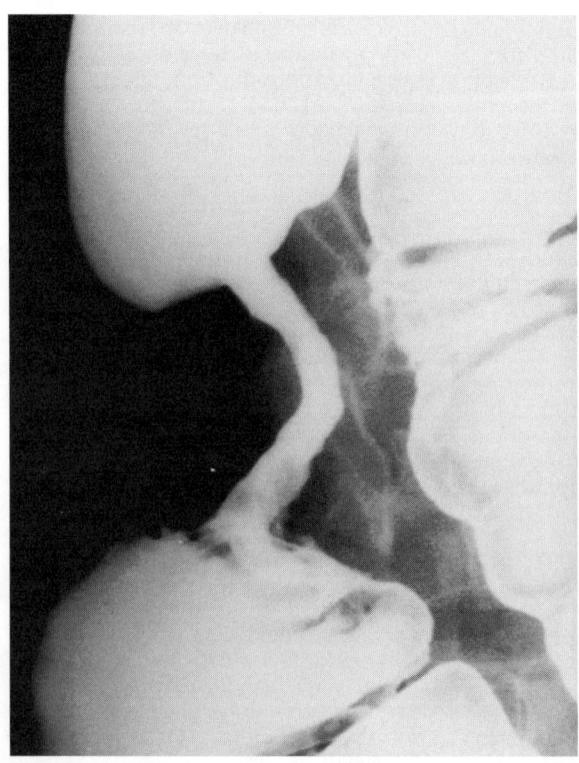

Fig. 1-105   Annular carcinoma of the colon, producing typical short-length, circumferential narrowing with "napkin ring" configuration. (From Halpert RD, Goodman R: *Gastrointestinal radiology: the requisites,* St Louis, 1993, Mosby.)

BASIC INFORMATION

■ DEFINITION
Condyloma acuminatum is a sexually transmitted viral disease of the vulva, vagina, and cervix that is caused by the human papillomavirus (HPV).

■ SYNONYMS
Genital warts
Venereal warts
Anogenital warts

ICD-9CM CODES
078.11 Condyloma acuminatum

■ EPIDEMIOLOGY & DEMOGRAPHICS
- Seen mostly in young adults with a mean age of onset of 16 to 25 yr
- A sexually transmitted disease spread by skin-to-skin contact
- Highly contagious, with 25% to 65% of sexual partners developing it
- Virus shed from both macroscopic and microscopic lesions
- Average incubation time 2 mo (range: 1 to 8 mo)
- Predisposing conditions: diabetes, pregnancy, local trauma, and immunosuppression (e.g., transplant patients, those with HIV infection).

■ PHYSICAL FINDINGS & CLINICAL PRESENTATION (Fig. 1-106)
- Usually found in genital area, but can be present elsewhere
- Lesions usually in similar positions on both sides of perineum
- Initial lesions pedunculated, soft papules about 2 to 3 mm in diameter, 10 to 20 mm long; may occur as single papule or in clusters
- Size of lesions varies from pinhead to large cauliflower-like masses
- Usually asymptomatic, but if infected, can cause pain, odor, or bleeding
- Vulvar condyloma more common than vaginal and cervical

■ ETIOLOGY
- HPV DNA types 6 and 11 usually found in exophytic warts and have no malignant potential
- HPV types 16 and 18 usually found in flat warts and are associated with increased risk of malignancy
- Recurrence associated with persisting viral infection of adjacent normal skin in 25% to 50% of cases

DIAGNOSIS

■ DIFFERENTIAL DIAGNOSIS
- Abnormal anatomic variants or skin tags around labia minora and introitus

- Dysplastic warts

■ WORKUP
- Colposcopic examination of lower genital tract from cervix to perianal skin with 3% to 5% acetic acid
- Biopsy of vulvar lesions that lack the classic appearance of warts and that become ulcerated or fail to respond to treatment
- Biopsy of flat white or ulcerated cervical lesions

■ LABORATORY TESTS
- Pap smear
- Cervical cultures for *N. gonorrhoeae* and *Chlamydia*
- Serologic test for syphilis
- HIV testing offered
- Wet mount for trichomoniasis, *Candida albicans,* and *Gardnerella vaginalis*
- Testing for diabetes (blood glucose)

TREATMENT

■ NONPHARMACOLOGIC THERAPY
- Keep genital area dry and clean.
- Keep diabetes, if present, well controlled.
- Advise use of condoms to prevent spread of infection to sexual partner.

■ ACUTE GENERAL Rx
Keratolytic agents:
- Podophyllin
  1. Acts by poisoning mitotic spindle and causing intense vasospasm
  2. Applied directly to lesion weekly and washed off in 6 hr
  3. Used in minimal vulvar or anal disease
  4. Applied cautiously to nonkeratinized epithelial surfaces
  5. Contraindicated in pregnancy
  6. Discontinued if lesions do not disappear in 6 wk; switch to other treatment
- Trichloroacetic acid (30% to 80% solution)

  1. Acts by precipitation of surface proteins
  2. Applied twice monthly to lesion
  3. Indicated for vulvar, anal, and vaginal lesions; can be used for cervical lesions.
  4. Less painful and irritating to normal tissue than podophyllin
- Fluorouracil
  1. Causes necrosis and sloughing of growing tissue
  2. Can be used intravaginally or for vulvar, anal, or urethral lesions
  3. Better tolerated; 3 g (two thirds of vaginal applicator) applied weekly for 12 wk
  4. Possible vaginal ulceration and erythema
  5. Patient's vagina examined after four to six applications
  6. 80% cure rate

Physical agents:
- Cryotherapy
  1. Can be used weekly for 3 to 6 wk
  2. 62% to 79% success rate
  3. Not suitable for large warts
- Laser therapy
  1. Done by physician with necessary expertise and equipment
  2. Painful; requires anesthesia
- Electrocautery or excision
  1. For recurrent, very large lesions
  2. Local anesthesia needed

Immunotherapy
- Interferon
  1. Injected intralesionally at a dose of 3 million U/m^2 three times weekly for 8 wk
  2. Side effects: fever, chills, malaise, headache
- Autologous vaccine
  1. Made from host's own condyloma acuminatum; not very effective

■ DISPOSITION
Follow closely with pelvic examinations and Pap smears every 3 mo for 6 mo, every 6 mo for 12 mo, and then yearly if no evidence of recurrence.

■ REFERRAL
Consult gynecologist in case of extensive lesions or lesions resistant to treatment with keratolytic agents (podophyllin and trichloroacetic acid).

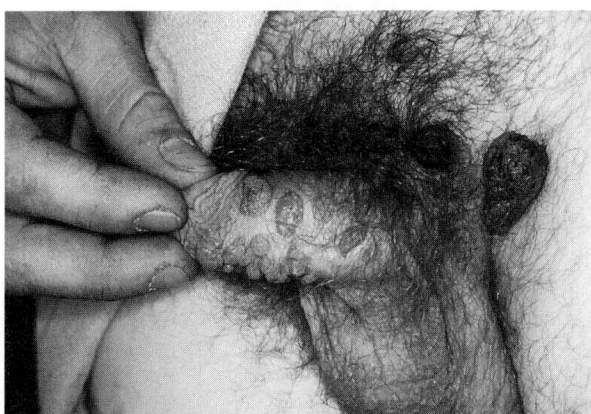

Fig. 1-106 Condylomata. Verrucoid pigmented lesions on the penis. (From Noble J: *Primary care medicine,* ed 3, St. Louis, 2001, Mosby.)

BASIC INFORMATION

■ DEFINITION
Congestive heart failure is a patho-physiologic state characterized by congestion in the pulmonary or systemic circulation. It is caused by the heart's inability to pump sufficient oxygenated blood to meet the metabolic needs of the tissues.

■ SYNONYMS
CHF
Cardiac failure
Heart failure

ICD-9CM CODES
428.0 Congestive heart failure

■ EPIDEMIOLOGY & DEMOGRAPHICS
CHF is the most common admission diagnosis in elderly patients.

■ PHYSICAL FINDINGS & CLINICAL PRESENTATION
The findings on physical examination in patients with CHF vary depending on the severity and whether the failure is right-sided or left-sided.
- Common clinical manifestations are:
  1. Dyspnea on exertion initially, then with progressively less strenuous activity, and eventually manifesting when patient is at rest; caused by increasing pulmonary congestion
  2. Orthopnea caused by increased venous return in the recumbent position
  3. Paroxysmal nocturnal dyspnea (PND) resulting from multiple factors (increased venous return in the recumbent position, decreased Pao_2, decreased adrenergic stimulation of myocardial function)
  4. Nocturnal angina resulting from increased cardiac work (secondary to increased venous return)
  5. Cheyne-Stokes respiration: alternating phases of apnea and hyperventilation caused by prolonged circulation time from lungs to brain
  6. Fatigue, lethargy resulting from low cardiac output
- Patients with failure of the left side of the heart will have the following abnormalities on physical examination: pulmonary rales, tachypnea, S_3 gallop, cardiac murmurs (AS, AR, MR), paradoxic splitting of S_2.
- Patients with failure of right side of the heart manifest with jugular venous distention, peripheral edema, perioral and peripheral cyanosis, congestive hepatomegaly, ascites, hepatojugular reflux.
- In patients with heart failure, elevated jugular venous pressure and a third heart sound are each independently associated with adverse outcomes.
- Acute precipitants of CHF exacerbations are: noncompliance with salt restriction, pulmonary infections, arrhythmias, medications (e.g., calcium channel blockers/antiarrhythmic agents), and inappropriate reductions in CHF therapy.

■ ETIOLOGY
LEFT VENTRICULAR FAILURE:
- Systemic hypertension
- Valvular heart disease (AS, AR, MR)
- Cardiomyopathy, myocarditis
- Bacterial endocarditis
- Myocardial infarction
- IHSS

Left ventricular failure is further differentiated according to systolic dysfunction (low ejection fraction) and diastolic dysfunction (normal or high ejection fraction), or "stiff ventricle." It is important to make this distinction because treatment is significantly different (see "Treatment").
- Common causes of systolic dysfunction are post-MI, cardiomyopathy, myocarditis.
- Causes of diastolic dysfunction are hypertensive cardiovascular disease, valvular heart disease (AS, AR, MR, IHSS), restrictive cardiomyopathy.

RIGHT VENTRICULAR FAILURE:
- Valvular heart disease (mitral stenosis)
- Pulmonary hypertension
- Bacterial endocarditis (right-sided)
- Right ventricular infarction

BIVENTRICULAR FAILURE:
- Left ventricular failure
- Cardiomyopathy
- Myocarditis
- Arrhythmias
- Anemia
- Thyrotoxicosis
- AV fistula
- Paget's disease
- Beriberi

DIAGNOSIS

■ DIFFERENTIAL DIAGNOSIS
- Cirrhosis
- Nephrotic syndrome
- Venous occlusive disease
- COPD, asthma
- Pulmonary embolism
- ARDS
- Heroin overdose
- Pneumonia

■ WORKUP
- Chest x-ray examination, electrocardiography, echocardiography, cardiac catheterization (selected patients)
- Standard 12-lead ECG is useful to diagnose ischemic heart disease and obtain information about rhythm abnormalities

■ LABORATORY TESTS
CBC (to rule out anemia, infections), BUN, creatinine, liver enzymes, TSH

■ IMAGING STUDIES
- Chest x-ray examination:
  1. Pulmonary venous congestion
  2. Cardiomegaly with dilation of the involved heart chamber
  3. Pleural effusions
- Two-dimensional echocardiography is useful to assess global and regional left ventricular function and estimate ejection fraction.
- Exercise stress testing may be useful for evaluating concomitant coronary disease and assess degree of disability. The decision to perform exercise stress testing should be individualized.
- Cardiac catheterization remains an excellent method to evaluate ventricular diastolic properties, significant coronary artery disease, or valvular heart disease; however, it is invasive. The decision to perform cardiac catheterization should be individualized.

TREATMENT

■ NONPHARMACOLOGIC THERAPY
- Determine if CHF is secondary to systolic or diastolic dysfunction and treat accordingly.
- Identify and correct precipitating factors (i.e., anemia, thyrotoxicosis, infections, increased sodium load, β-blockers, medical noncompliance).
- Decrease cardiac workload in patients with systolic dysfunction: restrict patients' activity only during periods of acute decompensation; the risk of thromboembolism during this period can be minimized by using heparin 5000 U SC q12h in hospitalized patients. In patients with mild to moderate symptoms aerobic training may improve symptoms and exercise capacity.
- Restrict sodium intake to ≤3 g/day.
- Restricting fluid intake to 2 L or less may be useful in patients with hyponatremia.

■ ACUTE GENERAL Rx
TREATMENT OF CHF SECONDARY TO SYSTOLIC DYSFUNCTION:

1. Diuretics: indicated in patients with systolic dysfunction and volume overload
   a. Furosemide: 20 to 80 mg/day produces prompt venodilation and diuresis. IV therapy may produce diuresis when oral therapy has failed; when changing from IV to oral furosemide, doubling the dose is usually necessary to achieve an equal effect.
   b. Thiazides are not as powerful as furosemide but are useful in mild to moderate CHF.
   c. The addition of metolazone to furosemide enhances diuresis.
   d. Blockade of aldosterone receptors by spironolactone (12.5 to 25 mg qd) used in conjunction with ACE inhibitors reduces both mortality and morbidity in patients with severe CHF and is generally not associated with hyperkalemia. It should be considered in patients with recent or recurrent class IV (NYHA) symptoms.
   e. Frequent monitoring of renal function and electrolytes is recommended in all patients receiving diuretics.
2. ACE inhibitors:
   a. They cause dilation of the arteriolar resistance vessels and venous capacity vessels, thereby reducing both preload and afterload.
   b. They are associated with decreased mortality and improved clinical status when used in patients with CHF caused by systolic dysfunction. They are also indicated in patients with ejection fraction <40%.
   c. They can be used as first-line therapy or they can be added to diuretics in patients with CHF poorly controlled with only diuretic therapy.
   d. Therapy with ACE inhibitors should be initiated at low dose (e.g., enalapril 2.5 mg qd or bid) to prevent hypotension and rapidly titrated up to high doses if tolerated.
3. β-blockers: All patients with stable NYHA class II or III heart failure caused by left ventricular systolic dysfunction should receive a β-blocker unless they have a contraindication to its use or are intolerant to it. β-Blockers are especially useful in patients who remain symptomatic despite therapy with ACE inhibitors and diuretics. Effective agents are carvedilol (Coreg) 3.125 mg bid, bisoprolol 1.25 mg qd, or metoprolol 12.5 mg qd.
4. Angiotensin II receptor blockers (ARBS) block the A-II type 1 (AT) receptor, which is responsible for many of the deleterious effects of angiotensin II. These receptors are potent vasoconstrictors that may contribute to the impairment of LV function. They are useful in patients unable to tolerate ACE inhibitors because of angioedema or intractable cough. They can also be used in combination with an ACE inhibitor or a β-blocker.
5. Digitalis is useful because of its positive inotropic and vagotonic effects in patients with CHF secondary to systolic dysfunction; it is of limited value in patients with mild CHF and normal sinus rhythm. It is more beneficial in patients with rapid atrial fibrillation, severe CHF, or ejection fraction of <30%; it can be added to diuretics and ACE inhibitors in patients with severe CHF. In patients with chronic heart failure and normal sinus rhythm, digoxin does not reduce mortality, but it does reduce the rate of hospitalization both overall and for worsening heart failure.
6. Direct vasodilating drugs (hydralazine, isosorbide) are useful in the therapy of systolic dysfunction with CHF because they can reduce the systemic vascular resistance and pulmonary venous pressure, especially when used in combination. They are less effective than ACE inhibitors, and tolerance develops for these agents. The combination of hydralazine and isosorbide is useful in patients who cannot tolerate ACE inhibitors or who have significant renal insufficiency, and in patients remaining symptomatic even while taking an ACE inhibitor. In hospitalized patients with class IV CAF, the combination of IV furosemide and IV vasodilators such as nitroglycerin or nitroprusside is generally effective, however tolerance can develop quickly to nitroglycerin and nitroprusside administration is associated with accumulation of toxic metabolites.
7. Continuous infusion of positive inotropic agents (e.g., dobuta-mine, milrinone) may improve quality of life in selected patients with refractory heart failure.
8. Anticoagulants:
   a. Anticoagulation is not recommended for patients in sinus rhythm and no prior history of stroke, left ventricular thrombi, or arteriolar emboli.
   b. Anticoagulation therapy is appropriate for patients with heart failure and atrial fibrillation or a history of embolism.
9. Surgical revascularization should be considered in patients with both heart failure and severe limiting angina.
10. Antiarrhythmic therapy with amiodarone has a modest effect in reducing mortality in patients with CHF; however, it is not recommended for general use in CHF. Its benefits must be weighed against the risk for adverse effects, especially potentially fatal pulmonary toxicity.
11. Nesiritide (Natrecor) is a recombinant human B-type natriuretic peptide (BNP) recently approved by the FDA for IV treatment of hospitalized class IV (NYHA) heart failure. It is very effective, but may result in prolonged hypotension in patients given concomitant high-dose diuretic therapy.
12. Atriobiventricular pacing significantly improves exercise tolerance and quality of life in patients with chronic heart failure and intraventricular conduction delay.

TREATMENT OF CHF SECONDARY TO DIASTOLIC DYSFUNCTION: Therapeutic options are determined by the cause

1. Hypertension
   a. Calcium channel blockers (verapamil)
   b. ACE inhibitors
   c. β-Blockers or verapamil to control heart rate and prolong diastolic filling
   d. Diuretics: vigorous diuresis should be avoided, because a higher filling pressure may be needed to maintain cardiac output in patients with diastolic dysfunction
   e. ARBs
2. Aortic stenosis
   a. Diuretics
   b. Contraindicated medications: ACE inhibitors, nitrates, digitalis (except to control rate of atrial fibrillation)
   c. Aortic valve replacement in patients with critical stenosis

3. Aortic insufficiency and mitral regurgitation
   a. ACE inhibitors increase cardiac output and decrease pulmonary wedge pressure. They are agents of choice along with diuretics.
   b. Hydralazine combined with nitrates can be used if ACE inhibitors are not tolerated.
4. IHSS
   a. β-Blockers or verapamil
   b. Contraindicated medications (they increase outlet obstruction by decreasing the size of the left ventricle in end systole): diuretics, digitalis, ACE inhibitors, hydralazine
   c. Restoration of intravascular volume with IV saline solution if necessary in acute pulmonary edema
   d. Septal myotomy in selected patients

TREATMENT OF CHF SECONDARY TO MITRAL STENOSIS:
1. Diuretics
2. Control of the heart rate and atrial fibrillation with digitalis, verapamil, and/or β-blockers is critical to allow emptying of left atrium and relief of pulmonary congestion.
3. Repairing or replacing the mitral valve is indicated if CHF is not readily controlled by the above measures.
4. Balloon valvuloplasty is useful in selected patients.

■ DISPOSITION
- Annual mortality ranges from 10% in stable patients with mild symptoms to >50% in symptomatic patients with advanced disease.
- Sudden death secondary to ventricular arrhythmias occurs in >40% of patients with heart failure.
- Cardiac transplantation has a 5-yr survival rate of >70% in many centers and represents a viable option in selected patients.
- The use of a left ventricular assist device in patients with advanced heart failure can result in a clinically meaningful survival benefit and improve quality of life. It is an acceptable alternative therapy in selected patients who are not candidates for cardiac transplantation.

REFERENCES
Cazean S et al: Effects of multisite biventricular pacing in patients with heart failure and intraventricular conduction delay, *N Engl J Med* 344:873, 2001.

Cohn JN et al: A randomized trial of the ARB valsartan in chronic heart failure, *N Engl J Med* 345:1667, 2001.

Gomberg-Maitland M et al: Treatment of congestive heart failure, *Arch Intern Med* 161:342, 2001.

Jamali AH et al: The role of ARBs in the management of chronic heart failure, *Arch Intern Med* 161:667, 2001.

Nesiritide for decompensated congestive heart failure, *Med Lett Drugs Ther* 43:100, 2001.

Packer M et al: Consensus recommendations for the management of chronic heart failure, *Am J Cardiol* 83:2A, 1999.

Rose EA et al: Long-term use of a left ventricular assist device for end space heart failure, *N Engl J Med* 345:1635, 2001.

Tsuyuki RT et al: Acute precipitants of CAF exacerbations, *Arch Intern Med* 161:2337, 2001.

Author: **Fred F. Ferri, M.D.**

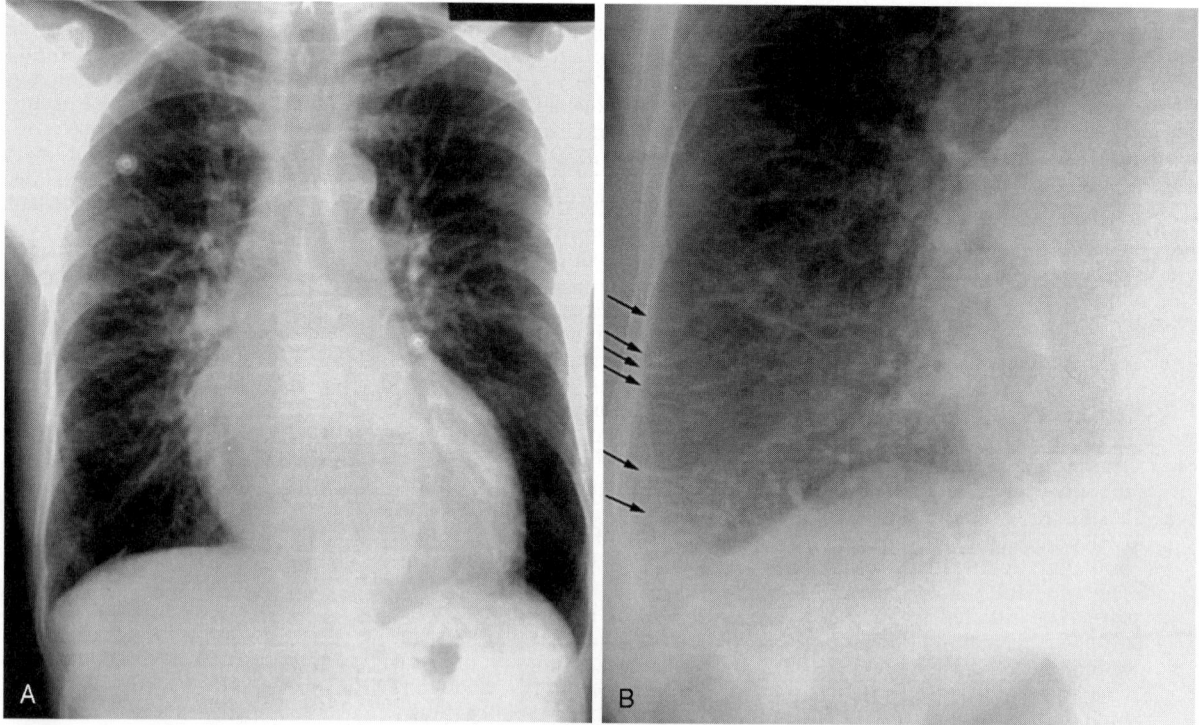

Fig. 1-107 Early findings of congestive heart failure. The major signs on upright PA chest radiograph **(A)** are cardiomegaly and redistribution of the pulmonary vascularity. Normally, the vessels to the lower lobes are more prominent than those in the upper lobes; however, here they appear at least equally prominent. On a close-up view in another patient **(B)**, small horizontal lines can be seen at the very periphery of the lung *(arrows)*. These are known as Kerley B lines and represent fluid in the interlobular septa. (From Mettler FA [ed]: *Primary care radiology*, Philadelphia, 2000, WB Saunders.)

BASIC INFORMATION

■ DEFINITION
The term *conjunctivitis* refers to an inflammation of the conjunctiva resulting from a variety of causes, including allergies and bacterial, viral, and chlamydial infections.

■ SYNONYMS
"Red eye"
Acute conjunctivitis
Subacute conjunctivitis
Chronic conjunctivitis
Purulent conjunctivitis
Pseudomembranous conjunctivitis
Papillary conjunctivitis
Follicular conjunctivitis
Newborn conjunctivitis

ICD-9CM CODES
372.30 Conjunctivitis, unspecified

■ EPIDEMIOLOGY & DEMOGRAPHICS
INCIDENCE (IN U.S.): Newborn 1.6% to 12%
PREVALENCE (IN U.S.):
- Very common
- Often seasonal and can be extremely contagious
PREDOMINANT AGE: Occurs at any age
PEAK INCIDENCE: More common in the fall when viral infections and pollens increase

■ PHYSICAL FINDINGS & CLINICAL PRESENTATION
- Injection and chemosis of conjunctivae with discharge (Fig. 1-108)
- Cornea clear
- Vision usually normal

■ ETIOLOGY
- Bacterial
- Viral
- Chlamydial
- Allergic

DIAGNOSIS

■ DIFFERENTIAL DIAGNOSIS
- Acute glaucoma
- Corneal lesions
- Acute iritis
- Episcleritis
- Scleritis
- Uveitis
- Canalicular obstruction
- Table 2-174 describes the differential diagnosis of red eye.

■ WORKUP
- History and physical examination
- Reports of itching, pain, visual changes

■ LABORATORY TESTS
Cultures are useful if not successfully treated with antibiotic medications; initial culture is usually not necessary.

TREATMENT

■ NONPHARMACOLOGIC THERAPY
- Warm compresses if infective conjunctivitis
- Cold compresses in irritative or allergic conjunctivitis

■ ACUTE GENERAL Rx
- Antibiotic drops (gentamicin, bacitracin, erythromycin, Polysporin, furoquinolone, etc. ophthalmic solution; one or two drops q2-4h)
- Caution: be careful with steroid treatment and avoid unless sure of diagnosis; steroids exacerbate infections

■ CHRONIC Rx
- Depends on cause
- If allergic, nonsteroidals such as Voltarin, mast cell stabilizers such as Alocril, Patanol, Zadator
- If infections, Polytrim or Occuflox

■ DISPOSITION
Follow carefully for the first 2 wk to make sure secondary complications do not occur.

■ REFERRAL
To ophthalmologist if symptoms refractory to initial treatment

PEARLS & CONSIDERATIONS

■ COMMENTS
Do not use steroids indiscriminately; use only when the diagnosis is certain.

REFERENCE
Morrow GL, Abbott RL: Conjunctivitis, *Am Fam Physician* 57:735, 1998.
Author: **Melvyn Koby, M.D.**

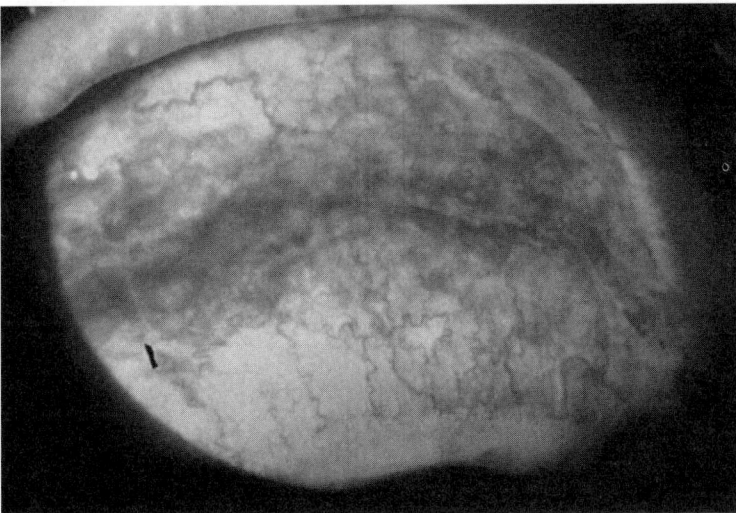

Fig. 1-108   Conjunctival injection from viral conjunctivitis. (From Rosen P [ed]: *Emergency medicine,* ed 4, St Louis, 1998, Mosby.)

BASIC INFORMATION

DEFINITION

Contraception refers to the various options that a sexually active couple have to prevent pregnancy. These options can be either medical or non-medical and used by men or women or both. The options are as follows:

- No contraception: failure rate 85% both typical and perfect
- Abstinence
  1. 12.4% of unmarried men
  2. 13.2% of unmarried women
  3. More frequently practiced before age 17 yr
  4. No intercourse experienced by 13% of women ages 30 to 34 yr old
  5. Failure rate 0%
- Withdrawal
  1. Used in only 2% of sexually active women
  2. Failure rate with perfect use, 4%; with typical use, 19%
- Rhythm method (natural family planning)
  1. Failure rate with perfect use, 1% to 9%; with typical use, 20%
  2. Symptothermal type: mucus method and ovulation pain combined with basal body temperature
  3. Ovulation (Billings' method): takes into account mucus quality
  4. Basal body temperature method: uses biphasic temperature chart
  5. Lactation amenorrhea method: effective in fully breast-feeding women, especially 70 to 100 days after delivery; depends on number of feedings per day
- Barriers
  1. Diaphragm and cervical cap: failure rate 5% to 9% in nulliparous women, 20% in multiparous women
  2. Female condom: failure rate with perfect use, 5.1%; with typical use, 12.4%; FDA labeling states 25% failure rate
  3. Male condom: failure rate with perfect use, 3%, with typical use, 12%
  4. Spermicides (aerosols, foam, jellies, creams, tabs): failure rate with perfect use, 3%; with typical use, 21%
- Oral contraceptives
  1. Failure rate with perfect use, <1%; with typical use, 3%
  2. Come in combinations of estrogen/progestin or as progestin only
- Hormonal implants and injectables
  1. Norplant
     a. Most typically used in U.S.
     b. Failure rate in first 5 yr: 1%
     c. Failure rate after 6 yr: 2%
  2. Depo-Provera: failure rate 0.3% in first year of use

3. Lunelle (approved October 2000): failure rate 0.2% in first year
4. Etonogestrel Implant: 2-year cumulative pregnancy rate 0%
- Mini pill (progesterone only pill)
  1. Failure rate with typical use, 1.1% to 13.2%
  2. With perfect use, 5 pregnancies/1000 women
- Emergency postcoital contraception
  1. Decreases pregnancy rate by 75% with women treated immediately postcoitally
  2. Involves hormonal use or IUD insertion
- IUD
  1. Progestasert: failure rate with perfect use, 2%; with typical use, 3%
  2. Copper T (380-A): failure rate with perfect use, 0.8%; with typical use, 3%
  3. Levonorgestrel Intrauterine System (Mirena)
     a. 1-year failure rate <1%
     b. 5-year cumulative failure rate is 0.71/100 women
- Female sterilization (tubal ligation): failure rate with perfect use, 0.2%; with typical use, 3%
- Male sterilization (vasectomy): failure rate of 0.1% in first year
- Vaginal ring: studies ongoing; failure rate not known
- Contraceptive patch: limited data published

■ SYNONYMS

Birth control
Family planning

ICD-9CM CODES

V25.01 Oral contraceptives
V25.02 Other contraceptive measures
V25.09 Family planning
V25.1 IUD
V25.2 Sterilization

■ EPIDEMIOLOGY & DEMOGRAPHICS

For women at risk for pregnancy, ranges for use of most commonly used birth control are dependent, as follows:
- Oral contraceptives: 3% (40 to 44 yr old) to 60% (20 to 24 yr old)
- Condoms: 9% (40 to 44 yr old) to 26% (15 to 19 yr old)
- Diaphragm: 0.8% (15 to 19 yr old) to 8% (30 to 34 yr old)
- Periodic abstinence: 0.7% (15 to 19 yr old) to 3% (35 to 39 yr old)
- Withdrawal: 1.1% (40 to 44 yr old) to 3% (20 to 30 yr old)
- IUD: 0% (15 to 19 yr old) to 3% (30 to 34 yr old)
- Spermicides: 0.8% (15 to 19 yr old) to 2.7% (35 to 39 yr old)
- No method: 6.3% (35 to 39 yr old) to 19.8% (15 to 19 yr old)

- Sterilization
  Female: 0.2% (15 to 19 yr old) to 47% (40 to 44 yr old)
  Male: 0.2% (15 to 19 yr old) to 21% (40 to 44 yr old)
Women are more likely to use contraception. The only two male forms available are condoms and vasectomy (sterilization).

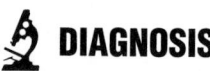 **DIAGNOSIS**

■ WORKUP

- Thorough medical history
- Thorough surgical history
- Obstetric history (fertility desired?)
- Gynecologic history, including:
  1. History of previous sexually transmitted diseases
  2. Number of partners
  3. Previous difficulties with contraception
  4. Frequency of intercourse
- Family history

■ LABORATORY TESTS

- Pap smear
- Cultures, aerobic and *Chlamydia*
- Pregnancy test if suspected pregnancy
- Lipid profile if family history of premature vascular event

TREATMENT

■ NONPHARMACOLOGIC THERAPY

- Male condoms
  1. 95% latex (rubber), 5% skin or natural membrane.
  2. Proper use: place on an erect penis and leave one-half inch empty space at the tip of the condom; use with non-oil-based lubricants.
  3. Effectiveness increased when used with spermicides.
- Female condoms
  1. Composed of polyurethane, with one end open and one end closed.
  2. Proper use: place closed end over cervix, open end hanging out of vagina to cover penis and scrotum.
  3. Highly effective against HIV.
- Spermicides
  1. Types: nonoxynol, octoxynol.
  2. Forms: jellies, creams, foams, suppositories, tablets, soluble films.
  3. Proper use: put in immediately before intercourse; may be used with other barrier methods.
- Diaphragm and cervical cap
  1. Must be fitted by practitioner, used with contraceptive gels, and refitted with weight gain or loss.

2. Diaphragm sizes: 50 to 95 mm; cervical cap sizes: 22, 25, 28, and 31 mm.
3. Proper use of diaphragm: put in immediately before intercourse and keep in for 6 hr after intercourse; must not remain in the vagina for longer than 24 hr.
4. Proper use of cervical cap: fit over the cervix exactly; must not remain in place for longer than 48 hr.

- Lactation amenorrhea method
  1. Depends on number of breast-feedings per day; effective as birth control for 6 mo if 15 or more feedings, lasting 10 min each, are accomplished daily.
  2. Not a common practice in the U.S.
- Withdrawal
  1. Withdrawal of the penis from the vagina before ejaculation
  2. Dependent on self-control
- Rhythm method
  1. Dependent on awareness of physiology of male and female reproductive tracts
  2. Sperm viable in vagina for 2 to 7 days
  3. Ovum life span 24 hr
- Sterilization
  1. Male:
     a. Vasectomy to interrupt vas deferens and block passage of sperm to seminal ejaculate
     b. Scalpel and nonscalpel techniques available
     c. More easily performed procedure than female sterilization and does not require general anesthesia
  2. Female:
     a. Leading method of birth control in U.S. in women older than 30 yr
     b. Interrupts fallopian tubes, blocking passage of ovum proximally and sperm distally through tube
     c. Several types; modified Pomeroy done during cesarean section or laparoscopic done in nonpregnant females most common

■ ACUTE GENERAL Rx
- Combination oral contraceptives
  1. Taken daily for 21 days, pill-free interval of 7 days
  2. Less than 50 μg ethynyl estradiol in most common combination oral contraceptives; progestins most commonly used in combination pills are norethindrone, levonorgestrel, norgestrel, norethindrone acetate, ethynodiol diacetate, norgestimate, or desogestrel; triphasic combination oral contraceptives (give varying doses of progestin and estrogens throughout cycle); monophasic oral contraceptives offer same

dose of progestin and estrogen throughout cycle, taken daily at same time; estrophasic pill (constant progesterone with variation of estrogen throughout the cycle)
  3. If pill taken with antibiotics, efficacy affected by inadequate gastrointestinal absorption in most cases; only rifampin truly reduces pill's effectiveness
- Mini pill
  1. Progestin only; taken without a break
  2. Causes much irregular bleeding because of the lack of estrogen effect on the lining of the uterus
- Hormonal implants and injectables
  1. Norplant
     a. Progestin only; inserted under the skin
     b. Six levonorgestrel implants placed subcutaneously in upper inner arm effective for 5 yr
  2. Depo-Provera
     a. Medroxyprogesterone acetate given every 3 mo in IM injection form
     b. Major side effect: irregular bleeding
     c. Fertility return possibly delayed up to 18 mo after discontinuation
  3. Lunelle: monthly injectable admistered intramuscularly. Contains 0.5 ml aqueous, 5 mg estradiol cypionate and 25 mg medroxyprogesterone acetate
  4. Etonogestrel Implant: single-rod release etonogestrel for 3 yr placed subdermally
- Postcoital contraception
  1. Done on emergency basis, usually secondary to noncompliance with birth control or failure of birth control (e.g., condom breakage) at the time of ovulation
  2. Methods:
     a. IUD insertion within 7 days of coitus
     b. Hormonal methods (combination pills and danazol) given within 48 hr of coitus
- IUD
  1. Device inserted into uterus to prevent sperm and ovum from uniting in fallopian tube
  2. Types available in the U.S.:
     a. Progestasert: A T-shaped device that is an ethylene vinyl acetate copolymer T; vertical stem contains 38 mg progesterone and must be changed yearly
     b. ParaGard (Copper T/380-A): a polyethylene T wrapped with a fine copper wire that is effective for 10 yr of use
     c Levonorgestrel Intrauterine System (LNGIUS): a T-shaped system with a chamber that contains LNG. Releases 20 μg per day; is effective for 5 yr

- Vaginal ring (brand name Nuvarine)
  1. Provides daily dose of 120 μg of etonogestrel and 15 μg ethinyl estradiol
  2. Stays in vagina 3 wk and removed the fourth. Not yet available for use
- Contraceptive patch (brand name Evra)
  1. Provides low daily dose of steroids
  2. Releases a progestin and estrogen (ethinyl estradiol)
  3. Different-sized patches determine daily dose
  4. Common dose 250 μg/day progestin and 25 μg/day estrogen
  5. Worn 3 of 4 wk. Not yet available

■ CHRONIC Rx
- With all of the above types of birth control, patient is followed at least yearly, or as necessary, if problems arise.
- Full history, physical examination, and Pap smear, including cultures when needed, are performed yearly.
- Patients with medical problems are followed about every 6 mo when taking hormonal therapy.

■ DISPOSITION
- Follow yearly or more frequently according to patient's side effects.
- Tailor birth control to patient according to different needs or side effects present at different times in life.

■ REFERRAL
With hormonal contraception, if neurologic or cardiac symptoms arise, stop method immediately, evaluate, and refer to internist when appropriate.

☼ PEARLS & CONSIDERATIONS

■ COMMENTS
- Patient education information available through American College of Obstetricians and Gynecologists (ACOG) at 1-800-673-8444 and through various drug companies representing and supplying the particular type of contraception.
- A clinical algorithm on the use of oral contraceptives is described in Fig. 3-42.

REFERENCES
Clinical proceedings: Association of Reproductive Health Professionals, February 2001.
Dickey R: *Managing contraceptive pill patients,* EMIS, 1998, Louisiana State University Press.
Hatcher RA: *Contraceptive technology,* ed 17, Emory University School of Medicine, 1998, Ardent Media.
Author: **Maria A. Corigliano, M.D.**

BASIC INFORMATION

■ DEFINITION

Conversion disorder is an alteration or loss of voluntary motor or sensory function suggestive of a physical disorder but without demonstrable physical cause and related to a psychologic stress or a conflict.

■ SYNONYMS

Hysteria
Hysterical conversion
Pseudoneurologic illness
Nondisease
Psychosomatic illness
Persistent somatization
Function illness

ICD-9CM CODES

300.11 Conversion disorder

■ EPIDEMIOLOGY & DEMOGRAPHICS

INCIDENCE (IN U.S.): 22 cases/100,000 persons/yr (in Iceland, 11 cases/100,000 persons/yr)
PREVALENCE (IN U.S.): 11 to 300 cases/100,000 persons
PREDOMINANT SEX: More common in women (2-10:1)
PREDOMINANT AGE: Generally a disease of adults
PEAK INCIDENCE: Older than 10 yr and younger than 35 yr
GENETICS: Monozygotic twins have increased risk, but dizygotic twins do not.

■ PHYSICAL FINDINGS & CLINICAL PRESENTATION

- Dysfunction of voluntary activity or sensation
- Most common symptoms: amnesia, difficulty swallowing, speech dysfunction, deafness, visual problems, loss of sensation, fainting, pseudoseizures, gait abnormalities, paresis, and paralysis
- In women: left side of the body more commonly affected
- Other presentations, such as hyperemesis
- In children <10 yr old: gait difficulties or pseudoseizures

- Physical abnormalities (if present) insufficient to explain the presentation
- Proximal psychologic issue identifiable

■ ETIOLOGY

The term *conversion* was coined by Freud and Breuer, who proposed that psychic energy of a conflict is converted into physical symptoms; this remains one of the best theoretical formulations.

DIAGNOSIS

■ DIFFERENTIAL DIAGNOSIS

- Malingering: dysfunction is consciously created for the purpose of secondary gain or avoidance of noxious duties
- Factitious disorder (e.g., Munchausen's syndrome): dysfunction is consciously created for the purpose of assuming the patient role
- Somatization: a related disorder in which psychologic difficulties present with a wide range of somatic complaints that affect several organ systems

■ WORKUP

Physical examination and laboratory evaluation must be sufficient to rule out a physical cause for the dysfunction.

■ LABORATORY TESTS

- No specific laboratory tests
- Goal of tests: to exclude physical cause for the dysfunction

■ IMAGING STUDIES

Goal of tests: to exclude physical cause for the dysfunction

TREATMENT

■ NONPHARMACOLOGIC THERAPY

- Psychotherapy that attempts to address the underlying psychologic conflicts is generally recommended.

- Affected individuals generally are not ideal psychotherapy candidates; supportive psychotherapy is possibly the only reasonable intervention.
- Patients are frequently suggestible, so interventions such as suggestion and hypnosis can be useful.

■ ACUTE GENERAL Rx

Amobarbital (Sodium Amytal) interviews are sometimes used both diagnostically and therapeutically; conversion may disappear under the influence of Amytal.

■ CHRONIC Rx

Conversion has a high recurrence rate, so ongoing psychotherapy may be cost effective.

■ DISPOSITION

- Among hospitalized patients with conversion disorder, remission typically occurs within 2 wk. However, recurrence may occur in 20% to 25% of patients within 1 yr. Recurrences foretell future recurrences.
- Symptoms of pseudoseizures and tremor are less likely to remit than symptoms of paralysis, aphonia, or blindness.

■ REFERRAL

If supportive interventions are not helpful, disability is extreme, or there is no improvement in 2 wk

PEARLS & CONSIDERATIONS

■ COMMENTS

Many patients "elaborate" on symptoms to convince the physician they are ill; this may considerably complicate appropriate diagnosis and therapy.
Author: **Rif S. El-Mallakh, M.D.**

BASIC INFORMATION

■ DEFINITION
A corneal abrasion is a loss of surface epithelial tissue of the cornea caused by trauma.

■ SYNONYMS
Corneal erosion
Corneal contusion

ICD-9CM CODES
918.1 Corneal abrasion

■ EPIDEMIOLOGY & DEMOGRAPHICS
INCIDENCE (IN U.S.): A universal problem
PREDOMINANT AGE: Any age
PEAK INCIDENCE: Childhood through active adulthood

■ PHYSICAL FINDINGS & CLINICAL PRESENTATION
- Haziness of the cornea
- Disruption of the corneal surface (Fig. 1-109)
- Redness and infection of the conjunctiva
- Pain
- Sensation of a foreign body

■ ETIOLOGY
Trauma (direct mechanical event)

DIAGNOSIS

■ DIFFERENTIAL DIAGNOSIS
- Acute angle glaucoma
- Herpes ulcers and other corneal ulcers
- Foreign body in the cornea (be certain it is not a keratitis)

■ WORKUP
- Fluorescein staining, slit lamp evaluation
- Assessment of visual acuity
- Intraocular pressure

TREATMENT

■ NONPHARMACOLOGIC THERAPY
- Warm compresses
- Pressure dressing (controversial)
- Removal of any foreign particles if present

■ ACUTE GENERAL Rx
- Topical antibiotics such as 10% sulfacetamide or Occuflox qid or q2hr
- Pressure patching of eye with eyelid closed
- Cycloplegics such as 5% homatropine

■ CHRONIC Rx
Topical antibiotics to prevent secondary infection

■ DISPOSITION
Follow-up in 24 hr and then every 3 days until abrasion has cleared and vision has returned to normal

■ REFERRAL
To ophthalmologist if patient experiences no relief within 24 hr

PEARLS & CONSIDERATIONS

■ COMMENTS
Never give patient topical anesthetic to use at home because these can cause decomposition of the cornea and permanent damage.

REFERENCE
Le Sage N et al: Efficiency of eye patching for traumatic corneal abrasions: a controlled clinical trial, *Ann Emerg Med* 78:129, 2001.
Author: **Melvyn Koby, M.D.**

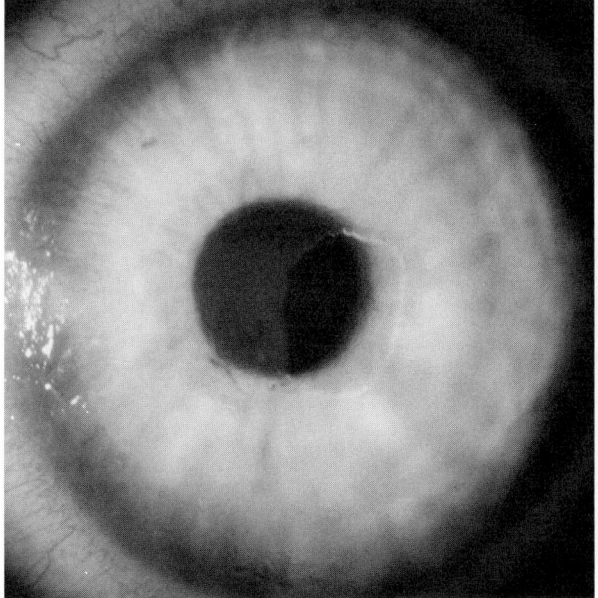
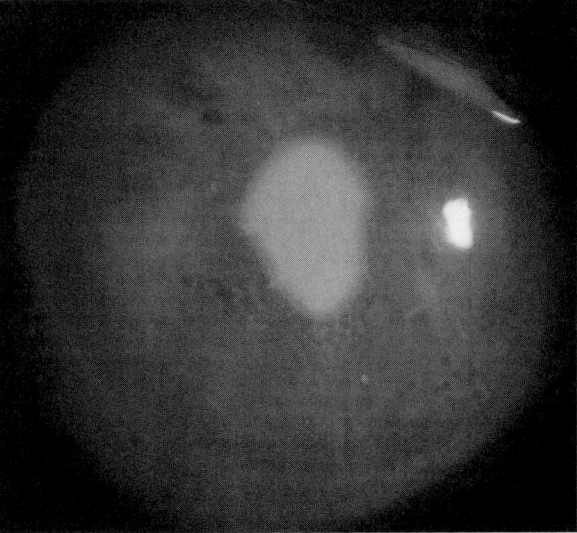

Fig. 1-109 Corneal epithelial abrasion. **A,** Epithelial defect without fluorescein highlighting the defect. An irregularity in the otherwise smooth corneal surface is the key to identifying the defect if no fluorescein is available. **B,** Classic fluorescein staining of an epithelial defect. (From Palay D [ed]: *Ophthalmology for the primary care physician,* St Louis, 1997, Mosby.)

BASIC INFORMATION

■ **DEFINITION**
Corneal ulceration refers to the disruption of the corneal surface and/or deeper layers caused by trauma or infection.

■ **SYNONYMS**
Infectious keratitis
Bacterial keratitis
Viral keratitis
Fungal keratitis

ICD-9CM CODES
370.0 Corneal ulcer NOS

■ **EPIDEMIOLOGY & DEMOGRAPHICS**
INCIDENCE (IN U.S.): 4 to 6 cases/mo seen by average general ophthalmologist
PREVALENCE (IN U.S.): Common
PREDOMINANT SEX: Either
PREDOMINANT AGE: All ages

■ **PHYSICAL FINDINGS**
• Localized, well-demarcated, infiltrative lesion with corresponding focal ulcer (Fig. 1-110) or oval, yellow-white stromal suppuration with thick mucopurulent exudate and edema

• Eye possibly painful, with conjunctival edema and infection

■ **ETIOLOGY**
• Complication of contact lens wear, trauma, or diseases such as herpes simplex keratitis, keratoconjunctivitis sicca
• Viral causes often contagious

 DIAGNOSIS

■ **DIFFERENTIAL DIAGNOSIS**
• *Pseudomonas* and pneumococcus infection—virulent
• *Moraxella, Staphylococcus, α-Streptococcus* infection—less virulent
• Herpes simplex infection or disease caused by other viruses

■ **WORKUP**
• Fluorescein staining, slit lamp
• Appearance often typical

■ **LABORATORY TESTS**
Microscopic examination and culture of scrapings

■ **TREATMENT**

■ **NONPHARMACOLOGIC THERAPY**
• Warm compresses
• Remove eyelid crusting

■ **ACUTE GENERAL Rx**
• An ophthalmic emergency
• Bacterial infection: subconjunctival cefazolin or gentamicin
• Fungal infection: hospitalization and topical application of antifungal agents

■ **DISPOSITION**
Ideally treated by an ophthalmologist if the patient does not rapidly respond to antibiotics (within 24 hr).

■ **PEARLS & CONSIDERATIONS**

■ **COMMENTS**
Do not use topical steroids because herpes, fungal, or other ulcers may be aggravated, leading to perforation of the cornea.
Author: **Melvyn Koby, M.D.**

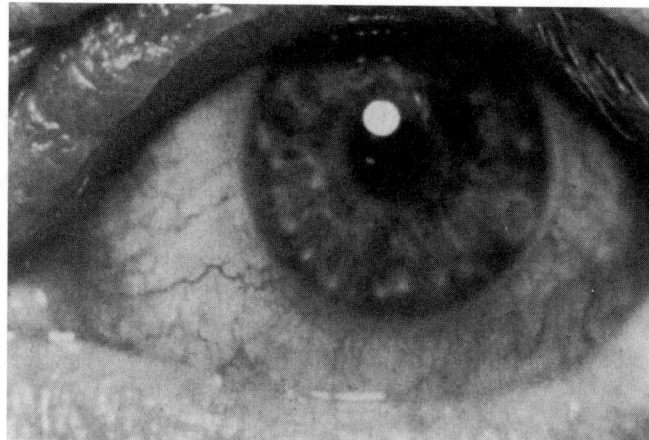

Fig. 1-110   Peripherally located corneal ulcer. (From Rosen P [ed]: *Emergency medicine,* ed 4, St Louis, 1998, Mosby.)

BASIC INFORMATION

■ DEFINITION
Cor pulmonale refers to the enlargement of the right ventricle caused by pulmonary hypertension. Cor pulmonale may be acute or chronic.

■ SYNONYMS
- Acute cor pulmonale
- Chronic cor pulmonale

ICD-9CM CODES
415.0 Cor pulmonale, acute
416.9 Cor pulmonale, chronic

■ EPIDEMIOLOGY & DEMOGRAPHICS
- Cor pulmonale is the third most common cardiac disorder after the age of 50.
- More common in men than in women.

■ PHYSICAL FINDINGS & CLINICAL PRESENTATION
No symptoms are specific for cor pulmonale. Typically cor pulmonale presents according to the underlying disease process, e.g., pulmonary embolism or COPD.
- Dyspnea, pleuritic chest pain, and cough
- Leg swelling
- Hemoptysis
- Wheezing and rales
- Tachypnea and tachycardia
- Cyanosis
- Jugular venous distention with large V waves
- Holosystolic murmur heard best along the left parasternal line, fourth intercostal space and is augmented during inspiration
- Pulsatile hepatomegaly

■ ETIOLOGY
- Cor pulmonale is caused by pulmonary hypertension.
- Mechanisms leading to pulmonary hypertension include:
  1. Pulmonary vasoconstriction resulting from any condition causing alveolar hypoxia and/or acidosis.
  2. Lung parenchymal disorders (e.g., emphysema, interstitial lung disease, pulmonary emboli).
  3. Conditions leading to increased bloom viscocity (e.g., polycythenia vera, Waldenstrom's macroglobulinemia).

4. Idiopathic primary pulmonary hypertension.

 DIAGNOSIS

The diagnosis of cor pulmonale is made in any patient with underlying evidence of pulmonary hypertension and findings of right-sided heart failure.

■ DIFFERENTIAL DIAGNOSIS
- Pulmonary thromboembolic disease
- Chronic obstructive pulmonary disease (COPD)
- Interstitial lung disease
- Neuromuscular diseases causing hypoventilation(e.g., ALS)
- Collagen vascular disease (e.g., SLE, CREST, systemic sclerosis)
- Pulmonary venous disease
- Primary pulmonary hypertension

■ WORKUP
Any patient suspected of cor pulmonale should undergo a workup consisting of blood tests, chest x-ray, echocardiogram, MRI, and occasionally right-side heart catheterization.

■ LABORATORY TESTS
- CBC may show erythrocytosis secondary to hypoxia
- Arterial blood gas (ABGs) confirming hypoxemia and acidosis or hypercapnia.

■ IMAGING STUDIES
- Chest x-ray may show evidence of COPD and pulmonary hypertension.
- Echocardiogram with continuous, pulse, and color Doppler can estimate pulmonary artery pressure. M-mode and 2D measures chamber size and wall thickness.
- Radionuclide ventriculography reveals depressed right ventricular ejection fraction.
- MRI is a sensitive test to measure right ventricular dimensions and detect hypertrophy.
- Right-side catheterization measures pulmonary artery pressures and vascular resistance. It also helps determine response to various therapies (e.g. oxygen, calcium blockers, angiotensin-converting enzyme inhibitors, etc.)

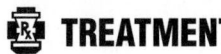 **TREATMENT**

The treatment of cor pulmonale is directed at the underlying etiology while at the same time reversing hypoxemia, hypercapnia, and acidosis.

■ NONPHARMACOLOGIC THERAPY
- Chest physiotherapy is beneficial in patients with COPD and infectious exacerbations.
- Continuous positive airway pressure (CPAP) is used in patients with obstructive sleep apnea.
- Long-term oxygen supplementation has improved survival in hypoxemic patients with COPD.

■ ACUTE GENERAL Rx
- Pulmonary embolism is the most common cause of acute cor pulmonale. Treatment includes:
  1. Thrombolytic therapy (urokinase, tPA, streptokinase) in the hemodynamically unstable patient.
  2. Heparin IV followed by warfarin therapy maintaining an INR between 2 and 3 is the standard therapy for pulmonary embolism (see pulmonary embolism).

■ CHRONIC Rx
- Treatment of chronic cor pulmonale is directed at:
  1. The underlying cause (e.g., COPD, the most common cause of chronic cor pulmonale)
  2. The underlying pathologic process (e.g., pulmonary hypertension)
  3. The underlying pathologic sequelae (e.g., right ventricular [RV] failure)
- Cause
  1. COPD is treated in the standard fashion with metered dose inhalers (see "Chronic Obstructive Pulmonary Disease")
- Rx of pulmonary hypertension
  1. Oxygen supplementation
  2. Vasodilators including nitroglycerine, calcium channel blockers, and angiotensin-converting enzyme inhibitors can be tried.
- Rx of RV failure with diuretics (e.g., furosemide 40 to 80 mg PO qd and digoxin 0.25 mg PO qd)

■ DISPOSITION
- Nearly 50,000 people die each year from acute pulmonary embolism.
- The prognosis of patients with severe COPD and cor pulmonale is poor (survival <2 yr).

✿ PEARLS & CONSIDERATIONS

■ COMMENTS
- Acute elevation of pulmonary artery pressures (30 to 40 mm Hg) results in:
  1. RV dilatation
  2. LV compression
  3. Decreased LV end-diastolic volume
  4. Decreased cardiac output
  5. Hypotension
  6. Mean pulmonary artery pressures >40 mm Hg usually signify a chronic underlying process.

REFERENCES
MacNee W: Pathophysiology of cor pulmonale in chronic obstructive pulmonary disease, *Am J Respir Crit Care Med* 150:833, 1994.

Palevsky HI, Fishman MD: Chronic cor pulmonale: etiology and management, *JAMA* 263(17):2347, 1990.

Author: **Peter Petropoulos, M.D.**

BASIC INFORMATION

■ DEFINITION
Costochondritis is a poorly defined chest wall pain of uncertain cause.

■ SYNONYMS
- Benign chest wall pain syndrome
- Costosternal syndrome
- Costosternal chondrodynia

ICD-9CM CODES
733.6 Costochondritis

■ EPIDEMIOLOGY & DEMOGRAPHICS
PREVALENCE: Unknown
PREVALENT SEX: Women > men
PREVALENT AGE: Over age 40 yr

■ PHYSICAL FINDINGS & CLINICAL PRESENTATION
- Tenderness of costochondral junctions (second through fifth) and/or sternum
- Pain with coughing and deep breathing
- Both sides of chest equal in frequency of involvement

■ ETIOLOGY
- Unknown
- May be a form of regional fibrositis
- May be referred pain from cervical or thoracic spine

DIAGNOSIS

■ DIFFERENTIAL DIAGNOSIS
- Tietze's syndrome
- Cardiovascular disease
- GI disease
- Pulmonary disease
- Osteoarthritis (see Table 1-22)
- Cervical disc syndrome

■ WORKUP
There are no laboratory or radiographic abnormalities.

TREATMENT

■ ACUTE GENERAL Rx
- Explanation, reassurance
- Tricyclic antidepressants for sleep disturbance
- Aerobic exercise program

■ DISPOSITION
- The duration of the disorder is variable
- Spontaneous remission is the rule.

PEARLS & CONSIDERATIONS

■ COMMENTS
In spite of the name, no inflammation is present. After other, more serious conditions are ruled out, the treatment is strictly symptomatic and supportive.
Author: **Lonnie R. Mercier, M.D.**

TABLE 1-22   Musculoskeletal Chest Pain

DISORDER	CLINICAL FEATURES	COMMENTS
Tietze's syndrome	Pain and swelling of sternoclavicular joint or second or third costochondral junctions (usually left). Worse with cough and deep breathing. Local tenderness.	Traumatic cause? Rare.
Costochondritis	Pain and tenderness but no swelling. Costochondral junctions of ribs 2-5. Increased pain with cough and sneeze.	Sometimes associated with headache and hyperventilation.
Seronegative spondyloarthropathy (ankylosing spondylitis)	Sternoclavicular or manubriosternal joint. Worse in AM. Relieved by activity. May be associated with swelling.	Local chest findings usually associated with other symptoms of ankylosing spondylitis such as sacroilitis. May need HLA-B27 antigen testing.
Cervical, thoracic disc disease	Referred regional pain from affected area. No local swelling. Often aggravated by spine motion and may be accompanied by radicular pain into arm if cervical or along intercostal nerve if thoracic.	May mimic chest disease if spinal complaints are minimal and referred or radicular symptoms predominate.
Fibromyalgia	Widespread pain with other sites involved. Symptoms often change in location. Local "tender points" but no swelling or objective findings.	Female:male ratio of 9:1. Prevalent age 30-50 yr
Osteoarthritis, sternoclavicular or manubriosternal joint	Dull, aching local pain with tenderness. Occsional bony joint enlargement with soft-tissue swelling.	Crepitus may rarely be present.

BASIC INFORMATION

■ DEFINITION
Craniopharyngiomas are tumors arising from squamous cell remnants of Rathke's pouch, located in the infundibulum or upper anterior hypophysis.

■ SYNONYMS
Subset of nonadenomatous pituitary tumors

ICD-9CM CODES
237.0 Craniopharyngioma

■ EPIDEMIOLOGY & DEMOGRAPHICS
PEAK INCIDENCE: Occurs at all ages; peak during the first two decades of life, with a second small peak occurring in the sixth decade.
PREDOMINANT SEX: Both sexes are usually equally affected. Craniopharyngiomas represent 2% to 4% of intracranial neoplasms and 10% of central nervous system tumors in childhood.

■ PHYSICAL FINDINGS & CLINICAL PRESENTATION
- Presenting symptoms are usually related to the effects of a sella turcica mass. Approximately 75% of patients complain of headache and have visual disturbances.
- The usual visual defect is bitemporal hemianopsia. Optic nerve involvement with decreased visual acuity and scotomas and homonymous hemianopsia from optic tract involvement may also occur.
- Other symptoms include mental changes, nausea, vomiting, somnolence, or symptoms of pituitary failure. In adults, sexual dysfunction is the most common endocrine complaint, with impotence in males and primary or secondary amenorrhea in females. Diabetes insipidus is found in 25% of cases. In children, craniopharyngiomas may present with dwarfism.

■ ETIOLOGY
Craniopharyngiomas are believed to arise from nests of squamous epithelial cells that are commonly found in the suprasellar area surrounding the pars tuberalis of the adult pituitary.

DIAGNOSIS

■ DIFFERENTIAL DIAGNOSIS
- Pituitary adenoma
- Empty sella syndrome
- Pituitary failure of any cause
- Primary brain tumors (e.g., meningiomas, astrocytomas)
- Metastatic brain tumors
- Other brain tumors
- Cerebral aneurysm

■ LABORATORY TESTS
- Hypothyroidism (low TT_4, TT_3, T_3RU, FT_4, FT_3) with low TSH
- Hypocortisolism (low cortisol) with low ACTH
- Low sex hormones (testosterone, estriol) with low FSH and LH
- Diabetes insipidus (see "Diabetes insipidus")
- Prolactin may be normal or slightly elevated
- Pituitary stimulation tests may be required in some cases

■ IMAGING STUDIES
- Visual field testing for bitemporal hemianopsia
- Skull film
  Enlarged or eroded sella turcica (50%)
  Suprasellar calcification (50%)
- Head CT scan or MRI (Fig. 1-111)

TREATMENT

- Surgical resection (curative or palliative)
  Transsphenoidal surgery for small intrasellar tumors
  Subfrontal craniotomy for most patients
- Postoperative radiation
- Intralesional ^{32}P irradiation or bleomycin for unresectable tumors

■ PROGNOSIS
- Operative mortality: 3% to 16% (higher with large tumors)
- Postoperative recurrence rate: 10% to 40%
- 5-yr and 10-yr survival: 88% and 76%, respectively, with surgery and radiation

REFERENCES
Asa SL, Horvath E, Kovacs K: Craniopharyngiomas. In Mazzaferri EL, Samaan NA (eds): *Endocrine tumors,* Boston, 1993, Blackwell Scientific Publications

Leavens ME et al: Nonadenomatous intrasellar and parasellar neoplasms. In Mazzaferri EL, Samaan NA (eds): *Endocrine tumors,* Boston, 1993, Blackwell Scientific Publications.
Author: **Tom J. Wachtel, M.D.**

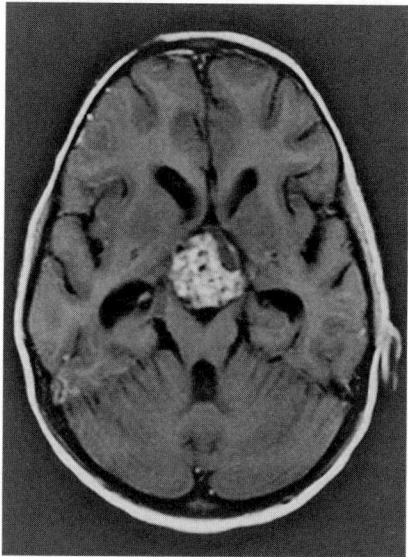

Fig. 1-111   MRI scan of a craniopharyngioma, demonstrating a cystic contrast-enhancing mass in the suprasellar area extending upward and compressing the hypothalamus. (From Goetz CG: *Textbook of clinical neurology,* Philadelphia, 1999, WB Saunders.)

BASIC INFORMATION

■ DEFINITION
Creutzfeldt-Jakob disease is a progressive, dementing process caused by an infectious agent known as a *prion*.

■ SYNONYMS
Subacute spongiform encephalopathy
Gerstmann-Sträussler syndrome

■ ICD-9CM CODES
046.1 Creutzfeldt-Jakob disease

■ EPIDEMIOLOGY & DEMOGRAPHICS
INCIDENCE (IN U.S.): 1 case/1 million persons/yr
PREVALENCE (IN U.S.): After diagnosis, death occurs in 6 mo to 1 yr
PREDOMINANT SEX: Men = women
PEAK INCIDENCE: Over 50 yr
PEAK AGE: 60 yr
GENETICS: 5% to 15% familial

■ PHYSICAL FINDINGS & CLINICAL PRESENTATION
Subacute dementia and *myoclonus* (Alzheimer's with movements like a cat going to sleep)

■ ETIOLOGY
Infectious "slow virus" prion

DIAGNOSIS

■ DIFFERENTIAL DIAGNOSIS
• Alzheimer's disease
• Other dementias (vascular, endocrine, vitamin deficiency, infectious syphilis)
A clinical algorithm for the evaluation of dementia is described in Fig. 3-49.

■ WORKUP
• Evaluate for curable causes of dementia (see Alzheimer's disease).
• Brain biopsy can be diagnostic, but it is usually not performed. The prion is transmitted, as far as is known, from brain to an open wound. For this reason, neurosurgeons and pathologists are reluctant to be involved with these cases, although there is no documented case of this having actually occurred (Table 1-23).

■ LABORATORY TESTS
• EEG may show burst-suppression pattern (Fig. 1-112).
• Rule out curable causes of dementia.

■ IMAGING STUDIES
CT scan to rule out NPH, space-occupying lesions

TREATMENT

■ NONPHARMACOLOGIC THERAPY
Constant caregiver usually necessary

■ ACUTE GENERAL Rx
No known therapy

■ CHRONIC Rx
No known therapy

■ DISPOSITION
Nursing home often required

■ REFERRAL
If NPH or brain tumor found

PEARLS & CONSIDERATIONS

■ COMMENTS
• Not known to be transmissible except through direct contact with brain.
• Autopsy important to confirm diagnosis.
• Only the patient's brain is infective.
• Closely related to "mad cow" disease.

REFERENCE
Johnson RT, Gibbs CJ: Creutzfeldt-Jakob disease and related transmissible spongiform encephalopathies, *N Engl J Med* 339:1994, 1998.
Author: **William H. Olson, M.D.**

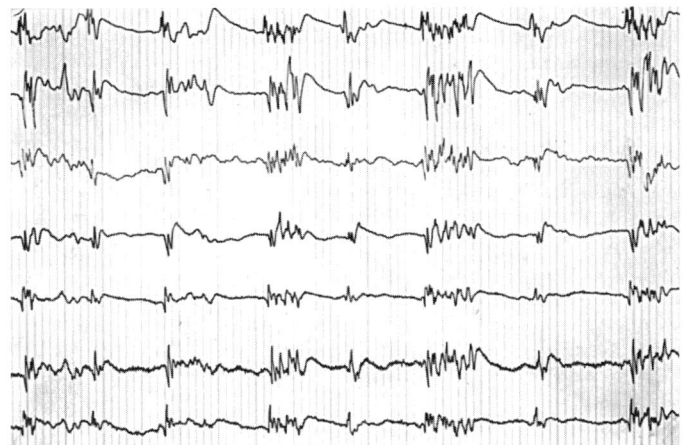

Fig. 1-112 Periodic electroencephalographic recordings in sporadic Creutzfeldt-Jakob disease. Tracing shows a "burst-suppression" pattern. (From Goetz CG: *Textbook of clinical neurology,* Philadelphia, 1999, WB Saunders.)

TABLE 1-23 **Iatrogenic Transmission of Creutzfeldt-Jakob Disease by Products of Human Origin**

| PRODUCT | NO. PATIENTS | INCUBATION | |
		MEAN	RANGE
Corneal transplants	2	17 mo	16-18 mo
Dura mater allograft*	48	7.4 yr	13-16 yr
Human pituitary extract			
Growth hormone	>95†	12 yr	5-30 yr
Gonadotropin	4	13 yr	12-16 yr

From Noble J: *Primary care medicine,* ed 3, St Louis, 2001, Mosby.
*Cases recently recognized in Japan are not included.
†Sixteen cases/≈8000 estimated recipients in United States.

BASIC INFORMATION

■ DEFINITION
Crohn's disease is an inflammatory disease of the bowel of unknown etiology, most commonly involving the terminal ileum and manifesting primarily with diarrhea, abdominal pain, fatigue, and weight loss.

■ SYNONYMS
Regional enteritis
Inflammatory bowel disease (IBD)

ICD-9CM CODES
555.9 Crohn's disease, unspecified site
555.0 Crohn's disease, small intestine
555.1 Crohn's disease involving large intestine

■ EPIDEMIOLOGY & DEMOGRAPHICS
PREVALENCE: 1 case/1000 persons; most common in Caucasians and Jews

■ PHYSICAL FINDINGS & CLINICAL PRESENTATION
- Abdominal tenderness, mass, or distention
- Hyperactive bowel sounds in patients with partial obstruction, bloody diarrhea
- Delayed growth and failure of normal development in children
- Perianal and rectal abscesses, mouth ulcers, and atrophic glossitis
- Extraintestinal manifestations: joint swelling and tenderness, hepatosplenomegaly, erythema nodosum, clubbing, tenderness to palpation of the sacroiliac joints

■ ETIOLOGY
Unknown

DIAGNOSIS

■ DIFFERENTIAL DIAGNOSIS
- Ulcerative colitis
- Infectious diseases (TB, *Yersinia, Salmonella, Shigella, Campylobacter*)
- Parasitic infections (amebic infection)
- Pseudomembranous colitis
- Ischemic colitis in elderly patients
- Lymphoma
- Colon carcinoma
- Diverticulitis
- Radiation enteritis
- Collagenous colitis
- Fungal infections (*Histoplasma, Actinomyces*)
- Gay bowel syndrome (in homosexual patient)
- Carcinoid tumors
- Celiac sprue
- Mesenteric adenitis

■ LABORATORY TESTS
- Decreased Hgb and Hct from chronic blood loss.
- Hypokalemia, hypomagnesemia, hypocalcemia, and low albumin from chronic diarrhea possible.
- Vitamin B_{12} and folate deficiency.
- Endoscopic features of Crohn's disease include asymmetric and discontinued disease, deep longitudinal fissures, cobblestone appearance, presence of strictures. Crypt distortion and inflammation are also present. Granulomas may be present.

■ IMAGING STUDIES
- Barium imaging studies reveal deep ulcerations (often longitudinal and transverse), segmental lesions (skip lesions, strictures, fistulas, cobblestone appearance of mucosa caused by submucosal inflammation); "thumbprinting" is common, "string sign" in terminal ileum may be noted.
- In 5% to 10% of patients with IBD, a clear distinction between ulcerative colitis and Crohn's disease cannot be made. Generally, Crohn's disease can be distinguished from ulcerative colitis by presence of transmural involvement and the frequent presence of noncaseating granulomas and lymphoid aggregates.

TREATMENT

■ NONPHARMACOLOGIC THERAPY
- Nutritional supplementation is needed in patients with advanced disease. TPN may be necessary in selected patients.
- Low-residue diet is necessary when obstructive symptoms are present.
- If diarrhea is prominent, increased dietary fiber and lowering of fat in the diet are sometimes helpful.
- Psychotherapy is useful for situational adjustment crises. A trusting and mutually understanding relationship and referral to self-help groups are very important because of the chronicity of the disease and the relatively young age of the patients.
- Avoid oral feedings during acute exacerbation to decrease colonic activity: a low-roughage diet may be helpful in early relapse.

■ ACUTE GENERAL Rx
- Sulfasalazine, 500 mg PO qid initially, increased qd or qod by 1 g until therapeutic dosages of 4 to 6 g/day are achieved. The oral salicylates, mesalamine (Asacol, Rowasa) are as effective as sulfasalazine and better tolerated but more expensive; they may be useful in patients allergic to the sulfa moiety of sulfasalazine molecule.
- Corticosteroids (prednisone) 40 to 60 mg/day are useful for acute exacerbation. Steroids are usually tapered over approximately 2 to 3 mo. Some patients require a low dose for prolonged period of maintenance.
- Immunosuppressive drugs, such as azathioprine (Imuran) 150 mg/day, methotrexate or cyclosporine can be used for severe, progressive disease. In patients with Crohn's disease who enter remission after treatment with methotrexate, a low dose of methotrexate maintains remission.
- Metronidazole (Flagyl) 50 mg qid is useful for colonic fistulas.
- Infliximab, a chimeric monoclonal antibody targeting tumor necrosis factor-alpha, is effective in the treatment of enterocutaneous fistulas.
- Hydrocortisone (Cortenema) enema bid or tid is useful for proctitis.
- Most patients who have anemia associated with Crohn's disease respond to intravenous iron alone. Erythropoietin is useful in patients with anemia refractory to treatment with iron and vitamins.

■ CHRONIC Rx
- Monitoring of disease activity with symptom review and laboratory evaluation (CBC and sedimentation rate)
- Liver tests and vitamin B_{12} levels monitored on a yearly basis

■ REFERRAL
- GI referral is needed for endoscopic procedures.
- Surgical referral is needed for complications such as abscess formation, obstruction, fistulas, toxic megacolon, refractory disease, or severe hemorrhage. A conservative surgical approach is necessary, because surgery is not curative. Multiple surgeries may also result in short bowel syndrome.

REFERENCES
Feagan BG et al: A comparison of methotrexate with placebo for the maintenance of remission in Crohn's disease, *N Engl J Med* 342:1627, 2000.
Schwartz D et al: Diagnosis and treatment of perianal fistulas in Crohn disease, *Ann Intern Med* 135(10):906, 2001.
Author: **Fred F. Ferri, M.D.**

BASIC INFORMATION

■ DEFINITION
Cryptococcosis is an infection caused by the fungal organism *Cryptococcus neoformans*.

ICD-9CM CODES
117.5 Cryptococcosis

■ EPIDEMIOLOGY & DEMOGRAPHICS
INCIDENCE (IN U.S.)
- 1 to 2 cases/1 million (non-HIV-infected) persons annually
- 6% to 7% in HIV-infected persons

PREDOMINANT SEX: Equal sex distribution when corrected for HIV status
PREDOMINANT AGE: Less than 2 yr of age; 20 to 40 yr of age
PEAK INCIDENCE: 20 to 40 yr (parallel to AIDS epidemic)
NEONATAL INFECTION: Very uncommon

■ PHYSICAL FINDINGS & CLINICAL PRESENTATION
- Over 90% present with meningitis; almost all have fever and headache.
- Meningismus, photophobia, mental status changes are seen in approximately 25%.
- Focal intracranial infection occurs in rare cases with focal deficit, increased intracranial pressure.
- Most common infections outside the CNS:
  1. In the lungs (fever, cough, dyspnea)
  2. In the skin (cellulitis, papular eruption)
  3. In the lymph nodes (lymphadenitis)
  4. Potential involvement of virtually any organ

■ ETIOLOGY
- Caused by the fungal organism *C. neoformans*
- Transmission by the respiratory route
- Disseminates to the CNS in most cases, usually without recognizable lung involvement
- Almost always in the setting of AIDS or other disorders of cellular immune function (hematologic malignancies, long-term corticosteroid therapy, immunosuppressive therapy following organ transplantation), or pregnancy

DIAGNOSIS

■ DIFFERENTIAL DIAGNOSIS
- Acute or subacute meningitis (caused by *Neisseria meningitidis, Streptococcus pneumoniae, Haemophilus influenzae, Listeria monocytogenes, Mycobacterium tuberculosis, Histoplasma capsulatum,* viruses)
- Intracranial mass lesion (neoplasms, toxoplasmosis, TB)
- Pulmonary involvement confused with *Pneumocystis carinii* pneumonia when diffuse or confused with TB or bacterial pneumonia when focal or involving the pleura
- Skin lesions confused with bacterial cellulitis or molluscum contagiosum

■ WORKUP
- Lumbar puncture to exclude cryptococcal meningitis; a differential diagnosis of common fungal infections in the CNS is described in Table 2-79.
- CT scan of the head when focal lesion or increased intracranial pressure are suspected.
- Biopsy of enlarged lymph nodes and skin lesions if feasible.

■ LABORATORY TESTS
- Culture and India ink stain (60% to 80% sensitive in culture-proven cases [Fig. 1-113]), examination of the CSF in all cases when CNS involvement is suspected
- Blood and serum cryptococcal antigen assay (>90% sensitivity and specificity)
- Culture and histologic examination of biopsy material

■ IMAGING STUDIES
- CT scan or MRI of the head if focal neurologic involvement is suspected
- Chest x-ray examination to exclude pulmonary involvement

TREATMENT

■ ACUTE GENERAL Rx
- Therapy is initiated with IV amphotericin B (0.5 mg/kg/day) with or without flucytosine.
- After stabilization (usually several weeks), consider fluconazole (200 to 400 mg qd PO) for additional 6 to 8 wk.
- Alternative: IV fluconazole for initial therapy in patients unable to tolerate amphotericin B.
- If symptomatic increased intracranial pressure, consider therapeutic lumbar taps or intraventricular shunt.

■ CHRONIC Rx
Fluconazole (200 mg PO qd) is highly effective in preventing a relapse in HIV-infected patients.

■ DISPOSITION
Without maintenance therapy, relapse rate is >50% among AIDS patients.

■ REFERRAL
- For consultation with infectious diseases specialist in all cases
- For neurologic consultation if level of consciousness is depressed or focal lesion is present

PEARLS & CONSIDERATIONS

■ COMMENTS
Cryptococcosis is considered an AIDS-defining infection when it occurs in the absence of other known causes of immunodeficiency; thus all patients should be advised to be HIV tested and, if positive, referred for evaluation and follow-up by a physician experienced in the management of HIV infection.

REFERENCE
Powderly WG: Current approach to the acute management of cryptococcal infections, *J Infect Dis* 41:18, 2000.
Author: **Joseph R. Masci, M.D.**

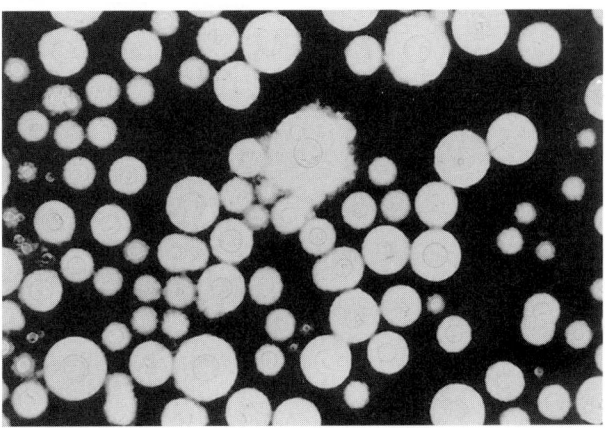

Fig. 1-113 India ink preparation of cerebrospinal fluid revealing encapsulated cryptococci. Note the large capsules surrounding the smaller organisms. (From Andreoli TE [ed]: *Cecil essentials of medicine*, ed 4, Philadelphia, 1997, WB Saunders.)

BASIC INFORMATION

■ DEFINITION
Cryptorchidism refers to a testis that neither resides in nor can be manipulated into the scrotum.

■ SYNONYMS
Undescended testis

ICD-9CM CODES
752.51 Cryptorchidism

■ EPIDEMIOLOGY & DEMOGRAPHICS
Cryptorchidism is the most common genitourinary disorder of male children. The incidence is 3% to 5% at birth, decreasing to about 1% at 3 mo of age (similar to the postpubertal rate). Increased rates are associated with premature birth, low birth weight, and twinning. Associations have been seen with Kallmann's and Prader-Willi syndromes, pituitary hypoplasia, testicular feminization, and Reifenstein syndrome.

■ PHYSICAL FINDINGS & CLINICAL PRESENTATION
- Typically asymptomatic and is noted incidentally on screening examination
- The testis may be impalpable or palpable in a location other than the scrotum but usually along the path of normal descent (Fig. 1-114)
- Associated with infertility and a 10- to 20-fold increase in risk of testicular cancer, which can occur in the contralateral descended testis

■ ETIOLOGY
Normal testicular descent is a complex interplay between differential growth and endocrine, gubernaculum, and genitofemoral nerve function. Developmental problems among some or all of these are postulated in causing cryptorchidism.

DIAGNOSIS

■ DIFFERENTIAL DIAGNOSIS
- Retractile testis
- Ascended testis
- Dislocated testis
- Anorchia

■ WORKUP
Physical examination, hormonal challenge, imaging studies

■ PHYSICAL EXAMINATION
When properly done in a warm room, an examination identifies presence or absence of palpable testis and location of palpable testes.

■ HORMONAL CHALLENGE
Administration of hCG will confirm the presence of testes that are not palpable by leading to testosterone production. hCG will cause retractile testes to remain in the scrotum.

■ IMAGING
CT scan or MRI can be used to identify impalpable testes, but the sensitivity is inadequate. Laparoscopy is preferred and can be used therapeutically.

TREATMENT

■ FOLLOW-UP
- Repeat examination at 3 mo of age, because many testes will descend spontaneously
- Lifelong testicular examination after puberty to screen for malignancy

■ HORMONAL Rx
GnRH and hCG alone or in succession

■ SURGICAL Rx
Orchiopexy alone or following hormonal therapy or orchiectomy is an alternative.

■ DISPOSITION
Prognosis is fair. Fertility and malignancy risks not greatly affected by treatment.
Author: **Michael Picchioni, M.D.**

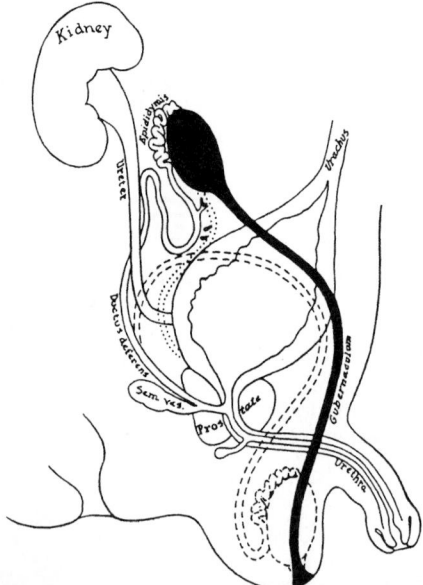

Fig. 1-114 Undescended testes are common in male neonates with neuromuscular disease already symptomatic at birth, regardless of the etiology. The gubernaculum is a cylinder of striated muscle surrounding a core of smooth muscle that actively pulls the testicle into the scrotum in late gestation. Weakness of the gubernaculum in a generalized myopathy of fetal life prevents or delays the descent of the testis. (Reproduced with permission from Sarnat HB, Sarnat MS: Disorders of muscle in the newborn. In Moss AJ, Stern L [eds]: *Pediatrics update,* ed 4, New York, 1983, Elsevier-North Holland.)

BASIC INFORMATION

■ **DEFINITION**

The intracellular protozoan parasite *Cryptosporidium parvum* is associated with gastrointestinal disease and diarrhea, especially in AIDS patients or immunocompromised hosts. It is also associated with waterborne outbreak in immunocompetent hosts.

■ **SYNONYMS**

Cryptosporidosis

ICD-9CM CODES

00.7.4 Cryptosporidia infection

■ **EPIDEMIOLOGY & DEMOGRAPHICS**

PREVALENCE: Worldwide, especially third world countries; associated with poor hygiene as a waterborne pathogen

TRANSMISSION:
• Person to person (daycare, family members)
• Animal to person (pets, farm animals)
• Environmental (water-associated outbreaks, including travel associated with swimming in or drinking contaminated water)
• May be significant pathogen causing diarrhea in AIDS

INCIDENCE (IN U.S.):
• Approximately 2% in industrial countries, 5% to 10% in third world countries
• 10% to 20% HIV patients may excrete cyst in U.S.

PREDOMINANT SEX: Male = female

■ **PHYSICAL FINDINGS & CLINICAL PRESENTATION**

• Usually limited to gastrointestinal tract
• Diarrhea, severe abdominal pain (2 to 28 days)
• Impaired digestion, dehydration
• Fever, malaise, fatigue, nausea, vomiting
• Pneumonia if aspirated

■ **ETIOLOGY**

Cryptosporidium parvum

 DIAGNOSIS

Clinical presentation of acute gastrointestinal illness, especially associated with HIV or with travel and waterborne outbreaks.

■ **DIFFERENTIAL DIAGNOSIS**
• *Campylobacter*
• *Clostridium difficile*
• *Entamoeba histolytica*
• *Giardia lamblia*
• *Salmonella*
• *Shigella*
• Microsporida
• Cytomegalovirus
• *Mycobacterium avium*

Disease may cause cholecystitis, reactive arthritis, hepatitis, pancreatitis, pneumonia in immunocompromised or HIV-infected patients.

■ **WORKUP**
• Stool evaluation looking for characteristic oocyst by modified acid-fast stain (Fig. 1-115)

• Serologic testing investigational
• May be seen in mucosal surfaces of GI lumen by biopsy

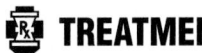 **TREATMENT**

May be self-limited in normal host—often requiring hydration. Antidiarrhea agents Pepto-Bismol, Kaopectate, or loperamide may give symptomatic relief.

Pharmacologic treatment with antibiotics have to date varying and usually poor response. Oocyst excretion reduction has been shown with paromomycin (1 g bid)/azithromycin (600 mg/day) therapy along with decreasing stool frequency. If treatment failure, consider metromidazole or bactrim.

REFERENCES

Manabe YC et al: Cryptosporidiosis in patients with AIDS: correlates of disease and survival, *Clin Infect Dis* 27:536, 1998.

Smith NH et al: Combination drug therapy for cryptosporidiosis in AIDS, *J Infect Dis* 178:900, 1998.

Tzipori S: Cryptosporidiosis: laboratory investigations and chemotherapy, *Adv Parasitol* 40:187, 1998.

Author: **Dennis J. Mikolich, M.D.**

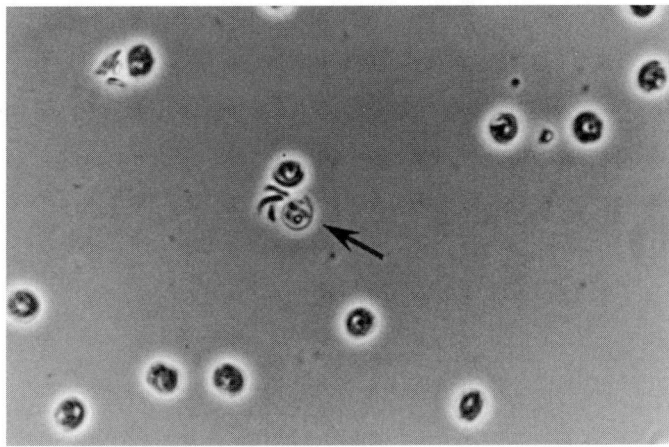

Fig. 1-115 Human stool–derived *Cryptosporidium* oocysts. Excysting oocyst *(arrow)* is releasing three of its four sporozoites. (Phase-control microscopy ×630.) (From Gorbach SL: *Infectious diseases,* ed 2, Philadelphia, 1998, WB Saunders.)

BASIC INFORMATION

■ DEFINITION
- Cushing's syndrome is the occurrence of clinical abnormalities associated with glucocorticoid excess secondary to exaggerated adrenal cortisol production or chronic glucocorticoid therapy.
- Cushing's disease is Cushing's syndrome caused by pituitary ACTH excess.

ICD-9CM CODES
255.0 Cushing's disease or syndrome

■ PHYSICAL FINDINGS & CLINICAL PRESENTATION
- Hypertension
- Central obesity with rounding of the facies (moon facies); thin extremities
- Hirsutism, menstrual irregularities, hypogonadism
- Skin fragility, ecchymoses, red-purple abdominal striae, acne, poor wound healing, hair loss, facial plethora, hyperpigmentation (when there is ACTH excess)
- Psychosis, emotional lability, paranoia
- Muscle wasting with proximal myopathy

NOTE: The above characteristics are not commonly present in Cushing's syndrome secondary to ectopic ACTH production. Many of these tumors secrete a biologically inactive ACTH that does not activate adrenal steroid synthesis. These patients may have only weight loss and weakness.

■ ETIOLOGY
- Iatrogenic from chronic glucocorticoid therapy (common)
- Pituitary ACTH excess (Cushing's disease; 60%)
- Adrenal neoplasms (30%)
- Ectopic ACTH production (neoplasms of lung, pancreas, kidney, thyroid, thymus; 10%)

DIAGNOSIS

■ DIFFERENTIAL DIAGNOSIS
- Alcoholic pseudo-Cushing's syndrome (endogenous cortisol overproduction)
- Obesity associated with diabetes mellitus
- Adrenogenital syndrome

■ WORKUP (see Fig. 1-116)
- In patients with a clinical diagnosis of Cushing's syndrome the initial screening test is the overnight dexamethasone suppression test:
  1. Dexamethasone 1 mg PO given at 11 PM

  2. Plasma cortisol level measured 9 hr later (8 AM)
  3. Plasma cortisol level <5 μg/100 ml excludes Cushing's syndrome
- Serial measurements (two or three consecutive measurements) of 24-hr urinary free cortisol and creatinine (to ensure adequacy of collection) are undertaken if overnight dexamethasone test is suggestive of Cushing's syndrome. Persistent elevated cortisol excretion (>300 μg/24 hr) indicates Cushing's syndrome.
- The low-dose (2 mg) dexamethasone suppression test is useful in order to exclude pseudo-Cushing's syndrome if the above results are equivocal. CRH stimulation after low-dose dexamethasone administration (dexamethasone-CRH test) is also used to distinguish patients with suspected Cushing's syndrome from those who have mildly elevated urinary free cortisol level and equivocal findings.
- The high-dose (8 mg) dexamethasone test and measurement of ACTH by RIA are useful to determine the etiology of Cushing's syndrome.
  1. ACTH undetectable or decreased and lack of suppression indicates adrenal etiology of Cushing's syndrome.
  2. ACTH normal or increased and lack of suppression indicate ectopic ACTH production.
  3. ACTH normal or increased and partial suppression suggest pituitary excess (Cushing's disease).
- A single midnight serum cortisol (normal diurnal variation leads to a nadir around midnight) >7.5 μg/dl has been reported as 96% sensitive and 100% specific for the diagnosis of Cushing's syndrome
- Fig. 1-116 describes a diagnostic approach to Cushing's syndrome

■ LABORATORY TESTS
- Hypokalemia, hypochloremia, metabolic alkalosis, hyperglycemia, hypercholesterolemia
- Increased 24-hr urinary free cortisol (>100 μg/24 hr)

■ IMAGING STUDIES
- CT scan of adrenal glands in suspected adrenal Cushing's syndrome
- MRI of pituitary gland with gadolinium in suspected pituitary Cushing's syndrome
- Additional imaging studies to localize neoplasms of the lung, pancreas, kidney, thyroid, or thymus in patients with ectopic ACTH production

TREATMENT

■ ACUTE GENERAL Rx
The treatment of Cushing's syndrome varies with its cause:

- Pituitary adenoma: transsphenoidal microadenomectomy is the therapy of choice in adults. Pituitary irradiation is reserved for patients not cured by transsphenoidal surgery. In children, pituitary irradiation may be considered as initial therapy, since 85% of children are cured by radiation. Stereotactic radiotherapy (photon knife or gamma knife) is effective and exposes the surrounding neuronal tissues to less irradiation than conventional radiotherapy. Total bilateral adrenalectomy is reserved for patients not cured by transsphenoidal surgery or pituitary irradiation.
- Adrenal neoplasm:
  1. Surgical resection of the affected adrenal
  2. Glucocorticoid replacement for approximately 9 to 12 mo after the surgery to allow time for the contralateral adrenal to recover from its prolonged suppression
- Bilateral micronodular or macronodular adrenal hyperplasia: bilateral total adrenalectomy
- Ectopic ACTH:
  1. Surgical resection of the ACTH-secreting neoplasm
  2. Control of cortisol excess with metyrapone, aminoglutethimide, mifepristone, or ketoconazole
  3. Control of the mineralocorticoid effects of cortisol and 11-deoxycorticosteroid with spironolactone
  4. Bilateral adrenalectomy: a rational approach to patients with indolent, unresectable tumors

■ CHRONIC Rx
Patient education regarding maintenance of proper weight and side effects of drug therapy

■ DISPOSITION
Prognosis is favorable in patients with surgically amenable disease.

PEARLS & CONSIDERATIONS

■ COMMENTS
Screening for MEN I should be considered in patients with Cushing's disease.

REFERENCES

Boscaro M et al: The diagnosis of Cushing's syndrome, *Arch Intern Med* 160:3045, 2000.

Papanicolaou DA et al: A single midnight serum cortisol measurement distinguishes Cushing's syndrome from pseudo-Cushing states, *J Clin Endocrinol Metab* 83:1163, 1998.

Author: **Fred F. Ferri, M.D.**

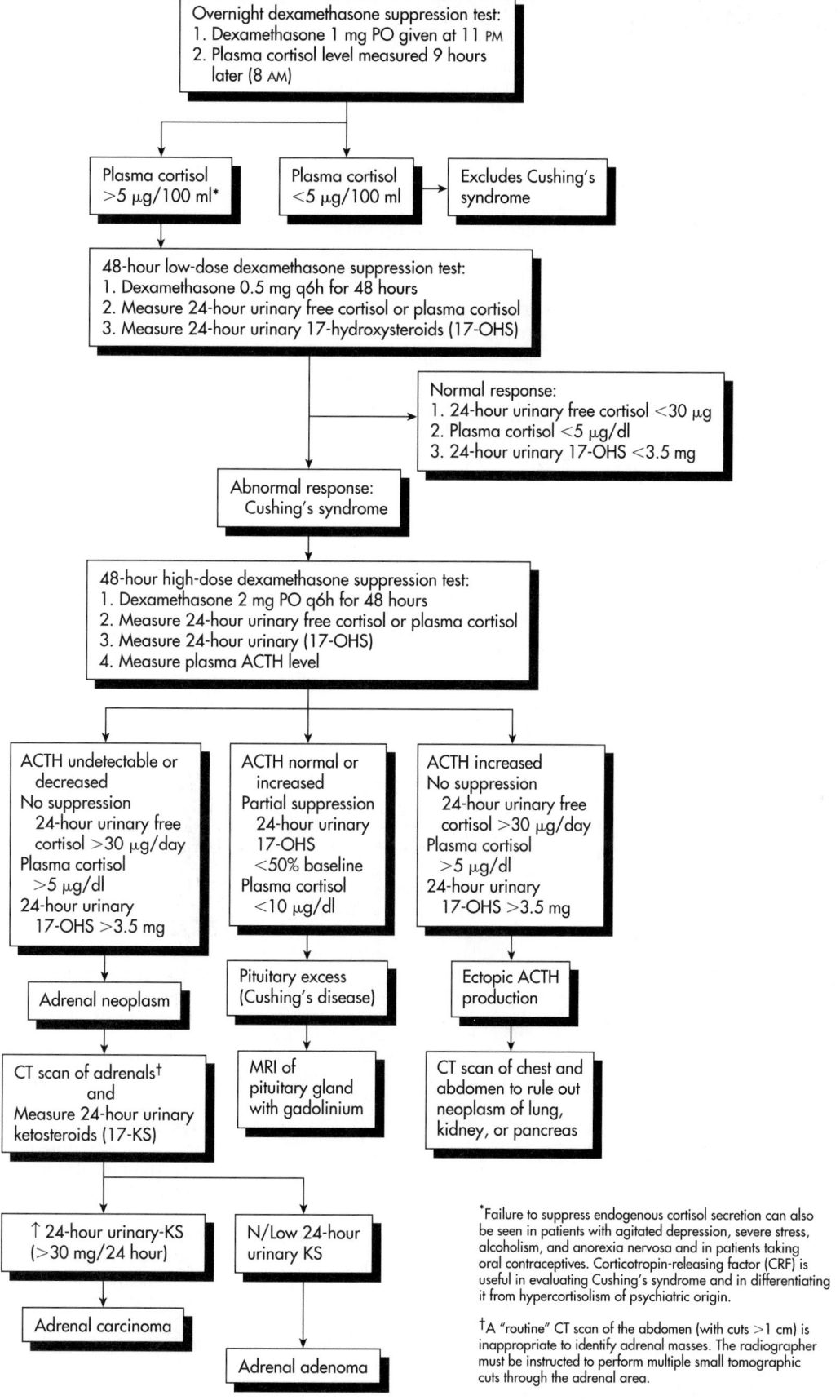

Fig. 1-116   Cushing's syndrome. *ACTH,* Adrenocorticotropic hormone; *CT,* computed tomography; *MRI,* magnetic resonance imaging; *PO,* by mouth. (From Ferri F: *Practical guide to the care of the medical patient,* ed 5, St Louis, 2001, Mosby.)

BASIC INFORMATION

■ DEFINITION
Cystic fibrosis (CF) is an autosomal recessive disorder characterized by dysfunction of exocrine glands.

■ ICD-9CM CODES
277.0 Cystic fibrosis

■ EPIDEMIOLOGY & DEMOGRAPHICS
• It is the most common fatal hereditary disorder of whites in the U.S. (1 case/2500 whites).
• Median survival is 30 yr.

■ PHYSICAL FINDINGS & CLINICAL PRESENTATION
• Failure to thrive in children
• Increased anterior/posterior chest diameter
• Basilar crackles and hyperresonance to percussion
• Digital clubbing
• Chronic cough
• Abdominal distention
• Greasy, smelly feces

■ ETIOLOGY
Chromosome 7 gene mutation (CFTR gene) resulting in abnormalities in chloride transport and water flux across the surface of epithelial cells; the abnormal secretions cause obstruction of glands and ducts in various organs and subsequent damage to exocrine tissue (recurrent pneumonia, atelectasis, bronchiectasis, diabetes mellitus, biliary cirrhosis, cholelithiasis, intestinal obstruction, increased risk of GI malignancies)

DIAGNOSIS

■ DIFFERENTIAL DIAGNOSIS
• Immunodeficiency states
• Celiac disease
• Asthma
• Recurrent pneumonia

■ WORKUP
A diagnosis of CF requires a positive quantitative pilocarpine iontophoresis test with one or more phenotypic features consistent with CF (e.g., chronic suppurative obstructive lung disease, pancreatic insufficiency) or documented CF in a sibling or first cousin.

■ LABORATORY TESTS
• Pilocarpine iontophoresis ("sweat test"): diagnostic of cystic fibrosis in children if sweat chloride is >60 mmol/L (>80 mmol/L in adults) on two separate tests on consecutive days

• DNA testing may be useful for confirming the diagnosis and providing genetic information for family members.
• Sputum C&S and Gram stain (frequent bacterial infections with *Staphylococcus aureus, Pseudomonas, Haemophilus influenzae*)
• Low albumin level, increased 72-hr fecal fat excretion
• ABGs: hypoxemia
• Pulmonary function studies: decreased TLC, forced vital capacity, pulmonary diffusing capacity

■ IMAGING STUDIES
• Chest x-ray examination: may reveal focal atelectasis, peribronchial cuffing, bronchiectasis, increased interstitial markings, hyperinflation
• High resolution chest CT scan: bronchial wall thickening, cystic lesions, ring shadows (bronchiectasis)

TREATMENT

■ NONPHARMACOLOGIC THERAPY
• Postural drainage and chest percussion
• Encouragement of regular exercise and proper nutrition
• Psychosocial evaluation and counseling of patient and family members

■ ACUTE GENERAL Rx
• Antibiotic therapy based on results of Gram stain and C&S of sputum (PO ciprofloxacin or floxacillin for *Pseudomonas*, cephalosporins for *S. aureus*, IV aminoglycosides plus ceftazidine for life-threatening *Pseudomonas* infections)
• Bronchodilators for patients with air flow obstruction
• Chronic pancreatic enzyme replacement
• Alternate-day prednisone (2 mg/kg) possibly beneficial in children with cystic fibrosis (decreased hospitalization rate, improved pulmonary function); routine use of corticosteroids not recommended in adults; among children with cystic fibrosis who have received alternate-day treatment with prednisone, boys, but not girls, have persistent growth impairment after treatment is discontinued
• Proper nutrition and vitamin supplementation
• Recombinant human deoxyribonuclease (DNase [Dornase alpha]) 2.5 mg qd or bid given by aerosol for patients with viscid sputum; useful but expensive (annual cost to the pharmacist is >$10,000); most bene-

ficial in patients with FVC values >40% of predicted
• Intermittent administration of inhaled tobramycin has been reported beneficial in CF
• Treatment of glucose intolerance and diabetes mellitus

■ CHRONIC Rx
Pneumococcal vaccination, yearly influenza vaccination

■ DISPOSITION
• More than 50% of children with cystic fibrosis live beyond age 20 yr.
• Lung transplantation is the only definitive treatment; 3-yr survival following transplantation exceeds 50%.
• Obstructive azoospermia is present in >98% of postpubertal males.

■ REFERRAL
• To regional ambulatory care cystic fibrosis center
• For lung transplantation in selected patients
• For screening of family members with DNA analysis

PEARLS & CONSIDERATIONS

■ COMMENTS
• Genetic testing for CF should be offered to adults with a positive family history of CF, to couples currently planning a pregnancy, and to couples seeking prenatal care. Patient education material can be obtained from Cystic Fibrosis Foundation, 6931 Arlington Road, Suite 2000, Bethesda, MD 20814.

REFERENCES
Lai H et al: Risk of persistent growth impairment after alternate-day prednisone treatment in children with cystic fibrosis, *N Engl J Med* 342:851, 2000.
National Institute of Health Consensus Development Conference Statement on Genetic Testing for Cystic Fibrosis, *Arch Intern Med* 159:1529, 1999.
Ramsey BW et al: Intermittent administration of inhaled tobramycin in patients with cystic fibrosis, *N Engl J Med* 340:23, 1999.
Rosenstein BJ, Cutting GR for the Cystic Fibrosis Foundation Consensus Panel: The diagnosis of cystic fibrosis: a consensus statement, *J Pediatr* 132:589, 1998.
Author: **Fred F. Ferri, M.D.**

BASIC INFORMATION

■ DEFINITION

Cysticerci, the larval form of the pork tapeworm *Taenia solium,* are so named because they are enclosed in bladderlike cysts. Cysticercosis represents a tissue infection with the cysts of *T. solium.* The mature tapeworm resides in the host intestine, but egg ingestion can lead to cysts being deposited in both soft tissue and, more important, the central nervous system; the latter condition is referred to as *neurocysticercosis.*

ICD-9CM CODES
123.1 Cysticercosis

■ EPIDEMIOLOGY & DEMOGRAPHICS

Neurocysticercosis, considered the most common parasitic disease of the CNS, affects thousands of people in Latin America, Asia, and Africa. Increasing numbers of immigrants from developing countries and improved diagnostic procedures have led to increased recognition of the entity in the United States. Neurocysticercosis is no longer an exotic disease in this country, and it accounts for up to 2% of neurologic and neurosurgical admissions in southern California and more than 1000 cases per year nationally. Cysticercosis is acquired by ingesting fecally contaminated food or water containing eggs of the pork tapeworm. Exposure to undercooked pork does not directly expose the host to cysticerci but to intestinal *Taenia;* excretion of eggs in the feces follows. Eggs can be ingested by the source patient or be transmitted via food handlers. Neurocysticercosis has been reported in AIDS patients; immunosuppression does not seem to increase the incidence of the infection.

■ PHYSICAL FINDINGS & CLINICAL PRESENTATION

- Soft tissue deposition of cysts can cause local inflammation, which results in only minor morbidity compared to the damage possible in neurocysticercosis.
- Epilepsy caused by intracerebral cysts is most common manifestation of neurocysticercosis (70% to 90% of cases).
- Less common: headache, nausea and vomiting resulting from increased intracranial pressure, and altered mental status, including psychosis.
- The patient with a seizure history often has no unusual physical findings.
- Inflammation around degenerating cysts can cause focal encephalitis, vasculitis, chronic meningitis, and cranial nerve palsies.

- Cysts can occur in the ventricles and cause hydrocephalus; more rarely, they can be found in the spinal cord and eye.

■ ETIOLOGY

While ingestion of the *Taenia solium* cysticerci in infected, undercooked pork results in human intestinal tapeworms, ingestion of the *Taenia solium* eggs leads to release of an oncosphere, which traverses the intestinal wall and enters the circulation. Oncospheres mature into cysticerci; these can be deposited in the soft tissue or the CNS. The presence of viable cysts in the CNS is usually asymptomatic. With time, inflammation around degenerating cysts causes symptoms dependent on the cysts' location, number, and size.

DIAGNOSIS

■ DIFFERENTIAL DIAGNOSIS
- Idiopathic epilepsy
- Migraine
- Vasculitides
- Primary neoplasia of CNS
- Toxoplasmosis
- Brain abscess
- Granulomatous disease such as sarcoidosis

■ WORKUP
- Comprehensive clinical history
- Stool examination for ova if intestinal tapeworms also suspected
- Imaging studies (precedes laboratory tests if CNS involvement suspected)
- CSF examination
- Laboratory tests (serology)

■ IMAGING STUDIES

Head CT scan can show living cysticerci (hypodense lesions) and degenerating cysts (isodense or hyperdense lesions). Typically, there are multiple lesions. CT scan is the best method for detecting calcification associated with prior infection. Brain MRI provides detailed images of living and degenerating cysts, but it may not detect destroyed lesions. MRI is the best means to diagnose intraventricular cysticerci noninvasively.

■ LABORATORY TESTS
- CSF examination: may show pleocytosis, with lymphocytic or eosinophilic predominance, low glucose, elevated protein with neurocysticercosis
- Immunotest: both serum and CSF can be studied for antibodies. ELISA sensitivity and specificity >90% when done in inflammatory CSF

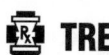

TREATMENT

A plan for treatment should follow a clear definition of the characteristics of the cysts and the degree of the immune response to the parasite.
- Inactive infection: patients with seizures and calcifications alone on neuroimaging studies are not thought to have viable parasites. Cysticidal therapy is usually not undertaken. Anticonvulsants can control seizures. For patients with hydrocephalus, ventriculoperitoneal shunting can resolve symptoms.
- Active parenchymal infection (most common form presentation): eradication of cysts is less controversial for active disease. Anticonvulsants should be given to control seizures. Some argue that only treatment of seizures, not antiparasitic therapy, is needed.
- Extraparenchymal neurocysticercosis: refer to a neurosurgeon.
  Ventricular: usually presents with obstructive hydrocephalus. The mainstay of therapy is the rapid correction of hydrocephalus.
  Subarachnoid: is associated with arachnoiditis. Diversion of CSF and steroid therapy may be needed.
- Cysticidal therapy: praziquantel has been the mainstay of therapy and is effective; albendazole is now being used more frequently, and it may have greater efficacy at a lesser cost than praziquantel.
  Dosage: PO praziquantel 50 mg/kg/day divided into three doses for 14 days. NOTE: Praziquantel is metabolized via P-450 and levels may be reduced when given in combination with anticonvulsants. Levels can increase with cimetidine.
  PO albendazole 15 mg/kg/day divided into three doses for 8 days. May add to steroid therapy, especially if treatment causes worsening of inflammation.

■ REFERRAL

Neurosurgical consultation if extraparenchymal neurocysticercosis or obstructive hydrocephalus suspected

PEARLS & CONSIDERATIONS

■ PREVENTION

Eradication of taeniasis/cysticercosis is possible, as demonstrated in countries that were endemic earlier in this century. The disease disappears with implementation of meat inspection, improvement of pig husbandry, and betterment of sociocultural conditions.

Authors: **Karoll Cortez, M.D., and Anne Spaulding, M.D.**

BASIC INFORMATION

■ DEFINITION
Infection with cytomegalovirus (CMV), a herpes virus, is common in the general population, with multiple mechanisms for transmission, often during childhood and adolescence. CMV is associated with pregnancy and can be a congenital disease. CMV is also associated with immunocompromised states and may be life threatening.

■ SYNONYMS
CMV
Cytomegalic inclusion disease virus

ICD-9CM CODES
078.5 CMV infection
771.1 Congenital or perinatal CMV infection
V01.7 Exposure to CMV

■ EPIDEMIOLOGY & DEMOGRAPHICS
- Seroprevalence is widespread: 40% to 100% antibody positivity in adults.
- Increased infection develops perinatally, in day care exposure, and then during reproductive age, related to sexual activity.

■ ROUTES OF TRANSMISSION
- Blood transfusions
- Sexually (STDs) via uterus, cervix, and semen
- Perinatally via breast milk
- Transplant of organs—kidneys, liver, heart, or lung

■ PHYSICAL FINDINGS & CLINICAL PRESENTATION
Children: Congenital—25% of infected children with symptoms if congenital:
- Jaundice
- Petechial rash
- Hepatosplenomegaly
- Lethargy
- Respiratory distress
- CNS involvement
- Seizures
Postnatal acquisition:
- CMV mononucleosis
- Pharyngitis
- Bronchitis
- Pneumonia
- Croup
Healthy adults:
- May be asymptomatic
- CMV mononucleosis similar to EBV mononucleosis
- Fever—lasting 9 to 30 days—mean of 19 days
- Rare lymphadenopathy—splenomegaly

- Interstitial pneumonia (rare)
- Hepatitis
- Guillain-Barré syndrome
- Meningoencephalitis
- Myocarditis
- Thrombocytopenia/hemolytic anemia
- Cervical adenopathy
- Granulomatous hepatitis
- Hemolytic anemia
Immunosuppressed patients:
- Febrile mononucleosis
- GI ulcerations, hepatitis, pneumonitis, retinitis, encephalopathy, meningoencephalopathy
- HIV associated—dementia, demyelination, retinitis (Fig. 1-117), acalculous cholecystitis, adrenalitis, diarrhea, enterocolitis, esophagitis
- Diabetes associated with pancreatitis
- Adrenalitis associated with HIV

■ ETIOLOGY
Cytomegalovirus infection can remain latent, reactive with immunosuppression.

DIAGNOSIS

■ DIFFERENTIAL DIAGNOSIS
Congenital:
- Acute viral, bacterial, parasitic infections including other congenitally transmitted agents (toxoplasmosis, rubella, syphilis, pertussis, croup, bronchitis).
Acquired:
- EBV mononucleosis
- Viral hepatitis—A, B, C
- Cryptosporidiosis
- Toxoplasmosis
- *Mycobacterium avium* infections

■ WORKUP
- Laboratory confirmation combined with clinical findings often with leukopenia, thrombocytopenia, lymphocytosis
- Demonstration of virus in tissue or serologic testing including rising titers of complement fixation (CF) and indirect fluorescent antibody (IFA) or anticomplement IFA
- Fundoscopic—necrotic patches with white granular component of retina
- Cultures—(viral) human fibroblast from urine, cervical swab, tissue buffy coat

■ IMAGING STUDIES
- Chest x-ray—if pneumonitis suspected, consider bronchoscopy
- Endoscopy—if GI involvement
- Fundoscopy—retinitis

- CT scan/MRI—if CNS involvement

TREATMENT

For compromised hosts with CMV retinitis or pneumonitis:
- Ganciclovir 5 mg/kg bid IV × 21 days, then 5 mg/kg/day IV, or 1 g PO tid or occular implant
- Foscarnet 60 mg/kg tid × 3 wk, then 90 mg/kg/day
- Cidofovir 5 mg/kg IV, repeat 1 wk later, then q2 wk IV
- Fomvirsen-salvage therapy for CMV retinitis 300 mcg injected into vitreous

REFERENCES
De Otoro J et al: CMV disease as a risk factor for graft loss and death after orthotopic liver transplantation, *Clin Infect Dis* 26:865, 1998.
MacDonald JC et al: High active antiretroviral therapy-related immune recovery in AIDS patients with cytomegalovirus retinitis, *Ophthalmology* 107:877, 2000.
Spector SA et al: Plasma CMV DNA load predicts CMV disease and survival in AIDS patients, *J Clin Invest* 101:497, 1998.
Author: **Dennis J. Mikolich, M.D.**

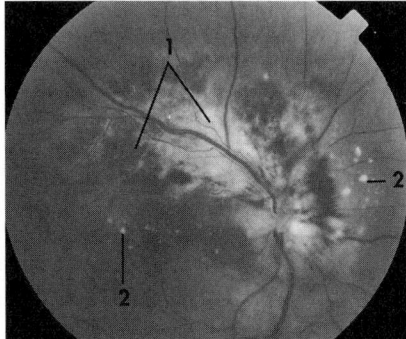

Fig. 1-117 Sight-threatening CMV retinitis involves the macula and optic nerve of this HIV-positive young man. White, infected retina with intraretinal hemorrhage is present in the arcuate distribution of the nerve fiber layer *(1)*. A small amount of lipid exudation near the fovea and nasal to the optic nerve is also seen *(2)*. (From Palay D [ed]: *Ophthalmology for the primary care physician,* St Louis, 1997, Mosby.)

BASIC INFORMATION

■ DEFINITION

Decubitus ulcers (pressure ulcers) are any damage to the skin and the underlying tissue or both that results from pressure, friction, or shearing forces that usually occur over bony prominences such as the sacrum or heels.

■ SYNONYMS

Pressure ulcers
Pressure sores
Bed sores
Sacral decubitus
Decubiti

■ ICD-9CM CODES

707.0 Decubitus ulcers

■ EPIDEMIOLOGY & DEMOGRAPHICS

Pressure ulcers are present in 5% to 10% of patients in all health care settings: hospitals, nursing homes, and home-confined. Pressure ulcers are associated with significant morbidity and mortality. Pain occurs in two thirds of patients with stage II or greater pressure ulcers. Cellulitis, osteomyelitis, abscesses, and sepsis are all associated with pressure ulcers. One-year mortality approaches 40%.

■ PHYSICAL FINDINGS & CLINICAL PRESENTATION

All pressure ulcers should be staged according to the depth and type of tissue damage.

Stage I	Nonblanchable erythema of intact skin
Stage II	Partial-thickness skin loss involving the epidemis, dermis, or both
Stage III	Full-thickness skin loss involving damage or necrosis of subcutaneous tissue that may extend down to, but not through, underlying fascia or muscle
Stage IV	Full-thickness skin loss with extensive destruction and tissue damage to muscle, bone, or supporting structures (e.g., tendons, joint capsule)

■ ETIOLOGY

- Impaired mobility leading to prolonged pressure
- Urinary or fecal incontinence
- Malnutrition
- Friction or shearing forces on skin

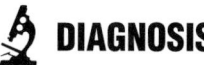 **DIAGNOSIS**

■ DIFFERENTIAL DIAGNOSIS

- Venous stasis ulcers
- Arterial ulcers
- Diabetic ulcers
- Skin cancer
- Cellulitis

■ WORKUP

All ulcers should have a description of the ulcer (i.e., stage, location, size), the wound bed (i.e., epithelialization, granulation tissue, necrotic tissue, eschar), the presence of any exudates, which includes type and amount, the wound edges (i.e., undermining, sinus tracts, tunneling, or fistulas), signs of infection, and pain. In addition, pressure ulcer risk factors and their causes should be reassessed.

■ LABORATORY TESTS

Directed at identifying the cause of risk factors or any complications arising from the pressure ulcer (e.g., abscess or osteomyelitis)

■ IMAGING STUDIES

MRI or bone scans can be used to help identify osteomyelitis.

TREATMENT

■ PREVENTION STRATEGIES

- Identify high-risk patients
- Routine skin inspection and good skin care for high-risk patients
- Minimize prolonged skin exposure to moisture, including urine and stool
- Avoid excessive drying and cracking of skin
- Reduce skin pressure through repositioning and pressure-reducing devices
- Proper positioning when in bed or chair
- Shear and friction reduction

■ MANAGEMENT STRATEGIES FOR PRESSURE ULCERS

- Pressure ulcers should be cleaned at each dressing change, and necrotic tissue should be debrided.
- Wound irrigation should not exceed 15 psi and is best done with an 18-gauge angiocatheter.
- Use dressing to keep ulcer bed moist and protect it from urine and stool.
- Avoid agents that are cytotoxic to epithelial cells (e.g., iodine, iodophor, sodium hypochlorite, hydrogen peroxide, acetic acid, and alcohol).
- Reduce pressure by using foam mattress, dynamic support surface (e.g., low-air-loss bed), and frequent repositioning (e.g., q2h).
- Hyperbaric oxygen, ultrasound, ultraviolet and low-energy radiation, and growth factors either are ineffective or have not been evaluated.
- Correct poor nutrition.
- Minimize urinary and fecal incontinence.

■ DISPOSITION

When systematic risk assessments are done and preventive measures are followed, most pressure ulcers can be prevented. Most pressure ulcers heal when appropriate management strategies are followed.

■ REFERRAL

- To physical and occupational therapists to improve bed and chair mobility
- Wounds with necrotic tissue to physicians, nurses, or physical therapists trained in sharp debridement
- To plastic surgeons for operative repair for large stage III or IV ulcers that do not respond to optimal care

REFERENCES

Pressure ulcers in adults: prediction and prevention, Clinical practice guideline No 3; Treatment of pressure ulcers, Clinical practice guideline No 4, AHCPR Publication No 92-0047 & 95-0652, Rockville, Md, 1994, US Department of Health and Human Services, Public Health Service, Agency for Health Care Policy and Research.
Author: **David R. Gifford, M.D., M.P.H.**

BASIC INFORMATION

■ DEFINITION
Delirium tremens refers to overactivity of the central nervous system after cessation of alcohol intake. The time interval is variable; it usually occurs within 1 wk after reduction or cessation of heavy alcohol intake and persists for 1 to 3 days (Fig. 1-118).

■ SYNONYMS
Alcohol withdrawal syndrome
DTs
Alcoholic delirium

ICD-9CM CODES
291.00 Alcohol withdrawal delirium

■ EPIDEMIOLOGY & DEMOGRAPHICS
INCIDENCE (IN U.S.): Up to 500,000 cases annually
PREDOMINANT SEX: Male
PEAK INCIDENCE: 30 yr and older
PEAK AGE: Teenage years and older
GENETICS: More common with patients who have relatives who are alcoholics

■ PHYSICAL FINDINGS & CLINICAL PRESENTATION
• Initially: anxiety, insomnia, tremulousness
• Early: tachycardia, sweating, anorexia, agitation, headache, GI distress
• Late: seizures, visual hallucinations, delirium

■ ETIOLOGY
Alcoholism

 DIAGNOSIS

■ DIFFERENTIAL DIAGNOSIS
Be alert for coexisting illness, trauma, and drug usage.

■ WORKUP
• Frequent rating of symptoms (hallucinations, tremor, sweating, agitation, orientation).
• The CIWA-Ar Scale can be used to measure the severity of alcohol withdrawal.

■ LABORATORY TESTS
• Electrolytes
• Close monitoring of glucose levels
• Drug screen

■ IMAGING STUDIES
CT scan of head if there is a history of head trauma

TREATMENT

■ NONPHARMACOLOGIC THERAPY
Refer to drug rehabilitation program after patient recovers.

■ ACUTE GENERAL Rx
• Prescribe diazepam 150 to 200 mg/day or chlordiazepoxide 400 to 600 mg/day.
• 100 mg thiamine IV daily.
• For severe withdrawal, consider adrenergic blockers (0.1 to 0.3 tid of clonidine).

■ CHRONIC Rx
Alcoholics Anonymous has the best record in breaking addiction, but the results are still disappointing.

■ DISPOSITION
Refer to drug rehabilitation program.

■ REFERRAL
If cardiac arrhythmias are prominent or respiratory distress develops

PEARLS & CONSIDERATIONS

■ COMMENTS
This is a potentially lethal disease if not carefully treated. Mortality is 15% in untreated patients.
Author: **William H. Olson, M.D.**

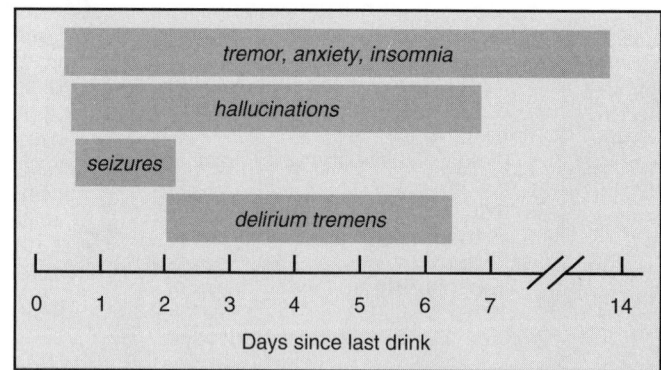

Fig. 1-118 Time course of alcohol withdrawal. (From Goldman L, Bennett JC [eds]: *Cecil textbook of medicine,* ed 21, Philadelphia, 2000, WB Saunders.)

BASIC INFORMATION

■ DEFINITION

Major depression is an episodic, frequently recurrent syndrome lasting at least 2 wk with five of the following symptoms: depressed mood; diminished interest, pleasure, energy, self-worth, ability to think and concentrate; altered sleep pattern, appetite, and level of psychomotor activity.

■ SYNONYMS

Unipolar depression
Depressive episode

ICD-9CM-CODES

296.2 Major depressive disorder, single episode

■ EPIDEMIOLOGY & DEMOGRAPHICS

INCIDENCE (IN U.S.): 10% of men; 20% of women
PREVALENCE (IN U.S.): 2.5% of men; 8% of women
PREDOMINANT SEX: Female > male
PREDOMINANT AGE: 25 to 44 yr
PEAK INCIDENCE: 30 to 40 yr
GENETICS:
• Clear evidence of familial predominance
• No established pattern of inheritance

■ PHYSICAL FINDINGS & CLINICAL PRESENTATION

• Psychomotor retardation with slowed thinking, slowed responses, slowed physical movements, depressed affect and mood, sleep disturbance, appetite disturbance
• May be associated with mood-congruent delusional thinking (paranoid and melancholic themes)
• May be associated with active or passive suicidal ideation

■ ETIOLOGY

• Unknown
• Several factors possible: neuroendocrine response to unremitting stress, hormones, social/developmental factors

DIAGNOSIS

■ DIFFERENTIAL DIAGNOSIS

• Hypothyroidism
• Neurosyphilis
• Major organ system disease (e.g., cardiovascular, liver, renal, neuronal diseases, and others) with depressive symptoms
• Elderly patients: frequently coexists with dementia

■ WORKUP

• History
• Physical examination
• Mental status examination
• A clinical approach to the treatment of depression in primary care is described in Fig. 1-119.

■ LABORATORY TESTS

All done to rule out other major organ system disease:
• Routine chemistries
• CBC with differential
• Sedimentation rate
• Thyroid function studies

■ IMAGING STUDIES

With unusual presentations (e.g., associated with new-onset severe headache, focal neurologic signs, a cognitive or sensory disturbance), the following are performed:
• EEG (diffuse slowing indicates metabolic encephalopathy)
• Anatomic brain imaging (CT scan or MRI)

TREATMENT

■ NONPHARMACOLOGIC THERAPY

• Many forms of psychotherapy are helpful.
• Behavioral, cognitive, and interpersonal psychotherapies have efficacy rates of 40% to 50%.

■ ACUTE GENERAL Rx

• Many antidepressants are available, all with efficacy rates of 60% to 65%.
• Serotonin reuptake inhibitors generally are first-line agents.
• Therapy should be continued for 6 to 12 mo.
• Several treatment-refractory strategies are available.

■ CHRONIC Rx

The risk of recurrence exceeds 90% in individuals having experienced three or more depressive episodes; for these individuals continuous prophylactic therapy is recommended.

■ DISPOSITION

• Course is variable.
• Additional episodes are experienced by >60% of individuals having one depressive episode.
• There can be increasing or decreasing numbers of episodes into old age.
• Depression associated with physical disorders generally does not resolve until physical disorder improves.

■ REFERRAL

• If treatment refractory
• If patient imminently suicidal (Box 1-14)

☼ PEARLS & CONSIDERATIONS

■ CAUTION

All threats of suicide should be taken very seriously.

REFERENCES

El-Mallakh RS et al: Clues to depression in primary care practice, *Postgrad Med* 100:85, 1996.
Irwin M et al: Screening for depression in the older adult, *Arch Intern Med* 159:1701, 1999.
Sampson SM: Treating depression with selective serotonin reuptake inhibitors: a practical approach, *Mayo Clin Proc* 76:739, 2001.
Whooler MA, Simon GE: Managing depression in medical outpatients, *N Engl J Med* 343:1842, 2000.
Author: **Rif S. El-Mallakh, M.D.**

BOX 1-14   Interview Protocol for Evaluating Suicidal Ideation

1. "You have said you are depressed; could you tell me what that's like for you?"
2. "Are there times you feel like crying?"
3. "When you feel that way, what sort of thoughts go through your mind?"
4. "Do you ever get to the point where you feel that if this is the way things are that it is not worth going on?"
5. "Have you gone so far as to think of taking your own life?"
6. "Have you made any plan?"
7. "Do you have the means to carry out such a plan?"
8. "Is there anything that would prevent you from carrying out the plan?"

From Goldberg RJ (ed): *Practical guide to the care of the psychiatric patient,* ed 2, St Louis, 1998, Mosby.

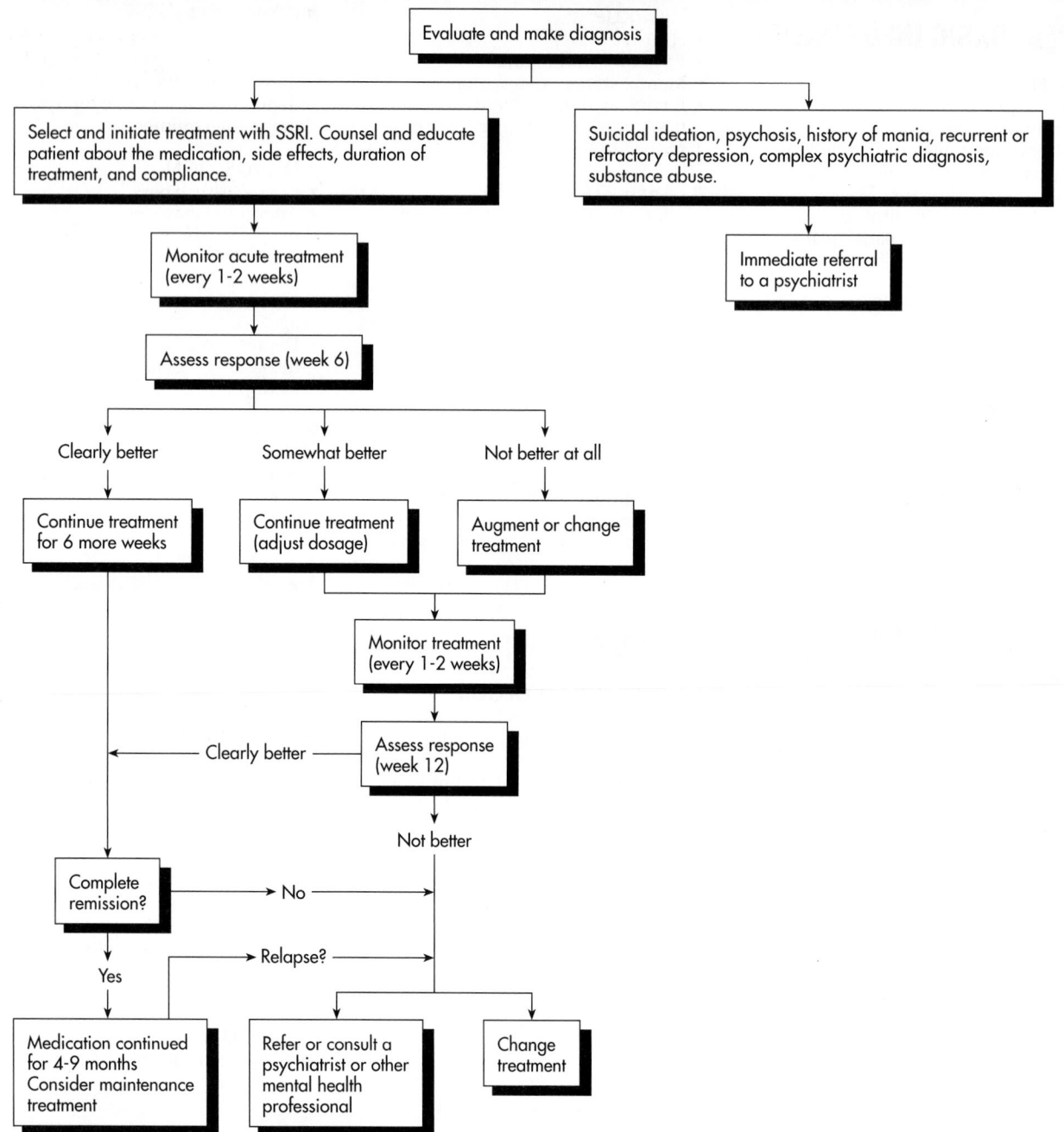

Fig. 1-119   Guidelines for the treatment of depression in the primary care setting. *SSRI,* Selective serotonin reuptake inhibitor. NOTE: Time of assessment (weeks 6 and 12) rests on very modest data. It may be necessary to revise the treatment plan earlier for patients who fail to respond. (From AHCPR Quick Reference Guide of Clinicians, No. 5: Depression in primary care: *Detection, diagnosis and treatment,* 1993; and American Psychiatric Association: *Diagnostic and statistical manual of mental disorders,* ed 4, Washington, DC, 1994, American Psychiatric Association.)

BASIC INFORMATION

■ **DEFINITION**
De Quervain's tenosynovitis refers to a stenosing inflammatory process of the first dorsal retinacular compartment containing the tendons of the abductor pollicis longus (APL) and extensor pollicis brevis (EPB).

■ **SYNONYMS**
Stenosing tenosynovitis of the radial styloid
Stenosing tenovaginitis of the first dorsal compartment

■ **ICD-9CM CODES**
727.04 Tenosynovitis radial styloid

■ **EPIDEMIOLOGY & DEMOGRAPHICS**
• More common in women than in men (10:1)
• Usually occurs between the ages of 30 to 50
• Associated with rheumatoid arthritis
• Seen in occupations (e.g., clerical, assembly, and manual labor)

■ **PHYSICAL FINDINGS & CLINICAL PRESENTATION**
• Pain over the styloid process of the radius.
• Swelling.
• Positive Finkelstein's test (Fig. 1-120): stretching the tendons of the APL and EPB by clasping the thumb with the fingers and passive deviation of the wrist to the ulnar side. Provocation of pain is a positive sign.
• Crepitance.

■ **ETIOLOGY**
• The cause is usually repetitive use or overuse of the hands.

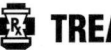 **DIAGNOSIS**

• The diagnosis of de Quervain's tenosynovitis is based on the clinical triad of:
  1. Tenderness over the radial styloid
  2. Swelling over the first dorsal retinacular compartment
  3. Positive Finkelstein's test (Fig. 1-120)
• Sometimes 1.5 cc of 1% xylocaine can be injected into the tenosynovial sac and if all three physical signs resolve, the diagnosis is confirmed

■ **DIFFERENTIAL DIAGNOSIS**
• Carpal tunnel syndrome
• Ostearthritis
• Gout
• Infiltrative tenosynovitis
• Radiculopathy
• Compression neuropathy (e.g., superficial branch of the radial nerve "bracelet syndrome")
• Infection (e.g., tuberculosis, bacterial)

■ **WORKUP**
The workup of suspected de Quervain's tenosynovitis requires laboratory testing and x-rays to exclude other causes of wrist and hand pain.

■ **LABORATORY TESTS**
• ESR is usually normal in patients with de Quervain's tenosynovitis. If elevated, a search for an infectious or infiltrative cause should be pursued.
• Aspiration with examination of the specimen under polarized microscope to rule out gout.
• Gram stain and culture of aspirate to rule out infectious etiology.

■ **IMAGING STUDIES**
• X-ray studies of the hand may show findings of osteoarthritis of the first carpometacarpal joint that can mimic de Quervain's tenosynovitis.

TREATMENT

■ **NONPHARMACOLOGIC THERAPY**
• Rest
• Splinting
• Physiotherapy

■ **ACUTE GENERAL Rx**
• Corticosteroid injection using 20 to 40 mg triamcinolone acetonide and 1% Xylocaine is effective in relieving pain.
• NSAIDs ibuprofen 800 mg tid or naproxen 500 mg bid can be tried in patients refusing steroid injection therapy.

■ **CHRONIC Rx**
• Surgical release is generally reserved for patients not responding to NSAIDs and corticosteroid injection therapy.

■ **DISPOSITION**
• Approximately 90% of patients have relief of symptoms with either single or multiple steroid injections.
• Complications of steroid injections include:
  1. Infection
  2. Tendon rupture
• Surgical control of symptoms occurs in 90% of cases.
• Complications of surgery include:
  1. Radial nerve damage
  2. Paresthesia (~10%)
  3. Neuroma

REFERRAL

Consultation with either a rheumatologist or an orthopedist is recommended in patients with de Quervain's tenosynovitis requiring injection therapy.

PEARLS & CONSIDERATIONS

■ COMMENTS

- Dr. Fritz de Quervain published the original article on stenosing tenovaginitis in 1895.
- Finkelstein's description of stenosing tenosynovitis was originally published in *J Bone Joint Surg* in 1930.

REFERENCES

Anderson BC, Manthey R, Brounds MC: Treatment of de Quervain's tenosynovitis with corticosteroids: a prospective study of the response to local injection, *Arthr Rheum* 34(7):793, 1991.

Conoso JJ: *Rheumatology in primary care,* Baltimore, 1997, Saunders.

Moore JS: De Quervain's tenosynovitis: stenosing tenosynovitis of the first dorsal compartment, *J Occup Environ Med* 39(10):990, 1997.

Author: **Peter Petropoulos, M.D.**

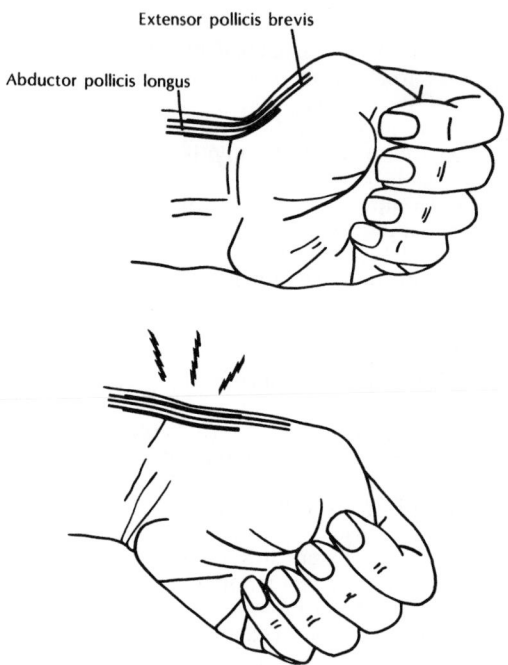

Extensor pollicis brevis

Abductor pollicis longus

Fig. 1-120   Finkelstein's test is positive in de Quervain's stenosing synovitis. Ulnar flexion of the wrist produces pain over the dorsal compartment containing the extensor policis brevis and abductor pollicis longus. (From Noble J [ed]: *Textbook of primary care medicine,* ed 2, St Louis, 1996, Mosby.)

BASIC INFORMATION

■ **DEFINITION**

Atopic dermatitis is a genetically determined eczematous eruption that is pruritic, symmetric, and associated with personal family history of allergic manifestations (atopy).

■ **SYNONYMS**

Eczema
Atopic neurodermatitis
Atopic eczema

ICD-9CM CODES
691.8 Atopic dermatitis

■ **EPIDEMIOLOGY & DEMOGRAPHICS**

- Incidence is between 5 and 25 cases/1000 persons.
- Highest incidence is among children (5%). It accounts for 4% of acute care pediatric visits.
- Onset of disease before age 5 yr in 85% of patients.
- Over 50% of children with generalized atopic dermatitis develop asthma and allergic rhinitis by age 13 yr.
- Concordance in monozygotic twins is 86%.

■ **PHYSICAL FINDINGS & CLINICAL PRESENTATION**

- There are no specific cutaneous signs for atopic dermatitis.
- The primary lesions are a result of itching caused by severe and chronic pruritus. The repeated scratching modifies the skin surface, producing lichenification, dry and scaly skin, and redness.
- The lesions are typically on the neck, face, upper trunk, and bends of elbows and knees (symmetric on flexural surfaces of extremities).
- There is dryness, thickening of the involved areas, discoloration, blistering, and oozing.
- Papular lesions are frequently found in the antecubital and popliteal fossae.
- In children, red scaling plaques are often confined to the cheeks and the perioral and perinasal areas.
- Inflammation in the flexural areas and lichenified skin is a very common presentation in children.
- Constant scratching may result in areas of hypopigmentation or hyperpigmentation (more common in blacks).
- In adults, redness and scaling in the dorsal aspect of the hands or about the fingers are the most common expression of atopic dermatitis; oozing and crusting may be present.
- Secondary skin infections may be present (*Staphylococcus aureus,* dermatophytosis, herpes simplex).

■ **ETIOLOGY**

Unknown; elevated T-lymphocyte activation, defective cell immunity, and B

cell IgE overproduction may play a significant role.

🔬 **DIAGNOSIS**

■ **DIFFERENTIAL DIAGNOSIS**

- Scabies
- Psoriasis
- Dermatitis herpetiform
- Contact dermatitis
- Photosensitivity
- Seborrheic dermatitis
- Candidiasis
- Lichen simplex chronicus
- Other: Wiskott-Aldrich syndrome, PKU, mycosis fungoides, ichthyosis, HIV dermatitis, nonnummular eczema, histiocytosis X

A comparison of the various types of dermatitis is described in Table 2-52.

■ **WORKUP**

Diagnosis is based on the presence of three of the following major features and three minor features.

MAJOR FEATURES:
- Pruritus
- Personal or family history of atopy: asthma, allergic rhinitis, atopic dermatitis
- Facial and extensor involvement in infants and children
- Flexural lichenification in adults

MINOR FEATURES:
- Elevated IgE
- Eczema-perifollicular accentuation
- Recurrent conjunctivitis
- Ichthyosis
- Nipple dermatitis
- Wool intolerance
- Cutaneous *S. aureus* infections or herpes simplex infections
- Food intolerance
- Hand dermatitis (nonallergic irritant)
- Facial pallor, facial erythema
- Cheilitis
- White dermographism
- Early age of onset (after 2 mo of age)

■ **LABORATORY TESTS**

- Tests are generally not helpful.
- Elevated IgE levels are found in 80% to 90% of atopic dermatitis.
- Blood eosinophilia correlates with disease severity.

💊 **TREATMENT**

■ **NONPHARMACOLOGIC THERAPY**

Avoidance of triggering factors:
- Sudden temperature changes, sweating, low humidity in the winter
- Contact with irritating substance (e.g., wool, cosmetics, some soaps and detergents, tobacco)
- Foods that provoke exacerbations (e.g., eggs, peanuts, fish, soy, wheat, milk)

- Stressful situations
- Allergens and dust
- Excessive hand washing
- Clip nails to decrease abrasion of skin

■ **ACUTE GENERAL Rx**

- Emollients can be used to prevent dryness. Severely affected skin can be optimally hydrated by occlusion in addition to application of emollients.
- Topical corticosteroids (e.g., 1% to 2.5% hydrocortisone) may be helpful. Consider intermediate-potency steroids (e.g., triamcinolone, fluocinolone) for more severe cases and limit potent corticosteroids (e.g., betamethasone, desoximetasone, clobetasol) to severe cases.
- Pimecrolimus cream (Elidel) 1% applied bid is a steroid-free compound with antiinflammatory effects secondary to blockage of activated T-cell cytokine production. It is highly effective in atopic dermatitis without having the adverse effects associated with topical corticosteroids.
- Tacrolimus (protopic) ointment (0.03% or 0.1%) applied bid represents an effective alternative to topical corticosteroids. It does not cause skin atrophy and may be particularly useful on the face and neck. It is a macrolide that decreases activation of T-lymphocytes, inhibits release of inflammatory mediators from cutaneous mast cells and basophils, and suppresses humoral and cell-mediated immune responses.
- Oral antihistamines (e.g., hydroxyzine, diphenhydramine) are effective in controlling pruritus and inducing sedation, restful sleep, and prevention of scratching during sleep. Doxepin and other tricyclic antidepressants also have antihistamine effect, induce sleep, and reduce pruritus.
- Oral prednisone, IM triamcinolone, Goeckerman regimen, PUVA are generally reserved for severe cases.
- Methotrezate, cyclosporine azathioprine, and systemic corticosteroids are sometimes tried for recalcitrant disease.

■ **DISPOSITION**

- Resolution occurs in approximately 40% of patients by adulthood.
- Most patients have a course characterized by remissions and intermittent flares.

🔆 **PEARLS & CONSIDERATIONS**

■ **COMMENTS**

Patients should be reassured that atopic dermatitis is not an emotional disorder and that prognosis is generally benign.

Author: **Fred F. Ferri, M.D.**

BASIC INFORMATION

■ DEFINITION
Contact dermatitis is an acute or chronic skin inflammation, usually eczematous dermatitis resulting from exposure to substances in the environment. It can be subdivided into "irritant" contact dermatitis (Fig. 1-122) (nonimmunologic physical and chemical alteration of the epidermis) and "allergic" contact dermatitis (delayed hypersensitivity reaction).

■ SYNONYMS
Irritant contact dermatitis
Allergic contact dermatitis

ICD-9CM CODES
692 Contact dermatitis and other eczema

■ EPIDEMIOLOGY & DEMOGRAPHICS
- 20% of all cases of dermatitis in children are caused by allergic contact dermatitis.
- Rhus dermatitis (poison ivy, poison oak, and poison sumac) is responsible for most cases of contact dermatitis.
- Frequent causes of irritant contact dermatitis are soaps, detergents, and organic solvents.

■ PHYSICAL FINDINGS & CLINICAL PRESENTATION
IRRITANT CONTACT DERMATITIS:
- Mild exposure may result in dryness, erythema, and fissuring of the affected area (e.g., hand involvement in irritant dermatitis caused by exposure to soap, genital area involvement in irritant dermatitis caused by prolonged exposure to wet diapers).
- Eczematous inflammation may result from chronic exposure.

ALLERGIC CONTACT DERMATITIS:
- Poison ivy dermatitis can present with vesicles and blisters; linear lesions (as a result of dragging of the resins over the surface of the skin by scratching) are a classic presentation.
- The pattern of lesions is asymmetric; itching, burning, and stinging may be present.
- The involved areas are erythematous, warm to touch, swollen, and may be confused with cellulitis.

■ ETIOLOGY
- Irritant contact dermatitis: cement (construction workers), rubber, ragweed, malathion (farmers), orange and lemon peels (chefs, bar-

tenders), hair tints, shampoos (beauticians), rubber gloves (medical, surgical personnel)
- Allergic contact dermatitis: poison ivy, poison oak, poison sumac, rubber (shoe dermatitis), nickel (jewelry), balsam of Peru (hand and face dermatitis), neomycin, formaldehyde (cosmetics)

DIAGNOSIS

■ DIFFERENTIAL DIAGNOSIS
- Impetigo
- Lichen simplex chronicus
- Atopic dermatitis
- Nummular eczema
- Seborrheic dermatitis
- Psoriasis
- Scabies

Table 2-52 describes the differential diagnosis of dermatitis.

■ WORKUP
- Medical history: gradual onset vs. rapid onset, number of exposures, clinical presentation, occupational history
- Physical examination: contact dermatitis in the neck may be caused by necklaces, perfumes, after-shave lotion; involvement of the axillae is often secondary to deodorants, clothing; face involvement can occur with cosmetics, airborne allergens, after-shave lotion

■ LABORATORY TESTS
- Patch testing (Fig. 1-121) is useful to confirm the diagnosis of contact dermatitis; it is indicated particularly when inflammation persists despite appropriate topical therapy and avoidance of suspected causative agent; patch testing should not be used for irritant contact dermatitis since this is a nonimmunologic-mediated inflammatory reaction.
- Gram stain and cultures are indicated only in cases of suspected secondary infection or impetigo.

TREATMENT

■ NONPHARMACOLOGIC THERAPY
Avoidance of suspected allergens

■ ACUTE GENERAL Rx
- Removal of the irritant substance by washing the skin with plain water or

mild soap within 15 min of exposure is helpful in patients with poison ivy, poison oak, or poison sumac dermatitis.
- Cold or cool water compresses for 20 to 30 min five to six times a day for the initial 72 hr are effective during the acute blistering stage.
- Oral corticosteroids (e.g., prednisone 20 mg bid for 6 to 10 days) are generally reserved for severe, widespread dermatitis.
- IM steroids (e.g., Kenalog) are used for severe reactions and in patients requiring oral corticosteroids but unable to tolerate PO.
- Oral antihistamines (e.g., hydroxyzine 25 mg q6h) will control pruritus, especially at night; calamine lotion is also useful for pruritus; however, it can lead to excessive drying.
- Colloidal oatmeal (Aveeno) baths can also provide symptomatic relief.
- Patients with mild to moderate erythema may respond to topical steroid gels or creams.
- Patients with shoe allergy should change their socks at least once a day; use of aluminum chloride hexahydrate in a 20% solution (Drysol) qhs will also help control perspiration.
- Use hypoallergenic surgical gloves in patients with rubber and surgical glove allergy.

■ DISPOSITION
Allergic contact dermatitis generally resolves within 2 to 4 wk if reexposure to allergen is prevented.

■ REFERRAL
For patch testing in selected patients (see "Laboratory Tests")

PEARLS & CONSIDERATIONS

■ COMMENTS
- Commercially available corticosteroid dose packs should be avoided, since they generally provide an inadequate amount of medication.
- Principles of treatment of hand dermatitis are described in Box 1-15.

Author: **Fred F. Ferri, M.D.**

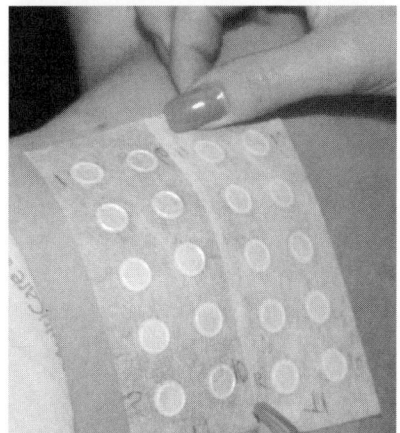

Fig. 1-121   Patch testing. Samples (patches) of standardized allergens are placed on the patient's back and worn for 48 hours. The patches are then removed, and each patch test site examined on at least two occasions for dermatitis, which could represent a positive response. Patch testing has a central role in the diagnosis of allergic contact dermatitis. (From Altman LV [ed]: *Allergy in primary care,* Philadelphia, 2000, WB Saunders.)

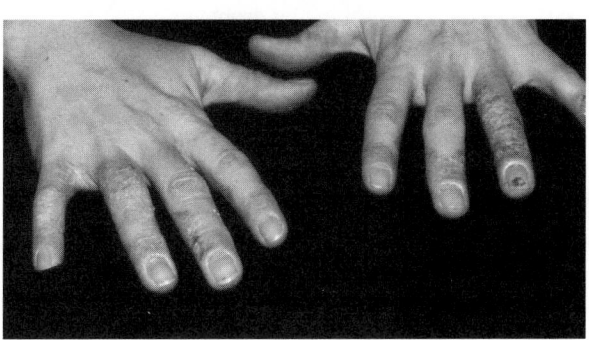

Fig. 1-122   Irritant contact dermatitis (ICD) superimposed on atopic hand dermatitis in a machinist. There is predominantly involvement of the dorsal aspects of the fingers, and also web space involvement, typical of ICD. The palms are relatively spared. All patch test results, including a panel of antigens specific for machinists, were negative. (From Altman LV [ed]: *Allergy in primary care,* Philadelphia, 2000, WB Saunders.)

BOX 1-15   Principles of Treatment of Hand Dermatitis

- Protect the hands from direct contact with soap, detergent, scouring powder, and similar harsh chemicals by wearing waterproof heavy-duty vinyl gloves, either lined or unlined. It is often beneficial to wear white cotton gloves under the vinyl gloves. The patient should have a sufficient number of white cotton gloves so that they can be washed frequently, and also a sufficient supply of heavy-duty vinyl gloves. Heavy-duty vinyl gloves are preferable to rubber gloves because patients occasionally become allergic to rubber gloves.
- Wear the gloves while cooking with acid foods (e.g., peeling or squeezing lemons, oranges, or grapefruit, peeling potatoes, and handling tomatoes).
- Wear leather or heavy-duty fabric gloves when doing dry work and especially when gardening. Dirty the gloves, not the hands. The patient should place a dozen pairs of cheap cotton gloves strategically about the home for dry housework. When dirty, put in the washing machine. Wash gloves, not hands.
- Dishwashers and automatic clothes washers are musts for people with hand dermatitis.
- Avoid direct contact with household products that contain irritating solvents (e.g., turpentine, paint, paint thinner, and various polishes [metal, floor, furniture, and shoe]).
- Wear heavy-duty waterproof gloves when using them.
- Use lukewarm water and very mild soap when washing the hands. Rinse the soap off thoroughly and dry gently. All soaps are irritating.
- Lubricate the hands immediately after washing. Place a lubricant strategically near any sink you use. Petrolatum is best. The patient should carry a small tube or bottle of lubricant.
- The patient should remove rings when doing housework and before washing the hands because rings often worsen dermatitis by trapping irritating materials beneath them.
- When outdoors in cold or windy weather, wear gloves to protect the hands from drying or chapping.
- Use only prescribed medicines and lubricants on the hands. Do not use other lotions, creams, or medications because some of these may irritate the skin.
- Suspected bacterial superinfection (often manifested by fissures and honey-colored crusts) should be treated aggressively with antistaphylococcal antibiotics.
- Topical corticosteroid ointments are preferable to topical corticosteroid creams or lotions for treatment of inflammation.
- The hands should be protected for *at least* 4 months after the dermatitis has healed and maybe longer. It takes a long time for skin to recover, and unless one is careful the dermatitis tends to recur.
- There is no fast "magic" treatment for hand dermatitis. The skin must be given a rest from irritation. Follow the above-listed instructions carefully.

From Altman LV (ed): *Allergy in primary care,* Philadelphia, 2000, WB Saunders.

BASIC INFORMATION

■ DEFINITION
Dermatomyositis (DM) refers to a chronic idiopathic inflammatory myopathy characterized by a skin rash and proximal muscle weakness.

■ SYNONYMS
Idiopathic inflammatory myopathy

ICD-9CM CODES
710.3 Dermatomyositis

■ EPIDEMIOLOGY & DEMOGRAPHICS
- Dermatomyositis (DM) occurs in children and in adults
- Incidence 1:100,000
- More common in females than males (2:1).
- DM can occur in children between the ages of 10 to 15 yr and adults between the ages of 45 to 60 yr.
- DM usually occurs alone but sometimes can be associated with systemic sclerosis and mixed connective tissue disease.
- Approximately 15% to 20% of patients with DM over the age of 50 have associated malignancies.

■ PHYSICAL FINDINGS & CLINICAL PRESENTATION
- Most patients with DM have a subacute onset, over weeks to months.
- Symmetrical proximal muscle weakness involving the shoulder and pelvic girdle.
- Difficulty getting up from a chair, climbing stairs, or combing hair.
- Distal muscle and ocular involvement is uncommon.
- Dysphagia and dysphonia resulting from proximal pharyngeal muscle involvement.
- Rales, dyspnea, and respiratory failure.
- Skin findings
  1. Heliotrope rash on the upper eyelids (Fig. 1-123)
  2. Erythematous rash on the face (see Fig. 1-123)
  3. Can also involve the back and shoulders (shawl sign), neck and chest (V-shape), knees and elbows.
  4. Photosensitive
  5. Gottron's sign (red scaly eruption of the knuckles)
  6. Nail cracking, thickening, and irregularity with periungual telangiectasia (Fig. 1-124)

■ ETIOLOGY
The cause of DM is not known but is believed to be an immune-related phenomenon.

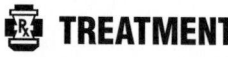

DIAGNOSIS

The diagnosis of DM requires the following:
- History and physical findings of proximal muscle weakness
- Elevated muscle enzymes
- EMG abnormalities suggesting a myopathic process
- Muscle biopsy confirmation
- Characteristic skin rash

■ DIFFERENTIAL DIAGNOSIS
- Polymyositis
- Inclusion body myositis
- Muscular dystrophies
- Amyotrophic lateral sclerosis
- Myasthenia gravis
- Eaton-Lambert syndrome
- Drug-induced myopathies
- Diabetic amyotrophy
- Guillain-Barré syndrome
- Hyperthyroidism or hypothyroidism

■ WORKUP
Patients suspected of having DM by clinical presentation should have an EMG, muscle biopsy, and specific blood tests to confirm the diagnosis.

■ LABORATORY TESTS
- ESR, although not specific, is elevated in the majority of cases.
- Creatine kinase is the most sensitive muscle enzyme test and can be elevated as much as 50 times above normal.
- Aldolase, AST, ALT, alkaline phosphatase, and LDH can be elevated.
- Anti-Jo-1 antibodies are more common in polymyositis than DM.
- Electrolytes, TSH, Ca, and Mg should be requested to exclude other causes.
- Electromyography (EMG) is abnormal in 90% of patients and distinguishes a myopathic from neuropathic process.
- Muscle biopsy is the definitive test. Characteristic findings separate DM from polymyositis, inclusion body myositis, and neuromuscular disorders mimicking DM.

■ IMAGING STUDIES
- A chest x-ray to rule out pulmonary involvement. If suspicious for pulmonary interstitial disease, a high-resolution CT scan of the chest may be helpful.
- A barium swallow to look for upper esophageal dysfunction in patients with dysphagia and DM.
- MRI can help to locate sites of muscle involvement.

TREATMENT

■ NONPHARMACOLOGIC THERAPY
- Sun-blocking agents with SF 15 or greater for skin lesions.
- Physical therapy is beneficial in increasing muscle tone and strength.
- Occupational therapy to assist with activities of daily living.
- Speech therapy for dysphagia and swallowing problems.

■ ACUTE GENERAL Rx
- Prednisone 1 to 2 mg/kg/day is the treatment of choice in patients with DM. The dose is continued until muscle strength improves and/or muscle enzymes have returned to normal for 4 wk. Thereafter taper by 10 mg/mo until off prednisone.
- Immunosuppresive agents (azathioprine, cyclophosphamide, or methotrexate) should be used if the patient fails to improve on prednisone or muscle enzymes begin rising when tapering off prednisone. See below for specific dosage.

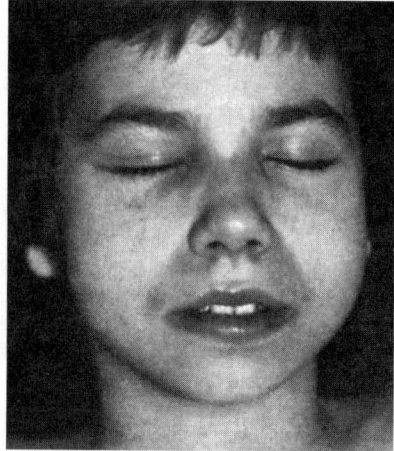

Fig. 1-123 The facial rash of juvenile dermatomyositis. There is erythema over the bridge of the nose and malar areas, with violaceous (heliotropic) discoloration of the upper eyelids. (From Behrman RE: *Nelson textbook of pediatrics,* ed 16, Philadelphia, 2000, WB Saunders.)

- Hydroxychloroquine is used to treat the cutaneous lesions of DM.

■ CHRONIC Rx
- Chronic prednisone therapy may be needed for years.
- Azathioprine (2.5 to 3.5 mg/kg/day) or methotrexate (0.5 mg/kg/wk) can be added as stated above.
- Azathioprine 2 to 3 mg/kg/day tapered to 1 mg/kg/day once steroid is tapered to 15 mg/day. Reduce dosage monthly by 25 mg intervals. Maintenance dosage is 50 mg/day.
- Methotrexate 7.5 to 10 mg PO per week, increased by 2.5 mg per week to total of 25 mg per week.
- Cyclophosphanide 1 to 3 mg/kg/day PO or 2 to 4 mg/kg/day in conjunction with prednisone.
- Other drugs considered in the chronic treatment of DM include mycophenolate, cyclosporine, hydroxychloroquine, and IV immunoglobulins.

■ DISPOSITION
- As treatment is initiated, the muscle enzymes should return to normal before symptoms improve.

- During exacerbations, enzymes will rise first before symptoms appear.
- Approximately 50% of the patients will go into remission and stop therapy within 5 yr. The remaining will either have active disease requiring ongoing treatment or inactive disease with permanent muscle atrophy and contractures.
- Poor prognostic indicators include:
  1. Delay in diagnosis
  2. Older age
  3. Recalcitrant disease
  4. Malignancy
  5. Interstitial pulmonary fibrosis
  6. Dysphagia
  7. Leukocytosis
  8. Fever
  9. Anorexia
- Infection, malignancy, and cardiac and pulmonary dysfunction are the most common causes of death.
- With early treatment 5 and 8 year survival rates of 80% and 73% have been reported.

■ REFERRAL
For any suspected cases of DM a rheumatology referral should be made to help establish the diagnosis and implement treatment.

☼ PEARLS & CONSIDERATIONS

■ COMMENTS
- When assessing response to treatment, it is best to follow clinical muscle strength over muscle enzyme tests.
- The concern of malignancies (ovary, lung, breast, GI) associated with myositis is legitimate and merits screening in patients over the age of 40.
- Malignancies can occur before, during, or after the diagnosis of dermatomyositis.

REFERENCES
Callen JP: Dermatomyositis, *Lancet* 355(9197):53, 2000.
Koler RA, Montemarano A: Dermatomyositis, *Am Fam Physician* 64(156):5, 2001.
Author: **Peter Petropoulos, M.D.**

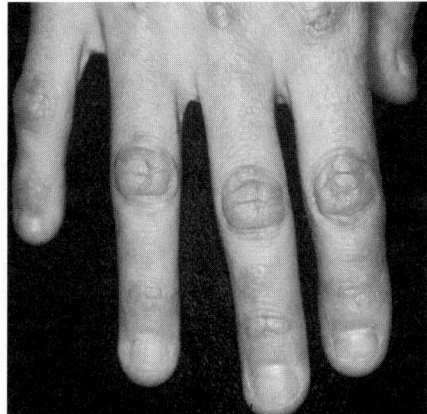

Fig. 1-124 Dermatomyositis (Gottron's papules). Note erythematous papules over joints and periungual telangiectasias. (From Noble J [ed]: *Textbook of primary care medicine,* ed 2, St Louis, 1996, Mosby.)

BASIC INFORMATION

■ DEFINITION

Diabetes insipidus is a polyuric disorder resulting from insufficient production of antidiuretic hormone (ADH) (pituitary [neurogenic] diabetes insipidus) or unresponsiveness of the renal tubules to ADH (nephrogenic diabetes insipidus).

■ ICD-9CM CODES
253.5 Diabetes insipidus

■ EPIDEMIOLOGY & DEMOGRAPHICS
GENETICS:
• Nephrogenic diabetes insipidus can be inherited as sex-linked recessive.
• There is also a rare autosomal dominant form of neurogenic diabetes insipidus.

■ PHYSICAL FINDINGS & CLINICAL PRESENTATION
• Polyuria: urinary volumes ranging from 2.5 to 6 L/day
• Polydipsia (predilection for cold or iced drinks)
• Neurologic manifestations (seizures, headaches, visual field defects)
• Evidence of volume contractions
NOTE: The above physical findings and clinical manifestations are generally not evident until vasopressin secretory capacity is reduced <20% of normal.

■ ETIOLOGY
NEUROGENIC DIABETES INSIPIDUS:
• Idiopathic
• Neoplasms of brain or pituitary fossa (craniopharyngiomas, metastatic neoplasms from breast or lung)
• Posttherapeutic neurosurgical procedures (e.g., hypophysectomy)
• Head trauma (e.g., basal skull fracture)
• Granulomatous disorders (sarcoidosis or TB)
• Histiocytosis (Hand-Schüller-Christian disease, eosinophilic granuloma)
• Familial (autosomal dominant)
• Other: interventricular hemorrhage, aneurysms, meningitis, postencephalitis, multiple sclerosis
NEPHROGENIC DIABETES INSIPIDUS:
• Drugs: lithium, amphotericin B, demeclocycline, methoxyflurane anesthesia
• Familial: X-linked
• Metabolic: hypercalcemia or hypokalemia
• Other: sarcoidosis, amyloidosis, pyelonephritis, polycystic disease, sickle cell disease, postobstructive

DIAGNOSIS

■ DIFFERENTIAL DIAGNOSIS
• Diabetes mellitus, nephropathies
• Primary polydipsia, medications (e.g., chlorpromazine)
• Osmotic diuresis (glucose, mannitol, anticholinergics)
• Psychogenic polydipsia, electrolyte disturbances
Box 2-206 describes the differential diagnosis of polyuria.

■ WORKUP
• The diagnostic workup is aimed at showing that the polyuria is caused by the inability to concentrate urine and determining whether the problem is secondary to decreased ADH or insensitivity to ADH. This is done with the water deprivation test:
  1. Following baseline measurement of weight, ADH, plasma sodium, and urine and plasma osmolarity, the patient is deprived of fluids under strict medical supervision.
  2. Frequent (q2h) monitoring of plasma and urine osmolarity follows.
  3. The test is generally terminated when plasma osmolarity is >295 or the patient loses ≥3.5% of initial body weight.
  4. Diabetes insipidus is confirmed if the plasma osmolarity is >295 and the urine osmolarity is <500.
  5. To distinguish nephrogenic from neurogenic diabetes insipidus, the patient is given 5 U of vasopressin (ADH) and the change in urine osmolarity is measured. A significant increase (>50%) in urine osmolarity following administration of ADH is indicative of neurogenic diabetes insipidus.
• Fig. 1-125 describes a diagnostic flowchart for diabetes insipidus.

■ LABORATORY TESTS
• Decreased urinary specific gravity (≤1.005)
• Decreased urinary osmolarity (usually <200 mOsm/kg) even in the presence of high serum osmolality
• Hypernatremia, increased plasma osmolarity, hypercalcemia, hypokalemia

■ IMAGING STUDIES
MRI of the brain if neurogenic diabetes insipidus is confirmed

TREATMENT

■ NONPHARMACOLOGIC THERAPY
• Patient education regarding control of fluid balance and prevention of dehydration with adequate fluid intake
• Daily weight

■ ACUTE GENERAL Rx
Therapy varies with the degree and type of diabetes insipidus:
NEUROGENIC DIABETES INSIPIDUS:
  1. Desmopressin acetate (DDAVP) 10 to 40 μg qd intranasally in one to three divided doses or in tablet form 0.05 mg bid. Usual oral dose is 0.1 to 1.2 mg/day in two to three divided doses. Desmopressin is also available in injectable form given as 2 to 4 μg/day SC or IV in two divided doses.
  2. Vasopressin tannate in oil: 2.5 to 5 U IM q24-72h; useful for long-term management because of its long life.
  3. In mild cases of neurogenic diabetes insipidus, the polyuria may be controlled with HCTZ 50 mg qd or chlorpropamide (Diabinese) 250 mg qd.
NEPHROGENIC DIABETES INSIPIDUS:
  1. Adequate hydration
  2. Low-sodium diet and chlorothiazide to induce mild sodium depletion
  3. Polyuria of diabetes insipidus secondary to lithium can be ameliorated by using amiloride (5 mg PO bid initially, increased to 10 mg bid after 2 wk)

■ CHRONIC Rx
Patients should be aware of the danger of dehydration and the need for liberal water intake.

■ REFERRAL
Endocrinology evaluation for diagnostic testing

PEARLS & CONSIDERATIONS

■ COMMENTS
Patients should be instructed to wear a medical identification tag or bracelet identifying their medical illness.

REFERENCE
Maghnie M et al: Central diabetes insipidus in children and young adults, *N Engl J Med* 343:998, 2000.
Author: **Fred F. Ferri, M.D.**

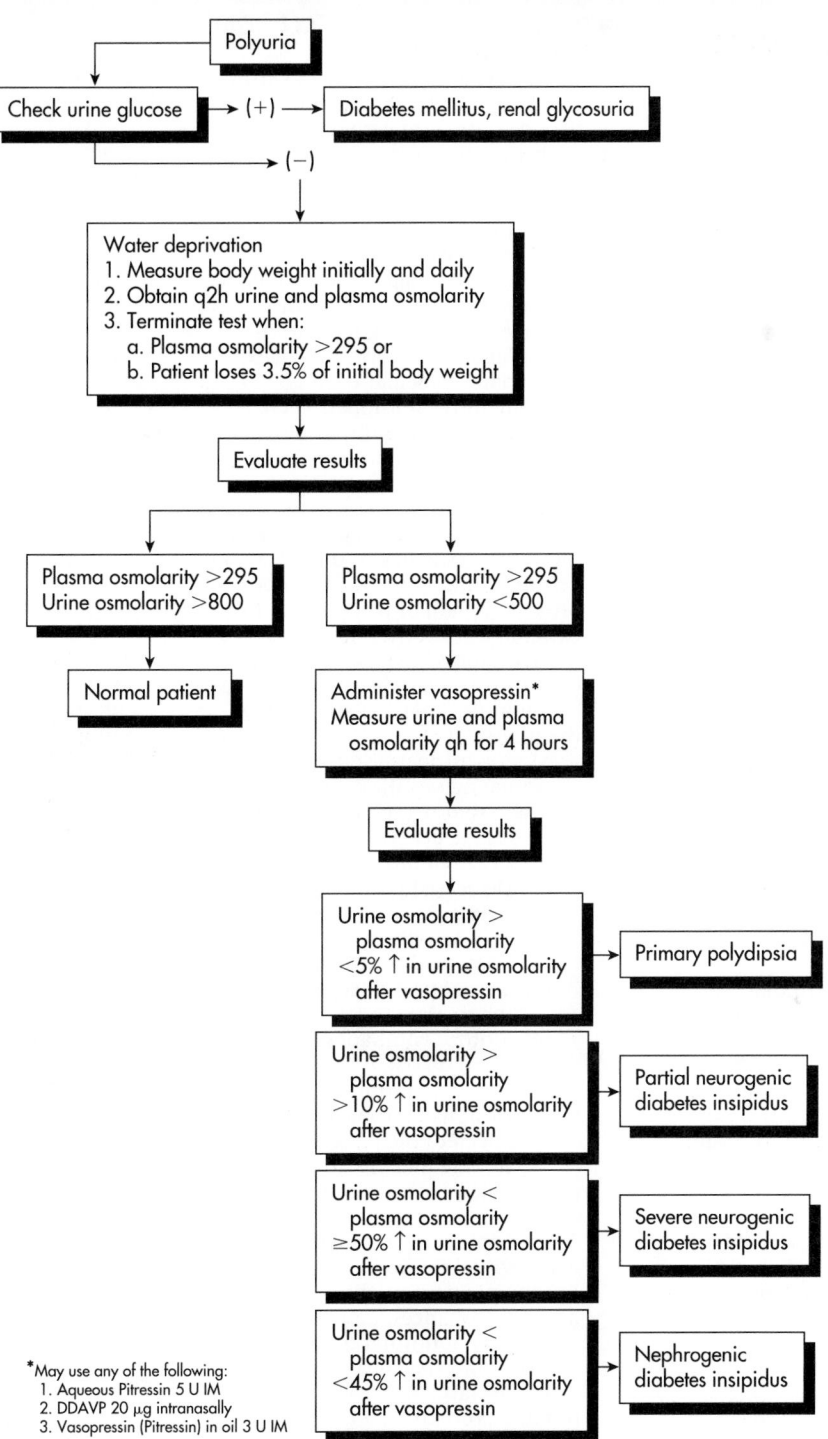

Fig. 1-125   Diagnostic flowchart for diabetes insipidus. (From Ferri F: *Practical guide to the care of the medical patient,* ed 5, St Louis, 2001, Mosby.)

BASIC INFORMATION

■ DEFINITION
- Diabetes mellitus (DM) refers to a syndrome of hyperglycemia resulting from many different causes (see "Etiology"). It can be classified into type 1 insulin-dependent (formerly IDDM) and type 2 non-insulin-dependent (formerly NIDDM) DM. Because "insulin-dependent" and "non-insulin-dependent" refer to stage at diagnosis, when a type 2 diabetic needs insulin, he remains classified as type 2 and does not revert to type 1. Table 1-24 provides a general comparison of the two most common types of diabetes mellitus.
- The American Diabetes Association (ADA) defines DM as (1) a fasting plasma glucose ≥ 126 mg/dl or (2) a nonfasting plasma glucose ≥ 200 mg/dl or (3) an oral glucose tolerance test (OGTT) ≥ 200 mg/dl in the 2-hr sample. Furthermore, the ADA also defines a value of 110 mg/dl on fasting blood sugar as the upper limit of normal for glucose. A fasting glucose between 110 mg/dl and 126 mg/dl is classified as "Impaired Fasting Glucose" (IFG). When results of the oral glucose test are between 110 mg/dl and 200 mg/dl, the patient is also classified as having IFG.

■ SYNONYMS
IDDM (insulin-dependent diabetes mellitus)
NIDDM (non-insulin-dependent diabetes mellitus)
Type 1 diabetes mellitus (insulin-dependent diabetes mellitus)
Type 2 diabetes mellitus (non-insulin-dependent diabetes mellitus)

ICD-9CM CODES
250.0 Diabetes mellitus (NIDDM)
250.1 Insulin-dependent diabetes mellitus without complication (IDDM)

■ EPIDEMIOLOGY & DEMOGRAPHICS
- DM affects 5% to 7% of the U.S. population. Prevalence in Pima Indians is 35%.
- Incidence increases with age, with 2% in persons ages 20 to 44 yr to 18% in persons 65 to 74 yr of age.
- Diabetes accounts for 8% of all legal blindness and is the leading cause of end-stage renal disease in the U.S.
- Patients with diabetes are twice as likely as nondiabetic patients to develop cardiovascular disease.

■ PHYSICAL FINDINGS & CLINICAL PRESENTATION
1. Physical examination varies with the presence of complications and may be normal in early stages.
2. Diabetic retinopathy:
   a. Nonproliferative (background diabetic retinopathy):
      (1) Initially: microaneurysms, capillary dilation, waxy or hard exudates, dot and flame hemorrhages, AV shunts
      (2) Advanced stage: microinfarcts with cotton wool exudates, macular edema
   b. Proliferative retinopathy: characterized by formation of new vessels, vitreal hemorrhages, fibrous scarring, and retinal detachment
3. Cataracts and glaucoma occur with increased frequency in diabetics.
4. Peripheral neuropathy: patients often complain of paresthesias of extremities (feet more than hands); the symptoms are symmetric, bilateral, and associated with intense burning pain (particularly during the night).
   a. Mononeuropathies involving cranial nerves III, IV, and VI, intercostal nerves, and femoral nerves are also common.
   b. Physical examination may reveal:
      (1) Decreased pinprick sensation, sensation to light touch, and pain sensation.
      (2) Decreased vibration sense.
      (3) Loss of proprioception (leading to ataxia).
      (4) Motor disturbances (decreased DTR, weakness and atrophy of interossei muscles); when the hands are affected, the patient has trouble picking up small objects, dressing, and turning pages in a book.
      (5) Diplopia, abnormalities of visual fields.
5. Autonomic neuropathy:
   a. GI disturbances: esophageal motility abnormalities, gastroparesis, diarrhea (usually nocturnal)
   b. GU disturbances: neurogenic bladder (hesitancy, weak stream, and dribbling), impotence.
   c. Orthostatic hypotension: postural syncope, dizziness, lightheadedness.
6. Nephropathy: pedal edema, pallor, weakness, uremic appearance.
7. Foot ulcers: occur frequently and are usually secondary to peripheral vascular insufficiency, repeated trauma (unrecognized because of sensory loss), and superimposed infections.
8. Neuropathic arthropathy (Charcot's joints): bone or joint deformities from repeated trauma (secondary to peripheral neuropathy).
9. Necrobiosis lipoidica diabeticorum: plaquelike reddened areas with a central area that fades to white-yellow found on the anterior surfaces of the legs; in these areas the skin becomes very thin and can ulcerate readily.

■ ETIOLOGY
IDIOPATHIC DIABETES:
Type 1 (IDDM)
- Hereditary factors:
  1. Islet cell antibodies (found in 90% of patients within the first year of diagnosis)
  2. Higher incidence of HLA types DR3, DR4
  3. 50% concordance in identical twins
- Environmental factors: viral infection (possibly coxsackie virus, mumps virus)
- Fig. 1-126 illustrates the natural history of type 1 DM
Type 2 (NIDDM)
- Hereditary factors: 90% concordance in identical twins
- Environmental factor: obesity
- Fig. 1-127 describes the natural history of type 2 DM
DIABETES SECONDARY TO OTHER FACTORS:
- Hormonal excess: Cushing's syndrome, acromegaly, glucagonoma, pheochromocytoma
- Drugs: glucocorticoids, diuretics, oral contraceptives
- Insulin receptor unavailability (with or without circulating antibodies)
- Pancreatic disease: pancreatitis, pancreatectomy, hemochromatosis
- Genetic syndromes: hyperlipidemias, myotonic dystrophy, lipoatrophy
- Gestational diabetes

🔬 DIAGNOSIS

Diagnosis is made on the basis of:
- Fasting glucose ≥126 mg/dl (ADA criteria)
- Glucose level 2 hr after 75 g glucose load (Glucola) ≥200 mg/dl
- Elevated glycosylated hemoglobin (Hb A1c) level (this test is not recommended for diagnosis at this time by the ADA)

■ DIFFERENTIAL DIAGNOSIS
- Diabetes insipidus
- Stress hyperglycemia
- Diabetes secondary to hormonal excess, drugs, pancreatic disease

℞ TREATMENT

■ NONPHARMACOLOGIC THERAPY
1. Diet
   a. Calories
      (1) The diabetic patient can be started on 15 calories/lb of ideal body weight; this number can be increased to 20 calories/lb for an active person and 25 calories/lb if the patient does heavy physical labor.
      (2) The calories should be distributed as 55% to 60% carbohydrates, 25% to 35% fat, and 15% to 20% protein.
      (3) The emphasis should be on complex carbohydrates rather than simple and refined starches and on polyunsaturated instead of saturated fats in a ratio of 2:1.
   b. Seven food groups
      (1) The exchange diet of the ADA includes protein, bread, fruit, milk, and low- and intermediate-carbohydrate vegetables.
      (2) The name of each exchange is meant to be all inclusive (e.g., cereal, muffins, spaghetti, potatoes, rice are in the bread group; meats, fish, eggs, cheese, peanut butter are in the protein group).
      (3) The *glycemic index* compares the rise in blood sugar after the ingestion of simple sugars and complex carbohydrates with the rise that occurs after the absorption of glucose; equal amounts of starches do not give the same rise in plasma glucose (pasta equal in calories to a baked potato causes less of a rise than the potato): thus it is helpful to know the glycemic index of a particular food product.
      (4) Fiber: insoluble fiber (bran, celery) and soluble globular fiber (pectin in fruit) delay glucose absorption and attenuate the postprandial serum glucose peak; they also appear to lower the elevated triglyceride level often present in uncontrolled diabetics.
2. Exercise increases the cellular glucose uptake by increasing the number of cell receptors. The following points must be considered:
   a. Exercise program must be individualized and built up slowly.
   b. Insulin is more rapidly absorbed when injected into a limb that is then exercised, and this can result in hypoglycemia.
3. Weight loss: to ideal body weight if the patient is overweight

■ ACUTE GENERAL Rx
- When the above measures fail to normalize the serum glucose, oral hypoglycemic agents (e.g., metformin, glitazones, or a sulfonylurea) should be added to the regimen in type 2 DM. Table 1-25 describes commonly used oral hypoglycemic agents.
- Because metformin does not produce hypoglycemia when used as a monotherapy, it is preferred for most patients. It is contraindicated in patients with renal insufficiency.
- Sulfonylureas and repaglinide work best when given before meals because they increase the postprandial output of insulin from the pancreas. All sulfonylureas are contraindicated in patients allergic to sulfa.
- Acarbose and miglitol work by competitively inhibiting pancreatic amylase and small intestinal glucosidases, thereby reducing alimentary hyperglycemia. The major side effects are flatulence, diarrhea, and abdominal cramps.
- Pioglitazone and rosiglitazone reduce insulin resistance and are useful in addition to other agents in type 2 diabetics whose hyperglycemia is inadequately controlled. Serum transaminase levels should be obtained before starting therapy and monitored periodically.
- Insulin is indicated for the treatment of all type 1 DM and type 2 DM patients who cannot be adequately controlled with diet and oral agents. Table 1-26 describes commonly used types of insulin.
- Low-dose ASA to decrease the risk of cerebrovascular disease is beneficial for diabetics over age 30 with other risk factors (hypertension, dyslipidemia, smoking, obesity).

■ DISPOSITION
The Diabetes Control and Complications Trial (DCCT) proved that intensive treatment decreases the development and progression of complications of DM. Each patient should be made aware of these findings.
- Retinopathy occurs in approximately 15% of diabetic patients after 15 yr and increases 1%/yr after diagnosis.
- The frequency of neuropathy in type 2 diabetics approaches 70% to 80%. Amitryptiline or gabapentin is effective for the symptomatic treatment of peripheral neuropathic pain.
- Nephropathy occurs in 35% to 45% of patients with type 1 DM and in 20% of type 2 DM. ACE inhibitors are highly effective in slowing the progression of renal disease in both type I and type II DM, independently of their reduction in blood pressure. ARBs are also effective in protecting against the progression of nephropathy in diabetics.
- Infections are generally more common in diabetics because of multiple factors, such as impaired leukocyte function, decreased tissue perfusion secondary to vascular disease, repeated trauma because of loss of sensation, and urinary retention secondary to neuropathy.
- Diabetic ketoacidosis and hyperosmolar coma are described in detail in Section I.

■ REFERRAL
- Diabetic patients should be advised to have annual ophthalmologic examination. In type 1 DM, ophthalmologic visits should begin within 3 to 5 years, whereas type 2 DM patients should be seen from disease onset.
- Podiatric care can significantly reduce the rate of foot infections and amputations in patients with DM.

☼ PEARLS & CONSIDERATIONS

■ COMMENTS

- Because normalization of serum glucose level is the ultimate goal, every patient should measure his blood glucose unless contraindicated by senility or blindness.
- For blood glucose monitoring, glucose oxidase strips are used in conjunction with a meter to give a digital reading. The testing can be done once day, but the time should be varied each day so that over a period of time the serum glucose level before meals and at bedtime can be assessed frequently without pricking the patient's fingers four times daily.
- Glycosylated hemoglobin should be measured at least twice yearly; measurement of microalbumin in the urine on a yearly basis is also recommended.

REFERENCES

Hanley CH: Diabetes mellitus. In Ferri FF: *Practical guide to the care of the medical patient,* ed 5, St Louis, 2001, Mosby.

Kaplan NM: Management of hypertension in patients with type 2 diabetes mellitus: guidelines based on current evidence, *Ann Intern Med* 135:1079, 2001.

Lenhard MJ, Reeves GD: Continuous subcutaneous insulin infusion, a comprehensive review of insulin pump therapy, *Arch Intern Med* 161:2243, 2001.

Report of the Expert Committee on the Diagnosis and Classification of Diabetes Mellitus, *Diabetes Care* 21:S5-19, 1998.

Van Den Berche C et al: Intensive insulin therapy in critically ill patients, *N Engl J Med* 345:1359, 2001.

Author: **Fred F. Ferri, M.D.**

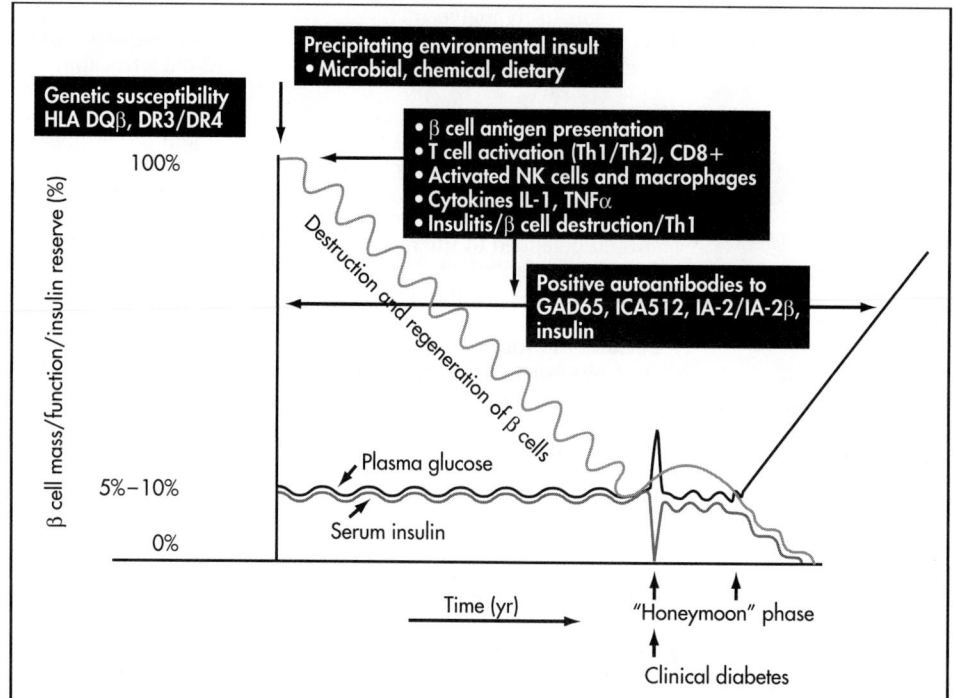

Fig. 1-126 Natural history of type 1 diabetes mellitus. The "honeymoon" period with temporary improvement in β-cell function occurs with the initiation of insulin therapy at the time of clinical diagnosis. *ICA512,* Islet cell autoantigen 512 (fragment of 1A-2); *1A-2/1A-2β,* tyrosine phosphatases; *GAD,* glutamic acid decarboxylase; *ICA,* islet cell antibody; *IAA,* insulin autoantibodies; *IL,* interleukin; *NK,* natural killer; *Th1,* subset of CD4+ T-helper cells, responsible for cell-mediated immunity; *Th2,* subset of CD4+ T-helper cells, responsible for humoral immunity; *TNF,* tumor necrosis factor. (From Andreoli TE [ed]: *Cecil essentials of medicine,* ed 5, Philadelphia, 2001, WB Saunders.)

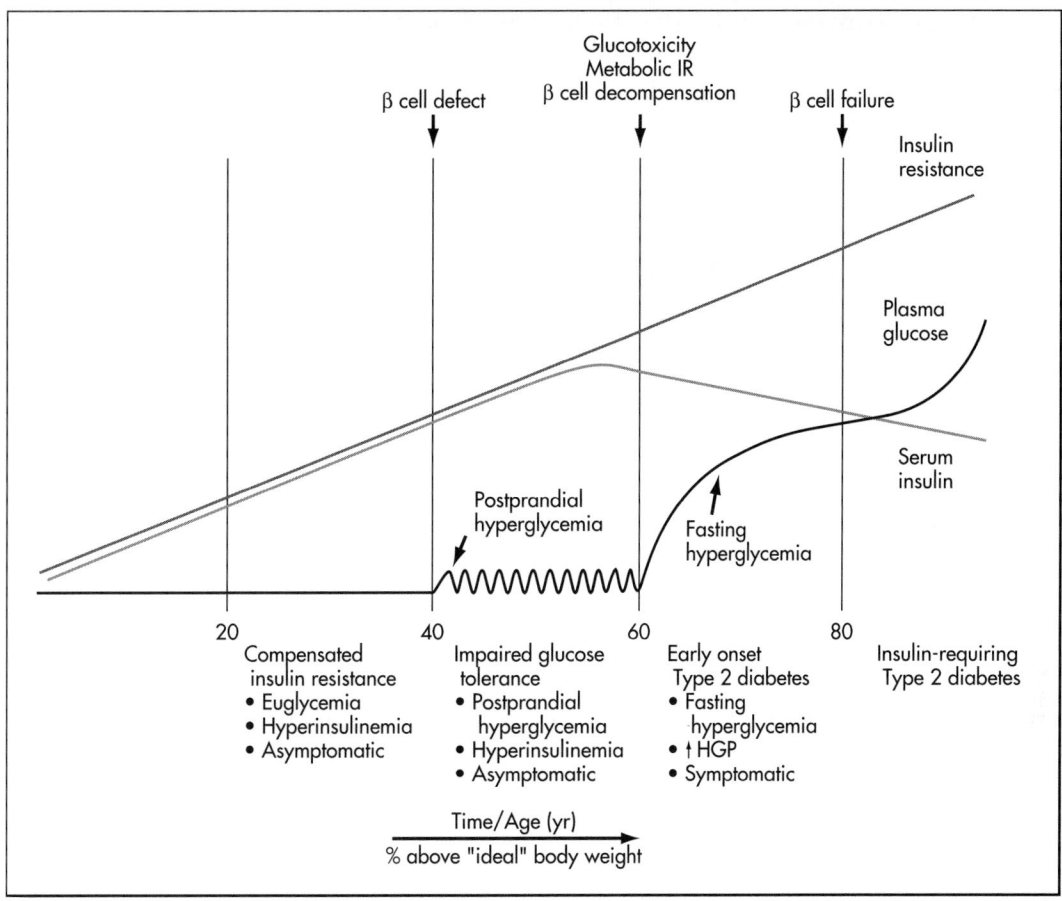

Fig. 1-127   Natural history of type 2 diabetes mellitus. The similar numbers for age and percentage greater than "ideal" body weight are only approximate. Likewise, the age markers for the different phases of β-cell decompensation toward overt diabetes and an insulin-requiring state are approximate guides. Certain groups are more insulin sensitive and require a greater loss of β-cell function to precipitate diabetes than obese insulin-resistant people who develop diabetes after small declines in β-cell function. Use of insulin in patients with type 2 diabetes varies considerably and is not age dependent. Insulin resistance increases proportionately to adiposity, represented here by weight. *HGP,* Hepatic glucose production; *IR,* insulin resistance. (From Andreoli TE [ed]: *Cecil essentials of medicine,* ed 5, Philadelphia, 2001, WB Saunders.)

TABLE 1-24 **General Comparison of the Two Most Common Types of Diabetes Mellitus**

	TYPE 1	TYPE 2
Previous terminology	Insulin-dependent diabetes mellitus (IDDM), type I, juvenile-onset diabetes	Non-insulin-dependent diabetes mellitus, type II, adult-onset diabetes
Age of onset	Usually <30 yr, particularly childhood and adolescence, but any age	Usually >40 yr, but any age
Genetic predisposition	Moderate; environmental factors required for expression; 35%-50% concordance in monozygotic twins; several candidate genes proposed	Strong; 60%-90% concordance in monozygotic twins; many candidate genes proposed; some genes identified in maturity-onset diabetes of the young
Human leukocyte antigen associations	Linkage to DQA and DQB, influenced by DRB(3 and 4) [DR2 protective]	None known
Other associations	Autoimmune; Graves' disease, Hashimoto's thyroiditis, vitiligo, Addison's disease, pernicious anemia	Heterogenous group, ongoing subclassification based on identification of specific pathogenic processes and genetic defects
Precipitating and risk factors	Largely unknown; microbial, chemical, dietary, other	Age, obesity (central), sedentary lifestyle, previous gestational diabetes
Findings at diagnosis	85%-90% of patients have one and usually more autoantibodies to ICA512/IA-2/IA-2β, GAD$_{65}$, insulin (IAA)	Possibly complications (microvascular and macrovascular) caused by significant preceeding asymptomatic period
Endogenous insulin levels	Low or absent	Usually present (relative deficiency), early hyperinsulinemia
Insulin resistance	Only with hyperglycemia	Mostly present
Prolonged fast	Hyperglycemia, ketoacidosis	Euglycemia
Stress, withdrawal of insulin	Ketoacidosis	Nonketotic hyperglycemia, occasionally ketoacidosis

From Andreoli TE (ed): *Cecil essentials of medicine*, ed 5, Philadelphia, 2001, WB Saunders.
GAD, Glutamic acid decarboxylase; *IA-2/IA-2β,* tyrosine phosphatases; *IAA,* insulin autoantibodies; *ICA,* islet cell antibody; *ICA512,* islet cell autoantigen 512 (fragment of IA-2).

TABLE 1-25 Oral Antidiabetic Agents as Monotherapy

	SULFONYLUREAS	BIGUANIDES	α-GLUCOSIDASE INHIBITORS	THIAZOLIDINEDIONES	MEGLITINIDES
Generic name	Glimepiride, gly-buride, glipizide, chlorpropamide, tolbutamide	Metformin	Acarbose, miglitol	Troglitazone, rosiglitazone, pioglitazone	Repaglinide, nateglinide
Mode of action	↑↑ Pancreatic insulin secretion chronically	↓↓ HGP; ↓ peripheral IR; ↓ intestinal glucose absorption	Delays PP digestion of carbohydrates and absorption of glucose	↓↓ Peripheral IR; ↑↑ glucose disposal; ↓ HGP	↑↑ Pancreatic insulin secretion acutely
Preferred patient type	Diagnosis age >30 yr, lean, diabetes <5 yr, insulinopenic	Overweight, IR, fasting hyperglycemia, dyslipidemia	PP hyperglycemia	Overweight, IR, dyslipidemia, renal dysfunction	PP hyperglycemia, insulinopenic
Therapeutic effects					
↓ HBA_{1c}* (%)	1-2	1-2	0.5-1	0.8-1	1-2
↓ FPG* (mg/dl)	50-70	50-80	15-30	25-50	40-80
↓ PPG* (mg/dl)	~90	80	40-50	—	30
Insulin levels	↑	—	—	—	↑
Weight	↑	–/↓	—	–/↑	↑
Lipids	—	↓ LDL ↓↓ TG		↑ Large "fluffy" LDL ↓↓ TG ↑ HDL	—
Side effects	Hypoglycemia	Diarrhea, lactic acidosis	Abdominal pain, flatulence, diarrhea	Idiosyncratic hepato-toxicity with trog-litazone; edema	Hypoglycemia (low-risk)
Dose(s)/day	1-3	2-3	1-3	1	1-4+
Maximum daily dose (mg)	Depends on agent	2550	150 (<60-kg bw) 300 (>60-kg bw)	Depends on agent	16 (repaglinide), 360 (nateglinide)
Range/dose (mg)	Depends on agent	500-1000	25-50 (<60-kg bw) 25-100 (>60-kg bw)	Depends on agent	0.5-4 (repaglinide), 60, 120 (nateglinide)
Optimal adminis-tration time	~30 min premeal (some with food, others on empty stomach)	With meal	With first bite of meal	With meal (breakfast)	Preferably <15 (0-30 min) premeals (omit if no meal)
Main site of metabolism/ excretion	Hepatic/renal, fecal	Not metabolized/ renal	Only 2% absorbed/fecal	Hepatic/fecal	Hepatic/fecal

Modified from Andreloi TE (ed): *Cecil essentials of medicine*, ed 5, Philadelphia, 2001, WB Saunders.
↑, Increased; ↓, decreased; —, unchanged; *bw*, body weight; *FPG*, fasting plasma glucose; *HDL*, high-density lipoprotein; *HGP*, hepatic glucose production; *IR*, insulin resistance; *LDL*, low-density lipoprotein; *PP*, postprandial; *PPG*, postprandial plasma glucose; *TG*, triglyceride.
*Values combined from numerous studies; values are also dose dependent.

TABLE 1-26 Types of Insulin

INSULIN TYPE	GENERIC NAME	PREPRANDIAL INJECTION TIMING* (HR)	ONSET* (HR)	PEAK* (HR)	DURATION* (HR)	BLOOD GLUCOSE (BG) NADIR* (HR)
Rapid acting	Lispro†	0-0.2	0.2-0.5	0.5-2	<5	2-4
Short acting	Regular Lente	0.5-(1)	0.3-1 1-2	2-6 4-12	4-8 (≤16)	3-7 (Pre-next meal)
Intermediate acting	NPH	0.5-(1)	1-3	6-15	16-26	6-13
Long acting‡	Ultralente	0.5-(1)	4-6	8-30	24-36	10-28
Mixed, short/intermediate acting	70/30					
	50/50	0.5-(1)	0.5-1	3-12	16-24	3-12

From Andreoli TE (ed): *Cecil essentials of medicine,* ed 5, Philadelphia, 2001, WB Saunders.
70/30, 70% NPH, 30% regular; *50/50,* 50% NPH, 50% regular; *NPH,* neutral protamine Hagedorn.
*Times depend on several factors including dose, anatomic site of injection, method (SQ, IM, IV), duration of diabetes, degree of insulin resistance, level of activity, and body temperature. Some time ranges are wide to include data from several separate studies. Preprandial injection depends on premeal BG values as well as insulin type. If BG is low, may need to inject insulin and eat immediately (carbohydrate portion of meal first). If BG is high, may delay meal after insulin injection and eat carbohydrate portion last.
†Insulin analogue with reversal of lysine and proline at positions 28 and 29 on the β chain.
‡Insulin glargine [rDNA origin] is a newer, once-daily insulin analog (Lantus) that provides 24-hour basal glucose-lowering with once-a-day bedtime dosing. Onset of action is 2-3 hr, duration of action is 24+ hr.

BASIC INFORMATION

■ **DEFINITION**

Diabetic ketoacidosis (DKA) is a life-threatening complication of diabetes mellitus resulting from severe insulin deficiency and manifested clinically by severe dehydration and alterations in the sensorium.

■ **SYNONYMS**

DKA

ICD-9CM CODES

250.1 Diabetic ketoacidosis

■ **EPIDEMIOLOGY & DEMOGRAPHICS**

INCIDENCE/PREVALENCE: 46 episodes/10,000 diabetics; cause of 14% of all hospital admissions of diabetic patients

PREDOMINANT AGE: 1 to 25 yr

■ **PHYSICAL FINDINGS & CLINICAL PRESENTATION**

- Evidence of dehydration (tachycardia, hypotension, dry mucous membranes, sunken eyeballs, poor skin turgor)
- Clouding of mental status
- Tachypnea with air hunger (Kussmaul's respiration)
- Fruity breath odor (caused by acetone)
- Lipemia retinalis in some patients
- Possible evidence of precipitating factors (infected wound, pneumonia)
- Abdominal or CVA tenderness in some patients

■ **ETIOLOGY**

Metabolic decompensation in diabetics usually precipitated by an infectious process (up to 40% of cases). Poor compliance with insulin therapy and severe medical illness (e.g., CVA, MI) are other common causes. Cocaine abuse has been reported as a risk factor for DKA, particularly in patients with multiple admissions.

🔬 **DIAGNOSIS**

■ **DIFFERENTIAL DIAGNOSIS**

- Hyperosmolar nonketotic state (Table 1-27)
- Alcoholic ketoacidosis
- Uremic acidosis
- Metabolic acidosis secondary to methyl alcohol, ethylene glycol
- Salicylate poisoning

■ **WORKUP**

- Laboratory evaluation (see below) to confirm diagnosis and evaluate precipitating factors
- Admission ECG to evaluate electrolyte abnormalities and rule out myocardial ischemia/infarction as a contributing factor

■ **LABORATORY TESTS**

- Glucose level reveals severe hyperglycemia (serum glucose generally >300 mg/dl).
- ABGs reveal acidosis: arterial pH usually <7.3 with P_{CO_2} <40 mm Hg.
- Serum electrolytes:
  1. Serum bicarbonate is usually <15 mEq/L.
  2. Serum potassium may be low, normal, or high. There is always significant total body potassium depletion regardless of the initial potassium level.
  3. Serum sodium is usually decreased as a result of hyperglycemia, dehydration, and lipemia. Assume 1.6 mEq/L decrease in extracellular sodium for each 100 mg/dl increase in glucose concentration.
  4. Calculate the anion gap (AG):

$$AG = Na^+ - (Cl^- + HCO_3^-)$$

In DKA the anion gap is increased; hyperchloremic metabolic acidosis may be present in unusual circumstances when both the glomerular filtration rate and the plasma volume are well maintained.

- CBC with differential, urinalysis, urine and blood cultures to rule out infectious precipitating factor.
- Serum calcium, magnesium, and phosphorus; the plasma phosphate and magnesium levels may be significantly depressed and should be rechecked within 24 hr because they may decrease further with correction of DKA.
- BUN and creatinine generally reveal significant dehydration.
- Amylase, liver enzymes should be checked in patients with abdominal pain.

■ **IMAGING STUDIES**

Chest x-ray examination is helpful to rule out infectious process. The initial chest x-ray may be negative if the patient has significant dehydration. Repeat chest x-ray examination after 24 hr if pulmonary infection is strongly suspected.

TABLE 1-27 **A Comparison of Diabetic Ketoacidosis (DKA) and Hyperosmolar Nonketotic Syndrome (HNKS)**

FEATURE	DKA	HNKS
Age of patient	Usually <40 yr	Usually >60 yr
Duration of symptoms	Usually <2 days	Usually >5 days
Serum glucose concentration	Usually <800 mg/dl	Usually >800 mg/dl
Serum sodium concentration (Na^+)	More likely to be normal or low	More likely to be normal or high
Serum bicarbonate concentration (HCO_3^-)	Low	Normal
Ketone bodies	At least 4 + in 1:1 dilution	<2 + in 1:1 dilution
pH	Low	Normal
Serum osmolality	Usually <350 mOsm/kg	Usually >350 mOsm/kg
Cerebral edema	Occasionally clinical symptoms	Rarely (never?) clinical
Prognosis	3% to 10% mortality	10% to 20% mortality
Subsequent course	Insulin therapy required in almost all cases	Insulin therapy not required in most cases

From Andreoli TE (ed): *Cecil essentials of medicine*, ed 4, Philadelphia, 1997, WB Saunders.

TREATMENT

■ NONPHARMACOLOGIC THERAPY

- Monitor mental status, vital signs, and urine output qh until improved, then monitor q2-4h.
- Monitor electrolytes, renal function, and glucose level (see below).

■ ACUTE GENERAL Rx

FLUID REPLACEMENT (THE USUAL DEFICIT IS 6 TO 8 L)

1. Do not delay fluid replacement until laboratory results have been received.
2. The initial fluid replacement should be with 0.9% NS. Careful monitoring for fluid overload is necessary in elderly patients and those with a history of CHF.
3. The rate of fluid replacement varies with the age of the patient and the presence of significant cardiac or renal disease.

- The usual rate of infusion is 500 ml to 1 L over the first hour; 300 to 500 ml/hr for the next 12 hr.
- Continue the infusion at a rate of 200 to 300 ml/hr, using 0.45% NS until the serum glucose level is <300 ml/dl, then change the hydrating solution to D_5W to prevent hypoglycemia, replenish free water, and introduce additional glucose substrate (necessary to suppress lipolysis and ketogenesis).

INSULIN ADMINISTRATION:

1. The patient should be given an initial loading IV bolus of 0.15 to 0.2 U/kg of regular insulin followed by a constant infusion at a rate of 0.1 U/kg/hr (e.g., 25 U of regular insulin in 250 ml of 0.9% saline solution at 70 ml/hr equals 7 U/hr for a 70-kg patient).
2. Monitor serum glucose qh for the first 2 hr, then monitor q2-4h.
3. The goal is to decrease serum glucose level by 80 mg/dl/hr (following an initial drop because of rehydration); if the serum glucose level is not decreasing at the expected rate, double the rate of insulin infusion.
4. When the serum glucose level approaches 250 mg/dl, decrease the rate of insulin infusion to 2 to 3 U/hr and continue this rate until the patient has received adequate fluid replacement, HCO_3^- is close to normal, and ketones have cleared.

5. Approximately 30 to 60 min before stopping the IV insulin infusion, administer an SC dose of regular insulin (dose varies with the patient's demonstrated insulin sensitivity); this SC dose of regular insulin is necessary because of the extremely short life of the insulin in the IV infusion.
6. When the patient is able to eat, regular insulin is administered before each meal and at hs. It is best to use sliding scale doses of regular insulin until maintenance doses are established. In newly diagnosed diabetics, the total daily dose to maintain metabolic control ranges from 0.5 to 0.8 U/kg/day. Split dose therapy with regular and NPH insulin may be given, with two thirds of the total daily dose administered in the morning and one third in the evening.

ELECTROLYTE REPLACEMENT:

Potassium Replacement: The average total potassium loss in DKA is 300 to 500 mEq.

- The rate of replacement varies with the patient's serum potassium level, degree of acidosis (decreased pH, increased potassium level), and renal function (potassium replacement should be used with caution in patients with renal failure).
- As a rule of thumb, potassium replacement may be started when there is no ECG evidence of hyperkalemia (tall, narrow, or tent-shaped T waves, decreased or absent P waves, short QT intervals, widening of QRS complex).
- In patients with normal renal function, potassium replacement can be started by adding 20 to 40 mEq KCl/L of IV hydrating solution if serum potassium is 4 to 5 mEq/L, more if serum potassium level is lower than 4 mEq/L.
- Monitor serum potassium level qh for the first 2 hr, then monitor q2-4h.

Phosphate Replacement: If the serum PO_4 is <1.5 mEq/L, give 2.5 mg/kg IV over 6 hr of elemental phosphate. Routine replacement of phosphate (in absence of laboratory evidence of significant hypophosphatemia) is not indicated. Rapid IV phosphate administration can cause hypocalcemia.

Magnesium Replacement: Replacement indicated only in the presence of significant hypomagnesemia or refractory hypokalemia.

BICARBONATE THERAPY: Routine use of bicarbonate in DKA is contraindicated, because it can worsen hypokalemia and intracellular acidosis and cause cerebral edema. Bicarbonate therapy should be used only if the arterial pH is <7. In these patients 44 to 88 mEq of sodium bicarbonate can be added to a liter of 0.45% NS q2-4h until pH increases >7. Use of bicarbonate therapy is particularly dangerous in the pediatric population. Children with DKA who have low partial pressures of arterial carbon dioxide and high serum urea nitrogen concentration at presentation and who are treated with bicarbonate are at increased risk for cerebral edema. Bicarbonate therapy in children with DKA should be limited to those with severe circulatory failure and a high risk of cardiac decompensation resulting from profound acidosis.

■ DISPOSITION

- Average mortality in DKA is 5% to 10%.
- In children <10 yr of age, DKA causes 70% of diabetes-related deaths.
- Cerebral edema occurs in 1% of episodes of DKA in children and is associated with a mortality rate of 40% to 90%.

■ REFERRAL

Patients with DKA should be admitted to the ICU.

☼ PEARLS & CONSIDERATIONS

■ COMMENTS

Potential complications of DKA therapy include hypoglycemia, cerebral edema, cardiac arrhythmias, shock, MI, and acute pancreatitis.

REFERENCES

Glaser N et al: Risk factor for cerebral edema in children with diabetic ketoacidosis, *N Engl J Med* 344:264, 2001.
Kitabchi AE, Wall BM: Management of diabetic ketoacidosis, *Am Fam Physician* 60:455, 1999.
Author: **Fred F. Ferri, M.D.**

Gwendolyn R. Lee, M.D.
Internal Medicine

BASIC INFORMATION

■ DEFINITION
Diffuse interstitial lung disease is a group of blood disorders involving the lung interstitium and characterized by inflammation of the alveolar structures and progressive parenchymal fibrosis.

■ SYNONYMS
Interstitial lung disease
ILD

ICD-9CM CODES
136.3 Acute interstitial lung disease
515 Chronic interstitial lung disease

■ EPIDEMIOLOGY & DEMOGRAPHICS
- The incidence of interstitial lung disease is 5 cases/100,000 persons
- There are >100 known disorders that can cause interstitial lung disease (see "Etiology").

■ PHYSICAL FINDINGS & CLINICAL PRESENTATION
- The patient generally presents with progressive dyspnea and nonproductive cough; other clinical manifestations vary with the underlying disease process.
- Physical examination typically shows end respiratory dry rales (Velcro rales), cyanosis, clubbing, and right-sided heart failure.

■ ETIOLOGY
- Occupational and environmental exposure: pneumoconiosis, asbestosis, organic dust, gases, fumes, berylliosis, silicosis
- Granulomatous lung disease: sarcoidosis, infections (e.g., fungal, mycobacterial)
- Drug-induced: bleomycin, busulfan, methotrexate, chlorambucil, cyclophosphamide, BCNU (carmustine), gold salts, tetrazolium chloride, amiodarone, tocainide, penicillin, zidovudine, sulfonamide
- Radiation pneumonitis
- Connective tissue diseases: SLE, rheumatoid arthritis, dermatomyositis
- Idiopathic pulmonary fibrosis: bronchiolitis obliterans, interstitial pneumonitis, DIP
- Infections: viral pneumonia, *Pneumocystis* pneumonia
- Others: Wegener's granulomatosis, Goodpasture's syndrome, eosinophilic granuloma, lymphangitic carcinomatosis, chronic uremia, chronic gastric aspiration, hypersensitivity pneumonitis, lipoid pneumonia, lymphoma, lymphoid granulomatosis

DIAGNOSIS

■ DIFFERENTIAL DIAGNOSIS
- CHF
- Chronic renal failure
- Lymphangitic carcinomatosis
- Sarcoidosis
- Allergic alveolitis

The differential diagnosis of granulomatous lung disease is described in Table 2-85.

■ WORKUP
Chest x-ray examination, ABGs, PFTs, bronchoscopy with bronchioloalveolar lavage, biopsy, laboratory evaluation

■ LABORATORY TESTS
- ABGs provide only limited information; initially ABGs may be normal but with progression of the disease, hypoxemia may be present.
- Antineutrophil cytoplasmic antibody (c-ANCA) is frequently positive in Wegener's granulomatosis.
- Antiglomerular basement membrane (anti-GBM) and anti-pulmonary basement membrane antibody are often present in Goodpasture's syndrome.

■ IMAGING STUDIES
Chest x-ray examination may be normal in 10% of patients.
- Ground-glass appearance is often an early finding.
- A coarse reticular pattern is usually a late finding.
- CHF causing interstitial changes on chest x-ray film must always be ruled out.
- Differential diagnosis of interstitial patterns include the following: pulmonary fibrosis, pulmonary edema, PCP, TB, sarcoidosis, eosinophilic granuloma, pneumoconiosis, and lymphangitic spread of carcinoma.
- Pulmonary function testing: findings are generally consistent with restrictive disease (decreased VC, TLC, and diffusing capacity).
- Bronchoscopy with bronchioloalveolar lavage is useful to characterize the pulmonary inflammatory response; the effector cell population in patients with interstitial lung disease consists of two major cell types:
  1. Lymphocytes (e.g., sarcoidosis, berylliosis, silicosis, hypersensitive pneumonitis)
  2. Neutrophils (e.g., asbestosis, collagen-vascular disease, idiopathic pulmonary fibrosis)
- Open lung biopsy or transbronchial biopsy is useful to identify the underlying disease process and exclude neoplastic involvement; transbronchial biopsy is less invasive but provides less tissue for analysis (this factor may be important in patients with irregular pulmonary involvement).
- Gallium-67 scanning plays a limited role in the evaluation of interstitial lung disease because it is not specific and a negative result does not exclude the disease (e.g., patients with end-stage fibrosis may have a negative scan).

TREATMENT

■ NONPHARMACOLOGIC THERAPY
Avoidance of tobacco (may adversely affect pulmonary function)

■ ACUTE GENERAL Rx
- Removal of offending agent (e.g., environmental exposure)
- Treatment of infectious process with appropriate antibiotic therapy
- Supplemental oxygen in patients with significant hypoxemia
- Corticosteroids in symptomatic patients with sarcoidosis
- Immunosuppressive therapy in selected cases (e.g., cyclophosphamide in patients with Wegener's granulomatosis)
- Treatment of any complications (e.g., pneumothorax, pulmonary embolism)

■ DISPOSITION
Overall mortality is 50% within 5 yr of diagnosis.

■ REFERRAL
- Surgical referral for biopsy
- Pulmonary referral for bronchoscopy and bronchoalveolar lavage (selected patients)
- Lung transplantation (selected patients)

PEARLS & CONSIDERATIONS

■ COMMENTS
Although open lung biopsy is the gold standard for diagnosis, it may be inappropriate in elderly patients; therefore individual consideration is advisable.
Author: **Fred F. Ferri, M.D.**

BASIC INFORMATION

■ DEFINITION
Acute or chronic consumption of digitalis leading to signs and symptoms of digitalis toxicity. May occur when serum levels are within the therapeutic range.

■ SYNONYMS
Digoxin
Digitoxin
Cardiac glycosides

ICD-9CM CODES
972.1 Digitalis overdose

■ PHARMACOKINETICS
After acute ingestion, peak effect occurs in 6 to 12 hr (before tissue distribution is complete)
BIOAVAILABILITY: (1) Digoxin 60% to 80%, (2) Digitoxin >90%
VOLUME OF DISTRIBUTION: (1) Digoxin 5 to 10 L/kg, (2) Digitoxin 0.5 L/kg
HALF-LIFE: (1) Digoxin 30 to 50 hr, (2) Digitoxin 5 to 8 days
THERAPEUTIC LEVEL: (1) Digoxin 0.5 to 2 ng/ml, (2) Digitoxin 10 to 30 ng/ml
Ingesting 3 mg of digoxin may result in serum levels above the therapeutic range in adults.

■ EPIDEMIOLOGY & DEMOGRAPHICS
- Digitalis toxicity occurs in 5% to 15% of individuals at some point during therapy.
- Factors that potentiate toxicity: advanced age, renal insufficiency, cardiac amyloidosis, drugs that interfere with digoxin elimination (amiodarone, indomethacin, quinidine, quinine, verapamil), hypokalemia, hypomagnesemia, hypercalcemia, hypoxemia, hypothyroidism, and volume depletion.

■ PHYSICAL FINDINGS & CLINICAL PRESENTATION
Cardiac, gastrointestinal, and central nervous systems are affected.
ACUTE TOXICITY: Vomiting, hyperkalemia, sinus bradycardia, second- and third-degree AV block, VT or VF, sinoatrial arrest.

CHRONIC TOXICITY: Anorexia, nausea, fatigue, visual disturbance (scotomas, color perception changes), confusion, almost any cardiac arrhythmia: most frequently accelerated junctional rhythm and paroxysmal atrial tachycardia with block but may have sinus bradycardia or ventricular arrhythmias.

■ ETIOLOGY
Cardiac glycosides reversibly inhibit the function of the sodium-potassium ATPase pump that increases myocardial contractility. Toxicity causes (1) increased vagal tone resulting in decreased conduction velocity in the sinus and AV nodes, (2) increased automaticity in the Purkinje fibers possibly because of increased delayed afterdepolarizations.

DIAGNOSIS

■ DIFFERENTIAL DIAGNOSIS
- β-Blockers
- Cyclic antidepressants
- Disopyramide
- Encainide and flecainide
- Phenothiazines
- Procainamide
- Propoxyphene
- Quinidine

■ WORKUP
History, physical examination, laboratory tests

■ LABORATORY TESTS
- Stat digoxin or digitoxin levels (may not correlate with severity of intoxication)
- Electrolytes, BUN, creatinine, magnesium
- ECG (Figs. 1-128 and 1-129)

TREATMENT

■ NONPHARMACOLOGIC THERAPY
- Ensure adequate airway
- EKG monitor for 12 to 24 hr after ingestion

■ ACUTE GENERAL Rx
DECREASE TOXICITY:
- Acute toxicity: 50 to 100 g activated charcoal and cathartic; repeat dose of activated charcoal q3-4h if needed. Gastric lavage is not needed if activated charcoal is given promptly.
- Treat hypokalemia and hypomagnesemia. (Often seen with chronic toxicity and may worsen tachyarrhythmias)
- Fab fragments of digoxin specific antibodies (Digibind):
  1. Specific antibodies that bind to digoxin and to a lesser extent digitoxin and other cardiac glycosides.
  2. Reversal of intoxication occurs in 30 to 60 min, and complete reversal occurs by 4 hr.
  3. Indications: severe hyperkalemia, persistent symptomatic arrhythmia, massive overdose with high serum levels.
  4. Dosing: 1 vial (40 mg) of Fab fragments binds 0.6 mg of digoxin. *Acute ingestion:* number of vials = [(ingested digoxin mg) × 0.8]/0.6, *Chronic ingestion:* number of vials = [(serum digoxin level ng/ml) × weight kg]/100. Average requirement for acute overdose is 10 vials and chronic toxicity usually requires 5 vials.
  5. After use of Fab fragments the digoxin level is falsely elevated; accurate measure of free digoxin level can be obtained by fluorescence polarization assay of protein-free ultrafiltrate.
  6. Inactive complex excreted in urine, half-life of complex is 16 to 20 hr. In renal insufficiency consider plasmapheresis to remove antigen-antibody complex since, theoretically, complexes may degrade before excreted.
  7. Class C for pregnancy.
  8. Adverse effects of treatment: May undo desirable action of drug and exacerbate heart failure and increased ventricular response in previously controlled atrial fibrillation, hypokalemia, hypersensitivity reaction, and serum sickness.
  9. Hemoperfusion: controversial, potentially useful for digitoxin, not useful for digoxin.

COMPLICATIONS:
Treat hyperkalemia if >5.5 (mild hyperkalemia may protect against tachy-arrhythmias)
- Sodium bicarbonate 1 mEq/kg
- Glucose 0.5 g/kg IV and insulin 0.1 U/kg IV
- Sodium polystyrene sulfonate (kayexalate) 0.5 g/kg PO
- Do not use calcium because it may worsen ventricular arrhythmias
Bradycardia and heart block:
- Atropine 0.5 to 2 mg IV
- Temporary pacemaker if there is persistent symptomatic bradycardia or supraventricular and ventricular tachycardia
- Lidocaine or phenytoin
- Avoid quinidine, bretylium, and procainamide
- Elective cardioversion is contraindicated since it may precipitate ventricular fibrillation.
- Rapid IV verapamil is contraindicated because both digoxin and verapamil inhibit the AV node. Verapamil and digoxin can be used together in the absence of digoxin toxicity and AV block.

■ **DISPOSITION**
Good with prompt treatment

REFERENCE
Carey CF, Lee HH, Woeltje KF: *The Washington manual of medical therapeutics*, ed 29, Philadelphia, 1998, Lippincott-Raven.
Author: **Sudeep K. Aulakh, M.D., F.R.C.P.C.**

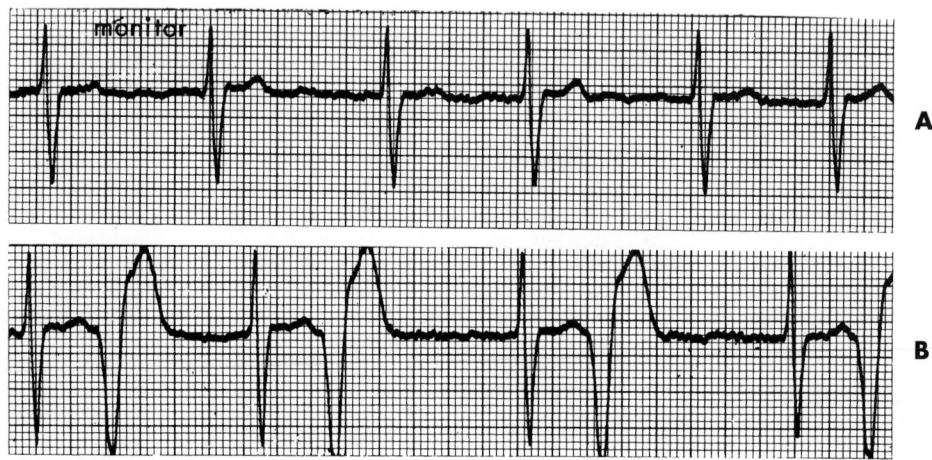

Fig. 1-128   Ventricular bigeminy caused by digitalis toxicity. Ventricular ectopy is one of the most common signs of digitalis toxicity. The underlying rhythm in **A** is atrial fibrillation. In **B**, each normal QRS is followed by a VPB. (From Goldberger AL [ed]: *Clinical electrocardiography*, ed 5, St Louis, 1994, Mosby.)

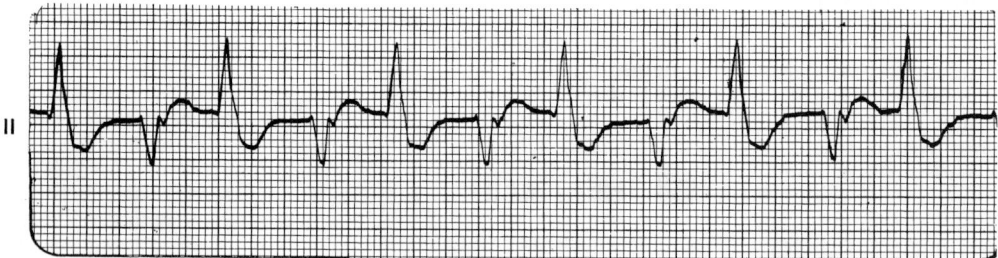

Fig. 1-129   This digitalis-toxic arrhythmia is a special type of ventricular tachycardia (bidirectional tachycardia) with QRS complexes that alternate in direction from beat to beat. No P waves are present. (From Goldberger AL [ed]: *Clinical electrocardiography*, ed 5, St Louis, 1994, Mosby.)

BASIC INFORMATION

■ DEFINITION
Diphtheria is an infection of the mucous membranes or skin caused by *Corynebacterium diphtheriae.*

■ ICD-9CM CODES
032.9 Diphtheria

■ EPIDEMIOLOGY & DEMOGRAPHICS
INCIDENCE (IN U.S.):
- Fewer than 5 cases/yr since 1980 (<0.002 cases/100,000 persons)
- Last culture-confirmed indigenous case in 1988

PREDOMINANT AGE: Adult years

■ PHYSICAL FINDINGS & CLINICAL PRESENTATION
RESPIRATORY DIPHTHERIA:
- Commonly presenting as pharyngitis, but any part of the respiratory tract may be involved, including the nasopharynx, larynx, trachea, or bronchi
- Areas of gray or white exudate coalescing to form a "pseudomembrane" that bleeds when removed
- Possible fever and dysphagia
- Complications: respiratory tract obstruction and pneumonia
- Systemic effects of the toxin: myocarditis and polyneuritis (frequently involving a bulbar distribution)
- Occurs mostly in nonimmune individuals; usually milder and less likely to be complicated in those adequately immunized

CUTANEOUS DIPHTHERIA:
- Usually complicates existing skin lesion (i.e., impetigo or scabies)
- Resembles the underlying condition

■ ETIOLOGY
- Caused by *C. diphtheriae,* an aerobic, gram-positive rod
- Transmitted by close contact through droplets of nasopharyngeal secretions
- Symptomatic disease of the respiratory system caused by toxin-producing strains (tox$^+$)
- Systemic effects of toxin: ranging from nausea and vomiting to polyneuropathy, myocarditis, and vascular collapse
- Presence of strains not producing toxin (tox$^-$) in the respiratory tract of asymptomatic carriers and in skin lesions of cutaneous diphtheria

DIAGNOSIS

■ DIFFERENTIAL DIAGNOSIS
- *Streptococcus* pharyngitis
- Viral pharyngitis
- Mononucleosis

■ WORKUP
- Presence of a pseudomembrane in the oropharynx suggestive of diagnosis (not always present)
- Gram stains of secretions to show club-shaped organisms, which appear as "Chinese letters"
- Nasolaryngoscopy to identify lesions in the nares, nasopharynx, larynx, or tracheobronchial tree
- Electrocardiogram
- Possible ICU monitoring

■ LABORATORY TESTS
- Cultures of mucosal lesions or of nasal discharge
  1. Positive culture for *C. diphtheriae* confirms the diagnosis.
  2. Laboratory is notified of the suspected diagnosis so that appropriate culture medium (Tinsdale agar) is used.
- Testing of all isolated organisms for toxin production

■ IMAGING STUDIES
- Chest x-ray examination to rule out pneumonia
- Bronchopneumonia has been described in fatal cases

TREATMENT

■ NONPHARMACOLOGIC THERAPY
- Intubation or tracheostomy if signs of respiratory distress occur
- Nasogastric or parenteral nutrition in those with bulbar signs
- ICU monitoring for patients with signs of systemic toxicity
- Cardiac pacing in patients with heart block
- Respiratory isolation

■ ACUTE GENERAL Rx
- Administration of diphtheria antitoxin once a clinical diagnosis is made
- If tests for hypersensitivity to horse serum are negative: 50,000 U given for mild to moderate disease or 60,000 to 120,000 U for critically ill patients
- IV infusion of antitoxin over 60 min

- Serum sickness in 10% of treated individuals; those with hypersensitivity to horse serum should be desensitized before administration of antitoxin
- Antibiotics to eradicate the organism in carriers or patients
- For respiratory diphtheria:
  1. Erythromycin 500 mg qid PO or IV or IM penicillin 600,000 U bid for 14 days
  2. Carriers or patients with cutaneous disease: erythromycin 500 mg PO qid or rifampin 600 mg PO qd for 7 days

■ CHRONIC Rx
Antibiotics to limit toxin production and eradicate carrier state, thereby preventing transmission

■ DISPOSITION
Complete recovery with adequate supportive measures and antitoxin

■ REFERRAL
- Hospitalization and referral to an infectious disease specialist for all suspected patients
- To an otolaryngologist for evaluation in cases of respiratory diphtheria
- All cases reported to the public health authorities

PEARLS & CONSIDERATIONS

■ COMMENTS
- Most cases are imported by travelers in epidemic areas, so recent epidemics in Europe are a cause for concern. A widespread epidemic of diphtheria began in 1990 in the former Soviet Union.
- Vaccination with diphtheria toxoid (attenuated toxin) is safe and effective in the form of DPT or Td; Td boosters should be given to adults every 10 yr.
- According to serologic studies, 20% to 60% of U.S. adults >20 yr of age are susceptible to diphtheria.

REFERENCES
Bisgard KM et al: Respiratory diphtheria in the United States: 1980 through 1995, *Am J Pub Health* 88:787, 1998.
Hadfield TL et al: The pathology of diphtheria, *J Infect Dis* 181:s116, 2000.
Markina SS et al: Diphtheria in the Russian Federation in the 1990s, *J Infect Dis* 181 (Suppl 1):S27, 2000.
Author: **Maurice Policar, M.D.**

BASIC INFORMATION

■ DEFINITION

Discoid lupus erythematosus (DLE) refers to a chronic cutaneous usually localized skin disorder sometimes associated with systemic lupus erythematosus (SLE). Erythematous plaque lesions with scaling, follicular plugging, atrophy, and scarring characterize DLE.

■ SYNONYMS

Chronic cutaneous lupus erythematosus

■ ICD-9CM CODES

695.4 Lupus erythematosus (local discoid)

■ EPIDEMIOLOGY & DEMOGRAPHICS

- Discoid lupus is more common in African-Americans.
- DLE is more common in females, with peak incidence in the fourth decade of life.
- Less than 5% of patients with DLE progress to SLE.
- Approximately 10% to 20% of patients with SLE will also have discoid lupus skin lesions.

■ PHYSICAL FINDINGS & CLINICAL PRESENTATION

History
- Appearance of single or multiple asymptomatic plaque lesions (Fig. 1-130)

Physical findings
- Anatomic distribution
  1. DLE commonly involves the scalp, face, and ears but is not limited to these areas.
- Lesion configuration
  1. Irregularly grouped
- Lesion morphology
  1. Plaque lesions with scales
  2. Follicular plugging
  3. Atrophy
  4. Scarring
  5. Telangiectasia
- Color
  1. Erythematous
  2. Red-to-violaceous
  3. Hyperpigmentation or hypopigmentation

- Alopecia can occur and is permanent.
- Urticaria (5%)
- May be associated with other criteria for SLE (e.g., oral ulcers, arthritis, pleuritis, pericarditis).

■ ETIOLOGY

The exact cause of DLE is not known, although an immune complex mediated mechanism is thought to be responsible.

DIAGNOSIS

Clinical inspection and skin biopsy usually establish the diagnosis of DLE.

■ DIFFERENTIAL DIAGNOSIS

- Psoriasis
- Lichen planus
- Secondary syphilis
- Superficial fungal infections
- Photosensitivity eruption
- Sarcoidosis
- Subacute cutaneous lupus erythematosus
- Rosacea
- Keratoacanthoma
- Actinic keratosis
- Dermatomyositis

■ WORKUP

The workup for isolated DLE includes laboratory tests and x-rays looking for diagnostic criteria for SLE.

■ LABORATORY TESTS

Laboratory tests are done to exclude criteria for SLE. Laboratory statements below refer to patients having SLE with DLE.
- CBC is usually normal in isolated DLE.
- BUN/creatinine is normal.
- ESR is elevated in active disease associated with SLE.
- Urinalysis looking for proteinuria and hematuria.
- ANA may be positive in 20% of patients with isolated DLE.
- Anti-Ro (SS-A) autoantibodies are present in approximately 1% to 3% of patients.
- dsDNA and antiSm antibodies are rarely present.

- Complement levels may be low in patients with SLE but not in DLE.
- Skin biopsy shows degeneration of the basal cell layer with follicular plugging and atrophy of the epidermis.

■ IMAGING STUDIES

CXR is not specific in the diagnosis of DLE; however, it is helpful when assessing for SLE.

TREATMENT

■ NONPHARMACOLOGIC THERAPY

- The goals of management are to control existing lesions and limit scarring, and to prevent development of further lesions.
- Avoid sun exposure from 10 AM to 4 PM.
- Use sunscreens with sun protective factor (SPF) of at least 15.

■ ACUTE GENERAL Rx

- Topical steroid is first-line therapy for DLE.
- Intradermal steroid triamcinolone acetonide, 3 mg/ml with 1% Xylocaine is injected into the lesion.
- Hydroxychloroquine 400 mg PO qd for 1 mo, then decrease the dose to 200 mg qd. Treatment is continued for 3 to 6 mo.

■ CHRONIC Rx

- Dapsone 100 mg/day can be used in patients who fail to respond to topical steroid or hydroxychloroquine.
- Other alternatives include
  1. Chloroquine 250-500 mg PO qd
  2. Auranofin 6 mg/day PO qd or divided bid; after 3 mo, may increase to 9 mg/day divided tid
  3. Thalidomide 100-300 mg PO hs, aq, and >1 hr pc
  4. Azathioprine 1 mg/kg/day PO for 6-8 wk, increase by 5 mg/kg q4wk until response is seen or dose reaches 2.5 mg/kg/day
  5. If all of the above fail, mycophenolate 1 g PO bid or interferon alpha-2b (2 million units/m^2 SQ 3 times/wk for 30 days) have been tried

■ DISPOSITION

- If left untreated, DLE is a chronic disorder that can lead to atrophy and scarring of the skin.
- A minority of patients with isolated cutaneous DLE progress to systemic lupus erythematosus. Prognosis is better in this group than unselected SLE patients.

■ REFERRAL

Patients with isolated DLE involving the face and scalp should be referred to a dermatologist. If associated with SLE, a rheumatology consultation is recommended.

☼ PEARLS & CONSIDERATIONS

■ COMMENTS

- Cutaneous lesions account for 4 of the 11 criteria in the diagnosis of SLE (e.g., malar rash, discoid rash, photosensitivity, and oral ulcers).
- Cutaneous lupus erythematosus is classified as:
  1. Chronic cutaneous lupus erythematosus (discoid lupus is included in this category).
  2. Subacute cutaneous lupus erythematosus
  3. Acute cutaneous lupus erythematosus

- DLE lesions are not as photosensitive as the subacute cutaneous lesions.
- Rarely does DLE degenerate into a malignant nonmelanotic skin cancer.

REFERENCES

Callen JP: Collagen vascular diseases, *Med Clin North Am* 82(6):1217, 1998.
Callen JP: Lupus erythematosus, discoid *e Medicine Journal,* 2(11) 2001 (www.emedicine.com).
Author: **Peter Petropoulos, M.D.**

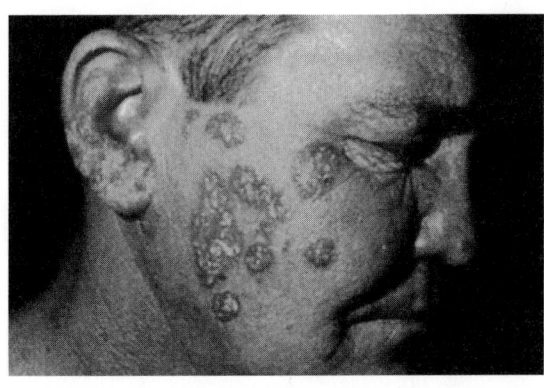

Fig. 1-130 Scaling plaques with thick scales on the ear and face of a patient who has discoid lupus. (Courtesy Department of Dermatology, University of North Carolina at Chapel Hill. In Goldstein BG, Goldstein AO [eds]: *Practical dermatology,* ed 2, St Louis, 1977, Mosby.)

BASIC INFORMATION

■ **DEFINITION**

Disseminated intravascular coagulation (DIC) is an acquired thromboembolic disorder characterized by generalized activation of the clotting mechanism, which results in the intravascular formation of fibrin and ultimately thrombotic occlusion of small and midsize vessels.

■ **SYNONYMS**

Consumptive coagulopathy
DIC
Defibrination syndrome

ICD-9CM CODES
286.6 Disseminated intravascular coagulation

■ **EPIDEMIOLOGY & DEMOGRAPHICS**

Greater than 50% of cases are associated with gram-negative sepsis or other septicemic infections.

■ **PHYSICAL FINDINGS & CLINICAL PRESENTATION**

- Wound site bleeding, epistaxis, gingival bleeding, hemorrhagic bullae
- Petechiae, ecchymosis, purpura
- Dyspnea, localized rales, delirium
- Oliguria, anuria, GI bleeding, metrorrhagia

■ **ETIOLOGY**

- Infections (e.g., gram-negative sepsis, Rocky Mountain spotted fever, malaria, viral or fungal infection)
- Obstetric complications (e.g., dead fetus, amniotic fluid embolism, toxemia, abruptio placentae, septic abortion, eclampsia)
- Tissue trauma (e.g., burns, hypothermia-rewarming)
- Neoplasms (e.g., adenocarcinomas [GI, prostate, lung, breast], acute promyelocytic leukemia)
- Quinine, cocaine-induced rhabdomyolysis
- Liver failure
- Acute pancreatitis
- Transfusion reactions
- Respiratory distress syndrome
- Other: SLE, vasculitis, aneurysms, polyarteritis, cavernous hemangiomas

 DIAGNOSIS

■ **DIFFERENTIAL DIAGNOSIS**

- Hepatic necrosis: normal or elevated Factor VIII concentrations
- Vitamin K deficiency: normal platelet count
- Hemolytic uremic syndrome
- Thrombocytopenic purpura
- Renal failure, SLE, sickle cell crisis, dysfibrinogenemias

■ **WORKUP**

Diagnostic workup includes laboratory screening to confirm the diagnosis and exclude conditions noted in the differential diagnosis.

■ **LABORATORY TESTS**

- Peripheral blood smear generally shows RBC fragments and low platelet count.
- Coagulation factors are consumed at a rate in excess of the capacity of the liver to synthesize them, and platelets are consumed in excess of the capacity of the bone marrow megakaryocytes to release them. Diagnostic characteristics of DIC are increased PT, PTT, TT, fibrin split products, D-dimer; decreased fibrinogen level, thrombocytopenia (Table 1-28).
- Coagulopathy secondary to DIC must be differentiated from that secondary to liver disease or vitamin K deficiency.
  1. Vitamin K deficiency manifests with prolonged PT and normal PTT, TT, platelet, and fibrinogen level; PTT may be elevated in severe cases.
  2. Patients with liver disease have abnormal PT and PTT; TT and fibrinogen are usually normal unless severe disease is present; platelets are usually normal unless splenomegaly is present.
  3. Factors V and VIII are low in DIC, but they are normal in liver disease with coagulopathy.

■ **IMAGING STUDIES**

Imaging studies are generally not useful. Chest x-ray examination may be helpful to exclude infectious processes in patients presenting with pulmonary symptoms such as dyspnea, cough, or hemoptysis.

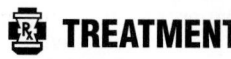 **TREATMENT**

■ **NONPHARMACOLOGIC THERAPY**

No specific precautions regarding activity level are necessary unless thrombocytopenia is severe.

■ **ACUTE GENERAL Rx**

- Correct and eliminate underlying cause (e.g., antimicrobial therapy for infection).
- Give replacement therapy with FFP and platelets in patients with significant hemorrhage:
  1. FFP 10 to 15 ml/kg can be given with a goal of normalizing INR.
  2. Platelet transfusions are given when platelet count is <10,000 (or higher if major bleeding is present).
  3. Cryoprecipitate 1 U/5 kg is reserved for hypofibrinogen states.
  4. Antithrombin III treatment may be considered as a supportive therapeutic option in patients with severe DIC. Its modest results and substantial cost are limiting factors.
- Heparin therapy at a dose lower than that used in venous thrombosis (300 to 500 U/hr) may be useful in selected cases to increase neutralization of thrombin (e.g., DIC associated with acute promyelocytic leukemia, purpura fulminans, acral ischemia).

■ **CHRONIC Rx**

Follow-up management includes coagulation screening to assess factor replacement therapy. Laboratory abnormalities generally correct with treatment of the underlying disorder. Chronic laboratory monitoring is not required.

■ DISPOSITION
Mortality in severe DIC exceeds 75%. Death generally results from progression of the underlying disease and complications such as acute renal failure, intracerebral hematoma, shock, or cardiac tamponade.

■ REFERRAL
Hematology consultation is recommended in all cases of DIC.

PEARLS & CONSIDERATIONS

■ COMMENTS
The treatment of chronic DIC is controversial. Low-dose SC heparin and/or combination antiplatelet agents such as aspirin and dipyridamole may·be useful.

REFERENCE
Levi M, Cate H: Disseminated intravascular coagulation, *N Engl J Med* 341:586, 1999.
Author: **Fred F. Ferri, M.D.**

TABLE 1-28   **Laboratory Findings in Disseminated Intravascular Coagulation, Vitamin K Deficiency, and Liver Disease**

	DISORDER		
TEST	**DIC**	**VITAMIN K DEFICIENCY**	**LIVER DISEASE**
PTT	P	P	P
PT	P	P	P
TT	P	N	P
Platelet count	L	N	N/L
FSPs	+	−	±
Fibrinogen	L	N	L
Factor VIII	L	N	N/L

From Behrman RE: *Nelson textbook of pediatrics*, ed 16, Philadelphia, 2000, WB Saunders.
DIC, Disseminated intravascular coagulation; *PTT*, partial thromboplasm time; *PT*, prothrombin time; *TT*, thrombin time, *FSPs*, fibrinolytic split products; *P*, prolonged; *N*, normal; *L*, low; *N/L*, normal or low; +, present; −, absent; ±, present or absent; *I*, increased.

BASIC INFORMATION

■ DEFINITION

- Colonic diverticula are herniations of mucosa and submucosa through the muscularis. They are generally found along the colon's mesenteric border at the site where the vasa recta penetrates the muscle wall (anatomic weak point).
- *Diverticulosis* is the asymptomatic presence of multiple colonic diverticula.
- *Diverticulitis* is an inflammatory process or localized perforation of diverticulum.

ICD-9CM CODES
562.10 Diverticulosis of colon
562.11 Diverticulitis of colon

■ EPIDEMIOLOGY & DEMOGRAPHICS

- Incidence of diverticulosis in the general population is 35% to 50%.
- Diverticulosis is more common in Western countries, affecting >30% of people >40 yr and >50% of people >70 yr.

■ PHYSICAL FINDINGS & CLINICAL PRESENTATION

- Physical examination in patients with diverticulosis is generally normal.
- Painful diverticular disease can present with LLQ pain, often relieved by defecation; location of pain may be anywhere in the lower abdomen because of the redundancy of the sigmoid colon.
- Diverticulitis can cause muscle spasm, guarding, and rebound tenderness predominantly affecting the LLQ.

■ ETIOLOGY

- Diverticular disease is believed to be secondary to low intake of dietary fiber.

DIAGNOSIS

■ DIFFERENTIAL DIAGNOSIS

- Irritable bowel syndrome
- IBD
- Carcinoma of colon
- Endometriosis
- Ischemic colitis
- Infections (pseudomembranous colitis, appendicitis, pyelonephritis, PID)
- Lactose intolerance

■ LABORATORY TESTS

- WBC count in diverticulitis reveals leukocytosis with left shift.

- Microcytic anemia can be present in patients with chronic bleeding from diverticular disease. MCV may be elevated in acute bleeding secondary to reticulocytosis.

■ IMAGING STUDIES

- Barium enema will demonstrate multiple diverticula and muscle spasm ("sawtooth" appearance of the lumen) in patients with painful diverticular disease. Barium enema can be hazardous and should not be performed in the acute stage of diverticulitis because it may produce free perforation.
- A CT scan of the abdomen can be used to diagnose acute diverticulitis; typical findings are thickening of the bowel wall, fistulas, or abscess formation.
- Evaluation of suspected diverticular bleeding:
  1. Arteriography if the bleeding is faster than 1 ml/min (advantage: the possible infusion of vasopressin directly into the arteries supplying the bleeding, as well as selective arterial embolization; disadvantages: its cost and invasive nature)
  2. Technetium-99m sulfa colloid
  3. Technetium-99m labeled RBC (can detect bleeding rates as low as 0.12 to 5 ml/min)

TREATMENT

■ NONPHARMACOLOGIC THERAPY

- Increase in dietary fiber intake and regular exercise to improve bowel function
- NPO and IV hydration in severe diverticulitis; NG suction if ileus or small bowel obstruction is present

■ ACUTE GENERAL Rx
TREATMENT OF DIVERTICULITIS:

- Mild case: broad-spectrum PO antibiotics (e.g., ciprofloxin and metronidazole) and liquid diet for 7 to 10 days
- Severe case: NPO and aggressive IV antibiotic therapy (e.g., triple antibiotic therapy with ampicillin, gentamicin, and metronidazole)
- Surgical treatment consisting of resection of involved areas and reanastomosis (if feasible); otherwise a diverting colostomy with reanastomosis performed when infection has been controlled; surgery should be considered in patients with:
  1. Repeated episodes of diverticulitis (two or more)
  2. Poor response to appropriate medical therapy (failure of conservative management)

  3. Abscess or fistula formation
  4. Obstruction
  5. Peritonitis
  6. Immunocompromised patients, first episode in young patient (<40 yr old)
  7. Inability to exclude carcinoma (10% to 20% of patients diagnosed with diverticulosis on clinical grounds are subsequently found to have carcinoma of the colon)

DIVERTICULAR HEMORRHAGE: 70% of diverticular bleeding occurs in the right colon.
  1. Bleeding is painless and stops spontaneously in the majority of patients (60%); it is usually caused by erosion of a blood vessel by a fecalith present within the diverticular sac.
  2. Medical therapy consists of blood replacement and correction of volume and any clotting abnormalities.
  3. Colonoscopic treatment with epinephrine injections, bipolar coagulation, or both may prevent recurrent bleeding and decrease the need for surgery.
  4. Surgical resection is necessary if bleeding does not stop spontaneously after administration of 4 to 5 U of PRBCs or recurs with severity within a few days; if attempts at localization are unsuccessful, total abdominal colectomy with ileoproctostomy may be indicated (high incidence of rebleeding if segmental resection is performed without adequate localization).

■ CHRONIC Rx
Asymptomatic patients with diverticulosis can be treated with a high-fiber diet or fiber supplements.

■ DISPOSITION

- Most patients with diverticulitis respond well to antibiotic management and bowel rest. Up to 30% of patients with diverticulitis will eventually require surgical management.
- Diverticular bleeding can recur in 15% to 20% of patients within 5 yr.

■ REFERRAL
Surgical referral when considering resection (see "Acute General Rx")

REFERENCE
Jensen DM et al: Urgent colonoscopy for the diagnosis and treatment of severe diverticular hemorrhage, *N Engl J Med* 342:78, 2000.
Author: **Fred F. Ferri, M.D.**

BASIC INFORMATION

■ DEFINITION
Down syndrome is a chromosomal abnormality causing mental retardation and multiple organ defects.

■ SYNONYMS
Trisomy 21

ICD-9CM CODES
758.0 Down syndrome

■ EPIDEMIOLOGY & DEMOGRAPHICS
INCIDENCE (IN U.S.): 1 in 700 births
PREVALENCE (IN U.S.): 300,000 persons
PREDOMINANT SEX: Male:female ratio of 1:3 to 1:0
PREDOMINANT AGE: Newborn to early adulthood
PEAK INCIDENCE: Newborn
GENETICS:
• Nondisjunction causing trisomy 21
• Increases with increasing maternal age

■ PHYSICAL FINDINGS
• Microcephaly
• Flattening of occiput and face
• Upward slant to eyes with epicanthal folds (Fig. 1-131)
• Brushfield spots in iris
• Broad stocky neck
• Small feet, hands, and digits
• Palmar crease
• Associated with congenital heart disease, malformations of the GI tract, cataracts, hypothyroidism, hip dysplasia

■ ETIOLOGY
Nondisjunction of chromosome 21

DIAGNOSIS

■ DIFFERENTIAL DIAGNOSIS
• Prenatal diagnosis is possible with ultrasound and amniocentesis.
• Anticipate associated congenital abnormalities.

■ LABORATORY TESTS
• CBC (transient leukemoid reaction)
• Chromosomal karyotype
• Thyroid screen
• Auditory brain stem responses

■ IMAGING STUDIES
Echocardiogram

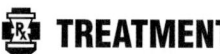 TREATMENT

■ NONPHARMACOLOGIC THERAPY
Usual outcome is that the patient remains at home until young adulthood, then enters a small group home.

■ CHRONIC Rx
• See "Nonpharmacologic Therapy."
• Frequent visits to pediatrician or special clinic are necessary.

■ DISPOSITION
Down syndrome clinics use a preventive checklist to anticipate many clinical challenges.

■ REFERRAL
Refer if not experienced in following children with Down syndrome.

PEARLS & CONSIDERATIONS

■ COMMENTS
• Most patients develop early Alzheimer's disease by age 40.
• This disease accounts for approximately one third of moderate to severe cases of mental retardation and presents many medical and ethical challenges.
• Median age at death in 1997 is 50 yr among whites, 25 yr among blacks, and 11 yr among people of other races.

REFERENCES
Haddow J: Antenatal screening for Down syndrome: where are we and where next? *Lancet* 352:336, 1998.
Racial disparities in median age at death of persons with Down syndrome—United States, 1968-97, *MMWR* 50:463, 2001.
Smith DS: Health care management of adults wtih Down syndrome, *Am Fam Physician* 64:1031, 2001.
Author: **William H. Olson, M.D.**

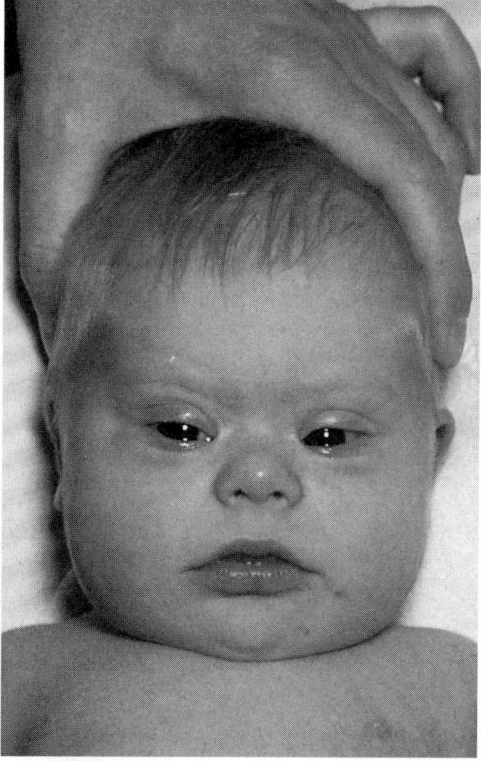

Fig. 1-131   Down syndrome. Note depressed nasal bridge, epicanthal folds, mongoloid slant of eyes, low set ears, and large tongue. (From Zitelli BJ, Davis HW: *Atlas of pediatric physical diagnosis,* ed 3, St Louis, 1997, Mosby.)

BASIC INFORMATION

■ DEFINITION
Dumping syndrome refers to the rapid transit of food products from the stomach to the small intestine seen after gastric surgery.

■ SYNONYMS
Early postgastrectomy syndrome

ICD-9CM CODES
564.2 Postgastric surgery syndromes

■ EPIDEMIOLOGY & DEMOGRAPHICS
Incidence is 10% of all patients having gastric surgery.
- Vagotomy and pyloroplasty (8.5% to 20%)
- Vagotomy and antrectomy (4% to 27%)
- Subtotal gastrectomy (10% to 40%)
- Parietal cell vagotomy (3% to 5%)
- Affects males and females equally

■ PHYSICAL FINDINGS & CLINICAL PRESENTATION
Early dumping
- Symptoms start within 1 hr after eating food
- No symptoms in fasting state
- Nausea, vomiting, and belching
- Epigastric fullness, cramping, and diarrhea
- Dizziness, flushing, diaphoresis, and syncope
- Palpitations and tachycardia
Late dumping
- Symptoms occurring 1 to 3 hr after eating
- Diaphoresis
- Irritability
- Difficulty concentrating
- Tremulous

■ ETIOLOGY
Dumping syndrome occurs almost exclusively in patients having gastric surgery.
- Systemic symptoms are thought to be due to hypovolemia caused by rapid shifts of fluid from the intravascular space into the lumen of the bowel.
- Increase in vasoactive substances is thought to play a role in dumping syndrome.
- Late dumping symptoms are thought to be due to reactive hypoglycemia.

DIAGNOSIS

A detailed clinical history and evidence of prior gastric surgery usually makes the diagnosis of dumping syndrome. Oral glucose challenge test and radiographic imaging studies aid in establishing the diagnosis.

■ DIFFERENTIAL DIAGNOSIS
- Pancreatic insufficiency
- Inflammatory bowel disease
- Afferent loop syndromes
- Bile acid reflux after surgery
- Bowel obstruction
- Gastroenteric fistula

■ WORKUP
Typically the diagnosis is made on clinical grounds. In certain clinical settings (e.g., symptoms in patients with no prior history of gastric surgery), a workup, including oral glucose challenge and imaging studies, may be pursued.

■ LABORATORY TESTS
Oral glucose challenge test:
- Oral intake of 50 g of glucose is followed by serial measurements of heart rate, serum glucose, and hydrogen breath test every 15 min for 6 hr.
- An increase in the heart rate >12 beats/min and a rise in hydrogen breath excretion had a sensitivity of 94% and specificity >92%. A nadir blood glucose <3.3 mmol/L was present in 75% of late dumpers.

■ IMAGING STUDIES
- Upper GI series properly defines anatomy.
- Scintigraphic imaging documents rapid gastric emptying and may be useful in patients with dumping syndrome and no prior history of gastric surgery.

TREATMENT

■ NONPHARMACOLOGIC THERAPY
- Diet modification
  1. Divide calorie intake over six small meals
  2. Limit fluid intake with meals
  3. Decrease carbohydrate intake
  4. Increase dietary fibers

■ ACUTE GENERAL Rx
- Acarbose 50 mg PO qd can be tried if dietary modification does not help.

- Octreotide 25 to 50 μg subcutaneously 30 min before meals is effective in relieving symptoms of dumping syndrome.

■ CHRONIC Rx
- Surgery is considered in patients with severe symptoms refractory to the above-mentioned dietary and acute general treatment.
- Surgical procedures include: reconstruction of the pylorus, converting Billroth II to a Billroth I anastomosis and a Roux-en-Y reconstruction.

■ DISPOSITION
- Dumping syndrome improves with time. Approximately 1% to 2% of patients will continue to have significant symptoms several months after surgery.
- Dietary modification effectively treats the majority of patients.

■ REFERRAL
- A GI consult is recommended in patients suspected of having dumping syndrome.
- If medical management is unsuccessful, a general surgical consultation is warranted.

PEARLS & CONSIDERATIONS

■ COMMENTS
- The majority of patients usually manifest with early dumping symptoms or combination of early and late symptoms. Few have late dumping symptoms alone.
- Octreotide has an inhibitory effect on the release of insulin and other vasoactive substances released by the gut. It also works by decreasing gastric emptying.

REFERENCES
Eagon JC, Miedema BW, Kelly KA: Postgastrectomy syndromes, *Surg Clin North Am* 72(2):445, 1992.
Vecht J, Masclee AAM, Lamers CBHW: The dumping syndrome: current insights into pathophysiology, diagnosis and treatment, *Scand J Gastroenterol* 32 (223):21, 1997.
Vecht J et al: Diagnostic value of dumping provocation in patients after gastric surgery, *Gastroenterology* 108(4):A704, 1995.
Author: **Peter Petropoulos, M.D.**

BASIC INFORMATION

■ DEFINITION

Dupuytren's contracture is a disease of the palmar fascia characterized by nodular fibroblastic proliferation that often results in progressive contractures of the fascia and flexion deformity of the fingers.

ICD-9CM CODES
728.6 Dupuytren's contracture

■ EPIDEMIOLOGY & DEMOGRAPHICS
PREVALENCE: Varies depending on nationality
PREVALENT AGE: 40 to 60 yr
PREVALENT SEX: Male:female ratio of 10:1

■ PHYSICAL FINDINGS & CLINICAL PRESENTATION
- Usually asymptomatic
- Most common complaints: deformity and interference with the use of the hand by the flexed, contracted fingers (Fig. 1-132)
- Process usually begins in the ulnar side of the hand, often starting at the ring finger
- Isolated painless nodules that eventually harden and mature into a longitudinal cord that extends into the finger

- Lesion often begins in the distal palmar crease
- Overlying skin adherent to the fascia
- Later stages: fibrous cord begins to contract and pull the finger into flexion
- Possible involvement of other fingers, particularly small finger

■ ETIOLOGY
Unknown

DIAGNOSIS

■ DIFFERENTIAL DIAGNOSIS
Soft tissue tumor, tendon cyst

TREATMENT

■ NONPHARMACOLOGIC THERAPY
- Stretching exercises
- Local heat

■ DISPOSITION
Rate of development is variable.

■ REFERRAL
- If joint contracture begins to develop
- For excision of rare nodule that is painful (at any stage)

PEARLS & CONSIDERATIONS

■ COMMENTS
- Dupuytren's contracture develops earlier and more often in certain families.
- The disorder is more common in Scandinavians, and some Northern Europeans have a 25% prevalence over age 60 yr.
- About 5% of patients develop a similar condition elsewhere, such as Peyronie's disease or Ledderhose disease (involvement of the plantar fascia).
- Soft tissue "pads" in the knuckles may also be present.
- Individuals with these additional findings are considered to have Dupuytren's diathesis, and their disease is generally more severe and recurrent.

Author: **Lonnie R. Mercier, M.D.**

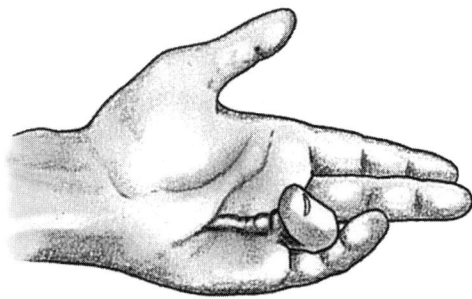

Fig. 1-132 Dupuytren's contracture. A flexion deformity of the finger is present, with nodular thickening of the fascia to the ring finger.

BASIC INFORMATION

■ DEFINITION

Dysfunctional uterine bleeding (DUB) describes abnormal uterine bleeding in the absence of disease in the pelvis, pregnancy, or medical illness. Specific types of abnormal bleeding include the following:

- Hypermenorrhea: excessive bleeding in amount during normal duration of regular menstrual cycles.
- Hypomenorrhea: decreased bleeding in amount in regular menstrual cycles.
- Menorrhagia: regular normal intervals, excessive flow and duration.
- Metrorrhagia: irregular intervals, excessive flow and duration.
- Menometrorrhagia: irregular or excessive bleeding during menstruation and between periods.
- Oligomenorrhea: intervals greater than 35 days.
- Polymenorrhea: intervals less than 21 days.

■ SYNONYMS

DUB

ICD-9CM CODES

626 Disorders of menstruation and other abnormal bleeding from female genital tract
626.2 Hypermenorrhea
626.1 Hypomenorrhea
626.2 Menorrhagia
626.6 Metrorrhagia
626.2 Menometrorrhagia
626.1 Oligomenorrhea
626.2 Polymenorrhea

■ EPIDEMIOLOGY & DEMOGRAPHICS

- Most cases of DUB occur in post-menarcheal and perimenopausal age groups.
- During reproductive age, <20% of abnormal bleeding results from anovulatory DUB.

■ PHYSICAL FINDINGS & CLINICAL PRESENTATION

- A clinical diagnosis of exclusion
- Thorough physical and pelvic examination to exclude the other causes of abnormal bleeding
  1. Includes thyroid, breasts, liver, presence or absence of ecchymotic lesions
  2. Patient possibly obese and hirsute (polycystic ovarian disease)
  3. No evidence of any vulvar, vaginal, cervical lesions, uterine (fibroid) or ovarian tumor, urethral caruncle, urethral diverticula, hemorrhoids, anal fissure, colorectal lesions
  4. Bimanual pelvic examination: normal-sized or slightly enlarged uterus

■ ETIOLOGY & PATHOGENESIS

- 90% is caused by anovulation.
- 10% is ovulatory in origin; can be caused by dysfunction of corpus luteum or mid-cycle bleeding.
- Box 2-230 describes the various causes of abnormal uterine bleeding.

DIAGNOSIS

■ DIFFERENTIAL DIAGNOSIS

- Pregnancy-related cause
- Anatomic uterine causes:
  1. Leiomyomas
  2. Adenomyosis

  3. Polyps
  4. Endometrial hyperplasia
  5. Cancer
  6. Sexually transmitted diseases
  7. Intrauterine contraceptive devices
- Anatomic nonuterine causes:
  1. Cervical neoplasia, cervicitis
  2. Vaginal neoplasia, adhesions, trauma, foreign body, atrophic vaginitis, infections, condyloma
  3. Vulvar trauma, infections, neoplasia, condyloma, dystrophy, varices
  4. Urinary tract: urethral caruncle, diverticulum, hematuria
  5. GI tract: hemorrhoids, anal fissure, colorectal lesions
- Systemic diseases:
  1. Exogenous hormone intake
  2. Coagulopathies: von Willebrand's disease, thrombocytopenia, hepatic failure
  3. Endocrinopathies: thyroid disorder, hypo- and hyperthyroidism, diabetes mellitus
  4. Renal diseases
- Table 2-206 describes a differential diagnosis of vaginal bleeding abnormalities.

■ WORKUP

- A detailed history and thorough physical examination, including a pelvic examination to exclude above causes.
- Fig. 3-26 describes clinical algorithms for the evaluation of vaginal bleeding.

■ LABORATORY TESTS

- CBC with platelets; possible iron deficiency anemia or thrombocytopenia
- Prothrombin (PT); partial thromboplastin and bleeding time if coagulopathy is suspected

- Serum human chorionic gonado-tropin (hCG)
- Chemistry profile, including liver function tests
- Thyroid profile
- Stool testing for occult blood
- Urinalysis for hematuria
- Pap smear
- Cultures for gonorrhea and *Chlamydia*
- Serum gonadotropins and prolactin
- Serum androgens
- Endometrial biopsy in women >30 yr old and barely >20 yr old
- Hysterogram and hysteroscopy

■ **IMAGING STUDIES**
Pelvic ultrasound, including measurement of endometrial thickness

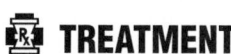 **TREATMENT**

■ **NONPHARMACOLOGIC THERAPY**
Increase iron intake in the form of pills and in a diet rich in iron.

■ **ACUTE GENERAL Rx**
- Progestational agents:
  1. Progesterone in oil, 100 to 200 mg
  2. Medroxyprogesterone acetate, 20 to 40 mg qd for 15 days
  3. Megestrol acetate, 40 to 120 mg qd
  4. Oral contraceptives: any oral contraceptive pill, one tablet qid for 5 to 7 days, followed by one tablet low-dose estrogen qd for 21 days; causes one heavy withdrawal

bleeding, should then be on cyclical Provera or continue on oral contraceptives
- Estrogens:
  1. Conjugated estrogen (Premarin) 25 mg IV q4h until bleeding is under control (in cases of severe or life-threatening bleeding); maximum three doses
  2. For prolonged bleeding that is not life-threatening: Premarin 1.25 mg (Estrace 2 mg) q4h for 24 hr, followed by Provera to bring on withdrawal bleeding; then sequential regimen of estrogen and progestin (Premarin 1.25 mg qd for 24 days; Provera 10 mg for 10 days) or oral contraceptives
- Surgical treatment:
  1. Dilatation and curettage
  2. Hysterectomy

■ **CHRONIC Rx**
- Progestational agents:
  1. Medroxyprogesterone acetate 10 mg qd for 12 days, then cyclically to induce monthly withdrawal bleeding
  2. Norethindrone 1 mg qd for 12 days
  3. Depo-Provera 150 mg IM and then 150 mg q3mo
  4. Oral contraceptives one tablet qd
- Clomiphene citrate: patients with anovulatory bleeding who want to become pregnant
- Others:
  1. Antiprostaglandins
  2. Danazol
  3. Gonadotropin-releasing hormone analogs (GNRH)

  4. Human menopausal gonadotropin (HMG)
- Surgical treatment:
  1. Dilatation and curettage (D&C)
  2. Endometrial ablation
  3. Hysterectomy

■ **DISPOSITION**
Cyclical treatment on birth control pills or Provera for several cycles, then discontinue pill and watch patient for onset of regular menses

■ **REFERRAL**
To gynecologist in case of failure of treatment

⚙ **PEARLS & CONSIDERATIONS**

■ **COMMENTS**
Patient education material may be obtained from the American College of Obstetricians and Gynecologists, 409 12th Street SW, Washington, DC 20024-2188; phone (202)638-5577.

REFERENCES
Mishell DR, Stenchever MA, Drogemuller W: *Comprehensive gynecology*, ed 3, St Louis, 1997, Mosby.
Speroff L: *Clinical gynecologic endocrinology and infertility*, ed 6, Baltimore, 1999, Williams & Wilkins.
Author: **Mandeep K. Brar, M.D.**

BASIC INFORMATION

■ DEFINITION

Dysmenorrhea is pain with menstruation, usually as cramping and usually centered in the lower abdomen. It is defined as *primary dysmenorrhea* when there is no associated organic pathology and *secondary dysmenorrhea* when there is demonstrable organic pathology.

■ SYNONYMS

Menstrual cramps
Painful periods

ICD-9CM CODES
625.3 Dysmenorrhea

■ EPIDEMIOLOGY & DEMOGRAPHICS

Approximately 50% of menstruating women are affected by dysmenorrhea, with approximately 10% of them having severe dysmenorrhea with incapacitation for 1 to 3 days/mo. Dysmenorrhea is most common in the age group from 20 to 24 yr, and primary dysmenorrhea usually appears within 6 to 12 mo after menarche.

■ PHYSICAL FINDINGS & CLINICAL PRESENTATION

- Sharp, crampy, midline, lower abdomen pain without a lower quadrant or adnexal component but possible radiation to the lower back and upper thighs
- Unremarkable pelvic examination in nonmenstruating patient
- Accompanying symptoms: nausea, vomiting, headaches, anxiety, fatigue, diarrhea, fainting, and abdominal bloating
- Cramps usually lasting <24 hr and seldom lasting >2 to 3 days
- Secondary dysmenorrhea: dyspareunia is a common complaint, and bimanual pelvic-abdominal examination may demonstrate uterine or adnexal tenderness, fixed uterine retroflexion, uterosacral nodularity, a pelvic mass, or an enlarged, irregular uterus

■ ETIOLOGY

Prostaglandin $F_{2}\alpha$ (PG $F_{2}\alpha$) is the agent responsible for dysmenorrhea. It stimulates uterine contractions, cervical stenosis or narrowing, and increased vasopressin release. Behavior and psychologic factors have also been implicated in the etiology of primary dysmenorrhea. Primary dysmenorrhea only occurs in ovulatory cycles. Secondary dysmenorrhea is usually caused by endometriosis, adenomyosis, leiomyomas and, less commonly, chronic salpingitis, IUD use, or congenital or acquired outflow tract obstruction, including cervical stenosis.

DIAGNOSIS

■ DIFFERENTIAL DIAGNOSIS

- Adenomyosis
- Adhesions
- Allen-Masters syndrome
- Cervical structures or stenosis
- Congenital malformation of müllerian system
- Ectopic pregnancy
- Endometriosis, endometritis
- Imperforate hymen
- IUD use
- Leiomyomas
- Ovarian cysts
- Pelvic congestion syndrome, pelvic inflammatory disease
- Polyps
- Transverse vaginal septum

■ WORKUP

- Primary dysmenorrhea: characteristic history, physical examination normal with the absence of an identifiable cause of pelvic pain
- Secondary dysmenorrhea: history of onset generally >2 yr after menarche, physical examination may reveal uterine irregularity, cul-de-sac tenderness, or nodularity or pelvic masses

■ LABORATORY TESTS

- No specific tests diagnostic for dysmenorrhea
- Elevated WBC count in the presence of infection
- hCG to rule out ectopic pregnancy

■ IMAGING STUDIES

- Ultrasound scan of the pelvis to evaluate the presence of leiomyomas, ovarian cysts, or ectopic pregnancy
- Hysterosalpingogram to assess the uterine cavity to rule out endometrial polyps, submucosal or intraluminal leiomyomas

TREATMENT

■ NONPHARMACOLOGIC THERAPY

- Applying heat to the lower abdomen with hot compresses, heating pads, or hot water bottles seems to offer some relief.
- Other reassurance that this is a treatable condition.

■ ACUTE GENERAL Rx

- Nonsteroidal antiinflammatory drugs such as ibuprofen 400 to 600 mg q4-6h or naproxen sodium 550 mg q12h, mefenamic acid 500 mg initial dose followed by 250 mg q6h PRN, aspirin 650 mg q4-6h, or oral contraceptives
- Nifedipine 30 mg qd in difficult cases of dysmenorrhea
- Secondary dysmenorrhea: treatment directed to the specific underlying condition; surgery plays a greater role
- Endometriosis: use of nonsurgical approaches, such as using danazol, gonadotropin-releasing hormone agonists, and oral contraceptives

■ CHRONIC Rx

Acupuncture and transcutaneous electrical nerve stimulation (TENS) may be tried. In cases where medical therapy has not worked, laparoscopy should be considered, as well as other surgical treatments depending on the secondary cause of the dysmenorrhea.

■ DISPOSITION

The majority of patients are satisfactorily treated with good outcomes. It is thought that primary dysmenorrhea generally improves with age and parity and that secondary dysmenorrhea usually has good results with adequate treatment. Possible chronic complications with primary dysmenorrhea that hasn't been adequately treated can lead to anxiety and depression. With certain causes of secondary dysmenorrhea infertility can become a problem.

■ REFERRAL

If a secondary cause of dysmenorrhea is revealed, refer to the appropriate specialist for further medical or surgical treatment (gynecologist, pain management center).

PEARLS & CONSIDERATIONS

■ COMMENTS

Patient education materials can be obtained through various pharmaceutical companies (e.g., booklet "Painful periods" from Warner Lambert, Inc.)
Author: **George T. Danakas, M.D.**

BASIC INFORMATION

■ DEFINITION
Dystonia is characterized by involuntary muscle contractions (sustained or spasmodic) that lead to abnormal body movements or postures. Dystonia can be generalized or focal.

■ ICD-9CM CODES
333.6 Dystonia musculorum deformans
335.7 Dystonia due to drugs
333.7 Dystonia, torsion, symptomatic

■ SYNONYMS
Blepharospasm
Oromandibular dystonia
Torticollis
Writer's cramp

■ EPIDEMIOLOGY & DEMOGRAPHICS
PREVALENCE: Estimated at 1 in 3000 persons.
PREDOMINANT SEX: Cervical dystonia has a 3:2 female preponderance.
PREDOMINANT AGE:
- Cervical dystonia usually has its onset in the fifth decade.
- Hereditary forms may have an onset in childhood or adulthood.
GENETICS: Autosomal dominant, autosomal recessive, and X-linked forms of dystonia have been identified.

■ PHYSICAL FINDINGS & CLINICAL PRESENTATION
Focal dystonias produce abnormal sustained muscle contractions in an area of the body:
- Neck: most commonly affected (torticollis); tendency for the head to turn to one side
- Eyelids (blepharospasm): involuntary closure of the eyelids
- Oromandibular dystonia, involuntary contraction of muscles of the mouth, tongue, or face
- Hand (writer's cramp) (Fig. 1-133)
Generalized dystonia affects multiple areas of the body and can lead to marked joint deformities.

■ ETIOLOGY
- Exact pathophysiology is unknown, thought to involve abnormalities of basal ganglia.
- Hereditary forms have been described, including the severe progressive form, dystonia musculorum deformans.
- Sporadic or idiopathic forms occur.
- Dystonia can occur secondary to other diseases such as CNS disease, hypoxia, kernicterus, Huntington's disease, Wilson's disease, Parkinson syndrome, lysosomal storage diseases.
- Acute dystonia can occur following treatment with drugs that block dopamine receptors, such as phenothiazines or butyrophenones.
- Tardive dyskinesia or dystonia can result from long-term treatment with antipsychotic drugs such as phenothiazines or butyrophenones.

DIAGNOSIS

■ DIFFERENTIAL DIAGNOSIS
- Parkinson's disease
- Progressive supranuclear palsy
- Wilson's disease
- Huntington's disease
- Drug effects

■ WORKUP
History (including family history, birth history, medication use) and physical examination

■ LABORATORY TESTS
- Usually not helpful for establishing diagnosis
- Serum ceruloplasmin if Wilson's disease is suspected

■ IMAGING STUDIES
CT scan or MRI of brain if a CNS lesion is suspected

℞ TREATMENT

■ NONPHARMACOLOGIC THERAPY
- Heat, massage, physical therapy to relieve pain
- Splints to prevent contractures

■ ACUTE GENERAL Rx
For acute dystonic reactions to phenothiazines or butyrophenones: diphenhydramine 50 mg IV or benztropine 2 mg IV

■ CHRONIC Rx
- Treatment is often ineffective.
- Diazepam, baclofen, or carbamazepine may be helpful.
- Trihexyphenidyl may be helpful in tardive dyskinesia or dystonia.
- Injections of botulinum toxin into the affected muscles can be used for refractory cases.
- Surgical procedures including myectomy, rhizotomy, or thalamotomy may be helpful for severe, refractory cases.

■ DISPOSITION
Spontaneous remission of focal cervical dystonia can occur, but dystonia is generally progressive and pharmacologic therapy is often ineffective.

■ REFERRAL
To neurologist for severe or refractory cases
Author: **Mark J. Fagan, M.D.**

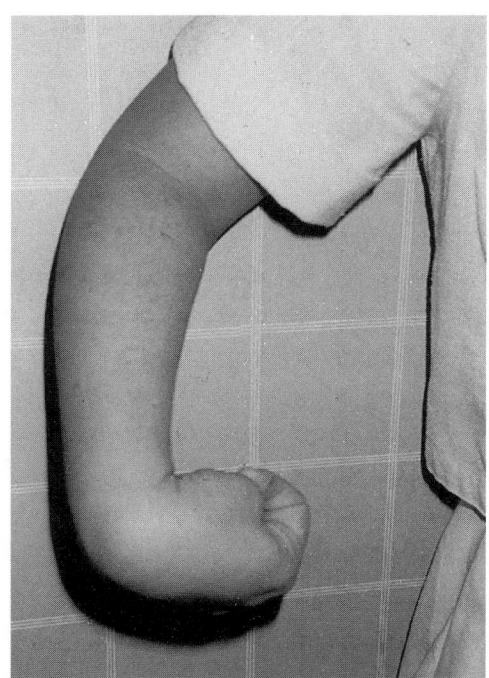

Fig. 1-133 Focal dystonia of the distal right arm. (From Goldman L, Bennett JC [eds]: *Cecil textbook of medicine,* ed 21, Philadelphia, 2000, WB Saunders.)

BASIC INFORMATION

■ DEFINITION
Echinococcosis is a chronic infection caused by the larval stage of several animal cestodes (flat worms) of the genus *Echinococcus*.

■ SYNONYMS
Hydatid disease

ICD-9-CM CODES
122.9 *Echinococcus* infection

■ EPIDEMIOLOGY & DEMOGRAPHICS
INCIDENCE (IN U.S.): Seen primarily in immigrants; varies widely depending on areas of origin.
PREVALENCE (IN U.S.): See "Incidence."
PREDOMINANT SEX: Male = female
PREDOMINANT AGE: 20 to 50 yr of age
PEAK INCIDENCE: Presumed to be acquired in childhood or early adulthood in most cases.

■ PHYSICAL FINDINGS & CLINICAL PRESENTATION
- Signs of an enlarging mass lesion in a visceral site such as the liver, lungs, kidneys, bone, or CNS
- Occasional cyst rupture causing allergic manifestations such as urticaria, angioedema, or anaphylaxis that bring the patient to medical attention
- Incidental discovery of cysts by abdominal or thoracic imaging studies performed for other reasons

■ ETIOLOGY
- Four species of *Echinococcus*: *E. granulosus*, *E. multilocularis*, *E. oligarthrus*, and *E. vogeli*.
  1. *E. granulosus* is the cause of cystic hydatid disease.
  2. *E. multilocularis* and *E. vogeli* are the causes of alveolar and polycystic disease.
- The disease is transmitted to humans by infected canines (domestic or wild dogs, wolves, foxes) and seen most commonly in livestock-producing areas of the Middle East, Africa, Australia, New Zealand, Europe, and the Americas, including the southwestern U.S.
- Eggs are present in the feces of infected canines; human infection occurs by ingestion of viable eggs in contamined food.
- It is common in many areas of the world, especially the Middle East.

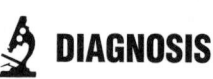

DIAGNOSIS

■ DIFFERENTIAL DIAGNOSIS
- Cystic neoplasms
- Abscess (amebic or bacterial)
- Congenital polycystic disease

- Table 2-25 describes the differential diagnosis of cestode tissue infections.

■ WORKUP
- Antibody assay
- Imaging study (CT scan, ultrasonography)
- Histologic examination of cyst or contents obtained by aspiration or resection (if possible) to confirm diagnosis

■ LABORATORY TESTS
Antibody assays (ELISA and Western blot): >90% sensitive and specific for liver cysts, but less accurate for cysts in other sites

■ IMAGING STUDIES
Ultrasonography and/or CT scan:
- Both are extremely sensitive for the detection of cysts, especially in the liver (Fig. 1-134).
- Both lack specificity and are inadequate to establish the diagnosis of echinococcosis with certainty.

TREATMENT

■ NONPHARMACOLOGIC THERAPY
- Treatment of choice for echinococcal cysts is surgical resection, when feasible.
- If resection is not feasible, perform percutaneous drainage with instillation of 95% ethanol to prevent dissemination of viable larvae.
- Surgical therapy is followed by medical therapy with albendazole (see "Acute General Rx").

■ ACUTE GENERAL Rx
For echinococcosis confined to the liver:
- Albendazole (400 mg twice daily for 28 days followed by 14 days of rest for at least three cycles)

- Mebendazole (50 to 70 mg/kg qd) if albendazole not available

■ CHRONIC Rx
See "Acute General Rx."

■ DISPOSITION
- Long-term follow-up is necessary following surgical or medical therapy because of the high incidence of late relapse.
- Antibody assays and imaging studies are repeated every 6 to 12 mo for several years following successful surgical or medical therapy.

■ REFERRAL
- All patients for evaluation for possible surgical resection of cysts
- For consultation with a physician experienced in the medical and surgical management of echinococcosis

✷ PEARLS & CONSIDERATIONS

■ COMMENTS
Surgical resection, if indicated, should be performed by surgeons experienced in the management of echinococcal cysts.

REFERENCES
Anadol D et al: Treatment of hydatid disease, *Paediatr Drugs* 3(2):123, 2001.
Eckert J, Conraths FJ, Tackman K: Echinococcosis: an emerging or reemerging zoonosis? *Int J Parasitol* 30(12-13):1283, 2000.
Pedrosa I et al: Hydatid disease: radiologic and pathologic features and complications, *Radiographics* 20(30):795, 2000.
Siles-Lucas MM, Gottstein BB: Molecular tools for the diagnosis of cystic and alveolar echinococcosis, *Trop Med Int Health* 6(6):463, 2001.
Author: **Joseph R. Masci, M.D.**

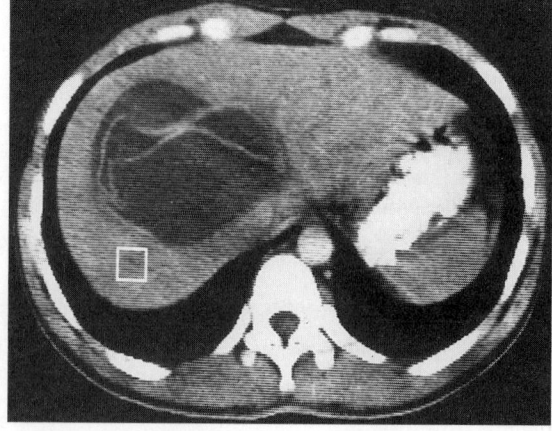

Fig. 1-134 Computed tomography scan of an echinococcal cyst in a 25-year-old man, demonstrating the complex structure of the wall and the interior. (From Goldman L, Bennett JC [eds]: *Cecil textbook of medicine,* ed 21, Philadelphia, 2000, WB Saunders.)

BASIC INFORMATION

■ DEFINITION
Eclampsia is the occurrence of seizures or coma in a woman with preeclampsia, occurring at >20 wk gestation or <48 hr postpartum. Atypical eclampsia occurs at <20 wk gestation or as much as 14 days postpartum.

■ SYNONYMS
Toxemia
Seizures of pregnancy

ICD-9CM CODES
642.6 Eclampsia

■ EPIDEMIOLOGY & DEMOGRAPHICS
INCIDENCE: 1 case/150 to 3000 pregnancies; 2% to 4% of those with preeclampsia
RISK FACTORS: Multifetal gestation (3.6% in twin gestation), molar pregnancy, nonimmune hydrops fetalis, uncontrolled hypertension, preexisting hypertension or renal disease
GENETICS: Increased incidence with first-degree relatives (sister or mother) having had eclampsia

■ PHYSICAL FINDINGS & CLINICAL PRESENTATION
• Seizure begins as facial twitching then spreads to generalized clonic-tonic state, with cessation of respiration, followed by a postictal period of amnesia, agitation, and confusion.
• 40% have severe hypertension, 40% have mild to moderate hypertension, and 20% are normotensive.
• Generalized edema with rapid weight gain (>2 lb/wk) may be one of the earliest signs of eclampsia.
• Persistent occipital headache and hyperreflexia with clonus occur in 80% of patients with eclampsia; epigastric pain exists in 20% of these patients.

■ ETIOLOGY
Although the exact etiology is unknown, the common pathway relates to abnormalities in autoregulation of cerebral blood flow. This may involve transient vasospasm, ischemia, cerebral hemorrhage, and edema, occurring by a mechanism involving hypertensive encephalopathy, decreased colloid osmotic pressure, and prostaglandin imbalance.

DIAGNOSIS

■ DIFFERENTIAL DIAGNOSIS
• Preexisting seizure disorder
• Metabolic abnormalities (hypoglycemia, hyponatremia, hypocalcemia)
• Substance abuse
• Head trauma, infection (meningitis, encephalitis)
• Intracerebral bleeding or thrombosis
• Amniotic fluid embolism
• Space-occupying brain lesions or neoplasms
• Pseudoseizure

■ WORKUP
• Rule out other causes of seizures during pregnancy.
• Atypical presentations such as prolonged postictal state, status epilepticus, gestational age <20 wk or >48 hr postpartum, or signs of meningitis, substance abuse, or severe uncontrolled hypertension should prompt a search for other seizure etiologies.

■ LABORATORY TESTS
• Proteinuria: severe (49%), mild to moderate (29%), absent (22%)
• Hct: elevated secondary to hemoconcentration
• Platelet count: decreased; LFTs elevated in HELLP syndrome
• BUN and creatinine: elevated with renal involvement
• Serum electrolytes, glucose, calcium, toxicology profile: to rule out other causes of seizures
• Hyperuricemia: >6.9 mg/dl found in 70% of eclamptics
• ABG: maternal acidemia and hypoxia

■ IMAGING STUDIES
• CT scan or MRI indicated in atypical presentation, suspected intracerebral bleeding, focal neurologic deficit.
• There are abnormal findings, including cerebral edema, hemorrhage, and infarction, in 50% of patients.

TREATMENT

■ NONPHARMACOLOGIC THERAPY
• Airway protection (risk of aspiration)
• Supportive care during acute event

■ ACUTE GENERAL Rx
• Maintain airway, adequate oxygenation, and IV access.
• Fetal resuscitation, involving maternal oxygenation, left lateral positioning, and continuous fetal heart rate monitoring, is needed.
• Give magnesium sulfate 6 g IV load over 20 min, then 3 g/hr maintenance, for recurrent seizure prophylaxis. If repeated convulsion, may give an additional 2 g IV over 3 to 5 min. About 10% to 15% of patients will have a second seizure after initial loading dose. Check magnesium level 1 hr after loading dose, then q6h (therapeutic range 4 to 6 mg/dl). Antidote for toxicity is calcium gluconate 10 ml of 10% solution. Phenytoin has been used as an alternative in patients in whom magnesium sulfate is contraindicated (renal insufficiency, heart block, myasthenia gravis, hypoparathyroidism).
• Give sodium amobarbital 250 mg IV over 3 min for persistent seizures.
• Treat blood pressure if >160 mm Hg/110 mm Hg, with labetalol 20- to 40-mg IV bolus, hydralazine 10 mg IV, or nifedipine 10 to 20 mg sublingual q20min.
• Evaluate patient for delivery.

■ CHRONIC Rx
• The first priority is stabilization of the mother in terms of adequate oxygenation, hemodynamics, and laboratory abnormalities, such as associated coagulopathies.
• Cervical status and gestational age should be assessed. If unfavorable cervix and <30 wk consider C-section, otherwise consider induction.
• Controlled epidural is the anesthesia of choice for labor or C-section.
• Avoid general anesthesia in uncontrolled hypertension to minimize risk of catastrophic cerebral events.

■ DISPOSITION
The maternal mortality rate for eclampsia averages 5% to 6%. Morbidity is 25%, including placental abruption (10%), maternal apnea with fetal asphyxia, aspiration pneumonia, pulmonary edema (4%), renal failure, cardiopulmonary arrest, and coma.

■ REFERRAL
Because of the potential for serious permanent maternal and fetal sequelae, all cases should be managed by a team approach of obstetrician, neonatologist, and intensivist.

PEARLS & CONSIDERATIONS

■ COMMENTS
• Eclampsia antepartum, 50%; intrapartum, 20%; and postpartum, 30%
• Postseizure there is an associated period of fetal bradycardia from 1 to 9 min; if there is evidence of fetal compromise beyond that time, consider alternative etiologies such as placental abruption (23% incidence).
Author: Scott J. Zuccala, D.O.

BASIC INFORMATION

■ DEFINITION

An ectopic pregnancy (EP) is one in which a fertilized ovum implants outside the endometrial lining of the uterus.

■ SYNONYMS

Abdominal pregnancy (1% to 2%)
Cervical pregnancy (0.5%)
Interstitial pregnancy (2% to 3%)
Ovarian pregnancy (1%)
Tubal pregnancy (97%)

ICD-9CM CODES
633 Ectopic pregnancy

■ EPIDEMIOLOGY & DEMOGRAPHICS

- 1% to 2% of pregnancies
- 13% of maternal deaths

PREVALENCE (IN U.S.): Increasing number of EP; 17,800 reported cases in 1970 and 108,000 reported cases in 1992.

RISK FACTORS: Previous salpingitis, previous EP, previous tubal ligation, previous tuboplasty, IUD use, progestin-only pill, and assisted reproductive techniques

■ PHYSICAL FINDINGS & CLINICAL PRESENTATION

- Abdominal tenderness: 95%
- Adnexal tenderness : 87% to 99%
- Peritoneal signs: 71% to 76%
- Adnexal mass: 33% to 53%
- Enlarged uterus: 6% to 30%
- Shock: 2% to 17%
- Amenorrhea or abnormal vaginal bleeding: 75%
- Shoulder pain: 10%
- Tissue passage: 6% to 7%

■ ETIOLOGY

- Anatomic obstruction to zygote passage
- Abnormalities in tubal motility
- Transperitoneal migration of the zygote

DIAGNOSIS

■ DIFFERENTIAL DIAGNOSIS

- Corpus luteum cyst
- Rupture or torsion of ovarian cyst
- Threatened or incomplete abortion
- PID
- Appendicitis
- Gastroenteritis
- Dysfunctional uterine bleeding
- Degenerating uterine fibroids
- Endometriosis

■ WORKUP

1. The classic presentation of EP includes the triad of abnormal vaginal bleeding, pelvic pain, and an adnexal mass. Consider in all women with abdominal-pelvic pain and a positive pregnancy test.
2. Culdocentesis is clinically useful when other diagnostic modalities are not readily available.
   - Positive tap means nonclotting blood with Hct >12%.
   - Negative tap means clear or blood-tinged fluid.
   - Nondiagnostic tap means clotted blood or no fluid.
3. Laparoscopy.

■ LABORATORY TESTS

- hCG: if normal IUP, 85% have doubling time of 2 days. If abnormal gestation, will show <66% increase of QhCG within 2 days. However, 13% of ectopic pregnancies have a normal doubling time (Fig. 1-135).
- Progesterone: decreased production in EP, <5 ng/ml strongly predictive of abnormal pregnancy. If >25 ng/ml, strongly predictive of normal IUP.
- Dropping Hct associated with tubal rupture.
- Leukocytosis.

■ IMAGING STUDIES

- Ultrasound: presence of an IUP rules out EP.
- If QhCG >6000 mIU/ml, should see IUP on abdominal scan, and QhCG >1500 mIU/ml for transvaginal scan.
- Findings on ultrasound in EP include:
  1. Empty uterus
  2. Adnexal mass
  3. Cul-de-sac fluid
  4. Fetal sac in tube
  5. Fetal cardiac activity in adnexa

TREATMENT

■ NONPHARMACOLOGIC THERAPY

Surgery: can be performed by laparoscopy if patient is stable or by laparotomy if patient is unstable. Salpingiosis: direct injection of chemotherapy into ectopic via laparoscopy, transvaginal ultrasound, or hysteroscopy.
- Conservative surgery-salpingostomy or segmental resection depends on tubal location and size of ectopic.
- Salpingectomy should be considered in the following circumstances:

1. Ruptured tube
2. Future fertility not desired
3. Recurrent ectopic in the same tube
4. Uncontrolled hemorrhage

■ ACUTE GENERAL Rx

- If the patient is stable and compliant may consider medical management with methotrexate. Patient should not have contraindications to methotrexate such as hepatic or renal disease, thrombocytopenia, leukopenia, or significant anemia. There should be no evidence of hemoperitoneum on transvaginal ultrasound. Ectopic should be <4 cm mass with QhCG <30,000 mIU/ml.
- Most common regimen is methotrexate 50 mg/m^2 body surface area. May require second dose or surgical intervention if QhCG increases or plateaus after 7 days.

■ CHRONIC Rx

Persistent EP results from residual trophoblastic tissue or secondary implantation after conservative surgery. There is a 5% incidence of persistent ectopic with conservative treatment.

■ DISPOSITION

If diagnosed and treated early (before rupture) prognosis is excellent for good recovery. Follow QhCG weekly until negative. Use reliable contraception until hCG negative. With subsequent pregnancies, follow QhCG and perform early ultrasound to confirm IUP. There is a 12% recurrence rate for EP.

■ REFERRAL

Should obtain gynecologic consultation if EP is suspected.

PEARLS & CONSIDERATIONS

■ COMMENTS

Patient information can be obtained through American College of Obstetricians and Gynecologists, 409 12th St SW, Washington, DC 20024-2188.

REFERENCES

Gracia CR, Barnhart KT: Diagnosing ectopic pregnancy: decision analysis comparing six strategies, *Obstet Gynecol* 97(3):464, 2001.

Lipscomb GH, Stovall TG, Ling FW: Nonsurgical treatment of ectopic pregnancy, *N Engl J Med* 343:1325, 2000.

Author: **George T. Danakas, M.D.**

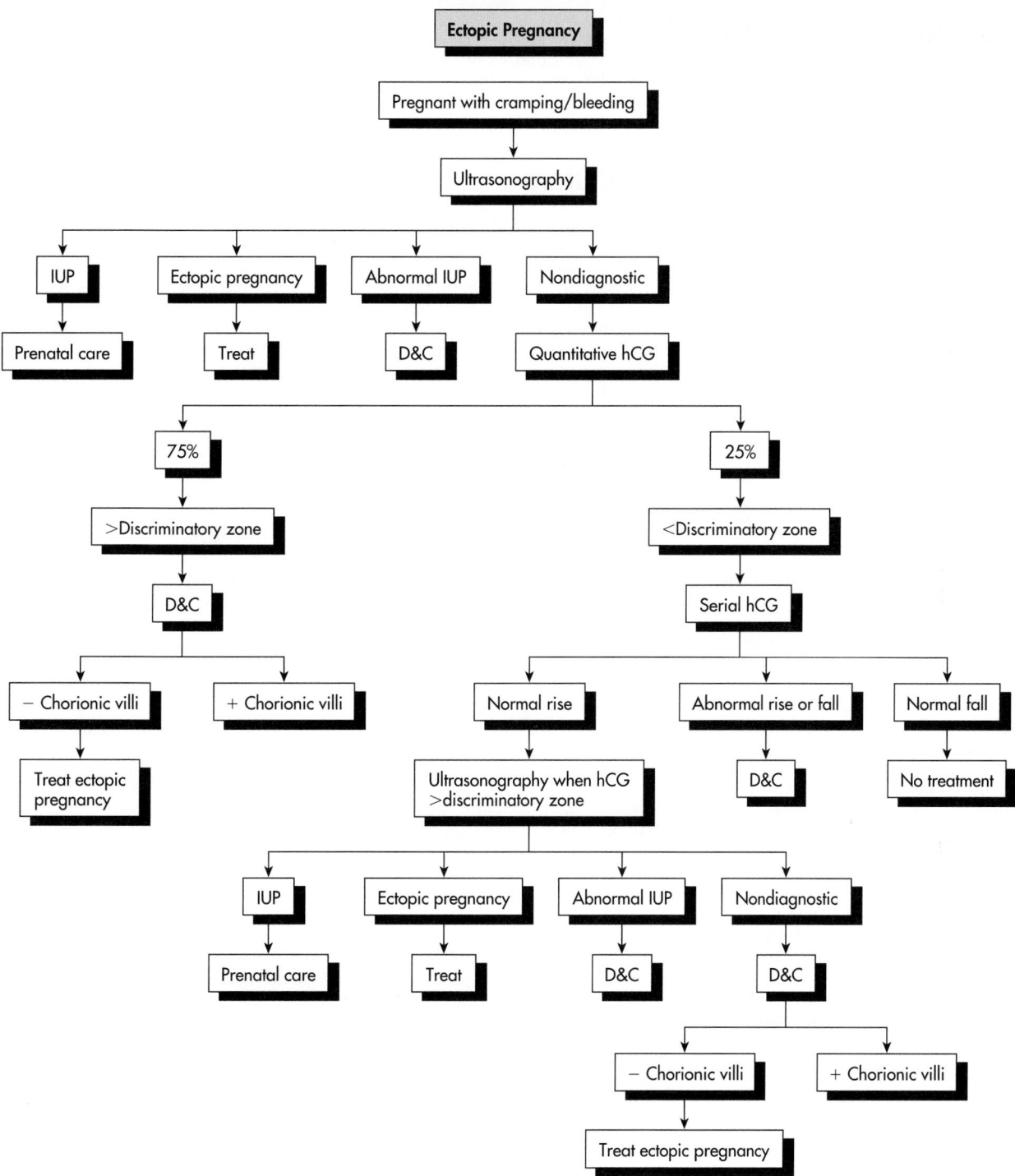

Fig. 1-135   Sample approach to ectopic pregnancy. *D&C,* Dilatation and curettage; *hCG,* human chorionic gonadotropin; *IUP,* intrauterine pregnancy. (From Gracia CR, Barnhart KT: *Obstet Gynecol* 97:465, 2001.)

BASIC INFORMATION

■ DEFINITION
Ehlers-Danlos syndrome (EDSs) are a group of genetically heterogeneous connective tissue disorders that are characterized by a variety of clinical abnormalities of the skin, ligaments, and internal organs. The revised classification scheme and diagnostic criteria (1998) are listed below.

ICD-9CM CODES
756.83 Ehlers-Danlos syndrome

■ EPIDEMIOLOGY & DEMOGRAPHICS
The prevalence of EDSs is estimated to be about 1 in 5000 births, although it is somewhat higher in African-Americans. Types I, II, and III are most prevalent. In most cases transmission is autosomal dominant except for V and IX (X-linked) and X and one strain (C) of VII (autosomal recessive).

■ PHYSICAL FINDINGS & CLINICAL PRESENTATION
See Fig. 1-136.
- Classic: (EDS I and II) hyperextensibility, easy scarring and bruising ("cigarette-paper scars").
- Hypermobility (EDS III): Joint hypermobility and some skin hypermobility with or without very smooth skin.
- Vascular (EDS IV): Thin, translucent skin with visible veins; marked bruising; pinched nose; acrogeria; spontaneous rupture of medium and large arteries and hollow organs especially large intestine and uterus.
- Kyphoscoliotic (EDS VI): Characterized by joint hypermobility, progressive scoliosis; ocular fragility and possible globe rupture, mitral valve prolapse and aortic dilation.
- Arthrochalasia (EDS VII A and B): Prominent joint hypermobility, with subluxations, congenital hip dislocation, skin hyperextensibility and tissue fragility.
- Dermatosperaxis (EDS VIIC): Severe skin fragility with decreased elasticity, bruising, hernias.
- Unclassified type:
  1. EDS V: Classic characteristics
  2. EDS VIII: Classic characteristics and periodontal disease.
  3. EDS IX: X-linked classic characteristics.
  4. EDS X: Mild classic characteristics, mitral valve prolapse.
  5. EDS XI: Joint instability.

■ ETIOLOGY
Genetically variable defects of collagen in extracellular matrices of multiple tissues (skin, tendons, blood vessels, and viscera).

DIAGNOSIS

■ DIFFERENTIAL DIAGNOSIS
Generally limited to types of EDSs. Some individuals with Marfan's syndrome have joint laxity. Some patients with osteogenesis imperfecta have joint laxity and easy bruising. Patients with joint hypermobility without skin changes are more likely to have familial joint hypermobility.

■ WORKUP
Diagnosis is based solely on clinical criteria.

■ LABORATORY TESTS
- Limited biochemical assays and gene analyses are performed for known molecular defects.
- It is important to identify patients with EDS type IV because of the grave consequences of the disease.

TREATMENT

- All patients should receive genetic counseling about the mode of inheritance of their EDSs and the risk of having children with EDSs.

- Surgical repair and tightening of joint ligaments require careful evaluation of individual patients because ligaments frequently will not hold sutures. Physical therapy to strengthen muscles is helpful.
- Vascular type requires special surgical care because of increased friability of tissues. Women with EDS type IV should be counseled to avoid pregnancy.
- Patients should be advised to avoid contact sports, and elevated blood pressure should be aggressively treated.

■ DISPOSITION
Prognosis varies according to type of EDSs.

■ REFERRAL
Referral to orthopedic, plastic surgery, and physical therapy as needed.

REFERENCES
Pepin M et al: Clinical and genetic features of Ehlers-Danlos syndrome type IV, the vascular type, *N Engl J Med* 342:673, 2000.
Pyeritz R: Ehlers-Danlos syndrome, *N Engl J Med* 342(10):730, 2000
Pyeritz RE: Ehlers-Danlos syndromes. In Goldman L, Bennett JC (eds): *Cecil textbook of medicine,* ed 21, vol 1, Philadelphia, 2000, WB Saunders.
Author: **Anne W. Moulton, M.D.**

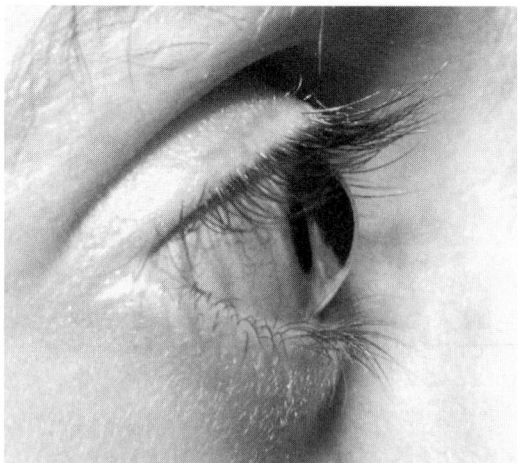

Fig. 1-136 Ehlers-Danlos syndrome is characterized by poor cross-linking of collagen. This results in joint hypermobility, skin hyperextensibility, easy bruising, and a propensity toward tissue rupture. A blue sclera (as seen here) results from thinning of the sclera. (From Palay D [ed]: *Ophthalmology for the primary care physician,* St Louis, 1997, Mosby.)

BASIC INFORMATION

■ DEFINITION
The three clinically significant disorders of ejaculation are ejaculatory failure, retrograde ejaculation, and premature ejaculation. Ejaculatory failure is the lack of production of seminal emission. Retrograde ejaculation is a backward flow of the emission into the bladder. Premature ejaculation is the inability to control ejaculation for sufficient time to allow adequate penetration and intercourse.

ICD-9CM CODES
606.9
302.75 Premature ejaculation (psychosexual)
302.74 Orgasm inhibited male psychosexual

■ EPIDEMIOLOGY & DEMOGRAPHICS
Ejaculatory failure and retrograde ejaculation are uncommon disorders seen predominantly with diseases affecting the autonomic nervous system. Premature ejaculation is a common functional problem seen mostly in younger men.

■ PHYSICAL FINDINGS & CLINICAL PRESENTATION
Varies with disorder:
- Ejaculatory failure: no ejaculate is expelled; physical findings may be normal or may show autonomic or central nervous system dysfunction (e.g., spinal cord injury); results in infertility.
- Retrograde ejaculation: no ejaculate is expelled at orgasm and subsequent bladder void reveals cloudy urine; physical examination is often normal but may reveal autonomic nervous system dysfunction; results in infertility.
- Premature ejaculation: ejaculation occurs quickly following excitation; physical examination is normal.

■ ETIOLOGY
- Ejaculatory failure: lumbar sympathectomy, spinal cord injury, duct obstruction, sympatholytic drugs, substance abuse, psychologic factors, aging
- Retrograde ejaculation: open or transurethral prostatectomy, urethral or bladder procedures, congenital urethral anomalies, lumbar sympathectomy, sympatholytic drugs (antihypertensives, psychotropics), diabetes
- Premature ejaculation: fears, sexual ignorance

 DIAGNOSIS

■ WORKUP
- History, physical examination, and laboratory analysis
- Imaging occasionally

■ HISTORY
Psychosexual history, medication and substance use, history of genitourinary surgeries or infections, and past medical and trauma history

■ PHYSICAL EXAMINATION
Neurologic and genitourinary examinations

■ LABORATORY TESTS
Postorgasmic urine should be evaluated for spermatozoa, viscosity, and fructose to differentiate ejaculatory failure from retrograde ejaculation.

■ IMAGING STUDIES
Transrectal ultrasound or vasography can show dilated seminal vesicles or ejaculatory ducts if obstruction is present.

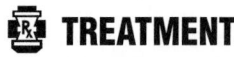 **TREATMENT**

■ NONPHARMACOLOGIC THERAPY
- Ejaculatory failure: vibratory or electrical stimulation of emission
- Retrograde ejaculation: viable sperm can be recovered from the bladder
- Premature ejaculation: sex therapy

■ GENERAL Rx
Offending drugs should be eliminated if possible. Alpha-adrenergic sympathomimetics such as pseudoephedrine, ephedrine, or phenylpropanolamine may convert retrograde to antegrade ejaculation. Psychotropic medications such as sertraline, fluoxetine, and clomipramine have shown success in delaying premature ejaculation. Topical anesthetics such as lidocaine cream have also been used.

■ SURGICAL Rx
Correction of anatomic abnormalities, such as relieving obstruction or improving the competence of the internal urethral sphincter apparatus

■ REFERRAL
All fertility issues and suspected anatomic problems should be referred to a urologist.
Author: **Michael Picchioni, M.D.**

BASIC INFORMATION

■ DEFINITION

Premature ejaculation is a persistent and recurrent problem in which a male experiences orgasm or ejaculation in the early phases of sexual contact and before he wishes it. Other definitions have emphasized elapsed time after intromission (with durations of 30 sec to several min), number of thrusts, or rate of partner satisfaction.

■ SYNONYMS

Rapid ejaculation
Early ejaculation
Inadequate ejaculatory control

ICD-9CM CODES

F52.4 Premature ejaculation (DSM-IV Code 302.75)

■ EPIDEMIOLOGY & DEMOGRAPHICS

INCIDENCE (IN U.S.): Reported as 21% in 1988; 46% in 1970
PREVALENCE (IN U.S.): 7% to 38%
PREDOMINANT SEX: Only males affected
PREDOMINANT AGE: None defined
PEAK INCIDENCE: Adolescence and young adulthood
GENETICS: No identifiable genetic factors

■ PHYSICAL FINDINGS & CLINICAL PRESENTATION

- Complaint of ejaculation before, upon, or shortly after penetration
- Frequently associated anxiety related to either sexual activity or more generalized anxiety disorder
- Premature ejaculation secondary to a medical condition frequently associated with low anxiety, low desire, and/or erectile insufficiency

■ ETIOLOGY

- Unclear etiology; different theoretical frameworks emphasizing anxiety related to performance or personal interactions, behavioral concepts of learned expectations related to early experience, or heightened penile sensitivity
- Organic factors in a small fraction of individuals (e.g., abdominal or pelvic trauma or surgery, neuropathies, or urologic pathology such as prostatic urethritis)

 DIAGNOSIS

■ DIFFERENTIAL DIAGNOSIS

- In as many as 25% of men with complaints of premature ejaculation, partner is anorgasmic.
- In young adolescents, premature ejaculation is normally experienced as a consequence of heightened excitation.

■ WORKUP

- History with a specific emphasis on sexual activities, beliefs, orientation, and gender identity
- History of relationships
- Collateral information from sexual partner when possible
- Additional history regarding surgery, trauma, and myologic symptoms
- History of prescribed and recreational drugs revealing contributory factors (e.g., tricyclic antidepressants, alcohol, opiates)

■ LABORATORY TESTS

Urinalysis and urine culture after prostatic massage may uncover a urinary or prostatic infection.

■ IMAGING STUDIES

None indicated

℞ TREATMENT

■ NONPHARMACOLOGIC THERAPY

- Behavioral and psychotherapeutic interventions: strongly guided by a specific theoretical framework; often inadequate data to suggest the superiority of any particular approach
- Use of condoms frequently recommended to reduce penile sensitivity
- Use of pause-squeeze technique, in which 4 sec of moderate pressure is applied to the frenulum to reduce ejaculatory urge

■ ACUTE GENERAL Rx

- Topical anesthetics (benzodiazepines) increase ejaculatory latency.
- Anxiolytics may be useful in individuals with anxiety.
- Serotonin reuptake inhibiting antidepressants, which frequently delay orgasm in both men and women, are a common intervention but have not been extensively studied.

■ DISPOSITION

- Premature ejaculation is frequently a chronic, lifelong problem.
- There is gradual improvement with age but few spontaneous remissions.
- Impact of successful therapy may be prolonged.

■ REFERRAL

If behavioral sex therapy or psychotherapy is indicated or if significant urologic abnormalities are discovered
Author: **Rif S. El-Mallakh, M.D.**

BASIC INFORMATION

DEFINITION
Electrical injuries are wounds occurring as a result of contact with an electrical current (Fig. 1-137).

SYNONYMS
None

ICD-9CM CODES
994.8 Electrical shock, nonfatal

EPIDEMIOLOGY & DEMOGRAPHICS
- Electrical injuries cause approximately 250 deaths per year in the U.S.
- Account for 4% to 6.5% of all admissions to burn units.
- Deaths typically occur in the young.
- Most electrical burns in adults are occupationally related.
- Children commonly experience oral burns from electrical appliances.

PHYSICAL FINDINGS & CLINICAL PRESENTATION
- Depending on the extent of injury the patient may be unconscious, seizing, or confused and unable to present a history.
- Extensive burns (~10% to 25% of the body surface)
  1. Located over the entry and exit sites.
  2. Most common entry sites are the hands and skull.
  3. Most common exit sites are the heels.
  4. "Kissing burns" over the flexor creases
  5. Superficial partial thickness
  6. Oral burns in children
  7. Bleeding from the labial artery may present 7 to 10 days after the injury.
- Cardiac arrest (asystole or ventricular fibrillation) may be the initial presenting rhythm.
- Pulseless extremities
- Fractures
- Compartment syndrome from severe muscle tissue damage
- Headaches
- Weakness and paresthesias
- Motor and sensory deficits

ETIOLOGY
- Electricity causes tissue injury by converting electrical energy into heat.
- The higher the electrical voltage, the greater the tissue destruction.
- The longer the duration of contact with the electrical source, the greater the damage.
  1. Direct current (DC) contact causes a single muscle contraction throwing the patient away from the source.
  2. Alternating current (AC) contact precipitates a tetanic contraction, not allowing the patient to withdraw from the source and prolonging the duration of contact.
  3. Therefore AC contact is more ominous than DC contact.
- Electrical injuries are arbitrarily divided into high voltage (1000 volts) and low voltage (500 volts).
- The entry and exit path the electrical current travels in the body determines which tissues are affected.

DIAGNOSIS

The diagnosis of electrical injury is based on history and physical examination.

WORKUP
A detailed workup is indicated in patients with electrical injuries because the physical examination may not reveal the extent of damage that has occurred.

LABORATORY TESTS
- CBC
- Electrolytes
- BUN/creatinine
- Arterial blood gases
- Myoglobin
- Creatinine kinase CPK with isoenzyme fractionation
- Urinalysis including screening for myoglobinuria
- Liver function tests
- Type and cross-match
- EKG

IMAGING STUDIES
- C-spine films in patients with suspected spinal injury
- X-ray any suspicious area for bone fractures
- CT scan of the head and skull in patients with major head injury
- Technetium pyrophosphate scanning may locate areas of myonecrosis

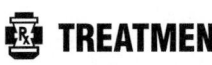 **TREATMENT**

NONPHARMACOLOGIC THERAPY
- If at the scene of the injury, make sure the power source is turned off before approaching the victim.
- Maintain urine output of at least 50 cc/hr with IV fluids
- Cardiac monitoring
- Oxygen
- Tetanus prophylaxis

ACUTE GENERAL Rx
- Alkalinization of the urine (sodium bicarbonate 50 mEq in 1 L of normal saline) is indicated in patients who are suspected of having myoglobinuria.
- Furosemide 20 to 40 mg PO or IV may be used to force diuresis.
- Mannitol 12.5 g/kg/hr assist in maintain diuresis.
- Seizures are treated in the standard fashion.
- Treat burns with sulfadiazine silver dressings.

CHRONIC Rx
- Aymptomatic patients with a normal physical examination, negative urinalysis, and normal EKG findings may be discharged home with close follow-up.

DISPOSITION
- Patients with severe burns should be transferred to the regional burn center.
- Complications of electrical injuries include:
  1. Infection
  2. Renal failure from rhabdomyolysis
  3. Seizure disorder
  4. Fasciotomies
  5. Amputation

- Delayed neurologic damage may present as ascending paralysis, amyotrophic lateral sclerosis, or transverse myelitis weeks to years after the injury.
- Vascular damage may also present in a delayed fashion.

■ REFERRAL

A general surgery consultation is recommended in any patient with significant electrical injuries and tissue damage. Plastic surgery is recommended in children with oral burns. Ophthalmology consultation is also recommended screening for cataract formation.

☼ PEARLS & CONSIDERATIONS

■ COMMENTS

- Electrical injuries are caused by:
  1. Direct contact with the electrical source.
  2. Conversion of electrical energy to heat.
  3. Blunt trauma after being thrown from the electrical source or from continuous muscle contraction (tetany).
- Electrical burns are the most frequent cause of amputation in burn units.
- Cataract formation has been shown to occur within 1 to 24 mo following a high-voltage electrical injury in approximately 5% to 20 % of patients.
- The absence of physical findings on the initial examination does not exclude extensive underlying tissue damage.

REFERENCES

Cooper MA: Electrical and lightning injuries. In Rosen P, Barkin R: *Emergency medicine: concepts and clinical practice,* ed 4, St Louis, 1998, Mosby.
Jeschke RJ, Herndon RE: Electrical injuries: a 30-year review, *J Trauma* 46(5):933, 1999.
Author: **Peter Petropoulos, M.D.**

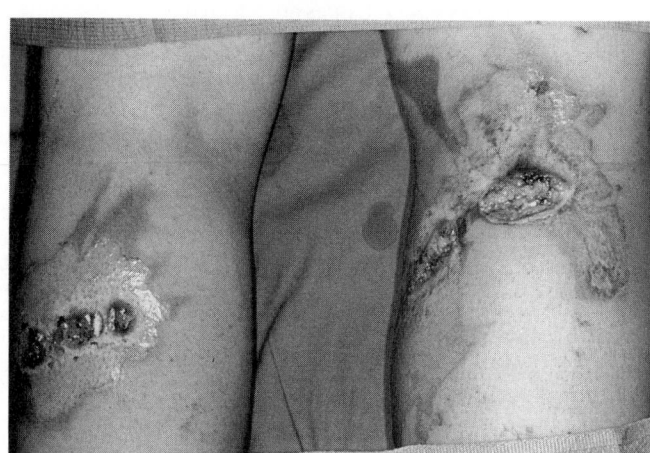

Fig. 1-137   Charring of the skin of both calves indicates points of contact with a high-voltage electrical current. These contact points are surrounded by full-thickness cutaneous burns caused by arcing of current. The extent of deep tissue destruction is often not related to the size of the cutaneous manifestations of the injury. (From Goldman L, Bennett JC [eds]: *Cecil textbook of medicine,* ed 21, Philadelphia, 2000, WB Saunders.)

BASIC INFORMATION

■ **DEFINITION**

Electromechanical dissociation (EMD) is the absence of effective cardiac output in the presence of organized electrical activity.

■ **SYNONYMS**

Pulseless electrical activity (PEA)

ICD-9CM CODES

426.89 Electromechanical dissociation

■ **EPIDEMIOLOGY & DEMOGRAPHICS**

- Less frequent than VT/VF, asystole
- May be last electrical activity of dying myocardium

■ **PHYSICAL FINDINGS & CLINICAL PRESENTATION**

PRIMARY EMD:
- Organized electrical activity
- No palpable pulse

SECONDARY EMD:
As above and may also have:
- Bradycardia: drug overdose
- Tachycardia: hypovolemia, massive PE
- Decreased JVP: hypovolemia
- Elevated JVP and no pulse with CPR: cardiac tamponade, massive PE, tension pneumothorax
- Absent unilateral breath sounds with mechanical ventilation and tracheal deviation: tension pneumothorax
- Cyanosis: hypoxia

■ **ETIOLOGY**

PRIMARY EMD: Myocardial excitation and contraction uncoupling secondary to advanced heart muscle disease

SECONDARY EMD: Because of changes in the loading conditions of the heart (significant decrease in preload or afterload, inflow or outflow obstruction), ischemia, myocardial depressors
- Hypovolemia
- Cardiac tamponade
- Tension pneumothorax
- Massive PE

- Massive MI
- Hypothermia/hyperthermia
- Hyperkalemia
- Hypoglycemia
- Hypocalcemia
- Hypoxia
- Acidosis
- Drug overdose: β-blockers, calcium channel blockers, digoxin, tricyclic antidepressants
- Shock: septic, anaphylactic, neurogenic
- Atrial myxoma
- Hypertrophic obstructive cardiomyopathy
- Severe pulmonary hypertension
- Severe aortic or pulmonary stenosis

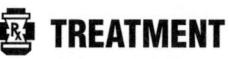 **DIAGNOSIS**

■ **DIFFERENTIAL DIAGNOSIS**

- Pseudo-EMD
- Idioventricular rhythm
- Postdefibrillation idioventricular rhythm
- Ventricular escape rhythm
- Bradyasystolic rhythm

■ **WORKUP**

- Stabilizing patient and workup to establish etiology of EMD should proceed simultaneously
- History, physical examination, laboratory tests, imaging studies

■ **LABORATORY TESTS**

- Potassium, calcium, glucose
- Arterial blood gas
- ECG (Fig. 1-138):
    Low voltage: tamponade
    Right heart strain: PE, pneumothorax
    Heart block: MI, metabolic abnormalities
    ST changes, Q waves: MI

■ **IMAGING STUDIES**

- Chest x-ray: rule out pneumothorax
- Pulmonary arteriogram: rule out PE
- Echocardiogram: rule out tamponade, valve dysfunction and atrial myxoma

- Abdominal x-ray: rule out rupture of abdominal aortic aneurysm

℞ TREATMENT

■ **NONPHARMACOLOGIC THERAPY**

Begin CPR
- Intubate and ventilate
- Obtain IV access
- Continuous cardiac monitor
- Confirm absence of blood flow with Doppler ultrasound, arterial line, or bedside echocardiogram

■ **ACUTE GENERAL Rx**

- Epinephrine 1 mg IV push, repeat q3-5min
- If bradycardic (<60 beats/min): atropine 1 mg IV q3-5min to a maximum of 0.04 mg/kg
- If preexisting hyperkalemia: sodium bicarbonate 1 mEq/kg
- Treat specific cause if known

PROBABLY HELPFUL:
Sodium bicarbonate 1 mEq/kg if:
- Preexisting bicarbonate responsive acidosis
- Tricyclic antidepressant overdose
- Drug overdoses that respond to alkalization of urine

POSSIBLY HELPFUL:
Sodium bicarbonate 1 mEq/kg if:
- Intubated and prolonged arrest
- Successful resuscitation after prolonged arrest

Epinephrine at higher doses:
- 2 to 5 mg IV push q3-5min
- 1 mg, 3 mg, 5 mg IV push, 3 min apart
- 0.1 mg/kg IV push q3-5min

■ **DISPOSITION**

- Poor overall. Of hospitalized patients who develop EMD, 4% survive to discharge.
- Prompt treatment may be successful in secondary EMD.

Author: **Sudeep K. Aulakh, M.D., F.R.C.P.C.**

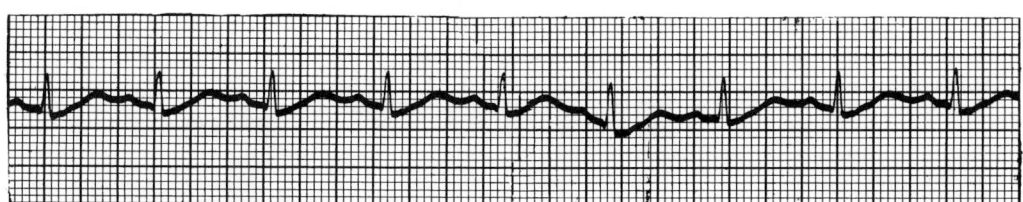

Fig. 1-138　Sinus rhythm with electromechanical dissociation (EMD). Although the ECG showed sinus rhythm, the patient had no pulse or blood pressure. In this case the EMD was a result of depressed myocardial function after a cardiac arrest. (From Goldberg AL: *Clinical electrocardiography,* ed 5, St Louis, 1994, Mosby.)

BASIC INFORMATION

■ DEFINITION
Acute viral encephalitis is an acute febrile syndrome with evidence of meningeal involvement and of derangement of the function of the cerebrum, cerebellum, or brain stem.

■ SYNONYMS
Arboviral encephalitis
Brain stem encephalitis
Acute necrotizing encephalitis
Rasmussen encephalitis
Encephalitis lethargica

■ ICD-9CM CODES
049.9 Viral encephalitis NOS

■ EPIDEMIOLOGY & DEMOGRAPHICS
INCIDENCE (IN U.S.): About 20,000 cases/yr are reported to the CDC.
PREVALENCE (IN U.S.): Unknown
PREDOMINANT SEX: Male = female
PREDOMINANT AGE: Any age
PEAK INCIDENCE: Any age
GENETICS: No specific genetic or congenital predisposition

■ ETIOLOGY
- Can be caused by a host of viruses, with herpes simplex the most common virus identified
- Arboviruses: agents causing Eastern equine encephalitis, Western equine encephalitis, St. Louis encephalitis, Venezuelan equine encephalitis, California virus encephalitis, Japanese B encephalitis, Murray Valley and West Nile encephalitis, Russian spring-summer encephalitis, as well as other less known agents
- Also implicated: rabies-causing agents, CMV, Epstein-Barr, varicella-zoster, echo virus, mumps, adenovirus, coxsackie, rubeola, and herpes viruses
- Meningoencephalitis: acute retroviral infection

■ PHYSICAL FINDINGS & CLINICAL PRESENTATION
- Initially, fever and evidence of meningeal irritation
- Headache and stiff neck
- Later, development of signs of cortical dysfunction: lethargy, coma, stupor, weakness, seizures, facial weakness, as well as brain stem findings
- Cerebellar findings: ataxia, nystagmus, hypotonia; myoclonus, cranial nerve palsies, and abnormal tendon reflexes
- Patients with rabies: hydrophobia, anxiety, facial numbness, psychosis, coma, or dysarthria
- Rarely, movement disorders, such as chorea, hemiballismus, or dystonia
- Recall of a prodromal viral-like illness (this finding is not at all uniform)

DIAGNOSIS

■ DIFFERENTIAL DIAGNOSIS
- Bacterial infections: brain abscess, toxic encephalopathies, TB
- Protozoal infections
- Behçet's disease
- Lupus encephalitis
- Sjögren's syndrome
- Multiple sclerosis
- Syphilis
- Cryptococcus
- Toxoplasmosis
- Brucellosis
- Leukemic or lymphomatous meningitis
- Other metastatic tumors
- Lyme disease
- Cat-scratch disease
- Vogt-Koyanagi-Harada syndrome
- Mollaret's meningitis

■ WORKUP
- Lumbar puncture to reveal pleocytosis, usually lymphocytic although neutrophils may be seen early on
- Usually, elevated CSF protein
- Normal or low CSF glucose
- In herpes simplex encephalitis: RBCs and xanthochromia
- EEG changes showing periodic high-voltage sharp waves in the temporal regions and slow wave complexes suggestive of herpes encephalitis
- CT scan and MRI to reveal edema and hemorrhage in the frontal and temporal lobes
- Arboviral infections suspected during outbreaks in specific areas
- Rising titers of neutralizing antibodies from the acute to the convalescent stage demonstrated but often not helpful in the acutely ill patient
- Polymerase chain reaction that amplifies DNA from the CSF for herpes simplex encephalitis
- Rarely, brain biopsy to assist in the diagnosis; viral culture of cerebral tissue obtained if biopsy done
- Classic herpetic skin lesions suggestive of herpes encephalitis
- In diagnosing arboviral encephalitis:
  1. Presence of antiviral IgM within the first few days of symptomatic disease; detected and quantified by ELISA
  2. Unusual to recover an arbovirus from the blood or CSF

■ LABORATORY TESTS
- Aside from the lumbar puncture, most other laboratory studies are nonspecific.
- Skin lesions and urine may be cultured for herpes simplex and CMV.

TREATMENT

■ ACUTE GENERAL Rx
- Supportive care, frequent evaluation, and neurologic examination
- Ventilatory assistance for patients who are moribund or at risk for aspiration
- Avoidance of infusion of hypotonic fluids to minimize the risk of hyponatremia
- For patients who develop seizures: anticonvulsant therapy and follow-up in a critical care setting
- For comatose patients:
  1. Aggressive care to avoid decubiti, contractures, and DVT
  2. Close attention to weights, input/output, and serum electrolytes
- Acyclovir 30 mg/kg/day IV for 14 days for herpes simplex encephalitis
- Short courses of corticosteroids to control brain edema and prevent herniation
- In patients with suspected rabies:
  1. Human rabies immune globulin (HRIG) should be given at a dose of 20 U/kg.
  2. Active immunization may be stimulated by recently developed rabies vaccine, which is grown on a human diploid cell line (HDCV) and has reduced the number of doses needed to five.
  3. If suspect animal can be found, observe closely for 10 days to detect rabid behavior.
  4. If signs are seen, animal should be euthanized and its brain examined for signs of rabies.
- No specific pharmacologic therapy for most other viral pathogens

■ CHRONIC Rx
Some patients may develop permanent neurologic sequelae; these patients will gain benefit from intensive rehabilitation programs, including physical, occupational, and speech therapy.

REFERENCE
Benjamin R, Chang G: Acute disseminated encephalomyelitis: a case based review, *Hosp Phys* 34:40, 1998.
Author: **Joseph J. Lieber, M.D.**

BASIC INFORMATION

■ DEFINITION
Encopresis is the voluntary or involuntary passage of stool into inappropriate places, in children over the developmental age of 4 yr, with the absence of direct physiologic causes.

■ SYNONYMS
Functional incontinence of stool

ICD-9CM CODES
787.6 Incontinence of feces
307.7 Encopresis

■ EPIDEMIOLOGY & DEMOGRAPHICS
INCIDENCE (IN U.S.): 1% of 5 yr olds
PREVALANCE (IN U.S.): 3% of the pediatric population
PREDOMINANT SEX: Male > female
PREDOMINANT AGE: 4 to 9 yr of age
PEAK INCIDENCE: 4 to 5 yr of age
GENETICS: Factors that contribute to slow gut motility may predispose to encopresis

■ PHYSICAL FINDINGS & CLINICAL PRESENTATION
- When constipation and overflow incontinence are causative, defecation is usually uncomfortable or painful, so patient avoids defecation with consequent stool retention.
- Stool is usually poorly formed and leakage is continuous (occurring during sleep and wakefulness).
- Encopresis resolves when the constipation is resolved.
- When there is no constipation with overflow incontinence, stool is more likely to be normal in character.
- Soiling is intermittent and usually in a prominent location.
- Coexisting oppositional-defiant or conduct disorders are frequent.

■ ETIOLOGY
- Approximately 96% of children will have bowel movements between three times daily to once every other day. When bowel movements are less frequent, stool becomes drier and harder and much more uncomfortable to pass. Children may avoid the discomfort by avoiding elimination, but this only results in worsening constipation.
- Soiling results from more liquid stool that leaks around the main stool mass.
- Constipation may begin gradually as a result of a slow decrease in elimination frequency or more acutely after an illness, dehydration, or prolonged bed rest.
- In encopresis without constipation and overflow incontinence, soiling is usually intentional. This frequently occurs in the setting of comorbid oppositional-defiant disorder or conduct disorder.
- Incontinence can also result from anal masturbation.

 DIAGNOSIS

■ DIFFERENTIAL DIAGNOSIS
- Hirschsprung's disease
- Cerebral palsy
- Myelomeningocele
- Pseudoobstruction
- Anorectal lesions
- Malformations
- Trauma
- Rectal prolapse
- Hypothyroidism
- Medications

■ WORKUP
- History: pay particular attention to frequency of elimination, character of the stool, associated pain, and presence of enuresis (with which it is frequently associated).
- Physical examination: pay particular attention to the abdomen, anus, rectum, and saddle sensation.

■ LABORATORY TESTS
- Thyroid profile
- Electrolytes (including calcium)
- Adrenal function
- Urinalysis and urine culture

■ IMAGING STUDIES
- Abdominal x-rays to determine extent of obstruction or megacolon
- Anorectal manometric studies to determine sphincter function if Hirschsprung's disease is suspected; if abnormal, followed up with a barium enema and rectal biopsy

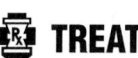 **TREATMENT**

■ NONPHARMACOLOGIC THERAPY
- Psychotherapy or family therapy in chronic encopresis
- Biofeedback to improve sphincter function

■ ACUTE GENERAL Rx
- Disimpaction with hypertonic phosphate (30 ml/5 kg body weight) or isotonic saline enemas
- Resistant cases: repeated instillation of 200 to 600 ml of milk of magnesia enemas
- If child does not permit enemas: oral disimpaction with large doses of mineral oil or lactulose until stool mass is cleared (NOTE: this is frequently more painful and more uncomfortable than an enema)

■ CHRONIC Rx
- Prevention of recurrence of constipation by increased dietary fiber and the use of laxatives
- In immediate postdisimpaction period (3 mo following acute treatment) laxatives needed because bowel tone remains low
- Laxatives possibly required for several years or indefinitely

■ DISPOSITION
In most cases encopresis is self-limited and of relatively brief duration; it is rarely chronic.

■ REFERRAL
If patient is resistant to treatment, complicated family factors are involved, or encopresis is purposeful
Author: **Rif S. El-Mallakh, M.D.**

BASIC INFORMATION

■ DEFINITION
Infective endocarditis is an infection of the endocardial surface of the heart or mural endocardium.
ACUTE ENDOCARDITIS: Usually caused by *Staphylococcus aureus, Streptococcus pyogenes,* pneumococcus, and *Neisseria* organisms; classic clinical presentation of fever, positive blood cultures, vascular and immunologic phenomenon
SUBACUTE ENDOCARDITIS: Usually caused by viridans streptococci in the presence of valvular pathology; less toxic, often indolent presentation with lower fevers, night sweats, fatigue
INFECTIVE ENDOCARDITIS IN INJECTION DRUG USERS: Often involving *S. aureus* or *Pseudomonas aeruginosa* with variation that may be geographically influenced; tricuspid or multiple valvular involvement; high mortality rate of 50% to 60%
EARLY PROSTHETIC VALVE ENDOCARDITIS: Usually caused by *S. epidermidis* within 2 mo of valve replacement; other organisms include *S. aureus,* gram-negative bacilli, diphtheroids, *Candida* organisms
LATE PROSTHETIC VALVE ENDOCARDITIS: Typically develops >60 days after valvular replacement; involved organisms similar to early prosthetic valve endocarditis, including viridans streptococci, enterococci, and group D streptococci
NOSOCOMIAL ENDOCARDITIS: Secondary to intravenous catheters, TPN lines, pacemakers; coagulase negative staphylococci, *S. aureus,* and streptococci most common

■ SYNONYMS
Bacterial endocarditis

ICD-9CM CODES
421.0 Infective endocarditis
996.61 Prosthetic valve endocarditis

■ EPIDEMIOLOGY & DEMOGRAPHICS
INCIDENCE (IN U.S.): 1.7 to 3.8 cases/100,000 persons/yr
NOSOCOMIAL ENDOCARDITIS: 14% to 28% of cases
PREVALENCE (IN U.S.): 0.3 to 3 cases/1000 hospital admissions

PREDOMINANT SEX: Male > female
PREDOMINANT AGE: 45 to 65 yr
PEAK INCIDENCE: Females: often <35 yr old; males: 45 to 65 yr old

■ PHYSICAL FINDINGS & CLINICAL PRESENTATION
- Fever may be variable in presentation; may be high, hectic, or absent.
- Fever, chills, fatigue, and rigors occur in 25% to 80% of patients.
- Heart murmur may be absent in right-sided endocarditis.
- Embolic phenomenon with peripheral manifestations are found in 50% of patients.
- Skin manifestations include petechiae, Osler nodes, splinter hemorrhages, Janeway lesions.
- Splenomegaly is more common with subacute course.

■ ETIOLOGY
Streptococcal and staphylococcal infections are the most common causes of infective endocarditis. Variation in incidence may occur that is influenced by the patient's risk for developing infection.
ACUTE ENDOCARDITIS:
- *S. aureus*
- *Streptococcus pneumoniae*
- Streptococcal species and groups A through G
- *Haemophilus influenzae*
SUBACUTE ENDOCARDITIS:
- Viridans streptococci (α-hemolytic)
- *Str. bovis*
- Enterococci
- *S. aureus*
ENDOCARDITIS IN IV DRUG ADDICTS:
- *S. aureus*
- *P. aeruginosa*
- *Candida* species
- Enterococci
PROSTHETIC VALVE (EARLY):
- *S. epidermidis*
- *S. aureus*
- Gram-negative bacilli
- Group D streptococci
PROSTHETIC VALVE (LATE):
- *S. epidermidis*
- Viridans streptococci
- *S. aureus*
- Enterococci and group D streptococci

NOSOCOMIAL ENDOCARDITIS:
- Coagulase negative *Staphylococcus*
- *S. aureus*
- Streptococci: viridans, group B, enterococcus
HACEK ORGANISMS:
- Fastidious gram-negative bacilli
- *Haemophilus parainfluenzae*
- *Haemophilus aphrophilus*
- *Actinobacillus actinomycetemcomitans*
- *Cardiobacterium homimis*
- *Eikenella corrodens*
- *Kingella kingae*

DIAGNOSIS

■ DIFFERENTIAL DIAGNOSIS
- Brain abscess
- FUO
- Pericarditis
- Meningitis
- Rheumatic fever
- Osteomyelitis
- Salmonella
- TB
- Bacteremia
- Pericarditis
- Glomerulonephritis

■ WORKUP
Physical examination to evaluate for the above physical findings followed by laboratory testing (see below)

■ LABORATORY TESTS
- Blood cultures: three sets in first 24 hr
- More culturing if patient has received prior antibiotic
- CBC (anemia possibly present, subacute)
- WBC (leukocytosis is higher in acute endocarditis)
- ESR (elevated)
- Positive rheumatoid factor (subacute endocarditis)
- False-positive VDRL
- Proteinuria, hematuria, RBC casts

■ IMAGING STUDIES
- Echocardiogram: two-dimensional
- Transesophageal echocardiography: more sensitive in detecting vegations if two-dimensional is negative, especially helpful with prosthetic valves or in detecting perivalvular disease

TREATMENT

Initial IV antibiotic therapy (before culture results) is aimed at the most likely organism:

- In patients with prosthetic valves or patients with native valves who are allergic to penicillin: vancomycin plus rifampin and gentamicin
- In IV drug users: nafcillin or oxacillin plus gentamicin; if MRSA, vancomycin plus gentamicin
- In native valve endocarditis: combination of penicillin and gentamicin; a penicillase-resistant penicillin (oxacillin or nafcillin) can be used if acute bacterial endocarditis is present or if *S. aureus* is suspected as one of the possible causative organisms; for Hacek organisms, treat with third-generation cephalosporin
- Ceftriaxone and an aminoglycoside for 2 wk can be used in streptococcus viridens endocarditis

Antibiotic therapy after identification of the organism should be guided by susceptibility testing.

PEARLS & CONSIDERATIONS

■ COMMENTS
For endocarditis prophylaxis refer to Boxes 5-1 to 5-3 and Tables 5-25 and 5-26.

REFERENCES
Heiro M et al: Diagnosis of infective endocarditis, *Arch Intern Med* 158:18, 1998.

Mylonakis E, Calderwood SB: Infective endocarditis in adults, *N Engl J Med* 345:1318, 2001.

Author: **Dennis J. Mikolich, M.D.**

BASIC INFORMATION

■ DEFINITION
Endometrial cancer is a malignant transformation of endometrial stroma and/or glands typified by irregular nuclear membranes, nuclear atypia, mitotic activity, loss of glandular pattern, irregular cell size (Fig. 1-139).

■ SYNONYMS
Uterine cancer (some forms)

ICD-9CM CODES
182 Malignant neoplasm of body of uterus

■ EPIDEMIOLOGY & DEMOGRAPHICS
INCIDENCE: 21.2 cases/100,000 persons; approximately 30,000 new cases annually
PREDOMINANCE: Median age at onset: 60 yr; only 5% occur in women <40 yr
RISK FACTORS: Obesity, diabetes, nulliparity, early menarche and late menopause, unopposed estrogen therapy, tamoxifen use, endometrial atypical hyperplasia

■ PHYSICAL FINDINGS & CLINICAL PRESENTATION
- Abnormal uterine bleeding or postmenopausal bleeding in 90%
- Pyometra or hematometra
- Abnormal Pap smear

■ ETIOLOGY
Endogenous or exogenous chronic unopposed estrogen stimulation of the endometrium

DIAGNOSIS

■ DIFFERENTIAL DIAGNOSIS
- Atypical hyperplasia
- Other genital tract malignancy
- Polyps
- Atrophic vaginitis
- Granuloma cell tumor
- Fibroid uterus

■ WORKUP
- Complete history and physical examination
- Endometrial biopsy or dilation and curettage
- Assessment of operative risk

■ LABORATORY TESTS
- CBC
- Chemistry profile including liver function tests
- Consider CA-125 level

■ IMAGING STUDIES
- Chest x-ray examination
- Possible CT scan, BE, and/or pelvic ultrasound
- Endovaginal ultrasound in postmenopausal women with vaginal bleeding

TREATMENT

■ NONPHARMACOLOGIC THERAPY
- Surgery is the mainstay of treatment, with or without radiation, depending on tumor stage and grade.
- Surgery consists of pelvic washings, total abdominal hysterectomy and bilateral salpingo-oophorectomy, omental biopsy, and selective pelvic and periaortic lymphadenectomy, depending on stage and grade.
- Brachytherapy and/or teletherapy are added in an advanced stage.
- Chemotherapy (cisplatin, Adriamycin) or tamoxifen may also be used.

■ ACUTE GENERAL Rx
- A thorough workup should be completed before any therapy for endometrial cancer.
- Surgery is the treatment of choice.

■ CHRONIC Rx
- Physical and pelvic examination every 3 mo for 2 yr, then every 6 mo for 2 yr, annually thereafter

- Yearly Pap smear
- Hormone replacement (combination) a consideration in low-risk patients

■ DISPOSITION
The majority of cases present early, where the 5-yr survival is generally good:

Stage I	75% to 100%
Stage II	60%
Stage III	50%
Stage IV	20%

Some histologic types (clear cell, serous papillary) have poorer survival rates.

■ REFERRAL
A gynecologist may manage early-stage disease, otherwise refer to a gynecologic oncologist.

■ COMMENTS
Estrogen replacement therapy (ERT) after surgery for endometrial cancer remains controversial. Recent data suggest that ERT does not increase endometrial cancer recurrence rates.

REFERENCES
Smith-Bindman R et al: Endovaginal ultrasound to exclude endometrial cancer and other endometrial abnormalities, *JAMA* 280:1510, 1998.
Suriano KA et al: Estrogen replacement therapy in endometrial cancer patients, *Obstet Gynecol* 97:555, 2001.
Author: **Gil Farkash, M.D.**

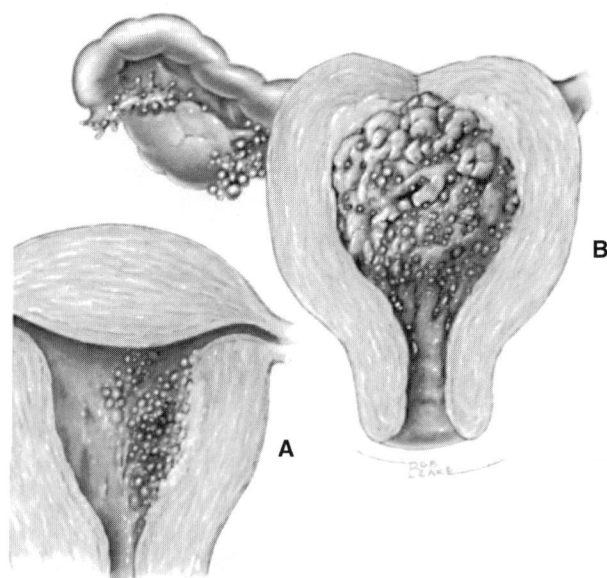

Fig. 1-139 Carcinoma of the endometrium. **A,** Stage I. **B,** Stage III, myometrial invasion. (From Sabiston D: *Textbook of surgery,* ed 15, Philadelphia, 1997, WB Saunders.)

BASIC INFORMATION

DEFINITION
Endometriosis is defined as the presence of functioning endometrial glands and stroma outside the uterine cavity (Fig. 1-140).

ICD-9CM CODES
617.9 Endometriosis

EPIDEMIOLOGY & DEMOGRAPHICS
PREVALENCE:
- Women of reproductive age: 2% to 5%
- Infertile women: 20% to 40%

MOST COMMON AGE AT DIAGNOSIS:
25 to 29 yr

GENETICS:
- Multifactorial inheritance pattern
- 6.9% occurrence rate in first-degree female relatives

PHYSICAL FINDINGS & CLINICAL PRESENTATION
- Classic triad is dysmenorrhea, dyspareunia, and infertility.
- Presence of pelvic pain *not correlated* with the total area of endometriosis, type of lesion, or volume of disease, but it *is correlated* with the depth of infiltration.
- Most severe discomfort is associated with lesions >1 cm in depth.
- Bimanual examination may reveal tender uterosacral ligaments, cul-de-sac nodularity, induration of the rectovaginal septum, fixed retroversion of the uterus, adnexal mass, and generalized or localized tenderness.

ETIOLOGY
- Reflux and direct implantation theory: retrograde menstruation with implantation of viable endometrial cells to surrounding pelvic structures
- Coelomic metaplasia theory: transformation of multipotential cells of the coelomic epithelium into endometrium-like cells
- Vascular dissemination theory: transport of endometrial cells to distant sites via the uterine vascular and lymphatic systems
- Autoimmune disease theory: disorder of immune surveillance allows growth of endometrial implants

DIAGNOSIS

DIFFERENTIAL DIAGNOSIS
- Ectopic pregnancy
- Acute appendicitis
- Chronic appendicitis
- PID
- Pelvic adhesions
- Hemorrhagic cyst
- Hernia
- Psychologic disorder
- Irritable bowel syndrome
- Uterine leiomyomata
- Adenomyosis
- Nerve entrapment syndrome
- Scoliosis
- Muscular/skeletal strain
- Interstitial cystitis

WORKUP
- Thorough history and physical examination, including inquiry about physical and emotional abuse
- Colonoscopy if rectal bleeding present
- Laparoscopy for definitive diagnosis
- Revised American Fertility Society (RAFS) scale to classify endometriosis (since 1985):

Stage I	minimal
Stage II	mild
Stage III	moderate
Stage IV	severe

LABORATORY TESTS
Cancer antigen 125 [CA125]
- Also elevated in ovarian epithelial neoplasm, myomas, adenomyosis, acute PID, ovarian cysts, pancreatitis, chronic liver disease, menstruation, and pregnancy
- CA 125 value >35 U/ml: positive predictive value of 0.58 and a negative predictive value of 0.96 for the presence of endometriosis

IMAGING STUDIES
- Ultrasound: for evaluating adnexal mass; cannot reliably distinguish endometriomas from other benign or malignant ovarian conditions
- MRI:
  1. Highly accurate in detecting endometriomas
  2. Limited sensitivity in detecting diffuse pelvic endometriosis

TREATMENT

NONPHARMACOLOGIC THERAPY
Expectant management (observation for 5 to 12 mo) for stage I or stage II endometriosis-associated infertility

ACUTE GENERAL Rx
NSAIDs for symptomatic relief of dysmenorrhea

CHRONIC Rx
PHARMACOLOGIC MANAGEMENT:
Estrogen-progesterone:
- State of "pseudopregnancy" created by continuous use of combination oral contraceptives for 6 to 12 mo
- Breakthrough bleeding treated by administering conjugated estrogens 1.25 mg/day for 2 wk

Danazol:
- Initial dose 200 mg PO bid
- If no improvement within 6 wk, dosage increased to 300 or 400 mg PO bid
- Treatment generally continued for 6 mo, after which up to 90% of patients with mild to moderate endometriosis experience alleviation of pelvic pain
- Treatment begun after menses to avoid fetal exposure

Progestins:
- Medroxyprogesterone acetate 10 to 30 mg PO qd and occasionally up to 100 mg PO qd
- Alternatively, 100 mg IM q2wk for four doses, followed by 200 mg IM monthly for 4 mo
- Breakthrough bleeding treated with ethinyl estradiol (20 µg/day) or conjugated estrogens (1.25 mg/day) for 1 to 2 wk
- Comparison with danazol: progestins cost less, have a more tolerable side-effect profile, and have comparable efficacy with regard to pain relief, so are often the first-line drug

Gonadotropin-releasing hormone (GnRH) agonists:
- Use usually limited to 6 mo
- Leuprolide acetate depot 3.75 mg IM monthly *or* 11.25 mg IM q3mo
- *or* nafarelin 200 µg nasal puffs bid
- *or* goserelin 3.6 mg SC monthly

I

- As effective as danazol for relief of pelvic pain
- Add-back therapy for protection against vasomotor symptoms and bone loss: norethindrone acetate 5 mg PO qd alone *or* in combination with conjugated estrogen 0.625 mg PO qd
- Add-back therapy allows GnRH agonist use to be extended to 1 yr

SURGICAL MANAGEMENT:

Conservative:
- Directed at enhancing fertility or treating pain unresponsive to first-line medical treatment
- Usually accomplished through laparoscopy
- Removal or destruction of endometriotic implants by excision, electrocautery, or laser
- Unless pregnancy is desired, patient is usually started on GnRH agonist therapy immediately after surgery
- For those desiring pregnancy, surgery alone results in significant increase in fertility

Definitive:
- Directed at relieving endometriosis-associated pain
- Total abdominal hysterectomy with bilateral salpingo-oophorectomy and complete excision or ablation of endometriosis
- Thorough abdominal exploration to ensure removal of all disease
- Must be prepared to manage possible GI and urinary tract endometriosis

- 90% effective in pain relief
- Estrogen replacement therapy (ERT) to be considered in all women undergoing definitive surgical management; after ERT, recurrence rate of 0% to 5% in women with endometriosis confined to the pelvis but 18% in women with bowel involvement

MANAGEMENT OF ENDOMETRIOSIS-ASSOCIATED INFERTILITY:

Conservative Surgery:
- Yields significantly increased pregnancy rate than does expectant management, in part because of correction of mechanical factors such as adhesions

Assisted Reproductive Technologies:
- Can be used to circumvent unknown mechanism of endometriosis-associated infertility
- Superovulation with clomiphene citrate or human menopausal gonadotropins; clomiphene citrate results in threefold pregnancy rate over either danazol or expectant management
- Further improvement with intrauterine insemination combined with superovulation
- In vitro fertilization if above unsuccessful

■ **DISPOSITION**

Tends to recur unless definitive surgery is performed

■ **REFERRAL**

To a reproductive endocrinologist for advanced surgical management or infertility management

☼ **PEARLS & CONSIDERATIONS**

■ **COMMENTS**

Patient information can be obtained through the following organizations: Endometriosis Association, 8585 North 76th Place, Milwaukee, WI 53223, 414-355-2200 or 800-992-ENDO; Women's Reproductive Health Network, P.O. Box 30167, Portland, OR 97230-9067; phone: 503-667-7757.

REFERENCES

Hornstein MD et al for the Lupron Addback Study Group: Leuprolide acetate depot and hormonal add-back in endometrosis: a 12-month study, *Obstet Gynecol* 91:16, 1998.

Johnson KM: Endometriosis: the immunoendocrine factor, *Female Patient* 21:15, 1996.

Olive DL, Pritts EA: Treatment of endometriosis, *N Engl J Med* 345:266, 2001.

Author: **Wan J. Kim, M.D.**

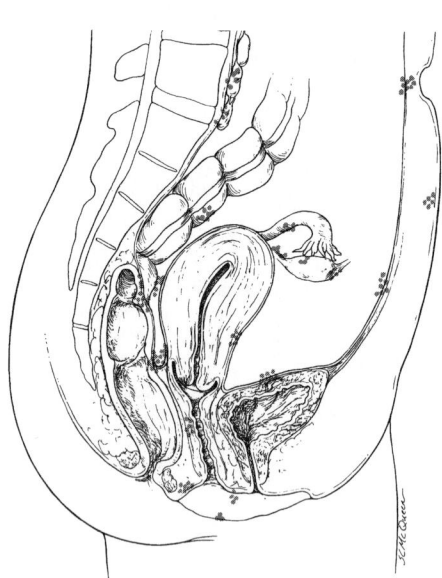

Fig. 1-140   Common pelvic sites of endometriosis. (From Mishell D [ed]: *Comprehensive gynecology*, ed 3, St Louis, 1997, Mosby.)

BASIC INFORMATION

■ DEFINITION
Endometritis is defined as a uterine infection following delivery or abortion.

■ SYNONYMS
Endomyometritis
Endoperimetritis
Metritis

ICD-9CM CODES
615.9 Endometritis

■ EPIDEMIOLOGY & DEMOGRAPHICS
- Overall rate of postpartum infection: estimated between 1% and 8%
- Most common genital tract infection following delivery
- Usually presents early in postpartum period; more commonly seen following C-section than vaginal delivery; also seen with an incomplete abortion (spontaneous abortion, legal abortion, or illegal abortion)
- Possible following any uterine manipulation in the presence of an undiagnosed cervicitis or vaginitis

■ PHYSICAL FINDINGS & CLINICAL PRESENTATION
- Postpartum oral temperature >37.8° C
- Localized uterine tenderness, purulent or foul lochia; physical exmination revealing uterine or parametrial tenderness
- Nonspecific signs and symptoms such as malaise, abdominal pain, chills, and tachycardia

■ ETIOLOGY
Endometritis is usually associated with multiple organisms: group A or B streptococci, *Staphylococcus aureus* and *Bacteroides* species, *Neisseria gonorrhoeae*, *Chlamydia trachomatis*, enterococci, *Gardnerella vaginalis, E. coli,* and *Mycoplasma.*

DIAGNOSIS

■ DIFFERENTIAL DIAGNOSIS
Causes of postoperative or postprocedural infections

■ WORKUP
Diagnosis based on symptoms of fever, malaise, abdominal pain, uterine tenderness, and purulent, foul vaginal discharge

■ LABORATORY TESTS
CBC, blood cultures, and uterine culture

■ IMAGING STUDIES
Ultrasound may be useful if retained products are considered a possible source of infection.

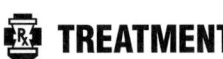

TREATMENT

■ ACUTE GENERAL Rx
- In treating endometritis after a vaginal delivery, ampicillin 2 g IV q6h plus gentamicin loading dose IV or IM (2 mg/kg of body weight), followed by a maintenance dose (1.5 mg/kg of body weight) q8h are used.
- Regimen should be continued for at least 48 hr after substantial clinical improvement. If response is not adequate, check cultures and treat with appropriate antibiotics (Table 1-29).
- Endometritis following C-section should be treated with ampicillin 2 g IV q6h plus gentamicin loading dose IV or IM (2 mg/kg of body weight), followed by a maintenance dose (1.5 mg/kg of body weight) q8h and clindamycin 900 mg IV q8h. If *Chlamydia* is one of the etiologic agents, add doxycycline 100 mg PO bid for completion of a 14-day course of therapy (if breast feeding, use erythromycin).

■ CHRONIC Rx
Watch for recurrent infection.

■ DISPOSITION
With appropriate antibiotic therapy, 95% to 98% cure rate.

■ REFERRAL
For patients who do not respond within 48 to 72 hr of appropriate antibiotic therapy, obtain an infectious disease consult or gynecologic consultation.

REFERENCE
Centers for Disease Control and Prevention: Sexually transmitted disease treatment guideline, *MMWR* 47(RR-1), 1998.
Author: **George T. Danakas, M.D.**

TABLE 1-29   Identified Causes of Poor Response to Antibiotic Therapy in Patients with Endometritis

CAUSE	APPROXIMATE PREVALENCE (%)
Infected mass, including abscess, hematoma, septic pelvic thrombophlebitis, pelvic cellulitis, retained placenta	40-50
Resistant organisms, commonly enterococci, in a patient receiving clindamycin-aminoglycoside or a cephalosporin	20
Additional cause, including catheter phlebitis, inadequate dose of antibiotics	10
No cause evident but response to empirical change in antibiotic therapy	20-30

From Gorbach SL: *Infectious diseases,* ed 2, Philadelphia, 1998, WB Saunders.

BASIC INFORMATION

■ DEFINITION
Enuresis refers to the voiding of urine into clothes or in bed that is usually involuntary but occasionally intentional in individuals who are expected to be continent (i.e., >5 yr of age). The diagnosis is made if voiding occurs at least twice a week for 3 mo.

■ SYNONYMS
Urinary incontinence
Bed-wetting
Self-wetting

■ ICD-9CM CODES
F98.0
DMS-IV Code 307.6

■ EPIDEMIOLOGY & DEMOGRAPHICS
PREVALENCE (IN U.S.):
- Age 5: 7% of males and 3% of females
- Age 10: 3% of males and 2% of females
- Age 18: 1% of males and even fewer females

PREDOMINANT SEX: Twice as many males as females
PREDOMINANT AGE: By definition, enuresis does not begin before age 5 yr, at which time the prevalence is highest, and decreases steadily through life.
PEAK INCIDENCE: Early childhood, ages 5 to 10 yr
GENETICS:
- Approximately 75% of children with enuresis have a first-degree relative with enuresis.
- Concordance rate may be higher in monozygotic twins than dizygotic twins.

■ PHYSICAL FINDINGS & CLINICAL PRESENTATION
Three subtypes are defined:
- Nocturnal only: usually occurs in first third of sleep, frequently during REM sleep; child may recall a dream with voiding.
- Diurnal only: more frequent in girls and rarely after age 9 yr; voiding occurs in early afternoon on school days.
- Combined nocturnal and diurnal enuresis.

■ ETIOLOGY
- No clear etiology
- Hypotheses: lax toilet training, stress, inability to concentrate urine, and altered smooth muscle physiology
- Diurnal enuresis associated with a higher rate of urinary tract infections

DIAGNOSIS

■ DIFFERENTIAL DIAGNOSIS
- May be associated with encopresis and sleep disorders such as sleep terrors
- Must rule out organic causes associated with polyuria or urgency but may coexist if enuresis was present before or after treatment of the associated medical condition

■ WORKUP
History and physical examination to rule out anatomic abnormalities
NOTE: Because children frequently experience shame, gentleness and care must be exercised when questioning or examining the child.

■ LABORATORY TESTS
- Urinalysis to determine specific gravity
- Urine culture to rule out urinary tract infection
- Serum studies to rule out diabetes and fluid balance abnormalities

■ IMAGING STUDIES
- In complicated cases: sleep studies possibly useful
- If an anatomic abnormality suspected: renal ultrasound or IVP possibly indicated

TREATMENT

■ NONPHARMACOLOGIC THERAPY
- Scheduled voiding to reduce the frequency of enuretic episodes
- Conditioning, psychotherapy, and bed alarms: all reported as useful but not found to be adequate by the children's caregivers

■ ACUTE GENERAL Rx
- Imipramine: used with mixed results; the use of tricyclic antidepressants in children is problematic because of the risk of sudden death.
- Serotonin reuptake inhibitors: lack of adequate trials is notable.

■ DISPOSITION
- After age 5 yr, the rate of spontaneous remissions is 5% to 10%/yr.
- Usually the disorder resolves by adolescence.
- Fewer than 1% will experience enuresis as adults.

■ REFERRAL
If coexisting psychiatric condition complicates the course of treatment
Author: **Rif S. El-Mallakh, M.D.**

BASIC INFORMATION

■ **DEFINITION**

Eosinophilic fasciitis is an inflammatory disease of the skin and subcutaneous tissue that is initially characterized by pain, swelling, and peripheral eosinophilia. This condition may progress to sclerosis and contractures.

■ **SYNONYMS**

Shulman's syndrome

ICD-9CM CODES

728.89 Eosinophilic fasciitis

■ **EPIDEMIOLOGY & DEMOGRAPHICS**

• Males and females are affected equally.
• The disease most commonly presents in the fourth and fifth decades.

■ **PHYSICAL FINDINGS & CLINICAL PRESENTATION**

• Initial presentation consists of swelling and pain with or without erythema.
• The extremities are usually symmetrically involved.
• Upper extremities are more commonly affected than lower extremities.
• The face, fingers, and toes tend to be spared.
• The skin may appear deeply rippled with an orange peel texture.
• Sunken veins may be seen when the extremity is elevated (Fig. 1-141).
• The groove sign marks the borders of different muscle groups.
• Arthritis is found in 40% of cases.
• Chronic complications are carpal tunnel syndrome and flexion contractures.
• Spontaneous resolution or improvement has been reported after 2 to 5 yr.

■ **ETIOLOGY**

• The etiology is unclear. A defect in humoral immunity has been hypothesized to cause the disease.
• Elevated polyclonal IgG levels and immune complexes have been associated with the disease.
• Eosinophilic fasciitis has been seen in association with myelodysplastic syndromes, aplastic anemia, thrombocytopenia, and Hodgkin's disease.

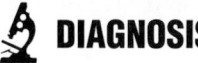 **DIAGNOSIS**

■ **DIFFERENTIAL DIAGNOSIS**

• Systemic sclerosis
• Chemical induced sclerosis
• Generalized lichen sclerosus et atrophicus
• Graft versus host disease
• Porphyria cutanea tarda
• Chronic Lyme borreliosis

■ **WORKUP**

• Physical examination to confirm characteristic distribution
• Some authorities suggest bone marrow biopsy to rule out hematologic malignancy

■ **LABORATORY TESTS**

• Peripheral eosinophilia in up to 70%
• Elevated erythrocyte sedimentation rate
• Hypergammaglobulinemia
• Occasionally thrombocytopenia and anemia

■ **DEEP TISSUE BIOPSY**

Skin biopsy that penetrates to muscle is optimal for diagnosis:
• Epidermis is usually normal.
• Dermis may demonstrate mild inflammation with lymphocytes, histiocytes, plasma cells, and eosinophils with some fibrosis.

• Subcutaneous tissue shows moderate inflammation and sclerosis of fat septa.
• Muscle demonstrates perivascular mixed inflammatory cell infiltrate.

■ **TREATMENT**

• Oral steroids are effective in most patients, but the duration and extent of symptom reduction are variable.
• Methotrexate and cimetidine have also been used.
• Surgery is sometimes required to reduce contractures and maintain function.

■ **DISPOSITION**

Prognosis is generally good with frequent spontaneous regression and response to steroids. However, 10% may develop blood dyscrasias and contractures are common.

■ **REFERRAL**

Dermatology referral may be needed for definitive diagnosis (biopsy). Functional impairment requires surgical evaluation.

Author: **James J. Ng, M.D.**

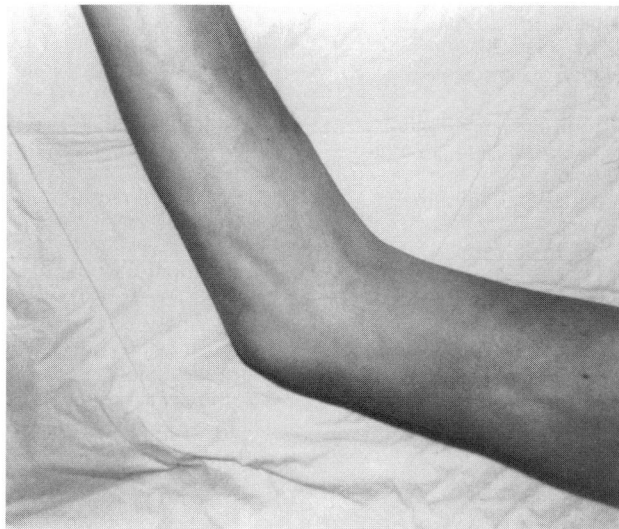

Fig. 1-141   Eosinophilic fasciitis. This 29-year-old butcher had to stop working because of generalized painful induration of his skin. Fingers were spared. As he raised his forearms the collapsed veins appeared as grooves (the "groove sign"), which is pathognomonic of eosinophilic fasciitis. Four years later his condition subsided, leaving joint contractures. (From Canoso J: *Rheumatology in primary care*, Philadelphia, 1997, WB Saunders.)

BASIC INFORMATION

■ DEFINITION
Eosinophilic pneumonias are a group of disorders characterized by infiltrates on chest radiographs (x-rays), pulmonary parenchymal eosinophilia, and peripheral blood eosinophilia.

ICD-9CM CODES
518.3 Eosinophilic pneumonia

■ EPIDEMIOLOGY & DEMOGRAPHICS
Varies depending on the specific cause of the pneumonia

■ PHYSICAL FINDINGS & CLINICAL PRESENTATION
- Usually a combination of fever, cough, and shortness of breath
- Varies depending on the specific cause

■ ETIOLOGY
SIMPLE PULMONARY EOSINOPHILIA (LÖFFLER'S SYNDROME):
- Transient infiltrates
- Symptoms range from asymptomatic to dyspnea and dry cough
- Usually idiopathic
- May be secondary to parasitic infection or drugs such as nitrofurantoin or penicillin
- Therapy consists of removing the offending agent
- If idiopathic and severe symptoms, then give glucocorticoid therapy

CHRONIC EOSINOPHILIC PNEUMONIA:
- Idiopathic disease
- Presents with productive cough, dyspnea, malaise, weight loss, night sweats, and fever
- Progressive peripheral pulmonary infiltrates
- Blood eosinophilia is not always present
- Diagnose by bronchoalveolar lavage (BAL) or lung biopsy
- Spontaneous remission in 10% of cases
- Treatment with glucocorticoids is rapidly effective
- Relapses are common

ALLERGIC BRONCHOPULMONARY ASPERGILLOSIS:
- Hypersensitivity reaction to *Aspergillus*

- Occurs most often in patients with asthma and atopy
- Fever, flulike symptoms, myalgias, and lassitude
- Chest x-ray: infiltrates (sometimes migratory) and atelectasis
- Blood and sputum eosinophilia
- Diagnosis by:
  1. *Aspergillus* isolation from multiple sputum samples
  2. Positive skin test to *Aspergillus* antigen
  3. Elevated serum IgE
  4. *Aspergillus*-specific IgE and IgG antibodies
- Treatment: systemic corticosteroids

TROPICAL PULMONARY EOSINOPHILIA:
- Onset of asthma, fever, marked blood eosinophilia
- Basilar reticulonodular and alveolar infiltrates
- Presumed etiology: filariasis

PULMONARY VASCULITIS (ALLERGIC GRANULOMATOSIS AND ANGIITIS):
- Vasculitis and necrotizing granulomatous inflammation that involves many organ systems
- Blood eosinophilia and elevated IgE levels

HYPEREOSINOPHILIC SYNDROME:
- A disease of elevated eosinophils with no known cause
- Cardiac problems are the prominent clinical feature
- Pulmonary involvement results in fever, cough, weight loss, and wheezing
- Diagnosis of exclusion
- Check echocardiogram
- Treat with steroids if symptoms or cardiac abnormalities

ACUTE EOSINOPHILIC PNEUMONIA:
- Acute onset of cough, dyspnea, fever, tachypnea, and rales
- Patients often require mechanical ventilation
- Tends to affect the young
- Often blood eosinophilia
- Chest radiographs show alveolar infiltrates
- BAL eosinophils often >20%
- Glucocorticoid therapy often leads to rapid improvement
- Relapses are rare

DIAGNOSIS

- Diagnosis varies depending on the specific cause of the eosinophilic pneumonia.
- Usually involves a combination of chest radiograph, peripheral eosinophil count, and BAL.

■ DIFFERENTIAL DIAGNOSIS
- Tuberculosis
- Brucellosis
- Fungal diseases
- Bronchogenic carcinoma
- Hodgkin's disease
- Immunoblastic lymphadenopathy
- Rheumatoid lung disease
- Sarcoidosis

■ WORKUP
Physical examination, laboratory tests, and bronchoscopy

■ LABORATORY TESTS
- WBC counts are often normal
- Often there is an increase in blood eosinophils
- BAL will often reveal an elevation in the eosinophil count

■ IMAGING STUDIES
Chest radiograph may show a variety of infiltrates depending on the cause of the eosinophilic pneumonia.

TREATMENT

- Varies depending on the cause of the pneumonia
- Remove or treat any offending agent
- Steroids may be helpful
- Supportive respiratory care

■ REFERRAL
Consultation with a pulmonologist may be necessary if a BAL is needed to establish the diagnosis.

Author: **Jennifer Clarke, M.D.**

BASIC INFORMATION

■ DEFINITION
Epicondylitis is an inflammation of the musculotendinous origin of the common extensors at the lateral elbow or the flexor pronator group at the medial elbow.

■ SYNONYMS
Tennis elbow (lateral epicondylitis)
Golfer's elbow (medial epicondylitis)

ICD-9CM CODES
726.31 Medial epicondylitis
726.32 Lateral epicondylitis

■ EPIDEMIOLOGY & DEMOGRAPHICS
PREVALENCE: 10% to 15% of regular (2 hr/wk) tennis players
PREVALENT AGE: 20 to 40 yr
The lateral side is involved 5 times more often than the medial.

■ PHYSICAL FINDINGS & CLINICAL PRESENTATION
- Local tenderness over affected epicondyle
- Reproduction of pain by resistance against wrist extension (lateral) (Fig. 1-142) or flexion (medial)

■ ETIOLOGY
- Unknown
- Overuse probably causing minor tendinous tears resulting in inflammation

🔬 DIAGNOSIS

■ DIFFERENTIAL DIAGNOSIS
- Cervical radiculopathy
- Intraarticular elbow pathology (osteoarthritis, osteochondritis dissecans, loose body)
- Radial nerve compression
- Ulnar neuropathy
- Medial collateral ligament instability

■ IMAGING STUDIES
Traction spur or minor soft-tissue calcification may be present on plain radiography. Other studies are not usually needed.

℞ TREATMENT

- Rest, restricted activities
- Ice after exercise
- Stretching exercise program
- NSAIDs

- Local steroid/lidocaine injection (Table 1-30), (Fig. 1-143)
- Counterforce brace
- Proper technique in sports activities
- Intermittent immobilization

■ DISPOSITION
Disorder is self-limited in most cases. Resolution of symptoms may take months to years.

■ REFERRAL
- If symptoms fail to respond to medical management
- For surgical consideration

REFERENCES
Chen FS, Rokito AS, Jobe FW: Medial elbow problems in the overhead-throwing athlete, *J Am Acad Orthop Surg* 9:99, 2001.
Hay EM et al: Pragmatic randomized controlled trial of local corticosteroid injection and naproxen for treatment of lateral epicondylitis of elbow in primary care, *BMJ* 319:964, 1999.
Author: **Lonnie R. Mercier, M.D.**

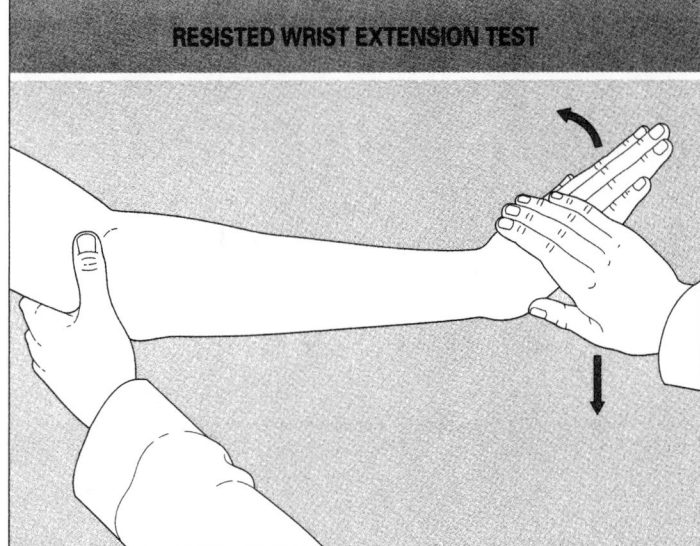

Fig. 1-142 Resisted wrist extension to test for lateral epicondylitis. The examiner asks the patient to try to extend the wrist, but prevents movement by fixing the wrist; this puts tension on the lateral epicondyle without moving the elbow and reproduces the pain of lateral epicondylitis. (From Klippel J, Dieppe P, Ferri F [eds]: *Primary care rheumatology,* London, 1999, Mosby.)

TABLE 1-30 **Guidelines for Common Steroid Injections**

Using 1 ml of the appropriate steroid, the volume is increased by the addition of local anesthetic. Injecting a "space" should not cause pain during the injection. If it does, the needle tip may be in the synovium, capsule, or fat pad, and the needle should be redirected or the shot may not be as effective. Injecting soft tissue should be performed slowly so as not to cause pain from the sudden volume pressure.

SITE	DIAGNOSIS	NEEDLE SIZE (GAUGE, INCHES)	ANESTHETIC VOLUME (ml)
Subacromial bursa	Rotator cuff tendinitis	22,1½	4 to 5
Bicipital groove	Biceps tendinitis	22,1½	2 to 3
A-C joint	Arthritis	25,1½	1 to 2
L, M epicondyle	Epicondylitis	25,⅝	1.5
First extensor sheath	De Quervain's disease	25,⅝	1.5
Trochanteric bursa	Tendinitis	22,spinal	4 to 5
Knee joint	Arthritis	22,1½	5 to 10
Knee, soft tissue	Tendinitis	25,1½	3 to 4
Plantar fascia	Fasciitis	25,1½	1.0
Toe MPJ	Arthritis	25,⅝	1.5

From Mercier LR: *Practical orthopedics,* ed 5, St Louis, 2000, Mosby.

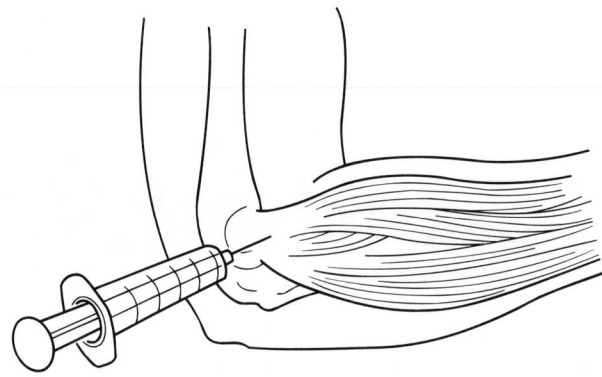

Fig. 1-143 Soft-tissue injection for lateral epicondylitis. The patient is supine, and the elbow is flexed 90 degrees. A 25-gauge needle is used to inject the tender spot, which is usually about 1 cm distal to the bony epicondyle. (From Mercier L: *Practical orthopedics,* ed 5, St Louis, 2000, Mosby.)

BASIC INFORMATION

■ DEFINITION
Epididymitis is an inflammatory reaction of the epididymis caused by either an infectious agent or local trauma.

■ SYNONYMS
Nonspecific bacterial epididymitis
Sexually transmitted epididymitis

ICD-9CM CODES
604.90 Nonvenereal epididymitis
098.0 Gonococcal epididymitis

■ EPIDEMIOLOGY & DEMOGRAPHICS
INCIDENCE (IN U.S.): Cause of >600,000 visits to physicians per year
PREDOMINANT SEX: Exclusive to males
PREDOMINANT AGE: All ages affected but usually in sexually active men or older males
PEAK INCIDENCE: Sexually active years
CONGENITAL: Congenital urologic structural disorders possibly predisposing to infections

■ PHYSICAL FINDINGS & CLINICAL PRESENTATION
- Tender swelling of the scrotum with erythema
- Dysuria and/or urethral discharge
- Fever and signs of systemic illness (less common)
- Pain and redness on scrotal examination
- Hydrocele or even epididymoorchitis, especially late
- Chronic draining scrotal sinuses with a "beadlike" enlargement of the vas deferens in tuberculous disease

■ ETIOLOGY
- In young, sexually active men, the most common infectious agents isolated are *N. gonorrhoeae* and *Chlamydia trachomatis.*
- In men >35 yr or with underlying urologic disease:
  1. Gram-negative aerobic rods are predominant.
  2. Similar organisms are found in men following invasive urologic procedures.
  3. Gram-positive cocci are rarely seen in these groups.
  4. Mycobacteria are also a cause of epididymitis.
- Young, prepubertal boys may present with epididymitis caused by coliform bacteria; almost always a complication of underlying urologic disease such as reflux.
- Recently, in AIDS patients, CMV and *Salmonella* epididymitis have been described. CMV may have a negative urine culture. Toxoplasmosis should also be considered as a cause of epididymitis in AIDS patients.

DIAGNOSIS

■ DIFFERENTIAL DIAGNOSIS
- Orchitis
- Testicular torsion, trauma, or tumor
- Epididymal cyst
- Hydrocele
- Varicocele
- Spermatocele

Box 2-222 describes the differential diagnosis of scrotal swelling.

■ WORKUP
- Consideration of a full assessment of the urologic tract in patients with bacterial infection, especially if recurrent
- Imaging with sonogram or IVP (possibly procedures of choice)
- If discharge is present: cultures and Gram stain
- In sexually active men: gonococcal cultures of the throat and rectum possibly of value
- If testicular torsion a consideration: radionuclear imaging

■ LABORATORY TESTS
- Urinalysis and urine culture if dysuria is present or if urinary tract infection is suspected
- VDRL in sexually active men
- PPD placed and chest x-ray viewed if TB suspected
- Rarely, biopsy to assure the diagnosis of tuberculous epididymitis

TREATMENT

■ ACUTE GENERAL Rx
- Ice packs and scrotal elevation for relief of pain
- Analgesia with acetaminophen with or without codeine or NSAIDs (such as ibuprofen or Naprosyn)
- Antibiotics to cover suspected pathogens
- In sexually active men, doxycycline 100 mg PO bid or tetracycline 500 mg PO qid for 10 days to cover both gonococci and chlamydiae; ceftriaxone 1 g IV or IM may be adequate for gonococci alone
- Best treatment for older men with gram-negative bacteria and leukocyturia: trimethoprim-sulfa DS PO bid or ciprofloxacin 500 mg PO bid, both for 10 to 14 days
- *Pseudomonas* covered by ciprofloxacin or ceftazidime (1 g IV q6-8h)
- Gentamicin in toxic-appearing patients (1 mg/kg IV q8h following a loading dose of 2 mg/kg): doses must be adjusted for renal function and these agents may be more toxic
- Vancomycin (1 g IV q12h) to cover suspected gram-positive infections
- Surgical aspiration of local abscesses or even open surgical drainage
- Diabetics: especially prone to develop more extensive scrotal infections, including Fournier's gangrene
- Reinforcement of compliance with antibiotics to avoid partial treatment

■ CHRONIC Rx
- Repair of underlying structural defects is considered especially if infections are severe or recur.
- Surgical repair of reflux in young boys should be undertaken promptly and at a young age when possible.

■ DISPOSITION
Usually self-limited

■ REFERRAL
- If abscess or chronic structural problems suspected
- If other diagnosis, such as testicular torsion, strongly considered

REFERENCE
Lott B: Epididymitis. In Rakel RE (ed): *Saunders manual of medical practice,* Philadelphia, 1996, WB Saunders.
Author: **Joseph J. Lieber, M.D.**

BASIC INFORMATION

■ DEFINITION
Epiglottitis is a rapidly progressive cellulitis of the epiglottis and adjacent soft tissue structures with the potential to cause abrupt airway obstruction.

■ SYNONYMS
Supraglottitis
Cherry-red epiglottitis

ICD-9CM CODES
464.30 Epiglottitis

■ EPIDEMIOLOGY
INCIDENCE (IN U.S.): Highest in young children, 2 to 4 yr old
INCIDENCE (IN U.S.): Unknown
PREDOMINANT SEX: Males
PEAK INCIDENCE: Peaks in young boys ages 2 to 4 yr, but it is reported in adults as well

■ PHYSICAL FINDINGS & CLINICAL PRESENTATION
• Irritability, fever, dysphonia, and dysphagia
• Respiratory distress, with child tending to lean up and forward
• Often, drooling or oral secretions
• Often, presence of tachycardia and tachypnea
• On visualization, edematous and cherry-red epiglottis
• Often, no classic barking cough as seen in croup
• Possibly fulminant course (especially in children), leading to complete airway obstruction

■ ETIOLOGY
• In children, *Haemophilus influenzae* type b is usual.
• In adults, *H. influenzae* can be isolated from blood and/or epiglottis (about 26% of cases).
• Pneumococci, streptococci, and staphylococci are also implicated.
• Role of viruses in epiglottitis unclear.

DIAGNOSIS

■ DIFFERENTIAL DIAGNOSIS
• Croup
• Angioedema
• Peritonsillar abscess
• Retropharyngeal abscess
• Diphtheria
• Foreign body aspiration
• Lingual tonsillitis

■ WORKUP
• Cultures of blood and urine
• Lateral neck radiograph to show an enlarged epiglottis, ballooning of the hypopharynx, and normal subglottic structures (Fig. 1-144)

1. Radiographs are of only moderate sensitivity and specificity and take time to perform.
2. Epiglottis should be visualized directly to secure diagnosis and only when prepared to urgently secure the airway.
3. Visualization of the epiglottis may be safer in adults than in children.
• Cultures of the epiglottis

■ LABORATORY TESTS
• CBC: may reveal a leukocytosis with a shift to the left
• Chest x-ray examination: may reveal evidence of pneumonia in close to 25% of cases
• Cultures of blood, urine, and the epiglottis, as noted above

TREATMENT

■ ACUTE GENERAL Rx
• Maintenance of adequate airway is critical.
• Early placement of an endotracheal or nasotracheal tube in a child is advised (Fig. 1-145).
• Closely follow adult patient and defer intubation, provided the airway reveals no signs of obstruction.
• In children, visualization and intubation are best done in the most controlled environment, such as an operating room; pay close attention to vital signs, oxygen saturation, respiratory rate, input, and output, since abrupt deterioration can occur.
• *H. influenzae* in children may be less common thanks to the HIB vaccine.
• Use antibiotics such as ceftriaxone (80 to 100 mg/kg/day in two divided doses), cefotaxime (50 to 180 mg/kg/day in four divided doses), or ampicillin (200 mg/kg/day in four divided doses) with chloramphenicol (75 to 100 mg/kg/day in four divided doses).
• If possible, obtain cultures before initiating antibiotics, but do not delay antibiotic therapy if cultures cannot be obtained quickly.
• Treat adult patients with similar antibiotic regimens.
• Give close family contacts of the patient who are <4 yr old rifampin 20 mg/kg/day for 4 days (up to 600 mg/day) for prophylaxis.
• Role of epinephrine or corticosteroids in the management of epiglottitis is not firmly established.

■ REFERRAL
For effective management:
• Close cooperation between the pediatrician or internist, anesthesiologist, and otorhinolaryngologist, especially when epiglottis is visualized and when the patient requires endotracheal intubation
• Best managed in a critical care setting or ICU
Author: **Joseph J. Lieber, M.D.**

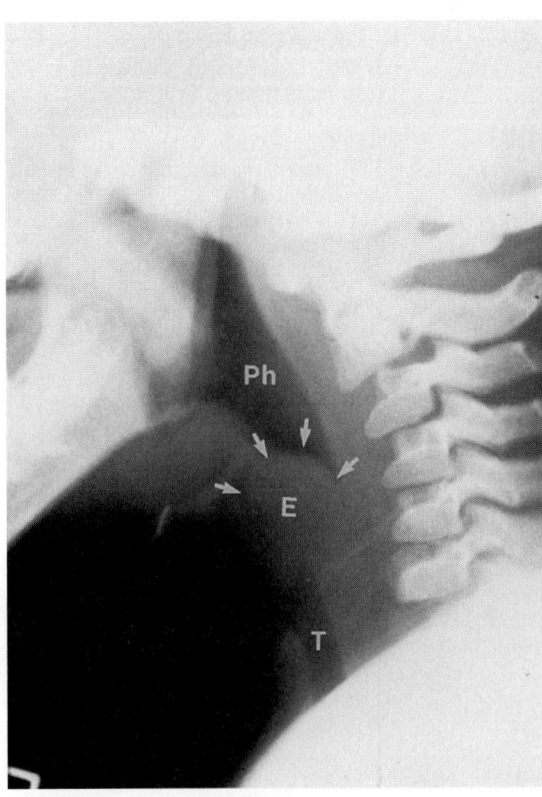

Fig. 1-144 Epiglottitis. A lateral soft tissue view of the neck shows a ballooned pharynx *(Ph)* with a swollen epiglottis *(E)* in the shape of a large thumbprint *(arrows)*. T, Trachea. (From Mettler FA [ed]: *Primary care radiology,* Philadelphia, 2000, WB Saunders.)

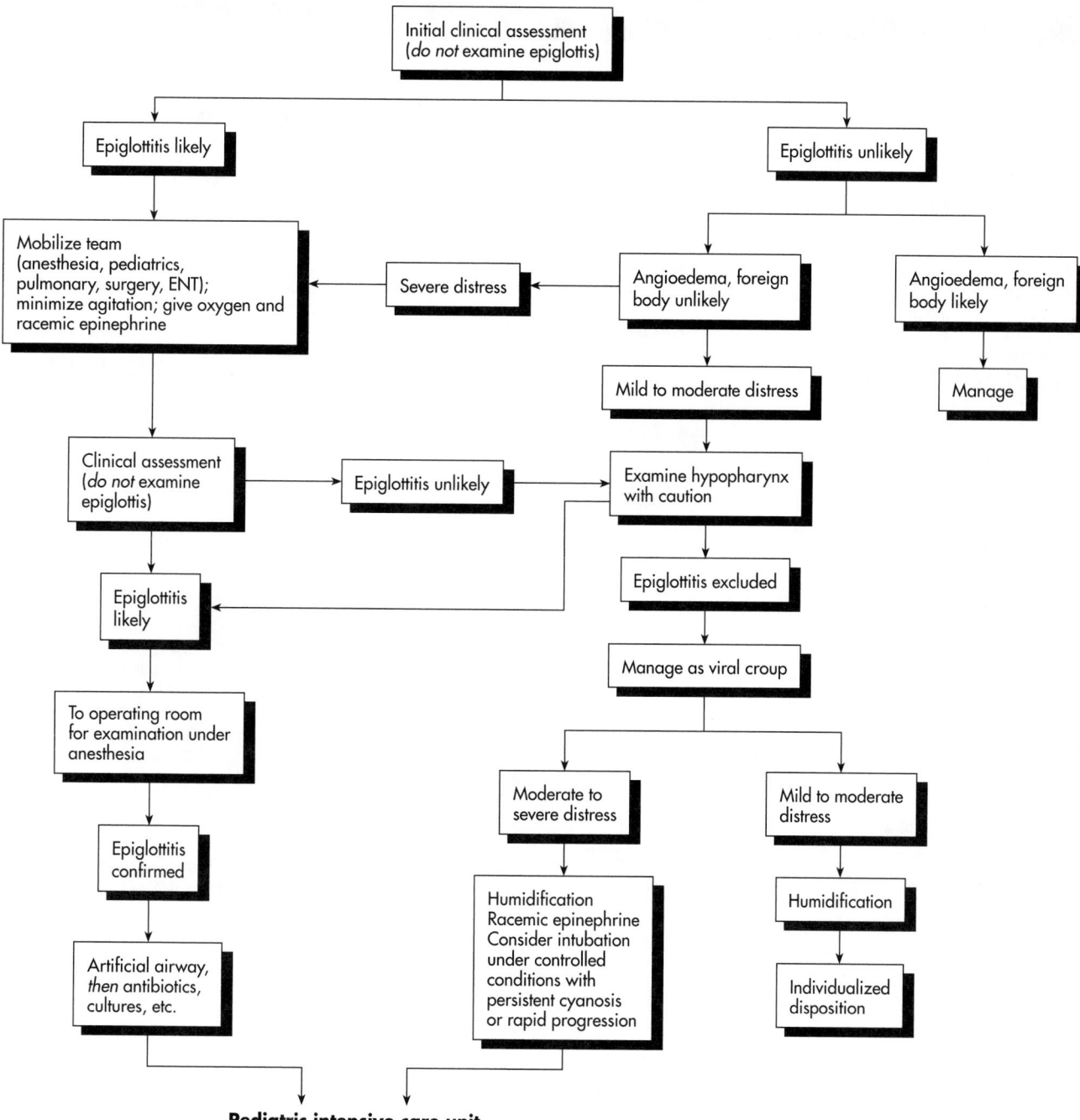

Fig. 1-145   Optimal assessment and management of upper airway obstruction caused by epiglottitis or severe croup. Care must be individualized to reflect resources and logistic issues within a given institution. *ENT,* Ear, nose, throat. (From Barkin RM, Rosen P: *Emergency pediatrics,* St Louis, 1999, Mosby.)

BASIC INFORMATION

■ DEFINITION

Episcleritis is an inflammation of the episclera, or thin layer of vascular elastic tissue between the sclera and conjunctiva.

ICD-9CM CODES
379.0 Scleritis and episcleritis

■ EPIDEMIOLOGY & DEMOGRAPHICS
INCIDENCE (IN U.S.): Relatively rare in an ophthalmologic practice
PREDOMINANT SEX: None
PREDOMINANT AGE: 43 yr
PEAK INCIDENCE: Most common in middle and old age

■ PHYSICAL FINDINGS & CLINICAL PRESENTATION
- Red, vascular injection of conjunctiva with engorged and enlarged blood vessels beneath the conjunctions (Fig. 1-146)
- Pain in area of inflammation

■ ETIOLOGY
Associated with collagen-vascular diseases

DIAGNOSIS

■ DIFFERENTIAL DIAGNOSIS
- Acute glaucoma
- Conjunctivitis
- Scleritis
- Subconjunctival hemorrhage
- Congenital or lymphoid masses
- Table 2-174 describes the differential diagnosis of "red eye."

■ WORKUP
Eye examination

■ LABORATORY TESTS
Studies for collagen-vascular disease

TREATMENT

■ NONPHARMACOLOGIC THERAPY
Warm compresses

■ ACUTE GENERAL Rx
Topical steroids, 1% prednisolone if no glaucoma; nonsteroidals if there is a tendency for glaucoma

■ CHRONIC Rx
NSAIDs such as Voltarin or Acular qid

■ DISPOSITION
Close follow-up needed

■ REFERRAL
To ophthalmologist if patient unresponsive to treatment after a few days

PEARLS & CONSIDERATIONS

■ COMMENTS
Usually related to systemic disease
Author: **Melvyn Koby, M.D.**

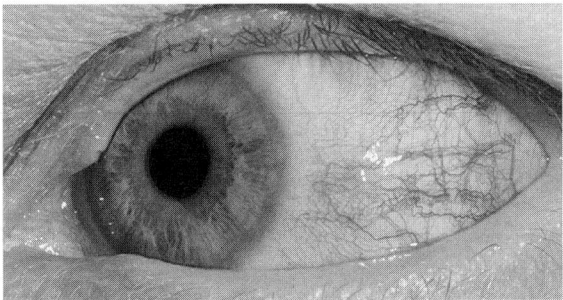

Fig. 1-146 Nodular episcleritis in a patient with gout. (From Palay D [ed]: *Ophthalmology for the primary care physician,* St Louis, 1997, Mosby.)

BASIC INFORMATION

■ DEFINITION
Epistaxis is defined as bleeding from the nose or nasal hemorrhage and is classified as either anterior or posterior.

■ SYNONYMS
Nosebleed

ICD-9CM CODES
784.7 Epistaxis

■ EPIDEMIOLOGY & DEMOGRAPHICS
- Epistaxis is usually anterior and occurs from Kiesselbach's plexus (Fig. 1-147)
- Only 5% of patients with epistaxis have posterior bleeds.

■ PHYSICAL FINDINGS & CLINICAL PRESENTATION
- Nosebleed
- Hypotension and hemodynamic instability with acute severe epistaxis.

■ ETIOLOGY
- The cause of epistaxis is multifactorial including:
  1. Cold, dry environment
  2. Trauma (nose picking, accidents, and physical altercations)
  3. Infection (sinusitis)
  4. Allergies
  5. Foreign bodies in the nasal cavity
  6. Tumors
  7. Irritants
  8. Hypertension
  9. Coagulopathy (hemophilia, von Willebrand's disease, thrombocytopenia)
  10. Osler-Weber-Rendu disease
  11. Renal failure
  12. Drugs: aspirin, nonsteroidal antiinflammatory drugs, warfarin, and alcohol

DIAGNOSIS

■ DIFFERENTIAL DIAGNOSIS
The differential diagnosis is as described under "Etiology."

■ WORKUP
The diagnosis of epistaxis is self-evident. The workup should include laboratory blood testing to exclude obvious causes and to prepare in case the bleeding cannot be stopped.

■ LABORATORY TESTS
- Hemoglobin and hematocrit
- Platelet count
- BUN/creatinine
- Coagulation studies (PT and PTT)
- Type and crossmatching of blood products

■ IMAGING STUDIES
X-ray studies are usually not helpful in the assessment of patients with epistaxis.

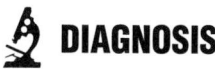

TREATMENT

■ NONPHARMACOLOGIC THERAPY
- Digital compression or pinching the nose for 4 to 5 min.
- Cotton or tissue plug.
- Bend forward at the waist allowing blood to flow out of the nostrils as opposed to bending backward, which would allow the blood to flow down the throat.
- Application of cold compresses to the bridge of the nose, causing a vasoconstrictive effect.

■ ACUTE GENERAL Rx
Anterior Epistaxis
- Local vasoconstriction is performed by moistening a cotton pledget with either:
  1. 4% lidocaine with 1:1000 epinephrine
  2. 4% lidocaine with 1% phenylephrine (Neo-Synephrine)
  3. 4% lidocaine with 0.05% oxymetazoline (Afrin)
  4. 4% cocaine

Then insert the pledget into the nasal cavity with bayonet forceps.
- Cauterization with silver nitrate is performed once hemostasis is achieved.

- Anterior nasal packing is needed when local measures are unsuccessful in controlling hemostasis. Nasal packing is done by inserting Vaseline gauze strips in layers from the floor of the nasal cavity to the front entrance of the nasal orifice. Enough pressure is placed to tamponade the epistaxis (Fig. 1-148).
- Other commercially available nasal packing using sponge packs that expand when exposed to blood or moisture can be used for anterior epistaxis.

Posterior Epistaxis
- Posterior nasal packing
  1. Commercially available nasal sponge packing can be applied.
  2. Rolled gauze technique (see reference)
- Foley catheter balloon insertion into the nasopharynx can be tried in patients with posterior epistaxis (for the proper technique, please refer to the reference).

■ CHRONIC Rx
- If acute treatment fails to stop the bleeding or the site of bleeding cannot be located, endoscopic cauterization can be used.
- Arterial ligation or embolization has been used in refractory posterior epistaxis.

■ DISPOSITION
- Most cases of anterior epistaxis from Kiesselbach's plexus can be stopped by nasal compression and local vasoconstriction or cauterization.
- Nasal packing with gauze or sponge can control 90% of anterior epistaxis.
- Anterior and posterior packs are removed in 2 to 3 days.
- Although rare, epistaxis can lead to death by aspiration of blood, hemodynamic compromise from rapid excessive blood loss, or toxic shock syndrome.

■ REFERRAL
- If epistaxis cannot be controlled in the acute setting by the above-mentioned nonpharmacologic and pharmacologic measures, ENT specialist should be called for assistance.

• ENT specialist should be consulted in any patient with posterior epistaxis requiring posterior packing.

PEARLS & CONSIDERATIONS

■ COMMENTS

• Silver nitrate cauterization, if done on both sides of the nasal septum, can lead to septal perforation and should be discouraged.

• If anterior nasal packing is done, broad-spectrum antibiotics (e.g., amoxicillin-clavulanate 250 mg PO tid or trimethoprim-sulfamethoxazole 1 tab PO bid) are used until the anterior packs are removed.
• Complications of nasal packing include
  1. Aspiration
  2. Dislodged packing
  3. Infection
  4. Nasal trauma

REFERENCES

Bentley B: Nasal emergencies. In Cline DM et al (eds): *Emergency medicine: a comprehensive study guide,* ed 4, American College of Emergency Physicians, New York, 1996, McGraw-Hill.

Kotecha B et al: Management of epistaxis: a national survey, *Ann R Coll Surg Engl* 78:444, 1996.

Tan LKS, Calhoun KH: Epistaxis, *Med Clin North Am* 83(1):43, 1999.

Viduich RA, Bland MP, Gerson LW: Posterior epistaxis: clinical features and acute complications, *Ann Emerg Med* 25:592, 1995.

Author: **Peter Petropoulos, M.D.**

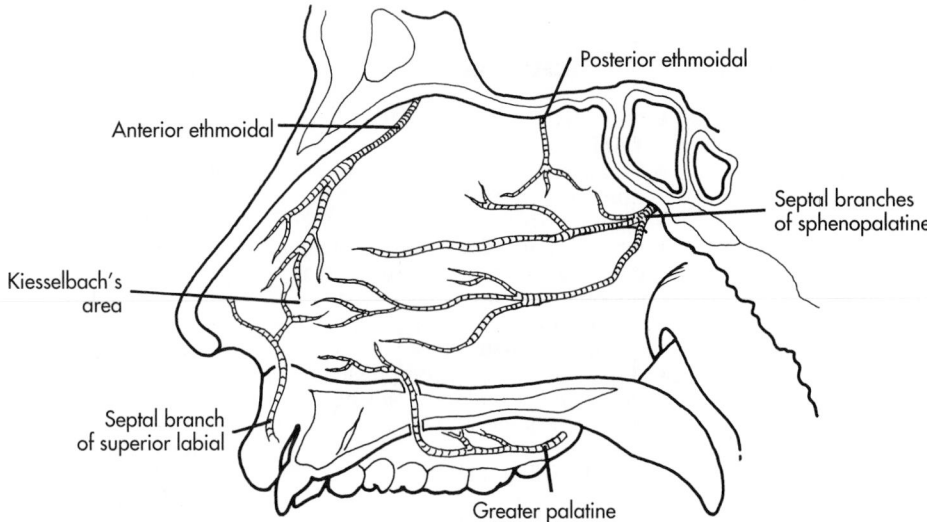

Fig. 1-147 Kiesselbach's plexus on the anterior septum derives blood supply from the superior labial, descending palatine, and sphenopalatine arteries. (From Noble J: *Primary care medicine,* ed 3, St Louis, 2001, Mosby.)

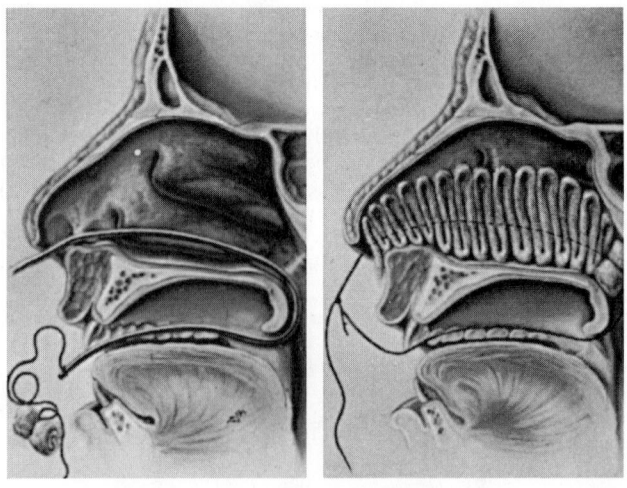

Fig. 1-148 Packing of the nose for epistaxis with a postnasal pack and an anterior nose pack. (From Boies LR et al: *Fundamentals of orolaryngology: a textbook of ear, nose, and throat diseases,* ed 4, Philadelphia, 1964, WB Saunders.)

BASIC INFORMATION

▪ DEFINITION
Epstein-Barr virus infection refers to a disease caused by Epstein-Barr virus (EBV), a human herpesvirus.

▪ SYNONYMS
Infectious mononucleosis

▪ ICD-9CM CODES
075 Mononucleosis

▪ EPIDEMIOLOGY & DEMOGRAPHICS
INCIDENCE (IN U.S.): 45 cases/100,000 persons/yr of infectious mononucleosis (IM)
PREDOMINANT SEX: Neither, although peak incidence occurs about 2 years earlier in women
PREDOMINANT AGE:
- Infectious mononucleosis: occurs most commonly between the ages of 15 and 24 yr.
- EBV infection: occurs earlier in life in lower socioeconomic groups.

▪ PHYSICAL FINDINGS
- Most EBV infections either are asymptomatic or cause a nonspecific illness.
- Incubation period is 1 to 2 mo, possibly followed by a prodrome of anorexia, malaise, headache, and chills; after several days, clinical triad of pharyngitis, fever, and adenopathy may appear, accompanied by fatigue and malaise.
- Pharyngitis is usually the most severe symptom; exudates are common.
- Lymphadenopathy is most prominent in the cervical region but may be diffuse.
- Splenomegaly is possible, most commonly during the second week of illness.
- Rash is uncommon, but will occur in nearly all patients who receive ampicillin.
- Possible IM presentation: fever and adenopathy without pharyngitis.
- Although complications may be severe, they are also uncommon and tend to resolve completely.
- Involvement of the hematologic, pulmonary, cardiac, or nervous systems possible; splenic rupture is rare.
- IM is usually a self-limited illness, but symptoms of malaise and fatigue may last months before resolving.
- Besides IM, EBV is also related to lymphoproliferative syndromes in transplant recipients and in AIDS patients.
- Increasing evidence showing an association between EBV infection and both African Burkitt's lymphoma and nasopharyngeal carcinoma.

▪ ETIOLOGY
- Ubiquitous virus
- Prevalence is higher in lower socioeconomic groups than in age-matched controls in more affluent groups.
- Infection during childhood is much less likely to cause significant illness.
- Frequency of IM in late adolescence is attributed to the onset of social contact between the sexes.
- Close personal contact is usually necessary for transmission, although EBV is occasionally transmitted by blood transfusion; transfer via saliva while kissing may be responsible for many cases.

DIAGNOSIS

▪ DIFFERENTIAL DIAGNOSIS
- Heterophile-negative infectious mononucleosis caused by CMV
- Although clinical presentation similar, CMV more frequently follows transfusion
- Bacterial and viral causes of pharyngitis
- Toxoplasmosis
- Acute retroviral syndrome of HIV
- Lymphoma

▪ WORKUP
Heterophile antibody and CBC

▪ LABORATORY TESTS
- Increased WBC common, with a relative lymphocytosis and neutropenia
- Hallmark of IM: atypical lymphocytes (not pathognomonic)
- Mild thrombocytopenia
- Falling Hct signaling splenic rupture
- Elevated hepatocellular enzymes and cryoglobulins in most cases
- Heterophile antibody
  1. As measured by the Monospot test, may be positive at presentation or may appear later in the course of illness.
  2. Negative test is repeated if clinical suspicion is high.
  3. A positive test has been reported with primary HIV infection.
- Virus-specific antibodies possibly responding to IM: determination of these EBV-specific antibodies is rarely necessary to diagnose IM

▪ IMAGING STUDIES
Chest x-ray examination:
- May rarely show infiltrates
- Possible elevated left hemidiaphragm with splenic rupture

☒ TREATMENT

▪ NONPHARMACOLOGIC THERAPY
- Supportive
- Rest advocated by some; impact on outcome not clear
- Splenectomy if rupture occurs
- Transfusions for severe anemia or thrombocytopenia

▪ ACUTE GENERAL Rx
- Pharmacologic therapy is not indicated in uncomplicated illness.
- Use of steroids:
  1. Suggested in patients who have severe thrombocytopenia or hemolytic anemia, or impending airway obstruction resulting from enlarged tonsils
  2. Prednisone 60 to 80 mg PO qd for 3 days, then tapered over 1 to 2 wk
- There is no role for antiviral agents such as acyclovir in the management of IM.

▪ CHRONIC Rx
An extremely rare, chronic form of IM with persistent fevers and other objective findings has been described and should be differentiated from chronic fatigue syndrome, which is not related to EBV.

▪ DISPOSITION
Eventual resolution of all symptoms

▪ REFERRAL
If more than mild illness

☼ PEARLS & CONSIDERATIONS

▪ COMMENTS
Avoidance of contact sports during the first month of illness, because splenic rupture can occur even in the absence of clinically detectable splenomegaly.

REFERENCES
Auwaerter PG: Infectious mononucleosis in middle age, *JAMA* 281:454, 1999.
Cohen JI: Epstein-Barr virus infection, *N Engl J Med* 343:481, 2000.
Vidrih JA et al: Positive Epstein-Barr virus heterophile antibody tests in patients with primary human immunodeficiency virus infection, *Am J Med* 111(3):237, 2001.
Author: **Maurice Policar, M.D.**

BASIC INFORMATION

■ DEFINITION
Erectile dysfunction is the inability to achieve or sustain an erection of adequate rigidity to make intercourse possible.

■ SYNONYMS
Impotence
Male erectile disorder
Sexual dysfunction (a nonspecific term)

■ ICD-9CM CODES
F52.2 Male erectile disorder (DSM-IV Code: 302.72 Male erectile disorder)

■ EPIDEMIOLOGY & DEMOGRAPHICS
INCIDENCE (IN U.S.): Unknown
PREVALENCE (IN U.S.):
- Increases with age
- Nearly 2% for men in their 40s, 25% for men in their 60s, 80% for men in their 80s

PREDOMINANT SEX: By definition, only in males
PREDOMINANT AGE: Increases with age
PEAK INCIDENCE: Over 70 yr old

■ PHYSICAL FINDINGS & CLINICAL PRESENTATION
- Psychogenic impotence: inability to obtain erection, inability to obtain or maintain an adequate erection, or the loss of erection before completion of sexual intercourse; nocturnal penile tumescence usually normal
- Organic impotence: inability to obtain an erection or inability to obtain an adequate erection; nocturnal penile tumescence usually abnormal

■ ETIOLOGY
- Psychogenic erectile dysfunction resulting from a wide range of experiential, historical, or even psychotic processes
- Organic impotence resulting from a wide variety of insults to neurologic, hormonal, or vascular structures
- Medications (antihypertensives, antidepressants, antipsychotics, histamine blockers, nicotine, alcohol, and others) commonly causative
- Endocrinopathies such as diabetes, hypogonadism, hypo- or hyperthyroidism, and hyperprolactinemia
- Neurogenic causes including spinal cord lesions, cortical lesions, and peripheral neuropathies

⚲ DIAGNOSIS

■ DIFFERENTIAL DIAGNOSIS
- Treatment dependent on the etiology
- Psychogenic dysfunction distinguished from organic
- Etiology of organic dysfunction to be determined
- Erectile dysfunction possible in the setting of another psychiatric condition (e.g., depression or obsessive-compulsive disorder)
- Box 2-145 describes the differential diagnosis of impotence.

■ WORKUP
- History (often including partner report) with a focus on risk factors (e.g., smoking, alcohol)
- Report of nocturnal erections
- Physical examination to rule out neuronal damage, direct penile damage (e.g., fibrosis), or testicular atrophy
- Fig. 3-150 describes a clinical algorithm for evaluation of sexual dysfunction.

■ LABORATORY TESTS
Screen for endocrinopathy with AM testosterone levels, fasting glucose, and thyroid profile.

■ IMAGING STUDIES
- Nocturnal penile tumescence very specific for distinguishing psychogenic and organic causes
- Vascular etiologies screened by the penile-brachial pressure index (measures the loss of systolic blood pressure between the arm and penis) or with Doppler studies
- Neurogenic etiolgies examined by the bulbocavernosus reflex or the pudendal-evoked response
- Intracorporeal injection of prostaglandin E_1 to distinguish vascular and nonvascular etiologies (erection is achieved in patients with nonvascular etiologies)

℞ TREATMENT

■ NONPHARMACOLOGIC THERAPY
- Various psychotherapeutic approaches: cognitive behavioral therapy preferred because it is the most focused; success rates decrease with advancing age and duration of symptoms.

- Sex therapy and couples' therapy are used to address technical or social issues that contribute to impotence.
- Vacuum devices (70% to 90% effective) work for many men, but they are difficult to use and cumbersome.

■ ACUTE GENERAL Rx
- Sildenafil (Viagra) 50 mg PO 1 hr before sexual activity; avoid concomitant use of nitrates
- Intracavernosal injections of vasodilators (e.g., papaverine or prostaglandin E_1 pellet)
- Oral medications such as pentoxifylline and yohimbine (limited success)

■ CHRONIC Rx
- Psychogenic impotence: open-ended, insight psychotherapies possibly curative but time-consuming and require extraordinary motivation
- Successful acute approaches maintained over time, but intracavernosal injections of papaverine associated with penile scarring
- For men failing other approaches: penile prosthesis (does not address issues of sexual drive or orgasm)
- Testosterone therapy in elderly hypogonadal males

■ DISPOSITION
- When erectile dysfunction is secondary to an organic cause, it does not remit unless the organic cause is corrected; therefore, it is usually a chronic condition.
- Psychogenic acquired erectile dysfunction will remit spontaneously in 15% to 30% of the cases.
- Lifelong erectile dysfunction is usually a chronic and unremitting condition.
- Situational erectile dysfunction may remit with changes in social environment, but it usually recurs.

■ REFERRAL
If psychotherapy, sex therapy, or invasive organic treatment required

REFERENCES
Goldstein I et al: Oral sildenafil in the treatment of erectile dysfunction, *N Engl J Med* 338:1197, 1998.
Miller TA: Diagnostic evaluation of erectile dysfunction, *Am Fam Physician* 61:95, 2000.
Author: **Rif S. El-Mallakh, M.D.**

BASIC INFORMATION

■ DEFINITION
Erysipelas is a type of cellulitis caused by infection of the superficial layers of the skin and cutaneous lymphatics. Erysipelas is characterized by redness, induration, and a sharply demarcated, raised border.

■ ICD-9CM CODES
035 Erysipelas

■ SYNONYMS
St. Anthony's fire

■ EPIDEMIOLOGY & DEMOGRAPHICS
Erysipelas occurs most often in the young or old, in patients with impaired lymphatic or venous drainage (mastectomy, saphenous vein harvesting), and in immunocompromised patients. Recurrence is relatively common.

■ PHYSICAL FINDINGS & CLINICAL PRESENTATION
- Distinctive red, warm, tender skin lesion with induration and a sharply defined, advancing, raised border is present (Fig. 1-149).
- Most common sites are lower extremities or face.
- Systemic signs of infection (fever) are often present.
- Vesicles or bullae may develop.
- After several days, lesions may appear ecchymotic.
- After 7 to 10 days desquamation of affected area may occur.

■ ETIOLOGY
- Usually group A β-hemolytic streptococci

- Less often group B, C, or G streptococci
- Rarely *Staphylococcus aureus*

■ COMPLICATIONS
- Abscess
- Necrotizing fasciitis
- Thrombophlebitis
- Gangrene
- Metastatic infection

DIAGNOSIS

■ DIFFERENTIAL DIAGNOSIS
- Other types of cellulitis
- Necrotizing fasciitis
- DVT
- Contact dermatitis
- Erythema migrans (Lyme disease)
- Insect bite
- Herpes zoster
- Erysipeloid
- Acute gout
- Pseudogout

■ WORKUP
History, physical examination, and laboratory evaluation

■ LABORATORY TESTS
Diagnosis is usually made by characteristic clinical setting and appearance.
- CBC and WBC often elevated
- Blood cultures positive in 5% of patients
- Gram stain and culture of any drainage from skin lesions
- Culture of aspirated fluid from leading edge of skin lesion has low yield

■ IMAGING STUDIES
- Duplex ultrasound for patients suspected of having DVT

- CT scan or MRI for patients with suspected necrotizing fasciitis

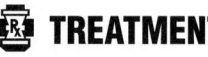

TREATMENT

■ NONPHARMACOLOGIC THERAPY
- Elevation of the affected limb
- Warm compresses

■ ACUTE GENERAL Rx
Typical erysipelas of extremity in non-diabetic patient:
- PO: penicillin V 250 mg to 500 mg qid
- IV: penicillin G (aqueous) 1 to 2 million units q6h

NOTE: Use erythromycin or cephalosporin in patients allergic to penicillin. Facial erysipelas (include coverage for *Staphylococcus aureus*):
- PO dicloxacillin 500 mg q6h
- IV nafcillin or oxacillin 2 g q4h

■ DISPOSITION
Prognosis is good with antibiotic treatment, but recurrence is common.

■ REFERRAL
For surgical debridement for patients with necrotizing fasciitis or for drainage of abscess

Author: **Mark J. Fagan, M.D.**

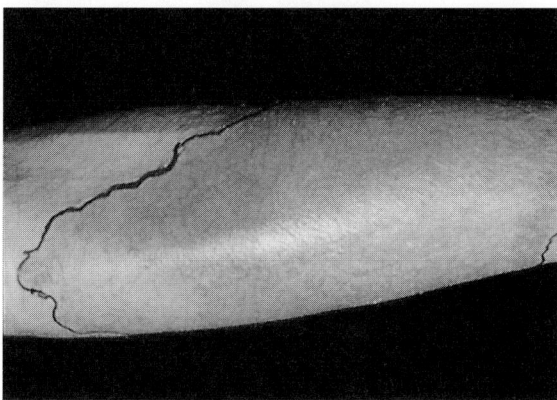

Fig. 1-149   Erysipelas. Note well-demarcated erythematous plaque on arm. (From Goldstein B [ed]: *Practical dermatology,* ed 2, St Louis, 1997, Mosby. Courtesy Department of Dermatology, University of North Carolina at Chapel Hill.)

BASIC INFORMATION

■ DEFINITION
Erythema multiforme is an inflammatory disease believed to be secondary to immune complex formation and subsequent deposition in the skin and mucous membranes.

■ SYNONYMS
EM

■ ICD-9CM CODES
695.1 Erythema multiforme

■ EPIDEMIOLOGY & DEMOGRAPHICS
- Predominant age: 20 to 40 yr
- Often associated with herpes simplex and other infectious agents, drugs, and connective tissue diseases

■ PHYSICAL FINDINGS & CLINICAL PRESENTATION
- Symmetric skin lesions with a classic "target" appearance (caused by the centrifugal spread of red maculopapules to circumference of 1 to 3 cm with a purpuric, cyanotic, or vesicular center) are present (Fig. 1-150).
- Lesions are most common in the back of the hands and feet and extensor aspect of the forearms and legs. Trunk involvement can occur in severe cases.
- Urticarial papules, vesicles, and bullae may also be present and generally indicate a more severe form of the disease.
- Individual lesions heal in 1 or 2 wk without scarring.
- Bullae and erosions may also be present in the oral cavity.

■ ETIOLOGY
- Immune complex formation and subsequent deposition in the cutaneous microvasculature may play a role in the pathogenesis of erythema multiforme.
- The majority of EM cases follow outbreaks of herpes simplex.
- In >50% of patients, no specific cause is identified.
- Erythema multiforme associated with bupropion use has been recently reported.

DIAGNOSIS

■ DIFFERENTIAL DIAGNOSIS
- Chronic urticaria
- Secondary syphilis
- Pityriasis rosea
- Contact dermatitis
- Pemphigus vulgaris
- Lichen planus
- Serum sickness
- Drug eruption
- Granuloma annulare

■ WORKUP
- Medical history with emphasis on drug ingestion
- Laboratory evaluation in patients with suspected collagen-vascular diseases
- Skin biopsy when diagnosis is unclear

■ LABORATORY TESTS
- CBC with differential
- ANA
- Serology for *Mycoplasma pneumoniae*
- Urinalysis

TREATMENT

■ NONPHARMACOLOGIC THERAPY
- Mild cases generally do not require treatment; lesions resolve spontaneously within 1 mo.
- Potential drug precipitants should be removed.

■ ACUTE GENERAL Rx
- Treatment of associated diseases (e.g., acyclovir for herpes simplex, erythromycin for *Mycoplasma* infection).
- Prednisone 40 to 80 mg/day for 1 to 3 wk may be tried in patients with many target lesions; however, the role of systemic steroids remains controversial.
- Levamisole, an immunomodulator, may be effective in treatment of patients with chronic or recurrent oral lesions (dose is 150 mg/day for 3 consecutive days used alone or in combination with prednisone).

■ DISPOSITION
The rash of EM generally evolves over a 2-wk period and resolves within 3 to 4 wk without scarring. A severe bullous form can occur (see "Stevens-Johnson syndrome").

■ REFERRAL
Hospital admission in patients with Stevens-Johnson syndrome

PEARLS & CONSIDERATIONS

■ COMMENTS
The risk of recurrence of erythema multiforme exceeds 30%.

REFERENCE
Lineberry TW et al: Bupropion-induced erythema multiforme, *Mayo Clin Proc* 76:664, 2001.
Author: **Fred F. Ferri, M.D.**

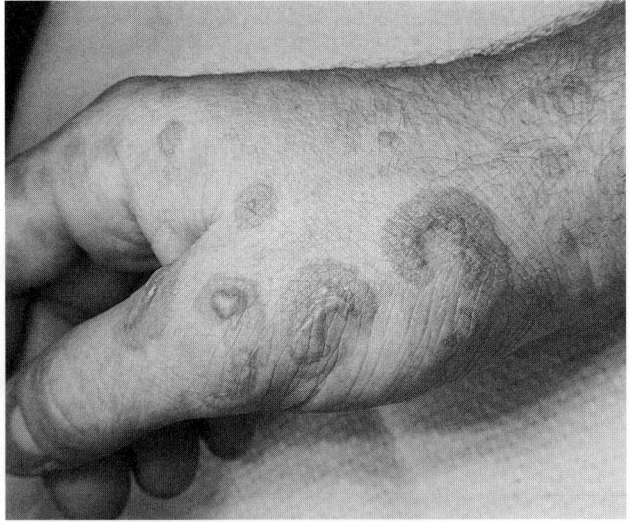

Fig. 1-150   Iris and arcuate lesions of erythema multiforme. Note erythematous lesions with multiform configurations—target, arcuate, and vesicles. (From Noble J et al: *Textbook of primary care medicine,* ed 2, St Louis, 1995, Mosby.)

BASIC INFORMATION

■ DEFINITION
Erythema nodosum is an acute, tender, erythematous, nodular skin eruption resulting from inflammation of subcutaneous fat, often associated with bruising.

ICD-9CM CODES
695.2 Erythema nodosum
017.10 Erythema nodosum, tuberculous, NOS

■ EPIDEMIOLOGY & DEMOGRAPHICS
INCIDENCE: 2 to 3 cases per 100,000 person per year
PEAK AGE: 25 to 40 yr
SEX DISTRIBUTION: Ratio of 3-4:1 (female:male)

■ PHYSICAL FINDINGS & CLINICAL PRESENTATION
- Acute onset of tender nodules typically located on shins (Fig. 1-151), occasionally seen on thighs and forearms.
- The nodules are usually ⅛ to 1 inch in diameter, but can be as large as 4 inches; they begin as light red lesions, then become darker and often ecchymotic. The nodules heal within 8 wk without ulceration.
- Associated findings:
  Fever
  Lymphadenopathy
  Arthralgia
  Signs of the underlying illness

■ ETIOLOGY
Cell-mediated hypersensitivity reaction seen more frequently in persons with HLA antigen B8. The lesion results from an exaggerated interaction between an antigen and cell-mediated immune mechanisms leading to granuloma formation.
Infections:
- Bacteria
  Streptococcal pharyngitis
  Salmonella enteritis
  Yersinia enteritis
  Psittacosis
  Chlamydia pneumoniae infection
  Mycoplasma pneumonia
  Meningococcal infection
  Gonorrhea
  Syphilis
  Lymphogranuloma venereum
  Tularemia
  Cat-scratch disease
  Leprosy
  Tuberculosis
- Fungi
  Histoplasmosis
  Coccidioidomycosis
  Blastomycosis
  Trichophyton verrucosum
- Viruses
  Cytomegalovirus
  Hepatitis B
  Epstein-Barr virus
- Drugs
  Sulfonamides
  Penicillins
  Oral contraceptives
  Gold salts
  Prazosin
  Aspirin
  Bromides
- Sarcoidosis
- Cancer, usually lymphoma
- Ankylosing spondylosis and reactive arthropathies (e.g., associated with inflammatory bowel disease)

DIAGNOSIS

■ DIFFERENTIAL DIAGNOSIS
- Insect bites
- Posttraumatic ecchymoses
- Vasculitis
- Weber-Christian disease
- Fat necrosis associated with pancreatitis

■ WORKUP
- Physical examination
- Diagnosis of underlying illness by history, physical examination, and laboratory tests as indicated

■ LABORATORY TESTS
- Erythrocyte sedimentation rate (ESR)
- Throat culture and antistreptolysin O titer
- PPD
- Others depending on index of suspicion

■ IMAGING STUDIES
- Chest x-ray for sarcoidosis and TB
- Skin biopsy in doubtful cases
  Early lesion: inflammation and hemorrhage in subcutaneous tissue
  Late lesion: giant cells and granulomata

TREATMENT

The disease is self-limited and treatment is symptomatic
- NSAIDs for pain
- Systemic steroids in severe cases

■ PROGNOSIS
Typical case:
- Pain for 2 wk
- Resolution within 8 wk

REFERENCE
Dixey J: Erythema nodosum. In Klippel JH et al (eds): *Rheumatology,* St Louis, 1994, Mosby.
Author: **Tom J. Wachtel, M.D.**

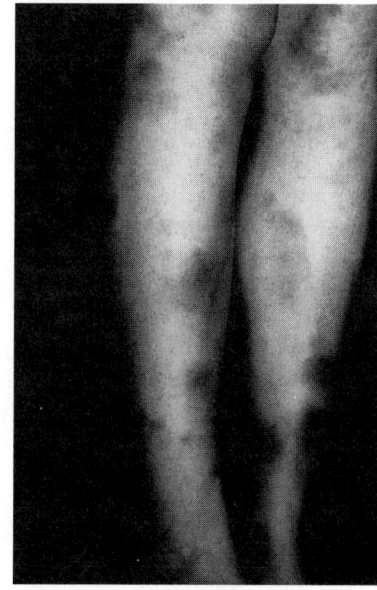

Fig. 1-151 Erythema nodosum. (From Arndt KA et al: *Cutaneous medicine and surgery,* vol 1, Philadelphia, 1997, WB Saunders.)

BASIC INFORMATION

■ DEFINITION

Esophageal tumors are defined as benign and malignant tumors arising from the esophagus. Approximately 15% of esophageal cancers arise in the cervical esophagus, 50% in the middle third of the esophagus, and 35% in the lower third. Eighty-five percent of esophageal tumors are squamous cell carcinoma (arising from squamous epithelium). Adenocarcinomas arise from columnar epithelium dysplastic in the distal esophagus secondary to chronic gastric reflux.

ICD-9CM CODES
150.9 Cancer, esophagus
230.1 Carcinoma of esophagus, in site

■ EPIDEMIOLOGY & DEMOGRAPHICS

Carcinomas of the esophageal epithelium, both squamous cell and adenocarcinoma, are by far the most common and important tumors of the esophagus. Benign neoplasms, leiomyoma, papilloma, and fibrovascular polyps are much less common. Prevalence of esophageal carcinoma varies widely in different parts of world, from 7.6 cases per 100,000 persons in the U.S. to 130 cases per 100,000 persons in China. It occurs frequently within the so-called Asian "esophageal cancer belt," extending from the southern shore of the Caspian Sea to northern China, with certain high-incidence pockets in Finland, Ireland, SE Africa, and NW France. In the U.S., it is more common among blacks than whites and males than females (male:female ratio of 3:1). It usually develops in the seventh and eighth decades of life and is an illness associated with lower socioeconomic status.

■ PHYSICAL FINDINGS & CLINICAL PRESENTATION

Symptoms and signs:
• Dysphagia: initially occurs with solid foods and gradually progresses to include semisolids and liquids; indicates incurable disease (60% or more involvement of the esophageal circumference with the tumor)
• Weight loss: usually of short duration
• Cervical adenopathy (supraclavicular lymph nodes)
• Clear cough suggesting tracheal involvement
• Aspiration pneumonia: caused by development of fistula with the trachea
• Massive hemoptysis or hematemesis resulting from the invasion of vascular structures
• Hoarseness suggesting recurrent laryngeal nerve involvement
• Odynophagia is an unusual symptom
• Advanced disease spreads to liver, lungs, and pleura
• Hypercalcemia is usually associated with squamous cell carcinoma because of the secretion of a tumor protein similar to the parathyroid hormone

■ ETIOLOGY

• Excess alcohol consumption accounts for 80% to 90% of esophageal cancer in the U.S., whiskey associated with higher incidence than wine or beer
• Cigarette smoking: ETOH and tobacco use combined together increase the risk substantially
• Other ingested carcinogens:
   Nitrates (converted to nitrites): South Asia, China
   Smoked opiates: Northern Iran
   Fungal toxins in pickled vegetables
• Mucosal damage
   Long-term exposure to extremely hot tea
   Lye ingestion
   Radiation-induced strictures
   Chronic achalasia: incidence is seven times higher
• Host susceptibility secondary to precancerous lesions
   Plummer-Vinson syndrome (Paterson-Kelly): glossitis with iron deficiency
   Congenital hyperkeratosis and pitting of palms and soles
   Caustic injury to esophagus
• Chronic GERD leading to Barrett's esophagus (whites are affected more than blacks).
• Possible association with dietary deficiencies of molybdenum, zinc, vitamin A; also associated with celiac sprue

DIAGNOSIS

■ DIFFERENTIAL DIAGNOSIS
• Achalasia of the esophagus
• Scleroderma of the esophagus
• Diffuse esophageal spasm
• Esophageal rings and webs

■ PHYSICAL EXAMINATION
• Findings are limited to cervical and supraclavicular lymph nodes

• Signs of lung consolidation from aspiration pneumonia

■ LABORATORY TESTS
Complete blood cell count, chemistries, liver enzymes

■ IMAGING STUDIES
• Double contrast esophagogram effectively identifies large esophageal lesions (Fig. 1-152).
• In contrast to benign esophageal leiomyomata, which cause esophageal narrowing with preservation of normal mucosal pattern, esophageal carcinomas cause ragged ulcerating changes in the mucosa in association with deeper infiltration.
• Smaller tumors can be missed by esophagogram, therefore esophagoscopy is recommended.
• Esophagoscopy is performed to visualize tumor and obtain histopathologic confirmation.
• Because same population is at risk for cancers of head, neck, and lung, endoscopic inspection of larynx, trachea, and bronchi should also be performed.
• Endoscopic biopsies may fail to recover enough tissue to confirm diagnosis, so cytologic examination of tumor should be routinely performed.
• Chest and abdominal CT scan should be performed to determine the extent of tumor spread to mediastinum, paraaortic lymph nodes, and liver.

TREATMENT

■ ACUTE GENERAL Rx
• Surgical resection of squamous cell and adenocarcinoma of lower third of the esophagus is done in most centers if there is no widespread metastasis.
• Less than 20% of patients who survive a total resection can be expected to survive after 5 yr. Usually stomach or colon is used for esophageal replacement.

POSSIBLE COMPLICATIONS OF SURGERY:
• Anatomic fistula (usually with colon interposition, subphrenic abscesses); respiratory complications are less common as a result of advances in surgical techniques, respiratory therapy, hyperalimentation, and anesthetic support during surgery. Cardiovascular complications are by far the most common including MI, CVA, and PE.

- Squamous cell carcinomas are more radiosensitive than adenocarcinoma, and radiation achieves good local control and is an excellent palliative modality for obstructive symptoms. Usually employed for tumors in upper third of esophagus, often for middle third tumors as well.
- About 40% of tumors cannot be destroyed even after 6000 rads.
- Palliative radiation therapy for bone metastasis is also effective.

COMPLICATIONS OF RADIATION THERAPY:

- Esophageal stricture, radiation-induced pulmonary fibrosis, transverse myelitis: less common with modern techniques, radiation-induced cardiomyopathy, and skin changes.

- Single agent resulted in significant tumor regression in 15% to 25% of patients and combination chemotherapy including cisplatin achieved significant tumor reduction in 30% to 60% of patients.
- Vary with agent used and include mucositis, GI toxicity, and myelosuppression in general. With cisplatin nephrotoxicity, ototoxicity and neurotoxicity can develop.

COMBINATION CHEMOTHERAPY, RADIATION Rx, AND SURGICAL Rx:

- Combination therapy has been found to be associated with increased mortality rate and does not confer a survival advantage.
- Palliative procedures such as repeated endoscopic dilatation, surgical placement of feeding tube, or polyvinyl prosthesis to bypass tumors have been used for surgically unresectable patients.

■ **DISPOSITION**

- Surgery: 5-yr survival rate is 48% in stages I and II, 20% in advanced stages
- Radiation therapy: 5-year survival rate is between 6% and 20%
- Chemotherapy: Simple agent response rate 15% to 38%; combination response rate 80%
- Combined modality: 18% response rate

Author: **Madhavi Yerneni, M.D.**

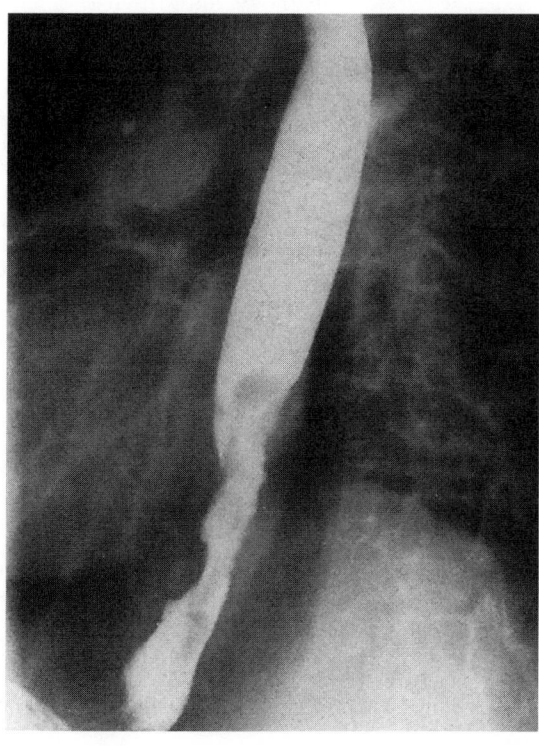

Fig. 1-152   Barium swallow demonstrating the classic findings in cancer of the distal third of the esophagus. (From Noble J [ed]: *Primary care medicine,* ed 2, St Louis, 1996, Mosby.)

BASIC INFORMATION

■ DEFINITION
Acute fatty liver of pregnancy (AFLP) is characterized histologically by microvesicular fatty cytoplasmic infiltration of hepatocytes with minimal hepatocellular necrosis.

■ SYNONYMS
Acute fatty metamorphosis
Acute yellow atrophy

ICD-9CM CODES
646.7 Liver disorders in pregnancy

■ EPIDEMIOLOGY & DEMOGRAPHICS
INCIDENCE:
- Approximately 1 in 10,000 pregnancies
- Equal frequencies in all races and at all maternal ages

AVERAGE GESTATIONAL AGE: 37 wk (range 28 to 42 wk)

RISK FACTORS:
- Primiparity
- Multiple gestation
- Male fetus

GENETICS: Some with a familial deficiency of long-chain 3-hydroxyacyl-CoA dehydrogenase (LCHAD)

■ PHYSICAL FINDINGS & CLINICAL PRESENTATION
- Initial manifestations:
  1. Nausea and vomiting (70%)
  2. Pain in RUQ or epigastrium (50% to 80%)
  3. Malaise and anorexia
- Jaundice often in 1 to 2 wk
- Late manifestations:
  1. Fulminant hepatic failure
  2. Encephalopathy
  3. Renal failure
  4. Pancreatitis
  5. GI and uterine bleeding
  6. Disseminated intravascular coagulation
  7. Seizures
  8. Coma
- Liver
  1. Usually small
  2. Normal or enlarged in preeclampsia, eclampsia, HELLP (hemolysis, elevated liver enzymes, and low platelets) syndrome, and acute hepatitis
  3. Coexistent preeclampsia in up to 46% of patients

■ ETIOLOGY
- Postulated that inhibition of mitochondrial oxidation of fatty acids may lead to microvesicular fatty infiltration of liver.
- Fatty metamorphosis of preeclamptic liver disease thought to be of different etiology.

DIAGNOSIS

■ DIFFERENTIAL DIAGNOSIS
- Acute gastroenteritis
- Preeclampsia or eclampsia with liver involvement
- HELLP syndrome
- Acute viral hepatitis
- Fulminant hepatitis
- Drug-induced hepatitis caused by halothane, phenytoin, methyldopa, isoniazid, hydrochlorothiazide, or tetracycline
- Intrahepatic cholestasis of pregnancy
- Gallbladder disease
- Reye's syndrome
- Hemolytic-uremic syndrome
- Budd-Chiari syndrome
- SLE
- Table 2-123 describes the differential diagnosis of liver disease in pregnancy.

■ WORKUP
- A clinical diagnosis is based predominantly on physical and laboratory findings.
- Most definitive diagnosis is through liver biopsy with oil red O staining and electron microscopy.
- Liver biopsy is reserved for atypical cases only and only after any existing coagulopathy corrected with FFP.

■ LABORATORY TESTS
Tests to determine the following:
- Hypoglycemia (often profound)
- Hyperammonemia
- Elevated aminotransferases (usually <500 U/ml)
- WBC count >15,000
- Hyperbilirubinemia (usually <10 mg/dl)
- Low albumin
- DIC (in 75%)

■ IMAGING STUDIES
- Ultrasound: best used to rule out other diseases in the differential diagnosis such as gallbladder disease
- CT scan: plays minimal role because of a high false-negative rate

TREATMENT

■ NONPHARMACOLOGIC THERAPY
- Patient is admitted to intensive care unit for stabilization.
- Fetus is delivered; spontaneous resolution usually follows delivery.
- Mode of delivery is based on obstetric indications and clinical assessment of disease severity.

■ ACUTE GENERAL Rx
- Decrease in endogenous ammonia through dietary protein restriction; neomycin 6 to 12 g/day PO to decrease presence of ammonia-producing bacteria; magnesium citrate 30 to 50 ml PO or enema to evacuate nitrogenous wastes from colon
- Administration of intravenous fluids with glucose to keep glucose levels >60 mg/dl
- Coagulopathy corrected with FFP
- Avoidance of drugs metabolized by liver
- Aggressive avoidance and treatment for nosocomial infections; consideration of prophylactic antibiotics

■ CHRONIC Rx
Orthotopic liver transplantation is the only treatment for irreversible liver failure.

■ DISPOSITION
- Before 1980, both maternal and fetal mortalities: approximately 85%
- After 1980, both maternal and fetal mortalities: below 20%
- Usually rapid return of liver function to normal after delivery
- Minimal risk of recurrence with future pregnancies

■ REFERRAL
To tertiary health care facility as soon as diagnosis is suspected

REFERENCES
Cunningham FG et al: Gastrointestinal disorders. In Cunningham FG et al (eds): *Williams' obstetrics,* ed 20, Stamford, Conn, 1997, Appleton & Lange.

Davidson KM: Acute fatty liver of pregnancy, *Postgrad Obstet Gynecol* 15:1, 1995.

Knox TA, Olans LB: Liver disease in pregnancy, *N Engl J Med* 335:569, 1996.

Sawai SK: Acute fatty liver of pregnancy. In Foley MR, Strong TH Jr: *Obstetric intensive care: a practical manual,* Philadelphia, 1997, WB Saunders.
Author: **Wan J. Kim, M.D.**

BASIC INFORMATION

■ **DEFINITION**
Felty's syndrome (FS) is defined as the triad of rheumatoid arthritis (RA), splenomegaly, and leukopenia. It is an extraarticular manifestation of seropositive RA in which recurrent local and systemic infections are the major source of morbidity and mortality.

ICD-9CM CODES
714.1 Felty's syndrome

■ **EPIDEMIOLOGY & DEMOGRAPHICS**
• FS occurs in less than 1% of patients with RA
• 60% to 70% are women
• Recognized in the fifth through seventh decades in patients who have had RA for 10 yr or more

■ **PHYSICAL FINDINGS & CLINICAL PRESENTATION**
• Rarely, splenomegaly and granulocytopenia are present before the arthritis.
• Articular involvement is usually more severe in patients with FS as compared to other patients with RA; however, one third may have relatively inactive synovitis with elevated ESR.
• Degree of splenomegaly varies and may be detectable only by imaging studies.
• The degree of splenomegaly has no correlation with the degree of granulocytopenia.
• FS patients have a greater frequency of extraarticular manifestations (nodules, weight loss, Sjögren's syndrome, etc.) than other patients with RA.
• Approximately 25% of patients have refractory leg ulcers, often associated with hyperpigmentation of the anterior tibia.
• Mild hepatomegaly is common (up to 68%).

■ **ETIOLOGY**
The pathogenesis of FS is probably multifactorial and no clear explanation has been elucidated.
Proposed mechanisms of the neutropenia:

• Splenic sequestration and peripheral destruction of granulocytes secondary to immune complexes and antineutrophil antibodies
• Impaired granulopoiesis as a result of decreased cytokine production, presence of inhibitors, or humoral and cell-mediated immune suppression
• Excessive margination

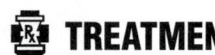 **DIAGNOSIS**

■ **DIFFERENTIAL DIAGNOSIS**
• Drug reaction
• Myeloproliferative disorders
• Lymphoma/reticuloendothelial malignancies
• Hepatic cirrhosis with portal hypertension
• Sarcoidosis
• Tuberculosis
• Amyloidosis
• Chronic infections

■ **WORKUP**
Physical examination and laboratory evaluation

■ **LABORATORY TESTS**
• Complete blood count with differential, looking for:
  1. Neutropenia
  2. Mild to moderate anemia
  3. Mild thrombocytopenia
• ESR
• Bone marrow biopsy in most patients will show myeloid metaplasia with an excess of immature granulocyte precursors ("maturation arrest")
• Rheumatoid factor: positive in 98%, usually high titer
• ANA: positive in 67%
• Antihistone antibody: positive in 83%
• HLA-DR4: positive in 95%
• Immunoglobulins: level usually high
• Complement: level usually low

■ **IMAGING STUDIES**
Ultrasonography or CT scan may be useful in diagnosing splenomegaly

TREATMENT

There is no uniformly effective therapy for FS.

■ **ACUTE GENERAL Rx**
Splenectomy
• Standard therapy since 1932
• Acutely reverses hematologic abnormalities
• 25% to 30% will have recurrent neutropenia
• Improvement in frequency of recurrent infection variable and not correlated with hematologic improvement
• Usually reserved for patients with profound neutropenia and severe recurrent infections
Lithium
• Stimulates granulopoiesis
• No demonstration of long-term benefit or conclusive reduction in rate of infection
• Used as short-term therapy while awaiting response to other measures
Parenteral testosterone
• Efficacy limited by toxicity, especially in women
Corticosteroids
• Pulse dosing is a potential alternative for short-term elevation of neutrophils
Antirheumatic drugs
• Gold salt injections
• Penicillamine
• Methotrexate
Recombinant G-CSF
• Improves neutrophil count but not arthritis and anemia of FS
• May be useful as adjunctive therapy during serious infection or in preparation for surgery
Infection
• Patients with FS have a 20 times increased frequency of infections as compared to other RA patients.
• There is usually an adequate response to appropriate antibiotic therapy.

■ **REFERRAL**
• To rheumatologist for treatment of RA
• To hematologist for treatment of leukopenia
Author: **Rebecca A. Griffith, M.D.**

BASIC INFORMATION

■ DEFINITION
A femoral neck fracture occurs within the capsule of the hip joint between the base of the head and the intertrochanteric line.

■ SYNONYMS
Intracapsular fracture

ICD-9CM CODES
820.8 Femoral neck fracture

■ EPIDEMIOLOGY & DEMOGRAPHICS
PREVALENCE: Lifetime risk in women approximately 16%
PREVALENT SEX: Female:male 3:1
PREVALENT AGE: 90% over age 60

■ PHYSICAL FINDINGS & CLINICAL PRESENTATION
- A hip or groin pain
- Affected limb usually shortened and externally rotated in displaced fractures
- Impacted fractures: possibly no deformity and only mild pain with hip motion
- Mild external bruising

■ ETIOLOGY
- Trauma
- Age-related bone weakness, usually caused by osteoporosis
- Increased risk fractures in elderly (decline in muscle function, use of psychotropic medication, etc.)

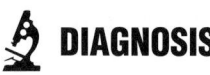

DIAGNOSIS

■ DIFFERENTIAL DIAGNOSIS
Pathologic fracture

■ WORKUP
Diagnosis usually obvious based on clinical and radiographic findings

■ IMAGING STUDIES
- Standard roentgenograms consisting of an AP of the pelvis and a cross-table lateral of the hip to confirm the diagnosis (Fig. 1-153)

- If initial roentgenograms negative and diagnosis of an occult femoral neck fracture suspected, hospital admission and further radiographic assessment with either bone scanning or MRI
- Bone scanning most sensitive after 48 to 72 hr.

TREATMENT

- Orthopedic consultation
- Surgery indicated in most cases, usually within 24 hr
- DVT prophylaxis

■ DISPOSITION
- Mortality rate within 1 yr in elderly patients is 25% to 30%.
- Dementia is a particularly poor prognostic sign.

PEARLS & CONSIDERATIONS

■ COMMENTS
- Complications: nonunion and avascular necrosis
- Intracapsular fractures: occasionally occur in nonambulatory patients
  1. Usually treated nonsurgically, especially in the patient with dementia and limited pain perception

2. Early bed-to-chair mobilization and vigilant nursing care to avoid skin breakdown
3. Fracture usually pain free in a short time even if solid bony healing does not occur
- As a result of the increasing life span of the female population, femoral neck fractures are becoming more common. The initial physical examination and roentgenographic studies may be completely negative. Groin pain, sometimes quite severe, may be the only early clue to the diagnosis.
- The rate of hip fracture could be reduced by:
  1. Elimination of environmental hazards (poor lighting, loose rugs)
  2. Regular exercise for balance and strength
  3. Patient education about fall prevention
  4. Medication review to minimize side effects
  5. Prevention and treatment of osteoporosis

REFERENCES
McClung MR et al: Effect of risedronate on the risk of hip fracture in elderly women. Hip Intervention Program Study Group, *N Engl J Med* 344(5):333, 2001.
Stevens JA, Olson S: Reducing falls and resulting hip fractures among older women, *Home Care Prov* 5(4)134, 2000.
Author: **Lonnie R. Mercier, M.D.**

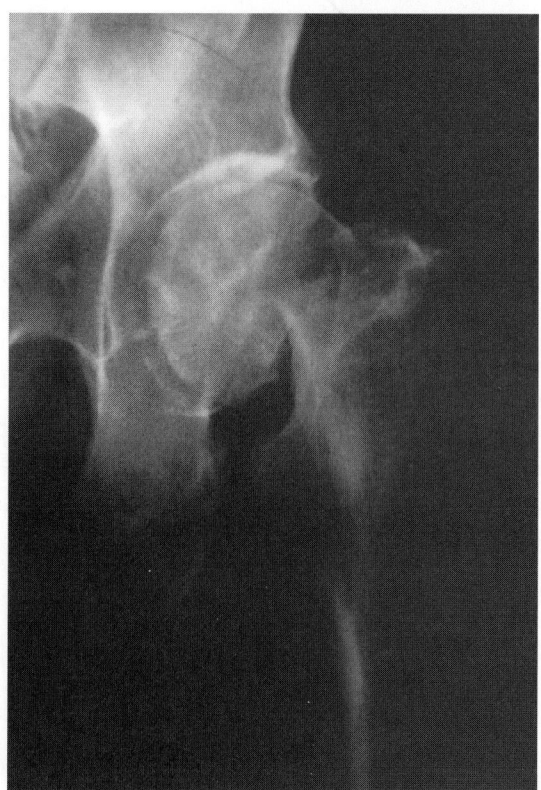

Fig. 1-153 Femoral neck fracture. (From Scudieri G [ed]: *Sports medicine: principles of primary care,* St Louis, 1997, Mosby.)

BASIC INFORMATION

■ DEFINITION

Fever of undetermined origin (FUO) was defined by Petersdorf in 1961 as an illness characterized by temperatures surpassing 101° F for more than 3 wk with no known cause despite extensive workup.

- Persistence for greater than 2 wk separates a FUO from an insignificant viral illness.
- Traditionally, diagnosis made only after at least a 1-wk inpatient workup.
- In contemporary practice, much of the workup is performed outpatient; taking time for a complete history and physical examination is still essential.
- Different settings—community vs. hospital vs. oncology ward—dictate duration needed for FUO designation.

ICD-9CM CODES

780.6 Pyrexia of undetermined origin

■ EPIDEMIOLOGY & DEMOGRAPHICS

Incidence is difficult to calculate because of inconsistent designation of febrile illnesses as FUO.

■ ETIOLOGY

Classic (1 wk workup after 2 wk persistently febrile): Divided among infection, malignancy, collagen-vascular, and other etiology; proportion for each dependent on age and geography. A partial list of eventual etiologies, with most common diagnoses in *italics*:

- *Factitious fever, Munchausen syndrome*
- *Abscess: dental, abdominal, pelvic*
- *Lymphoma and leukemia*
- Endocarditis
- Biliary tract infection
- Osteomyelitis
- Tuberculosis
- Whipple's disease
- Psittacosis
- Fungal: histoplasmosis, cryptomycosis
- Leishmaniasis
- Renal cell carcinoma, other solid malignancies
- Systemic lupus erythematosus
- Still's disease
- Hypersensitivity vasculitis
- Temporal arteritis
- Drug-induced fever
- Inflammatory bowel disease
- Sarcoidosis
- Granulomatous hepatitis
- Central fever (rare)

Neutropenic (PMN <500 and febrile >3 days): with blood cultures from onset negative, ruling out *Pseudomonas* and other gram-negative bacteremia, staphylococcal bacteremia from line infection; urinalysis and chest x-ray negative. Possible etiologies:

- Perianal infection
- Occult fungal infection
- Drug fever

HIV-associated: Etiology depends on CD4 count. HIV itself may be the cause. With low CD4 count—MAI bacteremia, lymphoma.

Nosocomial (febrile for 3 days in hospital): UTI, pneumonia, line-related bacteremia, *Clostridium difficile* diarrhea, or sinusitis secondary to intubation

- Noninfectious etiology: deep venous thrombosis, hematoma, drug fever

DIAGNOSIS

■ DIFFERENTIAL DIAGNOSIS

Factitious fever: body temperature not elevated when accurately measured.

■ WORKUP

- Accurate history and careful physical examination is essential.
- Laboratory tests and radiologic examinations dependent on historical clues, physical findings.
- "Shotgun" approach, ordering every test for every possibility, is rarely helpful.
- Tests and procedures should be thoughtful, directed toward localizing signs and symptoms (Fig. 1-154).
- When in doubt, perform another complete history and physical examination.

■ HISTORICAL CLUES

- Fever duration, tempo; inciting factors
- Associated symptoms: rash, myalgia, weight loss, pain
- Sick contacts
- Past medical history: HIV, malignancies, surgeries
- Medications
- Family history: tuberculosis in a relative, malignancies, familial Mediterranean fever
- Social history: daily routine, rural vs. urban, pets and animal contacts, arthropod bites, travel—recent and remote, socioeconomic status, occupation, military service, sexual history

■ PHYSICAL FINDINGS

- HEENT: rule out sinusitis, dental abscesses; examine eyes carefully
- Neck: check adenopathy
- Lungs: auscultate for rales
- Heart: listen for murmur
- Abdomen: check for organomegaly
- Rectal: examine for prostate tenderness
- Pelvic: rule out cervical motion tenderness
- Extremities: look for clubbing, splinter hemorrhages; examine IV access site
- Musculoskeletal: examine for joint effusions
- Skin: note any rashes, wounds

■ LABORATORY TESTS

- Base on historical clues and physical findings.
- Blood cultures, CBC, urinalysis, transaminases, PPD testing is important in most FUO workups.
- Base on leads from history, examination—whether need for serum antibody testing, lumbar puncture, thyroid function testing, stool culture and *C. difficile* assay, bone marrow biopsy, skin biopsy, ANA.
- May need to repeat laboratory examinations at regular intervals until diagnosis is established.

■ IMAGING STUDIES

- Base on historical clues and physical findings.
- Chest x-ray, abdominal CT scan are important eventually in most workups where diagnosis is elusive.

TREATMENT

■ PHARMACOTHERAPY

Antibiotics and other treatment are indicated only after definitive or highly probable diagnosis is established, unless patient appears severely ill or septic.

■ DISPOSITION

Diagnoses are found in majority of fevers with initially undetermined origin. Some will continue to defy diagnosis for years.

■ REFERRAL

To an infectious disease specialist if no diagnosis after thoughtful workup

REFERENCES

Mackowiak PA, Durack DT: Fever of unknown origin. In Mandel G, Bennett J, Dolin R (eds): *Principles and practice of infectious disease,* ed 5, Philadelphia, 2000, Churchill Livingstone.

Petersdorf R, Beeson P: Fever of unexplained origin: report of 100 cases, *Medicine* 40:1, 1961.

Author: **Anne Spaulding, M.D.**

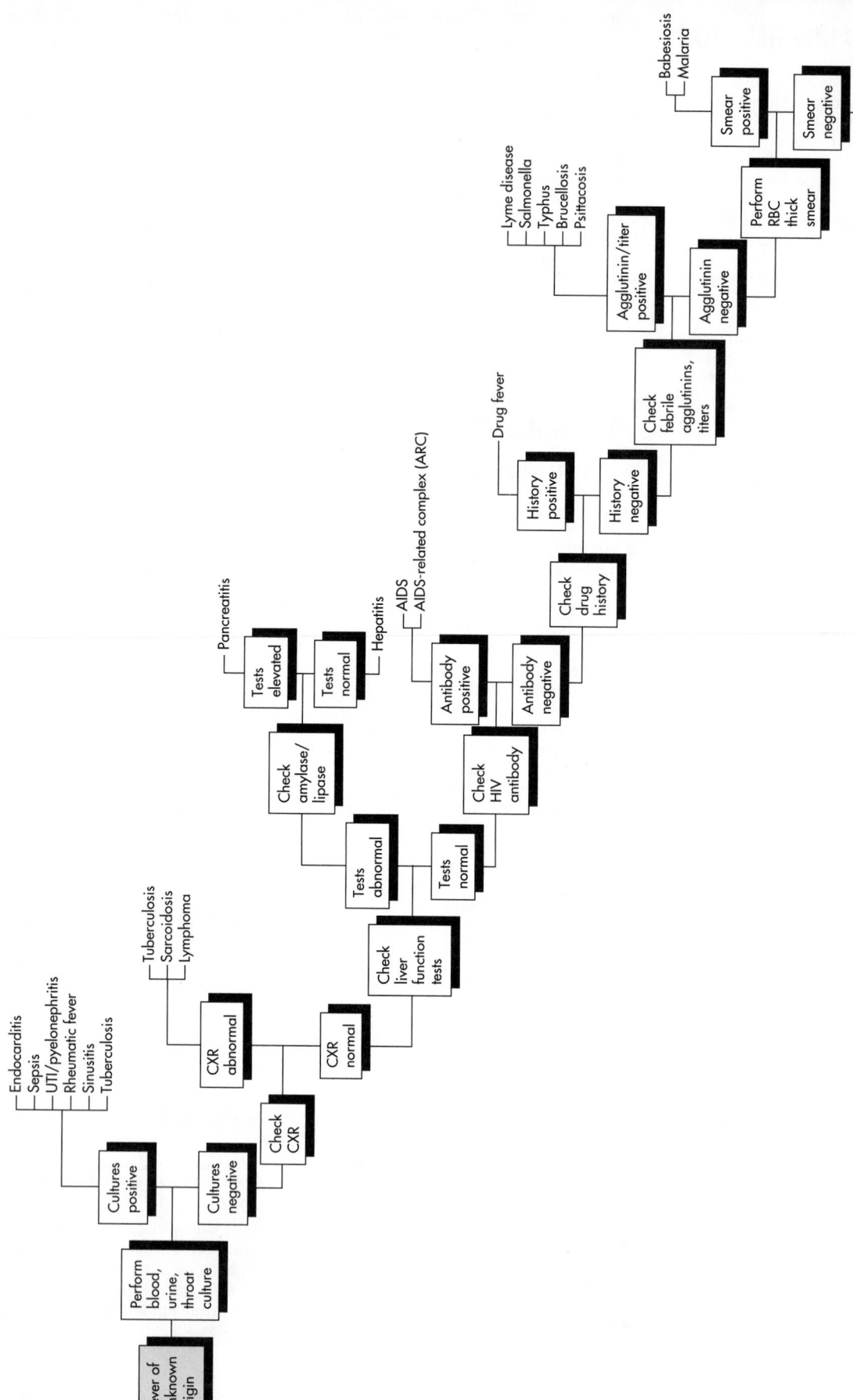

Fig. 1-154 **Approach to the patient with fever of undetermined origin.** *AIDS,* Acquired immunodeficiency syndrome; *ANA,* antinuclear antibody; *CT,* computed tomography; *CXR,* chest x-ray; *ESR,* erythrocyte sedimentation rate; *GI,* gastrointestinal; *HIV,* human immunodeficiency virus; *RBC,* red blood cell; *UTI,* urinary tract infection. (From Healey PM: *Common medical diagnosis: an algorithmic approach,* ed 3, Philadelphia, 2000, WB Saunders.)

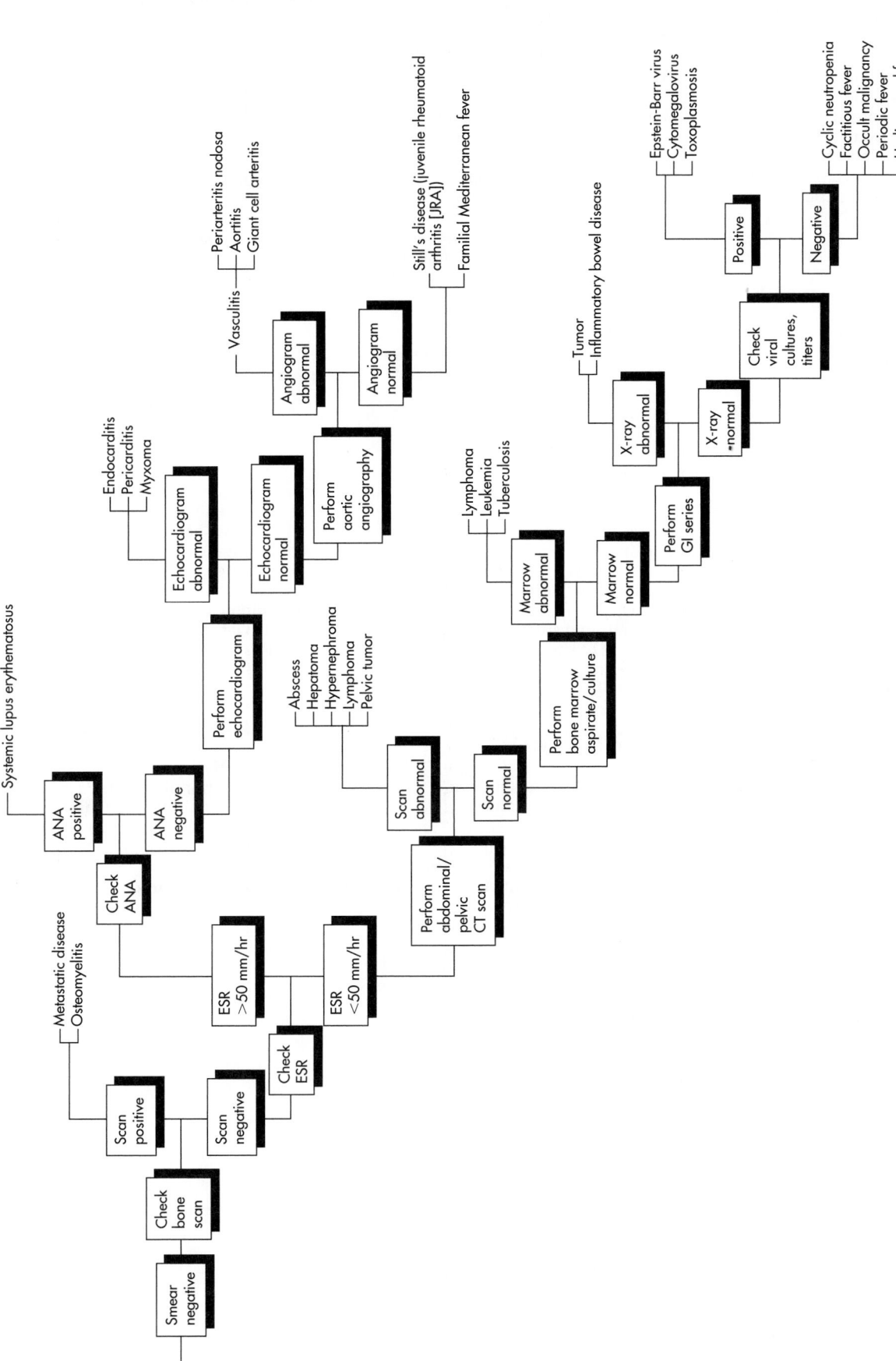

Fig. 1-154, cont'd *AIDS,* Acquired immunodeficiency syndrome; *ANA,* antinuclear antibody; *CT,* computed tomography; *CXR,* chest x-ray; *ESR,* erythrocyte sedimentation rate; *GI,* gastrointestinal; *HIV,* human immunodeficiency virus; *RBC,* red blood cell; *UTI,* urinary tract infection. (From Healey PM: *Common medical diagnosis: an algorithmic approach,* ed 3, Philadelphia, 2000, WB Saunders.)

BASIC INFORMATION

■ DEFINITION
Fibrocystic breast disease (FCD) is a "nondisease," which includes nonmalignant breast lesions such as microcystic and macrocystic changes, fibrosis, ductal or lobular hyperplasia, adenosis, apocrine metaplasia, fibroadenoma, papilloma, papillomatosis, and other changes. Atypical ductal or lobular hyperplasia is associated with a moderate increase in breast cancer risk.

■ SYNONYMS
Cystic changes
Chronic cystic mastitis
Mammary dysplasia

ICD-9CM CODES
610.0 Solitary cyst of the breast
610.1 Fibrocystic disease of the breast

■ EPIDEMIOLOGY & DEMOGRAPHICS
• Ubiquitous in premenopausal women after 20 yr of age
• Palpable nodular changes in the breast termed *FCD* clinically; such changes observable in more than half of adult women 20 to 50 yr of age

■ PHYSICAL FINDINGS & CLINICAL PRESENTATION
• Tender breasts
• Nodular areas
• Dominant mass
• Thickening
• Nipple discharge
• Can vary with menstrual cycle

■ ETIOLOGY
• Although frequently seen and diagnosed, mechanism of development not understood.
• Because found in majority of healthy breasts, regarded as nonpathologic process.
• With hormone replacement therapy, may be carried into menopausal age.

DIAGNOSIS

■ DIFFERENTIAL DIAGNOSIS
• If presenting as dominant mass or masses: exclude possible carcinoma.
• Carcinoma: detection is difficult with FCD, particularly among premenopausal women.
• If presenting with nipple discharge: differentiate from discharge of possible malignant origin. Fig. 3-32 describes breast nipple discharge evaluation. Box 2-46 describes the differential diagnosis of breast inflammatory lesions.

■ WORKUP
• Exclude breast carcinoma if breast mass, thickening, discharge, and pain present.
• Perform biopsy of suspected area for histologic confirmation.

■ IMAGING STUDIES
Mammography and ultrasound studies required:
• For mammographic changes (suspicious densities, microcalcifications, architectural distortion): careful evaluation, including possibly biopsy to exclude breast cancer
• Ultrasound study: to establish cystic nature of clinical or mammographic mass lesion

TREATMENT

■ NONPHARMACOLOGIC THERAPY
• Not considered a "disease" and does not require treatment
• Surgical intervention diagnostic to eliminate possibility of breast cancer
• Periodic physician examination to follow patients with FCD who have pronounced nodular features
• Aspiration for palpable cysts (NOTE: Cysts often recur; repeat aspiration is not always required unless pain is a problem.)

■ ACUTE GENERAL Rx
Majority of women require no treatment.

■ CHRONIC Rx
For breast pain:
• Danocrine (Danazol): limited success reported
• Bromocriptine or tamoxifen: used less frequently
• Limited caffeine intake: not as successful in controlling pain or nodularity as originally suggested

■ DISPOSITION
• Careful evaluation to exclude suspicious changes for breast cancer, then reassurance and periodic reevaluation as required
• Regular self-examination, annual physician examination, and annual mammograms for women with atypical ductal or lobular hyperplasia

■ REFERRAL
• For further evaluation and/or biopsy if there are suspicious changes that may be associated with FCD (including changing of dominant mass or thickening, persistent or spontaneous discharge, suspicious mammographic changes or lesions)
• To alleviate anxiety associated with breast symptoms or changes

PEARLS & CONSIDERATIONS

■ COMMENTS
Patient education material is available from American College of Obstetricians and Gynecologists, 408 12th Street SW, Washington, DC 20024-2188.

Author: **Takuma Nemoto, M.D.**

BASIC INFORMATION

■ DEFINITION
Fibromyalgia is a poorly defined disorder characterized by multiple trigger points and referred pain.

■ SYNONYMS
Myofascial pain syndrome
Fibrositis
Psychogenic rheumatism
Nonarticular rheumatism
Fibromyalgia syndrome (FS)

ICD-9CM CODES
729.0 Rheumatism, unspecified and fibrositis
729.1 Myalgia and myositis, unspecified

■ EPIDEMIOLOGY & DEMOGRAPHICS
PREVALENCE: 1% to 2% of the general population
PREVALENT SEX: Female:male ratio of 9:1
PREVALENT AGE: 30 to 50 yr

■ PHYSICAL FINDINGS
Tender "nodules" and tender points (Fig. 1-155)

■ ETIOLOGY
- Unknown
- Pain magnification may play a role

DIAGNOSIS

■ DIFFERENTIAL DIAGNOSIS
- Polymyalgia rheumatica
- Referred discogenic spine pain
- Rheumatoid arthritis
- Localized tendinitis
- Connective tissue disease
- Osteoarthritis
- Thyroid disease
- Spondyloarthropathies

■ WORKUP
- Subsets of this disorder are often described:
  1. If symptoms develop in conjunction with other conditions (rheumatoid disease or acute stress)
  2. If findings are more regionally distributed, such as those in the neck following motor vehicle accidents
- The primary condition is often suggested by the following criteria from the American College of Rheumatology:
  1. History of widespread pain
  2. Pain in eleven of eighteen selected tender spots on digital palpation (mainly in the spine, elbows, and knees)

■ LABORATORY TESTS
There are no abnormalities in fibromyalgia, but laboratory assessment may be required to rule out other conditions and may include:
- CBC, ESR, rheumatoid factor, ANA
- CPK, T_4

TREATMENT

■ ACUTE GENERAL Rx
- Self-management
- Explanation, reassurance
- Tricyclic antidepressants for sleep disturbance
- Aerobic and stretching exercise, particularly swimming
- Mild analgesics; avoidance of chronic narcotic use
- Trigger point injections
- Physical therapy

■ DISPOSITION
- Prognosis is uncertain.
- Symptoms come and go for years in spite of an aggressive multifaceted approach to treatment.

PEARLS & CONSIDERATIONS

■ COMMENTS
- Before making this diagnosis, all other more likely disorders should be ruled out.
- The term "fibrositis" is often used, but no inflammation has ever been found.
- The number of trigger points needed to establish the diagnosis is debated.

REFERENCES
Clauw DJ: Elusive syndromes: treating the biologic basis of fibromyalgia and related syndromes, *Cleve Clin J Med* 68:830, 2001.
Goldenberg DL: Fibromyalgia syndrome a decade later: what have we learned? *Arch Intern Med* 159:777,1999.
Leventhal LJ: Management of fibromyalgia, *Ann Intern Med* 131:850, 1999.
O'Malley PG et al: Treatment of fibromyalgia with antidepressants: a meta-analysis, *J Gen Intern Med* 15:659, 2000.
Worrel LM et al: Treating fibromyalgia with a brief interdisciplinary program: initial outcomes and predictors of response, *Mayo Clin Proc* 76:381, 2001.
Author: **Lonnie R. Mercier, M.D.**

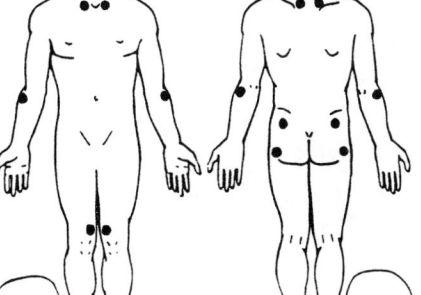

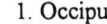

1. Occiput

2. Low cervical

3. Trapezius

4. Supraspinatus

5. Second rib

6. Lateral epicondyle

7. Gluteal

8. Greater trochanter

9. Knees

Fig. 1-155 The sites of the 18 tender points of the 1990 ACR criteria for the classification of fibromyalgia. (From Conn R: *Current diagnosis,* ed 9, Philadelphia, 1997, WB Saunders.)

BASIC INFORMATION

■ DEFINITION

Fifth disease is a viral exanthem of childhood affecting primarily school-age children, which is caused by parvovirus B-19. Erythema infectiosum was the "fifth" in a series of described viral exanthems of childhood and is the most common clinical syndrome associated with B-19.

■ SYNONYMS

Erythema infectiosum

ICD-9CM CODES
057.0 Fifth disease (eruptive)

■ EPIDEMIOLOGY & DEMOGRAPHICS
- Peak age range 5 to 18 yr old
- Peak incidence in late winter and spring, especially April and May
- Fifty to sixty percent of adults have demonstrated protective antibodies to parvovirus B-19

■ PHYSICAL FINDINGS & CLINICAL PRESENTATION
- Typical bright red nontender maxillary rash with circumoral pallor over cheeks, producing the classic "slapped cheek" appearance (Fig. 1-156).
- Reticular nonpruritic lacy, erythematous maculopapular rash over trunk and extremities lasting for up to several weeks after the acute episode. May be worsened by heat or sunlight.
- Polyarthritis and arthralgias are commonly seen in older patients; less common in children. Arthritis involves small joints of extremities in symmetric fashion.
- Mild fever seen in up to one third of patients.

■ ETIOLOGY
- Syndrome caused by parvovirus B-19, a single-stranded DNA virus

DIAGNOSIS

■ DIFFERENTIAL DIAGNOSIS
- Juvenile rheumatoid arthritis (Still's disease)
- Rubella, measles (rubeola), and other childhood viral exanthems
- Mononucleosis
- Lyme disease
- Acute HIV infection
- Drug eruption

■ WORKUP
- Diagnosis made by typical clinical picture
- Parvovirus B-19 IgM antibody seen in 90% of patients with acute illness

■ LABORATORY TESTS
- Complete blood count. Transient aplastic crisis is a syndrome distinct from fifth disease, which may be seen in patients with chronic hematologic illness (described with sickle cell disease, spherocytosis, and other hemolytic processes) infected with parvovirus B-19. It is usually self-limited and associated with prodrome of fever and malaise. Lasts for 1 to 2 wk followed by marrow recovery. Rash usually absent. These patients are highly infective.
- hCG in women of childbearing age. Infection during early pregnancy may result in fetal death (10%) or severe anemia but is usually asymptomatic and not associated with congenital malformations.
- Antibody testing usually not necessary.
- Lyme titers, monospot performed.
- Testing for other viral diseases as indicated by clinical picture.

TREATMENT

■ ACUTE GENERAL Rx
- Treatment is supportive only
- NSAIDs for arthralgias/arthritis

- Intravenous immunoglobulin and transfusion support may be used in patients with immunocompromised state with red cell aplasia.
- Consider immunoglobulin treatment or prophylaxis in pregnancy.

■ DISPOSITION & PROGNOSIS
- Self-limited illness lasting 1 to 2 wk
- Arthritis lasts for weeks. In some patients it may be chronic and develop into rheumatoid arthritis as adult.
- Pregnant women should avoid contact with patients who have marrow suppression.
- Patients with transient aplastic crisis or chronic B-19 infection pose a risk for nosocomial spread and, when hospitalized, should be isolated with contact and respiratory precautions.
- Children with fifth disease are not contagious and may attend school and day care.
- Vaccine is under development.

■ REFERRAL
- For signs of marrow suppression
- For signs of severe or erosive arthritis

Author: **Dominick Tammaro, M.D.**

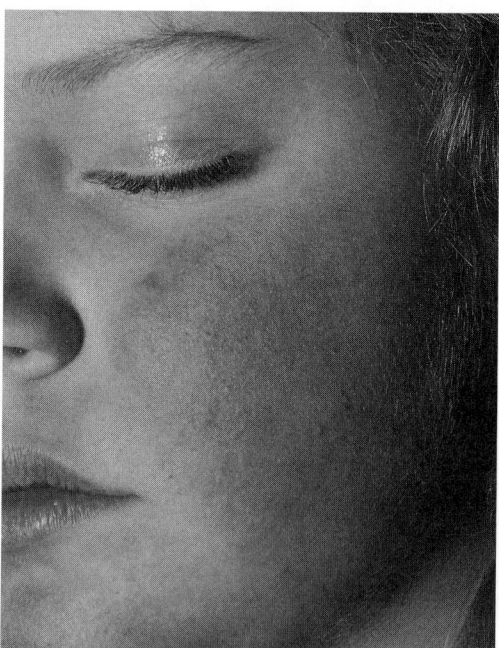

Fig. 1-156 Fifth disease (erythema infectiosum). Facial erythema "slapped cheek." The red plaque covers the cheek and spares the nasolabial and the circumoral region. (From Habif TP: *Clinical dermatology: a color guide to diagnosis and therapy,* ed 3, St Louis, 1996, Mosby.)

BASIC INFORMATION

◼ DEFINITION

Filariasis is a general term for an infection caused by nematodes (roundworms) of the genera *Wuchereria* and *Brugia,* found in the tropical and subtropical regions of the world. The disease is variably characterized by acute lymphatic inflammation or chronic lymphatic obstruction associated with intermittent fevers or recurrent episodes of dyspnea and bronchospasm.

◼ SYNONYMS

Lymphatic filariasis

◼ ICD-9CM CODES

125.0 Bancroftian
125.1 Brugian
125.9 Filariasis

◼ EPIDEMIOLOGY & DEMOGRAPHICS

INCIDENCE (IN U.S.): Unknown
PREDOMINANT SEX: Male
PREDOMINANT AGE: For both males and females, risk is greatest between the ages of 15 to 35 yr.
PEAK INCIDENCE: Unknown

◼ PHYSICAL FINDINGS & CLINICAL PRESENTATION

- Clinical manifestations result from acute lymphatic inflammation or chronic lymphatic obstruction.
- Many patients are asymptomatic despite the presence of microfilaremia.
- Episodes of lymphangitis and lymphadenitis are associated with fever, headache, and back pain.
- Acute funiculitis and epididymitis or orchitis may also be present; all usually resolve within days to weeks but tend to recur.
- Chronic infections may be associated with lymphedema, most commonly manifested by hydrocele.
- It is a progressive disease, leading to nonpitting edema and brawny changes that may involve a whole limb (Fig. 1-157).
- Elephantiasis occurs in about 10% of patients, with skin of the scrotum or leg becoming thickened and fissured; patient is thereafter plagued by recurrent ulceration and infection.
- Chyluria, a condition that develops when lymphatic vessels rupture into the urinary tract, may occur.

◼ ETIOLOGY

Caused by one of three types of nematode parasites, all of which are transmitted to humans by mosquitoes.
- *W. bancrofti:* distributed in Africa, areas of central and South America, the Pacific Islands, and the Caribbean Basin
- *B. malayi:* restricted to southeast Asia
- *B. timori:* confined to the Indonesian archipelago

After bite of an infected mosquito:
- Filarial larvae move into lymphatic vessels and nodes, settling and maturing over 3 to 15 mo into adult male and female worms.
- After fertilization, the female nematode produces large numbers of larvae or microfilariae that enter into the blood stream via the lymphatics.
- Nocturnal periodicity, characteristic of *B. malayi,* is an increased presence of microfilariae in the circulation during the night.
- Microfilariae of *W. bancrofti* are maximal during late afternoon.
- Most microfilariae remain in the body as immature forms for 6 mo to 2 yr.
- Infected larvae are ingested by mosquitoes, then transmitted to humans where the microfilariae mature into new adult worms.

Acute and chronic inflammatory and granulomatous changes in the lymphatic channels:
- Result from complex interaction of adult worms and host's immune systems
- Eventually lead to fibrosis and obstruction
- Most likely to develop into obstructive lymphatic disease with recurrent exposure over many years

DIAGNOSIS

◼ DIFFERENTIAL DIAGNOSIS

- Elephantiasis is distinguished from other causes of chronic lymphedema, including Milroy's disease, postoperative scarring, and lymphedema of malignancy.
- The differential diagnosis of nematode tissue infections is described in Table 2-140.

◼ WORKUP

Diagnosis is suspected in individuals who have resided in endemic areas for at least 3 to 6 mo or more and complain of recurrent episodes of lymphangitis, lymphadenitis, scrotal edema, or thrombophlebitis, with or without fever.

◼ LABORATORY TESTS

- Demonstration of microfilariae on a blood smear for definitive diagnosis
- For patients from southeastern Asia: blood sample drawn at night, especially between midnight and 2 AM
- Occasionally, microfilaremia in chylous urine or hydrocele fluid
- Prominent eosinophilia only during periods of acute lymphangitis or lymphadenitis
- Serologic tests for antibody, including enzyme-linked immunosorbent assay and indirect fluorescent antibody (often unable to distinguish among the various forms of filariasis or between acute and remote infection)
- Immunoassays (such as circulating filaria antigen [CFA]): more successful in antigen detection in patients who are microfilaremic than in those who are amicrofilaremic

◼ IMAGING STUDIES

- Chest x-ray examination: reticular nodular infiltrates (tropical pulmonary eosinophilia syndrome)
- In men proven to be microfilaremic, scrotal ultrasonography to aid in the detection of adult worms
- Compared with adults, children with FS have more sleep disturbances, fewer tender points, and a better prognosis.

TREATMENT

◼ NONPHARMACOLOGIC THERAPY

- Standard of care for elephantiasis:
  1. Elevation of the affected limb
  2. Use of elastic stockings
  3. Local foot care
- General wound care for chronic ulcers and prevention of secondary infection

◼ ACUTE GENERAL Rx

- Diethylcarbamazine citrate (DEC) to reduce microfilaremia by 90%
  1. Effect on adult worms, especially those of the *Wuchereria* species, less certain
  2. Given in an oral dose of 6 mg/kg qd for 12 to 14 days
- Ivermectin alone or in combination with diethylcarbamazine citrate to decrease microfilaremia

I

- Both drugs are similar in efficacy and tolerability; advantage of ivermectin: administration in a single oral dose of 200 μg/kg
- World Health Organization (WHO) recommendation: DEC given as a single dose, alone or (preferably) in combination with ivermectin as treatment in endemic areas

■ CHRONIC Rx
- Surgical drainage of hydroceles
- No satisfactory therapy for those patients with chyluria

■ DISPOSITION
Rarely fatal, but the psychologic impact of limb and scrotal deformities associated with elephantiasis are substantial.

■ REFERRAL
To a surgeon for management of hydrocele

☼ PEARLS & CONSIDERATIONS

- Studies in endemic areas suggest that filarial-specific IgG1 is associated with amicrofilaremic states highest in children, regardless of sex.
- Levels of IgE and IgG4 increase with age and are associated with increased levels of microfilaremia.

■ COMMENTS
Individuals who intend to travel or reside in endemic areas should be advised to institute preventive measures such as the use of netting and insect repellents, especially at night.

REFERENCES

Gupta S et al: Microfilariae in association with neoplastic lesions: report of five cases, *Cytopathology* 12(2):120, 2001.

Hassan MM et al: Circulating filarial antigens for monitoring the efficacy of ivermectin in treatment of filariasis, *J Egypt Soc Parasitol* 31(2):575, 2001.

Ismail MM et al: Long-term efficacy of single-dose combinations of albendazole, ivermectin, and diethylcarbamazine for the treatment of bancroftian filariasis, *Trans R Soc Trop Med Hyg* 95(3):332, 2001.

Mathai E et al: Intraocular filariasis, *Trans R Soc Trop Med Hyg* 94(3):317, 2000.

Terhell AJ et al: Adults acquire filarial infection more rapidly than children: a study in Indonesian transmigrants, *Parasitology* 122 (Pt 6):633, 2001.

Witt C: Lymphatic filariasis: an infection of childhood, *Trop Med Int Health* 6(8):582, 2001.

Author: **George O. Alonso, M.D.**

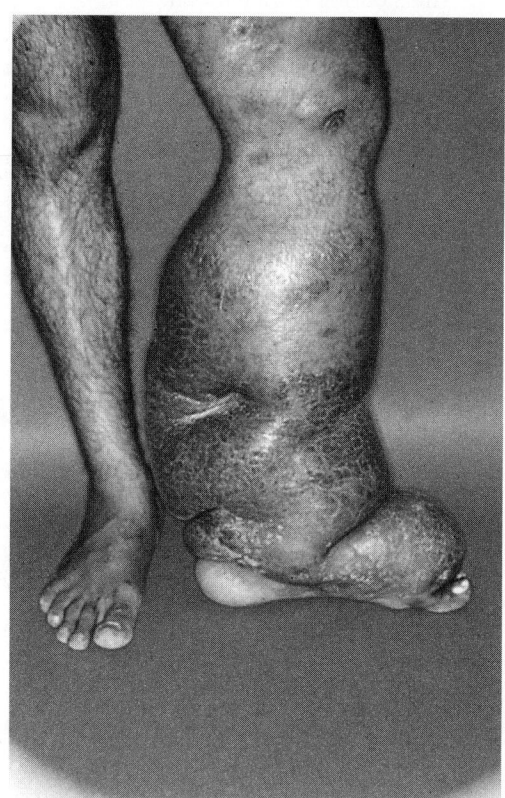

Fig. 1-157 Filariasis that eventually leads to elephantiasis. Note massive swelling of the extremity. (From Goldstein B [ed]: *Practical dermatology,* ed 2, St Louis, 1997, Mosby.)

BASIC INFORMATION

■ DEFINITION
Folliculitis is the inflammation of the hair follicle as a result of infection, physical injury, or chemical irritation.

■ SYNONYMS
Sycosis barbae

ICD-9CM CODES
704.8 Other specified diseases of hair and hair follicles

■ EPIDEMIOLOGY & DEMOGRAPHICS
- Staphylococcal folliculitis is the most common form of infectious folliculitis; it occurs most commonly in persons with diabetes.
- Sycosis barbae occurs most frequently in men who have commenced shaving.

■ PHYSICAL FINDINGS & CLINICAL PRESENTATION
- The lesions generally consist of painful yellow pustules surrounded by erythema; a central hair is present in the pustules.
- Patients with sycosis barbae may initially present with small follicular papules or pustules that increase in size with continued shaving; deep follicular pustules may occur surrounded by erythema and swelling; the upper lip is frequently involved (Fig. 1-158).
- "Hot tub" folliculitis occurs within 1 to 4 days following use of hot tub with poor chlorination, and it is characterized by pustules with surrounding erythema generally affecting torso, buttocks, and limbs.

■ ETIOLOGY
- *Staphylococcus* infection (e.g., sycosis barbae), *Pseudomonas aeruginosa* ("hot tub" folliculitis)
- Gram-negative folliculitis *(Klebsiella, Enterobacter, Proteus)* associated with antibiotic treatment of acne
- Chronic irritation of the hair follicle (use of cocoa butter or coconut oil, chronic irritation from workplace)
- Initial use of systemic corticosteroid therapy (steroid acne), eosinophilic folliculitis (AIDS patients), *Candida albicans* (immunocompromised patients)
- *Pityrosporum orbiculare*

DIAGNOSIS

■ DIFFERENTIAL DIAGNOSIS
- Pseudofolliculitis barbae (ingrown hairs)
- Acne vulgaris
- Dermatophyte fungal infections
- Keratosis biliaris
- Cutaneous candidiasis
- Superficial fungal infections
- Miliaris

■ WORKUP
Physical examination and medical history (e.g., use of hot tub: "hot tub" folliculitis; adolescent patients who have started shaving: sycosis barbae; use of occlusive topical steroid therapy: *Staphylococcus* folliculitis).

■ LABORATORY TESTS
Gram stain is useful to identify the infective organisms in infectious folliculitis and to differentiate infectious folliculitis from noninfectious.

TREATMENT

■ NONPHARMACOLOGIC THERAPY
- Prevention of chemical or mechanical skin irritation
- Glycemic control in diabetics
- Proper chlorination of hot tubs and spas
- Shaving with a clean razor

■ ACUTE GENERAL Rx
- Cleansing of the area with chlorhexidine and application of saline compresses to involved area
- Application of 2% mupirocin ointment (Bactroban) for bacterial folliculitis affecting a limited area (e.g., sycosis barbae)
- Treatment of severe cases of *Pseudomonas* folliculitis with ciprofloxacin
- Treatment of *S. aureus* folliculitis with dicloxacillin 250 mg qid for 10 days

■ CHRONIC Rx
- Chronic nasal or perineal *S. aureus* carriers with frequent folliculitis can be treated with rifampin 300 mg bid for 5 days.
- Mupirocin (Bactroban ointment 2%) applied to nares bid is also effective for nasal carriers.

■ DISPOSITION
- Most cases of bacterial folliculitis resolve completely with proper treatment.
- Steroid folliculitis responds to discontinuation of steroids.

PEARLS & CONSIDERATIONS

■ COMMENTS
Patients should be instructed in good personal hygiene and avoidance of sharing razors, towels, and washcloths.
Author: **Fred F. Ferri, M.D.**

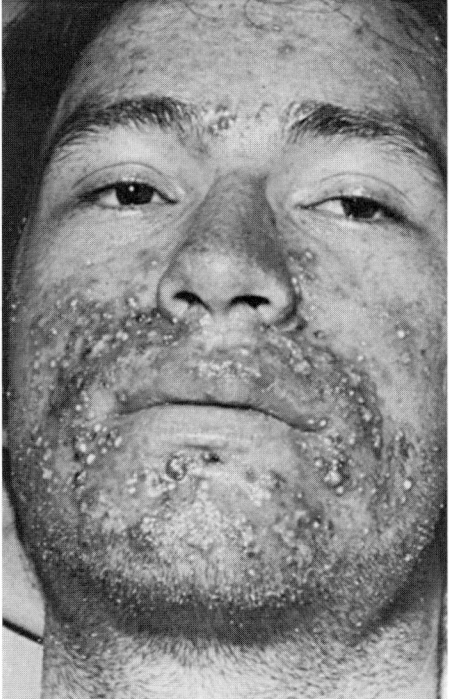

Fig. 1-158 Folliculitis. Note the pustular eruption with small abscess formation in the hair-bearing areas of the face. General symptoms usually are absent. (From Mandell GL: *Mandell, Douglas, and Bennett's principles and practice of infectious diseases,* ed 5, New York, 2000, Churchill Livingstone.)

BASIC INFORMATION

■ DEFINITION
Food poisoning is an illness caused by ingestion of food contaminated by bacteria and/or bacterial toxins.

ICD-9CM CODES
See specific illness.

■ EPIDEMIOLOGY & DEMOGRAPHICS
INCIDENCE (IN U.S.):
- Estimated range of 6 to 80 million cases/yr
- Majority of identifiable causes are bacterial

PREDOMINANT AGE: Varies with specific agent

PEAK INCIDENCE: Varies with specific organism
- Summer: *Staphylococcus aureus, Salmonella, Shigella*
- Summer and fall: *Clostridium botulinum, Vibrio parahaemolyticus*
- Spring and fall: *Campylobacter jejuni*
- Winter: *Clostridium perfringens, Yersinia*

NEONATAL INFECTION: Rare but severe with *Shigella*

■ PHYSICAL FINDINGS & CLINICAL PRESENTATION
- Any combination of GI symptoms and fever
- Specific organisms suspected on the basis of the incubation period and predominant symptoms, although a great deal of overlap exists
  1. Short incubation period (1 to 6 hr): involve the ingestion of preformed toxin; noninvasive
     a. *S. aureus:* nausea, profuse vomiting, and abdominal cramps common; diarrhea possible, but fever uncommon; usually resolves within 24 hr; foods implicated in outbreaks include meats, mayonnaise, and cream pastries
     b. *B. cereus:* two forms, a short incubation (emetic) form (characterized by vomiting and abdominal cramps in virtually all patients, diarrhea in one third of patients, fever uncommon) and a long incubation *(diarrheal)* form; illness usually mild, resolves within 12 hr; unrefrigerated rice most often implicated as vehicle

  2. Moderate incubation period (8 to 16 hr): involves the in vivo production of toxin; noninvasive
     a. *C. perfringens:* severe crampy abdominal pain and watery diarrhea common; fever and vomiting unlikely; symptoms usually resolving within 24 hr; outbreaks invariably related to cooked meat or poultry that is allowed to cool without refrigeration; most cases in the fall and winter months
     b. *B. cereus:* diarrheal (or long incubation) form most commonly beginning with diarrhea, abdominal cramps, and occasionally vomiting; fever uncommon; usually resolves within 24 hr; the responsible food is usually fried rice
  3. Long incubation period (>16 hr): some toxin-mediated, some invasive
     a. Toxin-producing organisms include:
        (1) *C. botulinum:* should be considered when a diarrheal illness coincides with or precedes paralysis; severity of illness related to the quantity of toxin ingested; characteristic cranial nerve palsies progressing to a descending paralysis; fever usually absent; usually associated with home-canned foods
        (2) Enterotoxigenic *E. coli* (ETEC): most common cause of travelers' diarrhea; after 1- to 2-day incubation period, abdominal cramps and copious diarrhea occur; vomiting and fever uncommon; usually resolves after 3 to 4 days; vehicle usually unbottled water or contaminated salad or ice
        (3) Enterohemorrhagic *E. coli* (EHEC): can cause severe abdominal cramps and watery diarrhea, which may eventually become bloody; bacteria (strain O157:H7) are noninvasive; no fever; illness may be complicated by hemolytic-uremic syndrome; associated with contamined beef
        (4) *V. cholerae:* varies from a mild, self-limited illness to

life-threatening cholera; diarrhea, nausea and vomiting, abdominal cramps, and muscle cramps; no fever; severe cases may progress to shock and death within hours of onset; survivors usually have resolution of symptoms in 1 wk; U.S. cases are either imported or result from ingestion of imported food
     b. Invasive organisms include:
        (1) *Salmonella:* associated most often with nontyphoidal strains; incubation period generally 12 to 48 hr; nausea, vomiting, diarrhea, and abdominal cramps typical; fever possible; outbreaks of gastroenteritis related to contaminated poultry, meat, and dairy products
        (2) *Shigella:* asymptomatic infection possible, but some with fever and watery diarrhea that may progress to bloody diarrhea and dysentery; with mild illness, usually self-limited, resolves in a few days; with severe illness, may develop complications; transmission usually from person to person but can occur via contaminated food or water
        (3) *C. jejuni:* the most common food-borne bacterial pathogen; incubation period is about 1 day, then a prodrome of fever, headache, and myalgias; intestinal phase marked by diarrhea associated with fever, malaise, and abdominal pain; diarrhea mild to profuse and bloody; usually resolves in about 7 days, but relapse is possible; associated with undercooked meats and poultry, unpasteurized dairy products, and drinking from freshwater streams
        (4) *Y. enterocolitica* and *Y. pseudotuberculosis:* infrequent causes of enteritis in U.S.; children affected more often than adults; fever, diarrhea, and abdom-

inal pain lasting 1 to 3 wk; some with mesenteric adenitis that mimics acute appendicitis; contaminated food or water is usually responsible
(5) *V. parahaemolyticus:* In U.S., most outbreaks in coastal states or on cruise ships during the summer months; incubation period usually <1 day, followed by explosive watery diarrhea in the majority of cases; nausea, vomiting, abdominal cramps, and headache also common; fever less common; usually resolves by 1 wk; related to ingestion of seafood
(6) Enteroinvasive *E. coli* (EIEC): a rare cause of disease in the U.S.; high incidence of fever and bloody diarrhea; may resemble bacillary dysentery
(7) *V. vulnificus:* may cause serious, often fatal illness in persons with chronic liver disease; GI symptoms usually absent, but fever, chills, hypotension, and hemorrhagic skin lesions possible; patients with liver disease or at increased risk of developing liver disease should avoid eating raw oysters

■ ETIOLOGY
Classically categorized as either inflammatory (invasive) or noninflammatory:
- Noninflammatory: *B. cereus, S. aureus, C. botulinum, C. perfringens, V. cholerae,* enterotoxigenic *E. coli* (ETEC), and enterohemorrhagic *E. coli* (EHEC); toxin-producing organisms that are noninvasive; fecal leukocytes are not seen.
- Inflammatory: *Campylobacter,* enteroinvasive *E. coli* (EIEC), *Salmonella, Shigella, V. parahaemolyticus,* and *Yersinia;* cause disease by invasion of intestinal tissue; fecal leukocytes are seen.

🔬 DIAGNOSIS

■ DIFFERENTIAL DIAGNOSIS
Gastroenteritis caused by viruses (Norwalk or rotavirus), parasites *(Amoeba histolytica, Giardia lamblia),* or toxins (ciguatoxins, mushrooms, heavy metals)

■ LABORATORY TESTS
- Test stool for fecal leukocytes to help narrow the differential diagnosis:
  1. Send stool for culture and for ova and parasites.
  2. Send stool for *C. difficile* toxin in patients with current or recent antibiotic use.
  3. NOTE: Some pathogens are not identified on routine stool culture; laboratory should be advised if *Yersinia, C. botulinum, Vibrio,* or enterohemorrhagic *E. coli* (O157:H7) are suspected.
  4. Finding *B. cereus, C. perfringens,* or *E. coli* in stool is of little value, since these may be part of the normal bowel flora.
- If botulism suspected, send food, serum, and stool for toxin assay.
- Blood cultures are needed for all febrile patients.

💊 TREATMENT

■ NONPHARMACOLOGIC THERAPY
Adequate rehydration is the mainstay of therapy.

■ ACUTE GENERAL Rx
- Gastroenteritis caused by the following organisms requires no antimicrobial treatment: *B. cereus, S. aureus, C. perfringens, V. parahaemolyticus, Yersinia,* and enterohemorrhagic and enteroinvasive *E. coli.*
- The usual cause of traveler's diarrhea is enterotoxigenic *E. coli.* Although usually a self-limited illness, antibiotics can shorten the course.
  1. SMX/TMP one DS tab bid for 3 days
  2. Ciprofloxacin 500 mg PO bid for 3 days
- The mainstay of therapy for cholera is fluid replacement. Antibiotics should be given to decrease shedding and duration of illness.
  1. Doxycycline 100 mg PO bid for 3 days
  2. SMX/TMP one DS tab bid for 3 days
- Treatment is not indicated for *Salmonella* gastroenteritis. Patients who are at high risk of developing bacteremia may be treated for 48 to 72 hr (see "Salmonellosis").
- Although shigellosis tends to be a self-limited illness, antibiotics shorten the course of illness and may limit transmission of the illness (see "Shigellosis").

- Those with moderate or severe *Campylobacter* diarrhea may benefit from treatment.
  1. Erythromycin 500 mg PO qid for 5 days
  2. Ciprofloxacin 500 mg PO bid for 5 days
- *V. vulnificus* sepsis should be treated with:
  1. Doxycycline 100 mg IV bid for 2 wk
  2. Ceftazidime 2 g IV q8h for 2 wk
- For suspected botulism, antitoxin should be administered early (see "Botulism").

■ CHRONIC Rx
Patients with *Salmonella* infections may become carriers and may require treatment (see "Salmonellosis").

■ DISPOSITION
- Most infections are self-limited and do not require therapy.
- In immunocompromised host or patient with underlying disease, serious complications are possible.
- Postinfectious syndromes are important with some infections:
  1. Reiter's syndrome: *Salmonella, Shigella, Campylobacter, Yersinia;* more common in genetically susceptible host (HLA-B27+)
  2. Guillain-Barré syndrome: *Campylobacter*

■ REFERRAL
If more than a mild illness

💡 PEARLS & CONSIDERATIONS

■ COMMENTS
- Grossly underreported and undiagnosed
- All cases to be reported to the local health department
- Table 2-74 compares incubation period, symptoms, and common vehicles for microbial causes of food poisoning.

REFERENCE
Centers for Disease Control and Prevention: Diagnosis and management of foodborne illnesses: a primer for physicians, *MMWR Recomm Rep* 50(RR-2):1, 2001.
Author: **Maurice Policar, M.D.**

BASIC INFORMATION

■ DEFINITION

Friedreich's ataxia is the term used for the most common of a group of hereditary early-onset ataxias caused by degeneration of multiple spinal cord pathways and peripheral nervous system axons.

■ ICD-9CM CODES
334.0 Friedreich's ataxia

■ EPIDEMIOLOGY & DEMOGRAPHICS
INCIDENCE (IN U.S.): Not reported
PREVALENCE (IN U.S.): Not reported
PREDOMINANT SEX: Male = Female
PREDOMINANT AGE: Second decade of life
PEAK INCIDENCE: 8 to 15 yr
GENETICS: Autosomal recessive, with gene localized to chromosome 9

■ PHYSICAL FINDINGS
- Onset of progressive limb and gait ataxia before age 25 yr and absent muscle stretch reflexes in the lower extremity
- With disease progression: dysarthria, areflexia, leg weakness, extensor plantar responses, distal loss of position and vibration sense
- Common findings: scoliosis, distal atrophy, pes cavus, and cardiomyopathy

■ ETIOLOGY
- Genetic: responsible gene is localized to the centromeric region of chromosome 9.
- Biochemical defect is unknown.

DIAGNOSIS

■ DIFFERENTIAL DIAGNOSIS
- Hereditary motor and sensory neuropathy type I (Charcot-Marie-Tooth disease type I)
- Abetalipoproteinemia
- Early-onset cerebellar ataxia with retained reflexes
- Box 2-37 describes the differential diagnosis of ataxia. Gait abnormalities are described in Table 2-80.

■ WORKUP
- Diagnostic criteria include electrophysiologic documentation of an axonal sensory neuropathy.
- ECG shows widespread T-wave inversion and evidence of left ventricular hypertrophy in 65% of patients.

■ LABORATORY TESTS
- EMG/NCS
- ECG
- Peripheral smear for acanthocytes
- Lipid profile

■ IMAGING STUDIES
MRI of the spinal cord may demonstrate atrophy (Fig. 1-159)

TREATMENT

■ NONPHARMACOLOGIC THERAPY
- Surgical correction of scoliosis and foot deformities in selected patients
- Physical therapy

■ ACUTE GENERAL Rx
None

■ CHRONIC Rx
None

■ DISPOSITION
- Loss of ambulation typically occurs within 15 yr of symptom onset, and 95% are wheelchair bound by age 45 yr.
- Life expectancy is reduced, particularly if heart disease is present.

■ REFERRAL
- If uncertain about diagnosis
- For genetic counseling (recommended if available)

Author: **Michael Gruenthal, M.D., Ph.D.**

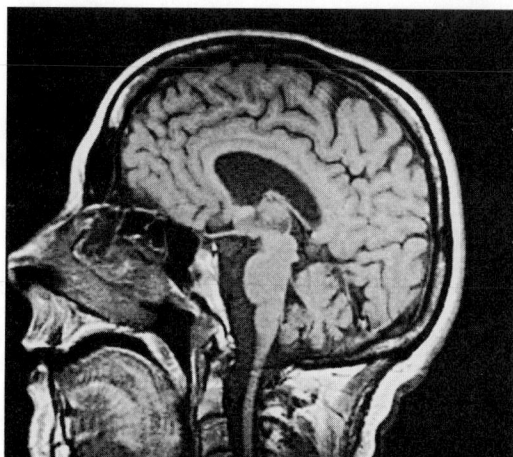

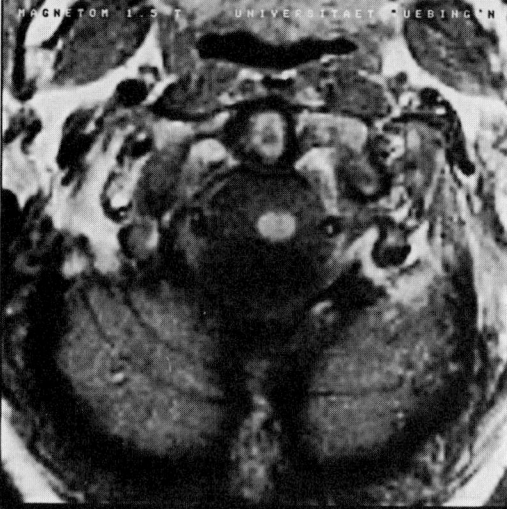

Fig. 1-159   T1-weighted MRIs of the brain and cervical spinal cord in Friedreich's ataxia. The images are, **A,** midsagittal plane of the head and, **B,** an axial slice at the level of the dens axis. There is severe shrinkage of the cervical spinal cord. In contrast, the cerebellum and brain stem are of normal size. (From Goetz CG: *Textbook of clinical neurology,* Philadelphia, 1999, WB Saunders.)

BASIC INFORMATION

■ DEFINITION
Frostbite represents tissue injury (or death) from freezing and vasoconstriction induced by severe environmental cold exposure.

■ SYNONYMS
Cold-induced tissue injury

ICD-9CM CODES
991.3 Frostbite

■ EPIDEMIOLOGY & DEMOGRAPHICS
- Environmental factors include wind chill factor, temperature, duration of exposure, altitude, and degree of wetness.
- Host factors include immobility, history of cold injuries, lack of acclimatization, skin damage, psychiatric illness, preexisting CNS or cardiovascular disease, diabetes, malnutrition, tobacco use, sedative drugs (especially alcohol), fatigue, hypothyroidism, anemia, and perhaps race (African Americans may be more susceptible).

■ PHYSICAL FINDINGS & CLINICAL PRESENTATION
- Frostbite may be classified into degrees of injury or, more practically, into *superficial* and *deep* groups.
- *Superficial* frostbite involves the skin and subcutaneous tissue. The frozen part is waxy white and firm but soft and resilient below the surface when gently depressed. After rewarming, the frostbitten area may appear mottled and swollen and superficial blisters may form within 6 to 24 hr (Fig.1-160). There is no ultimate tissue loss.
- *Deep* frostbite extends into subcutaneous tissues and may involve muscles, nerves, tendons, or bones. The skin may be hard or wooden, without tissue resilience. Edema, cyanosis, hemorrhagic bullae (after 3 to 7 days), tissue necrosis, and gangrene may develop. Affected tissue has a poor prognosis.
- Patients initially experience numbness, prickling, and itching. More severe injury can produce paresthesias, stiffness, and burning or throbbing pain on thawing.

DIAGNOSIS

- Diagnosis is clinically based on the appropriate environmental conditions.

- Other locally induced cold injuries include:
  Pernio (chilblains): cold-induced vasculitis of dermal vessels often affecting dorsum of hands and feet and seen with repeated cold exposure.
  Cold immersion (trench) foot: caused by ischemic injury resulting from sustained severe vasoconstriction in cold-immersed appendage.

■ WORKUP
- CBC.
- Wound and blood cultures in more severe cases.
- IV isotope studies and bone scans have been used with mixed results to predict subsequent tissue loss and demonstrate ischemic tissue at risk. Angiography may be used to evaluate for chronic vascular abnormalities.

TREATMENT

■ NONPHARMACOLOGIC THERAPY
- Remove constricting or wet clothing and gently insulate and immobilize the affected area.
- Avoid thawing if there is any risk of refreezing.
- Never rub or massage the affected area, and avoid dry heat.
- If there is associated hypothermia, core temperature must first be stabilized.

■ ACUTE GENERAL Rx
- Immerse affected area in circulating warm water that is 40° to 42° C for 20 to 30 min.
- Parenteral narcotics are often required for pain control.
- Topical aloe vera (Dermaide) q6h (thromboxane inhibitor)

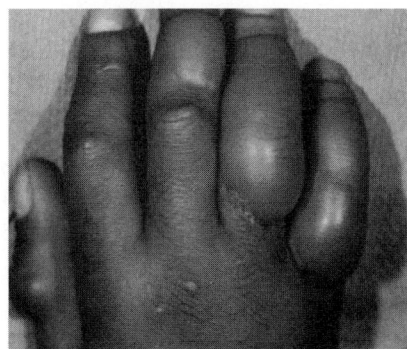

Fig. 1-160   Large, clear frostbite blisters on the right hand. (From Rosen P [ed]: *Emergency medicine,* ed 4, St Louis, 1998, Mosby.)

- Td prophylaxis
- Streptococcal prophylaxis for 48 to 72 hr with IV penicillin for severe cases
- Limb elevation to minimize edema
- Sterile dressing

■ CHRONIC Rx
- Ibuprofen 400 mg bid to tid (inhibits coagulation cascade and produces fibrinolysis).
- Blister management is controversial. Debride broken clear vesicles and aspirate hemorrhagic vesicles.
- Whirlpool hydrotherapy with an antiseptic for 20 to 30 min bid to tid for several weeks.
- Gentle, progressive physical therapy after edema resolves.
- Avoid all vasoconstrictors, including nicotine.

■ DISPOSITION
Long-term residual symptoms including neuropathic pain, sensory deficits, hyperhidrosis, secondary Raynaud's disease, edema, hair or nail deformities, and arthritis occur in 65% of patients.

■ REFERRAL
- Hospitalize if patient has systemic hypothermia or more than superficial frostbite.
- Surgical decisions regarding amputation should be deferred until there is clear demarcation of viable tissue (may take months) unless refractory pain, sepsis, or supervening gangrene occurs.

REFERENCES
Britt LD, Dascombe WH, Rodriguez A: New horizons in the management of hypothermia and frostbite injury, *Surg Clin North Am* 71:345, 1991.

Celestino F: Cold and heat injuries. In Mengel M, Schwiebert L (eds): *Ambulatory medicine: the primary care of families,* ed 2, Stamford, Conn, 1996, Appleton & Lange.

Danzl D: Frostbite. In Rosen P (ed): *Emergency medicine: concepts and clinical practice,* vol 1, ed 4, St Louis, 1998, Mosby.

Rabold M: Frostbite and other localized cold-related injuries. In Tintinelli J (ed): *Emergency medicine: a comprehensive study guide,* New York, 1996, McGraw-Hill.

Reamy B: Frostbite: review and current concepts, *J Am Board Fam Pract* 11(1):341, 1998.

Author: **Michael P. Johnson, M.D.**

BASIC INFORMATION

■ DEFINITION
Frozen shoulder is a condition unique to the shoulder and characterized by pain and restricted passive and active range of motion (Fig. 1-161).

■ SYNONYMS
Adhesive capsulitis
Periarthritis
Pericapsulitis
Check-rein shoulder

ICD-9CM CODES
726.0 Adhesive shoulder capsulitis

■ EPIDEMIOLOGY & DEMOGRAPHICS
PREVALENT AGE: Over 40 yr
PREVALENT SEX: Females > males

■ PHYSICAL FINDINGS & CLINICAL PRESENTATION
- Arm held protectively at the side with apprehension caused by pain
- Varying degrees of deltoid and spinatus atrophy
- Generalized shoulder tenderness
- Restricted active and passive shoulder motion of varying degrees

■ ETIOLOGY
- Unknown.
- Fig. 1-161 illustrates the sequence of events terminating in frozen shoulder.

DIAGNOSIS

■ DIFFERENTIAL DIAGNOSIS
- Secondary causes of shoulder stiffness (prolonged immobilization following trauma or surgery)
- Posterior shoulder dislocation
- Ruptured rotator cuff
- Glenohumeral osteoarthritis
- Rotator cuff inflammation
- Superior sulcus tumor
- Cervical disk disease
- Brachial neuritis

■ WORKUP
Laboratory and radiographic studies are generally normal.

TREATMENT

■ NONPHARMACOLOGIC THERAPY
Prevention is important. Shoulder motion should be maintained during those periods of time when the patient may be inactive as a result of illness or injury.

■ ACUTE GENERAL Rx
- Moist heat, sedation, and analgesics as needed
- A local steroid/lidocaine mixture injected into the subacromial space and joint (Table 1-30)
- Home exercise program
- Manipulation of shoulder under anesthesia (rarely needed)

■ DISPOSITION
- The initial stage of pain followed by stiffness may last several months; recovery phase may also last several months; complete recovery is usually the case.
- Recurrence in the same shoulder is rare, although the opposite limb may develop the same symptoms.
- Some patients have mild residual loss of movement but without any significant functional impairment.

■ REFERRAL
Orthopedic consultation in patients with resistant disease

☼ PEARLS & CONSIDERATIONS

■ COMMENTS
- "Capsulitis" with an inflammatory infiltrate is not consistently found pathologically.
- Frozen shoulder is increased in patients with diabetes, thyroid disease, and recent cardiopulmonary conditions.
- Some cases present with findings of reflex sympathetic dystrophy.

REFERENCES
Kivimaki J, Pohjolainen T: Manipulation for frozen shoulder with and without steroid injection, *Arch Phys Med Rehabil* 82:1188, 2001.
Tuten HR, Young DC et al: Adhesive capsulitis of the shoulder in male cardiac surgery patients, *Orthopedics* 23:693, 2000.
Author: **Lonnie R. Mercier, M.D.**

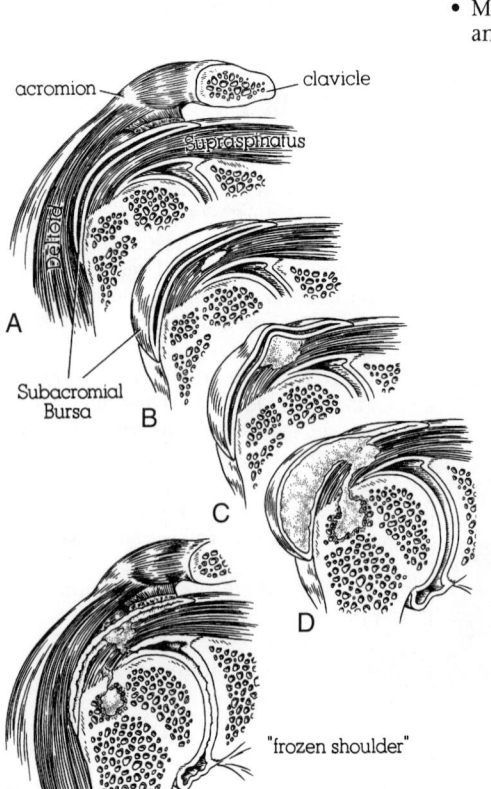

Fig. 1-161 Sequence of events terminating in frozen shoulder. **A,** Normal structures of the shoulder. **B,** Supraspinatus tendinitis, sometimes calcific, in the "critical zone." **C,** Spread of inflammation to the tendon sheath and a bulge into the floor of the subacromial bursa. **D,** Rupture into the subacromial bursa and extension of the inflammatory process as an osteitis into the humeral head and greater tuberosity. **E,** Frozen shoulder with involvement of tendons, bursa, capsule, synovium, and muscle with fibrous contracture and markedly diminished volume of the shoulder joint space. (From Noble J [ed]: *Primary care medicine,* ed 2, St Louis, 1996, Mosby.)

BASIC INFORMATION

■ DEFINITION
Ganglia are cystic structures thought to derive from a tendon sheath or joint capsule.

ICD-9CM CODES
727.43 Ganglion

■ EPIDEMIOLOGY & DEMOGRAPHICS
- Ganglia are more common in women than men (3:1).
- Can occur at any age but usually occurs between second and fourth decades of life.
- Most common soft tissue tumor of the hand and wrist.

■ PHYSICAL FINDINGS & CLINICAL PRESENTATION
- Most ganglia occur on the dorsum of the wrist (50% to 70%) (Fig. 1-162).
- Volar wrist (18% to 20%) is the next most common site.
- Ganglia can also involve the proximal digital flexor tendons and the distal interphalangeal joints.
- Left and right hands are equally affected.
- Ganglia are usually solitary, firm, smooth, round, and fluctulant.
- Pain from mass effect or compression up against nearby structure may be present (e.g., median nerve and radial nerve).
- Hand numbness may be present.
- Patient may experience hand muscle weakness.
- Ganglia usually develop over a period of months but may arise suddenly.

■ ETIOLOGY
- Ganglia are thought to derive from synovial herniation or expansion from the joint capsule or tendon sheath.

DIAGNOSIS

Direct inspection and localization of the cyst often is enough to make the diagnosis of ganglia.

■ DIFFERENTIAL DIAGNOSIS
- Lipoma
- Fibroma
- Epidermoid inclusion cyst
- Osteochondroma
- Hemangioma
- Infection (tuberculosis, fungi, and secondary syphilis)
- Gout
- Rheumatoid nodule
- Radial artery aneurysm

■ WORKUP
The workup of ganglia usually consists of history, physical examination, and x-ray imaging.

■ LABORATORY TESTS
Blood tests are not specific in the diagnosis of ganglia.

■ IMAGING STUDIES
- X-ray of the hand and wrist is done to rule out other bone or joint abnormalities.
- Ultrasound studies are helpful in the diagnosis of ganglia demonstrating smooth cystic walls that may be septated.
- CT scan can be done if the ultrasound is equivocal.

- MRI although not done often for the diagnosis of ganglia aids in differentiating malignant bone lesions from cystic structures.
- Arthrography may demonstrate a communication between the joint and ganglia (not commonly done).

TREATMENT

Treatment is indicated for pain, muscle weakness, and for cosmetic purposes.

■ NONPHARMACOLOGIC THERAPY
- Attempts to rupture the cyst by sharp blows with a book or with finger compression.
- Aspiration, heat, and sclerotherapy have been tried but met with high recurrence rates (60%).

■ ACUTE GENERAL Rx
- Aspiration with a large-bore needle (18-gauge) followed by injection of 20 to 40 mg of triamcinolone acetonide can be tried.
- This may be repeated if the ganglia recurs (35% to 40%).

■ CHRONIC Rx
- Total ganglionectomy is the surgical procedure of choice.

■ DISPOSITION
- Ganglia spontaneously resolve in approximately 40% to 50% of cases.
- Aspiration with steroid injection is successful in approximately 65% of cases.
- Surgery provides cure in 85% to 95% of the cases.

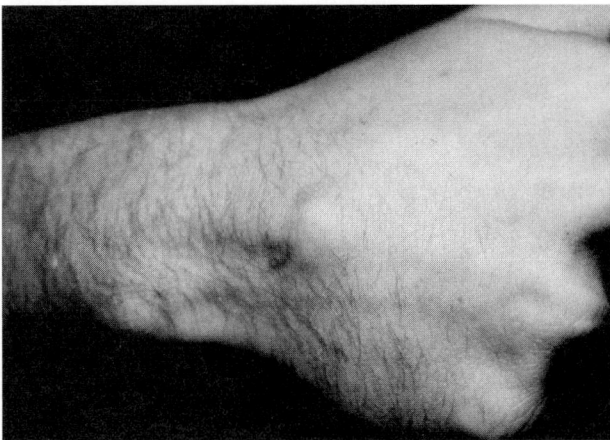

Fig. 1-162 Round and firm ganglion cyst bulging from the dorsal aspect of the hand. (From Kelly WN: *Textbook of rheumatology,* ed 5, Philadelphia, 1997, WB Saunders.)

- Complications of ganglia include:
  1. Carpal tunnel syndrome with pain and muscle atrophy
  2. Radial nerve impingement
  3. Radial artery compression
- Complications of ganglion surgery includes:
  1. Infection
  2. Recurrence (5% to 15%) usually secondary to inadequate excision
  3. Reflex sympathetic dystrophy
  4. Scar formation

■ REFERRAL
It is best to refer patients with symptomatic ganglia to a hand surgeon.

PEARLS & CONSIDERATIONS

■ COMMENTS
- Ganglia synovial membrane maintains its secretory function. Aspiration of ganglia often demonstrates a viscous, mucinous clear fluid containing albumin, globulin, and hyaluronic acid.
- Dorsal ganglia usually originate from the scapholunate ligament.
- Volar ganglia typically originate between the tendons of the flexor carpi radialis and brachioradialis.

REFERENCES
Rosson JW, Walker G: The natural history of ganglion in children, *J Bone Joint Surg* 71B:707, 1989.

Young L, Bartell T, Logan SE: Ganglions of the hand and wrist, *So Med J* 81(6):751, 1988.

Author: **Peter Petropoulos, M.D.**

BASIC INFORMATION

■ DEFINITION

Gardner's syndrome is an autosomal dominant condition characterized by (1) multiple adenomatous intestinal polyposis, (2) osteomas, and (3) soft tissue tumors (epidermoid cysts, fibromas, lipomas). It is a variant of familial adenomatous polyposis (FAP), which is characterized by prominent extraintestinal lesions (Fig. 1-163).

ICD-9CM CODES
211.3 Gardner's syndrome

■ EPIDEMIOLOGY & DEMOGRAPHICS

- FAP accounts for 1% of all colorectal cancers.
- The entire GI tract may have polyps, but the malignant potential is highest in the colon. Individuals with Gardner's syndrome develop hundreds to thousands of colonic adenomatous polyps.
- Polyps occur at a mean age of 16 yr.
- Cancer develops in 7% of individuals by age 21 yr, 50% by age 39 yr, and 90% by age 45 yr. There is 100% chance of developing colorectal cancer.
- Average age of symptomatic presentation in unscreened individuals is 35 yr, at which time about two thirds will have colon cancer.
- Soft tissue and bone abnormalities may precede intestinal disease by up to 10 yr. Osteomas typically appear at puberty and frequently involve the angle of the mandible, although any bone may be affected.

- Individuals with Gardner's syndrome are at increased risk for other cancers: about 10% develop desmoid tumors and 10% develop periampullary cancer. Risk for liver, adrenal, thyroid, and brain cancers is also increased.

■ CLINICAL PRESENTATION

- Congenital hypertrophy of the retinal pigment epithelium (often the first sign of the syndrome) is detected by indirect ophthalmoscopy.
- Supernumerary teeth
- Soft tissue lesions: epidermoid cysts, fibromas, lipomas
- Bony abnormalities of skull and long bones
- Abdominal mass, occult blood in stool

■ ETIOLOGY

- Both Gardner's syndrome and FAP are caused by mutations of the adenomatous polyposis coli (APC) gene on chromosome 5q21. It is hypothesized that a modifying gene is present that gives rise to the prominent extraintestinal lesions that differentiate Gardner's syndrome from FAP.
- Spontaneous mutations may also occur.

DIAGNOSIS

■ DIFFERENTIAL DIAGNOSIS
- FAP
- Turcot's syndrome
- Attenuated adenomatous polyposis coli
- Peutz-Jeghers syndrome
- Juvenile polyposis

■ WORKUP
History, physical examination, laboratory tests, imaging studies

■ LABORATORY TESTS
Genetic tests:
- Peripheral blood leukocyte in vitro synthesized protein assay (IVSP)
- Linkage testing

■ IMAGING STUDIES
Sigmoidoscopy, upper GI endoscopy

■ SCREENING
GENETIC TESTS:
In vitro synthesized protein assay (IVSP)
- Testing rules out the disorder in a person at risk only when no mutation is found in that person but a mutation has been identified in an affected family member.
- Able to identify a mutation in 80% of families with FAP. To ensure that the mutation affecting the family is identifiable, a family member known to have FAP should be tested first.
- If the test is positive in the affected individual, other family members can be screened and the test can differentiate with 100% accuracy affected and unaffected family members. If the family member with disease tests negative, screening family members will not be useful in determining disease status (because the pedigree represents the 20% of families whose mutation is not detected with IVSP).
- If there is no known family member with the disorder, screening the individual in question is reasonable. A positive test rules in the condition, but a negative test does not rule it out.

I

Linkage testing
- Two individuals in a family must already be diagnosed with FAP to diagnose other family members. Linkage testing has 98% accuracy and can identify about 95% of individuals at risk. It can be used if IVSP is not informative.

CONGENITAL HYPERTROPHY OF THE RETINAL PIGMENT EPITHELIUM (CHRPE): CHRPE lesions occur in some families and are a reliable indicator of affected status in these families.

SIGMOIDOSCOPY
- Sigmoidoscopy surveillance is sufficient to determine if the patient is expressing the syndrome.
- Yearly examination allows the detection of the syndrome before cancer develops.
- Annual sigmoidoscopy should begin at age 12 yr in all family members with positive genetic tests and in all family members in pedigrees with an unidentified APC mutation.

UPPER GASTROINTESTINAL ENDOSCOPY (INCLUDING VISUALIZATION OF THE AMPULLA OF VATER): Screening of the gastric and duodenum should begin once colonic polyps are detected and should continue every 2 to 4 yr. Observe for extraintestinal lesions.

☒ TREATMENT

- Colectomy is recommended once polyps are seen on sigmoidoscopy. Regular screening of remaining GI tract and extraintestinal manifestations must continue after colectomy.
- Treat other complications and cancers.

■ DISPOSITION
There is a 100% chance of colorectal cancer in untreated individuals. Many other neoplasms occur at higher rates.

■ REFERRAL
- GI for yearly sigmoidoscopy
- Surgery for prophylactic colectomy at detection of polyps
- Genetic counseling

☼ PEARLS & CONSIDERATIONS

- Sulindac (an NSAID) has been found to cause polyp regression in individuals with FAP. Whether cancer risk is changed is not clear. Sulindac does not replace colon resection for cancer prevention.
- Desmoid tumors have been induced and promoted by surgical procedures, OCP use, and pregnancy.

Author: **Sudeep K. Aulakh, M.D., F.R.C.P.C.**

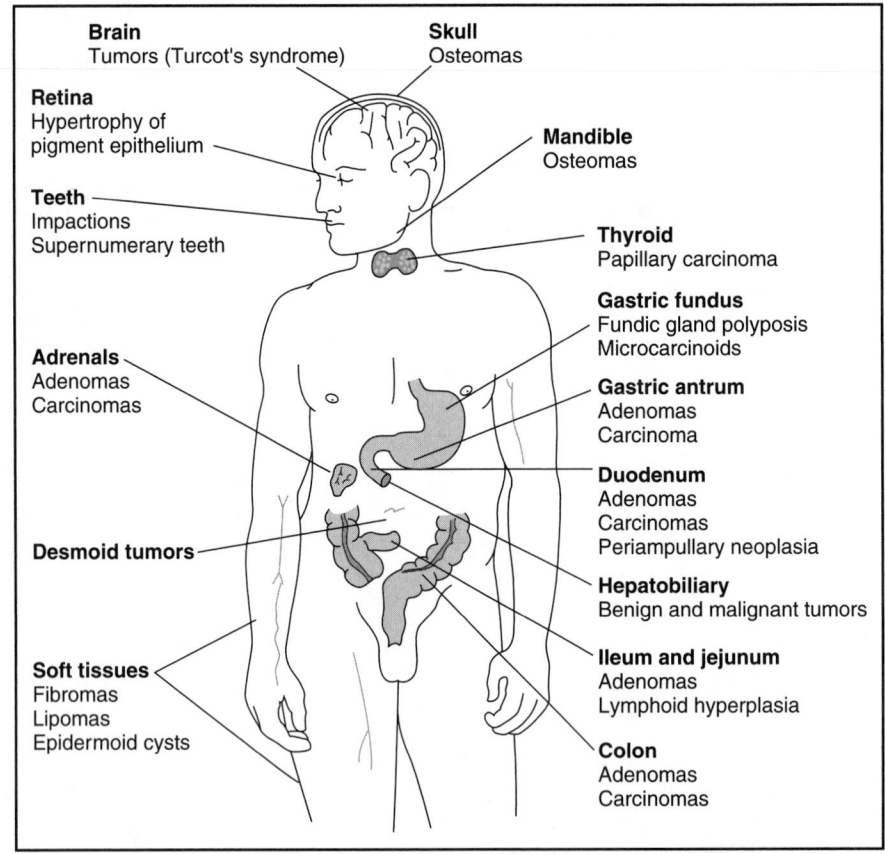

Fig. 1-163 Schematic representation of the intestinal and extraintestinal manifestations of familial adenomatous polyposis (FAP) and Gardner's syndrome. The primary features of Gardner's syndrome consist of a triad of colonic polyposis, bone tumors (particularly in the skull and mandible), and soft tissue tumors, but the phenotypic overlap between FAP and Gardner's syndrome is considerable. (From Feldman M, Scharschmidt BF, Sleisenger MH [eds]: *Sleisinger and Fordtran's gastrointestinal and liver disease: pathophysiology, diagnosis, management,* ed 6, Philadelphia, 1998, WB Saunders.)

BASIC INFORMATION

■ DEFINITION
Gastric cancer is an adenocarcinoma arising from the stomach.

■ SYNONYMS
Stomach cancer
Linitis plastica

ICD-9CM CODES
451 Malignant neoplasm of stomach

■ EPIDEMIOLOGY & DEMOGRAPHICS
- Annual incidence of gastric cancer in the U.S. is 7 cases/100,000 persons. The incidence is much higher in Japan, with rates as high as 80 cases/100,000 persons.
- Most gastric cancers arise in the antrum (35%).
- The incidence of proximal tumors of the cardia and fundus is on the rise.
- Gastric cancer occurs most commonly in male patients >65 yr (70% of patients are >50 yr).
- Incidence of gastric cancer has been declining over the past 30 yr.
- Male:female ratio is 3:2.
- Familiar diffuse gastric cancer is a disease with autosomal dominant inheritance in which gastric cancer develops at a young age. Germ-line truncating mutations in the E-cadherin gene (CDH1) is found in these families.

■ PHYSICAL FINDINGS & CLINICAL PRESENTATION
- Epigastric or abdominal mass (30% to 50%)
- Skin pallor secondary to anemia
- Hard, nodular liver: generally indicates metastatic disease to the liver
- Hemoccult-positive stools
- Ascites, lymphadenopathy, or pleural effusions: may indicate metastasis

■ ETIOLOGY
Risk factors:
- Chronic *H. pylori* gastritis Gastric cancer develops in persons infected with *H. pylori* but not in uninfected persons. Those with histologic findings of severe gastric atrophy, corpus-predominant gastritis, or intestinal metaplasia are at increased risk. Persons with *H. pylori* infection and duodenal ulcer are not at risk, whereas those with gastric ulcers, nonulcer dyspepsia, and gastric hyperplastic polyps are.
- Tobacco abuse, alcohol consumption
- Food additives (nitrosamines), smoked foods, occupational exposure to heavy metals, rubber, asbestos
- Chronic atrophic gastritis with intestinal metaplasia, hypertrophic gastritis, and pernicious anemia

DIAGNOSIS

■ DIFFERENTIAL DIAGNOSIS
- Gastric lymphoma (5% of gastric malignancies)
- Hypertrophic gastritis
- Peptic ulcer
- Reflux esophagitis

■ WORKUP
- Upper endoscopy with biopsy will confirm diagnosis.
- Medical history may reveal complaints of postprandial fullness with significant weight loss (70% to 80%), nausea/emesis (20% to 40%), dysphagia (20%), and dyspepsia, usually unrelieved by antacids; epigastric discomfort, usually lessened by fasting and exacerbated by food intake, is also common.

■ LABORATORY TESTS
- Microcytic anemia
- Hemoccult-positive stools
- Hypoalbuminemia
- Abnormal liver enzymes in patients with metastasis to the liver

- Mutation-specific predictive genetic testing by PCR amplification followed by restriction—enzyme digestion and DNA sequencing for truncating mutations in the E-cadherin gene (CDH1) is recommended in families of patients with familiar diffuse cancer because gastric cancer develops in three of every four carriers of a mutant CDH1 gene.

■ IMAGING STUDIES
- Upper GI series (Fig. 1-164) with air contrast (90% accurate) if endoscopy is not readily available
- Abdominal CT scan to evaluate for metastasis (70% accurate for regional node metastases)

TREATMENT

■ ACUTE GENERAL Rx
- Gastrectomy is performed in patients with curative potential (<30% of patients at time of diagnosis).
- Palliative resection may prolong duration and quality of life.
- Chemotherapy (FAM: 5-fluorouracil, Adriamycin, and mitomycin C) may provide some palliation; however, it generally does not prolong survival.

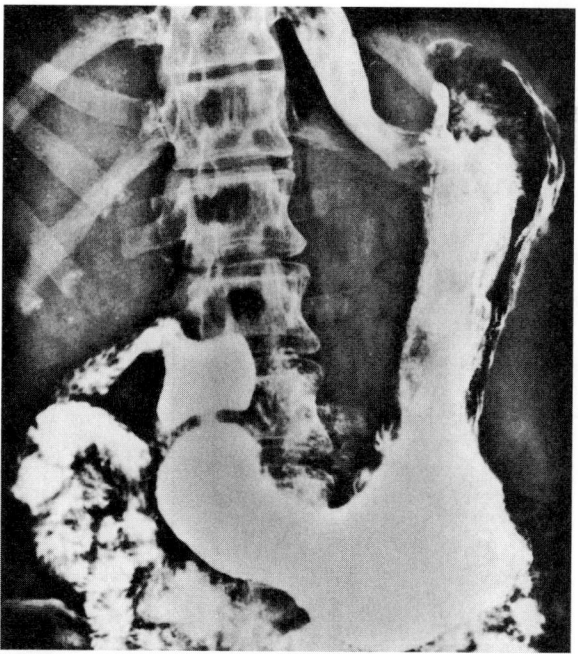

Fig. 1-164 Adenocarcinoma of the proximal stomach. Note the apparent rigidity and narrowing of the stomach with multiple filling defects. (From Stein J [ed]: *Internal medicine*, ed 5, St Louis, 1998, Mosby.)

- Postoperative chemoradiotherapy should be considered for all patients at high risk for recurrence of adenocarcinoma of the stomach or gastroesophageal junction who have undergone curative resection.

■ DISPOSITION
- 5-yr survival rate of gastric carcinoma is 12% overall.
- 5-yr survival for early gastric cancers (usually detected incidentally with endoscopy in populations where screening is recommended) is >35%.

■ REFERRAL
Surgical referral for resection

☼ PEARLS & CONSIDERATIONS

■ COMMENTS
- Gastrectomy patients will need vitamin B_{12} replacement. They are also at risk for dumping syndrome and should be advised to ingest frequent, small meals.
- Prophylactic gastrectomy should be considered in young asymptomatic carriers of germ-line truncating CDH1 mutations who belong to families with highly penetrant heredity diffuse gastric cancer.

REFERENCES

Huntsman DE et al: Early gastric cancer in young, asymptomatic carriers of germ-line E-cadherin mutations, *N Engl J Med* 344:1906, 2001.

Macdonald JS et al: Chemoradiotherapy after surgery compared with surgery alone for adenocarcinoma of the stomach or gastroesophageal junction, *N Engl J Med* 345:725, 2001.

Vemura N et al: *Helicobacter pylori* infection and the development of gastric cancer, *N Engl J Med* 345:784, 2001.

Author: **Fred F. Ferri, M.D.**

BASIC INFORMATION

■ DEFINITION
Histologically, gastritis refers to inflammation in the stomach. Endoscopically, "gastritis" refers to a number of abnormal features such as erythema, erosions, and subepithelial hemorrhages. Gastritis can also be subdivided into erosive, nonerosive, and specific types of gastritis with distinctive features both endoscopically and histologically.

■ SYNONYMS
Erosive gastritis
Hemorrhagic gastritis
Helicobacter pylori gastritis

ICD-9CM CODES
535.5 Gastritis (unless otherwise specified)
535.0 Gastritis, acute
535.3 Alcoholic gastritis
535.1 Atrophic (chronic) gastritis
535.4 Erosive gastritis
535.2 Hypertrophic gastritis

■ EPIDEMIOLOGY & DEMOGRAPHICS
• Erosive and hemorrhagic gastritis are most commonly seen in patients taking NSAIDs, alcoholics, and critically ill patients (usually on ventilator support).
• *H. pylori* infection with gastritis is believed to be present in 30% to 50% of the population; however, the majority are asymptomatic.
• The prevalence of *H. pylori* infection increases with age from <10% in Caucasians <40 yr old to >50% in patients >50 yr.

■ PHYSICAL FINDINGS & CLINICAL PRESENTATION
• Epigastric tenderness in acute alcoholic gastritis (may be absent in chronic gastritis)
• Foul-smelling breath
• Hematemesis ("coffee-ground" emesis)

■ ETIOLOGY
• Alcohol, NSAIDs, stress (critically ill patients usually on mechanical respiration), hepatic or renal failure, multiorgan failure
• Infection (bacterial, viral)
• Bile reflux, pancreatic enzyme reflux
• Gastric mucosal atrophy, portal hypertension gastropathy
• Irradiation

DIAGNOSIS

■ DIFFERENTIAL DIAGNOSIS
• Peptic ulcer disease
• GERD
• Nonulcer dyspepsia
• Gastric lymphoma or carcinoma
• Pancreatitis
• Gastroparesis

■ WORKUP
Patients with gastritis generally present with nonspecific clinical signs and symptoms (e.g., epigastric pain, abdominal tenderness, bloating, anorexia, nausea [with or without vomiting]). Symptoms may be aggravated by eating. Diagnostic workup includes a comprehensive history and endoscopy with biopsy.

■ LABORATORY TESTS
• Serologic (IgG antibody to *H. pylori*) or breath test (^{13}C urea breath tests) for *H. pylori;* patients should not receive proton pump inhibitors for 2 wk before undergoing urea breath test for *H. pylori* infection. Serum antibody tests are not reliable because of a high rate of false-positive results and the fact that antibodies persist even after treatment. The urea breath test is more sensitive and specific; however, it is not readily available. Histologic evaluation of endoscopic biopsy samples is currently the gold standard for accurate diagnosis of *H. pylori* infection.
• Stool antigen test for *H. pylori* is useful to confirm successful eradication of *H. pylori* following treatment.
• Vitamin B$_{12}$ level in patients with atrophic gastritis.
• Hct (low if significant bleeding has occurred).

■ IMAGING STUDIES
Upper GI series is generally insensitive for the detection of gastritis. Gastroscopy with biopsy is the gold standard diagnostic test and will also detect *H. pylori.*

TREATMENT

■ NONPHARMACOLOGIC THERAPY
• Avoidance of mucosal irritants such as alcohol and NSAIDs
• Lifestyle modifications with avoidance of tobacco and foods that trigger symptoms

■ ACUTE GENERAL Rx
• Eradication of infectious agents: *H. pylori* therapy with
  1. Proton pump inhibitors (PPI) bid (e.g., omeprazole 20 mg bid or lansoprazole 30 mg bid) *plus* clarithromycin 500 mg bid *and* amoxicillin 1000 mg bid for 7 to 10 days
  2. PPI bid *plus* amoxicillin 500 mg bid *plus* metronidazole 500 mg for 7 to 10 days
  3. PPI bid *plus* clarithromycin 500 mg bid *and* metronidazole 500 mg bid for 7 days
  4. Bismouth compound qid *plus* tetracycline 500 mg qid *and* metronidazole 500 mg qid for 14 days
• Prophylaxis and treatment of stress gastritis with sucralfate suspension 1 g orally q4-6h or H$_2$-receptor antagonists
• Misoprostol (Cytotec) in patients on chronic NSAIDs therapy

■ CHRONIC Rx
• Misoprostol 100 μg qid in patients receiving chronic NSAIDs
• Avoidance of alcohol, tobacco, and prolonged NSAID use
• Surveillance gastroscopy in patients with atrophic gastritis (increased risk of gastric cancer)

■ DISPOSITION
• Prognosis is good with most cases resolving with treatment. Successful eradication of *H. pylori* infection can be achieved in >80% of patients with appropriate therapy. Undetectable serum antibody levels beyond the first year of therapy accurately confirm cure of *H. pylori* infection in initially seropositive healthy subjects with reasonable sensitivity.
• Most patients with atrophic gastritis and intestinal metaplasia improve within 12 months following successful *H. pylori* eradication.

■ REFERRAL
• GI referral for endoscopy in selected cases
• Hospitalization of patients with significant bleeding

PEARLS & CONSIDERATIONS

■ COMMENTS
Patient education explaining the meaning of gastritis, reassuring the patient, and stressing the importance of lifestyle modifications.

REFERENCES
Feldman M et al: Role of seroconversion in confirming cure of *H. pylori* infection, *JAMA* 280:363, 1998.
Ohrusa T et al: Improvement in atrophic gastritis and intestinal metaplasia in patients in whom *H. pylori* was eradicated, *Ann Intern Med* 134:380, 2001.
Author: **Fred F. Ferri, M.D.**

BASIC INFORMATION

■ **DEFINITION**
Gastroesophageal reflux disease (GERD) is a motility disorder characterized primarily by heartburn and caused by the reflux of gastric contents into the esophagus.

■ **SYNONYMS**
Peptic esophagitis
Reflux esophagitis
GERD

■ **ICD-9CM CODES**
530.81 Gastroesophageal reflux disease
530.1 Esophagitis
787.1 Heartburn

■ **EPIDEMIOLOGY & DEMOGRAPHICS**
GERD is one of the most prevalent GI disorders. Nearly 7% of persons in the United States experience heartburn daily, 20% experience it monthly, and 60% experience it intermittently. Incidence in pregnant women exceeds 80%. Nearly 20% of adults use antacids or OTC H_2-blockers at least once a week for relief of heartburn.

■ **PHYSICAL FINDINGS & CLINICAL PRESENTATION**
• Physical examination: generally unremarkable
• Clinical signs and symptoms: heartburn, dysphagia, sour taste, regurgitation of gastric contents into the mouth
• Chronic cough and bronchospasm
• Chest pain, laryngitis, early satiety, abdominal fullness, and bloating with belching

■ **ETIOLOGY**
• Incompetent LES
• Medications that lower LES pressure (calcium channel blockers, β-adrenergic blockers, theophylline, anticholinergics)
• Foods that lower LES pressure (chocolate, yellow onions, peppermint)
• Tobacco abuse, alcohol, coffee
• Pregnancy
• Gastric acid hypersecretion
• Hiatal hernia (controversial) present in >70% of patients with GERD; however, most patients with hiatal hernia are asymptomatic

■ **DIAGNOSIS**

■ **DIFFERENTIAL DIAGNOSIS**
• Peptic ulcer disease
• Unstable angina
• Esophagitis (from infections such as herpes, *Candida*), medication induced (doxycycline, potassium chloride)
• Esophageal spasm (nutcracker esophagus)
• Cancer of esophagus
• Table 2-89 describes the differential diagnosis of heartburn and indigestion.

■ **WORKUP**
• Aimed at eliminating the conditions noted in the differential diagnosis and documenting the type and extent of tissue damage with upper endoscopy
• A clinical algorithm for evaluation of heartburn is described in Fig. 3-74.

■ **LABORATORY TESTS**
• 24-hr esophageal pH monitoring and Bernstein test are sensitive diagnostic tests; however, they are not very practical and generally not done. They are useful in patients with atypical manifestations of GERD, such as chest pain or chronic cough.
• Esophageal manometry is indicated in patients with refractory reflux in whom surgical therapy is planned.

■ **IMAGING STUDIES**
• Upper GI series can identify ulcerations and strictures; however, it may miss mucosal abnormalities. Only one third of patients with GERD have radiographic signs of esophagitis.
• Upper GI endoscopy is useful to document the type and extent of tissue damage in GERD and to exclude potentially malignant conditions such as Barrett's esophagus.

■ **TREATMENT**

■ **NONPHARMACOLOGIC THERAPY**
• Lifestyle modifications with avoidance of foods and drugs that decrease LES pressure (e.g., caffeine, β-blockers)
• Avoidance of tobacco and alcohol use
• Elevation of head of bed using blocks
• Avoidance of lying down directly after late or large evening meals
• Weight reduction, decreased fat intake

■ **ACUTE GENERAL Rx**
• Proton pump inhibitors (PPIs) (omeprazole 20 mg qd or lansoprazole 30 mg qd, or rabeprazole 20 mg qd, or pantoprazole 40 mg qd) are safe, tolerated, and very effective in most patients.
• H_2-Blockers (nizatidine 300 mg qhs, famotidine 40 mg qhs, ranitidine 300 mg qhs, or cimetidine 800 mg qhs) are generally much less effective than PPIs.

• Antacids (may be useful for relief of mild symptoms; however, they are generally ineffective in severe cases of reflux).
• Prokinetic agents (metoclopramide) are indicated only when PPIs are not fully effective. They can be used in combination therapy; however, side effects limit their use.
• For refractory cases: surgery with Nissen fundoplication. Although laparoscopic fundoplication is now widely used, surgery should not be advised with the expectation that patients with GERD will no longer need to take antisecretory medications or that the procedure will prevent esophageal cancer among those with GERD and Barrett's esophagus.

■ **CHRONIC Rx**
Lifestyle modification must be followed lifelong, since this is generally an irreversible condition.

■ **DISPOSITION**
• The majority of the patients respond well to therapy.
• Recurrence of reflux is common if treatment is discontinued.
• There is a strong and probably causal relation between symptomatic prolonged and untreated GERD and esophageal adenocarcinoma.

■ **REFERRAL**
• GI referral for upper endoscopy is needed when there are concerns about associated PUD, Barrett's esophagus, or esophageal cancer.
• Patients with Barrett's esophagus should undergo surveillance endoscopy with mucosal biopsy every 2 yr or less because the risk of developing adenocarcinoma of esophagus is at least 30 times greater than that of the general population.

☼ PEARLS & CONSIDERATIONS

■ **COMMENTS**
• Chronic GERD is the primary cause of Barrett's esophagus.
• The primary approach for most GERD patients is pharmacologic. Surgery is associated with up-front morbidity and mortality risk and generally eventual return to medical therapy.

■ **REFERENCES**
Eisen GM: The burning issue of chronic GERD, *Ann Intern Med* 133:227, 2000.
Spechler S et al: Long term outcome of medical and surgical therapies for GERD, *JAMA* 285:2331, 2001.
Author: **Fred F. Ferri, M.D.**

BASIC INFORMATION

■ DEFINITION
Giardiasis is an intestinal and/or biliary tract infection caused by the protozoal parasite *Giardia lamblia*.

ICD-9CM CODES
007.1 Giardiasis

■ EPIDEMIOLOGY & DEMOGRAPHICS
INCIDENCE (IN U.S.):
- Exact incidence unknown
- Frequently occurs in outbreaks

PREVALENCE (IN U.S.): 4%
PREDOMINANT SEX: Male = female
PREDOMINANT AGE:
- Preschool children, especially if in day care
- 20 to 40 yr old, especially among sexually active homosexual men

PEAK INCIDENCE:
- Varies with risk factors, outbreaks
- All age groups affected

GENETICS:
Familial Disposition: Patients with common variable immunodeficiency or X-linked agammaglobulinemia are at increased risk of infection.
Neonatal Infection: Rare; infection is common among preschool children in day care.

■ PHYSICAL FINDINGS & CLINICAL PRESENTATION
- More than 70% with one or more intestinal symptoms (diarrhea, flatulence, cramps, bloating, nausea)
- Fever in <20%
- Malaise, anorexia
- Chronic diarrhea, malabsorption, and weight loss
- GI bleeding is unusual

- Continuous or intermittent symptoms, lasting for weeks
- Of infected patients, 20% to 25% are asymptomatic

■ ETIOLOGY
Infection is acquired by ingestion of viable cysts of the organism, typically in contaminated water or by fecal-oral contact.

DIAGNOSIS

■ DIFFERENTIAL DIAGNOSIS
- Other agents of infective diarrhea (amebae, *Salmonella* sp., *Shigella* sp., *Staphylococcus aureus, Cryptosporidium*, etc.)
- Noninfectious causes of malabsorption
- Table 2-110 describes the differential diagnosis of infectious diseases in travelers

■ WORKUP
Stool specimen (three specimens yield 90% sensitivity) or duodenal aspirate for microscopic examination to establish diagnosis and exclude other pathogens (Fig. 1-165)

■ LABORATORY TESTS
- Serum albumin, vitamin B$_{12}$ levels, and stool fat test to exclude malabsorption
- Serum antibody test if desired for epidemiologic purposes

■ IMAGING STUDIES
- Not necessary unless biliary obstruction is suspected
- In detection of organism, possible interference by barium in stool from radiographic studies

TREATMENT

■ NONPHARMACOLOGIC THERAPY
Avoidance of milk products to reduce symptoms of transient lactase deficiency that occur in many patients

■ ACUTE GENERAL Rx
Adults:
- Metronidazole 250 mg PO three times daily for 7 days (metronidazole avoided in pregnancy) *or*
- Paromomycin 25 to 30 mg/kg/day in three doses for 5 to 10 days

■ CHRONIC Rx
May require retreatment

■ DISPOSITION
Reinfection is possible.

■ REFERRAL
For evaluation by gastroenterologist if malabsorption and weight loss do not resolve with therapy

PEARLS & CONSIDERATIONS

■ COMMENTS
Travelers to endemic areas (developing world, wilderness areas) should be cautioned to boil drinking water, or if this is impossible, use halogenated water purification tablets.

REFERENCE
Thompson RC: Giardiasis as a re-emerging infectious disease and its zoonotic potential, *Int J Parasitol* 30(12-13):1259, 2000.
Author: **Joseph R. Masci, M.D.**

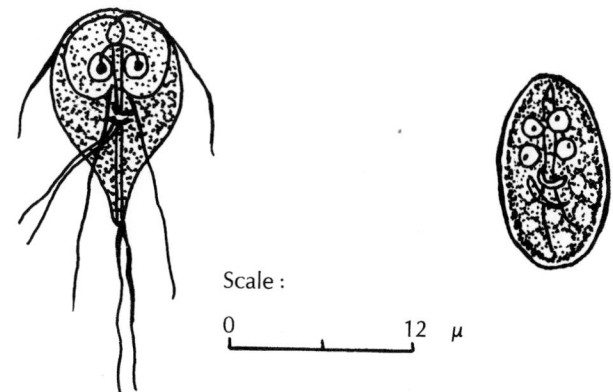

Fig. 1-165 *Giardia* organisms. The trophozoite *(left)* is 12 to 15 μm long and has four pairs of flagella. This form is not commonly seen in stools. Cysts *(right)* are 9 to 19 μm long and may have two to four nuclei. (From Hoekelman R [ed]: *Primary pediatric care*, ed 3, St Louis, 1997, Mosby.)

BASIC INFORMATION

■ DEFINITION
Gilbert's disease is an autosomal dominant disease characterized by indirect hyperbilirubinemia caused by impaired glucuronyl transferase activity.

■ SYNONYMS
Gilbert's syndrome

■ ICD-9CM CODES
277.4 Gilbert's syndrome

■ EPIDEMIOLOGY & DEMOGRAPHICS
- Probable autosomal dominant disease affecting >5% of the U.S. population
- Male:female ratio of 3:1

■ PHYSICAL FINDINGS & CLINICAL PRESENTATION
- No abnormalities on physical examination other than mild jaundice when bilirubin exceeds 3 mg/dl.
- A family history of unconjugated hyperbilirubinemia may be present.

■ ETIOLOGY
Decreased elimination of bilirubin in bile is caused by inadequate conjugation of bilirubin. Alcohol consumption and starvation diet can increase the bilirubin level. The pathogenesis of Gilbert's syndrome has been linked to a reduction in bilirubin UGT-1 gene (HUG-Brl) transcription resulting from a mutation in the promoter region.

DIAGNOSIS

■ DIFFERENTIAL DIAGNOSIS
- Hemolytic anemia
- Liver disease (chronic hepatitis, cirrhosis)
- Crigler-Najjar syndrome

■ WORKUP
- Most patients are diagnosed during or after adolescence, when isolated hyperbilirubinemia is detected as an incidental finding on routine biochemical testing.
- Laboratory evaluation to exclude hemolysis and liver diseases as a cause of the elevated bilirubin level (Table 1-31).

■ LABORATORY TESTS
Elevated indirect (unconjugated) bilirubin (rarely exceeds 5 mg/dl)

TREATMENT

■ ACUTE GENERAL Rx
Treatment is generally unnecessary. Phenobarbital (if clinical jaundice is present) can rapidly decrease serum indirect bilirubin level.

■ DISPOSITION
Prognosis is excellent. Treatment is generally unnecessary.

■ REFERRAL
Referral is generally not necessary.

PEARLS & CONSIDERATIONS

■ COMMENTS
- Patients should be reassured about the benign nature of their condition.
- Fasting for ≥2 days or significant dehydration may raise the bilirubin level and result in the clinical recognition of jaundice.

Author: **Fred F. Ferri, M.D.**

TABLE 1-31   Characteristic Patterns of Liver Function Tests

DISORDER	BILIRUBIN	ALKALINE PHOSPHATASE	AST	ALT	PROTHROMBIN TIME	ALBUMIN
Gilbert's syndrome (abnormal bilirubin metabolism)	↑	NL	NL	NL	NL	NL
Bile duct obstruction (pancreatic cancer)	↑↑↑	↑↑↑	↑	↑	↑-↑↑	NL
Acute hepatocellular damage (toxic, viral hepatitis)	↑-↑↑↑	↑-↑↑	↑↑↑	↑↑↑	NL-↑↑↑	NL-↓↓
Cirrhosis	NL-↑	NL-↑	NL-↑	NL-↑	NL-↑↑	NL-↓↓

From Andreoli TE (ed): *Cecil essentials of medicine,* ed 4, Philadelphia, 1997, WB Saunders.
ALT, Alanine aminotransferase; *AST,* aspartate aminotransferase; *NL,* normal; ↑, increase; ↓, decrease (arrows indicate extent of change: ↑-↑↑↑, slight to large).

BASIC INFORMATION

■ DEFINITION
Gingivitis refers to inflammation of the gums covering the maxilla and mandible.

■ ICD-9CM CODES
523.1 Gingivitis

■ EPIDEMIOLOGY & DEMOGRAPHICS
PREDOMINANT AGE: Adulthood

■ PHYSICAL FINDINGS & CLINICAL PRESENTATION
- Usually painless inflammation
- Possible bleeding with minor trauma such as brushing teeth
- Bluish discoloration of the gums; possible halitosis
- Subgingival plaque on close examination
- In time, detachment of soft tissue from the tooth surface
- Possible long-standing infection leading to destructive periodontal disease that may involve teeth and bones
- Acute necrotizing ulcerative gingivitis (ANUG or "trench mouth"): a dramatic form of gingivitis manifested by acute, painful, inflammation of the gingivae, with bleeding, ulceration, and halitosis. At times accompanied by fever and lymphadenopathy (Fig. 1-166).
- *Linear gingival erythema* ("HIV gingivitis") presents as a brightly inflamed band of marginal gingiva. It may be painful, with easy bleeding and rapid destruction.
- Possible severe periodontitis in patients with diabetes mellitus or HIV infection and in primary HIV infection (acute retroviral syndrome).

- Pregnancy: sometimes associated with an acute form of gingivitis
- Gingivae become inflamed and hypertrophic, possibly the result of hormonal shifts.

■ ETIOLOGY
- Various organisms found in the environment of plaque; anaerobes are predominant in periodontal disease.
- Improper hygiene and poorly fitting dentures contribute to development of gingivitis.
- Excessive use of tobacco and alcohol predispose individuals to gingival disease.
- In patients with HIV infection, gram-negative anaerobes, enteric organisms, and yeast predominate.
- Appropriate oral hygiene, such as flossing and tooth brushing, is preventative for the accumulation of bacterial plaque.
- Once plaque is present, adequate hygiene is more difficult.

DIAGNOSIS

■ DIFFERENTIAL DIAGNOSIS
Gingival hyperplasia, which may be caused by phenytoin or nifedipine

■ WORKUP
Oral examination

■ LABORATORY TESTS
Elevated serum glucose in diabetics

■ IMAGING STUDIES
Radiographs of the teeth and facial bones to reveal extension of infection to these structures

TREATMENT

■ NONPHARMACOLOGIC THERAPY
Removal of plaque and, at times, debridement of soft tissue

■ ACUTE GENERAL Rx
- Penicillin VK 500 mg PO qid for 1 to 2 wk *or*
- Clindamycin 300 mg PO qid for 1 to 2 wk
- For *linear gingival erythema* chlorhexidine rinses and nystatin rinses or troches may be used.

■ CHRONIC Rx
Periodic evaluation and debridement for extensive or recurrent infection

■ DISPOSITION
Continued inflammation, leading eventually to destruction of teeth and bone

■ REFERRAL
To a dentist or oral surgeon

PEARLS & CONSIDERATIONS

■ COMMENTS
- Presence of periodontal disease is associated with an increased incidence of anaerobic pleuropulmonary infections.

REFERENCE
Obernesser MS: Gingivitis and periodontitis syndromes. In *Up to date,* Clinical reference CD, vol 8:1, 2000.
Author: **Maurice Policar, M.D.**

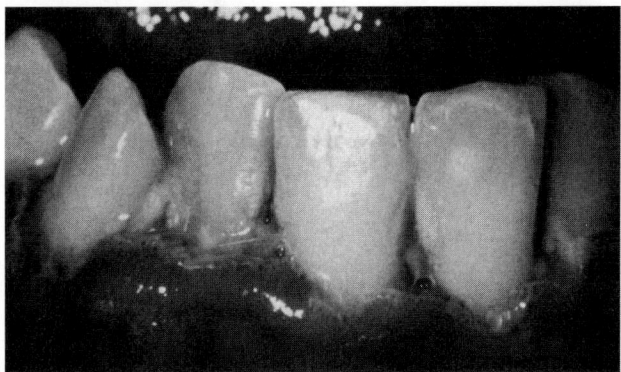

Fig. 1-166   Acute necrotizing ulcerative gingivitis involving lower anterior teeth. (From Rosen P [ed]: *Emergency medicine,* ed 4, St Louis, 1998, Mosby.)

BASIC INFORMATION

■ DEFINITION
Chronic open-angle glaucoma refers to optic nerve damage often associated with elevated intraocular pressure; it is a chronic, slowly progressive (Fig. 1-167), usually bilateral disorder associated with visual loss, eye pain, and optic nerve damage.

■ ICD-9CM CODES
365.1 Open-angle glaucoma

■ EPIDEMIOLOGY & DEMOGRAPHICS
INCIDENCE (IN U.S.): Third most common cause of visual loss (75% to 95% of all glaucomas are open angle.)
PREVALENCE (IN U.S.):
- 15,000,000 Americans may have glaucoma and 1,600,000 have visual field loss.
- 150,000 patients suffer bilateral blindness.
- Disease occurs in 2% of people >40 yr old.
- Prevalence is higher in diabetics, with high myopia, and among older persons.
PREDOMINANT AGE:
- Persons >50 yr old
- Can occur in 30s and 40s
PEAK INCIDENCE: Increases after 40 yr
GENETICS:
- Four to six times higher incidence in blacks than whites
- No clear-cut hereditary patterns but a strong hereditary tendency

■ PHYSICAL FINDINGS
- High intraocular pressures and large optic nerve cup (Fig. 1-167)
- Abnormal visual fields
- Open-angle gonioscopy

■ ETIOLOGY
- Uncertain hereditary tendency
- Topical steroids
- Trauma
- Inflammatory
- High-dose oral corticosteroids taken for prolonged periods

DIAGNOSIS

■ DIFFERENTIAL DIAGNOSIS
- Other optic neuropathies
- Secondary glaucoma from inflammation and steroid therapy

■ WORKUP
- Intraocular pressure
- Slit lamp examination
- Visual fields
- Gonioscopy

■ LABORATORY TESTS
Blood sugar

■ IMAGING STUDIES
- Optic nerve photography
- Visual field testing
- GDx (laser scan of nerve fiber layer)

TREATMENT

■ ACUTE GENERAL Rx
- β-Blockers (Timolol)
- Diamox or pilocarpine
- Hyperosmotic agents (mannitol)
- Prostaglandins

■ CHRONIC Rx
At least biannual checks of intraocular pressure and adjustment of medication

■ DISPOSITION
Usually followed by ophthalmologist

■ REFERRAL
Immediately to ophthalmologist

PEARLS & CONSIDERATIONS

■ COMMENTS
- Early diagnosis and treatment may minimize visual loss.
- Glaucoma is not solely caused by increased intraocular pressure, because approximately 20% of patients with glaucoma have normal intraocular pressure.

REFERENCE
Alward WL: Medical management of glaucoma, *N Engl J Med* 339:1298, 1998.
Author: **Melvyn Koby, M.D.**

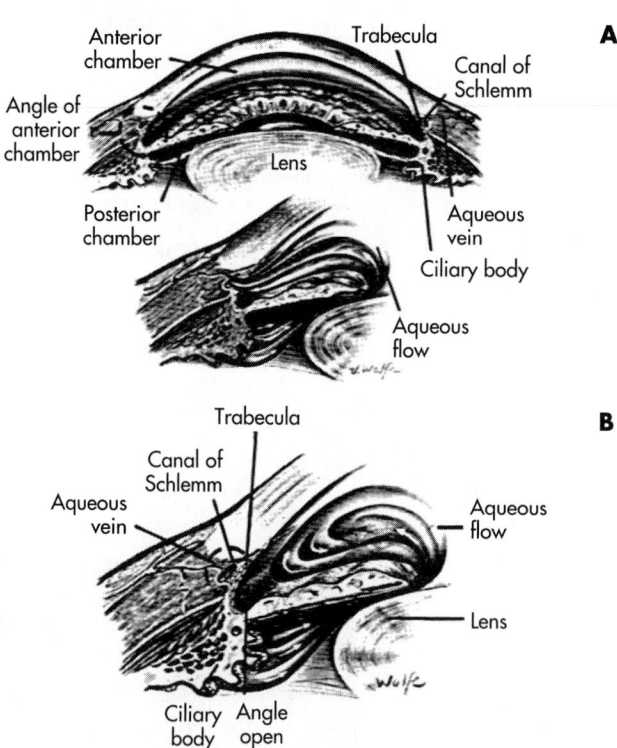

Fig. 1-167 **A,** Flow of aqueous from the ciliary body, leaving the eye through the trabecula and canal of Schlemm via a normal open, wide angle. **B,** Chronic open-angle glaucoma. (From Scheie HG, Albert DM: *Textbook of ophthalmology,* ed 9, Philadelphia, 1977, WB Saunders.)

BASIC INFORMATION

DEFINITION
Primary closed-angle glaucoma occurs when elevated intraocular pressure is associated with closure of the filtration angle.

SYNONYMS
Glaucoma
Pupillary block glaucoma

ICD-9CM CODES
365.2 Primary angle-closure glaucoma

EPIDEMIOLOGY & DEMOGRAPHICS
INCIDENCE (IN U.S.):
- In 2% to 8% of all patients with glaucoma
- Higher incidence among those with hyperopia

PREDOMINANT SEX: Females > males
PREDOMINANT AGE: 50 to 60 yr
PEAK INCIDENCE: Greater after 50 yr of age
GENETICS: High family history

PHYSICAL FINDINGS & CLINICAL FINDINGS
- Hazy cornea (Fig. 1-168)
- Narrow angle
- Red eyes
- Pain
- Injection of conjunctiva

ETIOLOGY
- Narrow angles with acute closure

- Topiramate (Topamax)

DIAGNOSIS

DIFFERENTIAL DIAGNOSIS
- Open-angle glaucoma
- Conjunctivitis
- Corneal disease
- Table 2-211 describes the differential diagnosis of acute painful loss of vision

WORKUP
- Intraocular pressure
- Gonioscopy
- Slit lamp examination
- Visual field examination
- GDx examination (laser scan of nerve fiber layer)

LABORATORY TESTS
Blood sugar and CBC (if diabetes or inflammatory disease is suspected)

IMAGING STUDIES
- Fundus photography
- Fluorescein angiography for neurovascular disease

TREATMENT

NONPHARMACOLOGIC THERAPY
Laser iridotomy early in disease process

ACUTE GENERAL Rx
- IV mannitol
- Pilocarpine
- β-Blockers
- Diamox

CHRONIC Rx
Iridotomy

DISPOSITION
Refer to ophthalmologist immediately.

REFERRAL
This is an emergency—refer immediately to an ophthalmologist.

PEARLS & CONSIDERATIONS

COMMENTS
- After iridotomy, the majority of patients will be totally cured and will need no further medication and have no visual loss.
- Lower socioeconomic status and higher levels of social deprivation are risk factors for delayed detection and probable worse outcomes in glaucoma.

REFERENCES
Alward WL: Medical management of glaucoma, *N Engl J Med* 339:1298, 1998.
Fraser S et al: Deprivation and late presentation of glaucoma: case control study, *BMJ* 322:638, 2001.
Author: **Melvyn Koby, M.D.**

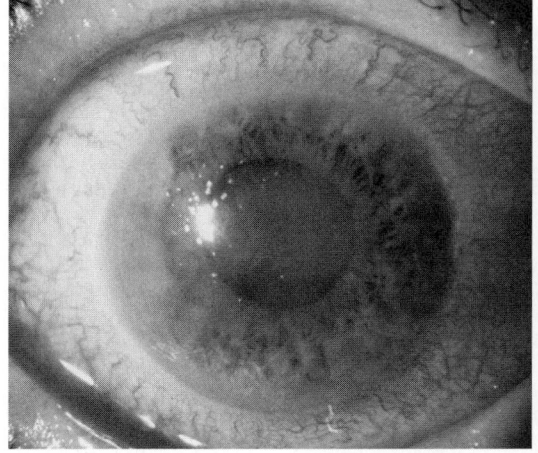
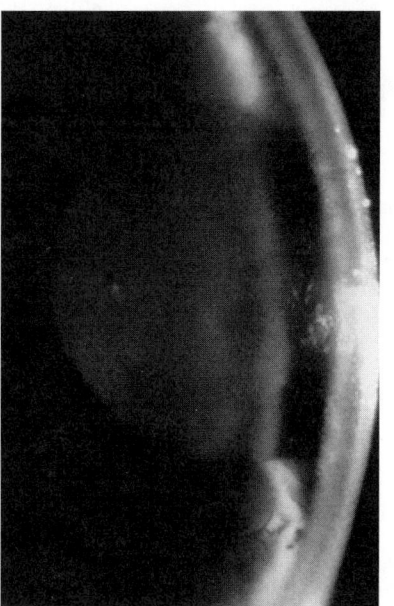

Fig. 1-168   Acute angle-closure glaucoma. **A,** Acutely elevated pressure produces an inflamed eye with corneal edema (note fragmented light reflex) and a middilated pupil. **B,** Slit lamp examination shows a very shallow central anterior chamber (space between cornea and iris) *(1)* and no peripheral chamber *(2)*. (From Palay D [ed]: *Ophthalmology for the primary care physician,* St Louis, 1997, Mosby.)

BASIC INFORMATION

■ DEFINITION

Acute glomerulonephritis is an immunologically mediated inflammation primarily involving the glomerulus that can result in damage to the basement membrane, mesangium, or capillary endothelium. Table 1-32 summarizes primary renal diseases that present as acute glomerulonephritis.

■ SYNONYMS

Postinfectious glomerulonephritis
Acute nephritic syndrome

■ ICD-9CM CODES

583.9 Glomerulonephritis, acute

■ EPIDEMIOLOGY & DEMOGRAPHICS

- Over 50% of cases involve children <13 yr old.
- Glomerulonephritis is the most common cause of chronic renal failure (25%).
- IgA nephropathy glomerulonephritis (Berger's disease) is the most common glomerulonephritis worldwide.

■ PHYSICAL FINDINGS & CLINICAL FINDINGS

- Edema (peripheral, periorbital, or pulmonary)
- Joint pains, oral ulcers, malar rash (frequently seen with lupus nephritis)
- Dark urine
- Hypertension
- Findings of palpable purpura in patients with Henoch-Schönlein purpura
- Heart murmurs may indicate endocarditis
- Impetigo, skin pallor, tenderness in the abdomen and/or back, pharyngeal erythema may be present

■ ETIOLOGY

Acute glomerulonephritis may be due to primary renal disease or a systemic disease. A number of pathogenic processes (e.g., antibody deposition, cell-mediated immune mechanisms, complement activation, hemodynamic alterations) have been implicated in the pathogenesis of glomerular inflammation. Medical disorders generally associated with glomerulonephritis are:

- Post group A β-hemolytic *Streptococcus* infection (other infectious etiologies including endocarditis and visceral abscess)
- Collagen-vascular diseases (SLE)
- Vasculitis (Wegener's granulomatosis, polyarteritis nodosa)
- Idiopathic glomerulonephritis (membranoproliferative, idiopathic, crescentic, IgA nephropathy)

- Goodpasture's syndrome
- Other cryoglobulinemia (Henoch-Schönlein purpura)
- Drug-induced (gold, penicillamine)
- Table 1-32 is a summary of primary renal diseases that present as acute glomerulonephritis

DIAGNOSIS

■ DIFFERENTIAL DIAGNOSIS

- Cirrhosis with edema and ascites
- CHF
- Acute interstitial nephritis
- Severe hypertension
- Hemolytic-uremic syndrome
- SLE, diabetes mellitus, amyloidosis, preeclampsia, sclerodermal renal crisis

■ WORKUP

- Initial evaluation of suspected glomerulonephritis consists of laboratory testing.

■ LABORATORY TESTS

- Urinalysis (hematuria [dysmorphic erythrocytes and red cell casts], proteinuria)
- Serum creatinine (to estimate GFR), BUN
- 24-hr urine for protein excretion and creatinine clearance (to document degree of renal dysfunction and amount of proteinuria). Proteinuria in acute glomerulonephritis typically ranges from 500 mg/day to 3 g/day but nephrotic-range proteinuria (>3.5 g/day) may be present
- Streptococcal tests (Streptozyme), antistreptolysin O (ASO) quantitative titer (highest in 3 to 5 wk); ASO titer, however, is not related to severity of renal disease, duration, or prognosis
- Additional useful tests depending on the history: Anti-DNA antibodies (rule out SLE), CH_{50} level (if elevated, obtain C_3, C_4 levels), triglycerides, cryoglobulins, hepatitis B and C serologies, ANCA (antineutrophil cytoplasmic antibody), c-ANCA (in suspected cases of Wegener's granulomatosis), p-ANCA found in pauci-immune (lack of immune deposits) idiopathic rapidly progressive glomerulonephritis with or without systemic vasculitis, anti-glomerular basement membrane (type alpha[3] IV collagen) antibodies
- Hct (decrease in glomerulonephritis), platelet count (thrombocytopenia in cases of lupus nephritis)
- Anti-GBM antibody (in Goodpasture's syndrome)
- Blood cultures are indicated in all febrile patients

■ IMAGING STUDIES

- Chest x-ray examination: pulmonary congestion, Wegener's granulomatosis, and Goodpasture's syndrome
- Renal ultrasound if GFR is depressed to evaluate renal size and determine extent of fibrosis. A kidney size of <9 cm is suggestive of extensive scarring and low likelihood of reversibility
- Echocardiogram in patients with new cardiac murmurs or positive blood cultures to rule out endocarditis and pericardial effusion
- Renal biopsy and light, electron, and immunofluorescent microscopy to confirm diagnosis
- Kidney biopsy: generally reveals a granular pattern in poststreptococcal glomerulonephritis, linear pattern in Goodpasture's syndrome (Fig. 1-169); absence of immune deposits suggests vasculitis; renal biopsy: although helpful to define the etiology of glomerulonephritis, is not usually essential. It is useful to determine the degree of inflammation and fibrosis. It is also especially important for patients with RPGN where prompt diagnosis and treatment is essential
- Immunofluorescence: generally reveals C3; negative immunofluorescence suggests Wegener's granulomatosis, idiopathic crescentic glomerulonephritis, or polyarteritis nodosa
- Angiography or biopsy of other affected organs if systemic vasculitis is suspected

TREATMENT

■ NONPHARMACOLOGIC THERAPY

- Avoidance of salt if edema or hypertension is present
- Low-protein intake (approximately 0.5 g/kg/day) in patients with renal failure
- Fluid restriction in patients with significant edema
- Avoidance of high-potassium foods

■ ACUTE GENERAL Rx

- Correction of electrolyte abnormalities (hypocalcemia, hyperkalemia) and acidosis (if present)
- Treatment of streptococcal infection with penicillin (or erythromycin in penicillin-allergic patients)
- Furosemide in patients with significant hypertension and/or edema; hydralazine or nifedipine in patients with hypertension
- Immunosuppressive treatment in patients with heavy proteinuria or rapidly decreasing glomerular

filtration rate (high-dose steroids, cyclosporin A, cyclophosphamide); corticosteroids generally not useful in poststreptococcal glomerulonephritis
- Fish oil (n-3 fatty acids) 12 g/day: may prevent or slow down loss of renal function in patients with IgA nephropathy
- Plasma exchange therapy and immunosuppressive drugs (prednisone and cyclophosphamide): effective in Goodpasture's syndrome

■ CHRONIC Rx
- Frequent monitoring of urinalysis, serum creatinine, and blood pressure in the initial 12 mo
- Monitoring for onset of hypertensive retinopathy, encephalopathy
- Aggressive treatment of infections, particularly streptococcal infections
- Dosage adjustment of all renally excreted medications

■ DISPOSITION
- Prognosis is generally related to histology with excellent prognosis in patients with minimal change glomerulonephritis and focal segmental proliferative glomerulonephritis; 25% to 30% of patients with mesangial IgA disease and membranous glomerulonephritis generally progress to chronic renal failure; >70% of patients with mesangial capillary glomerulonephritis will develop chronic renal failure.
- Generally prognosis is worse in patients with heavy proteinuria, severe hypertension, and significant elevations of creatinine.
- Recovery of renal function occurs within 8 to 12 wk in 95% of patients with poststreptococcal glomerulonephritis.

■ REFERRAL
- Nephrology consultation. The urgency for referral depends on the GFR. Urgent consultation is recommended if GFR is significantly abnormal, rapidly deteriorating, or if there are systemic symptoms.
- Surgical referral for biopsy in selected cases

◇ PEARLS & CONSIDERATIONS

■ COMMENTS
- Anticoagulation to prevent DVT should be considered in patients with a low level of physical activity.
- Monitoring of lipids and aggressive treatment of hyperlipidemias is recommended.
- Close monitoring of side effects of immunosuppressive drugs and complications of corticosteroids is necessary.

REFERENCES
Hricik D et al: Glomerulonephritis, *N Engl J Med* 339:888, 1998.
Madaio MP, Harrington JT: The diagnosis of glomerular diseases, *Arch Intern Med* 161:25, 2001.
Author: **Fred F. Ferri, M.D.**

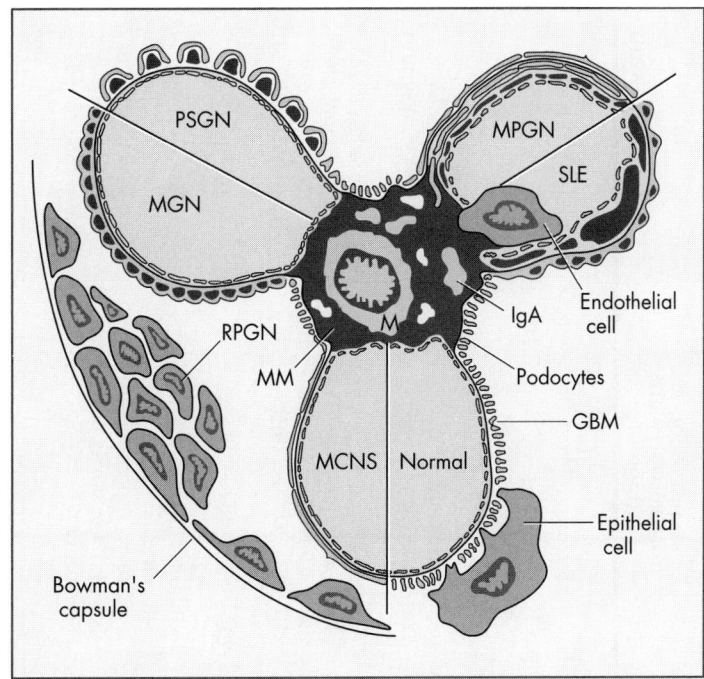

Fig. 1-169 Schematic drawing of a glomerulus illustrating the normal features as well as several diseases. *GBM,* Glomerular basement membrane; *IgA,* IgA deposits in IgA nephropathy; *M,* mesangial cell; *MCNS,* minimal change nephrotic syndrome; *MGN,* membranous glomerulopathy; *MM,* mesangial matrix; *MPGN,* membranoproliferative glomerulopathy; *PSGN,* poststreptococcal glomerulonephritis; *RPGN,* rapidly progressive glomerulonephritis; *SLE,* systemic lupus erythematosus. (From Andreoli TE [ed]: *Cecil essentials of medicine,* ed 4, Philadelphia, 1997, WB Saunders.)

TABLE 1-32 Summary of Primary Renal Diseases That Present as Acute Glomerulonephritis

DISEASES	POSTSTREPTOCOCCAL GLOMERULONEPHRITIS (PSGN)	IgA NEPHROPATHY	MEMBRANOPROLIFERATIVE GLOMERULONEPHRITIS	IDIOPATHIC RAPIDLY PROGRESSIVE GLOMERULONEPHRITIS (RPGN)
Clinical manifestations				
Age and sex	All ages, mean 7 yr, 2:1 male	15-35 yr, 2:1 male	15-30 yr, 6:1 male	Mean 58 yr, 2:1 male
Acute nephritic syndrome	90%	50%	90%	90%
Asymptomatic hematuria	Occasionally	50%	Rare	Rare
Nephrotic syndrome	10%-20%	Rare	Rare	10%-20%
Hypertension	70%	30%-50%	Rare	25%
Acute renal failure	50% (transient)	Very rare	50%	60%
Other	Latent period of 1-3 wk	Follows viral syndromes	Pulmonary hemorrhage; iron-deficiency anemia	None
Laboratory findings	↑ ASO titers (70%) Positive streptozyme (95%) ↓ C3-C9 Normal C1, C4	↑ Serum IgA (50%) IgA in dermal capillaries	Positive anti-GBM antibody	Positive ANCA
Immunogenetics	HLA-B12, D "EN" (9)*	HLA-Bw 35, DR4 (4)*	HLA-DR2 (16)*	None established
Renal pathology				
Light microscopy	Diffuse proliferation	Focal proliferation	Focal → diffuse proliferation with crescents	Crescentic GN
Immunofluorescence	Granular IgG, C3	Diffuse mesangial IgA	Linear IgG, C3	No immune deposits
Electron microscopy	Subepithelial humps	Mesangial deposits	No deposits	No deposits
Prognosis	95% resolve spontaneously 5% RPGN or slowly progressive	Slow progression in 25%-50%	75% stabilize or improve if treated early	75% stabilize or improve if treated early
Treatment	Supportive	None established	Plasma exchange, steroids, cyclophosphamide	Steroid pulse therapy

Modified from Couser WG: Glomerular disorders. In Wyngaarden JB, Smith LH, Bennett JC (eds): *Cecil textbook of medicine*, vol 1, ed 19, Philadelphia, 1992, WB Saunders. *ANCA*, Antineutrophil cytoplasm antibody; *GBM*, glomerular basement membrane; *GN*, glomerulonephritis; *Ig*, immunoglobulin.
*Relative risk.

BASIC INFORMATION

■ DEFINITION
Glossitis is an inflammation of the tongue that can lead to loss of filiform papillae.

■ ICD-9CM CODES
529.0 Glossitis

■ EPIDEMIOLOGY & DEMOGRAPHICS
Glossitis is seen more frequently in patients of lower socioeconomic status, malnourished patients, alcoholics, smokers, elderly patients, immunocompromised patients, and patients with dentures.

■ PHYSICAL FINDINGS & CLINICAL PRESENTATION
- The appearance of the tongue is variable depending on the etiology of the glossitis. Loss of filiform papillae results in red, smooth-surfaced tongue (Fig. 1-170).
- The tongue may appear pale in patients with significant anemia.
- Pain and swelling of the tongue may be present when glossitis is associated with infections, trauma, or lichen planus.
- Ulcerations may be present in patients with herpetic glossitis, pemphigus, or streptococcal infection.
- Excessive use of mouthwash may result in a "hairy" appearance of the tongue.

■ ETIOLOGY
- Nutritional deficiencies (vitamin E, riboflavin, niacin, vitamin B_{12}, iron deficiency)
- Infections (viral, candidiasis, TB, syphilis)
- Trauma (generally caused by poorly fitting dentures)
- Irritation of the tongue secondary to toothpaste, medications, alcohol, tobacco, citrus
- Lichen planus, pemphigus vulgaris, erythema multiforme
- Neoplasms

DIAGNOSIS

■ DIFFERENTIAL DIAGNOSIS
- Infections
- Use of chemical irritants
- Neoplasms
- Skin disorders (e.g., Behçet's syndrome, erythema multiforme)

■ WORKUP
- Laboratory evaluation to exclude infectious processes, vitamin deficiencies, and systemic disorders
- Biopsy of lesion only when there is no response to treatment

■ LABORATORY TESTS
- CBC: Decreased Hgb and Hct, low MCV (iron deficiency anemia), elevated MCV (vitamin B_{12} deficiency)
- Vitamin B_{12} level
- 10% KOH scrapings in patients with white patches suspect for candidiasis

TREATMENT

■ NONPHARMACOLOGIC THERAPY
Avoidance of primary irritants such as hot foods, spices, tobacco, and alcohol

■ ACUTE GENERAL Rx
Treatment varies with the etiology of the glossitis.
- Malnutrition with avitaminosis: multivitamins
- Candidiasis: fluconazole 200 mg on day 1, then 100 mg/day for at least 2 wk or nystatin 400,000 U suspension qid for 10 days or 200,000 pastilles dissolved slowly in the mouth four to five times qd for 10 to 14 days
- Painful oral lesions: rinsing of the mouth with 2% lidocaine viscous, 1 to 2 tablespoons q4h PRN; triamcinolone 0.1% applied to painful ulcers PRN for symptomatic relief

■ CHRONIC Rx
- Lifestyle changes with elimination of tobacco, alcohol, and other primary irritants
- Dental evaluation for correction of ill-fitting dentures
- Correction of associated metabolic abnormalities such as hyperglycemia from diabetes mellitus

■ DISPOSITION
Most patients experience prompt improvement with identification and treatment of the cause of the glossitis.

■ REFERRAL
Surgical referral for biopsy of solitary lesions unresponsive to treatment to rule out neoplasm

PEARLS & CONSIDERATIONS

■ COMMENTS
If the primary cause of glossitis is not identified or cannot be corrected, enteric nutritional replacement therapy should be considered in malnourished patients.

Author: **Fred F. Ferri, M.D.**

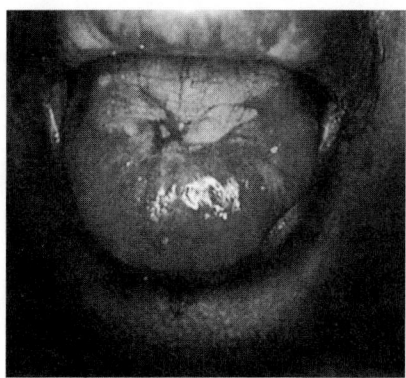

Fig. 1-170 Glossitis. (From Seidel HM [ed]: *Mosby's guide to physical examination,* ed 4, St Louis, 1999, Mosby.)

BASIC INFORMATION

■ DEFINITION

Gonorrhea is a sexually transmitted bacterial infection with a predilection for columnar and transitional epithelial cells. It commonly manifests as urethritis, cervicitis, or salpingitis. Infection may be asymptomatic. It differs in males and females in course, severity, and ease of recognition.

■ SYNONYMS

Gonococcal urethritis
Gonococcal vulvovaginitis
Gonococcal cervicitis
Gonococcal bartholinitis
Clap
GC

■ ICD-9CM CODES

098 Gonococcal infections

■ EPIDEMIOLOGY & DEMOGRAPHICS

- The disease is common worldwide, affects both sexes, all ages, especially younger adults; highest incidence is in inner-city areas, with an estimated 3 million new cases annually.
- Asymptomatic anterior urethral carriage may occur in 12% to 50% of cases in men.
- Asymptomatic in 50% to 80% of cases in women. Most common dissemination by mucosal passage to fallopian tubes, resulting in PID in 10% to 15% of infected women. Hematogenous spread may result in septic arthritis and skin lesions. Conjunctivitis rarely occurs but may result in blindness if not rapidly treated. Infection can occur in both men and women in oropharynx and anorectally.

■ PHYSICAL FINDINGS & CLINICAL PRESENTATION

- Males: purulent discharge from anterior urethra with dysuria appearing 2 to 7 days after infecting exposure. May have rectal infection causing pruritus, tenesmus, and discharge or may be asymptomatic.
- Females: initial urethritis, cervicitis may occur a few days after exposure, frequently mild. In about 20% of cases, uterine invasion occurs after menstrual period with signs and symptoms of endometritis, salpingitis, or pelvic peritonitis. The patient may have purulent discharge, inflamed Skene's or Bartholin's glands.

- Classic presentation of acute gonococcal PID is fever, abdominal and adnexal tenderness, often absence of purulent discharge. Physical examination may be normal if asymptomatic.

■ ETIOLOGY

Neisseria gonorrhoeae is the gonococcus. Plasmids coding for β-lactamase render some strains resistant to penicillin or tetracycline (PPNG, TRNG). There is an increasing frequency of chromosomally mediated resistance to penicillin, tetracycline, and cefoxitin. In the Far East, high-level resistance to spectinomycin is endemic.

There is a rising number of cases of quinolone-resistant *N. gonorrhoeae* (QRNG) worldwide, with the expected number to rise in the U.S. from importation. As long as the total number of QNRG strains remains less than 1% of strains isolated, fluoroquinolones may still be used with confidence.

DIAGNOSIS

■ DIFFERENTIAL DIAGNOSIS

- Nongonococcal urethritis (NGU)
- Nongonococcal mucopurulent cervicitis
- *Chlamydia trachomatis*

■ WORKUP

- Diagnosis is dependent on bacteriologic investigation.
- Gram-negative intracellular diplococci are diagnostic in male urethral smears. There is a false-negative rate of 60% to 70% in female cervical or urethral smears. Culture is essential in women.

■ LABORATORY TESTS

- Gonorrhea culture on Thayer-Martin medium (Organism is fastidious, requires aerobic conditions with increased carbon dioxide atmosphere. Incubate ASAP.)
- Serologic testing for syphilis on all patients
- *Chlamydia* testing on all patients
- Offer of HIV counseling and testing

TREATMENT

■ ACUTE GENERAL Rx

Uncomplicated infections of the cervix, urethra, and rectum:
- Cefixime 400 mg PO × 1 dose *or*
- Ceftriaxone 125 mg IM × 1 dose *or*
- Ciprofloxacin 500 mg PO × 1 dose *or*
- Ofloxacin 400 mg PO × 1 dose *plus* azithromycin 1 g PO × 1 dose *or*
- Doxycycline 100 mg PO bid × 7 days

Alternatives:
- Spectinomycin 2 g IM × 1 dose

Uncomplicated pharyngeal infection:
- Ceftriaxone 125 mg IM × 1 dose *or*
- Ciprofloxacin 500 mg PO × 1 dose *or*
- Ofloxacin 400 mg PO × 1 dose *plus* azithromycin 1 g PO × 1 dose *or*
- Doxycycline 100 mg PO bid × 7 days

Pregnancy: patients should not be treated with quinolones or tetracyclines. They should be treated with one of the above recommended or alternative cephalosporins.

■ DISPOSITION

- Pregnant patients require test of cure (as do those treated with regimens other than ceftriaxone/doxycycline); reculture 4 to 7 days after treatment.
- Treatment failure in nonpregnant patients is rare, and test of cure is not required. Rescreening in 1 to 2 mo detects treatment failures and re-infections.
- Sexual partners should all be identified, examined, cultured, and receive presumptive treatment.

■ REFERRAL

PID requiring hospitalization, disseminated gonococcal infection

PEARLS & CONSIDERATIONS

■ COMMENTS

- This is a reportable disease.

REFERENCE

Centers for Disease Control 1998 guidelines for treatment of sexually transmitted disease, *MMWR* 47(RR-1);1, 1998.

Author: **Eugene G. Louie-Ng, M.D.**

BASIC INFORMATION

■ DEFINITION

Goodpasture's syndrome is characterized by idiopathic recurrence of alveolar hemorrhage and rapidly progressive glomerulonephritis. It can also be defined by the triad of glomerulonephritis, pulmonary hemorrhage, and antibody to basement membrane antigens.

ICD-9CM CODES
446.2 Goodpasture's syndrome

■ EPIDEMIOLOGY & DEMOGRAPHICS
- Goodpasture's syndrome affects predominantly young white male smokers.
- Male:female ratio is 6:1.
- Goodpasture's syndrome accounts for 5% of all cases of rapidly progressive glomerulonephritis.
- 80% of patients are HLA-BR2 positive.

■ PHYSICAL FINDINGS & CLINICAL PRESENTATION
- Dyspnea, cough, hemoptysis
- Skin pallor, fever, arthralgias (may be mild or absent at the time of initial presentation)

■ ETIOLOGY
Presence of glomerular basement membranes (GBM) antibody deposition in kidneys and lungs with subsequent pulmonary hemorrhage and glomerulonephritis.

 DIAGNOSIS

■ DIFFERENTIAL DIAGNOSIS
- Wegener's granulomatosis
- SLE
- Systemic necrotizing vasculitis
- Idiopathic rapidly progressive glomerulonephritis
- Drug-induced renal pulmonary disease (e.g., penicillamine)

■ WORKUP
Laboratory evaluation, diagnostic imaging, immunofluorescence studies of renal biopsy

■ LABORATORY TESTS
- Presence of circulating serum anti-GBM antibodies

- Absence of circulating immunocomplexes, antineutrophils, cytoplasmic antibodies, and cryoglobulins
- Urinalysis revealing microscopic hematuria and proteinuria
- Elevated BUN and creatinine from rapidly progressive glomerulonephritis
- Immunofluoresence studies of renal biopsy material: linear deposits of anti-GBM antibody, often accompanied by C3 deposition
- Anemia from iron deficiency (secondary to blood loss and iron sequestration in the lungs)

■ IMAGING STUDIES
Chest x-ray examination: fluffy alveolar infiltrates, evidence of pulmonary hemorrhage (Fig. 1-171)

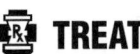 **TREATMENT**

■ ACUTE GENERAL Rx
- Plasma exchange therapy
- Immunosuppressive therapy with prednisone (1 mg/kg/day) and cyclophosphamide (2 mg/kg/day)

- Dialysis support in patients with renal failure

■ DISPOSITION
Life-threatening pulmonary hemorrhage and irreversible glomerular damage are the major causes of death.

■ REFERRAL
- Surgical referral for renal biopsy to guide the management
- Referral of patients with renal failure to dialysis center
- Consideration for renal transplantation in patients with end-stage renal failure

Author: **Fred F. Ferri, M.D.**

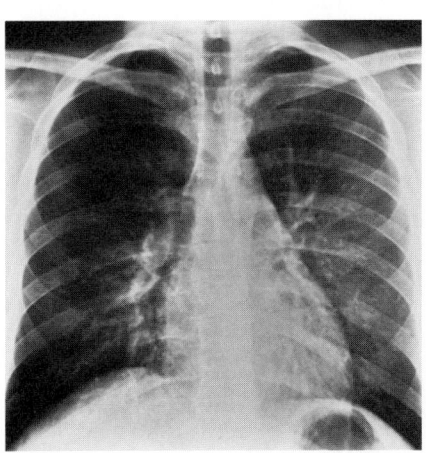
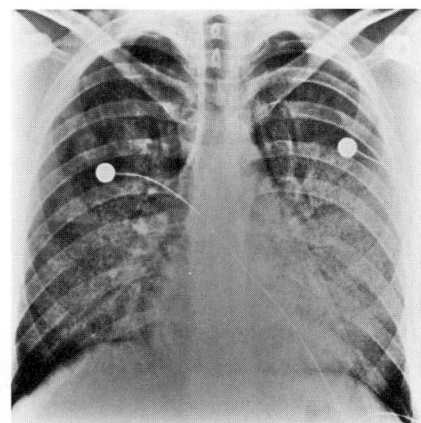

Fig. 1-171   Goodpasture's syndrome. PA chest radiographs several days apart demonstrate consolidation in the left lung, **A,** which progressed to diffuse alveolar disease (consolidation), **B.** (From McLoud TC: *Thoracic radiology: the requisites,* St Louis, 1998, Mosby.)

BASIC INFORMATION

■ DEFINITION

Gout is a clinical disorder in which crystals of monosodium urate become deposited in tissue as a result of hyper-uricemia. Gout and hyperuricemia can be classified as either primary or secondary if resulting from another disorder.

ICD-9CM CODES
274.9 Gout

■ EPIDEMIOLOGY & DEMOGRAPHICS
PREVALENCE: 3 cases/1000 persons
PREDOMINANT SEX: 95% males, rare in females before menopause
PREDOMINANT AGE: 30 to 50 yr

■ PHYSICAL FINDINGS & CLINICAL PRESENTATION

- Usually, initial attack in a single joint or an area of tenosynovium
- Mainly a disease of the lower extremities
- First site of involvement: classically, MP joint of the great toe
- Another common site of acute attack: extensor tenosynovium on the dorsum of the mid-foot
- Severe pain and inflammation, which may be precipitated by exercise, dietary indiscretions, and physical or emotional stress
- Attacks following illness or surgery
- Presence of swelling, heat, redness, and other signs of inflammation (the physical findings simulating cellulitis)
- Exquisite soft tissue tenderness
- Fever, tachycardia, and other constitutional symptoms
- Eventually, deposits of urate crystals (tophi) in the subcutaneous tissue

■ ETIOLOGY

- Hyperuricemia and gout develop from excessive uric acid production, a decrease in the renal excretion of uric acid, or both.
- Primary gout results from an inborn error of metabolism and may be attributed to several biochemical defects.
- Secondary hyperuricemia may develop as a complication of acquired disorders (e.g., leukemia) or as a result of the use of certain drugs (e.g., diuretics).

 DIAGNOSIS

■ DIFFERENTIAL DIAGNOSIS

- Pseudogout
- Rheumatoid arthritis
- Osteoarthritis
- Cellulitis
- Infectious arthritis

Box 2-33 describes the differential diagnosis of acute monoarticular and oligoarticular arthritis.

■ WORKUP

Hyperuricemia accompanying a typical history of monoarticular acute arthritis is usually sufficient to establish the diagnosis.

■ LABORATORY TESTS

- Mild leukocytosis
- Elevated ESR
- Hyperuricemia
- Synovial aspirate: usually cloudy and markedly inflammatory in nature; urate crystals in fluid: needle-shaped and birefringent under polarized light

■ IMAGING STUDIES

- Plain radiography to rule out other disorders
- No typical findings in early gouty arthritis but late disease possibly associated with characteristic punched-out lesions and joint destruction

📋 TREATMENT

■ NONPHARMACOLOGIC THERAPY

- Modification of diet (avoidance of foods high in purines [e.g., anchovies, organ meat, liver, spinach, mushrooms, asparagus, oatmeal, cocoa, sweetbreads]) and lifestyle
- Treatment for obesity
- Moderation in alcohol intake, no more than two drinks per day
- Hypertension and its management requiring careful assessment and possibly nondiuretic drugs

■ ACUTE GENERAL Rx

- Quick-acting NSAIDs such as ibuprofen
- Colchicine (given PO or IV)
- Corticosteroids or ACTH for those who are intolerant of NSAIDs or colchicine
- Intraarticular cortisone when oral medication cannot be given
- General measures, such as rest, elevation, and analgesics as needed

■ CHRONIC Rx

- Prevention is achieved through normalization of serum urate concentration.
- Uricosuric agents (e.g., probenecid) or xanthine oxidase inhibitors (allopurinol) are used in patients with recurrent attacks despite adequate dietary restrictions.
- A 24-hr urine collection is useful in deciding which antihyperuremic agent is indicated. Allopurinol is generally used if the uric acid output is >900 mg/day on a regular diet. However, hypourecemic therapy should not be started for at least 2 wk after the acute attack has resolved because it may prolong the acute attack and it can also precipitate new attacks by rapidly lowering the serum uric acid level.
- Urinary uric acid hypoexcretors (<700 mg/day) can be given probenecid (250 mg bid for 1 wk, then increased to 500 mg bid) to block absorption of uric acid. Probenecid should be started only after the acute attack of gout has completely subsided.
- Colchicine 0.6 mg bid is indicated for acute gout prophylaxis before starting hypouricemic therapy. It is generally discontinued 6 to 8 wk after normalization of serum urate levels. Long-term colchicine therapy (0.6 mg qd or bid) may be necessary in patients with frequent gout attacks despite the use of uricosuric agents.
- Surgery usually limited to excision of large tophi and, occasionally, arthroplasty.

■ DISPOSITION

- Musculoskeletal complications are usually limited to joint disease.
- Surgical intervention may occasionally be indicated.
- Renal disease is the most frequent complication of gout after arthritis;

most gouty patients develop renal disease as a result of parenchymal urate deposition but the involvement is only slowly progressive and often has no effect on life expectancy.
- Incidence of urolithiasis is increased, with 80% of calculi being uric acid stones.

■ REFERRAL
For orthopedic consultation when joint destruction has occurred

☼ PEARLS & CONSIDERATIONS

■ COMMENTS
- No significant correlation between coronary artery disease and gout
- No indication to treat asymptomatic hyperuricemia
- Acute attacks of gout occasionally associated with normal levels of uric acid

REFERENCES

Agudelo CA, Wise CM: Crystal-associated arthritis in the elderly, *Rheum Dis Clin N Am* 26:527, 2000.

Agudelo CA, Wise CM: Gout: diagnosis, pathogenesis, and clinical manifestations, *Curr Opin Rheumatol* 13:234, 2001.

Schlesinger N, Schumacher HR: Gout: can management be improved? *Curr Opin Rheumatol* 13:240, 2001.

Snaith ML: Gout: diet and uric acid revisited, *Lancet* 358:521, 2001.

Wortmann RL: Effective management of gout: an analogy, *Am J Med* 105:513, 1998.

Author: **Lonnie R. Mercier, M.D.**

BASIC INFORMATION

■ DEFINITION

Granuloma inguinale is caused by a gram-negative bacterium, *Calymmatobacterium granulomatis,* that may be sexually transmitted, possibly by anal intercourse. It can also be spread through close, chronic nonsexual contact.

■ SYNONYMS

Donovanosis

ICD-9CM CODES

099.2 Granuloma inguinale

■ EPIDEMIOLOGY & DEMOGRAPHICS

- Rare in the U.S. (<100 cases reported annually) and other developed countries
- Endemic in Australia, India, Caribbean, and Africa
- Can affect both males and females
- Incubation period is variable: 1 to 2 wk

■ PHYSICAL FINDINGS & CLINICAL PRESENTATION

- Indurated nodule is the primary lesion and is usually painless.
- Lesion erodes to granulomatous heaped ulcer (Fig. 1-172); progresses slowly.
- Pathogenic features are as follows:
  1. Large infected mononuclear cell containing many Donovan bodies
  2. Intracytoplasmic location

■ ETIOLOGY

Calymmatobacterium granulomatis is a gram-negative bacillus that reproduces within PMNs, plasma cells, and histiocytes, causing the infected cells to rupture 20 to 30 organisms.

DIAGNOSIS

■ DIFFERENTIAL DIAGNOSIS

- Carcinoma
- Secondary syphilis: condylomata lata
- Amebiasis: necrotic ulceration
- Concurrent infections
- Lymphogranuloma venereum
- Chancroid
- Genital herpes

■ WORKUP

- Check for clinical manifestations.
  1. Lesions bleed easily.
  2. Lesions sharply defined and painless.
  3. Secondary infection may ensue.
  4. Inguinal involvement may cause pseudobuboes.

5. Elephantiasis can result from obstruction of lymphatics.
6. Suppuration and sinus formation are rare in female patients.
- Screen for other sexually transmitted diseases.
- Exclude other causes of lesions.
- Obtain stained, crushed prep from lesion.
- A clinical algorithm for evaluation of genital ulcer disease is described in Fig. 3-69.

Table 2-84 describes the differential diagnosis of genital sores.

■ LABORATORY TESTS

Wright stain: observation of Donovan bodies (intracellular bacteria); organisms in vacuoles within macrophages

TREATMENT

■ ACUTE GENERAL Rx

- Tetracycline 500 mg, qid × 3 to 5 wk
- Trimethoprim/sulfamethoxazole, one double-strength tablet orally twice daily ×3 wk minimum or doxycycline 100 mg orally twice daily ×3 wk minimum
- Chloramphenicol 500 mg, q8h × 3 wk
- Gentamicin 1 mg/kg, bid × 3 wk
- Streptomycin 1 g IM, bid × 3 wk
- Ampicillin 500 g, qid × 12 wk

■ CHRONIC Rx

If there is a poor initial response, extend treatment. Treatment of relapses is often necessary. Patients should be counseled to avoid risky sex practices and not resume having sex until infection is cleared.

■ DISPOSITION

Routine annual or semiannual visits

■ REFERRAL

If response is poor, consider referral to infectious disease specialist.

PEARLS & CONSIDERATIONS

■ COMMENTS

Patient education material can be obtained from local and state health clinics and also from ACOG.

REFERENCES

Centers for Disease Control and Prevention: Sexually transmitted diseases treatment guidelines, *MMWR* 47(RR-1), 1998.

Mead PB et al: *Protocols for infectious diseases in obstetrics and gynecology,* ed 2, Cambridge, Mass, 2000, Blackwell Science.

Author: **George T. Danakas, M.D.**

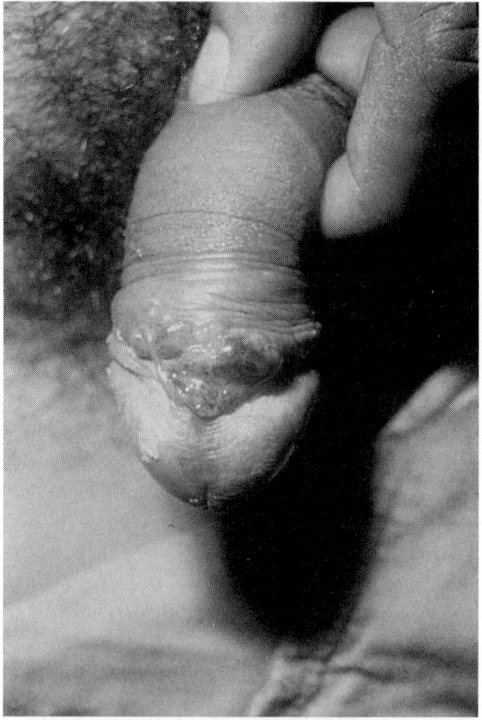

Fig. 1-172 Involvement of the penis, with a beefy red, granulomatous ulceration in a patient with granuloma inguinale. (From Goldstein B [ed]: *Practical dermatology,* ed 2, St Louis, 1997, Mosby.)

BASIC INFORMATION

■ DEFINITION

Graves' disease is a hypermetabolic state characterized by thyrotoxicosis, diffuse goiter, and infiltrative ophthalmopathy (edema and inflammation of the extraocular muscles and an increase in orbital connective tissue and fat); infiltrative dermopathy characterized by lymphocytic infiltration of the dermis, accumulation of glycosaminoglycans, and edema is occasionally present.

■ SYNONYMS

Thyrotoxicosis

ICD-9CM CODES

242.0 Toxic diffuse goiter

■ EPIDEMIOLOGY & DEMOGRAPHICS

INCIDENCE/PREVALENCE: Hyperthyroidism affects 2% of women and 0.2% of men in their lifetimes. More than 80% of these cases are caused by Graves' disease.
PREDOMINANT AGE: Most common before age 50 yr
GENETICS: Increased prevalence of HLA-B8 and HLA-DR3 in whites with Graves' disease. Concordance rate is 20% among monozygotic twins.

■ PHYSICAL FINDINGS & CLINICAL FINDINGS

- Tachycardia, palpitations, tremor, hyperreflexia
- Goiter, exophthalmos (50% of patients), lid retraction, lid lag
- Nervousness, weight loss, heat intolerance, atrial fibrillation
- Increased sweating, brittle nails, clubbing of fingers
- Nervousness, weight loss, heat intolerance, and atrial fibrillation
- Localized dermopathy (1% to 2% of patients) is most frequent over the anterolateral aspects of the skin but can be found at other sites (especially after trauma)

■ ETIOLOGY

Autoimmune etiology: the activity of the thyroid gland is stimulated by the action of T cells, which induce specific B cells to synthesize antibodies against TSH receptors in the follicular cell membrane.

DIAGNOSIS

■ DIFFERENTIAL DIAGNOSIS

- Anxiety disorder
- Premenopausal state
- Thyroiditis

- Other causes of hyperthyroidism (e.g., toxic multinodular goiter, toxic adenoma)
- Other: metastatic neoplasm, diabetes mellitus, pheochromocytoma

■ WORKUP

The diagnostic workup includes a detailed medical history followed by laboratory and imaging studies. Patients often present with anxiety, heat intolerance, menstrual dysfunction, increased appetite, and weight loss. Elderly patients can have an atypical presentation (apathetic hyperparathyroidism). For additional information, refer to the topic "Hyperthyroidism."

■ LABORATORY TESTS

- Increased free thyroxine (T_4) and free triiodothyronine (T_3)
- Decreased TSH
- Presence of thyroid autoantibodies (useful in selected patients to differentiate Graves' disease from toxic nodular goiter)
- A diagnostic approach to thyroid tests is described in Fig. 3-166

■ IMAGING STUDIES

- 24-hr radioactive iodine uptake (RAIU): increased homogeneous uptake
- CT or MRI of the orbits is useful if there is uncertainty about the cause of ophthalmopathy

TREATMENT

■ NONPHARMACOLOGIC THERAPY

Patient education and discussion of therapeutic options

■ ACUTE GENERAL Rx

- Antithyroid drugs (ATDs) to inhibit thyroid hormone synthesis or peripheral conversion of T_4 to T_3
  1. Propylthiouracil (PTU) 50 to 100 mg q8h or methimazole (Tapazole) 10 to 20 mg q8h for 6 to 24 mo
  2. Side effects: skin rash (3% to 5%), arthralgias, myalgias, granulocytopenia (0.5%); rare side effects: aplastic anemia, hepatic necrosis (PTU), cholestatic jaundice (methimazole)
- Radioactive iodine (RAI)
  1. Treatment of choice for patients >21 yr of age and younger patients who have not achieved remission after 1 yr of ATD therapy
  2. Contraindicated during pregnancy and lactation
- Surgery: near-total thyroidectomy is rarely performed; indications: obstructing goiters despite RAI and

ATD therapy, patients who refuse RAI and cannot be adequately managed with ATDs, and pregnant women inadequately managed with ATDs
- Adjunctive therapy: propranolol (20 to 40 mg q6h) to alleviate the β-adrenergic symptoms of hyperthyroidism (tachycardia, tremor); contraindicated in patients with CHF and bronchospasm
- Graves' ophthalmopathy: methylcellulose eye drops to protect against excessive dryness, sunglasses to decrease photophobia, systemic high-dose corticosteroids for severe exophthalmos; worsening of ophthalmopathy after RAI therapy often transient and can be prevented by the administration of prednisone

■ CHRONIC Rx

Patients undergoing treatment with ATDs should be seen every 1 to 3 mo until euthyroidism is achieved and every 3 to 4 mo while they are receiving ATDs.

■ DISPOSITION

- ATDs induce sustained remission in <60% of cases.
- The incidence of hypothyroidism post RAI is >50% within first year and 2%/yr thereafter.
- Complications of surgery include hypothyroidism (28% to 43% after 10 yr), hypoparathyroidism, and vocal cord paralysis (1%).
- Successful treatment of hyperthyroidism requires lifelong monitoring for the onset of hypothyroidism or the recurrence of thyrotoxicosis.
- RAI therapy is followed by the appearance or worsening of ophthalmopathy more often than is therapy with methimazole, particularly in patients who are cigarette smokers. It can be prevented with the administration of prednisone 0.5 mg/kg of body weight per day starting 2 to 3 days post RAI, continued for 1 mo, then tapered off over 2 mo.
- Mild to moderate ophthalmopathy often improves spontaneously. Severe cases can be treated with high-dose glucocorticoids, orbital irradiation, or both. Orbital decompression may be used in patients with optic neuropathy and exophthalmos.

REFERENCE

Weetman AP: Graves' disease, *N Engl J Med* 343:1236, 2000.
Author: **Fred F. Ferri, M.D.**

BASIC INFORMATION

■ **DEFINITION**
Guillain-Barré syndrome (GBS) is an acute inflammatory demyelinating polyradiculopathy (AIDP) predominantly affecting motor function.

■ **SYNONYMS**
Acute polyneuropathy
Ascending paralysis
GBS

■ **ICD-9CM CODES**
357.0 Guillain-Barré

■ **EPIDEMIOLOGY & DEMOGRAPHICS**
INCIDENCE/PREVALENCE: 1 to 2 cases/100,000 persons annually; incidence increases with age (0.8 cases/100,000 persons at age 18, 3.2 cases/100,000 persons at age 60)
RISK FACTORS: HIV, *Campylobacter jejuni* enteritis, upper respiratory infections, Epstein-Barr viral infection, CMV infection, immunizations, pregnancy, Hodgkin's lymphoma, mycoplasma infections, hepatitis B infections

■ **PHYSICAL FINDINGS & CLINICAL PRESENTATION**
• Symmetric weakness, initially involving proximal muscles, subsequently involving both proximal and distal muscles; difficulty in ambulating, getting up from a chair, or climbing stairs
• Depressed or absent reflexes bilaterally
• Initial manifestations involving the cranial musculature or the upper extremities (e.g., tingling of the hands) in some patients
• Minimal to moderate glove and stocking anesthesia
• Ataxia and pain in a segmental distribution in some patients (caused by involvement of posterior nerve roots)
• Autonomic abnormalities (bradycardia or tachycardia, hypotension, or hypertension)
• Respiratory insufficiency (caused by weakness of intercostal muscles)
• Facial paresis, difficulty swallowing (secondary to cranial nerve involvement)

■ **ETIOLOGY**
Infection with *C. jejuni* often precedes GBS and is associated with axonal degeneration, slow recovery, and severe residual disability.

🔬 **DIAGNOSIS**

■ **DIFFERENTIAL DIAGNOSIS**
• Neuropathy from heavy metals (lead, arsenic)
• Neuropathy from systemic diseases (uremia, diabetes, amyloidosis, lupus and other collagen-vascular disorders, porphyria)
• Poliomyelitis
• Botulism, diphtheria
• Hysterical paralysis
• Deficiency states (alcoholism, vitamin B_{12}, folic acid)
• Hereditary polyneuropathies

■ **WORKUP**
1. Rule out other causes of neuropathy (see above).
2. Lumbar puncture:
   • Typical findings include elevated CSF protein (especially IgG) and presence of few mononuclear leukocytes.
   • Normal values may be seen at the beginning of illness.
   • If the diagnosis is strongly suspected, a repeat lumbar puncture is indicated.
3. Electromyography reveals slowed conduction velocities; prolonged motor, sensory, and F-wave latencies are also present.

■ **LABORATORY TESTS**
• CBC may reveal early leukocytosis with left shift.
• Vitamin B_{12} level, folate, and heavy metal screening are indicated only in selected cases.

💊 **TREATMENT**

■ **NONPHARMACOLOGIC THERAPY**
• Close monitoring of respiratory function (frequent measurements of vital capacity and pulmonary toilet), because respiratory failure is the major complication in GBS
• Frequent repositioning of patient to minimize formation of pressure sores
• Prevention of thromboembolism with antithrombotic stockings and SC heparin (5000 U q12h)
• Emotional support and social counseling

■ **ACUTE GENERAL Rx**
• Infusion of IV immunoglobulins (0.4 mg/kg/day for 5 days) has replaced plasmapheresis as therapy of

choice at many centers. The addition of glucocorticoids (IV methylprednisolone) to IV immunoglobulins is controversial. It may result in additional improvement, but it is often associated with a high frequency of complications.
• Early therapeutic plasma exchange (TPE, plasmapheresis), started within 7 days of onset of symptoms, is beneficial in preventing paralytic complications in patients with rapidly progressive disease. It is contraindicated in patients with cardiovascular disease (recent MI, unstable angina), active sepsis, and autonomic dysfunction.
• Mechanical ventilation may be needed if FEV is <12 to 15 ml/kg, vital capacity is rapidly decreasing or is <1000 ml and Pao$_2$ is <70, or the patient is having significant difficulty clearing secretions and is aspirating.

■ **CHRONIC Rx**
• Ventilatory support: may be necessary in 10% to 20% of patients
• Aggressive nursing care to prevent decubiti, infections, fecal impactions, and pressure nerve palsies
• Monitoring and treatment of autonomic dysfunction (bradyarrhythmias or tachyarrhythmias, orthostatic hypotension, systemic hypertension, altered sweating)
• Treatment of back pain and dysesthesia with low-dose tricyclics
• Stress ulcer prevention in patients receiving ventilator support

■ **DISPOSITION**
• Mortality is approximately 3%.
• Prognosis for full recovery is very good. Only 15% to 20% of patients may have minor residual motor deficits.

■ **REFERRAL**
Tracheostomy may be necessary in patients with prolonged ventilatory support.

☼ **PEARLS & CONSIDERATIONS**

■ **COMMENTS**
Patient education information may be obtained from the Guillain-Barré Foundation International, Box 262, Wynnewood, PA 19096; phone: (610) 667-0131.
Author: **Fred F. Ferri, M.D.**

BASIC INFORMATION

■ DEFINITION

Hand-foot-mouth (HFM) disease is a viral illness that is characterized by superficial lesions of the oral mucosa and of the skin of the extremities. HFM is highly contagious. Although children are predominantly affected, adults are also at risk. This disease is usually self-limited and benign.

■ SYNONYMS

Vesicular stomatitis with exanthem
Coxsackievirus infection

■ ICD-9CM CODES

074.0 Hand-foot-mouth disease

■ EPIDEMIOLOGY & DEMOGRAPHICS

- Children under the age of 5 yr are at the highest risk.
- HFM is usually found in children below the age of 10 yr.
- Close contacts of affected children, including family members and health care workers, are the most commonly affected adults.
- Outbreaks tend to occur during the summer.

■ PHYSICAL FINDINGS & CLINICAL PRESENTATION

Symptoms:
- After a 3- to 5-day incubation period, patients may complain of odynophagia, sore throat, malaise, and fever.
- One to 2 days later the characteristic oral lesions appear.
- In 75% of cases, skin lesions on the extremities accompany these oral manifestations.
- Lesions appear over the course of 1 or 2 days.

Physical findings:
- Oral lesions, usually between five and ten, are commonly found on the tongue and buccal mucosa.
- Gingiva, palate, pharynx, and the floor of the mouth may also be involved.
- Oral lesions initially start as erythematous macules and evolve into gray vesicles on an erythematous base.
- Vesicles are frequently broken by the time of presentation and appear as superficial gray ulcers with surrounding erythema.
- Skin lesions of the hands and feet start as linear erythematous papules (3 to 10 mm in diameter) that evolve into gray vesicles that may be mildly painful (Fig. 1-173). These vesicles are usually intact at presentation and remain so until they desquamate within 2 wk.
- In rare cases, encephalitis, meningitis, myocarditis, and pulmonary edema may develop.
- Spontaneous abortion may occur if the infection takes place early in pregnancy.

■ ETIOLOGY

Coxsackievirus group A, type 16, was the first and is the most common viral agent isolated. Coxsackieviruses A5, A7, A9, A10, B2, and B5 have also been implicated.

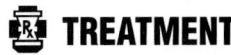

DIAGNOSIS

■ DIFFERENTIAL DIAGNOSIS

- Aphthous stomatitis
- Herpes simplex infection
- Herpangina
- Behçet's disease
- Erythema multiforme
- Pemphigus
- Gonorrhea
- Acute leukemia
- Lymphoma

■ WORKUP

The diagnosis is usually made on the basis of history and characteristic physical examination.

■ LABORATORY TESTS

Not indicated unless the diagnosis is in doubt

TREATMENT

■ ACUTE GENERAL Rx

- Palliative therapy is given for this usually self-limited disease.
- One small, uncontrolled case series reported a decrease in duration of symptoms in response to acyclovir.

■ DISPOSITION

Prognosis is excellent except in rare cases of CNS or cardiac involvement. Most are managed as outpatients.

■ REFERRAL

Not usually needed

REFERENCE

Chang LY et al: Clinical features and risk of pulmonary edema after enterovirus-related hand, foot, and mouth disease, *Lancet* 354(9191):1682, 1999.
Author: **James J. Ng, M.D.**

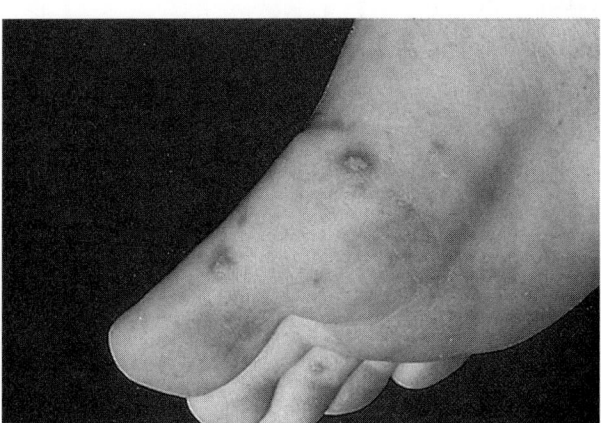

Fig. 1-173 Hand-foot-mouth disease. Note oval lesions on an erythematous base. (From Goldstein B [ed]: *Practical dermatology,* ed 2, St Louis, 1997, Mosby.)

BASIC INFORMATION

■ **DEFINITION**
The term *cluster headache* refers to recurrent episodes of intense, unilateral headache centered around the orbit and lasting 30 to 120 min. Headaches occur in clusters lasting 4 to 12 wk, during which one to three episodes occur per day at predictable times, typically during sleep. The episodes then remit for months to years.

■ **SYNONYMS (all obsolete terms)**
Horton's headache
Histaminic cephalgia
Vidian neuralgia
Sphenopalatine neuralgia

ICD-9CM CODES
346.2 Variants of migraine

■ **EPIDEMIOLOGY & DEMOGRAPHICS**
INCIDENCE (IN U.S.): Unknown
PREVALENCE (IN U.S.): Unknown
PREDOMINANT SEX: Male:female ratio of 10:1
PREDOMINANT AGE: Third to fourth decade, rarely in children
PEAK INCIDENCE: Age 30 yr
GENETICS:
• Unknown
• Association with hazel eye color and "masculine" facial features reported

■ **PHYSICAL FINDINGS & CLINICAL PRESENTATION**
• During attack: conjunctival injection, lacrimation, nasal congestion, rhinorrhea, facial sweating, myosis, ptosis, eyelid edema
• Typical avoidance of immobility, with patients pacing, stomping, or running
• Permanent partial Horner's syndrome in 5% of patients; otherwise examination normal
• Box 1-16 describes criteria for cluster headache

■ **ETIOLOGY**
Unknown

DIAGNOSIS

■ **DIFFERENTIAL DIAGNOSIS**
• Migraine
• Trigeminal neuralgia
• Arteritis
• Postherpetic neuralgia
• Intracranial mass
• Table 2-86 describes the differential diagnosis of headaches.

■ **WORKUP**
• Diagnosis is usually established by characteristic history.
• Imaging studies are sometimes warranted if diagnosis is uncertain.

■ **LABORATORY TESTS**
None

■ **IMAGING STUDIES**
None, unless history or examination suggests structural etiology.

TREATMENT

■ **NONPHARMACOLOGIC THERAPY**
• Avoidance of ethanol and tobacco during clusters

• Surgical ablation of components of the trigeminal nerve in rare instances

■ **ACUTE GENERAL Rx**
• Inhalation of 100% oxygen by face mask at 8 to 10 L/min for 15 min often aborts an attack.
• Sumatriptan 6 mg SC or ergotamines may abort an attack or prevent one if given just before a predictable episode.

■ **CHRONIC Rx**
Various medications have been tried without great success, although good responses may be obtained in up to 50% of cases. Examples include:
• Prednisone: 30 to 60 mg/day for 1 to 2 wk, then taper
• Lithium: 200 mg tid with frequent monitoring and adjustment to maintain therapeutic serum level
• Verapamil: up to 240 mg/day as tolerated
• Methysergide: 1 to 2 mg tid; requires familiarity with the potential adverse effects and use of "drug holidays" to decrease risk of fibrosis
• Topiramate: 25 mg/qd

■ **DISPOSITION**
• Most patients continue to have clusters with variable periods of remission.
• Response to medication is variable.

■ **REFERRAL**
• If unfamiliar with potential adverse effects or contraindications of medication
• If surgical opinion is desired for medication failure
Author: **Michael Gruenthal, M.D., Ph.D.**

BOX 1-16 Criteria for Cluster Headache

Severe unilateral orbital, supraorbital, or temporal pain peaking in 10 to 15 min and lasting 30 to 45 min (occasionally up to 180 min). Pain rapidly resolves. Cluster headaches have a propensity to occur at night and may lead to sleep deprivation. Cycles generally last for a few weeks or months but may last for more than 1 yr.
Headache is associated with at least one of the following on the painful side:
• Conjunctival injection
• Rhinorrhea
• Lacrimation
• Miosis
• Nasal congestion
• Ptosis
• Forehead and facial sweating
• Eyelid edema
Additionally:
• Frequency of attacks ranges from one to eight daily.
• There have been at least five episodes of headache.

From Graber MA: *The family practice handbook,* ed 4, St Louis, 2001, Mosby.

BASIC INFORMATION

■ DEFINITION
Migraine headaches are recurrent headaches of variable intensity and duration, often unilateral and associated with nausea and vomiting. Some headaches are preceded by, or associated with, neurologic or mood disturbances. Boxes 1-17 and 1-18 describe criteria for headache.

■ ICD-9CM CODES
346 Migraine

■ EPIDEMIOLOGY & DEMOGRAPHICS
INCIDENCE (IN U.S.): Females: 22 cases/1000 persons/yr, males: 5 cases/1000 persons/yr
PREVALENCE (IN U.S.): Females: 18%; males: 6%
PREDOMINANT SEX: Female:male ratio of 3:1
PREDOMINANT AGE: >10 yr
PEAK INCIDENCE: Teenage years
GENETICS:
- Familial predisposition, with up to 90% of migraineurs having an affected family member
- Autosomal dominant transmission with incomplete penetrance postulated

■ PHYSICAL FINDINGS & CLINICAL PRESENTATION
- Normal between episodes
- During migraine with aura, focal motor or sensory abnormalities possible (Fig. 1-174), but first episode of any headache associated with neurologic deficits requires thorough investigation

■ ETIOLOGY
- Unknown.
- Early theories of primary vascular mechanism have been replaced by proposals that primary neuronal event is responsible.

DIAGNOSIS

■ DIFFERENTIAL DIAGNOSIS
- Subarachnoid hemorrhage
- Tumor
- Aneurysm
- Arteriovenous malformation
- Meningitis
- Table 2-86 describes the differential diagnosis of headaches.

■ WORKUP
- Generally no additional investigation is needed with recurrent, typical attacks with typical age of onset, family history, and a normal physical examination.

- Diagnosis is not based on first headache.
- If there is an unusual presentation and/or unexpected findings on examination, investigation for other causes is required.

■ LABORATORY TESTS
None

■ IMAGING STUDIES
- Not routinely necessary for typical cases
- If diagnosis uncertain: MRI, MRA, or conventional angiography to detect other causes

TREATMENT

■ NONPHARMACOLOGIC THERAPY
- Avoid any identifiable provoking factors: caffeine, tobacco, and alcohol may trigger attacks, as may dietary or other environmental precipitants (less common).
- Try biofeedback (effective in some cases).

■ ACUTE GENERAL Rx
- Medications effective in aborting an attack include nonnarcotic analgesics (NSAIDs, acetaminophen), vasoactive drugs (ergotamine preparations, sumatriptan), and opioids (meperidine, butorphanol nasal spray) (Table 1-33).
- Early administration improves effectiveness.
- Fig. 1-175 describes an algorithm for the treatment of migraine.

■ CHRONIC Rx
- The prophylactic drugs of choice are gabapentin (Neurontin) 400 mg qd or tid, or topiramate (Topamax) 25 mg in evening. Less effective drugs used in the past include β-blockers, calcium channel blockers, antidepressants, anticonvulsants, and serotonin antagonists.
- Prophylactic treatment is generally indicated when headaches occur more than twice a week or when symptomatic treatments are contraindicated or not effective.

■ DISPOSITION
- After age 30 yr, 40% of patients are migraine free.
- Chronic daily headache is possible, sometimes representing rebound headache caused by overuse of analgesics.

■ REFERRAL
If uncertain about diagnosis or treatment not effective

PEARLS & CONSIDERATIONS

■ CAUTION
If there is no aura or, if during headache, patient does not have nausea or vomiting, then diagnosis of migraine is suspect.

REFERENCES
Bartleson JD: Treatment of migraine headaches, *Mayo Clin Proc* 74:702, 1999.
Pryse P et al: Guidelines for the nonpharmacologic management of migraine in clinical practice, *CMAJ* 159:47, 1998.
Author: **Michael Gruenthal, M.D., Ph.D.**

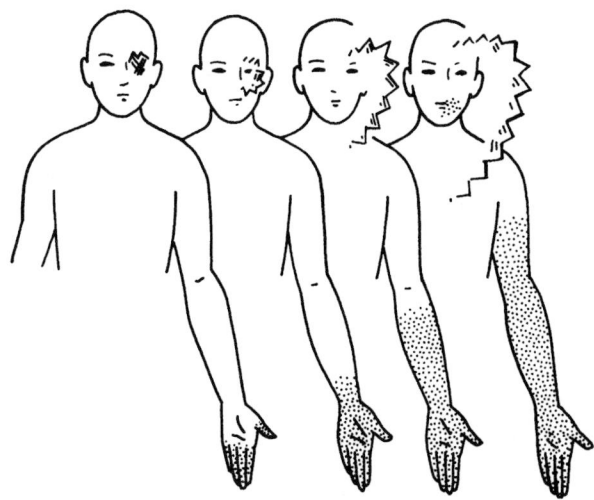

Fig. 1-174 The two most typical aura symptoms of migraine, the scintillating scotoma and digitolingual paresthesias, in their successive stages of development *(left to right).* (From Carlson K [ed]: *Primary care of women,* St Louis, 1995, Mosby.)

BOX 1-17   Criteria for Migraine without Aura

Migraine without aura must have at least five attacks meeting the following criteria:

Headache attacks last 4 to 72 hr

Headache has at least two of the following:

- Unilateral location
- Pulsating quality
- Moderate or severe intensity (inhibits daily activity)
- Aggravation by routine physical activity

During the headache, at least one of the following:

- Nausea or vomiting
- Photophobia and phonophobia

No organic etiology found by history, physical, or neurologic examination

From Graber MA: *The family practice handbook,* ed 4, St Louis, 2001, Mosby.

BOX 1-18   Criteria for Migraine with Aura

Migraine with aura must have at least two attacks fulfilling the following criteria:

At least three of the following are present:

- One or more fully reversible aura symptoms indicating focal cerebral cortical or brain stem dysfunction
- At least one aura symptom develops gradually over more than 4 min
- No aura symptom lasts more than 60 min (duration proportionally increases if more than one aura symptom present)
- HA follows the aura within 60 min (but HA may begin before or with the aura); HA usually lasts 4 to 72 hr but may have only the aura
- No organic etiology found by history, physical, or neurologic examination

Note: Common aura types include scintillating scotomata, multiple small dots, homonymous visual disturbance, hemisensory disturbance, difficulty communicating, and occasionally vertigo.

From Graber MA: *The family practice handbook,* ed 4, St Louis, 2001, Mosby.

HA, Headache.

TABLE 1-33 Abortive and Analgesic Therapy for Migraine*

DRUG	DOSE	ROUTE
Triptans (serotonin agonists)		
Sumatriptan	6 mg, repeat in 2 hr (max 2 doses/day)	Subcutaneous
Sumatriptan	25 mg, 50 mg, 100 mg, repeat in 2 hr (max 200 mg/day)	Oral
Sumatriptan	5 mg and 20 mg, repeat in 2 hr (max 200 mg/day)	Nasal Spray
Zolmitriptan	2.5 mg, 5 mg, repeat in 2 hr (max 10 mg/day)	Oral
Naratriptan	1 mg, 2.5 mg, repeat in 2 hr (max 5 mg/day)	Oral
Rizatriptan	5 mg, 10 mg, repeat in 2 hr (max 30 mg/day)	Oral
Ergotamine preparations		
Ergotamine and caffeine	2 tablets, repeat in 1 hr; max 4/day	Oral
Ergotamine and caffeine	1 suppository, repeat in 1 hr; max 2/day	Rectal
Ergotaminel	1 tablet, repeat in 1 hr; max 2/day	Sublingual
Dihydroergotamine	0.5-1.0 ml, repeat twice at 1-hr intervals (max 3 mg/attack)	Intramuscular
		Subcutaneous
		Intravenous
Sympathomimetics (with or without barbiturates or codeine)		
Isometheptene	2 capules, repeat in 1 hr, max 2/day	Oral
Acetaminophen	2 capsules, repeat in 1 hr, max 2/day	Oral
Dichloralphenazone	2 capsules, repeat in 1 hr, max 2/day	Oral
Nonsteroidal antiinflammatory drugs		
Naproxen	550-750 mg, repeat in 1 hr; max 3 times/wk	Oral
Meclofenamate	100-200 mg, repeat in 1 hr; max 3 times/wk	Oral
Flurbiprofen	50-100 mg, repeat in 1 hr; max 3 times/wk	Oral
Ibuprofen	200-300 mg, repeat in 1 hr; max 3 times/wk	Oral
Antiemetics		
Promethazine	50-125 mg	Oral
		Intramuscular
Prochlorperazine	1-25 mg	Oral
	2.5-25 mg (suppository)	Rectal
	5-10 mg	Intramuscular
Chlorpromazine	10-25 mg	Oral
	50-100 mg (suppository)	Rectal
	Up to 35 mg	Intravenous
Trimetobenzamide	250 mg	Oral
	200 mg	Rectal
Metoclopramide	5-10 mg	Oral
	10 mg	Intramuscular
	5-10 mg	Intravenous
Dimenhydrinate	50 mg	Oral

From Wiederholt WC: *Neurology for non-neurologists*, ed 4, Philadelphia, 2000, WB Saunders.
*For side effects and contraindications consult the manufacturer's drug insert before prescribing any of these drugs.

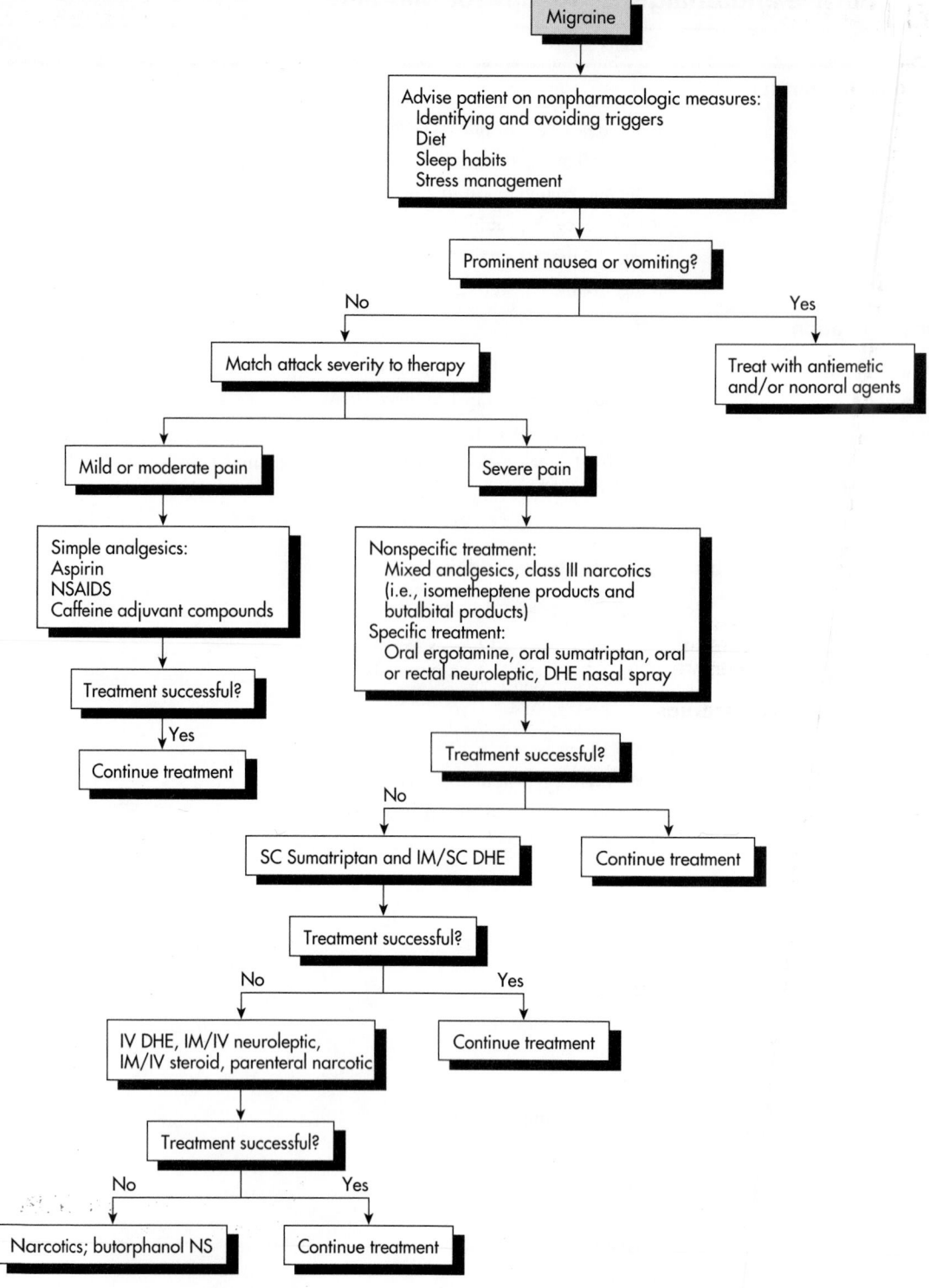

Fig. 1-175 The treatment of migraine. *DHE,* Dihydroergotamine; *IM,* intramuscular; *IV,* intravenous; *NS,* normal saline; *NSAIDs,* nonsteroidal antiinflammatory drugs; *SC,* subcutaneous. (From Silberstein SD, Young WB, Lipton RB: Migraine and cluster headaches. In Johnson RT, Griffin JW [eds]: *Current therapy in neurologic disease,* ed 5, St Louis, 1997, Mosby.)

BASIC INFORMATION

■ DEFINITION
Tension headaches are recurrent headaches lasting 30 min to 7 days without nausea or vomiting and with at least two of the following characteristics: pressing or tightening quality, mild or moderate intensity, bilateral, and not aggravated by routine physical activity.

■ SYNONYMS
Muscle contraction headache
Tension headache
Stress headache
Ordinary headache
Psychomyogenic headache
Psychogenic headache
Essential headache
Greater occipital neuralgia

ICD-9CM CODES
307.81 Tension headache

■ EPIDEMIOLOGY & DEMOGRAPHICS
INCIDENCE (IN U.S.):
• Undetermined
• Believed to be the most common type of headache; as high as 70% of all headaches presenting to primary care physician
PREVALENCE (IN U.S.): Males: 63%/yr; females: 86%/yr
PREDOMINANT SEX: Females > males
PREDOMINANT AGE: >10 yr
PEAK INCIDENCE: Occurs at all ages
GENETICS: Not established

■ PHYSICAL FINDINGS & CLINICAL PRESENTATION
Percussion tenderness high in cervical area, paracervical and trapezius muscle spasm, and decreased sensation in scalp. Patient may complain of scalp tenderness or hair "hurting."

■ ETIOLOGY
• Unknown
• There are no recent data to support the long-standing belief that these headaches arise from stress or other psychologic factors.
• These headaches respond poorly to standard migraine therapy.

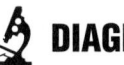 **DIAGNOSIS**

■ DIFFERENTIAL DIAGNOSIS
• Migraine
• Cervical spine disease
• Intracranial mass
• Idiopathic intracranial hypertension
• Rebound headache from overuse of analgesics
• Table 2-86 describes the differential diagnosis of headaches.

■ WORKUP
• Thorough history and physical examination for any new-onset headache
• Imaging studies to rule out intracranial abnormalities, especially in new-onset and severe headache

■ LABORATORY TESTS
• No routine tests
• ESR in elderly patients suspected of having cranial arteritis

■ IMAGING STUDIES
CT scan and/or MRI may be used to exclude intracranial pathology as cause of new-onset headaches

 TREATMENT

■ NONPHARMACOLOGIC THERAPY
• Relaxation training
• Biofeedback
• Heat
• Massage
• Ultrasound
• Stretching exercises

■ ACUTE GENERAL Rx
Nonnarcotic analgesics with limited frequency to prevent drug-induced headache

■ CHRONIC Rx
• Neurontin, 400 mg in evening; may increase to 400 tid.
• Antidepressants (e.g., amitriptyline 10 to 150 mg hs)
• Trigger point injections
• Occipital nerve blocks

■ DISPOSITION
Rarely responds fully to treatment

■ REFERRAL
If uncertain about diagnosis

REFERENCE
Holroyd KA et al: Management of chronic tension-type headache with tricyclic anti-depressant medication, stress management therapy, and their combination: a randomized controlled trial, *JAMA* 285(17):2208, 2001.
Author: **Michael Gruenthal, M.D., Ph.D.**

BASIC INFORMATION

■ DEFINITION
In complete heart block, there is complete blockage of all AV conduction. The atria and ventricles have separate, independent rhythms.

■ SYNONYMS
Third-degree AV block

ICD-9CM CODES
426.0 Complete heart block

■ EPIDEMIOLOGY & DEMOGRAPHICS
Over 100,000 permanent pacemakers are implanted worldwide each year for complete heart block.

■ PHYSICAL FINDINGS & CLINICAL PRESENTATION
Physical examination may be normal. Patients may present with the following clinical manifestations:
- Dizziness, palpitations
- Stokes-Adams syncopal attacks
- CHF
- Angina

■ ETIOLOGY
- Degenerative changes in His-Purkinje system
- Acute anterior wall MI
- Calcific aortic stenosis
- Cardiomyopathy
- Trauma
- Cardiovascular surgery
- Congenital

DIAGNOSIS

■ DIFFERENTIAL DIAGNOSIS
The differential diagnosis involves only the etiology. ECG will confirm diagnosis.

■ WORKUP
ECG:
- P waves constantly change their relationship to the QRS complexes (Fig. 1-176).
- Ventricular rate is usually <50 bpm (may be higher in congenital forms).
- Ventricular rate is generally lower than the atrial rate.
- QRS complex is wide.

TREATMENT

■ ACUTE GENERAL Rx
- Immediate pacemaker insertion unless the patient has congenital third-degree AV block and is completely asymptomatic
- Therapy of underlying etiology

■ CHRONIC Rx
Patients with permanent pacemakers need regular follow-up and pacemaker monitoring to ensure proper sensing.

■ DISPOSITION
Prognosis is favorable following insertion of pacemaker and related to the underlying etiology of complete AV block (e.g., MI, cardiomyopathy).

■ REFERRAL
Referral for implantation of permanent pacemaker

PEARLS & CONSIDERATIONS

■ COMMENTS
- Patients should be instructed on avoidance of activities that may damage the pacemaker (e.g., contact sports).
- Common environmental causes of pacemaker malformation are electrocautery, transthoracic defibrillation, MRI, extracorporeal shock wave lithotripsy, transcutaneous electrical nerve stimulation, therapeutic radiation, ECT, diathermy, radiofrequency ablation for treatment of tachyarrhythmias.

REFERENCE
Bayce M et al: Evolving indications for permanent pacemakers, *Ann Intern Med* 134:1130, 2001.
Author: **Fred F. Ferri, M.D.**

THIRD-DEGREE (COMPLETE) AV BLOCK

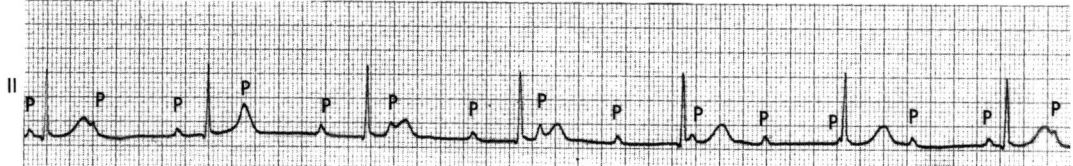

Fig. 1-176 Third-degree complete AV heart block is characterized by independent atrial *(P)* and ventricular (QRS) activity. The atrial rate is always faster than the ventricular rate. The PR intervals are completely variable. Some P waves fall on the T wave, distorting its shape. Others may fall in the QRS complex and be "lost." Notice that the QRS complexes are of normal width, indicating that the ventricles are being paced from the AV junction. (From Goldberger AL [ed]: *Clinical electrocardiography,* ed 5, St Louis, 1994, Mosby.)

BASIC INFORMATION

DEFINITION
Second-degree heart block is the blockage of some (but not all) impulses from the atria to the ventricles. There are two types of second-degree AV block:
MOBITZ TYPE I (WENCKEBACH):
- There is a progressive prolongation of the PR interval before an impulse is completely blocked; the cycle repeats periodically.
- Cycle with dropped beat is less than two times the previous cycle.
- Site of block is usually AV node (proximal to the bundle of His).
MOBITZ TYPE II:
- There is a sudden interruption of AV conduction without prior prolongation of the PR interval.
- Site of block is infranodal.

SYNONYMS
Wenckebach block (Mobitz type I block)
Mobitz type II block

ICD-9CM CODES
426.13 Mobitz type I
426.12 Mobitz type II

EPIDEMIOLOGY & DEMOGRAPHICS
Mobitz type I block is more common and may occur in individuals with heightened vagal tone or secondary to some medications such as β-blockers or calcium channel blockers.

PHYSICAL FINDINGS & CLINICAL PRESENTATION
- Patients with Mobitz type I are usually asymptomatic.
- Sudden loss of consciousness without warning (Adams-Stokes attack) can occur in patients with Mobitz type II; however, it is much more common in patients with complete heart block.
- Irregular pulse with dropped beats is present (Mobitz type I).
- Irregular pulse with occasional dropped beats is present (Mobitz type II).

ETIOLOGY
MOBITZ TYPE I:
- Vagal stimulation
- Degenerative changes in the AV conduction system
- Ischemia at the AV nodes (particularly in inferior wall MI)
- Drugs (digitalis, quinidine, procainamide, adenosine, calcium channel blockers, β-blockers)
- Cardiomyopathies
- Aortic regurgitation
- Lyme carditis
MOBITZ TYPE II:
- Degenerative changes in the His-Purkinje system
- Acute anterior wall MI
- Calcific aortic stenosis

DIAGNOSIS

DIFFERENTIAL DIAGNOSIS
The ECG will distinguish between Mobitz type I and Mobitz type II block and other conduction abnormalities.

WORKUP
ECG, 24-hr Holter monitor (selected patients)
MOBITZ TYPE I (Fig. 1-177): ECG shows:
- Gradual prolongation of PR interval leading to a blocked beat
- Shortened PR interval after dropped beat
MOBITZ TYPE II: ECG shows:
- Fixed duration of PR interval
- Sudden appearance of blocked beats

TREATMENT

NONPHARMACOLOGIC THERAPY
Elimination of drugs that may induce AV block

ACUTE GENERAL Rx
MOBITZ TYPE I:
- Treatment generally is not necessary. This type of block is usually transient.
- If symptomatic (e.g., dizziness), atropine 1 mg (may repeat once after 5 min) may be tried to increase AV conduction; if no response, insert temporary pacemaker.
- If block is secondary to drugs (e.g., digitalis), discontinue the drug.
- If associated with anterior wall MI and wide QRS escape rhythm, consider insertion of temporary pacemaker.
- Significant AV block post-MI may be caused by adenosine produced by the ischemic myocardium. These arrhythmias (which may be resistant to conventional therapy such as atropine) may respond to theophylline (adenosine antagonist).
MOBITZ TYPE II:
- Pacemaker insertion is needed, because this type of block is usually permanent and often progresses to complete AV block.

DISPOSITION
Prognosis is good with insertion of pacemaker in patients with Mobitz type II.

REFERRAL
Referral for pacemaker insertion (see "Acute General Rx")

PEARLS & CONSIDERATIONS

COMMENTS
Patients with Mobitz type I should be followed routinely for potential development of high-grade AV block.

REFERENCE
Barold S, Hayes D: Second-degree atrioventricular block: a reappraisal, *Mayo Clin Proc* 76:44, 2001.
Author: **Fred F. Ferri, M.D.**

WENCKEBACH (MOBITZ TYPE I) SECOND-DEGREE AV BLOCK

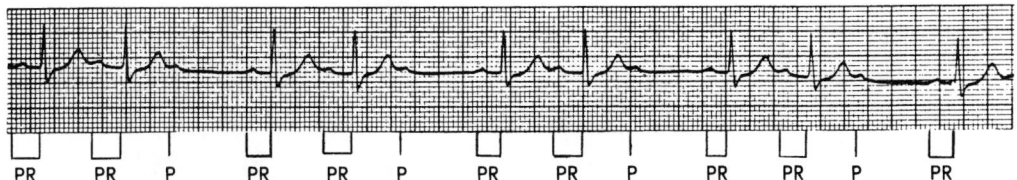

Fig. 1-177 Wenckebach (Mobitz type I) second-degree AV block. Notice the progressive increase in PR intervals, with the third P wave in each sequence not followed by a QRS. Wenckebach block produces a characteristically syncopated rhythm with grouping of the QRS complexes (group beating). (From Goldberger AL [ed]: *Clinical electrocardiography*, ed 5, St Louis, 1994, Mosby.)

BASIC INFORMATION

■ **DEFINITION**

HEAT EXHAUSTION: An illness resulting from prolonged heavy activity in a hot environment with subsequent dehydration, electrolyte depletion, and rectal temperature >37.8° C.
HEAT STROKE: A life-threatening heat illness characterized by extreme hyperthermia, dehydration, and neurologic manifestations.

■ **SYNONYMS**

Heat illness
Hyperthermia

ICD-9CM CODES
992.0 Heat stroke
992.5 Heat exhaustion

■ **EPIDEMIOLOGY & DEMOGRAPHICS**

Heat exhaustion and stroke occur more frequently in elderly patients, especially those taking diuretics or medications that impair heat dissipation (e.g., phenothiazines, anticholinergics, antihistamines, β-blockers).

■ **PHYSICAL FINDINGS & CLINICAL PRESENTATION**

HEAT EXHAUSTION: Profuse sweating, tachycardia, hypotension, hyperventilation, headache, nausea, vomiting, dizziness
HEAT STROKE: Elevated body temperature (usually >40° C), delirium, seizures, coma, skin pallor, anhidrosis, tachycardia, tachypnea

■ **ETIOLOGY**

- Exogenous heat gain (increased ambient temperature)
- Increased heat production (exercise, infection, hyperthyroidism, drugs)
- Impaired heat dissipation (high humidity, heavy clothing, neonatal or elderly patients, drugs [phenothiazines, anticholinergics, antihistamines, butyrophenones, amphetamines, cocaine, alcohol, β-blockers])

DIAGNOSIS

■ **DIFFERENTIAL DIAGNOSIS**

- Infections (meningitis, encephalitis, sepsis)
- Head trauma
- Epilepsy
- Thyroid storm
- Acute cocaine intoxication
- Malignant hyperthermia

- Heat exhaustion can be differentiated from heat stroke by the following:
  1. Essentially intact mental function and lack of significant fever in heat exhaustion
  2. Mild or absent increases in CPK, AST, LDH, ALT in heat exhaustion

■ **WORKUP**

- Heat stroke: comprehensive history, physical examination, and laboratory evaluation.
- Heat exhaustion: in most cases, laboratory tests are not necessary for diagnosis.

■ **LABORATORY TESTS**

Laboratory abnormalities may include the following:
- Elevated BUN, creatinine, Hct
- Hyponatremia or hypernatremia, hyperkalemia or hypokalemia
- Elevated LDH, AST, ALT, CPK, bilirubin
- Lactic acidosis, respiratory alkalosis (secondary to hyperventilation)
- Myoglobinuria, hypofibrinogenemia, fibrinolysis, hypocalcemia

TREATMENT

■ **NONPHARMACOLOGIC THERAPY**

- Treatment of **heat exhaustion** consists primarily of placing the patient in a cool, shaded area and providing rapid hydration and salt replacement.
  1. Fluid intake should be at least 2 L q4h in patients without history of CHF.
  2. Salt replacement can be accomplished by using ¼ teaspoon of salt or two 10-grain salt tablets dissolved in 1 L of water.
  3. If IV fluid replacement is necessary, young athletes can be given normal saline IV (3 to 4 L over 6 to 8 hr); in elderly patients, consider using $D_5\frac{1}{2}NS$ IV with rate titrated to cardiovascular status.
- Patients with **heat stroke** should undergo rapid cooling.
  1. Clothing should be removed.
  2. The patient should be placed in a cool, well-ventilated room.
  3. Monitor body temperature q5min.
  4. The goal is to reduce body temperature to 39° C (102.2° F) in 30 to 60 min.
  5. Spray the patient with a cool mist and use fans to enhance air flow over the body (rapid evaporation method).

6. Immersion of the patient in ice water, stomach lavage with iced saline solution, IV administration of cool fluids, and inhalation of cold air are advisable only when other means for rapid evaporation are not available.
7. Ice packs should not be used because they increase peripheral vasoconstriction and may induce shivering.
8. Antipyretics are ineffective because the hypothalamic set point during heat stroke is normal despite increased body temperature.
9. Immersion in tepid water (15° C, 59° F) is preferred over ice water immersion to minimize risk of shivering.
- Intubate comatose patients and insert Foley catheter.
- Continuous ECG monitoring is recommended.
- Begin IV hydration with NS or lactated Ringer's solution.

■ **ACUTE GENERAL Rx**

In addition to the treatment given above, the patient should be monitored and aggressively treated for the following complications:
- Hypotension: vigorous hydration with NS or LR solution
- Convulsions: diazepam 5 to 10 mg IV (slowly)
- Shivering: chlorpromazine 25 to 50 mg IV
- Acidosis: judicious use of bicarbonate (only in severe acidosis)
- Monitoring for evidence of rhabdomyolysis, hepatic, renal, or cardiac failure and treating accordingly

■ **DISPOSITION**

Most patients recover completely within 48 hr. Mortality can exceed 30% in patients with prolonged and severe hyperthermia.

PEARLS & CONSIDERATIONS

■ **COMMENTS**

Patients should be educated as to the precipitating factors leading to heat illness and should be instructed to acclimatize slowly in warm environments, drink adequate amounts of fluids in warm climate, and limit strenuous activities.

REFERENCE

Waters TA: Heat illness: tips for recognition and treatment, *Cleve Clin J Med* 68:685, 2001.
Author: **Fred F. Ferri, M.D.**

BASIC INFORMATION

■ DEFINITION
Hemochromatosis is an autosomal recessive disorder characterized by increased accumulation of iron in various organs (adrenals, liver, pancreas, heart, testes, kidneys, pituitary) and eventual dysfunction of these organs if not treated appropriately.

■ SYNONYMS
Bronze diabetes

ICD-9CM CODES
275.0 Hemochromatosis

■ EPIDEMIOLOGY & DEMOGRAPHICS
- Hemochromatosis is generally diagnosed in males in their fifth decade.
- Diagnosis in females is generally not made until 10 to 20 yr after menopause.
- Incidence in whites is approximately 1 in 300 persons.
- Most common genetic disorder in North European ancestry.

■ PHYSICAL FINDINGS & CLINICAL PRESENTATION
Examination may be normal; patient with advanced case may present with the following:
- Increased skin pigmentation
- Hepatomegaly, splenomegaly, hepatic tenderness, testicular atrophy
- Loss of body hair, peripheral edema, gynecomastia, ascites
- Amenorrhea (25% of females)
- Loss of libido (50% of males)
- Arthropathy
- Joint pain (44%)
- Fatigue (45%)

■ ETIOLOGY
- Autosomal recessive disease; the gene HFE, which contains two missense mutations (C 282Y and H 63D), was recently identified.

 DIAGNOSIS

■ DIFFERENTIAL DIAGNOSIS
- Hereditary anemias with defect of erythropoiesis
- Cirrhosis
- Repeated blood transfusions

■ WORKUP
Medical history, physical examination, and laboratory evaluation should be focused on affected organ systems (see "Physical Findings"); liver biopsy is the gold standard for diagnosis; it reveals iron deposition in hepatocytes, bile ducts, and supporting tissues.

■ LABORATORY TESTS
- Transferrin saturation is the best screening test. Plasma ferritin is also a good indicator of total body iron stores but may be elevated in many other conditions (inflammation, malignancy). Some authors recommend measurement of both fasting transferrin saturation and serum ferritin level as initial tests for population-based screening to detect and treat hemochromatosis before iron loading occurs.
- Elevated AST, ALT, alkaline phosphatase.
- Hyperglycemia.
- Endocrine abnormalities (decreased testosterone, LH, FSH).
- Measurement of hepatic iron index (hepatic iron concentration [HIC] divided by age) in liver biopsy specimen can confirm diagnosis (Fig. 1-179).

- Genetic testing (HFE genotyping for the C 282 Y and H63 D mutations) may be useful in selected patients with liver disease and suspected iron overload (e.g., patients with transferrin saturation >40%). Genetic testing should not be performed as part of initial routine evaluation for hereditary hemochromatosis. Once a patient has been identified, first-degree relatives of the index patient should also be screened.

■ IMAGING STUDIES
CT scan or MRI of the liver is useful to exclude other etiologies and may in some cases show iron overload in the liver (Fig. 1-178)

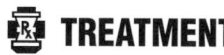 **TREATMENT**

■ NONPHARMACOLOGIC THERAPY
Weekly phlebotomies of 500 ml of blood should be continued for several months until depletion of iron stores is achieved. Subsequent phlebotomies can be performed on a PRN basis to maintain a normal transferrin saturation and a ferritin level <50 μg/L.

■ ACUTE GENERAL Rx
Deferoxamine (iron chelating agent) is generally reserved for patients with severe hemochromatosis with diffuse organ involvement (e.g., liver disease, heart disease) and when phlebotomy is not possible. It is administered in a dose of 0.5 to 1 g IM qd or 20 mg SC over a 12- to 24-hr period with a constant infusion pump.

■ CHRONIC Rx
Phlebotomy on a PRN basis depending on the Hct level; generally, Hct should not exceed 40%.

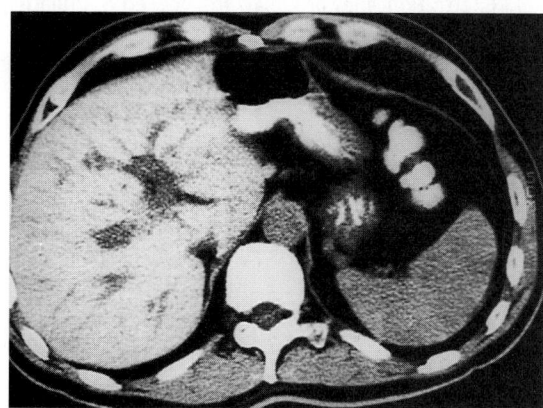

Fig. 1-178 Noncontrast CT of the liver of a patient with hemochromatosis. Note the markedly increased density of the liver parenchyma. (From Halpert RD, Goodman P: *Gastrointestinal radiology: the requisites,* St Louis, 1993, Mosby.)

■ DISPOSITION

Prognosis is good if phlebotomy is started early (before onset of cirrhosis or diabetes mellitus); women can have the full phenotypic expression of the disease, including cirrhosis, and should also be aggressively treated.

■ REFERRAL

For liver biopsy if diagnosis is uncertain.

☼ PEARLS & CONSIDERATIONS

■ COMMENTS

- Patient education material on hemochromatosis can be obtained from the Hemochromatosis Research Foundation, Inc., PO Box 8569, Albany, NY 12208.
- Cirrhotic patients must be periodically monitored (ultrasound or CT scan) because of their increased risk of hepatocellular carcinoma.
- HFE gene testing for C282Y mutation is a cost-effective method of screening relatives of patients with hereditary hemochromatosis.

REFERENCES

El-Serag H et al: Screening for hereditary hemochromatosis in siblings and children of affected patients, *Ann Intern Med* 132:261, 2000.

Steinberg K et al: Prevalence of $C_{282}Y$ and $H_{63}D$ mutations in the hemochromatosis (HFE) gene in the United States, *JAMA* 285:2216, 2001.

Author: **Fred F. Ferri, M.D.**

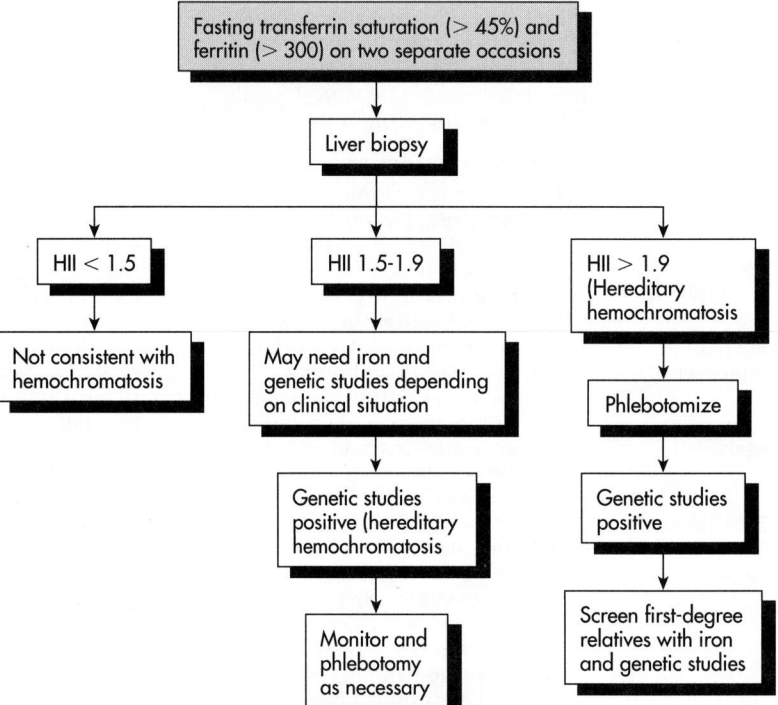

Fig. 1-179   Liver biopsy in hereditary hemochromatosis. *HII,* Hepatic iron index. (From Rakel RE [ed]: *Principles of family practice,* ed 6, Philadelphia, 2002, WB Saunders.)

BASIC INFORMATION

■ DEFINITION
Hemolytic-uremic syndrome refers to an acute syndrome characterized by hemolytic anemia, thrombocytopenia, and severe renal failure.

■ SYNONYMS
HUS

ICD-9CM CODES
283.11 Hemolytic-uremic syndrome

■ EPIDEMIOLOGY & DEMOGRAPHICS
- HUS affects mainly children younger than 10 yr old.
- Incidence is 2.6 cases/100,000 in people younger than 5 yr of age.
- Incidence is 0.97 cases/100,000 in people over the age of 18.
- May be epidemic, most commonly occurring during the summer months.
- Most common cause of acute renal failure in children.
- In the United States 300 to 700 new cases occur each year.

■ PHYSICAL FINDINGS & CLINICAL PRESENTATION
- HUS usually preceded by diarrhea in 90% of cases
- Bloody diarrhea (75%)
- Abdominal pain
- Vomiting
- Fever
- Irritability, lethargy, and seizures (10%)
- Hypertension
- Pallor
- Anuria or oliguria

■ ETIOLOGY
Pathologically the primary lesions of hemolytic-uremic syndrome are arteriolar and capillary microthrombi and red blood cell fragmentation result from endothelial cell damage specifically in the renal vasculature.
In children:
- *E. coli* serotye O157:H7 is the leading cause of HUS.
- The infection is acquired by eating undercooked red meat, especially hamburgers.

Other causes of HUS in children and adults are:
- Drugs (cyclosporin, mitomycin, cisplatin, quinine, penicillin, penicillamine, oral contraceptives)
- Infection (*Salmonella, Shigella, Yersinia, Campylobacter,* coxsackievirus, rubella, influenza virus, Epstein-Barr virus)
- Toxins
- Pregnancy (usually postpartum)

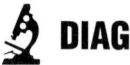

DIAGNOSIS

The triad of thrombocytopenia, acute renal failure, and microangiopathic hemolytic anemia establishes the diagnosis of HUS.

■ DIFFERENTIAL DIAGNOSIS
- The differential is vast, including all causes of bloody and nonbloody diarrhea because the GI symptoms usually precede the triad of HUS
- Thrombotic thrombocytopenic purpura
- Disseminated intravascular coagulation
- Prosthetic valve hemolysis
- Malignant hypertension
- Vasculitis

■ WORKUP
The workup for suspected HUS patients include blood tests and stool cultures.

■ LABORATORY TESTS
- CBC with hemoglobin <10 g/dl.
- Peripheral smear shows the hallmark microangiopathic hemolytic anemia with schistocytes, burr cells, and helmet cells.
- Thrombocytopenia (platelet counts usually <60,000/mm³).
- Reticulocyte count is high.
- LDH level is elevated.
- Haptoglobin is low.
- Indirect bilirubin is elevated.
- BUN and creatinine are elevated.
- Urinalysis reveals proteinuria, microscopic hematuria, and pyuria.
- Stool cultures for *E. coli* O157:H7 is positive in over 90% of cases if obtained during the first week of illness. After the first week only one third are positive.

■ IMAGING STUDIES
Imaging studies are not very helpful in the diagnosis of HUS.

TREATMENT

The treatment of HUS is primarily supportive.

■ NONPHARMACOLOGIC THERAPY
- Blood transfusions for severe anemia
- Antibiotics should be avoided and are not indicated for the treatment of *E. coli* O157:H7.
- Correction of electrolyte abnormalities

■ ACUTE GENERAL Rx
Hypertension control

■ CHRONIC Rx
For anuric or oliguric renal failure, dialysis may be required.

■ DISPOSITION
- Adults presenting with HUS have a worse prognosis than children do with HUS.
- Mortality rate is 5%.
- Morbidity includes:
  1. Proteinuria (31%)
  2. Renal insufficiency (31%)
  3. Hypertension (6%)

■ REFERRAL
- The local health department should be notified if the bacteria *E. coli* O157:H7 has been isolated.
- Consultation with hematology and nephrology specialist is recommended in patients with HUS.

PEARLS & CONSIDERATIONS

■ COMMENTS
- Hemolytic-uremic syndrome was first described by Gasser and colleagues in 1955.
- Children testing positive for the *E. coli* O157:H7 serotype should not return to school or day care facilities until two consecutive stools test negative for the microorganism.
- *E. coli* O157:H7 can be transmitted from person to person, therefore universal precautions and hand washing are recommended in preventing the spread of the infection.

REFERENCES
Begue RE, Mehta D, Blecker U: *Escherichia coli* and the hemolytic-uremic syndrome, *South Med J* 91(9):798, 1998.
Boyce TG, Swerdlow DL, Griffin PM: *Escherichia coli* O157:H7 and the hemolytic-uremic syndrome, *N Engl J Med* 333(6):364, 1995.
Gordjani N et al: Hemolytic uremic syndromes in childhood, *Semin Thromb Hem* 23(3):281,1997.
Lakkis FG, Campbell OC, Badr KF: Microvascular diseases of the kidney. In Brenner BM, Rector FC (eds): *Brenner & Rector's the kidney,* ed 5, Baltimore, 1996, WB Saunders.
Author: **Peter Petropoulos, M.D.**

BASIC INFORMATION

■ **DEFINITION**
Hemophilia is a hereditary bleeding disorder caused by low factor VIII coagulant activity (hemophilia A) or low levels of Factor IX coagulant activity (hemophilia B).

■ **SYNONYMS**
Hemophilia A: Classic hemophilia, factor VIII deficiency hemophilia
Hemophilia B: Christmas disease, factor IX hemophilia

ICD-9CM CODES
286.0 Hemophilia A
286.1 Hemophilia B

■ **EPIDEMIOLOGY & DEMOGRAPHICS**
INCIDENCE/PREVALENCE (IN U.S.):
Hemophilia A: 100 cases/1 million males, hemophilia B: 20 cases/1 million males
GENETIC FACTORS: Both hemophilias have an X-linked recessive pattern of inheritance with only males affected.

■ **PHYSICAL FINDINGS & CLINICAL PRESENTATION**
- The clinical features of hemophilia A and B are generally indistinguishable from each other.
- Bleeding is most commonly seen in joints (knees, ankles, elbows) resulting in hot, swollen, painful joints and subsequent crippling joint deformity.
- Bleeding can also occur into the muscles and the GI tract.
- Compartment syndromes can occur from large hematomas.
- Hematuria may be present.

■ **ETIOLOGY**
- Hemophilia A: low factor VIII coagulant (VIII:C) activity; can be classified as mild if factor VIII:C levels are >5%, moderate: levels are 1% to 5%, severe: levels are <1%.
- Hemophilia B: low levels of factor IX coagulant activity.
- Both disorders are congenital.
- Spontaneous acquisition of factor VIII inhibitors (acquired hemophilia) is rare.

■ **DIAGNOSIS**

■ **DIFFERENTIAL DIAGNOSIS**
- Other clotting factor deficiencies.
- Platelet function disorders.
- Vitamin K deficiency.
- Fig. 3-28 describes a clinical algorithm for evaluation of congenital bleeding disorders. Table 2-21 describes the presumptive diagnosis of common bleeding disorders based on routine screening tests.

■ **WORKUP**
Patients with mild hemophilia bleed only in response to major trauma or surgery and may not be diagnosed until young adulthood. Diagnostic workup includes laboratory evaluation (see "Laboratory Tests").

■ **LABORATORY TESTS**
- Partial thromboplastin time (PTT) is prolonged.
- Reduced factor VIII:C level distinguishes hemophilia A from other causes of prolonged PTT.
- Factor VIII antigen, PT, fibrinogen level, and bleeding time are normal.
- Factor IX coagulant activity levels are reduced in patients with hemophilia B.
- Coagulation factor activity measurement is useful to correlate with disease severity: normal range is 50 to 150 U/dl; 5 to 20 U/dl indicates mild disease, 2 to 5 U/dl indicates moderate disease, and <2 U/dl indicates severe disease with spontaneous bleeding episodes.

■ **TREATMENT**

■ **NONPHARMACOLOGIC THERAPY**
- Avoidance of contact sports
- Patient education regarding their disease; promotion of exercises such as swimming
- Avoidance of aspirin or other NSAIDs
- Orthopedic evaluation and physical therapy evaluation in patients with joint involvement
- Hepatitis vaccination

■ **ACUTE GENERAL Rx**
HEMOPHILIA A:
- Reversal and prevention of acute bleeding in hemophilia A and B are based on adequate replacement of deficient or missing factor protein.
- The choice of the product for replacement therapy is guided by availability, capacity, concerns, and cost. Recombinant factors cost two to three times as much as plasma-derived factors, and the limited capacity to produce recombinant factors often results in periods of shortage. In the U.S., 60% of patients with severe hemophilia use recombinant products.
- Factor VIII concentrates are effective in controlling spontaneous and traumatic hemorrhage in severe hemophilia. The new recombinant factor VIII is stable without added human serum albumin (decreased risk of transmission of infectious agents).
- A new recombinant activated factor VII is useful to stop spontaneous hemorrhages and prevent excessive bleeding during surgery in 75% of patients with inhibitors. Recommended dose is 90 μg/mg of body weight every 2-3 hr for treatment of life-threatening hemorrhage. It is, however, very expensive ($1 per μg).
- Desmopressin acetate 0.3 μg/kg q24h (causes release of factor VIII:C) may be used in preparation for minor surgical procedures in mild hemophiliacs.
- Aminocaproic acid (EACA, Amicar) 4 g PO q4h can be given for persistent bleeding that is unresponsive to factor VIII concentrate or desmopressin.
HEMOPHILIA B:
- Infuse factor IX concentrates. It is important to remember that factor IX concentrates contain other proteins that may increase the risk of thrombosis with recurrent use. Therefore factor IX concentrates must be used only when clearly indicated.
- Daily administration of oral cyclophosphamide and prednisone without empirical factor VIII therapy is an effective and well-tolerated treatment for acquired hemophilia.

■ CHRONIC Rx

- The aim of chronic treatment is to prevent spontaneous bleeding and to prevent excessive bleeding during any surgical intervention.
- Implantation of genetically altered fibroblasts that produce factor VIII is safe and well tolerated. This form is feasible in patients with severe hemophilia. Hemophilia will likely be the first common, severe genetic disease to be cured by gene therapy.

■ DISPOSITION

- Despite the advent of virally safe blood products and blood treatment programs, nearly 70% of hemophiliacs are HIV-seropositive. Survival is of normal expectancy in HIV-negative patients with mild disease.
- Intracranial bleeds are the second most common cause of death in hemophiliacs after AIDS. They are fatal in 30% of patients, occur in 10% of patients, and are generally secondary to trauma.

■ REFERRAL

- Outpatient home infusion therapy is preferred. However, significant bleeding episodes will require inpatient treatment for infusions.
- Orthopedic referral may be necessary in patients with severe joint deformity and crippling.

REFERENCES

Mannucci PM, Tuddenham E: The hemophilias, from royal genes to gene therapy, *N Engl J Med* 344:1773, 2001.

Roth DA et al: Non-viral transfer of the gene encoding coagulation factor VIII in patients with severe hemophilia, *N Engl J Med* 344:1735, 2001.

Author: **Fred F. Ferri, M.D.**

BASIC INFORMATION

■ DEFINITION
A hemorrhoid is a varicose dilation of a vein of the superior or inferior hemorrhoidal plexus, resulting from a persistent increase in venous pressure. External hemorrhoids are below the pectinate line (inferior plexus). Internal hemorrhoids are above the pectinate line (superior plexus) (Fig. 1-180).

■ SYNONYMS
Piles

ICD-9CM CODES
455.6 Hemorrhoids

■ EPIDEMIOLOGY & DEMOGRAPHICS
- Potential for development of symptomatic hemorrhoids in all adults
- Prevalence: estimated 50% of the adult population in the U.S.
- Males = females

■ PHYSICAL FINDINGS & CLINICAL PRESENTATION
- Painless bleeding with defecation; bleeding is bright red and staining on toilet paper
- Perianal irritation
- Mucofecal staining of underclothes
- Acute external hemorrhoids: painful, swollen, and often thrombosed (Fig. 1-181)
- Prolapse
- Constipation

■ ETIOLOGY
- Low-fiber, high-fat diet
- Chronic constipation and straining with defecation
- High resting anal sphincter pressures
- Pregnancy
- Obesity
- Rectal surgery (i.e., episiotomy)
- Prolonged sitting
- Anal intercourse

DIAGNOSIS

■ DIFFERENTIAL DIAGNOSIS
- Fissure
- Abscess
- Anal fistula
- Condylomata acuminata
- Hypertrophied anal papillae
- Rectal prolapse
- Rectal polyp
- Neoplasm

■ WORKUP
- Inspection
- Digital rectal examination
- Anoscopy
- Sigmoidoscopy

TREATMENT

■ NONPHARMACOLOGIC THERAPY
- Avoidance of constipation and straining with defecation
- Avoidance of prolonged sitting on toilet
- High-fiber diet (20 to 30 g/day)
- Increased fluid intake (six to eight glasses of water per day)
- Cleaning with mild soap and water after defecation
- Warm soaks or ice to soothe
- Sitz baths

■ ACUTE GENERAL Rx
- Fiber supplements to provide bulk (psyllium extracts or mucilloids)
- Medicated compresses with witch hazel
- Topical hydrocortisone (1% to 3% cream or ointment)
- Topical anesthetic spray
- Glycerin suppositories
- Stool softeners

■ CHRONIC Rx
- Rubber-band ligation
- Injection sclerotherapy
- Photocoagulation
- Cryodestruction
- Hemorrhoidectomy (Fig. 1-182)
- Anal dilatation
- Laser or cautery hemorrhoidectomy

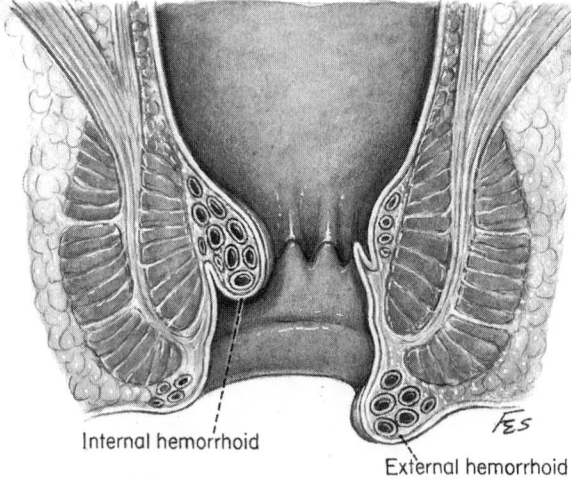

Internal hemorrhoid

External hemorrhoid

Fig. 1-180 Anatomy of internal and external hemorrhoids. (From Noble J [ed]: *Textbook of primary care medicine,* ed 2, St Louis, 1996, Mosby.)

- Observance for complications: thrombosis, bleeding, infection, anal stenosis or weakness

■ DISPOSITION
Should resolve, but there is a high rate of recurrence

■ REFERRAL
To colorectal or general surgeon for any hemorrhoid that does not respond to conservative therapy

☼ PEARLS & CONSIDERATIONS

■ COMMENTS
- Patients need to understand the importance of a healthy diet, regular exercise, and rectal hygiene.
- Stress the importance of avoiding prolonged sitting and straining on the toilet.
- Stress the need not to defer the urge to defecate.

Author: **Maria A. Corigliano, M.D.**

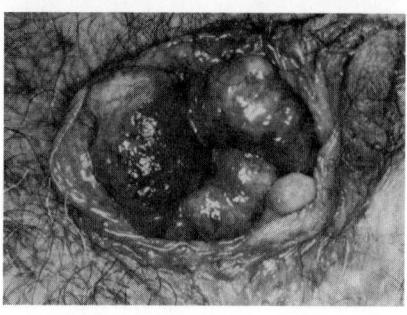

Fig. 1-181 Third-degree hemorrhoids. Note the squamous epithelial change and the darkened mucosa. (From Sabiston D: *Textbook of surgery,* ed 15, Philadelphia, 1997, WB Saunders.)

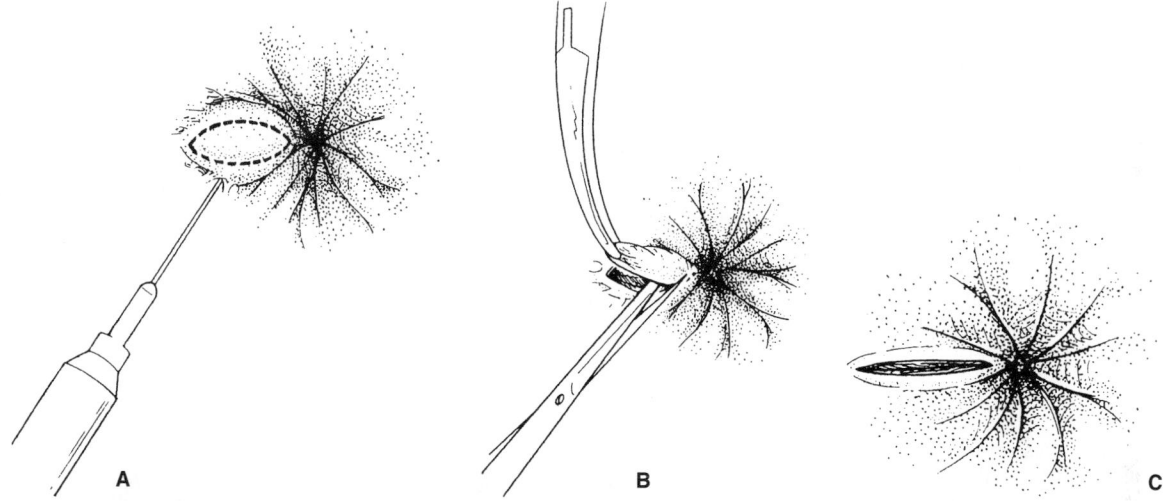

Fig. 1-182 Excision of thrombosed hemorrhoid. The area is infiltrated with local anesthetic, and the planned elliptical incision is outlined **(A)**. The thrombosed hemorrhoid is excised sharply wih scissors **(B)**, and the edges of the wound are left open after ensuring hemostasis **(C)**. (From Prager E: Common ailments of the anorectal region. In Block GE, Moosa AR [eds]: *Operative colorectal surgery,* Philadelphia, 1994, WB Saunders.)

BASIC INFORMATION

DEFINITION

Henoch-Schönlein purpura (HSP) is a systemic small vessel vasculitis characterized by palpable purpura in dependent areas (buttocks, legs), gastrointestinal bleeding and other symptoms, arthralgias, arthritis, and renal involvement.

SYNONYMS

Anaphylactoid purpura
Allergic purpura

ICD-9CM CODES

287.0 Henoch-Schönlein purpura

EPIDEMIOLOGY & DEMOGRAPHICS

HSP is the most common vasculitis seen in children and younger age groups. It is seen mostly from 4 to 15 yr of age, although it can also be seen in older adolescents and young adults. A 2:1 male to female ratio exists. Peak incidence is seen in spring, although cases are seen throughout the year.

PHYSICAL FINDINGS & CLINICAL PRESENTATION

- Palpable purpura of dependent areas, especially lower extremities (Fig. 1-183), and areas subjected to pressure such as the beltline
- Subcutaneous edema
- Arthralgias and arthritis in 80% of patients
- GI symptoms are seen in approximately one third of patients. Common findings are nausea, vomiting, diarrhea, cramping, abdominal pain, hematochezia, and melena
- Anecdotally may follow upper respiratory infection
- Renal insufficiency seen in 10% to 20% of patients

ETIOLOGY

The presumptive etiology is exposure to a trigger antigen that causes antibody formation. Antigen-antibody (immune) complex deposition then occurs in arteriole and capillary walls of skin, renal mesangium, and GI tract. IgA deposition is most common. Antigen triggers postulated include drugs, foods, immunization, and upper respiratory and other viral illnesses.

 DIAGNOSIS

Diagnosis is made on clinical grounds. Skin manifestations are most common. Palpable purpura is seen in 70% of adult patients and is less pronounced in children, in whom GI complaints are more common. Skin biopsy will show leukocytoclastic vasculitis.

DIFFERENTIAL DIAGNOSIS

Other forms of cutaneous or leukocytoclastic vasculitis:
- Polyarteritis nodosa
- Meningococcemia
- Thrombocytopenic purpura

WORKUP

History, physical examination, laboratory testing to rule out other diagnostic considerations, and skin biopsy

LABORATORY TESTS

- Electrolytes, blood urea nitrogen, and creatinine
- Urinalysis
- Complete blood count
- Prothrombin time, fibrinogen, and fibrin degradation products
- Blood cultures

Laboratory abnormalities are not specific for HSP. Leukocytosis and eosinophilia may be seen. IgA levels are elevated in approximately 50% of patients. Glomerulonephritis may be present and result in microscopic hematuria, proteinuria, and RBC casts.

IMAGING STUDIES

Imaging studies are not useful in diagnosis of HSP. Arteriography or magnetic resonance angiography may be helpful in distinguishing from polyarteritis nodosa.

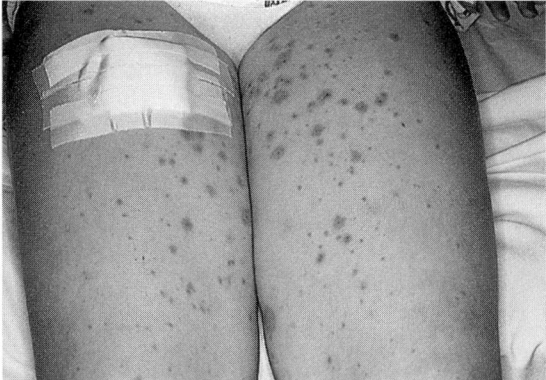

Fig. 1-183 Henoch-Schönlein purpura on the lower extremities of a child. (Courtesy Medical College of Georgia, Division of Dermatology. From Goldstein B [ed]: *Practical dermatology,* ed 2, St Louis, 1997, Mosby.)

TREATMENT

- Prednisone 1 mg/kg PO is given if renal or severe GI disease, although benefits are not clear.
- Corticosteroids and azathioprine may be beneficial if rapidly progressive glomerulonephritis present.
- Nonsteroidal antiinflammatory drugs for arthritis and arthralgias.

NONPHARMACOLOGIC THERAPY

Supportive care with pain management, adequate hydration and nutrition

DISPOSITION & PROGNOSIS

- Prognosis excellent with spontaneous recovery of most patients within 4 wk.
- End-stage renal disease occurs in 5% of patients. Chronic renal insufficiency is the most common long-term morbidity.
- GI complications include mesenteric infarction, perforation, and intussusception.
- Recurrences can occur.

REFERRAL

- For renal or gastrointestinal complications
- For severe clinical syndrome

Author: **Dominick Tammaro, M.D.**

BASIC INFORMATION

■ **DEFINITION**
Hepatic encephalopathy is an abnormal mental status occurring in patients with severe impairment of liver function and consequent accumulation of toxic products not metabolized by the liver.

■ **SYNONYMS**
Hepatic coma

ICD-9CM CODES
572.2 Hepatic encephalopathy

■ **EPIDEMIOLOGY & DEMOGRAPHICS**
INCIDENCE/PREVALENCE: Hepatic encephalopathy occurs in >50% of all cases of cirrhosis.

■ **PHYSICAL FINDINGS & CLINICAL PRESENTATION**
Hepatic encephalopathy can be classified in stages or grades 1 to 4:
- Grades 1 and 2: mild obtundation
- Grades 3 and 4: stupor to deep coma, with or without decerebrate posturing.

The physical examination in hepatic encephalopathy varies with the stage and may reveal the following abnormalities:
- Skin: jaundice, palmar erythema, spider angiomata, ecchymosis, dilated superficial periumbilical veins (caput medusae) in patients with cirrhosis
- Eyes: scleral icterus, Kayser-Fleischer rings (Wilson's disease)
- Breath: fetor hepaticus
- Chest: gynecomastia in men with chronic liver disease
- Abdomen: ascites, small nodular liver (cirrhosis), tender hepatomegaly (congestive hepatomegaly)
- Rectal examination: hemorrhoids (portal hypertension), guaiac-positive stool (alcoholic gastritis, bleeding esophageal varices, PUD, bleeding hemorrhoids)
- Genitalia: testicular atrophy in males with chronic liver disease
- Extremities: pedal edema from hypoalbuminemia
- Neurologic: flapping tremor (asterixis), obtundation, coma with or without decerebrate posturing

■ **ETIOLOGY**
- Precipitating factors in patients with underlying cirrhosis (UGI bleeding, hypokalemia, hypomagnesemia, analgesic and sedative drugs, sepsis, alkalosis, increased dietary protein)
- Acute fulminant viral hepatitis
- Drugs and toxins (e.g., isoniazid, acetaminophen, diclofenac, statins, methyldopa, loratadine, PTU, lisinopril, labetalol, halothane, carbon tetrachloride, erythromycin, nitrofurantoin, troglitazone)
- Reye's syndrome
- Shock and/or sepsis
- Fatty liver of pregnancy
- Metastatic carcinoma, hepatocellular carcinoma
- Other: autoimmune hepatitis, ischemic venoocclusive disease, sclerosing cholangitis, heat stroke, amebic abscesses

DIAGNOSIS

■ **DIFFERENTIAL DIAGNOSIS**
- Delirium secondary to medications or illicit drugs
- CVA, subdural hematoma
- Meningitis, encephalitis
- Hypoglycemia
- Uremia
- Cerebral anoxia
- Hypercalcemia
- Metastatic neoplasm to brain
- Alcohol withdrawal syndrome

■ **WORKUP**
Exclude other etiologies with comprehensive history (obtained from patient, relatives, and others), physical examination, laboratory and imaging studies. A pertinent history should include exposure to hepatitis, ethanol intake, drug history, exposure to toxins, IV drug abuse, measles or influenza with aspirin use (Reye's syndrome), history of carcinoma (primary or metastatic).

■ **LABORATORY TESTS**
- ALT, AST, bilirubin, alkaline phosphatase glucose, calcium, electrolytes, BUN, creatinine, albumin
- CBC, platelet count, PT, PTT
- Serum and urine toxicology screen in suspected medication or illegal drug use
- Blood and urine cultures, urinalysis
- Venous ammonia level
- ABGs

■ **IMAGING STUDIES**
CT scan of head may be useful in selected patients to exclude other etiologies.

TREATMENT

■ **NONPHARMACOLOGIC THERAPY**
- Identification and treatment of precipitating factors
- Restriction of protein intake (30 to 40 g/day) to reduce toxic protein metabolites

■ **ACUTE GENERAL Rx**
REDUCTION OF COLONIC AMMONIA PRODUCTION:
- Lactulose 30 ml of 50% solution qid initially, dose is subsequently adjusted depending on clinical response. Ornithine aspartate 9 g tid is also effective.
- Neomycin 1 g PO q4-6h or given as a 1% retention enema solution (1 g in 100 ml of isotonic saline solution); neomycin should be used with caution in patients with renal insufficiency; metronidazole may be as effective as neomycin and is not nephrotoxic.
- A combination of lactulose and neomycin can be used when either agent is ineffective alone.

TREATMENT OF CEREBRAL EDEMA:
Cerebral edema is often present in patients with acute liver failure, and it accounts for nearly 50% of deaths. Monitoring intracranial pressure by epidural, intraparenchymal, or subdural transducers and treatment of cerebral edema with mannitol (100 to 200 ml of 20% solution [0.3 to 0.4 g/kg of body weight]) given by rapid IV infusion is helpful in selected patients (e.g., potential transplantation patients).

■ **CHRONIC Rx**
- Avoidance of any precipitating factors (e.g., high-protein diet, medications)
- Consideration of liver transplantation in selected patients with progressive or recurrent encephalopathy

■ **DISPOSITION**
- Prognosis varies with the underlying etiology of the liver failure and the grade of encephalopathy (generally good for grades 1, 2; poor for grades 3, 4).
- Table 3-3 describes prognostic variables based on the Child-Pugh score.

■ **REFERRAL**
The early stages of hepatic encephalopathy can be managed in the outpatient setting, whereas stages 3 or 4 require hospital admission.

PEARLS & CONSIDERATIONS

■ **COMMENTS**
Patients not responding to supportive therapy should be evaluated for liver transplantation.
Author: **Fred F. Ferri, M.D.**

BASIC INFORMATION

■ DEFINITION
Hepatitis A is an acute, self-limited infection caused by hepatitis A virus (HAV), which leads to varying degrees of inflammation of liver parenchymal cells. Infection may range from asymptomatic to fulminant hepatitis.

■ SYNONYMS
Infectious hepatitis
Short incubation (15 to 45 days) hepatitis

ICD-9CM CODES
070.1 Hepatitis A

■ EPIDEMIOLOGY & DEMOGRAPHICS
- Hepatitis A is the most common cause of acute hepatitis in the U.S.
- In U.S. average disease rate is approximately 10 cases/100,000 persons/yr.
- Substantially higher rates in western U.S., from 20-48 cases/100,000 persons/yr.
- Highest incidence among children 5 to 14 yr; approximately one third of cases involve children <15 yr of age.
- Highest rates among American Indians and Alaskan natives, lowest among Asians. Rates among Hispanics higher than among non-Hispanics.
- At risk groups include:
  1. Residents and staff of group homes
  2. Children, employees of day care centers
  3. Persons who engage in oral-anal contact, regardless of sexual orientation
  4. Injecting and noninjecting drug users
  5. Travel to endemic areas
  6. Consumption of contaminated shellfish
  7. Areas of overcrowding, poor sanitation, inadequate sewage treatment
  8. Persons having contact with non-human primates that are born in the wild

PREVALENCE
- Approximately one third of U.S. population has serologic evidence of prior HAV infection.
- Anti-HAV prevalence has inverse relation to income and household size.
- Age-adjusted anti-HAV rates are 70% for Mexican-Americans, 39% for non-Hispanic African-Americans, 23% for non-Hispanic whites.

PREDOMINANT SEX
None, except higher infection rates seen in homosexual males who engage in oral-anal contacts.

PREDOMINANT AGE/PEAK INCIDENCE
- In areas of high rates of hepatitis A, 30% to 40% of children are infected by age 5, and almost all persons are infected before young adulthood.
- In areas with intermediate rates, disease occurs in a wider range of ages; children with asymptomatic HAV can be a source of infection for older persons.
- In areas of low rates of hepatitis A most cases occur in school-age children, adolescents, and young adults.

■ PHYSICAL FINDINGS & CLINICAL PRESENTATION
- Infection with HAV may have acute or subacute presentation, icteric or anicteric. Severity of illness seems to increase with age (90% of infections in children <5 yr may be subclinical).
- Incubation period is 15 to 50 days (mean of 30 days), typically followed by nonspecific symptoms.
- A preicteric, prodromal phase of approximately 1 to 14 days (average 5 to 7 days). 15% with no apparent prodrome. Symptoms are usually abrupt in onset and may include anorexia, malaise, nausea/vomiting, fever, headache, abdominal pain.
- Less common symptoms are chills, myalgias/arthralgias, upper respiratory symptoms, constipation, diarrhea, pruritus, urticaria.
- Jaundice occurs in >70% of patients.
- The icteric phase is preceded by dark urine. Constitutional symptoms may subside or persist.
- Bilirubinuria is typically followed a few days later by clay-colored stools and icterus.

PHYSICAL EXAM:
- Hepatomegaly (87%), splenomegaly (5% to 15%), RUQ tenderness, spider nevi on trunk.
- Rarely, rashes, petechiae, mild edema, cardiac arrythmias.
- Duration of illness varies, but the majority of infections are resolving by the third week.

■ COMPLICATIONS
- Cholestatic hepatitis: an occasional complication, manifested by fever, pruritus, and jaundice up to 18 wk.
- Prolonged infection: jaundice observed up to 17 wk, elevated aminotransferase levels.
- Relapsing infection: a second rise in liver enzymes, 15 to 90 days after resolution of initial illness. All of these processes have favorable resolution.
- Fulminant hepatitis: a rare complication. Occurs more often in adults, and mortality is correlated with age and presence of other comorbidities. Characterized by increasing jaundice, deterioration in liver enzymes, and prolongation of PT. Patients may exhibit confusion, irritability, insomnia, severe vomiting.
- Spontaneous recovery rate for all groups is 35%.
- Fatality rate for hepatitis A is 1.3%.
- Extrahepatic complications: acute cholecystitis, acute pancreatitis, autoimmune hemolytic anemia, thrombocytopenic purpura, pure red cell aplasia, aplastic anemia, acute reactive arthritis, pleural and pericardial effusions, Guillain-Barré syndrome, transverse myelitis, optic neuritis, acute renal failure.

■ ETIOLOGY
- Caused by HAV, a 27-nm picornavirus (nonenveloped, single-stranded RNA virus).
- Transmission is fecal-oral route, from person to person. Transmission requires close contact, usually occurs within families.
- Parenteral transmission was considered rare; however, there have been several cases reported of infection occurring from transfusion of blood, blood products, platelets, plasma, clotting factors, and anticancer immunotherapy agents.

DIAGNOSIS

■ DIFFERENTIAL DIAGNOSIS
ACUTE DISEASE:
- Other hepatitis viruses (B, C, D, E)
- Other viral illnesses producing systemic disease (e.g., yellow fever, EBV, CMV, HIV, rubella, rubeola, coxsackie B, adenovirus, HSV, HZV)
- Nonviral hepatitis (e.g., leptospirosis, toxoplasmosis, alcoholic hepatitis, drug-induced [e.g., acetaminophen, INH], toxic hepatitis [carbon tetrachloride, benzene])

HEPATITIS E:
- Similar to HAV (fecal-oral spread; short incubation period; no chronic disease)
- High mortality (fulminant hepatitis and DIC) in late pregnancy
- Rare in U.S.

■ WORKUP
- IgM antibody specific for HAV
- Liver function tests: ALT and AST elevations are sensitive for liver parenchymal damage, but not specific for HAV
- CBC: may find mild lymphocytosis
- Liver biopsy (for fulminant hepatitis); rarely indicated

■ LABORATORY TESTS
- Diagnosis confirmed by IgM anti-HAV; it is detectable in almost all infected patients at presentation and remains positive for 3 to 6 mo.

- IgG anti-HAV may be present at disease onset and peaks 6 to 12 mo after the acute illness. It may persist for years.
- A fourfold rise in titer of total antibody (IgM and IgG) to HAV confirms acute HAV infection, although in many patients the titers have already peaked at the time of presentation.
- HAV antigen or virus shed in the stool may be the first marker of infection, but usually begins 1 to 2 wk before onset of symptoms and peaks before patients seek medical attention.
- Liver function tests:
  1. ALT and AST usually more than eight times normal in acute infection
  2. Bilirubin usually five to fifteen times normal
  3. Alkaline phosphatase minimally elevated (one to three times normal) acutely; may be elevated in cholestasis
  4. Albumin and prothrombin time are generally normal; if elevated, may herald hepatic necrosis

■ IMAGING STUDIES
- Rarely useful
- Sonogram (fulminant hepatitis)

℞ TREATMENT

- Supportive care. Those with fulminant hepatitis may require hospitalization and treatment of associated complications.
- Activity as tolerated.
- No specific dietary restrictions. Although by convention patients are advised to avoid alcohol, there is no evidence that modest alcohol intake effects outcome.
- Patients with fulminant hepatitis should be assessed for liver transplantation; however, 60% of these patients will recover without intervention.
- Avoid hepatically metabolized drugs.
- Cholestyramine may ameliorate severe pruritus secondary to cholestasis.

■ CHRONIC Rx
- No chronic HAV and no chronic carrier state

■ DISPOSITION
- Follow-up as outpatient.
- Acute disease usually lasts <2 mo; 10% to 15% of infected persons will have prolonged or relapsing illness of up to 6 mo.

☼ PEARLS & CONSIDERATIONS

- HAV replicates in the liver, is excreted in bile and shed in the stool. Peak infectivity occurs when viral concentration in stool is highest, the 2 wk before onset of jaundice.
- HAV is transmitted via the fecal-oral route, by person-to-person contact or ingestion of contaminated food or water.
- Rarely, HAV has been transmitted in blood and blood products transfusions.
- HAV can survive in the environment for several months.
- Heating foods to >185° F (85° C) for 1 min and disinfecting surfaces with a 1:100 dilution of sodium hypochlorite (household bleach) in water will inactivate HAV.

■ PREVENTION
- Improvements in hygiene and sanitation.
- For hospitalized patients, enteric precautions are adequate. Only patients incontinent of stool require private rooms.

■ PASSIVE IMMUNIZATION
- Immune globulin provides protection against HAV through passive transfer of antibody. Immune globulin IM and IG both contain anti-HAV, but IGIM is the one used.
- Preexposure prophylaxis indicated for:
  Persons traveling to developing countries.
  Dose: 0.02 ml/kg given IM confers protection for <3 mo
  0.6 ml/kg given IM confers protection for ≤5 mo
  Persons residing in endemic areas for prolonged periods should receive IGIM every 5 mo.
- Postexposure prophylaxis with IG indicated for:
  Persons with recent exposure (within 2 wk) to HAV and who have not been previously vaccinated.

This includes household and sexual contacts of persons with serologically confirmed HAV and those who have shared illegal drugs with an infected person.
Close contacts who have received at least one dose of HAV vaccine at least one month before exposure do not need IG prophylaxis.
When given with 2 wk after exposure, IG is >85% effective in preventing HAV infection. Efficacy is greater the earlier postexposure that it is given.
  Dose: 0.02 ml/kg given IM

■ ACTIVE IMMUNIZATION
- There are several inactivated and attenuated hepatitis A vaccines; only the inactivated vaccines are currently available for use and they have been found to be safe and highly immunogenic.
- Protective antibody levels were reached in 94% to 100% of adults one mo after the first dose, and in 100% after the second dose. Similar results have been found for children and adolescents.
- Theoretic analyses of antibody levels estimate duration of immunity to be 10 to 20 yr.

INDICATIONS FOR HEPATITIS A VACCINE:
Note: the vaccine is licensed for use in adults and children ≥2 years of age.
- Should be considered for persons who are at risk: persons traveling to or working in endemic areas, men who engage in sex with men, illegal drug users, persons with occupational exposure (work with HAV-infected primates, HAV research lab, contact with sewage), persons with clotting factor disorders, persons with chronic liver disease, children in areas with high rates of hepatitis A infection.
- Vaccine may be administered simultaneously with IG as part of postexposure prophylaxis.
- Typically, the vaccine is administered in three doses, at 0, 1, 6 mo or 0, 1, 12 mo.

REFERENCES
Bell BP et al: Prevention of hepatitis A through active or passive immunization: recommendations of the advisory committee on immunization practices, *MMWR* 48(RR-12):1, 1999.
Cuthbert JA: Hepatitis A: old and new, *Clin Microbiol Rev* 14(1):38, 2001.
Author: **Jane V. Eason, MD**

BASIC INFORMATION

■ DEFINITION
Hepatitis B is an acute infection of the liver parenchymal cells caused by the hepatitis B virus (HBV).

■ SYNONYMS
Serum hepatitis
Long incubation (30 to 180 days) hepatitis

ICD-9CM CODES
070.3 Hepatitis B

■ EPIDEMIOLOGY & DEMOGRAPHICS
INCIDENCE (IN U.S.)
- Approximately 200,000 to 300,000 infections annually in U.S.
- Much higher incidence in Europe (approximately 1 million new cases annually) and in areas of high endemicity.
- In U.S. transmission mainly horizontal (percutaneous and mucous membrane exposure to infectious blood and other body fluids, [e.g., sexual transmission, either homosexual or heterosexual]); also from needle sharing amongst drug abusers; occupational exposure to contaminated blood and blood products; persons receiving transfusions of blood and blood products; hemodialysis patients.
Note: improved screening of blood and blood products has greatly reduced, although not eliminated, the risk of posttransfusion HBV infection.
- In areas of high endemicity, transmission is largely vertical (perinatal): HBV exists in the blood and body fluids. Perinatal transmission from HBsAg-positive mothers is as high as 90%.

PREVALENCE (IN U.S.):
- North America, Western Europe, and Australia are areas of low prevalence, <2%.
- Africa, Asia, and the Western Pacific region are areas of high prevalence, ≥8%.
- Southern and Eastern Europe have intermediate rates, 2% to 7%.
- Chronically infected persons, those with positive HBsAg for >6 months, represent the major source of infection.
- Up to 95% of infants and children <5 yr of age, who typically have subclinical acute infection, will become chronic HBV carriers.
- Adults are more likely to have clinical evident acute infection, but only 1% to 5% will develop chronic infection.
- Approximately 0.1% with acute infection will develop fulminant acute hepatitis resulting in death.

PREDOMINANT SEX:
- Predominant in males because of increased intravenous drug abuse, homosexuality
- Females more commonly terminate in chronic carrier state

PREDOMINANT AGE:
20 to 45 yr

PEAK INCIDENCE:
30 to 45 yr of age, at rates of 5% to 20%

GENETICS:
Neonatal infection:
- Rare in U.S.
- High (up to 90%) in areas of high endemicity (only 5% to 10% of perinatal infections occur in utero)

■ PHYSICAL FINDINGS & CLINICAL PRESENTATION (FIG. 1-140)
- Often nonspecific symptoms
- Profound malaise
- Many asymptomatic cases
- Prodrome:
  1. 15% to 20% serum sickness (urticaria, rash, arthralgia) during early HBsAg
  2. HBsAg-Ab complex disease (arthritis, arteritis, glomerulonephritis)
- Hepatomegaly (87%) with RUQ tenderness
  1. Hepatic punch tenderness
  2. Splenomegaly: rare (10% to 15%)
- Jaundice, dark urine, with occasional pruritus
- Variable fever (when present, generally precedes jaundice and rapidly declines following onset of icteric phase)
- Spider angiomata: rare; resolves during recovery
- Rare polyarteritis nodosa, cryoglobulinemia

■ ETIOLOGY
- Caused by hepatitis B virus (42-nm hepadnavirus with an outer surface coat [HBsAg], inner nucleocapsid core [HBcAg; HBeAg]; DNA polymerase; and partially double-stranded DNA genome)
- Transmission by parenteral route (needle use, tattooing, ear piercing, acupuncture, transfusion of blood and blood products, hemodialysis, sexual contact), perinatal transmission
- Infection may result from contact of infectious material with mucous membranes and open skin breaks (e.g., HBV is stable and can be transmitted from toothbrushes, utensils, razors, baby toys, various medical equipment [respirators, endoscopes])
- Oral intake of infectious material may result in infection through breaks in the oral mucosa
- Food or water virtually never found to be sources of HBV infection

- Infection occurring primarily in liver, where necrosis probably results from cytotoxic T-cell response, direct cytopathic effect of HBcAg (core antigen), high-level HBsAg (surface antigen) expression, or co-infection with delta (D) hepatitis virus (RNA delta core within HBsAg envelope)
- Recovery (>90%):
  1. Fulminant hepatitis occurring in <1% (especially if co-infected with hepatitis D); 80% fatal
  2. Unusual (5%) prolonged acute disease for 4 to 12 mo, with recovery
  3. Overall fatality increases with age and viral innoculation (e.g., transfusions)
- Chronic infection (1% to 2%):
  1. Persistent carrier state without hepatitis (HBsAg positive)
  2. Chronic persistent hepatitis (CPH) (clinically well), or chronic active hepatitis (CAH) (HBsAg positive and HBeAg positive)
  3. Cirrhosis
  4. Hepatocellular carcinoma (especially after neonatal infection)
  5. Chronic infection: more common following low-dose exposure and mild acute hepatitis, with earlier age of infection, in males, or if immunosuppressed
  6. One third to one quarter of chronically infected will develop progressive liver disease (cirrhosis, hepatocellular carcinoma)

DIAGNOSIS

■ DIFFERENTIAL DIAGNOSIS
- Acute disease confused with other viral hepatitis infections (A, C, D, E)
- Any viral illness producing systemic disease and hepatitis (e.g., yellow fever, EBV, CMV, HIV, rubella, rubeola, coxsackie B, adenovirus, herpes simplex or zoster)
- Nonviral etiologies of hepatitis (e.g., leptospirosis, toxoplasmosis, alcoholic hepatitis, drug-induced [e.g., acetominophen, INH], toxic hepatitis [carbon tetrachloride, benzene])

■ WORKUP
- Acute serum specimen for hepatitis B serology (HBsAg, HBsAb, HBcAb, HBeAg, HBeAb)
- Liver function tests (see Fig. 3-95)
- CBC
- Liver biopsy: rarely indicated for diagnosis of fulminant viral hepatitis, chronic hepatitis, cirrhosis, carcinoma

■ **LABORATORY TESTS**
- Diagnosis of acute HBV infection is best confirmed by IgM HBcAb in acute or early convalescent serum.
  1. Generally, IgM present during onset of jaundice
  2. Coexisting HBsAg
- HBsAg and IgG-HBcAb during acute jaundice are strongly suggestive of remote HBV infection and another etiology for current illness.
- HBsAb alone is suggestive of immunization response.
- With recovery, HBeAg is rapidly replaced by HBeAb in 2 to 3 mo, and HBsAg is replaced by HBsAb in 5 to 6 mo.
- In chronic HBV hepatitis, HBsAg and HBeAg are persistent without corresponding Ab.
- In chronic carrier state, HBsAg is persistent, but HBeAg is replaced by HBe AB.
- HBcAb develops in all outcomes.
- HBeAg correlation with highest infectivity; appearance of HBeAb heralds recovery.
- Liver function tests:
  1. ALT and AST: usually more than eight times normal (often 1000 U/L) at onset of jaundice (minimal acute ALT/AST rises often followed by chronic hepatitis or hepatocellular carcinoma)
  2. Bilirubin: variably elevated in icteric viral hepatitis
  3. Alkaline phosphatase: minimally elevated (one to three times normal) acutely
- Albumin and prothrombin time:
  1. Generally normal
  2. If abnormal, possible harbinger of impending hepatic necrosis (fulminant hepatitis)
- WBC and ESR: generally normal

■ **IMAGING STUDIES**
- Rarely useful
- Sonogram to document rapid reduction in liver size during fulminant hepatitis or mass in hepatocellular carcinoma

℞ TREATMENT

■ **NONPHARMACOLOGIC THERAPY**
- Symptomatic treatment as necessary
- Activity as tolerated
- High-calorie diet preferred; often best tolerated in morning

■ **ACUTE GENERAL Rx**
- In most cases of acute HBV infection no treatment necessary; >90% of adults will spontaneously clear infection

- Hospitalization advisable for any patient in danger from dehydration due to poor oral intake, whose PT is prolonged, who has rising bilirubin level >15 to 20 μg/dl, or who has any clinical evidence of hepatic failure
- IV therapy needed (rarely) for hydration during severe vomiting
- Avoid hepatically metabolized drugs
- No therapeutic measures are beneficial
- Steroids not shown helpful

■ **CHRONIC Rx**
The aim of therapy in chronic HBV infection is to eradicate the virus. The two modalities of therapy available to achieve this goal have been: immune modulators (interferon alpha) and antiviral agents in the form of nucleoside analogues (e.g., lamivudine, famciclovir).
- Until recently IFN-α has been the mainstay of therapy. Its mechanism of action is to stimulate the immune system to attack HBV-infected hepatocytes, thus inhibiting viral protein synthesis.
- A 4-month course of treatment results in a 30% to 40% response with significant reduction of serum HBV DNA, normalization of ALT, and loss of HBeAg. Seroconversion from HBeAg to HBeAb occurs in 15% to 20%.
- Factors that increase the likelihood of response to IFN-α therapy include:
  1. Adult onset of infection
  2. High baseline ALT
  3. Low baseline HBV DNA
  4. Absence of cirrhosis
  5. Female
  6. HBeAg positive
- Infrequent relapse after successful completion of therapy.
- 80% of patients who lose HBeAg during therapy lose HBsAg in the decade after therapy.
- >50% of patients who do not seroconvert after initial therapy develop a delayed HBeAg seroconversion months to years after therapy.
- Overall incidence of cirrhosis and hepatocellular carcinoma is decreased in those treated with IFN-α.
- IFN-α is successful only in patients with an active immune response; therefore it is not effective in patients with HIV infection and organ transplant patients.
- Asians respond poorly to IFN-α.
- Treatment with IFN-α in general is also poorly tolerated: side effects include flulike symptoms, injection-site reactions, rash, weight loss, anxiety, depression, alopecia, thrombocytopenia, granulocytopenia, thyroid dysfunction.

- Nucleoside analogues block viral replication by inhibiting HBV polymerase.
- Lamivudine is, to date, the only one of these agents approved for treatment of chronic HBV infection; it has been shown to rapidly reduce HBV replication and suppress HBV DNA to undetectable levels after a few weeks of treatment, and treatment for 1 yr is as effective as IFN-α with respect to loss of HBeAg seroconversion to HBeAb and loss of HBV DNA.
  1. It is better tolerated than IFN-α
  2. Easier administration: given orally
  3. Suppression of HBV replication regardless of sex, ethnicity, disease severity
- Other nucleoside agents under evaluation include famciclovir (found less effective than lamivudine), adefovir and adefovir dipivoxil, ganciclovir, lobucavir, entecavir, emtricitabine.
- A problem with the antiviral therapies is emergence of resistant HBV strains (YMDD variants [tyrosine-methionine-aspartate-aspartate]).
- Combination therapy with two or three nucleoside analogues or combination therapy with IFN-α currently under investigation.
- Liver transplantation (consider for fulminant hepatitis).

■ **DISPOSITION**
- Follow-up as outpatient
- Acute disease: usually <6 weeks
- Rare fatalities (fulminant hepatitis)
- Possible chronic carrier state, cirrhosis, hepatocellular carcinoma

■ **REFERRAL**
To infectious disease specialist and gastroenterologist for consultation regarding fulminant hepatitis or prolonged cholestasis, for cases of uncertain etiology, or for treatment of chronic active hepatitis

☼ PEARLS & CONSIDERATIONS

■ **COMMENTS**
- Virus and HBsAg in high titers in blood for 1 to 7 wk before jaundice and for a variable time thereafter.
- Transmission is possible during entire period of HBsAg (and especially during HBeAg) in serum.
- Universal precautions should be followed for all contacts with blood or secretions/excretions contaminated with blood.
- Preventing before exposure:
  1. Lifestyle changes
  2. Meticulous testing of blood supply (although B some chroni-

cally infected, infectious donors are HBsAg negative)
3. Sterilization via steam or hypochlorite
4. Hepatitis B vaccine for high-risk groups given IM in deltoid to induce HBsAb (response should be confirmed) is protective (>90% effective)
5. Recommendation for universal childhood immunization with doses at birth, 1 mo, and 6 mo

• Prevention after exposure:
1. HBV hyperimmune globulin (HBIG) given immediately after needlestick, within 14 days of sexual exposure, or at birth, followed by HBV vaccination
2. Standard immune globulin: nearly as effective as HBIG
Tables 5-23 and 5-24 describe hepatitis B prophylaxis.

REFERENCES

Maddrey WC: Hepatitis B: an important public health issue, *J Med Virol* 61:362, 2000.

Torresi J, Locarnini S: Antiviral chemotherapy for the treatment of hepatitis B virus infections, *Gastroenterol* 118:S83, 2000.

Weinberg MS et al: Preventing transmission of hepatitis B virus from people with chronic infection, *Am J Prev Med* 20(4):272, 2001.

Author: **Jane V. Eason, MD**

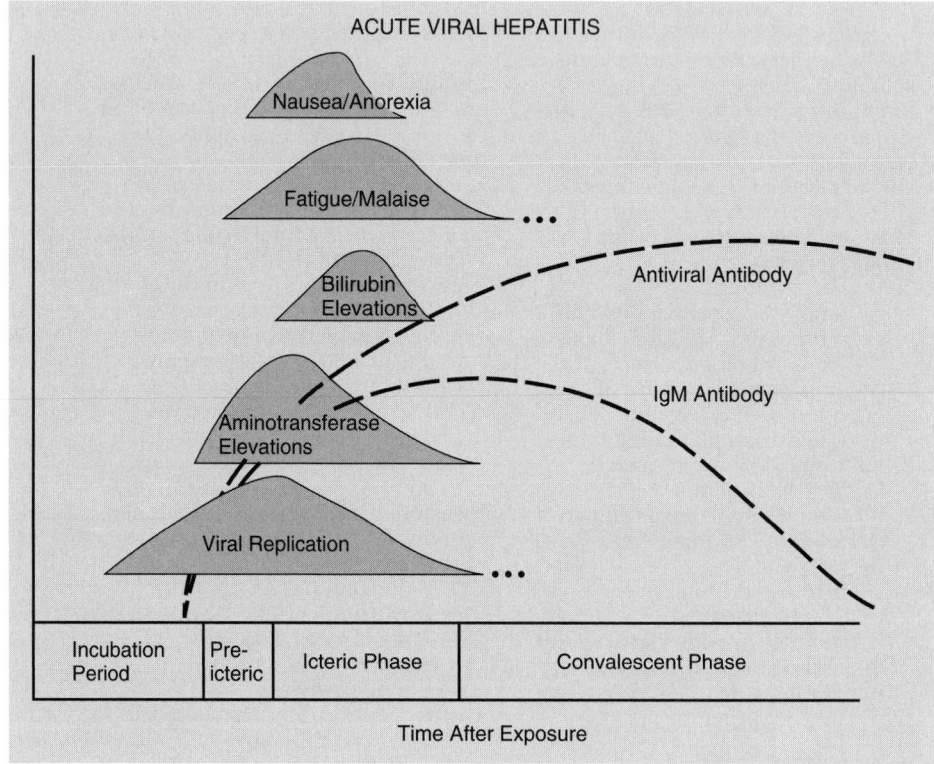

Fig. 1-184 The typical course of acute viral hepatitis. (From Goldman L, Bennett JC [eds]: *Cecil textbook of medicine,* ed 21, Philadelphia, 2000, WB Saunders.)

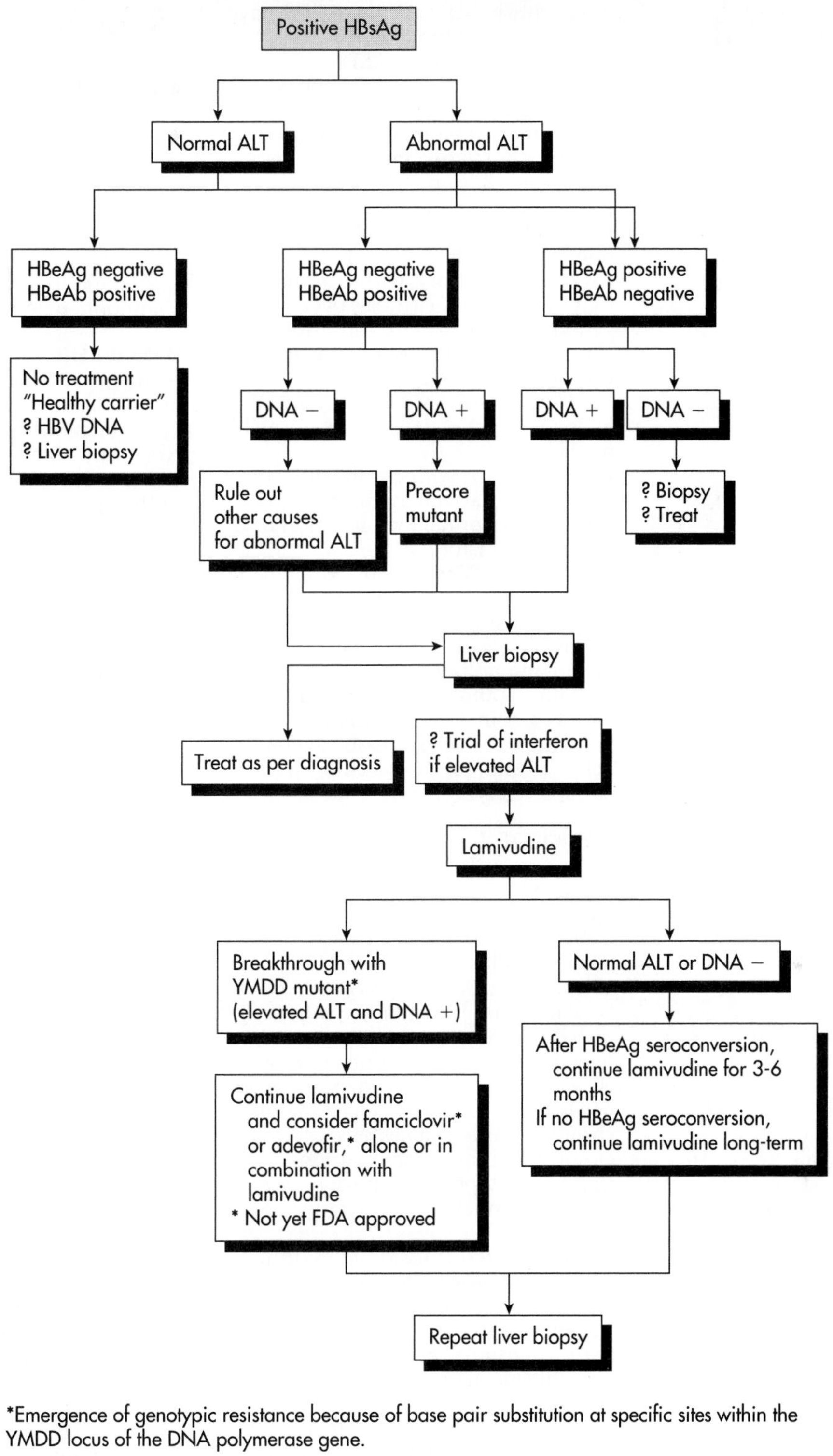

*Emergence of genotypic resistance because of base pair substitution at specific sites within the YMDD locus of the DNA polymerase gene.

Fig. 1-185   The management of patients with chronic hepatitis B virus infection. *ALT,* Alanine aminotransferase; *DNA,* deoxyribonucleic acid; *FDA,* Food and Drug Administration; *HBV,* hepatitis B virus. (From Mandell GL: *Mandell, Douglas, and Bennett's principles and practice of infectious diseases,* ed 5, New York, 2000, Churchill Livingstone.)

BASIC INFORMATION

■ DEFINITION
Hepatitis C is an acute liver parenchymal infection caused by hepatitis C virus (HCV).

■ SYNONYMS
Transfusion-related non-A, non-B hepatitis (incubation period averages 6 wk, intermediate between hepatitis A and B)

ICD-9CM CODES
070.51 Other viral hepatitis

■ EPIDEMIOLOGY & DEMOGRAPHICS
Hepatitis C infection is the most common chronic blood-borne infection in the U.S.
INCIDENCE (IN U.S.)
- 150,000 new cases/year (37,500, symptomatic; 93,000, later chronic liver disease; 30,700, cirrhosis)
- Approximately 9000 of these ultimately die of HCV infection; most common (40%) cause of nonalcoholic liver disease in U.S.
PREVALENCE (IN U.S.):
Overall prevalence of anti-HCV is 1.8% (an estimated 3.9 million persons nationwide)
Highest prevalence in hemophiliacs transfused before 1987 and injecting-drug users, 72% to 90%
Among low risk groups, prevalence 0.6%
PREDOMINANT SEX:
Slight male predominance
PREDOMINANT AGE:
Highest prevalence in 30 to 49 yr age group (65%)
PEAK INCIDENCE:
20 to 39 yr old
African-Americans and whites have similar incidence of acute disease; Hispanics have higher rates.
Prevalence substantially higher among non-Hispanic blacks than among non-Hispanic whites.
GENETICS:
Neonatal infection: Rare. Increased risk with maternal HIV-1 coinfection.

■ PHYSICAL FINDINGS & CLINICAL PRESENTATION
Symptoms usually develop 7 to 8 wk after infection (2 to 26 wk), but 70% to 80% of cases are subclinical.
10% to 20% report acute illness with jaundice and nonspecific symptoms (abdominal pain, anorexia, malaise). Fulminant hepatitis may rarely occur during this period.

After acute infection, 15% to 25% have complete resolution (absence of HCV RNA in serum, normal ALT). Progression to chronic infection is common, 50% to 84%. 74% to 86% have persistent viremia; spontaneous clearance of viremia in chronic infection is rare. 60% to 70% of patients will have persistent or fluctuating ALT levels, 30% to 40% with chronic infection have normal ALT levels.
15% to 20% of those with chronic HCV will develop cirrhosis over a period of 20 to 30 yr; in most others chronic infection leads to hepatitis and varying degrees of fibrosis.
0.4% to 2.5% of patients with chronic infection develop hepatocellular carcinoma.
25% of patients with chronic infection continue to have an asymptomatic course with normal liver function tests and benign histology.
In chronic HCV infection, extrahepatic sequelae include a variety of immunologic and lymphoproliferative disorders (e.g., cryoglobulinemia, membranoproliferative glomerulonephritis, and possibly Sjögren syndrome, autoimmune thyroiditis, polyarteritis nodosa, aplastic anemia, lichen planus, porphyria cutanea tarda, B-cell lymphoma, others).

■ ETIOLOGY
Caused by HCV (single-stranded RNA flavivirus).
Most HCV transmission is parenteral. In the U.S., advances in screening of blood and blood products in 1990 and 1992 have made transfusion-related HCV infection rare (the risk is estimated to be 0.001%/unit transfused). Injecting-drug use accounts for most HCV transmission in the U.S. (60% of newly acquired cases, 20% to 50% of chronically infected persons).
Occupational needlestick exposure from an HCV-positive source has a seroconversion rate of 1.8% (range 0% to 7%).
Nosocomial transmission rates (from surgery and procedures such as colonoscopy, hemodialysis) are extremely low.
Sexual transmission and maternal-fetal transmission are infrequent (estimated at 5%).
No identifiable risk in 40% to 50% of community-acquired HIV infection.
HCV infection may stimulate production of cytotoxic T lymphocytes and cytokines (INF-γ), which likely mediate hepatic necrosis.

DIAGNOSIS

■ DIFFERENTIAL DIAGNOSIS
- Other hepatitis viruses (A, B, D, E)
- Other viral illnesses producing systemic disease (e.g., yellow fever, EBV, CMV, HIV, rubella, rubeolae coxsackie B, adenovirus, HSV, HZV)
- Nonviral hepatitis (e.g., leptospirosis, toxoplasmosis, alcoholic hepatitis, drug-induced hepatitis [acetaminophen, INH], toxic hepatitis)

■ WORKUP
Acute hepatitis C antibody (Fig. 1-186 and Table 1-34)
Liver function tests; CBC
Note: ALT is an easy and inexpensive test to monitor infection and efficacy of therapy. However, ALT levels may fluctuate or even be normal in active or chronic infection and even with cirrhosis, and ALT may remain elevated even after clearance of viremia.
Liver biopsy with histologic staging is the gold standard for assessing the degree of disease activity and the likelihood of disease progression, and also help rule out other causes of liver disease.

■ LABORATORY TESTS
Diagnosis is often by exclusion, because it takes 6 wk to 12 mo to develop anti-HCV antibody (70% positive by 6 wk, 90% positive by 6 mo)
Diagnostic tests include serologic assays for antibodies and molecular tests for viral particles.
1. Enzyme immunoassay is the test for anti-HCV antibody:
   - The current version can detect antibody within 4 to 10 wk after infection
   - False negative rate in low-risk populations is 0.5% to 1%
   - False negatives also in immune-compromised persons, HIV-1, renal failure, HCV-associated essential mixed cryoglobulinemia
   - False positives in autoimmune hepatitis, paraproteinemia, and persons with no risk factors
2. Recombinant immunoblot is used to confirm positive enzyme immunoassays:
   - Recommended only in low-risk settings
3. Qualitative and quantitative HCV RNA tests using PCR:
   - Lower limit of detection is <100 copies HCV RNA/ml
   - Used to confirm viremia and to assess response to treatment

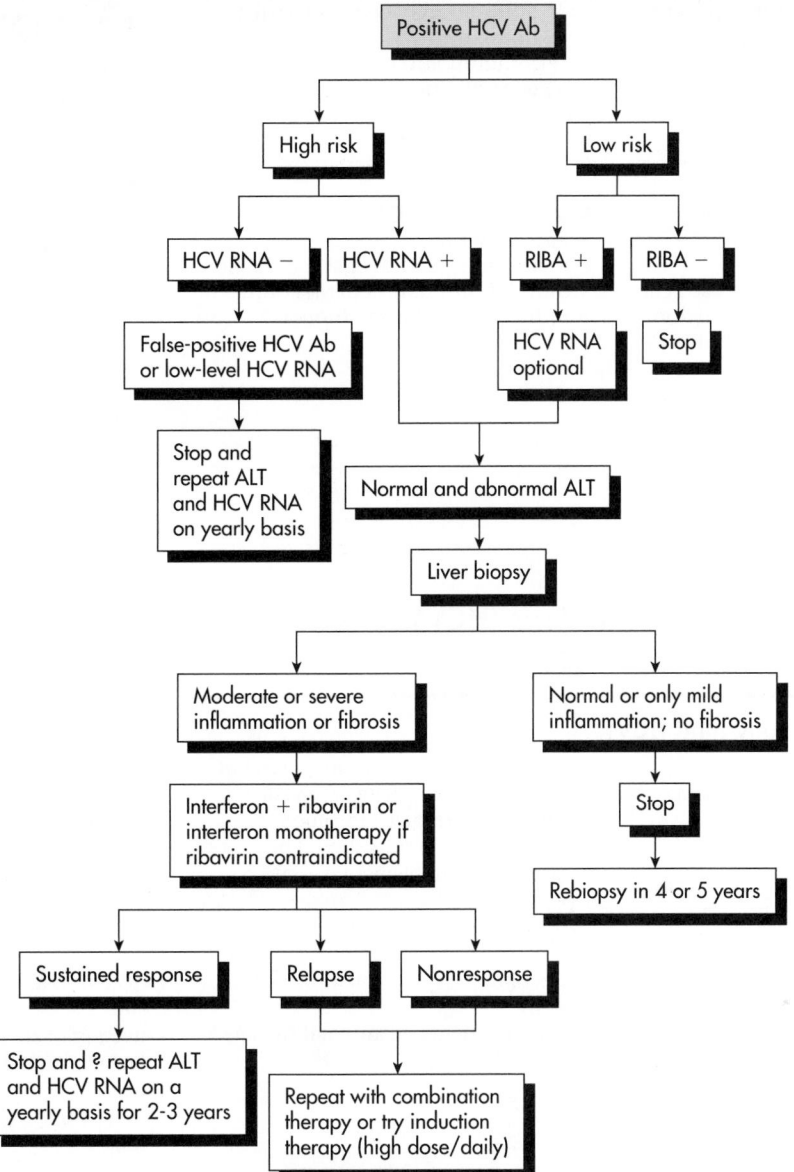

Fig. 1-186   The management of patients with chronic hepatitis C virus infection. *ALT,* Alanine aminotransferase; *HCV,* hepatitis C virus; *RIBA,* recombinant immunoblot assay; *RNA,* ribonucleic acid. (From Mandell GL: *Mandell, Douglas, and Bennett's principles and practice of infectious diseases,* ed 5, New York, 2000, Churchill Livingstone.)

- Qualitative PCR useful in patients with negative enzyme immunoassay in whom infection is suspected
- Quantitative tests use either branched-chain DNA or reverse transcription PCR; the latter is more sensitive
4. Viral genotyping can distinguish between genotypes 1, 2, and 3, which is helpful in choosing therapy; most of these tests use PCR (Note: genotype 1, 2, and 3 predominate in the U.S. and Europe [1 is especially common in North America])
5. Liver function tests:
  - ALT and AST may be elevated to more than eight times normal in acute infection; in chronic infection ALT may be normal or fluctuate

- Bilirubin may be 5 to 10 times normal
- Albumin and prothrombin time generally normal; if abnormal, may be harbinger of impending hepatic necrosis
6. WBC and ESR are generally normal

■ **IMAGING STUDIES**
- Rarely useful
- Sonogram: rapid liver size reduction during fulminant hepatitis or mass in hepatocellular carcinoma

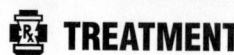 **TREATMENT**

■ **NONPHARMACOLOGIC THERAPY**
Activity and diet as tolerated

■ **ACUTE GENERAL Rx**
Supportive care
Avoid hepatically metabolized drugs

■ **SPECIFIC Rx FOR ACUTE HCV INFECTION**
- Recent studies demonstrate that *early* treatment with IFN-α-2b during acute HCV infection prevents chronic infection. The aim is to decrease viral load early in infection and allow the patient's immune system to control viral replication, thus preventing progression to

TABLE 1-34 Tests for Hepatitis C Virus (HCV) Infection

TEST/TYPE	APPLICATION	COMMENTS
Hepatitis C Virus Antibody (anti-HCV)		
EIA (enzyme immunoassay) Supplemental assay (i.e., recombinant immunoblot assay [RIBA])	Indicates past or present infection but does not differentiate among acute, chronic, or resolved infection All positive EIA results should be verified with a supplemental assay	Sensitivity ≥97% EIA alone has low-positive predictive value in low-prevalence populations
HCV RNA (Hepatitis C Virus Ribonucleic Acid) *Qualitative Tests**†		
Reverse transcriptase polymerase chain reaction (RT-PCR) amplification of HCV RNA by in-house or commercial assays (e.g., Amplicor HCV)	Detect presence of circulating HCV RNA Monitor patients on antiviral therapy	Detect virus as early as 1-2 wk after exposure Detection of HCV RNA during course of infection might be intermittent; a single negative RT-PCR is not conclusive False-positive and false-negative results might occur
Quantitative Tests*†		
RT-PCR amplification of HCV RNA by in-house or commercial assays (e.g., Amplicor HCV Monitor) Branched chain DNA‡ (bDNA) assays (e.g., Quantiplex HCV RNA Assay)	Determine concentration of HCV RNA Might be useful for assessing the likelihood of response to antiviral therapy	Less sensitive than qualitative RT-PCR Should not be used to exclude the diagnosis of HCV infection or to determine treatment endpoint
Genotype*†		
Several methodologies available (e.g., hybridization, sequencing)	Group isolates of HCV based on genetic differences, into 6 genotypes and >90 subtypes With new therapies, length of treatment might vary based on genotype	Genotype 1 (subtypes 1a and 1b) most common in U.S. and associated with lower response to antiviral therapy
Serotype*		
EIA based on immunoreactivity to synthetic peptides (e.g., Murex HCV Serotyping 1-6 Assay)	No clinical utility	Cannot distinguish among subtypes Dual infections often observed

From *MMWR* 47: RR-19, 1998.
*Currently not U.S. Food and Drug Administration approved; lack standardization.
†Samples require special handling (e.g., serum must be separated within 2-4 hours of collection and stored frozen [−20° C or −70° C]; frozen samples should be shipped on dry ice).
‡Deoxyribonucleic acid.

chronic infection. The primary end-point was sustained virologic response, with absence of HCV RNA in serum 24 wk after completion of therapy.

- Further investigations are in progress.

■ CHRONIC Rx

- Response to therapy is influenced by HCV genotype. Patients with genotype 1 rarely respond to interferon alone, and response to combination therapy with interferon and ribavarin is less than for genotypes 2 and 3.
- IFN-α alone or combined with ribavarin have been the mainstays of therapy.
- IFN-α monotherapy for 12 to 18 mo achieves initial response (normalization of transaminases and undetectable HCV RNA) in 40%, but most have relapse after therapy; sustained response in only 6% to 21%; those

with genotype 1 and those with cirrhosis at time of therapy have even lower response rates.

- Combination interferon alpha and ribavarin given thrice weekly has been shown to achieve sustained virologic response in up to 40% of patients. Those with genotype 1 and those with high viral loads required 48 wk of therapy to achieve optimal response (versus 24 wk for those with genotypes 2 and 3 and those with low viral loads).
- 49% of patients who relapse after IFN-α monotherapy have a sustained virologic response to IFN-α and ribavarin combination therapy. In those with contraindications to ribavarin, a more prolonged course of treatment with higher dose IFN-α or PEG-interferon may be an option.
- Both IFN-α and ribavarin have numerous contraindications (absolute and relative) to use and may cause a variety of side effects. IFN-α can

cause flulike symptoms, thrombocytopenia, granulocytopenia, rash, alopecia, anorexia, psychiatric disturbances, others. Ribvarin can cause hemolysis, nausea, anemia, nasal congestion, pruritus.

- In patients who fail to respond to IFN-α or combination therapy with ribavarin, <10% will respond to retreatment.
- Pegylated interferons are IFN-α with an attached polyethylene glycol molecule. The PEG molecule confers a longer half-life and extended therapeutic activity compared with IFN-α, and reduced dosing, once a week.
- Recent treatment trials have shown that pegylated interferon alone achieves higher response rates than does IFN-α alone in patients with chronic hepatitis C without cirrhosis, and in patients with chronic hepatitis C with cirrhosis or bridging fibrosis. Their enhanced efficacy over interferon-alpha may be the result of

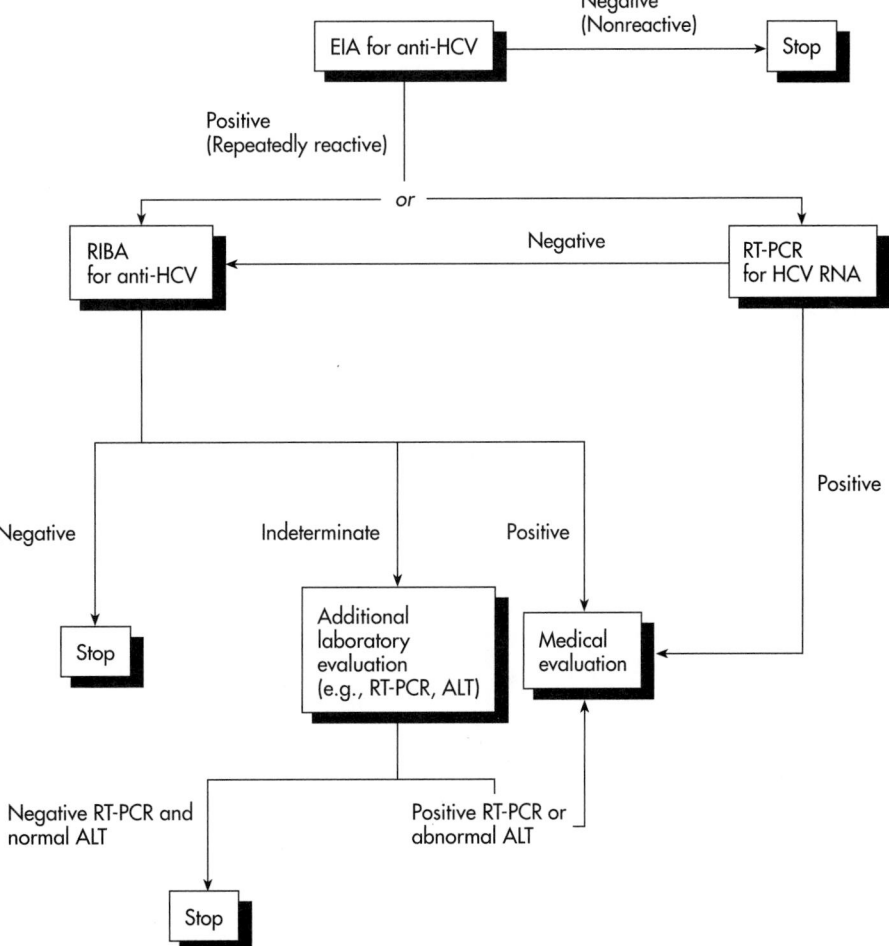

Fig. 1-187   Hepatitis C virus infection testing for asymptomatic persons. *ALT,* Alanine aminotransferase; *Anti-HCV,* antibody to HCV; *EIA,* enzyme immunoassay; *HCV,* hepatitis C virus; *RIBA,* recombinant immunoblot assay; *RT-PCR,* reverse transcriptase polymerase chain reaction. (From *MMWR:* 47: RR-19, 1998.)

a more vigorous immune response (e.g., increased hepatitis C-specific T-helper-1 response).

- Pegylated interferons can be used in the treatment of persons who cannot be treated with ribavarin.
- Optimal regimens with pegylated interferons have yet to be determined; currently trials are underway using pegylated interferon in combination with ribavarin.

LIVER TRANSPLANTATION:
- Hepatitis C is the main indication for liver transplantation in the U.S.
- It is the only option for patients with deteriorating HCV-related cirrhosis and for some patients with hepatocellular carcinoma.
- Recurrent infection occurs in almost all patients with progressive fibrosis and cirrhosis; up to 20% progress to cirrhosis within 5 yr posttransplant.

CO-INFECTION WITH HIV:
- These patients have a poor response to IFN-α alone.
- Consider initiating therapy for HCV before starting antiretrovirals, because immune reconstitution syndrome occurring with initiation of antiretrovirals may exacerbate HCV-related hepatitis.

■ DISPOSITION
- Follow-up as outpatient
- Monitor ALT levels as a clue for chronic disease
- Chronic carrier state, cirrhosis, hepatic carcinoma more common than with hepatitis A and B

☼ PEARLS & CONSIDERATIONS

- More rapid progression of disease in persons who drink alcohol regularly, persons of advanced age at time of infection, and those coinfected with other viruses (HIV, hepatitis B).
- No preventive vaccine available; post-exposure immune globulin may provide minimal protection.
- Preventive measures include use of universal precautions, careful screening of blood and blood products, lifestyle changes.

REFERENCES

Germer HH, Zein NN: Advances in the molecular diagnosis of hepatitis C and their implications, *Mayo Clin Proc* 76:911, 2001.

Jaeckel E et al: Treatment of acute hepatitis C with interferon alfa-2b, *N Engl J Med* 345(20):1452, 2001.

Lauer GM, Walker BD: Hepatitis C virus infection, *N Engl J Med* 345(1):41, 2001.

Author: **Jane V. Eason, M.D.**

BASIC INFORMATION

■ DEFINITION
Hepatocellular carcinoma is a malignant tumor of the liver, arising from hepatocytes.

■ ICD-9CM CODES
155.0 Hepatocellular carcinoma

■ SYNONYMS
Hepatoma

■ EPIDEMIOLOGY & DEMOGRAPHICS
Incidence of hepatocellular carcinoma varies widely in parts of the world:
- Areas with high rates of hepatitis B and hepatitis C (Asia, sub-Saharan Africa) have correspondingly high rates of hepatocellular carcinoma.
- Males are affected more commonly than females.
- Peak incidence is in fifth and sixth decades in Western countries, earlier in areas with perinatal transmission of hepatitis B.

■ RISK FACTORS
- Chronic liver disease
- Cirrhosis
- Chronic hepatitis B or C infection
- Hepatotoxins including alcohol, mycotoxins (aflatoxin B_1), high-dose anabolic steroids, vinyl chloride, possibly estrogen
- Systemic diseases affecting the liver such as alpha-1 antitrypsin deficiency, hemochromatosis, tyrosinemia

■ PHYSICAL FINDINGS & CLINICAL PRESENTATION
- One third of patients are asymptomatic.
- Signs of underlying cirrhosis are often present (e.g., weight loss, ascites).

DIAGNOSIS

■ DIFFERENTIAL DIAGNOSIS
- Metastatic tumor to liver
- Benign liver tumors such as adenomas, focal nodular hyperplasia, hemangiomas
- Focal fatty infiltration

■ WORKUP
- History with regard to above risk factors
- Physical examination with attention to signs of chronic liver disease
- Laboratory evaluation and imaging

■ LABORATORY TESTS
- Liver function tests.
- Elevated alpha-fetoprotein in 70% of patients.
- Paraneoplastic syndromes associated with hepatocellular carcinoma may cause abnormalities such as hypercalcemia, hypoglycemia, and polycythemia.

■ IMAGING STUDIES
Ultrasound, CT scan, or MRI (Fig. 1-188)

■ BIOPSY
Percutaneous biopsy under ultrasound or CT scan usually is diagnostic.

■ SCREENING
Screening high-risk patients with ultrasound and alpha-fetoprotein may identify hepatocellular carcinoma at an early stage.

TREATMENT

- Depends on size of lesion and severity of underlying liver disease.
- For patients with small solitary lesions less than 5 cm, good liver function, and no portal hypertension, surgical resection is the best option.
- For patients who are not candidates for surgical resection, percutaneous ethanol injection, transcatheter arterial chemotherapy with or without embolization of the tumor, or ultrasound-guided cryoablation can be used for local tumor control.
- Patients with advanced cirrhosis and small tumors should be considered for liver transplantation.

■ DISPOSITION
- For unresectable tumors, prognosis is poor.
- Five-year survival following surgical resection is 20% to 30%.

■ REFERRAL
For treatment planning

PEARLS & CONSIDERATIONS

Prevention:
- Hepatitis B vaccination
- Eliminate aflatoxin contamination of food
- Decrease alcohol consumption
- Identify and treat hemochromatosis
- Interferon therapy in patients with hepatitis C reduces the risk of hepatocellular carcinoma.

REFERENCES
Mor E et al: Treatment of hepatocellular carcinoma associated with cirrhosis in the era of liver transplantation, *Ann Intern Med* 129:643, 1998.

Yoshida H et al: Interferon therapy reduces the risk of hepatocellular carcinoma. National Surveillance program of cirrhotic and noncirrhotic patients with chronic hepatitis C in Japan, *Ann Intern Med* 131:174, 1999.
Author: **Mark J. Fagan, M.D.**

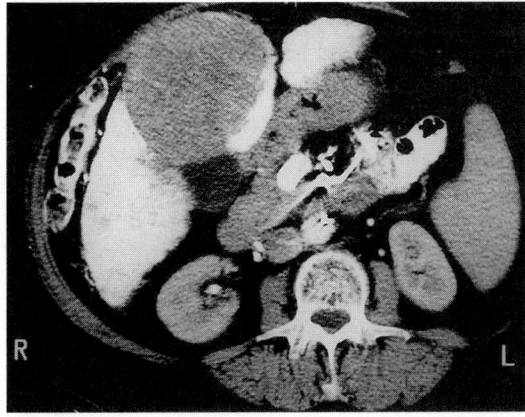 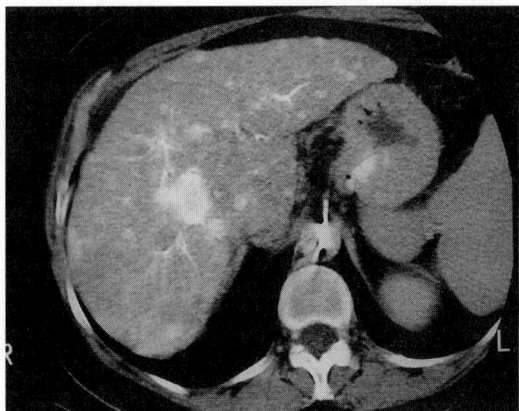

Fig. 1-188   **A,** CT scan through the lower portion of the liver obtained during the portal venous phase shows a single large hypodense lesion. Percutaneous biopsy confirmed a hepatoma. **B,** CT scan through the cranial portion of the liver during the arterial phase demonstrates multiple additional hypervascular lesions, suggesting an unresectable, multicentric hepatoma. (From Goldman L, Bennett JC [eds]: *Cecil textbook of medicine,* ed 21, Philadelphia, 2000, WB Saunders.)

 BASIC INFORMATION

■ **DEFINITION**
Hepatorenal syndrome (HRS) is a condition of intense renal vasoconstriction resulting from loss of renal autoregulation occurring as a complication of severe liver disease.

■ **SYNONYMS**
Hepatic nephropathy
Oliguric renal failure of cirrhosis
HRS

ICD-9CM CODES
572.4 Hepatorenal syndrome

■ **EPIDEMIOLOGY & DEMOGRAPHICS**
The probability of HRS in patients with cirrhosis is 18% at 1 yr, and 39% at 5 yr.

■ **PHYSICAL FINDINGS & CLINICAL PRESENTATION**
• Evidence of cirrhosis is usually present: jaundice, spider angiomas, splenomegaly, ascites, fetor hepaticus, pedal edema
• Hepatic encephalopathy: flapping tremor (asterixis), coma
• Tachycardia and bounding pulse
• Oliguria

■ **ETIOLOGY**
An exacerbation of end-stage liver disease, HRS may occur after significant reduction of effective blood volume (e.g., paracentesis, GI bleeding, diuretics) or in the absence of any precipitating factors.

 DIAGNOSIS

■ **DIFFERENTIAL DIAGNOSIS**
• Prerenal azotemia: response to sustained plasma expansion is good (prompt diuresis with volume expansion).
• Acute tubular necrosis: urinary sodium >30, FeNa >1.5%, urinary/plasma creatinine ratio <30, urine/plasma osmolality ratio = 1, urine sediment reveals casts and cellular debris, there is no significant response to sustained plasma expansion.

■ **WORKUP**
Patients with acute azotemia and oliguria in the setting of liver disease should undergo laboratory evaluation to differentiate HRS from acute tubular necrosis and volume challenge to differentiate HRS from prerenal azotemia if FeNa <1%.

■ **LABORATORY TESTS**
• Obtain serum electrolytes, BUN, creatinine, osmolality, urinalysis, urinary sodium, urinary creatinine, urine osmolality.
• Calculate fractional excretion of sodium (FeNa) (see "Clinical Formulas" in Section V).
• In HRS: urinary sodium <10 mEq/L, FeNa <1%, urinary plasma creatinine ratio >30, urinary-plasma osmolality ratio >1.5, urine sediment is unremarkable.

■ **IMAGING STUDIES**
Renal ultrasound may be indicated if renal obstruction is suspected.

 TREATMENT

■ **NONPHARMACOLOGIC THERAPY**
Avoidance of precipitating factors

■ **ACUTE GENERAL Rx**
• Volume challenge (to increase mean arterial pressure) followed by large-volume paracentesis (to increase cardiac output and decrease renal venous pressure) is recommended to distinguish HRS from prerenal azotemia in patients with FeNa <1%. In patients with prerenal azotemia, the increase in renal perfusion pressure and renal blood flow will result in prompt diuresis; the volume challenge can be accomplished by giving a solution of 100 g of albumin in 500 ml of isotonic saline.
• The only effective treatment of HRS is liver transplantation; low-dose dopamine or ornipressin is used in some liver units to avoid further deterioration of renal function in patients awaiting liver transplantation.

■ **DISPOSITION**
Mortality rate exceeds 80%; liver transplantation is the only curative treatment.

■ **REFERRAL**
Referral for liver transplantation when indicated (see below)

PEARLS & CONSIDERATIONS

■ **COMMENTS**
Liver transplantation may be indicated in otherwise healthy patients (age preferably <65 yr) with sclerosing cholangitis, chronic hepatitis with cirrhosis, or primary biliary cirrhosis; contraindications to liver transplantation are AIDS, most metastatic malignancies, active substance abuse, uncontrolled sepsis, uncontrolled cardiac or pulmonary disease.
Author: **Fred F. Ferri, M.D.**

BASIC INFORMATION

■ DEFINITION
Herpangina is a self-limited upper respiratory tract infection associated with a characteristic vesicular rash on the soft palate.

ICD-9CM CODES
074.0 Herpangina

■ EPIDEMIOLOGY & DEMOGRAPHICS
INCIDENCE (IN U.S.): Unknown
PREVALENCE (IN U.S.): Unknown
PREDOMINANT SEX: Male = female
PREDOMINANT AGE: 3 to 10 yr
PEAK INCIDENCE: Summer outbreaks common

■ PHYSICAL FINDINGS & CLINICAL PRESENTATION
- Characterized by ulcerating lesions typically located on the soft palate (Fig. 1-189)
- Usually fewer than six lesions that evolve rapidly from a diffuse pharyngitis to erythematous macules and subsequently to vesicles that are moderately painful
- Fever, vomiting, and headache in the first few days of illness but subsiding spontaneously
- Pharyngeal lesions typical for several more days

■ ETIOLOGY
- Most caused by coxsackie A viruses (A2, A4, A5, A6, A10)
- Occasional cases caused by other viruses

DIAGNOSIS

■ DIFFERENTIAL DIAGNOSIS
- Herpes simplex
- Bacterial pharyngitis
- Tonsillitis
- Aphthous stomatitis
- Hand-foot-mouth disease

■ WORKUP
Diagnosis is typically based on characteristic lesions on the soft palate.

■ LABORATORY TESTS
Viral and bacterial cultures of the pharynx to exclude herpes simplex infection and streptococcal pharyngitis if the diagnosis is in doubt

TREATMENT

- Symptomatic treatment for sore throat
- No antiviral therapy indicated

■ NONPHARMACOLOGIC THERAPY
Analgesic throat lozenges are helpful in some cases.

■ ACUTE GENERAL Rx
Antipyretics when indicated

■ CHRONIC Rx
Self-limited infection

■ DISPOSITION
- Generally, resolution of symptoms within 1 wk
- Persistence of fever or mouth lesions beyond 1 wk suggestive of an alternative diagnosis (see "Differential Diagnosis")

■ REFERRAL
For consultation with otolaryngologist or infectious disease specialist if the diagnosis is in doubt

PEARLS & CONSIDERATIONS

■ COMMENTS
Household outbreaks may occur, especially during the summer months.

REFERENCE
Ho M, Chen ER et al: An epidemic of enterovirus 71 infection in Taiwan: Taiwan Enterovirus Epidemic Working Group, *N Engl J Med* 341(13):929, 1999.
Author: **Joseph R. Masci, M.D.**

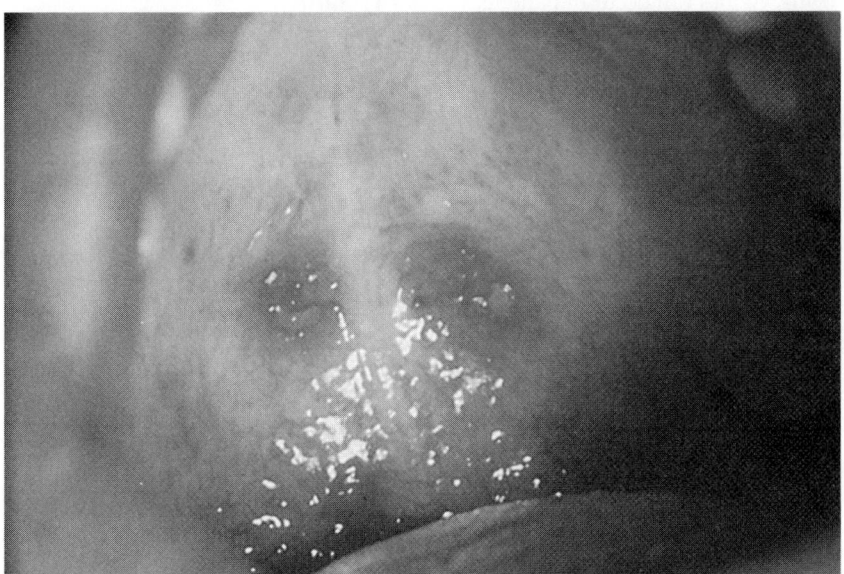

Fig. 1-189   Herpangina with shallow ulcers in the roof of the mouth. (Courtesy Marshall Guill, M.D. From Goldstein B [ed]: *Practical dermatology,* ed 2, St Louis, 1997, Mosby.)

BASIC INFORMATION

■ DEFINITION

Herpes simplex is a viral infection caused by the herpes simplex virus (HSV); HSV-1 is associated primarily with oral infections, whereas HSV-2 causes mainly genital infections; however, each type can infect any site; following the primary infection, the virus enters the nerve endings in the skin directly below the lesions and ascends to the dorsal root ganglia where it remains in a latent stage until it is reactivated.

■ SYNONYMS

Genital herpes
Herpes labialis
Herpes gladiatorum
Herpes digitalis

ICD-9CM CODES

054.10 Genital herpes
054.9 Herpes labialis

■ EPIDEMIOLOGY & DEMOGRAPHICS

- More than 85% of adults have serologic evidence of HSV-1 infection. The seroprevalence of adults with HSV-2 in the United States is 25%; however, only about 20% of these persons recall having symptoms of HSV infection.
- Most cases of eye or digital herpetic infections are caused by HSV-1.
- Frequency of recurrence of HSV-2 genital herpes is higher than HSV-1 oral labial infection.
- The frequency of recurrence is lowest for oral labial HSV-2 infections.
- The incidence of complications from herpes simplex (e.g., herpes encephalitis) is highest in immunocompromised hosts.

■ PHYSICAL FINDINGS

PRIMARY INFECTION:
- Symptoms occur from 3 to 7 days after contact (respiratory droplets, direct contact).
- Constitutional symptoms include low-grade fever, headache and myalgias, regional lymphadenopathy, and localized pain.
- Pain, burning, itching, and tingling last several hours.
- Grouped vesicles (Fig. 1-190) usually with surrounding erythema appear and generally ulcerate or crust within 48 hr.
- The vesicles are uniform in size (differentiating it from herpes zoster vesicles, which vary in size).
- During the acute eruption the patient is uncomfortable; involve-

ment of lips and inside of mouth may make it unpleasant for the patient to eat; urinary retention may complicate involvement of the genital area.
- Lesions generally last from 2 to 6 wk and heal without scarring.

RECURRENT INFECTION:
- Generally caused by alteration in the immune system; fatigue, stress, menses, local skin trauma, and exposure to sunlight are contributing factors.
- The prodromal symptoms (fatigue, burning and tingling of the affected area) last 12 to 24 hr.
- A cluster of lesions generally evolve within 24 hr from a macule to a papule and then vesicles surrounded by erythema; the vesicles coalesce and subsequently rupture within 4 days, revealing erosions covered by crusts.
- The crusts are generally shed within 7 to 10 days, revealing a pink surface.
- The most frequent location of the lesions is on the vermilion border of the lips (HSV-1), the penile shaft or glans penis and the labia (HSV-2), buttocks (seen more frequently in women), fingertips (herpetic whitlow), and trunk (may be confused with herpes zoster).
- Rapid onset of diffuse cutaneous herpes simplex (eczema herpeticum) may occur in certain atopic infants and adults. It is a medical emergency, especially in young infants, and should be promptly treated with acyclovir.
- Herpes encephalitis, meningitis, and ocular herpes can occur in patients with immunocompromised status and occasionally in normal hosts.

■ ETIOLOGY

HSV-1 and HSV-2 are both DNA viruses.

🔬 DIAGNOSIS

■ DIFFERENTIAL DIAGNOSIS

- Impetigo
- Behçet's syndrome
- Coxsackie virus infection
- Syphilis
- Stevens-Johnson syndrome
- Herpangina
- Aphthous stomatitis
- Varicella
- Herpes zoster

■ WORKUP

Diagnosis is based on clinical presentation. Laboratory evaluation will confirm diagnosis.

■ LABORATORY TESTS

- Direct immunofluorescent antibody slide tests will provide a rapid diagnosis.
- Viral culture is the most definitive method for diagnosis; results are generally available in 1 or 2 days; the lesions should be sampled during the vesicular or early ulcerative stage; cervical samples should be taken from the endocervix with a swab.
- Tzanck smear is a readily available test; it will demonstrate multinucleated giant cells. However, it is not a very sensitive test.
- Pap smear will detect HSV-infected cells in cervical tissue from women without symptoms.
- Serologic tests for HSV: IgG and IgM serum antibodies. Antibodies to HSV occur in 50% to 90% of adults. Routine tests do not discriminate between antibodies that are HSV-1 and HSV-2; the presence of IgM or a fourfold or greater rise in IgG titers indicates a recent infection (convalescent sample should be drawn 2 to 3 wk after the acute specimen is drawn).

💊 TREATMENT

■ NONPHARMACOLOGIC THERAPY

Application of topical cool compresses with Burow's solution for 15 min four to six times daily may be soothing in patients with extensive erosions on the vulva and penis (decrease edema and inflammation, debridement of crusts and purulent material).

■ ACUTE GENERAL Rx

- Acyclovir ointment (Zovirax) applied using finger-cot or rubber glove q3-6h (six times daily) for 7 days may be useful for the first clinical episode of genital herpes. Severe primary genital infections may be treated with IV acyclovir (5 mg/kg infused at a constant rate over 1 hr q8h for 7 days in patients with normal renal function) or oral acyclovir 200 mg five times daily for 7 to 10 days.

- Valacyclovir caplets (Valtrex) can also be used for the initial episode of genital herpes (1 g bid for 10 days).
- Acyclovir is not approved for primary or recurrent herpes labialis; however, it is frequently used for this purpose by many physicians.
- Penciclovir 1% cream (Denavir) can be used for recurrent herpes labialis on the lips and face. It should be applied q2h while awake for 4 days. Treatment should be started at the earliest sign or symptom.
- Docosanol 10% cream (Abreva), a long-chain saturated alcohol, inhibits fusion between the plasma membrane and the viral envelope, blocking viral entry and subsequent replication. It is available over the counter and, when applied at the first sign of recurrence of herpes labialis, may shorten the durations of the episode.

■ CHRONIC Rx

- Recurrent episodes of genital herpes can be treated with acyclovir (200 mg PO five times a day for 5 days, 400 mg PO tid for 5 days, or 800 mg PO bid for 5 days, generally started during the prodrome or within 2 days of onset of lesions; famciclovir (Famvir) is also useful for treatment of recurrent genital herpes (dose is 125 mg q12h for 5 days in patients with normal renal function) started at the first sign of symptoms, or valacyclovir (Valtrex) (dose is 500 mg q12h for 5 days in patients with normal renal function).

- Acyclovir-resistant mucocutaneous lesions in patients with HIV can be treated with foscarnet (40 to 60 mg/kg IV q8h in patients with normal renal function); HPMPC has also been reported to be effective in HSV infections resistant to acyclovir or foscarnet.
- Patients with ≥6 recurrences of genital herpes/year can be treated with valacyclovir 1 g qd, acyclovir 400 mg bid, or famciclovir 250 mg bid.

■ DISPOSITION
Most patients recover from the initial episode or recurrences without complications; immunocompromised hosts are at risk for complications (e.g., disseminated herpes simplex infection, herpes encephalitis).

■ REFERRAL
Hospital admission in patients with herpes encephalitis, herpes meningitis, and in immunocompromised hosts with diffuse herpes simplex infection Ophthalmology referral in patients with suspected ocular herpes

☼ PEARLS & CONSIDERATIONS

■ COMMENTS
- Provide patient education regarding transmission of HSV.
- Condom use offers significant protection against HSV-1 infection in susceptive women.
- Patients should be instructed on the use of condoms for sexual inter-

course and on avoiding kissing or sexual intercourse until lesions are crusted.
- Patients should also avoid contact with immunocompromised hosts or neonates while lesions are present.
- Proper hand-washing techniques should be explained.
- Patients with herpes gladiatorum (cutaneous herpes in athletes involved in contact sports) should be excluded from participation in active sports until lesions have resolved.
- For additional information on genital herpes simplex, refer to "Herpes Simplex, Genital" in Section I.
- Many new HSV-2 infections are asymptomatic, but new symptoms may result from old infections.

REFERENCES
Emmert D: Treatment of common cutaneous herpes simplex infections, *Am Fam Physician* 61:1697, 2000.
Langenberg AGM et al: A prospective study of new infections with herpes simplex virus type 1 and type 2, *N Engl J Med* 341:432, 1999.
Wald A: Effect of condoms on reducing the transmission of herpes simplex virus type 2 from men and women, *JAMA* 285:3100, 2001.
Author: **Fred F. Ferri, M.D.**

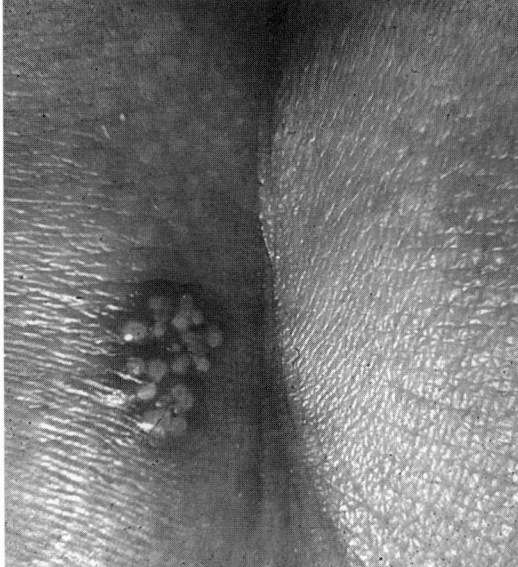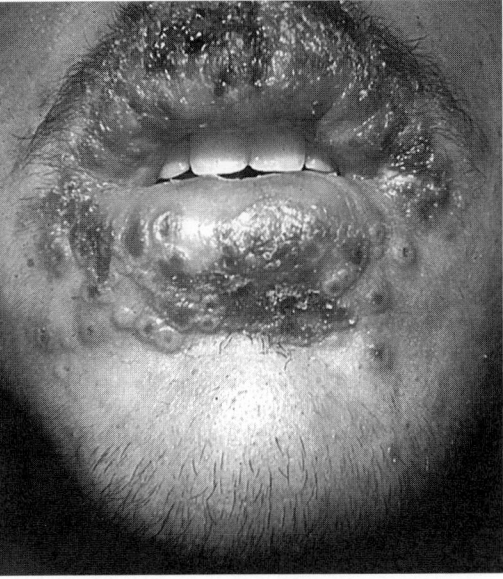

Fig. 1-190 Herpes simplex. (From Scuderi G [ed]: *Sports medicine: principles of primary care,* St Louis, 1997, Mosby.)

BASIC INFORMATION

■ DEFINITION
Herpes simplex infection is a sexually transmitted disease caused by a double-stranded DNA virus. Two forms of infection exist: HSV-1, or oral herpes (15% of genital cases), and HSV-2, or genital herpes.

ICD-9CM CODES
054.10 Genital herpes

■ EPIDEMIOLOGY & DEMOGRAPHICS
INCIDENCE:
- 1% to 2%, with 500,000 new cases/yr
- Antibodies to HSV-1 or HSV-2 in up to 80% of adults

RISK FACTORS:
- Promiscuity
- Highest frequency in 15- to 29-yr-old population
- Associated with other sexually transmitted diseases, such as syphilis, gonorrhea, or chlamydia

GENETICS: No associated genetic predisposition

■ PHYSICAL FINDINGS & CLINICAL PRESENTATION
Three separate syndromes, as follows:
- First episode primary:
  1. No antibodies to HSV-1 or HSV-2
  2. Severe local symptoms such as painful bilateral genital ulcers or vesicles, inguinal adenopathy
  3. Constitutional findings of fever, malaise, myalgia
  4. Lesions persisting >16 days, with extragenital symptoms on fingers, buttock, or mouth
- First episode nonprimary:
  1. Presence of antibodies to HSV-1 and HSV-2
  2. Milder clinical course with symptoms similar to those of recurrent disease
- Recurrent herpes:
  1. Shorter duration (5 to 10 days)
  2. Mild symptoms
  3. Unilateral distribution
  4. Few systemic symptoms
  5. Prodrome of itching or burning before lesions appear

■ ETIOLOGY
Double-stranded DNA virus with a lytic as well as a latent phase

DIAGNOSIS

- Classic appearance of vesicles or ulcers in various stages of development
- Clinical history of recurrent prodromal symptoms and recurrences

■ DIFFERENTIAL DIAGNOSIS
- Human papillomavirus
- Molluscum contagiosum
- HIV infection
- Fungal infections *(Candida)*
- Bacterial infections (syphilis, chancroid, granuloma inguinale)
- Follicular abscess
- Hidradenitis suppurativa
- Vulvar dystrophies
- Cancer of the vulva

Table 2-84 describes the differential diagnosis of genital sores.

■ WORKUP
- Clinical history, including a thorough search for other sexually transmitted diseases
- Complete physical examination, including culture of suspected sites
- Possibly antibody screening

■ LABORATORY TESTS
- Viral culture
  1. Gold standard
  2. Requires 48 to 72 hr in most cases, with a higher chance of a positive culture with more viral load (first episode or early vesicular lesions)
  3. Disease not excluded by a negative culture result
- Tzanck smear
  1. Low sensitivity
  2. Tests for presence of intranuclear inclusions or giant cells
- Immunoperoxidase stains
- Monoclonal antibody, ELISA

TREATMENT

■ NONPHARMACOLOGIC THERAPY
- Exposure of affected areas to dry environment, avoiding contact of early vesicles with noninfected tissue
- Avoidance of intercourse during outbreak or with prodromal symptoms, with consideration of condom use if there are frequent recurrent episodes

■ ACUTE GENERAL Rx
- First clinical episode: acyclovir 200 mg PO × 5 for 7 to 10 days or until resolution of symptoms

- Recurrent disease:
  1. Course of recurrence shortened if treatment begun during prodromal phase or within initial phase of disease
  2. Acyclovir 200 mg PO × 5 for 5 days, 400 mg × 3 for 5 days, or 800 mg PO × 2 for 5 days
- Severe disease (encephalitis, pneumonia, or hepatitis):
  1. Requires intravenous treatment
  2. Acyclovir 5 to 10 mg/kg q8h for 7 days

■ CHRONIC Rx
Suppressive therapy:
- Indicated for patients with >6 recurrences per year
- Acyclovir 400 mg PO bid, valacyclovir 500 mg qd, or famciclovir 250 mg bid
- Reevaluation after 1 yr of therapy to assess for continued suppression
- May reduce frequency of recurrences by 75%

■ DISPOSITION
Most cases responsive to initial therapy with acyclovir, but for those with recurrences, suppressive treatment (noted above) is indicated.

■ REFERRAL
To infectious disease specialist or obstetrician for patients with life-threatening diseases or who are pregnant, especially in third trimester

PEARLS & CONSIDERATIONS

■ COMMENTS
HSV infection during pregnancy requires consideration of fetus as well as mother:
- Culture of any lesion suspicious for herpes should be performed.
- If active disease is suspected at the time of delivery, C-section may be indicated to decrease chance of neonatal infection.

REFERENCES
Baker DA et al: Once-daily valcyclovir for suppression of recurrent genital herpes, *Obstet Gynecol* 94:103, 1999.

Dinz-Mitoma F et al: Oral famciclovir for the suppression of recurrent genital herpes, *JAMA* 280:887, 1998.

Author: **Scott J. Zuccala, D.O.**

BASIC INFORMATION

DEFINITION
Herpes zoster is a disease caused by reactivation of the varicella-zoster virus. Following the primary infection (chickenpox) the virus becomes latent in the dorsal root ganglia and re-emerges when there is a weakening of the immune system (secondary to disease or advanced age).

SYNONYMS
Shingles

ICD-9CM CODES
053.9 Herpes zoster

EPIDEMIOLOGY & DEMOGRAPHICS
- Herpes zoster occurs during lifetime in 10% to 20% of the population.
- There is an increased incidence in immunocompromised patients (AIDS, malignancy), the elderly, and children who acquired chickenpox when younger than 2 mo.

PHYSICAL FINDINGS & CLINICAL PRESENTATION
- Pain generally precedes skin manifestation by 3 to 5 days and is generally localized to the dermatome that will be affected by the skin lesions.
- Constitutional symptoms are often present (malaise, fever, headache).
- The initial rash consists of erythematous maculopapules generally affecting one dermatome (thoracic region in majority of cases); some patients (<50%) may have scattered vesicles outside of the affected dermatome.
- The initial maculopapules evolve into vesicles and pustules by the third or the fourth day.
- The vesicles have an erythematous base, are cloudy, and have various sizes (a distinguishing characteristic from herpes simplex in which the vesicles are of uniform size).
- The vesicles subsequently become umbilicated and then form crusts that generally fall off within 3 wk; scarring may occur.
- Pain during and after the rash is generally significant.
- Secondary bacterial infection with *Staphylococcus aureus* or *Streptococcus pyogenes* may occur.
- Regional lymphadenopathy may occur.
- Herpes zoster may involve the trigeminal nerve (most frequent cranial nerve involved); involvement of the geniculate ganglion can cause facial palsy and a painful ear, with the presence of vesicles on the pinna and external auditory canal (Ramsay Hunt syndrome).

ETIOLOGY
Reactivation of varicella virus (human herpesvirus III)

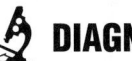

DIAGNOSIS

DIFFERENTIAL DIAGNOSIS
- Rash: herpes simplex and other viral infections
- Pain from herpes zoster: may be confused with acute myocardial infarction, pulmonary embolism, pleuritis, pericarditis, renal colic

LABORATORY TESTS
Laboratory tests are generally not necessary (viral cultures and Tzanck smear will confirm diagnosis in patients with atypical presentation).

TREATMENT

NONPHARMACOLOGIC THERAPY
- Wet compresses (using Burow's solution or cool tap water) applied for 15 to 30 min 5 to 10 times a day are useful to break vesicles and remove serum and crust.
- Care must be taken to prevent any secondary bacterial infection.

ACUTE GENERAL Rx
- Suppression of pain: an approach to herpetic and postherpetic neuralgia is described in Fig. 1-191. Gabapentin 300 to 1200 mg qd is effective in the treatment of pain and sleep interference associated with postherpetic neuralgia.
- Lidocaine patch 5% (Lidoderm) is also effective in relieving postherpetic neuralgia. Patches are applied to intact skin to cover the most painful area for up to 12 hr within a 24-hr period.
- Oral antiviral agents can decrease acute pain, inflammation, and vesicle formation when treatment is begun within 48 hr of onset of rash. Treatment options are:
  1. Acyclovir (Zovirax) 800 mg ×5 for 7 days
  2. Valacyclovir (Valtrex) 1000 mg tid for 7 days
  3. Famciclovir (Famvir) 500 mg tid for 7 days
- Immunocompromised patients should be treated with IV acyclovir 500 mg/m^2 or 10 mg/kg q8h in 1-hr infusions for 7 days, with close monitoring of renal function and adequate hydration; vidarabine (continuous 12-hr infusion of 10 mg/kg/day for 7 days) is also effective for treatment of disseminated herpes zoster in immunocompromised hosts.
- Patients with AIDS and transplant patients may develop acyclovir-resistant varicella-zoster; these patients can be treated with foscarnet (40 mg/kg IV q8h) continued for at least 10 days or until lesions are completely healed.
- Capsaicin cream (Zostrix) can be useful for treatment of postherpetic neuralgia. It is generally applied three to five times daily for several weeks.
- Sympathetic blocks (stellate ganglion or epidural) with 0.25% bupivacaine and rhizotomy are reserved for severe cases unresponsive to conservative treatment.
- Corticosteroids should be considered in older patients if there are no contraindications. Initial dose is prednisone 60 mg/day tapered over a period of 21 days.

DISPOSITION
- The incidence of postherpetic neuralgia increases with age (30% by age 40 yr, >70% by age 70 yr); antivirals reduce the risk of postherpetic neuralgia.
- Incidence of disseminated herpes zoster is increased in immunocompromised hosts (e.g., 15% to 50% of patients with active Hodgkin's disease).
- Immunocompromised hosts are also more prone to neurologic complications (mortality rate is 10% to 20% in immunocompromised hosts with disseminated zoster).
- Motor neuropathies occur in 5% of all cases of zoster; complete recovery occurs in >70% of patients.

REFERRAL
- Hospitalization for IV acyclovir in patients with disseminated herpes zoster
- Surgical referral for rhizotomy in patients with severe pain unresponsive to conventional treatment
- Sympathetic blocks in selected patients

REFERENCES
Helgason S et al: Prevalence of postherpetic neuralgia after a first episode of herpes zoster: prospective study with long term follow up, *BMJ* 321:794, 2000.
Rowbotham M et al: Gabapentin for the treatment of post-herpetic neuralgia, *JAMA* 280:1837, 1998.
Author: **Fred F. Ferri, M.D.**

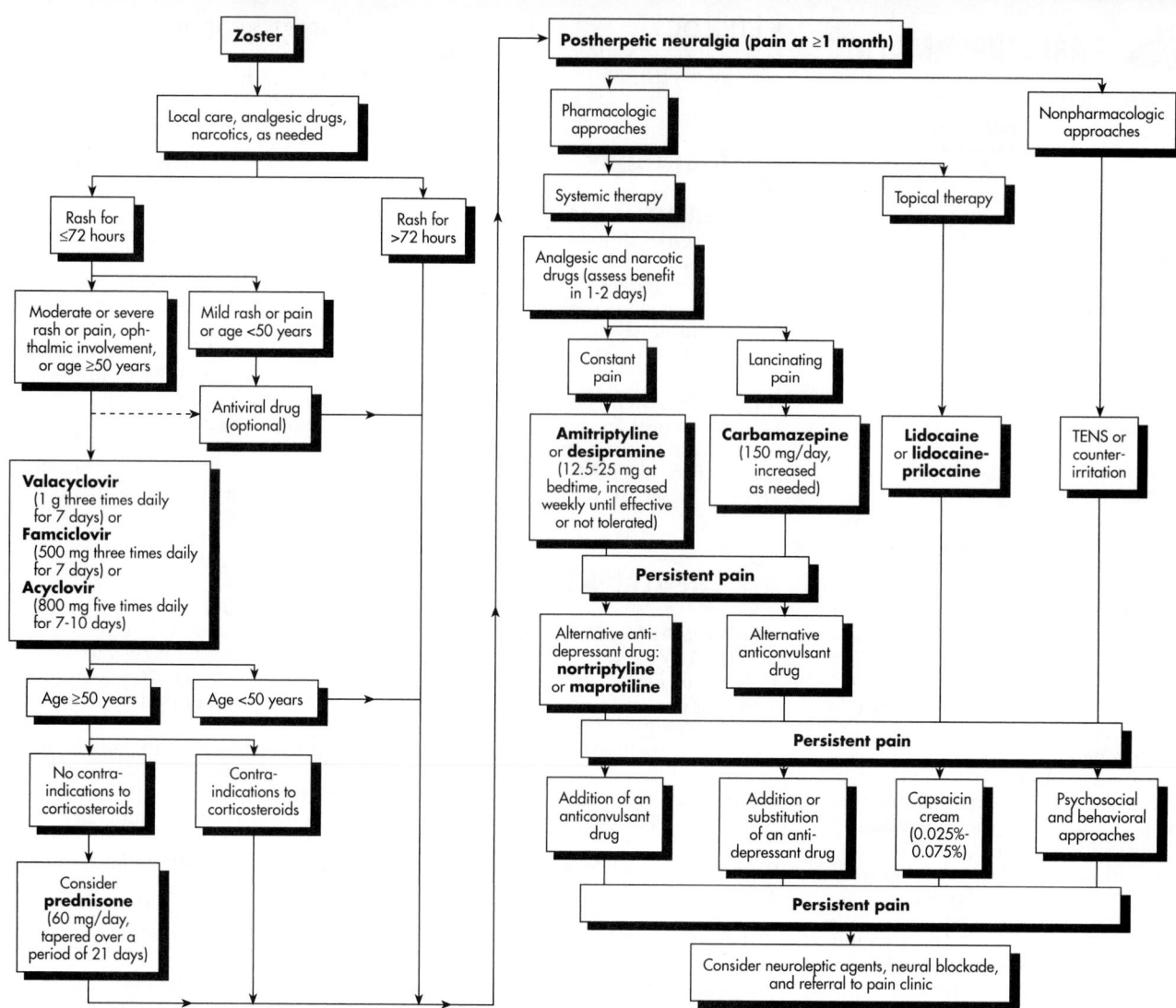

Fig. 1-191   Approaches to the treatment and prevention of acute zoster-associated pain and postherpetic neuralgia. Medications shown in bold have been demonstrated effective based on fairly convincing data from controlled trials. The decision to use antiviral drugs in patients with zoster must be individualized, but the prompt use of antiviral therapy in older patients or those with ophthalmic involvement is recommended. Younger patients with mild eruptions and little pain may not require antiviral therapy. Corticosteroids should be considered in older patients if there are no contraindications (e.g., diabetes mellitus, hypertension, or glaucoma). Patients with neuropathic pain within 1 month after the onset of zoster may be treated early, on an empiric basis. The therapeutic approaches for established postherpetic neuralgia are more numerous than those for acute zoster-associated pain, but their value is less well documented. Primary approaches include a topical anesthetic drug and trials of analgesic and narcotic drugs, with the addition of an antidepressant drug if the former prove ineffective, inadequate, or poorly tolerated. *TENS,* Transcutaneous electrical nerve stimulation. (From Kost RG, Straus SE: *N Engl J Med* 335:32, 1996.)

BASIC INFORMATION

■ DEFINITION
A hiatal hernia is the herniation of a portion of the stomach into the thoracic cavity through the diaphragmatic esophageal hiatus.

■ SYNONYMS
Diaphragmatic hernias

ICD-9CM CODES
750.6 Hiatal hernia

■ EPIDEMIOLOGY & DEMOGRAPHICS
• Found in 50% of patients over the age of 50.
• More prevalent in Western countries than in Africa and Asia.
• Sliding hiatal hernias are more common in women than men (4:1).
• Gastroesophageal reflux disease (GERD) is often associated with hiatal hernias.
• More than 90% of patients with documented endoscopic esophagitis have hiatal hernias.

■ PHYSICAL FINDINGS & CLINICAL PRESENTATION
Most patients with hiatal hernias are asymptomatic. Symptomatic patients present similar to patients with GERD.
• Heartburn
• Dysphagia
• Regurgitation
• Chest pain
• Postprandial fullness
• GI bleed
• Dyspnea
• Hoarseness
• Wheezing with bowel sounds heard over the left lung base

■ ETIOLOGY
• Hiatal hernias are classified as:
  1. Sliding (Fig. 1-192 and 1-193, *A*), axial or concentric hiatal hernia (most common type)
  2. Paraesophageal hernia (Fig. 1-193, *B*)
  3. Mixed

• Hiatal hernias are thought to develop from an imbalance between normal pulling forces of the esophagus through the diaphragmatic hiatus during swallowing and the supporting structures maintaining normal esophagogastric junction positioning.

 DIAGNOSIS

The diagnosis of hiatal hernia relies on history and imaging studies.

■ DIFFERENTIAL DIAGNOSIS
• Peptic ulcer disease
• Unstable angina
• Esophagitis (e.g., *Candida,* herpes, NSAIDs, etc.)
• Esophageal spasm
• Barrett's esophagus
• Schatzki's ring
• Achalasia
• Zenker's diverticulum
• Esophageal cancer

■ WORKUP
• The workup is directed at excluding conditions noted in the differential diagnosis and documenting the presence of a hiatal hernia. Upper endoscopy may also be needed to exclude abnormal metaplasia, dysplasia, or neoplasia.
• A clinical algorithm for evaluation of heartburn is described in Fig. 3-74.

■ LABORATORY TESTS
• Blood tests are not very specific in diagnosing hiatal hernias.
• Esophageal manometry, although not commonly done, can be used in establishing a diagnosis.

■ IMAGING STUDIES
• Barium contrast UGI series best defines the anatomic abnormality. A hiatal hernia is considered to be present if the gastric cardia is herniated 2 cm above the hiatus.
• Upper GI endoscopy is useful to document the presence of a hiatal hernia and also to exclude common associated findings of esophagitis and Barrett's esophagus.

TREATMENT

■ NONPHARMACOLOGIC THERAPY
• Lifestyle modifications with avoidance of foods and drugs that decrease lower esophageal pressure (e.g. caffeine, chocolate, mint, calcium channel blockers, and anticholinergics)
• Weight loss
• Avoid large quantities of food with meals
• Sleep with the head of the bed elevated 4 to 6 inches with blocks

■ ACUTE GENERAL Rx
• Antacids may be useful to relieve mild symptoms.
• H_2 antagonists (e.g., cimetidine 400 mg bid, ranitidine 150 mg bid, or famotidine 20 mg bid) can be used for symptomatic relief.
• If significant GERD is present with documented esophagitis by upper EGD, proton pump inhibitors (e.g., omeprazole 20 mg qd or lansoprazole 30 mg qd) are used.
• Prokinetic agents (e.g., metoclopramide 10 mg taken 30 min before each meal) can be added to an H_2 antagonist or proton pump inhibitor.

■ CHRONIC Rx
• Although rarely indicated, surgery can be done in patients with refractory symptoms impairing quality of life and causing both intestinal (e.g., recurrent GI bleeds) and extraintestinal complications (e.g., aspiration pneumonia, asthma, and ENT complications).
• Surgery is a consideration in all patients with paraesophageal hiatal hernias.

■ DISPOSITION
• Over 90% of patients with a hiatal hernia having GERD symptoms respond well to medical therapy.
• Complications of hiatal hernias are similar to complications occurring in patients with GERD:
  1. Erosive esophagitis
  2. Ulcerative esophagitis
  3. Barrett's esophagus
  4. Peptic stricture
  5. GI hemorrhage
  6. Extraintestinal complications

■ REFERRAL

All patients with documented hiatal hernia refractory to conventional H_2 antagonists, antacids, and proton pump inhibitors or having complications as mentioned above should be referred to a gastroenterology specialist.

☼ PEARLS & CONSIDERATIONS

■ COMMENTS

- Once in a lifetime upper endoscopy has been proposed in the literature to exclude Barrett's esophagus.
- Approximately 5% of patients with Barrett's esophagus go on to develop esophageal cancer.
- Yearly surveillance by upper EGD is recommended in patients with Barrett's esophagus.

REFERENCES

Epstein FH: The esophagogastric junction, *N Engl J Med* 336(13):924, 1997.

Mittal RK: Hiatal hernia: myth or reality? *Am J Med* 103(5A):33S, 1997.

Sloan S, Rademaker AW, Kahrilas PJ: Determinants of gastroesophageal junction incompetence: hiatal hernia, lower esophageal sphincter or both? *Ann Intern Med* 117:977, 1992.

Author: **Peter Petropoulos, M.D.**

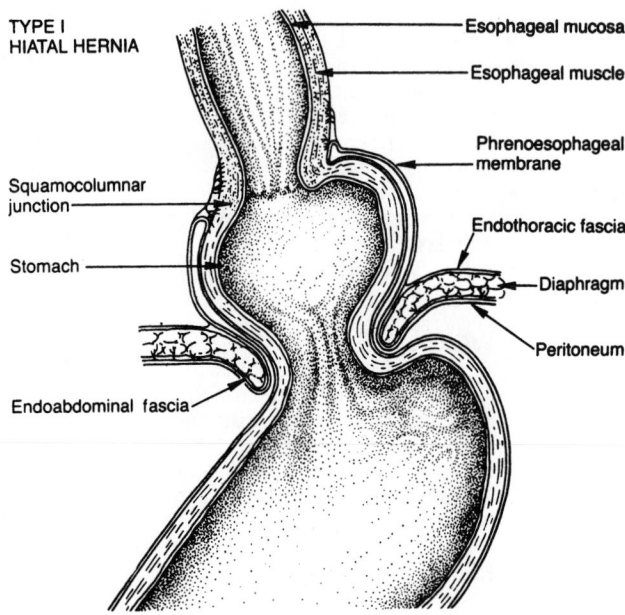

Fig. 1-192   Schematic diagram of a type I sliding hiatal hernia. (From Sabiston DC, Jr [ed]: *Textbook of surgery,* ed 13, Philadelphia, 1986, WB Saunders.)

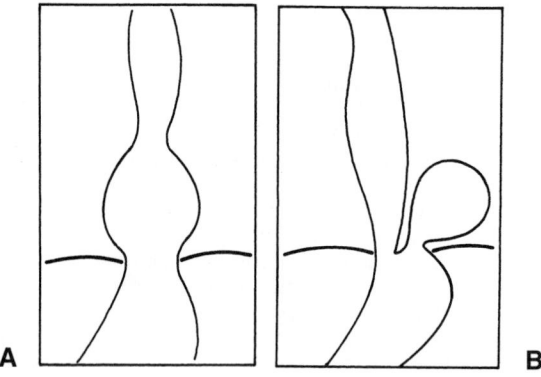

Fig. 1-193   Types of esophageal hiatal hernia. **A,** Sliding hiatal hernia, the most common type. **B,** Paraesophageal hiatal hernia. (From Behrman RE: *Nelson textbook of pediatrics,* ed 16, Philadelphia, 2000, WB Saunders.)

BASIC INFORMATION

■ DEFINITION
Histiocytosis X is a rare disorder characterized by the abnormal proliferation of pathologic Langerhans cells.

■ SYNONYMS
- Eosinophilic granuloma
- Hand-Schuller-Christian disease
- Letterer-Siwe disease
- Langerhans cell histiocytosis
- Langerhans cell granulomatosis

ICD-9CM CODES
277.8 Histiocytosis X

■ EPIDEMIOLOGY & DEMOGRAPHICS
- Histiocytosis X is a rare disease in adults.
- Peak incidence is from 1 to 3 yr.
- Incidence 4/1 million.
- Affects males more often than females—2:1.
- Disseminated histiocytosis X usually occurs before to 2 yr of age.
- Approximately 50% of isolated eosinophilic granuloma cases occur before the age of 5.

■ PHYSICAL FINDINGS & CLINICAL PRESENTATION
- A characteristic feature of histiocytosis X is its variable clinical presentation. The clinical spectrum ranges from:
  1. A benign isolated bony lesion (eosinophilic granuloma)
  2. Multiple bone lesions with soft tissue gingival and oral mucosal involvement (Hand-Schuller-Christian disease).
  3. An aggressive disseminated disease infiltrating organs and causing organ dysfunction (Letterer-Siwe disease).
- Bone lesions (80% to 100%)
  1. May be isolated or multiple
  2. Painful
  3. Skull most frequently involved, followed by long bones; lesions rarely seen in small bones of hands and feet
  4. Proptosis
  5. Mastoiditis
  6. Loose teeth
  7. Gingival hypertrophy
- Skin is involved in more than 80% of patients with disseminated disease and in 30% of patients with less extensive disease.
  1. Seborrhea-like scaling of scalp, petechial and purpuric lesions, ulcers, and bronzing of the skin may occur.
  2. Common sites: scalp, neck, trunk, groin, and extremities.

- Lymphadenopathy (10%): cervical and inguinal.
- Lung involvement may manifest with cough, tachypnea, cyanosis, inspiratory crackles, pleural effusions, or pneumothorax.
- Liver involvement manifesting with jaundice and hepatomegaly.
- Splenomegaly (5%)
- CNS involvement occurs in 1% to 4% of patients primarily manifesting as diabetes insipidus with insatiable thirst and urination.

■ ETIOLOGY
- The etiology of histiocytosis is unknown.
- Initially, histiocytosis was thought to represent an abnormal immune response to a virus or other stimulant resulting in the proliferation of pathologic Langerhans cells. More recent evidence suggests histiocytosis X as a monoclonal proliferative neoplastic disorder.

DIAGNOSIS

Tissue biopsy revealing pathologic Langerhans cells characterized by the presence of surface nucleoprotein, CD1a antigen, and "Birbeck granules" noted on electron microscopy establishes the diagnosis of histiocytosis X.

■ DIFFERENTIAL DIAGNOSIS
The differential diagnosis is extensive, including all causes of diabetes insipidus, lytic bone lesions, dermatitis, hepatomegaly, and lymphadenopathy.

■ WORKUP
The workup of patients suspected of having histiocytosis X includes blood tests and imaging studies to assess the extent of disease involvement.

■ LABORATORY TESTS
- CBC is not specific in the diagnosis of histiocytosis X but may reveal cytopenias in patients with bone marrow involvement.
- Electrolytes, BUN, creatinine, urinalysis, and urine and serum osmolality are helpful in the diagnosis of diabetes insipidus during fluid deprivation testing.
- Liver function tests may be elevated in patients with liver involvement.
- Bronchoalveolar lavage (BAL) may show increased numbers of CD1a-positive histiocytes or Langerhans cells in patients with pulmonary histiocytosis X.

■ IMAGING STUDIES
- X-ray studies of affected areas show lytic lesions with or without sclerotic

margins.
- X-ray bone survey is done searching for other lesions.
- Bone scan complements the bone survey studies.
- Panoramic dental view of the mandible and maxilla for children with oral involvement.
- Chest x-ray can show interstitial reticulonodular infiltrates (Fig. 1-194).
- High-resolution CT scan of the chest confirms interstitial lung scarring.
- CT scans of the temporal bone looking at the mastoid, and inner and middle ear.
- Ultrasound of the abdomen may show hepatosplenomegaly.
- MRI of the brain visualizing the hypothalamic-hypophyseal region in patients suspected of having diabetes insipidus.

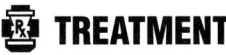

TREATMENT

Treatment is based on the extent of involvement:
- Single-system disease:
  1. Single site: single bone lesion, isolated skin disease, or solitary lymph node.
  2. Multiple site: multiple bone lesions, multiple lymph nodes.
- Multiple disease: Multiple organ involvement, with or without dysfunction.

■ ACUTE GENERAL Rx
Isolated bone lesions can be treated by:
- Curettage at the time of diagnosis
- Intralesional steroid injection
- Radiation therapy
Single skin lesions are treated with:
- Topical steroid (e.g., triamcinolone acetonide) applied bid
- Nitrogen mustard in 20% solution
Solitary lymph node
- Excision at the time diagnosis
- Systemic oral prednisone
Multisystem disease treatment includes:
- Vinblastine 6 mg/m^2 IV bolus qwk × 6 mo or etoposide 150 mg/m^2 IV for 3 days q3wk for 6 mo plus
- Methylprednisolone 30 mg/kg/day for 3 days

■ CHRONIC Rx
- High-risk patients not responding to initial treatment should be considered for salvage therapy, including either bone marrow transplantation or combination cyclosporin A, antithymocyte globulin, and prednisolone.
- Diabetes insipidus is treated with DDAVP 0.1 mg to 0.8 mg PO or 1 spray bid to tid.

■ DISPOSITION

- A poor prognostic feature in the multisystem treatment group is the failure to respond to therapy in the first 6 wk.
- Multisystem disease patients categorized as low-risk group were patients >2 yr of age with no evidence of organ involvement (e.g., bone marrow, liver, lung, or spleen).
- Age of onset (<2 yr) with organ involvement is considered a high-risk group.
- In patients with disseminated histiocytosis X and <2 yr of age, the mortality rate is 30%.
- The association of histiocytosis X with other malignancies (e.g., ALL, acute nonlymphoblastic leukemia, and solid tumors) has been cited. It remains unclear if the associated malignancies result from the treatment of histiocytosis X or chance events.

■ REFERRAL

Histiocytosis X patients require a multidisciplinary approach including pediatric oncologist, radiation oncologists, oral maxillary surgeons, ENT specialists, audiology, dermatology, endocrinology, and family counseling.

☼ PEARLS & CONSIDERATIONS

■ COMMENTS

- Dr. Alfred Hand, Jr. described the first case of histiocytosis X in 1893. Drs. Letterer, Siwe, Schuller, and Christian also described similar cases between 1915 to 1933.
- Dr. Louis Lichtenstein noted the similarities of the cases and coined the term name *histiocytosis X*.
- In 1987, the Histiocyte Society was formed and the disease was officially termed *Langerhans cell histiocytosis*.

REFERENCES

Arico M, Egeler RM: Clinical aspects of Langerhans cell histiocytosis, *Hematol/Oncol Clin North Am* 12(2):247, 1998.

Broadbent V, Gadner H: Current therapy for Langerhans cell histiocytosis, *Hematol/Oncol Clin North Am* 12(2):327, 1998.

Lamper F: Langerhans cell histiocytosis: historical perspectives, *Hematol/Oncol Clin North Am* 12(2):213, 1998.

Nicholson HS, Egeler RM, Nesbit ME: The epidemiology of Langerhans cell histiocytosis, *Hematol/Oncol Clin North Am* 12(2):379, 1998.

Schmitz L, Favara BE: Nosology and pathology of Langerhans cell histiocytosis, *Hematol/Oncol Clin North Am* 12(2):221, 1998.

Author: **Peter Petropoulos, M.D.**

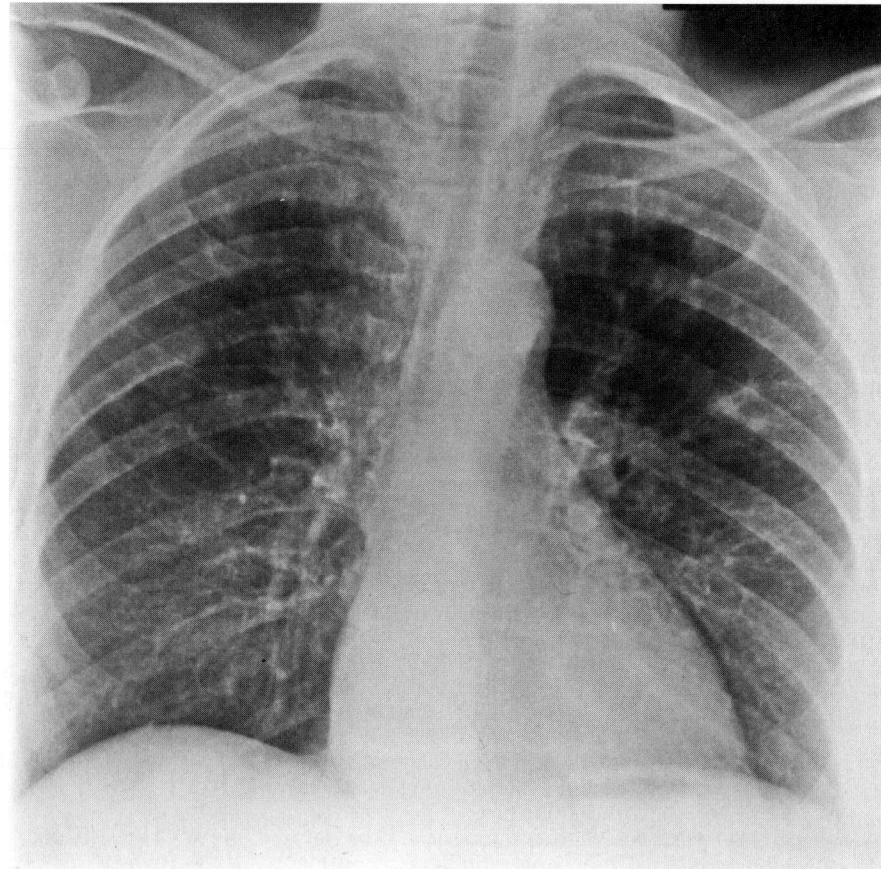

Fig. 1-194 Histiocytosis X. There is a reticular nodular pattern in the upper lobes. The lung volumes are preserved. (From McLoud TC [ed]: *Thoracic radiology, the requisites,* St Louis, 1998, Mosby.)

BASIC INFORMATION

■ DEFINITION

Histoplasmosis is an infectious disease caused by the fungus *Histoplasma capsulatum,* which is usually asymptomatic and characterized by a primary pulmonary focus with occasional progression to chronic pulmonary histoplasmosis (CPH) or various forms of dissemination. Progressive disseminated histoplasmosis (PDH) may present with a diverse clinical spectrum, including adrenal necrosis, pulmonary and mediastinal fibrosis, and ulcerations of the oropharynx and GI tract. In those patients who are concurrently infected with the human immunodeficiency virus (HIV), it is a defining disease for acquired immunodeficiency syndrome (AIDS).

ICD-9CM CODES
115.90 Histoplasmosis
115.94 Histoplasmosis with endocarditis
115.91 Histoplasmosis with meningitis
115.93 Histoplasmosis with pericarditis
115.95 Histoplasmosis with pneumonia
115.92 Histoplasmosis with retinitis

■ EPIDEMIOLOGY & DEMOGRAPHICS
INCIDENCE (IN U.S.):
- Unknown for acute pulmonary disease
- For CPH, estimated at 1/100,000 cases in endemic areas
- For PDH in immunocompetent adults, estimated at 1/2000 cases of histoplasmosis

PREVALENCE: Unknown
PREDOMINANT SEX: Clinically evident disease is most common in males; male:female ratio of 4:1
PREDOMINANT AGE:
- CPH is most often seen in males >50 yr old with an associated history of COPD.
- Presumed ocular histoplasmosis syndrome (POHS) is most commonly diagnosed between ages of 20 and 40 yr.

PEAK INCIDENCE: Unknown

■ PHYSICAL FINDINGS & CLINICAL PRESENTATION
- Conidia are deposited in alveoli, then fungus is converted to a yeast in the initial focus of bronchopneumonia and spreads to regional lymph nodes and other organs, especially liver and spleen, via lymphatics.
- From 7 to 18 days after onset, granulomatous inflammatory response marking host's cellular immunity begins to contain the yeast in the form of discrete granulomas.
- In normal host, fungistasis is achieved slowly as granulomas undergo contraction and, later, fibrosis with frequent calcification.
- With maturation of specific cellular immunity, there is development of delayed-type cutaneous hypersensitivity to *Histoplasma* antigens, usually 3 to 6 wk after exposure.
- Clinical disease manifests in various forms, depending on host cellular immunity and inoculum size:
  1. Acute primary pulmonary histoplasmosis
     a. Overwhelming number of patients are asymptomatic.
     b. Most clinically apparent infections manifest by complaints of fever, headache, malaise, pleuritic chest pain, nonproductive cough, and weight loss.
     c. Less than 10%, mainly women, complain of arthralgias, myalgias, and skin manifestations such as erythema multiforme or erythema nodosum.
     d. Acute pericarditis presents in smaller percentage of patients.
     e. On auscultation findings are minimal; hepatosplenomegaly, seen sometimes in adults, is most commonly observed in children.
     f. With particularly heavy exposure, there is severe dyspnea, marked hypoxemia, impending respiratory failure.
     g. Most patients are asymptomatic within 6 wk.
  2. CPH
     a. Presents insidiously with low-grade fever, malaise, weight loss, cough, sometimes with blood-streaked sputum or frank hemoptysis.
     b. Most patients with cavitary lesions present with associated COPD or chronic bronchitis, masking underlying fungal disease.
     c. Tends to worsen preexisting pulmonary disease and further contribute to eventual respiratory insufficiency.
  3. PDH
     a. In both acute and subacute forms, constitutional symptoms of fever, fatigue, malaise, and weight loss are common.
     b. Acute form (seen most commonly in infants and children) is distinguished by predominance of respiratory symptoms, fevers consistently >101° F (38.3° C), generalized lymphadenopathy, marked hepatosplenomegaly, and fulminant course resembling septic shock associated with a high fatality rate.
     c. Subacute form is more common in adults and associated with lower temperatures, hepatosplenomegaly, oropharyngeal ulceration, focal organ involvement (including Addison's disease secondary to adrenal destruction, endocarditis, chronic meningitis, and intracerebral mass lesions).
     d. Course of subacute form is relentless, with untreated patient dying within 2 yr.
     e. Chronic PDH is found in adults and marked by gradual, often intermittent, symptoms of weight loss, weakness, easy fatigability; fever only uncommonly and usually of low grade when present; oropharyngeal ulcerations and hepatomegaly and/or splenomegaly in one third of patients.
     f. Less clinical evidence of focal organ involvement in chronic form than in subacute form.
     g. Natural history of chronic form protracted and intermittent, spanning months to years.
- Histoplasmoma
  1. A healed area of caseation necrosis surrounded by a fibrous capsule
  2. Usually asymptomatic

- Mediastinal fibrosis
  1. A rare consequence of a fibroblastic process that encases caseating mediastinal lymph nodes after primary histoplasma bronchopneumonia
  2. Progressive fibrosis producing severe retraction, compression, and distortion of mediastinal structures
  3. Constriction of the bronchi resulting in bronchiectasis, also esophageal stenosis associated with dysphagia, and superior vena cava syndrome
- POHS
  1. Diagnosis characterized by distinct clinical features, including atrophic choroidal scars and maculopathy in patient with a history suggestive of exposure to the fungus (e.g., residence in an endemic area)
  2. Patient complains of distortion or loss of central vision without pain, redness, or photophobia
  3. Usually no evidence of systemic infection except for a positive skin reaction to histoplasmin
- In patients with AIDS
  1. Possible presentation as overwhelming infection similar to acute PDH seen in children
  2. Constitutional symptoms: fever, weight loss, malaise, cough, dyspnea
  3. About 10% with cutaneous maculopapular, erythematous eruptions or purpuric lesions on face, trunk, and extremities
  4. Up to 20% with CNS involvement, manifesting as intracerebral mass lesions, chronic meningitis, or encephalopathy
  5. Infrequent oropharyngeal ulceration

■ ETIOLOGY

- *H. capsulatum* is a dimorphic fungus present in temperate zones and river valleys around the world.
- In the U.S., it is highly endemic in southeastern, mid-Atlantic, and central states.
- Exists as mold at ambient temperature and favors surface soil enriched with bird or bat droppings.
- In endemic areas, contaminated dusty soil containing spores (microconidia) may be windswept or otherwise made airborne by sweeping, raking, or bulldozing, and then be inhaled.

🔬 DIAGNOSIS

■ DIFFERENTIAL DIAGNOSIS

- Acute pulmonary histoplasmosis
  1. *Mycobacterium tuberculosis*
  2. Community-acquired pneumonias caused by *Mycoplasma* and *Chlamydia*
  3. Other fungal diseases, such as *Blastomyces dermatitidis* and *Coccidioides immitis*
- Chronic cavitary pulmonary histoplasmosis: *M. tuberculosis*
- Yeast forms of histoplasmosis on tissue section: cysts of *Pneumocystis carinii*, which tend to be larger, extracellular, and do not display budding
- Intracellular parasites of *Leishmania* and *Toxoplasma* species: distinguishable by inability to take up methenamine silver
- Histoplasmomas: true neoplasms

■ WORKUP

- Suspect diagnosis in patients who present with an influenza-like illness and a history of residence or travel in an endemic area, especially if engaged in occupations (e.g., outside construction or street cleaning) or hobbies (e.g., cave exploring and aviary keeper) that increase the likelihood of exposure to fungal spores.
- Suspect diagnosis in immunosuppressed patients with remote history of exposure, especially if associated with characteristic calcifications on chest x-ray examination.

■ LABORATORY TESTS

- Demonstration of organism on culture from body fluid or tissues to make definitive diagnosis
  1. Especially high yield in patients with AIDS
  2. Characteristic oval yeast cells in neutrophils stained with Wright-Giemsa on peripheral smear
  3. Preparations of infected tissue with Gomori's silver methenamine for revealing yeast forms, especially in areas of caseation necrosis
- Serologic tests, including complement-fixing (CF) antibodies and immunodiffusion assays
  1. To establish previous infection and suggest active disease

  2. Possibly limited by inability to distinguish acute disease from remote infection and cross-reactivity with other fungi
- Detection of *Histoplasma* antigen in urine: may be influenced by infections with *Blastomyces* and *Coccidioides*
- Skin testing with histoplasmin: useful epidemiologically but essentially useless for diagnosis of acute disease
- In PDH
  1. Pancytopenia
  2. Marked elevations in alkaline phosphatase and alanine aminotransferase (ALT) common
  3. Most evident in acute and subacute forms and to a lesser extent in chronic form
- In chronic meningitis (majority of cases)
  1. CSF pleocytosis with either lymphocytes or neutrophils predominating
  2. Elevated CSF protein levels
  3. Hypoglycorrhachia

■ IMAGING STUDIES

- Chest x-ray examination in acute pulmonary histoplasmosis
  1. Singular or multiple patchy infiltrates, especially in the lower lung fields
  2. Hilar or mediastinal lymphadenopathy with or without pneumonitis
  3. Diffuse nodular or confluent bilateral miliary infiltrates characteristic of heavier exposure
  4. Infrequent pleural effusions, except when associated with pericarditis
- Chest x-ray examination in histoplasmoma: coin lesion displaying central calcification, ranging from 1 to 4 cm in diameter, predominantly located in the subpleural regions
- Chest x-ray examination in CPH:
  1. Upper lobe disease frequently associated with cavities (thick-walled, secondarily infected with an *Aspergillus* fungus ball)
  2. Preexisting calcifications in the hilum associated with peribronchial streaking extending to the parenchyma
- Chest x-ray examination in acute PDH: hilar adenopathy and/or diffuse nodular infiltrates (Fig. 1-195)
- CT scan of adrenals to reveal bilateral enlargement and low-attenuation centers

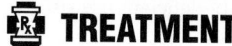 TREATMENT

■ NONPHARMACOLOGIC THERAPY

For life-threatening disease seen in acute disseminated disease or infection in patients with AIDS: supportive therapy with IV fluids

■ ACUTE GENERAL Rx

- No drug therapy is required for patients with asymptomatic pulmonary disease and most patients with mild symptomatic pulmonary disease.
- Brief course of therapy with ketoconazole 400 mg/day or itraconazole 200 mg/day PO for 3 to 6 wk may be beneficial in some patients with acute pulmonary distress.
- Same therapy appropriate for immunocompetent, mild to moderately symptomatic patients with CPH and subacute and chronic forms of PDH, but duration of therapy is longer, ranging for 6 to 12 mo.
- Use amphotericin B 0.7 to 1 mg/kg IV for 6 to 12 mo in patients hypersensitive to or intolerant of azole therapy.
- Do not give immunocompromised patients, especially those with AIDS, ketoconazole as primary therapy for disseminated histoplasmosis.

- Give amphotericin B for life-threatening disease or continued illness as a result of primary failure or relapse of adequate azole therapy.
  1. For acute pulmonary histoplasmosis associated with acute respiratory distress syndrome (ARDS), acute PDH, and histoplasma meningitis: dose of 0.7 to 1 mg/kg IV >4 hr
  2. End point of therapy for patient with complicated acute pulmonary disease: total dose of 500 mg
  3. End point for patient with acute PDH: total dose 35 mg/kg or 2.5 g total
  4. Concomitant administration of prednisone 60 to 80 mg/day beneficial for severe fungal hypersensitivity complicating acute pulmonary disease
- Endocarditis: surgical treatment is preferable, with excision of infected valve or graft combined with amphotericin for a total dose of 35 mg/kg or 2.5 g
- For pericardial disease:
  1. Antifungal therapy: no apparent benefit
  2. Best managed with NSAIDs
- For POHS:
  1. Antifungal therapy: no apparent benefit
  2. May respond to laser therapy

■ CHRONIC Rx

In patients with AIDS: lifelong suppressive therapy with either itraconazole, given 200 mg PO qd, or IV amphotericin B at a dose of 50 mg once weekly

■ DISPOSITION

- Most immunocompetent patients with acute histoplasmosis are asymptomatic.
- For those with chronic or progressive disease, especially if immunocompromised by virtue of disease or medication, outcome and favorable prognosis are dependent on prompt recognition of varied forms of disease and timely administration of appropriate antifungal drugs.

■ REFERRAL

- For consultation with infectious disease specialist in suspected cases of disseminated disease, especially if immunocompromised
- To a pulmonologist for patients with CPH form because progressive respiratory compromise usually results from chronic infection and underlying COPD
- For consultation with a thoracic surgeon for decompression procedures in patients symptomatic as a consequence of progressive mediastinal fibrosis

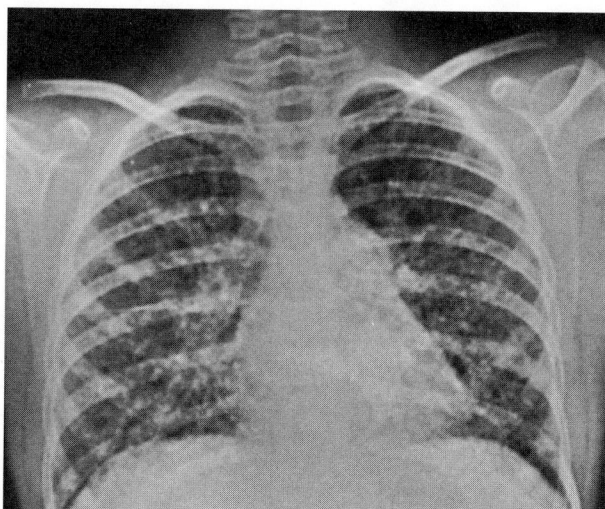

Fig. 1-195 Chest radiograph of a patient with disseminated histoplasmosis showing diffuse interstitial alveolar infiltrates. (From Gorbach SL: *Infectious diseases,* ed 2, Philadelphia, 1998, WB Saunders.)

☼ PEARLS & CONSIDERATIONS

- *H. capsulatum,* variety *duboisii,* also known as African histoplasmosis, is restricted to Senegal, Nigeria, Zaire, and Uganda.
- Unlike *H. capsulatum,* pulmonary forms of *duboisii* are not seen, and the disease is limited to the skin, soft tissues, and bone.

■ COMMENTS

- Patients living in endemic areas, especially if immunocompromised, should be advised to take appropriate respiratory precautions when sweeping or disposing of bird waste from rooftop or home aviaries.
- Appropriate respiratory precautions should also be taken when leisure traveling to areas that act as a natural haven for the fungus, such as bat caves.
- Immunocompetent hosts are generally unaware of fungal infection, but the immunocompromised suffer devastating consequences.

REFERENCES

Chemaly RF et al: Rapid diagnosis of *Histoplasma capsulatum* endocarditis using the AccuProbe on an excised valve, *J Clin Microbiol* 39(7):2640, 2001.

Hajjeh RA et al: Multicenter case control study of risk factors for histoplasmosis in human immunodeficiency virus-infected persons, *Clin Infect Dis* 32(8):1215, 2001.

Limaye AP et al: Transmission of *Histoplasma capsulatum* by organ transplantation, *N Engl J Med* 343(16):163, 2000.

Martin RC et al: Histoplasmosis as an isolated liver lesion: review and surgical therapy, *Am Surg* 67(5):430, 2001.

Rozenblit AM et al: Adrenal histoplasmosis manifested as Addison's disease: unusual CT features with magnetic resonance imaging correlation, *Clin Radiol* 56(8):682, 2001.

Author: **George O. Alonso, M.D.**

BASIC INFORMATION

■ DEFINITION
Hodgkin's disease is a malignant disorder of lymphoreticular origin, characterized histologically by the presence of multinucleated giant cells (Reed-Sternberg cells) usually originating from B lymphocytes in germinal centers of lymphoid tissue (Fig. 1-196).

ICD-9CM CODES
201.9 Hodgkin's disease, unspecified
201.4 Hodgkin's disease, lymphocyte predominance
201.5 Hodgkin's disease, nodular sclerosis
201.6 Hodgkin's disease, mixed cellularity
201.7 Hodgkin's disease, lymphocyte depletion

■ EPIDEMIOLOGY & DEMOGRAPHICS
• There is a bimodal age distribution (15 to 34 yr and >50 yr).
• Concordance for Hodgkin's disease in identical twins suggests that a genetic susceptibility underlies Hodgkin's disease in young adulthood.
• The disease is more common in males (in childhood Hodgkin's disease, >80% occurs in males), in Caucasians, and in higher socioeconomic groups.
• Overall incidence of Hodgkin's disease in the U.S. is approximately 4:100,000.

■ PHYSICAL FINDINGS & CLINICAL PRESENTATION
• Palpable lymphadenopathy, generally painless
• Most common site of involvement: neck region
• See "Workup" for description of common symptoms.

■ ETIOLOGY
Unknown; evidence implicating Epstein-Barr virus remains controversial.

DIAGNOSIS

■ DIFFERENTIAL DIAGNOSIS
• Non-Hodgkin's lymphoma
• Sarcoidosis
• Infections (e.g., CMV, Epstein-Barr virus, toxoplasma, HIV)
• Drug reaction
• Figs. 3-106 and 3-107 describe clinical algorithms for evaluation of lymph-adenopathy.
• Box 2-160 describes the differential diagnosis of lymphadenopathy.

■ WORKUP
Symptomatic patients with Hodgkin's disease usually present with the following manifestations:
• Fever and night sweats: fever in a cyclical pattern (days or weeks of fever alternating with afebrile periods) is known as Pel-Epstein fever
• Weight loss, generalized malaise
• Persistent, nonproductive cough
• Pain associated with alcohol ingestion, often secondary to heavy eosinophil infiltration of the tumor sites
• Pruritus
• Others: superior vena cava syndrome and spinal cord compression (rare)
Diagnosis can be made with lymph node biopsy. There are four main **histologic subtypes,** based on the number of lymphocytes, Reed-Sternberg cells, and the presence of fibrous tissue:
  1. Lymphocyte predominance
  2. Mixed cellularity
  3. Nodular sclerosis
  4. Lymphocyte depletion
Nodular sclerosis is the most common type and occurs mainly in young adulthood, whereas the mixed cellularity type is more prevalent after age 50 yr.
Staging for Hodgkin's disease follows the **Ann Arbor staging classification.**
  Stage I: Involvement of a single lymph node region
  Stage II: Two or more lymph node regions on the same side of the diaphragm
  Stage III: Lymph node involvement on both sides of diaphragm, including spleen
  Stage IV: Diffuse involvement of external sites
  Suffix A: No systemic symptoms
  Suffix B: Presence of fever, night sweats, or unexplained weight loss of 10% or more body weight over 6 mo
  Suffix X: Indicates bulky disease >⅓ widening of mediastinum or >10 cm maximum dimension of nodal mass on a chest film.
Proper **staging** requires the following:
• Detailed history (with documentation of "B symptoms" and physical examination)
• Surgical biopsy
• Laboratory evaluation (CBC, sedimentation rate, BUN, creatinine, alkaline phosphatase, liver function studies, albumin, LDH, uric acid)
• Chest x-ray studies (PA and lateral); see Fig. 2-5 for differential diagnosis of mediastinal masses or widening on chest x-ray examination (Fig. 1-197)
• Bilateral bone marrow biopsy

• CT scan of the chest (when abnormal findings are noted on chest x-ray examination) and of the abdomen and pelvis to visualize the mesenteric, hepatic, portal and splenic hilar nodes
• Bipedal lymphangiography in selected patients to define periaortic and iliac lymph node involvement
• Exploratory laparotomy and splenectomy (selected patients) (Fig. 1-198):
  1. Decision to perform staging laparotomy depends on the therapeutic plan; it is generally not indicated in patients who have a large mediastinal mass (these patients will generally be treated with combined chemotherapy and radiation). Staging laparotomy may also not be required in patients with clinical stage I or unlikely to have abdominal disease (e.g., females with supradiaphragmatic disease).
  2. Exploratory laparotomy and splenectomy may be used for patients with clinical stage I-IIA or IIB.
  3. It is useful in identifying patients who can be treated with irradiation alone with curative intent.
  4. Polyvalent pneumococcal vaccine should be given prophylactically to all patients before splenectomy (increased risk of sepsis from encapsulated organisms in splenectomized patients).
• Gallium scan

■ LABORATORY TESTS
See "Workup."

■ IMAGING STUDIES
See "Workup."

TREATMENT

■ ACUTE GENERAL Rx
The main therapeutic modalities are radiotherapy and chemotherapy; the indication for each vary with pathologic stage and other factors.
• Stage I and II: radiation therapy alone unless a large mediastinal mass is present (mediastinal to thoracic ratio ≥1.3); in the latter case, a combination of chemotherapy and radiation therapy is indicated.
• Stage IB or IIB: total nodal irradiation is often used, although chemotherapy is performed in many centers.
• Stage IIIA: treatment is controversial. It varies with the anatomic substage after splenectomy.
  1. III$_1$A and minimum splenic involvement: radiation therapy alone may be adequate.

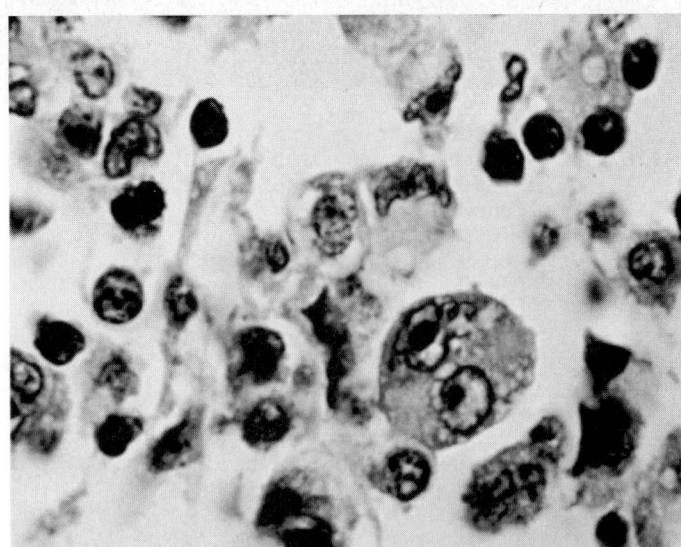

Fig. 1-196 Reed-Sternberg cell that contains two nuclei, each with a prominent nucleolus and distinct nuclear membrane. The cytoplasm of this cell is relatively abundant. Others cells present are lymphocytes, plasma cells, and tissue mononuclear cells. Presence of these cells in lymph node tissue is diagnostic of Hodgkin's disease. (From Behrman RE: *Nelson textbook of pediatrics,* Philadelphia, 1996, WB Saunders.)

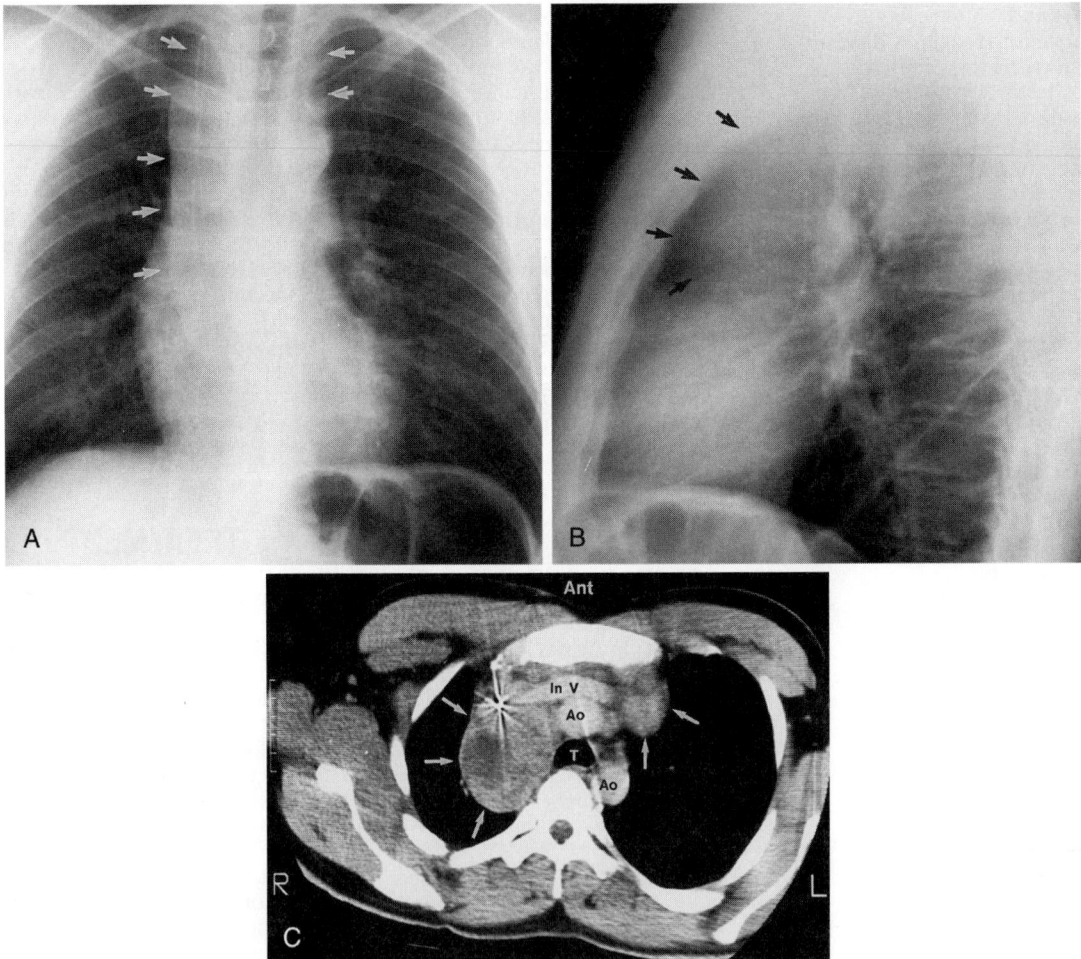

Fig. 1-197 Hodgkin's disease. In this 20-year-old male with low-grade fevers, a PA chest radiograph **(A)** shows marked widening of the middle and superior mediastinum *(arrows)*. On the lateral chest radiograph **(B)**, there is filling in of the retrosternal space by an ill-defined anterior mediastinal mass *(arrows)*. The transverse contrast-enhanced CT scan **(C)** through the upper portion of the chest shows the innominate vein, ascending and descending aorta, and trachea. They are all enveloped by a mass of nodes *(arrows)*. *CT,* Computed tomography; *PA,* posteroanterior. (From Mettler FA [ed]: *Primary care radiology,* Philadelphia, 2000, WB Saunders.)

2. III$_2$ or III$_1$A with extensive splenic involvement: there is disagreement whether chemotherapy alone or a combination of chemotherapy and radiation therapy is the preferred treatment modality.

3. IIIB and IVB: the treatment of choice is chemotherapy with or without adjuvant radiotherapy. Various regimens can be used for combination of chemotherapy; some commonly used regimens are MOPP, MOPP-ABV, ABVD, MOPP-ABVD, MOPP-BAP.

■ **DISPOSITION**
• The overall survival at 10 yr is approximately 60%.
• Poor prognostic features include presence of "B symptoms," advanced age, advanced stage at initial presentation, mixed-cellularity, and lymphocyte depletion histology.

• Chemotherapy significantly increases the risk of leukemia.
• The peak in risk of leukemia is seen approximately 5 yr after the initiation of chemotherapy.
• The risk of leukemia is greater for those who undergo splenectomy and for patients with advanced stages of Hodgkin's disease; the risk is unaffected by concomitant radiotherapy.
• Mediastinal irradiation increases the risk of subsequent death from heart disease caused by sclerosis of coronary artery secondary to irradiation. Risk increases with high mediastinal doses, minimal protective cardiac blocking, young age at irradiation, and increased duration of follow-up.
• Both chemotherapy and radiation therapy increase the risk of developing secondary solid tumors (e.g., carcinoma of the lung, breast, and stomach).

■ **REFERRAL**
• Surgical referral for lymph node biopsy
• Hematology/oncology referral

⚙ **PEARLS & CONSIDERATIONS**

■ **COMMENTS**
Young male patients should consider sperm banking before the initiation of therapy.

REFERENCE
Loeffler M et al: Metaanalysis of chemotherapy versus combined modality treatment trials in Hodgkin's disease, *J Clin Oncol* 16:818, 1998.
Author: **Fred F. Ferri, M.D.**

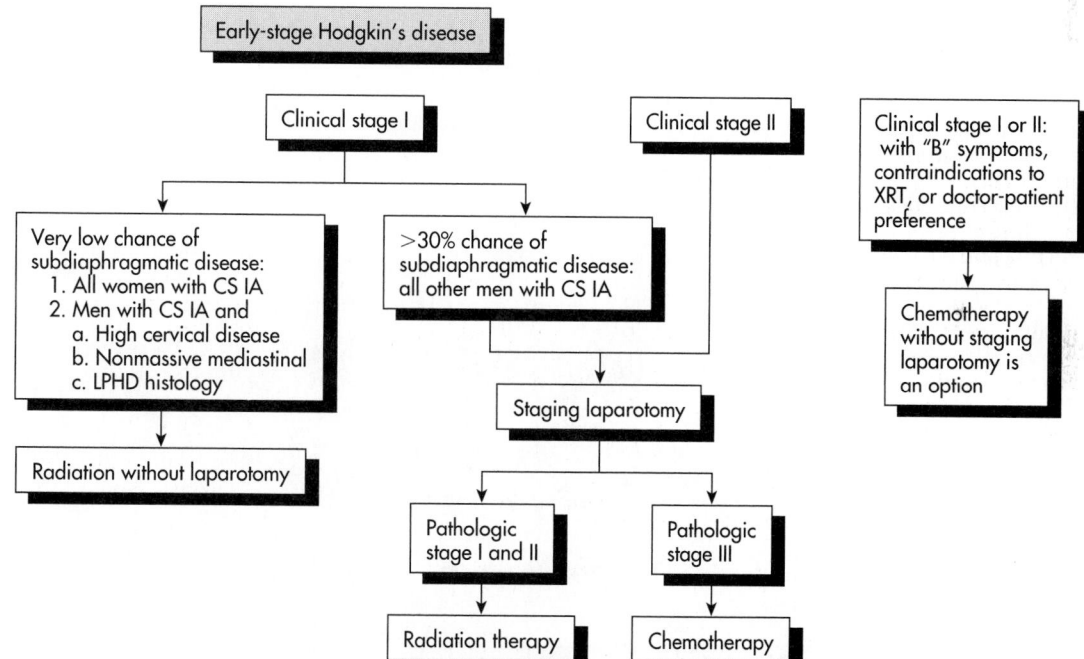

Fig. 1-198   Treatment of early-stage Hodgkin's disease. *CSIA,* Clinical stage IA; *LPHD,* lymphocyte predominance Hodgkin's disease; *XRT,* radiation therapy. (From Abeloff MD: *Clinical oncology,* ed 2, New York, 2000, Churchill Livingstone.)

BASIC INFORMATION

■ **DEFINITION**
Hookworm is a parasitic infection of the intestine caused by helminths (Fig. 1-199).

ICD-9CM CODES
126.35 Hookworm

■ **EPIDEMIOLOGY & DEMOGRAPHICS**
INCIDENCE (IN U.S.):
• Varies greatly in different areas of the U.S.
• Most common in rural areas of southeastern U.S.
• Increased likelihood in areas of poor sanitation and increased rainfall
PREVALENCE (IN U.S.): Varies from 10% to 90% in regions where it is found
PREDOMINANT AGE: Schoolchildren

■ **PHYSICAL FINDINGS & CLINICAL PRESENTATION**
• Most infections are asymptomatic
• Nonspecific abdominal complaints
• Because these organisms consume host RBCs, symptoms related to iron-deficiency anemia, depending on the amount of iron in the diet and the worm burden
• Fatigue, tachycardia, dyspnea, and high-output failure
• Hypoproteinemia and edema from loss of proteins into the intestinal tract
• Unusual for pulmonary manifestations to occur when the larvae migrate through the lungs
• Skin rash at sites of larval penetration in some individuals without prior exposure

■ **ETIOLOGY**
Two species are causative: *Necator americanus* and *Ancylostoma duodenale*. *N. americanus* is the predominant cause of hookworm in the U.S.
• Penetration of the skin by the larval form, with subsequent migration via the blood stream to the alveoli, up the respiratory tract, then into the GI tract

• Sharp mouth parts for attachment to intestinal mucosa

DIAGNOSIS

■ **DIFFERENTIAL DIAGNOSIS**
• Strongyloidiasis
• Ascariasis
• Table 2-113 describes the differential diagnosis of intestinal helminths.

■ **WORKUP**
Examine stool for hookworm eggs.

■ **LABORATORY TESTS**
CBC to show hypochromic, microcytic anemia; possible mild eosinophilia and hypoalbuminemia

■ **IMAGING STUDIES**
Chest x-ray examination: occasionally shows opacities

TREATMENT

■ **NONPHARMACOLOGIC THERAPY**
Prevention of disease by not walking barefoot and by improving sanitary conditions

■ **ACUTE GENERAL Rx**
• Mebendazole 100 mg PO bid for 3 days
• Iron supplementation possibly helpful

■ **DISPOSITION**
Easily treated.

■ **REFERRAL**
If diagnosis uncertain

PEARLS & CONSIDERATIONS

■ **COMMENTS**
Appropriate disposal of human wastes is important in controlling the disease in areas with a high prevalence of hookworm infestation.

REFERENCES
Biegel Y et al: Clinical problem-solving: letting the patient off the hook, *N Engl J Med* 342:1658, 2000.
Kitchen LW: Case studies in international travelers, *Am Fam Physician* 59:3040, 1999.
Author: **Maurice Policar, M.D.**

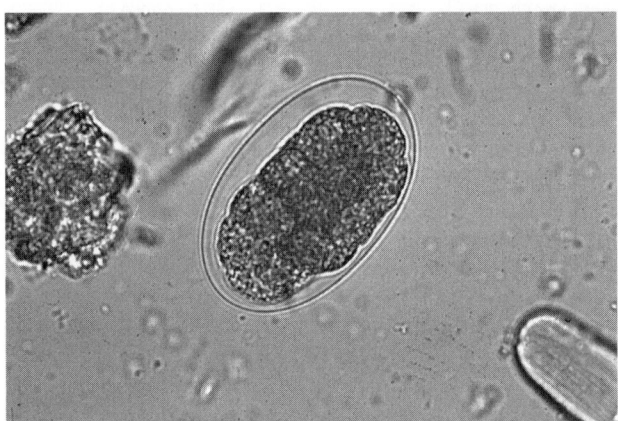

Fig. 1-199 Hookworm egg. Sixteen-cell stage of embryonation. (From Gorbach SL: *Infections diseases,* ed 2, Philadelphia, 1998, WB Saunders.)

BASIC INFORMATION

DEFINITION
A hordeolum is an acute inflammatory process affecting the eyelid and arising from the meibomian (posterior) or Zeis (anterior) glands. It is most often infectious and usually caused by *Staphylococcus aureus*.

SYNONYMS
Stye

ICD-9CM CODES
373.11 External hordeolum
373.12 Internal hordeolum

EPIDEMIOLOGY & DEMOGRAPHICS
INCIDENCE (IN U.S.): Unknown
PREVALENCE (IN U.S.): Unknown
PREDOMINANT SEX: No gender predilection
PREDOMINANT AGE: May occur at any age
PEAK INCIDENCE: May occur at any age
NEONATAL INFECTION: Rare in the neonatal period

PHYSICAL FINDINGS & CLINICAL PRESENTATION
• Abrupt onset with pain and erythema of the eyelid
• Localized, tender mass in the eyelid (Fig. 1-200)
• May be associated with blepharitis
• External hordeolum: points toward the skin surface of the lid and may spontaneously drain
• Internal hordeolum: can point toward the conjunctival side of the lid and may cause conjunctival inflammation

ETIOLOGY
• 75% to 95% of cases are caused by *S. aureus*.
• Occasional cases are caused by *Streptococcus pneumoniae*, other streptococci, gram-negative enteric organisms, or mixed bacterial flora.

DIAGNOSIS

DIFFERENTIAL DIAGNOSIS
• Eyelid abscess
• Chalazion
• Allergy or contact dermatitis with conjunctival edema
• Acute dacryocystitis
• Herpes simplex infection
• Cellulitis of the eyelid

LABORATORY TESTS
• Generally, none are necessary.
• If incision and drainage are performed, specimens should be sent for bacterial culture.

IMAGING STUDIES
None necessary

TREATMENT

NONPHARMACOLOGIC THERAPY
Usually responds to warm compresses

ACUTE GENERAL Rx
• Systemic antibiotics generally not necessary
• In refractory cases, an oral anti-staphylococcal agent (e.g., dicloxacillin 500 mg PO qid) possibly helpful
• Topical erythromycin ophthalmic ointment applied to the lid margins two to four times daily until resolution
• Incision and drainage: rarely needed but should be considered for progressive infections

CHRONIC Rx
None necessary

DISPOSITION
• Usually sporadic occurrence
• Possible relapse if resolution is not complete

REFERRAL
• For evaluation by an ophthalmologist if visual acuity or ocular movement is affected or if the diagnosis is in doubt
• For surgical drainage if necessary

PEARLS & CONSIDERATIONS

COMMENTS
Seborrheic dermatitis may coexist with hordeolum.
Author: **Joseph R. Masci, M.D.**

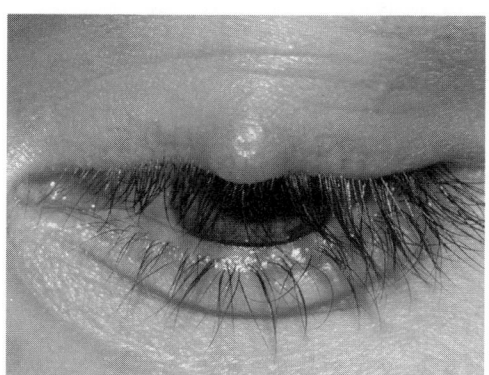

Fig. 1-200 External stye. (From Palay D [ed]: *Ophthalmology for the primary care physician,* St Louis, 1997, Mosby.)

BASIC INFORMATION

■ **DEFINITION**
Horner's syndrome is a cluster of physical findings including unilateral ptosis, miosis, and sometimes anhidrosis or hyperemia of the affected side of the face. These physical findings are the result of disruption of the cervical sympathetic pathway along its course from the hypothalamus to the eye. Disruption of any of the three neurons involved in the pathway (central, preganglionic, or postganglionic) can be the cause of Horner's syndrome.

ICD-9CM CODES
337.9 Horner's syndrome

■ **SYNONYMS**
Oculosympathetic paresis
Raeder's syndrome (painful Horner's syndrome of the postganglionic neuron)

■ **EPIDEMIOLOGY & DEMOGRAPHICS**
• May occur congenitally
• Associated with vascular disease and neoplasms

■ **PHYSICAL FINDINGS & CLINICAL PRESENTATION**
• Miosis on the affected side results from loss of sympathetic pupillodilator activity (Fig. 1-201).
• Affected pupil reacts normally to light and accommodation.
• Variable degree of ptosis results from loss of sympathetic tone to eyelid muscles.
• Anhidrosis may occur with lesions below the superior cervical ganglion (central or preganglionic neurons).

• Conjunctival or facial hyperemia may occur on the affected side because of loss of sympathetic vasoconstrictor activity.
• In congenital Horner's syndrome, the iris on the affected side may fail to become pigmented, resulting in heterochromia of the iris, with the affected iris remaining blue-gray.

■ **ETIOLOGY**
Lesions affecting any of the neurons involved in the sympathetic pathway can cause Horner's syndrome.
  Mechanical:
• Syringomyelia
• Trauma
• Benign tumors
• Malignant tumors (especially Pancoast tumor)
• Neurofibromatosis
• Metastatic tumor
• Cervical rib
• Lymphadenopathy
• Cervical disk prolapse
  Vascular:
• Posterior inferior cerebellar artery (Wallenberg) syndrome
• Internal carotid artery aneurysm, dissection, or surgery
• Angiography
• Cluster headache, migraine
• Congenital
• Idiopathic
  Miscellaneous:
• Pneumothorax
• Herpes zoster
• Radiation

 DIAGNOSIS

■ **DIFFERENTIAL DIAGNOSIS**
Causes of anisocoria:
• Normal variant
• Mydriatic use

• Prosthetic eye
• Unilateral cataract
• Iritis
• Disorders causing ptosis are described in Table 2-167.

■ **WORKUP**
History, physical examination, and imaging

■ **IMAGING STUDIES**
• Chest x-ray for patients with suspected apical lung (Pancoast) tumor
• CT scan or MRI of the head and neck to identify lesions affecting the cervical sympathetic pathway

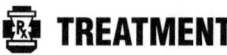 **TREATMENT**

Treatment depends on underlying cause.

■ **DISPOSITION**
Prognosis depends on underlying cause. Horner's syndrome is an uncommon presentation for malignancy. In one study, 60% of cases were idiopathic.

■ **REFERRAL**
• To vascular surgeon for carotid disease
• To oncologist for Pancoast tumor
Author: **Mark J. Fagan, M.D.**

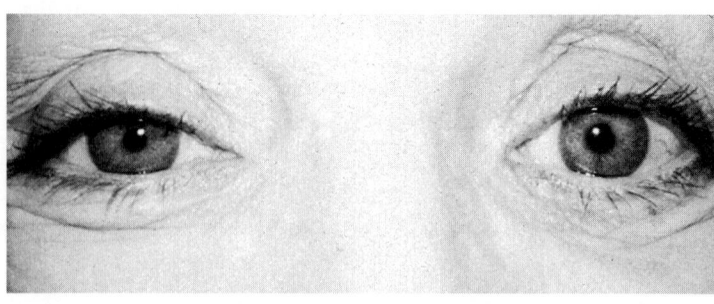

Fig. 1-201 Horner's syndrome. The mild ptosis (1 to 2 mm) and smaller pupil (in room light) can be seen on the affected right side. (From Palay D [ed]: *Ophthalmology for the primary care physician,* St Louis, 1997, Mosby.)

BASIC INFORMATION

■ DEFINITION

Human granulocytic ehrlichiosis (HGE) is a zoonotic infection of granulocytes, caused by an *Ehrlichia* species closely related to *E. phagocytophila, E. equi* and *E. ewingii,* with multisystem manifestations.

■ ICD-9CM CODES

082-8 other tick-borne rickettsiosis

■ EPIDEMIOLOGY & DEMOGRAPHICS

INCIDENCE (IN U.S.): Highest overall incidence in New York, New Jersey, Connecticut, Wisconsin, Minnesota, and northern California. >600 cases identified in the U.S. since 1990.
PREDOMINANT SEX: Males outnumber females by 2 to 1.
PREDOMINANT AGE: Most severe disease 50 to 70 yr.
PEAK INCIDENCE: Occurs throughout the year, with peak incidence between May and July and again in November.

■ PHYSICAL FINDINGS & CLINICAL PRESENTATION

- Most common initial symptoms:
  1. Fever
  2. Chills, rigor
  3. Headache
  4. Myalgia
- Subsequent symptoms
  1. Anorexia, nausea
  2. Arthralgia
  3. Cough
  4. Confusion
  5. Abdominal pain
  6. Rash (erythematous to pustular) rare (<11%)
- Complications
  1. Hepatitis
  2. Interstitial pneumonitis
  3. Noncardiogenic pulmonary edema
  4. Renal insufficiency
  5. Bilateral facial palsy
  6. Meningitis

■ ETIOLOGY

- Obligate intracellular gram-negative bacterium (family *Rickettsiaceae,* genus *Ehrlichia*), closely related to *E. phagocytophila, E. equi,* and *E. ewingii.*
- Vector:
  1. Almost certainly tick-borne, recently transmitted by infected blood.
  2. Transmitted by *Ixodes scapularis* in the northeastern and upper midwestern states and *Ixodes pacificus* in the Pacific western states.
  3. Tick exposure reported in >90% of patients, with approximately 60% reporting tick bite.

- Mammalian host: deer, horses, dogs, white-footed mice, cattle, sheep, goats, bison.
- Precise pathogenesis is unclear, although host inflammatory and immune responses may define final spectrum of disease beyond granulocytes, including hepatitis, interstitial pneumonitis, and nephritis with mild azotemia.
- Between 6% and 21% of patients with HGE also have serologic evidence of other infection, both transmitted by *Ixodes* spp. tick bites.
- Recovery is usual outcome; fatality rate of HGE is <1%.

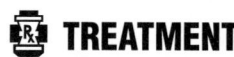

DIAGNOSIS

■ DIFFERENTIAL DIAGNOSIS

- Human monocytic ehrlichiosis (HME)
  1. Caused by *E. chaffeensis* (vector: tick *Amblyomma americanum,* possibly *Dermocenter variabilis*)
  2. Rash more common, sometimes petechial
  3. Morulae in monocytes
- Rocky Mountain spotted fever, Colorado tick fever, Q fever, relapsing fever
- Babesiosis
- Leptospirosis
- Typhus
- Lyme disease
- Legionnaire's disease
- Tularemia
- Typhoid fever, paratyphoid fever
- Brucellosis
- Viral hepatitis
- Enteroviral infections
- Meningococcemia
- Influenza
- Adenovirus pneumonia

■ WORKUP

- Acute blood samples for Giemsa-stained smears
- CBC
- Prothrombin time
- Acute serum samples for serology
- Chest x-ray examination
- Liver function and renal function tests
- MRI
- CSF analysis
- Bone marrow rarely needed

■ LABORATORY TESTS

- Giemsa-stained smear demonstrating morulae of *Ehrlichia* within granulocytes
- CBC progressive leukopenia and thrombocytopenia with nadir near day 7
- C reactive protein concentration is generally elevated

- Liver function test—twofold to fourfold increase in concentration of hepatic transaminases
- Serologic titer (IFA) >80 or fourfold increase in titer to *E. equi* antigen
- Polymerase chain reaction (PCR) to facilitate early diagnosis
- Culture on the first 7 days of illness
- Spinal tap for PCR analysis

■ IMAGING STUDIES

- Chest x-ray examination to show interstitial pneumonitis (unusual)
- MRI of the brain

TREATMENT

■ ACUTE GENERAL Rx

- Immediate therapy to limit extent of acute illness and complication.
- Tetracycline and doxycyclin have demonstrated marked activity against the HGE, although doxycyclin has been preferred because of a better pharmacokinetic profile and better toleration by patient.
- Rifampin is an alternative drug of choice.

■ CHRONIC Rx

Probably unnecessary; undefined

■ PROGNOSIS

Poor prognostic indicators include:
1. Advanced age
2. Concomitant chronic illness (such as diabetes mellitus, collagen vascular disease)
3. Lack of diagnosis recognition
4. Delayed onset of specific antibiotic therapy

■ DISPOSITION

- Follow-up as outpatient
- Repeat CBC every 2 to 4 wk until normal

■ REFERRAL

- For consultation with infectious diseases specialist and hematologist in suspected cases
- For coagulopathy

PEARLS & CONSIDERATIONS

■ COMMENTS

Duration of time tick must be attached to produce illness is at least 24 hr.

REFERENCE

Bakken JS, Dumler JS: Human granulocytic ehrlichiosis *Clin Infect Dis* 31:554, 2000.
Author: **Vasanthi Arumugam, M.D.**

BASIC INFORMATION

■ **DEFINITION**
The human immunodeficiency virus, type 1 (HIV) causes a chronic infection that culminates, usually after several years, in acquired immunodeficiency syndrome (AIDS).

■ **SYNONYMS**
Acquired immunodeficiency syndrome (AIDS) when a patient with HIV infection meets specific diagnostic criteria (see "Acquired Immunodeficiency Syndrome" in Section I)

ICD-9CM CODES
044.9 HIV, unspecified

■ **EPIDEMIOLOGY & DEMOGRAPHICS**
INCIDENCE (IN U.S.):
• No complete incidence data available.
• Greatest incidence is in metropolitan areas with population >500,000.
PREVALENCE (IN U.S.): Estimated at 1 to 2 million cases.
PREDOMINANT SEX:
• Adults: Most recently, estimated to be 74% males, 24% females, but is changing toward more women
• Children: male = female
PREDOMINANT AGE: 80% of cases occur between ages 20 and 40 yr
PEAK INCIDENCE: Age 30 to 35 yr
GENETICS:
Familial Disposition: No proven genetic predisposition
Congenital Infection:
• 80% of childhood cases are caused by peripartum infection, which may occur in utero, during delivery, or after delivery via breast-feeding.
• No specific congenital abnormalities are associated with HIV infection, although risk of spontaneous abortion and low birth weight is greater.
Neonatal Infection:
• May occur during delivery or via breast-feeding
• Typically asymptomatic

■ **PHYSICAL FINDINGS & CLINICAL PRESENTATION**
• Signs and symptoms variable with stage of disease (Boxes 2-127 to 2-131 and Tables 2-92 to 2-102)
• In acute infection:
  1. May cause a self-limited mononucleosis-like illness characterized by fever, sore throat, lymphadenopathy, headache, and a rash resembling roseola.
  2. In a minority of acute cases: frank aseptic meningitis, Bell's palsy, or peripheral neuropathy.

• Later in the course of infection, after a prolonged asymptomatic phase: nonspecific symptoms of lymphadenopathy, weight loss, diarrhea, and skin changes including seborrheic dermatitis, localized herpes zoster, or fungal infection.
• Advanced disease: characterized by the infections and malignancies associated with acquired immunodeficiency syndrome (see specific disorders).
• Table 2-102 describes rheumatic syndromes in HIV infection.

■ **ETIOLOGY**
• RNA retrovirus (Fig. 1-202)
• Transmitted by sexual contact, shared needles, blood transfusion, or from mother to child during pregnancy, delivery, or breast-feeding
• Primary target of infection: CD4 lymphocyte
• Direct CNS involvement: manifested as encephalopathy, myelopathy, or neuropathy in advanced cases
• Renal failure, rheumatologic disorders, thrombocytopenia, or cardiac abnormalities
• Table 2-102 describes rheumatic syndromes in HIV infection.

 DIAGNOSIS

■ **DIFFERENTIAL DIAGNOSIS**
• Acute infection: mononucleosis or other respiratory viral infections
• Late symptoms: similar to those produced by other wasting illnesses such as neoplasms, TB, disseminated fungal infection, malabsorption, or depression
• HIV-related encephalopathy: confused with Alzheimer's disease or other causes of chronic dementia (cognitive impairment in HIV infection is described in Box 2-128); myelopathy and neuropathy possibly resembling other demyelinating diseases such as multiple sclerosis

■ **WORKUP**
Diagnosis is established by voluntary testing for antibody to the virus, available through public health laboratories or private facilities.

■ **LABORATORY TESTS**
HIV antibody detected by a two-step technique:
• ELISA as a sensitive screening test
• Confirmation of positive ELISA tests with the more specific Western blot technique
• Fig. 1-203 describes the immunologic response to HIV infection

 TREATMENT

■ **NONPHARMACOLOGIC THERAPY**
Maintenance of adequate nutrition

■ **ACUTE GENERAL Rx**
• Acute management of opportunistic infections and malignancies (see AIDS-associated disorders, "*Pneumocystis carinii* Pneumonia," "Cryptococcosis," "Tuberculosis," "Toxoplasmosis" elsewhere in this text)
• Acute HIV syndrome:
  1. Treat with combination antiretroviral therapy, consisting of one or more nucleoside agents (zidovudine [AZT], didanosine [DDI], zalcitabine [DDC], lamivudine [3TC] abacavir) with a protease inhibitor (ritonavir, indinavir, saquinavir melfinavir aquerate), or nonnucleoside reverse transcriptase inhibitors (nevirapine, delavirdine, efavirenz)
  2. Recommended doses of these drugs and specific combinations are currently being assessed

■ **CHRONIC Rx**
• All HIV-infected patients should be considered candidates for therapy with two- or three-drug combinations of the agents listed above.
• Specific recommendations are evolving, dictated by clinical and immunologic stage, as well as measurements of viral load and genotypic resistance testing. See also "Acquired Immunodeficiency Syndrome."
• Patients with CD4 lymphocyte count <200/mm^3 should be given preventive therapy for *Pneumocystis carinii* pneumonia (PCP) (see "*Pneumocystis carinii* pneumonia").
• Evaluation of chronic diarrhea in patients with HIV is described in Fig. 3-53 and Table 3-5.
• Table 1-5 describes primary prophylaxis of opportunistic infections in adults and adolescents with HIV infection. Criteria for discontinuing and restarting opportunistic prophylaxis for adults with HIV infection is described in Table 1-6.

■ **DISPOSITION**
• Ongoing care consisting of frequent medical evaluations and T-lymphocyte subset analysis
• Long-term care focused on providing up-to-date antiretroviral therapy and prophylaxis of PCP and other opportunistic infections, as well as early detection of complications (see Figs. 3-80 to 3-82)

■ REFERRAL
To a physician knowledgeable and experienced in the management of HIV infection and its complications

REFERENCES
Carpenter C et al: Antiretroviral therapy in adults, updated recommendations of the International AIDS Society-USA Panel, *JAMA* 283:381, 2000.

Cohen OJ: Antiretroviral therapy: time to think strategically, *Ann Intern Med* 132(4):320, 2000.
Schacker TW et al: Biological and virologic characteristics of primary HIV infection, *Ann Intern Med* 128:613, 1998.
Author: **Joseph R. Masci, M.D.**

☼ PEARLS & CONSIDERATIONS

■ COMMENTS
• HIV chemoprophylaxis after occupational exposure is described in Box 5-10 and Tables 5-29 and 5-30.

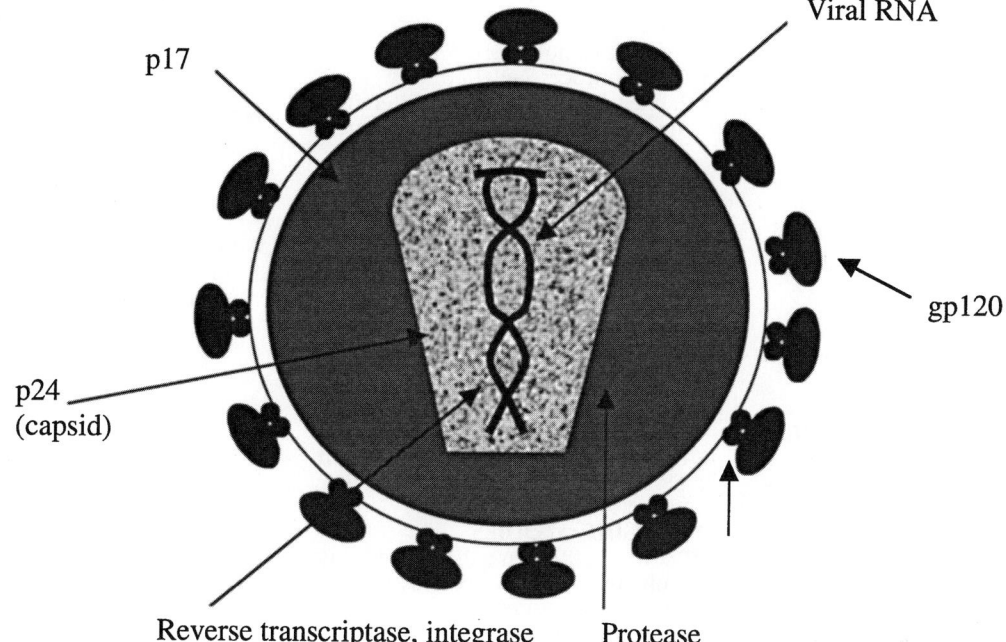

Fig. 1-202   Locations of viral proteins and nucleic acids in the HIV-1 virion. (From Mandell GL: *Mandell, Douglas, and Bennett's principles and practice of infectious diseases,* ed 5, New York, 2000, Churchill Livingstone.)

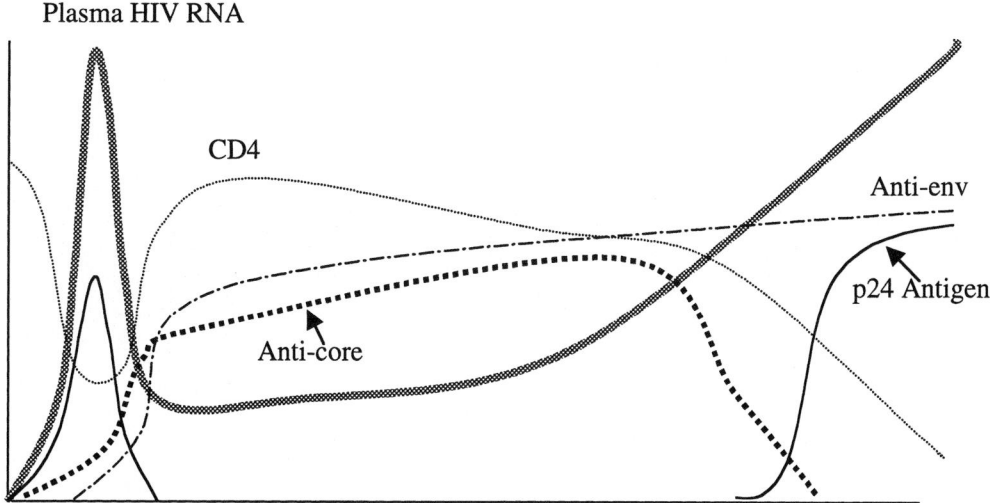

Fig. 1-203   Course of human immunodeficiency virus infection. (From Mandell GL: *Mandell, Douglas, and Bennett's principles and practice of infectious diseases,* ed 5, New York, 2000, Churchill Livingstone.)

BASIC INFORMATION

■ **DEFINITION**
Huntington's chorea is an inherited progressive neurodegenerative disorder characterized by choreoathetosis and neuropsychiatric dysfunction associated with pronounced neuronal loss in the caudate nucleus.

■ **SYNONYMS**
Huntington's disease

ICD-9CM CODES
333.4 Huntington's chorea

■ **EPIDEMIOLOGY & DEMOGRAPHICS**
PREVALENCE (IN U.S.): 4.1 to 5.4 cases/100,000 persons
PREDOMINANT SEX: Female = male
PREDOMINANT AGE: Early adulthood
PEAK INCIDENCE: Late 30s and 40s, with onsets from age 2 to 70 yr
GENETICS: Autosomal dominant; responsible gene an expanded trinucleotide repeat sequence located on the short arm of chromosome 4

■ **PHYSICAL FINDINGS & CLINICAL PRESENTATION**
• Initially, subtle disturbance of oculomotor function, small choreiform movements, or psychiatric dysfunction
• With progression, pronounced choreoathetotic movements, resulting in a characteristically erratic gait
• Juvenile onset variant: cognitive dysfunction, bradykinesia, and rigidity

■ **ETIOLOGY**
• Unknown
• Proposed cause: excitatory amino acid transmitter–mediated toxicity

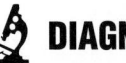 **DIAGNOSIS**

■ **DIFFERENTIAL DIAGNOSIS**
• Drug-induced chorea
• Sydenham's chorea
• Benign hereditary chorea
• Senile chorea
• Wilson's disease
• Neuroacanthocytosis
• Olivopontocerebellar atrophy
• Table 2-105 describes the differential diagnosis of hyperkinetic movement disorders.

■ **WORKUP**
Onset of symptoms in an individual with an established family history requires no additional investigation.

■ **LABORATORY TESTS**
• Confirm diagnosis by chromosome analysis.
• If normal, obtain CBC with smear, ESR, electrolytes, serum ceruloplasmin, 24-hr urinary copper excretion, TFT, ANA, VDRL, HIV, and ASO titer.

■ **IMAGING STUDIES**
CT scan or MRI scan will show caudate atrophy in more advanced cases.

 TREATMENT

■ **NONPHARMACOLOGIC THERAPY**
• Supportive counseling
• Physical and occupational therapy
• Home health care
• Genetic counseling

■ **CHRONIC Rx**
• Chorea may be diminished by low doses of neuroleptics (e.g., haloperidol 1 to 10 mg/day).
• Depression with suicidal ideation is common; may improve with tricyclic or SSRI antidepressants.

■ **DISPOSITION**
Relentless, progressive course of variable duration leading to progressive disability and death

■ **REFERRAL**
If uncertain about diagnosis or management
Author: **Michael Gruenthal, M.D., Ph.D.**

BASIC INFORMATION

■ **DEFINITION**
A hydrocele is a fluid collection in a serous scrotal space usually between the layers of the tunica vaginalis (Figs. 1-204 and 1-205)

ICD-9CM CODES
603.9 Hydrocele

■ **PHYSICAL FINDINGS & CLINICAL PRESENTATION**
Symptoms:
• Scrotal enlargement
• Scrotal heaviness or discomfort radiating to the inguinal area
• Back pain
Physical findings:
• Scrotal distention (testicle may be impossible to palpate)
• Transillumination

■ **ETIOLOGY & PATHOGENESIS**
Hydroceles may occur as a congenital abnormality where the processus vaginalis fails to close. In this case, an inguinal hernia is virtually always associated with the malformation. Congenital hydroceles are most common in infants and children. In adults, hydroceles are more frequently caused by infection, tumor, or trauma. Infection of the epididymis often results in the development of a secondary hydrocele. Tropical infections such as filariasis may produce hydroceles.

 DIAGNOSIS

■ **DIFFERENTIAL DIAGNOSIS**
• Spermatocele
• Inguinoscrotal hernia
• Testicular tumor
• Varicocele
• Epididymitis

■ **IMAGING**
Scrotal ultrasound (useful to rule out a testicular tumor as the cause of the hydrocele)

TREATMENT

• No treatment if asymptomatic and testicle is thought to be normal
• Surgical repair

REFERENCE
Rowland RG, Foster RS, Donohue JP: Scrotum and testis. In Gillenwater JY et al (eds): *Adult and pediatric urology,* ed 3, St Louis, 1996, Mosby.
Author: **Tom J. Wachtel, M.D.**

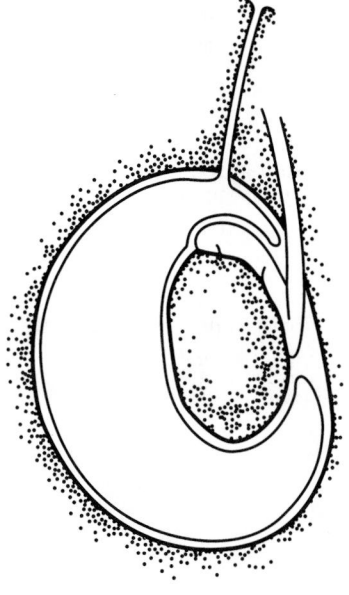

Fig. 1-204 A hydrocele is a fluid collection in the serous space between the layers of the tunica vaginalis. The tunica vaginalis may or may not remain patent, allowing the hydrocele to communicate with the peritoneum.

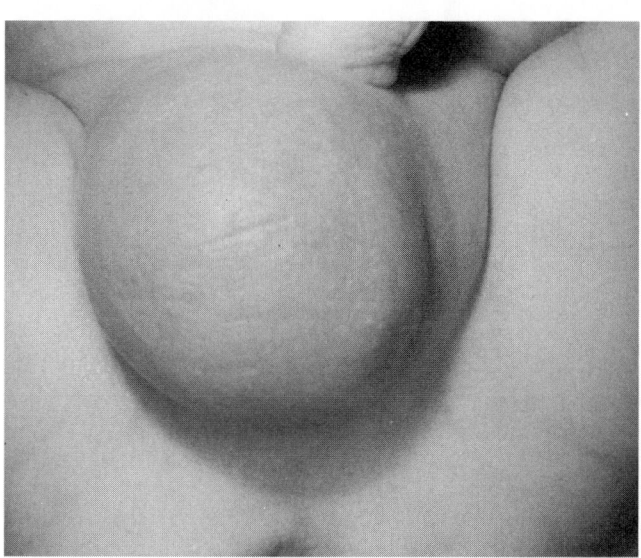

Fig. 1-205 Newborn with large right hydrocele. (From Behrman RE: *Nelson textbook of pediatrics,* ed 16, Philadelphia, 2000, WB Saunders.)

BASIC INFORMATION

■ DEFINITION
Normal pressure hydrocephalus (NPH) is marked by a clinical triad of gait disturbance, mental deterioration, and urinary incontinence associated with chronic hydrocephalus and normal CSF pressure as measured by routine lumbar puncture.

ICD-9CM CODES
742.3 Congenital hydrocephalus

■ EPIDEMIOLOGY & DEMOGRAPHICS
PREDOMINANT SEX: Males = females
PREDOMINANT AGE: Fourth to sixth decade

■ PHYSICAL FINDINGS & CLINICAL PRESENTATION
- Initial symptoms: gait difficulty
- Typical finding: difficulty initiating ambulation, with the appearance that the feet are stuck to the floor ("magnetic gait")
- Cognitive slowing, forgetfulness and inattention without agnosia, aphasia, or other "cortical" disturbances
- Later signs: urinary urgency and subsequent incontinence

■ ETIOLOGY
- Most cases: chronic communicating hydrocephalus (50% idiopathic)
- Other 50%: result from prior subarachnoid hemorrhage, meningitis, trauma, or intracranial surgery

DIAGNOSIS

■ DIFFERENTIAL DIAGNOSIS
Signs and symptoms are nonspecific and may be seen with any process causing bilateral periventricular white matter lesions.

■ WORKUP
- Lumbar puncture with accurate opening pressure measurement is essential; elevated opening pressure suggests more acute process, which must be investigated.
- Numerous attempts at establishing a confirming test have been disappointing.
- Clinical response to removal of CSF and isotope cisternography are popular, but lack sensitivity or specificity to confirm the diagnosis or predict improvement from shunting.

■ LABORATORY TESTS
CSF should be sent for routine fluid analyses to exclude other pathology.

■ IMAGING STUDIES
CT scan (Fig. 1-206), MRI, and isotope cisternography are popular but unreliable.

TREATMENT

■ NONPHARMACOLOGIC THERAPY
- Some patients (30% of those with idiopathic NPH and 60% of patients with a known etiology) show significant improvement from shunting.
- There is a better outcome with early shunting, before substantial cognitive decline or incontinence.

PEARLS & CONSIDERATIONS

■ CAUTION
This is a rare disease often overdiagnosed by radiologists.

■ ACUTE GENERAL Rx
Shunting in selected patients

■ REFERRAL
Neurosurgical referral for shunting in appropriate patients.
Author: **Michael Gruenthal, M.D., Ph.D.**

A   **B**   **C**

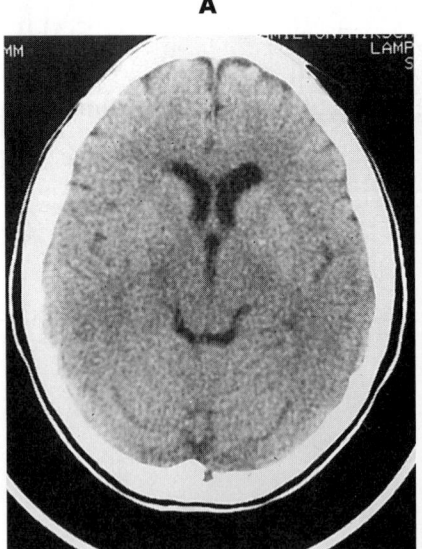
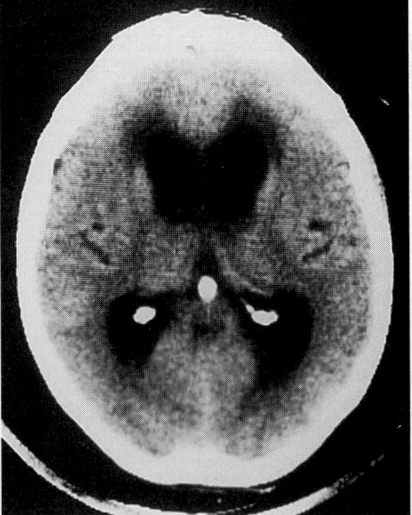
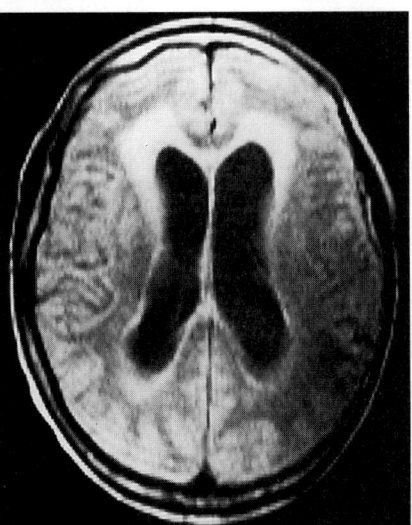

Fig. 1-206 Communicating hydrocephalus. A 61-year-old woman 7 years after uncomplicated removal of carcinoma of the lung developed symptoms of headache and depression of mood. Neurologic examination and CT scan evaluation **(A)** were considered unremarkable. Over the next 4 months she became increasingly withdrawn, occasionally incontinent, and finally disoriented. She developed a broad-based ataxic gait, and CT scan showed ventricular dilation **(B).** MRI confirmed the ventricular enlargement and showed periventricular increased signals typical of edema **(C).** Spinal fluid contained increased protein, glucose 25 mg/dl, and malignant cells. Cerebrospinal fluid pressure was 180 mm in the lateral recumbent position. Her alertness and gait temporarily improved following spinal drainage. (From Andreoli TE [ed]: *Cecil essentials of medicine,* ed 4, Philadelphia, 1997, WB Saunders.)

BASIC INFORMATION

■ DEFINITION
Hydronephrosis is dilation of the renal pyelocalyceal system, most often as a result of impairment of urinary flow.

■ SYNONYMS
Hydroureter (dilation of ureter, often seen with hydronephrosis when obstruction is in lower urinary tract)
Urinary tract obstruction

ICD-9CM CODES
591 Acquired hydronephrosis
753.2 Congenital hydronephrosis

■ EPIDEMIOLOGY & DEMOGRAPHICS
Children usually have congenital malformations, whereas adults tend to have acquired defects as etiologies.

■ PHYSICAL FINDINGS & CLINICAL PRESENTATION
HISTORY:
- Pain is caused by distention of collecting system or renal capsule and is more related to the rate of onset than the degree of obstruction. It can vary in location from flank to lower abdomen to testes/labia. Pain in flank occurring only on micturition is highly suggestive of vesicoureteral reflux.
- Anuria can occur with total obstruction of urinary flow (bilateral hydronephrosis or unilateral if only one kidney is present).
- Polyuria or nocturia can occur with chronic (incomplete) obstruction because of deleterious effects on renal concentrating ability (nephrogenic diabetes insipidus).
- Urinary frequency, hesitancy, postvoid dribbling, and difficulty initiating stream are all symptoms that can occur with obstruction at or below the bladder (e.g., prostatic hyperplasia).
- Chronic urinary infections can either result from chronic urinary obstruction (organisms favoring growth with stasis of urine) or lead to conditions (e.g., urine pH changes) that favor stone formation and subsequent obstruction.

PHYSICAL EXAMINATION:
- Hypertension can be caused by increased renin release in acute or subacute obstruction.
- Fever or CVA tenderness can suggest urinary tract infection.
- Distended bladder or kidneys present.
- Rectal examination should be done to evaluate prostate for size and nodularity and also to check rectal sphincter tone.
- Pelvic examination is done to assess for vaginal anatomy, pelvic mass, or PID.
- Penile examination performed to rule out meatal stenosis or phimosis.
- Bladder catheterization is needed to assess postvoid residual volume if urinary tract obstruction is considered. NOTE: Rule out postrenal obstruction in unexplained acute renal failure.

■ ETIOLOGY
MECHANICAL IMPAIRMENTS:
- Congenital: ureteropelvic junction narrowing, ureterovesical junction narrowing, ureterocele, retrocaval ureter, bladder neck obstruction, urethral valves, urethral stricture, meatal stenosis
- Acquired:
  1. Intrinsic to urinary tract: calculi, inflammation, trauma, sloughed papillae, ureteral tumor, blood clots, prostatic hypertrophy or cancer, bladder cancer, urethral stricture, phimosis
  2. Extrinsic to urinary tract: gravid uterus, retroperitoneal fibrosis or tumor (e.g., lymphoma), aortic aneurysm, uterine fibroids, trauma (surgical or nonsurgical), PID, pelvic malignancies (e.g., prostate, colorectal, cervical, uterine, bladder)

FUNCTIONAL IMPAIRMENTS:
- Neurogenic bladder (often with adynamic ureter) can occur with spinal cord disease or diabetic neuropathy.
- Pharmacologic agents such as α-adrenergic antagonists and anticholinergic drugs can inhibit bladder emptying.
- Vesicoureteral reflux may occur.
- Pregnancy causes hydroureter and hydronephrosis (right more often than left) as early as the second month. Hormonal effects on ureteral tone combine with mechanical factors.

DIAGNOSIS

■ DIFFERENTIAL DIAGNOSIS
- Urinary stones
- Neoplastic disease
- Prostatic hypertrophy

- Neurologic disease
- Urinary reflux
- Urinary tract infection
- Medication effects
- Trauma
- Congenital abnormality of urinary tract

■ LABORATORY TESTS
- Serum BUN and creatinine to assess for renal insufficiency (usually implies bilateral obstruction or unilateral obstruction of a solitary kidney).
- Electrolytes may reveal hypernatremia (if nephrogenic DI), hyperkalemia (from renal failure and effects on tubular function), or distal renal tubular acidosis.
- Urinalysis and examination of sediment may reveal WBCs, RBCs, or bacteria in the appropriate setting (e.g., infection, stones), but often the sediment is normal in obstructive renal disease.

■ IMAGING STUDIES
- Abdominal plain film of kidneys, ureters, and bladder is used to look for nephrocalcinosis or a radiopaque stone.
- Assess kidney and bladder size with ultrasound; contour of pyelocalyces and ureters (Fig. 1-207). Ultrasound is about 90% sensitive and specific for hydronephrosis and is noninvasive, so it will not worsen preexisting renal insufficiency.
- Intravenous pyelogram (IVP) helps localize the site of obstruction (Fig. 1-208) when hydronephrosis is seen on ultrasound, but the contrast may have deleterious effects on the kidneys if there is renal insufficiency.
- Antegrade or retrograde urograms can be performed if renal failure is a concern with IVP and either of these two procedures could be extended to provide relief of the obstruction.
- Abdominal CT scan can be done without IV contrast and provides excellent localization of the site of obstruction.
- Voiding cystourethrogram is helpful in diagnosing vesicoureteral reflux and obstructions of the bladder neck or urethra.

TREATMENT

- Urgent treatment is required if urinary tract obstruction is associated with urinary tract infection, acute renal failure, or uncontrollable pain.

- Conservative management of calculi with IV fluid, IV antibiotics (if evidence of infection), and aggressive analgesia may be enough to treat acute unilateral urinary tract obstruction depending on the size (90% of stones <5 mm will pass spontaneously).
- Urethral catheter is adequate to relieve most obstructions at or distal to the bladder, but occasionally a suprapubic catheter will be required (e.g., impassable urethral stricture or urethral injury). Neurogenic bladder may require intermittent clean catheterization if frequent voiding and pharmacologic treatments are ineffective.
- Nephrostomy tube can be placed percutaneously to facilitate urinary drainage.
- Extracorporeal shock wave lithotripsy (ESWL) is used to fragment large stones to facilitate spontaneous passage or subsequent extraction (NOTE: ESWL is contraindicated in pregnancy).
- Nephroscopy is performed for extraction of proximal stones under direct vision.
- Cystoscopy with ureteroscopy is used for removal of distal ureteral stones using a loop or basket with or without fragmentation by ultrasonic or laser lithotripsy.
- Ureteral stents can be used for extrinsic and some intrinsic ureteral obstructions.
- Urethral dilation or internal urethrotomy can be used for urethral strictures.
- Nephrectomy or ureteral diversion may be required in severe cases (e.g., malignancy).
- Ureterovesical reimplantation can be used for reflux disease.
- Transurethral retrograde prostatectomy (TURP) is used for severe obstruction from BPH.

- IV fluid and electrolyte replacement is needed; the patient must be monitored closely during the postobstructive diuresis (usually lasting several days to a week).

■ DISPOSITION
Aggressive treatment of infections and early relief of obstruction can usually prevent progressive loss of renal function; however, chronic bilateral obstruction (often from BPH) can lead to chronic renal failure.

■ REFERRAL
- Urologist consultation early for diagnostic and/or therapeutic procedures
- Oncologist if a neoplasm is diagnosed
- Gynecologist if pregnancy or female pelvic anatomy is involved

Author: **William F. Boyd, M.D.**

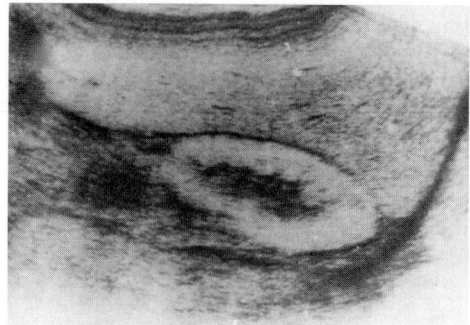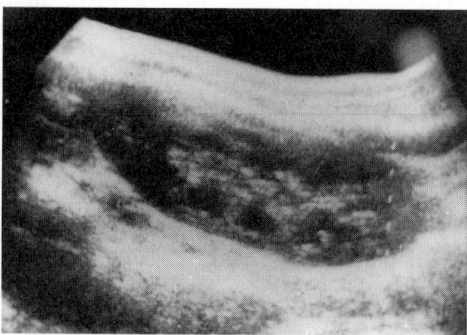

Fig. 1-207 Renal ultrasound. **A,** Normal features include peripheral homogeneous thick cortex (white) and central heterogeneous fluid-filled calyces (black). Note that individual calyces cannot be visualized. **B,** In acute hydronephrosis, features include normal cortex (gray) and dilated calyces (gray areas within central white). (From Harrington J [ed]: *Consultation in internal medicine,* ed 2, St Louis, 1997, Mosby.)

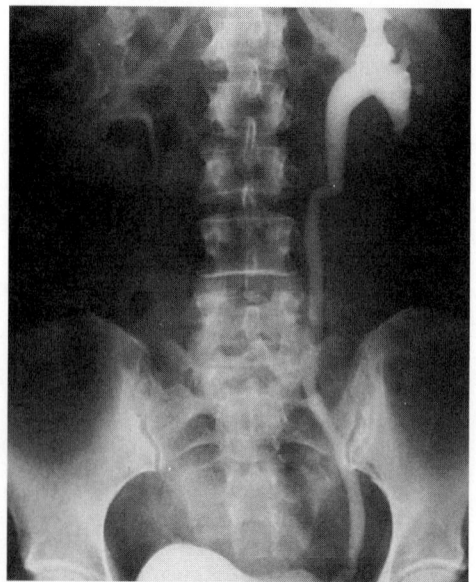

Fig. 1-208 Left-side obstruction demonstrating dense nephrogram-dilated collecting system and ureter. Calculus of the ureterovesicle junction *(open arrow),* is responsible for the obstruction. (From Stein JH [ed]: *Internal medicine,* ed 5, St Louis, 1998, Mosby.)

BASIC INFORMATION

■ DEFINITION

Hypercholesterolemia refers to a blood cholesterol measurement >200 mg/dl. A cholesterol level of 200 to 239 mg/dl is considered borderline high, and a level of ≥240 mg/dl is considered to be a high cholesterol measurement.

■ SYNONYMS

Hypercholesteremia
Hypercholesterinemia
Type II familial hyperlipoproteinemia

ICD-9CM CODES

272.0 Hypercholesterolemia

■ EPIDEMIOLOGY & DEMOGRAPHICS

INCIDENCE/PREVALENCE:

- There are well over 100 million Americans with a total serum cholesterol >200 mg/dl.
- Elevated cholesterol requires drug therapy in about 60 million Americans.
- Incidence of heterozygous familial hypercholesterolemia: about 1:500.
- Incidence of homozygous familial hypercholesterolemia: about 1:1 million.
- Prevalence of hypercholesterolemia increases with increasing age.

GENETICS:

- Familial hypercholesterolemia: autosomal dominant disorder
- Familial combined hyperlipidemia: possibly an autosomal dominant disorder
- Multifactorial predilection: apparent in majority of affected individuals

RISK FACTORS:

- Dietary intake
- Genetic predisposition
- Sedentary lifestyle
- Associated secondary causes

■ PHYSICAL FINDINGS & CLINICAL PRESENTATION

- Most patients: no physical findings
- Possible findings particularly in the familial forms
  1. Tendon xanthomas
  2. Xanthelasma
  3. Arcus corneae
  4. Arterial bruits (young adulthood)

■ ETIOLOGY

Primary
  1. Genetics
  2. Obesity
  3. Dietary intake
Secondary
  1. Diabetes mellitus
  2. Alcohol
  3. Oral contraceptives
  4. Hypothyroidism
  5. Glucocorticoid use
  6. Most diuretics
  7. Nephrotic syndrome
  8. Hepatoma
  9. Extrahepatic biliary obstruction
  10. Primary biliary cirrhosis

DIAGNOSIS

■ DIFFERENTIAL DIAGNOSIS

- No real differential diagnosis; however, consider underlying secondary causes/etiologies for the elevated cholesterol.

■ LABORATORY TESTS

PRIMARY PREVENTION WITHOUT ATHEROSCLEROSIS:

  1. Total cholesterol <200 mg/dl, and the HDL >35: repeat in 5 yr.
  2. Cholesterol 200 to 239 mg/dl and the HDL >35: discuss dietary modification, repeat in 1 to 2 yr.
  3. Total cholesterol >240 mg/dl or the HDL <35 mg/dl: need a fasting lipid profile (cholesterol, HDL, triglycerides, from which an LDL can be calculated).
  4. Fasting lipid profile with LDL <130 mg/dl: dietary guidance and repeat in 5 yr.
  5. Fasting lipid profile with LDL 130 to 159 mg/dl (borderline high risk), and less than two risk factors for CAD: diet and exercise modification, with repeat profile in 1 yr.
  6. Fasting lipid profile with LDL >160 mg/dl or borderline LDL and two or more risk factors for CAD: need drug therapy.

SECONDARY PREVENTION WITHOUT ATHEROSCLEROSIS OR DIABETES MELLITUS:

  1. All patients: fasting lipid profile
  2. If LDL <100 mg/dl: instruction on diet and exercise, and repeat annually
  3. If LDL >100 mg/dl: drug therapy required

TREATMENT

■ NONPHARMACOLOGIC THERAPY

- First line of treatment: dietary therapy (see Box 1-19)
- Dietary modifications
  1. Low-cholesterol, low-fat diet (fat intake to 30% or less of the total caloric intake)
  2. Saturated fats <7% of total calories
  3. No more than 200 mg/day of cholesterol
- Increased activity with aerobic exercise: encourage 20 to 30 min of aerobic exercise three to four times a week
- Smoking cessation encouraged
- Counseling on CAD risk factors

■ ACUTE GENERAL Rx

No acute treatment needed

■ CHRONIC Rx

- In primary prevention: needed for patients with LDL >160 mg/dl or LDL 130 to 159 mg/dl with two or more risk factors for CAD
- In secondary prevention: needed for patients with known CAD, vascular disease or diabetes mellitus, and LDL >100 mg/dl
- In primary prevention: considered in patients on dietary therapy with LDL >190 mg/dl with no risk factors, LDL >160 mg/dl with two or more risk factors, or HDL <30 mg/dl
- Medications that can be used (see Table 1-35):
  1. Bile acid sequestrants (poorly tolerated)
  2. Niacin (poorly tolerated)
  3. HMG-CoA reductase inhibitors ("statins")
  4. Fibric acids
  5. Medication tailored to the patient's lipid profile, life-style, and the medication's side effect profile
- Bile acid sequestrants to lower LDL
- Niacin to lower LDL and triglycerides and raise HDL
- HMG-CoA reductase inhibitors to lower LDL
- Fibric acids work to lower triglycerides more than LDL

I

■ DISPOSITION

- After initiation of therapy, repeat laboratory tests in 4 to 6 wk, with modifications as necessary.
- Once goal is achieved, lifelong medication and monitoring are needed at least three to four times a year.
- Dietary modification is needed to continue with drug therapy.
- Repeat review for additional CAD risk factors.

⚙ PEARLS & CONSIDERATIONS

■ COMMENTS

Figs. 1-209, 1-210 describe algorithms for hyperlipidemia.

REFERENCES

Cleeman JI: Detection and evaluation of dyslipoproteinemia, *Endocrinol Metab Clin North Am* 27(3):597, 1998.

Illingworth DR: Management of hypercholesterolemia, *Med Clin North Am* 84(1):23, 2000.

National Cholesterol Education Program: Second Report on the Expert Panel on Detection, Evaluation, and Treatment of High Cholesterol in Adults (adult treatment panel III), *JAMA* 285:2486, 2001.

Author: **Beth J. Wutz, M.D.**

TABLE 1-35 Drugs Affecting Lipoprotein Metabolism

DRUG CLASS	AGENTS AND DAILY DOSES	LIPID/LIPOPROTEIN EFFECTS		SIDE EFFECTS	CONTRAINDICATIONS
HMG-CoA reductase inhibitors (statins)	Lovastatin (20-80 mg) Pravastatin (20-80 mg) Simvastatin (20-80 mg) Fluvastatin (20-80 mg) Atorvastatin (10-80 mg)	LDL HDL TG	↓18%-55% ↑5%-15% ↓7%-30%	Myopathy Increased liver enzymes	Absolute: • Active or chronic liver disease Relative: • Concomitant use of certain drugs*
Bile acid sequestrants	Cholestyramine (4-16 g) Colestipol (5-20 g) Colesevelam (2.6-3.8 g)	LDL HDL TG	↓1.5%-30% ↑3%-5% No change or increase	Gastrointestinal distress Constipation Decreased absorption of other drugs	Absolute: • Dysbetalipoproteinemia • TG >400 mg/dl Relative: • TG >200 mg/dl
Nicotinic acid	Immediate release (crystalline) nicotinic acid (1.5-3 g), extended-release nicotinic acid (Niaspan) 1-2 g), sustained release nicotinic acid (1-2 g)	LDL HDL TG	↓5%-25% ↑15%-35% ↓20%-50%	Flushing Hyperglycemia Hyperuricemia (or gout) Upper GI distress Hepatotoxicity	Absolute: • Chronic liver disease • Severe gout Relative: • Diabetes • Hyperuricemia • Peptic ulcer disease
Fibric acids	Gemfibrozil (600 mg bid) Fenofibrate (160 mg qd) Clofibrate (1000 mg bid)	LDL *(may be increased in patients with high TG)* HDL TG	↓5%-20% ↑10%-20% ↓20%-50%	Dyspepsia Gallstones Myopathy	Absolute: • Severe renal disease • Severe hepatic disease

From The National Cholestrol Education Program, *JAMA* 285:2486, 2001.
CoA, Coenzyme A; *GI,* gastrointestinal; *HDL,* high-density lipoprotein; *HMG,* 3-hydroxy-3 methylglutanyl; *LDL,* low-density lipoprotein; *TG,* triglyceride.
*Cyclosporine, macrolide antibiotics, various antifungal agents, and cytochrome P-450 inhibitors (fibrates and niacin should be used with appropriate caution).

BASIC INFORMATION

■ DEFINITION

A hypercoagulable state is an inherited or acquired condition associated with an increased risk of thrombosis.

ICD-9CM CODES
289.8 Hypercoagulable state

■ EPIDEMIOLOGY & DEMOGRAPHICS (Table 1-36)
- Most people with a genetic defect or laboratory abnormality will not suffer thrombotic disease.
- More than half of patients with thrombosis have a predisposing hereditary or acquired blood protein or platelet defect.

■ HISTORY
- Spontaneous thrombosis: absence of other medical conditions associated with increased risk of thrombosis
- Less than 45 yr old at first episode of thrombosis
- Family history of thrombosis
- Recurrent thrombotic events
- Thrombosis in unusual anatomic location
- Thrombosis in pregnancy
- Second-trimester pregnancy loss
- Warfarin-associated skin necrosis

■ PHYSICAL FINDINGS & CLINICAL PRESENTATION
- Thrombosis
- Medical conditions associated with increased risk of thrombosis

■ ETIOLOGY (Table 1-36)
- Often a multifactorial process with genetic, environmental, and acquired factors
- Multiple genetic factor defects are not uncommon

COMMON INHERITED:
Factor V Leiden
- Mutation causing activated protein C resistance
- Most common genetic risk factor for venous thrombosis
- Heterozygous carrier has sevenfold increased risk and homozygous carrier has eightyfold increased risk of thrombosis
- Accounts for 20% of miscarriages in the second trimester

Protein C:
- Decreased level or abnormal function
- Strongly associated with warfarin skin necrosis

Protein S:
- Decreased level or abnormal function
- May be associated with warfarin skin necrosis
- Risk of hypercoagulable potential in question; recently one study found no increased thrombotic risk in individuals with PS deficiency

Antithrombin III:
- Decreased level or abnormal function
- Poses greater risk for thrombosis than protein C or protein S deficiency
- Can cause heparin resistance

Prothrombin Gene Defect-Factor II Sticky Platelet Syndrome

UNCOMMON INHERITED:
- Hyperhomocysteinemia, heparin cofactor II defect, tissue plasminogen activator (tPA) defect, plasminogen activator inhibitor (PAI-1) defect, dysfibrinogenemia, plasminogen defect, lipoprotein (a)

ACQUIRED:
Antiphospholipid Antibodies:
- Accounts for 12% of miscarriages in the second trimester
- Associated with thrombocytopenia

Lupus anticoagulant
Anticardiolipin antibodies
- Five times more common than lupus anticoagulant
- 50% to 70% chance of fetal wastage without treatment

Medical Conditions Associated with Increased Risk of Thrombosis:
- Chronic medical illness: CHF, DM, obesity, nephrotic syndrome
- Pregnancy, OCP, estrogen
- Immobilization, postoperative
- Myeloproliferative disorder
- Cancer: disease or treatment related
- Heparin-induced thrombocytopenia and thrombosis (HATT)

DIAGNOSIS

■ WORKUP
- Individuals with history suggestive of hypercoagulable state.
- History, physical examination, laboratory tests.

- Acute thrombosis, anticoagulation, and many medical conditions affect results and must be considered in interpretation of workup.

■ LABORATORY TESTS
- Lupus anticoagulant: PTT, dilute Russell viper venom test
- Anticardiolipin antibody: enzyme linked immunosorbent assay
- Factor V Leiden
DNA genotyping can be done while on anticoagulation or inhibitors are present.
- Protein C activity: level and activity
- Protein S activity: free and total level and activity (functional assay may be false positive if have factor V Leiden mutation)

If no etiology defined and suspicion is high proceed with these tests:
- Hyperhomocysteinemia: plasma homocysteine and RBC folate after 8-hr fast, plasma B_{12}, methylene tetrahydrofolate reductase by DNA
- Antithrombin III: heparin cofactor assay, DNA analysis
- Plasminogen activity
- Thrombin time/fibrinogen: activity and level

■ IMAGING STUDIES
As appropriate to diagnose thrombosis and to rule out medical conditions associated with increased thrombotic risk

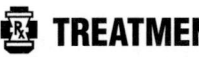# TREATMENT

■ NONPHARMACOLOGIC THERAPY
OCP use and smoking are contraindicated.

■ PROPHYLAXIS
- Asymptotic carriers should receive adjusted dose heparin or warfarin when immobilized for surgery or prolonged illness.
- Two or more spontaneous thromboses: oral anticoagulants for life.
- AT III: high-risk patients should receive perioperative and postoperative AT III concentrates. Dosing: 50 U/kg IV if baseline activity is about 50%. Repeat dose: 60% of loading dose every 24 hr to maintain levels >80%. AT III level increases 1.4%/U/kg given.

- Homocysteinemia: increase dietary intake of vitamins B_6, B_{12}, and folic acid; this may decrease risk of arterial and venous thrombosis by decreasing plasma homocysteine levels

Pregnancy prophylaxis
- AT III: heparin SC or LMWH throughout pregnancy; AT III concentrates during labor, delivery, and obstetric complications
- PC, PS, APC-R and history of thrombosis: adjusted dose heparin SC throughout pregnancy
- Antiphospholipid antibodies and recurrent abortion: treat with ASA 81 mg/day preconception and add heparin 5000 to 7500 SC bid postconception, continue both until term

■ ACUTE GENERAL Rx
Venous thrombosis
- Heparin for 5 to 7 days IV or SC. Begin warfarin when therapeutic on heparin, stop heparin when INR is 2 to 3 for 48 hr, continue warfarin for 3 to 6 months.
- Alternatives: low-molecular-weight heparin (enoxaprin or dalteparin 100 U/kg).
- Inferior vena cava filter if anticoagulation is contraindicated.

Arterial thrombosis
- Anticoagulation with heparin.
- Surgical consult for definitive procedure.

Protein C
- Protein C concentrates may be used for deficiency.

AT III deficiency
- Acute thrombosis: AT III concentrates in addition to usual care.
- Heparin resistance or thrombosis despite anticoagulation: treat with AT III concentrates.

Antiphospholipid antibodies
- Thrombosis requires long-term anticoagulation; stop only if anticardiolipin antibody test is negative for 4 to 6 months.

Lupus anticoagulant
- Acute thrombosis: LMWH or if using unfractionated heparin, follow heparin or factor Xa levels.
- Follow heparin levels or factor Xa.
- Warfarin INR 2 to 3 for venous thrombosis, INR 3 to 3.5 for arterial thrombosis.

Sticky platelet syndrome
- ASA 81 mg/day; if platelets fail to normalize, increase ASA to 325 mg/day or try ticlopidine.

HATT
- Stop heparin; use an alternate anticoagulant; definitive surgical procedure for thrombosis.

Warfarin skin necrosis
- Stop warfarin; give vitamin K, heparin anticoagulation.

■ DISPOSITION
Depends on underlying condition

■ REFERRAL
- Hematology
- Surgery

⚙ PEARLS & CONSIDERATIONS
Screen family members: may be able to decrease risk with lifestyle modification

INTERPRETING WORKUP: Many medical conditions cause acquired deficiency.
- Age: Neonates have low levels of protein C and protein S, reach adult levels by teenage years. AT III levels reach adult levels by 6 mo of age.
- Heparin therapy: Antithrombin III levels decrease.
- Warfarin therapy: Protein C, protein S levels decrease. After several weeks of therapy levels should be ≥60%, if less may have congenital deficiency.
- Protein C, protein S, antithrombin III levels decrease with acute thrombosis, postoperative state, liver disease, and DIC.
- Protein S levels also decrease with pregnancy, estrogen therapy (HRT, OCP), and nephrotic syndrome.
- Antithrombin III levels also decrease with nephrotic syndrome and OCP use. Wait 6 to 9 mo after thrombosis to rule out congenital deficiency.

REFERENCES
Bick RL, Kaplan H: Syndromes of thrombosis and hypercoagulability, congenital and acquired causes of thrombosis, *Med Clin North Am* 82(3):409, 1998.

Bucur SZ et al: Uses of antithrombin III concentrate in congenital and acquired deficiency states, *Transfusion* 38(5):481, 1998.

Author: **Sudeep K. Aulakh, M.D., F.R.C.P.C.**

TABLE 1-36 Common Hypercoagulable Conditions

	PREVALENCE IN NORMAL POPULATION	PREVALENCE IN POPULATION WITH THROMBOSIS	ARTERIAL (A)/VENOUS (V) EVENTS	FETAL LOSS
Factor V Leiden	• About 15% of whites • Rare in non-Europeans	20%-60%	A + V	Yes
PS	1%	1%-10%	A + V	
PC	0.4%	3%-5%	V > A	
AT III	0.2%	3%-8%	V > A	Yes
Prothrombin gene defect—Factor II	2%	6%	V	
Sticky platelet syndrome			A + V	Yes
Anticardiolipin antibody			A + V	Yes
Lupus anticoagulant		6%-8%	V > A	Yes

BASIC INFORMATION

■ DEFINITION

Hyperemesis gravidarum is the persistent nausea and vomiting with onset in the first trimester of pregnancy, resulting in weight loss and fluid and electrolyte and acid-base imbalances.

ICD-9CM CODES
643.1 Hyperemesis gravidarum

■ EPIDEMIOLOGY & DEMOGRAPHICS
INCIDENCE: 0.5 to 10 cases/1000 pregnancies
GENETICS: No genetic disposition
RISK FACTORS:
- Multiple pregnancy
- Molar pregnancy
- Previous history of unsuccessful pregnancy
- Nulliparity
- Hyperemesis gravidarum in a prior pregnancy
- No correlation with race, socioeconomic status, or marital status

PEAK ONSET: 8 to 12 wk of gestation

■ PHYSICAL FINDINGS & CLINICAL PRESENTATION
- Weight loss
- Rapid heart rate
- Fall in blood pressure
- Dry mucous membranes
- Loss of skin elasticity
- Ketotic odor
- In severe cases, Wernicke's encephalopathy as a result of thiamine deficiency

■ ETIOLOGY
Specific etiology is unknown.

DIAGNOSIS

■ DIFFERENTIAL DIAGNOSIS
- Pancreatitis, cholecystitis, hepatitis, pyelonephritis

■ WORKUP
Hyperemesis gravidarum is a diagnosis of exclusion. A detailed history and physical examination along with laboratory tests to rule out other causes of vomiting in early pregnancy are indicated.

■ LABORATORY TESTS
- Urinalysis to document ketonuria and proteinuria
- Urine C&S to rule out pyelonephritis
- Serum electrolytes to rule out electrolyte and acid-base imbalance
- Serum concentration of aminotransferases and bilirubin to rule out hepatitis.
- Serum amylase to rule out pancreatitis
- Free T_4 and TSH (elevated T_4 with suppressed TSH levels present in up to 60% of patients with hyperemesis gravidarum. This biochemical hyperthyroidism usually spontaneously resolves after 18 wk.)

■ IMAGING STUDIES
- Pelvic ultrasound examination to rule out multiple gestation and molar pregnancy
- Ultrasound of the gallbladder to rule out cholecystitis

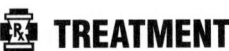 **TREATMENT**

■ NONPHARMACOLOGIC THERAPY
- Reassurance
- Psychologic support
- Avoidance of foods that trigger nausea
- Frequent small meals once oral intake has resumed

■ ACUTE GENERAL Rx
- NPO.
- Fluid and electrolyte replacement.
- Parenteral vitamin supplementation.
- Daily supplementation of thiamine 100 mg IM or IV to prevent Wernicke's encephalopathy.

- Antiemetics, such as promethazine (Phenergan) or droperidol (Inapsine), have not been found to be associated with fetal malformations when given in early pregnancy. Promethazine given as a low-dose continuous infusion of 25 mg in each liter of IV fluid has been shown to be very effective in controlling nausea and vomiting.
- Restart oral intake gradually no less than 48 hr after vomiting has ceased.

■ CHRONIC Rx
If the above acute therapy does not resolve vomiting and oral intake is not feasible, parenteral hyperalimentation may be necessary.

■ DISPOSITION
- Untreated hyperemesis gravidarum can result in maternal renal and hepatic damage or death from fluid and electrolyte imbalance.
- Hyperemesis gravidarum with severe weight loss has been associated with lower average birth weight and with CNS malformations in neonates.

■ REFERRAL
For parenteral hyperalimentation if required

PEARLS & CONSIDERATIONS

■ COMMENTS
Although the specific etiology of hyperemesis gravidarum is not known, psychogenic causes proposed in older literature have been largely discredited. "Behavioral therapies" for hyperemesis gravidarum are inappropriate.
Author: **Laurel White, M.D.**

BASIC INFORMATION

■ DEFINITION

Hypereosinophilic syndrome (HES) refers to a group of disorders of unknown cause characterized by sustained overproduction of eosinophils and organ dysfunction.

■ SYNONYMS

Idiopathic hyereosinophilic syndrome

ICD-9CM CODES

288.3 Hypereosinophilic syndrome

■ EPIDEMIOLOGY & DEMOGRAPHICS

- HES usually occurs between the ages of 20 and 50 yr.
- Occurs in men more often than women (9:1).

■ PHYSICAL FINDINGS & CLINICAL PRESENTATION

- Clinical presentation of patients with HES may vary from an incidental finding of eosinophilia on peripheral blood smear to sudden onset of cardiac or neurologic symptoms.
- *Cardiac manifestations* (58%) include dyspnea, orthopnea, signs and symptoms of congestive heart failure, murmurs of mitral regurgitation or tricuspid regurgitation.
  1. Symptoms are the result of endocardial infiltration of eosinophils leading to tissue necrosis. Thrombosis of the damaged tissue ensues and ultimately results in scarring and fibrosis.
  2. The pathologic process may result in a restrictive cardiomyopathy, dilated cardiomyopathy, and valvular heart disease.
- *Neurologic manifestations* (54%) may be of three types:
  1. Thromboembolic (e.g., cardiac emboli or local vascular thrombosis).
  2. CNS dysfunction—confusion, loss of memory, ataxia, upper motor neuron signs, Babinski's sign, seizures, and behavior changes. The cause is unknown.
  3. Peripheral neuropathy may be symmetric or asymmetric, sensory or mixed sensory and motor deficits.
- *Pulmonary manifestations* (40%) include a chronic persistent nonproductive cough, shortness of breath, and dyspnea on exertion.
- *Cutaneous manifestations* (56%) usually include urticaria, angioedema, or erythematous pruritic papules and nodules.
- *GI manifestations* (23%) include diarrhea but findings of gastritis, colitis, pancreatitis, and hepatitis can occur.
- *Ocular manifestations* (23%) are thought to be due to microemboli causing visual disturbances (e.g., blurring).

■ ETIOLOGY

- The etiology of HES is unknown.
- HES is thought to be a composite of many diseases.

DIAGNOSIS

Criteria for the diagnosis of idiopathic HES include:
- Persistent eosinophilia of >1500 eosinophils/mm^3 for more than 6 mo
- Exclusion of other conditions causing eosinophilia (e.g., parasites, allergies)
- Signs and symptoms of organ system dysfunction (e.g., heart, liver, lung)

■ DIFFERENTIAL DIAGNOSIS

The differential includes all causes of peripheral blood eosinophilia. Parasitic infections (filariasis, schistosomiasis, ascariasis, trichinosis, etc.), coccidioidomycosis, cat-scratch disease, asthma, Churg-Strauss syndrome, allergic rhinitis, atopic dermatitis, drug reactions, aspergillosis, eosinophilic pneumonia, hypersensitivity pneumonitis, HIV, eosinophilic gastroenteritis, inflammatory bowel disease.

■ WORKUP

The workup of a patient who is suspected of having HES should exclude other causes mentioned in the "Differential Diagnosis" leading to peripheral eosinophilia.

■ LABORATORY TESTS

- CBC with total eosinophil count. Often the total white cell count ranges from 10,000 to 30,000/mm^3 with eosinophilia of 30% to 70%.
- Erythrocyte sedimentation rate (ESR)
- Electrolytes, BUN, and creatinine
- Liver function tests
- Urinalysis
- HIV assay
- Stools for ova and parasites × 3
- Serologic blood tests for parasitic infections (e.g., *Strongyloides*)
- Total IgE level
- Rheumatoid factor
- Bone marrow aspirate and biopsy
- Duodenal aspirate
- ECG

■ IMAGING STUDIES

- Chest x-ray may be clear or show infiltrates, effusions, or fibrotic scarring.
- CT scan of chest, abdomen, and pelvis.
- Echocardiogram can assess for ventricular function, valvular pathology including regurgitation and thrombi formation.

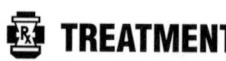

TREATMENT

Treatment is usually not initiated unless there is evidence of organ involvement and therapy is designed at controlling organ damage.

■ NONPHARMACOLOGIC THERAPY

- In patients with hypereosinophilia without organ involvement serial echocardiograms is recommended at 6-month intervals.

■ ACUTE GENERAL Rx

- In patients with organ involvement, initial therapy is with prednisone 1 mg/kg/day or 60 mg/day in adults.
- Patient's symptoms and peripheral eosinophil counts are monitored as a means of assessing response.
- Doses may be tapered to alternate day prednisone use in patients whose eosinophil counts have been suppressed.

■ CHRONIC Rx

- Patients not responding to corticosteroids, hydroxyurea 1 to 2 g/day may be tried.
- Hydroxyurea is aimed at reducing the total white blood cell count to <10,000/mm^3.
- If the disease continues to progress, vincristine, etopside, interferon-α, cyclosporine, and leukapheresis are alternative choices.
- Anticoagulation with warfarin and/or antiplatelet agents is often used in patients with HES.
- If all else fails, bone marrow transplantation may be considered.

■ DISPOSITION

- Before the use of cardiac imaging (echo) and cardiac surgeries (valve replacement), patients with HES had a poor prognosis with a mean survival of 9 mo and a 3-yr survival of 12%.
- Deaths usually resulted from congestive heart failure, valvular endocarditis, and systemic embolization.

- Patients responding to corticosteroids (reduction of eosinophil counts to normal range) have a better prognosis than patients who do not respond to corticosteroids.
- There are now reports of 5-, 10-, and 15-yr survival rates.

■ REFERRAL
- HES is a rare and complicated disorder requiring a multidisciplinary approach. Cardiology, neurology, pulmonary, ophthalmology, and hematology consultations should be requested in the appropriate clinical setting.

PEARLS & CONSIDERATIONS

■ COMMENTS
- There is still much to be learned about HES. The etiology and exact mechanism of organ damage caused by eosinophils remains unknown and research is ongoing to attempt to answer these and other questions.

REFERENCES
Ackerman SJ: *Hematology basic principles and practice,* ed 3, New York, 2000, Churchill Livingstone.

Weller PF, Bubley GJ: The idiopathic hypereosinophilic syndrome, *Blood* 83(10):2749, 1994.

Weller PF, Dvorak AM: The idiopathic hypereosinophilic syndrome, *Arch Dermatol* 132(5):583, 1996.

Author: **Dennis Mikolich, M.D.**

BASIC INFORMATION

■ DEFINITION
Primary hyperlipoproteinemia refers to a group of genetic disorders of the lipid transport proteins in the blood, which manifests as abnormally elevated levels of cholesterol, triglycerides, or both in the serum of affected patients (Table 1-37).

■ SYNONYMS
Hyperlipidemia

ICD-9CM CODES
272.4 Hyperlipoproteinemia
272.3 Fredrickson type I
272.0 Fredrickson type IIa
272.2 Fredrickson type IIb, III
272.1 Fredrickson type IV
272.3 Fredrickson type V

■ EPIDEMIOLOGY & DEMOGRAPHICS
INCIDENCE:
- Variable depending on the genetic defect
- Spectrum spans the common familial hypercholesterolemia, with an incidence of 1:500, to the rare familial lipoprotein lipase deficiency

PREDOMINANT SEX: None
GENETICS:
- Familial lipoprotein lipase deficiency: autosomal recessive, resulting in an elevation in the plasma chylomicrons and triglycerides
- Familial apoprotein CII deficiency: autosomal recessive, resulting in increased serum chylomicrons, VLDL, and hypertriglyceridemia
- Familial type 3 hyperlipoproteinemia: single-gene defect requiring contributory factors to manifest
- Familial hypercholesterolemia: autosomal dominant defect of the LDL receptor resulting in an elevated serum cholesterol level and normal triglycerides
- Familial hypertriglyceridemia: common, autosomal dominant defect resulting in elevated VLDL and triglycerides
- Multiple lipoprotein–type hyperlipidemia: autosomal dominant, manifesting as isolated hypercholesterolemia, isolated hypertriglyceridemia, or hyperlipidemia
- Polygenic hypercholesterolemia: multifactorial
- Polygenic hyperalphalipoproteinemia: autosomal dominant or polygenic, causing an elevated HDL

■ PHYSICAL FINDINGS & CLINICAL PRESENTATION
- Familial lipoprotein lipase deficiency: recurrent bouts of abdominal pain in infancy, eruptive xanthomas, hepatomegaly, splenomegaly, lipemia retinalis
- Familial apoprotein CII deficiency: occasional eruptive xanthomas
- Familial type 3 hyperlipoproteinemia: after age 20 yr see xanthoma striata palmaris or tuberoeruptive xanthomas, xanthelasmas, arterial bruits at a young age, gangrene of the lower extremities at a young age
- Familial hypercholesterolemia: tendon xanthomas, arcus corneae, xanthelasma

---

TABLE 1-37 Classification of Lipoprotein Disorders by Phenotypes, Genotypes, and Corresponding Clinical Manifestations

| PHENOTYPE | PLASMA LIPID LEVELS | | GENOTYPE | XANTHOMAS | OTHER CLINICAL MANIFESTATIONS |
	CHOLESTEROL	TRIGLYCERIDE			
I	Normal or elevated	Elevated lipemia	Familial lipoprotein lipase deficiency, Apo C-II deficiency	Eruptive, tubero-eruptive	Recurrent abdominal pain, other gastrointestinal symptoms, hepatosplenomegaly
IIA	Normal	Elevated	FHC, familial combined hyperlipidemia—polygenic and sporadic hypercholesterolemia	Tendinous, xanthelasma, tuberous; planar (homozygous)	Premature CAD, arcus corneae, aortic stenosis (homozygous FHC), arthritic symptoms
IIB	Elevated	Elevated	Familial combined hyperlipidemia, FHC		
III	Elevated	Elevated	Familial dysbetalipoproteinemia	Planar (especially palmar), tuberous	Premature CAD and peripheral vascular disease, male > female, obesity, abnormal glucose tolerance, hyperuricemia, aggravated by hypothyroidism, good response to therapy
IV	Normal or elevated	Elevated	Familial hypertriglyceridemia, familial combined hyperlipidemia, sporadic hypertriglyceridemia	Usually none; rarely eruptive or tubero-eruptive	CAD and peripheral vascular disease, obesity, abnormal glucose tolerance, hyperuricemia, arthritic symptoms, gallbladder disease
V	Normal or elevated	Elevated	Homozygous FHC	Eruptive, tubero-eruptive	Recurrent abdominal pain, other gastrointestinal symptoms, hepatosplenomegaly, peripheral paresthesia

From Graber MA: *The family practice handbook*, ed 4, St Louis, 2001, Mosby.
CAD, Coronary artery disease; *FHC*, familial hypercholesterolemia; *IDL*, intermediate-density lipoprotein; *LDL*, low-density lipoprotein, *VLDL*, very-low-density lipoprotein.

- Familial hypertriglyceridemia: associated obesity; with exacerbations eruptive xanthomas can develop
- Multiple lipoprotein type hyperlipidemia: no discerning physical findings
- Polygenic hypercholesterolemia: no discerning physical findings
- Polygenic hyperalphalipoproteinemia: no discerning physical findings

■ ETIOLOGY
Genetic defects causing lipid abnormalities

DIAGNOSIS

■ DIFFERENTIAL DIAGNOSIS
Secondary causes of hyperlipoproteinemias:
- Diabetes mellitus
- Glycogen storage diseases
- Lipodystrophies
- Glucocorticoid use/excess
- Alcohol
- Oral contraceptives
- Renal disease
- Hepatic dysfunction

■ WORKUP
- Detailed family history for premature cardiac disease
- Recurrent pancreatitis
- Thorough physical examination

■ LABORATORY TESTS
- Lipoprotein analysis
- Lipoprotein electrophoresis

℞ TREATMENT

■ NONPHARMACOLOGIC THERAPY
- Cornerstone of treatment: dietary therapy
- Familial lipoprotein lipase deficiency and familial apoprotein CII deficiency: fat-free diet
- Remainder of cases, except those with polygenic hyperalphalipoproteinemia: fat- and cholesterol-restricted diets

■ ACUTE GENERAL Rx
No acute treatment needed

■ CHRONIC Rx
- Familial lipoprotein lipase deficiency, polygenic hyperalphalipoproteinemia, or familial apoprotein CII deficiency: no chronic drug therapy
- Familial type 3 hyperlipoproteinemia: usually responds well to secondary causes being treated and diet therapy; if not, fibric acids may be tried
- Familial hypercholesterolemia: bile acid sequestrants, HMG-CoA reductase inhibitors, or niacin
- Familial hypertriglyceridemia: fibric acids
- Multiple lipoprotein type hyperlipidemia: drug therapy aimed at the predominant lipid abnormality noted

■ DISPOSITION
- Those with polygenic hyperalphalipoproteinemia: excellent prognosis for longevity
- Those with familial hypercholesterolemia, familial type 3 hypercholesterolemia, and multiple lipoprotein type hyperlipidemia: even with aggressive treatment, at high risk for accelerated atherosclerosis and CAD

☼ PEARLS & CONSIDERATIONS

■ COMMENTS
- Patient information is available through the American Heart Association.
- Fig. 1-209 describes an algorithm for hyperlipidemia.

REFERENCES
Cleeman JI: Detection and evaluation of dyslipoproteinemia, *Endocrinol Metab Clin North Am* 27(3):597, 1998.

Davignon J, Genesh J, Jr: Genetics of lipoprotein disorders, *Endocrinol Metab Clin North Am* 27(3):521, 1998.

National Cholesterol Education Program: Second Report on the Expert Panel on Detection, evaluation and treatment of high cholesterol in adults (adult treatment panel III), *JAMA* 285:2486, 2001.

Author: **Beth J. Wutz, M.D.**

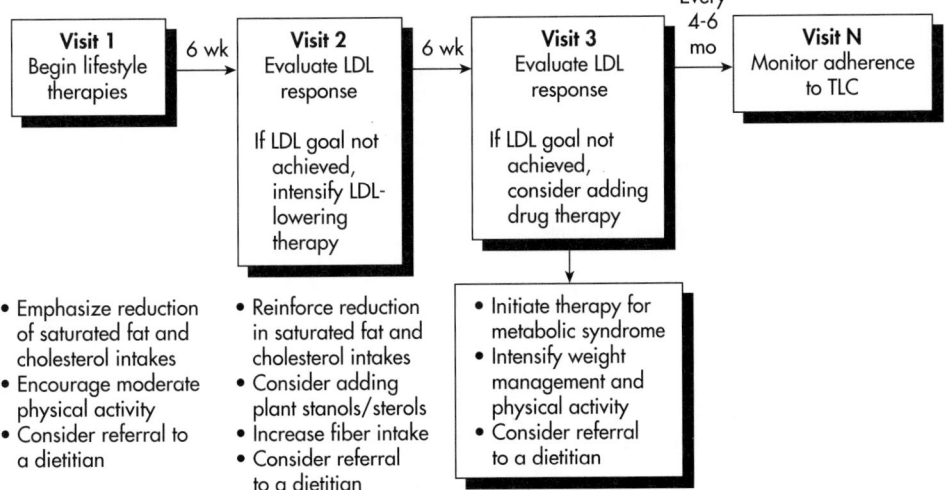

Fig. 1-209 Model of steps in therapeutic lifestyle changes (TLC). *LDL,* Low-density lipoprotein. (From National Cholesterol Education Program Expert Panel on Detection, Evaluation, and Treatment o High Blood Cholesterol in Adults [Adult Treatment Panel III], National Institutes of Health, *JAMA* 285:2486, 2001.)

BOX 1-19   Nutrient Composition of the Therapeutic Lifestyle Changes (TLC) Diet

NUTRIENT	RECOMMENDED INTAKE
Saturated fat*	<7% of total calories
Polyunsaturated fat	Up to 10% of total calories
Monounsaturated fat	Up to 20% of total calories
Total fat	25%-35% of total calories
Carbohydrate†	50%-60% of total calories
Fiber	20-30 g/day
Protein	Approximately 15% of total calories
Cholesterol	<200 mg/day
Total calories‡	Balance energy intake and expenditure to maintain desirable body weight/prevent weight gain

From National Cholesterol Education Program Expert Panel on Detection, Evaluation, and Treatment of High Blood Cholesterol in Adults (Adult Treatment Panel III), National Institutes of Health, *JAMA* 285:2486, 2001.
*Trans fatty acids are another LDL-raising fat that should be kept at a low intake.
†Carbohydrates should be derived predominantly from foods rich in complex carbohydrates, including grains, especially whole grains, fruits, and vegetables.
‡Daily energy expenditure should include at least moderate physical activity (contributing approximately 200 kcal/d).

BOX 1-20   ATP III Classification of LDL, Total, and HDL Cholesterol (mg/dl)

LDL cholesterol

<100	Optimal
100-129	Near or above optimal
130-159	Borderline high
160-189	High
≥190	Very high

Total cholesterol

<200	Desirable
200-239	Borderline high
≥240	High

HDL cholesterol

<40	Low
≥60	High

From National Cholesterol Education Program Expert Panel on Detection, Evaluation, and Treatment of High Blood Cholesterol in Adults (Adult Treatment Panel III), National Institutes of Health, *JAMA* 285:2486, 2001.
ATP, Adult treatment panel; *HDL,* high-density lipoprotein, *LDL,* low-density lipoprotein.

BOX 1-21   Major Risk Factors (Exclusive of LDL Cholesterol) That Modify LDL Goals*

Cigarette smoking
Hypertension (blood pressure ≥140/90 mm Hg or on antihypertensive medication)
Low HDL cholesterol (<40 mg/dL)†
Family history of premature CHD (CHD in male first-degree relative (<55 yr; CHD in female first-degree relative <65 yr)
Age (men ≥45 yr; women ≥55 yr)

From National Cholesterol Education Program Expert Panel on Detection, Evaluation, and Treatment of High Blood Cholesterol in Adults (Adult Treatment Panel III), National Institutes of Health, *JAMA* 285:2486, 2001.
HDL, High-density lipoprotein; *LDL,* low-density lipoprotein.
*Diabetes is regarded as a coronary heart disese (CHD) risk equivalent.
†HDL cholesterol ≥60 mg/dL counts as a "negative" risk factor; its presence removes 1 risk factor from the total count.

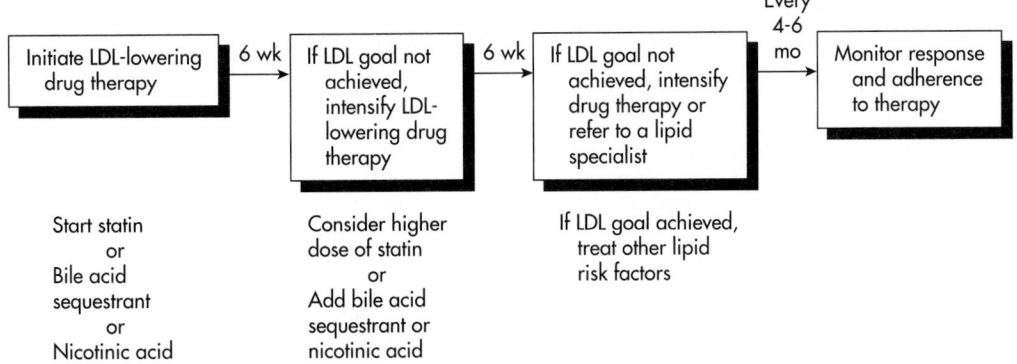

Fig. 1-210 Progression of drug therapy in primary prevention. *LDL,* Low-density lipoprotein. (From National Cholesterol Education Program Expert Panel on Detection, Evaluation, and Treatment of High Blood Cholesterol in Adults (Adult Treatment Panel III), National Institutes of Health, *JAMA* 285:2486, 2001.)

TABLE 1-38   LDL Cholesterol Goals and Cutpoints for Therapeutic Lifestyle Changes (TLC) and Drug Therapy in Different Risk Categories

RISK CATEGORY	LDL GOAL (mg/dl)	LDL LEVEL AT WHICH TO INITIATE THERAPEUTIC LIFESTYLE CHANGES (mg/dl)	LDLD LEVEL AT WHICH TO CONSIDER DRUG THERAPY (mg/dl)
CHD or CHD risk equivalents (10-yr risk >20%)	<100	≥100	≥130 (100-129: drug optional)*
2+ Risk factors (10-yr risk ≤20%)	<130	≥130	10-yr risk 10%-20%: ≥130 10-yr risk <10%: ≥160
0-1 Risk factor†	<160	≥160	≥190 (160-189: LDL-lowering drug optional)

From National Cholesterol Education Program Expert Panel on Detection, Evaluation, and Treatment of High Blood Cholesterol in Adults (Adult Treatment Panel III), National Institutes of Health, *JAMA* 285:2486, 2001.
CHD, Coronary heart disease; *LDL,* low-density lipoprotein.
*Some authorities recommend use of LDL-lowering drugs in this category if an LDL cholesterol level of <100 mg/dl cannot be achieved by therapeutic lifestyle changes. Others prefer use of drugs that primarily modify triglycerides and HDL (e.g., nicotinic acid or fibrate). Clinical judgment also may call for deferring drug therapy in this subcategory.
†Almost all people with 0-1 risk factor have a 10-year risk <10%; thus 10-year risk assessment in people with 0-1 risk factor is not necessary.

TABLE 1-39   Comparison of LDL Cholesterol and Non-HDL Cholesterol Goals for Three Risk Categories

RISK CATEGORY	LDL GOAL (mg/dl)	NON-HDL GOAL (mg/dl)
CHD and CHD risk equivalent (10-yr risk for CHD >20%)	<100	<130
Multiple (2+) risk factors and 10-yr risk ≤20%	<130	<160
0-1 Risk factor	<160	<190

From National Cholesterol Education Program Expert Panel on Detection, Evaluation, and Treatment of High Blood Cholesterol in Adults (Adult Treatment Panel III), National Institutes of Health, *JAMA* 285:2486, 2001.
CHD, Coronary heart disease; *HDL,* high-density lipoprotein; *LDL,* low-density lipoprotein.

BOX 1-22   Interventions to Improve Adherence

Focus on the Patient

Simplify medication regimens
Provide explicit patient instruction and use good counseling techniques to teach the patient how to follow the prescribed treatment
Encourage the use of prompts to help patients remember treatment regimens
Use systems to reinforce adherence and maintain contact with the patient
Encourage the support of family and friends
Reinforce and reward adherence
Increase visits for patients unable to achieve treatment goal
Increase the convenience and access to care
Involve patients in their care through self-monitoring

Focus on the Physician and Medical Office

Teach physicians to implement lipid treatment guidelines
Use reminders to prompt physicians to attend to lipid management
Identify a patient advocate in the office to help deliver or prompt care
Use patients to prompt preventive care
Develop a standardized treatment plan to structure care
Use feedback from past performance to foster change in future care
Remind patients of appointments and follow up missed appointments

Focus on the Health Delivery System

Provide lipid management through a lipid clinic
Utilize case management by nurses
Deploy telemedicine
Utilize the collaborative care of pharmacists
Execute critical care pathways in hospitals

From National Cholesterol Education Program Expert Panel on Detection, Evaluation, and Treatment of High Blood Cholesterol in Adults (Adult Treatment Panel III), National Institutes of Health, *JAMA* 285:2486, 2001.

BOX 1-23   Clinical Identification of the Metabolic Syndrome

RISK FACTOR	DEFINING LEVEL
Abdominal obesity* (waist circumference)†	
Men	>102 cm (>40 in)
Women	>88 cm (>35 in)
Triglycerides	≥150 mg/dl
High-density lipoprotein cholesterol	
Men	<40 mg/dl
Women	<50 mg/dl
Blood pressure	≥130/≥85 mm Hg
Fasting glucose	≥110 mg/dl

From National Cholesterol Education Program Expert Panel on Detection, Evaluation, and Treatment of High Blood Cholesterol in Adults (Adult Treatment Panel III), National Institutes of Health, *JAMA* 285:2486, 2001.
*Overweight and obesity are associated with insulin resistance and the metabolic syndrome. However, the presence of abdominal obesity is more highly correlated with the metabolic risk factors than is an elevated body mass index (BMI). Therefore, the simple measure of waist circumference is recommended to identify the body weight component of the metabolic syndrome.
†Some male patients can develop multiple metabolic risk factors when the waist circumference is only marginally increased, for example, 94-102 cm (37-40 in). Such patients may have strong genetic contribution to insulin resistance, and they should benefit from changes in life habits, similarly to men with categorical increases in waist circumference.

BASIC INFORMATION

■ DEFINITION
Hyperosmolar coma is a state of extreme hyperglycemia, marked dehydration, serum hyperosmolarity, altered mental status, and absence of ketoacidosis.

■ SYNONYMS
Nonketotic hyperosmolar coma
Hyperosmolar nonketotic state

ICD-9CM CODES
250.2 Hyperosmolar coma

■ PHYSICAL FINDINGS & CLINICAL PRESENTATION
- Evidence of extreme dehydration (poor skin turgor, sunken eyeballs, dry mucous membranes)
- Neurologic defects (reversible hemiplegia, focal seizures)
- Orthostatic hypotension, tachycardia
- Evidence of precipitating factors (pneumonia, infected skin ulcer)
- Coma (25% of patients), delirium

■ ETIOLOGY
- Infections, 20% to 25% (e.g., pneumonia, UTI, sepsis)
- New or previously unrecognized diabetes (30% to 50%)
- Reduction or omission of diabetic medication
- Stress (MI, CVA)
- Drugs: diuretics (dehydration), phenytoin, diazoxide (impaired insulin secretion)

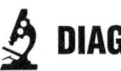

DIAGNOSIS

■ DIFFERENTIAL DIAGNOSIS
- Diabetic ketoacidosis
- The differential diagnosis of coma is described in Box 2-61.

■ LABORATORY TESTS
- Hyperglycemia: serum glucose usually >600 mg/dl.
- Hyperosmolarity: serum osmolarity usually >340 mOsm/L.
- Serum sodium: may be low, normal, or high; if normal or high, the patient is severely dehydrated, because an elevated glucose draws fluid from intracellular space decreasing the serum sodium; the corrected sodium can be obtained by increasing the serum sodium concentration by 1.6 mEq/dl for every 100 mg/dl increase in the serum glucose level over normal.

- Serum potassium: may be low, normal, or high; regardless of the initial serum level, the total body deficit is approximately 5 to 15 mEq/kg.
- Serum bicarbonate: usually >12 mEq/L (average is 17 mEq/L).
- Arterial pH: usually >7.2 (average is 7.26); both serum bicarbonate and arterial pH may be lower if lactic acidosis is present.
- BUN: azotemia (prerenal) is usually present (BUN generally ranges from 60 to 90 mg/dl).
- Phosphorus: hypophosphatemia (average deficit is 70 to 140 mm).
- Calcium: hypocalcemia (average deficit is 50 to 100 mEq).
- Magnesium: hypomagnesemia (average deficit is 50 to 100 mEq).
- CBC with differential, urinalysis, blood and urine cultures should be performed to rule out infectious etiology.

■ IMAGING STUDIES
- Chest x-ray examination is useful to rule out infectious process. The initial chest x-ray may be negative if the patient has significant dehydration. Repeat chest x-ray examination after 24 hr if pulmonary infection is suspected.
- CT scan of head should be performed in patients with suspected CVA.

TREATMENT

■ NONPHARMACOLOGIC THERAPY
- Monitor mental status, vital signs, urine output qh until improved, then monitor q2-4h.
- Monitor electrolytes, renal function, and glucose level (see "Acute General Rx").

■ ACUTE GENERAL Rx
- Vigorous fluid replacement: the volume and rate of fluid replacement are determined by renal and cardiac function. Typically, infuse 1000 to 1500 ml/hr for the initial 1 to 2 L; then decrease the rate of infusion to 500 ml/hr and monitor urinary output, blood chemistries, and blood pressure; use 0.9% NS (isotonic solution) if the patient is hypotensive or serum osmolarity is <320 mOsm/L; otherwise use 0.45% NS solution. Slower infusion rate may be used initially in patients with compromised cardiovascular or renal status.

- Replace electrolytes and monitor serum levels frequently (e.g., serum sodium and potassium q2h for the first 12 hr). Serum KCl replacement in patients with normal renal function and adequate urinary output is started when the serum potassium level is <5.2 mEq/L (e.g., 10 mEq KCl/hr if potassium level is 4 to 5.2 mEq/L). Continuous ECG monitoring and hourly measurement of urinary output are recommended.
- Correct hyperglycemia. The goal is for plasma glucose to decline by at least 75 to 100 mg/dl/hr.
  1. Vigorous IV hydration will decrease the serum glucose level in most patients by 80 mg/dl/hr; a regular insulin IV bolus (10 U) is often not necessary.
  2. Low-dose insulin infusion at 1 to 2 U/hr (e.g., 25 U of regular insulin in 250 ml of 0.9% saline solution at 20 ml/hr) until the serum glucose level approaches 300 mg/dl; then the patient is started on regular SC insulin with sliding scale coverage. If the plasma glucose does not decrease over 2 to 4 hr despite adequate fluid administration and urine output, consider doubling the hourly insulin dose.
  3. Glucose should be monitored q1-2h in the initial 12 hr.
- In the absence of renal failure, phosphate can be administered at a rate of 0.1 mmol/kg/hr (5 to 10 mmol/hr) to a maximum of 80 to 120 mmol in 24 hr. Magnesium replacement, in absence of renal failure, can be administered IM (0.05 to 0.10 ml/kg of 20% magnesium sulfate) or as IV infusion (4 to 8 ml of 20% magnesium sulfate [0.08 to 0.16 mEq/kg]). Repeat magnesium, phosphate, and calcium levels should be obtained after 12 to 24 hr.

■ DISPOSITION
Mortality in nonketotic hyperosmolar coma ranges from 20% to 50%.

PEARLS & CONSIDERATIONS

■ COMMENTS
The typical patient presenting with hyperosmolar coma is an elderly or bed-confined diabetic with impaired ability to communicate thirst who is evaluated after an interval of 1 to 2 wk of prolonged osmotic diuresis.
Author: **Fred F. Ferri, M.D.**

BASIC INFORMATION

■ DEFINITION

Primary hyperparathyroidism is an endocrine disorder caused by the excessive secretion of parathyroid hormone (PTH) from the parathyroid glands.

ICD-9CM CODES
252.0 Primary hyperparathyroidism
253.9 Ectopic hyperparathyroidism
588.8 Secondary hyperparathyroidism in chronic renal disease

■ EPIDEMIOLOGY & DEMOGRAPHICS
PREVALENCE: 1 case/1000 persons
PREDOMINANT AGE AND SEX:
Primary hyperparathyroidism occurs most frequently in postmenopausal women; prevalence in this group may be as high as 3%. The condition is asymptomatic in >50% of patients.
GENETICS: Hyperparathyroidism can occur in conjunction with MEN I or II.

■ PHYSICAL FINDINGS & CLINICAL PRESENTATION
Physical examination may be entirely normal. The presence of signs and symptoms varies with the rapidity of development and degree of hypercalcemia. The following abnormalities may be present:
- GI: constipation, anorexia, nausea, vomiting, pancreatitis, ulcers
- CNS: confusion, obtundation, psychosis, lassitude, depression, coma
- GU: nephrolithiasis, renal insufficiency, polyuria, decreased urine-concentrating ability, nocturia, nephrocalcinosis
- Musculoskeletal: myopathy, weakness, osteoporosis, pseudogout, bone pain
- Other: hypertension, metastatic calcifications, band keratopathy (found in medial and lateral margin of the cornea), pruritus

■ ETIOLOGY
- A single adenoma is found in 80% of patients; 90% of the adenomas are found within one of the parathyroid glands, the other 10% are in ectopic sites (lateral neck, thyroid, mediastinum, retroesophagus).
- Parathyroid gland hyperplasia occurs in 20% of patients.

DIAGNOSIS

■ DIFFERENTIAL DIAGNOSIS
Other causes of hypercalcemia:
- Malignancy: neoplasms of breast, lung, kidney, ovary, pancreas; myeloma, lymphoma
- Granulomatous disorders (e.g., sarcoidosis)
- Paget's disease
- Vitamin D intoxication, milk-alkali syndrome
- Thiazide diuretics
- Other: familial hypocalciuric hypercalcemia, thyrotoxicosis, adrenal insufficiency, prolonged immobilization, vitamin A intoxication, recovery from acute renal failure, lithium administration, pheochromocytoma, disseminated SLE

■ WORKUP
- The serum PTH level is the single best test for initial evaluation of confirmed hypercalcemia. The "intact" PTH (iPTH) is the best assay. The iPTH distinguishes primary hyperparathyroidism from hypercalcemia caused by malignancy when the serum calcium level is >12 mg/dl.
- A high level of urinary cyclic AMP is also suggestive of primary hyperparathyroidism.
- Parathyroid hormone–like protein (PLP) is increased in hypercalcemia associated with solid malignancies.
- ECG may reveal shortening of the QT interval secondary to hypercalcemia.
- Fig. 3-83 describes clinical algorithms for evaluation and treatment of hypercalcemia.

■ LABORATORY TESTS
- Elevated serum ionized calcium level, low serum phosphorus, and normal or elevated alkaline phosphatase.
- Elevated urine calcium level (in contrast with very low urinary calcium levels seen in patients with familial hypocalciuric hypercalcemia).
- Possibly elevated serum chloride levels, decreased serum CO_2, hyperchloremic metabolic acidosis.
- Table 2-103 describes the differential diagnosis of hypercalcemia.

■ IMAGING STUDIES
- A bone survey may show evidence of subperiosteal bone resorption (suggesting PTH excess). The classic bone disease of primary hyperparathyroidism is *osteitis fibrosa cystica*.
- Parathyroid localization with technetium-99m sestamibi has been shown to have a high sensitivity and specificity for single adenomas.
- Screen for osteopenia with measurement of bone mineral density in all postmenopausal women.

TREATMENT

■ NONPHARMACOLOGIC THERAPY
- Unless contraindicated, patients should maintain a high intake of fluids (3 to 5 L/day) and sodium chloride (>400 mEq/day) to increase renal calcium excretion. Calcium intake should be ≤1000 mg/day
- Potential hypercalcemic agents (e.g., thiazide diuretics) should be discontinued.
- Surgery is the only effective treatment for primary hyperparathyroidism. It is generally indicated in all patients under age 50 and patients with complications from hyperthyroidism, such as nephrolithiasis and osteopenia. The conventional surgical approach is bilateral neck exploration under general anesthesia. Minimally invasive adenomectomy guided by preoperative technetium-99-m sestamibi scanning or ultrasound plus spiral CT is an alternative to conventional neck exploration.
- Asymptomatic elderly patients can be followed conservatively with periodic monitoring of serum calcium level and review of symptoms. Serum creatinine and PTH levels should also be obtained at 6- to 12-month intervals, bone density (cortical and trabecular) yearly.

■ ACUTE GENERAL Rx
Acute severe hypercalcemia (serum calcium >13 mg/dl) or symptomatic patients can be treated with the following:
- Vigorous IV hydration with NS followed by IV furosemide. Use NS with caution in patients with cardiac or renal insufficiency to avoid fluid overload.
- Calcitonin 4 IU/kg q12h is indicated when saline hydration and furosemide are ineffective or contraindicated.
- Biphosphonates (pamidronate, etidronate), mithramycin, and gallium nitrate are also effective for severe hypercalcemia.

■ CHRONIC Rx
Hormone replacement therapy should be strongly considered in all postmenopausal women with primary hyperparathyroidism.

PEARLS & CONSIDERATIONS

■ COMMENTS
Patients with hyperparathyroidism should undergo further evaluation for the presence of MEN I or II.

REFERENCES
Marx SJ: Hyperparathyroid and hypoparathyroid disorders, *N Engl J Med* 343:1863, 2000.

Smit PC et al: Direct, minimally invasive adenomectomy for primary hyperparathyroidism: An alternative to conventional neck exploration? *Ann Surg* 231:559, 2000.
Author: **Fred F. Ferri, M.D.**

BASIC INFORMATION

■ DEFINITION

Hypersensitivity pneumonitis is an immunologically induced inflammation of the lung parenchyma, which is caused by intense or repeated inhalation of an organic agent.

■ SYNONYMS

Extrinsic allergic alveolitis
Specific examples:
- Bird fancier's lung
- Farmer's lung
- Chemical worker's lung
- Humidifier lung

ICD-9CM CODES
495.9 Pneumonitis, hypersensitivity

■ EPIDEMIOLOGY & DEMOGRAPHICS

Anyone with exposure to an offending antigen is susceptible. Diagnosis should be suspected when bronchitis and dyspnea occur without an obvious cause.

■ PHYSICAL FINDINGS & CLINICAL PRESENTATION

Vary depending on frequency and intensity of antigen exposure.
- *Acute:* Fever, cough, and dyspnea 4 to 6 hr after an intense exposure, lasting 18 to 24 hr
- *Subacute:* Insidious onset of productive cough, dyspnea on exertion, anorexia, and weight loss, usually from a heavy, sustained exposure
- *Chronic:* Gradually progressive cough, dyspnea, malaise, and weight loss, usually from low-grade or recurrent exposure

Physical examination: cyanosis and "crepitant rales," possible fever

■ ETIOLOGY
- Numerous environmental agents, often encountered in occupational settings
- Common sources of antigens: "moldy" hay, silage, grain, or vegetables; bird droppings or feathers; low-molecular-weight chemicals (i.e., isocyanates), pharmaceutical products

DIAGNOSIS

■ DIFFERENTIAL DIAGNOSIS
- Idiopathic pulmonary fibrosis
- Sarcoidosis
- Collagen-vascular disease
- Drug-induced interstitial lung disease
- Allergic bronchopulmonary mycoses
- Eosinophilic pneumonia

■ WORKUP
History (focusing on possible exposure to etiologic agents, changes in symptoms with exposure to versus avoidance of the agent), chest x-ray, pulmonary function tests; skin testing not helpful

■ LABORATORY TESTS
- Pulmonary function tests: acutely, decreased lung volumes, diffusing capacity, and compliance.
- Oximetry: exercise-induced hypoxemia.
- Chronic disease similarly associated with restrictive pattern, but may also show obstruction.
- Tests may be normal after an acute episode has resolved.

■ IMAGING STUDIES
Chest x-ray: Nonspecific; may be normal in early stage.
- *Acute/subacute:* Bilateral interstitial and alveolar nodular infiltrates (Fig. 1-211) in a patchy or homogeneous distribution. Apices are often spared.
- *Chronic:* Diffuse reticulonodular infiltrates and fibrosis. Honeycombing may develop.

High-resolution chest CT scan: No pathognomonic features.

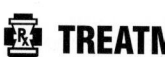 TREATMENT

■ NONPHARMACOLOGIC THERAPY
Recognition and avoidance of the causative antigen

■ ACUTE GENERAL Rx
- *Acute:* Usually recover without glucocorticoids; if severe, prednisone 1 mg/kg/day, tapered slowly after 2 wk
- *Subacute:* Prednisone 1 mg/kg/day for 1 to 2 wk, then tapered over 2 to 6 wk

■ CHRONIC RX
Prednisone 1 mg/kg/day for 2 to 4 wk, then tapered to lowest dosage to maintain patient's functional status

■ DISPOSITION
- *Acute:* Usually recover without glucocorticoids
- *Subacute:* May progress clinically despite antigen removal, thus requiring corticosteroids
- *Chronic:* May gradually recover following environmental control; can result in irreversible lung damage

■ REFERRAL
Laboratory inhalation challenge: testing to prove a direct relationship between a suspected antigen and disease; extract of antigen is inhaled via a nebulizer.
- Lung biopsy may be consistent with but not pathognomic for hypersensitivity pneumonitis

Author: **Jeanne M. Oliva, M.D.**

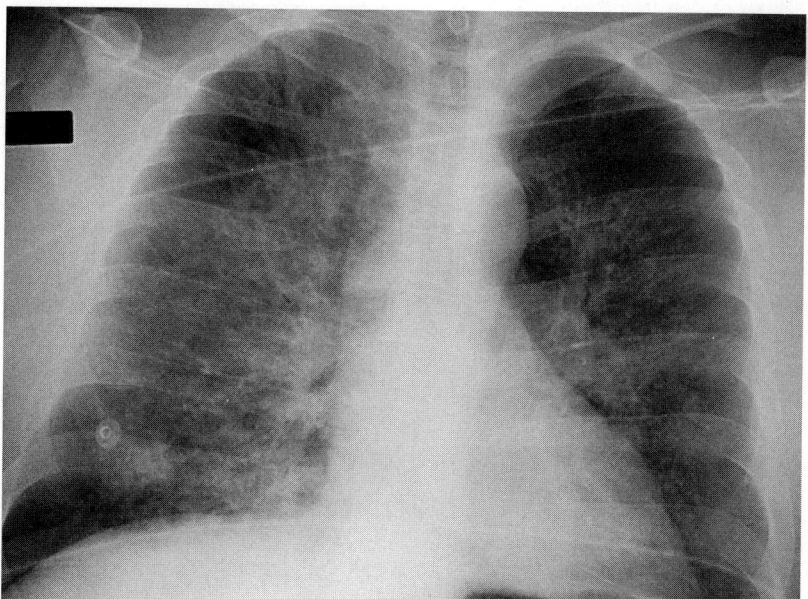

Fig. 1-211 Chest radiograph of a patient with acute hypersensitivity pneumonitis. Bilateral interstitial infiltrates are evident, more on the right side than the left. Note the absence of pleural effusion, hilar adenopathy, and hyperinflation. (From Altman LV [ed]: *Allergy in primary care,* Philadelphia, 2000, WB Saunders.)

BASIC INFORMATION

■ DEFINITION

Hypersplenism is a syndrome characterized by splenomegaly, cytopenia (decrease of one or more of the peripheral cell lines), and compensatory hyperplastic bone marrow.

ICD-9CM CODES

289.4 Hypersplenism

■ EPIDEMIOLOGY & DEMOGRAPHICS

- Most often seen in patients with chronic liver disease and congestive splenomegaly.
- Frequency of cytopenias: thrombocytopenia occurs most frequently, leukopenia occurs more often than anemia.

■ PHYSICAL FINDINGS & CLINICAL PRESENTATION

- History: early satiety, abdominal pain, left upper quadrant pleuritic pain, episodes of acute left upper quadrant pain (sequestration crisis)
- Physical examination: splenomegaly, presence of a rub in left upper quadrant (suggestive of a splenic infarct), stigmata of cytopenias

■ ETIOLOGY

Hypersplenism can be caused by splenomegaly of almost any cause.

- Splenomegaly increases the proportion of blood channeled through the red pulp, causing inappropriate splenic pooling of both normal and abnormal blood cells. Up to 25% of the RBC mass and up to 90% of platelets may be pooled in an enlarged spleen.
- Increased destruction of RBCs by the spleen. Platelets and WBCs have about normal survival time even when sequestered and may be available if needed.

- Cytopenia may be exacerbated by dilution because of plasma volume expansion resulting from splenomegaly.

DIAGNOSIS

■ DIFFERENTIAL DIAGNOSIS

- Infections: TB, malaria, infectious mononucleosis, subacute bacterial endocarditis, brucellosis, leishmaniasis, schistosomiasis
- Disordered immunoregulation: Felty syndrome, SLE
- Autoimmune cytopenias: hemolytic anemia, immune thrombocytopenia, and neutropenia
- Abnormal RBCs: sickle cell anemia, thalassemia, spherocytosis, elliptocytosis
- Infiltrative disease: Gaucher's disease, lymphoma, leukemia, metastatic tumors, myeloproliferative diseases, polycythemia vera, amyloidosis, Niemann-Pick disease, glycogen storage disease
- Altered splenic blood flow: hepatic cirrhosis, CHF, portal vein thrombosis, splenic vein obstruction, Budd-Chiari syndrome
- Miscellaneous: sarcoidosis

■ WORKUP

History, physical examination, laboratory tests, imaging studies

■ LABORATORY TESTS

- CBC
- Peripheral smear may be normal or may reveal spherocytosis, reticulocytosis
- Bone marrow biopsy: hyperplasia of corresponding cellular element

■ IMAGING STUDIES

- Abdominal ultrasound to determine splenic size
- CT scan, MRI to obtain structural information; rule out cysts, tumors, infarcts

TREATMENT

■ ACUTE GENERAL Rx

- Treat underlying disease
- Splenectomy is considered if
  1. Cannot treat underlying cause
  2. Have persistent symptomatic disease
  3. Necessary for diagnosis
  Risks:
  - Increase infections: can be decreased with pneumococcal vaccine
  - Rapid increase in platelet count may cause thromboembolic complications

■ DISPOSITION

- Cytopenias usually correctable with splenectomy, cell counts return to normal within a few weeks.
- Splenectomy may alleviate portal hypertension.
- Prognosis depends on the underlying disease.

■ REFERRAL

Hematology for bone marrow biopsy

REFERENCE

Barker LR, Burton JR, Zieve PD: *Principles of ambulatory medicine*, ed 5, Baltimore, 1999, Williams & Wilkins.
Author: **Sudeep K. Aulakh, M.D., F.R.C.P.C.**

BASIC INFORMATION

■ DEFINITION
Hypertension can be defined as a systolic blood pressure (BP) ≥140 mm Hg and/or diastolic BP >90 mm Hg (Table 1-40, Table 1-41).

■ SYNONYMS
Essential hypertension
Idiopathic hypertension
High blood pressure

ICD-9CM CODES
401.1 Essential hypertension
401.0 Malignant hypertension due to renal artery stenosis
642 Hypertension complicating pregnancy
405.01 Malignant hypertension secondary to renal artery stenosis
437.2 Hypertensive encephalopathy

■ EPIDEMIOLOGY & DEMOGRAPHICS
- Incidence of hypertension in adult population: 10% to 15%
- Increased incidence in males and in the elderly

■ PHYSICAL FINDINGS & CLINICAL PRESENTATION
Physical examination may be entirely within normal limits except for the presence of hypertension. A proper initial physical examination on a hypertensive patient should include the following:
- Measure height and weight.
- Evaluate skin for the presence of café-au-lait spots (neurofibromatosis), uremic appearance (CRF), striae (Cushing's syndrome).
- Perform careful funduscopic examination: check for papilledema, retinal exudates, hemorrhages, arterial narrowing, AV compression.
- Examine the neck for carotid bruits, distended neck veins, or enlarged thyroid gland.
- Perform extensive cardiopulmonary examination: check for loud aortic component of S_2, S_4, ventricular lift, murmurs, arrhythmias.
- Check abdomen for masses (pheochromocytoma, polycystic kidneys), presence of bruits over the renal artery (renal artery stenosis), dilation of the aorta.
- Obtain two or more BP measurements separated by 2 min with the patient either supine or seated and after standing for at least 2 min. Measure BP in both upper extremities (if values are discrepant, use the higher value).
- Examine arterial pulses (dilated or absent femoral pulses and BP greater in upper extremities than lower extremities suggest aortic coarctation).

TABLE 1-40   JNC VI Guidelines: Blood Pressure Classification and Recommended Follow-Up

CATEGORY	BLOOD PRESSURE (mm Hg)* SYSTOLIC		DIASTOLIC	RECOMMENDED FOLLOW-UP
Optimal	<120	and	<80	N/A†
Normal	<130	and	<85	Recheck in 2 yr
High-normal	130-139	or	85-89	Recheck in 1 yr; advise lifestyle modification
Hypertension				
Stage 1	140-159	or	90-99	Confirm within 2 mo; advise lifestyle modification
Stage 2	160-179	or	100-109	Evaluate or provide referral within 1 mo
Stage 3	≥180	or	≥110	Evaluate or provide referral within 1 wk

Modified from Joint National Committee on Prevention, Detection, Evaluation, and Treatment of High Blood Pressure and the National High Blood Pressure Education Program Coordinating Committee, *Arch Intern Med*, 57:2413, 1997.
*If systolic and diastolic readings fall into different categories, the higher category is selected (e.g., a blood pressure of 175/92 mm Hg is classified as stage 2 hypertension).
†Unusually low readings should be evaluated for clinical significance.

TABLE 1-41   Risk Stratification and Treatment*

BLOOD PRESSURE STAGES (mm Hg)	RISK GROUP A (NO RISK FACTORS; NO TOD/CCD)	RISK GROUP B (AT LEAST 1 RISK FACTOR, NOT INCLUDING DIABETES; NO TOD/CCD)	RISK GROUP C (TOD/CCD AND/OR DIABETES, WITH OR WITHOUT OTHER RISK FACTORS)
High-normal (130-139/85-89)	Lifestyle modification	Lifestyle modification	Drug therapy‡
Stage 1 (140-159/90-99)	Lifestyle modification (up to 12 mo)	Lifestyle modification† (up to 6 mo)	Drug therapy
Stages 2 and 3 (≥160/≥100)	Drug therapy	Drug therapy	Drug therapy

Modified from Joint National Committee on Prevention, Detection, Evaluation, and Treatment of High Blood Pressure and the National High Blood Pressure Education Program Coordinating Committee, *Arch Intern Med* 57:2413, 1997.
CCD, Clinical cardiovascular; *TOD*, target organ disease.
*NOTE: For example, a patient with diabetes and a blood pressure of 142/94 mm Hg plus LVH should be classified as having stage 1 hypertension with target organ disease LVH and with another major risk factor (diabetes). This patient would be categorized as "stage 1, risk group C" and recommended for immediate initiation of pharmacologic treatment. Lifestyle modification should be adjunctive therapy for all patients recommended for pharmacologic therapy.
†For patients with multiple risk factors, clinicians should consider drugs as initial therapy plus lifestyle modifications.
‡For those with heart failure, renal insufficiency, or diabetes.

- Note the presence of truncal obesity (Cushing's syndrome) and pedal edema (CHF, nephrosis).
- Perform full neurologic assessment.
- The clinical evaluation should help determine if the patient has primary or secondary (possibly reversible) hypertension, if there is target organ disease present, and if there are cardiovascular risk factors in addition to hypertension.

■ ETIOLOGY
- Essential (primary) hypertension (90%)
- Renal hypertension (5%)
  1. Renal parenchymal disease (3%)
  2. Renovascular hypertension (<2%)
- Endocrine (4% to 5%)
  1. Oral contraceptives (4%)
  2. Primary aldosteronism (0.5%)
  3. Pheochromocytoma (0.2%)
  4. Cushing's syndrome (0.2%)
- Coarctation of the aorta (0.2%)

🔬 DIAGNOSIS

■ WORKUP
Pertinent history:
- Age of onset of hypertension, previous antihypertensive therapy
- Family history of hypertension, stroke, cardiovascular disease
- Diet, salt intake, alcohol, drugs (e.g., oral contraceptives, NSAIDs, decongestants, steroids)
- Occupation, lifestyle, socioeconomic status, psychologic factors
- Other cardiovascular risk factors: hyperlipidemia, obesity, diabetes mellitus, carbohydrate intolerance
- Symptoms of secondary hypertension:
  1. Headache, palpitations, excessive perspiration (possible pheochromocytoma)
  2. Weakness, polyuria (consider hyperaldosteronism)
  3. Claudication of lower extremities (seen with coarctation of aorta)

■ LABORATORY TESTS
- Urinalysis: for evidence of renal disease.
- BUN, creatinine: to rule out renal disease. High-normal serum is a predictor of cardiovascular risk in essential hypertension.
- Serum electrolyte levels: low potassium is suggestive of primary aldosteronism, diuretic use.
- Screening for coexisting diseases that may adversely affect prognosis:
  1. Fasting serum glucose
  2. Serum cholesterol, HDL, triglycerides, uric acid, calcium

3. If pheochromocytoma is suspected: 24-hr urine for metanephrines

■ IMAGING STUDIES
- ECG: check for presence of left ventricular hypertrophy (LVH) with strain pattern.
- Ultrasound of the renal arteries: in suspected renovascular hypertension.

💊 TREATMENT

■ NONPHARMACOLOGIC THERAPY
Life-style modifications:
- Lose weight if overweight.
- Limit alcohol intake to ≤1 oz of ethanol per day.
- Exercise (aerobic) regularly.
- Reduce sodium intake to <100 mmol/day (<2.3 g of sodium).
- Maintain adequate dietary potassium, calcium, and magnesium intake.
- Stop smoking and reduce dietary saturated fat and cholesterol intake for overall cardiovascular health.

■ ACUTE GENERAL Rx
According to the Sixth Report of the Joint National Committee on Detection, Evaluation, and Treatment of High Blood Pressure:
- Diuretics or β-blockers are preferred by some clinicians for initial therapy because a reduction in morbidity and mortality has been demonstrated and because of their lower cost.
- ACE inhibitors, calcium antagonists, α-1 receptor blockers, and α-β blockers are also effective.
- When selecting drugs, also consider the cost of the medication, metabolic and subjective side effects, and drug-drug interactions.
- The major advantages and limitations of each class of drugs are described below:
  1. Diuretics
     a. Advantages: inexpensive, once per day dosing. Useful in blacks, edema states, CHF, chronic renal disease, elderly patients (decreased incidence of hip fractures in elderly patients).
     b. Disadvantages: significant adverse metabolic effects, increased risk of cardiac arrhythmias, sexual dysfunction, possible adverse effects on lipids and glucose levels.
  2. β-Blockers
     a. Advantages: ideal in hypertensive patients with ischemic heart disease or post-MI.

Favored in hyperkinetic, young patients (resting tachycardia, wide pulse pressure, hyperdynamic heart) and stable CHF patients.
  b. Disadvantages: adverse effect on quality of life (increased incidence of fatigue, depression, impotence, aggravation of CHF, bronchospasm, hypoglycemia, peripheral vascular disease, adverse effects on lipids, masking of signs and symptoms of hypoglycemia in diabetics; possible increased risk of sudden cardiac death.
  3. Calcium antagonists
     a. Advantages: helpful in hypertensive patients with ischemic heart disease. Generally favorable effect on quality of life; can be used in patients with bronchospastic disorders, renal disease, peripheral avascular disease, metabolic disorders, and salt sensitivity.
     b. Disadvantages: excessive cost; diltiazem and verapamil should be avoided in patients with CHF because of their chronotropic and inotropic effects; pedal edema may occur with nifedipine and amlodipine; constipation can be severe in elderly patients receiving verapamil.
  4. ACE inhibitors
     a. Advantages: well tolerated, favorable impact on quality of life; useful in hypertension complicated by CHF; helpful in prevention of diabetic renal disease; effective in decreasing LVH.
     b. Disadvantages: generally more expensive than generic diuretics and β-blockers, generic ACE inhibitors are available at lower cost; cough is a frequent side effect (5% to 20% of patients); hyperkalemia may occur in patients with diabetes or severe renal insufficiency; hypotension may occur in volume-depleted patients.
  5. Angiotensin II receptor blockers (ARB)
     a. Advantages: well tolerated, favorable impact on quality of life; useful in patients unable to tolerate ACE inhibitors because of persistent cough and in CHF and diabetic patients; single daily dose.
     b. Disadvantages: excessive cost; hypotension may occur in volume-depleted patients; contraindicated in pregnancy.

6. α-Adrenergic blockers
   a. Advantages: no adverse effect on blood lipids or insulin sensitivity; helpful in BPH.
   b. Disadvantages: frequent postural hypotension; syncope can be avoided by giving an initial low dose at bedtime.

TREATMENT OF RENOVASCULAR HYPERTENSION (RVH): The therapeutic approach varies with the cause of the RVH.
1. Young patients with fibromuscular dysplasia are best treated with percutaneous transluminal renal angioplasty (PTRA).
2. Medical therapy is advisable in elderly patients with atheromatous renal vascular hypertension; useful agents are:
   a. β-Blockers: very effective in patients with elevated plasma renin.
   b. ACE inhibitors: very effective; however, should be avoided in patients with bilateral renal artery stenosis or in patients with solitary kidney and renal stenosis.
   c. Diuretics: often used in combination with ACE inhibitors.
3. Surgical revascularization is generally reserved for atheromatous RVH in patients responding poorly to medical therapy (uncontrolled hypertension, deteriorating renal function).

HYPERTENSION DURING PREGNANCY:
1. Hypertension complicates 5% to 12% of all pregnancies.
2. The American Obstetrical Committee defines blood pressure of 130/80 mm Hg as the upper limit of normal at any time during pregnancy.
3. A rise of 30 mm Hg systolic or 15 mm Hg diastolic is also considered abnormal regardless of the absolute values obtained.
4. Chronic hypertension (occurring before pregnancy) must be distinguished from preeclampsia, because the risk to mother and fetus is much greater in the latter.
5. Treatment of chronic hypertension during pregnancy is as follows:
   a. Initial treatment with conservative measures (proper nutrition, limited physical activity).
   b. When drug therapy is necessary, initiation of one of the following agents—methyldopa, hydralazine, labetalol, or atenolol—is preferred.
   c. ACE inhibitors can cause fetal and neonatal complications; their use should be avoided in pregnancy.
   d. The safety of calcium channel blockers remains unclear.
   e. Diuretics should be used only if there is a specific reason for initiating and maintaining their use (e.g., hypertension associated with severe fluid overload or left ventricular dysfunction).

MALIGNANT HYPERTENSION, HYPERTENSIVE EMERGENCIES, AND HYPERTENSIVE URGENCIES:
• Definitions:
1. **Malignant hypertension** is a potentially life-threatening situation that is secondary to elevated BP.
   a. The rate of BP rise is a critical factor.
   b. The clinical manifestations are grade IV hypertensive retinopathy (exudates, hemorrhages, and papilledema), cardiovascular and/or renal compromise, and encephalopathy.
   c. It requires immediate BP reduction (not necessarily into normal ranges) to prevent or limit target organ disease.
2. **Hypertensive emergencies** are situations that require rapid (within 1 hr) lowering of BP to prevent end-organ damage.
3. **Hypertensive urgencies** are significant BP elevations that should be corrected within 24 hr of presentation.
• Therapy:
The choice of therapeutic agents in malignant hypertension varies with the cause.
1. Nitroprusside is the drug of choice in hypertensive encephalopathy, hypertension and intracranial bleeding, malignant hypertension, hypertension and heart failure, dissecting aortic aneurysm (used in combination with the propranolol); its onset of action is immediate.

2. The following are important points to remember when treating hypertensive emergencies:
   a. Introduce a plan for long-term therapy at the time of the initial emergency treatment.
   b. Agents that reduce arterial pressure can cause the kidney to retain sodium and water; therefore the judicious administration of diuretics should accompany their use.
   c. The initial goal of antihypertensive therapy is not to achieve a normal BP, but rather to gradually reduce the BP; cerebral hyperperfusion may occur if the mean BP is lowered >40% in the initial 24 hr.
3. Hypertensive urgencies can be effectively treated with oral clonidine 0.1 mg q20min (to a maximum of 0.8 mg); sedation is common.

☼ PEARLS & CONSIDERATIONS

■ COMMENTS
Fig. 1-213 describes an algorithm for primary hypertension; Fig. 1-212 describes an algorithm for evaluation of secondary hypertension.

REFERENCES
Deedwania PC: Hypertension and diabetes, new therapeutic options, *Arch Intern Med* 160:1585, 2000.
Papademetriou V: Selection of antihypertensive therapy for patients with hypertensive renal disease, *JAMA* 285:2774, 2001.
Vasan RS et al: Impact of high-normal blood pressure on the risk of cardiovascular disease, *N Engl J Med* 345:1291, 2001.
Zamorski M, Gaegon L: NHBPEP report on high blood pressure in pregnancy: a summary for family physicians, *Am Fam Physician* 64:263, 2001.
Author: **Fred F. Ferri, M.D.**

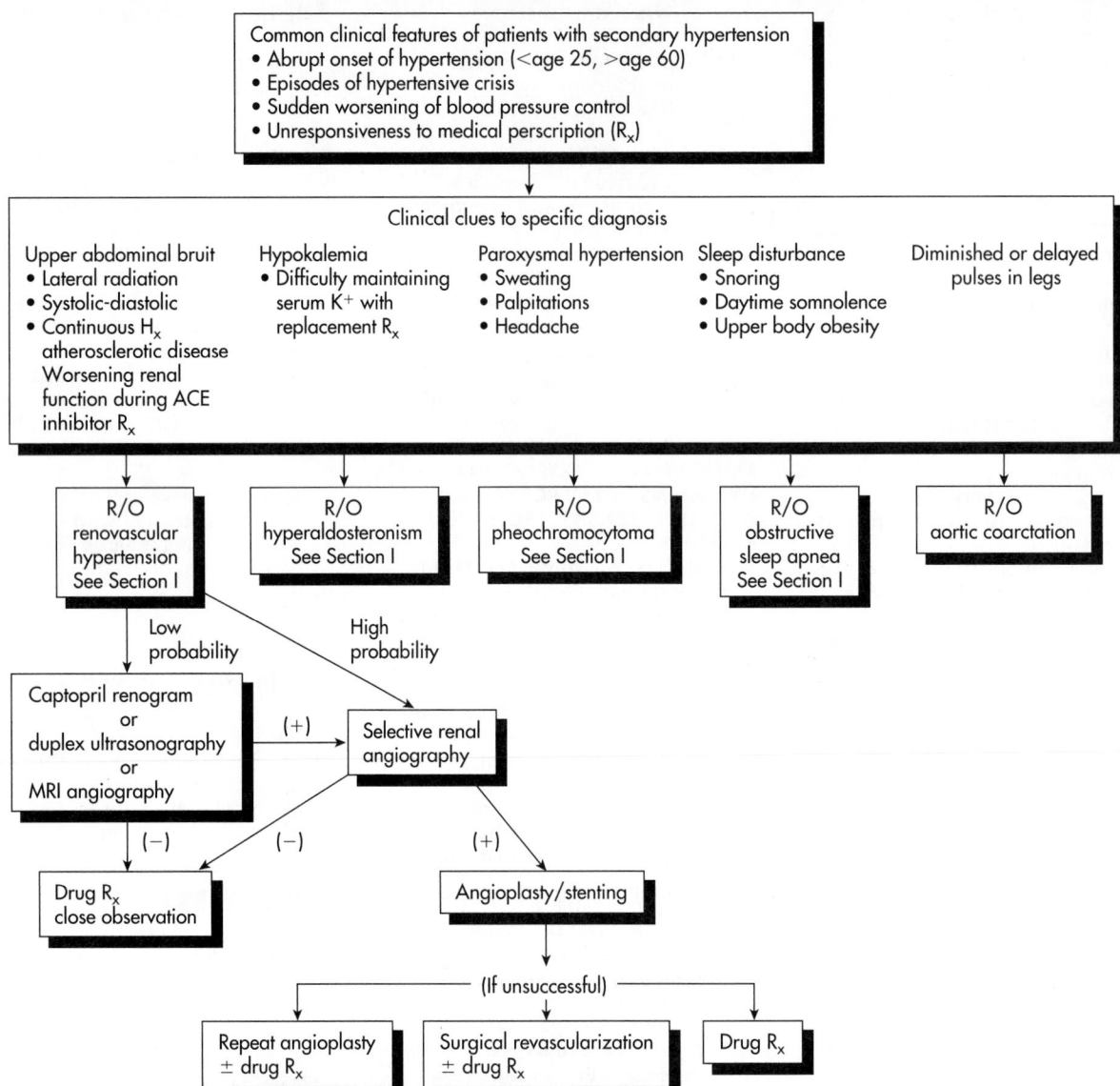

Fig. 1-212 Algorithm for identifying patients for evaluation of secondary causes of hypertension. *ACE,* Angiotension-converting enzyme; *Hx,* history; K^+, potassium; *R/O,* rule out. (From Goldman L, Bennett JC [eds]: *Cecil textbook of medicine,* ed 2, Philadelphia, 2000, WB Saunders.)

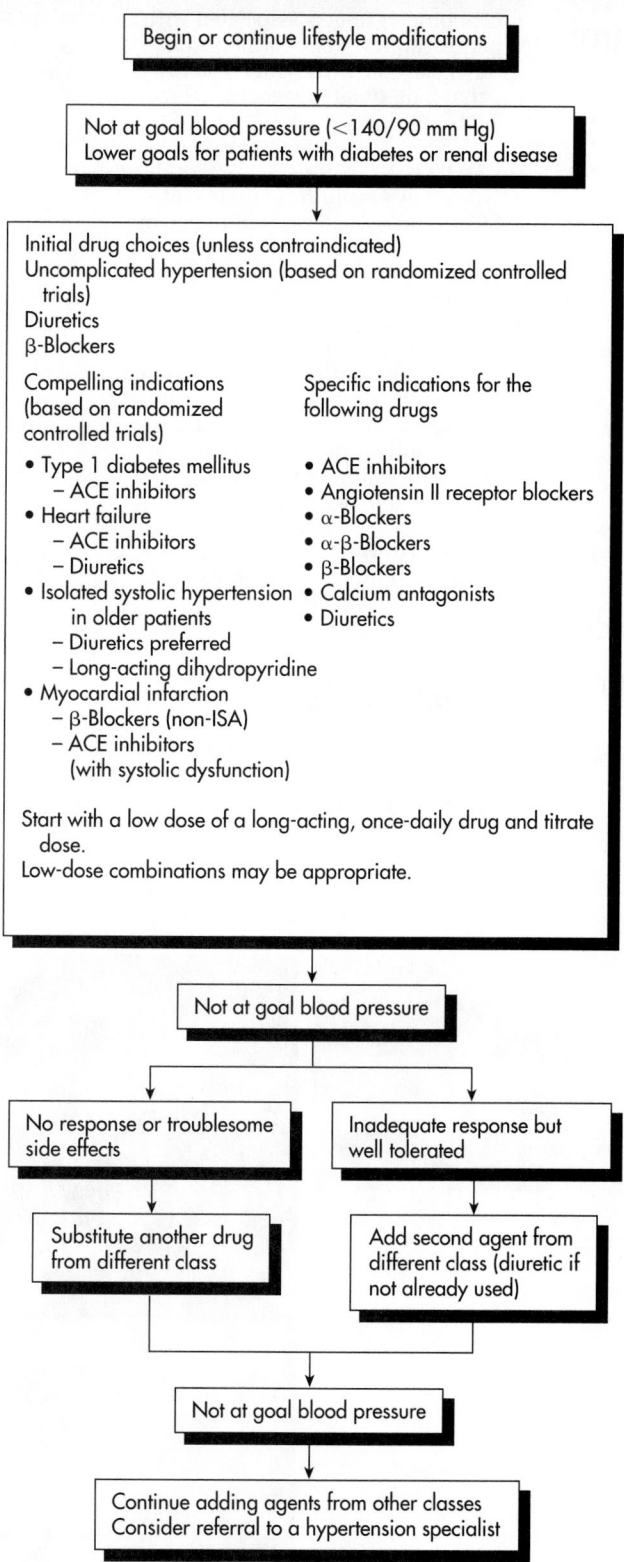

Fig. 1-213 JNC VI algorithm for the treatment of hypertension. *ACE,* Angiotensin-converting enzyme; *non-ISA,* nonintrinsic sympathomimetic activity. (Modified from Joint National Committee on Prevention, Detection, Evaluation, and Treatment of High Blood Pressure and the National High Blood Pressure Education Program Coordinating Commitee, *Arch Intern Med* 157:2413, 1997.)

BASIC INFORMATION

■ DEFINITION
Hyperthyroidism is a hypermetabolic state resulting from excess thyroid hormone.

■ SYNONYMS
Thyrotoxicosis

ICD-9CM CODES
242.9 Hyperthyroidism
242.0 Hyperthyroidism with goiter
242.2 Hyperthyroidism, multinodular
242.3 Hyperthyroidism, uninodular

■ EPIDEMIOLOGY & DEMOGRAPHICS
INCIDENCE/PREVALENCE: Hyperthyroidism affects 2% of women and 0.2% of men in their lifetimes.

■ PHYSICAL FINDINGS & CLINICAL PRESENTATION
- Tachycardia (resting rate >90 bpm), palpitations
- Tremor, hyperreflexia
- Increased sweating, warm and moist skin, onycholysis (brittle nails)
- Goiter, bruit over thyroid
- Exophthalmos, lid retraction (Fig. 1-214, *A*), lid lag (Graves' ophthalmopathy)
- Clubbing of fingers associated with periosteal new bone formation in other skeletal areas (Graves' acropachy), pretibial myxedema (Fig. 1-214, *B*)

■ ETIOLOGY
- Graves' disease (diffuse toxic goiter): 80% to 90% of all cases of hyperthyroidism
- Toxic multinodular goiter (Plummer's disease)
- Toxic adenoma
- Iatrogenic and factitious
- Transient hyperthyroidism (subacute thyroiditis, Hashimoto's thyroiditis)
- Rare causes: hypersecretion of TSH (e.g., pituitary neoplasms), struma ovarii, ingestion of large amount of iodine in a patient with preexisting thyroid hyperplasia or adenoma (Jod-Basedow phenomenon), hydatidiform mole, carcinoma of thyroid, amiodarone therapy

DIAGNOSIS

■ DIFFERENTIAL DIAGNOSIS
- Anxiety disorder
- Pheochromocytoma
- Metastatic neoplasm
- Diabetes mellitus
- Premenopausal state

■ WORKUP
Suspected hyperthyroidism requires laboratory confirmation and identification of its etiology, because treatment varies with its cause. A detailed medical history will often provide clues to the diagnosis and etiology of the hyperthyroidism:
- Patients with hyperthyroidism generally present with the following clinical manifestations: anxiety, irritability, emotional lability, panic attacks, heat intolerance, sweating, increased appetite, diarrhea, weight loss, menstrual dysfunction (oligomenorrhea, amenorrhea); the presentation may be different in elderly patients (see below).
- Patients with Graves' disease may present with the following signs and symptoms of ophthalmopathy: blurring of vision, photophobia, increased lacrimation, double vision, deep orbital pressure.
- Toxic multinodular goiter usually occurs in women >55 yr old and is more common than Graves' disease in the elderly.
- In the elderly the clinical signs of hyperthyroidism may be masked by manifestations of coexisting disease (e.g., new-onset atrial fibrillation, exacerbation of CHF).

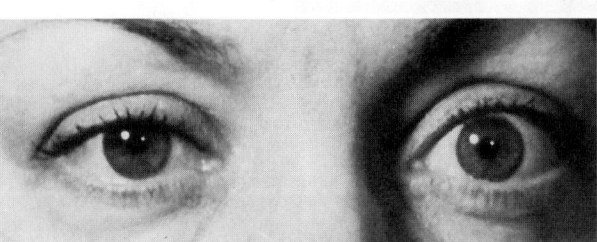

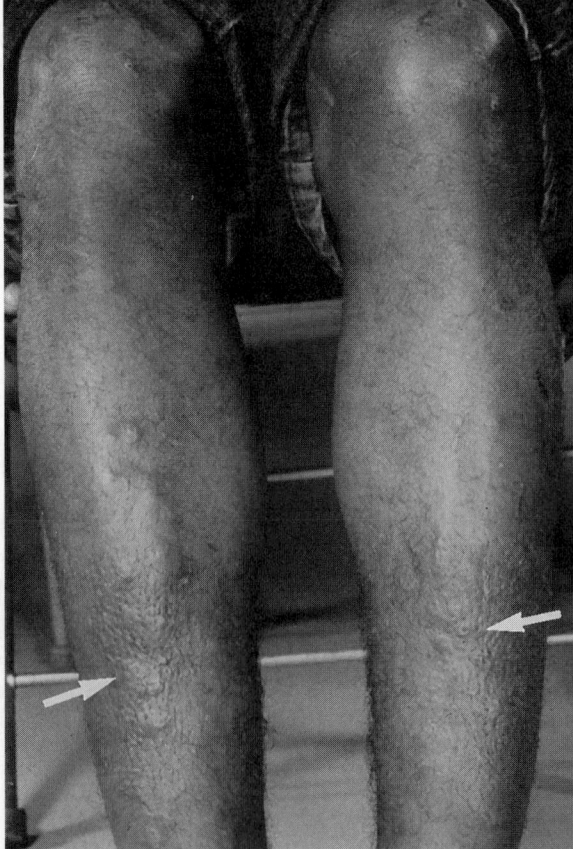

Fig. 1-214 **A,** Unilateral *(left)* lid retraction in a patient with hyperthyroidism. **B,** Pretibial myxedema *(arrows)* in a patient with Graves' disease. (From Noble J [ed]: *Textbook of primary care medicine,* ed 2, St Louis, 1996, Mosby.)

■ LABORATORY TESTS
- Elevated free thyroxine (T_4)
- Elevated free triiodothyronine (T_3): generally not necessary for diagnosis
- Low TSH (unless hyperthyroidism is a result of the rare hypersecretion of TSH from a pituitary adenoma)
- Thyroid autoantibodies useful in selected cases to differentiate Graves' disease from toxic multinodular goiter (absent thyroid antibodies)

■ IMAGING STUDIES
- 24-hr radioactive iodine uptake (RAIU) is useful to distinguish hyperthyroidism from iatrogenic thyroid hormone synthesis (thyrotoxicosis factitia) and from thyroiditis.
- An overactive thyroid shows increased uptake, whereas a normal underactive thyroid (iatrogenic thyroid ingestion, painless or subacute thyroiditis) shows normal or decreased uptake.
- The RAIU results also vary with the etiology of the hyperthyroidism: Graves' disease: increased homogeneous uptake. Multinodular goiter: increased heterogeneous uptake. Hot nodule: single focus of increased uptake.
- RAIU is also generally performed before the therapeutic administration of radioactive iodine to determine the appropriate dose.

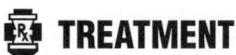

TREATMENT

■ NONPHARMACOLOGIC THERAPY
Patient education regarding thyroid disease and discussion of the therapeutic options (medications, radioactive iodine, and thyroid surgery)

■ ACUTE GENERAL Rx
ANTITHYROID DRUGS (THIONAMIDES): Propylthiouracil (PTU) and methimazole (Tapazole) inhibit thyroid hormone synthesis by blocking production of thyroid peroxidase (PTU and methimazole) or inhibit peripheral conversion of T_4 to T_3 (PTU).
1. Dosage: PTU 50 to 100 mg PO q8h; methimazole 10 to 20 mg PO q8h or 30 to 60 mg/day given as a single dose.
2. Antithyroid drugs can be used as the primary form of treatment or as adjunctive therapy before radioactive therapy or surgery or afterward if the hyperthyroidism recurs.
3. Side effects: skin rash (3% to 5% of patients), arthralgias, myalgias, granulocytopenia (0.5%). Rare side effects are aplastic anemia, hepatic necrosis from PTU, cholestatic jaundice from methimazole.
4. When antithyroid drugs are used as primary therapy, they are usually given for 6 to 24 mo; prolonged therapy may cause hypothyroidism.
5. The use of antithyroid drugs before radioactive iodine therapy is best reserved for patients in whom exacerbation of hyperthyroidism after radioactive iodine therapy is hazardous (e.g., elderly patients with coronary artery disease or significant coexisting morbidity). In these patients the antithyroid drug can be stopped 2 days before radioactive iodine therapy, resumed 2 days later, and continued for 4 to 6 wk.

RADIOACTIVE IODINE (RAI; ^{131}I):
1. RAI is the treatment of choice for patients >21 yr of age and younger patients who have not achieved remission after 1 yr of antithyroid drug therapy. Radioiodine is also used in hyperthyroidism caused by toxic adenoma or toxic multinodular goiter.
2. Contraindicated during pregnancy (can cause fetal hypothyroidism) and lactation. Pregnancy should be excluded in women of child-bearing age before radioactive iodine is administered.
3. A single dose of radioactive iodine is effective in inducing euthyroid state in nearly 80% of patients.
4. There is a high incidence of post-radioactive iodine hypothyroidism (>50% within first year and 2%/yr thereafter); therefore these patients should be frequently evaluated for the onset of hypothyroidism (see "Chronic Rx.").

SURGICAL THERAPY (SUBTOTAL THYROIDECTOMY):
1. Indicated in obstructing goiters, in any patient who refuses radioactive iodine and cannot be adequately managed with antithyroid medications (e.g., patients with toxic adenoma or toxic multinodular goiter), and in pregnant patients who cannot be adequately managed with antithyroid medication or develop side effects to them.
2. Patients should be rendered euthyroid with antithyroid drugs before surgery.
3. Complications of surgery include hypothyroidism (28% to 43% after 10 yr), hypoparathyroidism, and vocal cord paralysis (1%).
4. Hyperthyroidism recurs after surgery in 10% to 15% of patients.

ADJUNCTIVE THERAPY: Propranolol alleviates the β-adrenergic symptoms of hyperthyroidism; initial dose is 20 to 40 mg PO q6h; dosage is gradually increased until symptoms are controlled; major contraindications to use of propranolol are CHF and bronchospasm. Diagnosis and treatment of "thyroid storm" are discussed elsewhere in Section I.

■ CHRONIC Rx
Patients undergoing treatment with antithyroid drugs should be seen every 1 to 3 mo until euthyroidism is achieved and every 3 to 4 mo while they remain on antithyroid therapy. After treatment is stopped, periodic monitoring of thyroid function tests with TSH every 3 mo for 1 yr, then every 6 mo for 1 yr, then annually is recommended.

■ DISPOSITION
Successful treatment of hyperthyroidism requires lifelong monitoring for the onset of hypothyroidism or the recurrence of thyrotoxicosis.

■ REFERRAL
- Endocrinology referral is recommended at the time of initial diagnosis and during treatment.
- Surgical referral in selected patients (see "Surgical Therapy" above).
- Hospitalization of all patients with thyroid storm.

☼ PEARLS & CONSIDERATIONS

■ COMMENTS
- Elderly hyperthyroid patients may have only subtle signs (weight loss, tachycardia, fine skin, brittle nails). This form is known as *apathetic hyperthyroidism* and manifests with lethargy rather than hyperkinetic activity. An enlarged thyroid gland may be absent. Coexisting medical disorders (most commonly cardiac disease) may also mask the symptoms. These patients often have unexplained CHF, worsening of angina, or new-onset atrial fibrillation resistant to treatment. See "Graves' Disease" in Section I for additional information on the diagnosis and treatment of Graves' disease.
- Fig. 3-166 illustrates a diagnostic approach to thyroid disease.

REFERENCES
Toft AD: Sub-clinical hyperthyroidism, *N Engl J Med* 345:512, 2001.
Woeber KA: Update on the management of hyperthyroidism and hypothyroidism, *Arch Intern Med* 160:1067, 2000.
Author: **Fred F. Ferri, M.D.**

BASIC INFORMATION

■ DEFINITION

Hypertrophic osteoarthropathy (HOA) is a syndrome of clubbing of the digits, periostitis of long bones, and arthritis. HOA may be primary or secondary to other underlying disease processes.

■ SYNONYMS

- Primary hypertrophic osteo-arthropathy
  1. Pachydermoperiostosis
  2. Heredofamilial
  3. Idiopathic clubbing
  4. Touraine-Solente-Gole syndrome
- Secondary hypertrophic osteo-arthropathy

ICD-9CM CODES
731.2 Hypertrophic osteoarthropathy

■ EPIDEMIOLOGY & DEMOGRAPHICS

- Primary HOA is familial autosomal dominant disease affecting young children between ages 1 and 20.
- Secondary HOA typically occurs in adults and is associated with other illnesses including:
  1. Pulmonary: Bronchogenic carcinoma, lung abscess, bronchiectasis, cystic fibrosis, pulmonary fibrosis, mesothelioma, sarcoidosis.
  2. Gastrointestinal: Esophageal carcinoma, colon cancer, inflammatory bowel disease (Crohn's disease, ulcerative colitis), hepatocellular carcinoma, liver cirrhosis, amebiasis.
  3. Cardiac: Infective endocarditis, right-to-left cardiac shunts, aortic aneurysm.
  4. Thymoma
  5. Lymphoma
  6. Connective tissue diseases
  7. Thyroid acropachy

■ PHYSICAL FINDINGS & CLINICAL PRESENTATION

- Primary HOA typically presents with the insidious onset of clubbing of the hands and feet is and described as "spadelike." Other signs and symptoms include:
  1. Joint pain and swelling
  2. Decreased use of the fingers and hands
  3. Facial changes, coarse facial skin grooves
  4. Thickening of the arms and legs
  5. Oily skin, diaphoresis, gynecomastia, and acne

- Secondary HOA patients may present with clinical symptoms before the underlying disorder can be detected. Signs and symptoms are similar to the above mentioned in addition to findings related to the underlying disease (e.g., bronchogenic carcinoma, infective endocarditis).

■ ETIOLOGY

Unknown; immunologic, endocrine, and vascular etiologies have been suggested.

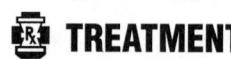

DIAGNOSIS

■ DIFFERENTIAL DIAGNOSIS

- Other causes of periostitis include Paget's disease, Reiter's syndrome, psoriasis, syphilis, osteoarthritis, rheumatoid arthritis, and osteomyelitis.
- Hypertrophic osteoarthropathy with the classic finding of clubbing of the digits warrants an investigation into any associated illnesses.

■ WORKUP

Primarily consists of blood tests, x-rays, and bone scans.

■ LABORATORY TESTS

- CBC, electrolytes, and urine studies will typically be normal in both primary and secondary HOA.
- ESR will be elevated in secondary HOA.

- Liver function tests may be abnormal in patients with secondary HOA from GI pathology.
- Alkaline phosphatase may be elevated secondary to periostitis of long bones.
- Analysis of the synovial fluid from joint effusions reveals a low white cell count with normal viscosity, color, and complement levels.

■ IMAGING STUDIES

- X-rays of the long bones show periosteal new bone formation (Fig. 1-215)
- A chest x-ray should be obtained to rule out underlying lung cancer.
- Bone scan with technetium-99m reveals uptake along the long bones, phalanxes, and periarticular joint spaces are common findings.

TREATMENT

■ ACUTE GENERAL Rx

- Treatment of primary HOA is symptomatic. Aspirin (acetylsalicylic acid) 325 mg PO q4-6 hr prn, salicylate 750 mg bid prn, ibuprofen 400 to 800 mg tid prn, naproxen 250 to 500 mg bid prn, indomethacin 25 to 50 mg qid prn will provide bone and joint pain relief.
- For secondary HOA the treatment of choice is to eradicate the underlying disease (e.g., antibiotics for infective endocarditis, surgery for bronchogenic carcinoma).

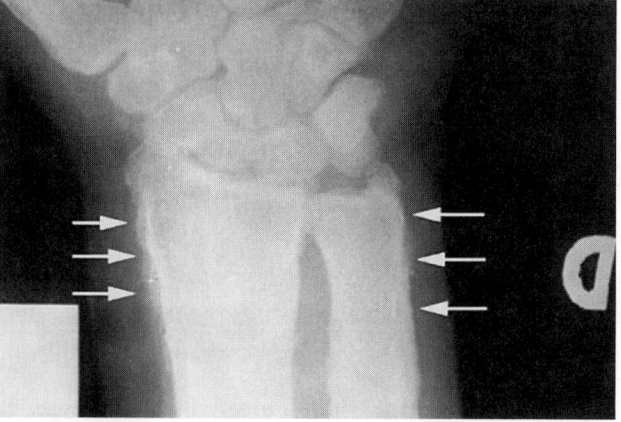

Fig. 1-215 Hypertrophic osteoarthropathy. Coarse periosteal new bone formation in the distal ulna and radius *(arrows)* in a patient with cyanotic congenital heart disease. (Courtesy Dr. Manuel Martinez Lavin, Mexico City. In Canoso J: *Rheumatology in primary care,* Philadelphia, 1997, WB Saunders.)

■ **CHRONIC Rx**
- In patients with secondary HOA refractory to NSAIDs and aspirin, vagotomy has been tried with some success. However, the definitive treatment is to treat the underlying disease.

■ **DISPOSITION**
- Patients with primary HOA typically will have symptoms of joint pains and swelling for the early part of their life, but thereafter the disease becomes quiescent.
- Prognosis and disease course in patients with secondary HOA will depend on the underlying cause. The insidious development of clubbing suggests infectious process, whereas the rapid progression of clubbing may suggest underlying malignancy.

■ **REFERRAL**
Referral should be made to rheumatology when the diagnosis of HOA is suspected and the cause remains unclear.

☼ PEARLS & CONSIDERATIONS

■ **COMMENTS**
- HOA may be a marker for an underlying serious illness and a thorough investigation should be pursued. Infections and intrathoracic malignancies are the most common causes of secondary HOA.

REFERENCES

Altman RD, Tenebaum J: *Hypertrophic osteoarthropathy.* In Kelly WN et al (eds): *Textbook of rheumatology,* ed 5, Baltimore, 1997, WB Saunders.

Pineda CF, Fonseca C, Martinenez-Lavin M: The spectrum of soft tissue and skeletal abnormalities of hypertrophic osteoarthropathy, *J Rheumatol* 17:773, 1990.

Author: **Peter Petropoulos M.D.**

BASIC INFORMATION

■ DEFINITION
Hypoaldosteronism is an aldosterone deficiency or impaired aldosterone function.

■ ICD-9CM CODES
255.4 Hypoadrenalism

■ EPIDEMIOLOGY AND DEMOGRAPHICS
• Selective hypoaldosteronism accounts for as many as 10% of cases of unexplained hyperkalemia.

■ PHYSICAL FINDINGS & CLINICAL PRESENTATION
• Physical examination may be entirely within normal limits.
• Hypertension may be present in some patients.
• Profound muscle weakness and cardiac arrhythmias may be present.

■ ETIOLOGY
• Hyporeninemic hypoaldosteronism (renin-angiotensin dependent): decreased aldosterone production secondary to decreased renin production; the typical patient has renal disease secondary to various factors (e.g., diabetes mellitus, interstitial nephritis, multiple myeloma).
• Hyperreninemic hypoaldosteronism (renin-angiotensin independent): renin production by the kidneys is intact; the defect is in aldosterone biosynthesis or in the action of angiotensin II. Common causes of this form of hypoaldosteronism are medications (ACE inhibitors, heparin), lead poisoning, aldosterone enzyme defects, and severe illness.

DIAGNOSIS

■ DIFFERENTIAL DIAGNOSIS
• Pseudohypoaldosteronism: renal unresponsiveness to aldosterone. In this condition, both renin and aldosterone levels are elevated. Pseudohypoaldosteronism can be caused by medications (spironolactone), chronic interstitial nephritis, systemic disorders (SLE, amyloidosis), or primary mineralocorticoid resistance.
• Box 2-136 describes the differential diagnosis of hyperkalemia.

■ WORKUP
Measurement of plasma renin activity following 4 hours of upright posture can differentiate hyporeninemic from hyperreninemic causes. Renin levels in the normal or low range identify cases that are renin-angiotensin dependent, whereas high renin levels identify cases that are renin-angiotensin independent. The diagnosis and etiology of hypoaldosteronism can be confirmed with the renin-aldosterone stimulation test:
• Hyporeninemic hypoaldosteronism: low stimulated renin and aldosterone levels
• End-organ refractoriness to aldosterone action: high stimulated renin and aldosterone levels
• Adrenal gland abnormality: high stimulated renin and low aldosterone levels
• Fig. 1-216 illustrates the normal function of the renal pressor system.

■ LABORATORY TESTS
• Increased potassium, normal or decreased sodium
• Hyperchloremic metabolic acidosis (caused by the absence of hydrogen-secreting action of aldosterone)
• Increased BUN and creatinine (secondary to renal disease)
• Hyperglycemia (diabetes mellitus is common in these patients)

TREATMENT

■ NONPHARMACOLOGIC THERAPY
• Low-potassium diet with liberal sodium intake (at least 4 g of sodium chloride per day)
• Avoidance of ACE inhibitors and potassium-sparing diuretics

■ ACUTE GENERAL Rx
• Judicious use of fludrocortisone (0.05 to 0.1 mg PO qAM) in patients with aldosterone deficiency associated with deficiency of adrenal glucocorticoid hormones
• Furosemide 20 to 40 mg qd to correct hyperkalemia of hyporeninemic hypoaldosteronism

■ DISPOSITION
Prognosis varies with the etiology of hypoaldosteronism and presence of associated disorders.

■ REFERRAL
Endocrinology referral for renin-aldosterone stimulation test

PEARLS & CONSIDERATIONS

■ COMMENTS
Treatment of pseudohypoaldosteronism is the same as for hypoaldosteronism; however, effect is limited because of impaired renal sensitivity.
Author: **Fred F. Ferri, M.D.**

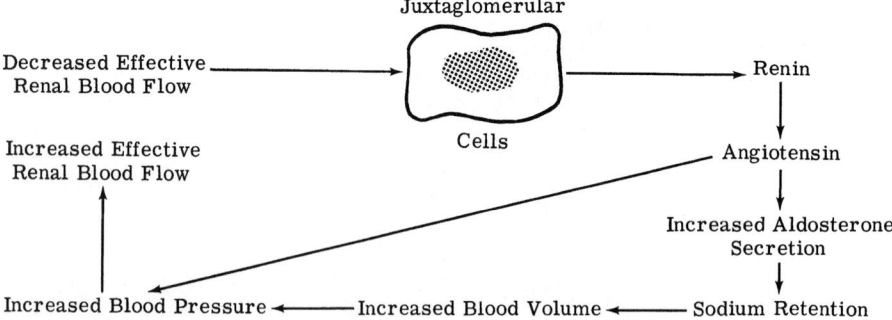

Fig. 1-216   Renal pressor system. (From Ravel R [ed]: *Clinical laboratory medicine,* ed 6, St Louis, 1995, Mosby.)

BASIC INFORMATION

■ DEFINITION

Hypopituitarism is the partial or complete loss of pituitary hormone secretion resulting from diseases of the hypothalamus or pituitary gland.

■ SYNONYMS

Panhypopituitarism
Pituitary insufficiency

■ ICD-9CM CODES

253.2 Panhypopituitarism

■ EPIDEMIOLOGY & DEMOGRAPHICS

- Pituitary tumors are the most common causes of hypopituitarism with an incidence of 0.2 to 2.8 cases per 100,000.
- Increased incidence of vascular or cerebrovascular disease in patients with panhypopituitarism.
- Predisposing factors for pituitary apoplexy (another cause of panhypopituitarism) include diabetes mellitus, anticoagulant therapy, head trauma, pituitary tumors, and radiation.
- Empty sella syndrome, a third cause of panhypopituitarism, can occur in both adults and children.

■ PHYSICAL FINDINGS & CLINICAL PRESENTATION

The onset of hypopituitarism is usually gradual, and symptoms are related to the lack of one or more hormones and/or mass effect if a pituitary tumor is the cause.
- Mass effect of a pituitary tumor can cause headaches and visual disturbances
- Corticotropin deficiency:
  1. Fatigue and weakness, no appetite, abdominal pain, nausea, and vomiting
  2. Hypotension, hair loss, and change in mental status
- Thyrotropin deficiency:
  1. Fatigue and weakness, weight gain, cold intolerance, and constipation
  2. Bradycardia, hung-up reflexes, pretibial edema, and hair loss
- Gonadotropin deficiency:
  1. Loss of libido, erectile dysfunction, amenorrhea, hot flashes, dyspareunia
  2. Gynecomastia with lack of hair growth and decreased muscle mass
- Growth hormone deficiency:
  1. Growth retardation in children
  2. Easy fatigue
  3. Decreased muscle mass and obesity

- Hyperprolactinemia
  1. Galactorrhea
  2. Hypogonadism
- Vasopressin deficiency:
  1. Polyuria, polydipsia and nocturia
  2. Hypotension and dehydration

■ ETIOLOGY

Hypopituitarism is the result of destruction of pituitary cells caused by:
- Pituitary tumors
  1. Macroadenomas >10 mm
  2. Microadenomas <10 mm
- Pituitary apoplexy caused by hemorrhage or infarction of the pituitary gland
- Pituitary radiation therapy
- Pituitary surgery
- Empty sella syndrome with enlargement of the sella turcica and flattening of the pituitary gland caused by extension of the subarachnoid space and filling of cerebrospinal fluid into the sella turcica
- Infiltrative disease including sarcoidosis, hemochromatosis, histiocytosis X, Wegener's granulomatosis, and lymphocytic hypophysitis
- Infection (tuberculosis, mycosis, and syphilis)
- Head trauma
- Internal carotid artery aneurysm

🔬 DIAGNOSIS

The diagnosis of hypopituitarism is suspected by clinical history and physical findings and is established by endocrine stimulation testing.

■ DIFFERENTIAL DIAGNOSIS

The differential diagnosis is as outlined under "Etiology." Other rare causes include postpartum necrosis (Sheehan's syndrome), hypopituitary tumors (e.g., craniopharyngiomas and meningioma), metastatic tumors, and developmental abnormalities.

■ WORKUP

Includes basal determination of each anterior pituitary hormone followed by provocative stimulation tests and x-ray imaging.

■ LABORATORY TESTS

- Corticotropin deficiency:
  1. Serum AM cortisol level usually is low.
  2. Corticotropin stimulation test using 250 μg of corticotropin given IV and measuring serum cortisol before and 30 and 60 min after administration. A normal response is an increase in serum cortisol level >20 μg/dl.

- Thyrotropin deficiency:
  1. TSH and free T_4 measurements.
  2. Primary hypothyroidism shows elevated TSH with low free T_4. Secondary hypothyroidism shows normal or low TSH with low free T_4.
- Gonadotropin deficiency:
  1. FSH, LH, estrogen, and testosterone measurements.
  2. In men, hypogonadotropic hypogonadism is seen with low testosterone levels and normal or low FSH and LH levels.
  3. In premenopausal women with amenorrhea, low estrogen with normal or low FSH and LH levels is typically seen.
- Growth hormone deficiency:
  1. Insulin-induced hypoglycemia stimulation test using 0.1 to 0.15 unit/kg regular insulin given IV and measuring growth hormone 30, 60, and 120 min after administration. A normal response is a growth hormone level >10 μg/dl.
  2. Serum insulin-like growth factor I can also be measured after provocative testing.
- Hyperprolactinemia:
  1. Prolactin levels may be elevated in prolactin-secreting pituitary adenomas.
- Vasopressin deficiency:
  1. Urinalysis shows low specific gravity.
  2. Urine osmolality is low.
  3. Serum osmolality is high.
  4. Fluid deprivation test over 18 hr with inability to concentrate the urine.
  5. Serum vasopressin level is low.
  6. Electrolytes may show hyponatremia and exclude hyperglycemia.

■ IMAGING STUDIES

- MRI is more sensitive than CT scan of the head in visualizing the pituitary fossa, sella turcica, optic chiasm, pituitary stalk, and cavernous sinuses. It is also more sensitive in detecting pituitary microadenomas.
- CT scan with coronal cuts through the sella turcica gives better images of bony structures.
- Skull films can be done but are not very sensitive.

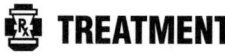 TREATMENT

Hormone replacement therapy and either surgery, radiation, or medications in patients with pituitary tumors.

■ NONPHARMACOLOGIC THERAPY

- IV fluid resuscitation with normal saline to maintain hemodynamic stability may be needed in some circumstances.
- Correction of electrolyte and metabolic abnormalities with potassium, bicarbonate, and oxygen therapy.

■ ACUTE GENERAL Rx

Acute situations like adrenal crisis or myxedema coma can occur in untreated hypopituitarism and should be treated accordingly with IV corticosteroids (e.g., hydrocortisone 100 mg IV q6h for 24 hr) and levothyroxine (e.g., 5 to 8 μg/kg IV over 15 min, then 100 μg IV q24h).

■ CHRONIC Rx

Treatment is lifelong and requires the following hormone replacement therapy:

- Hydrocortisone 20 mg PO qAM and 10 mg PO qPM or prednisone 5 mg PO qAM and 2.5 mg PO qPM.
- Testosterone enanthate or propionate 200 to 300 mg IM q2 to 3 wk or transdermal testosterone scrotal patches can be tried.

- Conjugated estrogen 0.3 to 1.25 mg/day and held the last 5 to 7 days of each month plus medroxyprogesterone 10 mg/day given during days 15 to 25.
- Levothyroxine 0.05 to 0.15 mg/day.
- Growth hormone is not used in adults; however, can be given at 0.04 to 0.08 mg/kg/day subcutaneously in children.
- Desmopressin (DDAVP) 10 to 20 μg via intranasal spray or 0.05 to 0.1 mg PO bid is used in patients with diabetes insipidus.

■ DISPOSITION

- Hormone replacement therapy is adjusted according to serum hormone blood monitoring.
- Hypopituitarism if untreated can lead to adrenal crisis, severe hyponatremia and hypothyroidism, metabolic abnormalities, and death.
- Life expectancy can be normal in patients with eradication of the pituitary disease and adequate hormone replacement therapy.

■ REFERRAL

Anyone suspected of having hypopituitarism should have an endocrine consultation. For patients with pituitary tumors, a radiation oncologist and neurosurgeon consultation should be consulted.

☼ PEARLS & CONSIDERATIONS

■ COMMENTS

- Thyroxine supplementation increases the rate of cortisol metabolism and can lead to adrenal crisis. It is therefore recommended to supplement corticosteroids first prior to administering thyroid hormone replacement therapy.
- Stress doses of corticosteroids are indicated before surgery or for any medical emergency (e.g., sepsis, acute myocardial infarction, etc.).

REFERENCES

Heshmann AM et al: Hypopituitarism caused by intracellular aneurysms, *Mayo Clin Proc* 76:789, 2001.

Lamberts SWJ, de Herder WW, van der Lely AJ: Pituitary insufficiency, *Lancet* 352:127, 1998.

Vance ML: Hypopituitarism, *N Engl J Med* 330(23):1651, 1994.

Author: **Peter Petropoulos, M.D.**

BASIC INFORMATION

■ DEFINITION

Hypothermia is a rectal temperature <35° C (95.8° F). *Accidental hypothermia* is unintentionally induced decrease in core temperature in absence of preoptic anterior hypothalamic conditions.

ICD-9CM CODES

991.6 Accidental hypothermia
780.9 Hypothermia not associated with low environmental temperature

■ EPIDEMIOLOGY & DEMOGRAPHICS

Hypothermia occurs most frequently in the following groups: alcoholics, learning-impaired, patients with cardiovascular, cerebrovascular, or pituitary disorders, those using sedatives or tranquilizers, and elderly patients.

■ PHYSICAL FINDINGS & CLINICAL PRESENTATION

• The clinical presentation varies with the severity of hypothermia (Table 1-42); shivering may be absent if body temperature is <33.3° C (92° F) or in patients taking phenothiazines.
• Hypothermia may masquerade as CVA, ataxia, or slurred speech, or the patient may appear comatose or clinically dead.
• Physiologic stages of hypothermia:
1. Mild hypothermia (32.2° to 35° C [90° to 95° F]): dysarthria, ataxia
2. Moderate hypothermia (28° to 32.2° C [82.4° to 90° F]):
    a. Progressive decrease of level of consciousness, pulse, cardiac output, and respiration
    b. Fibrillation, dysrhythmias (increased susceptibility to ventricular tachycardia)
    c. Elimination of shivering mechanism for thermogenesis
3. Severe hypothermia (≤28° C [82.4° F]):
    a. Absence of reflexes or response to pain
    b. Decreased cerebral blood flow, decreased CO_2
    c. Increased risk of ventricular fibrillation or asystole

■ ETIOLOGY

Exposure to cold temperatures for a prolonged period

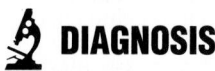

DIAGNOSIS

■ DIFFERENTIAL DIAGNOSIS

• CVA
• Myxedema coma
• Drug intoxication
• Hypoglycemia

■ LABORATORY TESTS

• ABGs: metabolic and respiratory acidosis; when blood cools, arterial pH increases, Po_2 increases, Pco_2 falls
• Electrolytes: hypokalemia initially, then hyperkalemia with increasing hypothermia
• CBC: elevated Hct (secondary to hemoconcentration), leukopenia, thrombocytopenia (secondary to splenic sequestration)
• Increased blood viscosity, increased clotting time

TABLE 1-42 Characteristics of the Four Zones of Hypothermia

STAGE	CORE TEMPERATURE °C	°F	CHARACTERISTICS
Mild	37.6	99.6 ± 1	Normal rectal temperature
	37.0	98.6 ± 1	Noraml oral temperature
	36.0	96.8	Increase in metabolic rate and blood pressure and preshivering muscle tone
	35.0	95.0	Urine temperature 34.8° C; maximum shivering thermogenesis
	34.0	93.2	Amnesia, dysarthria, and poor judgment develop; maladaptive behavior; normal blood pressure; maximum respiratory stimulation; tachycardia, then progressive bradycardia
	33.30	91.4	Ataxia and apathy develop; linear depression of cerebral metabolism; tachypnea, then progressive decrease in respiratory minute volume; cold diuresis
Moderate	32.0	89.6	Stupor; 25% decrease in oxygen consumption
	31.0	87.8	Extinguished shivering thermogenesis
	30.0	86.0	Atrial fibrillation and other arrhythmias develop; poikilothermia; pupils and cardiac output two thirds of normal; insulin ineffective
	29.0	85.2	Progressive decrease in level of consciousness, pulse, and respiration; pupils dilated; paradoxical undressing
Severe	28.0	82.4	Decreased ventricular fibrillation threshold; 50% decrease in oxygen consumption and pulse; hypoventilation
	27.0	80.6	Loss of reflexes and voluntary motion
	26.0	78.8	Major acid-base disturbances; no reflexes or response to pain
	25.0	77.0	Cerebral blood flow one third of normal; loss of cerebrovascular autoregulation; cardiac output 45% of normal; pulmonary edema may develop
	24.0	75.2	Significant hypotension and bradycardia
	23.0	73.4	No corneal or oculocephalic reflexes; areflexia
	22.0	71.6	Maximum risk of ventricular fibrillation; 75% decrease in oxygen consumption
Profound	20.0	68.0	Lowest resumption of cardiac electromechanical activity; pulse 20% of normal
	19.0	66.2	Electroencephalographic silencing
	18.0	64.4	Asystole
	13.7	56.8	Lowest adult accidental hypothermia survival
	15.0	59.2	Lowest infant accidental hypothermia survival
	10.0	50.0	92% decrease in oxygen consumption
	9.0	48.2	Lowest therapeutic hypothermia survival

From Auerbach PS: *Wilderness medicine,* ed 4, St Louis, 2001, Mosby.

■ **IMAGING STUDIES**
- Chest x-ray examination: generally not helpful; may reveal evidence of aspiration (e.g., intoxicated patient with aspiration pneumonia).
- ECG: prolonged PR, QT, and QRS segments, depressed ST segments, inverted T waves, AV block, hypothermic J waves (Osborn waves) may appear at 25° to 30° C; characterized by notching of the junction of the QRS complex and ST segments (Fig. 1-218).

℞ **TREATMENT**

■ **NONPHARMACOLOGIC THERAPY**
- Treatment of hypothermia varies with the following:
  1. Degree of hypothermia
  2. Existence of concomitant diseases (e.g., cardiovascular insufficiency)
  3. Patient's age and medical condition (e.g., elderly, debilitated patients vs. young, healthy patients)
- General measures:
  1. Secure an airway before warming all unconscious patients; precede endotracheal intubation with oxygenation (if possible) to minimize the risk of dysrhythmias during the procedure.
  2. Peripheral vasoconstriction may impede placement of a peripheral intravenous catheter; consider femoral venous access as an alternative to the jugular or subclavian sites to avoid ventricular stimulation.

  3. A Foley catheter should be inserted, and urinary output should be monitored and maintained above 0.5 to 1 ml/kg/hr with intravascular volume replacement.

■ **ACUTE GENERAL Rx**
- Continuous ECG monitoring of patients is recommended; ventricular arrhythmias can be treated with bretylium; lidocaine is generally ineffective, and procainamide is associated with an increased incidence of ventricular fibrillation in hypothermic patients.
- Correct severe acidosis and electrolyte abnormalities.
- Hypothyroidism, if present, should be promptly treated (refer to "Myxedema Coma").
- If clinical evidence suggests adrenal insufficiency, administer IV methylprednisolone.
- In patients unresponsive to verbal or noxious stimuli or with altered mental status, 100 mg of thiamine, 0.4 mg of naloxone, and 1 ampule of 50% dextrose may be given.
- Warm (104° to 113° F [40° to 45° C]), humidified oxygen should also be given if it is available.
- Specific treatment:
  1. Mild hypothermia (rectal temperature <32.3° C [90° F]): passive external rewarming is indicated. Place the patient in a warm room (temperature >21° C [69.8° F]), and cover with insulating material after gently removing wet clothing; recommended rewarming rates vary between 0.5° and 20° C/hr but should not exceed 0.55° C/hr in elderly persons.

  2. Moderate to severe hypothermia:
     a. Active core rewarming
        (1) Delivery of heat via fluids: warm GI irrigation (with saline enemas and via NG tube); IV fluids (usually D$_5$NS without potassium) warmed to 104° to 107.6° F (40° to 42° C), peritoneal dialysis with dialysate heated to 40.5° to 42.5° C.
        (2) Inhalation of heated humidified oxygen
     b. Active external rewarming: immersion in a bath of warm water (40° to 41° C); active external rewarming may produce shock because of excessive peripheral vasodilation. Ideal candidates are previously healthy, young patients with acute immersion hypothermia.
     c. Extracorporeal blood warming with cardiopulmonary bypass appears to be an efficacious rewarming technique in young, otherwise healthy persons.

☼ **PEARLS & CONSIDERATIONS**

■ **COMMENTS**
Fig. 1-217 describhes an algorithm for the treatment of hypothermia.
Author: **Fred F. Ferri, M.D.**

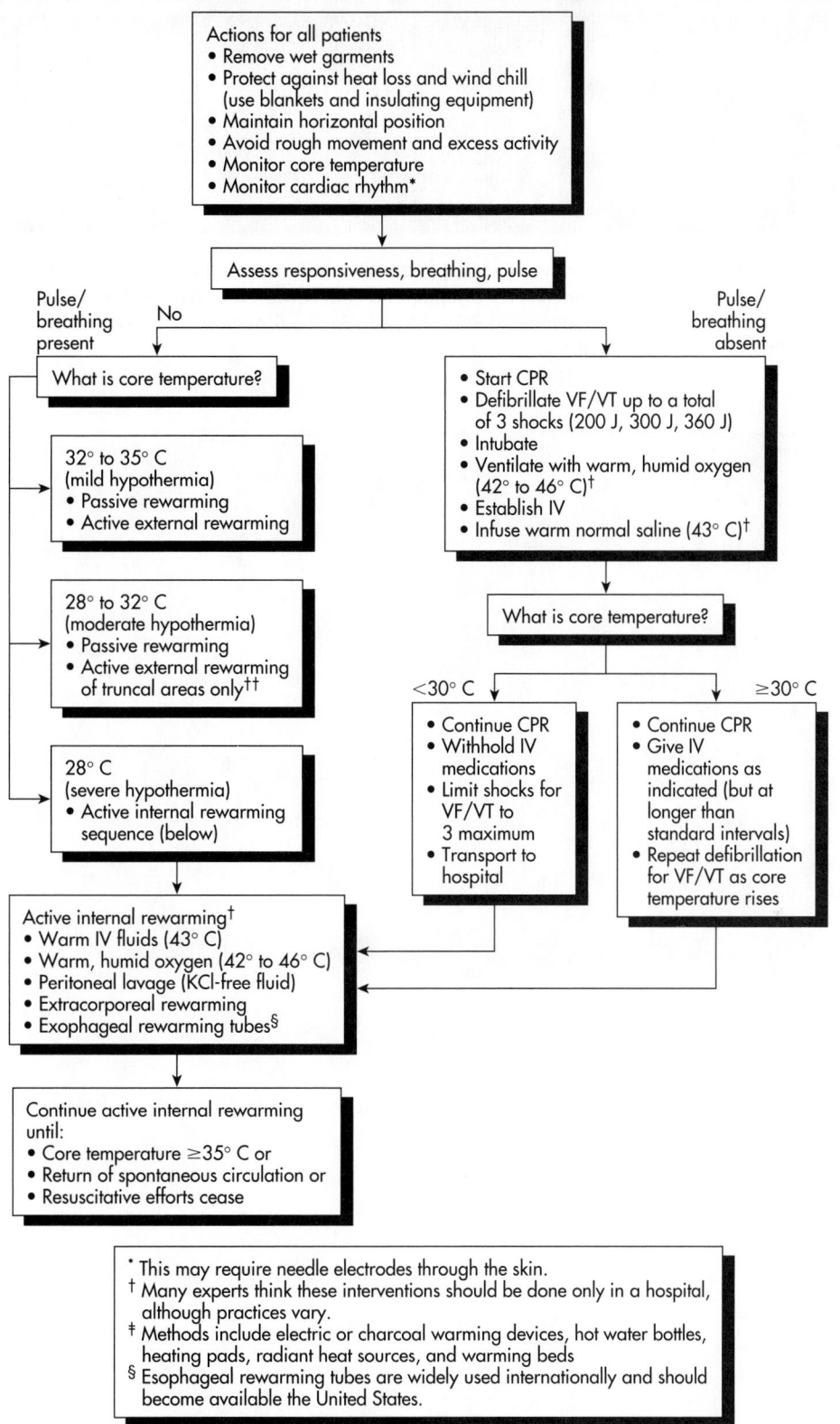

Fig. 1-217 **Treatment of hypothermia.** *CPR,* Cardiopulmonary resuscitation; *IV,* intravenous; *KCl,* potassium chloride; *VF/VT,* ventricular fibrillation/ventricular tachycardia. (Adapted from Standards and guidelines for cardiopulmonary resuscitation and emergency cardiac care, *JAMA* 268:2172, 1992.)

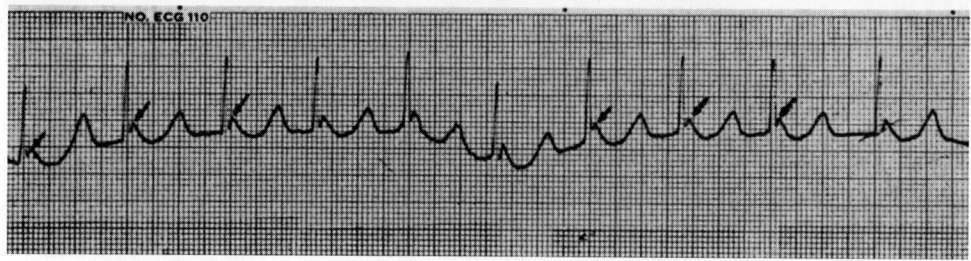

Fig. 1-218 Osborne waves *(arrows)* in an 80-year-old man with core temperature of 86°F (30°C). These waves disappeared with rewarming. (From Morse CD, Rial WY: Emergency medicine. In Rakel RE [ed]: *Textbook of family practice,* ed 4, Philadelphia, 1990, WB Saunders.)

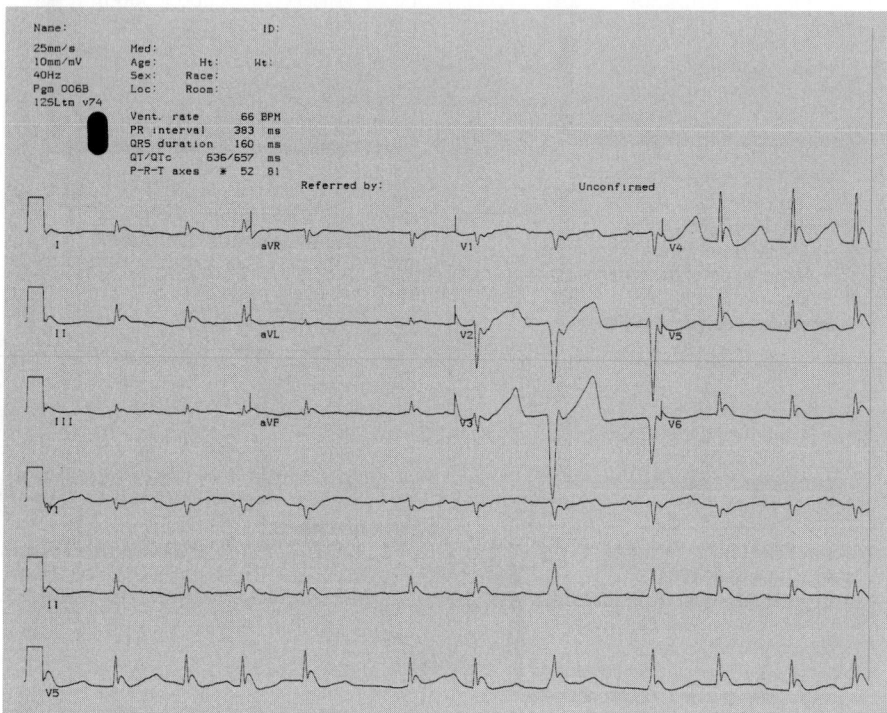

Fig. 1-219 The J or Osborn wave of hypothermia. (From Auerbach PS: *Wilderness medicine,* ed 4, St Louis, 2001, Mosby.)

BASIC INFORMATION

■ DEFINITION
Hypothyroidism is a disorder caused by the inadequate secretion of thyroid hormone.

■ SYNONYMS
Myxedema

ICD-9CM CODES
244 Acquired hypothyroidism
243 Congenital hypothyroidism
244.1 Surgical hypothyroidism
244.3 Iatrogenic hypothyroidism
244.8 Pituitary hypothyroidism
246.1 Sporadic goitrous hypothyroidism

■ EPIDEMIOLOGY & DEMOGRAPHICS
INCIDENCE/PREVALENCE: 1.5% to 2% of women and 0.2% of men
PREDOMINANT AGE: Incidence of hypothyroidism increases with age; among persons older than 60 yr, 6% of women and 2.5% of men have laboratory evidence of hypothyroidism (TSH > twice normal).

■ PHYSICAL FINDINGS & CLINICAL PRESENTATION
- Skin: dry, coarse, thick, cool, sallow (yellow color caused by carotenemia); nonpitting edema in skin of eyelids and hands (myxedema) secondary to infiltration of subcutaneous tissues by a hydrophilic mucopolysaccharide substance
- Hair: brittle and coarse; loss of outer one third of eyebrows
- Facies: dulled expression, thickened tongue, thick slow-moving lips
- Thyroid gland: may or may not be palpable (depending on the cause of the hypothyroidism)
- Heart sounds: distant, possible pericardial effusion
- Pulse: bradycardia
- Neurologic: delayed relaxation phase of the DTRs, cerebellar ataxia, hearing impairment, poor memory, peripheral neuropathies with paresthesia
- Musculoskeletal: carpal tunnel syndrome, muscular stiffness, weakness

■ ETIOLOGY
PRIMARY HYPOTHYROIDISM (THYROID GLAND DYSFUNCTION):
The cause of >90% of the cases of hypothyroidism
- Hashimoto's thyroiditis is the most common cause of hypothyroidism after 8 yr of age.
- Idiopathic myxedema (nongoitrous form of Hashimoto's thyroiditis).
- Previous treatment of hyperthyroidism (radioiodine therapy, subtotal thyroidectomy).
- Subacute thyroiditis.
- Radiation therapy to the neck (usually for malignant disease).
- Iodine deficiency or excess.
- Drugs (lithium, PAS, sulfonamides, phenylbutazone, amiodarone, thiourea).
- Congenital (approximately 1 case per 4000 live births).
- Prolonged treatment with iodides.
SECONDARY HYPOTHYROIDISM: Pituitary dysfunction, postpartum necrosis, neoplasm, infiltrative disease causing deficiency of TSH
TERTIARY HYPOTHYROIDISM: Hypothalamic disease (granuloma, neoplasm, or irradiation causing deficiency of TRH)
TISSUE RESISTANCE TO THYROID HORMONE: Rare

DIAGNOSIS

Hypothyroid patients generally present with the following signs and symptoms: fatigue, lethargy, weakness, constipation, weight gain, cold intolerance, muscle weakness, slow speech, slow cerebration with poor memory.

■ DIFFERENTIAL DIAGNOSIS
- Depression
- Dementia from other causes
- Systemic disorders (e.g., nephrotic syndrome, CHF, amyloidosis)

■ LABORATORY TESTS
- Increased TSH: TSH may be normal if patient has secondary or tertiary hypothyroidism, is receiving dopamine or corticosteroids, or the level is obtained following severe illness
- Decreased free T_4
- Other common laboratory abnormalities: hyperlipidemia, hyponatremia, and anemia
- Increased antimicrosomal and antithyroglobulin antibody titers: useful when autoimmune thyroiditis is suspected as the cause of the hypothyroidism

TREATMENT

■ NONPHARMACOLOGIC THERAPY
Patients should be educated regarding hypothyroidism and its possible complications. Patients should also be instructed about the need for lifelong treatment and monitoring of their thyroid abnormality.

■ ACUTE GENERAL Rx
Start replacement therapy with levothyroxine (Synthroid, Levothroid) 25 to 100 μg/day, depending on the patient's age and the severity of the disease. The dose may be increased every 6 to 8 wk, depending on the clinical response and serum TSH level. Elderly patients and patients with coronary artery disease should be started with 12.5 to 25 μg/day (higher doses may precipitate angina). The average maintenance dose of levothyroxine is 1.7 μg/kg/day (100 to 150 μg/day in adults). The elderly may require <1 μg/kg/day, whereas children generally require higher doses (up to 3 to 4 μg/kg/day). Pregnant patients also have increased requirements. Estrogen therapy may also increase the need for thyroxine.

■ CHRONIC Rx
Periodic monitoring of TSH level is an essential part of treatment. Patients should be evaluated initially with office visit and TSH levels every 6 to 8 wk until the patient is clinically euthyroid and the TSH level is normalized. The frequency of subsequent visits and TSH measurement can then be decreased to every 6 to 12 mo. Pregnant patients should be checked every trimester.

■ REFERRAL
Admission to the hospital ICU is recommended in all patients with myxedema coma. Additional information on the diagnosis and treatment of this life-threatening complication of hypothyroidism is available in the topic "Myxedema Coma" in Section I.

⚙ PEARLS & CONSIDERATIONS

■ COMMENTS
- *Subclinical hypothyroidism* occurs in as many as 15% of elderly patients and is characterized by an elevated serum TSH and a normal free T_4 level. Treatment is individualized. Generally, replacement therapy is recommended for all patients with serum TSH >10 mU/L and with presence of goiter or thyroid autoantibodies.
- Fig. 3-165 describes a diagnostic approach to thyroid function tests.

REFERENCES
Cooper DS: Sub-clinical hypothyroidism, *N Engl J Med* 345:260, 2001.
Woeber KA: Update on the management of hyperthyroidism and hypothyroidism, *Arch Intern Med* 160:1067, 2000.
Author: **Fred F. Ferri, M.D.**

BASIC INFORMATION

■ DEFINITION
Idiopathic thrombocytopenic purpura (ITP) is a disorder characterized by isolated low platelet count in absence of other causes of thrombocytopenia.

■ SYNONYMS
ITP
Immune thrombocytopenic purpura
Autoimmune thrombocytopenic
  purpura

ICD-9CM CODES
287.3 Idiopathic thrombocytopenic purpura (ITP)

■ EPIDEMIOLOGY & DEMOGRAPHICS
PREVALENCE: 5 to 10 cases/100,000 persons
PREDOMINANT SEX: 72% of patients >10 yr old are female; in children, males = females
PREDOMINANT AGE: Children age 2 to 4 yr and young women (70% are <40 yr old)

■ PHYSICAL FINDINGS & CLINICAL PRESENTATION
- The physical examination may be entirely normal.
- Patients with severe thrombocytopenia may have petechiae, purpura, epistaxis, or heme-positive stool from GI bleeding
- Splenomegaly is unusual; its presence should alert to the possibility of other etiologies of thrombocytopenia.
- The presence of dysmorphic features (skeletal anomalies, auditory abnormalities) may indicate a congenital disorder as the etiology of the thrombocytopenia.

■ ETIOLOGY
Increased platelet destruction caused by autoantibodies to platelet-membrane antigens

DIAGNOSIS

■ DIFFERENTIAL DIAGNOSIS
- Falsely low platelet count (resulting from EDTA-dependent or cold-dependent agglutinins)
- Viral infections (e.g., HIV, mononucleosis, rubella)
- Drug-induced (e.g., heparin, quinidine, sulfonamides)
- Hypersplenism resulting from liver disease
- Myelodysplastic and lymphoproliferative disorders

- Pregnancy, hypothyroidism
- SLE, TTP, hemolytic-uremic syndrome
- Congenital thrombocytopenias (e.g., Fanconi's syndrome, May-Hegglin anomaly, Bernard-Soulier syndrome)
- Box 2-244 describes differential diagnosis of thrombocytopenia.

■ WORKUP
The history should focus on bleeding symptoms and on excluding other potential causes of thrombocytopenia (e.g., medications, alcohol abuse, risk factors for HIV, family history of hematologic disorders). The presentation of ITP is different in children and adults.
- Children generally present with sudden onset of bruising and petechiae from severe thrombocytopenia.
- In adults the presentation is insidious; a history of prolonged purpura may be present; many patients are diagnosed incidentally on the basis of automated laboratories that now routinely include platelet counts.
- Fig. 3-163 describes a diagnostic approach to thrombocytopenia.

■ LABORATORY TESTS
- CBC, platelet count, and peripheral smear: platelets are decreased but are normal in size or may appear larger than normal. RBCs and WBCs have a normal morphology.
- Additional tests may be ordered to exclude other etiologies of the thrombocytopenia when clinically indicated (e.g., HIV, ANA, TSH, liver enzymes, bone marrow examination).

■ IMAGING STUDIES
CT scan of abdomen in patients with splenomegaly to exclude other disorders causing thrombocytopenia

TREATMENT

■ NONPHARMACOLOGIC THERAPY
- Minimize activity to prevent injury or bruising (e.g., contact sports should be avoided).
- Avoid medications that increase the risk of bleeding (e.g., aspirin and other NSAIDs).

■ ACUTE GENERAL Rx
- Treatment varies with the platelet count and bleeding status.
- Observation and frequent monitoring of platelet count are needed in asymptomatic patients with platelet counts >30,000/mm³.

- Prednisone 1 to 2 mg/kg qd, continued until the platelet count is normalized then slowly tapered off, is indicated in adults with platelet counts <20,000/mm³ and those who have counts <50,000/mm³ and significant mucous membrane bleeding.
- High-dose immunoglobulins (IgG 0.4 g/kg/day IV, infused on 3 to 5 consecutive days) or high-dose parenteral glucocorticoids (methylprednisolone 30 mg/kg/day) are used in children with platelet count <20,000/mm³ and significant bleeding or adults with severe thrombocytopenia or bleeding.
- Platelet transfusion is needed only in case of life-threatening hemorrhage.
- Splenectomy should be considered in adults with platelet count <30,000/mm³ after 6 wk of medical treatment. In children, splenectomy is generally reserved for persistent thrombocytopenia (>1 yr) and clinically significant bleeding. Appropriate immunizations (pneumococcal vaccine in adults and children, *H. influenzae* vaccine, meningococcal vaccine in children) should be administered before splenectomy.

■ CHRONIC Rx
Frequent monitoring of platelet count and symptom review in patients with chronic ITP

■ DISPOSITION
- Over 80% of children have a complete remission within a few weeks.
- In adults, the course of the disease is chronic and only 5% of adults have spontaneous remission.
- The principal cause of death from ITP is intracranial hemorrhage (1% of children, 5% of adults).

■ REFERRAL
- Surgical referral for splenectomy in selected cases (see above)
- Hospitalization in patients with platelet count <20,000/mm³ who have significant bleeding

PEARLS & CONSIDERATIONS

■ COMMENTS
In general, patients who have poor response to IV immune globulin are unlikely to have good response to splenectomy.
Author: **Fred F. Ferri, M.D.**

BASIC INFORMATION

■ DEFINITION

Impetigo is a superficial skin infection generally secondary to *Staphylococcus aureus* and/or *Streptococcus* spp. Common presentations are bullous impetigo (generally secondary to staphylococcal disease) and nonbullous impetigo (secondary to streptococcal infection and possible staphylococcal infection); the bullous form is caused by an epidermolytic toxin produced at the site of infection.

■ SYNONYMS

Impetigo vulgaris
Pyoderma

ICD-9CM CODES

684 Impetigo

■ EPIDEMIOLOGY & DEMOGRAPHICS

- Bullous impetigo is most common in infants and children. The nonbullous form is most common in children ages 2 to 5 yr with poor hygiene in warm climates.
- The overall incidence of acute nephritis with impetigo varies between 2% and 5%.

■ PHYSICAL FINDINGS & CLINICAL PRESENTATION

- Multiple lesions with golden yellow crusts and weeping areas often found on the skin around the nose, mouth, and limbs (nonbullous impetigo) (Fig. 1-220).
- Presence of vesicles that enlarge rapidly to form bullae with contents that vary from clear to cloudy; there is subsequent collapse of the center of the bullae; the peripheral areas may retain fluid, and a honey-colored crust may appear in the center; as the lesions enlarge and become contiguous with the others, a scaling border replaces the fluid-filled rim (bullous impetigo); there is minimal erythema surrounding the lesions.
- Regional lymphadenopathy is most common with nonbullous impetigo.
- Constitutional symptoms are generally absent.

■ ETIOLOGY

- *S. aureus* coagulase positive is the dominant microorganism.
- *S. pyogenes* (group A β-hemolytic streptococci): M-T serotypes of this organism associated with acute nephritis are 2, 49, 55, 57, and 60.

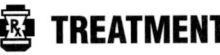 **DIAGNOSIS**

■ DIFFERENTIAL DIAGNOSIS

- Acute allergic contact dermatitis
- Herpes simplex infection
- Ecthyma
- Folliculitis
- Eczema
- Insect bites
- Scabies
- Tinea corporis
- Pemphigus vulgaris and bullous pemphigoid
- Chickenpox

■ WORKUP

Diagnosis is clinical.

■ LABORATORY TESTS

- Generally not necessary
- Gram stain and C&S to confirm the diagnosis when the clinical presentation is unclear
- Sedimentation rate parallel to activity of the disease
- Increased anti-DNAse B and anti-hyaluronidase
- Urinalysis revealing hematuria with erythrocyte casts and proteinuria in patients with acute nephritis (most frequently occurring in children between 2 and 4 yr of age in the southern part of the U.S.)

℞ TREATMENT

■ NONPHARMACOLOGIC THERAPY

Remove crusts by soaking with wet cloth compresses (crusts block the penetration of antibacterial creams).

■ ACUTE GENERAL Rx

- Application of 2% mupirocin ointment (Bactroban) tid for 10 days to the affected area or until all lesions have cleared.
- Oral antibiotics are used in severe cases: commonly used agents are dicloxacillin 250 mg qid for 7 to 10 days, cephalexin 250 mg qid for 7 to 10 days, or azithromycin 500 mg on day 1, 250 mg on days 2 through 5.

■ CHRONIC Rx

- Impetigo can be prevented by prompt application of mupirocin or triple antibiotic ointment (bacitracin, Polysporin, and neomycin) to sites of skin trauma.
- Patients who are carriers of *S. aureus* in their nares should be treated with mupirocin ointment applied to their nares bid for 5 days.

- Fingernails should be kept short, and patients should be advised not to scratch any lesions to avoid spread of infection.

■ DISPOSITION

Most cases of impetigo resolve promptly with appropriate treatment. Both bullous and nonbullous forms of impetigo heal without scarring.

■ REFERRAL

Nephrology referral in patients with acute nephritis

⚙ PEARLS & CONSIDERATIONS

■ COMMENTS

- Patients should be instructed on use of antibacterial soaps and avoidance of sharing of towels and washcloths, because impetigo is extremely contagious
- Children attending day care should be removed until 48 to 72 hr after initiation of antibiotic treatment.

REFERENCE

O'Dell ML: Skin and wound infection: an overview, *Am Fam Physician* 10:2424, 1998.
Author: **Fred F. Ferri, M.D.**

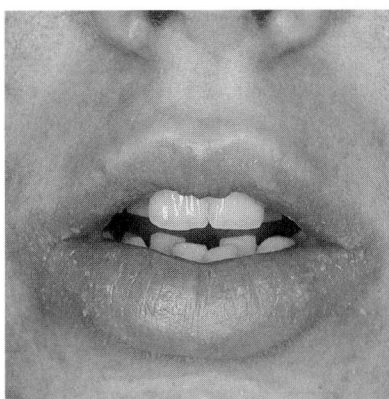

Fig. 1-220 Impetigo. Serum and crust at the angle of the mouth is a common presentation for impetigo. (From Habif TB: *Clinical dermatology: a color guide to diagnosis and therapy,* ed 3, St Louis, 1996, Mosby.)

I

BASIC INFORMATION

■ DEFINITION

Inappropriate secretion of antidiuretic hormone (SIADH) is a syndrome characterized by excessive secretion of ADH in absence of normal osmotic or physiologic stimuli (increased serum osmolarity, decreased plasma volume, hypotension).

■ SYNONYMS

SIADH

ICD-9CM CODES

276.9 Inappropriate secretion of antidiuretic hormone

■ EPIDEMIOLOGY & DEMOGRAPHICS

Nearly 50% of hyponatremia detected in the hospital setting is caused by SIADH.

■ PHYSICAL FINDINGS & CLINICAL PRESENTATION

- The patient is generally normovolemic or slightly hypervolemic; edema is absent.
- Delirium, lethargy, and seizures may be present if the hyponatremia is severe or of rapid onset.
- Manifestations of the underlying disease may be evident (e.g., fever from an infectious process or headaches and visual field defects from an intracranial mass).
- Diminished reflexes and extensor plantar responses may occur with severe hyponatremia.

■ ETIOLOGY

- Neoplasm: lung, duodenum, pancreas, brain, thymus, bladder, prostate, mesothelioma, lymphoma, Ewing's sarcoma
- Pulmonary disorders: pneumonia, TB, bronchiectasis, emphysema, status asthmaticus
- Intracranial pathology: trauma, neoplasms, infections (meningitis, encephalitis, brain abscess), hemorrhage, hydrocephalus
- Postoperative period: surgical stress, ventilators with positive pressure, anesthetic agents
- Drugs: chlorpropamide, thiazide diuretics, vasopressin, desmopressin, oxytocin, chemotherapeutic agents (vincristine, vinblastine, cyclophosphamide), carbamazepine, phenothiazines, MAO inhibitors, tricyclic antidepressants, narcotics, nicotine, clofibrate, haloperidol, SSRIs
- Other: acute intermittent porphyria, Guillain-Barré syndrome, myxedema, psychosis, delirium tremens, ACTH deficiency (hypopituitarism)

DIAGNOSIS

■ DIFFERENTIAL DIAGNOSIS

- Hyponatremia associated with hypervolemia (CHF, cirrhosis, nephrotic syndrome)
- Factitious hyponatremia (hyperglycemia, abnormal proteins, hyperlipidemia)
- Hypovolemia associated with hypovolemia (e.g., burns, GI fluid loss)

■ WORKUP

- Demonstration through laboratory evaluation (see "Laboratory Tests") of excessive secretion of ADH in absence of appropriate osmotic or physiologic stimuli
- Normal thyroid, adrenal, and cardiac function
- No recent or concurrent use of diuretics
- Fig. 1-185 illustrates a diagnostic approach to hyponatremia.

■ LABORATORY TESTS

- Hyponatremia
- Urinary osmolarity > serum osmolarity
- Urinary sodium usually >30 mEq/L
- Normal BUN, creatinine (indicative of normal renal function and absence of dehydration)
- Decreased uric acid

■ IMAGING STUDIES

Chest x-ray examination to rule out neoplasm or infectious process

TREATMENT

■ NONPHARMACOLOGIC THERAPY

Fluid restriction to 500 to 800 ml/day

■ ACUTE GENERAL Rx

In emergency situations (seizures, coma) SIADH can be treated with combination of hypertonic saline solution (slow infusion of 250 ml of 3% NaCl) and furosemide; this increases the serum sodium by causing diuresis of urine that is more dilute than plasma; the rapidity of correction varies depending on the degree of hyponatremia and if the hyponatremia is acute or chronic; generally the serum sodium should be corrected only halfway to normal in the initial 24 hr and serum sodium should be increased by <0.5 mEq/L/hr.

■ CHRONIC Rx

- Depending on the underlying etiology, fluid restriction may be needed indefinitely. Monthly monitoring of electrolytes is recommended in patients with chronic SIADH.
- Demeclocycline (Declomycin) 300 to 600 mg PO bid may be useful in patients with chronic SIADH (e.g., secondary to neoplasm), but use with caution in patients with hepatic disease; its side effects include nephrogenic DI and photosensitivity. This medication is expensive (cost to the pharmacist is >$300 for fifty 300-mg tablets).

■ DISPOSITION

- Prognosis varies depending on the cause. Generally prognosis is benign when SIADH is caused by an infectious process.
- Morbidity and mortality are high (>40%) when serum sodium concentration is <110 mEq/L.

■ REFERRAL

Hospital admission depending on severity of symptoms and degree of hyponatremia

PEARLS & CONSIDERATIONS

■ COMMENTS

- Use of hypertonic (3%) saline is contraindicated in patients with CHF, nephrotic syndrome, or cirrhosis
- Too rapid correction of hyponatremia can cause demyelination and permanent CNS damage

Author: **Fred F. Ferri, M.D.**

BASIC INFORMATION

■ DEFINITION
Inclusion body myositis (IBM) refers to a chronic idiopathic inflammatory myopathy with characteristics similar to polymyositis and dermatomyositis.

■ SYNONYMS
Idiopathic inflammatory myopathy

ICD-9CM CODES
729.1 Myositis

■ EPIDEMIOLOGY & DEMOGRAPHICS
- Incidence is 1/100,000 cases.
- More common in men than in women (3:1).
- More common in whites than in blacks.
- Usually affects persons over the age of 50 yr.
- Associated with autoimmune diseases in up to 15% of the cases.

■ PHYSICAL FINDINGS & CLINICAL PRESENTATION
- Most patients with IBM develop insidiously.
- Usually presents with symmetric proximal muscle weakness but can be asymmetric and involve distal muscles as well (e.g., foot extensors and finger flexors).
- Patients have difficulties with buttoning a shirt, sewing, and typing.
- IBM may specifically involve the quadriceps, iliopsoas, triceps, and biceps muscles.
- Early loss of patellar reflex
- Like polymyositis and dermatomyositis, IBM can involve the upper esophageal muscle leading to dysphagia, aspiration, and respiratory distress.

■ ETIOLOGY
The cause of IBM is not known but is believed to be a cell-mediated immune response directed against muscle fibers.

DIAGNOSIS

The diagnosis of inclusion body myositis is made by:
- History and physical findings of both proximal and distal muscle weakness
- Elevated muscle enzymes
- EMG abnormalities suggesting a myopathic process
- Muscle biopsy confirmation

■ DIFFERENTIAL DIAGNOSIS
- Polymyositis
- Muscular dystrophy
- Diabetic neuropathy
- Trichinosis
- AIDS
- Alcoholic myopathy
- Hypothyroidism
- Hypophosphatemia
- Myasthenia gravis, Eaton-Lambert syndrome
- Amyotrophic lateral sclerosis
- Guillain-Barré syndrome

■ WORKUP
Patients suspected of having IBM by clinical presentation should have an EMG, muscle biopsy, and specific blood tests to confirm the diagnosis.

■ LABORATORY TESTS
- ESR, although not specific, is elevated in the majority of cases.
- Creatine kinase is the most sensitive muscle enzyme test and can be elevated as much as 10 times above normal. In some cases of IBM, the CPK may be normal.
- Aldolase, AST, ALT, alkaline phosphatase, and LDH can be elevated.
- Anti-Jo-1 antibodies are more common in polymyositis than IBM.
- Electrolytes, TSH, Ca, and Mg should be requested to exclude other causes.
- Electromyography (EMG) is abnormal in 90% of patients and distinguishes a myopathic from neuropathic process.
- Muscle biopsy is the definitive test showing pathognomonic inclusion granules in the cytoplasm along with small "rimmed vacuoles."

■ IMAGING STUDIES
- A chest x-ray to rule out pulmonary involvement. If suspicious for pulmonary interstitial disease, a high-resolution CT scan of the chest may be helpful.
- A barium swallow to look for upper esophageal dysfunction in patients with dysphagia and IBM.
- MRI can help to locate sites of muscle involvement.

TREATMENT

What distinguishes IBM from the other two inflammatory myopathies (polymyositis and dermatomyositis) is its lack of responsiveness to immunosupressive treatment.

■ NONPHARMACOLOGIC THERAPY
- Physical therapy is beneficial in increasing muscle tone and strength.
- Occupational therapy to assist with activities of daily living.
- Speech therapy for dysphagia and swallowing problems.

■ ACUTE GENERAL Rx
- Up to 90% of patients with dermatomyositis and polymyositis respond to corticosteroids. Patients with IBM generally are resistant to therapy.
- Prednisone 1 to 2 mg/kg/day for 6 mo can still be given as a therapeutic trial in patients with IBM.

■ CHRONIC Rx
- Azathioprine, methotrexate, and immunoglobulins have all been tried in patients with IBM but with little effect, if any.

■ DISPOSITION
- Inclusion body myositis usually progresses slowly over years.

■ REFERRAL
Whenever the diagnosis of inflammatory myopathy is suspected and specifically inclusion body myositis, a rheumatologist and neurologist should be consulted for assistance.

PEARLS & CONSIDERATIONS

■ COMMENTS
- Inclusion body myositis is often incorrectly diagnosed as polymyositis.
- Features distinguishing IBM from polymyositis are:
  1. IBM involves distal as well as proximal muscles.
  2. IBM can be asymmetric and selectively involve quadriceps muscle.
  3. Inclusion bodies on muscle biopsy of patients with IBM.
  4. IBM is resistant to immunosuppressants.
- Unlike dermatomyositis, there is no associated increase risk of malignancy in patients with IBM.

REFERENCES
Amato AA et al: Inclusion body myositis: clinical and pathological boundaries, *Ann Neurol* 40:581, 1996.
Dalakas MC: Polymyositis, dermatomyositis, and inclusion body myositis, *N Engl J Med* 325:1487, 1991.
Griggs RC et al: Inclusion body myositis and myopathies, *Ann Neurol* 38:705, 1995.

Author: **Peter Petropoulos, M.D.**

BASIC INFORMATION

■ DEFINITION
Incontinence is the involuntary loss of urine.

ICD-9CM CODES
788.3 Incontinence
625.6 Stress incontinence
788.33 Mixed stress and urge incontinence
788.32 Male incontinence
788.39 Neurogenic incontinence
307.6 Nonorganic origin

■ EPIDEMIOLOGY & DEMOGRAPHICS
INCIDENCE AND PREVALENCE: In the general population between the ages of 15 and 64 yr, 1.5% to 5% of men and 10% to 25% of women will suffer from incontinence. In the nursing home population, 50% of the population suffers some degree of incontinence. Nearly 20% of children through the midteenage years have episodes of urinary incontinence.

■ CLINICAL, PSYCHOLOGIC, & SOCIAL IMPACT
Less than 50% of the individuals with incontinence living in the community consult health care providers, preferring to "suffer silently," turning to "home remedies," commercially available absorbent materials, and supportive aids. As their condition worsens, they become depressed, sacrifice their independence, suffer from recurrent urinary tract infection and its sequelae, limit their social interaction, refrain from sexual intimacy, and become homebound. In terms of costs, for all ages living in the community, it is estimated that $7 billion is spent for incontinence annually.

■ MAJOR TYPES OF INCONTINENCE
TRANSIENT INCONTINENCE: Incontinence occurring as a result or reaction to an acute medical problem affecting the lower urinary tract. Many of these problems can be reversed with treatment of the underlying problem.

URGE INCONTINENCE: Involuntary loss of urine associated with an abrupt and strong desire to void. It is usually associated with involuntary detrusor contractions on urodynamic investigation. In *neurologically impaired patients,* the involuntary detrusor contraction is referred to as *detrusor hyperreflexia.* In *neurologically normal patients* the involuntary contraction is called *detrusor instability.*

STRESS INCONTINENCE: The involuntary loss of urine with physical activities that increase abdominal pressure in the absence of a detrusor contraction or an overdistended bladder. Classification of stress incontinence:
Type 0: Complaint of incontinence without demonstration of leakage
Type I: Incontinence in response to stress but little descent of the bladder neck and urethra
Type II: Incontinence in response to stress with >2 cm descent of the bladder neck and urethra
Type III: Bladder neck and urethra wide open without bladder contraction; intrinsic sphincter deficiency; and denervation of the urethra. The most common causes: urethral hypermobility and displacement of the bladder neck with exertion, intrinsic sphincter deficiency from failed antiincontinence surgery, prostatectomy, radiation, cord lesions, epispadias, or myelomeningocele.

OVERFLOW INCONTINENCE: Loss of urine resulting from overdistention of the bladder with resultant "overflow" or "spilling" of the urine. Causes: hypotonic-to-atonic bladder resulting from drug effect, fecal impaction, or neurologic conditions such as diabetes, spinal cord injury, surgery, vitamin B_{12} deficiency. It is also caused by obstruction at the bladder neck and urethra. In this situation, prostatism, prostatic cancer, urethral stenosis, antiincontinence surgery, pelvic prolapse, and detrusor-sphincter dyssynergia cause the incontinence.

FUNCTIONAL INCONTINENCE: Involuntary loss of urine resulting from chronic impairments of physical and/or cognitive functioning. This is a diagnosis of exclusion. The condition can sometimes be improved or cured by improving the patient's functional status, treating comorbidities, changing medications, reducing environmental barriers, etc.

MIXED STRESS AND URGE INCONTINENCE
SENSORY URGENCY INCONTINENCE: Involuntary loss of urine as a result of decreased bladder compliance and increased intravesical pressures accompanied by severe urgency and bladder hypersensitivity without detrusor overactivity. This is seen with radiation cystitis, interstitial cystitis, eosinophilic cystitis, myelomeningocele, and radical pelvic surgery. Nephropathy can occur as a complication of this vesicoureteral reflux.

SPHINCTERIC INCONTINENCE:
Urethral Hypermobility: The basic abnormality is a weakness of pelvic floor support. Because of this weakness, during increases in abdominal pressure there is rotational descent of the vesical neck and proximal urethra. If the urethra opens concomitantly, stress urinary incontinence ensues. Urethral hypermobility is often present in women who are not incontinent. Its mere presence is not sufficient evidence to make the diagnosis of sphincteric abnormality unless incontinence is shown.
Intrinsic Sphincter Deficiency: There is an intrinsic malfunction of the sphincter itself. It is characterized by an open vesical neck at rest and a low leak point pressure (<65 cm water). Urethral hypermobility and intrinsic sphincter deficiency may coexist in the same patient. Causes of intrinsic sphincter deficiency are previous pelvic surgery, antiincontinence surgery, urethral diverticulectomy, radical hysterectomy, abdominoperineal resection of the rectum, urethrotomy, Y-V plasty of the vesical neck, myelodysplasia, anterior spinal artery syndrome, lumbosacral disease, aging, and hypoestrogenism.

DIAGNOSIS

■ HISTORY

- History of present illness, psychosocial factors, congenital disorders, access issues for the physically challenged, neurologic disorders, and disorders pertinent to the urologic tract
- Review of prescription and nonprescription medications
- Voiding diary to assess total voided volume, frequency of micturition, mean volume voided, largest single volume, diurnal distribution, nature and severity of incontinence

■ WORKUP

- Physical examination including general examination, gait of the patient (neuromuscular deficits), estrogen status, vaginal examination to include the periurethral region, evaluation for cystocele, rectocele, and enterocele
- Pelvic floor strength assessment
- Rectal examination to assess sphincter tone and bulbocavernosus reflex
- Neurologic examination
- Postvoid residual check using bladder scan or catheter

■ LABORATORY TESTS

Urinalysis, urine culture, urine cytology, BUN, and creatinine

■ IMAGING STUDIES

- KUB to assess bony skeleton
- IVP to rule out upper tract abnormalities, developmental anomalies, bladder configuration, and fistula
- Renal ultrasound if dye study is contraindicated

■ SPECIALIZED STUDIES

Simple cystometrogram, complex urodynamics including leak point pressures and uroflowmetry, endoscopic evaluation, and cystogram

℞ TREATMENT

■ TRANSIENT INCONTINENCE

Treatment of underlying medical conditions and behavioral therapy to include habit training and timed voiding

■ URGE INCONTINENCE

Bladder relaxants (i.e., tolterodine [Detrol], oxybutynin [Ditropan], imipramine), estrogen, biofeedback, Kegel exercises, and surgical removal of obstructing or other pathologic lesions

■ STRESS INCONTINENCE

- Pelvic floor exercises, Kegel exercises, α-adrenergic agonists (i.e., ephedrine), estrogen, biofeedback. CYSTOURETHROPEXY: Marshall-Marchetti-Krantz procedure, Burch procedure, Raz procedure, Stamey-Raz procedure, Gittes procedure, in situ transvaginal sling, pubovaginal sling with autologous or cadaver graft, laparoscopic Burch procedure, laparoscopic sling, tension-free vaginal tape (TVT)
  - For intrinsic sphincter deficiency: bulking agents (e.g., collagen), sling, and artificial sphincter

■ OVERFLOW INCONTINENCE

Surgical removal of any obstructing lesions, clean intermittent catheterization, and indwelling catheter

■ FUNCTIONAL INCONTINENCE

Behavioral training to include habit training and timed voiding, incontinence undergarments and pads, external collecting devices, and environmental manipulation

■ MIXED URGENCY AND STRESS INCONTINENCE

Use of measures recommended in the management of stress and urge incontinence

■ SENSORY URGENCY

Bladder relaxants (e.g., anticholinergics, muscle relaxants, and tricyclic antidepressants), behavior therapy to include habit training and timed voiding, cystoscopy and hydrodilatation

■ SPHINCTERIC DEFICIENCY

Urethral bulking agents, sling procedure, artificial sphincter, mechanical clamp, and external collection devices

☼ PEARLS & CONSIDERATIONS

■ COMMENTS

Other forms of incontinence:
NOCTURNAL ENURESIS: (ICD-9CM Code: 788.3) Can be caused by sphincter abnormalities and detrusor overactivity; can occur as idiopathic, neurogenic, and with outlet obstruction
POSTVOID DRIBBLE: (ICD-9CM Code: 599.2) A postsphincteric collection of urine that is seen with urethral diverticulum and can be idiopathic
EXTRAURETHRAL INCONTINENCE: Enterovesical (ICD-9CM Codes: 596.1 and 596.2), Urethral (ICD-9CM Code: 599.1), also known as fistula
CONDITIONS THAT PREDISPOSE TO SURGICAL FAILURE: Advanced age, postmenopausal state, hysterectomy, prior failed incontinence surgery, concurrent detrusor instability, abnormal perineal electromyography, pelvic radiation

REFERENCES

Burgio UL et al: Behavioral vs. drug treatment for urge urinary incontinence in older women: a randomized controlled trial, *JAMA* 280:1995, 1998.
US Department of Health and Human Services, Public Health Service, Agency for Health Care Policy and Research: *Clinical practice guideline: urinary incontinence in adults,* Rockville, Md, 1996, US Department of Health and Human Services.
Author: **Philip J. Aliotta, M.D., M.S.H.A.**

BASIC INFORMATION

■ DEFINITION
Influenza is an acute febrile illness caused by infection with influenza type A or B virus.

■ SYNONYMS
Flu

ICD-9CM CODES
487.1 Influenza

■ EPIDEMIOLOGY & DEMOGRAPHICS
INCIDENCE (IN U.S.): Annual incidence of influenza-related deaths is approximately 20,000 deaths/yr.
PREDOMINANT SEX: Male = female
PREDOMINANT AGE: Attack rates are higher among children than adults, although children are less prone to develop pulmonary complications.
PEAK INCIDENCE: Winter outbreaks lasting 5 to 6 wk

■ PHYSICAL FINDINGS & CLINICAL PRESENTATION
- "Classic flu" is characterized by abrupt onset of fever, headache, myalgias, anorexia, and malaise after a 1- to 2-day incubation period.
- Clinical syndromes are similar to those produced by other respiratory viruses, including pharyngitis, common colds, tracheobronchitis, bronchiolitis, croup.
- Respiratory symptoms such as cough, sore throat, and nasal discharge are usually present at the onset of illness, but systemic symptoms predominate.
- Elderly patients may experience fever, weakness, and confusion without any respiratory complaints.
- Acute deterioration to status asthmaticus may occur in patients with asthma.
- Influenza pneumonia: rapidly progressive cough, dyspnea, and cyanosis may occur after typical flu onset.

■ ETIOLOGY
- Variation in the surface antigens of the influenza virus, hemagglutinin (HA) and neuraminidase (NA), leading to infection with variants to which resistance is inadequate in the population at risk
- Transmitted by small-particle aerosols and deposited on the respiratory tract epithelium

DIAGNOSIS

■ DIFFERENTIAL DIAGNOSIS
- Respiratory syncytial virus, adenovirus, parainfluenza virus infection
- Secondary bacterial pneumonia or mixed bacterial-viral pneumonia

■ WORKUP
- Virus isolation from nasal or throat swab or sputum specimens is the most rapid diagnostic method in the setting of acute illness.
- Specimens are placed into virus transport medium and processed by a reference laboratory.
- For serologic diagnosis:
  1. Paired serum specimens, acute and convalescent, the latter obtained 10 to 20 days later
  2. Fourfold rises or falls in the titer of antibodies (various techniques) considered diagnostic of recent infection

■ LABORATORY TESTS
Septic syndrome presentation: CBC, ABG analysis, blood cultures

■ IMAGING STUDIES
- Chest x-ray examination to demonstrate findings of viral pneumonia: peribronchial and patchy interstitial infiltrates in multiple lobes with atelectasis
- Possible progression to diffuse interstitial pneumonitis

TREATMENT

■ NONPHARMACOLOGIC THERAPY
- Bed rest
- Hydration

■ ACUTE GENERAL Rx
- Supportive care: antipyretics—*Avoid use of aspirin in children because of the association with Reye's syndrome.*
- Antibiotics if bacterial pneumonia is proven or suspected.
- Amantadine (100 mg PO twice daily for children >10 yr and adults <65 yr; once daily in patients >65 yr) and rimantadine (same dose schedule as amantadine).
  1. Further dose adjustments needed with renal insufficiency
  2. Fewer CNS side effects with rimantadine

- Neuraminidase inhibitors block release of virions from infected cells, resulting in shortened duration of symptoms and decrease in complications; effective against both influenza A and B:
  1. Zanamivir, administered via inhaler, 10 mg twice daily
  2. Oseltamivir, administered orally

■ DISPOSITION
Patients are hospitalized if signs of pneumonia are present.

■ REFERRAL
Infectious disease and/or pulmonary consultation when influenza pneumonia is suspected

PEARLS & CONSIDERATIONS

■ COMMENTS
- Prevention of influenza in patients at high risk is an important goal of primary care.
- Vaccines reduce the risk of infection and the severity of illness.
  1. Antigenic composition of the vaccine is updated annually.
  2. Vaccination should be given at the start of the flu season (October) for the following groups:
     a. Adults ≥65 yr
     b. Adults and children with chronic cardiac or pulmonary disease, including asthma
     c. Adults and children with illness requiring frequent follow-up (e.g., hemoglobinopathies, diabetes mellitus)
     d. Children receiving long-term aspirin therapy
     e. Immunocompromised patients
     f. Household contacts of persons in the above groups
     g. Health-care workers
  3. Only contraindication to vaccination is hypersensitivity to hen's eggs.
  4. Special efforts should be made to vaccinate high-risk patients younger than 65 yr, only 10% to 15% of whom are vaccinated each year.
- Chemoprophylaxis:
  1. Amantadine and rimantadine approved for prophylaxis against influenza A; they are ineffective against influenza B.

2. Consider:
   a. For high-risk patients in whom vaccination is contraindicated
   b. When the available vaccine is known not to include the circulating strain
   c. To provide added protection to immunosuppressed patients likely to have a diminished response to vaccination
   d. In the setting of an outbreak, when immediate protection of unvaccinated or recently vaccinated patients is desired

3. Give for 2 wk in the case of late vaccination and for the duration of the flu season in all other patients.

REFERENCES

Carrat F et al: Evaluation of clinical case definitions of influenza: detailed investigation of patients during the 1995-1996 epidemic in France, *Clin Infect Dis* 28:283, 1999.

Demicheli V et al: Vaccines for preventing influenza in healthy adults, *Cochrane Database Syst Rev* 2000(2):CD001269.

MIST Study Group: Randomized trial of efficacy and safety of inhaled zaramivir in treatment of influenza A and B virus infections, *Lancet* 352:1877, 1998.

Author: **Claudia L. Dade, M.D.**

I

BASIC INFORMATION

■ DEFINITION
Insemination is a therapeutic intervention designed to overcome defects preventing achieving proper concentration of functional sperm cells in the vicinity of the egg.

■ SYNONYMS
Artificial insemination

ICD-9CM CODES
606.0 Irreversible azoospermia
Husband's carrier status for genetic disease such as:
303.1 Tay-Sachs
286.0 Hemophilia
333.4 Huntington's disease
758.9 Chromosomal abnormalities
773.0 Severe Rh disease
608.89.1 Husband's sperm frozen before orchidectomy
606.8 Husband's sperm frozen before radiation or chemotherapy

■ ETIOLOGY
See "ICD-9CM Codes" above.

 DIAGNOSIS

■ DIFFERENTIAL DIAGNOSIS
See "ICD-9CM Codes" above.

■ WORKUP
Male: refer to urologist; ascertain that azoospermia is indeed irreversible. Individuals who were considered intractable in the recent past can now produce pregnancies with intracyto-plasmic sperm injections (ICSI), even with cells obtained by testicular biopsy. Such an option should be offered to the patient before recommending a donor.

■ LABORATORY TESTS
- Testing of both partners for hepatitis, HIV, and other STDs is recommended before donor inseminations.
- Female: as described in the topic "Therapeutic Insemination (Husband/Partner)" for general infertility workup.

■ IMAGING STUDIES
As described in the topic "Therapeutic Insemination (Husband/Partner)" for general infertility workup.

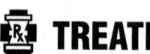 **TREATMENT**

■ NONPHARMACOLOGIC THERAPY
SPERM SOURCE: *Use of fresh donor semen is no longer acceptable.* Semen is obtained from state-certified "sperm banks" adhering to the proper routines of donor screening for genetic and infectious diseases, and quarantining the sperm for at least 6 mo. Sperm can be shipped from the bank in containers that will maintain the sample in a frozen state for 48 hr. After this time the sample has to be transferred to another liquid nitrogen storage tank.
SPERM PREPARATION: Sperm is removed from the liquid nitrogen and allowed to thaw at room temperature, or is thawed per sperm bank instruc-tions. Refer to "Therapeutic Insemination (Husband/Partner)" in Section I for insemination techniques. If sperm supply is not limited and the woman's age is not a factor (<35 yr), simple applications of thawed semen to the external cervical os are usually undertaken first.

■ DISPOSITION
In healthy women <34 yr of age, fecundity of approximately 10% per cycle can be expected. Fertility is age dependent. After 12 cycles, expect 75% pregnancy for women <34 yr of age.

☼ PEARLS & CONSIDERATIONS

■ COMMENTS
- Risks: infections with STDs, including AIDS, although rare, have been reported as a result of donor semen insemination.
- Caution: observe laws applicable in the state and obtain proper consents.
- Caution: before declaring the male azoospermic, centrifuge the semen and examine sediment; several sperm cells missed on "plain" microscopic examination may suffice for ICSI.

REFERENCE
Speroff L, Glass RH, Kase NG: *Clinical gynecologic endocrinology and infertility*, ed 6, Baltimore, 1999, Lippincott Williams & Wilkins.
Author: **John M. Wieckowski, M.D., Ph.D.**

BASIC INFORMATION

■ DEFINITION

Insemination is a therapeutic intervention designed to overcome defects preventing achieving proper concentration of functional sperm cells in the vicinity of the egg.

■ SYNONYMS

Artificial insemination

ICD-9CM CODES

628.9 Infertility (female unspecified)
606.9 Infertility (male unspecified)
302.7 Sexual/erectile dysfunction
625.1 Vaginismus
752.6 Hypospadias
792.2 Asthenospermia
606.1 Oligospermia

■ EPIDEMIOLOGY & DEMOGRAPHICS

Approximately 15% of couples experience infertility.

■ ETIOLOGY

MALE:
- Hypospadias: congenital
- Sexual/erectile dysfunction: psychogenic, vascular, neurogenic
- Asthenospermia: idiopathic, varicocele, status post vasectomy reversal, environmental (toxins, heavy metals, heat exposure, trauma to testicles)
- Antisperm antibodies, unknown, trauma to testicles, vasectomy

FEMALE:
- Cervical mucus hostility: unknown, infection
- Antisperm antibodies: unknown
- Idiopathic infertility: unknown

DIAGNOSIS

■ DIFFERENTIAL DIAGNOSIS

- Diagnosis of infertility is established by a history of 1 yr of unprotected intercourse without conception.
- Establish male vs. female infertility, or combined.
- Male: rule out congenital abnormalities, variocele, endocrine defects.
- Female: rule out ovulatory dysfunction, tubal factors, uterine defects, endometriosis.

■ WORKUP

- Male routine: urologic examination, semen analysis
- Specialized (if indicated): sonography, vasogram, Doppler studies, testicular biopsy
- Female routine: gynecologic examination, establish ovulatory pattern by basal body temperature or endometrial biopsy
- Postcoital test
- Specialized (if indicated): diagnostic/therapeutic laparoscopy

■ LABORATORY TESTS

- Male routine: semen analysis; specialized (if indicated): antisperm antibodies, endocrine studies, testicular biopsy
- Female routine: blood type, rubella immunity, hepatitis immunity
- Selectively (>35 yr or as indicated by history): day 3 of the cycle, test FSH, LH, and estradiol to rule out occult ovarian failure, polycystic ovarian syndrome (LH/FSH inversion); androgen levels if hirsutism present; prolactin level if galactorrhea;

thyroid studies if clinically indicated; anti-*Chlamydia* antibodies if tubal damage suspected or history of IUD use

■ IMAGING STUDIES

- Hysterosalpingogram: rule out hydrosalpinx, salpingitis isthmica nodosa, intramural tubal polyps, intrauterine synechiae, or polyps
- Pelvic sonography: in midcycle to rule out myomas, endometrial polyps, endometrial hypoplasia, ovarian pathology (cysts, endometriomas), or confirm dominant follicle formation
- Pituitary MRI if tumor suspected

TREATMENT

■ NONPHARMACOLOGIC THERAPY

Type of insemination depends on the nature of the fertility defect and varies in depth to which the sperm cells are delivered into the female genital tract. The following types of inseminations may be done:
- Cervical and endocervical insemination
- Intrauterine insemination
- Intratubal insemination
- Cul-de-sac insemination
- Intrafollicular insemination
- In vitro fertilization (IVF)
- IVF with intracytoplasmic sperm injection (ICSI)

Only the cervical and intrauterine inseminations can be done in a primary care setting.

CERVICAL AND INTRACERVICAL INSEMINATION: This method is indicated when normal coital sperm delivery to the cervix is prevented (e.g., coital dysfunction and hypospadias).
Semen Preparation: None; whole semen is used.
Technique: Semen is delivered to the external os or endocervical canal using a syringe with soft-tipped cannula. Cervical cap, which prolongs the contact of semen with the cervix, can be used to overcome high semen viscosity.
INTRAUTERINE INSEMINATION (IUI): This method is used for the following reasons (listed in order of decreasing effectiveness):
- Cervical mucus hostility caused by poor mucus production or quality (idiopathic or iatrogenic, such as status postcervical conization, laser treatment, etc.)
- Antisperm antibodies
- Empirical treatment for unexplained infertility
- Mild male factor defects, such as oligospermia, high semen viscosity, high or low seminal volume

Semen Preparation: Seminal fluid should not be introduced into the uterine cavity. Sperm cells have to be separated from the seminal fluid by the process of sperm "washing," and resuspended in a protein-containing medium (5% to 10% serum or synthetic serum substitute), to endow the cells with proper motility. Method that can be used without the necessity of having incubator involves centrifugation of semen through a density gradient and resuspending the pellet in the protein-containing medium. Media for the above procedures, with or without antibiotics, are commercially available from several sources.
Technique: Internal cervical os is negotiated with one of the various commercially available "insemination catheters" and the "washed" sperm

suspension is delivered to the endometrial cavity. Timing: basal body temperature graphs, cervical mucus observation, testing of urine for LH surge, or serial sonography is often used for detecting ovulation. Cervical insemination should be performed within 24 hr before anticipated ovulation. Timing of IUI should be within a few hours of ovulation, preferably before it. It is usually performed at 40 hr after the ovulation-inducing hCG injection.
ACUTE GENERAL Rx:
- Clomiphene citrate (Clomid, Serophene) is commonly used to correct ovulatory defects. It is given in doses of 50 to 200 mg qd, on days 5 through 9 after the onset of progesterone withdrawal bleeding. The higher the dose of clomiphene necessary to induce ovulation, the lower the pregnancy chance. Prolonged use of clomiphene may adversely affect the endometrium and cervical mucus.
- Tamoxifen (Nolvadex) 10 to 20 mg qd given on days 5 through 9 as described above is also a mild ovulation-inducing agent that improves endometrial formation and cervical mucus.
- Human chorionic gonadotropin (hCG, Pregnyl, Profasi, APL) can be used to trigger ovulation when the dominant follicle size reaches 20 mm diameter.
- Use of injectable FSH (Humegon, Fertinex) preparations is not advisable in primary care setting.
DISPOSITION: Majority of conceptions should occur within the first 6 mo of insemination. In healthy young women a 15% to 25% pregnancy rate per cycle can be expected. The great variety of results reported in the literature indicates that the practitioner's skill in performing ovarian stimulations and sperm preparation plays a significant role in the outcome.

REFERRAL: To specialist if:
- No result after six cycles of inseminations
- Ovulatory dysfunction does not promptly respond to a low dose (50 to 100 mg) of clomiphene citrate
- Woman's age >35 yr: efficiency of treatment becomes critical
- Poor semen parameters
- Pelvic pathology needs correction

☼ PEARLS & CONSIDERATIONS

■ COMMENTS
- Risks of insemination: flare-up of unsuspected pelvic infection, ovarian overstimulation with gonadotropins, multifetal pregnancy.
- Caution: if sperm is in limited supply (semen frozen before orchidectomy) or woman's age is an issue, a thorough fertility evaluation is indicated to make sure that no valuable time or valuable semen is wasted. If fertility defects are found, they should be corrected, or IVF should be offered.
- IVF combined with ICSI is the ultimate insemination technique and delivers pregnancy rates of 20% to 40% per cycle.
- Results of several studies suggest that ICSI is associated with a slightly increased risk for chromosomal abnormalities.

REFERENCES
Abulghar H et al: A prospective controlled study of karyotyping for 430 consecutive babies conceived through intracytoplasmic injection, *Fertil Steril* 76:249, 2001.
Speroff L, Glass RH, Kase NG: *Clinical gynecologic endocrinology and infertility,* ed 6, Baltimore, 1999, Lippincott Williams & Wilkins.
Author: **John M. Wieckowski, M.D., Ph.D.**

BASIC INFORMATION

■ DEFINITION
Insomnia refers to a disturbance of nocturnal sleep patterns that causes adverse daytime consequences.

■ SYNONYMS
Disorders of initiating and maintaining sleep (DIMS)

ICD-9CM CODES
780.50 Sleep disturbance, unspecified
780.51 Insomnia with sleep apnea
780.52 Other insomnia

■ EPIDEMIOLOGY & DEMOGRAPHICS
INCIDENCE (IN U.S.): 33 cases/100 persons/yr
PREVALENCE (IN U.S.): Up to 33% of the population
PREDOMINANT SEX: More common in women
PREDOMINANT AGE: >60 yr
PEAK INCIDENCE: Affects all age groups, but more common in those >60 yr old.
GENETICS:
• Primary insomnia with childhood onset may be familial.
• No known genetic basis for other causes.

■ PHYSICAL FINDINGS & CLINICAL PRESENTATION
• None
• Patients usually complain of:
  1. Difficulty initiating sleep, wakefulness during sleep cycle, or early awakening
  2. Daytime fatigue, drowsiness

■ ETIOLOGY
• Psychiatric disorders (35%)
• Psychophysiologic (15%)
• Drug and alcohol abuse (12%)
• Periodic leg movements (12%)
• Sleep apnea (6%)
• Medical and toxic conditions (4%)

DIAGNOSIS

■ DIFFERENTIAL DIAGNOSIS
Insomnia is a symptom that may have numerous underlying causes (see "Etiology").

■ WORKUP
• Thorough history and examination to identify possible etiology
• Sleep log

■ LABORATORY TESTS
Nighttime polysomnography in an accredited sleep laboratory may be needed to establish the etiology.

TREATMENT

■ NONPHARMACOLOGIC THERAPY
Rules of sleep hygiene may eliminate bad habits and adverse environmental factors (Box 1-24).

■ ACUTE GENERAL Rx
• Transient insomnia: benzodiazepines for no more that a week.
• Acute pain: analgesics.
• Zolpidem (Ambien), a nonbenzodiazepine agent, 5 to 10 mg qhs may be useful for the short-term treatment of insomnia.

■ CHRONIC Rx
• Antidepressants if appropriate for underlying etiology
• Choice of a particular agent, depending on precise nature of sleep disturbance (see "References" for details)
• Possible tolerance and dependence with prolonged use of benzodiazepines

■ DISPOSITION
Significant improvements in sleep can be achieved in many cases.

■ REFERRAL
• If etiology uncertain
• For assessment at a sleep disorders center (recommended)

REFERENCE
Edinger ID et al: Cognitive behavior therapy for treatment of chronic primary insomnia, *JAMA* 285:1856, 2001.
Author: **Michael Gruenthal, M.D., Ph.D.**

BOX 1-24   Sleep Hygiene

• Maintain a regular sleep-wake schedule. Get out of bed early in the morning whether or not you have slept well.
• Avoid naps. Exercise during the time that you might otherwise nap.
• Preserve your bed as a haven for sleep and sex. Avoid other waking activities in bed (such as reading or watching television in the evening).
• Minimize alcohol consumption and avoid caffeine during the afternoon and evening. Don't eat heavily shortly before bed.
• Make sure your bedroom environment is conducive to sleep. It should be cool, quiet, and dark.
• If your mind is preoccupied by something such that you can't fall asleep, put the problem to rest by writing it down in a sentence or two and set it aside until morning.
• Don't try too hard to fall asleep; it will only make things worse. If you can't fall asleep after 20 to 30 minutes, get out of bed, do something relaxing, and go back to bed when you feel sleepy.

From Johnson RT, Griffin JW: *Current therapy in neurologic disease,* ed 4, St Louis, 1997, Mosby.

BASIC INFORMATION

DEFINITION
Insulinoma is a pancreatic insulin-secreting tumor that causes symptoms associated with hypoglycemia.

ICD-9CM CODES
M8151/0 Insulinoma

EPIDEMIOLOGY & DEMOGRAPHICS
INCIDENCE: 1 case/250,000 patient-years
DEMOGRAPHICS: Insulinomas occur in both sexes (approximately 60% in women) and at all ages. In the Mayo Clinic series, the median age at diagnosis was 50 yr in sporadic cases but 23 yr in patients with multiple endocrine neoplasia (MEN), type 1.

PHYSICAL FINDINGS & CLINICAL PRESENTATION
Symptoms occur typically in the morning before breakfast (i.e., fasting hypoglycemia as opposed to reactive hypoglycemia, which is not commonly associated with insulinoma)

Neuroglycopenic symptoms	%
Various combinations of diplopia, blurred vision, sweating, palpitations, or weakness	85
Confusion or abnormal behavior	80
Unconsciousness or amnesia	53
Grand mal seizures	12
Adrenergic symptoms	**%**
Sweating	43
Tremulousness	23
Hunger, nausea	12
Palpitations	10

ETIOLOGY, PATHOLOGY, PATHOPHYSIOLOGY
- Insulinomas are almost always solitary. Malignant insulinomas account for 5% of the total; they tend to be larger (6 cm) and metastases are usually to the liver (47%), regional lymph nodes (30%), or both.
- Insulinomas are evenly distributed in the head, body, and tail of the pancreas; ectopic insulinomas are rare (1% to 3%). Tumor size: 5% 0.5 cm or less, 34% 0.5 to 1 cm, 53% 1 to 5 cm, 8% >5 cm.
- Histologic classification includes insulinoma in 86% of patients, adenomatosis in 5% to 15%, nesidioblastosis in 4%, and hyperplasia in 1%. Adenomatosis consists of multiple macroadenomas or microadenomas and occurs especially in patients with MEN-1. Nesidioblastosis is also a diffuse lesion, in which islet cells form as buds on ductular structures.

DIAGNOSIS

DIFFERENTIAL DIAGNOSIS (OF FASTING HYPOGLYCEMIA)
HYPERINSULINISM:
- Insulinoma
- Nonpancreatic tumors
- Severe congestive heart failure
- Severe renal insufficiency in non-insulin-dependent diabetes

HEPATIC ENZYME DEFICIENCIES OR DECREASED HEPATIC GLUCOSE OUTPUT (PRIMARILY IN INFANTS, CHILDREN):
- Glycogen storage diseases
- Endocrine hypofunction
- Hypopituitarism
- Addison's disease
- Liver failure
- Alcohol abuse
- Malnutrition

EXOGENOUS AGENTS:
- Sulfonylureas, biguanides
- Insulin
- Other drugs (aspirin, pentamidine)

FUNCTIONAL FASTING HYPO-GLYCEMIA: Autoantibodies to insulin receptor or insulin

LABORATORY TESTS
- An overnight fasting blood sugar level combined with a simultaneous plasma insulin, proinsulin, and/or C peptide level will establish the existence of fasting organic hypoglycemia in 60% of patients.
- If single overnight fasting glucose and insulin levels are nondiagnostic, a 72-hr fast is usually done with blood glucose and insulin levels determined at 2- to 4-hr intervals: 75% of patients with insulinoma develop symptoms and a blood sugar level of less than 40 mg/dl by 24 hr, 92% to 98% develop these by 48 hr, and virtually all patients develop them by 72 hr. The test is considered positive for insulinoma if the plasma insulin/glucose ratio is more than 0.3. If, at any point, the patient becomes symptomatic, plasma insulin and glucose values should be obtained and intravenous glucose should be administered.
- Plasma proinsulin, C-peptide, antibodies to insulin, and plasma sulfonylurea levels may be used to rule out factitious use of insulin or hypoglycemic agents or autoantibodies against the insulin receptor or insulin.
- See Fig. 3-91 for a description of the diagnostic approach to patients with documented hypoglycemia and elevated insulin.

IMAGING STUDIES
- Abdominal CT scan or MRI detects half to two thirds of insulinomas (abdominal ultrasound is not effective). Should be done only after laboratory tests for insulinoma have confirmed the diagnosis.
- Intraoperative ultrasound
- Arteriography
- Octreotide scan

TREATMENT

SURGICAL TREATMENT
- Enucleation of single insulinoma
- Partial pancreatectomy for multiple adenomas

MEDICAL TREATMENT
- Carbohydrate administration
- Diazoxide directly inhibits insulin release and has an extrapancreatic, hyperglycemic effect that enhances glycogenolysis
- Lanreotide and octreotide (somatostatin analogs)
- Streptozotocin

REFERRAL
At some point in the workup the patient will probably be referred to an endocrinologist and then to a surgeon. A combination of fasting hypoglycemia and elevated insulin level is probably a good point at which to refer.

REFERENCES
Axelrod L: Insulinoma: cost-effective care in patients with rare disease, *Ann Intern Med* 123:311, 1995.
Service FJ et al: Functioning insulinoma—incidence, recurrence and long-term survival of patients, *Mayo Clin Proc* 66:711, 1991.
Author: **Tom J. Wachtel, M.D.**

BASIC INFORMATION

■ DEFINITION
Interstitial nephritis refers to a group of disorders primarily affecting the interstitium and renal tubules. Interstitial nephritis may be acute or chronic.

■ SYNONYMS
Acute interstitial nephritis (AIN)
Chronic interstitial nephritis (CIN)
Tubulointerstitial diseases

ICD-9CM CODES
583.9 Nephritis
580.89 Acute
582.89 Chronic

■ EPIDEMIOLOGY & DEMOGRAPHICS
- Approximately 1% of patients being evaluated for hematuria and proteinuria will have interstitial nephritis.
- Interstitial nephritis accounts for 25% of all cases of chronic renal failure.
- Up to 15% of all renal biopsies performed on patients with renal diseases have acute interstitial nephritis.
- Drug-induced AIN is more common in adults.
- Infection-induced AIN is more common in children.

■ PHYSICAL FINDINGS & CLINICAL PRESENTATION
Acute interstitial nephritis (AIN)
- Patients usually asymptomatic and found to have a sudden decrease in renal function
- Characteristically occurs over several days to weeks after an infection or initiation of a new medication
- Classic triad—fever, rash, and eosinophilia
- Lumbar flank pain
- Gross hematuria
- Usually oliguric
Chronic interstitial nephritis (CIN)
- Usually present with symptoms related to the underlying cause (e.g., sarcoidosis, multiple myeloma, urate nephropathy)
- Symptoms of renal failure (e.g., weakness, nausea, pruritus)
- Hypertension

■ ETIOLOGY
- AIN is usually caused by drugs, infection, or for idiopathic reasons.
- Common drugs include penicillin, methicillin, rifampin, cephalosporins, trimethoprimsulfamethoxazole, ciprofloxacin, NSAIDs, thiazides, furosemide, triamterene, allopurinol, phenytoin, captopril, and cimetidine.
- Infection (e.g., *Streptococcus, Legionella, Corynebacterium diphtheriae, Yersinia, Salmonella,* HIV, EBV, CMV, *Mycoplasma, Rickettsia,* and *Mycobacterium tuberculosis*).
- Idiopathic AIN is uncommon.
- Common causes of CIN include polycystic kidney disease, urate nephropathy, analgesic nephropathy, sarcoidosis, multiple myeloma, lead nephropathy, hypercalcemia, and Balkan nephropathy.

 DIAGNOSIS

The diagnosis of interstitial nephritis relies on a thorough history and is usually confirmed by renal biopsy.

■ DIFFERENTIAL DIAGNOSIS
The differential diagnosis includes the diseases listed under "Etiology."

■ WORKUP
Any patient found to be in renal failure without evidence of prerenal or obstructive uropathy should be worked up for interstitial nephritis. Workup generally includes blood and urine studies, x-rays, and renal biopsy.

■ LABORATORY TESTS
- CBC showing anemia and eosinophilia
- BUN and creatinine are elevated and typically represent the first clue of interstitial nephritis
- Electrolytes, calcium, and phosphorus
- Uric acid
- Elevated IgE level
- Urinalysis reveals hematuria and pyuria
- Eosinophiluria by Hansen stain is suggestive of allergic interstitial nephritis
- Proteinuria <3 g/24 hr

■ IMAGING STUDIES
- Ultrasound of the kidneys shows normal size kidneys in AIN and small contracted kidneys in CIN.
- IVP findings are similar to ultrasound findings.
- Renal biopsy in AIN reveals infiltration of inflammatory cells into the interstitium with interstitial edema and sparing of the glomeruli (Fig. 1-221). In CIN fibrotic scar tissue replaces the cellular infiltrate.

TREATMENT

■ NONPHARMACOLOGIC THERAPY
- Low-protein, low-potassium, low-sodium diet
- Correction of underlying electrolyte abnormalities
- IV hydration for hypercalcemia

■ ACUTE GENERAL Rx
- Corticosteroids 1 mg/kg/day are used in patients with drug-induced AIN not responding to withdrawal of the medication within 3 to 4 days. Therapy is continued for a total of 4 to 6 wk.
- Cyclophosphamide 2 mg/kg/day is added as a second agent for patients not responding to corticosteroids.
- Combined therapy is continued for 6 wk.

■ CHRONIC Rx
- Treatment of chronic interstitial nephritis is directed at the underlying cause (e.g., corticosteroids for sarcoidosis, EDTA in lead nephropathy).
- Other therapeutic measures include blood pressure control, reducing uric acid and calcium levels if indicated.

■ DISPOSITION
- Most cases of AIN resolve by withdrawing the offending drug or agent within several days.
- Dialysis is required in up to one third of patients with drug-induced AIN.
- By the time most patients with chronic interstitial nephritis present, their creatinine clearance is <50 ml/min.

Gwendolyn R. Lee, M.D.
Internal Medicine

• Chronic interstitial nephritis patients usually have progressive deterioration in their renal function.

■ **REFERRAL**

Patients with acute renal failure or chronic renal failure from interstitial nephritis should be referred to a nephrologist.

PEARLS & CONSIDERATIONS

■ **COMMENTS**

• There are no randomized controlled trials comparing treatment of AIN with corticosteroids versus other forms of therapy.
• If AIN has resulted from penicillin, the use of another penicillin or cephalosporins has led to recurrence.
• Patients with chronic interstitial nephritis usually have advanced renal disease with no specific therapy.

REFERENCES

Kelly CJ, Neilson EG: Tubulointerstitial diseases. In Brenner BM, Rector FC (eds): *Brenner & Rector's the kidney,* ed 5, Philadelphia, 1996, WB Saunders.

Neilson EG: Pathogenesis and therapy of interstitial nephritis (clinical conference), *Kidney Int* 35:1257, 1989.

Paller MS: Drug-induced nephropathies, *Med Clin North Am* 74:909, 1990.

Author: **Peter Petropoulos, M.D.**

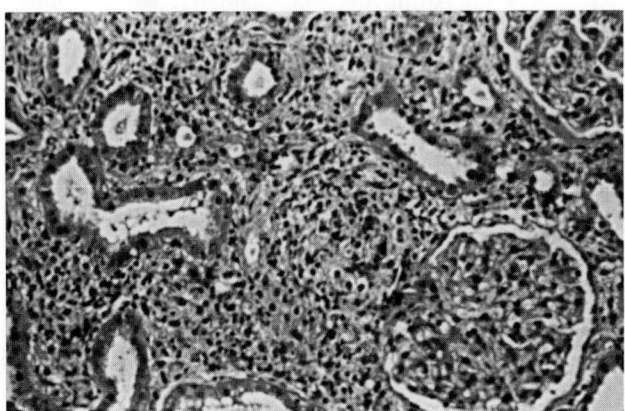

Fig. 1-221 Biopsy from a patient with acute interstitial nephritis. The tubules are widely separated by edema and an intense inflammatory infiltrate containing lymphocytes, plasma cells, eosinophils, and neutrophils. The glomeruli are preserved (×80). (From Behrman RE: *Nelson textbook of pediatrics,* Philadelphia, 1996, WB Saunders.)

BASIC INFORMATION

DEFINITION
Irritable bowel syndrome (IBS) is a chronic functional disorder manifested by alteration in bowel habits and recurrent abdominal pain and bloating.

SYNONYMS
Irritable colon
Spastic colon
IBS

ICD-9CM CODES
564.1 Irritable bowel syndrome

EPIDEMIOLOGY & DEMOGRAPHICS
- IBS occurs in 20% of population of industrialized countries and is responsible for >50% of GI referrals.
- Female:male ratio is 2:1.
- Nearly 50% of patients have psychiatric abnormalities, with anxiety disorders being most common.

PHYSICAL FINDINGS & CLINICAL PRESENTATION
- Physical examination is generally normal.
- Nonspecific abdominal tenderness and distention may be present.

ETIOLOGY
- Unknown
- Possible neurologic or muscular hypersensitivity of the colon, with resulting abnormal colon motility
- Risk factors: anxiety, depression, personality disorders, history of childhood sexual abuse, and domestic abuse in women

DIAGNOSIS

DIFFERENTIAL DIAGNOSIS
- IBD
- Diverticulitis
- Colon malignancy
- Endometriosis
- PUD
- Biliary liver disease
- Chronic pancreatitis

WORKUP
The clinical presentation of IBS consists of abdominal pain and abnormalities of defecation, which may include loose stools usually after meals and in the morning, alternating with episodes of constipation. Diagnostic workup is aimed primarily at excluding the conditions listed in the differential diagnoses. It is important to identify "red flags" of other diseases, such as weight loss, rectal bleeding, onset in patients >50 years of age, fever, nocturnal pain, family history of malignancy.

The criteria for diagnosis of IBS are: More than 3 months of symptoms *including* abdominal pain that is relieved by a bowel movement, *or* pain accompanied by a change in bowel pattern, *and* abnormality in bowel movement >25% of the time, characterized by ≥two of the following features:
  a. Abdominal distention
  b. Abnormal consistency
  c. Abnormal defecation (e.g., straining, sense of incomplete evacuation)
  d. Abnormal frequency
  e. Mucus with bowel movement

LABORATORY TESTS
- Blood work is generally normal. The presence of anemia should alert to the possibility of a colonic malignancy or IBD.
- Testing of stool for ova and parasites should be considered in patients with chronic diarrhea.

IMAGING STUDIES
- Small bowel series and barium enema are normal and not necessary for diagnosis.
- Sigmoidoscopy is generally normal except for the presence of some spasms.

TREATMENT

NONPHARMACOLOGIC THERAPY
- The patient should be encouraged to maintain a high-fiber diet and to eliminate foods that aggravate symptoms.
- Behavioral therapy is also recommended, particularly in younger patients.
- Importance of regular exercise and adequate fluid intake should be stressed.

ACUTE GENERAL Rx
- The mainstay of treatment of IBS is high-fiber diet. Because symptoms are chronic, the use of laxatives should be avoided.
- Fiber supplementation with psyllium 1 tablespoon bid or calcium polycarbophil (FiberCon) 2 tablets one to four times daily followed by 8 oz of water may be necessary in some patients.
- Patients should be instructed that there might be some increased bloating on initiation of fiber supplementation, which should resolve within 2 to 3 wk. It is important that patients take these fiber products on a regular basis and not only PRN.
- Antispasmodics-anticholinergics may be useful in refractory cases (e.g., dicyclomine [Bentyl] 10 to 20 mg up to three times daily).
- Patients who appear anxious can benefit from use of sedatives and anticholinergics such as chlordiazepoxide-clidinium (Librax) or SSRIs.
- Loperamide is effective for diarrhea.

CHRONIC Rx
Patient education regarding maintenance of high-fiber diet and elimination of stressors, which can precipitate attacks of IBS

DISPOSITION
Greater than 60% of patients respond successfully to treatment over the initial 12 mo; however, IBS is a chronic relapsing condition and requires prolonged therapy.

REFERRAL
GI referral is recommended in patients with rectal bleeding, fever, nocturnal diarrhea, anemia, weight loss, or onset of symptoms after age 40 yr.

PEARLS & CONSIDERATIONS

COMMENTS
- Patients should be reassured that their condition cannot lead to cancer.
- The modified ROME criteria define IBS as the presence of ≥12 wk of continuous or recurrent abdominal pain or discomfort that cannot be explained by structural or biochemical abnormalities and the presence of at least two of the following three features: Pain is relieved with defecation, its onset is associated with a change in the frequency of bowel movement, or its onset is associated with a change in the form of the stool.

REFERENCES
Horwitz BJ, Fisher RS: The irritable bowel syndrome, *N Engl J Med* 344:1846, 2001.
Jailwala J et al: Pharmacologic treatment of the irritable bowel syndrome: a systematic review of randomized, controlled trials, *Ann Intern Med* 133:136, 2000.
Author: **Fred F. Ferri, M.D.**

BASIC INFORMATION

■ DEFINITION
Kaposi's sarcoma (KS) is a vascular neoplasm most frequently occurring in AIDS patients. It can be divided into the following four subsets:
1. *Classic Kaposi's sarcoma:* most frequently found in elderly Eastern European and Mediterranean males. It consists initially of violaceous macules and papules with subsequent development of plaques and red/purple nodules. Growth is slow, and most of the patients die of unrelated causes.
2. *Epidemic or AIDS-related Kaposi's sarcoma:* most frequently occurs in homosexual men. Lesions are generally multifocal and widespread. Lymphadenopathy may be associated.
3. *Endemic Kaposi's sarcoma:* usually affects African children and adults. An aggressive lymphadenopathic form affects African children in particular.
4. *Immunosuppression-associated, or transplantation-associated, Kaposi's sarcoma:* usually associated with chemotherapy.

■ SYNONYMS
KS

ICD-9CM CODES
173.9 Malignant neoplasm of the skin

■ EPIDEMIOLOGY & DEMOGRAPHICS
- AIDS-related KS affects >35% of AIDS cases.
- Highest incidence is in homosexual men.

■ PHYSICAL FINDINGS & CLINICAL PRESENTATION
- AIDS-related KS: multifocal and widespread red-purple or dark plaques and/or nodules on cutaneous or mucosal surfaces (Fig. 1-222).
- Generalized lymphadenopathy at the time of diagnosis is present in >50% of patients with AIDS-related KS; the initial lesions have a rust-colored appearance; subsequent progression to red or purple nodules or plaques occurs.
- Most frequently affected areas are the face, trunk, oral cavity, and upper and lower extremities.

■ ETIOLOGY
A herpesvirus (HHV-8, Kaposi's sarcoma-associated herpesvirus KSHV) has been isolated from patients with most forms of KS and is believed to be the causative agent. It can be transmitted sexually (homosexual, heterosexual activities) and by other forms of nonsexual contact such as maternal-infant transmission (common in African countries).

DIAGNOSIS

■ DIFFERENTIAL DIAGNOSIS
- Stasis dermatitis
- Pyogenic granuloma
- Capillary hemangiomas
- Granulation tissue
- Postinflammatory hyperpigmentation
- Cutaneous lymphoma
- Melanoma
- Dermatofibroma
- Hematoma
- Prurigo nodularis

Table 2-96 describes the differential diagnosis of cutaneous lesions in patients with HIV infection.

■ WORKUP
Diagnosis can generally be made on clinical appearance; tissue biopsy will confirm diagnosis.

■ LABORATORY TESTS
HIV in patients suspected of AIDS

TREATMENT

■ NONPHARMACOLOGIC THERAPY
Observation is a reasonable option in patients with slowly progressive disease.

■ ACUTE GENERAL Rx
- Excisional biopsy often provides adequate treatment for single lesions and resected recurrences in classic Kaposi's sarcoma.
- Liquid nitrogen cryotherapy can result in complete response in 80% of lesions.
- Interlesional chemotherapy with vinblastine is useful for nodular lesions >1 cm in diameter. Intralesional injection of interferon alfa-2b has also been reported as effective and well tolerated.

- Radiation therapy is effective in non-AIDS KS and for large tumor masses that interfere with normal function.
- Systemic therapy with interferon is also effective in AIDS-related KS and is often used in combination with AZT.
- Systemic chemotherapy (vinblastine, bleomycin, doxorubicin, and dacarbazine) can be used for rapidly progressive disease and for classic and African endemic KS.
- Oral etoposide is also effective and has less myelosuppression than vinblastine.
- Paclitaxel is also effective in patients with advanced KS and represents an excellent second-line therapy.

■ DISPOSITION
- Prognosis is poor in AIDS-related KS. Death is often a result of other AIDS-defining illnesses.
- Prognosis is better in African cutaneous KS and classic sarcoma (patients usually die of unrelated causes).

■ REFERRAL
Surgical referral for biopsy of suspected lesions

PEARLS & CONSIDERATIONS

■ COMMENTS
Immunosuppression-associated Kaposi's sarcoma usually regresses with the cessation, reduction, or modification of immunosuppression therapy in most patients. Similarly in HIV patients, Kaposi's sarcoma responds concurrently with the decrease in serum HIV RNA and increase in the CD4 count.

REFERENCE
Antman K, Chang Y: Kaposi's sarcoma, *N Engl J Med* 342:1027, 2000.
Author: **Fred F. Ferri, M.D.**

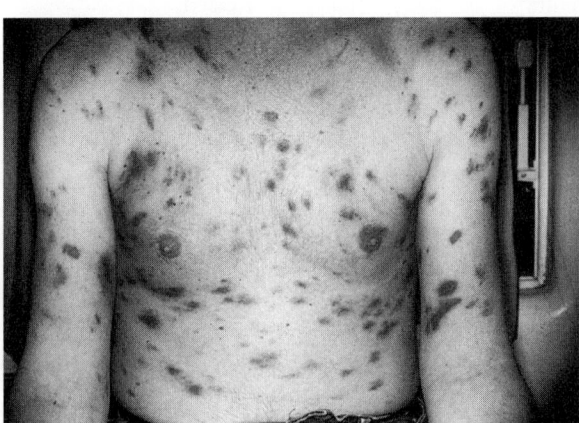

Fig. 1-222 Kaposi's sarcoma. More advanced lesions. Note widespread hemorrhagic plaques and nodules. (From Noble J et al: *Textbook of primary care medicine,* ed 2, St Louis, 1995, Mosby.)

BASIC INFORMATION

■ DEFINITION
Kawasaki disease (KD) refers to a generalized vasculitis of unknown etiology and characterized by cutaneous and mucous membrane edema, rash, lymphadenopathy, and involvement of multiple organs.

■ SYNONYMS
Mucocutaneous lymph node syndrome

ICD-9CM CODES
446.1 Kawasaki disease

■ EPIDEMIOLOGY & DEMOGRAPHICS
- KD is a leading cause of acquired heart disease in children.
- KD commonly occurs under the age of 5 (80%).
- KD is found more often in boys than in girls (1.5:1).
- In the United States the incidence of KD is 8.9 cases/100,000 children <5 years of age.
- Approximately 1900 new cases are diagnosed each year in the U.S.
- The incidence of KD in Japan is 80 to 90/100,000 under the age of 5.

■ PHYSICAL FINDINGS & CLINICAL PRESENTATION
A typical presentation is a young child with fever unresponsive to antibiotics for more than 5 days associated with:
- Bilateral conjunctivitis
- Erythema and edema of the hands and feet (Fig. 1-223, *B*)
- Periungual desquamation
- Fissuring of the lips
- Erythematous pharynx
- Strawberry tongue (Fig. 1-223, *A*)
- Cervical adenopathy
- Truncal scarlatiniform rash, usually nonvesicular
- Diarrhea
- Dyspnea
- Arthralgias and myalgia
- Sudden death from coronary artery involvement
- Myocardial infarction
- Congestive heart failure

■ ETIOLOGY
- The cause of KD is not known although evidence substantiates an infectious etiology precipitating an immune-mediated reaction.

DIAGNOSIS

The diagnosis of Kawasaki disease is based on a fever lasting more than 5 days along with four of the following five features:
- Bilateral conjunctival swelling
- Inflammatory changes of the lip, tongue, and pharynx
- Skin changes of the limbs
- Rash over the trunk
- Cervical lymphadenopathy

■ DIFFERENTIAL DIAGNOSIS
- Scarlet fever
- Stevens-Johnson syndrome
- Drug eruption
- Henoch-Schönlein purpura
- Toxic shock syndrome
- Measles
- Rocky Mountain spotted fever
- Infectious mononucleosis

■ WORKUP
Clinical findings in addition to lab and imaging studies are useful in searching for organ system involvement and complications (e.g., cardiac, lung, liver).

■ LABORATORY TESTS
- CBC commonly shows an elevated WBC and platelet count
- ESR is elevated
- C-reactive protein is positive
- Liver function tests (e.g., elevated SGOT and SGPT)
- Urinalysis may show sterile pyuria

■ IMAGING STUDIES
- Chest x-ray may reveal pulmonary infiltrates.
- Echocardiogram is very helpful and may show depressed left ventricular function with regional wall motion abnormalities, pericardial effusions (30%), and abnormal coronary artery aneurysms. The echocardiogram is also useful in the long-term follow-up of patients with KD.
- Intravascular ultrasound looking for coronary artery lumen irregularities.
- Exercise testing with myocardial perfusion studies can be done to assess for coronary blood flow.
- Cardiac catheterization with coronary angiography in the proper clinical setting is done to rule out significant obstructive coronary disease.

TREATMENT

■ NONPHARMACOLOGIC THERAPY
- Oxygen in selected patients
- Salt restriction in patients with CHF

■ ACUTE GENERAL Rx
- Intravenous immunoglobulin (IVIG) 2 mg/kg IV over 8 to 12 hours is the treatment of choice in children diagnosed with KD and ideally should be given within the first 10 days of the illness.
- Aspirin 80 to 100 mg/kg qid is given until the patient is no longer febrile.
- Prednisone and NSAIDs are not effective in the treatment of KD.

■ CHRONIC Rx
Interventional and surgical procedures can be tried in children who have developed cardiac complications of KD.
- Percutaneous transluminal coronary angioplasty
- Coronary bypass graft surgery using the internal mammary artery or the gastroepiploic artery has met with greater patency success than saphenous vein grafts.
- Cardiac transplantation is an option and is indicated in patients with:
  1. Severe left ventricular failure
  2. Malignant arrhythmias
  3. Multivessel distal coronary artery disease

■ DISPOSITION
- Mortality rate of children with KD is 0.5% to 2.8%, usually from coronary artery aneurysm, coronary thrombosis, myocarditis, and pancarditis.
- Death usually occurs in the third to fourth week of the illness.
- Before the use of IVIG, approximately 20% of all patients with KD develop coronary aneurysms.
- Treatment with IVIG has reduced the incidence of coronary aneurysms by 80%.
- IVIG has also been shown to improve left ventricular function during the acute stages of the disease.
- Risk factors for the development of coronary aneurysms or giant coronary aneurysms (>8 mm) are:
  1. Fever lasting >10 days
  2. Age <1 year
  3. Male
  4. Recurrence of fever
- Between 1% to 2% of patients have recurrences of KD.

■ REFERRAL

Multiple specialists may be consulted to assist in the diagnosis of KD including dermatology, rheumatology, and infectious disease. Cardiology consultation is recommended in any patient with cardiac involvement and in the long-term follow up of patients with KD.

○ PEARLS & CONSIDERATIONS

■ COMMENTS

- KD was first described by Dr. Tomasaku Kawasaki in 1967 and published in the *Journal of Allergology.*
- Kawasaki disease is not transmitted from person to person.
- The mechanism of action of intravenous gamma-globulin therapy for KD remains unknown.

REFERENCES

Barron KL et al: Report of the National Institutes of Health Workshop on Kawasaki Disease, *J Rheumatol* 26(1):170, 1999.

Kato H et al: Long-term consequences of Kawasaki disease. A 10-to 21-year follow-up study of 594 patients, *Circulation* 94:1379, 1996.

Rowley AH, Shulman ST: Kawasaki syndrome, *Pediatr Clin North Am* 46(2):313, 1999.

Taubert KA, Shulman ST: Kawasaki disease, *Am Fam Physician* 59(11):3093, 1999.

Author: **Peter Petropoulos, M.D.**

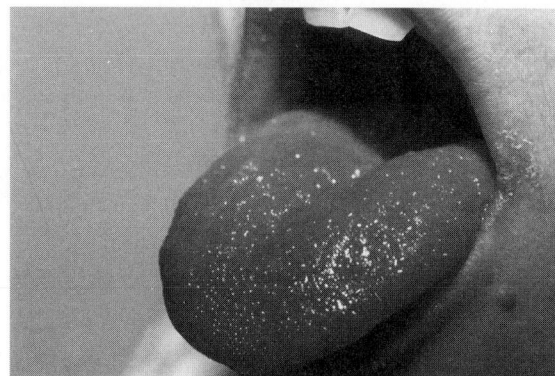 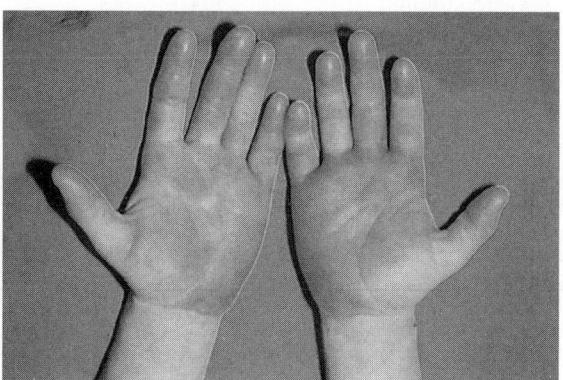

Fig. 1-223 **A,** Strawberry tongue in a patient with Kawasaki syndrome. **B,** Kawasaki syndrome. Note the erythema of the hands, to be followed by desquamation. (**A** Courtesy Marshall Guill, MD. In Goldstein B [ed]: *Practical dermatology,* ed 2, St Louis, 1997, Mosby. **B** Courtesy Department of Dermatology, University of North Carolina at Chapel Hill. In Goldstein B [ed]: *Practical dermatology,* ed 2, St Louis, 1997, Mosby.)

BASIC INFORMATION

■ DEFINITION
Klinefelter's syndrome is a congenital disorder in which a 47,XXY chromosome complement is associated with hypogonadism and infertility.

■ SYNONYMS
47,XXY Hypogonadism

■ ICD-9CM CODES
758.7 Klinefelter's syndrome

■ EPIDEMIOLOGY & DEMOGRAPHICS
INCIDENCE: 1 in 500 men (most common sex chromosome disorder)
GENETICS: The most common mosaic complement is 46,XY/47.XXY. 47,XXY karyotype and occasional 48,XXYY; 48,XXXY; or 49,XXXXY have been reported. The manifestations vary in severity in patients. It is this sex chromosome mosaicism that is thought to account for the variable presentation. Fertility, although very rare, has been reported in men with Klinefelter's syndrome.

■ PHYSICAL FINDINGS
CLASSIC TRIAD: Small firm testes, azoospermia, and gynecomastia
Prepubertal: Small testes, gonadal volume <1.5 ml is a result of loss of germ cells before puberty.
Postpubertal: Gynecomastia (periductal fat growth) with small, firm, pea-sized testes. Exaggerated growth of the lower extremities results in a decreased crown-to-pubis:pubis-to-floor ratio (Fig. 1-224). There are diminished strength, diminished ability to grow a full beard or mustache, infertility; decreased intellectual development and antisocial behavior are thought to occur with high frequency.

■ ETIOLOGY
- Several postulated mechanisms: nondisjunction during meiosis and mitosis and anaphase lag during mitosis or meiosis
- Reason: maternal age
  1. The incidence of Klinefelter's rises from 0.6% when the maternal age is 35 yr or less to 5.4% when the maternal age is in excess of 45 yr.
  2. It is of interest to note that the extra X chromosome has a paternal origin as often as a maternal origin.

DIAGNOSIS

■ LABORATORY TESTS
- Normal to low serum testosterone
- Elevated sex hormone binding globulin
- Increased sex hormone binding globin (acts to further suppress any available free testosterone)
- Normal to increased estradiol (a result of augmented peripheral conversion of testosterone to estradiol)
- Testis biopsy shows azoospermia, Leydig cell hyperplasia, hyalinization, and fibrosis of the seminiferous tubules. Mosaics may have focal areas of spermatogenesis, and, on rare occasions, a sperm may appear in the ejaculate. It is the extra X chromosome that is the pivotal factor controlling spermatogenesis as well as affecting neuronal function directly leading to the behavioral abnormalities related to decreased IQ.
- Buccal smear: one sex chromatin body
PREPUBERTAL MALE: Gonadotropin levels are normal.
POSTPUBERTAL MALE: Gonadotropin levels are elevated even when the testosterone level is normal.
DISEASE ASSOCIATIONS:
Malignancies: Breast cancer (20 times greater than XY men and 20% the rate of occurrence in women), nonlymphocytic leukemia, lymphomas, marrow dysplastic syndromes, extragonadal germ cell neoplasms
Autoimmune Disorders: Chronic lymphocytic thyroiditis, Takayasu arteritis, taurodontism (enlarged molar teeth), mitral valve prolapse, varicose veins, asthma, bronchitis, osteoporosis, and abnormal glucose tolerance testing
Others: Diabetes, varicose veins

TREATMENT

Revolves around three facets of Klinefelter's syndrome:
1. Hypogonadism: androgen replacement in the form of testosterone
2. Gynecomastia: cosmetic surgery
3. Psychosocial problems: androgen therapy and educational support
4. After extensive genetic counseling intracytoplasmic sperm insertion (ICSI) has been used to treat infertility with limited success.

PEARLS & CONSIDERATIONS

■ COMMENTS
- Androgen therapy should not be used in the case of severe mental retardation.
- Also, rule out breast and prostate cancer before initiating or continuing androgen therapy.
- Furthermore, androgen therapy will not improve infertility; it may suppress any spermatogenesis that is taking place within the testes.
- Other causes of primary hypogonadism:
  1. Myotonic muscular dystrophy
  2. Sertoli cell only syndrome
  3. Kartagener's syndrome
  4. Anorchia
  5. Acquired hypogonadism

REFERENCES
Palermo GD et al: Births after intracytoplasmic sperm insertion of sperm obtained by testicular extraction from men with non-mosaic Klinefelter's syndrome, *N Engl J Med* 338:588, 1998.
Smyth CM, Bremner WJ: Klinefelter syndrome, *Arch Intern Med* 158:1309, 1998.
Author: **Philip J. Aliotta, M.D., M.S.H.A.**

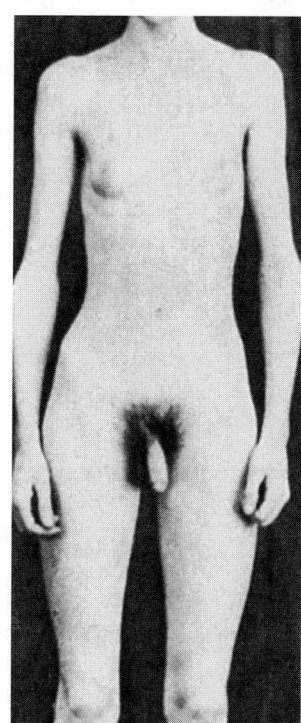

Fig. 1-224 Klinefelter's syndrome. (From Harrison JH et al: *Campbell's urology*, ed 4, Philadelphia, 1979, WB Saunders.)

BASIC INFORMATION

■ DEFINITION

Korsakoff's psychosis involves a disproportionate impairment in memory, relative to other cognitive function, resulting from a thiamine deficiency.

■ SYNONYMS

Korsakoff's syndrome
Wernicke-Korsakoff syndrome
Alcoholic polyneuritic psychosis

■ ICD-9CM CODES

291.1 Alcohol amnestic syndrome

■ EPIDEMIOLOGY & DEMOGRAPHICS

INCIDENCE (IN U.S.): Most common in alcoholics
PREVALENCE (IN U.S.): Slightly less than incidence
PREDOMINANT SEX: More common in males
PREDOMINANT AGE: Middle age
PEAK INCIDENCE: Middle age

■ PHYSICAL FINDINGS & CLINICAL PRESENTATION

- Impairment of ability to remember new material
- Relatively intact remote memory
- Possible confabulation

■ ETIOLOGY

Thiamine deficiency, usually but not always in alcoholics

 # DIAGNOSIS

■ DIFFERENTIAL DIAGNOSIS

- Brain tumor
- Cerebral anoxia
- Dementia from any cause

■ WORKUP

Consider in all alcoholics, in malnutrition, and in malabsorption.

■ LABORATORY TESTS

This is a chronic, permanent condition, and lab tests are normal once proper nutrition is maintained and alcohol intake ceases.

■ IMAGING STUDIES

MRI shows bilateral thalamic and mamillary body lesions in up to 30% of acute cases; ventricular enlargement and cerebral atrophy are common.

TREATMENT

■ NONPHARMACOLOGIC THERAPY

A supervised environment may be required.

■ ACUTE GENERAL Rx

Thiamine 100 mg IV or IM, given during Wernicke's phase (disorders of extraocular movements, confusion, and ataxia), is highly effective in preventing Korsakoff's symptoms.

■ CHRONIC Rx

No cure

■ DISPOSITION

Patient often must live in protected environment for rest of life.

■ REFERRAL

If there is doubt about the diagnosis; neuropsychologic tests may be helpful.

PEARLS & CONSIDERATIONS

■ COMMENTS

- This disease is probably underdiagnosed.
- Give thiamine if the disease is even suspected.
- A preventable cause is prolonged IV fluids without daily thiamine.

Author: **William H. Olson, M.D.**

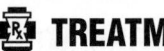 **BASIC INFORMATION**

■ **DEFINITION**
Labyrinthitis is an acute onset of vertigo, nausea, and vomiting not associated with auditory or other neurologic symptoms.

■ **SYNONYMS**
Acute labyrinthitis
Acute vestibular neuronopathy
Viral neurolabyrinthitis

■ **ICD-9CM CODES**
386.3 Labyrinthitis

■ **EPIDEMIOLOGY & DEMOGRAPHICS**
INCIDENCE (IN U.S.): Most common cause of transient vertigo, nausea, and vomiting at any age.
PREDOMINANT AGE: Any

■ **PHYSICAL FINDINGS**
• Nystagmus
• Nausea
• Vomiting
• Vertigo worsening with head movement
• Abnormal caloric tests
• Normal hearing

■ **ETIOLOGY**
Often preceded 1 wk by an upper respiratory illness

DIAGNOSIS

■ **DIFFERENTIAL DIAGNOSIS**
• Cholesteatoma
• Suppurative labyrinthitis
• Labyrinthine fistula
• Benign positional vertigo
• Meniere's syndrome
• Vascular insufficiency
• Drug-induced
Table 2-145 describes the differential diagnosis of nystagmus. Box 2-256 describes the differential diagnosis of vertigo.

■ **WORKUP**
• Caloric test if presentation is atypical
• Careful cranial nerve testing
Fig. 3-177 describes an algorithm for the evaluation of vertigo.

■ **LABORATORY TESTS**
• Routine laboratory tests are generally not helpful.
• CBC with sedimentation rate may be useful in selected patients.

■ **IMAGING STUDIES**
None are usually necessary, but enhancement of bony labyrinth may be seen by MRI after injection of contrast material.

TREATMENT

■ **NONPHARMACOLOGIC THERAPY**
Reassurance

■ **ACUTE GENERAL Rx** (Table 1-43)
• Compazine or other antiemetics are effective
• Meclizine 12.5 to 25 mg qid often used, but scopolamine patch is most effective.

■ **CHRONIC Rx**
None necessary

■ **DISPOSITION**
Referral usually not necessary

■ **REFERRAL**
If symptoms persist or cranial nerve abnormalities are present

PEARLS & CONSIDERATIONS

■ **COMMENTS**
"Labyrinthitis" covers a broad range of diseases; here we refer only to the acute, self-limited type.
Author: **William H. Olson, M.D.**

TABLE 1-43 Vestibular Suppressants

DRUG	DOSE	ADVERSE REACTIONS	PHARMACOLOGIC CLASS AND PRECAUTIONS
Meclizine (Antivert, Bonine)	12.5-50 mg q 4-6h	Sedating, precautions in prostatic enlargement, glaucoma	Antihistamine Anticholinergic
Lorazepam (Ativan)	0.5 mg bid	Mildly sedating Drug dependency	Benzodiazepine
Clonazepam (Klonopin)	0.5 mg bid	Mildly sedating Drug dependency	Benzodiazepine
Scopolamine (Transderm-Scop)	0.5 mg patch q3d	Topical allergy with chronic use. Precautions in glaucoma, tachyarrhythmias, prostatic enlargement	Anticholinergic
Dimenhydrinate (Dramamine)	50 mg q4-6h	Same as meclizine	Antihistamine
Diazepam (Valium)	2-10 mg (1 dose) given acutely orally, intramuscularly, or intravenously	Sedating Respiratory depressant Drug dependency Precaution in glaucoma	Anticholinergic Benzodiazepine

From Goetz CG: *Textbook of clinical neurology,* Philadelphia, 1999, WB Saunders.
Doses listed are used in adults. Drugs arranged in order of preference.

BASIC INFORMATION

■ **DEFINITION**
Lactose intolerance is the insufficient concentration of lactase enzyme, leading to fermentation of malabsorbed lactose by intestinal bacteria with subsequent production of intestinal gas and various organic acids.

■ **SYNONYMS**
Lactase deficiency
Milk intolerance

ICD-9CM CODES
271.3 Lactose intolerance

■ **EPIDEMIOLOGY & DEMOGRAPHICS**
Nearly 50 million people in the U.S. have partial or complete lactose intolerance. There are racial differences, with <25% of white adults being lactose intolerant, whereas >85% of Asian-Americans and >60% of blacks have some form of lactose intolerance.

■ **PHYSICAL FINDINGS & CLINICAL PRESENTATION**
• Abdominal tenderness and cramping, bloating, flatulence
• Diarrhea
• Physical examination: may be entirely within normal limits

■ **ETIOLOGY**
• Congenital lactase deficiency: common in premature infants; rare in full-term infants and generally inherited as a chromosomal recessive trait
• Secondary lactose intolerance: usually a result of injury of the intestinal mucosa (Crohn's disease, viral gastroenteritis, AIDS enteropathy, cryptosporidiosis, Whipple's disease, sprue)

DIAGNOSIS

■ **DIFFERENTIAL DIAGNOSIS**
• IBD
• IBS
• Pancreatic insufficiency
• Nontropical and tropical sprue
• Cystic fibrosis

■ **WORKUP**
Diagnostic workup includes confirming the diagnosis with hydrogen breath test and excluding other conditions listed in the differential diagnosis that may also coexist with lactase deficiency.

■ **LABORATORY TESTS**
• Lactose breath hydrogen test: A rise in breath hydrogen >20 ppm within 90 min of ingestion of 50 g of lactose is positive for lactase deficiency
• Diarrhea associated with lactase deficiency is osmotic in nature with an osmotic gap and a pH below 6.5.

■ **IMAGING STUDIES**
Imaging studies are generally not indicated. A small bowel series may be useful in patients with significant malabsorption.

TREATMENT

■ **NONPHARMACOLOGIC THERAPY**
A lactose-free diet generally results in prompt resolution of symptoms. Lactose is primarily found in dairy products but may be present as an ingredient or component of common foods and beverages. Possible sources of lactose are breads, candies, cold cuts, dessert mixes, cream soups, bologna, commercial sauces and gravies, chocolate, drink mixes, salad dressings, and medications. Labels should be read carefully to identify sources of lactose.

■ **ACUTE GENERAL Rx**
• Addition of lactase (Lactaid tablets) before the ingestion of milk products may prevent symptoms in some patients. However, it is not effective for all lactose-intolerant patients.
• Calcium supplementation is recommended to prevent osteoporosis.

■ **CHRONIC Rx**
Patient education regarding foods high in lactose, such as milk, cottage cheese, or ice cream, is recommended.

■ **DISPOSITION**
Clinical improvement with restriction or elimination of milk products

■ **REFERRAL**
GI referral for endoscopic procedures if concomitant GI disorders are suspected

PEARLS & CONSIDERATIONS

■ **COMMENTS**
There is great variability in signs and symptoms in patients with lactose intolerance depending on the degree of lactase deficiency.
Author: **Fred F. Ferri, M.D.**

BASIC INFORMATION

■ DEFINITION

Lambert-Eaton myasthenic syndrome is a disorder of neuromuscular transmission caused by antibodies directed against presynaptic voltage-gated calcium channels on motor nerve terminals.

■ SYNONYMS

Eaton-Lambert syndrome

ICD-9CM CODES

199.1 Malignant neoplasm without specification of site, other

■ EPIDEMIOLOGY & DEMOGRAPHICS

INCIDENCE (IN U.S.): Uncertain; estimated at 5 cases/1 million persons/yr
PREVALENCE (IN U.S.): Uncertain; estimated at 400 total cases
PREDOMINANT SEX: Male:female of 2:1
PREDOMINANT AGE: 60 yr
PEAK INCIDENCE: Sixth decade
GENETICS: Predisposition in people with a personal or family history of autoimmune disease

■ PHYSICAL FINDINGS & CLINICAL PRESENTATION

- Weakness with diminished or absent muscle stretch reflexes
- Proximal lower extremity muscles affected most
- Ocular and bulbar muscles possibly mildly affected
- Transient strength improvement with brief exercise
- Possible autonomic dysfunction

■ ETIOLOGY

- Antibodies directed against presynaptic voltage-gated calcium channels are present in most patients.

- The reduction in calcium permeability causes a reduction in acetylcholine release.
- Associated malignancy, usually small cell lung cancer, is present in 50% to 70% of patients.

DIAGNOSIS

■ DIFFERENTIAL DIAGNOSIS

- Myasthenia gravis
- Polymyositis
- Cachexia

Box 2-169 describes the differential diagnosis of muscle weakness.

■ WORKUP

Confirm diagnosis by characteristic electrodiagnostic (EMG/NCS) findings.

■ LABORATORY TESTS

As needed to screen for an underlying malignancy

■ IMAGING STUDIES

As needed to screen for an underlying malignancy

TREATMENT

■ NONPHARMACOLOGIC THERAPY

- Avoid elevated body temperature.
- Treat systemic illnesses promptly.

■ ACUTE GENERAL Rx

- Anticholinesterase agents (e.g., pyridostigmine 30 to 60 mg q4-6h) may yield some improvement.
- Guanidine hydrochloride: start at 5 to 10 mg/kg/day; may increase up to 30 mg/kg/day in 3-day or longer intervals.
- Plasma exchange or IV immunoglobulins (2 g/kg over 2 to 5 days) often produce significant, temporary improvement.

- Prednisone 60 to 80 mg/day can be gradually tapered over weeks or months to minimal effective dose.
- Azathioprine can be given alone or in combination with prednisone. Give 50 mg/day and increase by 50 mg every 3 days up to 150 to 200 mg/day.

■ CHRONIC Rx

- Treat underlying malignancy if present.
- Give pharmacotherapy as described in "Acute General Rx."

■ DISPOSITION

- Gradually progressive weakness leading to impaired mobility
- Possible substantial improvement with successful treatment of underlying malignancy

■ REFERRAL

To a neurologist (recommended) because of infrequency of this disease and risks associated with some treatments

PEARLS & CONSIDERATIONS

■ COMMENTS

- Many drugs may worsen weakness and should be used only if absolutely necessary. Included are succinylcholine, d-tubocurarine, quinine, quinidine, procainamide, aminoglycoside antibiotics, β-blockers, and calcium channel blockers.
- Watch for increased weakness when starting any new medication.

Author: **Michael Gruenthal, M.D., Ph.D.**

BASIC INFORMATION

■ **DEFINITION**
Laryngitis is an acute or chronic inflammation of the laryngeal mucous membranes.

■ **SYNONYMS**
Laryngotracheitis (although this includes inflammation of the trachea as well as the larynx)

ICD-9CM CODES
464.0 Acute laryngitis
476.0 Chronic laryngitis

■ **PHYSICAL FINDINGS & CLINICAL PRESENTATION**
ACUTE LARYNGITIS
- Usually associated with an upper respiratory infection, often the common cold or influenza
- Onset usually characterized by sore throat, cough, nasal congestion, and rhinorrhea, followed by hoarseness and occasionally aphonia
- Larynx with diffuse erythema, edema, and vascular engorgement of the vocal folds, and perhaps mucosal ulcerations (Fig. 1-225)
- In young children: subglottis is often affected, resulting in airway narrowing with marked hoarseness, inspiratory stridor, dyspnea, and restlessness
- Respiratory compromise rare in adults
CHRONIC LARYNGITIS
- Hoarseness is the most common complaint
- Tends to be indolent, with symptoms lasting several weeks
- Posterior laryngitis (a form of chronic laryngitis) includes one or more of the following: erythema/edema of arytenoid cartilage, erythema/edema of interarytenoid tissue, erythema of the posterior third of vocal cords, erythema/edema of the entire larynx, or pachyderma laryngis

■ **ETIOLOGY**
ACUTE LARYNGITIS:
- Most often associated with viral infections: influenza virus, rhinovirus, and adenovirus are the most common, but parainfluenza virus, myxovirus, paramyxovirus, coxsackievirus, coronavirus, respiratory syncytial virus, herpesvirus, Epstein-Barr virus, varicella zoster virus, and variola virus are sometimes implicated.

- Superinfection is possible with bacteria such as group A *streptococci*, *Staphylococcus aureus,* and *Streptococcus pneumoniae.*
- 50% to 55% of adults with laryngitis harbor *Moraxella catarrhalis* in the nasopharynx, compared with 6% to 14% of controls.
Corynebacterium diphtheriae is also a cause and may affect both the pharynx and larynx.
CHRONIC LARYNGITIS:
- Results from any of the following: Tuberculosis, usually through bronchogenic spread; leprosy, from nasopharyngeal or oropharyngeal spread; syphilis, in secondary and tertiary stages; rhinoscleroma, extending from the nose and nasopharynx; actinomycosis; histoplasmosis; blastomycosis; paracoccidiodomycosis; coccidiosis; candidiasis; aspergillosis; sporotrichosis; rhinosporidiosis; parasitic infections, including leishmaniasis.
- Nonspecific inflammation can occur as a result of exposure to irritants such as tobacco smoke and chemicals, air pollutants, and from vocal abuse (singers, cheerleaders).
- Gastroesophageal reflux disease (GERD) has a well-recognized association with posterior laryngitis.

 DIAGNOSIS

■ **DIFFERENTIAL DIAGNOSIS**
Young children with signs of airway obstruction:
- Supraglottitis (epiglottitis)
- Laryngotracheobronchitis
- Bacterial tracheitis
- Foreign body aspiration
ADULTS:
- Hoarseness from streptococcal pharyngitis
- With persistent hoarseness, consider laryngeal tumors, papillomatosis

■ **WORKUP**
- History and physical examination; diagnosis is usually apparent
- Laryngoscopy for severe or persistent cases
- Presence of mucosal exudate is consistent with streptococcal infection, diphtheria, mononucleosis, candidiasis
Patients with posterior laryngitis are the major group of patients with GERD-associated laryngitis. Most will have documented pharyngeal reflux by pH monitoring.

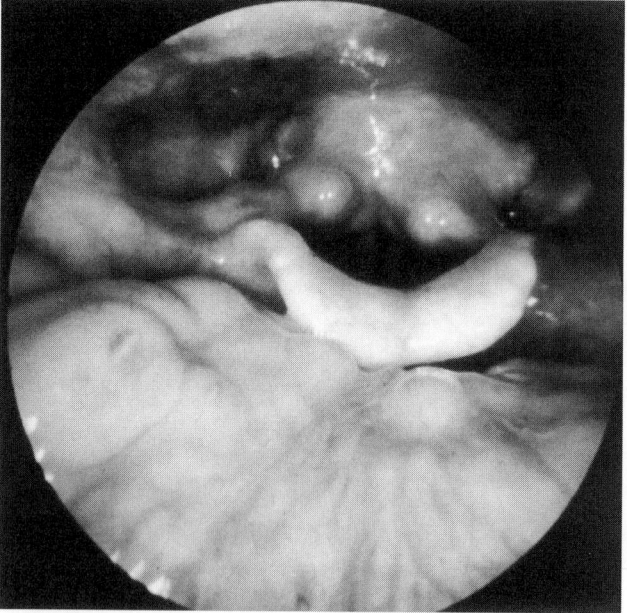
Fig. 1-225 Acute laryngitis: interarytenoid edema prevents complete glottal closure. (From Woodson GE: *Ear, nose and throat disorders in primary care,* Philadelphia, 2001, WB Saunders.)

■ LABORATORY TESTS

If etiology other than acute viral infection is suspected, obtain laryngeal cultures and biopsies

■ IMAGING STUDIES

- Not indicated unless evidence of airway compromise
- Plain radiographs of neck, anteroposterior and lateral, to differentiate laryngitis from acute laryngotracheobronchitis or supraglottitis.

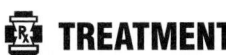 **TREATMENT**

■ NONPHARMACOLOGIC THERAPY

- Rest the voice
- Use an air humidifier

■ ACUTE GENERAL Rx

- Antibiotics and other antimicrobials: indicated only when a specific pathogen is isolated
- In GERD associated laryngitis:
    1. Acid suppressive therapy
        a. H_2 blockers (cimetidine, ranitidine)
        b. Proton pump inhibitors (omeprazole, lansoprazole)
    2. Nocturnal antireflux precautions
        a. Avoid oral intake 3 hr before bedtime
        b. Elevation of head of bed
    3. Surgery

■ DISPOSITION

Uncomplicated laryngitis is usually benign, with gradual resolution of symptoms.

■ REFERRAL

If symptoms persist for >2 wk, refer to otolaryngologist for laryngoscopy. Consider referral to gastroenterologist if suspect GERD.

REFERENCES

Nostrant TT: Gastroesophageal reflux and laryngitis: a skeptic's view, *Am J Med* 108(4A):149S, 2000.

Ulualp SO: Outcomes of acid suppressive therapy in patient with posterior laryngitis, *Otolaryngol Head Neck Surg* 124(1):16, 2001.

Author: **Jane V. Eason, M.D.**

BASIC INFORMATION

■ **DEFINITION**
Acute laryngotracheobronchitis is a viral infection of the upper and lower respiratory tract leading to erythema and edema of the tracheal walls and narrowing of the subglottic region.

■ **SYNONYMS**
Croup

■ **ICD-9CM CODES**
464.4 Croup

■ **EPIDEMIOLOGY & DEMOGRAPHICS**
• Croup is primarily a disease of children occurring between the ages of 1 and 6 yr.
• The peak incidence of croup is the second year of life (50 cases/1000 children).
• Most cases usually occur in the fall and represent parainfluenza type 1 viral infection.
• Winter outbreaks usually represent infection by influenza A and B viruses.
• Croup accounts for 10% to 15% of lower respiratory tract infections in young children.
• Boys are affected more often than girls.

■ **PHYSICAL FINDINGS & CLINICAL PRESENTATION**
• Most children with croup present with symptoms of an upper respiratory infection for several days.
• Rhinorrhea
• Cough
• Low-grade fever
• Barking cough that usually occurs at night and wakes the child up.
• Sore throat
• Stridor
• Apprehension
• Use of accessory muscles of respiration
• Tachypnea
• Tachycardia
• Wheezing

■ **ETIOLOGY**
• Parainfluenza viruses (types 1, 2, and 3) are the most common causes of croup in the U.S.
• Influenza A and B, although not a common cause of croup, does lead to more severe cases of the disease.
• Adenovirus
• Respiratory syncytial virus
• *Mycoplasma pneumoniae* (rare)

DIAGNOSIS

The diagnosis of croup is usually based on the characteristic clinical presentation of a young child between the ages of 1 to 6 yr waking up with a barking cough ("seal's bark") and stridor.

■ **DIFFERENTIAL DIAGNOSIS**
Spasmodic croup, epiglottitis, bacterial tracheitis, angioneurotic edema, diphtheria, peritonsillar abscess, retropharyngeal abscess, smoke inhalation, foreign body

■ **WORKUP**
• The workup of a child with croup is to differentiate viral laryngotracheobronchitis from noninfectious causes of stridor and epiglottitis caused by *H. influenzae.*
• The clinical presentation and plain films of the soft tissues of the neck assists in differentiating viral from nonviral and noninfectious causes.

■ **LABORATORY TESTS**
• Laboratory tests are not often used to make the diagnosis of viral tracheobronchitis.
• CBC, viral serology, and tissue cultures can be ordered and may detect the infecting agent in up to 65% of cases.
• Pulse oximetry and arterial blood gas determination for patients with tachypnea and respiratory distress.

■ **IMAGING STUDIES**
• Plain (AP and lateral) films of the soft tissues of the neck may show the classic radiographic finding of subglottic stenosis or "steeple" sign.
• CT scan of the soft tissues of the neck may be performed in the cases where the differential between croup, epiglottitis, and noninfectious is more difficult.
• Direct visualization via laryngoscopy may be useful in some situations under a controlled setting.

TREATMENT

Treatment of croup focuses on airway management.

■ **NONPHARMACOLOGIC THERAPY**
• Oxygen
• Cool mist
• Hot steam

■ **ACUTE GENERAL Rx**
• Use of 0.25 to 0.75 ml of 2.25% racemic epinephrine every 20 min is used in children with severe respiratory symptoms, rest stridor, and impending intubation.
• Corticosteroids (e.g., dexamethasone 0.6 mg/kg IV or PO, prednisone 2 mg/kg/day) have been shown to be effective.
• Budesonide, a nebulized corticosteroid given at 4 mg, has been shown to improve symptoms in patients with moderate to severe croup.

■ **CHRONIC Rx**
• Croup is an acute infectious disease with a short natural history; thus, chronic management is not usually an issue.

■ **DISPOSITION**
• Croup is usually benign and self-limited, resolving within 3 to 4 days.
• Complications include:
  1. Airway obstruction
  2. Otitis media
  3. Pneumonia
  4. Dehydration

■ **REFERRAL**
If intubation is needed (rarely), an emergency consultation with ENT and/or anesthesiology is recommended.

PEARLS & CONSIDERATIONS

■ **COMMENTS**
• Most patients with croup can be managed at home (e.g., patients without stridor and in no respiratory distress).
• Hospitalization and observation is required for children with moderate-to-severe croup (e.g., rest stridor, respiratory distress refractory to the above-mentioned acute treatments).

REFERENCES
Johnson DW, Jacobson S, Edney PC: A comparison of nebulized budesonide, intramuscular dexamethasone, and placebo for moderately severe croup, *N Engl J Med* 339(8):498, 1998.
Kadaitis AG, Ward ER: Viral croup: current diagnosis and treatment, *Pediatr Infect Dis J* 17(9):827, 1998.
Macdonald WBG: Management of childhood croup, *Thorax* 52:757, 1997.
Rosekrans JA: Viral croup: current diagnosis and treatment, *Mayo Clin Proc* 73:1102, 1998.
Author: **Dennis Mikolich, M.D.**

BASIC INFORMATION

■ **DEFINITION**

Lead poisoning refers to multisystem abnormalities resulting from excessive lead exposure.

■ **SYNONYMS**

Plumbism

ICD-9CM CODES
984.0 Lead poisoning

■ **EPIDEMIOLOGY & DEMOGRAPHICS**

- Lead poisoning is most common in children ages 1 to 5 yr (17,000 cases/100,000 persons). The highest rates are among blacks, those with low income, and urban children.
- In 1991 the Centers for Disease Control and Prevention lowered the definition of a safe blood lead level to <10 μg/dl of whole blood (a blood lead level of 25 μg/dl was considered acceptable before 1991).
- It is estimated that >15% of preschoolers in the U.S. have a blood lead level >15 μg/dl.

■ **PHYSICAL FINDINGS & CLINICAL PRESENTATION**

- Findings vary with the degree of toxicity. Examination may be normal in patients with mild toxicity.
- Myalgias, irritability, headache, and general fatigue may be present initially.
- Abdominal cramping, constipation, weight loss, tremor, paresthesias and peripheral neuritis, seizures, and coma may occur with severe toxicity.
- Motor neuropathy is common in children with lead poisoning; learning disorders are also frequent.

■ **ETIOLOGY**

Chronic repeated exposure to paint containing lead, plumbing, storage of batteries, pottery, lead soldering

DIAGNOSIS

■ **DIFFERENTIAL DIAGNOSIS**

- Polyneuropathies from other sources
- Anxiety disorder, attention deficit disorder
- Malabsorption, acute abdomen
- Iron deficiency anemia

■ **WORKUP**

Laboratory screening: all U.S. children should be considered to be at risk for lead poisoning and should be screened routinely starting at 1 yr of age for low-risk children and 6 mo of age for high-risk ones.

■ **LABORATORY TESTS**

- Venous blood lead level: normal level: <10 μg/dl; levels of 50 to 70 μg/dl: indicative of moderate toxicity; levels >70 μg/dl: associated with severe poisoning
- Mild anemia with basophilic stippling on peripheral smear
- Elevated zinc protoporphyrin levels or free erythrocyte protoporphyrin level
- An increased body burden of lead with previous high-level exposure in patients with occupational lead poisoning can be demonstrated by measuring the excretion of lead in urine after premedication with calcium EDTA or another chelating agent

■ **IMAGING STUDIES**

- Imaging studies are generally not necessary.
- A plain abdominal film can visualize lead particles in the gut.
- "Lead lines" may be noted on x-rays of long bones.

TREATMENT

■ **NONPHARMACOLOGIC THERAPY**

- Provide adequate amounts of calcium, iron, zinc, and protein in patient's diet.
- Family education on sources of lead exposure and potential adverse health effects

■ **ACUTE GENERAL Rx**

- For children with blood levels of 10 to 19 μg/dl the CDC recommends nonpharmacologic interventions (see above).
- For children with blood levels between 20-44 μg/dl the CDC recommendations include case management by a qualified social worker, clinical management, environmental assessment, and lead hazard control. Chelation therapy should be considered in children with refractory blood lead levels.

Chelation therapy is indicated in children with blood lead levels ≥45 μg/dl:
  a. Succimer (DMSA) 10 mg/kg PO q8h for 5 days then q12h for 2 wk can be used in patients with levels between 45 and 70 μg/dl.
  b. Edetate calcium disodium (EDTA) and dimercaprol (BAL) are effective in patients with severe toxicity.
  c. Use of both EDTA and DMSA is indicated in children with blood levels >70 μg/dl
  d. D-Penicillamine (Cuprimine) can also be used for lead poisoning, but it is not FDA approved for this condition.

■ **CHRONIC Rx**

- Reduce exposure, remove any potential lead sources.
- Correct iron deficiency and any other nutritional deficiencies.
- Recheck blood lead level 7 to 21 days after chelation therapy.

■ **DISPOSITION**

Patients with mild to moderate toxicity generally improve without any residual deficits. The presence of encephalopathy at diagnosis is a poor prognostic sign. Residual neurologic deficits may persist in these patients. Chelation therapy seems to slow the progression of renal insufficiency in patients with mildly elevated body lead burden.

■ **REFERRAL**

If exposure to lead is work related, it should be reported to the Office of the United States Occupational Safety and Health Administration (OSHA).

PEARLS & CONSIDERATIONS

■ **COMMENTS**

- Provide patient education regarding ways to prevent or decrease the risk of exposure.
- Screening of household members of affected individuals is recommended.
- In children with blood lead levels ≤45 mg/dl, treatment with succimer does not improve scores on tests of cognition, behavior, or neuropsychological function.

REFERENCES

Ellis MR, Kane KY: Lightening the lead load in children, *Am Fam Physician* 62:545, 2000.

Matte TD: Reducing blood lead levels, *JAMA* 281:2340, 1999.

Rogan WJ et al: The effect of chelation therapy with succimer of neuropsychological development in children exposed to lead, *N Engl J Med* 344:1421, 2001.

Staudinger KC, Roth VS: Occupational lead poisoning, *Am Fam Physician* 57:719, 1998.

Tong S et al: Declining blood lead levels and changes in cognitive function during childhood, *JAMA* 280:1915, 1998.

Author: **Fred F. Ferri, M.D.**

BASIC INFORMATION

■ DEFINITION
Legg-Calvé-Perthes disease is a self-limited disorder of unknown etiology caused by ischemia of the immature femoral head that leads to bone necrosis and variable amounts of collapse during the reparative process.

■ SYNONYMS
Coxa plana
Capital femoral osteochondrosis

ICD-9CM CODES
732.1 Perthes' disease

■ EPIDEMIOLOGY & DEMOGRAPHICS
PREVALENCE: 1 case/1300 children
PREDOMINANT SEX: Male:female ratio of 4:1
PREDOMINANT AGE: 3 to 10 yr

■ PHYSICAL FINDINGS & CLINICAL PRESENTATION
- Initial complaint: usually a mildly painful limp
- Pain referred down the inner aspect of the thigh to the knee
- Moderate restriction of motion resulting from hip synovitis (abduction and internal rotation are especially limited)
- Pain at the extremes of movement and tenderness over anterior hip joint

■ ETIOLOGY
Unknown

DIAGNOSIS

■ DIFFERENTIAL DIAGNOSIS
- Toxic synovitis
- Low-grade septic arthritis
- JRA

■ WORKUP
Diagnosis is usually based on the physical findings and eventual radiographic findings.

■ IMAGING STUDIES
- Plain roentgenography to establish the diagnosis (Fig. 1-226)
- AP and frog-leg lateral radiographs
- Technetium bone scanning to assist in making the diagnosis in early cases

TREATMENT

■ ACUTE GENERAL Rx
- A brief period of bed rest followed by bracing (except in mild cases)
- Bracing possibly required for 2 to 3 yr

■ DISPOSITION
- Prognosis depends on age of patient and degree of involvement of the femoral head at onset.
- Young patients (under 6 yr) with minimal involvement do well.
- Older patients (over 8 yr) often do poorly.
- A few patients eventually develop degenerative arthritis.

■ REFERRAL
For orthopedic consultation when diagnosis is suspected

PEARLS & CONSIDERATIONS

■ COMMENTS
- There is great uncertainty regarding treatment and its effect on outcome. It may be that bracing has no effect whatsoever on the end result.

REFERENCES
Adkins SB, Figler RA: Hip pain in athletes, *Am Fam Physician* 61:2109, 2000.
Guerado E, Garces G: Perthes disease, *J Bone Joint Surg* 83(B):569, 2001.
Joseph B, Mulpari K, Varghese G: Perthes disease in the adolescent, *J Bone Joint Surg* 83(B):715, 2001.
Stevens DB, Tao SS, Glueck CJ: Recurrent Legg-Calvé-Perthes disease: case report and long term follow up, *Clin Orthop* 385:124, 2001.
Author: **Lonnie R. Mercier, M.D.**

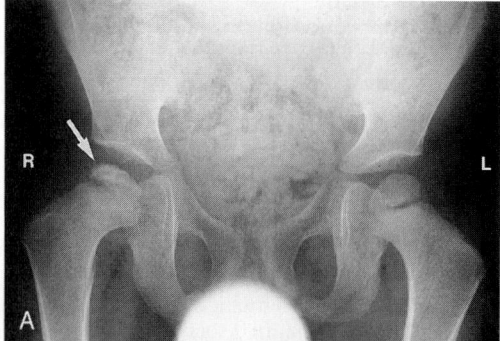
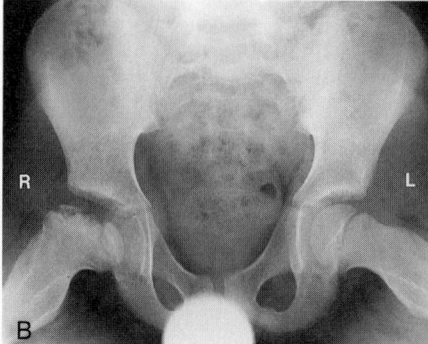
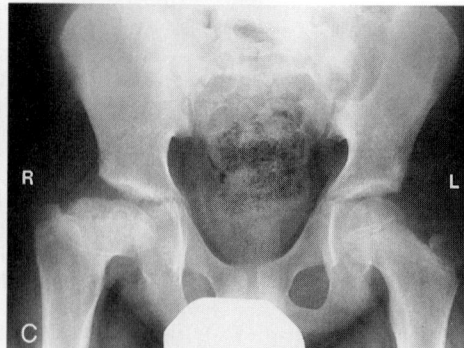

Fig. 1-226 Legg-Calvé-Perthes disease. **A,** An anteroposterior view of the pelvis demonstrates fragmentation and sclerosis of the right femoral epiphysis *(arrow)* in this 6-year-old male. **B,** A follow-up film obtained 8 years later shows continuing deformity resulting from the osteonecrosis. The patient developed significant degenerative arthritis **(C)** by the age of 12 years. (From Mettler FA [ed]: *Primary care radiology,* Philadelphia, 2000, WB Saunders.)

BASIC INFORMATION

■ DEFINITION
Leprosy is a chronic granulomatous infection of humans that primarily affects the skin and peripheral nerves.

■ SYNONYMS
Hansen's disease

ICD-9CM CODES
030.9 Leprosy

■ EPIDEMIOLOGY & DEMOGRAPHICS
- The number of cases worldwide has fallen from more than 5 million cases in 1985 to less than 1 million cases in 1998.
- Nearly 75% of the cases of leprosy are found in India, Brazil, Bangladesh, Indonesia, and Myanmar.
- More than 85% of the cases diagnosed in the United States are found among immigrants.
- Worldwide incidence is 650,000 new cases per year.
- Annual incidence in the U.S. is 150 new cases per year.
- Leprosy is more common in men than women (2:1).
- Can occur at any age but usually is found in young children.

■ PHYSICAL FINDINGS & CLINICAL PRESENTATION
- A skin lesion: most common initial presentation
- Sensory loss
- Anhidrosis
- Neuritic pain
- Palpable peripheral nerves
- Nerve damage (most commonly affected nerves are ulnar, median, common peroneal, posterior tibial, radial cutaneous nerve of the wrist, facial, and posterior auricular)
- Muscle atrophy and weakness
- Foot drop
- Claw hand and claw toes
- Lagophthalmos, nasal septal perforation, collapse of bridge of nose (Fig. 1-227, *A*), loss of eyebrows resulting in "leonine" facies

Leprosy can present along a spectrum from simple cutaneous skin lesions with minimal sensory loss (Fig. 1-227, *B*) to severe extensive skin involvement, painful neuritis, muscle wasting and contractures, and multiple peripheral nerve damage.

■ ETIOLOGY
- Leprosy is caused by *Mycobacterium leprae,* an obligate intracellular acid-fast rod.
- The mode of transmission remains elusive. Spread in humans is thought to occur via the respiratory route or entry through broken skin.
- Zoonotic transmission from armadillos has not been proven.
- The majority of people exposed to patients with leprosy do not develop the disease because of their natural immunity.
- Incubation period is 3 to 5 yr.

DIAGNOSIS

- The diagnosis of leprosy relies on a detailed history and physical examination and is established by the demonstration of acid-fast bacilli in skin smears or skin biopsies of the affected sites.
- Leprosy has been classified according to the WHO system into:
  1. Paucibacillary leprosy defined as fewer than five skin lesions with no bacilli on skin smear.
  2. Multibacillary leprosy defined as six or more skin lesions and may be skin-smear positive.
- Leprosy has also been classified more specifically according to the type of skin lesions, sensory and motor deficits, and biopsy into:
  1. Indeterminate leprosy
  2. Tuberculoid leprosy
  3. Borderline tuberculoid leprosy
  4. Borderline lepromatous leprosy
  5. Lepromatous leprosy

■ DIFFERENTIAL DIAGNOSIS
The differential diagnosis of leprosy includes: sarcoidosis, rheumatoid arthritis, systemic lupus erythematosus, lymphomatoid granulomatosis, carpal tunnel syndrome, cutaneous leishmaniasis, fungal infections and other causes of hypopigmented, hyperpigmented, and erythematous skin lesions.

■ WORKUP
Any patient who presents with skin lesions and a sensory or muscle deficit should have a workup for leprosy.

■ LABORATORY TESTS
- *Mycobacterium leprae* cannot be cultured on artificial media. The bacteria rapidly proliferate when injected into the footpads of mice or into armadillos and sometimes is used for drug-sensitivity testing.
- Serologic tests, including the antibody to phenolic glycolipid 1 (PGL-1), are available and used for diagnostic confirmation and research epidemiologic studies.
- Lepromin intradermal skin test is not diagnostic and not for commercial use.
- Skin smears are taken from active sites or most commonly from the earlobe, elbows, or knees and are stained for acid-fast bacilli.
- Skin biopsies of active sites are stained for acid-fast bacilli.
- Peripheral nerve biopsy can be done in patients with sensory loss and no skin lesions. Common nerves biopsied are the radial cutaneous nerve of the wrist and the sural nerve of the ankle.

■ IMAGING STUDIES
X-ray studies are usually of no benefit in the diagnosis or treatment of leprosy.

TREATMENT

■ NONPHARMACOLOGIC THERAPY
- Physical therapy for patients with upper and lower extremity deformities.
- Proper foot care and footwear to prevent ulcer formation.

■ ACUTE GENERAL Rx
For paucibacillary leprosy:
- Dapsone 100 mg PO qd for 6 mo in an unsupervised setting is the treatment of choice.
- Rifampin 600 mg PO qd for 6 mo in a supervised setting is the recommendation by WHO.
- Ofloxacin 400 mg qd or minocycline 100 mg qd are other alternatives.
For multibacillary leprosy:
- Rifampin 600 mg PO qd and clofazimine 300 mg PO qd for 24 mo in a supervised setting.
- Rifampin 100 mg PO qd and clofazimine 50 mg PO qd for 24 mo in an unsupervised setting.
- Dapsone 100 mg PO qd is sometimes added as triple therapy in this group of patients.

■ CHRONIC Rx
- If relapse occurs, the patient is treated with the same medical regimen because resistance is low.
- If relapse is from paucibacillary to multibacillary, the medical regimen for multibacillary should be used for therapy.

■ DISPOSITION

- Relapse is <1% for multibacillary and just over 1% in paucibacillary cases.
- Patients are initially followed up monthly and when treatment is completed every 3 to 6 mo for the next 5 to 10 yr.
- Some patients develop reactions known as erythema nodosum leprosum and reversal reaction, usually during treatment.
  1. Erythema nodosum leprosum results in tender nodules and is treated with either prednisolone 40 to 60 mg qd until the reaction is controlled and tapered or thalidomide 300 to 400 mg qd and tapered to 100 mg qd with monthly attempts to wean down further.
  2. Reactive reaction results in the development of new skin lesions with swelling and erythema of existing lesions. Treatment is with either NSAIDs or prednisolone.

REFERRAL

Any suspected case of leprosy merits an infectious disease consultation. Consultation with orthopedic, podiatry, ophthalmology, physical therapy, plastic surgery, and psychology are all in order for any of the potential sequelae of the disease.

〇 PEARLS & CONSIDERATIONS

■ COMMENTS

- The risk of transmission is low in patients with leprosy, and therefore no infection control precautions of patients hospitalized is needed.
- Family members and close contacts need to be examined frequently for the development lesions.
- Dapsone or rifampin prophylaxis is not recommended in the prevention of leprosy.
- BCG vaccination has a 50% protective effect in the prevention of leprosy and may be considered.

REFERENCES

Cambau E et al: Multidrug-resistance to dapsone, rifampicin, and ofloxacin in *Mycobacterium leprae*, *Lancet* 349:103,1997.
Jacobsen RR, Krahenbuhl JL: Leprosy, *Lancet* 353:655, 1999.
Author: **Peter Petropoulos, M.D.**

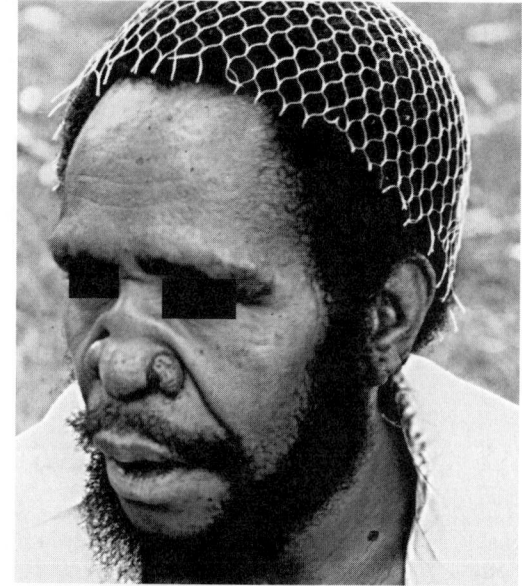

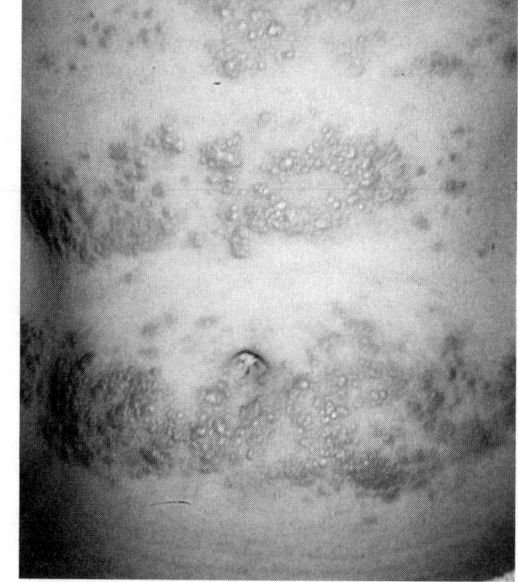

Fig. 1-227   A, Advanced lepromatous leprosy with collapse of the nasal septum. **B,** Lepromatous leprosy characterized by extensive papule formation over abdomen. Minimal or no sensory loss is present in the affected areas. (**A** From Gorbach SL: *Infectious diseases,* ed 2, Philadelphia, 1998, WB Saunders; **B** from Mandell GL: *Mandell, Douglas, and Bennett's principles and practice of infectious diseases,* ed 5, New York, 2000, Churchill Livingstone.)

BASIC INFORMATION

■ DEFINITION
Leptospirosis is a zoonosis caused by the spirochete *Leptospira interrogans*.

■ SYNONYMS
Weil's disease

ICD-9CM CODES
100.9 Leptospirosis

■ EPIDEMIOLOGY & DEMOGRAPHICS
INCIDENCE (IN U.S.):
- 0.05 cases/100,000 persons
- Significant underestimation because of underreporting

PREDOMINANT SEX: Male (4:1)
PREDOMINANT AGE: Teenagers and young adults
PEAK INCIDENCE: Summer months, into the fall
GENETICS:
Neonatal Infection: Can occur

■ PHYSICAL FINDINGS & CLINICAL PRESENTATION
ANICTERIC FORM:
- Milder and more common presentation of disease
- A self-limited systemic illness with two stages:
  1. Septicemic stage: presents abruptly with fevers, headache, severe myalgias, rigors, prostration, and sometimes circulatory collapse; conjunctival suffusion is common; skin rash, pharyngitis, lymphadenopathy, hepatomegaly, splenomegaly, or muscle tenderness is possible; lasts about 1 wk with complete resolution usual.
  2. Immune stage: occurs a few days after first stage with similar symptoms; hallmark is aseptic meningitis.

ICTERIC LEPTOSPIROSIS (WEIL'S SYNDROME):
  1. Denotes severe cases, with symptoms of hepatic, renal, and vascular dysfunction
  2. Biphasic course: persistence of fever, jaundice, and azotemia
  3. Complications: oliguria or anuria, hemorrhage, hypotension, vascular collapse

■ ETIOLOGY
Caused by a spirochete, *L. interrogans*
- Infects a variety of animals, including most mammals
- Specific serotypes associated with different hosts—*pomona* in livestock, *canicola* in dogs (Fig. 1-228), and *icterohaemorrhagiae* in rodents
- Exposure to animal urine or infected water method by which organism penetrates skin or mucous membranes; recently described cases in inner-city residents are related to exposure to rat urine

DIAGNOSIS

■ DIFFERENTIAL DIAGNOSIS
- Bacterial meningitis
- Viral hepatitis
- Influenza
- Legionnaire's disease

■ WORKUP
Culture of blood, CSF, and urine:
- Organism can be isolated from blood or CSF during first 10 days of illness.
- Urine should be cultured after first week and for up to 30 days after onset of illness.

■ LABORATORY TESTS
- Normal or elevated WBCs, at times up to 70,000/mm^3
- Elevated transaminases or bilirubin
- Anemia, azotemia, hypoprothrombinemia in those with icteric illness
- Elevated CK in first phase
- Meningitis in both phases, but aseptic in second phase

■ IMAGING STUDIES
Chest radiographs to show bilateral nonlobar infiltrates

TREATMENT

■ NONPHARMACOLOGIC THERAPY
- Supportive
- Observation for dehydration, hypotension, renal failure, hemorrhage

■ ACUTE GENERAL Rx
- IV penicillin G 1 million U q4h
- Doxycycline 100 mg PO bid for 7 days
- Vitamin K administration if hypoprothrombinemia present
- Possible Jarisch-Herxheimer reaction when treated with penicillin

■ DISPOSITION
- Anicteric leptospirosis is self-limited, but administration of antibiotics can decrease severity and duration of symptoms.
- Icteric leptospirosis, even with supportive therapy, has a mortality as high as 10%.

■ REFERRAL
- If more than mild disease
- If no response to treatment

PEARLS & CONSIDERATIONS

■ COMMENTS
Significantly underreported illness

REFERENCE
Centers for Disease Control and Prevention: Outbreak of acute febrile illness among athletes participating in triathlons—Wisconsin and Illinois, 1998, *MMWR* 280(17):1474, 1998.
Author: **Maurice Policar, M.D.**

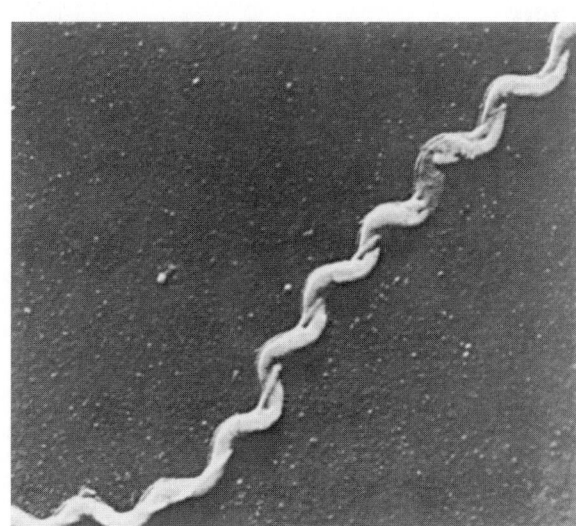

Fig. 1-228 Electron micrograph of *Leptospira interrogans* (serovar *canicola*) showing the tightly coiled helicoid rod with the periplasmic axial filament. (Courtesy Armed Forces Institute of Pathology, AFIP No. 60-10941. In Gorbach SL: *Infectious diseases,* ed 2, Philadelphia, 1998, WB Saunders.)

BASIC INFORMATION

■ DEFINITION
Acute lymphoblastic leukemia (ALL) is characterized by uncontrolled proliferation of abnormal, immature lymphocytes and their progenitors, ultimately replacing normal bone marrow elements.

■ SYNONYMS
Lymphoid leukemia
ALL

ICD-9CM CODES
204.0 Acute lymphoblastic leukemia

■ EPIDEMIOLOGY & DEMOGRAPHICS
- ALL is primarily a disease of children (peak incidence at ages 2 to 10 yr).
- It is diagnosed in 3000 to 4000 persons in the U.S. each year; two thirds are children.

■ PHYSICAL FINDINGS & CLINICAL PRESENTATION
- Skin pallor, purpura, or easy bruising
- Lymphadenopathy or hepatosplenomegaly
- Fever, bone pain, oliguria, weakness, weight loss, mental status changes

■ ETIOLOGY
- Unknown; increased risk in patients with a previous use of antineoplastic agents (e.g., chemotherapy of NHL, Hodgkin's disease, ovarian cancer, myeloma)
- Environmental factors (e.g., ionizing radiation), toxins (e.g., benzene)

DIAGNOSIS

■ DIFFERENTIAL DIAGNOSIS
Acute myeloid leukemia (AML): the distinction between ALL and AML and the classification of the various subtypes are based on the following factors:
- Cell morphology
  1. Lymphoblasts: a high nucleus/cytoplasmic ratio; usually, cytoplasmic granules are not present.
  2. Myeloblasts: abundant cytoplasm; often, cytoplasmic granules (Auer rods) are present.
- Histochemical stains
  1. Peroxidase and Sudan black stains: negative in ALL; useful to distinguish nonlymphoid from lymphoid cells
  2. Chloroacetate esterase: a pink cytoplasmic reaction identifies granulocytes; useful to distinguish granulocytes from monocytes in patients with AML

Lymphoblastic lymphoma
Aplastic anemia
Infectious mononucleosis
Leukemoid reaction to infection
Multiple myeloma

■ WORKUP
- Laboratory evaluation
- Bone marrow examination (with biopsy, cytochemistry, immunophenotyping, and cytogenetics)
- Lumbar puncture and imaging studies

■ LABORATORY TESTS
- CBC reveals normochromic, normocytic anemia, thrombocytopenia.
- Peripheral smear will reveal lymphoblasts.
- Initial blood work should also include BUN, creatinine, serum electrolytes, uric acid, LDH.
- Special diagnostic tests include immunophenotyping, cytogenetics, and cytochemistry.
- The French, American, British (FAB) Cooperative Study Group has classified ALL into three groups (L1-L3) based on cell size, cytoplasmic appearance, nucleus shape, and chromatin pattern; the most common form is the L2 type.
- Immunologic classification is on the basis of expression of surface antigens by blast cells: T lineage and B lineage.

■ IMAGING STUDIES
- Chest radiograph to evaluate for the presence of mediastinal mass
- CT scan or ultrasound of abdomen to assess splenomegaly or leukemic infiltration of abdominal organs

TREATMENT

■ ACUTE GENERAL Rx
- Emergency treatment is indicated in patients with intracerebral leukostasis. It consists of one or more of the following:
  1. Cranial irradiation of the whole brain in one- or two-dose fractions
  2. Leukapheresis
  3. Oral hydroxyurea (requires 48 to 72 hr to significantly lower the circulating blast count)
- Urate nephropathy can be prevented by vigorous hydration and lowering uric acid level with allopurinol and urine alkalization with acetazolamide.
- Infections must be aggressively treated with broad-spectrum antibiotics.
  1. Any febrile or neutropenic patients must have cultures taken

and be properly treated with IV antibiotics.
  2. If evidence of infection persists despite adequate treatment with antibiotics, amphotericin B may be added to provide coverage against fungal infections (Candida, Aspergillus).
- Correct significant thrombocytopenia (platelet counts <20,000/mm^3) with platelet transfusion.
- Bleeding secondary to DIC is treated with heparin and replacement of clotting factors.
- Induction therapy is intensive chemotherapy to destroy a significant number of leukemic cells and achieve remission; it usually consists of a combination of vincristine (Oncovin), prednisone, and L-asparaginase (ELSPAR) in children or an anthracine in adults.
- Consolidation therapy consists of an aggressive course of chemotherapy with or without radiotherapy shortly after complete remission has been obtained. Its purpose is to prolong the remission period or cure. Commonly used agents are VM-26, VP-16, HiDAC.
- Meningeal prophylactic therapy with intrathecal methotrexate with or without cranial irradiation is indicated to prevent meningeal sequestration of leukemic cells.
- The goal of maintenance therapy is to maintain a state of remission. In patients wtih ALL, intermittent therapy is continued for at least 3 yr with a combination of methotrexate and 6-mercaptopurine (Purinethol).
- Bone marrow transplantation: patients should receive allograft in the first complete remission if they are between ages 20 and 50 yr and have matched a sibling donor.

■ DISPOSITION
- Prognosis is generally poorer in adult disease compared with childhood disease (40% adult cure rate versus 80% cure rate in children).
- Five-year leukemia-free survival is <40%.
- The presence of Philadelphia chromosome (Ph$^+$), monosomy 5 and 7, and abnormalities of 11q23 are bad prognostic signs.

REFERENCE
Ching-Hon P, Evans W: Acute lymphocytic leukemia, *N Engl J Med* 339:605, 1998.
Author: **Fred F. Ferri, M.D.**

BASIC INFORMATION

■ DEFINITION

Acute myelogenous leukemia (AML) is a disorder characterized by uncontrolled proliferation of primitive myeloid cells (blasts), ultimately replacing normal bone marrow elements frequently resulting in hematopoietic insufficiency (granulocytopenia, thrombocytopenia, or anemia) with or without leukocytosis.

■ SYNONYMS

Acute nonlymphoblastic leukemia (ANLL)
Acute nonlymphocytic leukemia
Acute myeloid leukemia (AML)

ICD-9CM CODES
205.0 Acute myelogenous leukemia

■ EPIDEMIOLOGY & DEMOGRAPHICS

AML usually affects adults (most patients are 30 to 60 yr old; median age at presentation is 50 yr).
• Annual incidence is 2 to 4/100,000

■ PHYSICAL FINDINGS & CLINICAL PRESENTATION

Patients generally come to medical attention because of the effects of the cytopenias:
• Anemia manifests with weakness or fatigue.
• Thrombocytopenia can manifest with bleeding, petechiae, and ecchymosis.
• Neutropenia can result in infections and fever.
• Physical examination may reveal skin pallor, bruises, petechiae; abdominal examination may reveal hepatosplenomegaly; peripheral lymphadenopathy may also be present.
• Hyperleukocytosis can lead to symptoms of leukostasis, such as ocular and cerebrovascular dysfunction or bleeding.

■ ETIOLOGY

Risk factors are previous use of antineoplastic agents, chromosomal abnormalities, ionizing radiation, toxins, immunodeficiency states, and chronic myeloproliferative disorders.

DIAGNOSIS

■ DIFFERENTIAL DIAGNOSIS
• Acute lymphocytic leukemia
• Leukemoid reaction
• Myelodysplastic syndrome
• Infiltrative diseases of the bone marrow
• Epstein-Barr, other viral infection

■ LABORATORY TESTS

• CBC reveals anemia, thrombocytopenia. Peripheral WBC count varies from <5000/mm^3 to >100,000/mm^3.
• Additional laboratory findings may include elevated LDH and uric acid levels, decreased fibrinogen, and increased FDP secondary to DIC.
• Cytogenetic abnormalities are common (chromosome 8 is most frequently involved in AML).
• The distinction between ALL and AML and the classification of the various subtypes are based on the following factors:
  1. Cell morphology: myeloblasts reveal abundant cytoplasm; cytoplasmic granules are often present (Auer rods).
  2. Histochemical stains:
     a. Peroxidase and Sudan black stains are negative in ALL.
     b. Chloroacetate esterase: a pink cytoplasmic reaction identifies granulocytes; useful to distinguish granulocytes from monocytes in patients with AML.
• AML is diagnosed by the presence of at least 30% blast cells and positive peroxidase or Sudan black histochemical stain in the bone marrow aspirate.
• The French, American, British (FAB) Cooperative Study Group has classified AML into seven categories (M1-M7) based on the type and percentage of immature cells.

■ IMAGING STUDIES

• Chest x-ray examination is useful to evaluate for the presence of mediastinal masses.
• CT scan of the abdomen may reveal hepatosplenomegaly or leukemic involvement of other organs.

TREATMENT

■ ACUTE GENERAL Rx

• Emergency treatment consisting of one or more of the following is indicated in patients with intracerebral leukostasis:
  1. Cranial irradiation
  2. Leukapheresis
  3. Oral hydroxyurea
• Urate nephropathy can be prevented by vigorous hydration and lowering uric acid level with allopurinol and urine alkalinization with acetazolamide.
• Infections must be aggressively treated with broad-spectrum antibiotics.
• Correct significant thrombocytopenia with platelet transfusions.
• Bleeding secondary to DIC is treated with heparin and replacement of clotting factors.
• Intensive induction chemotherapy to destroy a significant number of

leukemic cells and achieve remission usually consists of cytarabine (Cytosar) and daunorubicin. All-trans-retinoic acid is effective for the induction of remission of AML M3 subtype (acute promyelocytic leukemia).
• High-dose cytarabine (ARA-C) (HiDAC) can be used in patients with refractory or relapsed AML. It usually takes 28 to 32 days from the start of therapy to achieve remission. The duration of remission is variable; the median duration of remission in an adult with AML is 1 yr.
• Consolidation therapy consists of an aggressive course of chemotherapy with or without radiation shortly after complete remission has been obtained; its purpose is to prolong the remission period or cure. Complications of consolidation therapy are usually secondary to severe bone marrow suppression (anemia, thrombocytopenia, granulocytopenia).
• Goal of therapy is to maintain a state of remission. A postinduction course of high-dose cytarabine can provide equivalent disease-free survival and somewhat better overall survival than autologous marrow transplantation in adults.
• Autologous bone marrow transplantation is indicated in patients <55 yr without a sibling donor. Allogeneic bone marrow transplantation is generally available to <20% of patients; usually performed only in patients <40 yr old because of higher incidence of GVHD with advancing age.

■ DISPOSITION

• Remission can be achieved in nearly 80% of patients <55 yr of age. Remission rates are highest in children.
• Cure for allogeneic bone marrow transplantation approaches 60%; cure rates with autologous transplantation are slightly lower.
• Favorable cytogenics are inv (16) (p13;q22) and t(8;21), t(15;17).

PEARLS & CONSIDERATIONS

■ COMMENTS

• The major complication of chemotherapy is profound marrow depression with pancytopenia lasting 3 to 4 wk. Treatment is aimed at RBC and platelet replacement and aggressive monitoring and treatment of suspected infections.
• Low doses of arsenic trioxide can induce complete remissions in patients with acute promyelocytic leukemia.

REFERENCE

Lowenberg B et al: Acute myeloid leukemia, *N Engl J Med* 341:1051, 1999.
Author: **Fred F. Ferri, M.D.**

BASIC INFORMATION

■ DEFINITION
Chronic lymphocytic leukemia (CLL) is a lymphoproliferative disorder characterized by proliferation and accumulation of mature-appearing neoplastic lymphocytes.

■ SYNONYMS
CLL

ICD-9CM CODES
204.1 Leukemia, chronic lymphocytic

■ EPIDEMIOLOGY & DEMOGRAPHICS
- Most frequent form of leukemia in Western countries (10,000 new cases/yr in the U.S.)
- Generally occurs in middle-aged and elderly patients (median age of 65 yr)
- Male:female ratio of 2:1

■ PHYSICAL FINDINGS & CLINICAL PRESENTATION
- Lymphadenopathy, splenomegaly, and hepatomegaly in the majority of patients
- Variable clinical presentation according to stage of the disease
- Abnormal CBC: many cases are diagnosed on the basis of laboratory results obtained after routine physical examination
- Some patients come to medical attention because of weakness and fatigue (secondary to anemia) or lymphadenopathy

■ ETIOLOGY
Unknown

DIAGNOSIS

■ DIFFERENTIAL DIAGNOSIS
- Hairy cell leukemia
- Adult T cell lymphoma
- Prolymphocytic leukemia
- Viral infections
- Waldenström's macroglobulinemia

■ WORKUP
- Laboratory evaluation
- Bone marrow aspirate
- Chromosome analysis

■ LABORATORY TESTS
- Proliferative lymphocytosis (≥15,000/dl) of well-differentiated lymphocytes is the hallmark of CLL.
- There is monotonous replacement of the bone marrow by small lymphocytes (marrow contains ≥30% of well-differentiated lymphocytes).

- Hypogammaglobulinemia and elevated LDH may be present at the time of diagnosis.
- Anemia or thrombocytopenia, if present, indicates poor prognosis.
- Trisomy-12 is the most common chromosomal abnormality, followed by 14 q+, 13 q, and 11 q; these all indicate a poor prognosis.

STAGING
- Rai et al divided CLL into five clinical stages:
  Stage 0—Characterized by lymphocytosis only (≥15,000/mm^3 on peripheral smear, bone marrow aspirate ≥40% lymphocytes). The coexistence of lymphocytosis and other factors increases the clinical stage.
  Stage 1—Lymphadenopathy
  Stage 2—Lymphadenopathy/hepatomegaly
  Stage 3—Anemia (Hgb <11 g/mm^3)
  Stage 4—Thrombocytopenia (platelets <100,000/mm^3)
- Another well-known staging system developed by Binet divides chronic lymphocytic leukemia into three stages:
  Stage A—Hgb ≥10 g/dl, platelets ≥100,000/mm^3, and fewer than three areas involved (the cervical, axillary, and inguinal lymph nodes [whether unilaterally or bilaterally]; the spleen; and the liver)
  Stage B—Hgb ≥10 g/dl, platelets ≥100,000/mm^3, and three or more areas involved
  Stage C—Hgb <10 g/dl, low platelets (<100,000/mm^3), or both (independent of the areas involved)

■ IMAGING STUDIES
CT scan of abdomen to evaluate for hepatomegaly and splenomegaly

TREATMENT

■ NONPHARMACOLOGIC THERAPY
- Treatment goals are relief of symptoms and prolongation of life.
- Observation is appropriate for patients in Rai Stage 0 or Binet Stage A.

■ ACUTE GENERAL Rx
- Symptomatic patients in Rai Stage I and II or Binet Stage B: chlorambucil; local irradiation for isolated symptomatic lymphadenopathy and lymph nodes that interfere with vital organs
- Fludarabine is an effective treatment for CLL that does not respond to initial treatment with chlorambucil. Recent reports indicate that when used as the initial treatment for CLL, fludarabine yields higher response

rates and a longer duration of remission and progression-free survival than chlorambucil; overall survival, however, is not enhanced.
- Rai Stages III and IV, Binet Stage C: chlorambucil chemotherapy with or without prednisone
  1. Fludarabine, CAP (cyclophosphamide, Adriamycin, prednisone), or cyclophosphamide, doxorubicin, vincristine, and prednisone (mini-CHOP) can be used in patients who respond poorly to chlorambucil.
  2. Splenic irradiation can be used in selected patients with advanced disease.

■ CHRONIC Rx
Treatment of systemic complications:
- Hypogammaglobulinemia is frequent in CLL and is the chief cause of infections. Immune globulin (250 mg/kg IV every 4 wk) may prevent infections but has no effect on survival. Infections should be treated with broad-spectrum antibiotics. Patients should be monitored for opportunistic infections.
- Recombinant hematopoietic cofactors (e.g., granulocyte-macrophage colony–stimulating factor and granulocyte colony–stimulating factor) may be useful to overcome neutropenia related to treatment.
- Erythropoietin may be useful to treat anemia that is unresponsive to other measures.

■ DISPOSITION
The patient's prognosis is directly related to the clinical stage (e.g., the average survival in patients in Rai Stage 0 or Binet Stage A is >120 mo, whereas for RAI Stage 4 or Binet Stage C it is approximaely 30 mo). Overall 5-yr survival is 60%.

PEARLS & CONSIDERATIONS

■ COMMENTS
Long-term follow-up and frequency of follow-up are generally determined by the pace of the disease.

REFERENCES
Dighiero G et al: Chlorambucil in indolent chronic lymphocytic leukemia, *N Engl J Med* 338:1506, 1998.
Rai KR et al: Fludarabine compared with chlorambucil as primary therapy for CLL, *N Engl J Med* 343:1750, 2000.
Author: **Fred F. Ferri, M.D.**

BASIC INFORMATION

DEFINITION
Chronic myelogenous leukemia (CML) is a malignant clonal disorder of hemopoietic stem cells characterized by abnormal proliferation and accumulation of immature granulocytes. CML is characterized by a chronic phase lasting months to years, followed by an accelerated myeloproliferative phase manifested by poor response to therapy, worsening anemia, or decreased platelet count; the second phase then evolves into a terminal phase (acute transformation), characterized by elevated number of blast cells and numerous complications (e.g., sepsis, bleeding).

SYNONYMS
CML
Chronic granulocytic leukemia
Chronic myeloid leukemia

ICD-9CM CODES
201.1 Chronic myelogenous leukemia

EPIDEMIOLOGY & DEMOGRAPHICS
- CML usually affects middle-aged patients (median age at presentation is 53 yr) and accounts for 15% of adult leukemias
- 4300 new cases/yr in the U.S.

PHYSICAL FINDINGS & CLINICAL PRESENTATION
- The chronic phase usually reveals splenomegaly; hepatomegaly is not infrequent, but lymphadenopathy is very unusual and generally indicates the accelerated proliferative phase of the disease.
- Common complaints at the time of diagnosis are weakness or discomfort secondary to an enlarged spleen (abdominal discomfort or pain). Splenomegaly is present in up to 40% of patients at time of diagnosis.
- Forty percent of patients are asymptomatic and diagnosis is based solely on an abnormal blood count.

ETIOLOGY
Current evidence strongly implicates the chromosome translocation t (9;22) (q34;q11.2) as the cause of chronic granulocytic leukemia. This translocation is present in >95% of patients. The remaining patients have a complex or variant translocation involving additional chromosomes that have the same end result (fusion of the BCR [break point cluster region] gene on chromosome 22 to ABL [Ableson leukemia virus] gene on chromosome 9).

 DIAGNOSIS

DIFFERENTIAL DIAGNOSIS
- Splenic lymphoma
- CLL
- Myelodysplastic syndrome

LABORATORY TESTS
- Elevated WBC count (generally >100,000/mm^3) with broad spectrum of granulocytic forms.
- Bone marrow demonstrates hypercellularity with granulocytic hyperplasia, increased ratio of myeloid cells to erythroid cells, and increased number of megakaryocytes. Blasts and promyelocytes constitute <10% of all cells.
- Philadelphia chromosome (which results from the reciprocal translocation between the long arms of chromosomes 9 and 22) is present in >95% of patients with CML; its presence (Ph^1) is a major prognostic factor because survival rate of patients with Philadelphia chromosome is approximately eight times better than that of those without it. Some believe that Ph$^+$ defines CML and that those who are Ph$^-$ have another disease.
- Leukocyte alkaline phosphatase (LAP) markedly decreased (used to distinguish CML from other myeloproliferative disorders).
- Anemia and thrombocytosis are often present.
- Additional laboratory results are elevated vitamin B$_{12}$ levels (caused by increased transcobalamin 1 from granulocytes) and elevated blood histamine levels (because of increased basophils).

IMAGING STUDIES
Chest x-ray examination and CT scan of abdomen

 TREATMENT

ACUTE GENERAL Rx
The therapeutic approach varies with the clinical phase and the degree of hyperleukocytosis.
- Symptomatic hyperleukocytosis (e.g., CNS symptoms) is treated with leukapheresis and hydroxyurea; allopurinol should be started to prevent urate nephropathy following the rapid lysis of the leukemia cells.
- Cytotoxic chemotherapy with hydroxyurea decreases WBC count and spleen size.
- Persistence of significant thrombocytosis may require treatment with thiotepa or melphalan.
- Long-term treatment of chromosome-positive CML with interferon alfa 2A can induce more karyotypic responses, delay disease progression longer, and prolong survival in patients with Philadelphia chromosome.
- Interferon-based therapy is generally used in patients over age 50 and in others when there is no HLA-matched related donor available.
- The combination of interferon and cytarabine as compared with interferon alone increases the rate of major cytogenic response and prolongs survival in patients in the chronic phase of CML.
- Allogeneic stem-cell transplantation (SCT) (following intense chemotherapy with busulfan and cyclophosphamide or combined chemotherapy with cyclophosphamide and fractionated total body irradiation to destroy residual leukemic cells) is the only curative treatment for CML in chronic phase. Generally only 20% of patients are candidates for SCT given the limitations of age or lack of HLA-matched related donors.
  1. It should be considered in "young" patients (increased survival in patients <55 yr) with compatible siblings.
  2. Early transplantation is also important for patient's survival.
- Transplantation of marrow from an HLA-matched, unrelated donor is also now recognized as safe and effective therapy for selected patients with chronic myelogenous leukemia.
- Imatinib mesylate (STI-571, Gleevec), an oral tyrosine kinase inhibitor, has been approved by the FDA for CML myeloid blast crisis, accelerated phase, or CML in its chronic phase after failure of interferon treatment. It is very effective, producing sustained remissions in most patients with CML. Cost is approximately $2400 per mo for 400 mg PO daily dose. Dose for accelerated phase or blast crisis is 600 mg PO qd or 400 mg bid. It should be considered in all patients for whom transplantation is not an option.

REFERENCES
Gleevec (STI-571) for chronic myeloid leukemia, *Med Lett Drugs Ther* 43(1106):49, 2001.
Vialidas M et al: Chronic myelogenous leukemia, *JAMA* 286:895, 2001.
Author: **Fred F. Ferri, M.D.**

BASIC INFORMATION

■ DEFINITION

Hairy cell leukemia is a lymphoid neoplasm characterized by the proliferation of mature B cells with prominent cytoplasmic projections (hairs).

■ SYNONYMS

Leukemic reticuloendotheliosis

ICD-9CM CODES

202.4 Hairy cell leukemia

■ EPIDEMIOLOGY & DEMOGRAPHICS

PREVALENCE: Occurs predominantly in men between 40 and 60 yr of age. About 2% of leukemia cases are of the hairy cell type.
PREDOMINANT SEX: Male:female ratio of 4:1

■ PHYSICAL FINDINGS & CLINICAL PRESENTATION

- Usually, splenomegaly (present in >90% of cases) secondary to tumor cell infiltration
- Pallor, ecchymosis, and evidence of infection if the pancytopenia is severe
- Weakness, lethargy, and fatigue
- Infections (resulting from impaired resistance secondary to neutropenia) and easy bruising (secondary to thrombocytopenia) also common

■ ETIOLOGY

Neoplastic disease of the lymphoreticular system of unknown etiology

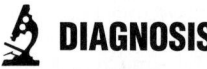

DIAGNOSIS

■ DIFFERENTIAL DIAGNOSIS

- Other forms of leukemia
- Lymphoma
- Viral syndrome

■ WORKUP

Comprehensive history, physical examination, and laboratory evaluation to confirm the diagnosis

■ LABORATORY TESTS

- Pancytopenia involving erythrocytes, neutrophils, and platelets is common; anemia is usually present and varies from minimal to severe.
- Hairy cells (Fig. 1-229) can account for 5% to 80% of cells in the peripheral blood. The cytoplasmic projections on the cells are redundant plasma membranes.
- Leukemic cells stain positively for tartrate-resistant acid phosphatase (TRAP) stain.
- Bone marrow may result in a "dry tap" (because of increased marrow reticulin).

TREATMENT

■ NONPHARMACOLOGIC THERAPY

Approximately 8% to 10% of patients are asymptomatic and have minimal splenomegaly and minor cytopenia. They are usually detected on routine laboratory evaluation and do not require initial therapy. They should, however, be frequently monitored for progression of their disease.

■ ACUTE GENERAL Rx

- Interferon alfa produces a partial remission in 30% to 70% of patients, and complete remission, often of short duration, in 5% to 10%.
- The purine analogues 2-deoxycoformycin (DCF, Pentostatin) and 2-chlorodeoxyadenosine (Cda, Cladribine) induce complete remissions in up to 85% of patients and partial responses in 5% to 25%.
- 2-Chloro-2 deoxyadenosine (CdA) 0.14 mg/kg qd for 7 days is emerging as the treatment of choice because of its minimal toxicity and its ability to induce complete durable responses with a single course of therapy.
- The anti-CD 22 recombinant immunotoxin BL 22 can induce complete remission in patients with hairy cell leukemia that is resistant to treatment with purine analogues.

■ CHRONIC Rx

Patients should be monitored with periodic examination and laboratory tests for progression of their disease.

■ DISPOSITION

Prognosis has become increasingly favorable with the newer agents. Approximately 90% of patients who are treated have a complete or partial response.

■ REFERRAL

Hematology consultation is recommended in all patients.

PEARLS & CONSIDERATIONS

■ COMMENTS

The diagnosis of hairy cell leukemia is occasionally missed and subsequently made by the histopathologist following removal of the spleen for diagnostic purposes.

REFERENCES

Kreitman RJ et al: Efficacy of the anti-CD 22 recombinant immunotoxin BL 22 in chemotherapy resistant hairy-cell leukemia, *N Engl J Med* 345:241, 2001.
Piro LD et al: Lasting remissions in hairy-cell leukemia induced by a single infusion of 2-chlorodeoxyadenosine, *N Engl J Med* 322:1117, 1990.
Author: **Fred F. Ferri, M.D.**

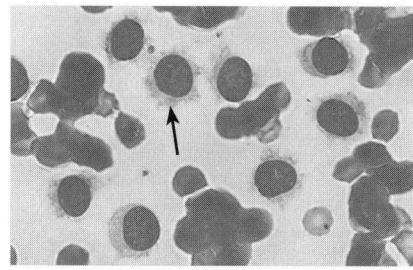

Fig. 1-229　Hairy cell leukemia. Note the lymphocytes with hairlike cytoplasmic projections surrounding the nucleus. (From Rodak BF: *Diagnostic hematology,* Philadelphia, 1995, WB Saunders.)

BASIC INFORMATION

■ DEFINITION
Oral hairy leukoplakia (OHL) is a painless, white, plaquelike lesion typically located on the lateral aspect of the tongue.

■ ICD-9CM CODES
528.6 Oral hairy leukoplakia

■ ETIOLOGY
Epstein-Barr virus (EBV) is implicated in its etiology, and OHL is a result of replication EBV in the epithelium of keratinized cells.

■ EPIDEMIOLOGY & DEMOGRAPHICS
OHL is usually found in human immunodeficiency virus (HIV) seropositive individuals but may also be identified in other immunocompromised patients such as transplant recipients (particularly renal) and patients taking steroids. A diagnosis of OHL is an indication to institute a workup to evaluate and manage HIV disease. Despite a high incidence of EBV seroprevalence in HIV-seropositive individuals, OHL occurs in only 25% of these cases.

■ PHYSICAL FINDINGS & CLINICAL PRESENTATION
- Varying morphology and appearance
- May be unilateral or bilateral
- White and can be small with fine vertical corrugations on the lateral margin of the tongue (Fig. 1-230)
- Irregular surface; may have prominent folds or projection, occasionally markedly resembling hairs
- May spread to cover the entire dorsal surface or spread onto the ventral surface of the tongue where they usually appear flat
- Rarely lesions manifest on the soft palate, buccal mucosa, and in the posterior oropharynx
- Usually asymptomatic, but some have mouth pain, soreness, or a burning sensation, impaired taste, or difficulty eating; others complain of its unsightly appearance

DIAGNOSIS

■ DIFFERENTIAL DIAGNOSIS
- *Candida albicans*
- Lichen planus
- Idiopathic leukoplakia
- White sponge nevus
- Dysplasia
- Squamous cell carcinoma

■ WORKUP
Requires physical examination and evaluation of HIV disease

■ LABORATORY TESTS
The *provisional* diagnosis is clinical and based on:
- Visual inspection
- Inability to scrape the lesion off the tongue with a blade
- Failure to respond to antifungal therapy

The *presumptive* diagnosis requires biopsy and histologic demonstration of:
- Epithelial hyperplasia with hairs
- Absence of inflammatory cell infiltrate

The *definitive* diagnosis requires:
- In situ hybridization of histologic or cytologic specimens revealing EBV DNA *or*
- Electron microscopy of specimens revealing herpeslike particles

NOTE: Specimens obtained from lesions may demonstrate hyphae of *Candida albicans*, which may coexist and potentiate EBV-induced OHL.

TREATMENT

■ NONPHARMACOLOGIC THERAPY
- OHL is usually asymptomatic and requires no specific therapy. It may resolve spontaneously and has no known premalignant potential.

■ ACUTE GENERAL Rx
- Highly active antiretroviral (HAART) therapy has considerably changed the frequency of oral lesions caused by opportunistic infections in HIV-seropositive individuals.
- Topical retinoids (0.1% vitamin A) may improve the appearance of OHL-affected oral surfaces through their dekeratinizing and immunomodulation effects; however, they are expensive and prolonged use may result in a burning sensation over the treated area.
- Topical podophyllin resin 25% solution has been reported to induce resolution.
- Surgical excision and cryotherapy may help, but the lesions may recur.
- High-dose acyclovir or ganciclovir will cause lesions to resolve, but only temporarily.

Author: **Sajeev Handa, M.D.**

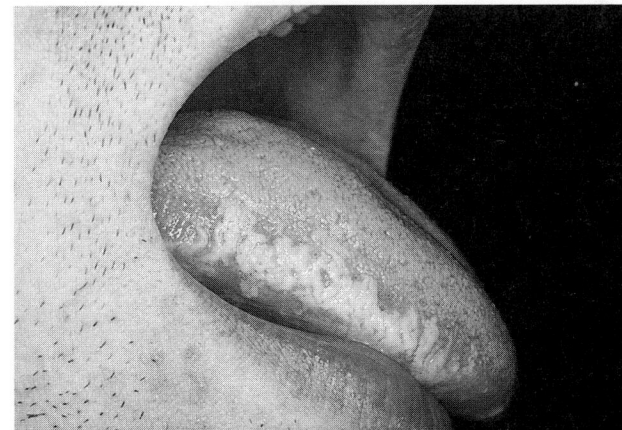

Fig. 1-230 Oral hairy leukoplakia. Note white verrucoid plaques on the lateral border of the tongue. (From Noble J: *Primary care medicine,* ed 3, St Louis, 2001, Mosby.)

BASIC INFORMATION

■ DEFINITION
Lichen planus refers to a papular skin eruption characteristically found over the flexor surfaces of the extremities, genitalia, and mucous membranes.

■ SYNONYMS
Lichen
Lichen planus et atrophicus

■ ICD-9CM CODES
697.0 Lichen planus

■ EPIDEMIOLOGY & DEMOGRAPHICS
- Incidence in the U.S. (440/100,000)
- Usually found in people between the ages of 30 to 60
- Found equally between males and females (1:1)
- Lichen planus associated with discoid lupus, SLE, pemphigus vulgaris, bullous pemphigoid, myasthenia gravis, and ulcerative colitis

■ PHYSICAL FINDINGS & CLINICAL PRESENTATION
History
- Usually starts on an extremity and may remain localized or it can spread to involve other areas over a 1- to 4-mo time period.
- Pruritic

Physical findings (Fig. 1-231)
- Anatomic distribution:
  1. Flexor surface of wrists, forearms, shins, and upper thighs
  2. Neck and back area
  3. Nails
  4. Scalp
  5. Oral mucosa, buccal mucosa, tongue, gingiva, and lips

Genital mucosa
- Lesion configuration:
  1. Linear
  2. Annular (more common)
  3. Reticular pattern noted on oral mucosa and genital area
- Lesion morphology:
  1. Papules (flat, smooth and shiny)—most common presentation
  2. Hypertrophic
  3. Follicular
  4. Vesicular

- Color:
  1. Dark red, bluish red, purplish-violaceous color is noted in cutaneous lichen planus.
  2. Individual lesions characteristically have white lines visible (Wickham's striae).
  3. Oral and genital lichen planus have a reticular network of white lines that may be raised or annular in appearance.
  4. Atrophic purplish violaceous color.
- Scalp lesions may result in alopecia.

■ ETIOLOGY
- The cause of lichen planus is unknown. Leading theory is cell-mediated immune response.
- Lichenlike reactions can occur from drugs (e.g., tetracycline, quinacrine, chloroquine, penicillamine, and hydrochlorothiazide).

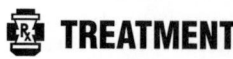 **DIAGNOSIS**

- Clinical history and physical findings usually establish the diagnosis of lichen planus.
- Skin biopsy can be done to confirm the diagnosis.

■ DIFFERENTIAL DIAGNOSIS
- Drug eruption
- Psoriasis
- Basal cell carcinoma
- Bowen's disease
- Leukoplakia
- Candidiasis
- Lupus rash
- Secondary syphilis
- Seborrheic dermatitis

■ WORKUP
No workup is necessary in patients with lichen planus. If the diagnosis is questionable, a skin biopsy is performed.

■ LABORATORY TESTS
Laboratory tests are not specific for the diagnosis of lichen planus.

■ IMAGING STUDIES
Imaging studies are not helpful in diagnosing lichen planus.

TREATMENT

There are no large, randomized trials published to date substantiating the benefit and effectiveness of treatment in lichen planus. Much of the therapeutic information is based on observational data and the personal preferences of experts.

■ NONPHARMACOLOGIC THERAPY
- Avoid scratching.
- Use mild soaps and emollients after bathing to prevent dryness.

■ ACUTE GENERAL Rx
For cutaneous lichen planus
- Topical steroids, triamcinolone acetonide 0.1% with occlusion.
- Acitretin 30 mg/day PO for 8 wk can be used.
- Systemic prednisone 30 to 60 mg/day as a starting dose and tapered to 15 to 20 mg/day maintenance for 6 wk has also been tried.
- Intradermal steroid triamcionolone acetonide 5 mg/ml can be tried for thick hyerkeratotic lesions.
- Hydroxyzine 25 mg PO q6h can be used for pruritus.
For oral lichen planus
- Topical steroid fluocinonide in an adhesive base used 6 times/day for 9 wk.
- Topical retinoids 0.1% retinoic acid in an adhesive base or gel can be used for oral or genital lesions.
- Etretinate 75 mg/day for 2 mo can also be used for oral lesions.

■ CHRONIC Rx
Refer to acute general treatment

■ DISPOSITION
- Spontaneous remissions of cutaneous lichen planus occur in over 65% of cases within the first year.

- Spontaneous remission of oral lichen planus usually occurs by 5 yr.
- Approximately 10% to 20% of patients will have recurrence.

■ **REFERRAL**

If the diagnosis of lichen planus is suspected, a dermatology consultation is recommended.

🔆 **PEARLS & CONSIDERATIONS**

■ **COMMENTS**
- Lichen planus can be remembered as purple, planar, pruritic, polygonal papules (5 Ps).
- Lesions can develop at the site of prior skin injury (Koebner's phenomenon).
- Although transformation to skin cancer has been seen in patients with lichen planus, it remains unclear if there is a true correlation.

REFERENCES

Boyd AS, Neldner KH: Lichen planus, *J Am Acad Dermatol* 25:593, 1991.
Cribier B, Rances C, Chosidow O: Treatment of lichen planus: an evidence-based medicine analysis of efficacy, *Arch Dermatol* 134(12):1521, 1998.
Fitzpatrick TB et al: *Dermatology in general medicine*, ed 4, New York, 1993, McGraw-Hill.
Author: **Peter Petropoulos, M.D.**

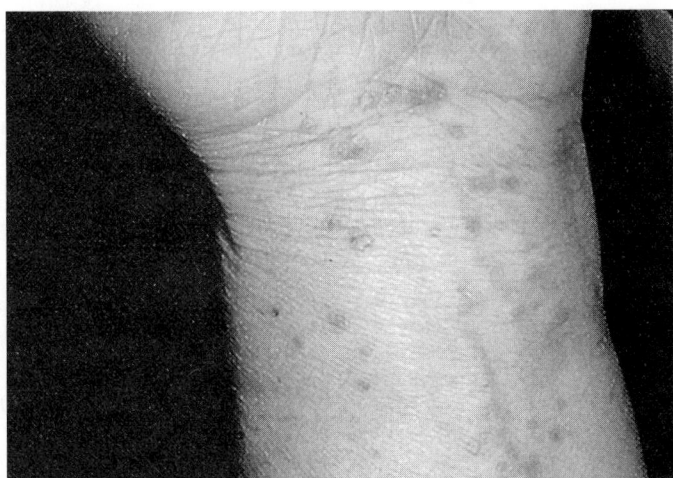

Fig. 1-231   Lichen planus. Note discrete polygonal scaling erythematous papules on the wrist. (Courtesy Department of Dermatology, Medical College of Georgia. In Goldstein BG, Goldstein AO: *Practical dermatology,* ed 2, St Louis, 1997, Mosby.)

BASIC INFORMATION

■ DEFINITION
Listeriosis is a systemic infection caused by the gram-positive aerobic bacterium *Listeria monocytogenes*.

ICD-9CM CODES
027.0 Listeriosis
771.2 Congenital listeriosis
771.2 Fetal listeriosis
665.4 Suspected fetal damage affecting management of pregnancy

■ EPIDEMIOLOGY & DEMOGRAPHICS
INCIDENCE (IN U.S.):
- Listeria meningitis: about 0.7 cases/100,000 persons (fourth most common cause of community-acquired bacterial meningitis in adults)
- Perinatal listeriosis: 8.6 cases/100,000 persons
- Nonperinatal listeriosis: 3 cases/1 million persons
PREDOMINANT SEX: Pregnant women are more susceptible to *Listeria* bacteremia, accounting for up to one third of reported cases.
PREDOMINANT AGE:
- Pregnant women
- Immunocompromised patients of any age
GENETICS
Congenital Infection:
- With transplacental transmission, syndrome termed *granulomatosis infantisepticum* in neonate
- Characterized by disseminated abscesses in multiple organs, skin lesions, conjunctivitis
- Mortality: 33% to 100%
Neonatal Infection:
- Infant becoming ill after 3 days of age; mother invariably asymptomatic
- Clinical picture of sepsis of unknown origin

■ PHYSICAL FINDINGS & CLINICAL PRESENTATION
- Infections in pregnancy
  1. More common in third trimester
  2. Usually present with fever and chills without localizing symptoms or signs of infection
- Meningoencephalitis
  1. More common in neonates and immunocompromised patients, but up to 30% of adults have no underlying condition
  2. In neonates: poor appetite with or without fever possibly the only presenting signs

  3. In adults: presentation often subacute, with low-grade fever and personality change as only signs
  4. Focal neurologic signs seen without demonstrable brain abscess on CT scan
- Cerebritis/rhomboencephalitis:
  1. Headache and fever may be only presenting complaints.
  2. Progressive cranial nerve palsies, hemiparesis, seizures, depressed level of consciousness, cerebellar signs, respiratory insufficiency may also be seen.
- Focal infections
  1. Ocular infections (purulent conjunctivitis) and skin lesions (granulomatosis infantisepticum) as a result of inadvertent inoculation by laboratory and veterinary personnel
  2. Others: arthritis, prosthetic joint infections, peritonitis, osteomyelitis, organ abscesses, cholecystitis

■ ETIOLOGY
- Direct invasion of skin and eye has been documented, but mechanism of GI entry is unclear.
- Organism's intracellular life cycle explanatory of:
  1. Importance of cell-mediated immunity in host defense
  2. Increased incidence of infection in neonates, pregnant women, and immunocompromised hosts

DIAGNOSIS

■ DIFFERENTIAL DIAGNOSIS
- Meningitis caused by other bacteria, mycobacteria, or fungi
- CNS sarcoidosis
- Brain neoplasm or abscess
- Tuberculous and fungal (especially cryptococcal) meningitis
- Cerebral toxoplasmosis
- Lyme disease
- Sarcoidosis

■ WORKUP
Dictated by age, end-organ involvement, and immune status

■ LABORATORY TESTS
- Cultures of blood and other appropriate body fluids
- Variable CSF findings, but neutrophils usually predominate
- Organisms uncommonly seen on Gram stain and may be difficult to identify morphologically
- Monoclonal antibodies, polymerase chain reaction, and DNA probe techniques to detect *Listeria* in foods

■ IMAGING STUDIES
- If focal cerebral involvement suspected: CT scan or MRI
- MRI most sensitive for evaluation of brainstem and cerebellum

TREATMENT

Empiric therapy should be administered when diagnosis is suspected because overall mortality is 23%.

■ ACUTE GENERAL Rx
- Drugs of choice:
  1. IV ampicillin 8 to 12 g/day in divided doses
  2. IV penicillin 12 to 24 million U/day in divided doses
- Continuation of therapy for 2 wk
- Alternative: trimethoprim/sulfamethoxazole
- Gentamicin added to provide synergy

■ CHRONIC Rx
Relapses reported, especially in immunocompromised hosts, after 2 wk of therapy

■ DISPOSITION
Long-term follow-up of immunodeficiency state

■ REFERRAL
Infectious disease consultation for all patients

PEARLS & CONSIDERATIONS

■ COMMENTS
- Foodborne cases have been linked to various products: coleslaw, soft cheese, pasteurized milk, vegetables, undercooked chicken, hot dogs.
- Complete decontamination of food products is difficult because *Listeria* is resistant to pasteurization and refrigeration.

REFERENCES
Jayaraj K, DiBisceglie AM, Gison S: Spontaneous bacteria peritonitis caused by infection with *Listeria monocytogenes*: a case report and review of the literature, *Am J Gastroenterol* 93(9):1556, 1998.
Taige AJ: Listeriosis: recognizing it, treating it, preventing it, *Cleve Clin J Med* 66:375, 1999.
Author: **Claudia L. Dade, M.D.**

BASIC INFORMATION

■ DEFINITION
Long QT syndrome is an electrocardiographic abnormality characterized by a corrected QT interval longer than 0.44 sec and associated with an increased risk of developing life-threatening ventricular arrhythmias (Fig. 1-232).

■ SYNONYMS
Congenital forms:
- Jervell and Lange-Nielsen syndrome (associated with deafness)
- Romano-Ward syndrome (associated with normal hearing)

Sporadic forms of long QT syndrome (nonfamilial)

ICD-9CM CODES
427.9 Unspecified cardiac dysrhythmia

■ EPIDEMIOLOGY & DEMOGRAPHICS
- Familial associated with deafness: autosomal recessive
- Familial associated with normal hearing: autosomal dominant (the incidence is unknown)

■ PHYSICAL FINDINGS & CLINICAL PRESENTATION
- Syncope caused by ventricular tachycardia
- Sudden death
- Abnormal ECG (prolonged QT) in asymptomatic relatives of known case
- Routine (baseline) ECG finding

■ ETIOLOGY
- Cardiac repolarization abnormality
- Congenital cause (chromosome 3 or chromosome 7 abnormality)
- Acquired causes:
  Drugs (quinidine, procainamide, sotalol, amiodarone, disopyramide, phenothiazines, tricyclic antidepressants, astemizole or cisapride given with ketoconazole or erythromycin, and antimalarials)
  Hypokalemia, hypomagnesemia
  Liquid protein diet
  CNS lesions
  Mitral valve prolapse

DIAGNOSIS

■ DIFFERENTIAL DIAGNOSIS
See "Syncope."

■ WORKUP
In relatives of known patients with long QT syndrome or in young patients with syncope:
- Stress test may prolong the QT interval or cause T-wave alternans
- Valsalva maneuver: may prolong the QT interval or cause T-wave alternans
- Prolonged ECG monitoring with various stimulations aimed at increasing catecholamines (perform in a setting that can provide resuscitation)

TREATMENT

- Asymptomatic sporadic forms with no complex ventricular arrhythmias: no treatment
- All others:
  Avoid competitive sports
  β-blocker at maximum tolerated dose
  Cardiology referral is recommended for all cases

REFERENCES
Ackerman MJ: The long QT syndrome: ion channel diseases of the heart, *Mayo Clin Proc* 73:250, 1998.
Rodriguez I et al: Drug-induced QT prolongation in women during the menstrual cycle, *JAMA* 285:1322, 2001.
Author: **Tom J. Wachtel, M.D.**

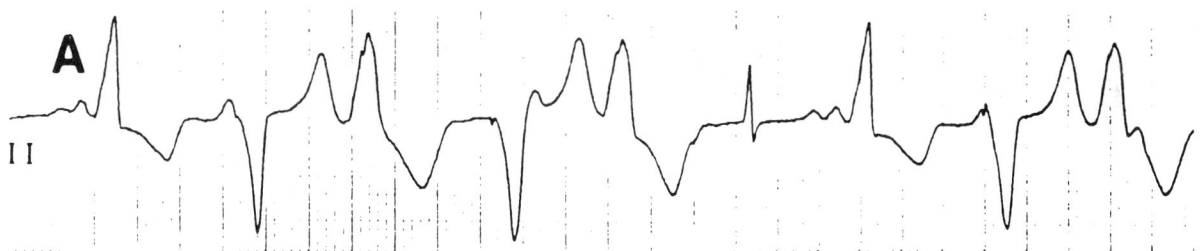

Fig. 1-232 Strips show multiform ventricular complexes in a patient treated with quinidine. Note that the normally conducted beat (narrow QRS complex) is associated with marked prolongation of the QT interval. (From Goldman L, Braunwald E [eds]: *Primary cardiology,* Philadelphia, 1998, WB Saunders.)

■ BASIC INFORMATION

■ DEFINITION
Lumbar disk syndromes are diseases resulting from disk disorder, either herniation or degenerative change (spondylosis). Massive disk protrusion may rarely lead to paralysis in the lower extremity, a condition termed *cauda equina syndrome*. Gradual narrowing of the spinal canal (lumbar stenosis), usually from spondylosis, may also cause lower extremity symptoms.

ICD-9CM CODES
722.10 Lumbar disk displacement
724.02 Lumbar stenosis
344.60 Cauda equina syndrome
721.3 Lumbar spondylosis

■ EPIDEMIOLOGY & DEMOGRAPHICS
PREVALENCE:
- Variable
- At least one episode in 80% of adults

PREVALENT AGE:
- Herniation: 20 to 40 yr
- Stenosis: >40 to 50 yr
- Disk symptoms: rare <20 yr

PREVALENT SEX: Approximately equal

■ PHYSICAL FINDINGS & CLINICAL PRESENTATION (Table 1-44)
- Overlapping clinical syndromes that may result:
  1. Mild herniation without nerve root compression
  2. Herniation with nerve root compression
  3. Cauda equina syndrome
  4. Chronic degenerative disease with or without leg symptoms
  5. Spinal stenosis
- Low back pain, often worsened by activity or coughing and sneezing
- Local lumbar or lumbosacral tenderness
- Paresthesias, usually unilateral
- Restricted low back motion
- Increased pain on bending toward affected side
- Weakness and reflex changes
- Sensory examination usually not helpful
- Lumbar stenosis that possibly produces symptoms (pseudoclaudica-

tion), which are often misinterpreted as being vascular
- Positive straight leg raising test if nerve root compression is present (see Fig. 1-233)

■ ETIOLOGY
Unknown

■ DIAGNOSIS

■ DIFFERENTIAL DIAGNOSIS
- Soft-tissue strain/sprain
- Tumor
- Degenerative arthritis of hip
Table 2-18 describes the differential diagnosis of common low back pain syndromes.

■ WORKUP
In most cases, the diagnosis can be established on a clinical basis alone.

■ IMAGING STUDIES
- Plain roentgenograms may be indicated within the first few weeks; they are usually normal in soft disk herniation, but with chronic degenerative disk disease, loss of height of the disk space and osteophyte formation can occur.
- Myelography, CT scanning, and MRI may be indicated in patients whose symptoms do not resolve or when other spinal pathology may be suspected.
- Electrodiagnostic studies may confirm the diagnosis or rule out peripheral nerve disorders.

■ TREATMENT

■ NONPHARMACOLOGIC THERAPY
- Short course (3 to 5 days) of bed rest for severe pain; prolonged rest for acute disk herniation with leg pain
- Physical therapy for modalities plus a careful gradual exercise program (Fig. 1-233)
- Lumbosacral corset brace during rehabilitation process in conjunction with exercise program
- Percutaneous electrical nerve stimulation (PENS) may be beneficial in selected patients with chronic back pain

■ PHARMACOLOGIC THERAPY
- NSAIDs
- "Muscle relaxants" for sedative effect
- Analgesics
- Epidural steroid injection for leg symptoms in selected patients

■ DISPOSITION
- Almost all lumbar disk syndromes improve with time.
- Recurrent episodes usually respond to medical management.
- Recovery from the rare paralytic event is often incomplete.

■ REFERRAL
For orthopedic or neurosurgical consultation for intractable pain or significant neurologic deficit

✿ PEARLS & CONSIDERATIONS

■ COMMENTS
A clinical algorithm for evaluation of back pain is described in Fig. 3-22.

REFERENCES
Ghoname EA et al: Percutaneous electrical nerve stimulation for low back pain: a randomized crossover study, *JAMA* 281:818, 1999.
Linton SJ: A review of psychological risk factors in back and neck pain, *Spine* 25:1148, 2000.
Paassilta P et al: Identification of a novel common genetic risk factor for lumbar disc disease, *JAMA* 285:1843, 2001.
Papagelopoulos PJ et al: Treatment of lumbrosacral radicular pain with epidural steroid injections, *Orthopedics* 24:145, 2001.
Robinson LR: Role of neurophysiologic evaluation in diagnosis, *J Am Acad Orthop Surg* 8:190, 2000.
Simotas AC: Non-operative treatment for lumbar spinal stenosis, *Clin Orthop* 384:153, 2001.
Vromen PC et al: Lack of effectiveness of bed rest for sciatica, *N Engl J Med* 340:418, 1999.
Author: **Lonnie R. Mercier, M.D.**

TABLE 1-44　Diagnosis of Lower Lumbar and Sacral Radiculopathy

	PAIN	WEAKNESS (SELECTED MUSCLES)	SENSORY LOSS	REFLEX LOSS
L4	Across thigh and medial leg to medial malleolus	Quadriceps, thigh adductors, tibialis anterior	Medial leg	Knee
L5	Posterior thigh and lateral calf, dorsum of foot	Extensor digitorum brevis and longus, peronei	Dorsum of foot	
S1	Buttock and posterior thigh, calf, and lateral foot	Extensor digitorum brevis, peronei, gastrocnemius, soleus	Sole or lateral border of foot	Ankle
S2-4	Posterior thigh, buttock, and genitalia	Gastrocnemius, soleus, abductor hallucis, abductor digiti quinti pedis, sphincter muscles	Buttocks, anal region, and genitalia	Bulbocavernosus, anal

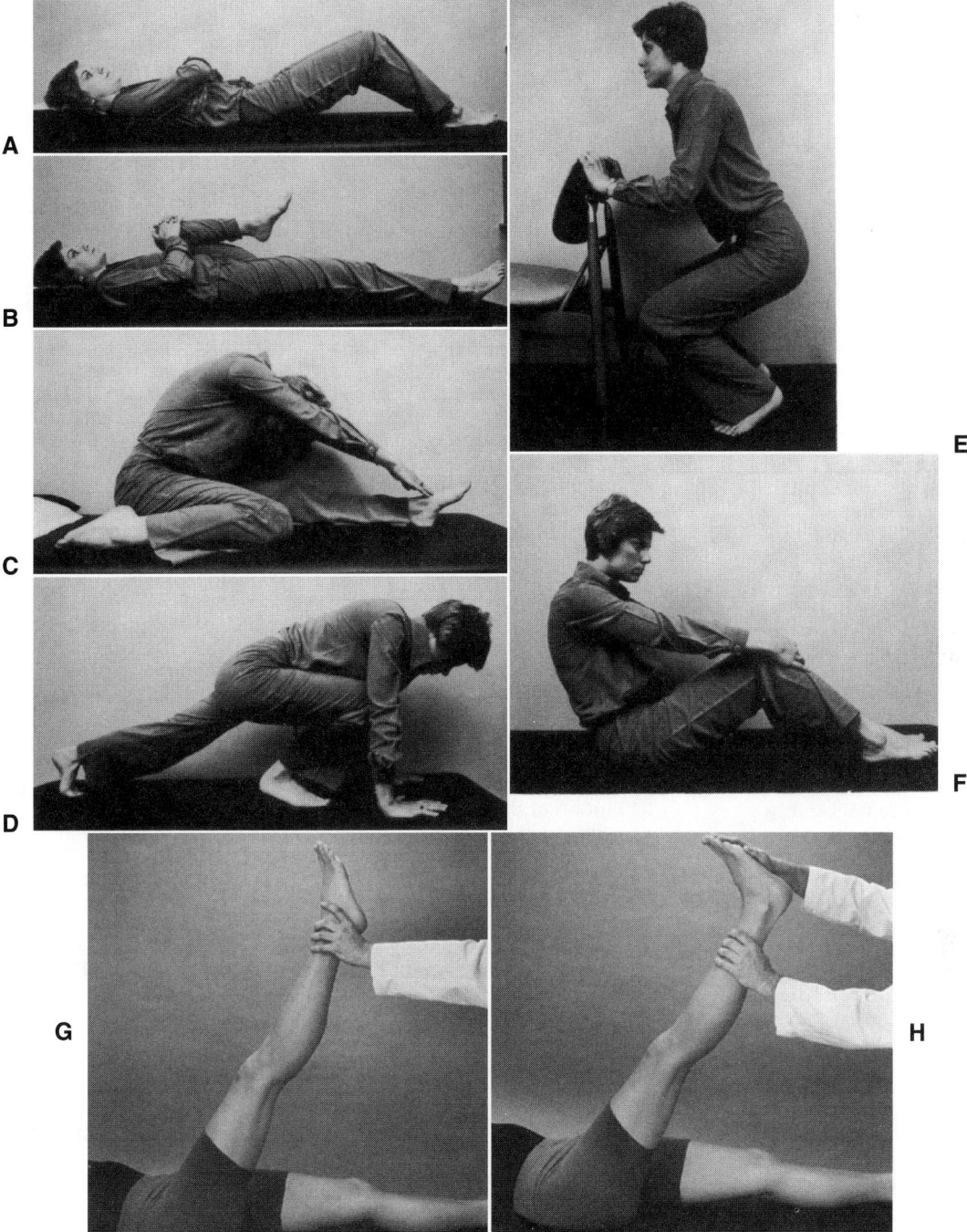

Fig. 1-233   Low back exercises. **A,** Pelvic tilt performed to decrease lumbar lordosis and raise the anterior aspect of the pelvis. The small of the back is pressed to the floor and the abdominal and buttock muscles are tightened. **B,** Hip flexion, performed to stretch the tight posterior spinal musculature and unload the posterior of the disk. Each knee is drawn up and pulled firmly to the chest several times and the position held for 10 to 20 seconds. The exercise is then repeated with both knees. After the acute pain has subsided, the remainder of the exercises are performed. **C,** Hamstring-stretching exercises; **D,** hip flexor–stretching exercises; **E,** quadriceps-strengthening and heel cord–stretching exercise; **F,** abdomen strengthening exercise (sit-ups, which may be partial). All exercises are performed on a carpeted floor and should be repeated in sets of 5 to 10 at least three times daily. **G,** Straight-leg raising test. **H,** Lasegue's test. (**A** to **F** from Mercier LR [ed]: *Practical orthopaedics,* ed 4, 1995, St Louis, Mosby; **G** and **H** from Reider B: *The orthopaedic physical examination,* Philadelphia, 1999, WB Saunders.)

BASIC INFORMATION

■ DEFINITION

A primary lung neoplasm is a malignancy arising from lung tissue. The World Health Organization distinguishes twelve types of pulmonary neoplasms. Among them, the major types are *squamous cell carcinoma, adenocarcinoma, small cell carcinoma,* and *large cell carcinoma.* However, the crucial difference in the diagnosis of lung cancer is between small cell and non–small cell types, because the therapeutic approach is different. Selective characteristics of lung carcinomas:

ADENOCARCINOMA: Represents 35% of lung carcinomas; frequently located in mid lung and periphery; initial metastases are to lymphatics, frequently associated with peripheral scars

SQUAMOUS CELL (EPIDERMOID): 20% to 30% of lung cancers; central location; metastasis by local invasion; frequent cavitation and obstructive phenomena

SMALL CELL (OAT CELL): 20% of lung carcinomas; central location; metastasis through lymphatics; associated with lesion of the short arm of chromosome 3; high cavitation rate

LARGE CELL: 15% to 20% of lung carcinomas; frequently located in the periphery; metastasis to CNS and mediastinum; rapid growth rate with early metastasis

BRONCHOALVEOLAR: 5% of lung carcinomas; frequently located in the periphery; may be bilateral; initial metastasis through lymphatic, hematogenous, and local invasion; no correlation with cigarette smoking; cavitation rare

■ SYNONYMS

Lung cancer

ICD-9CM CODES

162.9 Malignant neoplasm of bronchus and lung, unspecified

■ EPIDEMIOLOGY & DEMOGRAPHICS

- Lung cancer is responsible for >30% of cancer deaths in males and >25% of cancer deaths in females.
- Tobacco smoking is implicated in 85% of cases; second-hand smoke is responsible for approximately 20% of cases.
- There are >180,000 new cases of lung cancer yearly in the U.S., most occurring >age 50 yr (<4% in patients <40 yr of age).

■ PHYSICAL FINDINGS & CLINICAL PRESENTATION

- Weight loss, fatigue, fever, anorexia, dysphagia

- Cough, hemoptysis, dyspnea, wheezing
- Chest, shoulder, and bone pain
- Paraneoplastic syndromes:
  1. *Eaton-Lambert syndrome:* myopathy involving proximal muscle groups
  2. Endocrine manifestations: hypercalcemia, ectopic ACTH, SIADH
  3. Neurologic: subacute cerebellar degeneration, peripheral neuropathy, cortical degeneration
  4. Musculoskeletal: polymyositis, clubbing, hypertrophic pulmonary osteoarthropathy
  5. Hematologic or vascular: migratory thrombophlebitis, marantic thrombosis, anemia, thrombocytosis, or thrombocytopenia
  6. Cutaneous: acanthosis nigricans, dermatomyositis
- Pleural effusion (10% of patients), recurrent pneumonias (secondary to obstruction), localized wheezing
- Superior vena cava syndrome:
  1. Obstruction of venous return of the superior vena cava is most commonly caused by bronchogenic carcinoma or metastasis to paratracheal nodes.
  2. The patient usually complains of headache, nausea, dizziness, visual changes, syncope, and respiratory distress.
  3. Physical examination reveals distention of thoracic and neck veins, edema of face and upper extremities, facial plethora, and cyanosis.
- *Horner's syndrome:* constricted pupil, ptosis, facial anhidrosis caused by spinal cord damage between C8 and T1 secondary to a superior sulcus tumor (bronchogenic carcinoma of the extreme lung apex); a superior sulcus tumor associated with ipsilateral Horner's syndrome and shoulder pain is known as *"Pancoast" tumor*

■ ETIOLOGY

- Tobacco abuse
- Environmental agents (e.g., radon) and industrial agents (e.g., ionizing radiation, asbestos, nickel, uranium, vinyl chloride, chromium, arsenic, coal dust)

DIAGNOSIS

■ DIFFERENTIAL DIAGNOSIS

- Pneumonia
- TB
- Metastatic carcinoma to the lung
- Lung abscess
- Granulomatous disease
- Carcinoid tumor
- Mycobacterial and fungal diseases

- Sarcoidosis
- Viral pneumonitis

The differential diagnosis of solitary pulmonary nodules is described in Table 2-170.

■ WORKUP

- Workup includes chest x-ray examination, CT scan of chest, and/or PET scan, and tissue biopsy.
- A diagnostic approach to pulmonary nodules is described in Fig. 3-182.

■ LABORATORY TESTS

- Cytologic examination of at least three sputum specimens unless a positive cytology is obtained on the first or second specimen (inexpensive test; however, positive yield is low and this test is rarely ordered)
- Biopsy of any suspicious lymph nodes (e.g., supraclavicular node)
- Flexible fiberoptic bronchoscopy: brush and biopsy specimens are obtained from any visualized endobronchial lesions
- Transbronchial needle aspiration: done via a special needle passed through the bronchoscope; this technique is useful to sample mediastinal masses or paratracheal lymph nodes
- Transthoracic fine-needle aspiration biopsy with fluoroscopic or CT scan guidance to evaluate peripheral pulmonary nodules
- Mediastinoscopy and anteromedial sternotomy in suspected tumor involvement of the mediastinum
- Pleural biopsy in patients with pleural effusion

■ IMAGING STUDIES

- Chest x-ray examination:
  1. The radiographic presentation often varies with the cell type (see "Definition").
  2. Pleural effusion, lobar atelectasis, and mediastinal adenopathy can accompany any cell types.
  3. Benign lesions that simulate thoracic malignancy:
     a. Lobar atelectasis: pneumonia, TB, chronic inflammatory disease, allergic bronchopulmonary aspergillosis
     b. Multiple pulmonary nodules: septic emboli, Wegener's granulomatosis, sarcoidosis, rheumatoid nodules, fungal disease, multiple pulmonary AV fistulas
     c. Mediastinal adenopathy: sarcoidosis, lymphoma, primary TB, fungal disease, silicosis, pneumoconiosis, drug-induced (e.g., phenytoin, trimethadione)

d. Pleural effusion: CHF, pneumonia with parapneumonic effusion, TB, viral pneumonitis, ascites, pancreatitis, collagen-vascular disease
- Thoracentesis of pleural effusion and cytologic evaluation of the obtained fluid: may confirm diagnosis
- CT scan of chest: to evaluate mediastinal and pleural extension of suspected lung neoplasms. Positron emission tomography (PET) with 18F-fluorodeoxyglucose, a metabolic marker of malignant tissue, has been reported as superior to CT scan in detecting mediastinal and distant metastases in non–small cell lung cancer.

STAGING
- Following confirmation of diagnosis, patients should undergo staging:
  1. The international staging system is the most widely accepted staging system for non–small cell lung cancer. In this system, stage I (N0 [no lymph node involvement], stage II (N1 [spread to ipsilateral bronchopulmonary or hilar lymph nodes]) include localized tumors for which surgical resection is the preferred treatment. Stage 3 is subdivided into 3A (potentially resectable) and 3B. The surgical management of stage IIIA disease (N2 [involvement of ipsilateral mediastinal nodes] is controversial). Only 20% of N2 disease is considered minimal disease (involvement of only one node) and technically resectable. Stage 4 indicates metastatic disease. The pathologic staging system uses a tumor/nodal involvement/metastasis system.
  2. In patients with small cell lung cancer, a more practical accepted staging system is the one developed by the Veterans Administration Lung Cancer Study Group (VALG). This system contains two stages:
     a. Limited stage: disease confined to the regional lymph nodes and to one hemithorax (excluding pleural surfaces)
     b. Extensive stage: disease spread beyond the confines of limited stage disease
  3. Pretreatment staging procedures for lung cancer patients, in addition to complete history and physical examination, generally include the following tests:
     a. Chest x-ray examination (PA and lateral), ECG
     b. Laboratory evaluation: CBC, electrolytes, platelets, calcium, phosphorus, glucose, renal and liver function studies, ABGs, and skin tests for TB
     c. Pulmonary function studies
     d. CT scan of chest and/or PET scan

     e. Mediastinoscopy or anterior mediastinotomy in patients being considered for possible curative lung resection
     f. Biopsy of any accessible suspect lesions
     g. CT scan of liver and brain; radionuclide scans of bone in all patients with small cell carcinoma of the lung and patients with non–small cell lung neoplasms suspected of involving these organs
     h. Bone marrow aspiration and biopsy only in selected patients with small cell carcinoma of the lung. In the absence of an increased LDH or cytopenia, routine bone marrow examination is not recommended.

TREATMENT

NONPHARMACOLOGIC THERAPY
- Nutritional support
- Avoidance of tobacco or other substances toxic to the lungs
- Supplemental O_2 PRN

ACUTE GENERAL Rx
NON–SMALL CELL CARCINOMA:
- Surgery
  1. Surgical resection is indicated in patients with limited disease (not involving mediastinal nodes, ribs, pleura, or distant sites). This represents approximately 15% to 30% of diagnosed cases.
  2. Preoperative evaluation includes review of cardiac status (e.g., recent MI, major arrhythmias) and evaluation of pulmonary function (to determine if the patient can tolerate any loss of lung tissue). Pneumonectomy is possible if the patient has a preoperative FEV_1 ≥2 L or if the MVV is >50% of predicted capacity.
  3. Preoperative chemotherapy should be considered in patients with more advanced disease (stage 3A) who are being considered for surgery, because it increases the median survival time in patients with non–small cell lung cancer compared with the use of surgery alone.
- Treatment of unresectable non–small cell carcinoma of the lung:
  1. Radiotherapy can be used alone or in combination with chemotherapy; it is used primarily for treatment of CNS and skeletal metastases, superior vena cava syndrome, and obstructive atelectasis; although thoracic radiotherapy is generally considered standard therapy for stage 3 disease, it has limited effect on survival.

  2. Chemotherapy: various combination regimens are available (e.g., combinations of mitomycin, vinblastine, cisplatin, vindesine, ifosfamide, and paclitaxel; carboplatin, cyclophosphamide, and etoposide are also useful agents); however, the overall results are disappointing.
  3. The addition of chemotherapy to radiotherapy improves survival in patients with locally advanced, unresectable, non–small cell lung cancer. The absolute benefit is relatively small, however, and should be balanced against the increased toxicity associated with the addition of chemotherapy.

TREATMENT OF SMALL CELL LUNG CANCER:
- Limited stage disease: thoracic radiotherapy and chemotherapy (cisplatin and etoposide)
- Extensive stage disease: combination chemotherapy (cisplatin and etoposide or combination regimen of ifosfamide, carboplatin, and oral etoposide or monotherapy with oral etoposide in elderly patients in whom aggressive therapy is not desired)
- Prophylactic cranial irradiation for patients in complete remission to decrease the risk of CNS metastasis

DISPOSITION
- The 5-yr survival of patients with non–small cell carcinoma when the disease is resectable is approximately 30%.
- Median survival time in patients with limited stage disease and small cell lung cancer is 15 mo; in patients with extensive stage disease, it is 9 mo.

REFERRAL
Surgical referral for biopsy and resection (see "Acute General Rx")

PEARLS & CONSIDERATIONS

COMMENTS
Malignant pleural effusions associated with lung cancer are treated with therapeutic thoracentesis and pleurodesis.

REFERENCES
Adjei AA et al: Current guidelines for the management of small cell lung cancer, *Mayo Clin Proc* 74:809, 1999.
Auperin A et al: Prophylactic cranial irradiation for patients with small-cell lung cancer in complete remission, *N Engl J Med* 341:476, 1999.
Pieterman RM et al: Preoperative staging of non–small cell lung cancer with positron-emission tomography, *N Engl J Med* 343:254, 2000.
Author: **Fred F. Ferri, M.D.**

BASIC INFORMATION

■ DEFINITION
Lyme disease is a multisystem disorder caused by the transmission of a spirochete, *Borrelia burgdorferi*, from a tick. This disease often develops in summer months with the following types of presentation:
Early localized: early Lyme disease, erythema chronicum migrans (ECM); skin rash, often at site of tick bite; possible fever, myalgias 3 to 32 days after tick bite
Early disseminated: days to weeks later; multi–organ system involvement, including CNS, joints, cardiac; related to dissemination of spirochete
Late persistent: months to years after tick exposure; affects central and peripheral nervous system, cardiac, joints

■ SYNONYMS
Bannworth's syndrome
Acrodermatitis chronica atrophicans

ICD-9CM CODES
088.8 Lyme disease

■ EPIDEMIOLOGY & DEMOGRAPHICS
INCIDENCE (IN U.S.): Geographic variation, 4.4 cases/100,000 persons; reported in 43 states and District of Columbia
PREDOMINANT SEX: Male = female
PREDOMINANT AGE: Median age of 28 yr
PEAK INCIDENCE: May to November

■ PHYSICAL FINDINGS
• ECM (Fig. 1-234) frequently occurring at site of tick bite, can be followed by annular lesions (secondary).
• Lymphadenopathy, neck pains, pharyngeal erythema, myalgias, hepatosplenomegaly often present early in the disease.
• Patients will complain of malaise, fatigue, lethargy, headache, fever/chills, neck pain, myalgias, back pain.

■ ETIOLOGY
Borrelia burgdorferi transmitted from bite of an *Ixodes* tick (most commonly belonging to the species *Scapularis*).

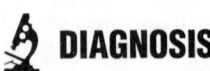

DIAGNOSIS

Clinical presentation, exposure to ticks in endemic area, and diagnostic testing for antibody response to *B. burgdorferi*

■ DIFFERENTIAL DIAGNOSIS
• Chronic fatigue/fibromyalgia
• Acute viral illnesses
• Babesiosis
• Ehrlichiosis

■ WORKUP
• ELISA testing—Western blot
• Immunofluorescent assay
• Early disease often difficult to diagnose serologically secondary to slow immune response
• Culturing of skin lesions (ECM) and polymerase chain reaction (PCR) of skin biopsy and blood to give definitive diagnosis (available only in reference laboratories)

■ IMAGING STUDIES
• Echocardiogram if conduction abnormalities are present with cardiac involvement
• CT scan, MRI of head for CNS involvement

TREATMENT

• Early Lyme disease
  1. Doxycycline 100 mg bid or amoxicillin 500 mg qid for 21 days (doxycycline should be avoided in children/pregnant females)
  2. Alternative treatments: cefuroxime axetil 500 mg bid for 21 days, azithromycin 500 mg PO qd for 1 day followed by 250 mg qd for 6 days
• Disseminated infection: 30 days of treatment necessary; doxycycline and ceftriaxone appear equally effective for acute disseminated Lyme disease
• Arthritis: 30 days of doxycycline or amoxicillin plus probenecid (repeated courses of therapy are often needed)
• Neurologic involvement
  1. Parenteral antibiotics
  2. Ceftriaxone 2 g/day for 21 to 28 days
  3. Alternative: cefotaxime 2 g q8h
  4. Alternative: penicillin G 5 million U qid
• Cardiac involvement: IV ceftriaxone or penicillin plus cardiac monitoring

PEARLS & CONSIDERATIONS

Vaccination is now available for prevention of Lyme disease in endemic areas in patients with high exposure risk.

REFERENCES
Gardener P: Lyme disease vaccines, *Ann Intern Med* 129:583, 1998.
Wormser GP et al: Practice guidelines for the treatment of Lyme disease, *Clin Infect Dis* 31(Suppl 1):1, 2000.
Author: **Dennis J. Mikolich, M.D.**

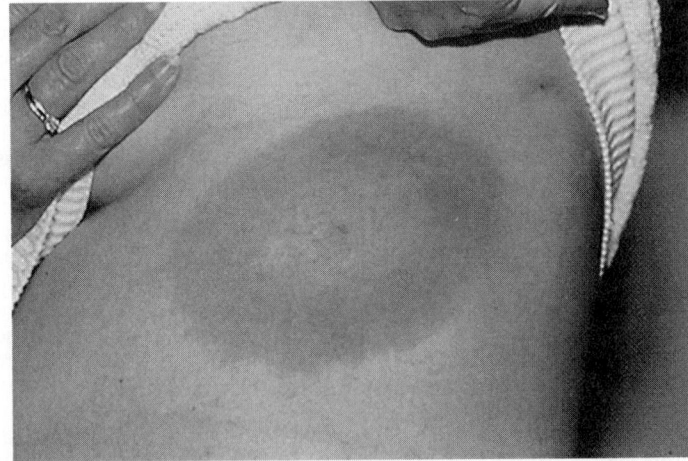

Fig. 1-234 Erythema migrans. Note expanding erythematous lesion with central clearing on trunk. (Courtesy John Cook, MD. From Goldstein B [ed]: *Practical dermatology,* ed 2, St Louis, 1997, Mosby.)

BASIC INFORMATION

DEFINITION
Lymphangitis refers to the inflammation of lymphatic vessels.

SYNONYMS
Nodular lymphangitis
Sporotrichoid lymphangitis

ICD-9CM CODES
457.2 Lymphangitis

PHYSICAL FINDINGS & CLINICAL PRESENTATION
ACUTE LYMPHANGITIS:
- Commonly associated with a bacterial cellulitis
- May or may not recognize site of skin trauma (i.e., laceration, puncture, ulcer)
- In hours to days, distal appearance of erythema, edema, and tenderness, with linear erythematous streaks extending proximally to regional lymph nodes
- Possible lymphadenitis and fever
- Predisposition to group A streptococcal infection of the skin in those with chronic lymphedema and superficial fungal infections (e.g., tinea pedis)

"SPOROTRICHOID" OR "NODULAR" LYMPHANGITIS:
- Includes subcutaneous nodules that develop along the path of involved lymphatics
- Most commonly results from inoculation of the skin of the hand
- Lesions apparent from one to several weeks after inoculation
- Initially, nodular or papular lesion; may ulcerate
- May have frank pus or a serosanguineous discharge
- Systemic complaints uncommon, but infection with certain microorganisms associated with fever, chills, myalgias, and headache

ETIOLOGY
- Acute lymphangitis: usually associated with *Streptococcus pyogenes* (group A streptococcus), but staphylococcal organisms also seen
- Nodular lymphangitis caused by one of several organisms
  1. *Sporothrix schenckii*
     a. Most common recognized cause in the U.S., usually in the Midwest
     b. Found in soil and plant debris
  2. *Nocardia brasiliensis:* found in soil
  3. *Mycobacterium marinum:* associated with trauma related to water (e.g., aquariums, swimming pools, fish)
  4. *Francisella tularensis*
     a. Most often in Midwestern states
     b. Associated with contact with infected mammals (e.g., rabbits) or tick bites

 DIAGNOSIS

DIFFERENTIAL DIAGNOSIS
- Nodular lymphangitis
- Insect or snake bites
- Filariasis

WORKUP
- Acute lymphangitis: blood cultures
- Nodular lymphangitis: various stains and cultures of drainage or biopsy specimens of inoculation sites to make definitive diagnosis

LABORATORY TESTS
- WBCs possibly elevated with cellulitis
- Eosinophilia common with helminthic infections

 TREATMENT

NONPHARMACOLOGIC THERAPY
Limb elevation

ACUTE GENERAL Rx
- Penicillin possibly sufficient, but 1 wk of dicloxacillin or cephalexin 500 mg PO qid commonly used to ensure antistaphylococcal coverage
- If allergic to penicillin:
  1. Clindamycin 300 mg PO qid for 7 days *or*
  2. Erythromycin 500 mg PO qid for 7 days
- Nodular lymphangitis: specific therapy directed at etiologic agent
- For superficial fungal infections: treatment may prevent recurrence of acute lymphangitis

DISPOSITION
- Acute lymphangitis: usually resolves with therapy
- Recurrent attacks: may lead to chronic lymphedema of limb, rarely resulting in elephantiasis nostras (nonfilarial elephantiasis)
- Nodular lymphangitis: usually responds to appropriate therapy

REFERRAL
- If acute lymphangitis is more than a mild disease or involves the face
- If nodular lymphangitis or filariasis is suspected

PEARLS & CONSIDERATIONS

COMMENTS
- Outside of the U.S., initial episodes of filariasis caused by *Brugia malayi* resemble acute lymphangitis.
- Chronic lymphedema or elephantiasis results from recurrent episodes.

Author: **Maurice Policar, M.D.**

BASIC INFORMATION

■ DEFINITION
Lymphedema is the result of impaired lymph drainage caused by obstruction, injury, or the abnormal development of the lymph vessels that leads to swelling of the extremities.

■ SYNONYMS
Elephantiasis

ICD-9CM CODES
457.1 Lymphedema: acquired (chronic), praecox, secondary
457.1 Elephantiasis (nonfilarial)

■ EPIDEMIOLOGY & DEMOGRAPHICS
PRIMARY LYMPHEDEMA:
- Found in 1.1:100,000 people <20 yr old.
- Females outnumber males 3.5:1.
- Incidence peaks between ages 12 to 16 yr old.

SECONDARY LYMPHEDEMA: See specific etiology (e.g., filariasis, breast cancer, prostate cancer)

■ PHYSICAL FINDINGS & CLINICAL PRESENTATION
Edema:
- Painless and progressive
  1. Initially, the edema is pitting and smooth; however, with advanced cases, the edema becomes nonpitting (this depends on the extent of fibrosis that has occurred).
  2. Elevation of the leg resolves the swelling in the early stages but not in the advanced stages.
- More often unilateral but depending on the etiology can be bilateral
- Not always restricted to the lower extremities but may involve the genitals, face, or upper extremities (e.g., arm swelling after mastectomy)
- Stemmer's sign (squaring of the toes caused by edema in the digits)
- "Buffalo hump" appearance of the dorsum of the foot
- Loss of the ankle contour, giving a "tree trunk" appearance of the leg (Fig. 1-235)
Skin:
- Hard, thick, leathery skin
- Occasional drainage of lymph
- Infections (cellulitis, lymphangitis, onychomycosis)

■ ETIOLOGY
Primary idiopathic lymphedema (thought to result from developmental abnormalities)
- Congenital lymphedema
  1. Detected at birth; involving one or both extremities, usually the entire leg
  2. May be familial (Milroy's disease)
- Lymphedema praecox
  1. Usually unilateral; occurring in the teenage years
  2. May be familial (Meige's disease)
- Lymphedema tarda
  1. Usually occurs after the age of 30 yr
- Browse describes a functional classification of the primary lymphedemas:
  1. Distal obliteration (found in 80% of cases)
  2. Proximal obliteration (found in 10% of cases)
  3. Hyperplasia (found in 10% of cases)
Secondary lymphedema
- Malignancy (breast, prostate, lymphoma)
- Inflammation (streptococci, filariasis)
- Trauma
- Radiation with lymph node removal

DIAGNOSIS

■ DIFFERENTIAL DIAGNOSIS
Exclude other causes of edema (e.g., cirrhosis, nephrosis, CHF, myxedema, hypoalbuminemia, chronic venous stasis, reflex sympathetic dystrophy, obstruction from abdominal or pelvic malignancy).

■ WORKUP
A detailed history and physical examination should help exclude most of the differential diagnosis.

■ LABORATORY TESTS
- BUN, Cr, liver function tests, albumin, urine analysis, TFTs are obtained to exclude possible systemic causes of edema.
- Noninvasive venous studies help exclude venous insufficiency.

■ IMAGING STUDIES
- Lymphoscintigraphy:
  1. Diagnostic image of choice
  2. Sensitivity and specificity of 100% in diagnosing lymphedema

- CT scan: to exclude malignancy leading to obstruction
- Lymphangiography:
  1. Available but rarely used
  2. May be requested by surgeons considering repair or excision of tissue for lymphedema
  3. Difficult to perform; most information can be obtained from the nuclear lymphoscintigram

TREATMENT

■ NONPHARMACOLOGIC THERAPY
Reduce leg swelling and size:
- Leg elevation
- Limb massage
- Pneumatic leg compression
Maintain edema-free state:
- Elastic support stockings that are properly fitted according to compression pressure and length are essential to prevent edema from returning.
- Compression pressures are graduated; most of the pressure is distal with less and less pressure from the stockings, moving proximally.
- Compression pressures range from 20 to 30 mm Hg, 30 to 40 mm Hg, 40 to 50 mm Hg, and 50 to 60 mm Hg. Most prefer 40 to 50 mm Hg for lymphedema.
- The length should cover the edematous site. Choices include below the knee, thigh-high, and pantyhose lengths.

■ ACUTE GENERAL Rx
- Diuretics, including furosemide 40 to 80 mg qd, may aid in reducing leg swelling but should be used only temporarily. Hydrochlorothiazide 25 mg qd can also be used for reducing edema or preventing leg swelling.
- Treat infections, such as lymphangitis (usually caused by group A streptococcus), with penicillin VK 250 mg qid for 10 days or erythromycin 250 mg qid in penicillin-allergic patients. If recurrent episodes of infection occur, many consider prophylaxis with penicillin VK 250 mg qid for 10 days at the beginning of each month. Clotrimazole 1% cream should be applied qd to dried fissured areas in between toes to prevent fungal infections.

- In secondary lymphedema, treating the underlying cause is indicated (e.g., prostate cancer, breast cancer). If the etiology is filariasis caused by the parasites *Wuchereria bancrofti* or *Brugia malayi,* treatment is diethyl-carbamazine citrate (DEC) 5 mg/kg in divided doses for 3 wk.

■ CHRONIC Rx
Surgery for chronic lymphedema is considered if:
- There is continued increase in leg size despite medical treatment.
- There is impaired leg function.
- There are recurrent infections.
- There is emotional lability secondary to the cosmetic appearance.
Surgical procedures are divided into two types:
- Those performed to improve lymph node drainage (e.g., anastomoses of the lymph system with the venous system)

- Those performed to excise the subcutaneous tissue (e.g., Charles' procedure, Thompson's procedure, and the modified Homans' procedure)

■ DISPOSITION
Lymphedema is a slowly progressive disorder that can lead to significant disfigurement of the extremities or other body parts.

■ REFERRAL
Consultation with vascular surgeons should be made if medical therapy for leg size reduction fails or if recurrent infections occur.

⚙ PEARLS & CONSIDERATIONS

■ COMMENTS
- It is important to remember that surgery is not a cure.

- Children and adolescents (along with parents and adults) should be encouraged to pursue a normal life, participating in school activities and sports (preferably noncontact, e.g., swimming).
- It should also be remembered that cases of lymphangiosarcomas have been associated, although rarely, with postmastectomy lymphedema.

REFERENCES
Lerner R: What's new in lymphedema therapy in America, *Int J Angioplasty* 7(3):191, 1998.

Rockson SG et al: American Cancer Society Lymphedema Workshop. Workgroup III: diagnosis and management of lymphedema, *Cancer* 83(12 suppl):2882, 1998.

Szuba A et al: Lymphedema classification, diagnosis, and therapy, *Vasc Med* 3(2):145, 1998.

Author: **Peter Petropoulos, M.D.**

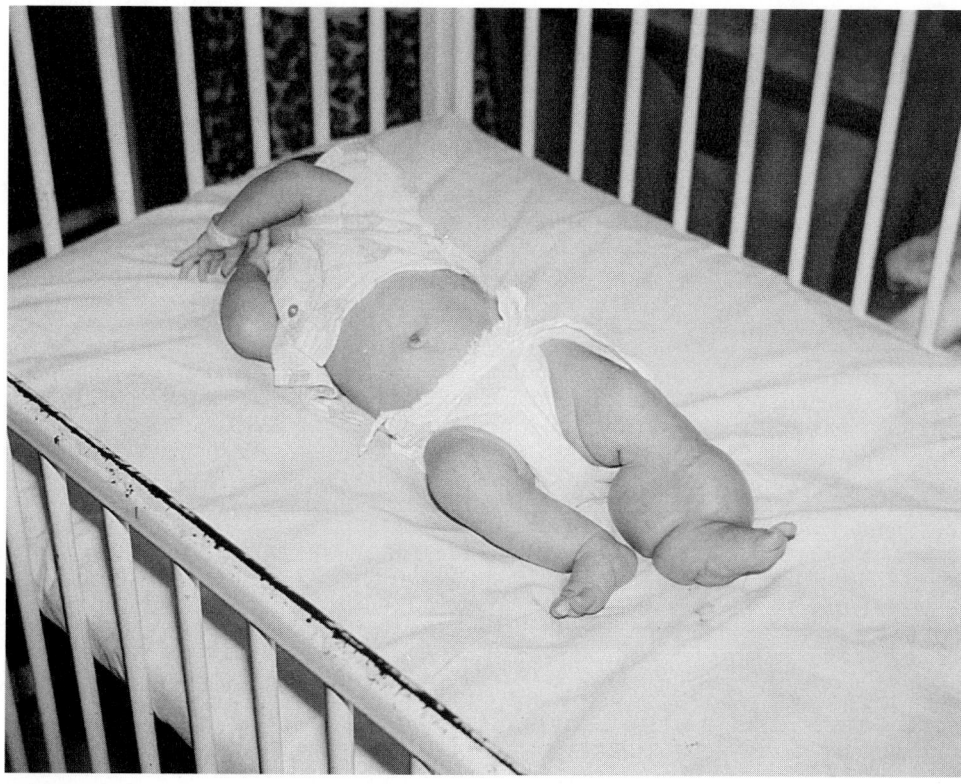

Fig. 1-235 Lymphedema. (From Seidel HM [ed]: *Mosby's guide to physical examination,* ed 4, St Louis, 1999, Mosby.)

BASIC INFORMATION

■ **DEFINITION**

Lymphogranuloma venereum (LGV) is a sexually transmitted, systemic disease caused by *Chlamydia trachomatis*.

■ **SYNONYMS**

Tropical bubo
Poradenitis inguinalis
LGV

ICD-9CM CODES

099.1 Lymphogranuloma venereum

■ **EPIDEMIOLOGY & DEMOGRAPHICS**

• Male:female ratio is 5:1
• LGV is rare in the U.S. (285 cases reported in 1993).
• LGV is endemic in Africa, India, parts of Southeast Asia, South America, and the Caribbean.

■ **PHYSICAL FINDINGS & CLINICAL PRESENTATION**

Primary stage:
• Primary lesion caused by multiplication of organism at site of infection
• Papule, shallow ulcer
• Herpetiform lesion at site of inoculation (most common)
• Incubation period of 3 to 21 days
• Most common site of lesion in women: posterior wall, fourchette, or vulva
• Spontaneous healing, without scarring

Second stage:
• Inguinal syndrome: characteristic inguinal adenopathy
• Begins 1 to 4 wk after primary lesion
• Syndrome is the most frequent clinical sign of the disease
• Unilateral inguinal adenopathy in 70% of cases
• Symptoms: painful, extensive adenitis (bubo) and suppuration may occur with numerous sinus tracts
• "Groove sign" signaling femoral and inguinal node involvement (20%); most often seen in men
• Involvement of deep iliac and retroperitoneal lymph nodes in women may present as a pelvic mass

Third stage (anogenital syndrome):
• Subacute: proctocolitis
• Late: tissue destruction or scarring, sinuses, abscesses, fistulas, strictures of perineum, elephantiasis

■ **ETIOLOGY**

Chlamydia trachomatis is the causative agent. There are three serotypes: L1, L2, and L3.

🔬 **DIAGNOSIS**

■ **DIFFERENTIAL DIAGNOSIS**

• Inguinal adenitis, suppurative adenitis, retroperitoneal adenitis, proctitis, schistosomiasis
• Table 2-84 describes the differential diagnosis of genital sores.

■ **WORKUP**

• Clinical manifestation
• Screening for other STDs
• A clinical algorithm for evaluation of genital ulcer disease is described in Fig. 3-85.

■ **LABORATORY TESTS**

• Positive Frei test:
  1. Intradermal chlamydial antigen
  2. Nonspecific for all *Chlamydia*
  3. No longer available (historical significance only)
• Complement fixation test:
  1. Titer >1:64 in active infection
  2. Convalescent titers no difference
• Cell culture of *Chlamydia*—aspiration of fluctuant node yields highest rates of recovery
• CBC—mild leukocytosis with lymphocytosis or monocytosis
• Elevated sedimentation rate
• VDRL and HIV screening to rule out other STDs

■ **IMAGING STUDIES**

• Barium enema: may reveal elongated structure of LGV
• CT scan for retroperitoneal adenitis

℞ **TREATMENT**

■ **NONPHARMACOLOGIC THERAPY**

• Avoid milk and milk products while taking medication.
• Practice sexual abstinence.
• Treat sexual partners.

■ **ACUTE GENERAL Rx**

• Doxycycline 100 mg PO bid × 21 days
• Erythromycin base 500 mg PO qid × 21 days
• Sulfisoxazole 500 mg PO qid × 21 days
• Surgical:
  1. Aspirate fluctuant nodes.
  2. Incise and drain abscesses.

■ **CHRONIC Rx**

• Longer course of therapy will be needed for chronic or relapsing cases, which may be caused by reinfection and/or inadequate treatment.
• A rectal stricture will require a colostomy.
• Surgery should be considered only after antibiotic treatment.

■ **DISPOSITION**

Good prognosis with early treatment, usually resulting in complete resolution of symptoms.

■ **REFERRAL**

Surgical consultation if patient develops obstruction, fistula, or rectal stricture. May need referral to plastic surgeon if patient has lymphatic obstruction.

☀ **PEARLS & CONSIDERATIONS**

■ **COMMENTS**

• Pregnant and lactating women should be treated with erythromycin regimen.
• Congenital transmission does not occur, but infection may be acquired through an infected birth canal.
• Patient education materials may be obtained through local and state health clinics.

REFERENCE

Centers for Disease Control and Prevention: Sexually transmitted diseases treatment guidelines, *MMWR* 47(RR-1), 1998.

Author: **George T. Danakas, M.D.**

BASIC INFORMATION

■ DEFINITION
Non-Hodgkin lymphoma is a heterogeneous group of malignancies of the lymphoreticular system.

■ SYNONYMS
NHL

■ ICD-9CM CODES
201.9 Lymphoma, non-Hodgkin

■ EPIDEMIOLOGY & DEMOGRAPHICS
- Median age at time of diagnosis: 50 yr
- Sixth most common neoplasm in the U.S. (56,000 new cases/yr)
- Increasing incidence with age

■ PHYSICAL FINDINGS & CLINICAL PRESENTATION
- Patients often present with asymptomatic lymphadenopathy.
- Approximately one third of NHL originates extranodally. Involvement of extranodal sites can result in unusual presentations (e.g., GI tract involvement can simulate PUD).
- NHL cases associated with HIV occur predominantly in the brain.
- Pruritus, fever, night sweats, weight loss are less common than in Hodgkin's disease.
- Hepatomegaly and splenomegaly may be present.

DIAGNOSIS

■ DIFFERENTIAL DIAGNOSIS
- Hodgkin's disease
- Viral infections
- Metastatic carcinoma
- A clinical algorithm for evaluation of lymphadenopathy is described in Figs. 3-106 and 3-107.
- Box 2-160 describes the differential diagnosis of lymphadenopathy.

■ WORKUP
Initial laboratory evaluation may reveal only mild anemia and elevated LDH and ESR. Proper staging of non-Hodgkin's lymphoma requires the following:
- A thorough history, physical examination, and adequate biopsy
- Routine laboratory evaluation (CBC, ESR, urinalysis, LDH, BUN, creatinine, serum calcium, uric acid, liver function tests, serum protein electrophoresis)
- Chest x-ray examination (PA and lateral)
- Bone marrow evaluation (aspirate and full bone core biopsy)

- CT scan of abdomen and pelvis; CT scan of chest if chest x-ray films abnormal
- Bone scan (particularly in patients with histiocytic lymphoma)
- Depending on the histopathology, the results of the above studies and the planned therapy, some other tests may be performed: gallium scan (e.g., in patients with high-grade lymphomas), liver/spleen scan, lymphangiography, lumbar puncture
- β-2 Microglobulin level, serum interleukin level

CLASSIFICATION: The Working Formulation of non-Hodgkin lymphoma for clinical usage subdivides lymphomas into low grade, intermediate grade, high grade, and miscellaneous (Table 1-45).
STAGING: The Ann Arbor classification is used to stage non-Hodgkin lymphomas (see "Hodgkin's Disease" in Section I). Histopathology has greater therapeutic implications in NHL than in Hodgkin's disease.

■ IMAGING STUDIES
See "Workup."

TREATMENT

■ ACUTE GENERAL Rx
The therapeutic regimen varies with the histologic type and pathologic stage. Following are the commonly used therapeutic modalities:
LOW-GRADE NHL (e.g., nodular, poorly differentiated):
1. Local radiotherapy for symptomatic obstructive adenopathy
2. Deferment of therapy and careful observation in asymptomatic patients
3. Single-agent chemotherapy with cyclophosphamide or chlorambucil and glucocorticoids
4. Combination chemotherapy alone or with radiotherapy: generally indicated only when the lymphoma becomes more invasive, with poor response to less aggressive treatment; commonly used regimens: CVP, CHOP, CHOP-BLEO, COPP, BACOP; addition of recombinant alpha interferon at low doses to chemotherapy prolongs remission duration in patients with low-grade NHL
5. New purine analogs (FLAMP, 2CDA): can be used in salvage treatment of refractory lymphomas
6. The anti-CD 20 monoclonal antibody rituximab is useful for treatment of relapsed or refractory low-grade or follicular B-cell non-Hodgkin lymphoma

INTERMEDIATE- AND HIGH-GRADE LYMPHOMAS (e.g., diffuse histiocytic lymphoma): Combination chemotherapy regimens (e.g., CHOP, PRO-MACE-CYTABOM, MACOP-B, M-BACOD)
1. High-dose sequential therapy is superior to standard-dose MACOP-B for patients with diffuse large-cell lymphoma of the B-cell type.
2. Dose-modified chemotherapy should be considered for most HIV-infected patients with lymphoma. As compared with treatment with standard doses of cytotoxic chemotherapy (M-BACOD), reduced doses cause significantly fewer hematologic toxic effects yet have similar efficacy in patients with HIV-related lymphoma.
- Three cycles of CHOP followed by involved-field radiotherapy may be superior to eight cycles of CHOP alone in patients with localized intermediate- and high-grade NHL.
- Granulocyte-colony stimulating factor (G-CSF): may be effective in reducing the risk of infection in patients with aggressive lymphoma undergoing chemotherapy
- Radioimmunotherapy with (^{131}I) anti-B1 antibody therapy for NHL either by itself or in combination with other treatments
- Treatment with high-dose chemotherapy and autologous bone marrow transplant: as compared with conventional chemotherapy, increases event-free and overall survival in patients with chemotherapy-sensitive non-Hodgkin lymphoma in relapse

■ DISPOSITION
- Patients with low-grade lymphoma, despite their long-term survival (6 to 10 yr average) are rarely cured, and the great majority (if not all) eventually die of the lymphoma, whereas patients with a high-grade lymphoma may achieve a cure with aggressive chemotherapy.
- Complete remission occurs in 35% to 50% of patients with intermediate- and high-grade lymphoma. Prognostic factors include the histologic subtype, age of patient, and bulk of disease.

REFERENCES
McCune SL et al: Monoclonal antibody therapy in the treatment of non-Hodgkin lymphoma, *JAMA* 286:1149, 2001.

Miller TP et al: Chemotherapy alone compared with chemotherapy plus radiotherapy for localized intermediate and high grade non-Hodgkin lymphoma, *N Engl J Med* 339:21, 1998.
Author: **Fred F. Ferri, M.D.**

TABLE 1-45   Classification Systems for Grading Lymphomas

KIEL CLASSIFICATION	WORKING FORMULATION	REVISED EUROPEAN-AMERICAN CLASSIFICATION
Low-grade malignancy	Low grade	B-cell lymphomas
Lymphocytic, CLL	A. Malignant lymphoma, small lymphocytic	
Lymphocytic, other	Consistent with chronic lymphocytic leukemia	B-CLL/SLL
Lymphoplasmacytoid		Lymphoplasmacytoid lymphoma
Centrocytic	B. Malignant lymphoma, follicular, predominantly small cleaved cell	Follicle center lymphomas
		Marginal zone lymphomas (MALT)
Centroblastic/Centrocytic		Mantle cell lymphoma
Follicular without sclerosis	Diffuse areas	
Follicular with sclerosis	Sclerosis	
Follicular and diffuse, without sclerosis	C. Malignant lymphoma, follicular mixed, small cleaved and large cell	
Follicular and diffuse, with sclerosis	Diffuse areas	Diffuse large B-cell lymphoma
Diffuse	Sclerosis	Primary mediastinal large B-cell lymphoma
Low-grade malignant lymphoma, unclassified	Intermediate grade	Burkitt's lymphoma
High-grade malignancy	D. Malignant lymphoma, follicular	T-cell lymphomas
Centroblastic	Diffuse areas	
Lymphoblastic, Burkitt's type	E. Malignant lymphoma, diffuse small cleaved cell	
Lymphoblastic, convoluted cell type		T-CLL
Lymphoblastic, other (unclassified) immunoblastic		Mycosis fungoides/Sézary syndrome
High-grade malignant lymphoma, unclassified	F. Malignant lymphoma, diffuse mixed, small and large cell sclerosis	
Malignant lymphoma unclassified (unable to specify high grade or low grade)	G. Malignant lymphoma diffuse	Peripheral T-cell lymphoma, unspecified
Composite lymphoma	Large cell	Angioimmunoblastic T-cell lymphoma
	Cleaved cell	Angiocentric lymphoma
	Noncleaved cell	Intestinal T-cell lymphoma
	Sclerosis	Adult T-cell lymphoma/leukemia
	High grade	Anaplastic large cell lymphoma
	H. Malignant lymphoma large cell, immunoblastic	Precursor T-lymphoid lymphoma/leukemia
	Plasmacytoid	
	Clear cell	
	Polymorphous	
	Epithelioid cell component	
	I. Malignant lymphoma lymphoblastic	
	Convoluted cell	
	Nonconvoluted cell	
	J. Malignant lymphoma small noncleaved cell	
	Burkitt's	
	Follicular areas	

From Abeloff MD: *Clinical oncology,* ed 2, New York, 2000, Churchill Livingstone.
B-CLL, B-cell chronic lymphoid leukemia; *MALT,* mucosa-associated lymphoid tumor; *SLL,* lymphoid leukemia; *T-CLL,* T-cell CLL.

BASIC INFORMATION

■ DEFINITION
Macular degeneration refers to a group of diseases associated with loss of central vision and damage to the macula. Degenerative changes occur in the pigment, neural, and vascular layers of the macula. The dry macular degeneration is usually ischemic in etiology, and a wet macular degeneration is associated with leakage of fluid from blood vessels.

ICD-9CM CODES
362.5 Degeneration of macula and posterior pole

■ EPIDEMIOLOGY & DEMOGRAPHICS
INCIDENCE (IN U.S.):
• Main cause of blindness in the U.S.
• Increases with age
PREVALENCE (IN U.S.): Varies, but approximately 5% of people <50 yr old have some signs of macular degeneration.
PREDOMINANT SEX: Male = female
PREDOMINANT AGE: >50 yr
PEAK INCIDENCE:
• 75 to 80 yr old
• Dramatic increases in incidence and prevalence with age until approximately 80% of people 75 yr or older have senile macular degeneration.
GENETICS:
• Different syndrome: senile macular degeneration is age related.
• Several rare neurologic syndromes are associated with macular degeneration.

■ PHYSICAL FINDINGS
• Decreased central vision.
• The most common abnormality seen in age-related macular degeneration (AMD) is the presence of drusen, or yellowish deposits deep to the retina (Fig. 1-236).

■ ETIOLOGY
• Pigmentary and vascular changes with exudate, edema, and scar tissue development
• Early in course, possible subretinal neovascularization

DIAGNOSIS

■ DIFFERENTIAL DIAGNOSIS
• Diabetic retinopathy
• Hypertension
• Histoplasmosis
• Trauma

■ WORKUP
Complete eye examination, including visual field and fluorescein angiography

■ LABORATORY TESTS
Evaluate for diabetes and other metabolic problems, as well as vascular diseases.

■ IMAGING STUDIES
None necessary

TREATMENT

■ NONPHARMACOLOGIC THERAPY
Laser treatment to stop progression of disease

■ ACUTE GENERAL Rx
Laser treatment

■ CHRONIC Rx
Repeated laser treatments

■ DISPOSITION
• Follow closely by ophthalmologist.
• If vision deteriorates, refer urgently to an ophthalmologist.

■ REFERRAL
To ophthalmologist early in the course of the disease if the sight is to be saved

PEARLS & CONSIDERATIONS

■ COMMENTS
The vision of only 1 out of 10 people can be saved, but the disease is so devastating that vigorous therapy should be attempted.

REFERENCE
Fine SL et al: Age-related macular degeneration, *N Engl J Med* 342:483, 2000.
Author: **Melvyn Koby, M.D.**

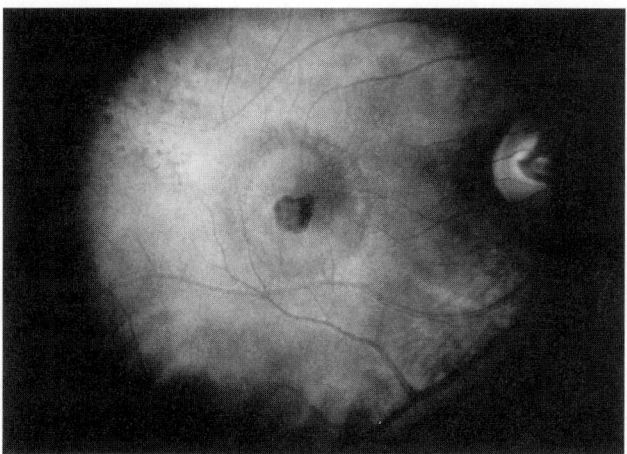

Fig. 1-236   Wet macular degeneration. (From Noble J: *Primary care medicine,* ed 3, St Louis, 2001, Mosby.)

BASIC INFORMATION

■ DEFINITION
Malaria is a febrile, flulike illness characterized by fever and chills and caused by one of the four species of the genus *Plasmodium,* which infect human RBCs and produce synchronous lysis.

ICD-9CM CODES
084.6 Malaria

■ EPIDEMIOLOGY & DEMOGRAPHICS
INCIDENCE (IN U.S.):
- Essentially none, although competent mosquito vectors are present (*Anopheles albimanus* in eastern U.S. and *A. freeborni* in western U.S.).
- Transmission is limited by absence of infected humans.
- Transmission at minimal levels, because imported cases of malaria provide the plasmodia for mosquito transmission.
  1. Following return of troops from endemic areas
  2. Following arrival of Southeast Asian refugees

PREVALENCE:
- Essentially none in the U.S.
- Possible for approximately 10% of population in hyperendemic areas to be infected at single time

PREDOMINANT AGE: <5 yr old (in Africans), any age in travelers.

GENETICS:
Familial Disposition: In sub-Saharan Africa, where *P. falciparum* kills 1 million children annually, survival is enhanced by the selective advantage afforded by sickle cell gene:
- Homozygous (HbSS) sickle cell anemia is often fatal.
- Heterozygous state (HbAS):
  1. Occurs with 25% prevalence
  2. Associated with diminished severe or complicated malaria, compared with normal (HbAA) peers, despite infection (probably caused by parasite growth within distorted SS-RBCs trapped in the hypoxic microvasculature)
- Duffy factor is absent from human RBCs in most of West Africa, conferring resistance to *P. vivax.*
- Other potential protective factors:
  1. Glucose-6-phosphate deficiency
  2. Thalassemia
  3. HLA-Bw53

■ PHYSICAL FINDINGS & CLINICAL PRESENTATION
ALL SPECIES:
- Fever (generally daily until synchronization of infection after several weeks, when periodic fevers may result)
- Rigors (especially non-*falciparum* strains)
- Diaphoresis
- Fatigue and malaise
- Nausea, vomiting

P. FALCIPARUM:
- Diarrhea (often bloody)
- Headache
- Seizures
- Coma
- Pulmonary edema
- Cardiogenic shock with hypotension
- Other metabolic complications

OTHER FINDINGS:
- Mild jaundice (from hemolysis)
- Liver tenderness
- Splenomegaly (especially with chronic infection)
- Pulmonary edema
- Nephrotic syndrome
- Uremia

■ ETIOLOGY
Four species of *Plasmodium:*
  1. *P. falciparum*
  2. *P. vivax*
  3. *P. malariae*
  4. *P. ovale*

GEOGRAPHIC DISTRIBUTION:
1. *P. falciparum*
   - Haiti
   - Papua New Guinea
   - Sub-Saharan Africa
   - India
2. *P. vivax*
   - Central America
   - Indian subcontinent
3. *P. vivax* and *P. falciparum*
   - South America
   - Eastern Asia
   - Oceania
4. *P. malariae*
   - Rare
   - Exists in most areas (especially Central and West Africa)
5. *P. ovale*
   - Africa

All are transmitted by the bite of the female anopheline mosquito.

LIFE CYCLE (FIG. 1-237):
- Sporozoites (formed in the mosquito following sexual maturation of ingested gametocytes to produce gametes, and ultimately to zygotes and sporozoites within salivary glands) are injected into humans with mosquito saliva during a bite.
- Sporozoites travel to the human liver via the bloodstream, enter hepatocytes (by binding parasite ligand and circumsporozoite protein), and mature to schizonts that rupture and release merozoites into the bloodstream, beginning the symptomatic, asexual erythrocytic (RBC) phase.
- Within the liver, an alternative maturation pathway allows some sporozoites of *P. vivax* and *P. ovale* to remain dormant as hypnozoites, which become active 6 to 11 mo later, generating hepatic schizonts, completing the hepatic cycle, and producing relapsing malaria.
- After attaching (via the parasite ligands Pv135 or EBA175) to specific RBC surface receptors (Duffy factor or glycophorin A), merozoites enter RBCs, utilize and degrade RBC intracellular proteins (including Hgb, which is reduced to malarial pigment in the parasitic food vacuole), and mature to rings to trophozoites to schizonts (containing multiple merozoites), which rupture, lysing the RBC and releasing merozoites (some of which reenter uninfected RBCs to amplify and perpetuate the infection, while others mature into gametocytes).
- While the gametocytes of *P. vivax, P. malariae,* and *P. ovale* appear as similar round forms, the banana-shaped gametocyte of *P. falciparum* is distinctive and diagnostic.

PATHOGENESIS:
- Parasites that evade splenic filtration induce a variety of cellular host defenses, including macrophage activation and release of tumor necrosis factor (TNF) and interleukins (IL 1, 6, 8).
- Microvascular disease is produced only by *P. falciparum,* resulting from cytoadherence of parasitized RBCs, via knobs that appear on their surface membranes, to endothelial cells (utilizing TNF-alpha-induced host receptor molecules thrombospondin, CD36, ICAM-1, VCAM-1, and ELAM-1), especially in capillaries of brain, kidneys.
- The nondeformable RBCs become sequestered and produce microvascular obstruction, accounting for the severe cerebral, renal, and occasional GI complications of *P. falciparum,* as well as the absence of its mature forms (schizonts, merozoites) on peripheral blood smears, and sheltering from splenic removal.
- Glucose consumption and lactate production (enhanced by the hypoglycemia effects of quinine or quinidine therapy, TNF-alpha, and probably IL-1 and TNF-beta) contribute to tissue acidosis.
- RBC lysis results from parasite and TNF-alpha effects and exposes glycosylphosphatidylinositol (GPI) anchors that stimulate TNF-alpha.
- Pulmonary edema may result from TNF-alpha-induced lung damage.
- These events, unique to *P. falciparum,* are consistent with clinical complications (cerebral malaria [seizures, coma], acute renal failure, severe anemia, pulmonary edema, diarrhea, hypoglycemia, lactic acidosis, cardiogenic shock, DIC) accompanying this species.

- *P. malariae* may cause nephrotic syndrome in children.
- *P. vivax* may produce late splenic rupture.

DIAGNOSIS

■ DIFFERENTIAL DIAGNOSIS
- Typhoid fever (both produce leukopenia and splenomegaly without localizing symptoms)
- Meningitis
- Pneumonia
- Influenza
- Cerebrovascular accidents
- Dengue
- Leishmaniasis
- Hepatitis
- Gastroenteritis
- Lymphoma
- Miliary tuberculosis

■ WORKUP
- CBC
- Blood smears for malaria parasites
- Blood cultures to rule out other causes of febrile illness (especially typhoid fever)

■ LABORATORY TESTS
- Careful, competent examination of Giemsa-stained peripheral blood smears (multiple over 3 days if initial smears are negative) for malarial parasites (Fig. 1-238)
  1. *P. falciparum*
     a. Produces monotony of ring trophozoites (fine, delicate rings with sparse cytoplasm opposite the dot [nucleus])
     b. Produces heavy (>5%) infestation with many parasitized RBCs of all ages, multiple rings/RBCs, double-chromatin dots/ring, peripheral (applique) adherence of ring to inside of RBC cell membrane
     c. Generally, schizonts and merozoites absent
     d. Occasionally diagnostic banana-shaped gametocytes
  2. *P. vivax*
     a. Produces rings with thicker cytoplasm opposite the dot (signet shaped)
     b. Produces lighter overall infestation
     c. Produces infection primarily of macrocytes (reticulocytes) and presence of all forms (including schizonts and merozoites)
  3. *P. malariae*
     a. Produces band forms (across the equator of the RBC)
     b. Produces rosette-formed schizonts
     c. Appears as *P. vivax*

  4. *P. ovale*
     a. Parasitizes senescent RBC with fringed edges
     b. Produces forms similar to *P. vivax*
- Fluorescent staining with Acridine Orange and DNA probes promises efficient and accurate future diagnostic tools.
- Leukopenia is common (its absence argues strongly against malaria as a diagnosis), as is thrombocytopenia, especially with *P. falciparum*.
- Possible associations with *P. falciparum*:
  1. Uremia (elevated creatinine)
  2. Severe anemia
  3. Proteinuria
  4. Hemoglobinuria
  5. Abnormal liver function tests
  6. Evidence of DIC (generally made worse with heparin therapy)
- Serologic testing is of limited value.

■ IMAGING STUDIES
- Generally not necessary
- Occasionally, brain CT scan to rule out other causes of coma or seizures

TREATMENT

■ NONPHARMACOLOGIC THERAPY
- DDT is no longer effective in most of the world, as a result of widespread mosquito resistance.
- Particularly in hyperendemic areas (e.g., Africa), increased efforts (especially including DEET repellents and insecticide [pyrethrin]-impregnated bed netting) are focused on diminishing anopheline mosquito exposure to gametocytes.

■ ACUTE GENERAL Rx
Adults
- Consult infectious disease expert.
- All strains of *P. vivax*, *P. malariae*, and *P. ovale* are sensitive to chloroquine.
- For *P. falciparum*, chloroquine resistance is the rule in most countries, with chloroquine-sensitive strains distributed only in Haiti/Dominican Republic, Central America west and north of the Panama Canal Zone, Paraguay and northern Argentina, Egypt, and the Middle East.
- *P. falciparum* strains are resistant to chloroquine plus Fansidar (sulfapyrimethamine) in Thailand, Myanmar (Burma), Cambodia, the Amazon Basin, and sub-Saharan Africa.
- Strains in Thailand are additionally resistant to mefloquine, leaving only tetracycline as an effective prophylactic agent.

- Chloroquine, quinine, and mefloquine are effective against RBC phase organisms.
- Primaquine eliminates persistent hepatic-phase forms (only *P. vivax* and *P. ovale*) and gametocytes (which produce no symptoms and need not be treated, except for epidemiologic reasons during massive epidemics).
- Chloroquine and primaquine doses often given in two rather confusing units:
  1. Weight of the compound (chloroquine phosphate or primaquine phosphate)
  2. Lesser weight of the base alone (chloroquine or primaquine)

TREATMENT OF *P. VIVAX, P. OVALE*:
  1. Chloroquine phosphate 1 g (600 mg base) PO at T_o, then 500 mg (300 mg base) at 6, 24, 48 hr (total dose = 2.5 g)
  2. Thereafter, primaquine phosphate 26.3 mg (15 mg base) PO qd × 14 days
     a. First dose given on the same day as last dose of chloroquine
     b. May induce severe hemolysis in G6PD-deficient individuals (test all recipients before treatment)

TREATMENT OF *P. MALARIAE* AND CHLOROQUINE-SENSITIVE *P. FALCIPARUM*:
  1. Chloroquine phosphate 1 g (600 mg base) PO at T_o, then 500 mg (300 mg base) at 6, 24, 48 hr (total dose 2.5 g)
  2. No primaquine needed, since no persistent liver phase exists

TREATMENT OF CHLOROQUINE-RESISTANT *P. FALCIPARUM*:
  1. Quinine sulfate 600 mg (500 mg base) PO tid × 3 to 7 days (10 days if malaria acquired in Southeast Asia) plus either doxycycline 100 mg PO bid × 7 days, or clindamycin 900 mg PO tid × 5 days. Quinine:
     a. May be difficult to obtain, and tablets may weigh only 260 mg
     b. Causes tinnitus, optic atrophy, delirium, hemolysis, diarrhea
  2. Alternative regimen: mefloquine 1250 mg PO in a single dose (25 mg/kg in Southeast Asia)
     a. Causes GI (abdominal pain, diarrhea), CNS (seizures, psychosis), and cardiac (arrhythmias; do not use if patient on β-blockers) toxicities
     b. Consultation with infectious disease expert
  3. Treatment if severely ill:
     a. Quinidine gluconate IV continuous infusion
     b. Loading dose 10 mg/kg over 1 to 4 hr; then maintenance dose 0.02 mg/kg/min by infu-

sion pump for 72 hr or until patient can swallow; then quinine PO to complete 7-day course
  c. Do not use loading dose if patient received quinine, quinidine, or mefloquine in past 24 hr
  d. Contraindication for steroids, as they prolong coma
  e. If no improvement in 24 hr, consider exchange transfusion
  f. Consultation with infectious disease expert

■ PREVENTIVE Rx
Adults
P. VIVAX, P. OVALE, P. MALARIAE, AND P. FALCIPARUM FROM CHLOROQUINE-SENSITIVE AREAS:
See regions above, "Acute General Rx"; *P. vivax, P. malariae, P. ovale*

- Chloroquine phosphate 500 mg (300 mg base [if >70 kg, 5 mg/kg]) PO once weekly
- Begin 1 wk before, and continue 4 wk after exposure
- In highly malarious areas, 100 mg base PO qd

P. FALCIPARUM **FROM CHLOROQUINE-RESISTANT AREAS:**
See regions above, "Acute General Rx"
- Consult infectious disease expert
- Mefloquine 250 mg PO weekly (duration: 1 wk before to 4 wk after exposure) *or*
- Doxycycline 100 mg PO qd (sole effective regimen for Thailand) *or*
- Chloroquine phosphate 500 mg (300 mg base) PO weekly plus proguanil 200 mg PO qd (if >70 kg, 3 mg/kg/day)

■ DISPOSITION
Follow-up blood smears to confirm cure if resistant *P. falciparum* was possibly the etiologic agent

■ REFERRAL
To infectious disease expert:
- Species identification requires experience.
- Differential diagnosis is often complex.
- Therapy requires precise knowledge of changing global sensitivity patterns of *P. falciparum* and familiarity with complexities and toxicities of drug therapy.
- All travels to malaria-endemic areas should see a travel medicine expert to correct chemoprophylaxis.

Author: **Peter Nicholas, M.D.**

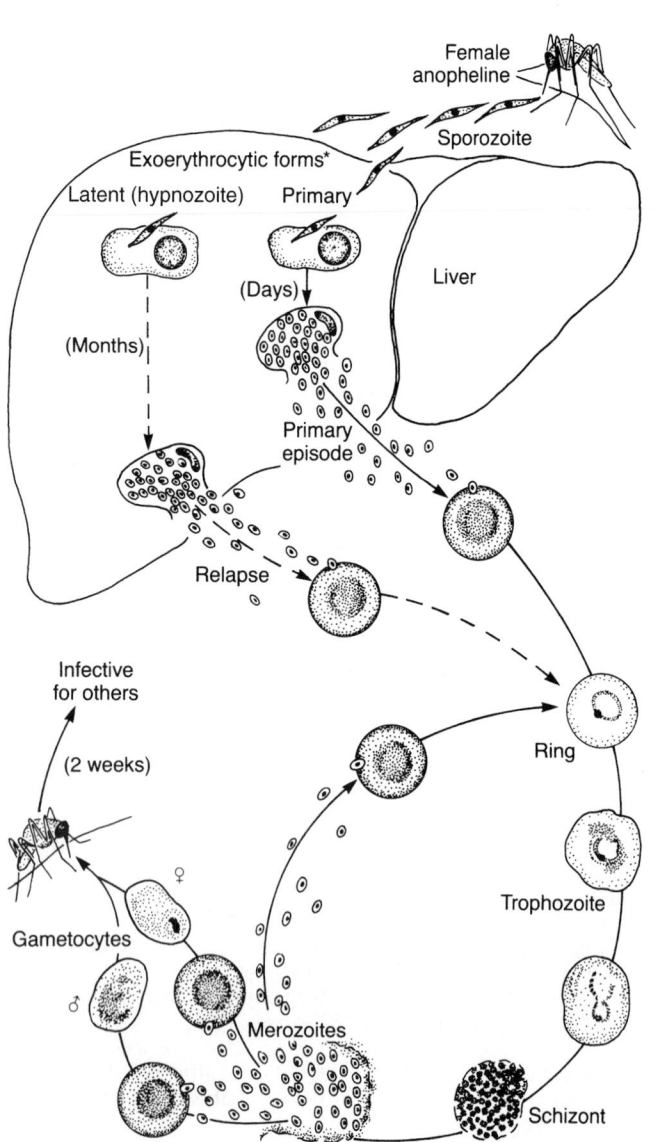

Fig. 1-237   Life cycle of plasmodia in humans. *Exoerythrocytic forms are also called tissue schizonts. (From Gorbach SL: *Infectious diseases,* ed 2, Philadelphia, 1998, WB Saunders.)

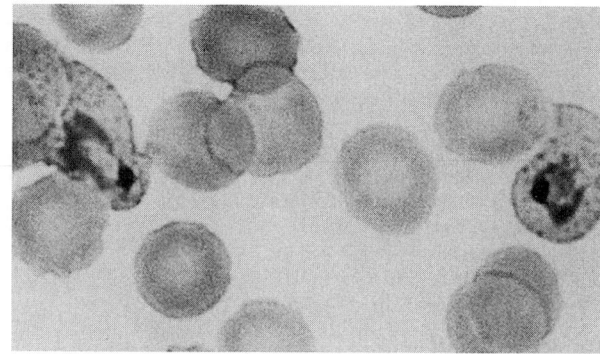

Fig. 1-238   Giemsa-stained blood smear in *Plasmodium vivax* malaria. Asexual parasites. Note that the parasites are large and ameboid, the infected erythrocytes are the largest cells in the field (because they are reticulocytes), and the erythrocytes contain numerous pink dots (Schüffner's dots) (×2000). (From Klippel JH et al [eds]: *Internal medicine,* ed 5, St Louis, 1998, Mosby.)

BASIC INFORMATION

■ **DEFINITION**
Marfan's syndrome is an inherited disorder of connective tissue involving skeleton, cardiovascular system, eyes, lungs, and central nervous system.

ICD-9CM CODES
759.82 Marfan's syndrome

■ **EPIDEMIOLOGY & DEMOGRAPHICS**
PREVALENCE: 1 case/10,000 persons
• Both sexes are affected equally by this autosomal dominant syndrome.
• Approximately 30% of cases are a new mutation.

■ **PHYSICAL FINDINGS & CLINICAL PRESENTATION**
Diagnostic criteria for Marfan's syndrome (Fig. 1-239):
• Skeleton
  Joint hypermobility, tall stature, pectus excavatum, reduced thoracic kyphosis, scoliosis, arachnodactyly, dolichosternomelia, pectus carinatum, and erosion of the lumbosacral vertebrae from dural ectasia†
• Eye
  Myopia, retinal detachment, elongated globe, ectopia lentis†
• Cardiovascular
  Mitral valve prolapse, endocarditis, dysrhythmia, dilated mitral annulus, mitral regurgitation, tricuspid valve prolapse, aortic regurgitation, aortic dissection,† dilation of the aortic root†
• Pulmonary
  Apical blebs, spontaneous pneumothorax
• Skin and integument
  Inguinal hernias, incisional hernias, striae atrophicae
• Central nervous system
  Attention deficit disorder, hyperactivity, verbal-performance discrepancy, dural ectasia, anterior pelvic meningocele†
  If the family history is positive for a close relative clearly affected by Marfan's syndrome, manifestations should be present in the skeleton and one of the other organ systems, and the diagnosis confirmed by linkage analysis or mutation detection.
  If the family history is negative or unknown, the patient should have manifestations in the skeleton, the cardiovascular system, and one other system, and at least one of the manifestations indicated by †.
  Manifestations are listed within each organ system in increasing speci-

ficity for Marfan's syndrome; although none is completely specific, those indicated by † are the most specific.

■ **ETIOLOGY**
Mutations in the gene that encodes fibrillin-1, the major constituent of microfibrils, which form the frame for elastic fibers. All the manifestations of Marfan's syndrome can be explained by the defective microfibrils.

🔬 **DIAGNOSIS**

■ **DIFFERENTIAL DIAGNOSIS**
Each of the clinical manifestations of the syndrome may have other causes; however, if the diagnostic criteria are met, the diagnosis is made.

■ **WORKUP**
• Echocardiography to establish:
  Mitral valve prolapse
  Mitral regurgitation
  Tricuspid valve prolapse
  Aortic regurgitation
  Dilation of the aortic root
• Chest x-ray

• Transesophageal echocardiography, chest CT scan, chest MRI, or aortography for suspected aortic dissection
• Chest x-ray for pulmonary apical bullae
• Ophthalmologic examination by ophthalmologist

💊 **TREATMENT**

• Regular cardiac and aorta monitoring by physical examination and echocardiography
• Endocarditis prophylaxis
• Restriction of contact sports, weight lifting, and overexertion
• β-Blockers
• Genetic counseling
• Monitor aorta during pregnancy (because of increased risk of dissection)

REFERENCE
Pyertiz ER: Marfan's syndrome. In Braunwald E (ed): *Heart disease: a textbook of cardiovascular medicine*, ed 5, Philadelphia, 1997, WB Saunders.
Author: **Tom J. Wachtel, M.D.**

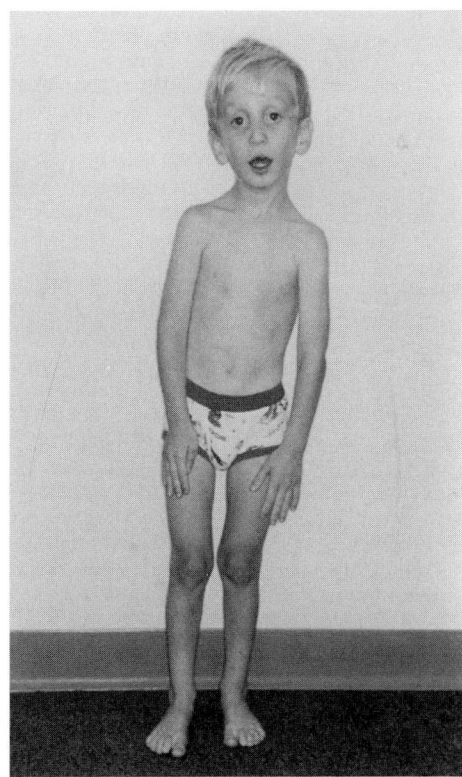

Fig. 1-239 Marfan's syndrome. Note the elongated facies, droopy lids, apparent dolichostenomelia, and mild scoliosis. (From Behrman RE: *Nelson's textbook of pediatrics*, Philadelphia, 1996, WB Saunders.)

BASIC INFORMATION

■ **DEFINITION**
Mastoiditis is inflammation of the mastoid process and air cells, a complication of acute otitis media.

ICD-9CM CODES
383.00 Mastoiditis, acute or subacute
383.1 Mastoiditis, chronic

■ **EPIDEMIOLOGY & DEMOGRAPHICS**
INCIDENCE (IN U.S.): Widespread use of broad-spectrum antibiotics has led to a marked decline in the incidence of acute mastoiditis
PREDOMINANT SEX: More common in males
PREDOMINANT AGE: 2 mo to 18 yr
PEAK INCIDENCE: Early childhood

■ **PHYSICAL FINDINGS & CLINICAL PRESENTATION**
- Acute mastoiditis is usually a complication of acute otitis media.
- Most common presenting symptom: pain and tenderness in the postauricular region.
- Other signs or symptoms include:
  1. Fever
  2. Postauricular erythema and edema
  3. Protrusion of the pinna inferiorly and anteriorly
  4. Tympanic membrane usually intact with signs of acute otitis media (occasionally ruptured with otorrhea)
- Complications of acute mastoiditis include:
  1. Subperiosteal abscess (most common complication)
  2. Hearing loss
  3. Facial nerve palsy
  4. Labrynthitis
  5. Intracranial complications such as hydrocephalus, meningitis, encephalitis, intracranial abscess, and lateral sinus thrombosis
- Chronic mastoiditis (which follows a long course of recurrent otitis media, treated but never controlled completely) is characterized by chronic otorrhea and chronic tympanic membrane perforation.

■ **ETIOLOGY**
- All patients with otitis media exhibit some degree of mastoid inflammation because of the continuity between the middle air space and the mastoid cavity.
- Initial hyperemia and edema of the mucosal lining of the air cells results in accumulation of purulent exudate.
- Dissolution of calcium from bony septae and osteoclastic activity in the inflamed periosteum lead to bone necrosis and coalescence of air cells. This process can result in the development of a subperiosteal abscess.
- Most common bacterial isolates:
  1. *Streptococcus pneumoniae*
  2. *Streptococcus pyogenes*
  3. *Haemophilus influenzae*
  4. *Moraxella catarrhalis*
  5. *Staphylococcus aureus*
- Often, multiple organisms in chronic mastoiditis, with predominance of anaerobes and gram-negative bacteria.
- *Mycobacterium tuberculosis* as well as nontuberculous mycobacteria have been isolated in cases of mastoiditis.
- Unusual organisms such as *Aspergillus* and *Rhodococcus equi* have been reported in cases of mastoiditis in severely immunocompromised individuals.

 DIAGNOSIS

■ **DIFFERENTIAL DIAGNOSIS**
- Children
  1. Rhabdomyosarcoma
  2. Histiocytosis X
  3. Leukemia
  4. Kawasaki syndrome
- Adults
  1. Fulminant otitis externa
  2. Histiocytosis X
  3. Metastatic disease

■ **WORKUP**
Thorough history and physical examination are important in establishing diagnosis.

■ **LABORATORY TESTS**
- Fluid for Gram stain and culture may be obtained by myringotomy.
- If there is a perforation in the tympanic membrane with drainage, cultures of this may be taken after carefully cleaning the external canal.

■ **IMAGING STUDIES**
- Plain x-rays of the mastoid region may demonstrate clouding or opacification in areas of pneumatization resulting from inflammatory swelling of the air cells.
- CT scan is the best radiologic modality for evaluating inflammation in this region.
- CT scan can demonstrate early involvement of bone (mastoiditis with bone destruction).
- MRI is more sensitive than CT scan in evaluating soft tissue involvement and is useful in conjunction with CT scan to investigate other complications of mastoiditis.

 TREATMENT

■ **NONPHARMACOLOGIC THERAPY**
Myringotomy, if the ear is not already draining

■ **ACUTE GENERAL Rx**
- Initiated with IV antibiotics directed against the common organisms *S. pneumoniae* and *H. influenzae*. If the disease in the mastoid has had a prolonged course, coverage for *Staphylococcus aureus* with gram-negative enteric bacilli may be considered for initial therapy until results of cultures become available.
- Continued until all signs of mastoiditis have resolved
- Directed against enteric gram-negative organisms and anaerobes in chronic mastoiditis
- Indications for mastoidectomy:
  1. Failure to improve after 24 to 72 hr of therapy
  2. Persistent fever
  3. Imminent or overt signs of intracranial complications
  4. Evidence of a subperiosteal abscess in the mastoid bone

■ **DISPOSITION**
Proceed with mastoidectomy when medical therapy fails.

■ **REFERRAL**
- To otorhinolaryngologist:
  1. If diagnosis in doubt
  2. If aural complications present
  3. To evaluate for surgical intervention
- To neurosurgeon if intratemporal or intracranial extension of infection suspected.
  1. Aural complications: bone destruction, subperiosteal abscess, petrositis, facial paralysis, labyrinthitis
  2. Intracranial complications: extradural abscess, lateral sinus thrombophlebitis or thrombosis, subdural abscess, meningitis, brain abscess, otitic hydrocephalus

REFERENCES

Carrasco VN, Pillsbury HC, Workman JR: Mastoiditis. In Johnston JT, Yu VL (eds): *Infectious disease and antimicrobial therapy of the ears, nose and throat,* Philadelphia, 1997, WB Saunders.
Lee ES et al: Clinical experiences with acute mastoiditis, 1988 through 1998, *Ear, Nose Throat J* 79(11):884, 2000.
Wang NE, Burg JM: Mastoiditis: a case-based review, *Pediatr Emerg Care* 14(4):290, 1998.
Author: **Marilyn Fabbri, M.D., and Jane V. Eason, M.D.**

BASIC INFORMATION

■ DEFINITION
Measles is a childhood exanthem, caused by an RNA virus called *Morbillivirus*, belonging to the family *Paramyxoviridae*.

■ SYNONYMS
Rubeola

ICD-9CM CODES
055.9 Measles
055.0 Encephalitis
055.1 Pneumonia
V04.2 Vaccination

■ EPIDEMIOLOGY & DEMOGRAPHICS
• Before the introduction of an effective vaccine in 1963, measles was one of the most common childhood illnesses, and in developing countries, where it strikes mostly children under age 5 yr, it remains a leading cause of childhood mortality.
• In developed countries, measles outbreaks occur occasionally in adolescents and young adults who have not been immunized.

■ PHYSICAL FINDINGS & CLINICAL PRESENTATION
• Incubation: 10 to 14 days (up to 3 wk in adults)
• Prodrome: 2 to 4 days; malaise, fever, rhinorrhea, conjunctivitis, cough
• Exanthem phase: 7 to 10 days
The fever increases and peaks at 104° to 105° F together with the rash; it persists for 5 or 6 days. The patient's fever decreases over 24 hr.
Rash: Erythematous maculopapular eruption begins behind the ears, progresses to the forehead and neck (Fig. 1-240), then spreads to face, trunk, upper extremities, buttocks, and lower extremities in that order. After 3 days the rash fades in the same sequence by becoming copper brown and then desquamates.
Enanthem: Koplik spots are white papules of 1 to 2 mm in diameter or an erythematous base. They first appear on the buccal mucosa opposite the lower molar 2 days before the rash and spread over 24 hours to involve most of the buccal and lower labial mucosa. They fade after 3 days.

Other symptoms and signs: malaise, anorexia, vomiting, diarrhea, abdominal pain, pharyngitis, lymphadenopathy, and occasional splenomegaly
• Atypical measles (in vaccinated persons)
Incubation: 10 to 14 days
Prodrome: 1 to 3 days; high fever and headache
Rash: maculopapular, urticarial, or petechial rash that begins peripherally and progresses centrally
• Modified measles applies to patients who have received immune serum globulin and develop a milder illness
• Complications:
Otitis media
Laryngitis, tracheitis
Pneumonia (accounts for 90% of measles deaths)
Encephalitis with lethargy, irritability, and seizures; 60% recover completely, 25% have neurologic sequelae (mental retardation, hemiplegia, paraplegia, epilepsy, deafness), and 15% die.
Myocarditis, pericarditis, and hepatitis
Complications more common in immunocompromised hosts and persons with AIDS

■ ETIOLOGY & PATHOGENESIS
• The measles virus is transmitted through the respiratory tract by airborne droplets.
• It initially infects the respiratory epithelium; the patient becomes viremic during the prodromal phase and the virus is disseminated to skin, respiratory tract, and other organs.
• Viral clearance is achieved via cellular immunity.

DIAGNOSIS

■ DIFFERENTIAL DIAGNOSIS
• Other viral infections by enteroviruses, adenoviruses, human parvovirus B-19, rubella
• Scarlet fever
• Allergic reaction
• Kawasaki disease

■ WORKUP
Knowledge of outbreak, history and physical findings (Koplik spots are diagnostic), laboratory tests

■ LABORATORY TESTS
• CBC: leukopenia
• ELISA for measles antibodies, which appear shortly after the onset of the rash and peak 3 to 4 wk later
• CSF analysis in encephalitis may reveal a pleocytosis (lymphocytes) and an elevated protein

■ IMAGING STUDIES
Chest x-ray if pneumonia is suspected

TREATMENT

• Supportive
• Vitamin A
• Ribavirin for severe measles pneumonitis

■ PREVENTION
• Passive immunization: Human immunoglobulin 0.25 ml/kg IM within 6 days of exposure. Double the dose for immunocompromised persons.
• Active immunization (see Table 5-6).

REFERENCES
Bernstein DI, Schiff GM: Measles. In Gorbach SL, Bartlett JG, Blacklow NR (eds): *Infectious diseases,* ed 2, Philadelphia, 1998, Saunders.
Epidemiology of measles—United States, *MMWR* 48:749, 1998.
Author: **Tom J. Wachtel, M.D.**

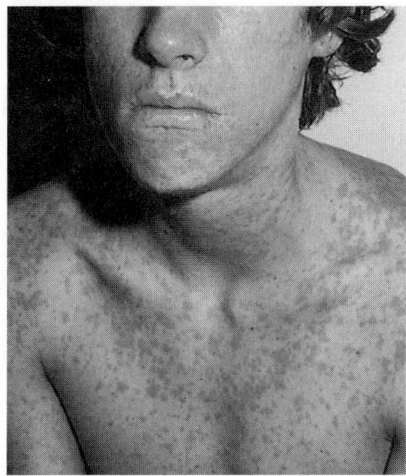
Fig. 1-240   Rubeola. (From Zitelli BJ, Davis HW: *Atlas of pediatric physical diagnosis,* ed 3, St Louis, 1997, Mosby.)

BASIC INFORMATION

■ **DEFINITION**

Meckel's diverticulum is an ileal diverticulum located 100 cm proximal to the cecum. It results from failure of the omphalomesenteric duct to obliterate completely (as it should by the eighth week of gestation). (Fig. 1-241)

ICD-9CM CODES
751.0 Meckel's diverticulum

■ **EPIDEMIOLOGY & DEMOGRAPHICS**

Meckel's diverticulum, based on autopsy studies, occurs in 1% to 3% of the population. Complications occur more frequently in males.

■ **PHYSICAL FINDINGS & CLINICAL PRESENTATION**

- Painless lower GI bleeding (4%)
- Intestinal obstruction secondary to intussusception, volvulus, herniation, or entrapment of a loop of bowel through a defect in the diverticular mesentery (6%)
- Meckel's diverticulitis mimics acute appendicitis (5%)
- Rare primary tumor arising from diverticulum (carcinoid, sarcoma, leiomyoma, adenocarcinoma)
- Asymptomatic (80% to 95%)

■ **ETIOLOGY & PATHOGENESIS**

As a remnant of the omphalomesenteric duct, Meckel's diverticulum contains all layers of the intestinal wall and has its own mesentery and blood supply (branch of the superior mesenteric artery). The mucosa is usually ileal or gastric.

 DIAGNOSIS

■ **DIFFERENTIAL DIAGNOSIS**

- Appendicitis
- Crohn's disease
- All causes of lower GI bleeding (polyp, colon cancer, AV malformation, diverticulosis, hemorrhoids)

Diagnosis is often made intraoperatively when the preoperative diagnosis is appendicitis. In the case of GI bleeding of unknown sources, a technetium scan will identify Meckel's diverticulum (sensitivity: 85% in children, 62% in adults; specificity: 95% in children, 9% in adults) (Fig. 1-242)

 TREATMENT

Surgical resection

REFERENCES

Keljo DJ, Squires RH: Meckel's diverticulum. In Feldman M, Scharschmidt BF, Sleisenger MH (eds): *Gastrointestinal and liver disease,* ed 6, Philadelphia, 1998, WB Saunders.

Martin JP et al: Meckel's diverticulum, *Am Fam Physician* 61:1037, 2000.

Author: **Tom J. Wachtel, M.D.**

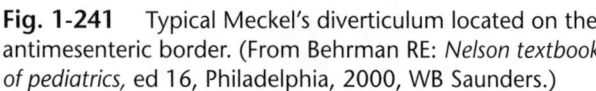 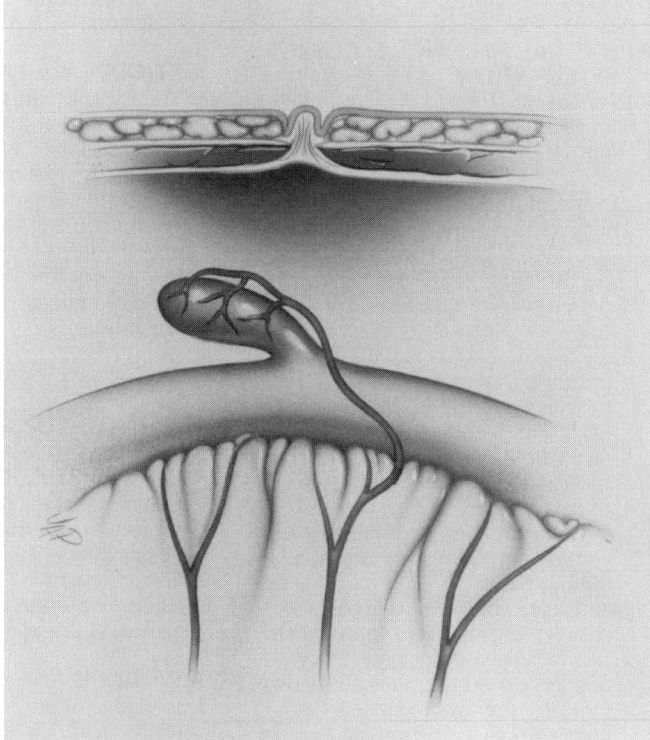

Fig. 1-241   Typical Meckel's diverticulum located on the antimesenteric border. (From Behrman RE: *Nelson textbook of pediatrics,* ed 16, Philadelphia, 2000, WB Saunders.)

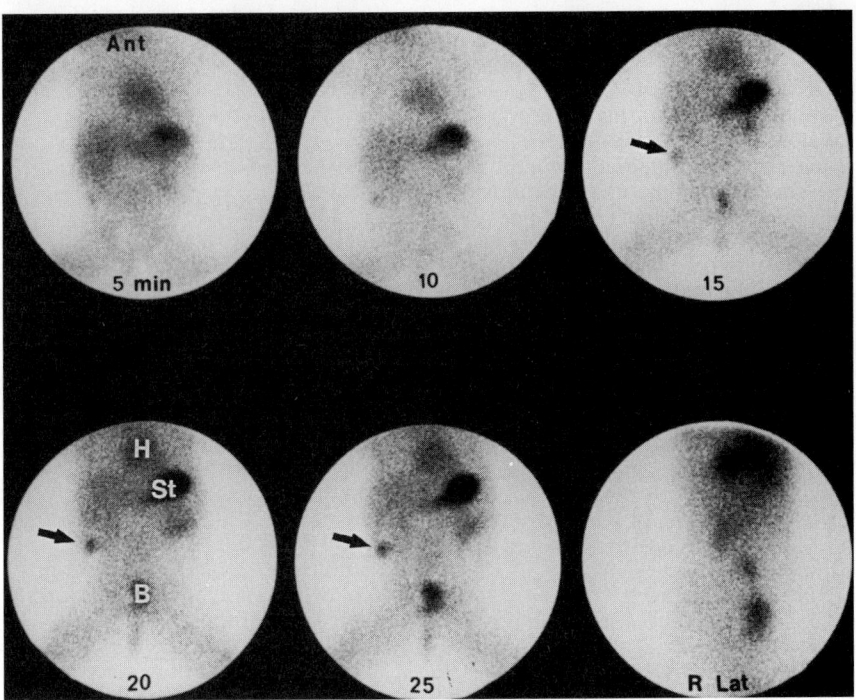

Fig. 1-242   Meckel's diverticulum. In this 2-year-old child who had unexplained rectal bleeding, a nuclear medicine study was performed using radioactive material that concentrates in gastric mucosa (technetium-99m pertechnetate). Sequential 5-minute images of the abdomen are obtained. On the 20-minute image, the heart (H), stomach (St), and bladder (B) are clearly seen, in addition to an ectopic focus of activity *(arrow)* representing a Meckel diverticulum. (From Mettler FA [ed]: *Primary care radiology,* Philadelphia, 2000, WB Saunders.)

BASIC INFORMATION

DEFINITION
Meigs' syndrome is characterized by the presence of a benign solid ovarian tumor associated with ascites and right hydrothorax that disappear after tumor removal.

ICD-9CM CODES
620.2 Ovarian mass (unspecified)
220.0 Benign ovarian lesion
789.5 Ascites
511.9 Pleural effusion

EPIDEMIOLOGY & DEMOGRAPHICS
- Occurs in <1% of ovarian fibromas (associated with approximately 0.004% of ovarian tumors)
- Most frequently encountered during middle age (average age, approximately 48 yr)

PHYSICAL FINDINGS & CLINICAL PRESENTATION
- Asymptomatic pelvic mass on bimanual examination
- Intermittent pelvic pain (intermittent torsion)
- Acute pelvic tenderness
- Acute abdominal tenderness
- Abdominal pelvic mass
- Abdominal bloating
- Fluid wave
- Shifting dullness
- "Puddle sign"
- Hyperresonance or flatness to chest percussion, absence of tactile and vocal fremitus
- Absent or loud bronchial breath sounds, rales, mediastinal displacement, tracheal shift
- Weight loss and emaciation

ETIOLOGY
- Not specifically known
- Usually associated with "edematous" fibromas (or other benign ovarian solid tumor) in excess of 10 cm
- Plausible that large fibroma with narrow stalk has inadequate lymphatic drainage; when coupled with intermittent torsion, results in back flow transudation into the peritoneal cavity; accumulated peritoneal ascites then passes to the right pleural cavity via lymphatics (overloaded thoracic duct) or via abdominal pleural commutation (i.e., foramen of Bochdalek)

DIAGNOSIS

DIFFERENTIAL DIAGNOSIS
- Abdominal ovarian malignancy
- Various gynecologic disorders:
  1. Uterus; endometrial tumor, sarcoma, leiomyoma ("pseudo-Meigs' syndrome")
  2. Fallopian tube: hydrosalpinx, granulomatous salpingitis, fallopian tube malignancy
  3. Ovary: benign, serous, mucinous, endometrioid, clear cell, Brenner tumor, granulosa, stromal, dysgerminoma, fibroma, metastatic tumor
- Nongynecologic (GI tract or GU tract tumor or pathology) causes of pelvic mass
  1. Ascites
  2. Portal vein obstruction
  3. IVC obstruction
  4. Hypoproteinemia
  5. Thoracic duct obstruction
  6. TB
  7. Amyloidosis
  8. Pancreatitis
  9. Neoplasm
  10. Ovarian hyperstimulation
  11. Pleural effusion
  12. CHF
  13. Malignancy
  14. Collagen-vascular disease
  15. Pancreatitis
  16. Cirrhosis

WORKUP
- Clinical condition characterized by ovarian mass, ascites, and right-sided pleural effusion
- Ovarian malignancy and the other causes (see "Differential Diagnosis") of pelvic mass, ascites, and pleural effusion to be considered
- History of early satiety, weight loss with increased abdominal girth, bloating, intermittent abdominal pain, dyspnea, nonproductive cough

LABORATORY TESTS
- CBC to rule out inflammatory process
- Tumor markers (CA-125, Hcg, AFP, CEA) to evaluate malignancy
- Chemical/LFT profile to evaluate metabolic or hepatic involvement

IMAGING STUDIES
- Pelvic sonography (color flow Doppler evaluation of adnexal mass)

to evaluate pelvic pathology (CT scan or MRI if etiology indeterminate)
- Chest x-ray examination
- ABG if respiratory compromise

TREATMENT

NONPHARMACOLOGIC TREATMENT
- Informed consent and proper preparation of patient for possible staging laparotomy (TAHBSO, omentectomy, possible bowel resection, pelvic/periaortic lymphadenectomy)
- Bowel prep if considering pelvic malignancy

ACUTE GENERAL Rx
Depending on clinical presentation, size of pelvic mass, amount of ascites, and pleural effusion:
- If pelvic mass <10 cm, minimal ascites/pleural effusion: consider diagnostic open laparoscopy (possible exploratory laparotomy) and salpingo-oophorectomy with removal of ovarian fibroma (tumor).
- If pelvic mass >10 cm, moderate/large amount ascites/pleural effusion: consider pleurocentesis if respiratory compromise (cytology: AFB) and exploratory laparotomy with salpingo-oophorectomy and removal of ovarian fibroma (tumor).
- Treat pelvic malignancy, GI or GU tumor as indicated.

CHRONIC Rx
- Resolution of ascites and right-sided pleural effusion after removal of ovarian fibroma
- No long-term follow-up for benign ovarian fibroma

DISPOSITION
Excellent progress and complete survival are expected.

REFERRAL
To gynecologist or gynecologic oncologist for evaluation and treatment, especially if malignancy considered or encountered
Author: **Dennis M. Weppner, M.D.**

BASIC INFORMATION

■ DEFINITION

Melanoma is a skin neoplasm arising from the malignant degeneration of melanocytes. It is classically subdivided in four types:
- Superficial spreading melanoma (70%) (Fig. 1-243, *A*)
- Nodular melanoma (15% to 20%) (Fig. 1-243, *B*)
- Lentigo maligna melanoma (5% to 10%)
- Acral lentiginous melanoma (7% to 10%)

■ SYNONYMS

Malignant melanoma

ICD-9CM CODES

172.9 Melanoma of the skin, site unspecified

■ EPIDEMIOLOGY & DEMOGRAPHICS

- Annual incidence of melanoma is 13 cases/100,000 persons.
- Lifetime risk of cutaneous melanoma for white Americans is 1/90.
- Melanoma is the leading cause of death from skin disease.
- Median age at diagnosis is 53 yr.
- Superficial spreading melanoma occurs most often in young adults on sun-exposed areas.
- Acral lentiginous melanoma is most often found in Asian-Americans and black Americans and is not related to sun exposure.
- Death rate for white men with melanoma is 3/100,000.

■ PHYSICAL FINDINGS & CLINICAL PRESENTATION

Variable depending on the subtype of melanoma:
- *Superficial spreading melanoma* is most often found on the lower legs, arms, and upper back. It may have a combination of many colors or may be uniformly brown or black.
- *Nodular melanoma* can be found anywhere on the body, but it most frequently occurs on the trunk on sun-exposed areas. It has a dark-brown or red-brown appearance, can be dome shaped or pedunculated; they are frequently misdiagnosed because they may resemble a blood blister or hemangioma and may also be amelanotic.
- *Lentigo maligna melanoma* is generally found in older adults in areas continually exposed to the sun and frequently arising from lentigo maligna (Hutchinson's freckle) or melanoma in situ. It might have a complex pattern and variable shape; color is more uniform than in superficial spreading melanoma.
- *Acral lentiginous melanoma* frequently occurs in soles, subungual mucous membranes, and palms (sole of the foot is the most prevalent site). Unlike other types of melanoma, it has a similar incidence in all ethnic groups.
- The warning signs that the lesion may be a melanoma can be summarized with the ABCD rules:
  A: Asymmetry (e.g., lesion is bisected and halves are not identical)
  B: Border irregularity (uneven, ragged border)
  C: Color variegation (presence of various shades of pigmentation)
  D: Diameter enlargement (>6 mm)

■ ETIOLOGY

- UV light is the most important cause of malignant melanoma.
- There is a modest increase in melanoma risk in patients with small nondysplastic nevi and a much greater risk in those with dysplastic lesions.

DIAGNOSIS

■ DIFFERENTIAL DIAGNOSIS

- Dysplastic nevi
- Solar lentigo
- Vascular lesions
- Blue nevus
- Basal cell carcinoma
- Seborrheic keratosis

■ WORKUP

- Perform excisional biopsy with elliptical excision that includes 1 to 2 mm of normal skin surrounding the lesion and extends to the subcutaneous tissue; incisional punch biopsy is sometimes necessary in surgically sensitive areas (e.g., digits, nose).
- The sentinel lymph node dissection (SLND) should be considered in patients with intermediate (1 to 4 mm) melanomas or high-risk skin tumors (Clark's level III or greater) to obtain information regarding a patient's subclinical lymph node status with minimal morbidity. It involves the use of radiologic lymphoscintigraphy to map lymphatic drainage from the site of the primary melanoma to the first "sentinel" lymph node in the region (Fig. 1-245). When properly performed, if the sentinel node is negative, the remaining lymph nodes in the region will not have metastages in more than 98% of cases.

■ LABORATORY TESTS

The pathology report should indicate the following:
- Tumor thickness (Breslow microstage)
- Tumor depth (Clark level [Fig. 1-244])
- Mitotic rate
- Radial growth rates vs. vertical growth rate
- Tumor infiltrating lymphocyte

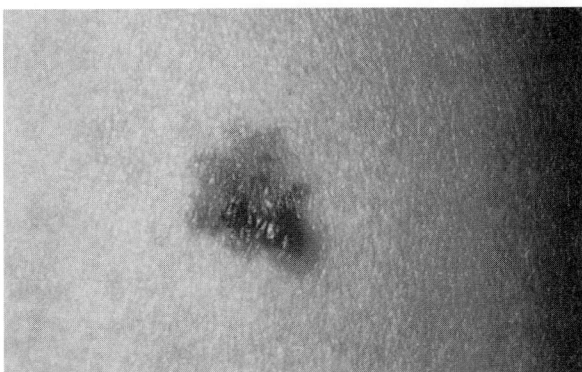
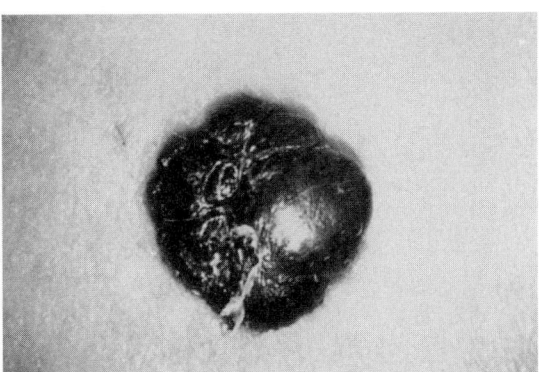

Fig. 1-243   A, Superficial spreading melanoma. **B,** Nodular melanoma. (From Abeloff MD: *Clinical oncology,* ed 2, New York, 2000, Churchill Livingstone.)

- Histologic regression
- Reverse transcriptase-polymerase chain reaction (RT-PCR) assay for tyrosine messenger RNA is a useful marker for the presence of melanoma cells. It is performed on sentinel lymph node biopsy and is useful for detection of submicroscopic metastases.

℞ TREATMENT

■ NONPHARMACOLOGIC THERAPY
Avoid excessive sun exposure; liberal use of sunscreens with UBV and UVA protection (recent laboratory data suggest that melanoma is promoted by UVA; therefore UVB sunscreens may not be effective in preventing melanoma).

■ ACUTE GENERAL Rx
- Initial excision of the melanoma
- Reexcision of the involved area after histologic diagnosis:
  1. The margins of reexcision depend on the thickness of the tumor.
  2. Low-risk or intermediate-risk tumors require excision of 1 to 3 cm.
  3. Melanomas of moderate thickness (0.9 to 2.0 mm) can be excised safely with 2-cm margins.
- Lymph node dissection: recommended in all patients with enlarged lymph nodes.
  1. Elective lymph node dissection remains controversial.
  2. It is indicated with positive sentinel node. It may be considered in those with a primary melanoma that is between 1 and 4 mm thick (especially in patients <60 yr old).

- Adjuvant therapy with interferon alfa-2b (intron A) is considered controversial in patients with metastatic melanoma. It is approved by the FDA for AJCC stages IIb and III melanoma; however, its statistical benefit remains unclear.

■ CHRONIC Rx
Patients with a history of melanoma should be followed with skin examinations every 6 mo or sooner if patient detects any new lesions; the assessments usually consist of medical history, physical examination, chest x-ray examination, and laboratory evaluation.

■ DISPOSITION
- Prognosis varies with the stage of the melanoma. Five-yr survival related to thickness is as follows: <0.76 mm, 99% survival; 0.6 to 1.49 mm, 85%; 1.5 to 2.49 mm, 84%; 2.5 to 3.9 mm, 70%; >4 mm, 44%.

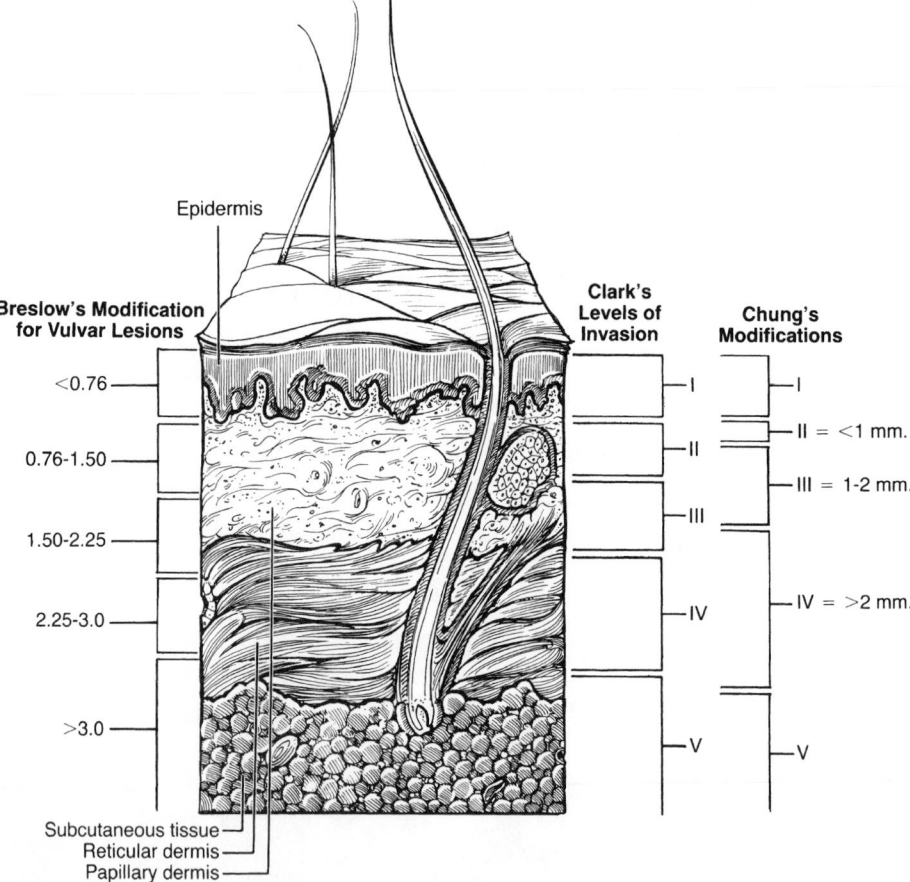

Fig. 1-244 Schematic comparison of the different levels of invasion for melanoma. (From Copeland LJ: *Textbook of gynecology,* ed 2, Philadelphia, 2000, WB Saunders.)

- The 5-yr survival in patients with distant metastasis is <10%.
- Treatment of advanced disease consists (in addition to surgical excision and lymph node dissection) of chemotherapy, immunotherapy, and radiation therapy.

REFERENCES

Cohn-Cederman et al: Long-term results of randomized study by the Swedish Melanoma Study Group on 2-cm versus 5-cm resection margins for patients with cutaneous melanoma with tumor thickness of 0.9-2 mm, *Cancer* 89:1495, 2000.

Goldstein BG, Goldstein AD: Diagnosis and management of malignant melanoma, *Am Fam Physician* 63:1359, 2001.

Jerant AF et al: Early detection and treatment of skin cancer, *Am Fam Physician* 62:357, 2000.

Kanzler MH, Mraz-Gernhard S: Treatment of primary cutaneous melanoma, *JAMA* 285:1819, 2001.

Shivers S et al: Molecular staging of malignant melanoma, *JAMA* 280:1410, 1998.

Whited JD, Grichnik JM: Does this patient have a mole or a melanoma? *JAMA* 279:696, 1998.

Author: **Fred F. Ferri, M.D.**

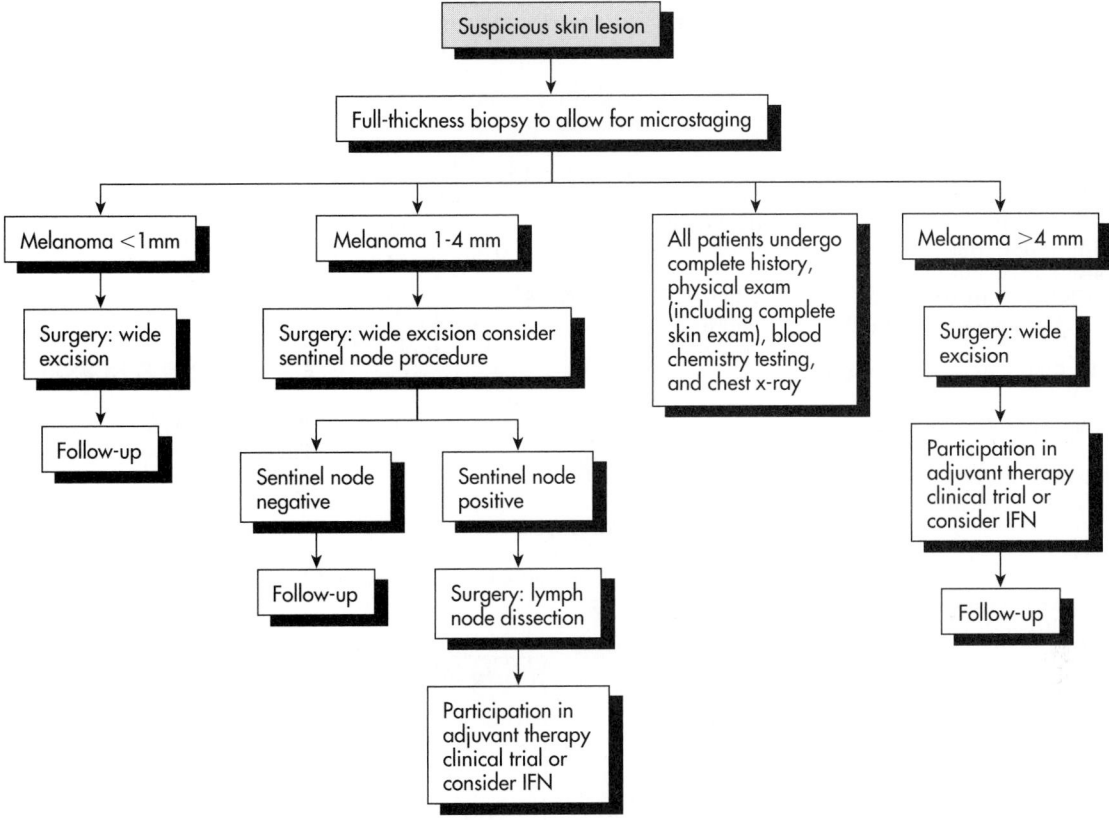

Fig. 1-245 Approach to the work-up and treatment of patients with newly diagnosed malignant melanoma. *IFN,* Interferon. (From Abeloff MD: *Clinical oncology,* ed 2, New York, 2000, Churchill Livingstone.)

BASIC INFORMATION

DEFINITION
Meniere's disease is a syndrome characterized by hearing loss, roaring noises in ear, and episodic dizziness associated with nausea and vomiting.

SYNONYMS
Endolymphatic hydrops
Lermoyez's syndrome
Meniere's syndrome or vertigo

ICD-9CM CODES
386.00 Meniere's disease, syndrome, or vertigo

EPIDEMIOLOGY & DEMOGRAPHICS
INCIDENCE (IN U.S.): 100 cases/100,000 persons
PREVALENCE (IN U.S.): 15 cases/100,000 persons
PREDOMINANT SEX: Male = female
PREDOMINANT AGE: Adults
PEAK INCIDENCE: 20 to 50 yr
GENETICS: Not known to be genetic

PHYSICAL FINDINGS & CLINICAL PRESENTATION
- Hearing may be unilaterally decreased.
- Pallor, sweating, and nausea may occur during a severe attack.

ETIOLOGY
- Unknown; viral and autoimmune etiologies have been suggested.
- Associated with endolymphatic hydrops.

DIAGNOSIS

DIFFERENTIAL DIAGNOSIS
- Acoustic neuroma
- Migrainous vertigo
- Multiple sclerosis
- Autoimmune inner ear syndrome
- Otitis media
- Vertebrobasilar disease
- Viral labyrinthitis
Box 2-75 describes the differential diagnosis of dizziness.

WORKUP
- Glycerol test and electrocochleography are used by some ENT specialists.
- A clinical algorithm for evaluation of hearing loss is described in Fig. 3-73.

LABORATORY TESTS
Audiometry suggests cochlear-type hearing loss and unilateral peripheral vestibular hypofunction (Fig. 1-246).

IMAGING STUDIES
MRI to rule out acoustic neuroma, especially if cerebellar or CNS dysfunction is present

TREATMENT

NONPHARMACOLOGIC THERAPY
Limit activity during attacks

ACUTE GENERAL Rx
- Prochlorperazine 5 to 10 mg PO q6h or 25 mg PO bid
- Promethazine 12.5 to 25 mg PO q4-6h
- Diazepam 5 to 10 mg IV/PO for acute attack
- Meclizine 25 mg q6h
- Scopolamine patch

CHRONIC Rx
No proven treatment, but diuretics, salt restriction, and avoidance of caffeine are traditional.

DISPOSITION
- Usually followed by ENT specialist.
- Usual course of disease consists of alternating attacks and remissions.
- Majority of patients can be managed medically. Less than 10% of patients will undergo surgical intervention for persistent incapacitating vertigo.

REFERRAL
If attacks persist

PEARLS & CONSIDERATIONS

COMMENTS
There is no proven medical or surgical therapy.
Author: **William H. Olson, M.D.**

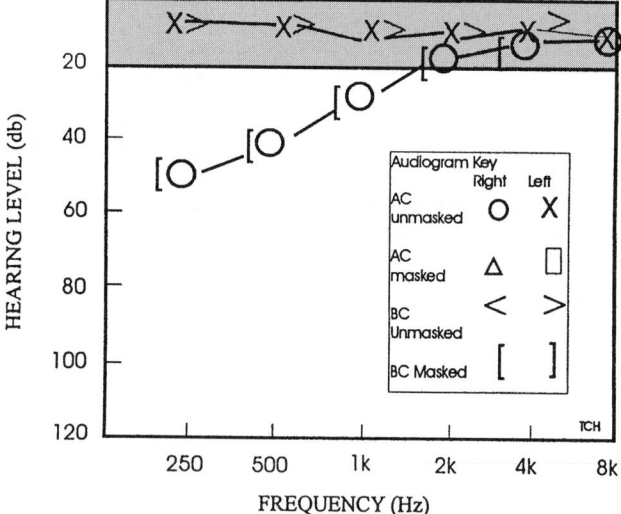

Fig. 1-246 Audiogram depicting the low tone sensorineural loss typical of Meniere's disease. The gray shaded area indicates the normal range. The left ear *(X)* is normal at all frequencies. The right ear *(circles)* has decreased hearing on both air and bone for lower frequencies. (From Goetz CG: *Textbook of clinical neurology,* Philadelphia, 1999, WB Saunders.)

BASIC INFORMATION

■ **DEFINITION**

A meningioma is an intracranial tumor arising from arachnoid cells.

ICD-9CM CODES
225.2 Cerebral meninges

■ **EPIDEMIOLOGY & DEMOGRAPHICS**

INCIDENCE (IN U.S.): 2 cases/100,000 persons/yr
PREVALENCE (IN U.S.): Not reported
PREDOMINANT SEX: Female:male ratio of 3:2 in adults; female = male in childhood
PREDOMINANT AGE: Males: sixth decade, females: seventh decade
PEAK INCIDENCE: >50 yr of age; rare in childhood
GENETICS: Associated with a missing sequence on chromosome 22

■ **PHYSICAL FINDINGS & CLINICAL PRESENTATION**

• Varies with location and size
• May be asymptomatic
• Seizures and hemiparesis common

■ **ETIOLOGY**

• Most are associated with an abnormality on chromosome 22.
• Cranial radiation may be responsible for some cases.
• Trauma and viruses are possible precipitants.

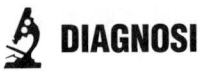 **DIAGNOSIS**

■ **DIFFERENTIAL DIAGNOSIS**

Other well-circumscribed intracranial tumors

■ **WORKUP**

Imaging studies followed by surgical removal with histologic confirmation if clinically indicated

■ **IMAGING STUDIES**

CT scan with contrast (Fig. 1-247) or MRI with contrast

■ **TREATMENT**

■ **NONPHARMACOLOGIC THERAPY**

Surgical removal if symptomatic

■ **ACUTE GENERAL Rx**

• Generally none
• Anticonvulsants to control seizures

■ **CHRONIC Rx**

• Radiation therapy may be beneficial in patients with incomplete resections or inoperable tumors.
• Hormonal treatments are under investigation.

■ **DISPOSITION**

• Estimated surgical mortality is 7%.
• Long-term outcome is variable, based on location and completeness of resection.
• Most incidentally discovered meningiomas remain asymptomatic. Calcified tumors may be less likely to progress than noncalcified ones.

■ **REFERRAL**

Neurosurgical consultation for all cases

REFERENCE

Gor S et al: The natural history of asymptomatic meningiomas in Olmsted County, Minnesota, *Neurology* 51:1718, 1998.
Author: **Michael Gruenthal, M.D., Ph.D.**

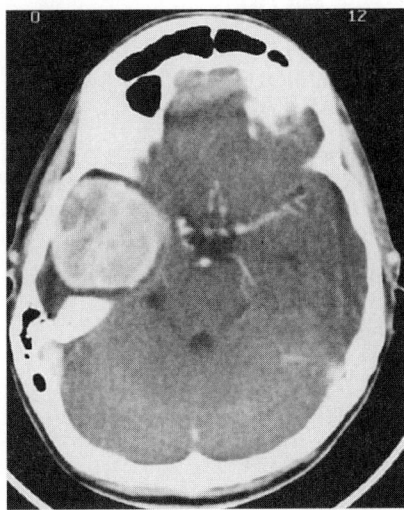

Fig. 1-247   Contrast-enhanced CT scan demonstrates a large contrast-enhancing right sphenoid wing meningioma. (From Specht N [ed]: *Practical guide to diagnostic imaging,* St Louis, 1998, Mosby.)

BASIC INFORMATION

■ DEFINITION
Bacterial meningitis is an inflammation of meninges with increased intracranial pressure, and pleocytosis or increased WBCs in CSF secondary to bacteria in the pia-subarachnoid space and ventricles, leading to neurologic sequelae and abnormalities.

■ ICD-9CM CODES
320 Bacterial meningitis

■ EPIDEMIOLOGY & DEMOGRAPHICS
INCIDENCE (IN U.S.): 3 cases/100,000 persons
PREDOMINANT SEX: Male = female
PREDOMINANT AGE: All ages, neonate to geriatric

■ PHYSICAL FINDINGS & CLINICAL PRESENTATION
- Fever
- Headache
- Neck stiffness, nuchal rigidity, meningismus
- Altered mental state, lethargy
- Vomiting, nausea
- Photophobia
- Seizures
- Coma; lethargy, stupor
- Rash: petechial associated with meningococcal infection
- Myalgia
- Cranial nerve abnormality (unilateral)
- Papilledema
- Dilated, nonreactive pupil(s)
- Posturing: decorticate/decerebrate

■ ETIOLOGY
Neisseria meningitidis is now more common than *Haemophilus influenzae* as a cause of bacterial meningitis in children as well as adults. *H. influenzae* is the cause of >30% of cases of meningitis (usually in infants and children <6 yr old). It is associated with sinusitis, otitis media.
- Neonates: group B streptococci, *Escherichia coli, Klebsiella* sp., *Listeria monocytogenes*
- Infants through adolescence:
  1. *N. meningitidis*
  2. *H. influenzae*
  3. *Streptococcus pneumoniae*
- Adults
  1. *N. meningitidis*
  2. *S. pneumoniae*
- Elderly
  1. *S. pneumoniae*
  2. *N. meningitidis*
  3. *L. monocytogenes*
  4. Gram-negative bacilli

DIAGNOSIS

Diagnostic approach is based on patient presentation and physical examination. Key elements to diagnosis are CSF evaluation and CT scan or MRI if the patient is in a coma or has focal neurologic deficits, pupillary abnormalities, or papilledema.

■ DIFFERENTIAL DIAGNOSIS
- Endocarditis, bacteremia
- Intracranial tumor
- Lyme disease
- Brain abscess
- Partially treated bacterial meningitis
- Medications
- SLE
- Seizures
- Acute mononucleosis
- Other infectious meningitides
- Neuroleptic malignant syndrome
- Subdural empyema
- Rocky Mountain spotted fever
- Table 2-38 describes CSF abnormalities in various CNS conditions.

■ WORKUP
CSF examination:
- Opening pressure >100 to 200 mm Hg
- WBC count: <5 to >100
- Neutrophilic predominance: >80%
- Gram stain of CSF: positive in 60% to 90% patients
- CSF protein: >50 mg/dl
- CSF glucose: <40 mg/dl
- Culture: positive in 65% to 90% cases
- CSF bacterial antigen: 50% to 100% sensitivity
- E-test for susceptibility of pneumococcal isolates

■ LABORATORY TESTS
Blood culturing, WBC with differential, and CSF examination (see "Workup")

■ IMAGING STUDIES
- CT scan or MRI of head: necessary with increased intracranial pressure, coma, neurologic deficits
- Sinus CT: if sinusitis suspected

TREATMENT

- Empiric therapy is necessary with IV antibiotic treatment if patient has purulent CSF fluid at time of lumbar puncture, is asplenic, or has signs of DIC/sepsis pending Gram stain and culture results. Therapy after Gram stain pending cultures is recommended for the following age and patient risk groups:
  1. Neonates: ampicillin plus cefotaxime
  2. Infants/children: ampicillin or third-generation cephalosporin (plus chloramphenicol if purulent or patient compromised)
  3. Adults (18 to 50 yr): third-generation cephalosporin
  4. Older adults (>50 yr): ampicillin plus third-generation cephalosporin
- Penicillin-resistant pneumococcus: because of an increasing incidence of this organism, empiric treatment with ceftriaxone or cefotaxime plus vancomycin (60 mg/kg/day) has been recommended.
- Table 1-46 describes common pathogens of bacterial meningitis and their empiric treatment based on age.
- Table 1-47 describes specific antibiotic treatments for unknown pathogens.
- Steroids: dexamethasone 0.15 mg/kg q6h for first 4 days of therapy should be used in adults with bacterial meningitis and mental status changes or acute neurologic phenomenon. Decreased mortality and neurologic sequelae are seen with adjunct therapy.
- Dexamethasone also benefits children with Hib or pneumococcal meningitis and should be given within the first 2 days of illness.

■ COMMENTS
Prevention of meningitis can be achieved through chemoprophylaxis of close contacts (household members and anyone exposed to oral secretions). Effective medications are rifampin 10 mg/kg PO bid for 2 days or ceftriaxone 250 mg IM single dose in patients over age 12; 125 mg IM if age 12 and under.
- Vaccines with antibodies against serogroup A, C, Y, W-135 capsular polysaccharides are available for adults and children over the age of 2 yr.

REFERENCE
Aronin SI et al: Community-acquired bacterial meningitis: risk stratification for adverse clinical outcome and effect of antibiotic timing, *Ann Intern Med* 129:862, 1998.
Author: **Dennis J. Mikolich, M.D.**

TABLE 1-46   **Common Pathogens of Bacterial Meningitis and Their Empiric Treatment Based on Age**

AGE	COMMON PATHOGENS	TREATMENT*	DURATION (DAYS)
0-1 mo	Group B streptococcus	Ampicillin + third-generation cephalosporin†	14-21
	Listeria monocytogenes	or ampicillin + aminoglycoside	14-21
	Escherichia coli		21
	Streptococcus pneumoniae		10-14
1-3 mo	Group B streptococcus,	Ampicillin + third-generation cephalosporin†	14-21
	E. coli, L. monocytogenes		14-21
	S. pneumoniae		10-14
	Neisseria meningitidis,		7-10
	Haemophilus influenzae		
3 mo-18 yr	*H. influenzae, H. meningitidis,*	Third-generation cephalosporin† or	7-10 (*N. influenzae* and
	S. pneumoniae	meropenem or chloramphenicol	*N. meningitidis*)
			10-14 (*S. pneumoniae*)
18-50 yr	*H. influenzae, N. meningitidis,*	Third-generation cephalosporin† or	Same as above
	S. pneumoniae	meropenem or ampicillin + chloramphenicol	
>50 yr	*S. pneumoniae, L. monocyto-*	Ampicillin + third-generation cephalosporin†	10-14 (*S. pneumoniae*)
	genes, gram-negative bacilli	or ampicillin + fluoroquinolone‡ or	14-21 (*L. monocytogenes*)
		Meropenem	21 Gram-negative bacilli
			other than *H. influenzae*

From Rakel RE (ed): *Principles of family practice,* ed 6, Philadelphia, 2002, WB Saunders.
*Add vancomycin in areas where there is greater than 2% incidence of highly drug resistant *S. pneumoniae.*
†Ceftriaxone or cefotaxime.
‡Ciprofloxacin or levofloxacin.

TABLE 1-47   **Specific Antibiotic Treatments for Known Pathogens**

PATHOGEN	PRIMARY THERAPY	ALTERNATIVE*
Group B streptococcus	Penicillin G or ampicillin	Vancomycin or third-generation cephalosporin†
Streptococcus pneumoniae (MIC < 0.1)	Third-generation cephalosporin†	Meropenem, penicillin
S. pneumoniae (MIC > 0.1)	Vancomycin + Third-generation cephalosporin*	Substitute rifampin for vancomycin; or meropenem; or vancomycin as monotherapy if highly allergic to other alternatives
Haemophilus influenzae (β-lactamase-negative)	Ampicillin	Third-generation cephalosporin† or chloramphenicol or aztreonam
H. influenzae (β-lactamase-positive)	Third-generation cephalosporin†	Chloramphenicol or aztreonam or fluoroquinolones‡
Listeria monocytogenes	Ampicillin + gentamicin	Trimethoprim-sulfamethoxazole
Neisseria meningitidis	Penicillin G or ampicillin	Third-generation cephalosporin†
Enterobacteriaccae	Third-generation cephalosporin† + aminoglycoside	Trimethoprim-sulfamethoxazole or aztreonam or fluoroquinolones or antipseudomonal penicillin (or ampicillin) + aminoglycoside
Pseudomonas aeruginosa	Ceftazidine + aminoglycoside	Aminoglycoside + aztreonam or aminoglycoside + antipseudomonal penicillin§
Staphylococcus aureus (methicillin-sensitive)	Antistaphylococcal penicillin¶ ± rifampin	Vancomycin + rifampin or trimethoprim-sulfamethoxazole + rifampin
S. aureus (methicillin-resistant)	Vancomycin + rifampin	
Staphylococcus epidermidis	Vancomycin + rifampin	

From Rakel RE (ed): *Principles of family practice,* ed 6, Philadelphia, 2002, WB Saunders.
MIC, Minimum inhibitory concentration.
*If patient is highly allergic or intolerant of primary therapy.
†Ceftriaxone or cefotaxime.
‡Ciprofloxacin or levofloxacin.
§Piperacillin, mezlocillin, or ticarcillin.
¶Nafcillin, oxacillin, or methicillin.

BASIC INFORMATION

■ DEFINITION
Viral meningitis is an acute aseptic meningitis usually with lymphocytic pleocytosis and negative CSF stains and cultures.

■ SYNONYMS
Aseptic meningitis

ICD-9CM CODES
047.8 Meningitis, aseptic

■ EPIDEMIOLOGY & DEMOGRAPHICS (TABLE 1-48)
INCIDENCE (IN U.S.): 11 cases/100,000 persons
PREDOMINANT SEX: Male = female
GENETICS: Those with abnormal humoral immunity and agammaglobulinemia have associated difficulty with viral clearance.

■ PHYSICAL FINDINGS & CLINICAL PRESENTATION
- Fever
- Headache
- Nuchal rigidity
- Photophobia
- Myalgias
- Vomiting
- Rash
- Diarrhea
- Pharyngitis

■ ETIOLOGY
- Enterovirus
- Mumps virus
- Measles
- Enteroviruses
- Arboviruses
- Herpes (simplex and zoster)
- HIV
- Lymphocytic choriomeningitis virus
- Adenovirus
- CMV
- Arthropod-borne viruses
- West Nile virus

DIAGNOSIS

The diagnostic approach is similar to bacterial meningitis (see "Bacterial Meningitis"); the foremost need is to rule out bacterial meningitis with CSF evaluation. Presentation may be similar to that of meningitis with bacterial involvement.

■ DIFFERENTIAL DIAGNOSIS
- Bacterial meningitis
- Meningitis secondary to Lyme disease, TB, syphilis, amebiasis, leptospirosis
- Rickettsial illnesses: Rocky Mountain spotted fever
- Migraine headache
- Medications
- SLE
- Acute mononucleosis/Epstein-Barr virus
- Seizures
- Carcinomatous meningitis
- Table 2-38 describes CSF abnormalities in various CSF conditions

■ WORKUP
CSF examination:
- Usually shows pleocytosis
- Lymphocytic predominance (polys in early stages)
- Opening pressure: 200 to 250 mm Hg
- WBC count: 100 to 1000
- Increased CSF protein
- Decreased or normal CSF glucose
- Negative Gram stain, cultures, CIE, latex agglutination
- No viral cultures routinely available; if patient is suspected of having mumps, serologic testing may be diagnostic; complement fixation used
- PCR for HSV, West Nile

■ LABORATORY TESTS
CBC with differential, blood culturing, and CSF examination (see "Workup")

■ IMAGING STUDIES
CT scan or MRI: if cerebral edema, focal neurologic findings develop

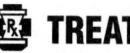

TREATMENT

No specific antiviral therapy for enterovirus, arbovirus, mumps virus; lymphocytic choriomeningitis virus is available. Treatment is supportive unless HSV is detected, which would be treated with IV acyclovir.

REFERENCE
Attia J et al: Does this adult patient have acute meningitis? *JAMA* 282:175, 1999.
Author: **Dennis J. Mikolich, M.D.**

TABLE 1-48 Epidemiology of Acute Viral Meningitis

	EPIDEMIOLOGIC FACTORS*			
SEASON	**PATIENT'S AGE (yr)**	**PATIENT'S SEX**	**RISK FACTOR**	**SUGGESTED VIRAL AGENT**
Summer-fall	Infant	—	Infected mother	Coxsackievirus B
	1-15	—	Swimming pools, closed communities	Enteroviruses
			Geographic area: California, southeastern United States	California serogroup virus
Winter	1-15	—	School exposure	Varicella virus, measles virus
		Male/female 3:1		Mumps virus
	16-21	—	College exposure	Measles virus
		Male/female 3:1		Mumps virus
		—		Epstein-Barr virus (mononucleosis)
	Any	—	Mice, rats, hamsters	Lymphocytic choriomeningitis virus
	Adults	—	Varicella-zoster	Varicella-zoster virus
Any	Any	—	Immunocompromise	Adenovirus
		—	Acquired immunodeficiency syndrome	Human immunodeficiency virus

From Gorbach SI: *Infectious diseases*, ed 2, Philadelphia, 1998, WB Saunders.
*Epidemiologic factors are suggestive but should not be used to exclude diagnoses in individual cases.

BASIC INFORMATION

■ DEFINITION
Meningomyelocele is a defective fusion of embryonal tissues resulting in a saclike protrusion containing meninges and spinal cord.

■ SYNONYMS
Meningocele (meninges only)

ICD-9CM CODES
741.9 Spina bifida without mention of hydrocephalus
741.9 Meningomyelocele

■ EPIDEMIOLOGY & DEMOGRAPHICS
INCIDENCE (IN U.S.): 2 cases/1000 births
PREVALENCE (IN U.S.): 50% death if untreated
PREDOMINANT SEX: Male = female
PREDOMINANT AGE: Infancy
PEAK INCIDENCE: Infancy
GENETICS: Autosomal recessive with possible environmental contribution

■ PHYSICAL FINDINGS & CLINICAL PRESENTATION
- Evident at birth—a sac protruding in lumbar region (Fig. 1-248)
- Usually, paralysis of lower extremity
- Relaxed rectal sphincter
- Constant urinary dribbling

DIAGNOSIS

■ DIFFERENTIAL DIAGNOSIS
Teratoma

■ WORKUP
Evaluate for other congenital abnormalities: heart, intestinal malformation, club foot, skeletal deformities.

■ LABORATORY TESTS
α-Fetoprotein in amniotic fluid or maternal serum

■ IMAGING STUDIES
- Lumbar x-rays (show spina bifida)
- Cervical spine films (Arnold-Chiari malformation)
- CT scan or MRI to show anatomy more precisely

TREATMENT

■ NONPHARMACOLOGIC THERAPY
- Surgical reduction
- Control of hydrocephalus (shunt)
- Management of urinary incontinence
- Correction of deformities
- Counseling of parents

■ ACUTE GENERAL Rx
Early correction is recommended.

■ CHRONIC Rx
Follow closely for development of hydrocephalus.

■ DISPOSITION
Usually followed by a team of specialists

■ REFERRAL
To neurosurgery for evaluation

PEARLS & CONSIDERATIONS

■ COMMENTS
- The decision for vigorous therapy in severely handicapped infants is beset with serious ethical considerations.
- Intrauterine repair of myelomeningocele decreases the incidence of hindbrain herniation and shunt-dependent hydrocephalus in infants with spina bifida, but increases the incidence of premature delivery.
- Folate during pregnancy may reduce incidence.

REFERENCE
Bruner JP et al: Fetal surgery for myelomeningocele and the incidence of shunt-dependent hydrocephalus, *JAMA* 282:1819, 1999.
Author: **William H. Olson, M.D.**

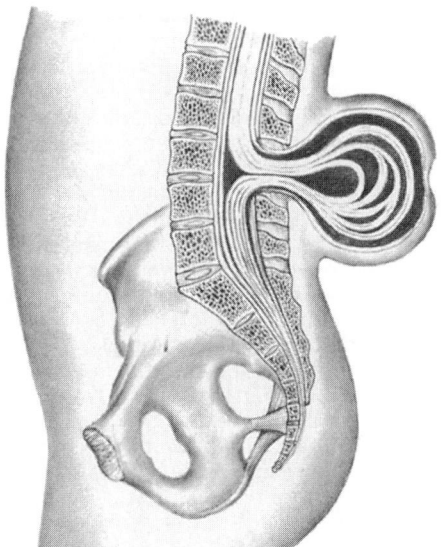
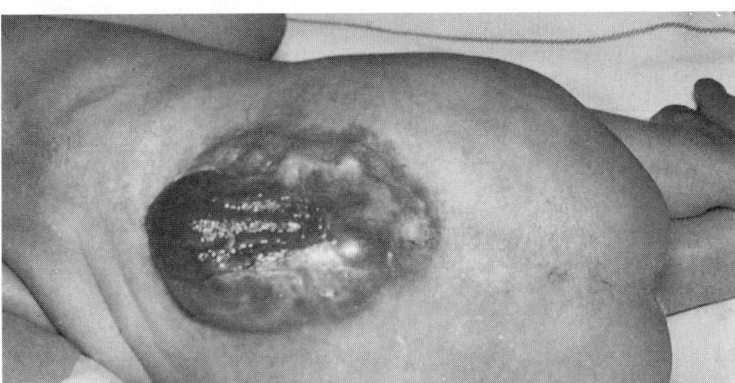

Fig. 1-248 Myelomeningocele. (From Wong DL: *Whaley's and Wong's nursing care of infants and children,* ed 5, St Louis, 1995, Mosby.)

BASIC INFORMATION

■ DEFINITION

Menopause is the occurrence of no menstrual periods for 1 yr after age 40 yr or permanent cessation of ovulation following lost ovarian activity. It is a climacteric reproductive stage of life marked by waxing and waning estrogen levels followed by decreasing ovarian function. Premature ovarian failure and no menstrual periods may also occur because of depletion of ovarian follicles before the age of 40 yr.

■ SYNONYMS

Change of life
Climacteric ovarian failure

ICD-9CM CODES

627 Premenopausal menorrhagia
627.2 Menopausal or female climacteric states
627.4 States associated with artificial menopause
716.3 Climacteric arthritis

■ EPIDEMIOLOGY & DEMOGRAPHICS

- Average age of menopause in the U.S. is 51 yr.
- Age at which menopause occurs is genetically determined.
- Smokers experience menopause an average of 1.5 yr earlier than non-smokers.
- More than one third of a woman's life will be spent after menopause.
- Onset of perimenopause is usually in a woman's mid- to late-40s.
- Approximately 4000 women each day begin menopause.

■ PHYSICAL FINDINGS & CLINICAL PRESENTATION

- Atrophic vaginitis, which can cause burning, itching, bleeding, dyspareunia
- Either complete cessation of menses or a period of irregular cycles and diminished or heavier bleeding
- Osteoporosis
- Psychologic dysfunction:
  1. Anxiety
  2. Depression
  3. Insomnia
  4. Nervousness
  5. Irritability
  6. Inability to concentrate
- Sexual changes, decreased libido, dyspareunia
- Urinary incontinence
- Vasomotor symptoms (hot flashes, flushes), night sweats, cardiovascular disease, coronary artery disease, atherosclerosis, headaches, tiredness, and lethargy

■ ETIOLOGY

- The most common etiology: physiologic, caused by degenerating theca cells that fail to react to endogenous gonadotropins, producing less estrogen; decreased negative feedback in the hypothalamic pituitary access, increased follicle-stimulating hormone (FSH), and increased luteinizing hormone (LH), which leads to stromal cells that continue to produce androgens as a result of the LH stimulation
- Surgical castration
- Family history of early menopause, cigarette smoking, blindness, abnormal chromosomal karyotype (Turner's syndrome, gonadal dysgenesis), precocious puberty, and left-handedness

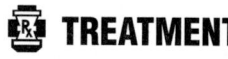

DIAGNOSIS

■ DIFFERENTIAL DIAGNOSIS

- Asherman's syndrome
- Hypothalamic dysfunction
- Hypothyroidism
- Pituitary tumors
- Adrenal abnormalities
- Ovarian abnormalities
- Polycystic ovarian syndrome
- Pregnancy
- Ovarian neoplasm
- TB

■ WORKUP

- If the clinical picture is highly suggestive of menopause, estrogen can be prescribed. If all symptoms resolve, then diagnosis has essentially been made. Before estrogen is prescribed, a complete history and physical examination are needed. If a patient has estrogen-dependent malignancy, unexplained abnormal uterine bleeding, history of thrombophlebitis, or acute liver disease, estrogen therapy is contraindicated.
- Progesterone challenge test: progesterone 100 mg is given IM to induce withdrawal bleeding. If no withdrawal bleeding is obtained, it would be safe to assume that a hypoestrogenic state is present.

- Physical examination, height, weight, blood pressure, breast examination, and pelvic examination are needed.
- Assess risk for coronary artery disease, osteoporosis, cigarette smoking, personal history, history of breast cancer, liver disease, active coagulation disorder, or any unexplained vaginal bleeding.

■ LABORATORY TESTS

- FSH, LH, and estrogen levels: if the FSH is markedly elevated and the estrogen level is markedly depressed, constitutes laboratory diagnosis of ovarian failure; LH only if polycystic ovarian disease is to be ruled out in a younger patient
- TSH to rule out thyroid dysfunction and prolactin level if patient has symptoms of galactorrhea and if suspicion of pituitary adenoma exists
- A general chemistry profile to check for any systemic diseases
- Pap smear, endometrial biopsy, or D&C in patients who have had irregular periods or intermenstrual or postmenopausal bleeding
- Mammogram

■ IMAGING STUDIES

- CT scan or MRI of head if pituitary tumor is suspected
- Bone density studies
- Pelvic ultrasound to check endometrial stripe

TREATMENT

■ NONPHARMACOLOGIC THERAPY

- A balanced diet: low in fat, with total fat intake being <30% of calories; total calories sufficient to maintain body weight or to produce weight loss if that is needed
- Avoidance of smoking, excessive alcohol or caffeine intake
- Exercise: weight-bearing exercise for osteoporosis prevention
- Kegel exercises for strengthening the pelvic floor
- Adequate calcium intake: 1500 mg qd is necessary to maintain zero calcium balance in postmenopausal women
- Change in the ambient temperature (may ameliorate hot flashes and reduce night sweats)

- Vitamin E
- Avoidance of caffeine, alcohol, and spicy foods if they trigger hot flashes
- Vaginal lubricants to help with the dyspareunia secondary to vaginal dryness (e.g., Replens, K-Y Jelly, or Gyne-Moistrin cream)

■ ACUTE GENERAL Rx
Estrogen replacement, which can be done in a variety of forms, including oral estrogen and transdermal estrogen patch.
- Examples of oral estrogen would include conjugated estrogens:
  1. Premarin: start with 0.625 mg qd and increase up to 1.25 mg qd, depending on symptoms. Cenestin (synthetic conjugated estrogens, A) available in 0.625-, 0.9-, and 1.25-mg doses.
  2. Estradiol (Estrace): start with 1 mg qd and increase to 2 mg qd; also available in 0.5 mg tablet for patients who experience side effects from the estrogen.
  3. Esterified estrogens (Estratab): start with 0.3 to 1.25 mg qd.
  4. Estropipate (Ogen, Ortho-Est): start with 0.625 to 1.25 mg qd.
  5. Esterified estrogen/testosterone combination: give 1.25 mg and methyltestosterone 2.5 mg (Estratest) and esterified estrogen 0.625 mg and methyltestosterone 1.25 mg (Estratest HS).
- If the patient has had a hysterectomy for benign disease, estrogen alone is sufficient. However, if she still has her uterus, progestin should be added for its protective effect against endometrial cancer. Medroxyprogesterone acetate (Provera) is the most commonly prescribed progestin. It can be prescribed in a continual daily dose of 2.5 mg or of 5 mg if continual breakthrough bleeding is encountered. This can also be prescribed in a 5-mg cyclic fashion for the first 14 days of the month or as 10-mg tablets for the first 10 days of the month. Patients need to be advised that this generally will cause withdrawal bleeding but in a fairly regular fashion. Continuous hormone replacement therapy is preferred, because after a period of time the patient should be amenorrheic. Patients should be counseled that they may experience some irregular spotting for the first 6 to 9 mo after starting the hormone replacement therapy.
- Combination oral preparations Femhrt ⅕ (1 mg norethindrone acetate/5 μg ethinyl estradiol) one pill daily.

Ortho—Prefest 1 mg 17β-estradiol (white pill) alternating with 1 mg 17β-estradiol and 0.9 mg norgestinate (pink pill) q3d
Prempro 0.625 mg conjugated estrogen/2.5 mg medroxyprogesterone one pill daily
Prempro 0.625 mg conjugated estrogen/5.0 mg medroxyprogesterone one pill daily
Activella 1 mg estradiol and 0.5 mg norethindrone acetate
Premphase 0.625 mg conjugated estrogen with 5 mg medroxyprogesterone last 14 days.
- Transdermal patches can be either estradiol (Estraderm, Vivelle, Fempatch) 0.025 to 0.1 mg applied twice weekly or Climara 0.025 to 0.1 mg used once a week. With these preparations, progesterone should be used in a similar fashion. Combipatch—apply twice weekly (combination estrogen and progesterone).
- Vaginal creams can be used, and these should be reserved for local therapy of atrophic vaginitis. Systemic absorption does occur; however, blood levels are unpredictable. Start with a loading dose of 2 to 4 g of estrogen-containing cream nightly for 1 to 2 wk. When symptoms improve, once to twice weekly is adequate maintenance.
- Vagifem estradiol vaginal tablets. Initial dosage: one Vagifem tablet, inserted vaginally, once daily for 2 wk. Maintenace dose: one Vagifem tablet, inserted vaginally, twice weekly.
- For women in whom estrogen is contraindicated or for those who do not wish to take estrogen, the following regimens can be used:
  1. Depo-Provera 150 mg IM every month (may be helpful in alleviating hot flashes)
  2. Clonidine 0.05 to 0.15 mg qd
  3. Bellergal-S
  4. Fosamax (alendronate sodium) 5 mg qd or 35 mg weekly is approved for prophylactic prevention of osteoporosis. Fosamax should be taken on an empty stomach; wait at least 30 min before ingesting any substance, including liquids, because this decreases its absorption into the body. Fosamax should be swallowed on arising for the day with a full glass of water, 6 to 8 oz, and patients should not lie down for at least 30 min and until after their first food of the day.
  5. Evista (Raloxifene) 60 mg daily PO has positive bone effect, a total cholesterol–lowering effect, and LDL cholesterol–lowering effect; it is a selective estrogen receptor agonist; it does not affect

estrogen receptors in the breast or uterus. It does not ameliorate vasomotor symptoms or vaginal atrophy.

■ CHRONIC Rx
Hormone replacement therapy should be lifelong unless the patient develops a contraindication to receiving hormone replacement therapy.

■ DISPOSITION
If treated, the patient should have resolution of her symptoms, reduced incidence of coronary artery disease, osteoporosis, and, most recently, reduction in the risk of developing Alzheimer's disease. Lifelong medical supervision is necessary to monitor adequacy of treatment and prevention of complications. This should include annual Pap smears, pelvic examinations, breast examinations, mammography, and endometrial sampling of any type of abnormal bleeding. If untreated, the vasomotor symptoms will eventually disappear; however, this takes many years, and some women who are in their 80s have experienced hot flashes. Urogenital atrophy will continue to worsen. Osteoporosis and coronary artery disease risks will increase with every passing year.

■ REFERRAL
Most menopausal women are managed by their gynecologist. However, this condition can be managed adequately by the patient's primary care physician who has an interest in treating menopausal women.

☼ PEARLS & CONSIDERATIONS

■ COMMENTS
Patient education materials can be obtained through the American College of Obstetricians and Gynecologists, 409 12th Street SW, Washington, DC 20024, and Menopause News, 2074 Union Street, San Francisco, CA 94123; phone: 1-800-241-MENO. Multiple patient educational brochures are produced by pharmacologic companies.

REFERENCES
Manson JE, Martin KA: Postmenopausal hormone-replacement therapy, N Engl J Med 345:34, 2001.
Soares C et al: Efficacy of estradiol for the treatment of depressive disorders in perimenopausal women: a double-blind randomized, placebo-controlled trial, Arch Gen Psychiatry 58:529, 2001.
Author: George T. Danakas, M.D.

BASIC INFORMATION

■ DEFINITION
Mesenteric adenitis is a painful enlargement of mesenteric lymph nodes.

ICD-9CM CODES
289.2 Mesenteric adenitis

■ EPIDEMIOLOGY & DEMOGRAPHICS
- Incidence unknown
- Affects mostly children (under age 18 yr) with no sex preference
- When *Yersinia* enterocolitis is the cause, boys are more frequently involved

■ PHYSICAL FINDINGS & CLINICAL PRESENTATION
- Abdominal pain of variable severity (mild ache to severe colic) beginning in upper abdomen or right lower quadrant, eventually localizes in right side but not in a precise location (unlike appendicitis)
- In *Yersinia* infection outbreaks, the symptoms include abdominal pain (84%), diarrhea (78%), fever (43%), anorexia (22%), nausea (13%), and vomiting (8%)

- Physical findings:
  Other lymphadenopathy (20% of cases)
  Right lower quadrant tenderness (site of maximum tenderness may vary from one examination to the next)
  Guarding (rare)
  Mild fever

■ ETIOLOGY & PATHOGENESIS
- Reactive hyperplasia of lymph nodes that drain the ileocecal region, similar to that seen in inflammatory or allergic conditions.
- *Yersinia enterocolitica, Yersinia pseudotuberculosis, Salmonella* species, *E. coli,* streptococci have been implicated with mesenteric adenitis.

DIAGNOSIS

■ DIFFERENTIAL DIAGNOSIS
- Acute appendicitis (5% to 10% of patients admitted to hospitals with a diagnosis of appendicitis are discharged with a diagnosis of mesenteric adenitis)
- Crohn's disease
Box 2-2 describes the differential diagnosis of abdominal pain.

■ LABORATORY TESTS
- CBC may show leukocytosis
- Abdominal sonography and helical appendiceal CT scan may be useful.
- Laparotomy if appendicitis is suspected

■ PROGNOSIS
Recurrent bouts are common; therefore, if laparotomy is performed and a normal appendix is found, it should be removed.

REFERENCES
Adam JT: Nonspecific mesenteric lymphadenitis. In Schwartz SE et al (eds): *Principles of surgery,* ed 6, New York, 1994, McGraw-Hill.
Pearson RD, Guerrant RL: Enteric fever and other causes of abdominal symptoms with fever. In Mandell GL (ed): *Mandell, Douglas, and Bennett's principles and practice of infectious diseases,* ed 5, New York, 2000, Churchill Livingstone.
Author: **Tom J. Wachtel, M.D.**

BASIC INFORMATION

DEFINITION
Mesenteric venous thrombosis (MVT) is a thrombotic occlusion of the mesenteric venous system involving major trunks or smaller branches and leading to intestinal infarction in its acute form.

ICD-9CM CODES
557.0 Mesenteric venous thrombosis

EPIDEMIOLOGY & DEMOGRAPHICS
Between 5% and 10% of patients with acute mesenteric infarction have mesenteric venous thrombosis. MVT is slightly more common in men than women. The typical age of occurrence is 50 to 60 yr.

PHYSICAL FINDINGS & CLINICAL PRESENTATION
Acute MVT
- Symptoms: abdominal pain in 90% of patients, typically out of proportion to the physical findings. Nausea and vomiting occur in 50% and GI bleeding occurs in 50% (occult), 15% (gross).
- Physical findings:
  Early: abdominal tenderness, decreased bowel sounds, abdominal distention
  Later: guarding and rebound tenderness, fever, and septic shock
Subacute MVT
- Symptoms: nonspecific abdominal pain for weeks or months
- Physical findings: none
Chronic MVT
- Symptoms: upper GI hemorrhage from bleeding varices
- Physical findings: none other than signs of blood loss if significant

ETIOLOGY & PATHOGENESIS
Hypercoagulable states (see "Hypercoagulable States" in Section I)
- Peripheral deep venous thrombosis
- Neoplasms
- Antithrombin III, protein C, protein S deficiencies
- Lupus anticoagulant (antiphospholipid antibody)
- Oral contraceptive use, pregnancy
- Polycythemia vera
- Thrombocytosis
Portal hypertension
- Cirrhosis
Inflammation
- Pancreatitis
- Peritonitis (e.g., appendicitis, diverticulitis, perforated viscus)
- Inflammatory bowel disease
- Pelvic or intraabdominal abscess
- Intraabdominal cancer
Postoperative state or trauma
- Blunt abdominal trauma
- Postoperative states (abdominal surgery)
Thrombosis may begin in small mesenteric branches (e.g., in hypercoagulable states) and propagate to the major venous mesenteric trunks, or begin in large veins (e.g., in cirrhosis, intraabdominal cancer, surgery) and extend distally. If collateral drainage is inadequate, the intestine becomes congested, edematous, cyanotic, and hemorrhagic and eventually may infarct.

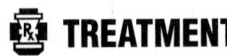 **DIAGNOSIS**

DIFFERENTIAL DIAGNOSIS
All other causes of abdominal pain (e.g., peritonitis, intestinal obstruction, pancreatitis, peptic ulcer disease, gastritis, inflammatory bowel disease, perforated viscus). Also to be considered in the differential diagnosis of GI hemorrhage.

WORKUP
Laboratory tests and imaging studies

LABORATORY TESTS
- CBC: leukocytosis
- Electrolytes: metabolic acidosis (lactic)
- Elevated amylase

IMAGING STUDIES
- Abdominal plain x-ray: ileus, ascites, bowel dilation, bowel wall thickening, loop separation, and thumbprinting
- Abdominal CT scan (diagnostic in 90%) (Fig. 1-249): bowel wall thickening, venous dilation, venous thrombus
- Arteriography if CT scan is not diagnostic
Occasionally the diagnosis is made by a laparotomy.

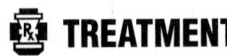 **TREATMENT**

- Anticoagulation or thrombolytic therapy
- Laparotomy if intestinal infarction is suspected
  Short ischemic segment: resection
  Long ischemic segment:
  1. Nonviable: resection or close
  2. Viable: intraarterial papaverine, and/or thrombectomy followed by "second look" intervention

PROGNOSIS
- Mortality of acute mesenteric venous thrombosis: 20% to 50%
- Recurrence rate: 15% to 25%

REFERENCE
Brandt LJ, Smithline AE: Ischemic lesions of the bowel. In Feldman M, Scharsachmidt BF, Sleisenger MH (eds): *Gastrointestinal and liver disease*, ed 6, Philadelphia, 1998, WB Saunders.
Author: **Tom J. Wachtel, M.D.**

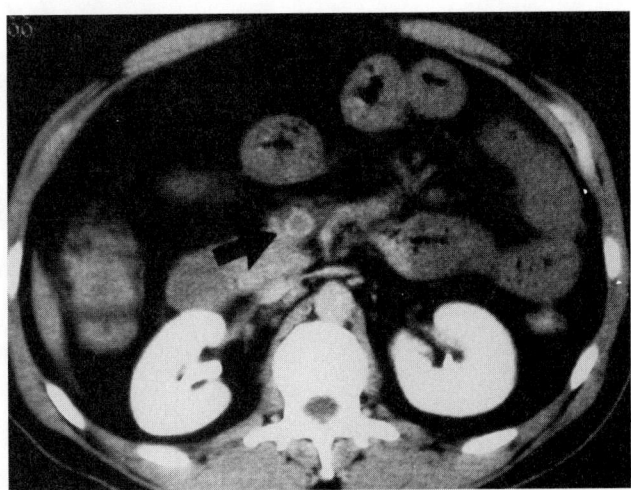

Fig. 1-249   This CT scan demonstrates thrombus within a dilated superior mesenteric vein *(arrow)*. Abdominal imaging techniques such as CT scan or duplex ultrasonography provide a direct examination of the mesenteric and portal veins. (From Sabiston D: *Textbook of surgery,* ed 15, Philadelphia, 1997, WB Saunders.)

BASIC INFORMATION

■ DEFINITION
Metatarsalgia refers to pain of the metatarsus, especially of the MTP articulation (Fig. 1-250). This is a nonspecific symptom usually involving the lesser toes.

ICD-9CM CODES
726.7 Metatarsalgia

■ PHYSICAL FINDINGS & CLINICAL PRESENTATION
- Pain beneath the metatarsal heads with ambulation
- Plantar callus formation beneath the metatarsal heads, usually involving one of the middle three toes
- Local tenderness
- Deformity
- Joint stiffness

■ ETIOLOGY
- Splayfoot
- Osteoarthritis, rheumatoid arthritis
- Freiberg's disease (avascular necrosis of second metatarsal head)
- Cavus foot (high arch)
- Bunion deformity
- Hallux rigidis
- MTP synovitis
- Morton's neuroma
- Often, no obvious cause

DIAGNOSIS

■ DIFFERENTIAL DIAGNOSIS
See "Etiology."

■ WORKUP
Underlying cause should always be sought.

■ LABORATORY TESTS
Rheumatoid factor may be required to rule out rheumatoid synovitis.

■ IMAGING STUDIES
Plain radiography to determine presence or absence of joint disease or deformity

TREATMENT

■ NONPHARMACOLOGIC THERAPY
- Metatarsal bar or pad proximal to heads to redistribute weight
- Extra-depth shoe for contracture or deformity, if present

- Soft orthotic or well-padded liner to diffuse pressure around metatarsal heads
- Relief pads for plantar keratoses
- Soaks and pumice stone abrasion to decrease callus volume
- Rocker bottom shoe for resistant cases

■ CHRONIC Rx
- NSAIDs
- Intraarticular injection in selected cases with joint involvement

■ DISPOSITION
Prognosis is variable, depending on etiology.

■ REFERRAL
Failure to respond to medical management

Author: **Lonnie R. Mercier, M.D.**

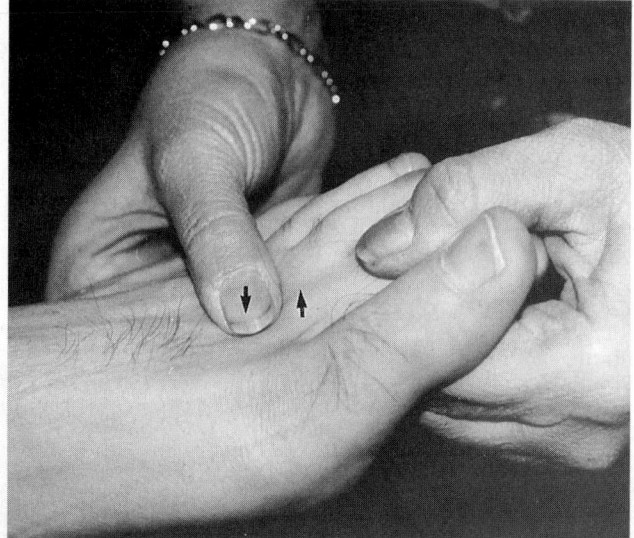

Fig. 1-250 Vertical stress test for metatarsophalangeal stability. One of the examiner's hands stabilizes the metatarsal head, whereas the other grasps the proximal phalanx. Examiner attempts to displace the proximal phalanx dorsally. A positive test result is the ability to displace dorsally while reproducing symptoms. (From Scuderi G [ed]: *Sports medicine: principles of primary care,* St Louis, 1997, Mosby.)

BASIC INFORMATION

DEFINITION

Mitral regurgitation (MR) is retrograde blood flow through the left atrium secondary to an incompetent mitral valve. Eventually there is an increase in left atrial and pulmonary pressures, which may result in right ventricular failure.

SYNONYMS

Mitral insufficiency
MR

ICD-9CM CODES

424.0 Mitral regurgitation

EPIDEMIOLOGY & DEMOGRAPHICS

The incidence of MR has increased over the past 30 yr; however, this may be because of increasing availability of echocardiography rather than any real increases in this condition.

PHYSICAL FINDINGS & CLINICAL PRESENTATION

- Hyperdynamic apex, often with palpable left ventricular lift and apical thrill
- Holosystolic murmur at apex with radiation to base or to left axilla; poor correlation between the intensity of the systolic murmur and the degree of regurgitation
- Apical early- to mid-diastolic rumble (rare)

ETIOLOGY

- Papillary muscle dysfunction (as a result of ischemic heart disease)
- Ruptured chordae tendineae
- Infective endocarditis
- Calcified mitral valve annulus
- Left ventricular dilation
- Rheumatic valvulitis
- Primary or secondary mitral valve prolapse
- Hypertrophic cardiomyopathy
- Idiopathic myxomatous degeneration of the mitral valve
- Myxoma
- SLE
- Fenfluramine, dexfenfluramine

DIAGNOSIS

DIFFERENTIAL DIAGNOSIS

- Hypertrophic cardiomyopathy
- Pulmonary regurgitation
- Tricuspid regurgitation
- VSD

- Table 2-35 describes the differential diagnosis of heart murmurs.

WORKUP

- Patients with MR generally present with the following symptoms:
  1. Fatigue, dyspnea, orthopnea, frank CHF
  2. Hemoptysis (caused by pulmonary hypertension)
  3. Possible systemic emboli in patients with left atrial mural thrombi associated with atrial fibrillation

  Diagnostic workup consists of echocardiography, ECG, and chest x-ray examination.

IMAGING STUDIES

- Echocardiography: enlarged left atrium, hyperdynamic left ventricle (erratic motion of the leaflet is seen in patients with ruptured chordae tendineae); Doppler electrocardiography will show evidence of MR. The most important aspect of the echocardiographic examination is the quantification of left ventricular systolic performance.
- Chest x-ray study:
  1. Left atrial enlargement (usually more pronounced in mitral stenosis)
  2. Left ventricular enlargement
  3. Possible pulmonary congestion
- ECG:
  1. Left atrial enlargement
  2. Left ventricular hypertrophy
  3. Atrial fibrillation

TREATMENT

NONPHARMACOLOGIC THERAPY

Salt restriction

ACUTE GENERAL Rx

- Medical: Medical therapy is primarily directed toward treatment of complications (e.g., atrial fibrillation) and prevention of bacterial endocarditis.
  1. Digitalis (for inotropic effect and to control ventricular response if atrial fibrillation with fast ventricular response is present)
  2. Afterload reduction (to decrease the regurgitant fraction and to increase cardiac output): may be accomplished with nifedipine, hydralazine plus nitrates or ACE inhibitors
  3. Anticoagulants if atrial fibrillation occurs

  4. Antibiotic prophylaxis before dental and surgical procedures (see Boxes 5-1 to 5-3 and Tables 5-25 and 5-26)
- Surgery: Surgery is the only definitive treatment for MR. Transesophageal echocardiography allows accurate assessment of the feasibility of valve repair and is indicated before surgical intervention. The timing of surgical repair is controversial; generally surgery should be considered early in symptomatic patients despite optimal medical therapy and in patients with moderate to severe MR and minimal symptoms if there is echocardiographic evidence of rapidly progressive increase in left ventricular end-diastolic and end-systolic dimension (echocardiographic evidence of systolic failure includes end-systolic dimension >55 mm and fractional shortening <31%). Surgery is also indicated in asymptomatic patients with preserved ventricular function if there is a high likelihood of valve repair or if there is evidence of pulmonary hypertension or recent atrial fibrillation.

DISPOSITION

Prognosis is generally good unless there is significant impairment of left ventricle or significantly elevated pulmonary artery pressures. Most patients remain asymptomatic for many years (average interval from diagnosis to onset of symptoms is 16 yr.)

REFERRAL

Surgical referral in selected patients (see "Acute General Rx"); emergency surgery may be necessary in patients with MR caused by ruptured chordae tendineae following MI.

PEARLS & CONSIDERATIONS

COMMENTS

Patients should be counseled regarding weight reduction (if obese), avoidance of tobacco, and maintenance of normal (nonstrenuous) activities.

REFERENCE

Otto CM: Evaluation and management of chronic mitral regurgitation, *N Engl J Med* 345:740, 2001.
Author: **Fred F. Ferri, M.D.**

BASIC INFORMATION

■ DEFINITION

Mitral stenosis is a narrowing of the mitral valve orifice. The cross section of a normal orifice measures 4 to 6 cm^2. A murmur becomes audible when the valve orifice becomes smaller than 2 cm^2. When the orifice approaches 1 cm^2, the condition becomes critical, and symptoms become more evident.

■ SYNONYMS

MS

■ ICD-9CM CODES

394.0 Mitral stenosis

■ EPIDEMIOLOGY & DEMOGRAPHICS

- The occurrence of mitral valve stenosis has decreased worldwide over the past 30 yr (particularly in developed countries) as a result of declining incidence of rheumatic fever.
- The incidence of mitral stenosis is higher in women.

■ PHYSICAL FINDINGS & CLINICAL PRESENTATION

- Prominent jugular A waves are present in patients with normal sinus rhythm.
- Opening snap occurs in early diastole; a short (<0.07-second) A$_2$ to opening snap interval indicates severe mitral stenosis.
- Apical middiastolic or presystolic rumble that does not radiate is present.
- Accentuated S$_1$ (because of delayed and forceful closure of the valve) is present.
- If pulmonary hypertension is present, there may be an accentuated P$_2$ and/or a soft, early diastolic decrescendo murmur (Graham Steell murmur) caused by pulmonary regurgitation (it is best heard along the left sternal border and may be confused with aortic regurgitation).
- A palpable right ventricular heave may be present at the left sternal border.
- Patients with mitral stenosis usually have symptoms of left-sided heart failure: dyspnea on exertion, PND, orthopnea.
- Right ventricular dysfunction (in late stages) may be manifested by peripheral edema, enlarged and pulsatile liver, and ascites.

■ ETIOLOGY

- Progressive fibrosis, scarring, and calcification of the valve
- Rheumatic fever (still a common cause in underdeveloped countries); heart valves most frequently affected in rheumatic heart disease (in descending order of occurrence): mitral, aortic, tricuspid, and pulmonary
- Congenital defect (parachute valve)
- Rare causes: endomyocardial fibroelastosis, malignant carcinoid syndrome, SLE

DIAGNOSIS

■ DIFFERENTIAL DIAGNOSIS

- Left atrial myxoma
- Other valvular abnormalities (e.g., tricuspid stenosis, mitral regurgitation)
- Atrial septal defect
- Table 2-35 describes the differential diagnosis of heart murmurs.

■ WORKUP

Physical examination and echocardiography; significant clinical findings:
- Exertional dyspnea initially, followed by orthopnea and PND
- Acute pulmonary edema (may develop after exertion)
- Systemic emboli (caused by stagnation of blood in the left atrium; may occur in patients with associated atrial fibrillation)
- Hemoptysis (may be present as a result of persistent pulmonary hypertension)

■ IMAGING STUDIES

- Echocardiography:
  1. The characteristic finding on echocardiogram is a markedly diminished E to F slope of the anterior mitral valve leaflet during diastole; there is also fusion of the commissures, resulting in anterior movement of the posterior mitral valve leaflet during diastole (calcification in the valve may also be noted).
  Two-dimensional echocardiogram can accurately establish valve area.
- Chest x-ray study:
  1. Straightening of the left cardiac border caused by dilated left atrial appendage
  2. Left atrial enlargement on lateral chest x-ray film (appearing as double density of PA chest x-ray film)
  3. Prominence of pulmonary arteries
  4. Possible pulmonary congestion and edema (Kerley B lines)
- ECG:
  1. Right ventricular hypertrophy; right axis deviation caused by pulmonary hypertension
  2. Left atrial enlargement (broad notched P waves)
  3. Atrial fibrillation

- Cardiac catheterization to help establish the severity of mitral stenosis and diagnose associated valvular and coronary lesions. Findings on cardiac catheterization include:
  1. Normal left ventricular function
  2. Elevated left atrial and pulmonary pressures

TREATMENT

■ NONPHARMACOLOGIC THERAPY

Decrease level of activity in symptomatic patients.

■ ACUTE GENERAL Rx

- Medical:
  1. If the patient is in atrial fibrillation, control the rate response with diltiazem, digitalis, or esmolol. Although digitalis is the drug of choice for chronic heart rate control, IV diltiazem or esmolol may be acutely preferable when a rapid decrease in heart rate is required.
  2. If the patient has persistent atrial fibrillation (because of large left atrium), permanent anticoagulation is indicated to decrease the risk of serious thromboembolism.
  3. Treat CHF with diuretics and sodium restriction.
  4. Give antibiotic prophylaxis with dental and surgical procedures (see Boxes 5-1 to 5-3, and Tables 5-18 and 5-19).
- Surgical: valve replacement is indicated when the valve orifice is <0.7 to 0.8 cm^2 or if symptoms persist despite optimal medical therapy; commissurotomy may be possible if the mitral valve is noncalcified and if there is pure mitral stenosis without significant subvalvular disease.
- Percutaneous transvenous mitral valvotomy (PTMV) is becoming the therapy of choice for many patients with mitral stenosis responding poorly to medical therapy, particularly those who are poor surgical candidates and whose valve is not heavily calcified; balloon valvotomy gives excellent mechanical relief, usually resulting in prolonged benefit.

■ DISPOSITION

- Prognosis is generally good except in patients wtih chronic pulmonary hypertension.
- Operative mortality rates for mitral valve replacement are 1% to 5% in most institutions.

Author: **Fred F. Ferri, M.D.**

BASIC INFORMATION

DEFINITION
Mitral valve prolapse (MVP) is the posterior bulging of interior and posterior leaflets in systole. Mitral valve prolapse syndrome refers to a constellation of MVP and associated symptoms (e.g., autonomic dysfunction, palpitations) or other physical abnormalities (e.g., pectus excavatum).

SYNONYMS
MVP
Mitral click murmur syndrome

ICD-9CM CODES
424.0 Mitral valve disorders
394.9 Other and unspecified mitral valve diseases

EPIDEMIOLOGY & DEMOGRAPHICS
- MVP can be found by 2-D echocardiogram in 4% of the general population (females > males).
- Increased incidence is seen with autoimmune thyroid disorders, Ehlers-Danlos syndrome, Marfan's syndrome, pseudoxanthoma elasticum, pectus excavatum, anorexia nervosa, and bulimia.

PHYSICAL FINDINGS & CLINICAL PRESENTATION
- Usually, young female patient with narrow AP chest diameter, low body weight, low blood pressure
- Mid to late click, heard best at the apex
- Crescendo mid to late diastolic murmur
- Findings accentuated in the standing position
- Most patients with MVP are asymptomatic; symptoms (if present) consist primarily of chest pain and palpitations.
- Neurologic abnormalities (e.g., TIA or stroke) are rare.
- Patients may also complain of anxiety, fatigue, and dyspnea

ETIOLOGY
- Myxomatous degeneration of connective tissue of mitral valve
- Congenital deformity of mitral valve and supportive structures
- Secondary to other disorders (e.g., Ehlers-Danlos, pseudoxanthoma elasticum)

DIAGNOSIS

DIFFERENTIAL DIAGNOSIS
- Other valvular abnormalities
- Constrictive pericarditis
- Ventricular aneurysm
- Table 2-35 describes the differential diagnosis of heart murmurs.

WORKUP
- Medical history and physical examination.
- Workup consists primarily of echocardiography in patients with a systolic click or murmur on careful auscultation.

IMAGING STUDIES
Echocardiography shows the anterior and posterior leaflets bulging posteriorly in systole.

TREATMENT

NONPHARMACOLOGIC THERAPY
Avoidance of stimulants (e.g., caffeine, nicotine) in patients with palpitations

ACUTE GENERAL Rx
- The empiric use of antiarrhythmic drugs to prevent sudden death in patients with uncomplicated MVP is not advisable; β-blockers may be tried in symptomatic patients (e.g., palpitations, chest pain); they decrease the heart rate, thus decreasing the stretch on the prolapsing valve leaflets.
- Antibiotic prophylaxis for infective endocarditis when undergoing dental, GI, or GU procedures is indicated only in patients with MVP who have a systolic murmur and echocardiographic evidence of mitral regurgitation (see Boxes 5-1 to 5-3 and Tables 5-25 and 5-26).

CHRONIC Rx
Monitoring for complications:
- Bacterial endocarditis (risk is three to eight times that of the general population)
- TIA or stroke secondary to embolic phenomena (from fibrin and platelet thrombi); risk in young patients: <0.05%/yr
- Cardiac arrhythmias (usually supraventricular)
- Sudden death (rare occurrence, most often caused by ventricular arrhythmias)
- Mitral regurgitation (most common complication of MVP)

DISPOSITION
The incidence of complications of MVP is very low (<1%/yr) and generally associated with an increase in mitral leaflet thickness to ≥5 mm; young patients (age <45) with absence of mitral systolic murmur or mitral regurgitation on Doppler echocardiography are at low risk for any complications.

REFERRAL
Surgical referral may be necessary in patients who develop symptomatic progressive mitral regurgitation.

PEARLS & CONSIDERATIONS

COMMENTS
- Patient education material may be obtained from the American Heart Association, 7320 Green Mill Avenue, Dallas, TX 75231.
- Recent studies suggest that the prevalence of MVP and its propensity to cause symptoms and serious complications have been overestimated in the past.
- Asymptomatic patients with MVP and mild or no mitral regurgitation can be evaluated clinically every 3 to 5 years. High-risk patients should undergo a follow-up exam once a year.

REFERENCES
Bouknight DP, O'Rourke RA: Current management of mitral valve prolapse, *Am Fam Physician* 61:3343, 2000.
Freed LA: Prevalence and clinical outcome of mitral valve prolapse, *N Engl J Med* 341:1, 1999.
Gilon D et al: Lack of evidence of an association between MVP and stroke in young patients, *N Engl J Med* 341:8, 1999.
Author: **Fred F. Ferri, M.D.**

BASIC INFORMATION

■ **DEFINITION**
The term *mixed connective tissue disease* describes a set of connective tissue symptoms that sometimes overlap with other known connective tissue diseases (SLE, progressive systemic sclerosis, polymyositis) but whose exact significance remains under debate. The disorder is sometimes referred to as an "overlap syndrome," but many prefer the term *undifferentiated connective tissue disease.*

ICD-9CM CODES
710.9 Diffuse connective tissue disease

■ **EPIDEMIOLOGY & DEMOGRAPHICS**
PREVALENCE: Approximately 10 to 15 cases/100,000 persons
PREDOMINANT SEX: Female:male ratio of 8:1
PREDOMINANT AGE: 4 to 80 yr

■ **PHYSICAL FINDINGS & CLINICAL PRESENTATION**
- Polyarthritis, polyarthralgia
- Raynaud's phenomenon, hand swelling, or sclerodactyly
- Esophageal hypomotility, myalgia, and muscle weakness
- Other: pericarditis, facial erythema, psychosis

■ **ETIOLOGY**
Autoimmune disorder

DIAGNOSIS

■ **DIFFERENTIAL DIAGNOSIS**
Other connective tissue disorders (SLE, progressive systemic sclerosis, polymyositis)

■ **WORKUP**
- Diagnosis is not well defined.
- Commonly used diagnostic tests are described below.

■ **LABORATORY TESTS** (BOX 1-25)
- Rheumatoid factor is often present in low titers.
- If myositis is present, muscle enzyme (CPK) levels increase.
- Positive ANA is often present with a speckled pattern.
- ESR is elevated.
- Anti-RNP antibodies may be present.

TREATMENT

- Except for pulmonary and scleroderma-like symptoms, response to corticosteroids is excellent in most cases.
- Rheumatoid symptoms may respond to NSAIDs, but other cases may not even respond to gold or penicillamine.
- Immunosuppressive agents are used on occasion, but the best therapeutic options remain uncertain.

■ **DISPOSITION**
- Initially, this disorder was thought to be a mild variant of SLE, sometimes called "benign lupus," with excellent prognosis.
- Further studies suggested, however, that this was not always the case and serious renal, vascular, and neurologic complications were noted.

- Pulmonary involvement is a common clinical manifestation that may even lead to pulmonary hypertension and sometimes death.
- Whether MCTD is a separate entity continues under debate as concepts about the disorder evolve.
- Long-term outcomes remain uncertain.

PEARLS & CONSIDERATIONS

■ **COMMENTS**
A clinical algorithm for evaluation of a positive ANA titer is described in Fig. 3-14.

REFERENCES
Fernandes C et al: Mixed connective tissue disease presenting with pneumonitis and pneumatosis intestinalis, *Arthritis Rheum* 43:704, 2000.
Kozaka T et al: Pulmonary involvement in mixed connective tissue disease: high-resolution CT findings in 41 patients, *J Thorac Imaging* 16:94, 2001.
Ling TC, Johnson BT: Esophageal investigations in connective tissue disease: which tests are most appropriate? *J Clin Gastroenterol* 32:33, 2001.
Lopez-Longo FJ et al: Does mixed connective tissue disease have a less favorable prognosis than systemic lupus erythematosis? *Arthritis Rheum* 44(suppl):119, 2001.
Lowe D, Kredich DW, Schanberg Durham LE: Thalidomide: an effective and safe agent for the treatment of pediatric mixed connective tissue disease, *Arthritis Rheum* 43(suppl):117, 2000.
Author: **Lonnie R. Mercier, M.D.**

BOX 1-25   Guidelines for Diagnosing Mixed Connective Tissue Disease

General
Clinical features of a diffuse connective tissue disorder

Serologic
1. Positive ANA, speckled pattern, titer >1:1000
2. Antibodies to U1 RNP
3. Absence of antibodies to dsDNA, histones, Sm, Scl-70, and other specificities
4. Commonly: Hypergammaglobulinemia and positive rheumatoid factor

Clinical
1. Sequential evolution of overlap features over course of several years, including Raynaud's phenomenon, serositis, gastrointestinal dysmotility, myositis, arthritis, sclerodactyly, skin rashes, and an abnormal DL$_{co}$ on pulmonary function tests
2. Absence of truncal scleroderma, severe renal disease, and severe central nervous system involvement
3. A nail fold capillary pattern identical to that seen in systemic sclerosis (dropout and dilated vessels)

From Bennett RM: Mixed connective tissue disease and other overlap syndromes. In Kelley WN et al (eds): *Textbook of rheumatology,* ed 3, Philadelphia, 1989, WB Saunders.
ANA, Antinuclear antibodies; *dsDNA,* double-stranded DNA; *MCTD,* mixed connective tissue disease; *RNP,* ribonucleoprotein.

BASIC INFORMATION

■ DEFINITION
Mononucleosis is a symptomatic infection caused by Epstein-Barr virus.

■ SYNONYMS
Infectious mononucleosis (IM)

ICD-9CM CODES
075 Infectious mononucleosis

■ EPIDEMIOLOGY & DEMOGRAPHICS
INCIDENCE (IN U.S.): 45 cases/100,000 persons/yr
PREDOMINANT SEX:
- Male = female
- Occurs earlier in females
PREDOMINANT AGE: Most common between the ages of 15 and 24 yr

■ PHYSICAL FINDINGS & CLINICAL PRESENTATION
- Incubation period of 1 to 2 mo
- Prodrome
  1. Fever
  2. Chills
  3. Malaise
  4. Anorexia
  5. Lasts several days
- Classic triad
  1. Pharyngitis
  2. Fever
  3. Adenopathy
- Fatigue and malaise prominent
- Pharyngitis usually most severe symptom
- Exudates common
- Lymphadenopathy
  1. Most prominent in cervical region
  2. May be diffuse
- Splenomegaly, most commonly during the second week of illness
- Rash
  1. Uncommon
  2. Occurs in nearly all patients who receive ampicillin
- Can present as fever and adenopathy without pharyngitis
- Complications
  1. May be severe
  2. Uncommon
  3. Tend to resolve completely
- Involvement of other systems
  1. Hematologic
  2. Pulmonary
  3. Cardiac
  4. Nervous
- Splenic rupture rare
- Illness usually self-limited
- Malaise and fatigue may last months before resolving

■ ETIOLOGY
- Primary infection with Epstein-Barr virus (EBV)

1. During childhood
   a. Causes few or no symptoms
   b. More common in lower socioeconomic groups
2. During late adolescence: frequency attributed to the onset of social contact between the sexes
- Transmission
  1. Close personal contact usually necessary for transmission
  2. Transfer via saliva while kissing (responsible for many cases)
  3. Occasionally transmitted by blood transfusion

DIAGNOSIS

■ DIFFERENTIAL DIAGNOSIS
- Heterophile-negative infectious mononucleosis caused by cytomegalovirus (CMV)
- Bacterial and viral causes of pharyngitis
- Toxoplasmosis
- Acute retroviral syndrome of HIV
- Lymphoma

■ WORKUP
- Heterophile antibody (Monospot)
- CBC

■ LABORATORY TESTS
- Commonly, increased WBCs with relative lymphocytosis and neutropenia
- Hallmark: atypical lymphocytes, but not pathognomonic
- Mild thrombocytopenia
- Falling Hct (possible signal of splenic rupture)
- Elevated hepatocellular enzymes and cryoglobulins
- Heterophile antibody:
  1. Measured by the Monospot test
  2. Positive at presentation
  3. May appear later in the course of illness
  4. Negative test repeated if clinical suspicion high
  5. If test negative for 8 wk, other causes likely
  6. Monospot usually positive for 3 to 6 mo, but can last for 1 yr
  7. A positive test has been reported with primary HIV infection
- Virus-specific antibodies in response to IM
  1. Determination of EBV-specific antibodies is rarely necessary.
  2. Early diagnosis in Monospotnegative cases is made by isolating IgM to the viral capsid antigen (VCA) (usually positive during acute illness).

■ IMAGING STUDIES
Chest radiograph:
- Rarely shows infiltrates
- Possible elevated left hemidiaphragm in cases of splenic rupture

TREATMENT

■ NONPHARMACOLOGIC THERAPY
- Supportive
- Rest advocated by some, but impact on outcome not clear
- Splenectomy if rupture occurs
- Transfusions for severe anemia or thrombocytopenia

■ ACUTE GENERAL Rx
- Pharmacologic therapy is not indicated in uncomplicated illness.
- Steroids are suggested in patients who have the following:
  1. Severe thrombocytopenia
  2. Hemolytic anemia
  3. Impending airway obstruction caused by enlarged tonsils
- Prednisone 60 to 80 mg PO is given qd for 3 days, then tapered over 1 to 2 wk.
- There is no role for antiviral agents such as acyclovir.

■ DISPOSITION
Eventual resolution of all symptoms

■ REFERRAL
More than mild illness

PEARLS & CONSIDERATIONS

■ COMMENTS
- Contact sports should be avoided during the first month of illness, because splenic rupture can occur, even in the absence of clinically detectable splenomegaly.
- An extremely rare, chronic form of IM with persistent fevers and other objective findings has been described; this should be differentiated from chronic fatigue syndrome, which is not related to EBV.

REFERENCES
Auwaerter PG: Infectious mononucleosis in middle age, *JAMA* 281:454, 1999.
Godshall SE, Kirchner JT: Infectious mononucleosis: complexities of a common syndrome, *Postgrad Med* 107:175, 2000.
Author: **Maurice Policar, M.D.**

BASIC INFORMATION

■ DEFINITION
Morton's neuroma refers to an inflammatory fibrosing process of the plantar digital nerve characterized by pain in the sole of the foot.

■ SYNONYMS
Morton's metatarsalgia
Morton's toe
Interdigital neuroma

ICD-9CM CODES
355.6 Morton's neuroma

■ EPIDEMIOLOGY & DEMOGRAPHICS
- Morton's neuroma most commonly involves the plantar digital nerve between the heads of the third and fourth metatarsals.
- May also involve the second and third metatarsal and can involve both simultaneously.
- Commonly occurs in people wearing tight-fitting shoes in toe region and high heels.
- Morton's neuroma is usually unilateral.
- Morton's neuroma is found more often in women than in men.
- Can occur in both young and old.

■ PHYSICAL FINDINGS & CLINICAL PRESENTATION
- Pain is usually located in a specific region, usually in the sole of the foot between the third and fourth metatarsal area (Fig. 1-251).
- Numbness may occur.
- Pain is exacerbated with exercise and relieved with rest and may radiate to the toes and to the ankle.
- Point tenderness is noted on examination, and palpation reveals fullness at the site of discomfort.
- An audible, painful click called "Murder's click" is noted in patients with Morton's neuroma after compressing and releasing the forefoot.

■ ETIOLOGY
- Morton's neuroma is thought to be caused by nerve thickening from repeated injury.
- The typical finding is swelling of the plantar digital nerve that pathologically resembles other nerve entrapment syndromes (e.g., median nerve compression in carpal tunnel syndrome).

DIAGNOSIS

- The diagnosis of Morton's neuroma is strictly made on clinical grounds alone as there are no laboratory tests or x-ray imaging studies that are specific for this disorder.

■ DIFFERENTIAL DIAGNOSIS
- Diabetic neuropathy
- Alcoholic neuropathy
- Nutritional neuropathy
- Toxic neuropathy
- Osteoarthritis
- Trauma (e.g., fracture)
- Gouty arthritis
- Rheumatoid arthritis

■ WORKUP
Exclude other causes as mentioned above in the "Differential Diagnosis."

■ LABORATORY TESTS
- Laboratory studies are not specific for the diagnosis of Morton's neuroma.
- CBC and ESR are usually normal.
- Blood glucose
- B_{12} and folic acid level.

■ IMAGING STUDIES
- X-ray imaging is primarily done to exclude other causes of foot pain (e.g., fractures, ostearthritis, gouty arthritis).
- MRI can detect and localize a neuroma but is rarely needed to make the diagnosis. An MRI can also be performed in patients with recurrent pain after surgical excision of a Morton's neuroma.

- Ultrasound imaging is also being used to locate Morton's neuromas but is rarely needed to make the diagnosis.

TREATMENT

■ NONPHARMACOLOGIC THERAPY
- Changing the type of footwear is the first line of treatment.
- Use open footwear and custom shoe inserts and avoid weight-bearing activities.
- Metatarsal pad with arch support is helpful.
- Participate in ultrasound therapy.

■ ACUTE GENERAL Rx
- If conservative measures are unsuccessful, injection of the intermetatarsal bursa with hydrocortisone may help.
- Nonsteroidal antiinflammatory agents (e.g., ibuprofen 400 to 800 mg PO tid or naproxen 250 to 500 mg bid).

■ CHRONIC Rx
- If nonpharmacologic and acute treatments do not give sufficient relief, surgical excision of the nerve has been successful in 95% of the cases.
- Surgery can be performed in the physician's office using local anesthesia.
- Numbness in the area where the nerve was excised is a common postoperative finding.

■ DISPOSITION
- Postoperative patients return to their normal activities by 3 to 6 weeks.
- In cases where pain persists after surgery a "stump neuroma" may be present.
- Approximately 80% of patients who failed to have relief with the initial surgery did find relief with a second procedure.

■ **REFERRAL**
- If surgery is being considered, a consultation with either a podiatrist or an orthopedic surgeon is indicated.

💡 **PEARLS & CONSIDERATIONS**

■ **COMMENTS**
- Dr. Thomas G. Morton is given credit for describing this disorder in 1876.
- Morton's neuroma occurs just before the nerve bifurcates at the metatarsal area to innervate sides of two adjacent toes.

REFERENCES

Wu J, Chin DT: Painful neuromas: a review of treatment modalities, *Ann Plast Surg* 43(6):661, 1999.

Wu KK: Morton's interdigital neuroma: a clinical review of its etiology, treatment and results, *J Foot Ankle Surg* 35(2):112, 1996.

Author: **Dennis J. Mikolich, M.D.**

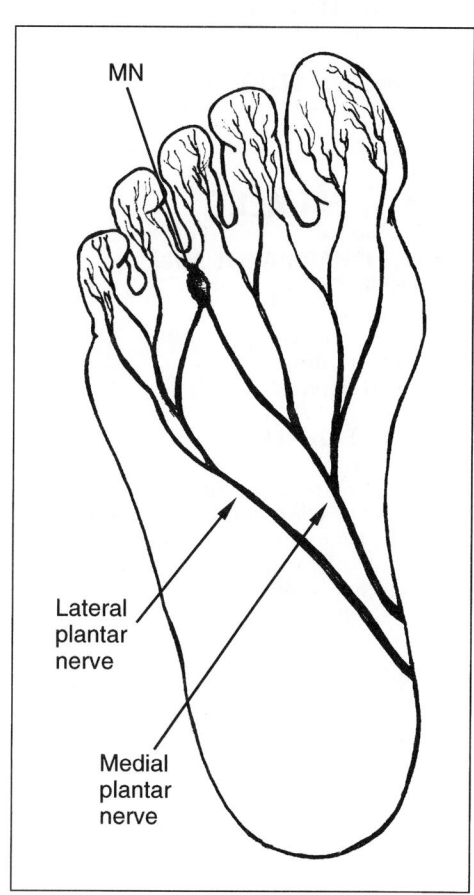

Fig. 1-251   Morton's neuroma *(MN).* The common digital nerve of the third space, site of most cases of MN, is formed by branches of the medial and lateral digital nerves. (From Canoso J: *Rheumatology in primary care,* Philadelphia, 1997, WB Saunders.)

BASIC INFORMATION

■ DEFINITION

Patients with motion sickness suffer perspiration, nausea, vomiting, increased salivation, and generalized malaise in response to movement.

■ SYNONYMS

Physiologic vertigo

ICD-9CM CODES

994.6 Motion sickness

■ EPIDEMIOLOGY & DEMOGRAPHICS

INCIDENCE (IN U.S.): Common
PREVALENCE (IN U.S.): Common
PREDOMINANT SEX: Male = female
PREDOMINANT AGE: Any age
PEAK INCIDENCE: Any age
GENETICS: Not known to be genetic

■ PHYSICAL FINDINGS & CLINICAL PRESENTATION

• Vomiting
• Sweating
• Pallor

■ ETIOLOGY

• Motion (e.g., amusement rides, rides in automobiles or planes)
• Exacerbated by anxiety, fumes (e.g., industrial pollutants), visual stimuli

DIAGNOSIS

■ DIFFERENTIAL DIAGNOSIS

• Acute labyrinthitis
• Gastroenteritis
• Metabolic disorders
• Viral syndrome

■ WORKUP

None necessary in routine case

■ LABORATORY TESTS

None necessary

■ IMAGING STUDIES

None necessary

TREATMENT

■ NONPHARMACOLOGIC THERAPY

• Fixate on far object.
• Cease motion.
• Avoid reading.
• Avoid alcohol.

■ ACUTE GENERAL Rx

• Scopolamine patches (where available) are most effective.
• Over-the-counter oral preparations (e.g., Dramamine) are less effective.
• Meclizine (Antivert) 12.5 to 25 mg q6h may be effective.

■ CHRONIC Rx

• Rarely chronic
• Symptoms generally resolve completely with cessation of motion exposure.

■ DISPOSITION

Follow-up is not needed.

■ REFERRAL

If another diagnosis is suspected (e.g., purulent ear, fever, cranial nerve abnormalities)

PEARLS & CONSIDERATIONS

■ COMMENTS

• Many patients with migraine report having severe motion sickness as a child.
• Improved ventilation, avoidance of large meals before travel, semirecumbent sitting, and avoidance of reading while in motion will minimize the risk of motion sickness.

Author: **William H. Olson, M.D.**

BASIC INFORMATION

DEFINITION
Mucormycosis is a fungal infection by *Zygomycetes* fungi, which include *Mucorales* spp. (*Mucor, Rhizopus, Absidia, Cunninghamella, Mortierella, Saksenaea, Syncephalastrum, Apophysomyces,* and *Thamnidium*) and *Entomorphthorales* spp. (*Conidiobolus* and *Basidiobolus*).

ICD-9CM CODES
117.7 Mucormycosis

EPIDEMIOLOGY & DEMOGRAPHICS
Infection by these ubiquitous organisms occurs in association with underlying conditions including diabetes mellitus, lymphoma, severe burns or trauma, prolonged postoperative course, multiple myeloma, hepatitis, cirrhosis, renal failure, steroid treatment, immunodeficiency states (e.g., AIDS), and use of contaminated Elastoplast bandages. Immunocompetent hosts may become infected in tropical climates.

PHYSICAL FINDINGS & CLINICAL PRESENTATION
- Rhinocerebral-rhinoorbital-paranasal syndrome may present with fever, facial and orbital pain, headache, diplopia, loss of vision, facial or orbital cellulitis, facial anesthesia, cranial nerve dysfunction, black nasal discharge, epistaxis, and seizure. Physical findings in this situation include proptosis, chemosis, nasal, palatal (Fig. 1-252), or pharyngeal necrotic ulcerations, and retinal infarction. Thrombosis of the cavernous sinus or internal carotid artery may occur.
- Pulmonary mucormycosis can present with pneumonia, lung abscess, pulmonary infarction, pleurisy, pleural effusion, hemoptysis, chills, and fever.
- Gastrointestinal zygomycosis presents with abdominal pain, diarrhea, GI hemorrhage, ulcers, peritonitis, and bowel infarction.
- Cutaneous zygomycosis presents as nodular lesions (hematogenous seeding) or a wound infection.
- Cardiac mucormycosis is a form of endocarditis.
- Septic arthritis and osteomyelitis
- Brain abscess.
- Disseminated zygomycosis (rare but uniformly fatal).
- Physical findings depend on the location of the infection.

ETIOLOGY & PATHOGENESIS
The cause of mucormycosis is infection by a fungus of the *Zygomycetes* class (see "Definition"). Normal host defenses include leukocytes and pulmonary macrophages. Quantitative (e.g., neutropenia) or qualitative (e.g., diabetes mellitus or steroid treatment) disruption in the host defenses predisposes the patient to infection

DIAGNOSIS

DIFFERENTIAL DIAGNOSIS
- Infection of the sites described above by other organisms (bacterial [including TB and leprosy], viral, fungal, or protozoan)
- Noninfectious tissue necrosis (e.g., neoplasia, vasculitis, degenerative) of the sites described above

WORKUP
- Biopsy of infected tissue with direct light microscopy examination establishes the diagnosis within minutes of the biopsy in the case of nasopharyngeal infection
- Bronchoalveolar lavage or bronchoscopy with biopsy for smear, culture, and histologic examination
- X-rays and other imaging studies of symptomatic sites may be required before infection is suspected and tissue specimens are obtained

TREATMENT

Amphotericin B given IV at a daily dose of 0.5 to 1.5 mg/kg infused over 2 to 4 hr for a total of 1 to 4 g. Adverse reactions may be managed as follows:
- Fever, chills, headache, myalgias, nausea, and vomiting: premedicate with aspirin (650 mg PO), acetaminophen (650 mg PO), diphenhydramine (25 to 50 mg IV), hydrocortisone (25 to 100 mg IV), or meperidine (25 to 50 mg IV).
- Hypokalemia and hypomagnesemia are treated with potassium and magnesium replacement.
- Nephrotoxicity and renal tubular acidosis can be mitigated to some extent with 500 ml of normal saline infusion 30 min before and after each dose of amphotericin. Amphotericin dose reduction may also be necessary.
- Renal function and electrolytes should be monitored twice a week during the entire course of amphotericin.
- Lipid preparations of amphotericin B may be less toxic (i.e., amphotericin B lipid complex, amphotericin B colloidal dispersion, and liposomal amphotericin B).
- The role of flucytosine, rifampin, and tetracycline is controversial.
Surgical debridement or radical resection

PROGNOSIS
- Sinus infection with no underlying disease: 75% survival.
- Sinus infection with diabetes: 60% survival.
- Sinus infection with renal disease: 25% survival.
- Surgery may increase survival by 5% to 20%.
- Early diagnosis improves survival as well as control of the underlying condition.

REFERENCE
Meyers BR, Gurtman AC: Phycomycetes. In Gorbach SL, Bartlett JG, Blacklow NR (eds): *Infectious diseases,* ed 2, Philadelphia, 1998, WB Saunders.
Author: **Tom J. Wachtel, M.D.**

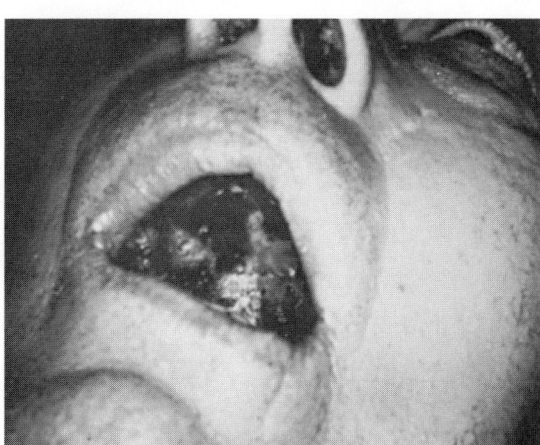

Fig. 1-252 Necrosis of the hard palate secondary to invasion by *Rhizopus* species in a renal transplant patient taking corticosteroids. (From Gorbach SL: *Infectious diseases,* ed 2, Philadelphia, 1998, WB Saunders.)

BASIC INFORMATION

■ DEFINITION

Multifocal atrial tachycardia is a supraventricular, moderately rapid arrhythmia (rate 100 to 140 bpm) with P waves having at least three or more different morphologies.

■ SYNONYMS

Chaotic atrial rhythm; the term "wandering pacemaker" is used for a similar arrhythmia associated with a normal or slow heart rate.

ICD-9CM CODES

427.89 Multifocal atrial tachycardia

■ EPIDEMIOLOGY & DEMOGRAPHICS

Same as chronic lung disease (obstructive or restrictive), which the arrhythmia may complicate

■ PHYSICAL FINDINGS & CLINICAL PRESENTATION

Symptoms:
• Palpitation
• Lightheadedness
• Syncope
• Symptoms of the underlying pulmonary disease
• Physical findings associated with the underlying pulmonary disease

■ ETIOLOGY

• Exact mechanism unknown
• Associated abnormalities include hypoxia, hypercarbia, acidosis, electrolyte disturbances, digitalis toxicity

DIAGNOSIS

■ DIFFERENTIAL DIAGNOSIS

• Atrial fibrillation
• Atrial flutter
• Sinus tachycardia
• Paroxysmal atrial tachycardia
• Extrasystoles

■ WORKUP

• ECG (Fig. 1-253)
• Pulmonary function tests
• Electrolytes
• Arterial blood gases
• Digoxin level (if patient on digoxin)

TREATMENT

• Improve the pulmonary or metabolic dysfunction if possible
• Calcium blockers
• β-Blockers if not contraindicated by obstructive lung disease
• If the arrhythmia is asymptomatic, it can be left untreated

REFERENCE

Myerburg RJ, Kessler KM, Castellanos A: Recognition, clinical assessment, and management of arrhythmias and conduction disturbances. In Alexander RW et al (eds): *Hurst's: the heart, arteries, and veins,* ed 9, New York, 1998, McGraw-Hill.
Author: **Tom J. Wachtel, M.D.**

MULTIFOCAL ATRIAL TACHYCARDIA

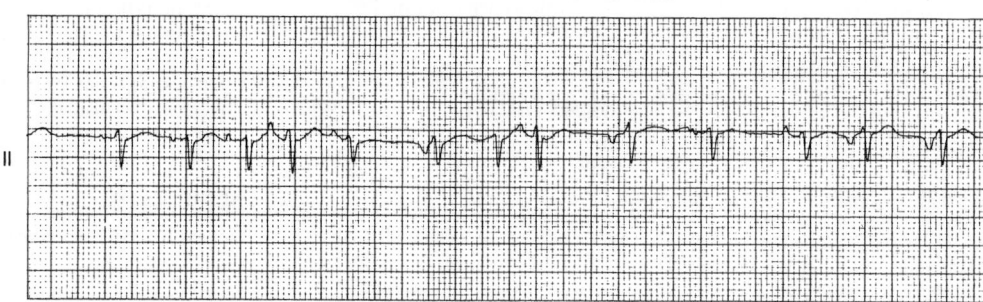

Fig. 1-253   The P waves show variable shapes or variable PR intervals, or both. (From Goldberger AL: *Clinical electrocardiography,* ed 5, St Louis, 1994, Mosby.)

BASIC INFORMATION

■ DEFINITION
Multiple myeloma is a malignancy of plasma cells characterized by overproduction of intact monoclonal immunoglobulin or free monoclonal kappa or lambda chains.

■ SYNONYMS
Plasma cell myeloma

ICD-9CM CODES
203.0 Multiple myeloma

■ EPIDEMIOLOGY & DEMOGRAPHICS
ANNUAL INCIDENCE: 4 cases/100,000 persons (blacks affected twice as frequently as whites)
PREDOMINANT AGE: Peak incidence in the seventh decade at a median age of 69 yr

■ PHYSICAL FINDINGS & CLINICAL PRESENTATION
- Pallor and generalized weakness from anemia
- Purpura, epistaxis from thrombocytopenia
- Evidence of infections from impaired immune system
- Bone pain, weight loss
- Swelling on ribs, vertebrae, and other bones

DIAGNOSIS

The patient usually comes to medical attention because of one or more of the following:
- Bone pain (back, thorax) or pathologic fractures caused by osteolytic lesions
- Fatigue or weakness because of anemia secondary to bone marrow infiltration with plasma cells
- Recurrent infections as a result of impaired neutrophil function and deficiency of normal immunoglobulins
- Nausea and vomiting caused by constipation and uremia
- Delirium secondary to hypercalcemia
- Neurologic complications, such as spinal cord or nerve root compression, blurred vision from hyperviscosity

■ DIFFERENTIAL DIAGNOSIS
- Metastatic carcinoma
- Lymphoma
- Bone neoplasms (e.g., sarcoma)
- Monoclonal gammopathy of undetermined significance (MGUS)

■ LABORATORY TESTS
- Normochromic, normocytic anemia; rouleaux formation on peripheral smear
- Hypercalcemia
- Elevated BUN, creatinine, uric acid, and total protein
- Proteinuria secondary to overproduction and secretion of free monoclonal kappa or lambda chains (Bence Jones protein)
- Tall homogeneous monoclonal spike (M spike) on protein immunoelectrophoresis (IEP) in approximately 75% of patients; decreased levels of normal immunoglobulins; <2% of patients have nonsecreting myeloma (no increase in immunoglobulins and no light chains in the urine)
- Reduced ion gap, hyponatremia, elevated LDH, serum hyperviscosity
- Bone marrow examination: usually demonstrates nests or sheets of plasma cells, which comprise >30% of the bone marrow, and ≥10% are immature

■ IMAGING STUDIES
X-ray films of painful areas usually demonstrate punched-out lytic lesions or osteoporosis. Bone scans are not useful, because lesions are not blastic.

TREATMENT

■ NONPHARMACOLOGIC THERAPY
- Prevention of renal failure with adequate hydration and avoidance of nephrotoxic agents and dye contrast studies
- Consideration of autologous bone marrow transplantation in younger patients (see "Acute General Rx")

■ ACUTE GENERAL Rx
Chemotherapy may be withheld until symptoms develop or complications are imminent; frequently used regimen includes:
- Melphalan and prednisone: the rates of response to this treatment range from 40% to 60%. Adding continuous low-dose interferon to standard melphalan-prednisone therapy does not improve response rate or survival; however, response duration and plateau phase duration are prolonged by maintenance therapy with interferon.
- Vincristine, doxorubicin (Adriamycin), and dexamethasone (VAD) can be used in patients not responding or relapsing after treatment with melphalan and prednisone.
- High-dose chemotherapy (HDCT) with vincristine, melphalan, cyclophosphamide, and prednisone (VMCP) alternating with vincristine, carmustine, doxorubicin, and prednisone (BVAP) combined with bone marrow transplantation improves the response rate, event-free survival, and overall survival in patients with myeloma.
- Current HDCT regimen with autologous stem-cell support achieve complete response in approximately 20% to 30% of patients, with best results seen in good-risk patients, defined as young patients (<50 yr of age) with good performance status and a low tumor burden (β_2 microglobulin ≤2.5 mg/L).
- Thalidomide is useful to induce responses in patients with multiple myeloma refractory to chemotherapy.

■ CHRONIC Rx
- Promptly diagnose and treat infections.
- Control hypercalcemia and hyperuricemia.
- Control pain with analgesics; radiation therapy and surgical stabilization may also be indicated.
- Treat anemia with epoetin alfa.
- Monthly infusions of the biphosphonate pamidronate provide significant protection against skeletal complications and improve the quality of life of patients with advanced multiple myeloma. Zoledronic acid (Zometa) can be infused over 15 min and is more effective than pamidronate for treatment of hypercalcemia of malignancy. Biphosphonates (pamidronate, zoledranate, and ibandronate) also appear to have an antitumor effect.

■ DISPOSITION
- The median survival time is approximately 30 mo with standard therapy and depends on the stage of the disease, histologic subtype, and various other factors (e.g., elevated LDH levels or β_2 microglobulin >8 mg/L at the time of diagnosis indicates poor prognosis).
- Prognosis is much better in asymptomatic patients with indolent or smoldering myeloma: median survival time is approximately 10 yr in persons with no lytic bone lesions and a serum myeloma protein concentration <3 g/dl.

REFERENCES
Kyle RA: The role of biphosphonates in multiple myeloma, *Ann Intern Med* 132:734, 2000.
Singhal S et al: Antitumor activity of thalidomide in refractory multiple myeloma, *N Engl J Med* 341:1565, 1999.
Author: **Fred F. Ferri, M.D.**

BASIC INFORMATION

■ **DEFINITION**

Multiple sclerosis (MS) is a chronic demyelinating disease of unknown etiology characterized pathologically by zones of demyelinization (plaques) scattered throughout the white matter.

■ **SYNONYMS**

MS
Disseminated sclerosis

■ **ICD-9CM CODES**

340 Multiple sclerosis

■ **EPIDEMIOLOGY & DEMOGRAPHICS**

PREVALENCE: 50 to 100 cases/100,000 persons, increasing in higher latitudes. It is the most common demyelinating disease in humans.
GENETICS: Increased prevalence with haplotypes DR2, DQW1, DQA1, DQB1, A3, and B7 of the major histocompatibility complex
Predominant Age: Young adults (17 to 35 yr)

■ **PHYSICAL FINDINGS & CLINICAL PRESENTATION**

• Visual abnormalities:
  1. Paresis of medial rectus muscle on lateral conjugate gaze (internuclear ophthalmoplegia) and horizontal nystagmus of the adducting eye
  2. Central scotoma, decreased visual acuity (optic neuritis)
  3. Nystagmus
• Abnormalities of reflexes: increased DTRs, positive Hoffmann's and Babinski's signs, decreased abdominal skin reflex, decreased cremasteric reflex
• Lhermitte's sign: flexion of the neck while the patient is lying down elicits an electrical sensation extending bilaterally down the arms, back, and lower trunk
• Charcot's triad: nystagmus, scanning speech, and intention tremor

■ **ETIOLOGY**

The etiology of MS is unknown. It is currently believed that it is the result of an autoimmune process triggered by infection or other environmental factors in individuals with genetic predisposition. There is some evidence that Epstein-Barr virus (EBV) infection may increase the risk of MS.

🔬 **DIAGNOSIS**

MS is primarily a clinical diagnosis based on evidence of CNS white matter lesions disseminated in time and space (two distinct episodes of neurologic symptoms affecting two distinct areas of the CNS). The clinical signs vary with the location of the plaques. In relapsing-remitting MS (80% of patients), signs and symptoms evolve over a period of several days, stabilize, and then improve spontaneously or in response to corticosteroids. In primary progressive MS, manifestations gradually worsen from disease onset without relapses. In secondary progressive MS, after an initial relapsing remitting course, manifestations worsen gradually with or without superimposed acute relapses. In progressive relapsing MS, manifestations gradually worsen from disease onset with subsequent superimposed relapses. The following are the more common manifestations:
• Weakness: usually involving the lower extremities; complaints of difficulty ambulating, tendency to drop things, easy fatigability
• Sensory disturbances: numbness, tingling, "pins and needles" sensation
• Visual disturbances: diplopia, blurred vision, visual loss
• Incoordination: gait impairment, clumsiness of upper extremities
• Other: vertigo, incontinence, loss of sexual function, slurred speech

■ **DIFFERENTIAL DIAGNOSIS**

• Systemic disorders: sarcoidosis, SLE, pernicious anemia, vasculitis
• Ruptured intervertebral disk
• Infections: CNS infections, syphilis
• Small cerebral infarctions
• Neoplasms: brainstem, cerebellar, spinal cord
• Other: ALS, syringomyelia, neurofibromatosis, Friedreich's ataxia
• Box 2-193 describes the differential diagnosis of paresthesias.

■ **WORKUP**

• Lumbar puncture
  1. In MS the CSF may show increased gamma globulin (mostly IgG, but often IgA and IgM).
  2. Agarose electrophoresis discloses discrete "oligoclonal" bands in the gamma region in approximately 90% of patients, including some with normal IgG levels.
  3. Other frequent CSF abnormalities are increased total protein, increased mononuclear WBCs, presence of myelin basic protein (elevated in acute attacks, indicates active myelin destruction).

• Measurement of visual evoked response (VER) to assess nerve fiber conduction (myelin loss or destruction will slow conduction velocity)

■ **IMAGING STUDIES**

MRI of the head can identify lesions as small as 3 to 4 mm and is frequently diagnostic in suspected cases; can also be used to assess disease load, activity, and progression; however, a normal MRI cannot be used conclusively to exclude MS.

💊 **TREATMENT**

■ **NONPHARMACOLOGIC THERAPY**

Patient education regarding the disease and prognosis and the need for the entire family to accept and understand the disease

■ **ACUTE GENERAL Rx**

• Corticosteroids can be used to treat relapses. There is no consensus about optimal dose or duration of corticosteroid therapy. Typically, high-dose IV methylprednisolone (5-day course at a dose of 1000 mg/day can be used; an alternative dose is 15 mg/kg/day).
• Currently available disease-modifying drugs for MS are interferon beta 1a (Avonex), interferon beta 1b (Betaseron), and glatiramer acetate (Copaxone). All three drugs have been shown to slow the progression of the disease. Interferon is effective in both secondary-progressive and relapsing-remitting phases of MS. Initiating treatment with interferon beta-1a at the time of a first demyelinating event is beneficial for patients with brain lesions on MRI that indicate a high risk of clinically definite multiple sclerosis, and it delays the appearance of other symptoms, thus delaying progression of the disease.

■ **CHRONIC Rx**

• Fatigue is a common complaint; it can be treated with amantadine 100 mg bid. Treatment should continue for 2 to 3 wk before deciding whether it is effective. Pemoline and fluoxetine can also be used when amantadine is not effective.
• Spasticity may be controlled with baclofen or lorazepam.
• Pain is a frequent complaint and can be treated with carbamazepine. Tricyclic antidepressants, misoprostol, and NSAIDs are also effective.

- Depression is frequent (20% of patients) and can be treated with antidepressants and referral to a psychiatrist.
- Urinary urgency can be treated with oxybutynin or propantheline.
- Tremor can generally be controlled with clonazepam 0.5 mg bid.

■ DISPOSITION

The majority of patients experience clinical improvement in weeks to months after the initial manifestations. The disease may be of the exacerbating-remitting type or may follow a chronic progressive course. The average interval from the initial clinical presentation to death is 35 yr. Premature death is usually secondary to infection.

■ REFERRAL

- Initial neurology referral is recommended in all patients with MS.
- Referral to a physician specializing in rehabilitation or to PT/OT is also recommended following exacerbations.

REFERENCES

Ascherio A et al: Epstein-Barr virus antibodies and risk of multiple sclerosis, *JAMA* 286:3083, 2001.

Jacobs LD et al: Intramuscular interferon beta-1a therapy, initiated during a first demyelinating event in multiple sclerosis, *N Engl J Med* 343:898, 2000.

Lublin FD, Reingold SC: Defining the clinical course of multiple sclerosis: results of an international survey, *Neurology* 46:907, 1996.

Noseworthy JH et al: Multiple sclerosis, *N Engl J Med* 343:938, 2000.
Author: **Fred F. Ferri, M.D.**

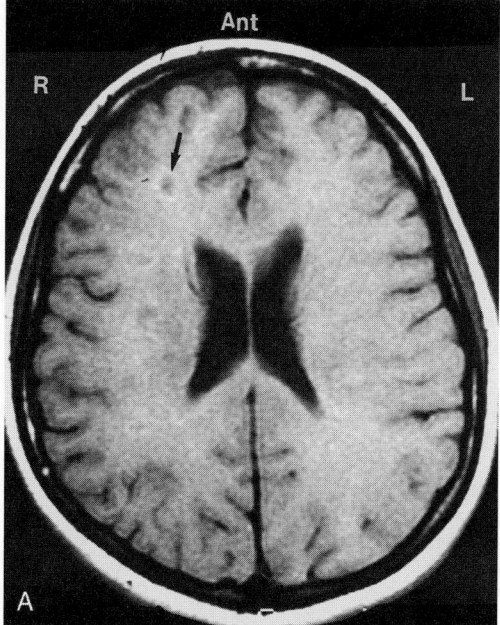

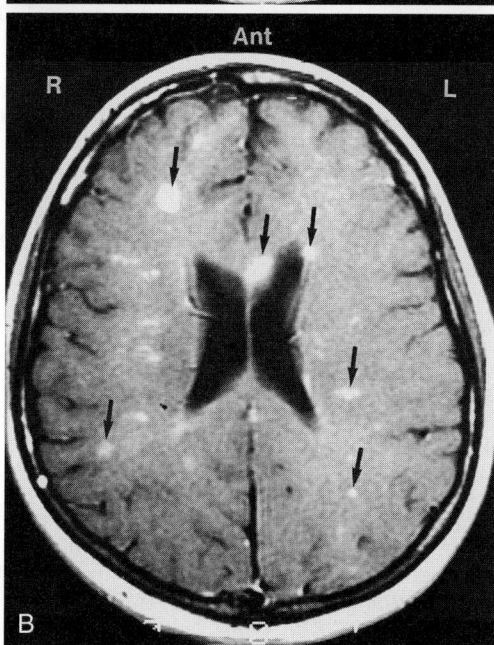

Fig. 1-254   Multiple sclerosis. The noncontrasted T1-weighted magnetic resonance scan **(A)** is generally unremarkable with the exception of one lesion *(arrow)* in the right frontal lobe. A gadolinium-enhanced scan **(B)** is much better and shows many enhancing lesions, only some of which are indicated *(arrows)*. (From Mettler FA [ed]: *Primary care radiology,* Philadelphia, 2000, WB Saunders.)

BASIC INFORMATION

■ DEFINITION

Mumps is an acute generalized viral infection that is usually characterized by nonsupportive swelling and tenderness of one or both parotid glands. It is caused by mumps virus, a paramyxovirus and member of the Paramyxoviridae family.

ICD-9CM CODES
072.9 Mumps

■ EPIDEMIOLOGY & DEMOGRAPHICS

INCIDENCE (IN U.S.):
- About 1600 infections/yr
- More than 150,000 cases/yr before licensure of mumps vaccine in 1967

PREDOMINANT SEX: Males = females

PREDOMINANT AGE: 75% of disease in teenage yr

PEAK INCIDENCE: Late winter and early spring months

GENETICS:

Congenital Infection:
- First-trimester infection is associated with excessive fetal deaths.
- Second- and third-trimester infection is not associated with increased fetal mortality.

Neonatal Infection:
- Uncommon
- Uncommon in infants <1 yr because of passive immunity conferred by placental transfer of maternal antibody

■ PHYSICAL FINDINGS & CLINICAL PRESENTATION

- Prodromal period:
  1. Low-grade fever
  2. Malaise
  3. Anorexia
  4. Headache
- Parotid swelling and tenderness are often first signs of infection.
  1. Progresses over 2 to 3 days, then opposite side may become involved
  2. Unilateral parotitis in 25% of cases

3. Considerable pain with parotid swelling, causing trismus and difficulty with mastication and pronunciation
4. Pain exacerbated by eating or drinking citrus and other acidic foods
5. Possible fever with parotid swelling, ranging up to 40° C
6. Parotid swelling usually resolving within 1 wk
- CNS involvement:
  1. May occur from 1 wk before to 2 wk after the onset of parotitis or even in its absence
  2. Meningitis
     a. Occurs in 1% to 10% of persons with mumps parotitis
     b. Symptoms: headache, fever, nuchal rigidity, and vomiting
     c. Full recovery with no sequelae
  3. Encephalitis
     a. May develop early, as a result of direct viral invasion of neurons, or late, around the second week after onset of parotitis, and is a postinfectious demyelinating process
     b. Symptoms: fever, alterations in the level of consciousness, possible seizures, paresis, and aphasia. Fever can be quite high (40° C to 41° C).
     c. May result in permanent sequelae or death
  4. Other rare neurologic complications
     a. Cerebellar ataxia
     b. Transverse myelitis
     c. Guillain-Barré syndrome
- Epididymoorchitis:
  1. Most common extrasalivary gland complication of mumps in adult men
  2. Occurs in 20% to 30% of postpubertal males who have mumps
  3. Most often unilateral, but is bilateral in 17% of males who develop this complication
  4. May precede development of parotitis
  5. May be only manifestation of mumps
  6. Two thirds of cases develop during first week of parotitis
  7. One quarter of cases develop in second week

8. Symptoms:
   a. Severe pain, swelling, and tenderness of the testes and scrotal erythema
   b. Fever and chills
   c. Fever and severity of testicular involvement parallel
9. Epididymitis
   a. Precedes orchitis
   b. Occurs in 85% of cases
10. Some degree of testicular atrophy in 50% of cases, months to years later
11. Sterility from bilateral orchitis is rare
- Involvement of pancreas and ovaries:
  1. Abdominal pain
  2. Fever
  3. Vomiting
  4. Oophoritis
     a. Occurs in 5% of postpubertal women with mumps
     b. Symptoms include fever, nausea, vomiting, and lower abdominal pain.
     c. May rarely result in decreased fertility and premature menopause
- Transient renal impairment:
  1. Common
  2. Manifest by hematuria, polyuria, and viruria
- Joint involvement:
  1. Migratory polyarthritis is most frequent
  2. Infrequently affects adults with mumps
  3. Rarely affects children
  4. Self-limited, with complete resolution
- Pancreatitis
  1. Uncommon as a severe illness
  2. Mild degree of upper abdominal discomfort
- Deafness:
  1. Most often unilateral and of high frequencies
  2. Most patients recover
  3. Permanent unilateral deafness reported in 1 in 20,000 cases

■ ETIOLOGY
- Virus is spread via direct contact, droplet nuclei or secretions through the nose and mouth
- Patients are contagious from 48 hr before to 9 days after parotid swelling.

DIAGNOSIS

DIFFERENTIAL DIAGNOSIS

- Other viruses that may cause acute parotitis:
  1. Parainfluenza types 1 and 3
  2. Coxsackie viruses
  3. Influenza A
  4. Cytomegalovirus
- Suppurative parotitis:
  1. Most often caused by *Staphylococcus aureus*
  2. May be differentiated from mumps
     a. Extreme induration, tenderness, and erythema overlying the gland
     b. Ability to express pus from Stensen's duct or massage of parotid
- Other conditions that may occur with parotid enlargement or swelling:
  1. Sjögren's syndrome
  2. Leukemia
  3. Uveoparotid sarcoidosis
  4. Diabetes mellitus
  5. Uremia
  6. Malnutrition
  7. Cirrhosis
- Drugs that cause parotid swelling:
  1. Phenothiazines
  2. Phenylbutazone
  3. Thiouracil
  4. Iodides
- Conditions that cause unilateral parotid swelling:
  1. Tumors
  2. Cysts
  3. Stones causing obstruction
  4. Strictures causing obstruction

WORKUP

- Diagnosis is based on history of exposure and physical findings of parotid tenderness with mild to moderate constitutional symptoms.
- Diagnosis is confirmed by a variety of serologic tests or isolation of the virus.

LABORATORY TESTS

- Diagnosis is confirmed by fourfold rise between acute and convalescent sera, by CF, HAI, ELISA, or neutralization tests.
- Virus can be isolated from the saliva, usually from 2 to 3 days before to 4 to 5 days after the onset of parotitis.
- Virus also can be isolated from CSF in patients with meningitis, during the first 3 days of meningeal findings.
- Virus can be detected in urine during the first 2 wk of infection.
- Viremia is rarely detected.
- WBCs:
  1. May be normal
  2. Possible mild leukopenia with a relative lymphocytosis
  3. Leukocytosis with left shift with extrasalivary gland involvement, such as meningitis, orchitis, or pancreatitis
- Serum amylase:
  1. Elevated in the presence of parotitis
  2. Sometimes elevated without clinical parotitis
  3. May remain elevated for 2 to 3 wk
  4. Elevated in mumps pancreatitis
  5. May be differentiated from mumps and parotitis by isoenzyme analysis or serum pancreatic lipase
- Mumps meningitis:
  1. CSF WBCs from 10 to 2000 WBC/mm^3, with a predominance of lymphocytes
  2. In 20% to 25% of patients, predominance of polymorphonuclear cells
  3. CSF protein normal or mildly elevated
  4. CSF glucose low, >40 mg/100 ml, in 6% to 30% of patients

TREATMENT

NONPHARMACOLOGIC THERAPY

- Supportive treatment
- Adequate hydration and nutrition

ACUTE GENERAL Rx

- Analgesics and antipyretics to relieve pain and fever
- Narcotic analgesics, along with bed rest, ice packs, and a testicular bridge, to relieve pain associated with mumps orchitis
- IV fluids for patients with frequent vomiting associated with mumps pancreatitis or meningitis

DISPOSITION

Most patients recover without incident.

PEARLS & CONSIDERATIONS

COMMENTS

Prevention:

- Attenuated live mumps virus vaccine has been available since 1967.
  1. Usually given in combination with measles and rubella vaccines
  2. Should be given at 15 mo of age, and again at 5 to 12 yr
  3. Seroconversion in about 98% of infants given the vaccine
  4. Contraindicated in pregnant women and immunocompromised patients
- Infected patients should be isolated until parotid swelling resolves.
- Because virus may be shed before the onset of parotid swelling, isolation possibly not of great value in limiting spread of infection.

Author: **Zeena Lobo, M.D.**

BASIC INFORMATION

■ DEFINITION

Munchausen syndrome is marked by the willful, and often active, production of symptoms or feigning of disease, usually associated with exaggerated lying (pseudologia fantastica) and with the apparent purpose of inducing medical testing, procedures, and treatment, or assuming the patient role.

■ SYNONYMS

Factitious disorder
Munchausen syndrome
Munchausen by proxy
Deliberate disability
Hospital addiction syndrome
Artifactual illness
Artefaktkrankheit
Dermatitis artefacta
Surreptitious illness

ICD-9CM CODES

300.19 Factitious disorder

■ EPIDEMIOLOGY & DEMOGRAPHICS

INCIDENCE (IN U.S.): Unknown
PREVALENCE (IN U.S.): Unknown
PREDOMINANT SEX: Male:female ratio of 2:1
PREDOMINANT AGE: 30 to 40 yr
PEAK INCIDENCE: 30s
GENETICS: No genetic predisposition known

■ PHYSICAL FINDINGS & CLINICAL PRESENTATION

- False complaints or self-inflicted injury or symptoms without clear secondary gain
- Presentation often acute and dramatic
- Workup usually negative but a predisposing condition often present

■ ETIOLOGY

- Unknown
- Personality disorders and psychodynamic factors: thought to play a role

DIAGNOSIS

■ DIFFERENTIAL DIAGNOSIS

- Malingering: a clear secondary gain (e.g., financial gain or avoidance of unwanted duties) is present.
- Somatoform disorders or hypochondriasis: similar presentations, but disorder is not under the patient's control.
- Self-injurious behavior is common in many other psychiatric conditions (e.g., borderline personality disorder, psychoses, or nonfatal suicide attempt as may occur in depression); in those conditions the patients confess the intentional self-harm and describe motivating factors.

■ WORKUP

- Workup is often dictated by the presenting complaints.
- No specific tests for Munchausen syndrome although Minnesota Multiphasic Personality Inventory (MMPI) may show an unreliable profile.
- Diagnosis is invariably made when the patient is caught in the act of lying or inducing an injury.

■ LABORATORY TESTS

No specific tests are required.

TREATMENT

■ NONPHARMACOLOGIC THERAPY

- Therapy is difficult, because patients nearly always terminate the physician-patient relationship (usually in an angry manner) when discovered.
- Only one case of successful psychiatric therapy exists in the literature.

■ ACUTE GENERAL Rx

None

■ DISPOSITION

- Ultimate course is unknown.
- After confronted with their behavior, patients seek other physicians or hospitals.
- Extensive medical workups and exploratory surgery are frequent.

■ REFERRAL

Always when diagnosis is made
Author: **Rif S. El-Mallakh, M.D.**

BASIC INFORMATION

■ DEFINITION
The term *muscular dystrophy* (MD) refers to a group of inherited diseases primarily affecting muscle.

■ SYNONYMS
Distal MD
Duchenne's MD
Erb's MD
Facioscapulohumeral disease
Gower's syndrome
Landouzy-Dejerine disease
Limb-girdle MD
Myotonic MD
Ocular MD
Oculopharyngeal MD

ICD-9CM CODES
359 Muscular dystrophies and other myopathies
359.1 Hereditary progressive muscular dystrophy

■ EPIDEMIOLOGY & DEMOGRAPHICS
INCIDENCE (IN U.S.): Duchenne's: 1 in 3500 male births
PREVALENCE (IN U.S.): Boys with Duchenne's are usually younger than 12 yrs old. Many other types of dystrophies are possible.
PREDOMINANT SEX: Male (for Duchenne's)
PREDOMINANT AGE:
• Depends on type of dystrophy
• Most commonly diagnosed in children
PEAK INCIDENCE: Childhood (Duchenne's)
GENETICS: Duchenne's: X-linked recessive (Xp21)

■ PHYSICAL FINDINGS & CLINICAL PRESENTATION
• Proximal muscle weakness.
• Late atrophy.
• Contracture of Achilles tendon.
• Difficulty in rising from a supine to a standing position (Gower's sign [Fig. 1-255]) as a result of truncal and hip-girdle weakness. Affected patients push themselves on all fours and then quickly grab their thighs and walk up the thighs to a standing position.

■ ETIOLOGY
Genetic abnormality; specifically, a muscle protein, dystrophin, is absent (Duchenne's dystrophy).

DIAGNOSIS

■ WORKUP
• Muscle biopsy with histochemistry
• ECG/EMG
• Muscle biopsy with dystrophin analysis
• Box 2-169 describes the differential diagnosis of muscle weakness.

■ LABORATORY TESTS
• Serum creatine kinase
• Possible DNA analysis

■ IMAGING STUDIES
Muscle biopsy with histochemistry

TREATMENT

■ NONPHARMACOLOGIC THERAPY
• Genetic counseling
• Physical therapy

■ ACUTE GENERAL Rx
None

■ CHRONIC Rx
• Be alert for development of contractures, respiratory distress, and cardiac complications.

• No cure is known for Duchenne's MD.

■ DISPOSITION
Usually, follow-up in a muscular dystrophy specialty clinic

■ REFERRAL
• See "Disposition."
• For family anxiety with the diagnosis.

PEARLS & CONSIDERATIONS

■ COMMENTS
"Muscular dystrophy" refers to many diseases; Duchenne's, limb-girdle, and myotonic dystrophy are the most common, but many other dystrophies have been described.
Author: **William H. Olson, M.D.**

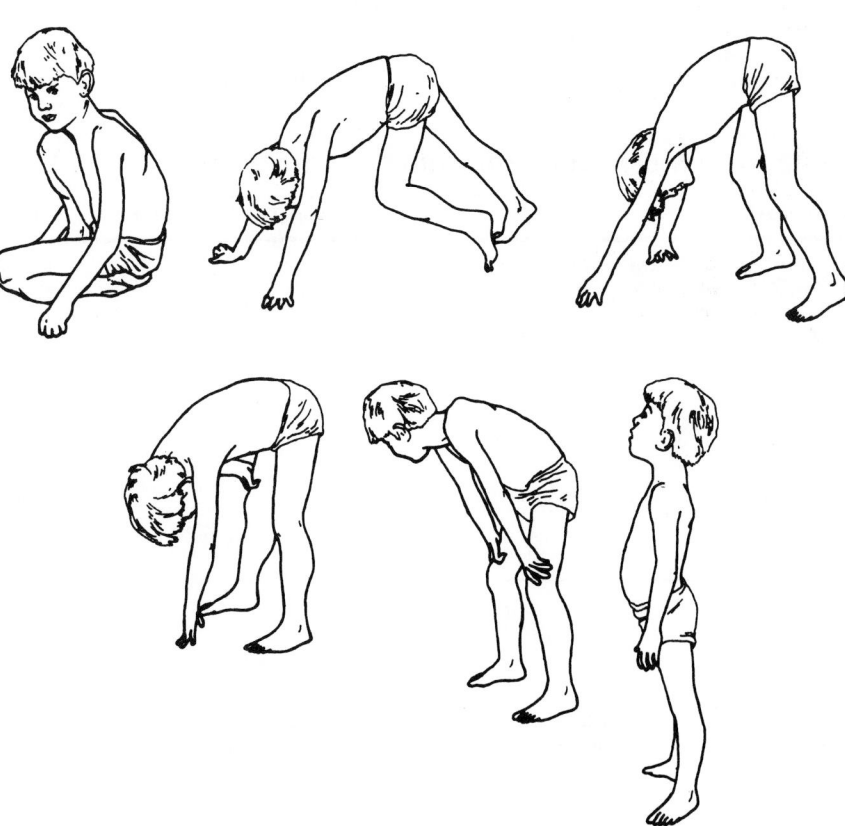

Fig. 1-255 Gower's sign in Duchenne's muscular dystrophy. (From Siegel IM: *Muscle and its diseases: an outline primer of basic science and clinical method,* Chicago, 1986, Year Book Medical.)

BASIC INFORMATION

■ DEFINITION
Mushroom poisoning is intoxication resulting from ingestion of poisonous mushrooms.

■ ICD-9CM CODES
988.1 Mushroom poisoning

■ EPIDEMIOLOGY & DEMOGRAPHICS
- Five percent of all mushrooms are poisonous. Distinction between poisonous and edible mushrooms may be difficult even by experienced persons.
- Common poisonous species include *Amanita, Russula, Gyromitra,* and *Omphalotus.*

■ PHYSICAL FINDINGS & CLINICAL PRESENTATION (TABLE 1-49)
- *Russula* causes confusion, delirium, visual disturbance, tachycardia, and diarrhea within a few hours of ingestion. Prognosis: spontaneous recovery (mortality <1%).
- *Amanita* and *Gyromitra* intoxication begins with symptoms of gastroenteritis (nausea, vomiting, diarrhea, abdominal cramps) approximately 10 hr following ingestion. *Amanita* then goes on to cause cardiomyopathy and hepatic and renal failure. *Gyromitra* produces jaundice and seizures. Both mushrooms are associated with a 50% mortality rate.
- *Omphalotus* causes symptoms of gastroenteritis that subside spontaneously within 24 hr.

■ PATHOPHYSIOLOGY
- *Amanita* contains cytotoxic substances and isoxazoles that are gamma-aminobutyric acid neurotransmitter analogs.
- *Gyromitra* contains a pyridoxine antagonist that disrupts the GI mucosa and causes hemolysis.
- *Russula* contains a cholinergic substance.

DIAGNOSIS

■ DIFFERENTIAL DIAGNOSIS
- Food poisoning
- Overdose of prescription or illegal drug
- Other intoxications
- See topic on specific organ failure (e.g., renal or hepatic failure) for differential diagnosis of those conditions.

■ WORKUP
- History
- Inspection and identification of suspected mushrooms
- Mushroom or gastric content analysis (by thin-layer chromatography or radioimmunoassay)

TREATMENT

- Gastric lavage
- Repeated administration of activated charcoal
- Supportive care as needed (may require respiratory assistance, hemodialysis, or emergency liver transplantation)

REFERENCE
Haubrich WS: Mushroom poisoning. In Haubrich WS, Schaffner F, Berk JE (eds): *Gastroenterology,* ed 5, Philadelphia, 1995, WB Saunders.
Author: **Tom J. Wachtel, M.D.**

TABLE 1-49   Mushroom Poisoning Syndromes

SYNDROME	INCUBATION PERIOD (hr)	SPECIES	TOXIN
Confusion, restlessness, visual disturbances, lethargy	2	*Amanita muscaria* *Amanita pantherina*	Ibotenic acid, muscimol
Parasympathetic activity	2	*Inocybe* sp. *Clitocybe* sp.	Muscarine
Hallucinations	2	*Psilocybe* sp. *Panacolus* sp.	Psilocybin Psilocin
Disulfiram	2	*Coprinus atramentarius*	Disulfiram-like substances
Gastroenteritis	2	Many	Unknown
Hepatorenal failure	6-24	*Amanita phalloides* *Amanita virosa* *Amanita verna* *Galerina autumnalis* *Galerina marginata* *Galerina venenata*	Amatoxins Phallotoxins
Hepatic failure	6-24	*Gyromitra* sp.	Gyromitrin

From Gorbach SL: *Infectious diseases,* ed 2, Philadelphia, 1998, WB Saunders.

BASIC INFORMATION

■ DEFINITION

Myasthenia gravis (MG) is a disorder of neuromuscular transmission characterized by the presence of a gamma globulin antibody (AChR-ab) directed against the nicotinic acetylcholinic receptor (AChR) of the neuromuscular junction, resulting in postsynaptic response to ACh.

■ ICD-9CM CODES
358.0 Myasthenia gravis

■ EPIDEMIOLOGY & DEMOGRAPHICS
INCIDENCE (IN U.S.): 2 to 5 cases/yr/1,000,000 persons
PREVALENCE (IN U.S.): 1/20,000 persons
PREDOMINANT SEX: Female > male (3:2) in adults; female = male in elderly
PREDOMINANT AGE: 20 to 40 yr
PEAK INCIDENCE: Female: third decade; male: fifth decade
GENETICS: Increased frequency of HLA-B8, DR3
Familial Predisposition: 5% of adult and juvenile cases
Congenital MG: Autosomal recessive; permanent condition
Neonatal MG: Occurs in 15% to 20% of infants born to mothers with MG. This condition is only temporary and is caused by transplacental passage of AChR-ab. Spontaneous recovery often occurs within 1 mo.

■ PHYSICAL FINDINGS & CLINICAL PRESENTATION
- The hallmark of MG is weakness made worse with exercise and improved with rest.
- More than 50% of patients are initially seen with ptosis, ocular muscle weakness, or both.
- Difficulty in chewing, abnormal smile, dysarthria, and dysphagia are also common.
- Pain may occur in fatigued muscles (e.g., neck muscles).
- Clinical manifestations are reproducible with exercise.
- Physical examination may be normal at rest.

■ ETIOLOGY
Injury of the acetylcholine receptors in the postsynaptic neuromuscular junction on an autoimmune basis (AChR-ab directed against the nicotinic acetylcholinic receptor of the neuromuscular junction)

DIAGNOSIS

■ DIFFERENTIAL DIAGNOSIS
Polymyositis, multiple sclerosis, chronic fatigue syndrome, myopathies, neurasthenia, polymyositis, cranial nerve lesions, pernicious anemia, thyrotoxic ophthalmopathy
Box 2-169 describes the differential diagnosis of muscle weakness.

■ WORKUP
- Improvement of symptoms after use of anticholinesterase medications: Edrophonium chloride (Tensilon), 2 mg IV; useful in MG patients with ocular symptoms; it has rapid onset (30 sec) and short duration of action (5 min).
  Pyridostigmine bromide (Mestinon), 60 mg PO; has longer duration of action and is often used in patients with generalized symptoms.
- Single-fiber electromyography (SFEMG); highly accurate in confirming MG in suspected patients with normal conventional repetitive stimulation.

■ LABORATORY TESTS
Elevated level of AChR-ab (present in 90% of patients with generalized MG and 60% of patients with ocular myasthenia): this serologic test must be performed only if testing with anticholinesterase drugs supports the diagnosis of MG.
- TSH, free T_4: to rule out thyroid disease (found in 5% to 15% of patients with MG)
- Vitamin B_{12} level to rule out pernicious anemia
- ANA, RF (increased association with SLE, rheumatoid arthritis)

■ IMAGING STUDIES
CT scan of anterior chest to rule out thymoma (found in 12% of patients with MG)

TREATMENT

■ NONPHARMACOLOGIC THERAPY
Prevention of exacerbations:
- Avoidance of temperature extremes; prompt treatment of infections, stress reduction
- Avoidance of selected drugs known to provoke exacerbations of MG (penicillamine, aminoglycoside antibiotics, tetracyclines, class I antiarrhythmics)

■ ACUTE GENERAL Rx
- Cholinesterase inhibitors: pyridostigmine 30 to 60 mg PO q4-6h initially; onset of effects is 30 min, duration 4 hr. A longer-acting preparation (Mestinon Timespan, 180 mg) can be given qd or bid; however, absorption may be erratic; major side effects are GI upset and increased salivary and bronchial secretions.
- Corticosteroids: prednisone doses range from 5 mg qod to 100 mg qd, depending on patient response; most patients require steroid therapy indefinitely. Slowly tapering steroids once control is achieved and switching to alternate day doses should be attempted.
- Immunosuppressants: azathioprine (Imuran) 2 to 3 mg/kg/day or cyclosporine 5 mg/kg/day is often used in patients with severe generalized weakness and may reduce the need for corticosteroids. Most patients require lifelong immunosuppressive therapy.
- Plasmaspheresis and leukoplasmapheresis are effective in severely ill patients and preoperatively in thymectomy candidates.

■ CHRONIC Rx
- Thymectomy is indicated in all patients with thymoma.
- Thymectomy in absence of thymoma is more controversial—generally recommended for MG patients aged 18 (postpubertal) to 50 yr, particularly patients not responding well to medical treatment.
- Drug therapy (cholinesterase inhibitors, corticosteroids, and immunosuppressants) may be useful.
- Prevent exacerbations (see above).

■ DISPOSITION
Course of disease is highly variable, with exacerbations and remissions.

■ REFERRAL
Surgical referral for thymectomy in selected cases (see above)

PEARLS & CONSIDERATIONS

■ COMMENTS
Patients must be closely monitored for onset of respiratory complications (acute respiratory arrest, aspiration pneumonia, chronic respiratory insufficiency).
Author: **Fred F. Ferri, M.D.**

BASIC INFORMATION

■ **DEFINITION**

Myocosis fungoides refers to a T-cell lymphoproliferative disorder with characteristic cutaneous skin lesions and with the potential to disseminate into lymph nodes and viscera (Fig. 1-256).

■ **SYNONYMS**

Cutaneous T-cell lymphoma

ICD-9CM CODES

202.1 Mycosis fungoides

■ **EPIDEMIOLOGY & DEMOGRAPHICS**

- Incidence of mycosis fungoides is 4/1 million.
- Approximately 1000 new cases are diagnosed annually in the United States.
- More commonly affects males than females (2:1).
- Blacks >whites (2:1).
- Usually found in males 40 to 60 years of age.

■ **PHYSICAL FINDINGS & CLINICAL PRESENTATION**

Mycosis fungoides characteristically progresses through 3 phases:

- A premycotic phase featuring scaly, erythematous patches that can last from months to years. During this stage the diagnosis can only be suspected, because the histopathological features are not definitive for mycosis fungoides. Lesions are pruritic and can appear anywhere but usually found in sun-shielded areas. Parapsoriasis en plaques, poikilodermatous parapsoriasis, parapsoriasis lichenoides, and variegata are skin lesions suspicious of representing premycotic cutaneous T-cell lymphoma.
- The infiltrative plaque phase features raised, indurated erythematous palpable plaques that are pruritic and may be associated with alopecia.
  1. Stage IA disease is defined as a patch or plaque skin disease involving <10% of the skin surface area.
  2. Stage IB disease is defined as a patch or plaque skin disease involving ≥10% of the skin surface area.
- The tumor phase is characterized by large, lumpy nodules arising from a premycotic patch, plaque, or unaf-

fected skin and represents systemic infiltration and spreading. The tumors can be pruritic and large (>10 cm) and ulceration can occur.
  1. Stage II disease is defined by the presence of tumors.
- In approximately 5% of cases of mycosis fungoides, the presentation may be a diffuse, painful, pruritive erythroderma known as Sézary syndrome.
  1. Stage III disease is defined by the presence of generalized erythroderma.
- Lymphadenopathy can occur during the plaque or tumor stages and may be regional or diffuse.
  1. Stage IVA disease is defined by a lymph node biopsy showing large clusters of atypical cells, more than six cells, or showing total effacerent by atypical cells.
- Infiltration of the liver, spleen, lungs, bone marrow, kidney, stomach, and brain can occur.
  1. Stage IVB disease is defined by the presence of visceral involvement.

■ **ETIOLOGY**

The specific cause of mycosis fungoides is not known. Infection with the retrovirus HTLV-1 has been suspected, given the association of HTLV-1 infected individuals and T-cell leukemia. Other considerations listed but unsubstantiated include environmental toxins (e.g., tobacco, pesticides, herbicides, and solvents) and genetic predisposition.

DIAGNOSIS

The diagnosis of mycosis fungoides is established by skin biopsy. This may be difficult to differentiate from other skin lesions in the early phases of the disease (e.g., premycotic patch or early plaque lesions) and therefore the diagnosis can only be suspected.

■ **DIFFERENTIAL DIAGNOSIS**

- Contact dermatitis
- Atopic dermatitis
- Nummular dermatitis
- Parapsoriases
- Superficial fungal infections
- Drug eruptions
- Psoriasis
- Photodermatitis
- Alopecia mucinosa
- Lymphomatoid papulosis

■ **WORKUP**

- Any patient who is suspected of having mycosis fungoides should have a staging workup done. Prognosis in patients with mycosis fungoides depends on the type of skin lesions and the extent of disease.
- The workup should focus on identifying:
  1. The type of skin lesion and the extent of skin involvement of the body (e.g., skin involvement is > or <10% of the skin surface).
  2. Presence of lymphadenopathy.
  3. Visceral involvement (e.g., lungs, liver).
  4. Presence of Sézary cells in the blood.
- A TNM staging classification has been proposed by the Cutaneous T-Cell Lymphoma Workshop in 1979 and continues to be used today in guiding therapy.

■ **LABORATORY TESTS**

- CBC with differential.
- Total lymphocyte count.
- Measure the percentage of Sézary cells present (normal <5%).
- BUN/creatinine.
- Electrolytes, calcium, and phosphorus.
- Liver function test.
- Multiple skin biopsies over suspected areas are done to confirm the diagnosis.
- If lymph nodes are present, excisional lymph node biopsy is performed.
- Bone marrow and liver biopsies can be done if initial laboratory screening suggests organ involvement.

■ **IMAGING STUDIES**

- Chest x-ray to rule out pulmonary involvement
- Chest, abdominal, and pelvic CT-scan looking for mediastinal, abdominal, and pelvic lymphadenopathy.

TREATMENT

Treatment is guided according to the stage of disease.

■ **NONPHARMACOLOGIC THERAPY**

- For dry cracking skin, emollients (e.g., lanolin and petrolatum) are applied bid.
- Moisturizing lotion (e.g., ammonium lactate) applied bid.

- Topical antibiotics (e.g., bacitracin) are used on ulcerative tumors.

■ ACUTE GENERAL Rx
- Treatment of patients with premycotic limited patch or plaque phase include:
  1. Psoralen ultraviolet light (PUVA) therapy where 0.6 mg/kg of 8-methoxypsoralen is ingested 1 to 2 hr before exposure of the skin to UV light (320 to 400 nm). This is done three times per week and tapered to two times per week until all the lesions have cleared. This is typically continued for 6 mo.
  2. Remissions can be retreated with PUVA.
- Treatment of patients with cutaneous patch and plaque lesions involving >10% of the skin surface includes:
  1. Topical chemotherapy using nitrogen mustard, carmustine, or mechlorethamine hydrochloride applied to the affected body areas.
  2. PUVA is an alternative treatment option.
- Treatment of patients with tumor phase disease includes:
  1. Total skin electron beam therapy in doses of 3000 to 3600 cGy given over 8 to 10 wk.
  2. Total skin electron beam therapy with PUVA is an alternative in recurrence tumor phase disease.

■ CHRONIC Rx
- In patients developing diffuse erythroderma (e.g., Sézary syndrome, extracorporeal photophoresis) where 8-methoxypsoralen is ingested and peripheral blood is exposed to UVA through a membrane filter.
- Interferon and other systemic chemotherapeutic agents (e.g., methotrexate, cyclophosphamide, doxorubicin, vincristine, and prednisone) are considered in disseminated mycosis fungoides.

■ DISPOSITION
- The median survival in patients with early patch or plaque phase disease and no extradermal involvement is 12 yr.
- The median survival of patients with skin involvement, lymph node involvement, but no visceral involvement is approximately 5 yr.
- The median survival in patients with visceral involvement is 2.5 yr.

■ REFERRAL
Any patient with suspected mycosis fungoides should be referred to a dermatologist for definitive diagnosis and initial therapy. Oncology consultation is also indicated in patients with more advanced disease.

☼ PEARLS & CONSIDERATIONS

■ COMMENTS
- Mycosis fungoides is thought to represent one class of the spectrum of cutaneous T cell lymphomas. Sézary syndrome, reticulum-cell sarcoma, and histiocytic lymphoma are also classified as T cell neoplasias.

- Alibert was the first to describe mycosis fungoides in 1806 and named it so because of its resemblance to mushrooms.

REFERENCES
Abel EA, Wood GS, Hopps RT: Mycosis fungoides: clinical and histologic features, staging, evaluation, and approach to treatment, *CA Cancer J* 43:93, 1993.

Diamandidoue E, Coner PR, Kurzrock R: Mycosis fungoides and Sézary syndrome, *Blood* 88(7):2385, 1996.

Kim YH, Hoppe RT: Mycosis fungoides and the Sézary syndrome, *Semin Oncol* 26(3):276, 1999.

Koh HK, Charif M, Weinstock MA: Epidemiology and clinical manifestations of cutaneous T-cell lymphonia, *Hematol Oncol Clin North Am* 9(5):1031, 1995.

Lorincz AL: Cutaneous T-cell lymphoma (mycosis fungoides), *Lancet* 347(9005):871, 1996.

Author: **Peter Petropoulos, M.D.**

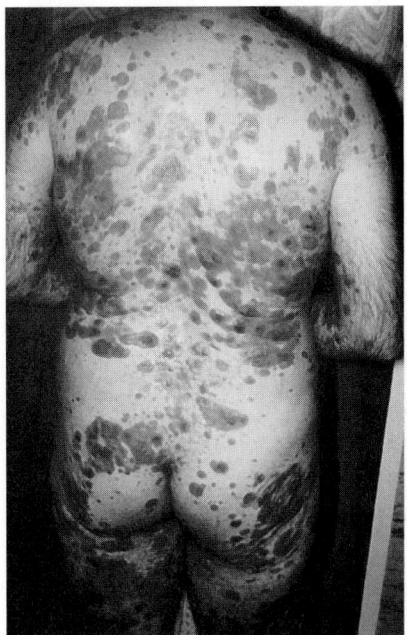

Fig. 1-256 Cutaneous T-cell lymphoma (mycosis fungoides). Note patch, plaque, and tumor stages. (From Noble J [ed]: *Textbook of primary care medicine,* ed 2, St Louis, 1996, Mosby.)

BASIC INFORMATION

■ DEFINITION
Myelodysplastic syndromes (MDS) are a group of acquired clonal disorders affecting the hemopoietic stem cells and characterized by cytopenias with hypercellular bone marrow and various morphologic abnormalities in the hemopoietic cell lines. Myelodysplastic syndromes show abnormal (dysplastic) hemopoietic maturation. Marrow cellularity is increased, reflecting an effective hematopoiesis, but inadequate maturation results in peripheral cytopenias. Myelodysplasia encompasses several heterogenous syndromes. The French-American-British classification of myelodysplastic syndromes includes the following: refractory anemia, refractory anemia with ringed sideroblasts, refractory anemia with excess blasts, chronic myelomonocytic leukemia, and refractory anemia with excess blasts in transformation.

■ SYNONYMS
MDS
Preleukemia
Dysmyelopoietic syndrome

■ ICD-9CM CODES
238.7 Myelodysplastic syndrome

■ EPIDEMIOLOGY & DEMOGRAPHICS
INCIDENCE (IN U.S.): Approximately 82 cases/100,000 persons/yr
PREDOMINANT AGE: More common in elderly patients, with a median age of >65 yr

■ PHYSICAL FINDINGS & CLINICAL PRESENTATION
- Splenomegaly, skin pallor, mucosal bleeding, ecchymosis may be present.
- Patients often present with fatigue.
- Fever, infection, and dyspnea are common.

■ ETIOLOGY
Unknown. However, exposure to radiation, chemotherapeutic agents, benzene, or other organic compounds is associated with myelodysplasia.

DIAGNOSIS

■ DIFFERENTIAL DIAGNOSIS
- Hereditary dysplasias (e.g., Fanconi's anemia, Diamond-Blackfan syndrome)
- Vitamin B_{12}/folate deficiency
- Exposure to toxins (drugs, alcohol, chemotherapy)
- Renal failure
- Irradiation
- Autoimmune disease
- Infections (TB, viral infections)
- Paroxysmal nocturnal hemoglobinuria

■ WORKUP
- Diagnostic workup includes laboratory evaluation and bone marrow examination.
- Fig. 1-257 describes an algorithmic approach to patients with suspected myelodysplastic syndromes.

■ LABORATORY TESTS
- Anemia with variable MCV (normal or increased)
- Reduced reticulocyte count (in relation to the degree of anemia)
- Hypogranular or agranular neutrophils
- Thrombocytopenia or normal platelet count
- Hypogranular platelets may be present
- Hypercellular bone marrow, with frequent clonal chromosomal abnormalities

■ IMAGING STUDIES
Abdominal CT scan may reveal hepatosplenomegaly.

TREATMENT

■ NONPHARMACOLOGIC THERAPY
RBC transfusions in patients with severe symptomatic anemia

■ ACUTE GENERAL Rx
- Results of chemotherapy are generally disappointing.
- The role of myeloid growth factors (granulocyte colony–stimulating factor, granulocyte-macrophage colony–stimulating factor) and immunotherapy is undefined.

- Allogeneic stem-cell transplantation should be considered in patients <60 yr old since this is the established procedure with cure potential.

■ CHRONIC Rx
Monitor for infections, bleeding, and complications of anemia.

■ DISPOSITION
- Cure rates in young patients with allogeneic bone marrow transplantations approach 30% to 50%.
- The risk of transformation to acute myelogenous leukemia varies with the percentage of blasts in the bone marrow.
- Advanced age, male sex, and deletion of chromosomes 5 and 7 are associated with a poor prognosis.
- According to the International Myelodysplastic Syndrome Risk Analysis Workshop, the most important variables in disease outcome are the specific cytogenetic abnormalities, the percentage of blasts in the bone marrow, and the number of hematopoietic lineages involved in the cytopenias.

■ REFERRAL
Hematology referral in all patients with myelodysplastic syndromes

PEARLS & CONSIDERATIONS

■ COMMENTS
Erythropoietin (epoetin alfa) SC three times weekly may be effective in increasing the Hgb and reducing the RBC transfusion requirement in some patients.
- Patients with cytogenetic abnormalities associated with poor prognosis should be considered for aggressive treatment with high-dose chemotherapy and stem-cell transplantation.

REFERENCE
Heaney ML, Golde DW: Myelodysplasia, *N Engl J Med* 340:1649, 1999.
Author: **Fred F. Ferri, M.D.**

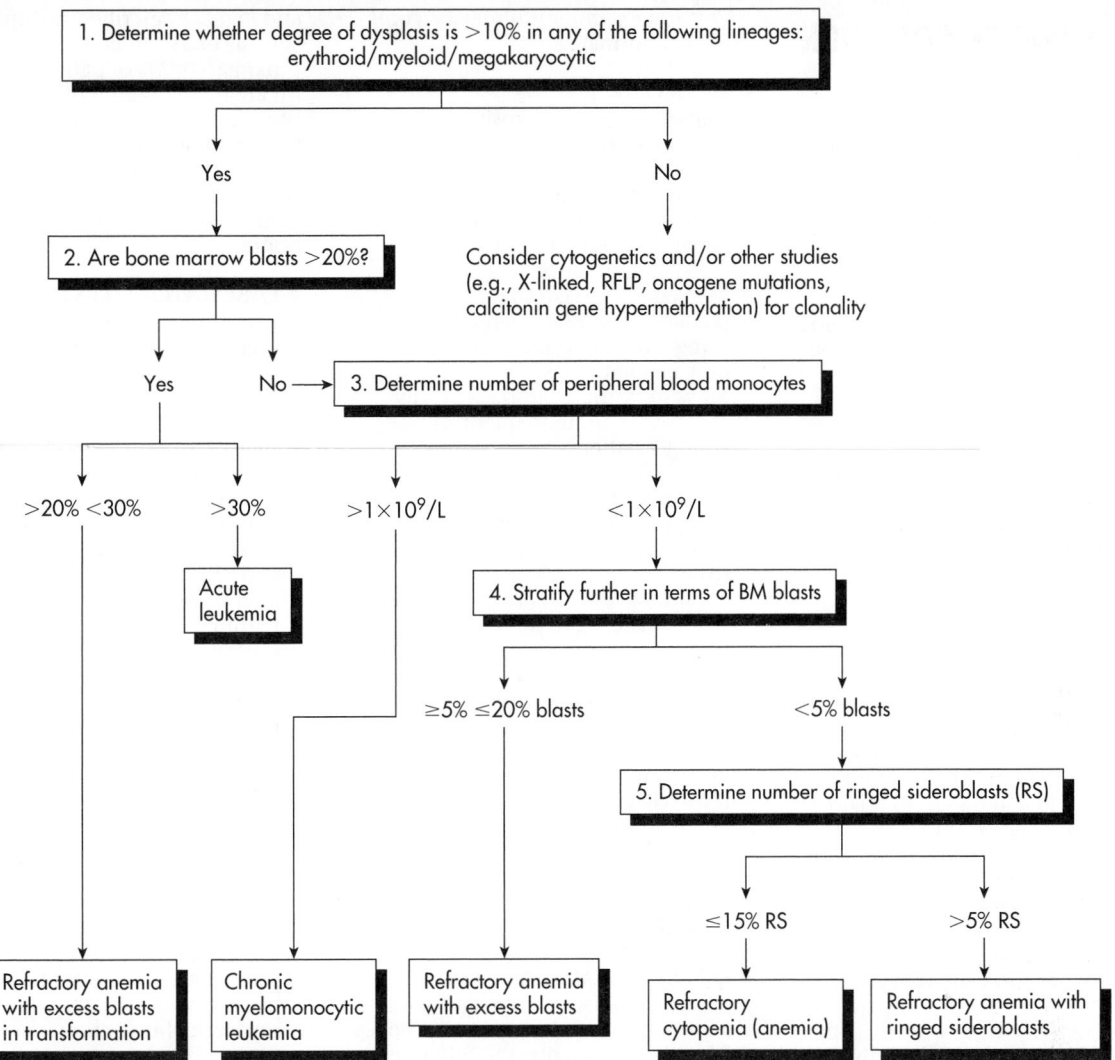

Fig. 1-257   Myelodysplastic syndromes. *BM blasts,* Bone marrow blastocyst; *RFLP,* restriction fragment length polymorphism. (From Abeloff MD: *Clinical oncology,* ed 2, New York, 2000, Churchill Livingstone.)

BASIC INFORMATION

■ DEFINITION

Myocardial infarction (MI) is characterized by necrosis resulting from an insufficient supply of oxygenated blood to an area of the heart.
- *Non–Q wave:* Area of ischemic necrosis is limited to the inner one third to half of the myocardial wall.
- *Q wave:* Area of ischemic necrosis penetrates the entire thickness of the ventricular wall.

■ SYNONYMS

MI
Heart attack
Coronary thrombosis
Coronary occlusion

■ ICD-9CM CODES

410.9 Acute myocardial infarction, unspecified site

■ EPIDEMIOLOGY & DEMOGRAPHICS

INCIDENCE/PREVALENCE (IN U.S.):
- >500 cases/100,000 persons.
- >500,000 MIs in the U.S. yearly.
- More prominent in males between the ages of 40 and 65 yr; no predominant sex after age 65 yr.
- Women experience more lethal and severe first acute MIs than men, regardless of comorbidity, previous angina, or age.
- At least one fourth of all myocardial infections are clinically unrecognized.

■ PHYSICAL FINDINGS & CLINICAL PRESENTATION

Clinical presentation:
- Crushing substernal chest pain usually lasts longer than 30 min.
- Pain is unrelieved by rest or sublingual nitroglycerin or is rapidly recurring.
- Pain radiates to the left or right arm, neck, jaw, back, shoulders, or abdomen and is not pleuritic in character.
- Pain may be associated with dyspnea, diaphoresis, nausea, or vomiting.
- There is no pain in approximately 20% of infarctions (usually in diabetic or elderly patients).
Physical findings:
- Skin may be diaphoretic, with pallor (because of decreased oxygen).
- Rales may be present at the bases of lungs (indicative of CHF).
- Cardiac auscultation may reveal an apical systolic murmur caused by mitral regurgitation secondary to papillary muscle dysfunction; S_3 or S_4 may also be present.

- Physical examination may be completely normal.

■ ETIOLOGY

- Coronary atherosclerosis.
- Coronary artery spasm.
- Coronary embolism (caused by infective endocarditis, rheumatic heart disease, intracavitary thrombus).
- Periarteritis and other coronary artery inflammatory diseases.
- Dissection into coronary arteries (aneurysmal or iatrogenic).
- Congenital abnormalities of coronary circulation.
- MI with normal coronaries (MINC syndrome): more frequent in younger patients and cocaine addicts. The risk of acute MI is increased by a factor of 24 during the 60 min after the use of cocaine in persons who are otherwise at relatively low risk. Most patients with cocaine-related MI are young, non-white, male cigarette smokers without other risk factors for ASHD who have a history of repeated cocaine use. Blood and urine toxicology screen for cocaine is recommended in all young patients who present with acute MI.
- Hypercoagulable states, increased blood viscosity (polycythemia vera).

 DIAGNOSIS

■ DIFFERENTIAL DIAGNOSIS

The various causes of myocardial ischemia are described in Box 2-173. Boxes 2-57 and 2-58 describe the differential diagnosis of chest pain. Table 2-189

and Fig. 2-7 describe the differential diagnosis of ST segment elevation. Approximately 2% of patients with acute MI are inadvertently discharged from the emergency department. A normal ECG is the most likely predictor of inadvertent discharge of these patients (the 30-day mortality rate is 10.5%) among patients with acute MI sent home.

■ LABORATORY TESTS

- Creatine kinase MB isoenzyme is a useful marker for myocardial infarction. It is released in the circulation in amounts that correlate with the size of the infarct.
- Cardiac troponin levels: cardiac-specific troponin T (cTnT) and cardiac-specific troponin I (cTnI) are highly specific for myocardial injury. Increases in serum levels of cTnT and cTnI may occur relatively early after muscle damage (3-12 hr), peak within 24 hr, and may be present for several days after MI (up to 7 days for cTnI and up to 10 to 14 days for cTnT). Troponin T tests can be falsely positive in patients with renal failure. The threshold level of troponin T considered positive for MI is 0.1 ng/ml in patients with normal renal function or 0.5 ng/ml in patients with renal impairment.
- Neither CK-MB nor troponin consistently appear in the blood within 6 hr after an ischemic event; therefore, serial testing (e.g., on presentation and after 8 hr) is necessary to definitely rule out myocardial infarction.
- ECG:
  1. In Q wave infarction (Table 1-50), there is development of:

TABLE 1-50   **Electrocardiographic Location of Q Wave Infarct**

AREA OF INFARCTION	ECG ABNORMALITY	ARTERY INVOLVED
Anterior wall	Q waves in V_1-V_4	LAD
Anteroseptal	Q waves in V_1-V_2	Proximal LAD
Anteroapical	Q waves in V_2-V_3	LAD or branches of LAD
Anterolateral	Q waves in V_4-V_6, I, aVL	Mid-LAD or CFX
Lateral wall	Q waves in I, aVL	CFX
Inferior wall	Q waves in II, III, aVF	RCA
Posterior wall	R > S in V_1 Q wave in V_6	PDA

From Ferri F: *Practical guide to the care of the medical patient,* ed 5, St Louis, 2001, Mosby.
CFX, Left circumflex artery; *ECG,* electrocardiographic; *LAD,* left anterior descending; *PDA,* posterior descending artery; *RCA,* right coronary artery.

a. Inverted T waves, indicating an area of ischemia
b. Elevated ST segment, indicating an area of injury
c. Q waves, indicating an area of infarction (usually develop over 12 to 36 hr)
2. In non–Q wave infarction, Q waves are absent, but:
   a. History and myocardial enzyme elevations are compatible with MI.
   b. ECG shows ST segment elevation, depression, or no change followed by T wave inversion.

■ IMAGING STUDIES
- Chest radiography is useful to evaluate for pulmonary congestion and exclude other causes of chest pain.
- Echocardiography can evaluate wall motion abnormalities and identify mural thrombus or mitral regurgitation, which can occur acutely after MI.

 ## TREATMENT

■ NONPHARMACOLOGIC THERAPY
- Limit patient's activity: bed rest for the initial 24 hr; if the patient remains stable, gradually increase activity.
- Diet: NPO until stable, then no added salt and a low-cholesterol diet.
- Patient education to decrease the risk of subsequent cardiac events (proper diet, cessation of smoking, regular exercise) should be initiated when the patient is medically stable.

■ ACUTE GENERAL Rx
- Any patient with suspected acute MI should immediately receive the following:
  1. Nasal oxygen: administer at 2 to 4 L/min.
  2. Nitrates: they increase the supply of oxygen by reducing coronary vasospasm and decrease consumption of oxygen by reducing ventricular preload. Sublingual nitroglycerin can be administered immediately on suspicion of MI (unless systolic blood pressure is <90 mm Hg or heart rate is <50 bpm or >100 bpm); IV nitroglycerin can be subsequently used. Nitroglycerin should be used with great caution in patients with inferior wall MI; nitrate usage can result in hypotension because these patients are sensitive to change in preload.
  3. Adequate analgesia: morphine sulfate 2 mg IV q5min PRN can be given for severe pain unre-

lieved by nitroglycerin.
  4. Aspirin: give 160 to 325 mg orally unless true aspirin allergy is suspected. If the first dose is chewed, a blood level is achieved more rapidly than if it is swallowed.
- If readily available without delay, primary angioplasty with adjunctive glycoprotein II b/III a is preferred over thrombolytic therapy. It is effective and generally results in more favorable outcomes than thrombolytic therapy. Prompt access to emergency coronary artery bypass graft (CABG) surgery is mandatory if primary PTCA is to be undertaken. When primary PTCA is performed, use of IV heparin is recommended. Coronary stents are useful to decrease ischemia, improve long-term patency, and lower the rate of restenosis of the infarct-related artery.
- Thrombolytic therapy (Fig. 1-258): if the duration of pain has been <6 hr and primary angioplasty is not readily available, recanalization of the occluded arteries should be attempted with thrombolytic agents, possibly in combination with glyco-

protein IIb/IIIa inhibition. When tPA or rPA is used, IV heparin is given to increase the likelihood of patency in the infarct-related artery. In patients receiving streptokinase or APSAC, IV heparin is not indicated, because it does not offer any additional benefit and can result in increased bleeding complications. Teneteplase and reteplase are comparable with accelerated infusion recombinant TPA in terms of efficacy and safety, but are more convenient because they are administered by bolus injection. Lanoplase and heparin bolus plus infusion is as effective as TPA with regard to mortality, but the rate of intracranial hemorrhage is significantly higher.
- β-adrenergic blocking agents should be given to all patients with evolving acute MI, provided that there are no contraindications (see below). β-Blockers are useful to reduce myocardial oxygen consumption and prevent tachyarrhythmias. Early IV β-blockage (in the inital 24 hr) followed by institution of an oral maintenance regimen is also effective in

---

General selection criteria
1. Chest pain consistent with MI of ≥30 min duration
2. Electrocardiographic evidence of acute Q wave MI:
   - ST elevation (≥0.1 mV) in at least 2 leads in anterior, inferior, or lateral locations
   - Acute ST depression with prominent R wave in leads V_1-V_2 (posterior MI)
   - New left bundle branch block
3. Time since symptoms began:
   <6 hours: greatest benefit
   >12 hours: less benefit, but still useful if chest pain continues

⬇

Exclusion criteria
- Major surgery or trauma in preceding 6 wk
- Gastrointestinal or genitourinary bleeding within 6 mo
- Systemic bleeding disorder
- Acute pericarditis or aortic dissection
- Cardiopulmonary resuscitation for >10 min
- Intracranial tumor or previous intracranial surgery
- Cerebrovascular accident within previous 6 mo
- Severe hypertension (>200/120)
- Pregnancy

⬇

Administer adjunctive therapy:
1. Heparin to maintain aPTT = 2 × control for 2-3 days
2. Aspirin 160-325 mg PO qd

⬇

Subsequent coronary arteriography reserved for:
- Spontaneous recurrent ischemia
- Positive exercise test before discharge

Fig. 1-258 Approach to thrombolytic therapy in acute Q wave MI. *MI,* Myocardial infarction; *ST,* sinus tachycardia. (From Noble J [ed]: *Primary care medicine,* ed 3, St Louis, 2001, Mosby.)

reducing recurrent infarction and ischemia. Frequently used agents are:

1. Metoprolol (Lopressor): IV 5 mg q2min × 3 doses, then PO 25 to 50 mg q6h, given 15 min after last IV dose, continued for 48 hr; maintenance dosage is 50 to 100 mg bid.
2. Atenolol (Tenormin): IV 5 mg over 5 min, repeat in 10 min if initial dose is well tolerated, then start PO dose 10 min after the last IV dose; PO 50 mg qd, increasing to 100 mg as tolerated.
3. Before using β-blockers, some of the contraindications and side effects (i.e., exacerbation of CHF, exacerbation of asthma, CNS effects, hypertension, bradycardia) must be carefully assessed.

- ACE inhibitors reduce left ventricular dysfunction and dilation and slow the progression of CHF during and after acute MI. They should be initiated within hours of hospitalization, provided that the patient does not have hypotension or a contraindication (bilateral renal stenosis, renal failure, or history of angioedema caused by previous treatment with ACE inhibitors).
  1. Commonly used agents are captopril 12.5 mg PO bid, enalapril 2.5 mg bid, or lisinopril 2.5 to 5 mg qd initially, with subsequent titration as needed.
  2. ACE inhibitors may be stopped in patients without complications and no evidence of left ventricular dysfunction after 6 to 8 wk.
  3. ACE inhibitors should be continued indefinitely in patients with impaired left ventricular function (ejection fraction <40%) or clinical CHF.
- Glycoprotein IIb receptor inhibitors (tirofiban, eptifibatide), when administered with heparin and aspirin, further reduce the incidence of ischemic events in patients with non-Q wave MI. The use of IV glycoprotein IIb/IIIa inhibitors (e.g., abciximab) before and during PTCA also reduces the risk of closure postangioplasty.

■ **CHRONIC Rx**
Evaluation of post-MI patients (also see Fig. 1-259)
- Submaximal (low level) treadmill test (can be done 1 to 3 wk after MI) in stable patients without any clinical evidence of significant left ventricular dysfunction or post-MI angina
  1. Useful to assess the patient's functional capacity and formulate an at-home exercise program
  2. Helpful to determine the patient's prognosis

- Radionuclide angiography or two-dimensional echocardiography
  1. To evaluate patient's left ventricular ejection fraction
  2. To evaluate ventricular size and segmental wall motion
  3. Echocardiography to rule out presence of mural thrombi in patients with anterior wall infarction; transesophageal echo is preferred if mural thrombosis is suspected
- A 24-hr Holter monitor study to evaluate patients who have demonstrated significant arrhythmias during their hospital stay; selected patients with complex ventricular ectopy may be candidates for programmed electrical stimulation studies and antiarrhythmic therapy and/or implanted defibrillator, depending on the results of these studies

■ **DISPOSITION**
The prognosis after MI depends on multiple factors:
- Use of β-blockers: the mortality of patients on a regular regimen of β-blockers is significantly decreased when compared with that of control groups.
- Presence of arrhythmias, frequent ventricular ectopy (≥10/hr), or repetitive forms of ventricular ectopic beats (couplets, triplets) indicates an increased risk (two to three times greater) of sudden cardiac death. New bundle-branch block, Mobitz II second-degree block, and third-degree heart block also adversely affect outcome.
- Size of infarct: the larger it is, the higher the post-MI mortality rate. Significant myocardial stunning with subsequent improvement of ventricular function occurs in most patients after Q wave anterior MI. A lower level of creatine kinase, an estimate of the extent of necrosis, is independently predictive of recovery of function.
- Site of infarct: inferior wall MI carries a better prognosis than anterior wall MI; however, patients with inferior wall MI and right ventricular involvement have a high risk for arrhythmic complications and cardiac shock.
- Type of infarct: although the in-hospital mortality rate is higher for patients with Q wave infarcts, the long-term prognosis for non–Q wave MI may be worse because these patients have a higher incidence of sudden cardiac death after hospital discharge.
- Ejection fraction after MI: the lower the left ventricular ejection fraction, the higher the mortality after MI.

- Presence of post-MI angina indicates a high mortality rate.
- Performance on low-level exercise test: the presence of ST segment changes during the test is a predictor of high mortality during the first year.
- Presence of pericarditis during the acute phase of MI increases mortality at 1 yr.
- Type A behavior (competitive drive, ambitiousness, hostility) is associated with a lower mortality rate after symptomatic MI.
- Self-reported moderate alcohol consumption in the year before acute MI is associated with reduced 1-yr mortality.
- Use of lipid-lowering agents in patients with hyperlipidemia unresponsive to exercise and dietary restrictions is beneficial. Statins may also lower vascular inflammation and damage by mechanisms other than reduction of LDL cholesterol. Early initiation of statin treatment in patients with acute MI is associated with reduced 1-yr mortality.
- Additional poor prognostic factors include the following: cigarette smoking, history of hypertension or prior MI, presence of ST segment depression in acute MI, increasing age, diabetes mellitus, and female sex (especially women >50 yr of age).

REFERENCES
Lange RA, Hillis LD: Cardiovascular complications of cocaine use, *N Engl J Med* 345:351, 2001.
Llevadot J et al: Bolus fibrinolytic therapy in acute myocardial infarction, *JAMA* 286:442, 2001.
Mukamal KJ: Prior alcohol consumption and mortality following acute myocardial infarction, *JAMA* 285:1965, 2001.
Sheifer S et al: Unrecognized myocardial infarction, *Ann Intern Med* 135:801, 2001.
Solomon SD et al: Recovery of ventricular function after MI in the reperfusion era: the healing and early afterload reducing therapy study, *Ann Intern Med* 134:451, 2001.
Stenestrand U, Wallentin L: Early statin treatment following acute MI and 1-year survival, *JAMA* 285:430, 2001.
Welch RD et al: Prognostic value of normal or non-specific initial ECG in acute MI, *JAMA* 286:1977, 2001.
Wu WC et al: Blood transfusion in elderly patients with acute myocardial infarction, *N Engl J Med* 345:1230, 2001.
Author: **Fred F. Ferri, M.D.**

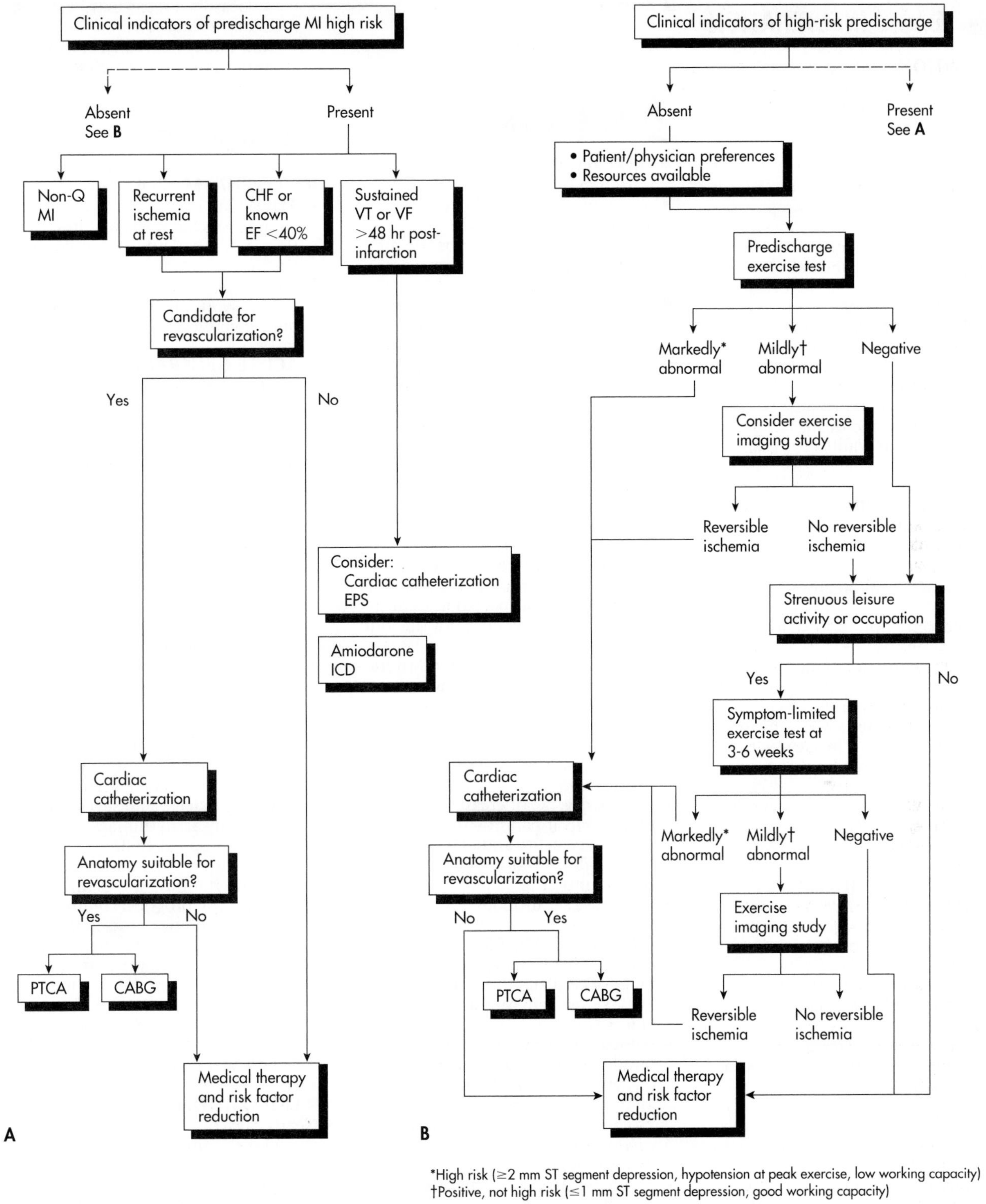

*High risk (≥2 mm ST segment depression, hypotension at peak exercise, low working capacity)
†Positive, not high risk (≤1 mm ST segment depression, good working capacity)

Fig. 1-259 **Management algorithm for risk stratification after acute myocardial infarction** *(MI)*. **A,** Patients with clinical indicators of high risk at hospital discharge, such as recurrent ischemia at rest or depressed left ventricular function, should be considered candidates for revascularization and referral to cardiac catheterization for ultimate triage to either percutaneous transluminal coronary angioplasty *(PTCA)*/coronary artery bypass graft surgery *(CABG)* or medical therapy and risk factor reduction. Patients with life-threatening arrhythmias, such as sustained ventricular tachycardia *(VT)* or ventricular fibrillation *(VF)*, should be considered for diagnostic cardiac catheterization, electrophysiology study *(EPS)*, and management with either amiodarone or an implantable cardioverter-defibrillator *(ICD)*, or both. *CHF,* Congestive heart failure; *EF,* ejection fraction. **B,** Patients without indicators of high risk at hospital discharge can be evaluated either with a submaximal exercise test before discharge (at least 5 to 7 days) or with a symptom-limited exercise at 14 to 21 days. Patients with either a markedly abnormal exercise test or no evidence of reversible ischemia on an exercise imaging study can be managed with medical therapy and risk factor reduction. (From Antman EM, Braunwald E: Acute myocardial infarction. In Braunwald E [ed]: *Heart disease,* ed 5, Philadelphia, 1997, WB Saunders.)

BASIC INFORMATION

■ DEFINITION
Myocarditis is an inflammatory condition of the myocardium.

ICD-9CM CODES
429.0 Myocarditis, nonspecific
391.2 Myocarditis, rheumatic
422.91 Myocarditis, viral (except coxsackie)
074.23 Myocarditis, coxsackie
422.92 Myocarditis, bacterial

■ EPIDEMIOLOGY & DEMOGRAPHICS
- The incidence of focal myocarditis reported at autopsy is 1% to 7% in asymptomatic patients.
- Myocarditis is a major cause of sudden unexpected death (15% to 20% of cases) in adults <40 years of age.

■ PHYSICAL FINDINGS & CLINICAL PRESENTATION
- Persistent tachycardia out of proportion to fever
- Faint S_1, S_4 sound on auscultation
- Murmur of mitral regurgitation
- Pericardial friction rub if associated with pericarditis
- Signs of biventricular failure (hypotension, hepatomegaly, peripheral edema, distention of neck veins, S_3)
- Patients may present with a history of recent flulike syndrome (fever, arthralgias, malaise)

■ ETIOLOGY
- Infection
  1. Viral (coxsackie B virus, CMV, echovirus, polio virus, adenovirus, mumps, HIV, EBV)
  2. Bacterial (*Staphylococcus aureus, Clostridium perfringens,* diphtheria, and any severe bacterial infection)
  3. Mycoplasma
  4. Mycotic *(Candida, Mucor, Aspergillus)*
  5. Parasitic (*Trypanosoma cruzi, Trichinella, Echinococcus,* amoeba, *Toxoplasma)*
  6. *Rickettsia rickettsii*
  7. Spirochetal *(Borrelia burgdorferi—* Lyme carditis)
- Rheumatic fever
- Secondary to drugs (e.g., cocaine, emetine, doxorubicin, sulfonamides, isoniazid, methyldopa, amphotericin B, tetracycline, phenylbutazone, lithium, 5-FU, phenothiazines, interferon alfa, tricyclic antidepressants, cyclophosphamides)
- Toxins (carbon monoxide, ethanol, diphtheria toxin, lead, arsenicals)
- Collagen-vascular disease (SLE, scleroderma, sarcoidosis, Kawasaki syndrome)
- Sarcoidosis
- Radiation
- Postpartum

DIAGNOSIS

■ DIFFERENTIAL DIAGNOSIS
- Cardiomyopathy
- Acute myocardial infarction
- Valvulopathies

Boxes 2-61 and 2-62 describe the differential diagnosis of chest pain.

■ WORKUP
- Medical history: the clinical presentation of myocarditis is nonspecific and can consist of fatigue, palpitations, dyspnea, precordial discomfort, myalgias.
- Diagnostic workup includes chest x-ray examination, ECG, laboratory evaluation, echocardiogram, cardiac catheterization, and endomyocardial biopsy (selected patients).

■ LABORATORY TESTS
- Elevated cardiac troponin T (TnT) is suggestive of myocarditis in patients with clinically suspected myocarditis. A normal level does not rule out the diagnosis.
- Increased CK (with elevated MB fraction, LDH), and AST secondary to myocardial necrosis.
- Increased ESR (nonspecific but may be of value in following the progress of the disease and the response to therapy).
- Increased WBC (increased eosinophils if parasitic infection).
- Viral titers (acute and convalescent).
- Cold agglutinin titer, ASLO titer, blood cultures.
- Lyme disease antibody titer.

■ IMAGING STUDIES
- Chest x-ray examination: enlargement of cardiac silhouette
- ECG: sinus tachycardia with nonspecific ST-T wave changes; interventricular conduction defects and bundle-branch block may be present
  1. Lyme disease and diphtheria cause all degrees of heart block.
  2. Changes of acute MI can occur with focal necrosis.
- Echocardiogram:
  1. Dilated and hypokinetic chambers
  2. Segmental wall motion abnormalities
- Cardiac catheterization and angiography:
  1. To rule out coronary artery disease and valvular disease.
  2. A right ventricular endomyocardial biopsy can confirm the diagnosis, although a negative biopsy result does not exclude myocarditis. Recent studies have shown that myocardial biopsy may be unnecessary, becauase immunosuppression therapy based on biopsy results is generally ineffective.

TREATMENT

■ NONPHARMACOLOGIC THERAPY
- Supportive care is the first line of therapy for patients with myocarditis.
- Restrict physical activity (to decrease cardiac work). Bed rest is advisable during viremia.

■ ACUTE GENERAL Rx
- Treat underlying cause (e.g., use specific antibiotics for bacterial infection).
- Treat CHF with diuretics, ACE inhibitors, and salt restriction. A β-blocker may be added once clinical stability has been achieved. Digoxin should be used wtih caution and only at low doses.
- If ventricular arrhythmias are present, treat with quinidine or procainamide.
- Provide anticoagulation to prevent thromboembolism.
- Use preload and afterload reducing agents for treating cardiac decompensation.
- Corticosteroid use is contraindicated in early infectious myocarditis; it may be justified in only selected patients with intractable CHF, severe systemic toxicity, and severe life-threatening arrhythmias.
- Immunosuppressive drugs (prednisone with cyclosporine or azathioprine) do not have any significant effect on the prognosis of myocarditis and should not be used in the routine treatment of patients with myocarditis. Immunosuppression may have a role in the treatment of myocarditis from systemic autoimmune disease (e.g., SLE, scleroderma) and in patients with idiopathic giant cell myocarditis.

■ DISPOSITION
Nearly 50% of patients with myocarditis will die within 5 yr of diagnosis.

■ REFERRAL
Consider heart transplant if patient develops intractable CHF.

REFERENCES
Feldman AM, McNamara D: Myocarditis. *N Eng J Med* 343:1388, 2000.
Wu LA et al: Current role of endomyocardial biopsy in the management of dilated cardiomyopathy and myocarditis, *Mayo Clin Proc* 76:1030, 2001.
Author: **Fred F. Ferri, M.D.**

BASIC INFORMATION

■ DEFINITION
Myotonia is a type of muscular dystrophy in which relaxation of a muscle after contraction is delayed or prolonged. The most common type of muscular dystrophy with myotonia is myotonic dystrophy, which is described below.

■ SYNONYMS
Myotonic dystrophy

ICD-9CM CODES
359.2 Myotonic disorders
728.85 Muscle spasm

■ EPIDEMIOLOGY & DEMOGRAPHICS
PREVALENCE: 3 to 5 cases/100,000 persons
- Genetic disorder inherited as an autosomal dominant illness
- Symptoms usually manifest during adolescence or early adulthood. Cases of infantile myotonic dystrophy have been described.

■ PHYSICAL FINDINGS & CLINICAL PRESENTATION
- Usual first complaint is distal extremity weakness sometimes associated with muscle stiffness, cramps, or difficulty relaxing the grasp.
- Weakness spreads to eventually involve all muscle groups. Flexor neck muscle weakness and masseter and temporal wasting are often prominent features, as is dysarthria.
- Percussion of a muscle produces a slow contraction followed by prolonged relaxation. The "myotonic reflex" is best tested by percussing the thenar muscles and observing a slow flexion followed by slow relaxation of the thumb.
- As the disease progresses, generalized weakness becomes more pronounced and myotonia becomes less evident.
- Extramuscular involvement:
  Mental retardation of variable severity (may be absent)
  Frontal baldness (Fig. 1-260)
  Cataracts
  Diabetes mellitus
  Hypogonadism
  Adrenal failure
  Cardiomyopathy
- Infantile myotonic dystrophy presents as neonatal extreme hypotonia with "shark mouth" deformity (upper lip forming an inverted V).

■ ETIOLOGY & PATHOGENESIS
Genetic disorder encoded on chromosome 19 leading to sustained firing of the muscle membrane, causing prolonged muscle contraction

DIAGNOSIS

■ DIFFERENTIAL DIAGNOSIS
- Myotonia congenita (Thomsen's disease)
  May be autosomal dominant or recessive (two distinct varieties)
  The disease is limited to muscles and causes hypertrophy and stiffness after rest. Muscle function normalizes with exercise. There is no weakness. Symptoms are exacerbated by exposure to cold.
- Paramyotonia congenita
  Autosomal dominant disease
  Weakness and stiffness of facial muscles and distal upper extremities, especially or exclusively on cold exposure
- Muscular dystrophies
- Inflammatory myopathies (polymyositis)
- Metabolic muscle diseases
- Myasthenic syndromes
- Motor neuron disease

■ WORKUP
- History and physical examination usually sufficient
- Muscle enzymes usually abnormal (CPK, aldolase, AST)
- EMG: typical myotonic "dive bomber" bursts
- Muscle biopsy: type I fiber atrophy, ring fibers, and increased central nucleation

TREATMENT

- Phenytoin
- Quinine
- Quinidine
- Procainamide
- Acetazolamide
- Genetic counseling
- Assistive devices, orthotics

■ REFERRAL
To neurologist

REFERENCE
Rose M, Griggs R: Inherited muscle, neuromuscular, and neuronal disorders. In Goetz CG (ed): *Textbook of clinical neurology*, Philadelphia, 1999, WB Saunders.
Author: **Tom J. Wachtel, M.D.**

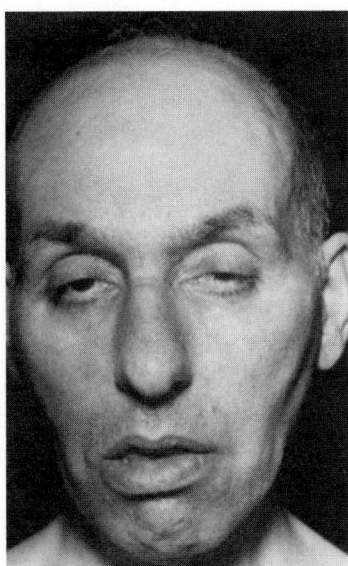
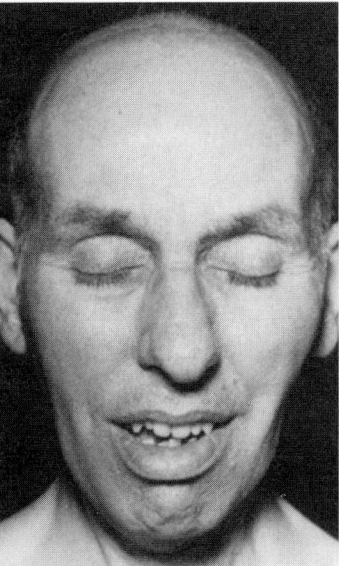

Fig. 1-260   Myotonic dystrophy with typical myopathic facies, frontal balding, and sunken cheeks. (From Dubowitz V: *Muscle disorders in childhood,* London, 1995, WB Saunders.)

BASIC INFORMATION

■ DEFINITION

Myxedema coma is a life-threatening complication of hypothyroidism characterized by profound lethargy or coma and usually accompanied by hypothermia.

ICD-9CM CODES
244.8 Myxedema, pituitary
244.1 Myxedema, primary

■ PHYSICAL FINDINGS & CLINICAL PRESENTATION
- Profound lethargy or coma
- Hypothermia (rectal temperature <35° C [95° F]); often missed by using ordinary thermometers graduated only to 34.5° C or because the mercury is not shaken below 36° C
- Bradycardia, hypotension (secondary to circulatory collapse)
- Delayed relaxation phase of DTR, areflexia
- Myxedema facies (Fig. 1-261)
- Alopecia, macroglossia, ptosis, periorbital edema, nonpitting edema, doughy skin
- Bladder dystonia and distention

■ ETIOLOGY
Decompensation of hypothyroidism secondary to:
- Sepsis
- Exposure to cold weather
- CNS depressants (sedatives, narcotics, antidepressants)
- Trauma, surgery

DIAGNOSIS

■ DIFFERENTIAL DIAGNOSIS
- Severe depression, primary psychosis
- Drug overdose
- CVA, liver failure, renal failure
- Hypoglycemia, CO_2 narcosis, encephalitis

■ WORKUP
Diagnosis of hypothyroidism and exclusion of contributing factors (e.g., sepsis, CVA) with laboratory and radiographic studies (see below)

■ LABORATORY TESTS
- Markedly increased TSH (if primary hypothyroidism), decreased serum free T_4
- CBC with differential, urine and blood cultures to rule out infectious process
- Electrolytes, BUN, creatinine, liver function tests, calcium, glucose
- ABGs to rule out hypoxemia and carbon dioxide retention
- Cortisol level to rule out adrenal insufficiency
- Elevated CPK
- Hyperlipidemia

■ IMAGING STUDIES
- CT scan of head in suspected CVA
- Chest x-ray examination to rule out infectious process

TREATMENT

■ NONPHARMACOLOGIC THERAPY
Prevent further heat loss; cover the patient but avoid external rewarming because it may produce vascular collapse.
Support respiratory function; intubation and mechanical ventilation may be required.
Monitor patients in the ICU.

■ ACUTE GENERAL Rx
- Give levothyroxine 5 to 8 µg/kg (300 to 500 µg) IV infused over 15 min, then 100 µg IV q24h.
- Glucocorticoids should also be administered until coexistent adrenal insufficiency can be ruled out. Hydrocortisone hemisuccinate 100 mg IV bolus is initially given, followed by 50 mg IV q12h or 25 mg IV q6h until initial plasma cortisol level is confirmed normal.
- IV hydration with D_5NS is used to correct hypotension and hypoglycemia (if present); avoid overhydration and possible water intoxication because clearance of free water is impaired in these patients.
- Rule out and treat precipitating factors (e.g., antibiotics in suspected sepsis).

■ CHRONIC Rx
Refer to "Hypothyroidism" in Section I.

■ DISPOSITION
Mortality rate in myxedema coma is 20% to 50%.

■ REFERRAL
Endocrinology consultation is appropriate in patients with myxedema coma.

PEARLS & CONSIDERATIONS

■ COMMENTS
If the diagnosis is suspected, initiate treatment immediately without waiting for confirming laboratory results.

REFERENCE
Wall CR: Myxedema coma: diagnosis and treatment, 62:2485, 2000.
Author: **Fred F. Ferri, M.D.**

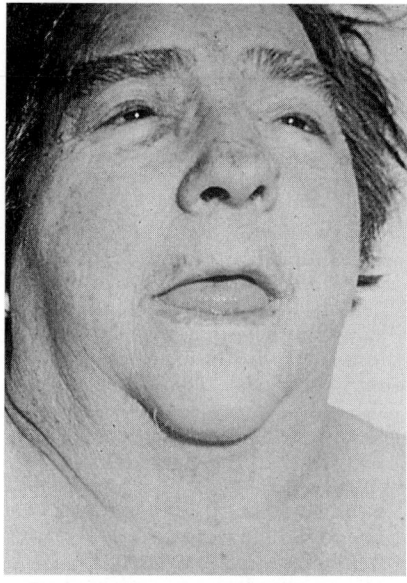

Fig. 1-261 Myxedema facies. Note dull, puffy, yellowed skin; coarse, sparse hair; temporal loss of eyebrows; periorbital edema; prominent tongue. (Courtesy Paul W. Ladenson, MD. The Johns Hopkins University and Hospital, Baltimore: In Seidel HM [ed]: *Mosby's guide to physical examination,* ed 4, St Louis, 1999, Mosby.)

BASIC INFORMATION

■ **DEFINITION**
Narcolepsy is a sleep disorder in which REM sleep occurs suddenly during wakefulness. It is characterized by the tetrad of excessive daytime sleepiness, irresistible sleep attacks, cataplexy, hypnagogic hallucinations, and sleep paralysis.

ICD-9CM CODES
347 Cataplexy and narcolepsy

■ **EPIDEMIOLOGY & DEMOGRAPHICS**
INCIDENCE (IN U.S.): 1 case/1000 persons/yr; more than 50-fold increased incidence in families with a positive history
PREVALENCE (IN U.S.): 50 to 60 cases/100,000 persons
PREDOMINANT SEX: Males = females
PREDOMINANT AGE: Second decade
PEAK INCIDENCE: Age 15 to 25 yr
GENETICS: Strong association with HLA-DR2 and HLA-DOw1 antigens

■ **PHYSICAL FINDINGS & CLINICAL PRESENTATION**
• Sleep attacks last from a few seconds to 30 min, during which patients are easily awakened by tactile stimuli.
• Cataplexy, which occurs in 80% of patients, is an abrupt loss of voluntary muscle control precipitated by a strong emotion. Consciousness is preserved.
• Sleep paralysis, which occurs in 60% of patients, is a loss of muscle tone during the transition between sleep and wakefulness. It may be interrupted by tactile stimuli.

• Hypnagogic hallucinations may be experienced during the transition from wakefulness to sleep.

■ **ETIOLOGY**
Unknown

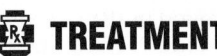 **DIAGNOSIS**

■ **DIFFERENTIAL DIAGNOSIS**
• Sleep apnea
• Periodic movements in sleep
• Hypothyroidism
• Sedative drugs
• Encephalopathic states
• Seizures

■ **WORKUP**
Nocturnal polysomnography followed by a multiple sleep latency test

■ **LABORATORY TESTS**
Some 90% to 95% of patients are HLA-DR2 positive, so a negative test is evidence against the diagnosis, although a positive test does not establish the diagnosis, because HLA-DR2 is found in the normal population.

TREATMENT

■ **NONPHARMACOLOGIC THERAPY**
Short, scheduled daytime naps

■ **CHRONIC Rx**
• For hypersomnolence:
  1. Medafinil (Provigil) 200 mg PO qAM
  2. Methylphenidate (Ritalin) 10 mg bid initially
  3. Pemoline (Cylert) 37.5 mg/day in the morning initially; increase until desired response is obtained
• For cataplexy:
  1. Clomipramine (Anafranil) 25 mg/day initially
  2. Protriptyline (Vivactil) 5 mg tid initially
  3. Imipramine (Tofranil) 25 to 50 mg/day initially
  4. Desipramine (Norpramine) 10 mg bid initially
  5. Fluoxetine (Prozac) 20 mg qd initially

■ **DISPOSITION**
A chronic sleep disorder without periods of remission

■ **REFERRAL**
If sleep studies are needed, they should be performed in an accredited sleep disorders laboratory.

PEARLS & CONSIDERATIONS

■ **COMMENTS**
True narcolepsy is a relatively rare cause of daytime sleepiness.

REFERENCE
Krahn LE et al: Narcolepsy: new understanding of irresistable sleep, *Mayo Clin Proc* 76:185, 2001.
Author: **Michael Gruenthal, M.D., Ph.D.**

BASIC INFORMATION

■ DEFINITION
Nephrotic syndrome is characterized by high urine protein excretion (>3.5g/1.73 m^3/24 hr), peripheral edema, and metabolic abnormalities (hypoalbuminemia, hypercholesterolemia).

■ ICD-9CM CODES
581.9 Nephrotic syndrome

■ EPIDEMIOLOGY & DEMOGRAPHICS
- Nephrotic syndrome occurs predominantly in children ages 2 to 6 yr (2 new cases/100,000 persons/yr) and in adults of all ages (3 to 4 new cases/100,000 persons/yr).
- Membranous glomerulonephritis is the most common cause of nephrotic syndrome.

■ PHYSICAL FINDINGS & CLINICAL PRESENTATION
- Peripheral edema
- Ascites, anasarca
- Hypertension
- Pleural effusion
- Typically patients present with severe peripheral edema, exertional dyspnea, and abdominal fullness secondary to ascites. There is a significant amount of weight gain in most patients.

■ ETIOLOGY
- Idiopathic (may be secondary to the following glomerular diseases: minimal change disease [nil disease, lipoid nephrosis], focal segmental glomerular sclerosis, membranous nephropathy, membranoproliferative glomerular nephropathy).
- Associated with systemic diseases (diabetes mellitus, SLE, amyloidosis). Amyloidosis and dysproteinemias should be considered in patients older than 40 years.
- Majority of children with nephrotic syndrome have minimal change disease (this form also associated with allergy, nonsteroidals, and Hodgkin's disease).
- Focal glomerular disease: can be associated with HIV infection, heroin abuse. A more severe form of nephrotic syndrome associated with rapid progression to end-stage renal failure within months can also occur in HIV seropositive patients and is known as "collapsing glomerulopathy."
- Membranous nephropathy: can occur with Hodgkin's lymphoma, carcinomas, SLE, gold therapy.
- Membranoproliferative glomerulonephropathy: often associated with upper respiratory infections.
- Table 1-51 describes primary renal diseases that present as idiopathic nephrotic syndrome.

■ DIAGNOSIS

■ DIFFERENTIAL DIAGNOSIS
- Other edema states (CHF, cirrhosis)
- Primary renal disease (e.g., focal glomerulonephritis, membranoproliferative glomerulonephritis). Table 1-51 summarizes primary renal diseases that present as idiopathic nephrotic syndrome.
- Carcinoma, infections
- Malignant hypertension
- Polyarteritis nodosa
- Serum sickness
- Toxemia of pregnancy

■ WORKUP
- Diagnostic workup consists of family history and history of drug use or toxin exposure and laboratory evaluation. Renal biopsy is generally performed in individuals with persistent proteinuria in whom the etiology of the proteinuria is unclear.

■ LABORATORY TESTS
- Urinalysis reveals proteinuria. The presence of hematuria, cellullar casts, and pyuria is suggestive of nephritic syndrome. Oval fat bodies (tubular epithelial cells with cholesterol esters) are also found in the urine in patients with nephrotic syndrome.
- 24-hr urine protein excretion is >3.5 g/1.73 m^3/24 hr.
- Abnormalities of blood chemistries include serum albumin <3 g/dl, decreased total protein, elevated serum cholesterol, glucose, azotemia.
- Additional tests in patients with nephrotic syndromes depending on the history and physical examination are ANA, serum and urine immunoelectrophoresis, C3, C4, CH-50, LDH, liver enzymes, alkaline phosphatase, hepatitis B and C screening, and HIV.

■ IMAGING STUDIES
- CT scan or ultrasound of kidneys
- Chest x-ray

■ TREATMENT

■ NONPHARMACOLOGIC THERAPY
- Bed rest as tolerated, avoidance of nephrotoxic drugs, low-fat diet, fluid restriction in hyponatremic patients; normal protein intake unless urinary protein loss exceeds 10 g/24 hr (some patients may require additional dietary protein to prevent negative nitrogen balance and significant protein malnutrition).
- Improved urinary protein excretion and serum lipid changes have been observed with a low-fat soy protein diet providing 0.7 g of protein/kg/day. However, because of increased risk of

malnutrition, many nephrologists recommend normal protein intake.
- Strict sodium restriction to help manage peripheral edema.
- Close monitoring of patients for development of peripheral venous thrombosis and renal vein thrombosis because of hypercoagulable state secondary to loss of antithrombin III and other proteins involved in the clotting mechanism.

■ ACUTE GENERAL Rx
- Furosemide is useful for severe edema.
- Use of ACE inhibitors to reduce proteinuria is generally indicated even in normotensive patients.
- Anticoagulant therapy should be administered as long as patients have nephrotic proteinuria, an albumin level <20 g/L, or both.

The mainstay of therapy is treatment of the underlying disorder:
- Minimal change disease generally responds to prednisone 1 mg/kg/day. Relapses can occur when steroids are discontinued. In these individuals, cyclophosphamide and chlorambucil may be useful.
- Focal and segmental glomerulosclerosis: steroid therapy is also recommended. However, response rate is approximately 35% to 40%, and most patients progress to end-stage renal disease within 3 yr.
- Membranous glomerulonephritis: prednisone 2 mg/kg/day may be useful in inducing remission. Cytotoxic agents can be added if there is poor response to prednisone.
- Membranoproliferative glomerulonephritis: most patients are treated with steroid therapy and antiplatelet drugs. Despite treatment, the majority of patients will progress to end-stage renal disease within 5 yr.

■ CHRONIC Rx
- Patients should be monitored for azotemia and should be aggressively treated for hypertension and hyperlipidemia. Furosemide is useful for severe edema. Anticoagulants may be necessary for thromboembolic events. Prophylactic anticoagulation should be considered in patients with membranous glomerulonephritis.
- Oral vitamin D is useful in the treatment of hypocalcemia (because of vitamin D loss).

■ REFERRAL
Nephrology consultation is recommended.

REFERENCE
Madaio MP, Harrington JT: The diagnosis of glomerular diseases, *Arch Intern Med* 161:25, 2001.
Author: **Fred F. Ferri, M.D.**

NEPHROTIC SYNDROME

TABLE 1-51 Summary of Primary Renal Diseases That Present as Idiopathic Nephrotic Syndrome

	MINIMAL-CHANGE NEPHROTIC SYNDROME (MCNS)	FOCAL SEGMENTAL SCLEROSIS	MEMBRANOUS NEPHROPATHY	MEMBRANOPROLIFERATIVE GLOMERULONEPHRITIS (MPGN) TYPE I	TYPE II
Frequency*					
Children	75%	10%	<5%	10%	10%
Adults	15%	15%	50%	10%	10%
Clinical Manifestations					
Age (yr)	2-6, some adults	2-10, some adults	40-50	5-15	5-15
Sex	2:1 male	1.3:1 male	2:1 male	Male-female	Male-female
Nephrotic syndrome	100%	90%	80%	60%	60%
Asymptomatic proteinuria	0	10%	20%	40%	40%
Hematuria	10%-20%	60%-80%	60%	80%	80%
Hypertension	10%	20% early	Infrequent	35%	35%
Rate of progression to renal failure	Does not progress	10 years	50% in 10-20 yr	10-20 yr	5-15 yr
Associated conditions	Allergy? Hodgkin's disease, usually none	None	Renal vein thrombosis, cancer, SLE, hepatitis B	None	Partial lipodystrophy
Laboratory Findings	Manifestations of nephrotic syndrome ↑ BUN in 15%-30%	Manifestations of nephrotic syndrome ↑ BUN in 20%-40%	Manifestations of nephrotic syndrome	Low C1, C4, C3-C9	Normal C1, C4, low C3-C9
Immunogenetics	HLA-B8, B12 (3.5)†	Not established	HLA-DRW3 (12-32)†	Not established	C3 nephritic factor
Renal Pathology					
Light microscopy	Normal	Focal sclerotic lesions	Thickened GBM, spikes	Thickened GBM, proliferation	Lobulation
Immunofluorescence	Negative	IgM, C3 in lesions	Fine granular IgG, C3	Granular IgG, C3	C3 only
Electron microscopy	Foot process fusion	Foot process fusion	Subepithelial deposits	Mesangial and subendothelial deposits	Dense deposits
Response of Steroids	90%	15%-20%	May be slow progression	Not established	Not established

Modified from Couser WG: Glomerular disorders. In Wyngaarden JB, Smith LH, Bennett JC (eds): *Cecil textbook of medicine*, ed 19, Philadelphia, 1992, WB Saunders.
*Approximate frequency as a cause of idiopathic nephrotic syndrome. About 10% of adult nephrotic syndrome is due to various diseases that usually present with acute glomerulonephritis.
†Relative risk.
BUN, Blood urea nitrogen; *C*, complement; *GBM*, glomerular basement membrane; *HLA*, human leukocyte antigen; *Ig*, immunoglobulin; *SLE*, systemic lupus erythematosus; *hepatitis B*, hepatitis B virus; ↑, elevated.

BASIC INFORMATION

■ **DEFINITION**
Neuroblastomas are neural tumors and abnormalities that have cell origins from the neural crest.

ICD-9CM CODES
194.0 Neuroblastoma, unspecified site

■ **EPIDEMIOLOGY & DEMOGRAPHICS**
INCIDENCE (IN U.S.): 8% of all solid tumors of childhood; 10 cases/ 1 million children <15 yr
PREDOMINANT SEX: Male:female ratio of 1:1.3
PEAK INCIDENCE: Childhood
PEAK AGE: Infants and children
GENETICS: N-*myc* protooncogene; loss of short arm chromosome 1 (1p36) found in some children

■ **PHYSICAL FINDINGS & CLINICAL PRESENTATION**
- Mass in abdomen, neck, or chest (Fig. 1-262)
- Spinal cord compression
- Dancing eyes
- Chronic pain
- Ecchymosis around eyes
- Weight loss
- Fever
- Irritability

■ **ETIOLOGY**
Tumor arises from neural crest, so gene abnormality is likely.

 DIAGNOSIS

■ **DIFFERENTIAL DIAGNOSIS**
- Other childhood tumors
- Wilms' tumor

■ **WORKUP**
- Careful general physical examination
- Biopsy of tumor when possible
- Staging (Evans classification)
  - I. Confined to single organ
  - II. Extension beyond organ of origin but not past midline
  - III. Extension across midline
  - IV. Distant metastases

■ **LABORATORY TESTS**
- Urinary catecholamines
- Bone marrow aspiration

■ **IMAGING STUDIES**
CT scan or MRI of suspected affected area

■ **TREATMENT**

■ **NONPHARMACOLOGIC THERAPY**
Assure patient that there is hope for recovery with aggressive treatment.

■ **ACUTE GENERAL Rx**
- Surgery
- Multiagent chemotherapy (e.g., cyclophosphamide, vincristine, dacarbazine, melphalan, doxorubicin, cisplatin)
- Radiotherapy

■ **CHRONIC Rx**
- The condition results in either death or cure.
- Overall survival is >40%.
- Survival in stage I is >95%, whereas survival in stage II is <20%.

■ **DISPOSITION**
Refer immediately to oncology team.

■ **REFERRAL**
A multidisciplinary team is necessary.

PEARLS & CONSIDERATIONS

■ **COMMENTS**
Children <1 yr with low-stage disease have 80% chance of survival; those with stage IV have 20% chance of survival.
Author: **William H. Olson, M.D.**

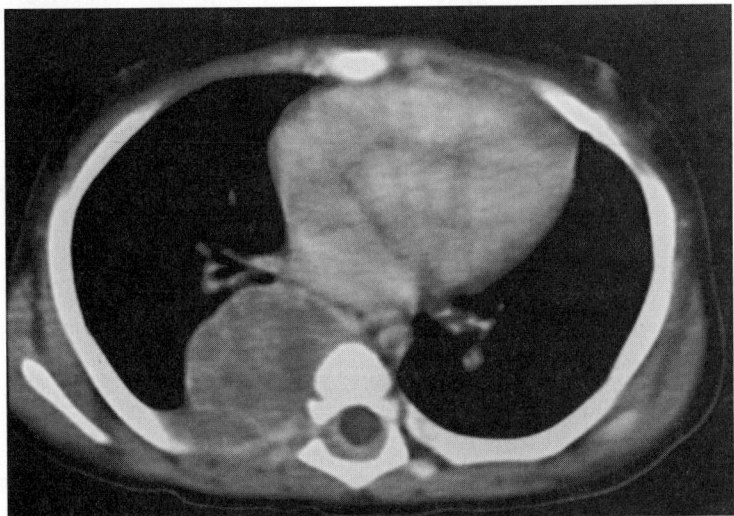
Fig. 1-262 CT scan of a thoracic neuroblastoma with intraspinal extension at diagnosis. (From Behrman RE: *Nelson textbook of pediatrics,* Philadelphia, 1996, WB Saunders.)

BASIC INFORMATION

■ DEFINITION

Neurofibromatosis (NF) is an autosomal dominant inherited neurocutaneous disorder. There are two types of neurofibromatosis disorders: NF type 1 (NF1) and NF type 2 (NF2).

■ SYNONYMS

- NF1 is also called von Recklinghausen disease
- NF2 is also called bilateral acoustic neurofibromatosis

ICD-9CM CODES

237.71 Type 1, von Recklinghausen's
237.72 Type 2 acoustic

■ EPIDEMIOLOGY & DEMOGRAPHICS

- Incidence of NF1 (1/3000), NF2 (1/33,000).
- Prevalence of NF1 (1/5000), NF2 (1/210,000).
- NF1 and NF2 are autosomal dominant with approximately 50% of cases having no family history.
- The two disorders affect approximately 100,000 people in the United States.
- Equally affects males and females.
- NF1 may be associated with optic gliomas, astrocytomas, spinal neurofibromas, pheochromocytomas, and chronic myeloid leukemia.
- NF2 may be associated with meningiomas, spinal schwannomas, and cataracts.

■ PHYSICAL FINDINGS & CLINICAL PRESENTATION

- Common features of NF1 include:
  1. Café-au-lait macules (100% of children by age 2)
     a. Hyperpigmented skin lesions occurring anywhere on the body except the face, palms, and soles
     b. Appear early in life and increase in size and number during puberty
     c. Focal or diffuse
  2. Axillary and inguinal freckling (70%)
  3. Multiple cutaneous and subcutaneous neurofibromas (95%) (Fig. 1-263)
     a. Firm, varying in size from mm to cm
     b. Vary in number from a few to thousands
     c. May be sessile, pedunculated, regular or irregular in shape

  4. Lisch nodule (small hamartoma of the iris) found in >90% of adult cases
  5. Visual defects possibly related to optic gliomas (2% to 5%)
  6. Neurodevelopment problems (30% to 40%)
- Common features of NF2 include:
  1. Hearing loss and tinnitus related to bilateral acoustic neuromas (>90% of adults)
  2. Cataracts (81%)
  3. Headache
  4. Unsteady gait
  5. Cutaneous neurofibromas but less than NF1
  6. Café-au-lait macules (1%)

■ ETIOLOGY

- NF1 is caused by DNA mutations located on the long arm of chromosome 17 responsible for encoding the protein neurofibromin.
- NF2 is caused by DNA mutations located in the middle of the long arm of chromosome 22 responsible for encoding the protein merlin.

DIAGNOSIS

- NF1 is diagnosed if the person has two or more of the following features:
  1. Six or more café-au-lait macules over 5 mm in prepubertal patients and greater than 15 mm in postpubertal patients
  2. Two or more neurofibromas of any type or one plexiform neurofibroma
  3. Axillary or inguinal freckling
  4. Optic glioma
  5. Two or more Lisch nodules (iris hamartomas)
  6. Sphenoid wing dysplasia or cortical thinning of long bones, with or without pseudarthrosis
  7. A first-degree relative (parent, sibling, or child) with NF1 based on the above criteria
- NF2 is diagnosed if the person has either of the following two criteria:
  1. Bilateral eighth nerve masses seen by appropriate imaging studies
  2. A first-degree relative with NF2 and either a unilateral eighth nerve mass or two of the following: neurofibroma, meningioma, glioma, schwannoma, or juvenile posterior subcapsular lenticular opacity

■ WORKUP

The diagnosis of neurofibromatosis is usually self-evident. Workup is dictated by clinical symptoms in NF1 and usually includes MRI evaluation of the head and spine in NF2.

■ LABORATORY TESTS

- Genetic testing is possible in individuals who desire prenatal diagnosis for NF1. There is no single standard test and multiple tests are required. Results can only tell if an individual is affected but cannot predict the severity of the disease.
- In NF2, linkage analysis testing provides a >99% certainty the individual has NF2.

■ IMAGING STUDIES

- MRI with gadolinium is the imaging study of choice in both NF1 and NF2 patients. MRI increases detection of optic gliomas, tumors of the spine, acoustic neuromas, and "bright spots" thought to represent hamartomas.
- MRI of the spine is recommended in all patients diagnosed with NF2 to exclude intramedullary tumors.

TREATMENT

Treatment is directed primarily at symptoms and complications of NF1 and NF2.

■ NONPHARMACOLOGIC THERAPY

- Counseling addressing prognosis, genetic, psychological, and social issues.
- Slit-lamp examination by an ophthalmologist searching for cataracts and hamartomas.
- Hearing testing and speech pathology evaluation.

■ ACUTE GENERAL Rx

- Surgery is usually not done on skin tumors unless cosmetically requested or if suspicion of malignant transformation exists.
- Surgery may be indicated for spinal or cranial neurofibromas, gliomas, or meningiomas.
- Acoustic neuromas can be treated by surgical excision.

■ **CHRONIC Rx**
• Radiation may be indicated in NF1 patients with optic nerve gliomas.
• Stereotactic radiosurgery using gamma knife may be an alternative approach to surgery for acoustic neuromas.

■ **DISPOSITION**
• Prognosis varies according to the severity of involvement.
• There is no cure for neurofibromatosis.

■ **REFERRAL**
A multidisciplinary team of consultants is needed in patients with neurofibromatosis including neurosurgeon, otolaryngologist, dermatologist, neurologist, audiologist, speech pathologist, and neuropsychologist.

PEARLS & CONSIDERATIONS

■ **COMMENTS**
• Friedrich Daniel von Recklinghausen first reported his cases in 1882, although there had been similar accounts dating back to the 1600s.
• The first report in the literature of NF2 was by Wishart in 1822.
• For additional information refer to the National Neurofibromatosis Foundation (141 Fifth Avenue, Suite 7-S, New York, NY 10010, 800-322-7838) or Neurofibromatosis Inc. (3401 Woodbridge Court, Mitchellville, MD 20716, 301-577-8984).

REFERENCES
Gutmann DH et al: The diagnostic evaluation and multidisciplinary management of neurofibromatosis 1 and neurofibromatosis 2, *JAMA* 278(1):51, 1997.
Huson SM: What level of care for the neurofibromatoses? *Lancet* 353(9159): 1114, 1999.
Karnes PS: Neurofibromatosis: a common neurocutaneous disorder, *Mayo Clin Proc* 73(11):1071, 1998.
Mulvihill JJ et al: Neurofibromatosis 1 (Recklinghausen disease) and neurofibromatosis 2 (bilateral acoustic neurofibromatosis): an update, *Ann Intern Med* 113(1):39, 1990.
Author: **Peter Petropoulos, M.D.**

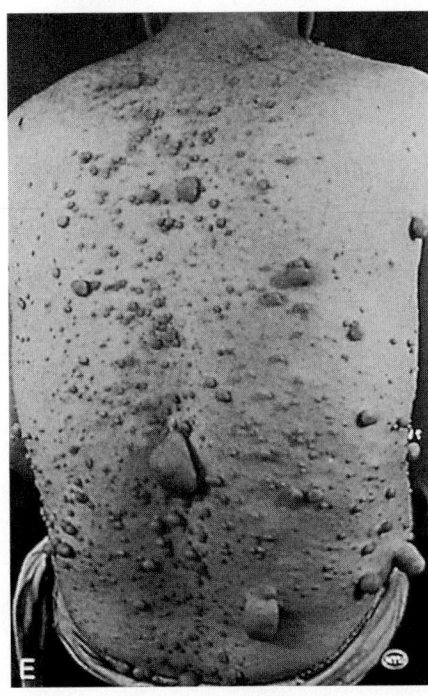

Fig. 1-263 Nodules. Solid, large (>1 cm), deep-seated mass in dermal or subcutaneous tissues. These nodules are neurofibromas in a patient with neurofibromatosis. (From Goldman L, Bennett JC [eds]: *Cecil textbook of medicine,* ed 21, Philadelphia, 2000, WB Saunders.)

BASIC INFORMATION

■ **DEFINITION**

Neuroleptic malignant syndrome is an adverse reaction to dopamine-blocking neuroleptics characterized by hyperthermia, muscular rigidity, autonomic dysfunction, and altered consciousness.

■ **SYNONYMS**

Malignant hyperthermia

ICD-9CM CODES

333.92 Neuroleptic malignant syndrome

■ **EPIDEMIOLOGY & DEMOGRAPHICS**

INCIDENCE (IN U.S.): 0.5% to 1% of patients receiving neuroleptics
PREDOMINANT SEX: More than two thirds of patients are male.
PREDOMINANT AGE: Young and middle-aged adults
PEAK INCIDENCE: 42 yr
GENETICS:
• Not applicable
• Malignant hyperthermia a familial disorder

■ **PHYSICAL FINDINGS & CLINICAL PRESENTATION**

• "Lead pipe" rigidity
• Hyperthermia (38.6° to 42.3° C)
• Profuse sweating
• Tachycardia
• Labile BP
• Semicomatose

■ **ETIOLOGY**

• History of haloperidol use in 65% of cases
• History of combination drug therapy in 34% of cases
• Rare cases after withdrawal of dopamine agonists

DIAGNOSIS

■ **DIFFERENTIAL DIAGNOSIS**

• Heat stroke
• Catatonia
• Similar syndrome: possible complication of anesthesia, thyroid storm, toxins

■ **WORKUP**

Careful drug history

■ **LABORATORY TESTS**

• Elevated CPK
• Urinary myoglobin
• Leukocytosis
• Electrolytes
• Renal function
• Blood gases
• Drug levels

■ **IMAGING STUDIES**

None specific for this disease

TREATMENT

■ **NONPHARMACOLOGIC THERAPY**

• Respiratory support
• Careful intake and output monitoring
• Stop all neuroleptic agents

■ **ACUTE GENERAL Rx**

• Bromocriptine, a dopamine receptor agonist, is the mainstay of therapy for patients with neuroleptic malignant syndrome. Initial doses of 2.5 to 10 mg are given IV q8h and are increased by 5 mg/day until clinical improvement is seen. The drug should be continued for at least 10 days after the syndrome has been controlled and then tapered slowly.

• Dantrolene therapy is also effective. Initially, patients can be given 0.25 mg/kg IV q6-12h, followed by a maintenance dose up to 3 mg/kg/day. After 2 to 3 days, patients may be given the drug orally (25 to 600 mg/day in divided doses). Oral dantrolene therapy may need to be continued for several days.

■ **CHRONIC Rx**

• This is a potentially fatal disease, but most patients recover.
• Mortality rate is currently 10% to 20% despite above therapeutic measures.
• Factors adversely affecting mortality are development of renal failure and core temperature >104° F (40° C).

■ **DISPOSITION**

Monitor closely for future complications of pharmacologic therapy.

■ **REFERRAL**

If patient's condition is critical; most patients are treated in ICU.

PEARLS & CONSIDERATIONS

■ **COMMENTS**

Early detection and diagnosis lead to a more favorable outcome. Treatment is a medical emergency.
Author: **William H. Olson, M.D.**

BASIC INFORMATION

■ DEFINITION

Nocardiosis is an infection caused by aerobic actinomycetes found in soil and characterized by lung, soft tissue, or CNS involvement.

ICD-9CM CODES

039 Actinomycotic infections
039.9 Nocardiosis NOS, of unspecified site

■ EPIDEMIOLOGY & DEMOGRAPHICS

- *Nocardia* species are found worldwide in the soil.
- Nocardiosis is found most commonly in patients who are compromised (e.g., receiving steroids, immunosuppressive therapy, lymphoma, leukemia, lung cancer, and other pulmonary infections [Fig. 1-264]).
- Other underlying conditions associated with nocardiosis are pemphigus vulgaris, Whipple's disease, Goodpasture's syndrome, Cushing's disease, cirrhosis, ulcerative colitis, and rheumatoid arthritis.
- Between 500 to 1000 new cases are diagnosed each year in the United States.
- Approximately 2% of patients with AIDS develop nocardiosis.
- Occur more commonly in men than in women (2:1).
- Adults > children.

■ PHYSICAL FINDINGS & CLINICAL PRESENTATION

- The most common presentation of nocardiosis is pneumonia (75%) with fever, chills, dyspnea, and a productive cough.
  1. Presentation can be acute, subacute, or chronic.
  2. Nocardiosis should be suspected if soft tissue abscesses or CNS tumors or abscesses form in conjunction with the pulmonary infection.
  3. Pulmonary infection may spread into the pericardium, mediastinum, and superior vena cava.
- Infection can follow skin puncture by a thorn or splinter with inoculation and introduction of the microorganism and lead to:
  1. Cellulitis.
  2. Lymphocutaneous nodules appearing along lymphatic sites draining the infected puncture wound.
  3. Mycetoma (Madura foot), a chronic deep nodular infection usually involving the hands or feet that can cause skin breakdown, fistula formation, and spread along the fascial planes to infect surrounding skin, subcutaneous tissue and bone.
- The CNS system is infected in approximately one third of all cases. Brain abscesses is the most common pathologic finding.
- Dissemination of nocardiosis may infect other tissues and organs including kidney, heart, skin, and bone.

■ ETIOLOGY

- The most common *Nocardia* species leading to infection in humans are:
  1. *N. asteroides* (causing over 80% of the cases of pulmonary nocardiosis).
  2. *N. brasiliensis* (most common cause of mycetoma)
  3. *N. otitidiscaviarum*
- *N. asteroides* has two subgroups
  1. *N. farcinica*
  2. *N. nova*

DIAGNOSIS

- The diagnosis of nocardiosis requires a high index of suspicion in the proper clinical setting and is confirmed by bacteriologic staining and growth of the organism in culture.

■ DIFFERENTIAL DIAGNOSIS

- There are no pathognomonic findings separating nocardiosis pneumonia from other infectious etiologies of the lung. Diagnoses presenting in a similar manner and often confused for nocardiosis are:
  1. Tuberculosis
  2. Lung abscess
  3. Lung tumor
  4. Other causes of pneumonia
  5. Actinomycosis
  6. Mycosis
  7. Cellulitis
  8. Coccidioidomycosis
  9. Histoplasmosis
  10. Aspergillosis
  11. Kaposi's sarcoma

■ WORKUP

All patients with suspected nocardiosis need laboratory identification of the microorganism by obtaining sputum in the case of pneumonia, cultures of the infected skin lesions in mycetoma or lymphocutaneous disease, or the sampling of any purulent material (e.g., brain abscess, lung abscess, and pleural effusion).

■ LABORATORY TESTS

- Blood tests are not very sensitive in the diagnosis of nocardiosis.
- Gram stain shows gram-positive beaded filaments with multiple branches.
- Gomori methenamine silver staining may detect the organism.
- *Nocardia* species are acid-fast on a modified Ziehl-Neelsen stain.
- Colony growth in cultures may take up to 7 days.

■ IMAGING STUDIES

- Chest x-ray may demonstrate infiltrates, densities, nodules, cavitary masses, or multiple abscesses.
- CT scan of the brain is indicated in the appropriate clinical setting to exclude CNS brain abscesses.

TREATMENT

■ NONPHARMACOLOGIC THERAPY

- Supportive therapy with oxygen in patients with pneumonia
- Chest physiotherapy
- For any abscess formation, surgical drainage indicated (e.g., skin, lung, or brain)

■ ACUTE GENERAL Rx

- The treatment of choice is sulfonamides. Sulfadiazine 6 to 10 g is given in 4 to 6 divided oral doses.
- Trimethoprim-sulfamethoxazole (160 mg/800 mg) given orally every 6 to 8 hr.
- Amikacin has been the IV antibiotic of choice.
- Alternative drug treatment includes:
  1. Minocycline 100 to 200 mg bid
  2. Erythromycin 500 mg qid and ampicillin 1 g qid for *N. nova* species.
  3. Amoxicillin 500 mg and clavulanate 125 mg tid.
  4. Ofloxacin 400 mg bid.
  5. Clarithromycin 500 mg bid.

■ CHRONIC Rx

- Long-term therapy is generally recommended for all infections caused by *Nocardia*.
- Patients with cellulitis and lyphocutaneous syndrome are treated for 2 to 4 mo depending on whether there is bone involvement or not.
- Mycetomas are best treated with antibiotics for 6 to 12 mo but may required surgical drainage.
- Pulmonary and systemic nocardiosis excluding the CNS is treated for 6 to 12 mo.

- CNS involvement is treated with drainage and antibiotics for 12 mo.
- All immunosuppressed patients should receive 12 mo of antibiotic therapy.

■ DISPOSITION
- Patients with pulmonary nocardiosis have a mortality rate of 15% to 30%.
- CNS involvement carries a >40% mortality rate.
- Isolated skin lesions have a low mortality rate.

■ REFERRAL
Whenever the diagnosis of nocardiosis is suspected, consultation with infectious disease is indicated. Pulmonary evaluation and assistance may be needed in pulmonary nocardiosis. Neurosurgery consultation is indicated in patients with single or multiple brain abscesses.

✦ PEARLS & CONSIDERATIONS

■ COMMENTS
- Tuberculosis and nocardiosis may coexist in the same patient.

- Nocardiosis does not spread from infected animal to humans.
- Nocardiosis is not transmitted from person to person.
- Nocardiosis tends to relapse, justifying long-term therapy.

REFERENCES
Boiron P et al: Nocardia, nocardiosis and mycetoma, *Med Mycol* 36(Suppl 1):26, 1998.
Lerner PI: Nocardiosis, *Clin Infect Dis* 22(6):891, 1996.
Wallace RJ et al: Taxonomy of *Nocardia* species, *Clin Infect Dis* 18:476, 1994.
Author: **Peter Petropoulos, M.D.**

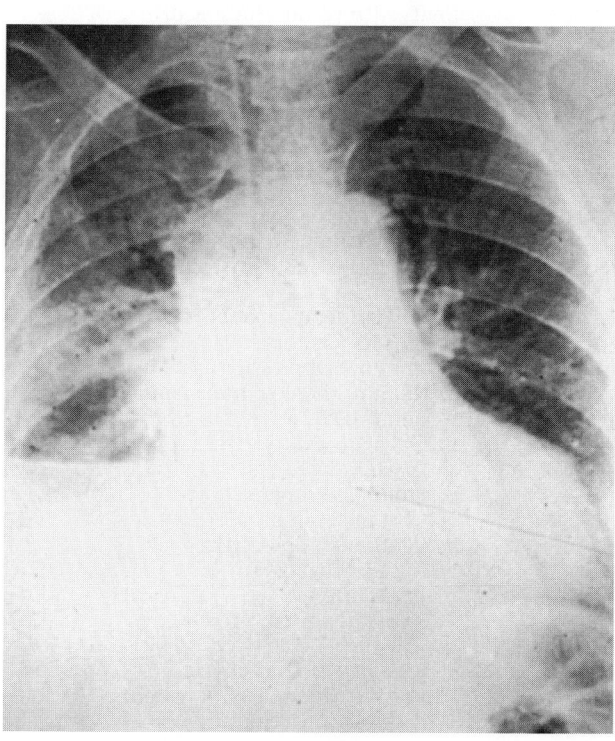

Fig. 1-264   Right lower lobe *Nocardia* pneumonia in a renal transplant recipient. (From Gorbach SL: *Infectious diseases,* ed 2, Philadelphia, 1998, WB Saunders.)

BASIC INFORMATION

■ **DEFINITION**

Nosocomial infections (NI) are infections acquired as a result of hospitalization, generally after 48 hr of admission.

■ **SYNONYMS**

Hospital-acquired infections

■ **EPIDEMIOLOGY & DEMOGRAPHICS**

INCIDENCE (IN U.S.):
- Develop in at least 5% of hospitalized patients
- Account for 88,000 deaths/yr

In 1992 these infections were estimated to add $45 billion to the annual expenditures for health care in the U.S.

PREVALENCE (IN U.S.): 2 to 4 million cases/yr

PREDOMINANT SEX:
- Overall, approximately equal
- Elderly women: predominantly nosocomial urinary tract infections

PREDOMINANT AGE:
- Elderly patients (>60 yr old) at highest risk
- High-risk patients who may develop NI at any age:
  1. ICU
  2. Intubation
  3. Chronic lung disease
  4. Renal disease
  5. Comatose
  6. Chronic urethral or vascular catheterization
  7. Malnutrition
  8. Postoperative state

PEAK INCIDENCE: Varies widely with infection site

■ **PHYSICAL FINDINGS & CLINICAL PRESENTATION**

Vary with specific NI

■ **ETIOLOGY**

- Bacteria
- Fungi
- Viruses

SOURCES AND MODES OF TRANSMISSION:
1. Patient's own flora
   a. Comprises resistant organisms acquired during hospitalization
   b. Frequently maintained thereafter by persistent GI colonization

2. Unwashed hands of staff
   a. Physicians
   b. Nurses
3. Invasion of protective defenses (intact skin, respiratory cilia, urinary sphincters, and mucosa)
   a. IV lines
   b. Catheters
   c. Respiratory equipment
   d. Surgical wounds
   e. Scopes and other imaging devices
4. Failure to provide adequate negative pressure, high-volume air flow chambers for respiratory isolation of patients with TB
5. Failure to rapidly identify and provide appropriate care (with isolation or precautions) for patients with communicable diseases
6. Inanimate environment
7. Food
8. Fomites

RISKS AMPLIFIED:
1. Use of broad-spectrum antibiotics
   a. Select highly resistant bacteria
   b. Establish highly resistant bacteria as endemic flora in microenvironments within the hospital
2. Highly vulnerable patients with specific risk factors
   a. Immunosuppression (as a result of therapy, transplantation, AIDS)
   b. Old age
   c. Postsurgery
   d. Prolonged surgery
   e. Chronic lung disease
   f. Ventilator dependence
   g. Antacid therapy
   h. Vascular lines
   i. Hyperalimentation
   j. ICU stay
   k. Recent antibiotic therapy
3. Clustering of seriously ill patients
   a. Often with wounds or drainage of contaminated materials
   b. Intensifying probability of cross-infection

HAND WASHING BETWEEN ALL PATIENT CONTACTS: Single most important method of decreasing NI
1. Regular soap
2. Chlorhexidine for methicillin-resistant *Staphylococcus aureus* (MRSA) and other resistant gram-positive organisms
3. Iodophor for resistant gram-negative organisms

4. Purpose
   a. Degrease hand surfaces
   b. Wash away oils and associated bacteria
5. Procedure
   a. Lukewarm water
   b. Must include all surfaces
   c. Special attention to areas between fingers and to the dirtier dominant hand (most people reflexively wash their cleaner, nondominant hand more vigorously)

VANCOMYCIN-RESISTANT *ENTEROCOCCUS FAECIUM* (VREF):
1. The percentage of nosocomial infections caused by VREF increased more than twentyfold between 1989 and 1993, rising from 0% to 3% to 7% to 9%.
2. A high percentage of VREF isolated, 80% are also ampicillin resistant.
3. Factors predisposing to VREF colonization or infection include percentage of hospital days receiving antimicrobial therapy, use of IV, underlying disease, immunosuppression, and abdominal surgery.
4. Evidence suggests that vehicle is the hands of medical personnel.
5. Control measures
   a. Aggressive isolation of colonized and infected patients
   b. Restraint in using broad-spectrum antibiotics

CLOSTRIDIUM DIFFICILE:
1. Causes diarrhea as a result of pseudomembranous colitis
2. May be transmitted among hospitalized patients
3. Warrants stool (contact) precautions

SURVEILLANCE:
1. Crucial for early identification of infections
   a. Enabling immediate intervention
   b. Education
2. Prospective, concurrent, total hospital surveillance
   a. Provides most complete data
   b. Feasible with sophisticated computerized data collection and analysis
3. Daily plotting of all infections on comprehensive wall maps
   a. Including all beds on all wards
   b. Enhances immediate recognition of microclusters of infections by body site and by organism
   c. Facilitates proper early control of potential outbreaks

🔬 DIAGNOSIS

■ MOST COMMON NOSOCOMIAL INFECTIONS:
- Urinary tract infections (40% to 45%)
- Surgical wound and other soft tissue infections (25% to 30%)
- Pneumonia (15% to 20%)
- Bacteremia (5% to 12%)

NOSOCOMIAL URINARY TRACT INFECTIONS:
- General associations:
  1. Foley catheters
  2. Inappropriate catheter care (including opening catheter junctions)
  3. Female sex
  4. Absence of systemic antibiotics
- Physical findings:
  1. Fever
  2. Dysuria
  3. Leukocytosis
  4. Pyuria
  5. Flank or costovertebral angle tenderness
- Usual organisms:
  1. *E. coli*
  2. *Klebsiella*
  3. *Enterobacter*
  4. *Pseudomonas*
  5. *Enterococcus*
- Sepsis in 1% to 3% of nosocomial UTIs
- Prevention:
  1. Meticulous technique during insertion and daily perineal care
  2. Never open the catheter-collection tubing junction
  3. Obtain all specimens using sterile syringe
  4. Substitute intermittent catheterization for Foley catheters

NOSOCOMIAL BACTEREMIAS:
- General associations:
  1. IV lines
  2. Arterial lines
  3. CVP lines
  4. Phlebitis
  5. Hyperalimentation
- Fever possibly only presenting sign
- Exit site of all vascular lines carefully evaluated for:
  1. Erythema
  2. Induration
  3. Tenderness
  4. Purulent drainage
- Usual organism for device-associated bacteremia
  1. *S. aureus*
  2. *Staphylococcus epidermidis* for long-term IV lines
  3. *Enterobacter*
  4. *Klebsiella*
  5. *Candida* spp.
  6. *Pseudomonas aeruginosa* may come from a water source or reflect cutaneous bacteria

- Phlebitis in 1.3 million patients yearly
- Approximately 10,000 annual deaths from IV sepsis
- Prevention:
  1. Meticulous sterile technique during IV insertion.
  2. Emphasis should be placed on attention to detail, include hand washing, adherence to guidelines for catheter insertion and maintenance, appropriate use of antiseptic solutions such as chlorhexidine or iodine to prepare the skin around the catheter insertion site, and use of sterile technique for central catheter insertion.
  3. Modified catheter may reduce risk for endoluminal colonization and catheter-related sepsis in subclavian lines.
  4. Decrease use of routine IVs (patients would rather drink).

NOSOCOMIAL PNEUMONIAS:
- More common in ICUs
- General associations:
  1. Aspiration
  2. Intubation
  3. Altered consciousness
  4. Old age
  5. Chronic lung disease
  6. Postsurgery
  7. Antacids
- Signs of pneumonia common among patients on general wards:
  1. Cough
  2. Sputum
  3. Fever
  4. Leukocytosis
  5. New infiltrate on chest x-ray examination
- Signs more subtle in ICUs, because many patients have purulent sputum because of chronic intubation
  1. Change in sputum character or volume
  2. Small changes on chest x-ray examination
- Usual organisms:
  1. *Klebsiella*
  2. *Acinetobacter*
  3. *Enterobacter*
  4. *Pseudomonas aeruginosa*
  5. *S. aureus*
- Less common organisms:
  1. MRSA
  2. *Legionella, Flavobacterium*
  3. Respiratory syncytial virus (infants)
  4. Adenovirus
- 1% of hospitalized patients affected
- Mortality rate high (40%)
- Prevention:
  1. Meticulous sterile technique during suctioning and handling airway

  2. Do not routinely change ventilator breathing circuits and components more frequently than q48h
  3. Drain respirator tubing without allowing fluid to return to respirator
  4. Hand washing routinely to prevent colonization of patients and transfer of organisms among patients

NOSOCOMIAL SOFT TISSUE INFECTIONS:
- Associations:
  1. Decubitus ulcers
  2. Surgical wound classification (contaminated or dirty-infected)
  3. Abdominal surgery
  4. Presence of drain
  5. Preoperative length of stay
  6. Duration of surgery >2 hr
  7. Surgeon
  8. Presence of other infection
- Physical findings:
  1. Decubitus ulcer with fluctuance at margin or under firm eschar
  2. Erythema extending >2 cm beyond margin of surgical wound
  3. Tenderness
  4. Induration
  5. Erythema
  6. Fluctuance
  7. Purulent drainage
  8. Dehiscence of sutures
- Usual organisms:
  1. *S. aureus*
  2. *Enterococcus*
  3. *Enterobacter*
  4. *Acinetobacter*
  5. *E. coli*
- Prevention:
  1. Careful skin care and frequent, proper positioning of patient to prevent decubitus ulcer
  2. Meticulous sterile surgical technique
  3. Hand washing to decrease colonization when handling postoperative wound
  4. Limit prophylactic antibiotics to 24 hr perioperatively
  5. Double-wrap contaminated dressings (hold in gloved hand and evert gloves over dressings) before disposal

■ LABORATORY TESTS
- Appropriate to specific NI and specific patient's condition
- Cultures generally indicated for proper confirmation of responsible pathogens
  1. Urine
  2. Blood
  3. Sputum
  4. Soft tissue infection
- Molecular analysis of nosocomial epidemics
  1. Plasmid fingerprinting

2. Restriction endonuclease digestion (plasmid and genomic DNA)
3. Peptide analysis by SDS-PAGE
4. Immunoblotting
5. Ribosomal (rRNA) typing
6. DNA probes
7. Multilocus enzyme electrophoresis
8. Restriction fragment length polymorphism (RFLP)
9. Polymerase chain reaction (PCR)
10. Provide confirmation of point-source or common strains
11. Offer occasionally indispensable corroboration of hypotheses reached utilizing classic epidemiology

■ IMAGING STUDIES
Rarely needed for diagnosis of NI

■ TREATMENT

■ ACUTE GENERAL Rx
- Appropriate to etiologic organism:
  1. Antibiotic
  2. Antifungal
  3. Antiviral
- Specific therapy determined after careful consideration of resident flora within the microenvironment in which the patient was hospitalized
  1. Empiric therapy
     a. Frequently difficult to fashion accurately
     b. Often undesirable, unless the patient's clinical condition requires urgent treatment
  2. Consultation for expert advice regarding antibiotic selection in view of known epidemiologic risks within the hospital
     a. Nosocomial infection control nurses
     b. Hospital epidemiologist
- Avoid unnecessary treatment for organisms that are colonizing but not infecting patients

- Prevention of spread of communicable diseases often requiring Isolation or Precautions
  1. Classic Schema (Strict, Respiratory Isolation and Contact [Skin and Wound] Precautions) being replaced by more streamlined Revised Guidelines (Airborne, Droplet, Contact Isolation Precautions)
  2. Less careful response to some diseases (e.g., hemorrhagic fevers) inadvertently induced by removal of strict isolation category
  3. Universal/Standard Precautions and Body Substance Isolation continue within a new Standard Isolation Precautions Guideline
- Universal Precautions used for all patients during all contacts with blood, body fluids, or secretions
  1. Gloves
  2. Goggles
  3. Impermeable gowns if aerosol or splash is likely
- Consider aggressive isolation to restrict spread of resistant organisms and their plasmids
  1. MRSA
  2. VREF
  3. Highly resistant gram-negative organisms

■ REFERRAL
- To nosocomial infection control nurses
- To hospital epidemiologist

☼ PEARLS & CONSIDERATIONS

■ COMMENTS
- Sharps and splash injuries to staff relatively are rare, but nearly all are preventable.
  1. Nurses incur most injuries.
  2. Usual causes:
     a. Needle sticks
     b. Scalpel and surgical needle injuries
     c. Blood splashes

3. Prevention:
   a. Never recap needles
   b. Needle disposal only in rigid, impermeable plastic containers
   c. Clearly announce instrument passes in operating room or during procedures and use passing trays
   d. Gloves and goggles if aerosol or splash is likely
   e. Never leave needles or other sharp items in beds
   f. Never dispose of sharp items in regular trash bags
4. Infection control staff should be consulted immediately after exposure to determine need for prophylaxis for hepatitis B or HIV.
5. All staff should be immune to hepatitis B (natural or vaccine).
- Fungi previously considered to be contaminants now risks for patients with cancer and organ transplantation
  1. *Candida* spp.
     a. *C. guilliermondi*
     b. *C. krusei*
     c. *C. parapsilosis*
     d. *C. tropicalis*
  2. *Aspergillus* spp.
  3. *Curvularia* spp.
  4. *Bipolaris* spp.
  5. *Exserohilum* spp.
  6. *Alternaria* spp.
  7. *Fusarium* spp.
  8. *Scopulariopsis* spp.
  9. *Pseudallescheria boydii*
  10. *Trichosporon beigelii*
  11. *Malassezia furfur*
  12. *Hensenula* spp.
  13. *Microsporum canis*
- Focused, committed efforts by the entire health care staff continuously directed toward prevention
  1. Each NI addressed as an opportunity to improve the organization and delivery of care
  2. Essential that individual staff members understand that small risks applied to large populations result in a large number of total events (i.e., NI)

Author: **Zeena Lobo, M.D.**

BASIC INFORMATION

■ DEFINITION
- Obesity refers to excess body fat defined as a body mass index (BMI) ≥30 kg/m². Overweight is defined as BMI of 25 to 29.9 kg/m².

■ SYNONYMS
Overweight

ICD-9CM CODES
278.0 Obesity

■ EPIDEMIOLOGY & DEMOGRAPHICS
- Approximately 97 million adults in the U.S. are overweight or obese.
- Between 1960 and 1994 the prevalence of obese people has increased from 12.8% to 22.5%.
- The Third National Health and Nutrition Examination Survey (NHANES III) estimated that 13.7% of children and 11.5% of adolescents are overweight.
- According to NHANES III data, 54.9% of U.S. adults aged 20 yr and older are either overweight or obese (32.6% are overweight with BMI 25 to 29.9; 22.3% are obese with BMI ≥30).
- Overweight and obesity is defined as stated above on the basis of epidemiologic data showing increased mortality with BMIs above 25 kg/m².
- For persons with a BMI of ≥30 kg/m², all-cause mortality is increased by 50% to 100% above that of persons with BMIs in the range of 20 to 25 kg/m².
- Obesity is more prevalent in black and Hispanic women compared to non-Hispanic white women and men.
- Women in the U.S. with low incomes or low education are more likely to be obese than those of higher socioeconomic status.
- In 1993 the Deputy Assistant Secretary for Health (J. Michael McGinnis) and the former Director of the Centers for Disease Control and Prevention (CDC) (William Foege) co-authored a journal article, "Actual Causes of Death in the U.S." It concluded that a combination of dietary factors and sedentary activity patterns accounts for at least 300,000 deaths each year, and obesity is the second leading cause of preventable death in the United States.

■ PHYSICAL FINDINGS & CLINICAL PRESENTATION
- Obesity is self-evident on examination.
- Measuring the height in meters and weight in kilograms determines your BMI.
- Increased waist circumference (>40 inches in men and >35 inches in women) are apparent.
- Hypertension is related to obesity.
- Symptoms of diabetes (e.g., polyuria, polydipsia, retinopathy, and neuropathy) may be present.
- Joint pain and swelling are associated with osteoarthritis and obesity.
- Dyspnea may be present.

■ ETIOLOGY
- The cause of obesity is multifactorial, involving social, cultural, behavioral, physiologic, metabolic, and genetic factors.
- Supporting genetic factors come from identical twins reared apart and "obesity genes" encoding for the appetite-suppressant hormone leptin.
- Environmental factors are a major determinant of obesity with the underlying theme of excess calorie intake and lack of physical activity.

DIAGNOSIS

- Determination of the BMI establishes the diagnosis of obesity according to the definition given above and assesses the individual's risk for disease.
- BMI is defined as the weight in kilograms divided by the square of the height in meters ($W \div H^2$).

■ DIFFERENTIAL DIAGNOSIS
- Hypothalamic disorders, hypothyroidism, Cushing's syndrome, insulinoma, and chronic corticosteroid use can cause obesity.

■ WORKUP
The workup of an obese patient typically requires laboratory work to assess for risks and complications.

■ LABORATORY TESTS
- Lab tests are not specific in diagnosing obesity; however, they are used to identify diabetes and hyperlipidemia commonly related to excess weight.

- In the proper clinical setting thyroid function studies (TSH, free T_4) will exclude hypothyroidism as a cause of obesity.

■ IMAGING STUDIES
- X-ray imaging studies are not specific in the diagnosis of obesity.
- Several methods are available for determining or calculating total body fat but offer no significant advantage over the BMI.
  1. Total body water
  2. Total body potassium
  3. Bioelectrical impedance
  4. Dual-energy x-ray absorptiometry

TREATMENT

- Treatment is aimed at weight reduction and risk factor modification (e.g., diabetes, lipids, hypertension).
- Once a joint decision between patient and clinician has been made to lose weight, the expert panel recommends as an initial goal the loss of 10% of baseline weight, to be lost at a rate of 1 to 2 lb/wk over a 6-mo period.

■ NONPHARMACOLOGIC THERAPY
- The three major components of weight loss therapy are:
  1. Dietary therapy establishing an energy deficit of 500 to 1000 kcal/d. NCEP's step I or II diet is used in patients with hyperlipidemia.
  2. Increased physical activity initially by walking 30 min 3 times/wk and gradually build up to intense walking 45 min 5 days/wk. The eventual goal is at least 30 min of moderate intense walking.
  3. Behavioral therapy is also necessary.

■ ACUTE GENERAL Rx
- Pharmacotherapy may be useful as an adjunct to diet and physical activity for patients with a BMI of ≥30 with no concomitant obesity-related risk factors or diseases, and for patients with a BMI ≥27 with concomitant obesity-related risk factors or diseases.

- In 1997 both dexfenfluramine and fenfluramine have been withdrawn from the market secondary to side effects of valvular heart lesions.
- FDA has approved Sibutramine (10 mg qd) for the management of obesity.
- Orlistat, one 120-mg capsule tid with each meal that includes fat, has recently been approved by the FDA. Major side effects are oily spotting, flatus with discharge, and fecal urgency.

■ CHRONIC Rx
- Surgery is a consideration in clinically severe obesity (e.g., BMI ≥ 40 or ≥ 35 with comorbid conditions).
- Gastroplasty, gastric partitioning, and gastric bypass are the surgical procedures performed.

■ DISPOSITION
- Obesity increases the risk of developing hypertension, hyperlipidemia, type 2 diabetes, coronary artery disease, cerebrovascular disease, osteoarthritis, sleep apnea, and endometrial, breast, prostate, and colon cancers.
- All-cause mortality is increased in obese patients.

■ REFERRAL
Obesity is commonly seen in the primary care setting. If pharmacologic therapy is considered, consultation with physicians specializing in obesity and experienced with the use of the drug is recommended. In addition, consultation with nutritionists and behavioral therapists is helpful. A consultation with general surgery is indicated in patients being considered surgical intervention.

☼ PEARLS & CONSIDERATIONS

■ COMMENTS
- The National Heart, Lung, and Blood Institute's (NHLBI) Obesity Education Initiative in cooperation with the National Institute of Diabetes convened the Expert Panel on the Identification, Evaluation, and Treatment of Overweight and Obesity in Adults in May 1995 and have since published evidence-based clinical guidelines.
- The total cost attributable to obesity in 1995 was $99.2 billion dollars or 5.7% of the national health expenditure within the U.S.

REFERENCES
Blanck HM et al: Use of non-prescription weight loss products: results from a multistate survey, *JAMA* 286:930, 2001.

Clinical Guidelines on the Identification, Evaluation, and Treatment of Overweight and Obesity in Adults. The Evidence Report. National Institute of Health, National Heart, Lung, and Blood Institute. *www.nhlbi.nih.gov/guidelines/obesity/ob_gdlns.pdf*

Executive Summary of the Clinical Guidelines on the Identification, Evaluation, and Treatment of Overweight and Obesity in Adults, *Arch Intern Med* 158(17):1855, 1867, 1998.

Lyznicki JM et al: Obesity: assessment and management in primary care, *Am Fam Physician* 63:2185, 2001.

Author: **Peter Petropoulos, M.D.**

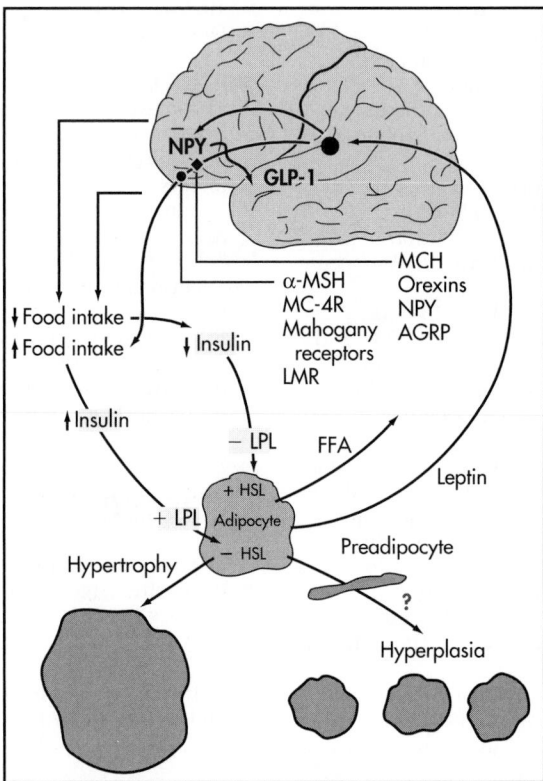

Fig. 1-265 Pathogenesis of obesity. Increased food intake stimulates insulin secretion. Insulin, in turn, stimulates lipoprotein lipase (+LPL), permitting uptake of circulating triglyceride by the adipocyte, and insulin simultaneously inhibits hormone-sensitive lipase (−HSL) and the release of adipocyte free fatty acids (FFA). The overfed adipocyte may hypertrophy, or a stimulus, currently unknown, may trigger differentiation of preadipocytes. The well-fed adipocyte secretes leptin, which circulates and binds to receptors in the hypothalamus, causing glucagon-like peptide-1 (GLP-1) release and inhibiting neuropeptide-Y (NPY), a powerful stimulator of appetite and feeding. Reduced food intake, in contrast, lowers insulin, leading to LPL suppression (−LPL), activation of HSL (+HSL), and FFA release. (From Andreoli TE [ed]: *Cecil essentials of medicine,* ed 5, Philadelphia, 2001, WB Saunders.)

BASIC INFORMATION

■ **DEFINITION**
Obsessive-compulsive disorder (OCD) involves recurrent obsessions (intrusive and inappropriate thoughts, impulses, or images) or compulsions (behaviors or mental acts performed in response to obsessions or rigid application of rules) that consume >1 hr/day or cause impairment or distress.

■ **SYNONYMS**
Abortive insanity

ICD-9CM CODES
F42.8 Obsessive-compulsive disorder (DSM-IV 300.3)

■ **EPIDEMIOLOGY & DEMOGRAPHICS**
PREVALENCE (IN U.S.): 1% to 2% of adults
PREDOMINANT SEX: Approximately equal distribution between sexes.
PREDOMINANT AGE:
• Modal age of onset for females is between 20 and 29 yr.
• Modal age of onset for males is between 6 and 15 yr.
• Condition is chronic.
PEAK INCIDENCE: Mean age at onset is 19.6 yr.
GENETICS:
• There is no clear genetic pattern.
• Rate of concordance is higher in monozygotic (33%) vs. dizygotic (7%) twins.
• Rate of disorder is also higher in first-degree relatives of individuals with OCD and Tourette's disorder than the general population.

■ **PHYSICAL FINDINGS & CLINICAL PRESENTATION**
• Persistent and recurrent intrusive and ego-dystonic obsessive ideas, thoughts, impulses, or images that are perceived as alien and beyond one's control.
• Frequent experiencing of obsessions related to contamination (e.g., when using the telephone), excessive doubt (e.g., was the door locked?), organization (the need for a particular order), violent impulses (e.g., to yell obscenities in church), or intrusive sexual imagery.
• Obsessions possibly leading to compulsive behaviors (e.g., repeated hand washing, checking, rearranging), or mental tasks (e.g., counting, repeating phrases).
• Obsessions and compulsions almost always accompanied with high anxiety and subjective distress.

■ **ETIOLOGY**
• In the past, OCD was seen in context of the psychoanalytic theory in which obsessions and compulsions were viewed as arrest of psychosexual development in the anal stage, perhaps secondary to excessively restrictive or punitive parenting.
• Disorder now seen as a biologic condition closely linked with learning disabilities and Tourette's disorder.
• Serotoninergic pathways believed important in some ritualistic instinctual behaviors, with dysfunction of these pathways possibly giving rise to OCD.

 DIAGNOSIS

■ **DIFFERENTIAL DIAGNOSIS**
• Other psychiatric disorders in which obsessive thoughts occur (e.g., body dysmorphic disorder or phobias).
• Other conditions in which compulsive behaviors are seen (e.g., trichotillomania).
• Major depression, hypochondriasis, and several anxiety disorders with predominant obsessions or compulsions; however, in these disorders the thoughts are not anxiety provoking or are extremes of normal concern.
• Delusions or psychosis, which may be mistaken for obsessive thoughts; distinguished from OCD in that the individual recognizes the ideas are not real.
• Tics and stereotypic movements that appear compulsive but are not driven by the desire to neutralize an obsession.
• Paraphilias or pathologic gambling; distinguished from compulsions in that they are usually enjoyable.

■ **WORKUP**
• Careful history leading to diagnosis
• Neurologic examination to rule out concomitant Tourette's or other tic disorder
• In adolescents and children: psychologic testing to reveal learning disabilities

■ **LABORATORY TESTS**
No specific tests are indicated.

■ **IMAGING STUDIES**
• No specific studies are indicated.
• There have been research reports of reversible abnormalities on PET scans.

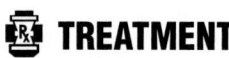 **TREATMENT**

■ **NONPHARMACOLOGIC THERAPY**
Behavioral therapies are often quite helpful, but success is often greater for compulsions than for obsessions.

■ **ACUTE GENERAL Rx**
None

■ **CHRONIC Rx**
• Antidepressants with serotonergic reuptake blockade, including fluoxetine, clomipramine, fluvoxamine, paroxetine, and sertraline
• No response in only 15% of patients
• Indefinite treatment

■ **DISPOSITION**
• OCD is a chronic condition with a waxing and waning course.
• Exacerbations are usually associated with stress.
• When untreated, 15% of patients progressively deteriorate in function.

■ **REFERRAL**
• If distinction from other psychiatric conditions, particularly delusional disorder, is not clear
• If patient refractory to treatment
• If treatment with antidepressants is problematic (e.g., when comorbid with bipolar illness)
Author: **Rif S. El-Mallakh, M.D.**

BASIC INFORMATION

■ **DEFINITION**
The term *ocular foreign body* refers to a foreign body on the surface of the corneal epithelium.

ICD-9CM CODES
930 Foreign body in external eye

■ **EPIDEMIOLOGY & DEMOGRAPHICS**
INCIDENCE (IN U.S.): Universal, with a predominance in active people
PREDOMINANT SEX: Perhaps slightly more common in men
PREDOMINANT AGE: Childhood through active adult years
PEAK INCIDENCE: Childhood through active adult years

■ **PHYSICAL FINDINGS & CLINICAL PRESENTATION**
Most common foreign bodies:
• Grinding (Fig. 1-266)
• Drilling
• Auto mechanics
• Working beneath cars
• Airborne particles blown by fans, etc.

DIAGNOSIS

■ **DIFFERENTIAL DIAGNOSIS**
• Corneal abrasion
• Corneal ulceration
• Glaucoma
• Herpes ulcers
• Infection
• Other keratitis

■ **WORKUP**
Fluorescein stain, slit lamp examination if no foreign body is found

■ **LABORATORY TESTS**
Intraocular pressure to make certain that eye has not been penetrated

■ **IMAGING STUDIES**
Occasionally, MRI of the orbits to identify foreign bodies not found by other means

TREATMENT

■ **NONPHARMACOLOGIC THERAPY**
Remove foreign body.

■ **ACUTE GENERAL Rx**
• Saline irrigation
• Removal of foreign body with moist cotton-tipped applicator after instillation of topical anesthetic drops
• Cycloplegics, antibiotics, and pressure dressing after removal of foreign body

■ **DISPOSITION**
If symptoms persist 24 hr after examination, refer to an ophthalmologist.

■ **REFERRAL**
To ophthalmology within 24 hr if patient not completely comfortable.

PEARLS & CONSIDERATIONS

■ **COMMENTS**
Alkaline or acidic chemical foreign bodies can be dangerous, and pH test must be performed if either of these is suspected (for all chemical foreign bodies).
Author: **Melvyn Koby, M.D.**

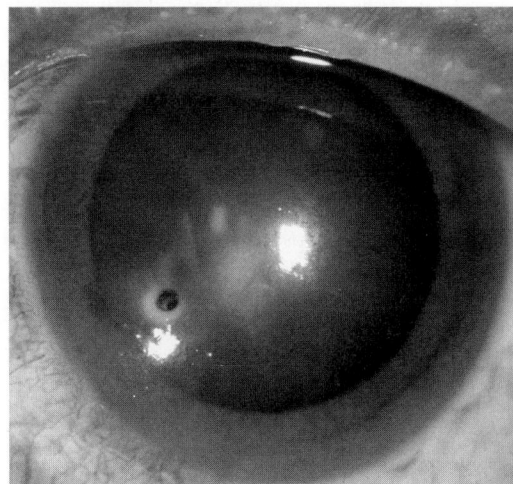

Fig. 1-266 A small, iron foreign body may be seen on external examination. (Courtesy Department of Dermatology, University of North Carolina at Chapel Hill. In Goldstein BG, Goldstein AO: *Practical dermatology,* ed 2, St Louis, 1997, Mosby.)

BASIC INFORMATION

■ DEFINITION

Onychomycosis is defined as a persistent fungal infection affecting the toenails and fingernails.

■ SYNONYMS

Tinea unguium
Ringworm of the nails

■ ICD-9CM CODES

110.1 Onychomycosis

■ EPIDEMIOLOGY & DEMOGRAPHICS

- Onychomycosis is most commonly found in people between the ages of 40 to 60 yr.
- Onychomycosis rarely occurs before puberty.
- Incidence: 20 to 100 cases/1000 population.
- Toenail infection is four to six times more common than fingernail infections.
- Onychomycosis affects men more often than women.
- Occurs more frequently in patients with diabetes, peripheral vascular disease, and any conditions resulting in the suppression of the immune system.
- Occlusive footwear, physical exercise followed by communal showering, and incompletely drying the feet predisposes the individual to developing onychomycosis.

■ PHYSICAL FINDINGS & CLINICAL PRESENTATION

- Onychomycosis causes nails to become thick, brittle, hard, distorted, and discolored (yellow to brown color). Eventually, the nail may loosen, separate from the nail bed and fall off (Fig. 1-267).
- Onychomycosis is frequently associated with tinea pedis (athlete's foot).

■ ETIOLOGY

- The most common causes of onychomycosis are dermatophyte, yeast, and nondermatophyte molds.
- The dermatophyte *Trichophyton rubrum* accounts for 80% of all nail infections caused by fungus.
- *Trichophyton interdigitale* and *Trichophyton mentagrophytes* are other fungi causing onychomycosis.

- The yeast *Candida albicans* is responsible for 5% of the cases of onychomycosis.
- Nondermatophyte molds *Scopulariopsis brevicaulis* and *Aspergillus niger*, although rare, can also cause onychomycosis.
- Onychomycosis is classified according to the clinical pattern of nail bed involvement. The main types are:
  1. Distal and lateral subungual onychomycosis (DLSO)
  2. Superficial onychomycosis
  3. Proximal subungual onychomycosis
  4. Endonyx onychomycosis
  5. Total dystrophic onychomycosis

DIAGNOSIS

The diagnosis of onychomycosis is based on the clinical nail findings and confirmed by direct microscopy and culture.

■ DIFFERENTIAL DIAGNOSIS

- Psoriasis
- Contact dermatitis
- Lichen planus
- Subungual keratosis
- Paronychia
- Infection(e.g., *Pseudomonas*)
- Trauma
- Peripheral vascular disease
- Yellow nail syndrome

■ WORKUP

The workup of suspected onychomycosis is directed at confirming the diagnosis of onychomycosis by visualizing hyphae under the microscope or by growing the organism in culture.

■ LABORATORY TESTS

- Blood tests are not specific in the diagnosis of onychomycosis.
- KOH prep.
- Fungal cultures on Sabouraud medium.

■ IMAGING STUDIES

- Imaging studies are not very specific in making the diagnosis of onychomycosis.
- If an infection is present and osteomyelitis is a consideration, an x-ray of the specific area and a bone scan may help establish the diagnosis.

TREATMENT

■ NONPHARMACOLOGIC THERAPY

- Surgical removal of the nail plate is a treatment option; however, the relapse rate is high.
- Prevention of reinfection by wearing properly fitted shoes, avoiding public showers, and keeping feet and nails clean and dry.

■ ACUTE GENERAL Rx

- Topical antifungal creams are used for early superficial nail infections.
  1. Miconazole 2% cream applied over the nail plate bid.
  2. Clortrimazole 1% cream bid.
- Oral agents
  1. *Itraconazole*
     a. For toenails: 200 mg qd × 3 mo.
     b. For fingernails: 200 mg PO bid × 7 days, followed by 3 wk of no medicine, for two pulses.
  2. *Terbinafine*
     a. For toenails: 250 mg/day for 3 mo
     b. For fingernails: 250 mg/day for 6 wk
  3. *Fluconazole*
     a. For toenails: 150 to 300 mg once weekly, until infection clears.
     b. For fingernails: 150 to 300 mg once weekly until infection clears.
- All oral agents used for onychomycosis require periodic monitoring of liver function blood tests.
- Itraconazole is contraindicated in patients taking cisapride, astemizole, triazolam, midazolam, and terfenadine. Lovastatin and simvastatin should be discontinued during itraconazole therapy.
- Fluconazole is contraindicated in patients taking cisapride and terfenadine.
- Oral antifungal agents should not be initiated during pregnancy.
- Ciclopirox, a topical nail lacquer anti-fungal agent, is FDA-approved for treatment of mild to moderate disease not involving the lunula.

■ CHRONIC Rx

- See under "Acute General Rx."

■ DISPOSITION

- Spontaneous remission of onychomycosis is rare.

- A disease-free toenail is reported to occur in approximately 25% to 50% of patients treated with the oral antifungal agents mentioned above.

■ **REFERRAL**
- Podiatry consultation is indicated in diabetic patients for proper instruction in foot care, footwear, and nail debridement or surgical removal of the toenail.
- Dermatology consultation is indicated in patients refractory to treatment or if another diagnosis is considered (e.g., psoriasis).

✪ **PEARLS & CONSIDERATIONS**

■ **COMMENTS**
- The growth of fungus on an infected nail typically begins at the end of the nail and spreads under the nail plate to infect the nail bed as well.
- Please review informational insert regarding drug-drug interactions and contraindications before initiating oral antifungal agents.

REFERENCES

Elewski BE, Hay RJ: Update on the management of onychomycosis: highlights of the Third International Summit on Cutaneous Antifungal Therapy, *Clin Infect Dis* 23:305, 1996.

Epstein E: How often does oral treatment of toenail onychomycosis produce a disease-free nail? an analysis of published data, *Arch Dermatol* 134(12):1551, 1998.

Gupta AK: The new oral antifungal agents for onychomycosis of the toenails, *J Eur Acad Dermatol Venereol* 13(1):1, 1999.

Rodgers P, Bassler M: Treating onychomycosis, *Am Fam Physician* 63:663, 2001.

Scher RK, Coppa LM: Advances in the diagnosis and treatment of onychomycosis, *Hosp Med* 34(4):11, 1998.

Author: **Dennis Mikolich, M.D.**

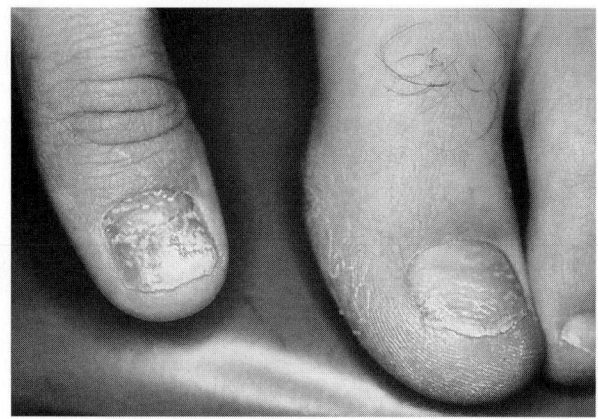 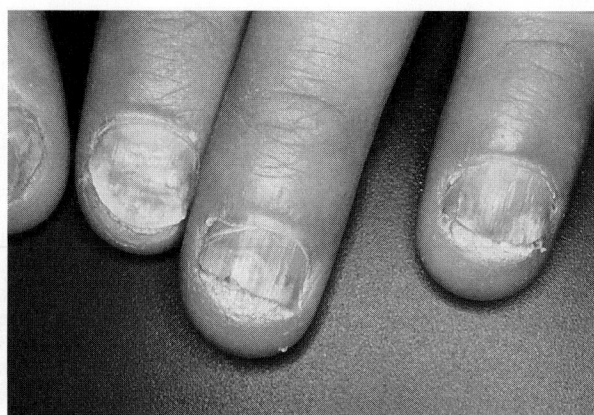

Fig. 1-267 **A,** Superficial white onychomycosis. **B,** Distal subungual onychomycosis. (From Noble J [ed]: *Textbook of primary care medicine,* ed 2, St Louis, 1996, Mosby.)

BASIC INFORMATION

■ DEFINITION
Optic atrophy refers to the degeneration of the optic nerve, which can have many causes.

■ SYNONYMS
Bilateral optic atrophy
Unilateral optic atrophy

ICD-9CM CODES
377.10 Atrophy, optic nerve

■ EPIDEMIOLOGY & DEMOGRAPHICS
PREDOMINANT SEX: From head injury, most common in males
PREDOMINANT AGE: 21 to 40 yr
PEAK INCIDENCE: All ages, depending on etiology

■ PHYSICAL FINDINGS & CLINICAL PRESENTATION
- At first, the temporal part of optic disc is pale (Fig. 1-268); later it appears "porcelain white."
- Unilateral lesion produces a Marcus Gunn pupil (relative afferent pupillary defect [RAPD]: swing flashlight eye to eye; abnormal pupil appears to dilate to direct light)
- Decreased visual acuity and central scotoma are noted.

■ ETIOLOGY
- Optic neuritis
- Ischemia (embolus, temporal arteritis)
- Compression
- Inflammation
- Hereditary
- Toxic metabolic
- Head injury

DIAGNOSIS

■ DIFFERENTIAL DIAGNOSIS
- Nutritional, toxic, and hereditary causes are usually bilateral.
- Unilateral optic atrophy in a young person is usually MS.
- Postviral atrophy is seen in childhood.

■ WORKUP
- Skin examination for evidence of phakomatoses
- Visual evoked responses

■ LABORATORY TESTS
- Depends on suspect etiology: none for trauma, tumor, MS
- Autoimmune diseases: ESR, ANA, etc.

■ IMAGING STUDIES
MRI with special cuts through orbits to identify compressive lesions or MS

TREATMENT

■ ACUTE GENERAL Rx
Treatment underlying cause (e.g., operation is indicated if tumor is identified).

■ CHRONIC Rx
The optic nerve does not regenerate.

■ DISPOSITION
- Visual loss occurs over weeks to months.
- Usually, follow-up by neurologist or ophthalmologist

■ REFERRAL
If tumor is found

PEARLS & CONSIDERATIONS

■ COMMENTS
- Every physician should be able to identify pale optic discs and Marcus Gunn pupil, which are important in identifying this condition.
- Patient education material can be obtained from the National Eye Institute, Department of Health and Human Services, 9000 Rockville Pike, Bethesda, MD 20892.

Author: **William H. Olson, M.D.**

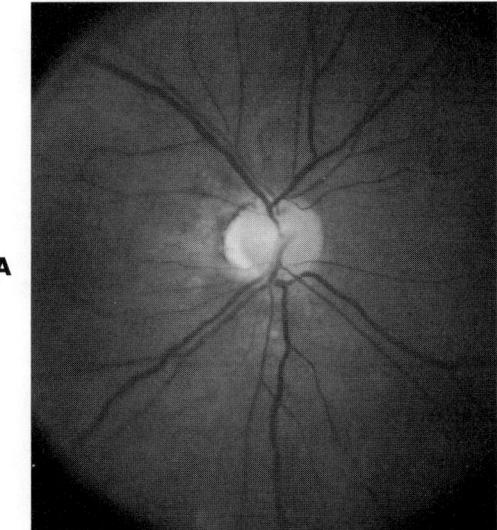 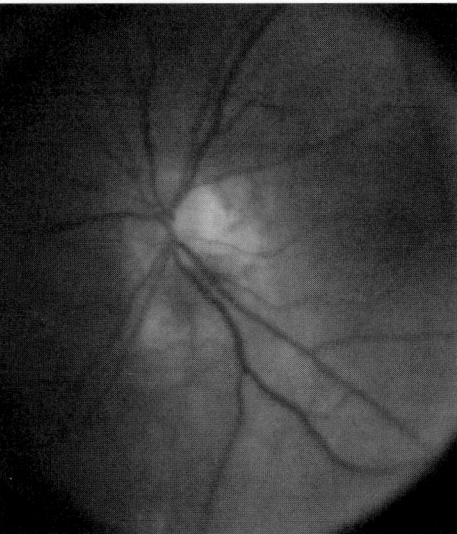

Fig. 1-268 Optic atrophy. **A,** Patient's right eye shows atrophy. **B,** Left eye is unaffected. (Courtesy John W. Payne, MD, The Wilmer Ophthalmological Institute, The Johns Hopkins University and Hospital, Baltimore. From Seidel HM [ed]: *Mosby's guide to physical examination,* ed 4, St Louis, 1999, Mosby.)

BASIC INFORMATION

■ **DEFINITION**
Optic neuritis is an inflammation of one or both optic nerves resulting in a temporary reduction of visual function.

■ **SYNONYMS**
Optic neuropathy
Optic papillitis
Retrobulbar neuritis

ICD-9CM CODES
377.3 Optic neuritis

■ **EPIDEMIOLOGY & DEMOGRAPHICS**
INCIDENCE (IN U.S.): Relatively common
PREVALENCE (IN U.S.): Common in patients with multiple sclerosis (MS)
PREDOMINANT SEX: Female
PEAK INCIDENCE: Rare in children and patients >45 yr old
PEAK AGE: 20s and 30s
GENETICS: MS more common in patients with certain HLA blood type

■ **PHYSICAL FINDINGS & CLINICAL PRESENTATION**
• Marcus Gunn pupil (swing flashlight eye to eye—abnormal pupil appears to dilate to direct light)
• Decreased visual acuity
• Visual field abnormalities
• Normal optic disc
• Pain on movement of affected eye

■ **ETIOLOGY**
MS develops in 80% of patients.

🔬 **DIAGNOSIS**

■ **DIFFERENTIAL DIAGNOSIS**
• Giant cell arteritis
• Ischemic optic atrophy
• Diabetic papillopathy
• Leber's optic neuropathy
• Optic drusen
• Acute papilledema
• Toxic/nutritional optic neuropathy

■ **WORKUP**
General physical examination should be normal.

■ **LABORATORY TESTS**
• Depends on history
• CBC, ANA, ESR, VDRL
• Possibly HIV testing
• Possibly Lyme disease testing
• Possibly sarcoidosis testing (chest x-ray examination, ABS)

■ **IMAGING STUDIES**
If MS suspected, MRI may show evidence of other lesions (Fig. 1-269).

℞ **TREATMENT**

■ **NONPHARMACOLOGIC THERAPY**
Assure patient that most vision will return.

■ **ACUTE GENERAL Rx**
A short course of methylprednisolone 10 mg IV for 10 days hastens recovery and outcome.

■ **CHRONIC Rx**
Full visual acuity usually returns in 6 mo.

■ **DISPOSITION**
Follow visual acuity weekly until vision improves.

■ **REFERRAL**
If patient has other neurologic signs, such as proptosis or tender temporal artery, if onset is gradual, and if vision does not improve after several weeks

💡 **PEARLS & CONSIDERATIONS**

■ **COMMENTS**
• Unilateral optic neuritis is a major risk factor for multiple sclerosis; one third of patients will develop MS in 15 yr.
• Patient education materials can be obtained from the National Eye Institute, Department of Health and Human Services, 9000 Rockville Pike, Bethesda, MD 20892.
Author: **William H. Olson, M.D.**

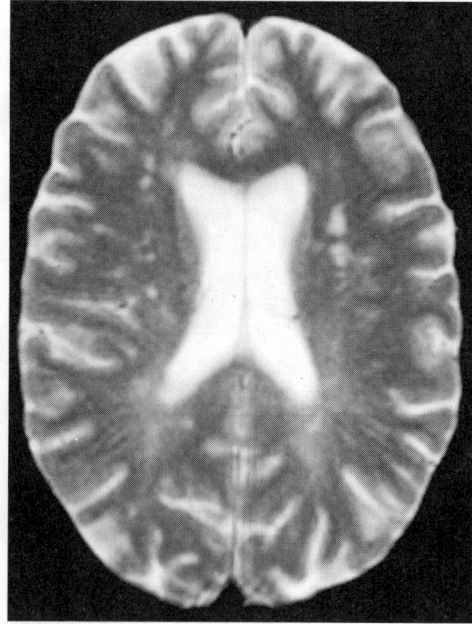

Fig. 1-269 Optic neuritis. A 32-year-old woman noted progressive decline in the vision of her right eye over 5 days as well as pain with eye movement. The optic discs and fundus were normal, but a large relative afferent pupillary defect was present in the right eye. MRI revealed periventricular white matter plaques *(1)* characteristic of multiple sclerosis. (From Palay D [ed]: *Ophthalmology for the primary care physician,* St Louis, 1997, Mosby.)

I

 BASIC INFORMATION

■ **DEFINITION**

Orchitis is an inflammatory process (usually infectious) involving the testicles. Infection may be viral or bacterial and can be associated with infection of other male sex organs (prostate, epididymis, bladder) or lower urogenital tract or sexually transmitted diseases often via hematogenous spread. Common causes are:

- Viral: Mumps—20% postpubertal; coxsackie B virus
- Bacterial: Pyogenic via spread from involving epididymis; bacteria include *Escherichia coli, Klebsiella pneumoniae, Staphylococcus, Streptococcus, P. aeruginosa, Rickettsia, Brucella*
- Other:
  HIV associated
  CMV
  Toxoplasmosis
  Fungi
  1. Cryptococcosis
  2. Histoplasmosis
  3. *Candida*
  4. Blastomycosis
  Mycobacteria

ICD-9CM CODES
0.72 Mumps
098.13 Acute gonococcal orchitis
095.8 Syphilitic orchitis
016.50 Tuberculous orchitis, unspecified

■ **EPIDEMIOLOGY & DEMOGRAPHICS**
PREDOMINANT SEX: Male
PREDOMINANT ORGANISM: The leading cause of viral orchitis is mumps. The mumps virus rarely causes orchitis in prepubertal males but involves one or both testicles in nearly 30% of postpubertal males.

■ **PHYSICAL FINDINGS & CLINICAL PRESENTATION**
- Testicular pain, swelling
- Unilateral or bilateral
- May have associated epididymitis, prostatitis, fever, scrotal edema, erythema cellulitis
- Inguinal lymphadenopathy
- Nausea, vomiting
- Acute hydrocele (bacterial)
- Rare development—abscess formation, pyocele of scrotum, testicular infarction
- Spermatic cord tenderness may be present

 DIAGNOSIS

Clinical presentation as described above with possible history of acute viral illness or concomitant epididymitis.

■ **DIFFERENTIAL DIAGNOSIS**
- Epididymoorchitis—gonococcal
- Autoimmune disease
- Vasculitis

- Epididymyosis
- Mumps—with or without parotitis
- Neoplasm
- Hematoma
- Spermatic cord torsion

■ **LABORATORY TESTS**
- CBC with differential
- Urinalysis
- Viral titer—mumps
- Urine culture
- Ultrasound of testicle to rule out abscess

■ **IMAGING STUDIES**
Ultrasound if abscess suspected

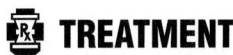 **TREATMENT**

- Dependent on etiology
- Viral (mumps)—observation
- Bacterial—empiric antibiotic treatment with parenteral antibiotic treatment for identified pathogen, including gram-negative rods, staphylococci, streptococci
- Surgery for abscess, pyogenic process

Author: **Dennis J. Mikolich, M.D.**

BASIC INFORMATION

■ **DEFINITION**
Osgood-Schlatter disease is a painful swelling of the tibial tuberosity that occurs in adolescence.

ICD-9CM CODES
732.4 Osgood-Schlatter disease

■ **EPIDEMIOLOGY & DEMOGRAPHICS**
PREVALENCE: 4 cases/100 adolescents
PREDOMINANT AGE: 11 to 15 yr (bilateral in 20%)
PREDOMINANT SEX: Male:female ratio of 3:1

■ **PHYSICAL FINDINGS & CLINICAL PRESENTATION**
• Pain at the tibial tubercle that is aggravated by activity, especially stair-walking and squatting
• Tender swelling and enlargement of the tibial tubercle
• Increased pain with knee extension against resistance

■ **ETIOLOGY**
• Unknown
• May be traumatically induced inflammation

 DIAGNOSIS

■ **DIFFERENTIAL DIAGNOSIS**
• Referred hip pain (any child with hip pain should have a thorough clinical hip examination)
• Patellar tendinitis

■ **WORKUP**
In most cases, the diagnosis is obvious on a clinical basis.

■ **IMAGING STUDIES**
• Lateral roentgenogram of the upper portion of the tibia with the leg slightly internally rotated may reveal variable degrees of separation and fragmentation of the upper tibial epiphysis (Fig. 1-270).
• Occasionally, fragmented area fails to unite to the tibia and persists into adulthood.

 TREATMENT

■ **ACUTE GENERAL Rx**
• Ice, especially after exercise
• NSAIDs
• Gentle hamstring and quadriceps stretching exercises
• Abstinence from physical activity

• Temporary immobilization in a knee splint for 2 to 4 wk in resistant cases

■ **DISPOSITION**
• Prognosis for complete restoration of function and relief from pain is excellent.
• Condition usually heals when the epiphysis closes.
• Complications are rare.
• Symptoms in the adult:
  1. Although unusual, prominence of the tibial tubercle is usually permanent
  2. May be more susceptible to local irritation, especially when kneeling
  3. Rarely, nonunion of the epiphyseal fragment, but it is usually asymptomatic
  4. Surgery rarely required

■ **REFERRAL**
For orthopedic consultation when diagnosis is uncertain or when symptoms persist.

■ **COMMENTS**
Larsen-Johansson disease is a similar disorder that can develop where either the quadriceps or patellar tendon inserts into the patella. Treatment and prognosis are the same as with Osgood-Schlatter disease.
Author: **Lonnie R. Mercier, M.D.**

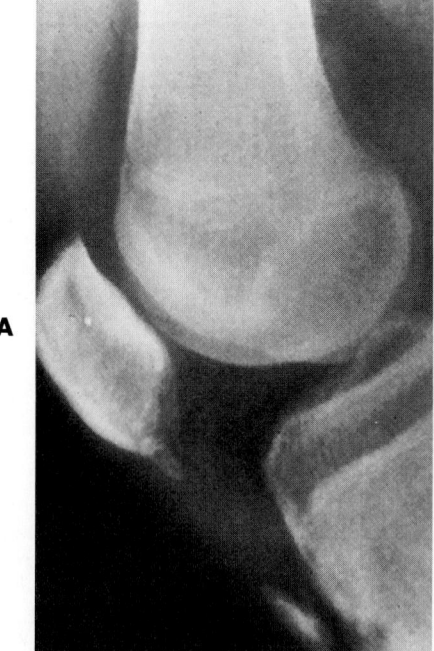
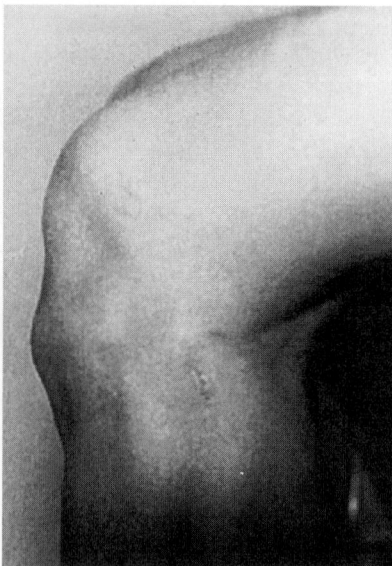

Fig. 1-270 **A,** Radiograph of Osgood-Schlatter disease demonstrating thickening of patella tendon, fragmentation of the tibial tubercle, and soft tissue swelling. **B,** Clinical picture of bony prominence anteriorly at the tibial tubercle. (From Scuderi G [ed]: *Sports medicine: principles of primary care,* St Louis, 1997, Mosby.)

BASIC INFORMATION

■ DEFINITION
Osteoarthritis is a joint condition in which degeneration and loss of articular cartilage occur, leading to pain and deformity. Two forms are usually recognized: primary (idiopathic) and secondary. The primary form may be localized or generalized.

■ SYNONYMS
Degenerative joint disease
Osteoarthrosis
Arthrosis

ICD-9CM CODES
715.0 Osteoarthrosis and allied disorders

■ EPIDEMIOLOGY & DEMOGRAPHICS
PREVALENCE: 2% to 6% of general population
PREDOMINANT SEX: Female = male
PREDOMINANT AGE: >50 yr

■ PHYSICAL FINDINGS & CLINICAL PRESENTATION
- Similar symptoms in most forms: stiffness, pain, and crepitus
- Joint tenderness, swelling
- Decreased range of motion
- Crepitus with motion
- Bony hypertrophy
- Pain with range of motion
- DIP joint involvement possibly leading to development of nodular swellings called Heberden's nodes (Fig. 1-271)
- PIP joint involvement possibly leading to development of nodular swellings called Bouchard's nodes

■ ETIOLOGY
Primary osteoarthritis is of unknown cause. Secondary osteoarthritis may result from a number of disorders including trauma, metabolic conditions, and other forms of arthritis.

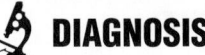 # DIAGNOSIS

■ DIFFERENTIAL DIAGNOSIS
- Bursitis, tendinitis
- Radicular spine pain
- Inflammatory arthritides
- Infectious arthritis

■ WORKUP
- No diagnostic test exists for degenerative joint disease.
- Laboratory evaluation is normal.
- Rheumatoid factor, ESR, CBC, and ANA tests may be required if inflammatory component is present.
- Synovial fluid examination is generally normal.

■ IMAGING STUDIES
- Roentgenographic evaluation reveals:
    1. Joint space narrowing
    2. Subchondral sclerosis
    3. New bone formation in the form of osteophytes
- When knee is involved, standing AP x-ray on any patient over 40.

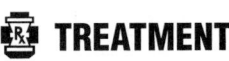 # TREATMENT

■ ACUTE GENERAL Rx
- Rest, restricted use or weight bearing, and heat
- Walking aids such as a cane (often helpful for weight-bearing joints)
- Suitable footwear
- Gentle range of motion and strengthening exercise
- Local creams and liniments to provide a counterirritant effect
- Education, reassurance

■ PHARMACOLOGIC THERAPY
- Mild analgesics for joint pain
- NSAIDs if inflammation is present
- Occasional local corticosteroid injections (see Table 1-18)

- Mild antidepressants, especially at night, if depression is present
- Viscosupplementation (injection of hyaluronic acid products into the degenerative joint) is of uncertain benefit.
- Nutritional supplements (glucosamine and chondroitin) are unproven.

■ DISPOSITION
Progression is not always inevitable, and the prognosis is variable depending on the site and extent of the disease.

■ REFERRAL
Surgical consultation for patients not responding to medical management

⚙ PEARLS & CONSIDERATIONS

■ COMMENTS
Surgical intervention is generally helpful in degenerative joint disease. Arthroplasty, arthrodesis, and realignment osteotomy are the most common procedures performed.

REFERENCES
Brander VA: Osteoarthritis of the knee: pathogenesis, pathophysiology, and radiographic progression, *Am J Orthop* 30:6, 2001.

Brief AA, Maurer SG, Dicesare PE: Use of glucosamine and chondroitin sulfate in the management of osteoarthritis, *J Am Acad Orthop Surg* 9:71, 2001.

Buckwalter JA et al: The increasing need for nonoperative treatment of patients with osteoarthritis, *Clin Orthop* 385:36, 2001.

Chard J, Dieppe P: Glucosamine for osteoarthritis: magic, hype, or confusion? *BMJ* 322:1439, 2001.

Hoaglund FT, Steinbach LS: Primary osteoarthritis of the hip: etiology and epidemiology, *J Am Acad Orthop Surg* 9:320, 2001.

Manek NJ: Medical management of osteoarthritis, *Mayo Clin Proc* 76:533, 2001.

NIH Conference, Felson DT, chair: Osteoarthritis: new insights. Part 1: The disease and its risk factors, *Ann Intern Med* 133:635, 2000.

NIH Conference, Felson DT, chair: Osteoarthritis: new insights. Part 2: Treatment approaches, *Ann Intern Med* 133:726, 2000.

Watterson JR, Esdaile JM: Viscosupplementation: therapeutic mechanisms and clinical potential in osteoarthritis of the knee, *J Am Acad Orthop Surg* 8:277, 2000.

Wright KE, Maurer SG, DiCesare PE: Viscosupplementation of osteoarthritis, *Am J Orthop* 29:80, 2000.
Author: **Lonnie R. Mercier, M.D.**

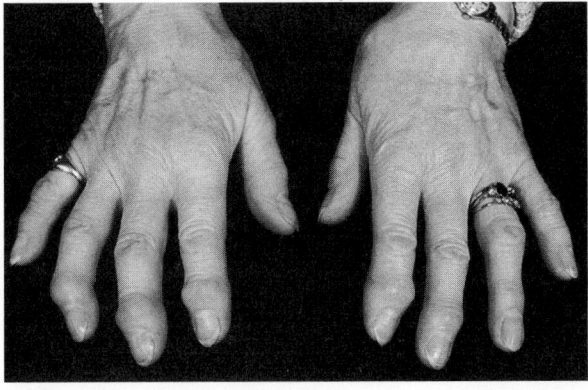

Fig. 1-271   Osteoarthritis of the distal interphalangeal (DIP) joints. This patient has the typical clinical findings of advanced osteoarthritis of the DIP joints, including large, firm swellings (Heberden's nodes), some of which are tender and red because of associated inflammation of the periarticular tissues as well as of the joint. (From Klippel J, Dieppe P, Ferri F [eds]: *Primary care rheumatology,* London, 1999, Mosby.)

BASIC INFORMATION

■ DEFINITION
Osteochondritis dissecans is a disorder in which a portion of cartilage and underlying subchondral bone separates from a joint surface and may even become detached.

■ SYNONYMS
Osteochondrosis
Talar dome fracture: commonly used in describing the lesion of the talus

ICD-9CM CODES
732.7 Osteochrondritis dissecans

■ EPIDEMIOLOGY & DEMOGRAPHICS
PREVALENCE: 0.3 cases/1000 persons
PREVALENT AGE: Onset at 10 to 30 yr
PREVALENT SEX: Male:female ratio of 3:1
The most common joint affected is the knee, with the lateral surface of the medial femoral condyle the most frequent area involved. The capitellum of the humerus, dome of the talus, shoulder, and hip may also be affected.

■ PHYSICAL FINDINGS & CLINICAL PRESENTATION
- Pain, stiffness, and swelling
- Intermittent locking if the fragment becomes detached
- Occasionally palpable loose body
- Tenderness at the site of the lesion
- When the knee is involved, positive Wilson's sign (pain with knee extension and internal rotation)
- Some asymptomatic cases

■ ETIOLOGY
Unknown

DIAGNOSIS

■ DIFFERENTIAL DIAGNOSIS
- Acute fracture
- Neoplasm

■ IMAGING STUDIES
- Plain roentgenography to confirm the diagnosis (Fig. 1-272)
- "Tunnel view" helpful in knee cases
- Typical finding: radiolucent, semilunar line outlining the oval fragment of bone (but findings variable, depending on the amount of healing and stability)
- MRI or bone scanning usually not necessary in establishing diagnosis but helpful in determining prognosis and management, especially with regards to the stability of the lesion

TREATMENT

■ ACUTE GENERAL Rx
- Observation every 4 to 6 mo for patients in whom the lesion is asymptomatic
- Symptomatic patients who are skeletally immature:
  1. Observation with an initial period of non–weight-bearing for 6 to 8 wk (in knee cases)
  2. When symptoms subside, gradual resumption of activities

■ DISPOSITION
- Juvenile cases with open epiphyses have a favorable prognosis.
- Cases developing after skeletal maturity are more likely to develop osteoarthritis.
- Large fragments, especially those in weight-bearing areas, have a more unfavorable prognosis, especially if they involve the lateral femoral condyle.
- Loose body formation and degenerative joint disease are more common when condition develops after age 20 yr.

■ REFERRAL
For orthopedic consultation:
- For most adults with unstable lesions
- If a loose body is present
- If symptomatic care has failed

PEARLS & CONSIDERATIONS

■ COMMENTS
- Although inflammation is suggested by the name, it has not been shown to be of significance in this disorder. "Osteochondral lesion" or "osteochondrosis dissecans" may be more appropriate term to describe these disorders.
- Repetitive trauma with ischemic necrosis is the most likely cause.
- The condition is often bilateral, especially in the knee, which could suggest the possibility of an endocrine or genetic basis.
- This condition should always be considered in the patient whose "sprained ankle" does not improve over the usual course of treatment.

REFERENCE
Hixon AL, Gibbs LM: Osteochondritis dissecans: a diagnosis not to miss, *Am Fam Physician* 61:151, 2000.
Author: **Lonnie R. Mercier, M.D.**

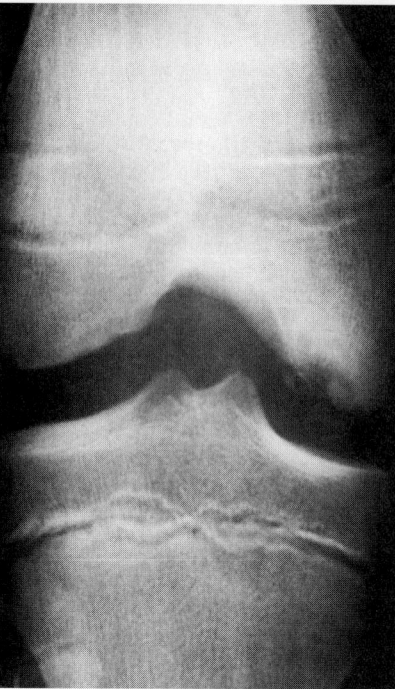

Fig. 1-272 Osteochondritis dissecans of the knee. The "tunnel" view is often helpful in visualizing the defect. This fragment may become detached and form a loose body. This area should not be confused with the normal irregularity of the distal femoral epiphysis in young children.

BASIC INFORMATION

■ **DEFINITION**
Osteomyelitis is an acute or chronic infection of the bone secondary to the hematogenous or contiguous source of infection or direct traumatic inoculation, which is usually bacterial.

■ **SYNONYMS**
Bone infection

■ **ICD-9CM CODES**
730.1 Chronic osteomyelitis
730.2 Acute or subacute osteomyelitis

■ **EPIDEMIOLOGY & DEMOGRAPHICS**
PREDOMINANT SEX: Male > female
PREDOMINANT AGE: All ages

■ **PHYSICAL FINDINGS**
HEMATOGENOUS OSTEOMYELITIS:
Usually occurs in tibia/fibula (children).
• Localized inflammation: often secondary to trauma with accompanying hematoma or cellulitis
• Abrupt fever
• Lethargy
• Irritability
• Pain in involved bone
VERTEBRAL OSTEOMYELITIS: Usually hematogenous.
• Fever: 50%
• Localized pain/tenderness
• Neurologic defects: motor/sensory
CONTIGUOUS OSTEOMYELITIS: Direct inoculation.
• Associated with trauma, fractures, surgical fixation
• Chronic infection of skin/soft tissue
• Fever, drainage from surgical site

CHRONIC OSTEOMYELITIS:
• Bone pain
• Sinus tract drainage, nonhealing ulcer
• Chronic low-grade fever
• Chronic localized pain

■ **ETIOLOGY**
• *Staphylococcus aureus*
• *S. aureus* (methicillin-resistant)
• *Pseudomonas aeruginosa*
• Enterobacteriaceae
• *Streptococcus pyogenes*
• *Enterococcus*
• Mycobacteria
• Fungi
• Coagulase-negative staphylococci
• *Salmonella* (in sickle cell disease)

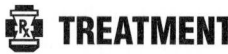 **DIAGNOSIS**

■ **DIFFERENTIAL DIAGNOSIS**
• Brodie's abscess
• Gaucher's disease
• Bone infarction
• Charcot's joint
• Gout
• Fracture

■ **WORKUP**
• ESR, C-reactive protein
• Blood culturing
• Bone culture
• Pathologic evaluation of bone biopsy for acute/chronic changes consistent with necrosis or acute inflammation

■ **IMAGING STUDIES**
• Bone x-ray examination
• Bone scan (Fig. 1-273)
• Gallium scan
• Indium scan
• MRI (most accurate imaging study)

• Doppler studies: useful in patients with peripheral vascular disease to determine vascular adequacy

■ **TREATMENT**

Surgical debridement in biopsy-positive cases will give direction for antibiotic therapy. This will vary with type of osteomyelitis. Duration of therapy is usually 6 wk for acute osteomyelitis; chronic osteomyelitis may need a longer course of medication.
• *S. aureus:* cefazolin IV, nafcillin IV, vancomycin IV (in patient allergic to penicillin)
• *S. aureus* (methicillin resistant): vancomycin IV
• *Streptococcus* spp.: cefazolin or ceftriaxone
• *P. aeruginosa:* piperacillin plus aminoglycoside or ceftazidime plus aminoglycoside
• Enterobacteriaceae: ceftriaxone or fluoroquinolone
• Hyperbaric oxygen therapy: may be useful in treatment of chronic osteomyelitis, especially with associated wound healing
• Surgical debridement of all devitalized bone and tissue
• Immobilization of affected bone (plaster, traction) if bone is unstable
• Bone grafts using a vascularized or open graft may be necessary if the remaining bone is inadequate

REFERENCE
Boutin RD et al: Update on imaging of orthopedic infections, *Orthop Clin North Am* 29:41, 1998.
Author: **Dennis J. Mikolich, M.D.**

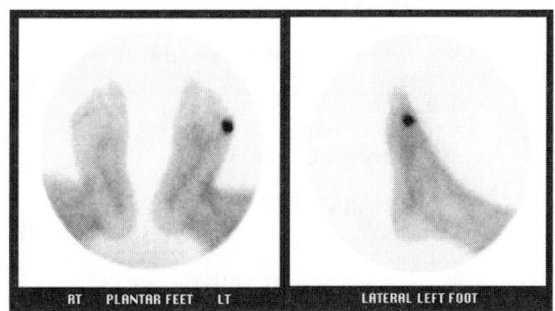

Fig. 1-273 Osteomyelitis. Intense accumulation of Tc-99m WBC in proximal phalanx of fifth digit of left foot at 4 hours after injection. (From Specht N [ed]: *Practical guide to diagnostic imaging,* St Louis, 1998, Mosby.)

BASIC INFORMATION

■ **DEFINITION**
Osteonecrosis refers to the death of bone marrow, cortex, and medullary bone caused by interruption of blood supply to the bone.

■ **SYNONYMS**
Aseptic necrosis
Avascular necrosis
Ischemic necrosis

ICD-9CM CODES
730.1 Osteonecrosis

■ **EPIDEMIOLOGY & DEMOGRAPHICS**
- Osteonecrosis accounts for 10% of all hip surgeries performed annually in the U.S.
- Osteonecrosis involves the femoral head most frequently followed by the humeral head, femoral condyles, and distal femur.
- Between 5% to 25% of patients on chronic corticosteroid use develop osteonecrosis.
- Incidence of osteonecrosis in alcoholics is 2% to 5%.
- Osteonecrosis is found in 10% of patients with sickle cell anemia.

■ **CLINICAL PRESENTATION & PHYSICAL FINDINGS**
- May be clinically silent
- Pain in the affected bone (hip, knee or shoulder)
- Pain at rest or with use
- Decreased range of motion of the affected joint
- Joint pain with passive motion

■ **ETIOLOGY**
The etiology of osteonecrosis can be divided into:
- Atraumatic
  1. Idiopathic
  2. Alcohol
  3. Hemoglobinopathy (e.g., sickle cell disease)
  4. Connective tissue disorders (SLE, rheumatoid arthritis, vasculitis, antiphospholipid syndrome)
  5. Corticosteroid use
  6. Pregnancy
  7. Estrogen use
  8. Gaucher's disease
  9. Dysbarism
  10. Radiation therapy
- Traumatic
  1. Femoral neck fracture
  2. Septic

■ **DIAGNOSIS**

The diagnosis of avascular necrosis should be suspected in any patient with focal bone pain on corticosteroids or with any of the above mentioned comorbid conditions.

■ **DIFFERENTIAL DIAGNOSIS**
The differential diagnosis of osteonecrosis is as stated under "Etiology" and includes hyperlipidemias, pancreatitis, renal transplantation, chronic liver disease, obesity, and chemotherapy.

■ **WORKUP**
Radiographic imaging is the mainstay for confirming the clinical suspicion of osteonecrosis.

■ **LABORATORY TESTS**
CBC, electrolytes, BUN, creatinine, liver function tests, ESR, ANA, RF, lipid profile, and other serologic tests are used as adjuncts in supporting the diagnosis of avascular necrosis.

■ **IMAGING STUDIES**
- Plain films help define and classify the disease course. Staging systems have been developed for osteonecrosis of the femoral head:
  1. Stage I: Initial x-rays are normal, but bone scan is positive.
  2. Stage II: Abnormal radiolucency is noted.
  3. Stage III: Deformity with collapse and sclerosis.
  4. Stage IV: Early osteoarthritis.
- Bone scan reveals decreased uptake at the affected site with a "doughnut sign" and can detect avascular necrosis before the plain x-rays.
- MRI scan is more sensitive and specific than bone scan, especially when looking for osteonecrosis of the femoral head.
- If a MRI is not available, CT scan of the involved bone is efficacious.

■ **TREATMENT**

Treatment of osteonecrosis of the hip can be directed at three stages:
- Before bone collapse
- After bone collapse
- After arthritic formation

■ **NONPHARMACOLOGIC THERAPY**
- Immobilization
- Non-weight bearing with the use of crutches
- Special muscle strengthening exercise

■ **ACUTE GENERAL Rx**
- Nonsteroidal antiinflammatory agents, ibuprofen 800 mg PO tid, naproxen 500 mg bid, or acetaminophen 500 mg (2 tabs) PO q6h can be used for symptom relief.
- For displaced hip fractures, prompt surgical reduction is indicated in attempt to reperfuse the femoral head.

■ **CHRONIC Rx**
- For patients with stage I or II osteonecrosis (before bone collapse occurs), core decompression treatment is tried to prevent bone collapse.
- In stage III osteonecrosis (after bone collapse), a hemiarthroplasty or total joint replacement is required.
- In stage IV osteonecrosis (arthritis setting in after bone collapse), a total joint replacement is usually required.

■ **DISPOSITION**
- There is no therapy to prevent avascular necrosis from occurring in patients predisposed to getting the disease.
- Patients diagnosed with avascular necrosis have a slow progressive course.
- Patients with symptoms and diagnosed by x-ray imaging to be at stage I or II (pre-bone collapse) can expect within 18 to 36 mo to develop bone collapse of the affected site.

■ **REFERRAL**
Whenever the diagnosis of avascular necrosis is suspected clinically or detected radiographically, a rheumatology and/or orthopedic consultation should be made.

☼ **PEARLS & CONSIDERATIONS**

■ **COMMENTS**
- The pathogenesis of osteonecrosis is secondary to decrease perfusion of the bone elements leading to necrosis. Interruption of blood supply can occur either by arterial or venous occlusion, traumatic vascular injury, or extravascular compression.
- How each specific cause (e.g., alcohol, corticosteroids, SLE) leads to vascular interruption remains elusive.
- In approximately 70% of all patients with displaced hip fractures, there is near total loss of blood supply to the femoral head.

REFERENCES
Jones JP: Concepts of etiology and early pathogenesis of osteonecrosis. Instructional course lectures, *Am Acad Orthop Surg* 43:499, 1994.
Koo K-H et al: Preventing collapse in early osteonecrosis of the femoral head, *J Bone Joint Surg* 77B: 870, 1995.
Mankin HJ: Nontraumatic necrosis of bone (osteonecrosis), *N Engl J Med* 326(22):1473, 1992.
Author: **Peter Petropoulos, M.D.**

BASIC INFORMATION

■ DEFINITION
Osteoporosis is characterized by a progressive decrease in bone mass that results in increased bone fragility and a higher fracture risk. The various types are as follows:
PRIMARY OSTEOPOROSIS: 80% of women and 60% of men with osteoporosis
- Idiopathic osteoporosis: unknown pathogenesis; may occur in children and young adults
- Type I osteoporosis: may occur in postmenopausal women (age range: 51 to 75 yr); characterized by accelerated and disproportionate trabecular bone loss and associated with vertebral body and distal forearm fractures (estrogen withdrawal effect)
- Type II osteoporosis (involutional): occurs in both men and women >70 yr of age; characterized by both trabecular and cortical bone loss, and associated with fractures of the proximal humerus and tibia, femoral neck, and pelvis
SECONDARY OSTEOPOROSIS: 20% of women and 40% of men with osteoporosis; osteoporosis that exists as a common feature of another disease process, heritable disorder of connective tissue, or drug side effect (see "Differential Diagnosis")

ICD-9CM CODES
733.0 Osteoporosis

■ EPIDEMIOLOGY & DEMOGRAPHICS
PREVALENCE (IN U.S.):
- Approximately 25 million men and women
- Twice as common in women
- Results in 1.5 million fractures annually (70% women)
- Osteoporosis-related fractures in 50% women and 20% men >65 yr
- Results: institutionalization, mortality, and costs in excess of $10 billion annually
RISK FACTORS:
- Age: each decade after 40 yr associated with a fivefold increase risk
- Genetics:
  1. Ethnicity (white/Asian > black > Polynesian)
  2. Gender (female > male)
  3. Family history
- Environmental factors: poor nutrition, calcium deficiency, physical inactivity, medication (steroids/heparin), tobacco use, ETOH, traumatic injury
- Chronic disease states: estrogen deficiency, androgen deficiency, hyperthyroidism, hypercortisolism, cirrhosis, gastrectomy

■ PHYSICAL FINDINGS & CLINICAL PRESENTATION
- Most commonly silent with no signs and symptoms
- Insidious and progressive development of dorsal kyphosis (dowager's hump), loss of height, and skeletal pain typically associated with fracture (Fig. 1-274); other physical findings related to other conditions with associated increased risk for osteoporosis (see "Risk Factors")

■ ETIOLOGY
- Primary osteoporosis; multifactorial resulting from a combination of factors including nutrition, peak bone mass, genetics, level of physical activity, age of menopause (spontaneous vs. surgical), and estrogen status
- Secondary osteoporosis: associated decrease in bone mass resulting from an identified cause, including endocrinopathies—hypogonadism, hyperthyroidism, hyperparathyroidism, Cushing's syndrome, hyperprolactinemia, acromegaly, diabetes mellitus, gastrointestinal disease, malabsorption, primary biliary cirrhosis, gastrectomy, malnutrition (including anorexia nervosa)

DIAGNOSIS

■ DIFFERENTIAL DIAGNOSIS
- Malignancy (multiple myeloma, lymphoma, leukemia, metastatic carcinoma)
- Primary hyperparathyroidism
- Osteomalacia
- Paget's disease
- Osteogenesis imperfecta: types I, III, and IV (see also "Epidemiology and Demographics" and "Etiology")

■ WORKUP
- History and physical examination (20% of women with type I osteoporosis have associated secondary cause), with appropriate evaluation for identified risk factors and secondary causes
- Diagnosis of osteoporosis made by bone mineral density (BMD) determination (BMD should ideally evaluate the hip, spine, and wrist):
  1. Dual-energy x-ray absorptiometry (DEXA)
  2. Single-energy x-ray
  3. Peripheral dual-energy x-ray
  4. Single-photon absorptiometry
  5. Dual-photon absorptiometry
  6. Quantitative CT scan
  7. Radiographic absorptiometry

■ LABORATORY TESTS
- Biochemical profile to evaluate renal and hepatic function, primary hyperparathyroidism, and malnutrition
- CBC for nutritional status and myeloma
- TSH to rule out the presence of hyperthyroidism
- Consideration of 24-hr urine collection for calcium (excess skeletal loss, vitamin D malabsorption/deficiency), creatinine, sodium, and free cortisol (to detect occult Cushing's disease); no need to measure calcitropic hormones (PTH, calcitriol, calcitonin) unless specifically indicated
- Biochemical markers of bone remodeling; may be useful to predict rate of bone loss and/or follow therapy response; specific biochemical markers followed (e.g., 3-mo interval) to document normalization as a response to therapy
  1. High turnover osteoporosis: high levels of resorption markers (lysyl pyridinoline [LP], deoxylysyl pyridinoline [DPD], n-telopeptide of collagen cross-links [NTX], C-telopeptide of collagen cross-links [PICP]) and formation markers (osteocalcin [OCN], bone-specific alkaline phosphatase [BSAP], carboxy-terminal extension peptide of type I procollagen [PICP]); accelerated bone loss responding best to antiresorptive therapy
  2. Low-normal turnover osteoporosis: normal or low levels of the markers of resorption and formation (see "high turnover osteoporosis" above); no accelerated bone loss; responds best to drugs that enhance bone formation

■ IMAGING STUDIES
- BMD determination (see "Workup") should be performed on all women with determined risk factors and/or associated secondary causes; accepted screening criteria are currently being investigated.
  1. Normal: BMD <1 SD of the young adult reference mean
  2. Osteopenia: BMD <1 to 2.5 SD below the young adult reference mean
  3. Osteoporosis: BMD >2.5 SD below the young adult reference mean
- For patient undergoing treatment: annual BMD to follow response to therapy
- X-ray examination of appropriate part of skeleton to evaluate clinical osteoporotic fracture only

℞ TREATMENT

■ NONPHARMACOLOGIC THERAPY
Prevention:
- Identification and minimization of risk factors
- Appropriate diagnosis and treatment of secondary causes
- Behavioral modification: proper nutrition (dietary calcium >800 mg/day, vitamin D 400 to 800 U/day), physical activity, fracture prevention strategies

■ ACUTE GENERAL Rx
- Vitamin D supplement: 400 U/day
- Calcium supplement: 1000 to 1500 mg/day
- Estrogen (conjugated equine estrogen or equivalent): 0.3 to 0.625 mg/day
- Progestin: continuous (e.g., 2.5 mg medroxyprogesterone acetate/day or equivalent) or cyclic (e.g., 10 mg medroxyprogesterone acetate days 16 to 25 each month or equivalent) coadministered in nonhysterectomized women
- Alendronate: 10 mg/day on awakening with 8 oz water on empty stomach with no oral intake for at least 30 min
- Alendronate: 70 mg once weekly for treatment of postmenopausal osteoporosis and a 35-mg tablet for the prevention of osteogenesis in postmenopausal women
- Synthetic salmon calcitonin: 100 U/day SC or 200 U/day intranasally
- Raloxifene: 60 mg qd
- Risedronate: 5 mg/day on awakening with 8 oz water or empty stomach

with no oral intake for at least 30 min
- Other FDA-approved drugs (without osteoporosis indication) used to treat osteoporosis:
  1. Calcitriol
  2. Etidronate
  3. Thiazide
- Combination estrogen/alendronate or estrogen-progestin/alendronate may be considered in individualized patients on HRT with identified osteoporosis
- BMD baseline obtained before onset of therapy and at 1 yr; decrease of 2% or greater results in dosage adjustment or medication change
- Baseline biochemical markers of remodeling baseline considered; identified high turnover osteoporosis patients rescreened at 3 mo to document marker return to normal

■ CHRONIC Rx
- Lifelong disorder requiring lifelong attention to behavior modification issues (nutrition, physical activity, fracture prevention strategies) and compliance with pharmacologic intervention
- Continuing need to eliminate high-risk factors where possible and to diagnose and optimally manage secondary causes of osteoporosis

■ DISPOSITION
Goal for diagnosis and treatment: identification of women at risk, initiation of preventive measures for all women lifelong, institution of treatment modalities that will result in a decrease in fracture risk, and reduction of morbidity, mortality, and unnecessary institutionalization, thereby improving

quality of independent life and productivity.

■ REFERRAL
- To reproductive endocrinologist, endocrinologist, gynecologist, or rheumatologist if unfamiliar with diagnosis and management of osteoporosis
- If multidisciplinary management is required, to other specialties depending on presence of acute fracture and/or secondary associated disorders

☼ PEARLS & CONSIDERATIONS

■ COMMENTS
Patient information is available from American College of Obstetricians and Gynecologists.

REFERENCES
Kleerekoper M: Detecting osteoporosis: beyond the history and physical examination, *Postgrad Med* 103:45, 1998.

NIH consensus development panel on osteoporosis prevention, diagnosis, and therapy, *JAMA* 285:785, 2001.

Prestwood KM: Osteoporosis: pathogenesis, diagnosis, and treatment in older adults, *Clin Geriatr Med* 14:577, 1998.

South-Paul JE: Osteoporosis: part I. Evaluation and assessment, *Am Fam Physician* 63(5):897, 2001.

South-Paul JE: Osteoporosis: part II. Nonpharmacologic and pharmacologic treatment, *Am Fam Physician* 63(6):1121, 2001.

Author: **Dennis M. Weppner, M.D.**

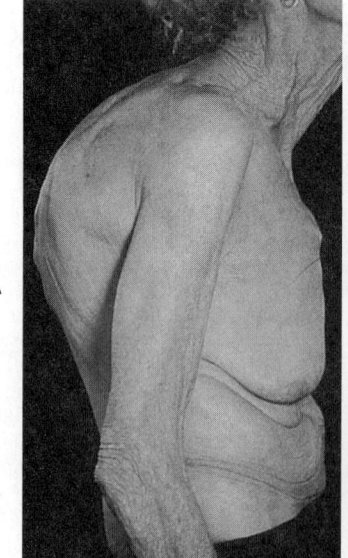
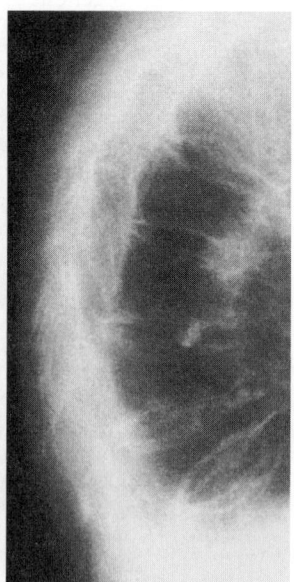

Fig. 1-274 Dowager's hump. **A,** Marked thoracic kyphosis resulting from multiple osteoporotic fractures in an elderly woman with, **B,** the corresponding radiograph. (From Klippel J, Dieppe P, Ferri F [eds]: *Primary care rheumatology,* London, 1999, Mosby.)

BASIC INFORMATION

■ DEFINITION

Otitis externa is a term encompassing a variety of conditions causing inflammation and/or infection of the external auditory canal (and/or auricle and tympanic membrane). There are six subgroups of otitis externa:

- Acute localized otitis externa (furunculosis)
- Acute diffuse bacterial otitis externa (swimmer's ear)
- Chronic otitis externa
- Eczematous otitis externa
- Fungal otitis externa (otomycosis)
- Invasive or necrotizing (malignant) otitis externa

■ SYNONYMS

See "Definition" above

ICD-9CM CODES
38.10 Otitis externa

■ EPIDEMIOLOGY & DEMOGRAPHICS
INCIDENCE (IN U.S.)
- Among the most common disorders
- Affects 3% to 10% of patients seeking otologic care
PREVALENCE (IN U.S.)
- Diffuse otitis externa (swimmer's ear) is most often seen in swimmers and in hot, humid climates, conditions that lead to water retention in the ear canal.
- Necrotizing otitis externa is more common in elderly, diabetics, immunocompromised patients.
PREDOMINANT SEX: None
PREDOMINANT AGE:
- Occurs at all ages
- Necrotizing otitis externa: typically occurs in elderly: mean age >65 years

■ PHYSICAL FINDINGS & CLINICAL PRESENTATION
The two most common symptoms are otalgia, ranging from pruritus to severe pain exacerbated by motion (e.g., chewing), and otorrhea. Patients may also experience aural fullness and hearing loss secondary to swelling with occlusion of the canal. More intense symptoms may occur with bacterial otitis externa, with or without fever, and lymphadenopathy (anterior to tragus). There are also findings unique to the various forms of the infection:
- Acute localized otitis externa (furunculosis):
  1. Occurs from infected hair follicles, usually in the outer third of the ear canal, forming pustules and furuncles
  2. Furuncles are superficial and pointing or deep and diffuse

- Impetigo:
  1. In contrast to furunculosis, this is a superficial spreading infection of the ear canal that may also involve the concha and the auricle
  2. Begins as a small blister that ruptures, releasing straw-colored fluid that dries as a golden crust
- Erysipelas:
  1. Caused by group A *Streptococcus*
  2. May involve the concha and canal
  3. May involve the dermis and deeper tissues
  4. Area of cellulitis, often with severe pain
  5. Fever chills, malaise
  6. Regional adenopathy
- Eczematous otitis externa:
  1. Stems from a variety of dermatologic problems that can involve the external auditory canal
  2. Severe itching, erythema, scaling, crusting, and fissuring possible
- Acute diffuse otitis externa (swimmers's ear):
  1. Begins with itching and a feeling of pressure and fullness in the ear that becomes increasingly tender and painful
  2. Mild erythema and edema of the external auditory canal, which may cause narrowing and occlusion of the canal, leading to hearing loss
  3. Minimal serous secretions, which may become profuse and purulent
  4. Tympanic membrane may appear dull and infected

5. Usually absence of systemic symptoms such as fever, chills
- Otomycosis:
  1. Chronic superficial infection of the ear canal and tympanic membrane
  2. In primary fungal infection, major symptom is intense itching
  3. In secondary infection (fungal infection superimposed on bacterial infection), major symptom is pain
  4. Fungal growth of variety of colors
- Chronic otitis externa:
  1. Dry and atrophic canal
  2. Typically, lack of cerumen
  3. Itching, often severe, and mild discomfort rather than pain
  4. Occasionally, mucopurulent discharge
  5. With time, thickening of the walls of the canal, causing narrowing of the lumen
- Necrotizing otitis externa (also known as malignant otitis externa):
  1. Redness, swelling, and tenderness of the ear canal
  2. Classic finding of granulation tissue on the floor of the canal and the bone-cartilage junction
  3. Small ulceration of necrotic soft tissue at bone-cartilage junction
  4. Most common complaints: pain (often severe) and otorrhea
  5. Lessening of purulent drainage as infection advances
  6. Facial nerve palsy often the first and only cranial nerve defect
  7. Possible involvement of other cranial nerves

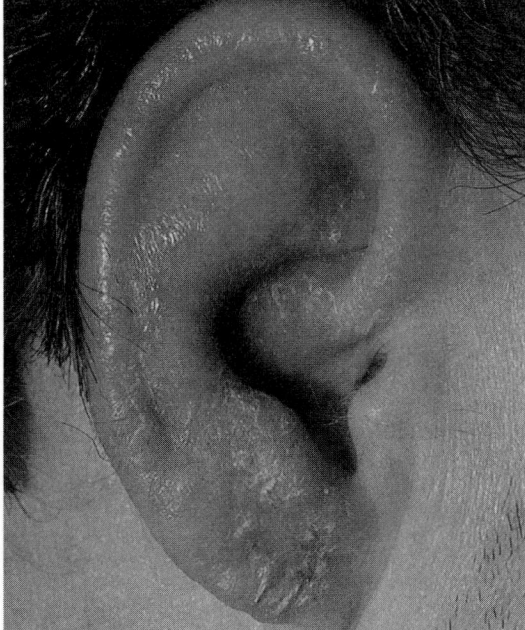

Fig. 1-275 Malignant external otitis. Severe infection of the ear has occurred after months of chronic inflammation of the pinna. (From Habif TP: *Clinical dermatology: a color guide to diagnosis and therapy*, ed 3, St Louis, 1996, Mosby.)

■ ETIOLOGY
- Acute localized otitis externa: *Staphylococcus aureus*
- Impetigo:
  1. *S. aureus*
  2. *Streptococcus pyogenes*
- Erysipelas: *S. pyogenes*
- Eczematous otitis externa:
  1. Seborrheic dermatitis
  2. Atopic dermatitis
  3. Psoriasis
  4. Neurodermatitis
  5. Lupus erythematosus
- Acute diffuse otitis externa:
  1. Swimming
  2. Hot, humid climates
  3. Tightly fitting hearing aids
  4. Use of ear plugs
  5. *Pseudomonas aeruginosa*
  6. *S. aureus*
- Otomycosis:
  1. Prolonged use of topical antibiotics and steroid preparations
  2. Aspergillus (80% to 90%)
  3. Candida
- Chronic otitis externa: persistent low-grade infection and inflammation
- Necrotizing otitis externa (NOE):
  1. Complication of persistent otitis externa
  2. Extends through Santorini's fissures, small apertures at the bone-cartilage junction of the canal, into the mastoid and along the base of the skull
  3. *P. aeruginosa*

▲ DIAGNOSIS

■ DIFFERENTIAL DIAGNOSIS
- Acute otitis media
- Bullous myringitis
- Mastoiditis
- Foreign bodies
- Neoplasms

■ WORKUP
Thorough history and physical examination

■ LABORATORY TESTS
- Cultures from the canal are usually not necessary unless the patient is refractory to treatment.
- Leukocyte count normal or mildly elevated.
- ESR is often quite elevated in malignant otitis externa.

■ IMAGING STUDIES
- CT scan is the best technique for defining bone involvement and extent of disease in malignant otitis externa.
- MRI is slightly more sensitive in evaluation of soft tissue changes.
- Gallium scans are more specific than bone scans in diagnosing NOE.

- Follow-up scans are helpful in determining efficacy of treatment.

Note: Expert opinion supports history and physical examination as the best means of diagnosis. Persistent pain that is constant and severe should raise the question of NOE (particularly in elderly, diabetics, and immunocompromised).

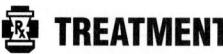

■ TREATMENT

■ NONPHARMACOLOGIC THERAPY
- Cleansing and debridement of the ear canal with cotton swabs and hydrogen peroxide or other antiseptic solution allows for a more thorough examination of the ear.
- If the canal lumen is edematous and too narrow to allow adequate cleansing, a cotton wick or gauze strip inserted into the canal serves as a conduit for topical medications to be drawn into the canal. Usually remove wick after 2 days.
- Local heat is useful in treating deep furunculosis.
- Incision and drainage is indicated in treatment of superficial pointing furunculosis.

■ ACUTE GENERAL Rx
Topical medications:
- An acidifying agent, such as 2% acetic acid, inhibits growth of bacteria and fungi.
- Topical antibiotics (in the form of otic or ophthalmic solutions) or antifungals, often in combination with an acidifying agent and a steroid preparation.
- The following are some of the available preparations:
  1. Neomycin otic solutions and suspensions:
     a. with polymyxin-B-hydrocortisone (Corticosporin)
     b. with hydrocortisone-thonzonium (Coly-Mycin S)
  2. Polymyxin-B-hydrocortisone (Otobiotic)
  3. Quinolone otic solutions:
     a. Ofloxacin 0.3% solution (Floxin Otic)
     b. Ciprofloxacin 0.3% with hydrocortisone (Cipro HC)
  4. Quinolone ophthalmic solutions:
     a. Ofloxacin 0.3% (Ocuflox)
     b. Ciprofloxacin 0.3% (Ciloxan)
  5. Aminoglycoside ophthalmic solutions
     a. Gentamicin sulfate 0.3% (Garamycin)
     b. Tobramycin sulfate 0.3% (Tobrex)
     c. Tobramycin 0.3% and dexamethasone 0.1% (TobraDex)
  6. Chloramphenicol 0.5% otic solution or 0.25% ophthalmic solution (Chloromycetin)

  7. Gentian violet (methylrosaniline chloride 1%, 2%)
  8. Antifungals:
     a. Amphotericin B 3% (Fungizone lotion)
     b. Clotrimazole 1% solution (Lotrimin)
     c. Tolnaftate 1% (Tinactin)
- Topical preparations should be applied qid (bid for quinolones, antifungals), generally for 3 days after cessation of symptoms (average 10 to 14 days total).

Systemic antibiotics:
- Reserved for severe cases, most often infections with *Pseudomonas aeruginosa* or *Staphylococcus aureus*
- Treatment usually for 10 days with ciprofloxacin 750 mg q12h or ofloxacin 400 mg q12h, or with anti-staphylococcal agent (e.g., dicloxacillin or cephalexin 500 mg q6h)

Treatment for NOE:
- Requires prolonged therapy up to 3 mo. Whether to use oral parenteral therapy is based on clinical judgment.
- Oral quinolones, ciprofloxacin 750 mg q12h or ofloxacin 400 mg q12h may be appropriate initial therapy or used to shorten the course of IV therapy.
- Intravenous antipseudomonals with or without aminoglycosides are also appropriate.
- Local debridement.

Pain control:
- May require NSAIDs or opioids
- Topical corticosteroids to reduce swelling and inflammation

■ CHRONIC Rx
- Patients prone to recurrent infections should try to identify and avoid precipitants to infection.
- Swimmers should try tight-fitting ear plugs or tight-fitting bathing caps, and remove all excess water from the ears after swimming.
- Treat underlying systemic diseases and dermatologic conditions that predispose to infection.

■ DISPOSITION
Inadequate treatment of otitis externa may lead to NOE and mastoiditis.

■ REFERRAL
To an otolaryngologist:
- NOE
- Treatment failure
- Severe pain

REFERENCES
Holten KB, Gick J: Management of the patient with otitis externa, *J Fam Practice* 50(4):353, 2001.

Sander R: Otitis externa: a practical guide to treatment and prevention, *Am Fam Physician* 63(5):927, 2001.
Author: **Jane V. Eason, M.D.**

BASIC INFORMATION

■ DEFINITION

Otitis is media is the presence of fluid in the middle ear accompanied by signs and symptoms of infection.

■ SYNONYMS

Acute suppurative otitis media
Purulent otitis media

ICD-9CM CODES

382.9 Acute or chronic otitis media
382.10 381.00 Otitis media with effusion

■ EPIDEMIOLOGY & DEMOGRAPHICS

INCIDENCE (IN U.S.)

- Affects patients of all ages, but is largely a disease of infants and young children.
- Occurs once in about 75% of all children.
- Occurs three or more times in one third of all children by 3 yr of age.
- The diagnosis of acute otitis media increased from 9.9 million in 1975 to 25.5 million in 1990.
- From 1975 to 1990 office visits for acute otitis media increased three-fold for children <2 yr, doubled for children ages 2 to 5, and almost doubled for children ages 6 to 10 yr.

PREDOMINANT SEX: Males
PREDOMINANT AGE:

- 47% to 60% of all children have their first episode of OM during their first year of life, 60% to 70% by their fourth birthday.
- Incidence of infection declines with age; seen infrequently in adults.

PEAK INCIDENCE:

- Between 6 and 36 mo
- Second peak between ages 4 and 6 yr
- Fall, winter, early spring

GENETICS:

Familial Disposition:
- Native Americans
- Eskimos
- Australian aborigines
- Those with a strong family history

Congenital Infection: High incidence in children born with cleft palates and other craniofacial abnormalities

■ PHYSICAL FINDINGS & CLINICAL PRESENTATION

- Fluid in the middle ear along with signs and symptoms of local inflammation (Figs. 1-276 and 1-277).
  1. Erythema with diminished light reflex
- Erythema of the tympanic membrane without other abnormalities is not a diagnostic criterion for acute otitis media because it may occur with any inflammation of the upper respiratory tract, crying, or nose blowing.
- As infection progresses, middle ear exudation occurs (exudative phase);

the exudate rapidly changes from serous to purulent (suppurative phase).
  1. Retraction and poor motility of the tympanic membrane, which then becomes bulging and convex
- At any time during the suppurative phase the tympanic membrane may rupture, releasing the middle ear contents
- Symptoms:
  1. Otalgia, ranging from slight discomfort to severe, spreading to the temporal region
  2. Ear stuffiness and hearing loss may precede or follow otalgia
  3. Otorrhea
  4. Vertigo
  5. Nystagmus
  6. Tinnitus
  7. Fever
  8. Lethargy
  9. Irritability
  10. Nausea, vomiting
  11. Anorexia
- After an episode of acute otitis media:
  1. Persistence of effusion for weeks or months (called secretory, serous, or nonsuppurative otitis media)
  2. Fever and otalgia usually absent
  3. Hearing loss possible (10 to 50 dB, with predominant involvement of the low frequencies)

■ ETIOLOGY

- Most common etiologic factor is an upper respiratory tract infection (often viral), which causes inflammation and obstruction of the eustachian tube. Bacterial colonization of the nasopharynx in conjunction with eustachian tube dysfunction leads to infection.
- May occasionally develop as a result of hematogenous spread or via direct invasion from the nasopharynx.
- Most common bacterial pathogens:
  1. *Streptococcus pneumoniae* causes 40% to 50% of cases and is the least likely of the major pathogens to resolve without treatment
  2. *Haemophilus influenzae* causes 20% to 30% of cases
  3. *Moraxella catarrhalis* causes 10% to 15% of cases
  4. Of increasing importance, infection caused by penicillin-nonsusceptible *S. pneumoniae* (MIC ≥0.1 μg/ml), ranging from 8% to 34%. About 50% of PNSSP isolates are penicillin-intermediate (MIC 0.1 to 1.0 μg/ml)
- Viral pathogens:
  1. Respiratory syncytial virus
  2. Rhinovirus
  3. Adenovirus
  4. Influenza
- Others:
  1. *Mycoplasma pneumoniae*
  2. *Chlamydia trachomatis*

DIAGNOSIS

■ DIFFERENTIAL DIAGNOSIS

- Otitis externa
- Referred pain
  1. Mouth
  2. Nasopharynx
  3. Tonsils
  4. Other parts of the upper respiratory tract
- Table 2-56 describes the differential diagnosis of earache.

■ WORKUP

Thorough otoscopic examination; adequate visualization of the tympanic membrane requires removal of cerumen and debris.
- Tympanometry
  1. Measures compliance of the tympanic membrane and middle ear pressure
  2. Detects the presence of fluid
- Acoustic reflectometry
  1. Measures sound waves reflected from the middle ear
  2. Useful in infants >3 mo
  3. Increased reflected sound correlated with the presence of effusion

■ LABORATORY TESTS

- Tympanocentesis
  1. Not necessary in most cases as the microbiology of middle ear effusions has been shown to be quite consistent
  2. May be indicated in:
     a. Highly toxic patients
     b. Patients who fail to respond to treatment in 48 to 72 hr
     c. Immunocompromised patients
- Cultures of the nasopharynx: sensitive but not specific
- Blood counts: usually show a leukocytosis with polymorphonuclear elevation
- Plain mastoid radiographs: generally not indicated; will reveal haziness in the periantral cells that may extend to entire mastoid
- CT or MRI may be indicated if serious complications suspected (meningitis, brain abscess)

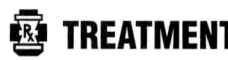

TREATMENT

■ ACUTE GENERAL Rx

Hydration, avoidance of irritants (e.g., tobacco smoke), nasal systemic decongestants, cool mist humidifier
Antimicrobials:
Note: Most uncomplicated cases of acute otitis media resolve spontaneously, without complications. Studies have demonstrated limited therapeutic benefit from antibiotic therapy. However, when opting to employ antibiotic therapy:

- Amoxicillin remains the drug of choice for first-line treatment of uncomplicated acute otitis media, despite increasing prevalence of drug-resistant *S. pneumoniae.*
- Treatment failure is defined by lack of clinical improvement of signs or symptoms after 3 days of therapy.
- With treatment failure, in the absence of an identified etiologic pathogen, therapy should be redirected to cover.
  1. Drug-resistant *S. pneumoniae*
  2. β-lactamase–producing strains of *H. influenzae* and *M. catarrhalis*
- Agents fulfilling these criteria include amoxicillin/clavulanate, second-generation cephalosporins (e.g., cefuroxime axetil, cefaclor); ceftriaxone (given IM). Cefaclor, cefixime, loracarbef and ceftibuten are active against *H. influenzae* and *M. catarrhalis,* but less active against *pneumococci,* especially drug resistant strains, than the agents listed above.
- Trimethoprim/sulfamethoxazole and macrolides have been used as first- and second-line agents, but pneumococcal resistance to these agents is rising (up to 25% resistance to trimethoprim/sulfamethoxazole, and up to 10% resistance to erythromycin).
- Cross-resistance between these drugs and the β-lactams exist, therefore patients who are treatment failures on amoxicillin are more likely to have infections resistant to trimethoprim/sulfamethoxazole and macrolides.
- Newer fluoroquinolones (grepafloxacin, levofloxacin, sparfloxacin, trovafloxacin) have enhanced activity against *pneumococci* as compared with older agents (ciprofloxacin, ofloxacin).
- Treatment should be modified according to cultures and sensitivities.
- Generally treatment course is 10 to 14 days.
- Follow-up approximately 4 wk after discontinuation of therapy to verify resolution of all symptoms, return to normal otoscopic findings, and restoration of normal hearing.
Note: Effusions may persist for 2 to 6 wk or longer in many cases of adequately treated otitis media.

■ SURGICAL Rx
- No evidence to support the routine of myringotomy, but in severe cases it provides prompt pain relief and accelerates resolution of infection.
- Purulent secretions retained in the middle ear lead to increased pressure that may lead to spread of infection to contiguous areas. Myringotomy to decompress the middle ear is necessary to avoid complications.
- Complications include mastoiditis, facial nerve paralysis, labyrinthitis, meningitis, brain abscess.
- Other procedures used for drainage

of the middle ear include insertion of a ventilation tube and/or simple mastoidectomy.

■ CHRONIC Rx
- Myringotomy and tympanostomy tube placement for persistent middle ear effusion unresponsive to medical therapy for ≥3 mo if bilateral or ≥6 mo if unilateral.
- Adenoidectomy, with or without tonsillectomy, often advocated for treatment of recurrent otitis media, although indications for this procedure are controversial.
- Chronic complications include tympanic membrane perforations, cholesteatoma, tympanosclerosis, ossicular necrosis, toxic or suppurative labyrinthitis, and intracranial suppuration.

■ REFERRAL
- To otorhinolaryngologist if:
  1. Medical treatment failure
  2. Diagnosis uncertain: adults with ≥1 episode of otitis media should be referred for ENT evaluation to rule out underlying process (e.g., malignancy)
  3. Any of the above acute and chronic complications

◯ PEARLS & CONSIDERATIONS

■ COMMENTS
Prevention:
- Multiple component conjugate vaccines hold promise for decreasing recurrent episodes of acute otitis media
- Breast-feeding, bottle-feeding infants in an upright position
- Avoidance of irritants (e.g., tobacco smoke)

REFERENCES
Dowell SF et al: Acute otitis media: management and surveillance in an era of pneumococcal resistance—a report from the Drug-resistant *Streptococcus pneumoniae* Therapeutic Working Group, *Pediatr Infect Dis J* 18(1):1, 1999.

Heikkinen T et al: Prevalence of various respiratory viruses in the middle ear during acute otitis media, *N Engl J Med* 340:260, 1999.

Takata GS et al: Evidence assessment of management of acute otitis media: I. The role of antibiotics in treatment of uncomplicated acute otitis media, *Pediatrics* 108(2):239, 2001.
Author: **Jane V. Eason, M.D.**

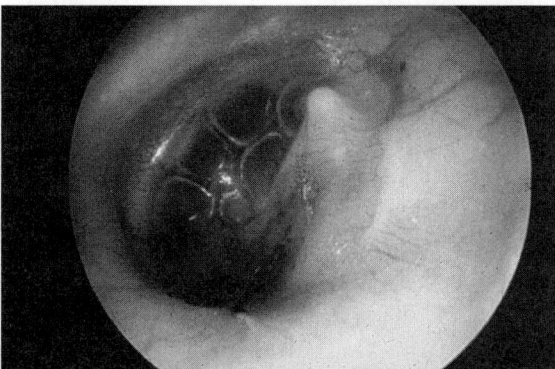

Fig. 1-276 Otitis media with effusion of left ear. Retracted eardrum, prominent short process of malleus, and air bubbles seen anteriorly through the tympanic membrane. (From Behrman RE: *Nelson textbook of pediatrics,* ed 16, Philadelphia, 1996, WB Saunders.)

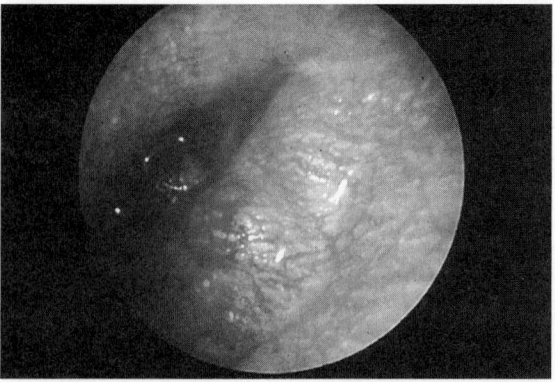

Fig. 1-277 Acute left otitis media. (From Behrman RE: *Nelson textbook of pediatrics,* ed 16, Philadelphia, 1996, WB Saunders.)

BASIC INFORMATION

■ DEFINITION

Otosclerosis is a conductive hearing loss secondary to fixation of the stapes resulting in gradual hearing loss. About 15% of cases affect only one ear.

ICD-9CM CODES
387.9 Otosclerosis

■ EPIDEMIOLOGY & DEMOGRAPHICS

INCIDENCE (IN U.S.): Most common cause of hearing loss in young adults
PREVALENCE (IN U.S.): 5 cases/1000 persons
PREDOMINANT SEX: Male:female ratio of 2:1
PREDOMINANT AGE: Symptoms start between 15 and 30 yr, with slowly progressive hearing loss.
PEAK INCIDENCE: Middle age
GENETICS: One half of cases are dominantly inherited.

■ PHYSICAL FINDINGS & CLINICAL PRESENTATION

- Tympanic membrane is normal in most cases (tested with tuning fork).
- Bone conduction is greater than air conduction.
- Weber localizes to affected ear.

■ ETIOLOGY

- A disease where vascular type of spongy bone is laid down
- Unknown

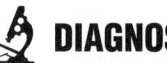

DIAGNOSIS

■ DIFFERENTIAL DIAGNOSIS

- Hearing loss from any cause: cochlear otosclerosis, polyps, granulomas, tumors, osteogenesis imperfecta, chronic ear infections, trauma
- A clinical algorithm for evaluation of hearing loss is described in Fig. 3-90.

■ WORKUP

Audiometry

■ LABORATORY TESTS

None, unless infection suspected

■ IMAGING STUDIES

MRI with specific cuts through inner ear

TREATMENT

■ NONPHARMACOLOGIC THERAPY

Hearing aid only of temporary use

■ CHRONIC Rx

Progresses to deafness without surgical intervention

■ DISPOSITION

Referral to ENT specialist

■ REFERRAL

To ENT specialist for surgery if moderate hearing loss suspected

⚡ PEARLS & CONSIDERATIONS

■ COMMENTS

- A full ENT evaluation in a young or middle-aged person with hearing loss is mandatory unless cause is obvious (such as trauma or repeated infection).

Author: **William H. Olson, M.D.**

BASIC INFORMATION

■ DEFINITION

Ovarian tumors can be benign, requiring operative intervention but not recurring or metastasizing; malignant, recurring, metastasizing, and having decreased survival; or borderline, having a small risk of recurrence or metastases but generally having a good prognosis.

■ SYNONYMS

Epithelial ovarian cancer
Germ cell tumor
Sex cord stromal tumor
Ovarian tumor of low malignant potential

ICD-9CM CODES
183.0 Malignant neoplasm of ovary

■ EPIDEMIOLOGY & DEMOGRAPHICS

INCIDENCE: 12.9 to 15.1 cases/100,000 persons; approximately 25,000 new cases annually
PREDOMINANCE: Median age of 61 yr, peaks at age 75 to 79 yr (54/100,000)
GENETICS: Familial susceptibility has been shown with the BRCA1 gene located on 17q12 to 21. This correlates with breast-ovarian cancer syndrome.
RISK FACTORS: Low parity, delayed childbearing, use of talc on the perineum, high-fat diet, fertility drugs (possibly), Lynch II syndrome (non-polyposis colon cancer, endometrial cancer, breast cancer, and ovarian cancer clusters in first- and second-degree relatives), breast-ovarian familial cancer syndrome, site-specific familial ovarian cancer (NOTE: Use of oral contraceptives appears to have a protective effect.)

■ PHYSICAL FINDINGS & CLINICAL PRESENTATION

- 60% present with advanced disease
- Abdominal fullness, early satiety, dyspepsia
- Pelvic pain, back pain, constipation
- Pelvic or abdominal mass
- Lymphadenopathy (inguinal)
- Sister Mary Joseph nodule (umbilical mass)

■ ETIOLOGY

- Can be inherited as site-specific familial ovarian cancer (two or more first-degree relatives have ovarian cancer)
- Breast-ovarian cancer syndrome (clusters of breast and ovarian cancer among first- and second-degree relatives)
- Lynch syndrome

- No family history and unknown etiology in the majority of ovarian cancer cases

DIAGNOSIS

■ DIFFERENTIAL DIAGNOSIS

- Primary peritoneal cancer
- Benign ovarian tumor
- Functional ovarian cyst
- Endometriosis
- Ovarian torsion
- Pelvic kidney
- Pedunculated uterine fibroid
- Primary cancer from breast, GI tract, or other pelvic organ metastasized to the ovary

■ WORKUP

- Definitive diagnosis made at laparotomy
- Careful physical and history including family history
- Exclusion of nongynecologic etiologies
- Observation of small, cystic masses in premenopausal women for regression for 2 mo

■ LABORATORY TESTS

- CBC
- Chemistry profile
- CA-125 or lysophosphatidic acid level
- Consider: hCG, Inhibin, AFP, neuron-specific enolase (NSE), and LDH in patients at risk for germ cell tumors

■ IMAGING STUDIES

- Ultrasound (has not been shown to be effective as a screening mechanism but is useful in the evaluation of a pelvic mass)
- Chest x-ray examination
- Mammogram
- CT scan to help evaluate extent of disease
- Other studies (BE, MRI, IVP, etc.) as clinically indicated

TREATMENT

■ NONPHARMACOLOGIC THERAPY

Virtually all cases of ovarian cancer involve surgical exploration. This includes:
- Abdominal cytology
- Total abdominal hysterectomy and bilateral salpingo-oophorectomy (except in early stages where fertility is an issue)
- Omentectomy
- Diaphragm sampling

- Selective lymphadenectomy
- Primary cytoreduction with a goal of residual tumor diameter <2 cm
- Bowel surgery, splenectomy if needed to obtain optimal (<2 cm) cytoreduction

■ ACUTE GENERAL Rx

- Optimal cytoreduction is generally followed by chemotherapy (except in some early-stage disease).
- Cisplatin-based combination chemotherapy is used for stage II or greater.
- Chemotherapy regimens continue to change as research continues.
- Consider second-look surgery when chemotherapy is complete.

■ CHRONIC Rx

- Physical and pelvic examinations every 3 mo for 2 yr, every 4 mo during third year, then every 6 mo
- CA-125 every visit
- Yearly Pap smear

■ DISPOSITION

- Overall 5-yr survival rates remain low because of the preponderance of late-stage disease:
  Stage I and II 80% to 100%
  Stage III 15% to 20%
  Stage IV 5%
- Younger patients (<50 yr) in all stages have a considerably better 5-yr survival than older patients (40% vs. 15%).

■ REFERRAL

- Studies have shown that optimal cytoreduction is most likely to occur in the hands of a gynecologic oncologist.
- Have gynecologic/oncology backup available if suspicious of malignancy.
- Always refer advanced disease.

REFERENCES

Modan B et al: Parity, oral contraceptives and the risk of ovarian cancer among carriers and noncarriers of a brca1 or brca2 mutation, *N Engl J Med* 345:235, 2001.
Olson SH et al: Symptoms of ovarian cancer, *Obstet Gynecol* 98:212, 2001.
Xu Y et al: Lysophosphatidic acid as a potential biomarker for ovarians or other gynecologic cancers, *JAMA* 280:719, 1998.
Author: **Gil Farkash, M.D.**

BASIC INFORMATION

■ **DEFINITION**

Benign ovarian neoplasms are clinically indistinguishable from their malignant counterparts. Therefore all persistent adnexal masses must be considered malignant until proven otherwise. Nonneoplastic tumors are as follows:
- Germinal inclusion cyst
- Follicle cyst
- Corpus luteum cyst
- Pregnancy luteoma
- Theca lutein cysts
- Sclerocystic ovaries
- Endometrioma

Neoplastic tumors that are derived from coelomic epithelium are as follows:
- Cystic tumors: serous cystoma, mucinous cystoma, mixed forms
- Tumors with stromal overgrowth: fibroma, adenofibroma, Brenner tumor

Tumors derived from germ cells are dermoids (benign cystic teratomas).

ICD-9CM CODES
220 Benign neoplasm of ovary

■ **EPIDEMIOLOGY & DEMOGRAPHICS**
- Reproductive years:
  1. Most common benign ovarian neoplasms: serous cystadenoma and benign cystic teratoma
  2. Most common adnexal mass: functional cyst
- Risk of malignancy increases after age 40 yr.
- Infants: adnexal masses are usually follicular cysts secondary to maternal hormone stimulation that regress during first few months of life.
- Childhood:
  1. Adnexal masses are rare.
  2. 8% are malignant.
  3. Almost always dysgerminomas or teratomas (germ cell origin).
  4. Frequency of malignancy is inversely correlated with age.
- Adolescence:
  1. Most common adnexal mass is a functional cyst.
  2. Most common neoplastic ovarian tumor is a benign cystic teratoma.
  3. Solid/cystic adnexal tumors are rare and almost always dysgerminomas or malignant teratomas.

■ **PHYSICAL FINDINGS & CLINICAL PRESENTATION**
- Usually asymptomatic
- Pelvic pain/pressure
- Dyspareunia
- Abdominal pain ranging from mild to severe peritoneal irritation
- Increasing abdominal girth/distention
- Adnexal mass of pelvic examination
- Children: abdominal/rectal mass

■ **ETIOLOGY**
- Physiologic
- Endometriosis
- Unknown

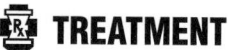 **DIAGNOSIS**

■ **DIFFERENTIAL DIAGNOSIS**
- Ovarian torsion
- Malignancy: ovary, fallopian tube, colon
- Uterine fibroid
- Diverticular abscess/diverticulitis
- Appendiceal abscess/appendicitis (especially in children)
- Tuboovarian abscess
- Paraovarian cyst
- Distended bladder
- Pelvic kidney
- Ectopic pregnancy
- Retroperitoneal cyst/neoplasm

■ **WORKUP**
- Complete history and physical examination
- Pelvic examination/rectrovaginal examination to reveal firm, irregular, mobile mass
- Laparoscopy/laparotomy to establish diagnosis

■ **LABORATORY TESTS**
- Pregnancy test
- Serum tumor markers:
  1. Cancer antigen 125 (CA 125)
  2. α-Fetoprotein (AFP) (endodermal sinus tumor, immature teratoma)
  3. β-Human chorionic gonadotropin (hCG)
  4. Lactic dehydrogenase (LDH) (dysgerminoma)

■ **IMAGING STUDIES**
Ultrasound:
- May differentiate adnexal mass from other pelvic masses

- Features that increase risk of malignancy include solid component, papillae, multiple septations/solitary thick septa, ascites, matted bowel, bilaterality, irregular borders
- CT scan with contrast or IVP
- Colonoscopy/barium enema, if symptomatic

TREATMENT

■ **NONPHARMACOLOGIC THERAPY**
Repeat pelvic examination for premenopausal women in 4 to 6 wk.

■ **ACUTE GENERAL Rx**
Indications for surgery:
- Postmenopausal or premenarcheal palpable adnexal mass
- Adnexal mass with suspicious ultrasound features
- Premenopausal woman with persistent cyst >5 cm
- Any adnexal mass >10 cm
- Suspected torsion or rupture

■ **CHRONIC Rx**
- Depends on diagnosis
- Possible suppression of formation of new cysts by oral contraceptives

■ **DISPOSITION**
- Depends on diagnosis

■ **REFERRAL**
- If malignancy suspected
- If surgery required

REFERENCE
Copeland LJ, Jarrell JF: *Textbook of gynecology*, ed 2, Philadelphia, 1999, WB Saunders.
Author: **Maria Elena Soler, M.D.**

BASIC INFORMATION

■ DEFINITION
Paget's disease of the bone is a non-metabolic disease of bone characterized by repeated episodes of osteolysis and excessive attempts at repair that results in a weakened bone of increased mass. Monostotic (solitary lesion) and polyostotic (numerous lesions) disease are both described.

■ SYNONYMS
Osteitis deformans

ICD-9CM CODES
731.0 Paget's disease (osteitis deformans)

■ EPIDEMIOLOGY & DEMOGRAPHICS
PREVALENCE: Localized lesions in 3% of patients >50 yr
PREVALENT AGE: Rare before 40 yr
PREVALENT SEX: Male:female ratio of 2:1

■ PHYSICAL FINDINGS & CLINICAL PRESENTATION
- Many lesions are asymptomatic.
- Onset is variable.
- Symptoms result mainly from the effects of complications:
  1. Skeletal pain, especially hip and pelvis
  2. Bowing of long bones, sometimes leading to pathologic fracture
  3. Increased heat of extremity (resulting from increased vascularity)
  4. Skull enlargement and spinal involvement caused by characteristic bone enlargement, which can produce neurologic complications (vision, hearing loss, radicular pain, and cord compression)
  5. Thoracic kyphoscoliosis
  6. Secondary osteoarthritis, especially of hip
  7. Heart failure as a result of chest and spine deformity and blood shunting

■ ETIOLOGY
Unknown

DIAGNOSIS

■ DIFFERENTIAL DIAGNOSIS
- Fibrous dysplasia
- Skeletal neoplasm (primary or metastatic)
- Osteomyelitis
- Hyperparathyroidism
- Vertebral hemangioma

■ LABORATORY TESTS
- Increased serum alkaline phosphatase (SAP)
- Normal serum calcium and phosphorus levels
- Increased urinary excretion of pyridinoline cross-links, although test is expensive and not usually required in routine cases
- Other: bone biopsy only in uncertain cases or if sarcomatous degeneration is suspected

■ IMAGING STUDIES
- Appropriate radiographs reflect the characteristic radiolucency and opacity (Fig. 1-278).
- Bone scanning usually reflects the activity and extent of the disease.

TREATMENT

■ ACUTE GENERAL Rx
- Counseling regarding home environment to prevent falls
- Cane for balance and weight-bearing pain

■ PHARMACOLOGIC THERAPY
- Calcitonin
- Biphosphonates
- NSAIDs for pain relief

■ DISPOSITION
- Many monostotic lesions probably remain asymptomatic.
- Progression of the disease is common.
- Malignant degeneration occurs in <1% of patients and should be considered when there is a sudden increase in pain.
- Sarcomatous change carries a grave prognosis.

■ REFERRAL
- For dental evaluation if there is involvement of the mandible or maxilla
- For ENT evaluation if there is hearing loss
- For ophthalmologic evaluation if there is impaired vision
- For orthopedic consultation for assessment of pain in bone or joint

PEARLS & CONSIDERATIONS

■ COMMENTS
Surgical intervention is often required for neurologic complications or joint symptoms
- Often associated with profuse blood loss
- Elective cases: benefit from preoperative treatment to suppress bone activity and vascularity

REFERENCES
Crandall C: Risedronate: a clinical review, *Arch Intern Med* 161:353, 2001.
Roodman GD: Studies in Paget's disease and their relevance to oncology, *Semin Oncol* 28:15, 2001.
Russell G et al: Clinical disorders of bone resorption, *Novartis Found Symp* 232:251, 2001.
Theriault RL, Hortobagyi GN: The evolving role of bisphosphonates, *Semin Oncol* 28:284, 2001.
Author: **Lonnie R. Mercier, M.D.**

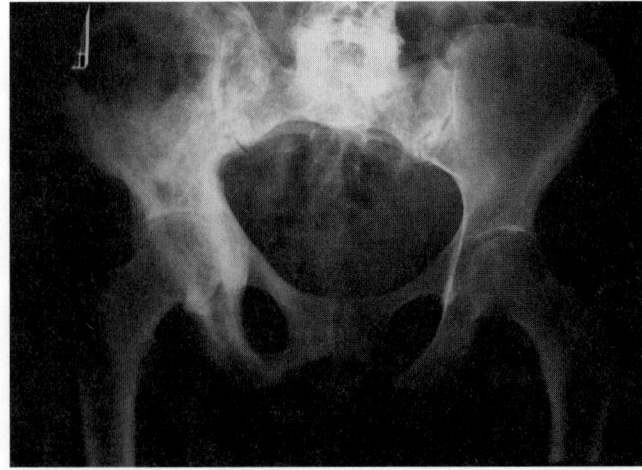

Fig. 1-278 Frontal radiograph of the pelvis shows marked prominence to the trabeculae in the right ilium, ischium, and pubic bones with small lytic areas identified compatible with the later stages of Paget's disease. (From Specht N [ed]: *Practical guide to diagnostic imaging*, St Louis, 1998, Mosby.)

BASIC INFORMATION

■ DEFINITION
Paget's disease of the breast is a malignant disease that presents itself as a scaly, sore, eroding, bleeding ulcer of the nipple. Microscopically, typical large clear cells (Paget's cells) with pale and abundant cytoplasm and hyperchromatic nuclei with prominent nucleoli are found in the epidermal layer. Paget's disease is more often associated with primary invasive or in situ carcinoma of the breast.

ICD-9CM CODES
174.0 Malignant neoplasm of female breast, nipple, and areola

■ EPIDEMIOLOGY & DEMOGRAPHICS
• Not common
• Found in 1 in 100 to 200 breast cancer patients

■ PHYSICAL FINDINGS & CLINICAL PRESENTATION
• Variable
• Itching or burning nipple and/or reported lump
• Very minimal scaly lesion that may bleed when scales are lifted
• Typical ulcer located on nipple with serous fluid weeping or small amount of bleeding coming from it (Fig. 1-279)
• Palpable carcinoma in the breast of some patients

■ ETIOLOGY
• Exact origin unknown
• Possibly migration of either in situ or invasive carcinoma cells in breast to nipple skin to produce Paget's disease

DIAGNOSIS

■ DIFFERENTIAL DIAGNOSIS
• Chronic dermatitis
• Florid papillomatosis of the nipple or nipple adenoma
• Eczema

■ WORKUP
• Clinically apparent
• Careful breast examination with diagnosis in mind
• Palpable mass or mammographic lesions in 60% to 70% of patients
• A clinical algorithm for the evaluation of nipple discharge is described in Fig. 3-32.

■ LABORATORY TESTS
Biopsy of nipple lesion

■ IMAGING STUDIES
Mammograms to search for possible primary carcinoma

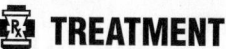

TREATMENT

■ NONPHARMACOLOGIC THERAPY
• Fewer patients:
 1. Paget's disease of nipple only finding when mammographically negative breast
 2. Consideration of wide excision of nipple with or without radiation
• Other patients: additional invasive or in situ carcinoma recognized
• Either modified mastectomy or breast conservation treatment
• Presence of underlying in situ or invasive carcinoma in mastectomy specimen of majority of patients

■ ACUTE GENERAL Rx
Systemic adjuvant therapy, depending on extent of invasive carcinoma found

■ DISPOSITION
• Parallel prognosis to that of breast cancer patient without Paget's disease
• Regular follow-up as in other invasive or in situ carcinoma patients

■ REFERRAL
At outset, all suspicious nipple lesions should be referred for evaluation and treatment.
Author: **Takuma Nemoto, M.D.**

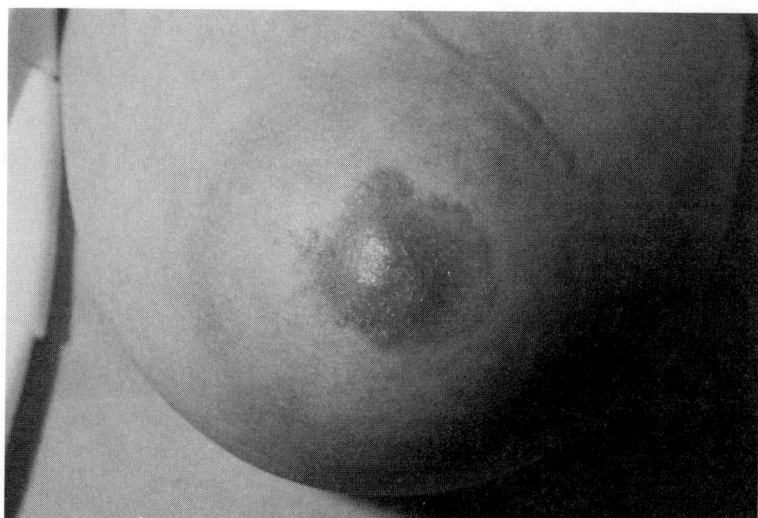

Fig. 1-279 Paget's disease of the breast. The lesion has insidiously spread for 1 year to infiltrate the areola and surrounding skin. (From Habif TP: *Clinical dermatology: a color guide to diagnosis and therapy,* ed 3, St Louis, 1996, Mosby.)

BASIC INFORMATION

■ DEFINITION
Pancreatic cancer is an adenocarcinoma derived from the epithelium of the pancreatic duct.

ICD-9CM CODES
157.9 Pancreatic cancer
157.0 (head)
157.1 (body)
157.2 (tail)
157.3 (duct)
230.9 (in situ)

■ EPIDEMIOLOGY & DEMOGRAPHICS
INCIDENCE: 1 case/10,000 persons/yr
PEAK AGE: Seventh and eighth decades of life
PREDOMINANT SEX: Male:female ratio of 2:1

■ PHYSICAL FINDINGS & CLINICAL PRESENTATION
Presenting symptoms:
• Jaundice
• Abdominal pain
• Weight loss
• Anorexia/change in taste
• Nausea
• Uncommonly: depression, GI bleeding, acute pancreatitis, back pain
Physical findings:
• Icterus
• Cachexia
• Excoriations from scratching pruritic skin

■ ETIOLOGY
Unknown, but several conditions have been associated with pancreatic cancer:
• Smoking
• Alcoholism
• Gallstones
• Diabetes mellitus
• Chronic pancreatitis
• Diet rich in animal fat
• Occupational exposures: oil refining, paper manufacturing, chemical industry

DIAGNOSIS

■ DIFFERENTIAL DIAGNOSIS
• Common duct cholelithiasis
• Cholangiocarcinoma
• Common duct stricture
• Sclerosing cholangitis
• Primary biliary cirrhosis
• Drug-induced cholestasis (e.g., phenothiazines)
• Chronic hepatitis
• Sarcoidosis
• Other pancreatic tumors (islet cell tumor, cystadenocarcinoma, epidermoid carcinoma, sarcomas, lymphomas)

■ WORKUP

Routine laboratory tests	% abnormal
Alkaline phosphatase	80
Bilirubin	55
Total protein	15
Amylase	15
Hematocrit	60

■ IMAGING STUDIES

Noninvasive imaging	% abnormal
Abdominal ultrasonography	60
Abdominal CT scan (Fig. 1-280) (without or with contrast [IV or oral])	90
Abdominal MRI scan	90
Invasive imaging	
Endoscopic retrograde cholangiopancreatography (ERCP)	90
CT scan or ultrasonography-guided needle aspiration cytology	90-95

TREATMENT

• Surgery
Curative pancreatectomy (Whipple's procedure) appropriate for only 10% to 20% of patients whose lesion is <5 cm, solitary, and without metastases. Surgical mortality is 5%.
Palliative surgery (for biliary decompression/diversion)
Palliative therapeutic endoscopic retrograde cholangiopancreatography (ERCP) using stents
• Chemotherapy
The best combination chemotherapy using streptozotocin, mitomycin C, and 5-FU provides only a 19-wk median survival.
• Radiation
External beam radiation for palliation of pain.
• Combined chemotherapy and radiation provides a median survival of 11 mo.
• Celiac plexus block by an experienced anesthesiologist provides pain relief in 80% to 90% of cases.

REFERENCES
Cello JP: Pancreatic cancer. In Feldman M, Scharschmidt BF, Sleisenger MH (eds): *Gastrointestinal and liver disease,* ed 6, Philadelphia, 1998, WB Saunders.
Michaud DS et al: Physical activity, obesity, height, and the risk of pancreatic cancer, *JAMA* 286:821, 2001.
Author: **Tom J. Wachtel, M.D.**

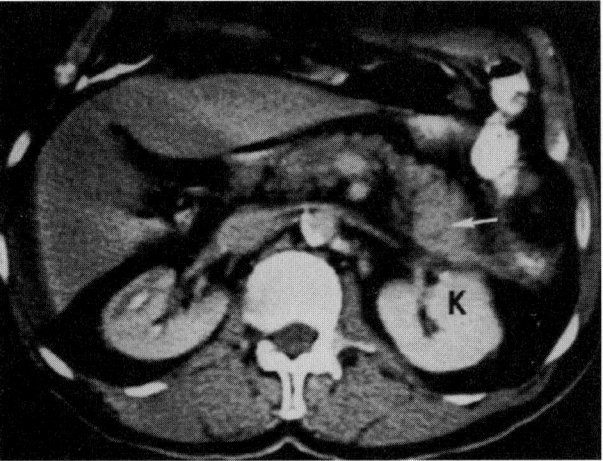

Fig. 1-280   CT scan of a patient with adenocarcinoma of the body and tail of the pancreas. The tumor *(arrow)* is seen anterior and adjacent to the left kidney *(K).* At operation, the tumor was invading Gerota's fascia. (From Sabiston D: *Textbook of surgery,* ed 15, Philadelphia, 1997, WB Saunders.)

BASIC INFORMATION

■ **DEFINITION**
Acute pancreatitis is an inflammatory process of the pancreas with intrapancreatic activation of enzymes that may also involve peripancreatic tissue and/or remote organ systems.

ICD-9CM CODES
577.0 Acute pancreatitis

■ **EPIDEMIOLOGY & DEMOGRAPHICS**
- Acute pancreatitis is most often secondary to biliary tract disease and alcohol.
- Incidence in urban areas is twice that of rural areas (20 cases/100,000 persons in urban areas)
- 20% of patients have necrotizing pancreatitis; the remainder have interstitial pancreatitis.

■ **PHYSICAL FINDINGS & CLINICAL PRESENTATION**
- Epigastric tenderness and guarding; pain usually developing suddenly, reaching peak intensity within 10 to 30 min, severe and lasting several hours without relief
- Hypoactive bowel sounds (secondary to ileus)
- Tachycardia, shock (secondary to decreased intravascular volume)
- Confusion (secondary to metabolic disturbances)
- Fever
- Tachycardia, decreased breath sounds (atelectasis, pleural effusions, ARDS)
- Jaundice (secondary to obstruction or compression of biliary tract)
- Ascites (secondary to tear in pancreatic duct, leaking pseudocyst)
- Palpable abdominal mass (pseudocyst, phlegmon, abscess, carcinoma)
- Evidence of hypocalcemia (Chvostek's sign, Trousseau's sign)
- Evidence of intraabdominal bleeding (hemorrhagic pancreatitis):
  1. Gray-bluish discoloration around the umbilicus (Cullen's sign)
  2. Bluish discoloration involving the flanks (Grey Turner's sign)
- Tender subcutaneous nodules (caused by subcutaneous fat necrosis)

■ **ETIOLOGY**
- In >90% of cases: biliary tract disease (calculi or sludge) or alcohol
- Drugs (e.g., thiazides, furosemide, corticosteroids, tetracycline, estrogens, valproic acid, metronidazole, azathioprine, methyldopa, pentamidine, ethacrynic acid, procainamide, sulindac, nitrofurantoin, ACE inhibitors, danazol, cimetidine, piroxicam, gold, ranitidine, sulfasalazine, isoniazid, acetaminophen, cisplatin, opiates, erythromycin)
- Abdominal trauma
- Surgery
- ERCP
- Infections (predominantly viral infections)
- Peptic ulcer (penetrating duodenal ulcer)
- Pancreas divisum (congenital failure to fuse of dorsal or ventral pancreas)
- Idiopathic
- Pregnancy
- Vascular (vasculitis, ischemic)
- Hypolipoproteinemia (types I, IV, and V)
- Hypercalcemia
- Pancreatic carcinoma (primary or metastatic)
- Renal failure
- Hereditary pancreatitis
- Occupational exposure to chemicals: methanol, cobalt, zinc, mercuric chloride, creosol, lead, organophosphates, chlorinated naphthalenes
- Others: scorpion bite, obstruction at ampulla region (neoplasm, duodenal diverticula, Crohn's disease), hypotensive shock

🔬 **DIAGNOSIS**

■ **DIFFERENTIAL DIAGNOSIS**
- PUD
- Acute cholangitis, biliary colic
- High intestinal obstruction
- Early acute appendicitis
- Mesenteric vascular obstruction
- DKA
- Pneumonia (basilar)
- Myocardial infarction (inferior wall)
- Renal colic
- Ruptured or dissecting aortic aneurysm

■ **LABORATORY TESTS**
Pancreatic enzymes
- Amylase is increased, usually elevated in the initial 3 to 5 days of acute pancreatitis. Isoamylase determinations (separation of pancreatic cell isoenzyme components of amylase) are useful in excluding occasional cases of salivary hyperamylasemia. The use of isoamylase rather than total serum amylase reduces the risk of erroneously diagnosing pancreatitis and is preferred by some as initial biochemical test in patients suspected of having acute pancreatitis.
- Urinary amylase determinations are useful to diagnose acute pancreatitis in patients with lipemic serum, to rule out elevated serum amylase secondary to macroamylasemia, and to diagnose acute pancreatitis in patients whose serum amylase is normal.
- Serum lipase levels are elevated in acute pancreatitis; the elevation is less transient than serum amylase; concomitant evaluation of serum amylase and lipase increases diagnostic accuracy of acute pancreatitis. An elevated lipase/amylase ratio is suggestive of alcoholic pancreatitis.
- Elevated serum trypsin levels are diagnostic of pancreatitis (in absence of renal failure); measurement is made by radioimmunoassay. Although not routinely available, the serum trypsin level is the most accurate laboratory indicator for pancreatitis.
- Rapid measurement of urinary trypsinogen-2 (if available) is useful in the ER as a screening test for acute pancreatitis in patients with abdominal pain; a negative dipstick test for urinary trypsinogen-2 rules out acute pancreatitis with a high degree of probability, whereas a positive test indicates need for further evaluation.
Additional tests:
- CBC: reveals leukocytosis; Hct may be initially increased secondary to hemoconcentration; decreased Hct may indicate hemorrhage or hemolysis.
- BUN is increased secondary to dehydration.
- Elevation of serum glucose in previously normal patient correlates with the degree of pancreatic malfunction and may be related to increased release of glycogen, catecholamines, and glucocorticoid release and decreased insulin release.
- Liver profile: AST and LDH are increased secondary to tissue necrosis; bilirubin and alkaline phosphatase may be increased secondary to common bile duct obstruction. A threefold or greater rise in serum ALT concentrations is an excellent indicator (95% probability) of biliary pancreatitis.
- Serum calcium is decreased secondary to saponification, precipitation, and decreased PTH response.
- ABGs: Pao_2 may be decreased secondary to ARDS, pleural effusion(s); pH may be decreased secondary to lactic acidosis, respiratory acidosis, and renal insufficiency.
- Serum electrolytes: potassium may be increased secondary to acidosis or renal insufficiency, sodium may be increased secondary to dehydration.

■ IMAGING STUDIES

- Abdominal plain film is useful to distinguish other conditions that may mimic pancreatitis (perforated viscus); it may reveal localized ileus (sentinel loop), pancreatic calcifications (chronic pancreatitis), blurring of left psoas shadow, dilation of transverse colon, calcified gallstones.
- Chest x-ray film may reveal elevation of one or both diaphragms, pleural effusions, basilar infiltrates, platelike atelectasis.
- Abdominal ultrasonography is useful in detecting gallstones (sensitivity of 60% to 70% for detecting stones associated with pancreatitis). It is also useful for detecting pancreatic pseudocysts; its major limitation is the presence of distended bowel loops overlying the pancreas.
- CT scan is superior to ultrasonography in identifying pancreatitis and defining its extent, and it also plays a role in diagnosing pseudocysts (they appear as a well-defined area surrounded by a high-density capsule); GI fistulation or infection of a pseudocyst can also be identified by the presence of gas within the pseudocyst. Sequential contrast-enhanced CT is useful for detection of pancreatic necrosis. The severity of pancreatitis can also be graded by CT scan.
- ERCP should not be performed during the acute stage of disease unless it is necessary to remove an impacted stone in the ampulla of Vater; patients with severe or worsening pancreatitis but without obstructive jaundice (biliary obstruction) do not benefit from early ERCP and papillotomy.

℞ TREATMENT

■ NONPHARMACOLOGIC THERAPY

- Bowel rest with avoidance of PO liquids or solids during the acute illness
- Avoidance of alcohol and any drugs associated with pancreatitis

■ ACUTE GENERAL Rx

General measures:
- Maintain adequate intravascular volume with vigorous IV hydration.
- Patient should remain NPO until clinically improved, stable, and hungry.
- Nasogastric suction is useful in severe pancreatitis to decompress the abdomen in patients with ileus.
- Control pain: oral analgesics may cause spasms of the sphincter of

Oddi (meperidine may produce less constriction than other analgesics; however, clear evidence regarding this claim is lacking and metabolites may cause significant neurotoxic effects such as seizures, myoclonus, or tremors).
- Correct metabolic abnormalities (e.g., replace calcium and magnesium as necessary).
- TPN may be necessary in prolonged pancreatitis.

Specific measures:
- IV antibiotics should not be used prophylactically; their use is justified if the patient has evidence of septicemia, pancreatic abscess, or pancreatitis secondary to biliary calculi. Appropriate empiric antibiotic therapy should cover:
  1. *B. fragilis* and other anaerobes (cefotetan, cefoxitin, metronidazole, or clindamycin plus aminoglycoside)
  2. *Enterococcus* (ampicillin)
- Surgical therapy has a limited role in acute pancreatitis; it is indicated in the following:
  1. Gallstone-induced pancreatitis: cholecystectomy when acute pancreatitis subsides
  2. Perforated peptic ulcer
  3. Excision or drainage of necrotic or infected foci
- Identification and treatment of complications:
  1. Pseudocyst: round or spheroid collection of fluid, tissue, pancreatic enzymes, and blood.
     a. Diagnosed by CT scan or sonography
     b. Treatment: CT scan or ultrasound-guided percutaneous drainage (with a pigtail catheter left in place for continuous drainage) can be used, but the recurrence rate is high; the conservative approach is to reevaluate the pseudocyst (with CT scan or sonography) after 6 to 7 wk and surgically drain it if the pseudocyst has not decreased in size. Generally pseudocysts <5 cm in diameter are reabsorbed without intervention whereas those >5 cm require surgical intervention after the wall has matured.
  2. Phlegmon: represents pancreatic edema. It can be diagnosed by CT scan or sonography. Treatment is supportive measures, because it usually resolves spontaneously.
  3. Pancreatic abscess: diagnosed by CT scan (presence of bubbles in the retroperitoneum); Gram staining and cultures of fluid obtained from guided percutaneous

aspiration (GPA) usually identify bacterial organism. Therapy is surgical (or catheter) drainage and IV antibiotics.
  4. Pancreatic ascites: usually caused by leaking of pseudocyst or tear in pancreatic duct. Paracentesis reveals very high amylase and lipase levels in the pancreatic fluid; ERCP may demonstrate the lesion. Treatment is surgical correction if exudative ascites from severe pancreatitis does not resolve spontaneously.
  5. GI bleeding: caused by alcoholic gastritis, bleeding varices, stress ulceration, or DIC.
  6. Renal failure: caused by hypovolemia resulting in oliguria or anuria, cortical or tubular necrosis (shock, DIC), or thrombosis of renal artery or vein.
  7. Hypoxia: caused by ARDS, pleural effusion, or atelectasis.

■ DISPOSITION

Prognosis varies with the severity of pancreatitis; overall mortality in acute pancreatitis is 5% to 10%; poor prognostic signs are the following:
- Age >55 yr.
- Fluid sequestration >6000 ml.
- Laboratory abnormalities on admission: WBC >16,000, blood glucose >200 ml/dl, serum LDH >350 IU/L, AST >250 IU/L.
- Laboratory abnormalities during the initial 48 hr: decreased Hct >10% with hydration or Hct <30%, BUN rise >5 mg/dl, serum calcium <8 mg/dl, arterial Po_2 <60 mm Hg, and base deficit >4 mEq/L.

■ REFERRAL

- Hospitalization is indicated in moderate/severe cases of pancreatitis.
- Surgical consultation is needed in suspected gallstone pancreatitis, perforated peptic ulcer, or presence of necrotic or infected foci.

REFERENCES

Baron TH, Morgan DE: Acute necrotizing pancreatitis, *N Engl J Med* 340:1412, 1999.

Morrow JB, Conwell D: Idiopathic recurrent pancreatitis, *Cleve Clin J Med* 66:84, 1999.

Munoz A, Katerndahl D: Diagnosis and management of acute pancreatitis, *Am Fam Physician* 62:164, 2000.

Spigel B: Meperidine or morphine in acute pancreatitis? *Am Fam Physician* 64:219, 2001.

Author: **Fred F. Ferri, M.D.**

BASIC INFORMATION

■ DEFINITION
Chronic pancreatitis is a recurrent or persistent inflammatory process of the pancreas characterized by chronic pain and by pancreatic exocrine and/or endocrine insufficiency.

ICD-9CM CODES
577.1 Chronic pancreatitis

■ EPIDEMIOLOGY & DEMOGRAPHICS
- Chronic pancreatitis occurs in approximately 5 to 10/100,000 persons in industrialized countries.
- Male:female ratio is 5:1.

■ PHYSICAL FINDINGS & CLINICAL PRESENTATION
- Persistent or recurrent epigastric and LUQ pain, may radiate to the back
- Tenderness over the pancreas, muscle guarding
- Significant weight loss
- Bulky, foul-smelling stools, greasy in appearance
- Epigastric mass (10% of patients)
- Jaundice (5% to 10% of patients)

■ ETIOLOGY
- Chronic alcoholism
- Obstruction (ampullary stenosis, tumor, trauma, pancreas divisum, annular pancreas)
- Hereditary pancreatitis
- Severe malnutrition
- Idiopathic
- Untreated hyperparathyroidism (hypercalcemia)
- Mutations of the cystic fibrosis transmembrane conductance regulator (CFTR) gene and the TF genotype
- Sclerosing pancreatitis: A form of chronic pancreatitis characterized by infrequent attacks of abdominal pain, irregular narrowing of the pancreatic duct, and swelling of the pancreatic parenchyma; these patients have high levels of serum immunoglobins (IgG4)

DIAGNOSIS

■ DIFFERENTIAL DIAGNOSIS
- Pancreatic cancer
- PUD
- Cholelithiasis with biliary obstruction
- Malabsorption from other etiologies
- Recurrent acute pancreatitis

■ WORKUP
Medical history with focus on alcohol use, laboratory tests, diagnostic imaging

■ LABORATORY TESTS
- Serum amylase and lipase may be elevated (normal amylase levels, however, do not exclude the diagnosis).
- Hyperglycemia, glycosuria, hyperbilirubinemia, and elevated serum alkaline phosphatase may also be present.
- 72-hr fecal fat determination reveals excess fecal fat.
- Bentiromide test or secretin stimulation test can confirm pancreatic insufficiency.
- Elevated levels of serum IgG4 are found in sclerosing pancreatitis, but not in other disorders of the pancreas.

■ IMAGING STUDIES
- Plain abdominal radiographs may reveal pancreatic calcifications (95% specific for chronic pancreatitis) (Fig. 1-281).
- Ultrasound of abdomen may reveal duct dilation, pseudocyst, calcification, and presence of ascites.
- CT scan of abdomen is useful for the detection of calcifications, to evaluate for ductal dilation, and for ruling out pancreatic cancer.
- ERCP can be used to evaluate for the presence of dilated ducts, strictures, pseudocysts, and intraductal stones.

TREATMENT

■ NONPHARMACOLOGIC THERAPY
- Avoidance of alcohol
- Frequent, small-volume, low-fat meals

■ ACUTE GENERAL Rx
- Avoidance of narcotics if possible (simple analgesics or NSAIDs can be used)
- Treatment of steatorrhea with pancreatic supplements (e.g., Pancrease, Creon, Pancrealipase titrated PRN

based on the amount of steatorrhea and patient's weight loss)
- Octreotide 200 μg SC tid may be useful for pain secondary to idiopathic chronic pancreatitis
- Treatment of complications (e.g., IDDM)
- Glucocorticoid therapy in patients with sclerosing pancreatitis can induce clinical remission and significantly decrease serum concentrations of IgG4, immune complexes, and the IgG4 subclass of immune complexes

■ CHRONIC Rx
- Surgical intervention may be necessary to eliminate biliary tract disease and improve flow of bile into the duodenum by eliminating obstruction of pancreatic duct.
- ERCP with endoscopic sphincterectomy and stone extraction is useful in selected patients.
- Transduodenal sphincteroplasty or pancreaticojejunostomy in selected patients. Surgery should also be considered in patients with intractable pain.

■ DISPOSITION
- Long-term survival is poor (50% of patients die within 10 hr from chronic pancreatitis or malignancy).
- Prognosis is best in patients with recurrent acute pancreatitis resulting from cholelithiasis, hyperparathyroidism, or stenosis of the sphincter of Oddi.

■ REFERRAL
GI referral for ERCP, surgical referral in selected patients (see "Chronic Rx").

REFERENCE
Hamano H et al: High serum IgG4 concentrations in patients with sclerosing pancreatitis, *N Engl J Med* 344:732, 2001.
Author: **Fred F. Ferri, M.D.**

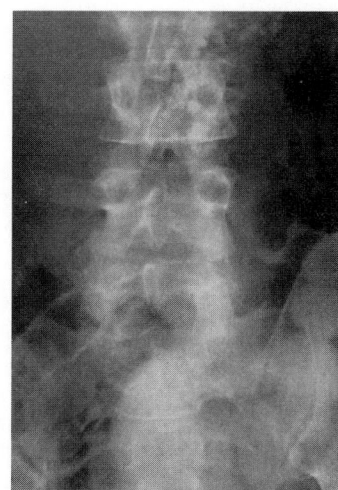

Fig. 1-281 Calcification in pancreas. (From Noble J: *Primary care medicine*, ed 3, St Louis, 2001, Mosby.)

BASIC INFORMATION

■ DEFINITION
Parkinson's disease is a progressive neurodegenerative disorder characterized pathologically by cytoplasmic eosinophilic inclusions (Lewy bodies) in neurons of the substantia nigra and locus ceruleus and by depigmentation of the brain stem nuclei (Fig. 1-282).

■ SYNONYMS
Paralysis agitans

ICD-9CM CODES
332.0 Idiopathic Parkinson's disease, primary
332.1 Parkinson's disease, secondary

■ EPIDEMIOLOGY & DEMOGRAPHICS
INCIDENCE: 40,000 to 50,000 cases/yr
PREVALENCE:
- 0.3% of general population
- 3% of population over age 65
- Highest incidence in whites, lowest incidence in Asians and black Africans

■ PHYSICAL FINDINGS & CLINICAL PRESENTATION
Rigidity—increased muscle tone (>20% of patients at initial diagnosis):
- Involves both agonist and antagonist muscle groups
- Widespread resistance to passive movement, which is more prominent at large joints ("cogwheeling" rigidity is noted)
Tremor—resting tremor, with a frequency of 4 to 7 movements/sec (>70% of patients at initial diagnosis):
- Usually noted in the hands and often involves the thumb and forefinger ("pill-rolling" tremor)
- Improves or disappears with purposeful function

Akinesia—inability to initiate or execute a movement:
- Sitting immobile, because even the simple task of getting up from a chair seems impossible
- Face may reveal a marked absence of movement (masked facies); usually open mouth, drooling
Gait disturbance (10% to 20% at initial diagnosis):
- Stooped posture (head bowed, trunk bent forward, shoulders drooped; knees and arms flexed, "soccer goalie stance")
- Difficulty initiating the first step; small shuffling steps that increase in speed (festinating gait) as if the patient is chasing his or her center of gravity (steps become progressively faster and shorter while the trunk inclines further forward)
- Abnormal reflexes
- Palmomental reflex: stroking the palm of the hand near the base of the thumb results in contraction of the ipsilateral mentalis muscle, causing wrinkling of the skin on the chin
- Glabellar relex: repeated gentle tapping on the glabella evokes blinking of both eyes
Others: orthostatic hypotension, micrographia

■ ETIOLOGY
- Unknown
- Mutations in the *parkin* gene are a major cause of early-onset autosomal recessive familial Parkinson's disease and isolated juvenile-onset Parkinsons' disease (at or before age 20).

DIAGNOSIS

There are no formal criteria for making the diagnosis of Parkinson's disease. A presumptive clinical diagnosis can be made based on a comprehensive history and physical examination. The disease often begins insidiously in pa-

tients >60 yr of age with resting tremor, generalized slowness, and slight loss of motor dexterity. It is important to exclude other conditions that may also present with signs of parkinsonism (see "Differential Diagnosis").

■ DIFFERENTIAL DIAGNOSIS
- Multisystem degenerative diseases (e.g., striatonigral degeneration, olivopontocerebellar atrophy)
- Alzheimer's disease with extrapyramidal features
- Essential tremor
- Secondary (acquired) parkinsonism:
  1. Iatrogenic (e.g., phenothiazines, butyrophenones)
  2. Postencephalitic (sequela of encephalitis lethargica)
  3. Toxins (e.g., MPTP, manganese, carbon monoxide)
  4. Hypoparathyroidism, hyperparathyroidism
  5. Cerebrovascular disease (Binswanger's disease, basal ganglia lacunae)

■ WORKUP
Identification of clinical signs and symptoms associated with Parkinson's disease (see "Physical Findings") and elimination of conditions that may mimic it with a comprehensive history, physical examination, and diagnostic imaging

■ IMAGING STUDIES
CT scan or MRI of head to eliminate conditions that may present with signs of parkinsonism (see "Differential Diagnosis")

TREATMENT

■ NONPHARMACOLOGIC THERAPY
- Physical therapy, patient education and reassurance, treatment of associated conditions (e.g., depression)

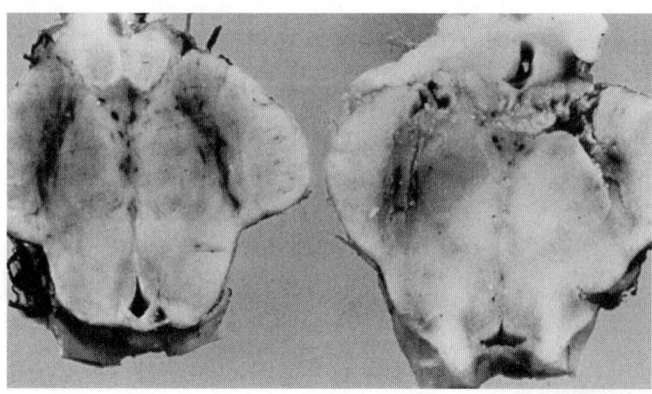
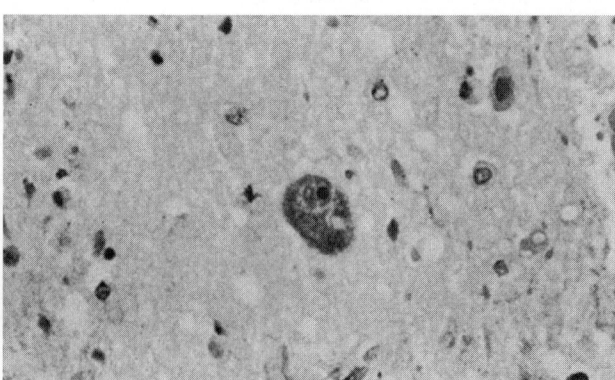

Fig. 1-282   A and **B,** An isolated Lewy body, a distinctive eosinophilic cytoplasmic inclusion body found in the substantia nigra in Parkinson's disease. (From Goetz CG: *Textbook of clinical neurology,* Philadelphia, 1999, WB Saunders.)

- Avoidance of drugs that can induce or worsen parkinsonism: neuroleptics (especially haloperidol), certain antiemetics (prochlorperazine, trimethobenzamide), metoclopramide, nonselective MAO inhibitors (may induce hypertensive crisis), reserpine, methyldopa

■ ACUTE GENERAL Rx

- The optimal treatment sequence of levodopa and dopamine receptor agonists remains controversial. Many neurologists advocate that drug therapy should be delayed until symptoms significantly limit the patient's daily activities, because tolerance and side effects to antiparkinsonian agents are common. Medications used in the therapy of Parkinson's disease are discussed under "Chronic Rx."
- Fig. 1-283 describes an approach to the patient with symptoms of parkinsonism.

■ CHRONIC Rx

- Selegiline (Eldepryl), an inhibitor of MAO B, is favored by some as initial treatment for younger patients with early disease because of its possible neuroprotective effect; usual dose, 5 mg bid with breakfast and lunch. Selegiline also inhibits catabolism of dopamine in the brain and can be added to levodopa in patients experiencing deterioration while taking it. When it is added to levodopa, a smaller dose should be used (2.5 mg/day) to avoid increasing levodopa toxicity. Concurrent use of fluoxetine or meperidine should be avoided (toxic reaction).
- Levodopa therapy, the cornerstone of symptomatic therapy, is commonly used with a peripheral dopa decarboxylase inhibitor (carbidopa) to minimize side effects (nausea, mood changes, cardiac arrhythmias, postural hypotension). The combination of the two drugs is marketed under the trade name Sinemet; usual starting dose is 25/100 mg tid 1 hr before meals. It is most effective in the first 2 to 5 yr of therapy. Controlled-release preparations (Sinemet CR [200 mg levodopa/50 mg of carbidopa, or 100 mg levodopa/25 mg carbidopa] given bid) produce fewer fluctuations in the plasma concentration of levodopa and result in a smoother therapeutic response. Their major problem is slower onset of action. This can be corrected by adding half of the standard Sinemet dose (25/100) with each morning dose of Sinemet CR. Levodopa-induced psychosis and hallucinosis can be treated with clozapine (Clozaril) or risperidone. Clozapine use carries a 1% risk of

agranulocytosis and requires frequent monitoring of white blood cell differential.

- Dopamine receptor agonists are not as potent as levodopa, but they are often used as initial treatment in younger patients to attempt to delay the tolerance and onset of complications (dyskinesias, motor fluctuations) associated with levodopa therapy; these medications are generally expensive and poorly tolerated by elderly patients with cognitive impairment:
  1. Bromocriptine (Parlodel): initial dose, 1.25 mg qhs. Bromocriptine may be beneficial in delaying motor complications and dyskinesias with effects similar to levodopa therapy on impairment and disability.
  2. Pergolide (Permax): initial dose, 0.05 mg for first 2 days increased by 0.1 mg every third day over next 12 days.
  3. Ropinirole (Requip): initial dose is 0.25 mg tid.
  4. Pramipexole (Mirapex): initial dose of 0.125 mg tid, when used as initial treatment in patients with early Parkinson's disease, is better than levodopa at decreasing the development of dopaminergic motor complications but is associated with more side effects (somnolence, hallucinations, peripheral edema).
- Amantadine (Symmetrel) is an antiviral agent that may increase dopamine in the brain and improve rigidity and bradykinesia; it can be used alone early in the disease or in combination with levodopa; dosage is 100 mg qd (50 mg qd in elderly and renally impaired patients); side effects include delirium and pedal edema.
- Anticholinergic agents are helpful in treating the tremor and drooling in patients with Parkinson's disease and can be used alone or in combination with levodopa; potential side effects (particularly in the elderly) include constipation, urinary retention, memory impairment, and hallucinations:
  1. Trihexyphenidyl (Artane): initial dose, 1 mg PO tid pc
  2. Benztropine (Cogentin): usual dose, 0.5 to 1 mg qd or bid
- Current research involves transplantation of fetal tissues, ventrolateral thalamotomy (for control of tremor, rigidity, dystonia), medial pallidotomy (to control akinesia or "on-off" effects), and development of new synthetic dopamine agonists.
- Thalamic stimulation and thalamotomy are equally effective for the suppression of drug-resistant tremor, but thalamic stimulation has fewer

adverse effects and results in a greater improvement in function. Bilateral stimulation of the subthalamic nucleus or pars interna of the globus pallidus is associated wtih significant improvement in motor function in patients with Parkinson's disease whose function cannot be further improved with medical therapy.

- Human embryonic dopamine-neuron transplants survive in patients with severe Parkinson's disease and result in some clinical benefit in younger but not in older patients.

■ DISPOSITION

Parkinson's disease usually follows a slowly progressive course leading to eventual disability over the course of several years.

■ REFERRAL

- Neurology consultation is recommended on initial diagnosis of Parkinson's disease.
- Rehabilitation medicine referral to a physiatrist or physical therapist for outpatient physical therapy is recommended for most patients with disabling symptoms.

☼ PEARLS & CONSIDERATIONS

■ COMMENTS

Additional patient information on Parkinson's disease can be obtained from the internet at www.parkinson.org and from the National Parkinson Foundation, Inc., 1501 Ninth Avenue NW, Miami, FL 33136; phone: (800) 327-4545.

REFERENCES

The Deep-Brain Stimulation for Parkinson's Disease Study Group: Deep brain stimulation of the subthalamic nucleus or the pars interna of the globus pallidus in Parkinson's disease, *N Engl J Med* 345:956, 2001.

Freed CR et al: Transplantation of embryonic dopamine neurons for severe Parkinson's disease, *N Engl J Med* 344:710, 2001.

Lang AE, Lozano AM: Parkinson's disease, *N Engl J Med* Part I 339:1130, Part II 339:1044, 1998.

Lucking C et al: Association between early-onset Parkinson's disease and mutations in the Parkin gene, *N Engl J Med* 342:1560, 2000.

Schurman PR et al: A comparison of continuous thalamic stimulation and thalamotomy for suppression of severe tremor, *N Engl J Med* 342:461, 2000.

Author: **Fred F. Ferri, M.D.**

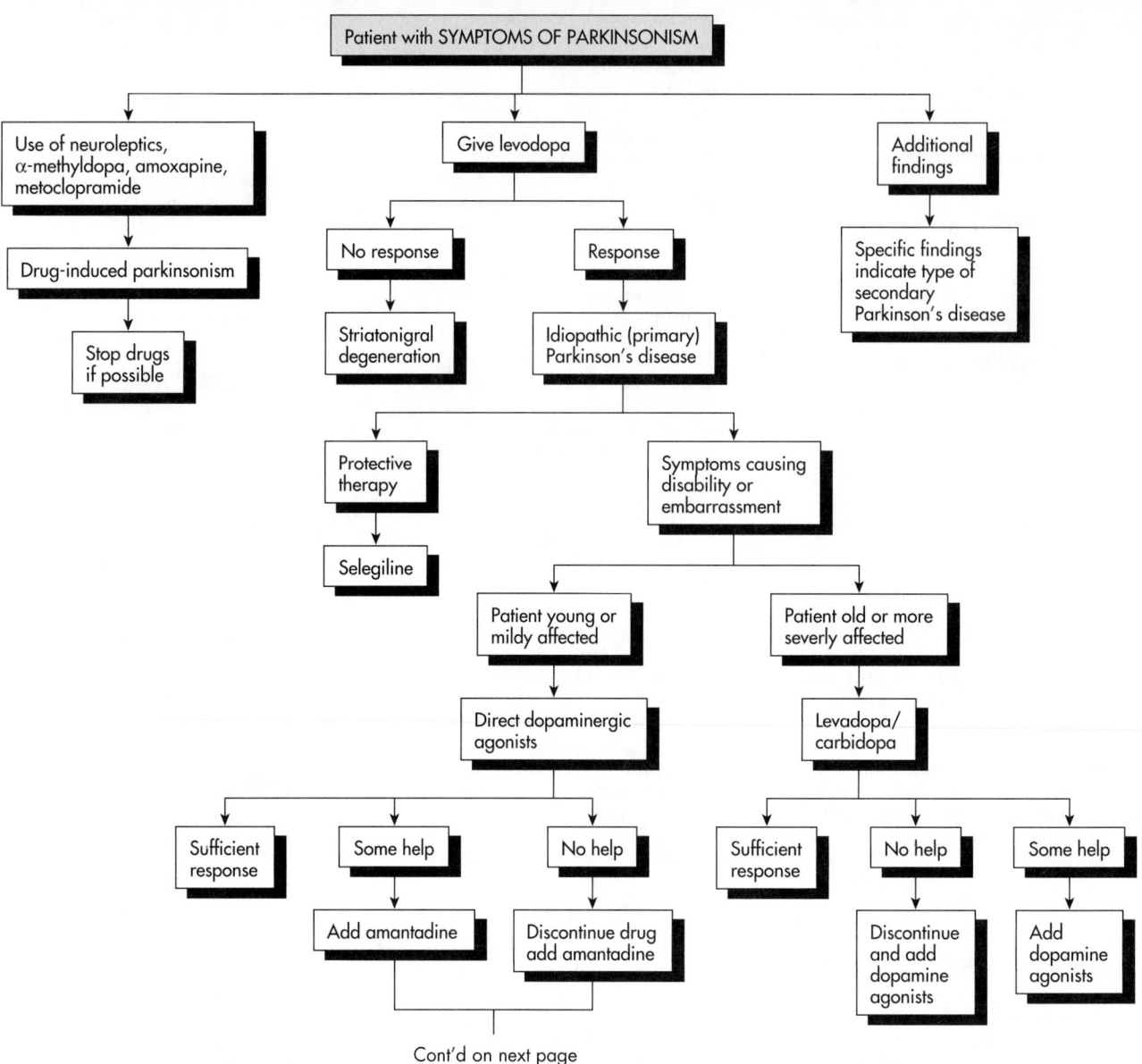

Fig. 1-283   Approach to the patient with symptoms of parkinsonism. (From Greene HL, Johnson WP, Lemcke DL: *Decision making in medicine,* ed 2, St Louis, 1998, Mosby.)

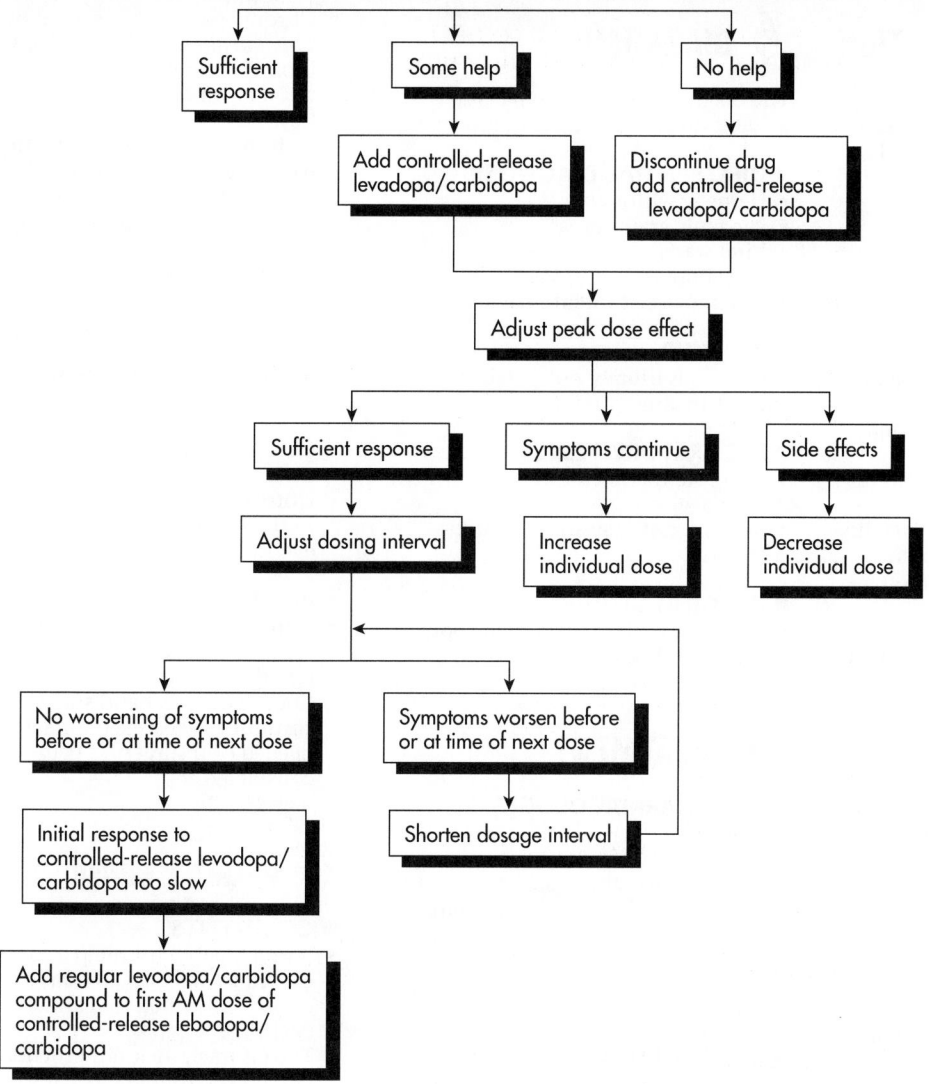

Fig. 1-283, cont'd   Approach to the patient with symptoms of parkinsonism. (From Greene HL, Johnson WP, Lemcke DL: *Decision making in medicine,* ed 2, St Louis, 1998, Mosby.)

BASIC INFORMATION

■ DEFINITION
Paronychia is a localized superficial infection or abscess of the lateral and proximal nail fold. Paronychia may be acute or chronic.

ICD-9CM CODES
681.9 Paronychia

■ EPIDEMIOLOGY & DEMOGRAPHICS
- Acute paronychia affects male and females equally.
- Chronic paronychia more common in females than males (9:1).
- Acute paronychia most often occurs in children.
- Chronic paronychia usually presents in the fifth or sixth decade of life.
- Paronychia is the most common infection of the hand.

■ PHYSICAL FINDINGS & CLINICAL PRESENTATION
- Acute paronychia usually presents with the sudden onset of redness, swelling, and pain with abscess or cellulitis formation in the nail fold.
- Chronic paronychia is insidious, presenting with mild swelling and erythema of the nail folds.
- Acute paronychia usually involves only one finger.
- Chronic paronychia may involve more than one finger.
- Acute paronychia usually involves the thumb.
- Chronic paronychia commonly involves the middle finger.

■ ETIOLOGY
- Any disruption of the seal between the proximal nail fold and the nail plate can cause paronychial infections.
- Acute paronychia is almost always bacterial in origin (e.g., *Staphylococcus aureus* [most common], *Streptococcus pyogenes*, *Streptococcus faecalis*, *Proteus* and *Pseudomonas* species, and anaerobes).
- Chronic paronychia is commonly caused by *Candida albicans* (70%) with bacterial organisms accounting for the remaining 30%.
- Trauma, nail biting, hangnails, diabetes, and chronic exposure to water are common predisposing features of paronychia.

DIAGNOSIS

The diagnosis of paronychia is self-evident on physical examination.

■ DIFFERENTIAL DIAGNOSIS
- Herpetic whitlow
- Pyogenic granuloma
- Viral warts
- Ganglions
- Squamous cell carcinoma

■ WORKUP
A workup is usually not pursued unless there is treatment failure.

■ LABORATORY TESTS
- Gram stain and culture any purulent drainage.
- KOH mount may show pseudohyphae.

■ IMAGING STUDIES
- X-ray the digit if concerned about osteomyelitis.

TREATMENT

■ NONPHARMACOLOGIC THERAPY
- For acute paronychia without purulent drainage, warm soaks tid or qid are helpful. If pus is present, surgical drainage in required.
- For chronic paronychia, avoid chronic immersion in water or exposure to moisture.

■ ACUTE GENERAL Rx
- First-generation cephalosporin (e.g., cephalexin 250 to 500 mg qid) or penicillinase-resistant penicillin (e.g., dicloxacillin 250 to 500 mg qid) are usually the antibiotics of choice for acute paronychia.
- Alternative antibiotic choices include clindamycin and amoxacillin-clavulanate potassium
- Surgical drainage is indicated if purulent discharge is noted.
- A No. 11 blade scalpel is used to lift the lateral paronychium and proximal eponychium off the nail, facilitating drainage.
- If the pus is located beneath the nail, the lateral edge of the nail can be lifted off the nail bed and excised.

■ CHRONIC Rx
- If no fungal organism is found, tincture of iodine (2 drops bid) helps keep the nail and skin dry.
- Chronic paronychia caused by *Candida albicans* is treated with topical antifungal agents (e.g., miconazole or ketoconazole applied tid).
- Unresponsive cases may be treated with itraconazole or fluconazole but should be done in consultation with dermatology and/or infectious disease.
- Surgery may be needed in refractory cases.

■ DISPOSITION
- Most acute paronychias with appropriate treatment resolve within 7 to 10 days.
- Osteomyelitis is a potential complication of paronychia.
- Untreated chronic paronychia leads to thickening and discoloration with eventual nail loss.

■ REFERRAL
- Chronic paronychia refractory to topical medical therapy is best referred to dermatology and/or infectious disease. A hand surgeon is consulted if abscess drainage is needed or if surgery is being considered.

PEARLS & CONSIDERATIONS

■ COMMENTS
- Women with chronic paronychia caused by *Candida albicans* should also be examined for candidal vaginitis.
- The GI tract, including the mouth and bowel, were the usual sources of *Candida albicans* in chronic paronychia.

REFERENCES
Black JR: Paronychia, *Clin Podiatr Med Surg* 12(2):183, 1995.
Brook I: Aerobic and anaerobic microbiology of paronychia, *Ann Emerg Med* 19:994, 1990.
Jebson PJ: Infections of the fingertip. paronychias and felons, *Hand Clin* 14(4):547, 1998.
Rich P: Nail disorders. Diagnosis and treatment of infectious, inflammatory, and neoplastic conditions, *Med Clin North Am* 82:1171, 1998.
Rockwell PG: Acute and chronic paronychia, *Am Fam Physician* 63:1113, 2001.
Author: **Peter Petropoulos, M.D.**

BASIC INFORMATION

■ DEFINITION

Paroxysmal atrial tachycardia (PAT) is a group of arrhythmias that generally originate as reentrant rhythm from the AV node and are characterized by sudden onset and abrupt termination.

■ SYNONYMS

PAT
SVT
Supraventricular tachycardia

ICD-9CM CODES

427.0 Paroxysmal atrial tachycardia

■ PHYSICAL FINDINGS & CLINICAL PRESENTATION

- Patient is usually asymptomatic.
- Patient may be aware of "fast" heartbeat.
- Persistent tachycardia may precipitate CHF or hypotension during acute MI.

■ ETIOLOGY

- Preexcitation syndromes (Wolff-Parkinson-White [WPW] syndrome)
- Atrial septal defect
- Acute MI

DIAGNOSIS

■ WORKUP

ECG:

- Absolutely regular rhythm at rate of 150 to 220 bpm is present.
- P waves may or may not be seen (the presence of P waves depends on the relationship of atrial to ventricular depolarization).
- Wide QRS complex (>0.12 sec) with initial slurring (delta wave) during sinus rhythm and short PR (≤0.12 sec) is characteristic of WPW syndrome; this syndrome is a result of an accessory AV pathway (bundle of Kent) that preexcites the ventricular muscle earlier than would be expected if the impulse reached the ventricles by way of normal conduction system; arrhythmias associated with WPW are narrow-complex SVT, atrial fibrillation, and ventricular fi-

brillation; digoxin and verapamil use should be avoided because they can lead to arrhythmia acceleration through the accessory pathway. Radiofrequency catheter ablation of accessory pathways (performed in conjunction with diagnostic electrophysiology testing) is a safe and effective treatment of patients with WPW syndrome.

- A clinical algorithm for the evaluation of narrow-complex tachycardia is described in Fig. 3-160. Evaluation of wide-complex tachycardia is described in Fig. 3-161.

TREATMENT

■ NONPHARMACOLOGIC THERAPY

- Valsalva maneuver in the supine position is the most effective way to terminate SVT; carotid sinus massage (after excluding occlusive carotid disease) is also commonly used to elicit vagal efferent impulses.
- Synchronized DC shock is used if patient shows signs of cardiogenic shock, angina, or CHF.

■ ACUTE GENERAL Rx

- Adenosine (Adenocard), an endogenous nucleoside, is useful for treatment of paroxysmal SVT, particularly that associated with WPW; it is considered by many the first choice of therapy for treatment of almost all episodes of SVT unresponsive to vagal maneuvers; the dose is 6 mg given as a rapid IV bolus; tachycardia is usually terminated within a few seconds; if necessary, may repeat with 12 mg IV bolus. Contraindications are second- or third-degree AV block, sick sinus syndrome (SSS), atrial fibrillation, and ventricular tachycardia. Adenosine may cause bronchospasm in asthmatics. Patients receiving theophylline (a competitive antagonist of adenosine receptors) are usually refractory to treatment. Dipyridamole enhances the effect of adenosine; therefore patients receiving dipyridamole should be started at lower doses.

- Verapamil 5 to 10 mg IV is given over 5 min; if no effect, may repeat in 30 min.
  1. Verapamil should be used cautiously in patients with SVT associated with hypotension.
  2. Slow injection of calcium chloride (10 ml of a 10% solution given over 5 to 8 min before verapamil administration) decreases the hypotensive effect without compromising its antiarrhythmic effect.
- Repeat carotid massage after IV verapamil if SVT persists.
- Metoprolol (IV 5 mg/2 min up to 15 mg) or esmolol (500 μg/kg IV bolus, then 50 μg/kg/min) may be effective in the treatment of SVT.
- IV digitalization (0.75 to 1 mg slow IV loading)
  1. Repeat carotid massage 30 min later; if not successful, give additional 0.25 mg IV digoxin and repeat carotid sinus massage 1 hr later.
  2. Digoxin should be avoided in patients with WPW syndrome and narrow QRS tachycardia (increased risk of atrial fibrillation during AV reentrant tachycardia).

■ DISPOSITION

Most patients respond well with resolution of the paroxysmal atrial tachycardia with treatment (see "Acute General Rx").

■ REFERRAL

Radiofrequency ablation is the procedure of choice in patients with accessory pathways and recurrent symptomatic episodes.

PEARLS & CONSIDERATIONS

■ COMMENTS

Accessory pathways occur in 0.1% to 0.3% of the general population.
Author: **Fred F. Ferri, M.D.**

BASIC INFORMATION

■ DEFINITION
Paroxysmal nocturnal hemoglobinuria (PNH) is a rare disease characterized by episodes of intravascular hemolysis and hemoglobinuria usually occurring at night. Thrombocytopenia, leukopenia, and recurrent venous thrombosis are also associated with PNH.

■ SYNONYMS
PNH

ICD-9CM CODES
283.2 Paroxysmal nocturnal hemoglobinuria

■ EPIDEMIOLOGY & DEMOGRAPHICS
- Affects patients of any age (reported spectrum 6 to 82 yr) but most common in patients aged 30 to 50 yr
- Affects both sexes (slight female predominance) and all races

■ PHYSICAL FINDINGS & CLINICAL PRESENTATION
Initial manifestations
- Anemia symptoms (35%)
- Hemoglobinuria (25%)
- Bleeding (20%)
- Aplastic anemia (15%)
- GI symptoms (10%)
- Hemolytic anemia (10%)
- Iron deficiency anemia (5%)
- Venous thrombosis (5%)
- Infections (5%)
- Neurologic symptoms
Hemoglobinuria
- Typically the first morning void reveals dark urine with progressive clearing during the day. The cause for the circadian rhythm is unknown.
Hemolysis
- In addition to the circadian hemolysis and resulting hemoglobinuria, episodes of hemolytic exacerbations can accompany infections, menstruation, transfusion, surgery, iron therapy, and vaccinations. Symptoms of severe hemolysis include chest, back, or abdominal pain, headache, fever, malaise, and fatigue.
Aplastic anemia
- Aplastic anemia may be the presenting manifestation of PNH (therefore PNH must be in the differential diagnosis of aplastic anemia) or may develop as a later complication of PNH.
Thrombosis
- Lower extremity DVT
- Subclavian thrombosis
- Portal or mesenteric vein thrombosis
- Hepatic vein thrombosis (Budd-Chiari syndrome)
- Cerebrovascular thromboses
Renal failure
- Acute renal failure associated with massive hemoglobinuria (acute tubular necrosis)
- Progressive renal failure associated with thrombosis within renal small veins
Dysphagia
Infections (associated with leukopenia or steroid treatment)
Physical findings include:
- Pallor (anemia)
- Jaundice (hemolysis)
- Splenomegaly
- Unilateral extremity swelling (DVT)
- Ascites (Budd-Chiari syndrome)

■ ETIOLOGY & PATHOGENESIS
- Complement-mediated hemolysis; the erythrocytes are abnormally sensitive to acidified serum.
- Patients have two populations of RBCs, some sensitive to hemolysis (PNH III cells) and others not (PNH I cells) in variable proportions (10% to 75% PNH III cells). About 20% PNH III are required for hemoglobinuria to be detectable.
- The RBC defects in PNH are in the membrane proteins as follows:
  Acetylcholinesterase deficiency
  Decay-accelerating factor deficiency
  Membrane inhibitor of reactive lysis deficiency.
  C-8 binding protein deficiency
- These protein deficiencies are the result of an acquired mutation located in the X chromosome, which regulates glycosylphosphatidylinositol (GPI). GPI anchors the above-mentioned proteins in the RBC membrane; GPI-deficient RBCs proliferate as an abnormal clone. Because women are affected at least as frequently as men are, the mutation must be expressed as dominant gene. The mechanism whereby the mutant stem cells can dominate hematopoiesis in PNH is unknown.
- The pathophysiology of the relationship of PNH and aplastic anemia is unknown.

DIAGNOSIS

Clinical situations:
- Intravascular hemolysis
- Hemoglobinuria
- Pancytopenia associated with hemolysis
- Iron deficiency associated with hemolysis
- Recurrent venous thrombosis
- Recurrent episodes of abdominal pain, headache, or back pain associated with hemolysis

■ DIFFERENTIAL DIAGNOSIS
- See "Hemolytic Anemia" in Section I.
- See "Aplastic Anemia" in Section I.
- See "Anemia" algorithm in Section III.

■ LABORATORY TESTS
- CBC: anemia, leukopenia, thrombocytopenia
- Reticulocytosis
- RBC smear: spherocytes
- Negative Coombs' test
- Low leukocyte alkaline phosphatase
- Elevated LDH
- Low serum haptoglobin
- Low serum iron saturation, low ferritin
- Elevated urine hemoglobin
- Elevated urine urobilinogen
- Elevated urine hemosiderin
- Positive Ham test (acidified serum RBC lysis)
- Normoblastic hyperplasia on bone marrow aspirate or biopsy
- Identification of GPI-anchored protein deficiency on hematopoietic cells using monoclonal antibodies or flow cytometry
- Cytogenetic studies are not diagnostic

TREATMENT

- Androgenic steroids
- Prednisone (15 to 40 mg qod)
- Iron replacement
- Transfusions
- Treatment and prevention of thrombosis (heparin, coumarin)
- Avoidance of oral contraceptives
- Bone marrow transplantation

■ REFERRAL
To hematologist

■ PROGNOSIS
- 50% survival to 10 to 15 yr
- 25% survival to 25 yr
- If thrombosis at presentation, only 40% survival to 4 yr
- 1% incidence of leukemia
- 5% incidence of myelodysplastic syndrome

REFERENCE
Parker CJ, Lee GR: Paroxysmal nocturnal hemoglobinuria. In Lee GR et al (eds): *Wintrobe's clinical hematology,* ed 10, Baltimore, 1999, Williams & Wilkins.
Author: **Tom J. Wachtel, M.D.**

BASIC INFORMATION

■ DEFINITION

Pediculosis is lice infestation. Humans can be infested with three kinds of lice: *Pediculus capitis* (head louse) [Fig. 1-284], *Pediculus corporis* (body louse), and *Phthirus pubis* (pubic, or crab, louse). Lice feed on human blood and deposit their eggs (nits) on the hair shafts (head lice and pubic lice) and along the seams of clothing (body lice). Nits generally hatch within 7 to 10 days. Lice are obligate human parasites and cannot survive away from their hosts for longer than 7 to 10 days.

■ SYNONYMS

Lice

ICD-9CM CODES

132.9 Pediculosis

■ EPIDEMIOLOGY & DEMOGRAPHICS

- There are 6 million to 12 million cases of head lice in the U.S. yearly.
- Lice infestation of the scalp is most common in children (girls > boys).
- Infestation of the eyelashes is most frequently seen in children and may indicate sexual abuse.
- The chance of acquiring pubic lice from one sexual exposure with an infested partner is >90% (most contagious STD known).
- Body lice is most common in conditions of poor hygiene.

■ PHYSICAL FINDINGS & CLINICAL PRESENTATION

- Pruritus with excoriation may be caused by hypersensitivity reaction, inflammation from saliva, and fecal material from the lice.
- Nits can be identified by examining hair shafts.
- The presence of nits on clothes is indicative of body lice.
- Lymphadenopathy may be present (cervical adenopathy with head lice, inguinal lymphadenopathy with pubic lice).
- Head lice is most frequently found in the back of the head and neck, behind the ears.
- Scratching can result in pustules and crusting.
- Pubic lice may affect the hair around the anus.

■ ETIOLOGY

Lice are transmitted by close personal contact or use of contaminated objects (e.g., combs, clothing, bed linen, hats).

DIAGNOSIS

■ DIFFERENTIAL DIAGNOSIS

- Seborrheic dermatitis
- Scabies
- Eczema
- Other: pilar casts, trichonodosis (knotted hair), monilethrix
- A clinical evaluation of generalized pruritus is described in Fig. 3-135.
- Box 2-210 describes the differential diagnosis of pruritus.

■ WORKUP

Diagnosis is made by seeing the lice or their nits.

■ LABORATORY TESTS

Wood's light examination is useful to screen a large number of children: live nits fluoresce, empty nits have a gray fluorescence, nits with unborn louse reveal white fluorescence.

TREATMENT

■ NONPHARMACOLOGIC THERAPY

- Patients with body lice should discard infested clothes and improve their hygiene.
- Personal items such as combs and brushes should be soaked in hot water for 15 to 30 min.
- Close contacts and household members should also be examined for the presence of lice.

■ ACUTE GENERAL Rx

The following products are available for treatment of lice:

- Permethrin: available over the counter (1% permethrin [Nix]) or by prescription (5% permethrin [Elimite]); should be applied to the hair and scalp and rinsed out after 10 min. A repeat application is generally not necessary in patients with head lice.

- Lindane 1% (Kwell), pyrethrin S (Rid): available as shampoos or lotions; they are applied to the affected area and washed off in 5 min; treatment should be repeated in 7 to 10 days to destroy hatching nits.
- Eyelash infestation can be treated with the application of petroleum jelly rubbed into the eyelashes three times a day for 5 to 7 days. The application of baby shampoo to the eyelashes and brows three or four times a day for 5 days is also effective. The use of fluorescein drops applied to the lids and eyelashes is also toxic to lice.
- In patients who have previously failed treatment or in whom resistance with 1% permethrin cream rinse occurs, a 10-day course of trimethoprim-sulfamethoxazole (TMP-SMX) 8 mg/kg/day of trimethoprin in divided doses is an effective treatment for head lice infestation.
- Ivermectin (Mectizan), an antiparasitic drug, given in a single oral dose of 200 μg/kg is effective for head lice resistant to other treatments (currently not FDA approved for pediculosis).

PEARLS & CONSIDERATIONS

■ COMMENTS

- Patients with pubic lice should notify their sexual contacts.
- Parents of patients should also be educated that head lice infestation (unlike body lice) does not indicate poor hygiene.

REFERENCE

Hipolito RB et al: Head lice infestation: single drug versus combination therapy with one percent permethrin and TMP-SMX, *Pediatrics* 107:30, 2001.

Author: **Fred F. Ferri, M.D.**

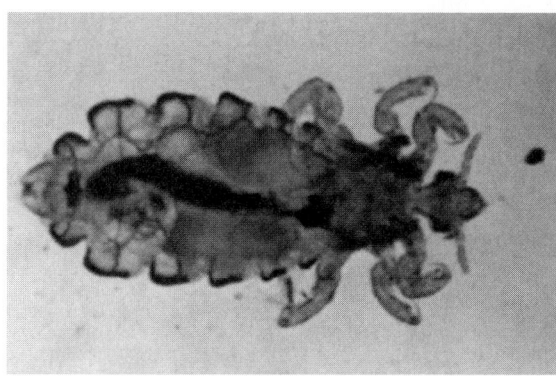

Fig. 1-284 *Pediculus humanus* var. *capitis* (head louse). (From Mandell GL: *Mandell, Douglas, and Bennett's principles and practice of infectious diseases*, ed 5, New York, 2000, Churchill Livingstone.)

BASIC INFORMATION

■ DEFINITION
Pedophilia is a sexual disorder of at least 6 mo of recurrent, intense, distressing sexual urges and/or fantasies involving prepubescent children.

■ SYNONYMS
Pedophilia erotica
Acts referred to as child sexual abuse or child molestation
One of the paraphilias

ICD-9CM CODES
302.2 Pedophilia

■ EPIDEMIOLOGY & DEMOGRAPHICS
INCIDENCE (IN U.S.): Accurate data are unavailable.
PREVALENCE (IN U.S.): Prevalence of victimization is variable, ranging from 5% to 60% of all adults reporting at least one case of sexual abuse (not necessarily penetration) before age 13 yr.
PREDOMINANT SEX:
- Majority are men: nearly 75% attracted to females exclusively; nearly 25% attracted to males exclusively; small minority attracted to both sexes
- Females: 5% to 20%
PREDOMINANT AGE: No available data
PEAK INCIDENCE:
- No available data
- Usually, onset in adolescence
GENETICS: No genetic factor has been identified.

■ PHYSICAL FINDINGS & CLINICAL PRESENTATION
- Often shy, passive, and with social and interpersonal difficulties
- Frequently, has experienced early abuse himself/herself
- Sexually excited by young children and adults with the build that resembles young children
- Do not all act on their sexual fantasies; may occasionally seek help before any sexual acts with children
- Some "belief" among those who actually molest children that their behavior is good for or welcomed by the child

■ ETIOLOGY
- Etiology is unclear.
- Personal experience with early molestation may be important, but clearly only a minority of molested children develop pedophilia.
- Influence of personality factors is possible.

DIAGNOSIS

■ DIFFERENTIAL DIAGNOSIS
- Psychosis: may present with unusual ideas or statements that may rarely be confused with pedophilia; but statements or behaviors of psychotic individuals are usually disorganized and relatively short lived.
- Incest: some is not based in pedophilia, but may instead reflect a dysfunctional family unit.
- Paraphilic sexual behavior in the setting of another condition such as mental retardation, brain injury, or drug intoxication.

■ WORKUP
- History is essential for diagnosis; however, most pedophiles are less than forthcoming even to direct questions by a physician.
- Collateral information should be obtained from family members, suspected victims, or legal and social organizations; but even experienced interviewers may be unable to diagnose pedophilia consistently.

■ LABORATORY TESTS
- Hormone profile (total testosterone, free testosterone, luteinizing hormone, follicle-stimulating hormone, prolactin, and progesterone) is sometimes recommended, but results do not guide diagnosis or treatment.
- If a medical condition with secondary CNS dysfunction is suspected, tailor laboratory investigation accordingly.

■ IMAGING STUDIES
Useful only if pedophilic behavior is believed to be a consequence of CNS damage (e.g., head trauma or mental retardation), then a head CT scan or MRI may document extent of anatomic damage.

TREATMENT

■ NONPHARMACOLOGIC THERAPY
- Usually obtain treatment under legal coercion after child molestation charge.
- Rarely, may initiate treatment request.
- Behavioral approaches are centered on aversion conditioning in which an aversive stimulus is paired with the pedophilic fantasy; when outcome is measured by repeat child molestation charges, these methods are moderately successful.
- For incestuous adult-child relationships not based in pedophilia, intensive family systems investigation and therapy are needed.

■ ACUTE GENERAL Rx & CHRONIC Rx
- Castration is an effective method of control of paraphilic behaviors, including child molestation. However, the irreversibility of the surgery and the subjective aversion to the procedure make it less than desirable.
- Chemical castration with antiandrogen compounds is more acceptable to the public; although research into the optimal dosage and the efficacy of these compounds is far from complete, they are generally believed to be safe, effective, and reversible.
- Medroxyprogesterone acetate (Provera) can be administered PO (60 mg/day) or in a depot IM form (200 to 400 mg IM once weekly).

■ DISPOSITION
- Untreated, child molesters are highly likely to be repeat offenders.
- Pedophiles who do not act on their fantasies are likely to continue these fantasies.
- NOTE: Contrary to popular belief, the majority of sexual acts are committed in the absence of alcohol.

■ REFERRAL
If pedophilia is highly suspected.
Author: Rif S. El-Mallakh, M.D.

BASIC INFORMATION

■ DEFINITION
Pelvic inflammatory disease (PID) is a spectrum of inflammatory disorders of the upper genital tract including a combination of any of the following:
- Endometritis, salpingitis, tuboovarian abscess, or pelvic peritonitis
- Resulting from an ascending lower genital tract infection
- Not related to obstetric or surgical intervention

■ SYNONYMS
Adnexitis
Pyosalpinx
Salpingitis
Tuboovarian abscess

ICD-9CM CODES
614.9 Unspecified inflammatory disease of female pelvic organs and tissue

■ EPIDEMIOLOGY & DEMOGRAPHICS
INCIDENCE/PREVALENCE:
- Estimated 600,000 to 1 million cases annually (U.S.)
- Diagnosed in 2% to 5% of women seen in STD clinics
- Most common cause of female infertility and ectopic pregnancy
RISK FACTORS:
- Adolescent sexually active in females <20 yr old (1:8)
- Previous episode of gonococcal PID
- Multiple sexual partners
- Vaginal douching
- Use of intrauterine device (threefold to fivefold increased risk of developing acute PID)

■ PHYSICAL FINDINGS & CLINICAL PRESENTATION
- Lower abdominal pain
- Abnormal vaginal discharge
- Abnormal uterine bleeding
- Dysuria
- Dyspareunia
- Nausea and vomiting (suggestive of peritonitis)
- Fever
- RUQ tenderness (perihepatitis): 5% of PID cases
- Cervical motion tenderness and adnexal tenderness
- Adnexal mass

■ ETIOLOGY
- *Chlamydia trachomatis*
- *Neisseria gonorrhoeae*
- Polymicrobial infection—*Bacteroides fragilis, Escherichia coli, Gardnerella vaginalis, Haemophilus influenzae, Mycoplasma hominis*
- *Mycobacterium tuberculosis* (an important cause in developing countries)

DIAGNOSIS

■ DIFFERENTIAL DIAGNOSIS
- Ectopic pregnancy
- Appendicitis
- Ruptured ovarian cyst
- Endometriosis
- Urinary tract infection (cystitis or pyelonephritis)
- Renal calculus
- Adnexal torsion
- Proctocolitis

■ WORKUP
DIAGNOSTIC CONSIDERATIONS:
- Clinical diagnosis is difficult and imprecise. A clinical algorithm for the evaluation of pelvic pain in the reproductive-age woman is described in Fig. 3-129; evaluation of vaginal discharge is described in Fig. 3-172.
- Clinical diagnosis of symptomatic PID has a positive predictive value of 65% to 90% when compared with laparoscopy as the standard.
- No single historical, physical, or laboratory finding is both sensitive and specific for the diagnosis of PID.

1998 CDC DIAGNOSTIC CRITERIA FOR PID:
- Empiric treatment is based on the presence of all of the following minimum criteria:
  1. Lower abdominal pain
  2. Adnexal tenderness
  3. Cervical motion tenderness
- Additional criteria to increase the specificity of the diagnosis of PID in women with severe clinical signs:
  1. Oral temperature >38.3° C
  2. Abnormal cervical or vaginal discharge
  3. Elevated ESR
  4. Elevated C-reactive protein
  5. Laboratory documentation of cervical infection with *N. gonorrhoeae* or *C. trachomatis*
- Definitive criteria for diagnosing PID, which are warranted in selected cases:
  1. Laparoscopic abnormalities consistent with PID
  2. Histopathologic evidence of endometritis on biopsy
  3. Transvaginal sonography or other imaging techniques showing thickened fluid-filled tubes with or without free pelvic fluid or tuboovarian complex

■ LABORATORY TESTS
- Leukocytosis
- Elevated acute phase reactants: ESR >15 mm/hr, C-reactive protein
- Gram stain of endocervical exudate: >30 PMNs per high-power field correlates with chlamydial or gonococcal infection
- Endocervical cultures for *N. gonorrhoeae* and *C. trachomatis*
- Fallopian tube aspirate or peritoneal exudate culture if laparoscopy performed
- hCG to rule out ectopic pregnancy

■ IMAGING STUDIES

- Transvaginal ultrasound to look for adnexal mass has sensitivity for PID of 81%, specificity 78%, accuracy 80%.
- MRI has sensitivity for PID of 95%, specificity 89%, accuracy 93%. It is useful not only for establishing the diagnosis of PID, but also for detecting other processes responsible for the symptoms. Disadvantages are its higher cost and unavailability in certain areas.

℞ TREATMENT

■ NONPHARMACOLOGIC THERAPY

- Most patients are treated as outpatients.
- Criteria for hospitalization (1998 CDC) as follows:
  1. Surgical emergencies such as appendicitis cannot be excluded
  2. Tuboovarian abscess
  3. Pregnant patient
  4. Patient is immunodeficient
  5. Severe illness, nausea, or vomiting precluding outpatient management
  6. Patient unable to follow or tolerate outpatient regimens
  7. No clinical response to outpatient therapy

■ ACUTE GENERAL Rx
REGIMENS FOR TREATMENT OF PID RECOMMENDED BY THE CDC, 1998:

- Outpatient treatment: Regimen A:
  1. Ofloxacin 400 mg PO bid × 14 days plus metronidazole 500 mg PO bid × 14 days
- Outpatient treatment: Regimen B:
  1. Cefoxitin 2 g IM plus probenecid 1 g PO *or*
  2. Ceftriaxone 250 mg IM *or*
  3. Equivalent cephalosporin (ceftizoxime or cefotaxime) plus doxycycline 100 mg PO bid × 10 to 14 days
- Inpatient treatment: Regimen A:
  1. Cefoxitin 2 g IV q6h or cefotetan 2 g IV q12h plus doxycycline 100 mg IV or PO q12h
  2. Continuation of regimen for at least 24 hr after substantial clinical improvement, after which doxycycline 100 mg PO bid is continued for a total of 14 days

- Inpatient treatment: Regimen B:
  1. Clindamycin 900 mg IV q8h plus gentamicin loading dose IV or IM (2 mg/kg of body weight), followed by a maintenance dose (1.5 mg/kg) q8h
  2. Continuation of regimen for at least 24 hr after substantial clinical improvement, followed by doxycycline 100 mg PO bid or clindamycin 450 mg PO qid to complete a total of 14 days of therapy

■ CHRONIC Rx
Hospitalized patients receiving IV therapy:
  1. Significant clinical improvement is characterized by defervescence, decreased abdominal tenderness, and decreased uterine, adnexal, and cervical motion tenderness within 3 to 5 days.
  2. If no clinical improvement occurs, further diagnostic workup is necessary, including possible surgical intervention.

■ DISPOSITION
- Long-term sequelae of PID: recurrent PID, chronic pelvic pain, ectopic pregnancy, infertility, Fitz-Hugh–Curtis syndrome (Fig. 1-285).
- Risk of tubal infertility related to episodes of PID: first episode, 8%; second episode, 20%; third episode, 40%.
- Essential to evaluate and treat male sex partners.

■ REFERRAL
If there is no clinical improvement with outpatient therapy observed within 72 hr, patient should be hospitalized and gynecology consult requested.

☼ PEARLS & CONSIDERATIONS

■ COMMENTS
Patient education material is available from local and state health departments or from the American College of Obstetricians and Gynecologists.

REFERENCES

Centers for Disease Control and Prevention: 1998 Sexually transmitted diseases treatment guidelines, *MMWR* 47(RR-1), 1998.

Tukeva TA et al: MR imaging in pelvic inflammatory disease: comparison with laparoscopy and ultrasound, *Radiology* 210:209, 1999.

Author: **George T. Danakas, M.D.**

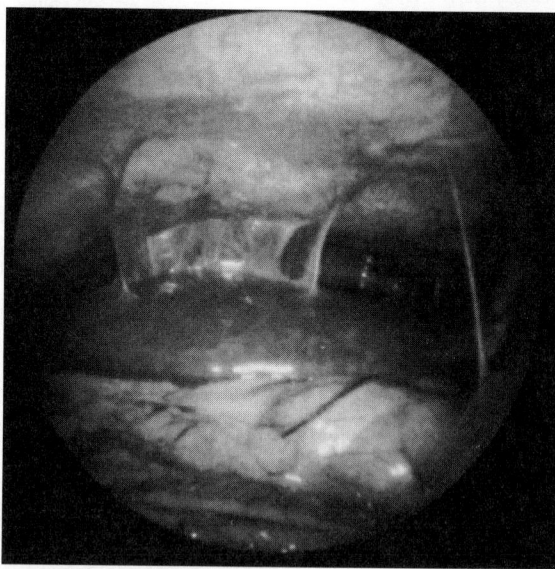

Fig. 1-285 "Violin string" adhesions are visualized in this patient with Fitz-Hugh–Curtis syndrome. (From Copeland LJ: *Textbook of gynecology,* ed 2, Philadelphia, 2000, WB Saunders.)

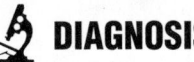 **BASIC INFORMATION**

DEFINITION
- Pemphigus refers to a group of chronic, autoimmune diseases resulting in intraepidermal blister formation.
- Pemphigus has four subtypes:
  1. Pemphigus vulgaris (Fig. 1-286)
  2. Pemphigus vegetans
  3. Pemphigus foliaceus
  4. Pemphigus erythematosus
- Pemphigus vulgaris refers to an intraepidermal blistering skin disorder characterized by the formation of the flaccid blister.

SYNONYMS
Pemphigus

ICD-9CM CODES
694.4 Pemphigus

EPIDEMIOLOGY & DEMOGRAPHICS
- Incidence is 1/100,000
- More common in Ashkenazi Jews
- Typically occurs in the fourth and fifth decades of life
- Male = females
- Can occur in the young

PHYSICAL FINDINGS & CLINICAL PRESENTATION
- History
  1. Oral mucosa lesions typically occur first, followed by a generalized bullous eruption within a few months.
  2. Lesions are fragile and rupture easily, leaving painful denuded lesions.
  3. Usually not pruritic.
- Physical findings
  1. Anatomic distribution
     a. Oral mucosa
     b. Can also involve the pharynx, larynx, vagina, penis, anus, and conjunctival mucosa
     c. Generalized cutaneous involvement
  2. Lesion configuration
     a. All stratified squamous epithelium can become involved.
  3. Lesion morphology
     a. Bullae
     b. Denuded crusting and erosion commonly occurs

ETIOLOGY
Pemphigus vulgaris, like all subtypes of pemphigus, is an autoimmune disease caused by autoantibodies binding to antigens within the epithelial layer of the skin.

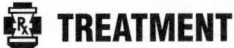 **DIAGNOSIS**

The diagnosis of pemphigus vulgaris should be suspected in patients with oral lesion and flaccid bullae on the skin.

DIFFERENTIAL DIAGNOSIS
- Bullous pemphigoid (see Table 1-52)
- Cicatricial pemphigoid
- Behçet's disease
- Erythema multiforme
- Systemic lupus erythematosus
- Aphthous stomatitis
- Dermatitis herpetiformis
- Drug eruptions

WORKUP
The workup for patients with suspected pemphigus vulgaris requires specific laboratory tests and special histology and immunofluorescence testing to establish the diagnosis.

LABORATORY TESTS
- Autoantibodies can be detected in the serum by indirect immunofluorescence assays.
- Skin biopsy reveals intraepidermal bulla formation, also called acantholysis (loss of cell adhesion between the epidermal cells).
- Direct and indirect immunofluorescence studies of the lesion show deposits of IgG and C3 in the epidermal layers of the skin.

IMAGING STUDIES
X-ray imaging is not useful in the diagnosis of pemphigus vulgaris.

TREATMENT

NONPHARMACOLOGIC THERAPY
- Use mild soaps.
- Soak lesions with Burow's solution.
- Soft diet and viscous lidocaine can be used in patients with oral lesions.

ACUTE GENERAL Rx
- For mild cases, topical intralesional steroids using triamcinolone acetonide 5 to 10 mg/ml can be used for individual lesions.
- For more severe cases, systemic corticosteroids are indicated at high dosages:
  1. Prednisone 200 to 400 mg/day for 6 to 8 wk, tapered to 15 mg/day.
  2. Alternative approaches include prednisone 80 to 120 mg PO qd increasing the dose rapidly by 50% every 7 days until no new lesions appear; then proceed with tapering over a 6-mo period.

CHRONIC Rx
- Adjuvant therapy is tried in patients in an attempt to decrease the amount of steroids required.
  1. Azathioprine 100 to 150 mg qd given concurrently with prednisone
  2. Cyclophosphamide 1 to 3 mg/kg/day
  3. Dapsone 25 to 100 mg/day
  4. Nicotinamide 500 mg PO qd plus tetracycline 1.5 to 3 g/day
  5. Plasmapheresis

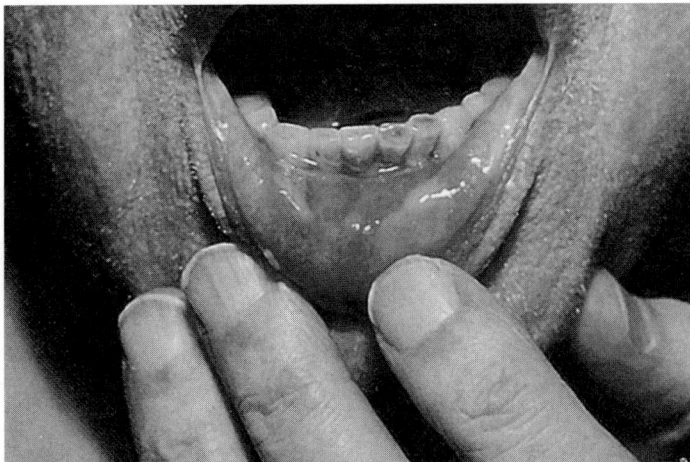

Fig. 1-286 Pemphigus vulgaris with oral lesions and no intact bullae. (Courtesy Department of Dermatology, University of North Carolina at Chapel Hill. In Goldstein BG, Goldstein AO: *Practical dermatology,* ed 2, St Louis, 1997, Mosby.)

■ DISPOSITION

- Before the use of corticosteroids, approximately 75% of patients died of pemphigus.
- Combined corticosteroids and adjuvant therapy has decreased mortality rates to <10%.
- Pemphigus vulgaris patients usually die from sepsis or complications from therapy.

■ REFERRAL

A dermatology consult is recommended for any patient with pemphigus vulgaris.

☼ PEARLS & CONSIDERATIONS

■ COMMENTS

- Pemphigus vulgaris, unlike bullous pemphigus, rarely occurs in the elderly population.

- It is important to diagnose pemphigus vulgaris early in its course.

REFERENCES

Bystryn JC, Steinman NM: The adjuvant therapy of pemphigus: an update, *Arch Dermatol* 132(2):203, 1996.

Scott JE, Ahmed AR: The blistering diseases, *Med Clin North Am* 82(6):1239,1998.

Stanley JR: Therapy of pemphigus vulgaris, Editorial, *Arch Dermatol* 135(1):76, 1999.

Author: **Peter Petropoulos, M.D.**

TABLE 1-52   Differentiation of Pemphigus Vulgaris and Bullous Pemphigoid

CHARACTERISTICS	PEMPHIGUS VULGARIS	BULLOUS PEMPHIGOID
Age	≥50 years	≥60 years
Site	Oral mucosa, face, chest, groin	Flexural areas, groin, axilla, less often oral
Findings	Flaccid bullae, intraepidermal blisters, IgG autoantibodies	Intact bullae, subepidermal blisters, IgG and complement autoantibodies
Treatment	Prednisone 40-60 mg/day, immunosuppressant agents; often chronically steroid-dependent	Prednisone 1 mg/kg/day or higher initially; taper over months to years
Prognosis	>90% respond; steroid side effects significant	>90% respond; remissions and recurrences common

From Goldstein BG: *Practical dermatology,* ed 2, St Louis, 1997, Mosby.

BASIC INFORMATION

■ **DEFINITION**

Peptic ulcer disease (PUD) is an ulceration in the stomach or duodenum resulting from an imbalance between mucosal protective factors and various mucosal damaging mechanisms (see "Etiology").

■ **SYNONYMS**

PUD
Duodenal ulcer (DU)
Gastric ulcer (GU)

■ **ICD-9CM CODES**

536.8 Peptic ulcer disease
531.3 Peptic ulcer, stomach, acute
531.7 Peptic ulcer, stomach, chronic
532.3 Peptic ulcer, duodenum, acute
532.7 Peptic ulcer, duodenum, chronic

■ **EPIDEMIOLOGY & DEMOGRAPHICS**

• Incidence: 250,000 to 500,000 (200,000 to 400,000 DU; 50,000 to 100,000 GU) annually; duodenal ulcer:gastric ulcer ratio is 4:1.
• Anatomic location: >90% of DUs occur in the first portion of the duodenum; GU occurs most frequently in the lesser curvature near the incisura angularis.

■ **PHYSICAL FINDINGS & CLINICAL PRESENTATION**

• Physical examination is often unremarkable.
• Patient may have epigastric tenderness, tachycardia, pallor, hypotension (from acute or chronic blood loss), nausea and vomiting (if pyloric channel is obstructed), boardlike abdomen and rebound tenderness (if perforated), and hematemesis or melena (with a bleeding ulcer).

■ **ETIOLOGY**

Often multifactorial; the following are common mucosal damaging factors:
• *Helicobacter pylori* infection
• Medications (NSAIDs, glucocorticoids)
• Incompetent pylorus or LES
• Bile acids
• Impaired proximal duodenal bicarbonate secretion
• Decreased blood flow to gastric mucosa
• Acid secreted by parietal cells and pepsin secreted as pepsinogen by chief cells
• Cigarette smoking
• Alcohol

■ **DIAGNOSIS**

■ **DIFFERENTIAL DIAGNOSIS**

• GERD
• Cholelithiasis syndrome
• Pancreatitis
• Gastritis
• Nonulcer dyspepsia
• Neoplasm (gastric carcinoma, lymphoma, pancreatic carcinoma)
• Angina pectoris, MI, pericarditis
• Dissecting aneurysm
• Other: high small bowel obstruction, pneumonia, subphrenic abscess, early appendicitis

■ **WORKUP**

• Comprehensive history and physical examination to exclude other diagnoses. Diagnostic modalities include endoscopy or UGI series. Endoscopy (Fig. 1-287) is invasive and more expensive; however, it is preferred for the following reasons:
  1. Highest accuracy (approximately 90% to 95%)
  2. Useful to identify superficial or very small ulcerations
  3. Essential to diagnose gastric ulcers (1% to 4% of gastric ulcers diagnosed as benign by UGI series are eventually diagnosed as gastric carcinoma)
  4. Additional advantages over UGI series include:
  Biopsy of suspicious looking ulcers
  Electrocautery of bleeding ulcers
  Measurement of gastric pH in suspected gastrinoma (e.g., patient with multiple ulcers)
  Diagnosis of esophagitis, gastritis, duodenitis
  Endoscopic biopsy for *H. pylori*

■ **LABORATORY TESTS**

• Routine laboratory evaluation is usually unremarkable.
• Anemia may be present in patients with significant GI bleeding.
• *H. pylori* testing via endoscopic biopsy, urea breath test, stool antigen test (HpSA), or specific antibody test is recommended:
  1. Serologic testing for antibodies to *H. pylori* is easy and inexpensive; however, the presence of antibodies demonstrates previous but not necessarily current infection. Antibodies to *H. pylori* can remain elevated for months to years after infection has cleared; therefore antibody levels must be interpreted in light of patient's symptoms and other test results (e.g., PUD seen on UGI series).
  2. The urea breath test documents active infection. The patient ingests a small amount of urea labeled with carbon 13 (^{13}C) or

carbon 14. If urease is present (produced by the organism), the urea is hydrolyzed and the patient exhales labeled carbon dioxide that is then collected and measured. This test is more expensive and not as readily available. Patients should not receive proton pump inhibitors for 2 wk before undergoing the urea breath test.
  3. Histologic evaluation of endoscopic biopsy samples is currently the gold standard for accurate diagnosis of *H. pylori* infection.
  4. Stool antigen test is as accurate as the urea breath test for follow-up evaluation of patients treated for *H. pylori*.
• Additional laboratory evaluation is indicated only in specific cases (e.g., amylase level in suspected pancreatitis, serum gastrin level in suspected Zollinger-Ellison [Z-E] syndrome).

■ **IMAGING STUDIES**

Conventional UGI barium studies identify approximately 70% to 80% of PUD; accuracy can be increased to approximately 90% by using double contrast.

■ **TREATMENT**

■ **NONPHARMACOLOGIC THERAPY**

• Stop cigarette smoking; cigarette smoking increases the risk of PUD, decreases the healing rate, and increases the frequency of recurrence.
• Avoid NSAIDs and alcohol.
• Special diets have been proved *unrelated* to ulcer development and healing; however, avoid foods that cause symptoms.

■ **ACUTE GENERAL Rx**

Eradication of *H. pylori,* when present, can be accomplished with various regimens:
  1. Proton pump inhibitors (PPI) bid (e.g., omeprazole 20 mg bid or lansoprazole 30 mg bid) *plus* clarithromycin 500 mg bid *and* amoxicillin 1000 mg bid for 7 to 10 days
  2. PPI bid *plus* amoxicillin 500 mg bid *plus* metronidazole 500 mg for 7 to 10 days
  3. PPI bid *plus* clarithromycin 500 mg bid *and* metronidazole 500 mg bid for 7 days
  4. Bismouth compound qid *plus* tetracycline 500 mg qid *and* metronidazole 500 mg qid for 14 days

PUD patients testing negative for *H. pylori* should be treated with antisecretory agents:
- Histamine-2 receptor antagonists (H_2RAs): cimetidine, ranitidine, famotidine, and nizatidine are all effective; they are usually given in split dose or at nighttime.
- Proton pump inhibitors (PPIs): can also induce rapid healing; they are usually given 30 min before meals.

Antacids and sucralfate are also effective agents for the treatment and prevention of PUD.

■ CHRONIC Rx
Maintenance therapy in duodenal ulcer patients is indicated in the following situations:
- Persistent smokers
- Recurrent ulcerations
- Chronic treatment with NSAIDs, glucocorticoids
- Elderly or debilitated patients
- Aggressive or complicated ulcer disease (e.g., perforation, hemorrhage)
- Asymptomatic bleeders

Misoprostol therapy (100 μg qid with food, increased to 200 μg qid if well tolerated) should be considered for the prevention of NSAID-induced gastric ulcers in all patients on long-term NSAID therapy; it is contraindicated in women of childbearing age because of its abortifacient properties. Proton pump inhibitors are also effective at healing ulcers and maintaining remission in patients on long-term NSAIDs.

■ DISPOSITION
- The recurrence rate for untreated PUD is approximately 60% (>70% in smokers). Treatment decreases the recurrence rate by nearly 30%.
- Patients with recurrent ulcers should be retreated for an additional 8 wk and then placed on maintenance therapy with H_2RAs, PPIs, sucralfate, or antacids.
- An ulcer is considered refractory to tratment if healing is not evident after 8 wk for duodenal ulcers and 12 wk for gastric ulcers. In these patients maximum acid inhibition (e.g., omeprazole 40 mg qd) is preferred over continued therapy with standard antiulcer therapy.
- Eradication of *H. pylori* (when present) is indicated in all patients. Undetectable serum antibody levels beyond the first year of therapy accurately confirm cure of *H. pylori* infection with reasonable sensitivity in initially seropositive healthy subjects.
- Screening for Zollinger-Ellison (Z-E) syndrome should also be considered in patients with multiple recurrent ulcers; in patients with Z-E, the serum gastrin level is >1000 pg/ml and the basal acid output is usually >15 mEq/hr.
- Surgery for refractory ulcers is now only rarely performed; it consists of highly selective vagotomy for duodenal ulcers or ulcer removal with antrectomy or hemigastrectomy without vagotomy for gastric ulcers.

■ REFERRAL
- GI referral for patients requiring endoscopy
- Surgical referral for patients with nonhealing ulcers despite appropriate medical therapy

✷ PEARLS & CONSIDERATIONS

■ COMMENTS
- Patients with gastric ulcers should have repeat endoscopy after 4 to 6 wk of therapy to document healing and test exfoliative cytology for gastric carcinoma.
- After endoscopic treatment of bleeding peptic ulcers, bleeding recurs in up to 20% of patients. A high-dose infusion of omeprazole (80 mg IV bolus followed by an infusion of 8 mg/hr for 72 hours) substantially reduces the risk of recurrent bleeding.

REFERENCES
Lau JYW et al: Effect of IV omeprazole on recurrent bleeding after endoscopic treatment of bleeding peptic ulcers, *N Engl J Med* 343:310, 2000.

Vaira D et al: Noninvasive antigen-based assay for assessing *H. pylori* eradication: a European multicenter study, *Am J Gastroenterol* 95:925, 2000.

Author: **Fred F. Ferri, M.D.**

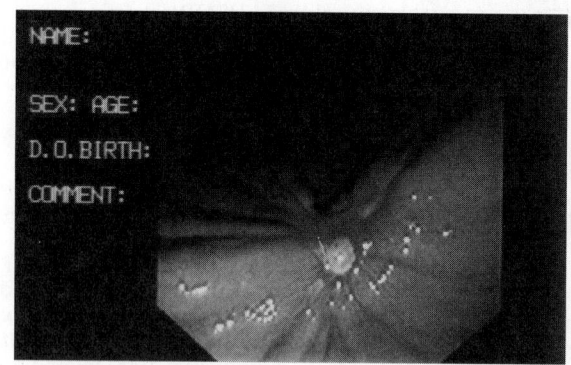 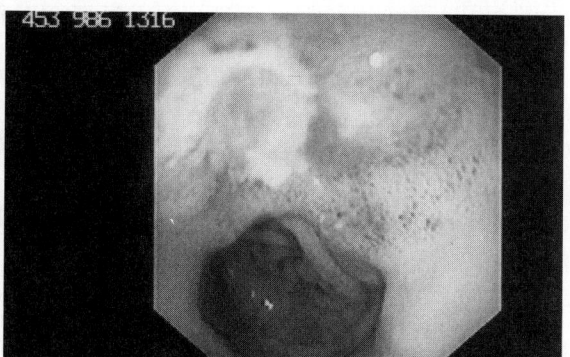

Fig. 1-287 A, Endoscopic view of gastric ulcer located on the angularis. Note radiating folds emanating from the ulcer crater. **B,** Endoscopic view of 1 cm duodenal ulcer. Note punctate erosions in duodenal bulb with associated duodenitis. (From Noble J [ed]: *Textbook of primary care medicine,* ed 2, St Louis, 1996, Mosby.)

I

BASIC INFORMATION

■ DEFINITION
Pericarditis is the inflammation (or infiltration) of the pericardium associated with a wide variety of causes (see "Etiology").

ICD-9CM CODES
420.91 Pericarditis

■ EPIDEMIOLOGY & DEMOGRAPHICS
- The incidence of acute pericarditis is 2% to 6%.
- Increased incidence in males and in adults compared with children.
- Most common cause (>40%) of constrictive pericarditis is idiopathic.
- The use of thrombolytic agents has greatly reduced the incidence of both early postinfarction pericarditis and Dressler's syndrome.

■ PHYSICAL FINDINGS & CLINICAL PRESENTATION
- Severe constant pain that localizes over the anterior chest and may radiate to arms and back; it can be differentiated from myocardial ischemia, because the pain intensifies with inspiration and is relieved by sitting up and leaning forward (the pain of myocardial ischemia is not pleuritic).
- Pericardial friction rub is best heard with patient upright and leaning forward and by pressing the stethoscope firmly against the chest; it consists of three short, scratchy sounds:
  1. Systolic component
  2. Diastolic component
  3. Late diastolic component (associated with atrial contraction)
- Cardiac tamponade may be occurring if the following are observed:
  1. Tachycardia
  2. Low blood pressure and pulse pressure
  3. Distended neck veins
  4. Paradoxical pulse

■ ETIOLOGY
- Idiopathic (possibly postviral)
- Infectious (viral, bacterial, tuberculous, fungal, amebic, toxoplasmosis)
- Collagen-vascular disease (SLE, rheumatoid arthritis, scleroderma, vasculitis, dermatomyositis)
- Drug-induced lupus syndrome (procainamide, hydralazine)
- Acute MI
- Trauma or posttraumatic
- After MI (Dressler's syndrome)
- After pericardiotomy
- After mediastinal radiation (e.g., patients with Hodgkin's disease)
- Uremia
- Sarcoidosis
- Neoplasm (primary or metastatic)
- Leakage of aortic aneurysm in pericardial sac
- Familial Mediterranean fever
- Rheumatic fever
- Leukemic infiltration
- Other: anticoagulants, amyloidosis, ITP

DIAGNOSIS

■ DIFFERENTIAL DIAGNOSIS
- Angina pectoris
- Pulmonary infarction
- Dissecting aneurysm
- GI abnormalities (e.g., hiatal hernia, esophageal rupture)
- Pneumothorax
- Hepatitis
- Cholecystitis
- Pneumonia with pleurisy

■ WORKUP
ECG, laboratory tests, and echocardiogram

■ LABORATORY TESTS
The following tests may be useful in absence of an obvious cause:
- CBC with differential
- Viral titers (acute and convalescent)
- ESR (not specific but may be of value in following the course of the disease and the response to therapy)
- ANA, rheumatoid factor
- PPD, ASLO titers
- BUN, creatinine
- Blood cultures
- Cardiac isoenzymes (usually normal, but mild elevations of CK-MB may occur because of associated epicarditis)

■ IMAGING STUDIES
- Echocardiogram to detect and determine amount of pericardial effusion; absence of effusion does not rule out the diagnosis of pericarditis
- ECG: varies with the evolutionary stage of pericarditis
  1. Acute phase: diffuse ST-segment elevations (particularly evident in the precordial leads), which can be distinguished from acute MI by:
     a. Absence of reciprocal ST-segment depression in oppositely oriented leads (reciprocal ST-segment depression may be seen in aV_R and VI)
     b. Elevated ST segments concave upward
     c. Absence of Q waves
  2. Intermediate phase: return of ST segment to baseline, and T wave inversion in leads previously showing ST-segment elevation (Fig. 1-222)
  3. Late phase: resolution of the T wave changes
- Table 2-190 and Fig. 2-12 describe the differential diagnosis of ST-segment elevation.

TREATMENT

■ NONPHARMACOLOGIC THERAPY
- Limitation of activity until the pain abates
- Patient education regarding potential complications (e.g., cardiac tamponade, constrictive pericarditis)

■ ACUTE GENERAL Rx
- Antiinflammatory therapy (NSAIDs, [e.g., naproxen 500 mg bid, indomethacin 25 to 50 mg tid])
- Prednisone 30 mg bid for severe forms of acute pericarditis (before use of prednisone, tuberculous pericarditis must be excluded)
- Codeine 15 to 60 mg PO qid for pain refractory to salicylates, indomethacin, or prednisone
- Close observation of patients for signs of cardiac tamponade
- Avoidance of anticoagulants (increased risk of hemopericardium)

TREATMENT OF UNDERLYING CAUSE:
1. Bacterial pericarditis
   a. Commonly caused by streptococci, meningococci, staphylococci, *Haemophilus*, gram-negative bacteria, anaerobic bacteria
   b. Therapy: systemic antibiotics and surgical drainage of pericardium
2. Fungal pericarditis
   a. Caused by histoplasmosis, coccidioidomycosis, candidiasis, blastomycosis, or aspergillosis
   b. Therapy: IV amphotericin B and drainage of pericardial space (if necessary)
3. Tuberculous endocarditis
   a. Therapy: antituberculous drugs for a minimum of 9 mo; concomitant corticosteroid therapy early in treatment may decrease inflammatory response and improve prognosis.
   b. Pericardiectomy may be necessary 2 to 4 wk after antituberculous drugs have been started.

POTENTIAL COMPLICATIONS FROM PERICARDITIS:

1. Pericardial effusion: the time required for pericardial effusion to develop is of critical importance; if the rate of accumulation is slow, the pericardium can gradually stretch and accommodate a large effusion (up to 1000 ml), whereas rapid accumulation can cause tamponade with as little as 200 ml of fluid.
2. Chronic constrictive pericarditis:
   a. Physical examination reveals jugular venous distention, Kussmaul's sign (increase in jugular venous distention during inspiration as a result of increased venous pulse), pericardial knock (early diastolic filling sound heard 0.06 to 0.1 sec after S_2), clear lungs, tender hepatomegaly, pedal edema, ascites.
   b. Chest x-ray: clear lung fields, normal or slightly enlarged heart, pericardial calcification
   c. ECG: low-voltage QRS complex
   d. Echocardiography: may show pericardial thickening or may be normal
   e. Cardiac catheterization: M or W contour of the central venous pattern caused by both systolic (x) and diastolic (y) dips (this differs from cardiac tamponade, which does not display a prominent diastolic descent; in chronic constrictive pericarditis, there is also increased right ventricular and pulmonary arterial pressures)
   f. Therapy: surgical stripping or removal of both layers of the constricting pericardium

3. Cardiac tamponade:
   a. Signs and symptoms: dyspnea, orthopnea, interscapular pain
   b. Physical examination: distended neck veins, distant heart sounds, decreased apical impulse, diaphoresis, tachypnea, tachycardia, Ewart's sign (an area of dullness at the angle of the left scapula caused by compression of the lungs by the pericardial effusion), pulsus paradoxus (decrease in systolic blood pressure >10 mm Hg during inspiration), hypotension, narrowed pulse pressure
   c. Chest x-ray: cardiomegaly (water bottle configuration of the cardiac silhouette may be seen) with clear lungs; the chest x-ray film may be normal when acute tamponade occurs rapidly in the absence of prior pericardial effusion.
   d. ECG reveals decreased amplitude of the QRS complex, variation of the R wave amplitude from beat to beat (electrical alternans). This results from the heart's oscillating in the pericardial sac from beat to beat and frequently occurs with neoplastic effusions.
   e. Echocardiography: detects effusions as small as 30 ml; a paradoxical wall motion may also be seen.
   f. Cardiac catheterization: equalization of pressures within chambers of the heart, elevation of right atrial pressure with a prominent x but no significant y descent.

   g. MRI can also be used to diagnose pericardial effusions.
   h. Therapy for pericardial tamponade consists of immediate pericardiocentesis; in patients with recurrent effusions (e.g., neoplasms), placement of a percutaneous drainage catheter or pericardial window draining in the pleural cavity may be necessary. Aspirated fluid should be sent for analysis (protein, LDH, cytology, CBC, Gram stain, AFB stain) and cultures for AFB, fungi, and bacterial C&S.

■ **DISPOSITION**
- Complete resolution of pain and other signs and symptoms during the initial 3 wk of therapy.
- Recurrence in 10% to 15% of patients within the initial 12 mo.
- Recurrent pericarditis in 28% of patients.
- Relapsing acute pericarditis and idiopathic chronic large pericardial effusion without tamponade may respond to treatment with colchicine.
- Recurrence of large effusion after pericardiocentesis is common in patients with idiopathic chronic pericardial effusion. Pericardiectomy should be considered in these patients.

REFERENCES

Adler Y et al: Colchicine for large pericardial effusion, *Clin Cardiol* 21:143, 1998.

Sagrista-Sauleda J et al: Long-term follow-up of idiopathic chronic pericardial effusion, *N Engl J Med* 341:2054, 1999.

Author: **Fred F. Ferri, M.D.**

PERICARDITIS, EVOLVING PATTERN

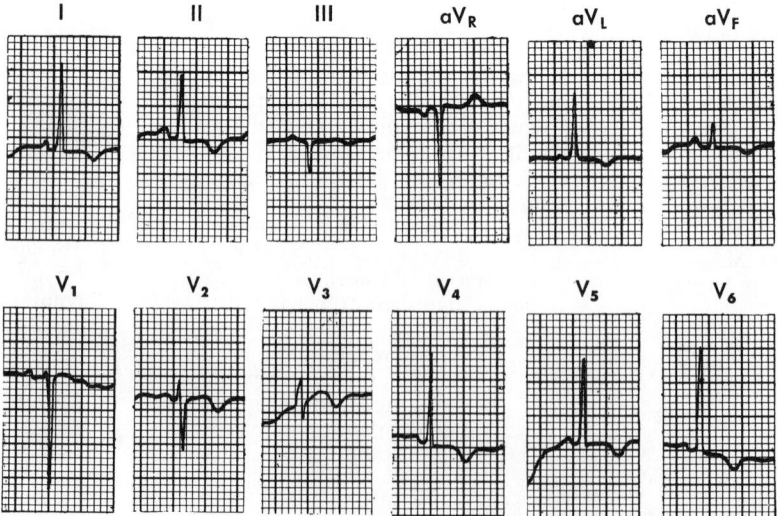

Fig. 1-288 Notice the diffuse T wave inversions in leads I, II, III, aV$_L$, aV$_F$, and V$_2$ to V$_6$. (From Goldberger AL [ed]: *Clinical electrocardiography*, ed 5, St Louis, 1994, Mosby.)

BASIC INFORMATION

■ DEFINITION

- *Peripheral neuropathy* is any disorder involving the peripheral nerves.
- *Polyneuropathy (symmetric polyneuropathy)* is a generalized process resulting in widespread and symmetric effects on the nervous system.
- *Focal or multifocal neuropathy (mononeuropathy, mononeuropathy multiplex)* is the local involvement of one or more individual peripheral nerves.
- *Paresthesias* are spontaneous aberrant sensations (e.g., pins and needles).

ICD-9CM CODES
356.9 Peripheral nerve neuropathy
355.10 Lower extremity neuropathy
354.11 Upper extremity neuropathy

■ PHYSICAL FINDINGS & CLINICAL PRESENTATION
Vary with the etiology of the neuropathy (see below); the most common presentation of peripheral neuropathy is distal symmetric sensorimotor dysfunction; the following findings may be present:
- Sensory ataxia
- Reduced or absent tendon reflexes
- Muscle weakness and wasting
- Progressive distal weakness and wasting
- Foot and hand deformities
- Neuropathic ulcers and arthropathy with prolonged peripheral neuropathy
- Autonomic neuropathy (postural hypotension, anhidrosis)

■ ETIOLOGY
HEREDITARY NEUROPATHIES:
- Charcot-Marie-Tooth syndrome
  1. Most common familial motor and sensory abnormality
  2. Foot deformity is common
- Others: Dejerine-Sottas disease, Refsum's disease, Riley-Day syndrome

ACQUIRED NEUROPATHIES:
- Neuropathy associated with systemic disase
  1. Diabetes mellitus: paresthesias of extremities (feet more than hands); the symptoms are symmetric, bilateral, and associated with intense burning pain (particularly at night).
  2. Mononeuropathies involving the cranial nerves III, IV, and VI, intercostal nerves, and femoral nerves are also common. A mononeuropathy involving a segmental nerve of the trunk can cause pain that mimics herpes zoster; but there is no rash.
  3. Myxedema: distal sensory neuropathy manifested by burning sensation and paresthesias of the limbs; delayed relaxation phase of DTR is common.
  4. Uremia: symmetric distal mixed motor and sensory disturbances.
  5. Sarcoidosis: cranial nerve palsies (most common in facial nerve).
  6. Alcohol: pain numbness and weakness of extremities.
  7. Neoplasms: sensory and sensorimotor neuropathies.
  8. Nutritional deficiencies: thiamine, folic acid, vitamin B_{12}; vitamin B_{12} deficiency affects the posterior and lateral columns of the spinal cord; it manifests with numbness and paresthesias of the extremities, weakness, ataxia, and loss of vibration sense.
- Guillain-Barré neuropathy (see "Guillain-Barré Syndrome" in Section I)
- Toxic neuropathies
  1. Drugs: chloramphenicol, lithium, isoniazid, pyridoxine, nitrofurantoin, disulfiram, dapsone, ethionamide, cisplatin, vincristine, metronidazole, gold, hydralazine, amiodarone, phenytoin, penicillamine, indomethacin, amphotericin B, amitriptyline, sulfonamides, colchicine, antiretrovirals (didanosine, stavudine, zalcitabine)
  2. Toxic chemicals: lead, arsenic, cyanide, thallium, carbon disulfide, mercury, organophosphates, trichloroethylene
- Neuropathies associated with infection: leprosy, herpes zoster, TB, diphtheria, Lyme disease, HIV
- Entrapment neuropathy (e.g., carpal tunnel syndrome)

DIAGNOSIS

■ DIFFERENTIAL DIAGNOSIS
- Polyradiculopathy
- Combined systems degeneration
- Table 2-141 describes the differential diagnosis of neuropathies.

■ WORKUP
- Inquire about the following:
  1. Family history of neuropathies: to rule out hereditary neuropathies
  2. Current and past employment: to rule out exposure to toxic agents
  3. Current or recent medications: to rule out neuropathy secondary to drugs
  4. Any systemic diseases, such as diabetes, renal failure, hypothyroidism, sarcoidosis
  5. Ethanol abuse: to rule out alcoholic neuropathy
  6. Any special diets (e.g., food faddists): to rule out nutritional deficiencies
  7. History of trauma: to rule out compression-entrapment neuropathies
  8. Risk factors for AIDS
  9. History of tick bite or ECM: to rule out Lyme disease
- Electromyography: in neurogenic lesions there are spontaneous fibrillation potentials and positive sharp waves at rest.
- Nerve conduction studies: slowing of motor or sensory conduction velocities and decrease in sensory action potential amplitude may be present.
- Lumbar puncture should be performed in suspected Guillain-Barré syndrome.
- Nerve biopsy may be needed in selected cases.
- Fig. 1-289 describes an approach to the patient with peripheral neuropathy.

■ LABORATORY TESTS
- CBC, glucose, electrolytes, BUN, creatinine, LFTs, calcium, magnesium, phosphate
- ESR, urinalysis
- HIV in patients with risk factors
- Lyme titer in endemic areas or in patients with suggestive history
- TSH level in suspected hypothyroidism
- Vitamin B_{12} and folate levels in suspected nutritional deficiencies
- Heavy metal screening in suspected toxic neuropathy

■ IMAGING STUDIES
- Chest x-ray examination to rule out sarcoidosis and lung carcinoma
- X-ray study in suspected trauma or peripheral nerve compression

TREATMENT

■ NONPHARMACOLOGIC THERAPY
- Stop offending agent
- Physical therapy
- Surgical referral for entrapment neuropathy

■ ACUTE GENERAL Rx
Therapy is tailored to the symptoms and to the causative agents:
- Diffuse pain and paresthesias may be treated with amitriptyline 25 to 75 mg at hs.
- Topical capsaicin (Zostrix) is effective in postherpetic neuralgia.
- Fludrocortisone is useful in autonomic neuropathy with postural hypotension.
- Vitamin B supplements should be used in alcoholic neuropathy.

Author: **Fred F. Ferri, M.D.**

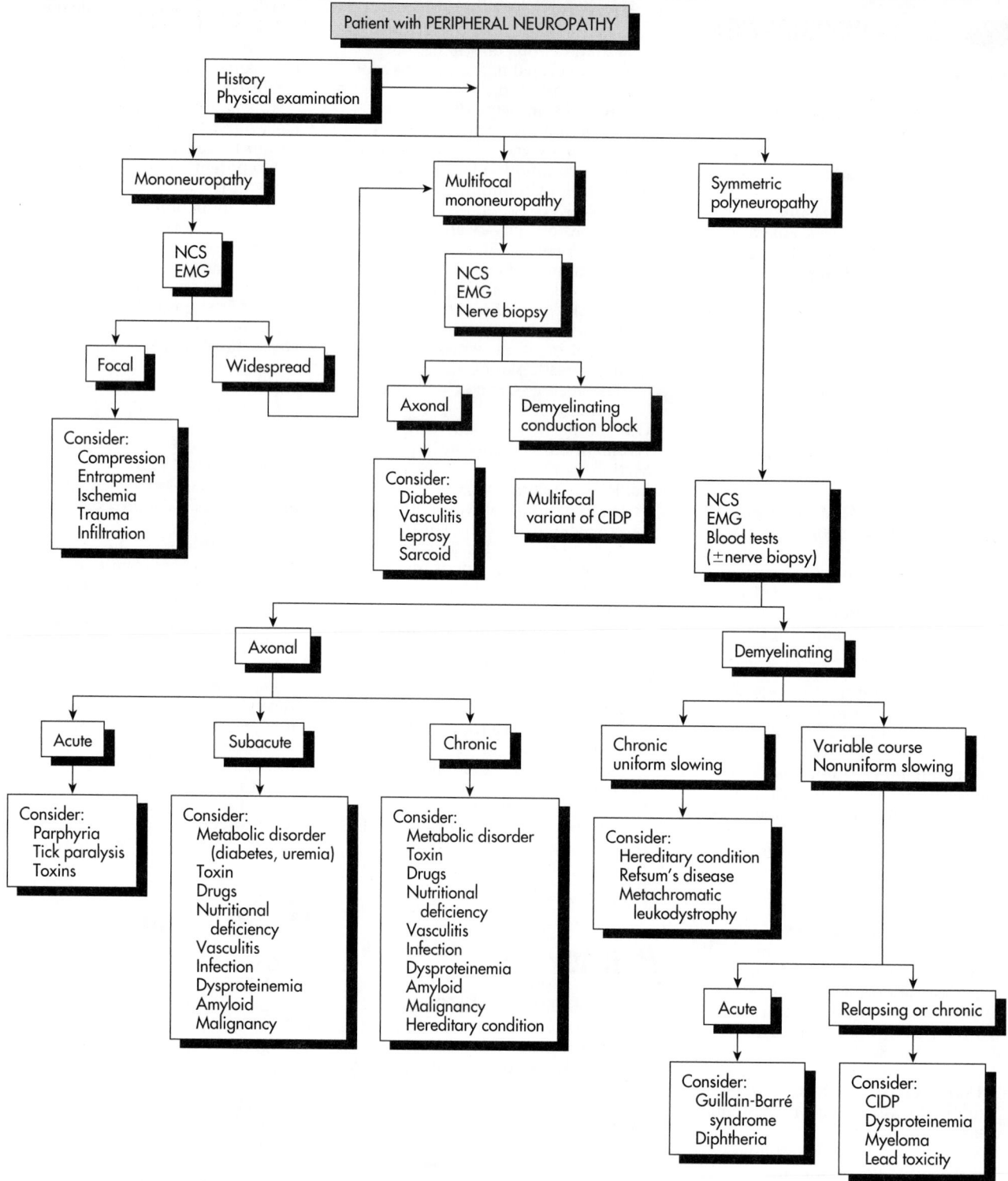

Fig. 1-289 **Approach to the patient with peripheral neuropathy.** *CIDP,* Chronic inflammatory demyelinating polyradioneuropathy; *EMG,* electromyogram; *NCS,* nerve conduction studies. (From Greene HL, Johnson WP, Lemcke DL: *Decision making in medicine,* ed 2, St Louis, 1998, Mosby.)

BASIC INFORMATION

DEFINITION
Peritonitis refers to the acute onset of severe abdominal pain secondary to peritoneal inflammation.

SYNONYMS
Acute abdomen
Surgical abdomen

ICD-9CM CODES
567.2 Peritonitis

EPIDEMIOLOGY & DEMOGRAPHICS
Common presentation as a result of diverse etiologies; for example, 5% to 10% of the population have acute appendicitis at some point in their life.

PHYSICAL FINDINGS
- Acute abdominal pain
- Abdominal distention and ascites
- Abdominal rigidity, rebound, and guarding
- Fever, chills
- Exacerbation with movement
- Anorexia, nausea, and vomiting
- Constipation
- Decreased bowel sounds
- Hypotension and tachycardia
- Tachypnea, dyspnea

ETIOLOGY
Although acute peritonitis can be caused by a wide variety of problems, similar clinical presentation is a result of stimulation of pain receptors within the peritoneum by purulent exudates, bleeding, inflammation, or the release of caustic materials such as pancreatic juice, bile, and gastric secretions.

DIAGNOSIS

DIFFERENTIAL DIAGNOSIS
- Postoperative: abscess, sepsis, bowel obstruction, injury to internal organs
- Gastrointestinal: perforated viscus, appendicitis, IBD, infectious colitis, diverticulitis, acute cholecystitis, peptic ulcer perforation, pancreatitis, bowel obstruction
- Gynecologic: ruptured ectopic pregnancy, PID, ruptured hemorrhagic ovarian cyst, ovarian torsion, degenerating leiomyoma
- Urologic: nephrolithiasis, interstitial cystitis
- Miscellaneous: abdominal trauma, penetrating wounds, infections secondary to intraperitoneal dialysis

WORKUP
- Acute peritonitis is mainly a clinical diagnosis based on patient history and physical examination.
- Laboratory and imaging studies (see below) assist in determining the need for and type of intervention.
- If patient is hemodynamically unstable, immediate diagnostic laparotomy should be performed in lieu of adjuvent diagnostic studies.

LABORATORY TESTS
- CBC: leukocytosis, left shift, anemia
- SMA7: electrolyte imbalances, kidney dysfunction
- LFT: ascites secondary to liver disease, cholelithiasis
- Amylase: pancreatitis
- Blood cultures: bacteremia, sepsis
- Peritoneal cultures: infectious etiology
- Blood gas: respiratory vs. metabolic acidosis
- Ascitic fluid analysis: exudate vs. transudate
- Urinalysis and culture: urinary tract infection
- Cervical cultures for gonorrhea and *Chlamydia*
- Urine/serum hCG

IMAGING STUDIES
- Abdominal series: free air secondary to perforation, small or large bowel dilatation secondary to obstruction, identification of fecalith
- Chest x-ray examination: elevated diaphragm, pneumonia
- Pelvic/abdominal ultrasound: abscess formation, abdominal mass, intrauterine vs. ectopic pregnancy, identify free fluid suggestive of hemorrhage or ascites
- CT: mass, ascites

TREATMENT

NONPHARMACOLOGIC THERAPY
- IV hydration to correct dehydration, hypovolemia
- Blood transfusion to correct anemia secondary to hemorrhage
- Nasogastric decompression, especially if obstruction is present
- Oxygen: intubation if necessary
- Bed rest

ACUTE GENERAL Rx
- Surgery to correct underlying pathology, such as controlling hemorrhage, correct perforation, drain abscess, etc.
- Broad-spectrum antibiotics:
  1. Single agent: ceftriaxone 1 to 2 g IV q24h, cefotaxime 1 to 2 g IV q4-6h
  2. Multiple agents:
     a. Ampicillin 2 g IV q4-6h; gentamicin 1.5 mg/kg/day; clindamycin 600 to 900 mg IV q8h
     b. Ampicillin 2 g IV q4-6h; gentamicin 1.5 mg/kg/day; metronidazole 500 mg IV q6-8h
- Pain control: morphine or meperidine as needed (hold until diagnosis confirmed)

DISPOSITION
Dependent on etiology of peritonitis, age of patient, coexisting medical disease, and duration of process before presentation

REFERRAL
Surgical consultation is required in all cases of acute peritonitis.

Author: **Matthew L. Withiam-Leitch, M.D., Ph.D.**

BASIC INFORMATION

■ **DEFINITION**
Spontaneous bacterial peritonitis (SBP) is an inflammatory reaction of the peritoneum secondary to the presence of bacteria or other microorganisms, most commonly associated with alcoholic cirrhosis and ascites in adults.

■ **SYNONYMS**
Primary peritonitis
SBP

■ **ICD-9CM CODES**
567.2 Peritonitis

■ **EPIDEMIOLOGY & DEMOGRAPHICS**
PREDOMINANT SEX: Male > female

■ **PHYSICAL FINDINGS & CLINICAL PRESENTATION**
• Acute fever with accompanying abdominal pain/ascites, nausea, vomiting, diarrhea
• In cirrhotic patients, presentation may be subtle when low-grade temperature (100° F) with or without abdominal abnormalities
• In patients with ascites, a heightened degree of awareness is necessary for detection
• Jaundice and encephalopathy
• Deterioration of mental status and/or renal function

■ **ETIOLOGY**
• *Escherichia coli*
• *Klebsiella pneumoniae*
• *Streptococcus pneumoniae*
• *Streptococcus* spp., including *Enterococcus*
• *Staphylococcus aureus*
• Anaerobic pathogens: *Bacteroides*, *Clostridium* organisms
• Other: fungal, mycobacterial, viral

■ **DIAGNOSIS**

■ **DIFFERENTIAL DIAGNOSIS**
• Appendicitis (in children)
• Perforated peptic ulcer
• Secondary peritonitis
• Peritoneal abscess
• Splenic, hepatic, or pancreatic abscess
• Cholecystitis
• Cholangitis

■ **WORKUP**
• Paracentesis and ascitic fluid analysis (see "Laboratory Tests" below) will confirm diagnosis.
• Laparotomy may be life threatening in end-stage cirrhosis.
• Positive blood cultures in an individual with ascites requires exclusion of a peritoneal source by paracentesis.

■ **LABORATORY TESTS**
Ascitic fluid analysis reveals the following:
• Polymorphonuclear (PMN) cell count: >250/mm^3
• Presence of bacteria on Gram stain
• pH: <7.31
• Lactic acid: >32/dl
• Protein: <1 g/dl
• Glucose: >50 mg/dl
• LDH: <225 mU/ml
• Positive culture of peritoneal fluid

■ **IMAGING STUDIES**
• Abdominal ultrasound: if there is clinical difficulty in performing paracentesis
• CT scan: to rule out secondary peritonitis (if indicated) and to exclude abscess, mass

■ **TREATMENT**

■ **ACUTE GENERAL Rx**
Cefotaxime 1 to 2 g IV q8h or ceftriaxone 2 g IV q24h in patients with normal renal function; duration of treatment is generally 7 to 10 days. Oral quinolone therapy (ofloxacin 400 to 800 mg/day) or ciprofloxacin may be an acceptable alternative in selected patients.

■ **PROPHYLAXIS**
Give double-strength trimethoprim/sulfamethoxazole qd 5 days/wk or ciprofloxacin 750 mg/wk PO. Both have been shown to decrease occurrence of SBP in patients with cirrhosis.

■ **COMMENTS**
Renal failure is a major cause of morbidity in cirrhotic patients with SBP. The use of IV albumin (1.5 g/kg at the time of diagnosis and 1 g/kg on day 3) may lower the rate of renal failure and mortality in patients with SBP.

REFERENCES
Navassa M et al: Randomized, comparative study of oral ofloxacin versus intravenous cefotoxin in spontaneous bacterial peritonitis, *Gastroenterology* 111:1011, 1996.
Sort P et al: Effects of intravenous albumin on renal impairment and mortality in patients with cirrhosis and SBP, *N Engl J Med* 341:403, 1999.
Such J, Runyon BA: Spontaneous bacterial peritonitis, *Clin Infect Disease* 27:669, 1998.
Author: **Dennis J. Mikolich, M.D.**

BASIC INFORMATION

■ DEFINITION

Pertussis is a prolonged bacterial infection of the upper respiratory tract characterized by paroxysms of an intense cough.

■ SYNONYMS

Whooping cough

ICD-9CM CODES

033.9 Pertussis

■ EPIDEMIOLOGY

INCIDENCE (IN U.S.): Approximately 5000 new cases/yr (Fig. 1-290)
PREDOMINANT AGE:
• 50% in children <1 yr of age
• 20% in children >15 yr of age
PEAK INCIDENCE:
• Childhood
• Usually affects children <1 yr of age

■ PHYSICAL FINDINGS & CLINICAL PRESENTATION

• Usually begins with a 1- to 2-wk prodrome that resembles a common cold.
• Following this initial phase, increased production of mucus is noted.
• Increased mucus production is followed by an intense, paroxysmal cough, ending with gasps and an inspiratory whoop.
• In some children, cyanosis and anoxia are noted.
• When prolonged, frank exhaustion and even apnea occur.
• Pertussis is characterized by the finding of intense cough with a marked lymphocytosis.
• Improvement during the later stage is possible.
• High fever may be an indication of secondary bacterial pneumonia, which may be a later complication of pertussis.

■ ETIOLOGY

Gram-negative rod, *Bordetella pertussis,* which adheres to human cilia

DIAGNOSIS

■ DIFFERENTIAL DIAGNOSIS

• Croup
• Epiglottitis
• Foreign body aspiration
• Bacterial pneumonia

■ WORKUP

• Blood cultures
• Chest x-ray examination
• Culture of bacteria, usually from nasopharynx
• Immunofluorescent staining of nasopharyngeal secretions
• ELISA for detection of antibody to pertussis

■ LABORATORY TESTS

CBC, which usually demonstrates marked lymphocytosis:
  1. Up to 18,000 WBCs
  2. 70% to 80% lymphocytes

■ IMAGING STUDIES

Chest x-ray examination is of value if secondary bacterial pneumonia is suspected.

TREATMENT

■ ACUTE GENERAL Rx

• Intensive supportive care:
  1. Adequate hydration
  2. Control of secretions
  3. Maintenance of airway
• Antibiotics are indicated even though their ability to alter the course of the disease is controversial.
  1. Erythromycin 50 mg/kg/day for 14 days. Recent literature reports indicate that a 7-day treatment regimen may be as effective as a 14-day course of erythromycin.
  2. Although unproved, dexamethasone 1 mg/kg/day in 4 doses for severe, life-threatening paroxysms

  3. Ceftriaxone 75 mg/kg/day in 2 doses for broad coverage of secondary bacterial pneumonias
  4. Nafcillin or vancomycin when staphylococcal pneumonia is suspected
• Vaccination is successful in preventing the disease: universal vaccination is advised for all children <7 yr of age.
• Erythromycin is recommended for all close contacts in the household: trimethoprim/sulfamethoxazole in two oral doses per day for those intolerant to erythromycin.

■ DISPOSITION

Close attention to accepted vaccination schedules is the best prevention.

■ REFERRAL

To intensive care setting for life-threatening infections:
  1. Pulmonologist
  2. Infectious disease specialist

REFERENCES

He Q et al: Whooping cough caused by *Bordetella pertussis* and *Bordetella parapertussis* in an immunized population, *JAMA* 280:635, 1998.
Yaari E et al: Clinical manifestations of *Bordetella pertussis* infection in immunized children and young adults, *Chest* 115:1254, 1999.
Author: **Joseph J. Lieber, M.D.**

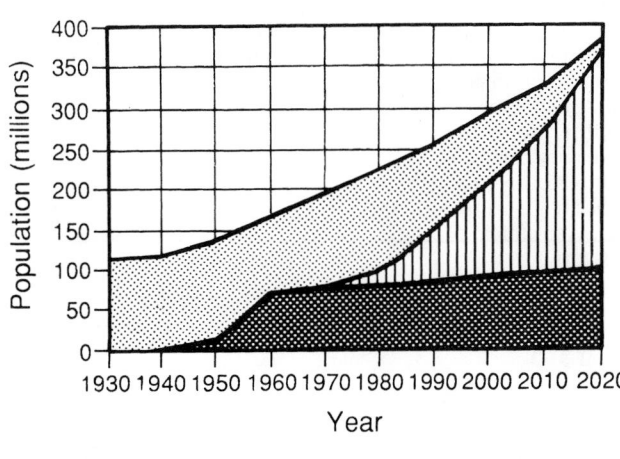

Fig. 1-290   Projected pertussis epidemiology in the United States through the year 2020 with continued use of present-day whole-cell pertussis vaccines. (Modified from Bass JW, Stephenson SR: *Pediatr Infect Dis J* 6:141, 1987.)

BASIC INFORMATION

■ DEFINITION
Peyronie's disease is an abnormal curvature and shortening of the penis during an erection (Fig. 1-291). This is caused by scarring of the tunica albuginea of the corpora cavernosa.

■ SYNONYMS
Plastic induration of the penis
Penile fibromatosis

■ ICD-9CM CODES
607.89 Peyronie's disease

■ EPIDEMIOLOGY & DEMOGRAPHICS
- Peyronie's disease occurs in approximately 1% of men (7:700).
- It is commonly seen between the ages of 45 to 60.
- A genetic predisposition has been suggested.
- There is no incidence and prevalence data available in the literature.

■ PHYSICAL FINDINGS & CLINICAL PRESENTATION
- Painful erections
- Tenderness over the scar tissue area
- Erectile dysfunction
- Curvature of the erected penis interfering with penetration
- Dupuytren's contracture is a commonly associated finding in patients with Peyronie's disease

■ ETIOLOGY
- The specific cause of the disease is not known. It is thought that scar tissue forms on either the dorsal or ventral midline surface of the penile shaft. The scar restricts expansion at the involved site, causing the penis to bend or curve in one direction.
- The precipitating factor appears to be trauma either from repetitive microvascular injury caused by vigorous sexual intercourse, accidents, or prior surgeries (e.g., transurethral prostatectomy or radical prostatectomy, cystoscopy).

DIAGNOSIS

■ DIFFERENTIAL DIAGNOSIS
- The history differentiates congenital from acquired curvature of the penis.
- Other causes of erectile dysfunction must be excluded including metabolic, diabetes, thyroid, renal, hypogonadism, and hyperprolactinemia.

■ WORKUP
History and physical examination alone usually will establish the diagnosis of Peyronie's disease.

■ LABORATORY TESTS
There are no specific blood tests to diagnose Peyronie's disease. Electrolytes, BUN, creatinine, glucose, thyroid function tests (TSH, T_3U, T_4), testosterone, and prolactin level are blood tests to obtain to exclude other medical causes of erectile dysfunction.

■ IMAGING STUDIES
Imaging studies are not specific.

TREATMENT

■ NONPHARMACOLOGIC THERAPY
A conservative approach of reassurance and observation is taken at first because the disease process may be self-limiting.

■ ACUTE GENERAL Rx
Although not substantiated by direct randomized, controlled clinical trials, the following treatment modalities have been tried:
- Vitamin E 400 mg bid
- Paraaminobenzoic acid 12 g/day
- Colchicine 0.6 mg bid for 2 to 3 wk
- Fexofenadine 60 mg bid for 3 mo
- Steroid injection into the scar tissue
- Collagenase injection into the scar tissue
- Radiation to the scar tissue area

■ CHRONIC Rx
In patients who have progressed to intractable pain with erection or erectile dysfunction, surgical treatment with excision of the plaque and skin grafting may be indicated.

■ DISPOSITION
Peyronie's disease evolves slowly and in some cases can resolve on its own.

Waiting for 1 yr before proceeding with surgical attempts is recommended.

■ REFERRAL
A urologic consultation is recommended in patients with progressive symptoms and erectile dysfunction.

✸ PEARLS & CONSIDERATIONS

■ COMMENTS
- Peyronie's disease is not commonly seen in younger patients because they are able to sustain intracorporeal pressures high enough to stretch the scar tissue, preventing it from deforming the penis during erection.
- Trauma from buckling of the erected penis is thought to be the precipitant cause of scar formation and Peyronie's disease. It is found more often in men who are sexually very active and vigorous, having sexual intercourse daily or almost daily.
- Sexual positions with the women being on top or thrusting the penis into the anterior vaginal wall is thought to increase the chances of developing Peyronie's disease.

REFERENCES
Carrieri MP et al: A case-control study on risk factors for Peyronie's disease, *J Clin Epidemiol* 51(6):511, 1998.
International Conference on Peyronie's Disease: Advances in basic and clinical research, March 17-19, 1993, *J Urol* 157(1):271, 1997.
Jordan GH, Schlossberg SM, Devine CJ: Surgery of the penis and urethra. In Walsh PC et al (eds): *Campbell's urology*, ed 7, Philadelphia, 1998, WB Saunders.
Author: **Peter Petropoulos, M.D.**

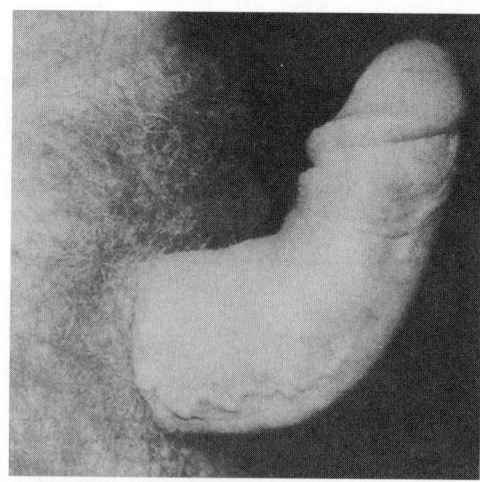

Fig. 1-291 Peyronie's disease. (Courtesy Patrick C, Walsh, MD, The Johns Hopkins University School of Medicine, Baltimore. In Seidel HM [ed]: *Mosby's guide to physical examination*, ed 4, St Louis, 1999, Mosby.)

BASIC INFORMATION

■ DEFINITION
Pharyngitis/tonsillitis is inflammation of the pharynx or tonsils.

■ SYNONYMS
Sore throat

ICD-9CM CODES
462 Pharyngitis

■ EPIDEMIOLOGY & DEMOGRAPHICS
PREDOMINANT SEX: Female = male
PREDOMINANT AGE:
- All ages affected
- Streptococcal pharyngitis most common among school-age children

PEAK INCIDENCE: Late winter/early spring (group A streptococcal infections)
GENETICS:
Neonatal Infection: Pharyngitis below the age of 3 yr is almost always of viral etiology.

■ PHYSICAL FINDINGS & CLINICAL PRESENTATION
- Pharynx (Fig. 1-292):
  1. May appear normal to severely erythematous
  2. Tonsillar hypertrophy and exudates commonly seen but do not indicate etiology
- Viral infection:
  1. Rhinorrhea
  2. Conjunctivitis
  3. Cough
- Bacterial infection, especially group A *Streptococcus:*
  1. High fever
  2. Systemic signs of infection
- Herpes simplex or enterovirus infection: vesicles
- Streptococcal infection:
  1. Rare complications:
     a. Scarlet fever
     b. Rheumatic fever
     c. Acute glomerulonephritis
  2. Extension of infection: tonsillar, parapharyngeal, or retropharyngeal abscess presenting with severe pain, high fever, trismus

■ ETIOLOGY
- Viruses:
  1. Respiratory syncytial virus
  2. Influenza A and B
  3. Epstein-Barr virus
  4. Adenovirus
  5. Herpes simplex
- Bacteria:
  1. *Streptococcus pyogenes*
  2. *Neisseria gonorrhoeae*
  3. *Arcanobacterium haemolyticum*
- Other organisms:
  1. *Mycoplasma pneumoniae*
  2. *Chlamydia pneumoniae*

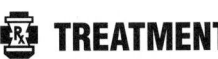

DIAGNOSIS

■ DIFFERENTIAL DIAGNOSIS
- Sore throat associated with granulocytopenia, thyroiditis
- Tonsillar hypertrophy associated with lymphoma
- Table 2-188 describes the differential diagnosis of sore throat.

■ WORKUP
- Throat swab for culture to exclude *S. pyogenes, N. gonorrhoeae* (requires specific transport medium)
- Rapid streptococcal antigen test (culture should be performed if rapid test negative)
- Monospot

■ LABORATORY TESTS
- CBC with differential
  1. May help support diagnosis of bacterial infection
  2. Streptococcal infection suggested by leukocytosis >15,000/mm^3
- Viral cultures, serologic studies rarely needed

■ IMAGING STUDIES
Seldom indicated

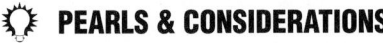

TREATMENT

■ NONPHARMACOLOGIC THERAPY
- Fluids
- Salt water gargles

■ ACUTE GENERAL Rx
- Aspirin (acetaminophen culture)
- If streptococcal infection proven or suspected:
  1. Penicillin V 500 mg PO bid for 10 days or benzathine penicillin 1.2 million U IM once (adults)
  2. Erythromycin 500 mg PO bid or 250 mg qid for 10 days if penicillin allergic
- If gonococcal infection proven or suspected: ceftriaxone 125 mg IM once

■ CHRONIC Rx
Recurrent streptococcal infections are common and may represent reinfection from other household members.

■ REFERRAL
- To otolaryngologist:
  1. If peritonsillar or other abscess is suspected
  2. If tonsillar hypertrophy persists
- To infectious diseases expert if unusual pathogen is suspected

PEARLS & CONSIDERATIONS

■ COMMENTS
Antibiotic therapy should be avoided unless bacterial etiology is suspected or proven, especially in adults.

REFERENCES
Bisno AL: Acute pharyngitis, *N Engl J Med* 344:205, 2001.
Snow V et al: Principles of appropriate antibiotic use for acute pharyngitis in adults, *Ann Intern Med* 134:506, 2001.
Woods WA et al: Group A streptococcal pharyngitis in adults 30 to 65 years of age, *South Med J* 92(5):491, 1999.
Author: **Joseph R. Masci, M.D.**

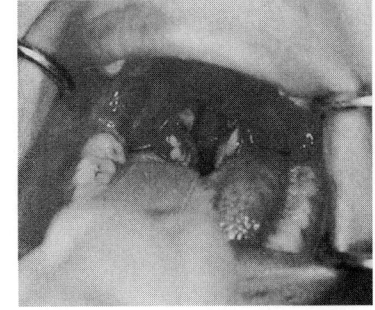
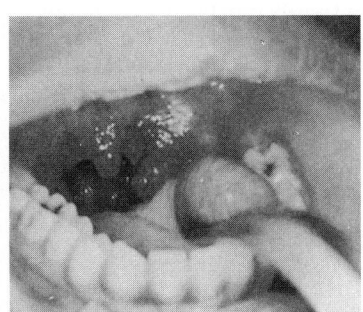

Fig. 1-292 Findings of the oropharynx. **A,** Tonsillitis and pharyngitis. **B,** Acute viral pharyngitis. (Courtesy Edward L. Applebaum, MD, Head, Department of Otolaryngology, University of Illinois Medical Center, Chicago. In Barkauskas VH et al: *Health and physical assessment,* ed 2, St Louis, 1998, Mosby.)

BASIC INFORMATION

■ DEFINITION
Pheochromocytomas are catecholamine-producing tumors that originate from chromaffin cells of the adrenergic system. They generally secrete both norepinephrine and epinephrine, but norepinephrine is usually the predominant amine.

■ SYNONYMS
Paraganglioma

ICD-9CM CODES
194.0 Pheochromocytoma

■ EPIDEMIOLOGY & DEMOGRAPHICS
- Incidence: 0.05% of population; peak incidence in 30s and 40s.
- "Rough" rule of 10: 10% are extra-adrenal, 10% are malignant, 10% are familial, 10% occur in children, 10% involve both adrenals, 10% are multiple (other than bilateral adrenal).
- Pheochromocytoma is a feature of two disorders with autosomal dominant pattern of inheritance:
  1. Multiple endocrine neoplasia II
  2. Von Hippel-Lindau disease: angioma of the retina, hemangioblastoma of the CNS, renal cell carcinoma, pancreatic cysts, and epididymal cystoadenoma
- Pheochromocytomas occur in 5% of patients with neurofibromatosis type 1.

■ PHYSICAL FINDINGS & CLINICAL PRESENTATION
- Hypertension: can be sustained (55%) or paroxysmal (45%).
- Headache (80%): usually paroxysmal in nature and described as "pounding" and severe.
- Palpitations (70%): can be present with or without tachycardia.
- Hyperhidrosis (60%): most evident during paroxysmal attacks of hypertension.
- Physical examination may be entirely normal if done in a symptom-free interval; during a paroxysm the patient may demonstrate marked increase in both systolic and diastolic pressure, profuse sweating, visual disturbances (caused by hypertensive retinopathy), dilated pupils (secondary to catecholamine excess), paresthesias in the lower extremities (caused by severe vasoconstriction), tremor, tachycardia.

■ ETIOLOGY
- Catecholamine-producing tumors that are usually located in the adrenal medulla.
- Specific mutations of the RET proto-oncogene cause familial predisposition to pheochromocytoma in MEN II.
- Mutations in the von Hippel-Lindau tumor suppressor gene cause familial disposition to pheochromocytoma in von Hippel-Lindau disease.

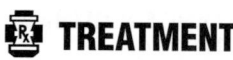

DIAGNOSIS

■ DIFFERENTIAL DIAGNOSIS
- Anxiety disorder
- Thyrotoxicosis
- Amphetamine or cocaine abuse
- Carcinoid
- Essential hypertension

■ WORKUP
Laboratory evaluation and imaging studies to locate the neoplasm; a diagnostic approach to adrenal mass is described in Fig. 3-5.

■ LABORATORY TESTS
- Measurements of plasma levels of free metanephrines is an effective initial test to diagnose pheochromocytomas. Plasma concentrations of normetanephrines >2.5 pmol/ml or metanephrine levels >1.4 pmol/ml indicate a pheochromocytoma with 100% specificity.
- 24-hr urine collection for metanephrines (100% sensitive) will also show increased metanephrines; the accuracy of the 24-hr urinary levels for metanephrines can be improved by indexing urinary metanephrine levels by urine creatinine levels.
- The clonidine suppression test is useful for distinguishing between high levels of plasma norepinephrine caused by release from sympathetic nerves and those caused by release from a pheochromocytoma. A decrease <50% in plasma norepinephrine levels after clonidine administration is normal, whereas persistent elevations are indicative of pheochromocytoma.

■ IMAGING STUDIES
- Abdominal CT scan (88% sensitivity) is useful in locating pheochromocytomas >0.5 inch in diameter (90% to 95% accurate).
- MRI: pheochromocytomas demonstrate a distinctive MRI appearance (100% sensitivity); MRI may become the diagnostic imaging modality of choice.
- Scintigraphy with ^{131}I-MIBG (100% sensitivity): this norepinephrine analog localizes in adrenergic tissue; it is particularly useful in locating extraadrenal pheochromocytomas.
- 6 [^{18}F] Fluorodopamine positron emission tomography is reserved for cases in which clinical symptoms and signs suggest pheochromocytoma and results of biochemical tests are positive but conventional imaging studies cannot locate the tumor. An alternative approach is to use vena caval sampling for plasma cathecholamines and metanephrines.

TREATMENT

■ ACUTE GENERAL Rx
Laparoscopic removal of the tumor (surgical resection for both benign and malignant disease):
1. Preoperative stabilization with combination of phenoxybenzamine, β blocker, metyrosine, and liberal fluid and salt intake starting 10 to 14 days before surgery.
   a. Volume expansion is done to prevent postoperative hypotension.
   b. α-Blockade to control hypertension: phenoxybenzamine (Dibenzyline) 5 mg PO bid initially, gradually increased to 10 mg q3d up to 50-100 mg bid; prazosin may be used when phenoxybenzamine therapy alone is not effective or not well tolerated.
   c. β-Blockade with propranolol 20 to 40 mg PO q6h (to be used only after α-blockade) is useful to prevent catecholamine-induced arrhythmias and tachycardia.
   d. Metyrosine reduces tumor stores of catecholamines, decreases need for intraoperative medication to control blood pressure, and lowers intraoperative fluid requirements.

2. Hypertensive crisis preoperatively and intraoperatively should be controlled with phentolamine (Regitine) 2 to 5 mg IV q1-2h PRN or nitroprusside used in combination with β-adrenergic blockers.
3. Combination chemotherapy with cyclophosphamide, vincristine, and dacarbazine is useful for symptomatic advanced malignant pheochromocytoma.

■ DISPOSITION
- The 5-yr survival rate is approximately 95% with benign disease, 40% for malignant pheochromocytoma (malignancy is determined by metastasis).
- Pheochromocytomas are three times more likely to be malignant in women.

- Postoperative follow-up of patients with sporadic and familial forms should include plasma metanephrine levels after 6 wk, 6 mo, and then annually.

⚙ PEARLS & CONSIDERATIONS

■ COMMENTS
- Screening for pheochromocytoma should be considered in patients with any of the following:
  1. Malignant hypertension
  2. Poor response to antihypertensive therapy
  3. Paradoxical hypertensive response
  4. Hypertension during induction of anesthesia, parturition, surgery, or thyrotropin-releasing hormone testing

  5. Hypertension associated with imipramine or desipramine
  6. Neurofibromatosis (increased incidence of pheochromocytoma)
- All patients with pheochromocytoma should be screened for MEN-II and von Hippel-Lindau disease with pentagastrin test, serum PTH, ophthalmoscopy, MRI of the brain, CT scan of the kidneys and pancreas, and ultrasonography of the testes.

REFERENCE
Pacak R: Recent advances in genetics, diagnosis, localization, and treatment of pheochromocytoma, *Ann Intern Med* 134:315, 2001.
Author: **Fred F. Ferri, M.D.**

BASIC INFORMATION

■ DEFINITION

A phobia is severe anxiety that is elicited by a specific object or situation and that often leads to avoidance behavior. The provoking stimuli may be social or performance situations (social phobia) or any other stimulus (specific phobia of animals, natural environments, blood, or situational).

■ SYNONYMS

Simple phobia (obsolete name for specific phobia)
Phobias named according to the inducing stimulus, e.g., arachnophobia (fear of spiders), claustrophobia (fear of tight spaces), kneebophobia (fear of knee bending backward)
Social anxiety disorder (obsolete name for social phobias)

ICD-9CM CODES

F40.2 Specific phobia (DSM-IV: 300.29)
F40.1 Social phobia (DMS-IV: 300.23)

■ EPIDEMIOLOGY & DEMOGRAPHICS

PREVALENCE (IN U.S.):
- For specific phobias, the 1-yr prevalence rate is 9% and the lifetime rates range from 10% to 11.3%.
- For social phobias, prevalence rates of 3% to 13% have been reported, but only about 2% experience a significant degree of impairment to warrant clinical concern or intervention.

PREDOMINANT SEX:
- Females with specific phobias outnumber males.
- Rates vary according to the phobia (e.g., of individuals with animal or nature phobias, 75% to 90% are female; of individuals who fear blood, 55% to 70% are female; of people with situational fears, 75% to 70% are female). Similarly, more women are affected with social phobia; however, men are more likely to seek treatment.

PREDOMINANT AGE:
- Onset of most specific phobias is in childhood.
- Major exceptions: situational phobias, which have two peaks—the first in childhood and the second in the mid-20s.
- Once developed, fears are stable.
- Roots of social phobia may be in childhood, with described shyness or social inhibition, but onset usually in the midteens or into late adulthood; disorder is generally lifelong.

PEAK INCIDENCE:
- Specific phobias: lifelong condition
- Social phobia: may alternate in mid-to-late adulthood

GENETICS: Both specific phobias and social phobias are more common in first-degree relatives than the general population; however, this does not necessarily mean a genetic etiology.

■ PHYSICAL FINDINGS & CLINICAL PRESENTATION

- Specific phobias: frequently have other anxiety disorders, particularly panic and agoraphobias; most phobias are associated with sinus tachycardia on exposure to the stimulus, although blood phobias frequently (in 75% of those afflicted) are associated with sinus bradycardia, hypotension, and fainting.
- Social phobias: usually have low self-esteem and fear of evaluation from others; avoid or are fearful of any situation in which others may assess or evaluate them directly or indirectly; concurrent anxiety disorders are common, but these persons are less likely to develop panic than panic disorder patients when challenged with panicogenic lactate infusion or CO_2 inhalation.

■ ETIOLOGY

- Unknown
- Biologic features probably a relatively small component

DIAGNOSIS

■ DIFFERENTIAL DIAGNOSIS

- Panic attacks: anxiety symptoms seen in specific phobia may resemble panic attacks, but the stimulus in specific phobias or social phobias is clear, whereas panic attacks seem more random.
- Generalized anxiety disorder: difficult to distinguish from social phobia, but in social phobia the cognitive focus is fear of embarrassment or humiliation, whereas in generalized anxiety disorder the focus is more internal on the subjective sensations of discomfort.

■ WORKUP

- History: usually diagnostic
- Physical examination: to confirm absence of cardiovascular abnormalities (e.g., a chronic sinus arrhythmia)

■ LABORATORY TESTS

No specific laboratory tests are indicated.

■ IMAGING STUDIES

If phobias are associated with fainting, a cardiac workup (EEG, Holter) may be indicated.

TREATMENT

■ NONPHARMACOLOGIC THERAPY

- Treatment of choice for specific phobias is desensitization.
- Cognitive-behavioral therapy and other psychotherapeutic approaches are effective.
- Success rates are higher when the phobia is not complicated by other anxiety disorders.
- Social phobia is more problematic to treat because the psychologic difficulties are more pervasive, but cognitive-behavioral therapy and other psychotherapies are quite effective.
- For social phobia, psychotherapy is almost always required, at least as adjunct.

■ ACUTE GENERAL Rx

- Benzodiazepines: provide rapid, effective relief of anxiety associated with exposure to fearful stimuli
- Alprazolam or lorazepam: both administered sublingually to increase rate of absorption
- β-Blockers: given before exposure to the fearful stimulus (e.g., before a public speech); the lipophilic β-blockers are preferred
- Acute management of anxiety symptoms: not advisable in view of chronicity of the symptoms of social phobia

■ CHRONIC Rx

- If the phobic stimulus is encountered rarely and unexpectedly, benzodiazepines may be appropriate long-term treatment.
- If the phobic stimulus can be anticipated, β-blockers may be appropriate long-term treatment.
- Social phobia is a chronic condition. Individuals with social phobia often underachieve, drop out of school, avoid seeking work as a result of anxiety about interviews, refrain from dating and remain with family of origin, and are less likely to marry. In addition to this social and occupational dysfunction, these individuals lead very unfulfilled lives.
- Paroxetine is effective in social anxiety disorder.

■ REFERRAL

If psychotherapy advised

Authors: **Rif S. El-Mallakh, M.D., and Peggy L. El-Mallakh, B.S.N.**

BASIC INFORMATION

■ DEFINITION
A *pilonidal sinus* is a short tract that extends from the skin surface, is most commonly found in the intergluteal fold, and most likely represents a distended hair follicle. An *acute pilonidal abscess*, which consists of pus and a wall of edematous fat, results from rupture of an infected follicle into fat. A *chronic pilonidal abscess* results when an infected follicle ruptures directly into surround tissues; the wall of a chronic pilonidal abscess consists of fibrous tissue. A *pilonidal cyst* develops from a chronic abscess of long duration as a thin and flat lining of epithelium grows into the cavity from the skin surface.

■ SYNONYMS
Jeep disease

ICD-9CM CODES
685.1 Pilonidal cyst

■ EPIDEMIOLOGY & DEMOGRAPHICS
INCIDENCE: 26 cases/100,000 persons
PREDOMINANT SEX: Male > female (2.2:1)
AVERAGE AGE OF PRESENTATION: 21 yr
GENETICS: Theory of congenital origin is now disfavored.
RISK FACTORS:
- Male sex
- Caucasian race
- Family predisposition
- Obesity
- Sedentary lifestyle
- Occupation requiring prolonged sitting
- Local hirsutism
- Poor hygiene
- Increased sweat activity

■ PHYSICAL FINDINGS & CLINICAL PRESENTATION
- May manifest as asymptomatic pits or pores in the natal cleft
- Tenderness after physical activity or prolonged sitting
- Acute pilonidal abscess in 20% of patients with pilonidal disease
- Presents as a hot, tender, fluctuant swelling just lateral to the midline over the sacrum that may exude pus through the midline pit
- Chronic pilonidal abscess in 80% of patients with pilonidal disease
- Acute suppuration, tenderness, swelling, and heat
- Infrequently, systemic reaction: occasionally fever, leukocytosis, and malaise

■ ETIOLOGY
- Currently, thought to be acquired rather than congenital.
- Drilling of hair shed from the perineum or the head into sebaceous or hair follicles in the natal cleft.
- Drilling is facilitated by the friction of the natal cleft.
- Subsequent infection by skin organisms leads to pilonidal abscess.

DIAGNOSIS

■ DIFFERENTIAL DIAGNOSIS
- Perianal abscess arising from the posterior midline crypt
- Hidradenitis suppurativa
- Carbuncle
- Furuncle
- Osteomyelitis
- Anal fistula
- Coccygeal sinus

■ WORKUP
- Diagnosis is based on history and physical exmaination.
- Midline pits present behind the anus overlying the sacrum and coccyx.
- Broken hairs are often seen extruding from the midline pits.
- Insert probe in pilonidal sinus in path away from the anus.
- Complicated anal fistula may be angulating posteriorly before passing into a retrorectal abscess, but thorough examination of the anal cavity usually discloses point of origin.

■ LABORATORY TESTS
CBC

■ IMAGING STUDIES
CT scan in advanced recurrent cases

TREATMENT

■ NONPHARMACOLOGIC THERAPY
Prevention of exacerbations:
1. Local hygiene
2. Avoidance of prolonged sitting position
3. Weight reduction

■ ACUTE GENERAL Rx
- Procedure of choice for first-episode acute abscess: simple incision and drainage in an outpatient setting
- Cure rate of 76% after 18 mo
- Antibiotics: generally not indicated unless the patient has a medical condition such as rheumatic heart disease or is immunosuppressed

■ CHRONIC Rx
Elective treatment of pilonidal disease:
1. Minimal surgery
   a. Remove hair from midline pits and shave buttocks.
   b. May use a fine wire brush with local anesthesia to clear the pits and any lateral openings of granulation tissue and hair.
   c. Keep area clean.
2. Opening of sinus tracts
   a. Used when minimal surgery does not control episodes of suppuration.
   b. Pass probe to outline the pilonidal sinus and open tract surgically.
   c. Curette granulation tissue at the base of the sinus and excise edges of the skin.
   d. Keep open granulating wound meticulously clean and allow to heal.
   e. If complete healing does not take place, use a skin graft or advancement flap to close the defect.
3. Excision
   a. This is the treatment of choice for chronic pilonidal disease.
   b. Wide excision of the pilonidal area is performed, including all affected skin and subcutaneous tissues down to the presacral fascia.
   c. Wound is left open, allowed to marsupialize, or closed as a primary procedure.
   d. Give antibiotics for 24 hr (particularly those directed against *Staphylococcus* and *Bacteroides* spp).

■ DISPOSITION
Recurrence rate for excision (most definitive procedure): 1% to 6%

■ REFERRAL
- Emergency room for incision and drainage for an acute abscess
- To a surgeon for elective treatment or management of chronic or recurrent disease.

PEARLS & CONSIDERATIONS

■ COMMENTS
Because of significant associated morbidity, the elective surgical procedures outlined are performed only after the potential risks vs. benefits are carefully weighed.

REFERENCES
Nyhus LM, Baker RJ, Fischer JE (eds): *Mastery of surgery*, ed 3, vol 2, Boston, 1997, Little, Brown.
Sebastian MW: Pilonidal cysts and sinuses. In Sabiston DC Jr (ed): *Textbook of surgery: the biologic basis of modern surgical practice*, Philadelphia, 1997, WB Saunders.
Spivak H et al: Treatment of chronic pilonidal disease, *Dis Colon Rectum* 39:1136, 1996.
Author: **Wan J. Kim, M.D.**

BASIC INFORMATION

■ DEFINITION
Pinworms are a noninvasive infestation of the intestinal tract by *Enterobius vermicularis,* a helminth of the nematode family.

■ SYNONYMS
Enterobiasis

ICD-9CM CODES
127.4 Enterobiasis

■ EPIDEMIOLOGY & DEMOGRAPHICS
- Most common intestinal nematode with approximately 30,000 cases/year in the U.S.
- Worldwide distribution, but most common in temperate climates.
- Highest infection rate in school-age children.
- Clusters are found in families, institutionalized persons, and homosexual men.

■ PHYSICAL FINDINGS & CLINICAL PRESENTATION
- Most infested persons are asymptomatic.
- Perianal itching is the most common reported symptom, with scratching leading to excoriation and sometimes secondary infection.
- Rarely insomnia, irritability, anorexia, and weight loss are described.
- Granulomas have been described in various organs resulting from worms wandering outside the intestines and dying there.

■ ETIOLOGY & PATHOGENESIS
Humans are the only host for this worm. Infestation is by fecal-oral route; ingested eggs hatch in the stomach and the larvae migrate to the colon where they mature. Gravid female worms migrate to the perianal skin at night, lay their eggs there, and die. The eggs cause itching; scratching causes egg deposition under fingernails, from which they can contaminate food or lead to autoreinfection.

DIAGNOSIS

■ DIFFERENTIAL DIAGNOSIS
- Perianal itching related to poor hygiene.
- Hemorrhoidal disease and anal fissures.
- Perineal yeast/fungal infections.
- Box 2-211 describes the causes of pruritus ani.

■ WORKUP
Identification of adult worms or eggs (Fig. 1-293) on transparent tape placed on the perianal skin upon awakening (NOTE: Five consecutive negative tests rule out the diagnosis).

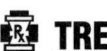

TREATMENT

Single dose of mebendazole or pyrantel pamoate repeated after 2 to 3 wk

REFERENCE
Hamer DH, Despommier DD: Intestinal nematodes. In Gorbach SL, Bartlett JG, Blacklow NR (eds): *Infectious diseases,* ed 2, Philadelphia, 1998, WB Saunders.
Author: **Tom J. Wachtel, M.D.**

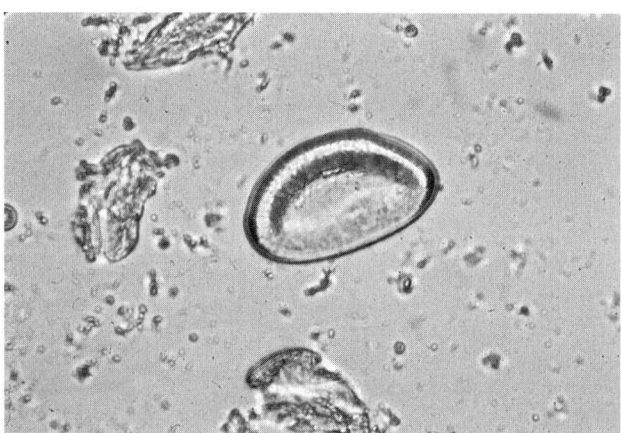

Fig. 1-293 *Enterobius vermicularis* embryonated egg. Note larva inside (40 × 10 μm). (From Gorbach SL, Bartlett JG, Blacklow NR (eds): *Infectious diseases,* ed 2, Philadelphia, 1998, WB Saunders.)

BASIC INFORMATION

■ **DEFINITION**

Pituitary adenoma is a benign neoplasm of the anterior lobe of the pituitary that causes symptoms, either by excess secretion of hormones or by a local mass effect as the tumor impinges on other, nearby structures (e.g., optic chiasm, hypothalamus, pituitary stalk). Pituitary adenomas are classified by their size, function, and features that characterize their appearance. Microadenomas are <10 mm in size, and macroadenomas are >10 mm in size.

- *Acromegaly* is the disease state characterized by a pituitary adenoma that secretes growth hormone (GH).
- A *prolactinoma* secretes prolactin (PRL).
- *Cushing's disease* is a disease state in which there is hypersecretion of adrenocorticotropic hormone (ACTH).
- *Thyrotropin-secreting pituitary adenomas* secrete primarily thyroid-stimulating hormone (TSH).
- *Nonsecretory pituitary adenomas* are those in which the neoplasm is a space-occupying lesion whose secretory products do not cause a specific disease state.

ICD-9CM CODES

253 Pituitary adenoma
253.0 Acromegaly
253.1 Prolactinoma

■ **EPIDEMIOLOGY & DEMOGRAPHICS**

CLASSIFICATION (BY HORMONE SECRETED):

- PRL only ~35%
- No hormone ~30%
- GH only −20%
- PRL and GH ~7%
- ACTH ~7%
- LF/FSH/TSH ~1%

PREVALENCE/INCIDENCE:

Pituitary Adenomas: Up to 10% to 15% of all intracranial neoplasms; 3% to 27% autopsy series

Prolactinomas: Up to 20% in women with unexplained primary or secondary amenorrhea

Growth Hormone–Secreting Pituitary Adenoma: 50 to 60 cases/1,000,000 persons

Thyrotropin-Secreting Pituitary Adenoma: 2.8% of pituitary adenomas with a slight female:male predominance of 1.7:1

Corticotropin-Secreting Pituitary Adenomas: Female:male predominance of 8:1

■ **PHYSICAL FINDINGS**
PROLACTINOMAS:

- Females:
  1. Galactorrhea
  2. Amenorrhea
  3. Oligomenorrhea with anovulation
  4. Infertility
  5. Estrogen deficiency leading to hirsutism
  6. Decreased vaginal lubrication
  7. Osteopenia
- Males:
  1. Large tumors more common secondary to delayed diagnosis
  2. Possible impotence or decreased libido or hypogonadism
  3. Galactorrhea rare because males lack the estrogen-dependent breast growth and differentiation

GROWTH HORMONE–SECRETING PITUITARY ADENOMA: Acromegaly

- Coarse facial features
- Oily skin
- Prognathism
- Carpal tunnel syndrome
- Osteoarthritis
- History of increased hat, glove, or shoe size
- Decreased exercise capacity
- Visual field deficits
- Diabetes mellitus

CORTICOTROPIN-SECRETING PITUITARY ADENOMA: Cushing's disease

- Usually present when the tumor is small (1 to 2 mm)
- 50% of the tumors <5 mm
- Other symptoms:
  1. Truncal obesity
  2. Round facies (moon face)
  3. Dorsocervical fat accumulation (buffalo hump)
  4. Hirsutism
  5. Acne
  6. Menstrual disorders
  7. Hypertension
  8. Striae
  9. Bruising
  10. Thin skin
  11. Hyperglycemia

THYROTROPIN-SECRETING PITUITARY ADENOMA:

- In males, larger, more invasive, and more rapidly growing tumors that present later in life
- Other symptoms: thyrotoxicosis, goiter, visual impairment

NONSECRETORY PITUITARY ADENOMAS (ENDOCRINE INACTIVE PITUITARY ADENOMA):

- Usually large at the time of diagnosis
- Symptoms:
  1. Bitemporal hemianopia secondary to compression of the optic chiasm
  2. Hypopituitarism secondary to compression of the pituitary gland

  3. Hypogonadism in men and in premenopausal women
  4. Cranial nerve deficits, secondary to extension into the cavernous sinus
  5. Hydrocephalus, secondary to extension into the third ventricle, compressing the foramen of Monro
  6. Diabetes insipidus, secondary to compression of the hypothalamus or pituitary stalk (a rare complication)

■ **ETIOLOGY**

Benign neoplasms of epithelial origin

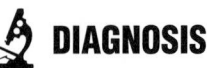 **DIAGNOSIS**

■ **DIFFERENTIAL DIAGNOSIS**
PROLACTINOMA:

- Pregnancy
- Postpartum puerperium
- Primary hypothyroidism
- Breast disease
- Breast stimulation
- Drug ingestion (especially phenothiazines, antidepressants, haloperidol, methyldopa, reserpine, opiates, amphetamines, and cimetidine)
- Chronic renal failure
- Liver disease
- Polycystic ovarian disease
- Chest wall disorders
- Spinal cord lesions
- Previous cranial irradiation

ACROMEGALY: Ectopic production of growth hormone–releasing hormone from a carcinoid or other neuroendocrine tumor

CUSHING'S DISEASE:

- Diseases that cause ectopic sources of ACTH overproduction (including small cell carcinoma of the lung, bronchial carcinoid, intestinal carcinoid, pancreatic islet cell tumor, medullary thyroid carcinoma, or pheochromocytoma)
- Adrenal adenomas, adrenal carcinoma
- Nelson's syndrome

THYROTROPIN-SECRETNG PITUITARY ADENOMAS: Primary hypothyroidism
NONSECRETORY PITUITARY ADENOMA: Nonneoplastic mass lesions of various etiologies (e.g., infectious, granulomatous)

■ **WORKUP** (FIG. 1-294)

PROLACTINOMA: First step: Measurement of basal PRL levels

- Elevated PRL levels are correlated with tumor size.
- Levels >200 ng/ml are diagnostic, with levels of 100 to 200 ng/ml being equivocal.

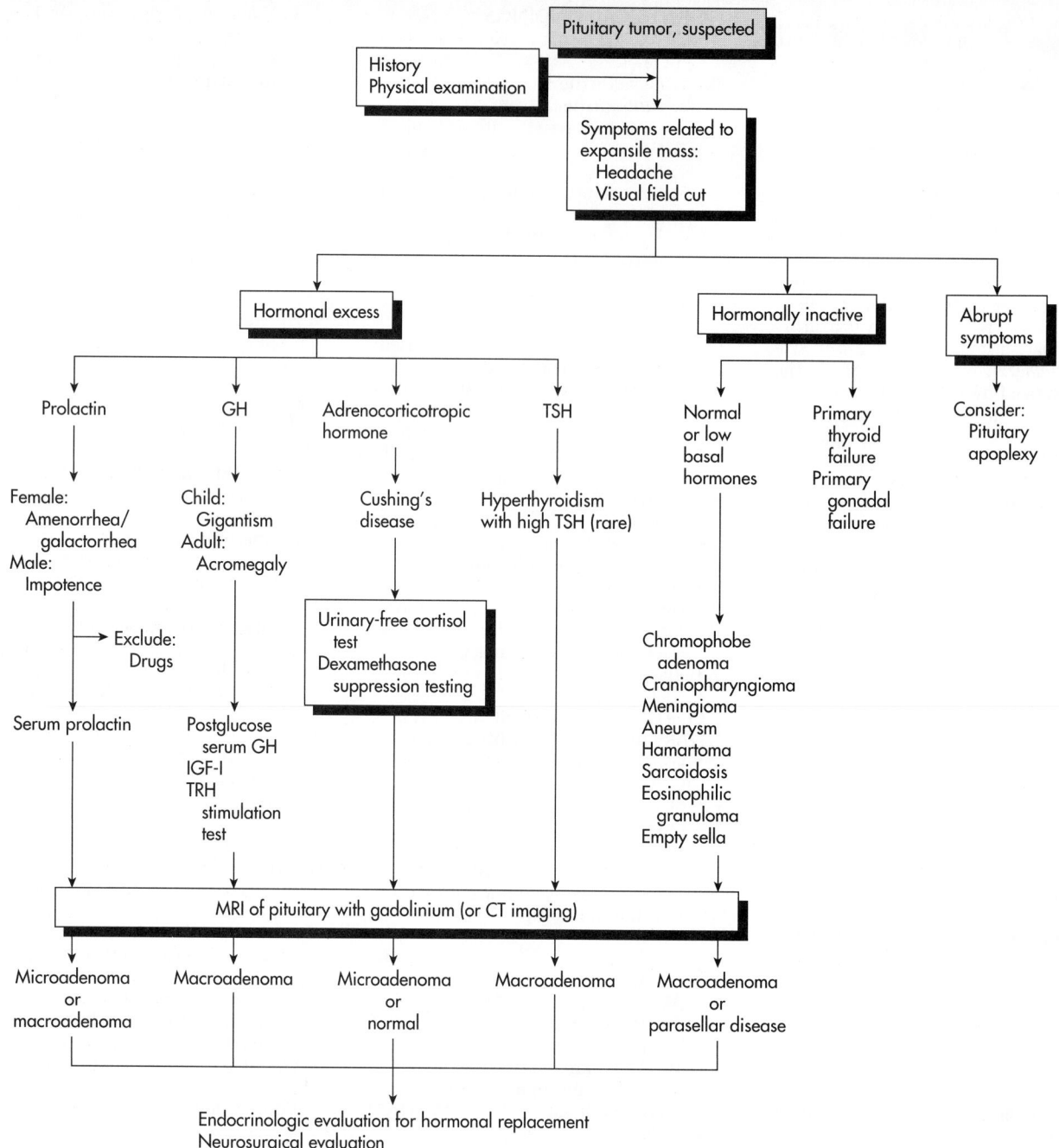

Fig. 1-294   Evaluation of suspected pituitary tumor. *CT,* Computed tomography; *GH,* growth hormone; *IGF-I,* one of the insulin-like growth factors; *MRI,* magnetic resonance imaging; *TRH,* thyrotropin-releasing hormone; *TSH,* thyroid-stimulating hormone. (From Greene HL, Johnson WP, Lemcke D: *Decision making in medicine,* ed 2, St Louis, 1998, Mosby.)

- Basal PRL levels between 20 and 100 suggest a microprolactinoma, as well as other conditions such as drug ingestion
- Basal level <20 is normal.

ACROMEGALY:
- First screening test is the measurement of the serum IGF-I level, post serum GH, TRH stimulation test.
- Follow with an oral glucose tolerance test.
- Failure to suppress serum GH to <2 ng/ml with an oral load of 100 g glucose is considered conclusive.
- A GHRH level >300 ng/ml is indicative of an ectopic source of GH.

CUSHING'S DISEASE:
- Normal or slightly elevated corticotropin levels ranging from 20 to 200 pg/ml; normal is 10 to 50 pg/ml.
- Levels <10 pg/ml usually indicate an autonomously secreting adrenal tumor.
- Levels >200 pg/ml suggest an ectopic corticotropin-secreting neoplasm.
- Cushing's disease is confirmed by demonstration of low-dose dexamethasone, which shows presence of abnormal cortisol suppressibility.
- 24-hr urine collection should demonstrate an increased level of cortisol excretion.

THYROTROPIN-SECRETING PITUITARY ADENOMA:
- Highly sensitive thyrotropin assays, which evaluate the presence of thyrotoxicosis, are one way to detect a thyrotropin-secreting tumor.
- Free alpha subunit is secreted by >80% of tumors with the ratio of the alpha subunit to thyrotropin >1.
- With central resistance to thyroid hormone, ratio is <1 and the sella is normal.
- Laboratory tests show elevated serum levels of both T_3 and T_4.

NONSECRETORY PITUITARY ADENOMA:
- Visual field testing
- Assessment of the pituitary and organ function to determine if there is hypopituitarism or hypersecretion of hormones (even if the effects of hypersecretion are subclinical)
- TRH to provoke secretion of FSH, LH, and LH-beta-subunit; will not elicit response in normal persons
- Exclusion of Klinefelter's syndrome in patient with long-standing primary hypogonadism, elevated gonadotropin levels, and enlargement of the sella

■ IMAGING STUDIES
- Study of choice: MRI of the pituitary and hypothalamus
  1. When evaluating Cushing's disease, small size at the onset of symptoms noted
- MRI, in this case, only 60% sensitive at best and may yield false positive results
- CT scan only when MRI is unavailable or is otherwise contraindicated

℞ TREATMENT

■ NONPHARMACOLOGIC THERAPY
SURGERY:
- Selective transsphenoidal resection of the adenoma is the treatment of choice for prolactinoma, acromegaly, Cushing's disease, and thyrotropin-secreting pituitary adenomas, which all tend to be microadenomas at the time of onset of symptoms.
- Macroadenomas, such as the nonsecretory pituitary adenoma, may also be surgically removed, but risk of recurrence is greater with these tumors, and adjunctive therapy such as irradiation may also be necessary.
- Radiotherapy is reserved for patients who have failed surgical treatment and who still experience the symptoms of their adenoma.
- Bilateral adrenalectomy has been done in patients with Cushing's disease on failure of other therapies; complications requiring lifelong hormone replacement or Nelson's syndrome may occur.

RADIOTHERAPY:
- Generally reserved for patients who have failed surgical treatment
- Used with varying degrees of success in all of the different pituitary adenomas

■ PHARMACOLOGIC THERAPY
PROLACTINOMA:
- Bromocriptine, a dopamine analog, is generally given orally in divided doses of 1.5 to 10 mg.
- Side effects include orthostatic hypotension, nausea, and dizziness; avoided by beginning with low-dose therapy.
- Other compounds under investigation include pergolide mesylate, a long-acting ergot derivative with dopaminergic properties, as well as other nonergot derivatives.

ACROMEGALY:
- Octreotide, a somatostatin analog, 100 µg SC, is the medical therapy of choice but is limited by side effects such as biliary sludge and gallstones, nausea, cramps, steatorrhea, and its parenteral administration.
- Bromocriptine 10 to 69 mg PO tid-qid is less effective than octreotide, but has the advantage of oral administration.

CUSHING'S DISEASE:
- Ketoconazole, which inhibits the cytochrome P-450 enzymes involved in steroid biosynthesis, is effective in managing mild to moderate disease in daily oral dosages of 600 to 1200 mg.
- Metyrapone and aminoglutethimide can be used to control hypersecretion of cortisol but are generally used when preparing a patient for surgery or while waiting for a response to radiotherapy.

THYROTROPIN-SECRETING PITUITARY ADENOMA:
- Ablative therapy with either radioactive iodide or surgery is indicated.
- Treatment directed to the thyroid alone may accelerate growth of the pituitary adenoma.
- Octreotide has been shown to be effective in doses similar to those used for acromegaly.

NONSECRETORY PITUITARY ADENOMA:
- There is no role for medical therapy at this time
- Surgery and radiotherapy are indicated.

■ CHRONIC Rx
For all pituitary adenomas:
- Careful follow-up is important. Patients undergoing transsphenoidal microsurgical resection should be seen in 4 to 6 wk to ensure that the adenoma has been completely removed and that the endocrine hypersecretion is resolved.
- If there is good clinical response, patient should be monitored yearly for recurrence and to follow the level of the hypersecreted hormone.
- Patients who have undergone irradiation should have close follow-up with backup medical therapy because response to radiotherapy may be delayed; incidence of hypopituitarism also increases with time.

REFERENCE
Shimon I, Melmed S: Management of pituitary tumors, *Ann Intern Med* 129:472, 1998.
Author: **Beth J. Wutz, M.D.**

BASIC INFORMATION

■ DEFINITION
Pityriasis is a common self-limiting skin eruption of unknown etiology.

■ ICD-9CM CODES
696.3 Pityriasis rosea

■ EPIDEMIOLOGY & DEMOGRAPHICS
- Most cases of pityriasis rosea occur between ages 10 and 35 yr; mean age is 23 yr.
- The incidence of disease is highest in the fall and spring.
- Female:male ratio is 1.5:1.

■ PHYSICAL FINDINGS & CLINICAL PRESENTATION
- Initial lesion (herald patch) precedes the eruption by approximately 1 to 2 wk; typically measures 3 to 6 cm; it is round to oval in appearance and most frequently located on the trunk.
- Eruptive phase follows within 2 wk and peaks after 7 to 14 days.
- Lesions are most frequently located in the lower abdominal area. They have a salmon-pink appearance in whites and a hyperpigmented appearance in blacks.
- Most lesions are 4 to 5 mm in diameter; center has a "cigarette paper" appearance; border has a characteristic ring of scale (collarette).
- Lesions occur in a symmetric distribution and follow the cleavage lines of the trunk (Christmas tree pattern [Fig. 1-295]).

- The number of lesions varies from a few to hundreds.
- Most patients are asymptomatic; pruritus is the most common symptom.
- History of recent fatigue, headache, sore throat, and low-grade fever is present in approximately 25% of cases.

■ ETIOLOGY
Unknown, possibly viral (picornavirus)

DIAGNOSIS

■ DIFFERENTIAL DIAGNOSIS
- Tinea corporis (can be ruled out by potassium hydroxide examination)
- Secondary syphilis (absence of herald patch, positive serologic test for syphilis)
- Psoriasis
- Nummular eczema
- Drug eruption
- Viral exanthem (see Table 2-61)
- Eczema
- Lichen planus
- Tinea versicolor (the lesions are more brown and the borders are not as ovoid)

■ WORKUP
Presence of herald lesion and characteristic rash are diagnostic. Skin biopsy is generally reserved for atypical cases.

■ LABORATORY TESTS
Generally not necessary; serologic test for syphilis if clinically indicated

TREATMENT

■ NONPHARMACOLOGIC THERAPY
The disease is self-limited and generally does not require any therapeutic intervention.

■ ACUTE GENERAL Rx
- Use calamine lotion or oral antihistamines in patients with significant pruritus.
- Use prednisone tapered over 2 wk in patients with severe pruritus.
- Direct sun exposure or use of ultraviolet light within the first week of eruption is beneficial in decreasing the severity of disease.

■ DISPOSITION
- Spontaneous complete resolution of the rash within 4 to 8 wk.
- Recurrence rare (<2% of cases)

PEARLS & CONSIDERATIONS

■ COMMENTS
Reassure patient that the disease is not contagious and its course is benign.
Author: **Fred F. Ferri, M.D.**

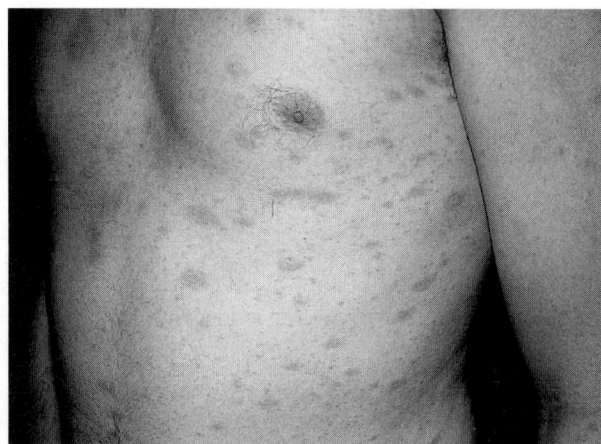

Fig. 1-295 Scale (pityriasis rosea). Shows example of how unique scaling (collarette of fine scale within several lesions), distribution and shape of lesions (oval lesions with long axis paralleling natural skin cleavage lines), and color (salmon-pink) help in diagnosing skin disease. (From Noble J et al: *Textbook of primary care medicine,* ed 2, St Louis, 1995, Mosby.)

BASIC INFORMATION

■ DEFINITION
Aspiration pneumonia is a lung infection caused by bacterial organisms aspirated from nasopharyngeal space.

ICD-9CM CODES
507.0 Aspiration pneumonia

■ EPIDEMIOLOGY & DEMOGRAPHICS
INCIDENCE (IN U.S.):
- Few reliable data
- 20% to 35% of all pneumonias

PREVALENCE (IN U.S.): Unreliable data
PREDOMINANT SEX: Equal
PREDOMINANT AGE: Elderly
PEAK INCIDENCE: Elderly patients in hospitals or nursing homes

■ PHYSICAL FINDINGS & CLINICAL PRESENTATION
- Shortness of breath, tachypnea, cough, sputum, fever after vomiting, or difficulty swallowing
- Rales, rhonchi, often diffusely throughout lung

■ ETIOLOGY
Complex interaction of etiologies, ranging from chemical (often acid) pneumonitis following aspiration of sterile gastric contents (generally not requiring antibiotic treatment) to bacterial aspiration

COMMUNITY-ACQUIRED ASPIRATION PNEUMONIA:
- Generally results from predominantly anaerobic mouth bacteria (anaerobic and microaerophilic streptococci, fusobacteria, gram-positive anaerobic non–spore-forming rods) and less common *Bacteroides* species *(melaninogenicus, intermedius, oralis, ureolyticus)*
- Rarely caused by *Bacteroides fragilis* (of uncertain validity in published studies) or *Eikenella corrodens*
- High-risk groups: elderly, alcoholics, IV drug users, patients who are obtunded, those with esophageal disorders, seizures, poor dentition, or recent dental manipulations

HOSPITAL-ACQUIRED ASPIRATION PNEUMONIA:
- Often occurs among elderly patients and others with diminished gag reflex; those with nasogastric tubes, intestinal obstruction, or ventilator support; and especially those exposed to contaminated nebulizers or unsterile suctioning
- High-risk groups: seriously ill hospitalized patients (especially patients with coma, acidosis, alcoholism, uremia, diabetes mellitus, nasogastric intubation, or recent antimicrobial therapy, who are frequently colonized with aerobic gram-negative

rods); patients undergoing anesthesia; those with strokes, dementia, swallowing disorders; the elderly; and those receiving antacids or H_2 blockers (but not sucralfate)
- Hypoxic patients receiving concentrated O_2 have diminished ciliary activity, encouraging aspiration
- Causative organisms:
  1. Anaerobes listed previously, although in many studies gram-negative aerobes (60%) and gram-positive aerobes (20%) predominate
  2. *E. coli, P. aeruginosa, S. aureus, Klebsiella, Enterobacter, Serratia,* and *Proteus* spp. *Haemophilus influenzae, S. pneumoniae, Legionella,* and *Acinetobacter* spp. (sporadic pneumonias) in two thirds of cases
  3. Fungi, including *Candida albicans,* in fewer than 1%

 DIAGNOSIS

■ DIFFERENTIAL DIAGNOSIS
- Other necrotizing or cavitary pneumonias (especially tuberculosis, gram-negative pneumonias)
- See "Pulmonary Tuberculosis"

■ WORKUP
- Chest x-ray examination
- CBC, blood cultures
- Sputum Gram stain and culture
- Consideration of tracheal aspirate

■ LABORATORY TESTS
- CBC: leukocytosis often present
- Sputum Gram stain
  1. Often useful when carefully prepared immediately after obtaining suctioned or expectorated specimen, examined by experienced observer.
  2. Only specimens with multiple WBCs and rare or absent epithelial cells should be examined.
  3. Unlike nonaspiration pneumonias (e.g., pneumococcal), multiple organisms may be present.
  4. Long, slender rods suggest anaerobes.
  5. Sputum from pneumonia caused by acid aspiration may be devoid of organisms.
  6. Cultures should be interpreted in light of morphology of visualized organisms.

■ IMAGING STUDIES
- Chest x-ray examination often reveals bilateral, diffuse, patchy infiltrates.
- Aspiration pneumonias of several days' or longer duration may reveal necrosis (especially community-acquired anaerobic pneumonias)

and even cavitation with air-fluid levels, indicating lung abscess.

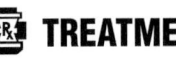 **TREATMENT**

■ NONPHARMACOLOGIC THERAPY
- Airway management to prevent repeated aspiration
- Ventilatory support if necessary

■ ACUTE GENERAL Rx
Acute aspiration of acidic gastric contents without bacteria may not require antibiotic therapy; consult infectious diseases or pulmonary expert.

FOR COMMUNITY-ACQUIRED ANAEROBIC ASPIRATION PNEUMONIA:
- Often successfully treated with penicillin G (12 to 18 million U/day IV), although some *Bacteroides* and *Fusobacterium* spp. may be resistant to penicillin, responding instead to clindamycin 600 mg q8h.
- Treat nursing home aspirations like hospital aspirations in general.

HOSPITAL-ACQUIRED ASPIRATION PNEUMONIA:
- Often responds to vancomycin 15 mg/kg q12h (<2 g/day), plus ceftazidime 1 to 2 g q8-12h, or to imipenem 500 mg q6h, or ampicillin/sulbactam 1.5 to 3 q6h.
- Knowledge of resident flora in the microenvironment of the aspiration within the hospital is crucial to intelligent antibiotic selection; consult infection control nurses or hospital epidemiologist.
- Confirmed *Pseudomonas* pneumonia should be treated with antipseudomonal β-lactam agent plus an aminoglycoside until antimicrobial sensitivities confirm that less toxic agents may replace aminoglycoside.
- Clindamycin may be added for improved anaerobic coverage.
- Do not use metronidazole alone for anaerobes.

■ CHRONIC Rx
Generally not indicated, except for lung abscess (usually anaerobic)

■ DISPOSITION
Repeat chest x-ray examination in 6 to 8 wk.

■ REFERRAL
For consultation with infectious disease and/or pulmonary experts for patients with respiratory distress, hypoxia, ventilatory support, pneumonia in more than one lobe, necrosis or cavitation on x-ray examination, or not responding to antibiotic therapy within 2 to 3 days.

Author: Beth J. Wutz, M.D.

BASIC INFORMATION

■ DEFINITION
Bacterial pneumonia is an infection involving the lung parenchyma

ICD-9CM CODES
486.0 Pneumonia, acute
507.0 Pneumonia, aspiration
482.9 Pneumonia, bacterial
481 Pneumonia, pneumococcal
482.1 Pneumonia, *Pseudomonas*
482.4 Pneumonia, staphylococcal
428.0 Pneumonia, *Klebsiella*
482.2 Pneumonia, *Haemophilus influenzae*

■ EPIDEMIOLOGY & DEMOGRAPHICS
- Incidence of community-acquired pneumonia is 1/100 persons.
- Incidence of nosocomial pneumonia is 8 cases/1000 persons/yr.
- Primary care physicians see an average of 10 cases of pneumonia annually.
- Hospitalization rate for pneumonia is 15% to 20%.
- Most cases of pneumonia occur in the winter and in elderly patients.

■ PHYSICAL FINDINGS & CLINICAL PRESENTATION
- Fever, tachypnea, chills, tachycardia, cough
- Presentation varies with the cause of pneumonia, the patient's age, and the clinical situation:
  1. Patients with streptococcal pneumonia usually present with high fever, shaking chills, pleuritic chest pain, cough, and copious production of purulent sputum.
  2. Elderly or immunocompromised hosts may initially present with only minimal symptoms (e.g., low-grade fever, confusion); respiratory and nonrespiratory symptoms are less commonly reported by older patients with pneumonia.
  3. Generally, auscultation reveals crackles and diminished breath sounds.
  4. Percussion dullness is present if the patient has pleural effusion.

■ ETIOLOGY
- *Streptococcus pneumoniae*
- *Haemophilus influenzae*
- *Legionella pneumophila* (1% to 5% of adult pneumonias)
- *Klebsiella, Pseudomonas, E. coli*
- *Staphylococcus aureus*
- Pneumococcal infection is responsible for 50% to 75% of community-acquired pneumonias, whereas gram-negative organisms cause >80% of nosocomial pneumonias.
- Predisposing factors are:
  1. COPD: *H. influenzae, S. pneumoniae, Legionella*
  2. Seizures: aspiration pneumonia
  3. Compromised hosts: *Legionella,* gram-negative organisms
  4. Alcoholism: *Klebsiella, S. pneumoniae, H. influenzae*
  5. HIV: *S. pneumoniae*
  6. IV drug addicts with right-sided bacterial endocarditis: *S. aureus*

DIAGNOSIS

■ DIFFERENTIAL DIAGNOSIS
- Exacerbation of chronic bronchitis
- Pulmonary embolism or infarction
- Lung neoplasm
- Bronchiolitis
- Sarcoidosis
- Hypersensitivity pneumonitis
- Pulmonary edema
- Drug-induced lung injury
- Viral pneumonias
- Fungal pneumonias
- Parasitic pneumonias
- Atypical pneumonia
- Tuberculosis

■ WORKUP
Laboratory evaluation (in hospitalized patients) and chest x-ray examination

■ LABORATORY TESTS
- In hospitalized patients obtain an adequate sputum specimen for Gram stain and cultures.
  1. An expectorated sputum sample is often inadequate because of many false positive results (secondary to contamination from oral flora) and many false negative results; a specimen may be considered adequate if the Gram stain shows >25 PMNs and <10 epithelial cells per low-power field.
  2. Aerosol induction with hypertonic saline solution (3% to 10%) may increase the diagnostic yield of sputum.

3. The use of fiberoptic bronchoscopy to obtain a sputum sample is generally reserved for critically ill patients responding poorly to initial antimicrobial therapy.
- WBC count is elevated, usually with left shift.
- Blood cultures: positive in approximately 20% of cases of pneumococcal pneumonia.
- ABGs: hypoxemia with partial pressure of oxygen <60 mm Hg while the patient is breathing room air is a standard criterion for hospital admission.
- Direct immunofluorescent examination of sputum (e.g., direct fluorescent antibody [DFA] stain is a highly specific and rapid test for detecting legionellae in clinical specimen).
- Serologic testing for HIV is advocated by the CDC for hospitalized patients between the ages of 15 and 54 yr who are treated in hospitals with a high prevalence of AIDS (≥1:1000 discharges).
- Gram stain of sputum:
  1. Lancet-shaped, gram-positive cocci indicate streptococcal pneumonia.
  2. Pleomorphic, small coccobacillary, gram-negative organisms indicate *H. influenzae.*
  3. Encapsulated gram-negative bacilli: *K. pneumoniae*

■ IMAGING STUDIES
Chest x-ray study: findings vary with the stage and type of pneumonia and the hydration of the patient (Fig. 1-296).
- Classically, pneumococcal pneumonia presents with a segmental lobe infiltrate.
- Diffuse infiltrates on chest x-ray can be seen with *L. pneumophila, M. pneumoniae,* viral pneumonias, *P. carinii,* miliary TB, aspiration, aspergillosis.
- An initial chest x-ray film is also useful to rule out the presence of any complications (pneumothorax, empyema, abscesses).

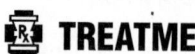

TREATMENT

■ NONPHARMACOLOGIC THERAPY
- Avoidance of tobacco use
- Oxygen to maintain partial oxygen pressure in arterial blood >60 mm Hg

- IV hydration, correction of dehydration
- Assisted ventilation in patients with significant respiratory failure

■ ACUTE GENERAL Rx
- Initial antibiotic therapy should be based on clinical, radiographic, and laboratory evaluation; if the clinical diagnosis is substantiated by an adequate Gram stain, the choice of initial therapy is relatively simple. In otherwise healthy adult patients with community-acquired pneumonia and insidious presentation, azithromycin is the antibiotic of choice. Clarithromycin is also effective. Levofloxacin (Levaquin) is a quinolone with excellent activity against organisms commonly encountered in community-acquired pneumonia. In patients who require hospitalization, cefotaxime or ceftriaxone is a reasonable choice pending culture results. A macrolide (e.g., azithromycin) can be added to cover mycoplasma, legionella, and chlamydia.
- In immunocompromised patients with negative Gram stain, the initial antibiotic treatment should be broad spectrum but with emphasis on gram-negative organisms, *Legionella,* and *S. aureus.* In these patients, the following antibiotics should be considered:
  1. Patients with AIDS: high-dose TMP-SMX plus azithromycin.

2. Neutropenic patients: ticarcillin-piperacillin 3 to 4 g IV q4-6h plus tobramycin 2 mg/kg IV q12h or ceftazidine plus aminoglycoside.
3. Immunocompromised, non-AIDS, nonneutropenic patients (e.g., diabetes mellitus, elderly, COPD): cefuroxime plus aminoglycoside (if pneumonia is hospital or nursing home acquired).
4. Most hospitalized and immunocompromised patients with legionnaires' disease can be effectively treated with levofloxacin (500 mg/day for 7 to 10 days) or azithromycin (500 mg qd for 5 days).

■ CHRONIC Rx
Parapneumonic effusion-empyema can be managed with chest tube placement for drainage. Instillation of fibrinolytic agents (streptokinase, urokinase) via the chest tube may be necessary in resistant cases.

■ DISPOSITION
Most patients respond well to antibiotic therapy. Hospitalization is recommended in immunocompromised patients and patients with hypoxemia with partial pressure oxygen <60 mm Hg while the patient is breathing room air.

☼ PEARLS & CONSIDERATIONS

■ COMMENTS
Causes of slowly resolving or nonresolving pneumonia:
- Difficult to treat infections: viral pneumonia, *Legionella,* pneumococci, or staphylococci with impaired host response, TB, fungi
- Neoplasm: lung, lymphoma, metastasis
- CHF
- Pulmonary embolism
- Immunologic or idiopathic: Wegener's granulomatosis, pulmonary eosinophilic syndromes, SLE
- Drug toxicity (e.g., amiodarone)

Author: **Fred F. Ferri, M.D.**

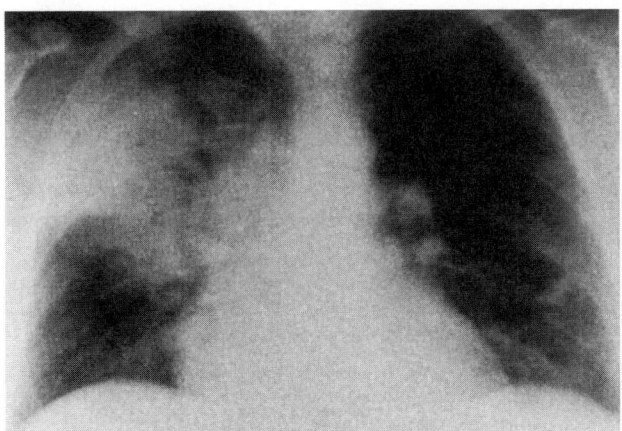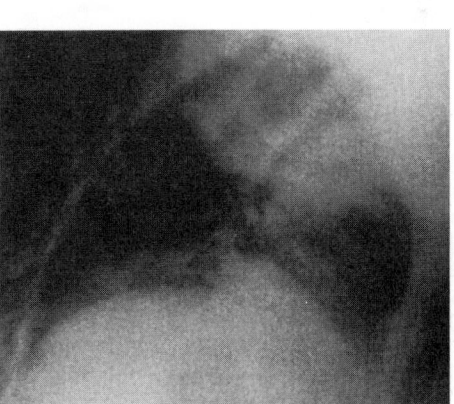

Fig. 1-296   **A,** PA and, **B,** lateral chest radiographs reveal right upper lobe pneumonia and patchy left lower lobe infiltrate. A variety of organisms can produce this pattern, including *S. pneumoniae* and *H. influenzae.* (From Rosen P [ed]: *Emergency medicine,* ed 4, St Louis, 1998, Mosby.)

BASIC INFORMATION

■ **DEFINITION**

Mycoplasma pneumonia is an infection of the lung parenchyma caused by *Mycoplasma pneumoniae*.

■ **SYNONYMS**

Primary atypical pneumonia
Eaton's pneumonia
Walking pneumonia

ICD-9CM CODES
483 *Mycoplasma* pneumonia

■ **EPIDEMIOLOGY & DEMOGRAPHICS**

INCIDENCE (IN U.S.):
- Hard to determine incidence precisely because of difficulty in making the diagnosis, but it is a frequent cause of community-acquired pneumonia.
- Probably many cases resolve without coming to medical attention.
- Incidence is estimated at 1 case/1000 persons/yr.
- Incidence is estimated to at least triple every (approximately) 5 yr during epidemics.

PREVALENCE (IN U.S.):
- Estimated to be present in 1 of 5 patients hospitalized for pneumonia (generally a self-limited disease, so its true prevalence is unknown)
- Estimated to cause 7% of all pneumonias and about half in those age 5 to 20 yr

PREDOMINANT SEX: Equal distribution

PREDOMINANT AGE:
- Most commonly affected: school-age children and young adults (ages 5 to 20 yr)
- Occurs in older adults as well, especially with household exposure to a young child
- More severe infections in affected elderly patients

PEAK INCIDENCE:
- Some increased incidence in fall to early winter
- Seems more prevalent in temperate climates

GENETICS:
Familial Disposition:
- None known
- May be more severe in patients with sickle cell anemia

Neonatal Infection: Severe respiratory distress, sometimes requiring intubation, attributed to this disease in infants.

■ **PHYSICAL FINDINGS & CLINICAL PRESENTATION**
- Nonexudative pharyngitis (common)
- Rhonchi or rales, without evidence of consolidation (common) in lower lung zones
- Associated with bullous myringitis (perhaps no more frequently than in other pneumonias)
- Skin rashes in up to one fourth of patients
  1. Morbilliform
  2. Urticaria
  3. Erythema nodosum (unusual)
  4. Erythema multiforme (unusual)
  5. Stevens-Johnson syndrome (rare)
- Muscle tenderness (<50% of the patients)
- On examination (and confirmed with testing):
  1. Mononeuritis or polyneuritis
  2. Transverse myelitis
  3. Cranial nerve palsies
  4. Meningoencephalitis
- Lymphadenopathy and splenomegaly
- Conjunctivitis

■ **ETIOLOGY**
Infection is spread by droplet infection from respiratory tract secretions.

🔬 **DIAGNOSIS**

■ **DIFFERENTIAL DIAGNOSIS**
- *Chlamydia pneumoniae*
- *C. psittaci*
- *Legionella* spp.
- *Coxiella burnetii*
- Several viral agents
- Q fever
- *Pneumococcus pneumoniae*
- Pleuritic pain
- Pulmonary embolism/infarction

■ **WORKUP**
- Chest x-ray examination
- Thorough history and physical examination
- Laboratory tests

- Evaluation guided by symptoms and findings

■ **LABORATORY TESTS**
- WBC:
  1. WBC count >10,000/mm^3 in about a quarter of patients
  2. Differential count nonspecific
  3. Leukopenia rare
- Cold agglutinins:
  1. Detected in about half of the patients
  2. Also may be found in:
     a. Lymphoproliferative diseases
     b. Influenza
     c. Mononucleosis
     d. Adenovirus infections
     e. Occasionally, legionnaires' disease
  3. Titers typically >1:64
     a. May be detectable with bedside testing
     b. Appear between days 5 and 10 of the illness (so may be demonstrable when patient is first examined) and disappear within about 1 mo
- Uncommonly, hemolysis
- Complement fixation testing of paired sera (fourfold rise) in patients with pneumonia and a compatible history:
  1. Considered diagnostic
  2. Not specific for the disease
- Culture of the organism from specimens
  1. Only truly specific test for infection
  2. Technically difficult and done reliably by few laboratories
  3. May require weeks to get results
- Sputum
  1. Often no sputum produced for laboratory testing
  2. When present, gram-stained specimens show polyps without organisms
- Infection occasionally complicated by pancreatitis or glomerulitis
- Disseminated intravascular coagulation is a rare complication.
- Electrocardiographic evidence of pericarditis or myocarditis may be present.

■ **IMAGING STUDIES**
- Predilection for lower lobe involvement (upper lobes involved in less than a fourth), with radiographic ab-

normalities frequently out of proportion to those on physical examination (Fig. 1-297)

- Small pleural effusions in about 30% of patients
- Large effusions: rare
- Infiltrates: patchy, unilateral, and with a segmental distribution, although multilobe involvement may be seen
- Evidence of hilar adenopathy on chest films in 20% to 25%
- Rare cases reported:
  1. Associated lung abscess
  2. Residual pneumatoceles
  3. Lobar collapse
  4. Hyperlucent lung syndrome

TREATMENT

■ ACUTE GENERAL Rx
- Therapy (10 to 14 days) with erythromycin (500 mg qid), azithromycin (500 mg daily), or clarithromycin (500 mg bid) is preferred to tetracycline, especially in young children or women of childbearing age.
- Therapy shortens the duration and severity of symptoms and may hasten radiographic clearing, but the disease is self-limiting.

■ CHRONIC Rx
- Effective antimicrobial therapy does not eliminate the organism from the respiratory secretions, which may be positive for weeks.
- Serum antibody response does not necessarily provide lifelong immunity.
- Chronic symptoms do not occur, although clinical relapses may occur 7 to 10 days following the initial response and may be associated with new areas of infiltration.

■ DISPOSITION
- Clinical improvement is almost universal within 10 days.
- Infiltrates generally clear within 5 to 8 wk.
- Rare deaths are likely attributable to underlying medical diseases.
- Person-to-person spread can be minimized by avoiding open coughing, especially in enclosed areas.

■ REFERRAL
- Not responding to treatment
- Severe infection
- Severe extrapulmonary manifestations
- Multilobe involvement accompanied by respiratory embarrassment (very rare)

☼ PEARLS & CONSIDERATIONS

■ COMMENTS
X-ray resolution complete by 8 wk in about 90% of patients.

REFERENCES
Ewig S, Torres A: Severe community-acquired pneumonia, *Clin Chest Med* 20:575, 1999.

Foy HM: *Mycoplasma pneumoniae* pneumonia: current perspectives, *Clin Infect Dis* 28:237, 1999.

Reittner P et al: *Mycoplasma pneumoniae* pneumonia: radiographic and high-resolution CT features in 28 patients, *Am J Roentgenol* 174:37, 2000.

Ruiz M et al: Etiology of community-acquired pneumonia: impact of age, comorbidity, and severity, *Am J Respir Crit Care Med* 160:397, 1999.

Tan JS: Role of 'atypical' pneumonia pathogens in respiratory tract infections, *Can Respir J* (Suppl 6) A:15A, 1999.

Author: **Harvey M. Shanies, M.D., Ph.D.**

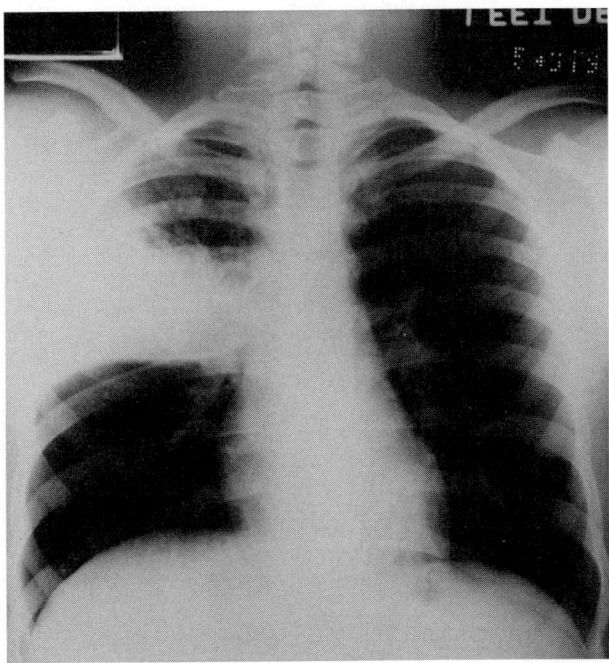

Fig. 1-297   Localized airspace opacification secondary to *Mycoplasma pneumoniae*. (From Specht N [ed]: *Practical guide to diagnostic imaging,* St Louis, 1998, Mosby.)

BASIC INFORMATION

■ DEFINITION
Pneumocystis carinii pneumonia is a serious respiratory infection caused by the fungal or protozoal organism *Pneumocystis carinii*.

■ SYNONYMS
PCP

ICD-9CM CODES
136.3 *Pneumocystis carinii* pneumonia

■ EPIDEMIOLOGY & DEMOGRAPHICS
INCIDENCE (IN U.S.):
- Seen primarily in the setting of acquired immunodeficiency syndrome (AIDS)
- Approximately 11 cases/100 patient-years among HIV-infected patients with CD4 lymphocyte counts $<100/mm^3$

PREDOMINANT SEX: Equal incidence when corrected for HIV status
PREDOMINANT AGE:
- <2 yr
- 20 to 40 yr

PEAK INCIDENCE: 20 to 40 yr (parallel to AIDS epidemic)
GENETICS:
Neonatal Infection:
- Most frequent opportunistic infection among HIV-infected children, occurring in approximately 30%
- Neonatal occurrence unusual

■ PHYSICAL FINDINGS & CLINICAL PRESENTATION
- Fever, cough, shortness of breath present in almost all cases
- Lungs frequently clear to auscultation, although rales occasionally present
- Cyanosis and pronounced tachypnea in severe cases
- Hemoptysis unusual
- Spontaneous pneumothorax

■ ETIOLOGY
- *Pneumocystis carinii*, recently reclassified as a fungal organism
- Reactivation of dormant infection
- Extrapulmonary involvement rare

DIAGNOSIS

■ DIFFERENTIAL DIAGNOSIS
- Other opportunistic respiratory infections:
  1. Tuberculosis
  2. Histoplasmosis
  3. Cryptococcosis

- Nonopportunistic infections:
  1. Bacterial pneumonia
  2. Viral pneumonia
  3. Mycoplasmal pneumonia
  4. Legionellosis
- Occurs virtually exclusively in the setting of profound depression of cellular immunity

■ WORKUP
- Chest x-ray examination
- ABG
- Sputum examination for cysts of PCP and to exclude other pathogens
- Bronchoscopy with bronchoalveolar lavage or lung biopsy for diagnosis if sputum examination is negative or equivocal

■ LABORATORY TESTS
- ABG monitoring
- Elevated lactate dehydrogenase (LDH) in majority of cases
- HIV antibody test if cause of underlying immune deficiency state is unclear

■ IMAGING STUDIES
Diffuse uptake on gallium scanning of the lungs is suggestive but not diagnostic.

TREATMENT

■ NONPHARMACOLOGIC THERAPY
- Supplemental oxygen
- Ventilatory support if needed
- Prompt thoracotomy if pneumothorax develops

■ ACUTE GENERAL Rx
For confirmed or suspected PCP:
- Trimethoprim-sulfamethoxazole (20 mg/kg trimethoprim and 100 mg/kg sulfamethoxazole qd) PO or IV
- Pentamidine (4 mg/kg IV qd)
- Either regimen with prednisone (40 mg PO bid):
  1. If arterial oxygen pressure <70 mm Hg
  2. If arterial-alveolar oxygen pressure difference >35 mm Hg
  3. Dose tapered to 20 mg bid after 5 days and 20 mg qd after 10 days
- Therapy continued for 3 wk
- Alternative therapies available for patients unable to tolerate conventional therapy:
  1. Dapsone/trimethoprim
  2. Clindamycin/primaquine
  3. Atovaquone
- Alternative therapies should be given in consultation with a physician experienced in the management of PCP

■ CHRONIC Rx
- After completion of therapy, lifelong prophylaxis should be maintained with trimethoprim-sulfamethoxazole (one single-strength tablet PO qd or double-strength three times weekly).
- Patients intolerant of this therapy should be treated with dapsone (50 mg PO qd) plus pyrimethamine (50 mg PO weekly) plus leucovorin (25 mg PO weekly).
- Inhaled pentamidine (300 mg monthly by standardized nebulizer) is less effective and is reserved for patients intolerant to other forms of prophylaxis.
- Same approach taken to all HIV-infected patients with CD4 lymphocyte counts <200 to $250/mm^3$ or <20% of the total lymphocyte count because of their high risk of PCP.

■ DISPOSITION
- Patients should be hospitalized unless infection mild.
- After completion of therapy, long-term ambulatory follow-up is mandatory to provide secondary prevention of PCP (above) and management of the underlying immunodeficiency syndrome.

■ REFERRAL
To pulmonologist for bronchoscopy if diagnosis cannot be confirmed by sputum examination

PEARLS & CONSIDERATIONS

■ COMMENTS
All patients, especially those with severe infection or intolerant of conventional therapy, should be followed by a physician experienced in the management of PCP and, if appropriate, in the long-term management of HIV infection or other underlying disease.

REFERENCES
Kaplan JE et al: Epidemiology of human immunodeficiency virus: associated opportunistic infections in the United States in the era of highly active antiretroviral therapy, *Clin Infect Dis* 30(suppl 1):S5, 2000.
Russian DA, Levine SJ: *Pneumocystis carinii* pneumonia in patients without HIV infection, *Am J Med Sci* 321(1):56, 2001.
Author: **Joseph R. Masci, M.D.**

BASIC INFORMATION

■ **DEFINITION**
Viral pneumonia is infection of the pulmonary parenchyma caused by any of a large number of viral agents. The most important viruses are discussed below.

■ **SYNONYMS**
Nonbacterial pneumonia
Atypical pneumonia

ICD-9CM CODES
480.9 Viral pneumonia

■ **EPIDEMIOLOGY & DEMOGRAPHICS**
INCIDENCE (IN U.S.):
• Influenza virus:
  1. 10% to 20% of population in temperate zones infected during 1- to 2-mo epidemics occurring yearly during winter months.
  2. Up to 50% infected during pandemics.
  3. Pneumonia develops in small percentage of infected persons.
• Incidence of other important viral pneumonias is not known precisely.
PREVALENCE (IN U.S.):
• Often related to immune status of the population or presence of an epidemic
• Normal hosts (estimates):
  1. 86% of cases of pneumonia resulting in hospitalization in American adults
  2. 16% of pediatric pneumonias managed as outpatients
  3. 49% of hospitalized infants with pneumonia
• Important problem in hosts with impaired immunity
PREDOMINANT SEX:
• None generally
• Male sex may predispose to more severe respiratory disease in respiratory syncytial virus (RSV) infection
PREDOMINANT AGE:
Influenza:
• Overall incidence greatest at age 5 yr
• Falls with increasing age
• The most serious sequelae in those with chronic medical illnesses, especially cardiopulmonary disease
• Hospitalizations greatest in infants and adults >64 yr of age
RSV:
• Young children (as the major cause of pneumonia)
• Occurs throughout life

Adenoviruses:
• Young children
• Adults, primarily military recruits
Varicella:
• About 16% of adults (not infected in childhood) who contract chickenpox
• Acute varicella during pregnancy more likely to be complicated by severe pneumonia
• 90% of reported varicella pneumonia cases are in adults (highest incidence 20 to 60 yr old)
Measles:
• Young adults and older children who received a single vaccination (5% failure rate)
• Measles during pregnancy more likely to be complicated by pneumonia
• Underlying cardiopulmonary diseases and immunosuppression predispose to serious pneumonia complicating measles
• Before availability of measles vaccine, 90% of pneumonias in those <10 yr
• Currently over a third of U.S. patients >14 yr old
• 3% to 50% of measles cases are complicated by pneumonia
CMV:
• Neonatal through adult
• Immunosuppression is key predisposing factor
PEAK INCIDENCE:
Influenza:
• Winter months for influenza A
• Year round for influenza B
• Peak of pneumonia seen weeks into the outbreak of infection
RSV: Winter and spring
Adenovirus: Endemic (military)
Varicella: Spring in temperate zones
Measles: Year round
CMV: Year round
GENETICS:
Familial Disposition:
• Close contact, not genetics, is important in acquisition.
• Congenital anomalies and immunosuppression worsen course of RSV pneumonia.
Congenital Infection:
• CMV is the most common intrauterine infection in the U.S.
• Pneumonia occurs occasionally in infants with symptomatic congenital infection.
Neonatal Infection:
• Severe RSV pneumonia
• Adenovirus pneumonia
  1. 5% to 20% fatality rate
  2. Can lead to residual restrictive or obstructive functional abnormalities

• "Varicella neonatorum"
  1. Disseminated visceral disease including pneumonia
  2. May develop in neonates whose mothers develop peripartum chickenpox
• CMV pneumonia
  1. Generally fatal
  2. Associated with severe cerebral damage in this population

■ **PHYSICAL FINDINGS & CLINICAL PRESENTATION**
INFLUENZA:
• Fever
• Uncomfortable or lethargic appearance
• Prominent dry cough (rarely hemoptysis)
• Flushed integument and erythematous mucous membranes
• Rales or rhonchi
RSV:
• Fever
• Tachypnea
• Prolonged expiration
• Wheezes and rales
ADENOVIRUSES:
• Hoarseness
• Pharyngitis
• Tachypnea
• Cervical adenitis
MEASLES:
• Conjunctivitis
• Rhinorrhea
• Koplik's spots
• Exanthem
• Pneumonitis
  1. May occur as a complication in 3% to 4% of adolescents and young adults
  2. Coincident with rash
  3. May also develop following apparent recovery from measles
• Fever
• Dry cough
VARICELLA:
• Fever
• Maculopapular or vesicular rash
  1. Becomes encrusted
  2. Pneumonia typical 1 to 6 days after rash appears
  3. Pneumonia accompanied by cough, and occasionally hemoptysis
• Few auscultatory abnormalities noted on examination of the lungs
CMV:
• Fever
• Paroxysmal cough
• Occasional hemoptysis
• Diffuse adenopathy when pneumonia occurs after transfusion

■ ETIOLOGY
Viral infection can lead to pneumonia in both immunocompetent and immunocompromised hosts.

 DIAGNOSIS

■ DIFFERENTIAL DIAGNOSIS
- Bacterial pneumonia, which frequently complicates (i.e., can follow or be simultaneous with) viral (especially influenza) pneumonia
- Other causes of atypical pneumonia:
  1. *Mycoplasma*
  2. *Chlamydia*
  3. *Coxiella*
  4. Legionnaires' disease
- ARDS
- Physical findings and associated hypoxemia confused with pulmonary emboli

■ WORKUP
- Information about the prevalent strain of influenza virus can be obtained from local health departments or from the Centers for Disease Control and Prevention.
- Viral diagnostic tests are usually not necessary once an outbreak has been defined.
- Influenza and other viruses can be cultured from respiratory secretions during the initial few days of the illness (special media and techniques necessary).
- Paired sera antibody titers are also useful.
- Monoclonal antibody tests are available for influenza and other respiratory viruses.
- Measles and adenovirus pneumonia are usually diagnosed clinically.
- Polymerase chain reaction may be able to rapidly detect and identify viral nucleic acid.
- Open lung biopsy is required for definite diagnosis of CMV pneumonia.

■ LABORATORY TESTS
- Sputum Gram stain (usually produced in scanty amounts) typically shows few polymorphonuclear leukocytes and few bacteria.
- WBC count may vary from leukopenic to modest elevation, usually without a leftward shift.
- Disseminated intravascular coagulation has occasionally complicated adenovirus type 7 pneumonia.

- Multinucleated giant cells on Tzanck preparation of an unroofed vesicular lesion are useful in diagnosing varicella in a patient with an infiltrate (also found in herpes simplex).
- Severe immunosuppression is associated with symptomatic CMV pneumonia (usually reactivation of latent infection, or in previously seronegative recipients from the donor).
- Hypoxemia may be profound.
- Cultures may be helpful in identifying superinfecting bacterial pathogens.
- When they occur, parapneumonic pleural effusions are exudative.

■ IMAGING STUDIES
- Chest x-ray examination may demonstrate a spectrum of findings from ill-defined, patchy, or generalized interstitial infiltrates, which can be associated with the acute respiratory distress syndrome (ARDS).
- A localized dense alveolar infiltrate suggests a superimposed bacterial pneumonia.
- Small calcified nodules may develop as a radiographic residual of varicella pneumonia (Fig. 1-298).

 TREATMENT

■ NONPHARMACOLOGIC THERAPY
GENERAL:
- Measures to diminish person-to-person transmission
- Modified bed rest
- Maintenance of adequate hydration
- Possible ventilatory support for severe pneumonia or ARDS

INFLUENZA:
- Yearly prophylactic strain-specific influenza vaccination (only subvirion vaccine should be used in children <13 yr) can be given to prevent infection.
- Live, attenuated influenza vaccines administered by nose drops may be more effective than the injected inactivated viral vaccines now available (under investigation).

RSV:
- Isolation techniques are important in limiting spread of RSV infections.
- Immunoglobulins with a high RSV-neutralizing antibody titer are beneficial in treamtent.

ADENOVIRUSES:
- Intestinal inoculation of respiratory adenoviruses has been used to successfully immunize military recruits.
- Although they produce no disease in recipients, the viruses may be shed chronically and may infect others at a later date.
- These vaccines are not available for civilian populations.

VARICELLA:
- Live, attenuated varicella vaccine has been successfully used in clinical trials.
- Varicella-zoster immune globulin should be administered within 4 days of exposure to prevent or modify the disease in susceptible persons.
- Nonimmunized persons exposed to varicella are potentially infectious between 10 and 21 days after exposure.

MEASLES:
- Effective measles vaccine is available:
  1. The vaccine should be administered at 15 mo.
  2. A second dose should be administered at the time of school entry.
- Live, attenuated vaccine or γ-globulin can prevent measles in unvaccinated persons if administered early following exposure.
- Vitamin A given PO for 2 days reduces morbidity and mortality from measles in exposed children.

■ ACUTE GENERAL Rx
GENERAL: Administer appropriate antibiotics for bacterial superinfections.

INFLUENZA:
- Amantadine and rimantadine (not commercially available) for influenza A. Early use can speed recovery from small airways dysfunction, but whether it influences the development or course of pneumonia is uncertain.
- Amantadine is also effective prophylactically during the time it is administered.
- Aerosolized ribavirin or amantadine may have a role in severe influenza pneumonia but have not been approved for this indication.

RSV: Ribavirin aerosol is effective for severe RSV pneumonia.

ADENOVIRUSES: No effective antiadenovirus agent.

VARICELLA:
- Varicella pneumonia can be treated with IV acyclovir.

- Adults who develop chickenpox should be considered for acyclovir treatment, which may prevent the development of pneumonia.

MEASLES: No effective antimeasles agent.

CMV:
- Acyclovir can prevent CMV infection in renal transplant recipients.
- Ganciclovir and foscarnet, with or without CMV hyperimmune globulin, show promise in the treatment of serious CMV infection, including pneumonia, in compromised hosts.

■ DISPOSITION
- Supportive therapy is useful.
- Deaths are possible during acute illness.
- Residual functional abnormalities may be persistent, develop into, or predispose to chronic respiratory diseases in later life.

- Morbidity and mortality following most viral pneumonias are increased by bacterial superinfection.

■ REFERRAL
- Uncertainty about the diagnosis in a compromised host
- Symptoms or findings progressive
- Severe respiratory compromise, diffuse infiltrates, or the development of ARDS

✷ PEARLS & CONSIDERATIONS

■ COMMENTS
- Influenza spreads by close contact and by small droplets transmitted by cough, which typifies the illness.

- RSV is effectively transmitted by fomites and by direct contact (little by aerosol).
- Varicella is transmitted by direct contact or by aerosol.
- Measles is transmitted by aerosol and possibly by fomites.

REFERENCES
Chien JW, Johnson JL: Viral pneumonias: multifaceted approach to an elusive diagnosis, *Postgrad Med* 107:67, 2000.

Colacino JM, Staschke KA, Laver WG: Approaches and strategies for the treatment of influenza virus infections, *Antivir Chem Chemother* 10:155, 1999.

Glezen WP et al: Impact of respiratory virus infections on persons with chronic underlying conditions, *JAMA* 283:499, 2000.

Author: **Harvey M. Shanies, M.D., Ph.D.**

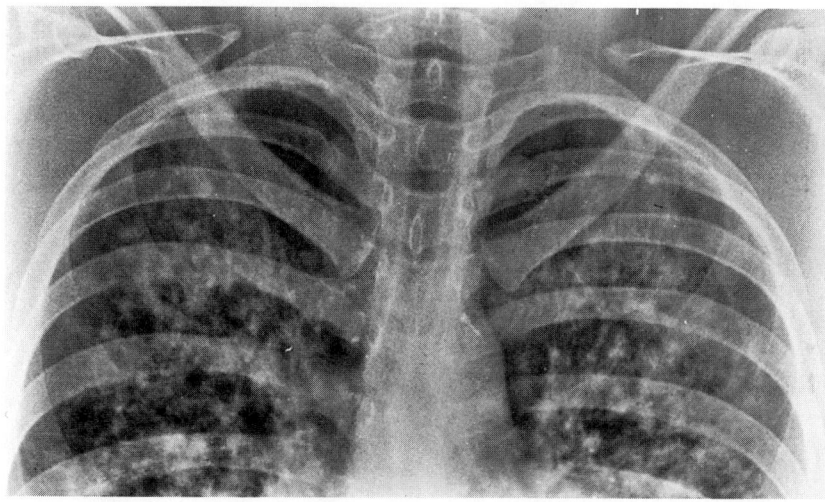

Fig. 1-298 Chickenpox—varicella pneumonia. Coned-down view of the upper lobes shows multiple ill-defined nodules in both upper lobes. (From McLoud TC: *Thoracic radiology: the requisites,* St Louis, 1998, Mosby.)

BASIC INFORMATION

■ DEFINITION
A pneumothorax is defined as the accumulation of air into the pleural space, collapsing the lung (Fig. 1-299). A spontaneous pneumothorax (SP) is a pneumothorax occurring without any obvious cause.

■ SYNONYMS
Primary spontaneous pneumothorax
Secondary spontaneous pneumothorax

ICD-9CM CODES
512.0 Spontaneous tension pneumothorax
512.8 Other spontaneous pneumothorax

■ EPIDEMIOLOGY & DEMOGRAPHICS
• Primary SP occurs in healthy individuals whereas secondary SP occurs in patients who have underlying lung disease.
• Approximately 20,000 new cases of spontaneous pneumothoraces occur each year in the U.S.
• SP is more common in men than women (6:1).
• Incidence of primary SP is 7.4/100,000 in men and 1.2/100,000 in women.
• Incidence of secondary SP 6.3/100,000 in men and 2.0/100,000 in women.
• Commonly seen in tall, thin young men 20 to 40 yr of age.
• Tobacco increases the risk of SP.

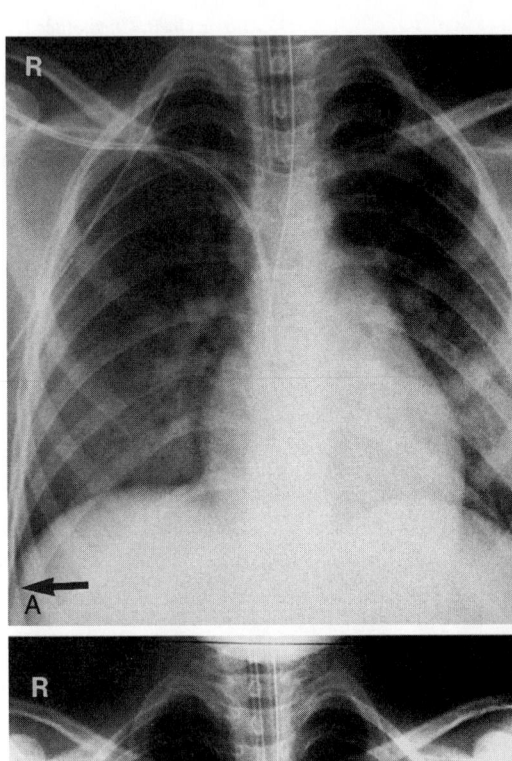

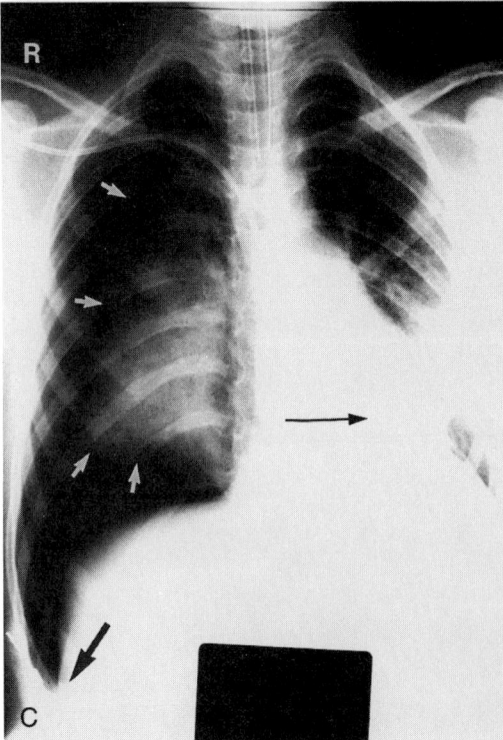

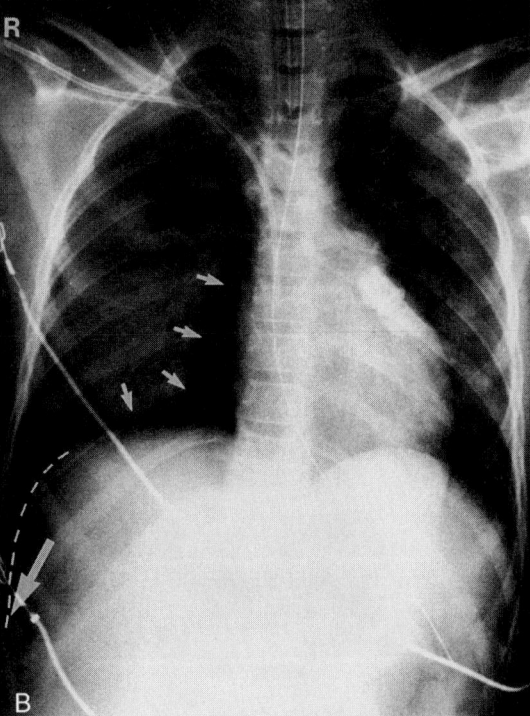

Fig. 1-299 Deep sulcus sign of pneumothorax. On a PA chest radiograph **(A)**, the costophrenic angle is normally acute *(arrow)*. In a supine patient, a pneumothorax will often be anterior, medial, and basilar. On a subsequent supine film **(B)** the dark area along the right cardiac border and lung base got bigger *(small arrows)*, and the costophrenic angle became much deeper and more acute than normal *(large arrow)*. These findings were not recognized, and, as a result, the same patient developed a tension pneumothorax **(C)** with an extremely deep costophrenic angle *(large black arrow)* and almost completely collapsed right lung *(small white arrows)* and shift of the mediastinum to the left. (From Mettler FA [ed]: *Primary are radiology*, Philadelphia, 2000, WB Saunders.)

■ PHYSICAL FINDINGS & CLINICAL PRESENTATION

- Sudden onset of pleuritic chest pain (90%)
- Dyspnea (80%)
- Tachycardia
- Diminished breath sounds
- Decreased tactile fremitus
- Hyperresonance

■ ETIOLOGY

- In primary SP, rupture of small blebs usually located near the apex of the upper lobes is a common cause.
- In secondary SP, COPD is the most common cause but can also be associated with pneumonia, bronchogenic carcinoma, mesothelioma, sarcoidosis, tuberculosis, cystic fibrosis, and many other lung diseases.

 # DIAGNOSIS

Established by the chest x-ray

■ DIFFERENTIAL DIAGNOSIS

- Pleurisy
- Pulmonary embolism
- Myocardial infarction
- Pericarditis
- Asthma
- Pneumonia

■ WORKUP

Includes arterial blood gases, chest x-ray, and in some cases, CT scan of the chest

■ LABORATORY TESTS

ABGs may show hypoxemia and hypocapnia secondary to hyperventilation.

■ IMAGING STUDIES

- Spontaneous pneumothorax is usually confirmed by chest x-ray. X-ray findings include:
  1. Pleural line with absence of vessel markings peripheral to this line.
  2. Expiratory films are better at demarcating the pneumothorax pleural line.
  3. Films should be done with patient standing and not supine.

- CT scan can be done in suspected but difficult-to-visualize pneumothoraces.

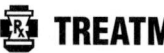 # TREATMENT

■ NONPHARMACOLOGIC THERAPY

- Supplemental oxygen increases the rate of pneumothorax absorption.
- Cautious observation in the asymptomatic patient with <15% pneumothorax can be done but requires close daily outpatient monitoring.

■ ACUTE GENERAL Rx

- Aspiration using a small IV catheter in the second intercostal space midclavicular line attached to a three-way stopcock and a large syringe. Air is aspirated until resistance, excess cough by the patient, or >2.5 L is taken out. Repeat films are done immediately after aspiration and again in 24 hr.
- Chest tube insertion has been recommended for patients with primary SP who failed observation and simple aspiration and for all patients with secondary SP.

■ CHRONIC Rx

- Chest tube with pleurodesis has been used to prevent recurrence of both primary and secondary SP. Sclerosing agents commonly instilled through the chest tube into the pleural cavity are minocycline 5 mg/kg in 50 ml of normal saline or doxycycline 500 mg in 50 ml of normal saline.
- Talc has also been used as a sclerosing agent.
- Thoracoscopy or video-assisted thoracoscopy (VAT) is indicated in patients who have not responded to chest tube suctioning in 7 days, patients who have persistent bronchopleural fistula, and patients who have recurrent pneumothorax after chemical pleurodesis.
- Open thoracotomy is done in patients who fail VAT.

■ DISPOSITION

- Approximately 25% of patients with primary SP will have recurrence within 2 yr.
- The rate of recurrence after the second and third episode of spontaneous pneumothorax is 60% and 80% respectively, with the majority of recurrences occurring on the same side as the first pneumothorax.
- Death from primary SP is uncommon. In patients with secondary SP and COPD, mortality ranges from 1% to 16%.
- Recurrence rates after open thoracotomy is <2%.

■ REFERRAL

A pulmonary specialist and general surgeon consultation is recommended.

☼ PEARLS & CONSIDERATIONS

■ COMMENTS

- The rate of pleural air absorption is about 1.25%/day.
- Patients with AIDS and *Pneumocystis carinii* infection have a high incidence of SP. Treatment typically requires chest tube placement and either thoracoscopy or open thoracotomy.

REFERENCES

Baumann MH, Strange C: Treatment of spontaneous pneumothorax: a more aggressive approach, *Chest* 112(3):789, 1997.

Jantz MA, Pierson DJ: Pneumothorax and barotrauma, *Clin Chest Med* 15.1:75, 1994.

Light RW: Management of spontaneous pneumothorax, *Am Rev Respir Dis* 148(1):245, 1993.

Miller AC, Harvey JE: Guidelines for the management of spontaneous pneumothorax, *BMJ* 307(6896):114, 1993.
Author: **Peter Petropoulos, M.D.**

BASIC INFORMATION

■ DEFINITION
Poliomyelitis is a symptomatic infection caused by poliovirus, which (on rare occasions) may result in paralysis.

■ SYNONYMS
Polio
Infantile paralysis

ICD-9CM CODES
045.9 Poliomyelitis

■ EPIDEMIOLOGY & DEMOGRAPHICS
INCIDENCE (IN U.S.):
- Approximately 8 cases/yr.
- All cases in the U.S. and Western Hemisphere are now vaccine associated (because of oral polio vaccine [OPV]).

PREDOMINANT AGE: Almost always infants or young children
GENETICS:
Neonatal Infection: Most cases occur in otherwise healthy infants who receive OPV, or their contacts.

■ PHYSICAL FINDINGS & CLINICAL PRESENTATION
- Exposure of a nonimmune host to poliovirus usually results in asymptomatic infection.
- A small percentage of individuals may have one of three presentations:
  1. Abortive poliomyelitis: a flulike illness
     a. Fever
     b. Malaise
     c. Headache
     d. Sore throat
  2. Nonparalytic poliomyelitis: an aseptic meningitis that correlates with invasion of the CNS
     a. Headache
     b. Neck stiffness
     c. Change in mental status
  3. Paralytic poliomyelitis
     a. Most commonly affects the lumbar or bulbar regions
     b. Following paralysis, a period of variable degrees of recovery, the majority of which occurs in 2 to 6 mo
     c. Paralysis from involvement of motor neurons in the spinal cord
     d. Flaccid paralysis without sensory defects
     e. Postpolio syndrome late sequela, which may occur many years after the acute illness
     f. Functional deterioration of muscle groups that had recovered from initial paralysis thought to result from failure of reinnervation, which initially was able to restore function to weakened or paralyzed areas

■ ETIOLOGY
- Virus of genus *Enterovirus*
- Classic endemic and epidemic disease caused by wild-type poliovirus
- All cases in the U.S. currently caused by a live, attenuated virus in the OPV
  1. Extremely rare complication that occurs in vaccine recipients or their contacts
  2. Paralysis from lower motor neuron damage caused by viral infection

DIAGNOSIS

■ DIFFERENTIAL DIAGNOSIS
- Guillain-Barré syndrome
- CVA
- Spinal cord compression
- Other enteroviruses:
  1. Aseptic meningitis
  2. Paralysis (rare)

■ WORKUP
- Isolation of virus:
  1. Stool or a rectal swab
  2. Throat swabs
  3. Rarely CSF
- Paired sera for antibody titer determinations

■ LABORATORY TESTS
CSF:
- Aseptic meningitis
- Elevated WBCs
- Elevated protein
- Normal glucose

■ IMAGING STUDIES
MRI may show involvement of anterior horn of the spinal cord.

TREATMENT

■ NONPHARMACOLOGIC THERAPY
- Maintenance of respiration and hydration
- Early mobilization and exercise once fever subsides

■ ACUTE GENERAL Rx
- Aimed at reduction of pain and muscle spasm
- No agent to alter the course of disease

■ CHRONIC Rx
Physical therapy

■ DISPOSITION
- In the abortive and nonparalytic forms, complete recovery
- Paralytic disease:
  1. Variable degrees of recovery
  2. 80% usually in the first 6 mo following illness

■ REFERRAL
To an infectious disease consultant

PEARLS & CONSIDERATIONS

■ COMMENTS
- Risk of disease in recipients of OPV is approximately 1 in 2.5 million.
- Use of inactivated polio vaccine (IPV) is not associated with disease:
  1. Does not confer local (mucosal) immunity
  2. Will not immunize nonvaccinated contacts
  3. Requires boosters
  4. Is given by injection
- To decrease the incidence of vaccine-associated polio, the routine childhood vaccination schedule has been changed. A recent recommendation for use of a sequential IPV-OPV schedule has again been modified. Exclusive use of IPV is now recommended. OPV use is limited to unvaccinated persons with plans for imminent (<4 wk) travel to polio-endemic areas.
- Cases should be reported to public health agencies.

REFERENCES
Centers for Disease Control and Prevention: Recommendations of the Advisory Committee on Immunization Practices: Revised recommendations for routine poliomyelitis vaccination, *MMWR* 48:590, 1999.
Halstead LS: Post-polio syndrome, *Sci Am* 278:42, 1998.
Author: **Maurice Policar, M.D.**

BASIC INFORMATION

DEFINITION
Polyarteritis nodosa is a vasculitic syndrome involving medium-size to small arteries, characterized histologically by necrotizing inflammation of the arterial media and inflammatory cell infiltration.

SYNONYMS
Periarteritis nodosa
PAN
Necrotizing arteritis

ICD-9CM CODES
446.0 Polyarteritis nodosa

EPIDEMIOLOGY & DEMOGRAPHICS
- Incidence is 1:100,000 annually.
- Male:female ratio is 2:1.
- Increased incidence in patients with hepatitis B surface antigen, hepatitis C virus.

PHYSICAL FINDINGS & CLINICAL PRESENTATION
- Weight loss, nausea, vomiting
- Testicular pain or tenderness
- Myalgias, weakness, or leg tenderness
- Neuropathy (mononeuritis multiplex), foot drop
- Livedo reticularis, ulceration of digits, abdominal pain after meals, hematemesis, hematochezia, hypertension, asymmetric polyarthritis (tending to involve large joints of lower extremities)
- Fever may be present (polyarteritis nodosa is often a cause of fever of unknown origin)

ETIOLOGY
- Unknown
- Immune complexes have been implicated

DIAGNOSIS

DIFFERENTIAL DIAGNOSIS
Cryoglobulinemia, SLE, infections (e.g., SBE, trichinosis, *Rickettsia*), lymphoma

WORKUP
- Laboratory evaluation, arteriography, and biopsy of small or medium-size arteries can confirm diagnosis. Clinical manifestations are variable and depend on the arteries involved and the organs affected (e.g., kidney involvement occurs in >80% of cases).
- The presence of any three of the following ten items allows the diagnosis of periarteritis nodosa with a sensitivity of 82% and a specificity of 86%:
  1. Weight loss >4 kg
  2. Livedo reticularis
  3. Testicular pain or tenderness
  4. Myalgias, weakness, or leg tenderness
  5. Neuropathy
  6. Diastolic blood pressure >90 mm Hg
  7. Elevated BUN or creatinine
  8. Positive test for hepatitis B virus
  9. Arteriography revealing small or large aneurysms and focal constrictions between dilated segments
  10. Biopsy of small or medium-size artery containing WBC

LABORATORY TESTS
- Elevated BUN or creatinine, positive test for hepatitis B virus or hepatitis C.
- Elevated ESR, anemia, elevated platelets, eosinophilia, proteinuria, RBC casts in the urine
- Biopsy of small or medium-size artery of symptomatic sites (muscle, nerve) is >90% specific.

IMAGING STUDIES
Arteriography can be done in patients with negative biopsies or if there are no symptomatic sites. Visceral angiography will reveal aneurysmal dilatation of the renal, mesenteric, or hepatic arteries (Fig. 1-300).

TREATMENT

NONPHARMACOLOGIC THERAPY
Low-sodium diet in hypertensive patients

ACUTE GENERAL Rx
Prednisone 1 to 2 mg/kg/day; cyclophosphamide in refractory cases

CHRONIC Rx
Monitoring for infections and potential complications such as thrombosis, infarction, or organ necrosis

DISPOSITION
The 5-yr survival is <20% in untreated patients. Treatment with corticosteroids increases survival to approximately 50%. Usage of both corticosteroids and immunosuppressive drugs may increase 5-yr survival >80%. Poor prognostic signs are severe renal or GI involvement.

REFERRAL
Surgical referral for biopsy
Author: **Fred F. Ferri, M.D.**

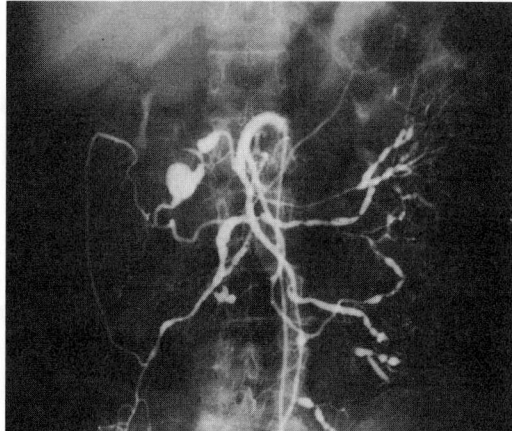

Fig. 1-300 Mesenteric arteriogram in a patient with polyarteritis. Characteristic multiple microaneurysms, as well as scattered luminal irregularities, are evident. (From Stein J [ed]: *Internal medicine,* ed 5, St Louis, 1998, Mosby.)

BASIC INFORMATION

■ DEFINITION
Polycystic kidney disease refers to a systemic hereditary disorder characterized by the formation of cysts in the cortex and medulla of both kidneys (Fig. 1-301).

■ SYNONYMS
Autosomal dominant polycystic kidney disease (ADPKD)

ICD-9CM CODES
753.1 Polycystic kidney, unspecified type
753.13 Polycystic kidney, autsomal dominant

■ EPIDEMIOLOGY & DEMOGRAPHICS
- Occurs in 1:400 to 1:1000 people
- Incidence: 6000 new cases per year
- Approximately 500,000 people with ADPKD in the U.S.
- Found in all ages
- Accounts for 10% of end-stage renal disease
- Associated with liver cysts (50% to 70%), pancreatic cysts (10%), splenic cysts (5%), and CNS arachnoid cysts (5%)
- Also associated with cerebral aneurysms (20%); 6% of patients with berry aneurysms have polycystic kidney disease
- Increased incidence of diverticular disease and mitral valve prolapse

■ PHYSICAL FINDINGS & CLINICAL PRESENTATION
- Usually presents in the third to fourth decade of life
- Pain (abdominal, flank or back)
- Palpable flank mass
- Hypertension
- Headache
- Nocturia
- Hematuria
- Nephrolitiasis (20%)
- Urinary tract infection

■ ETIOLOGY
- Approximately 90% of cases are inherited as an autosomal dominant trait.
- Spontaneous mutations occur in 10% of cases.
- The abnormal gene in the majority of cases has been located to the short arm of chromosome 16. In the minority of cases the defect is located on chromosome 4.
- All cysts develop from preexisting renal tubules segments and only a small portion of the nephrons (1%) undergoes cystic formation.

 DIAGNOSIS

A person is considered to have polycystic kidney disease if three or more cysts are noted in both kidneys and there is a positive family member with ADPKD.

■ DIFFERENTIAL DIAGNOSIS
- Simple cysts
- Autosomal recessive polycystic kidney disease in children
- Tuberous sclerosis
- Von Hippel-Lindau syndrome
- Acquired cystic kidney disease

■ WORKUP
The workup to establish the diagnosis of ADPKD includes a detailed family history and either an ultrasound or a CT scan of the abdomen to visualize bilateral renal cysts.

■ LABORATORY TESTS
- Hemoglobin and hematocrit is elevated because of increased secretion of erythropoietin from functioning renal cysts. This also explains the relatively mild anemia found in patients with ADPKD and renal insufficiency.
- Electrolyte abnormalities commonly seen in any patients with renal insufficiency may be present.
- BUN and creatinine can be elevated.
- Urinalysis can show microscopic hematuria, WBC casts in pyelonephritis, or proteinuria (seldom >1 g/24 hr).
- Increased erythropoietin level.
- Patients with a strong positive family history of ADPKD and no cysts detected by imaging studies can undergo genetic linkage analysis.

■ IMAGING STUDIES
- Abdominal renal ultrasound is the easiest and more cost-efficient test for renal cysts. Renal ultrasound can detect cysts from 1 to 1.5 cm.
- Abdominal CT scan is more sensitive than ultrasound and can detect cysts as small as 0.5 cm.
- Both studies can detect associated hepatic, splenic, and pancreatic cysts.
- MRI is more sensitive than ultrasound and may help in distinguishing renal cell carcinomas from simple cysts.

 TREATMENT

■ NONPHARMACOLOGIC THERAPY
- Nephrolithiasis is treated in a similar manner with either IV or PO hydration. If stones remain lodged, lithotripsy or percutaneous nephrostolithotomy can be done.
- Hypertension treatment is initiated with salt restriction, weight loss, and daily walking exercise.
- Avoidance of physical contact sports is advised.

■ ACUTE GENERAL Rx
- Kidney infections should be treated with antibiotics known to penetrate the cyst (e.g., trimethoprim-sulfamethoxazole 1 tablet PO bid or ciprofloxacin 250 mg PO bid).
- Angiotensin-converting enzyme inhibitors (e.g., captopril 25 mg bid or tid, lisinopril 10 mg PO qd, fosinopril 10 mg PO qd, or enalapril 10 mg qd) are effective in the treatment of hypertension associated with ADPKD.
- Calcium channel blockers (e.g., nifedipine 30 to 90 mg PO qd, amlodipine 5 to 10 mg PO qd, or felodipine 5 to 10 mg PO qd) can be used with or without ACE inhibitors in the treatment of hypertension.
- α-blockers and diuretics can be added as adjunctive therapy for hypertension.
- Blood pressure <130/85 is the goal for patients with renal disease. If there is >1 g of urinary protein per 24 hr, the target blood pressure is <125/75 mm Hg.

■ CHRONIC Rx
- Dialysis for end-stage renal failure
- Renal transplantation
- Cystic decompression in patients with intractable pain caused by enlarging cysts

■ DISPOSITION
- Approximately half the patients with ADPKD will progress to renal failure.
- Gross hematuria is usually self-limited.
- Complications of ADPKD include:
  1. End-stage renal failure
  2. Infected cysts and urinary tract infections
  3. Pyelonephritis
  4. Nephrolithiasis
  5. Electrolyte abnormalities
  6. Cerebral aneurysm rupture
  7. Intractable pain from enlarging cysts

■ REFERRAL
Nephrology consultation should be made in patients with renal insufficiency, difficult-to-control hypertension, recurrent infections, or renal stones. Urology can also be consulted in patients with nephrolithiasis, recurrent episodes of gross hematuria, or consideration for nephrectomy before transplantation.

PEARLS & CONSIDERATIONS

■ COMMENTS

- A cyst is considered to be present if it measures >2 mm in diameter.
- A positive family history of ADPKD is found in approximately 60% of the cases. Renal ultrasound performed on patient's parents reveals ADPKD in about 30% of the cases.
- Up to 25% of patients may not have cysts present before the age of 30.

- Screening patients with ADPKD for cerebral aneurysms is not recommended unless there is a positive family history of cerebral aneurysms or family member with ruptured cerebral aneurysm.

REFERENCES

Beebe DK: Autosomal dominant polycystic kidney disease, *Am Fam Physician* 53(3):925, 1996.

Chapman AB, Johnson AM, Gabow PA: Intracranial aneurysms in patients with autosomal dominant polycystic kidney disease: how to diagnose and who to screen, *Am J Kidney Dis* 22:526, 1993.

Gabow PA: Autosomal dominant polycystic kidney disease, *N Engl J Med* 329(5):332, 1993.

Welling LW, Grantham JJ: Cystic and developmental diseases of the kidney. In Brenner BM, Rector FC: *Brenner & Rector's the kidney,* ed 5, Philadelphia, 1996, WB Saunders.

Author: **Peter Petropoulos, M.D.**

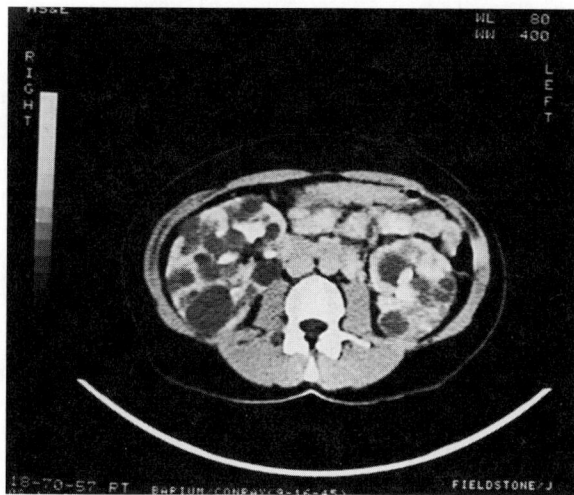

Fig. 1-301   Tomogram of autosomal dominant polycystic kidney disease. Kidney cysts. (From Stein JH [ed]: *Internal medicine,* ed 5, St Louis, 1998, Mosby.)

BASIC INFORMATION

■ DEFINITION
Polycystic ovary syndrome (PCOS) in its complete form associates polycystic ovaries, amenorrhea, hirsutism, and obesity.

■ SYNONYMS
Stein-Leventhal syndrome
PCOS

ICD-9CM CODES
256.4 Polycystic ovary syndrome

■ EPIDEMIOLOGY & DEMOGRAPHICS
PREVALENCE: 3% of adolescent and adult women.
Symptoms usually begin around the time of menarche, and the diagnosis is often made during adolescence or young adulthood.

■ PHYSICAL FINDINGS & CLINICAL PRESENTATION
- Oligomenorrhea or amenorrhea
- Dysfunctional uterine bleeding
- Infertility
- Hirsutism
- Acne
- Obesity (40% only)
- Insulin resistance (type 2 diabetes mellitus)

■ ETIOLOGY & PATHOGENESIS
- PCOS is probably a genetic disorder, but in most cases no family history is evident. Whether transmission is autosomal or X-linked is still unclear.
- Elevated serum LH concentrations and an increased serum LH:FSH ratio result either from an increased GnRH hypothalamic secretion or less likely from a primary pituitary abnormality. This results in dysregulation of androgen secretion and increased intraovarian androgen, the effect of which in the ovary is follicular atresia, maturation arrest, polycystic ovaries, and anovulation. Hyperinsulinemia is a contributing factor to ovarian hyperandrogenism, independent of LH excess. A role for insulin growth factor (IGF) receptors has been postulated for the association of PCOS and diabetes.

DIAGNOSIS

Clinical:
- PCOS is the most common cause of chronic anovulation with estrogen present. A positive progesterone withdrawal test establishes the presence of estrogen. Medroxyprogesterone (Provera) 10 mg qd is administered for 5 days and bleeding occurs if estrogen is present.
- The presence of oligomenorrhea, hirsutism, obesity, and documentation of polycystic ovaries establishes the diagnosis.

■ DIFFERENTIAL DIAGNOSIS
Causes of amenorrhea:
- Primary (unusual in PCOS)
  Genetic disorder (Turner's syndrome)
  Anatomic abnormality (e.g., imperforate hymen)
- Secondary
  Pregnancy
  Functional (cause unknown, anorexia nervosa, stress, excessive exercise, hyperthyroidism, less commonly hypothyroidism, adrenal dysfunction, pituitary dysfunction, severe systemic illness, drugs such as oral contraceptives, estrogens, or dopamine agonists)
  Abnormalities of the genital tract (uterine tumor, endometrial scarring, ovarian tumor)

■ LABORATORY TESTS
Fasting blood glucose to rule out diabetes

■ IMAGING STUDIES
Pelvic ultrasound (or CT scan) reveals the presence of twofold to fivefold ovarian enlargement with a thickened tunica albuginea, thecal hyperplasia, and 20 or more subcapsular follicles from 1 to 15 mm in diameter (Fig. 1-302).

TREATMENT

The goal is to interrupt the self-perpetuating abnormal hormone cycle:

- Reduction of ovarian androgen secretion by laparoscopic ovarian wedge resection
- Reduction of ovarian androgen secretion by using oral contraceptives or LHRH analogs
- Weight reduction for all obese women with PCOS
- FSH stimulation with clomiphene HMG, or pulsatile LHRH
- Urofollitropin (pure FSH) administration
- Glitazones may improve ovulation and hirsutism in the polycystic ovary syndrome

Choice of treatment:
- The management of hirsutism without risking pregnancy includes oral contraceptives, glucocorticoids, LHRH analogs, or spironolactone (an antiandrogen)
- Pregnancy can be achieved with clomiphene (alone or with glucocorticoids, hCG, or bromocriptine), HMG, urofollitropin, pulsatile LHRH, or ovarian wedge resection

■ REFERRAL
Gynecologist or endocrinologist

REFERENCES
Azziz R et al: Troglitazone improves ovulation and hirsutism in the polycystic ovary syndrome: a multicenter, double blind, placebo-controlled trial, *J Clin Endocrinol Metab* 86:1626, 2001.
Carr BR: Polycystic ovary syndrome. In Wilson JD et al (eds): *Williams' textbook of endocrinology*, ed 9, Philadelphia, 1998, WB Saunders.
Kazer RR: The polycystic ovary, *Semin Reprod Endocrinol* 15(2):193, 1997.
Author: **Tom J. Wachtel, M.D.**

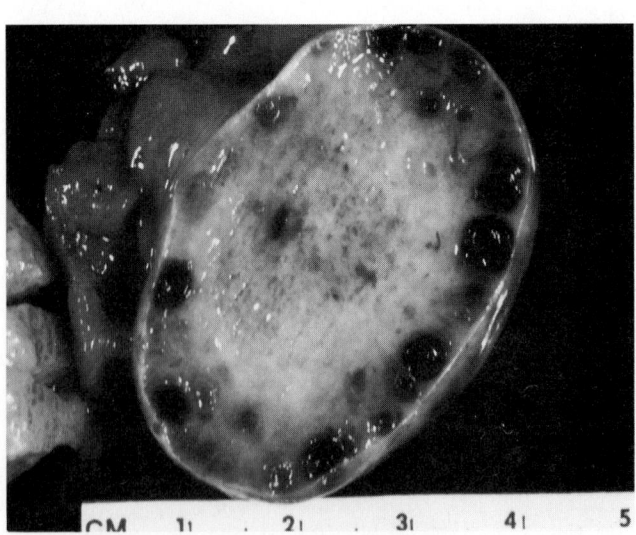

Fig. 1-302 Sagittal section of a polycystic ovary illustrating large number of follicular cysts and thickened stroma. (From Mishell DR: *Comprehensive gynecology*, ed 3, St Louis, 1997, Mosby.)

BASIC INFORMATION

■ **DEFINITION**
Polycythemia vera is a rare hematologic disorder characterized by clonal proliferation of bone marrow progenitors.

■ **SYNONYMS**
Primary polycythemia
Vaquez disease

■ **ICD-9CM CODES**
238.4 Polycythemia vera

■ **EPIDEMIOLOGY & DEMOGRAPHICS**
INCIDENCE/PREVALENCE: 0.5 cases/100,000 persons; mean age at onset is 60 yr; men are more effected than women

■ **PHYSICAL FINDINGS & CLINICAL PRESENTATION**
- Facial plethora, congestion of oral mucosa, ruddy complexion
- Enlargement and tortuosity of retinal veins
- Splenomegaly (found in >75% of patients)
- Symptoms include headache, transient neurologic or ocular complaints, paresthesias, pruritus after bathing

 DIAGNOSIS

■ **DIFFERENTIAL DIAGNOSIS**
1. SMOKING:
- Polycythemia is secondary to increased carboxyhemoglobin, resulting in left shift in the Hgb dissociation curve.
- Laboratory evaluation shows increased Hct, RBC mass, erythropoietin level, and carboxyhemoglobin.
- Splenomegaly is not present on physical examination.
2. HYPOXEMIA (SECONDARY POLYCYTHEMIA): Living for prolonged periods at high altitudes, pulmonary fibrosis, congenital cardiac lesions with right-to-left shunts
- Laboratory evaluation shows decreased arterial oxygen saturation and elevated erythropoietin level.
- Splenomegaly is not present on physical examination.
3. ERYTHROPOIETIN-PRODUCING STATES: Renal cell carcinoma, hepatoma, cerebral hemangioma, uterine fibroids, polycystic kidneys
- The erythropoietin level is elevated in these patients; the arterial oxygen saturation is normal.
- Splenomegaly may be present with metastatic neoplasms.

4. STRESS POLYCYTHEMIA (GAISBÖCK'S SYNDROME, RELATIVE POLYCYTHEMIA):
- Laboratory evaluation demonstrates normal RBC mass, arterial oxygen saturation, and erythropoietin level; plasma volume is decreased.
- Splenomegaly is not present on physical examination.
5. HEMOGLOBINOPATHIES ASSOCIATED WITH HIGH OXYGEN AFFINITY:
An abnormal oxyhemoglobin-dissociation curve (P50) is present.

■ **WORKUP**
The patient generally comes to medical attention because of symptoms associated with increased blood volume and viscosity or impaired platelet function:
- Impaired cerebral circulation resulting in headache, vertigo, blurred vision, dizziness, TIA, CVA
- Fatigue, poor exercise tolerance
- Pruritus, particularly following bathing (caused by overproduction of histamine)
- Bleeding: epistaxis, UGI bleeding (increased incidence of PUD)
- Abdominal discomfort secondary to splenomegaly; hepatomegaly may be present
- Hyperuricemia may result in nephrolithiasis and gouty arthritis
In patients with a presumptive diagnosis of polycythemia vera, the following diagnostic approach is useful:
- Measure RBC mass by isotope dilution using ^{51}Cr-labeled autologous RBCs; a high value eliminates stress polycythemia.
- Measure arterial saturation; a normal value eliminates polycythemia secondary to smoking.
- Measure erythropoietin level; if elevated, obtain IVP and abdominal CT to rule out renal cell carcinoma.
- The diagnosis of hemoglobinopathy with high affinity is ruled out by a normal oxyhemoglobin dissociation curve.
- Use of serum erythropoietin level and endogenous erythroid colony assay is a potential alternative method in the diagnosis of polycythemia vera.

■ **LABORATORY TESTS**
- Elevated RBC count (>6 million/mm³), elevated Hgb (>18 g/dl in men, >16 g/dl in women), elevated Hct (>54% in men, >49% in women)
- Increased WBC (often with basophilia); thrombocytosis in the majority of patients
- Elevated leukocyte alkaline phosphatase, serum vitamin B_{12}, and uric acid levels
- A low serum erythropoietin level highly suggestive of polycythemia vera
- Bone marrow aspiration revealing RBC hyperplasia and absent iron stores

 TREATMENT

■ **NONPHARMACOLOGIC THERAPY**
Phlebotomy to keep Hct <45% in men and <42% in women is the mainstay of therapy.

■ **ACUTE GENERAL Rx**
- Hydroxyurea can be used in conjunction with phlebotomy to decrease the incidence of thrombotic events.
- Interferon alfa-2b is also effective in controlling RBC values without significant side effects.
- Myelosuppressive therapy with chlorambucil is effective but not routinely used because of its leukemogenic potential.

■ **CHRONIC Rx**
- Patient education regarding need for lifelong monitoring and treatment
- Adjunctive therapy: treatment of pruritus with antihistamines, control of significant hyperuricemia with allopurinol, reduction of gastric hyperacidity with antacids of H_2 blockers, low-dose aspirin to treat vasomotor symptoms in patients without bleeding diathesis

■ **DISPOSITION**
- The median survival time without treatment is 6 to 18 mo following diagnosis; phlebotomy extends the average survival time to 12 yr.
- Prognosis is worse in patients >60 yr of age and those who have a history of thrombosis.

 PEARLS & CONSIDERATIONS

■ **COMMENTS**
The diagnosis of polycythemia vera generally requires the following three major criteria or the first two major criteria plus two minor criteria:
- Major criteria
  1. Increased RBC mass (>36 ml/kg in men, >32 ml/kg in women)
  2. Normal arterial oxygen saturation (>92%)
  3. Splenomegaly
- Minor criteria
  1. Thrombocytosis (>400,000/mm³)
  2. Leukocytosis (>12,000/mm³)
  3. Elevated leukocyte alkaline phosphatase (>100)
  4. Elevated serum vitamin B_{12} (>900 pg/ml) or vitamin B_{12} binding protein (>2200 pg/ml)

REFERENCE
Tefferi A et al: A clinical update in polycythemia vera and essential thrombocytopenia, *Am J Med* 109:141, 2000.
Author: **Fred F. Ferri, M.D.**

BASIC INFORMATION

■ DEFINITION
Polymyalgia rheumatica is a disorder of unknown cause affecting older patients. It is characterized by shoulder and hip stiffness and an elevated erythrocyte sedimentation rate (ESR).

■ SYNONYMS
Anarthritic rheumatoid syndrome

ICD-9CM CODES
725.0 Polymyalgia rheumatica

■ EPIDEMIOLOGY & DEMOGRAPHICS
PREVALENCE: 1 case/2000 persons >50 yr old
PREDOMINANT SEX: Female:male ratio of 2:1
PREDOMINANT AGE: Rare under age 50 yr; average age at onset: 70 yr

■ PHYSICAL FINDINGS & CLINICAL PRESENTATION
- Symptoms are frequently of sudden onset but are often present for months before the diagnosis is made.
- Neck, shoulder, low back, and thigh pain are common complaints.
- Morning stiffness lasting 2 to 3 hr is typical, and patients often have difficulty getting out of bed.
- Malaise, weight loss, depression, and a low-grade fever are common constitutional symptoms and may suggest systemic inflammation.
- Physical findings are usually limited. Synovitis may be present in peripheral joints and may also be responsible for the proximal girdle symptoms in spite of the fact that they appear to be "muscular" in nature.
- Mild soft tissue tenderness may be present.
- Distal extremity manifestations (knee, wrist, metacarpophalangeal joints) may occur in 25% to 45% of patients.
- The temporal arteries should be carefully examined because of the strong relation of polymyalgia rheumatica with temporal or giant cell arteritis.

■ ETIOLOGY
Unknown

DIAGNOSIS

■ DIFFERENTIAL DIAGNOSIS
(TABLE 1-53)
- Rheumatoid arthritis: rheumatoid factor is negative in polymyalgia.
- Polymyositis: enzyme studies are negative in polymyalgia.

■ WORKUP
The diagnosis of polymyalgia rheumatica is suggested by the following findings:

- Pain and stiffness of pectoral and pelvic musculature
- Patient >50 yr old
- Morning stiffness
- Normal motor strength
- Symptoms for at least 4 to 6 wk
- Elevated ESR (>45)
- Rapid clinical response to low-dose corticosteroid therapy

■ LABORATORY TESTS
- CBC, ESR, and rheumatoid factor should be performed.
- Mild anemia may be present.

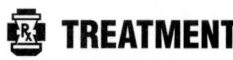

TREATMENT

■ ACUTE GENERAL Rx
- Prednisone 10 to 20 mg/day is given. The response is often so dramatic that it can be used to confirm the diagnosis. Improvement is usually noted within 24 to 48 hr. Generally, if the initial prednisone dose is 20 mg/day, reduce by 2.5 mg every wk to 10 mg/day, then by 1 mg/day every month if tolerated.
- Steroids are gradually tapered over the next few weeks as soon as symptoms permit, but small doses (5 mg/day) may be needed for 2 yr.
- NSAIDs may be tried in mild cases.
- Physical therapy is usually unnecessary.

TABLE 1-53 Differential Features in Polymyalgia Rheumatica and Similar Disorders

SIGNS/SYMPTOMS	POLYMYALGIA RHEUMATICA	GIANT CELL ARTERITIS	RHEUMATOID ARTHRITIS	DERMATOMYOSITIS	FIBROMYALGIA
Morning stiffness >30 min	+	±	+*	±	Variable
Headache and/or scalp tenderness	0	+	0	0	Variable
Pain with active joint movement	+	0	+*	0	Inconstant
Tender joints	±	0	+*	0	Tender spots
Swollen joints	±	±	+	0	0
Muscle weakness	±†	0	+*	+	0
Normochromic anemia	+	+	+	0	0
Elevated erythrocyte sedimentation rate	+	+	+	±	0
Elevated serum creatine kinase	0	0	0	+	0
Serum rheumatoid factor	0	0	70%	0	0
Distinct electromyographic abnormality	0	0	0	+	0
Response to nonsteroidal antiinflammatory drug	±	0	+	0	0

From Goldman L, Bennett JC, (eds): *Cecil textbook of medicine,* ed 21, Philadelphia, 2000, WB Saunders.
0, Absent; +, present; ±, present in minority of cases.
*Associated with affected joints
†Pain inhibits movement. Disuse atrophy may occur.

PEARLS & CONSIDERATIONS

■ COMMENTS
The prognosis is generally favorable. Relapse occasionally occurs in several years, but again responds well to prednisone.

REFERENCES

Cohen MD, Abril A: Polymyalgia rheumatica revisited, *Bull Rheum Dis* 50:1, 2001.

De Jager JP: Polymyalgia rheumatica and giant cell arteritis: avoiding management traps, *Aust Fam Physician* 30:643, 2001.

Meskimen S, Cook TD, Blake RL: Management of giant cell arteritis and polymyalgia rheumatica, *Am Fam Physician* 61:2061, 2000.

Salvarani C et al: Distal musculoskeletal manifestations in PMR, *Arthritis Rheum* 41:1221, 1998.

Weyland CM et al: Corticosteroid requirements in polymyalgia rheumatica, *Arch Intern Med* 159:577, 1999.

Author: **Lonnie R. Mercier, M.D.**

BASIC INFORMATION

■ DEFINITION
Polymyositis is a chronic idiopathic inflammatory myopathy.

■ SYNONYMS
Primary idiopathic polymyositis

ICD-9CM CODES
710.4 Polymyositis

■ EPIDEMIOLOGY & DEMOGRAPHICS
- Incidence: 5 cases/1 million/yr
- More common in females than males (2:1)

■ PHYSICAL FINDINGS & CLINICAL PRESENTATION
- Most patients with polymyositis have a subacute onset, over weeks to months.
- Symmetric proximal muscle weakness involving initially the shoulders and pelvic girdle resulting in difficulty rising from a chair, walking up stairs, or combing one's hair.
- Dysphagia and dysphonia result from pharyngeal muscle involvement.
- Dyspnea.
- Nonproductive cough.
- Rales.
- Aspiration pneumonia.
- Respiratory failure.
- Fever.
- "Mechanic's hand" (fissured and coarse skin over the area between the thumb and the index finger).
- Raynaud's phenomenon.

■ ETIOLOGY
- The exact cause of polymyositis is not known.
- An immunologic cause is suggested with increased frequency of HLA-DR3 and DRw52 antigens in patients with polymyositis.
- A viral etiology has been proposed secondary to the presence of autoantibodies to histidyl transferase antibody, anti-Jo-1 antibody, and signal recognition particle.

DIAGNOSIS

The diagnosis of polymyositis is made by:
- History and physical findings of proximal muscle weakness
- Elevated muscle enzyme tests
- EMG
- Muscle biopsy

■ DIFFERENTIAL DIAGNOSIS
- Dermatomyositis
- Muscular dystrophies
- Amyotrophic lateral sclerosis
- Myasthenia gravis or Eaton-Lambert syndrome
- Guillain-Barré syndrome
- Alcoholic myopathy
- Fibromyalgia
- Drug induced myopathies (e.g., HMG-reductase inhibitors, gemfibrozil)
- Diseases associated with polymyositis (e.g., sarcoidosis, HIV)
- Inclusion body myositis

■ WORKUP
Patients suspected of having polymyositis by clinical presentation should have an EMG, muscle biopsy, and specific blood tests to confirm the diagnosis.

■ LABORATORY TESTS
- ESR although not specific is elevated in the majority of cases.
- Creatine kinase is the most sensitive muscle enzyme test and can be elevated as much as 50 times above normal.
- Aldolase, AST, ALT, alkaline phosphatase, and LDH can be elevated.
- Anti-Jo-1 antibodies are more common in polymyositis.
- Electrolytes, TSH, Ca, and Mg should be requested to exclude other causes.
- Electromyography (EMG) is abnormal in 90% of patients and distinguishes a myopathic from a neuropathic process.
- Muscle biopsy is the definitive test. Characteristic findings separate polymyositis from dermatomyositis, inclusion body myositis, and neuromuscular disorders mimicking polymyositis.

■ IMAGING STUDIES
- A chest x-ray to rule out pulmonary involvement. If suspicious for pulmonary interstitial disease, a high-resolution CT scan of the chest may be helpful.
- A barium swallow to look for upper esophageal dysfunction in patients with dysphagia and polymyositis.
- MRI can help to locate sites of muscle involvement.

TREATMENT

■ NONPHARMACOLOGIC THERAPY
- Physical therapy is beneficial in increasing muscle tone and strength.
- Occupational therapy to assist with activities of daily living.
- Speech therapy for dysphagia and swallowing problems.

■ ACUTE GENERAL Rx
- Prednisone 1 to 2 mg/kg/day is the treatment of choice in patients with polymyositis. The dose is continued until muscle enzymes have returned to normal for 4 wk. Thereafter taper by 10 mg/mo until off of prednisone.
- Immunosuppresive agents (azathioprine, cyclophosphamide, or methotrexate) should be used if the patient fails to improve on prednisone or muscle enzymes begin rising when tapering off prednisone. See below for specific dosage.

■ CHRONIC Rx
- Chronic prednisone therapy may be needed for years.
- Azathioprine (2.5 to 3.5 mg/kg/day) or methotrexate (0.5 mg/kg/wk) can be added as stated above.

■ DISPOSITION
- As treatment is initiated, one should see the muscle enzymes return to normal before symptoms improve.
- During exacerbations enzymes will rise first before symptoms appear.
- Approximately 50% of patients will go into remission and stop therapy within 5 yr. The remaining will either have active disease requiring ongoing treatment or inactive disease with permanent muscle atrophy and contractures.
- The 5-year mortality rate is 20%.

■ REFERRAL
For any suspected cases of polymyositis a rheumatology referral should be made to help establish the diagnosis and implement treatment.

PEARLS & CONSIDERATIONS

■ COMMENTS
- When assessing response to treatment, it is best to follow clinical muscle strength over muscle enzyme tests.
- The concern of malignancies (ovary, lung, breast, GI) associated with myositis is legitimate and merits screening patients over the age of 40, particularly patients with dermatomyositis.

REFERENCES
Callen JP: Relationship of cancer to inflammatory muscle diseases: dermatomyositis, polymyositis, and inclusion body myositis, *Rheum Dis Clin North Am* 20(4):943, 1994.

Medsger TA et al: Classification and diagnostic criteria for polymyositis and dermatomyositis. *J Rheumatol* 22:581, 1995.

Tanimoto K et al: Classification criteria for polymyositis and dermatomyositis, *J Rheumtol* 22:668, 1995.

Dalakas MC: Polymyositis, dermatomyositis, and inclusion-body myositis, *N Engl J Med* 325(21):1487, 1991.
Author: **Peter Petropoulos, M.D.**

BASIC INFORMATION

■ **DEFINITION**
Portal vein thrombosis is thrombotic occlusion of the portal vein.

■ **SYNONYMS**
Pylethrombosis

ICD-9CM CODES
452 Portal vein thrombosis
572.1 Septic portal vein thrombosis

■ **EPIDEMIOLOGY & DEMOGRAPHICS**
Occurs with equal frequency in children (peak age: 6 yr) and adults (peak age: 40 yr)

■ **PHYSICAL FINDINGS & CLINICAL PRESENTATION**
Upper GI hemorrhage (hematemesis and/or melena) caused by esophageal varices. If abdominal pain is present, mesenteric venous thrombosis should be suspected (see "Mesenteric Venous Thrombosis" in Section I).

■ **ETIOLOGY AND PATHOPHYSIOLOGY**
In children: umbilical sepsis (pathophysiology unknown)
In adults:
1. Hypercoagulable states
• Antiphospholipid syndrome
• Neoplasm (common cause)
• Paroxysmal nocturnal hemoglobinuria
• Myeloproliferative diseases
• Oral contraceptives
• Polycythemia vera
• Pregnancy
• Protein S or C deficiency
• Sickle cell disease
• Thrombocytosis
2. Inflammatory diseases
• Crohn's disease
• Pancreatitis
• Ulcerative colitis
3. Complications of medical intervention
• Ambulatory dialysis
• Chemoembolization
• Liver transplantation
• Partial hepatectomy
• Sclerotherapy
• Splenectomy
• Transjugular intrahepatic portosystemic shunt
4. Infections
• Appendicitis
• Diverticulitis
• Cholecystitis
5. Miscellaneous
• Cirrhosis (common cause)
• Bladder cancer
Pathophysiology: portal vein thrombosis results in portal hypertension leading to esophageal and gastrointestinal varices. The liver sustained by the hepatic artery maintains normal function.

 DIAGNOSIS

■ **DIFFERENTIAL DIAGNOSIS**
All causes of upper GI hemorrhage (see Box 2-37).

■ **WORKUP**
• Esophagogastroscopy shows esophageal varices.
• Abdominal ultrasound (Fig. 1-303) or MRI may show the portal vein thrombosis.

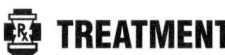 **TREATMENT**

• Variceal sclerotherapy or banding
• Surgical mesocaval or splenorenal shunt

■ **REFERRAL**
To gastroenterologist, surgeon, or both

REFERENCE
Schafter DF, Sorrell MF: Vascular diseases of the liver. In Feldman M et al (eds): *Gastrointestinal and liver disease,* ed 6, Philadelphia, 1998, WB Saunders.
Author: **Tom J. Wachtel, M.D.**

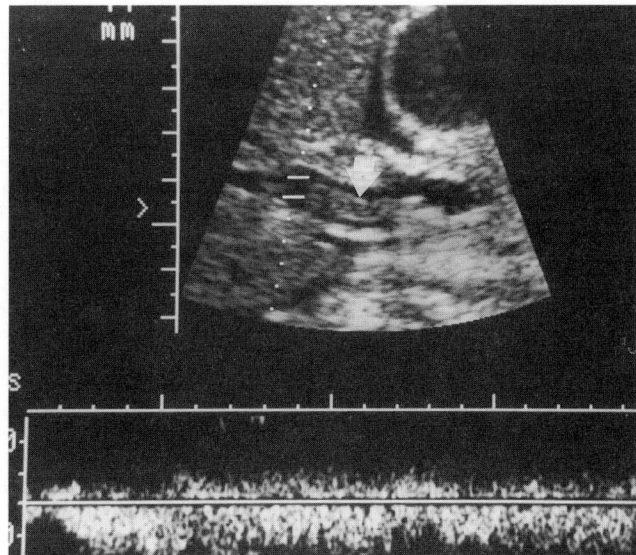

Fig. 1-303   Thrombus in portal vein evident on pulsed Doppler ultrasonography. An echogenic thrombus *(arrow)* is within the lumen of the portal vein. Doppler tracing indicates flow within portal vein. (From Sabiston D: *Textbook of surgery,* ed 15, Philadelphia, 1997, WB Saunders.)

BASIC INFORMATION

■ DEFINITION

- Postconcussive syndrome (PCS) refers to persistent neurologic symptoms that result from mild traumatic brain injury or concussion.
- Concussion may be defined as an acute trauma-induced alteration of mental function lasting fewer than 24 hr, with or without preceding loss of consciousness.
- Concussion is graded by the Colorado Medicine Society (Table 1-54) as:
  1. Grade 1 concussion (mild): No loss of consciousness (LOC), no posttraumatic amnesia but with confusion.
  2. Grade 2 concussion (moderate): No LOC, but posttraumatic amnesia and confusion.
  3. Grade 3 concussion (severe): LOC of any duration along with post-traumatic amnesia and confusion.

ICD-9CM CODES
310.2 Postconcussive syndrome

■ EPIDEMIOLOGY & DEMOGRAPHICS

- PCS incidence is 27/100,000.
- Approximately 15% of patients with mild traumatic brain injury will have persistent neurologic symptoms 1 yr after the injury.
- More often seen in men than in women.
- Usually seen in the young 20 to 30 yr of age.

■ PHYSICAL FINDINGS & CLINICAL PRESENTATION

- PCS patients usually present with neurologic symptoms and no focal neurologic deficits on examination. Symptoms start within a few days after the head injury with 15% of patients having persistent symptoms 1 yr later.
- Symptoms include:
  1. Headache (migraine type)
  2. Neck pain
  3. Dizziness and vertigo
  4. Paresthesias
  5. Difficulty in concentrating and with memory
  6. Insomnia
  7. Irritability

■ ETIOLOGY

- PCS by definition is caused by traumatic brain injury from falls, motor vehicle accidents, contact sports, etc.

- Postmortem findings reveal diffuse axonal injury as the primary pathologic finding along with small petechial hemorrhages and local edema.
- Diffuse axon injury is thought to lead to altered neurotransmitters and possibly to clinical manifestations.

DIAGNOSIS

A careful history, a nonfocal neurologic examination, and normal neurologic testing usually will establish the diagnosis of postconcussive syndrome.

■ DIFFERENTIAL DIAGNOSIS

- Headache (vascular or tension)
- Epidural hematoma
- Subdural hematoma
- Skull fracture
- Cervical spine disk disease
- Whiplash
- Seizure
- Cerebrovascular accident
- Depression
- Anxiety

■ WORKUP

A patient presenting with PCS merits a workup to exclude other causes of neurologic symptoms following traumatic brain injury.

■ LABORATORY TESTS

Blood tests are not very specific in diagnosing PCS.

■ IMAGING STUDIES

- CT scan of the head is normal.
- MRI of the head is often normal but may show petechial hemorrhages or cerebral contusions.
- EEG is normal.
- Evoked potentials are normal.
- Neuropsychologic testing may reveal difficulties in concentration, memory, and executive function but are not very specific for PCS.

TREATMENT

Postconcussive syndrome must be recognized as a physiologic and psychologic problem and treated accordingly.

■ NONPHARMACOLOGIC THERAPY

- Heat
- Physical therapy
- Avoidance of alcohol, narcotics, and sleep deprivation

■ ACUTE GENERAL Rx

- Headaches can be treated with NSAIDs, ibuprofen 800 mg tid or naproxen 500 mg bid.
- Neck pain can be treated in a similar fashion.

■ CHRONIC Rx

- Psychotherapy.
- Behavioral therapy.
- Vocational rehabilitation.
- Depression can be treated with SSRIs but may not respond as well when compared to non-PCS patients with depression.

■ DISPOSITION

- Most patients after mild traumatic brain injury improve without any residual deficits.
- Neuropsychological testing may be abnormal but usually improves during the first 6 mo after injury.
- If related to contact sports, see Table 1-54.
- Predictors for the development of persistent postconcussive syndrome (>1 yr) include:
  1. Female
  2. Ongoing litigation
  3. Low socioeconomic status
  4. Prior headaches
  5. Prior mild traumatic brain injury
  6. Prior psychiatry illnesses

■ REFERRAL

Postconcussive syndrome patients may benefit from consultations with psychologists, psychiatrists, and neurologists.

PEARLS & CONSIDERATIONS

■ COMMENTS

- PCS syndrome starts within a few days after the injury. Recognizing depression and treating pain symptoms early in the course may help prevent the development of persistent postconcussive syndrome (>1 yr).
- The severity of the fall, duration of unconsciousness, and amnesia helps assess the severity of axonal injury.
- Attempts to determine how much of a role psychologic and neurologic factors play in the PCS are important but very difficult.

REFERENCES

Alexander MP: Mild traumatic brain injury: pathophysiology, natural history, and clinical management, *Neurology* 45:1253, 1995.

Evans RW: Mild traumatic brain injury, *Phys Med Rehabil Clin North Am* 3:427, 1992.

Evans RW: The postconcussive syndrome: 130 years of controversy, *Semin Neurol* 14:32, 1994.

Koshner DS: Concussion in sports: minimizing the risk for complications, *Am Fam Physician* 64:1007, 2001.

Author: **Peter Petropoulos, M.D.**

TABLE 1-54 Concussion Guidelines and Recommendations

Acute head injuries are usually divided into two categories:
1. Diffuse brain injuries—concussion and diffuse axonal injuries.
2. Focal brain injuries—all fractures and intracranial injuries.

It is not necessary to have loss of consciousness to have a concussion.* Several severity grading scales for concussion exist; one that is commonly used is the following:

COLORADO MEDICAL SOCIETY GUIDELINES

GRADE	CONFUSION	AMNESIA	LOSS OF CONSCIOUSNESS
I	+	−	−
II	+	+	−
III	+	+	+

Return-to-Play Criteria

Return-to-play criteria are based on prevention of the *second impact syndrome*. This syndrome is characterized by a loss of autoregulation of cerebral blood flow, manifest as a rapid increased intracranial pressure following a second head injury before full recovery from the initial head injury has occurred. Return to contact sports is based on the grade of the injury.

RECOMMENDATIONS FOR RETURN TO CONTACT SPORTS FOLLOWING A CONCUSSION†

GRADE	MINIMUM TIME TO RETURN	TIME ASYMPTOMATIC‡
I	20 min	When examined
II	1 wk	1 wk
III	1 mo	1 wk

RECOMMENDATIONS FOR RETURN TO CONTACT SPORTS FOLLOWING REPEATED CONCUSSIONS

GRADE	MINIMUM TIME TO RETURN	TIME ASYMPTOMATIC‡
I (second time)	2 wk	1 wk
II (second time)	1 mo	1 wk
I (× 3), II (× 2), III (× 2)	Season over	1 wk

From Behrman RE: *Nelson textbook of pediatrics,* ed 16, Philadelphia, 2000, WB Saunders.

*In animal studies, there is evidence that there are microscopic changes in the brain after a concussion. These may not be evident in imaging studies, so the clinician must rely on history and neuropsychologic examination to follow a patient's progress. In college football players who experienced their first concussion, the neuropsychologic testing normalized in 5 days and symptoms of headache and memory resolved in 10 days.

The chronic effects of repetitive boxing injuries include cortical atrophy and a cavum septum pellucidum (identified radiographically). Whether this occurs in other sports in which head injuries are common (football, ice hockey, wrestling) or in which the head is used as part of the game (soccer) is debatable. However, there appears to be no danger in the young soccer player occasionally heading the ball.

†Contact sports means any situation in which contact is possible, including practice.

‡A symptomatic athlete should not return to contact sports regardless of the initial diagnosis. Athletes with focal brain injuries are excluded from contact sports indefinitely. Patients with a neck injury can return to contact sports when they have full, pain-free range of motion, strength and sensation, and normal lordosis of the cervical spine.

BASIC INFORMATION

■ DEFINITION

Posttraumatic stress disorder (PTSD) is an anxiety disorder that arises when an individual has witnessed or experienced a potentially fatal or serious injurious condition during which he or she felt helpless or horrified. After resolution of the event the individual continues to experience the event in the form of flashbacks (reliving the trauma), intrusive recollections, dreams, or physiologic reactivity or psychologic distress in response to cues symbolizing the event. These responses are associated with persistent hyperarousal (e.g., hypervigilance, exaggerated startle, sleep disturbance, irritability, and difficulty concentrating) and avoidance (both physically and cognitively) of stimuli associated with the traumatic event.

■ SYNONYMS

Soldier's heart
Effort syndrome
Shell shock
Irritable heart
Traumatic necrosis
Survivor syndrome
Concentration camp syndrome
Gross stress reaction (DSM-I, published in 1952)

ICD-9CM CODES

308.3 Posttraumatic stress syndrome, acute
309.81 Posttraumatic stress syndrome, chronic

■ EPIDEMIOLOGY & DEMOGRAPHICS
INCIDENCE (IN U.S.):
Occurs in some 50% of people experiencing a severe life-threatening event (e.g., PTSD was diagnosed in 85% of Nazi concentration camp survivors, 57% of Coconut Grove fire survivors, 67% of WWII prisoners of war, and 50% of Cambodian children subjected to various atrocities).
PREVALENCE (IN U.S.):
• Lifetime prevalence estimates range from 1% to 15% of the American population.
• Prevalence estimates among high-risk populations (e.g., combat veterans or victims of violent crimes) range from 3% to 58%.
PREDOMINANT SEX: No specific gender predisposition has been identified.
PREDOMINANT AGE:
• Development in children is possible, but presentation may be slightly different.
• No predisposing age factors have been identified.

PEAK INCIDENCE: Symptoms may begin immediately after the trauma and peak within 4 to 5 mo of the event.
GENETICS: No specific factors have been identified.

■ PHYSICAL FINDINGS & CLINICAL PRESENTATION
• After severe life-threatening event, complaints of derealization, depersonalization, detachment, dissociation, or being dazed, in association with a marked increase in anxiety and arousal
• Within 3 mo, signs of persistent hyperarousal, anxiety, and distressing memories or reexperiences of the traumatic event in most patients; symptoms may be disabling

■ ETIOLOGY
• There is a "dose-response" relationship between intensity and duration of the stress and severity of PTSD, with duration of the stress the most important factor.
• Man-made disasters cause more intense reactions than natural disasters.
• Premorbid factors (dysthymia, introversion, personality types, alcohol abuse, and family psychiatric history) may predispose to PTSD.
• Symptoms are mediated, in part, by the autonomic nervous system and the hypothalamic-pituitary-adrenal system.

 DIAGNOSIS

■ DIFFERENTIAL DIAGNOSIS
• Diagnosis is made when a dysfunctional response occurs to any stress, so although most people with PTSD technically suffer from an adjustment disorder, the stress to which they are responding is usually extreme.
• Acute stress disorder is similar to PTSD but occurs within the first 4 wk of the stress.
• If symptoms of acute stress disorder persist longer than 4 wk, PTSD is possible.
• Malingering is sometimes difficult to rule out when there is secondary gain.

■ WORKUP
• History to determine symptoms.
• Physical examination to look for signs of autonomic hyperactivity.
• NOTE: Only the history is required for diagnosis.

℞ TREATMENT

■ NONPHARMACOLOGIC THERAPY
• Various forms of individual psychotherapy are effective in reducing severity of symptoms.
• Group therapy is the mainstay treatment for many PTSD victims, particularly in the combat veterans population.

■ ACUTE GENERAL Rx
• Purely symptomatic and generally aimed at alleviating distress
• Benzodiazepines for reducing the symptoms of anxiety
• β-Blockers to alleviate some of the autonomic symptoms
• Sedating antidepressants (e.g., amitriptyline) to treat initial insomnia and suppress nightmares; in low doses may also alleviate daytime anxiety

■ CHRONIC Rx
• Antidepressants (both tricyclic and serotonin reuptake inhibitor) and nonbenzodiazepine anxiolytic buspirone are mainstay of chronic pharmacologic management.
• Although these agents provide relief, they frequently have persisting residual and often troubling symptoms.
• Alternative approaches:
  1. Monoamine oxidase inhibiting antidepressants
  2. Chronic use of β-blockers or α_2-agonists (e.g., clonidine)
  3. Anticonvulsants such as carbamazepine

■ DISPOSITION
• Spontaneous remission in 6 mo for nearly half of patients
• Possible chronic symptoms for years
• Predictors of chronic course:
  1. Premorbid psychiatric function
  2. Acute response to stress (e.g., individuals who experience an acute stress disorder immediately after the trauma do better in the long term)

■ REFERRAL
Because early intervention improves outcome, referral made for all patients to psychotherapy as soon as diagnosis made

REFERENCES
Davidson J: Recognition and treatment of posttraumatic stress disorder, *JAMA* 286:584, 2001.
Krakow B et al: Imagery rehearsal for chronic nightmares in sexual assault survivors with posttraumatic stress disorder, *JAMA* 286:537, 2001.
Author: **Rif S. El-Mallakh, M.D.**

BASIC INFORMATION

■ DEFINITION
Precocious puberty is defined as sexual development occurring before 8 yr of age in males and 9 yr of age in females.

■ SYNONYMS
Pubertas praecox

■ ICD-9CM CODES
259.1 Precocious puberty

■ EPIDEMIOLOGY & DEMOGRAPHICS
INCIDENCE: Estimated to be between 1:5000 and 1:10,000
PREDOMINANT SEX: Females > males for the idiopathic variant; for other causes, dependent on the underlying etiology.
GENETICS: The genetics for some of the etiologies of precocious puberty are known.

■ PHYSICAL FINDINGS & CLINICAL PRESENTATION
- In females: breast development, pubic hair development, accelerated growth, and menarche
- In males: increase in testicular volume and penile length, pubic hair development, accelerated growth, muscular development, acne, change in voice, and penile erections

■ ETIOLOGY
- Idiopathic or true: diagnosis of exclusion
- CNS pathology: tumors, hydrocephalus, ventricular cysts, benign lesions
- Severe hypothyroidism
- Posttraumatic head injury
- Genetic disorders: neurofibromatosis, tuberous sclerosis, McCune-Albright syndrome, congenital adrenal hyperplasia
- Gonadal tumors
- Nongonadal tumors: hepatoblastoma
- Exposure to exogenous sex steroids
- Box 2-214 describes the various causes of precocious puberty.

DIAGNOSIS

■ DIFFERENTIAL DIAGNOSIS
- Most common diagnoses to consider: premature thelarche and premature adrenarche

- Gonadotropin hormone–releasing hormone (GnRH)–dependent precocious puberty: idiopathic, CNS tumors, hypothalamic hamartomas, neurofibromatosis, tuberous sclerosis, hydrocephalus, post acute head injury, ventricular cysts, post CNS infection.
- GnRH-independent precocious puberty: congenital adrenal hyperplasia, adrenocortical tumors (males), McCune-Albright syndrome (females), gonadal tumors, ectopic hCG-secreting tumors (chorioblastoma, hepatoblastoma), exposure to exogenous sex steroids, severe hypothyroidism.

■ WORKUP
Thorough history and physical examination are essential to determine if the patient has true precocious puberty. Particular attention should be paid to growth, development, order of appearance of the secondary sexual characteristics, pubertal development in family members, medications, neurologic symptoms, Tanner staging, abdominal and neurologic examination. Fig. 3-138 describes a clinical approach to precocious puberty.

■ LABORATORY TESTS
- GnRH testing will help determine if dependent or independent cause
- Sex hormone studies: LH, FSH, hCG, testosterone (males), estrogen (females)
- T_4, TSH

■ IMAGING STUDIES
- CT scan or MRI of the brain to evaluate for CNS pathology
- Consideration of pelvic ultrasound in female patients to evaluate for cysts/tumors
- Abdominal imaging with CT scan if intraabdominal pathology suspected

TREATMENT

■ NONPHARMACOLOGIC THERAPY
- Good communication with the parents is essential to care.
- Psychologic support for the child may be needed with regard to self-image and problems with peer acceptance.

■ ACUTE GENERAL Rx
There is no acute therapy for precocious puberty.

■ CHRONIC Rx
Therapy depends on the etiology of precocious puberty:
- For true precocious puberty and some CNS lesions, the treatment of choice is leuprolide 0.25 to 0.3 mg/kg with a 7.5 mg minimum IM every 4 wk.
- For other CNS lesions and extragonadal tumors, therapy is dependent on the type of lesion, location of the lesion, and the overall prognosis of the underlying problem.
- For severe hypothyroidism, treatment with thyroid hormone will result in regression of the sexual development. The child will subsequently undergo appropriate pubertal development later in life.
- For familial male gonadotropin-independent precocious puberty, ketoconazole can be used at doses of 600 mg/day divided tid or a combination of testolactone and spironolactone can be used.

■ DISPOSITION
- For true precocious puberty and some CNS lesions, long-term outcome is usually very good. When drug therapy is instituted, it is continued until a time when further pubertal development is appropriate. It is then discontinued, allowing the child to progress through puberty.
- For other cases, long-term outcomes are dependent on the prognosis of the underlying cause.

■ REFERRAL
- Initial workup can be instituted by the primary care provider.
- Referral to an endocrinologist is indicated for most children because they will need long-term management, monitoring, and treatment.

REFERENCE
Root AW: Precocious puberty, *Pediatr Rev* 21(1):10, 2000.
Author: **Beth J. Wutz, M.D.**

BASIC INFORMATION

■ DEFINITION

Preeclampsia involves a triad of hypertension, proteinuria, and edema that develops after the twentieth week of gestation. Mild preeclampsia is defined as a blood pressure of <140/90 mm Hg. Severe preeclampsia is associated with a blood pressure >160/110 mm Hg, proteinuria >5 g in a 24-hr urine collection, oliguria (<400 ml/24 hr), cerebral or visual disturbances, epigastric pain, pulmonary edema, thrombocytopenia, hepatic dysfunction, or severe intrauterine growth retardation.

■ SYNONYMS

Pregnancy-induced hypertension
Toxemia of pregnancy

ICD-9CM CODES

642.6 Preeclampsia

■ EPIDEMIOLOGY & DEMOGRAPHICS

INCIDENCE: 10% to 14% in primigravidas, 5.7% to 7.3% in multigravidas
RISK FACTORS: Increased incidence and severity with multiple gestations, renal or collagen-vascular diseases. Extremes of reproductive age, <20 or >35 yr of age.
GENETICS: Positive correlation with maternal and paternal family history.

■ PHYSICAL FINDINGS & CLINICAL PRESENTATION

- Generalized swelling or nondependent edema, possibly manifested by rapid weight gain (>4 lb/wk) even in the absence of edema
- Auscultation of pulmonary rales
- RUQ pain (HELLP syndrome or subcapsular liver hematoma)
- Hyperreflexia or clonus
- Vaginal bleeding (placental abruption)
- Acute or chronic fetal compromise manifested by intrauterine growth restriction or fetal tachycardia with late decelerations, respectively
- Wide range of symptoms attributable to multiorgan system dysfunction, involving hepatic, hematologic, renal, pulmonary, and CNS
- Possibility of severe disease despite "normal" blood pressure readings, so a high index of suspicion must be maintained in high-risk situations

■ ETIOLOGY

- Exact etiology or toxic substance is unknown.
- Theories
  1. Imbalance between thromboxane A_2 (vasoconstrictor and platelet aggregator) and prostacyclin (vasodilator).
  2. Abnormal trophoblastic invasion of spiral arteries.
  3. Increased sensitivity to angiotensin II by the muscular walls of the arteries.

DIAGNOSIS

■ DIFFERENTIAL DIAGNOSIS

- Acute fatty liver of pregnancy
- Appendicitis
- Diabetic ketoacidosis
- Gallbladder disease
- Gastroenteritis
- Glomerulonephritis
- Hemolytic-uremic syndrome
- Hepatic encephalopathy
- Hyperemesis gravidarum
- Idiopathic thrombocytopenia
- Thrombotic thrombocytopenic purpura
- Nephrolithiasis
- Pyelonephritis
- PUD
- SLE
- Viral hepatitis

■ WORKUP

- Two blood pressure measurements in lateral recumbent position 6 hr apart, with an absolute pressure >140/90 mm Hg or an increase of 30 mm Hg systolic or 15 mm Hg diastolic from baseline, an increase in the mean arterial pressure (MAP) of 20 mm Hg, or an absolute MAP >105 mm Hg
- Evaluation for proteinuria as defined by >0.1 g/L on urine dipstick or >300 mg protein on a 24-hr urine collection
- Evaluation of fetal status for evidence of intrauterine growth restriction, oligohydramnios, alteration in umbilical or uterine artery Doppler flow, or acute compromise, such as abruption
- Because of the insidious nature of the disease with potential for multiple organ involvement, complete evaluation for preeclampsia in any pregnant patient presenting with CNS derangement or GI complaints after 20 wk of gestation
- Evaluation for associated conditions such as disseminated intravascular coagulation, hepatic dysfunction, or subcapsular hematoma

■ LABORATORY TESTS

- High-risk patients: baseline assessment of renal function (24-hr urine collection for protein and creatinine clearance), platelets, BUN, creatinine, liver function tests, and uric acid should be obtained at the first prenatal visit.
- CBC (Hgb, Hct, platelets) may show signs of volume contraction or HELLP syndrome.
- Liver function tests (AST, ALT, LDH) are useful in evaluation for HELLP syndrome or to exclude important differentials.
- Hyperuricemia or increased creatinine may indicate decreasing renal function.
- PT, PTT, and fibrinogen should be checked to rule out disseminated intravascular coagulation.
- Peripheral smear may demonstrate microangiopathic hemolytic anemia.
- Complement levels can be used to differentiate from an acute exacerbation of a collagen-vascular disease.

■ IMAGING STUDIES

- CT scan of head if atypical presentation of eclampsia, possibility of intracerebral bleed, or prolonged postictal state
- Sonogram of fetus to evaluate for IUGR, amniotic fluid, placenta
- Sonogram of maternal liver if suspect subcapsular hematoma

℞ TREATMENT

■ NONPHARMACOLOGIC THERAPY

Bed rest in left lateral decubitus position

■ ACUTE GENERAL Rx

Delivery is the treatment of choice and the only cure for the disease. This must be taken in the context of the gestational age of the fetus, severity of the preeclampsia, and the likelihood of a successful induction and reliability of patient.

- Administer magnesium sulfate 6 g IV loading dose, with 2 to 3 g maintenance or phenytoin at 10 to 15 mg/kg loading dose, then 200 mg IV q8h starting 12 hr after loading dose.
- Hydralazine 10 mg IV, labetalol hydrochloride 20 to 40 mg IV, nifedipine 20 mg SL can be used for acute blood pressure control.
- Continuous fetal monitoring is needed.
- Epidural is anesthesia of choice for pain management in labor or C-section.
- All patients undergoing induction of labor should receive antiseizure medications regardless of severity of disease.

■ CHRONIC Rx

- Mild preeclampsia <37 wk: close observation for worsening maternal or fetal condition, with delivery at ≥37 wk with favorable cervix or at 40 wk regardless of cervical status.
- Severe preeclampsia: delivery in the presence of maternal or fetal compromise, labor, or >34 wk; at 28 to 34 wk consider steroids with close monitoring, and at <24 wk consider termination of pregnancy.
- Aldomet is drug of choice for chronic blood pressure control during pregnancy.

■ DISPOSITION

Preeclampsia is a progressive and unpredictable disease process; a course of expectancy should be managed with caution. Up to 20% of patients who have seizures are normotensive.

■ REFERRAL

Obstetric management is indicated because of the insidious nature of the disease, with transfer of all cases <34 wk to a facility with a level three nursery.

⚙ PEARLS & CONSIDERATIONS

■ COMMENTS

- Low-dose aspirin 80 mg qd and calcium supplementation 1500 mg qd can be considered in high-risk patients to decrease the risk of recurrence.
- Begin after first trimester.

REFERENCES

Creasy RT, Resnik R: *Maternal-fetal medicine,* ed 4, Philadelphia, 1999, WB Saunders.

Duley L et al: Antiplatelet drugs for prevention of pre-eclampsia and its consequences: systematic review, *BMJ* 322:329, 2001.

Esplin MS et al: Paternal and maternal components of the predisposition to preeclampsia, *N Engl J Med* 344:867, 2001.

Author: **Scott J. Zuccala, D.O.**

BASIC INFORMATION

■ DEFINITION
Premenstrual syndrome (PMS) is a cyclic recurrence during the luteal phase of the menstrual cycle of somatic, affective, and behavioral disturbances that are of sufficient severity to affect interpersonal relationships adversely or interfere with normal activities (Fig. 1-304).

■ SYNONYMS
PMS
PMDD

ICD-9CM CODES
625.4 Premenstrual tension syndromes

■ EPIDEMIOLOGY & DEMOGRAPHICS
• PMS is thought to be extremely prevalent, intermittently affecting approximately one third of all premenopausal women.
• Severe cases occur in approximately 2% to 10% of women with PMS.
• Those seeking treatment for PMS are usually in their 30s or 40s.
• The natural history of PMS has not been clearly elucidated.

■ PHYSICAL FINDINGS & CLINICAL PRESENTATION
• Diverse and potentially disabling symptoms
• Associated with >150 psychologic, physical, and behavioral symptoms
• Most frequent reason for seeking treatment: emotional symptoms

• Most common emotional symptoms: depression, irritability, anxiety, labile moods, anger, crying easily, sadness, overly sensitive, nervous tension
• Most common physical complaints: headache, bloating, cramps, breast tenderness, migraines, fatigue, weight gain, aches and pains, palpitations
• Most common behavior symptom: food cravings
• Other behavioral symptoms: increased appetite, increased alcohol intake, decreased motivation, decreased efficiency, avoidance of activities, staying home, sleep changes, libido changes, forgetfulness, decreased concentration

■ ETIOLOGY
• Etiology remains obscure.
• Because of multifactorial-multiorgan nature of PMS, a single etiologic cause is unlikely.

DIAGNOSIS

■ DIFFERENTIAL DIAGNOSIS
• A diagnosis of exclusion, so other medical or psychologic disorders should be ruled out
• Most common disorders: depression or anxiety, thyroid disease
• Table 2-109 describes the differential diagnosis of menstrual pain

■ WORKUP
• History
• Physical examination
• Laboratory studies to rule out alternative diagnosis
• If no alternative diagnosis confirms diagnosis of PMS, basal body temperature charting is used to determine if the patient is ovulating:
  1. If she is not ovulating, it is not PMS.
  2. If she is ovulating, symptoms should be charted for at least two cycles to determine if the symptoms occur in the luteal phase.
  3. If symptoms are not occurring in the luteal phase, it is not PMS, and further investigation is needed.
     a. If symptoms occur in the follicular phase, patient has premenstrual exacerbation of another condition.
     b. If symptoms do not occur in the follicular phase, diagnosis of PMS is confirmed.

■ LABORATORY TESTS
• None available to specifically confirm the diagnosis of PMS
• Thyroid function tests to rule out thyroid disease

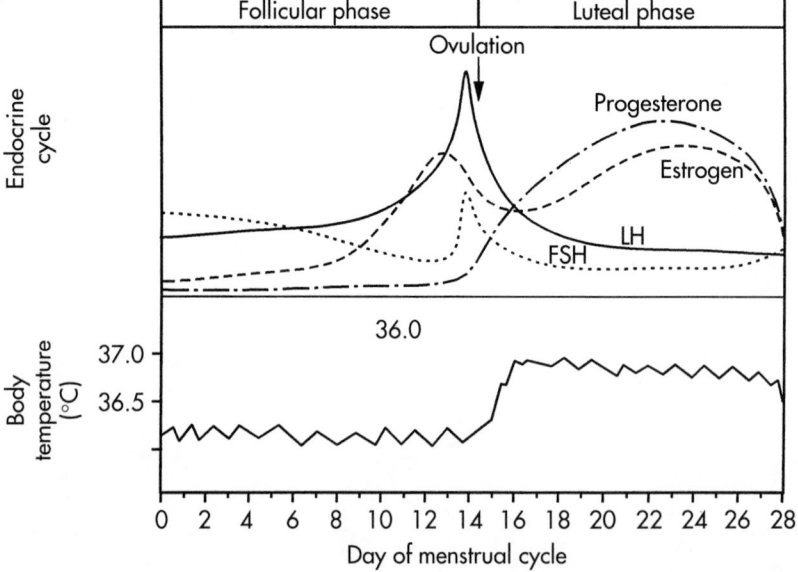

Fig. 1-304 The female hormonal cycle. (From Noble J [ed]: *Textbook of primary care medicine,* ed 2, St Louis, 1996, Mosby.)

TREATMENT

NONPHARMACOLOGIC THERAPY
- Individualization of the treatment plan to maximize therapeutic response
- Psychosocial intervention:
  1. Education
  2. Stress management
  3. Environmental changes
  4. Adequate rest and sleep
  5. Regular exercise
- Nutritional recommendations:
  1. Regularly eaten, well-balanced meals
  2. Adequate amounts of protein, fiber, and complex carbohydrates; low fat
  3. Avoidance of foods that are high in salt and simple sugars; may promote water retention, weight gain, and physical discomfort
  4. Avoidance of caffeine-containing beverages; stimulant effects of caffeine may worsen tension, irritability, and insomnia
  5. Avoidance of alcohol and illicit drugs; may worsen emotional lability
  6. Calcium supplementation (1000 mg/day for women 19 to 50 yr, 1300 mg/day for girls 14 to 18 yr) to reduce the physical and emotional symptoms
  7. Magnesium (360 mg/day) to reduce water retention and the negative affect associated with PMS.
  8. Pyridoxine (vitamin B_6) 50 mg bid to improve depression, fatigue, irritability and natural diuretic ability; neurotoxicity observed at higher dosages

ACUTE GENERAL Rx
SUPPRESSION OF OVULATION:
- Oral contraceptives—one pill per day
- Progestin-only oral contraceptive—one pill per day
- Oral micronized progesterone—100 mg qAM and 200 mg qPM on days 17 through 28 of menstrual cycle
- Progestin suppository—200 to 400 mg bid on days 17 through 28 of menstrual cycle
- Medroxyprogesterone (depot)—150 mg IM every 3 mo
- Levonorgestrel implants—surgical insertion every 5 yr
- Transdermal estradiol—one or two 100-μg patches every 3 days
- Danazol—100 to 200 mg/day (ovulation not suppressed at this dose)
- Gonadotropin-releasing hormone (GnRH) agonists—daily by intranasal spray or monthly by depot injection

SUPPRESSION OF PHYSICAL SYMPTOMS:
- Spironolactone—25 to 50 mg bid on days 14 through 28 of menstrual cycle
- Mefenamic acid
  1. For fluid retention: 250 mg tid on days 24 through 28 of cycle
  2. For pain: 500 mg tid on days 19 through 28 of cycle
- Bromocriptine—5 mg/day on days 10 through 26 of cycle
- Danazol—200 mg/day on days 19 through 28 of cycle
- Naproxen (Anaprox)—550 mg bid on days 17 through 28 of cycle; Naprosyn—500 mg bid on days 17 through 28 of cycle.

SUPPRESSION OF PSYCHOLOGIC SYMPTOMS:
- Nortriptyline—50 to 125 mg/day
- Fluoxetine (Prozac)—20 mg/day (this medication has indications for premenstrual dysphoric disorder)
- Buspirone—10 mg bid or tid on days 16 through 28 of cycle, then taper drug
- Alprazolam—25 mg tid on days 16 through 28 of cycle, then taper drug
- Clonidine—0.1 mg bid
- Naltrexone—0.25 mg/day on days 9 through 18 of cycle
- Atenolol—50 mg/day
- Paroxetine (Paxil)—20 mg/day
- Sertraline (Zoloft)—50 to 100 mg/day
- Nefazodone (Serzone)—Initial dosage 100 mg bid; after 1 wk increase to 150 mg bid
- Propranolol—20 to 40 mg bid
- Verapamil—100 to 320 mg qd

CHRONIC Rx
- Therapy is largely trial and error, with the goal of providing effective treatment with the safest and most simple therapy.
- For severe intractable PMS: hysterectomy with bilateral oophorectomy; give trial of GnRH therapy or danazol before surgery.
- Estrogen replacement therapy recommended postoperatively to reduce the risk of osteoporosis, heart disease, and genitourinary atrophy.

DISPOSITION
Improved symptoms in 90% of women over time.

REFERRAL
- For counseling with a psychologist or psychiatrist if underlying psychiatric disorder is discovered
- To a gynecologist if surgical therapy is contemplated

PEARLS & CONSIDERATIONS

COMMENTS
Patient educational material is available through bookstores and pharmaceutical companies.

REFERENCES
Dimmock PW et al: Efficacy of selective serotonin-reuptake inhibitors in premenstrual syndrome: a systematic review, *Lancet* 356:1131, 2000.
Thys-Jacobs S et al: Calcium carbonate and the premenstrual syndrome: effects on premenstrual and menstrual symptoms, *Am J Obstet Gynecol* 179:444, 1998.
Wyatt KM et al: Efficacy of vitamin B-6 in the treatment of premenstrual syndrome: systematic review, *BMJ* 318:1375, 1999.
Author: **George T. Danakas, M.D.**

BASIC INFORMATION

■ **DEFINITION**

Priapism is the persistent, usually painful, erection associated or unassociated with sexual stimulation.

ICD-9CM CODES

607.3 Priapism

■ **EPIDEMIOLOGY & DEMOGRAPHICS**

- Incidence and prevalence unavailable because of relative rarity
- Can affect male of any age, including children

■ **PHYSICAL FINDINGS & CLINICAL PRESENTATION**

- In idiopathic priapism the initial erection is associated with prolonged sexual excitement. Previous transient episodes are frequently reported. The erection involves the corpora cavernosa alone. Detumescence does not occur spontaneously.
- In secondary priapism, sexual excitement need not be involved. Otherwise the clinical picture is the same as in idiopathic priapism.
- Table 1-55 compares normal erection and priapism.

■ **ETIOLOGY**

Idiopathic: prolonged sexual arousal
Secondary or associated causes:
- Sickle cell disease
- Diabetes
- Leukemia
- Solid tumor penile infiltration
Iatrogenic
- TPN, which includes a fat emulsion

- Anticoagulant therapy
- Phenothiazines
- Trazodone
- Intracorporeal injection therapy for impotence
- Sildenafil (Viagra)

■ **PATHOPHYSIOLOGY**

- Low-flow priapism: prolonged erection leads to edema of the cavernosal trabeculae, resulting in a sequence of statis, thrombosis, venous occlusion, fibrosis, scarring, and possibly impotence
- High-flow priapism: cavernosal artery rupture leading to an arteriocavernous fistula

 DIAGNOSIS

■ **WORKUP**

None if the associated underlying causes are known to be present. Otherwise they should be ruled out.

TREATMENT

Goal: achieve detumescence with preservation of potency
1. Medical therapies:
- Ice packs
- Ice water enemas
- Hot water enemas
- Pressure dressing
- Sedatives
- Analgesics
- Antispasmodic/anticholinergic drugs

- Estrogens
- Anticoagulants
- Procaine
- Amyl nitrate
- Local or general anesthesia
- Ketamine (1 mg/lb)
2. In the patient with sickle cell disease: intravenous hydration, alkalinization, transfusion or exchange-transfusion, oxygen
3. Corpora cavernosa aspiration followed by injection of an α-adrenergic agonist (e.g., phenylephrine 50 μg)
4. Surgery
- Cavernospongiosum shunt
- Glans-cavernosum shunt
- Cavernosaphenous shunt
- In the less common situation of high-flow priapism (diagnosed by the finding of bright red arterial blood on aspiration), arterial embolization or surgical ligation is recommended.

■ **PROGNOSIS**

Impotence is associated with the duration of priapism, with 36 hr being an important threshold

■ **REFERRAL**

To urologist

REFERENCE

Benson GS, Boileau MA: Priapism. In Gillenwater JY et al (eds): *Adult and pediatric urology*, St Louis, 1996, Mosby.
Author: **Tom J. Wachtel, M.D.**

TABLE 1-55 Comparison of Normal Erection and Priapism

FACTOR	NORMAL ERECTION	PRIAPISM
Portion of penis involved	Corpora cavernosa and corpus spongiosum and glans	Corpora cavernosa
Cause	Vasodilatation of penile arteries	Obstruction of venous outflow
		Disturbance of neuroarterial mechanism (imbalance between it and adrenergic activity)
		Increased viscosity
Sexual desire	Present	Absent
Pain	Absent	Present
Duration	Minutes to hours	Hours to days

From Nseyo UO (ed): *Urology for primary care physicians*, Philadelphia, 1999, WB Saunders.

BASIC INFORMATION

■ DEFINITION
Prolactinomas are monoclonal tumors that secrete prolactin.

ICD-9CM CODES
253.1 Forbes-Albright syndrome

■ EPIDEMIOLOGY & DEMOGRAPHICS
INCIDENCE: Most common pituitary tumor; nearly 30% of all pituitary adenomas secrete enough prolactin to cause hyperprolactinemia.
PREDOMINANT SEX: Microadenomas are more common in women; macroadenomas are more frequent in men.

■ PHYSICAL FINDINGS & CLINICAL PRESENTATION
MEN: Decreased facial and body hair, small testicles; may also have decreased libido, impotence, and delayed puberty (caused by decreased testosterone secondary to inhibition of gonadotropin secretion).
WOMEN: Physical examination may be normal; history may reveal amenorrhea, galactorrhea, oligomenorrhea, and anovulation.
BOTH SEXES: Visual field defects and headache may occur depending on size of tumor and its expansion.

■ ETIOLOGY
Prolactin-secreting pituitary adenomas: microadenomas (<10 mm diameter) or macroadenomas (>10 mm diameter)

DIAGNOSIS

■ DIFFERENTIAL DIAGNOSIS
Hyperprolactinemia may be caused by the following:
- Drugs: phenothiazines, methyldopa, reserpine, MAO inhibitors, androgens, progesterone, cimetidine, tricyclic antidepressants, haloperidol, meprobamate, chlordiazepoxide, estrogens, narcotics, metoclopramide, verapamil, amoxapine, cocaine, oral contraceptives
- Hepatic cirrhosis, renal failure, primary hypothyroidism
- Ectopic prolactin-secreting tumors (hypernephroma, bronchogenic carcinoma)
- Infiltrating diseases of the pituitary (sarcoidosis, histiocytosis)
- Head trauma, chest wall injury, spinal cord injury
- Polycystic ovary disease, pregnancy, nipple stimulation
- Idiopathic hyperprolactinemia, stress, exercise

■ WORKUP
- Demonstration of an elevated serum prolactin level:
  1. Normal mean levels are 8 ng/ml in women and 5 ng/ml in men.
  2. Levels >300 ng/ml are virtually diagnostic of prolactinomas.
  3. Prolactin levels can vary with time of day, stress, sleep cycle, and meals. More accurate measurements can be obtained 2 to 3 hr after awakening, preprandially, and when patient is not distressed.
  4. Serial measurements are recommended in patients with mild prolactin elevations.
- TRH stimulation test may be useful in equivocal cases. The normal response is an increase in serum prolactin levels by 100% within 1 hr of TRH infusion; failure to demonstrate an increase in prolactin level is suggestive of pituitary lesion.

■ IMAGING STUDIES
- MRI with gadolinium enhancement is the procedure of choice in the radiographic evaluation of pituitary disease.
- In absence of MRI, a radiographic diagnosis is best accomplished with a high-resolution CT scanner and special coronal cuts through the pituitary region.

TREATMENT

Management of prolactinomas depends on their size and encroachment on the optic chiasm and other vital structures.

■ NONPHARMACOLOGIC THERAPY
Pregnancy and breast-feeding should be avoided, because they can encourage tumor growth.

■ ACUTE GENERAL Rx
- Transsphenoidal resection: the success rate depends on the location of the tumor (entirely intrasellar), experience of the neurosurgeon, and size of the tumor (<10 mm in diameter); the recurrence rate may reach 80% within 5 yr. Possible complications of transsphenoidal surgery include transient diabetes insipidus, hypopituitarism, CSF rhinorrhea, and infections (meningitis, wound infection).
- Medical therapy is preferred when fertility is an important consideration.
  1. Bromocriptine (Parlodel): dosage is 2.5 to 10 mg/day; it decreases

size of the tumor and generally lowers the prolactin level into the normal range when the initial serum prolactin is <500 ng/ml. Side effects of bromocriptine are nausea, constipation, dizziness, and nasal stuffiness.
  2. Pergolide (Permax) is an alternative medication when bromocriptine is not well tolerated.
  3. Cabergoline (Dostinex) is a newer, longer-acting dopamine agonist that may be more effective and better tolerated than bromocriptine; initial dose is 0.25 mg twice weekly.
- Pituitary irradiation is useful as adjunctive therapy of macroadenomas (>10 mm in diameter) and in patients with persistent hypersecretion following surgery. Potential complications include cranial nerve damage, radionecrosis, and cognitive abnormalities.
- Stereotactic radiosurgery (gamma knife) is a newer modality in the treatment of prolactinomas. A high dose of ionizing radiation is delivered to the tumor through multiple ports. Its advantage is minimal irradiation to surrounding tissues. Proximity of the tumor to the optic chiasm limits this therapeutic modality.

■ CHRONIC Rx
- Patients on medical therapy require periodic measurement of prolactin levels.
- Evaluation and monitoring of pituitary function are recommended following transsphenoidal surgery.

■ DISPOSITION
- Transsphenoidal surgery will result in a cure in nearly 50% to 75% of patients with microadenomas and 10% to 20% of patients with macroadenomas.
- Nearly 20% of microprolactinomas resolve during long-term dopamine agonist treatment.

PEARLS & CONSIDERATIONS

■ COMMENTS
Patients must be monitored for several years after surgery, since up to 50% of microadenomas and nearly 90% of macroadenomas can recur.
Author: **Fred F. Ferri, M.D.**

BASIC INFORMATION

■ DEFINITION AND CLASSIFICATION

Prostate cancer is a neoplasm involving the prostate; various classifications have been developed to evaluate malignancy potential and prognosis:
- The degree of malignancy varies with the stage (Fig. 1-305):
  Stage A: Confined to the prostate, no nodule palpable
  Stage B: Palpable nodule confined to the gland
  Stage C: Local extension
  Stage D: Regional lymph nodes or distant metastases
- In the Gleason classification, histologic patterns are independently assigned numbers 1 to 5 (best to least differentiated). These numbers are added to give a total tumor score:
  1. Prognosis is generally good if score is <5.
  2. Score 6 to 10 carries an intermediate prognosis.
  3. Score >10 correlates with anaplastic lesions with poor prognosis.
- Another commonly used classification is the Tumor-Node-Metastasis (TNM) classification of prostate cancer.

ICD-9CM CODES
185 Malignant neoplasm of prostate

■ EPIDEMIOLOGY & DEMOGRAPHICS
- Prostate cancer has surpassed lung cancer as the most common nonskin cancer in men.
- More than 100,000 cases are diagnosed yearly, and nearly 30,000 males die from prostate cancer each year (second leading cause of death from cancer in U.S. men).
- Incidence of prostate cancer increases with age: uncommon <50 yr; 80% of new cases are diagnosed in patients ≥65 yr.
- Average age at time of diagnosis is 72 yr.
- Blacks in the U.S. have the highest incidence of prostate cancer in the world (1 in every 9 males).
- Incidence is low in Asians.
- Approximately 9% of all prostate cancers may be familial.

■ PHYSICAL FINDINGS & CLINICAL PRESENTATION
- Generally silent disease until it reaches advanced stages.
- Bone pain and pathologic fractures may be initial symptoms of prostate cancer.

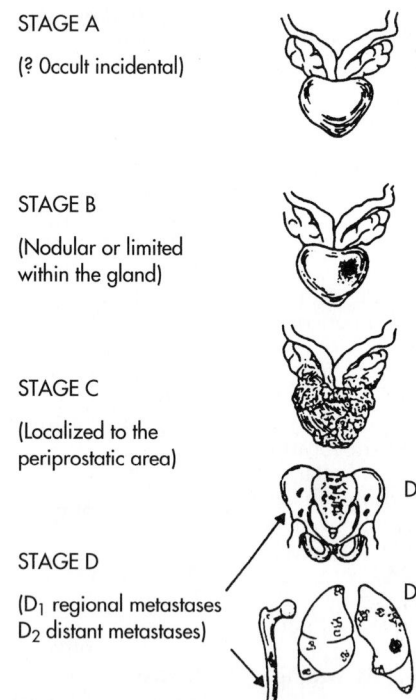

STAGE A

(? Occult incidental)

STAGE B

(Nodular or limited within the gland)

STAGE C

(Localized to the periprostatic area)

D₁

STAGE D

(D₁ regional metastases
D₂ distant metastases)

D₂

Fig. 1-305   Clinical staging of prostatic cancer. (From Rakel RE [ed]: *Principles of family practice,* ed 6, Philadelphia, 2002, WB Saunders.)

- Local growth can cause symptoms of outflow obstruction.
- Digital rectal examination (DRE) may reveal an area of increased firmness; 10% of patients will have a negative DRE.
- Prostate may be hard, fixed, with extension of tumor to the seminal vesicles in advanced stages.

DIAGNOSIS

■ DIFFERENTIAL DIAGNOSIS
- Benign prostatic hypertrophy
- Prostatitis
- Prostate stones

■ LABORATORY TESTS
- Measurement of PSA is useful in early diagnosis of prostate cancer and in monitoring efficacy of therapy. Normal PSA is found in >20% of patients with prostate cancer. For discussion of "free" PSA, refer to "Prostatic Hyperplasia." The American Cancer Society recommends offering the PSA test and digital rectal examination yearly to men 50 years or older who have a life expectancy of at least 10 years. Earlier testing, starting at age 45, is recommended for men at high risk (e.g., blacks, men with family history of prostate cancer).
- Prostatic acid phosphatase (PAP) can be used for evaluation of nonlocalized disease.
- Transrectal biopsy and fine-needle aspiration of prostate can confirm the diagnosis.

■ IMAGING STUDIES
- Bone scan (Fig. 1-306) is useful to evaluate bone metastasis (present or eventually develops in almost 80% of patients). However, according to the American Urological Association (AUA), the routine use of bone scanning is not required for staging of prostate cancer in asymptomatic men with clinically localized cancer if the PSA level is ≤20 ng/ml.
- CT scan, MRI, and transrectal ultrasonography may be useful in selected patients to assess extent of prostate cancer. However, according to the AUA, transrectal ultrasonography adds little to the combination of PSA and digital rectal examination. Similarly, CT and MRI imaging are generally not indicated for cancer staging in men with clinically localized cancer and PSA <25 ng/ml. With regard to pelvic lymph node dissection in staging, the AUA states that it may not be required in patients with PSA levels <10 ng/ml and when PSA level is <20 ng/ml and the Gleason score is <6.

℞ TREATMENT

■ NONPHARMACOLOGIC THERAPY
Watchful waiting is reasonable in patients with early stage (T-IA) and projected life expectancy <10 yr or in patients with focal and moderately differentiated carcinoma.

■ ACUTE GENERAL RX
- Therapeutic approach varies with the following:
  1. Stage of the tumor
  2. Patient's life expectancy
  3. General medical condition
  4. Patient's treatment preference (e.g., patient may be opposed to orchiectomy)
- The optimal treatment of clinically localized prostate cancer is unclear.
  1. Radical prostatectomy is generally performed in patients with localized prostate cancer and life expectancy >10 yr.
  2. Radiation therapy (external beam irradiation or implantation of radioactive pellets [seeds]) represents an alternative in patients with localized prostate cancer, especially poor surgical candidates or patients with a high-grade malignancy.
- Patients with advanced disease and projected life expectancy <10 yr are candidates for radiation therapy and hormonal therapy (DES, LHRH analogs, antiandrogens, bilateral orchiectomy).
- Recommended treatment of patients with regional metastatic prostate cancer with projected life expectancy ≥10 yr includes radical prostatectomy, radiation therapy, hormonal therapy.
- Androgen-deprivation therapy with a gonadotropin-releasing hormone agonist is the mainstay of treatment for metastatic prostate cancer. Adjuvant treatment with GnRH analog goserelin (Zoladex), when started simultaneously with external irradiation, improves local control and survival in patients with locally advanced prostate cancer. Pamidronate inhibits osteoclast-mediated bone resorption and prevents bone loss in the hip and lumbar spine in men receiving treatment for prostate cancer with a GnRH.

■ CHRONIC Rx
- Patients should be monitored at 3- to 6-mo intervals with clinical examination, and PSA for the first year, then every 6 mo for the second year, then yearly if stable. For patients who have undergone radical prostatectomy, a rising PSA level suggests evidence of residual or recurrent prostate cancer.
- Chest x-ray examination, bone scan should be performed yearly or sooner if patient develops symptoms.

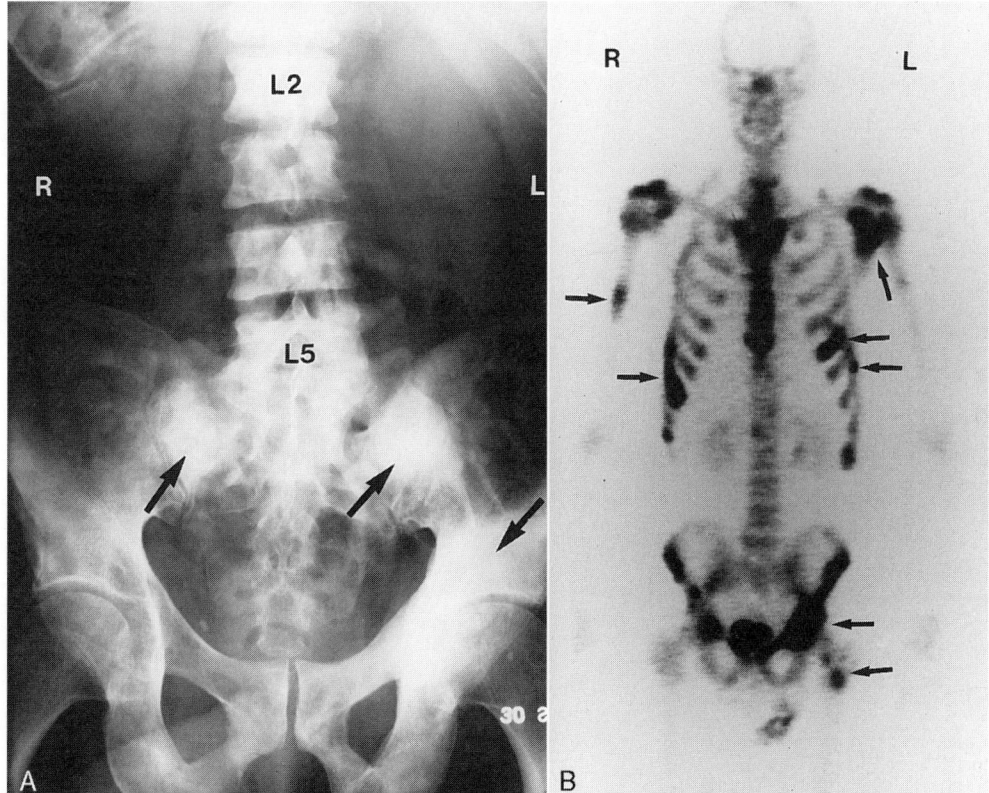

Fig. 1-306 Metastatic prostate cancer. **A,** An anteroposterior view of the pelvis and lumbar spine demonstrates multiple areas of increased density *(arrows)* in a patchy distribution. Vertebrae L2 and L5 are also abnormally white or increased in density. **B,** A nuclear medicine whole-body bone scan most commonly shows the metastatic deposits as areas of increased activity *(arrows)*. (From Mettler FA [ed]: *Primary care radiology,* Philadelphia, 2000, WB Saunders.)

Gwendolyn R. Lee, M.D.
Internal Medicine

■ DISPOSITION

- Prognosis varies with the stage of the disease (see "Definition") and the Gleason classification (see "Definition").
- The ploidy of the tumor also has prognostic value: prognosis is better with diploid tumor cells, worse with aneuploid tumor cells.
- For grade 1 tumors, the extended 10-yr, disease-specific survival is similar for patients with prostatectomy (94%), radiotherapy (90%), and conservative management (93%); survival rate is better with surgery than with radiotherapy or conservative management in patients with grade 2 or 3 localized prostate cancer.

REFERENCES

Barry MJ: Clinical practice: prostate-specific-antigen testing for early diagnosis of prostate cancer, *N Engl J Med* 344:1373, 2001.

Smith MR: Pamidronate to prevent bone loss during androgen-deprivation therapy for prostate cancer, *N Engl J Med* 345:948, 2001.

Author: **Fred F. Ferri, M.D.**

BASIC INFORMATION

■ **DEFINITION**

Benign prostatic hyperplasia is the benign growth of the prostate, generally originating in the periureteral and transition zones, with subsequent obstructive and irritative voiding symptoms.

■ **SYNONYMS**

BPH
Prostatic hypertrophy

ICD-9CM CODES

600 Benign prostatic hyperplasia

■ **EPIDEMIOLOGY & DEMOGRAPHICS**

- 80% of men have evidence of benign prostatic hypertrophy by age 80 yr.
- Medical and surgical intervention for problems caused by BPH is required in >20% of males by age 75 yr.
- Transurethral resection of the prostate (TURP) is the tenth most common operative procedure (>400,000/yr in U.S.).

- 10% to 30% of men with BPH have occult prostate cancer.

■ **PHYSICAL FINDINGS & CLINICAL PRESENTATION**

- Digital rectal examination (DRE) reveals enlargement of the prostate.
- Focal enlargement may be indicative of malignancy.
- There is poor correlation between size of prostate and symptoms (BPH may be asymptomatic if it does not encroach on the urethral lumen).
- Most patients with BPH complain of difficulty in initiating urination (hesitancy), decrease in caliber and force of stream, incomplete emptying of bladder often resulting in double voiding (need to urinate again a few minutes after voiding), postvoid "dribbling," and nocturia.

■ **ETIOLOGY**

Multifactorial; a functioning testicle is necessary for development of BPH (as evidenced by the absence in males who were castrated before puberty).

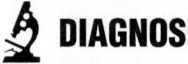

DIAGNOSIS

■ **DIFFERENTIAL DIAGNOSIS**

- Prostatitis
- Prostate cancer
- Strictures (urethral)
- Medication interfering with the muscle fibers in the prostate and also with bladder function

■ **WORKUP**

- Symptom assessment (use of American Urological Association [AUA] Symptom Index for BPH [Table 1-56]), laboratory tests, and imaging studies
- Fig. 1-307 describes a clinical pathway for patients with benign prostatic hypertrophy.

■ **LABORATORY TESTS**

- Prostate specific antigen (PSA): protease secreted by epithelial cells of the prostate; elevated in 30% to 50% of patients with BPH. Testing for PSA increases detection rate for prostate

---

TABLE 1-56 **International Prostate Symptom Score (I-PSS)**

SYMPTOM	NOT AT ALL	LESS THAN 1 TIME IN 5	LESS THAN HALF THE TIME	ABOUT HALF THE TIME	MORE THAN HALF THE TIME	ALMOST ALWAYS	TOTAL SCORE
Incomplete emptying: Over the past month, how often have you had a sensation of not emptying your bladder completely after you finished urinating?	0	1	2	3	4	5	
Frequency: Over the past month, how often have you had to urinate again <2 hr after you finished urinating?	0	1	2	3	4	5	
Intermittency: Over the past month, how often have you found you stopped and started again several times when you urinated?	0	1	2	3	4	5	
Urgency: Over the past month, how often have you found it difficult to postpone urination?	0	1	2	3	4	5	
Weak stream: Over the past month, how often have you had a weak urinary stream?	0	1	2	3	4	5	
Straining: Over the past month, how often have you had to push or strain to begin urination?	0	1	2	3	4	5	
	NONE	1 TIME	2 TIMES	3 TIMES	4 TIMES	5 OR MORE TIMES	
Nocturia: Over the past month, how many times did you most typically get up to urinate from the time you went to bed at night until the time you got up in the morning?	0	1	2	3	4	5	

Total I-PSS score =

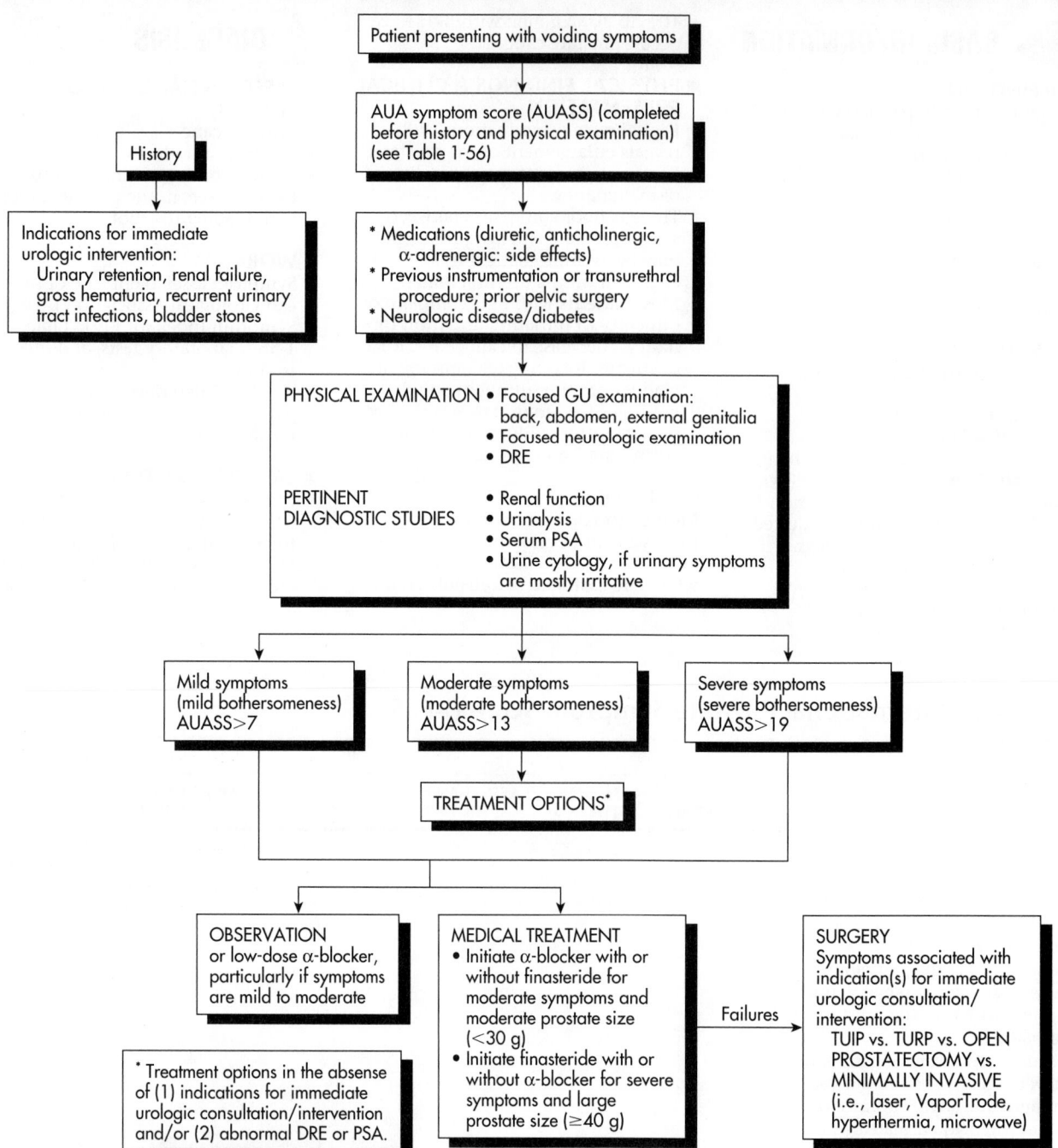

Fig. 1-307 **Critical pathway for patients with benign prostatic hypertrophy.** *AUA,* American Urological Association; *DRE,* digital rectal examination; *GU,* genitourinary; *PSA,* prostate-specific antigen; *TUIP,* transurethral incision of the prostate; *TURP,* transurethral resection of the prostate. (From Nseyo UO [ed]: *Urology for primary care physicians,* Philadelphia, 1999, WB Saunders.)

cancer and tends to detect cancer at an earlier stage. However, the PSA test does not discriminate well between patients with symptomatic BPH and those with prostate cancer, particularly if the cancers are pathologically localized and curable. The test may also trigger additional evaluation, including ultrasound biopsy of the prostate. Recent data indicate that asymptomatic men with PSA levels <2 ng/ml do not need annual testing. According to the AUA policy report published in the February 2000 issue of *Oncology,* PSA testing and digital rectal examination should be offered to any asymptomatic man older than 50 years of age with a life expectancy of ≥10 years. PSA testing can also be offered at an earlier age in men at higher risk of prostatic cancer (e.g., first-degree relatives with prostate cancer; black men).

- Measurement of "free" PSA is useful to assess the probability of prostate cancer in patients with normal digital rectal examination and total PSA between 4 and 10 ng/ml. In these patients the global risk of prostate cancer is 25%; however, if the free PSA is >25%, the risk of prostate cancer decreases to 8%, whereas if the free PSA is <10%, the risk of cancer increases to 56%. Free PSA is also useful to evaluate the aggressiveness of prostate cancer. A low free PSA percentage generally indicates a high-grade cancer, whereas a high free PSA percentage is generally associated with a slower growing tumor.
- Urinalysis, urine C&S to rule out infection (if suspected).
- BUN and creatinine to rule out postrenal insufficiency.

■ IMAGING STUDIES

- Transrectal ultrasound may be indicated in patients with palpable nodules or significant elevation of PSA. It is also useful to estimate prostate size.
- Uroflowmetry may be used to determine relative impact of obstruction on urine flow. Urethral pressure profile is useful to predict prostatic hypertrophy within the urethral lumen.
- Pressure flow studies, although invasive, are particularly helpful in patients whose history and/or examination suggest primary bladder dysfunction as a cause of symptoms of prostatism. They are also useful in patients for whom a distinction between prostatic obstruction and impaired detrusor contractility may affect the choice of therapy. However, pressure flow studies may not be useful in the workup of the usual patient with symptoms of prostatism.

- Postvoid residual urine measurement has not been proved useful in predicting the need for or response to treatment; may be useful in monitoring the course of the disease in patients who elect nonsurgical treatment.
- Urethral cystoscopy is an option during later evaluation if invasive treatment is being planned.

℞ TREATMENT

■ NONPHARMACOLOGIC THERAPY

- Avoidance of caffeine or any other foods that may exacerbate symptoms
- Avoidance of medications that may exacerbate symptoms (e.g., cold and allergy remedies)

■ ACUTE GENERAL Rx

- Asymptomatic patients with prostate enlargement caused by BPH generally do not require treatment. Patients with mild to moderate symptoms are candidates for pharmacologic treatment. For those patients who have specific complications from BPH, prostate surgery is usually the most appropriate form of treatment. However, surgery may result in significant complications (e.g., incontinence, infection).
- TURP is the most commonly used surgical procedure for BPH. Transurethral incision of the prostate (TUIP), a procedure almost equivalent in efficacy, is limited to patients whose estimated resection tissue weight would be 30 g or less. TUIP can be performed in an ambulatory setting or during a 1-day hospitalization. Open prostatectomy is typically performed on patients with very large prostates.
- Laser therapy for BPH is a less invasive alternative to TURP; however, recent studies indicate that at least in the initial 7 months after surgery, TURP is moderately more effective than laser therapy in relieving symptoms of BPH.
- Surgery need not be treatment of last resort for most patients; that is, patients need not undergo other treatments for BPH before they can have surgery. However, recommending surgery on the grounds that a patient's surgical risk will "only increase with age" is generally inappropriate.
- Balloon dilation of the prostatic urethra is less effective than surgery for relieving symptoms but is associated with fewer complications. It is a reasonable treatment option for patients with smaller prostates and no middle lobe enlargement.

- α-blockers (e.g., tamsulosin, doxazosin, prazosin, and terazosin) relax smooth muscle of the bladder neck and prostate and can increase peak urinary flow rate. They are useful in symptomatic patients.
- Hormonal manipulation with finasteride (Proscar), a 5α-reductase inhibitor that blocks conversion of testosterone to dihydrotestosterone, can reduce the size of the prostate. Treatment requires 6 mo or more for maximal effect.

■ CHRONIC Rx

- Avoid medications and foods that exacerbate symptoms.
- Symptomatic improvement occurs in >70% of patients with proper treatment.

■ DISPOSITION

With appropriate therapy, symptoms improve or stabilize in >70% of patients with BPH.

■ REFERRAL

Urology referral for patients with severe or intolerable symptoms and for any patient suspected of having prostate cancer (10% to 30% of men with BPH).

☼ PEARLS & CONSIDERATIONS

■ COMMENTS

Emerging technologies for treating BPH include lasers, coils, stents, thermal therapy, and hyperthermia. Laser prostatectomy appears promising; however, long-term effectiveness has not yet been demonstrated.

- The increase in the use of pharmacological management has resulted in over 30% reduction in the total number of transurethral resections of the prostate.

REFERENCES

Catalona WJ et al: Use of the percentage of free PSA to enhance differentiation of prostate cancer from benign prostatic disease: a prospective multicenter clinical trial, *JAMA* 279:1542, 1998.

Donovan JL et al: A randomized trial comparing TURP, laser therapy, and conservative treatment of men with symptoms associated with benign prostatic enlargement: the CLASP study; *J Urol* 164:65, 2000.

McConnell JD et al: *Benign prostatic hyperplasia: diagnosis and treatment—quick reference guide for clinicians,* AHCPR Publication No 94-0583, Rockville, Md, 1994, Agency for Health Care Policy and Research, Public Health Service, US Department of Health and Human Services.

Author: **Fred F. Ferri, M.D.**

BASIC INFORMATION

■ **DEFINITION**

Pruritus ani refers to an intense chronic itching of the anus and peri-anal skin.

ICD-9CM CODES
698.0 Pruritus ani

■ **EPIDEMIOLOGY & DEMOGRAPHICS**
• Any age can be affected.
• Occurs in 1% to 5% of the population.
• Male to female predominance of 4:1.

■ **PHYSICAL FINDINGS & CLINICAL PRESENTATION**
• Anal itching
• Anal fissures
• Hemorrhoids
• Excoriations
• Pinworms
• Fecal incontinence

■ **ETIOLOGY**
ANORECTAL DISEASES AND FECAL CONTAMINATION:
• Diarrhea
• Anal incontinence
• Hemorrhoids
• Fissures
• Fistulae
• Rectal prolapse
• Malignancy: Bowen's disease, epidermoid cancer, perianal Paget's disease
INFECTIONS:
• Fungal: candidiasis, dermatophytes
• Parasitic: pinworms, scabies
• Bacterial: *Staphylococcus aureus,* erythrasma
• Venereal: herpes, gonococcal syphilis, human papillomavirus
LOCAL IRRITANTS:
• Moisture, obesity, excessive perspiration
• Soaps, hygiene products
• Toilet paper: perfumed, dyed
• Underwear: irritating fabrics, detergents
• Anal creams, suppositories

• Dietary: coffee, beer, acidic foods
• Drugs: mineral oil, ascorbic acid, hydrocortisone sodium succinate, quinine, colchicine
DERMATOLOGIC DISEASES:
• Psoriasis
• Atopic dermatitis
• Seborrheic dermatitis
Box 2-211 also describes the various causes of pruritus ani.

🔬 **DIAGNOSIS**

■ **DIFFERENTIAL DIAGNOSIS**
• Allergies
• Anxiety
• Dermatologic conditions
• Infections
• Parasites
• Diabetes mellitus
• Chronic liver disease
• Neoplasia

■ **WORKUP**
• Detailed history regarding bowel habits, hygiene, use of perfumed products, and medical history
• Inspection of perianal area
• Possible biopsy to exclude neoplasia
• Microscopic inspection of scrapings
• Colposcopy of perineum

■ **LABORATORY TESTS**
• Chemistry profile
• Urinalysis
• Cultures
• Stool for ova and parasites
• Tape test
• Glucose tolerance test, if necessary

💊 **TREATMENT**

■ **NONPHARMACOLOGIC THERAPY**
• Avoidance of tight, nonporous clothing and underclothing
• Discontinuation or curtailment of coffee, beer, citrus fruits, tomatoes, chocolate, and tea

• Cleansing of anal area after bowel movements with a premoistened pad or tissue and avoidance of perfumes and dyes present in toilet paper and soaps
• Avoidance of excessive perspiration
• Aggressive management of fecal leakage or incontinence to avoid soiling of perianal skin

■ **ACUTE GENERAL Rx**
• Minimization of frequent loose stools with antidiarrheals and fiber agents if appropriate
• Use of a 1% hydrocortisone cream sparingly bid during the acute phase of pruritus ani but not for >2 wk to avoid atrophy
• Treatment of predisposing factors, such as parasites, diabetes, liver disease, hemorrhoids, and other infections

■ **CHRONIC Rx**
• Possible complications: excoriation and secondary bacterial infection; must be treated aggressively
• Long-standing, intractable pruritus ani: good response to intracutaneous injections of methylene blue and other agents, steroid injection

■ **DISPOSITION**
• Usually good results with total resolution of symptoms
• In some, persistent and recurrent symptoms

■ **REFERRAL**
To colorectal specialist if conservative measures fail

REFERENCE
Yamada T, Alpers DH, Laine L: *Textbook of gastroenterology,* ed 3, Baltimore, 1999, Lippincott Williams & Wilkins.
Author: **Maria A. Corigliano, M.D.**

BASIC INFORMATION

■ DEFINITION
Pruritus vulvae refers to intense itching of the female external genitalia.

■ SYNONYMS
Vulvodynia

ICD-9CM CODES
698.1 Pruritus of genital organs

■ EPIDEMIOLOGY & DEMOGRAPHICS
- A female disorder that can affect women at any age
- Young girls: infection is usually causative
- Postmenopausal women: frequently affected because of hypoestrogenic state

■ PHYSICAL FINDINGS & CLINICAL PRESENTATION
Constant intense itching or burning of the vulva

■ ETIOLOGY
- About 50% are caused by monilial infection or trichomoniasis.
- Other infectious causes are herpes simplex, condylomata acuminata, and molluscum contagiosum.
- Other causes:
  1. Infestations with scabies, pediculosis pubis, and pinworms
  2. Dermatoses such as hypertrophic dystrophy, lichen sclerosus, lichen planus, and psoriasis
  3. Neoplasms such as Bowen's disease, Paget's disease, and squamous cell carcinoma
  4. Allergic or chemical dermatitis caused by dyes in clothing or toilet paper, detergents, contraceptive gels, vaginal medications, douches, or soaps
  5. Vulva or vaginal atrophy
- Severe pruritus is probably caused by degeneration and inflammation of terminal nerve fibers.
- Most intense itching occurs with hyperplastic lesions.

DIAGNOSIS

■ DIFFERENTIAL DIAGNOSIS
- Vulvitis
- Vaginitis
- Lichen sclerosus
- Squamous cell hyperplasia
- Pinworms
- Vulvar cancer

■ WORKUP
- Inspection of vulva, vagina, and perianal area looking for infection, fissures, ulcerations, induration, or thick plaques
- Must rule out trichomoniasis, candidiasis, allergy, vitamin deficiencies, diabetes

■ LABORATORY TESTS
- Wet prep of saline and KOH of vaginal discharge
- Tape test to look for pinworms
- Vaginal cultures
- Biopsy when needed

TREATMENT

■ NONPHARMACOLOGIC THERAPY
- Keep vulva clean and dry.
- Wear white cotton panties.
- Avoid perfumes and body creams over vulvar area because they can cause irritation.
- Reduce stress.
- Apply wet dressings with aluminum acetate (Burow's) solution frequently.
- Avoid coffee and caffeine-containing beverages, chocolate, tomatoes.
- Sitz baths may be helpful.

■ ACUTE GENERAL Rx
Need to treat underlying problem:
- Yeast infection: any of the vaginal creams or Diflucan 150-mg one-time dose
- Trichomoniasis or *Gardnerella vaginalis:* Flagyl 500 mg or 375 mg PO bid for 7 days
- Urinary tract infection: treatment of specific organism

- Estrogen replacement therapy if atrophy is the cause of pruritus
- Pinworms: mebendazole (Vermox) 100 mg one tablet at diagnosis and repeated in 1 to 2 wk; also treat other members in family >2 yr of age
- Squamous cell hyperplasia: local application of corticosteroids
  1. One of the high- or medium-potency corticosteroids (0.025% or 0.01% fluocinolone acetonide or 0.01% triamcinolone acetonide) can be used to relieve itching.
  2. Rub into vulva bid or tid for 4 to 6 wk.
  3. Once itching is controlled, fluorinated steroid can be discontinued and patient can be switched to hydrocortisone preparation.
- Lichen sclerosus: topical 2% testosterone in petrolatum massaged into the vulvar tissue bid or tid; Temovate (clobetasol propionate gel 0.05%) cream tid × 5 days is very effective

■ CHRONIC Rx
- If not relieved by topical measures: intradermal injection of triamcinolone (10 mg/ml diluted 2:1 saline) 0.1 ml of the suspension injected at 1-cm intervals and tissue gently massaged
- If symptoms still uncontrollable: SC injection of absolute alcohol 0.1 ml at 1-cm intervals

■ DISPOSITION
Usually controlled with conservative measures and topical steroids

■ REFERRAL
To a gynecologist for further workup if conservative measures do not give relief

REFERENCES
Copeland L: *Textbook of gynecology,* ed 2, Philadelphia, 1999, WB Saunders.
Mead P: *Protocols for infectious diseases in obstetrics and gynecology,* ed 2, Cambridge, Mass, 2000, Blackwell Science.
Author: **Maria A. Corigliano, M.D.**

BASIC INFORMATION

■ DEFINITION
Pseudogout is one of the clinical patterns associated with a crystal-induced synovitis resulting from the deposition of calcium pyrophosphate dehydrate (CPPD) crystals in joint hyaline and fibrocartilage. The cartilage deposition is termed *chrondrocalcinosis*.

■ SYNONYMS
Calcium pyrophosphate dehydrate crystal deposition disease (CPDD)
Chondrocalcinosis
Pyrophosphate arthropathy

ICD-9CM CODES
275.4 Chondrocalcinosis

■ EPIDEMIOLOGY & DEMOGRAPHICS
PREVALENCE:
• Uncertain
• Probably similar to gout (3/1000 persons)
• Chondrocalcinosis is present in >20% of all people at age 80 yr, but most are asymptomatic.
PREDOMINANT SEX: Female:male ratio of approximately 1.5:1
PREVALENT AGE: 60 to 70 yr at onset

■ PHYSICAL FINDINGS & CLINICAL PRESENTATION
• Symptoms are similar to those of gouty arthritis with acute attacks and chronic arthritis
• Knee joint is most commonly affected
• Swelling, stiffness, and increased heat in affected joint

■ ETIOLOGY
• Unknown
• Often associated with various medical conditions, including hyperparathyroidism and amyloidosis

DIAGNOSIS

■ DIFFERENTIAL DIAGNOSIS
• Gouty arthritis
• Rheumatoid arthritis
• Osteoarthritis
• Neuropathic joint
Box 2-33 describes the differential diagnosis of acute monoarticular and oligoarticular arthritis. Table 2-14 compares crystal-induced arthritides. An algorithm for evaluation of arthralgia limited to one or few joints is described in Fig. 3-18.

■ WORKUP
• Variable clinical presentation
• Diagnosis dependent on the identification of CPPD crystals
• The American Rheumatism Association revised diagnostic criteria for CPPD crystal deposition disease (pseudogout) are often used:
1. Criteria
   I. Demonstration of CPPD crystals (obtained by biopsy, necroscopy, or aspirated synovial fluid) by definitive means (e.g., characteristic "fingerprint" by x-ray diffraction powder pattern or by chemical analysis)
   II. (a) Identification of monoclinic and/or triclinic crystals showing either no or only a weakly positive birefringence by compensated polarized light microscopy
   (b) Presence of typical calcifications in roentgenograms
   III. (a) Acute arthritis, especially of knees or other large joints, with or without concomitant hyperuricemia
   (b) Chronic arthritis, especially of knees, hips, wrists, carpus, elbow, shoulder, and metacarpophalangeal joints, especially if accompanied by acute exacerbations; the following features are helpful in differentiating chronic arthritis from osteoarthritis:
   1. Uncommon site—e.g., wrist, MCP, elbow, shoulder
   2. Appearance of lesion radiologically—e.g., radiocarpal or patellofemoral joint space narrowing, especially if isolated (patella "wrapped around" the femur)
   3. Subchondral cyst formation
   4. Severity of degeneration—progressive, with subchondral bony collapse (microfractures), and fragmentation, with formation of intraarticular radiodense bodies
   5. Osteophyte formation—variable and inconstant
   6. Tendon calcifications, especially Achilles, triceps, obturators
2. Categories
   Definite—Criteria I or II (a) plus (b) must be fulfilled.
   Probable—Criteria II(a) or II(b) must be fulfilled.
   Possible—Criteria III(a) or (b) should alert the clinician to the possibility of underlying CPPD deposition.

■ LABORATORY TESTS
Crystal analysis of the synovial fluid aspirate to reveal rhomboid calcium pyrophosphate crystals

■ IMAGING STUDIES
Plain radiographs to reveal the following:
• Stippled calcification in bands running parallel to the subchondral bone margins
• Crystal deposition in menisci, synovium, and ligament tissue; triangular wrist cartilage and symphysis pubis are often affected

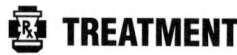

TREATMENT

■ NONPHARMACOLOGIC THERAPY
General measures such as heat, rest, and elevation as needed

■ ACUTE GENERAL Rx
• NSAIDs (as for gout)
• Colchicine
• Aspiration/steroid injection

■ DISPOSITION
Structural joint damage may occasionally occur, requiring arthroplasty in rare cases.

■ REFERRAL
For orthopedic consultation for destructive joint changes

PEARLS & CONSIDERATIONS

■ COMMENTS
As with gout, acute attacks may be triggered by various surgical or medical events.

REFERENCES
Agudelo CA, Wise CM: Crystal-associated arthritis in the elderly, *Rheum Dis Clin North Am* 26:527, 2000.
Canhao H et al: Cross-sectional study of 50 patients with calcium pyrophosphate dihydrate crystal arthropathy, *Clin Rheumatol* 20:119, 2001.
Halverson PB, Derfus BA: Calcium crystal-induced inflammation, *Curr Opin Rheumatol* 13:221, 2001.
Sagarin MJ: Pseudogout, *Emerg Med* 18:373, 2000.
Author: **Lonnie R. Mercier, M.D.**

BASIC INFORMATION

■ DEFINITION

Pseudomembranous colitis is the occurrence of diarrhea and bowel inflammation associated with antibiotic use.

■ SYNONYMS

Antibiotic-induced colitis

■ ICD-9CM CODES

008.45 *Clostridium difficile*, pseudomembranous colitis

■ EPIDEMIOLOGY & DEMOGRAPHICS

- Cephalosporins are the most frequent offending agent in pseudomembranous colitis because of their high rates of use.
- The antibiotic with the highest incidence is clindamycin (10% incidence of pseudomembranous colitis with its use).
- *Clostridium difficile* causes more than 250,000 cases of diarrhea and colitis in the U.S. every year.

■ PHYSICAL FINDINGS & CLINICAL PRESENTATION

- Abdominal tenderness (generalized or lower abdominal).
- Fever.
- In patients with prolonged diarrhea, poor skin turgor, dry mucous membranes, and other signs of dehydration may be present.

■ ETIOLOGY

Risk factors for *C. difficile* (the major identifiable agent of antibiotic-induced diarrhea and colitis):

- Administration of antibiotics: can occur with any antibiotic, but occurs most frequently with clindamycin, ampicillin, and cephalosporins.
- Prolonged hospitalization.
- Abdominal surgery.
- Hospitalized, tube-fed patients are at risk for *C. difficile*–associated diarrhea. Clinicians should consider testing for *C. difficile* in tube-fed patients with diarrhea unrelated to the feeding solution.

DIAGNOSIS

The clinical signs of pseudomembranous colitis generally include diarrhea, fever, and abdominal cramps following use of antibiotics.

■ DIFFERENTIAL DIAGNOSIS

- GI bacterial infections (e.g., *Salmonella, Shigella, Campylobacter, Yersinia*)
- Enteric parasites (e.g., *Cryptosporidium, Entamoeba histolytica*)
- IBD
- Celiac sprue
- Irritable bowel syndrome

■ WORKUP

- All patients with diarrhea accompanied by current or recent antibiotic use should be tested for *C. difficile* (see "Laboratory Tests").
- Sigmoidoscopy (without cleansing enema) may be necessary when the clinical and laboratory diagnosis is inconclusive and the diarrhea persists.
- In antibiotic-induced pseudomembranous colitis, the sigmoidoscopy often reveals raised white-yellow exudative plaques adherent to the colonic mucosa (Fig. 1-308).

■ LABORATORY TESTS

- *C. difficile* toxin can be detected by cytotoxin tissue-culture assay (gold standard for identifying *C. difficile* toxin in stool specimen) and by enzyme-linked immunoassay (EIA) for *C. difficile* toxins A and B.
- Fecal leukocytes (assessed by microscopy or lactoferrin assay) are generally present in stool samples.
- CBC usually reveals leukocytosis.

■ IMAGING STUDIES

Abdominal film (flat plate and upright) is useful in patients with abdominal pain or evidence of obstruction on physical examination.

TREATMENT

■ NONPHARMACOLOGIC THERAPY

- Discontinue offending antibiotic.
- Fluid hydration and correct electrolyte abnormalities.

■ ACUTE GENERAL Rx

- Metronidazole 250 mg PO qid for 10 to 14 days.

- Vancomycin 125 mg PO qid for 10 to 14 days in cases resistant to metronidazole.
- Cholestyramine 4 g PO qid for 10 days in addition to metronidazole to control severe diarrhea (avoid use with vancomycin).
- When parenteral therapy is necessary (e.g., patient with paralytic ileus), IV metronidazole 500 mg qid can be used. It can also be supplemented with vancomycin 500 mg via NG tube or enema.

■ CHRONIC Rx

Judicious future use of antibiotics to prevent recurrences (e.g., avoid prolonged antibiotic therapy)

■ DISPOSITION

Most patients recover completely with appropriate therapy; mortality exceeds 10% in untreated patients.

■ REFERRAL

Hospital admission and IV hydration in severe cases.

PEARLS & CONSIDERATIONS

■ COMMENTS

Possible complications of pseudomembranous colitis include dehydration, bowel perforation, toxic megacolon, electrolyte imbalance, and reactive arthritis.

REFERENCES

Mylonakis E et al: *Clostridium difficile*–associated diarrhea: a review, *Arch Intern Med* 161:525, 2001.
Yassin S et al: *Clostridium difficile*–associated diarrhea and colitis, *Mayo Clin Proc* 76:725, 2001.

Author: **Fred F. Ferri, M.D.**

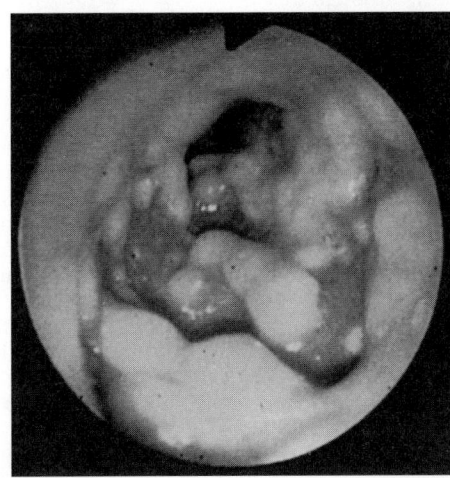

Fig. 1-308 Pseudomembranous plaques seen with colonoscopy in a patient with *C. difficile*–associated PMC. (From Gorbach SL: *Infectious diseases,* ed 2, Philadelphia, 1998, WB Saunders.)

BASIC INFORMATION

■ DEFINITION

Psittacosis is a systemic infection caused by *Chlamydia psittaci*.

■ SYNONYMS

Ornithosis

ICD-9CM CODES

073.9 Psittacosis

■ EPIDEMIOLOGY & DEMOGRAPHICS

INCIDENCE (IN U.S.):
- 45 cases reported in 1996
- True incidence possibly higher because infections may be subclinical
- Highest incidence among pet owners and people working in contact with birds

PREVALENCE (IN U.S.):
- Low among humans
- Organism carried in 5% to 8% of birds

PREDOMINANT SEX: Equal sex distribution

PREDOMINANT AGE: More common in adults

PEAK INCIDENCE: 30 to 60 yr of age

■ PHYSICAL FINDINGS & CLINICAL PRESENTATION

- Incubation period of 5 to 15 days
- Subclinical infection
- Onset abrupt or insidious
- Most common symptoms:
  1. Fever
  2. Myalgias
  3. Chills
  4. Cough
- Most common clinical syndrome: atypical pneumonia with fever, headache, dry cough, and a chest x-ray more dramatically abnormal than the physical examination
- Ranges from mild disease to respiratory failure and death, although this is extremely unusual
- Other clinical presentations:
  1. Mononucleosis-like syndrome
  2. Typhoidal form
- Most frequent physical findings:
  1. Fever
  2. Pharyngeal erythema
  3. Rales
  4. Hepatomegaly
- Less common findings:
  1. Somnolence
  2. Confusion
  3. Relative bradycardia
  4. Pleural rub
  5. Adenopathy
  6. Splenomegaly
  7. Horder's spots (pink blanching maculopapular rash)

- Besides the lungs, other specific end-organ involvement:
  1. Pericarditis
  2. Myocarditis
  3. Endocarditis
  4. Hepatitis
  5. Joints
  6. Kidneys (glomerulonephritis)
  7. CNS

■ ETIOLOGY

- *Chlamydia psittaci* is an obligate intracellular bacterium.
- Infection is usually spread by the respiratory route from infected birds.
- There is a history of exposure to birds in 85% of patients.
- Strains from turkeys and psittacine birds are most virulent for humans.
- Cows, goats, and sheep are occasionally implicated.

DIAGNOSIS

■ DIFFERENTIAL DIAGNOSIS

- *Legionella*
- *Mycoplasma*
- *Chlamydia pneumoniae* (TWAR)
- Viral respiratory infections
- Bacterial pneumonia
- Typhoid fever
- Viral hepatitis
- Aseptic meningitis
- Fever of unknown origin
- Mononucleosis

■ WORKUP

- CBC, renal and liver function tests
- *Chlamydia* serology
- Chest x-ray examination
- Special immunostaining of respiratory secretions

■ LABORATORY TESTS

- WBC count is normal or slightly elevated.
- Mild liver function abnormalities are common (50%).
- Blood cultures are almost always negative.
- Studies on respiratory secretions:
  1. Direct immunofluorescent antibody (DFA) of respiratory secretions with monoclonal antibodies to chlamydial antigens
  2. Chlamydial LPS (lipopolysaccharide) antigen by enzyme immunoassay (EIA)
  3. Polymerase chain reaction (PCR)
- Serologic studies:
  1. Complement-fixing antibodies
  2. Microimmunofluorescence
  3. Possible false-negative results and cross-reaction with other chlamydial species with both techniques

■ IMAGING STUDIES

- Chest x-ray examination is abnormal in 50% to 90% with a variety of patterns.
- Pleural effusions are common.

TREATMENT

■ NONPHARMACOLOGIC THERAPY

Oxygen supplementation as needed

■ ACUTE GENERAL Rx

- Tetracycline (500 mg PO qid) *or*
- Doxycycline (100 mg PO bid) *or*
- Erythromycin (500 mg PO qid): less effective

■ CHRONIC Rx

In the rare cases of endocarditis, combination of heart valve replacement and prolonged antibiotic course may be the treatment of choice.

■ DISPOSITION

- Mortality low (0.7%)
- Poor prognostic factors:
  1. Advanced age
  2. Leukopenia
  3. Severe hypoxemia
  4. Renal failure
  5. Confusion
  6. Multilobe pulmonary involvement
- Possible reinfection

■ REFERRAL

- To infectious disease expert:
  1. Complicated atypical pneumonia or other end-organ involvement
  2. Suspicion of an outbreak
- To pulmonologist for diagnostic bronchoscopy

PEARLS & CONSIDERATIONS

■ COMMENTS

- Hospitalized patients do not require specific isolation precautions.
- Any confirmed or suspected case of psittacosis should be reported to public health authorities.

REFERENCES

Centers for Disease Control and Prevention: Compendium of measures to control *Chlamydia psittaci* and pet birds (avian chlamydiosis), 1998, *MMWR* 47(RR-10):1, 1998.
Elliott JH: Psittacosis: a flu-like syndrome, *Aust Fam Physician* 30(8):739, 2001.
Author: **Michele Halpern, M.D.**

BASIC INFORMATION

■ DEFINITION

Psoriasis is a chronic skin disorder characterized by excessive proliferation of keratinocytes, resulting in the formation of thickened scaly plaques, itching, and inflammatory changes of the epidermis and dermis. The various forms of psoriasis include guttate, pustular, and arthritis variants.

ICD-9CM CODES

696.0 Psoriasis, arthritis, arthropathic
696.1 Psoriasis, any type except arthropathic

■ EPIDEMIOLOGY & DEMOGRAPHICS

- Psoriasis affects 1% to 3% of the world's population. Most patients have limited psoriasis involving <5% of their body surface.
- There is a strong association between psoriasis and HLA B13, B17, and B27 (pustular psoriasis).
- Peak age of onset is bimodal (adolescents and at 60 yr of age).
- Men and women are equally affected.

■ PHYSICAL FINDINGS & CLINICAL PRESENTATION

- The primary psoriatic lesion is an erythematous papule topped by a loosely adherent scale. Scraping the scale results in several bleeding points (Auspitz sign).
- Chronic plaque psoriasis generally manifests with symmetric, sharply demarcated, erythromatous, silver-scaled patches affecting primarily the intergluteal folds, elbows, scalp, fingernails, toenails, and knees (Fig. 1-309, *A*). This form accounts for 80% of psoriasis cases.
- Psoriasis can also develop at the site of any physical trauma (sunburn, scratching). This is known as Koebner's phenomenon.
- Nail involvement is common (pitting of the nail plate), resulting in hyperkeratosis, onychodystrophy with onycholysis (Fig. 1-309, *B*).
- Pruritus is variable.
- Joint involvement can result in sacroiliitis and spondylitis.

- Guttate psoriasis is generally preceded by streptococcal pharyngitis and manifests with multiple droplike lesions on the extremities and the trunk (Fig. 1-309, *C*).

■ ETIOLOGY

- Unknown
- Familial clustering (genetic transmission with a dominant mode with variable penetrants)
- One third of persons affected have a positive family history.

DIAGNOSIS

■ DIFFERENTIAL DIAGNOSIS

- Contact dermatitis
- Atopic dermatitis
- Stasis dermatitis
- Tinea
- Nummular dermatitis
- Candidiasis
- Mycosis fungoides
- Cutaneous SLE
- Secondary and tertiary syphilis
- Drug eruption

■ WORKUP

- Diagnosis is clinical.
- Skin biopsy is rarely necessary.

■ LABORATORY TESTS

Generally not necessary for diagnosis

TREATMENT

■ NONPHARMACOLOGIC THERAPY

- Sunbathing generally leads to improvement.
- Eliminate triggering factors (e.g., stress, certain medications [e.g., lithium, β-blockers, antimalarials]).
- Patients with psoriasis benefit from a daily bath in warm water followed by application of a cream or ointment moisturizer. Regular use or an emollient moisturizer limits evaporation of water from the skin and allows the stratum corneum to rehydrate itself.

■ ACUTE GENERAL Rx

Therapeutic options vary according to the extent of disease.
- Patients with limited disease (<20% of the body) can be treated with the following:
  1. Topical steroids: disadvantages are brief remissions, expense, and decreased effect with continued use.

  Salicylic acid can be compounded by pharmacist in concentrations of 2% to 10% and used in combination with a corticosteroid to decrease amount of scale.
  2. Calcipotriene (Dovonex): a vitamin D analogue, is effective for moderate plaque psoriasis; adults should comb the hair, apply solution to the lesions, and rub it in, avoiding uninvolved skin; disadvantages are its cost and potential burning and skin irritation. It should not be used concurrently with salicylic acid because calcipotriene is inactivated by the acidic nature of salicylic acid.
  3. Tar products (Estar, LCD, psoriGel) can be used overnight and are most effective when combined with UVB light (Goeckerman regimen).
  4. Anthralin (Drithocreme): useful for chronic plaques, can result in purple/brown staining; best used with UVB light.
  5. Retinoids such as tazarotene 0.05%, 0.1% cream or gel, are effective in thinning plaques but are expensive and can produce irritation.
  6. Other useful measures include tape or occlusive dressing, UVB and lubricating agents, interlesional steroids.
- Therapeutic options for persons with generalized disease (affecting >20% of the body):
  1. UVB light exposure three times a week.
  2. Oral PUVA (psoralen plus ultraviolet A) administered 2 to 3 times weekly is effective for generalized disease. However, many treatments are required, necessitating frequent office visits, and it may be associated with phototoxicity, such as erythema and blistering, and increased risk of skin cancer.
- Systemic treatments include methotrexate 25 mg every week for severe psoriasis. Etretinate (Tegison) (a synthetic retinoid) is most effective for palmar-plantar pustular psoriasis. Dose is 0.5 to 1 mg/kg/day. It can cause liver enzyme and lipid abnormalities and is teratogenic.
- Cyclosporine is also effective in severe psoriasis; however, relapses are common.

- Chronic plaque psoriasis may be treated with alefacept, a recombinant protein that selectively targets T lymphocytes. Treatment with alefacept for 12 wk (0.025, 0.075, or 0.150 mg/kg of body weight IV weekly) may result in significant improvement. Some patients also experience a sustained clinical response after the cessation of treatment.

■ **CHRONIC Rx**
See "Acute General Rx."

■ **DISPOSITION**
The course of psoriasis is chronic, and the disease may be refractory to treatment.

■ **REFERRAL**
- Dermatology referral is recommended in all patients with generalized disease.
- Hospital admission may be necessary for severe diffuse or poorly responsive psoriasis. The Goeckerman regimen combines daily application of tar with UVB exposure and can result in prolonged remissions.

⚡ **PEARLS & CONSIDERATIONS**

■ **COMMENTS**
Psoriasis is more emotionally than physically disabling for most patients.

Counseling may be indicated, particularly when it affects younger patients.

REFERENCES

Ellis CN et al: Treatment of chronic plaque psoriasis by selective targeting memory effector T lymphocytes, *N Engl J Med* 345:248, 2001.
Granstein RD: New treatments for psoriasis, *N Engl J Med* 345:284, 2001.
Witman PM: Topical therapies for localized psoriasis, *Mayo Clin Proc* 76:943, 2001.
Author: **Fred F. Ferri, M.D.**

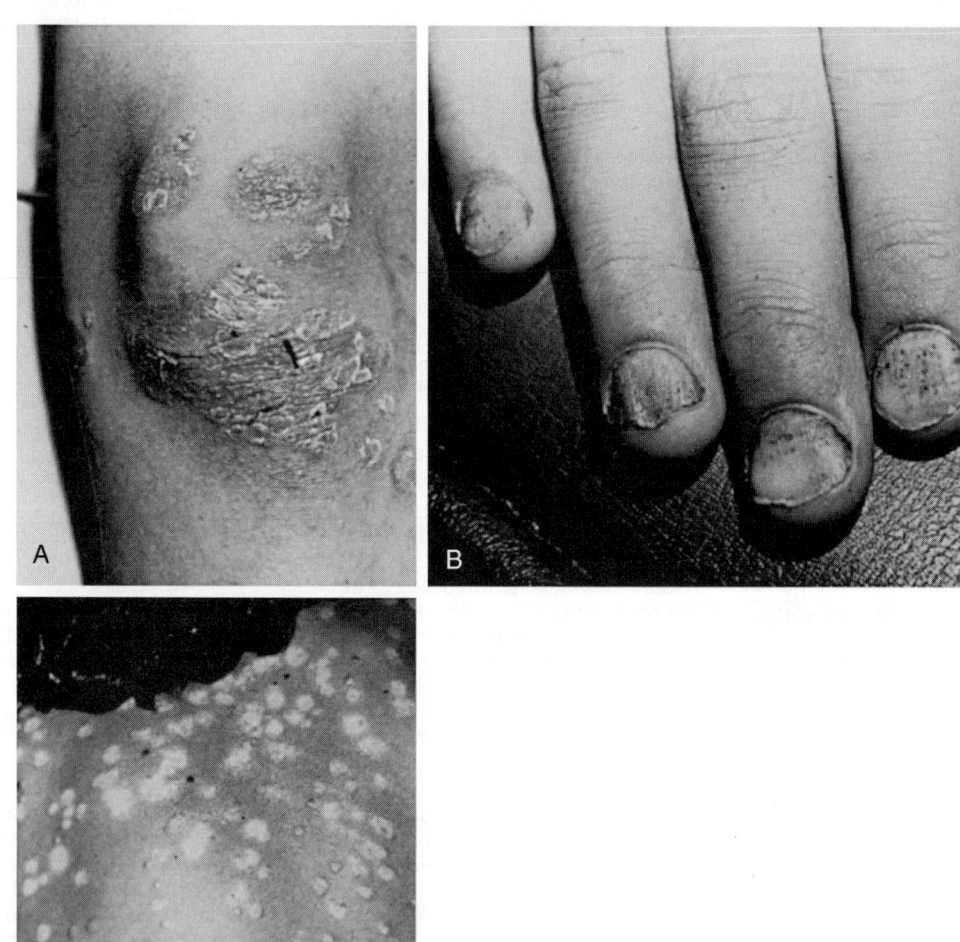

Fig. 1-309   A, Chronic psoriatic plaques on the knee. **B,** Psoriatic nail changes of pitting and dystrophy. **C,** Guttate psoriasis in widespread distribution over the trunk. (From Behrman RE: *Nelson textbook of pediatrics,* ed 16, Philadelphia, 2000, WB Saunders.)

BASIC INFORMATION

DEFINITION

Cardiogenic pulmonary edema is a life-threatening condition caused by severe left ventricular decompensation.

SYNONYMS

Cardiogenic pulmonary edema

ICD-9CM CODES

428.1 Acute pulmonary edema with heart disease

PHYSICAL FINDINGS & CLINICAL PRESENTATION

- Dyspnea with rapid, shallow breathing
- Diaphoresis, perioral and peripheral cyanosis
- Pink, frothy sputum
- Moist, bilateral pulmonary rales
- Increased pulmonary second sound, S_3 gallop (in association with tachycardia)
- Bulging neck veins

ETIOLOGY

Increased pulmonary capillary pressure secondary to
- Acute myocardial infarction
- Exacerbation of CHF
- Valvular regurgitation
- Ventricular septal defect
- Severe myocardial ischemia
- Mitral stenosis
- Other: cardiac tamponade, endocarditis, myocarditis, arrhythmias, cardiomyopathy, hypertensive crisis

DIAGNOSIS

DIFFERENTIAL DIAGNOSIS

- Noncardiogenic pulmonary edema
- Pulmonary embolism
- Exacerbation of asthma
- Exacerbation of COPD
- Sarcoidosis
- Pulmonary fibrosis
- Viral pneumonitis and other pulmonary infections

LABORATORY TESTS

ABGs: respiratory and metabolic acidosis, decreased Pao_2, increased Pco_2, low pH. NOTE: The patient may initially show respiratory alkalosis secondary to hyperventilation in attempts to maintain Pao_2.

IMAGING STUDIES

- Chest x-ray examination:
  1. Pulmonary congestion with Kerley B lines; fluffy perihilar infiltrates in the early stages; bilateral interstitial alveolar infiltrates
  2. Pleural effusions
- Echocardiogram:
  1. Useful to evaluate valvular abnormalities, diastolic vs. systolic dysfunction
  2. Can aid in differentiation of cardiogenic vs. noncardiogenic pulmonary edema
  3. Can also estimate pulmonary capillary wedge pressure and rule out presence of myxoma or atrial thrombus
- Right heart catheterization (selected patients): cardiac pressures and cardiogenic pulmonary edema reveal increased PADP and PCWP ≥25 mm Hg

TREATMENT

NONPHARMACOLOGIC THERAPY

Patients should be placed in a sitting position with legs off the side of the bed to improve breathing and decrease venous return.

ACUTE GENERAL Rx

All the following steps can be performed concomitantly:
- 100% oxygen by face mask. Both CPAP and BiPAP systems can improve oxygenation and lower carbon dioxide tensions. Check ABGs; if marked hypoxemia or severe respiratory acidosis, intubate the patient and place on a ventilator. Positive end-expiratory pressure (PEEP) increases functional capacity and improves oxygenation.
- Furosemide 40 to 100 mg IV bolus to rapidly establish diuresis and decrease venous return through its venodilator action; may double the dose in 30 min if no effect.
- Vasodilator therapy:
  1. Nitrates: particularly useful if the patient has concomitant chest pain.
     a. Nitroglycerin: 150 to 600 µg SL or nitroglycerin spray (Nitrolingual) may be given immediately on arrival and repeated multiple times if the patient remains symptomatic and blood pressure remains stable.
     b. 2% nitroglycerin ointment: 1 to 3 inches out of the tube applied continuously; absorption may be erratic.
     c. IV nitroglycerin: 100 mg in 500 ml of D_5W solution; start at 6 µg/min (2 ml/hr).
  2. Nitroprusside: useful for afterload reduction in hypertensive patients with decreased cardiac index (CI).
     a. Increases the CI and decreases left ventricular filling pressure.
     b. Vasodilator and diuretic therapy should be tailored to achieve PCWP ≤18 mm Hg, RAP ≤8 mm Hg, systolic blood pressure >90 mm Hg, SVR >1200 dynes/sec/cm^{-5}. The use of nitroprusside in patients with acute MI is controversial because it may intensify ischemia by decreasing the blood flow to the ischemic left ventricular myocardium.
- Morphine: 3 to 10 mg IV/SC/IM initially. May repeat q15min PRN. It decreases venous return, anxiety, and systemic vascular resistance (naloxone should be available at bedside to reverse the effects of morphine if respiratory depression occurs). Morphine may induce hypotension in volume-depleted patients.
- Dobutamine: parenteral inotropic agent of choice in severe cases of cardiogenic pulmonary edema. It can be administered at a dosage of 2.5 to 10 µg/kg/min IV. IV phosphodiesterase inhibitors (amrinone, milrinone) may be useful in refractory cases.
- Afterload reduction with ACE inhibitors. Captopril 25 mg PO tablet can be used for SL administration (placing a drop or two of water on the tablet and placing it under the tongue helps dissolve it), onset of action is <10 min, peak effect can be reached in 30 min. ACE inhibitors can also be given IV (e.g., enalaprilat 1 mg IV given q2h prn).
- Aminophylline: useful only if patient has concomitant severe bronchospasm.
- Digitalis: limited use in acute pulmonary edema caused by MI, but it is useful in pulmonary edema resulting from atrial fibrillation or flutter with a fast ventricular response.
- Acute cardiogenic pulmonary edema caused by IHSS must be treated with IV normal saline solution and negative inotropic agents such as verapamil and β-blockers.

DISPOSITION

- Mortality for cardiogenic pulmonary edema is approximately 60% to 80%.

REFERENCE

Gandhi SU et al: The pathogenesis of acute pulmonary edema associated with hypertension, *N Engl J Med* 344:17, 2001.
Author: **Fred F. Ferri, M.D.**

BASIC INFORMATION

■ DEFINITION
Pulmonary embolism (PE) refers to the lodging of a thrombus or other embolic material from a distant site in the pulmonary circulation.

■ SYNONYMS
Pulmonary thromboembolism
PE

ICD-9CM CODES
415.1 Pulmonary embolism and infarction

■ EPIDEMIOLOGY & DEMOGRAPHICS
- 650,000 cases of PE occur in the U.S. each year; 50,000 result in death (increased incidence in women and with advanced age).
- More than 90% of pulmonary emboli originate in the deep venous system of the lower extremities.
- Pulmonary thromboembolism is associated with >200,000 hospitalizations each year in the U.S.
- 8% to 10% of victims of PE die within the first hour.

■ PHYSICAL FINDINGS & CLINICAL PRESENTATION
- Most common symptom: dyspnea
- Chest pain: may be nonpleuritic or pleuritic (infarction)
- Syncope (massive PE)
- Fever, diaphoresis, apprehension
- Hemoptysis, cough
- Evidence of DVT may be present (e.g., swelling and tenderness of extremities)
- Cardiac examination: may reveal tachycardia, increased pulmonic component of S_2, murmur of tricuspid insufficiency, right ventricular heave, right-sided S_3
- Pulmonary examination: may demonstrate rales, localized wheezing, friction rub
- Most common physical finding: tachypnea

■ ETIOLOGY
- Thrombus, fat, or other foreign material
- Risk factors for PE:
  1. Prolonged immobilization
  2. Postoperative state
  3. Trauma to lower extremities
  4. Estrogen-containing birth control pills
  5. Prior history of DVT or PE
  6. CHF
  7. Pregnancy and early puerperium
  8. Visceral cancer (lung, pancreas, alimentary and genitourinary tracts)
  9. Trauma, burns
  10. Advanced age
  11. Obesity
  12. Hematologic disease (e.g., antithrombin III deficiency, protein C deficiency, protein S deficiency, lupus anticoagulant, polycythemia vera, dysfibrinogenemia, paroxysmal nocturnal hemoglobinuria, factor V Leiden mutation, G20210A prothrombin mutation)
  13. COPD, diabetes mellitus
  14. Prolonged air travel

DIAGNOSIS

■ DIFFERENTIAL DIAGNOSIS
- Myocardial infarction
- Pericarditis
- Pneumonia
- Pneumothorax
- Chest wall pain
- GI abnormalities (e.g., peptic ulcer, esophageal rupture, gastritis)
- CHF
- Pleuritis
- Anxiety disorder with hyperventilation
- Pericardial tamponade
- Dissection of aorta
- Asthma

■ WORKUP
- Evaluation of suspected pulmonary embolism is described in Fig. 1-311. It is important to remember that no single noninvasive test has both high sensitivity and high specificity for PE. Consequently, in addition to clinical assessment, most patients will require several noninvasive tests or pulmonary angiography to diagnose PE.
- Lung scan or pulmonary angiogram will confirm the diagnosis.
- Serial compressive duplex ultrasonography of lower extremities can be used in patients with "low-probability" lung scan and high clinical suspicion (see "Imaging Studies"). It is useful if positive, negative results do not exclude pulmonary embolism.

■ LABORATORY TESTS
- ABGs generally reveal decreased Pao_2 and $Paco_2$ and increased pH; normal results do not rule out PE.
- Alveolar-arteriolar (A-a) oxygen gradient, a measure of the difference in oxygen concentration between alveoli and arterial blood, is a more sensitive indicator of the alteration in oxygenation that Pao_2; it can easily be calculated using the information from ABGs (see Section VI, "Clinical Formulas"); a normal A-a gradient among patients without history of PE or DVT makes the diagnosis of PE unlikely.
- Plasma D-dimer measurement: D-dimer assays detect the presence of plasmin-mediated degradation products of fibrin that contain cross-linked D fragments in the whole blood or plasma. A normal plasma D-dimer level is useful to exclude pulmonary embolism in patients with a nondiagnostic lung scan and a low pretest probability of PE. However, it cannot be used to "rule in" the diagnosis because it increases with many other disorders (e.g., metastatic cancer, trauma, sepsis, postoperative state).

■ IMAGING STUDIES
- Chest x-ray film may be normal; suggestive findings include elevated diaphragm, pleural effusion, dilation of pulmonary artery, infiltrate or consolidation, abrupt vessel cut-off, or atelectasis. A wedge-shaped consolidation in the middle and lower lobes is suggestive of a pulmonary infarction and is known as "Hampton's hump."
- Lung scan (Fig. 1-310):
  1. A normal lung scan rules out PE.
  2. A ventilation-perfusion mismatch is suggestive of PE, and a lung scan interpretation of high probability is confirmatory.
  3. If the clinical suspicion of PE is high and the lung scan is interpreted as low probability, moderate probability, or indeterminate, a pulmonary arteriogram is indicated; a positive arteriogram confirms diagnosis; a positive compressive duplex ultrasonography for DVT obviates the need for an arteriogram, because treatment with IV anticoagulants is indicated in these patients; the overall sensitivity of compressive ultrasonography for DVT in patients with PE is 29%, specificity 97%; adding ultrasonography in patients with a nondiagnostic lung scan prevents 9% of angiographies; however, this improvement in efficacy is achieved at the cost of unnecessary anticoagulant therapy in 26% of patients who have false-positive ultrasonography results.
- Pulmonary angiography is the gold standard; however, it is invasive, expensive, and not readily available in some clinical settings. False-positive pulmonary angiograms may result from mediastinal disorders such as radiation fibrosis and tumors.
- CT angiography is an accurate, noninvasive tool in the diagnosis of PE at the main, lobar, and segmental pulmonary artery levels. A major

advantage of CT angiography over standard pulmonary angiography is its ability to diagnose intrathoracic disease other than PE that may account for the patient's clinical picture. It is also less invasive, less costly, and more widely available. Its major shortcoming is its poor sensitivity for subsegmental emboli.
- Gadolinium-enhanced magnetic resonance angiography of the pulmonary arteries has a high sensitivity and specificity for the diagnosis of PE; this new technique shows promise as a method of diagnosing PE; however, additional studies are necessary before it can be used to safely exclude PE.
- ECG is abnormal in 85% of patients with acute PE. Frequent abnormalities are sinus tachycardia, nonspecific ST-segment or T wave changes, S-I, Q-III, T-III pattern (10% of patients), S-I, S-II, S-III pattern, T wave inversion in V_1 to V_6, acute RBBB, new-onset atrial fibrillation, ST segment depression in lead II, right ventricular strain.

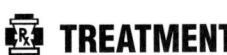 TREATMENT

■ NONPHARMACOLOGIC THERAPY
Correction of risk factors (see "Etiology") to prevent future PE

■ ACUTE GENERAL Rx
- Heparin by continuous infusion for at least 5 days; many experts recommend a larger initial IV heparin bolus (15,000 to 20,000 U) to block

platelet aggregation and thrombi and subsequent release of vasoconstrictive substances.
- Thrombolytic agents (urokinase, tPA, streptokinase): provide rapid resolution of clots; thrombolytic agents are the treatment of choice in patients with massive PE who are hemodynamically unstable and with no contraindication to their use. Thrombolytic therapy is not recommended for hemodynamically stable patients with large PE and right ventricular strain because the efficacy of thrombolytic therapy and treatment with heparin are similar but the risk of serious bleeding is greater with thrombolytics.
- Long-term treatment is generally carried out with warfarin therapy started on day 1 or 2 and given in a dose to maintain the INR at 2 to 3.
- If thrombolytics and anticoagulants are contraindicated (e.g., GI bleeding, recent CNS surgery, recent trauma) or if the patient continues to have recurrent PE despite anticoagulation therapy, vena caval interruption is indicated by transvenous placement of a Greenfield vena caval filter.
- Acute pulmonary artery embolectomy may be indicated in a patient with massive pulmonary emboli and refractory hypotension.

■ CHRONIC Rx
Elimination of risk factors (see "Etiology") and monitoring of warfarin dose with INR on a routine basis

■ DISPOSITION
- Mortality can be reduced to <10% by rapid and effective treatment.

- Mortality from recurrent pulmonary emboli is 8% with effective treatment and >30% in patients with untreated pulmonary emboli.

■ REFERRAL
Acute pulmonary embolectomy in selected patients (see "Acute General Rx")

⚙ PEARLS & CONSIDERATIONS

■ COMMENTS
- The duration of oral anticoagulant treatment is 6 mo in patients with reversible risk factors and indefinitely in patients with persistence of risk factors that caused the initial PE.
- Patients should be educated about the need for compliance with long-term anticoagulation therapy.

REFERENCES
Bates SM, Ginsberg JS: Helical computed tomography and the diagnosis of pulmonary embolism, *Ann Intern Med* 132:240, 2000.
Goldhaber SZ: Pulmonary embolism, *N Engl J Med* 339:93, 1998.
Oger E et al: Evaluation of a new, rapid, and quantitative D-dimer test in patients with suspected pulmonary embolism, *Am J Respir Crit Care Med* 158:65, 1998.
Ryu JH et al: Diagnosis of pulmonary embolism with use of computed tomographic angiography, *Mayo Clin Proc* 76:59, 2001.
Author: **Fred F. Ferri, M.D.**

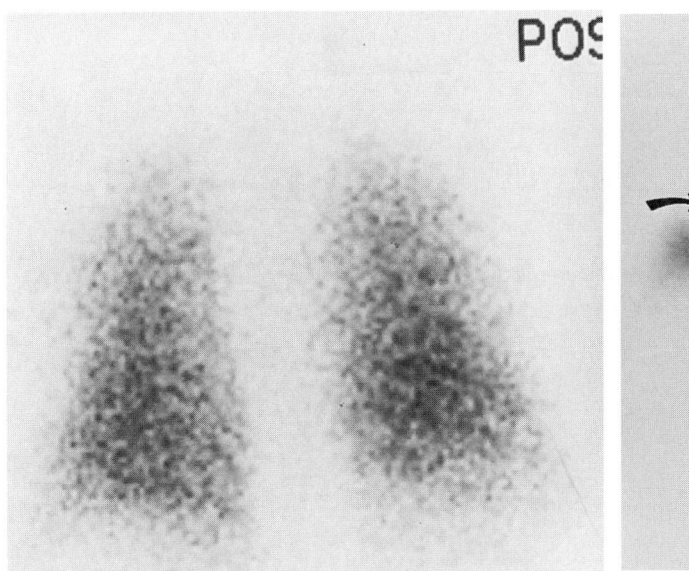
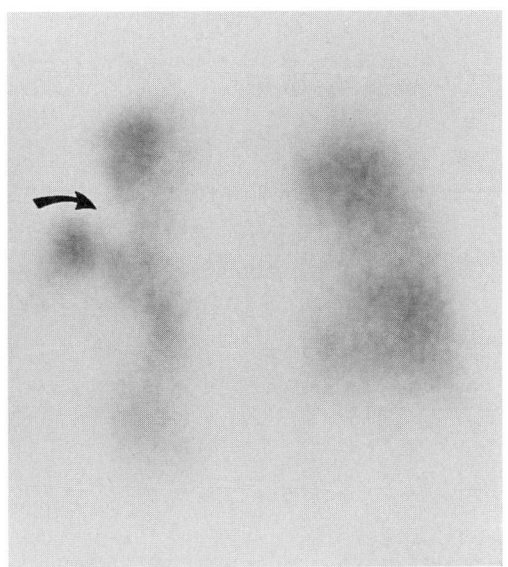

Fig. 1-310 A high-probability ventilation **(A)** and perfusion **(B)** scan. Note the nonmatched areas of segmental perfusion. There are no corresponding defects of the ventilation component of the scan. The arrow in **B** points to an area of nonperfused lung. (From Sabiston D: *Textbook of surgery,* ed 15, Philadelphia, 1997, WB Saunders.)

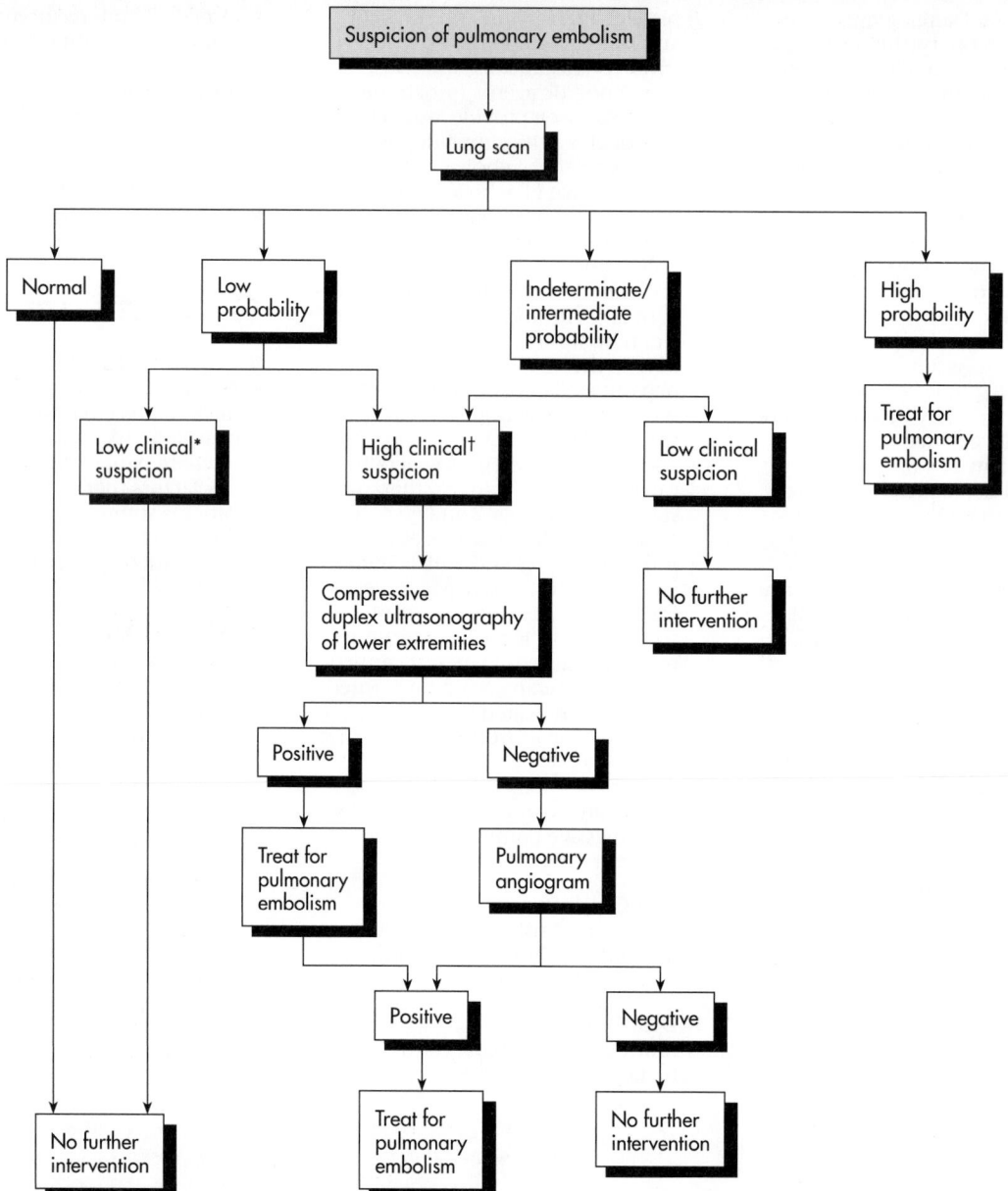

*Low clinical suspicion: after appropriate clinical evaluation, a diagnosis other than pulmonary embolism is evident in explaining the patient's presentation (e.g., heart failure, pneumonia).
†High clinical suspicion: after appropriate clinical evaluation there is no alternative diagnosis other than pulmonary embolism that can explain the patient's clinical presentation.

Fig. 1-311   Evaluation of suspected pulmonary embolism. (From Ferri F: *Practical guide to the care of the medical patient,* ed 5, St Louis, 2001, Mosby.)

BASIC INFORMATION

■ DEFINITION
Pulmonary hypertension is defined as the elevation of intravascular pressure within the pulmonary circulation. Pulmonary hypertension may be primary or secondary, acute or chronic. Systolic pulmonary artery pressures >30 mm Hg are considered elevated.

■ SYNONYMS
Primary pulmonary hypertension (PPH)
Secondary pulmonary hypertension

ICD-9CM CODES
416.0 Primary pulmonary hypertension
416.8 Secondary pulmonary hypertension

■ EPIDEMIOLOGY & DEMOGRAPHICS
- Primary pulmonary hypertension (PPH) is rare, occurring in 2 cases per 1 million people.
- PPH is more common in women than men (1.7:1), usually presenting in the third to fourth decade of life.
- PPH can be associated with portal hypertension and liver cirrhosis, appetite-suppressant drugs, and HIV disease.
- PPH may be familial.
- Secondary pulmonary hypertension is more common than PPH.
- Secondary pulmonary hypertension is the common pathophysiologic mechanism leading to cor pulmonale in patients with underlying pulmonary disease (e.g., COPD, pulmonary embolism).

■ PHYSICAL FINDINGS & CLINICAL PRESENTATION
Primary pulmonary hypertension:
- PPH is insidious and may go undetected for years.
- Dyspnea is the most common presenting symptom (60%).
- Syncope
- Chest pain
- Loud P_2 component of the second heart sound
- Right-sided S_4
- Jugular venous distinction
- Prominent parasternal (RV) impulse
- Holosystolic tricuspid regurgitation murmur heard best along the left fourth parasternal line that increases in intensity with inspiration.
- Peripheral edema
Secondary pulmonary hypertension:
- Similar to PPH but depends on the underlying cause (e.g., left-sided CHF, mitral stenosis, COPD).

■ ETIOLOGY
- The etiology of PPH is unknown.
- Secondary pulmonary hypertension is primarily caused by underlying pulmonary and cardiac conditions including:
  1. Pulmonary thromboembolic disease
  2. Chronic obstructive pulmonary disease (COPD)
  3. Interstitial lung disease
  4. Obstructive sleep disorder
  5. Neuromuscular diseases causing hypoventilation (e.g., ALS)
  6. Collagen vascular disease (e.g., SLE, CREST, systemic sclerosis)
  7. Pulmonary venous disease
  8. Left ventricular failure resulting from hypertension, CAD, aortic stenosis, and cardiomyopathy
  9. Valvular heart disease (e.g., mitral stenosis, mitral regurgitation)
  10. Congenital heart disease with left to right shunting (e.g., ASD)

DIAGNOSIS

Primary pulmonary hypertension is a diagnosis of exclusion; all secondary causes as mentioned under "Etiology" must be excluded.

■ DIFFERENTIAL DIAGNOSIS
The differential diagnosis is as listed under "Etiology."

■ WORKUP
The workup of a patient suspected of having PPH includes a detailed evaluation of the heart and lungs. Blood tests, chest x-ray, pulmonary function tests, CT scan of the chest, radionuclide studies of the heart and lungs, echocardiogram, electrocardiograms, pulmonary angiogram, and right and left heart catheterization are all required to exclude secondary causes of pulmonary hypertension.

■ LABORATORY TESTS
- CBC is usually normal in PPH but may show secondary polycythemia.
- ABGs show low PO_2 and oxygen saturation.
- PFT is done to exclude obstructive or restrictive lung disease.
- EKG may show evidence of both right atrial enlargement (tall P wave >2.5 mV in leads II, III, aVF) and right ventricular enlargement (right axis deviation >100 and R wave > S wave in lead V1).

■ IMAGING STUDIES
- Chest x-ray shows increase in central arteries with rapid tapering of the distal vessels (Fig. 1-312).
- Lung perfusion scan (V/Q scan) aids in excluding chronic pulmonary embolism.
- Echocardiogram including M-mode, 2 D, pulse, continuous and color Doppler assesses ventricular function, excludes significant valvular pathology, and visualizes abnormal shunting of blood between heart chambers if present.
- Pulmonary angiogram is done in patients with suspicious V/Q scans.
- Cardiac catheterization is performed to directly measure pulmonary artery pressures and to detect any shunting of blood.

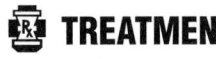

TREATMENT

■ NONPHARMACOLOGIC THERAPY
- Oxygen therapy to improve alveolar oxygen flow in both primary and secondary pulmonary hypertension
- Avoidance of vigorous exercise
- Chest physiotherapy

■ ACUTE GENERAL Rx
- PPH
  1. Diuretics (e.g., furosemide 40 mg to 80 mg qd) improves dyspnea and peripheral edema.
  2. Digoxin 0.25 mg qd has been used in patients with PPH.
  3. Vasodilator treatment is usually done with hemodynamic monitoring and include IV adenosine, prostacyclin, or nitric oxide.
- Secondary pulmonary hypertension treatment is aimed at the underlying cause (see specific disease in text for treatment).

■ CHRONIC Rx
- Chronic anticoagulation with warfarin is recommended to prevent thromboses and has been shown to prolong life in patients with PPH.
- Calcium channel blockers may alleviate pulmonary vasoconstriction and prolong life in about 20% of patients with PPH.
- Continuous infusion of epoprostenol, or prostacylin, a short-acting vasodilator and inhibitor of platelet aggregation, improves exercise capacity, quality of life, hemodynamics, and long-term survival in patients with class III or IV function.
- Lung transplantation and heart-lung transplantation are other options in end-stage class IV patients.

- Lung transplant recipients with PPH had survival rates of 73% at one yr, 55% at 3 yr, and 45% at 5 yr.

■ DISPOSITION
- Class II and III patients with PPH have a mean survival of 3.5 yr.
- Class IV patients have a mean survival of 6 mo.

■ REFERRAL
If the diagnosis of PPH is suspected, a consultation with a pulmonary specialist is recommended. Secondary causes of pulmonary hypertension may require consultations with rheumatology, neurology, and cardiology.

✦ PEARLS & CONSIDERATIONS

■ COMMENTS
Factors contributing to pulmonary arterial hypertension are:
- Alveolar hypoxia
- Acidosis
- Thromboemboli occluding arterial blood vessels (e.g., pulmonary embolism)
- Scarring or destruction of alveolar walls (e.g., COPD, infiltrative disease)
- Primary thickening of arterial walls as occurs in PPH.

REFERENCES
Krowka MJ: Pulmonary hypertension: diagnosis and therapeutics, *Mayo Clin Proc* 75:625, 2000.

Loscalzo J: Genetic clues to the cause of primary pulmonary hypertension, *N Engl J Med* 345:367, 2001.

Nauser T, Stites S: Diagnosis and treatment of pulmonary hypertension, *Am Fam Physician* 63:1789, 2001.

Rubin LJ: ACCP consensus statement. Primary pulmonary hypertension, *Chest* 104:236, 1993.

Rubin LJ: Primary pulmonary hypertension, *N Engl J Med* 336:111, 1997.

Author: **Peter Petropoulos, M.D.**

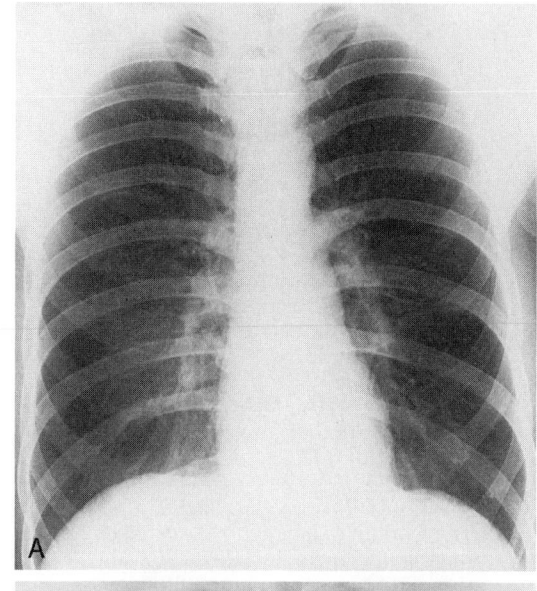
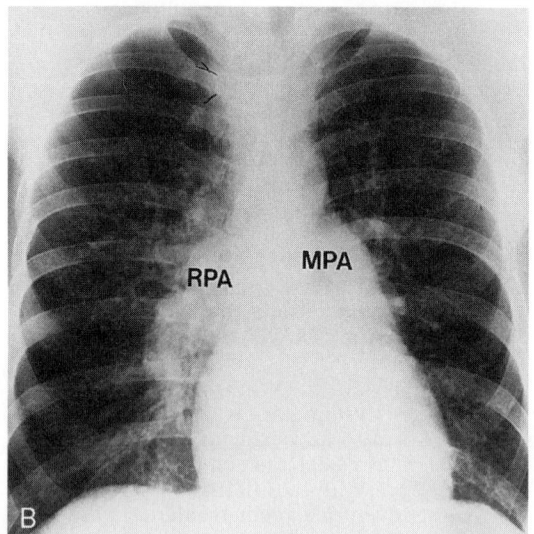

Fig. 1-312 Progressive pulmonary arterial hypertension. This patient initially presented with a relatively normal chest radiograph **(A).** However, several years later **(B),** there is increasing heart size as well as marked dilatation of the main pulmonary artery *(MPA)* and right pulmonary artery *(RPA)*. Rapid tapering of the arteries as they proceed peripherally is suggestive of pulmonary hypertension and is sometimes referrred to as *pruning.* (From Mettler FA [ed]: *Primary care radiology,* Philadelphia, 2000, WB Saunders.)

BASIC INFORMATION

■ **DEFINITION**

Pyelonephritis is an infection, usually bacterial in origin, of the upper urinary tract.

■ **SYNONYMS**

Acute pyelonephritis
Pyonephrosis
Renal carbuncle
Lobar nephronia
Acute bacterial nephritis

ICD-9CM CODES

590.81 Pyelonephritis
599.0 Urinary tract infection
595.9 Cystitis

■ **EPIDEMIOLOGY & DEMOGRAPHICS**

INCIDENCE (IN U.S.): Extremely common
PREDOMINANT SEX: Female
PREDOMINANT AGE:
• Sexually active years in women
• Usually >50 yr of age in men
PEAK INCIDENCE: See above.
GENETICS:
Congenital Infection: Congenital urologic structural disorders may predispose to infections at an early age.

■ **PHYSICAL FINDINGS & CLINICAL PRESENTATION**

• Fever
• Rigors
• Chills
• Flank pain
• Dysuria
• Polyuria
• Hematuria
• Toxic feeling and appearance
• Nausea and vomiting
• Headache
• Diarrhea
• Physical examination notable
  1. Costovertebral angle tenderness
  2. Exquisite flank pain

■ **ETIOLOGY**

• Gram-negative bacilli such as *E. coli* and *Klebsiella* spp. in more than 95% of cases
• Other, more unusual gram-negative organisms, especially if instrumentation of the urinary system has occurred
• Resistant gram-negative organisms or even fungi in hospitalized patients with indwelling catheters
• Gram-positive organisms such as enterococci
• *Staphylococcus aureus:* presence in urine indicates hematogenous origin
• Viruses: rarely, but these are usually limited to the lower tract

■ **DIAGNOSIS**

■ **DIFFERENTIAL DIAGNOSIS**

• Nephrolithiasis
• Appendicitis
• Ovarian cyst torsion or rupture
• Acute glomerulonephritis
• PID
• Endometritis
• Other causes of acute abdomen
• Perinephric abscess
• Hydronephrosis

■ **WORKUP**

• No workup in sexually active women
• Poorly responding infections, especially with azotemia and frank bacteremia
  1. Renal sonogram
  2. IVP
  3. To assess for underlying urologic pathology such as hydronephrosis
• Urologic imaging studies in all young men and boys
• Prostate assessment in older men

■ **LABORATORY TESTS**

• CBC with differential
• Renal panel
• Blood cultures
• Urine cultures
• Urinalysis
• Gram stain of urine
• Urgent renal sonography if obstruction or closed space infection suspected
• CT scans may better define the extent of collections of pus.
• Helical CT scans excellent to detect calculi

■ **TREATMENT**

■ **ACUTE GENERAL Rx**

• Hospitalization for:
  1. Toxic patients
  2. Complicated infections
  3. Diabetes
  4. Suspected bacteremia
• Keep patients well hydrated.
• IV fluids are indicated for those unable to take adequate amounts of liquids.
• Give antipyretics such as acetaminophen when necessary.
• Antibiotic therapy should be initiated after cultures are obtained and guided by the results of culture and sensitivity testing.

1. Oral trimethoprim-sulfamethoxazole DS (bid for 10 days) or ciprofloxacin (500 mg orally bid for 10 days): adequate for stable patients who can tolerate oral medications with sensitive pathogens
2. Trimethoprim-sulfamethoxazole or ciprofloxacin IV for more toxic patients
3. Ceftazidime 1 g IV q6-8h
4. Aminoglycosides such as gentamicin (2 mg/kg IV load followed by 1 mg/kg IV q8h adjusted for renal function) added but nephrotoxic especially in diabetics with azotemia
5. Vancomycin 1 g IV q12h to cover gram-positive cocci such as enterococci or staphylococci
6. Ampicillin 1 to 2 g IV q4-6h to cover enterococci, but an aminoglycoside is needed for synergy
7. Oral ampicillin or amoxicillin: no longer adequate for therapy of gram-negative infections because of resistance
• Prompt drainage with nephrostomy tube placement for obstruction
• Surgical drainage of large collections of pus to control infection
• Diabetic patients, as well as those with indwelling catheters, are especially prone to complicated infections and abscess formation.

■ **CHRONIC Rx**

• Repair underlying structural problems, especially when renal function is compromised.
  1. Reflux
  2. Obstruction
  3. Nephrolithiasis should be considered
• Patients with diabetes mellitus and indwelling urinary catheters are at particular risk of severe and complicated infections.
• When possible, remove catheters.

■ **REFERRAL**

• To surgeon: surgical correction of underlying urologic problems, such as reflux and hydronephrosis
• To pediatrician: in young children, prompt correction of reflux to avoid recurrent infections as well as loss of renal function
• To internist: aggressive metabolic as well as urologic evaluation and treatment for patients with nephrolithiasis

REFERENCE

Pomeroy C: Urinary tract infection. In Glassock RJ (ed): *Current therapy in nephrology and hypertension,* ed 4, St Louis, 1998, Mosby.
Author: **Joseph J. Lieber, M.D.**

BASIC INFORMATION

■ DEFINITION
Q fever is a systemic febrile illness caused by *Coxiella burnetti* that may be acute or chronic.

■ SYNONYMS
C. burnetti infection

ICD-9CM CODES
083.0 Q fever

■ EPIDEMIOLOGY & DEMOGRAPHICS
- *C. burnetti* is found worldwide.
- Common animal reservoirs are cattle, sheep, and goats.
- Most cases are found in individuals who have direct contact with infected animals (e.g., farmers, veterinarians) or who are exposed to contaminated animal urine, feces, milk, or placental tissues.
- Q fever is seen more in men than in women (3:1).

■ PHYSICAL FINDINGS & CLINICAL PRESENTATION
Acute Q fever presentation:
- Fever
- Pneumonia
- Hepatitis
- Meningoencephalitis

Chronic Q fever presentation:
- Endocarditis

Most common clinical symptoms:
- Chills
- Sweats
- Nausea
- Vomiting
- Cough, nonproductive
- Headache
- Fatigue

Most frequent physical findings:
- Fever
- Inspiratory rales
- Purpuric rash
- Hepatomegaly
- Splenomegaly

■ ETIOLOGY
- Q fever is caused by the rickettsial organism *C. burnetti*.
- *C. burnetti* is a gram-negative coccobacillus that is transmitted from arthropods to animals to humans.
- The disease is acquired most often via inhalation of aerosols. In the lungs, it proliferates in macrophases and then gains access to the blood, producing a transient bacteria. Thereafter it can invade many organs, but most commonly invades the lungs and liver.

- There is an incubation period between 3 to 30 days before systemic symptoms manifest.

DIAGNOSIS

■ DIFFERENTIAL DIAGNOSIS
Q fever can have various presentations and must be in the differential diagnosis of fever, hepatitis, pneumonia, endocarditis, and meningitis.

■ WORKUP
- CBC, ESR, and liver function tests
- Urinalysis
- Serology
- Chest x-ray

■ LABORATORY TESTS
In acute Q fever:
- CBC and white blood cell count is usually normal.
- Thrombocytopenia can occur (25%)
- Elevation of hepatic transaminases (2 to 3 times the abnormal range) may be seen
- Complement fixation (CF) shows a fourfold rise in titer between acute and convalescent samples.

In chronic Q fever (almost always endocarditis):
- ESR is elevated
- Anemia is present
- Microscopic hematuria
- Blood cultures are almost always negative
- Complement fixation (CF) titer of >1:200 to phase I antigen is diagnostic.

■ IMAGING STUDIES
- Chest x-ray examination is abnormal, showing segmental lobe consolidation
- Pleural effusions (35%)

TREATMENT

■ NONPHARMACOLOGIC THERAPY
Oxygen as needed in patients with pneumonia

■ ACUTE GENERAL Rx
- Acute Q fever can be treated with doxycycline (100 mg bid) for 14 to 21 days *or*
- Erythromycin (500 mg qid) for 14 days *or*
- Ofloxacin 200 mg PO q8h for 14 to 21 days

■ CHRONIC Rx
- Chronic Q fever is treated with a combination of two antibiotics, doxycylcine 100 mg bid and rifampin 300 mg qd *or*
- Doxycycline 100 mg bid and Ofloxacin 200 mg PO q8h *or*
- Doxycycline 100 mg bid and hydroxychloroquine 200 mg PO tid
- Duration of treatment: 2 to 3 yr.

■ DISPOSITION
- Patients with acute Q fever respond well with antibiotics with rare deaths reported.
- Mortality rates in chronic Q fever endocarditis is high (24%). Most patients will come to valve replacement surgery.

■ REFERRAL
Referral to an infectious disease expert is recommended in any cases of suspected acute or chronic Q fever.

PEARLS & CONSIDERATIONS

■ COMMENTS
- No vaccines are available.
- Infected patients do not require specific isolation precautions.
- Q fever derived its name in 1935 from Derrick, who was suspicious of a new disease during a series of acute febrile illness in abbatois workers of Queensland, Australia, justifying the name of Q fever (for query).

REFERENCES
Caron F et al: Acute Q fever pneumonia: a review of 80 hospitalized patients, *Chest* 114(3):808, 1998.

Dupont HT et al: Epidemiologic features and clinical presentation of acute Q fever in hospitalized patients: 323 French cases, *Am J Med* 93:427, 1992.

Marrie TJ: *Coxiella burnetti* (Q fever). In Mandell GL, Bennett JE, Dolin R: *Mandell, Douglas, and Bennett's principles and practice of infectious diseases*, ed 4, New York, 1995, Churchill Livingstone.
Author: **Peter Petropoulos, M.D.**

BASIC INFORMATION

■ DEFINITION

Rabies is a fatal illness caused by the rabies virus and transmitted to humans by the bite of an infected animal.

■ SYNONYMS

Hydrophobia

ICD-9CM CODES

071 Rabies

■ EPIDEMIOLOGY & DEMOGRAPHICS

INCIDENCE (IN U.S.): Approximately 2 cases/yr
PREDOMINANT SEX: Men (70% of cases)
PREDOMINANT AGE: <16 yr and >55 yr

■ PHYSICAL FINDINGS & CLINICAL PRESENTATION

- Incubation period of 10 to 90 days
  1. Shorter with bites of the face
  2. Longer if extremities involved
- Prodrome
  1. Fever
  2. Headache
  3. Malaise
  4. Pain or anesthesia at exposure site
  5. Sore throat
  6. GI symptoms
  7. Psychiatric symptoms
- Acute neurologic period, with objective evidence of CNS involvement
  1. Extreme hyperactivity and bizarre behavior alternating with periods of relative calm
  2. Hallucinations
  3. Disorientation
  4. Seizures
  5. Paralysis may occur
  6. Spasm of the pharynx and larynx, accompanied by severe pain, caused by drinking
  7. Fear elicited by seeing water
  8. Paralysis
  9. Coma
- Possible death from respiratory arrest

■ ETIOLOGY

- Rabies virus
- Cases in U.S. are associated with:
  1. Bats
  2. Raccoons
  3. Foxes
  4. Skunks
- In 8 of the 32 cases occurring in the U.S. since 1980, there was a history of exposure to bats without an actual bite or scratch.

- Imported cases are usually associated with dogs.
- Unusual acquisition:
  1. Via corneal transplantation
  2. Via aerosol transmission in laboratory workers and spelunkers

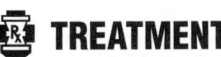

DIAGNOSIS

■ DIFFERENTIAL DIAGNOSIS

- Delirium tremens
- Tetanus
- Hysteria
- Psychiatric disorders
- Other viral encephalitides
- Guillain-Barré syndrome
- Poliomyelitis

■ WORKUP

- Rabies antibody
  1. Serum
  2. CSF
- Viral isolation
  1. Saliva
  2. CSF
  3. Serum
- Rabies fluorescent antibody: skin biopsy from the hair-covered area of the neck
- Characteristic eosinophilic inclusions (Negri bodies) in infected neurons

■ LABORATORY TESTS

See "Workup."

TREATMENT

■ NONPHARMACOLOGIC THERAPY

- Isolation of the patient to prevent transmission to others
- Supportive therapy (although this has not been shown to change outcome except in three cases in which the patients had received prophylaxis before onset of symptoms)

■ ACUTE GENERAL Rx

- No beneficial therapy
- Emphasis placed on prophylaxis of potentially exposed individuals as soon as possible following an exposure:
  1. Thorough wound cleansing
  2. Both active and passive immunization is most effective when used within 72 hr of exposure

- Vaccinations:
  1. Human diploid cell vaccine (HDCV) or rhesus monkey diploid cell vaccine (RVA), 1 ml IM (deltoid) on days 0, 3, 7, 14, and 28
  2. Human rabies hyperimmune globulin (RIG) 20 IU/kg, administered to persons not previously vaccinated. If anatomically feasible, the full dose should be infiltrated around the wounds and any remaining volume should be administered IM at an anatomically distant site from vaccine administration.
- Preexposure prophylaxis using HDCV or RVA (1 ml IM days 0, 7, and 21 or 28) in individuals at high risk for acquisition:
  1. Veterinarians
  2. Laboratory workers working with rabies virus
  3. Spelunkers
  4. Visitors to endemic areas

■ DISPOSITION

Virtually always fatal

■ REFERRAL

- To infectious disease consultant
- To local health authorities

PEARLS & CONSIDERATIONS

■ COMMENTS

- Most cases in the U.S. are caused by:
  1. Wild animal bites (bats)
  2. Dog bites occurring outside the U.S.
  3. Some unknown exposure
- Rare cases can be transmitted by mucous membrane contact of aerosolized virus.

REFERENCES

National Association of State Public Health Veterinarians, Inc.: Compendium of animal rabies prevention and control, 2001, *MMWR* 50(RR-8):1, 2001.

Noah DL et al: Epidemiology of human rabies in the United States, 1980 to 1996, *Ann Intern Med* 128:922, 1998.

Plotkin SA: Rabies, *Clin Infect Dis* 30:4, 2000.

U.S. Department of Health: Human rabies prevention, *MMWR* 48:RR-1, 1999.
Author: **Maurice Policar, M.D.**

I

BASIC INFORMATION

■ DEFINITION
Ramsay Hunt syndrome is a localized herpes zoster infection involving the seventh nerve and geniculate ganglia, resulting in hearing loss, vertigo, and facial nerve palsy.

■ SYNONYMS
Herpes zoster oticus
Geniculate herpes
Herpetic geniculate ganglionitis

■ ICD-9CM CODES
053.11 Ramsay Hunt syndrome

■ EPIDEMIOLOGY & DEMOGRAPHICS
PREDOMINANT SEX: Equal sex distribution
PREDOMINANT AGE:
- Increasingly common with advancing age
- Rare in childhood

■ PHYSICAL FINDINGS & CLINICAL PRESENTATION
- Characteristic vesicles:
  1. On pinna
  2. In external auditory canal
  3. In distribution of the facial nerve and, occasionally, adjacent cranial nerves
- Facial paralysis on the involved side

■ ETIOLOGY
Reactivation of dormant infection with varicella-zoster virus following primary varicella (usually in childhood)

DIAGNOSIS

- Usually made by recognition of the clinical features detailed above

- Viral culture and/or microscopic examination of specimens taken from active vesicles

■ DIFFERENTIAL DIAGNOSIS
- Herpes simplex
- External otitis
- Impetigo
- Enteroviral infection
- Bell's palsy of other etiologies
- Acoustic neuroma (before appearance of skin lesions)
- The differential diagnosis of headache and facial pain is described in Box 2-111.

■ WORKUP
If the diagnosis is in doubt, confirmation of varicella-zoster virus infection should be sought.

■ LABORATORY TESTS
- Viral culture of specimens of vesicular fluid and scrapings of the vesicle base
- Tzanck preparation, which may reveal multinucleated giant cells
- Direct immunofluorescent staining of scrapings

■ IMAGING STUDIES
MRI may demonstrate enhancement of the facial and vestibulocochlear nerves before appearance of vesicles.

TREATMENT

■ ACUTE GENERAL Rx
- Prednisone (40 mg PO for 2 days; 30 mg for 7 days; followed by tapering course) is recommended by some authors.

- Acyclovir (800 mg PO five times qd for 10 days), famciclovir (500 mg tid for 7 days), or valacyclovir (1 g every 8 hr for 7 days) may hasten healing.
- Analgesics should be used as indicated.

■ CHRONIC Rx
- Amitriptyline is effective in some cases of postherpetic pain.
- Narcotic analgesics may occasionally be necessary.

■ DISPOSITION
Recurrences are unusual.

■ REFERRAL
To otolaryngologist: patients with persistent facial paralysis for potential surgical decompression of the facial nerve

PEARLS & CONSIDERATIONS

■ COMMENTS
Immunodeficiency states, particularly infection with the human immunodeficiency virus (HIV), should be considered in:
- Younger patients
- Severe cases
- Patients with a history of specific risk behavior

REFERENCES
Hato N et al: Ramsay Hunt syndrome in children, *Ann Neurol* 48(2):254, 2000.
Ko JY, Sheen TS, Hsu MM: Herpes zoster oticus treated with acyclovir and prednisolone: clinical manifestations and analysis of prognostic factors, *Clin Otolaryngol* 25(2):139, 2000.
Author: **Joseph R. Masci, M.D.**

BASIC INFORMATION

■ DEFINITION

Raynaud's phenomenon is a vasospastic disorder usually affecting the digital arteries precipitated by exposure to cold temperatures or emotional distress and manifesting in a triphasic discoloration of the fingers or toes.

■ SYNONYMS

Primary Raynaud's phenomenon or Raynaud's disease
Secondary Raynaud's phenomenon

■ ICD-9CM CODES

443.0 Raynaud's syndrome, Raynaud's disease, Raynaud's phenomenon (secondary)
785.4 If gangrene present

■ EPIDEMIOLOGY & DEMOGRAPHICS

• Raynaud's phenomenon (either primary [idiopathic] or secondary [see "Etiology"]) is found in 5% to 20% of the population.
• Primary Raynaud's phenomenon is more common than secondary Raynaud's and occurs in women more often than men (4:1) and in the young (<40 yr of age) more than the old.
• Between 5% to 15% of patients thought to have primary Raynaud's will develop a secondary cause (commonly scleroderma or CREST syndrome).

■ PHYSICAL FINDINGS & CLINICAL PRESENTATION

• The classic manifestation is the triphasic color response to cold exposure (Fig. 1-313):
  1. Pallor of the digit resulting from vasospasm.
  2. Blue discoloration (cyanosis) secondary to desaturated venous blood.
  3. Red (rubor) along with pain and paresthesia when vasospasm resolves and blood returns to the digit.
• Color changes are well delineated, symmetric, and usually bilateral.
• Fingertips are most often involved, but feet, ears, and nose can be affected.
• Ulcerations and rarely gangrene may occur.
• Secondary Raynaud's phenomenon may be associated with typical findings of the underlying disease (e.g., sclerodactyly and telangiectasia in CREST syndrome).

■ ETOLOGY

• Primary Raynoud's phenomenon is generally referred to as Raynaud's disease when no cause can be found.
• Secondary Raynaud's phenomenon has many causes:
  1. CREST syndrome (calcinosis, Raynaud's phenomenon, esophageal dysmotility, sclerodactyly, and telangiectasia)
  2. Scleroderma
  3. Mixed connective tissue disease, polymyositis, and dermatomyositis
  4. SLE
  5. Rheumatoid arthritis
  6. Thromboangiitis obliterans (Buerger's disease)
  7. Drug induced (β-blockers, ergotamine, methysergide, vinblastine, bleomycin, oral contraceptives)
  8. Polycythemia, cryoglobulinemia, and certain vasculitides
  9. Carpal tunnel syndrome
  10. Tools causing vibration
  11. Estrogen replacement therapy without progesterone

DIAGNOSIS

• The diagnosis of Raynaud's phenomenon can be made by a history of well-demarcated digit discoloration induced by cold exposure and a physical examination looking for possible secondary causes.
• The digit triphasic color changes can sometimes be induced in the office by placing the hand in an ice bath.
• Color photos and questionnaires may be useful in assisting in the diagnosis.

■ DIFFERENTIAL DIAGNOSIS

See "Etiology."

■ WORKUP

• Once the diagnosis of Raynaud's phenomenon is established, differentiating primary from secondary is helpful in treatment and prognosis. History and physical examination usually make this distinction, whereas certain laboratory studies may predict secondary causes (see "Laboratory Tests").
• A test available but not commonly used is the nailfold microscopy; if

positive, it may be associated with certain collagen-vascular diseases.

■ LABORATORY TESTS

• CBC, electrolytes, BUN, Cr, ESR, ANA, urinalysis should be included in the initial evaluation.
• If the history, physical examination, and initial laboratory tests suggest a possible secondary cause, specific serologic testing (e.g., anticentromere antibodies, anti-Scl 70, cryoglobulins, complement testing, and protein electrophoresis) may be indicated.

■ IMAGING STUDIES

• Chest x-ray examination may be helpful if a secondary cause, such as scleroderma, is suggested.
• Barium swallow may be helpful if CREST syndrome is suspected.
• Angiography is rarely needed for Raynaud's phenomenon but may be helpful in diagnosing Buerger's disease as a possible etiology.

TREATMENT

■ NONPHARMACOLOGIC THERAPY

• Avoid medications that may precipitate Raynaud's phenomenon (see "Etiology").
• Avoid cold exposure. Use warm gloves, hats, and garments during the winter months or before going into cold environments (e.g., air-conditioned rooms).
• Avoid stressful situations.
• Avoid nicotine, caffeine, and over-the-counter decongestants.

■ ACUTE GENERAL Rx

• Typically, patients with Raynaud's phenomenon respond well to nonpharmacologic measures.
• Medications should be used if the above-mentioned treatment does not work.
• Goal is to prevent digital ulcers and gangrene.
• Medications commonly used are described in "Chronic Rx."

■ CHRONIC Rx

• Calcium channel blockers are the most effective treatment for Raynaud's phenomenon.
  1. Nifedipine is most often prescribed at a dose of 10 to 20 mg 30 min before going outside. If

symptoms occur with long duration, nifedipine XL 30 to 90 mg PO qd is effective.

2. If side effects occur with nifedipine, other calcium blockers can be used (e.g., diltiazem 30 mg qid and gradually increased to a maximum dose of 120 mg qid). Felodipine 2.5 mg qd up to 10 mg qd can also be used.

3. Verapamil has not been shown to be effective with Raynaud's phenomenon.

- Prazosin 1 mg bid up to 4 mg bid has been effective with Raynaud's phenomenon.
- Reserpine and guanethidine, although effective, have a high side effect profile.
- Other agents that have been tried with limited results include aspirin, pentoxifylline, captopril, and topical nitrates.
- IV prostaglandins, although not available in the U.S., may be promising in severe secondary Raynaud's phenomenon.

■ DISPOSITION
The prognosis of patients with Raynaud's phenomenon depends on the etiology.

- Primary Raynaud's phenomenon is fairly benign, usually remaining stable and controlled with nonpharmacologic medical treatment.
- Patients with secondary Raynaud's phenomenon, specifically those with scleroderma, CREST syndrome, and thromboangiitis obliterans, may develop severe ischemic digits with ulceration, gangrene, and autoamputation.

■ REFERRAL
- Rheumatology consult is indicated if secondary collagen-vascular disease is diagnosed.
- Vascular surgery consult is indicated if ulcers, gangrene, or threatened digit loss is noted.

⚙ PEARLS & CONSIDERATIONS

■ COMMENTS
Most patients with Raynaud's phenomenon can be managed by the primary care provider; however, it is important to differentiate primary from secondary forms. Secondary forms may become manifest as far out as 10 yr from the diagnosis of Raynaud's phenomenon. Periodic follow-up visits and reassessment to exclude secondary forms are important toward future treatment options and outcome.

REFERENCES

Spencer-Green G: Outcomes in primary Raynaud's phenomenon, *Arch Intern Med* 158:595, 1998.
Sturgill MG, Seibold JR: Rational use of calcium-channel antagonists in Raynaud's phenomenon, *Curr Opin Rheumatol* 10:584, 1998.
Wigley FM, Flavahan NA: Raynaud's phenomenon, *Rheum Dis Clin North Am* 22(4):765, 1996.
Author: **Peter Petropoulos, M.D.**

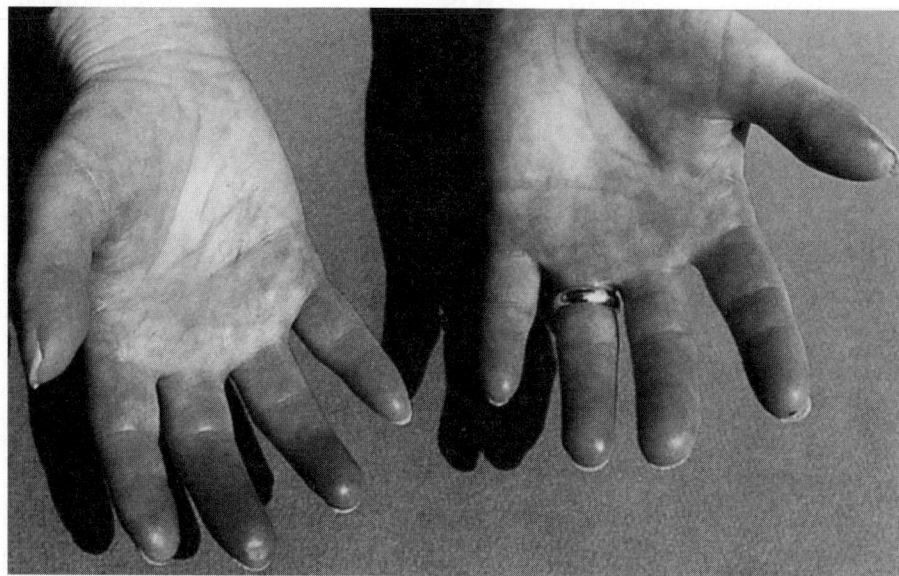

Fig. 1-313   Raynaud's phenomenon. Sharply demarcated cyanosis of the fingers with proximal venular congestion (livedo reticularis) is seen. (From Klippel J, Dieppe P, Ferri F [eds]: *Primary care rheumatology,* London, 1999, Mosby.)

BASIC INFORMATION

■ DEFINITION

Reflex sympathetic dystrophy (RSD) refers to a painful neuropathic symptom complex affecting an extremity following trauma, surgery, or nerve injury to that limb.

■ SYNONYMS

Causalgia
Shoulder-hand syndrome
Sudeck's atrophy
Posttraumatic pain syndrome

ICD-9CM CODES

337.20 Dystrophy sympathetic (post-traumatic) (reflex)

■ EPIDEMIOLOGY & DEMOGRAPHICS

- The incidence and prevalence of RSD is not known.
- RSD is usually initiated by trauma.
- RSD can occur in adults and children.
- RSD is often associated with psychiatric emotional lability, anxiety, and depression.

■ PHYSICAL FINDINGS & CLINICAL PRESENTATION

RSD is divided into three stages:
- Acute stage (occurring within hours to days after the injury)
  1. Burning or aching pain occurring over the injured extremity
  2. Hyperalgesia (exquisitely sensitive to touch)
  3. Edema
  4. Dysthermia
  5. Increased hair and nail growth
- Dystrophic stage (3 to 6 mo after the injury)
  1. Burning pain radiating both distal and proximally from the site of injury
  2. Brawny edema
  3. Hyperhidrosis
  4. Hypothermia and cyanosis
  5. Muscle tremors and spasms
  6. Increase muscle tone and reflexes

- Atrophic stage (6 mo after injury)
  1. Spread of pain proximally
  2. Cold, pale cyanotic skin
  3. Trophic skin changes with subcutaneous atrophy
  4. Fixed joints
  5. Contractures

■ ETIOLOGY

- The cause of RSD is unknown. It is thought to represent dysfunction of the sympathetic nervous system.
- Any injury can precipitate RSD including:
  1. Crush blunt trauma, burns, frostbite
  2. Surgery (Fig. 1-314)
  3. Parkinson's disease
  4. Cerebrovascular accident
  5. Myocardial infarction
  6. Osteoarthritis, cervical and lumbar disk disease
  7. Carpal tunnel and tarsal tunnel syndrome
  8. Diabetes
  9. Hyperthyroidism
  10. Isoniazid therapy

DIAGNOSIS

The diagnosis of RSD is primarily clinical, based on the patient's history and physical presentation.

■ DIFFERENTIAL DIAGNOSIS

The differential diagnosis includes all the causes mentioned under "Etiology."

■ WORKUP

In patients with RSD, no workup is needed because there are no specific diagnostic tests establishing the diagnosis.

■ LABORATORY TESTS

Blood tests are not specific in the diagnosis of RSD.

■ IMAGING STUDIES

- No imaging studies are diagnostic of RSD. Three-phase bone imaging may be helpful.
- Autonomic testing, although not commonly done, has been proposed.
  1. Measuring resting sweat output
  2. Measuring resting skin temperature
  3. Quantitative sudomotor axon reflex test
- X-ray studies of the affected limb may show osteoporosis from disuse.

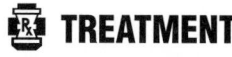

TREATMENT

Treatment is aimed at relieving the pain and improving disuse atrophy with physical therapy.

■ NONPHARMACOLOGIC THERAPY

- Physical therapy
- Transcutaneous nerve stimulation

■ ACUTE GENERAL Rx

- The following has been tried for neuropathic pain relief:
- Amitriptyline 10 mg to 150 mg qd
- Phenytoin 300 mg qd
- Carbamazepine 100 mg bid
- Calcium channel blockers, nifedipine extended release 30 to 60 mg qd
- Prednisone 60 to 80 mg qd × 2 wk and then tapered over 1 to 2 wk to a maintenance dose of 5 mg qd for 2 to 3 mo.

■ CHRONIC Rx

- Stellate ganglion and lumbar sympathetic blocks can be tried.
- IV qd α-adrenergic blockade with phentolamine is thought to be a good predictor of response to subsequent sympatholytic treatment.
- Surgical sympathectomy.

■ DISPOSITION
- Spontaneous remission can occur after several weeks to months.
- Patients with RSD variably will progress through all stages leading to atrophy and contractures.

■ REFERRAL
RSD is a very difficult diagnosis to make and referral to either rheumatology, neurology, orthopedic, or physiatry is recommended.

⚙ PEARLS & CONSIDERATIONS

■ COMMENTS
- RSD is a common clinical entity without clear definition, pathophysiologic features, or treatment.
- Pain is the most disabling symptom for most patients with RSD and is usually out of proportion to the extent of the injury.

REFERENCES
Ochoa JL: Reflex sympathetic dystrophy: a disease of medical understanding, *Clin J Pain* 8:363, 1992.

Schwartzman RJ: New treatments for reflex sympathetic dystrophy, *N Engl J Med* 343:654, 2000.

Schwartzman RJ, Maleki J: Postinjury neuropathic pain syndromes, *Med Clin North Am* 83(3):597, 1999.

Schwartzman RJ, McLellan TL: Reflex sympathetic dystrophy: a review, *Arch Neurol* 44:555, 1987.

Author: **Peter Petropoulos, M.D.**

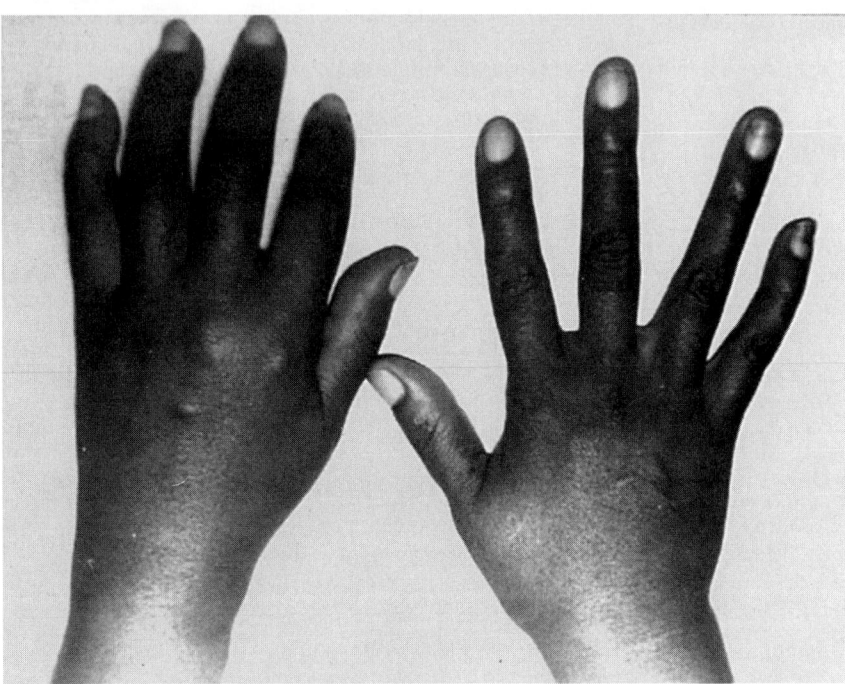

Fig. 1-314   Sympathetic dystrophy. Swollen, painful left hand after carpal tunnel release. This patient, a 40-year-old woman, had open release of the left carpal tunnel for idopathic carpal tunnel syndrome 1 month prior. She was treated with several stellate ganglion blocks and intensive physiotherapy. She was well 3 months later. (From Canoso J: *Rheumatology in primary care,* Philadelphia, 1997, WB Saunders.)

BASIC INFORMATION

■ DEFINITION
Reiter's syndrome is one of the seronegative spondyloarthropathies, so called because serum rheumatoid factor is not present in these forms of inflammatory arthritis. Reiter's syndrome is an asymmetric polyarthritis that affects mainly the lower extremities and is associated with one or more of the following:
- Urethritis
- Cervicitis
- Dysentery
- Inflammatory eye disease
- Mucocutaneous lesions

■ SYNONYMS
Reiter's disease
Reactive arthritis
Seronegative spondyloarthropathy

ICD-9CM CODES
099.3 Reiter's syndrome

■ EPIDEMIOLOGY & DEMOGRAPHICS
INCIDENCE (IN U.S.): 0.0035% annually of men <50 yr
PREDOMINANT SEX: Male
PREDOMINANT AGE: 20 to 40 yr
PEAK INCIDENCE: Most common in the third decade
GENETICS:
Familial Disposition: Strongly associated with HLA-B27 (63% to 96%)

■ PHYSICAL FINDINGS & CLINICAL PRESENTATION
- Polyarthritis
  1. Affecting the knee and ankle
  2. Commonly asymmetric
- Heel pain and Achilles tendinitis, especially at the insertion of the Achilles tendon
- Plantar fasciitis
- Large effusions
- Dactylitis or "sausage toe"
- Urethritis
- Uveitis or conjunctivitis; uveitis can progress to blindness without treatment
- Keratoderma blennorrhagicum
  1. Hyperkeratotic lesions on soles of the feet, toes, penis, hands
  2. Closely resembles psoriasis
- Aortic regurgitation similar to that seen in ankylosing spondylitis

■ ETIOLOGY
- Epidemic Reiter's syndrome following outbreaks of dysentery has been well described.
- Genetically susceptible HLA-B27–positive individuals are at risk for developing Reiter's syndrome following infection with certain pathogens:
  1. *Salmonella*
  2. *Shigella*
  3. *Yersinia enterocolitica*
  4. *Chlamydia trachomatis*
  5. Molecular mimicry mechanism suspected
- Symptom complex indistinguishable from Reiter's syndrome has been described in association with HIV infection.

 DIAGNOSIS

■ DIFFERENTIAL DIAGNOSIS
- Ankylosing spondylitis
- Psoriatic arthritis
- Rheumatoid arthritis
- Gonococcal arthritis-tenosynovitis
- Rheumatic fever

■ WORKUP
- X-ray examination of affected joints
- Synovial fluid examination and culture
- Careful examination of eyes and skin
- Cultures for gonococcus (urethral, cervical, stool)

■ LABORATORY TESTS
- Elevated but nonspecific ESR
- No specific laboratory tests to diagnose Reiter's syndrome

■ IMAGING STUDIES
Plain radiographs:
- Juxtaarticular osteopenia of affected joints
- Erosions and joint space narrowing in more advanced disease
- Periostitis and reactive new bone formation at the insertions of the Achilles tendon and the plantar fascia
- Sacroiliitis:
  1. Unilateral or bilateral
  2. Indistinguishable from ankylosing spondylitis
- Vertebral bridging osteophytes

TREATMENT

■ NONPHARMACOLOGIC THERAPY
Physical therapy to maintain range of motion of the back and other joints

■ ACUTE GENERAL Rx
Flares treated with NSAIDs such as indomethacin (25 to 50 mg PO tid)
- Enteric or urethral infection should be treated with appropriate antibiotic coverage.

- Uveitis should be treated with steroid eye drops in consultation with an ophthalmologist.
- Achilles tendinitis and plantar fasciitis should be treated with injections of methylprednisolone (40 to 80 mg).
- Sulfasalazine (2 to 3 g PO tid) may be effective.
- Careful monitoring for the following is essential:
  1. GI toxicity
  2. Hypersensitivity
  3. Bone marrow suppression
- Persistent and uncontrolled disease should be managed with cytotoxic drugs (methotrexate, azathioprine) in consultation with a rheumatologist.

■ CHRONIC Rx
Chronic disease is best managed by a team approach with the collaboration of a rheumatologist or other experienced physician and physical therapist.

■ DISPOSITION
- Recurrences are frequent, even with treatment.
- Long-term sequelae:
  1. Persistent polyarthritis
  2. Chronic back pain
  3. Heel pain
  4. Progressive iridocyclitis
  5. Aortic regurgitation

■ REFERRAL
- To ophthalmologist if uveitis is suspected
- To rheumatologist if arthritis and tendinitis fail to improve rapidly after a course of NSAIDs

PEARLS & CONSIDERATIONS

■ COMMENTS
- Infection with HIV is associated with particularly severe cases of Reiter's syndrome.
- HIV testing is recommended, especially if risk factors such as unprotected sexual activity or IV drug use are identified.

REFERENCES
Al-Arfaj A: Profile of Reiter's disease in Saudi Arabia, *Clin Exp Rheumatol* 19(20):184, 2001.
Amor B: Reiter's syndrome: diagnosis and clinical features, *Rheum Dis Clin North Am* 24(4):677, 1998.
Author: **Deborah L. Shapiro, M.D.**

BASIC INFORMATION

■ DEFINITION
Renal artery stenosis is the narrowing or occlusion of a renal artery, which can occur acutely (thrombosis or embolism) and cause renal infarction or progressively (e.g., atheroma or fibromuscular dysphasia) and cause renovascular hypertension and/or lead to ischemic nephropathy. In addition, renal atheroembolism caused by showers of cholesterol microemboli can lead to progressive renal failure if sustained or recurrent.

■ SYNONYMS
Acute:
　Renal artery thrombosis
　Renal artery embolism
Chronic:
　Renovascular hypertension

ICD-9CM CODES
593.81 Renal artery occlusion
440.1 Renal artery stenosis
405.01 Renovascular hypertension, secondary
447.9 Renal artery hyperplasia

■ EPIDEMIOLOGY & DEMOGRAPHICS
- In acute renal artery occlusion, the epidemiology depends on the underlying cause (see below).
- Renovascular hypertension: Prevalence of 0.2% to 5% of all hypertensive patients.
　The prevalence is higher in patients with severe hypertension, reaching 43% of white patients and 7% of black patients with malignant hypertension.
- Approximately 1 in 6 patients with end-stage renal disease has ischemic nephropathy, and survival of patients with end-stage renal disease associated with ischemic nephropathy is half that of patients with end-stage renal disease from other causes.
- The demographics of atheromatous renal artery stenosis mirrors the pattern seen in other arteriosclerotic conditions (coronary artery disease, cerebrovascular disease, peripheral vascular disease) and is influenced by the usual risk factors (smoking, family history, diabetes, hyperlipidemia). Fibromuscular dysplasia is most likely to be seen in young adult women. Takayasu's arteritis can involve the renal arteries and is also seen in young to middle-aged women.

■ PHYSICAL FINDINGS & CLINICAL PRESENTATION
Acute renal artery occlusion
- Flank or abdominal pain
- Fever
- Nausea or vomiting
- Leukocytosis
- Hematuria (microscopic or gross)
- Elevated AST, LDH, and alkaline phosphatase
- Oliguric renal failure if occlusion is bilateral; normal or near normal renal function in unilateral occlusion
Cholesterol emboli
- Multisystem manifestations resembling vasculitis (visual disturbance, painful distal extremities, abdominal pain, signs of organ or limb ischemia). Laboratory findings include eosinophiluria, proteinuria, renal failure, elevated ESR.
Progressive renal artery stenosis
- Hypertension in a young, white woman without a family history of such (fibromuscular dysplasia)
- Hypertension in a middle-aged man with other evidence of atheromatous disease
- Abdominal bruit (40% of cases)
- Renal failure
- Hypertensive retinopathy
- Pulmonary edema in a hypertensive patient
- Hypokalemia
- Renal failure following the administration of an angiotensin-converting enzyme inhibitor (if bilateral renal artery stenosis)

■ ETIOLOGY & PATHOGENESIS
Etiology of renal artery thrombosis
- Atherosclerosis
- Fibromuscular dysphasia
- Arteritis
- Aneurysm
- Arteriography
- Syphilis
- Hypercoagulable state
- Complication of renal transplantation (role of cyclosporine)
Etiology of renal artery embolism (cardiac conditions [90%])
- Myocardial infarction
- Atrial fibrillation
- Cardiomyopathy
- Endocarditis
- Paradoxical emboli from DVT in patient with cardiac septal defect
- Atheromatous plaques (cholesterol emboli).
PATHOGENESIS: Renal hypoperfusion or ischemia produces an increase in plasma renin that stimulates the conversion of angiotensin I to angiotensin II, causing vasoconstriction and aldosterone secretion, sodium retention, and potassium wasting. Hypertension results and can be self-sustaining after some time, even in the case of unilateral renal artery stenosis because of hypertensive damage to the other kidney.

■ WORKUP
- Documentation of hypertension
- Hypertensive workup (see "Hypertension" in Section I)

■ LABORATORY TESTS
- Creatinine
- Potassium level
- Urinalysis
- Peripheral plasma renin activity
- Captopril test (stimulation of excessive renin secretion)

■ IMAGING STUDIES
- Renal scan (70% sensitivity and 79% specificity)
- Captopril renal scan (92% sensitivity and 93% specificity)
- Hypertensive IVP (75% sensitivity and 85% specificity)
- Intravenous digital substraction angiography (88% sensitivity and 90% specificity)
- Magnetic resonance angiography
- Exercise renal scan (still being evaluated)
- Renal artery ultrasound (still being evaluated)

■ INVASIVE STUDIES
- Renal arteriography
- Selective renal vein renin measurements
- Renal biopsy for cholesterol emboli

TREATMENT

Acute renal artery thrombosis or embolism
- Thrombolytic therapy
- Anticoagulation
- Revascularization (surgery)
- Blood pressure control
Cholesterol emboli
- No treatment
Renal artery stenosis
- Blood pressure control (role of ACE inhibitors and angiotensin receptor blockers is controversial, but neither should be continued if renal function worsens).
- Angioplasty or revascularization should be reserved for patients whose blood pressure control with medication is difficult and for patients with progressive renal failure.

■ NATURAL HISTORY
- Renal artery stenosis caused by fibromuscular dysplasia does not progress.
- Renal artery stenosis associated with atherosclerosis is progressive. Of patients with >60% stenosis, 5% progress to total occlusion in 1 yr and 11% progress in 2 yr.

REFERENCES
Chabova V et al: Outcomes of atherosclerotic renal artery stenosis managed without revascularization, *Mayo Clinic Proc* 75:437, 2000.
Pickering TG, Glumenfeld JD, Laragh JH: Renovascular hypertension and ischemic nephropathy. In Brenner BM (ed): *The kidney*, ed 5, Philadelphia, 1996, WB Saunders.
Safian RD, Textor SC: Renal artery stenosis, *N Engl J Med* 344:431, 2001.
Vasbinder GB et al: Diagnostic tests for renal artery stenosis in patients suspected of having renovascular hypertension: a meta-analysis, *Ann Intern Med* 135:401, 2001.
Author: **Tom J. Wachtel, M.D.**

BASIC INFORMATION

■ DEFINITION

Renal cell adenocarcinoma (RCA) is a primary adenocarcinoma originating in the renal parenchyma from the malignant transformation of proximal renal tubular epithelial cells.

■ SYNONYMS

Hypernephroma
Clear cell carcinoma of the kidney
Grawitz tumor

■ ICD-9CM CODES

189.0 adenocarcinoma of kidney
189.1 (renal pelvis)

■ EPIDEMIOLOGY & DEMOGRAPHICS

INCIDENCE: Approximately 1:10,000 persons/yr (3% of all adult malignancies)
AGE: Peak in age 50 to 70 yr
SEX: Male:female ratio of 2:1

■ PHYSICAL FINDING & CLINICAL PRESENTATION

Presenting findings in RCA patients:

Hematuria	50% to 60%
Elevated erythrocyte sedimentation rate	50% to 60%
Abdominal mass	25% to 45%
Anemia	20% to 40%
Flank pain	35% to 40%
Hypertension	20% to 40%
Weight loss	30% to 35%
Fever	5% to 15%
Hepatic dysfunction	10% to 15%
Classic triad (hematuria, abdominal mass, flank pain)	5% to 10%
Hypercalcemia	3% to 6%
Erythrocytosis	3% to 4%
Varicocele	2% to 3%

■ ETIOLOGY

Hereditary forms
• Familial renal carcinoma
• Renal carcinoma associated with von Hippel-Lindau disease
• Hereditary papillary renal cell carcinoma

Risk factors
• Cigarette smoking
• Obesity
• Use of diuretics
• Phenacetin-containing analgesics
• Asbestos exposure
• Gasoline and other petroleum products
• Lead
• Cadmium
• Thorotrast
• Role of the VHL gene located on chromosome 3

DIAGNOSIS

■ DIFFERENTIAL DIAGNOSIS

• Transitional cell carcinomas of the renal pelvis (8% of all renal cancers)
• Wilms' tumor
• Other rare primary renal carcinomas and sarcomas
• Renal cysts
• All causes of hematuria (see Box 2-140)
• Retroperitoneal tumors

■ WORKUP

• Laboratory tests and imaging studies
• Fig. 3-144 describes the evaluation of patients with a renal mass

■ LABORATORY TESTS

• CBC: anemia or erythrocytosis
• Elevated sedimentation rate
• Nonmetastatic hepatic dysfunction with elevated alkaline phosphatase, prolonged prothrombin time, and hypoalbuminemia

• Hypercalcemia (secondary to parathyroid related protein)
• Other: elevated ferritin, elevated insulin and glucagon levels, elevated alpha-fetoprotein, and elevated beta-human chorionic gonadotropin

■ IMAGING STUDIES

• Intravenous pyelography (IVP)
• Renal ultrasound
• Abdominal CT scan with contrast (Fig. 1-315)
• MRI
• Renal arteriogram

■ STAGING

See Table 1-57.

■ COMMON SITES OF METASTASES

Lung	50% to 60%
Bone	30% to 40%
Regional nodes	15% to 30%
Main renal vein	15% to 20%
Perirenal fat	10% to 20%
Adrenal (ipsilateral)	10% to 15%
Vena cava	10% to 15%
Brain	10% to 15%
Adjacent organs (colon, pancreas)	10%
Kidney (contralateral)	2%

TREATMENT

• Surgery
  Surgical nephrectomy is the only effective management for stages I, II, and some stage III tumors.
  Various forms of partial nephrectomy may be available for patients with bilateral cancers or with a solitary kidney.
  The role of nephrectomy in patients with metastatic renal cell carcinoma is controversial and should probably be reserved for patients who have a solitary metastasis amenable to surgical resection.

- Angioinfarction (for palliation)
- Radiotherapy (for palliation)
- Chemotherapy (only 5% response rate)
- Hormonal therapy (high-dose progesterone may achieve a 15% to 20% response rate)
- Immunotherapy (interleukin-2 may achieve a 15% to 30% response rate; alpha, beta, and gamma interferons are somewhat less effective)

■ **PROGNOSIS**
Prognosis of surgically treated patients

TNM stage	5-year survival (%)
I	80 to 100
II	70 to 80
III (renal vein or vena cava)	50 to 60
III (nodal involvement)	15 to 25
IV	5 to 10

■ **REFERRAL**
To urologist

REFERENCE
Jennings SB, Linehan WM: Renal, perirenal, and ureteral neoplasms. In Gillenwater JY et al: *Adult and pediatric urology,* ed 3, St Louis, 1996, Mosby.
Author: **Tom J. Wachtel, M.D.**

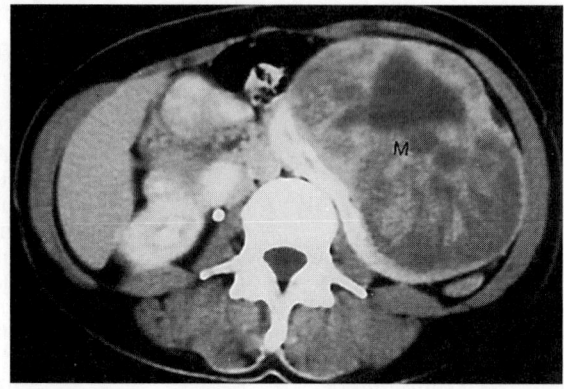

Fig. 1-315   Large renal cell carcinoma. Large mass *(M)* containing areas of high enhancement, low enhancement, and necrosis. (From Stein JH [ed]: *Internal medicine,* ed 5, St Louis, 1998, Mosby.)

TABLE 1-57   **Comparison of Conventional and TNM Staging Classification of RCC**

ROBSON STAGE	T	N	M
I: Tumor confined by capsule	T_1 (tumor 2.5 cm or less) T_2 (tumor >2.5 cm, limited to kidney)		
II: Tumor extension to perirenal fat or ipsilateral adrenal but confined by Gerota's fascia	T_3a (tumor invades adrenal gland or perinephric fat but not beyond Gerota's fascia)		
IIIa: Renal vein or inferior vena caval involvement	T_3b (renal vein or caval involvement below diaphragm) T_3c (caval involvement above diaphragm)	N_0 (nodes negative)	M_0 (no distant metastases)
IIIb: Lymphatic involvement	T_{1-4}	N_1 (single lymph node 2 cm or less) N_2 (single node between 2 and 5 cm, or multiple nodes <5 cm) N_3 (single or multiple nodes >5 cm)	
IIIc: Combination of IIIa and IIIb	$T_{3, 4}$		
IVa: Spread to contiguous organs except ipsilateral adrenal	T_4 (tumor extends beyond Gerota's fascia)		
IVb: Distant metastases	T_{1-4}		M_1 (distant metastases)

BASIC INFORMATION

■ DEFINITION
Acute renal failure (ARF) is the rapid impairment in renal function resulting in retention of products in the blood that are normally excreted by the kidneys.

■ SYNONYMS
ARF

■ ICD-9CM CODES
584.9 Acute renal failure, unspecified

■ EPIDEMIOLOGY & DEMOGRAPHICS
- ARF requiring dialysis develops in 5/100,000 persons annually.
- >10% of ICU patients develop ARF.
- >40% of hospital ARF is iatrogenic.
- The most common cause of ARF in hospitalized patients is intrinsic renal failure caused by acute tubular necrosis (ATN).

■ PHYSICAL FINDINGS & CLINICAL PRESENTATION
- Peripheral edema
- Skin pallor, ecchymoses
- Oliguria (however, patients can have nonoliguric renal failure)
- Delirium, lethargy, myoclonus, seizures
- Back pain, fasciculations, muscle cramps
- Tachypnea, tachycardia
- Weakness, anorexia, generalized malaise, nausea

■ ETIOLOGY
- Prerenal: inadequate perfusion caused by hypovolemia, CHF, cirrhosis, sepsis. Sixty percent of community-acquired cases of ARF are due to prerenal conditions.
- Postrenal: outlet obstruction from prostatic enlargement, ureteral obstruction (stones), bilateral renal vein occlusion. Postrenal causes account for 5% to 15% of community-acquired ARF.
- Intrinsic renal: glomerulonephritis, acute tubular necrosis, drug toxicity, contrast nephropathy
- Causes of acute renal failure are described in Fig. 1-316.

DIAGNOSIS

■ DIFFERENTIAL DIAGNOSIS
Refer to "Etiology."

■ WORKUP
A thorough review of the patient's history is necessary to identify contributing factors (e.g., nephrotoxin exposure, hypertension, diabetes mellitus). Laboratory evaluation to quantify degree of abnormality; radiographic studies to exclude prerenal and postrenal factors. Categorization of renal failure into oliguric (urinary output <400 ml/day) or nonoliguric is important. Anuria is common in obstructive uropathy and acute cortical necrosis.

■ LABORATORY TESTS
- Elevated serum creatinine: the rate of rise of creatinine is approximately 1 mg/dl/day in complete renal failure.
- Elevated BUN: BUN/creatinine ratio is >20:1 in prerenal azotemia, postrenal azotemia, and acute glomerulonephritis; it is <20:1 in acute interstitial nephritis and acute tubular necrosis (Table 1-58).
- Electrolytes (potassium, phosphorus) are elevated; bicarbonate level and calcium are decreased.
- CBC may reveal anemia because of decreased erythropoietin production, hemoconcentration, or hemolysis.
- Urinalysis may reveal the presence of hematuria (GN), proteinuria (nephrotic syndrome), casts (e.g., granular casts in ATN, RBC casts in acute GN, WBC casts in acute interstitial nephritis), eosinophiluria (acute interstitial nephritis).
- Urinary sodium and urinary creatinine should also be obtained to calculate the fractional excretion of sodium (FE_{Na}) (FE_{NA} = Urine sodium/plasma sodium × Plasma creatinine/urine creatinine × 100). The fractional excretion of sodium is <1 in prerenal failure, >1 in intrinsic renal failure.
- Urinary osmolarity is 250 to 300 mOsm/kg in ATN, <400 mOsm/kg

---

TABLE 1-58   Serum and Radiographic Abnormalities in Renal Failure

	PRERENAL	POSTRENAL (ACUTE)	INTRINSIC RENAL (ACUTE)	INTRINSIC RENAL (CHRONIC)
BUN	↑10:1 > Cr	↑ 20-40/d	↑ 20-40/d	Stable, ↑ varies with protein intake
Serum creatinine	N/moderate ↑	↑ 2-4/d	↑ 2-4/d	Stable ↑ (production equals excretion)
Serum potassium	N/moderate ↑	↑ varies with urinary volume	↑↑ (particularly when patient is oliguric) ↑↑↑ with rhabdomyolysis	Normal until end stage, unless tubular dysfunction (type 4 RTA)
Serum phosphorus	N/moderate ↑	Moderate ↑ ↑↑ with rhabdomyolysis	↑ Poor correlation with duration of renal disease	Becomes significantly elevated when serum creatinine level surpasses 3 mg/dl
Serum calcium	N	N/↓ with PO_4^{-3} retention	↓ (poor correlation with duration of renal failure)	Usually ↓
Renal size				
By ultrasound	N/↑	↑ and dilated calyces	N/↑	↓ and with ↑ echogenicity
FE_{Na}*	<1	<1 → >1	>1	>1

From Grant J: Renal failure. In Ferri FF (ed): *Practical guide to the care of the medical patient,* ed 5, St Louis, 2001, Mosby.
↑, Increase; ↓, decrease; ↑↑, large increase, *Cr*, creatinine; *N*, normal; *Na*, sodium; *P*, plasma; *RTA*, renal tubular acidosis; *U*, urine.
*$FE_{Na} = U_{Na}/P_{Na}U_{Cr}/P_{cr}$ × 100.

in postrenal azotemia, and >500 mOsm/kg in prerenal azotemia and acute glomerulonephritis (Table 1-59).
- Additional useful studies are blood cultures for patients suspected of sepsis, liver function studies, immunoglobulins, and protein electrophoresis in patients suspected of myeloma, creatinine kinase in patients with suspected rhabdomyolysis.
- Renal biopsy may be indicated in patients with intrinsic renal failure when considering specific therapy; major uses of renal biopsy are differential diagnosis of nephrotic syndrome, separation of lupus vasculitis from other vasculitis and lupus membranous from idiopathic membranous, confirmation of hereditary nephropathies on the basis of the ultrastructure, diagnosis of rapidly progressing glomerulonephritis, separation of allergic interstitial nephritis from ATN, separation of primary glomerulonephritis syndromes. The biopsy may be performed percutaneously or by open method. The percutaneous approach is favored and generally yields adequate tissue in >90% of cases. Open biopsy is generally reserved for uncooperative patients, those with solitary kidney, and patients at risk for uncontrolled bleeding.

■ IMAGING STUDIES
- Chest x-ray examination is useful to evaluate for CHF and for pulmonary renal syndromes (Goodpasture's syndrome, Wegener's granulomatosis).
- Ultrasound of kidneys is used to evaluate for kidney size (useful to distinguish ARF from CRF), to evaluate for the presence of obstruction, and to evaluate renal vascular status (with Doppler evaluation).
- Anterograde and/or retrograde pyelogram can be used for ruling out

obstruction; useful in patients at high risk of obstruction.

℞ TREATMENT

■ NONPHARMACOLOGIC THERAPY
- Dietary modification to supply adequate calories while minimizing accumulation of toxins; appropriate control of fluid balance. Physicians should recommend a nutrition program with an energy prescription of 120 to 150 KJ/kg per day and restriction of potassium (60 mEq/day), sodium (90 mEq/day), and phosphorus (800 mg/day). Ideal protein supplementation ranges from 0.6 to 1.4 g/kg depending on whether dialysis is required.
- Daily weight
- Modifications of dosage of renally excreted drugs

■ ACUTE GENERAL Rx
Treatment is variable with etiology of ARF:
- Prerenal: IV volume expansion in hypovolemic patients
- Intrinsic renal: discontinuation of any potential toxins and treatment of condition causing the renal failure
- Postrenal: removal of obstruction

■ CHRONIC Rx
- Monitoring of renal function and electrolytes
- Prevention of further insults to the kidneys with proper hydration, especially before contrast studies, and avoidance of nephrotoxic agents

■ DISPOSITION
- Prognosis is variable depending on the etiology of the renal failure, degree of renal failure, multiorgan involvement, and patient's age.

- Renal function recovery (ability to discontinue dialysis) varies from 50% to 75% in survivors of ARF.

■ REFERRAL
- Nephrology consultation is recommended in renal failure.
- General indications for initiation of dialysis are:
  1. Florid symptoms of uremia (encephalopathy, pericarditis)
  2. Severe volume overload
  3. Severe acid-base imbalance
  4. Significant derangement in electrolyte concentrations (e.g., hyperkalemia, hyponatremia)
- Surgical consult may be necessary in patients with obstruction.

✵ PEARLS & CONSIDERATIONS

■ COMMENTS
- It is important for physicians to recognize the growing list of medications that can result in ARF.
- Patient education material can be obtained from the National Kidney and Neurologic Disease Information Clearinghouse, Box NKUDIC, Bethesda, MD 20893.
- Booklet entitled *What Everyone Should Know About Kidneys and Kidney Disease* is available from the National Kidney Foundation, Inc., 30 East 33rd Street, New York, NY 10016.

REFERENCE
Albright RC: Acute renal failure: a practical update, *Mayo Clin Proc* 76:67, 2001.
Author: **Fred F. Ferri, M.D.**

TABLE 1-59   Urinary Abnormalities in Renal Failure

	PRERENAL	POSTRENAL (ACUTE)	INTRINSIC RENAL (ACUTE)	INTRINSIC RENAL (CHRONIC)
Urinary volume	↓	Absent-to-wide fluctuation	Oliguric or nonoliguric	1000 ml + until end stage
Urinary creatinine	↑ (U/P Cr ±40)	↓ (U/P Cr ±20)	↓ (U/P Cr <20)	↓ (U/P Cr <20)
Osmolarity	↑ (±400 mOsm/kg)	(<350 mOsm/kg)	(<350 mOsm/kg)	(<350 mOsm/kg)
Degree of proteinuria	Minimum	Absent	Varies with cause of renal failure: Modest with ATN Nephrotic range common with acute glomerulopathies, usually <2 g/24 hr with interstitial disease*	Varies with cause of renal disease (from 1-2 g/d to nephrotic range)
Urinary sediment	Negative, or occasional hyaline cast	Negative or hematuria with stones or papillary necrosis Pyuria with infectious prostatic disease	ATN: muddy brown Interstitial nephritis: lymphocytes, eosinophils (in stained preparations), and WBC casts RPGN: RBC casts Nephrosis: oval fat bodies	Broad casts with variable renal "residual" acute findings

From Grant J: Renal failure. In Ferri FF (ed): *Practical guide to the care of the medical patient,* ed 5, St Louis, 2001, Mosby.
*Except NSAID-induced allergic interstitial nephritis with concomitant "nil disease."

↑, Increased; ↓, decreased; *ATN,* acute tubular necrosis; *clearance* = $\dfrac{\text{Urinary concentration} \times \text{Urinary volume}}{\text{Plasma concentration}}$; *Cr,* creatinine; *RBC,* red blood cell;

RPGN, rapidly progressive glomerulonephritis; *U/P,* urine/plasma; *WBC,* white blood cell.

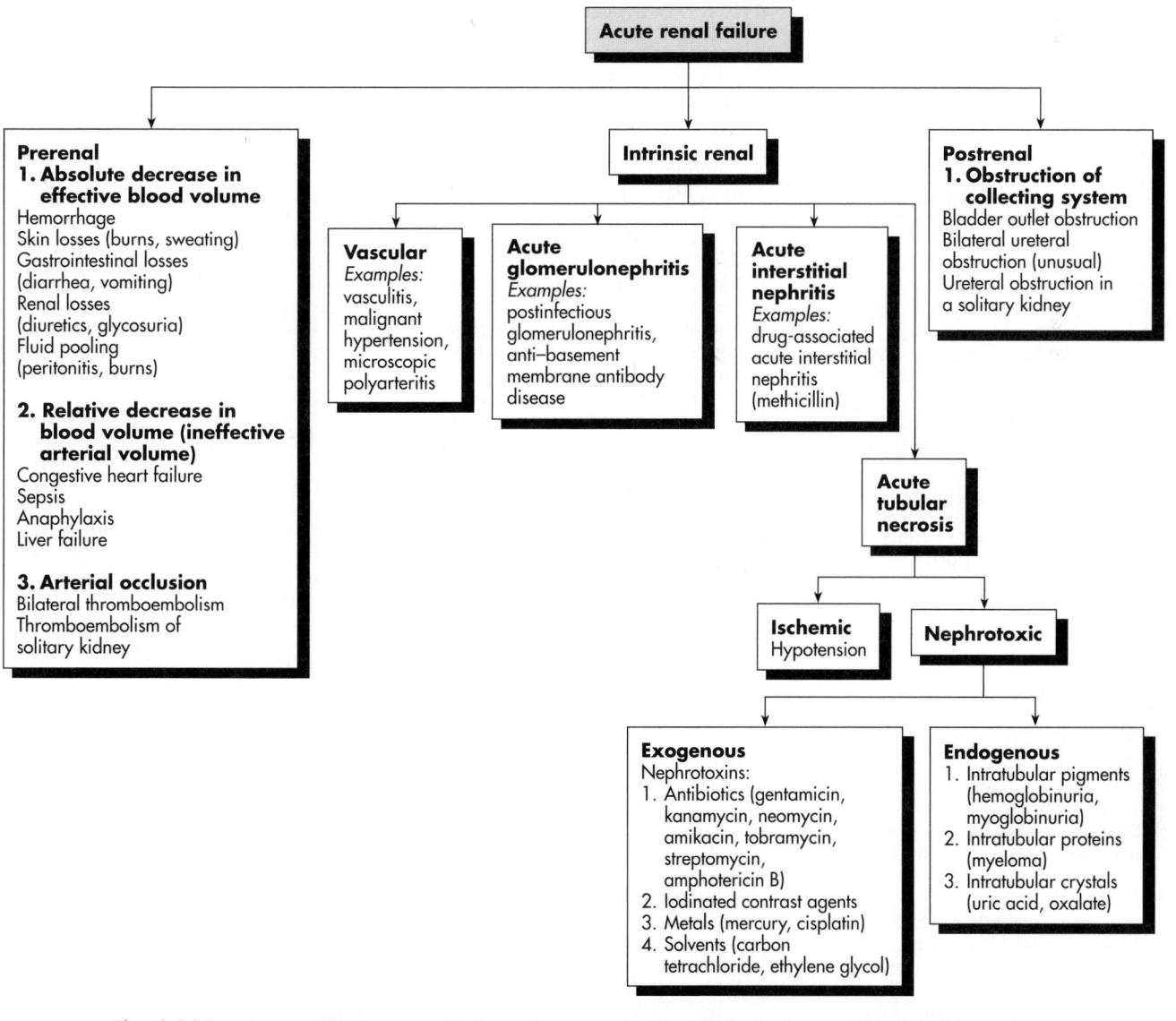

Fig. 1-316   Causes of acute renal failure. (From Andreoli TE [ed]: *Cecil essentials of medicine,* ed 4, Philadelphia, 1997, WB Saunders.)

BASIC INFORMATION

■ **DEFINITION**

Chronic renal failure (CRF) is a progressive decrease in renal function (>3 mo in duration) with subsequent accumulation of waste products in the blood, electrolyte abnormalities, and anemia.

■ **SYNONYMS**

CRF
End-stage renal disease

■ **ICD-9CM CODES**

585 Chronic renal failure

■ **EPIDEMIOLOGY & DEMOGRAPHICS**

- The number of patients with ESRD is increasing at the rate of 7% to 9%/yr in the U.S. Each year 2/10,000 persons develop end-stage CRF.
- In the U.S., >250,000/yr receive dialysis treatment for ESRD.

■ **PHYSICAL FINDINGS & CLINICAL PRESENTATION**

- Skin pallor, ecchymoses
- Edema
- Hypertension
- Emotional lability and depression
- The clinical presentation varies with the degree of renal failure and its underlying etiology. Common symptoms are generalized fatigue, nausea, anorexia, pruritus, insomnia, taste disturbances.

■ **ETIOLOGY**

- Diabetes (37%), hypertension (30%), chronic glomerulonephritis (12%)
- Polycystic kidney disease
- Tubular interstitial nephritis (e.g., drug hypersensitivity, analgesic nephropathy), obstructive nephropathies (e.g., nephrolithiasis, prostatic disease)
- Vascular diseases (renal artery stenosis, hypertensive nephrosclerosis)

DIAGNOSIS

■ **DIFFERENTIAL DIAGNOSIS**

- See "Etiology."
- CRF is primarily distinguished from ARF by the duration (progression over several months).
- Sonographic evaluation of the kidneys reveals smaller kidneys with increased echogenicity in CRF.

■ **WORKUP**

- Laboratory evaluation and imaging studies aimed at identifying reversible causes of acute decrements in GFR (e.g., volume depletion, urinary tract obstruction, CHF) superimposed on chronic renal disease

- Kidney biopsy: generally not performed in patients with small kidneys or with advanced disease

■ **LABORATORY TESTS**

- Elevated BUN, creatinine, creatinine clearance
- Urinalysis: may reveal proteinuria, RBC casts
- Serum chemistry: elevated BUN and creatinine, hyperkalemia, hyperuricemia, hypocalcemia, hyperphosphatemia, hyperglycemia, decreased bicarbonate
- Special studies: serum and urine immunoelectrophoresis (in suspected multiple myeloma), ANA (in suspected SLE)

■ **IMAGING STUDIES**

Ultrasound of kidneys to measure kidney size and to rule out obstruction

TREATMENT

■ **NONPHARMACOLOGIC THERAPY**

- Provide adequate nutrition and calories (147 to 168 kJ/kg/day in energy intake, chiefly from carbohydrate and polyunsaturated fats).
- Restrict sodium (approximately 100 mmol/day), potassium (≤60 mmol/day), and phosphate (<800 mg/day).
- Adjust drug doses to correct for prolonged half-lives.
- Restrict fluid if significant edema is present.
- Protein restriction (≤0.8 g/kg/day) may slow deterioration of renal function; however, recent studies have not confirmed this benefit.
- Resistance exercise training can preserve lean body mass, nutritional status, and muscle function in patients with moderate chronic kidney disease.
- Avoid radiocontrast agents.
- Initiate hemodialysis or peritoneal dialysis (see "Acute General Rx").
- Kidney transplantation in selected patients.

■ **ACUTE GENERAL Rx**

- ACE inhibitors and ARBs are useful in slowing the progression of chronic renal disease, especially in hypertensive diabetic patients.
- Initiation of dialysis
  1. Urgent indications: uremic pericarditis, neuropathy, neuromuscular abnormalities, CHF, hyperkalemia, seizures.
  2. Judgmental indications: creatinine clearance 10 to 15 ml/min; progressive anorexia, weight loss, reversal of sleep pattern, pruritus, uncontrolled fluid gain with hypertension and signs of CHF.
- Erythropoietin for anemia: 2000 to

3000 U three times a week IV/SC to maintain Hct 30% to 33%.
- Diuretics for significant fluid overload (loop diuretics are preferred).
- Correction of hypertension to at least 130/85 mm Hg with ACE inhibitors (avoid in patients with significant hyperkalemia) or calcium channel blockers.
- Correction of electrolyte abnormalities (e.g., calcium chloride, glucose, sodium polystyrene sulfonate for hyperkalemia), sodium bicarbonate in patients with severe metabolic acidosis.
- Control of renal osteodystrophy with calcium supplementation and vitamin D. Starting dose of calcium carbonate is 0.5 g with each meal, increased until the serum phosphorus concentration is normalized (most patients require 5 to 10 g/day). Calcitriol 0.125 to 0.25 µg/day PO is effective in increasing serum calcium concentration.
- Sevelamer (Renagel) is a useful phosphate binder to reduce serum phosphate levels.

■ **CHRONIC Rx**

Routine monitoring of renal function, Hct, and electrolytes

■ **DISPOSITION**

- Prognosis is influenced by comorbidity of multisystem diseases.
- Kidney transplantation in selected patients improves survival. The 2-yr kidney graft survival rate for living related donor transplantations is >80%, whereas the 2-yr graft survival rate for cadaveric donor transplantation is approximately 70%.

PEARLS & CONSIDERATIONS

■ **COMMENTS**

- Additional information on patient education can be obtained from the National Kidney and Urological Diseases Information Clearinghouse, Box NKUDIC, Bethesda, MD 20893 and from the National Kidney Foundation, Inc., 30 East 33rd Street, New York, NY 10016.
- Serum, radiographic, and urinary abnormalities in renal failure are described in Tables 1-58 and 1-59.

REFERENCES

Castaneda C et al: Resistance training to counteract the catabolism of a low-protein diet in patients with chronic renal insufficiency, *Ann Intern Med* 135:965, 2001.

Pastan S, Baley J: Dialysis therapy, *N Engl J Med* 338:1428, 1998.

Rahman M, Smith MC: Chronic renal insufficiency, *Arch Intern Med* 158:1743, 1998.

Author: **Fred F. Ferri, M.D.**

BASIC INFORMATION

■ DEFINITION

Renal tubular acidosis (RTA) is a disorder characterized by inability to excrete H^+ or inadequate generation of new HCO_3^-. There are four types of renal tubular acidosis:

- Type I (classic, distal RTA): abnormality in distal hydrogen secretion resulting in hypokalemic hyperchloremic metabolic acidosis
- Type II (proximal RTA): decreased proximal bicarbonate reabsorption resulting in hypokalemic hyperchloremic metabolic acidosis
- Type III (RTA of glomerular insufficiency): normokalemic hyperchloremic metabolic acidosis as a result of impaired ability to generate sufficient NH_3 in the setting of decreased glomerular filtration rate (<30 ml/min). This type of RTA is described in older textbooks and is considered by many not to be a distinct entity.
- Type IV (hyporeninemic hypoaldosteronemic RTA): aldosterone deficiency or antagonism resulting in decreased distal acidification and decreased distal sodium reabsorption with subsequent hyperkalemic hyperchloremic acidosis

■ SYNONYMS

RTA

ICD-9CM CODES

588.8 Renal tubular acidosis

■ EPIDEMIOLOGY & DEMOGRAPHICS

RTA type IV affects mostly adults, whereas RTA type I and II are more frequent in children.

■ PHYSICAL FINDINGS & CLINICAL PRESENTATION

- Examination may be normal.
- Poor skin turgor may be present from dehydration.
- Muscle weakness and muscle aches from hypokalemia may occur.
- Low back pain and bone pain may be present in patients with abnormalities of calcium metabolism (RTA II).
- There is failure to thrive in children (RTA II).

■ ETIOLOGY

- Type I RTA: primary biliary cirrhosis and other liver diseases, medications (amphotericin, nonsteroidals), SLE, Sjögren's syndrome
- Type II RTA: Fanconi's syndrome, primary hyperparathyroidism, multiple myeloma, medications (acetazolamide)
- Type IV RTA: diabetes mellitus, sickle cell disease, Addison's disease, urinary obstruction

DIAGNOSIS

■ DIFFERENTIAL DIAGNOSIS

- Diarrhea with significant bicarbonate loss
- Other causes of metabolic acidosis
- Respiratory acidosis

■ WORKUP

Detection of hyperchloremic metabolic acidosis with ABGs and serum electrolytes and evaluation of potential causes (see "Etiology")

■ LABORATORY TESTS

- ABGs reveal metabolic acidosis; serum potassium is low in RTA types I and II, normal in type III, and high in type IV.
- Minimal urine pH is >5.5 in RTA type I, <5.5 in types II, III, and IV.
- Urinary anion gap is 0 or positive in all types of RTA.
- Additional useful studies include serum calcium level and urine calcium.
- Anion gap is normal.
- PTH measurement is useful in patients suspected of primary hyperparathyroidism (may be associated with type II RTA).

■ IMAGING STUDIES

- Plain abdominal radiography is useful to evaluate for nephrocalcinosis.
- Renal sonogram can be used to evaluate renal size or presence of stones.
- IVP in patients with nephrocalcinosis or nephrolithiasis.

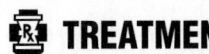 TREATMENT

■ ACUTE GENERAL Rx

- Type I and type II are treated with oral sodium bicarbonate (1 to 2 mEq/kg/day in RTA 1, 2 to 4 mEq/kg/day in RTA type II) titrated to correct acidosis.
- Potassium supplementation is needed in hypokalemic patients.
- Type IV RTA can be treated with furosemide to lower elevated potassium levels and sodium bicarbonate to correct significant acidosis. Fludrocortisone 100 to 300 µg/day can be used to correct mineralocorticoid deficiency.

■ CHRONIC Rx

- Frequent monitoring of potassium levels in type IV RTA
- Monitoring for bone disease in RTA type II
- Monitoring for nephrocalcinosis and nephrolithiasis in RTA type I

■ DISPOSITION

- Prognosis varies with the presence of associated conditions (see "Etiology").
- Untreated distal RTA may result in hypercalcemia, hyperphosphaturia, nephrolithiasis, and nephrocalcinosis.

PEARLS & CONSIDERATIONS

■ COMMENTS

Patient education material can be obtained from the National Kidney and Urologic Diseases Information Clearinghouse, Box NKUDIC, Bethesda, MD 20893.

Author: **Fred F. Ferri, M.D.**

BASIC INFORMATION

■ DEFINITION
Renal vein thrombosis is the thrombotic occlusion of one or both renal veins.

ICD-9CM CODES
453.3 Renal vein thrombosis

■ EPIDEMIOLOGY & DEMOGRAPHICS
- Incidence unknown, probably an underdiagnosed condition
- May occur at any age with no gender preference
- Epidemiology tied to the underlying cause

■ PHYSICAL FINDINGS & CLINICAL PRESENTATION
Acute bilateral renal vein thrombosis
- Back and bilateral flank pain
- Acute renal failure

Acute unilateral renal vein thrombosis
- Flank pain
- Decline in renal function
- Hematuria
- Increase in the amount of proteinuria if associated with nephrotic syndrome

Chronic unilateral renal vein thrombosis
- May be silent
- Pulmonary emboli and hemolysis
- Back pain
- DVT in lower extremities
- Edema
- Glycosuria
- Hyperchloremic acidosis
- Left varicocele (if the left renal vein is thrombosed)
- Dilated abdominal veins

■ ETIOLOGY & PATHOGENESIS
- Extrinsic compression by a tumor or retroperitoneal mass
- Invasion of the renal vein or inferior vena cava by tumor (almost always renal cell cancer)
- Trauma
- Hypercoagulable states
- Dehydration
- Glomerulopathies (membranous glomerulonephritis, crescenting glomerulonephritis, SLE, amyloidosis) especially in the presence of nephrotic syndrome when the serum albumin is lower than 2 g/dl.
- NOTE: For unknown reasons, diabetic nephropathy is not commonly associated with renal vein thrombosis even if the nephrotic syndrome is present.

A controversy has existed as to whether the renal vein thrombosis association with nephrotic syndrome is a complication of nephrotic syndrome or whether renal vein thrombosis occurring in the setting of increased renal vein pressure (e.g., with congestive heart failure, constrictive pericarditis, or extrinsic compression) can independently cause proteinuria. Current evidence is that renal vein thrombosis does not cause nephrotic syndrome.

DIAGNOSIS

■ DIFFERENTIAL DIAGNOSIS
The diagnosis of renal vein thrombosis does not include any differential consideration. The differential diagnosis is that of proteinuria. Renal vein thrombosis should be considered if proteinuria worsens or if renal function worsens in a patient with glomerulonephritis. Renal vein thrombosis should also be considered in patients with pulmonary emboli and no lower-extremity DVT.

■ WORKUP
Clinical suspicion (see differential diagnosis) and imaging studies

■ IMAGING STUDIES
- Abdominal ultrasound.
- Abdominal MRI.
- Renal arteriography (delayed films during venous phase).
- Selective renal vein venography (inferior venacavogram images should be obtained before advancing the catheter in the vena cava because clots, if present, could be dislodged).
- Renal biopsy may be indicated if evidence of nephritis is present (e.g., active urinary sediment).

TREATMENT

- Anticoagulation in acute renal vein thrombosis to prevent pulmonary emboli and in attempt to improve renal function and decrease proteinuria.
- The value of thrombolytic therapy or surgical thrombectomy has not been established.
- The value of anticoagulation in chronic renal vein thrombosis is dubious except in nephrotic patients with membranous glomerulonephritis with profound hypoalbuminemia where prolonged prophylactic anticoagulation may be of benefit even if renal vein thrombosis has not been documented.

■ PROGNOSIS
Probable worsening of the underlying glomerulonephritis by acute renal vein thrombosis; the effect of chronic renal vein thrombosis is unclear.

REFERENCE
Glassock RJ, Cohen AH, Adler SG: Renal vein thrombosis. In Brenner BM (ed): *The kidney*, ed 5, Philadelphia, 1996, WB Saunders.
Author: **Tom J. Wachtel, M.D.**

BASIC INFORMATION

■ DEFINITION

Acute respiratory distress syndrome (formerly called *adult respiratory distress syndrome*) (ARDS) is a form of noncardiogenic pulmonary edema that results from acute damage to the alveoli. It is characterized by acute diffuse infiltrative lung lesions with resulting interstitial and alveolar edema, severe hypoxemia, and respiratory failure. The definition of ARDS includes the following three components:
1. A ratio of Pao_2 to Fio_2 ≤200 regardless of the level of PEEP
2. The detection of bilateral pulmonary infiltrates on frontal chest x-ray
3. Pulmonary artery wedge pressure (PAWP) ≤18 mm Hg or no clinical evidence of elevated left atrial pressure on the basis of chest radiograph or other clinical data

■ SYNONYMS

ARDS
Adult respiratory distress syndrome

ICD-9CM CODES

518.82 Acute respiratory distress syndrome

■ EPIDEMIOLOGY & DEMOGRAPHICS

In the U.S. there are 75,000 to 100,000 ARDS cases/yr.
• Incidence is 1.5 to 8.3 cases/ 100,000/yr.

■ PHYSICAL FINDINGS & CLINICAL PRESENTATION

• Signs and symptoms
1. Dyspnea
2. Chest discomfort
3. Cough
4. Anxiety
• Physical examination
1. Tachypnea
2. Tachycardia
3. Hypertension
4. Coarse crepitations of both lungs
5. Fever may be present if infection is the underlying etiology.

■ ETIOLOGY

• Sepsis (>40% of cases)
• Aspiration: near drowning, aspiration of gastric contents (>30% of cases)
• Trauma (>20% of cases)
• Multiple transfusions, blood products
• Drugs (e.g., overdose of morphine, methadone, heroin, reaction to nitrofurantoin)
• Noxious inhalation (e.g., chlorine gas, high O_2 concentration)
• Postresuscitation
• Cardiopulmonary bypass
• Pneumonia
• Burns
• Pancreatitis
• A history of chronic alcohol abuse significantly increases the risk of developing ARDS in critically ill patients

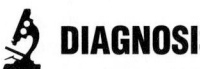

DIAGNOSIS

■ DIFFERENTIAL DIAGNOSIS

• Cardiogenic pulmonary edema
• Viral pneumonitis
• Lymphangitic carcinomatosis

■ WORKUP

The search for an underlying cause should focus on treatable causes (e.g., infections such as sepsis or pneumonia)
• ABGs
• Hemodynamic monitoring
• Bronchoalveolar lavage (selected patients)

■ LABORATORY TESTS

• ABGs:
1. Initially: varying degrees of hypoxemia, generally resistant to supplemental oxygen
2. Respiratory alkalosis, decreased Pco_2
3. Widened alveolar-arterial gradient
4. Hypercapnia as the disease progresses
• Bronchoalveolar lavage:
1. The most prominent finding is an increased number of polymorphonucleocytes.
2. The presence of eosinophilia has therapeutic implications, since these patients respond to corticosteroids.
• Blood and urine cultures

■ IMAGING STUDIES

Chest x-ray examination (Fig. 1-317).
• The initial chest radiogram might be normal in the initial hours after the precipitating event.
• Bilateral interstitial infiltrates are usually seen within 24 hr; they often are more prominent in the bases and periphery.
• "White out" of both lung fields can be seen in advanced stages.
Hemodynamic monitoring
• Hemodynamic monitoring can be used for the initial evaluation of ARDS (in ruling out cardiogenic pulmonary edema) and its subsequent management.
• Although no dynamic profile is diagnostic of ARDS, the presence of pulmonary edema, a high cardiac output, and a low PAWP is characteristic of ARDS.

• It is important to remember that partially treated intravascular volume overload and flash pulmonary edema can have the hemodynamic features of ARDS; filling pressures can also be elevated by increased intrathoracic pressures or with fluid administration; cardiac function can be depressed by acidosis, hypoxemia, or other factors associated with sepsis.

TREATMENT

■ NONPHARMACOLOGIC THERAPY

Ventilatory support: mechanical ventilation is generally necessary to maintain adequate gas exchange (Fig. 1-318); assist-control is generally preferred initially with the following ventilator settings:
• Fio_2 1.0 (until a lower value can be used to achieve adequate oxygenation).
• Tidal volume: conventional tidal volume (10 to 15 ml/kg of body weight) has been used in ARDS; however, recent evidence shows that it may be detrimental to patients with ARDS; the American College of Chest Physicians has recommended that the alveolar plateau should not exceed 35 cm H_2O, which in ARDS corresponds to a tidal volume of <5 ml/kg. Recently, a new strategy of mechanical ventilation, the "open lung approach," has been shown to have better oxygenation and a tendency toward decreased mortality in patients with ARDS. In addition to a low tidal volume and pressure-controlled inverse-ratio ventilation, the open-lung approach protocol included raising the level of PEEP above the lower inflection point on a pressure-volume curve to ensure adequate recruitment of atelectatic lung.
• PEEP <5 cm H_2O to increase lung volume and keep alveoli open. Recent data, however, raise questions about the use of minimal PEEP (5 to 10 cm H_2O) in patients with ARDS. The data suggest that the use of more liberal PEEP (10 to 20 cm H_2O) might be warranted even without a determination of the lower inflection point.
• Inspiratory flow: 60 L/min.
• Ventilatory rate: high ventilatory rates of 20 to 25 breaths/min are often necessary in patients with ARDS because of their increased physiologic deadspace and smaller lung volumes. Patients must be monitored for excessive intrathoracic gas trapping ("auto-PEEP" or "intrinsic-PEEP") that can depress cardiac output.

■ ACUTE GENERAL Rx

Identify and treat precipitating conditions:

- Blood and urine cultures and trial of antibiotics in presumed sepsis (routine administration of antibiotics in all cases of ARDS is not recommended)
- Prompt repair of bone fractures in patients with major trauma
- Bowel rest and crystalloid resuscitation in pancreatitis
- Fluid management: optimal fluid and hemodynamic management of patients with ARDS is patient specific; generally, administration of crystalloids is recommended if a downward trend in pulmonary capillary wedge pressures (PCWP) is associated with diminished cardiac index, resulting in prerenal azotemia, oliguria, and relative tachycardia; on the other hand, if PCWP increases with little or no change in cardiac index, one should begin diuretic therapy and use low-dose dopamine (2 to 4 μg/kg/min) to maintain natriuresis and support adequate renal flow.
- Positioning the patient: changes in position can improve oxygenation by improving the distribution of perfusion to ventilated lung regions; repositioning (lateral decubitus positioning) should be attempted in patients with hypoxemia that is not responsive to other medical interventions.

- Corticosteroids: routine use of corticosteroids in ARDS is not recommended; corticosteroids may be beneficial in patients with many eosinophils in the bronchoalveolar lavage fluid; systemic infections should be ruled out or adequately treated before administration of corticosteroids.
- Nutritional support: nutritional support is necessary to maintain adequate colloid oncotic pressure and intravascular volume.
- Tracheostomy: tracheostomy is warranted in patients requiring >2 wk of mechanical ventilation; discussion regarding tracheostomy should begin with patient (if alert and oriented) and family members/legal guardian, after 5 to 7 days of ventilatory support.

■ DISPOSITION

- Prognosis for ARDS varies with the underlying cause. Prognosis is worse in patients with chronic liver disease, nonpulmonary organ dysfunction, sepsis, and advanced age.
- Overall mortality varies between 40% and 60%. The majority of deaths is attributable to sepsis or multiorgan dysfunction rather than primary respiratory causes.

■ REFERRAL

Surgical referral for tracheostomy (see "Acute General Rx").

✺ PEARLS & CONSIDERATIONS

■ COMMENTS

DVT prophylaxis and stress ulceration prophylaxis are recommended.

REFERENCES

Acute Respiratory Distress Syndrome Network: Ventilation with lower tidal volumes as compared wtih traditional tidal volumes for acute lung injury and the acute respiratory distress syndrome, *N Engl J Med* 342:1301, 2000.

Amato MB et al: Effect of a protective-ventilation strategy on mortality in the acute respiratory distress syndrome, *N Engl J Med* 338:347, 1998.

Sadikot RT, Christman JW: ARDS: how and when does it develop? *J Respir Dis* 20:438, 1999.

Stewart T et al: Evolution of a ventilation strategy to prevent barotrauma in patients at high risk for ARDS, *N Engl J Med* 338:355, 1998.

Ware LB, Matthay MA: The acute respiratory distress syndrome, *N Engl J Med* 342:1334, 2000.

Author: **Fred F. Ferri, M.D.**

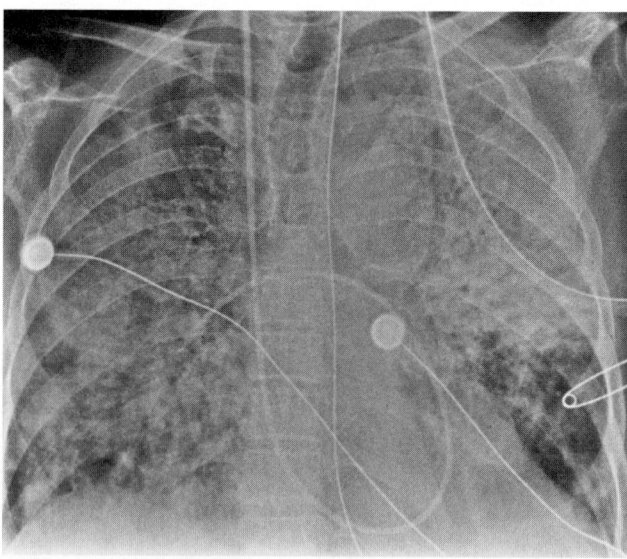

Fig. 1-317 ARDS. AP radiograph in an elderly woman reveals widespread consolidation with air bronchograms. The heart size is normal. There are no pleural effusions. (From McLoud TC: *Thoracic radiology: the requisites,* St Louis, 1998, Mosby.)

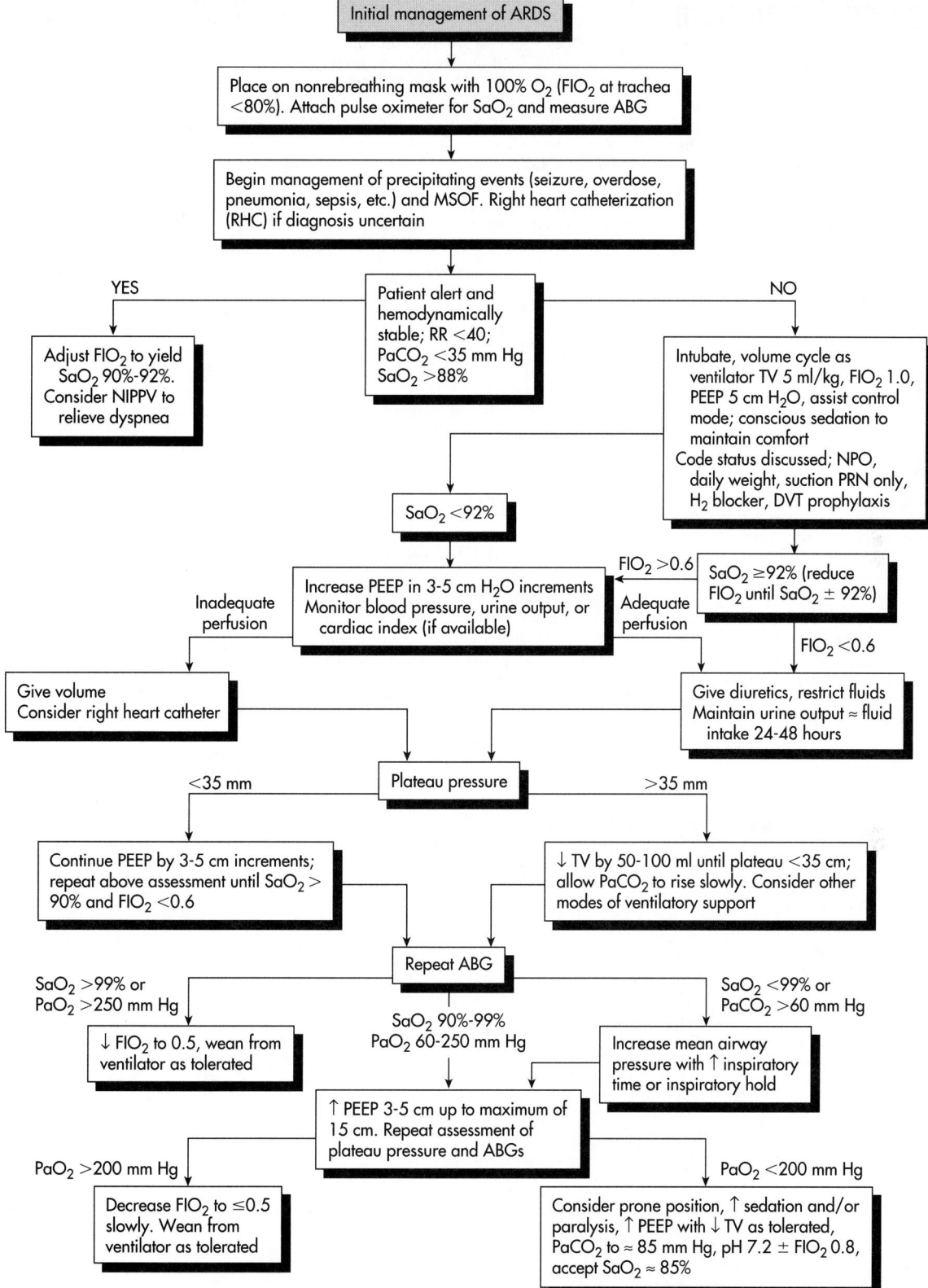

Fig. 1-318　Initial management of acute respiratory distress syndrome (ARDS). *ABG,* Arterial blood gas analysis; *CO₂,* carbon dioxide; *DVT,* deep venous thrombosis; *FIO₂,* inspired oxygen concentration; *MSOF,* multisystem organ failure; *NIPPV,* noninvasive intermittent positive-pressure ventilation; *O₂,* oxygen; *PaCO₂,* arterial partial pressure of carbon dioxide; *PaO₂,* arterial partial pressure of oxygen; *PEEP,* positive end-expiratory pressure; *RR,* respiratory rate; *SaO₂,* arterial oxygen saturation; *V_T,* tidal volume. (From Goldman L: *Cecil textbook of medicine,* ed 21, Philadelphia, 2000, WB Saunders.)

BASIC INFORMATION

■ DEFINITION
Restless legs syndrome is a primary neurologic disorder of unknown cause that manifests with both sensory and motor symptoms usually involving the lower extremities and disrupting sleep.

■ SYNONYMS
"Crazy legs" (lay term)
Nocturnal myoclonus

ICD-9CM CODES
333.99 Nocturnal myoclonus

■ EPIDEMIOLOGY & DEMOGRAPHICS
PREVALENCE: 5% to 15%
DEMOGRAPHICS: Age 2 yr to no upper limit
- Age 18 to 29: 3%
- Age 30 to 79: 10%
- Age 80 and above: 19%
- Prevalence increases with age (may explain a slight female overrepresentation)
- Symptoms worsen with age

■ PHYSICAL FINDINGS & CLINICAL PRESENTATION
- Sensory nocturnal complaints usually affecting both lower extremities:
  Crawly feeling or fizzle under the skin
  Itching under the skin
  Pain or ache
  Electric shocks
  Irresistible urge to move the symptomatic leg
- Other words used by patients to describe the leg symptoms: creeping, burning, searing, tugging, pulling, drawing, like water flowing, worms or bugs under the skin, restless, undescribable.
- Consistent symptom relief or improvement with leg movement or walking.
- Sleep disruption.
- Leg movements during sleep may occur but are not the prevailing complaint (unlike the urge to move). These movements are short bursts lasting less than 5 sec.
- Physical examination is normal.

■ ETIOLOGY
- Unknown/idiopathic
- Hereditary (30% to 60%)
- Associated with iron deficiency
- Associated with renal failure (end-stage)
- Associated with pregnancy
- Associated with peripheral neuropathy or radiculopathy
- Associated with rheumatologic conditions (rheumatoid arthritis, fibromyalgia)
- Medication induced (selective serotonin reuptake inhibitors)

DIAGNOSIS

■ DIFFERENTIAL DIAGNOSIS
- Periodic limb movement disorder (PLMD) (repetitive limb movements [lower extremities > upper extremities] occurring during sleep; associated with arousals from sleep and daytime sleeping; patient is typically unaware, but bed partner reports restlessness or kicking during sleep)
- Peripheral neuropathy and radiculopathy
- Anxiety and mood disorders
- Chronic fatigue
- Other sleep disorders
- Neuroleptic-induced akathisia
- Dyskinesias while awake
- Nocturnal leg cramps with or without peripheral artery disease.

■ WORKUP
- History is typically diagnostic with sensitivity and specificity both >90%
- Sleep logs
- Polysomnography
- Ambulatory recording of leg activity

TREATMENT

- Dopaminergic drugs are first line: Levodopa/carbidopa (Sinemet) Pergolide or pramipexole
- Benzodiazepines
- Trazodone
- Opioids
- Gabapentin (Neurontin)

■ PROGNOSIS
Tendency to worsen with age

REFERENCES
Allen RP: Restless legs syndrome: epidemiology and diagnosis, *Med Behav* 1:36, 1998.

Lin SC et al: Effect of pramipexole in treatment of resistant restless legs syndrome, *Mayo Clin Proc* 73:497, 1998.

National Heart, Lung, and Blood Institute Working Group on Restless Legs Syndrome: Restless legs syndrome: detection and management in primary care, *Am Fam Physician* 62:108, 2000.

Phillips B, Young T, Finn L, et al: Epidemiology of restless legs symptoms in adults, *Arch Intern Med* 160:2137, 2000.
Author: **Tom J. Wachtel, M.D.**

BASIC INFORMATION

■ DEFINITION
Retinal detachment is a retinal separation where the inner or neural layer of the retina separates from the pigment epithelial layer and results from numerous causes.

■ SYNONYMS
Inflammatory lesions of choroid
Uveitis
Tumor
Vascular lesions
Congenital disorders

ICD-9CM CODES
361 Retinal detachment and defects

■ EPIDEMIOLOGY & DEMOGRAPHICS
INCIDENCE (IN U.S.):
• 0.02% of the population
• Particularly common in patients with high myopia of 5 diopters or more
PREVALENCE (IN U.S.): Busy ophthalmologist may see one or two acute retinal detachments per month
PREDOMINANT SEX: None
PREDOMINANT AGE:
• Congenital in younger patients
• Usually trauma in patients 30 to 40 yr and older
• High myopia a predisposition
PEAK INCIDENCE: Incidence increases with increasing age or increasing myopia.

■ PHYSICAL FINDINGS & CLINICAL PRESENTATION
Elevation of retina and vessels associated with tears in the retina, with fluid, and/or with hemorrhage beneath the retina and changes in the vitreous (Fig. 1-319).
• Complaints of flashing lights and floaters

■ ETIOLOGY
• Trauma
• Tears in the retina
• Uveitis
• Fluid accumulation beneath the retina
• Tumors
• Scleritis
• Inflammatory disease
• Diabetes
• Collagen-vascular disease
• Vascular abnormalities

DIAGNOSIS

■ DIFFERENTIAL DIAGNOSIS
• Detachment
• Hemorrhage
• Tumors

■ WORKUP
• Full eye examination
• Fluorescein angiography
• Visual fields
• Ultrasonography to show the retinal detachment or tumors beneath it
• Medical workup only when inflammation or systemic disease considered

■ LABORATORY TESTS
Usually not necessary

■ IMAGING STUDIES
B scan of the eye

TREATMENT

■ NONPHARMACOLOGIC THERAPY
Immediate surgery

■ ACUTE GENERAL Rx
• Early surgery to repair the detachment
• Treatment of the underlying disorder

■ CHRONIC Rx
Occasionally, steroids or other treatment of underlying disease is indicated.

■ DISPOSITION
• Make an immediate referral to an ophthalmologist.
• Early intervention improves outcomes.

■ REFERRAL
Immediately

PEARLS & CONSIDERATIONS

■ COMMENTS
If treated early, most patients will recover a substantial portion of their vision.
Author: **Melvyn Koby, M.D.**

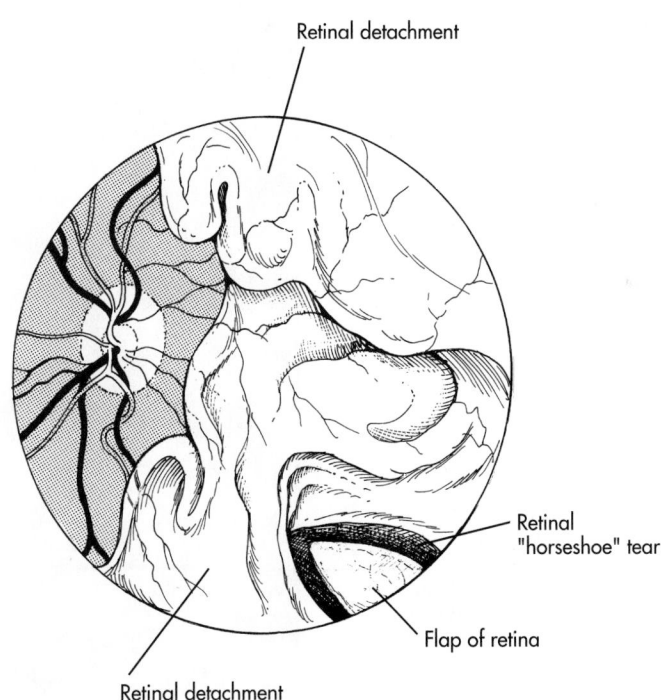

Fig. 1-319 Retinal detachment. (From Scuderi G [ed]: *Sports medicine: principles of primary care,* St Louis, 1997, Mosby.)

BASIC INFORMATION

■ DEFINITION
In a retinal hemorrhage, blood accumulates in the retinal and subretinal areas.

■ SYNONYMS
Pseudoxanthoma elasticum
Coats' disease
Retinal trauma
High-altitude retinopathy

ICD-9CM CODES
362.81 Retinal hemorrhage

■ EPIDEMIOLOGY & DEMOGRAPHICS
INCIDENCE (IN U.S.): Busy ophthalmologist sees one or two cases a month.
PREDOMINANT AGE: Degenerative disease in older patients
PEAK INCIDENCE:
• Children—associated primarily with trauma and hematologic disorders
• Increases with age

■ PHYSICAL FINDINGS & CLINICAL PRESENTATION
• Hemorrhage within the retina or subretinal area (Fig. 1-320)
• Evidence of retinal tears, tumors, and inflammation

■ ETIOLOGY
• Diabetes
• Hypertension
• Trauma
• Inflammation
• Tumors
• Subretinal neovascularization
• Associated with diabetes and aging

DIAGNOSIS

■ DIFFERENTIAL DIAGNOSIS
• Evaluate patients for local and systemic diseases.
• Either venous or arterial occlusion may cause retinal hemorrhage, and such occlusion is associated with atherosclerotic or heart disease, so look for these.
• Rule out malignant melanoma, trauma, hypertensive cardiovascular disease.
Table 2-212 describes the differential diagnosis of acute painless loss of vision.

■ WORKUP
Complete general physical examination

■ LABORATORY TESTS
• Minimum: CBC, sedimentation rate, and complete blood chemistries
• Fluorescein
• Angiography
• Visual field testing

■ IMAGING STUDIES
Usually not necessary

TREATMENT

■ NONPHARMACOLOGIC THERAPY
Laser or treatment of underlying disorder

■ ACUTE GENERAL Rx
• Laser is often indicated.
• Steroids may be indicated, depending on etiology.
• Treat underlying disease.
• Repair damage if from trauma.

■ CHRONIC Rx
Laser if hemorrhage is recurrent

■ DISPOSITION
Consider this an emergency.

■ REFERRAL
• Immediate referral to an ophthalmologist
• An emergency, with early treatment significantly affecting outcome

PEARLS & CONSIDERATIONS

■ COMMENTS
• Vision may return substantially.
• Complete recovery dependent on amount of scar tissue formed.
Author: **Melvyn Koby, M.D.**

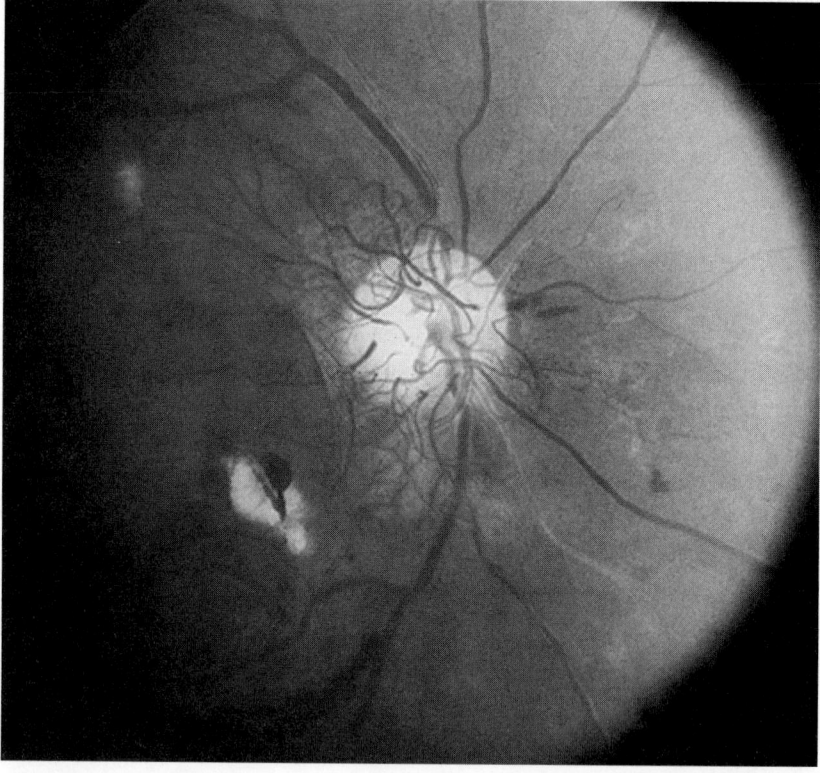

Fig. 1-320 Fronds of neovascularization *(1)* on the disc are present in this right eye. Temporally, two cotton-wool spots have adjacent intraretinal hemorrhage and preretinal hemorrhage. Native retinal arteries are narrowed and show evidence of sclerosis *(2)*. (From Palay D [ed]: *Ophthalmology for the primary care physician,* St Louis, 1997, Mosby.)

BASIC INFORMATION

■ DEFINITION

Retinitis pigmentosa is a generalized retinal pigment degeneration associated with a variety of inheritance patterns resulting in decreased vision. A simple recessive pattern is most severe. It may be associated with some rare neurologic syndromes.

ICD-9CM CODES

362.74 Retinitis pigmentosa, pigmentary retinal dystrophy

■ EPIDEMIOLOGY & DEMOGRAPHICS

PREVALENCE (IN U.S.): 1 in 4000 people
PREDOMINANT SEX: Depends on inheritance
PREDOMINANT AGE: 60 yr
PEAK INCIDENCE:
- Recessive incidence: in the 20s
- Dominant form: in the 40s
GENETICS:
- 19% dominant
- 19% recessive
- 8% X-linked
- 46% not known to be genetically related (mutations)
- 8% undetermined cause

■ PHYSICAL FINDINGS & CLINICAL PRESENTATION

- Deposition of retinal pigment in midperiphery and centrally in the retina with a pale optic nerve and narrowing of blood vessels (Fig. 1-321)
- Possible cataracts and macular edema
- Decrease in night vision and peripheral vision

■ ETIOLOGY

Usually hereditary

DIAGNOSIS

■ DIFFERENTIAL DIAGNOSIS

- Syphilis
- Old inflammatory scars
- Old hemorrhage
- Diabetes
- Toxic retinopathies (phenothiazines, chloroquine)

■ WORKUP

- Electrophysiologic studies
- Dark adaptation studies
- Visual fields

■ LABORATORY TESTS

- Usually not necessary
- VDRL, glucose (selected patients)

■ IMAGING STUDIES

Usually not necessary

TREATMENT

■ CHRONIC Rx

- No proven effective therapy
- Sometimes vitamin E or vitamin A may be helpful

■ DISPOSITION

Disease may be either mild or severe, but if the patient is expected to progress to total blindness, counseling and early education are important.

■ REFERRAL

To ophthalmologist to confirm diagnosis

PEARLS & CONSIDERATIONS

■ COMMENTS

- The spiderweb-like appearance of macular degeneration should not be confused with the extra pigments sometimes seen in dark-skinned individuals.
- Patient education material can be obtained from the Retinitis Pigmentosa Foundation Fighting Blindness, 1401 Mt. Royal Avenue, 4th Floor, Baltimore, MD 21217.

Author: **Melvyn Koby, M.D.**

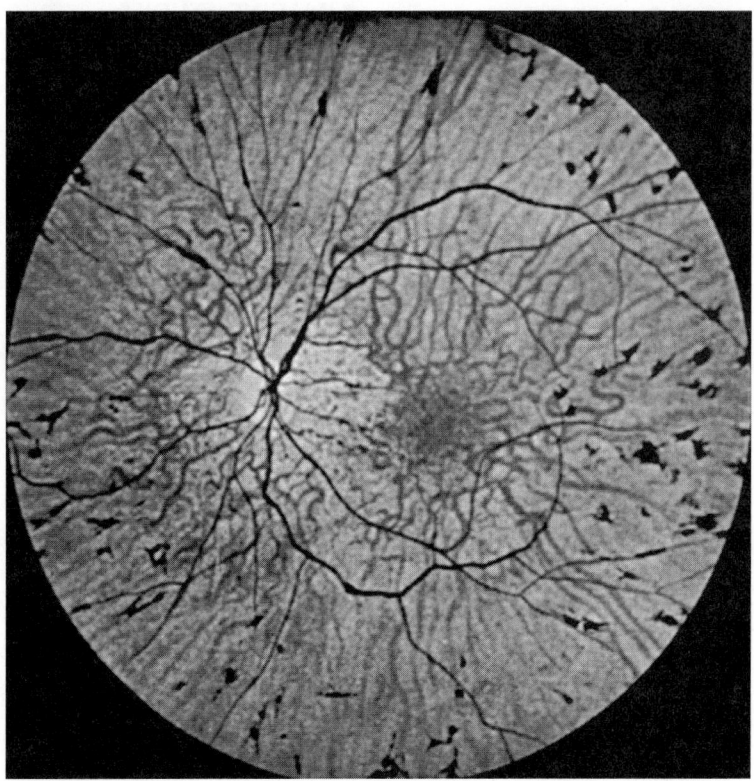

Fig. 1-321 Retinitis pigmentosa. (From Behrman RE: *Nelson textbook of pediatrics,* Philadelphia, 1996, WB Saunders.)

BASIC INFORMATION

■ **DEFINITION**
Retinoblastoma is an inherited, highly malignant congenital neoplasm arising from the neural layers of the retina.

■ **ICD-9CM CODES**
190.5 Retinoblastoma, malignant neoplasm of eyes, retina

■ **EPIDEMIOLOGY & DEMOGRAPHICS**
INCIDENCE (IN U.S.): 1 in every 23,000 to 34,000 births
PREDOMINANT AGE: 8 mo
PEAK INCIDENCE:
• 6 to 13 mo
• 72% diagnosed by 3 yr of age
• 90% diagnosed by 4 yr of age
GENETICS:
• Gene mutation or an autosomal dominant gene with 80% to 95% penetration
• 5% mutations

■ **PHYSICAL FINDINGS & CLINICAL PRESENTATION**
• White pupils (Fig. 1-322)
• White elevated retinal masses
• Strabismus
• Glaucoma
• Uveitis

■ **ETIOLOGY**
Genetic

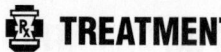 **DIAGNOSIS**

■ **DIFFERENTIAL DIAGNOSIS**
• Strabismus
• Retinal detachment
• Uveitis
• Other tumors
• Glaucoma
• Endophthalmitis
• Cataract

■ **WORKUP**
Ophthalmologic examination

■ **IMAGING STUDIES**
• MRI: may show calcifications in retina
• Ultrasonography: good delineation of mass

■ **TREATMENT**

■ **NONPHARMACOLOGIC THERAPY**
• Surgical enucleation of the eye
• Radiation and chemotherapy

■ **DISPOSITION**
Usually treated by an ophthalmologist/oncologist

■ **REFERRAL**
To ophthalmologist/oncologist

PEARLS & CONSIDERATIONS

■ **COMMENT**
With early aggressive treatment, some patients may survive.
Author: **Melvyn Koby, M.D.**

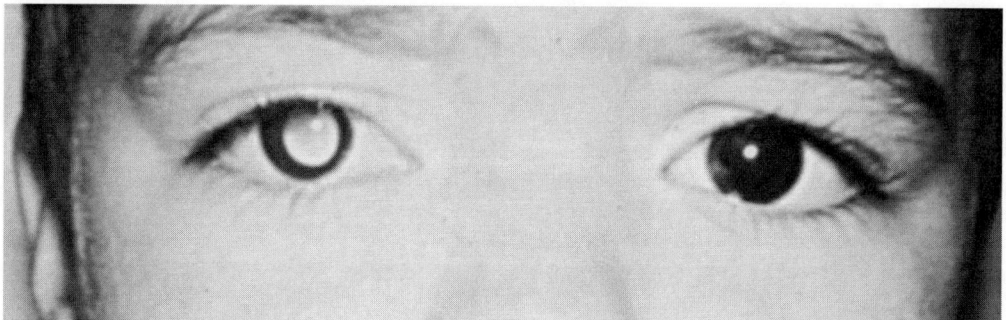

Fig. 1-322   Leukocoria. White pupillary reflex in a child with retinoblastoma. (From Behrman RE: *Nelson textbook of pediatrics,* Philadelphia, 1996, WB Saunders.)

BASIC INFORMATION

■ **DEFINITION**

Diabetic retinopathy is an eye abnormality associated with diabetes and consisting of microaneurysms, punctate hemorrhages, white and yellow exudates, flame hemorrhages, and neovascular vessel growth (Fig. 1-323).

■ **SYNONYMS**

NPDR—nonproliferative diabetic retinopathy
PDR—proliferative (advanced) diabetic retinopathy

ICD-9CM CODES

250.5 Diabetes with ophthalmic manifestations
362.1 Retinopathy, diabetic, background
362.02 Retinopathy, diabetic, proliferative

■ **EPIDEMIOLOGY & DEMOGRAPHICS**

INCIDENCE (IN U.S.):

- Affects 11 million persons
- A leading cause of blindness in people 20 to 70 yr old
- 5000 new cases annually

PREVALENCE (IN U.S.): Prevalence of retinopathy increases with duration of diabetes. Found in 18% of people diagnosed with diabetes for 3- to 4-yr duration and in up to 80% of diabetics with a diagnosis of 15 yr or more.

PREDOMINANT SEX: Male = female
PREDOMINANT AGE: 30 yr or older
PEAK INCIDENCE: Begins 10 yr after onset of diabetes
GENETICS: Diabetes is usually hereditary.

■ **PHYSICAL FINDINGS & CLINICAL PRESENTATION**

- See "Definition"
- Microaneurysms
- Hemorrhages
- Exudates
- Macular edema
- Neovascularization
- Retinal detachment
- Hemorrhages in the vitreous
- In early cases, patient may not complain of a visual disturbance

■ **ETIOLOGY**

Associated with diabetes mellitus

🔬 **DIAGNOSIS**

■ **DIFFERENTIAL DIAGNOSIS**

- Retinal inflammatory diseases
- Tumor
- Trauma
- Arteriosclerotic vascular disease

■ **WORKUP**

Fluorescein angiogram

■ **LABORATORY TESTS**

Those appropriate for diabetes mellitus

℞ **TREATMENT**

■ **NONPHARMACOLOGIC THERAPY**

Laser treatment

■ **ACUTE GENERAL Rx**

- Laser therapy
- Vitrectomy
- Repair of retinal detachment

■ **CHRONIC Rx**

Repeated laser treatments may be necessary.

■ **DISPOSITION**

- Retinal examination should be performed on all routine medical visits.
- Prognosis is improved with early diagnosis and treatment.

■ **REFERRAL**

If diabetic retinopathy is severe enough to interfere with vision, follow-up is best done by an ophthalmologist.

💡 **PEARLS & CONSIDERATIONS**

■ **COMMENTS**

- Early laser treatment of severe, nonproliferative and proliferative retinopathy may minimize complications and visual loss.
- Patient education information can be obtained from the American Academy of Ophthalmology (655 Beach Street, San Francisco, CA 94109-1336) and from the American Diabetes Association (1-800-232-3472).

Author: **Melvyn Koby, M.D.**

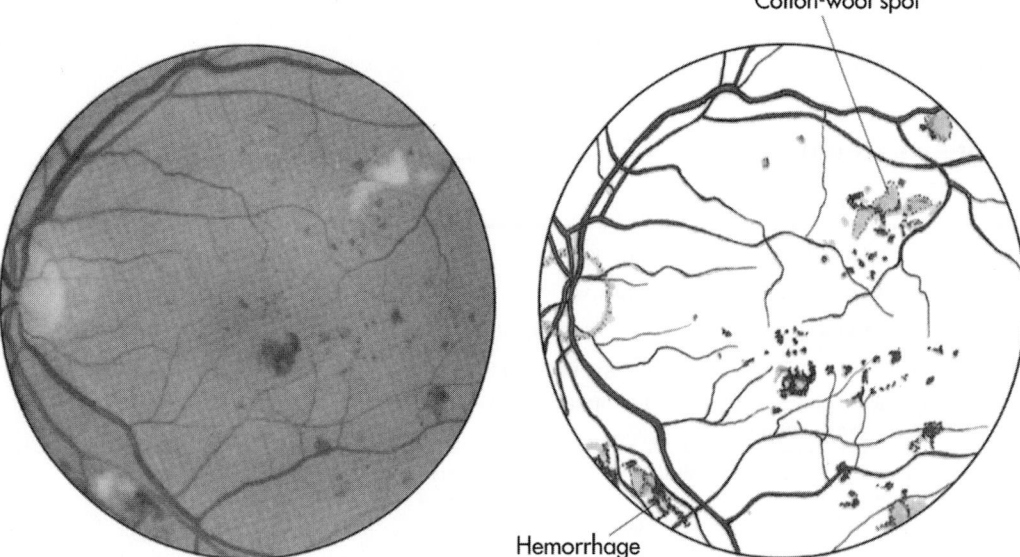

Cotton-wool spot

Hemorrhage

Fig. 1-323 Background diabetic retinopathy. Note flame-shaped and dot-blot hemorrhages, cotton-wool spots, and microaneurysms. (From Barkauskas VH et al: *Health and physical assessment,* ed 2, St Louis, 1998, Mosby.)

BASIC INFORMATION

■ DEFINITION

Reye's syndrome is a postinfectious triad consisting of encephalopathy, fatty liver degeneration, and transaminase elevation.

■ ICD-9CM CODES

331.81 Reye's syndrome

■ EPIDEMIOLOGY & DEMOGRAPHICS

- During the 1970s, 300 to 600 cases were being reported yearly in the U.S.
- Since the mid-1980s, following the understanding that aspirin is associated with Reye's syndrome, the yearly count has fallen to less than 20 cases.
- Seasonal relation with influenza and varicella outbreaks
- Age: rare in persons over age 18 yr; peak age (in the U.S.) is 6 to 8 yr
- Case fatality rate: 25% to 50%

■ PHYSICAL FINDINGS & CLINICAL PRESENTATION

Shortly following recovery from a viral infection (flu or chicken pox) an afebrile child begins to vomit intractably. Hepatomegaly is often present. The vomiting can lead to dehydration. Occasionally, symptoms of hypoglycemia are present. After 2 days, symptoms of encephalopathy dominate the clinical picture (lethargy, confusion, stupor, coma, seizures, decorticate or decerebrate posture) (Table 1-60).

■ ETIOLOGY

- Temporal association with influenza and varicella infection
- Epidemiologic association with aspirin or other salicylate use to treat the above viral infection
- Possible association with aflatoxin and pesticides
- Pathology
  Liver: no inflammation; the striking finding is panlobular microvesicular hepatocyte infiltration on light microscopy and mitochondrial injury on electron microscopy.
  Brain: no inflammation; there are cerebral edema and anoxic degeneration.
- Pathogenesis: not fully understood but mitochondrial dysfunction is clearly at the center stage

DIAGNOSIS

■ DIFFERENTIAL DIAGNOSIS

- Inborn errors of metabolism
  Carnitine deficiency
  Ornithine transcarbamylase deficiency
  Others
- Salicylate or amiodarone intoxication
- Jamaican vomiting sickness
- Hepatic encephalopathy of any cause

■ WORKUP

According to the CDC's case definition, the following conditions must be met for consideration as a Reye's syndrome case:

- Acute noninflammatory encephalopathy documented by:
  Alteration in the level of consciousness and, if available, a record of cerebrospinal fluid containing ≤8 leukocytes per mm^3 *or*
  Histologic specimen demonstrating cerebral edema without perivascular or meningeal inflammation
- Hepatopathy documented either by a liver biopsy or autopsy considered to be diagnostic of Reye's syndrome

or by a threefold or greater rise in the levels of serum aspartate aminotransferase, serum alanine aminotransferase, or serum ammonia *and*
- No more reasonable explanation for the cerebral and hepatic abnormalities

■ LABORATORY TESTS

- Elevated transaminase (ALT and AST)
- Elevated ammonia level
- Occasional elevation of CPK, LDH, and bilirubin and prolongation of prothrombin time
- Occasional hypoglycemia (in patients under the age of 4 yr)
- Cerebrospinal fluid is normal or contains fewer than 8 WBCs/ml
- Rarely a liver biopsy is indicated (in infants or in recurrent cases)

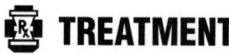

TREATMENT

- Supportive
- Mannitol, glycerol, or hyperventilation for cerebral edema if present
- Interferon alfa (experimental)
- Prevention
  Influenza vaccine
  Varicella vaccine
  Avoidance of aspirin in children, especially during influenza and varicella outbreaks

REFERENCES

Gellin BG, LaMontagne JR: Reye's syndrome. In Gorbach SL, Bartlett JG, Blacklow NR (eds): *Infectious diseases,* ed 2, Philadelphia, 1998, WB Saunders.
Reye syndrome—United States, 1985, *MMWR* 35:66, 1986.
Author: **Tom J. Wachtel, M.D.**

TABLE 1-60 Clinical Staging of Reye's Syndrome

GRADE	SYMPTOMS AT TIME OF ADMISSION
I	Usually quiet, **lethargic** and sleepy, vomiting, laboratory evidence of liver dysfunction
II	Deep lethargy, **confusion,** delirium, combative, hyperventilation, hyperreflexic
III	Obtunded, **light coma,** seizures, decorticate rigidity, intact pupillary light reaction
IV	Seizures, deepening coma, **decerebrate rigidity,** loss of oculocephalic reflexes, fixed pupils
V	Coma, loss of deep tendon reflexes, respiratory arrest, fixed dilated pupils, **flaccidity/decerebrate** intermittent isoelectric electroencephalogram

From Behrman RE: *Nelson textbook of pediatrics,* ed 15, Philadelphia, 1996, WB Saunders.

BASIC INFORMATION

■ DEFINITION
Rh incompatibility occurs when an absence of the D antigen on maternal RBCs and its presence on fetal RBCs causes risk of Rh isoimmunization.

ICD-9CM CODES
656.1 Rh incompatibility

■ EPIDEMIOLOGY & DEMOGRAPHICS
INCIDENCE:
- The absence of the D antigen (Rh$^-$ blood type) occurs in 15% of whites, 8% of blacks, and virtually no Asians or Native Americans. If the father's blood type is not known, the chance that an Rh$^-$ pregnant woman is bearing an Rh$^+$ fetus is about 60%.
- Of those pregnancies complicated by Rh incompatibility, the risk of maternal isoimmunization to the D antigen is about 8% for each ABO compatible pregnancy *if no prophylaxis is given.*
- Maternal-fetal ABO incompatibility is somewhat protective against Rh isoimmunization.

GENETICS: Five major loci determine Rh status: C, D, E, c, e. The presence of the D antigen results in an Rh$^+$ individual. Its absence results in an Rh$^-$ individual. Of Rh$^+$ fathers, 45% are homozygotes, 55% are heterozygotes. For homozygous Rh$^+$ fathers, the probability of an Rh$^+$ offspring is 100%. The probability for heterozygotes is about 50%.

RISK FACTORS FOR ISOIMMUNIZATION:
- Antepartum: fetal-to-maternal transfusion
- Intrapartum: fetal-to-maternal transfusion, spontaneous abortion, ectopic pregnancy, abruptio placentae, abdominal trauma, chorionic villus sampling, amniocentesis, percutaneous umbilical blood sampling (PUBS), external cephalic version, manual removal of the placenta, therapeutic abortion, autologous blood product administration

■ ETIOLOGY
The initial response to D antigen exposure is production of IgM (MW 900,000) that does not cross the placenta. With a repeated exposure, IgG (MW 160,000) is produced. IgG can cross the placenta and enter the fetal circulation, producing hemolysis in the fetus. This may produce erythroblastosis fetalis or hemolytic disease in the newborn, resulting in antepartum or neonatal death or neurologic damage to the fetus because of hyperbilirubinemia and kernicterus.

🔬 DIAGNOSIS

■ LABORATORY TESTS
ABO and Rh blood type and an antibody screen as part of the initial prenatal profile
- If antibody screen negative:
  1. Repeat antibody screen at 28 wk gestation.
  2. Obtain neonatal blood type after delivery.
  3. If Rh incompatibility is confirmed by the neonatal blood type, a Kleihauer-Betke or rosette test should be performed to determine the amount of fetomaternal transfusion in the following high-risk circumstances: abruptio placentae, placenta previa, cesarean delivery, intrauterine manipulation, manual removal of the placenta.
- If anti-D antibody screen is positive:
  1. Maternal indirect Coombs' test is needed to determine antibody titer.
  2. Determine paternal Rh status and zygosity.
  3. If father is heterozygous, PUBS or amniotic fluid is needed to determine fetal Rh status.

■ IMAGING STUDIES
Ultrasound evaluation can diagnose hydrops fetalis, but it cannot predict it.

💊 TREATMENT

■ PREVENTION OF D ISOIMMUNIZATION
- Give 50 μg of D immunoglobulin: after spontaneous or induced abortion or ectopic pregnancy <13 wk gestation.
- Give 300 μg of D immunoglobulin (protects against 30 ml of fetal blood):
  1. After spontaneous or induced abortion >13 wk gestation, amniocentesis, CVS, PUBS, external cephalic version or other intrauterine manipulation.
  2. As antepartum prophylaxis at 28 wk gestation.
  3. At delivery if the neonate is D- or Du-positive.
  4. If Kleihauer-Betke or rosette test confirms >30 ml of fetal red blood in maternal circulation, additional D immunoglobulin is indicated. Confirm adequacy of therapy by a maternal indirect Coombs' test 48 to 72 hr after Rh immune globulin is given.

■ MANAGEMENT OF D ISOIMMUNIZED PREGNANCIES
- Serial amniocentesis for assessment of OD$_{450}$ after 25 wk gestation with interpretation of the Delta OD$_{450}$ according to criteria established by Liley
- PUBS if ultrasonographic evidence of hydrops, rising zone II Delta OD$_{450}$ values on amniocentesis, maternal history of a severely affected child
- Intrauterine exchange transfusion if severe anemia is documented remote from term
- Initiation of steroids for lung maturation at 28 wk in severely affected pregnancies with delivery at lung maturity
- Delivery as soon as lung maturation is achieved in mild to moderately affected pregnancies

■ DISPOSITION
Survival of nonhydropic infants is 90%. Of infants with hydrops, 82% survive.

■ REFERRAL
Refer all Rh isoimmunized pregnancies to a tertiary care center before 18 to 20 wk gestation.
Author: **Laurel M. White, M.D.**

BASIC INFORMATION

■ DEFINITION
Rhabdomyolysis is the dissolution or disintegration of muscle, which causes membrane lysis and leakage of muscle constituents, resulting in the excretion of myoglobin in the urine.

ICD-9CM CODES
728.89 Rhabdomyolysis

■ EPIDEMIOLOGY & DEMOGRAPHICS
PREDOMINANT AGE: Rare in children

■ PHYSICAL FINDINGS & CLINICAL PRESENTATION
- Variable muscle tenderness
- Weakness
- Muscular rigidity
- Fever
- Altered consciousness
- Muscle swelling
- Malaise
- Dark urine

■ ETIOLOGY
- Exertion (exercise-induced)
- Electrical injury
- Drug-induced (statins, combination of statins with fibrates, amphetamines, haloperidol)
- Compartment syndrome
- Multiple trauma
- Malignant hyperthermia
- Limb ischemia
- Reperfusion after revascularization procedures for ischemia
- Extensive surgical (spinal) dissection
- Tourniquet ischemia
- Prolonged static positioning during surgery
- Infectious and inflammatory myositis
- Metabolic myopathies
- Hypovolemia and urinary acidification are important precipitating causes in the development of acute renal failure.

DIAGNOSIS

■ DIFFERENTIAL DIAGNOSIS
Fig. 3-46 describes a clinical algorithm for the evaluation of CPK elevation.

■ LABORATORY TESTS
- Screening for myoglobinuria with a simple urine dipstick test using orthotoluidine or benzidine
- BUN, creatinine
- Increased CPK (Fig. 1-324)
- Hyperkalemia
- Hypocalcemia
- Hyperphosphatemia
- Increased urinary myoglobin
- Pigmented granular casts
- Hyperuricemia

TREATMENT

■ ACUTE GENERAL Rx
- Aggressive high-volume IV fluid replacement with mannitol, to induce diuresis to prevent acute renal failure
- Treatment of electrolyte imbalances
- Alkalinization of urine is controversial but appears helpful in research models

■ DISPOSITION
The condition is easily treatable, but early diagnosis and management are necessary to avoid renal failure, which occurs in 30% of cases.

PEARLS & CONSIDERATIONS

■ COMMENTS
A clinical algorithm for the evaluation of muscle cramps and aches is described in Fig. 3-115.

REFERENCES
Garcia-Valdecasas-Campelo E et al: Acute rhabdomyolysis associated with cerivastatin therapy, *Arch Intern Med* 161:893, 2001.
Halachanova V, Sansone RA, McDonald S: Delayed rhabdomyolysis after ecstasy use, *Mayo Clin Proc* 76:112, 2001.
Schenk MR et al: Continuous venovenous hemofiltration for the immediate management of massive rhabdomyolysis after fulminant malignant hyperthermia in a bodybuilder, *Anesthesiology* 94:1139, 2001.
Wappler F et al: Evidence for susceptibility to malignant hyperthermia in patients with exercise-induced rhabdomyolysis, *Anesthesiology* 94:95, 2001.
Author: **Lonnie R. Mercier, M.D.**

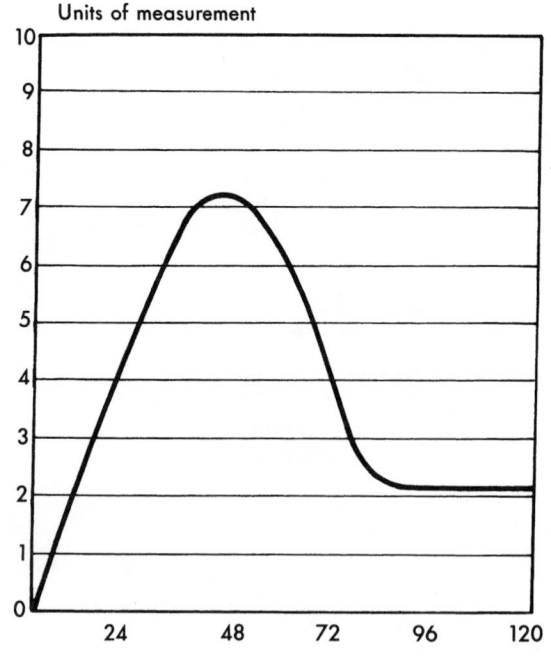

Fig. 1-324 Typical CK elimination curve. (From Rosen P [ed]: *Emergency medicine,* ed 4, St Louis, 1998, Mosby.)

BASIC INFORMATION

■ DEFINITION

Rheumatic fever is a multisystem inflammatory disease that occurs in the genetically susceptible host after a pharyngeal infection with group A streptococci.

■ SYNONYMS

Acute rheumatic fever
Rheumatic carditis

ICD-9CM CODES

390; 716.9 Rheumatic fever

■ EPIDEMIOLOGY & DEMOGRAPHICS

INCIDENCE (IN U.S.):
- 0.1% to 3% in patients with untreated streptococcal pharyngitis
- Higher incidence of streptococcal pharyngitis with:
  1. Crowding
  2. Poverty
  3. Young age

PREDOMINANT AGE:
- Age 5 to 15 yr for first attack
- Possible relapses later

PEAK INCIDENCE: School-age children
GENETICS:
Familial Disposition: Predisposition to the disease is likely to be genetically determined.

■ PHYSICAL FINDINGS & CLINICAL PRESENTATION

- Acute streptococcal pharyngitis, which may be subclinical and not reported by the patient
- After latent period of 1 to 5 wk (average, 19 days), acute rheumatic attack
- Patient is febrile, with a migratory polyarthritis of knees, ankles, wrists, elbows; typically severe for 1 wk, remits by 3 to 4 wk.
- Carditis
  1. New heart murmur
     a. Mitral regurgitation
     b. Aortic insufficiency
     c. Diastolic mitral murmur
  2. Cardiomegaly
  3. CHF
  4. Pericardial friction rub or effusion
- Rarely, pancarditis is severe and fatal.
- Subcutaneous nodules can be palpated over extensor tendon surfaces or bony prominences, such as the skull.
- Chorea (Sydenham's chorea) is characterized by rapid involuntary movements affecting all muscles.
  1. Muscular weakness
  2. Emotional lability
  3. Rarely seen after adolescence and almost never in adult males
- Erythema marginatum
  1. Evanescent, pink, well-demarcated spreading to trunk and proximal extremities

  2. Not specific
- Arthralgias (joint pain without swelling)
- Abdominal pain

■ ETIOLOGY

- Group A streptococci not recovered from tissue lesions.
- Does not occur in the absence of a streptococcal antibody response.
- Immunologic cross-reactivity between certain streptococcal antigens and human tissue antigens, suggests an autoimmune etiology.
- Both initial attacks and recurrences can be completely prevented by prompt treatment of streptococcal pharyngitis with penicillin.

DIAGNOSIS

■ DIFFERENTIAL DIAGNOSIS

- Rheumatoid arthritis
- Juvenile rheumatoid arthritis (Still's disease)
- Bacterial endocarditis
- Systemic lupus
- Viral infections
- Serum sickness

■ WORKUP

- "Jones Criteria (revised) for Guidance in the Diagnosis of Rheumatic Fever" published by the American Heart Association

One major and two minor criteria if supported by evidence of an antecedent group A streptococcal infection
- Major criteria
  1. Increased titer of antistreptococcal antibodies such as ASO
  2. Positive throat culture
  3. Recent scarlet fever
- Minor criteria
  1. Previous rheumatic fever or rheumatic heart disease
  2. Fever
  3. Arthralgia
  4. Increased acute-phase reactants
     a. ESR
     b. C-reactive protein
     c. Leukocytosis
  5. Prolonged P-R interval

■ LABORATORY TESTS

- Throat cultures are usually negative.
- Streptococcal antibody tests are more useful in establishing the diagnosis.
  1. Peak at the beginning of the attack
  2. Can document a recent streptococcal infection
- ASO (antistreptolysin O) titers peak:
  1. 4 to 5 wk after a streptococcal throat infection
  2. During the second or third week of illness

- Anti-DNase B (Streptozyme) is also commonly used but is less reliable.
- High-titer streptococcal antibodies:
  1. Are supportive of diagnosis, but not proof
  2. Should be interpreted in the context of clinical criteria

■ IMAGING STUDIES

- Chest x-ray to assess heart size
- Echocardiogram:
  1. To evaluate murmurs
  2. To rule out pericardial effusion

TREATMENT

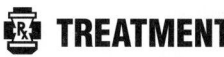

■ ACUTE GENERAL Rx

- Course of penicillin to eradicate throat carriage of group A streptococci
- Arthralgia or arthritis without carditis: aspirin 40 mg/lb/day for 2 wk, followed by 20 mg/lb/day for 4 to 6 wk
- Carditis and heart failure:
  1. Prednisone 40 to 60 mg/day
  2. IV corticosteroids, such as methylprednisolone, 10 to 40 mg/day for severe carditis

■ CHRONIC Rx

Secondary prevention (prevention of recurrences):
- Monthly treatment with benzathine penicillin 1.2 million U IM
- Erythromycin in patients with penicillin allergy

■ DISPOSITION

- Damage of heart valves because of fibrosis
  1. Late sequela of recurrent attacks
  2. Frequent cause of valvular heart disease in developing countries
- May progress to heart failure

■ REFERRAL

To cardiologist for management of severe carditis

REFERENCES

Carapetis JR, Currie BJ: Rheumatic fever in a high incidence population: the importance of monoarthritis and low grade fever, *Arch Dis Child* 85(30):223, 2001.

Figueroa FE et al: Prospective comparison of clinical and echocardiographic diagnosis of rheumatic carditis: long term follow up of patients with subclinical disease, *Heart* 85(40):407, 2001.

Thatai D, Turi ZG: Current guidelines for the treatment of rheumatic fever, *Drugs* 57(4):545, 1999.

Author: **Deborah L. Shapiro, M.D.**

BASIC INFORMATION

■ **DEFINITION**
Allergic rhinitis is an IgE-mediated hypersensitivity response to nasally inhaled allergens that causes sneezing, rhinorrhea, nasal pruritus, and congestion.

■ **SYNONYMS**
Hay fever
IgE-mediated rhinitis

ICD-9CM CODES
477.9 Allergic rhinitis

■ **EPIDEMIOLOGY & DEMOGRAPHICS**
• Allergic rhinitis affects approximately 10% to 20% of the U.S. population.
• Mean age of onset is 8 to 12 yr.

■ **PHYSICAL FINDINGS & CLINICAL FINDINGS**
• Pale or violaceous mucosa of the turbinates caused by venous engorgement (this can distinguish it from erythema present in viral rhinitis)
• Nasal polyps
• Lymphoid hyperplasia in the posterior oropharynx with cobblestone appearance
• Erythema of the throat, conjunctival and scleral injection
• Clear nasal discharge
• Clinical presentation: usually consists of sneezing, nasal congestion, cough, postnasal drip, loss of or alteration of smell, and sensation of plugged ears

■ **ETIOLOGY**
• Pollens in the springtime, ragweed in fall, grasses in the summer
• Dust, mites, animal allergens
• Smoke or any irritants
• Perfumes, detergents, soaps
• Emotion, changes in atmospheric pressure or temperature

DIAGNOSIS

■ **DIFFERENTIAL DIAGNOSIS**
• Infections (sinusitis; viral, bacterial, or fungal rhinitis)
• Rhinitis medicamentosa (cocaine, sympathomimetic nasal drops)
• Vasomotor rhinitis (e.g., secondary to air pollutants)
• Septal obstruction (e.g., deviated septum), nasal polyps, nasal neoplasms

• Systemic diseases (e.g., Wegener's granulomatosis, hypothyroidism [rare])
• Table 2-177 describes the differential diagnosis of chronic rhinitis.

■ **WORKUP**
• Workup is often unnecessary if the diagnosis is apparent. A detailed medical history is useful in identifying the culprit allergen.
• Allergy testing can be performed using skin testing or radioallergosorbent (RAST) testing. In vitro tests also can assess serum levels of specific IgE antibodies. Overall, skin tests show greater sensitivity than serum assays. In vitro tests should be considered in rare patients who fear skin tests, must take medication that interferes with skin testing, or have generalized dermatographism.
• Examination of nasal smears for the presence of neutrophils to rule out infectious causes and the presence of eosinophils (suggestive of allergy) may be useful in selected patients.
• Peripheral blood eosinophil counts are not useful in allergy diagnosis.
• Fig. 3-147 describes the evaluation and treatment of rhinorrhea.

■ **LABORATORY TESTS**
See "Workup."

■ **IMAGING STUDIES**
Sinus films only when sinusitis is suspected

TREATMENT

■ **NONPHARMACOLOGIC THERAPY**
• Maintain allergen-free environment by covering mattresses and pillows with allergen-proof casings, eliminating carpeting, eliminating animal products, and removing dust-collecting fixtures.
• Use of air purifiers and dust filters is helpful.
• Maintain humidity in the environment below 50% to prevent dust mites and mold.
• Use air conditioners, especially in the bedroom.
• Remove pets from homes of patients with suspected sensitivity to animal allergens.

■ **ACUTE GENERAL Rx**
• Determine if the patient is troubled by swollen turbinates (best treated with decongestants) or blockages secondary to mucus (effectively treated by antihistamines).

• Most first-generation antihistamines are available without a prescription and can cause considerable sedation and anticholinergic symptoms. The second-generation antihistamines (loratidine, fexofenadine, cetirizine) do not have any significant anticholinergic or sedative effects; however, they are much more expensive.
• Azelastine (Astelin) is an antihistamine nasal spray effective for seasonal allergic rhinitis.
• Topical nasal steroids are very effective and are preferred by many as first-line treatment for allergic rhinitis in adults. Patients should be instructed on proper use and informed that improvement might not occur for at least 1 wk after initiation of therapy. Commonly available inhalers are:
  1. Beclomethasone dipropionate (Beconase AQ): one to two sprays in each nostril bid
  2. Fluticasone (Flonase): initially two sprays in each nostril qd or one spray in each nostril bid, decreasing to one spray in each nostril qd based on response
  3. Flunisolide (Nasalide): initially two sprays in each nostril bid
  4. Budesonide (Rhinocort): two sprays in each nostril bid or four sprays in each nostril qAM

■ **CHRONIC Rx**
• Cromolyn sodium (Nasalcrom): one spray to each nostril three to four times daily can be used for prophylaxis (mast cell stabilizer).
• Immunotherapy is generally reserved for patients responding poorly to the above treatments.

■ **DISPOSITION**
Most patients experience significant relief with avoidance of allergens and proper use of medications.

■ **REFERRAL**
Allergy testing in patients with severe symptoms that are unresponsive to therapy or when the diagnosis is uncertain

PEARLS & CONSIDERATIONS

■ **COMMENTS**
Desloratadine (Clarinex) is a newer, nonsedating antihistamine. It is an active metabolite of loratidine recently approved for treatment of seasonal and perennial rhinitis and chronic idiopathic urticaria. Usual dose is 5 mg qd.
Author: **Fred F. Ferri, M.D.**

BASIC INFORMATION

■ DEFINITION

Rickets is a systemic disease of infancy and childhood in which mineralization of growing bone is deficient as a result of abnormal calcium, phosphorus, or vitamin D metabolism. *Osteomalacia* is the same condition in the adult. *Renal osteodystrophy* is a term used to describe a similar condition in patients with chronic kidney disease. Certain forms of the disorder may respond only to high doses of vitamin D and are referred to as *vitamin D–resistant rickets* (VDRR).

■ ICD-9CM CODES
268.0 Active rickets
275.3 Vitamin D–resistant rickets
588.0 Renal rickets (renal osteodystrophy)
268.2 Osteomalacia

■ PHYSICAL FINDINGS & CLINICAL PRESENTATION
The child with classic rickets usually develops a number of specific abnormalities:
- Softening of the skull bones (craniotabes) early in the disorder
- Enlargement of the ribs at the costochondral junctions, producing the "rachitic rosary"
- Limb deformities and epiphyseal swelling (Fig. 1-325)
- Height below normal range
- Irritability and easy fatigability
- Pigeon breast deformity and an indentation of the lower ribcage at the insertion of the diaphragm, sometimes referred to as Harrison's groove; possible decrease in thoracic volume, resulting in diminished pulmonary ventilation

Physical findings in the adult with osteomalacia are more subtle:
- Possible malaise and bone pain
- Many patients presumed to have osteoporosis but may also have osteomalacia

■ ETIOLOGY
- Deficiency states
  1. True classic VDDR is rare in Western society.
  2. Absorption of vitamin D, however, may be blocked in several GI disorders.
  3. Similar disorders may also prevent absorption of calcium and phosphorus, but in the absence of these other diseases, deficiencies of calcium and phosphorus are also rare.
- Acquired or inherited renal tubular abnormalities that cause resorptive defects and result in rickets and osteomalacia; syndromes include classical VDRR (probably the most common form of rickets seen in general practice)
- Chronic renal failure:
  1. Can produce renal rickets or renal osteodystrophy
  2. Results in the retention of phosphate

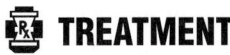

DIAGNOSIS

■ DIFFERENTIAL DIAGNOSIS
- Osteoporosis
- Hyperparathyroidism
- Hyperthyroidism

■ LABORATORY TESTS
- Requires a high degree of interest because many of the conditions are so similar that only a complicated laboratory evaluation may establish the diagnosis
- BUN, creatinine, alkaline phosphatase, calcium, and phosphorus levels in any patient suspected of having metabolic bone disease

■ IMAGING STUDIES
- In rickets:
  1. Characteristic radiographic changes in the ends of growing long bones caused by the lack of calcification of the cartilage matrix
  2. Typically widening and irregularity of the epiphyseal plate
- Radiographs in the adult with osteomalacia:
  1. More subtle and often confused with osteoporosis
  2. Possible pseudofractures (Looser's zones) where major arteries cross bone
  3. Insufficiency compression deformities in the vertebral bodies

TREATMENT

- Because of the complex nature of many of these disorders, a qualified endocrinologist and nephrologist should be consulted for treatment.
- The need for orthopedic intervention is rare.
- Surgical care is indicated for slipped capital femoral epiphysis, which is fairly common in renal rickets.
- Deformity may require bracing.

Author: **Lonnie R. Mercier, M.D.**

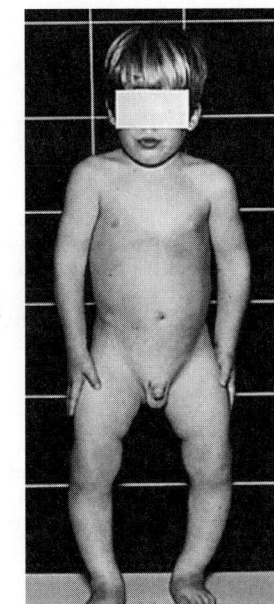 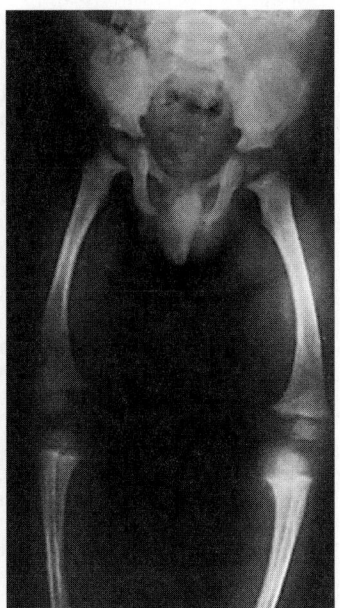

Fig. 1-325   A, Clinical and, **B,** radiographic appearance of a young boy with X-linked hypophosphatemic rickets. Note the striking bowing of the legs, apparent in both femora and tibiae, with flaring of the ends of the bones at the knee. (Courtesy Dr. Sara B. Arnaud. From Bikle DB: Osteomalacia and rickets. In Wyngaarden JB, Smith LH Jr, Bennett JB [eds]: *Cecil textbook of medicine,* ed 19, Philadelphia, 1992, WB Saunders.)

BASIC INFORMATION

■ **DEFINITION**

Rocky Mountain spotted fever (RMSF) is a febrile illness caused by infection with *Rickettsia rickettsii.*

ICD-9CM CODES

082.0 Rocky Mountain spotted fever

■ **EPIDEMIOLOGY & DEMOGRAPHICS**

INCIDENCE: 0.18 to 0.32 cases/100,000 person-years

DEMOGRAPHICS: Affects both genders equally and occurs at any age, but more likely in children aged 5 to 14 yr

GEOGRAPHY: Most prevalent in the Southeast, followed by the South Central states, but seen anywhere

■ **PHYSICAL FINDINGS & CLINICAL PRESENTATION**

• Incubation: 3 to 12 days
• First symptoms: fever, headache, malaise, and myalgias

Common history, signs, or symptoms	%
Tick bite	65
Fever	100
Rash	90
Rash on palms and soles	80
Headache	90
Myalgia	75
Nausea or vomiting	60
Abdominal pain	40
Conjunctivitis	30
Edema	20
Pneumonitis	15
Any severe neurologic complication (including stupor, delirium, seizures, ataxia, papilledema, focal neurologic deficits, and coma)	30

Rash:
• Appears during first 3 days in 50%; by day 5, 80% have it. No rash in 10%.
• Initial appearance: blanching erythematous macules on wrists and ankles that then spread to trunk, palms, and soles.
• Lesions may evolve into papules and eventually become nonblanching (petechiae or palpable purpura).

Gastrointestinal symptoms:
• Nausea, vomiting, and abdominal pain are common.
• Occasionally may mimic an "acute abdomen" (e.g., appendicitis, cholecystitis)
• Mild hepatitis

Cardiopulmonary involvement:
• Interstitial pneumonitis
• Myocarditis

Renal problems:
• Prerenal azotemia
• Interstitial nephritis
• Glomerulonephritis

Neurologic involvement:
• Encephalitis (confusion, lethargy, delirium)
• Ataxia
• Convulsion
• Cranial nerve palsy
• Speech impediment
• Hemiparesis or paraparesis
• Spasticity

Fulminant Rocky Mountain spotted fever
• Early, widespread vascular necrosis leading to multisystem illness and death

■ **ETIOLOGY & PATHOGENESIS**

• Infectious agent: *Rickettsia rickettsii* (an intracellular bacterium).
• Vector: dog tick and wood tick (vertical transmission exists in ticks, but horizontal transmission involving rodents represents an important reservoir for the agent).
• Pathogenesis: the spread of *R. rickettsii* is hematogenous with attachment to the vascular endothelium, causing a vasculitis. The manifestations of this illness are caused by increased vascular permeability.

 DIAGNOSIS

■ **DIFFERENTIAL DIAGNOSIS**

Influenza A, enteroviral infection, typhoid fever, leptospirosis, infectious mononucleosis, viral hepatitis, sepsis, ehrlichiosis, gastroenteritis, acute abdomen, bronchitis, pneumonia, meningococcemia, disseminated gonococcal infection, secondary syphilis, bacterial endocarditis, toxic shock syndrome, scarlet fever, rheumatic fever, measles, rubella, typhus, rickettsialpox, Lyme disease, drug hypersensitivity reactions, idiopathic thrombocytopenic purpura, thrombotic thrombocytopenic purpura, Kawasaki disease, immune complex vasculitis, connective tissue disorders

■ **WORKUP**

Consider RMSF in any patient with an acute febrile illness with headache and myalgia, especially with an associated history of tick exposure. Absence of rash does not rule the diagnosis.

■ **LABORATORY TESTS**

Routine tests	%
White cell count	
<10,000/mm^3	72
>10% bands	69
Platelet count	
<150,000/mm^3	52
<99,000/mm^3	32
Serum sodium value <132 mEq/L	56
Aspartate aminotransferase ≥2× normal	62
Alanine aminotransferase ≥2× normal	39
Bilirubin value >1.4 mg/dl	30
Cerebrospinal fluid	
Opening pressure ≥250 mm H$_2$O	14
Glucose value ≤50 mg/dl	8
Protein value ≥50 mg/dl	35
White cell count ≥5/mm^3	38
Mononuclear cell predominance	46
Polymorphonuclear cell predominance	50

Etiologic tests
• Antibody titers to *R. rickettsii* (by indirect fluorescent antibody test). The diagnosis of RMSF requires a fourfold increase 2 wk apart and thus is not helpful in the care of the patients despite a sensitivity and specificity of near 100%.
• The only test that can provide a timely diagnosis is the immunohistologic demonstration of *R. rickettsii* in skin biopsy specimens.

 TREATMENT

• Oral or intravenous doxycycline, 200 mg/day in two divided doses
• Oral tetracycline, 25 to 50 mg/kg/day in four divided doses
• Chloramphenicol, 50 to 75 mg/kg/day in four divided doses; therapy continued for at least 2 days after defervescence

■ **PROGNOSIS**

Fatality rate: 1% to 4% (five times greater if treatment is initiated after day 5 of illness, which is more likely in absence of rash and during seasonal nonpeak tick activity). Long-term sequelae seen in patients who recover from severe RMSF: paraparesis, hearing loss; peripheral neuropathy; bladder and bowel incontinence; cerebellar, vestibular, and motor dysfunction; language disorders; limb amputation; and scrotal pain after cutaneous necrosis.

REFERENCE

Dumler JS: Rocky Mountain spotted fever. In Gorbach SL, Bartlett JG, Blacklow NR (eds): *Infectious diseases,* ed 2, Philadelphia, 1998, WB Saunders.
Author: **Tom J. Wachtel, M.D.**

BASIC INFORMATION

■ **DEFINITION**

Rosacea is a chronic skin disorder characterized by papules and pustules affecting the face and often associated with flushing and erythema.

■ **SYNONYMS**

Acne rosacea

ICD-9CM CODES
695.3 Rosacea

■ **EPIDEMIOLOGY & DEMOGRAPHICS**

• Rosacea occurs in 1 in 20 Americans
• Onset often between age 30 and 50 yr
• More common in people of Celtic origin
• Female:male ratio of 3:1

■ **PHYSICAL FINDINGS & CLINICAL PRESENTATION**

• Facial erythema, presence of papules, pustules, and telangiectasia (Fig. 1-326).
• Excessive facial warmth and redness.
• Comedones are absent (unlike acne).
• Women are more likely to show symptoms on the chin and cheeks, whereas in men the nose is commonly involved.
• Ocular findings (conjunctival injection, burning, stinging, tearing, eyelid inflammation, swelling, and redness) are present in >20% of patients.

■ **ETIOLOGY**

• Unknown.
• Hot drinks, alcohol, and sun exposure may accentuate the erythema by causing vasodilation of the skin.
• Flare-ups may also result from reactions to medications (e.g., simvastatin, ACE inhibitors, vasodilators, fluorinated corticosteroids), stress, extreme heat or cold, spicy drinks.

DIAGNOSIS

■ **DIFFERENTIAL DIAGNOSIS**

• Drug eruption
• Acne vulgaris
• Contact dermatitis
• SLE
• Carcinoid flush
• Idiopathic facial flushing
• Seborrheic dermatitis
• Facial sarcoidosis

■ **WORKUP**

Diagnosis is based on clinical findings.

■ **LABORATORY TESTS**

Not indicated

TREATMENT

■ **NONPHARMACOLOGIC THERAPY**

• Avoid alcohol, excessive sun exposure, and hot drinks of any type.
• Use of mild, nondrying soap is recommended; local skin irritants should be avoided.
• Reassure patient that rosacea is completely unrelated to poor hygiene.

■ **ACUTE GENERAL Rx**

• Systemic antibiotics: tetracycline 250 mg qid until symptoms diminish, then taper off; doxycycline 100 mg bid is also effective.
• Minocycline 50 to 100 mg qd should be used only in resistant cases, because this medication is expensive.
• Isotretinoin (Accutane) 0.5 to 1 mg/kg/day in two divided doses for 15 to 20 wk can be used for refractory rosacea.
• Topical therapy with metronidazole aqueous gel (MetroGel) applied bid is effective as initial therapy for mild cases or following the use of oral antibiotics. A new 1% formulation of metronidazole (Noritate) applied qd may improve patient compliance. Clindamycin lotion (Cleocin) and sulfacetamide may also be effective.

■ **CHRONIC Rx**

See "Acute General Rx."

■ **DISPOSITION**

Rosacea is often resistant to initial treatment and recurrent. Periods of remission and relapse are common.

PEARLS & CONSIDERATIONS

■ **COMMENTS**

• Patients with resistant cases may have *Demodex folliculorum* mite infestation or tinea infection (diagnosis can be confirmed with potassium hydroxide examination); the role of *D. folliculorum* in rosacea is unclear. These mites can sometimes be found in large numbers in the lesions; however, their numbers do not generally decline with treatment.
• Patient education material may be obtained from the National Rosacea Society, 800 S Northwest Hwy, Suite 200, Barrington, IL 60010. Phone: 888-662-5874. Website: *www.Rosacea.org*

Author: **Fred F. Ferri, M.D.**

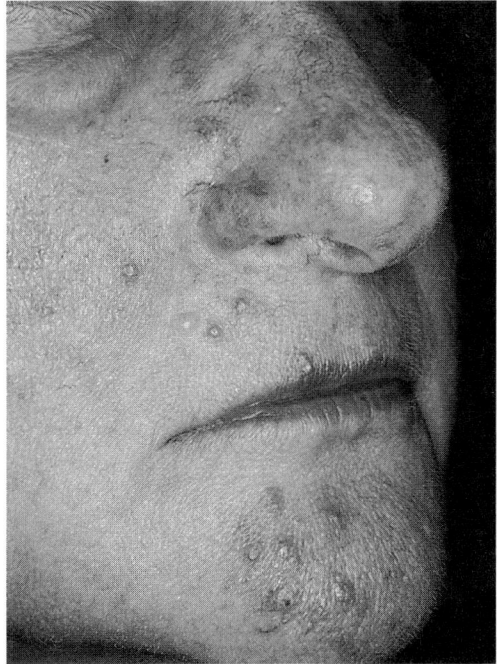

Fig. 1-326 Pustules (rosacea). Note also the presence of telangiectasia. (From Noble J et al: *Textbook of primary care medicine,* ed 2, St Louis, 1995, Mosby.)

BASIC INFORMATION

■ DEFINITION
Roseola is a benign viral illness found in infants and is characterized by high fevers, followed by a rash.

■ SYNONYMS
Exanthem subitum
Sixth disease
Roseola infantum

ICD-9CM CODES
057.8 Roseola

■ EPIDEMIOLOGY & DEMOGRAPHICS
- Nearly one third of all infants develop roseola before the age of 2 yr.
- More than 90% of children older than 2 yr of age are seropositive for the virus causing roseola.
- Roseola is spread from person to person, but it is not known how.
- It is not known how contagious roseola is.
- There is no predilection for gender or time of year.

■ PHYSICAL FINDINGS & CLINICAL PRESENTATION
- Typically the child develops a high fever, usually up to 104° F (40° C) that lasts for 3 to 5 days.
- Fever may be associated with a runny nose, irritability, and fatigue.
- A rash appears within 48 hr of defervescence, mainly on the face, neck, trunk, arms, and legs (Fig. 1-327).
- The rash is a faint pink maculopapular rash that blanches when palpated.
- The rash usually fades away within 48 hr.
- Anorexia
- Seizures
- Cervical adenopathy

■ ETIOLOGY
- Roseola is caused by human herpesvirus-6 (HHV-6).
- The incubation period is between 5 to 15 days.

DIAGNOSIS

- The diagnosis of roseola is usually made by the clinical presentation as stated above.

■ DIFFERENTIAL DIAGNOSIS
- Measles
- Rubella
- Fifth disease
- Drug eruption
- Mononucleosis
- All causes of fever (e.g., otitis media, pneumonia, and urinary tract infection).
- Meningitis
- Other causes of seizures

■ WORKUP
- If unsure of the diagnosis of roseola in a febrile infant, a fever workup is done to rule out other infectious causes.
- The decision to proceed with a fever workup is a clinical judgment call.

■ LABORATORY TESTS
- CBC with differential
- Erythrocyte sedimentation rate (ESR)
- Blood cultures
- Urinalysis and urine cultures
- Stool cultures if diarrhea is present
- Lumbar puncture

■ IMAGING STUDIES
- Chest x-ray to rule out pneumonia

TREATMENT

■ NONPHARMACOLOGIC
- Supportive care
- Maintain hydration by drinking clear fluids: water, fruit juice, lemonade, etc.
- Sponge bathe with lukewarm water if febrile.

■ ACUTE GENERAL Rx
- Acetaminophen 10 to 15 mg/kg per dose at 4-hr intervals for fever
- Ibuprofen 5 to 10 mg/kg per dose at 6-hr intervals (maximal dose 600 mg)

■ CHRONIC Rx
- Roseola is viral disease that is short lasting; chronic treatment is usually not an issue.

■ DISPOSITION
- Roseola is generally a benign, self-limited disease that usually lasts approximately 1 wk.
- Complications, although rare, can occur and include:
  1. Febrile seizures
  2. Meningitis
  3. Encephalitis
  4. Pneumonitis
  5. Hepatitis

■ REFERRAL
- Subspecialty consultation is made with the appropriate discipline if any of the above-mentioned complications occur (e.g., neurology for seizures)

PEARLS & CONSIDERATIONS

■ COMMENTS

- A child with fever and rash should be excluded from daycare.
- Human herpesvirus 6 is named accordingly because it is the sixth herpesvirus discovered after herpes simplex 1 (HSV-1), HSV-2, cytomegalovirus (CMV), Epstein-Barr virus (EBV), and varicella-zoster virus (VZV).

- Roseola is called sixth disease because it represents one of six "exanthems" that occurs during childhood. The other five exanthems included in this old classification are measles, scarlet fever, rubella, Dukes disease, and erythema infectiosum (fifth disease).

REFERENCES

Asano Y et al: Clinical features of infants with primary human herpesvirus 6 infection (exanthem subitum, roseola infantum), *Pediatrics* 93:104, 1994.

Dockrell DH, Smith TF, Paya C: Human herpesvirus 6, *Mayo Clin Proc* 74:163, 1999.

Author: **Dennis Mikolich, M.D.**

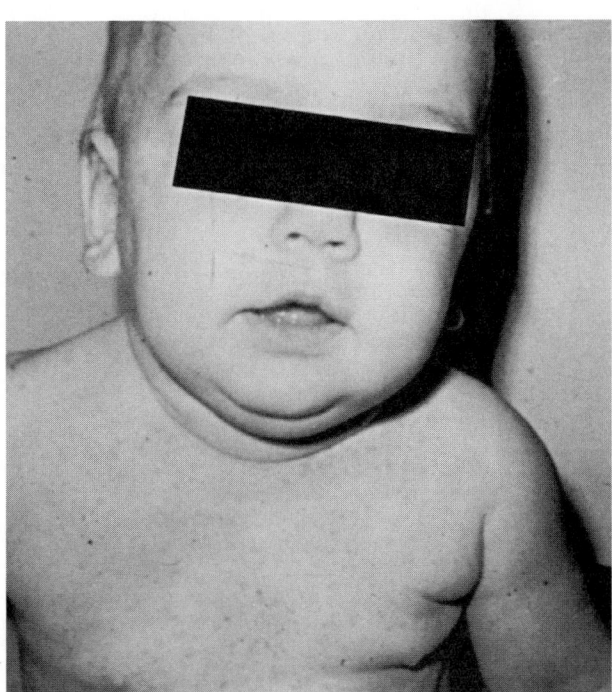

Fig. 1-327   Scattered maculopapular rash of roseola is most evident on the trunk, the face being relatively spared. (From Gorbach SL: *Infectious diseases,* ed 2, Philadelphia, 1998, WB Saunders.)

BASIC INFORMATION

■ DEFINITION

Rotator cuff syndrome refers to a spectrum of afflictions involving the tendons of the rotator cuff (primarily the supraspinatus), ranging from simple strains and tendinitis to complete rupture with cuff-tear arthropathy.

■ SYNONYMS

Impingement syndrome
Painful arc syndrome
Internal derangement of the subacromial joint
Supraspinatus syndrome

ICD-9CM CODES
726.10 Rotator cuff syndrome
727.61 Rotator cuff rupture

■ EPIDEMIOLOGY & DEMOGRAPHICS
PREVALENCE: 5% to 10% of the general population
PREDOMINANT AGE: Uncommon under 20 yr of age
PREDOMINANT SEX: More common in males than females

■ PHYSICAL FINDINGS & CLINICAL PRESENTATION
- Pain, often at night
- Rotator cuff tenderness
- Referred pain down deltoid, especially with abduction between 70 and 120 degrees ("the painful arc") (Fig. 1-328)
- Weakness in abduction or forward flexion
- Increased pain with overhead activities
- Atrophy in long-standing cases of complete tear
- Positive "drop-arm" test

■ ETIOLOGY
- Microtrauma from repetitive use
- Abnormally shaped acromion
- Shoulder instability
- Worsening of process by the overhead throwing motion

DIAGNOSIS

■ DIFFERENTIAL DIAGNOSIS
- Shoulder instability
- Degenerative arthritis
- Cervical radiculopathy
- Avascular necrosis
- Suprascapular nerve entrapment

■ WORKUP
- In chronic tendinitis, clinical findings similar to those seen in partial rupture

- Even with complete rupture, may have full, active range of motion in shoulder

■ IMAGING STUDIES
- Plain radiography to rule out other causes of shoulder pain; special views (if needed) to detect abnormally shaped acromion
- Shoulder arthrogram to diagnose full-thickness rotator cuff tear
- Ultrasonography to diagnose full-thickness rotator cuff tears
- MRI to evaluate full- or partial-thickness tears, chronic tendinitis, and other causes of shoulder pain

TREATMENT

■ ACUTE GENERAL Rx
- Rest to avoid overhead activity
- Ice or heat for comfort
- Carefully supervised program of stretching and strengthening
- Medication: NSAIDs, subacromial corticosteroid injection (see Table 1-18)

■ DISPOSITION
- All forms are likely to respond to nonsurgical management.
- Even many complete rotator cuff tears have minimal pain and little loss of function.

■ REFERRAL
For orthopedic consultation in cases that fail to respond to medical management or in which rotator cuff tear is suspected

PEARLS & CONSIDERATIONS

■ COMMENTS
- There is considerable disagreement regarding the likelihood of recovery once a significant rotator cuff rupture has developed.
- Indications for surgery vary among surgeons.

REFERENCES
Goldberg BA, Nolvinski RJ, Matsen FA: Outcome of nonoperative management of full-thickness rotator cuff tears, *Clin Orthop* 382:99, 2001.

Granger AJ et al: MR anatomy of the subcoracoid bursa and the association of subcoracoid effusion with tears of the anterior rotator cuff and the rotator interval, *Am J Roentgenol* 174:1377, 2000.

Murrell GA, Walton JR: Diagnosis of rotator cuff tears, *Lancet* 357:769, 2001.

Pradhan RL, Itoi E: Rotator interval lesions of the shoulder joint, *Orthopedics* 24:798, 2001.

Author: **Lonnie R. Mercier, M.D.**

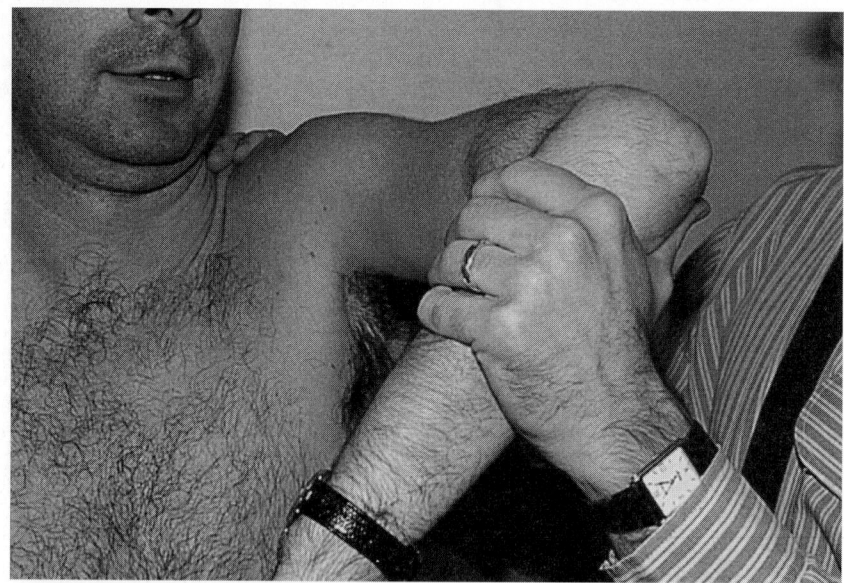

Fig. 1-328 Rotator cuff lesions are often accompanied by painful impingement of the upwardly subluxating humerus onto the acromion. Evidence for this as a cause of pain is elicited by impingement tests, for example, by forced, passive, internal rotation and abduction of the shoulder, as shown here. (From Klippel J, Dieppe P, Ferri F [eds]: *Primary care rheumatology,* London, 1999, Mosby.)

BASIC INFORMATION

■ DEFINITION

Rubella is a mild illness caused by the rubella virus that can cause severe congenital problems via in vitro transmission to the fetus when a pregnant woman becomes infected.

■ SYNONYMS

German measles

ICD-9CM CODES
056.9 Rubella
771.0 (congenital)
V04.3 (vaccination)

■ EPIDEMIOLOGY & DEMOGRAPHICS

- Before vaccination (i.e., before 1969) 28 reported cases per 100,000 persons-years, eight of which were in persons over age 15 yr
  Four cases of congenital rubella syndrome per 100,000 live births
- After mass vaccination (i.e., after 1980) most cases have occurred in unimmunized people with fewer than 1 case/100,000 person-years (acquired and congenital).
- Currently, 10% to 20% of childbearing-age women are susceptible.
- The highest risk of developing long-term complications of congenital infection exists during the first trimester of gestation; both risk of congenital infection and long-term complications drop during the second trimester, and while the risk of congenital infection increases during the third trimester, there is no risk of long-term complication at that point.

■ PHYSICAL FINDINGS & CLINICAL PRESENTATION

Acquired infection
- Incubation: 14 to 21 days
- Prodrome: 1 to 5 days; low-grade fever, headache, malaise, anorexia, mild conjunctivitis, coryza, pharyngitis, cough, and cervical, suboccipital, and postauricular lymphadenopathy
- Rash: 1 to 5 days
  Enanthema: palatal macules
  Exanthema (rash): blotchy eruption beginning on face and neck and then spreading to trunk and limbs
- Occasional splenomegaly and hepatitis (during rash)
- Complications: arthritis (15%, mostly in adult women), thrombocytopenia, myocarditis, optic neuritis, encephalitis (all less than 0.1%)

Congenital infection
- Deafness: 85%
- Intrauterine growth retardation: 70%
- Cataracts: 35%
- Retinopathy: 35%
- Patent ductus arteriosus: 30%
- Pulmonary artery hypoplasia: 25%
- In utero death: 20%
- Mental retardation: 10% to 20%
- Meningoencephalitis: 10% to 20%
- Behavior disorder: 10% to 20%
- Hepatosplenomegaly: 10% to 20%
- Bone radiolucencies: 10% to 20%
- Diabetes mellitus (type 1): 10% to 20% by age 35 yr
- Other congenital heart defects: 2% to 5%

■ ETIOLOGY & PATHOGENESIS

Acquired infection
- Viral portal of entry is upper respiratory tract.
- Viral replication occurs in lymph nodes, then hematogenous dissemination occurs to many organs, including placenta if present.
- Immune complexes may be cause of rash and arthritis.
Congenital infection
- Fetus is infected via placenta during maternal acquired infection.
- Cellular damage in the fetus results from cytolysis of fetal cells, mostly via a fetal vasculitis or from an immune-mediated inflammation and damage.

DIAGNOSIS

■ DIFFERENTIAL DIAGNOSIS

Acquired rubella syndrome
- Other viral infections by enteroviruses, adenoviruses, human parvovirus B-19, measles
- Scarlet fever
- Allergic reaction
- Kawasaki disease
Congenital rubella syndrome
- Congenital syphilis, toxoplasmosis, herpes simplex, cytomegalovirus, and enterovirus can cause a similar set of problems.

■ WORKUP

Acquired infection
- Serologic test (hemagglutination inhibition, neutralization tests, complement fixation tests, passive agglutination, enzyme immunoassay [EIA], enzyme-linked immunosorbent assay [ELISA])
- IgM antibodies (by EIA) are detected early: 2nd to 4th week
- IgG antibodies (by ELISA) can be measured as acute phase (7 days after rash onset) and convalescent phase (14 days later)
Congenital infection
- Viral culture (from nasopharynx)
- Serologic studies: IgM antirubella virus detection by EIA is the method of choice (after the newborn is 5 mo old)

■ IMMUNIZATION

Four existing vaccines provide persisting immunity in 92% of vaccinees. Indications:
- All children 12 mo or older (as part of the measles-mumps-rubella vaccine)
- Postpubertal women
  Vaccinate if not known to be immunized (advise not to become pregnant within 3 mo of vaccination)
  Premarital serologic screening for rubella immunity
  Prenatal or antepartum serologic screening for rubella
  Vaccinate susceptible women postpartum
  Serologic screening for female workers likely to be exposed to rubella (e.g., teachers, child care employees, health care workers)
Contraindications
- Pregnancy
- Recent receipt of immune globulin or blood transfusion (2 wk before to 3 mo after)
- Immunodeficiency (except AIDS)
Adverse reaction
- Fever, rash, or lymphadenopathy: 5% to 15%
- Arthralgias: 0.5% in children; 25% in adult women
- Transient peripheral neuropathy (rare)

TREATMENT

- No known effective antiviral therapy
- Management of specific congenital problems as appropriate

REFERENCESS

Rakowsky A, Sever JL: Rubella. In Gorbach SL, Bartlett JG, Blacklow NR (eds): *Infectious diseases*, ed 2, Philadelphia, 1998, WB Saunders.
U.S. Department of Health: Control and prevention of rubella: evaluation and management of suspected outbreaks, rubella in pregnant women, and surveillance for congenital rubella syndrome, *MMWR* 50(RR-12):1, 2001.
Author: **Tom J. Wachtel, M.D.**

BASIC INFORMATION

DEFINITION
Salivary gland neoplasms are benign or malignant tumors of a salivary gland (parotid, submandibular, or sublingual).

SYNONYMS
These tumors are often named according to their histologic type (see below).

ICD-9CM CODES
142.9 salivary gland neoplasm
142.0 (parotid)
142.1 (submandibular)
142.2 (sublingual)

EPIDEMIOLOGY & DEMOGRAPHICS
INCIDENCE: 1 to 2 cases/100,000 person-years (1% of all head and neck tumors)
DISTRIBUTION:
- Parotid gland 85% (80% are benign)
- Submandibular gland 10% (55% are benign)
- Sublingual and minor glands 5% (35% are benign)

PHYSICAL FINDINGS & CLINICAL PRESENTATION
- Parotid gland (Fig. 1-329):
  1. Painless swelling overlying the masseter muscle (under the temporomandibular joint)
  2. Pain
  3. Facial nerve palsy
  4. Cervical lymph nodes
  5. Mass in oral cavity
- Submandibular gland: swelling under anterior portion of the mandible
- Sublingual gland: intraoral swelling under the tongue, medial to the mandible

PATHOLOGY
History
BENIGN TUMORS:
- Mixed tumor (usually parotid)
- Adenolymphoma (Warthin's tumor)
- Adenoma
- Hemangioma, lymphangioma (in children)
- Other

MALIGNANT TUMORS:
- Mucoepidermoid carcinoma
- Adenoid cystic carcinoma
- Adenocarcinoma
- Malignant mixed tumor
- Squamous cell carcinoma
- Other

Stage (TNM)
T_0 No evidence of primary tumor
T_1 Tumor <2 cm
T_2 Tumor 2 to 4 cm
T_3 Tumor 4 to 6 cm
T_4 Tumor >6 cm
All subdivided into
- Without local extension
- With local extension
N_0 No lymph node metastasis
N_1 Single ipsilateral node <3 cm
N_2 Ipsilateral, contralateral, or bilateral node <6 cm
N_3 Any node >6 cm
M_0 No distant metastasis
M_1 Distant metastasis
Stage I T_{1a} or $_{2a}N_0M_0$
Stage II $T_{1b,2b,3a}\ N_0M_0$
Stage III $T_{3b,4a}\ N_0M_0$ or any T except $_{4b}N_1M_0$
Stage IV T_{4b} any N any M or any T $N_{2,3}M_0$ or any T, any N_1M_1

WORKUP
- Fine-needle aspiration
- Imaging by CT scan or MRI
- Open biopsy (rarely indicated)

TREATMENT

Malignant tumors:
- Surgery is the mainstay of treatment; gland resection and neck dissection if lymph nodes are involved
- Postoperative radiation
- Chemotherapy
Benign tumors: surgery for tumor resection

PROGNOSIS OF MALIGNANT TUMORS
Five-year survival rates:
- Mucoepidermoid carcinoma: 75% to 95%
- Adenoid cystic carcinoma: 40% to 80%
- Adenocarcinoma: 20% to 75%
- Malignant mixed tumor: 35% to 75%
- Squamous cell carcinoma: 25% to 60%

REFERENCE
Kaplan MJ, Johns ME: Malignant salivary neoplasms. In Cummings CW (ed): *Otolaryngology: head and neck surgery,* St Louis, 1992, Mosby.
Author: **Tom J. Wachtel, M.D.**

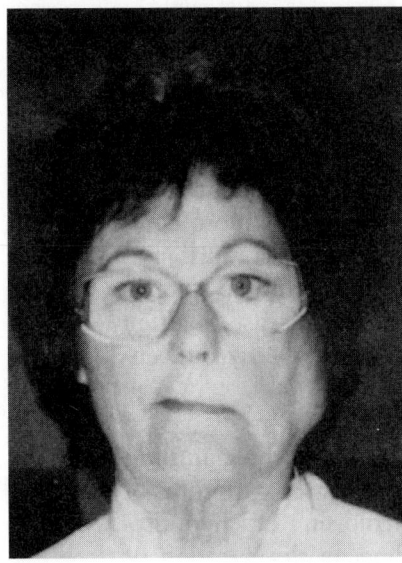

Fig. 1-329 Parotid gland tumor. This woman has a tumor in the left parotid gland, characterized by enlargement of the gland and asymmetry of the left jaw. There appear to be additional lesions present in the left mandible and below the left zygomatic arch. The patient also has paresis of the left facial nerve with drooping of the mouth. That finding raises the concern that the tumor has invaded facial nerve as it passes through the parotid gland. (Courtesy John P. Saunders, Jr., MD. Department of Surgery, Johns Hopkins University and Hospital, Baltimore. In Seidel HM [ed]: *Mosby's guide to physical examination,* ed 4, St Louis, 1999, Mosby.)

BASIC INFORMATION

■ **DEFINITION**
Salmonellosis is an infection caused by one of several serotypes of *Salmonella*.

■ **SYNONYMS**
Typhoid
Typhoid fever
Enteric fever

ICD-9CM CODES
003.0 Salmonellosis

■ **EPIDEMIOLOGY & DEMOGRAPHICS**
INCIDENCE (IN U.S.):
• Estimated 1 million cases/yr of nontyphoidal salmonellosis
• Approximately 500 cases of *S. typhi* infection reported each year
• Largest outbreak: 200,000 persons who ingested contaminated milk
PREDOMINANT AGE:
• <20 yr old
• >70 yr old
• Highest rates of infection in infants, especially neonates
PEAK INCIDENCE: Summer and fall
GENETICS:
Neonatal Infection: Highly susceptible to infection with nontyphoidal *Salmonella*

■ **PHYSICAL FINDINGS & CLINICAL PRESENTATION**
• Infections
  1. Localized to GI tract (gastroenteritis)
  2. Systemic (typhoid fever)
  3. Localized outside of GI tract
• Gastroenteritis
  1. Accounts for majority of disease in humans
  2. Incubation period: generally 12 to 48 hr
  3. Nausea
  4. Vomiting
  5. Diarrhea
  6. Abdominal cramps
  7. Fever
  8. Bacteremia
    a. Uncommon
    b. Occurs mostly in the immunocompromised host or those with underlying conditions
  9. Self-limited illness lasting 3 or 4 days
  10. Colonization of GI tract persistent for months, especially in those treated with antibiotics
• Typhoid fever
  1. Incubation period of few days to several months, usually several weeks
  2. Prolonged fever
  3. Myalgias
  4. Headache

  5. Cough
  6. Sore throat
  7. Malaise
  8. Anorexia
  9. Abdominal pain
  10. Hepatosplenomegaly
  11. Diarrhea or constipation early in the course of illness
  12. Rose spots (faint, maculopapular, blanching lesions) sometimes seen on chest or abdomen
• Untreated disease
  1. Fever lasting 1 to 2 mo
  2. Main complication of untreated disease: GI bleeding caused by perforation from ulceration of Peyer's patches in the ileum (Fig. 1-330)
  3. Rare complications:
    a. Mental status changes
    b. Shock
  4. Relapse rate of approximately 10%
• Infections outside GI tract
  1. Can occur in virtually any location.
  2. Rare.
  3. Usually occur in patients with underlying diseases.
  4. Endovascular infections are caused by seeding of atherosclerotic plaques or aneurysms.
  5. Endocarditis is a rare complication.
  6. Hepatic or splenic abscesses in patients with underlying disease in these organs.
  7. Urinary tract infections in patients with renal TB or schistosomiasis.
  8. Salmonellae are a frequent cause of gram-negative meningitis in neonates.
  9. Osteomyelitis in children with hemoglobinopathies may be caused by these organisms.

■ **ETIOLOGY**
• More than 2000 serotypes of *Salmonella* exist, but only a few cause disease in humans.
• Some found only in humans are the cause of enteric fever.
  1. *S. typhi*
  2. *S. paratyphi*
• Some responsible for gastroenteritis and frequently isolated from raw meat and poultry and uncooked or undercooked eggs.
  1. *S. typhimurium*
  2. *S. enteritidis*
• *S. cholerae-suis* is a prototype organism that causes extraintestinal nontyphoidal disease.
• Transmission generally via ingestion of contaminated food or drink.
• Outbreaks of gastroenteritis related to contaminated poultry, meat, and dairy products.

• Typhoid fever is a systemic illness caused by serotypes exclusive to humans.
  1. Acquisition by ingestion of food or water contaminated by other humans
  2. Most cases in the U.S. are:
    a. Acquired during foreign travel
    b. Acquired by ingestion of food prepared by chronic carriers, many of whom have acquired the organism outside of the U.S.

🔬 **DIAGNOSIS**

■ **DIFFERENTIAL DIAGNOSIS**
• Other causes of prolonged fever:
  1. Malaria
  2. TB
  3. Brucellosis
  4. Amebic liver abscess
• Other causes of gastroenteritis:
  1. Bacterial: *Shigella, Yersinia, Campylobacter*
  2. Viral: Norwalk virus, rotavirus
  3. Parasitic: *Amoeba histolytica, Giardia lamblia*
  4. Toxic: enterotoxigenic *E. coli, Clostridium difficile*

■ **WORKUP**
• Typhoid fever
  1. Cultures of blood, stool, urine; repeat if initially negative.
  2. Blood cultures are more likely to be positive early in the course of illness.
  3. Stool and urine cultures are more commonly positive in the second and third week of illness.
  4. Highest yield with bone marrow biopsy cultures:
    a. 90% positive
    b. Usually not necessary
  5. Serology using Widal's test is helpful in retrospect, showing a fourfold increase in convalescent titers.
• Gastroenteritis: stool cultures
• Extraintestinal localized infection:
  1. Blood cultures
  2. Cultures from the site of infection

■ **LABORATORY TESTS**
• Neutropenia is common.
• Transaminitis is possible.
• Culture to grow organism: blood, body fluids, biopsy specimens

■ **IMAGING STUDIES**
• Radiographs of bone may be suggestive of osteomyelitis.
• CT scan or sonogram of abdomen:
  1. May reveal hepatic or splenic abscesses
  2. May reveal aortic aneurysm

℞ TREATMENT

■ NONPHARMACOLOGIC THERAPY
Adequate hydration and electrolyte replacement in persons with diarrhea

■ ACUTE GENERAL Rx
- Typhoid fever:
  1. Ciprofloxacin 500 mg PO bid or 400 mg IV bid for 14 days
  2. Ceftriaxone 2 g IV qd for 14 days
  3. If sensitive, may switch therapy to TMP/SMX 1 to 2 DS tabs PO bid or amoxicillin 2 g PO q8h to complete 14 days
  4. Dexamethasone 3 mg IV initially, followed by 1 mg IV q6h for eight doses for patients with shock or mental status changes
- Gastroenteritis:
  1. Usually not indicated for gastroenteritis alone because this illness usually self-limited
  2. May prolong the carrier state
  3. Prophylactic treatment for patients who are at high risk of developing complications from bacteremia
     a. Neonates
     b. Patients with hemoglobinopathies
     c. Patients with atherosclerosis
     d. Patients with aneurysms
     e. Patients with prosthetic devices
     f. Immunocompromised patients
  4. Treatment can be oral or parenteral, with the same regimens used for typhoid, but only for 48 to 72 hr
- Intravascular infections require 6 wk of parenteral therapy.

■ CHRONIC Rx
- Carrier states are possible in those with typhoid fever.
- More common in persons >60 yr of age and in persons with gallstones.
- Usual site of colonization is the gallbladder.
- Treatment should be considered for those with persistently positive stool cultures and for food handlers.
- Suggested regimens for eradication of carrier state:
  1. Ciprofloxacin 500 mg PO bid for 4 wk
  2. SMX/TMP one to two DS tabs PO bid for 6 wk (if susceptible)
  3. Amoxicillin 2 g PO q8h for 6 wk (if susceptible)
- Cholecystectomy may be required in carriers with gallstones who fail medical therapy.
- Prolonged course of oral therapy or lifetime suppression for:
  1. Patients with AIDS who have chronic infection
  2. Patients with AIDS who relapse after therapy

■ DISPOSITION
- Typhoid fever
  1. Treated patients usually respond to therapy; small percentage of chronic carriers.
  2. Untreated patients may have serious complications.
- Gastroenteritis
  1. Usually self-limited
  2. May be recurrent or persistent in AIDS patients

■ REFERRAL
- If gastroenteritis is persistent or recurrent
- If there is evidence of extraintestinal infection
- For typhoid fever
- For chronic carriers

☼ PEARLS & CONSIDERATIONS

■ COMMENTS
- Quinolones should not be used in children or pregnant women.
- Infections should be reported to local health departments.

REFERENCES
Benenson S et al: The risk of vascular infections in adult patients with nontyphi *Salmonella bacteremia*, *Am J Med* 110(1):60, 2001.

Outbreaks of multi-drug resistant *Salmonella* typhimurium associated with veterinary facilities. *MMWR* 50(33):701, 2001.

Soravia-Dunand VA et al: Aortitis due to Salmonella: report of 10 cases and comprehensive review of the literature, *Clin Infect Dis* 29:862, 1999.

Author: **Maurice Policar, M.D.**

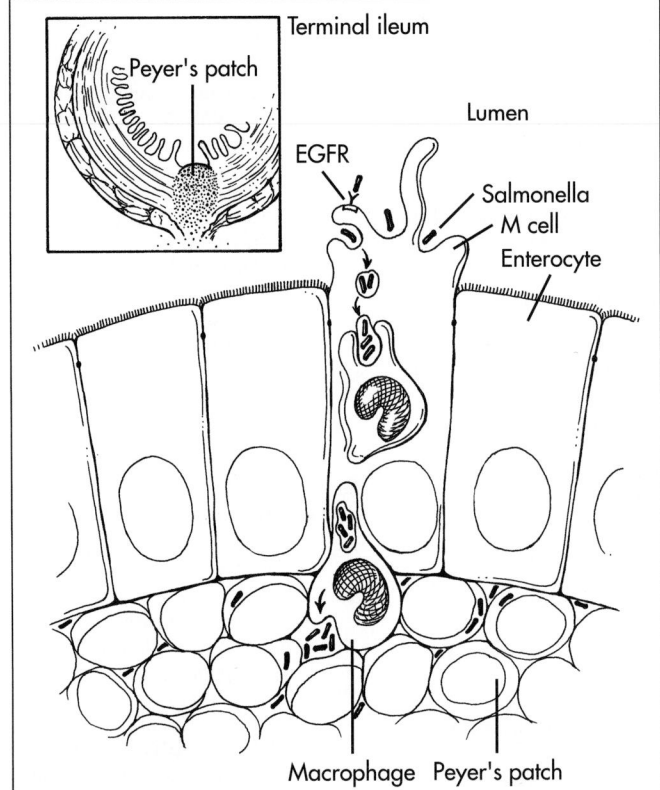

Fig. 1-330 *Salmonella typhi* invade M cells through membrane ruffling and EGF receptor-dependent pathways. Macrophages originating from Peyer's patch take up *S. typhi* in close association with M cells. *S. typhi* replicate in Peyer's patches and then enter the lymphatic system; leading to bacteremia. Replication in Peyer's patches causes hypertrophy followed by necrosis, which can cause intestinal perforation. (From Stein JH [ed]: *Internal medicine*, ed 5, St Louis, 1998, Mosby.)

BASIC INFORMATION

■ DEFINITION

Sarcoidosis is a chronic systemic granulomatous disease of unknown cause, characterized histologically by the presence of nonspecific, noncaseating granulomas.

■ SYNONYMS

Boeck's sarcoid

ICD-9CM CODES

135.0 Sarcoidosis

■ EPIDEMIOLOGY & DEMOGRAPHICS

- Incidence in U.S.: 10.9/100,000 whites, 35.5/100,000 blacks
- Increased incidence in females and patients 20 to 40 yr old
- Presents most commonly in the winter and early spring

■ PHYSICAL FINDINGS & CLINICAL PRESENTATION

- Clinical manifestations often vary with the stage of the disease and degree of organ involvement; patients may be asymptomatic, but a chest x-ray film may demonstrate findings consistent with sarcoidosis (see "Imaging Studies").
- Frequent manifestations:
  1. Pulmonary manifestations: dry, nonproductive cough, dyspnea, chest discomfort
  2. Constitutional symptoms: fatigue, weight loss, anorexia, malaise
  3. Visual disturbances: blurred vision, ocular discomfort, conjunctivitis, iritis, uveitis
  4. Dermatologic manifestations: erythema nodosum, macules, papules, subcutaneous nodules, hyperpigmentation, lupus pernio
  5. Myocardial disturbances: arrhythmias, cardiomyopathy
  6. Splenomegaly, hepatomegaly
  7. Rheumatologic manifestations: arthralgias have been reported in up to 40% of patients
  8. Neurologic and other manifestations: cranial nerve palsies, diabetes insipidus, meningeal involvement, parotid enlargement, hypothalamic and pituitary lesions, peripheral adenopathy

DIAGNOSIS

■ DIFFERENTIAL DIAGNOSIS

- TB
- Lymphoma
- Hodgkin's disease
- Metastases
- Pneumoconioses
- Enlarged pulmonary arteries
- Infectious mononucleosis
- Lymphangitic carcinomatosis
- Idiopathic hemosiderosis
- Alveolar cell carcinoma
- Pulmonary eosinophilia
- Hypersensitivity pneumonitis
- Fibrosing alveolitis
- Collagen disorders
- Parasitic infection

Table 2-85 describes the differential diagnosis of granulomatous lung disease; a classification of granulomatous disorders is described in Box 2-106.

■ WORKUP

- Chest x-ray examination and biopsy
- Biopsy should be done on accessible tissues suspected of sarcoid involvement (conjunctiva, skin, lymph nodes); bronchoscopy with transbronchial biopsy is the procedure of choice in patients without any readily accessible site.

■ LABORATORY TESTS

Laboratory abnormalities:

- Hypergammaglobulinemia, anemia, leukopenia
- Liver function test abnormalities
- Hypercalcemia, hypercalciuria (secondary to increased GI absorption, abnormal vitamin D metabolism, and increased calcitriol production by sarcoid granuloma)
- Cutaneous anergy to *Trichophyton, Candida,* mumps, and tuberculin
- Angiotensin-converting enzyme (ACE): elevated in approximately 60% of patients with sarcoidosis; nonspecific and generally not useful in following the course of the disease

■ IMAGING STUDIES

- Chest x-ray film (Fig. 1-331): adenopathy of the hilar and paratracheal nodes is a frequent finding; parenchymal changes may also be present, depending on the stage of the disease (stage 0, normal x-ray; stage I, bilateral hilar adenopathy; stage II, stage I plus pulmonary infiltrate; stage III, pulmonary infiltrate without adenopathy); stage IV, advanced fibrosis with evidence of honey-combing, hilar retraction, bullae, cysts, and emphysema.

TABLE 1-61 Indications for Use of Corticosteroids in Sarcoidosis

DISORDER	TREATMENT
Iridocyclitis	Corticosteroid eyedrops Local subjunctival deposit of cortisone
Posterior uveitis	Oral prednisone
Pulmonary involvement	Steroids rarely recommended for stage I; usually employed if infiltrate remains static or worsens over 3-mo period or the patient is symptomatic
Upper airway obstruction	Rare indication for intravenous steroids
Lupus pernio	Oral prednisone shrinks the disfiguring lesions
Hypercalcemia	Responds well to corticosteroids
Cardiac involvement	Corticosteroids usually recommended if patient has arrhythmias or conduction disturbances
CNS involvement	Response is best in patients with acute symptoms
Lacrimal/salivary gland involvement	Corticosteroids recommended for disordered function, *not* gland swelling
Bone cysts	Corticosteroids recommended if symptomatic

From Andreoli TE (ed): *Cecil essentials of medicine*, ed 5, Philadelphia, 2001, WB Saunders.
CNS, Central nervous system.

- PFTs: may be normal or may reveal a restrictive pattern and/or obstructive pattern.
- Gallium-67 scan: will localize in areas of granulomatous infiltrates; however, it is not specific. The "panda" sign (localization in the lacrimal and salivary glands, giving a "panda" appearance to the face) is suggestive of sarcoidosis.

 TREATMENT

■ ACUTE GENERAL Rx
- Corticosteroids (Table 1-61) remain the mainstay of therapy when treatment is required (e.g., prednisone 40 mg qd for 8 to 12 wk with gradual tapering of the dose to 10 mg qod over 8 to 12 mo); corticosteroids should be considered in patients with severe symptoms (e.g., dyspnea, chest pain), hypercalcemia, ocular,

CNS, or cardiac involvement, and progressive pulmonary disease.
- Patients with progressive disease refractory to corticosteroids may be treated with methotrexate 7.5 to 15 mg once/week or azathioprine.
- Hydroxychloroquine is effective for chronic disfiguring skin lesions.

■ CHRONIC Rx
- NSAIDs are useful for musculoskeletal symptoms and erythema nodosum.
- Pulmonary rehabilitation in patients with significant respiratory insufficiency.

■ DISPOSITION
The majority of patients with sarcoidosis have spontaneous remission within 2 yr and do not require treatment. Their course can be followed by periodic clinical evaluation, chest x-ray studies, and PFTs.

■ REFERRAL
Ophthalmologic examination is indicated in all patients with suspected sarcoidosis, because ocular findings (iridocyclitis, uveitis, conjunctivitis, and keratopathy) are found in >25% of documented cases.

PEARLS & CONSIDERATIONS

■ COMMENTS
Approximately 15% to 20% of patients with lung involvement advance to irreversible lung impairment (bronchiectasis, cavitation, progressive fibrosis, pneumothorax, and respiratory failure). Death from pulmonary failure occurs in 5% to 7% of patients with sarcoidosis.
Author: **Fred F. Ferri, M.D.**

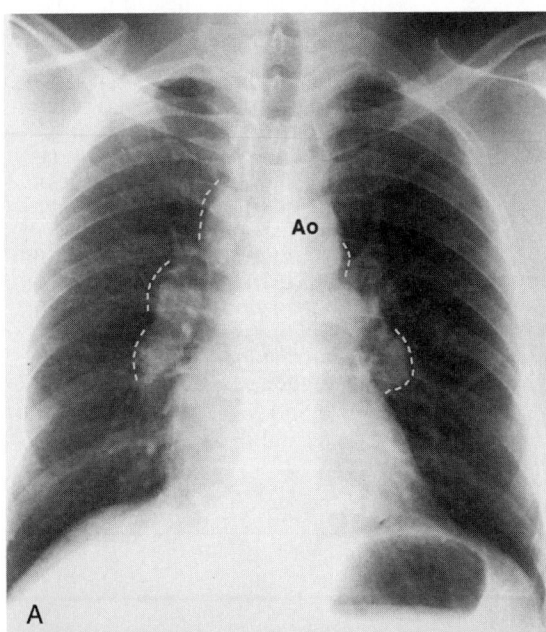
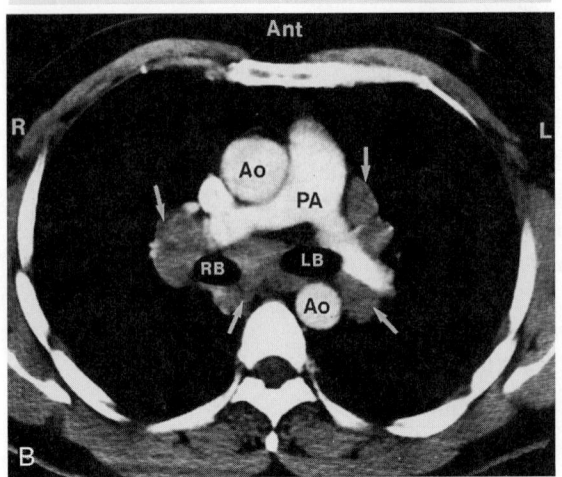

Fig. 1-331 Sarcoid. Marked lymphadenopathy *(dotted lines)* is seen in the region of both hila in the right paratracheal region **(A).** The transverse contrast-enhanced CT scan of the upper chest **(B)** clearly shows the ascending and descending aorta *(Ao)* as well as the pulmonary artery *(PA)* and superior vena cava. The right and left mainstem bronchus area is also seen. The *arrows* indicate the extensive lymphadenopathy. *LB,* Left bronchus; *RB,* right bronchus. (From Mettler FA [ed]: *Primary care radiology,* Philadelphia, 2000, WB Saunders.)

BASIC INFORMATION

■ DEFINITION

Scabies is a contagious disease caused by the mite *Sarcoptes scabiei*.

ICD-9CM CODES
133.0 Scabies

■ EPIDEMIOLOGY & DEMOGRAPHICS

- Scabies is generally acquired by sleeping with or in the bedding of infested individuals.
- It is generally associated with poor living conditions and is also common in hospitals and nursing homes.

■ PHYSICAL FINDINGS & CLINICAL PRESENTATION

- Primary lesions are caused when the female mite burrows within the stratum corneum, laying eggs within the tract she leaves behind; burrows (linear or serpiginous tracts) end with a minute papule or vesicle.
- Primary lesions are most commonly found in the web spaces of the hands, wrists, buttocks, scrotum, penis, breasts, axillae, and knees.
- Secondary lesions result from scratching or infection.
- Intense pruritus, especially nocturnal, is common; it is caused by an acquired sensitivity to the mite or fecal pellets and is usually noted 1 to 4 wk after the primary infestation.
- Examination of the skin may reveal burrows, tiny vesicles, excoriations, inflammatory papules.
- Widespread and crusted lesions (Norwegian or crusted scabies) may be seen in elderly and immunocompromised patients.

■ ETIOLOGY

Human scabies is caused by the mite *Sarcoptes scabiei*, var. *hominis* (Fig. 1-332).

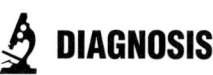

DIAGNOSIS

■ DIFFERENTIAL DIAGNOSIS

- Pediculosis
- Atopic dermatitis
- Flea bites
- Seborrheic dermatitis
- Dermatitis herpetiformis
- Contact dermatitis
- Nummular eczema
- Syphilis
- Other insect infestation
- The differential diagnosis of pruritus is described in Box 2-210.
- A clinical algorithm for the evaluation of generalized pruritus is described in Fig. 3-135.

■ WORKUP

Diagnosis is made on the clinical presentation and on the demonstration of mites, eggs, or mite feces.

■ LABORATORY TESTS

- Microscopic demonstration of the organism, feces, or eggs: a drop of mineral oil may be placed over the suspected lesion before removal; the scrapings are transferred directly to a glass slide; a drop of potassium hydroxide is added and a cover slip is applied.
- Skin biopsy is rarely necessary to make the diagnosis.

TREATMENT

■ NONPHARMACOLOGIC THERAPY

Clothing, underwear, and towels used in the 48 hr before treatment must be laundered.

■ ACUTE GENERAL Rx

- Following a warm bath or shower, Lindane (Kwell, Scabene) lotion should be applied to all skin surfaces below the neck (can be applied to the face if area is infested); it should be washed off 8 to 12 hr after application. Repeat application 1 wk later is usually sufficient to eradicate infestation.
- Pruritus generally abates 24 to 48 hr after treatment, but it can last up to 2 wk; oral antihistamines are effective in decreasing postscabietic pruritus.
- Topical corticosteroid creams may hasten the resolution of secondary eczematous dermatitis.
- If the patient is a resident of an extended care facility, it is important to educate the patients, staff, family, and frequent visitors about scabies and the need to have full cooperation in treatment. Scabicide should be applied to all patients, staff, and frequent visitors, whether symptomatic or not; symptomatic family members of staff and visitors should also receive treatment.
- Permethrin 5% cream (Elimite) is also effective with usually one treatment; it should be massaged into the skin from head to soles of feet; remove 8 to 14 hr later by washing. If living mites are present after 14 days, treat again.
- A single dose (150-200 mg/kg in 6-mg tablets) of ivermectin, an antihelminthic agent, is as effective as topical lindane for the treatment of scabies.

■ DISPOSITION

Refractory cases usually are seen with immunocompromised hosts or patients with underlying skin diseases.

PEARLS & CONSIDERATIONS

■ COMMENTS

- Lindane is potentially neurotoxic and should not be used for infants and pregnant women (permethrin is safe and effective in these situations).
- Sexual partners should be notified and treated.

REFERENCE

Chouela EN et al: Equivalent therapeutic efficacy and safety of ivermectin and lindane in the treatment of human scabies, *Arch Dermatol* 135:651, 1999.
Author: **Fred F. Ferri, M.D.**

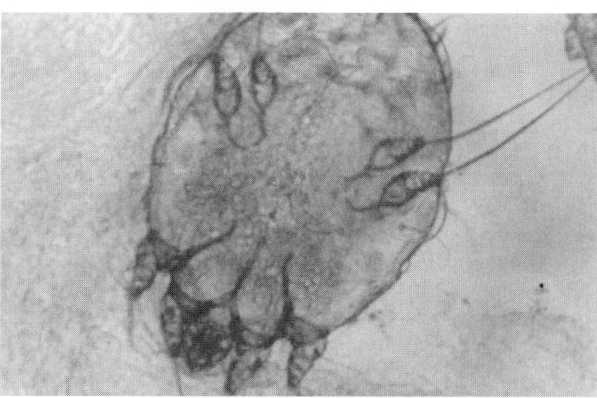

Fig. 1-332   Scabies organism in a wet mount preparation. (From Mandell GL: *Mandell, Douglas, and Bennett's principles and practice of infectious diseases,* ed 5, New York, 2000, Churchill Livingstone.)

BASIC INFORMATION

■ DEFINITION
Scarlet fever is a rash involving skin and tongue and complicating a streptococcal group A pharyngitis.

ICD-9CM CODES
034.1 Scarlet fever

■ EPIDEMIOLOGY & DEMOGRAPHICS
Same as streptococcal pharyngitis; namely, children aged 5 to 15 yr. May also complicate impetigo.

■ PHYSICAL FINDINGS & CLINICAL PRESENTATION
CLINICAL PRESENTATION:
- Febrile illness with headache, malaise, anorexia, and pharyngitis begins after a 2- to 4-day incubation period.
- Scarlatinal rash begins 1 or 2 days after the onset of pharyngitis (Fig. 1-333).

PHYSICAL FINDINGS:
- Diffuse erythema, beginning on face and spreading to neck, back, chest, rest of trunk, and extremities. Most intense on inner aspects of arms and thighs

- Erythema blanches, but nonblanching petechiae may be present or produced by a tourniquet
- Strawberry or raspberry tongue
- Rash lasts about 1 wk and then desquamates

■ ETIOLOGY
Caused by group A β-hemolytic *Streptococcus* infection, which produces one of three erythrogenic toxins (NOTE: Some streptococcal species have the ability to cause both scarlet fever and rheumatic fever)

DIAGNOSIS

■ DIFFERENTIAL DIAGNOSIS
- Viral exanthems (Table 2-50)
- Kawasaki disease
- Toxic shock syndrome
- Drug rashes
See differential diagnosis of pharyngitis in Section I.

■ WORKUP
- Identification of group A *Streptococcus* by throat culture
- SLO antibody titers

TREATMENT

- Penicillin 250 mg PO qid for 10 days or erythromycin 250 mg PO qid for 10 days in penicillin-allergic patients
- Benzathine penicillin 1 to 2 million U IM once; may be used for a patient who cannot swallow

■ COMPLICATIONS (RARE)
- Peritonsillar abscess
- Mastoiditis
- Otitis media
- Pneumonia
- Sepsis and distant foci of infection
- Acute rheumatic fever
- Inability to swallow liquids or upper airway obstruction require hospitalization

NOTE: Failure to respond to penicillin should raise doubt about the diagnosis because *Streptococcus* may be carried in the pharynx without causing infection.

REFERENCE
Stollerman GH: *Streptococcus pyogenes* (group A streptococci). In Gorbach SL, Bartlett JG, Blacklow NR (eds): *Infectious diseases,* ed 2, Philadelphia, 1998, WB Saunders.
Author: **Tom J. Wachtel, M.D.**

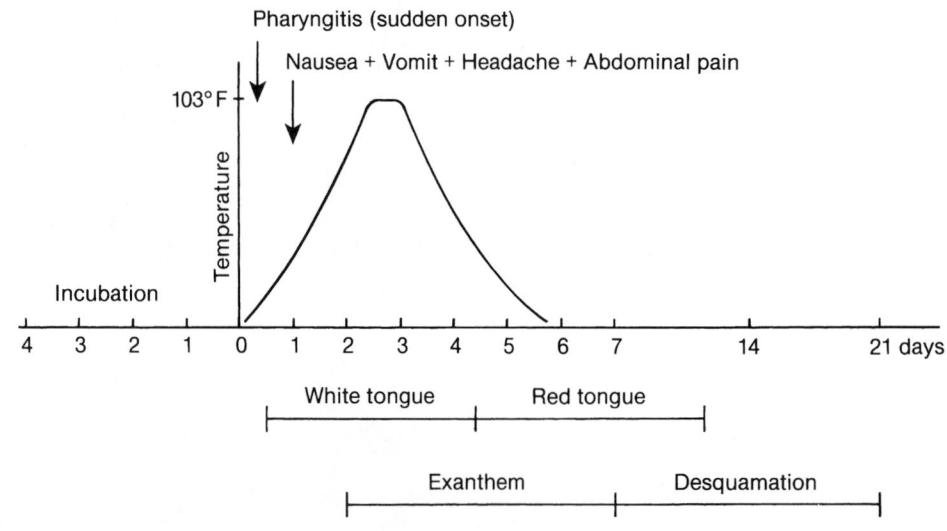

Fig. 1-333 Scarlet fever. Evolution of signs and symptoms. (From Habif TP: *Clinical dermatology: a color guide to diagnosis and therapy,* ed 3, St Louis, 1996, Mosby.)

BASIC INFORMATION

■ DEFINITION

Schizophrenia is diagnosed when an individual has experienced at least 1 mo of hallucinations, delusions, thought disorder, or catatonia and at least 6 mo of decreased function and negative symptoms (avolition, anhedonia, social isolation, affective flattening).

■ SYNONYMS

Dementia praecox

ICD-9CM CODES

295.9 Schizophrenia

■ EPIDEMIOLOGY & DEMOGRAPHICS

PREVALENCE: World: 0.2% to 2%, U.S.: 1%
PREDOMINANT SEX: Males have a more severe illness and therefore skew the gender distribution toward higher in males; however, distribution is probably equal.
PREDOMINANT AGE:
- Age at onset of psychotic symptoms is in the early 20s for males and late 20s for females.
- Age of onset of the negative symptoms is usually earlier (midteenage years).
PEAK INCIDENCE: 20 to 40 yr
GENETICS:
- First-degree relatives of schizophrenics have 10 times greater chance of becoming schizophrenic than the general population.
- Discordant rates among identical twins are higher than expected with simple inheritance pattern.
- Associations with several chromosomes have been described, but none have been replicated.

- Evidence exists that triplet nucleotide repeat expansion (such as seen with Huntington's disease) may play a role in inheritance of the disease.

■ PHYSICAL FINDINGS & CLINICAL PRESENTATION

- Best defined as a dementing illness beginning in early life and progressing slowly throughout the lifetime.
- Initial "negative" symptoms of adolescence—cognitive decline, social withdrawal and awkwardness, loss of motivation and pleasure, and loss of emotional expressiveness—begin after a period of normal development.
- In early adulthood, positive symptoms of psychosis and thought disturbance occur; psychotic symptoms then wax and wane throughout life; treatment ameliorates positive symptoms but generally does little for negative ones.
- Greatest chunk of occupational and social desirability is secondary to negative symptoms.

■ ETIOLOGY

- Unknown.
- Basic distinction of whether this is a degenerative or a developmental condition is not settled.
- Loss of cortical tissue has been established in a series of landmark studies of discordant identical twins.
- Major hypothesis: generation of the mesocortical pathways produce the hypofrontality and negative symptoms, along with a compensatory hyperactivation of the mesolimbic pathways, which produce the positive symptoms of psychosis.

 DIAGNOSIS

■ DIFFERENTIAL DIAGNOSIS

- Any medical condition, medicine, or substance of abuse that can affect brain homeostasis and cause psychosis: distinguished from schizophrenia by their relatively brief course and the alteration in mental status that could suggest an underlying delirium
- Other neurologic conditions (e.g., Huntington's) that have psychosis as the initial presentation
- Other psychiatric disorders: source of greatest confusion
- Mood disorders with psychosis: indistinguishable from schizophrenia cross-sectionally, but have a longitudinal course that includes full recovery
- Delusional disorder: has nonbizarre delusions and lacks the thought disturbance, hallucinations, and negative symptoms of schizophrenia
- Autism in the adult: has an early age at onset and lacks significant hallucinations or delusions

■ WORKUP

- History and physical examination to aid in determining if psychosis is secondary or primary
- Neurologic examination to uncover soft neurologic signs (clumsy, cortical thumb, loss of fine motor movements) common in schizophrenia

■ LABORATORY TESTS

- No laboratory tests are specific for schizophrenia.
- Laboratory examinations (chemistry profile, blood count, sedimentation rate, toxicology screen, and urinalysis) are geared toward excluding a primary medical condition.

■ IMAGING STUDIES

- CT scan or MRI of brain during initial workup; repeated if the course of the illness varies from expected
- Sometimes EEG to reveal slowing when psychosis is secondary to an encephalopathy
- Chest x-ray examination during initial workup to rule out a primary medical condition

▣ TREATMENT

■ NONPHARMACOLOGIC THERAPY

- Significant social support is required by most schizophrenic patients; available support services are grossly inadequate, and schizophrenia patients constitute nearly one third of all homeless individuals. They usually require help with basic social, occupational, and interactive skills.
- For schizophrenic patients who continue to live with their families, relapse rates are related to the degree of emotionality in the family (i.e., schizophrenics living in families with high expressed emotion levels relapse with greater rates), so family interventions can sometimes reduce morbidity.
- Traditional psychotherapy is usually not useful in schizophrenia, but supportive psychotherapy may reduce suicide rate.

■ ACUTE GENERAL Rx

- Acute psychosis is usually adequately controlled by antipsychotic agents.
- Mainstay of therapy is traditional neuroleptics (e.g., haloperidol, perphenazine, fluphenazine, chlorpromazine) and the newer atypical antipsychotics (e.g., risperidone, olanzapine, clozapine), which usually block dopamine and can cause a parkinsonian state; antiparkinsonian drugs (benztropine, amantadine) can frequently ameliorate these side effects.
- Sedatives (benzodiazepines, and to a lesser degree, barbiturates) can be used transiently if there is an agitated state.

■ CHRONIC Rx

- Compliance is long-term focus of treatment; relapse rates are quite high in noncompliant patients. Antipsychotic agents usually must be continued at the same doses that controlled psychosis. For noncompliant patients, depot preparations that are given biweekly or monthly can be used.
- Antiparkinsonian agents may also need to be continued chronically.
- Tardive dyskinesia (choreoathetoid movements of the muscles of tongue, face, and occasionally other muscle groups) can occur in as many as 30% of patients with long-term use of the neuroleptics.
- The negative symptoms of schizophrenia can resemble depression. Additionally, depressive disorders may occur in schizophrenic patients. Antidepressant treatment of the negative symptoms is usually without effect. However, antidepressants can improve the symptoms of a discrete comorbid depressive episode.
- Mood stabilizers, such as lithium, valproate, or carbamazepine, are of little use unless there is a comorbid impulse control disorder.
- Substance abuse is a major problem in more than one third of schizophrenics. Unfortunately, these patients do poorly in traditional substance abuse treatment programs. Specialized "dual diagnosis" programs with highly structured aftercare are required.

■ DISPOSITION

- The positive symptoms of as many as 20% to 30% of schizophrenic patients do not respond to available treatments. A much higher fraction relapse as a result of poor compliance.
- The negative symptoms are responsible for the 50% to 70% of cases in which deterioration in occupational and social function continues.
- More than 10% of patients will complete suicide.

■ REFERRAL

- If hospitalization is required
- If patient is noncompliant
- If patient is resistant to treatment

REFERENCE

Mortensen PB et al: Effects of family history and place and season of birth on the rise of schizophrenia, *N Engl J Med* 340:603, 1999.

Authors: **Rif S. El-Mallakh, M.D., and Peggy L. El-Mallakh, B.S.N.**

BASIC INFORMATION

■ **DEFINITION**

Scleritis is inflammation of the sclera.

■ **SYNONYMS**

Anterior scleritis
Diffuse nodular, necrotizing scleritis
Scleromalacia perforans

■ **ICD-9CM CODES**

379.0 Scleritis and episcleritis

■ **EPIDEMIOLOGY & DEMOGRAPHICS**

INCIDENCE (IN U.S.): Busy ophthalmologist may see one or two cases a year
PREVALENCE (IN U.S.): Relatively rare
PREDOMINANT SEX: 61% women
PREDOMINANT AGE: 52 yr
PEAK INCIDENCE: Increases with increasing age

■ **PHYSICAL FINDINGS & CLINICAL PRESENTATION**

• Deep, boring eye pain
• Photophobia
• Tearing
• Conjunctival injection (Fig. 1-334)
• Thinning of the sclera

■ **ETIOLOGY**

• Inflammatory
• Allergic
• Toxic

 DIAGNOSIS

■ **DIFFERENTIAL DIAGNOSIS**

• Most common causes are rheumatoid arthritis and collagen-vascular disease.
• Occasionally, there are allergic, infectious, or traumatic causes.
• Conjunctivitis, iritis, and episcleritis should be considered in the differential diagnosis.

■ **WORKUP**

• Fluorescein angiography
• Eye examination
• Visual field examination
• Workup for autoimmune disease

■ **LABORATORY TESTS**

• Usually not necessary
• RF, ANA, ESR may be useful

■ **IMAGING STUDIES**

Usually not necessary; CT scan of orbit may be useful in selected patients

TREATMENT

■ **NONPHARMACOLOGIC THERAPY**

• Patching
• Bandage lenses
• Surgery if thinning of the sclera is severe

■ **ACUTE GENERAL Rx**

• Steroids (topical, periocular, and systemic)
• Cycloplegic drops
• NSAIDs (topical and systemic)
• Other immunosuppressive drugs

■ **CHRONIC Rx**

• Systemic steroids can be given for the underlying disease.
• Local steroids may be helpful.

■ **DISPOSITION**

Urgent referral to ophthalmologist

■ **REFERRAL**

If not referred to an ophthalmologist early, patients may develop uveitis and other complications.

PEARLS & CONSIDERATIONS

■ **COMMENTS**

An ominous diagnosis because these patients often have other severe underlying debilitating disease processes.
Author: **Melvyn Koby, M.D.**

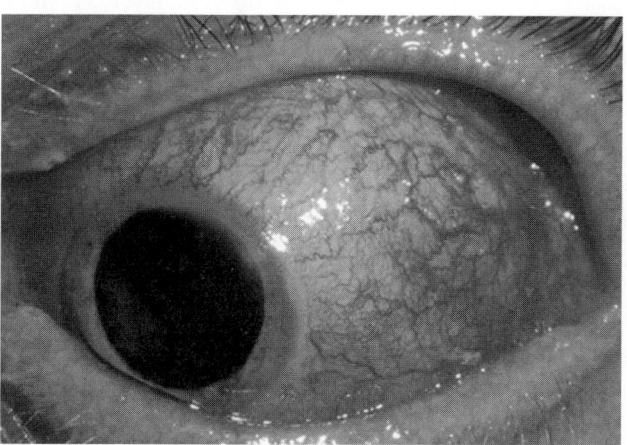

Fig. 1-334 In diffuse anterior scleritis, widespread injection of the conjunctival and deep episcleral vessels occurs. (From Palay D [ed]: *Ophthalmology for the primary care physician,* St Louis, 1997, Mosby.)

BASIC INFORMATION

■ DEFINITION
Scleroderma is a connective tissue disorder characterized by thickening and fibrosis of the skin and variably severe involvement of diverse internal organs.

■ SYNONYMS
Systemic sclerosis; morphea applies to localized scleroderma affecting only the skin. Scleredema is a disease of the skin distinct from scleroderma.

■ ICD-9CM CODES
710.1 (morphea: 701.0)

■ EPIDEMIOLOGY & DEMOGRAPHICS
INCIDENCE: 4 to 12 cases/million persons per year, but many mild cases go unrecognized
DEMOGRAPHICS: Female:male ratio of 4:1
PEAK AGE: 30 to 50 yr
DISTRIBUTION: Worldwide

■ PHYSICAL FINDINGS & CLINICAL PRESENTATION
CLINICAL PRESENTATION:
- Raynaud's phenomenon: initial complaint in 70% (NOTE: The prevalence of Raynaud's is 5% to 10% of the general population; most do not progress to scleroderma)
- Finger or hand swelling, sometimes associated with carpal tunnel syndrome
- Arthralgias/arthritis
- Internal organ involvement

PHYSICAL FINDINGS:
Skin
- Begins on hands, then face; skin is shiny, taut, sometimes red with loss of creases and hair
- Later skin tightening may limit movement
- Pigmentary changes occur
- Skin atrophy occurs in late stages
Musculoskeletal
- Symmetric inflammatory arthritis
- Myopathy
GI involvement
- Esophageal dysmotility with heartburn, dysphagia, odynophagia
- Delayed gastric emptying
- Small bowel dysmotility with abdominal cramps and diarrhea
- Colon dysmotility with constipation
- Primary biliary cirrhosis (see "Primary Biliary Cirrhosis" in Section I)
Pulmonary manifestations
- Pulmonary fibrosis with symptoms of dyspnea and nonproductive cough and fine inspiratory crackles on examination
- Pulmonary hypertension
Cardiac involvement
- Myocardial fibrosis leading to congestive heart failure
Renal involvement
- Malignant hypertension
- Rapidly progressive renal failure
Other organ involvement
- Hypothyroidism
- Erectile dysfunction
- Sjögren's syndrome
- Entrapment neuropathies
CREST syndrome
- Calcinosis, Raynaud's syndrome, esophageal dysmotility, sclerodactyly, telangiectasias (in CREST scleroderma is limited to distal extremities)

■ ETIOLOGY
Etiology is unknown. Unifying features exist in spite of heterogenous patterns of organ involvement and disease progression:
- Extracellular connective tissue activation
- Frequent immunologic abnormalities
- Inflammation
- Vasoconstriction

DIAGNOSIS

■ DIFFERENTIAL DIAGNOSIS
Dermatologic
- Mycosis fungoides
- Amyloidosis
- Porphyria cutanea tarda
- Eosinophilic fasciitis
- Reflex sympathetic dystrophy
Systemic
- Idiopathic pulmonary fibrosis
- Primary pulmonary hypertension
- Primary biliary cirrhosis
- Cardiomyopathies
- GI dysmotility problems
- SLE and overlap syndromes

■ WORKUP
Laboratory tests and imaging studies

■ LABORATORY TESTS
- Antinuclear antibodies (homogeneous, speckled, or nucleolar patterns)
- Negative antibody to native DNA
- Negative anti-Sm antibody
- Anti-nRNP positive in 20%
- Rheumatoid factor positive in 30%
- Anticentromere antibodies in fewer than 10% with systemic illness and in 50% to 95% with limited scleroderma (i.e., good prognosis if positive)
- Positive extractable nuclear antibody to SCL 70 in 30%
- Routine biochemistry tests may indicate specific organ involvement (e.g., liver, kidney, muscle)

■ IMAGING AND OTHER STUDIES
Arthritis: joint x-rays
GI
- Barium swallow
- Cine esophagography
- Endoscopy
- Esophageal manometry
Pulmonary
- Chest x-ray
- PFTs
- Chest CT scan
- Bronchoscopy with biopsy
- Gallium lung scan
- Bronchoalveolar lavage
Heart
- ECG
- Ambulatory (Holter) ECG monitoring
- Echocardiography
- Cardiac catheterization
Kidney: renal biopsy
Skin: skin biopsy

TREATMENT

D-penicillamine; recombinant human relaxin; supportive therapies used.
Raynaud's syndrome:
- Calcium channel blockers
- Peripheral α_1-adrenergic blockers
Arthralgias: NSAIDs
Skin: moisturizing agents
Esophageal reflux
- H_2-receptor blockers
- Proton pump inhibitors
Pulmonary hypertension and fibrosis
- Oxygen
- Lung transplant
Renal involvement
- Angiotensin-converting enzyme inhibitors
- Dialysis
- Renal transplantation

■ REFERRAL
To rheumatologist

REFERENCES
Seibold JR: Scleroderma. In Kelley WN et al (eds): *Textbook of rheumatology,* ed 5, Philadelphia, 1997, WB Saunders.
Seibold JR, Koan JH, Simms R, et al: Recombinant human relaxin in the treatment of scleroderma, *Ann Intern Med* 132:871, 2000.
Author: **Tom J. Wachtel, M.D.**

BASIC INFORMATION

■ DEFINITION

Scoliosis is a lateral curvature of the spine in the upright position, usually 10 degrees or greater. Scoliosis may be classified as either structural (fixed, nonflexible) or nonstructural (flexible, correctable).

ICD-9CM CODES

737.30 Idiopathic scoliosis
737.39 Paralytic scoliosis
754.2   Congenital scoliosis
724.3   Sciatic scoliosis
737.43 Associated with neuro-fibromatosis

■ EPIDEMIOLOGY & DEMOGRAPHICS (IDIOPATHIC FORM)

PREVALENCE: 4 cases/1000 persons
PREVALENT AGE:
- Onset is variable.
- Most curves are found in adolescents (age 11 yr and over).

PREDOMINANT SEX: Females > male (7:1)

■ PHYSICAL FINDINGS & CLINICAL PRESENTATION

- Record patient age (in years plus months) and height.
- Perform neurologic examination to rule out neuromuscular disease.
- Inspect the shoulders and iliac crests to determine if they are level.
- Palpate the spinous processes to determine their alignment.
- Have the patient bend forward symmetrically at the waist with the arms hanging free (Adams' position); observe from the back or front to detect abnormal spine rotation (Fig. 1-335).

■ ETIOLOGY

- 90% unknown, usually referred to as idiopathic (genetic)
- Congenital spine deformity
- Neuromuscular disease
- Leg length inequality
- Local inflammation or infection
- Acute pain (disk disease)
- Chronic degenerative disc disease with a symmetric disc narrowing

Curves of an idiopathic nature or those accompanying congenital deformity or neuromuscular disease are those associated with structural changes. The nonstructural types (leg length discrepancy, inflammation, or acute pain) disappear when the offending disorder is corrected.

DIAGNOSIS

■ WORKUP

- Curvatures associated with congenital spine abnormalities, neuromuscular disease, and the other less common forms of scoliosis can usually be identified by history or associated radiographic or physical findings.
- Fig. 1-336 describes an approach to scoliosis screening.

■ IMAGING STUDIES

- Diagnosis of idiopathic scoliosis is confirmed by a standing roentgenogram of the spine.
- Severity of the curve is measured in degrees, usually by the Cobb method.
- MRI is usually not indicated unless there is: (1) pain, (2) a neurologic deficit, or (3) a left thoracic curve (which is often associated with an underlying spinal disorder).

TREATMENT

■ ACUTE GENERAL Rx

- Treatment or correction of cause if curve is nonstructural
- Early detection is key in treating genetic curve
- Regular observation for curves <20 degrees
- Bracing for idiopathic curves of 20 to 40 degrees to prevent progression
- Surgery for idiopathic curves >40 degrees in immature patient

■ DISPOSITION

- The larger the curve at detection, the greater the chance of progression.
- Progression is more common in young children who are beginning their growth spurt.

- Curves in females are more likely to progress.
- Curves <20 degrees will improve spontaneously more than 50% of the time.
- Failure to diagnose and treat these curves may produce progressive deformity, pain, and cardiopulmonary compromise.
- Spinal deformities >50 degrees in adults may progress and eventually become painful.

■ REFERRAL

For orthopedic consultation if structural curve is present

PEARLS & CONSIDERATIONS

■ COMMENTS

Congenital scoliosis has a high incidence of cardiac and urinary tract abnormalities.

REFERENCES

Lenke LG et al: Adolescent idiopathic scoliosis, *J Bone Joint Surg* 83(A):1169, 2001.
Reamy BV, Slakey JB: Adolescent idiopathic scoliosis: review and current concepts, *Am Fam Physician* 64:111, 2001.
Yawn BP: Population-based study of school scoliosis screening; *JAMA* 282:1427, 1999.

Author: **Lonnie R. Mercier, M.D.**

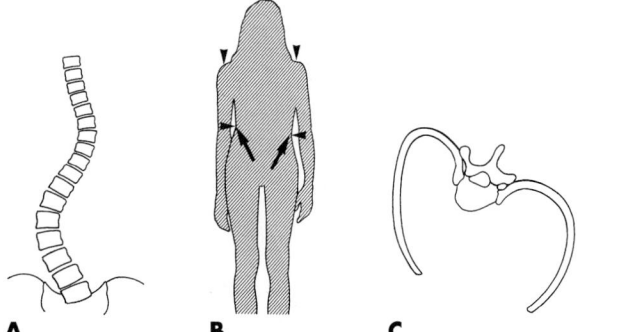

Fig. 1-335   Structural changes in idiopathic scoliosis. **A,** As curvature increases, alterations in body configuration develop in both the primary and compensatory curve regions. **B,** Asymmetry of shoulder height, waistline, and the elbow-to-flank distance are common findings. **C,** Vertebral rotation and associated posterior displacement of the ribs on the convex side of the curve are responsible for the characteristic deformity of the chest wall in scoliosis patients. **D,** In the school screening examination for scoliosis, the patient bends forward at the waist. Rib asymmetry of even a small degree is obvious. (From Scoles PV: Spinal deformity in childhood and adolescence. In Behrman RE, Vaughn VC III [eds]: *Nelson textbook of pediatrics,* ed 5, Philadelphia, 1989, WB Saunders.)

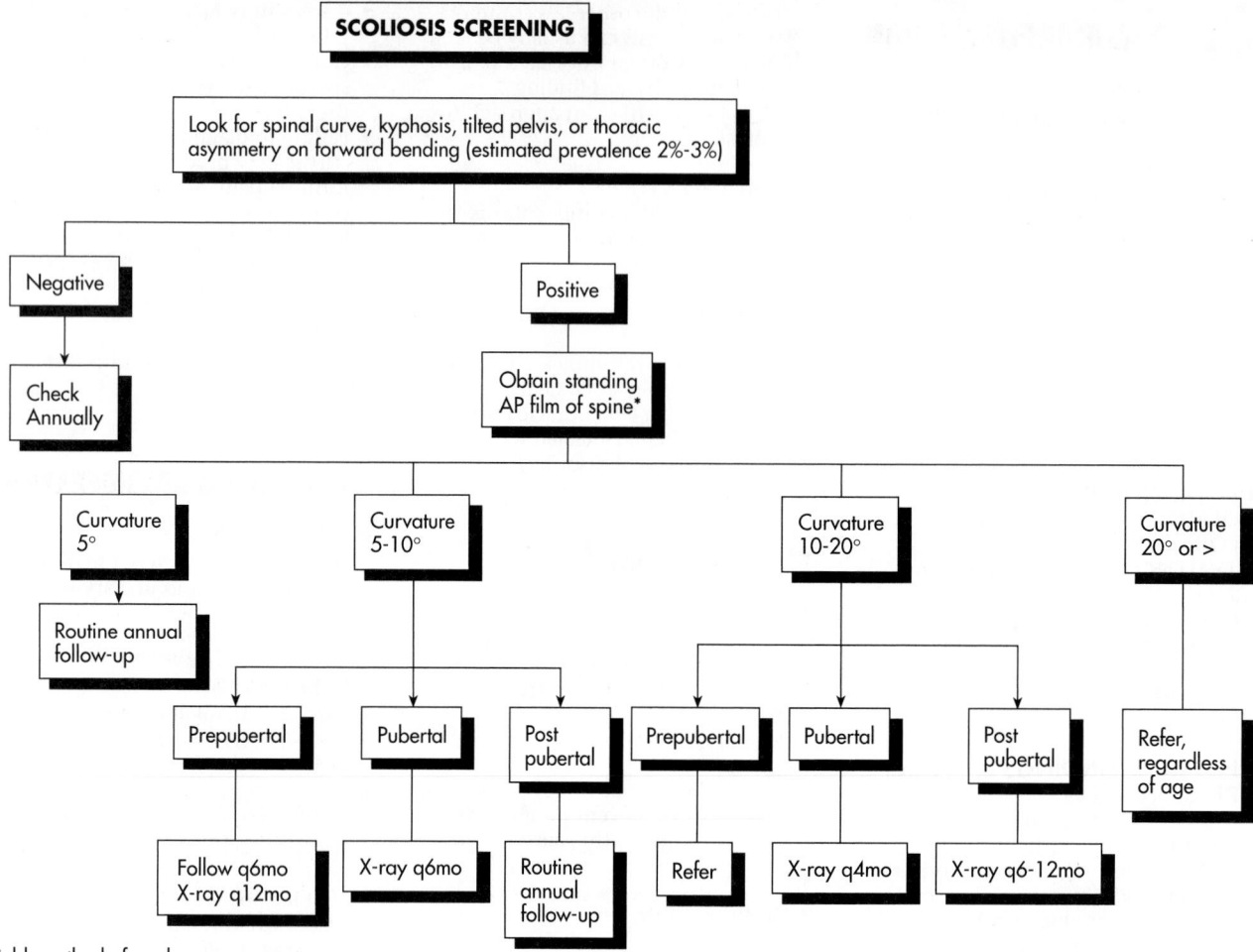

*Cobb method of angle measurement

1. Find the lowest vertebra whose bottom tilts toward concavity of curve.
2. Erect a perpendicular line from extension of bottom surface.
3. Find highest vertebra as in #1 and erect perpendicular from extension of top surface.
4. Measure intersecting angle = angle of scoliosis.

Fig. 1-336   Scoliosis screening and follow-up. *AP,* Anteroposterior. (From Driscoll C [ed]: *The family practice desk reference,* ed 3, St Louis, 1996, Mosby.)

BASIC INFORMATION

DEFINITION
Absence seizures are a type of generalized nonconvulsive seizure characterized by brief loss of consciousness (typically ≤15 sec) associated with a 3-sec generalized spike and slow wave EEG pattern, followed by abrupt return to full consciousness.

SYNONYMS
Petit mal seizures (obsolete)

ICD-9CM CODES
345.0 Generalized nonconvulsive epilepsy

EPIDEMIOLOGY & DEMOGRAPHICS
INCIDENCE (IN U.S.): 11 cases/100,000 persons from ages 1 through 10 yr, rare after age 14 yr
PREVALENCE (IN U.S.): 6.5 cases/1000 persons for all types of epilepsy
PREDOMINANT SEX: Female:male ratio of 2:1
PREDOMINANT AGE: 1 to 10 yr
PEAK INCIDENCE: 5 to 10 yr
GENETICS: Clear genetic predisposition; undetermined mode of inheritance

PHYSICAL FINDINGS & CLINICAL PRESENTATION
- Findings are normal between seizures in children with typical absence epilepsy.
- During seizure, patient typically appears awake but abruptly ceases ongoing activity and does not respond to or recall stimuli.

- More prolonged episodes may be associated with automatisms and therefore mistaken for complex partial seizures.

ETIOLOGY
- Unknown
- Experimental data: seizures arise from impaired regulation of rhythmic thalamic discharges

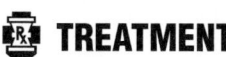

DIAGNOSIS

DIFFERENTIAL DIAGNOSIS
- Complex partial seizures
- Fatigue
- Daydreaming
- Psychogenic unresponsiveness
- Table 1-62 describes the differential diagnosis of epilepsy.

WORKUP
- EEG is the most powerful tool for identification of this seizure type.
- In the vast majority of untreated individuals, vigorous hyperventilation for 3 to 5 min provokes characteristic EEG finding.

IMAGING STUDIES
None needed for typical presentation

TREATMENT

NONPHARMACOLOGIC THERAPY
- Avoid sleep deprivation.
- Some patients are photosensitive.

ACUTE GENERAL Rx
Not indicated for individual seizures

CHRONIC Rx
- Drug of choice is ethosuximide. Initial dose for adults and children >6 yr is 500 mg/day.
- Sodium valproate is also effective.

DISPOSITION
- Favorable prognosis in typical childhood absence epilepsy without other seizure types
- Excellent response to medication
- Subsidence of seizures with advancing age in 70% to 90% of patients

REFERRAL
If uncertain about diagnosis

PEARLS & CONSIDERATIONS

COMMENTS
- Absence seizures may be mistakenly diagnosed as complex partial seizures based on clinical descriptions. The EEG is essential for making this distinction.
- Administering other anticonvulsants (particularly carbamazepine or phenytoin) to patients with typical absence epilepsy may exacerbate seizures.
- Patient education information can be obtained from the Epilepsy Foundation of America, 4351 Garden City Drive, Landover, MD 20785; phone: (800) EFA-1000.

REFERENCE
Quality Standards Subcommittee of the American Academy of Neurology: Practice parameter: management issues for women with epilepsy, *Neurology* 51:944, 1998.
Author: **Michael Gruenthal, M.D., Ph.D.**

TABLE 1-62 **Comparison of Childhood Absence, Juvenile Absence, and Juvenile Myoclonic Epilepsy**

	CHILDHOOD ABSENCE	JUVENILE ABSENCE	JUVENILE MYOCLONIC
Age of onset	3-12 yr	Puberty	Puberty
Frequency	Multiple daily	Rarely daily	Variable
EEG epileptiform activity	3 Hz spike wave	3.5-4 Hz spike wave	3.5-6 Hz spike wave
Generalized tonic-clonic	≤40	60%-80% (adolescence)	80%-85%
Medications	Ethosuximide, valproate	Valproate, ethosuximide	Valproate
Therapy length	Short*	Short or prolonged	Lifelong
Genetic	+	+	Chromosome 6p21.3
Prognosis	Favorable	Favorable	Favorable

From Johnson RT, Griffin JW: *Current therapy in neurologic disease,* ed 5, St Louis, 1997, Mosby.
*Generally short duration of treatment would be 2 years seizure free. Specific duration of treatment is variable; average age of cessation is 10.6 years.

BASIC INFORMATION

■ **DEFINITION**
Generalized tonic-clonic seizure disorder is marked by paroxysmal hypersynchronous neuronal activity involving both cerebral hemispheres and resulting in loss of consciousness and tonic muscle contraction followed by rhythmic clonic contractions.

■ **SYNONYMS**
All obsolete:
Grand mal seizure
Major motor seizure

ICD-9CM CODES
345.1 Generalized convulsive epilepsy

■ **EPIDEMIOLOGY & DEMOGRAPHICS**
INCIDENCE (IN U.S.): 10 cases/100,000 persons/yr between ages 10 and 65 yr; higher in older age groups
PREVALENCE (IN U.S.): 6.5 cases/1000 persons for all types of epilepsy
PREDOMINANT SEX: Males slightly higher than females
PREDOMINANT AGE: 80 yr
PEAK INCIDENCE: >65 yr old
GENETICS: Genetic predisposition exists for many of the primary generalized epilepsies; mode of transmission varies with the particular epilepsy syndrome.

■ **PHYSICAL FINDINGS & CLINICAL PRESENTATION**
• Generally normal
• Possible focal deficits in patients with secondary generalized tonic-clonic seizures, depending on underlying etiology

■ **ETIOLOGY**
• Seizures are a symptom of an underlying abnormality affecting the CNS, not a disease.
• In idiopathic generalized tonic-clonic seizures, the postulated inherited cellular abnormality remains undetermined.
• Secondary (symptomatic) generalized tonic-clonic seizures may result from several underlying causes, including inborn errors of metabolism, acquired metabolic abnormalities, CNS infection, and neuronal migration abnormalities.
• Secondary generalized tonic-clonic seizures (i.e., with partial onset) may be caused by tumors, infection, trauma, vascular malformations, or genetic predisposition.

 DIAGNOSIS

■ **DIFFERENTIAL DIAGNOSIS**
• Syncope
• Psychogenic events
• Table 2-58 describes the differential diagnosis of epilepsy.

■ **WORKUP**
New-onset seizures: a detailed history and physical examination with the goal of determining the underlying etiology

■ **LABORATORY TESTS**
• Serum glucose and electrolytes
• Additional blood studies as indicated by history and physical examination
• EEG: most valuable diagnostic tool for identifying seizure type and predicting the likelihood of recurrence

■ **IMAGING STUDIES**
• Generally not necessary in well-documented cases of idiopathic generalized tonic-clonic seizures
• MRI: modality of choice if history, examination, or EEG suggest partial (focal) onset

TREATMENT

■ **NONPHARMACOLOGIC THERAPY**
Avoid sleep deprivation or environmental precipitants (e.g., photosensitive epilepsy).

■ **ACUTE GENERAL Rx**
• Individual seizures lasting <5 min generally require no acute pharmacologic intervention.
• See "Status Epilepticus" in Section I for management of recurrent seizures.

■ **CHRONIC Rx**
• A single seizure with an identifiable and easily correctable provoking factor (e.g., hyponatremia) does not warrant long-term use of anticonvulsants.
• If there is significant risk of recurrence (Table 1-63) or more than one unprovoked seizure, treatment is indicated.
• The appropriate medication depends on several factors. In general, sodium valproate is the drug of choice for patients >4 yr of age with idiopathic generalized tonic-clonic epilepsy.

■ **DISPOSITION**
• Varies with underlying etiology
• Excellent outcome for most patients with idiopathic generalized tonic-clonic seizures

■ **REFERRAL**
If uncertain about diagnosis or seizure type

PEARLS & CONSIDERATIONS

■ **CAUTION**
• EEG is normal in as many as 50% of patients; thus diagnosis is primarily by history. Usually, a single seizure is not treated wtih chronic anticoagulants.

REFERENCES
Browne TR, Holmes GL: Epilepsy, *N Engl J Med* 344:1145, 2001.
Quality Standards Subcommittee of the American Academy of Neurology: Practice parameter: management issues for women with epilepsy, *Neurology* 51:944, 1998.
Author: **Michael Gruenthal, M.D., Ph.D.**

TABLE 1-63 **Risk of Recurrence After a First Tonic-Clonic Seizure**

HIGH	LOW
Abnormal neurologic findings	Febrile seizure in a child
Mental retardation	Febrile status epilepticus (child)
Abnormal EEG findings	Transient metabolic and toxic states
Myoclonic jerks, absences, or atonic seizures	Benign rolandic seizures
Structural brain lesions	Impact seizures in early nonsevere head trauma
Family history of epilepsy	
Elderly individuals	

From Johnson RT, Griffin JW: *Current therapy in neurologic disease,* ed 5, St Louis, 1997, Mosby. *EEG,* Electroencephalogram.

BASIC INFORMATION

DEFINITION
In partial seizure disorder, seizures occur in which the onset of abnormal electrical activity is confined to one hemisphere. Clinical manifestations may involve sensory, motor, autonomic, or psychic symptoms. Consciousness may be preserved (simple partial seizures) or impaired (complex partial seizures).

SYNONYMS
All obsolete:
Minor motor seizures
Jacksonian seizures
Psychomotor seizures

ICD-9CM CODES
345.5 Partial epilepsy, without mention of impairment of consciousness

EPIDEMIOLOGY & DEMOGRAPHICS
INCIDENCE (IN U.S.): 20 cases/100,000 persons through age 65 yr, then rises sharply
PREVALENCE (IN U.S.): 6.5 cases/1000 persons for all types of epilepsy
PREDOMINANT SEX: Males slightly higher than females
PREDOMINANT AGE: >60 yr
PEAK INCIDENCE: >65 yr
GENETICS: Most acquired, but several distinct inherited syndromes have been identified.

PHYSICAL FINDINGS & CLINICAL PRESENTATION
Range from normal to focal neurologic deficits, depending on underlying cause

ETIOLOGY
- Seizures are a symptom of an underlying abnormality affecting the CNS, not a disease.
- Partial-onset seizures may be caused by underlying disorders, including stroke, tumor, infection, trauma, vascular malformations, or genetic factors.

DIAGNOSIS

DIFFERENTIAL DIAGNOSIS
- Migraine
- TIA
- Presyncope
- Psychogenic phenomena
- Table 2-58 describes the differential diagnosis of epilepsy.

WORKUP
Because partial seizures are manifestations of an underlying focal CNS disturbance that must be identified if possible, imaging studies, preferably MRI, are essential.

LABORATORY TESTS
EEG is the most powerful tool for localization of the seizure focus.

IMAGING STUDIES
- MRI with contrast: modality of choice because of its high sensitivity for stroke, tumor, abscess, atrophy, and vascular malformations
- CT scan without contrast if hemorrhage is suspected

TREATMENT

NONPHARMACOLOGIC THERAPY
Avoid sleep deprivation.

ACUTE GENERAL Rx
- Individual seizures lasting <5 min generally require no acute pharmacologic intervention.
- For management of recurrent seizures, see "Status Epilepticus" in Section I.

CHRONIC Rx
Carbamazepine or phenytoin are common first-line therapeutic agents (Table 1-64).

- Sodium valproate may also be effective.
- For each patient, choice is influenced by factors such as effectiveness, cost, adverse effects, and ease of administration.

DISPOSITION
- Determined by underlying cause
- Approximately 70% of patients controlled with medication

REFERRAL
If uncertain about diagnosis or patient fails to respond to appropriate medication

PEARLS & CONSIDERATIONS

COMMENTS
- Patient education information can be obtained from the Epilepsy Foundation of America, 4351 Garden City Drive, Landover, MD 20785; phone: (800) EFA-1000.
- This is the most underdiagnosed, yet the most common, type of seizures in adults.

REFERENCE
Wiebe S et al: A randomized controlled trial of surgery for temporal-lobe epilepsy, *N Engl J Med* 345:311, 2001.
Author: **Michael Gruenthal, M.D., Ph.D.**

TABLE 1-64 Drugs of Choice in Treatment of Epilepsy

SEIZURE TYPE	DRUGS OF CHOICE*
Generalized tonic clonic, simple, and complex partial	Phenytoin, valproic acid
	Carbamazepine
	Primidone
	Phenobarbital, levetiracetam, zonisamide
Absence	Ethosuximide
	Valproic acid
Benign centrotemporal epilepsy	Phenytoin, gabapentin
	Phenobarbital
Neonatal seizures	Phenobarbital
Febrile seizures	Phenobarbital
	Valproic acid
Infantile spasms	ACTH, vigabatrin
Lennox-Gastaut syndrome	Felbamate
	Clonazepam, lamotrigine, topiramate
Newer drugs	
Generalized tonic clonic, simple, partial, and complex partial	Lamotrigine
	Tigabine
	Topiramate
	Zonisamide
	Oxcarbazepine
	Levetiracetam
	Gabapentin

*Drugs are listed in order of preference.

BASIC INFORMATION

■ **DEFINITION**
A febrile seizure is a single tonic or tonic-clonic seizure without focal features, lasting <15 min, provoked by a fever from a source outside the CNS.

■ **SYNONYMS**
Benign febrile seizure

ICD-9CM CODES
780.3 Convulsions

■ **EPIDEMIOLOGY & DEMOGRAPHICS**
INCIDENCE (IN U.S.): Not reported
PREVALENCE (IN U.S.): 2% to 4% in children <5 yr of age
PREDOMINANT SEX: Male = female
PREDOMINANT AGE: 18 to 22 mo
PEAK INCIDENCE: 6 mo to 5 yr; 90% occur by age 3 yr
GENETICS:
• Family history increases risk two to three times.
• Mode of inheritance is unknown.

■ **PHYSICAL FINDINGS & CLINICAL PRESENTATION**
• Typically occur early in the course of an illness when temperature is rising.
• Most commonly associated with a viral upper respiratory infection.
• Physical and neurologic examination and developmental history may be normal.

■ **ETIOLOGY**
Unknown

 DIAGNOSIS

■ **DIFFERENTIAL DIAGNOSIS**
• Epilepsy
• Meningitis
• Encephalitis
• Intracranial mass
The differential diagnosis of pediatric seizures is described in Box 2-225.

■ **WORKUP**
• Typical presentation: child between 6 mo and 5 yr with a family history of simple febrile seizures; no further evaluation is usually required
• Atypical presentations: seizures lasting >15 min, focal features or recurrent seizures with an interval of <24 hr; requires investigation

■ **LABORATORY TESTS**
• Signs or symptoms of intracranial infection require CSF examination.
• Atypical presentation may warrant EEG, toxicology screening, assessment of electrolytes, etc., depending on history and examination findings.

■ **IMAGING STUDIES**
• Typical presentation: not needed
• Atypical presentation: may warrant CT scan or MRI, depending on history and examination findings

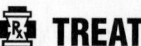 **TREATMENT**

■ **NONPHARMACOLOGIC THERAPY**
• Avoid excessive clothing.
• Encourage fluids.
• Apply tepid sponge bath to control fever.

■ **ACUTE GENERAL Rx**
• Antipyretics
• Possibly rectal diazepam in some instances of recurrent febrile seizures

■ **CHRONIC Rx**
• Prophylactic treatment with anticonvulsants is not indicated in children with typical benign febrile seizures.
• Use anticonvulsants prophylactically for other presentations of seizures associated with fever.

■ **DISPOSITION**
• Risk of recurrent benign febrile seizures is 30% up to the age of 5 yr.
• Risk of subsequent epilepsy is estimated at 1% to 2.5%.
• Available data: there is no risk reduction with prophylactic anticonvulsants.

■ **REFERRAL**
If uncertain about diagnosis or with atypical presentation
Author: **Michael Gruenthal, M.D., Ph.D.**

BASIC INFORMATION

■ DEFINITION
Septicemia is a systemic illness caused by generalized bacterial infection and characterized by evidence of infection, fever or hypothermia, hypotension, and evidence of end-organ compromise.

■ SYNONYMS
Sepsis
Sepsis syndrome
Systemic inflammatory response syndrome
Septic shock

ICD-9CM CODES
038.9 Sepsis
038.40 Sepsis, gram-negative bacteremia
038.1 Sepsis, *Staphylococcus*

■ EPIDEMIOLOGY & DEMOGRAPHICS
INCIDENCE (IN U.S.):
- Exact incidence is unknown
- Approximately 300,000 cases of gram-negative bacteremia among hospitalized patients each year
- Complicates a minority of bacteremia cases and may occur in the absence of documented bacteremia
PREDOMINANT SEX: Male = female
PREDOMINANT AGE:
- Neonatal period
- Patients >70 yr of age
GENETICS:
Familial Disposition: A great variety of congenital immunodeficiency states and other inherited disorders may predispose to septicemia.
Neonatal Infection: Incidence is high in neonatal period.

■ PHYSICAL FINDINGS & CLINICAL PRESENTATION
- Fever or hypothermia
- Hypotension
- Tachycardia
- Tachypnea
- Altered mental status
- Bleeding diathesis
- Skin rashes
- Symptoms that reflect primary site of infection: urinary tract, GI tract, CNS, respiratory tract

■ ETIOLOGY
- Disseminated infection with a great variety of bacteria:
  1. Gram-negative bacteria
  2. *E. coli*
  3. *Klebsiella* spp.
  4. *Pseudomonas aeruginosa*
  5. *Proteus* spp.
  6. *Staphylococcus aureus*
  7. *Streptococcus* spp.
  8. *Neisseria meningitidis*
- Less common infections:
  1. Fungal
  2. Viral
  3. Rickettsial
  4. Parasitic

- Activation of coagulation, complement, and kinin cascades with release of a variety of vasoactive endogenous mediators
- Predisposing host factors:
  1. General medical condition
  2. Age
  3. Immunosuppressive therapy
  4. Recent surgery
  5. Granulocytopenia
  6. Hyposplenism
  7. Diabetes
  8. Instrumentation

DIAGNOSIS

■ DIFFERENTIAL DIAGNOSIS
- Cardiogenic shock
- Acute pancreatitis
- Pulmonary embolism
- Systemic vasculitis
- Toxic ingestion
- Exposure-induced hypothermia
- Fulminant hepatic failure
- Collagen-vascular diseases

■ WORKUP
- Evaluation should focus on identifying a specific pathogen and localizing the site of primary infection.
- Hemodynamic, metabolic, coagulation disorders should be carefully characterized.
- Intensive monitoring, including the use of central venous or Swan-Ganz catheters, may be necessary.

■ LABORATORY TESTS
- Cultures of blood and examination and culture of sputum, urine, wound drainage, stool, CSF
- CBC with differential, coagulation profile
- Routine chemistries, liver function tests
- ABGs
- Urinalysis

■ IMAGING STUDIES
- Chest x-ray examination
- Other radiographic and radioisotope procedures according to suspected site of primary infection

TREATMENT

■ NONPHARMACOLOGIC THERAPY
- Tissue oxygenation: oxygen saturation maintained as high as possible; early mechanical ventilation
- Focal infection drained, if possible

■ ACUTE GENERAL Rx
- Blood pressure support
  1. IV hydration
  2. Therapy with pressors (e.g., dopamine) if mean blood pressure of 70 to 75 mm Hg cannot be maintained by hydration alone

- Correction of acidosis
  1. IV bicarbonate
  2. Mechanical ventilation
- Antibiotics
  1. Directed at the most likely sources of infection.
  2. Should generally provide broad coverage of gram-positive and gram-negative bacteria.
  3. Typical regimens:
     a. For hospital-acquired septicemia (pending culture results): vancomycin plus ceftazidime, imipenem, aztreonam, quinolones, or an aminoglycoside
     b. For community-acquired infection in the absence of granulocytopenia: above or single-drug therapy with third-generation cephalosporin
     c. For infection in the granulocytopenic host: above or dual gram-negative coverage (e.g., cephalosporin and aminoglycoside)
  4. Biological treatment
     Drotrecogin alfa (Xigris), a genetically engineered form of activated protein C, has recently been approved for use in patients with severe sepsis; when combined with conventional therapy, there may be a reduction in mortality.

■ CHRONIC Rx
- Adjust antibiotic therapy on the basis of culture results.
- In general, continue therapy for a minimum of 2 wk.

■ DISPOSITION
All patients with suspected septicemia should be hospitalized and given access to intensive monitoring and nursing care.

■ REFERRAL
- To infectious diseases expert
- To physician experienced in critical care

PEARLS & CONSIDERATIONS

■ COMMENTS
Mortality rises quickly if antibiotic therapy is not instituted promptly and metabolic derangements are not treated aggressively.

REFERENCES
Angus DC and Wax RS: Epidemiology of sepsis: an update, *Crit Care Med* 29(7 Suppl):S109, 2001.
Balk RA: Severe sepsis and septic shock: definitions, epidemiology, and clinical manifestations, *Crit Care Clin* 16(2):179, 2000.
Author: **Joseph R. Masci, M.D.**

BASIC INFORMATION

■ DEFINITION
Serotonin syndrome (SS) refers to a group of symptoms resulting from increased activity of serotonin (5-hydroxytryptamine) in the central nervous system. Serotonin syndrome is a drug-induced disorder that is characterized by a change in mental status and alteration in neuromuscular activity and autonomic function.

■ SYNONYMS
SS

ICD-9CM CODES
333.99 Syndrome serotonin

■ EPIDEMIOLOGY & DEMOGRAPHICS
- The incidence of serotonin syndrome is not known.
- Serotonin syndrome affects males and females from ages 20 to 70 yr.
- Serotonin syndrome commonly occurs in patients receiving two or more serotonergic drugs.
- Concomitant use of a selective serotonin reuptake inhibitor (SSRI) with a monoamine oxidase inhibitor (MAOI) poses the greatest risk of developing SS.
- Combination of SSRIs with other serotonergic drugs (e.g., tryptophan) or drugs with serotonin properties (e.g., lithium, meperidine) can also lead to SS.

■ PHYSICAL FINDINGS & CLINICAL PRESENTATION
- Symptoms usually start within minutes to hours after starting a new psychopharmacologic treatment or after administering a second serotonergic drug.
- Confusion, agitation, hypomania
- Fever, tachycardia, and tachypnea
- Nausea, vomiting, abdominal pain, and diaphoresis
- Diarrhea, tremors, shivering, and seizures
- Ataxia, myoclonus, and hyperreflexia

■ ETIOLOGY
- Hyperstimulation of the brainstem and spinal cord serotonin receptors due to blocking reuptake of serotonin and catecholamines is believed to be the underlying mechanism leading to the neuromuscular and autonomic symptoms seen in SS.
- Psychopharmacologic drugs, in particular, fluoxetine and sertraline coadministered with MAOI (e.g., tranylcypromine and phenelzine), have been cited in the literature as a common cause of SS.

DIAGNOSIS

- The diagnosis of SS is made on clinical grounds. There are no specific laboratory tests for SS. A high index of suspicion along with a detailed medication history is the mainstay of diagnosis.

■ DIFFERENTIAL DIAGNOSIS
Neuroleptic malignant syndrome, substance abuse (e.g., cocaine, amphetamines), thyroid storm, infection, alcohol and opioid withdrawal

■ WORKUP
- Other causes described in the differential diagnosis must be excluded to make the diagnosis of SS. Thus all patients should have blood tests and diagnostic imaging studies to rule out infectious, toxic, and metabolic etiologies.
- Additional laboratory tests are performed to exclude complicating features of SS (e.g., renal failure secondary to rhabdmyolysis).

■ LABORATORY TESTS
- CBC with differential to rule out sepsis
- Electrolytes, BUN, and creatinine to rule out acidosis and renal failure
- Blood and urine toxicology screen
- Thyroid function tests
- CPK with isoenzymes
- Urine and blood cultures
- EKG, because ventricular rhythm disturbance is a potentially fatal complication

■ IMAGING STUDIES
Imaging studies are not very specific in the diagnosis of SS and are only ordered to exclude other causes with similar clinical presentations as SS.

TREATMENT

There is no specific antidote for excess serotonin.

■ NONPHARMACOLOGIC THERAPY
- Discontinuation of the drug is the mainstay of therapy.
- Treatment is supportive: maintaining oxygenation and blood pressure and monitoring respiratory status.
- Cooling blankets for patients with hyperthermia.
- Mechanical intubation for patients unable to protect their airways as a result of mental status changes or seizures.

■ ACUTE GENERAL Rx
- Cyproheptadine 4 mg tablet is given in 4- to 8-mg doses q1-4h (up to 32 mg for adults, 12 mg in children) until a therapeutic response is achieved.
- Benzodiazepines—lorazepam 1 to 2 mg IV q30min has been used effectively in treating muscle rigidity, myoclonus, and seizure complications. Diazepam is an alternative choice.
- Methysergide has also been reported to be effective.
- Propranolol has serotonin blocking properties and is given 1 to 3 mg q5min up to 0.1 mg/kg.

■ CHRONIC Rx
For patients not requiring hospital admission, cyproheptadine, lorazepam, or propranolol can be given in an oral dose on a prn basis with close follow-up.

■ DISPOSITION
- Serotonin syndrome is a potentially life-threatening condition if not recognized early.
- Prompt diagnosis and withdrawal of the medication results in improvement of symptoms within 24 hours.
- Seizures, rhabdomyolysis, hyperthermia, ventricular arrhythmia, respiratory arrest, and coma are all complicating features of SS.

■ REFERRAL
All cases of SS secondary to psychotropic medications should be referred to a psychiatrist.

PEARLS & CONSIDERATIONS

■ COMMENTS
- The use of SSRIs and MAOIs is contraindicated.
- The use of SSRIs and other serotonergic agents is not an absolute contraindication; however, prompt withdrawal of the medication is recommended if any symptoms suggesting SS occur.
- Serotonin syndrome is usually found in patients being treated for depression, bipolar disorders, obsessive-compulsive disorder, attention-deficit disorder, and Parkinson's disease.

REFERENCES
Gillman PK: The serotonin syndrome and its treatment, *J Psychopharmacol* 13(1):100, 1999.
LoCurto MJ: The serotonin syndrome, *Emerg Med Clin North Am* 15(3):665, 1997.
Mills KC: Serotonin syndrome, *Am Fam Physician* 52(5):1475, 1995.
Author: **Peter Petropoulos, M.D.**

BASIC INFORMATION

■ **DEFINITION**
Sheehan's syndrome is a state of hypopituitarism resulting from an infarct of the pituitary secondary to postpartum hemorrhage or shock, causing partial or complete loss of the anterior pituitary hormones (i.e., ACTH, FSH, LH, GH, PRL, TSH) and their target organ functions.

ICD-9CM CODES
253.2 Sheehan's syndrome

■ **EPIDEMIOLOGY & DEMOGRAPHICS**
INCIDENCE: 1 case/10,000 deliveries (perhaps more rare in the U.S.)
PREDOMINANT SEX: Affects only females
RISK FACTORS:
• Hypovolemic shock
• Type I (insulin-dependent) diabetes mellitus (secondary to microvascular disease)
• Sickle cell anemia (secondary to occlusion of the small vessels in the pituitary)
ONSET OF SYMPTOMS: Average delay of 5 to 7 yr between onset of symptoms and diagnosis of disease.

■ **PHYSICAL FINDINGS & CLINICAL PRESENTATION**
• Failure of lactation
• Infertility
• Failure to resume menses after delivery
• Failure to regrow shaved pubic or axillary hair
• Skin depigmentation (including areola)
• Rapid breast involution
• Superinvolution of the uterus
• Hypothyroidism
• Adrenal cortical insufficiency
• Diabetes insipidus (rare)

■ **ETIOLOGY**
• Compromise of the blood supply to the low-pressure pituitary sinusoidal system may occur with postpartum hemorrhage or shock, resulting in pituitary infarct and/or necrosis.
• It is hypothesized that locally released factors may mediate vascular spasm of the pituitary blood supply.
• Severity of postpartum hemorrhage does not always correlate with the presence of Sheehan's syndrome.

DIAGNOSIS

■ **DIFFERENTIAL DIAGNOSIS**
• Chronic infections
• HIV
• Sarcoidosis
• Amyloidosis
• Rheumatoid disease
• Hemachromatosis
• Metastatic carcinoma
• Lymphocytic hypophysitis

■ **WORKUP**
• Target gland deficiency should be investigated by measuring levels of ACTH, FSH, LH, TSH (which may be normal or low), and T_4. Cortisol and estradiol (which may be low) should also be measured.
• Provocative testing of pituitary hormone reserves (e.g., metyrapone test, insulin tolerance test, and cosyntropin test): normal, subnormal, or delayed responses may suggest the presence of islands of pituitary cells that no longer have the support of the hypothalamic-portal circulation.
• Measurement of IGF-I to screen for GH deficiency: subnormal levels suggest decreased GH.
• Impaired prolactin response to TRH or dopamine antagonist stimulation is frequently found.
• During pregnancy, adjustments must be made in interpreting both hormone levels and responses to various stimuli because of normal physiologic changes.

■ **IMAGING STUDIES**
• Study of choice: MRI of the pituitary
  1. Sella turcica partially or totally empty
  2. Rules out mass lesion
• CT scan of the pituitary when MRI is unavailable or contraindicated

TREATMENT

■ **ACUTE GENERAL Rx**
• Acute form can be lethal, presenting with hypotension, tachycardia, failure to lactate, and hypoglycemia.

• A high degree of suspicion is required with any woman who has undergone postpartum hemorrhage and shock.
• Intravenous corticosteroids and fluid replacement should be given initially.
• Diagnosis is confirmed with a full endocrinologic workup as noted above.
• Thyroid hormone is replaced as L-thyroxin in doses of 0.1 to 0.2 mg qd.

■ **CHRONIC Rx**
• With late-onset disease (symptoms of general hypopituitarism, such as oligomenorrhea or amenorrhea, vaginal atrophic changes, and loss of libido): a full endocrinologic workup and replacement of the appropriate hormones are needed.
• With symptoms of adrenal insufficiency: corticosteroids should be given.
  1. A maintenance dose of cortisone acetate or prednisone may be given.
  2. Because adrenal production of cortisol is not entirely dependent on ACTH, replacement of mineralocorticoids is rarely necessary.
  3. Stress doses of glucocorticoids should be administered during surgery or during labor and delivery.

■ **DISPOSITION**
Patients who receive early diagnosis and adequate hormonal replacement may expect favorable outcomes, including subsequent pregnancy.

■ **REFERRAL**
Patients should have yearly examinations by endocrinologist.

REFERENCE
Dejagter S et al: Sheehan's syndrome: differential diagnosis in the acute phase, *J Intern Med* 244(3):261, 1998.
Author: **Beth J. Wutz, M.D.**

BASIC INFORMATION

■ **DEFINITION**
Shigellosis is an inflammatory disease of the bowel caused by one of several species of *Shigella.* It is the most common cause of bacillary dysentery in the U.S.

■ **SYNONYMS**
Bacillary dysentery

■ **ICD-9CM CODES**
004.9 Shigellosis

■ **EPIDEMIOLOGY & DEMOGRAPHICS**
INCIDENCE (IN U.S.): Approximately 15,000 cases/yr
PREDOMINANT SEX: Male homosexuals at increased risk
PREDOMINANT AGE: Young children
PEAK INCIDENCE: Summer
GENETICS:
Neonatal Infection: Rare but severe

■ **PHYSICAL FINDINGS & CLINICAL PRESENTATION**
• Possibly asymptomatic
• Mild illness that is usually self-limited, resolving in a few days
• Fever
• Watery diarrhea
• Bloody diarrhea
• Dysentery (abdominal cramps, tenesmus, and numerous, small-volume stools with blood, mucus, and pus)
• Descending intestinal tract illness, reflecting infection of small bowel first and then the colon (Fig. 1-337)

• Severe disease is more common in children and elderly
• Complications of severe illness:
  1. Seizures
  2. Megacolon
  3. Intestinal perforation
  4. Death
• Extraintestinal manifestations are rare
• Bacteremia described in patients with AIDS
• Hemolytic-uremic syndrome: usually occurs as the initial illness seems to be resolving
• Reactive arthritis, sometimes as part of Reiter's syndrome

■ **ETIOLOGY**
• *Shigella*
  1. *S. flexneri*
  2. *S. dysenteriae*
  3. *S. sonnei*
  4. *S. boydii*
• *S. sonnei* is the most commonly isolated species in the U.S., and it usually causes a mild watery diarrhea.
• Direct person-to-person transmission is thought to be the most common route.
• Contaminated food or water may transmit disease.

 DIAGNOSIS

■ **DIFFERENTIAL DIAGNOSIS**
• May mimic any bacterial or viral gastroenteritis
• Dysentery also caused by *Entamoeba histolytica*
• Bloody diarrhea may resemble disease caused by enterotoxigenic *E. coli*

■ **LABORATORY TESTS**
• Total WBCs may be low, normal, or high.
• Stool should be cultured from fresh samples, because the yield is increased by processing the specimen soon after passage.
• Serology is available but rarely useful.
• Polymerase chain reaction may be diagnostic.
• Fecal leukocyte preparation may show WBCs.

■ **IMAGING STUDIES**
Abdominal radiographs may suggest megacolon or perforation in rare, severe cases.

TREATMENT

■ NONPHARMACOLOGIC THERAPY
- Adequate hydration
- Electrolyte replacement

■ ACUTE GENERAL Rx
Antibiotics:
- To shorten course of illness
- To limit transmission of illness

- SMX/TMP, one DS tablet PO bid for 5 days
- Ciprofloxacin 500 mg PO bid for 5 days

■ DISPOSITION
- Most disease is self-limited.
- Severe illness may be fatal.

■ REFERRAL
For severe illness or complications.

PEARLS & CONSIDERATIONS

■ COMMENTS
- *Shigella* is one cause of "gay bowel syndrome."
- Illness is worsened by agents that decrease intestinal motility.
- A clinical algorithm for acute diarrhea is described in Fig. 3-66.

Author: **Maurice Policar, M.D.**

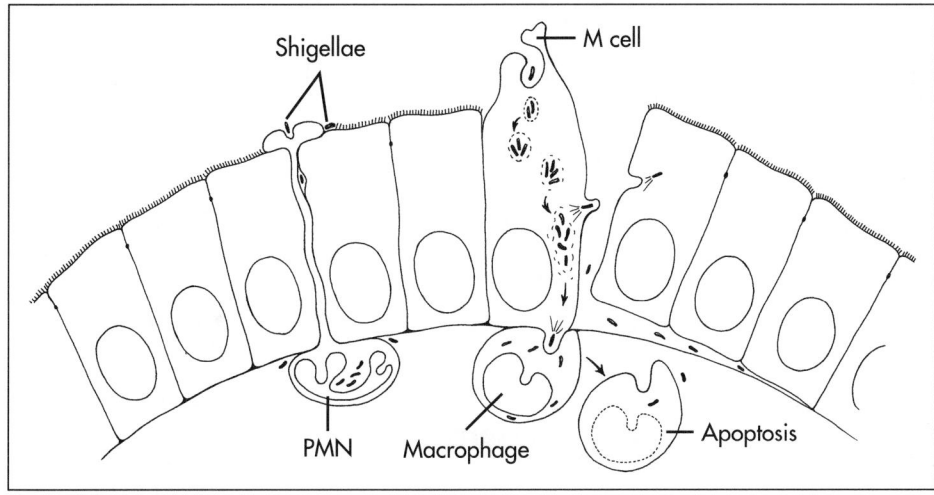

Fig. 1-337   Shigellae infect M cells, followed by uptake in macrophages. After infection, macrophages undergo apoptosis, which releases shigellae to infect the basolateral surfaces of intestinal epithelium. Shigellae also gain entry to basolateral surfaces by polymorphonuclear (PMN) intrusion through tight junctions in response to chemotactic signals. An intracellular actin motor drives transcytosis between cells. (From Stein JH [ed]: *Internal medicine,* ed 5, St Louis, 1998, Mosby.)

BASIC INFORMATION

■ DEFINITION
Short bowel syndrome is a malabsorption syndrome that results from extensive small intestinal resection.

■ SYNONYMS
Short bowel

ICD-9CM CODES
579.3 (postsurgical malabsorption)

■ EPIDEMIOLOGY & DEMOGRAPHICS
- Parallels Crohn's disease (see "Crohn's Disease" in Section I), which is the most common cause of the syndrome in adults
- In children, two thirds of short bowels are related to congenital abnormalities (intestinal atresia, gastroschisis, volvulus, aganglionosis) and one third are related to necrotizing enterocolitis
- Prevalence: 10,000 to 20,000 cases are estimated to exist in the U.S.

■ PHYSICAL FINDINGS & CLINICAL PRESENTATION
- Diarrhea and steatorrhea
- Weight loss
- Anemia related to iron or vitamin B_{12} absorption
- Bleeding diathesis related to vitamin K malabsorption
- Osteoporosis/osteomalacia related to vitamin D and calcium malabsorption
- Hyponatremia, hypokalemia
- Hypovolemia
- Other macronutrient or micronutrient deficiency states

■ ETIOLOGY
- Extensive bowel resection for treatment of the conditions mentioned above (see "Epidemiology")
- Pathogenesis (Fig. 1-338)

The human intestine is 3 to 8 m in length. Removal of up to one half of the small intestine produces no disruption in nutrient absorption, and most patients can maintain nutritional balance on oral feeding if they have more than 100 cm (3 ft) of jejunum. Similarly, 100 cm of intact jejunum can maintain a normal water, sodium, and potassium balance under normal circumstances. The presence of an intact colon can compensate for some small intestine loss.
Site-specific functions:
- Calcium, magnesium, phosphorus, iron, and vitamins are absorbed in the duodenum and proximal jejunum.
- Vitamin B_{12} and bile acids are absorbed in the ileum. The resection of more than 60 cm of ileum results in vitamin B_{12} malabsorption. The loss of more than 100 cm results in fat malabsorption (from the loss of bile acids).
- The loss of gastrointestinal endocrine hormones can affect intestinal motility.
- Intestinal bacterial overgrowth may also occur, especially if the ileocecal valve is lost.

DIAGNOSIS

Presence of macronutrient and/or micronutrient loss in a patient with a known history of bowel resection

■ DIFFERENTIAL DIAGNOSIS
Because the history of significant bowel resection is typically known, there is no differential diagnosis. If that history is not known, all causes of weight loss, malabsorption, and diarrhea must be considered (see respective chapters).

TREATMENT

Extensive small bowel resection with colectomy (less than 100 cm of jejunum)
- Rx: long-term parenteral nutrition (TPN). Some patients can switch to oral intake after 1 to 2 yr of TPN. In jejunostomy patients, excessive fluid loss can be reduced with H_2 blockers, proton pump inhibitors, or octreotide. Micronutrients are supplemented.

Extensive small bowel resection with partial colectomy (usually patients with Crohn's disease)
- Rx: oral intake alone is possible in all patients with >100 cm of jejunum. In addition to vitamin B_{12} deficiency, these patients often have diarrhea. Consider lactose malabsorption and bacterial overgrowth treated, respectively, with lactose restriction and antibiotics (tetracycline 250 mg tid or metronidazole 500 mg tid for 2 wk). Nonspecific antidiarrheal agents may also be indicated (e.g., Imodium or codeine). The patient must be monitored for micronutrient losses.

■ COMPLICATIONS
- Oxalate kidney stones
- Cholesterol gallstones
- D-Lactic acidosis

■ PROGNOSIS
Directly dependent on the extent of the bowel resection and in the case of Crohn's disease by the underlying illness

REFERENCE
Westergaard H: Short bowel syndrome. In Feldman M, Scharschmidt BF, Sleisenger MH (eds): *Gastrointestinal and liver disease*, ed 6, Philadelphia, 1998, WB Saunders.
Author: **Tom J. Wachtel, M.D.**

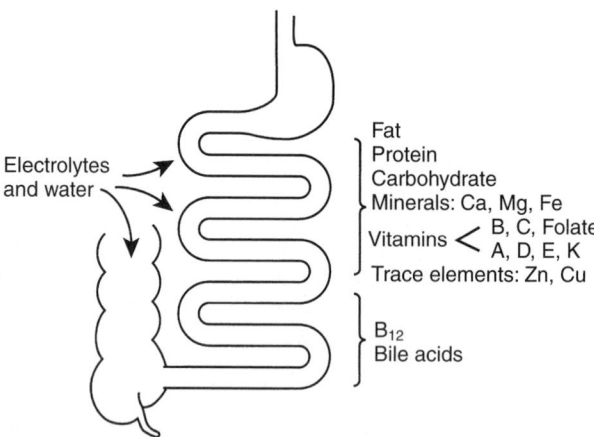

Fig. 1-338 Specific areas of absorption of constituents of diet and secretions in the gastrointestinal tract. Macronutrients and micronutrients are predominantly absorbed in the proximal jejunum. Bile acids and vitamin B_{12} are only absorbed in the ileum. Electrolytes and water are absorbed in both the small and the large intestine. (From Feldman M, Scharschmidt BF, Sleisenger MH [eds]: *Sleisenger and Fordtran's gastrointestinal and liver disease: pathophysiology, diagnosis, and management*, ed 6, Philadelphia, 1998, WB Saunders.)

BASIC INFORMATION

■ **DEFINITION**
Sialadenitis is an inflammation of the salivary glands.

ICD-9CM CODES
527.2 Sialadenitis

■ **EPIDEMIOLOGY & DEMOGRAPHICS**
Parotid or submandibular glands are most frequently affected (Fig. 1-339).

■ **PHYSICAL FINDINGS & CLINICAL PRESENTATION**
- Pain and swelling of the affected salivary gland
- Increased pain with meals
- Erythema, tenderness at the duct opening
- Purulent discharge from duct orifice
- Induration and pitting of the skin with involvement of the masseteric and submandibular spatial planes in severe cases

■ **ETIOLOGY**
- Ductal obstruction is generally secondary to a mucus plug caused by stasis of saliva with increased viscosity with subsequent stasis and infection.
- Most frequent infecting organisms are *Staphylococcus aureus, Pseudomonas, Enterobacter, Klebsiella, Enterococcus, Proteus,* and *Candida* spp.

- Sjögren's syndrome, trauma, radiation therapy, chemotherapy, dehydration, and chronic illness are predisposing factors.

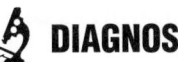 **DIAGNOSIS**

■ **DIFFERENTIAL DIAGNOSIS**
- Salivary gland neoplasm
- Ductal stricture
- Sialolithiasis
- Decreased salivary secretion secondary to medications (e.g., amitriptyline, diphenhydramine, anticholinergics)

■ **WORKUP**
- Generally not necessary
- Ultrasound or CT scan in patients not responding to medical treatment (see "Imaging Studies")

■ **LABORATORY TESTS**
- Generally not indicated
- CBC with differential to possibly reveal leukocytosis with left shift

■ **IMAGING STUDIES**
- Ultrasound or CT scan may be needed in patients not responding to medical therapy.
- Sialography should not be performed during the acute phase.

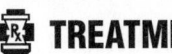 **TREATMENT**

■ **NONPHARMACOLOGIC THERAPY**
- Massage of the gland: may express pus and relieve some of the pressure
- Rehydration
- Warm compresses
- Oral cavity irrigations

■ **ACUTE GENERAL Rx**
- Amoxicillin clavulanate (Augmentin) 500 to 875 mg or cefuroxime (Ceftin) 250 mg bid should be given for 10 days. Clindamycin is an alternative choice in patients allergic to penicillin.
- IV antibiotics (e.g., cefoxitin, nafcillin) can be given in severe cases.

■ **DISPOSITION**
Complete recovery unless the patient has underlying obstruction (e.g., ductal stricture, tumor, or stone)

■ **REFERRAL**
- To ENT for nonresolving cases despite appropriate antibiotic therapy
- For salivary gland incision and drainage, which may be necessary in resistant cases

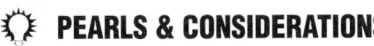 **PEARLS & CONSIDERATIONS**

■ **COMMENTS**
Prevention of dehydration will decrease the risk of sialadenitis.
Author: **Fred F. Ferri, M.D.**

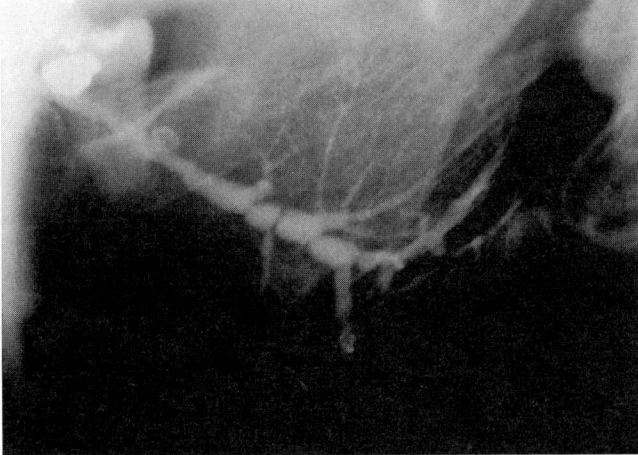

Fig. 1-339 Sialogram of patient with chronic sialadenitis showing sausage link–like patterns and massive duct dilation. (From Blitzer CE, Lawson W, Reino A: Sialadenitis. In Johnson JT, Yu VL [eds]: *Infectious diseases and antimicrobial therapy of the ears, nose, and throat,* Philadelphia, 1997, WB Saunders.)

BASIC INFORMATION

■ DEFINITION
Sialolithiasis is the existence of hardened intraluminal deposits in the ductal system of a salivary gland.

■ SYNONYMS
Salivary gland stone
Salivary calculus

ICD-9CM CODES
527.5 Sialolithiasis

■ EPIDEMIOLOGY & DEMOGRAPHICS
Affects patients mostly in their fifth to eighth decade and occurs most commonly in the submandibular gland (80%); only 14% are located in a parotid gland.

■ PHYSICAL FINDINGS & CLINICAL PRESENTATION
- Symptoms: colicky postprandial pain and swelling of a salivary gland. Tends to have a remitting/relapsing course.
- Signs: swelling and tenderness of a salivary gland. The stone may be felt by palpation of the floor of the mouth (Fig. 1-340).

■ ETIOLOGY
- The cause is unknown. Contributing factors include saliva stagnation, sialadenitis (inflammation of a salivary gland), ductal inflammation or injury.
- Salivary calculus composition is mainly calcium phosphate and carbonate, often combined with small proportions of magnesium, zinc, ammonium salts, and organic materials/debris.

DIAGNOSIS

■ DIFFERENTIAL DIAGNOSIS
- Lymphadenitis
- Salivary gland tumor
- Salivary gland bacterial (*Staphylococcus* or *Streptococcus*), viral (mumps), or fungal infection (sialadenitis)
- Noninfectious salivary gland inflammation (e.g., Sjögren's syndrome, sarcoidosis, lymphoma)
- Salivary duct stricture
- Dental abscess

■ IMAGING
- Plain x-ray
- Sialography

TREATMENT

- Warm soaks to area
- Antibiotics if associated bacterial sialadenitis is present
- Bland diet—avoid citrus fruit and spices
- Manual stone extraction sometimes associated with incisional enlargement of the ductal orifice
- Surgical salivary gland removal for retained hilar calculi

■ REFERRAL
To otorhinolaryngologist

REFERENCE
Kane WJ, McCaffrey TV: Sialolithiasis. In Cummings CW (ed): *Otolaryngology: head and neck surgery*, ed 2, St Louis, 1992, Mosby.
Author: **Tom J. Wachtel, M.D.**

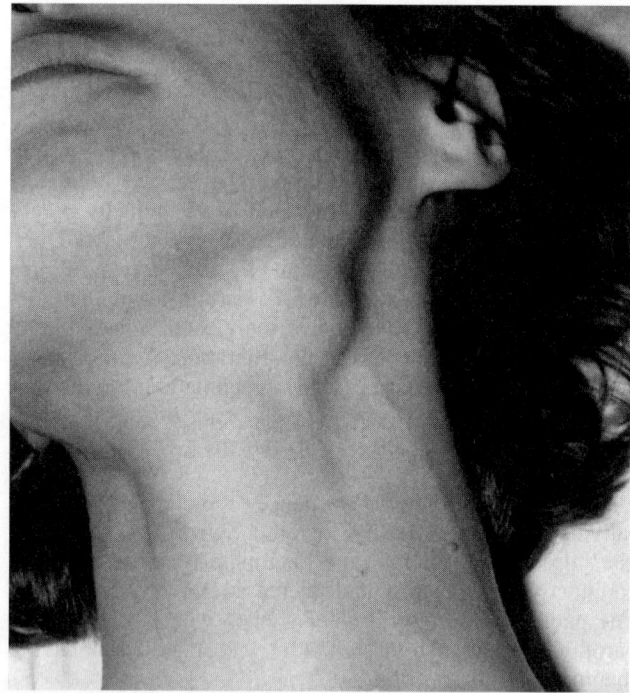

Fig. 1-340   Patient with large calculus and obstruction of the left submandibular gland. (From Blitzer CE, Lawson W, Reino A: Sialadenitis. In Johnson JT, Yu VL [eds]: *Infectious diseases and antimicrobial therapy of the ears, nose and throat*, Philadelphia, 1997, WB Saunders.)

BASIC INFORMATION

■ DEFINITION
Sick sinus syndrome is a group of cardiac rhythm disturbances characterized by abnormalities of the sinus node including (1) sinus bradycardia, (2) sinus arrest or exit block, (3) combinations of sinoatrial or atrioventricular conduction defects, and (4) supraventricular tachyarrhythmias. These abnormalities may coexist in a single patient so that a patient may have episodes of bradycardia and episodes of tachycardia.

■ SYNONYMS
Bradycardia-tachycardia syndrome

ICD-9CM CODES
427.81 Sick sinus syndrome

■ EPIDEMIOLOGY & DEMOGRAPHICS
- In children: associated with congenital heart disease
- In adults: typically associated with ischemic heart disease but may occur in the presence of a normal heart

■ PHYSICAL FINDINGS & CLINICAL PRESENTATION
- Lightheadedness, dizziness, syncope, palpitation
- Arterial embolization (e.g., stroke) associated with atrial fibrillation
- Physical examination may be normal or reveal abnormalities (e.g., heart murmurs or gallop sounds) associated with the underlying heart disease

■ ETIOLOGY
- Fibrosis or fatty infiltration involving the sinus node, atrioventricular node, the His bundle, or its branches
- In addition, inflammatory or degenerative changes of the nerves and ganglia surrounding the sinus nodes and other sclerodegenerative changes may be found

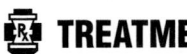 **DIAGNOSIS**

■ DIFFERENTIAL DIAGNOSIS
- Bradycardia: atrioventricular block
- Tachycardia: atrial fibrillation
- Atrial flutter
- Paroxysmal atrial tachycardia
- Sinus tachycardia
- Syncope (see "Syncope" in Section I)

■ WORKUP
- ECG
- Ambulatory cardiac rhythm monitoring
- 24-hour ambulatory ECG (Holter) (Fig. 1-341)
- Event recorder
- Electrophysiologic testing including sinus nodal recovery time and sinoatrial conduction time

TREATMENT

- Permanent pacemaker placement if symptoms are present
- The drug treatment of the tachycardia (e.g., with digitalis or calcium channel blockers) may worsen or bring out the bradycardia and become the reason for pacemaker requirement

■ REFERRAL
To cardiologist

REFERENCE
Zipes DP: Sick sinus syndrome. In Braunwald E (ed): *Heart disease: a textbook of cardiovascular medicine,* ed 5, Philadelphia, 1997, WB Saunders.
Author: **Tom J. Wachtel, M.D.**

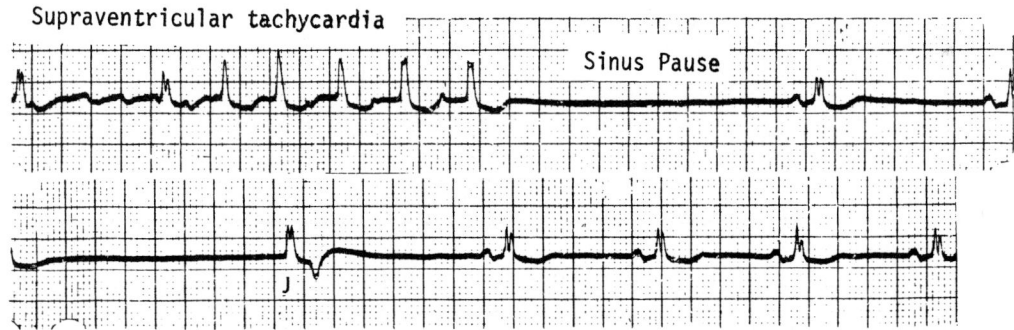

Fig. 1-341 Brady-tachy (sick sinus) syndrome. This rhythm strip shows a narrow-complex tachycardia (probably atrial flutter) followed by a sinus pause, an AV junctional escape beat *(J)*, and then sinus rhythm. (From Goldberger AL: *Clinical electrocardiography,* ed 5, St Louis, 1994, Mosby.)

BASIC INFORMATION

■ DEFINITION
Silicosis is a lung disease attributable to the inhalation of silica (silicon dioxide) in crystalline form (quartz) or in cristobalite or tridymite forms.

■ SYNONYMS
Pneumoconiosis caused by silica

ICD-9CM CODES
502 Silicosis, occupational
503 Pneumoconiosis due to other inorganic dust

■ EPIDEMIOLOGY & DEMOGRAPHICS
- Occupational disease affecting men and women involved in gathering, milling, processing, or using silica-containing rock or sand
- An estimated 1 million Americans are exposed (Table 1-65)

■ PHYSICAL FINDINGS & CLINICAL PRESENTATION
- Dyspnea
- Cough
- Wheezing
- Abnormal chest x-ray in an asymptomatic person
- See Table 1-66 for clinicopathologic types of silicoses

■ PATHOGENESIS
- Silica particles are ingested by alveolar macrophages, which in turn release oxidants causing cell injury and cell death, attract fibroblasts, and activate lymphocytes, increasing immunoglobulins in the alveolar space.
- Hyperplasia of alveolar epithelial cells occurs.
- Collagen accumulates in the interstitium.
- Neutrophils also accumulate and secrete proteolytic enzymes, which leads to tissue destruction and emphysema.
- Silica dust may be carcinogenic (not proven).
- Exposure to silicosis predisposes to tuberculosis.
- Some patients develop rheumatoid silicotic pulmonary nodules and may have arthritic symptoms of rheumatoid arthritis (Caplan's syndrome). Scleroderma has also been associated with silicosis.

DIAGNOSIS

■ DIFFERENTIAL DIAGNOSIS
- Other pneumoconiosis, berylliosis, hard metal disease, asbestosis
- Sarcoidosis
- Tuberculosis
- Interstitial lung disease
- Hypersensitivity pneumonitis
- Lung cancer
- Langerhans' cell granulomatosis (histiocytosis X)
- Granulomatous pulmonary vasculitis

■ WORKUP
- History of occupational exposure
- Chest x-ray (Fig. 1-342)
Chronic silicosis
- Characteristic finding: small, rounded lung parenchymal opacities
- Hilar lymphadenopathy with "eggshell" calcifications
- Pleural plaques (uncommon)
Accelerated silicosis (progressive massive fibrosis)
- Large parenchymal lesions resulting from coalesced small nodules
Acute silicosis
- Ground-glass appearance of the lung fields
- Chest CT scan
- Pulmonary function tests
Combination of obstructive and restrictive changes with or without reduction in diffusing capacity
- Bronchoscopy with lung biopsy in uncertain cases

■ COURSE
CHRONIC SILICOSIS:
- May not progress with absence of further exposure
- Accelerated silicosis: progressive respiratory failure and cor pulmonale
ACUTE SILICOSIS: Fatal course from respiratory failure over several months to a few years

TABLE 1-65   Industries and Occupations

INDUSTRIES	OCCUPATIONS
Mining, tunneling, and excavating	
Underground: gold, copper, iron, tin, uranium, civil engineering projects	Miner, driller, tunneler, developer, stoper
Surface: coal, iron, excavation of foundations	Mobile rig drill operator
Quarrying	
Granite, sandstone, slate, sand, china, stone/clay	Driller, hammer, digger
Stonework	
Granite sheds, monumental masonry	Cutter, dresser, driller, polisher, grinder, mason
Foundries	
Ferrous and nonferrous metals	Molder, knockout man, fettler, coremaker, caster
Abrasives	
Production: silica flour, metal polish, sandpapers, fillers in paint, rubber, and plastics	Crusher, pulverizer, and mixer; workers in the manufacture of abrasives
Sandblasting: oil rigs, tombstones	Operators of high-speed jets
Ceramics	
Manufacture of pottery, stoneware, refractory bricks for ovens and kilns	Workers at any stage of process if products are dry
Others	
Glass making, boiler scaling, traditional crafts, stone grinders, gemstone workers, dental technicians	

TABLE 1-66   Clinicopathologic Types of Silicosis

TYPE	EXPOSURE	PATHOLOGIC FEATURES	CLINICAL FEATURES
Chronic	Usually over 20 yr, often to dust containing <30% quartz	Mainly the classic silicotic islet or nodule; usually involving hilar nodes first, then upper lobes to which it may be limited	Small, rounded opacities on roentgenogram not necessarily associated with increased morbidity or mortality; impairment of pulmonary function may occur
Accelerated	5-15 yr, usually to fiber dusts of higher quartz content	Numerous nodules at various stages of development, sometimes with irregular interstitial fibrosis	Irregular upper zone fibrosis with a nodular component; symptomatic with impairment and often progression to respiratory failure and death; cavitation with infection by atypical mycobacteria not unusual
Acute	Several months, usually to very fine dusts of high quartz content	Alveoloproteinosis (airspaces filled with neutrophils, epithelial cells, and proteinaceous materials) with interstitial reactions and early, loosely organized nodules	Resembles acute airspace disease on chest roentgenogram, rapid progression to acute respiratory failure; fulminating tuberculosis is a possible terminal complication

℞ TREATMENT

- Prevention (industrial hygiene)
- Treatment of associated tuberculosis if present
- Supportive measures (oxygen, bronchodilators)
- Lung transplant

REFERENCE

Becklake MR: Silicosis. In Murray JF, Nadel JA (eds): *Textbook of respiratory medicine,* ed 2, Philadelphia, 1994, WB Saunders.
Author: **Tom J. Wachtel, M.D.**

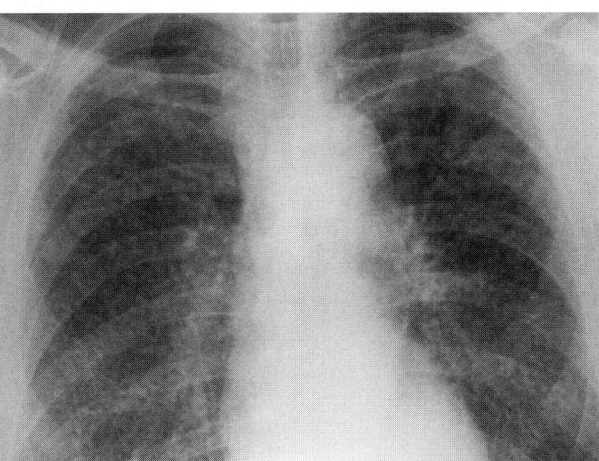

Fig. 1-342 Simple silicosis. There are multiple small (2- to 4- mm) nodules distributed throughout the lungs, with an upper lobe predominance. (From McLoud TC: *Thoracic radiology: the requisites,* St Louis, 1998, Mosby.)

BASIC INFORMATION

■ DEFINITION

Sinusitis is inflammation of the mucous membranes lining one or more of the paranasal sinuses. The various presentations are:

- Acute sinusitis: infection lasting <30 days, with complete resolution of symptoms.
- Subacute infection: lasts from 30 to 90 days, with complete resolution of symptoms.
- Recurrent acute infection: episodes of acute infection lasting <30 days, with resolution of symptoms, which recur at intervals at least 10 days apart.
- Chronic sinusitis: inflammation lasting >90 days, with persistent upper respiratory symptoms.
- Acute bacterial sinusitis superimposed on chronic sinusitis: new symptoms that occur in patients with residual symptoms from prior infection(s). With treatment, the new symptoms resolve but the residual ones do not.

ICD-9CM CODES
473.9 Sinusitis (accessory) (nasal) (hyperplastic) (nonpurulent) (purulent) (chronic)
461.9 Acute sinusitis

■ SYNONYMS

Rhinosinusitis: Sinusitis is almost always accompanied by inflammation of the nasal mucosa; thus it is now the preferred term.

■ EPIDEMIOLOGY & DEMOGRAPHICS
INCIDENCE (IN U.S.): Seems to correlate with the incidence of upper respiratory tract infections
PEAK INCIDENCE: Fall, winter, spring: September through March

■ PHYSICAL FINDINGS & CLINICAL PRESENTATION

- Patients often give a history of a recent upper respiratory illness with some improvement, then a relapse
- Mucopurulent secretions in the nasal passage
  1. Purulent nasal and postnasal discharge lasting >7 to 10 days
  2. Facial tightness, pressure, or pain
  3. Nasal obstruction
  4. Headache
  5. Decreased sense of smell
  6. Purulent pharyngeal secretions, brought up with cough, often worse at night
- Erythema, swelling, and tenderness over the infected sinus in a small proportion of patients
  1. Diagnosis cannot be excluded by the absence of such findings
  2. These findings are not common, and do not correlate with number of positive sinus aspirates

- Intermittent low-grade fever in about half of adults with acute bacterial sinusitis
- Toothache is a common complaint when the maxillary sinus is involved
- Periorbital cellulitis and excessive tearing with ethmoid sinusitis
  1. Orbital extension of infection: chemosis, proptosis, impaired extraocular movements
- Characteristics of acute sinusitis in children with upper respiratory tract infections:
  1. Persistence of symptoms
  2. Cough
  3. Bad breath
- Symptoms of chronic sinusitis (may or may not be present)
  1. Nasal or postnasal discharge
  2. Fever
  3. Facial pain or pressure
  4. Headache
- Nosocomial sinusitis typically seen in patients with nasogastric tubes or nasotracheal intubation

■ ETIOLOGY

- Each of the four paranasal sinuses is connected to the nasal cavity by narrow tubes (ostia), 1 to 3 mm diameter; these drain directly into the nose through the turbinates. The sinuses are lined with a ciliated mucous membrane (mucoperiosteum).
- Acute viral infection
  1. Infection with the common cold or influenza
  2. Mucosal edema and sinus inflammation
  3. Decreased drainage of thick secretions/obstruction of the sinus ostia
  4. Subsequent entrapment of bacteria
     a. Multiplication of bacteria
     b. Secondary bacterial infection
- Other predisposing factors
  1. Tumors
  2. Polyps
  3. Foreign bodies
  4. Congenital choanal atresia
  5. Other entities that cause obstruction of sinus drainage
  6. Allergies
  7. Asthma
- Dental infections lead to maxillary sinusitis
- Viruses recovered alone or in combination with bacteria (in 16% of cases):
  1. Rhinovirus
  2. Coronavirus
  3. Adenovirus
  4. Parainfluenza virus
  5. Respiratory syncytial virus
- The principal bacterial pathogens in sinusitis are *Streptococcus pneumoniae*, nontypeable *Haemophilus influenzae*, and *Moraxella catarrhalis*
- In the remainder of cases find *Streptococcus pyogenes, Staphylococcus aureus,* α-hemolytic streptococci, and mixed anaerobic infections (*Peptostreptococcus, Fusobacterium, Bacteroides, Prevotella*)

- Infection is polymicrobial in about one third of cases
- Anaerobic infections seen more often in cases of chronic sinusitis and in cases associated with dental infection; anaerobes are unlikely pathogens in sinusitis in children
- Fungal pathogens are isolated with increasing frequency in immunocompromised patients:
  1. *Aspergillus*
  2. *Pseudoallescheria*
  3. *Sporothrix*
  4. Phaeohyphomycoses
  5. Hyalohyphomycoses
  6. Zygomycetes
- Nosocomial infections: occur in patients with nasogastric tubes, nasotracheal intubation, cystic fibrosis, immunocompromised
  1. *S. aureus*
  2. *Pseudomonas aeruginosa*
  3. *Klebsiella pneumoniae*
  4. *Enterobacter spp.*
  5. *Proteus mirabilis*

Organisms typically isolated in chronic sinusitis:
  1. *S. aureus*
  2. *S. pneumoniae*
  3. *H. influenzae*
  4. *P. aeruginosa*
  5. Anaerobes

DIAGNOSIS

■ DIFFERENTIAL DIAGNOSIS
- Temporomandibular joint disease
- Migraine headache
- Cluster headache
- Dental infection
- Trigeminal neuralgia

■ WORKUP
- In the normal healthy host the paranasal sinuses should be sterile. Although the contiguous structures are colonized with bacteria and likely contaminate the sinuses, the mucociliary lining functions to remove these bacteria.
- Gold standard for diagnosis: recovery of bacteria in high density ($\geq 10^4$ colony-forming units/ml) from a paranasal sinus, in the setting of a patient with history of upper respiratory infection and symptoms persisting >7 to 10 days. Sinus aspiration is the best method for obtaining cultures; however, it must be performed by an otorhinolaryngologist and is not practical for the primary care practitioner. Therefore most diagnoses are based on the clinical history and presentation, possibly supported by radiologic evaluations.
  1. Standard four-view sinus radiographs (Fig. 1-343)
     a. Complete opacification and air-fluid levels are most specific findings (average 85% and 80%, respectively)

b. Mucosal thickening has low specificity (40% to 50%)

c. Absence of all three of the above findings has estimated sensitivity of 90%

d. Overall, standard radiographs are of limited use in diagnosis, although negative films are strong evidence against the diagnosis

2. CT scans:

a. Much more sensitive than plain radiographs in detecting acute changes and disease in the sinuses

b. Recommended for patients requiring surgical intervention, including sinus aspiration; it is a useful adjunct to guide therapy

3. Transillumination:

a. Used for diagnosis of frontal and maxillary sinusitis

b. Place transilluminator in the mouth or against cheek to assess maxillary sinuses, under medial aspect of the supraorbital ridge to assess frontal sinuses

c. Absence of light transmission indicates that sinus is filled with fluid

d. Dullness (decreased light transmission) is less helpful in diagnosing infection

4. Endoscopy:

a. Used to visualize secretions coming from the ostia of infected sinuses

b. Culture collection via endoscopy often contaminated by nasal flora; not nearly as good as sinus puncture

5. Sinus puncture:

a. Gold standard for collecting sinus cultures

b. Generally reserved for treatment failures, suspected intracranial extension, and nosocomial sinusitis

![Rx] TREATMENT

■ NONPHARMACOLOGIC THERAPY

To help promote sinus drainage:

- Air humidification with vaporizers (for steam) or humidifiers (for a cool mist)
- Application of hot, wet towel over the face
- Sipping hot beverages
- Hydration

■ ACUTE GENERAL Rx

- Sinus drainage:
  1. Nasal vasoconstrictors, such as phenylephrine nose drops, 0.25% or 0.5 %
  2. Topical decongestants should not be used for more than a few days

because of the risk of rebound congestion

3. Systemic decongestants

4. Nasal or systemic corticosteroids, such as nasal beclomethasone, short course oral prednisone

5. Nasal irrigation, with hypertonic or normal saline (saline may act as a mild vasoconstrictor of nasal blood flow)

6. Use of antihistamines has no proven benefit, and the drying effect on the mucous membranes may cause crusting, which blocks the ostia, thus interfering with sinus drainage

- Analgesics, antipyretics

Antimicrobial therapy:

- Most cases of acute sinusitis have a viral etiology and will resolve within 2 wk without antibiotics.
- Current treatment recommendations favor symptomatic treatment for those with mild symptoms.
- Antibiotics should be reserved for those with moderate to severe symptoms who meet the criteria for diagnosis of sinusitis.
- Antibiotic therapy is usually empiric, targeting the common pathogens:
  1. First-line antibiotics include amoxicillin, erythromycin, trimethoprim/sulfamethoxazole
  2. Second-line antibiotics include the newer macrolides: clarithromycin, azithromycin, amoxicillin/clavulanate, cefuroxime axetil, cefprozil, cefaclor, lorcarbef, ciprofloxacin, levofloxacin, clindamycin, metronidazole, others
  3. For patients with uncomplicated acute sinusitis the less-expensive first-line agents appear to be as effective as the costlier second-line agents
- Hospitalization and IV antibiotics may be required for more severe infection and those with suspected intracranial complications. Broader-spectrum antibiotic coverage may be indicated in severe cases, to cover for MRSA, *Pseudomonas,* and fungal pathogens

Duration of therapy generally 10 to 14 days, although some have success with much shorter regimens

Surgery:

- Surgical drainage indicated
  1. If intracranial or orbital complications suspected
  2. Many cases of frontal and sphenoid sinusitis
  3. Chronic sinusitis recalcitrant to medical therapy
- Surgical debridement imperative in the treatment of fungal sinusitis

Complications:

- Untreated, sinusitis may lead to a number of serious, life-threatening complications
- Intracranial complications include meningitis, brain abscess, epidural and subdural empyema

- Intracranial sequelae are more common with frontal and ethmoid infections
- Extracranial complications include orbital cellulitis, blindness, orbital abscess, osteomyelitis
- Extracranial sequelae more commonly seen with ethmoid sinusitis

■ CHRONIC Rx

- Broad-spectrum antibiotics that cover both aerobes and anaerobes
- Duration of therapy not clearly established: range 3 to 6 wk
- Adjunctive therapy: one or more of the various options listed above
- Surgical intervention may be necessary in nonresponders

■ DISPOSITION

Appropriate diagnosis and treatment necessary to avoid the various sequelae that can occur without proper therapy

■ REFERRAL

- To infectious disease specialist if failure to respond to initial therapy
- To otorhinolaryngologist for:
  1. Failure to respond to therapy
  2. Fungal infection suspected
  3. Intracranial or orbital complications suspected

REFERENCES

Incaudo GA, Wooding LG: Diagnosis and treatment of acute and subacute sinusitis in children and adults, *Clin Rev Allergy Immunol* 16(1-2):157, 1998.

Piccirillo JF et al: Impact of first-line vs second-line antibiotics for the treatment of acute uncomplicated sinusitis, *JAMA* 286(15):1849, 2001.

Snow V et al: Principles of appropriate antibiotic use for acute sinusitis in adults, *Ann Intern Med* 134(6):495, 2001.

Author: **Jane V. Eason, M.D.**

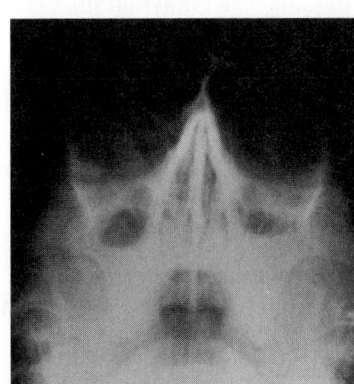

Fig. 1-343 Waters' view of maxillary sinus with air-fluid level. (From Noble J: *Primary care medicine,* ed 3, St Louis, 2001, Mosby.)

BASIC INFORMATION

■ DEFINITION
Sjögren's syndrome (SS) is an autoimmune disorder characterized by lymphocytic and plasma cell infiltration and destruction of salivary and lacrimal glands with subsequent diminished lacrimal and salivary gland secretions.
- *Primary:* dry mouth (xerostomia) and dry eyes (xerophthalmia) develop as isolated entities.
- *Secondary:* associated with other disorders.

■ SYNONYMS
SS
Sicca syndrome

ICD-9CM CODES
710.2 Sjögren's syndrome

■ EPIDEMIOLOGY & DEMOGRAPHICS
INCIDENCE/PREVALENCE: 1 case/2500 persons; secondary SS is just as common and can affect up to one third of SLE patients and nearly 20% of RA patients.
PREDOMINANT AGE: Peak incidence is in the sixth decade.
PREDOMINANT SEX: Female > male

■ PHYSICAL FINDINGS & CLINICAL PRESENTATION
- Dry mouth with dry lips (cheilosis), erythema of tongue, (Fig. 1-344) and other mucosal surfaces, carious teeth
- Dry eyes (conjunctival injection, decreased luster, and irregularity of the corneal light reflex)
- Possible salivary gland enlargement
- Purpura (nonthrombocytopenic, hyperglobulinemic, vasculitic) may be present
- Evidence of associated conditions (e.g., RA or other connective disease, lymphoma, hypothyroidism, COPD, trigeminal neuropathy, chronic liver disease, polymyopathy)

■ ETIOLOGY
Autoimmune disorder

DIAGNOSIS

■ DIFFERENTIAL DIAGNOSIS
- Medication-related dryness (e.g., anticholinergics)
- Age-related exocrine gland dysfunction
- Mouth breathing
- Anxiety
- Other: sarcoidosis, primary salivary hypofunction, radiation injury, amyloidosis

■ WORKUP
Workup involves the demonstration of the following criteria for diagnosis of primary and secondary Sjögren's syndrome:
PRIMARY:
- Symptoms and objective signs of ocular dryness:
  1. Schirmer's test: <8 mm wetting per 5 min
  2. Positive rose bengal or fluorescein staining of cornea and conjunctiva to demonstrate keratoconjunctivitis sicca
- Symptoms and objective signs of dry mouth:
  1. Decreased parotid flow using Lashley cups or other methods
  2. Abnormal biopsy result of minor salivary gland (focus score >2 based on average of four assessable lobules)
- Evidence of systemic autoimmune disorder:
  1. Elevated titer of rhematoid factor >1:320
  2. Elevated titer of ANA >1:320
  3. Presence of anti-SS A (Ro) or anti-SS B (La) antibodies
SECONDARY:
- Characteristic signs and symptoms of SS (described in "Physical Findings")
- Clinical features sufficient to allow a diagnosis of RA, SLE, polymyositis, or scleroderma

■ LABORATORY TESTS
- Positive ANA (>60% of patients) with autoantibodies anti-SS A and anti-SS B may be present.
- Additional laboratory abnormalities may include elevated ESR, anemia (normochromic, nomocytic), abnormal liver function studies, elevated serum β_2 microglobulin levels, rheumatoid factor.

- A definite diagnosis SS can be made with a salivary gland biopsy.

TREATMENT

■ NONPHARMACOLOGIC THERAPY
- Adequate fluid replacement
- Proper oral hygiene to reduce the incidence of caries

■ ACUTE GENERAL Rx
- Use artificial tears frequently.
- Pilocarpine 5 mg PO qid is useful to improve dryness.
- Cevimeline (Evoxac) 30 mg PO tid is effective for the treatment of dry mouth in patients with Sjögren's syndrome.

■ CHRONIC Rx
Periodic dental and ophthalmology evaluations to screen for complications

■ DISPOSITION
Prognosis is variable and depends on the presence of associated conditions.

PEARLS & CONSIDERATIONS

■ COMMENTS
Unusual presentations of SS may occur in association with polymyalgia rheumatica, chronic fatigue syndrome, FUO, and inflammatory myositis.

REFERENCE
Vivino FB et al: Pilocarpine tablets for the treatment of dry mouth and dry eye symptoms in patients with Sjögren's syndrome, *Arch Intern Med* 159:174, 1999.
Author: **Fred F. Ferri, M.D.**

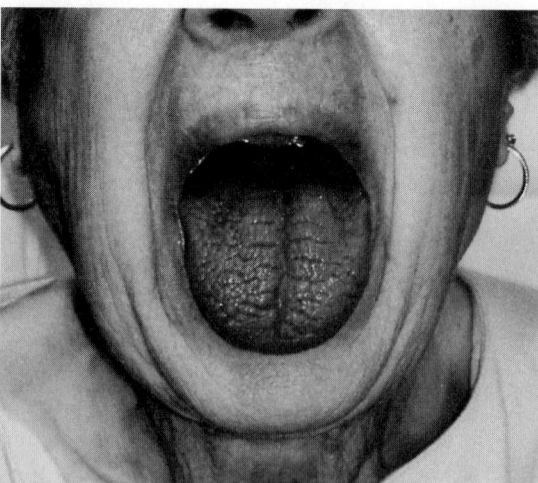

Fig. 1-344   "Crocodile tongue" in SS patient. (From Noble J: *Primary care medicine,* ed 3, St Louis, 2001, Mosby.)

BASIC INFORMATION

■ DEFINITION
Obstructive sleep apnea refers to upper airway occlusion usually accompanied by oxygen desaturation occurring repeatedly during sleep.

■ SYNONYMS
Sleep apnea syndrome

■ ICD-9CM CODES
780.53 Sleep apnea with hypersomnia
780.51 Sleep apnea with hyposomnia
780.57 Sleep apnea with sleep disturbance
306.1 Psychogenic apnea

■ EPIDEMIOLOGY & DEMOGRAPHICS
Obstructive sleep apnea occurs most frequently in obese, middle-aged men (4%) and women (2%).

■ PHYSICAL FINDINGS & CLINICAL PRESENTATION
- History of snoring and excessive daytime somnolence
- Obesity with body mass >20% of normal
- Memory impairment, inability to concentrate, personality changes
- Examination of oropharynx may reveal narrowing secondary to large tonsils, pendulous uvula, excessive soft tissue, prominent tongue.
- Patient's bed partner usually reports loud, cyclic snoring, disrupted sleep with repetitive awakenings, thrashing movements of extremities during sleep.
- Decreased libido and depression
- Systemic hypertension

■ ETIOLOGY
Narrowing of upper airway secondary to:
- Obesity
- Macroglossia
- Tonsillar hypertrophy
- Micrognathia
- Hypothyroidism
- Use of alcohol or sedatives at bedtime

DIAGNOSIS

■ DIFFERENTIAL DIAGNOSIS
- Narcolepsy
- Psychiatric: depression
- CHF
- COPD
- GERD
- Seizure disorder
- Parasomnias

Fig. 3-153 in Section III describes the diagnostic approach to sleep disorders

■ WORKUP
- Medical history should include questions about snoring because, essentially, all patients with obstructive sleep apnea snore when they sleep; other important signs of sleep apnea are daytime somnolence and higher frequency of accidents (automobile or work-related).
- Sleep apnea can be confirmed by all-night polysomnography. Testing is performed during a full night at the patient's habitual sleep hours and ideally includes all stages and positions of sleep: patient with sleep apnea has >15 apneic episodes per hour with desaturation of at least 4% by oximetry. Syndrome can be ruled out by normal overnight oximetry test or if saturation of oxygen level is <90%, <1% for a total sleep time.

■ LABORATORY TESTS
- TSH level is indicated in suspected hypothyroidism.
- CBC generally reveals erythrocytosis.

■ IMAGING STUDIES
Radiography of soft tissues in the neck in patients with suspected anatomic abnormalities

TREATMENT

■ NONPHARMACOLOGIC THERAPY
- Weight loss in overweight patients
- Avoidance of sedating medications and alcohol
- Treatment of nasal congestion
- Sleep hygiene training
- Elimination of the supine sleeping position
- Nighttime treatment with continuous positive airway pressure (CPAP) to overcome desaturation. Treatment with CPAP is, however, not effective in patients with sleep apnea but no daytime sleepiness.
- An oral appliance that attaches to the upper teeth and pushes the mandible forward, enlarging the upper airway, is also available as an initial treatment for mild obstructive sleep apnea

■ ACUTE GENERAL Rx
Patients who are unresponsive to CPAP and weight loss may be candidates for surgical therapy:
- Uvulopalatopharyngoplasty (UPPP, both standard and laser-assisted [LAUP]) in patients with significant obstruction of retropalatal airway

- Nasal septoplasty in patients with nasoseptal deformity
- Tracheostomy: reserved for life-threatening cases that are unresponsive to other treatments
- Radiofrequency ablation creates controlled coagulative lesions at specific locations within the upper airway. It is performed in the outpatient setting under local anesthesia and represents the newest approach to reducing upper-airway obstruction.

■ CHRONIC Rx
See "Acute General Rx."

■ DISPOSITION
- Most patients improve with weight loss and CPAP.
- Overall success rate for UPPP is about 40%.
- Pharmacologic therapy with protriptyline 10 to 20 mg PO qhs can provide improvement in a limited number of patients.

■ REFERRAL
Surgical referral for patients unresponsive to weight loss and CPAP

PEARLS & CONSIDERATIONS

■ COMMENTS
- The Epsworth sleepiness scale is a helpful office guide to gauge the degree of sleepiness. Patients with scores >10 have been shown to be more likely to have obstructive sleep apnea.
- The 16-item Berlin questionnaire is also a useful tool to identify patients at risk for sleep apnea.
- Nasal glucocorticoid therapy (e.g., fluticasone nasal inhaler) is beneficial in children with mild-to-moderate obstructive sleep apnea.

REFERENCES
Brouilette RT et al: Efficacy of fluticasone nasal spray for pediatric obstructive sleep apnea, *J Pediatr* 138:838, 2001.
Li KK et al: Radiofrequency volumetric reduction of the palate, *Otolaryngol Head Neck Surg* 122:410, 2000.
Piccirillo JF et al: Obstructive sleep apnea, *JAMA* 284:1492, 2000.
Netzer NC et al: Using the Berlin questionnaire to identify patients at risk for the sleep apnea syndrome, *Ann Intern Med* 131:485, 1999.
Author: **Fred F. Ferri, M.D.**

BASIC INFORMATION

■ **DEFINITION**

Smallpox infection is due to the variola virus, a DNA virus member of the genus *Orthopoxvirus*. It is a human virus with no known nonhuman reservoir of disease. Natural infection occurs following implantation of the virus on the oropharyngeal or respiratory mucosa.

ICD-9CM CODES

050.9 Smallpox NOS
V01.3 Smallpox exposure
050.0 Smallpox, hemorrhagic (pustular)
050.1 Variola minor (alastrim)
050.0 Variola major

■ **EPIDEMIOLOGY & DEMOGRAPHICS**

- Smallpox infection was eliminated from the world in 1977. The last cases of smallpox, from laboratory exposure, occurred in 1978. The threat of bioterrorism has brought on renewed interest in smallpox virus.
- Routine vaccination against smallpox ended in 1972.
- Smallpox is spread from one person to another by infected saliva droplets that expose a susceptible person who has face-to-face contact with the ill person.
- Persons with smallpox are most infectious during the first wk of illness, when the largest amount of virus is present in saliva; however, some risk of transmission lasts until all scabs have fallen off.
- The incubation period is about 12 days (range: 7 to 17 days) following exposure.
- Contaminated clothing or bed linen could also spread the virus. Special precautions need to be taken to ensure that all bedding and clothing of patients are cleaned appropriately with bleach and hot water. Disinfectants such as bleach and quaternary ammonia can be used for cleaning contaminated surfaces.

■ **PHYSICAL FINDINGS & CLINICAL PRESENTATION**

- Initial symptoms include high fever, fatigue, and headaches and back aches. A characteristic rash, most prominent on the face, arms, and legs, follows in 2 to 3 days (Fig. 1-345).
- The rash starts with flat red lesions that evolve at the same rate. The rash follows a centrifugal pattern.
- Lesions are firm to the touch, domed, or umbilicated. They become pus-filled and begin to crust early in the second wk.

- Scabs develop and then separate and fall off after about 3 to 4 wk. Depigmentation persists at the base of the skin lesions for 3 to 6 mo after illness. Scarring is usually most extensive on the face.
- Associated with the rash may be fever, headache, generalized malaise, vomiting, and colicky abdominal pain.
- Variola major may produce a rapidly fatal toxemia in some patients.
- Complications of smallpox include dehydration, pneumonia, blepharitis, conjunctivitis, and corneal ulcerations.

■ **ETIOLOGY**

Smallpox is caused by the variola virus. There are at least two strains of the virus, the most virulent known as *variola major* and a less virulent strain known as *variola minor* (elastrim).

DIAGNOSIS

■ **DIFFERENTIAL DIAGNOSIS**

Rash from other viral illnesses (e.g., hemorrhagic chicken pox)
Abdominal pain may mimic appendicitis
Meningococcemia

■ **WORKUP & LABORATORY TESTS**

- Laboratory examination requires high-containment (BL-4) facilities.
- Electron microscopy of vesicular scrapings can be used to distinguish poxvirus particles from varicella-zoster virus or herpes simplex. To obtain vesicular or pustular fluid it may be necessary to open lesions with the blunt edge of a scalpel. A cotton swab may be used to harvest the fluid.
- In absence of electron microscopy, light microscopy can be used to visualize variola viral particles (Guarnieri bodies) following Giemsa staining.
- Polymerase chain reaction (PCR) techniques and restriction fragment-length polymorphisms can rapidly identify variola.

■ **IMAGING STUDIES**

Chest x-ray in patients with suspected pneumonia

TREATMENT

■ **NONPHARMACOLOGIC THERAPY**

- Supportive therapy
- IV hydration in severe cases

■ **ACUTE GENERAL Rx**

- There is no proven treatment for smallpox. Vaccination administered within 3 to 4 days may prevent or significantly ameliorate subsequent illness. Vaccinia immune globulin can be used for treatment of vaccine complications and for administration with vaccine to those for whom vaccine is otherwise contraindicated.
- Patients can benefit from supportive therapy (e.g., IV fluids, acetaminophen for pain or fever).
- Antibiotics are indicated only if secondary bacterial infections occur.

■ **CHRONIC Rx**

None

■ **DISPOSITION**

Mortality for variola major is 20% to 50%. Variola minor has a mortality rate of <1%.

■ **REFERRAL**

ID consultation and notification of local health authorities is mandatory in all cases of smallpox.

PEARLS & CONSIDERATIONS

- The smallpox virus is fragile and in the event of an aerosol release of smallpox, all viruses will be inactivated or dissipated within 1 to 2 days. Buildings exposed to the initial aerosol release of the virus do not need to be decontaminated. By the time the first cases are identified, typically 2 wk after release, the virus in the building will be gone. Infected patients, however, will be capable of spreading the virus and possibly contaminating surfaces while they are sick. Standard hospital-grade disinfectants such as quaternary ammonias are effective in killing the virus on surfaces and should be used for disinfecting hospitalized patients' rooms or other contaminated surfaces. In the hospital setting, patients' linens should be autoclaved or washed in hot water with bleach added. Infectious waste should be placed in biohazard bags and autoclaved before incineration.
- Symptomatic patients with suspected or confirmed smallpox are capable of spreading the virus. Patients should be placed in medical isolation to avoid spread the virus. In addition, people who have come into close contact with smallpox patients should be vaccinated immediately and closely watched for symptoms of smallpox.

■ COMMENTS

- In people exposed to smallpox, the vaccine can lessen the severity of or even prevent illness if given within 4 days of exposure.
- Vaccine against smallpox contains another live virus called vaccinia. The vaccine does ot contain smallpox virus.

REFERENCES

Henderson DA et al: Smallpox as a biological weapon, *JAMA* 281:2127, 1999. www.bt.cdc.gov/Agent/Smallpox/SmallpoxGen.asp

Author: **Fred F. Ferri, M.D.**

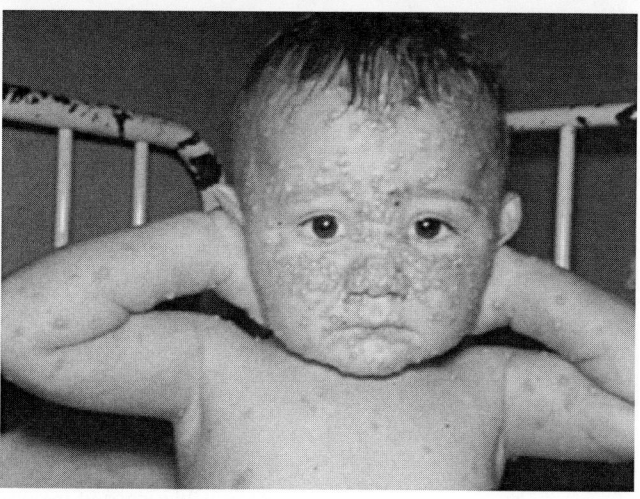

Fig. 1-345 Appearance of the rash of smallpox on day 6 to 7. All of the lesions are in the same stage of development. (From Gorbach SL: *Infectious diseases,* ed 2, Philadelphia, 1998, WB Saunders.)

BASIC INFORMATION

■ DEFINITION
Somatization disorder refers to a pattern of recurring multiple somatic complaints that begin before the age of 30 yr and persist over several years. Patients complain of multiple sites of pain (a minimum of four), GI symptoms (a minimum of two), a sexual or reproductive symptom, and a pseudoneurologic symptom. These cannot be explained by a medical condition or are in excess to expected disability from a coexisting medical condition.

■ SYNONYMS
Briquet's syndrome
Nonorganic physical symptoms
Medically unexplained symptoms
Functional somatic symptoms

ICD-9CM CODES
300.81 Somatization disorder

■ EPIDEMIOLOGY & DEMOGRAPHICS
PREVALENCE (IN U.S.): Lifetime rates of 0.25% to 2% in women, <0.2% in men
PREDOMINANT SEX:
- Women are more commonly affected in the U.S.
- Males of other cultures (e.g., Greece and Puerto Rico) are more commonly affected.
PREDOMINANT AGE: By definition, onset occurs before age 30 yr.
PEAK INCIDENCE: Typically before age 25 yr
GENETICS:
- Genetic and environmental factors may be involved.
- There is a high risk of associated substance abuse or antisocial personality disorder.

■ PHYSICAL FINDINGS & CLINICAL PRESENTATION
- Typical patient is unmarried, non-white, poorly educated, and from rural setting.
- Onset is frequently in the teens; course is marked by frequent, unexplained, and frequently disabling pain and physical complaints.
- Patient frequently undergoes multiple procedures and seeks treatment from multiple physicians.
- Patient meets criteria for at least one other psychiatric condition, most

commonly substance abuse disorders and personality disorders (antisocial disorder is the most common); anxiety and depressive disorders are also common.

■ ETIOLOGY
- Believed to be the physical expression of psychologic distress
- May be more common in individuals without sufficient verbal or intellectual capacity to communicate psychologic distress, individuals with alexithymia (inability to describe emotional states), or individuals from cultural backgrounds that consider emotional distress as an undesirable weakness
- Some aspects of somatization behavior possibly learned from somatizing patients

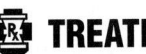

DIAGNOSIS

■ DIFFERENTIAL DIAGNOSIS
- Undifferentiated somatoform disorder (ICD-10 F45.1, DMS-IV 300.81): one or more physical complaints that cannot be explained by a medical condition are present for at least 6 mo (NOTE: Somatization is more severe and less common).
- Conversion disorder: there is an alteration or loss of voluntary motor or sensory function with demonstrable physical cause and related to a psychologic stress or a conflict (NOTE: With multiple complaints, the diagnosis of conversion is not made).
- Pain disorder: distinguished from somatization disorder by the presence of other somatic complaints.
- Munchausen's (factitious disorder) and malingering: the psychologic basis of the complaints in somatization disorder is not conscious as in factitious disorder (Munchausen's) and malingering, in which symptoms are produced intentionally.

■ WORKUP
- Rule out a general medical condition.
- If somatization is suspected on the basis of a history of repeated, multiple, unexplained complaints, restraint in ordering tests is recommended.

■ LABORATORY TESTS
No specific laboratory tests are required.

■ IMAGING STUDIES
No specific imaging studies are required.

TREATMENT

■ NONPHARMACOLOGIC THERAPY
- Legitimize patient's complaints; when this is not done, there is frequently an increase in complaints and associated disability.
- Minimize diagnostic investigation and symptomatic treatment.
- Set attainable treatment goals.
- Treat coexisting psychiatric conditions.

■ ACUTE GENERAL Rx
- No specific pharmacologic therapy is available.
- Antidepressants may be useful for coexisting anxiety and depression.

■ CHRONIC Rx
- A trusting relationship based on mutual respect between the patient and the physician is the best long-term treatment.
- If there is coexisting anxiety or depression, chronic use of antidepressants may be warranted.

■ DISPOSITION
A chronic condition with frequent exacerbations

■ REFERRAL
If therapy is required and the patient has the psychologic mindedness to participate

REFERENCE
Epstein RC et al: Somatization reconsidered, *Arch Intern Med* 159:215, 1999.
Author: **Rif S. El-Mallakh, M.D.**

BASIC INFORMATION

■ DEFINITION

Spinal cord compression is the neurologic loss of spine function. Lesions may be complete or incomplete and develop gradually or acutely. Incomplete lesions often present as distinct syndromes, as follows:
- Central cord syndrome (Fig. 1-346)
- Anterior cord syndrome
- Brown-Séquard syndrome
- Conus medullaris syndrome
- Cauda equina syndrome

ICD-9CM CODES
344.89 Brown-Séquard syndrome
344.60 Cauda equina syndrome
336.8 Conus medullaris syndrome
Other lesions listed by site

■ PHYSICAL FINDINGS & CLINICAL PRESENTATION
Clinical features reflect the amount of spinal cord involvement:
- Motor loss and sensory abnormalities
- Babinski testing usually positive
- Clonus
- Gradual compression, often manifested by progressive difficulty walking, clonus with weight bearing, and involuntary spasm; development of sensory symptoms; bladder dysfunction (late)
- Central cord syndrome: results in a variable quadriparesis with the upper extremities more severely involved than the lower extremities; some sensory sparing

- Anterior cord syndrome: results in motor, pain, and temperature loss below the lesion
- Brown-Séquard syndrome:
  1. Spinal cord syndrome caused by injury to either half of the spinal cord and resulting in the loss of motor function, position, vibration, and light touch on the affected side
  2. Pain and temperature sense lost on the opposite side
- Conus medullaris syndrome: results in variable motor loss in the lower extremities with loss of bowel and bladder function
- Cauda equina syndrome: typical low back pain, weakness in both lower extremities, saddle anesthesia, and loss of voluntary bladder and bowel control

■ ETIOLOGY
- Trauma
- Tumor
- Infection
- Inflammatory processes
- Degenerative disk conditions with spinal stenosis
- Acute disk herniation
- Cystic abnormalities

DIAGNOSIS

■ DIFFERENTIAL DIAGNOSIS
- See "Etiology."
- Box 2-192 describes the differential diagnosis of paraplegia.

■ WORKUP
- Spinal cord compression: requires an immediate referral for radiographic and neurologic assessment
- Laboratory results usually unremarkable unless infectious or inflammatory causes suspected

■ IMAGING STUDIES
- Depend on the suspected etiology
- MRI usually required

TREATMENT

Urgent surgical decompression is usually indicated as soon as the etiology is established.

■ DISPOSITION
Important indicators regarding prognosis (Leventhal):
- The greater the distal motor and sensory sparing, the greater the expected recovery.
- When a plateau of recovery is reached, no further improvement is expected.
- The quicker the recovery, the greater the recovery

■ REFERRAL
Immediate referral for radiographic and neurologic evaluation and treatment in all suspected cases of spinal cord compression
Author: **Lonnie R. Mercier, M.D.**

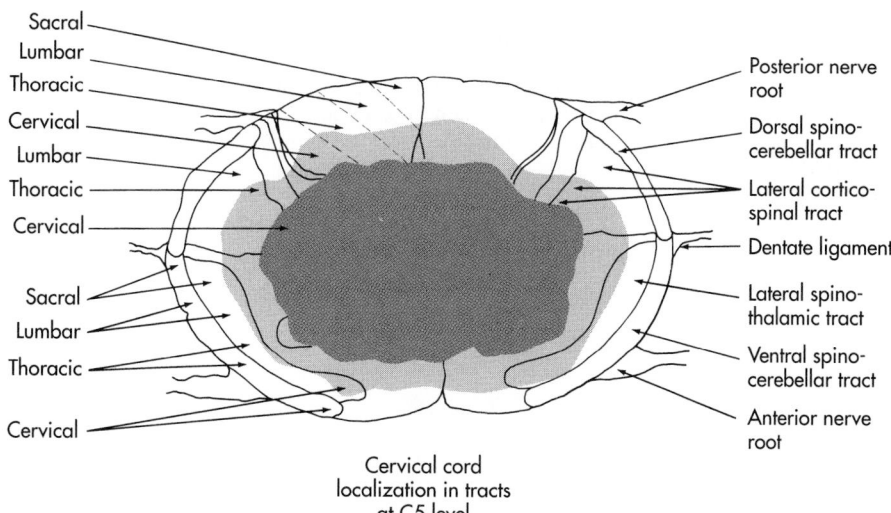

Fig. 1-346 Diagrammatic description of the spinal pathways at the lower cervical level showing the usual distribution of the contusion hemorrhage that causes a central cord syndrome. (From Goldman L, Bennett JC [eds]: *Cecil textbook of medicine,* ed 21, Philadelphia, 2000, WB Saunders.)

BASIC INFORMATION

■ DEFINITION
Spinal stenosis is the pathologic condition compressing or narrowing the spinal canal, nerve root canal, or intervertebral foramina.

■ SYNONYMS
Central spinal stenosis
Lateral spinal stenosis
Spondylosis

■ ICD-9CM CODES
724.02 Spinal stenosis lumbar, lumbosacral

■ EPIDEMIOLOGY & DEMOGRAPHICS
- More common in the elderly >65 yr
- More than 30,000 patients underwent surgery for spinal stenosis in 1994

■ CLINICAL PRESENTATION & PHYSICAL FINDINGS
- Neurogenic claudication: leg, buttock, or back pain precipitated by walking and relieved by sitting
- Radicular leg pain
- Paresthesias
- Difficulty standing or lying in an erect position
- Decreased lumbar extension
- Normal peripheral pulses
- Positive Romberg
- Wide-based gait
- Reduced knee and ankle reflex
- Urine incontinence

■ ETIOLOGY
Spinal stenosis may be primary or secondary
- Primary stenosis (congenital or developmental narrowing) (Fig. 1-347)
  1. Idiopathic
  2. Achondroplasia
  3. Morquio-Ullrich syndrome
- Secondary stenosis (acquired)
  1. Degenerative (hypertrophy of the articular processes, disk degeneration, ligamentum flavum hypertrophy, spondylolisthesis)
  2. Fracture/trauma
  3. Postoperative (postlaminectomy)
  4. Paget's disease
  5. Ankylosing spondylitis
  6. Tumors
  7. Acromegaly

■ DIAGNOSIS

■ DIFFERENTIAL DIAGNOSIS
Spinal stenosis must be differentiated from other common causes of back and leg pain; osteoarthritis of the knee or hip, osteomyelitis, epidural abscess, metastatic tumors, multiple myeloma, intermittent claudication secondary to peripheral vascular disease, neuropathy, scoliosis, herniated nucleus pulposus, spondylolisthesis, acute cauda equina syndrome, ankylosing spondylitis, Reiter's syndrome, fibromyalgia.

■ WORKUP
The workup of spinal stenosis consists of a detailed history, physical examination, and specific imaging studies.

■ IMAGING STUDIES
- Lumbar spine film.
- CT scan of the lumbosacral spine: sensitivity (75% to 85%), specificity (80%).
- MRI of the lumbosacral spine: sensitivity (80% to 90%), specificity (95%).
- Myelogram: sensitivity (77%), specificity (72%). Absolute stenosis is defined as the anterior-posterior (AP) diameter of the spinal canal <10 mm. Relative stenosis: 10 to 12 mm AP diameter.
- CT and MRI can visualize both the central and lateral canals.
Electromyography (EMG) and nerve conduction velocity (NCV) are additional studies particularly useful in differentiating peripheral neuropathy from lumbar spinal stenosis.

■ TREATMENT

■ NONPHARMACOLOGIC THERAPY
- Physiotherapy
- Lumbar corsets
- Back exercises
- Abdominal muscle strengthening
- Aquatic exercises

■ ACUTE GENERAL Rx
- Surgery is indicated in patients with significant compression of nerve roots as determined by MRI or CT and incapacitating symptoms limiting activities of daily living or bladder and bowel incontinence.
- Surgical procedures include decompressive laminectomy, arthrodesis, hemilaminectomy, and medial facetectomy.

■ CHRONIC Rx
- Conservative therapy with NSAIDs, (ibuprofen 800 mg PO tid, naproxen 500 mg PO bid) may be tried for symptomatic relief in addition to acetaminophen 1 g PO qid.
- Epidural steroid injections may provide temporary relief.

■ DISPOSITION
- Approximately 20% of patients having surgery require repeat surgery within 10 yr. Nearly a third of the patients continue to experience pain.
- The natural history of spinal stenosis is one of slow progression. In some cases symptoms improve. Although not very common, cord compression with resultant bowel and bladder incontinence and paresis can occur.

■ **REFERRAL**
- Patients who have spinal stenosis should be referred to an orthopedic surgeon specializing in back surgery or to a neurosurgeon.
- Pain clinic referrals should be made if surgery is contraindicated or if the patient does not want surgery.

⚙ **PEARLS & CONSIDERATIONS**

■ **COMMENTS**
Approximately a third of the patients with neurogenic claudication have co-existing peripheral vascular disease. Spinal stenosis not only is found in the elderly but also can be a common cause of chronic low back pain in the young and merits an evaluation.

REFERENCES

Fritz JM et al: Lumbar spinal stenosis: a review of current concepts in evaluation, management, and outcome measurements, *Arch Phys Med Rehabil* 79:700, 1998.

Katz JN et al: Degenerative spinal stenosis, diagnostic value of the history and physical examination, *Arthritis Rheum* 38:1236, 1995.

Katz JN et al: Seven to ten years outcome of decompressive surgery for degenerative lumbar spinal stenosis, *Spine* 21:92, 1996.

Postacchini F: Management of lumbar spinal stenosis, *J Bone Joint Surg* 78-B(1):154, 1996.

Author: **Peter Petropoulos, M.D.**

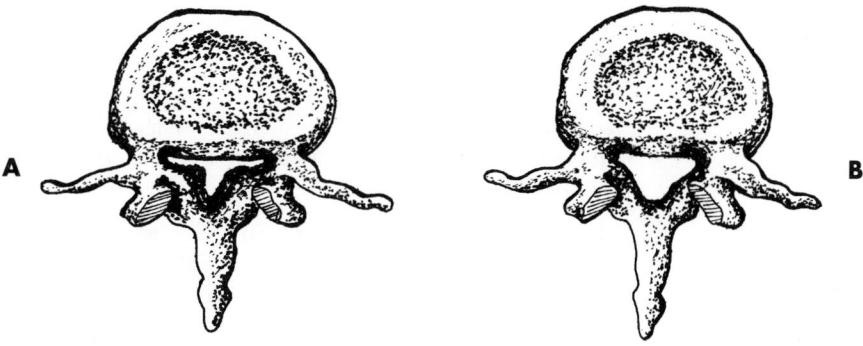

Fig. 1-347 Spinal stenosis. **A,** A trefoil spinal canal, with reduced diameters, is a frequent predisposing factor of spinal stenosis. Trefoil changes are present through development and become magnified from facet joint hypertrophy, ligamentum flavum hypertrophy, or other impingement mechanism(s). **B,** A normal spinal canal. (From Canoso J: *Rheumatology in primary care,* Philadelphia, 1997, WB Saunders.)

BASIC INFORMATION

■ DEFINITION

Spontaneous miscarriage is fetal loss before wk 20 of pregnancy, calculated from the patient's last menstrual period or the delivery of a fetus weighing <500 g. *Early loss* is before menstrual wk 12, while *late loss* refers to losses from 12 to 20 wk.

Miscarriage can also be classified as *incomplete* (partial passage of fetal tissue through partially dilated cervix), *complete* (spontaneous passage of all fetal tissue), *threatened* (uterine bleeding without cervical dilation or passage of tissue), *inevitable* (bleeding with cervical dilation without passage of fetal tissue), or *missed abortion* (intrauterine fetal demise without passage of tissue). *Recurrent miscarriage* involves three or more spontaneous pregnancy losses before wk 20.

ICD-9CM CODES

634.0 Spontaneous abortion

■ SYNONYMS

Abortion

■ EPIDEMIOLOGY & DEMOGRAPHICS

INCIDENCE: 15% to 20% of clinically recognized pregnancies, with 80% of miscarriages occurring in the first trimester

RISK FACTORS: Prior pregnancy history (risk after live birth = 5%, prior pregnancy aborted = 20% subsequent risk) is the most significant risk factor. Vaginal bleeding, especially >3 days, carries with it a 15% to 20% chance of miscarriage.

GENETICS:

- Distribution of abnormal karyotypes: autosomal trisomy (50%), monosomy 45,X (20%), triploidy (15%), tetraploidy (10%), structural chromosomal abnormalities (5%).
- With two or more spontaneous miscarriages, a karyotype should be performed to evaluate for balanced translocation, which has 80% risk for abortion, and, if the pregnancy is carried to term, has 3% to 5% risk for unbalanced karyotype.
- After 9 wk, the later in gestation, the greater the chance of a normal karyotype.

■ PHYSICAL FINDINGS & CLINICAL PRESENTATION

- Profuse bleeding and cramping has a higher association with miscarriage than bleeding without cramping, which is more consistent with a threatened miscarriage.
- Cervical dilation with history or finding of fetal tissue at cervical os may be present.
- In cases of missed abortion, uterine size may be smaller than menstrual dating, in contrast to molar gestation, where size may be greater than dates.

■ ETIOLOGY

- In a general overview the etiology can be classified in terms of maternal (environmental) and fetal (genetic) factors, with the majority of miscarriages being related to genetic or chromosomal causes.
- Causes: uterine anomalies (unicornuate uterus risk = 50%, bicornuate or septate uterus risk = 25% to 30%), incompetent cervix (iatrogenic or congenital, associated with 20% of midtrimester losses), diethylstilbestrol exposure in utero (T-shaped uterus), submucous leiomyomas, intrauterine adhesions or synechiae, luteal phase or progesterone deficiency, autoimmune disease such as anticardiolipin antibodies, uncontrolled diabetes mellitus, HLA associations between mother and father, infections such as TB, *Chlamydia*, *Ureaplasma*, smoking and alcohol use, irradiation, and environmental toxins

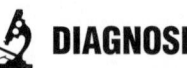 **DIAGNOSIS**

■ DIFFERENTIAL DIAGNOSIS

- Normal pregnancy
- Hydatidiform molar gestation
- Ectopic pregnancy
- Dysfunctional uterine bleeding
- Pathologic endometrial or cervical lesions

■ WORKUP

- Because of the potential for morbid maternal sequelae, all patients with bleeding in the first trimester should have an evaluation for possible ectopic pregnancy.
- Prior pregnancy history guides the workup, such that if there are three early, prior pregnancy losses a workup and treatment for recurrent miscarriage should begin before next conception, or if there is a strong history for second-trimester loss, consideration for cerclage should be given.
- Many of the treatments require preconceptual therapy, including control of disease processes, such as diabetes, and thus a careful workup can begin after the prior pregnancy loss but before conception.

■ LABORATORY TESTS

- Type and antibody screen is used to evaluate for the need for Rh immune globulin.
- In circumstances in which an ectopic gestation is considered, quantitative serum hCG can be used with transvaginal sonogram to assign a level of risk; 2000 mIU/ml (third reference standard) is the discriminatory zone above which an intrauterine gestational sac should be demonstrated.
- During the preconception period, Hgb A1C, anticardiolipin antibody, lupus anticoagulant, karyotyping, endometrial biopsy with progesterone level, and cervical cultures or serum antibodies can be checked for suspected disease processes.
- Progesterone level <5 mg/dl indicates nonviable gestation vs. >25 mg/dl, which confers a good prognosis.

■ IMAGING STUDIES

Transabdominal or transvaginal sonogram can be used in combination with menstrual dating and serum quantitative hCG to document pregnancy location, fetal heart presence, gestational sac size, and adnexal pathology and, if used serially, can help confirm a missed abortion.

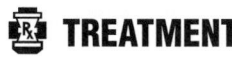

TREATMENT

■ NONPHARMACOLOGIC THERAPY

Depending on the patient's clinical status, desire to continue the pregnancy, and certainty of the diagnosis, expectancy can be considered. In pregnancies <6 wk or >14 wk, complete expulsion of fetal tissue occurs and surgical intervention such as dilation and curettage (D&C) can be avoided.

■ ACUTE GENERAL Rx

- *Incomplete miscarriage* between 6 and 14 wk can be associated with large amounts of blood loss, and thus these patients should undergo D&C.
- In cases of *missed abortion,* if fetal demise has occurred >6 wk before or gestational age is >14 wk, there is an increased risk of hypofibrinogenemia with disseminated intravascular coagulation, and thus D&C should be performed early in the disease course.
- *Threatened abortions* may be managed expectantly, watching for signs of cervical dilation or sonographic evidence of missed abortion. Hormonal therapy, such as progesterone, is contraindicated during this time because it may increase the chance of missed abortion.
- If surgical intervention is required, preoperative use of 40 U of oxytocin (Pitocin) in 1000 ml lactated Ringer's solution may be used to decrease the amount of bleeding and shorten the operative time.
- Postoperatively all patients undergoing a D&C should receive antibiotics (doxycycline 100 mg bid for 7 days), methylergonovine (Methergine) 0.2 mg q6h for four doses, and Motrin or NSAIDs PRN for pain.
- Preoperative laminaria is useful in cases of nondilated or primigravida cervices.

- In all cases of first- or second-trimester bleeding in Rh-negative patients, Rh immune globulin 300 μg should be given to prevent Rh sensitization.

■ CHRONIC Rx

Expectancy may be considered for those pregnancies <6 menstrual weeks depending on the clinical situation and the patient's desire.

■ DISPOSITION

In most cases it is important to document the resolution of the pregnancy, in terms of either a pathology specimen from a D&C or documentation of decreasing quantitative hCGs. If the pathology report does not confirm a miscarriage or the quantitative hCG value plateaus or rises after evacuation, the diagnosis of ectopic or molar gestation must be examined.

■ REFERRAL

In cases of ectopic gestation, incomplete or missed abortion, surgical evacuation of the uterus and possible laparoscopic evaluation of the adnexa should be undertaken by qualified personnel.

REFERENCE

Ness RB et al: Cocaine and tobacco use and the risks of spontaneous abortion, *N Engl J Med* 340:333, 1999.
Author: **Scott J. Zuccala, D.O.**

BASIC INFORMATION

■ DEFINITION
Sporotrichosis is a granulomatous disease caused by *Sporothrix schenckii.*

■ ICD-9CM CODES
117.1 Sporotrichosis

■ EPIDEMIOLOGY & DEMOGRAPHICS
PREDOMINANT SEX: Male in pulmonary sporotrichosis
PREDOMINANT AGE: 30 to 60 yr of age in pulmonary sporotrichosis
GENETICS:
Neonatal Infection: At least one case of transmission from the cheek lesion of the mother to the skin of the infant has been reported.

■ PHYSICAL FINDINGS & CLINICAL PRESENTATION
- Cutaneous disease
  1. Arises at the site of inoculation
  2. Initial lesion usually located on the distal part of an extremity, although any area may be affected, including the face
  3. Variable incubation period of approximately 3 wk once introduced into the skin
  4. Granulomatous reaction provoked
  5. Lesion becomes papulonodular, erythematous, elastic, variable in size
  6. Subsequently, nodule becomes fluctuant, undergoes central necrosis, breaks down, discharges mucoid pus from which fungus may be isolated
  7. Indolent ulcer with raised erythematous or violaceous borders
  8. Secondary lesions:
     a. Develop along superficial lymphatic channels
     b. Evolve in the same manner as the primary lesion, with subsequent inflammation, induration, and suppuration
- Fixed, or plaque form
  1. Erythematous verrucous, ulcerated, or crusted lesions
  2. Does not spread locally
  3. Does not involve lymphatic vessels
  4. Rarely undergoes spontaneous resolution
  5. More often persists for years without systemic symptoms and

within a setting of normal laboratory examinations
- Osteoarticular involvement
  1. Most common extracutaneous form
  2. Usually presents as monoarticular arthritis
  3. Left untreated, may progress to:
     a. Synovitis
     b. Osteitis
     c. Periostitis
     d. All involving elbows, knees, wrists, and ankles
  4. Joint inflamed
     a. Associated with an effusion
     b. Painful on motion
- Early pulmonary disease
  1. Usually associated with a paucity of clinical findings
     a. Low-grade fever
     b. Cough
     c. Fatigue
     d. Malaise
     e. Weight loss
  2. Untreated
     a. Cavitary pulmonary disease
     b. Frank pulmonary dysfunction
  3. Meningitis uncommon
     a. Except perhaps in the immunocompromised patient
     b. Presents with few signs or symptoms of neurologic involvement
  4. Few reported cases
     a. Infection of the ocular adnexa
     b. Endophthalmitis without antecedent trauma
     c. Infection of the testes and epididymis

■ ETIOLOGY
- *Sporothrix schenckii*
  1. Global in distribution
  2. Often isolated from soil, plants, and plant products
  3. Majority of case reports from tropical and subtropical regions of the Americas
- Occupational or recreational exposure
  1. Hay
  2. Straw
  3. Sphagnum moss
  4. Timber
  5. Thorny plants (e.g., roses and barberry bushes)
- Animal contact
  1. Armadillos
  2. Cats
  3. Squirrels
- Human-to-human transmission
- Tattooing

 DIAGNOSIS

■ DIFFERENTIAL DIAGNOSIS
- Fixed, or plaque, sporotrichosis
  1. Bacterial pyoderma
  2. Foreign body granuloma
  3. Tularemia
  4. Anthrax
  5. Other mycoses: blastomycosis, chromoblastomycosis
- Lymphocutaneous sporotrichosis
  1. *Nocardia brasiliensis*
  2. *Leishmania braziliensis*
  3. Atypical mycobacterial disease: *M. marinum, M. kansasii*
- Pulmonary sporotrichosis
  1. Pulmonary TB
  2. Histoplasmosis
  3. Coccidioidomycoses
- Osteoarticular sporotrichosis
  1. Pigmented villonodular synovitis
  2. Gout
  3. Rheumatoid arthritis
  4. Infection with *M. tuberculosis*
  5. Atypical mycobacteria: *M. marinum, M. kansasii, M. avium-intracellulare*
- Meningitis
  1. Histoplasmosis
  2. Cryptococcosis
  3. TB

■ WORKUP
- The diagnosis should be considered in individuals who are occupationally exposed to soil, decaying plant matter, and thorny plants (gardeners, horticulturists, farmers) who present with chronic nonhealing ulcers or lesions with or without associated arthritis or pulmonary symptoms.
- Diagnosis is made by culture:
  1. Pus
  2. Joint fluid
  3. Sputum
  4. Blood
  5. Skin biopsy
- Isolation of the fungus from any site is considered diagnostic of infection.
- Saprophytic colonization of the respiratory tract has been described.
- A positive blood culture may indicate infection in an immunocompromised host.
- Increasingly sensitive laboratory culturing systems may detect the fungus in the normal host.
- Biopsy specimens are diagnostic if characteristic cigar-shaped, round, oval, or budding yeast forms are seen.

- Despite special staining, the yeast may remain difficult to detect unless multiple sections are examined.
- No standard method of serologic testing is available.
- Previously described techniques have been hampered by the presence of antibody in the absence of infection.

■ LABORATORY TESTS

- CBCs and serum chemistries are generally normal.
- Elevated ESR is seen with extracutaneous disease.
- CSF analysis in meningeal disease reveals:
  1. Lymphocytic pleocytosis
  2. Elevated protein
  3. Hypoglycorrhachia

■ IMAGING STUDIES

- Chest x-ray examination: unilateral or bilateral upper lobe cavitary or noncavitary lesions
- Radiographic findings of affected joints:
  1. Loss of articular cartilage
  2. Periosteal reaction
  3. Periarticular osteopenia
  4. Cystic changes

TREATMENT

■ NONPHARMACOLOGIC THERAPY

Local heat and prevention of bacterial superinfection in cutaneous or plaque form

■ ACUTE GENERAL Rx

CUTANEOUS AND LYMPHOCUTANEOUS SPOROTRICHOSIS:

- Itraconazole at doses of 100 to 200 mg/day is the drug of choice and should be given for 3 to 6 mo.
- Use saturated solution of potassium iodide (SSKI) 5 to 10 drops PO tid or 1.5 ml PO tid, gradually increasing to 40 to 50 drops PO tid or 3 ml PO tid after meals.
- Maximum tolerated dose should be continued until cutaneous lesions have resolved, approximately 6 to 12 wk.
- Adjunctive therapy with heat is useful and occasionally curative.
- Side effects:
  1. Nausea
  2. Anorexia
  3. Diarrhea
  4. Parotid or lacrimal gland hypertrophy
  5. Acneiform rash

■ DEEP-SEATED MYCOSES (e.g., ostoarticular, noncavitary pulmonary disease)

- Itraconazole
  1. Appropriate initial chemotherapy
  2. Probably as effective as amphotericin B
  3. Less toxic than amphotericin B
  4. Better tolerated than ketoconazole
  5. 100 to 200 mg bid for 1 to 2 yr with continued lifelong suppressive therapy in selected patients
  6. Absence of relapses from 40 to 68 mo has been documented when at least 200 mg/day administered for 24 mo.
  7. Insufficient data for use in disseminated disease (e.g., fungemia and meningitis)
- Parenteral amphotericin B, total course of 2 to 2.5 g or more, results in cure in approximately two thirds of cases
  1. Relapses are common.
  2. Amphotericin B–resistant isolates of *Sporothrix schenkii* have been reported.
  3. Remains the drug of choice for severely ill patients with disseminated disease.
  4. In cavitary pulmonary disease, given perioperatively as an adjunct to surgical resection.
  5. In meningitis, amphotericin B may be used alone or in combination with 5-fluorocytosine.

Fluconazole
  1. Less effective than itraconazole
  2. Requires daily doses of 400 mg/day for lymphocutaneous disease and 800 mg/day for visceral or osteoarticular disease

■ CHRONIC Rx

For lymphocutaneous and visceral disease, therapy with itraconazole 200 mg/day for periods of 24 mo or greater

■ DISPOSITION

- Prognosis for cutaneous disease is good.
- Prognosis is less satisfactory for extracutaneous disease, especially if associated with abnormal immunologic states or other underlying systemic diseases.

■ REFERRAL

To surgeon; with an established diagnosis of pulmonary sporotrichosis, cavitary lesions require resection of involved tissue

☼ PEARLS & CONSIDERATIONS

■ COMMENTS

- In patients with underlying immunosuppression (e.g., hematologic malignancy or infection with HIV), progression of the initial infection may develop into multifocal extracutaneous sporotrichosis.
- In this subset of patients, dissemination of cutaneous lesions is accompanied by hematogenous spread to lungs, bone, mucous membranes, CNS.
- Osteoarticular and pulmonary manifestations predominate with the development of polyarticular arthritis and osteolytic bone lesions.
- In the absence of therapy, the infection is ultimately fatal.
- Patients with underlying immunosuppressive states should be carefully evaluated even when presenting with single cutaneous lesions.
- Diagnostic modalities should include:
  1. Radiographic examination of chest
  2. Technetium pyrophosphate bone scan
  3. Culture of synovial fluid, blood, skin lesion(s)
- In patients with AIDS, itraconazole appears to be the drug of choice, although meningitis and pulmonary disease may warrant the use of amphotericin B.
- In patients with AIDS, lifetime suppressive therapy with itraconazole should follow initial therapy given the potential for relapse and dissemination.

REFERENCES

Aaerstrup FM et al: Oral manifestation of sporotrichosis in AIDS patients, *Oral Dis* 7(2):134, 2001.

Burch JM et al: Unsuspected sporotrichosis in childhood, *Pediatr Infect Dis J* 20(4):442, 2001.

Edwards C et al: Disseminated osteoarticular sporotrichosis: treatment in a patient with acquired immunodeficiency syndrome, *South Med J* 93(8):803, 2000.

Fleury RN et al: Zoonotic sporotrichosis: transmission to humans by infected domestic cat scratching: report of four cases in Sao Paulo, Brazil, *Int J Dermatol* 40(5):318, 2001.

Habte G et al: Cutaneous sporotrichosis: the old iodide treatment remains effective, *Clin Microbiol Infect* 61(1):53, 2000.

Kauffman CA et al: Practice guidelines for the management of patients with sporotrichosis. For the Mycoses Study Group. Infectious Diseases Society of America, *Clin Infect Dis* 30(4):684, 2000.

Author: **George O. Alonso, M.D.**

BASIC INFORMATION

■ DEFINITION
Squamous cell carcinoma (SCC) is a malignant tumor of the skin arising in the epithelium.

■ SYNONYMS
SCC
Skin cancer

■ ICD-9CM CODES
173.9 Skin neoplasm, site unspecified

■ EPIDEMIOLOGY & DEMOGRAPHICS
• SCC is the second most common cutaneous malignancy, comprising 20% of all cases of non-melanoma skin cancer.
• Incidence is highest in lower latitudes (e.g., southern U.S., Australia).
• Male:female ratio of 2:1.
• Incidence increases with age and sun exposure.
• Average age at diagnosis is 66 yr.

■ PHYSICAL FINDINGS & CLINICAL PRESENTATION
• SCC commonly affects scalp, neck region, back of hands, superior surface of the pinna, and the lip.
• The lesion may have a scaly, erythematous macule or plaque.
• Telangiectasia, central ulceration may also be present (Fig. 1-348).
• Most SCC present as exophytic lesions that grow over a period of months.

■ ETIOLOGY
Risk factors include UVB radiation and immunosuppression (renal transplant recipients have a threefold increased risk).

DIAGNOSIS

■ DIFFERENTIAL DIAGNOSIS
• Keratoacanthomas
• Actinic keratosis
• Amelanotic melanoma
• Basal cell carcinoma
• Benign tumors
• Healing traumatic wounds
• Spindle cell tumors
• Warts

■ WORKUP
Diagnosis is made with full-thickness skin biopsy (incisional or excisional).

TREATMENT

■ ACUTE GENERAL Rx
• Electrodesiccation and curettage for small SCCs (<2 cm in diameter), superficial tumors and lesions located in extremity and trunk.
• Tumors thinner than 4 mm can be managed by simple local removal.
• Lesions between 4 and 8 mm thick or those with deep dermal invasion should be excised.
• Tumors penetrating the dermis can be treated with several modalities, including excision and Mohs' surgery, radiation therapy, and chemotherapy.
• Metastatic SCC can be treated with cryotherapy and combination of chemotherapy using 13-*cis*-retinoic acid and interferon α-2A.

■ DISPOSITION
• Survival is related to size, location, degree of differentiation, immunologic status of the patient, depth of invasion, and presence of metastases. Risk factors for metastasis include lesions on the lip or ear, increasing lesion depth, and poor cell differentiation.
• Patients whose tumors penetrate through the dermis or exceed 8 mm in thickness are at risk of tumor recurrence.
• The most common metastatic locations are regional lymph nodes, liver, and lung.
• Tumors on the scalp, forehead, ears, nose, and lips also carry a higher risk.
• SCCs originating in the lip and pinna metastasize in 10% to 20% of cases.
• Five-year survival for metastatic squamous cell carcinoma is 34%.

■ REFERRAL
Oncology referral for metastatic SCC

PEARLS & CONSIDERATIONS

■ COMMENTS
• SCC arising in areas of prior radiation, thermal injury, and areas of chronic ulcers or chronic draining sinuses are more aggressive and have a higher frequency of metastases than those originating in actinic damaged skin.

REFERENCES
Jerant AF et al: Early detection and treatment of skin cancer, *Am Fam Physician* 62:357, 2000.
Martinez JC, Otley CC: The management of melanoma and nonmelanoma skin cancer: a review for the primary care physician, *Mayo Clin Proc* 76:1253, 2001.
Author: **Fred F. Ferri, M.D.**

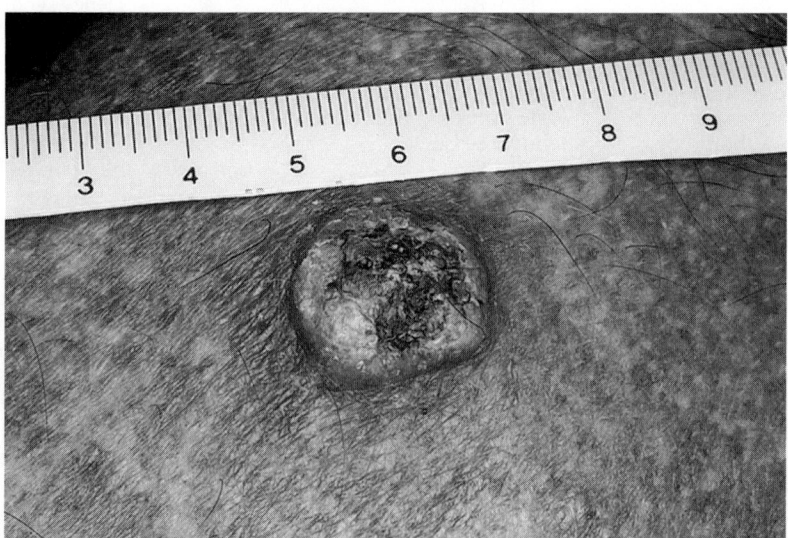

Fig. 1-348 Squamous cell carcinoma. Nodular hyperkeratotic lesion with central erosion. (From Noble J et al: *Textbook of primary care medicine,* ed 2, St Louis, 1995, Mosby.)

BASIC INFORMATION

■ DEFINITION
The term *status epilepticus* refers to >30 min of (1) continuous seizure activity or (2) two or more sequential seizures without full recovery of consciousness between seizures.

ICD-9CM CODES
345.3 Grand mal status

■ EPIDEMIOLOGY & DEMOGRAPHICS
INCIDENCE (IN U.S.): 61 cases/100,000 persons/yr
PREDOMINANT SEX: Male = female
PREDOMINANT AGE: >60 yr
PEAK INCIDENCE: <1 yr and >60 yr
GENETICS: Familial predisposition is rare.

■ PHYSICAL FINDINGS & CLINICAL PRESENTATION
- Findings depend on underlying etiology and duration.
- Convulsive seizures may evolve into subtle face or eye movements or into an appearance of coma despite ongoing electrographic seizure activity.

■ ETIOLOGY
- Stroke
- Systemic infection
- Low antiepileptic drug levels
- Remote CNS insult

DIAGNOSIS

■ DIFFERENTIAL DIAGNOSIS
- Coma
- Encephalopathic states
- Psychogenic unresponsiveness

■ WORKUP
Because convulsive and complex partial status epilepticus are emergencies with substantial morbidity and mortality, treatment must be early and aggressive, not postponed until an etiology is determined.

■ LABORATORY TESTS
- While treatment is being initiated: glucose, electrolytes, BUN, ABG, drug levels, CBC, UA
- Lumbar puncture in children with fever and adults suspected to have meningitis

■ IMAGING STUDIES
Unless the etiology is known, CT scan is recommended as soon as possible after seizures have been controlled.

TREATMENT

■ NONPHARMACOLOGIC THERAPY
- Give oxygen by nasal cannula.
- Maintain blood pressure.
- Maintain body temperature.
- Monitor ECG.
- Obtain IV access.

■ ACUTE GENERAL Rx
- Thiamine 100 mg IV and glucose 50 mg D_{50} by IV push (2 ml/kg D_{25} in children) unless hyperglycemic
- Lorazepam 0.1 mg/kg IV at 2 mg/min
- If seizures persist, phosphenytoin 20 mg/kg IV at 150 mg/min (if not available, use phenytoin at up to 50 mg/min as tolerated)
- If seizures persist, phenobarbital 20 mg/kg IV at 100 mg/min; will likely require intubation
- If seizures persist, emergency neurologic consultation

■ CHRONIC Rx
- A single episode with an identifiable and easily correctable provoking factor (e.g., hyponatremia) does not warrant long-term use of anticonvulsants.
- Treatment is indicated if there is significant risk of recurrence (e.g., known epilepsy, brain lesion, epileptiform EEG abnormalities).

■ DISPOSITION
- Favorable if status is treated promptly and no acute brain lesion is present
- Overall mortality of 22%; higher in the elderly (38%) and substantially lower in children (2.5%)

■ REFERRAL
If seizures do not respond to initial management as outlined

PEARLS & CONSIDERATIONS

■ COMMENTS
- Because of varied clinical presentations of status epilepticus, there are no clinical grounds of certainty that seizures have stopped unless the patient regains full consciousness.
- EEG provides definitive information about seizure cessation. If available, use of EEG in the management of status epilepticus is recommended highly.

REFERENCES
Alldredge BR et al: A comparison of lorazepam, diazepam, and placebo for the treatment of out-of-hospital status epilepticus, *N Engl J Med* 345:631, 2001.
Lowenstein DH, Alldredge B: Status epilepticus, *N Engl J Med* 338:970, 1998.
Treiman DM et al: A comparison of four treatments for generalized convulsive status epilepticus, *N Engl J Med* 339:792, 1998.
Author: **Michael Gruenthal, M.D., Ph.D.**

Gwendolyn R. Lee, M.D.
Internal Medicine

BASIC INFORMATION

■ DEFINITION
Stevens-Johnson syndrome (SJS) is a severe vesiculobullous form of erythema multiforme affecting skin, mouth, eyes, and genitalia.

■ SYNONYMS
SJS
Herpes iris
Febrile mucocutaneous syndrome

ICD-9CM CODES
695.1 Stevens-Johnson syndrome

■ EPIDEMIOLOGY & DEMOGRAPHICS
- SJS affects predominantly children and young adults.
- Male:female ratio of 2:1.

■ PHYSICAL FINDINGS & CLINICAL PRESENTATION
- The cutaneous eruption is generally preceded by vague, nonspecific symptoms of low-grade fever and fatigue occurring 1 to 14 days before the skin lesions. Cough is often present. Fever may be high during the active stages.
- Bullae generally occur on the conjunctiva, mucous membranes of the mouth, nares, and genital regions.
- Corneal ulcerations may result in blindness.
- Ulcerative stomatitis results in hemorrhagic crusting.
- Flat, atypical target lesions or purpuric maculae may be distributed on the trunk or be widespread (Fig. 1-349).
- The pain from oral lesions may compromise fluid intake and result in dehydration.
- Thick, mucopurulent sputum and oral lesions may interfere with breathing.

■ ETIOLOGY
- Drugs (e.g., phenytoin, penicillins, phenobarbital, sulfonamides) are the most common cause.
- Upper respiratory tract infections (e.g., *Mycoplasma pneumoniae*) and herpes simplex viral infections have also been implicated in SJS.

DIAGNOSIS

■ DIFFERENTIAL DIAGNOSIS
- Toxic erythema (drugs or infection)
- Pemphigus
- Pemphigoid
- Urticaria
- Hemorrhagic fevers
- Serum sickness
- *Staphylococcus* scalded-skin syndrome
- Behçet's syndrome

■ WORKUP
- Diagnosis is generally based on clinical presentation and characteristic appearance of the lesions.
- Skin biopsy is generally reserved for when classic lesions are absent and diagnosis is uncertain.

■ LABORATORY TESTS
CBC with differential, cultures in cases of suspected infection

■ IMAGING STUDIES
Chest x-ray examination may show patchy changes in patients with pulmonary involvement.

TREATMENT

■ NONPHARMACOLOGIC THERAPY
- Withdrawal of any potential drug precipitants
- Careful skin nursing to prevent secondary infection

■ ACUTE GENERAL Rx
- Treatment of associated conditions, (e.g., acyclovir for herpes simplex virus infection, erythromycin for mycoplasma infection)
- Antihistamines for pruritus
- Treatment of the cutaneous blisters with cool, wet Burow's compresses
- Relief of oral symptoms by frequent rinsing with lidocaine (Xylocaine Viscous)
- Liquid or soft diet with plenty of fluids to ensure proper hydration
- Treatment of secondary infections with antibiotics
- Corticosteroids: use remains controversial; when used, prednisone 20 to 30 mg bid until new lesions no longer appear, then rapidly tapered
- Topical steroids: may use to treat papules and plaques; however, should not be applied to eroded areas
- Vitamin A: may be used for lacrimal hyposecretion

■ DISPOSITION
- Prognosis varies with severity of disease. It is generally good in patients with limited disease; however, mortality may approach 10% in patients with extensive involvement.
- Oral lesions may continue for several months.
- Scarring and corneal abnormalities may occur in 20% of patients.

■ REFERRAL
- Hospital admission in a unit used for burn care is recommended in severe cases.
- Urethral involvement may necessitate catheterization.
- Ocular involvement should be monitored by an ophthalmologist.

PEARLS & CONSIDERATIONS

■ COMMENTS
Risk of recurrence of SJS is 30% to 40%.
Author: **Fred F. Ferri, M.D.**

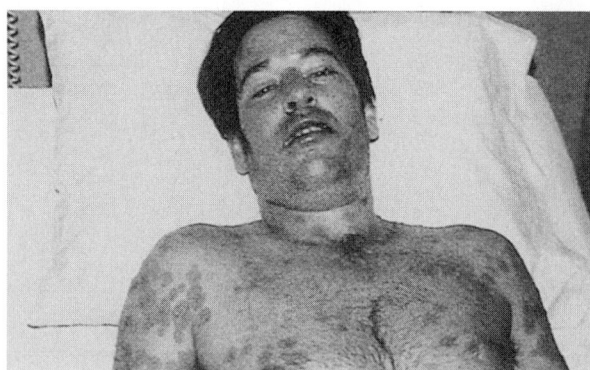

Fig. 1-349 Stevens-Johnson syndrome. (From Stein JH: *Internal medicine,* ed 5, St Louis, 1998, Mosby.)

BASIC INFORMATION

■ DEFINITION

Stomatitis is inflammation involving the oral mucous membranes.

■ SYNONYMS

Heterogeneous grouping of unrelated illnesses, each with their own designation(s)

ICD-9CM CODES

528.0 Stomatitis
054.2 (herpetic)
528.2 (aphthous)
112.0 (monilial)

■ CLASSIFICATION

WHITE LESIONS: Candidiasis (thrush)
Caused by yeast infection *(Candida albicans)*
Examination: white, curdlike material that when wiped off leaves a raw bleeding surface
Epidemiology: seen in the very young and the very old, those with immunodeficiency (AIDS, cancer), persons with diabetes, and patients treated with antibacterial agents
Diagnosis: Ovoid yeast and hyphae seen in scrapings treated with KOH culture
Treatment: Topical with nystatin or clotrimazole
Systemic with ketoconazole or fluconazole
Other
- Leukoedema: filmy opalescent-appearing mucosa, which can be reverted to normal appearance by stretching. This condition is benign.
- White sponge nevus: thick, white corrugated folds involving the buccal mucosa. Appears in childhood as an autosomal dominant trait. Benign condition.
- Darier's disease (keratosis follicularis): white papules on the gingivae, alveolar mucosa, and dorsal tongue. Skin lesions also present (erythematous papules). Inherited as an autosomal dominant trait.
- Chemical injury: white sloughing mucosa.
- Nicotine stomatitis: whitened palate with red papules.
- Lichen planus: linear, reticular, slightly raised striae on buccal mucosa. Skin is involved by pruritic violaceous papules on forearms and inner thighs.
- Discoid lupus erythematosus: lesion resembles lichen planus.
- Leukoplakia: white lesions that cannot be scraped off; 20% are premalignant epithelial dysplasia or squamous cell carcinoma.
- Hairy leukoplakia: shaggy white surface that cannot be wiped off; seen in HIV infection, caused by EBV.

RED LESIONS:
- Candidiasis may present with red instead of the more frequent white lesion (see above). Median rhomboid glossitis is a chronic variant.
- Benign migratory glossitis (geographic tongue): area of atrophic depapillated mucosa surround by a keratotic border. Benign lesion, no treatment required.
- Hemangiomas.
- Histoplasmosis: ill-defined irregular patch with a granulomatous surface, sometimes ulcerated.
- Allergy.
- Anemia: atrophic reddened glossal mucosa seen with pernicious anemia.
- Erythroplakia: red patch usually caused by epithelial dysplasia or squamous cell carcinoma.
- Burning tongue (glossopyrosis): normal examination; sometimes associated with denture trauma, anemia, diabetes, vitamin B_{12} deficiency, psychogenic problems.

DARK LESIONS (BROWN, BLUE, BLACK):
- Coated tongue: accumulation of keratin; harmless condition that can be treated by scraping
- Melanotic lesions: freckles, lentigines, lentigo, melanoma, Peutz-Jeghers syndrome, Addison's disease
- Varices
- Kaposi's sarcoma: red or purple macules that enlarge to form tumors; seen in patients with AIDS

RAISED LESIONS:
- Papilloma
- Verruca vulgaris
- Condyloma acuminatum
- Fibroma
- Epulis
- Pyogenic granuloma
- Mucocele
- Retention cyst

BLISTERS:
- Primary herpetic gingivostomatitis
Caused by herpes simplex virus type 1 or less frequently type 2
Course: day 1—malaise, fever, headache, sore throat, cervical lymphadenopathy; days 2 and 3—appearance of vesicles that develop into painful ulcers of 2 to 4 mm in diameter; duration of up to 2 wk
Diagnosis:
Exfoliative cytology
Viral culture
Immunofluorescence for herpes antigen
Treatment:
Supportive
Consider acyclovir
Recurrent intraoral herpes: rare, recurrences typically involve only the keratinized epithelium (lips)
- Pemphigus and pemphigoid
- Hand-foot-mouth disease: caused by coxsackievirus group A
- Erythema multiforme
- Herpangina: caused by echovirus
- Traumatic ulcer
- Primary syphilis
- Perlèche (or angular cheilitis)
- Recurrent aphthous stomatitis (canker sores)
- Behçet's syndrome (aphthous ulcers, uveitis, genital ulcerations, arthritis, and aseptic meningitis)
- Reiter's syndrome (conjunctivitis, urethritis, and arthritis with occasional oral ulcerations)
- Unknown cause

Course: solitary or multiple painful ulcers may develop simultaneously and heal over 10 to 14 days. The size of the lesions and the frequency of recurrences are variable.
Treatment: topical corticosteroids or systemic steroids for severe cases.

REFERENCE

Allen CM, Blozis GG: Oral mucosal lesions. In Cummings CW (ed): *Otolaryngology: head and neck surgery,* ed 2, St Louis, 1992, Mosby.
Author: **Tom J. Wachtel, M.D.**

BASIC INFORMATION

■ **DEFINITION**
Strabismus is a condition of the eyes in which the visual axes of the eyes are not straight in the primary position or in which the eyes do not follow each other in the different positions of gaze.

■ **SYNONYMS**
Esotropia
Exotropia
Restrictive eye movement

ICD-9CM CODES
378.9 Strabismus

■ **EPIDEMIOLOGY & DEMOGRAPHICS**
INCIDENCE (IN U.S.): 2% of all children
PREDOMINANT SEX: None
PREDOMINANT AGE: Birth to 5 yr of age
PEAK INCIDENCE: Childhood
GENETICS: None known

■ **PHYSICAL FINDINGS & CLINICAL PRESENTATION**
Conjugate gaze loss in both eyes with the eyes focusing independently (Fig. 1-350)

■ **ETIOLOGY**
• Most cases are congenital.
• Rarely, there is neurologic disease or severe refractive errors.

 DIAGNOSIS

■ **DIFFERENTIAL DIAGNOSIS**
• Refractive errors
• CNS tumors
• Orbital tumors
• Brain and CNS dysfunction

■ **WORKUP**
• Eye examination
• Visual field

■ **LABORATORY TESTS**
Generally not needed

■ **IMAGING STUDIES**
Necessary only if other neurologic findings are found

TREATMENT

■ **NONPHARMACOLOGIC THERAPY**
• Glasses
• Patching
• Prisms

■ **CHRONIC Rx**
• Glasses
• Alternate eye patching
• Surgery

■ **DISPOSITION**
• The earlier the condition is treated, the more likely it is that the child will have normal vision in both eyes.
• After age 5 yr, visual loss is usually permanent.

■ **REFERRAL**
• If surgery is contemplated
• To an ophthalmologist for management (usually)

PEARLS & CONSIDERATIONS

■ **COMMENTS**
• If properly treated, this easily recognizable and treatable condition results in normal vision.
• If not treated, this condition can result in decrease in vision in one eye (amblyopia).
Author: **Melvyn Koby, M.D.**

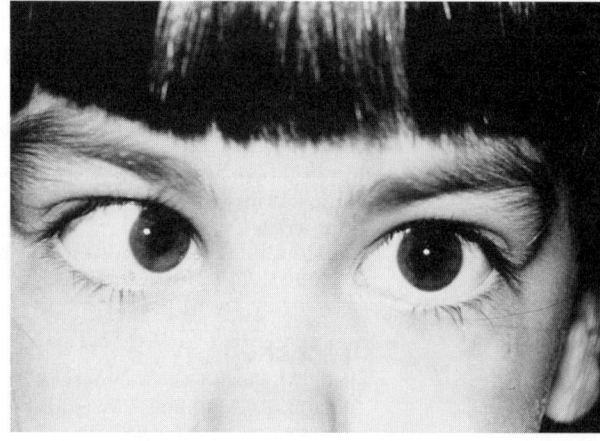
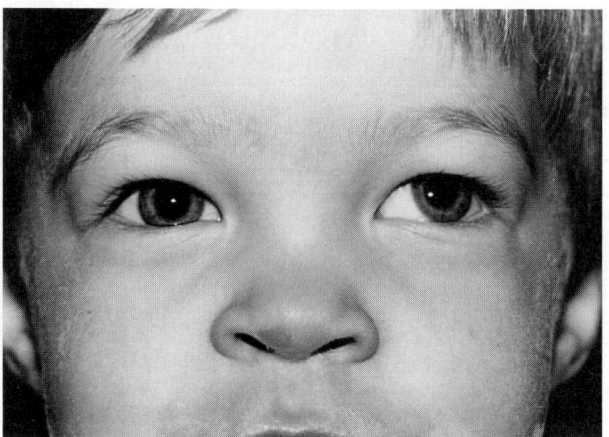

Fig. 1-350 A, Note the nasal deviation of the right eye with the corneal light reflection temporally displaced on the right eye and centered in the left pupil, indicating an esotropia. **B,** Divergent strabismus of the left eye, defining an exotropia. (From Hoekelman R [ed]: *Primary pediatric care,* ed 3, St Louis, 1997, Mosby.)

BASIC INFORMATION

DEFINITION
Subarachnoid hemorrhage is a mechanical disruption of an intracranial portion of the vascular system resulting in entry of blood into the subarachnoid space.

ICD-9CM CODES
430 Subarachnoid hemorrhage

EPIDEMIOLOGY & DEMOGRAPHICS
INCIDENCE (IN U.S.): 6 to 28 cases/100,000 persons/yr
PREDOMINANT SEX: Males > females in persons <40 yr of age; then female:male ratio of 3:2 in persons >40 yr old
PREDOMINANT AGE: >50 yr
PEAK INCIDENCE: 50 to 60 yr
GENETICS:
- Familial predisposition to multiple aneurysms
- Increased incidence in some inherited systemic diseases

PHYSICAL FINDINGS & CLINICAL PRESENTATION
- Patients typically present with abrupt onset of a severe headache of maximal intensity ("the worst headache of my life"), accompanied by nuchal rigidity, nausea, and vomiting.
- Transient loss of consciousness occurs in 45% of patients.
- Focal neurologic deficits may be present.
- Funduscopic examination may reveal subhyaloid hemorrhage.

ETIOLOGY
- Two thirds of cases: rupture of saccular ("berry") aneurysms
- Others: fusiform, mycotic, traumatic, dissecting, and tumor-related aneurysms

DIAGNOSIS

DIFFERENTIAL DIAGNOSIS
- Intraparenchymal hemorrhage
- Meningitis

WORKUP
- CT scan without contrast is initial test of choice, with a sensitivity of about 90%.
- If CT scan is unavailable, transfer patient immediately to a facility that has one.

LABORATORY TESTS
PT, PTT, platelet count at a minimum for clotting abnormality.

IMAGING STUDIES
CT scan (Fig. 1-351) followed by cerebral angiography if hemorrhage is confirmed

TREATMENT

NONPHARMACOLOGIC THERAPY
- Intubation as necessary
- Bed rest

ACUTE GENERAL Rx
- Short-acting analgesics (e.g., morphine 1 to 4 mg IV)
- Sedation (e.g., midazolam 1 to 5 mg IV)
- Stool softeners
- Neurosurgical or interventional neuroradiologic referral mandatory if aneurysm or arteriovenous malformation demonstrated by angiography

CHRONIC Rx
- Seizure prophylaxis (phenytoin 15 to 20 mg/kg IV)
- Vasospasm prophylaxis (nimodipine 60 mg PO q4h)
- BP control (e.g., labetalol 10 to 40 mg IV q30min)

DISPOSITION
Approximately 35% early mortality, 45% at 1 mo

REFERRAL
Transfer as soon as possible to a facility with neurosurgical care.

PEARLS & CONSIDERATIONS

COMMENTS
About 20% of patients experience warning signs within 3 mo before aneurysm rupture, including moderate or severe headache ("sentinel headache"), dizziness, nausea and vomiting, transient motor or sensory deficits, loss of consciousness, or visual disturbances.

REFERENCES
Bederson JB et al: Recommendations for the management of patients with unruptured intracranial aneurysms: a statement for healthcare professionals from the Stroke Council of the American Heart Association, *Circulation* 102(18):2300, 2000.

Edlow JA, Caplan LR: Avoiding pitfalls in the diagnosis of subarachnoid hemorrhage, *N Engl J Med* 342:29, 2000.

Morgenstern LB et al: Worst headache and subarachnoid hemorrhage: prospective modern computed tomography and spinal fluid analysis, *Ann Emerg Med* 32:297, 1998.
Author: **Michael Gruenthal, M.D., Ph.D.**

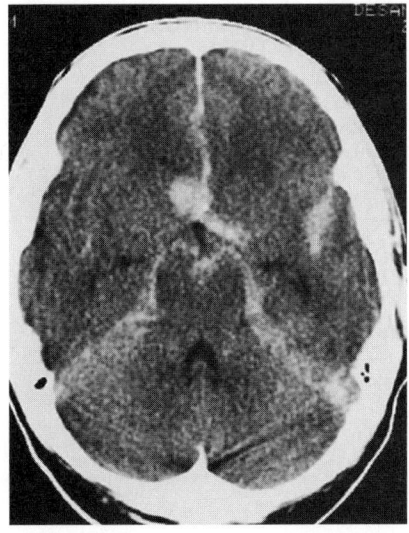

Fig. 1-351 Noncontrast CT demonstrates diffuse subarachnoid hemorrhage. The rounded area of hyperdensity anterior to the suprasellar cistern represents an aneurysm of the anterior communicating artery. (From Specht N [ed]: *Practical guide to diagnostic imaging,* St Louis, 1998, Mosby.)

BASIC INFORMATION

■ **DEFINITION**

Subclavian steal syndrome is an occlusion or severe stenosis of the proximal subclavian artery leading to decreased antegrade flow or retrograde flow in the ipsilateral vertebral artery and neurologic symptoms referable to the posterior circulation.

■ **SYNONYMS**

Proximal subclavian (or innominate) artery stenosis or occlusion

■ **ICD-9CM CODES**

435.2 Subclavian steal syndrome

■ **EPIDEMIOLOGY & DEMOGRAPHICS**

• Similar to that of other manifestations of atherosclerosis (coronary artery disease, cerebrovascular disease, or peripheral vascular disease)

• Affects middle-aged persons (men somewhat younger than women on average) with arteriosclerotic risk factors including family history, smoking, diabetes mellitus, hyperlipidemia, hypertension, sedentary lifestyle

■ **PHYSICAL FINDINGS & CLINICAL PRESENTATION**

Symptoms:

• Many patients are asymptomatic.

• Upper extremity ischemic symptoms: fatigue, exercise-related aching, coolness, numbness of the involved upper extremity.

• Neurologic symptoms are reported by 25% of patients with known unilateral subclavian steal. These include brief spells of:
  1. Vertigo
  2. Diplopia
  3. Decreased vision
  4. Oscillopsia
  5. Gait unsteadiness

These spells are only occasionally provoked by exercising the ischemic upper extremity (classic subclavian steal). Left subclavian steal is more common than right, but the latter is more serious.

• Posterior circulation stroke related to subclavian steal is rare.

• Innominate artery stenosis can cause decreased right carotid artery flow and cerebrovascular symptoms of the anterior cerebral circulation, but this is uncommon.

Physical findings:

• Delayed and smaller volume pulse (wrist or antecubital) in the affected upper extremity

• Lower blood pressure in the affected upper extremity

• Supraclavicular bruit

NOTE: Inflating a blood pressure cuff will increase the bruit if it originates from a vertebral artery stenosis and decrease the bruit if it originates from a subclavian artery stenosis.

■ **ETIOLOGY & PATHOGENESIS**

Etiology:

• Atherosclerosis

• Arteritis (Takayasu's disease and temporal arteritis)

• Embolism to the subclavian or innominate artery

• Cervical rib

• Chronic use of a crutch

• Occupational (baseball pitchers and cricket bowlers)

Pathogenesis: The vertebral artery originates from the subclavian artery. For subclavian steal to occur, the occlusion must be proximal to the takeoff of the vertebral artery. On the right side, only a small distance separates the bifurcation of the innominate artery and the takeoff of the vertebral artery, explaining why the condition occurs less commonly on the right side. Occlusion of the innominate artery must affect right carotid artery flow.

 DIAGNOSIS

• History (see above), physical findings (see above), and imaging studies.

• The carotid arteries should be evaluated at least noninvasively in all cases.

■ **DIFFERENTIAL DIAGNOSIS**

• Posterior circulation TIA (and stroke)

• Upper extremity ischemia
  1. Distal subclavian artery stenosis/occlusion
  2. Raynaud's syndrome
  3. Thoracic outlet syndrome

■ **IMAGING STUDIES**

• Noninvasive upper extremity arterial flow studies

• Doppler sonography of the vertebral, subclavian, and innominate arteries

• Arteriography

TREATMENT

• In most patients the disease is benign and requires no treatment other than atherosclerosis risk factor modification and aspirin. Symptoms tend to improve over time as collateral circulation develops.

• Vascular surgical reconstruction requires a thoracotomy; it may be indicated in innominate artery stenosis or when upper extremity ischemia is incapacitating.

REFERENCE

Caplan LR: Large-vessel occlusive disease of the posterior circulation. In Caplan LR (ed): *Stroke: a clinical approach,* ed 2, New York, 1993, Butterworth-Heinemann.

Author: **Tom J. Wachtel, M.D.**

BASIC INFORMATION

■ DEFINITION
Suicide refers to successful and unsuccessful attempts to kill oneself.

■ SYNONYMS
Self-murder

■ ICD-9CM CODES
Categorized by method (e.g., poisoning)

■ EPIDEMIOLOGY & DEMOGRAPHICS
INCIDENCE (IN U.S.):
- 11.4 cases/100,000 persons; 1.4% of total deaths
- 18.8/100,000 men
- 4.3/100,000 women

PREDOMINANT AGE: Increases with age (e.g., 13.1 cases/100,000 persons aged 15 to 24 yr, 16.9 cases/100,000 persons aged 65 to 74 yr, and 23.5 cases/100,000 persons aged 75 to 84 yr)
PEAK INCIDENCE: >65 yr of age
GENETICS:
- Biologic factors may increase the risk of suicide directly (e.g., by increasing impulsivity) or indirectly (e.g., by predisposing to a mental illness).
- Family history of suicide is associated with suicidal behavior.

■ PHYSICAL FINDINGS & CLINICAL PRESENTATION
Methods used in attempted (unsuccessful) suicides differ from those used in completed suicides.
- Overdose used in >70% of attempted suicides. Cutting of wrists or other parts of the body is the second most common form.
- About 60% of completed suicides are accomplished with firearms. Hanging is the second most common method for completed suicides. Suffocation (e.g., carbon monoxide) and overdose are also relatively common forms of completing suicide.
- Several risk factors are usually present concurrently, including a psychiatric illness such as depression or anxiety, middle age or advanced age, white race, male gender, a recent divorce or separation, comorbid substance abuse (particularly when intoxicated), previous history of suicide attempts, fatal plan (e.g., firearms or hanging), history of violence, and family history of suicide. Concurrent chronic physical illness increases the risk for suicide greatly (e.g., the risk for suicide among AIDS or renal dialysis patients is nearly 30 times that of the general population).

■ ETIOLOGY
- Individuals with a mental or a substance abuse disorder are responsible for >90% of all suicides.
- The concurrence of more than one condition (e.g., depression and alcohol abuse) greatly increases the risk of suicide.
- Hopelessness is a strong predictor of suicide potential.

DIAGNOSIS

■ DIFFERENTIAL DIAGNOSIS
- Some disorders are associated with self-injurious behavior that is not suicidal. Borderline personality disorder (e.g., manifests with self-mutilation without active suicidal intent). Eating disorders are harmful and may be fatal, but death is never the goal.
- Some suicidal behavior is intended as a "call for help." In these situations individuals usually design the suicide so that they will be discovered before significant damage has been done.

■ WORKUP
- Suicidal patients present in one of four ways:
  1. Covert suicidal ideation
  2. Overt suicidal ideation
  3. After a suicide attempt
  4. Dead from a suicide attempt
- Covert suicidal ideation occurs in patients primarily with multiple vague physical complaints, depression, anxiety, or substance abuse.
- As part of the history, the physician must directly inquire into the presence of suicidal ideation.
- The concurrence of multiple psychiatric problems, substance abuse, and multiple physical problems increases the risk.

TREATMENT

■ NONPHARMACOLOGIC THERAPY
- Major immediate intervention: placement of the patient in a safe environment (usually hospitalization in a psychiatric unit or a medical unit with continuous observation)
- Long-term: psychotherapy aimed at factors that underlie the decision to pursue suicide or at the risk factors contributing to suicidal behavior
- Substance abuse treatment (e.g., AA, NA) when substance abuse is present

■ ACUTE GENERAL Rx
- Benzodiazepines are useful in reducing the extreme anxiety and dysphoria in a suicidal patient; however, these agents are depressive and should be used only when patient is in safe environment.
- Antipsychotics can be used if psychosis is present (e.g., voices telling patient to hurt self).
- Mood stabilizers and antidepressants should be started in the acute setting but may have up to a 2-wk latency period.

■ CHRONIC Rx
- Therapy should be aimed at the underlying condition (e.g., antidepressants for depression, anxiolytics or antidepressants for anxiety, ongoing substance abuse treatment for substance abuse history, or psychotherapy for chronic low self-esteem, hopelessness).
- In elderly, loneliness and medical disability are major reasons for suicide and therefore major targets for intervention.

■ DISPOSITION
- Prior suicide attempt is the best predictor for completed suicides (i.e., patients who attempt suicide once are at high risk for completing suicide in the future).
- Conditions associated with suicide (e.g., depression, physical ailments) are usually chronic and recurring.

■ REFERRAL
If patient is acutely suicidal and requires protection in hospital

REFERENCE
Gould MS et al: Psychopathology associated with suicidal ideation and attempts among children and adolescents, *J Am Acad Child Adolesc Psychiatry* 37:915, 1998.
Author: **Rif S. El-Mallakh, M.D.**

BASIC INFORMATION

■ DEFINITION

Superior vena cava syndrome is a set of symptoms that results when a mediastinal mass compresses the superior vena cava (SVC) or the veins that drain into it (Fig. 1-352).

ICD-9CM CODES

453.2 (vena cava thrombosis)

■ EPIDEMIOLOGY & DEMOGRAPHICS

Mirrors lung cancer (especially small-cell carcinoma) and lymphoma: see "Lung Neoplasm" and "Lymphoma" in Section I

■ PHYSICAL FINDINGS & CLINICAL PRESENTATION

Symptoms:
• Shortness of breath
• Chest pain
• Cough
• Dysphagia
• Headache
• Syncope
• Visual trouble
Signs:
• Chest wall vein distention
• Neck vein distention
• Facial edema
• Upper extremity swelling
• Cyanosis

■ ETIOLOGY

• Lung cancer (80% of all cases, of which half are small cell lung cancer)
• Lymphoma (15%)
• Tuberculosis
• Goiter
• Aortic aneurysm (arteriosclerotic or syphilitic)
• SVC thrombosis
  1. Primary: associated with a central venous catheter
  2. Secondary: as a complication of SVC syndrome associated with one of the above causes

 DIAGNOSIS

■ DIFFERENTIAL DIAGNOSIS

The syndrome is characteristic enough to exclude other diagnoses. The differential diagnosis concerns the underlying etiologies listed above.

■ WORKUP

• Chest x-ray
• Venography
• Chest CT scan or MRI
• Ultrasonography
• Sputum cytology
• Bronchoscopy
• Mediastinoscopy
• Thoracotomy

 TREATMENT

Although invasive procedures such as mediastinoscopy or thoracotomy are associated with higher than usual risk of bleeding, a tissue diagnosis is usually needed before commencing therapy.
Emergency empiric radiation is indicated in critical situations such as respiratory failure or central nervous system signs associated with increased intracranial pressure.
• Treatment of the underlying malignancy
  1. Radiation
  2. Chemotherapy
• Anticoagulant or fibrinolytic therapy in patients who do not respond to cancer treatment within a week or if an obstructing thrombus has been documented.
• Diuretics
• Steroids

■ REFERRAL

To a thoracic surgeon, pulmonary specialist, and/or oncologist

REFERENCE

Markman M: Diagnosis and management of superior vena cava syndrome, *Cleveland Clin J Med* 66:59, 1999.
Author: **Tom J. Wachtel, M.D.**

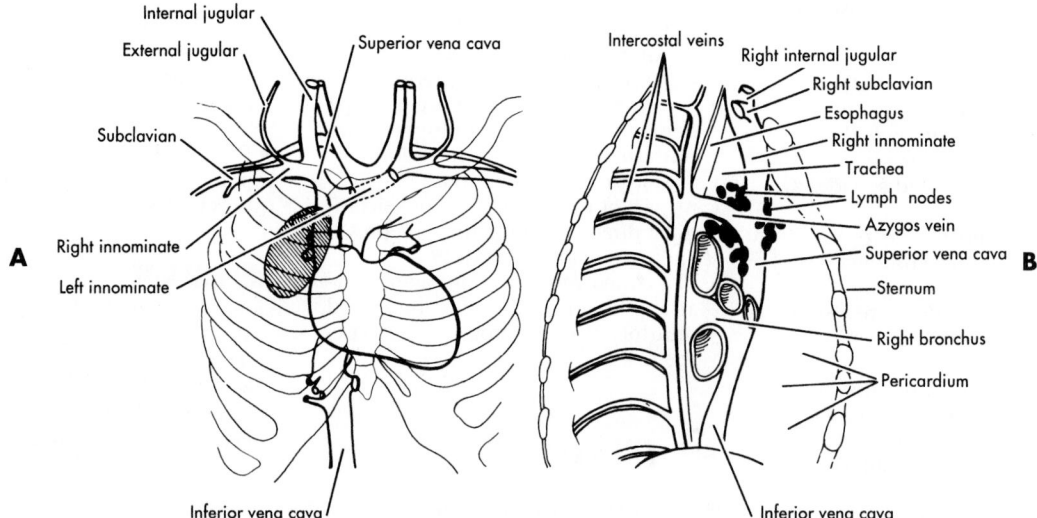

Fig. 1-352 **A,** Frontal and, **B,** sagittal sections of thorax showing relationship of azygos vein to superior vena cava (SVC), coalescence of innominates to form SVC at right second rib, and encasement of SVC by nodal structures. Shaded area indicates classic site of obstruction. (From Lokich JL, Goodman R: *JAMA* 231:58, 1975.)

BASIC INFORMATION

■ DEFINITION
Syncope is the temporary loss of consciousness resulting from an acute global reduction in cerebral blood flow.

ICD-9CM CODES
720.2 Syncope

■ EPIDEMIOLOGY & DEMOGRAPHICS
- Syncope accounts for 3% to 5% of emergency room visits.
- 30% of the adult population will experience at least one syncopal episode during their lifetime.
- Incidence of syncope is highest in elderly men and young women.

■ PHYSICAL FINDINGS & CLINICAL PRESENTATION
- Blood pressure: if low, consider orthostatic hypertension; if unequal in both arms (difference >20 mm Hg), consider subclavian steal or dissecting aneurysm. (NOTE: Blood pressure and heart rate should be recorded in the supine, sitting, and standing positions.)
- Pulse: if patient has tachycardia, bradycardia, or irregular rhythm, consider dysrhythmia.
- Mental status: if patient is confused after the "syncopal episode," consider postictal state.
- Heart: if there are murmurs present suggestive of AS or IHSS, consider syncope secondary to left ventricular outflow obstruction; if there are JVD and distal heart sounds, consider cardiac tamponade.
- Carotid sinus pressure: can be diagnostic if it reproduces symptoms and other causes are excluded; a pause >3 sec or a systolic BP drop >50 mm Hg without symptoms or <30 mm Hg with symptoms when sinus pressure is applied separately on each side for <5 sec is considered abnormal. This test should be avoided in patients with carotid bruits or cerebrovascular disease; ECG monitoring, IV access, and bedside atropine should be available when carotid sinus pressure is applied.

■ ETIOLOGY
- Vasovagal (vasodepressor)
  1. Psychophysiologic (panic disorders, hysteria)
  2. Visceral reflex
  3. Carotid sinus
  4. Glossopharyngeal neuralgia
  5. Reduction of venous return caused by Valsalva maneuver, cough, defecation, or micturition

- Orthostatic hypotension
  1. Hypovolemia
  2. Antihypertensive drugs
  3. Neurogenic, idiopathic
  4. Pheochromocytoma
  5. Systemic mastocytosis
- Cardiac
  1. Reduced cardiac output
     a. Left ventricular outflow obstruction (aortic stenosis, hypertrophic cardiomyopathy)
     b. Obstruction to pulmonary flow (pulmonary embolism, pulmonic stenosis, primary pulmonary hypertension)
     c. MI with pump failure
     d. Cardiac tamponade
     e. Mitral stenosis
  2. Dysrhythmias or asystole
     a. Extreme tachycardia (>160 to 180 bpm)
     b. Severe bradycardia (<30 to 40 bpm)
     c. Sick sinus syndrome
     d. AV block (second- or third-degree)
     e. Ventricular tachycardia or fibrillation
     f. Long QT syndrome
     g. Pacemaker malfunction
- Cardiovascular
  1. Vertebrobasilar TIA, spasm
  2. Subclavian steal
  3. Basilar migraine
  4. Colloid cyst of the third ventricle
- Other causes
  1. Mechanical reduction of venous return (atrial myxoma, valve thrombus)
  2. Not related to decreased blood flow: hypoxia, hypoglycemia, anemia, hyperventilation, seizure disorder, drug or alcohol abuse

DIAGNOSIS

■ DIFFERENTIAL DIAGNOSIS
See "Workup."

■ WORKUP
The history is crucial to diagnosing the cause of syncope and may suggest a diagnosis that can be evaluated with directed testing.
- Sudden loss of consciousness: consider cardiac arrhythmias, vertebrobasilar TIA.
- Gradual loss of consciousness: consider orthostatic hypotension, vasodepressor syncope, hypoglycemia.
- Patient's activity at the time of syncope:
  1. Micturition, coughing, defecation: consider syncope secondary to decreased venous return.
  2. Turning head while shaving: consider carotid sinus syndrome.

  3. Physical exertion in a patient with murmur: consider aortic stenosis.
  4. Arm exercise: consider subclavian steal syndrome.
  5. Assuming an upright position: consider orthostatic hypotension.
- Associated events:
  1. Chest pain: consider MI, pulmonary embolism.
  2. Palpitations: consider dysrhythmias.
  3. History of aura, incontinence during episode, and transient confusion after syncope: consider seizure disorder.
  4. Psychologic stress: syncope may be vasovagal.
- Review current medications, particularly antihypertensive drugs.

■ LABORATORY TESTS
Routine blood tests rarely yield diagnostically useful information and should be done only if they are specifically suggested by the results of the history and physical examination. Listed below are commonly ordered tests.
- Pregnancy test should be considered in women of childbearing age.
- CBC to rule out anemia, infection.
- Electrolytes, BUN, creatinine, magnesium, calcium to rule out electrolyte abnormalities and evaluate fluid status.
- Cardiac isoenzymes should be obtained if the patient gives a history of chest pain before the syncopal episode.
- ABGs to rule out pulmonary embolus, hyperventilation (when suspected).
- Evaluate drug and alcohol levels when suspecting toxicity.

■ IMAGING STUDIES
- Echocardiogram is useful in patients with a heart murmur to rule out AS, IHSS, or atrial myxoma.
- If seizure is suspected, CT scan of the head and EEG are indicated.
- If pulmonary embolism is suspected, ventilation-perfusion scan should be done.
- If arrhythmias are suspected, a 24-hr Holter monitor and admission to a telemetry unit is appropriate; loop recorders that can be activated after syncopal episode to retrieve information about the cardiac rhythm during the preceding 4 min add considerable diagnostic yield in patients with unexplained syncope. Generally Holter monitoring is rarely useful, revealing a cause for syncope in <3% of cases.

- Electrophysiologic studies may be indicated in patients with structural heart disease and/or recurrent syncope.
- ECG to rule out arrhythmias; may be diagnostic in 5% to 10% of patients

■ TILT-TABLE TESTING

- Useful to support a diagnosis of neurocardiogenic syncope. Patients older than age 50 should have stress testing before tilt-table testing. Positive results would preclude tilt-table testing.
- Indicated in patients with recurrent episodes of unexplained syncope as well as for patients in high-risk occupations (e.g., pilots, bus drivers) (Fig. 1-353)
- It is performed by keeping the patient in an upright posture on a tilt table with footboard support. The angle of the tilt table varies from 60 to 80 degrees. The duration of upright posture during tilt-table testing varies from 25 to 45 min. Pharmacologic provocation with graded isoproterenol infusions can be used in selected patients.
- The hallmark of neural cardiogenic syncope is severe hypotension associated with a paradoxical bradycardia after a period of symptomatic excitation. The diagnosis of neurocardiogenic syncope is likely if upright tilt testing without the infusion of isoproterenol reproduces these hemodynamic changes in <15 min and causes presyncope or syncope.

■ PSYCHIATRIC EVALUATION

- May be indicated in young patients without heart disease who have frequently recurring syncope and other somatic symptoms.
- Generalized anxiety disorder, pain disorder, and major depression predispose patients to neurally mediated reactions and may result in syncope.
- Alcohol and drug dependence can also lead to syncope.

℞ TREATMENT

■ NONPHARMACOLOGIC THERAPY

- Ensure proper hydration.
- Eliminate medications that may induce hypotension.

■ ACUTE GENERAL Rx

- Varies with the underlying etiology of syncope (e.g., pacemaker in patients with syncope secondary to complete heart block).

- Metoprolol or isopropamide may be useful in the treatment of neurocardiogenic syncope.
- Syncope caused by orthostatic hypotension is treated with volume replacement in patients with intravascular volume depletion. Drugs responsible for the orthostasis should be discontinued.

■ DISPOSITION

Prognosis varies with the age of the patient and the etiology of the syncope. Generally:

- Benign prognosis (very low 1-yr morbidity) in patients:
  1. Age <30 yr and having noncardiac syncope
  2. Age <70 yr and having vasovagal/psychogenic syncope or syncope of unknown cause
- Poor prognosis (high mortality and morbidity) in patients with cardiac syncope
- Patients with the following risk factors have a higher 1-year mortality: abnormal ECG, history of ventricular arrhythmia, history of CHF

■ REFERRAL

Hospital admission in elderly patients without prior history of syncope or unknown etiology of their syncope and in any patients suspected of having cardiac syncope.

☼ PEARLS & CONSIDERATIONS

■ COMMENTS

- Fig. 1-354 describes an algorithmic approach to the patient with syncope.
- The etiology of syncope is identified in <50% of cases during the initial evaluation.
- A thorough history and physical examination are the most productive means of establishing diagnosis in patients with syncope.

REFERENCES

Fenton AM et al: Vasovagal syncope, *Ann Intern Med* 133:722, 2000.
Kapoor WN: Syncope, *N Engl J Med* 343:1856, 2000.
Author: **Fred F. Ferri, M.D.**

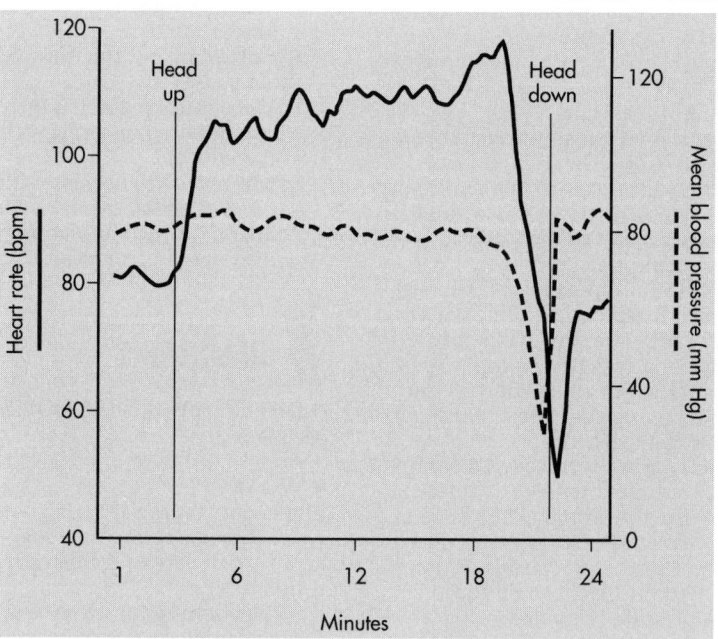

Fig. 1-353 Head-up tilt test performed on an 18-year-old woman with a history of syncope associated with pain, preceded by a prodrome of dizziness, graying vision, and diaphoresis. A similar prodrome preceded syncope during the test. Note the precipitous, nearly simultaneous, decline of heart rate and blood pressure after an initial rise in heart rate. Vital signs returned to normal rapidly after the head was lowered. (Courtesy Robert F. Sprung, University of Utah. In Goldman L, Bennett JC [eds]: *Cecil textbook of medicine*, ed 21, Philadelphia, 2000, WB Saunders.)

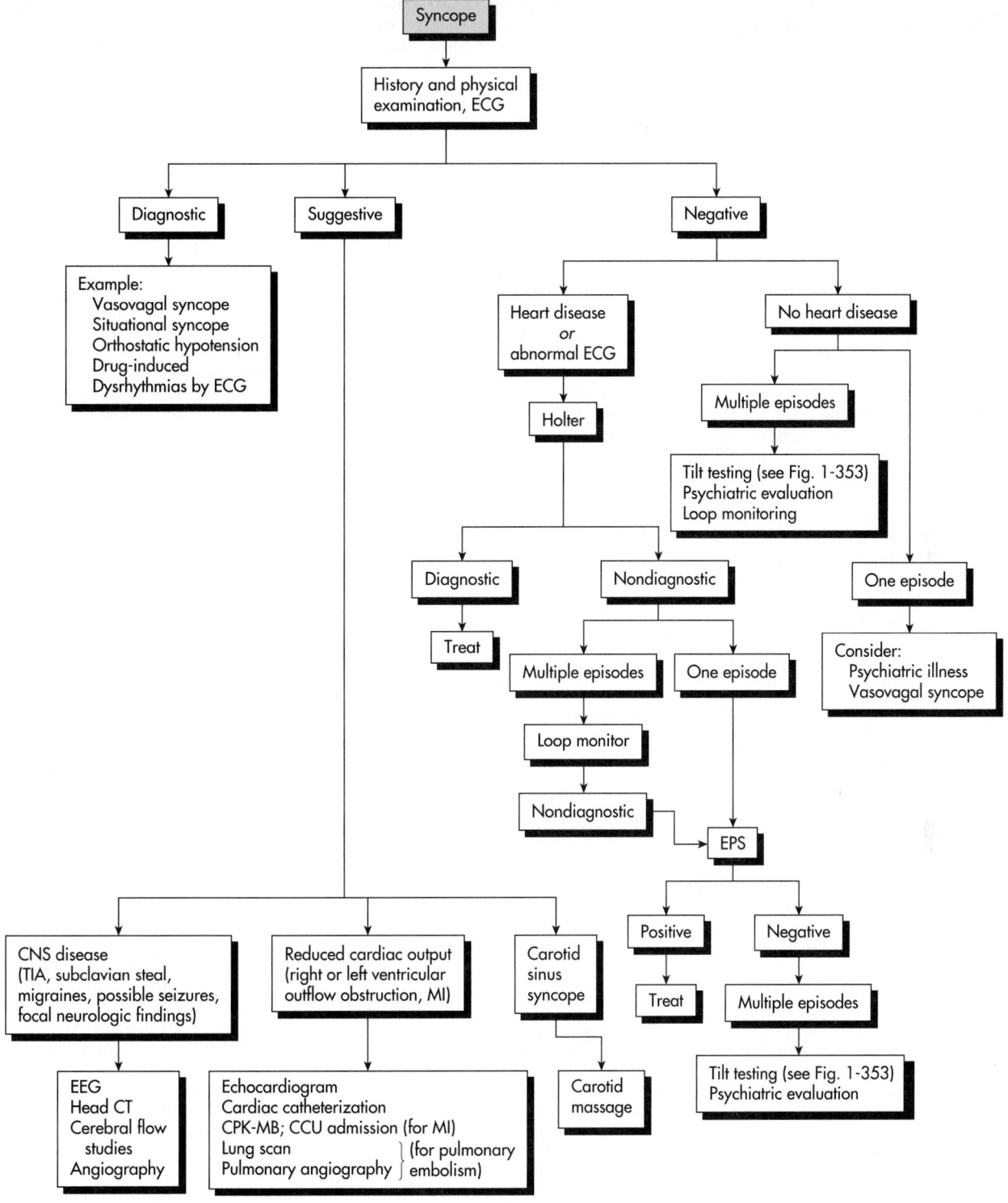

Fig. 1-354   Algorithm summarizing the diagnostic approach to syncope. *CCU,* Critical care unit; *CNS,* central nervous system; *CPK-MB,* isoenzyme of creatine kinase containing M and B subunits; *CT,* computed tomography; *ECG,* electrocardiogram; *EEG,* electroencephalogram; *EPS,* electrophysiologic studies; *MI,* myocardial infarction; *TIA,* transient ischemic attack. (From Noble J: *Primary care medicine,* ed 3, St Louis, 2001, Mosby.)

BASIC INFORMATION

■ DEFINITION

Syphilis is a sexually transmitted treponemal disease, acute and chronic, characterized by primary skin lesion, secondary eruption involving skin and mucous membranes, long periods of latency, and late lesions of skin, bone, viscera, CNS, and cardiovascular system.

■ SYNONYMS

Lues

ICD-9CM CODES

097.9 Syphilis, acquired unspecified

■ EPIDEMIOLOGY & DEMOGRAPHICS

- Widespread, primarily involving ages 20 to 35 yr. Racial differences in incidence are related to social factors. Usually more prevalent in urban areas. Estimated annual incidence of 90,000 cases in the U.S. Increase in incidence in the late 1980s to 1990s, likely related to illicit drug use and prostitution. Increase occurred primarily in lower socioeconomic groups.
- Communicability is indefinite and variable. Communicable during primary, secondary, and latent mucocutaneous lesions in up to first 4 yr of latency. Most probable congenital transmission occurs in early maternal syphilis. Adequate penicillin treatment ends infectivity within 24 to 48 hr.

■ PHYSICAL FINDINGS & CLINICAL PRESENTATION

PRIMARY SYPHILIS: Characteristic lesion is a painless chancre on genitalia, mouth, or anus; atypical primary lesions may occur. Usually appears 3 wk after exposure and may spontaneously involute.

SECONDARY SYPHILIS:
- Localized or diffuse mucocutaneous lesions and generalized lymphadenopathy. Common to have constitutional symptoms, flulike symptoms. May begin about 4 to 6 wk after appearance of primary lesion. Manifestations may resolve in 1 wk to 12 mo.
- 60% to 80% of patients have maculopapular lesions on their palms and soles.
- Condylomata lata intertriginous papules form at areas of friction and moisture, such as the vulva.
- 21% to 58% have mucocutaneous or mucosal lesions (pharyngitis, tonsillitis, "mucous patch" lesion on oral and genital mucosa).

EARLY LATENT (<1 YR): Generally asymptomatic.

LATE LATENT (>1 YR):
- Characterized by gummas (nodular, ulcerative lesions) that can involve the skin, mucous membranes, skeletal system, and viscera.
- Manifestations of cardiovascular syphilis include aortitis, aneurysm, or aortic regurgitation.
- Neurosyphilis may be asymptomatic or symptomatic. Tabes dorsalis, meningovascular syphilis, general paralysis of the insane. Iritis, choroidoretinitis, and leukoplakia may also occur.

■ ETIOLOGY

- *Treponema pallidum,* a spirochete
- Spread by sexual intercourse or by intrauterine transfer

DIAGNOSIS

■ DIFFERENTIAL DIAGNOSIS

- Other genitoulcerative diseases such as herpes, chancroid (see Table 2-84).
- See Fig. 3-69 for a clinical algorithm for the evaluation of genital ulcer disease.

■ WORKUP

Confirmation is primarily through laboratory diagnosis.

■ LABORATORY TESTS

- Dark-field microscopy of fluid from lesion to look for treponeme
- Serologic testing, both nontreponemal (VDRL, RPR) and treponemal (FTA, MHA)
- Lumbar puncture for CSF VDRL in patients with evidence of latent syphilis

TREATMENT

■ ACUTE GENERAL Rx

- Early (primary, secondary, early latent): penicillin G benzathine 2.4 million U IM × 1 or doxycycline 100 mg PO bid × 14 days.
- Late (late latent, cardiovascular, gumma): penicillin G benzathine 2.4 million U IM qwk × 3 wk or doxycycline 100 mg PO bid × 4 wk.
- Neurosyphilis: aqueous crystalline penicillin G 18 to 24 million U/day, administered as 3 to 4 million U IV q4h × 10 to 14 days or procaine penicillin 2.4 million U IM/day plus probenecid 500 mg PO qid, both for 10 to 14 days.
- Congenital syphilis: aqueous crystalline penicillin G 50,000 U/kg/dose IV q12h × first 7 days of life and q8h after that for total of 10 days or procaine penicillin G 50,000 U/kg/dose IM/day × 10 days.
- Tetracyclines are contraindicated in pregnancy. If pregnant and penicillin allergic, must be desensitized.

■ DISPOSITION

- Repeat quantitative nontreponemal tests at 3, 6, and 12 mo. Pregnancy requires monthly tests until delivery.
- If a fourfold increase in titer occurs, if initial high titer fails to drop by fourfold within a year, or persistent signs, retreatment may be indicated. Use treatment regimen for late syphilis.
- Pregnant women without a fourfold drop in titer in a 3-mo period need to be retreated.
- Cases should be reported to local or state health department for referral, follow-up, and partner notification.

■ REFERRAL

- Pregnant and possible congenital syphilis
- Pregnant and allergic to penicillin, with need to be desensitized
- Late latent syphilis with serious CNS, cardiovascular, or other organ system compromise

PEARLS & CONSIDERATIONS

■ COMMENTS

- Jarisch-Herxheimer reaction (fever, myalgia, tachycardia, hypotension) may occur within 24 hr of treatment.
- One third of untreated patients develop CNS and/or cardiovascular sequelae.
- Up to 80% of those treated during late stages remain seropositive indefinitely.
- Treponemal tests remain positive even after adequate therapy.

REFERENCES

Centers for Disease Control and Prevention: Sexually transmitted diseases treatment guidelines, *MMWR* 47(RR-1):1, 1998.

Centers for Disease Control: Primary and secondary syphilis—United States, 1999, *MMWR* 50(7):113, 2001.

Author: **Eugene J. Louie-Ng, M.D.**

BASIC INFORMATION

■ DEFINITION
Syringomyelia is a disease of the spine characterized by the formation of fluid-filled cavities within the spinal cord, sometimes extending into the brainstem.

ICD-9CM CODES
336.0 Syringomyelia

■ EPIDEMIOLOGY & CLINICAL PRESENTATION
- Often a history of birth injury exists.
- Onset is usually insidious, with symptoms often not beginning until the third or fourth decade.
- Cervical spine is the most commonly affected area.
  1. Intrinsic hand atrophy, weakness, and anesthetic sensory loss may develop.
  2. The latter may lead to unnoticed burns or other injuries in the hand.
  3. Loss of pain and temperature sensation may occur, but tactile sense in the upper extremity is preserved.
  4. Sharp testing elicits no pain, but patient often perceives the sharpness of the object.
  5. A Charcot joint in the shoulder or elbow may develop.
- Reflexes are absent in the upper extremity.
- Spasticity and hyperreflexia are present in the lower extremity.
- Scoliosis is common.
- Nystagmus and Horner's syndrome may also occur.
- Trophic skin changes eventually develop in many cases.

■ ETIOLOGY
- Cause is unknown, but condition is thought to result from obstruction of the outlet of the fourth ventricle, often associated with a Chiari I malformation, which causes fluid to be diverted down the central cord.
- Syrinxes later in life may be the result of trauma or an intramedullary tumor.

DIAGNOSIS

■ DIFFERENTIAL DIAGNOSIS
- ALS
- MS
- Spinal cord tumor
- Tabes dorsalis
- Progressive spinal muscular atrophy

■ IMAGING STUDIES
- Plain radiographs usually reveal widening of the bony canal in the region of involvement.
- Bony anomalies are often present at the base of the skull and at the C1-C2 spinal segments.
- Myelography, MRI (Fig. 1-355), and other imaging studies are recommended.

TREATMENT

Drainage and operative repair of any bony anomalies are undertaken, often with decompression laminectomy of C1 and C2.

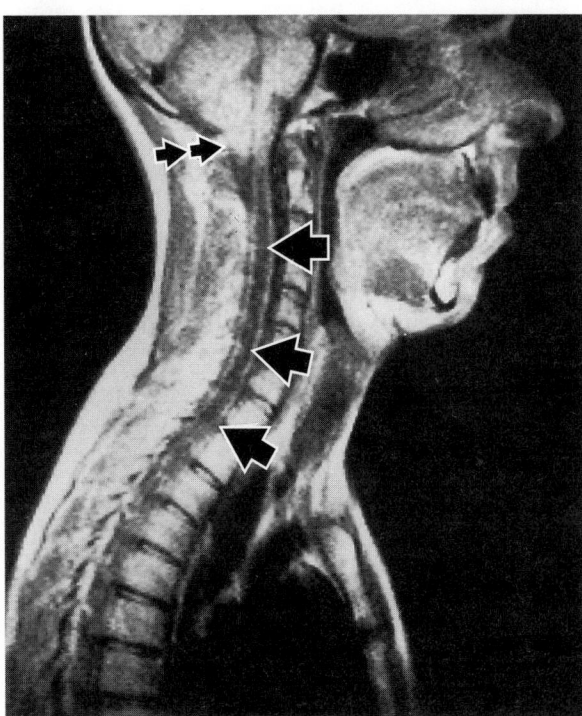

Fig. 1-355   Midsagittal magnetic resonance image of Arnold-Chiari malformation *(small black arrows)* and syringomyelia *(three white-block arrows)* in a 31-year-old man. Note the cerebellar tonsils extending below the posterior rim of the foramen magnum *(dark structure immediately above the black arrow).* The syrinx extends from the medulla well into the thoracic cord. (From Andreoli TE [ed]: *Cecil essentials of medicine,* ed 4, Philadelphia, 1997, WB Saunders.)

■ DISPOSITION
- Condition is slowly progressive in most cases, but course may be quite variable, ranging from death in a few months to slow incapacitation over several years: progression may halt at any time.
- Surgical intervention often stops progression but frequently does not lead to improvement in neurologic findings.

■ REFERRAL
For neurosurgical consultation when diagnosis is suspected
Author: **Lonnie R. Mercier, M.D.**

BASIC INFORMATION

■ DEFINITION

Systemic lupus erythematosus (SLE) is a chronic multisystemic disease characterized by production of autoantibodies and protean clinical manifestations.

■ SYNONYMS

SLE

ICD-9CM CODES

710.0 Systemic lupus erythematosus

■ EPIDEMIOLOGY & DEMOGRAPHICS

PREVALENCE: 20 cases/100,000 persons
PREDOMINANT SEX: Female:male ratio of 7:1
PREDOMINANT AGE: 20 to 45 yr (childbearing years)

■ PHYSICAL FINDINGS & CLINICAL PRESENTATION

- Skin: erythematous rash over the malar eminences (Fig. 1-356), generally with sparing of the nasolabial folds (butterfly rash), alopecia, raised erythematous patches with subsequent edematous plaques and adherent scales (discoid lupus), leg, nasal, or oropharyngeal ulcerations, livedo reticularis, pallor (from anemia), petechiae (from thrombocytopenia)
- Joints: tenderness, swelling, or effusion, generally involving peripheral joints
- Cardiac: pericardial rub (in patients with pericarditis), heart murmurs (if endocarditis or valvular thickening or dysfunction)
- Other: fever, conjunctivitis, dry eyes, dry mouth (sicca syndrome), oral ulcers, abdominal tenderness, decreased breath sounds (pleural effusions)

■ ETIOLOGY

Unknown

DIAGNOSIS

■ DIFFERENTIAL DIAGNOSIS

- Other connective tissue disorders (e.g., RA, MCTD, progressive systemic sclerosis)
- Metastatic neoplasm
- Infection

■ WORKUP

The diagnosis of SLE can be made by demonstrating the presence of any four or more of the following criteria of the American Rheumatism Association:

1. Butterfly rash
2. Discoid rash
3. Photosensitivity (particularly leg ulcerations)
4. Oral ulcers
5. Arthritis
6. Serositis (pleuritis, pericarditis)
7. Renal disorder (persistent proteinuria >0.5 g/day or 3+ if quantitation not performed, cellular casts)
8. Neurologic disorder (seizures, psychosis [in absence of offending drugs or metabolic derangement])
9. Hematologic disorder:
   a. Hemolytic anemia with reticulocytosis
   b. Leukopenia (<4000/mm^3 total on two or more occasions)
   c. Lymphopenia (<1500/mm^3 on two or more occasions)
   d. Thrombocytopenia (<100,000/mm^3 in the absence of offending drugs)
10. Immunologic disorder:
    a. Positive SLE cell preparation
    b. Anti-DNA (presence of antibody to native DNA in abnormal titer)
    c. Anti-Sm (presence of antibody to Smith nuclear antigen)
    d. False-positive STS known to be positive for at least 6 mo and confirmed by negative TPI or FTA tests
11. ANA: an abnormal titer of ANA by immunofluorescence or equivalent assay at any time in the absence of drugs known to be associated with "drug-induced lupus" syndrome

■ LABORATORY TESTS

Suggested initial laboratory evaluation of suspected SLE:

- Immunologic evaluation: ANA, anti-DNA antibody, anti-Sm antibody
- Other laboratory tests: CBC with differential, platelet count (Coombs' test if anemia detected), urinalysis (24-hr urine collection for protein if proteinuria is detected), PTT and anticardiolipin antibodies in patients with thrombotic events, BUN, creatinine to evaluate renal function

■ IMAGING STUDIES

- Chest x-ray examination for evaluation of pulmonary involvement (e.g., pleural effusions, pulmonary infiltrates)
- Echocardiogram to screen for significant valvular heart disease (present in 18% of patients with SLE); echocardiography can identify a subset of lesions (valvular thickening and dysfunction) other than verrucous (Libman-Sacks) endocarditis that are prone to hemodynamic deterioration

TREATMENT

■ NONPHARMACOLOGIC THERAPY

Patients with photosensitivity should avoid sunlight and use high-factor sunscreen.

■ ACUTE GENERAL Rx

- Joint pain and mild serositis are generally well controlled with NSAIDs; antimalarials are also effective (e.g., hydroxychloroquine [Plaquenil]).
- Cutaneous manifestations can be treated with topical corticosteroids and antimalarials.
- Renal disease: prednisone can be used for patients with mesangial and mild focal proliferative glomerulonephritis, whereas patients with diffuse proliferative or severe focal proliferative glomerulonephritis are candidates for immunosuppressive therapy (e.g., high-pulsed doses of cyclophosphamide given at monthly intervals). Combination therapy with pulse cyclophosphamide plus pulse methylprednisolone improves long-term renal outcome without adding toxicity in patients with lupus nephritis.
- CNS involvement: treatment generally consists of corticosteroid therapy; however, its efficacy is uncertain, and it is generally reserved for organic brain syndrome. Anticonvulsants and antipsychotics are also indicated in selected cases; headaches are treated symptomatically.
- Hemolytic anemia: treatment of Coombs'-positive hemolytic anemia consists of high doses of corticosteroids; nonhemolytic anemia (secondary to chronic disease) does not require specific therapy.
- Thrombocytopenia: initial treatment consists of corticosteroids. In patients with poor response to steroids, encouraging results have been reported with the use of danazol, vincristine, and immunoglobulins;

splenectomy generally does not cure the thrombocytopenia of SLE, but it may be necessary as an adjunct in managing selected cases.
- Infections are common because of compromised immune function secondary to SLE and the use of corticosteroid, cytotoxic, and antimetabolite drugs; pneumococcal bacteremia is associated with high mortality rate.

■ CHRONIC Rx
Close monitoring for exacerbation of the disease and for potential side effects from medications (corticosteroids, cytotoxic agents) with frequent laboratory evaluation and office visits

■ DISPOSITION
- Most patients with lupus experience remissions and exacerbations.
- The leading cause of death in SLE is infection (one third of all deaths);

active nephritis causes approximately 18% of deaths, and CNS disease causes 7% of deaths; the survival rate is 75% over the first 10 yr. Blacks and Hispanics generally have a worse prognosis.
- Symptomatic pericarditis occurs in $\frac{1}{4}$ of patients with SLE at some point during the course of the disease. Asymptomatic involvement is estimated to be more than 60% based on autopsy reports.
- Renal histologic studies and evaluation of renal function are useful in determining disease activity and predicting disease outcome (e.g., serum creatinine levels >3 mg/dl or evidence of diffuse proliferative involvement on renal biopsy are poor prognostic factors).

■ REFERRAL
- Rheumatology consultation in all patients with SLE
- Hematology consultation in patients with significant hematologic abnor-

malities (e.g., severe hemolytic anemia or thrombocytopenia)
- Nephrology consultation in patients with significant renal involvement

✿ PEARLS & CONSIDERATIONS

■ COMMENTS
Patient information on lupus can be obtained from the Lupus Foundation of America, Inc., No. 4 Research Place, Suite 180, Rockville, MD 20850-3226; phone: (800) 558-0121.

REFERENCES
Illei GG et al: Combination therapy with pulse cyclophosphamide plus methylprednisolone improves long-term renal outcome without adding toxicity in patients with lupus nephritis, *Ann Intern Med* 135:248, 2001.

Moder KG et al: Cardiac involvement in SLE, *Mayo Clin Proc* 74:275, 1999.

Petri M: Treatment of systemic lupus erythematosus: an update, *Am Fam Physician* 57:2753, 1998.

Author: **Fred F. Ferri, M.D.**

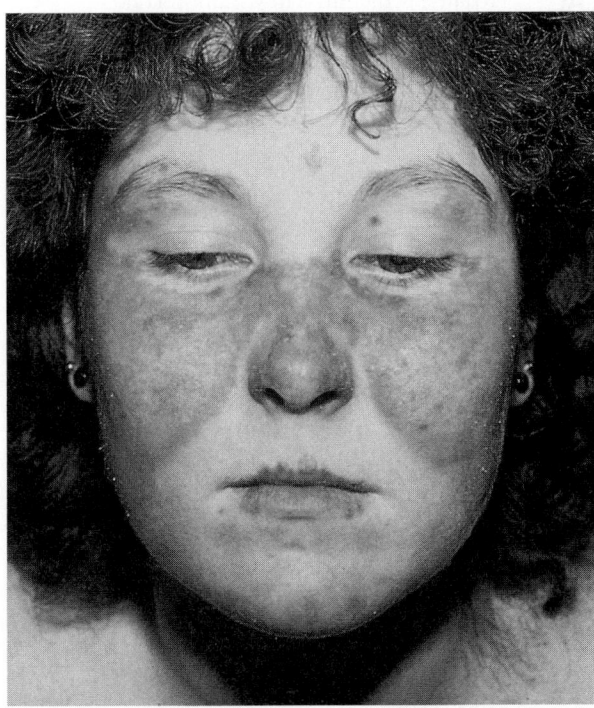

Fig. 1-356 Acute cutaneous LE (systemic LE). The classic butterfly rash occurs in 10% to 50% of patients with acute LE. (From Habif TP: *Clinical dermatology: a color guide to diagnosis and therapy,* ed 3, St Louis, 1996, Mosby.)

BASIC INFORMATION

■ DEFINITION
Tabes dorsalis is a form of tertiary neurosyphilis characterized by paroxysmal pain, particularly in the abdomen and legs; ataxia caused by posterior-column dysfunction; and Argyll Robertson pupils. Charcot's joint may also be present, indicating severe degenerative osteoarthritis.

■ SYNONYMS
Locomotor ataxia
Posterior spinal sclerosis
Tabetic neurosyphilis

ICD-9CM CODES
094.0 Tabes dorsalis, ataxia, locomotor

■ EPIDEMIOLOGY & DEMOGRAPHICS
INCIDENCE (IN U.S.): Rare, but increasing with AIDS
PREVALENCE (IN U.S.): Rare; more common with AIDS epidemic
PREDOMINANT SEX: Male
PREDOMINANT AGE: 50 yr or older
PEAK INCIDENCE: 50 to 60 yr

■ PHYSICAL FINDINGS & CLINICAL PRESENTATION
- Argyll Robertson pupil (reacts poorly to light but well to accommodation)
- Loss of position and vibration at ankles (wide-based gait; inability to walk in the dark)
- Loss of deep pain sensation
- Degenerative joint disease, especially in knees

■ ETIOLOGY
Infectious (*Treponema pallidum*)

DIAGNOSIS

■ DIFFERENTIAL DIAGNOSIS
- Combined system disease (vitamin B_{12} deficiency)
- Spinal cord neoplasm

■ WORKUP
Thorough neurologic examination

■ LABORATORY TESTS
- Lumbar puncture for VDRL and FTA-ABS
- Serum studies

■ IMAGING STUDIES
Not necessary if diagnosis confirmed

TREATMENT

■ ACUTE GENERAL Rx
Procaine penicillin 2 to 4 million U IM qd, along with 500 mg of probenecid PO qid, both for 14 days. Some experts also recommend subsequent administration of 2 to 4 million U of benzathine penicillin IM every week for 3 wk.

■ CHRONIC Rx
- Refer to rehabilitation center for physical therapy.
- Analgesics, carbamazepine, gabapentin, or steroids may help "lightning" pain.

■ DISPOSITION
Follow closely until CSF reverts to normal.

■ REFERRAL
If a spinal cord tumor persists

PEARLS & CONSIDERATIONS

■ COMMENTS
Many of the symptoms—degenerative joint disease, lightning pains—persist after treatment.
- Occurs years after initial infection (Fig. 1-357)

REFERENCE
Centers for Disease Control and Prevention: Sexually transmitted diseases treatment guidelines, *MMWR* 47(RR-1), 1998.
Author: **William H. Olson, M.D.**

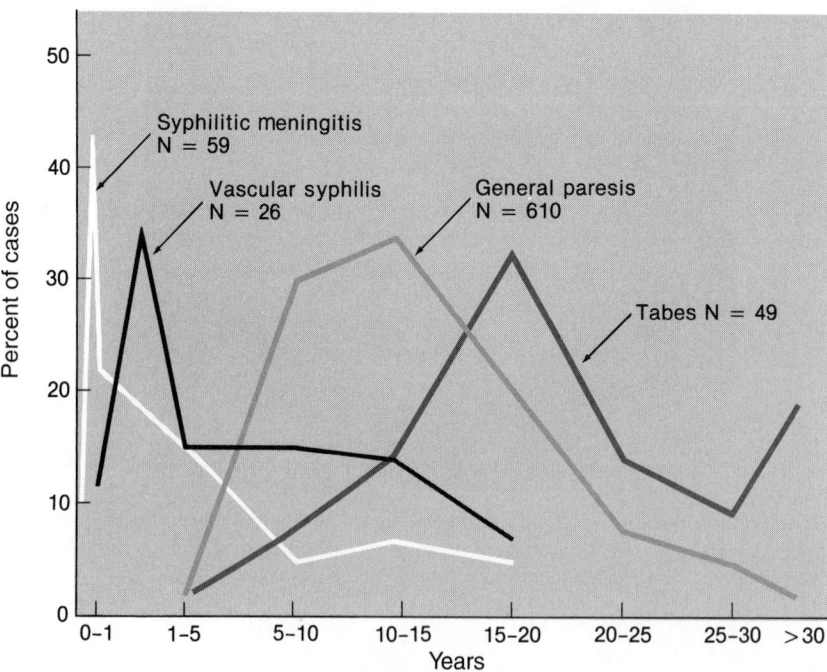

Fig. 1-357 Interval between primary and symptomatic neurosyphilis by type (meningeal, vascular, paretic, tabetic), abstracted from the literature and presented as percentage of total cases within type. (From Simon RP: *Arch Neurol* 42:606, 1985.)

BASIC INFORMATION

■ DEFINITION

Takayasu's arteritis refers to a chronic systemic granulomatous vasculitis primarily affecting large arteries (aorta and its branches).

■ SYNONYMS

Pulseless disease
Aortitis syndrome
Aortic arch arteritis

ICD-9CM CODES

446.7 Takayasu disease or syndrome

■ EPIDEMIOLOGY & DEMOGRAPHICS

- Most cases have been reported from Japan, China, India, and Mexico.
- Exact incidence and prevalence is not known.
- Incidence in the U.S. 2.6/1 million.
- Females > males 9:1.
- Seen predominantly in patients <30 yr old.

■ PHYSICAL FINDINGS & CLINICAL PRESENTATION

Takayasu's arteritis most frequently involves the aortic arch and its branches and can manifest as:
- Arm claudication, weakness, and numbness
- Amaurosis fugax, diplopia, headache, and dizziness
- Systemic symptoms
  1. Low-grade fever
  2. Malaise
  3. Weight loss
  4. Fatigue
- Vascular bruits of the carotid artery, subclavian artery, and aorta
- Discrepancy of blood pressures between the upper extremities
- Absence pulses
- Hypertension
- Retinopathy
- Aortic insufficiency murmur

■ ETIOLOGY

- The cause of Takayasu's arteritis is unknown. A delayed hypersensitivity to mycobacteria and spirochetes is a theory but remains to be substantiated.
- Infiltration of inflammatory cells into the vasa vasorum and media leads to thickening of the aorta and narrowing or obliteration of its branches.

 DIAGNOSIS

Criteria have been established for the diagnosis of Takayasu's arteritis by the American College of Rheumatology in 1990 and include:
- Age of disease <40 yr
- Claudication of extremities
- Decreased brachial artery pulse
- BP difference >10 mm Hg
- Bruit over subclavian arteries or aorta
- Abnormal arteriogram
- Takayasu's arteritis is diagnosed if at least three of the above six criteria are present, giving a sensitivity of 90% and a specificity of 98%.

■ DIFFERENTIAL DIAGNOSIS

Other causes of inflammatory aortitis must be excluded: giant cell arteritis, syphilis, tuberculosis, SLE, rheumatoid arthritis, Buerger's disease, Behçet's disease, Cogan's syndrome, Kawasaki disease, and spondyloarthropathies.

■ WORKUP

Any young patient with findings of absence pulses and loud bruits merits a workup for Takayasu's arteritis. The workup generally includes blood testing to look for signs of inflammation and imaging studies with the angiogram being the diagnostic gold standard.

■ LABORATORY TESTS

- CBC may reveal an elevated WBC count
- ESR is elevated in active disease

■ IMAGING STUDIES

- Ultrasound: Carotid, thoracic, and abdominal ultrasound are useful adjunctive imaging studies in diagnosing occlusive disease resulting from Takayasu's arteritis (Fig. 1-358).
- Doppler and noninvasive upper and lower extremity studies are helpful in assessing blood flow and absent pulses.
- CT scan is used to assess the thickness of the aorta.
- Angiogram can show narrowing of the aorta and/or branches of the aorta, aneurysm formation, and poststenotic dilation. Angiographic findings are classified as four types:
  1. Type I: Lesions involve only the aortic arch and its branches.
  2. Type II: Lesions only involving the abdominal aorta and its branches.
  3. Type III: Lesions involving the aorta above and below the diaphragm.
  4. Type IV: Lesions involving the pulmonary artery.

 TREATMENT

■ ACUTE GENERAL Rx

- Corticosteroids are the treatment of choice. Prednisone 40 to 60 mg PO qd or 1 mg/kg/day is used for 3 mo.
- Patients are monitored for symptoms and by following the ESR. If symptoms have resolved and the ESR is normal, attempts to taper prednisone are made.

■ CHRONIC Rx

- Patients who cannot be tapered off the corticosteroids or who have relapse of the disease are given methotrexate 0.15 to 0.35 mg/kg or approximately 15 mg/wk.
- Cyclophosphamide 1 to 2 mg/kg/day can be given with glucocorticoids as adjunctive therapy in relapse or treatment-resistant patients.

■ DISPOSITION

- Treatment improves symptoms within days with relief of ischemic claudication, return of pulses on examination, and reversal of lumen narrowing on angiograms. However, some patients may continue to have progression of arterial lesions despite therapy.

- With the addition of a second agent in patients with treatment resistance or relapse, 50% remission has been seen.
- Mortality results are mixed, showing high rates in reports from Asia and lower rates in studies done in the U.S. (2%).
- Death can occur suddenly from ruptured aneurysms, myocardial infarctions, and strokes.

■ REFERRAL

Whenever the diagnosis of vasculitis is suspected, a rheumatology consult is appropriate. Vascular surgery and cardiology consultations are recommended for any evidence of carotid, peripheral, and coronary artery disease or if a large abdominal aneurysm is found.

☼ PEARLS & CONSIDERATIONS

■ COMMENTS

Overall the long-term prognosis of treated patients with Takayasu's disease is good, with >90% of patients surviving more than 15 yr.

REFERENCES

Arend WP et al: American College of Rheumatology 1990 criteria for the classification of Takayasu's arteritis, *Arthr Rheum* 33:1129, 1990.

Ishikawa K, Maetani S: Long-term outcome for 120 Japanese patients with Takayasu's disease: clinical and statistical analyses of related prognostic factors, *Circulation* 90:1855, 1994.

Kerr GS et al: Takayasu arteritis, *Ann Intern Med* 120:919, 1994.

Author: **Peter Petropoulos, M.D.**

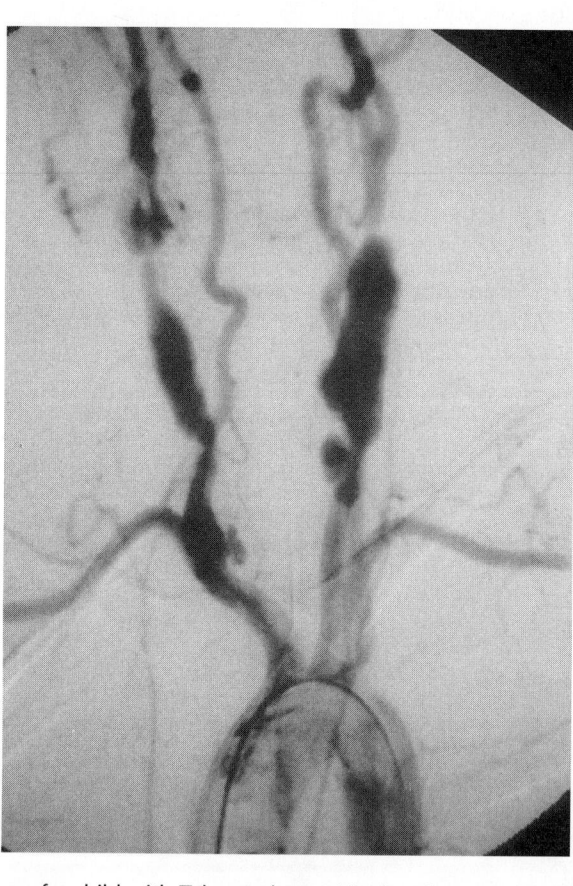

Fig. 1-358   Angiogram of a child with Takayasu's arteritis showing massive bilateral carotid dilation, stenosis, and poststenotic dilation. (From Behrman RE: *Nelson textbook of pediatrics,* ed 16, Philadelphia, 2000, WB Saunders.)

BASIC INFORMATION

■ DEFINITION
Four species of adult tapeworm may infect humans as the definitive host: *Taenia saginata* (beef tapeworm), *Taenia solium* (pork tapeworm), *Diphyllobothrium latum* (fish tapeworm), and *Hymenolepis nana*. In addition, *T. solium* may infect humans in its larval form (cysticercosis), and several animal tapeworms (see "Echinococcosis" in Section I) may cause infection in an analogous manner.

■ SYNONYMS
Cysticercosis (larval infection by *T. solium*)

ICD-9CM CODES
123.9 Tapeworm infestation

■ EPIDEMIOLOGY & DEMOGRAPHICS
INCIDENCE (IN U.S.):
- Diagnosed primarily in immigrants
- Varies widely by country of origin and dietary practices

PREVALENCE (IN U.S.):
- *T. saginata:* <0.1%
- *D. latum:* <0.05%
- *T. solium:* <0.1%
- *H. nana:* sporadic, often in setting of outbreak

PREDOMINANT SEX: Equal sex distribution

PREDOMINANT AGE:
- *T. saginata, T. solium, D. latum:* 20 to 39 yr of age
- *H. nana* in setting of institution outbreaks: children

■ PHYSICAL FINDINGS & CLINICAL PRESENTATION
- Adult worms
  1. Attach to bowel mucosa
  2. Feed and grow
  3. Cause minimal or no symptoms or sequelae
- Cysticercosis
  1. Mass lesions of brain (neurocysticercosis), soft tissue, viscera
  2. Neurocysticercosis may cause seizures, hydrocephalus
- Prolonged infection with *D. latum*
  1. Vitamin B_{12} deficiency
  2. Megaloblastic anemia

■ ETIOLOGY
TAPEWORM:
- Adult worm resides in small or large bowel; proglottids and eggs passed in stool.
- Eggs are ingested by the animal intermediate host.
- Eggs hatch into larvae.
- Larvae disseminate largely in skeletal muscle, brain, viscera.
- Humans eat infected beef *(T. saginata),* infected pork *(T. solium),* or infected fish *(D. latum).*
- Larvae mature into adults within the GI lumen.
- *H. nana* infection is acquired by ingesting eggs in human or rodent feces.

CYSTICERCOSIS:
- Humans ingest eggs of *T. solium* in food contaminated with human feces that contain the eggs.
- Eggs hatch into larvae in gut.
- Larvae disseminate widely through tissues (particularly soft tissue and CNS) forming cystic lesions containing either viable or nonviable larvae.

DIAGNOSIS

■ DIFFERENTIAL DIAGNOSIS
Table 2-113 describes the differential diagnosis of intestinal helminths.

■ WORKUP
- Stool examination for eggs or proglottids (tapeworm)
- Cerebral CT scan (neurocysticercosis)
- Serum antibody (neurocysticercosis)

■ IMAGING STUDIES
- Tapeworm: incidental finding on upper GI series
- Neurocysticercosis:
  1. Cerebral cysts are readily demonstrated by CT scan or MRI.
  2. Calcified lesions are an incidental finding.

TREATMENT

■ ACUTE GENERAL Rx
- All patients with intestinal tapeworm infections should be treated with a single oral dose of praziquantel.
  1. *T. solium:* 5 mg/kg
  2. *T. saginata:* 20 mg/kg
  3. *D. latum:* 10 mg/kg
  4. *H. nana:* 25 mg/kg
- Therapy that may be considered for symptomatic cysticercosis:
  1. May regress spontaneously
  2. Surgery
  3. Albendazole 15 mg/kg PO qd in three doses for 28 days
  4. Praziquantel 50 mg/kg PO qd in three doses for 15 days
- Therapy contraindicated with:
  1. Ocular infections
  2. Cerebral infections in which local inflammation caused by destruction of the parasite may cause significant damage

■ CHRONIC Rx
- Retreatment if required
- Avoidance of undercooked pork, meat, or fish
- Cysticercosis: proper hand washing, proper disposal of human waste

■ DISPOSITION
- Neurologic follow-up for patients with neurocysticercosis
- Ophthalmologic follow-up for patients with ocular involvement

■ REFERRAL
Patients treated for neurocysticercosis should be evaluated by a physician experienced in managing this infection, if possible.

PEARLS & CONSIDERATIONS

■ COMMENTS
T. solium is the most dangerous of the tapeworms because of the potential for cysticercosis by means of autoinfection.

REFERENCE
Garcia HH, Del Brutto OH: *Taenia solium* cysticercosis, *Infect Dis Clin North Am* 14(1):97, 2000.
Author: **Joseph R. Masci, M.D.**

BASIC INFORMATION

■ DEFINITION
Tarsal tunnel syndrome is a rare entrapment neuropathy that develops as a result of compression of the posterior tibial nerve in the tunnel formed by the flexor retinaculum behind the medial malleolus of the ankle (Fig. 1-359).

■ ICD-9CM CODES
355.5 Tarsal tunnel syndrome

■ EPIDEMIOLOGY & DEMOGRAPHICS
PREVALENCE: Unknown
PREDOMINANT SEX: Female = male

■ PHYSICAL FINDINGS & CLINICAL PRESENTATION
- Neuritic symptoms along the course of the posterior tibial nerve in the sole and heel
- Swelling over tarsal tunnel
- Possible positive Tinel's sign
- Possible reproduction of symptoms with sustained eversion of hindfoot or digital compression of tunnel
- Sensory and motor changes unusual

■ ETIOLOGY
Space-occupying lesions (ganglia, varicosities, lipomas, synovial hypertrophy)

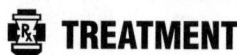

DIAGNOSIS

■ DIFFERENTIAL DIAGNOSIS
- Plantar fasciitis
- Peripheral neuropathy
- Proximal radiculopathy
- Local tendinitis
- Peripheral vascular disease
- Morton's neuroma

■ ELECTRICAL STUDIES
Electrodiagnostic testing is often inconclusive. Delayed sensory conduction or increased motor latency may be seen.

TREATMENT

- NSAIDs
- Immobilization
- Medial heel wedge or orthotic to minimize heel eversion
- Local steroid injection into tunnel

■ REFERRAL
For surgical decompression if needed
Author: **Lonnie R. Mercier, M.D.**

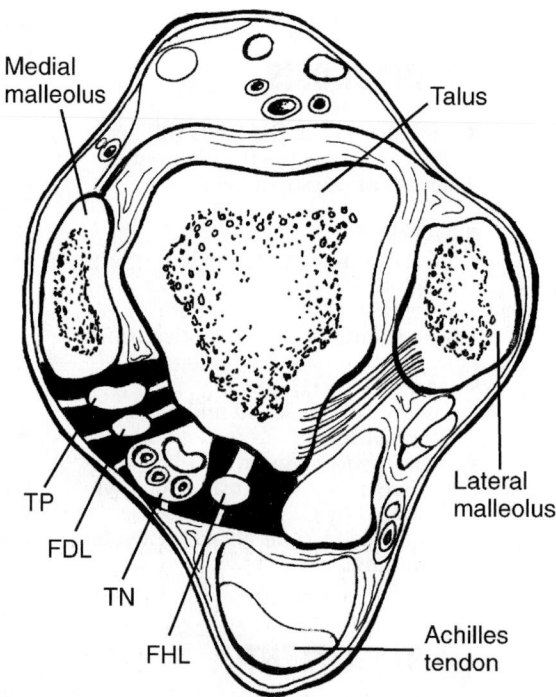

Fig. 1-359   Anatomy of tarsal tunnel syndrome. Transverse view of ankle. *FHL,* Flexor hallucis longus tendon; *TN,* tibial nerve (single contour), posterior tibial artery, veins; *FDL,* flexor digitorum longus; *TP,* tibialis posterior tendon. Tendons and neurovascular elements are included into individual fibrous septa that connect periosteum with the deep fascia. (From Canoso J: *Rheumatology in primary care,* Philadelphia, 1997, WB Saunders.)

BASIC INFORMATION

■ DEFINITION
Temporal arteritis is a systemic segmental granulomatous inflammation predominantly involving the arteries of the carotid system in patients >50 yr; however, it can involve any large- or medium-sized arteries.

■ SYNONYMS
Giant cell arteritis
Cranial arteritis

ICD-9CM CODES
446.5 Temporal arteritis

■ EPIDEMIOLOGY & DEMOGRAPHICS
PREVALENCE: 200 cases/100,000 persons
INCIDENCE: 17 to 23.3 new cases/100,000 persons >50 yr

■ PHYSICAL FINDINGS & CLINICAL PRESENTATION
- Tenderness, decreased pulsation, and nodulation of temporal arteries
- Visual disturbances: visual field cuts, diplopia, amaurosis fugax, ophthalmoplegia
- Diminished or absent pulses in upper extremities

■ ETIOLOGY
Vasculitis of unknown etiology

DIAGNOSIS

■ DIFFERENTIAL DIAGNOSIS
- Other vasculitic syndromes
- Primary amyloidosis
- TIA, CVA
- Infections
- Occult neoplasm, multiple myeloma

■ WORKUP
Temporal arteritis can present with the following clinical manifestations:
- Headache, often associated with marked scalp tenderness
- Constitutional symptoms (fever, weight loss, anorexia, fatigue)
- Polymyalgia syndrome (aching and stiffness of the trunk and proximal muscle groups)
- Visual disturbances, intermittent claudication of jaw and tongue on mastication

The presence of any three of the following five items allows the diagnosis of temporal arteritis with a sensitivity of 94% and a specificity of 91%:
- Age of onset >50 yr
- New-onset or new type of headache
- Temporal artery tenderness or decreased pulsation on physical examination
- Westergren ESR >50 mm/hr
- Temporal artery biopsy with vasculitis and mononuclear cell infiltrate or granulomatous changes. NOTE: Because of the presence of "skip lesions" in the artery, the biopsy segment of the temporal artery should be at least 2 cm long.

■ LABORATORY TESTS
- Elevated ESR (usually >50 mm/hr; however, a normal ESR does not exclude the diagnosis)
- Mild-to-moderate normochromic normocytic anemia, elevated platelets
- Liver function test abnormalities (most common: elevation of alkaline phosphatase)

■ IMAGING STUDIES
- Temporal arteritis is associated with a markedly increased risk for the development of aortic aneurysm, which is often a late complication and may cause death.
- Patients with a history of temporal arteritis may benefit from an annual radiograph of the chest, including a lateral view, and an examination that includes palpation of the abdominal aorta.
- Color duplex ultrasonography of the temporal arteries reveals a dark halo (which may be caused by edema of the artery wall) in patients with temporal arteritis. Patients with typical clinical signs and a halo on ultrasonography may be started on treatment without performing a temporal artery biopsy.

TREATMENT

■ ACUTE GENERAL Rx
- In stable patients without significant ocular involvement, therapy is usually started with prednisone 40 to 60 mg/day in divided doses and is continued for a few weeks until symptoms resolve and ESR returns to

normal. If the ESR remains normal, prednisone can be reduced by 5 mg every other week until a dose of 20 mg/day is reached. Subsequent dose reductions should be by 2.5 mg/day every 2 to 4 wk. When the total dose reaches 5 mg/day, reduction should be by 1 mg every 2 to 4 wk as tolerated. Usual duration of prednisone treatment is 6 mo to 2 yr.
- In very ill patients and those with significant ocular involvement (e.g., visual loss in one eye) rapid aggressive treatment with large doses of IV steroids (e.g., IV Solu-Medrol 250-1000 mg qd for 3 days before starting oral prednisone) is indicated to provide optimal protection to the uninvolved eye and offer any chance of recovery of the involved eye.

■ CHRONIC Rx
Patients should be instructed and monitored regarding the potential toxicity from prednisone (e.g., hypertension, diabetes, cataracts, dyspepsia, osteoporosis, psychosis). A baseline bone-density study in female patients is recommended.

■ DISPOSITION
Prognosis is generally good; complete blindness is rare with treatment.

■ REFERRAL
- Surgical referral for biopsy of temporal artery
- Ophthalmology referral in patients with visual disturbances and following initiation of corticosteroid therapy

PEARLS & CONSIDERATIONS

■ COMMENTS
The decision to continue tapering prednisone or to resume it after it has been discontinued should not be based solely on the sedimentation rate but on the clinical picture. A rising ESR in a clinically asymptomatic patient with normal Hct should raise suspicion for alternate explanations (e.g., infections, neoplasms).
Author: **Fred F. Ferri, M.D.**

BASIC INFORMATION

■ DEFINITION

Temporomandibular joint (TMJ) syndrome refers to a group of disorders leading to symptoms of the temporomandibular joint.

■ SYNONYMS

Temporomandibular dysfunction
Painful temporomandibular joint

ICD-9CM CODES

524.60 Temporomandibular joint pain-dysfunction syndrome

■ EPIDEMIOLOGY & DEMOGRAPHICS

- 15% of the population have TMJ disorders
- Females > males 4:1
- Occurs between the second and fourth decades of life
- Usually unilateral, affecting either side with equal frequency

■ PHYSICAL FINDINGS & CLINICAL PRESENTATION

- Otalgia
- Odontalgia
- Headaches (frontal, temporal, retroorbital)
- Tinnitus
- Dizziness
- Clicking or popping sounds with movement of the TMJ
- Joint locking
- Tender to palpation
- Limited range of motion of the TMJ

■ ETIOLOGY

Causes of TMJ syndrome are multifactorial, encompassing local anatomic anomalies to familiar disease processes that can involve the TMJ.

- Myofascial pain-dysfunction syndrome (MPD): the most common cause of TMJ syndrome and results from teeth grinding and clenching the jaw (bruxism)
- Internal TMJ derangement: abnormal connection of the articular disk to the mandibular condyle
- Degenerative joint disease
- Rheumatoid arthritis
- Gouty arthritis
- Pseudogout
- Ankylosing spondylitis
- Trauma
- Prior surgery (orthodontic, intraarticular steroid injection)
- Tumors

DIAGNOSIS

■ DIFFERENTIAL DIAGNOSIS

The differential diagnosis of TMJ syndrome is thought of in terms of etiology and includes the list as mentioned above under Etiology. Myofascial pain-dysfunction syndrome, internal TMJ derangement, and degenerative joint disease represent greater than 90% of all causes of TMJ syndrome.

■ WORKUP

Includes a detailed history and physical examination, followed by radiographic imaging evaluation.

■ LABORATORY TESTS

Laboratory examination is not very helpful in the diagnosis of TMJ syndrome

■ IMAGING STUDIES

- Plain x-rays: The most common x-rays are the panoramic, transorbital, and transpharyngeal views in both opened and closed positions.
- Arthrography helpful in looking for meniscus involvement.
- CT scan is very accurate in diagnosing meniscal and osseous derangements of the TMJ.
- MRI can better visualize soft tissue inflammation, if present.

TREATMENT

■ NONPHARMACOLOGIC THERAPY

- Soft diet to rest the muscles of mastication
- Heat 15 to 20 minutes 4 to 6 times per day
- Massage of the masseter and temporalis muscles
- Formed splints or bite appliances
- Range-of-motion exercises

■ ACUTE GENERAL Rx

- Nonsteroidal antiinflammatory drugs (NSAIDs): ibuprofen 800 PO mg tid prn, naproxen 500 PO mg bid prn, titrated to relieve symptoms.
- Muscle relaxants: diazepam 2.5 to 5 mg PO tid prn.
- In degenerative joint disease of the TMJ, intraarticular steroid injection can be tried.

■ CHRONIC Rx

- Most of the above-mentioned treatment is used for myofascial pain-dysfunction syndrome; however, it can be applied to other causes of TMJ syndrome. Surgery is usually a measure of last resort in patients who are refractory to nonpharmacologic and acute general treatment.
- Surgical procedures include:
  1. Meniscoplasty
  2. Meniscectomy
  3. Subcondylar osteotomy
  4. TMJ reconstruction

■ DISPOSITION

The course depends on the underlying etiology; however, a lengthy course with exacerbations of symptoms can be expected.

■ REFERRAL

All patients with TMJ syndrome refractory to conservative nonpharmacologic and acute therapy should be referred to a periodontist, oral maxillofacial surgeon, or ENT surgeon.

PEARLS & CONSIDERATIONS

■ COMMENTS

- Patients with rheumatoid arthritis involving the TMJ usually will have bilateral involvement.
- Frequently emotional stress initiates the myofascial pain-dysfunction, which accounts for 85% of all cases of TMJ syndrome.

REFERENCES

Blank LW: Clinical guidelines for managing mandibular dysfunction, *Gen Dentist* 46(6):592, 1998.

Dierks EJ: Temporomandibular disorders and facial pain syndromes. In Kelly WN et al: *Textbook of rheumatology,* ed 5, Philadelphia, 1997, WB Saunders.

Pankhurst CL: Controversies in the aetiology of temporomandibular disorders. Part I. Temporomandibular disorders: all in the mind? *Prim Dent Care* 4(1):25, 1997.

Author: **Peter Petropoulos, M.D.**

BASIC INFORMATION

■ DEFINITION
Testicular neoplasms are primary cancers originating in a testis (Fig. 1-360).

■ SYNONYMS
Testis tumor
Testicular cancer

ICD-9CM CODES
186.9 Testicular neoplasm
M906/3 (seminoma)
M9101/3 (embryonal carcinoma or teratoma)
M9100/3 (choriocarcinoma)

■ EPIDEMIOLOGY & DEMOGRAPHICS
- Incidence: 2 to 3 cases/100,000 men/yr
- 1% to 2% of all cancers in males
- Age: can occur in any age but most common in young adults; average age for embryonal cell carcinoma: 30 yr; average age for seminoma: 36 yr

■ PHYSICAL FINDINGS & CLINICAL PRESENTATION
- Any mass within the testicle should be considered cancer until proven otherwise. It may be found by the patient who brings it to the attention of a physician or it may be found by a physician on a routine examination.
- Symptoms other than scrotal or testicular swelling are typically absent unless the cancer has metastasized. Occasionally a patient may complain of scrotal fullness or heaviness.
- Testicular palpation should be performed with two hands. Transillumination may distinguish a solid mass (e.g., cancer) and a fluid-filled lesion (e.g., hydrocele or spermatocele). The mass is nontender, indeed less sensitive than a normal testicle.

■ ETIOLOGY & PATHOLOGY
- Cryptorchidism (undescended testes) even if corrected by orchiopexy
- Pathology

Cell type	Frequency %
Seminoma	42
Embryonal cell carcinoma	26
Teratocarcinoma	26
Teratoma	5
Choriocarcinoma	1

Other rare types:
  Yolk sac carcinoma
  Mixed germ cell tumors
  Carcinoid tumor
  Sertoli cell tumors
  Leydig cell tumors
  Lymphoma
  Metastatic cancer to the testes

- TNM staging system for testicular cancer

T_0	No apparent primary
T_1	Testis only (excludes rete testis)
T_2	Beyond the tunica albuginea
T_3	Rete testis or epididymal involvement
T_4	Spermatic cord
	1. Spermatic cord
	2. Scrotum
N_0	No nodal involvement
N_1	Ipsilateral regional nodal involvement
N_2	Contralateral or bilateral abdominal or groin nodes
N_3	Palpable abdominal nodes or fixed groin nodes
N_4	Juxtaregional nodes
M_0	No distant metastases
M_1	Distant metastases present

The clinical stages consist of stage A, with tumor confined to the testis and cord structures; stage B, with tumor confined to the retroperitoneal lymph nodes; and stage C, with tumor involving the abdominal viscera or disease above the diaphragm

DIAGNOSIS

■ DIFFERENTIAL DIAGNOSIS
- Spermatocele
- Varicocele
- Hydrocele
- Epididymitis
- Epidermoid cyst of the testicle
- Epididymis tumors

■ WORKUP
Physical examination, laboratory tests, and imaging studies (Fig. 1-361)

■ LABORATORY TESTS
- Serum human chorionic gonadotropin (hCG)
- Serum alpha-fetoprotein (AFP)
One of both of these tumor markers will be elevated in 70% of cases of testicular cancer
- Testicular biopsy is contraindicated

■ IMAGING STUDIES
- Ultrasound (Fig. 1-362)
- CT scan or MRI of pelvis and abdomen
- Chest x-ray

TREATMENT

- Surgical exploration of the testicle through an inguinal incision with a noncrushing clamp placed on the cord before direct testicular examination. If a mass is confined within the body of the testicle, an orchiectomy is performed.
- Retroperitoneal lymph node dissection for clinical stage A and low stage B (lymph nodes under 6 cm in greatest diameter) provides cure in 70%.
- Chemotherapy: cisplatin, vinblastine, and bleomycin
  1. Not indicated in clinical stage A
  2. Controversial in low stage B
  3. Cornerstone of treatment in high stage B or stage C
- Radiation therapy for stage A and low stage B seminoma provides cure in 85%.
- Fig. 1-363 describes therapeutic options for patients with clinical stage I germ cell tumors.

■ REFERRAL
To urologist

REFERENCE
Rowland RG, Foster RS, Donohue JP: Testis tumors. In Gillenwater JY et al (eds): *Adult and pediatric urology,* vol 2, ed 3, St Louis, 1998, Mosby.
Author: **Tom J. Wachtel, M.D.**

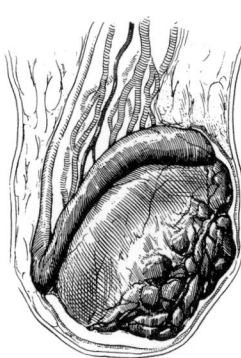

Fig. 1-360 Testicular tumor causing an irregular mass intrinsic to the testis. (From Sabiston D: *Textbook of surgery,* ed 15, Philadelphia, 1997, WB Saunders.)

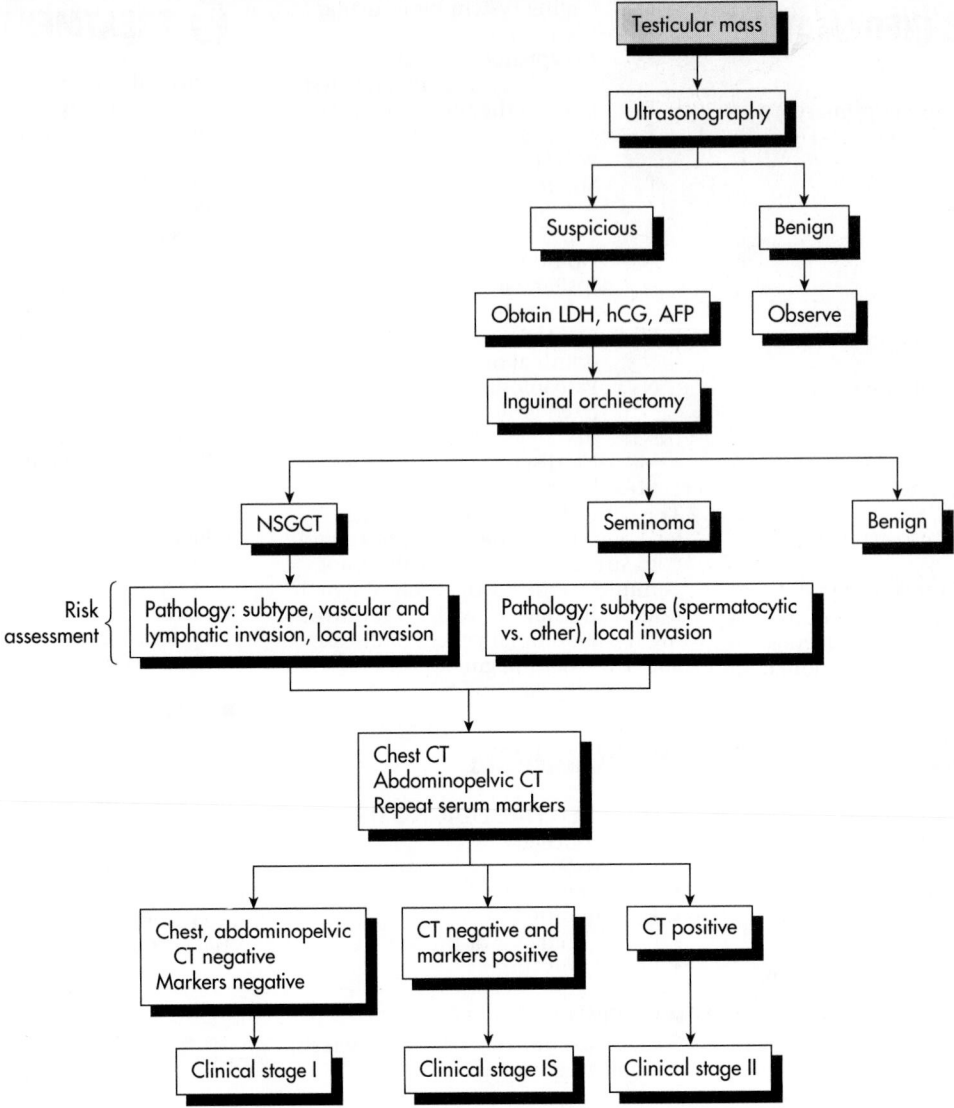

Fig. 1-361   Diagnosis, staging, and risk assessment of patients with testicular germ cell tumor.
AFP, Alpha-fetoprotein; *CT,* computed tomography; *hCG,* human chorionic gonadotropin; *LDH,* lactic dehydrogenase; *NSGCT,* nonseminoma germ cell tumor. (From Abeloff MD: *Clinical oncology,* ed 2, New York, 2000, Churchill Livingstone.)

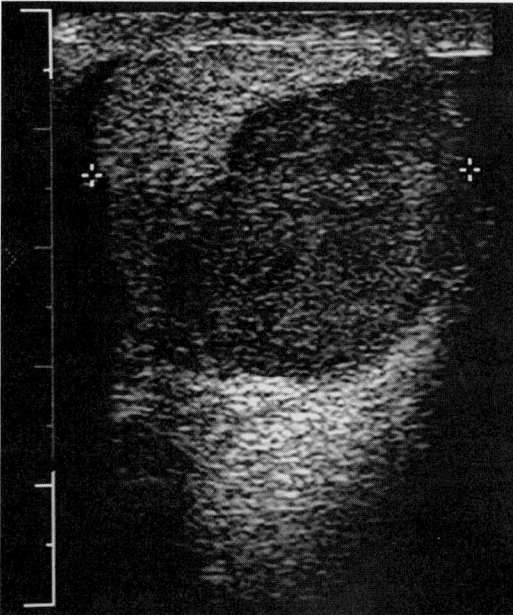

Fig. 1-362   Testicular ultrasound showing an intratesticular solid neoplasm. (From Nseyo UO [ed]: *Urology for primary care physicians,* Philadelphia, 1999, WB Saunders.)

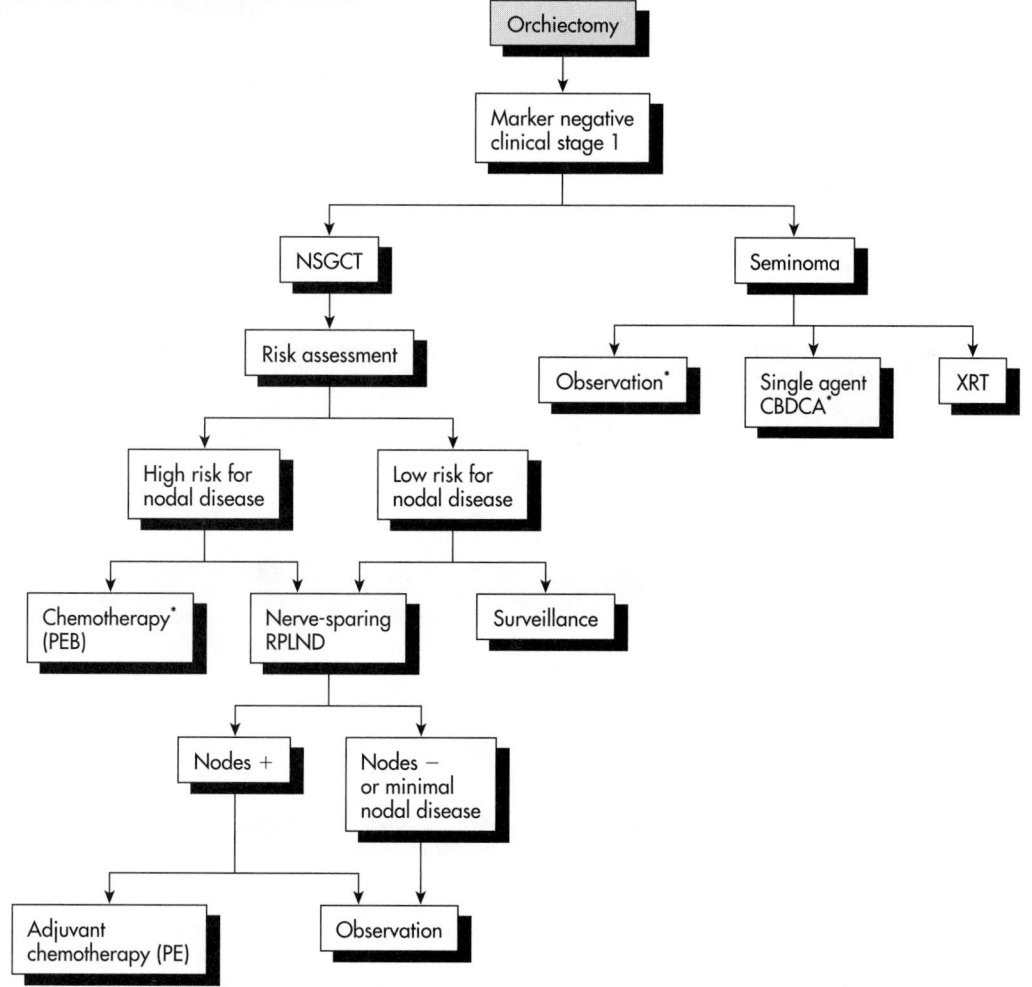

Fig. 1-363   Therapeutic options for patients with cinical stage I germ cell tumors.
*Investigational.
CBDCA, Carboplatin; *NSGCT,* nonseminoma germ cell tumor; *PE,* platinum, etoposide; *PEB,* platinum, etoposide, bleomycin; *RPLND,* retroperitoneal pelvic lymph node dissection; *XRT,* radiation therapy. (From Abeloff MD: *Clinical oncology,* ed 2, New York, 2000, Churchill Livingstone.)

BASIC INFORMATION

■ **DEFINITION**
Testicular torsion is a twisting of the spermatic cord leading to cessation of testicular blood flow, ischemia, and infarction if left untreated (Fig. 1-364).

■ **SYNONYMS**
Spermatic cord torsion

ICD-9CM CODES
608.2 Testicular torsion

■ **EPIDEMIOLOGY & DEMOGRAPHICS**
• Affects 1:4000 males
• Two thirds of all cases occur between the ages of 12 and 18 yr, but may occur at any age, including antenatally

■ **PHYSICAL FINDINGS & CLINICAL PRESENTATION**
• Typical sequence is sudden onset of hemiscrotal pain, then swelling, nausea, and vomiting without fever or urinary symptoms.
• Painless testicular swelling occurs in 10%.
• One out of three patients reports previous episodes of spontaneously remitting scrotal pain.
• In the neonate, testicular torsion should be presumed in patients with a painless, discolored hemiscrotal swelling.
• In rare cases, torsion may involve an undescended testicle. In such situations an empty hemiscrotum is palpated together with a tender lump in the inguinal area.

■ **ETIOLOGY**
Testicular torsion may occur without any underlying abnormality but is more likely when the tunica vaginalis extends high on the spermatic cord (bell-clapper deformity).

 DIAGNOSIS

■ **DIFFERENTIAL DIAGNOSIS**
(see Table 2-195)
• Torsion of the testicular appendages
• Testicular tumor
• Epididymitis
• Incarcerated inguinoscrotal hernia
• Orchitis
• Spermatocele
• Hydrocele

■ **WORKUP**
The diagnosis is usually based on history and physical examination.

■ **IMAGING STUDIES**
• Radionuclide scrotal scanning (technetium-99m): cold testicle
• Doppler ultrasonic stethoscope (Doppler flowmetry)

TREATMENT

Surgical derotation of the spermatic cord followed by bilateral testicular fixation with nonabsorbable sutures

■ **PROGNOSIS**
• There is an 80% testicular salvage rate if detorsion occurs within 12 hr of onset.
• After 24 hr, irreversible testicular infarction is expected.
• Because the contralateral testes can be affected (immunologic process), when treatment is delayed and return of blood flow does not occur after detorsion, some recommend orchiectomy of the infarcted testicle.

■ **REFERRAL**
To urologist

REFERENCE
Kogan S et al: Spermatic cord torsion. In Gillenwater JY et al (eds): *Adult and pediatric urology,* ed 3, St Louis, 1996, Mosby.
Author: **Tom J. Wachtel, M.D.**

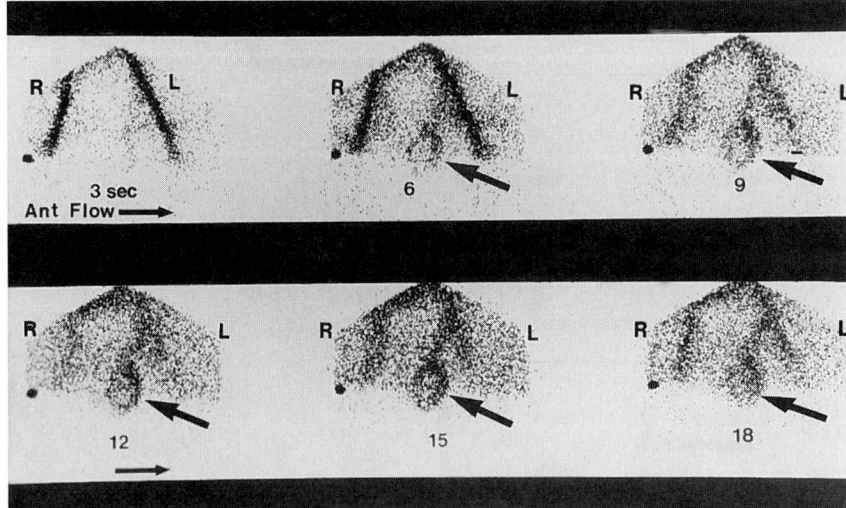

Fig. 1-364   Testicular torsion. Evaluation of blood flow to the testicle has been done by giving an intravenous bolus of radioactive material. The right and left iliac vessels are clearly identified, and sequential images are obtained every 3 sec. Here, increased flow is seen to the rim of the left testicle *(arrows),* and there is no blood flow centrally. This is the appearance of a testicular torsion in which the torsion has been present for more than approximately 24 hr. (From Mettler FA [ed]: *Primary care radiology,* Philadelphia, 2000, WB Saunders.)

BASIC INFORMATION

■ DEFINITION

Tetanus is a life-threatening illness manifested by muscle rigidity and spasms; it is caused by a neurotoxin (tetanospasmin) produced by *Clostridium tetani*.

ICD-9CM CODES
037 Tetanus

■ EPIDEMIOLOGY & DEMOGRAPHICS

INCIDENCE (IN U.S.): 48 to 64 cases reported annually since 1986
PREDOMINANT AGE: >60 yr of age
GENETICS:
Neonatal Infection:
• Rare in U.S.
• Among the leading causes of neonatal mortality in many parts of the world (caused by infection of the umbilical cord stump)

■ PHYSICAL FINDINGS & CLINICAL PRESENTATION
• Trismus ("lockjaw")
• Risus sardonicus (peculiar grin), characteristic grimace that results from contraction of the facial muscles
• Generalized muscle spasms causing severe pain and, at times, respiratory compromise and death
• Rigid abdominal muscles, flexed arms, and extended legs
• Autonomic dysfunction several days after onset of illness
• Leading cause of death: fluctuations in heart rate and blood pressure
• Usually, absence of fever
• Localized tetanus
  1. Rigidity of muscles near the injury
  2. Weakness as a result of lower motor neuron injury
  3. May be self-limited and resolve spontaneously
  4. More often progresses to generalized tetanus
  5. Cephalic tetanus:
     a. May occur with head injuries
     b. Can manifest as cranial nerve dysfunction

■ ETIOLOGY
• *C. tetani* is a gram-positive, spore-forming bacillus that resides primarily in the soil.

• Majority of cases are caused by punctures and lacerations.
• Toxin is elaborated from organisms in a contaminated wound.
• Local symptoms are caused by inhibition of neurotransmitter at presynaptic sites.
  1. Over the next 2 to 14 days, the toxin travels up the neurons to the CNS, where it acts on inhibitory neurons to prevent neurotransmitter release.
  2. Unopposed motor activity results in tonic contractions of muscles.

DIAGNOSIS

■ DIFFERENTIAL DIAGNOSIS
• Strychnine poisoning
• Dystonic reaction caused by neuroleptic agents
• Local infection (dental or masseter muscle) causing trismus
• Severe hypocalcemia
• Hysteria

■ WORKUP
• Positive wound culture is not helpful in diagnosis.
• Isolation of organism is possible in patients without the illness.

■ LABORATORY TESTS
• Usually, normal blood counts and chemistries
• Toxicology of serum and urine to rule out strychnine poisoning

TREATMENT

■ NONPHARMACOLOGIC THERAPY
• Monitoring in a hospital ICU: keep surroundings dark and quiet
• Intubation or tracheostomy for severe laryngospasm
• Debridement of wound

■ ACUTE GENERAL Rx
• Human tetanus immunoglobulin (HTIg) 500 U via IM injection
• Tetanus toxoid (Td) 0.5 ml by IM injection at a different site

• Metronidazole 500 mg IV q6h, or penicillin G 1 million U IV q4h for 10 days
• IV diazepam to control muscle spasms
• Neuromuscular blockade if necessary

■ CHRONIC Rx
• Supportive care
• Possible mechanical ventilation
• Minimal external stimuli
• Control of heart rate and blood pressure:
  1. Labetalol for sympathetic hyperactivity
  2. Pacemaker for sustained bradycardia
  3. Physical therapy once spasms subside

■ DISPOSITION
Full recovery over weeks to months if complications can be avoided

■ REFERRAL
• To emergency department
• To infectious disease specialist

PEARLS & CONSIDERATIONS

■ COMMENTS
• Illness is preventable.
• Boosters of Td should be given every 10 yr to maintain immune status.
• Passive as well as active immunization (HTIg + Td) should be given for patients with tetanus-prone wounds who have not been adequately immunized in the previous 5 yr.

REFERENCES
Centers for Disease Control and Prevention: Neonatal tetanus—Montana, 1998, *MMWR* 47(43), 1998.
Hsu SS et al: Tetanus in the emergency department: a current review, *J Emerg Med* 20(4):357, 2001.
O'Malley CD et al: Tetanus associated with body piercing, *Clin Infect Dis* 27:1343, 1998.
Talan DA, Moran GT: Tetanus among injecting-drug users—California, 1997, *Am Emerg Med* 32:385, 1998.
Author: **Maurice Policar, M.D.**

BASIC INFORMATION

■ DEFINITION
Thalassemias are a heterogeneous group of disorders of hemoglobin synthesis that have in common a deficient synthesis of one or more of the polypeptide chains of the normal human hemoglobin, resulting in a quantitative abnormality of the hemoglobin thus produced. There are no qualitative changes such as those encountered in the hemoglobinopathies (e.g., sickle cell disease).

■ SYNONYMS
Mediterranean anemia
Cooley's anemia

ICD-9CM CODES
282.4 Thalassemia

■ EPIDEMIOLOGY & DEMOGRAPHICS
- Thalassemia is the most common genetic disorder worldwide.
- The highest concentration of alpha-thalassemia is found in Southeast Asia and the African west coast. For example, in Thailand the prevalence is 5% to 10%. It is also common among blacks, with a prevalence of approximately 5%.
- The worldwide prevalence of beta-thalassemia is approximately 3%; in certain regions of Italy and Greece the prevalence reaches 15% to 30%. This high prevalence can be found in Americans of Italian or Greek descent.
- The distribution of thalassemia in Europe and Africa parallels that of malaria, suggesting that thalassemic persons are more resistant to the parasite, thus permitting evolutionary survival advantage.

■ CLASSIFICATION
BETA THALASSEMIA:
- Beta (+) thalassemia (suboptimal beta-globin synthesis)
- Beta (o) thalassemia (total absence of beta-globin synthesis)
- Delta-beta thalassemia (total absence of both delta-globin and beta-globin synthesis)
- Lepore hemoglobin (synthesis of small amounts of fused delta-beta-globin and total absence of delta- and beta-globin)
- Hereditary persistence of fetal hemoglobin (HPHF) (increased hemoglobin F synthesis and reduced or absence of delta- and beta-globin)

ALPHA THALASSEMIA:
- Silent carrier (three alpha-globin genes present)
- Alpha thalassemia trait (two alpha-globin genes present)
- Hemoglobin H disease (one alpha-globin gene present)
- Hydrops fetalis (no alpha-globin gene)
- Hemoglobin Constant Sprint (elongated alpha-globin chain)

THALASSEMIC HEMOGLO-BINOPATHIES: Hb Terre Haute, Hb Quong Sze, HbE, Hb Knossos

■ PHYSICAL FINDINGS & CLINICAL PRESENTATION
BETA THALASSEMIA:
- Heterozygous beta thalassemia (thalassemia minor): no or mild anemia, microcytosis and hypochromia, mild hemolysis manifested by slight reticulocytosis and splenomegaly
- Homozygous beta thalassemia (thalassemia major): intense hemolytic anemia; transfusion dependency; bone deformities (skull and long bones); hepatomegaly; splenomegaly; iron overload leading to cardiomyopathy, diabetes mellitus, and hypogonadism; growth retardation; pigment gallstones; susceptibility to infection
- Thalassemia intermedia caused by combination of beta and alpha thalassemia or beta thalassemia and Hb Lepore: resembles thalassemia major but is milder

ALPHA THALASSEMIA:
- Silent carrier: no symptoms.
- Alpha thalassemia trait: microcytosis only.
- Hemoglobin H disease: moderately severe hemolysis with microcytosis and splenomegaly.
- The loss of all four alpha-globin genes is incompatible with life (stillbirth of hydropic fetus). NOTE: Pregnancies with hydrops fetalis are associated with a high incidence of toxemia.

■ PATHOGENESIS
- Beta thalassemia: The reduction of beta-globin synthesis results in redundant alpha-globin chains (Heinz bodies), which are cytotoxic and cause intramedullary hemolysis and ineffective erythropoiesis. More than 100 mutations have been identified. Fetal hemoglobin may be increased.
- Alpha thalassemia: Several mutations can result in insufficient amounts of alpha globin available for combination with non–alpha globins.

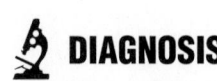

DIAGNOSIS

■ DIFFERENTIAL DIAGNOSIS
Usually the diagnosis is straightforward; iron deficiency must be ruled out in the presence of microcytosis; if iron deficiency is not present, the cause of microcytosis is probably thalassemia.

■ LABORATORY TESTS
BETA THALASSEMIA:
- Microcytosis (MCV: 55 to 80 FL)
- Normal RDW (RBC distribution width)
- Smear: nucleated RBCs, anisocytosis, poikilocytosis, polychromatophilia, Pappenheimer and Howell-Jolly bodies
- Hemoglobin electrophoresis: absent or reduced hemoglobin A, increased fetal hemoglobin, variable increase in the amount of hemoglobin A_2
- Markers of hemolysis: elevated indirect bilirubin and LDH, decreased haptoglobin

ALPHA THALASSEMIA:
- Microcytosis in the absence of iron deficiency
- Hemoglobin electrophoresis is normal, except for the presence of hemoglobin H in hemoglobin H disease

TREATMENT

- Thalassemia minor: no treatment but avoid iron administration for incorrect diagnosis of iron deficiency
- Beta thalassemia major (and hemoglobin H disease)
  1. Transfusion as required together with chelation of iron with desferrioxamine (by intravenous or subcutaneous administration, 8 to 12 hr nightly, 5 to 6 days a week at a dose of 2 to 6 g/day using a portable infusion pump)
  2. Splenectomy for hypersplenism if present
  3. Bone marrow transplantation
  4. Hydroxyurea may increase the level of hemoglobin F

■ REFERRAL
To hematologist

REFERENCE
Olivieri NF: The beta-thalassemias, *N Engl J Med* 341:99, 1999.
Author: **Tom J. Wachtel, M.D.**

BASIC INFORMATION

■ DEFINITION

Thoracic outlet syndrome is the term used to describe a condition producing upper extremity symptoms thought to result from neurovascular compression at the thoracic outlet. Three types are described based on the point of compression: (1) cervical rib and scalenus syndrome, in which abnormal scalene muscles or the presence of a cervical rib may cause compression; (2) costoclavicular syndrome, in which compression may occur under the clavicle; and (3) hyperabduction syndrome, in which compression may occur in the subcoracoid area.

ICD-9CM CODES
353.0 Thoracic outlet syndrome

■ EPIDEMIOLOGY & DEMOGRAPHICS
PREVALENCE: Varies from source to source; presence of cervical ribs in 0.5% to 1% of population (50% bilateral), but most are asymptomatic
PREDOMINANT AGE: Rare under 20 yr of age
PREDOMINANT SEX: Female > male (3.5:1)

■ PHYSICAL FINDINGS & CLINICAL PRESENTATION
- Symptoms and signs are related to the degree of involvement of each of the various structures at the level of the first rib.
- True venous or arterial involvement is rare.
- Diagnosis is most often used in the consideration of neural pain affecting the arm, which would suggest involvement of the brachial plexus.
  1. *Arterial compression:* pallor, paresthesias, diminished pulses, coolness, digital gangrene, and a supraclavicular bruit or mass
  2. *Venous compression:* edema and pain; thrombosis causing superficial venous dilation about the shoulder
  3. *"True" neural compression:* lower trunk (C8, T1) findings with intrinsic weakness and diminished sensation to the finger and small fingers and ulnar aspect of the forearm
  4. Possible supraclavicular tenderness
  5. Provocative tests (Adson's, Wright's): may reproduce pain but are of disputed usefulness

■ ETIOLOGY
- Congenital cervical rib or fibrous extension of cervical rib (Fig. 1-365)
- Abnormal scalene muscle insertion

- Drooping of shoulder girdle resulting from generalized hypotonia or trauma
- Narrowed costoclavicular interval as a result of downward and backward pressure on shoulder (sometimes seen in individuals who carry heavy backpacks)
- Acute venous thrombosis with exercise (effort thrombosis)
- Bony abnormalities of first rib
- Abnormal fibromuscular bands

DIAGNOSIS

■ DIFFERENTIAL DIAGNOSIS
- Carpal tunnel syndrome
- Cervical radiculopathy
- Brachial neuritis
- Ulnar nerve compression
- Reflex sympathetic dystrophy
- Superior sulcus tumor

■ WORKUP
Except for venous or arterial pathology, no ancillary diagnostic tests are reliable for diagnostic confirmation.

■ IMAGING STUDIES
- Arteriography or venography when vascular pathology is strongly suspected clinically
- Cervical spine radiographs to rule out cervical disk disease
- Chest film to rule out lung tumor
- EMG, NCV studies to rule out carpal tunnel syndrome, cervical radiculopathy

TREATMENT

■ ACUTE GENERAL Rx
- Sling for pain relief
- Physical therapy modalities plus shoulder girdle–strengthening exercises
- Postural reeducation
- NSAIDs

■ DISPOSITION
- Surgery: generally successful for vascular disorders
- Nonsurgical treatment: often successful for patients with pain as the primary symptom

■ REFERRAL
For vascular surgery consultation when venous or arterial impairment is present

PEARLS & CONSIDERATIONS

■ COMMENTS
- True thoracic outlet syndrome is probably an uncommon condition.
- Diagnosis is often used to describe a wide variety of clinical symptoms.
- Considerable disagreement exists regarding the frequency of this disorder.

Author: **Lonnie R. Mercier, M.D.**

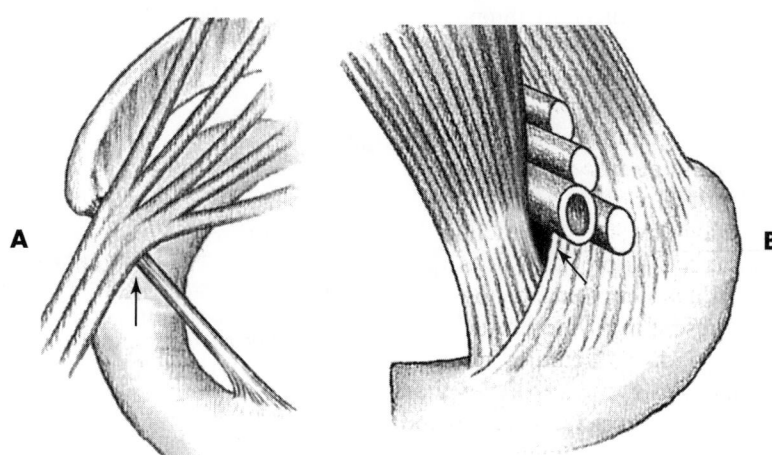

Fig. 1-365   A, Compression caused by a cervical rib *(arrow).* **B,** Abnormal scalene muscle insertions that may cause compression at the cervicobrachial region *(arrow).* (From Mercier LR: *Practical orthopedics,* ed 5, St Louis, 2000, Mosby.)

BASIC INFORMATION

■ DEFINITION
Thromboangiitis obliterans (Buerger's disease) is an occlusive inflammatory disease of the small- to medium-size arteries of the upper and lower extremities.

■ SYNONYMS
Buerger's disease
Presenile gangrene

ICD-9CM CODES
443.1 Thromboangiitis obliterans (Buerger's disease)

■ EPIDEMIOLOGY & DEMOGRAPHICS
- Since 1950, the incidence of thromboangiitis obliterans has fallen significantly.
- The prevalence of thromboangiitis obliterans is higher in Japan, India, and Southeast Asia when compared with the U.S.
- Thromboangiitis obliterans is rare in women.
- The disease typically occurs before the age of 50 yr and is found predominantly in men who smoke.

■ PHYSICAL FINDINGS & CLINICAL PRESENTATION
- Paresthesias, coldness, skin ulcers, gangrene, along with pain at rest or with walking (claudication)
- Prolonged capillary refill with dependent rubor
- Necrotic skin ulcers at the tips of the digits
- Pathognomonic migratory thrombophlebitis

■ ETIOLOGY
- Unknown.
- The remarkable feature is the close association between tobacco smoking and disease exacerbation. If abstinence from tobacco is adhered to, thromboangiitis obliterans takes a favorable course. If smoking is continued, the disease progresses, leading to gangrene and small-digit amputations.
- There is some thought of a genetic predisposition because the prevalence is higher in the Far East.

▲ DIAGNOSIS

■ DIFFERENTIAL DIAGNOSIS
Thromboangiitis obliterans must be distinguished from arteriosclerotic pe-

ripheral vascular disease by the criteria mentioned in "Workup."

■ WORKUP
The diagnosis of thromboangiitis obliterans is made on:
- Clinical criteria
  1. Peripheral vascular disease occurring predominantly in men before the age of 50 yr
  2. Typically, affects the arms and the legs and not just the lower extremities as arteriosclerosis does
  3. Found solely in tobacco smokers, with improvement in those who abstain
  4. Associated with migratory thrombophlebitis
  5. No other atherosclerotic risk factors (e.g., diabetes, cholesterol, or hypertension)
- Angiographic criteria (see "Imaging Studies")
- Pathologic criteria: fresh inflammatory thrombus within both small- and medium-size arteries and veins, along with giant cells around the thrombus

■ IMAGING STUDIES
- Noninvasive vascular studies help differentiate proximal occlusive disease characteristic of arteriosclerosis from distal disease typical of thromboangiitis obliterans.
- Angiography findings in thromboangiitis obliterans include:
  1. Involvement of distal small- and medium-size vessels.
  2. Occlusions are segmental, multiple, smooth, and tapered.
  3. Collateral circulation gives a "tree root" or "spider leg" appearance.
  4. Both upper and lower extremities are involved.

℞ TREATMENT

■ NONPHARMACOLOGIC THERAPY
Abstaining from smoking is the only way to stop the progression of the disease. Medical and surgical treatments will prove to be futile if the patient continues to smoke. Exacerbation of ischemic ulcers is directly related to tobacco use.

■ ACUTE GENERAL Rx
- The goal of medical treatment is to provide relief of ischemic pain and healing of ischemic ulcers. If the patient does not completely abstain from tobacco, medical measures will not be helpful.

- Prostaglandin vasodilator therapy given IV or intraarterially provides some relief of pain but does not change the course of the disease.
- Epidural anesthesia and hyperbaric oxygen have a vasodilator effect and have been shown to aid in pain relief from ischemic ulcers.

■ CHRONIC Rx
- Surgical bypass procedures and sympathectomy, as with medical treatment, will not be efficacious unless the patient stops smoking.
- Surgical bypass may be difficult because the occlusions of thromboangiitis obliterans are distal. Nevertheless, if successfully done, this can lead to rapid healing of ischemic ulcers.
- Sympathectomy leads to increased flow by decreasing the vasoconstriction of distal vessels and also has been shown to aid in the healing and relief of pain from ischemic ulcers.
- Debridement must be done on necrotic ulcers if needed.
- Amputation is frequently required for gangrenous digits; however, below-knee or above-knee amputations are rarely necessary.

■ DISPOSITION
The course of thromboangiitis obliterans can be dramatically changed by the cessation of tobacco smoking. If the patient continues to smoke, recurrent exacerbation of ischemic ulcers, necrosis, and gangrene leading to small digit amputations will be inevitable.

■ REFERRAL
Vascular surgical consultation is recommended in any young smoker with claudication and ischemic ulcers, especially if both the upper and lower extremities are involved.

☼ PEARLS & CONSIDERATIONS

■ COMMENTS
Smoking cessation is mandatory. In individuals who quit smoking, prognosis is markedly improved.

REFERENCES
Agarwal VK: Buerger's disease, *J Indian Med Assoc* 97(7):291, 1999.
Szuba A et al: Thromboangiitis obliterans: an update on Buerger's disease, *West J Med* 168(4):255, 1998.
Author: **Peter Petropoulos, M.D.**

BASIC INFORMATION

■ **DEFINITION**
Superficial thrombophlebitis is inflammatory thrombosis in subcutaneous veins.

■ **SYNONYMS**
Phlebitis

ICD-9CM CODES
451.0 Thrombophlebitis, superficial

■ **EPIDEMIOLOGY & DEMOGRAPHICS**
• 20% of superficial thrombophlebitis cases are associated with occult DVT.
• Catheter-related thrombophlebitis incidence is 100:100,000.

■ **PHYSICAL FINDINGS & CLINICAL PRESENTATION**
• Subcutaneous vein is palpable, tender; tender cord is present with erythema and edema of the overlying skin and subcutaneous tissue.
• Induration, redness, and tenderness are localized along the course of the vein. This linear appearance rather than circular appearance is useful to distinguish thrombophlebitis from other conditions (cellulitis, erythema nodosum).
• There is no significant swelling of the limb (superficial thrombophlebitis generally does not produce swelling of the limb).
• Low-grade fever may be present. High fever and chills are suggestive of septic phlebitis.

■ **ETIOLOGY**
• Trauma to preexisting varices
• Intravenous cannulation of veins (most common cause)

• Abdominal cancer (e.g., carcinoma of pancreas)
• Infection (*Staphylococcus* is the most common pathogen)
• Hypercoagulable state
• DVT

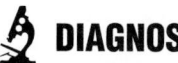 **DIAGNOSIS**

■ **DIFFERENTIAL DIAGNOSIS**
• Lymphangitis
• Cellulitis
• Erythema nodosum
• Panniculitis
• Kaposi's sarcoma

■ **WORKUP**
Laboratory evaluation to exclude infectious etiology and imaging studies to rule out DVT in suspected cases

■ **LABORATORY TESTS**
CBC with differential, blood cultures, culture of IV catheter tip (when secondary to intravenous cannulation)

■ **IMAGING STUDIES**
• Serial ultrasound or venography in patients with suspected DVT
• CT scan of abdomen in patients with suspected malignancy (Trousseau's syndrome: recurrent migratory thrombophlebitis)

TREATMENT

■ **NONPHARMACOLOGIC THERAPY**
• Warm, moist compresses
• It is not necessary to restrict activity; however, if there is extensive throm-

bophlebitis, bed rest with the leg elevated will limit the thrombosis and improve symptoms.

■ **ACUTE GENERAL Rx**
• NSAIDs to relieve symptoms
• Treatment of septic thrombophlebitis with antibiotics with adequate coverage of *Staphylococcus*
• Ligation and division of the superficial vein at the junction to avoid propagation of the clot in the deep venous system when the thrombophlebitis progresses toward the junction of the involved superficial vein with deep veins

■ **DISPOSITION**
Clinical improvement within 7 to 10 days

■ **REFERRAL**
Surgical referral in selected cases (see "Acute General Rx")

PEARLS & CONSIDERATIONS

■ **COMMENTS**
• Patients with positive cultures should be evaluated and treated for endocarditis.
• Septic thrombophlebitis is more common in IV drug addicts.
Author: **Fred F. Ferri, M.D.**

BASIC INFORMATION

■ DEFINITION
Deep vein thrombosis (DVT) is the development of thrombi in the deep veins of the extremities or pelvis.

■ SYNONYMS
DVT
Deep venous thrombophlebitis

ICD-9CM CODES
451.1 Thrombosis of deep vessels of lower extremities
451.83 Thrombosis of deep veins of upper extremities
541.9 Deep vein thrombosis of unspecified site

■ EPIDEMIOLOGY & DEMOGRAPHICS
Annual incidence in urban population is 1.6 cases/1000 persons.

■ PHYSICAL FINDINGS & CLINICAL PRESENTATION
• Pain and swelling of the affected extremity
• In lower extremity DVT, leg pain on dorsiflexion of the foot (Homans' sign)
• Physical examination may be unremarkable

■ ETIOLOGY
The etiology is often multifactorial (prolonged stasis, coagulation abnormalities, vessel wall trauma). The following are risk factors for DVT:
• Prolonged immobilization (≥3 days)
• Postoperative state
• Trauma to pelvis and lower extremities
• Birth control pills, high-dose estrogen therapy
• Visceral cancer (lung, pancreas, alimentary tract, GU tract)
• Age >60 yr
• History of thromboembolic disease
• Hematologic disorders (e.g., antithrombin III deficiency, protein C deficiency, protein S deficiency, sticky platelet syndrome, G20210A prothrombin mutation, lupus anticoagulant, dysfibrinogenemias, anticardiolipin antibody, hyperhomocystinemia, concurrent homocystinuria, high levels of factors VIII, XI, and factor V Leiden mutation)

• Pregnancy and early puerperium
• Obesity, CHF
• Surgery, fracture, or injury involving lower leg or pelvis
• Surgery requiring >30 min of anesthesia
• Gynecologic surgery (particularly gynecologic cancer surgery)
• Recent travel (within 2 wk, lasting >4 hr)
• Smoking and abdominal obesity

DIAGNOSIS

■ DIFFERENTIAL DIAGNOSIS
• Postphlebitic syndrome
• Superficial thrombophlebitis
• Ruptured Baker's cyst
• Cellulitis, lymphangitis, Achilles tendinitis
• Hematoma
• Muscle or soft tissue injury, stress fracture
• Varicose veins, lymphadema
• Arterial insufficiency

■ WORKUP
The clinical diagnosis of DVT is inaccurate. Pain, tenderness, swelling, or color changes are not specific for DVT. Commonly used diagnostic tests are described below in Table 1-67 and in Fig. 1-366. An initial negative test on compression ultrasonography or IPG should be repeated after 3 to 5 days (if the clinical suspicion of DVT persists) to detect propagation of any thrombosis to the proximal veins.

■ LABORATORY TESTS
• Laboratory tests are not specific for DVT. Baseline PT (INR), PTT, and platelet count should be obtained on all patients before starting anticoagulation.
• Laboratory evaluation of young patients with DVT, patients with recurrent thrombosis without obvious causes, and those with a family history of thrombosis should include protein S, protein C, fibrinogen, antithrombin III level, lupus anticoagulant, anticardiolipin antibodies, factor V Leiden, factor VIII, factor IX, and plasma homocysteine levels.

■ IMAGING STUDIES
• Contrast venography is the "gold standard" for evaluation of DVT of the lower extremity. It is, however, invasive and painful. Additional disadvantages are the increased risk of phlebitis, new thrombosis, renal failure, and hypersensitivity reaction to contrast media; it also gives poor visualization of deep femoral vein in the thigh and internal iliac vein and its tributaries.
• Compression ultrasonography is generally preferred as the initial study because it is noninvasive and can be repeated serially (useful to monitor suspected acute DVT); it offers good sensitivity for detecting proximal vein thrombosis (in the popliteal or femoral vein). Its disadvantages are poor visualization of deep iliac and pelvic veins and poor sensitivity in isolated or nonocclusive calf vein thrombi.

TREATMENT

■ NONPHARMACOLOGIC THERAPY
• Initial bed rest for 1 to 4 days followed by gradual resumption of normal activity
• Patient education on anticoagulant therapy and associated risks

■ ACUTE GENERAL Rx
• Traditional treatment consists of IV unfractionated heparin for 4 to 7 days followed by warfarin therapy. Low–molecular-weight heparin enoxaparin (Lovenox) is also effective for initial management of DVT and allows outpatient treatment. Recommended dose is 1 mg/kg q12h SC and continued for a minimum of 5 days and until a therapeutic INR (2 to 3) has been achieved with warfarin. Warfarin therapy should be initiated when appropriate (usually within 72 hr of initiation of heparin). Initial loading dose for warfarin should not exceed 5 mg/day.
• Low–molecular-weight heparin, when used, should be overlapped with warfarin for at least 5 days and until the INR has exceeded 2 for 2 consecutive days.

- Exclusions from outpatient treatment of DVT include patients with potential high complication risk (e.g., HB <7, platelet count <75,000, guaic-positive stool, recent CVA or noncutaneous surgery, noncompliance).

■ **CHRONIC Rx**
The optimal duration of anticoagulant therapy varies with the cause of DVT and the patient's risk factors:
1. Therapy for 3 to 6 mo is generally satisfactory in patients with reversible risk factors.
2. Anticoagulation for at least 6 mo is recommended for patients with idiopathic venous thrombosis.
3. Indefinite anticoagulation is necessary in patients with DVT associated with active cancer; long-term anticoagulation is also indicated in patients with inherited thrombophilia (e.g., deficiency of protein C or S antibody), antiphospholipid, and those with recurrent episodes of idiopathic DVT.

☼ **PEARLS & CONSIDERATIONS**

■ **COMMENTS**
Prophylaxis of DVT is recommended in all patients at risk (e.g., low–molecular-weight heparin after major trauma, post surgery of hip and knee; gradient elastic stockings alone or in combination with intermittent pneumatic compression [IPC] boots following neurosurgery).

REFERENCES
Agnelli G et al: Three months versus one year of oral anticoagulant therapy for idiopathic deep venous thrombosis, *N Engl J Med* 345:165, 2001.
Merli G et al: Subcutaneous enoxaparin once or twice daily compared with intravenous unfractionated heparin for treatment of venous thromboembolic disease, *Ann Intern Med* 134:191, 2001.
Seligsohn U, Lubetsky A: Genetic susceptibility to venous thrombosis, *N Engl J Med* 344:1222, 2001.
Thomas RH: Hypercoagulability syndromes, *Arch Intern Med* 161:2433, 2001.
Yusen R et al: Criteria for out-patient management of proximal lower extremity DVT, *Chest* 115:975, 1999.
Author: **Fred F. Ferri, M.D.**

TABLE 1-67 Diagnostic Tests for Venous Thromboembolism

DIAGNOSTIC METHOD	ADVANTAGES	DISADVANTAGES
Contrast venography	"Gold standard" for evaluation of DVT of lower extremity	Invasive, painful Increased risk of phlebitis, new thrombosis, renal failure, and hypersensitivity reaction to contrast media Poor visualization of deep femoral vein in thigh and internal iliac vein and its tributaries
Compressive duplex ultrasonography	Noninvasive Can be repeated serially (useful to monitor suspected acute DVT) Good sensitivity for proximal thrombosis and thrombosis of lower popliteal vein Fewer false-positive results than with IPG in patients with failure of right side of heart or receiving mechanical ventilation Positive predictive value of serial compressive ultrasonography is generally higher than that of classic IPG	Poor visualization of deep femoral, iliac, and pelvic veins Requires skilled operator Poor sensitivity in isolated or nonocclusive calf vein thrombi
Impedance plethysmography (IPG)	Noninvasive Can be performed repeatedly (useful to monitor suspected acute DVT) Good correlation with contrast venography for proximal DVT	Poor sensitivity in calf vein thrombi and nonobstructive proximal thrombi False-positive results in patients with peripheral vascular disease, failure of right side of heart, postoperative lower extremity swelling, and excessive leg tension and in patients receiving mechanical ventilation

From Ferri F: *Practical guide to the care of the medical patient*, ed 5, St Louis, 2001, Mosby.

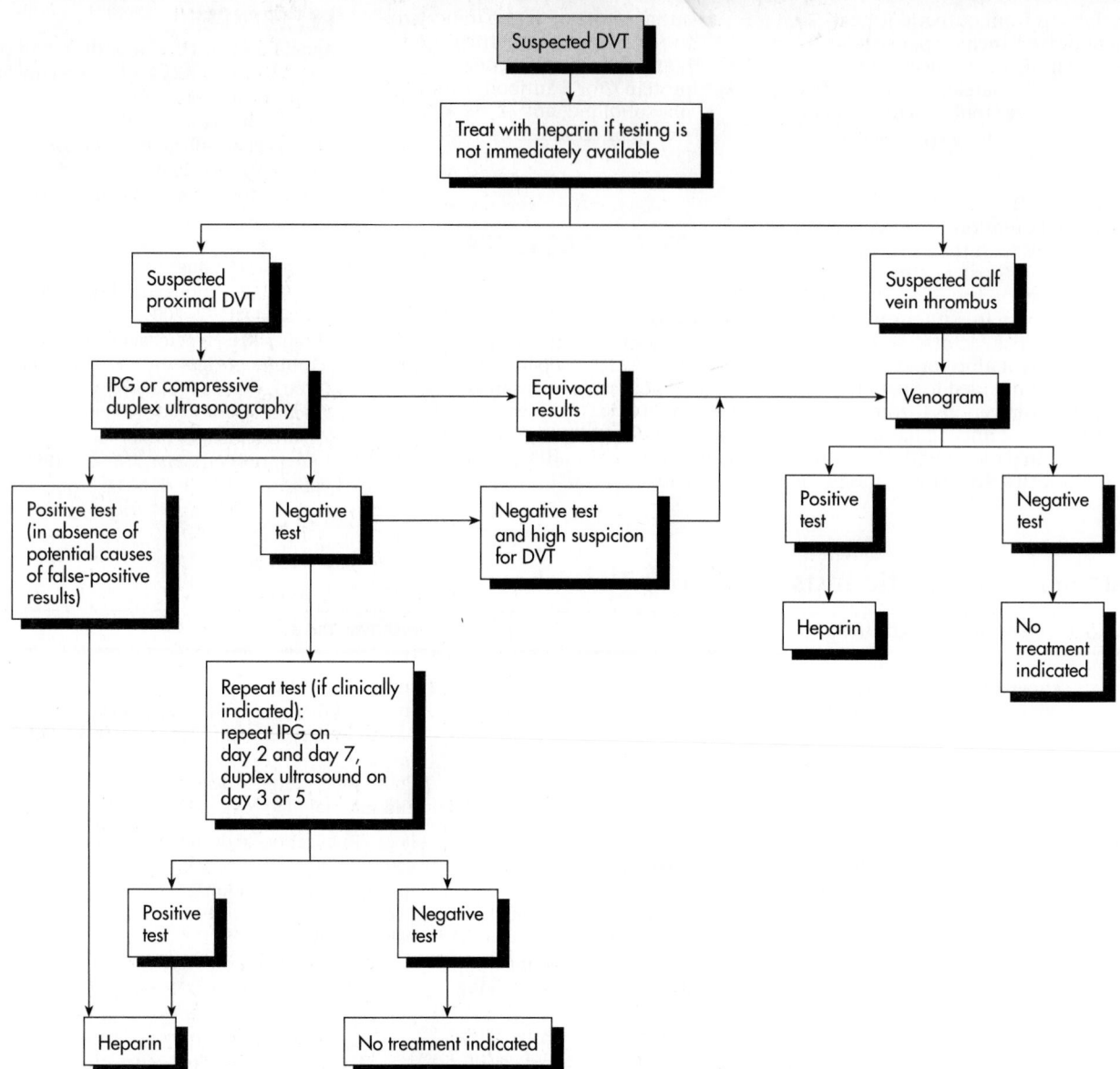

Fig. 1-366   **Evaluation of suspected deep venous thrombosis.** Repeat noninvasive testing (when clinically indicated) may be useful to diagnose patients with calf vein who subsequently develop proximal thrombosis. *DVT,* Deep venous thrombosis; *IPG,* intravenous pyelogram; *IV,* intravenous. (From Ferri F: *Practical guide to the care of the medical patient,* ed 5, St Louis, 2001, Mosby.)

BASIC INFORMATION

◼ DEFINITION
Thrombotic thrombocytopenic purpura (TTP) is a rare disorder characterized by thrombocytopenia (often accompanied by purpura) and microangiopathic hemolytic anemia; neurologic impairment, renal dysfunction, and fever may also be present.

◼ SYNONYMS
TTP

ICD-9CM CODES
446.6 Thrombotic thrombocytopenic purpura

◼ EPIDEMIOLOGY & DEMOGRAPHICS
- TTP primarily affects females between 10 and 50 yr of age.
- Frequency is 3.7 cases/yr/1 million persons.

◼ PHYSICAL FINDINGS & CLINICAL PRESENTATION
- Purpura (secondary to thrombocytopenia)
- Jaundice, pallor (secondary to hemolysis)
- Mucosal bleeding
- Fever
- Fluctuating levels of consciousness (secondary to thrombotic occlusion of the cerebral vessels)

◼ ETIOLOGY
- The exact cause of TTP remains unknown. Recent studies reveal that there is platelet aggregation as a result of abnormalities in circulating von Willebrand factor caused by endothelial injury.
- Many drugs, including clopidogrel, penicillin, antineoplastic agents, oral contraceptives, quinine, and ticlopidine, have been associated with TTP. Other precipitating causes include infectious agents, pregnancy, malignancies, allogenic bone marrow transplantation, and neurologic disorders.

DIAGNOSIS

◼ DIFFERENTIAL DIAGNOSIS
- DIC
- Malignant hypertension
- Vasculitis

- Eclampsia or preeclampsia
- Hemolytic-uremic syndrome (typically encountered in children, often following a viral infection)
- Gastroenteritis as a result of a serotoxin-producing serotype of *Escherichia coli*
- Medications: clopidogrel, ticlopidine, penicillin, antineoplastic chemotherapeutic agents, oral contraceptives

◼ WORKUP
- A comprehensive history, physical examination, and laboratory evaluation usually confirms the diagnosis.
- The disease often begins as a flulike illness ultimately followed by clinical and laboratory abnormalities.
- See Fig. 3-163 for a clinical algorithm for the evaluation of thrombocytopenia.

◼ LABORATORY TESTS
- Severe anemia and thrombocytopenia
- Elevated BUN and creatinine
- Evidence of hemolysis: elevated reticulocyte count, indirect bilirubin, LDH, decreased haptoglobin
- Urinalysis: hematuria (red cells and red cell casts in urine sediment) and proteinuria
- Peripheral smear: severely fragmented RBCs (schistocytes)
- No laboratory evidence of DIC (normal FDP, fibrinogen)

TREATMENT

◼ ACUTE GENERAL Rx
- Plasmapheresis with fresh frozen plasma (FFP) replacement; cryosupernatant may be substituted for FFP in patients who fail to respond to this treatment. Daily plasma exchange is generally performed until hemolysis has ceased and the platelet count has normalized.
- Corticosteroids (prednisone 1 to 2 mg/kg/day) may be effective alone in patients with mild disease or may be administered concomitantly with plasmapheresis plus plasma exchange with FFP.
- Vincristine has been used in patients refractory to plasmapheresis.

- Use of antiplatelet agents (ASA, dipyridamole) is controversial.
- Platelet transfusions are contraindicated except in severely thrombocytopenic patients with documented bleeding.
- Splenectomy is performed in refractory cases.

◼ CHRONIC Rx
- Relapsing TTP may be treated with plasma exchange.
- Splenectomy done while the patients are in remission has been used in some centers to decrease the frequency of relapse in TTP.

◼ DISPOSITION
- Survival of patients with TTP currently exceeds 80% with plasma exchange therapy.
- Relapse occurs in 20% to 40% of patients who have TTP in remission.

◼ REFERRAL
Surgical referral for splenectomy in selected patients (see "Acute General Rx" and "Chronic Rx")

PEARLS & CONSIDERATIONS

◼ COMMENTS
Thrombotic microangiopathy can also be associated with administration of cyclosporine and mitomycin C, and with HIV infection.

REFERENCES
Bennett CL et al: Thrombotic thrombocytopenic purpura associated with clopidogrel, *N Engl J Med* 342:1773, 2000.

Chen DK et al: Thrombotic thrombocytopenic purpura associated with ticlopidine use, *Arch Intern Med* 159:311, 1999.

Elliot MA, Nichols WL: Thrombotic thrombocytopenic purpura and hemolytic uremic syndrome, *Mayo Clin Proc* 76:1154, 2001.

Kojouri K et al: Quinine-associated thrombotic thrombocytopenic purpura-hemolytic uremic syndrome: frequency, clinical features, and long-term outcomes, *Ann Intern Med* 135:1047, 2001.
Author: **Fred F. Ferri, M.D.**

BASIC INFORMATION

■ **DEFINITION**

Thyroid carcinoma is a primary neoplasm of the thyroid. There are four major types of thyroid carcinoma: papillary, follicular, anaplastic, and medullary.

■ **SYNONYMS**

Papillary carcinoma of thyroid
Follicular carcinoma of thyroid
Anaplastic carcinoma of thyroid
Medullary carcinoma of thyroid

ICD-9CM CODES
193 Malignant neoplasm of thyroid

■ **EPIDEMIOLOGY & DEMOGRAPHICS**
• Thyroid cancer is the most common endocrine cancer, with an annual incidence of 14,000 new cases in the U.S. and about 1100 deaths.
• Female:male ratio of 3:1.
• Most common type (50% to 60%) is papillary carcinoma.
• Median age at diagnosis: 45 to 50 yr.

■ **PHYSICAL FINDINGS & CLINICAL PRESENTATION**
• Presence of thyroid nodule
• Hoarseness and cervical lymphadenopathy
• Painless swelling in the region of the thyroid

■ **ETIOLOGY**
• Risk factors: prior neck irradiation
• Multiple endocrine neoplasia II (medullary carcinoma)

DIAGNOSIS

■ **DIFFERENTIAL DIAGNOSIS**
• Multinodular goiter
• Lymphocytic thyroiditis
• Ectopic thyroid

■ **WORKUP**
The workup of thyroid carcinoma includes laboratory evaluation and diagnostic imaging. However, diagnosis is confirmed with fine-needle aspiration (FNA) or surgical biopsy. The characteristics of thyroid carcinoma vary with the type:
• Papillary carcinoma
1. Most frequently occurs in women during second or third decades.
2. Histologically, psammoma bodies (calcific bodies present in papillary projections) are pathognomonic; they are found in 35% to 45% of papillary thyroid carcinomas.
3. Majority are not papillary lesions but mixed papillary follicular carcinomas.
4. Spread is via lymphatics and by local invasion.
• Follicular carcinoma
1. More aggressive than papillary carcinoma.
2. Incidence increases with age.
3. Tends to metastasize hematogenously to bone, producing pathologic fractures.
4. Tends to concentrate iodine (useful for radiation therapy).
• Anaplastic carcinoma
1. Very aggressive neoplasm.
2. Two major histologic types: small cell (less aggressive, 5-yr survival approximately 20%) and giant cell (death usually within 6 mo of diagnosis).
• Medullary carcinoma
1. Unifocal lesion: found sporadically in elderly patients.
2. Bilateral lesions: associated with pheochromocytoma and hyperparathyroidism; this combination is known as MEN-II and is inherited as an autosomal dominant disorder.

■ **LABORATORY TESTS**
• Thyroid function studies are generally normal. TSH, T_4, and serum thyroglobulin levels should be obtained before thyroidectomy in patients with confirmed thyroid carcinoma.
• Increased plasma calcitonin assay in patients with medullary carcinoma (tumors produce thyrocalcitonin)

■ **IMAGING STUDIES**
• Thyroid scanning with iodine-123 or technetium-99m can identify hypofunctioning (cold) nodules, which are more likely to be malignant. However, warm nodules can also be malignant.
• Thyroid ultrasound can detect solitary solid nodules that have a high risk of malignancy. However, a negative ultrasound does not exclude diagnosis of thyroid carcinoma.
• FNA biopsy is the best method to assess a thyroid nodule (refer to "Thyroid Nodule" in Section I).

TREATMENT

■ **ACUTE GENERAL Rx**
• Papillary carcinoma
1. Total thyroidectomy is indicated if the patient has:
   a. Extrapyramidal extension of carcinoma
   b. Papillary carcinoma limited to thyroid but a positive history of irradiation to the neck
   c. Lesion >2 cm
2. Lobectomy with isthmectomy may be considered in patients with intrathyroid papillary carcinoma <2 cm and no history of neck or head irradiation; most follow surgery with suppressive therapy with thyroid hormone because these tumors are TSH responsive. The accepted practice is to suppress serum TSH concentrations to <0.1 μU/ml.
3. Radiotherapy with iodine-131 (after total thyroidectomy), followed by thyroid suppression therapy with triiodothyronine, can be used in metastatic papillary carcinoma.
• Follicular carcinoma
1. Total thyroidectomy followed by TSH suppression as noted previously
2. Radiotherapy with iodine-131 followed by thyroid suppression therapy with triiodothyronine is useful in patients with metastasis.
• Anaplastic carcinoma
1. At diagnosis, this neoplasm is rarely operable; palliative surgery is indicated for extremely large tumor compressing the trachea.
2. Management is usually restricted to radiation therapy or chemotherapy (combination of doxorubicin, cisplatin, and other antineoplastic agents); these measures rarely provide significant palliation.
• Medullary carcinoma
1. Thyroidectomy should be performed.
2. Patients and their families should be screened for pheochromocytoma and hyperparathyroidism.

■ **DISPOSITION**
Prognosis varies with the type of thyroid carcinoma: 5-yr survival approaches 80% for follicular carcinoma and is approximately 5% with anaplastic carcinoma.

PEARLS & CONSIDERATIONS

■ **COMMENTS**
Family members of patients with medullary carcinoma should be screened; DNA analysis for the detection of mutations in the RET gene structure permits the identification of MEN IIA gene carriers.

REFERENCE
Schlumberger MJ: Papillary and follicular thyroid carcinoma, *N Engl J Med* 338:297, 1998.
Author: **Fred F. Ferri, M.D.**

BASIC INFORMATION

■ DEFINITION
A thyroid nodule is an abnormality found on physical examination of the thyroid gland; nodules can be benign (70%) or malignant.

ICD-9CM CODES
241.0 Nodule, thyroid

■ EPIDEMIOLOGY & DEMOGRAPHICS
- Thyroid nodules can be found in 50% of autopsies; however, only 1 in 10 is palpable.
- Malignancy is present in 5% to 30% of palpable nodules.
- Incidence of thyroid nodules increases after 45 yr of age. They are found more frequently in women.
- History of prior head and neck irradiation increases the risk of thyroid cancer.
- Increased likelihood that nodule is malignant: nodule increasing in size or >2 cm, regional lymphadenopathy, fixation to adjacent tissues, age <40 yr, male sex.

■ PHYSICAL FINDINGS & CLINICAL PRESENTATION
- Palpable, firm, and nontender nodule in the thyroid area should prompt suspicion of carcinoma. Signs of metastasis are regional lymphadenopathy, inspiratory stridor.
- Signs and symptoms of thyrotoxicosis can be found in functioning nodules.

■ ETIOLOGY
- History of prior head and neck irradiation
- Family history of pheochromocytoma, carcinoma of the thyroid, and hyperparathyroidism (medullary carcinoma of the thyroid is a component of MEN-II)

 DIAGNOSIS

■ DIFFERENTIAL DIAGNOSIS
- Thyroid carcinoma
- Multinodular goiter
- Thyroglossal duct cyst
- Epidermoid cyst
- Laryngocele
- Nonthyroid neck neoplasm
- Branchial cleft cyst

■ WORKUP
- Fine-needle aspiration (FNA) biopsy is the best diagnostic study; the accuracy can be >90%, but it is directly related to the level of experience of the physician and the cytopathologist interpreting the aspirate.
- FNA biopsy is less reliable with thyroid cystic lesions; surgical excision should be considered for most thyroid cysts not abolished by aspiration.
- A diagnostic approach to thyroid nodule is described in Fig. 1-367.

■ LABORATORY TESTS
- TSH, T_4, and serum thyroglobulin levels should be obtained before thyroidectomy in patients with confirmed thyroid carcinoma on FNA biopsy.
- Serum calcitonin at random or after pentagastrin stimulation is useful when suspecting medullary carcinoma of the thyroid.
- Serum thyroid autoantibodies (see "Thyroiditis" in Section I) are useful when suspecting thyroiditis.

■ IMAGING STUDIES
- Thyroid ultrasound is done in some patients to evaluate the size of the thyroid and the number, composition (solid vs. cystic), and dimensions of the thyroid nodule; solid thyroid nodules have a higher incidence of malignancy, but cystic nodules can also be malignant.
- The introduction of high-resolution ultrasonography has made it possible to detect many nonpalpable nodules (incidentalomas) in the thyroid (found at autopsy in 30% to 60% of cadavers). Most of these lesions are benign. For most patients with nonpalpable nodules that are incidentally detected by thyroid imaging, simple follow-up neck palpation is sufficient.
- Thyroid scan with technetium-99m pertechnetate:
  1. Classifies nodules as hyperfunctioning (hot), normally functioning (warm), or nonfunctioning (cold); cold nodules have a higher incidence of malignancy; the differential diagnosis of cold thyroid nodules is described in Box 2-247.
  2. Scan has difficulty evaluating nodules near the thyroid isthmus or at the periphery of the gland.
  3. Normal tissue over a nonfunctioning nodule might mask the nodule as "warm" or normally functioning.
- Both thyroid scan and ultrasound provide information about the risk of malignant neoplasia based on the characteristics of the thyroid nodule, but their value in the initial evaluation of a thyroid nodule is limited because neither one provides a definite tissue diagnosis.

TREATMENT

■ ACUTE GENERAL Rx
- Evaluation of results of FNA
  1. Normal cells: may repeat biopsy during present evaluation or reevaluate patient after 3 to 6 mo of suppressive therapy (L-thyroxine, 100 to 200 μg PO qd)
     a. Failure to regress indicates increased likelihood of malignancy
     b. Reliance on repeat needle biopsy is preferable to routine surgery for nodules not responding to thyroxine.
  2. Malignant cells: surgery
  3. Hypercellularity: thyroid scan
     a. Hot nodule: ^{131}I therapy if the patient is hyperthyroid
     b. Warm or cold nodule: surgery (rule out follicular adenoma vs. carcinoma)

■ DISPOSITION
Variable with results of FNA biopsy. Refer to "Thyroid Carcinoma" in Section I for prognosis in patients with malignant nodules diagnosed with biopsy.

■ REFERRAL
Surgical referral for FNA biopsy

PEARLS & CONSIDERATIONS

■ COMMENTS
Surgery is indicated in hard or fixed nodule, presence of dysphagia or hoarseness, and rapidly growing solid masses regardless of "benign" results on FNA.

REFERENCE
Hermus AR, Huysmans DA: Treatment of benign nodular thyroid disease, *N Engl J Med* 338:1438, 1998.
Author: **Fred F. Ferri, M.D.**

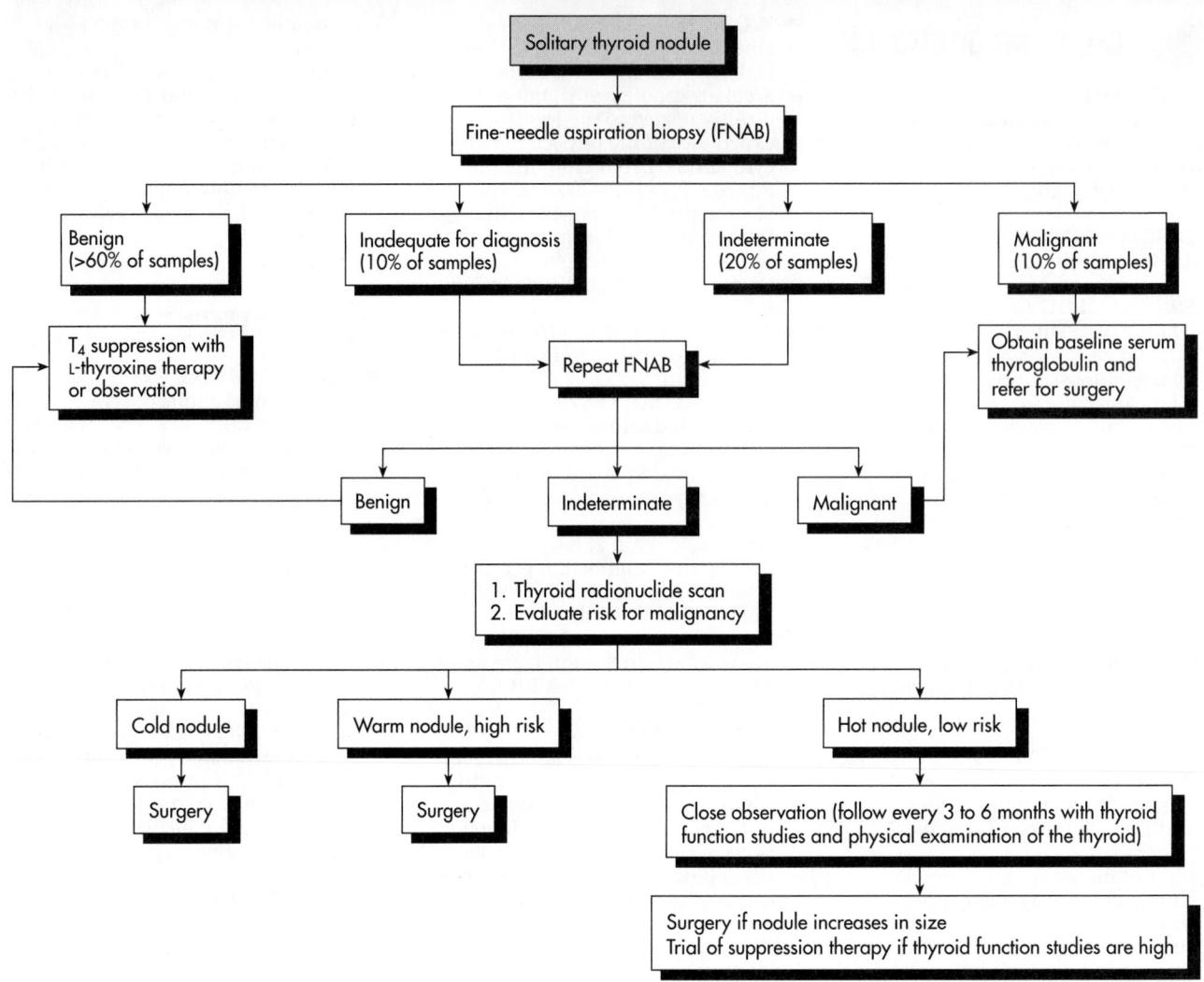

Fig. 1-367   Diagnostic evaluation of solitary thyroid nodule. High risk for malignancy: nodule >2 cm, age <40 yr, male sex, regional lymphadenopathy, fixation to adjacent tissues, history of prior head and neck irradiation. (From Ferri F: *Practical guide to the care of the medical patient,* ed 5, St Louis, 2001, Mosby.)

BASIC INFORMATION

■ DEFINITION

Thyroiditis is an inflammatory disease of the thyroid. It is a multifaceted disease with varying etiology, different clinical characteristics (depending on the stage), and distinct histopathology. Thyroiditis can be subdivided into three common types (Hashimoto's, subacute, silent) and two rare forms (suppurative, Riedel's). To add to the confusion, there are various synonyms for each form, and there is no internationally accepted classification of autoimmune thyroid disease.

■ SYNONYMS

Hashimoto's thyroiditis: chronic lymphocytic thyroiditis, chronic autoimmune thyroiditis
Subacute thyroiditis: granulomatous thyroiditis, de Quervain's thyroiditis
Silent thyroiditis: lymphocytic thyroiditis, painless thyroiditis, postpartum thyroiditis
Suppurative thyroiditis: acute thyroiditis, bacterial thyroiditis microbial inflammatory thyroiditis
Riedel's thyroiditis: invasive fibrous thyroiditis

ICD-9CM CODES

245.2 Hashimoto's thyroiditis
245.1 Subacute thyroiditis
245.9 Silent thyroiditis
245.0 Suppurative thyroiditis
245.3 Riedel's thyroiditis

■ PHYSICAL FINDINGS & CLINICAL PRESENTATION

- Hashimoto's: patients may have signs of hyperthyroidism (tachycardia, diaphoresis, palpitations, weight loss) or hypothyroidism (fatigue, weight gain, delayed reflexes) depending on the stage of the disease. Usually there is diffuse, firm enlargement of the thyroid gland; thyroid gland may also be of normal size (atrophic form with clinically manifested hypothyroidism).
- Subacute: exquisitely tender, enlarged thyroid, fever; signs of hyperthyroidism are initially present; signs of hypothyroidism can subsequently develop.
- Silent: clinical features are similar to subacute thyroiditis except for the absence of tenderness of the thyroid gland (painless thyroiditis).
- Suppurative: patient is febrile with severe neck pain, focal tenderness of the involved portion of the thyroid, erythema of the overlying skin.
- Riedel's: slowly enlarging hard mass in the anterior neck; often mistaken for thyroid cancer; signs of hypothyroidism occur in advanced stages.

■ ETIOLOGY

- Hashimoto's: autoimmune disorder that begins with the activation of CD4 (helper) T-lymphocytes specific for thyroid antigens. The etiologic factor for the activation of these cells is unknown.
- Subacute: possibly postviral; usually follows a respiratory illness; it is not considered to be a form of autoimmune thyroiditis.
- Silent: autoimmune thyroiditis; it frequently occurs postpartum.
- Suppurative: infectious etiology, generally bacterial, although fungi and parasites have also been implicated; it often occurs in immunocompromised hosts or following a penetrating neck injury.
- Riedel's: fibrous infiltration of the thyroid; etiology is unknown.

DIAGNOSIS

■ DIFFERENTIAL DIAGNOSIS

- The hyperthyroid phase of Hashimoto's, subacute, or silent thyroiditis can be mistaken for Graves' disease.
- Riedel's thyroiditis can be mistaken for carcinoma of the thyroid.
- Subacute thyroiditis can be mistaken for infections of the oropharynx and trachea or for suppurative thyroiditis.
- Factitious hyperthyroidism can mimic silent thyroiditis.

■ WORKUP

- The diagnostic workup includes laboratory and radiologic evaluation to rule out other conditions that may mimic thyroiditis (see "Differential Diagnosis") and to differentiate the various forms of thyroiditis.
- The patient's medical history may be helpful in differentiating the various types of thyroiditis (e.g., presentation following childbirth is suggestive of silent [postpartum, painless] thyroiditis; occurrence following a viral respiratory infection suggests subacute thyroiditis; history of penetrating injury to the neck indicates suppurative thyroiditis).
- Fig. 3-165 describes the approach to patients with painful thyroid.

■ LABORATORY TESTS

- TSH, free T_4: may be normal, or indicative of hypo- or hyperthyroidism depending on the stage of the thyroiditis.

- WBC with differential: increased WBC with "shift to the left" occurs with subacute and suppurative thyroiditis.
- Antimicrosomal antibodies: detected in >90% of patients with Hashimoto's thyroiditis and 50% to 80% of patients with silent thyroiditis.
- Serum thyroglobulin levels are elevated in patients with subacute and silent thyroiditis; this test is nonspecific but may be useful in monitoring the course of subacute thyroiditis and distinguishing silent thyroiditis from factitious hyperthyroidism (low or absent serum thyroglobulin level).

■ IMAGING STUDIES

24-hr radioactive iodine uptake (RAIU) is useful to distinguish Graves' disease (increased RAIU) from thyroiditis (normal or low RAIU).

TREATMENT

■ ACUTE GENERAL Rx

- Treat hypothyroid phase with levothyroxine 25 to 50 μg/day initially and monitor serum TSH initially every 6 to 8 wk.
- Control symptoms of hyperthyroidism with β-blockers (e.g., propranolol 20 to 40 mg PO q6h).
- Control pain in patients with subacute thyroiditis with NSAIDs. Prednisone 20 to 40 mg qd may be used if NSAIDs are insufficient, but it should be gradually tapered off over several weeks.
- Use IV antibiotics and drain abscess (if present) in patients with suppurative thyroiditis.

■ DISPOSITION

- Hashimoto's thyroiditis: long-term prognosis is favorable; most patients recover their thyroid function.
- Subacute thyroiditis: permanent hypothyroidism occurs in 10% of patients.
- Silent thyroiditis: 6% of patients have permanent hypothyroidism.
- Suppurative thyroiditis: there is usually full recovery following treatment.
- Riedel's thyroiditis: hypothyroidism occurs when fibrous infiltration involves the entire thyroid.

■ REFERRAL

Surgical referral in patients with compression of adjacent neck structures and in some patients with suppurative thyroiditis
Author: **Fred F. Ferri, M.D.**

BASIC INFORMATION

■ DEFINITION
Thyrotoxic storm is the abrupt and severe exacerbation of thyrotoxicosis.

ICD-9CM CODES
242.9 Thyrotoxic storm
242.0 With goiter
242.2 Multinodular
242.3 Adenomatous
242.8 Thyrotoxicosis factitia

■ PHYSICAL FINDINGS & CLINICAL PRESENTATION
- Goiter
- Tremor, tachycardia, fever
- Warm, moist skin
- Lid lag, lid retraction, proptosis
- Altered mental status (psychosis, coma, seizures)
- Other: evidence of precipitating factors (infection, trauma)

■ ETIOLOGY
- Major stress (e.g., infection, MI, DKA) in an undiagnosed hyperthyroid patient
- Inadequate therapy in a hyperthyroid patient

DIAGNOSIS

The clinical presentation is variable. The patient may present with the following signs and symptoms:
- Fever
- Marked anxiety and agitation, psychosis
- Hyperhidrosis, heat intolerance
- Marked weakness and muscle wasting
- Tachyarrhythmias, palpitations
- Diarrhea, nausea, vomiting
- Elderly patients may have a combination of tachycardia, CHF, and mental status changes

■ DIFFERENTIAL DIAGNOSIS
- Psychiatric disorders
- Alcohol or other drug withdrawal
- Pheochromocytoma
- Metastatic neoplasm

■ WORKUP
- Laboratory evaluation to confirm hyperthyroidism (elevated free T_4, decreased TSH)
- Evaluation for precipitating factors (e.g., ECG and cardiac enzymes in suspected MI, blood and urine cultures to rule out sepsis)
- Elimination of disorders noted in the differential diagnosis (e.g., psychi-

atric history, evidence of drug and alcohol abuse)

■ LABORATORY TESTS
- Free T_4, TSH
- CBC with differential
- Blood and urine cultures
- Glucose
- Liver enzymes
- BUN, creatinine
- Serum calcium
- CPK

■ IMAGING STUDIES
Chest x-ray examination to exclude infectious process, neoplasm, CHF in suspected cases

TREATMENT

■ NONPHARMACOLOGIC THERAPY
- Nutritional care: replace fluid deficit aggressively (daily fluid requirement may reach 6 L); use solutions containing glucose and add multivitamins to the hydrating solution.
- Monitor for fluid overload and CHF in the elderly and in those with underlying cardiovascular or renal disease.
- Treat significant hyperthermia with cooling blankets.

■ ACUTE GENERAL Rx
- Inhibition of thyroid hormone synthesis
  1. Administer propylthiouracil (PTU) 300 to 600 mg initially (PO or via NG tube), then 150 to 300 mg q6h.
  2. If the patient is allergic to PTU, use methimazole (Tapazole) 80 to 100 mg PO or PR followed by 30 mg PR q8h.
- Inhibition of stored thyroid hormone
  1. Iodide can be administered as sodium iodine 250 mg IV q6h, potassium iodide (SSKI) 5 gtt PO q8h, or Lugol's solution, 10 gtt q8h. It is important to administer PTU or methimazole 1 hr *before* the iodide to prevent the oxidation of iodide to iodine and its incorporation in the synthesis of additional thyroid hormone.
  2. Corticosteroids: dexamethasone 2 mg IV q6h or hydrocortisone 100 mg IV q6h for approximately 48 hr is useful to inhibit thyroid hormone release, impair peripheral conversion of T_3 from T_4, and provide additional adrenocortical

hormone to correct deficiency (if present).
- Suppression of peripheral effects of thyroid hormone
  1. β-Adrenergic blockers: Administer propranolol 80 to 120 mg PO q4-6h. Propranolol may also be given IV 1 mg/min for 2 to 10 min under continuous ECG and blood pressure monitoring. β-Adrenergic blockers must be used with caution in patients with CHF or bronchospasm. Cardioselective β-blockers (e.g., esmolol or metoprolol) may be more appropriate for patients with bronchospasm, but these patients must be closely monitored for exacerbation of bronchospasm because these agents lose their cardioselectivity at high doses.
- Control of fever with acetaminophen 325 to 650 mg q4h; avoidance of aspirin because it displaces thyroid hormone from its binding protein
- Digitalization of patients with CHF and atrial fibrillation (these patients may require higher than usual digoxin doses)
- Treatment of any precipitating factors (e.g., antibiotics if infection is strongly suspected)

■ CHRONIC Rx
Refer to "Hyperthyroidism" in Section I.

■ DISPOSITION
Patients with thyrotoxic crisis should be treated and appropriately monitored in the ICU.

■ REFERRAL
Endocrinology referral is appropriate in patients with thyrotoxic crisis.

PEARLS & CONSIDERATIONS

■ COMMENTS
If the diagnosis is strongly suspected, therapy should be started immediately without waiting for laboratory confirmation.

Author: **Fred F. Ferri, M.D.**

BASIC INFORMATION

■ DEFINITION
Tinea corporis is a dermatophyte fungal infection caused by the genera *Trichophyton* or *Microsporum*.

■ SYNONYMS
Ringworm
Body ringworm
Tinea circinata

ICD-9CM CODES
110.5 Tinea corporis

■ EPIDEMIOLOGY & DEMOGRAPHICS
• The disease is more common in warm climates.
• There is no predominant age or sex.

■ PHYSICAL FINDINGS & CLINICAL PRESENTATION
• Annular lesions with an advancing scaly border; the margin is slightly raised, reddened, and may be pustular.
• The central area becomes hypopigmented and less scaly as the active border progresses outward (Fig. 1-368).
• The trunk and legs are primarily involved.

■ ETIOLOGY
Trichophyton rubrum is the most common pathogen.

DIAGNOSIS

■ DIFFERENTIAL DIAGNOSIS
• Pityriasis rosea
• Erythema multiforme
• Psoriasis
• SLE
• Syphilis
• Nummular eczema
• Eczema
• Granuloma annulare

■ WORKUP
Diagnosis is usually made on clinical grounds. It can be confirmed by direct visualization under the microscope of a small fragment of the scale using wet mount preparation and potassium hydroxide solution; dermatophytes appear as translucent branching filaments (hyphae) with lines of separation appearing at irregular intervals.

■ LABORATORY TESTS
• Microscopic examination of hyphae.
• Culture is usually not necessary.

TREATMENT

■ NONPHARMACOLOGIC THERAPY
Affected areas should be kept clean and dry.

■ ACUTE GENERAL Rx
• Various creams are effective:
  1. Miconazole 2% cream (Monistat-Derm) applied bid for 2 wk
  2. Clotrimazole 1% cream (Mycelex) applied and gently massaged into the affected areas and surrounding areas bid for up to 4 wk
  3. Naftifine 1% cream (Naftin) applied qd
  4. Econazole 1% (Spectazole) applied qd
• Systemic therapy is reserved for severe cases and is usually given up to 4 wk; commonly used agents:
  1. Ketoconazole (Nizoral), 200 mg qd
  2. Itraconazole (Sporanox), 100 to 200 mg qd for 2 to 4 wk
  3. Fluconazole (Diflucan), 200 mg qd
  4. Terbinafine (Lamisil), 250 mg qd
  5. Griseofulvin (Fulvicin, Grisactin, Gris-Peg), 250 to 500 mg bid is the oldest oral treatment. It is used primarily in tinea infections not involving the nails.

■ DISPOSITION
Majority of cases resolve without sequelae within 3 to 4 wk of therapy.

■ REFERRAL
Dermatology referral in patients with persistent or recurrent infections
Author: **Fred F. Ferri, M.D.**

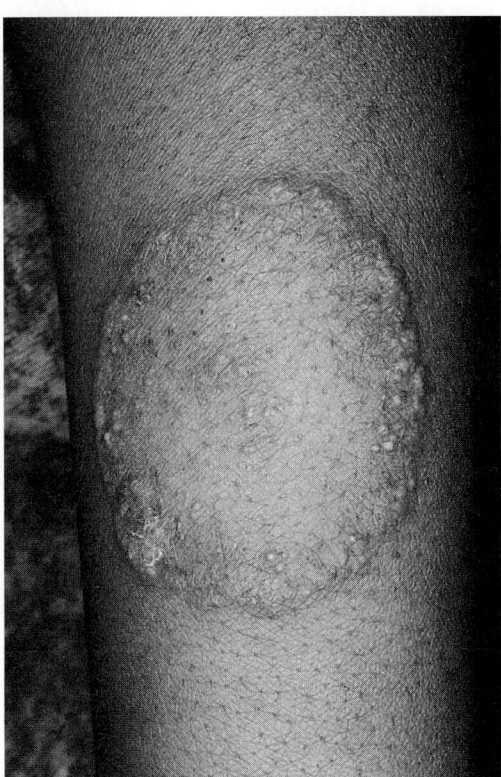

Fig. 1-368   Annular lesion (tinea corporis). Note raised erythematous scaling border and central clearing. (From Noble J et al: *Textbook of primary care medicine,* ed 2, St Louis, 1995, Mosby.)

BASIC INFORMATION

■ DEFINITION
Tinea cruris is a dermatophyte fungal infection of the groin.

■ SYNONYMS
Jock itch
Ringworm

ICD-9CM CODES
110.3 Tinea cruris

■ EPIDEMIOLOGY & DEMOGRAPHICS
• Most common during the summer.
• Men are affected more frequently than women.

■ PHYSICAL FINDINGS & CLINICAL PRESENTATION
• Erythematous plaques have a half-moon shape and a scaling border.
• The acute inflammation tends to move down the inner thigh and usually spares the scrotum; in severe cases the fungus may spread onto the buttocks.
• Itching may be severe.
• Red papules and pustules may be present.
• An important diagnostic sign is the advancing well-defined border with a tendency toward central clearing (Fig. 1-369).

■ ETIOLOGY
• Dermatophytes of the genera *Trichophyton, Epidermophyton,* and *Microsporum. T. rubrum* and *E. floccosum* are the most common causes.
• Transmission from direct contact (e.g., infected persons, animals).

DIAGNOSIS

■ DIFFERENTIAL DIAGNOSIS
• Intertrigo
• Psoriasis
• Seborrheic dermatitis
• Erythrasma
• Candidiasis
• Tinea versicolor

■ WORKUP
Diagnosis is based on clinical presentation and demonstration of hyphae microscopically using potassium hydroxide.

■ LABORATORY TESTS
• Microscopic examination
• Cultures are generally not necessary

TREATMENT

■ NONPHARMACOLOGIC THERAPY
• Keep infected area clean and dry.
• Use of boxer shorts is preferred to regular underwear.

■ ACUTE GENERAL Rx
• Drying powders (e.g., Miconazole nitrate [Zeasorb AF]) may be useful in patients with excessive perspiration.

• Various topical antifungal agents are available: miconazole (Lotrimin), terbinafine (Lamisil), sulconazole nitrate (Exelderm), betamethasone dipropionate/clotrimazole (Lotrisone).
• Oral antifungal therapy is generally reserved for cases unresponsive to topical agents. Effective medications are itraconazole (Sporonax) 100 mg/day for 2 to 4 wk, ketoconazole (Nizoral) 200 mg qd, fluconazole (Diflucan) 200 mg qd, and terbinafine (Lamisil) 250 mg qd.

■ DISPOSITION
Most cases respond promptly to therapy with complete resolution within 2 to 3 wk.
Author: **Fred F. Ferri, M.D.**

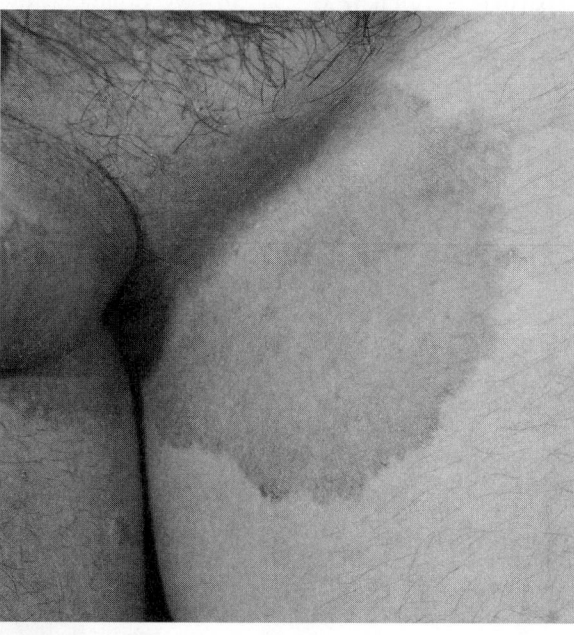

Fig. 1-369   Tinea cruris. A halfmoon-shaped plaque has a well-defined, scaling border. (From Habif TB: *Clinical dermatology: a color guide to diagnosis and therapy,* ed 3, St Louis, 1996, Mosby.)

BASIC INFORMATION

■ DEFINITION

Tinea versicolor is a fungal infection of the skin caused by the yeast *Pityrosporum orbiculare (Malassezia furfur)*.

■ SYNONYMS

Pityriasis versicolor

ICD-9CM CODES

111.0 Tinea versicolor

■ EPIDEMIOLOGY & DEMOGRAPHICS

- Increased incidence in adolescence and young adulthood
- More common during the summer (hypopigmented lesions are more evident when the skin is tanned)

■ PHYSICAL FINDINGS & CLINICAL PRESENTATION

- Most lesions begin as multiple small, circular macules of various colors.
- The macules may be darker or lighter than the surrounding normal skin and will scale with scraping.
- Most frequent site of distribution is trunk.
- Facial lesions are more common in children (forehead is most common facial site).
- Eruption is generally of insidious onset and asymptomatic.
- Lesions may be hyperpigmented in blacks.
- Lesions may be inconspicuous in fair-complexioned individuals, especially during the winter.
- Most patients become aware of the eruption when the involved areas do not tan (Fig. 1-370).

■ ETIOLOGY

The infection is caused by the lipophilic yeast *P. orbiculare* (round form) and *P. ovale* (oval form); these organisms are normal inhabitants of the skin flora; factors that favor their proliferation are pregnancy, malnutrition, immunosuppression, oral contraceptives, and excess heat and humidity.

DIAGNOSIS

■ DIFFERENTIAL DIAGNOSIS

- Vitiligo
- Pityriasis alba
- Secondary syphilis
- Pityriasis rosea
- Seborrheic dermatitis

■ WORKUP

Diagnosis is based on clinical appearance; identification of hyphae and budding spores (spaghetti and meatballs appearance) with microscopy confirms diagnosis.

■ LABORATORY TESTS

Microscopic examination using potassium hydroxide confirms diagnosis when in doubt.

TREATMENT

■ NONPHARMACOLOGIC THERAPY

Sunlight accelerates repigmentation of hypopigmented areas.

■ ACUTE GENERAL Rx

- Topical treatment: selenium sulfide 2.5% suspension (Selsun or Exsel) applied daily for 10 min for 7 consecutive days results in a cure rate of 80% to 90%.
- Antifungal topical agents (e.g., miconazole, ciclopirox, clotrimazole) are also effective but generally expensive.

- Oral treatment is generally reserved for resistant cases. Effective agents are ketoconazole (Nizoral) 200 mg qd for 5 days, or single 400-mg dose (cure rate >80%), fluconazole (Diflucan) 400 mg given as a single dose (cure rate >70% at 3 wk after treatment), or itraconazole 200 mg/day for 5 days.

■ DISPOSITION

The prognosis is good, with death of the fungus usually occurring within 3 to 4 wk of treatment; however, recurrence is common.

PEARLS & CONSIDERATIONS

■ COMMENTS

Patients should be informed that the hypopigmented areas will not disappear immediately after treatment and that several months may be necessary for the hypopigmented areas to regain their pigmentation.

Author: **Fred F. Ferri, M.D.**

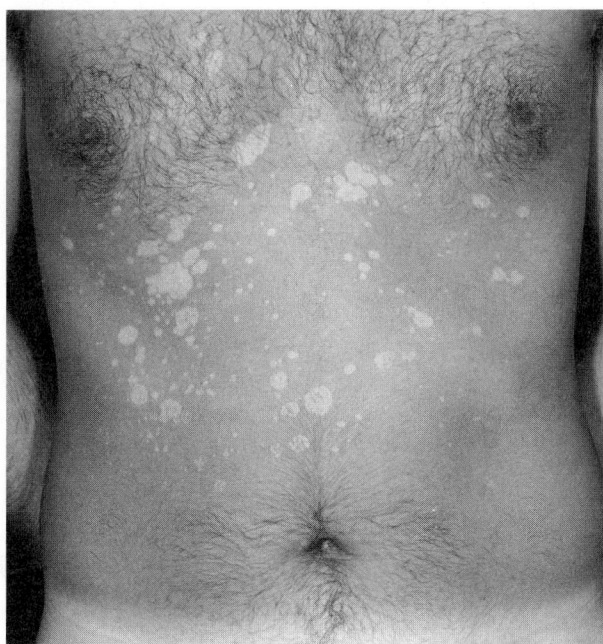

Fig. 1-370   The classic presentation of tinea versicolor with white, oval, or circular patches on tan skin. (From Habif TB: *Clinical dermatology: a color guide to diagnosis and therapy,* ed 3, St Louis, 1996, Mosby.)

BASIC INFORMATION

■ DEFINITION

Torticollis is a contraction or contracture of the muscles of the neck that causes the head to be tilted to one side (Fig. 1-371). It is usually accompanied by rotation of the chin to the opposite side with flexion. Usually it is a symptom of some underlying disorder. This term is often used incorrectly in cases when the torticollis may simply be positional.

■ SYNONYMS

Twisted neck
"Wry neck"

ICD-9CM CODES

723.5 Spastic (intermittent) torticollis
754.1 Congenital muscular (sternocleidomastoid)
300.11 Hysterical
714.0 Rheumatoid
333.83 Spasmodic

■ PHYSICAL FINDINGS & CLINICAL PRESENTATION

- Congenital muscular torticollis:
  1. Palpable soft tissue "mass" in the sternocleidomastoid shortly after birth
  2. Mass gradually subsides, leaving a shortened, contracted sternocleidomastoid muscle
  3. Head characteristically tilted toward the side of the mass and rotated in the opposite direction (Fig. 1-372)
  4. Facial asymmetry and other secondary changes persisting into adulthood

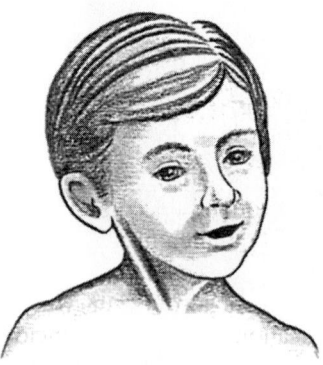

Fig. 1-371 Congenital muscular torticollis.

- Spasmodic torticollis:
  1. "Spasms" in the cervical musculature; may be bilateral and uncontrollable
  2. Head often tilted toward the affected side
- Findings in other cases depend on etiology.

■ ETIOLOGY

Torticollis has been attributed to over 50 different causes:
- Localized fibrous shortening of unknown cause involving the sternocleidomastoid, leading to the condition termed *congenital muscular torticollis*
- Spasmodic torticollis: of uncertain etiology, possibly a variant of dystonia musculorum deformans
- Infection, specifically pharyngitis, tonsillitis, retropharyngeal abscess
- Miscellaneous rare causes: congenital musculoskeletal deformities, trauma, inflammation from rheumatoid arthritis, vestibular disturbances, posterior fossa tumor, syringomyelia, neuritis of spinal accessory nerve, and drug reactions

DIAGNOSIS

■ DIFFERENTIAL DIAGNOSIS

- Usually involves separating each disorder from the others
- Acquired positional disorders (e.g., ocular disturbances, acute disk herniation)

■ WORKUP

- Workup is dependent on the clinical situation.
- Laboratory studies are usually not helpful unless infection or rheumatoid disease is suspected.
- Fig. 3-119 describes a clinical algorithm for the evaluation and therapy of neck pain.
- Any child with a gradually increasing torticollis should have a complete eye examination.

■ IMAGING STUDIES

- Plain radiographs in cases of trauma or to rule out congenital abnormalities
- MRI in appropriate cases
- Electrodiagnostic studies: only rarely indicated to rule out neurologic causes

TREATMENT

- Congenital muscular torticollis: gentle stretching exercises carried out by the parent
- Spasmodic torticollis: physical therapy, psychotherapy, cervical braces, biofeedback, and pain control
- Other forms: treated according to etiology

■ DISPOSITION

- Most patients with congenital muscular torticollis respond well to conservative treatment.
- Spasmodic torticollis is often resistant to normal conservative treatment.
- Prognosis of other forms of torticollis is dependent on etiology.

■ REFERRAL

- Torticollis often requires a multidisciplinary approach unless the etiology is obvious.
- Children usually do not require any specific studies; however, an orthopedic consultation is recommended.

REFERENCES

Cheng JC et al: Clinical determinants of the outcome of manual stretching in the treatment of congenital muscular torticollis infants, *J Bone Joint Surg* 83(A):679, 2001.
Duane DD: Spasmodic torticollis, *Adv Neurol* 49:135, 1988.
Author: **Lonnie R. Mercier, M.D.**

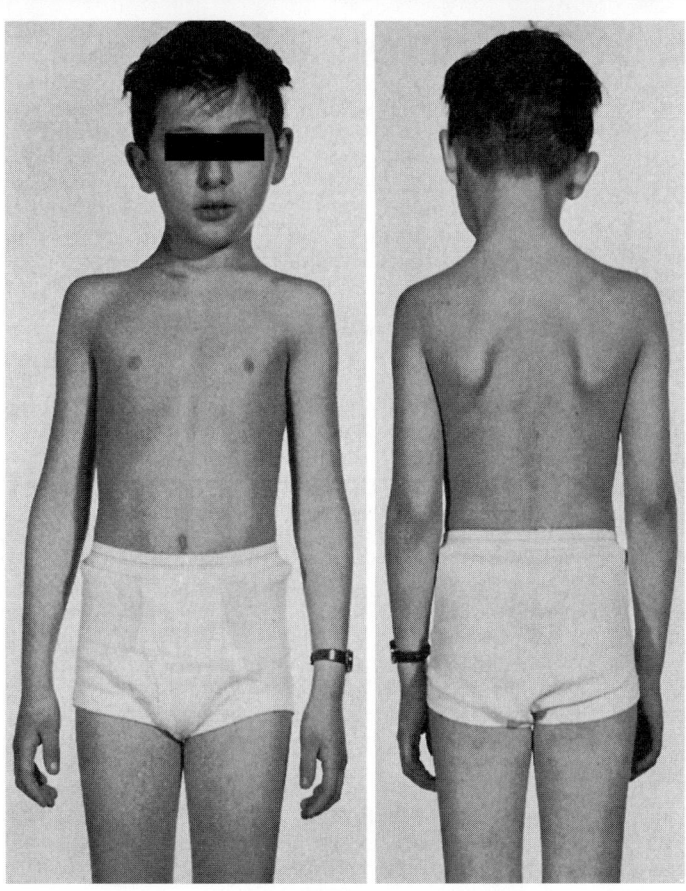

Fig. 1-372   Torticollis. In this child, the right sternocleidomastoid muscle is contracted. (From Brinker MR, Miller MD: *Fundamentals of orthopaedics,* Philadelphia, 1999, WB Saunders.)

BASIC INFORMATION

■ DEFINITION
The onset of Tourette's syndrome is in childhood, with axial motor (body or facial) tics or vocal tics (barking or coprolalia) (Box 1-26).

■ SYNONYMS
Gilles de la Tourette syndrome
Motor-verbal tic disorder

ICD-9CM CODES
307.23 Gilles de la Tourette disorder

■ EPIDEMIOLOGY & DEMOGRAPHICS
INCIDENCE (IN U.S.): Chronic, nonfatal disease
PREVALENCE (IN U.S.): 5 to 10 cases/10,000 persons
PREDOMINANT SEX: Male:female ratio of 9:1
PREDOMINANT AGE: <21 yr of age
PEAK INCIDENCE: Lifetime
GENETICS: Autosomal dominant, but variability in symptoms

■ PHYSICAL FINDINGS & CLINICAL PRESENTATION
- Vocal tics (clearing of throat, repetitive short phrases, e.g., "You bet," swearing [coprolalia])
- Axial tics (grimacing, blinking, head jerking)
- Tics that wax and wane (worse with emotional stress) and change over lifetime

■ ETIOLOGY
Genetic, associated with obsessive-compulsive disorder (OCD).

■ DIAGNOSIS

■ DIFFERENTIAL DIAGNOSIS
- Other idiopathic tic disorders
- Sydenham's chorea
- Transient tic disorders
- Head trauma
- Drug intoxication
- Postinfectious encephalitis

■ WORKUP
Clinical observation to confirm diagnosis

■ LABORATORY TESTS
No definitive laboratory tests

■ IMAGING STUDIES
CT scan and MRI of brain are normal.

■ TREATMENT

■ NONPHARMACOLOGIC THERAPY
Multidisciplinary: parents, teachers, psychologists, school nurses (educational)

■ ACUTE GENERAL Rx
- Dopamine-blocking agents may be used to reduce severity of tics (e.g., haloperidol 0.25 mg PO qhs initially).
- Clonidine 0.05 mg PO qd initially may be effective in patients with attention deficit disorder (ADD).
- Fluoxetine 20 mg PO qd initially is useful in patients with obsessive-compulsive symptoms.

■ CHRONIC Rx
Low-dose dopamine-blocking neuroleptic agents only if tics interfere with activities of daily living

■ DISPOSITION
- Usually live relatively normal life if psychologic consequences of tic minimized.
- More than 30% of patients develop OCD or ADD.

■ REFERRAL
To neurologist to confirm initial diagnosis

■ PEARLS & CONSIDERATIONS

■ COMMENTS
- Once thought rare, now recognized as common because of recognition of milder forms.
- Patient education may be obtained from the Tourette's Syndrome Association (TSA), 4240 Bell Blvd., Bayside, NY, 11361-2864; phone: (800) 237-0717.

REFERENCES
Jankovic J: Tourette's syndrome, *N Engl J Med* 345:1184, 2001.
Lechman LF et al: Course of tic severity in Tourette's syndrome: the first two decades, *Pediatrics* 102:14, 1998.
Author: **William H. Olson, M.D.**

BOX 1-26   Evaluation of Tourette's Syndrome

Core clinical manifestations
    Axial motor and vocal tics
    Obsessions and compulsions
Common clinical manifestations
    Distractibility, hyperactivity, and impulsivity
    Learning difficulties or disorders
Psychiatric manifestations
    Mood disorders, especially depression
    Anxiety disorders, especially separation and/or phobias

From Johnson RT, Griffin JW: *Current therapy in neurologic disease,* ed 5, St Louis, 1997, Mosby.

BASIC INFORMATION

■ DEFINITION

Toxic shock syndrome is an acute febrile illness resulting in multiple organ system dysfunction caused most commonly by a bacterial exotoxin. Disease characteristics also include hypotension, vomiting, myalgia, watery diarrhea, vascular collapse, and an erythematous sunburnlike cutaneous rash that desquamates during recovery.

ICD-9CM CODES
040.89 Toxic shock syndrome

■ EPIDEMIOLOGY & DEMOGRAPHICS
- Case reported incidence peak: 14 cases/100,000 menstruating women/yr in 1980; has since fallen to 1 case/100,000 persons
- Occurs most commonly between ages 10 and 30 yr in healthy, young menstruating white females
- Case fatality ratio of 3%

■ ETIOLOGY (Fig. 1-373)
- Menstrually associated TSS: 45% of cases associated with tampons, diaphragm, or vaginal sponge use
- Nonmenstruating associated TSS: 55% of cases associated with puerperal sepsis, post–cesarean section endometritis, mastitis, wound or skin infection, insect bite, pelvic inflammatory disease, and postoperative fever
- Causative agent: *S. aureus* infection of a susceptible individual (10% of population lacking sufficient levels of antitoxin antibodies), which liberates the disease mediator TSST-1 (exotoxin)
- Other causative agents: coagulase-negative streptococci producing enterotoxins B or C, and exotoxin A producing group A β-hemolytic streptococci

■ PHYSICAL FINDINGS & CLINICAL PRESENTATION
- Fever (≥38.9° C)
- Diffuse macular erythrodermatous rash that desquamates 1 to 2 wk after disease onset in survivors
- Orthostatic hypotension
- GI symptoms: vomiting, diarrhea, abdominal tenderness
- Constitutional symptoms: myalgia, headache, photophobia, rigors, altered sensorium, conjunctivitis, arthralgia
- Respiratory symptoms: dysphagia, pharyngeal hyperemia, strawberry tongue
- Genitourinary symptoms: vaginal discharge, vaginal hyperemia, adnexal tenderness

- End-organ failure
- Severe hypotension and acute renal failure
- Hepatic failure
- Cardiovascular symptoms: DIC, pulmonary edema, ARDS, endomyocarditis, heart block

DIAGNOSIS

■ DIFFERENTIAL DIAGNOSIS
- Staphylococcal food poisoning
- Septic shock
- Mucocutaneous lymph node syndrome
- Scarlet fever
- Rocky Mountain spotted fever
- Meningococcemia
- Toxic epidermal necrolysis
- Kawasaki's syndrome
- Leptospirosis
- Legionnaires' disease
- Hemolytic-uremic syndrome
- Stevens-Johnson syndrome
- Scalded skin syndrome
- Erythema multiforme
- Acute rheumatic fever

■ WORKUP
Broad-spectrum syndrome with multiorgan system involvement and variable but acute clinical presentation, including the following:
1. Fever ≥38.1° C
2. Classic desquamating (1 to 2 wk) rash
3. Hypotension/orthostatic SBP 90 or less
4. Syncope
5. Negative throat/CSF cultures
6. Negative serologic test for Rocky Mountain spotted fever, rubeola, and leptospirosis
7. Clinical involvement of three or more of the following:
   a. Cardiopulmonary: ARDS, pulmonary edema, endomyocarditis, second- or third-degree AV block
   b. CNS: altered sensorium without focal neurologic findings
   c. Hematologic: thrombocytopenia (PLT <100 k)
   d. Liver: elevated liver function test results
   e. Renal: >5/HPF, negative urine cultures, azotemia, and increased creatinine double normal
   f. Mucous membrane involvement: vagina, oropharynx, conjunctiva
   g. Musculoskeletal: myalgia, CPK twice normal
   h. GI: vomiting, diarrhea

■ LABORATORY TESTS
- Pan culture (cervix/vagina, throat, nasal passages, urine, blood, CSF, wound) for *Staphylococcus*, *Streptococcus*, or other pathogenic organisms
- Electrolytes to detect hypokalemia, hyponatremia
- CBC with differential and clotting profile for anemia (normocytic/normochromic), thrombocytopenia, leukocytosis, coagulopathy, and bacteremia
- Chemistry profile to detect decreased protein, increased AST, increased ALT, hypocalcemia, elevated BUN/creatinine, hypophosphatemia, increased LDH, increased CPK
- Urinalysis to detect WBC (>5/HPF), proteinemia, microhematuria
- ABGs to assess respiratory function and acid-base status
- Serologic tests considered for Rocky Mountain spotted fever, rubeola, and leptospirosis

■ IMAGING STUDIES
- Chest x-ray examination to evaluate pulmonary edema
- ECG to evaluate arrhythmia
- Sonography/CT scan/MRI considered if pelvic abscess or TOA suspected

TREATMENT

■ NONPHARMACOLOGIC THERAPY
- For optimal outcome: high index of suspicion and early and aggressive supportive management in an ICU setting
- Aggressive fluid resuscitation (maintenance of circulating volume, CO, SBP)
- Thorough search for a localized infection or nidus: incision and drainage, debridement, removal of tampon or vaginal sponge
- Central hemodynamic monitoring, Swan-Ganz catheter and arterial line for surveillance of hemodynamic status and response to therapy
- Foley catheter to monitor hourly urine output
- Possible MAST trousers as temporary measure
- Acute ventilator management if severe respiratory compromise
- Renal dialysis for severe renal impairment
- Surgical intervention for indicated conditions (i.e., ruptured TOA, wound abscess, mastitis)

■ ACUTE GENERAL Rx
- Isotonic crystalloid (normal saline solution) for volume replacement following "7-3" rule

I

- Electrolyte replacement (K⁺, Ca⁺)
- PRBC/coagulation factor replacement/FFP to treat anemia or D&C
- Vasopressor therapy for hypotension refractory to fluid volume replacement (i.e., dopamine beginning at 2 to 5 µg/kg/min)
- Naloxone infusion (i.e., 0.5 mg/kg/hr) to improve SBP by blocking endogenous endorphin effects
- Parenteral antibiotic therapy; β-lactamase resistant antibiotic (methicillin, nafcillin, or oxacillin) initiated early
- Broad-spectrum antibiotic added if concurrent sepsis suspected
- Tetracycline added if considering Rocky Mountain spotted fever

■ CHRONIC Rx
- Severely ill patient: may require prolonged hospitalization and supportive management with gradual recovery and/or sequelae from severe end-organ involvement (ARDS or renal failure requiring dialysis)
- Majority of patients: complete recovery
- Early late-onset complications (within 2 wk):

1. Skin desquamation
2. Impaired digit sensation
3. Denuded tongue
4. Vocal cord paralysis
5. ATN
6. ARDS
- Late-onset complications (after 8 wk):
  1. Nail splitting/loss
  2. Alopecia
  3. CNS sequelae
  4. Renal impairment
  5. Cardiac dysfunction
- Recurrent TSS:
  1. More common in menstrually related cases
  2. Less common in patient treated with β-lactamase–resistant antistaphylococcal antibiotics
  3. Patients with history of TSS: if suspect signs and symptoms occur, should have high index of suspicion and low threshold for evaluation and treatment

■ PREVENTION
- Avoidance of tampons or use of low-absorbency tampons only (<4 hr in situ) and alternate with napkins

- Education for patients concerning signs and symptoms of TSS
- Avoidance of tampons for patients with history of TSS

■ DISPOSITION
- Complete recovery for most patients
- Long-term management of early- and late-onset complications for minority of patients

■ REFERRAL
- For multidisciplinary management, involving primary physician, gynecologist, internist, infectious disease specialist, and other supportive care specialists
- To tertiary level hospital

☼ PEARLS & CONSIDERATIONS

■ COMMENTS
Patient information available from American College of Gynecologists and Obstetricians.
Author: **Dennis M. Weppner, M.D.**

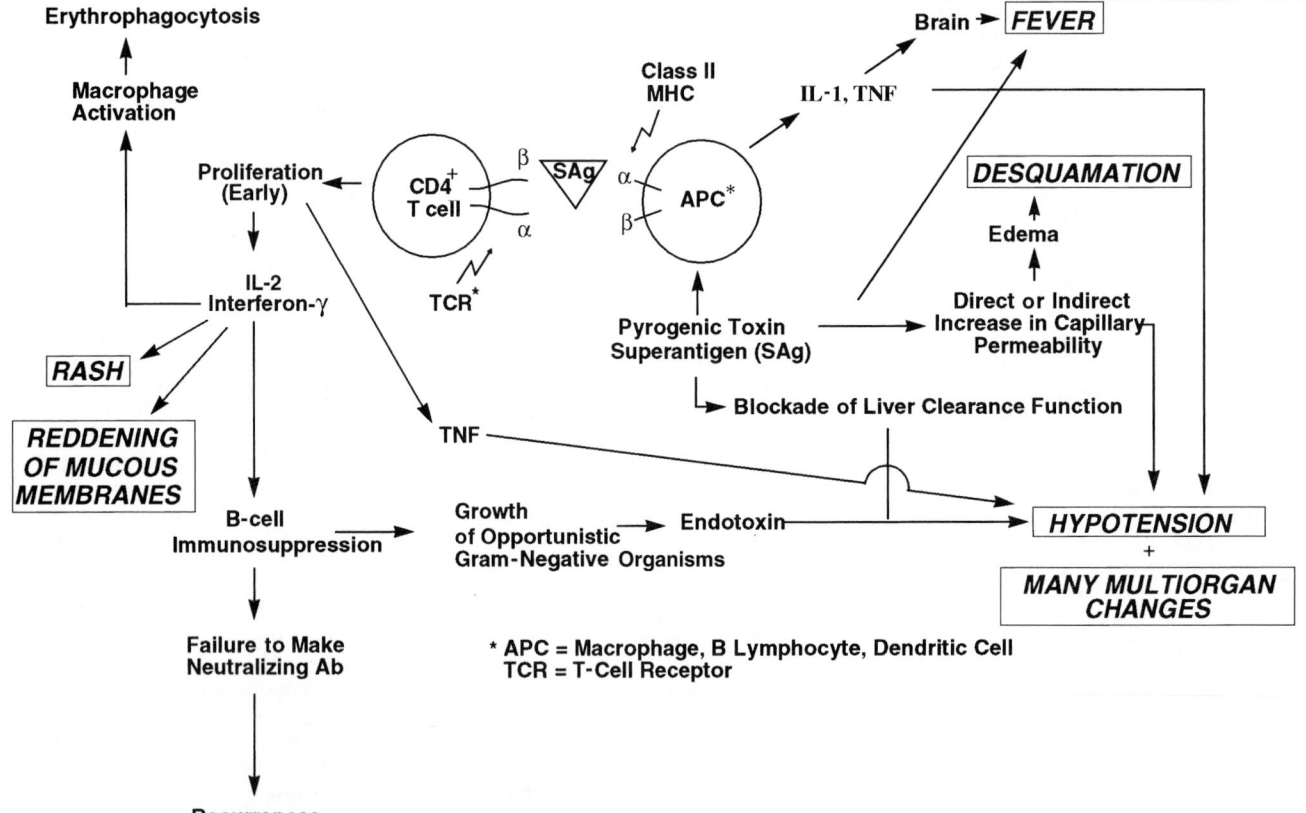

Fig. 1-373 Model for the development of toxic shock syndrome and related illnesses. *Ab,* Antibody; *IL1* interleukin-1; *IL2,* interleukin-2; *MHC,* major histocompatibility complex; *SAg,* superantigen; *TNF,* tumor necrosis factor. (From Gorbach SL, Bartlett JG, Blacklow NR [eds]: *Infectious diseases,* ed 2, Philadelphia, 1998, WB Saunders.)

BASIC INFORMATION

■ **DEFINITION**

Toxoplasmosis is an infection caused by the protozoal parasite *Toxoplasma gondii*.

ICD-9CM CODES
130.9 Toxoplasmosis

■ **EPIDEMIOLOGY & DEMOGRAPHICS**
INCIDENCE (IN U.S.):
• Increases with age
• Increases with certain activities
  1. Slaughterhouse workers
  2. Cat owners
• Increases with certain geographic locations: high prevalence of cats
INCIDENCE (IN U.S.): 3% to 70% of healthy adults
PREDOMINANT SEX: Equal gender distribution
PREDOMINANT AGE:
• Infancy (congenital infection)
• Prevalence increases with age
PEAK INCIDENCE: Temperate climates
GENETICS:
Congenital Infection:
• Incidence and severity vary with the trimester of gestation during which the mother acquired infection.
  1. 10% to 25% (first trimester)
  2. 30% to 54% (second trimester)
  3. 60% to 65% (third trimester)
• Congenital infection occurring in the first trimester is the most severe.
• 89% to 100% of infections in the third trimester are asymptomatic.
• Risk to the fetus is not correlated with symptoms in the mother.

■ **PHYSICAL FINDINGS & CLINICAL PRESENTATION**
• Acquired (immunocompetent host)
  1. 80% to 90% asymptomatic
  2. Adenopathy (usually cervical)
  3. Fever
  4. Myalgias
  5. Malaise
  6. Sore throat
  7. Maculopapular rash
  8. Hepatosplenomegaly
  9. Chorioretinitis rare
• Acquired (in patients with AIDS)
  1. 89% of symptomatic cases
    a. Encephalitis
    b. Intracerebral mass lesions
  2. Pneumonitis
  3. Chorioretinitis
  4. Other end-organ
• Acquired (immunocompromised patients)
  1. Encephalitis
  2. Myocarditis (especially in heart transplant patients)
  3. Pneumonitis

• Ocular infection in the immunocompetent host
  1. Congenital infection
  2. Blurred vision
  3. Photophobia
  4. Pain
  5. Loss of central vision if macula involved
  6. Focal necrotizing retinitis
  7. Typically presents in second or third decade
• Congenital
  1. Results from acute infection acquired by the mother within 6 to 8 wk before conception or during gestation
  2. Usually, asymptomatic mother
  3. No sign of disease
  4. Chorioretinitis
  5. Blindness
  6. Epilepsy
  7. Psychomotor or mental retardation
  8. Intracranial calcifications
  9. Hydrocephalus
  10. Microcephaly
  11. Encephalitis
  12. Anemia
  13. Thrombocytopenia
  14. Hepatosplenomegaly
  15. Lymphadenopathy
  16. Jaundice
  17. Rash
  18. Pneumonitis
  19. Most infected infants are asymptomatic at birth

■ **ETIOLOGY**
• *Toxoplasma gondii*
  1. Ubiquitous intracellular protozoan
  2. Present worldwide
  3. Cat is definitive host
• Human infection
  1. Ingestion of oocysts shed by cats
  2. Ingestion of meat containing tissue cysts
  3. Vertical transmission

 DIAGNOSIS

■ **DIFFERENTIAL DIAGNOSIS**
• Lymphadenopathy
  1. Infectious mononucleosis
  2. CMV mononucleosis
  3. Cat-scratch disease
  4. Sarcoidosis
  5. Tuberculosis
  6. Lymphoma
  7. Metastatic cancer
• Cerebral mass lesions in immunocompromised host
  1. Lymphoma
  2. Tuberculosis
  3. Bacterial abscess

• Pneumonitis in immunocompromised host
  1. *Pneumocystis carinii* pneumonia
  2. Tuberculosis
  3. Fungal infection
• Chorioretinitis
  1. Syphilis
  2. Tuberculosis
  3. Histoplasmosis (competent host)
  4. CMV
  5. Syphilis
  6. Herpes simplex
  7. Fungal infection
  8. Tuberculosis (AIDS patient)
• Myocarditis
  1. Organ rejection in heart transplant recipients
• Congenital infection
  1. Rubella
  2. CMV
  3. Herpes simplex
  4. Syphilis
  5. Listeriosis
  6. Erythroblastosis fetalis
  7. Sepsis

■ **WORKUP**
• Acute infection, immunocompetent host
  1. CBC
  2. *Toxoplasma* serology (IgG, Ig) in serial blood specimens 3 wk apart
  3. Lymph node biopsy if diagnosis uncertain
• Immunocompromised host
  1. CNS symptoms
    a. Cerebral CT scan or MRI if CNS symptoms present
    b. Spinal tap, if safe
    c. Brain biopsy if no response to empiric therapy
  2. Ocular symptoms
    a. Funduscopic examination
    b. Serologic studies
    c. Rarely, vitreous tap
  3. Pulmonary symptoms
    a. Chest x-ray examination
    b. Bronchoalveolar lavage
    c. Transbronchial or open lung biopsy
  4. Myocarditis
    a. Cardiac enzymes
    b. Electrocardiogram
    c. Endomyocardial biopsy for definitive diagnosis
• Toxoplasmosis in pregnancy
  1. Initial maternal screening with IgM and IgG
    a. If negative, mother at risk of acute infection and should be retested monthly
    b. If both IgG and IgM positive, obtain IgA and IgE ELISA, AC/HS test
    c. IgA and IgE ELISA, AC/HS test elevated in acute infection
    d. Ig high for 1 yr or more
    e. IgG repeated 3 to 4 wk later to determine if titer is stable

2. Acute maternal infection not excluded or documented
   a. Fetal blood sampling (for culture, Ig, IgA, IgE)
   b. Amniotic fluid PCR
3. Fetal ultrasound every other week if maternal infection documented
- Congenital toxoplasmosis
  1. Placental histology
  2. Specific IgM or IgA in infant's blood

■ LABORATORY TESTS
- Antibody studies
  1. More than one test necessary to establish diagnosis of acute toxoplasmosis
  2. IgM antibody
     a. Appears 5 days into infection
     b. Peaks at 2 wk
     c. Falls to low level or disappears within 2 mo
     d. May persist at low levels for 1 yr or more
  3. Antibody not measurable
     a. Ocular toxoplasmosis
     b. Reactivation
     c. Immunocompromised hosts
  4. IgA ELISA, IgE ELISA, and IgE ASAGA
     a. More sensitive tests
     b. Disappear more rapidly than Ig, establishing diagnosis of acute infection
  5. IgG antibody
     a. Appears 1 to 2 wk after infection
     b. Peaks at 6 to 8 wk
     c. Gradually declines over months to years

■ IMAGING STUDIES
- Chest x-ray examination if pulmonary involvement suspected
- Cerebral CT scan or MRI if encephalitis suspected

℞ TREATMENT

■ NONPHARMACOLOGIC THERAPY
- Selected cases of ocular infection
  1. Photocoagulation
  2. Vitrectomy
  3. Lentectomy
- Selected cases of congenital cerebral infection
  1. Ventricular shunting

■ ACUTE GENERAL Rx
- Acute infection, immunocompetent host
  1. No treatment, unless severe and persistent symptoms or vital organ damage
- Acute infection, immunocompromised host, non-AIDS
  1. Treat even if asymptomatic

2. Duration
   a. Until 4 to 6 wk after resolution of all signs and symptoms
   b. Usually 6 mo or longer
- Reactivated infection, immunocompromised host, non-AIDS
  1. Treat if symptomatic
- Acute or reactivated infection, AIDS
  1. Treat in all cases
  2. Induction course
     a. 3 to 6 wk
     b. Maintenance therapy continued for life
  3. Empiric therapy
     a. AIDS with positive IgG
     b. Multiple ring-enhancing lesions on cerebral CT scan or MRI
     c. Response seen by day 7 in 71% and day 14 in 91%
- Ocular infection
  1. Treat in all cases
  2. Therapy continued for 1 mo or longer if needed
  3. Response seen in 70% within 10 days
  4. Retreat as needed
  5. Steroids may be indicated
  6. Surgical treatment in selected cases
- Treatment regimens
  1. Pyrimethamine 100 to 200 mg loading dose once PO, then 25 mg PO qd (50 to 75 mg in AIDS) *plus*
  2. Leucovorin 10 to 20 mg PO qd *plus*
  3. Sulfadiazine 1 to 1.5 g PO q6h
- Acute infection in pregnancy
  1. Treat immediately
  2. Risk of fetal infection reduced by 60% with treatment
     a. First trimester
        i. Spiramycin 3 g PO qd in two to four divided doses
        ii. Sulfadiazine 4 g PO qd in four divided doses
     b. Second and third trimester
        i. Sulfadiazine as above *plus*
        ii. Pyrimethamine 25 mg PO qd *plus*
        iii. Leucovorin 5 to 15 mg PO qd
        iv. Spiramycin as above
- Congenital infection
  1. Sulfadiazine 50 mg/kg PO bid *plus*
  2. Pyrimethamine 2 mg/kg PO for 2 days, then 1 mg/kg PO, three times weekly *plus*
  3. Leucovorin 5 to 20 mg PO three times weekly
  4. Minimum duration of treatment: 12 mo

■ CHRONIC Rx
- Maintenance therapy in AIDS patients because of the high risk (80%) of relapse
  1. Pyrimethamine 25 mg PO qd
  2. Sulfadiazine 500 mg PO qid

3. Leucovorin 10 to 20 mg PO qd

■ DISPOSITION
- Prognosis
  1. Excellent in the immunocompetent host
  2. Good in ocular infection (although relapses are common)
- Treatment of acute infection in pregnancy
  1. Reduces incidence and severity of congenital toxoplasmosis
- Treatment of congenital infection
  1. Improvement in intellectual function
  2. Regression of retinal lesions
- AIDS
  1. 70% to 95% response to therapy

■ REFERRAL
- To infectious disease expert:
  1. Immunocompromised hosts
  2. Pregnant women
  3. Difficulty in making a diagnosis or deciding on treatment
- To pediatric infectious disease expert:
  1. Congenital infection
- To obstetrician:
  1. Pregnant seronegative mother
  2. Acute seroconversion
- To ophthalmologist:
  1. Congenital infection
  2. Any case of ocular infection

☼ PEARLS & CONSIDERATIONS

■ COMMENTS
- Prevention of toxoplasmosis is most important in seronegative pregnant women and immunocompromised hosts.
- Patient instructions:
  1. Cook meat to 66° C.
  2. Cook eggs.
  3. Do not drink unpasteurized milk.
  4. Wash hands thoroughly after handling raw meat.
  5. Wash kitchen surfaces that come in contact with raw meat.
  6. Wash fruits and vegetables.
  7. Avoid contact with materials potentially contaminated with cat feces.

REFERENCES

Beazley DM, Egerman RS: Toxoplasmosis, *Semin Perinatol* 22(4):332, 1998.
Boyer KM: Diagnostic testing for congenital toxoplasmosis, *Pediatr Infect Dis J* 20(1):59, 2001.
Jones JL et al: Congenital toxoplasmosis: a review, *Obstet Gynecol Surv* 56(50):296, 2001.
Author: **Michele Halpern, M.D.**

BASIC INFORMATION

■ DEFINITION

Bacterial tracheitis is an acute infectious disease affecting the trachea and large conducting airways. Tracheal inflammation may be caused by a large number of inhaled stimuli, but bacterial infection is a life-threatening illness associated with viscous purulent secretions and subglottic edema.

■ SYNONYMS

Bacterial tracheobronchitis
Pseudomembranous croup
Membranous laryngotracheobronchitis

ICD-9CM CODES
464.10 Tracheitis

■ EPIDEMIOLOGY & DEMOGRAPHICS
INCIDENCE (IN U.S.):
- Uncommon
- May be the most common cause of acute upper airway obstruction requiring admission to pediatric ICUs

PREDOMINANT SEX: Boys > girls in one series

PREDOMINANT AGE:
- 1 mo to 8 yr
- Almost all <13 yr (most <3 yr)

PEAK INCIDENCE: Three fourths of cases reported in winter

GENETICS: Down syndrome is a possible predisposing factor.

Congenital Infection: Some cases found in those with anatomic abnormalities of the upper airways.

■ PHYSICAL FINDINGS & CLINICAL PRESENTATION
- Croupy or "brassy" cough
- Inspiratory stridor (frequent)
- Wheezing (unusual)
- Fever (often >102° F)
- Thick, purulent secretions expectorated
  1. Minority of patients expectorate "rice-like" pellets.
  2. Most patients are unable to mobilize secretions.
     a. Become inspissated
     b. Form pseudomembranes

■ ETIOLOGY
- *Staphylococcus aureus*
- *Haemophilus influenzae*
- β-Hemolytic streptococcal infection
- Secondary to viral infections of the respiratory tract
  1. Primary influenza
  2. RSV
  3. Parainfluenza
- Many cases follow measles
  1. Especially when accompanied by chest radiographic infiltrates
  2. Sometimes fatal outcome

DIAGNOSIS

■ DIFFERENTIAL DIAGNOSIS
- Viral croup
- Epiglottitis
- Diphtheria
- Necrotizing herpes simplex infection in the elderly
- CMV in immunocompromised patients
- Invasive *Aspergillosis* in immunocompromised patients

■ WORKUP
- Direct laryngoscopy
  1. Typical secretions
     a. May form pseudomembranes
     b. Airway obstruction
  2. Normal epiglottis rules out epiglottitis
  3. Possible subglottic edema

■ LABORATORY TESTS
- WBC is sometimes elevated.
- On differential, left shift is almost universal.
- Gram stain and culture of tracheal secretions confirm diagnosis.
- Blood cultures are positive in a minority.

■ IMAGING STUDIES
- Lateral x-ray examination of neck
  1. Normal epiglottis
  2. Vague density or a "dripping candle" appearance of tracheal mucosa
     a. Secretions
     b. Pseudomembranes
- Films
  1. Not diagnostic
  2. Should not be performed on patients in acute respiratory distress, since severe or fatal upper airway obstruction can develop suddenly
- Pneumonic infiltrates frequent
- Atelectasis
  1. Unusual
  2. May involve an entire lung

TREATMENT

■ NONPHARMACOLOGIC THERAPY
- Aggressive maintenance of a patent airway
  1. Laryngoscopy or bronchoscopy used diagnostically and therapeutically to strip away pseudomembranes
  2. Voluminous and tenacious secretions suctioned from the underlying friable mucosa
     a. May extend from between the vocal cords to the main carina
     b. Larger channels of rigid instruments for more effective suctioning

- Prevention of complete large airway obstruction
  1. Nasotracheal intubation
  2. Humidification of inspired gas
  3. Frequent saline instillation and suctioning
  4. Intubation with general anesthesia, performed in the operating room, is preferred by some
- Ventilatory support necessary
- Initial management in ICU

■ ACUTE GENERAL Rx
- Antibiotic therapy
  1. Start immediately
  2. Continue for 2 wk
- Initial therapy
  1. β-Lactamase–producing *H. influenzae*
  2. β-Lactamase–producing staphylococci
- Oral therapy is usually sufficient after 5 or 6 days of IV administration

■ DISPOSITION
- Most patients are extubated in 5 to 6 days after initiating antibiotic therapy.
- Anoxic encephalopathy is reported in 7% of survivors.

■ REFERRAL
Suspected diagnosis

PEARLS & CONSIDERATIONS

■ COMMENTS
- Infants are at increased risk of airway obstruction because of the small transverse area of the upper airway.
- Presence of pneumonia and a staphylococcal etiology are thought to worsen prognosis.
- Reported complications:
  1. Toxic shock syndrome
  2. Persistent postextubation stridor
  3. Pneumothorax
  4. Volutrauma

REFERENCES
Ahmed QA, Niederman MS: Respiratory infection in the chronically critically ill patient, *Clin Chest Med* 22(10):71, 2001.

Bernstein T, Brilli R, Jacobs B: Is bacterial tracheitis changing? A 14-month experience in a pediatric intensive care unit, *Clin Infect Dis* 27:458, 1998.

Brook I: Aerobic and anaerobic microbiology of bacterial tracheitis in children, *Pediatr Emerg Care* 13:16, 1997.

Stroud RH, Friedman NR: An update on inflammatory disorders of the pediatric airway: epiglottitis, croup and tracheitis, *Am J Otolaryngol* 22(40):268, 2001.
Author: **Harvey M. Shanies, M.D., Ph.D.**

BASIC INFORMATION

■ DEFINITION
Hemolytic transfusion reaction is an acute intravascular hemolysis caused by mismatches in the ABO system. It is caused by complement-fixing Ig and IgG antibodies to group A and B RBCs. Hemolytic transfusion reactions can also be caused by minor antigen systems; however, they are usually less severe. In delayed serologic transfusion reactions, hemolysis with hemoglobinemia is unusual; in these delayed reactions the only manifestations may be the development of a newly positive Coombs' test and fever.

ICD-9CM CODES
999.8 Other transfusion reaction

■ EPIDEMIOLOGY & DEMOGRAPHICS
Acute intravascular hemolysis occurs in <1 in 50,000 transfusions.

■ PHYSICAL FINDINGS & CLINICAL PRESENTATION (Table 1-68)
• Hypotension
• Pain at the infusion site
• Fever, tachycardia, chest or back pain, dyspnea
• Often, severe reactions occur in surgical patients under anesthesia who are unable to give any warning signs

■ ETIOLOGY
Most fatal hemolytic reactions are caused by clerical errors and mislabeled specimens.

DIAGNOSIS

■ DIFFERENTIAL DIAGNOSIS
• Bacterial contamination of blood
• Hemoglobinopathies

■ WORKUP
The transfusion must be stopped immediately. The blood bank must be notified, and the donor transfusion bag must be returned to the blood bank along with a freshly drawn posttransfusion specimen.

■ LABORATORY TESTS
• Positive Coombs' test, elevated BUN, creatinine, and bilirubin
• Hemoglobinuria (wine-colored urine), hemoglobinemia (pink plasma)
• Decreased Hct, decreased serum haptoglobin

TREATMENT

■ NONPHARMACOLOGIC THERAPY
• Stop transfusion immediately. Test anticoagulated blood from the recipient for the presence of free Hgb in the plasma.
• Monitor vital signs.

■ ACUTE GENERAL Rx
• Vigorous IV hydration to maintain urine flow at >100 ml/hr until hypotension is corrected and hemoglobinuria clears. IV furosemide may be necessary to maintain adequate renal flow.
• The addition of mannitol may prevent renal damage (controversial).
• Monitor for the presence of DIC.
• Use of IV steroids is controversial.

■ DISPOSITION
Mortality exceeds 50% in severe transfusion reactions.

PEARLS & CONSIDERATIONS

■ COMMENTS
Hemolysis caused by minor antigen systems is generally less severe and may be delayed 5 to 10 days after transfusion.

REFERENCES
Goodnough LT et al: Transfusion medicine: blood transfusion, *N Engl J Med* 340:438, 1999.

Willimson LM et al: Serious hazards of transfusion (SHOT) initiative: analysis of the first two annual reports, *BMJ* 319:16, 1999.
Author: **Fred F. Ferri, M.D.**

TABLE 1-68 **Signs and Symptoms of Acute Adverse Reactions to Blood Transfusion**

REACTION	FEVER	CHILLS/ RIGORS	NAUSEA/ VOMITING	CHEST DISCOMFORT/ PAIN	FACIAL FLUSHING	WHEEZING/ DYSPNEA	BACK/ LUMBAR PAIN	DISCOMFORT AT INFUSION SITE	HYPOTENSION
Acute hemolytic	X	X	X	X	X	X	X	X	X
Febrile nonhemolytic	X	X		X	X				
Nonimmune hemolysis									
Acute lung injury	X			X		X			X
Allergic									
Massive transfusion complications									
Anaphylaxis	X	X	X	X	X	X	X	X	X
Passive cytokine infusion	X	X	X						
Hypervolemia						X			
Bacterial sepsis	X	X	X				X	X	X
Air embolus				X		X			

From Goldman L, Bennett JC (eds): *Cecil textbook of medicine,* ed 21, Philadelphia, 2000, WB Saunders.

BASIC INFORMATION

■ DEFINITION

The term *transient ischemic attack* (TIA) refers to a transient focal neurologic deficit caused by cerebrovascular compromise that typically lasts <60 min but always <24 hr and is followed by a full recovery of function.

■ SYNONYMS

TIA

ICD-9CM CODES

435.9 Unspecified transient cerebral ischemia

■ EPIDEMIOLOGY & DEMOGRAPHICS

INCIDENCE (IN U.S.): 49 cases/100,000 persons/yr
PREDOMINANT SEX: Males > females
PREDOMINANT AGE: >60 yr
PEAK INCIDENCE: >60 yr
GENETICS:
- There is no distinct genetic etiology.
- Family history is a risk factor.

■ PHYSICAL FINDINGS & CLINICAL PRESENTATION

- During an episode, neurologic abnormalities are confined to discrete vascular territory.
- Typical carotid territory symptoms are ipsilateral monocular visual disturbance, contralateral homonymous hemianopsia, contralateral hemimotor or sensory dysfunction, and language dysfunction (dominant hemisphere) alone or in combination.
- Typical vertebrobasilar territory symptoms are binocular visual disturbance, vertigo, diplopia, dysphagia, dysarthria, and motor or sensory dysfunction involving the ipsilateral face and contralateral body.

■ ETIOLOGY

Multiple, including emboli from extracranial or intracranial sources.

🔬 DIAGNOSIS

■ DIFFERENTIAL DIAGNOSIS

- Seizures
- Hypoglycemia
- Labyrinthine disease
- Migraine
- Mass lesions
- Boxes 2-181 and 2-182 describe the differential diagnosis of focal neurologic deficits.

■ WORKUP

- Thorough history and physical examination
- Ancillary investigations aimed at identifying the etiology

■ LABORATORY TESTS

- CBC
- Platelet count
- PT (INR)
- PTT
- ESR
- Glucose
- VDRL
- Lipid profile
- Urinalysis
- Chest x-ray examination
- ECG
- Other tests as dictated by suspected etiology

■ IMAGING STUDIES

- Head CT scan to exclude hemorrhage.
- MRI and MRA (the former identifies lacunar infarcts, the latter aneurysms, vasculitis).
- Carotid Doppler studies very helpful in identifying carotid stenosis; if greater than 70%, angiography should be considered.

- Echocardiography if cardiac source is suspected.
- 24-hr Holter monitoring if history suggests arrhythmia.
- Four-vessel cerebral angiogram if considering carotid endarterectomy.

💊 TREATMENT

■ NONPHARMACOLOGIC THERAPY

- Carotid endarterectomy for carotid territory TIA associated with an ipsilateral stenosis of 70% to 99%: should be done by a surgeon who is experienced with this procedure and who does them frequently
- Modification of risk factors

■ ACUTE GENERAL Rx

- Depends on etiology
- Acute anticoagulation possibly beneficial in patients with documented cardiogenic emboli. Patients with atrial fibrillation or demonstrated cardiac thrombi will benefit from long-term warfarin therapy.
- Fig. 1-374 describes an algorithm for the treatment of transient ischemic attacks.

■ CHRONIC Rx

- No data support the use of long-term anticoagulation in the management of TIA, although subpopulations may emerge in which this is found to be more effective than antiplatelet therapy.
- First line of treatment is with aspirin. No significant benefit of high-dose aspirin (up to 1500 mg/day) has been conclusively found over lower doses (75 mg to 325 mg/day).
- Plavix (clopidogrel) 75 mg PO qd or ticlopidine (Ticlid) 250 mg PO bid should be used for patients whose TIAs continue (aspirin failures).

■ **DISPOSITION**
- Stroke risk is 4.4% in the first month and 11.6% in the first year.
- The annual risk of myocardial infarction is 2.4%.
- One-year and 3-yr survival rates are 98% and 94%, respectively.

■ **REFERRAL**
If uncertain about diagnosis or management

 PEARLS & CONSIDERATIONS

■ **CAVEAT**
Many TIAs are simply lacunar infarcts secondary to hypertension; control the hypertension!

REFERENCES
Alamowitch S et al: Risk, causes, and prevention of ischaemic stroke in elderly patients with symptomatic internal-carotid-artery stenosis, *Lancet* 357:1154, 2001.
Gorelick PB et al: Prevention of a first stroke, *JAMA* 281:1112, 1999.
Author: **Michael Gruenthal, M.D., Ph.D.**

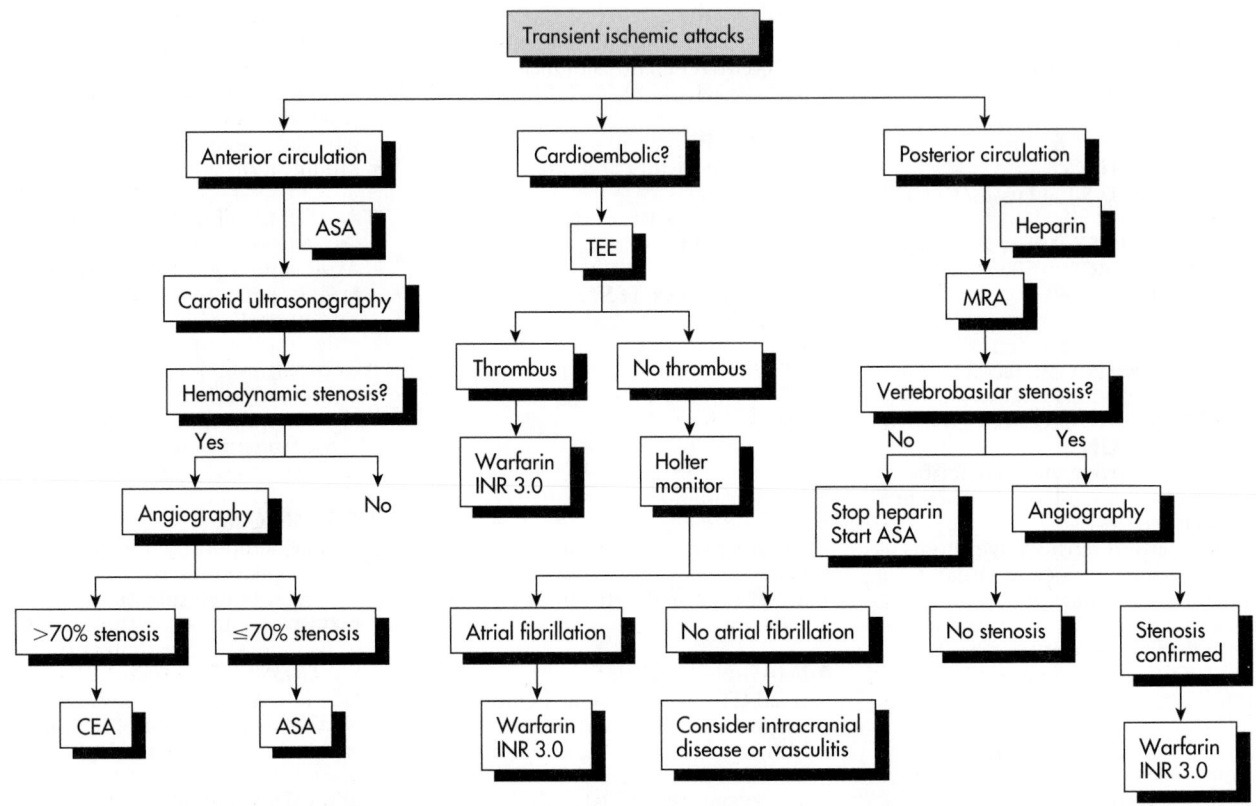

Fig. 1-374   The treatment of transient ischemic attacks (TIAs). *ASA,* Aspirin; *CEA,* carotid endarterectomy; *INR,* International Normalized Ratio; *MRA,* magnetic resonance angiography; *TEE,* transesophageal echocardiography. (Modified from Morgenstern LB, Grotta JC: Transient ischemic attacks. In Johnson RT, Griffin JW [eds]: *Current therapy in neurologic disease,* ed 5, St Louis, 1997, Mosby.)

BASIC INFORMATION

DEFINITION
Trichinosis is an infection by one of various species of *Trichinella*.

ICD-9CM CODES
124 Trichinosis

EPIDEMIOLOGY & DEMOGRAPHICS
INCIDENCE (IN U.S.): <100 cases/yr
GENETICS:
Congenital Infection:
- Abrupt delivery of stillbirths in infected pregnant women
- Vertical infection of the fetus

PHYSICAL FINDINGS
- Symptoms
  1. May vary widely depending on the time from ingestion of contaminated meat and on worm burden
  2. Most persons asymptomatic
- Enteral phase
  1. Correlates with penetration of ingested larvae into the intestinal mucosa
  2. May last from 2 to 6 wk
  3. Mild, transient diarrhea and nausea
  4. Abdominal pain
  5. Diarrhea or constipation
  6. Vomiting
  7. Malaise
  8. Low-grade fevers
- Migratory or parenteral phase
  1. In the intestine, maturation and mating
  2. Newborn larvae
     a. Penetrate into lymphatic and blood vessels
     b. Migrate to muscles where they penetrate into muscle cells, enlarge, coil, and develop a cyst wall
  3. Patients may present with
     a. Fever
     b. Myalgias
     c. Periorbital or facial edema
     d. Headache
     e. Skin rash
     f. Other symptoms caused by the penetration of tissues by the newborn migrating larvae

  4. Peak in symptoms 2 to 3 wk after infection, then slowly subside
- Severe complications
  1. Brain damage by granulomatous inflammation or occlusion of arteries
  2. Cardiac involvement
  3. Can lead to death

ETIOLOGY
- The nematode responsible for this illness is an obligate intracellular parasite belonging to the genus *Trichinella*.
- It is one of the most ubiquitous parasites in the world and may be found in virtually all warm-blooded animals.
- Infection in humans occurs by the ingestion of contaminated animal meat that is raw or partially cooked and contains viable cysts.
- Most cases are now related to the consumption of poorly processed pork or wild game (bear, wild boar, cougar, and walrus).

DIAGNOSIS

DIFFERENTIAL DIAGNOSIS
- Different presentations have different differential diagnoses.
- Early illness may resemble gastroenteritis.
- Later symptoms may be confused with:
  1. Measles
  2. Dermatomyositis
  3. Glomerulonephritis
- The differential diagnosis of nematode tissue infections is described in Table 2-140.

WORKUP
- Antibody assay of serum is usually positive by approximately 2 wk after infection.
- Muscle biopsy is used to detect the larva in muscle tissue if diagnosis unclear; best done by placing the tissue between two slides.

LABORATORY TESTS
- CBC: leukocytosis with prominent eosinophilia
- ESR: usually normal
- Elevation of muscle enzymes common (i.e., CPK, aldolase)

IMAGING STUDIES
Soft-tissue radiographs may show calcified cyst walls.

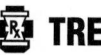

TREATMENT

NONPHARMACOLOGIC THERAPY
Bed rest for myalgias

ACUTE GENERAL Rx
- Thiabendazole to treat persons within 24 hr of ingesting contaminated meat, at the dose of 25 mg/kg/day for 1 wk.
- Salicylates to decrease muscle discomfort.
- Steroids in critically ill patients.
- A recent study showed clinical improvement of myositis significantly more often in patients treated with thiabendazole or mebendazole versus those treated with fluconazole or placebo.

DISPOSITION
- Most symptoms subside over time.
- Reports of long-term sequelae:
  1. Myalgias
  2. Headaches
- Occasionally, death occurs.

REFERRAL
Diagnosis uncertain

PEARLS & CONSIDERATIONS

COMMENTS
- Prevention by thorough cooking of meats
- Inadequate to smoke, cure, or dry meats

REFERENCES
Moorhead A et al: Trichinellosis in the United States, 1991-1996: declining but not gone, *Am J Trop Med Hyg* 60:66, 1999.
Watt G et al: Blinded, placebo-controlled trial of antiparasitic drugs for trichinosis myositis, *J Infect Dis* 182:371, 2000.
Author: **Maurice Policar, M.D.**

BASIC INFORMATION

■ DEFINITION

Tricuspid regurgitation (TR) refers to abnormal flow of blood from the right ventricle to the right atrium during systole (Fig. 1-375).

■ SYNONYMS

Tricuspid insufficiency

ICD-9CM CODES

397.0 Disease of the tricuspid valve
424.2 Tricuspid valve insufficiency (nonrheumatic)

■ EPIDEMIOLOGY & DEMOGRAPHICS

- Isolated TR is more common than tricuspid stenosis (TS).
- In patients with rheumatic heart disease, TR rarely occurs alone and is usually associated with mitral and/or aortic valve disease.
- Trivial TR is frequently detected by echocardiogram and is considered a normal variant.
- Functional TR is more common than structural valvular TR.

■ PHYSICAL FINDINGS & CLINICAL PRESENTATION

- Symptoms of TR are determined by the underlying cause (e.g., pulmonary hypertension, left ventricular failure, and mitral stenosis).
- Dyspnea
- Orthopnea
- Paroxysmal nocturnal dyspnea
- Signs of right-sided heart failure:
  1. Elevated jugular venous distention with large V waves
  2. Right ventricular lift
  3. Right-sided S_3
  4. Holosystolic murmur heard best along the left parasternal line and fourth intercostal space and is louder during inspiration.
  5. Pulsatile liver
  6. Hepatomegaly
  7. Ascites
  8. Edema

■ ETIOLOGY

- TR is usually functional rather than structural.

- Functional TR refers to conditions leading to dilation of the right ventricle and include:
  1. Any cause of pulmonary hypertension(e.g., COPD, pulmonary embolism, restrictive lung disease, collagen vascular disease, and primary pulmonary hypertension).
  2. Coronary artery disease with right ventricular infarction.
  3. Left-sided congestive heart failure leading to right-sided heart failure.
  4. Dilated cardiomyopathy (e.g., alcohol, idiopathic).
- Structural TR refers to conditions directly affecting the tricuspid valve and include:
  1. Rheumatic fever
  2. Infective endocarditis
  3. Congenital (e.g., Ebstein's anomaly)
  4. Carcinoid
  5. Marfan's syndrome
  6. Tricuspid valve prolapse
  7. Traumatic (e.g., pacemaker insertion)
  8. Right atrial myxoma
  9. Collagen-vascular disease (e.g., SLE)
  10. Radiation

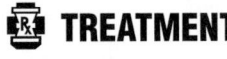

DIAGNOSIS

The diagnosis of TR is made by clinical history, physical examination, and adjunctive studies including ECG, chest x-ray, echocardiography, and rarely right-sided heart catheterization.

■ DIFFERENTIAL DIAGNOSIS

The differential diagnosis of TR is as stated above under "Etiology."

■ WORKUP

- Any patient suspected of having significant TR should undergo the following:
  1. Chest x-ray
  2. Electrocardiogram
  3. Echocardiogram
  4. Right-sided cardiac catheterization

■ LABORATORY TESTS

- Blood tests are not very specific in diagnosing TR.
- ECG may show evidence of:
  1. Right atrial enlargement (e.g., P-wave height in leads II, III, aVF >2.5 mV).
  2. Right ventricular enlargement/hypertrophy (e.g., R wave > S wave in lead V_1).
  3. Right axis deviation >100 degrees.
  4. Atrial fibrillation.

■ IMAGING STUDIES

- Chest x-ray can show:
  1. Evidence of COPD with flattened diaphragms, barrel chest, dilated pulmonary arteries, and increased retrosternal air space
  2. Enlarged right atrium
  3. Enlarged right ventricle
- Echocardiogram, M-mode, 2-D with continuous wave, pulse wave, and color Doppler will:
  1. Detect TR
  2. Estimate the severity of TR
  3. Estimate the pulmonary artery pressure
  4. Exclude vegetation, mass, or prolapse
  5. Assess overall ventricular function
- Right-sided catheterization shows:
  1. Elevated right atrial and right ventricular end-diastolic pressures
  2. Large V waves

TREATMENT

Treatment of TR is directed at the underlying cause.

■ NONPHARMACOLOGIC THERAPY

Oxygen therapy is beneficial in all patients with functional TR secondary to underlying pulmonary hypertension provoked by alveolar hypoxia.

■ ACUTE GENERAL Rx

- Functional TR caused by left-sided heart failure is treated in similar fashion with preload, inotrope, and afterload therapy:
  1. Digoxin 0.25 mg PO qd

2. Furosemide 40 to 80 mg PO qd for edema
3. Angiotensin-converting enzyme inhibitors (e.g., lisinopril 10 to 40 mg PO qd, fosinopril 10 to 40 mg PO qd, enalapril 10 mg PO bid, and captopril 50 mg PO tid).

- Structural TR treatment depends on the underlying cause(e.g., antibiotics for infective endocarditis).

■ CHRONIC Rx
- Tricuspid valve surgery is considered in patients with severe TR from rheumatic mitral stenosis and pulmonary hypertension, structural valve damage from carcinoid, congenital anomalies, or infective endocarditis.
- Surgical procedures may include:
1. Total valve replacement
2. Annuloplasty
3. Converting the tricuspid valve from three leaflets to two leaflets

■ DISPOSITION
- The natural history to tricuspid regurgitation will depend on the underlying etiology.
- Patients with rheumatic valve disease requiring replacement of both the mitral and tricuspid valve have a high 30-day morbidity/mortality rate of 15% to 20%.

■ REFERRAL
For patients with significant symptomatic TR, a cardiology consultation is recommended.

☼ PEARLS & CONSIDERATIONS

■ COMMENTS
- Antibiotic prophylaxis for dental, GI, or GU procedures is recommended in patients with tricuspid valve abnormalities.

- TR secondary to tricuspid valve prolapse may also be associated with mitral valve prolapse.

REFERENCES
Braunwald E: Valvular heart disease. In Braunwald E: *Heart disease: A textbook of cardiovascular medicine,* ed 6, Philadelphia, 2001, WB Saunders.

Waller BF et al: Pathology of tricuspid valve stenosis and pure tricuspid regurgitation—Part I, *Clin Cardiol* 18(2):97, 1995.

Waller BF et al: Pathology of tricuspid valve stenosis and pure tricuspid regurgitation—Part II, *Clin Cardiol* 18(3):167, 1995.

Author: **Peter Petropoulos, M.D.**

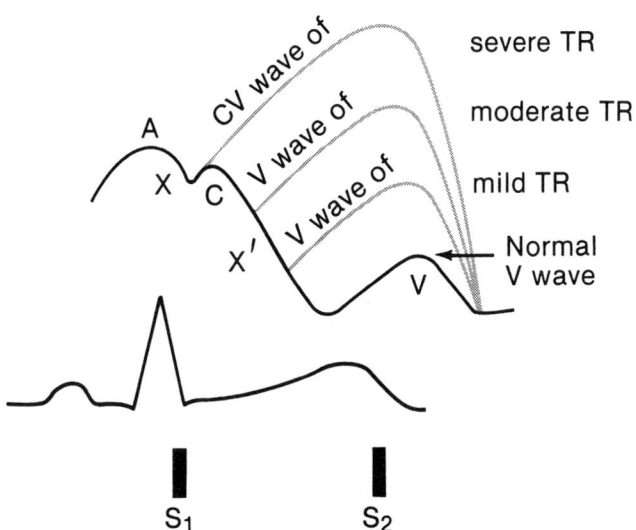

Fig. 1-375   The jugular venous pulse in tricuspid regurgitation. The jugular venous pulse wave normally drops during ventricular systole. As TR becomes more severe, the CV wave becomes more obvious during ventricular systole. (From Conn R: *Current diagnosis,* ed 9, Philadelphia, 1997, WB Saunders.)

BASIC INFORMATION

■ DEFINITION

Tricuspid stenosis (TS) is narrowing of the orifice of the tricuspid valve, resulting in a diastolic pressure gradient between the right atrium and right ventricle restricting right atrial emptying (Fig. 1-376).

■ SYNONYMS

Tricuspid valve stenosis
TS

ICD-9CM CODES

397.0 Disease of the tricuspid valve

■ EPIDEMIOLOGY & DEMOGRAPHICS

- TS is more common in women than in men and is seen in patients between the ages of 20 to 60.
- TS is more common in India than in the U.S.
- In patients who have rheumatic heart disease, tricuspid stenosis is present at autopsy in 15%, but was clinically significant in only 5%.
- TS very seldom occurs alone; it is usually associated with mitral valve disease and/or aortic valve disease.

■ PHYSICAL FINDINGS & CLINICAL PRESENTATION

- Patients with severe symptomatic TS usually present with symptoms fatigue, abdominal swelling, and anasarca. They may complain of right upper quadrant abdominal pain secondary to passive congestive hepatomegaly from elevated systemic venous pressures.
- Jugular venous distention with a prominent a wave is noted along with a palpable hepatic pulsation.
- Right atrial pulsation may be palpated to the right of the sternum and a diastolic thrill may be felt over the left sternal edge that is increased with inspiration.

- An opening snap and diastolic murmur is best heard along the left sternal border of the fourth intercostal space and is augmented by inspiration.

■ ETIOLOGY

Rheumatic heart disease is the primary cause of TS, resulting in scarring of the valve leaflets and fusion of the commissures. This along with shortening of the chordae tendineae and immobility of the valve leaflets results in narrowing of the tricuspid valve orifice.

DIAGNOSIS

■ DIFFERENTIAL DIAGNOSIS

- Congenital tricuspid atresia
- Right atrial myxoma
- Metastatic tumor
- Carcinoid syndrome
- Systemic lupus endocarditis
- Tricuspid valve vegetations from endocarditis
- Endomyocardial fibrosis
- Right atrial thrombi
- Constrictive pericarditis

■ WORKUP

- ECG
- Chest x-ray examination
- Echocardiography
- Cardiac angiography in selected patients

■ IMAGING STUDIES

- Chest x-ray reveals an enlarged heart with a prominent right border.
- ECG in many cases will show atrial fibrillation secondary to an enlarged right atrium. However, in patients who are in normal sinus rhythm, the ECG will show criteria for right atrial enlargement (tall peaked P waves >2.5 mm in height in leads II, III, or aVF).
- Echocardiography reveals doming of the anterior tricuspid leaflet with re-

striction of movement of the leaflet tip along with reduced excursion of the posterior and septal leaflets. Doppler is used to calculate the diastolic gradient across the tricuspid.
- Cardiac catheterization will measure simultaneous pressures in the right atrium and right ventricle giving you the gradient across the valve (normal gradient <1 mm Hg). Tricuspid valve area can also be determined (severe 1 cm^2).

TREATMENT

■ NONPHARMACOLOGIC THERAPY

Most patients with severe TS will have peripheral edema and therefore salt restriction is essential.

■ ACUTE GENERAL Rx

- Furosemide 40 mg qd; gradually increased according to symptoms and edema.
- Digoxin 0.25 mg qd and warfarin (maintaining the INR between 2 to 3) is used in patients who develop atrial fibrillation.

■ CHRONIC Rx

- It must be remembered that TS seldom occurs alone. It is usually associated with mitral disease. The decision to proceed with surgery for TS typically occurs in the setting of significant symptomatic mitral valve disease.
- Surgery for TS is considered if mitral surgery is going to be done and there is a mean diastolic gradient across the tricuspid valve of 5 mm Hg and the tricuspid valve area is <2 cm^2.
- Surgical procedures for significant tricuspid stenosis include closed commissurotomy, open commissurotomy, and tricuspid valve replacement. This is usually determined during surgery.

- Tricuspid valve replacement carries a high 30-day operative morbidity/mortality of 15% to 20% in addition to the high risk of thrombus formation.

■ DISPOSITION
The natural course of severe TS is not very well known.

■ REFERRAL
TS is difficult to diagnose and therefore consultation with a cardiology specialist is recommended.

⚙ PEARLS & CONSIDERATIONS

■ COMMENTS
- TS almost always occurs in association with either mitral valve disease and/or aortic valve disease.
- Unlike mitral stenosis patients, TS patients typically do not complain of dyspnea, orthopnea, or paroxysmal nocturnal dyspnea.

REFERENCES
Braunwald E: Valvular heart disease. In Braunwald E: *Heart disease: a textbook of cardiovascular medicine,* ed 6, Philadelphia, 2001, WB Saunders.

Roguin A et al: Long-term follow-up of patients with severe rheumatic tricuspid stenosis, *Am Heart J* 136(1):103, 1998.

Waller BF et al: Pathology of tricuspid valve stenosis and pure tricuspid regurgitation—Part I, *Clin Cardiol* 18(2):97, 1995.

Waller BF et al: Pathology of tricuspid valve stenosis and pure tricuspid regurgitation—Part II, *Clin Cardiol* 18(3):167, 1995.

Author: **Peter Petropoulos, M.D.**

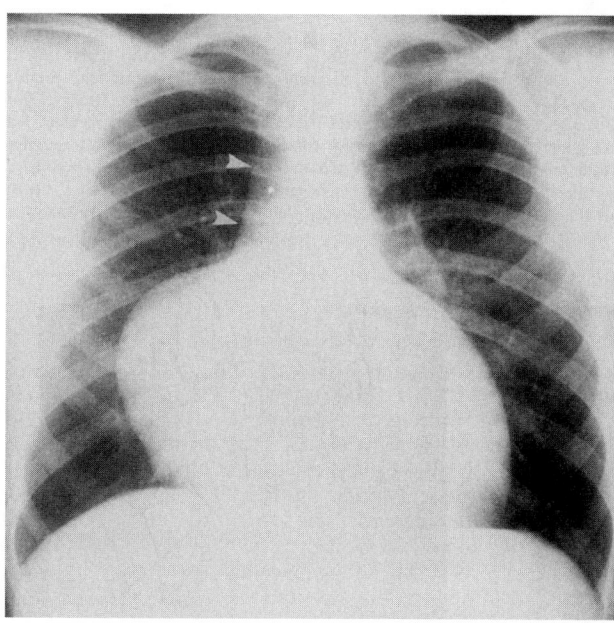

Fig. 1-376   Right atrial enlargement in congenital tricuspid stenosis. The right heart border is prominent; the superior vena cava is dilated *(arrowheads).* (From Rubens MB: Chest x-ray in adult heart disease. In Julian DG et al [eds]: *Diseases of the heart,* ed 2, London, 1996, WB Saunders.)

BASIC INFORMATION

■ DEFINITION
Tricyclic antidepressants (TCAs) are secondary or tertiary amines that have variable abilities to inhibit reuptake of neurotransmitters (norepinephrine, dopamine, and serotonin) and to be anticholinergic, antihistaminic, and sedating. These properties are important to consider when prescribing these agents and when managing an intentional or accidental overdose.

■ SYNONYMS
Tricyclic antidepressant intoxication or poisoning
TCA OD

■ ICD-9CM CODES
969.0

■ EPIDEMIOLOGY & DEMOGRAPHICS
- TCAs are the most common cause of death resulting from prescription drug overdose in the U.S.
- Available TCAs: amitriptyline, imipramine, desipramine, nortriptyline, doxepin, amoxapine, clomipramine, protriptyline, and others

■ PHYSICAL FINDINGS & CLINICAL PRESENTATION
Cardiovascular
- Intraventricular conduction delay (QRS prolongation)
- Sinus tachycardia
- Atrioventricular block
- Prolongation of the QT interval (Fig. 1-377)
- Ventricular tachycardia
- Wide complex tachycardia without P waves
- Refractory hypotension (the most common cause of death from TCA OD)
- Late arrhythmias or sudden death (in addition to the above, which occur during the first 24 to 48 hr: late problems can occur up to 5 days after the OD)

Central nervous system
- Coma
- Delirium
- Myoclonus
- Seizures

Other
- Hyperthermia
- Ileus
- Urinary retention
- Pulmonary complications (e.g., aspiration pneumonitis)
- Life-threatening overdose exists with the ingestion of more than 1 g of TCA. Among patients who reach a hospital, most deaths occur within the first 24 hr; lack of initial symptoms can be deceptive.

■ PATHOGENESIS
Mechanisms of tricyclic antidepressant cardiovascular toxicity (Table 1-69)
CNS toxicity
- Cholinergic blockade is believed to cause hyperthermia, ileus, urinary retention, pupillary dilation, delirium, and coma.
- The mechanism of myoclonus and seizures is not fully understood.

DIAGNOSIS

■ DIFFERENTIAL DIAGNOSIS
Cardiotoxicity from TCA can be confused with intoxication by drugs that cause QRS prolongation. These include class Ia antiarrhythmic agents (disopyramide, procainamide, quinidine), class Ic antiarrhythmic agents (encainide, flecainide, propafenone), cocaine, propranolol, quinine, chloroquine, neuroleptics, propoxyphene, and digoxin. Other causes of QRS prolongation include hyperkalemia, ischemic heart disease, cardiomyopathy, and cardiac conduction system dysfunction.

■ WORKUP
- Clinical presentation
- Knowledge of the overdose
- Serum drug levels (TCA concentration >1 μg/ml is life threatening and TCA concentration >3 μg/ml is often fatal)
- Baseline CBC, prothrombin time, BUN, creatinine, and electrolytes

■ MANAGEMENT
Initial measures
- Hospitalization with cardiac monitoring as well as monitoring of vital signs and temperature
- Initiate intravenous access
- Administer activated charcoal with sorbitol
- Large-bore tube gastric lavage is of unproven benefit
- Ipecac is contraindicated
- 12-Lead ECG
- If no evidence of cardiotoxicity has been noted during the first 6 hr of observation, further monitoring is not necessary; if there is evidence of cardiotoxicity, monitoring should continue for 24 hr after all signs of toxicity have resolved.

Treatment of specific complications of TCA toxicity: See Table 1-70
When the patient is medically stable, psychiatric evaluation should be obtained.

REFERENCES
Glauser J: Tricyclic antidepressant poisoning, *Cleve Clin J Med* 67:704, 2000.
Pentel PR, Keyler DE, Haddad LM: Tricyclic antidepressants. In Haddad LM, Shannon MW, Winchester JF (eds): *Clinical management of poisoning and drug overdose*, ed 3, Philadelphia, 1998, WB Saunders.
Author: **Tom J. Wachtel, M.D.**

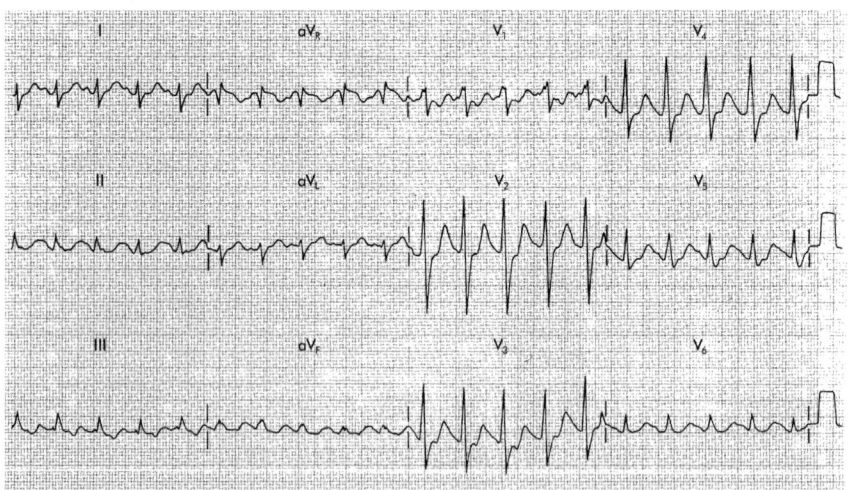

Fig. 1-377   The ECG from a patient with tricyclic antidepressant overdose shows three major findings: sinus tachycardia (from anticholinergic and adrenergic effects), prolongation of the QRS (from slowed ventricular conduction), and prolongation of the QT (from delayed repolarization). (From Goldberger AL: *Clinical electrocardiography*, ed 5, St Louis, 1994, Mosby.)

TABLE 1-69   **Mechanism of Tricyclic Antidepressant Cardiovascular Toxicity**

TOXIC EFFECT	MECHANISM
Conduction Delays, Arrhythmias	
QRS prolongation atrioventricular block	Cardiac sodium channel → slowed depolarization in atrioventricular node, His-Purkinje fibers, and ventricular myocardium
Sinus tachycardia	Cholinergic blockade, inhibition of norepinephrine reuptake
Ventricular tachycardia	
Monomorphic	Cardiac sodium channel inhibition → reentry
Torsades de pointes	Cardiac potassium channel inhibition → prolonged repolarization
Ventricular bradycardia	Impaired cardiac automaticity
Hypotension	
Vasodilation	Vascular α-adrenergic receptor blockade
Decreased cardiac contractility	Cardiac sodium channel inhibition → impaired excitation-contraction coupling

TABLE 1-70   **Treatment of Complications of Tricyclic Antidepressant Toxicity**

TOXIC EFFECT	TREATMENT
Cardiovascular	
QRS prolongation	Hypertonic $NaHCO_3$ if QRS prolongation is marked or progressing; not clear if treatment is needed in the absence of hypotension or arrhythmias
Hypotension	Intravascular volume expansion, $NaHCO_3$
	Vasopressors (norepinephrine) or inotropic agents (dopamine)
	Correct hyperthermia, acidosis, seizures
	Consider mechanical support
Ventricular tachycardia	$NaHCO_3$, lidocaine, overdrive, pacing
	Correct hypotension, hypothermia, acidosis, seizures
Torsades de pointes	Overdrive pacing
Ventricular bradycardia	Chronotropic agent (epinephrine), pacemaker
Sinus tachycardia	Treatment rarely needed
Atrioventricular block type II second or third degree	Pacemaker
Hypertension	Rapidly titratable antihypertensive agent (nitroprusside)
Central Nervous System	
Delirium	Restraints, benzodiazepine
	Neuromuscular blockade for hyperthermia, acidosis
Seizures	Benzodiazepine
	Neuromuscular blockade for hyperthermia, acidosis
Coma	Intubation, ventilation if needed
Other	
Hyperthermia	Control seizures, agitation
	Cooling measures
Acidosis	$NaHCO_3$
	Correct hypotension, hypoventilation

BASIC INFORMATION

■ DEFINITION
Trigeminal neuralgia is paroxysmal brief but intense lancinating pain in the distribution of one or more divisions of the trigeminal nerve. Pain may occur spontaneously but is often provoked by mild sensory stimuli. Involvement of the second and third divisions is common.

■ SYNONYMS
Tic douloureux

ICD-9CM CODES
350.1 Trigeminal neuralgia

■ EPIDEMIOLOGY & DEMOGRAPHICS
INCIDENCE (IN U.S.):
- Females: 5.9 cases/100,000 persons/yr
- Males: 3.4 cases/100,000 persons/yr

PREVALENCE (IN U.S.): 155/1 million persons
PREDOMINANT SEX: Females > males
PREDOMINANT AGE: >50 yr
PEAK INCIDENCE: Sixth to seventh decade
GENETICS: Family clustering rarely occurs

■ PHYSICAL FINDINGS & CLINICAL PRESENTATION
- Primary (idiopathic) cases: none
- Secondary (symptomatic) cases: possibly a fixed sensory loss in the distribution of the affected trigeminal nerve, as well as involvement of adjacent cranial nerves
- Multiple sclerosis in 3% of patients

■ ETIOLOGY
- Symptomatic cases: lesions in the vicinity of the nerve or nucleus, such as cerebellopontine angle tumors
- Some "idiopathic" cases: vascular compression of root of trigeminal nerve

DIAGNOSIS

■ DIFFERENTIAL DIAGNOSIS
- Dental pathology
- Posterior fossa masses
- Vascular malformations
- The differential diagnosis of headache and facial pain is described in Box 2-111.

■ WORKUP
MRI scans (CT scan with thin posterior fossa cuts if MRI not available) for all patients to exclude mass lesions

■ IMAGING STUDIES
See "Workup."

TREATMENT

■ NONPHARMACOLOGIC THERAPY
- In refractory cases, surgical options, including percutaneous radiofrequency gangliolysis and microvascular decompression
- Gamma-knife radiosurgery is an increasingly popular alternative to conventional surgery for trigeminal neuralgia

■ ACUTE GENERAL Rx
None, episodes are too brief

■ CHRONIC Rx
- Carbamazepine is the treatment of choice, providing relief to at least 75% of patients. Begin with 100 mg bid and increase gradually as tolerated using a tid regimen.
- If carbamazepine is not tolerated or effective, use gabapentin, 400 mg PO tid. Doses as high as 3600 mg/day are easily tolerated. Topiramate (Topamax) 25 mg qhs gradually titrated up to 100 mg bid is also effective.

■ DISPOSITION
Spontaneous remissions occur after months to years.

■ REFERRAL
If uncertain about diagnosis or if surgical treatment is necessary

PEARLS & CONSIDERATIONS

■ COMMENTS
Since prolonged remission may occur, drug tapering at yearly intervals is recommended.

REFERENCE
Maesawa S et al: Clinical outcomes after stereotactic radiosurgery for idiopathic trigeminal neuralgia, *J Neurosurg* 94:16, 2001.
Author: **Michael Gruenthal, M.D., Ph.D.**

BASIC INFORMATION

■ DEFINITION
Digital stenosing tenosynovitis refers to an inflammatory process of the digital flexor tendon sheath.

■ SYNONYMS
Trigger finger

ICD-9CM CODES
727.03 Trigger finger (acquired)

■ EPIDEMIOLOGY & DEMOGRAPHICS
- Trigger finger can be found in all age groups but is commonly found in patients older than 45 yr.
- More frequently affects females (4:1).
- Occupational risk groups: meat cutters, seamstress, tailors, and dentists.
- In adults the middle finger is most often affected (Fig. 1-378).
- In children the thumb is most often affected.

■ PHYSICAL FINDINGS & CLINICAL PRESENTATION
- Hand pain
- Painful triggering or snapping with flexion and extension of the affected digit
- Locking or loss of active digital extension is the most common symptom
- The digit possibly fixed in flexion (trapped or incarcerated)
- Usually affects one digit
- If more digits are involved, a systemic cause most likely present (e.g., diabetes, rheumatoid arthritis)
- A palpable tender nodule noted at the MCP joint of the affected digit
- Pain over the flexor tendon with resisted flexion
- Pain with passive stretching

■ ETIOLOGY
Trigger finger is described as being primary or secondary:
- Primary (idiopathic)
- Secondary
  1. Diabetes
  2. Rheumatoid arthritis
  3. Hypothyroidism
  4. Histiocytosis
  5. Amyloidosis
  6. Gout

DIAGNOSIS

The diagnosis of trigger finger is usually made by the clinical historical presentation and by physical examination.

■ DIFFERENTIAL DIAGNOSIS
- Dupuytren's contracture
- De Quervain's tenosynovitis
- Acute digital tenosynovitis
- Proliferative tenosynovitis
- Carpal tunnel syndrome
- Flexion tendon rupture
- Trauma

■ WORKUP
If a secondary cause of trigger finger is suspected, a workup should be pursued.

■ LABORATORY TESTS
- CBC with differential
- Electrolytes, BUN, and creatinine
- Blood glucose
- Thyroid function tests
- Uric acid
- Rheumatoid factor

■ IMAGING STUDIES
X-ray studies are not very helpful unless a secondary cause has affected other organs (e.g., rheumatoid lung).

TREATMENT

■ NONPHARMACOLOGIC THERAPY
- Splinting can be tried early in the course but has been very successful.

■ ACUTE GENERAL Rx
- In primary idiopathic trigger finger steroid injection, 15 to 20 mg depomethylprenisolone acetate in 1 ml 1% Xylocaine has been used with success.
- Triamcinolone 10 mg with 1 ml of 1% Xylocaine is an alternative steroid choice to be used in patients who do not respond to the first injection.
- If symptoms do not resolve in 3 wk, a repeat injection can be tried.

■ CHRONIC Rx
- Surgical release is indicated in patients with refractory symptoms (e.g., locked digits) despite nonpharmacologic and acute treatment.
- Surgery is also indicated in patients with recurrent symptoms despite steroid injection therapy.

■ DISPOSITION
- Following steroid injection, symptoms usually resolve in 3 to 5 days and locking resolves in 60% of the cases in 2 to 3 wk.
- If symptoms recur, a repeat steroid injection improves the symptoms in >80% of patients.
- Diabetic patients do not have the same success rate with steroid injections as the primary idiopathic group.

■ REFERRAL
If steroid injection therapy is considered, a rheumatology consult is requested.

PEARLS & CONSIDERATIONS

■ COMMENTS
If more than one digit is involved, a workup for a secondary systemic causes is in order.

REFERENCES
Anderson B, Kaye S: Treatment of flexor tenosynovitis of the hand ("trigger finger") with corticosteroids: a prospective study of the response to local injection, *Arch Intern Med* 151:153, 1991.

Canoso JJ: Trigger finger. In *Rheumatology in primary care*, Philadelphia, 1997, Saunders.

Kalb RL: Evaluation and treatment of wrist and hand pain, *Hosp Pract* 33(3):129, 1998.

Turowski GA, Zdankiewicz PD, Thomson JG: The results of surgical treatment of trigger finger, *Hand Surg Am* 22(1):145, 1997.

Author: **Peter Petropoulos, M.D.**

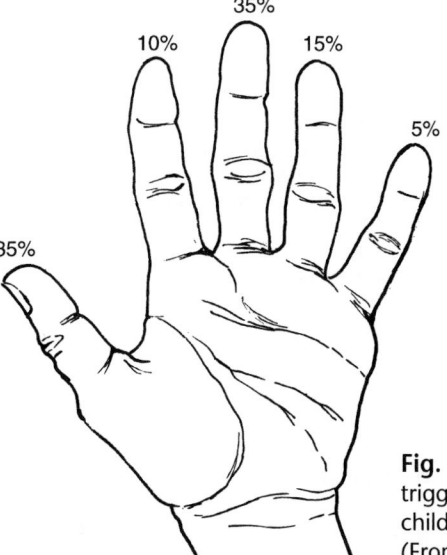

Fig. 1-378   Trigger finger. Frequency of trigger finger according to digit in adults. In children, virtually all cases occur in the thumb. (From Canoso J: *Rheumatology in primary care*, Philadelphia, 1997, WB Saunders.)

BASIC INFORMATION

■ DEFINITION

Trochanteric bursitis is a presumed inflammation or irritation of the gluteus maximus bursa or the bursa separating the greater trochanter from the gluteus medius and gluteus minimus (Fig. 1-379).

■ SYNONYMS

Greater trochanteric pain syndrome

ICD-9CM CODES

726.5 Bursitis trochanteric area

■ EPIDEMIOLOGY & DEMOGRAPHICS

- Trochanteric bursitis is commonly associated with other conditions:
  1. Osteoarthritis of the hip
  2. Lumbar spinal degenerative joint disease
  3. Rheumatoid arthritis
- Incidence peaks between the fourth and sixth decades of life but can occur at any age group.
- Occurs in females > males (4:1).

■ PHYSICAL FINDINGS & CLINICAL PRESENTATION

- Hip pain is the most common complaint. The pain is chronic, intermittent, and located over the lateral thigh.
- Numbness is present.
- Pain is precipitated with prolonged lying or standing on the affected side.
- Walking, climbing, and running exacerbate the pain.
- Point tenderness over the greater trochanter is noted.
- Pain is reproduced with resisted hip abduction.

■ ETIOLOGY

- The specific cause of trochanteric bursitis is not known although repetitive high-intensity use of the hip joint, trauma, infection (tuberculosis and bacterial), and crystal deposition can precipitate the disease.
- Trochanteric bursitis can occur when other conditions such as osteoarthritis of the knee and hip and bunions of the feet cause changes in the patient's gait, placing excess stress on the hip joint.

DIAGNOSIS

A detailed physical examination and clinical presentation usually make the diagnosis of trochanteric bursitis. Laboratory tests and x-ray images are helpful adjunctive studies used to exclude other conditions either associated with or mimicking trochanteric bursitis.

■ DIFFERENTIAL DIAGNOSIS

- Osteoarthritis of the hip
- Osteonecrosis of the hip
- Stress fracture of the hip
- Osteoarthritis of the lumbar spine
- Fibromyalgia
- Iliopsoas bursitis
- Trochanteric tendonitis
- Gout
- Pseudogout
- Trauma
- Neuropathy

■ WORKUP

A workup is indicated if suspected associated conditions exist; otherwise treatment can be started on clinical grounds alone.

■ LABORATORY TESTS

CBC with differential may show elevated white count if infection is present.
ESR is elevated in an infectious process.
Uric acid may be elevated in patients with gout.

■ IMAGING STUDIES

- Plain x-rays of the hip are not very helpful in diagnosing trochanteric bursitis. Sometimes calcifications may be seen around the greater trochanter.
- Bone scan can be done but is usually not necessary.
- CT and MRI may show bursitis but are usually not warranted because it will not alter treatment.

TREATMENT

■ NONPHARMACOLOGIC THERAPY

- Heat 15 to 20 min 4 to 6 times per day
- Ultrasound therapy
- Rest
- Partial weight bearing
- Physical therapy to strengthen back, hip, and knee muscles.

■ ACUTE GENERAL Rx

- Nonsteroidal antiinflammatory drugs (NSAIDs), ibuprofen 800 mg PO tid or naproxen 500 mg PO bid is used for pain relief.
- Acetaminophen 500-mg tablet, 1 to 2 tablets PO q6h prn can be used with NSAIDs or alternating with NSAIDs.
- Corticosteroid injection (30 to 40 mg depo-methylprednisolone acetate mixed with 3 ml 1% Xylocaine)

■ CHRONIC Rx

- Although rarely done, surgical removal of the bursa is possible for patients with refractory symptoms or infection.

■ DISPOSITION

- Most patients respond to NSAIDs and/or nonpharmacologic therapy.
- If steroid injection is used, approximately 70% of patients respond after the first injection and over 90% respond to two injections.
- 25% of patients receiving steroid injection may develop a relapse.

■ REFERRAL

A rheumatology or orthopedic referral is made if steroid injection therapy is needed or if the etiology is thought to be infectious.

PEARLS & CONSIDERATIONS

■ COMMENTS

- The absence of pain with flexion and extension differentiates trochanteric bursitis from degenerative joint disease of the hip.
- Localization of pain over the lateral thigh differentiates trochanteric bursitis from pain caused by meralgia paresthetica located over the anterolateral thigh and pain from osteoarthritis located over the inner thigh groin area.

REFERENCES

Canoso JJ: Hip pain. In Canoso JJ, Kersey R (eds): *Rheumatology in primary care.* Philadelphia, 1997, WB Saunders.

Caruso FA, Toney MA: *Trochanteric bursitis:* a case report of plain film, scintigraphic, and MRI correlation, *Clin Nucl Med* 19:393, 1994.

Schapira D, Nahir M, Scharf Y: Trochanteric bursitis: a common clinical problem, *Arch Phys Med Rehabil* 67:815, 1986.

Shebeeb MI, Matteson EL: Trochanteric bursitis (greater trochanter pain syndrome), *Mayo Clin Proc* 71:565, 1996.

Author: **Peter Petropoulos, M.D.**

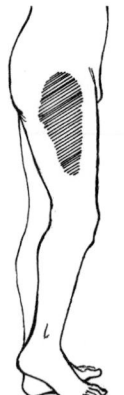

Fig. 1-379 Typical location of pain in trochanteric bursitis syndrome. This is also a frequent pain radiation site for a lumbar spine lesion, various nerve compression syndromes, and hip disease, particularly in osteonecrosis of the femoral head. (From Canoso J: *Rheumatology in primary care,* Philadelphia, 1997, WB Saunders.)

BASIC INFORMATION

■ **DEFINITION**
Tropical sprue is a malabsorption syndrome occurring primarily in tropical regions, including Puerto Rico, India, and Southeast Asia.

■ **SYNONYMS**
"Tropical enteropathy" refers to a subclinical form of tropical sprue.

ICD-9CM CODES
579.1 Tropical sprue

■ **EPIDEMIOLOGY & DEMOGRAPHICS**
Tropical sprue is endemic in tropical regions, the Middle East, the Far East, the Caribbean, and India.

■ **PHYSICAL FINDINGS & CLINICAL PRESENTATION**
• Diffuse, nonspecific abdominal tenderness and distention
• Low-grade fever
• Glossitis, cheilosis, hyperkeratosis, hyperpigmentation
• Diarrhea

■ **ETIOLOGY**
• Unknown
• Associated with overgrowth of predominantly coliform bacteria in the small intestine

DIAGNOSIS

The clinical features of tropical sprue include anorexia, diarrhea, weight loss, abdominal pain, and steatorrhea; these symptoms can develop in expatriates even several months after immigrating to temperate regions.

■ **DIFFERENTIAL DIAGNOSIS**
• Celiac disease
• Parasitic infestation
• Inflammatory bowel disease
• Other causes of malabsorption (e.g., Whipple's disease). A classification of malabsorptive disorders is described in Box 2-161.

■ **WORKUP**
• Diagnostic workup includes a comprehensive history (especially travel history), physical examination, laboratory evidence of malabsorption (see below), and jejunal biopsy; the biopsy results are nonspecific, with blunting, atrophy, and even disappearance of the villi and subepithelial lymphocytic infiltration.
• A clinical algorithm for the evaluation of malabsorption is described in Fig. 3-109.

■ **LABORATORY TESTS**
• Megaloblastic anemia (>50% of cases)
• Vitamin B_{12} deficiency, folate deficiency
• Steatorrhea, abnormal D-xylose absorption

■ **IMAGING STUDIES**
GI series with small bowel follow-through may reveal coarsening of the jejunal folds.

TREATMENT

■ **NONPHARMACOLOGIC THERAPY**
Monitoring of weight and calorie intake

■ **ACUTE GENERAL Rx**
• Folic acid therapy (5 mg bid for 2 wk followed by a maintenance dose of 1 mg tid) will improve anemia and malabsorption in over two thirds of patients.
• Tetracycline 250 mg qid for 4 to 6 wk in individuals who have returned to temperate zones, up to 6 mo in patients in endemic areas; ampicillin 500 mg bid for at least 4 wk in patients intolerant to tetracycline.
• Correction of vitamin B_{12} deficiency: vitamin B_{12} 1000 μg IM weekly for 4 wk, then monthly for 3 to 6 mo.
• Correction of other nutritional deficiencies (e.g., calcium, iron).

■ **DISPOSITION**
Complete recovery with appropriate therapy

■ **REFERRAL**
GI referral for jejunal biopsy

PEARLS & CONSIDERATIONS

■ **COMMENTS**
Additional patient education information can be obtained from National Digestive Diseases Information Clearinghouse, Box NDDIC, Bethesda, MD 20892; phone: (301) 654-3810.
Author: **Fred F. Ferri, M.D.**

BASIC INFORMATION

■ **DEFINITION**
Miliary tuberculosis (TB) is an infection of disseminated hematogenous disease, caused by the bacterium *Mycobacterium tuberculosis,* and is often characterized as resembling millet seeds on examination. Extrapulmonary disease may occur in virtually every organ site.

■ **SYNONYMS**
Disseminated TB

ICD-9CM CODES
018.94 Miliary tuberculosis

■ **EPIDEMIOLOGY & DEMOGRAPHICS**
INCIDENCE (IN U.S.):
- >38% of AIDS patients with TB have disseminated disease, often with concurrent pulmonary and extrapulmonary active sites. (See "Pulmonary Tuberculosis" in Section I.)

PREVALENCE (IN U.S.):
- Undetermined
- Highest prevalence
  1. AIDS patients
  2. Minorities
  3. Children
  4. Foreign-born persons
  5. Elderly

PREDOMINANT SEX:
- No specific predilection
- Male predominance in AIDS, shelters, and prisons reflected in disproportionate male TB incidence

PREDOMINANT AGE: Predominantly among 24- to 45-yr-olds
PEAK INCIDENCE: HIV-positive patients, regardless of age

■ **PHYSICAL FINDINGS & CLINICAL PRESENTATION**
- See also "Etiology"
- Common symptoms
  1. High intermittent fever
  2. Night sweats
  3. Weight loss
- Symptoms referable to individual organ systems may predominate
  1. Meninges
  2. Pericardium
  3. Liver
  4. Kidney
  5. Bone
  6. GI tract
  7. Lymph nodes
  8. Serous spaces
     a. Pleural
     b. Pericardial
     c. Peritoneal
     d. Joint
  9. Skin
  10. Lung: cough, shortness of breath

- Adrenal insufficiency possible due to infection of adrenal gland.
- Pancytopenia
  1. With fever and weight loss *or*
  2. Without other localizing symptoms or signs *or*
  3. With only splenomegaly
- TB hepatitis
  1. Tender liver
  2. Obstructive enzymes (alkaline phosphatase) elevated out of proportion to minimal hepatocellular enzymes (SGOT, SGPT) and bilirubin
- TB meningitis
  1. Gradual-onset headache
  2. Minimal meningeal signs
  3. Malaise
  4. Low-grade fever (may be absent)
  5. Sudden stupor or coma
  6. Cranial nerve VI palsy
- TB pericarditis
  1. Effusions resembling TB pleurisy
  2. Cardiac tamponade
- Skeletal TB
  1. Large joint arthritis (with effusions resembling TB pericarditis)
  2. Bone lesions (especially ribs)
  3. Pott's disease
     a. TB spondylitis, especially of lower thoracic spine
     b. Paraspinous TB abscess
     c. Possible psoas abscess
     d. Frequent cord compression (often relieved by steroids)
- Genitourinary TB
  1. Renal TB
     a. Papillary necrosis
     b. Destruction of renal pelvis
     c. Strictures of upper third of ureters
     d. Hematuria
     e. Pyuria with misleading bacterial cultures
     f. Preserved renal function
  2. TB orchitis or epididymitis
     a. Scrotal mass
     b. Draining abscess
  3. Chronic prostatic TB
- Gastrointestinal TB
  1. Diarrhea
  2. Pain
  3. Obstruction
  4. Bleeding
  5. Especially common with AIDS
  6. Bowel lesions
     a. Circumferential ulcers
     b. Short strictures
     c. Calcified granulomas
     d. TB mesenteric caseous adenitis
     e. Abscess, but rare fistula formation
     f. Often difficult to distinguish from granulomatous bowel disease (Crohn's disease)
- TB peritonitis
  1. Fluid resembles TB pleurisy
  2. PPD often negative
  3. Tender abdomen
  4. Doughy peritoneal consistency, often with ascites

  5. Peritoneal biopsy indicated for diagnosis
- TB lymphadenitis (scrofula)
  1. May involve all node groups
  2. Common adenopathies
     a. Cervical
     b. Supraclavicular
     c. Axillary
     d. Retroperitoneal
  3. Biopsy generally needed for diagnosis
  4. Surgical resection of nodes may be necessary
  5. Especially common with AIDS
- Cutaneous TB
  1. Skin infection from autoinoculation or dissemination
  2. Nodules or abscesses
  3. Tuberculids (possibly allergic reactions)
  4. Erythema nodosum
- Miscellaneous presentations
  1. TB laryngitis
  2. TB otitis
  3. Ocular TB
     a. Choroidal tubercles
     b. Iritis
     c. Uveitis
     d. Episcleritis
  4. Adrenal TB
  5. Breast TB

■ **ETIOLOGY**
- See also "Pulmonary Tuberculosis" in Section I.
- *Mycobacterium tuberculosis* (Mtb), a slow-growing, aerobic, non–spore-forming, nonmotile bacillus
- Humans are the only reservoir for Mtb.
- Pathogenesis:
  1. AFB (Mtb) are ingested by macrophages in alveoli, then transported to regional lymph nodes where spread is contained.
  2. Some AFB reach the bloodstream and disseminate widely.
  3. Immediate active disseminated disease may ensue or a latent period may develop.
  4. During latent period, T-cell immune mechanisms contain infection in granulomas until later reactivation occurs as a result of immunosuppression or other undefined factors in conjunction with reactivated pulmonary TB or alone.
- Miliary TB may occur as a consequence of the following:
  1. Primary infection: inability to contain primary infection leads to a hematogenous spread and progressive disseminated disease.
  2. In late chronic TB and in those with advanced age or poor immunity, a continuous seeding of the blood may develop and lead to disseminated disease.

🔬 DIAGNOSIS

■ DIFFERENTIAL DIAGNOSIS
- Widespread sites of possible dissemination associated with myriad differential diagnostic possibilities
- Lymphoma
- Typhoid fever
- Brucellosis
- Other tumors
- Collagen-vascular disease

■ WORKUP
- Prompt evaluation is essential
- Sputum for AFB stain and culture
- Chest x-ray examination
- PPD
- Fluid analysis and culture wherever available
  1. Sputum
  2. Blood: particularly helpful in patients with AIDS
  3. Urine
  4. CSF
  5. Pleural
  6. Pericardial
  7. Peritoneal
  8. Gastric aspirates
- Biopsy of any involved tissue is advisable to make immediate diagnosis
  1. Transbronchial biopsy preferred and easily accessible
  2. Bone marrow
  3. Lymph node
  4. Scrotal mass if present
  5. Any other involved site
  6. Positive granuloma or AFB on biopsy specimen is diagnostic
- Imaging studies as needed

■ LABORATORY TESTS
- Culture and fluid analysis as above
- Smear-negative sputum often is positive weeks later on culture
- CBC is usually normal
- ESR is usually elevated

■ IMAGING STUDIES
- Chest x-ray examination (may or may not be positive) (See "Pulmonary Tuberculosis" in Section I)
- CT scan or MRI of brain
  1. Tuberculoma
  2. Basilar arachnoiditis
- Barium studies of bowel

℞ TREATMENT

■ NONPHARMACOLOGIC THERAPY
- Bed rest during acute phase of treatment
- High-calorie, high-protein diet to reverse malnutrition and enhance immune response to TB
- Isolation in negative-pressure rooms with high-volume air replacement and circulation (with health care provider wearing proper protective 0.5- to 1-micron filter respirators)
  1. Until three consecutive sputum AFB smears are negative, if pulmonary disease coexists
  2. Isolation not required for closed-space TB infections

■ ACUTE GENERAL Rx
- See "Pulmonary Tuberculosis" in Section I.
- Therapy should be initiated immediately. Do not wait for definitive diagnosis.
- More rapid response to chemotherapy by disseminated TB foci than cavitary pulmonary TB.
- Treatment for 6 mo with INH plus rifampin plus PZA.
  1. Treatment for 12 mo often required for bone and renal TB.
  2. Prolonged treatment often required for CNS and pericardial.
  3. Prolonged treatment often required for all disseminated TB in infants.
- Compliance (rigid adherence to treatment regimen) is the chief determinant of success.
  1. Supervised DOT is recommended for all patients.
  2. Supervised DOT is mandatory for unreliable patients.
- Steroids are often helpful additions in fulminant miliary disease with the hypoxemia and DIC.

■ CHRONIC Rx
- Generally not indicated beyond treatment described above
- Prolonged treatment supervised by ID expert required in a few complicated infections caused by resistant organisms

■ DISPOSITION
- Monthly follow-up by physician experienced in TB treatment
- Confirm sensitivity testing, and alter treatment appropriately (see "Pulmonary Tuberculosis" in Section I)

■ REFERRAL
- To infectious disease expert for:
  1. HIV-positive patient
  2. Patient with suspected drug-resistant TB
  3. Patients previously treated for TB
  4. Patients whose fever has not decreased and sputum (if positive) has not converted to negative in 2 to 4 wk
  5. Patients with overwhelming pulmonary or extrapulmonary tuberculosis
- To pulmonary, orthopedic, or GI physicians for examinations or biopsy

💡 PEARLS & CONSIDERATIONS

■ COMMENTS
- All contacts (especially close household contacts and infants) should be properly tested for PPD conversions >3 mo following exposure.
- Those with positive PPD should be evaluated for active TB and properly treated or given prophylaxis.

REFERENCES

American Thoracic Society: Diagnostic standards and classification of tuberculosis in adults and children, *Am J Respir Crit Care Med* 161:1376, 2000.

Del-Giudice P et al: Unusual cutaneous manifestations of miliary tuberculosis, *Clin Infect Dis* 30(1):201, 2000.

Goto S et al: A successfully treated case of disseminated tuberculosis-associated hemophagocytic syndrome and multiple organ dysfunction syndrome, *Am J Kidney Dis* 38(4):E19, 2001.

Kuo PH et al: Severe immune hemolytic anemia in disseminated tuberculosis with response to antituberculosis therapy, *Chest* 119(6):1961, 2001.

Mert A et al: Spontaneous pneumothorax: a rare complication of miliary tuberculosis, *Ann Thorac Cardiovasc Surg* 7(1):45, 2001.

Small P, Fujiwara P: Management of tuberculosis in the United States, *N Engl J Med* 345:189, 2001.

Author: **George O. Alonso, M.D.**

BASIC INFORMATION

■ **DEFINITION**
Pulmonary tuberculosis (TB) is an infection of the lung and, occasionally, surrounding structures, caused by the bacterium *Mycobacterium tuberculosis*.

■ **SYNONYMS**
TB

■ **ICD-9CM CODES**
011.9 Pulmonary tuberculosis

■ **EPIDEMIOLOGY & DEMOGRAPHICS**
INCIDENCE (IN U.S.):
• Approximately 7 cases/100,000 persons—lowest in reported history
• >90% of new cases each year from reactivated prior infections
• 9% newly infected
• Only 10% of patients with PPD conversions (higher [8%/yr] in HIV-positive patients) will develop TB, most within 1 to 2 yr
• Two thirds of all new cases in racial and ethnic minorities
• 80% of new cases in children in racial and ethnic minorities
• Occurs most frequently in geographic areas and among populations with highest AIDS prevalence
   1. Urban blacks and Hispanics between 25 and 45 yr old
   2. Poor, crowded urban communities
• Nearly 36% of new cases from new immigrants
PREVALENCE (IN U.S.):
• Estimated 10 million people infected
• Varies widely among population groups
PREDOMINANT SEX:
• No specific predilection
• Male predominance in AIDS, shelters, and prisons reflected in disproportionate male incidence
PREDOMINANT AGE:
• 24 to 45 yr old
• Childhood cases common among minorities
• Nursing home outbreaks among elderly
PEAK INCIDENCE:
• Infancy
• Teenage years
• Pregnancy
• Elderly
• HIV-positive patients, regardless of age, at highest risk
GENETICS:
• Populations with widespread low native resistance have been intensely infected when initially exposed to TB.

• Following elimination of those with least native resistance, incidence and prevalence of TB tend to decline.

■ **PHYSICAL FINDINGS & CLINICAL PRESENTATION**
• See "Etiology"
• Primary pulmonary TB infection generally asymptomatic
• Reactivation pulmonary TB
   1. Fever
   2. Night sweats
   3. Cough
   4. Hemoptysis
   5. Scanty nonpurulent sputum
   6. Weight loss
• Progressive primary pulmonary TB disease: same as reactivation pulmonary TB
• TB pleurisy
   1. Pleuritic chest pain
   2. Fever
   3. Shortness of breath
• Rare massive, suffocating, fatal hemoptysis secondary to erosion of pulmonary artery within a cavity (Rasmussen's aneurysm)
• Chest examination
   1. Not specific
   2. Usually underestimates extent of disease
   3. Rales accentuated following a cough (posttussive rales)

■ **ETIOLOGY**
• *Mycobacterium tuberculosis* (Mtb), a slow-growing, aerobic, non–spore-forming, nonmotile bacillus, with a lipid-rich cell wall
   1. Lacks pigment
   2. Produces niacin
   3. Reduces nitrate
   4. Produces heat-labile catalase
   5. Mtb staining, acid-fast and acid-alcohol fast by Ziehl-Neelsen method, appearing as red, slightly bent, beaded rods 2 to 4 microns long (acid-fast bacilli [AFB]), against a blue background
   6. Polymerase chain reaction (PCR) to detect <10 organisms/ml in sputum (compared with the requisite 10,000 organisms/ml for AFB smear detection)
   7. Culture
      a. Growth on solid media (Lowenstein-Jensen; Middlebrook 7H11) in 2 to 6 wk
      b. Growth in liquid media (BACTEC, utilizing a radioactive carbon source for early growth detection) often in 9 to 16 days
      c. Enhanced in a 5% to 10% carbon dioxide atmosphere

   8. DNA fingerprinting (based on restriction fragment length polymorphism [RFLP])
      a. Facilitates immediate identification of Mtb strains in early growing cultures
      b. False-negatives possible if growth suboptimal
   9. Humans are the only reservoir for Mtb
   10. Transmission
      a. Facilitated by close exposure to high-velocity cough (unprotected by proper mask or respirators) from patient with AFB-positive sputum and cavitary lesions, producing aerosolized droplets containing AFB, which are inhaled directly into alveoli
      b. Occurs within prisons, nursing homes, and hospitals
• Pathogenesis
   1. AFB (Mtb) ingested by macrophages in alveoli, then transported to regional lymph nodes where spread is contained
   2. Some AFB may reach bloodstream and disseminate widely
   3. Primary TB (asymptomatic, minimal pneumonitis in lower or midlung fields, with hilar lymphadenopathy) essentially an intracellular infection, with multiplication of organisms continuing for 2 to 12 wk after primary exposure, until cell-mediated hypersensitivity (detected by positive skin test reaction to tuberculin purified protein derivative [PPD]) matures, with subsequent containment of infection
   4. Local and disseminated AFB thus contained by T-cell–mediated immune responses
      a. Recruitment of monocytes
      b. Transformation of lymphocytes with secretion of lymphokines
      c. Activation of macrophages and histiocytes
      d. Organization into granulomas, where organisms may survive within macrophages (Langhans' giant cells), but within which multiplication essentially ceases (95%) and from which spread is prohibited
   5. Progressive primary pulmonary disease
      a. May immediately follow the asymptomatic phase
      b. Necrotizing pulmonary infiltrates

c. Tuberculous bronchopneumonia
d. Endobronchial TB
e. Interstitial TB
f. Widespread miliary lung lesions
6. Postprimary TB pleurisy with pleural effusion
   a. Develops after early primary infection, although often before conversion to positive PPD
   b. Results from pleural seeding from a peripheral lung lesion or rupture of lymph node into pleural space
   c. May produce a large (sometimes hemorrhagic) exudative effusion (with polymorphonuclear cells early, rapidly replaced by lymphocytes), frequently without pulmonary infiltrates
   d. Generally resolves without treatment
   e. Portends a high risk of subsequent clinical disease, and therefore must be diagnosed and treated early (pleural biopsy and culture) to prevent future catastrophic TB illness
   f. May result in disseminated extrapulmonary infection
7. Reactivation pulmonary TB
   a. Occurs months to years following primary TB
   b. Preferentially involves the apical posterior segments of the upper lobes and superior segments of the lower lobes
   c. Associated with necrosis and cavitation of involved lung, hemoptysis, chronic fever, night sweats, weight loss
   d. Spread within lung occurs via cough and inhalation
8. Reinfection TB
   a. May mimic reactivation TB
   b. Ruptured caseous foci and cavities, which may produce endobronchial spread
9. Mtb in both progressive primary and reactivation pulmonary TB
   a. Intracellular (macrophage) lesions (undergoing slow multiplication)
   b. Closed caseous lesions (undergoing slow multiplication)
   c. Extracellular, open cavities (undergoing rapid multiplication)
   d. INH and rifampin are cidal in all three sites
   e. PZA especially active within acidic macrophage environment
   f. Extrapulmonary reactivation disease also possible
10. Rapid local progression and dissemination in infants with dev-astating illness before PPD conversion occurs
11. Most symptoms (fever, weight loss, anorexia) and tissue destruction (caseous necrosis) from cytokines and cell-mediated immune responses
12. Mtb has no important endotoxins or exotoxins
13. Granuloma formation related to tumor necrosis factor (TNF) secreted by activated macrophages

🔬 DIAGNOSIS

■ DIFFERENTIAL DIAGNOSIS
- Necrotizing pneumonia (anaerobic, gram-negative)
- Histoplasmosis
- Coccidioidomycosis
- Melioidosis
- Interstitial lung diseases (rarely)
- Cancer
- Sarcoidosis
- Silicosis
- Paragonimiasis
- Rare pneumonias
  1. *Rhodococcus equi* (cavitation)
  2. *Bacillus cereus* (50% hemoptysis)
  3. *Eikenella corrodens* (cavitation)

■ WORKUP
- Sputum for AFB stains
- Chest x-ray examination
- PPD
  1. Recent conversion from negative to positive within 3 mo of exposure is highly suggestive of recent infection.
  2. Single positive PPD is not helpful diagnostically.
  3. Negative PPD never rules out acute TB.
  4. Be certain that positive PPD does not reflect "booster phenomenon" (prior positive PPD may become negative after several years and return to positive only after second repeated PPD; repeat second PPD within 1 wk), which thus may mimic skin test conversion.
  5. Positive PPD reaction is determined as follows:
     a. Induration after 72 hr of intradermal injection of 0.1 ml of 5 TU-PPD
     b. 5-mm induration if HIV-positive, close contact of active TB, fibrotic chest lesions
     c. 10-mm induration if in high–medical risk groups (immunosuppressive disease or therapy, renal failure, gastrectomy, silicosis, diabetes),

foreign-born high-risk group (Southeast Asia, Latin America, Africa, India), low socioeconomic groups, IV drug addict, prisoner, health care worker
     d. 15-mm induration if low risk
  6. Anergy antigen testing (using mumps, *Candida*, tetanus toxoid) may identify patients who are truly anergic to PPD and these antigens, but results are often confusing. Not recommended.
  7. Patients with TB may be selectively anergic only to PPD.
  8. Positive PPD indicates prior infection but does not itself confirm active disease.

■ LABORATORY TESTS
- Sputum for AFB stains and culture
  1. Induced sputum if patient not coughing productively
- Sputum from bronchoscopy if high suspicion of TB with negative expectorated induced sputum for AFB
  1. Positive AFB smear is essential before or shortly after treatment to ensure subsequent growth for definitive diagnosis and sensitivity testing
  2. Consider lung biopsy if sputum negative, especially if infiltrates are predominantly interstitial
- AFB stain-negative sputum may grow Mtb subsequently
- Gastric aspirates reliable, especially in HIV-negative patients
- CBC
  1. Variable values
     a. WBCs: low, normal, or elevated (including leukemoid reaction: >50,000)
     b. Normocytic, normochromic anemia often
  2. Rarely helpful diagnostically
- ESR usually elevated
- Thoracentesis
  1. Exudative effusion
     a. Elevated protein
     b. Decreased glucose
     c. Elevated WBCs (polymorphonuclear leukocytes early, replaced later by lymphocytes)
     d. May be hemorrhagic
  2. Pleural fluid usually AFB-negative
  3. Pleural biopsy often diagnostic—may need to be repeated for diagnosis.
  4. Culture pleural biopsy tissue for AFB
- Bone marrow biopsy is often diagnostic in difficult-to-diagnose cases, especially miliary tuberculosis

■ IMAGING STUDIES
- Chest x-ray examination
  1. Primary infection reflected by calcified peripheral lung nodule with calcified hilar lymph node

2. Reactivation pulmonary TB
   a. Necrosis
   b. Cavitation (especially on apical lordotic views)
   c. Fibrosis and hilar retraction
   d. Bronchopneumonia
   e. Interstitial infiltrates
   f. Miliary pattern
   g. Many of above may also accompany progressive primary TB
3. TB pleurisy
   a. Pleural effusion, often rapidly accumulating and massive
4. TB activity not established by single chest x-ray examination
5. Serial chest x-ray examinations are excellent indicators of progression or regression

℞ TREATMENT

■ NONPHARMACOLOGIC THERAPY
- Bed rest during acute phase of treatment
- High-calorie, high-protein diet to reverse malnutrition and enhance immune response to TB
- Isolation in negative-pressure rooms with high-volume air replacement and circulation, with health care provider wearing proper protective 0.5- to 1-micron filter respirators, until three consecutive sputum AFB smears are negative

■ ACUTE GENERAL Rx
- Compliance (rigid adherence to treatment regimen) chief determinant of success
   1. Supervised directly observed therapy (DOT) recommended for all patients and mandatory for unreliable patients
- Preferred adult regimen: DOT
   1. Isoniazid (INH) 15 mg/kg (max 900 mg) + rifampin 600 mg + ethambutol (EMB) 30 mg/kg (max 2500 mg) + pyrazinamide (PZA) (2 g [<50 kg]; 2.5 g [51 to 74 kg]; 3 g [>75 kg]) thrice weekly for 6 mo
   2. Alternative, more complicated DOT regimens
- Short-course daily therapy: adult
   1. HIV-negative patient: 6 mo total therapy (2 mo INH 300 mg + rifampin 600 mg + EMB 15 mg/kg [max 2500 mg]) + PZA (1.5 g [<50 kg]; 2 g [51 to 74 kg]; 2.5 g [>75 kg]) daily and until smear negative and sensitivity confirmed; then INH + rifampin daily × 4 mo)
   2. HIV-positive patient: 9 mo total therapy (2 mo INH + rifampin + EMB + PZA daily until smear negative and sensitivity confirmed; then INH + rifampin qd × 7 mo)

3. Continue treatment at least 3 mo following conversion to negative cultures
- Drug resistance (often multiple drug resistance [MDRTB]) increased by:
   1. Prior treatment
   2. Acquisition of TB in developing countries
   3. Homelessness
   4. AIDS
   5. Prisoners
   6. IV drug addicts
   7. Known contact with MDRTB
- Never add single drug to failing regimen
- Never treat TB with fewer than two to three drugs or two to three new additional drugs
- Monitor for clinical toxicity (especially hepatitis)
   1. Patient and physician awareness that anorexia, nausea, RUQ pain, and unexplained malaise require immediate cessation of treatment
   2. Evaluation of liver function tests
      a. Minimal SGOT/SGPT elevations without symptoms generally transient and not clinically significant
- Preventive treatment for PPD conversion only (infection without disease)
   1. Must be certain that chest x-ray examination is negative and patient has no symptoms of TB
   2. INH 300 mg daily for 6 to 12 mo; at least 12 mo if HIV-positive
   3. Most important groups:
      a. HIV-positive
      b. Close contact of active TB
      c. Recent converter
      d. Old TB on chest x-ray examination
      e. IV drug addict
      f. Medical risk factor
      g. High-risk foreign country
      h. Homeless
- Infants generally given prophylaxis immediately if recent contact of active TB (even if infant PPD negative), then retested with PPD in 3 mo (continuing INH if PPD becomes positive and stopping INH if PPD remains negative)
- Chronic, stable PPD (several years) given INH prophylaxis generally only if patient is <35 yr old
   1. INH toxicity may outweigh benefit
   2. Individualize decision
- Preventive therapy for suspected INH-resistant organisms is unclear

■ CHRONIC Rx
- Generally not indicated beyond treatment described above
- Prolonged treatment, supervised by infectious disease expert, in a few very complicated infections caused by resistant organisms

■ DISPOSITION
- Monthly follow-up by physician experienced in TB treatment
- Confirm sensitivity testing and alter treatment appropriately
- Frequent sputum samples until culture is negative
- Confirm chest x-ray regression at 2 to 3 mo

■ REFERRAL
- To infectious disease expert for:
   1. HIV-positive patient
   2. Patient with suspected drug-resistant TB
   3. Patients previously treated for TB
   4. Patients whose fever has not decreased and sputum has not converted to negative in 2 to 4 wk
   5. Patients with overwhelming pulmonary or extrapulmonary tuberculosis
- To pulmonologist for bronchoscopy or pleural biopsy

☼ PEARLS & CONSIDERATIONS

■ COMMENTS
- All contacts (especially close household contacts and infants) should be properly tested for PPD conversions during 3 mo following exposure.
- Those with positive PPD should be evaluated for active TB and properly treated or given prophylaxis.

REFERENCES

Espinal MA et al: Infectiousness of *Mycobacterium tuberculosis* in HIV-1-infected patients wtih tuberculosis: a prospective study, *Lancet* 355(9200):275, 2000.

Kanaya AM, Glidden DV, Chambers HF: Identifying pulmonary tuberculosis in patients with negative sputum smear results, *Chest* 120(2):349, 2001.

Karcic AA et al: An elderly woman with chronic knee pain and abnormal chest radiography, *Postgrad Med* 77(911):600, 2001.

Mulder K: Tuberculosis: a case history, *Lancet* 358(9283):776, 2001.

Salazar GE et al: Pulmonary tuberculosis in children in a developing country, *Pediatrics* 108(2):448, 2001.

Small P, Fujiwara P: Management of tuberculosis in the United States, *N Engl J Med* 345:189, 2001.

Tudo G et al: Detection of unsuspected cases of nosocomial transmission of tuberculosis by use of a molecular typing method, *Clin Infect Dis* 33(4):453, 2001.

Author: **George O. Alonso, M.D.**

BASIC INFORMATION

■ **DEFINITION**
Tularemia is a systemic infection primarily of animals, and occasionally humans, caused by the bacterium *Francisella tularensis*.

■ **SYNONYMS**
Rabbit fever
Deer-fly fever
Market men's disease (U.S.)
Wild hare disease
Ohara's disease (Japan)
Water-rat trapper's disease (Russia)

ICD-9CM CODES
021.9 Tularemia

■ **EPIDEMIOLOGY & DEMOGRAPHICS**
INCIDENCE (IN U.S.):
- 0.05 to 0.15 cases/100,000 persons
- Varies greatly among states
- Most cases (55%)
  1. Arkansas
  2. Oklahoma
  3. Missouri
- Fewer cases
  1. Texas
  2. Oklahoma
- Total reported cases/yr = about 200
PREVALENCE (IN U.S.):
- Varies widely
- Most commonly affected:
  1. Laboratory workers
  2. Farmers
  3. Veterinarians
  4. Sheep workers
  5. Hunters
  6. Trappers
  7. Meat handlers
PREDOMINANT SEX: Male
PREDOMINANT AGE: >30 yr
PEAK INCIDENCE: Summer

■ **PHYSICAL FINDINGS & CLINICAL PRESENTATION**
- 2- to 5-day incubation period (range 1 to 21 days)
- Fever
- Chills
- Headache
- Myalgias
- Diarrhea
- Vomiting
- Cough (pulmonic form)
- Relative bradycardia (40% of patients)

- Ulceroglandular (UG) tularemia
  1. 80% of cases
  2. Follows skin inoculation
     a. Papule
     b. Sharp ulcer with necrotic base (absent in 20%)
     c. Large, tender regional lymph nodes
  3. Pharyngeal variant
     a. Exudative pharyngitis
     b. Ulceration
     c. Occasional membrane
  4. Adenopathy
     a. Rabbit-associated is predominantly axillary
     b. Tickborne is predominantly inguinal
- Oculoglandular (OG) tularemia
  1. Up to 5%
  2. Follows eye inoculation
     a. Conjunctivitis
     b. Regional adenopathy
- Pulmonic tularemia
  1. High mortality
  2. May coexist with other forms
  3. Nonproductive cough
  4. Bilateral rales
  5. Consolidation
  6. Pleuritic chest pain
  7. Hemoptysis rare
- Typhoidal form
  1. 5% to 30%
  2. Often concomitant with pulmonic form
  3. Fever
  4. Malaise
  5. Sore throat
  6. Abdominal discomfort
  7. Diarrhea
  8. Myalgias
  9. Absence of skin lesions
  10. Absence of adenopathy
  11. Hepatomegaly
  12. Splenomegaly
- Secondary skin rash
  1. Maculopapular
  2. Urticarial
  3. Erythema nodosum (especially in pulmonic form)
  4. Erythema multiforme

■ **ETIOLOGY**
- Gram-negative coccobacilli, *Francisella tularensis*
  1. Two biogroups
     a. *F. tularensis* biogroup *tularensis* type A (North America; most virulent)
     b. *F. tularensis* biogroup *palaearctica* type B (Asia, Europe > North America; less virulent)

  2. Encapsulated strains are more virulent
  3. Overall mortality <5%
- Most frequent during June to August
- Predominantly a disease of Northern Hemisphere
  1. 30° to 71° latitude
  2. Absent in United Kingdom
- Ecology
  1. Infection of rabbits
  2. Infection of rodents
     a. Squirrels
     b. Muskrats
     c. Beaver
- Human infection
  1. Insect bite
  2. Contact with contaminated animal (usually rabbit) products
  3. Contact with contaminated water
- Vectors
  1. Blood-feeding arthropods
     a. Ticks in Rocky Mountain states
  2. Biting flies
     a. California
     b. Southwest
  3. Most common tick vectors in U.S.
     a. Dog tick (*Dermacentor variabilis*)
     b. Wood tick (*D. andersoni*)
     c. Lone Star tick (*Amblyomma americanum*) (organism present in tick feces, saliva)
     d. Deer flies
  4. Most childhood disease in U.S. from tick bites
- Pathogenesis
  1. Primary infection (required dose: cutaneous much less than ingestion)
  2. Papule
     a. Develops locally over 3 to 5 days after cutaneous inoculation
     b. Followed by ulceration, spreading to lymph nodes, and dissemination (also via bacteremia)
  3. Granulomas (some caseating)
  4. Cell-mediated immunity required for recovery
  5. Antibodies not completely protective
  6. Pulmonic form
     a. May follow inhalation (often occupational)
     b. May follow hematogenous spread
  7. Pleural effusion usually lymphocytic; granulomas on biopsy

- Complications
  1. Disseminated suppurative adenitis
  2. Intravascular coagulation
  3. Hepatitis with jaundice
  4. Renal failure
  5. Rhabdomyolysis
  6. Rarely, meningitis (lymphocytic)
  7. Incidence of the following is decreased owing to antibiotic therapy:
     a. Osteomyelitis
     b. Encephalitis
     c. Splenic rupture

DIAGNOSIS

DIFFERENTIAL DIAGNOSIS
- UG form
  1. Pyogenic bacterial infections
  2. Cat-scratch disease
  3. Disseminated bacillary angiomatosis
  4. Syphilis
  5. Chancroid
  6. Lymphogranuloma venereum
  7. Tuberculosis
  8. Other mycobacteria
  9. Toxoplasmosis
  10. Sporotrichosis
  11. Rat-bite fever
  12. Anthrax
  13. Plague
  14. Diphtheria
  15. Streptococcal pharyngitis
  16. Mononucleosis
  17. Adenovirus
- OG form
  1. Cat-scratch disease
  2. Adenovirus conjunctivitis
  3. Syphilis
  4. Herpes simplex conjunctivitis
- Pulmonic form
  1. Tuberculosis
  2. *Mycoplasma*
  3. *Legionella*
  4. Q fever
  5. Psittacosis
  6. Mycoses
- Typhoidal form
  1. Typhoid fever
  2. Brucellosis
  3. *Legionella*
  4. Rickettsioses
  5. Malaria
  6. Endocarditis
  7. Histoplasmosis

WORKUP
- Cultures
  1. Blood
  2. Sputum
  3. Skin
  4. See warning under "Laboratory Tests"

- Serum for serology
- Chest x-ray examination
- Skin or other biopsy for fluorescent staining
- Liver function tests
- Renal function tests

LABORATORY TESTS
- CBC
  1. Usually nonspecific
  2. Thrombocytopenia common
  3. ESR variable
- Cultures
  1. Pose extreme danger to laboratory personnel; warn laboratory upon submission
  2. Often unsuccessful except on extremely supportive media containing cystine, thioglycolate, or Thayer-Martin; CO_2 atmosphere
- Serology
  1. More sensitive; especially ELISA, hemagglutination
  2. Both IgM and IgG may persist >10 yr
     a. Need serial rising titers for confirmation
     b. Cross-reaction with *Brucella, Yersinia, Proteus* OX19, heterophile titers
- Direct fluorescent antibody staining of tissue is definitive
- Severe disease
  1. Myoglobinuria
  2. Elevated CPK
  3. Hyponatremia
  4. Elevated creatinine
  5. Hepatitis with elevated ALT
  6. Decreased fibrinogen
  7. Elevated fibrin split products

IMAGING STUDIES
- Chest x-ray examination
  1. Lobar, apical, or miliary infiltrates
  2. Hilar adenopathy
  3. Pleural effusion
  4. Rare cavitation

TREATMENT

ACUTE GENERAL Rx
- Streptomycin is drug of choice (at least 7.5 to 10 mg/kg IM q12h × 7 to 14 days)
- Gentamicin is a suitable alternative
- For meningitis:
  1. Streptomycin plus chloramphenicol

2. Failures reported with
   a. Ceftriaxone
   b. Imipenem
   c. Quinolones
- Higher relapse rates with:
  1. Tetracycline
  2. Chloramphenicol (bacteriostatic)

CHRONIC Rx
Surgical drainage is required for chronic suppurative adenitis.

DISPOSITION
Careful follow-up until adenopathy, pneumonitis, pleural effusions, meningitis completely resolve

REFERRAL
- To infectious disease specialist for all aspects of diagnosis and treatment
- To surgeon for suppurative adenitis, empyema drainage

PEARLS & CONSIDERATIONS

COMMENTS
- Prevention
  1. Avoid exposure
     a. Skinning or handling animals with bare hands (use masks, eyecovers, gloves)
  2. Thoroughly cook wild game before ingestion
  3. Avoid tick and deer-fly exposure
     a. Repellents
     b. Clothing fitting tightly at wrists and ankles
- Person-to-person transmission does not occur
- Live attenuated vaccine
  1. Usually prevents typhoidal form
  2. Modifies but does not prevent other forms
- Streptomycin probably effective for postexposure prophylaxis following definite exposure (e.g., laboratory accidents)
- Considerable protective immunity induced by natural disease

REFERENCE
Ohara Y, Sato T, Homma M: Arthropod-borne tularemia in Japan: clinical analysis of 1,374 cases observed between 1924 and 1996, *J Med Entomol* 35(4):471, 1998.

Author: **Peter Nicholas, M.D.**

BASIC INFORMATION

■ **DEFINITION**

Turner's syndrome refers to a pattern of malformation characterized by short stature, ovarian hypofunction, loose nuchal skin, and cubitus valgus as described by Turner in 1938. An associated 45,X chromosome constitution was recognized by Ford et al in 1959.

■ **SYNONYMS**

All obsolete:
Ullrich-Turner syndrome
Bonnevie-Ullrich-Turner syndrome

ICD-9CM CODES
758.6 Syndrome, Turner's

■ **EPIDEMIOLOGY & DEMOGRAPHICS**

INCIDENCE: 1 case out of every 2500 to 5000 live births

■ **PHYSICAL FINDINGS & CLINICAL PRESENTATION**

- Turner's phenotype is recognizable at any point on the developmental spectrum.
- In spontaneous abortuses the most common sex chromosome abnormality detected (45,X chromosome constitution) is found in 75% of affected individuals and accounts for 20% of such cases.
- In fetuses, it is suspected because of such ultrasonographic manifestations as thickening of the nuchal folds, frank nuchal cystic hygromas, or mild shortness of the femora at midtrimester.
- In infants:
  1. At birth may display loose nuchal skin (pterygium colli) and edema on the dorsa of hands and feet
  2. Canthal folds reflecting midface hypoplasia and redundant skin in the periorbital region
  3. Nipples appearing widely spaced
  4. Heart and cardiovascular system: murmur of aortic stenosis or bicuspid aortic valve or diminished femoral pulses suggestive of aortic coarctation

  5. Renal ultrasonography: renal ectopia such as pelvic kidney or horseshoe kidneys
- In older children:
  1. Slow linear growth
  2. Short stature—may be improved with growth hormone therapy (Fig. 1-380)
  3. Delayed or absent menses—secondary sex characteristics possibly normalized with estrogen replacement therapy
  4. Intelligence is often normal, but delays in spatial perception or visual motor integration are commonly observed; frank mental retardation is rare

■ **ETIOLOGY**

- Phenotype caused by absence of the second sex chromosome, whether X or Y
- 45,X chromosome constitution in about 50% of affected individuals
- Other chromosome aberrations (40% of cases): isochromosome Xq (46,X,i[Xq]) or mosaicism (XX/X)
- With deletions involving the short (or "p") arm of the X chromosome: short stature but little ovarian hypofunction
- Deletions involving Xq13-q27: ovarian failure
- Usually a deficiency of paternal contribution of sex chromosome, reflecting paternal nondisjunction

 DIAGNOSIS

■ **DIFFERENTIAL DIAGNOSIS**

- Noonan syndrome, an autosomally dominant inherited disorder also characterized by loose nuchal skin, midface hypoplasia, canthal folds, and stenotic cardiac valvular defects and affecting males and females equally; also have normal chromosome constitutions
- Other conditions in the differential diagnosis of loose skin, whether or not associated with edema:
  1. Fetal hydantoin syndrome (loose nuchal skin, midface hypoplasia, distal digital hypoplasia)

  2. Disorders of chromosome constitution (trisomy 21, tetrasomy 12p mosaicism)
  3. Congenital lymphedema (Milroy edema)

■ **WORKUP**

- Giemsa banded karyotype to confirm clinical diagnosis
- Once diagnosis is established: cardiologic consultation for evaluation for cardiac valvular abnormalities or aortic coarctation
- Renal ultrasonography
- Endocrine evaluations in older patients with short stature or amenorrhea
- Psychometrics to document known or suspected learning disabilities

■ **LABORATORY TESTS**

- As noted, routine Giemsa banded karyotype on peripheral lymphocytes to confirm the clinical impression in all suspected cases of Turner's syndrome
- Recognition of associated medical problems, such as hypergonadotropic hypogonadism or autoimmune thyroiditis prompting periodic evaluation of these potential areas

■ **IMAGING STUDIES**

- Echocardiogram
- Renal ultrasonography
- Abdominal ultrasonography for evaluation of ovarian and uterine size and morphology
- MRI of brain (especially in cases with known or suspected neurologic impairment)
- Radiographs (for evaluation of carpal/metacarpal abnormalities, radioulnar synostosis)
- Bone age (for evaluation of short stature)

TREATMENT

Recognition of the multisystem involvement of Turner's syndrome necessitates multiple medical specialists working in concert with the primary care provider to maximize and improve outcome while minimizing unnecessary or redundant testing.

■ NONPHARMACOLOGIC THERAPY
General medical care guided by normal medical standards with special attention paid to identifying such age-related problems as developmental delays, learning disabilities, slow growth, or amenorrhea.

■ ACUTE GENERAL Rx
Specific treatment geared to the specific medical problem (e.g., cardiac or renal dysfunction)

■ CHRONIC Rx
- Estrogen replacement therapy in early adolescence
- Some benefit from recombinant human growth hormone therapy

■ REFERRAL
- To geneticist: clinical diagnosis, differential diagnosis, recurrence risk counseling, cytogenetic tests
- To endocrinologist (pediatric): evaluation of short stature, estrogen or growth hormone replacement therapy
- To cardiologist

☼ PEARLS & CONSIDERATIONS

■ COMMENTS
- Although newer studies are optimistic regarding outcomes, previous reports suffered from retrospective observations, case reports, and ascertainment bias, contributing to a generally poor interaction between physician and patient.

- Affected individuals and families often benefit from the contemporary experiences and expertise of members of genetic support groups. The Turner Syndrome Association (phone: 612-379-3607 or 800-365-9944; Internet: http://www.turner-syndrome-us.org) and the Alliance of Genetic Support Groups (phone: 800-336-4363; Internet: http://medhelp.org/www/agsg.htm) are valuable resources.
Author: **Luther K. Robinson, M.D.**

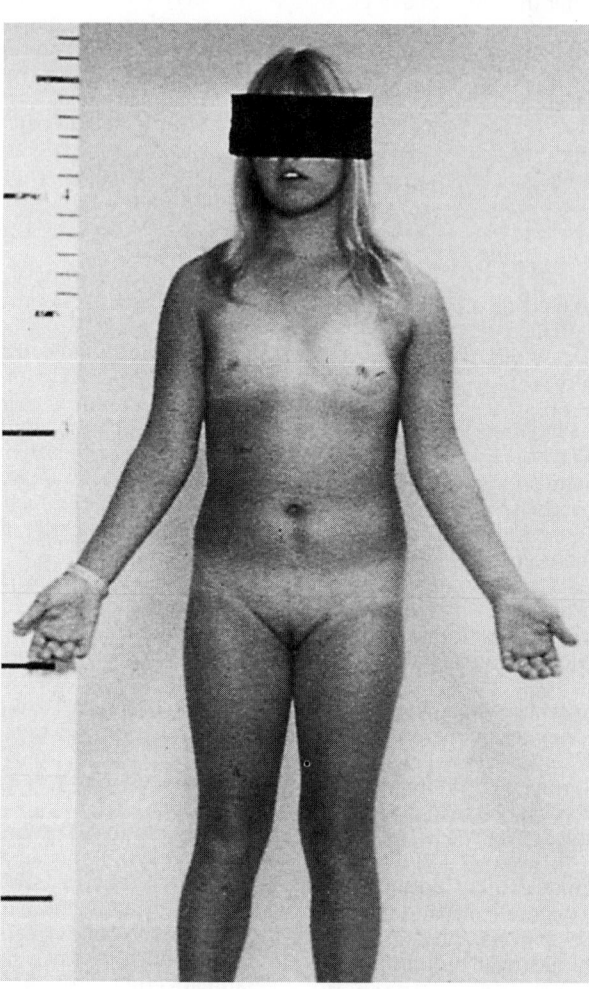

Fig. 1-380 A 17-year-old patient with Turner's syndrome demonstrating short stature, poor sexual development, and increased carrying angles at elbows. Patient also has webbing of the neck. (From Mishell D [ed]: *Comprehensive gynecology,* ed 3, St Louis, 1997, Mosby.)

BASIC INFORMATION

■ **DEFINITION**
Typhoid fever is a systemic infection caused by *Salmonella typhi*.

■ **SYNONYMS**
Typhoid
Enteric fever

■ **ICD-9CM CODES**
002.0 Typhoid fever

■ **EPIDEMIOLOGY & DEMOGRAPHICS**
INCIDENCE (IN U.S.): Approximately 500 cases of *S. typhi* infections are reported annually.

■ **PHYSICAL FINDINGS & CLINICAL PRESENTATION**
• Incubation period of a few days to several weeks
• Usual manifestations
  1. Prolonged fever
  2. Myalgias
  3. Headache
  4. Cough
  5. Sore throat
  6. Malaise
  7. Anorexia, at times with abdominal pain and hepatosplenomegaly
  8. Diarrhea or constipation may occur early in the course of illness.
  9. Rose spots, which are faint, maculopapular, blanching lesions, may sometimes be seen on the chest or abdomen.
• In the untreated patient, fever may last 1 to 2 mo. The main complication of untreated disease is GI bleeding as a result of perforation from ulceration of Peyer's patches in the ileum. Mental status changes and shock are rare complications. The relapse rate is approximately 10%.

■ **ETIOLOGY**
• *Salmonella typhi*
• *S. paratyphi*
• *S. typhi* or *S. paratyphi* found only in humans
• Acquisition of disease by ingestion of food or water contaminated by other humans
• In the U.S. most cases are acquired either during foreign travel or by ingestion of food prepared by chronic carriers, many of whom acquired the organism outside of the U.S.

DIAGNOSIS

■ **DIFFERENTIAL DIAGNOSIS**
• Malaria
• Tuberculosis
• Brucellosis
• Amebic liver abscess

■ **WORKUP**
• Blood, stool, and urine cultures are helpful.
• Cultures should be repeated if initially negative.
• Blood cultures are more likely to be positive early in the course of illness.
• Stool and urine cultures are more commonly positive in the second and third weeks of illness.
• Bone marrow biopsy cultures are 90% positive, although this procedure is usually not necessary.
• Serology using Widal test is helpful in retrospect, showing a fourfold increase in convalescent titers.

■ **LABORATORY TESTS**
• Neutropenia is common.
• Transaminitis is possible.
• Culture:
  1. Blood
  2. Body fluids
  3. Biopsy specimens

TREATMENT

■ **ACUTE GENERAL Rx**
• Ciprofloxacin 500 mg PO bid or 400 mg IV bid for 14 days
• Ceftriaxone 2 g IV qd for 14 days
• If organism sensitive
  1. SMX/TMP, 1 to 2 DS tabs PO bid *or*
  2. Amoxicillin, 2 g PO q8h to complete 14 days
• Dexamethasone, 3 mg IV initially, followed by 1 mg IV q6h for 8 doses for patients with shock or mental status changes

■ **CHRONIC Rx**
• Carrier states possible
• More common in age >60 yr and in persons with gallstones
• Usual site of colonization: gallbladder
• Treatment in those with persistently positive stool cultures and in food-handlers
• Suggested regimens for eradication of carrier state
  1. Ciprofloxacin 500 mg PO bid for 4 wk
  2. SMX/TMP 1 to 2 tabs PO bid for 6 wk (if susceptible)

  3. Amoxicillin, 2 g PO q8h for 6 wk (if susceptible)
• Cholecystectomy possibly required in carriers with gallstones who fail medical therapy

■ **DISPOSITION**
• Treated patients usually respond to therapy, with a small percentage becoming chronic carriers.
• The relapse rate is approximately 10%.
• Untreated patients may have serious complications.

■ **REFERRAL**
• Failure of therapy
• Chronic carrier

PEARLS & CONSIDERATIONS

■ **COMMENTS**
• Oral and parenteral vaccines are available for travelers to areas of high risk.
• Vaccines are about 70% effective.
• Immunity wanes after several years.
• Parenteral preparations are accompanied by frequent side effects:
  1. Pain at injection site
  2. Fever
  3. Malaise
  4. Headaches

REFERENCES
Ackers ML et al: Laboratory-based surveillance of *Salmonella* serotype *typhi* infections in the United States: antimicrobial resistance on the rise, *JAMA* 283(20):2668, 2000.

Guerrant RL, Kosek M: Polysaccharide conjugate typhoid vaccine, *N Engl J Med* 344(17):1322, 2001.

Hoffer RJ et al: Emergency department presentations of typhoid fever, *J Emerg Med* 19(4):317, 2000.

Koul PA: A *Salmonella typhi* Vi conjugate vaccine, *N Engl J Med* 345(7):545, 2001.

O'Brien D et al: Fever in returned travelers: review of hospital admissions for a 3-year period, *Clin Infect Dis* 33(50):603, 2001.

Yang HH et al: An outbreak of typhoid fever, Xing-An County, People's Republic of China, 1999: estimation of the field effectiveness of Vi polysaccharide typhoid vaccine, *J Infect Dis* 183(15):1775, 2001.

Author: **Maurice Policar, M.D.**

BASIC INFORMATION

■ DEFINITION
Ulcerative colitis is a chronic inflammatory bowel disease of undetermined etiology.

■ SYNONYMS
Inflammatory bowel disease (IBD)
Idiopathic proctocolitis

■ ICD-9CM CODES
556.9 Ulcerative colitis

■ EPIDEMIOLOGY & DEMOGRAPHICS
INCIDENCE:
- 50 to 150 cases/100,000 persons; most common between age 14 and 38 yr.
- Appendectomy for an inflammatory condition (appendicitis or lymphadenitis) but not for nonspecific abdominal pain is associated with a low risk of subsequent ulcerative colitis. This inverse relation is limited to patients who undergo surgery before the age of 20 yr.

■ PHYSICAL FINDINGS & CLINICAL PRESENTATION
- Abdominal distention and tenderness
- Bloody diarrhea
- Fever, evidence of dehydration
- Evidence of extraintestinal manifestations may be present: liver disease, sclerosing cholangitis, iritis, uveitis, episcleritis, arthritis, erythema nodosum, pyoderma gangrenosum, aphthous stomatitis

DIAGNOSIS

■ DIFFERENTIAL DIAGNOSIS
- Crohn's disease
- Bacterial infections
  1. Acute: *Campylobacter, Yersinia, Salmonella, Shigella, Chlamydia, Escherichia coli, Clostridium difficile,* gonococcal proctitis
  2. Chronic: Whipple's disease, TB, enterocolitis
- Irritable bowel syndrome
- Protozoal and parasitic infections (amebiasis, giardiasis, cryptosporidiosis)
- Neoplasm (intestinal lymphoma, carcinoma of colon)
- Ischemic bowel disease
- Diverticulitis
- Celiac sprue, collagenous colitis, radiation enteritis, endometriosis, gay bowel syndrome

■ WORKUP
Patients with ulcerative colitis often present with bloody diarrhea accompanied by tenesmus, fever, dehydration, weight loss, anorexia, nausea, and abdominal pain. Diagnostic workup includes:
- Comprehensive history, physical examination
- Laboratory and radiographic studies
- Sigmoidoscopy to establish the presence of mucosal inflammation: typical endoscopic findings in ulcerative colitis are friable mucosa, diffuse, uniform erythema replacing the usual mucosal vascular pattern, and pseudopolyps; rectal involvement is invariably present if the disease is active

■ LABORATORY TESTS
- Anemia, high sedimentation rate (in severe colitis) are common.
- Potassium, magnesium, calcium, albumin may be decreased.
- Antineutrophil cytoplasmic antibodies (ANCA) with a perinuclear staining pattern (pANCA) can be found in >45% of patients; there is an increased frequency in treatment-resistant left-sided colitis, suggesting a possible association between these antibodies and a relative resistance to medical therapy in patients with ulcerative colitis.

■ IMAGING STUDIES
Air-contrast barium enema may reveal continuous involvement (including the rectum), pseudopolyps, decreased mucosal pattern, and fine superficial ulcerations.

TREATMENT

■ NONPHARMACOLOGIC THERAPY
- Correct nutritional deficiencies; TPN with bowel rest may be necessary in severe cases; folate supplementation may reduce the incidence of dysplasia and cancer in chronic ulcerative colitis.
- Avoid oral feedings during acute exacerbation to decrease colonic activity; a low-roughage diet may be helpful in *early* relapse.
- Psychotherapy is useful in most patients. Referral to self-help groups is also important because of the chronicity of the disease and the young age of the patients.

■ ACUTE GENERAL Rx
The therapeutic options vary with the degree of disease (mild, severe, fulminant) and areas of involvement (distal, extensive):
- Mild or moderate disease can be treated with an oral aminosalicylate (e.g., sulfasalazine 500 mg PO bid initially, increased qd or qod by 1 g until therapeutic doses of 4 to 6 g/day are achieved); distal colitis can be treated with mesalamine (5-aminosalicylic acid) enemas 4 g (60 ml) at hs or steroid retention enemas.
- Severe disease usually responds to oral corticosteroids (e.g., prednisone 40 to 60 mg/day); corticosteroid suppositories or enemas are also useful for distal colitis.
- Fulminant disease generally requires hospital admission and parenteral corticosteroids (e.g., IV hydrocortisone 100 mg q6h); when bowel movements have returned to normal and the patient is able to eat normally, oral prednisone is resumed. IV cyclosporine can also be used in severe refractory cases; renal toxicity is a potential complication.
- Surgery is indicated in patients who fail to respond to intensive medical therapy. Colectomy is usually curative in these patients and also eliminates the high risk of developing adenocarcinoma of the colon (10% to 20% of patients develop it after 10 yr with the disease); newer surgical techniques allow for the preservation of the sphincter.

■ CHRONIC Rx
- Colonoscopic surveillance and multiple biopsies should be instituted approximately 10 yr after diagnosis because of the increased risk of colon carcinoma.
- Erythropoietin is useful in patients with anemia refractory to treatment with iron and vitamins.

■ DISPOSITION
The clinical course is variable; 15% to 20% of patients will eventually require colectomy; >75% of patients treated medically will experience relapse.

■ REFERRAL
- GI consultation for initial diagnostic sigmoidoscopy/colonoscopy in suspected cases
- Surgical referral for patients with severe disease unresponsive to medical therapy

REFERENCES
Andersson RG et al: Appendectomy and protection against ulcerative colitis, *N Engl J Med* 344:808, 2001.
D'Haens G et al: IV Cyclosporine versus IV corticosteroids as single therapy for severe attacks of ulcerative colitis, *Gastroenterology* 120:1323, 2001.
Author: **Fred F. Ferri, M.D.**

BASIC INFORMATION

■ DEFINITION
Urethritis is a well-defined clinical syndrome manifested by dysuria, a urethral discharge, or both.

■ ICD-9CM CODES
597.80 Urethritis, unspecified
098.20 Gonococcal

■ EPIDEMIOLOGY & DEMOGRAPHICS
• The major single specific etiology of acute urethritis is *Neisseria gonorrhoeae,* producing GCU. Urethritis of all other etiologies is called *nongonococcal urethritis* (NGU).
• NGU is twice as common as GCU in the U.S. NGU is the most common STD syndrome occurring in men, accounting for 6 million office visits annually. NGU is more frequently encountered in higher socioeconomic groups. GCU is more common in homosexual males than heterosexual males with acute urethritis.
• The gonococcus is a gram-negative, kidney-shaped diplococcus with flattened opposed margins. The urethra is the most common site of infection in all men. In heterosexual men, the pharynx is infected in 7%, and in homosexual men, the pharynx is infected in 40% and the rectum in 25%. A single episode of intercourse with an infected partner carries a transmission risk of 20% for males; female partners of an infected male will contract the disease 80% of the time.

■ PHYSICAL FINDINGS & CLINICAL PRESENTATION
SYMPTOMS OF GONOCOCCAL URETHRITIS: Urethral discharge (see Fig. 1-381 in "Urethritis, Nongonococcal") and dysuria are the most common symptoms. There is complaint of urethral itching. Prostatic involvement can cause frequency, urgency, and nocturia. It can involve the epididymis through spreading down the vas deferens, causing acute epididymitis.
INCUBATION PERIOD: 3 to 10 days. Without treatment urethritis persists for 3 to 7 wk, with 95% of men becoming asymptomatic after 3 mo. GCU is asymptomatic in up to 60% of contacts.

SIGNS OF GONOCOCCAL URETHRITIS: Yellow-brown discharge, meatal edema, urethral tenderness to palpation. Rectal bleeding with pus is seen with gonococcal proctitis. Periurethritis leading to urethral stenosis can occur. Disseminated infection can occur. Tenosynovitis and arthritis can occur. Rarely, hepatitis, myocarditis, endocarditis, and meningitis can occur.

DIAGNOSIS

■ DIFFERENTIAL DIAGNOSIS
• NGU
• Herpes simplex virus

■ LABORATORY TESTS
• Calcium alginate or rayon swab on a metal shaft (*not* cotton-tipped swabs, which are bactericidal) of the urethra should be done anywhere from 2 to 4 hr after voiding to prevent bacterial washout with voiding.
• Cultures of the pharynx and rectum when indicated.
• Gram staining should be done. Modified Thayer-Martin media is used.
• On examination of the urethral smear, the presence of small numbers of PMNs provides objective evidence of urethritis. The complete absence of PMNs on a urethral smear argues against urethritis. If in addition to the PMNs there are gram-negative, intracellular diplococci, the diagnosis of gonorrhea is established.

TREATMENT

■ NONPHARMACOLOGIC THERAPY
BEHAVIORAL MANAGEMENT: Avoid intercourse until cure has been attained and sexual partners have been evaluated and treated.

■ ACUTE GENERAL RX
FOR UNCOMPLICATED URETHRAL, CERVICAL, AND RECTAL GCU: Ceftriaxone 125 mg IM + doxycycline 100 mg bid × 7 days. Alternative therapy: ciprofloxacin 500 mg PO × 1 day; ofloxacin 400 mg PO × 1 day (all of these to be followed by 7 days of doxycycline 100 mg PO bid).

• In uncomplicated gonococcal infections, single-drug regimens using selected fluoroquinolones, selected cephalosporins, or spectinomycin are highly effective and safe.
• Resistance to penicillins, sulphonamides, and tetracyclines is now widespread.
• Dual treatment for gonococcal and chlamydial infections is based on theory and expert opinion rather than on evidence from clinical trials.
FOR EPIDIDYMITIS: Ceftriaxone 250 mg IM followed by doxycycline 100 mg PO bid × 10 days. Alternative therapy: ofloxacin 300 mg PO bid × 10 days.

■ CHRONIC Rx
POSTGONOCOCCAL URETHRITIS (PGU): Reinfection is the most common cause of recurrence. Repeat swab and culture of the urethra, pharynx, and rectum (where applicable) are mandatory. Persistence of PMNs with the absence of gram-negative intracellular diplococci suggests a diagnosis of postgonococcal urethritis. This occurs when GCU is treated with a regimen that is ineffective against coincident chlamydial infection; it represents NGU following GCU. The syndrome should be treated as NGU. Persistence of *N. gonorrhoeae* by smear or culture requires treatment for *N. gonorrhoeae.*

PEARLS & CONSIDERATIONS

■ COMMENTS
• CAUTION: Tetracyclines and fluoroquinolones are *contraindicated* in pregnancy. *Chlamydia* infection in pregnancy can be treated with amoxicillin 500 mg PO tid for 7 days or with clindamycin 450 mg PO tid for 10 days.
• *Posttreatment cultures are required.*

REFERENCE
Centers for Disease Control and Prevention: Sexually transmitted diseases treatment guidelines, *MMWR* 47(RR-1), 1998.
Author: **Philip J. Aliotta, M.D., M.S.H.A.**

BASIC INFORMATION

■ DEFINITION
Nongonococcal urethritis is urethral inflammation caused by any of several organisms.

■ SYNONYMS
NGU

ICD-9CM CODES
099.40 Nongonococcal
099.41 Chlamydial

■ EPIDEMIOLOGY & DEMOGRAPHICS
- Occurrence is 50% in STD clinics.
- Most commonly affects men in higher socioeconomic class, affecting heterosexual men more frequently than homosexual men.
- NGU carries a greater morbidity than GCU.

■ ETIOLOGY
- Most common agent is *Chlamydia* spp., an obligate intracellular parasite possessing both DNA and RNA, replicating by binary fission. It causes 20% to 50% of NGU cases. Two species exist:
  1. *Chlamydia psittaci*
  2. *Chlamydia trachomatis* with its 15 serotypes
     a. Serotypes A-C cause hyperendemic blinding trachoma.
     b. Serotypes D-K cause genital tract infection.
     c. Serotypes L1-L3 cause lymphogranuloma venereum.
- Other causes of NGU: *Ureaplasma urealyticum* causing 15% to 30% of the cases of NGU, *Trichomonas vaginalis,* and herpes simplex virus. The cause of 20% of the cases of NGU has not been identified.
- Asymptomatic infection occurs in 28% of the contacts of women with chlamydial cervical infection.

INCUBATION PERIOD: 2 to 35 days
SYMPTOMS: Dysuria, whitish-to-clear urethral discharge (Fig. 1-381), and urethral itching. The onset of symptoms in NGU is less acute than GCU.
SIGNS: Whitish-to-clear urethral discharge, meatal edema, and erythema. Infected women manifest pyuria, and the disease can present as acute urethral syndrome.
COMPLICATIONS: Epididymitis in heterosexual men may be linked to nonbacterial prostatitis, proctitis in homosexual men, and Reiter's syndrome.

DIAGNOSIS

■ DIFFERENTIAL DIAGNOSIS
- GCU
- Herpes simplex virus
- Trichomoniasis

■ LABORATORY TESTS
- Requires demonstration of urethritis and exclusion of infection with *N. gonorrhoeae.*
- The appearance of PMNs on urethral smear confirms the diagnosis of urethritis. Because *Chlamydia* is an intracellular parasite of the columnar epithelium, the best specimen for culture is an endourethral swab taken from an area 2 to 4 cm inside the urethra. The organism can only be grown in tissue culture, which is expensive.
- New techniques have been developed and are useful in making the diagnosis: nucleic acid hybridization, enzyme-linked immunosorbent assay (ELISA), and direct immunofluorescence.
- For culture, a Dacron-tipped swab is used; avoid calcium alginate or cotton swabs.

TREATMENT

Because it is impossible to differentiate among the common etiologies of NGU, the condition is treated syndromically, including in the initial treatment regimen those drugs effective against the common causative agents.
- Recommended: doxycycline 100 mg PO bid for 7 days
- Other drugs: tetracycline 500 mg PO qid for 7 days
- Alternative regimens: azithromycin 1000 mg as a single dose, erythromycin 500 mg PO qid for 7 days, ofloxacin 300 mg PO bid for 7 days
In pregnant women:
- Both amoxicillin and erythromycin are likely effective in achieving microbiological cure

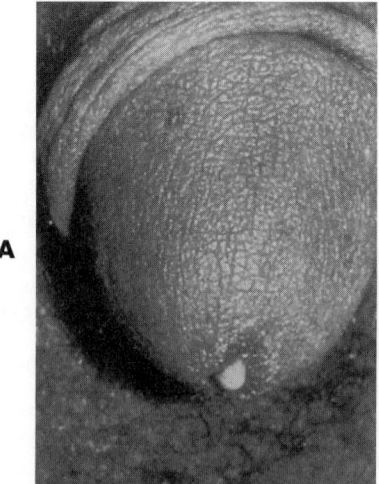
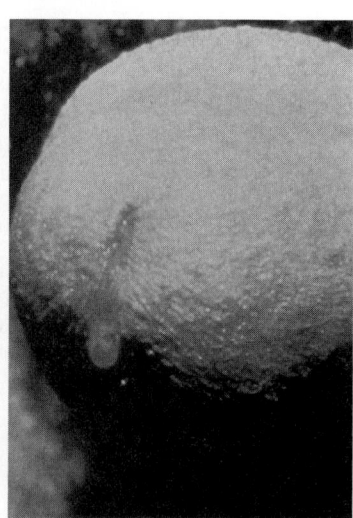

Fig. 1-381 Urethritis in men. Gonococcal urethritis classically produces a profuse and purulent discharge **(A),** whereas nongonococcal urethritis more often results in scant mucoid discharge **(B).** (From Noble J [ed]: *Primary care medicine,* ed 2, St Louis, 1996, Mosby.)

- Clindamycin and erythromycin have a similar effect on cure rates
- A single dose of azithromycin is more effective in achieving microbiological cure of *C. trachomatis* than a 7-day course of erythromycin

In men and nonpregnant women:
- Multiple-dose regimens of tetracyclines and macrolides achieve microbiological cure in at least 95% of patients
- Erythromycin daily dose of 2 g is likely beneficial
- Ciprofloxacin is less effective in the treatment of *C. trachomatis* infection when compared with doxycycline
- A single dose of azithromycin is as successful at curing *C. trachomatis* as a 7-day course of doxycycline

PEARLS & CONSIDERATIONS

COMMENTS
- CAUTION: Tetracyclines and fluoroquinolones are *contraindicated* in pregnancy. *Chlamydia* infection in pregnancy can be treated with amoxicillin 500 mg PO tid for 7 days or with clindamycin 450 mg PO tid for 10 days.
- *Posttreatment cultures are required.*

REFERENCE
Gaydos CA et al: *Chlamydia trachomatis* infections in female military recruits, *N Engl J Med* 339:739, 1998.
Author: **Philip J. Aliotta, M.D., M.S.H.A.**

I

BASIC INFORMATION

■ DEFINITION

Urinary tract infection (UTI) is a term that encompasses a broad range of clinical entities that have in common a positive urine culture. A conventional threshold is growth of >100,000 colony-forming units per ml from a midstream-catch urine sample. In symptomatic patients, a smaller number of bacteria (between 100 and 10,000 colony-forming units per ml of midstream urine) is recognized as an infection.

■ SYNONYMS

UTI

ICD-9CM CODES

595.0 Acute cystitis
595.3 Trigonitis
595.2 Chronic cystitis
590.1 Acute pyelonephritis
590.0 Chronic pyelonephritis
590.8 Nonspecific pyelonephritis

■ CLASSIFICATION

FIRST INFECTION: The first documented UTI; tends to be uncomplicated and is easily treated.

UNRESOLVED BACTERIURIA: UTI in which the urinary tract is not sterilized during therapy. Main causes are bacterial resistance, patient noncompliance with medication, resistance, mixed bacterial infection, rapid reinfection, azotemia, and infected stones.

BACTERIAL PERSISTENCE: UTI in which the urine cultures become sterile during therapy but a persistent source of infection from a site within the urinary tract that was excluded from the high urinary concentrations gives rise to reinfection by the same organism. Causes: infected stone, chronic bacterial prostatitis, atrophic infected kidney, vesicovaginal or enterovesical fistulas, obstructive uropa-

thy, infected pyelocalyceal diverticula, infected ureteral stump following nephrectomy, infected necrotic papillae from papillary necrosis, infected urachal cysts, infected medullary sponge kidney, urethral diverticula, and foreign bodies.

REINFECTION: UTI in which a new infection occurs with new pathogens at variable intervals after a previous infection has been eradicated.

Relapse: the less common form of recurrent infection; occurs within 2 wk of treatment when the same organism reappears in the same site as the previous infection. Relapsing infections of the urinary tract most commonly occur in pyelonephritis, kidney obstruction from a stone, and prostatitis.

■ EPIDEMIOLOGY & DEMOGRAPHICS

INCIDENCE:

In Neonates: More common in boys as a result of anatomic abnormalities.

In Preschool Children: More common in girls (4.5% vs. 0.5% for boys).

In Adulthood: More common in women, with a 1% to 3% prevalence in nonpregnant women. In pregnancy at 12 wk, the incidence of asymptomatic bacteriuria is similar to nonpregnant women, at 2% to 10%. However, 70% to 80% of women with asymptomatic bacteriuria develop acute pyelonephritis, especially in the second and third trimesters, and suffer a pyelonephritic recurrence rate of 10%. In adults, 65 yr and older, at least 10% of men and 20% of women have bacteriuria.

PATHOGENESIS:

- Four major pathways:
  1. Ascending from the urethra
  2. Lymphatic
  3. Hematogenous
  4. Direct extension from another organ system.
- Other risk factors: neurologic diseases, renal failure, diabetes; anatomic abnormalities: bladder

outlet obstruction, urethral stricture, vesicoureteral reflux, fistula, urinary diversion, megacystis, and infected stones; age; pregnancy; instrumentation, poor patient compliance, poor hygiene, infrequent voider, diaphragm contraceptives, tampon use, douches, and catheters

Catheters: All patients who require a long-term Foley catheter eventually develop significant levels of bacteriuria. Treatment is reserved for those individuals who become symptomatic (i.e., leukocytosis, fever, chills, malaise, loss of appetite, etc.) Using prophylactic antibiotics to treat patients who have chronic catheters is to be discouraged because of the risk of acquiring bacteria that are resistant to antibiotic therapy.

- Once bacteria reach the urinary tract, three factors determine whether the infection occurs (Box 1-27):
  1. Virulence of the microorganism
  2. Inoculum size
  3. Adequacy of the host defense mechanisms
- These factors also determine the anatomic level of the UTI.

Urinary Pathogens: In >95% of UTIs the infecting organism is a member of the Enterobacteriaceae, *Pseudomonas aeruginosa,* enterococci, or, in young women, *Staphylococcus saprophyticus.* In contrast, the organisms that commonly colonize the distal urethra and skin of both men and women and the vagina of women are *Staphylococcus epidermidis,* diphtheroids, lactobacilli, *Gardnerella vaginalis,* and a variety of anaerobes that rarely cause UTI. Generally, the isolation of two or more bacterial species from a urine culture signifies a contaminated specimen, unless the patient is being managed with a indwelling catheter or urinary diversion or has a chronic complicated infection.

BOX 1-27 Bacterial Factors

1. The size of the inoculum
2. The virulence of the infecting organism:
   a. Virulence factors:
      i. P-fimbriae facilitate the adherence of bacteria to biologic surfaces.
      ii. K-antigens facilitate adherence and protect the organisms from the host-immune response.
      iii. O-antigens are an important source of the systemic reactions, such as fever and shock, that occur with bacterial infections.
      iv. H antigens are associated with flagella and are related to bacterial locomotion.
      v. Hemolysin may potentiate tissue damage and facilitate local bacterial growth.
      vi. Urease alkalinizes the urine and facilitates stone formation, thus potentiating infection.
   b. Biofilms harbor bacteria on prosthetic devices and may be a source of recurrent infections.
   c. The presence of sialosyl galactosyl globoside (SGG) on the surface of kidney cells. This compound is a highly powerful receptor for *E. coli* bacteria.
   d. Women with a deficiency in human beta-defensin-1 (HBD-1) are at greater risk for urinary tract infection.
3. Adequacy of host defense mechanisms

Defense Mechanisms Against Cystitis:
Low pH and high osmolarity, mucopolysaccharide glycosaminoglycan protective layer, normal bladder that empties completely and has no incontinence, and the presence of estrogen

■ PHYSICAL FINDINGS
- UTI presentation is inconsistent and cannot be relied upon to diagnose UTI accurately or to localize the site of infection. Patients complain of:
  1. Urinary frequency, urgency
  2. Dysuria
  3. Urge incontinence
  4. Suprapubic pain
  5. Gross or microscopic hematuria
- When negative cultures are associated with significant pyuria, vaginal discharge, or hematuria, infections with *Chlamydia trachomatis, Neisseria gonorrhoeae,* and *Trichomonas vaginalis* should be considered.
- Acute pyelonephritis (PN) presents with fever, flank or abdominal pain, chills, malaise, vomiting, and diarrhea. It is these systemic symptoms that distinguish pyelonephritis from cystitis. Complications of acute pyelonephritis are renal abscess, perinephric abscess, emphysematous pyelonephritis, and pyonephrosis.

DIAGNOSIS

■ DIFFERENTIAL DIAGNOSIS
- Interstitial cystitis
- Vaginitis
- Urethritis (gonococcal, nongonococcal, *Trichomonas*)
- Frequency-urgency syndrome, prostatitis (acute and chronic)
- Obstructive uropathy
- Infected stones
- Fistulas
- Papillary necrosis
- Vesicoureteral reflux

■ LABORATORY TESTS
- Urinalysis with microscopic evaluation of clean-catch urine for bacteria and pyuria
- Urine C&S
- CBC with differential (shows leukocytosis)
- Antibody-coated bacteria are seen with pyelonephritis

■ IMAGING STUDIES
- Warranted only if renal infection or genitourinary abnormality is suspected
- KUB, VCUG, renal sonogram, IVP, CT scan, and nuclear scan
- Specialty examination: cystoscopy with occasional retrograde pyelography to rule out obstructive uropathy; stenting the obstruction possibly required

℞ TREATMENT

■ NONPHARMACOLOGIC THERAPY
- Hot sitz baths, anticholinergics, urinary analgesics
- For pyelonephritis: bed rest, analgesics, antipyretics, and IV hydration

■ ACUTE GENERAL Rx
- Conventional therapy of 7 days; short-term therapy of 1, 3, or 5 days.
- Agents of choice: amoxicillin/clavulanate, cephalosporins, fluoroquinolones, nitrofurantoin, and trimethoprim with sulfonamide.
- For pyelonephritis: hospitalization until afebrile and stable, then at home via home care agency with IV antibiotic comprised of aminoglycoside plus cephalosporin × 1 wk followed by oral agents (based on sensitivity) for 2 wk. Moderate forms of pyelonephritis have been successfully treated with fluoroquinolone therapy for 21 days, without requiring hospitalization. Most important, complicating factors such as obstructive uropathy or infected stones must be identified and treated.
- Fig. 1-382 describes an approach to the management of UTI.

☼ PEARLS & CONSIDERATIONS

■ COMMENTS
- *Asymptomatic bacteriuria:* occurs in both anatomically normal and abnormal urinary tracts. This can clear spontaneously, persist, or lead to symptomatic kidney infection. Treatment is recommended in patients with vesicoureteral reflux, stones, obstructive uropathy, parenchymal renal disease, diabetes mellitus, and pregnant or immunocompromised patients.
- *Pregnancy:* 20% to 40% of pregnant women with untreated bacteriuria develop pyelonephritis. This is associated with prematurity and low-birth-weight infants. Confirmed significant bacteriuria should be treated with an aminopenicillin and cephalosporin.
- *Recurrent UTI:* caused by an unresolved infection, vaginal colonization of the originally infecting organism, or reinfection with a new strain. Management of recurrent UTI includes continuous antibiotic prophylaxis, intermittent self-treatment, and postcoital prophylaxis. Prophylaxis is recommended for women who experience two or more symptomatic UTIs over a 6-mo period or three or more episodes over a 12-mo period.
  1. Changes after menopause: lower levels of lactobacilli, decreased estrogen, senile atrophy of the genitalia, and loss of bladder elasticity (compliance).

2. Biologic factors altering defense systems: the presence of sialosyl galactosyl globoside (SGG) on the surface of the kidney acts as a powerful receptor for *E. coli* and increases the risk for UTI; the presence of the blood group P1 causes increased binding of *E. coli* that is resistant to normal infection-fighting mechanisms in the body and it is believed that some individuals are deficient in a compound called *human beta-defensin-1* (HBD-1), a naturally occurring antibiotic that fights *E. coli* within the urinary tract.

Resistance:
- Because of the overuse of antibiotics, organisms once sensitive to a number of agents are now increasingly more resistant, making effective management of UTI and pyelonephritis more difficult and potentially more dangerous. Most important has been the increasing resistance to trimethoprim sulfamethoxazole (TMP-SMX), the current primary care provider drug of choice for acute uncomplicated UTI in women.
- Facts about bacterial resistance:
  1. Given enough antibiotic and time, resistance will develop
  2. Organisms that are resistant to one antibiotic will likely become resistant to others
  3. Resistance is progressive, moving from low to intermediate to high levels
  4. Once selected, drug resistance will not disappear; because of poorly reversible genetic and environmental factors, it may decline slowly
  5. When antibiotics are used by any patient, this use affects other people by changing the immediate and extended environment
  6. No counterselective steps against resistant bacteria now exist
- When choosing a treatment regimen physicians should consider such factors as:
  1. In-vitro susceptibility
  2. Adverse effects
  3. Cost effectiveness
  4. Resistance rates in the respective communities

REFERENCES
Gupta K et al: Increasing antimicrobial resistance and the management of uncomplicated community-acquired urinary tract infections, *Ann Int Med* 135:41, 2001.

Levy SB: Multidrug resistance—a sign of the times, *N Engl J Med* 338:1376, 1998 [editorial].

Saint S et al: The effectiveness of a clinical practical guideline for the management of presumed uncomplicated UTI in women, *Am J Med* 106:636, 1999.
Author: **Philip J. Aliotta, M.D., M.S.H.A.**

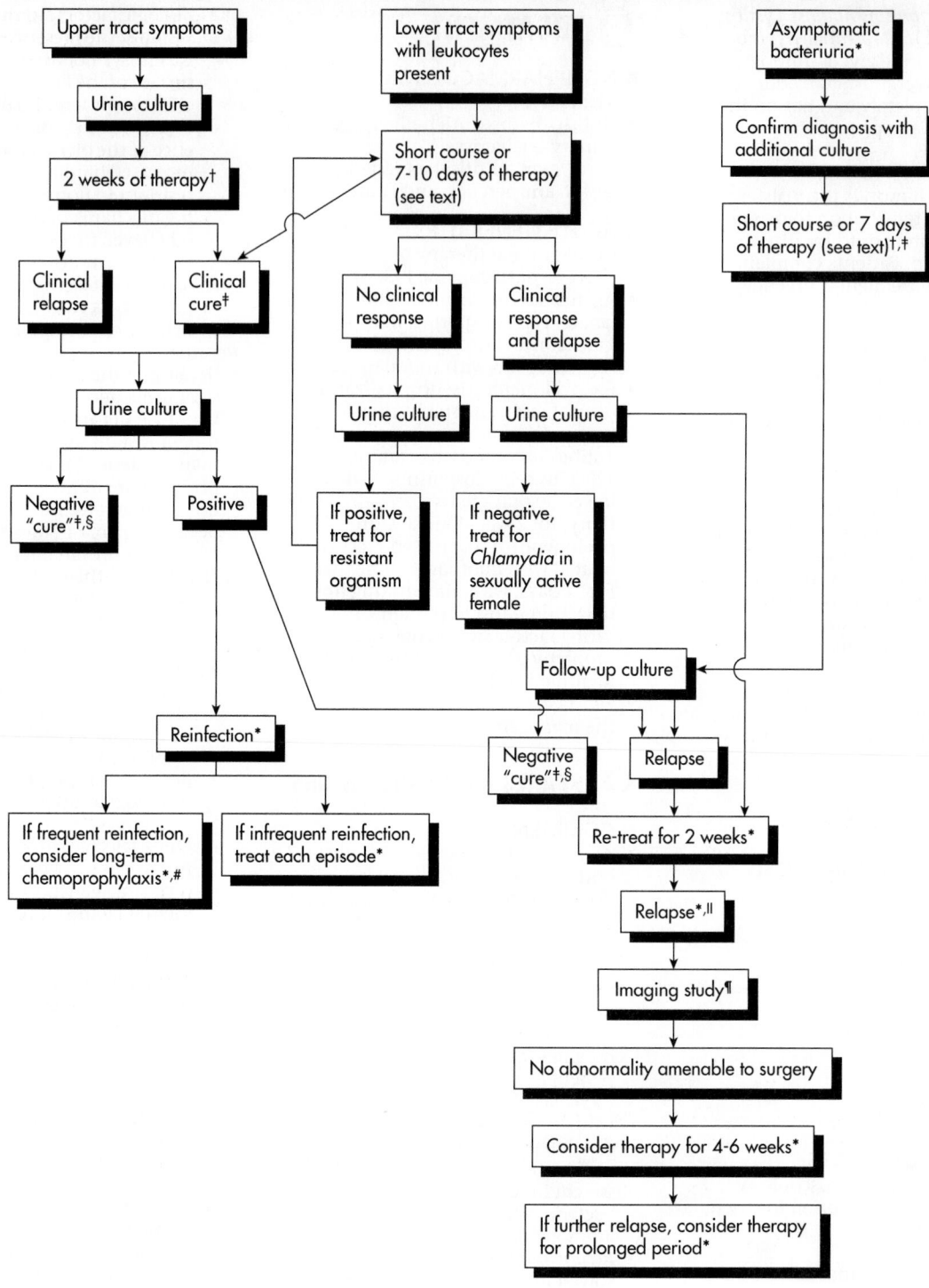

* Consider no therapy in nonpregnant adults without obstructive uropathy or symptoms of urinary tract infection.
† Consider imaging studies in all children and men with correction of significant lesions.
‡ Follow-up culture is required only in pregnancy, in children, and in adults with obstructive uropathy.
§ Obtain follow-up cultures monthly in pregnant women and at 6 weeks and 6 months in children.
‖ Evaluate men for chronic bacterial prostatitis.
¶ Delay 2 months postpartum in pregnant women.
# Consider imaging studies after three to four reinfections in women.

Fig. 1-382   Approach to the management of urinary tract infection. (From Mandell GL: *Mandell, Douglas, and Bennett's principles and practice of infectious diseases,* ed 5, New York, 2000, Churchill Livingstone.)

BASIC INFORMATION

■ DEFINITION
Urolithiasis is the presence of calculi within the urinary tract. The five major types of urinary stones are calcium oxalate (>50%), calcium phosphate (10% to 20%), uric acid (8%), struvite (15%), and cystine (3%).

■ SYNONYMS
Nephrolithiasis
Renal colic

ICD-9CM CODES
592.9 Urinary calculus

■ EPIDEMIOLOGY & DEMOGRAPHICS
- Urinary stone disease afflicts 250,000 to 750,000 Americans/yr.
- Male:female ratio is 4:1. After the sixth decade, the ratio is 1.5:1.
- Incidence of symptomatic nephrolithiasis is greatest during the summer (resulting from increased humidity and temperatures with increased risk of dehydration and concentrated urine).
- Calcium oxalate or mixed calcium oxalate/calcium phosphate stones account for 70% of urolithiasis.

■ PHYSICAL FINDINGS & CLINICAL PRESENTATION
Stones may be asymptomatic or may cause the following signs and symptoms from obstruction:
- Sudden onset of flank tenderness
- Nausea and vomiting
- Patient in constant movement, attempting to lessen the pain (patients with an acute abdomen are usually still because movement exacerbates the pain)
- Pain may be referred to the testes or labium (progression of stone down the urinary ureter)
- Fever and chills accompanying the acute colic if there is superimposed infection
- Pain may radiate anteriorly over to the abdomen and result in intestinal ileus

■ ETIOLOGY
- Increased absorption of calcium in the small bowel: type I absorptive hypercalciuria (independent of calcium intake)
- Increased dietary calcium: type II absorptive hypercalciuria
- Increased vitamin D synthesis (e.g., secondary to renal phosphate loss: type III absorptive hypercalciuria)
- Renal tubular malfunction with inadequate reabsorption of calcium and resulting hypercalciuria

- Hyperparathyroidism with resulting hypercalcemia
- Elevated uric acid level (metabolic defects, dietary excess)
- Chronic diarrhea (e.g., inflammatory bowel disease) with increased oxalate absorption
- Type I (distal tubule) renal tubular acidosis (<1% of calcium stones)
- Chronic hydrochlorothiazide treatment
- Chronic infections with urease-producing organisms (e.g., *Proteus, Providencia, Pseudomonas, Klebsiella*). Struvite, or magnesium ammonium phosphate crystals, are produced when the urinary tract is colonized by bacteria, producing elevated concentrations of ammonia
- Abnormal excretion of cystine
- Chemotherapy for malignancies
- Box 1-28 describes past medical history significant for urolithiasis

DIAGNOSIS

■ DIFFERENTIAL DIAGNOSIS
- Urinary tract infection
- Pyelonephritis
- Diverticulitis
- Pelvic inflammatory disease
- Ovarian pathology
- Factitious (drug addicts)
- Appendicitis
- Small bowel obstruction
- Ectopic pregnancy
- The differential diagnosis of obstructive uropathy is described in Box 2-250

■ WORKUP
- Laboratory and imaging studies (Box 1-28). Stone analysis should be performed on recovered stones.
- Fig. 1-383 is a clinical algorithm for evaluation of nephrolithiasis.

■ LABORATORY TESTS
- Urinalysis: hematuria may be present; however, its absence does not exclude urinary stones. Evaluation of urinary pH is of value in identification of type of stone (pH >7.5 is associated with struvite stones, whereas pH <5 generally is seen with uric acid or with cystine stones).
- Urine C&S should be obtained for all patients.
- Serum chemistries should include calcium, electrolytes, phosphate, and uric acid.
- Additional tests: 24-hr urine collection for calcium, uric acid, phosphate, oxalate, and citrate excretion is generally reserved for patients with recurrent stones.

■ IMAGING STUDIES
- Plain films of the abdomen can identify radioopaque stones (calcium, uric acid stones).
- Renal sonogram may be helpful.
- IVP demonstrates the size and location of the stone, as well as degree of obstruction.
- Unenhanced (noncontrast) helical CT scan does not require contrast media and can visualize the calculus (identified by the "rim sign" or "halo" representing the edematous ureteral wall around the stone). It is fast, accurate (sensitivity 15% to 100%, specificity 94% to 96%), and readily identifies all stone types in all locations. This modality is being used increasingly in the initial assessment of renal colic.

TREATMENT

■ NONPHARMACOLOGIC THERAPY
- Increase in water or other fluid intake (doubling of previous fluid intake unless patient has a history of CHF or fluid overload)
- Low-calcium diet in patients with type II absorptive hypercalciuria
- Sodium restriction (to decrease calcium excretion), decreased protein intake to 1 g/kg/day (to decrease uric acid, calcium, and oxalate excretion)
- Increase in bran (may decrease bowel transit time with increased binding of calcium and subsequent decrease in urinary calcium)

■ ACUTE GENERAL Rx
- Pain control (use of narcotics is generally indicated because of the severity of pain)
- Specific therapy tailored to the stone type:
  1. Uric acid calculi: control of hyperuricemia with allopurinol 100 to 300 mg/day; increase urinary pH with potassium citrate, 10-mEq tablets tid
  2. Calcium stones:
     a. HCTZ 25 to 50 mg qd in patients with type I absorptive hypercalciuria
     b. Decrease bowel absorption of calcium with cellulose phosphate 10 g/day in patients with type I absorptive hypercalciuria
     c. Orthophosphates to inhibit vitamin B synthesis in patients with type III absorptive hypercalciuria
     d. Potassium citrate supplementation in patients with hypocitraturic calcium nephrolithiasis

e. Purine dietary restrictions or allopurinol in patients with hyperuricosuric calcium nephrolithiasis
3. Struvite stones:
   a. Most of the stones are large and cause obstruction and bleeding.
   b. ESWL and percutaneous nephrolithotomy are generally necessary.
   c. Prolonged use of antibiotics directed against the predominant urinary tract organism may be beneficial to prevent recurrence.
4. Cystine stones: Penicillamine and tiopronin can be used to reduce the formation of cystine
- Surgical treatment in patients with severe pain unresponsive to medication and patients with persistent fever or nausea or significant impediment of urine flow:
  a. Ureteroscopic stone extraction
  b. Extracorporeal shock wave lithotripsy (ESWL) for most renal stones
- In 1997 the American Urological Association issued the following guidelines for the treatment of ureteral stones:
  1. Proximal ureteral stones <1 cm in diameter: options are ESWL, percutaneous nephroureterolithotomy, and ureteroscopy
  2. Proximal ureteral stones >1 cm in diameter: options are ESWL, percutaneous nephroureterolithotomy, and ureteroscopy. Placement of a ureteral stent should be considered if the stone is causing high-grade obstruction
  3. Distal ureteral stones <1 cm in diameter: most of these pass spontaneously. ESWL and ureteroscopy are two accepted modes of therapy
  4. Distal ureteral stones >1 cm in diameter: watchful waiting, ESWL, ureteroscopy (following stone fragmentation)
- Fig. 1-384 describes an approach to the management of ureteral calculi.

■ **CHRONIC Rx**
Maintenance of proper hydration and dietary restrictions (see "Acute General Rx").

■ **DISPOSITION**
- >50% of patients will pass the stone within 48 hr.
- Stones will recur in approximately 50% of patients within 5 yr if no medical treatment is provided.

■ **REFERRAL**
Urology referral in complicated or recurrent urolithiasis; most patients with small uncomplicated ureteral or renal calculi can be followed as outpatient, whereas patients with persistent vomiting, suspected UTI, pain unresponsive to oral analgesics, or obstructing calculus associated with solitary kidney should be admitted

☼ **PEARLS & CONSIDERATIONS**

■ **COMMENTS**
- Early identification and aggressive treatment of urinary tract infections is indicated in all patients with struvite stones.
- Alkalinization of urine (pH >7.5 with penicillamine) is useful in patients with recurrent cystine stones.
- An algorithmic approach to the management of ureteral calculi is described in Fig. 1-384.

REFERENCE
Portis AJ, Sundaram CP: Diagnosis and initial management of kidney stones, *Am Fam Physician* 63:1329, 2001.
Author: **Fred F. Ferri, M.D.**

BOX 1-28   Past Medical History Significant for Urolithiasis

Diseases associated with disturbances of calcium metabolism: primary hyperparathyroidism, Wilson's disease, medullary sponge kidney, osteoporosis, immobilization, sarcoidosis, osteolytic metastases, plasmacytoma, neuroendocrine tumors, Paget's disease
  Dietary history: purine gluttony, calcium excess, milk alkali, oxalate excess, sodium excess, low citrus fruit intake
  Medications: uricosurics, diuretics, analgesics, vitamins C and D, antacids (especially phosphorus-binding agents), acetazolamide, calcium channel blockers, triamterene, theophylline, protease inhibitors (indinavir), sulfonamides
Diseases associated with disturbances of oxalate metabolism: primary hyperoxaluria types I and II, Crohn's disease, ulcerative colitis, intestinal bypass surgery (especially jejunoileal bypass), ileal resection
Diseases associated with disturbances of purine metabolism
  Intrinsic metabolic disorders—anemia, neoplastic disorders (especially leukemias), intoxication, myocardial infarction, irradiation, cytotoxic chemotherapy
  Enzyme deficiency—primary gout, Lesch-Nyhan syndrome
  Altered excretion—renal insufficiency, metabolic acidosis
Infectious history: organisms (particularly *Proteus* and *Klebsiella*), febrile upper tract involvement and dates if hospitalized.

From Nseyo UO (ed): *Urology for primary care physicians,* Philadelphia, 1999, WB Saunders.

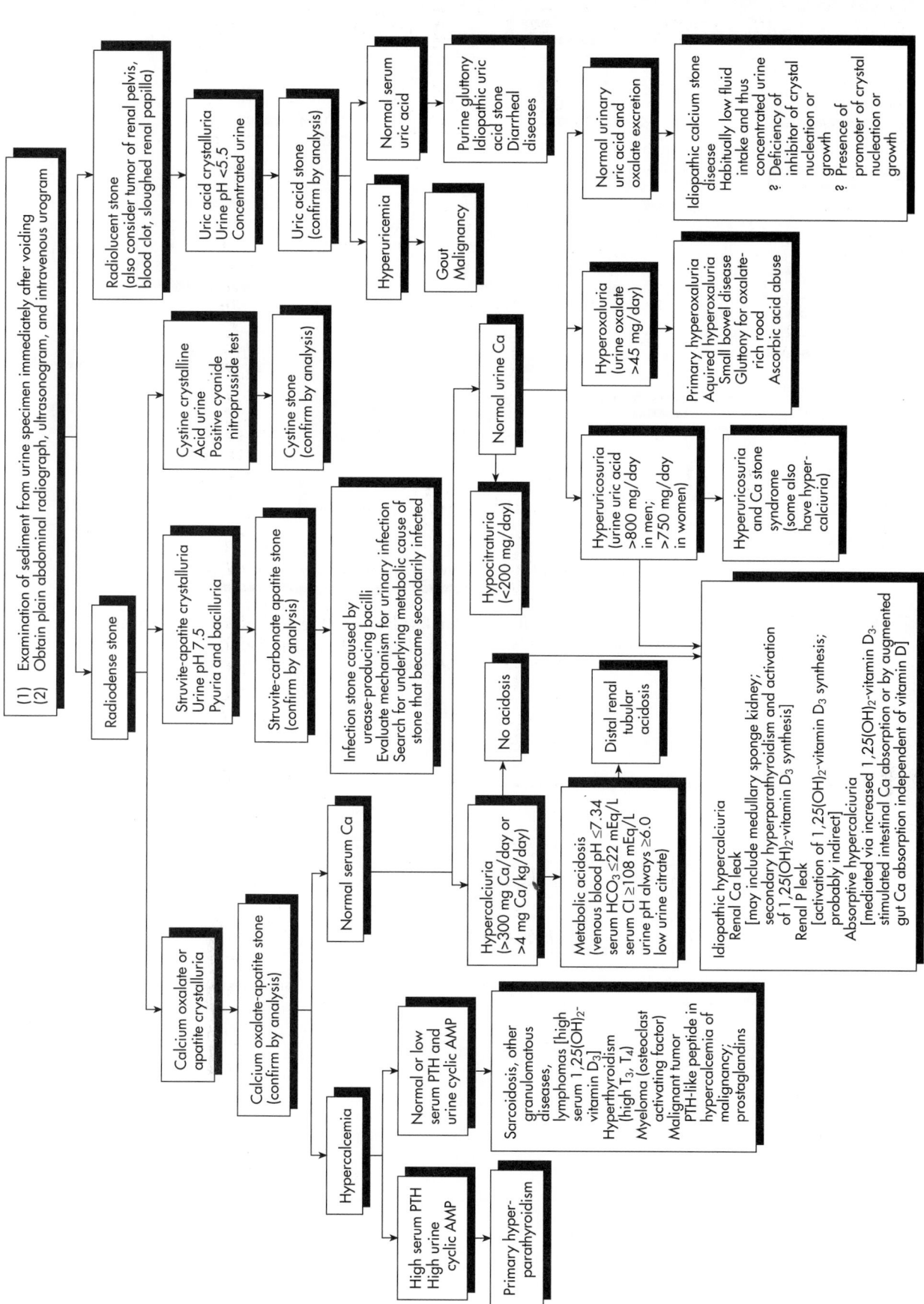

Fig. 1-383 Evaluation of patients with suspected nephrolithiasis (flank pain, ureteral colic, hematuria, fever). *AMP,* Adenosine monophosphate; *PTH,* parathyroid hormone. (From Stein JH [ed]: *Internal medicine,* ed 5, St Louis, 1998, Mosby.)

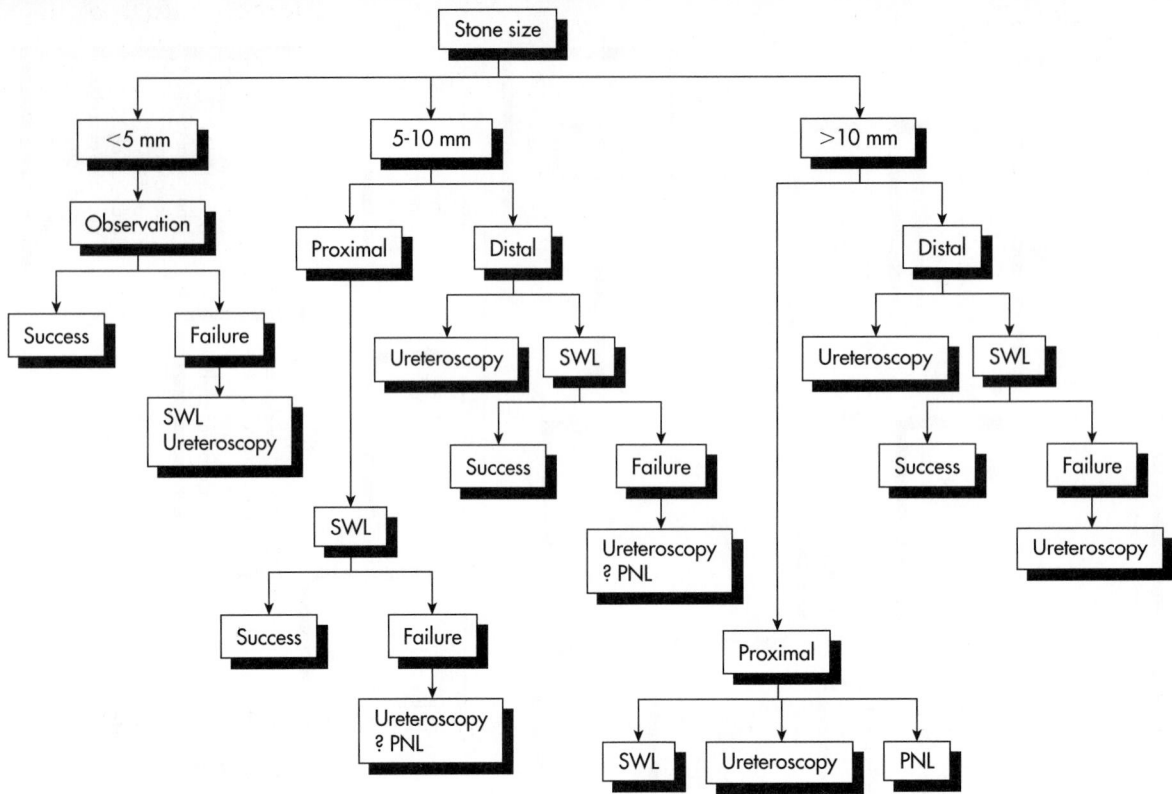

Fig. 1-384 **Management of ureteral calculi.** *PNL,* Percutaneous nephrostolithotomy; *SWL,* shock wave lithotripsy. (From Noble J: *Primary care medicine,* ed 3, St Louis, 2001, Mosby.)

BASIC INFORMATION

■ DEFINITION
Urticaria is a pruritic rash involving the epidermis and the upper portions of the dermis, resulting from localized capillary vasodilation and followed by transudation of protein-rich fluid in the surrounding tissue and manifesting clinically with the presence of hives.

■ SYNONYMS
Hives
Wheals

ICD-9CM CODES
708.8 Other unspecified urticaria

■ EPIDEMIOLOGY & DEMOGRAPHICS
- At least 20% of the population will have one episode of hives during their lifetime.
- Incidence is increased in atopic patients.
- The etiology of chronic urticaria (hives lasting longer than 6 wk) is determined in only 5% to 20% of cases.

■ PHYSICAL FINDINGS & CLINICAL PRESENTATION
- Presence of elevated, erythematous, or white nonpitting plaques that change in size and shape over time; they generally last a few hours and disappear without a trace.
- Annular configuration with central pallor (Fig. 1-385).

■ ETIOLOGY
- Foods (e.g., shellfish, eggs, strawberries, nuts)
- Drugs (e.g., penicillin, aspirin, sulfonamides)
- Systemic diseases (e.g., SLE, serum sickness, autoimmune thyroid disease, polycythemia vera)
- Food additives (e.g., salicylates, benzoates, sulfites)
- Infections (viral infections, fungal infections, chronic bacterial infections)
- Physical stimuli (e.g., pressure urticaria, exercise-induced, solar urticaria, cold urticaria)
- Inhalants (e.g., mold spores, animal danders, pollens)
- Contact (nonimmunologic) urticaria (e.g., caterpillars, plants)
- Other: hereditary angioedema, urticaria pigmentosa, pregnancy, cold urticaria, hair bleaches, chemicals, saliva, cosmetics, perfumes, pemphigoid, emotional stress

DIAGNOSIS

■ DIFFERENTIAL DIAGNOSIS
- Erythema multiforme
- Erythema marginatum
- Erythema infectiosum
- Urticarial vasculitis
- Herpes gestationis
- Drug eruption
- Multiple insect bites
- Bullous pemphigoid

■ WORKUP
- It is useful to determine whether hives are acute or chronic; a medical history focused on various etiologic factors is necessary before embarking on extensive laboratory testing.
- A diagnostic approach to chronic urticaria is described in Fig. 1-386.

■ LABORATORY TESTS
- CBC with differential
- Stool for ova and parasites in patients with suspected parasitic infestations
- ANA, ESR, TSH, liver function tests, eosinophil count are indicated only in selected patients

TREATMENT

■ NONPHARMACOLOGIC THERAPY
- Remove suspected etiologic agents (e.g., stop aspirin and all nonessential drugs), restrict diet (e.g., elimination of tomatoes, nuts, eggs, shellfish).
- Elimination of yeast should be attempted in patients with chronic urticaria (*Candida albicans* sensitivity may be a factor in patients with chronic urticaria).

■ ACUTE GENERAL Rx
- Oral antihistamines: use of nonsedating antihistamines (e.g., loratadine [Claritin] 10 mg qd or cetirizine [Zyrtec] 10 mg qd) is preferred over first-generation antihistamines (e.g., hydroxyzine, diphenhydramine).
- Doxepin (a tricyclic antidepressant) 25 to 75 mg qhs may be effective in patients with chronic urticaria.
- Oral corticosteroids should be reserved for refractory cases (e.g., prednisone 20 mg qd or 20 mg bid).

■ CHRONIC Rx
Use of nonsedating antihistamines, doxepin, and/or oral corticosteroids (see "Acute General Rx")

■ DISPOSITION
- Most cases of urticaria resolve within 6 wk.
- Only 25% of patients with a history of chronic urticaria are completely cured after 5 yr.

PEARLS & CONSIDERATIONS

■ COMMENTS
Local treatment (e.g., starch baths or Aveeno baths) may be helpful in selected patients; however, local treatment is generally not rewarding.

REFERENCE
Kozel MMA et al: The effectiveness of a history-based diagnostic approach in chronic urticaria and angioedema, *Arch Dermatol* 134:1575, 1998.
Author: **Fred F. Ferri, M.D.**

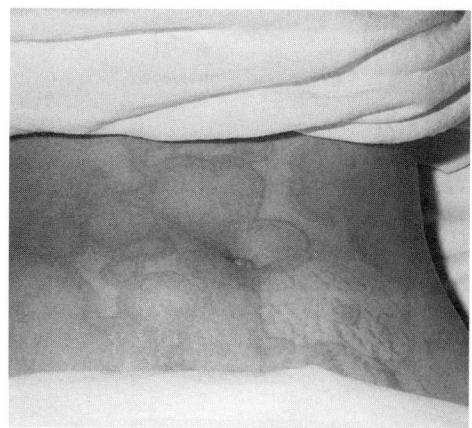

Fig. 1-385   Wheal (urticaria). Note central cleaning, giving annular configuration. (From Noble J et al: *Textbook of primary care medicine,* ed 2, St Louis, 1995, Mosby.)

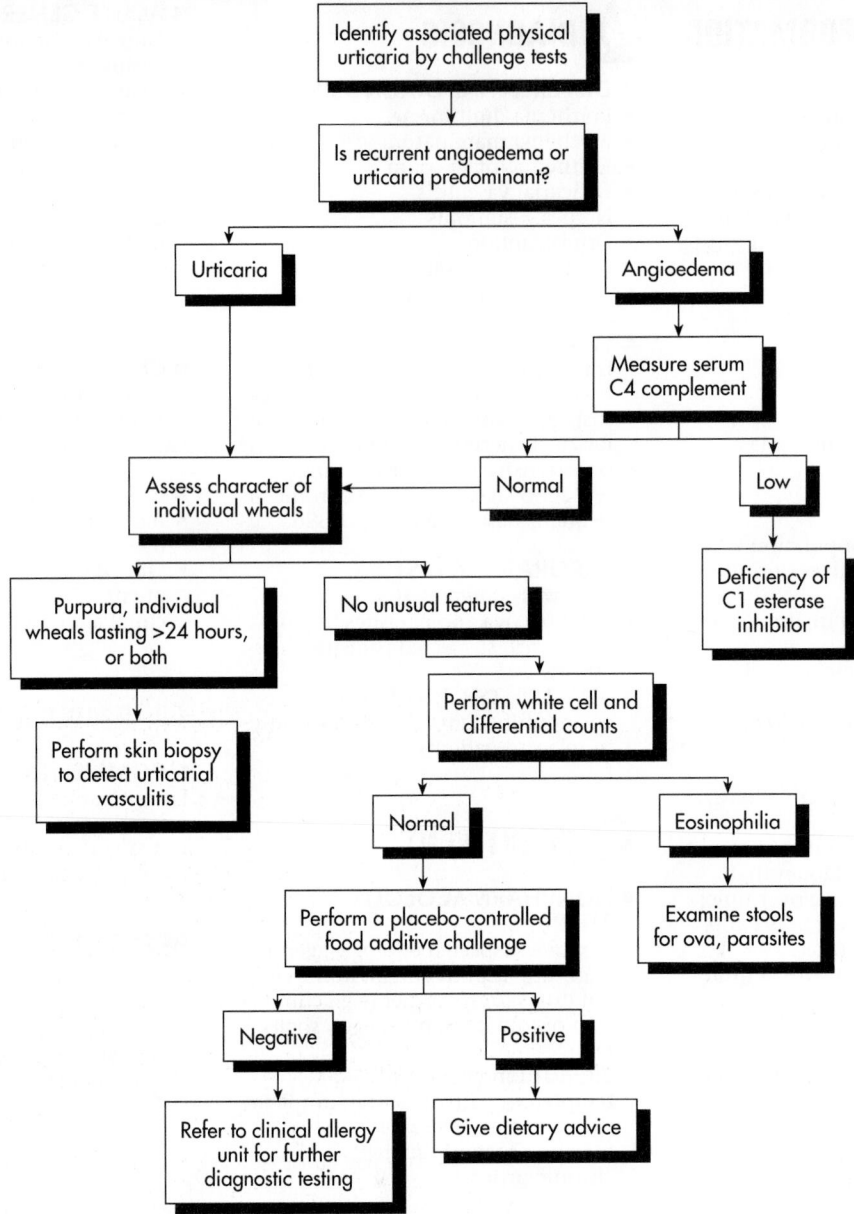

Fig. 1-386   Investigation and diagnosis of chronic urticaria. (From Greaves MW: *N Engl J Med* 332:1767, 1995.)

BASIC INFORMATION

■ DEFINITION
Uterine malignancy includes tumors from the endometrium (discussed elsewhere in this text) and sarcomas. Uterine sarcoma is an abnormal proliferation of cells originating from the mesenchymal, or connective tissue, elements of the uterine wall.

■ SYNONYMS
Leiomyosarcomas
Endometrial stromal sarcoma
Malignant mixed mullerian tumors
Adenosarcomas

ICD-9CM CODES
182.0 Malignant neoplasm of body of uterus (corpus uteri), except isthmus
182.1 Malignant neoplasm of body of uterus, isthmus
182.8 Malignant neoplasm of body of uterus, other specified sites of body of uterus

■ EPIDEMIOLOGY & DEMOGRAPHICS
PREVALENCE: Uterine sarcoma accounts for 4.3% of all cancers of the uterine corpus and is the most lethal gynecologic malignancy.
INCIDENCE: 17.1 cases/1 million females
MEAN AGE AT DIAGNOSIS: The age at diagnosis is variable. Mean age at diagnosis is 52 yr.
RISK FACTORS: Similar to endometrial carcinoma

■ PHYSICAL FINDINGS & CLINICAL PRESENTATION
- Abnormal vaginal bleeding is the most common symptom.
- May also present as pelvic pain or pressure and pelvic mass on examination.
- May appear as tumor protruding through the cervix
- Vaginal discharge may also be a presenting symptom.
- Rapidly enlarging uterus

■ ETIOLOGY
- The exact etiology is unknown.
- Prior pelvic radiation is a risk factor for sarcoma.
- Black women may be at higher risk.

DIAGNOSIS

■ DIFFERENTIAL DIAGNOSIS
Leiomyoma

■ WORKUP
Diagnosis is made histologically by biopsy for abnormal bleeding.

■ LABORATORY TESTS
Chest radiography, CT scans, and MRI are used to evaluate spread.

■ IMAGING STUDIES
- Chest radiography is usually done as routine preoperative testing.
- CT scans and MRI are good for assessing tumor spread once diagnosis is made.

TREATMENT

■ NONPHARMACOLOGIC THERAPY
- Surgery excision is the mainstay of treatment.
- Grade and stage of tumor affect prognosis (Fig. 1-387).

- Adjuvant radiotherapy may improve pelvic disease control, but it does not improve survival.
- Chemotherapeutic agents have produced only partial and short-term responses.

■ DISPOSITION
- Survival varies with each type of sarcoma but is generally very poor.
- Five-year survival for leiomyosarcoma ranges from 48% for stage I to 0% for stage IV.
- Five-year survival for malignant mixed mesodermal tumor ranges from 36% for stage I to 6% for stage IV.

■ REFERRAL
Uterine sarcoma should be managed by a gynecologic oncologist and radiation oncologist.
Author: **Gil Farkash, M.D.**

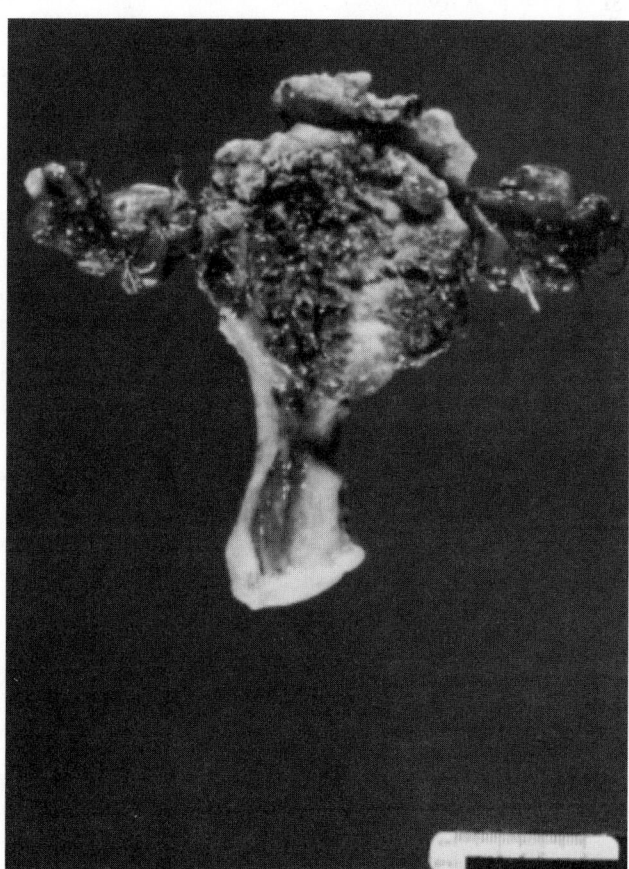

Fig. 1-387 This grade 3 adenocarcinoma demonstrates extensive myometrial invasion. The tumor has penetrated the uterine serosa and extends onto the fundus and into the upper left broad ligament. (From Copeland LJ: *Textbook of gynecology,* ed 2, Philadelphia, 2000, WB Saunders.)

BASIC INFORMATION

DEFINITION
Uterine myomas are discrete nodular tumors that vary in size and number and that may be found subserosal, intramucosal, or submucosal within the uterus or may be found in the cervix or broad ligament or on a pedicle.

SYNONYMS
Leiomyomas, fibroids

ICD-9CM CODES
218.9 Leiomyomas, fibroids

EPIDEMIOLOGY & DEMOGRAPHICS
- Estimated presence in at least 20% of all reproductive age women.
- The most common benign uterine tumor.
- More common in black than in white women.
- Asymptomatic fibroids may be present in 40% to 50% of women >40 yr of age.
- May occur singly but are often multiple.
- Fewer than half of all fibroids are estimated to produce symptoms.
- Frequently diagnosed incidentally on pelvic examination.
- There is increased familial incidence.
- Potential to enlarge during pregnancy, as well as to regress after menopause.
- Infrequent primary cause of infertility in <3% of infertile patients.

PHYSICAL FINDINGS & CLINICAL PRESENTATION
- Enlarged, irregular uterus on pelvic examination.
- Presenting symptoms:
  1. Menorrhagia (most common)
  2. Chronic pelvic pain (dysmenorrhea, dyspareunia, pelvic pressure)
  3. Acute pain (torsion of pedunculated myoma, infarction, and degeneration)
  4. Urinary symptoms (frequency from bladder pressure, partial ureteral obstruction, complete ureteral obstruction)
  5. Rectosigmoid compression with constipation or intestinal obstruction
  6. Prolapse through cervix of pedunculated submucosal tumor
  7. Venous stasis of lower extremities
  8. Polycythemia
  9. Ascites

ETIOLOGY
Unknown. It is suggested that myomas arise from a single neoplastic smooth muscle cell in the myometrium. Malignant degeneration of preexisting leiomyoma is extremely uncommon (<0.5%).

DIAGNOSIS

DIFFERENTIAL DIAGNOSIS
Leiomyosarcoma, ovarian mass (neoplastic, nonneoplastic, endometrioma), inflammatory mass, pregnancy

WORKUP
- Complete pelvic examination, rectovaginal examination, Pap test.
- Estimation of size of mass in centimeters.
- Endometrial sampling may be indicated (biopsy or D&C) when abnormal bleeding and pelvic mass are present.
- If urinary symptoms are prominent, cystometry, cystoscopy to rule out bladder lesions, IVP to rule out impingement on urinary system.

LABORATORY TESTS
- Pregnancy test
- Pap smear
- CBC, ESR
- Fecal occult blood

IMAGING STUDIES
- Pelvic ultrasound (transvaginal may have higher diagnostic accuracy) is useful.
- CT scan is helpful in planning treatment if malignancy is strongly suspected.
- Hysteroscopy may provide direct evidence of intrauterine pathology or submucosal leiomyoma that distorts uterine cavity.

TREATMENT

Management should be based on primary symptoms and may include observation with close follow-up, temporizing surgical therapies, medical management, or definitive surgical procedures.

NONSURGICAL Rx
- Patient observation and follow-up with periodic repeat pelvic examinations to ensure that tumors are not growing rapidly.

- GnRH agonist use results in 40% to 60% reduction in uterine volume. Hypoestrogenism, reversible bone loss, hot flushes associated with use. Limit to short-term use and consider low-dose hormonal replacement to minimize hypoestrogenic effects.
- Regrowth occurs in about 50% of women treated a few months after cessation.
- Indications for GnRH:
  1. Fertility preservation in women with large myomas before attempting conception or preoperative myectomy treatment.
  2. Anemia treatment to normalize hemoglobin before surgery.
  3. Women approaching menopause to avoid surgery.
  4. Preoperative for large myomas to make vaginal hysterectomy, hysteroscopic resection/ablation, or laparoscopic destruction more feasible.
  5. Women with medical contraindications for surgery.
  6. Personal or medical indications for delaying surgery.
- Progestational agents may also result in decrease in uterine size and amenorrhea, allowing iron therapy to treat anemia with limited success.

SURGICAL Rx
- Indications
  1. Abnormal uterine bleeding with anemia, refractory to hormonal therapy
  2. Chronic pain with severe dysmenorrhea, dyspareunia, or lower abdominal pressure/pain
  3. Acute pain, torsion, or prolapsing submucosal fibroid
  4. Urinary symptoms or signs such as hydronephrosis
  5. Rapid uterine enlargement premenopausal or any postmenopausal increase in size
  6. Infertility with leiomyoma as only finding
  7. Enlarged uterus with compression symptoms or discomfort
- Procedures
  1. Hysterectomy (definitive procedure)
  2. Abdominal myomectomy (to preserve fertility)
  3. Vaginal myomectomy for prolapsed pedunculated submucous fibroid
  4. Hysteroscopic resection
  5. Laparoscopic myomectomy

REFERRAL
Consultation with gynecologic oncologist if suspicion of malignancy

Author: **Eugene J. Louie-Ng, M.D.**

BASIC INFORMATION

■ DEFINITION
Uterine prolapse refers to the protrusion of the uterus into or out of the vaginal canal. In a *first-degree uterine prolapse,* the cervix is visible when the perineum is depressed. In a *second-degree uterine prolapse,* the uterine cervix has prolapsed through the vaginal introitus, with the fundus remaining within the pelvis proper. In a *third-degree uterine prolapse* (i.e., *complete uterine prolapse, uterine procidentia*), the entire uterus is outside the introitus.

■ SYNONYMS
Genital prolapse
Uterine descensus
Pelvic organ prolapse

ICD-9CM CODES
618.8 Genital prolapse
618.1 Uterine descensus
618.8 Pelvic organ prolapse

■ EPIDEMIOLOGY & DEMOGRAPHICS
Most prevalent in postmenopausal multiparous women.
RISK FACTORS;
• Pregnancy
• Labor
• Vaginal childbirth
• Obesity
• Chronic coughing
• Constipation
• Pelvic tumors
• Ascites
• Strenuous physical exertion
• Caucasian race
GENETICS: Increased incidence in women with spina bifida occulta.

■ PHYSICAL FINDINGS & CLINICAL PRESENTATION
• Pelvic pressure
• Bearing-down sensation
• Bilateral groin pain
• Sacral backache
• Coital difficulty
• Protrusion from vagina
• Spotting
• Ulceration
• Bleeding
• Examination of patient in lithotomy, sitting, and standing positions and before, during, and after a maximum Valsalva effort
• Erosion or ulceration of the cervix possible in the most dependent area of the protrusion

■ ETIOLOGY
• Vaginal childbirth and chronic increases in intraabdominal pressure leading to detachments, lacerations, and denervations of the vaginal support system

• Further weakening of pelvic support system by hypoestrogenic atrophy
• Some cases from congenital or inherited weaknesses within the pelvic support system
• Neonatal uterine prolapse mostly coexistent with congenital spinal defects

 DIAGNOSIS

■ DIFFERENTIAL DIAGNOSIS
Occasionally, elongated cervix; body of the uterus remains undescended

■ WORKUP
• Diagnosis is based on history and physical examination.
• If erosion or ulceration of the cervix is present, a Pap smear followed by a cervical biopsy should be performed if indicated.
• If urinary symptoms are significant, further urodynamic workup is indicated, looking for concurrent cystourethrocele, cystocele, enterocele, or rectocele.

■ LABORATORY TESTS
Urine culture

■ IMAGING STUDIES
Ultrasound if concurrent fibroids need further evaluation

 TREATMENT

■ NONPHARMACOLOGIC THERAPY
• Prophylactic measures
  1. Diagnosis and treatment of chronic respiratory and metabolic disorders
  2. Correction of constipation
  3. Weight control, nutrition, and smoking cessation counseling
  4. Teaching of pelvic muscle exercises
• Supportive pessary therapy
  1. Ring-type pessary useful for first- or second-degree prolapse
  2. Gellhorn pessary preferred for more advanced prolapse
  3. Use of pessaries in conjunction with continuous hormone replacement therapy, unless contraindicated
  4. Perineorrhaphy under local anesthesia possibly needed to support the pessary if the vaginal outlet is very relaxed

■ ACUTE GENERAL Rx
• Patients who are only infrequently symptomatic: insertion of a tampon

or diaphragm for temporary relief when prolonged standing is anticipated
• Neonatal uterine prolapse: simple digital reduction or the use of a small pessary

■ CHRONIC Rx
• Hormone replacement therapy at the time of menopause helps preserve tissue strength, maintain elasticity of the vagina, and promote the durability of surgical repairs.
• Gold standard for therapy is vaginal hysterectomy.
• Vaginal apex should be well suspended, but a prophylactic sacrospinous ligament fixation is not routinely required.
• If occult enterocele present, McCall culdoplasty performed.
• If vaginal approach to hysterectomy is contraindicated, abdominal hysterectomy is performed; vaginal apex likewise well supported.
• Colpocleisis is considered for the elderly patient who is sexually inactive and is a high-risk patient from a surgical point of view; can be done rapidly under local anesthesia with mild sedation if necessary.
• For symptomatic women who desire childbearing: management with pessaries or pelvic muscle exercises is recommended; if surgical correction is required, transvaginal sacrospinous fixation is the preferred method.
• Other surgical options are sling operations and sacral cervicopexy.

■ DISPOSITION
If untreated, uterine prolapse progressively worsens.

■ REFERRAL
To a gynecologist if pessary fitting or surgical intervention is needed

 PEARLS & CONSIDERATIONS

■ COMMENTS
Surgery contraindicated in mild or asymptomatic uterine prolapse because the patient will seldom benefit from the operation although exposed to its risks.

REFERENCE
Glass RH, Curtis MG, Hopkins MP: *Glass' office gynecology,* ed 5, Baltimore, 1999, Lippincott Williams & Wilkins.
Author: **Wan J. Kim, M.D.**

BASIC INFORMATION

■ DEFINITION
Uveitis is inflammation of the uveal tract, including the iris, ciliary body, and choroid. It may also involve other closed structures such as the sclera, retina, and vitreous humor.

■ SYNONYMS
Anterior uveitis
Posterior uveitis
Acute or chronic uveitis
Granulomatous or nongranulomatous uveitis

ICD-9CM CODES
364.3 Unspecified iridocyclitis, uveitis

■ EPIDEMIOLOGY & DEMOGRAPHICS
INCIDENCE (IN U.S.): Common; busy ophthalmologist will see two or more cases per week
PREVALENCE (IN U.S.): 17 cases/100,000 persons
PREDOMINANT SEX: None
PREDOMINANT AGE: 38 yr
PEAK INCIDENCE: Middle age or older

■ PHYSICAL FINDINGS & CLINICAL PRESENTATION
• Photophobia
• Blurred visual acuity
• Irregular pupil
• Hazy cornea
• Abnormal cells and flare in anterior chamber or vitreous humor
• Retinal hemorrhage, vascular sheathing (Fig. 1-388)
• Conjunctival injection
• Ciliary flush
• Keratitic precipitates (precipitates on the cornea)
• Hazy vitreous
• Retinal inflammation
• Iris nodules
• Glaucoma

DIAGNOSIS

■ DIFFERENTIAL DIAGNOSIS
• Glaucoma
• Conjunctivitis
• Retinal detachment
• Retinopathy
• Keratitis
• Scleritis
• Episcleritis

■ WORKUP
• Associated with arthritis, syphilis, tuberculosis, granulomatous disease, collagen-vascular disease, allergies, AIDS, sarcoid, Behçet's disease, histoplasmosis, and toxoplasmosis
• Slit lamp examination, indirect ophthalmoscopy

■ LABORATORY TESTS
• CBC
• Laboratory tests for specific inflammatory causes cited above in "workup" (e.g., ANA, ESR, VDRL, HLA-B27 PPD, Lyme titer)

■ IMAGING STUDIES
• Chest x-ray examination in suspected sarcoidosis, TB, histoplasmosis
• Sacroiliac x-ray examination in suspected ankylosing spondylitis

TREATMENT

■ NONPHARMACOLOGIC THERAPY
Treat the underlying disease.

■ ACUTE GENERAL Rx
• Cycloplegic drops (cyclopentolate [Cyclogyl]) or cycloplegic agents (homatropine hydrobromide [Optic] 1gtt q3-4h while awake) and topical steroids (prednisone acetate 1% 1 gtt qh during day, PRN at night until favorable response, then q4-6h); avoid topical corticosteroids in infectious uveitis
• Antibiotics when infection is suspected
• Systemic steroids if appropriate for the underlying disease.

■ CHRONIC Rx
Topical steroids and cycloplegics

■ DISPOSITION
Urgent referral to ophthalmologist

■ REFERRAL
• Eye problem should be followed early on by an ophthalmologist.
• Underlying medical disease should be treated by the primary care physician.

PEARLS & CONSIDERATIONS

■ COMMENTS
• In 90% of cases, the condition is idiopathic.
• Associated causes are found approximately 10% of the time, usually chronic and recurrent.

Author: **Melvyn Koby, M.D.**

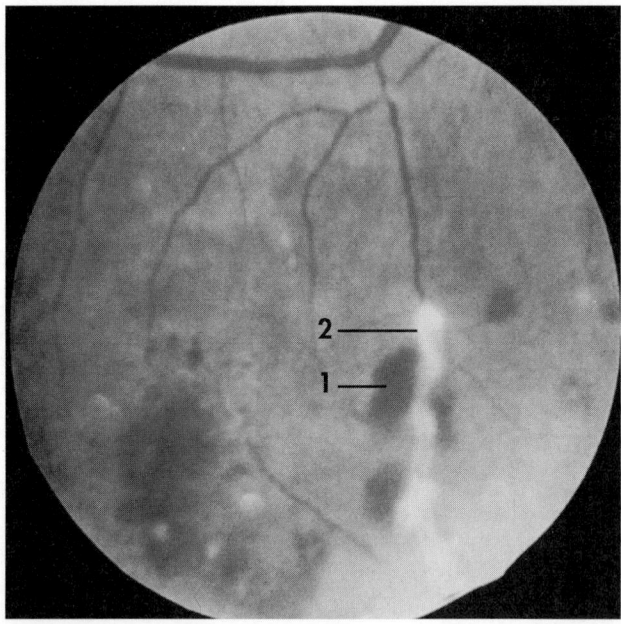

Fig. 1-388   Sarcoid posterior uveitis showing retinal hemorrhage *(1)* and vascular sheating *(2).* (From Palay D [ed]: *Ophthalmology for the primary care physician,* St Louis, 1997, Mosby.)

BASIC INFORMATION

■ DEFINITION

Bleeding per vagina at any time during pregnancy must be regarded as abnormal and is associated with an increased likelihood of pregnancy complications.

■ SYNONYMS

Hemorrhage

ICD-9CM CODES

634.9 Spontaneous abortion
633.9 Ectopic pregnancy
630/631 Molar pregnancy
622.7 Cervical polyps
180.9/180.0/180.8 Cervical dysplasia/cancer
616.0 Cervicitis
616.10 Vulvovaginitis
184.0 Vaginal cancer
644.2 Premature labor term labor
641.1 Placenta previa
641.2 Placental abruption

■ EPIDEMIOLOGY & DEMOGRAPHICS

- Common in U.S.; 20% to 25% of patients have vaginal spotting/bleeding in first trimester; of those, miscarriage occurs in 50%.
- Occurs in women of childbearing age.
- Between 1% and 2% of all pregnancies in the U.S. are ectopic.
- After one ectopic pregnancy, the chance of another is 7% to 15%.
- Ectopic pregnancy is the leading cause of maternal mortality in the first trimester.
- Average reported frequency for placental abruption is about 1 in 150 deliveries (0.3%).
- Incidence of placenta previa is <1 in 200 deliveries (0.5%).

■ PHYSICAL FINDINGS & CLINICAL PRESENTATION

- Bleeding: ranges from scant to life-threatening with hemodynamic instability
- Color: brown to bright red
- Can be painless or painful (cramps, back pain, severe abdominal pain)
- Fetal compromise: ranges from none to fetal demise

■ ETIOLOGY

- Influenced by gestational age
- Vaginal
- Cervical
- Uterine

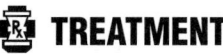

DIAGNOSIS

■ DIFFERENTIAL DIAGNOSIS

- Any gestational age:
  1. Cervical lesions: polyps, decidual reaction, neoplasia
  2. Vaginal trauma
  3. Cervicitis/vulvovaginitis
  4. Postcoital trauma
  5. Bleeding dyscrasias
- Gestation <20 wk:
  1. Spontaneous abortion
  2. Presence of intrauterine device
  3. Ectopic pregnancy
  4. Molar pregnancy
  5. Implantation bleeding
  6. Low-lying placenta
- Gestation >20 wk:
  1. Molar pregnancy
  2. Placenta previa
  3. Placental abruption
  4. Vasa previa
  5. Marginal separation of the placenta
  6. Bloody show at term
  7. Preterm labor
- Box 2-252 describes the differential diagnosis of vaginal bleeding in pregnancy.

■ WORKUP

- Gestation <20 wk (Fig. 3-24 describes a clinical algorithm for evaluation of vaginal bleeding in early pregnancy.)
  1. Pelvic examination
  2. Culdocentesis
  3. Laparoscopy
  4. Laparotomy
- Gestation >20 wk:
  1. Ultrasound to locate placenta before pelvic examination
  2. If placenta previa, no speculum or bimanual examination
  3. If preterm labor, appropriate evaluation done

■ LABORATORY TESTS

- Urine pregnancy test: if positive, get quantitative β human chorionic gonadotropin (hCG)
  1. Early pregnancy: follow serially every 48 hr
  2. Normal pregnancy: hCG doubles approximately every 48 hr
  3. Spontaneous abortion: hCG levels will fall
  4. Ectopic pregnancy: hCG level will rise inappropriately
  5. Molar pregnancy: hCG level is extremely high
- CBC
- Blood type and screen (Rh-negative patients need RhoGAM)
- Coagulation profile (useful in missed abortion and abruption)
- Cervical cultures/wet mount
- Pap smear for cervical malignancy; caution with biopsy, since cervix can bleed extensively

■ IMAGING STUDIES

Ultrasound:
- 5 to 6 wk: gestational sac (transvaginally); hCG >2500 mIU/ml (third IS) or >1000 mIU/ml (second IS)
- 8 to 9 wk: fetal cardiac activity
- Molar pregnancy: characteristic cluster of cysts
- Location of placenta
- Degree of placental separation: difficult to assess

TREATMENT

■ NONPHARMACOLOGIC THERAPY

- Pelvic rest: no coitus, douching, or tampons
- Bed rest, if >20 wk
- Counseling: genetic, bereavement

■ ACUTE GENERAL Rx

- Hemodynamic stabilization
- Emergency D&C, laparotomy, or cesarean section as necessary

■ CHRONIC Rx

Depends on diagnosis

■ DISPOSITION

Depends on diagnosis

■ REFERRAL

- If patient is unstable and needs emergency ob/gyn management and/or surgery
- If patient has diagnosis of ectopic or molar pregnancy, since immediate surgical treatment is indicated
- Perinatal consultation for high-risk pregnancy

Author: **Maria Elena Soler, M.D.**

BASIC INFORMATION

■ DEFINITION
Vaginal malignancy is an abnormal proliferation of vaginal epithelium demonstrating malignant cells below the basement membrane.

■ SYNONYMS
Squamous cell carcinoma of the vagina
Adenocarcinoma of the vagina
Melanoma of the vagina
Sarcoma of the vagina
Endodermal sinus tumor

ICD-9CM CODES
184.0 Vagina, vaginal neoplasm

■ EPIDEMIOLOGY & DEMOGRAPHICS
PREVALENCE: Vaginal cancer is the second rarest gynecologic cancer. It comprises 2% of malignancies of the female genital tract.
INCIDENCE: 0.42 cases/100,000 persons
MEAN AGE AT DIAGNOSIS: Predominantly a disease of menopause. Mean age at diagnosis is 60 yr old.

■ PHYSICAL FINDINGS & CLINICAL PRESENTATION
• Majority of cases are asymptomatic.
• Postmenopausal vaginal bleeding and/or vaginal discharge are the most common symptoms.
• May also present as pelvic pain or pressure, dyspareunia, dysuria, malodor, or postcoital bleeding.
• May present as a vaginal lesion or abnormal Pap smear.

■ ETIOLOGY
• The exact etiology is unknown.
• Vaginal intraepithelial neoplasia is thought to be a precursor for squamous cell carcinoma of the vagina.
• Chronic pessary use has been associated with vaginal malignancy.
• Prior pelvic radiation may be a risk factor.
• Clear-cell adenocarcinoma is related to in utero diethylstilbestrol exposure.

DIAGNOSIS

■ DIFFERENTIAL DIAGNOSIS
• Extension from other primary carcinoma; more common than primary vaginal cancer
• Vaginitis

■ WORKUP
• Diagnosis is made histologically by biopsy.
• Colposcopy and biopsy should follow suspicious Pap smear.
• Cystoscopy, proctosigmoidoscopy, chest radiography, IV urography, and barium enema may be used for clinical staging.
• CT scan and MRI are being used to evaluate spread.
• Staging I-IV (Fig. 1-389)

■ IMAGING STUDIES
• Chest radiography, IV urography, and barium enema are used for staging.
• CT scan and MRI are good for assessing tumor spread.

TREATMENT

■ NONPHARMACOLOGIC THERAPY
• Radiation therapy is the mainstay of treatment.
• Stage I tumors that are small and confined to the posterior, upper third of the vagina may be treated with radical surgery.
• Other stages require a whole-pelvis, interstitial, and/or intracavitary radiation therapy.
• Chemotherapy is used in conjunction with radiotherapy in rare select cases.

■ DISPOSITION
Five-year survival ranges from 80% for stage I to 17% for stage IV.

■ REFERRAL
Vaginal cancer should be managed by a gynecologic oncologist and radiation oncologist.
Author: **Gil Farkash, M.D.**

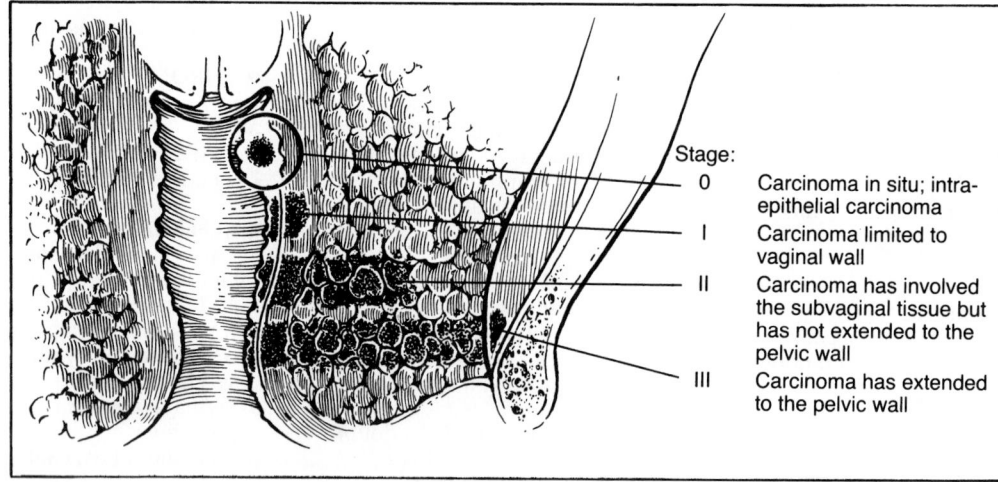

Fig. 1-389   Staging system for vaginal cancer. Metastatic disease that involves the bladder or rectum is stage IV-a. Metastatic disease beyond the pelvis is stage IV-b. (From Copeland LJ: *Textbook of gynecology,* ed 2, Philadelphia, 2000, WB Saunders.)

BASIC INFORMATION

■ DEFINITION

Vaginismus refers to the involuntary spasm of the vaginal, introital, and/or levator ani muscles, preventing penetration or causing painful intercourse.

ICD-9CM CODES

300.11 Hysterical vaginismus
306.51 Psychogenic or functional vaginismus
625.1 Reflex vaginismus

■ EPIDEMIOLOGY & DEMOGRAPHICS

PREVALENCE: Affects approximately 1:200 women
INCIDENCE: Estimated at about 11.7% to 42% of women presenting to sexual dysfunction clinics
RISK FACTORS: Any previous sexual trauma, including incest or rape
PREDOMINANT SEX: Affects only females

■ PHYSICAL FINDINGS & CLINICAL PRESENTATION

- Fear of pain with coitus
- Dyspareunia
- Orgasmic dysfunction

■ ETIOLOGY

- Learned conditioned response to real or imagined painful vaginal experience (e.g., traumatic speculum examination, incest, rape)
- Vaginitis
- PID
- Endometriosis
- Anatomic anomalies
- Atrophic vaginitis

- Mucosal tears
- Inadequate lubrication
- Focal vulvitis
- Painful hymenal tags
- Scarring secondary to episiotomy
- Skin disorders
- Topical allergies
- Postherpetic neuralgia

DIAGNOSIS

■ WORKUP

- Thorough history (including sexual history)
- Careful pelvic examination
- Behavioral therapy

TREATMENT

■ NONPHARMACOLOGIC THERAPY

- Deconditioning the response by systematic self-administered progressive dilation techniques using fingers or dilators
- Behavioral and/or psychosexual therapy

■ ACUTE GENERAL Rx

- Botulinum toxin therapy given locally has been shown to relieve the perineal muscle spasms associated with vaginismus, allowing resumption of intercourse.
  1. Acts by preventing neuromuscular transmission, causing muscle weakness
  2. Considered experimental treatment for vaginismus at this time

- Cause should be determined by history and explained to the patient so that she understands the mechanics of the muscle spasms.
- Patient must be motivated to desire painless vaginal insertion for such reasons as pleasurable coitus, tampon insertion, or gynecologic examination.
- Patient (and her partner) must be willing to patiently undergo the process of systematic desensitization and counseling.

■ DISPOSITION

A high percentage of successfully treated patients

■ REFERRAL

To a gynecologist or sex therapist

PEARLS & CONSIDERATIONS

■ COMMENTS

- May uncover early sexual abuse or an aversion to sexuality in general.
- To American Association of Sex Educators, Counselors and Therapists, 11 Dupont Circle, NW, Washington, DC, 20036.
- To Sex Information and Education Council of the U.S. (SIECUS), 85th Avenue, New York, NY 10022.

REFERENCE

Brin MF, Vapnek JM: Treatment of vaginismus with botulinum toxin injections, *Lancet* 349:252, 1997.
Author: **Beth J. Wutz, M.D.**

BASIC INFORMATION

■ DEFINITION
Bacterial vaginosis (BV) is a thin, gray, homogenous, malodorous vaginal discharge that results from an overgrowth of several bacterial species.

■ PREVIOUS NAMES
Before 1955: nonspecific vaginitis
1955: *Haemophilus vaginalis* vaginitis
1963: *Corynebacterium vaginalis* vaginitis
1980: *Gardnerella vaginalis* vaginitis
1990: Bacterial vaginosis

ICD-9CM CODES
616.10 Vaginitis, bacterial

■ EPIDEMIOLOGY & DEMOGRAPHICS
- Most common vaginal infection
- Studies by Thomason et al report that BV is present in:
  1. 16% of private patients
  2. 10% to 25% of obstetric clinic patients
  3. 38% to 64% of STD clinic patients
- *Gardnerella, Mycoplasma,* and *Mobiluncus* are harbored in the urethra of male partners; however,
  1. Male partners are asymptomatic.
  2. With a woman's first episode of BV, there is no improved cure rate or lower reinfection rate if her male partner is treated.
  3. If the woman has recurrent episodes of BV, treating the male partner with an oral regimen may help her achieve cure.
  4. Abstinence from intercourse or condom use while the patient completes her treatment regimen may improve cure rates and lessen recurrences.

■ PHYSICAL FINDINGS & CLINICAL PRESENTATION
- 50% of patients are asymptomatic
- A thin, dark, or dull gray homogenous discharge that adheres to the vaginal walls
- An offensive, "fishy" odor that is accentuated after intercourse or menses
- Pruritus (only in 13%)

■ ETIOLOGY & PATHOGENESIS
- *Gardnerella vaginalis* is detected in 40% to 50% of vaginal secretions
  1. Increase in vaginal pH caused by decrease in hydrogen peroxide–producing lactobacilli
  2. Anaerobes predominate and produce amines
- Amines, when alkalinized by semen, menstrual blood, the use of alkaline douches, or the addition of 10% KOH, volatilize and cause the unpleasant "fishy" odor.

- In BV:
  1. *Bacteroides* (anaerobes) species are increased 1000× the usual concentration
  2. *G. vaginalis* are 100× normal
  3. *Streptococcus* are 10× normal
  4. *Mycoplasma hominis* and Enterobacteriaceae members are present in increased concentrations.

■ ASSOCIATIONS WITH OTHER DISORDERS
Bacterial vaginosis has been associated with PID, cystitis, posthysterectomy vaginal cuff cellulitis, postabortal infection, preterm delivery, premature rupture of membranes (PROM), amnionitis, chorioamnionitis, and postpartum endometritis.

DIAGNOSIS

Detecting three of the four following signs will diagnose 90% correctly, with <10% false positives:
1. Thin, gray, homogenous, malodorous discharge that adheres to the vaginal walls
2. Elevated pH >4.5
3. Positive KOH whiff test
4. Clue cells present on wet mount
- Cultures are unnecessary.
- Pap smear will not identify *G. vaginalis*.
- Gram stain of vaginal secretions will reveal clue cells and abnormal mixed bacteria (Fig. 1-390).

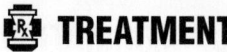

TREATMENT

■ TOPICAL REGIMENS
1. 0.75% metronidazole gel in vagina bid for 5 days
2. 2% clindamycin cream qd for 7 days

Both have about a 93% cure rate if used properly

■ ORAL REGIMENS
1. Metronidazole 500 mg PO bid for 7 days (95% cure rate)
2. Metronidazole ER 750 mg PO qd for 7 days
3. Metronidazole 2 g PO single dose (86% cure with higher relapse rate)
4. Clindamycin 300 mg PO bid for 7 days (increased incidence of diarrhea)

■ TREATMENT IN PREGNANCY
All pregnant patients proven to have BV should be treated because of its association with preterm labor, chorioamnionitis, and PROM.
FIRST TRIMESTER: 2% clindamycin cream × 7 days or oral clindamycin 300 mg bid × 7 days
SECOND & THIRD TRIMESTERS: Clindamycin vaginal/oral regimens *or* metronidazole vaginal/oral regimens may be used

REFERENCE
Mead P: *Protocols for infectious diseases in obstetrics and gynecology,* ed 2, New York, 2000, Blackwell Science.
Author: **Tiffany B. Genewick, M.D.**

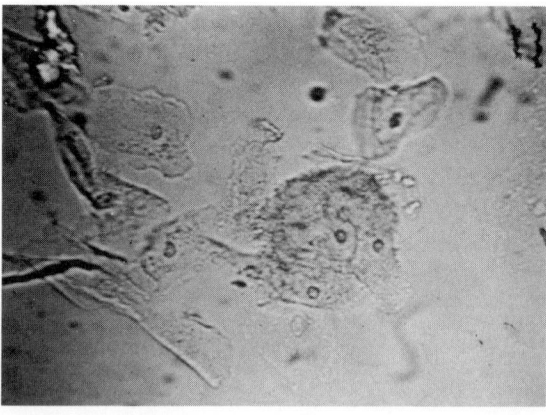

Fig. 1-390 Clue cells characteristic of bacterial vaginosis, squamous epithelial cells whose borders are obscured by bacteria. (From Carlson K [ed]: *Primary care of women,* St Louis, 1995, Mosby.)

BASIC INFORMATION

■ DEFINITION
Varicose veins are dilated networks of the subcutaneous venous system that result from valvular incompetence.

■ SYNONYMS
Chronic venous insufficiency
Stasis skin changes

ICD-9CM CODES
454.9 Varicose veins

■ EPIDEMIOLOGY & DEMOGRAPHICS
PREVALENCE:
- Approximately 30% of adults, with increasing incidence with age
- Increased incidence during pregnancy, especially with advanced maternal age

GENETICS:
- Familial tendency
- Evidence for dominant, recessive, and multifactorial types of inheritence

PREDOMINANT SEX: Female > male
RISK FACTORS:
- Advancing age
- Prolonged standing
- Pregnancy
- Obesity
- Use of oral contraceptives

■ PHYSICAL FINDINGS & CLINICAL PRESENTATION
- Dull ache, burning, or cramping in leg muscles
- Worsening discomfort with standing, warm temperatures, or menses
- Tortuous dilation of superficial veins
- Edema
- Varicose ulcer, sometimes with superficial infection
- Dermatitis pigmentation

■ ETIOLOGY
- Normally, blood flow directed from the superficial venous system to the deep venous system via communication of perforating vessels
- Best thought of as "venous hypertension"
- Valvular incompetence in perforator veins of lower extremity leading to reverse flow of fluid from high-pressure deep venous system to low-pressure superficial venous system, resulting in dilation of superficial veins, leg edema, and pain
- Rarely associated with deep vein thrombophlebitis
- Exacerbated by restrictive clothing

🔬 DIAGNOSIS

■ DIFFERENTIAL DIAGNOSIS
Conditions that can lead to superficial venous stasis other than primary valvular insufficiency include:
- Arterial occlusive disease
- Diabetes
- Deep vein thrombophlebitis
- Peripheral neuropathies
- Unusual infections
- Carcinoma

■ WORKUP
- Mainly a clinical diagnosis
- Arterial studies to rule out arterial insufficiency before initiating therapy for venous insufficiency

■ LABORATORY TESTS
Not useful

■ IMAGING STUDIES
Duplex ultrasound
- Gold standard for evaluation of varicose veins
- Quantitation of flow through venous valves under direct visualization
- Allows precise anatomic identification of source of venous reflux

💊 TREATMENT

■ NONPHARMACOLOGIC THERAPY
- Leg elevation and rest
- Graded compression stockings: used early in morning before edema accumulates and removed before going to bed
- Weight loss
- Avoidance of occlusive clothing

■ ACUTE GENERAL Rx
- For associated stasis dermatitis: topical corticosteroids
- Treatment of secondary infection with appropriate antibiotics

■ CHRONIC Rx
- Sclerotherapy: injection of 1% to 3% solution of sodium tetradecyl sulfate
- Surgery: indications include the following:
  1. Persistent varicosities with conservative treatment
  2. Failed sclerotherapy
  3. Previous or impending bleeding from ulcerated varicosities
  4. Disabling pain
  5. Cosmetic concerns
- Surgical methods include (must be combined with compressive therapy):
  1. Saphenous vein ligation
  2. Ligation of incompetent perforating veins
  3. Saphenous vein stripping with or without avulsion of varicosities
  4. Ambulatory "miniphlebectomies": avulsion of superficial varicosities with saphenous vein stripping

■ DISPOSITION
A chronic condition in which a combination of compressive and surgical therapy can adequately control varicosities

■ REFERRAL
- To dermatologist for dermatitis complications
- To surgeon for failed conservative management

REFERENCE
Bradbury A et al: What are the symptoms of varicose veins? Edinburgh Vein Study cross sectional population survey, *BMJ* 318:353, 1999.
Author: **Matthew L. Withiam-Leitch, M.D., Ph.D.**

BASIC INFORMATION

■ DEFINITION
- Ventricular septal defect (VSD) refers to an abnormal hole or opening in the septum separating the right and left ventricles.
- VSDs may be large or small, single or multiple.
- VSDs are located at various anatomic regions of the septum and classified as:
  1. Membranous (75% to 80%): Most common defect that can extend into the vascular septum.
  2. Canal or inlet defects (8%): Commonly lie beneath the septal leaflet of the tricuspid valve and often seen in patients with Down syndrome.
  3. Muscular or trabecular defects (5% to 20%): Can be single or multiple, small or large.
  4. Subarterial defect (5% to 7%): Least common and also called outlet, infundibular, or supracristal defect. Commonly found beneath the aortic valve, leading to aortic valve prolapse and regurgitation.
  5. Supracristal.

■ SYNONYMS
VSD

ICD-9CM CODES
745.4 Ventricular septal defect

■ EPIDEMIOLOGY & DEMOGRAPHICS
- Isolated VSD is the most common congenital heart abnormality found at birth and accounts for 30% of all congenital cardiac defects.
- Prevalence is 1.17 per 1000 live births and at 0.5 per 1000 adults.
- Found equally in males and females.
- Approximately 25% of all congenital heart defects found in children are VSDs.
- Approximately 10% of all congenital heart defects found in adults are VSDs.
- VSDs may be associated with:
  1. Coarctation of the aorta (17%)
  2. Patent ductus arteriosus (22%)
  3. Subvalvular aortic stenosis (4%)
  4. Subpulmonic stenosis
  5. Atrial septal defect (35%)
- Multiple VSDs are more prevalent in patients with tetralogy of Fallot and double outlet right ventricular defects.

■ PHYSICAL FINDINGS & CLINICAL PRESENTATION
- Clinical presentation is dictated by the direction and volume of the VSD shunt along with the ratio of the pulmonary to systemic vascular resistance
- Infants at birth may be asymptomatic because of elevated pulmonary artery pressures and resistance. Over the next few weeks, pulmonary arterial pressure decreases, allowing more blood flow through the VSD into the right ventricle, lungs, left atrium, and left ventricle and causing LV volume overload. Tachypnea, failure to thrive, and congestive heart failure ensue.
- In adults with VSDs the shunt is left to right in the absence of pulmonary stenosis and pulmonary hypertension and patients typically manifest with symptoms of heart failure (e.g., shortness of breath, orthopnea, and dyspnea on exertion).
- A spectrum of physical findings may be seen including:
  1. Holosystolic murmur heard best along the left sternal border
  2. Systolic thrill
  3. Mid-diastolic rumble heard at the apex
  4. S_3
  5. Rales
- With the development of pulmonary hypertension:
  1. Augmented pulmonic component of S_2
  2. Cyanosis and clubbing (seen in Eisenmenger's complex with reversal of the shunt in a right to left direction)

■ ETIOLOGY
Usually congenital, but may occur postmyocardial infarction.

DIAGNOSIS

The diagnosis of VSD is suspected by physical examination. Imaging studies, particularly transthoracic echocardiography, establishes the diagnosis.

■ DIFFERENTIAL DIAGNOSIS
Based on physical examination the diagnosis of VSD may be confused with other causes of systolic murmurs such as mitral regurgitation, aortic stenosis, asymmetric septal hypertrophy, and pulmonary stenosis.

■ WORKUP
Any person that is suspected of having a VSD should have an ECG, a chest x-ray, and an echocardiogram and be considered for a cardiac catheterization and angiography.

■ LABORATORY TESTS
- Laboratory tests are not specific but may offer insight into the severity of the disease.
- CBC may show polycythemia, especially in patients with Eisenmenger's complex.
- Arterial blood gases showing hypoxemia.

■ IMAGING STUDIES
- Chest x-ray findings in patients with VSDs include: Cardiomegaly resulting from volume overload directly related to the magnitude of the shunt.
- Enlargement of the proximal pulmonary arteries along with redistribution and pruning of the pulmonary vessels resulting from pulmonary hypertension (Fig. 1-391, A).
- ECG findings vary according to the size of the VSD and if pulmonary hypertension is present or not. In large VSDs with pulmonary hypertension, right axis deviation is seen along with evidence of right ventricular hypertrophy.
- Echocardiography is the noninvasive procedure of choice in the diagnosis of VSD.
  1. Two-dimensional echo and pulse wave Doppler displays the size and location of the VSD (Fig. 1-391, B).
  2. Continuous wave Doppler not only approximates the gradient between the left and right ventricle but also estimates the pulmonary artery pressure.
- Cardiac catheterization detects the shunt and estimates the pulmonary and systemic blood flow and pressures.
- Angiography also locates the VSD.

TREATMENT

The decision to treat a VSD depends on its type, size, shunt severity, pulmonary vascular resistance, functional capacity, and associated valvular abnormalities.

■ NONPHARMACOLOGIC THERAPY
- In young children, small asymptomatic VSDs with a pulmonary to systemic blood flow ratio of 1.5:1 and no evidence of pulmonary hypertension can be observed.
- Oxygen and low-salt diet in patients with congestive heart failure.

■ ACUTE GENERAL Rx
Surgery is indicated in:
- Infants with large VSDs and congestive heart failure
- Children between the ages of 1 to 6 with moderate to large VSD not closing over time and with pulmonary to systemic blood flow ratios >2:1

- Adults with VSD and flow ratios ~1.5:1
- Patients with VSD and elevated pulmonary vascular resistance up to 10 units per square meter

■ CHRONIC Rx
See "Acute General Rx."

■ DISPOSITION
- The natural history of isolated VSD depends on the type of defect, its size, and associated abnormalities.
- Approximately 75% to 80% of small VSDs close spontaneously by age 10 yr.
- In patients with large VSDs, only 10% to 15% will close spontaneously.
- Large VSDs left untreated may lead to arrhythmias, congestive heart failure, pulmonary hypertension, and Eisenmenger's complex.

- Eisenmenger's complex carries a poor prognosis, with most patients dying before the age of 40 yr.

■ REFERRAL
All infants and children diagnosed with VSD should be referred to a pediatric cardiologist. Adults with VSD should be referred to a cardiologist. Cardiothoracic surgeons experienced in congenital heart disease surgery should be consulted if surgery is indicated.

🔆 PEARLS & CONSIDERATIONS

■ COMMENTS
- Ventricular septal defect was first described by Dalrymple in 1847.
- Risk of patients with VSD developing infective endocarditis is 4%. The risk is higher if aortic insufficiency is present.

- Bacterial endocarditis prophylaxis is recommended in all patients with VSD.
- Postoperatively, if no shunt remains, endocarditis prophylaxis is not indicated after 6 mo.

REFERENCES
Ammash NM, Warnes CA: Ventricular septal defects in adults, *Ann Intern Med* 135:812, 2001.

Merrick AF et al: Management of ventricular septal defect: a survey of practice in the United Kingdom, *Ann Thorac Surg* 68(3):983, 1999.

Turner SW, Hunter S, Wyllie JP: The natural history of ventricular septal defects, *Arch Dis Child* 81(5):413, 1999.
Author: **Peter Petropoulos, M.D.**

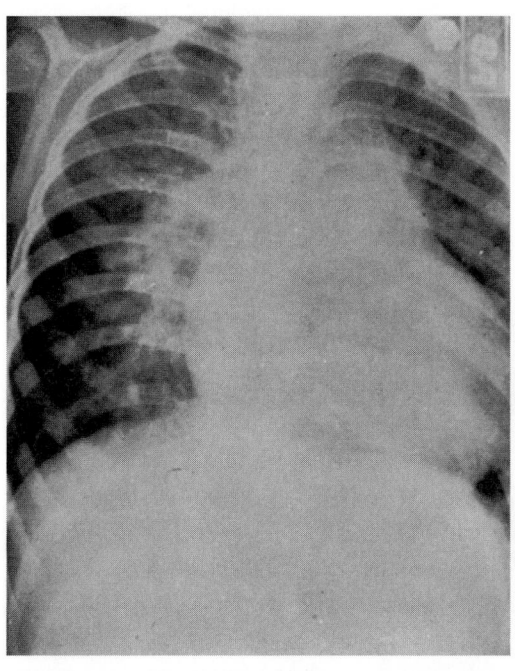
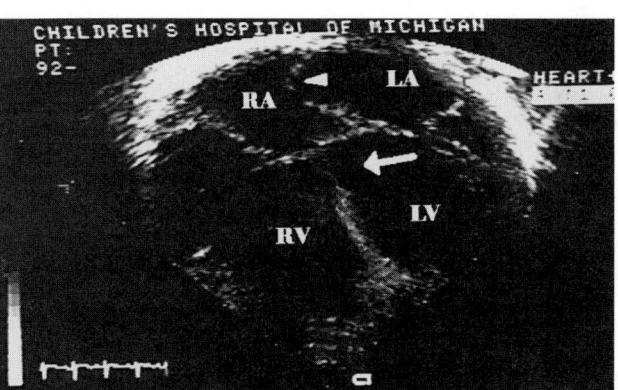

Fig. 1-391   A, Chest roentgenogram of a child with a large VSD, large pulmonary blood flow, and pulmonary hypertension, but only mild elevation of PVR. This is reflected in the evidence of left and right ventricular enlargement, enlargement of the main pulmonary artery, and marked increase in pulmonary blood flow. **B,** Apical four-chamber echocardiographic view of ventricular septal defect *(large arrow).* Small arrow points to interatrial septum. *RA,* Right atrium; *LA,* left atrium, *RV,* right ventricle; *LV,* left ventricle. (**A** From Pacifico AD, Kirklin JW, Kirklin JK: Surgical treatment of ventricular septal defect. In Sabiston DC, Jr, Spencer FC [eds]: *Surgery of the chest,* ed 5, Philadelphia, 1990, WB Saunders. **B** Courtesy Richard Humes, MD, Associate Professor of Pediatrics, Director of Echocardiography Laboratory, Children's Hospital of Michigan, Detroit.)

BASIC INFORMATION

■ DEFINITION
Vitiligo is the acquired loss of epidermal pigmentation characterized histologically by the absence of epidermal melanocytes.

ICD-9CM CODES
709.1 Vitiligo

■ EPIDEMIOLOGY & DEMOGRAPHICS
- Prevalence: 1% of the population
- Positive family history in 25% to 30%
- Can begin at any age, but age at onset is under 20 yr for half the patients

■ CLINICAL PRESENTATION & PHYSICAL FINDINGS
- Hypopigmented and depigmented lesions (Fig. 1-392) favor sun-exposed regions, intertriginous areas, genitalia, and sites over bony prominences (type A vitiligo).
- Areas around body orifices are also frequently involved.
- The lesions tend to be symmetric.
- Occasionally the lesions are linear or pseudodermatomal (type B vitiligo).
- Vitiligo lesions may occur at trauma sites (Koebner's phenomenon).
- The hair in affected areas may be white.
- The margins of the lesions are usually well demarcated, and when a ring of hyperpigmentation is seen, the term *trichrome vitiligo* is used.
- The term *marginal inflammatory vitiligo* is used to describe lesions with raised borders.
- Initially the disease is limited, but the lesions tend to become more extensive over the years.
- Type B vitiligo is more common in children.
- Vitiligo may begin around pigmented nevi, producing a halo (Sutton's nevus); in such cases the central nevus often regresses and disappears over time.

■ ETIOLOGY & PATHOGENESIS
Three pathophysiologic theories:
- Autoimmune theory (autoantibodies against melanocytes)
- Neural theory (neurochemical mediator selectively destroys melanocytes)
- Self-destructive process whereby melanocytes fail to protect themselves against cytotoxic melanin precursors

Although vitiligo is considered to be an acquired disease, 25% to 30% is familial; the mode of transmission is unknown (polygenic or autosomal dominant with incomplete penetrance and variable expression)

Associated disorders:
- Alopecia areata
- Type 1 diabetes mellitus
- Adrenal insufficiency
- Hyper- and hypothyroidism
- Mucocutaneous candidiasis
- Pernicious anemia
- Polyglandular autoimmune syndromes
- Melanoma

DIAGNOSIS

■ DIFFERENTIAL DIAGNOSIS (OTHER HYPOPIGMENTATION DISORDERS)
Acquired:
- Chemical-induced
- Halo nevus
- Idiopathic guttate hypomelanosis
- Leprosy
- Leukoderma associated with melanoma
- Pityriasis alba
- Postinflammatory hypopigmentation
- Tinea versicolor
- Vogt-Koyanagi syndrome (vitiligo, uveitis, and deafness)

Congenital:
- Albinism, partial (piebaldism)
- Albinism, total
- Nevus anemicus
- Nevus depigmentosus
- Tuberous sclerosis

■ WORKUP
- Physical examination
- Wood's light examination may enhance lesions in light-skinned individuals

TREATMENT

- Treatment indicated primarily for cosmetic purposes when depigmentation causes emotional or social distress. Depigmentation is more noticeable in darker complexions.
- Cosmetic masking agents (Dermablend, Covermark) or stains (Dy-O-Derm, Vita-Dye).
- Sunless tanning lotions (dihydroxyacetone).
- Repigmentation (achieved by activation and migration of melanocytes from hair follicles; therefore skin with little or no hair responds poorly to treatment).
- PUVA (psoralen phototherapy): oral or topical psoralen administration followed by phototherapy with UVA (150 to 200 treatments required over 1 to 2 yr).
- Psoralens and sunlight (Puvasol).
- Topical midpotency steroids (e.g., triamcinolone 0.1% or desonide 0.05% cream qd for 3 to 4 mo).
- Intralesional steroid injection.
- Systemic steroids (betamethasone 5 mg qd on two consecutive days per wk for 2 to 4 mo).
- Total depigmentation (in cases of extensive vitiligo) with 20% monobenzyl ether or hydroquinone. This is a permanent procedure, and patients will require lifelong protection from sun exposure.

REFERENCE
Habif TP: Vitiligo. In Habif TP (ed): *Clinical dermatology*, ed 3, St Louis, 1996, Mosby.
Author: **Tom J. Wachtel, M.D.**

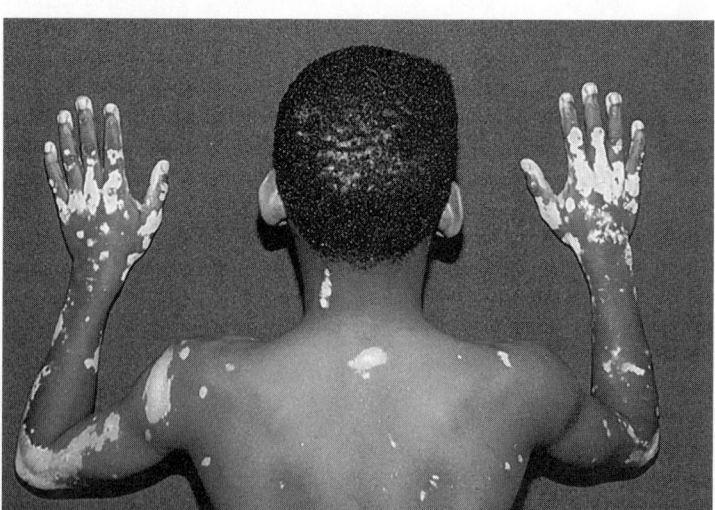

Fig. 1-392 Mutliple, sharply demarcated, symmetric, depigmented areas of vitiligo. (From Behrman RE: *Nelson textbook of pediatrics,* Philadelphia, 1996, WB Saunders.)

BASIC INFORMATION

■ **DEFINITION**

Von Hipppel-Lindau disease (VHL) is an autosomal dominant inherited disease characterized by the formation of hemangioblastomas, cysts, and malignancies involving multiple organs and systems.

■ **SYNONYMS**

Hippel-Lindau syndrome
Cerebelloretinal hemangioblastomatosis
Retinocerebellar angiomatosis

ICD-9CM CODE

759.6 von Hippel-Lindau disease

■ **EPIDEMIOLOGY & DEMOGRAPHICS**
- The incidence of VHL is 1 case/36,000 people.
- Age of onset varies but usually presents between the ages of 25 to 40 yr.
- In the U.S. approximately 7000 people are affected.
- Affected individuals are at risk of developing renal cell carcinoma, pheochromocytoma, pancreatic islet cell tumor, endolymphatic sac tumor, and hemangioblastomas of the cerebellum and retina.

■ **PHYSICAL FINDINGS & CLINICAL PRESENTATION**

The most common manifestations of VHL disease are:
- Retinal angiomas (59%)
  1. Most common presentation usually occurs by age 25.
  2. Multiple angiomas
  3. Detached retina
  4. Glaucoma
  5. Blindness
- CNS hemangioblastomas (59%)
  1. Cerebellum is the most common site followed by the spine and medulla.
  2. Usually multiple and occurs by the age of 30.
  3. Headache, ataxia, slurred speech, nystagmus, vertigo, nausea, and vomiting.
- Renal cysts (~60%) and clear cell renal cell carcinoma (25% to 45%).
  1. Usually occurs by the age of 40.
  2. May be asymptomatic or cause abdominal and flank pain.
  3. Renal cell carcinoma is bilateral in 75% of patients.
- Pancreatic cysts
  1. Usually asymptomatic
  2. Large cysts can cause biliary obstructive symptoms
  3. Diarrhea and diabetes may develop if enough of the pancreas is replaced by cysts.

- Pheochromocytoma (7% to 18%)
  1. Bilateral in 50% to 80% of cases
  2. Hypertension, palpitations, sweating, and headache
  3. Commonly occurs with pancreatic islet cell tumors
- Papillary cystadenoma of the epididymis (10% to 25% of men with VHL)
  1. Palpable scrotal mass
  2. May be unilateral or bilateral
- Endolymphatic sac tumors
  1. Ataxia
  2. Loss of hearing
  3. Facial paralysis

■ **ETIOLOGY**

VHL disease is primarily caused by a mutation of the von Hippel-Lindau gene located on chromosome 3. The VHL disease gene codes for a cytoplasmic protein that functions in tumor suppression.

 DIAGNOSIS

- The diagnosis of VHL disease is established if in the presence of a positive family history, a single retinal or cerebellar hemangioblastoma is noted or a visceral lesion is found (e.g., renal cell carcinoma, pheochromocytoma, pancreatic cysts or tumor).
- If no clear family history is present, two or more hemangioblastomas or one hemangioblastoma with a visceral lesion are required to make the diagnosis.
- Screening family members is essential in the early detection of VHL disease.

■ **WORKUP**

All patients with VHL disease or patients at risk for the disease should have screening laboratory, ophthalmoscopic, and imaging studies performed to look for sites of involvement.

■ **LABORATORY TESTS**
- CBC may reveal erythrocytosis requiring periodic phlebotomies.
- Electrolytes, BUN, and creatinine.
- Urine for norepinephrine, epinephrine, and vanillylmandelic acid looking for pheochromocytoma.

■ **IMAGING STUDIES**
- Indirect and direct ophthalmoscopy, fluorescein angioscopy, and tonometry are studies used in screening for retinal angiomas and glaucoma.

- CT scan of the abdomen is used in the screening, detection, and monitoring of patients with renal cysts renal tumors, pheochromocytomas, pancreatic cysts, and tumors (Fig. 1-393).
  1. Renal cysts grow on average 0.5 cm/yr.
  2. Renal tumors grow on average 1.5 cm/yr
  3. CT scans are done every 6 mo for the first 2 yr and every year for life in patients who have had surgery for renal cell carcinoma.
- MRI with gadolinium is used for screening and evaluation of CNS and spinal hemangioblastomas, endolymphatic sac tumors, and pheochromocytomas.
- Angiography may be done prior to CNS surgery.

 TREATMENT

■ **NONPHARMACOLOGIC THERAPY**

Genetic counseling is essential in patients diagnosed with VHL and in family members at risk.

■ **ACUTE GENERAL Rx**
- Laser photocoagulation and cryotherapy is used in patients with retinal angiomas to prevent blindness.
- For cerebellar hemangioblastomas the treatment is surgical removal. External-beam radiation and stereotaxic radiosurgery can also be done.
- For renal tumors, surgery is delayed until one of the renal tumors reaches 3 cm in diameter. Nephron-sparing surgery is the preferred surgical approach.
- Nephrectomy is indicated in patients with end-stage renal disease requiring dialysis because of the malignant potential of the disease.
- Pancreatic islet cell tumors usually require surgical removal.
- Adrenalectomy for pheochromocytoma.

■ **CHRONIC Rx**
- Dialysis has been delayed in many patients because of nephron-sparing surgery.
- Renal transplantation is usually delayed for 1 year after bilateral nephrectomy for renal tumors so as to ensure that no metastases occur.

■ **DISPOSITION**
- Median life expectancy is 49 yr of age.
- The most common cause of death in VHL disease is from renal cell carcinoma.

Gwendolyn R. Lee, M.D.
Internal Medicine

■ REFERRAL

- A coordinated team of physicians is needed in the management of patients with VHL disease including: geneticist, neurosurgeon, urologist, nephrologist, ophthalmologist, otolaryngologist, neurologist, endocrinologist, and radiation oncologist.
- Patients, family members, and physicians interested in learning more about VHL disease can contact: von Hippel-Lindau Family Alliance (171 Clinton Road, Brookline, MA 02146. Tel: 1-800-767-4VHL).

☼ PEARLS & CONSIDERATIONS

■ COMMENTS

- VHL disease is named after the German ophthalmologist, Eugen von Hippel, who described patients with retinal angiomas in 1904, and Arvid Lindau, a Swedish pathologist who associated the hereditary nature of patients with cerebellar hemangioblastomas and angiomas in 1927.
- Latif et al were the first to discover the VHL gene in 1993.
- Genetic testing is available but should be done under the guidance and expertise of a geneticist.

REFERENCES

Couch V, Lindor NM, Karnes PS, Michels VV: von Hippel-Lindau Disease, *Mayo Clin Proc* 75:265, 2000.

Zbar B et al: Third International meeting on von Hippel-Lindau disease, *Cancer Res* 59:2251, 1999.

Author: **Peter Petropoulos, M.D.**

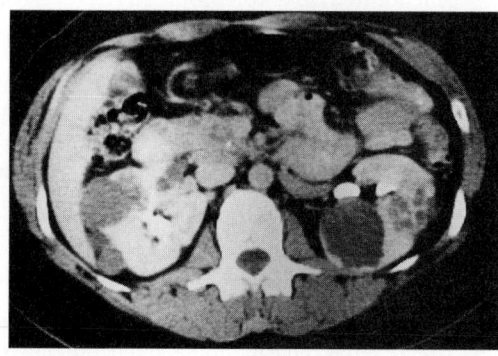

Fig. 1-393   Von Hippel-Lindau syndrome. Contrast CT demonstrates cystic and solid renal masses bilaterally. (From Barbaric ZL: *Principles of genitourinary radiology,* ed 2, New York, 1994, Thieme Medical.)

BASIC INFORMATION

■ DEFINITION
Von Willebrand's disease is a congenital disorder of hemostasis characterized by defective or deficient von Willebrand factor (vWF). There are several subtypes of von Willebrand's disease. The most common type (80% of cases) is type I, which is caused by a quantitative decrease in von Willebrand factor; type IIA and type IIB are results of qualitative protein abnormalities; type III is a rare autosomal recessive disorder characterized by a near complete quantitative deficiency of vWF.

■ SYNONYMS
Pseudohemophilia

ICD-9CM CODES
286.4 von Willebrand's disease

■ EPIDEMIOLOGY & DEMOGRAPHICS
- Autosomal dominant disorder
- Most common inherited bleeding disorder
- Occurs in >100/1 million persons

■ PHYSICAL FINDINGS & CLINICAL PRESENTATION
- Generally normal physical examination
- Mucosal bleeding (gingival bleeding, epistaxis) and GI bleeding may occur
- Easy bruising
- Postpartum bleeding, bleeding after surgery or dental extraction, menorrhagia

■ ETIOLOGY
Quantitative or qualitative deficiency of vWF (see "Definition")

DIAGNOSIS

■ DIFFERENTIAL DIAGNOSIS
- Platelet function disorders, clotting factor deficiencies
- A clinical algorithm for evaluation of congenital bleeding disorders is described in Fig. 3-28

■ WORKUP
- Laboratory evaluation (see "Laboratory Tests")
- Initial testing includes PTT (increased), platelet count (normal), and bleeding time (prolonged)
- Subsequent tests include vWF level (decreased), factor VIII:C (decreased), and ristocetin agglutination (increased in type II B) (Table 1-71)

■ LABORATORY TESTS
- Normal platelet number and morphology
- Prolonged bleeding time
- Decreased factor VIII coagulant activity
- Decreased von Willebrand factor antigen or ristocetin cofactor
- Normal platelet aggregation studies
- Type II A von Willebrand can be distinguished from type I by absence of ristocetin cofactor activity and abnormal multimer
- Type IIB von Willebrand is distinguished from type I by abnormal multimer

TREATMENT

■ NONPHARMACOLOGIC THERAPY
- Avoidance of aspirin and other NSAIDs

- Evaluation for likelihood of bleeding (with measurement of bleeding time) before surgical procedures

■ ACUTE GENERAL Rx
- Desmopressin acetate (DDAVP) is useful to release stored vWF from endothelial cells. It is used to cover minor procedures and traumatic bleeding in mild type I von Willebrand's disease. Dose is 0.3 μg/kg in 100 ml of normal saline solution IV infused >20 min. DDAVP is also available as a nasal spray (dose of 150 μg spray administered to each nostril) as a preparation for minor surgery and management of minor bleeding episodes. DDAVP is not effective in type IIA von Willebrand's disease and is potentially dangerous in type IIB (increased risk of bleeding and thrombocytopenia).
- In patients with severe disease, replacement therapy in the form of cryoprecipitate is the method of choice. The standard dose is 1 bag of cryoprecipitate per 10 kg of body weight.
- Factor VIII concentrate rich in vWF (Humate-P, Armour) is useful to correct bleeding abnormalities.
- Life-threatening hemorrhage unresponsive to therapy with cryoprecipitate or factor VIII concentrate may require transfusion of normal platelets.

■ DISPOSITION
Prognosis is very good; most patients have minor bleeding complications and are able to lead a normal life.
Author: **Fred F. Ferri, M.D.**

TABLE 1-71 Genetic and Laboratory Findings in von Willebrand's Disease

TYPE	BT	VIII-C	vW-Ag	R-Cof	RIPA	MULTIMER STRUCTURE	MODE OF INHERITANCE
I (classic)	P	R	R	R	R	N	AD
II							
A	P	N/R	N/R	R	R	Abn	AD
B	P	N/R	N/R	N/R	I	Abn	AD
III	P	R	R	R	R	Variable	AR

From Behrman RE: *Nelson textbook of pediatrics,* ed 15, Philadelphia, 1996, WB Saunders.
Abn, Abnormal; *AD,* autosomal dominant; *AR,* autosomal recessive; *BT,* bleeding time; *I,* increased; *N,* normal; *N/R,* normal or reduced; *P,* prolonged; *R,* reduced; *R-Cof,* ristocetin cofactor; *RIPA,* ristocetin-induced platelet aggregation (agglutination); *vW-Ag,* von Willebrand antigen (protein); *VIII-C,* factor VIII coagulant activity.

BASIC INFORMATION

DEFINITION

Vulvar cancer is an abnormal cell proliferation arising on the vulva and exhibiting malignant potential. The majority are of squamous cell origin; however, other types include adenocarcinoma, basal cell carcinoma, sarcoma, and melanoma (Fig. 1-394).

SYNONYMS

Squamous cell carcinoma of the vulva (90%)
Basal cell carcinoma of the vulva
Adenocarcinoma of the vulva
Melanoma of the vulva
Bartholin gland carcinoma
Verrucous carcinoma of the vulva
Vulvar sarcoma

ICD-9CM CODES
184.4 Vulvar neoplasm

EPIDEMIOLOGY & DEMOGRAPHICS

PREVALENCE: Vulvar cancer is uncommon. It comprises 4% of malignancies of the female genital tract. It is the fourth most common gynecologic malignancy.
INCIDENCE: 1.8 cases/100,000 persons
MEAN AGE AT DIAGNOSIS: Predominantly a disease of menopause. Mean age at diagnosis is 65 yr.

PHYSICAL FINDINGS & CLINICAL PRESENTATION

- Vulvar pruritus or pain is present.
- May produce a malodor or discharge or present as bleeding.
- Raised lesion, may have fleshy, ulcerated, leukoplakic, or warty appearance; may have multifocal lesions.
- Lesions are usually located on labia majora, but may be seen on labia minora, clitoris, and perineum.
- The lymph nodes of groin may be palpable.

ETIOLOGY

- The exact etiology is unknown.
- Vulvar intraepithelial neoplasia has been reported in 20% to 30% of invasive squamous cell carcinoma of the vulva, but the malignant potential is unknown.
- Human papillomavirus is found in 30% to 50% of vulvar carcinoma, but its exact role is unclear.
- Chronic pruritus, wetness, industrial wastes, arsenicals, hygienic agents, and vulvar dystrophies have been implicated as causative agents.

DIAGNOSIS

DIFFERENTIAL DIAGNOSIS

- Lymphogranuloma inguinale
- Tuberculosis
- Vulvar dystrophies
- Vulvar atrophy
- Paget's disease

WORKUP

- Diagnosis is made histologically by biopsy.
- Thorough examination of the lesion and assessment of spread.
- Possible colposcopy of adjacent areas.
- Cytologic smear of vagina and cervix.
- Cystoscopy and proctosigmoidoscopy may be necessary.

IMAGING STUDIES

- Chest radiography
- CT scan and MRI for assessing local tumor spread

TREATMENT

NONPHARMACOLOGIC THERAPY

- Treatment is individualized depending on the stage of the tumor.
- Stage I tumors with <1 mm stromal invasion are treated with complete local excision without groin node dissection.
- Stage I tumors with >1 mm stromal invasion are treated with complete local excision with groin node dissection.
- Stage II tumors require radical vulvectomy with bilateral groin node dissection.
- Advanced-stage disease may require the addition of radiation and chemotherapy to the surgical regimen.
- Fig. 1-395 describes a treatment algorithm for management of vulvar cancer.

DISPOSITION

Five-year survival ranges from 90% for stage I to 15% for stage IV.

REFERRAL

Vulvar cancer should be managed by a gynecologic oncologist and radiation oncologist.

Author: **Gil Farkash, M.D.**

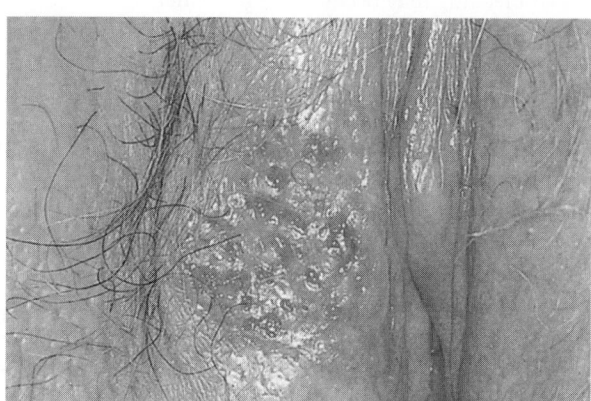

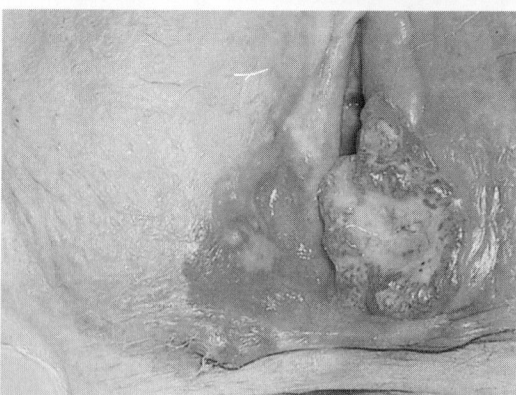

Fig. 1-394 **A,** Basal cell carcinoma of the vulva. **B,** Ulcerative squamous cell carcinoma of the vulva. (From Symonds EM, Macpherson MBA: *Color atlas of obstetrics and gynecology,* St Louis, 1994, Mosby.)

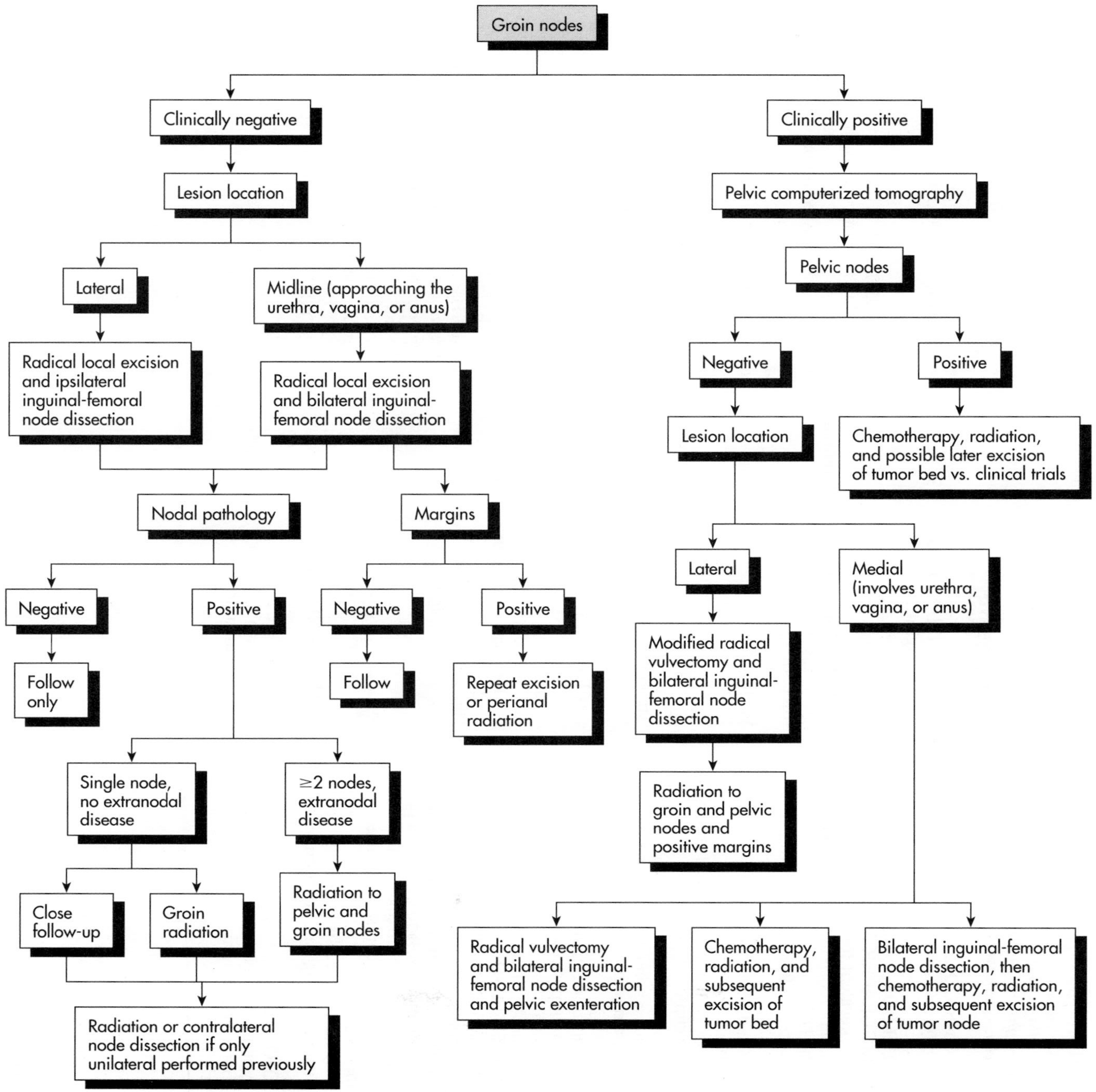

Fig. 1-395   Treatment algorithm for management of patients with vulvar cancer. (From Copeland LJ: *Textbook of gynecology,* ed 2, Philadelphia, 2000, WB Saunders.)

BASIC INFORMATION

■ **DEFINITION**
Bacterial vulvovaginitis is inflammation affecting the vagina, only rarely affecting the vulva, caused by anaerobic and aerobic bacteria.

■ **SYNONYMS**
Bacterial vaginosis
Gardnerella vaginalis
Haemophilus vaginalis
Corynebacterium vaginalis

ICD-9CM CODES
616.10 Vulvovaginitis

■ **EPIDEMIOLOGY & DEMOGRAPHICS**
• Most prevalent form of vaginal infection of reproductive age women in the U.S.
• 32% to 64% in patients visiting STD clinics
• 12% to 25% in other clinic populations
• 10% to 26% in patients visiting obstetric clinics
• Associated with adverse pregnancy outcomes: premature rupture of membranes, preterm labor, preterm birth
• Organisms frequently found in postpartum or postcesarean endometritis

■ **PHYSICAL FINDINGS & CLINICAL PRESENTATION**
• >50% of all women may be without symptoms.
• Unpleasant, fishy, or musty vaginal odor in about 50% to 70% of all patients. Odor exacerbated immediately after intercourse or during menstruation.
• Vaginal discharge is increased.
• Vaginal itching and irritation occur.

■ **ETIOLOGY**
• Synergistic polymicrobial infection characterized by an overgrowth of

bacteria normally found in the vagina
• Anaerobics: *Bacteroides* spp., *Peptostreptococcus* spp., *Mobiluncus* spp.
• Facultative anaerobes: *G. vaginalis*, *Mycoplasma hominis*
• Concentration of anaerobic bacteria increased to 100 to 1000 times normal
• Lactobacilli are absent or greatly reduced

DIAGNOSIS

■ **DIFFERENTIAL DIAGNOSIS**
• Fungal vaginitis
• *Trichomonas* vaginitis
• Atrophic vaginitis
• Cervicitis
• Table 2-207 describes the differential diagnosis of vaginal discharges and infections.

■ **WORKUP**
• Pelvic examination
• Speculum examination
• Normal saline and 10% KOH slide of discharge
• Amsel criteria for diagnosis (three of four should be present):
  1. pH >4.5
  2. Clue cells (epithelial cells covered with bacteria) on saline solution slide
  3. Positive whiff test on 10% KOH
  4. Homogeneous, white, adherent discharge
• Fig. 3-173 describes the evaluation of vaginal discharge.

TREATMENT

■ **ACUTE GENERAL Rx**
• Metronidazole 500 mg PO bid × 7 days, >90% cure rate
• Metronidazole 2 g PO × 1 day, 67% to 92% cure rate

• Metronidazole gel 5 g, intravaginal bid × 5 days
• Clindamycin 2% cream 5 g, intravaginal qd × 7 days
• Clindamycin 300 mg PO bid × 7 days in pregnancy

■ **CHRONIC Rx**
Clindamycin 300 mg PO bid × 7 days; cure rate similar to those achieved with metronidazole
Related to adverse pregnancy outcomes
• Metronidazole 250 mg PO bid × 7 days
• Metronidazole zympoxidase
• Clindamycin 300 mg PO bid × 7 days

■ **DISPOSITION**
• Reevaluate if not cured with treatment
• Recurrence fairly common

■ **REFERRAL**
Refer to obstetrician/gynecologist for recurrence or pregnant patient with bacterial vaginosis

PEARLS & CONSIDERATIONS

■ **COMMENTS**
Treating sexual partners has failed to demonstrate a benefit.

REFERENCES
Mead P, Hager WD, Faro S: *Protocols for infectious diseases in obstetrics and gynecology,* ed 2, New York, 2000, Blackwell Science.
1998 Guidelines for treatment of sexually transmitted diseases, *MMWR,* 47 (RR-1):1, 1998.
Author: **Julie Anne Szumigala, M.D.**

BASIC INFORMATION

■ DEFINITION
Estrogen-deficient vulvovaginitis is the irritation and/or inflammation of the vulva and vagina because of progressive thinning and atrophic changes secondary to estrogen deficiency (Fig. 1-396).

■ SYNONYMS
Atrophic vaginitis

ICD-9CM CODES
616.10 Vulvovaginitis

■ EPIDEMIOLOGY & DEMOGRAPHICS
• Seen most often in postmenopausal women
• Average age of menopause is 52 yr
• In 1990, there were 36 million women 50 yr of age or older

■ PHYSICAL FINDINGS & CLINICAL PRESENTATION
• Thinning of pubic hair, labia minora and majora
• Decreased secretions from the vestibular glands, with vaginal dryness
• Regression of subcutaneous fat
• Vulvar and vaginal itching
• Dyspareunia
• Dysuria and urinary frequency
• Vaginal spotting

■ ETIOLOGY
Estrogen deficiency

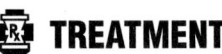

DIAGNOSIS

■ DIFFERENTIAL DIAGNOSIS
• Infectious vulvovaginitis
• Squamous cell hyperplasia
• Lichen sclerosus
• Vulva malignancy
• Vaginal malignancy
• Cervical and endometrial malignancy

■ WORKUP
• Pelvic examination
• Speculum examination
• Pap smear
• Possible endometrial biopsy if bleeding

■ LABORATORY TESTS
FSH and estradiol: generally after menopause, estradiol <15 pg and FSH >40 mIU/ml

TREATMENT

■ ACUTE GENERAL Rx
• Premarin 0.625 mg PO qd.
• Estraderm patch 0.05 mg × 2 per week.
• If uterus present:
  1. Estrogen + 2.5 mg PO Provera qd *or*
  2. Estrogen + 10 mg PO Provera × 10 days each mo
• Conjugated estrogen vaginal cream intravaginally. Estradiol vaginal cream 0.01%.
  2 to 4 g/day × 2 wk then
  1 to 2 g/day × 2 wk then
  1 to 2 g × 3 days/wk
• Vagifen (estradial vaginal tablets) 25 mg inserted intravaginally daily for

2 wk then twice weekly. May take up to 12 wk to feel the full benefits of the medication.
• Conjugated estrogen vaginal cream: 2-4 g qd (3 wk on, 1 wk off) for 3-5 months.

■ CHRONIC Rx
See "Acute General Rx." May discontinue vaginal estrogen cream once symptoms alleviate.

■ DISPOSITION
The symptoms should be improved with the therapy. Caution for vaginal bleeding if uterus present.

■ REFERRAL
To obstetrician/gynecologist if vaginal bleeding
Author: **Julie Anne Szumigala, M.D.**

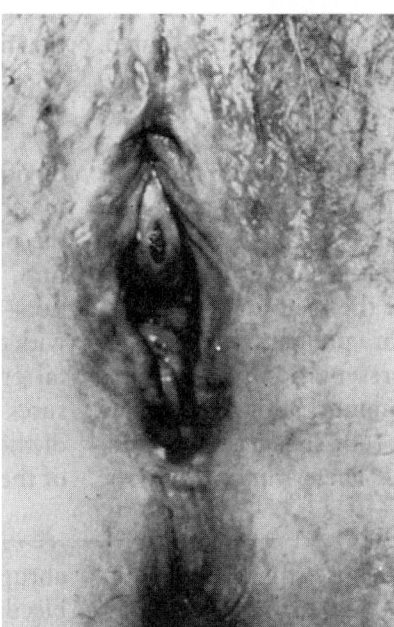

Fig. 1-396 Advanced postmenopausal atrophy of the vulva in a 72-year-old woman. (From Symonds EM, Macpherson MBA: *Color atlas of obstetrics and gynecology,* St Louis, 1994, Mosby.)

BASIC INFORMATION

■ **DEFINITION**
Fungal vulvovaginitis is the inflammation of vulva and vagina caused by *Candida* spp.

■ **SYNONYMS**
Monilial vulvovaginitis

ICD-9CM CODES
112.1 Vulvovaginitis, monilial

■ **EPIDEMIOLOGY & DEMOGRAPHICS**
• Second most common cause of vaginal infection.
• Approximately 13 million people were affected in 1990.
• 75% of women will have at least one episode during their child-bearing years, and approximately 40% to 50% of these will experience a second attack.
• No symptoms in 20% to 40% of women who have positive cultures.

■ **PHYSICAL FINDINGS & CLINICAL PRESENTATION**
• Intense vulvar and vaginal pruritus
• Edema and erythema of vulva
• Thick, curdlike vaginal discharge
• Adherent, dry, white, curdy patches attached to vaginal mucosa

■ **ETIOLOGY**
• *Candida albicans* is responsible for 80% to 95% of vaginal fungal infections.
• *Candida tropicalis* and *Torulopsis glabrata (Candida glabrata)* are the most common nonalbicans *Candida* species that can induce vaginitis.

■ **PREDISPOSING HOST FACTORS**
• Pregnancy
• Oral contraceptives (high-estrogen)
• Diabetes mellitus
• Antibiotics
• Immunosuppression
• Tight, poorly ventilated, nylon underclothing, with increased local perineal moisture and temperature

DIAGNOSIS

■ **DIFFERENTIAL DIAGNOSIS**
• Bacterial vaginosis
• *Trichomonas* vaginitis
• Atrophic vaginitis
• Table 2-207 describes the differential diagnosis of vaginal discharges and infections.

■ **WORKUP**
• Pelvic examination
• Speculum examination
• Hyphae or budding spores on 10% KOH preparation (positive in 50% to 70% of individuals with yeast infection)
• Fig. 3-173 describes the evaluation of vaginal discharge

■ **LABORATORY TESTS**
Culture, especially recurrence for identification

TREATMENT

■ **ACUTE GENERAL Rx**
• Cure rate of the various azole derivatives 85% to 90%; little evidence of superiority of one azole agent over another
• Cure rate of polyene (Nystatin) cream and suppositories, 75% to 80%
• Miconazole 200-mg suppository (Monistat 3), one suppository × 3 or 2% vaginal cream (Monistat 7), one applicator full intravaginally qhs × 7
• Clotrimazole 200-mg vaginal tablet, one tablet intravaginally qhs × 3 or 100-mg vaginal tablet (Gyne-Lotrimin, Mycelex-G) one tablet intravaginally qhs × 7, or 1% vaginal cream intravaginally qhs × 7
• Butoconazole 2% cream (Femstat) one applicator intravaginally qhs × 3
• Terconazole 80-mg suppository or 0.8% vaginal cream (Terazol 3), one suppository or one applicator intravaginally qhs × 3 or 0.4% vaginal cream (Terazol 7), one applicator intravaginally qhs × 7
• Tioconazole 6.5% ointment (Vagistat), one applicator intravaginally × 1
• Fluconazole (Diflucan) 150 mg PO × 1

■ **CHRONIC Rx**
• Resistance or recurrence
  1. 14- to 21-day course of 7-day regimens mentioned in "Acute General Rx"
  2. Fluconazole (Diflucan) 150 mg PO × 1

  3. Ketoconazole (Nizoral) 200 mg PO bid × 5 to 14 days
  4. Itraconazole (Sporanox) 200 mg PO qd × 3 days
  5. Boric acid 600-mg capsule intravaginally bid × 14 days
• Prophylactic regimens
  1. Clotrimazole one 500-mg vaginal tablet each month
  2. Ketoconazole 200 mg PO bid × 5 days each month
  3. Fluconazole 150 mg PO × 1 each month
  4. Miconazole 100-mg vaginal tablet × 2 weekly

■ **DISPOSITION**
• Approximately 40% of adult women experience more than one lifetime episode of fungal vulvovaginitis.
• If symptoms do not resolve completely with treatment, or if they recur within a 2- to 3-mo period, further evaluation is indicated.
• Reexamination and possibly culture are necessary.
• Positive culture in absence of symptoms should not lead to treatment. Approximately 30% of women harbor *Candida* spp. and other species in the vagina.

■ **REFERRAL**
To obstetrician/gynecologist for recurrence

PEARLS & CONSIDERATIONS

■ **COMMENTS**
Treatment of sexual partner is not recommended.
• Treatment of sex partners may be considered for women who have recurrent infection.
• Sex partners might benefit from treatment with topical antifungal agents.

REFERENCES
Nyirjesy P: Chronic vulvovagial candidiasis, *Am Fam Physician* 63:687, 2001.
Spinius A et al: Effect of antibiotic use on the prevalence of symptomatic vulvovaginal candidiasis, *Am J Obstet Gynecol* 180:14, 1999.
Author: **Julie Anne Szumigala, M.D.**

BASIC INFORMATION

■ DEFINITION

Prepubescent vulvovaginitis is an inflammatory condition of vulva and vagina.

ICD-9CM CODES

616.10 Vulvovaginitis

■ EPIDEMIOLOGY & DEMOGRAPHICS

- Most common gynecologic problem of the premenarcheal female.
- Prepubertal girl is susceptible to irritation and trauma because of the absence of protective hair and labial fat pads and the lack of estrogenization with atrophic vaginal mucosa.
- Symptoms of vulvovaginitis and introital irritation and discharge account for 80% to 90% of gynecologic visits.
- Nonspecific etiology in approximately 75% of children with vulvovaginitis.
- Majority of vulvovaginitis in children involves a primary irritation of the vulva with secondary involvement of the lower one third of the vagina.

■ PHYSICAL FINDINGS & CLINICAL PRESENTATION

- Vulvar pain, dysuria, pruritus
  1. Discharge is not a primary symptom.
  2. If present, vaginal discharge may be foul smelling or bloody.

■ ETIOLOGY

- Infections
  1. Bacterial
  2. Protozoal
  3. Mycotic
  4. Viral

- Endocrine disorders
- Labial adhesions
- Poor hygiene
- Sexual abuse
- Allergic substance
- Trauma
- Foreign body
- Masturbation
- Box 2-253 describes the differential diagnosis of vaginal discharge in prepubertal girls.

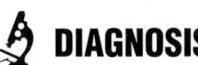 **DIAGNOSIS**

■ DIFFERENTIAL DIAGNOSIS

- Physiologic leukorrhea
- Foreign body
- Bacterial vaginosis
- Gonorrhea
- Fungal vulvovaginitis
- *Trichomonas* vulvovaginitis
- Sexual abuse
- Pinworms

■ WORKUP

- Pelvic, genital examination
- Speculum examination
- Rectal examination
- KOH and normal saline preparation of discharge
- Fig. 3-173 describes the evaluation of vaginal discharge

■ LABORATORY TESTS

- Urinalysis to rule out UTI and diabetes
- Cultures including STDs

TREATMENT

■ NONPHARMACOLOGIC THERAPY

- Avoid tight clothing
- Perineal hygiene
- Avoid irritant chemicals
- Reassurance

■ ACUTE GENERAL Rx

- Group A β *Streptococcus* and *Streptococcus pneumoniae*: penicillin V potassium 125 to 250 mg PO qid × 10 days
- *Chlamydia trachomatis*: erythromycin 50 mg/kg/day PO × 10 days
  1. Children >8 yr of age, doxycycline 100 mg bid PO × 7 days
- *Neisseria gonorrhoeae*: ceftriaxone 125 mg IM × 1 day
  1. Children >8 yr of age should also be given doxycycline 100 mg bid PO × 7 days
- *Staphylococcus aureus*: amoxicillin-clavulanate 20 to 40 mg/kg/day PO × 7 to 10 days
- *Haemophilus influenzae*: amoxicillin 20 to 40 mg/kg/day PO × 7 days
- *Trichomonas*: metronidazole 125 mg (15 mg/kg/day) tid PO × 7 to 10 days
- Pinworms: mebendazole 100-mg tablet chewable, repeat in 2 wk
- Labial agglutination: spontaneous resolution or topical estrogen cream for 7-10 days

■ CHRONIC Rx

See "Referral."

■ DISPOSITION

Further education:
- Young child: hygiene
- Adolescent: pregnancy prevention and "safe sex"

■ REFERRAL

- To obstetrician/gynecologist
- To pediatrician

Author: **Julie Anne Szumigala, M.D.**

BASIC INFORMATION

■ DEFINITION
Trichomonas vulvovaginitis is the inflammation of vulva and vagina caused by *Trichomonas* spp.

■ SYNONYMS
Trichomonas vaginalis

ICD-9CM CODES
131.01 Vulvovaginitis, trichomonal

■ EPIDEMIOLOGY & DEMOGRAPHICS
• Acquired through sexual contact
• Diagnosed in:
  1. 50% to 75% of prostitutes
  2. 5% to 15% of women visiting gynecology clinics
  3. 7% to 32% of women in STD clinics
  4. 5% of women in family planning clinics

■ PHYSICAL FINDINGS & CLINICAL PRESENTATION
• Profuse, yellow, malodorous vaginal discharge and severe vaginal itching
• Vulvar itching
• Dysuria
• Dyspareunia
• Intense erythema of the vaginal mucosa
• Cervical petechiae ("strawberry cervix")
• Asymptomatic in approximately 50% of women and 90% of men

■ ETIOLOGY
Single-cell parasite known as *trichomonad*

■ RISK FACTORS
• Multiple sexual partners
• History of previous STDs

DIAGNOSIS

■ DIFFERENTIAL DIAGNOSIS (Table 1-72)
• Bacterial vaginosis
• Fungal vulvovaginitis
• Cervicitis
• Atrophic vulvovaginitis

■ WORKUP
• Pelvic examination
• Speculum examination
• Mobile trichomonads seen on normal saline preparation: 70% to 90% sensitivity when symptomatic
• Elevated pH (>5) of vaginal discharge
• A large number of inflammatory cells on normal saline preparation
• Fig. 3-213 describes the evaluation of vaginal discharge

■ LABORATORY TESTS
• Culture (modified Diamond media): 90% sensitivity
• Direct enzyme immunoassay
• Fluorescein-conjugated monoclonal antibody test
• Pap test 40% detected

TREATMENT

■ NONPHARMACOLOGIC THERAPY
Condom use

■ ACUTE GENERAL Rx
Metronidazole (Flagyl) 2 g PO × 1 or 500 mg PO bid × 7 days

■ CHRONIC Rx
Metronidazole, 500 mg PO bid × 14 days or 2 g PO qd × 3 days accompanied by:
• Metronidazole gel (MetroGel-Vaginal), 5 g intravaginally bid × 5 days *or*
• Povidone-iodine suppository (Betadine), one suppository intravaginally bid × 14 to 28 days
Allergy, intolerance, or adverse reactions
• Alternatives to metronidazole are not available. Patients who are allergic to metronidazole can be managed by desensitization.

■ DISPOSITION
Trichomonas infection is considered an STD; therefore, treatment of the sexual partner is necessary.

■ REFERRAL
To obstetrician/gynecologist for recurrence and pregnancy

REFERENCE
1998 Guideline for treatment of sexually transmitted disease *MMWR* 47(RR-1):1, 1998.
Author: **Julie Anne Szumigala, M.D.**

TABLE 1-72   Differential Diagnosis of Vaginitis

CHARACTERISTICS OF VAGINAL DISCHARGE	C. ALBICANS VAGINITIS	T. VAGINALIS VAGINITIS	BACTERIAL VAGINOSIS
pH	4.5	>5.0	>5.0
White curd	Usually	No	No
Odor with KOH	No	Yes	Yes
Clue cells	No	No	Usually
Motile trichomonads	No	Usually	No
Yeast cells	Yes	No	No

From Goldman L, Bennett JC (eds): *Cecil textbook of medicine*, ed 21, Philadelphia, 2000, WB Saunders.

BASIC INFORMATION

DEFINITION
Waldenström's macroglobulinemia (WM) is a plasma cell dyscrasia characterized by the presence of IgM monoclonal macroglobulins.

SYNONYMS
WM
Monoclonal macroglobulinemia

ICD-9CM CODES
273.3 Waldenstrom's macroglobulinemia

EPIDEMIOLOGY & DEMOGRAPHICS
- Accounts for 2% of all hematologic cancers
- 1500 people diagnosed each year in the U.S.
- Incidence: 0.61/100,00 in men; 0.36/100,000 in women.
- Usually occurs in people over age 65 but can occur in younger people.
- More common among men than women and among whites than blacks.

PHYSICAL FINDINGS & CLINICAL PRESENTATION
- Weakness
- Fatigue
- Weight loss
- Headache, dizziness, vertigo, deafness, and seizures (hyperviscocity syndrome)
- Easy bleeding (e.g., epistaxis)
- Retinal vein link sausage shaped
- Lymphadenopathy
- Hepatomegaly
- Splenomegaly
- Purpura
- Peripheral neuropathy

ETIOLOGY
- The exact cause of WM is not known.
- Genetic predisposition, radiation exposure, occupational chemicals, and chronic inflammatory stimulation have been suggested but there is insufficient evidence to substantiate these hypotheses.

DIAGNOSIS

The diagnosis of WM is usually established by laboratory blood tests and by bone marrow biopsy.

DIFFERENTIAL DIAGNOSIS
- Monoclonal gammopathy of unknown significance (MGUS)
- Multiple myeloma
- Chronic lymphocytic leukemia
- Hairy-cell leukemia
- Lymphoma

WORKUP
In any patient suspected of having WM, specific blood tests (CBC, ESR, SPEP, IPEP, UPEP, IgM level, serum viscosity) and bone marrow biopsy will confirm the diagnosis.

LABORATORY TESTS
- CBC with differential:
  1. Anemia is a common finding. White blood cell count is usually normal; thromboctyopenia can occur.
  2. Peripheral smear may reveal malignant lymphoid cells in terminal patients.
- Elevated ESR
- Serum protein electrophoresis (SPEP): homogeneous M spike
- Immunoelectrophoresis: proves IgM
- Urine immunoelectrophoresis: monoclonal light chain usually kappa chains. Bence Jones protein can be seen but is not the typical finding in WM.
- IgM levels are high with symptoms usually occurring when the IgM concentration is 30 g/L or greater.
- Serum viscosity: symptoms usually occur when the serum viscosity is four times the viscosity of normal serum.
- Cryoglobulins, rheumatoid factor, or cold agglutinins may be present.
- Bone marrow biopsy: Characteristically reveals lymphoplasmacytoid cells that have infiltrated the bone marrow.

IMAGING STUDIES
- Chest x-ray can be obtained to rule out pulmonary involvement.

TREATMENT

NONPHARMACOLOGIC THERAPY
Asymptomatic patients do not require treatment, and these patients should be monitored periodically for the onset of symptoms or changes in blood tests (e.g., worsening anemia, thrombocytopenia, rising IgM, and serum viscosity).

ACUTE GENERAL Rx
Symptomatic patients with WM usually receive chemotherapy.
- Chlorambucil and prednisone are given daily for 10 days and repeated at 6-wk intervals until a response is seen in the IgM concentration. Approximately 60% of patients respond to chemotherapy as defined by a 75% reduction in IgM concentration.
- Combination melphalan, cyclophosphamide, and prednisone chemotherapy given for 7 days at 4- to 6-wk intervals for 12 courses followed by continuous therapy with chlorambucil and prednisone until relapse has shown promising results.

CHRONIC Rx
- Refractory patients can be tried on fludarabine or 2-CdA (2-chloro-deoxyadenosine).
- New treatment approaches include high-dose therapy with stem cell support and administration of monoclonal anti-CD 20 antibodies.

DISPOSITION
- The onset of WM is slow and insidious. Most patients die from progression of the disease with hyperviscocity, hemorrhage, and infection or from congestive heart failure.
- Some patients develop acute myelogenous leukemia, immunoblastic sarcoma, or chronic myelogenous leukemia as a preterminal event.
- Median survival in patients with WM is about 4 yr.
- Approximately 10% of patients will achieve complete remission with prognosis being more favorable (median survival 11 yr).

REFERRAL
If WM is suspected, a hematology consultation is helpful in guiding future workup, treatment, and monitoring.

PEARLS & CONSIDERATIONS

COMMENTS
- Waldenström's macroglobulinemia was first described in 1944 by the Swedish physician Jan Gosta Waldenström.
- Patients with MGUS carry a higher risk of developing WM.
- Amyloidosis is rare, occurring in 5% of patients with WM.

REFERENCES
Dimopoulos MA, Galani E, Matsouka C: Waldenström's macroglobulinemia, *Hematol Oncol Clin North Am* 13(6):1351, 1999.
Owen RG, Johnson SA, Morgan GJ: Waldenström's macroglobulinemia: laboratory diagnosis and treatment, *Hematol Oncol* 18(2):41-9, 2000.
Author: **Peter Petropoulos, M.D.**

BASIC INFORMATION

■ DEFINITION
Warts are benign epidermal neoplasms caused by human papillomavirus (HPV).

■ SYNONYMS
Verruca vulgaris (common warts)
Verruca plana (flat warts)
Condyloma acuminatum (venereal warts)
Verruca plantaris (plantar warts)
Mosaic warts (cluster of many warts)

ICD-9CM CODES
0.78.10 Viral warts
0.79.19 Venereal wart (external genital organs)

■ EPIDEMIOLOGY & DEMOGRAPHICS
- Common warts occur most frequently in children and young adults.
- Anogenital warts are most common in young, sexually active patients. Genital warts are the most common viral STD in the U.S., with up to 24 million Americans carrying the virus that causes them.
- Common warts are longer lasting and more frequent in immunocompromised patients (e.g., lymphoma, AIDS, immunosuppressive drugs).
- Plantar warts occur most frequently at points of maximal pressure (over the heads of the metatarsal bones or on the heels).

■ PHYSICAL FINDINGS & CLINICAL PRESENTATION
- Common warts (Fig. 1-398) have an initial appearance of a flesh-colored papule with a rough surface; they subsequently develop a hyperkera-

totic appearance with black dots on the surface (thrombosed capillaries); they may be single or multiple and are most common on the hands
- Warts obscure normal skin lines (important diagnostic feature). Cylindrical projections from the wart may become fused, forming a mosaic pattern.
- Flat warts generally are pink or light yellow, slightly elevated, and often found on the forehead, back of hands, mouth, and beard area; they often occur in lines corresponding to trauma (e.g., a scratch); are often misdiagnosed (particularly when present on the face) and inappropriately treated with topical corticosteroids.
- Filiform warts have a fingerlike appearance with various projections; they are generally found near the mouth, beard, or periorbital and paranasal regions.
- Plantar warts (Fig. 1-397) are slightly raised and have a roughened surface; they may cause pain when walking; as they involute, small hemorrhages (caused by thrombosed capillaries) may be noted.
- Genital warts are generally pale pink with several projections and a broad base. They may coalesce in the perineal area to form masses with a cauliflower-like appearance.
- Genital warts on the cervical epithelium can produce subclinical changes that may be noted on Pap smear or colposcopy.

■ ETIOLOGY
Human papillomavirus infection; >60 types of viral DNA have been identified. Transmission of warts is by direct contact.

DIAGNOSIS

■ DIFFERENTIAL DIAGNOSIS
- Molluscum contagiosum
- Condyloma latum
- Acrochordon (skin tags) or seborrheic keratosis
- Epidermal nevi
- Hypertrophic actinic keratosis
- Squamous cell carcinomas
- Acquired digital fibrokeratoma
- Varicella zoster virus in patients with AIDS
- Recurrent infantile digital fibroma
- Plantar corns (may be mistaken for plantar warts)

■ WORKUP
- Diagnosis is generally based on clinical findings.
- Suspect lesions should be biopsied.

■ LABORATORY TESTS
Colposcopy with biopsy of patients with cervical squamous cell changes

TREATMENT

■ NONPHARMACOLOGIC THERAPY
- Importance of use of condoms to reduce transmission of genital warts should be emphasized.
- Watchful waiting is an acceptable option in the treatment of warts, because many warts will disappear without intervention over time.
- Plantar warts that are not painful do not need treatment.

■ ACUTE GENERAL Rx
- Common warts:
  1. Application of topical salicylic acid 17% (e.g., Duofilm). Soak

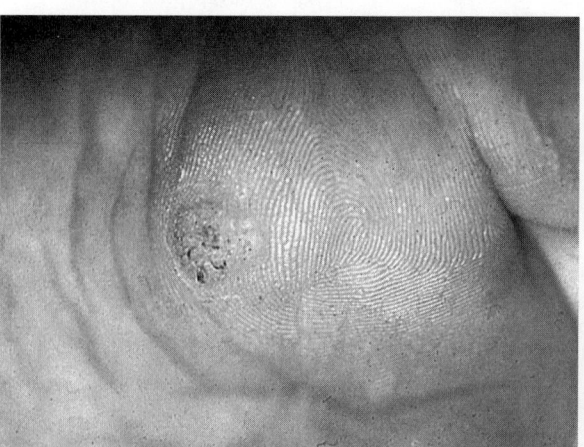
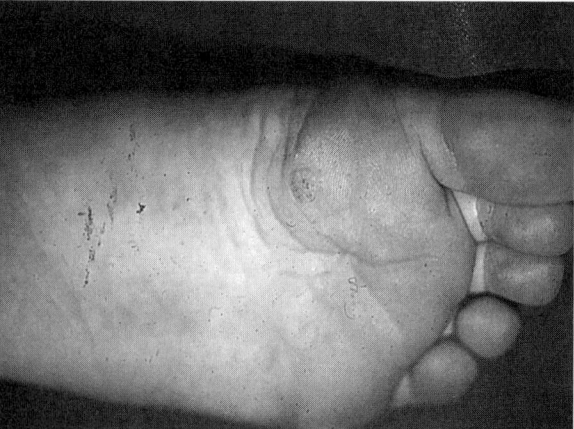

Fig. 1-397 Plantar wart. (From Scuderi G [ed]: *Sports medicine: principles of primary care,* St Louis, 1997, Mosby.)

area for 5 min in warm water and dry. Apply thin layer once or twice daily for up to 12 wk, avoiding normal skin. Bandage.
2. Liquid nitrogen, electrocautery are also excellent methods of removal.
3. Blunt dissection can be used in large lesions or resistant lesions.
- Filiform warts: surgical removal is necessary.
- Flat warts: generally more difficult to treat.
1. Tretinoin cream applied at hs over the involved area for several weeks may be effective.
2. Application of liquid nitrogen
3. Electrocautery
4. 5-Fluorouracil cream (Efudex 5%) applied once or twice a day for 3 to 5 wk is also effective. Persistent hyperpigmentation may occur following Efudex use.
- Plantar warts:
1. Salicylic acid therapy (e.g., Occlusal-HP). Soak wart in warm water for 5 min, remove loose tissue, dry. Apply to area, allow to dry, reapply. Use once or twice daily; maximum 12 wk. Use of 40% salicylic acid plasters (Mediplast) is also a safe, nonscarring treatment; it is particularly useful in treating mosaic warts covering a large area.

2. Blunt dissection is also a fast and effective treatment modality.
3. Laser therapy can be used for plantar warts and recurrent warts; however, it leaves open wounds that require 4 to 6 wk to fill with granulation tissue.
4. Interlesional bleomycin is also effective but generally used when all other treatments fail.
- Genital warts:
1. Can be effectively treated with 20% podophyllin resin in compound tincture of benzoin applied with a cotton tip applicator by the treating physician.
2. Podofilox (Condylox 0.5% gel) is now available for application by the patient. Local adverse effects include pain, burning, and inflammation at the site.
3. Cryosurgery with liquid nitrogen delivered with a probe or as a spray is effective for treating smaller genital warts.
4. Carbon dioxide laser can also be used for treating primary or recurrent genital warts (cure rate >90%).
5. Imiquimod (Aldara) cream, 5% is a new patient-applied immune response modifier effective in the treatment of external genital and perianal warts (complete clearing of genital warts in >70% of females and >30% of males in 4 to 16 wk). Sexual contact should

be avoided while the cream is on the skin. It is applied three times/wk before normal sleeping hours and is left on the skin for 6-10 hr.

■ DISPOSITION
- Warts can be effectively treated with the above modalities, with complete resolution in the majority of patients; however, recurrence rate is high.
- Cervical carcinomas and precancerous lesions in women are associated with genital papillomavirus infection.
- Squamous cell anal cancer is also associated with a history of genital warts.

■ REFERRAL
- Dermatology referral for warts resistant to conservative therapy
- Surgical referral in selected cases
- STD counseling for patients with anogenital warts

☼ PEARLS & CONSIDERATIONS

■ COMMENTS
Subungual and periungual warts are generally more resistant to treatment. Dermatology referral for cryosurgery is recommended in resistant cases.
Author: **Fred F. Ferri, M.D.**

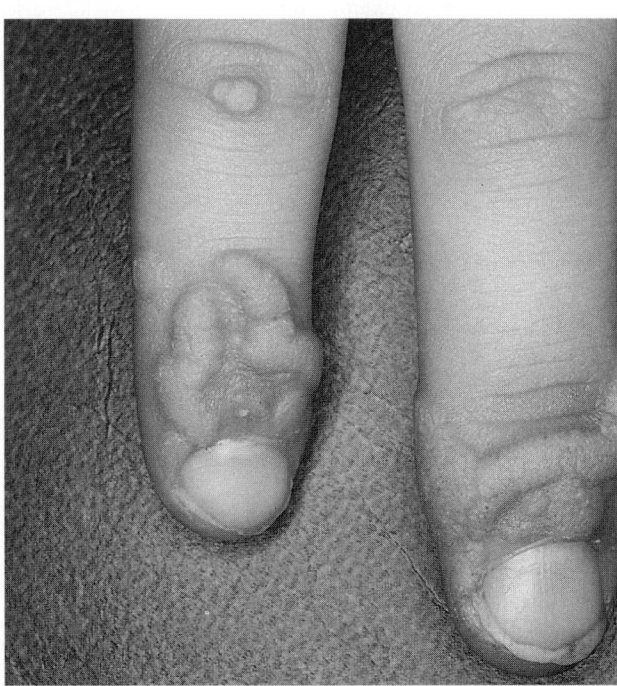

Fig. 1-398 Verruca vulgaris or common viral warts. These papules often have verrucous surface changes. (From Callen JP: *Color atlas of dermatology,* ed 2, Philadelphia, 2000, WB Saunders.)

BASIC INFORMATION

■ **DEFINITION**
Wegener's granulomatosis is a multi-system disease generally consisting of the classic triad of:
1. Necrotizing granulomatous lesions in the upper or lower respiratory tracts
2. Generalized focal necrotizing vasculitis involving both arteries and veins
3. Focal glomerulonephritis of the kidneys

"Limited forms" of the disease can also occur and may evolve into the classic triad; Wegener's granulomatosis can be classified using the "ELK" classification, which identifies the three major sites of involvement: *E*, ears, nose, and throat or respiratory tract; *L*, lungs; *K*, kidneys.

ICD-9CM CODES
446.4 Wegener's granulomatosis

■ **EPIDEMIOLOGY & DEMOGRAPHICS**
• The incidence of Wegener's granulomatosis is 0.5/100,000 persons.
• Mean age at onset is 40 yr.

■ **PHYSICAL FINDINGS & CLINICAL PRESENTATION**
• Clinical manifestations often vary with the stage of the disease and degree of organ involvement.
• Frequent manifestations are:
1. Upper respiratory tract: chronic sinusitis, chronic otitis media, mastoiditis, nasal crusting, obstruction and epistaxis, nasal septal perforation, nasal lacrimal duct stenosis, saddle nose deformities (resulting from cartilage destruction)

2. Lung: hemoptysis, multiple nodules, diffuse alveolar pattern
3. Kidney: renal insufficiency, glomerulonephritis
4. Skin: necrotizing skin lesions
5. Nervous system: mononeuritis multiplex, cranial nerve involvement
6. Joints: monarthritis or polyarthritis (nondeforming), usually affecting large joints
7. Mouth: chronic ulcerative lesions of the oral mucosa, "mulberry" gingivitis
8. Eye: proptosis, uveitis, episcleritis, retinal and optic nerve vasculitis

■ **ETIOLOGY**
Unknown

DIAGNOSIS

■ **DIFFERENTIAL DIAGNOSIS**
• Other granulomatous lung diseases (e.g., lymphomatoid granulomatosis, Churg-Strauss syndrome, necrotizing sarcoid granulomatosis, bronchocentric granulomatosis, sarcoidosis); Table 2-85 describes the differential diagnosis of granulomatous lung disease
• Neoplasms
• Goodpasture's syndrome
• Bacterial or fungal sinusitis
• Midline granuloma
• Viral infections

■ **WORKUP**
Chest x-ray examination, laboratory evaluation, PFTs, and tissue biopsy

■ **LABORATORY TESTS**
• Positive test for cytoplasmic pattern of ANCA (c-ANCA)
• Anemia, leukocytosis
• Urinalysis: may reveal hematuria, RBC casts, and proteinuria
• Elevated serum creatinine, decreased creatinine clearance
• Increased ESR, positive rheumatoid factor, and elevated C-reactive protein may be found.

■ **IMAGING STUDIES**
• Chest x-ray film: may reveal bilateral multiple nodules, cavitated mass lesions, pleural effusion (20%) (Fig. 1-399)
• PFTs: useful in detecting stenosis of the airways.
• Biopsy of one or more affected organs should be attempted; the most reliable source for tissue diagnosis is the lung. Lesions in the nasopharynx (if present) can be easily biopsied.

TREATMENT

■ **NONPHARMACOLOGIC THERAPY**
• Ensure proper airway drainage.
• Give nutritional counseling.

■ **ACUTE GENERAL Rx**
• Prednisone 60 to 80 mg/day and cyclophosphamide 2 mg/kg are generally effective and are used to control clinical manifestations; once the disease comes under control, prednisone is tapered and cyclophosphamide is continued.

- TMP-SMX therapy may represent a useful alternative in patients with lesions limited to the upper and/or lower respiratory tracts in absence of vasculitis or nephritis. Treatment with TMP-SMX (160 mg/800 mg bid) also reduces the incidence of relapses in patients with Wegener's granulomatosis in remission.

■ **DISPOSITION**
Five-year survival with aggressive treatment is approximately 80%; without treatment 2-yr survival is <20%.

■ **REFERRAL**
Surgical referral for biopsy

⚙ **PEARLS & CONSIDERATIONS**

■ **COMMENTS**
- Methotrexate (20 mg/wk) represents an alternative to cyclophosphamide in patients who do not have immediately life-threatening disease.
- C-ANCA levels should not dictate changes in therapy, since they correlate erratically with disease activity.

Author: **Fred F. Ferri, M.D.**

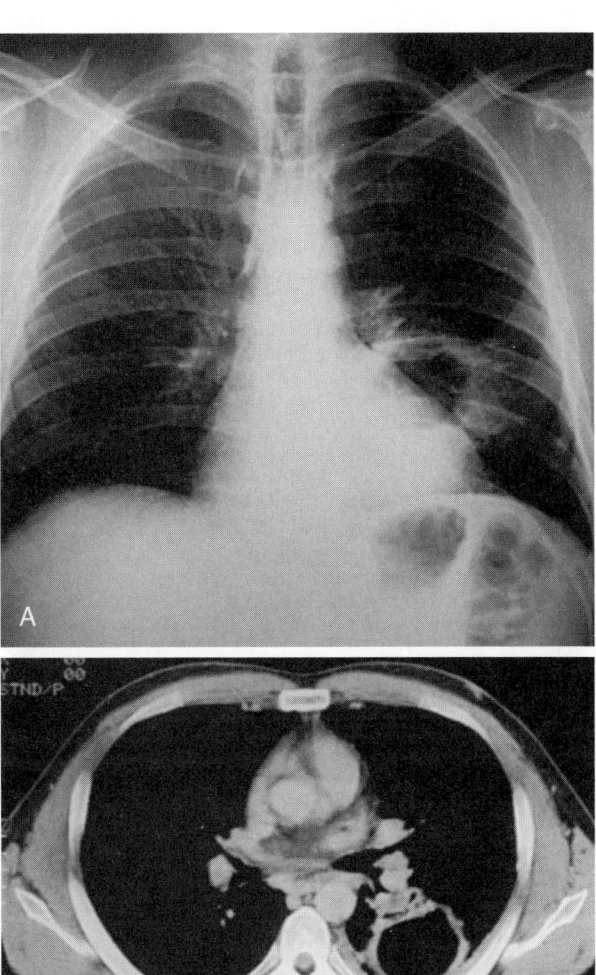

Fig. 1-399 **A,** Wegener's granulomatosis in a 35-year-old cattle farmer with a 2-month illness manifested by fever, malaise, weight loss, pleurisy, polyarthralgias, and palpable purpura of the lower extremities. Laboratory studies included a markedly elevated erythrocyte sedimentation rate, a positive test result for antineutrophil cytoplasmic autoantibody, and an abnormal urine sediment. Note the large cavitary mass lesion of the left lower lobe. **B,** A chest computed tomography scan demonstrates the lower lobe cavitary lesion and a small pleural effusion but no other pulmonary parenchymal abnormalities. (From Mandell GL: *Mandell, Douglas, and Bennett's principles and practice of infectious diseases,* ed 5, New York, 2000, Churchill Livingstone.)

BASIC INFORMATION

■ DEFINITION
Wernicke's encephalopathy is marked by an acute onset of extraocular muscle disorder associated with confusion and ataxia as a result of thiamine disturbance.

■ SYNONYMS
Wernicke-Korsakoff syndrome or psychosis

ICD-9CM CODES
265.1 Wernicke's encephalopathy, disease, or syndrome

■ EPIDEMIOLOGY & DEMOGRAPHICS
INCIDENCE (IN U.S.): Highest incidence in alcoholics
PREVALENCE (IN U.S.): Highest prevalence in alcoholics
PREDOMINANT SEX: Male most common
PEAK INCIDENCE: Early adulthood and upward
PEAK AGE: Adults
GENETICS: None proved

■ PHYSICAL FINDINGS & CLINICAL PRESENTATION
- Almost any disturbance of extraocular motility from nystagmus to paralysis
- Mental confusion
- Ataxia from cerebellar dysfunction
- Peripheral neuropathy

■ ETIOLOGY
Thiamine deficiency

 DIAGNOSIS

■ DIFFERENTIAL DIAGNOSIS
- Give all patients with the triad 100 mg thiamine immediately.
- Consider other diagnoses (such as multiple sclerosis) if symptoms do not dramatically improve in 12 hr.

■ WORKUP
When suspected, treat immediately.

■ LABORATORY TESTS
- CBC
- Serum chemistries

■ IMAGING STUDIES
- MRI shows bilateral thalamic and mammillary body lesions in some cases.
- CT scan may show cerebral atrophy from chronic alcoholism.

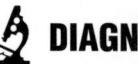 **TREATMENT**

■ NONPHARMACOLOGIC THERAPY
Alcoholics Anonymous

■ ACUTE GENERAL Rx
- 100 mg thiamine IV or IM daily for at least a week
- Prophylactic treatment for delirium tremens

■ CHRONIC Rx
Attempt to treat alcoholism.

■ DISPOSITION
Enter substance abuse program after acute phase.

■ REFERRAL
If symptoms do not resolve after thiamin therapy

 PEARLS & CONSIDERATIONS

■ COMMENTS
The syndrome may occur in malnutrition in malabsorption states, and in patients on prolonged IV therapy without vitamins.
Author: **William H. Olson, M.D.**

BASIC INFORMATION

■ **DEFINITION**
Whiplash refers to a hyperextension injury to the neck, often the result of being struck from behind by a fast-moving vehicle. It is an acceleration-deceleration injury to the neck.

■ **SYNONYMS**
• Cervical strain
• Soft tissue cervical hyperextension injury
• Acceleration flexion-extension neck injury

ICD-9CM CODES
847.0 Whiplash injury or syndrome

■ **EPIDEMIOLOGY & DEMOGRAPHICS**
• Whiplash occurs in more than 1 million people each year.
• Most injuries (40%) are the result of rear-end motor vehicle accidents.
• Whiplash occurs at all ages, in both sexes, and at all socioeconomic levels.
• Incidence is 4 per 1000 persons and is higher in women than men.
• Nearly 50% of patients with whiplash seek legal advice.
• Whiplash is also seen in shaken baby syndrome.

■ **PHYSICAL FINDINGS & CLINICAL PRESENTATION**
• Most present with a history of being involved in a motor vehicle accident and rear-ended by another vehicle
• Pain not present initially but usually develops hours to a few days later
• Neck tightness and stiffness
• Occipital headache
• Shoulder, arm, and back pain
• Numbness in the arms
• Tinnitus
• TMJ pain
• Dysphagia (retropharyngeal hematoma)
• Decreased range of motion of the neck

■ **ETIOLOGY**
• The mechanism of injury is due to the sudden acceleration of the body forward, forcing the neck to hyperextend backward, causing injury to ligaments, muscles, bone, and/or intervertebral disk. At the end of the accident the head is thrust forward in a flexion position, sometimes causing injury to C5-C6-C7.
• Motor vehicle accidents, trauma from falls, contact sports, physical abuse, and altercations are all possible causes of whiplash.

 DIAGNOSIS

The clinical presentation and physical examination determine both the diagnosis and clinical classification of whiplash-associated disorders (Table 1-73).

■ **DIFFERENTIAL DIAGNOSIS**
The differential diagnosis of cervical strain is:
• Osteoarthritis
• Cervical disk disease
• Fibrositis
• Neuritis
• Torticollis
• Spinal cord tumor
• TMJ syndrome
• Tension headache
• Migraine headache

■ **WORKUP**
Any patient who presents with symptoms of whiplash and musculoskeletal or neurologic signs merits a workup to exclude cervical spine fractures or herniated disk disease.

■ **LABORATORY TESTS**
Laboratory studies are not helpful in the diagnosis of whiplash or in excluding complications of acute neck injuries.

■ **IMAGING STUDIES**
• Plain C-spine films (AP, lateral, and odontoid views) to exclude cervical spine fractures
• Flexion/extension x-rays looking for C-spine instability
• CT scan to exclude fracture if suspected by plain films
• MRI to look for cervical disk bulging or herniation

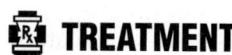 **TREATMENT**

■ **NONPHARMACOLOGIC THERAPY**
• Bed rest
• Soft cervical collar for no longer than 72 hr
• Moist heat 15 to 20 min 4 to 6 times per day

■ **ACUTE GENERAL Rx**
• Analgesics
1. Ibuprofen 800 mg PO tid
2. Naproxen 500 mg PO bid
3. Acetaminophen 1 g PO qid
• Muscle relaxants (short-term use)
1. Cyclobenzaprine 10 mg PO tid
2. Methocarbamol 1 g PO qid
3. Carisoprodol 350 mg PO qid

■ **CHRONIC Rx**
• NSAIDs as described above can be used long term.
• Intraarticular corticosteroids has been tried in the past; however, recently they were found not to be effective for pain relief in patients with chronic whiplash syndrome.

■ **DISPOSITION**
• Most patients recover from the acute whiplash injury within weeks.
• 20% to 40% may develop chronic whiplash syndrome (symptoms of headache, neck pain, and psychiatric complaints that persist for 6 mo).

■ **REFERRAL**

If symptoms are not relieved with conservative nonpharmacologic and acute treatments within 1 to 2 mo, a referral to orthopedic or rheumatology may be helpful.

☼ **PEARLS & CONSIDERATIONS**

■ **COMMENTS**

• The entity of chronic whiplash syndrome remains elusive. Some authorities argue that financial motivation is a factor leading to persistent neck symptoms. Other studies do not substantiate this, countering a true chronic injury to the soft tissues of the neck.
• Nearly one third of all personal injury cases involve cervical injuries.

REFERENCES

Barnsley L et al: Lack of effect of intraarticular corticosteroids for chronic pain in the cervical-zygapophyseal joints, *N Engl J Med* 330(15):1047, 1994.

Eck JC, Hodges SD, Humphreys SC: Whiplash: a review of a commonly misunderstood injury, *Am J Med* 110(8):651, 2001.

Livingston M: Whiplash injury, *J Rheumatol* 26(5):1206, 1999.

Sptizer WO et al: Scientific monograph of the Quebec Task Force on whiplash-associated disorders, *Spine* 208S:1S, 1995.

Author: **Peter Petropoulos, M.D.**

TABLE 1-73 **Proposed Clinical Classification of Whiplash-Associated Disorders**

GRADE	CLINICAL PRESENTATION
0	No complaint about the neck No physical sign(s)
I	Neck complaint of pain, stiffness, or tenderness only No physical sign(s)
II	Neck complaint and musculoskeletal sign(s)*
III	Neck complaint and neurologic sign(s)[†]
IV	Neck complaint and fracture or dislocation

From the Scientific Monograph of the Quebec Task Force on Whiplash Associated Disorders: *Spine* 20(8S):1S, 1995.
*Musculoskeletal signs include decreased range of motion and point tenderness.
[†]Neurologic signs include decreased or absent deep tendon reflexes, weakness, and sensory deficits.
Symptoms and disorders that can be manifest in all grades include deafness, dizziness, tinnitus, headache, memory loss, dysphagia, and temporomandibular joint pain.

BASIC INFORMATION

■ DEFINITION

Whipple's disease is a multisystem illness characterized by malabsorption and its consequences, lymphadenopathy, arthritis, cardiac involvement, ocular symptoms and neurologic problems, caused by the gram-positive bacillus *Tropheryma whippelii.*

■ SYNONYMS

Intestinal lipodystrophy (name used by Dr. Whipple in 1907)

ICD-9CM CODES

040.2 Whipple's disease

■ EPIDEMIOLOGY & DEMOGRAPHICS

- Uncommon illness
- Peak age: 30 to 60 yr of age
- More frequent in men than women

■ PHYSICAL FINDINGS & CLINICAL PRESENTATION

PRESENTATION: The disease may present with extraintestinal symptoms (e.g., arthralgia), but few clinicians will suspect the diagnosis unless or until GI symptoms are present.

The GI manifestations are those seen in malabsorption of any cause:
- Diarrhea: 5 to 10 semiformed, malodorous steatorrheic stools per day
- Abdominal bloating and cramps
- Anorexia

Extraintestinal manifestations of malabsorption:
- Weight loss, fatigue
- Anemia
- Bleeding diathesis
- Edema and ascites
- Osteomalacia

Extraintestinal involvement:
- Arthritis (intermittent, migratory, affecting small, large, and axial joints)
- Pleuritic chest pain and cough
- Pericarditis, endocarditis
- Dementia, ophthalmoplegia, myoclonus, and many other symptoms, because any portion of the central nervous system may be a disease site
- Fever

PHYSICAL FINDINGS:
- Abdominal distention, sometimes with tenderness and less commonly fullness or mass, which represents enlarged mesenteric lymph nodes

- Signs of weight loss, cachexia
- Clubbing
- Lymphadenopathy
- Inflamed joints
- Heart murmur or rub
- Sensory loss or motor weakness related to peripheral neuropathy
- Abnormal mental status examination
- Pallor

■ ETIOLOGY & PATHOGENESIS

- Infectious disease caused by *Tropheryma whippelii*, an actinobacter
- The bacillus has never been cultured, nor has direct transmission from patient to patient ever been documented; however, the agent can be seen in tissue samples by electron microscopy and identified by polymerase chain reaction (PCR).
- Predictable response to appropriate antibiotic therapy confirms the pathogenic role of the infection.
- Tissue infiltration by macrophages is believed to be the mechanism of specific organ dysfunction and symptoms.

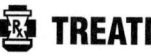

DIAGNOSIS

■ DIFFERENTIAL DIAGNOSIS

Malabsorption/maldigestion:
- Celiac disease
- *Mycobacterium avium-intracellulare* intestinal infection in patients with AIDS
- Intestinal lymphoma
- Abetalipoproteinemia
- Amyloidosis
- Systemic mastocytosis
- Radiation enteritis
- Crohn's disease
- Short bowel syndrome
- Pancreatic insufficiency
- Intestinal bacterial overgrowth
- Lactose deficiency
- Postgastrectomy syndrome
- Other cause of diarrhea (see Fig. 3-52 and Fig. 3-53)

Seronegative inflammatory arthritis (see Table 2-189)

Pericarditis and pleuritis

Lymphadenitis

Neurologic disorders

■ WORKUP

Laboratory tests and imaging studies

■ LABORATORY TESTS

- Anemia (iron, folate, and/or vitamin B_{12} deficiency)
- Hypokalemia
- Hypocalcemia
- Hypomagnesemia
- Hypoalbuminemia
- Prolonged prothrombin time
- Low serum carotene
- Low cholesterol
- Leukocytosis
- Steatorrhea demonstrated by a Sudan fecal fat stain
- 72-Hr stool collection demonstrating more than 7 g/24 hr of fat in the stool is impractical to perform, especially in ambulatory patients
- Defective D-xylose absorption

■ IMAGING STUDIES

Small bowel x-rays after barium ingestion often show thickening of mucosal folds

■ BIOPSY

Infiltration of the intestinal lamina propria by PAS-positive macrophages containing gram-positive, acid-fast negative bacilli, associated with lymphatic dilation (diagnostic); PCR of the involved tissue in uncertain cases

TREATMENT

- Antibiotics: trimethoprim/sulfamethoxazole DS bid for 6 to 12 mo
- Alternative antibiotics: penicillin alone, penicillin plus streptomycin, ampicillin, tetracycline, chloramphenicol, ceftriaxone
- Treat specific vitamin, mineral, and nutrient deficiencies

REFERENCES

Malwald M et al: *Tropheryma whippelii* DNA is rare in the intestinal mucosa of patients wtihout other evidence of whipple disease, *Ann Intern Med* 136:115, 2001.

Trier JS: Whipple's disease. In Feldman M, Scharschmidt BF, Sleisenger MH (eds): *Sleisenger and Fordtran's gastrointestinal and liver disease,* ed 6, Philadelphia, 1998, WB Saunders.

Author: **Tom J. Wachtel, M.D.**

BASIC INFORMATION

■ DEFINITION
Wilson's disease is a disorder of copper transport with inadequate biliary copper excretion, leading to an accumulation of the metal in liver, brain, kidneys, and corneas.

ICD-9CM CODES
275.1 Wilson's disease

■ EPIDEMIOLOGY & DEMOGRAPHICS
- Prevalence: 1 in 30,000
- Affects men and women equally (autosomal recessive gene)
- Onset of symptoms: 3 to 40 yr of age

■ CLINICAL PRESENTATION & PHYSICAL FINDINGS
Hepatic presentation:
- Acute hepatitis with malaise, anorexia, nausea, jaundice, elevated transaminase, prolonged prothrombin time; rarely fulminant hepatic failure
- Chronic active (or autoimmune) hepatitis with fatigue, malaise, rashes, arthralgia, elevated transaminase, elevated serum IgG, positive ANA and anti–smooth muscle antibody
- Chronic liver disease/cirrhosis with hepatosplenomegaly, ascites, low serum albumin, prolonged prothrombin time, portal hypertension
Neurologic presentation:
- Movement disorder: tremors, ataxia
- Spastic dystonia: masklike facies, rigidity, gait disturbance, dysarthria, drooling, dysphagia
Psychiatric presentation:
- Depression, obsessive-compulsive disorder, psychopathic behaviors
Other organs:
- Hemolytic anemia
- Renal disease (i.e., Fanconi's syndrome with hematuria, phosphaturia, renal tubular acidosis, vitamin D–resistant rickets)
- Cardiomyopathy
- Arthritis
- Hypoparathyroidism
- Hypogonadism
PHYSICAL FINDINGS:
- Ocular: the Kayser-Fleischer ring is a gold-yellow ring seen at the periphery of the iris (Fig. 1-400)
- Stigmata of acute or chronic liver disease
- Neurologic abnormalities: see above

■ ETIOLOGY & PATHOGENESIS
- Dietary copper is transported from the intestine to the liver where normally it is metabolized into ceruloplasmin. In Wilson's disease, defective incorporation of copper into ceruloplasmin and a decrease of biliary copper excretion lead to accumulation of this mineral.
- The gene for Wilson's disease is located in chromosome 3.

DIAGNOSIS

■ DIFFERENTIAL DIAGNOSIS
- Hereditary hypoceruloplasminemia
- Menke's disease
- Consider the diagnosis of Wilson's disease in all cases of acute or chronic liver disease where another cause has not been established.
- Consider Wilson's disease in patients with movement disorders or dystonia even without symptomatic liver disease.

■ LABORATORY TESTS
- Abnormal liver function tests (note that AST may be higher than ALT)
- Low serum ceruloplasmin level (under 200 mg/L)
- Low serum copper (less than 65 μg/L)
- 24-hr urinary copper excretion greater than 100 μg (normal <30 μg); increases to greater than 1200 μg/24 hr after 500 mg of D-penicillamine (normal <500 μg/24 hr)
- Low serum uric acid and phosphorus
- Abnormal urinalysis (hematuria)

■ BIOPSY
- Early:
  Steatosis, focal necrosis, glycogenated hepatocyte nuclei
  May reveal inflammation and piecemeal necrosis
- Late: cirrhosis
- Hepatic copper content (greater than 250 μg/g of dry weight) (normal is 20 to 50 μg)

TREATMENT

- Penicillamine: (chelator therapy) 0.75 to 1.5 g/day divided bid (with pyridoxine 25 mg/day)
  Monitor CBC and urinalysis weekly
- Trientine: (triethylene tetramine) (chelator therapy)
  1 to 1.2 g/day divided bid
  Monitor CBC
- Zinc: (inhibits intestinal copper absorption)
  50 mg tid
  Monitor zinc level
- Ammonium tetrathiomolybdate for neurologic symptoms
- Antioxidants
- Liver transplant (for severe hepatic failure unresponsive to chelation)

■ PROGNOSIS
Good with early chelation treatment

■ REFERRAL
To gastroenterologist

REFERENCE
Cox DW, Roberts EA: Wilson's disease. In Feldman M, Scharschmidt BF, Sleisenger MH (eds): *Sleisenger & Fordtran's gastrointestinal and liver disease,* ed 6, Philadelphia, 1998, WB Saunders.
Author: **Tom J. Wachtel, M.D.**

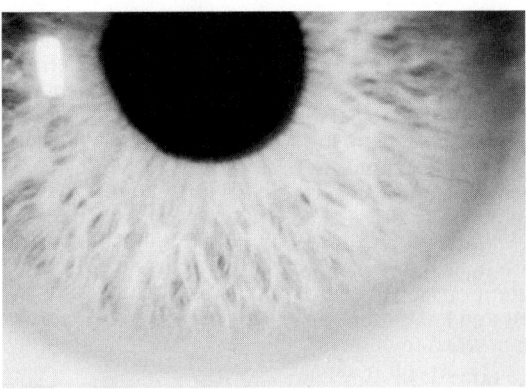

Fig. 1-400   Wilson's disease. A Kayser-Fleischer ring, which is a gold-yellow ring, extends to the limbus without a clear interval. (From Palay D [ed]: *Ophthalmology for the primary care physician,* St Louis, 1997, Mosby.)

BASIC INFORMATION

■ DEFINITION
Wolff-Parkinson-White syndrome is an electrocardiographic abnormality associated with earlier than normal ventricular depolarization following the atrial impulse and predisposing the affected person to tachyarrhythmias.

■ SYNONYMS
Preexcitation syndrome

ICD-9CM CODES
426.7 Wolff-Parkinson-White syndrome
426.81 Lown-Ganong-Levine syndrome

■ EPIDEMIOLOGY & DEMOGRAPHICS
- Prevalence: 1.5 cases/1000 persons
- Prevalence higher in males and decreases with age
- Most patients with WPW syndrome have normal hearts, but associations with mitral valve prolapse, cardiomyopathies, and Ebstein's anomaly have been reported.

■ PHYSICAL FINDINGS & CLINICAL PRESENTATION
Paroxysmal tachycardias
- 10% of WPW patients aged 20 to 40 yr
- 35% of WPW patients aged over 60 yr

The type of tachycardia is:
- Reciprocating tachycardia at 150 to 250 beats per minute (80%)
- Atrial fibrillation (15%)
- Atrial flutter (5%)
- Ventricular tachycardia: rare
- Sudden death is rare (less than 1/1000 cases)

■ PATHOPHYSIOLOGY
- Existence of accessory pathways (Kent bundles)
- If the accessory pathway is capable of anterograde conduction, two parallel routes of AV conduction are possible, one subject to delay through the AV mode, the other without delay through the accessory pathway. The resulting QRS complex is a fusion beat with the "delta" wave representing ventricular activation through the accessory pathway (Fig. 1-401).
- Tachycardias occur when, because of different refractory periods, conduction is anterograde in one pathway (usually the normal AV pathway) and retrograde in the other (usually the accessory pathway). Some patients (5% to 10%) with WPW syndrome have multiple accessory pathways.

DIAGNOSIS

Three basic features characterize the ECG abnormalities in WPW syndrome (Fig. 1-402):
- PR interval <120 msec
- QRS complex >120 msec with a slurred, slowly rising onset of QRS in some lead (delta wave)
- ST-T wave changes

Variants
- Lown-Ganong-Levine syndrome: atriohisian pathway with short PR interval and normal QRS complex on ECG (no delta wave)

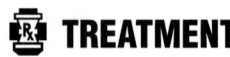

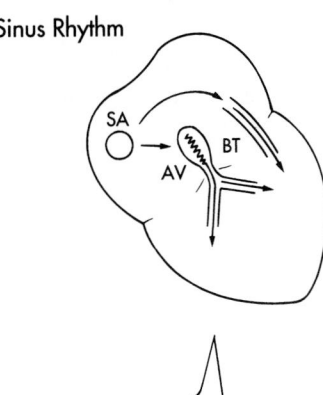

Fig. 1-401 With Wolff-Parkinson-White syndrome an abnormal accessory conduction pathway called a *bypass tract (BT)* connects the atria and ventricles. (From Goldberger AL [ed]: *Clinical electrocardiography: a simplified approach,* ed 6, St Louis, 1999, Mosby.)

- Atriofascicular accessory pathways: duplication of the AV node, with normal baseline ECG

TREATMENT

- No treatment in the absence of tachyarrhythmias.
- Symptomatic tachyarrhythmias.
- Acute episode: adenosine, verapamil, or diltiazem can be used to terminate an episode of reciprocal tachycardia.
- Digitalis should not be used because it can reduce refractoriness in the accessory pathway and accelerate the tachycardia. Cardioversion should be used in the presence of hemodynamic impairment.
- Prevention:
  Empiric trials or serial electrophysiologic drug testing of:
  1. Quinidine and propranolol
  2. Procainamide and verapamil
  3. Amiodarone
  4. Sotalol
  Electrical or surgical ablation of the accessory pathway

REFERENCES
Gollob MH et al: Identification of a gene responsible for familial Wolff-Parkinson-White syndrome, *N Engl J Med* 366:1823, 2001.
Zipes DP: Preexcitation syndrome. In Braunwald E (ed): *Heart disease: a textbook of cardiovascular medicine,* ed 5, vol 2, Philadelphia, 1997, WB Saunders.
Author: **Tom J. Wachtel, M.D.**

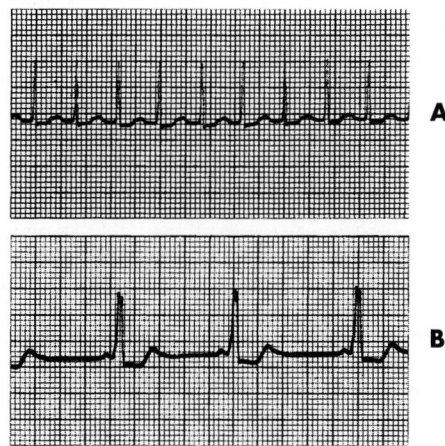

Fig. 1-402 **A,** SVT in a child with Wolff-Parkinson-White (WPW) syndrome. Note the normal QRS complexes during the tachycardia. **B,** Later the typical features of WPW syndrome are apparent (short P-R interval, δ wave, and wide QRS). (From Behrman RE: *Nelson textbook of pediatrics,* ed 16, Philadelphia, 2000, WB Saunders.)

BASIC INFORMATION

■ DEFINITION
Yellow fever is an infection, primarily of the liver, with systemic manifestations caused by the yellow fever virus (YFV).

ICD-9CM CODES
060.9 Yellow fever

■ EPIDEMIOLOGY & DEMOGRAPHICS
INCIDENCE (IN U.S.):
- None
- Approximate attack rates of 3% in Africa and Amazon

PREVALENCE (IN U.S.):
- None
- Endemic areas: 20% of population

PREDOMINANT SEX: In Africa and Amazon, male agricultural workers

PREDOMINANT AGE: 20 to 40 yr

PEAK INCIDENCE: Variable with outbreaks

■ PHYSICAL FINDINGS & CLINICAL PRESENTATION
- Clinical illness with jaundice in about 5% to 20% of infections
- Most subclinical
- Onset sudden after incubation period of 3 to 6 days
- Viremic (early) phase
  1. Fever, chills
  2. Severe headache
  3. Lumbosacral pain
  4. Myalgias
  5. Nausea
  6. Severe malaise
  7. Conjunctivitis
  8. Relative bradycardia
- After brief recovery, toxic phase:
  1. Jaundice
  2. Oliguria
  3. Albuminuria
  4. Hemorrhage (especially hematemesis)
  5. Encephalopathy
  6. Shock
  7. Acidosis

■ ETIOLOGY
- Yellow fever virus (*L. flavus*)
  1. Prototype flavivirus
  2. Infects primarily hepatic cells
  3. Replication
     a. Exclusively intracellular and intracytoplasmic
     b. Primarily in the endoplasmic reticulum
  4. Late in infection, cytopathic effects (antibody- and cell-mediated) produce pathology

- Vector
  1. *Aedes aegypti* (urban)
  2. *Aedes* spp., *Haemagogus* (especially in Amazon) mosquitos (sylvan)
  3. Primary hosts humans and simian species
  4. Virus maintained in mosquito ova during dry season
  5. Sylvan cycle interrupted by humans: agriculture, forest clearing
- Geographic distribution
  1. South American and Africa, in countries between +15 and −15 degrees latitude
  2. Not in Asia
- Recent increase in epidemics in Africa (especially Nigeria)
  1. Several hundred thousand cases between 1987 and 1991
  2. Fatality rate approximately 20% in jaundiced patients
  3. Death between days 7 and 10
- Pathogenesis
  1. Unclear
  2. Probably involves Kupffer cell, followed by hepatocyte infection
  3. Renal failure accompanied by viral antigen in glomeruli
  4. Shock and lactic acidosis accompanied by release of vasoactive mediators from liver, nodes, spleen
  5. Myocarditis contributes to shock and collapse
  6. Hemorrhage
     a. Decreased synthesis of clotting factors
     b. Disseminated intravascular coagulation
  7. Encephalopathy secondary to cerebral edema

DIAGNOSIS

■ DIFFERENTIAL DIAGNOSIS
- Viral hepatitis
- Leptospirosis
- Malaria
- Typhoid fever
- Hemorrhagic fevers (HF) with jaundice
  1. Dengue (HF)
  2. Rift Valley fever
  3. Crimean-Congo (HF)

■ WORKUP
- CBC
- Liver function tests
- Serum for serology (YFV, viral isolation)
- Coagulation studies
  1. Prothrombin time
  2. Fibrinogen
  3. Fibrin split products

- Liver biopsy contraindicated (death from bleeding)

■ LABORATORY TESTS
- CBC
  1. Generally nonspecific
  2. Mild leukopenia
  3. Thrombocytopenia
  4. Anemia
- Liver function tests
  1. Mildly to severely abnormal ALT, AST, and bilirubin
- Elevated creatinine and BUN
- Coagulation studies
  1. Normal *or*
  2. Demonstrate abnormal prothrombin time *or*
  3. Reveal disseminated intravascular coagulation (DIC)
- Terminal hypoglycemia
- Specific diagnosis confirmed by viral isolation from blood
- Serologic diagnosis
  1. Viral antigen in serum (ELISA)
  2. Viral RNA by PCR
  3. IgM by:
     a. Antibody-capture ELISA
     b. Hemagglutination inhibition
     c. Complement fixation
     d. Neutralization assays
  4. Appear within 5 to 7 days
     a. IgM
     b. HI
     c. N Ab
  5. Appear within 7 to 14 days
     a. CF Ab
  6. Rising Ab confirmed by paired sera
  7. CF persists up to 1 yr

TREATMENT

■ ACUTE GENERAL Rx
- Treatment symptomatic
- Acetaminophen (headache and fever)
- Antacids, cimetidine (GI bleeding)
- Blood transfusion, volume replacement for hemorrhage and shock
- Dialysis for renal failure
- No clearly useful antiviral agents

■ DISPOSITION
Follow-up until hepatic, renal, CNS disease resolved

■ REFERRAL
To infectious diseases expert for accurate diagnosis and management

☼ PEARLS & CONSIDERATIONS

■ COMMENTS
- Yellow fever is preventable.
- Recovery from yellow fever confers lasting immunity.
- Live, attenuated yellow fever vaccine provides protective immunity in 95% of vaccinees within 10 days of vaccination.
- Reimmunization at 10-yr intervals is required for travel.

- Vaccine contraindicated in:
  1. Infants <6 mo (postvaccinal encephalitis)
  2. Immunosuppressed patients
  3. Pregnant women (congenital infection may result, although generally without adverse effects on the fetus)
  4. Patients with egg hypersensitivity
- Cases of multiple organ system failure have been associated with recent administration of yellow fever vaccine. More data is needed to clearly define a causal association. Health care providers should provide vaccine only to persons planning to travel to areas reporting yellow fever activity or areas in the yellow fever endemic zone.

Author: **Marilyn Fabbri, M.D.**

BASIC INFORMATION

■ **DEFINITION**
Zenker's diverticulum refers to an acquired abnormality of the upper esophagus resulting in the herniation of the hypopharyngeal mucosa through a weakness in the posterior hypopharyngeal wall (Fig. 1-403).

■ **SYNONYMS**
• Pharyngoesophageal diverticulum
• Pulsion diverticulum

ICD-9CM CODES
530.6 Zenker's diverticulum (esophagus)

■ **EPIDEMIOLOGY & DEMOGRAPHICS**
• Rare disease: <1% of all barium swallows
• Commonly seen in people over 50 yr of age

■ **PHYSICAL FINDINGS & CLINICAL PRESENTATION**
Small Zenker's diverticulum may be asymptomatic. As they become larger, symptoms include:
• Dysphagia to solids and liquids
• Regurgitation of undigested food
• Sensation of globus or fullness in the neck
• Cough
• Halitosis
• Aspiration pneumonia
• Weight loss

■ **ETIOLOGY**
The specific cause of Zenker's diverticulum is not known; however, the leading hypothesis suggests the following:
• During swallowing there is raised intraluminal pressures secondary to the incomplete opening of the cricopharyngeus muscle before the bolus of food can be driven forward into the stomach.
• The elevated pressure leads to posterior protrusion of the hypopharyngeal mucosa and submucosa, thus forming a diverticulum where food may become lodged causing symptoms as mentioned above.

 DIAGNOSIS

Clinical presentation and barium swallow typically make the diagnosis of Zenker's diverticulum.

■ **DIFFERENTIAL DIAGNOSIS**
The differential diagnosis is similar to anyone presenting with dysphagia:
• Achalasia
• Esophageal spasm
• Esophageal carcinoma
• Esophageal webs
• Peptic stricture
• Lower esophageal (Schatzki) ring
• Foreign bodies
• CNS disorders (stroke, Parkinson's disease, ALS, multiple sclerosis, myasthenia gravis, muscular dystrophies)
• Dermatomyositis
• Infection

■ **WORKUP**
The workup for suspected Zenker's diverticulum should include a barium swallow. Upper endoscopy runs the risk of perforation. Manometry motility studies are usually not indicated because they will not change the course of treatment.

■ **LABORATORY TESTS**
There are no specific laboratory tests to diagnose Zenker's diverticulum.

■ **IMAGING STUDIES**
• Radiographically Zenker's diverticulum is easily demonstrated with a barium contrast study (Fig. 1-404).
• Barium swallow characteristically demonstrates a herniated sac with a narrow diverticular neck that typically originates just proximal to the cricopharyngeus at the level of C5-C6.
• A chest x-ray is performed in cases of suspected aspiration pneumonia.

TREATMENT

■ **NONPHARMACOLOGIC THERAPY**
• Soft mechanical diet can be tried in patients with symptoms of dysphagia.
• Avoid seeds, skins, and nuts.

■ **ACUTE GENERAL Rx**
• Surgery is the recommended treatment for symptomatic patients with Zenker's diverticulum.
• Surgical treatment relieves symptoms (dysphagia, cough, aspiration) in nearly all patients with Zenker's diverticulum.
• Surgical procedures include:
  1. Cervical diverticulectomy with cricopharyngeal myotomy (most common approach).
  2. Diverticulopexy or diverticular inversion with cricopharyngeal myotomy.
  3. Diverticulectomy alone
  4. Cricopharyngeal myotomy alone
• Surgical mortality <1.5%.

■ **CHRONIC Rx**
In patients not having surgery, treatment is directed toward any complications that may occur:
• Antibiotics for aspiration pneumonia
• H_2 antagonists for ulcerations that can develop within the diverticulum.

■ **DISPOSITION**
• The natural history of Zenker's diverticulum if left untreated is one of progressive enlargement of the diverticulum.
• As the diverticulum enlarges, the risk of complications, including aspiration pneumonia, increases.
• Recurrence of Zenker's diverticulum (4%) postoperatively can occur; however, patients are usually not symptomatic.

■ **REFERRAL**
Any patient with dysphagia requires a gastroenterology consultation. A thoracic surgical consultation is needed if surgery is considered for the Zenker's diverticulum.

☼ PEARLS & CONSIDERATIONS

■ COMMENTS
• The association of cancer with Zenker's diverticulum is rare (0.4%).

• Zenker's diverticulum forms in "Killian's triangle," the point between the oblique fibers of the inferior pharyngeal muscle and the horizontal fibers of the cricopharyngeus muscle.

REFERENCES
Achkar E: Zenker's diverticulum, *Dig Dis* 16(3):144, 1998.
Bremner CG: Zenker's diverticulum, *Arch Surg* 133(10):1131, 1998.
Siddiq MA, Sood S, Strachan D: Pharyngeal pouch (Zenker's diverticulum), *Postgrad Med J* 77(910):506, 2001.
Author: **Peter Petropoulos, M.D.**

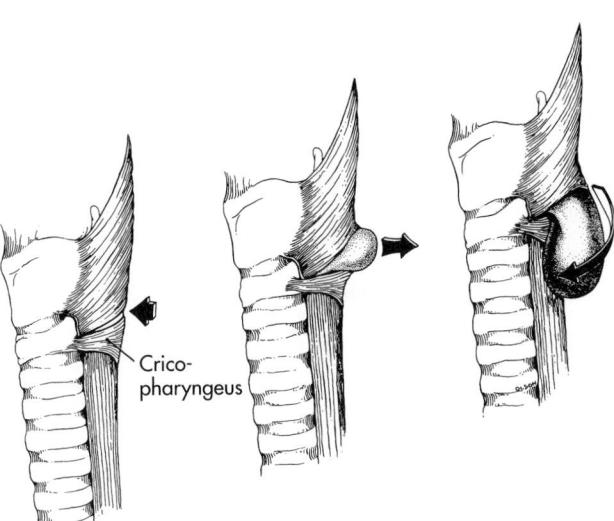

Fig. 1-403   Formation of pharyngoesophageal (Zenker's) diverticulum. *Left,* Herniation of the pharyngeal mucosa and submucosa occurs at the point of transition *(arrow)* between the oblique fibers of the thyropharyngeus muscle and the more horizontal fibers of the cricopharyngeus muscle. *Center* and *right,* As the diverticulum enlarges, it dissects toward the left side and downward into the superior mediastinum in the prevertebral space. (From Sabiston D: *Textbook of surgery,* ed 15, Philadelphia, 1997, WB Saunders.)

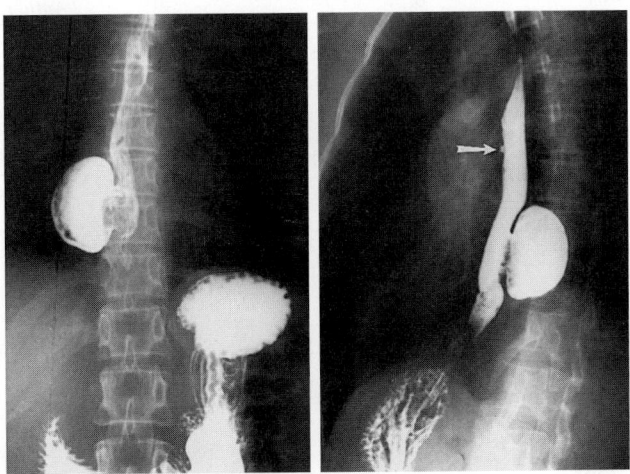

Fig. 1-404   Posteroanterior *(left)* and oblique *(right)* views from barium esophagogram showing both a typical diverticulum of the junction of the mid and distal esophagus and a small traction diverticulum *(arrow)* of the mid-esophagus. (From Sabiston D: *Textbook of surgery,* ed 15, Philadelphia, 1997, Saunders.)

BASIC INFORMATION

■ DEFINITION
Zollinger-Ellison (ZE) syndrome is a hypergastrinemic state caused by a pancreatic or extrapancreatic non–beta islet cell tumor (gastrinoma) and resulting in peptic acid disease.

■ SYNONYMS
Gastrinoma

ICD-9CM CODES
251.5 Zollinger-Ellison syndrome

■ EPIDEMIOLOGY & DEMOGRAPHICS
- Incidence is unknown, but 0.1% of all duodenal ulcers are believed to be caused by ZE.
- Occurs in both genders and at any age (most common in 30 to 50 yr of age).
- Two thirds of gastrinomas are sporadic, and one third are associated with multiple endocrine neoplasia type 1 (MEN-1), an autosomal dominant genetic disorder that also includes hyperparathyroidism and pituitary tumors.
- About 60% of gastrinomas are malignant.

■ PHYSICAL FINDINGS & CLINICAL PRESENTATION
- The vast majority of patients (95%) present with symptoms of peptic ulcer (see Section I)
- 60% of patients have symptoms related to gastroesophageal reflux disease (see Section I)
- One third of patients with ZE have diarrhea and, less commonly, steatorrhea.

The following circumstances warrant suspicion of ZE syndrome:
- Ulcers distal to the first portion of the duodenum
- Multiple peptic ulcers
- Ineffective treatment for peptic ulcer disease with the usual drug doses and schedules
- Peptic ulcer and diarrhea
- Familial history of peptic ulcer
- Patients with a personal or family history suggesting parathyroid or pituitary tumors of dysfunction
- Peptic ulcer and urinary tract calculi
- Patients with peptic ulcer who are negative for *H. pylori* and do not have a history of NSAID use

■ ETIOLOGY
- The pathophysiologic manifestations of ZE syndrome are related to the effects of hypergastrinemia. Gastrin stimulates gastric acid secretion, which in turn is responsible for the development of duodenal ulcers and diarrhea. Gastrin also promotes gastric mucosal epithelial cell growth and resulting parietal cell hyperplasia.
- Gastrinomas are usually small (0.1 to 2 cm) but sometimes large (>20 cm) tumors.
- 60% of gastrinomas are malignant, with liver and regional lymph nodes the most common site of metastases. Histology is not a good predictor of the biology of gastrinomas.
- 60% of patients with MEN-1 have gastrinomas.
- 10% of patients with ZE syndrome have islet cell hyperplasia rather than gastrinomas; in 10% to 20% of patients with gastrinoma the tumors cannot be located because of small size.

DIAGNOSIS

■ DIFFERENTIAL DIAGNOSIS
- Peptic ulcer disease (see Section I)
- Gastroesophageal reflux disease (see Section I)
- Diarrhea (see Fig. 3-52)

■ WORKUP
- Diagnosis of peptic ulcer
  UGI series (may also show prominent gastric rugal folds)
  Endoscopy
- Gastric acid secretion
- Serum gastrin level (fasting) >150 pg/ml (causes of false positive: pernicious anemia, renal failure, retained gastric antrum syndrome, diabetes mellitus, rheumatoid arthritis)
- Provocative gastrin level tests
  Secretin stimulation
  Calcium stimulation
  Standard test meal stimulation
- Gastrinoma localization
  Arteriography (Fig. 1-405)

Abdominal sonography
Abdominal CT scan
Abdominal MRI
Selective portal vein branch gastrin level
Octreotide scan

TREATMENT

- Surgical resection of the gastrinoma (NOTE: 90% of gastrinomas can be located, resulting in a 40% overall cure rate)
- Total gastrectomy or vagotomy (palliative in some patients)
- Medical treatment
  Proton pump inhibitors (e.g., omeprazole or lansoprazole)
  Somatostatin or octreotide
  Chemotherapy for metastatic gastrinoma with streptozotocin, 5-FU, and doxorubicin

■ PROGNOSIS
Five-year survival:
- Two thirds of all patients
- 20% with liver metastases
- 90% without liver metastases

■ REFERRAL
To gastroenterologist

REFERENCES
McGuigan JE: Zollinger-Ellison syndrome. In Feldman M, Scharschmidt BF, Sleisenger MH (eds): *Sleisenger & Fordtran's gastrointestinal and liver disease,* ed 6, St Louis, 1998, WB Saunders.

Norten JA et al: Surgery to cure Zollinger-Ellison syndrome, *N Engl J Med* 341:635, 1999.
Author: **Tom J. Wachtel, M.D.**

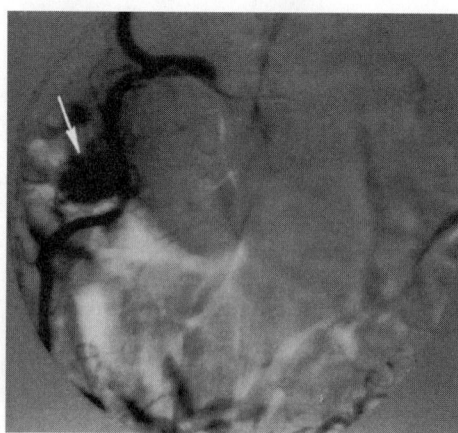

Fig. 1-405 Selective celiac arteriogram in a patient with Zollinger-Ellison syndrome. The hepatic artery injection fills the gastroduodenal artery, which reveals a tumor blush *(arrow)* in the region of the duodenum or head of the pancreas. At exploration, a 2-cm benign duodenal gastrinoma was identified and locally resected. (From Sabiston D: *Textbook of surgery,* ed 15, Philadelphia, 1997, WB Saunders.)

Differential Diagnosis, Etiology, and Classification of Common Signs and Symptoms

ABDOMINAL DISTENTION

BOX 2-1   Abdominal Distention

Nonmechanical Obstruction

Excessive intraluminal gas
Intraabdominal infection
Trauma
Retroperitoneal irritation (renal colic, neoplasms, infections)
Vascular insufficiency (thrombosis, embolism)
Mechanical ventilation
Extraabdominal infection (sepsis, pneumonia, empyema, osteomyelitis of spine)
Metabolic/toxic (hypokalemia, uremia, lead poisoning)
Chemical irritation (perforated ulcer, bile, pancreatitis)
Peritoneal inflammation
Severe pain, pain medications

Mechanical Obstruction

Neoplasm (intraluminal, extraluminal)
Adhesions, endometriosis
Infection (intraabdominal abscess, diverticulitis)
Gallstones
Foreign body, bezoars
Pregnancy
Hernias
Volvulus
Stenosis at surgical anastomosis, radiation stenosis
Fecaliths
Inflammatory bowel disease
Hematoma
Other: parasites, superior mesenteric artery (SMA) syndrome, pneumatosis intestinalis, annular pancreas, Hirschsprung's disease, intussusception, meconium

ABDOMINAL PAIN, BY LOCATION

BOX 2-2   Abdominal Pain, by Location

Diffuse

Early appendicitis
Aortic aneurysm
Gastroenteritis
Intestinal obstruction
Diverticulitis
Peritonitis
Mesenteric insufficiency or infarction
Pancreatitis
Inflammatory bowel disease
Irritable bowel
Mesenteric adenitis
Metabolic: toxins, lead poisoning, uremia, drug overdose, DKA, heavy metal poisoning
Sickle cell crisis
Pneumonia (rare)
Trauma
Urinary tract infection, PID
Other: acute intermittent porphyria, tabes dorsalis, periarteritis nodosa, Henoch-Schönlein purpura, adrenal insufficiency

Epigastric

Gastric: PUD, gastric outlet obstruction, gastric ulcer
Duodenal: PUD, duodenitis
Biliary: cholecystitis, cholangitis
Hepatic: hepatitis
Pancreatic: pancreatitis
Intestinal: high small bowel obstruction, early appendicitis
Cardiac: angina, MI, pericarditis
Pulmonary: pneumonia, pleurisy, pneumothorax
Subphrenic abscess
Vascular: dissecting aneurysm

Suprapubic

Intestinal: colon obstruction or gangrene, diverticulitis, appendicitis
Reproductive system: ectopic pregnancy, mittelschmerz, torsion of ovarian cyst, PID, salpingitis, endometriosis, rupture of endometrioma
Cystitis, rupture of urinary bladder

Right Upper Quadrant (RUQ)

Biliary: calculi, infection, inflammation, neoplasm
Hepatic: hepatitis, abscess, hepatic congestion, neoplasm, trauma
Gastric: PUD, pyloric stenosis, neoplasm, alcoholic gastritis, hiatal hernia
Pancreatic: pancreatitis, neoplasm, stone in pancreatic duct or ampulla
Renal: calculi, infection, inflammation, neoplasm, rupture of kidney
Pulmonary: pneumonia, pulmonary infarction, right-sided pleurisy
Intestinal: retrocecal appendicitis, intestinal obstruction, high fecal impaction
Cardiac: myocardial ischemia (particularly involving the inferior wall), pericarditis
Cutaneous: herpes zoster
Trauma
Fitz-Hugh–Curtis syndrome (perihepatitis)

Abdominal pain, by location
ICD-9CM # 789.60 Unspecified site
789.61 Upper right quadrant
789.62 Upper left quadrant
789.63 Lower right quadrant
789.64 Lower left quadrant
789.65 Periumbilic
789.66 Epigastric
789.67 Generalized

Continued

BOX 2-2 Abdominal Pain, by Location—cont'd

Left Upper Quadrant (LUQ)

Gastric: PUD, gastritis, pyloric stenosis, hiatal hernia

Pancreatic: pancreatitis, neoplasm, stone in pancreatic duct or ampulla

Cardiac: MI, angina pectoris

Splenic: splenomegaly, ruptured spleen, splenic abscess, splenic infarction

Renal: calculi, pyelonephritis, neoplasm

Pulmonary: pneumonia, empyema, pulmonary infarction

Vascular: ruptured aortic aneurysm

Cutaneous: herpes zoster

Trauma

Intestinal: high fecal impaction, perforated colon

Periumbilical

Intestinal: small bowel obstruction or gangrene, early appendicitis

Vascular: mesenteric thrombosis, dissecting aortic aneurysm

Pancreatic: pancreatitis

Metabolic: uremia, DKA

Trauma

Right Lower Quadrant (RLQ)

Intestinal: acute appendicitis, regional enteritis, incarcerated hernia, cecal diverticulitis, intestinal obstruction, perforated ulcer, perforated cecum, Meckel's diverticulitis

Reproductive: ectopic pregnancy, ovarian cyst, torsion of ovarian cyst, salpingitis, tuboovarian abscess, mittelschmerz, endometriosis, seminal vesiculitis

Renal: renal and ureteral calculi, neoplasms, pyelonephritis

Vascular: leaking aortic aneurysm

Psoas abscess

Trauma

Cholecystitis

Left Lower Quadrant (LLQ)

Intestinal: diverticulitis, intestinal obstruction, perforated ulcer, inflammatory bowel disease, perforated descending colon, inguinal hernia, neoplasm, appendicitis

Reproductive: ectopic pregnancy, ovarian cyst, torsion of ovarian cyst, tuboovarian abscess, mittelschmerz, endometriosis; seminal vesiculitis

Renal: renal or ureteral calculi, pyelonephritis, neoplasm

Vascular: leaking aortic aneurysm

Psoas abscess

Trauma

ABDOMINAL PAIN, POORLY LOCALIZED

Abdominal pain, poorly localized
ICD-9CM # 789.67 Abdominal tenderness, generalized

BOX 2-3 Causes of Poorly Localized Acute Abdominal Pain

Extraabdominal

Metabolic

DKA, acute intermittent porphyria, hyperthyroidism, hypothyroidism, hypercalcemia, hypokalemia, uremia, hyperlipidemia, hyperparathyroidism

Hematologic

Sickle cell crisis, leukemia or lymphoma, Henoch-Schönlein purpura

Infectious

Infectious mononucleosis, Rocky Mountain spotted fever, acquired immunodeficiency syndrome (AIDS), streptococcal pharyngitis (in children), herpes zoster

Drugs and Toxins

Heavy metal poisoning, black widow spider bites, withdrawal syndromes, mushroom ingestion

Referred Pain

Pulmonary: pneumonia, pulmonary embolism, pneumothorax

Cardiac: angina, myocardial infarction, pericarditis, myocarditis

Genitourinary: prostatitis, epididymitis, orchitis, testicular torsion

Musculoskeletal: rectus sheath hematoma

Functional

Somatization disorder, malingering, hypochondriasis, Munchausen syndrome

Intraabdominal

Early appendicitis, gastroenteritis, peritonitis, pancreatitis, abdominal aortic aneurysm, mesenteric insufficiency or infarction, intestinal obstruction, volvulus, ulcerative colitis

From Rosen P, Barkin R (eds): *Emergency medicine: concepts and clinical practice*, ed 5, St Louis, 2002, Mosby.
DKA, Diabetic ketoacidosis.

Abdominal pain, by age groups
ICD-9CM # 789.60 Unspecified site
          789.61 Upper right quadrant
          789.62 Upper left quadrant
          789.63 Lower right quadrant
          789.64 Lower left quadrant
          789.65 Periumbilic
          789.66 Epigastric
          789.67 Generalized

ABDOMINAL PAIN, BY AGE GROUPS

BOX 2-4   Common Causes of Acute Abdominal Pain by Age Groups

Infancy

Acute gastroenteritis
Appendicitis
Intussusception
Volvulus
Meckel's diverticulum
Other
  Colic
  Trauma

Childhood

Acute gastroenteritis
Appendicitis
Constipation

Cholecystitis, acute
Intestinal obstruction
Pancreatitis
Neoplasm
Inflammatory bowel disease
Other
  Functional abdominal pain
  Pyelonephritis
  Pneumonia
  Diabetic ketoacidosis
  Heavy metal poisoning
  Sickle cell crisis
  Trauma

Adolescence

Acute gastroenteritis
Appendicitis
Inflammatory bowel disease
Peptic ulcer disease
Cholecystitis
Neoplasm
Other
  Functional abdominal pain
  Pelvic inflammatory disease
  Pregnancy
  Pyelonephritis
  Renal stone
  Trauma

From Rosen P, Barkin R (eds): *Emergency medicine: concepts and clinical practice,* ed 5, St Louis, 2002, Mosby.

ABDOMINAL PAIN, IN PREGNANCY

TABLE 2-1   Differential Diagnosis of Abdominal Pain in Pregnancy

DIAGNOSIS	GESTATIONAL AGE	COMMENTS
Gynecologic		
Miscarriage	<20 wk; 80% <12 wk	Ultrasonography to confirm location
Septic abortion	<20 wk	Fever, uterine tenderness
Ectopic pregnancy	<14 wk	Must always consider in first trimester until intrauterine pregnancy confirmed
Corpus luteum cyst rupture	<12 wk	Sudden focal peritoneal pain; no fever
Ovarian torsion	Especially <24 wk	Large ovary; ischemic pain
Pelvic inflammatory disease	<12 wk	Very rare
Chorioamnionitis	>16 wk	Tender uterus, fever; amniocentesis reveals white blood cell counts
Abruptio placentae	>16 wk	Focal uterine tenderness, fetal distress, variable bleeding; possible disseminated intravascular coagulation
Nongynecologic		
Appendicitis	Throughout	Guarding may be less prominent; location changes
Cholecystitis	Throughout	Confirm with sonography
Hepatitis	Throughout	Confirm with liver function tests
Pyelonephritis	Throughout	Flank pain, fever, positive catheterized urinalysis
Preeclampsia	>20 wk	Hypertension, proteinuria, edema; right upper quadrant pain

From Rosen P, Barkin R (eds): *Emergency medicine: concepts and clinical practice,* ed 5, St Louis, 2002, Mosby.

Abdominal pain, in pregnancy
ICD-9CM # 789.60 Unspecified site
          789.61 Upper right quadrant
          789.62 Upper left quadrant
          789.63 Lower right quadrant
          789.64 Lower left quadrant
          789.65 Periumbilic
          789.66 Epigastric
          789.67 Generalized

ABORTION, RECURRENT

Abortion, recurrent
ICD-9CM # 761.8

BOX 2-5   Potential Causes of Recurrent Abortion

Parental chromosomal abnormalities
Congenital anatomic abnormalities
   Incomplete müllerian fusions or septum resorption
     defects
   DES exposure
   Uterine artery abnormalities
Acquired anatomic abnormalities
   Uterine synechiae (adhesions)
   Uterine fibroids
   Endometriosis
Endocrinologic abnormalities
   Luteal phase insufficiency

Hypothyroidism
Diabetes mellitus
Maternal infections
   Cervical mycoplasma, ureaplasma, and chlamydia
Other causes
   Heavy metal and chemical exposures
   Chronic medical illness
   Thrombocytosis
Immunologic phenomena
   Allogenic immunity
   Autoimmunity

From Carlson KJ et al: *Primary care of women,* ed 5, St Louis, 2002, Mosby.
DES, Diethylstilbestrol.

ABSCESSES, INTRAABDOMINAL

Abscesses, intraabdominal
ICD-9CM # 567.2 Abscess, abdominopelvic

TABLE 2-2   Intraabdominal Abscesses

SITE	PREDISPOSING FACTORS	LIKELY PATHOGENS	DIAGNOSIS	EMPIRIC TREATMENT*
Solid Organs				
Hepatic	GI or biliary sepsis, trauma	Gram-negative bacilli, anaerobes, streptococci, amebae	CT, MRI, ultrasound	Ampicillin/sulbactam, drainage; metronidazole for amebic abscess
Splenic	Trauma, hemoglobinopathy, endocarditis	Staphylococci, streptococci, gram-negative bacilli	CT	Ampicillin/sulbactam or vancomycin/tobramycin, splenectomy
Pancreatic	Pancreatitis, pseudocyst	Gram-negative bacilli, streptococci	CT	Ampicillin/sulbactam or clindamycin/tobramycin, drainage
Extravisceral				
Subphrenic	Abdominal surgery, peritonitis	Gram-negative bacilli, streptococci, anaerobes	CT	Ampicillin/sulbactam or clindamycin/tobramycin, drainage
Pelvic	Abdominal surgery, peritonitis, pelvic or GI inflammatory disease	Gram-negative bacilli, streptococci, anaerobes	CT	Ampicillin/sulbactam or clindamycin/tobramycin, drainage
Perinephrenic	Renal infection/obstruction, hematogenous	Gram-negative bacilli, staphylococci	CT	Ampicillin/sulbactam or vancomycin/tobramycin, drainage
Psoas	Vertebral osteomyelitis, hematogenous	Staphylococci, gram-negative bacilli, mycobacteria	CT	Ampicillin/sulbactam or vancomycin/tobramycin, drainage

From Andreoli TE (ed): *Cecil essentials of medicine,* ed 5, Philadelphia, 2001, WB Saunders.
CT, Computed tomography; *GI,* gastrointestinal; *MRI,* magnetic resonance imaging.
*Ampicillin/sulbactam, 2 g/1 g given intravenously (IV) q8h; vancomycin, 1 g IV q12h; tobramycin, 1.7 mg/kg IV q8h; clindamycin, 600 mg IV q8h.

ACHES AND PAINS, DIFFUSE

**BOX 2-6   Differential Diagnosis
of Diffuse Aches and Pains**

Postviral arthralgias/myalgias
Bilateral soft tissue rheumatism
Overuse syndromes
Fibrositis
Hypothyroidism
Metabolic bone disease
Paraneoplastic syndrome
Myopathy (polymyositis, dermatomyositis)
Rheumatoid arthritis
Sjögren's syndrome
Polymyalgia rheumatica with or without temporal
    arteritis
Hypermobility
Benign arthralgias/myalgias
Chronic fatigue syndrome
Hypophosphatemia

From Klippel J (ed): *Practical rheumatology,* London, 1995, Mosby.

BOX 2-7   Diffuse Aches and Pains—Red Flags

Clinical Feature	**Significance**
Age >50 years	Polymyalgia rheumatica, paraneoplastic syndrome
Constitutional symptoms	Inflammatory disease, vasculitis, sepsis, malignancy
Weakness	Myopathy, endocrinopathy
Gelling	Inflammatory rheumatic disorder
New headache	Temporal arteritis
Claudication	
Visual symptoms	
Tender, nodular, thickened or reddened temporal artery	
Bilateral symptoms	Systemic or metabolic cause

From Klippel J (ed): *Practical rheumatology,* London, 1995, Mosby.

**BOX 2-8   Laboratory Evaluation
of Diffuse Aches and Pains**

Complete blood count
Westergren erythrocyte sedimentation rate
Thyroid function tests (TSH)
Creatine phosphokinase or aldolase (if weakness)
Ca, PO_4

From Klippel J (ed): *Practical rheumatology,* London, 1995, Mosby.

ACIDOSIS, ANION GAP

Acidosis, anion gap
ICD-9CM # 276.2

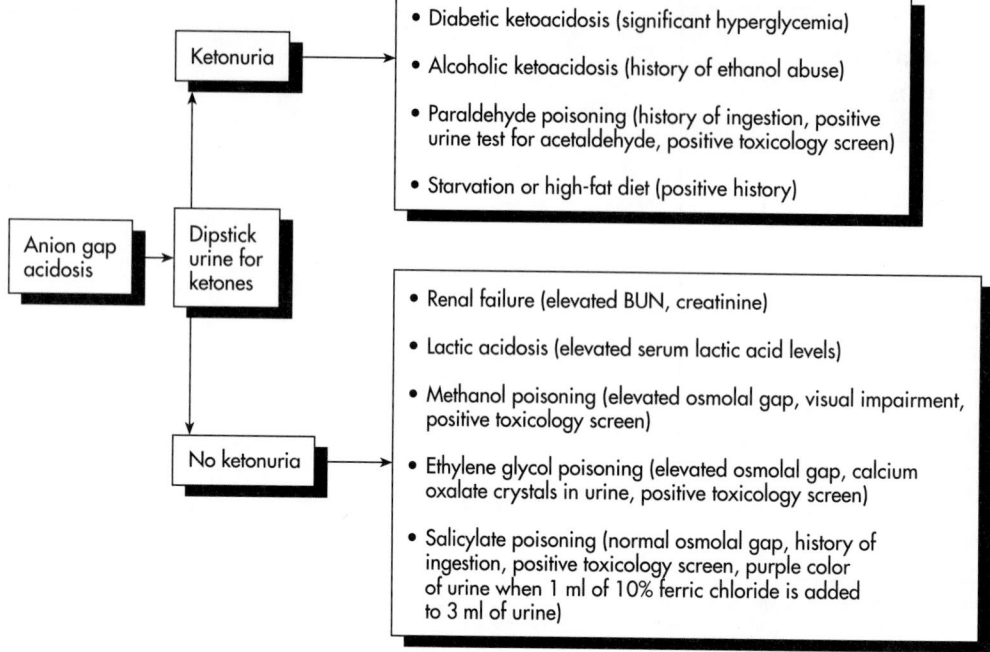

- Diabetic ketoacidosis (significant hyperglycemia)
- Alcoholic ketoacidosis (history of ethanol abuse)
- Paraldehyde poisoning (history of ingestion, positive urine test for acetaldehyde, positive toxicology screen)
- Starvation or high-fat diet (positive history)

- Renal failure (elevated BUN, creatinine)
- Lactic acidosis (elevated serum lactic acid levels)
- Methanol poisoning (elevated osmolal gap, visual impairment, positive toxicology screen)
- Ethylene glycol poisoning (elevated osmolal gap, calcium oxalate crystals in urine, positive toxicology screen)
- Salicylate poisoning (normal osmolal gap, history of ingestion, positive toxicology screen, purple color of urine when 1 ml of 10% ferric chloride is added to 3 ml of urine)

Ketonuria

Anion gap acidosis → Dipstick urine for ketones

No ketonuria

Fig. 2-1   Differential diagnosis of anion gap acidosis.

ACIDOSIS, LACTIC

Acidosis, lactic
ICD-9CM # 276.2

BOX 2-9   Etiology of Lactic Acidosis

Tissue Hypoxia

Shock (hypovolemic, cardiogenic, endotoxic)
Respiratory failure (asphyxia)
Severe congestive heart failure
Severe anemia
Carbon monoxide or cyanide poisoning

Associated with Systemic Disorders

Neoplastic diseases (e.g., leukemia, lymphoma)
Liver or renal failure
Sepsis
Diabetes mellitus
Seizure activity
Abnormal intestinal flora (D-lactic acidosis)

Alkalosis
Human immunodeficiency virus

Secondary to Drugs or Toxins

Salicylates
Ethanol, methanol, ethylene glycol
Fructose and sorbitol
Biguanides (phenformin, metformin [usually occurring in patients with renal insufficiency])
Isoniazid
Streptozocin

Hereditary Disorders

G6PD deficiency and others

ACIDOSIS, METABOLIC

Acidosis, metabolic
ICD-9CM # 276.2

BOX 2-10   Metabolic Acidosis

1. Metabolic acidosis with increased anion gap (AG acidosis)
   a. Lactic acidosis
   b. Ketoacidosis (diabetes mellitus, ethanol intoxication, starvation)
   c. Uremia (chronic renal failure)
   d. Ingestion of toxins (paraldehyde, methanol, salicylate, ethylene glycol)
   e. High-fat diet (mild acidosis)
2. Metabolic acidosis with normal anion gap (hyperchloremic acidosis)
   a. Renal tubular acidosis (including acidosis of aldosterone deficiency)
   b. Intestinal loss of bicarbonate (diarrhea, pancreatic fistula)
   c. Carbonic anhydrase inhibitors (e.g., acetazolamide)
   d. Dilutional acidosis (as a result of rapid infusion of bicarbonate-free isotonic saline)
   e. Ingestion of exogenous acids (ammonium chloride, methionine, cystine, calcium chloride)
   f. Ileostomy
   g. Ureterosigmoidostomy
   h. Drugs: amiloride, triamterene, spironolactone, β-blockers

ACIDOSIS, RESPIRATORY

Acidosis, respiratory
ICD-9CM # 276.2

BOX 2-11   Causes of Respiratory Acidosis

Disorders of ventilatory control
  Central nervous system
    Depression of respiratory center
      Anesthetics
      Drug intoxication
      Primary central hypoventilation
      Myxedema
      Oxygen therapy in chronic hypercapnic patients
      Sleep
  Peripheral neuromuscular disease
    Disorders of peripheral nerves
      Spinal cord injury
      Phrenic nerve palsy
      Guillain-Barré syndrome
      Myasthenia gravis
      Paralytic agents
      Botulism
  Disorders of muscle
    Myositis, myopathy, muscular dystrophies
    Fatigue in hypokalemia, hypophosphatemia
    Fatigue in obstructive airways disease
Disorders of pulmonary function
  Restrictive lung disease
    Kyphoscoliosis
    Flail chest
  Airways obstruction
    Upper airways obstruction (trachea, larynx, bronchi)
    Asthma and chronic obstructive pulmonary disease
Shunts
  Congenital heart disease with left-to-right shunt
  Intrapulmonary shunt
    Arteriovenous malformation
    Severe pneumonia, large emboli
Errors of ventilator management

From Stein JH (ed): *Internal medicine,* ed 5, St Louis, 1998, Mosby.

ACUTE SCROTUM

Acute scrotum
ICD-9CM # 608.9

TABLE 2-3   Acute Scrotum: Differential Diagnosis

	TORSION*	EPIDIDYMITIS	TUMOR
Age	Birth to 20 yr	Puberty to old age	15-35 yr
Pain			
Onset	Sudden	Rapid	Gradual
Degree	Severe	Increasing severity	Mild or absent†
Nausea/vomiting	Yes	No	No
Examination			
Testis	Swollen together and both tender	Normal early	Mass
Epididymis		Swollen, tender	Normal
Spermatic Cord	Shortened	Thickened, often tender as high as inguinal canal	Normal
Urinalysis	Normal	Often infection	Normal

From Nseyo UO (ed): *Urology for primary care physicians,* Philadelphia, 1999, WB Saunders.
*Testis and appendices of testis and epididymis.
†Present in 30% of patients with testis tumor.

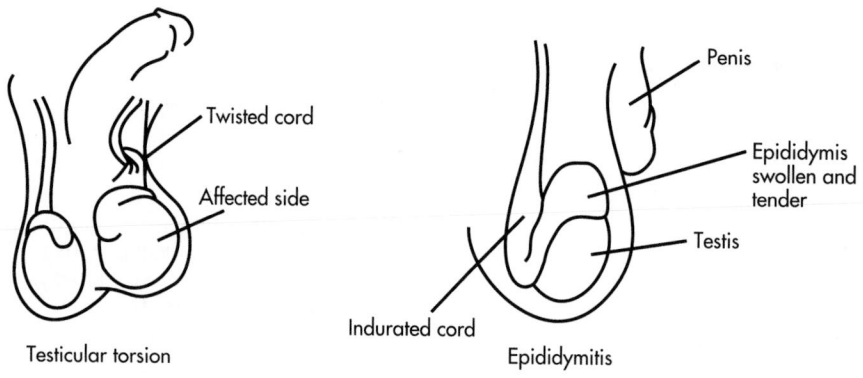

Testicular torsion

Epididymitis

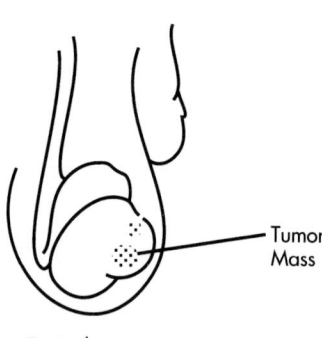

Testicular tumor

Fig. 2-2   Physical findings in acute scrotum: *Upper left,* Testicular torsion; *Upper right,* epididymitis; *Lower,* testicular tumor. Scrotal examination, which begins with palpation of the scrotal contents, should be performed in the following order: (1) testes; (2) epididymides; (3) spermatic cord structures; and (4) inguinal ring. (From Nseyo UO [ed]: *Urology for primary care physicians,* Philadelphia, 1999, WB Saunders.)

ADNEXAL MASS

Adnexal mass
ICD-9CM # Varies with specific disorder

TABLE 2-4   Differential Diagnosis of an Adnexal Mass

SITE	MASS
Ovary	Functional cyst
	Benign neoplasm
	Malignant neoplasm
	Endometriosis
Fallopian tube	Tuboovarian abscess
	Hydrosalpinx
	Paratubal cyst
	Ectopic pregnancy
	Benign neoplasm (rare)
	Malignant neoplasm
Uterus	Fibroid (pedunculated, interligamentous)
Gastrointestinal tract	Bowel loops with feces
	Diverticular disease
	Appendicitis
	Inflammatory bowel disease
	Benign small bowel neoplasm (leiomyoma)
	Colon cancer
Urinary tract	Distended bladder
	Pelvic kidney
	Urachal cyst
Retroperitoneum	Benign neoplasm (myxoid tumor)
	Sarcoma, lymphoma, or teratoma
	Abdominal wall hematoma or abscess

From Noble J: *Primary care medicine*, ed 3, St Louis, 2001, Mosby.

ADRENAL MASSES

BOX 2-12   Adrenal Masses

Unilateral Adrenal Masses
Functional Lesions

Adrenal adenoma
Adrenal carcinoma
Pheochromocytoma
Primary aldosteronism, adenomatous
   type

Nonfunctional Lesions

Adrenal adenoma
Adrenal carcinoma

Ganglioneuroma
Myelolipoma
Hematoma
Adrenolipoma
Metastasis

Bilateral Adrenal Masses
Functional Lesions

ACTH-dependent Cushing's syn-
   drome
Congenital adrenal hyperplasia
Pheochromocytoma

Conn's syndrome, hyperplastic
   variety
Micronodular adrenal disease
Idiopathic bilateral adrenal hypertrophy

Nonfunctional Lesions

Infection (tuberculosis, fungi)
Infiltration (leukemia, lymphoma)
Replacement (amyloidosis)
Hemorrhage
Bilateral metastases

From Stein JH (ed): *Internal medicine*, ed 5, St Louis, 1998, Mosby.

Adrenal masses
ICD-9CM # 194.0 Adrenal cortical carcinoma, site NOS M8370/3
          255.8 Adrenal hyperplasia

ADRENOCORTICAL HYPERFUNCTION

BOX 2-13   Etiologic Classification of Adrenocortical Hyperfunction

Excess androgen
  Congenital adrenal hyperplasia
    21-Hydroxylase (P450c21) deficiency
    11β-Hydroxylase (p450c11) deficiency
    3β-Hydroxysteroid dehydrogenase defect
  Tumor
    Carcinoma
    Adenoma
Excess cortisol (Cushing's syndrome)
  Bilateral adrenal hyperplasia
    Hypersecretion of corticotropin (Cushings disease)
    Ectopic secretion of corticotropin
    Exogenous corticotropin
  Adrenocortical nodular dysplasia
  Pigmented nodular adrenocortical diseases (Carney complex)
  Tumor
    Carcinoma
    Adenoma
Excess mineralocorticoid (hypertensive hypokalemic syndrome)
  Primary hyperaldosteronism
    Aldosterone-secreting adenoma
    Bilateral micronodular adrenocortical hyperplasia
    Glucocorticoid-suppressible aldosteronism
    Tumor
        Adenoma
        Carcinoma
  Desoxycorticosterone excess
    Congenital adrenal hyperplasia
        11β-Hydroxylase (P450c11)
        17α-Hydroxylase (P450c17)
    Tumor (carcinoma)
  Apparent mineralocorticoid excess
        11β-Hydroxysteroid dehydrogenase deficiency
  Excess estrogen (adrenal feminization syndrome)
    Carcinoma
    Adenoma
  Mixed hypercorticism—tumor

From Behrman RE: *Nelson textbook of pediatrics,* ed 16, Philadelphia, 2000, WB Saunders.

Adrenocortical hyperfunction
ICD-9CM # 255.3 (Cortical)
**   255.6 (Medulloadrenal)**

ADRENOCORTICAL HYPOFUNCTION

BOX 2-14   Etiologic Classification of Adrenocortical Hypofunction

Corticotropin-releasing hormone deficiency
  Isolated deficiency
  Multiple deficiencies
    Congenital defects (e.g., anencephaly, septo-optic dysplasia)
    Destructive lesions (e.g., tumor)
    Idiopathic (e.g., idiopathic hypopituitarism)
Corticotropin deficiency
  Isolated
  Autosomal recessive
  Multiple deficiencies
    Pituitary hypoplasia or aplasia
    Destructive lesions (e.g., craniopharyngioma)
    Autoimmune hypophysitis
Primary adrenal hypoplasia or aplasia
  X-linked
    With Duchenne muscular dystrophy and glycerol kinase deficiency (Xp21 deletion)
    With hypogonadotropic hypogonadism (DAX-1 mutation)
Familial glucocorticoid deficiency
  Corticotropin-receptor mutations
    With alacrima, achalasia, and neurologic disorders (triple A syndrome)
Defects of steroid biosynthesis
  Lipoid adrenal hyperplasia (StAR mutation)
  3β-Hydroxysteroid dehydrogenase deficiency
    Classic
      Salt loser
      Non–salt loser
    Mild or nonclassic
  21-Hydroxylase (P450C21) deficiency
    Classic
      Salt loser
      Non–salt loser
    Nonclassic or mild
  Isolated aldosterone (P450C18) deficiency
Pseudohypoaldosteronism (aldosterone unresponsiveness)
Adrenoleukodystrophy (peroxisomal membrane protein defect)
  Isolated adrenal involvement
  With neurologic involvement
Acid lipase deficiency
  Wolman disease, fatal neonatal form
Destructive lesions of adrenal cortex
  Granulomatous lesions (e.g., tuberculosis)
Autoimmune adrenalitis (idiopathic Addison disease)
  Isolated
  Associated with hypoparathyroidism or mucocutaneous candidiasis (type I autoimmune
    polyglandular syndrome), or both
  Associated with autoimmune thyroid disease and insulin-dependent diabetes (type II
    autoimmune polyglandular syndrome)
Neonatal hemorrhage
Acute infection (Waterhouse-Friderichsen syndrome)
Mitochondrial disorders
Acquired immunodeficiency syndrome
Iatrogenic
  Abrupt cessation of exogenous corticosteroids or corticotropin
  Removal of functioning adrenal tumor
  Adrenalectomy for Cushing's disease
  Drugs
    Aminoglutethimide
    Mitotane (o, p-DDD)
    Metyrapone
    Ketoconazole
Fetal adrenal suppression-maternal hypercortisolism
  Endogenous
  Therapeutic

From Behrman RE: *Nelson textbook of pediatrics*, ed 16, Philadelphia, 2000, WB Saunders.

Adrenocortical hypofunction
ICD-9CM # 255.4

AIRWAY OBSTRUCTION

Airway obstruction
ICD-9CM # 519.8

TABLE 2-5   Causes of Airway Obstruction

CAUSE	INTERVENTION
Aspiration of foreign body	Heimlich maneuver
	Removal by direct visualization and extraction
	Cricothyrotomy
Unconsciousness	Positioning
	Consider airway adjuncts
	Consider cricoid pressure
Apnea	Open airway
	Initiate rescue breathing
	Check for obstruction
	Consider airway adjuncts
Facial or neck trauma	Careful physical examination
	Remove debris in mouth
	Account for teeth
	Assess potential for swelling
	Positioning
	Secretion assistance
Allergic reactions	Remove from source of allergy
	Epinephrine if available
	Consider cool mist
	Consider topical or sprayed vasoconstrictors
	Consider inhaled β-agonists
	Consider airway adjuncts
Seizures	Pad environment
	Consider padded stick between side molars (no fingers)
	If possible, turn on side to facilitate gravity drainage of saliva or vomit

From Auerbach PS: *Wilderness medicine*, ed 4, St Louis, 2001, Mosby.

AIRWAY OBSTRUCTION, PEDIATRIC AGE

BOX 2-15   **Causes of Airway Obstruction**

Congenital Causes

Craniofacial dysmorphism
Hemangioma
Laryngeal cleft/web
Laryngoceles, cysts
Laryngomalacia
Macroglossia
Tracheal stenosis
Vascular ring
Vocal cord paralysis

Acquired Infectious Causes

Acute laryngotracheobronchitis
Diphtheria
Epiglottitis
Laryngeal papillomatosis
Membranous croup (bacterial tracheitis)
Mononucleosis
Retropharyngeal abscess
Spasmodic croup

Acquired Noninfectious Causes

Anaphylaxis
Angioneurotic edema
Foreign body aspiration
Supraglottic hypotonia
Thermal/chemical burn
Trauma
Vocal cord paralysis

From Hoekelman R (ed): *Primary pediatric care,* ed 3, St Louis, 1997, Mosby.

Airway obstruction, pediatric age
ICD-9CM # 496   Obstruction due to bronchospasm
934.9   Obstruction due to foreign body
478.75   Obstruction due to laryngospasm
506.9   Obstruction due to inhalation of fumes or vapors

AKINETIC/RIGID SYNDROME

BOX 2-16   **Differential Diagnosis of the Akinetic/Rigid Syndrome**

Idiopathic Parkinson's disease
Drug-induced parkinsonism
Diffuse Lewy body disease
Progressive supranuclear palsy
Multisystem atrophy
    Olivopontocerebellar atrophy; striatonigral degeneration; Shy-Drager syndrome
Vascular parkinsonism
Other hereditary neurodegenerative disorders: Huntington's disease; Hallervorden-Spatz disease
Toxic parkinsonism: carbon monoxide; manganese; MPTP
Catatonia (psychosis)

From Andreoli TE (ed): *Cecil essentials of medicine,* ed 5, Philadelphia, 2001, WB Saunders.

Akinetic/rigid syndrome
ICD-9CM # not available

ALKALOSIS, METABOLIC

Alkalosis, metabolic
ICD-9CM # 276.3

BOX 2-17   Metabolic Alkalosis

1. Chloride-responsive (urinary chloride <15 mEq/L)
   a. Vomiting
   b. Nasogastric suction
   c. Diuretics
   d. Post–hypercapnic alkalosis
   e. Stool losses (laxative abuse, cystic fibrosis, villous adenoma)
   f. Massive blood transfusion
   g. Exogenous alkali administration

2. Chloride-unresponsive (urinary chloride >15 mEq/L)
   a. Hyperadrenocorticoid states (Cushing's syndrome, primary hyperaldosteronism, secondary mineralo-corticoidism [licorice, chewing tobacco])
   b. Hypomagnesemia
   c. Hypokalemia
   d. Bartter's syndrome

ALKALOSIS, RESPIRATORY

Alkalosis, respiratory
ICD-9CM # 276.3

BOX 2-18   Causes of Respiratory Alkalosis

Hypoxemia
  Most pulmonary disease
  Organic heart disease
    Congenital heart disease with right-to-left shunts
    Congestive heart failure
  Altitude
Stimulation of respiratory center
  Drugs
    Salicylates
    Catecholamines

Theophylline
Doxapram
Progesterone excess
  Pregnancy
  Cirrhosis
Central nervous system disease
  Subarachnoid hemorrhage
  Disease of respiratory center
  Cheyne-Stokes respirations
Fever

Sepsis
Anxiety
Stimulation of peripheral pulmonary receptors
  Pneumonia
  Asthma
  Embolism
  Pulmonary edema
  Pulmonary fibrosis
  Pleural disease
Errors of ventilator management

From Stein JH (ed): *Internal medicine,* ed 5, St Louis, 1998, Mosby.

Alopecias
ICD-9CM # 704.00 Alopecia NOS
            704.01 Alopecia, androgenic
            704.01 Alopecia areata
            757.4 Alopecia, congenital
            316   Alopecia, psychogenic

ALOPECIAS

TABLE 2-6   Differential Diagnosis of Alopecias

DISEASE	HISTORY	PHYSICAL	LABORATORY	MANAGEMENT
Scarring Alopecia				
Congenital (aplasia cutis)	Present at birth	Alopecia Ulceration occasionally	None	Plastic surgery
Tinea capitis with inflammation (kerion)	Pruritic, scaly patches Pain and tenderness	Alopecia, scales Boggy patches Pustules	KOH positive Fungal culture	Oral antifungals
Bacterial folliculitis	Pruritic pustules	Pustules, papules Some alopecia	Gram's stain Bacterial culture	Antibiotics
Discoid lupus erythematosus	Pruritus occasionally Lesions other than scalp common	Erythema Scaly thick plaques Pigmentation	Skin biopsy DIF occasionally	Topical steroids Intralesional steroids Antimalarial agents
Lichen planopilaris	Pruritus occasionally	Alopecia Peripheral erythema Follicular accentuation	Skin biopsy	Topical steroids Intralesional steroids
Folliculitis decalvans	Rare Asymptomatic alopecia, inflammation	Patchy alopecia Follicular erythema at periphery	Skin biopsy	No effective Rx
Neoplasm	Asymptomatic alopecia	Evidence of tumor on the scalp	Skin biopsy	Treat tumor
Trauma	Traction, excessive hair treatments	Distribution where traction is most severe	None	Eliminate trauma
Nonscarring Alopecia *Breakage of Hairs*				
Cosmetic treatment	Frequent or excessive hair Rx	Broken hairs	None	Eliminate trauma
Tinea capitis	Pruritic scaly patches	Erythema, scales	KOH positive Fungal culture	Oral antifungals
Structural hair shaft disease	Unmanageable hair Childhood onset usual	Kinky hair Broken hairs	Microscopic hair examination	No effective Rx
Trichotillomania (hair pulling)	Children Frequently no history	Hair loss in irregular, bizarre pattern	Skin biopsy in difficult to diagnose cases	Counseling Behavior modification Clomipramine

TABLE 2-6   Differential Diagnosis of Alopecias—cont'd

DISEASE	HISTORY	PHYSICAL	LABORATORY	MANAGEMENT
Nonscarring Alopecia—cont'd				
Breakage of Hairs—cont'd				
Anagen arrest	Chemotherapy Radiation Rx Rapid fallout	Widespread shedding	None	Self-correcting
Shedding by Roots				
Telogen effluvium (telogen arrest)	Occurs 3 months after physical insult	Diffuse alopecia or thinning	Hair pull >5-10 hairs Forced hair pull analysis for anagen:telogen ratio	Reassurance Correct any identified causes Eliminate offending drug
Alopecia areata	Asymptomatic patches of alopecia	Round patches Noninflammatory May be diffuse	Skin biopsy in difficult cases	Topical steroids Intralesional steroids Induce contact dermatitis (DNCB) Ultraviolet therapy
Thinning Without Increased Shedding				
Androgenetic alopecia (male pattern balding)	Gradual thinning	Men: temporal and vertex Women: thinning over crown area	None usually Skin biopsy occasionally Rule out other causes	Topical minoxidil Hair transplant

From Noble J (ed): *Primary care medicine,* ed 3, St Louis, 2001, Mosby.
DIF, Direct immunofluorescence; *DNCB,* dinitrochlorobenzene; *KOH,* potassium hydroxide.

ALVEOLAR HEMORRHAGE

BOX 2-19   Causes of Alveolar Hemorrhage

Anti–basement membrane antibody disease (Goodpasture's syndrome)
Immune complex–mediated vasculitides
Wegener's vasculitis
Other antineutrophil cytoplasmic antibody (ANCA)–associated vasculitides
Pauciimmune-associated vasculitides
Idiopathic pulmonary hemosiderosis
Hematologic disorders (e.g., coagulopathies, thrombocytopenia, bone marrow transplantation)
Other agents (e.g., penicillamine, trimellitic anhydride, lymph-angiogram contrast)

From Noble J: *Primary care medicine,* ed 3, St Louis, 2001, Mosby.

**Alveolar hemorrhage
ICD-9CM # 770.3**

AMENORRHEA

TABLE 2-7 Differential Diagnosis of Amenorrhea

SITE OF ABNORMAL FUNCTION	DISORDER	PRIMARY OR SECONDARY AMENORRHEA	GONADOTROPIN LEVELS	ESTRADIOL LEVELS	CLINICAL FINDINGS	CONFIRMATORY TESTS
Uterus or outflow tract	Müllerian anomalies or agenesis	Primary	LH, FSH normal	Normal	May have cyclic pelvic pain	
	Testicular feminization	Primary	LH increased, FSH normal	Increased	Minimal body hair, good breast development, blind vagina	Elevated testosterone karyotype
	Uterine synechiae (Asherman's syndrome)	Secondary	LH, FSH normal	Normal	History of instrumentation or infection	Hysteroscopy or hysterosalpingo-gram
Ovary	Turner's syndrome (or mosaic)	Primary; sometimes secondary in mosaic form	FSH increased	Decreased	Short stature, webbed neck, shield chest, cardiac abnormalities and hypothyroidism (mosaics may be atypical)	Karyotype
	Premature ovarian failure	Secondary	FSH increased	Decreased	May have history of autoimmune disorder	
	Resistant ovary syndrome	Primary	FSH increased	Decreased		

From Carlson KJ et al: *Primary care of women,* ed 2, St Louis, 2002, Mosby.
LH, Luteinizing hormone; *FSH,* follicle-stimulating hormone.

Continued

TABLE 2-7   Differential Diagnosis of Amenorrhea—cont'd

SITE OF ABNORMAL FUNCTION	DISORDER	PRIMARY OR SECONDARY AMENORRHEA	GONADOTROPIN LEVELS	ESTRADIOL LEVELS	CLINICAL FINDINGS	CONFIRMATORY TESTS
Pituitary gland	Prolactinoma	Secondary	FSH, LH decreased or normal	Decreased	May have galactorrhea	Prolactin, cranial imaging
	Other tumors	Secondary	FSH, LH decreased or normal	Decreased	Signs of Cushing's syndrome or acromegaly	Urine free cortisol, growth hormone, cranial imaging
	Pituitary infarction	Secondary	FSH, LH decreased or normal	Decreased	Usually occurs postpartum	
Hypothalamus	Hypothalamic amenorrhea	Primary or secondary	FSH, LH decreased or normal	Decreased	Sometimes associated with stress, exercise, weight loss, chronic illness	
	Pituitary tumors	Primary or secondary	FSH, LH decreased or normal	Decreased	May manifest headache, visual symptoms	Cranial imaging
	Traumatic: head injury or irradiation	Secondary	FSH, LH decreased or normal	Decreased	History of head trauma or cranial irradiation	
Other	Polycystic ovarian syndrome	Secondary	Increased LH:FSH ratio	Decreased or normal	Signs of androgen excess	Testosterone, dehydroepiandrosterone sulfate, ultrasound

From Carlson KJ et al: *Primary care of women,* ed 2, St Louis, 2002, Mosby.
FSH, Follicle-stimulating hormone; *LH,* luteinizing hormone.

AMNESIA

BOX 2-20   Causes of Amnesia

Cerebrovascular events
  Hippocampal lesions
  Thalamic lesions
  Basal forebrain lesions
Wernicke-Korsakoff syndrome
Head trauma
Hypoxia
Hypoglycemia

Herpes simplex encephalitis
Degenerative diseases
  Alzheimer's disease
  Pick's disease
  Huntington's disease
Creutzfeldt-Jakob disease
Transient global amnesia
Neoplasms

Limbic encephalitis
Postsurgery
  Bilateral temporal lobectomy
  Bilateral fornix section
  Mammillary body surgery
  Cingulectomy

From Stein JH (ed): *Internal medicine,* ed 5, St Louis, 1998, Mosby.

Amnesia
ICD-9CM # 292.83 Drug induced
            300.12 Hysterical
            300.12 Psychogenic
            780.9   Retrograde
            437.7   Transient global

ANDROGEN RESISTANCE SYNDROMES

Androgen resistance syndromes
ICD-8CM # 257.8 Testicular feminization syndrome
257.2 Reifenstein syndrome
606.9 Male infertility, unspecified

TABLE 2-8   Androgen Resistance Syndromes

	EXTERNAL PHENOTYPE	INTERNAL PHENOTYPE	KARYOTYPE	INHERITANCE	SERUM TESTOSTERONE	SERUM ESTRADIOL	LH	FSH	PATHOGENESIS			
										Androgen Receptor Defects		
									Inability to form dihydrotestosterone	Absent	Qualitatively abnormal	Decreased amount
5-Alpha-reductase deficiency	Female genitalia at birth; variable virilization at expected time of puberty	Testes, epididymides, vasa deferentia present	46,XY	Autosomal recessive	Normal	Normal	Normal or slightly increased	Normal	Inability to form dihydrotestosterone			
Complete testicular feminization	Female external genitalia with a blind-ending vagina, female habitus and breast development, paucity of axillary and pubic hair	Testes present, absent wolffian and müllerian derivatives	46,XY	X-linked recessive	Normal or high male plasma levels	Higher than in normal men	Elevated	Normal		+++	+	+
Incomplete testicular feminization	Female habitus and breast development, normal axillary and pubic hair, clitoromegaly, and partial fusion of the labioscrotal folds	Testes present, under-developed wolffian duct derivatives	46,XY	X-linked recessive	Normal or high	Higher than in normal men	Elevated	Normal			++	
Reifenstein syndrome	Male with perineoscrotal hypospadias, normal axillary and pubic hair	Testes and wolffian duct structure present, varying in degree of male development	46,XY	X-linked recessive	Normal or high	Higher than in normal men	Elevated	Normal			+	++
Infertile male syndrome		Testes with oligospermia or azoospermia	46,XY	Probably X-linked	Normal	Higher than in normal men	Elevated (usually)	Normal			++	++

From Moore WT, Eastman RC: *Diagnostic endocrinology*, ed 2, St Louis, 1996, Mosby.
+, Frequency; *FSH*, follicle-stimulating hormone; *LH*, luteinizing hormone.

ANEMIA, DRUG-INDUCED

Anemia, drug induced
ICD-9CM # 283.0

BOX 2-21 Drugs That May Result in Anemia

Drugs That May Interfere with Red Cell Production by Inducing Marrow Suppression or Aplasia

Alcohol
Antineoplastic drugs
Antithyroid drugs
Antibiotics
Oral hypoglycemic agents
Phenylbutazone
Azidothymidine (AZT)

Drugs That Interfere with Vitamin B_{12}, Folate, or Iron Absorption or Utilization

Nitrous oxide
Anticonvulsant drugs
Antineoplastic drugs
Isoniazid, cycloserin A

Drugs Capable of Promoting Hemolysis
Immune Mediated

Penicillins
Quinine
Alpha-methyldopa
Procainamide
Mitomycin C

Oxidative Stress

Antimalarials
Sulfonamide drugs
Nalidixic acid

Drugs That May Produce or Promote Blood Loss

Aspirin
Alcohol
Nonsteroidal antiinflammatory agents
Corticosteroids
Anticoagulants

From Harrington J (ed): *Consultation in internal medicine*, ed 2, St Louis, 1997, Mosby.

ANEMIA, LOW RETICULOCYTE COUNT

Anemia, low reticulocyte count
ICD-9CM # 285.9

BOX 2-22 Differential Diagnosis of Anemia with Low Reticulocyte Count

Microcytic Anemia (MCV <80)

Iron deficiency
Thalassemia minor
Sideroblastic anemia
Lead poisoning

Macrocytic Anemia (MCV >100)

Megaloblastic anemias
  Folate deficiency
  Vitamin B_{12} deficiency
  Drug-induced megaloblastic anemia
Nonmegaloblastic macrocytosis
  Liver disease
  Hypothyroidism

Normocytic Anemia (MCV 80-100)

Early iron deficiency
Aplastic anemia
Myelophthysic disorders
Endocrinopathies
Anemia of chronic disease
Uremia
Mixed nutritional deficiency

From Andreoli TE (ed): *Cecil essentials of medicine*, ed 5, Philadelphia, 2001, WB Saunders.
MCV, Mean corpuscular volume.

Anemia, megaloblastic
ICD-9CM # 281.0 Pernicious deficiency
         281.1 B_{12} deficiency
         281.2 Folate deficiency
         281.3 B_{12} with folate deficiency
         281.4 Protein or amino acid deficiency
         281.8 Nutritional
         281.9 NOS

ANEMIA, MEGALOBLASTIC

BOX 2-23   Megaloblastic Anemias

I. Etiopathophysiologic classification of cobalamin (Cbl) deficiency
   A. Nutritional Cbl deficiency (insufficient Cbl intake) vegetarians, vegans, breast-fed infants of mothers with pernicious anemia
   B. Abnormal intragastric events (inadequate proteolysis of food Cbl), atrophic gastritis, partial gastrectomy with hypochlorhydria
   C. Loss/atrophy of gastric oxyntic mucosa (deficient IF molecules), total or partial gastrectomy, pernicious anemia (PA), caustic destruction (lye)
   D. Abnormal events in small bowel lumen
      1. Inadequate pancreatic protease (R-Cbl not degraded, Cbl not transferred to IF)
         a. Insufficiency of pancreatic protease—pancreatic insufficiency
         b. Inactivation of pancreatic protease—Zollinger-Ellison syndrome
      2. Usurping of luminal Cbl (inadequate Cbl binding to IF)
         a. By bacteria—stasis syndromes (blind loops, pouches of diverticulosis, strictures, fistulas, anastomoses); impaired bowel motility (scleroderma, pseudoobstruction), hypogammaglobulinemia
         b. By *Diphyllobothrium latum*
   E. Disorders of ileal mucosa/IF receptors (IF-Cbl not bound to IF receptors)
      1. Diminished or absent IF receptors—ileal bypass/resection/fistula
      2. Abnormal mucosal architecture/function—tropical/nontropical sprue, Crohn's disease, TB ileitis, infiltration by lymphomas, amyloidosis
      3. IF-/post IF-receptor defects—Imerslund-Graesbeck syndrome, TC II deficiency
      4. Drug-induced effects (slow K, biguanides, cholestyramine, colchicine, neomycin, PAS)
   F. Disorders of plasma Cbl transport (TC II-Cbl not delivered to TC II receptors)
      1. Congenital TC II deficiency, defective binding of TC II-Cbl to TC II receptors (rare)
   G. Metabolic disorders (Cbl not utilized by cell)
      1. Inborn enzyme errors (rare)
      2. Acquired disorders: (Cbl oxidized to cob[III]alamin)—N_2O inhalation
II. Etiopathophysiologic classification of folate deficiency
   A. Nutritional causes
      1. Decreased dietary intake—poverty and famine (associated with kwashiorkor, marasmus), insti-

tutionalized individuals (psychiatric/nursing homes), chronic debilitating disease/goats' milk (low in folate), special diets (slimming), cultural/ethnic cooking techniques (food folate destroyed) or habits (folate-rich foods not consumed)
      2. Decreased diet and increased requirements
         a. *Physiologic:* pregnancy and lactation, prematurity, infancy
         b. *Pathologic:* intrinsic hematologic disease (autoimmune hemolytic disease), drugs, malaria; hemoglobinopathies (SS, thalassemia), RBC membrane defects (hereditary spherocytosis, paroxysmal nocturnal hemoglobinopathy); abnormal hematopoiesis (leukemia/lymphoma, myelodysplastic syndrome, agnogenic myeloid metaplasia with myelofibrosis); infiltration with malignant disease; dermatologic (psoriasis)
   B. Folate malabsorption
      1. With normal intestinal mucosa
         a. Some drugs (controversial)
         b. Congenital folate malabsorption (rare)
      2. With mucosal abnormalities—tropical and nontropical sprue, regional enteritis
   C. Defective cellular folate uptake—familial aplastic anemia (rare)
   D. Inadequate cellular utilization
      1. Folate antagonists (methotrexate)
      2. Hereditary enzyme deficiencies involving folate
   E. Drugs (multiple effects on folate metabolism)—alcohol, sulfasalazine, triamterine, pyrimethamine, trimethoprim-sulfamethoxazole, diphenylhydantoin, barbiturates
   F. Acute folate deficiency
III. Miscellaneous megaloblastic anemias (not caused by Cbl or folate deficiency)
   A. Congenital disorders of DNA synthesis (rare)—orotic aciduria, Lesch-Nyhan syndrome, congenital dyserythropoietic anemia
   B. Acquired disorders of DNA synthesis
      1. Thiamine-responsive megaloblastosis (rare)
      2. Malignancy—erythroleukemia
                     —refractory sideroblastic anemias
                     —*all* antineoplastic drugs that inhibit DNA synthesis
      3. Toxic—alcohol

From Stein JH (ed): *Internal medicine,* ed 5, St Louis, 1998, Mosby.
DNA, Deoxyribonucleic acid; *IF,* intrinsic factor; *TC,* transcobalamin.

ANERGY, CUTANEOUS

Anergy, cutaneous
ICD-9CM # 279.9 Immune mechanism disorder

BOX 2-24   Causes of Cutaneous Anergy

I. Immunologic
  A. Acquired
    1. Acquired immunodeficiency syndrome (AIDS)
    2. Acute leukemia
    3. Carcinoma
    4. Chronic lymphocytic leukemia
    5. Hodgkin's disease
    6. Non-Hodgkin's lymphoma
  B. Congenital
    1. Ataxia telangiectasia
    2. Di George's syndrome
    3. Nezelof's syndrome
    4. Severe combined immunodeficiency
    5. Wiskott-Aldrich syndrome
II. Infections
  A. Bacterial
    1. Bacterial pneumonia
    2. Brucellosis
  B. Disseminated mycotic infections
  C. Mycobacterial
    1. Lepromatous leprosy
    2. Miliary and active tuberculosis
  D. Viral
    1. Varicella
    2. Hepatitis
    3. Influenza
    4. Infectious mononucleosis
    5. Measles
    6. Mumps
III. Immunosuppressive medications
  A. Cyclophosphamide
  B. Methotrexate
  C. Rifampin
  D. Systemic corticosteroids
IV. Other
  A. Alcoholic cirrhosis
  B. Anemia
  C. Biliary cirrhosis
  D. Burns
  E. Crohn's disease
  F. Diabetes
  G. Malnutrition
  H. Old age
  I. Pregnancy
  J. Pyridoxine deficiency
  K. Rheumatic disease
  L. Sarcoidosis
  M. Sickle cell anemia
  N. Surgery
  O. Uremia

From Stein JH (ed): *Internal medicine,* ed 5, St Louis, 1998, Mosby.

ANISOCORIA

Anisocoria
ICD-9CM # 379.41

BOX 2-25   Anisocoria

Mydriatic or miotic drugs
Prosthetic eye
Inflammation (keratitis, iridocyclitis)
Infections (herpes zoster, syphilis, meningitis, encephalitis, tuberculosis, diphtheria, botulism)
Subdural hemorrhage
Cavernous sinus thrombosis
Intracranial neoplasm
Cerebral aneurysm
Glaucoma
Central nervous system degenerative diseases
Internal carotid ischemia
Toxic polyneuritis (alcohol, lead)
Adie's syndrome
Horner's syndrome
Diabetes mellitus
Trauma
Congenital

APHASIA SYNDROMES

TABLE 2-9   Aphasia Syndromes

Aphasia syndromes
ICD-9CM # 784.3   Aphasia, unspecified
315.31   Aphasia, developmental expressive
315.32   Aphasia, developmental expressive
438.11   Aphasia, late effect cerebrovascular disease
784.3   Aphasia, unknown etiology

SYNDROME	SPONTANEOUS SPEECH	REPETITION	COMPRE-HENSIVE	NAMING	READING	WRITING	HEMIPARESIS	HEMISENSORY DEFECT	VISUAL FIELD DEFECT	NEUROPATHOLOGY IN LEFT HEMISPHERE
Broca's	Non-fluent	Poor	Good	Poor	Poor	Poor	Common	Rare	Rare	Posterior inferior frontal lobe
Wernicke's	Fluent, paraphasic	Poor	Poor	Poor	Poor	Poor	Rare	Variable	Variable	Posterior superior temporal lobe
Conduction	Fluent, paraphasic	Poor	Good	Variable	Good	Variable	Rare	Variable	Rare	Arcuate fasciculus region
Global	Nonfluent	Poor	Poor	Poor	Poor	Poor	Common	Common	Common	Combinations of the above three
Transcortical										
Motor	Nonfluent	Good	Good	Poor	Good	Poor	Common	Rare	Rare	Frontal, beyond Broca's area
Sensory	Fluent	Good	Poor	Poor	Poor	Poor	Rare	Common	Common	Parietal-temporal junction
Mixed	Nonfluent	Good	Poor	Poor	Poor	Poor	Common	Common	Common	Combination of the above two
Anomic	Fluent	Good	Good	Poor	Variable	Variable	Variable	Variable	Rare	Multiple sites
Subcortical										
Anterior	Nonfluent, paraphasic	Good	Good	Poor	Poor	Poor	Common	Rare	Rare	Putamen, globus pallidus
Posterior	Fluent, paraphasic	Good	Poor	Poor	Poor	Poor	Rare	Common	Variable	Thalamus

From Goldman L, Bennett JC (eds): *Cecil textbook of medicine*, ed 21, Philadelphia, 2000, WB Saunders.

Appetite loss in infants and children
ICD-9CM # 783.0   Appetite loss
                  307.59 Appetite loss, psychogenic origin

APPETITE LOSS IN INFANTS AND CHILDREN

BOX 2-26   Causes of Loss of Appetite in Infants and Children

Organic Disease

Infectious (acute or chronic)
Neurologic
   Congenital degenerative disease
   Hypothalamic lesion
   Increased intracranial pressure (including a brain
     tumor)
   Swallowing disorders (neuromuscular)
Gastrointestinal
   Oral lesions (e.g., thrush or herpes simplex)
   Gastroesophageal reflux
   Obstruction (especially with gastric or intestinal dis-
     tention)
   Inflammatory bowel disease
   Celiac disease
   Constipation
Cardiac
   Congestive heart failure (especially associated with
     cyanotic lesions)
Metabolic
   Renal failure and/or renal tubule acidosis
   Liver failure
   Congenital metabolic disease
   Lead poisoning
Nutritional
   Marasmus
   Iron deficiency
   Zinc deficiency

Fever
   Rheumatoid arthritis
   Rheumatic fever
Drugs
   Morphine
   Digitalis
   Antimetabolites
   Methylphenidate
   Amphetamines
Miscellaneous
   Prolonged restriction of oral feedings, beginning in the
     neonatal period
   Systemic lupus erythematosus
   Tumor

Psychologic Factors

Anxiety, fear, depression, mania (limbic influence on the
   hypothalamus)
Avoidance of symptoms associated with meals (abdominal pain, diarrhea, bloating, urgency, dumping syndrome)
Anorexia nervosa
Excessive weight loss and food aversion in athletes, simulating anorexia nervosa

From Hoekelman R (ed): *Primary pediatric care*, ed 3, St Louis, 1997, Mosby.

ARTERIAL OCCLUSION, ACUTE

TABLE 2-10   **Clinical Features of Acute Arterial Occlusion**

DIAGNOSIS	CAUSE AND SOURCE OF OCCLUSION	LOCATION OF OCCLUSION	TREATMENT
Arterial embolism			
Thromboembolism	85% originate in the heart 60%-70% are due to left ventricular thrombus post-MI Mitral stenosis Rheumatic valve disease Atrial fibrillation	Femoral and popliteal arteries	1. Fogarty's catheter thrombectomy 2. Heparinization 3. Treat underlying rhythm
Atheroembolism	Microemboli composed of cholesterol, calcium, and platelets from proximal atherosclerotic plaques	Cortical vessels Lower-extremity digits ("blue toe syndrome")	1. Treat underlying cause 2. Local and conservative care 3. Anticoagulation is contraindicated
Arterial thrombosis	In situ blood clot formation caused by endothelial injury, altered arterial blood flow, acute vasculitis, trauma, severe atherosclerosis	Based on mechanism	1. Heparinization 2. Direct arterial thrombolytic therapy 3. Surgical thromboebolectomy/bypass
Inflammation			
Miscellaneous	Drugs, irradiation, trauma, infectious, necrotizing (noninfectious)	Peripheral extremities	1. Reduce exposure to drug 2. Treat underlying infection 3. NSAIDs
Vasculitides	Possible immune complex mediated	Small vessels, retina, kidney, multiple organ dysfunction	1. Immunosuppression
Vasospasm	Mechanism unknown, possible autonomic dysfunction	Distal small arteries	1. Vasodilator* 2. Sympathectomy†
Trauma	In situ blood clot formation caused by endothelial injury, altered arterial blood flow, acute vasculitis	Location of trauma	1. Thromboembolectomy/bypass

From Goldman L, Braunwald E (eds): *Primary cardiology,* Philadelphia, 1998, WB Saunders.
MI, Myocardial infarction; *NSAIDs,* nonsteroidal antiinflammatory drugs.
*Recommended agents: prazosine, nifedipine, reserpine, phenoxybenzamine, and pentoxifylline.
†Limited to Buerger's disease.

Arterial occlusion, acute
ICD-9CM # 444.22 Arterial occlusion, lower extremities with thrombus or embolus
            444.21 Arterial occlusion, upper extremities with thrombus or embolus

ARTHRITIDES

Arthritides
ICD-9CM # Code varies with specific diagnosis

TABLE 2-11 Differentiating Features of Common Arthritides

DISEASE	DEMOGRAPHICS	JOINTS INVOLVED	SPECIAL FEATURES	LABORATORY FINDINGS
Gout	Men, postmenopausal women	Monoarticular or oligoarticular	Podagra, rapid onset of attack, polyarticular gout, tophi	SF: crystals, high WBC, >80% PMN
Septic arthritis	Any age	Usually large joints	Fever, chills	SF: high WBC, >90% PMN, culture
Osteoarthritis	Increases with age	Weight-bearing, hands		Noninflammatory SF
Rheumatoid arthritis	Any age, predominantly women ages 20-50 yr	Symmetric, small joints	Rheumatoid nodules, extra-articular disease	SF: high WBC, >70% PMN
Reiter's syndrome	Young males	Oligoarticular, asymmetric	Urethritis, conjunctivitis, skin and mucous membranes	SF: moderate WBC, >50% PMN
Spondyloarthropathy	Young to middle-aged males	Axial skeleton, pelvis (sacroiliac joints)	Uveitis, aortic insufficiency, enthesopathy	
Systemic lupus erythematosus	Females in childbearing years	Hands, knees	Nonerosive joint disease, autoantibodies, multiorgan disease	SF: low-moderate WBC, mostly mononuclear; almost 100% have antinuclear antibodies

From Andreoli TE (ed): *Cecil essentials of medicine,* ed 5, Philadelphia, 2001, WB Saunders.
PMN, Neutrophils; *SF,* synovial fluid; *WBC,* white blood cells.

ARTHRITIS AND EYE LESIONS

Arthritis and eye lesions
ICD-9CM # Code varies with specific diagnosis

TABLE 2-12 Differential Diagnosis of Conditions That Cause Arthritis and Eye Lesions

	CONJUNCTIVITIS	KERATITIS	SCLERITIS	IRITIS	POSTERIOR UVEITIS	RETINAL LESIONS
Rheumatoid arthritis		+	+			
JRA*				+		
Sjögren		+				
Lupus						+
Scleroderma						+
Necrotizing vasculitides						+
Wegener's granulomatosis		+		+	+	+
Giant cell arteritis						+
Takayasu						+
Reactive arthritis	+			+		
Ankylosing spondylitis				+		
Psoriatic arthritis				+		
Ulcerative colitis				+		
Crohn's†				+	+	
Behçet's†				+	+	+
Sarcoidosis†		+		+	+	+
Microbial endocarditis†						+
Syphilis		+		+		
Lyme disease				+		
Whipple's				+	+	

From Canoso J: *Rheumatology in primary care,* Philadelphia, 1997, WB Saunders.
JRA, Juvenile rheumatoid arthritis: oligoarthritis of lower extremities, chronic anterior uveitis, positive ANA.
†With or without arthritis.

ARTHRITIS AND HEART MURMUR

Arthritis and heart murmur
ICD-9CM # Code varies with specific diagnosis

BOX 2-27 **Arthritis and Heart Murmur**

- Subacute bacterial endocarditis
- Cardiac myxoma
- Ankylosing spondylitis
- Reactive arthritis
- Acute rheumatic fever
- Rheumatoid arthritis
- Systemic lupus erythematosus with Libman-Sack endocarditis
- Relapsing polychondritis

From Canoso J: *Rheumatology in primary care*, Philadelphia, 1997, WB Saunders.

ARTHRITIS AND MUSCLE WEAKNESS

Arthritis and muscle weakness
ICD-9CM # Code varies with specific diagnosis

BOX 2-28 **Arthritis and Muscle Weakness**

- Rheumatoid arthritis
- Ankylosing spondylitis
- Polymyositis
- Dermatomyositis
- Systemic lupus erythematosus, scleroderma, mixed connective tissue disease
- Sarcoidosis
- Human immunodeficiency virus–associated arthritis
- Whipple's disease

From Canoso J: *Rheumatology in primary care*, Philadelphia, 1997, WB Saunders.

ARTHRITIS AND RASH

Arthritis and rash
ICD-9CM # Code varies with specific diagnosis

BOX 2-29 **Arthritis and Rash**

- Chronic urticaria
- Vasculitic urticaria
- Systemic lupus erythematosus
- Dermatomyositis
- Polymyositis
- Psoriatic arthritis
- Reactive arthritis
- Chronic sarcoidosis
- Sweet's syndrome
- Leprosy

From Canoso J: *Rheumatology in primary care*, Philadelphia, 1997, WB Saunders.

ARTHRITIS AND SUBCUTANEOUS NODULES

BOX 2-30 Arthritis and Subcutaneous Nodules

- Rheumatoid arthritis
- Gout
- Pseudogout (rare)
- Sarcoidosis
- Light chain (LA) amyloidosis (primary, multiple myeloma)
- Acute rheumatic fever
- Hemochromatosis
- Whipple's disease
- Multicentric reticulohistiocytosis

From Canoso J: *Rheumatology in primary care,* Philadelphia, 1997, WB Saunders.

ARTHRITIS AND WEIGHT LOSS

BOX 2-31 Arthritis and Weight Loss

- Severe rheumatoid arthritis (RA)
- RA with vasculitis
- Reactive arthritis
- RA or psoriatic arthritis or ankylosing spondylitis with amyloidosis
- Cancer
- Enteropathic arthritis (Crohn's, ulcerative colitis)
- Human immunodeficiency virus
- Whipple's disease
- Blind loop syndrome
- Scleroderma with intestinal bacterial overgrowth

From Canoso J: *Rheumatology in primary care,* Philadelphia, 1997, WB Saunders.

Arthritis, axial skeleton
ICD-9CM # 720.0 Arthritis, rheumatoid, spine
         696.0 Arthritis, psoriatic
         715.9 Arthritis, degenerative NOS
         720.0 Ankylosing spondylitis

ARTHRITIS, AXIAL SKELETON

TABLE 2-13   Arthritis of the Axial Skeleton

	INTERVERTEBRAL DISK SPACE NARROWING	VACUUM PHENOMENA	INTERVERTEBRAL DISK SPACE CALCIFICATION	BONE OUTGROWTHS	APOPHYSEAL JOINT EROSION	APOPHYSEAL JOINT ANKYLOSIS	ATLANTOAXIAL SUBLUXATION
Rheumatoid arthritis	+	−	−	−	+	±	+
Psoriatic arthritis, Reiter's syndrome	±	−	−	Paravertebral ossification	±	±	+
Ankylosing spondylitis	±	−	±	Syndesmophytes	+	+	+
Juvenile rheumatoid arthritis	+	−	±	−	+	+	+
Degenerative disease of the nucleus pulposus	+	+	−	−	−	−	−
Spondylosis deformans	−	−	−	Osteophytes	−	−	−
Diffuse idiopathic skeletal hyperostosis	−	−	±	Flowing anterolateral ossification	−	−	−
Alkaptonuria	+	+	+	Syndesmophytes (rare)	−	−	−
Infection	+	−	−	−	−	−	−

From Stein JH (ed): *Internal medicine,* ed 5, St Louis, 1998, Mosby.
+, Common presentation; ±, uncommon; −, rare or absent.

ARTHRITIS, CRYSTAL-INDUCED

Arthritis, crystal-induced
ICD-9CM # 274.0   Gout
             275.49 Chondrocalcinosis (pseudogout)

TABLE 2-14   Comparison of Crystal-Induced Arthritides

CRYSTAL-INDUCED ARTHRITIS	CHARACTERISTICS OF CRYSTALS (FROM JOINT ASPIRATION)	COMMONLY INVOLVED JOINTS	COMMENTS AND THERAPY
Gouty arthritis	Monosodium urate crystals	First metatarsophalangeal, ankles, midfoot	See Section I
Calcium pyrophosphate deposition disease (pseudogout)	Calcium pyrophosphate dihydrate crystals Rhomboid or polymorphic-shaped, weakly positive, birefringent crystals	Knees, wrists	X-ray films of involved joint may reveal linear calcifications (chondrocalcinosis) on articular cartilage Possible associated conditions must be ruled out: Hyperparathyroidism Hypothyroidism Hemochromatosis Hypomagnesemia Therapy: NSAIDs, joint immobilization, intraarticular steroids
Hydroxyapatite arthropathy	Calcium hydroxyapatite crystals Crystals from nonbirefringent clumps with synovial fluid when placed on slide Diagnosis often requires electron microscopy because of small size of the crystals	Knees, hips, shoulders	Usually affects younger patients than the other crystal-induced arthritides Therapy: NSAIDs, joint immobilization, intraarticular steroids
Calcium oxalate–induced arthritis	Calcium oxalate crystals Bipyramidal-shaped, positive birefringent crystals	DIP, PIP joints of hands	Often seen in dialysis patients taking large doses of ascorbic acid (metabolized to oxalate) Therapy: NSAIDs, joint immobilization, intraarticular steroids

ARTHRITIS, FEVER, AND RASH

Arthritis, fever, and rash
ICD-9CM # Code varies with specific diagnosis

BOX 2-32   Arthritis, Fever, and Rash

- Rubella
- Parvovirus B-19
- Gonococcemia
- Meningococcemia
- Lyme borreliosis
- Secondary syphilis
- Adult acute rheumatic fever
- Adult Kawasaki disease?
- Vasculitic urticaria
- Acute sarcoidosis
- Adult Still's disease
- Familial Mediterranean fever
- Hyperimmunoglobulinemia D and periodic fever syndrome

From Canoso J: *Rheumatology in primary care*, Philadelphia, 1997, WB Saunders.

ARTHRITIS, MONOARTICULAR AND OLIGOARTICULAR

BOX 2-33   Differential Diagnosis of Acute Monoarticular and Oligoarticular Arthritis

Septic arthritis
Crystalline-induced arthritis
   Gout
   Pseudogout (calcium pyrophosphate arthropathy)
   Hydroxyapatite and other basic calcium/phosphate
     crystals
   Calcium oxalate

Traumatic joint injury
Hemarthrosis
Monoarticular or oligoarticular flare of an inflammatory
   polyarticular rheumatic disease (rheumatoid arthritis,
   psoriatic arthritis, Reiter's syndrome, systemic lupus
   erythematosus)

From Noble J (ed): *Primary care medicine*, ed 3, St Louis, 2001, Mosby.

Arthritis, monoarticular and oligoarticular
ICD-9CM # 715.3 Osteoarthritis, localized
          711.9 Infectious arthritis
          716.6 Monoarticular arthritis
               5th digit to be added to the above depending on site of arthritis
                0. Site unspecified
                1. Shoulder region
                2. Upper arm
                3. Forearm
                4. Hand
                5. Pelvic region and thigh
                6. Lower leg
                7. Ankle and/or foot
                8. Other specified except spine

II

ARTHRITIS, PEDIATRIC AGE

Arthritis, pediatric age
ICD-9CM # 711.9   Infectious arthritis
714.30 Juvenile chronic or unspecified
714.31 Juvenile rheumatoid polyarticular acute
714.32 Juvenile rheumatoid pauciarticular
714.33 Juvenile rheumatoid monoarticular

BOX 2-34   Differential Diagnosis of Juvenile Arthritis

Rheumatic Diseases of Childhood

Acute rheumatic fever
Systemic lupus erythematosus
Juvenile ankylosing spondylitis
Polymyositis and dermatomyositis
Vasculitis
Scleroderma
Psoriatic arthritis
Mixed connective tissue disease and overlap syndromes
Kawasaki disease
Behçet's syndrome
Familial Mediterranean fever
Reiter's syndrome
Reflex sympathetic dystrophy
Fibromyalgia (fibrositis)

Infectious Diseases

Bacterial arthritis
Viral or postviral arthritis
Fungal arthritis
Osteomyelitis
Reactive arthritis

Neoplastic Diseases

Leukemia
Lymphoma
Neuroblastoma
Primary bone tumors

Noninflammatory Disorders

Trauma
Avascular necrosis syndromes
Osteochondroses
Slipped capital femoral epiphysis
Diskitis
Patellofemoral dysfunction (chondromalacia patellae)
Toxic synovitis of the hip
Overuse syndromes

Genetic or Congenital Syndromes

Hematologic Disorders

Sickle cell disease
Hemophilia

Inflammatory Bowel Disease

Miscellaneous

Growing pains
Psychogenic arthralgias (conversion reactions)
Hypermobility syndrome
Villonodular synovitis
Foreign body arthritis

From Hoekelman R (ed): *Primary pediatric care*, ed 3, St Louis, 1997, Mosby.

ARTHRITIS, POLYARTICULAR

Arthritis, polyarticular
ICD-9CM # 715.09 Generalized osteoarthritis, multiple sites
716.89 Arthritis, multiple sites
714.31 Juvenile rheumatoid, polyarticular, acute

TABLE 2-15 Causes of Polyarthritis: Inflammatory Joint Diseases

CAUSE	COURSE			DISTRIBUTION	
	ACUTE	INTERMITTENT	CHRONIC	SYMMETRIC	ASYMMETRIC
Rheumatoid arthritis*		±	+	+	±
Systemic lupus erythematosus*		±	±	+	
Other connective tissue diseases		±	±	+	
Crystal deposition diseases		±	+	+	±
Neisserial infection	+			±	+
Hepatitis B	+		±	+	
Rubella	+			+	
Lyme arthritis	±	+	±		+
Bacterial endocarditis	+			+	±
Rheumatic fever	+			+	±
Erythema nodosum	+	±		+	±
Sarcoidosis	+	+	±	+	+
Hypersensitivity to serum or drugs	+	±		+	±
Henoch-Schönlein purpura	+			±	+
Relapsing polychondritis	±	+	±	+	+
Juvenile (rheumatoid) polyarthritis	±	±	+	+	+
Hypertrophic pulmonary osteoarthropathy	±		+	+	
Ankylosing spondylitis*		±	+	±	+
Reiter's disease*	±	±	±	±	+
Enteropathic arthropathy*	±	+	±	±	+
Psoriatic arthritis*		±	+	+	+
Reactive arthritis	+	±	±	±	+
Behçet's disease	±	+	±		+
Familial Mediterranean fever	±	+	±		+
Whipple's disease	±	+	±	±	+
Palindromic rheumatism	±	+		±	+

From Stein JH (ed): *Internal medicine*, ed 5, St Louis, 1998, Mosby.
+, Most common; ±, less common.
*The most important diagnoses.

ARTHROPOD-TRANSMITTED DISEASES

Arthropod-transmitted disease
ICD-9CM # 088.9

BOX 2-35   Diseases Transmitted to Humans By Biting Arthropods

Mosquitoes

Eastern equine encephalitis*
Western equine encephalitis*
St. Louis encephalitis*
La Crosse encephalitis*
Japanese encephalitis
Venezuelan equine encephalitis
Malaria
Yellow fever
Dengue fever
Bancroftian filariasis
Epidemic polyarthritis (Ross River virus)
Chikungunya fever
Rift Valley fever

Ticks

Lyme disease*
Rocky Mountain spotted fever*
Colorado tick fever*
Relapsing fever*
Ehrlichiosis*
Babesiosis*
Tularemia*
Tick paralysis*
Tick typhus

Flies

Tularemia*
Leishmaniasis*
African trypanosomiasis (sleeping sickness)
Onchocerciasis
Bartonellosis
Loa loa

Chigger Mites

Scrub typhus (tsutsugamushi fever)
Rickettsial pox*

Fleas

Plague*
Murine (endemic) typhus

Lice

Epidemic typhus
Relapsing fever

Kissing Bugs

American trypanosomiasis (Chagas' disease)

From Auerbach PS: *Wilderness medicine,* ed 4, St Louis, 2001, Mosby.
*May be found in the United States.

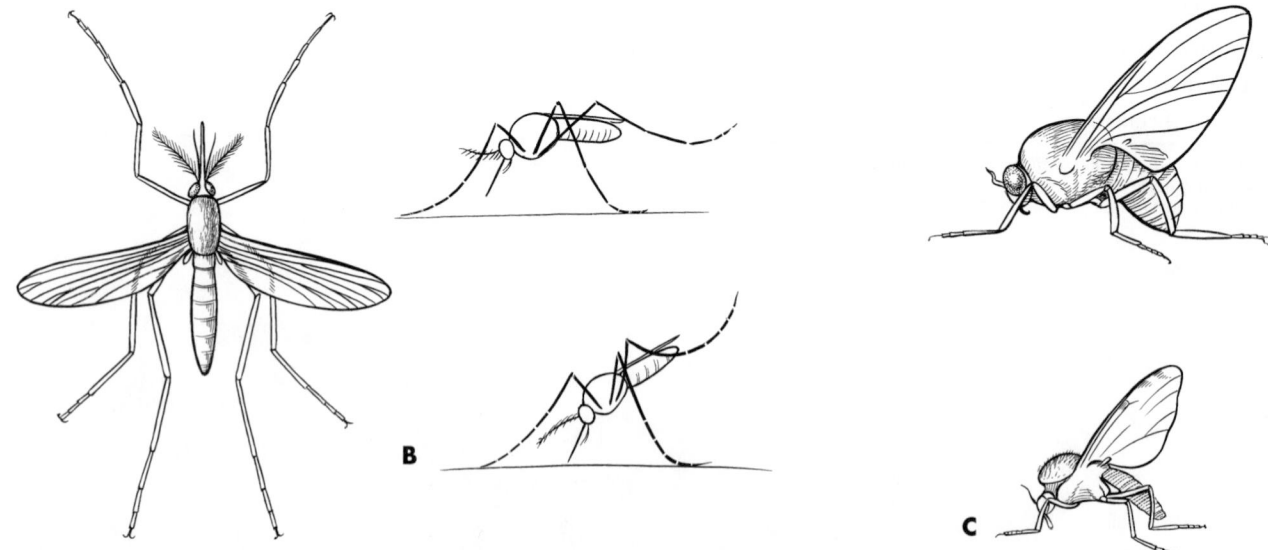

Fig. 2-3 Blood-feeding arthropods. **A,** Mosquito: Culex and Anopheles. **B,** Blackfly. **C,** Biting midge. (From Auerbach PS: *Wilderness medicine,* ed 4, St Louis, 2001, Mosby.)

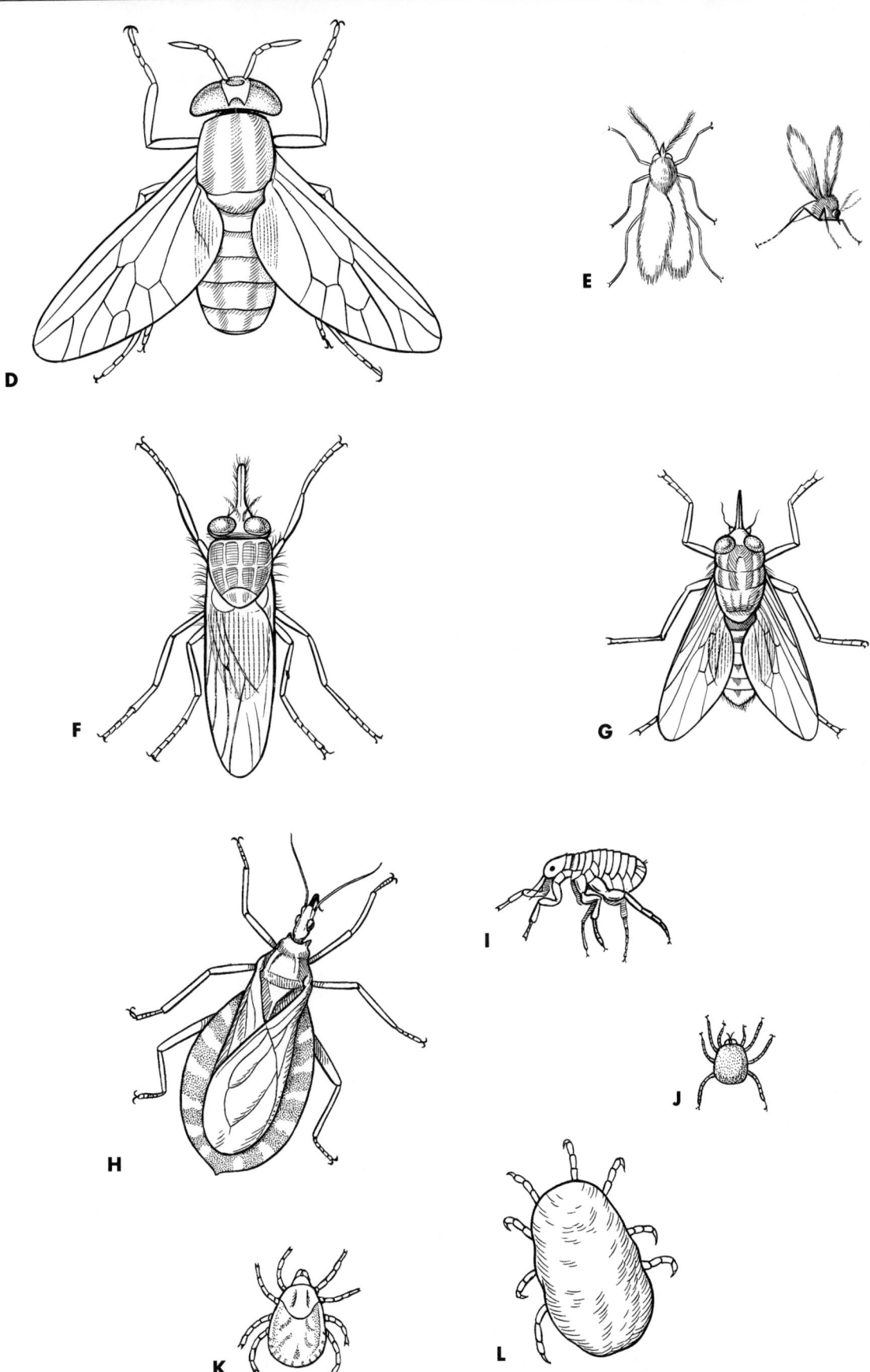

Fig. 2-3, cont'd   Blood-feeding arthropods. **D,** Tabanid fly. **E,** Sand fly. **F,** Tsetse fly. **G,** Stable fly. **H,** Kissing bug. **I,** Flea.
J, Chigger mite. **K,** Hard tick. **L,** Soft tick. (From Auerbach PS: *Wilderness medicine,* ed 4, St Louis, 2001, Mosby.)

ASCITES

Ascites
ICD-9CM # 789.5 Ascites NOS
197.6 Ascites, cancerous (malignant)
457.8 Ascites, chylous

BOX 2-36 Ascites

Hypoalbuminemia: nephrotic syndrome, protein-losing gastroenteropathy, starvation
Cirrhosis
Hepatic congestion: congestive heart failure, constrictive pericarditis, tricuspid insufficiency, hepatic vein obstruction (Budd-Chiari syndrome), inferior vena cava or portal vein obstruction

Peritoneal infections: tuberculosis and other bacterial infections, fungal diseases, parasites
Neoplasms: primary hepatic neoplasms, metastases to liver or peritoneum, lymphomas, leukemias, myeloid metaplasia
Lymphatic obstruction: mediastinal tumors, trauma to the thoracic duct, filariasis

Ovarian disease: Meigs' syndrome, struma ovarii
Chronic pancreatitis or pseudocyst: pancreatic ascites
Leakage of bile: bile ascites
Urinary obstruction or trauma: urine ascites
Myxedema
Chylous ascites

ASTHMA, CHILDHOOD

Asthma, childhood
ICD-9CM # 493.0
Use 5th digit 0. Without mention of status asthmaticus
1. With status asthmaticus

TABLE 2-16   Differential Diagnosis of Childhood Asthma

DISEASE	COMMENT
Infections	
Bronchiolitis (RSV)	Atopic individuals may have predisposition to wheeze with RSV
Pneumonia	Acute febrile illness
Croup	Barking cough, stridor, more than wheezing
Tuberculosis, histoplasmosis	Lymphadenopathy compresses bronchi with wheezing
Bronchiectasis	Congenital, acquired, first- or second-degree infections
Bronchiolitis obliterans	Postinfections process (influenza, adenovirus, measles)
Bronchitis	Probably asthma
Sinusitis	Cough usually worse at night; may trigger asthma
Anatomic, Congenital	
Cystic fibrosis	Persistent symptoms, clubbing, *Staphylococcus aureus, Pseudomonas aeruginosa, P. cepacia*
Vascular rings	Associated esophageal abnormalities
Ciliary dyskinesia	Chronic, recurrent infections, situs inversus
B lymphocyte immune defect	Recurrent sinopulmonary infection
Congestive heart failure	Murmur, large left-to-right shunt
Laryngotracheomalacia	Stridor, noisy respirations form birth
Tumor, lymphoma	Bronchial obstruction
H-type tracheoesophageal fistula	Rare, difficult to diagnose, recurrent aspiration pneumonia from birth
Repaired tracheoesophageal fistula	Patients have increased risk of reflux and wheezing, possibly asthma
Gastroesophageal reflux	May also exacerbate true asthma
Vasculitis, Hypersensitivity	
Allergic bronchopulmonary aspergillosis	Marked eosinophilia, high serum IgE levels; sputum positive for aspergillosis
Allergic alveolitis, hypersensitivity pneumonitis	Reaction to foreign antigen (fungi, bird protein, plants); occupational
Churg-Strauss syndrome	Allergic angitis and granulomatosis, eosinophilia
Periarteritis nodosa	Multisystem (kidney, lung, nerves), eosinophilia
Other	
Foreign body aspiration	Sudden cough, gagging, *localized* wheezing and diminished breath sounds
Pulmonary thromboembolism	Acute chest pain, hypoxia
Psychogenic cough	Absent during sleep
Sarcoidosis	Lymphadenopathy-induced bronchial obstruction
Bronchopulmonary dysplasia	History of prematurity, may predispose to asthma
Vocal cord dysfunction	Recurrent, severe shortness of breath and wheezing; flow-volume loop shows inspiratory obstruction; may mimic or complicate asthma; visualization of vocal cords necessary for diagnosis; oxygen saturation and spirometry normal during exacerbations.

From Behrman RE: *Nelson textbook of pediatrics*, ed 16, Philadelphia, 2000, WB Saunders.
IgE, Immunoglobulin E; *RSV*, respiratory syncytial virus.

ATAXIA

BOX 2-37   Ataxia

Vertebral-basilar artery ischemia
Diabetic neuropathy
Tabes dorsalis
Vitamin B_{12} deficiency
Multiple sclerosis and other demyelinating diseases
Meningomyelopathy
Cerebellar neoplasms, hemorrhage, abscess, infarct
Nutritional (Wernicke's encephalopathy)
Paraneoplastic syndromes
Parainfectious: Guillain-Barré syndrome, acute ataxia of
    childhood and young adults
Toxins: phenytoin, alcohol, sedatives, organophosphates

Wilson's disease (hepatolenticular degeneration)
Hypothyroidism
Myopathy
Cerebellar and spinocerebellar degeneration:
    ataxia/telangiectasia, Friedreich's ataxia
Frontal lobe lesions: tumors, thrombosis of anterior cere-
    bral artery, hydrocephalus
Labyrinthine destruction: neoplasm, injury, inflamma-
    tion, compression
Hysteria
Acquired immunodeficiency syndrome

Ataxia
ICD-9CM # **781.3**   **Ataxia NOS**
          303.0   **Alcoholic, acute**
          303.9   **Alcoholic, chronic**
          334.3   **Cerebellar**
          331.89 Cerebral
          334.0   **Friedreich's**
          300.11 Hysterical

ATAXIA, HEREDITARY

Ataxia, hereditary
ICD-9CM # 781.3

TABLE 2-17   Hereditary Ataxias

DISEASE	ONSET	ASSOCIATED SIGNS
Autosomal Recessive Inheritance		
Ataxia-telangiectasia	Childhood	Telangiectasia, recurrent sinus and pulmonary infection, choreoathetosis, mental retardation in 30%, neoplasms (lymphoma, lymphocytic leukemia)
Abetalipoproteinemia (Bassen-Kornzweig syndrome or acanthocytosis)	Childhood	Absent serum apolipoprotein B leads to fat malabsorption with decreased vitamins A, E, and K; retinitis pigmentosa; nystagmus
Friedreich's ataxia	Childhood	Scoliosis, cardiomyopathy, dysarthria, areflexia, Babinski signs, loss of joint position and vibration sense in legs, dysmetria
Autosomal Dominant Inheritance		
Spinocerebellar ataxia types 1-8	Adulthood	Variable combinations of long-tract signs, parkinsonism, dementia
Dentatorubral-palidoluysian atrophy		Sensory loss, myoclonus, chorea
Other forms of olivopontocerebellar atrophy		Dystonia and seizures

From Andreoli TE (ed): *Cecil essentials of medicine,* ed 5, Philadelphia, 2001, WB Saunders.

AXIS DEVIATION

Axis deviation
ICD-9CM # 794.31 EKG abnormal

BOX 2-38   Cause of Axis Deviation

Right

Normal variation
Mechanical shifts: inspiration, emphysema
Right bundle-branch block
Right ventricular hypertrophy
Left posterior hemiblock
Dextrocardia
Left ventricular ectopic rhythms
Some right ventricular ectopic rhythms
Pulmonary hypertension
Pulmonary embolus

Left

Normal variation
Mechanical shifts: expiration, high diaphragm (e.g., pregnancy)
Left anterior hemiblock
Left bundle-branch block
Congenital lesions
Wolff-Parkinson-White syndrome, hyperkalemia, right ventricular ectopic beats

---

Modified from Driscoll CE et al: *Family practice desk reference,* ed 3, St Louis, 1996, Mosby.

II

BACK PAIN

TABLE 2-18   Differential Diagnosis of Common Low Back Pain Syndromes

Back pain
ICD-9CM # 724.5   Back pain (postural)
724.2   Low back pain
307.89   Back pain, psychogenic
724.8   Stiff back
847.9   Back strain
724.6   Backache, sacroiliac

CLINICAL ENTITY	HISTORY	PHYSICAL EXAMINATION	SUPPORTING STUDIES
Mechanical low back pain	Pain in back, buttocks ± thigh; may be severe Onset after new or unusual exertion No history of major trauma, systemic infection or malignancy Relief of pain in supine position	Paravertebral tenderness/spasm Scoliosis or loss of lumbar lordosis common No neurologic signs	None necessary
Herniated intervertebral disk	Acutely, pain in back is severe and lancinating Antecedent flexion strain injury or trauma Sciatica Relief of pain in supine position with hip flexed Bilateral weakness with bowel and/or bladder dysfunction may be present with massive central disk prolapse With chronic disk herniation, pain, usually dull, may be confined to leg	Striking paravertebral tenderness/spasm with splinting in awkward postures Signs of radicular irritation/injury usually present in acute setting	MRI, CT, or myelogram Electromyography may provide supporting documentation of level of denervation
Referred visceral or vascular pain	Patient writhes in discomfort, with no relief in any position Pain may occur in waves	Abdominal findings usually predominate Fever or incipient shock often present	Imaging studies directed at abdomen and retroperitoneum may visualize aortic aneurysm or abnormality of viscera (e.g., ureteral calculus, pancreatitis)
Metastatic malignancy (or multiple myeloma)	Unremitting or progressive pain at rest Known or suspected malignancy Weight loss, fever, or other systemic symptoms History of weakness, bowel and/or bladder dysfunction may be present	Tender spinous process at level of involvement Variable neurologic findings, up to full paraplegia	Standard radiographs may reveal destructive bony lesions Radionuclide bone scan sensitive for metastatic carcinoma but not for myeloma Epidural impingement of spinal cord or roots best delineated by MRI, myelography, and/or CT Erythrocyte sedimentation rate elevated

Epidural abscess, vertebral osteomyelitis, or septic diskitis	Unremitting or progressive pain at rest Fever Drug abuse, diabetes mellitus, immunosuppression Suspected or known systemic infection Previous spinal or genitourinary surgery History of weakness, bowel and/or bladder dysfunction may be present	Tender spinous process at level of involvement Variable neurologic findings, up to full paraplegia Stigmata of systemic infection	Standard radiographs may reveal destructive bony lesions Radionuclide scans may suggest abscess Blood cultures often positive MRI probably best imaging modality to delineate extent of lesion and neural impingement Erythrocyte sedimentation rate elevated
Ankylosing spondylitis	Insidious onset Progressive morning back pain and stiffness over several months Relief with exercise Age at onset ≤40 yr	Painful or ankylosed sacroiliac joints Reduced mobility of spine Reduced chest wall expansion Possible associated uveitis	Sacroiliac joints and lumbosacral spine ankylosed on standard radiographs Erythrocyte sedimentation rate elevated HLA-B27 confirmatory Uveitis may be confirmed on ophthalmologic examination
Reactive spondyloarthropathies	As with ankylosing spondylitis Antecedent urethritis, rash, or colitis	As with ankylosing spondylitis Conjunctivitis, balanitis, urethritis, and/or keratoderma blennorrhagicum Psoriasis	As with ankylosing spondylitis Bowel studies may reveal infectious or idiopathic inflammatory bowel disease Infectious urethritis may be confirmed
Spinal stenosis	Back pain may vary from severe to absent Pseudoclaudication often prominent, often involving L4 root (anterior thigh) Pain worsens during the day, is aggravated by standing and relieved by rest Weakness, bladder and/or bowel dysfunction may be present	Neurologic findings vary, but often there is evidence of impairment at multiple spinal levels Findings of osteoarthritis may be prominent	Standard radiographs generally show extensive vertebral osteophytes and degenerative disk disease Imaging with MRI or CT ± myelography supports diagnosis if neurologic and imaging findings are concordant

From Noble J (ed): *Primary care medicine*, ed 3, St Louis, 2001, Mosby.
CT, Computed tomography; *MRI,* magnetic resonance imaging.

II

BEDSIDE-BALLOON FLOW-DIRECTED (SWAN-GANZ) CATHETER

Bedside balloon flow-directed (Swan-Ganz) catheter differential diagnosis
ICD-9CM # not available

TABLE 2-19 **Differential Diagnosis Using a Bedside Balloon Flow-Directed (Swan-Ganz) Catheter**

DISEASE STATE	THERMODILUTION CARDIAC OUTPUT	PCW PRESSURE	RA PRESSURE	COMMENTS
Cardiogenic shock	↓	↑	nl or ↓	↑ Systemic vascular resistance
Septic shock (early)	↑	↓	↓	↑ Systemic vascular resistance; myocardial dysfunction can occur late
Volume overload	nl or ↑	↑	↑	
Volume depletion	↓	↓	↓	
Noncardiac pulmonary edema	nl	nl	nl	
Pulmonary heart disease	nl or ↓	nl	↑	↑ PA pressure
RV infarction	↓	↓ or nl	↑	
Pericardial tamponade	↓	nl or ↑	↑	Equalization of diastolic RA, RV, PA, and PCW pressure
Papillary muscle rupture	↓	↑	nl or ↑	Large v waves in PCW tracing
Ventricular septal rupture	↑	↑	nl or ↑	Artifact due to RA → PA sampling of thermodilution technique; O_2 saturation higher in PA than RA; may have large v waves in PCW tracing

From Andreoli TE (ed): *Cecil essentials of medicine,* ed 5, Philadelphia, 2001, WB Saunders.
↑, Increased; ↓, decreased; *nl*, normal; *PA*, pulmonary artery; *PCW*, pulmonary capillary wedge; *RA*, right atrium; *RV*, right ventricle.

BELCHING, BLOATING, AND FLATULENCE

Belching, bloating, and flatulence
ICD-9CM # 787.3 Eructation
306.4 Eructation nervous or psychogenic
787.3 Bloating, abdominal
787.3 Flatulence

TABLE 2-20   Differential Diagnosis of Belching, Bloating, and Flatulence

CONDITION	NATURE OF PATIENT	NATURE OF SYMPTOMS	ASSOCIATED SYMPTOMS	PRECIPITATING AND AGGRAVATING FACTORS	AMELIORATING FACTORS	PHYSICAL FINDINGS	DIAGNOSTIC STUDIES
Belching							
Aerophagia	Nursing infants Nervous, anxious, and tense children and adults	Occurs with eating or drinking Conscious or unconscious nervous habit	Abdominal distention	*Infants:* nursing while in horizontal position Mouth breathing Gum chewing Orthodontic appliances Emotional stress Poorly fitting dentures Supine position Gastric or biliary disorders	Behavior modification: avoidance of gum chewing, eating quickly, smoking, and drinking carbonated beverages Upright position	Those of gas in stomach	
Bloating and flatulence							
Excessive intestinal bacterial fermentation causing increased gas	Most common cause at any age, especially in elderly adults	Flatulence Bloating	Abdominal discomfort or pain	Ingestion of nonabsorbable carbohydrates	Avoidance of all carbohydrates, particularly nonabsorbable ones Passage of flatus		
Increased awareness of normal amount of gas							

From Seller RH (ed): *Differential diagnosis of common complaints*, ed 4, Philadelphia, 2000, WB Saunders.
GI, Gastrointestinal; *LUQ,* left upper quadrant; *RUQ,* right upper quadrant.

Continued

TABLE 2-20 Differential Diagnosis of Belching, Bloating, and Flatulence—cont'd

CONDITION	NATURE OF PATIENT	NATURE OF SYMPTOMS	ASSOCIATED SYMPTOMS	PRECIPITATING AND AGGRAVATING FACTORS	AMELIORATING FACTORS	PHYSICAL FINDINGS	DIAGNOSTIC STUDIES
Bloating and flatulence—cont'd							
Malabsorption	Pancreatic insuffiency Pancreatic carcinoma Biliary disease Celiac disease Bacterial overgrowth in small intestine	Increased flatulence	Diarrhea	Nonabsorbable carbohydrates		Greasy, foul-smelling stools	Stool analysis GI radiographs
Lactase deficiency	Common in patients of African or Mediterranean descent and Native Americans	Bloating Excess flatulence	Diarrhea	Lactose load (from dairy products)	Avoidance of lactose Lactase supplement		Mucosal biopsy Lactose load Hydrogen breath test
Giardiasis	Campers and hikers at higher risk	Increased flatulence	Abdominal distention Watery diarrhea, often foul-smelling	Drinking water infested with *Giardia*			Stool analysis for *Giardia* Duodenal aspirate for *Giardia*
Gas entrapment Splenic flexure			Pseudoangina	Abdominal pain worsened by bending or wearing tight garments	Passage of flatus	LUQ pain on palpation Pain worsened by flexion of left leg on abdomen	Fluoroscopy for trapped gas
Hepatic flexure			Pain resembling gallbladder discomfort		Passage of flatus	RUQ pain on palpation Pain worsened by flexion of right leg on abdomen	

From Seller RH (ed): *Differential diagnosis of common complaints*, ed 4, Philadelphia, 2000, WB Saunders.
GI, Gastrointestinal; *LUQ*, left upper quadrant; *RUQ*, right upper quadrant.

BLADDER DYSFUNCTION

Bladder dysfunction
ICD-9CM # 596.9

BOX 2-39   Causes of the Poorly Functioning Bladder

A. Neurologic disorders (neurogenic bladder)
  1. Central diseases
     a. Parkinson's syndrome
     b. Dementia
     c. Multiple sclerosis
     d. Stroke
  2. Peripheral diseases
     a. Cord injury
     b. Spinal dysraphism
  3. Diabetes mellitus
  4. Myasthenia gravis
  5. Guillain-Barré syndrome
B. Pelvic surgery, especially abdominoperineal resection
C. Infectious disorders
  1. Pathogens with neurologic sequelae
     a. Varicella/herpes zoster
     b. Syphilis
     c. Poliomyelitis
  2. Pathogens with obstructive sequelae
     a. *Neisseria gonorrhoeae*
D. Medications
  1. Agents that increase outlet resistance
     a. α-agonists, especially nasal Neo-Synephrine
     b. Tricyclic antidepressants, especially imipramine

  2. Agents that decrease bladder contractility (negative cystotropes)
     a. Anticholinergics
        i. Sedatives, especially diphenhydramine (Benadryl)
        ii. Antispasmodics, especially dicyclomine HCl (Bentyl)
        iii. Tricyclic antidepressants, especially imipramine
     b. Other neurotropic drugs
  3. Calcium channel blockers, especially diltiazem
  4. Beta blockers, especially propranolol
  5. Dietary agents that can increase bladder irritability
     a. Caffeine (substituted xanthines)
     b. Ethanol
     c. Nicotine
     d. Food coloring (F.D. & C. Red #40, amaranth, tartrazine)
     e. Food additives (paprika, oleoresin, capsaicin)

From Nseyo UO (ed): *Urology for primary care physicians,* Philadelphia, 1999, WB Saunders.

BLEEDING DISORDERS

Bleeding disorders
ICD-9CM # 286.9 Bleeding disorder, familial
790.92 Abnormal bleeding time
286.7 Acquired coagulation defect

TABLE 2-21   Presumptive Diagnosis of Common Bleeding Disorders Based on Routine Screening Tests

PLATELET COUNT	BLEEDING TIME	PT	PTT	TT	MISCELLANEOUS	PRESUMPTIVE PROBLEM
↓	N-↑	N	N	N		Thrombocytopenia
N	↑	N	N	N		Platelet function defect or vascular defect
N	↑	N	↑	N	↓ VIII$_e$, ↓ VIII$_{ag}$, ↓ VIII$_{vWF}$	von Willebrand's disease
N	N	↑	N	N		Extrinsic pathway defect (VII)
N	N	N	↑	N		Intrinsic pathway defect (VIII, IX, XI, XII, prekallikrein, high molecular weight kininogen, inhibitor)
N	N	↑	↑	N		Common pathway or multiple pathway defects excluding fibrinogen
N	N	↑	↑	↑	High levels of FDP	Fibrinogen deficiency or dysfunction, vitamin K deficiency, liver disease, primary fibrinolysis
↓	N-↑	↑	↑	↑	High levels of FDP	DIC
N	N	N	N	N	Positive clot solubility	XIII deficiency

From Noble J (ed): *Primary care medicine,* ed 3, St Louis, 2001, Mosby.
↓, Decreased; ↑, increased; *DIC,* disseminated intravascular coagulation; *FDP,* fibrin(ogen) degradation products; *N,* normal.

BLEEDING, GASTROINTESTINAL: BY LOCATION

Bleeding, gastrointestinal: location
ICD-9CM # 578.9 GI bleeding, cause unspecified

BOX 2-40   Gastrointestinal Bleeding, by Location

Upper GI Bleeding (Originating Above the Ligament of Treitz)

Oral or pharyngeal lesions: swallowed blood from nose or oropharynx
Swallowed hemoptysis
Esophageal: varices, ulceration, esophagitis, Mallory-Weiss tear, carcinoma, trauma
Gastric: peptic ulcer (including Cushing and Curling's ulcers), gastritis, angiodysplasia, gastric neoplasms, hiatal hernia, gastric diverticulum, pseudoxanthoma elasticum, Rendu-Osler-Weber syndrome
Duodenal: peptic ulcer, duodenitis, angiodysplasia, aortoduodenal fistula, duodenal diverticulum, duodenal tumors, carcinoma of ampulla of Vater, parasites (e.g., hookworm), Crohn's disease
Biliary: hematobilia (e.g., penetrating injury to liver, hepatobiliary malignancy, endoscopic papillotomy)

Lower GI Bleeding (Originating Below the Ligament of Treitz)
Small Intestine

Ischemic bowel disease (mesenteric thrombosis, embolism, vasculitis, trauma)
Small bowel neoplasm: leiomyomas, carcinoids
Hereditary hemorrhagic telangiectasia (Rendu-Osler-Weber syndrome)
Meckel's diverticulum and other small intestine diverticula
Aortoenteric fistula
Intestinal hemangiomas: blue rubber-bleb nevi, intestinal hemangiomas, cutaneous vascular nevi
Hamartomatous polyps: Peutz-Jeghers syndrome (intestinal polyps, mucocutaneous pigmentation)
Infections of small bowel: tuberculous enteritis, enteritis necroticans
Volvulus
Intussusception
Lymphoma of small bowel, sarcoma, Kaposi's sarcoma
Irradiation ileitis

AV malformation of small intestine
Inflammatory bowel disease
Polyarteritis nodosa
Other: pancreatoenteric fistulas, Schönlein-Henoch purpura, Ehler-Danlos syndrome, systemic lupus erythematosus, amyloidosis, metastatic melanoma

Colon

Carcinoma (particularly left colon)
Diverticular disease
Inflammatory bowel disease
Ischemic colitis
Colonic polyps
Vascular abnormalities: angiodysplasia, vascular ectasia
Radiation colitis
Infectious colitis
Uremic colitis
Aortoenteric fistula
Lymphoma of large bowel
Hemorrhoids
Anal fissure
Trauma, foreign body
Solitary rectal/cecal ulcers
Long-distance running

BLEEDING, GASTROINTESTINAL: DIAGNOSTIC CONSIDERATIONS BY AGE

TABLE 2-22   **Gastrointestinal Hemorrhage: Diagnostic Consideration by Age**

INFANT (<3 MO)	TODDLER (<2 YR)	PRESCHOOLER (<5 YR)	SCHOOL-AGE CHILD (≥5 YR)
Upper Gastrointestinal Bleeding			
Swallowed maternal blood	Esophagitis	Esophagitis	Esophagitis
Gastritis	Gastritis	Gastritis	Gastritis
Ulcer, stress	Ulcer	Ulcer	Ulcer
Bleeding diathesis	Pyloric stenosis	Esophageal varices	Esophageal varices
Foreign body (NG tube)	Mallory-Weiss syndrome	Foreign body	Mallory-Weiss syndrome
Vascular malformation	Vascular malformation	Mallory-Weiss syndrome	Inflammatory bowel disease*
Duplication	Duplication	Hemophilia	Hemophilia
		Vascular malformation	Vascular malformation
Lower Gastrointestinal Bleeding			
Swallowed maternal blood	Anal fissure	Infectious colitis*	Infectious colitis*
Infectious colitis*	Infectious colitis*	Anal fissure	Inflammatory bowel disease*
Milk allergy	Milk allergy	Polyp	Pseudomembranous enterocolitis*
Bleeding diathesis*	Colitis	Intussusception*	Polyp
Intussusception*	Intussusception*	Meckel's diverticulum	Hemolytic-uremic syndrome
Midgut volvulus*	Meckel's diverticulum	Henoch-Schönlein purpura*	Hemorrhoid
Meckel's diverticulum	Polyp	Hemolytic uremic syndrome*	
Necrotizing enterocolitis (NEC)*	Duplication	Inflammatory bowel disease*	
	Hemolytic uremic syndrome*	Pseudomembranous enterocolitis*	
	Inflammatory bowel disease*		
	Pseudomembranous enterocolitis*		

From Barkin RM, Rosen P: *Emergency pediatrics: a guide to ambulatory care,* ed 5, St Louis, 1998, Mosby.
*Commonly associated with systemic illness involving multiple organ systems either primarily or secondarily.

Bleeding, gastrointestinal: diagnostic considerations by age
ICD-9CM # 578.9 GI bleeding, cause unspecified

BLEEDING, GENITAL TRACT

Bleeding, genital tract
ICD-9CM # 626.9 Menstrual disorder
626.7 Postcoital
623.8 Vaginal NOS
626.8 Uterine dysfunctional
627.1 Postmenopausal
626.2 Uterine unrelated to menstrual cycle

BOX 2-41   Abnormal Female Genital Tract Bleeding

Premenarcheal

1. Trauma
2. Genital tract neoplasm
   a. Cervical
   b. Vaginal
   c. Uterine
3. Foreign body
4. Exogenous estrogen
5. Sporadic gonadotropin surge
6. Precocious puberty
7. Pseudopuberty
8. Neoplasm, hormone secreting
   a. Estrogen–granulosa cell tumor
   b. Human chorionic gonadotropin (HCG)-embryonal carcinoma
   c. Choriocarcinoma
9. Adrenal tumors
10. Craniopharyngioma
11. Albright's syndrome
12. von Recklinghausen's disease
13. Adrenal hyperplasia
14. Hypothyroidism
15. Idiopathic, gastrointestinal bleeding
16. Urinary tract bleeding

Reproductive Age

1. Menorrhagia
2. Hypermenorrhea
3. Metrorrhagia
4. Oligomenorrhea
5. Polymenorrhea
6. Hypomenorrhea

Pregnancy

1. Intrauterine pregnancy with bleeding
   a. Placenta previa
   b. Vasa previa
   c. Abruptio placentae
   d. Spontaneous abortion
2. Ectopic pregnancy

Neoplasia

1. Genital tract
   a. Cervical
   b. Endometrial
   c. Gestational trophoblastic disease (GTD)
   d. Ovary: hormone producing
   e. Vaginal
   f. Vulvar
   g. Fallopian tube
2. Metastatic or contiguous involvement
3. Other
   a. Central nervous system (CNS)
   b. Adrenal
   c. Thyroid

Polyp

1. Cervical, endometrial
2. Leiomyoma: submucosal
3. Adenomyosis
4. Ectropion

Infection

Cervicitis: *Chlamydia trachomatis*

Endocrine Dysfunction

1. Hypothalamic or pituitary
2. Polycystic ovaries (PCO)
3. Adrenal
4. Hypothyroidism or hyperthyroidism

Blood Dyscrasias

1. von Willebrand's
2. Thrombocytopenia
3. Disseminated intravascular coagulation (DIC)
4. Chronic anticoagulation
   a. Heparin
   b. Coumadin

From Danakas G (ed): *Practical guide to the care of the gynecologic/obstetric patient,* St Louis, 1997, Mosby.

BOX 2-41　Abnormal Genital Tract Bleeding—cont'd

Dysfunctional Uterine Bleeding

1. Ovulatory
   a. Midcycle: inadequate proliferative estrogen
   b. Late cycle: inadequate progesterone production
2. Altered prostaglandin metabolism: increased PGI
3. Anovulatory
   a. Disturbance
      (1) Hypothalamic
      (2) Pituitary
      (3) Ovarian axis
   b. Emotional stress
   c. Anorexia
   d. Strenuous exercise
   e. Weight gain

Postmenopausal Bleeding

1. Neoplasm
   a. Endometrial hyperplasia
   b. Endometrial cancer
   c. Other tumors of uterus
2. Other pelvic neoplasm
   a. Direct extension or metastatic
      (1) Vulva
      (2) Vagina
      (3) Cervix
      (4) Fallopian tube
      (5) Ovary
   b. Endometrial or cervical polyp
   c. Unopposed estrogen
      (1) Exogenous
      (2) Endogenous
         (a) Peripheral conversion
         (b) Tumor production
            i. Granulosa cell tumor
            ii. Thecoma
3. Trauma: vaginal
4. Infection
   a. Vaginitis
   b. Endometritis
   c. Vulvar dystrophy
   d. Vaginal atrophy
   e. Idiopathic
   f. Urinary tract bleeding
      (1) Urinary tract infection (UTI)
      (2) Cystitis
      (3) Bladder tumor
   g. Gastrointestinal (GI) tract bleeding

Iatrogenic

1. Intrauterine device (IUD)
2. Drug use
   a. Estrogens
   b. Progestins
   c. Androgens
3. Nonhormonal drugs
   a. Phenothiazines
   b. Tricyclic antidepressants
   c. Reserpine
   d. Alpha-methyldopa

II

BLINDNESS, PEDIATRIC AGE

BOX 2-42   Etiologies of Childhood Amaurosis (Blindness)

Congenital

Optic nerve hypoplasia or aplasia
Optic coloboma
Congenital hydrocephalus
Hydranencephaly
Porencephaly
Micrencephaly
Encephalocele, particularly occipital type
Morning glory disc
Aniridia
Anterior microphthalmia
Peter's anomaly
Persistent pupillary membrane
Glaucoma
Cataracts
Persistent hyperplastic primary vitreous

Phakomatoses

Tuberous sclerosis
Neurofibromatosis (special association with optic glioma)
Sturge-Weber syndrome
von Hippel–Lindau disease

Tumors

Retinoblastoma
Optic glioma
Perioptic meningioma
Craniopharyngioma
Cerebral glioma
Posterior and intraventricular tumors when complicated by hydrocephalus
Pseudotumor cerebri

Neurodegenerative Diseases

Cerebral storage disease
Gangliosidoses, particularly Tay-Sachs disease (infantile amaurotic familial idiocy), Sandhoff's variant, generalized gangliosidosis
Other lipidoses and ceroid lipofuscinoses, particularly the late-onset amaurotic familial idiocies such as those of Jansky-Bielschowsky and of Batten-Mayou-Spielmeyer-Vogt
Mucopolysaccharidoses, particularly Hurler's syndrome and Hunter's syndrome
Leukodystrophies (dysmyelination disorders), particularly metachromatic leukodystrophy and Canavan's disease

Demyelinating sclerosis (myelinoclastic diseases), especially Schilder's disease and Devic's neuromyelitis optica
Special types: Dawson's disease, Leigh's disease, Bassen-Kornzweig syndrome, Refsum's disease
Retinal degenerations: retinitis pigmentosa and its variants, and Leber's congenital type
Optic atrophies: congenital autosomal recessive type, infantile and congenital autosomal dominant types, Leber's disease, and atrophies associated with hereditary ataxias—the types of Behr, of Marie, and of Sanger-Brown

Infectious Processes

Encephalitis, especially in the prenatal infection syndromes caused by *Toxoplasma gondii*, cytomegalovirus, rubella virus, *Treponema pallidum*, herpes simplex
Meningitis; arachnoiditis
Chorioretinitis
Endophthalmitis
Keratitis

Hematologic Disorders

Leukemia with central nervous system involvement

Vascular and Circulatory Disorders

Collagen vascular diseases
Arteriovenous malformations—intracerebral hemorrhage, subarachnoid hemorrhage
Central retinal occlusion

Trauma

Contusion or avulsion of optic nerves, chiasm, globe, cornea
Cerebral contusion or laceration
Intracerebral, subarachnoid, or subdural hemorrhage

Drugs and Toxins
Other

Retinopathy of prematurity
Sclerocornea
Conversion reaction
Optic neuritis
Osteopetrosis

Modified from Kliegman R: *Practical strategies in pediatric diagnosis and therapy*, Philadelphia, 1996, WB Saunders.

BLISTERS, SUBEPIDERMAL

Blisters, subepidermal
ICD-9CM # 919.2

TABLE 2-23 Differential Diagnosis of Subepidermal Blisters

INFLAMMATION	INTACT BLISTER ROOF	DYSKERATOSIS/NECROSIS PRESENT
None/sparse	Porphyria cutanea tarda	Toxic epidermal necrolysis
	Pseudoporphyria	Acute radiodermatitis
	Variegate porphyria	Burn
	Epidermolysis bullosa—junctional or dystrophic or acquired variants	Pressure necrosis (coma or surgery)
	Bullous pemphigoid	
	Amyloidosis	
Predominantly lymphocytes	Lichen sclerosus et atrophicus	Erythema multiforme
	Polymorphous light eruption	Fixed drug eruption
	Lupus erythematosus	Acute-graft-versus host reaction
Predominantly neutrophils	Dermatitis herpetiformis	Septic emboli
	Lupus erythematosus	Leukocytoclastic vasculitis
	Linear IgA disease of adults or children (Chronic bullous dermatosis of childhood) or drug-induced	
	Epidermolysis bullosa acquisita	
Predominantly eosinophils	Bullous pemphigoid	Arthropod bite reaction
	Herpes gestationis	
	Bullous drug reaction	
Predominantly mast cells	Urticaria pigmentosa	

From Callen JP (ed): *Color atlas of dermatology,* ed 2, Philadelphia, 2000, WB Saunders.
IgA, Immunoglobulin A.

BONE LESIONS, PREFERENTIAL SITE OF ORIGIN

Bone lesions, preferential site of origin
ICD-9CM # 170.0 Skull and face
170.1 Mandible
170.2 Vertebral column
170.3 Ribs, sternum, clavicle
170.4 Scapula, long bones upper limb
170.5 Short bones upper limb
170.6 Pelvic bones, sacrum, coccyx
170.7 Long bones lower limb
170.8 Short bones lower limb
170.9 Bone cancer NOS
198.5 Bone cancer, metastatic

BOX 2-43 Preferential Site of Origin of Various Bone Lesions

Epiphysis

Chondroblastoma
Giant-cell tumor—after fusion of growth plate
Langerhans' cell histiocytosis
Clear cell chondrosarcoma

Metaphysis

Osteosarcoma
Parosteal sarcoma
Chondrosarcoma
Fibrosarcoma
Nonossifying fibroma
Giant-cell tumor—before fusion of growth plate
Unicameral bone cyst
Aneurysmal bone cyst

Diaphysis

Myeloma
Ewing's tumor
Reticulum cell sarcoma

Metadiaphyseal

Fibrosarcoma
Fibrous dysplasia
Enchondroma
Osteoid osteoma
Chondromyofibroma

From Specht N (ed): *Practical guide to diagnostic imaging,* St Louis, 1998, Mosby.

BONE MARROW FAILURE SYNDROMES, INHERITED

TABLE 2-24   Inherited Bone Marrow Failure Syndromes

FEATURE	FANCONI ANEMIA	DYSKERATOSIS CONGENITA	SHWACHMAN-DIAMOND SYNDROME	AMEGAKARYOCYTIC THROMBOCYTOPENIA
Cases reported	1000	225	200	45
Male/female	1.3	4.3	1.7	1.6
Genetics	Autosomal recessive	X linked; autosomal recessive, dominant	Autosomal recessive	X linked, or autosomal recessive
Physical abnormalities (%)	80	100	40	60
Hand/arm anomalies (%)	48	15	<2	0
Median age (yr) at diagnosis of initial hematologic disease	7.5	16	4 mo	<1 wk
First hematologic manifestation	Pancytopenia	Pancytopenia	Neutropenia	Thrombocytopenia
Bone marrow	Aplastic	Aplastic	Hypocellular or myeloid arrest	Absent or small megakaryocytes
Aplastic anemia (%)	>95	50		
Leukemia (%)	12	0.4	20	45
Liver disease (%)	4	0	5	5
Cancer	5	10	0	0
Hb F	Increased	Increased	0	0
Chromosomes	Breaks increased with clastogens	Bleomycin sensitive	Increased	Increased
Spontaneous remissions	Very rare	None	Normal	Normal
Treatment, responses	BMT, androgens, 50%, transient	Androgens, 50%, transient	Rare G-CSF, BMT, 80%	BMT None
Prognosis	Poor	Poor	Fair	Poor
Prenatal diagnosis	Chromosome breaks, FAC	Xq28 RFLP	Neutropenia	Thrombocytopenia
Predicted median survival age (yr)	30	33	35	3

Modified from Alter BP, Young NS: The bone marrow failure syndromes. In Nathan DG, Orkin FA (eds): *Nathan and Oski's hematology of infancy and children,* ed 5, Philadelphia, 1998, WB Saunders.
BMT, Bone marrow transplantation; *G-CSF,* granulocyte colony-stimulating factor; *RFLP,* restriction fragment length polymorphism.

Bone marrow failure syndromes, inherited
ICD-9CM # 289.9

BONE METASTASES

TABLE 2-25   **Clinical, Radiologic, and Biochemical Features of Common Skeletal Disorders That May Mimic Bone Metastases**

DIAGNOSIS	CLINICAL FEATURES	RADIOLOGIC	BIOCHEMICAL
Bone metastases	Pain common Usually multiple sites Axial skeletal involvement typical	Bone scan very rarely completely normal Discrete lytic or sclerotic lesions on radiographs Fracture/vertebral pedicle destruction common Soft tissue extension on CT/MRI	Alkaline phosphatase usually elevated Increased urinary markers of bone resorption Hypercalcemia common
Degenerative disease	Elderly Limb involvement common Pain and stiffness Long history	Spinal involvement results in symmetric increased tracer uptake on scan Radiographs usually confirmatory	Usually normal
Osteoporosis	Elderly female Painless unless fracture or vertebral collapse	Normal scan unless recent fracture or vertebral collapse Diffuse osteopenia on radiographs Normal marrow on MRI	Usually normal serum parameters Slight elevation of urinary indices of bone resorption
Paget's disease of bone	Elderly Bony deformity common Involved site warm because of increased blood flow Skull often involved and enlarged	Diffuse involvement of bone on scan Sclerotic expanded appearance on radiographs Intense linear uptake on scan Rib lesions typically aligned, not randomly distributed	No hypercalcemia Alkaline phosphatase greatly elevated Increase in urinary hydroxyproline excretion Hypercalcemia very rare
Traumatic fractures	History of trauma usual Spontaneous rib fractures after chest wall irradiation common	No evidence of destruction of destruction around fracture site on radiographs (unless radiation induced)	Usually normal

From Abeloff MD: *Clinical oncology,* ed 2, New York, 2000, Churchill Livingstone.
CT, Computed tomography; *MRI,* magnetic resonance imaging.

**Bone metastases
ICD-9CM # 198.5**

BONE PAIN

Bone pain
ICD-9CM # not available

> ### BOX 2-44   Causes of Bone Pain
>
> **Focal pain**
>
> - Fracture or trauma
> - Infection
> - Malignancy
> - Paget's disease
> - Osteoid osteoma
>
> **Diffuse pain**
>
> - Malignancy
> - Paget's disease
> - Osteomalacia
> - Osteoporosis
> - Metabolic bone disease

From Epstein O (ed): *Clinical examination*, ed 2, London, 1997, Mosby.

BONE RESORPTION

Bone resorption
ICD-9CM # 733.90 Bone disorder

> ### BOX 2-45   Causes of Bone Resorption at Various Sites
>
> **Distal Clavicle**
>
> Hyperparathyroidism
> Rheumatoid arthritis
> Scleroderma
> Posttraumatic osteolysis
> Progeria
> Pycnodysostosis
> Cleidocranial dysplasia
>
> **Inferior Aspect of Ribs**
>
> Vascular impression, associated with but not limited
>   to coarctation of the aorta
> Hyperparathyroidism
> Neurofibromatosis
>
> **Terminal Phalangeal Tufts**
>
> Scleroderma
> Raynaud's phenomenon
> Vascular disease
> Frostbite, electrical burns
> Psoriasis
> Tabes dorsalis
> Hyperparathyroidism
>
> **Generalized Resorption**
>
> Paraplegia
> Myositis ossificans
> Osteoporosis

From Specht N (ed): *Practical guide to diagnostic imaging*, St Louis, 1998, Mosby.

BONE TUMORS AND CYSTS, BENIGN

TABLE 2-26 Benign Bone Tumors and Cysts

DISEASE	CHARACTERISTICS	ROENTGENOGRAPHY	TREATMENT	PROGNOSIS
Osteochondroma (osteocartilaginous exostosis)	Common: distal metaphysis of femur, proximal humerus, proximal tibia: painless, hard, nontender mass	Bony outgrowth, sessile or pedunculated	Excision, if symptomatic	Excellent; malignant transformation rare
Multiple hereditary exostoses	Osteochondroma of long bones; bone growth disturbances	As above	As above	Recurrences
Osteoid ostoma	Point tenderness: pain relieved by aspirin; femur and tibia; predominantly found in boys	Osteosclerosis surrounds small radiolucent nidus, 1 cm	As above	Excellent
Giant osteoid osteoma (osteoblastoma)	As above, but more destructive	Oseolytic component; size greater than 1 cm	As above	Excellent
Enchondroma	Tubular bones of hands and feet: pathologic fractures, swollen bone; Ollier disease if multiple lesions are present	Radiolucent diaphyseal or metaphyseal lesion; may calcify	Excision or curettage	Excellent; malignant transformation rare
Nonossifying fibroma	Silent; rare pathologic fracture; late childhood adolescence	Incidental roentgenographic fiding; thin sclerotic border, radiolucent lesion	None or curettage with fractures	Excellent; heals spontaneously
Eosinophilic granuloma	Age 5–10 yr: skull, jaw, long bones; pathologic fracture; pain	Small, radiolucent without reactive bone; punched-out lytic lesion	Biopsy, excision rare; irradiation	Excellent; may heal spontaneously
Brodie abscess	Insidious local pain; limp; suspected as malignancy	Circumscribed metaphyseal osteomyelitis; lytic lesions with sclerotic rim	Biopsy; antibiotics	Excellent
Unicameral bone cyst (simple bone cyst)	Metaphysis of long bone (femur, humerus): pain, pathologic fracture	Cyst in medullary canal, expands cortex; fluid-filled unilocular or multilocular cavity	Curettage; steroid injection into lesion	Excellent, some heal spontaneously
Aneurysmal bone cyst	As above; contains blood, fibrous tissue	Expands beyond metaphyseal cartilage	Curettage, bone graft	Excellent

From Behrman R, Kliegman R (eds): *Nelson essentials of pediatrics,* ed 2, Philadelphia, 1994, WB Saunders.

Bone tumors and cysts, benign
ICD-9CM # 733.20 Bone cyst, unspecified (localized)
733.21 Bone cyst solitary
733.22 Bone cyst aneurysmal
213.0 Bone neoplasm, benign, skull, face, upper jaw
213.1 Bone neoplasm, benign, lower jaw
213.2 Bone neoplasm, benign, spine
213.3 Bone neoplasm, benign, rib, sternum, clavicle
213.4 Bone neoplasm, benign, upper limb, long bones, scapula
213.5 Bone neoplasm, benign, upper limb, short bones
213.6 Bone neoplasm, benign, pelvis, sacrum, coccyx
213.7 Bone neoplasm, lower limb long bone
213.8 Bone neoplasm, lower limb short bone

BRAIN DISEASE, FOCAL

TABLE 2-27   Frontal Lobe Syndromes

SYMPTOMS	SITE OF LESION
Contralateral spastic weakness	Primary motor/premotor cortex
Broca's aphasia	Dominant inferior frontal lobe
Forced eye deviation	Frontal eye fields
Executive dysfunction/poor sequencing	Dorsolateral prefrontal lobe
Akinetic mutism/urinary incontinence	Medial frontal cortex
Disinhibition/emotional lability	Orbiofrontal cortex

From Andreoli TE (ed): *Cecil essentials of medicine,* ed 5, Philadelphia, 2001, WB Saunders.

TABLE 2-28   Parietal Lobe Syndromes

SYMPTOMS	SITE OF LESION
Contralateral sensory loss	Postcentral gyrus
Contralateral sensory neglect	Postcentral gyrus (non-dominant)
Wernicke's aphasia, apraxia	Inferior parietal/superior temporal cortex
Acalculia, finger agnosia, right-left confusion, agraphia (Gerstmann's syndrome)	Angular gyrus

From Andreoli TE (ed): *Cecil essentials of medicine,* ed 5, Philadelphia, 2001, WB Saunders.

TABLE 2-29   Syndromes of Temporal Lobe Lesions

SYMPTOMS	LESION SITE
Anomic/sensory aphasia	Lateral temporal lobe (dominant)
Contralateral superior quadratic anopsia	Superior lateral temporal lobe
Amnesia	Hippocampus
Oral-exploratory behavior, passivity, hypersexuality (Klüver-Bucy syndrome)	Amygdala (bilateral)
Visual delusions (déjà vu, jamais vu), olfactory hallucinations	Inferomedial temporal lobe

From Andreoli TE (ed): *Cecil essentials of medicine,* ed 5, Philadelphia, 2001, WB Saunders.

TABLE 2-30   Occipital Lobe Syndrome

SYMPTOMS	LESION SITE
Contralateral homonymous hemianopia	Striate cortex
Alexia without agraphia	Primary visual cortex (dominant) and splenium of corpus callosum
Visual agnosia, denial of blindness (Anton's syndrome), visual hallucinations	Medial occipital lobe
Optic apraxia, absent optokinetic nystagmus	Lateral (visual association) cortex

From Andreoli TE (ed): *Cecil essentials of medicine,* ed 5, Philadelphia, 2001, WB Saunders.

BREAST INFLAMMATORY LESION

Breast inflammatory lesion
ICD-9CM # 611.0 Acute mastitis
                610.1 Chronic cystic mastitis
                771.5 Neonatal infective mastitis
                778.7 Neonatal noninfective mastitis

BOX 2-46   Breast Inflammatory Lesion

1. Acute mastitis
   a. Infectious agent
      (1) *Staphylococcus aureus*
      (2) Streptococci
      (3) Foreign body
   b. Trauma
2. Chronic mastitis
3. Granuloma
   a. Tuberculosis
   b. Actinomycosis
   c. Blastomycosis
   d. Cryptococcosis
4. Foreign body mastitis
   a. Suture
   b. Silicone mammoplasty
5. Plasma cell mastitis
   a. Duct ectasia
6. Fat necrosis
   a. Postbiopsy
   b. Trauma
   c. Injection
   d. Mammoplasty
7. Necrosis or infarction
   a. Anticoagulant therapy
   b. Pregnancy
   c. Lactation
   d. Atherosclerosis in elderly
8. Breast malignancy

From Danakas G (ed): *Practical guide to the care of the gynecologic/ obstetric patient,* St Louis, 1997, Mosby.

II

BREAST LUMP

TABLE 2-31   Differential Diagnosis of Breast Lumps

Breast lump
ICD-9CM # 611.72 Breast mass or lump

CONDITION	NATURE OF PATIENT	NATURE OF SYMPTOMS	ASSOCIATED SYMPTOMS	PRECIPITATING AND AGGRAVATING FACTORS	AMELIORATING FACTORS	PHYSICAL FINDINGS	DIAGNOSTIC STUDIES
Fibroadenoma	Usually age 20-40 Rare in post-menopausal women unless taking estrogen	Usually asymptomatic	May enlarge, especially during adolescence and pregnancy			Usually solitary Multiple or bilateral in 15%-25% Firm, mobile, smooth, rubbery	Mammography Biopsy
Fibrocystic breasts	Frequency increases with age, peaks around menopause, then resolves	Cyclic breast pain, especially around menstruation Usually bilateral	Rare nipple discharge, usually not bloody	Pain and tenderness worsen premenstrually	Menopause Reduction in ingestion of methylxanthines in tea, coffee, cola, and chocolate Oral contraceptives	Multiple tender breast lumps Usually bilateral and in upper outer quadrants Occasionally single or unilateral	Mammography Ultrasonograpy
Cancer	Usually over age 40 1 in 10 women	Usually none until late in disease	Occasional pain in one breast in postmenopausal patient Bloody nipple discharge Axillary adenopathy	Increased incidence if mother and/or sister had breast cancer Early menarche Late menopause Over age 50 Nulliparous	Decreased incidence in users of oral contraceptives	Hard, irregular, fixed lump	Mammography Biopsy Fine-needle aspiration
Fat necrosis	Older women More common in large pendulous breasts	Painful, tender to palpation		Trauma; surgical trauma		Firm, solitary, irregular lump May be attached to skin	
Gynecomastia	Males, especially pubertal and elderly Alcoholics	Breast enlargement Unilateral or bilateral, often tender	Adrenogenital syndrome	Drugs: oral and topical estrogens, marijuana, spironolactone, methyldopa, phenytoin, cimetidine, digitalis, finasteride		Under nipple	

From Seller RH (ed): *Differential diagnosis of common complaints*, ed 4, Philadelphia, 2000, WB Saunders.

BREATH ODOR

Breath odor
ICD-9CM # 784.9 Halitosis

BOX 2-47   Breath Odor

Auscultation of the lungs makes it possible (occasionally uncomfortably so) to become aware of a patient's breath odor. Smelling the breath may provide a significant clue:

Sweet, fruity	Diabetic ketoacidosis; starvation ketosis
Fishy, stale	Uremia (trimethylamines)
Ammonia-like	Uremia (ammonia)
Musty fish, clover	Fetor hepaticus: hepatic failure, portal vein thrombosis, portacaval shunts
Foul, feculent	Intestinal obstruction/diverticulum
Foul, putrid	Nasal/sinus pathology: infection, foreign body, cancer; respiratory infections: empyema, lung abscess, bronchiectasis
Halitosis	Tonsillitis, gingivitis, respiratory infections, Vincent's angina, gastroesophageal reflux
Cinnamon	Pulmonary tuberculosis

Modified from Seidel HM (ed): *Mosby's guide to physical examination,* ed 4, St Louis, 1999, Mosby.

BREATHING, NOISY

Breathing, noisy
ICD-9CM # 786.09 Breathing labored, snoring, wheezing
786.1   Stridor

BOX 2-48   Some Causes of "Noisy Breathing" (Stridor, Wheezing, Snoring, Gurgling)

Infection

Upper respiratory infection
Peritonsillar abscess
Retropharyngeal abscess
Epiglottitis
Laryngitis
Tracheitis
Bronchitis
Bronchiolitis

Irritants and Allergens

Hyperactive airway
Asthma (reactive airway disease)
Rhinitis
Angioneurotic edema

Compression (from the Outside of the Airway)

Esophageal cysts or foreign body
A variety of tumors
Lymphadenopathy

Congenital Malformation and Abnormality

Vascular rings
Laryngeal webs
Laryngomalacia
Tracheomalacia
Hemangiomas within the upper airway

Stenoses within the upper airway
Cystic fibrosis

Acquired Abnormality (at Every Level of the Airway)

Nasal polyps
Hypertrophied adenoids and/or tonsils
Foreign body
Intraluminal tumors
Bronchiectasis

Neurogenic Disorder

Vocal cord paralysis

The exact nature and location of the stimulus to noisy breathing will determine the type of noise. Snoring and gurgling tend to arise in the nasopharynx, stridor in the area of the glottis, and wheezing much lower in the respiratory tree.

From Seidel HM (ed): *Mosby's guide to physical examination,* ed 4, St Louis, 1999, Mosby.

Bullous diseases
ICD-9CM # 694.9 Bullous dermatoses
694.5 Bullous pemphigoid
694.4 Pemphigus vulgaris
694.4 Pemphigus foliaceus

BULLOUS DISEASES

TABLE 2-32   Differential Diagnosis of Selected Bullous Diseases

DISEASE	HISTORY	PHYSICAL	LABORATORY	MANAGEMENT
Bullous Pemphigoid (BP)				
BP	Elderly population; intense pruritus; tense bullae; hives common	Widespread bullae; urticarial lesions; distribution not diagnostic	Skin biopsy; DIF linear IgG along basement membrane	Systemic oral corticosteroids; occasionally azathioprine or cyclophosphamide
Cicatricial pemphigoid	Elderly; mucous membranes and conjunctivae	Erosive blisters on mucous membranes and conjunctivae; skin lesions in 20%	Skin biopsy; DIF	Corticosteroids; tetracyclines
Herpes gestationis	Pregnancy; intense pruritus; hives and blisters	Urticaria; vesicles and bullae	Skin biopsy; DIF	Resolves after delivery; may require systemic corticosteroids
Epidermolysis bullosa acquisita (EBA)	Adult onset; skin fragility and blisters, extensor areas; pruritus	Bullae and vesicles; erosions; healed areas with scars and milia	Skin biopsy, DIF similar to BP; differentiation requires split skin DIF	Corticosteroids; immunosuppressive agents; difficult to treat
Dermatitis herpetiformis (DH)	Intense pruritus; extensor areas; GI symptoms occasionally	Grouped (herpetiform) vesicles; elbows, knees, back, buttocks	Skin biopsy; DIF; GI if diarrhea	Dapsone; gluten-free diet
Linear IgA bullous dermatosis	Pruritus; any age; vesicles and bullae	May be similar to DH or BP	Skin biopsy; DIF	Corticosteroids; immunosuppressive agents
Pemphigus Vulgaris				
Pemphigus vulgaris	Widespread erosions: oral lesions	Oral and cutaneous bullae and erosions	Skin biopsy; DIF; indirect IF agents; gold	Systemic corticosteroids: immunosuppressive
BP	Elderly; intense pruritus; blisters	Bullae widespread; urticaria common	Skin biopsy; DIF	Corticosteroids
Cicatricial pemphigoid	Elderly; mucous membranes and conjunctivae	Bullae, erosions, and scarring on mucous membranes and conjunctivae	Skin biopsy; DIF	Systemic corticosteroids: tetracyclines
Erythema multiforme (oral)	Oral mucosal lesions; painful	Oral erosions; may have target lesions on skin	Skin biopsy occasionally helpful; DIF to exclude pemphigus	Supportive; eliminate or treat underlying cause
Erosive lichen planus	Oral mucosal and tongue lesions	Erosions; white lacy mucosal changes	Skin biopsy helpful; DIF to exclude pemphigus	Topical and systemic steroids; retinoids; cyclosporin
Pemphigus Foliaceus				
Pemphigus foliaceus	Widespread crusted erosions; adult onset	Crusted plaques	Skin biopsy; DIF	Systemic corticosteroids
Impetigo	Crusted lesions; face; children	Crusted plaques; honey crusts; serous oozing	Culture	Antibiotics
Paraneoplastic Pemphigus				
Paraneoplastic pemphigus	Erosions; mucous membranes; associated malignancy	Oral and cutaneous erosions	Skin biopsy; DIF	Treat malignancy; systemic corticosteroids; immunosuppressive agents
Erythema multiforme (major Stevens-Johnson syndrome)	Mouth, conjunctivae, ears, and widespread; drug, viral infection	Erosions on mucous membranes; target lesions on skin	Skin biopsy	Supportive; treat or eliminate underlying cause

Modified from Noble J (ed): *Primary care medicine*, ed 3, St Louis, 2001, Mosby.
DIF, Direct immunofluorescence.

BURSITIS SYNDROMES

Bursitis syndromes
ICD-9CM # 727.3

TABLE 2-33 **Bursitis Syndromes**

LOCATION	SYMPTOM	FINDING
Subacromial	Shoulder pain	Tender subacromial space
Olecranon	Elbow pain	Tender olecranon swelling
Iliopectineal	Groin pain	Tender inguinal region
Trochanteric	Lateral hip pain	Tender at greater trochanter
Prepatellar	Anterior knee pain	Tender swelling over patella
Infrapatellar	Anterior knee pain	Tender swelling lateral or medial to patellar tendon
Anserine	Medial knee pain	Tender medioproximal tibia (below joint line of knee)
Ischiogluteal	Buttock pain	Tender ischial spine (at gluteal fold)
Retrocalcaneal	Heel pain	Tender swelling between Achilles tendon insertion and calcaneus
Calcaneal	Heel pain	Tender central heel pad

From Andreoli TE (ed): *Cecil essentials of medicine,* ed 5, Philadelphia, 2001, WB Saunders.

II

CARDIAC ARREST, NONTRAUMATIC

Cardiac arrest, nontraumatic
ICD-9CM # 427.5 Cardiac arrest NOS

BOX 2-49 Common Etiologies of Nontraumatic Cardiac Arrest

Cardiac
  Coronary artery disease
  Cardiomyopathies
  Structural abnormalities
  Valve dysfunction
Respiratory
  Hypoventilation
    CNS dysfunction
    Neuromuscular disease
    Toxic and metabolic en-
      cephalopathies
  Upper airway obstruction
    CNS dysfunction
    Foreign body
    Infection
    Trauma
    Neoplasm
  Pulmonary dysfunction
    Asthma and COPD

Pulmonary edema
Pulmonary embolus
Pneumonia
Circulatory
  Mechanical obstruction
    Tension pneumothorax
    Pericardial tamponade
    Pulmonary embolus
  Hypovolemia
    Hemorrhage
  Vascular tone
    Sepsis
    Neurogenic
Metabolic
  Electrolyte abnormalities
    Hypokalemia or hyperkalemia
    Hypermagnesemia
    Hypomagnesemia
    Hypocalcemia

Toxic
  Prescription medications
    Antidysrhythmics
    Digitalis
    β-Blockers
    Calcium channel blockers
    Tricyclic antidepressants
  Drugs of abuse
    Cocaine
    Heroin
  Toxins
    Carbon monoxide
    Cyanide
Environmental
  Lightning
  Electrocution
  Hypothermia or hyperthermia
  Drowning/near drowning

From Rosen P (ed): *Emergency medicine*, ed 5, St Louis, 2002, Mosby.
CNS, Central nervous system; *COPD*, chronic obstructive pulmonary disease.

CARDIAC DEATH, SUDDEN

Cardiac death, sudden
ICD-9CM # 427.5 Cardiac arrest NOS

BOX 2-50 Differential Diagnosis of Sudden Cardiac Death

1. Syncope
   a. Syncope caused by bradyarrhythmia
   b. Syncope caused by tachyarrhythmia
   c. Nonarrhythmic syncope (including neurocar-
      diogenic syncope)
2. Seizure
3. Hemodynamic causes of abrupt cardiovascular collapse
   a. Myocardial rupture after myocardial infarction
   b. Papillary muscle rupture
   c. Massive pulmonary emboli
   d. Acute aortic dissection
4. Arrhythmia
   a. Tachycardias
      (i) Ventricular tachycardia/ventricular fibrilla-
          tion
      (ii) Rapid supraventricular arrhythmias (e.g.,
          atrial fibrillation in Wolff-Parkinson-White
          syndrome)
   b. Bradycardias
      (i) Atrioventricular block
      (ii) Sick sinus syndrome
5. Central nervous system vascular catastrophes
   a. Massive stroke
   b. Hemorrhage

From Stein J (ed): *Internal medicine*, ed 5, St Louis, 1998, Mosby.

CARDIAC DEFECTS, CONGENITAL

Cardiac defects, congenital
ICD-9CM # 746.9 Heart disease, congenital NOS
746.9 Heart disease, congenital specified type necessary

TABLE 2-34   Findings in Selected Uncomplicated Congenital Cardiac Defects*

TYPE	PHYSICAL FINDINGS	ECG	CHEST RADIOGRAPH
Atrial septal defect	Ejection murmur across pulmonic valve Widely and fixed split S_2 Diastolic flow murmur across tricuspid valve Parasternal (RV) impulse	rSr′ or rSr′s′; left axis with ostium primum defect	Large pulmonary artery and increased pulmonary vascular markings (pulmonary plethora)
Ventricular septal defect	Holosystolic left parasternal murmur ± thrill Normal or moderately split S_2 Diastolic flow murmur and S_3 Apical impulse prominent and displaced laterally; also parasternal impulse	Biventricular or left ventricular hypertrophy	Cardiomegaly Prominent pulmonary artery and pulmonary plethora
Patent ductus arteriosus	Widened arterial pulse pressure Hyperdynamic apical impulse Continuous "machinery" murmur	LV hypertrophy	Prominent pulmonary artery and pulmonary plethora; enlarged LA, LV; occasionally calcified ductus
Congenital valvular aortic stenosis	Decreased pulse pressure and carotid upstroke Sustained apical impulse S_4; systolic ejection murmur ± thrill Single or paradoxical splitting of S_2 Concomitant aortic regurgitation common	LV hypertrophy	Poststenotic aortic dilation Prominent LV
Valvular pulmonic stenosis	Large jugular A-wave RV parasternal impulse Pulmonic ejection sound Systolic ejection murmur ± thrill at second left intercostal space Widely split S_2 with soft (or inaudible) P_2 Right ventricular S_4	RV hypertrophy RA abnormality	Pulmonary blood flow normal or reduced Poststenotic dilation of main or left pulmonary artery RA and RV enlargement
Coarctation of aorta	Reduced lower extremity blood pressure; delayed, diminished femoral pulses Mid-systolic coarctation murmur at left sternal border or posterior left intrascapular area Continuous murmur from collaterals Sustained apical impulse; S_4 Evidence of associated bicuspid aortic valve common	LV hypertrophy	Prominent ascending aorta; LV enlargement Poststenotic aortic dilation notching of inferior rib surfaces from collateral flow in intercostal arteries
Ebstein's anomaly	Acyanotic or cyanotic (right-to-left shunt owing to increased RA pressure) Increased jugular pressure and regurgitant wave Systolic murmur of tricuspid regurgitation increased with inspiration Wide splitting of S_2; S_4 and S_3	RA abnormality Right bundle branch block PR prolongation Ventricular preexcitation	Enlarged RA Pulmonary vascularity normal or decreased
Tetralogy of Fallot	Usually cyanotic Clubbing may be present Prominent ejection murmur at left sternal border Soft or absent P_2	RV hypertrophy RA abnormality	"Boot"-shaped heart owing to RV hypertrophy, small pulmonary artery, and small LV Pulmonary vascularity normal or reduced

From Andreoli TE et al: Congenital heart disease. In Andreoli TE (ed): *Cecil essentials of medicine*, ed 5, Philadelphia, 2001, WB Saunders.
ECG, Electrocardiogram; *LA*, left atrium; *LV*, left ventricle; *P₂*, second pulmonic heart sound; *RA*, right atrium; *RV*, right ventricle; *S₂*, second heart sound; *S₃*, third heart sound; *S₄*, fourth heart sound.
*Findings vary depending on severity of lesions and associated abnormalities.

II

CARDIAC ENLARGEMENT

Cardiac enlargement	
ICD-9CM # 429.3	Cardiomegaly, idiopathic
746.89	Cardiomegaly, congenital
402.0	Cardiomegaly, malignant
402.1	Cardiomegaly, benign

BOX 2-51   Cardiac Enlargement: Differential Diagnosis

Cardiac chamber enlargement
  Chronic volume overload
    Mitral or aortic regurgitation
    Left-to-right shunt (PDA, VSD, AV fistula)
  Cardiomyopathy
    Ischemic
    Nonischemic
  Decompensated pressure overload
    Aortic stenosis
    Hypertension
  High-output states
    Severe anemia
    Thyrotoxicosis
  Bradycardia
    Severe sinus bradycardia
    Complete heart block
  Left atrium
    LV failure of any cause
    Mitral valve disease
    Myxoma
  Right ventricle
    Chronic LV failure of any cause
    Chronic volume overload
      Tricuspid or pulmonic regurgitation
      Left-to-right shunt (ASD)
    Decompensated pressure overload
      Pulmonic stenosis
      Pulmonary artery hypertension
        Primary
        Secondary (PE, COPD)
      Pulmonary veno-occlusive disease
  Right atrium
    RV failure of any cause
    Tricuspid valve disease
    Myxoma
    Ebstein's anomaly
  Multichamber enlargement
    Hypertrophic cardiomyopathy
    Acromegaly
    Severe obesity
  Pericardial disease
    Pericardial effusion with or without tamponade
    Effusive constrictive disease
    Pericardial cyst, loculated effusion
  Pseudocardiomegaly
    Epicardial fat
    Chest wall deformity (pectus excavatum, straight back syndrome)
    Low lung volumes
    AP chest x-ray
    Mediastinal tumor, cyst

From Goldman L, Braunwald E (eds): *Primary cardiology*, Philadelphia, 1998, WB Saunders.
AP, Anteroposterior; *ASD*, atrial septal defect; *AV*, arteriovenous; *COPD*, chronic obstructive pulmonary disease; *LV*, left ventricular; *PDA*, patent ductus arteriosus; *PE*, pulmonary embolism; *RV*, right ventricular; *VSD*, ventricular septal defect.

CARDIAC MURMURS

TABLE 2-35   **Some Common Causes of Heart Murmurs**

	USUAL LOCATION	COMMON ASSOCIATED FINDINGS
Systolic		
Holosystolic		
Mitral regurgitation (MR)	Apex → axilla	↑ with handgrip; S_3 if marked MR; LV dilation common
Tricuspid regurgitation (TR)	LLSB	↑ with inspiration; RV dilation common
Ventricular septal defect (VSD)	LLSB → RLSB	Often with thrill
Early-midsystolic		
Aortic valvular stenosis (AS)	RUSB	
Fixed supravalvular or subvalvular	RUSB	Ejection click if mobile valve; soft or absent A_2 if valve immobile; later peak associated with more severe stenosis
Dynamic infravalvular	LLSB → apex + axilla	Hypertrophic obstructive cardiomyopathy; murmur louder if LV volume lower or contractility increased, softer if LV volume increased*; can be later in systole if obstruction delayed
Pulmonic valvular stenosis (PS)	LUSB	↑ with inspiration
Infravalvular (infundibular)	LUSB	↑ with inspiration
Supravalvular	LUSB	↑ with inspiration
"Flow murmurs"	LUSB	Anemia, fever, increased flow of any cause†
Mid-late Systolic		
Mitral valve prolapse (MVP)	LLSB or apex → axilla	Preceded by click; murmur lengthens with maneuvers that ↓ LV volume*
Papillary muscle dysfunction	Apex → axilla	Ischemic heart disease
Diastolic		
Early Diastolic		
Aortic regurgitation (AR)	RUSB, LUSB	High-pitched, blowing quality; endocarditis, diseases of the aorta, associated AS; signs of low peripheral vascular resistance
Pulmonic valve regurgitation (PR)	LUSB	Pulmonary hypertension as a causative factor
Mid-late Diastolic		
Mitral stenosis (MS), tricuspid stenosis (TS)	Apex, LLSB	Low-pitched; in rheumatic heart disease, opening snap commonly precedes murmur; can be due to increased flow across normal valve†
Atrial myxomas	Apex (L), LLSB (R)	"Tumor plop"
Continuous		
Venous hum	Over jugular or hepatic vein or breast	Disappears with compression of vein or pressure of stethoscope
Patent ductus arteriosus (PDA)	LUSB	
Arteriovenous (AV) fistula		
Coronary	LUSB	
Pulmonary, bronchial, chest wall	Over fistula	
Ruptured sinus of Valsalva aneurysm	RUSB	Sudden onset

From Goldman L, Bennett, JC (eds): *Cecil textbook of medicine,* ed 21, Philadelphia, 2000, WB Saunders.
LLSB, Left lower sternal border (4th intercostal space); *LUSB,* left upper sternal border (2nd-3rd intercostal spaces); *RLSB,* right lower sternal border (4th intercostal space); *RUSB,* right upper sternal border (2nd-3rd intercostal spaces).
*LV (left ventricular) volume is decreased by standing or during prolonged, forced expiration against a closed glottis (Valsalva maneuver); it is increased by squatting or by elevation of the legs; contractility is increased by adrenergic stimulation or in the beat after a postextrasystolic beat.
†Including a left-to-right shunt through an atrial septal defect for tricuspid or pulmonic flow murmurs and a ventricular septal defect for pulmonic or mitral flow murmurs.

CARDIAC SHUNT DISEASES, UNCOMPLICATED

Cardiac shunt diseases, uncomplicated
ICD-9CM # code not available

TABLE 2-36   **Findings in Uncomplicated Shunt Lesions**

TYPE	PHYSICAL FINDINGS	ELECTROCARDIOGRAM	CHEST RADIOGRAPH
Atrial septal defect	Parasternal RV impulse Widely and fixed split S_2 Ejection murmur across pulmonic valve	Right bundle branch block Left axis deviation with ostium primum defect	Large pulmonary artery Increased pulmonary markings
Ventricular septal defect	Hyperdynamic precordium Holosystolic left parasternal murmur, ± thrill	LV and RV hypertrophy	Cardiomegaly Prominent pulmonary vasculature
Patent ductus arteriosus	Hyperdynamic apical impulse Continuous "machinery" murmur	LV hypertrophy	Prominent pulmonary artery Enlarged LA and LV

From Andreoli TE (ed): *Cecil essentials of medicine*, ed 5, Philadelphia, 2001, WB Saunders.
LA, Left atrium; *LV*, left ventricle; *RV*, right ventricle.

CAROTID ARTERIAL PULSE ABNORMALITIES

Carotid arterial pulse abnormalities
ICD-9CM # code not available

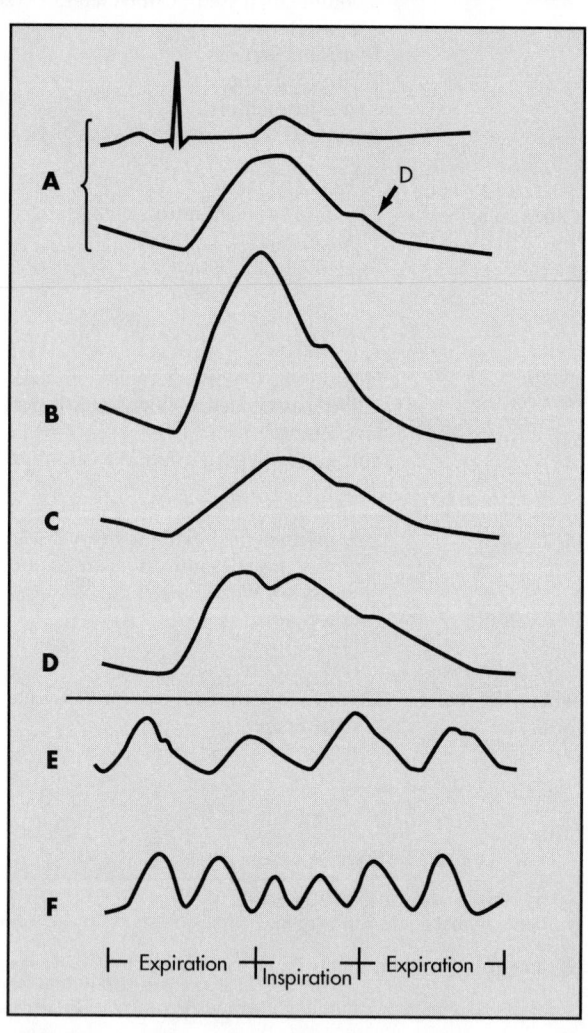

Fig. 2-4   Normal and abnormal carotid arterial pulse contours. **A,** Normal arterial pulse with simultaneous ECG. The dicrotic wave *(D)* occurs just after aortic valve closure. **B,** Wide pulse pressure in aortic insufficiency. **C,** Pulsus parvus et tardus (small amplitude with a slow upstroke) associated with aortic stenosis. **D,** Bisferious pulse with two systolic peaks, typical of hypertrophic obstructive cardiomyopathy or aortic insufficiency, especially if concomitant aortic stenosis is present. **E,** Pulsus alternans characteristic of severe left ventricular failure. **F,** Paradoxical pulse (systolic pressure decrease of greater than 10 mm Hg with inspiration), most characteristic of cardiac tamponade. (From Andreoli TE [ed]: *Cecil essentials of medicine,* ed 5, Philadelphia, 2001, WB Saunders.)

CATARACTS, PEDIATRIC AGE

BOX 2-52   Pediatric Cataracts: Causes and Associated Conditions

Intrauterine Infection
  Rubella
  Toxoplasmosis
  Herpes simplex
  Cytomegalovirus
  Varicella
Metabolic Disorders
  Galactosemia
  Galactokinase deficiency
  Hypoparathyroidism
  Pseudohypoparathyroidism
  Diabetes mellitus
  Hypoglycemia
  Hyperalimentation (vacuoles)
  Mannosidosis
Drug-induced
  Cortiocosteroids
  Chlorpromazine
  Ergot
  Naphthalene
  Triparanol
Inflammatory
  Juvenile rheumatoid arthritis
  Sarcoidosis
  Pars plana
  Atopic dermatitis
Trauma
Genetic/Syndromes
  Autosomal dominant
  Autosomal recessive
  X-linked recessive
  Down syndrome (trisomy 21)
  Trisomy 13
  Trisomy 18

Genetic Syndromes—cont'd
  Lowe syndrome
  Dubovitz syndrome
  Hallerman-Streiff syndrome
  Alport's syndrome
  Cri du chat syndrome
  Cerebrotendinous xanthomatosis
  Marinesco-Sjögren syndrome
  Myotonic dystrophy
  Rothmund-Thomson syndrome
  Cockayne's syndrome
  Incontinentia pigmenti
  Stickler syndrome
  Craniofacial syndromes
  Zellweger syndrome
  Wilson's syndrome
  Hallgren syndrome
  Laurence-Moon-Bardet-Biedl syndrome
  Chondrodysplasia punctata
  Refsum's disease
  Congenital ichthyosis
  Sclerodactyly
  G-6-PD deficiency
  Rubinstein-Taybi syndrome
Radiation Injury
Ocular Disease
  Retinitis pigmentosa
  Aniridia
  Persistent
    Hyperplastic
    Primary vitreous
  Leber's congenital amaurosis
  Retinopathy of prematurity
  Retinoblastoma

From Rakel RE (ed): *Principles of family practice,* ed 6, Philadelphia, 2002, WB Saunders.

II

Cardiomyopathy
ICD-9CM # 425.4 Cardiomyopathy NOS
425.4 Congestive
425.4 Hypertrophic
425.4 Restrictive

CARDIOMYOPATHY

TABLE 2-37   **Classification of Cardiomyopathy**

	DILATED (CONGESTIVE)	HYPERTROPHIC	RESTRICTIVE
Symptoms	Dyspnea, orthopnea, fatigue, leg edema	Dyspnea, angina, syncope after exertion, palpitations	Dyspnea, fatigue, leg edema
Characteristic cardiac physical findings	Cardiomegaly; S_3 and S_4 common; murmur of mitral and tricuspid regurgitation	Bifid apical impulse with palpable S_4, ejection murmur at LSB (increased with Valsalva); often associated mitral regurgitation murmur	Normal size or slightly enlarged heart; S_3 common; S_4; murmur of tricupsid or mitral regurgitation; elevated jugular venous pressure, inspiratory increase in venous pressure
Electrocardiogram	Sinus tachycardia; left bundle-branch block common	Left ventricular hypertrophy; abnormal Q waves	Low voltage; abnormal Q waves; conduction abnormalities
Echocardiogram	Dilated cardiac chambers; generalized reduced ventricular wall motion and systolic function	Normal or small left ventricular cavity; left ventricular hypertrophy; asymmetric septal thickening; systolic anterior motion of anterior mitral valve leaflet	Thick walls, reduced systolic function; glistening appearance of left ventricular in amyloid
Treatment	Diuretics; unloading agents; digoxin	β-adrenergic–blocking drugs or selected calcium channel–blocking drugs; sequential atrioventricular (DDD) pacing for selected patients with refractory symptoms; surgical septal myectomy for refractory obstructive symptoms	Treatment of underlying cause; diuretics

From Andreoli TE (ed): *Cecil essentials of medicine,* ed 5, Philadelphia, 2001, WB Saunders.
DDD, Atrial synchronous ventricular pacemaker; *LSB,* left sternal border.

CAVITARY LESION ON CHEST X-RAY

Cavitary lesion on chest x-ray
ICD-9CM # 793.1 Chest x-ray lung shadow

BOX 2-53 Differential Diagnosis of a Cavitary Lesion on Chest Radiograph

Necrotizing infections
  Bacteria: anaerobes *Staphylococcus aureus*, enteric gram-negative bacteria, *Pseudomonas aeruginosa*, *Legionella* spp., *Haemophilus influenzae*, *Streptococcus pyogenes*, *Streptococcus pneumoniae* (?), *Rhodococcus*, *Actinomyces*
  Mycobacteria: *Mycobacterium tuberculosis*, *Mycobacterium kansasii*, *Mycobacterium avium-intracellulare*
  Bacteria-like: *Nocardia* spp.
  Fungi: *Coccidioides immitis*, *Histoplasma capsulatum*, *Blastomyces hominis*, *Aspergillus* spp., *Mucor* spp.
  Parasitic: *Entamoeba histolytica*, *Paragonimus westermani*, *Echinococcus*
Cavitary infarction
  Bland infarction (with or without superimposed infection)
Septic embolism
  S. aureus, anaerobes, others
Vasculitis
  Wegener granulomatosis, periarteritis
Neoplasms
  Bronchogenic carcinoma, metastatic carcinoma, lymphoma
Miscellaneous lesions
  Cysts, blebs, bullae, or pneumatocele with or without fluid collections
  Sequestration
  Empyema with air-fluid level
  Bronchiectasis

From Gorbach SL: *Infectious diseases,* ed 2, Philadelphia, 1998, WB Saunders.

CEREBROVASCULAR DISEASE, ISCHEMIC

Cerebrovascular disease, ischemic
ICD-9CM # 437.9

BOX 2-54 Cerebrovascular Disease, Ischemic

Vascular disorders
  Large-vessel atherothrombotic disease
  Lacunar disease
  Arterial-to-arterial embolization
  Carotid or vertebral artery dissection
  Fibromuscular dysplasia
  Migraine
  Venous thrombosis
  Radiation
  Complications of arteriography
  Multiple, progressive intracranial arterial occlusions
Inflammatory disorders
  Giant cell arteritis
  Polyarteritis nodosa
  Systemic lupus erythematosus
  Granulomatous angiitis
  Takayasu's disease
  Arteritis associated with amphetamine, cocaine, or
    phenylpropanolamine
  Syphilis, mucormycosis

Sjögren syndrome
Behçet syndrome
Cardiac disorders
  Rheumatic heart disease
  Mural thrombus
  Arrhythmias
  Mitral valve prolapse
  Prosthetic heart valve
  Endocarditis
  Myxoma
  Paradoxical embolus
Hematologic disorders
  Thrombotic thrombocytopenic purpura
  Sickle cell disease
  Hypercoagulable states
  Polycythemia
  Thrombocytosis
  Leukocytosis
  Lupus anticoagulant

From Wiederholt WC: *Neurology for non-neurologists,* ed 4, Philadelphia, 2000, WB Saunders.

CEREBROSPINAL FLUID ABNORMALITIES

Cerebrospinal fluid abnormalities
ICD-9CM # 792.0

TABLE 2-38   Cerebrospinal Fluid Findings in Central Nervous System Disorders

CONDITION	PRESSURE (MM H₂O)	LEUKOCYTES (MM³)	PROTEIN (MG/DL)	GLUCOSE (MG/DL)	COMMENTS
Normal	50-80	<5, ≥75% lymphocytes	20-45	>50 (or 75% serum glucose)	
Common Forms of Meningitis					
Acute bacterial meningitis	Usually elevated (100-300)	100-10,000 or more; usually 300-2000; PMNs predominate	Usually 100-500	Decreased, usually <40 (or <66% serum glucose)	Organisms usually seen on Gram stain and recovered by culture. Latex agglutination of CSF usually positive
Partially treated bacterial meningitis	Normal or elevated	5-10,000; PMNs usual but mononuclear cells may predominate if pretreated for extended period of time	Usually 100-500	Normal or decreased	Organisms may be seen on Gram stain. Latex agglutination CSF may be positive. Pretreatment may render CSF sterile
Viral meningitis or meningoencephalitis	Normal or slightly elevated (80-150)	Rarely >1000 cells. Eastern equine encephalitis and lymphocytic choriomeningitis (LCM) may have cell counts of several thousand. PMNs early but mononuclear cells predominate through most of the course	Usually 50-200	Generally normal; may be decreased to <40 in some viral diseases, particularly mumps (15%-20% of cases)	HSV encephalitis is suggested by focal seizures or by focal findings on CT or MRI scans or EEG. Enteroviruses and HSV infrequently recovered from CSF. HSV and enteroviruses may be detected by PCR of CSF
Uncommon Forms of Meningitis					
Tuberculous meningitis	Usually elevated	10-500; PMNs early, but lymphocytes predominate through most of the course	100-3000; may be higher in presence of block	<50 in most cases; decreases with time if treatment is not provided	Acid-fast organisms almost never seen on smear. Organisms may be recovered in culture of large volumes of CSF. *Mycobacterium tuberculosis* may be detected by PCR of CSF
Fungal meningitis	Usually elevated	5-500; PMNs early but mononuclear cells predominate through most of the course. Cryptococcal meningitis may have no cellular inflammatory response	25-500	<50; decreases with time if treatment is not provided	Budding yeast may be seen. Organisms may be recovered in culture. Cryptococcal antigen (CSF and serum) may be positive in cryptococcal infection
Syphilis (acute) and leptospirosis	Usually elevated	50-500; lymphocytes predominate	50-200	Usually normal	Positive CSF serology. Spirochetes not demonstrable by usual techniques of smear or culture; darkfield examination may be positive
Amebic (*Naegleria*) meningoencephalitis	Elevated	1000-10,000 or more; PMNs predominate	50-500	Normal or slightly decreased	Mobile amebae may be seen by hanging-drop examination of CSF at room temperature

Brain and Parameningeal Abscesses

Condition	Pressure	Leukocytes	Protein	Glucose	Comments
Brain abscess	Usually elevated (100-300)	5-200; CSF rarely acellular; lymphocytes predominate; if abscess ruptures into ventricle, PMNs predominate and cell count may reach >100,000	75-500	Normal unless abscess ruptures into ventricular system	No organisms on smear or culture unless abscess ruptures into ventricular system
Subdural empyema	Usually elevated (100-300)	100-5000; PMNs predominate	100-500	Normal	No organisms on smear or culture of CSF unless meningitis also present; organisms found on tap of subdural fluid
Cerebral epidural abscess	Normal to slightly elevated	10-500; lymphocytes predominate	50-200	Normal	No organisms on smear or culture of CSF
Spinal epidural abscess	Usually low, with spinal block	10-100; lymphocytes predominate	50-400	Normal	No organisms on smear or culture of CSF
Chemical (drugs, dermoid cysts, myelography dye)	Usually elevated	100-1000 or more; PMNs predominate	50-100	Normal or slightly decreased	Epithelial cells may be seen within CSF by use of polarized light in some children with dermoids
Noninfectious Causes					
Sarcoidosis	Normal or elevated slightly	0-100; mononuclear	40-100	Normal	No specific findings
Systemic lupus erythematosus with CNS involvement	Slightly elevated	0-500; PMNs usually predominate; lymphocytes may be present	100	Normal or slightly decreased	No organisms on smear or culture. LE preparation may be positive. Positive neuronal and ribosomal P protein antibodies in CSF
Tumor, leukemia	Slightly elevated to very high	0-100 or more; mononuclear or blast cells	50-1000	Normal to decreased (20-40)	Cytology may be positive

From Behrman RE: *Nelson textbook of pediatrics*, ed 16, Philadelphia, 2000, WB Saunders.
CSF, Cerebrospinal fluid; *EEG*, electroencephalogram; *HSV*, herpes simplex virus; *PCR*, polymerase chain reaction; *PMN*, polymorphonuclear neutrophils.

II

CESTODE TISSUE INFECTIONS

Cestode tissue infections
ICD-9CM # 123.0 *Taenia solium* infection
          122.4 *Echinococcus granulosus* infection
          122.7 *Echinococcus multilocularis* infection

TABLE 2-39   Cestode Tissue Infections

SPECIES	EPIDEMIOLOGY	TRANSMISSION	MAJOR CLINICAL PRESENTATION	DIAGNOSIS	TREATMENT
Taenia solium (cysticercosis)	Worldwide	Ingestion of eggs or autoinfection from tapeworm	Seizures, focal neurologic symptoms, hydrocephalus	Serology, characteristic CT scan of head, radiograph of soft tissues	Albendazole 5 mg/kg tid for 8-28 days, repeated as necessary or praziquantel 20 mg/kg tid for 15 days; both treatments with or without steroids
Echinococcus granulosus (hydatid disease)	Sheep- and cattle-raising areas of world	Association with dogs, ingestion of contaminated dog excreta	Single mass in liver or lungs, anaphylactic shock after blunt trauma	Characteristic abdominal CT scan, serology	Surgery or surgery and/or albendazole 400 mg bid for 28 days, repeated as necessary or albendazole plus praziquantel†
Echinococcus multilocularis	Northern latitudes; North America, Europe, and Asia	Associated with infected animals or ingestion of food contaminated with dog excreta	Alveolar mass in liver	Characteristic abdominal CT scan, serology	Surgery or surgery plus albendazole*† 400 mg bid for 28 days

From Stein JH (ed): *Internal medicine,* ed 5, St Louis, 1998, Mosby.
bid, Twice a day; *CT,* computed tomography; *tid,* three times a day.
*Considered an investigational drug for this indication by the U.S. Food and Drug Administration.
†Effectiveness not clearly established.

CHANNELOPATHIES

Channelopathies
ICD-9CM # code not available

TABLE 2-40   Channelopathies and Related Disorders

DISORDER	CLINICAL FEATURES	INHERITANCE	CHROMOSOME	GENE
Chloride channelopathies				
Myotonia congenita				
Thomsen's disease	Myotonia	Autosomal dominant	7q35	CLC-1
Becker disease	Myotonia and weakness	Autosomal recessive	7q35	CLC-1
Sodium channelopathies				
Paramyotonia congenita	Paramyotonia	Autosomal dominant	17q13.1-13.3	SCNA4A
Hyperkalemic periodic paralysis	Periodic paralysis, myotonia, and paramyotonia	Autosomal dominant	17q13.1-13.3	SCNA4A
Calcium channelopathies				
Hypokalemic periodic paralysis	Periodic paralysis	Autosomal dominant	1q31-32	Dihydropyridine receptor
Malignant hyperthermia (some cases)	Anesthetic-induced delayed relaxation	Autosomal dominant	19q13.1	Ryanodine receptor
Rippling muscle disease	Muscle mounding/stiffness	Autosomal dominant	1q41	Unknown
Andersen's syndrome	Periodic paralysis, cardiac arrhythmia, distinctive facies	Autosomal dominant	Unknown	Unknown
Brody's disease	Delayed relaxation, no electromyographic myotonia	Autosomal recessive	16p12	Calcium-ATPase

From Andreoli TE (ed): *Cecil essentials of medicine,* ed 5, Philadelphia, 2001, WB Saunders.
ATP, Adenosine triphosphate.

CHEST PAIN IN CHILDREN

Chest pain in children
ICD-9CM # 786.50 Chest pain NOS
786.59 Chest pressure
786.52 Chest pain, pleuritic

BOX 2-55 Cardiac and Noncardiac Causes of Chest Pain in Children

Cardiac

I. Congenital cardiac structural diseases
   A. Obstruction of the outflow tract of the left ventricle
   B. Mitral valve prolapse
   C. Anomalous origin of the coronary artery (from the pulmonary artery)
   D. Cardiomyopathy
II. Dysrhythmias
   A. Supraventricular tachycardia
   B. Ventricular ectopy or tachycardia
III. Acquired cardiopulmonary diseases
   A. Inflammation of myocardium, pericardium—viral, bacterial, rheumatic
   B. Coronary arteritis, Kawasaki syndrome, systemic lupus erythematosus
   C. Pulmonary embolism
   D. Local tumor, inflammation, toxin related (cocaine)

Noncardiac

I. Psychogenic
   A. Hyperventilation
   B. Depression
   C. Conversion reaction
II. Rib cage
   A. Costochondritis
   B. Muscle-skeletal trauma and strains
   C. Mastalgia
   D. Pleuritis, bronchitis, bronchospasm
   E. Pneumothorax
III. Gastrointestinal
   A. Gastroesophageal reflux
   B. Peptic ulcer

From Rosen P, Barkin R (eds): *Emergency medicine: concepts and clinical practice,* ed 3, St Louis, 1992, Mosby.

Gwendolyn R. Lee, M.D.
Internal Medicine

CHEST PAIN IN CHILDREN

Chest pain in children
ICD-9CM # 786.50 Chest pain NOS
786.59 Chest pressure
786.52 Chest pain, pleuritic

BOX 2-56 Differential Diagnosis of Chest Pain in Pediatric Patients

Musculoskeletal (Common)

Trauma (accidental, abuse)
Exercise, overuse injury (strain, bursitis)
Costochondritis (Tietze's syndrome)
Herpes zoster (cutaneous)
Pleurodynia
Fibrositis
Slipping rib
Sickle cell anemia vaso-occlusive crisis
Osteomyelitis (rare)
Primary or metastatic tumor (rare)

Pulmonary (Common)

Pneumonia
Pleurisy
Asthma
Chronic cough
Pneumothorax
Infarction (sickle cell anemia)
Foreign body
Embolism (rare)
Pulmonary hypertension (rare)
Tumor (rare)

Gastrointestinal (Less Common)

Esophagitis (gastroesophageal reflux)
Esophageal foreign body

Esophageal spasm
Cholecystitis
Subdiaphragmatic abscess
Periheptatitis (Fitz-Hugh-Curtis syndrome)
Peptic ulcer disease

Cardiac (Less Common)

Pericarditis
Postpericardiotomy syndrome
Endocarditis
Mitral valve prolapse
Aortic or subaortic stenosis
Arrhythmias
Marfan's syndrome (dissecting aortic aneurysm)
Anomalous coronary artery
Kawasaki disease
Cocaine, sympathomimetic ingestion
Angina (familial hypercholesterolemia)

Idiopathic (Common)

Anxiety, hyperventilation
Panic disorder

Other (Less Common)

Spinal cord or nerve root compression
Breast-related pathologic condition
Castelman's disease (lymph node neoplasm)

From Behrman RE: *Nelson textbook of pediatrics,* ed 16, Philadelphia, 2000, WB Saunders.

CHEST PAIN, NONCARDIAC

Chest pain, noncardiac
ICD-9CM # Code varies with specific disorder

TABLE 2-41   Noncardiac Causes of Chest Pain

CONDITION	LOCATION	QUALITY	DURATION	AGGRAVATING OR RELIEVING FACTORS	ASSOCIATED SYMPTOMS OR SIGNS
Pulmonary embolism (chest pain often not present)	Substernal or over region of pulmonary infarction	Pleuritic (with pulmonary infarction) or angina-like	Sudden onset; minutes to <1 hr	May be aggravated by breathing	Dyspnea, tachypnea, tachycardia; hypotension, signs of acute right heart failure, and pulmonary hypertension with large emboli; rales, pleural rub, hemoptysis with pulmonary infarction
Pulmonary hypertension	Substernal	Pressure; oppressive		Aggravated by effort	Pain usually associated with dyspnea; signs of pulmonary hypertension
Pneumonia with pleurisy	Localized over involved area	Pleuritic localized		Painful breathing	Dyspnea, cough, fever, dull to percussion bronchial breath sounds, rales, occasional pleural rub
Spontaneous pneumothorax	Unilateral	Sharp, well localized	Sudden onset, lasts many hours	Painful breathing	Dyspnea; hyperresonance and decreased breath and voice sounds over involved lung
Musculoskeletal disorders	Variable	Aching	Short or long duration	Aggravated by movement; history of muscle exertion or injury	Tender to pressure or movement
Herpes zoster	Dermatomal in distribution		Prolonged	None	Vesicular rash appears in area of discomfort
Esophageal reflux	Substernal, epigastric	Burning, visceral discomfort	10-60 min	Aggravated by large meal, postprandial recumbency; relief with antacid	Water brash
Peptic ulcer	Epigastric, substernal	Visceral burning, aching	Prolonged	Relief with food, antacid	
Gallbladder disease	Epigastric, right upper quadrant	Visceral	Prolonged	May be unprovoked or follows meal	Right upper quadrant tenderness may be present
Anxiety states	Often localized over precordium	Variable; often location moves from place to place	Varies; often fleeting	Situational	Sighing respirations, often chest wall tenderness

From Andreoli TE (ed): *Cecil essentials of medicine,* ed 5, Philadelphia, 2001, WB Saunders.

CHEST PAIN, NONPLEURITIC

Chest pain, nonpleuritic
ICD-9CM # 786.50 Chest pain NOS
786.59 Chest discomfort

BOX 2-57 Nonpleuritic Chest Pain

Cardiac: myocardial ischemia/infarction, myocarditis
Esophageal: spasm, rupture, esophagitis, ulceration, neoplasm, achalasia, diverticula, foreign body
Referred pain from subdiaphragmatic GI structures
  Gastric and duodenal: hiatal hernia, neoplasm, PUD
  Gallbladder and biliary: cholecystitis, cholelithiasis, impacted stone, neoplasm
  Pancreatic: pancreatitis, neoplasm

Dissecting aortic aneurysm
Pain originating from skin, breasts, and musculoskeletal structures: herpes zoster, mastitis, cervical spondylosis
Mediastinal tumors: lymphoma, thymoma
Pulmonary: neoplasm, pneumonia, pulmonary embolism/infarction
Psychoneurosis
Chest pain associated with mitral valve prolapse

CHEST PAIN, PLEURITIC

Chest pain, pleuritic
ICD-9CM # 786.52 Chest pain, pleuritic

BOX 2-58 Pleuritic Chest Pain

Cardiac: pericarditis, postpericardiotomy/Dressler's syndrome
Pulmonary: pneumothorax, hemothorax, embolism/infarction, pneumonia, empyema, neoplasm, bronchiectasis, TB, carcinomatous effusion
GI: liver abscess, pancreatitis, Whipple's disease with associated pericarditis or pleuritis
Subdiaphragmatic abscess

Pain originating from skin and musculoskeletal tissues: costochondritis, chest wall trauma, fractured rib, interstitial fibrositis, myositis, strain of pectoralis muscle, herpes zoster, soft tissue and bone tumors
Collagen-vascular diseases with pleuritis
Psychoneurosis
Familial Mediterranean fever (FMF)

CHOREOATHETOSIS

Choreoathetosis
ICD-9CM # 275.1 Choreoathetosis-agitans syndrome
33.5 Choreoathetosis paroxysmal

BOX 2-59 Choreoathetosis

A. Causes of Choreoathetosis

Drugs and toxins
Systemic diseases
  Systemic lupus erythematosus
  Polycythemia
  Thyrotoxicosis
  Rheumatic fever
  Cirrhosis of the liver (acquired hepatocerebral degeneration)
  Diabetes mellitus
  Wilson's disease
Primary degenerative brain diseases
  Huntington's chorea
  Olivopontocerebellar atrophies
  Neuroacanthocytosis
Focal brain diseases
  Hemichorea
  Stroke
  Tumor
  Arteriovenous malformation

B. Drug-Induced Choreoathetosis

Parkinson's disease drugs
  Levodopa
Epilepsy drugs
  Phenytoin
  Carbamazepine
  Phenobarbital
  Gabapentin
  Valproate
Psychostimulant drugs
  Cocaine
  Amphetamine
  Methamphetamine
  Dextroamphetamine
  Methylphenidate
  Pemoline
Psychotropic drugs
  Lithium
  Tricyclic antidepressant drugs
Oral contraceptive drugs
Cimetidine

From Noble J: *Primary care medicine*, ed 3, St Louis, 2001, Mosby.

CLUBBING

Clubbing
ICD-9CM # 781.5 Clubbing finger

BOX 2-60   Clubbing

Pulmonary neoplasm (lung, pleura)
Other neoplasm (GI, liver, Hodgkin's, thymus)
Pulmonary infectious process (empyema, abscess,
  bronchiectasis, TB, chronic pneumonitis)
Extrapulmonary infectious process (subacute bacterial
  endocarditis, intestinal TB, bacterial or amebic
  dysentery)
Pneumoconiosis
Cystic fibrosis
Sarcoidosis

Cyanotic congenital heart disease
Endocrine (Graves' disease, hyperparathyroidism)
Inflammatory bowel disease
Sprue
Chronic liver disease
Congenital heart disease
Idiopathic
Hereditary (pachydermoperiostitis)
Chronic trauma (jackhammer operators, machine
  workers)

COAGULOPATHY, CONGENITAL

Coagulopathy, congenital
ICD-9CM # 286.9 Factor deficiency, congenital

TABLE 2-42   Congenital Disorders of Blood Coagulation

COAGULATION FACTOR	INHERITANCE	INCIDENCE (PER MILLION)	BLEEDING SYMPTOMS	ABNORMAL SCREENING TESTS	BIOLOGIC HALF-LIFE OF PROTEIN (HR)	TREATMENT
I (fibrinogen)	Autosomal recessive	1	Umbilical bleeding at birth, posttrauma hemorrhage	PT, PTT, TT	100	Cryoprecipitate
II (prothrombin)	Autosomal recessive	1	Similar to hemophilia	PT, PTT	72	FFP, rarely prothrombin complex concentrates
V	Autosomal recessive	1	Similar to hemophilia	PT, PTT	24	FFP, possibly platelet concentrates
VII	Autosomal recessive	1	Similar to hemophilia	PT	4-6	VII concentrates
VIII (hemophilia)	Sex-linked recessive	100 (milder disease is much more common)	Hemarthrosis, hematoma, bruising, severe postoperative bleeding	PTT	12	VIII concentrates
vWf (von Willebrand's factor)	Autosomal dominant or recessive	Probably as frequent as hemophilia A	Epistaxis, gingival bleeding, bruising, menorrhagia, severe postoperative bleeding	PTT	4-6, for correction of bleeding time	DDAVP, WF-rich VII concentrates

Continued

TABLE 2-42   Congenital Disorders of Blood Coagulation—cont'd

COAGULATION FACTOR	INHERITANCE	INCIDENCE (PER MILLION)	BLEEDING SYMPTOMS	ABNORMAL SCREENING TESTS	BIOLOGIC HALF-LIFE OF PROTEIN (HR)	TREATMENT
IX (hemophilia B)	Sex-linked recessive	20	Identical to hemophilia	PT, PTT	24	IX concentrates
X	Autosomal recessive	1	Similar to hemophilia	PT, PTT	50	FFP, rarely prothrombin complex concentrates
XI	Autosomal recessive	1	Mild; however, severe postoperative hemorrhage can occur	PTT	60	FFP, level of 25% adequate for hemostasis
XII	Autosomal recessive	1	None	PTT	60	None
XIII	Autosomal recessive	1	Umbilical bleeding at birth, posttrauma hemorrhage, poor wound healing	—	120	FFP monthly, because level of 2% is adequate for hemostasis
Alpha₂ antiplasmin	Autosomal recessive	Unknown	Similar to hemophilia	—	Unknown	FFP
Plasminogen activator inhibitor (PAI-I)	Unknown	Unknown	Severe postoperative and posttrauma bleeding	—	Unknown	EACA
Passovoy	Autosomal dominant	Unknown	Similar to factor XI	PTT	Unknown	FFP

From Stein JH (ed): *Internal medicine*, ed 5, St Louis, 1998, Mosby.
DDAVP, 1-Deamino-8-D-arginine vasopressin; *EACA*, ε-aminocaproic acid; *FFP*, fresh-frozen plasma; *PT*, prothrombin time; *PTT*, partial thromboplastin time; *TT*, thrombin (clotting) time.

COLDS, FLU, AND STUFFY NOSE

TABLE 2-43   Differential Diagnosis of Colds, Flu, and Stuffy Nose

Colds, flu, and stuffy nose
ICD-9CM # 460   Common cold
487.1 Influenza
477.9 Rhinitis allergic

CONDITION	NATURE OF PATIENT	NATURE OF SYMPTOMS AND ASSOCIATED SYMPTOMS	COMPLICATIONS	PRECIPITATING AND AGGRAVATING FACTORS	PHYSICAL FINDINGS	DIAGNOSTIC STUDIES
Common cold/viral upper respiratory tract infections	Anyone	Constitutional symptoms worse in children; Incubation period 1-3 days; Profuse nasal drainage; Nasal congestion; Sneezing; Postnasal drip; Cough; Sore throat; Headache; Fever (<102° F); Hoarseness; General malaise	Lower RTI, especially in adults with history of bronchitis, allergies, asthma, heavy cigarette smoking, immune incompetence; Sinusitis, especially in patients with history of recurrent sinusitis; Bronchitis in smokers and patients with pulmonary disease; Pneumonia in elderly and diabetic patients; Nasal airway obstruction; Streptococcal pharyngitis; Meningitis		Mucopurulent nasal discharge; Nasopharyngeal mucosal infection and swelling; Temperature usually <102° F; Pharyngeal exudates less frequent than with bacterial infections; Lymphadenopathy	Throat culture (to rule out streptococcal infection and pharyngitis); Monospot (to rule out infectious mononucleosis)
	Children	Vomiting; Diarrhea; Abdominal pain; Wheezing	Lower RTI in children with history of recurrent bronchitis, allergies, cystic fibrosis; Otitis media		Fever, may be >102° F; Wheezing when bronchiolitis is associated	
Allergic rhinitis Perennial	Onset before age 20; Family history of allergic disease	Nasal airway blockage; Persistent watery nasal discharge; No seasonal variation			Pale boggy nasal turbinates; Watery nasal discharge	Nasal smear: eosinophils
Seasonal		Sneezing; Itchy eyes; Lacrimation; Watery nasal discharge; Seasonal variation		Allergens; Dust; Pollen; Spores	Pale boggy nasal turbinates	

Condition	Nature of symptoms	History / predisposing factors	Precipitating / aggravating factors	Complications	Physical findings	Diagnostic tests
Chronic (idiopathic) rhinitis	Persistent nasal obstruction; May alternate sides; Profuse watery rhinorrhea; Sneezing not common		Allergy; Stress; Hormonal changes; Marked temperature changes; Chemical irritants		Swollen nasal turbinates	
Sinusitis		Prior history of sinusitis				Sinus CT scan; Transillumination of sinuses
Maxillary	Often recurrent pain over sinuses; Early: unilateral dull; Later: bilateral severe; May present as toothache		Coughing; Sneezing; Percussion of involved sinuses		Pain with percussion of teeth	
Ethmoid	Retro-orbital pain; Mucopurulent nasal discharge (may be bloody)		Coughing and sneezing may cause retro-orbital pain	Visual loss; Cavernous sinus thrombosis; Brain abscess	Chemosis; Proptosis; Extraocular muscle palsy; Orbital fixation	
Rhinitis medicamentosa	Nasal congestion; Nasal stuffiness	Frequent users of nasal drips, sprays, or inhalants; Hypertensive patients taking certain antihypertensive drugs	Nasal medications; Reserpine; β-blockers; Clonidine; Hydralazine; Methyldopa; Prazosin; Estrogens; Oral contraceptives; Chlordiazepoxide; Amitriptyline		Mucosa injected	Nasal smear: no eosinophils

From Seller RH (ed): *Differential diagnosis of common complaints*, ed 4, Philadelphia, 2000, WB Saunders. *CT*, Computed tomography; *RTI*, respiratory tract infection.

II

COLOR CHANGES, CUTANEOUS

Color changes, cutaneous
ICD-9CM # 709.00 Pigmentation anomaly

TABLE 2-44 Cutaneous Color Changes

COLOR	CAUSE	DISTRIBUTION	SELECT CONDITIONS
Brown	Darkening of melanin pigment	Generalized	Pituitary, adrenal, liver disease
		Localized	Nevi, neurofibromatosis
White	Absence of melanin	Generalized	Albinism
		Localized	Vitiligo
Red (erythema)	Increased cutaneous blood flow	Localized	Inflammation
		Generalized	Fever, viral exanthems, urticaria
	Increased intravascular red blood cells	Generalized	Polycythemia
Yellow	Increased bile pigmentation (jaundice)	Generalized	Liver disease
	Increased carotene pigmentation	Generalized (except sclera)	Hypothyroidism, increased intake of vegetables containing carotene
	Decreased visibility of oxyhemoglobin	Generalized	Anemia, chronic renal disease
Blue	Increased unsaturated hemoglobin secondary to hypoxia	Lips, mouth, nail beds	Cardiovascular and pulmonary diseases

From Seidel HM (ed): *Mosby's guide to physical examination,* ed 4, St Louis, 1999, Mosby.

COMA

Coma
ICD-9CM # 780.01

BOX 2-61 Common Differential Diagnoses of Coma

Bihemispheric dysfunction
  Functional
    Metabolic
      Hypoxia*
      Hypoglycemia*
      Hepatic dysfunction (hyperammonemia)
      Uremia
      Hyponatremia, hypernatremia
      Hyperglycemic hyperosmolar nonketotic coma
      Hypothyroidism (myxedema coma)
    Toxic
      Drug overdose
        Drugs of abuse: narcotics, barbiturates, benzo-
          diazepines, etc.
        Therapeutic drugs: anticholinergics,
          tricyclics, etc.
    Infectious
      Meningitis/meningoencephalitis
    Others
      Nonconvulsive status epilepticus
  Structural
    Infarction
      Bilateral hemispheric infarcts

Mass lesions
  Bilateral hemispheric
  Unilateral or bilateral hemispheric with elevated
    intracranial pressure* or local mass effect
Brainstem dysfunction
  Functional
  Structural
    Infarction
    Mass lesion
Mimics
  Organic
    Bilateral pontine infarcts ("locked-in" syndrome)
    Neuromuscular weakness
      Acute inflammatory demyelinating polyneuropathy
      Myasthenia gravis
      Botulism
      Drug-induced neuromuscular blockade
  Psychiatric
    Malignant catatonia
    Psychogenic unresponsiveness

From Johnson RT, Griffin JW: *Current therapy in neurologic disease,* ed 5, St Louis, 1997, Mosby.
*These possibilities need to be treated immediately.

COMA, NEUROLOGIC SIGNS

Coma, neurologic signs
ICD-9CM # 780.01

TABLE 2-45 Major Neurologic Signs Reflecting Anatomic Levels of Rostral-Caudal Progression in Coma

	MOTOR RESPONSE TO DEEP PAIN STIMULI	PUPILS	EXTRAOCULAR MOVEMENT	RESPIRATIONS
Diencephalic	Spontaneous movements: limbs/face/eye to loud hand clap Limb withdrawal to deep pain Decorticate posturing	Small/reactive Unilateral dilation in uncal herniation	Overly facile (brisk) Doll's eye reflexes May need cold-calories to elicit doll's eye reflex	Normal or Cheyne-Stokes
Mesencephalic	Decerebrate posturing, or fragments of it, to deep pain	Unresponsive	Need cold-calories to elicit Doll's eye reflexes	Central neurogenic Hyperventilation
Pontine	Flaccid tone/lack of motor response to deep pain	Unresponsive	No response to oculocephalic stimulation	Return of "normal" apneustic respiratory rhythm
Medullary	Flaccid tone/lack of motor response to deep pain	Unresponsive	No response to oculocephalic stimulation	Ataxic/irregular respiration Respiratory arrest

From Noble J: *Primay care medicine,* ed 3, St Louis, 2001, Mosby.

COMA, NORMAL COMPUTED TOMOGRAPHY

Coma, normal computed tomography
ICD-9CM # 780.01

BOX 2-62 Causes of Coma with Normal Computed Tomography Scan

Meningeal Disorders
Subarachnoid hemorrhage (uncommon)
Bacterial meningitis
Encephalitis
Subdural empyema

Exogenous Toxins
Sedative drugs and barbiturates
Anesthetics and γ-hydroxybutyrate*
Alcohols
Stimulants
  Phencyclidine†
  Cocaine and amphetamine‡
Psychotropic Drugs
  Cyclic antidepressants
  Phenothiazines
  Lithium
Anticonvulsants
Opioids
Clonidine§
Penicillins
Salicylates
Anticholinergics
Carbon monoxide, cyanide, and methemoglobinemia

Endogenous Toxins/Deficiencies/Derangements
Hypoxia and ischemia
Hypoglycemia
Hypercalcemia
Osmolar
  Hyperglycemia
  Hyponatremia
  Hypernatremia
Organ system failure
  Hepatic encephalopathy
  Uremic encephalopathy
  Pulmonary insufficiency (carbon dioxide narcosis)

Seizures
Prolonged postictal state
Spike-wave stupor

Hypothermia or Hyperthermia

Brainstem Ischemia

Basilar Artery Stroke

Brainstem or Cerebellar Hemorrhage

Conversion or Malingering

From Andreoli TE (ed): *Cecil essentials of medicine,* ed 5, Philadelphia, 2001, WB Saunders.
*General anesthetic, similar to γ-aminobutyric acid; recreational drug and body building aid. Rapid onset, rapid recovery often with myoclonic jerking and confusion. Deep coma (2-3 hr; Glasgow Coma Scale = 3) with maintenance of vital signs.
† Coma associated with cholinergic signs: lacrimation, salivation, bronchorrhea, and hyperthermia.
‡ Coma after seizures or status (i.e., a prolonged postictal state).
§ An antihypertensive agent active through the opiate receptor system; frequent overdose when used to treat narcotic withdrawal.

COMA, PEDIATRIC POPULATION

BOX 2-63   Causes of Coma in the Pediatric Population

Anoxia

Birth asphyxia
Carbon monoxide poisoning
Croup/epiglottitis
Meconium aspiration
Infection
Hemolysis
Blood loss
Hydrops fetalis

Infection

Meningoencephalitis
Sepsis
Postimmunization encephalitis

Increased intracranial pressure

Anoxia
Inborn metabolic errors
Toxic encephalopathy
Reye's syndrome
Head trauma/intracranial bleed
Hydrocephalus
Posterior fossa tumors

Hypertensive encephalopathy

Coarctation of aorta
Nephritis
Vasculitis
Pheochromocytoma

Ischemia

Hypoplastic left heart
Shunting lesions
Aortic stenosis
Cardiovascular collapse (any cause)

Purpuric causes

Disseminated intravascular coagulation
Hemolytic-uremic syndrome
Leukemia
Thrombotic purpura

Hypercapnia

Cystic fibrosis
Bronchopulmonary dysplasia
Congenital lung anomalies

Neoplasm

Medulloblastoma
Glioma of brain stem
Posterior fossa tumors

Drugs/toxins

Maternal sedation
Alcohol
Any drug
Lead
Salicylism
Arsenic
Pesticides

Electrolyte abnormalities

Hypernatremia (diarrhea, dehydration, salt poisoning)
Hyponatremia (SIADH, androgenital syndrome, gastroen-
 teritis)
Hyperkalemia (renal failure, salicylism, androgenitalism)
Hypokalemia (diarrhea, hyperaldosteronism, salicylism,
 DKA)
Hypocalcemia (vitamin D deficiency, hyperparathy-
 roidism)
Severe acidosis (sepsis, cold injury, salicylism, DKA)

Hypoglycemia

Birth injury or stress
Diabetes
Alcohol
Salicylism
Hyperinsulinemia
Iatrogenic

Postseizure

Renal causes

Nephritis
Hypoplastic kidneys

Hepatic causes

Acute hepatitis
Fulminant hepatic failure
Inborn metabolic errors
Bile duct atresia

From Rakel RE (ed): *Principles of family practice*, ed 6, Philadelphia, 2002, WB Saunders.
DKA, Diabetic ketoacidosis; *SIADH*, syndrome of inappropriate antidiuretic hormone.

COMPLEMENT DEFICIENCY STATES

Complement deficiency states
ICD-9CM # 279.8

TABLE 2-46   Complement Deficiency States

COMPONENT	NUMBER OF REPORTED PATIENTS	MODE OF INHERITANCE	FUNCTIONAL DEFECTS	DISEASE ASSOCIATIONS
Classic pathway			Impaired IC handling, delayed C´ activation, impaired immune response	CVD, 48%; infection (encaps bact), 22%; both, 18%; healthy, 12%
C1qrs	31	ACD		
C4	21	ACD		
C2	109	ACD		
Alternative pathway			Impaired C´ activation in absence of specific antibody	Infection (meningococcal), 74%; healthy, 26%
D	3	ACD		
P	70	XL		
Junction of classic and alternative pathways			Impaired IC handling, opson/phag; granulocytosis, CTX, immune response and absent SBA	CVD, 79%; recurrent infection (encaps bact), 71%
C3	19	ACD		
Terminal components			Impaired CTX; absent SBA	Infection (*Neisseria*, primarily meningococcal), 58%; CVD, 4%
C5	27	ACD		
C6	77	ACD	Absent SBA	Both, 1%
C7	73	ACD		Healthy, 25%
C8	73	ACD		
C9	165	ACD	Impaired SBA	Healthy, 91%; infection, 9%
Plasma proteins regulating C´ activation				
C1-INH	Many	AD Acq	Uncontrolled generation of an inflammatory mediator on C´ activation	Hereditary angioedema
H	13	ACD	Uncontrolled AP activation → low C3	CVD, 40%; CVD plus infection (encaps bact), 40%; healthy, 20%
I	14	ACD	Uncontrolled AP activation → low C3	Infection (encaps bact), 100%
Membrane proteins regulating C´ activation				
Decay-accelerating factor Homologous restriction factor CD59	Many	Acq	Impaired regulation of C3b and C8 deposited on host RBC; PMN, platelets → cell lysis	Paroxysmal nocturnal hemoglobinuria
CR3	>20	ACD	Impaired PMN adhesive functions (i.e., margination), CTX, C3bi-mediated opson/phag	Infection (*Staphylococcus aureus, Pseudomonas* spp.), 100%
Autoantibodies				
C3 nephritic factors	>59	Acq	Stabilize AP, convertase → low C3	MPGN, 41%; PLD, 25%; infection (encaps bact), 16%; MPGN plus PLD, 10%; PLD plus infection, 5%; MPGN plus PLD plus infection, 3%; MPGN plus infection, 2%
C4 nephritic factor		Acq	Stabilize CP, C3 convertase → low C3	Glomerulonephritis, 50%; CVD, 50%

From Mandell GL: *Mandell, Douglas, and Bennett's principles and practice of infectious diseases,* ed 5, New York, 2000, Churchill Livingstone.
ACD, Autosomal codominant; *Acq,* acquired; *AD,* autosomal dominant; *AP,* alternative pathway; *C´,* complement; *CP,* classic pathway; *CTX,* chemotaxis; *CVD,* collagen vascular disease; *encaps bact,* encapsulated bacteria; *IC,* immune complex, *MPGN,* membranoproliferative glomerulonephritis; *PLD,* partial lipodystrophy; *PMN,* polymorphonuclear neutrophil; *RBC,* red blood cells; *SBA,* serum bactericidal activity; *XL,* X-linked.

CONNECTIVE TISSUE FIBRILLAR PROTEINS HERITABLE DISORDERS

Connective tissue fibrillar proteins hereditable disorders
ICD-9CM # 710.9

TABLE 2-47   Heritable Disorders of Connective Tissue Fibrillar Proteins

DISORDER	INCIDENCE PER 100,000 BIRTHS	GENETIC ABNORMALITY	MAJOR CLINICAL MANIFESTATIONS
Abnormalities of Fibrous Proteins			
Osteogenesis imperfecta	~5	Mutations alter ability of α_1 or α_2 chains of type I collagen to be secreted, to form fibrils, or to be mineralized	Blue sclerae; thin, easily fractured bones; short stature; defective teeth and hearing loss common
Ehlers-Danlos syndrome	~20		
Classical type		α_1 and α_2 chains of type V collagen	Hyperextensible skin and joints
Hypermobility type		Unknown	Same as in classical type
Vascular type		α_1 chain of type III collagen	Thin, translucent skin; typical facies; arterial, intestinal, and uterine rupture; easy bruising
Kyphoscoliosis type		Lysyl hydroxyl deficiency	Severe muscle hypotaxia at birth; progressive scoliosis; rupture of ocular globe
Arthrocholasia type		Processing of α_1 and α_2 chains of type I collagen	Recurrent joint subluxations; congenital hip displacement
Dermatosparaxis type		N-terminal peptidase of type I collagen	Severe skin fragility; sagging redundant skin
Others			
Marfan's syndrome	~10	Abnormal synthesis, secretion, or accumulation of fibrillin I, a major microfibril component of elastic tissue and the zonular fibrils of the lens	Tall stature, long fingers and toes (arachnodactyly), long arms and legs (dolichostenomelia); inward displacement of sternum (pectus excavatum); dislocation of lens (ectopia lentis); lax joints; aortic dilatation, dissection, and rupture
Pseudoxanthoma elasticum	~0.6	Unknown; causes increased calcification and disruption of elastin	Redundant, lax, inelastic skin on face, neck, axilla, abdomen, and groin; hypertension; coronary and cerebral artery occlusion; gastrointestinal and urinary tract bleeding

From Andreoli TE (ed): *Cecil essentials of medicine,* ed 5, Philadelphia, 2001, WB Saunders.

CONSTIPATION

Constipation
ICD-9CM # 564.0

BOX 2-64   Constipation

Intestinal obstruction
  Fecal impaction
  GI neoplasm
  Gallstone ileus
  Adhesions
  Volvulus
  Intussusception
  Inflammatory bowel disease
  Diverticular disease
  Strangulated femoral hernia
  Tuberculous stricture
  Ameboma
  Hematoma of bowel wall secondary to trauma or anticoagulants
Poor dietary habits: insufficient bulk in diet, inadequate fluid intake

Change from daily routine: travel, hospital admission, physical inactivity
Acute abdominal conditions: renal colic, salpingitis, biliary colic, appendicitis
Hypercalcemia or hypokalemia, uremia
Irritable bowel syndrome, pregnancy, anorexia nervosa, depression
Painful anal conditions: hemorrhoids, fissure, stricture
Decreased intestinal peristalsis: old age, spinal cord injuries, myxedema, diabetes, multiple sclerosis, parkinsonism, and other neurologic diseases
Drugs: codeine, morphine, antacids with aluminum, verapamil, anticonvulsants, anticholinergics, disopyramide, cholestyramine, iron supplements
Hirschsprung's disease, meconium ileus, congenital atresia in infants

CORNIFICATION DISORDERS

TABLE 2-48 **Characteristics of More Common Disorders of Cornification**

TYPE	INHERITANCE PATTERN	ONSET	CUTANEOUS FEATURES	ASSOCIATIONS	COMMENTS
Ichthyosis vulgaris	AD	3-12 mo	Fine white scales, especially legs Palmoplantar keratoderma Seasonal variation	Atopy	Decreased granular layers and filaggrin protein
X-linked ichthyosis	X-LR	0-3 mo	Brown, adherent scales "Dirty neck" Usually normal	Corneal opacities May have genital defect	Deficiency of steroid sulfatase Increased epidermal cholesterol sulfate
Classic lamellar ichthyosis	AR	Usually birth; collodion	Large, platelike dark scales Ectropion, alopecia		Deficiency of transglutaminase I
Nonbullous congenital ichthyosiform erythroderma	AR	Usually birth; collodion	Fine, white scales Overlying variable erythema Mild ectropion Alopecia		
Bullous congenital ichthyosiform erythroderma	AD	Birth	Superficial blisters, especially in infancy Verrucous scaling, specifically at joints	Pyogenic infections	Epidermolytic hyperkeratosis on biopsy Keratin 1,2e,10 mutations
Erythrokeratoderma variabilis	AD	Up to 3 yr	Erythematous plaques Hyperkeratotic polycyclic plaques		Connexon gene GJB3
Sjögren-Larsson syndrome	AR	Birth or infancy	Resembles nonbullous congenital ichthyosiform erythroderma	Spasticity Retardation Retinal degeneration Speech defects Seizures	Defect in fatty alcohol cycle
Chrondrodysplasia punctata	AR AD X-D	Birth	Scaling plaques, overlying whorls, erythema, clears in first 6 months Residual follicular atrophoderma, cicatricial alopecia	Cataracts Shortened femora, humeri Epiphyseal stippling, other skeletal changes	
Netherton's syndrome	AR	Usually birth	Serpiginous, double edge scale (ichthyosis linearis circumflexa) Congenital ichthyosiform erythroderma Short, brittle hair (trichorrhexis invaginata)	Atopy	
Ichthyosis, brittle hair, impaired intelligence, decreased fertility, short stature (IBIDS) syndrome	AR	Birth, early infancy	Resembles nonbullous congenital ichthyosiform erythroderma Hypoplastic nails Brittle hair with trichothiodystrophy	Retardation Decreased fertility Short stature	May be photosensitive (PIBIDS)

From Callen JP (ed): *Color atlas of dermatology,* ed 2, Philadelphia, 2000, WB Saunders.
AD, Autosomal dominant; *AR,* autosomal recessive; *X-D,* X-linked, dominant; *X-LR,* X-linked, recessive.

COUGH

Cough
ICD-9CM # 786.2

BOX 2-65   Cough

Infectious process (viral, bacterial)
Postinfectious
"Smoker's cough"
Rhinitis (allergic, vasomotor, postinfectious)
Asthma
Exposure to irritants (noxious fumes, smoke, cold air)
Drug-induced (especially ACE inhibitors, β-blockers)
GERD
Interstitial lung disease
Lung neoplasms
Lymphomas, mediastinal neoplasms

Bronchiectasis
Cardiac (CHF, pulmonary edema, mitral stenosis, pericardial inflammation)
Recurrent aspiration
Inflammation of larynx, pleura, diaphragm, mediastinum
Cystic fibrosis
Anxiety
Other: pulmonary embolism, foreign body inhalation, aortic aneurysm, Zenker's diverticulum, osteophytes

ACE, Angiotensin converting enzyme; *CHF,* congestive heart failure; *GERD,* gastroesophageal reflux disease.

CRANIAL NERVE SYNDROMES, INFECTIOUS CAUSES

Cranial nerve syndromes, infectious causes
ICD-9CM # 951.9

TABLE 2-49   Cranial Nerve Syndromes

NERVE	FUNCTIONS	DISTRIBUTION	NEURONAL LOCATION	PERIPHERAL NERVES OR DIVISIONS	SIGNS OF PERIPHERAL NERVE DYSFUNCTION	COMMON INFECTIOUS CAUSES OF FINDINGS
III *Oculomotor*	Somatic motor	Superior, inferior, and medial rectus muscles Inferior oblique muscle Levator of lid	Brain stem	Oculomotor	*Abducted eye at rest* *Inability to rotate eye up, down, or medially* *Ptosis*	*Herpes zoster (gasserian)* *Meningitis* *Mononeuritis* *Cavernous sinus syndrome*
	Visceral motor	Sphincter pupillae Ciliary body			*Dilated nonreactive pupil* *Paralysis of accommodation*	
IV *Trochlear*	Motor	Superior oblique muscle	Brain stem	Trochlear	*Extortion of eye* *Weak downward gaze*	*Herpes zoster (gasserian)* *Meningitis* *Cavernous sinus syndrome*
V *Trigeminal*	Sensory	Skin: face, scalp (anterior two thirds) Mucosa: nose, mouth, cornea, conjunctiva	Gasserian ganglion	Ophthalmic n. Maxillary n. Mandibular n.	*Pain*	*Herpes zoster* *Petrositis* *Cavernous sinus syndrome*
	Motor	Masseter muscles Pterygoid muscles	Midpons	Mandibular n.	*Trismus*	*Central:* tetanus *Local:* adjacent inflammation
VI *Abducens*	Motor	External rectus muscles	Brain stem	Abducens	*Paralysis of abduction* *Partially abducted eye at rest*	*Herpes zoster (gasserian)* *Meningitis* *Mononeuritis* *Cavernous sinus syndrome* *Petrositis*
VII *Facial*	Sensory	Tongue (anterior two thirds): taste Ear (anterior wall, external auditory canal): all sensations	Geniculate ganglion	Nervus intermedius and branches Lingual n. Mandibular n.	*Loss of taste on hemitongue*	*Herpes zoster (Ramsay Hunt syndrome)*
	Secretomotor	Lacrimal gland Sublingual glands Submaxillary glands	Brain stem	Chorda tympani n.	*Reduced lacrimation* *Reduced salivary mucus*	*Herpes zoster (Ramsay Hunt syndrome)*

From Gorbach SL: *Infectious diseases,* ed 2, Philadelphia, 1998, WB Saunders.

TABLE 2-49   Cranial Nerve Syndromes—cont'd

NERVE	FUNCTIONS	DISTRIBUTION	NEURONAL LOCATION	PERIPHERAL NERVES OR DIVISIONS	SIGNS OF PERIPHERAL NERVE DYSFUNCTION	COMMON INFECTIOUS CAUSES OF FINDINGS
	Motor	Facial muscles Stylomastoid muscle Posterior belly, diagastric muscle Stapedius muscle	Brain stem (adjacent to VI n. nuclei)	Facial n. and branches	*Facial palsy or paralysis Eyelids will not close, eye rolls up Creaseless brows Recovery: weeks to months Late complications Hemifacial spasm Crocodile tears*	Otitis media, mastoiditis *Bell palsy pattern* (no vesicles) *of mononeuritis or bilateral neuritis* Brucellosis Cat scratch disease Human immunodeficiency virus infection Lyme borreliosis Relapsing fever
VIII *Cochleovestibular*	Sensory	Spiral organ of Corti Semicircular canal Saccule Utricle	Spiral ganglion (in cochlea) Scarpa vestibular ganglion (internal auditory meatus)	Cochlear n. Vestibular n.	*Deafness Vertigo Nystagmus Absent response to caloric stimulation*	*Otitis media* Meningitis Mastoiditis *Mastoiditis Meningitis*
IX *Glossopharyngeal*	Sensory Secretory	Tonsils, soft palate, posterior pharynx Pharyngeal mucosa	Petrosal ganglion Superior ganglion Medulla	Glossopharyngeal n.	*Anesthetic posterior pharynx Palatal paralysis (deviation) Hoarseness Dysphagia*	*Herpes zoster* (rare) *Herpes zoster* (rare) *Meningitis*
	Motor	Pharyngeal striated muscle	Medulla		*Weakness upper trapezoid and sternomastoid*	*Skull base infections*
X *Vagus*	Sensory	Ear (posterior wall of canal, concha and pinna) Pharynx, larynx, trachea, esophagus	Jugular ganglion Nodose ganglion	Posterior auricular n. Pharyngeal branch of vagus n.	*Decreased sensation in auditory canal and back of pinna Loss of gag reflex (affected side)*	*Herpes zoster* (infrequent)
	Somatic motor	Thoracic and abdominal viscera	Medulla	Thoracoabdominal branch of vagus n.	*Palatal paralysis: complete Loss of curtain movement of lateral pharyngeal walls*	*Herpes zoster* (infrequent) *Skull base infections*
		Larynx, pharynx, and palate (striated muscle)		Pharyngeal branch of vagus n.	*Nasal regurgitation Voice nasal, hoarse Abducted vocal cord*	
	Visceral motor	Heart, other thoracic organs Abdominal viscera	Medulla	Thoracoabdominal branch of vagus n.		
XI *Accessory*	Motor	Sternocleidomastoid muscle Trapezius muscle	High cervical cord (C1-5)	Accessory n.	*Partial paralysis: trapezius and sternocleidomastoid muscles Wing scapula*	*Skull base infections*
XII *Hypoglossal*	Motor	Tongue muscles Genioglossus Styloglossus Hypoglossus	Medulla	Hypoglossal n.	*Hemiparalysis of tongue (deviation to affected side) Progression to wrinkling, atrophy, fibrillary twitches*	*Basilar meningitis* *Skull base infections*

From Gorbach SL: *Infectious diseases*, ed 2, Philadelphia, 1998, WB Saunders.

CUTANEOUS ERUPTIONS, DRUG-INDUCED

Cutaneous eruptions, drug-induced
ICD-9CM # 782.1 Skin eruption, nonspecific

BOX 2-66 Drug-Induced Cutaneous Eruptions

Acneiform eruptions
  ACTH
  Bromides
  Corticosteroids
  Cyanocobalamin (vitamin B$_{12}$)
  Dactinomycin
  Iodides
  Isoniazid (INH)
  Lithium
  Oral contraceptives
  Phenytoin
Alopecia
  Allopurinol
  Amphetamines
  Anticoagulants (coumarin,
    heparin)
  Antithyroid drugs (carbimazole,
    thiouracil)
  Chemotherapeutic agents
  Heavy metals
  Hypocholesterolemic drugs
  Levodopa
  Oral contraceptives
  Propranolol
  Retinoids
Eczematous eruptions (topical
  sensitizer/systemic medication)
  Ampicillin
  Chlorbutanol/chloral hydrate
  Diphenhydramine (Caladryl/
    Benadryl)
  Disulfiram (Antabuse)
  Ethylenediamine/aminophylline,
    antihistamines
  Iodine/iodides
  Neomycin sulfate/streptomycin,
    kanamycin
  Paraamino aromatic benzenes/
    paraaminobenzoic acid, sulfon-
    amides, tolbutamide
  Penicillin
Erythema multiforme
  Allopurinol
  Barbiturates
  Chlorpropamide
  Griseofulvin
  Hydantoins
  Nonsteroidal antiinflammatory
    agents (meclofenamate,
    piroxicam, sulindac)
  Penicillin
  Phenothiazines

Sulfonamides
Thiazide diuretics
Erythema nodosum
  Bromides
  Codeine
  Iodides
  Oral contraceptives
  Penicillin
  Salicylates
  Sulfonamides
Exanthematous eruptions
  Allopurinol
  Antibiotics
  Anticonvulsants
  Barbiturates
  Benzodiazepines
  Captopril
  Chlorpropamide
  Gold salts
  Isoniazid
  Nonsteroidal antiinflammatory
    agents (meclofenamate,
    naproxen, phenylbutazone,
    piroxicam)
  Paraaminosalicylic acid
  Penicillamine
  Phenothiazines
  Quinidine
  Thiazide diuretics
Exfoliative dermatitis
  Allopurinol
  Carbamazepine
  Gold salts
  Hydantoins
  Isoniazid
  Paraaminosalicylic acid
  Phenindione
  Phenylbutazone
  Streptomycin
  Sulfonamides
Fixed drug eruptions
  Allopurinol
  Barbiturates
  Chlordiazepoxide
  Nonsteroidal antiinflammatory
    agents (naproxen, phenacetin,
    phenylbutazone, salicylates,
    sulindac, tolmetin)
  Phenolphthalein
  Sulfonamides
  Tetracycline

Leukocytoclastic vasculitis
  Allopurinol
  Cimetidine
  Gold salts
  Hydantoins
  Nonsteroidal antiinflammatory
    agents (ibuprofen, meclofena-
    mate, piroxicam)
  Phenothiazine
  Sulfonamides
  Thiazide diuretics
  Thiouracils
Lichenoid and lichen planus–like
  eruptions
  Antimalarials (chloroquine,
    hydroxychloroquine, quinacrine)
  Captopril
  Chlordiazepoxide
  Hydroxyurea
  Paraaminosalicylic acid
  Penicillamine
  Quinidine
  Thiazide diuretics
Photosensitivity eruptions
  Griseofulvin
  Nonsteroidal antiinflammatory
    agents
  Phenothiazines
  Sulfonamides
  Sulfonylureas
  Tetracycline
  Thiazide diuretics
Toxic epidermal necrolysis
  Allopurinol
  Aminopenicillins
  Anticonvulsant agents
  Imidazole antifungal agents
  Nonsteroidal antiinflammatory
    agents (oxicam derivatives)
  Sulfonamides
  Tetracycline
Urticaria
  Enzymes (L-asparaginase)
  Indomethacin
  Opiates
  Penicillin and related antibiotics
  Salicylates
  Sulfonamides
  X-ray contrast media

From Stein JH (ed): *Internal medicine*, ed 5, St Louis, 1998, Mosby.

CUTANEOUS SIGNS OF INTERNAL MALIGNANCY

Cutaneous signs of internal malignancy
ICD-9CM # 709.9 Skin disorder
709.9 Skin lesion

TABLE 2-50 Cutaneous Reactions to Internal Malignancy

DISEASE	HISTORY	PHYSICAL	MALIGNANCY
Acanthosis nigricans	Thickening of skin on hands and intertriginous areas	Hyperpigmented, velvety hyperkeratotic changes	Gastric carcinoma
Acquired hypertrichosis lanuginosa	Increased hair on face or other areas	Fine hypertrichosis; face common	Lymphoma
Acquired ichthyosis	Thickening, scaling on palms, soles, or other areas	Hyperkeratotic changes	Lymphoma
Bazex's syndrome (hyperkeratosis paraneoplastica)	Thickening of skin on nose, hands, feet	Focal hyperkeratotic plaques	Squamous cell carcinoma in the upper respiratory tract
Dermatomyositis	Muscle weakness; photoaccentuated dermatitis	Erythema, telangiectasia, atrophy, Gottron's papules, heliotrope rash (eyelids)	Multiple associated malignancies have been reported
Erythema gyratum repens	Rare; pruritus, scaling	Characteristic swirls of erythema, scaling	Lung carcinoma
Erythroderma	Rapid-onset total erythema	Erythema, some scaling	Cutaneous T-cell lymphoma
Flushing	Episodic head and neck flushing	Erythema (transient)	Carcinoid
Necrolytic migratory erythema (NME)	Periorificial shallow erosions; sore tongue; weight loss	Superficial blisters and erosions, perioral, perineal; glossitis	Glucagonoma
Herpes zoster	Pain and blisters; pain may precede lesions by 72 hr	Dermatomal; vesicles, papules, pustules	Any malignancy; immunosuppression
Leser-Trélat sign (multiple seborrheic keratoses)	Rapid onset of large numbers of asymptomatic small lesions	Multiple (>100) small to medium seborrheic keratoses	Breast carcinoma; GI carcinomas
Migratory thrombophlebitis	Painful swelling on an extremity; occasionally generalized hypercoagulability	Firm, linear, cordlike lesions involving superficial vessels	Visceral carcinomas, prostate carcinoma
Pruritus	Total body pruritus; sometimes worse after shower	No primary skin findings	Multiple malignancies; lymphomas
Pyoderma gangrenosum	Enlarging painful ulcers	Pustules, ulcerations; erythematous rolled edge	Leukemia, lymphoma; adenocarcinoma
Sweet's syndrome (acute febrile neutrophilic dermatosis)	High fever; malaise, arthralgias; skin rash	Erythematous nodules, plaques; lesions are tender; arthritis	Hematologic; AML most common
Urticaria	Pruritic hives	Urticaria	Multiple

From Noble J (ed): *Primary care medicine*, ed 3, St Louis, 2001, Mosby.

CYANOSIS

Cyanosis
ICD-9CM # 782.5 Cyanosis NOS
          770.8 Cyanosis, newborn

BOX 2-67   Cyanosis

Congenital heart disease with right-to-left shunt
Pulmonary embolism
Hypoxia
Pulmonary edema
Pulmonary disease (oxygen diffusion and alveolar venti-
   lation abnormalities)

Hemoglobinopathies
Decreased cardiac output
Vasospasm
Arterial obstruction
Pulmonary AV fistulas

DELIRIUM

BOX 2-68   Differential Diagnosis of Delirium

Toxic Etiologies

Steroids
Lithium
Salicylates
Anticholinergics
Sympathomimetics (cocaine, amphetamines)
Phencyclidine
Mushrooms containing muscimol and ibutinic acid:
   Amanita pantherina, Amanita muscaria
Monoamine oxidase inhibitors
Solvents
Carbon monoxide
Sedative-hypnotic withdrawal

Metabolic Etiologies

Sodium disorders
Hypoglycemia
Hypercarbia
Hypoxia, severe anemia
Calcium disorders

Uremia
Thyrotoxicosis
Hepatic encephalopathy
Hypertensive encephalopathy
Shock
Sepsis

Infectious and Inflammatory Etiologies

Meningoencephalitis
Meningitis
Vasculitis

Neurologic and Neurosurgical Abnormalities

Cerebrovascular accident
Subarachnoid hemorrhage
Subdural and epidural hematoma
Frontal contusion
Postictal state
Temporal lobe seizures

From Rosen P, Barkin R (eds): *Emergency medicine: concepts and clinical practice,* ed 5, St Louis, 2002, Mosby.

Delirium
ICD-9CM # 780.09 Delirium NOS
          293.0 Acute delirium

DELIRIUM, DIALYSIS PATIENT

Delirium, dialysis patient
ICD-9CM # 293.0 Acute delirium
293.9 Encephalopathy from dialysis

BOX 2-69   Differential Diagnosis of Altered Mental Status in Dialysis Patients

Structural

Cerebrovascular accident (particularly hemorrhage)
Subdural hematoma
Intracerebral abscess
Brain tumor

Metabolic

Disequilibrium syndrome
Uremia
Drug effects
Meningitis
Hypertensive encephalopathy
Hypotension
Postictal state
Hypernatremia or hyponatremia
Hypercalcemia
Hypermagnesemia
Hypoglycemia
Severe hyperglycemia
Hypoxemia
Dialysis dementia

From Rosen P (ed): *Emergency medicine,* ed 4, St Louis, 1998, Mosby.

DEMYELINATING DISEASES

Demyelinating diseases
ICD-9CM # 341.9

BOX 2-70   Demyelinating Diseases

Multiple sclerosis
  Relapsing and chronic progressive forms
  Acute multiple sclerosis
  Neuromyelitis optica (Devic's disease)
Diffuse cerebral sclerosis
  Schilder's encephalitis periaxialis diffusa
  Balo's concentric sclerosis
Acute disseminated encephalomyelitis
  After measles, chickenpox, rubella, influenza,
    mumps
  After rabies or smallpox vaccination
Necrotizing hemorrhagic encephalitis
  Hemorrhagic leukoencephalitis
Leukodystrophies
  Krabbe's globoid leukodystrophy
  Metachromatic leukodystrophy
  Adrenoleukodystrophy
  Adrenomyeloneuropathy
  Pelizaeus-Merzbacher leukodystrophy
  Canavan's disease
  Alexander's disease

From Wiederholt WC: *Neurology for non-neurologists,* ed 4, Philadelphia, 2000, WB Saunders.

DEMENTIA

Dementia
ICD-9CM # 290.10 Presenile dementia
290.0 Senile dementia
290.40 Arteriosclerotic dementia NOS
331.0 Alzheimer's dementia

TABLE 2-51 **Causes of Dementia**

DISEASE	LABORATORY AIDS TO DIAGNOSIS	DISEASE	LABORATORY AIDS TO DIAGNOSIS
Primary Neurologic Disease		**Toxic Encephalopathies**	
Alzheimer's disease and senile dementia	—	Alcohol-related dementia	Alcohol level, aspartate aminotransferase, mean corpuscular volume (MCV)
Pick's disease	CT or MRI, SPECT		
Huntington's disease	CT or MRI	Heavy metals (lead, arsenic, mercury)	24-hr urine collection
Progressive supranuclear palsy	—	Dialysis dementia	—
Olivopontocerebellar degeneration	MRI	Psychiatric drugs	Blood levels where available
Parkinsonism	—	Barbiturates, bromides, benzodiazepines, phenothiazines, haloperidol, lithium, especially certain combinations (e.g., thioridazine/lithium, haloperidol/methyldopa)	Urine toxicology screening
Brain tumors	CT with contrast or MRI		
Multiple sclerosis	CSF γ-globulin, oligoclonal banding, basic myelin protein, evoked potentials		
Wilson's disease	Serum ceruloplasmin, urinary copper, slit-lamp examination for Kayser-Fleischer rings	Drugs used in general medicine	
		Analgesics, antihypertensives, antidiabetic agents, digitalis preparations, cimetidine, methyldopa, propranolol, reserpine, OTC medications	
Ceroid lipofuscinosis	Brain biopsy		
Vascular Disease			
Multiinfarct dementia	MRI	**Infectious-Inflammatory**	
Lacunar state	CT or MRI	General paralysis	Blood and CSF tests for syphilis
Binswanger encephalopathy	CT or MRI		
Cerebral vasculitis (as in systemic lupus)	Erythrocyte sedimentation rate, specific antibodies (e.g., antinuclear antibody)	Chronic basilar meningitis (with/without hydrocephalus)	—
Traumatic CNS Lesions		Fungal (especially cryptococcal)	CSF cryptococcal antigen and fungal cultures
Multiple contusions	MRI	Syphilitic	Blood and CSF tests for syphilis
Dementia pugilistica ("punch-drunk" syndrome)	—	Sarcoid	Angiotensin-converting enzyme level, lymph node biopsy
Chronic subdural hematoma	CT or MRI		
Normal-Pressure Hydrocephalus		Carcinomatous-leukemic	CSF cytology
Idiopathic or following meningitis or subarachnoid hemorrhage	CT or MRI, isotope cisternography, high-volume lumbar puncture	Whipple disease of brain	Brain biopsy, periodic acid–Schiff staining of CSF cells, small bowel biopsy
Seizures		Creutzfeldt-Jakob disease	EEG, brain biopsy
Nonconvulsive status	EEG	Brain abscess	CT with contrast or MRI
Metabolic Disturbances		Progressive multifocal leukoencephalopathy	MRI
Anoxia-hypoxia	Arterial blood gases	Limbic encephalitis	Search for occult carcinoma (usually small cell carcinoma of lung)
Chronic hypercapnia	Arterial blood gases		
Hyperammonemic encephalopathy	Liver function studies, serum-ammonia, CSF glutamine	AIDS encephalopathy	HIV antibodies
Chronic electrolyte-calcium or acid-base imbalance	Serum Na, K, Cl, CO_2, Ca, pH, alkaline phosphatase	**Psychiatric**	
Endocrine dysfunction, hypothyroidism, apathetic form of hyperthyroidism, Cushing's disease, Addison's disease	Thyroid-stimulating hormone, timed serum cortisol levels	Pseudodementia of depression	Neuropsychologic testing Dexamethasone suppression test
Vitamin B_{12} deficiency	Serum B_{12} level, methylmalonic acid	Sensory deprivation	Hearing/vision testing
Thiamine or niacin deficiency	—		
Azotemia	Serum creatinine, blood urea nitrogen		

From Noble J (ed): *Primary care medicine*, ed 3, St Louis, 2001, Mosby.
AIDS, Acquired immunodeficiency syndrome; *CSF*, cerebrospinal fluid; *CT*, computed tomography; *EEG*, electroencephalography; *HIV*, human immunodeficiency virus; *MRI*, magnetic resonance imaging; *SPECT*, single photon emission computed tomography.

DERMATITIS

Dermatitis
ICD-9CM # 692.9 Dermatitis, unspecified

TABLE 2-52   Differential Diagnosis of Dermatitis

DIAGNOSIS	HISTORY	PHYSICAL EXAMINATION	LABORATORY	MANAGEMENT

Atopic dermatitis	Onset by age 5 yr
	Family Hx of atopy
	Pruritus
	Exacerbating factors
	Coexistent hay fever, asthma
		Flexural distribution
		Lichenification
		Papules, erythema
		Pustules if secondary *Staphylococcus*
			Routine: none
			Consider:
			  Culture/pustule
			  IgE
				Topical corticosteroids
				Control environment
				Antihistamines
				Emollients

Contact dermatitis Irritant type	Predisposing Hx of atopy Frequent water exposure Solvents Job description	Hands commonly Erythema, scale, fissuring	None	Topical steroid ointments Protect from wet exposures Gloves Emollients

Allergic type	Rapid onset
	Pruritus
	Exposures:
	  Plants
	  Cosmetics
		Erythema, vesicles, oozing
		Location corresponds to exposure
			None	Wet to dry dressings
				Topical or systemic corticosteroids
				Identify and avoid allergen

Stasis dermatitis	Gradual onset Distal legs Previous history Varicosities, leg trauma, etc.	Erythema Pigmentation Edema Fibrosis	None	Acute: steroid ointments Long-term: compression, leg elevation, emollient ointments
Xerotic dermatitis	Winter Low humidity Frequent baths Soap use Pretibial common	Patchy, erythema, scale Extensor areas Spares folds	None	Decrease soap and water exposure Liberal use of thick emollients, especially after bath Steroids short-term prn
Dyshidrosis	Pruritic papules and vesicles on hands Recurrent	Papules and small vesicles on hands	None Exclude fungus with KOH Exclude allergen	Systemic or topical steroids Antibiotics
Nummular dermatitis	Gradual onset Pruritic Frequent history Exposure to drying	Round patches Erythema Scaling occasional Oozing occasional	None KOH to exclude fungus	Steroid ointments Tar cream, gel Ultraviolet light

From Noble J (ed): *Primary care medicine*, ed 3, St Louis, 2001, Mosby.
Hx, History; *KOH*, potassium hydroxide.

DIARRHEA, CLASSIFICATION

TABLE 2-53   Classification of Diarrhea

TYPE	MECHANISM	EXAMPLES	CHARACTERISTICS
Secretory	Increased secretion and/or decreased absorption of Na^+ and Cl^-	Cholera Vasoactive intestinal peptide–secreting tumor Bile salt enteropathy Fatty acid-induced diarrhea	Large volume, watery diarrhea No gas or pus No solute gap Little or no response to fasting
Osmotic	Nonabsorbable molecules in gut lumen	Lactose intolerance (lactase deficiency) Generalized malabsorption (particularly carbohydrates) Mg^{2+}-containing laxatives	Watery stool, no blood or pus Improves with fasting Stool may contain fat globules or meat fibers and may have an increased solute gap
Inflammatory	Destruction of mucosa Impaired absorption Outpouring of blood, mucus	Ulcerative colitis Shigellosis Amebiasis	Small frequent stools with blood and pus Fever Variable
Decreased absorptive surface	Impaired reabsorption of electrolytes and/or nutrients Increased motility with decreased time for absorption of electrolytes and/or nutrients	Bowel resection Enteric fistula Hyperthyroidism Irritable bowel syndrome Scleroderma	Variable Malabsorption
Motility disorder	Decreased motility with bacterial overgrowth	Diabetic diarrhea	

From Andreoli TE (ed): *Cecil essentials of medicine,* ed 5, Philadelphia, 2001, WB Saunders.

DIARRHEA, DRUG-INDUCED

Diarrhea, drug-induced
ICD-9CM # 787.91 Diarrhea NOS
787.91 Diarrhea, noninfectious

BOX 2-71   Drugs Associated with Diarrhea

Laxatives (e.g., cascara sagrada, bisacodyl, phenol-
  phthalein, ricinoleic acid, lactulose)
Magnesium-containing antacids
Antibiotics: clindamycin, lincomycin, ampicillin,
  cephalosporin; may be associated with *Clostridium diffi-*
  cile toxin and pseudomembranes
Antiarrhythmic drugs: quinidine, propranolol
Digitalis

Antihypertensive drugs: guanethidine, propranolol
Potassium supplements
Artificial sweeteners: sorbitol, mannitol
Chenodeoxycholic acid
Cholestyramine*
Sulfasalazine
Anticoagulants

From Stein JH (ed): *Internal medicine,* ed 5, St Louis, 1998, Mosby.
*In patients with extensive ileal resection, bile salt depletion can result in malabsorption and diarrhea.

DIARRHEA IN PATIENTS WITH AIDS

BOX 2-72   Causes of Diarrhea in Patients with AIDS

FREQUENCY	ORGANISM
Most common	*Cryptosporidium* Cytomegalovirus
Common	*Entamoeba histolytica* (probably commensal, not causative) *Giardia lamblia* *Mycobacterium avium-intracellulare* *Salmonella* spp., especially *tymphimurium* *Aeromonas hydrophila* Microsporidia Astrovirus/picornavirus *Clostridium difficile*
Less common	*Campylobacter jejuni* Viruses—herpes simplex, rotovirus, adenovirus, Norwalk agent *Cyclospora*
Rare	*Isospora belli* *Enteromonas hominis* *Strongyloides stercoralis* *Blastocystis hominis* *Shigella* spp. *Yersinia enterocolitica*

From Rosen P, Barkin R (eds): *Emergency medicine: concepts and clinical practice,* ed 5, St Louis, 2002, Mosby.

Diarrhea in patients with AIDS
ICD-9CM # 007.4 Cryptosporidial
009.2 Infectious

II

DIARRHEA, OSMOTIC

Diarrhea, osmotic
ICD-9CM # 787.91

BOX 2-73   Some Causes of Osmotic Diarrhea

Laxatives Containing Poorly Absorbed Anion

Sodium phosphate (Phospho-soda)

Laxatives Containing Poorly Absorbed Cation

Magnesium hydroxide (Philips Milk of Magnesia), magnesium citrate (Citrate of Magnesia)

Disaccharidase Deficiency

Lactose intolerance

Poorly Absorbed Carbohydrate

Lactulose, sorbitol ("sugar free" gum), mannitol, congenital glucose-galactose or fructose malabsorption

General Malabsorption Syndromes

From Andreoli TE (ed): *Cecil essentials of medicine,* ed 5, Philadelphia, 2001, WB Saunders.

DIARRHEA, SECRETORY

Diarrhea, secretory
ICD-9CM # 787.91

BOX 2-74   Some Causes of Secretory Diarrhea

Infections

Bacterial toxins (enterotoxigenic *Escherichia coli*)

Stimulant Laxatives

Ricinoleic acid (castor oil), senna (Senekot), bisacodyl (Dulcolax)

Bile Acid and Fatty Acid Malabsorption

Intestinal Resection

Neuroendocrine Tumors

Zollinger-Ellison syndrome (gastrin)

Carcinoid syndrome (serotonin, substance P, prostaglandins)

Medullary carcinoma of the thyroid (calcitonin, prostaglandins)

Pancreatic cholera syndrome (vasoactive intestinal peptide)

From Andreoli TE (ed): *Cecil essentials of medicine,* ed 5, Philadelphia, 2001, WB Saunders.

DIPLOPIA, BINOCULAR

Diplopia, binocular
ICD-9CM # 368.2

TABLE 2-54   Disorders That May Cause Binocular Diplopia

ADDITIONAL HISTORY	KEY EXAM FEATURES
Third Nerve Palsy Third nerve palsy may be associated with aneurysm, microvascular infarct (particularly with diabetes or hypertension), tumor, trauma, and uncal herniation. Some patients may experience pain.	A droopy eyelid is seen on the involved side. The pupil may be fixed and dilated. If the pupil is involved, the cause of the disorder is probably an aneurysm (of the posterior communicating artery). If the pupil is not involved, microvascular ischemia is usually the cause. Because the third nerve controls superior, inferior, and medial movements, the eye is usually pointed down and out.
Fourth Nerve Palsy The fourth nerve controls vertical eye movement, so fourth nerve palsy causes vertical diplopia. Some patients report difficulty reading but may have no symptoms. This palsy may occur with trauma, microvascular infarct (particularly with diabetes or hypertension), tumor, and aneurysm.	The involved eye is higher than the uninvolved eye. The deviation may be so slight that detecting the difference on gross examination is difficult. Patients may have a head tilt that eliminates the double vision.
Sixth Nerve Palsy The sixth nerve controls lateral eye movements. Patients therefore complain of horizontal diplopia. Sixth nerve palsy may be associated with trauma, microvascular infarct (from diabetes or hypertension), increased intracranial pressure, temporal arteritis, cavernous sinus tumor, and aneurysm.	An inability to move the eye outward with the involved eye pointing in (esotropia) is significant.
Decompensated Strabismus The patient may report a history of strabismus or previous eye muscle surgery.	Horizontal (esotropia/exotropia) or vertical deviation may be present depending on the muscles involved.
Myasthenia Gravis Patients may have the typical symptoms of myasthenia gravis, including fatigue, weakness, and difficulty swallowing, chewing, and breathing; these symptoms may fluctuate during the day. The double vision also tends to fluctuate during the day and worsens with fatigue.	Droopy eyelids that become worse toward the end of the day or when the individual is fatigued are significant. With sustained upgaze, the droopy eyelids may worsen. Systemic edrophonium chloride (Tensilon) often improves the eyelid droop and/or double vision. Weakness of the facial muscles and limb muscles may occur, but no pupil abnormalities are present.
Thyroid Eye Disease Eye disease is usually associated with hyperthyroidism; however, patients may have a normal-functioning thyroid gland. The eye disease may be present even when the systemic disease is under good control.	Unilateral or bilateral proptosis may be present, and the conjunctiva can be injected or filled with fluid (chemosis). Eye movement may be limited, particularly up and out. When the patient looks down slowly, the upper eyelids may lag behind the eye movement such that the superior sclera is visible (lid lag). The proptosis may lead to an inability to fully close the lids, causing dry eye signs and symptoms.
Orbital Pseudotumor Patients report severe pain and redness, usually in one eye.	The conjunctiva is usually injected, and swelling of the conjunctiva (chemosis) may occur. The eyelids are often red and swollen. Proptosis and restriction of movement in one eye occur, and a palpable orbital mass may be present. The vision in the involved eye may be decreased.
Blow-Out Fracture Blow-out fracture is associated with a history of blunt trauma to the orbit.	Restricted eye movement, particularly in upgaze and/or lateral gaze, is significant. Subcutaneous air (crepitus) and numbness in the distribution of the infraorbital nerve, which involves the cheek and upper lip, are possible.

From Palay D (ed): *Ophthalmology for the primary care physician,* St Louis, 1997, Mosby.

DIZZINESS

Dizziness
ICD-9CM # 780.4 Dizziness NOS
            300.11 Dizziness, hysterical
            306.9 Dizziness, psychogenic

BOX 2-75 Differential Diagnosis of Dizziness

1. Vertigo

ACUTE	RECURRENT	POSITIONAL
Vertebrobasilar event	Ménière's disease	Benign positional vertigo
Toxic (illness or drug)	Migraine	Postinfectious
Infectious	Hypothyroid	Posttrauma
Trauma	Multiple sclerosis	Cervical
Tumor	Seizure	Central causes
Seizure	Syphilis	
	Vertebrobasilar transient ischemic attacks	

2. Presyncope (Impending Faint)

Orthostasis or near syncope
Hyperventilation

3. Imbalance

Medication toxicity
Multiple sensory impairments
Cervical spine disease
Muscle weakness, unstable joints
Neurologic disease (previous stroke, cerebellar degeneration, peripheral neuropathy, myelopathy, parkinsonism)

4. Ill-Defined Lightheadedness

Medications, visual disorders, previous stroke
Hyperventilation, psychiatric disorders
Carbon monoxide exposure

From Yoshikawa TT, Cobbs EL, Brummel-Smith K: *Practical ambulatory geriatrics*, St Louis, 1997, Mosby.

Dysentery and inflammatory enterocolitis
ICD-9CM # 009.2 Dysentery, unspecified
         008.45 Enterocolitis, pseudomembranous
         557.0 Enterocolitis, hemorrhagic

DYSENTERY AND INFLAMMATORY ENTEROCOLITIS

BOX 2-76   **Differential Diagnosis of Acute Dysentery and Inflammatory Enterocolitis**

Specific infectious processes

Bacillary dysentery (*Shigella dysenteriae, Shigella flexneri, Shigella sonnei, Shigella boydii;* invasive *Escherichia coli*)
Campylobacteriosis (*Campylobacter jejuni*)
Amebic dysentery (*Entamoeba histolytica*)
Ciliary dysentery (*Balantidium coli*)
Bilharzial dysentery (*Schistosoma japonicum, Schistosoma mansoni*)
Other parasitic infections (*Trichinella spiralis*)
Vibriosis (*Vibrio parahaemolyticus*)
Salmonellosis (*Salmonella typhimurium*)
Typhoid fever (*Salmonella typhi*)
Enteric fever (*Salmonella choleraesuis, Salmonella paratyphi*)
Yersiniosis (*Yersinia enterocolitica*)
Spirillar dysentery (*Spirillum* spp.)

Proctitis

Gonococcal (*Neisseria gonorrhoeae*)
Herpetic (herpes simplex virus)
Chlamydial (*Chlamydia trachomatis*)
Syphilitic (*Treponema pallidum*)

Other syndromes

Necrotizing enterocolitis of the newborn
Enteritis necroticans
Pseudomembranous enterocolitis (*Clostridium difficile*)
Diverticulitis
Typhlitis

Syndromes without known infectious etiology

Idiopathic ulcerative colitis
Crohn's disease
Radiation enteritis
Ischemic colitis
Allergic enteritis

From Mandell GL: *Mandell, Douglas, and Bennett's principles and practice of infectious diseases,* ed 5, New York, 2000, Churchill Livingstone.

DYSPAREUNIA

BOX 2-77   Dyspareunia

Introital

Vaginismus
Intact or rigid hymen
Clitoral problems
Vulvovaginitis
Vaginal atrophy: hypoestrogen
Vulvar dystrophy
Bartholin or Skene gland infection
Inadequate lubrication
Operative scarring

Midvaginal

Urethritis
Trigonitis
Cystitis
Short vagina
Operative scarring
Inadequate lubrication

Deep

Endometriosis
Pelvic infection
Uterine retroversion
Ovarian pathology
Gastrointestinal
Orthopedic
Abnormal penile size or shape

From Danakas G (ed): *Practical guide to the care of the gynecologic/obstetric patient,* St Louis, 1997, Mosby.

Dyspareunia
ICD-9CM # 625.0   Dyspareunia
608.89 Dyspareunia, male
302.76 Dyspareunia, psychogenic

Dysuria
ICD-9CM # 788.1   Dysuria
306.53 Dysuria, psychogenic

DYSURIA

BOX 2-78   Differential Diagnosis of Dysuria

I. Urinary tract infection
  A. Enterobacteriaceae
  B. Gram-positive organisms
  C. *Chlamydia trachomatis*
  D. *Mycobacterium tuberculosis*
II. Vaginitis
  A. Fungi *(Candida albicans)*
  B. Bacterial
    1. *Gardnerella vaginalis*
      (Haemophilus vaginalis)
    2. *Neisseria gonorrhoeae*
    3. *Treponema pallidum*
      (endourethral chancre)
    4. *Chlamydia trachomatis*
  C. Protozoa *(Trichomonas vaginalis)*

III. Genital infection
  A. Herpes simplex (genitalis)
  B. Condyloma acuminatum
  C. Paraurethral glands
IV. Estrogen deficiency
V. Interstitial cystitis (Hunner's ulcer)
VI. Reiter's syndrome
VII. Chemical irritants
  A. Douches
  B. Deodorant aerosols
  C. Contraceptive jellies
  D. Bubble bath

VIII. Impedance to flow
  A. Urethral caruncle or diverticula
  B. Meatal stenosis or stricture
  C. Transient urethral edema
  D. Chronic fibrosis after trauma
  E. Impaired synergy: bladder contraction and sphincter relaxation
IX. Regional disease
  A. Crohn's disease
  B. Diverticulitis
  C. Cervical radium implant
X. Bladder tumor

From Stein JH (ed): *Internal medicine,* ed 5, St Louis, 1998, Mosby.

EAR INFECTION

Ear infection
ICD-9CM # 380.10 external ear
386.30 inner ear
382.9 middle ear

TABLE 2-55   Ear Infection

A. External ear infection

	ETIOLOGY	CLINICAL FINDINGS	COMMON MICROBIOLOGIC AGENTS	MANAGEMENT
Bacterial Diffuse otitis externa	Swimming; trauma; metabolic disorders (diabetes)	Severe otalgia; tragal tenderness; diffuse inflammation of ear canal	*Pseudomonas; Staphylococcus aureus; Streptococcus; Escherichia coli*	Aural cleansing; topical antibiotic; Burow's solution
Localized otitis externa	Furuncles	Otalgia; otorrhea; localized tenderness; furuncle in outer third of ear canal	*Staphylococcus*	Aural cleansing; topical antibiotic; Burow's solution oral anti-*Staphylococcus*
Malignant otitis externa	Diabetes; immunosuppression	Diffuse external otitis; necrotizing granulation tissue; facial nerve paralysis	*Pseudomonas*	Systemic antibiotic; necrotic tissue debridement
Viral	Unknown	Otalgia; vesicles on ear canal; facial nerve paralysis	Herpes zoster (Ramsay Hunt syndrome); varicella; measles	Analgesics
Fungal	Diabetes; tropical climate	Pruritus; minimal otalgia; black, white, or yellow spores	*Aspergillus; Candida*	Aural cleansing; Burow's solution

B. Middle ear infection

	ETIOLOGY	CLINICAL FINDINGS	COMMON MICROBIOLOGIC AGENTS	MANAGEMENT
Acute suppurative otitis media	Bacterial contamination with possible eustachian tube dysfunction	Bulging or retracted TM; air-fluid level; pulsatile discharge	*H. influenzae; S. pneumoniae; Mycoplasma;* Grp. A strep.; *C. diphtheria;* gram-negative bacilli; parainfluenza virus; RSV	Aural cleansing; oral antibiotic; analgesia
Acute and serous otitis media	Eustachian tube dysfunction; barotrauma; nasopharyngeal tumor	Thickened, retracted TM; gray or amber fluid in middle ear; impaired mobility of TM; conductive hearing loss	Rare	Nasal decongestant autoinflation exercises
Chronic suppurative otitis media	Bacterial contamination	Mucopurulent otorrhea; perforated TM; conductive hearing loss; cholesteatoma	Mixed aerobic and anaerobic flora: *S. aureus; E. coli; Pseudomonas; B. fragilis*	Aural cleansing; topical antibiotic; surgical management

C. Inner ear infection

LABYRINTHITIS	ETIOLOGY	CLINICAL FINDINGS	COMMON MICROBIOLOGIC AGENTS	MANAGEMENT
Viral	Middle ear infection Meningitis	Unilateral inflammation of cochlea; sensorineural hearing loss; vertigo	Mumps	Symptomatic
Bacterial	Acute or chronic otitis media Meningitis	Severe vertigo; nausea; vomiting; hearing loss	Agents causing acute and chronic otitis media	Myringotomy; Intravenous antibiotic; mastoidectomy
Vascular	Occlusion of anteroinferior cerebellar artery or labyrinthine artery	Severe vertigo; hearing loss	Vascular insult	Symptomatic; possibly antiplatelet medications

From Noble J (ed): *Primary care medicine,* ed 3, St Louis, 2001, Mosby.
RSV, Respiratory syncytial virus; *TM,* tympanic membrane.

EARACHE

Earache
ICD-9CM # 388.70 Earache
388.72 Ear pain, referred

TABLE 2-56   Differential Diagnosis of Earache

CONDITION	NATURE OF PATIENT	NATURE OF SYMPTOMS	ASSOCIATED SYMPTOMS	PRECIPITATING AND AGGRAVATING FACTORS	PHYSICAL FINDINGS AND DIAGNOSTIC STUDIES
Otitis media	Children, especially <8 years	Pain is unilateral, deep, and severe	Irritability Restlessness Fever Poor feeding Ear feels full	URI	Tympanic membrane inflamed and bulging Decreased light reflex
Serous otitis media Eustachitis	Children and adults	Not usually painful Unilateral	Decreased hearing Crackling and gurgling sounds	URI	Fluid behind tympanic membrane Tympanic membrane shows decreased mobility Decreased conductive hearing Impedance tympanometry
Otitis externa	Adults Diabetic patients Patients with seborrhea "Ear pickers" Swimmers	Often bilateral			Pain on manipulation of pinna
Otitic barotrauma		Pain may be severe	URI Nasal stuffiness	Worse on airplane descent	Tympanic membrane retracted
Mastoiditis		Pain in and behind ear	Fever Drainage from middle ear >10 days	Otitis media 10-14 days previously	Exquisite pain with pressure on mastoid process Swelling behind ear Radiograph of mastoid
Foreign body Impacted cerumen	Children	Pain or vague discomfort	May impair hearing Recurrent problem		Foreign body or cerumen in ear
Referred otalgia, as with TMJ dysfunction, dental problems, and tumors	Adults Adults (increases with age)	Rarely bilateral TMJ dysfunction intermittent and often worse in morning	Resemble those of TMJ dysfunction: vertigo, tinnitus, jaw click Pain referred from infected tooth may be worse with hot or cold foods	TMJ arthritis Malocclusion or bruxism Impacted molar	Normal ear examination

From Seller RH (ed): *Differential diagnosis of common complaints,* ed 4, Philadelphia, 2000, WB Saunders.
TMJ, Temporomandibular joint; *URI,* upper respiratory infection.

ECG, ATRIAL ABNORMALITIES AND VENTRICULAR HYPERTROPHY

ECG, atrial abnormalities and ventricular hypertrophy
ICD-9CM # 794.31

BOX 2-79   ECG Manifestations of Atrial Abnormalities and Ventricular Hypertrophy

Left Atrial Abnormality

P wave duration ≥0.12 sec
Notched, slurred P wave in leads I and II
Biphasic P wave in V_1 with a wide, deep, negative terminal component

Right Atrial Abnormality

P wave duration ≤0.11 sec
Tall, peaked P waves of ≥2.5 mm in leads II, III, and aV_F

Left Ventricular Hypertrophy

Voltage criteria
R wave in AV_L ≥12 mm
R wave in I ≥15 mm
S wave in V_1 or V_2 + R wave in V_5 or V_6 ≥35 mm
Depressed ST segments with inverted T waves in the lateral leads
Left-axis deviation
QRS duration ≥0.09 sec
Left atrial enlargement

Right Ventricular Hypertrophy

Tall R waves over right precordium (R:S ratio in lead V_1 >1.0)
Right-axis deviation
Depressed ST segments with inverted T waves in V_1-V_3
Normal QRS duration (if no right bundle branch block)

From Andreoli TE (ed): *Cecil essentials of medicine,* ed 5, Philadelphia, 2001, WB Saunders.

ECG, FASCICULAR AND BUNDLE BRANCH BLOCKS

ECG, fascicular and bundle branch blocks
ICD-9CM # 794.31

BOX 2-80   ECG Manifestations of Fascicular and Bundle Branch Blocks

Left Anterior Fascicular Block

QRS duration ≤0.1 sec
Left-axis deviation (more negative than −45 degrees)
rS pattern in II, III, and aV_F
qR pattern in leads I and aV_L

Right Posterior Fascicular Block

QRS duration ≤0.1 sec
Right-axis deviation (+90 degrees or greater)
qR pattern in II, III, and aV_F
rS pattern in I and aV_L
Exclusion of other causes of right-axis deviation (chronic obstructive pulmonary disease, right ventricular hypertrophy)

Left Bundle Branch Block

QRS duration ≥0.12 sec
Broad, slurred or notched R waves in lateral leads (I, aV_L, V_5-V_6)
QS or rS pattern in anterior precordium
ST-T wave vectors opposite to terminal QRS vectors

Right Bundle Branch Block

QRS duration ≥0.12 sec
Large R' wave in lead V_1 (rsR')
Deep terminal S wave in V_6
Normal septal Q waves
Inverted T waves in V_1-V_2

From Andreoli TE (ed): *Cecil essentials of medicine,* ed 5, Philadelphia, 2001, WB Saunders.

ECG, METABOLIC AND DRUG INFLUENCES

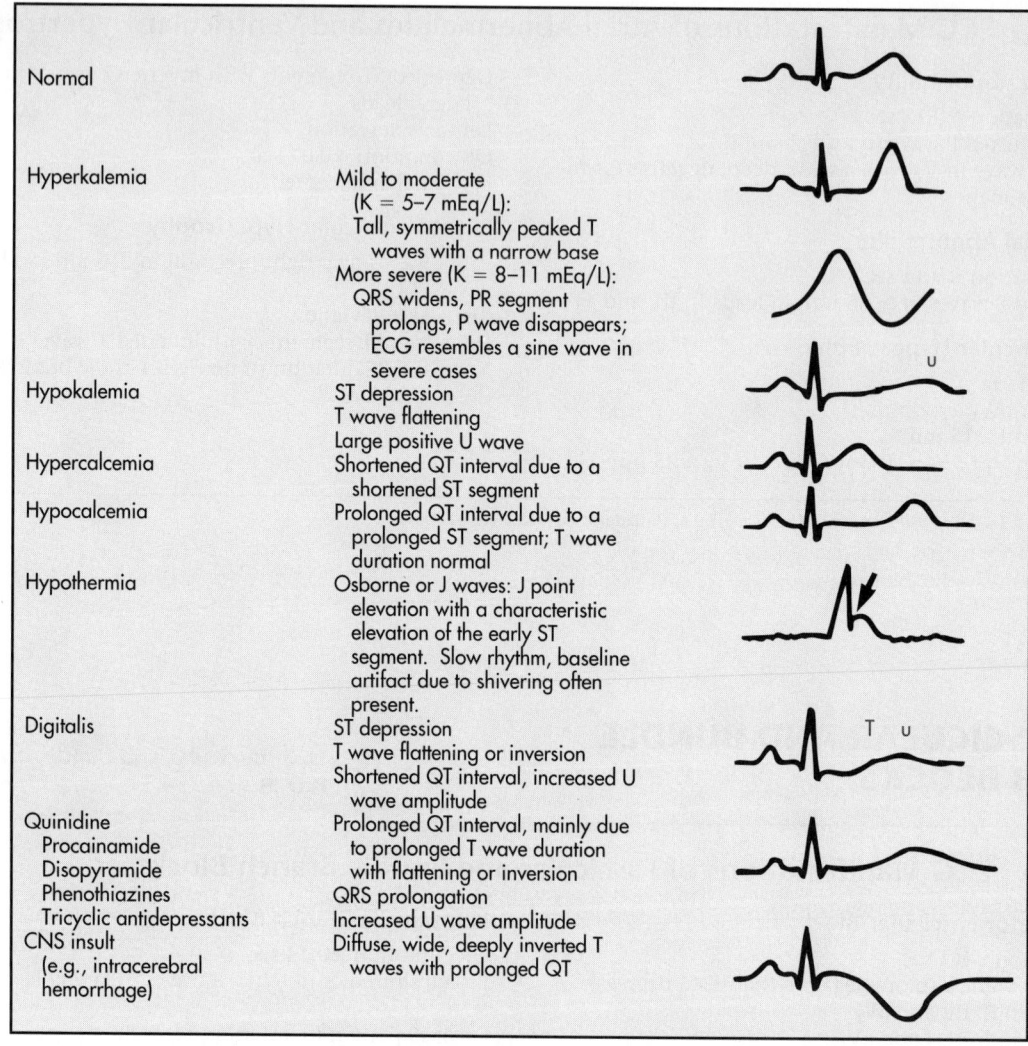

Normal	
Hyperkalemia	Mild to moderate (K = 5–7 mEq/L): Tall, symmetrically peaked T waves with a narrow base More severe (K = 8–11 mEq/L): QRS widens, PR segment prolongs, P wave disappears; ECG resembles a sine wave in severe cases
Hypokalemia	ST depression T wave flattening Large positive U wave
Hypercalcemia	Shortened QT interval due to a shortened ST segment
Hypocalcemia	Prolonged QT interval due to a prolonged ST segment; T wave duration normal
Hypothermia	Osborne or J waves: J point elevation with a characteristic elevation of the early ST segment. Slow rhythm, baseline artifact due to shivering often present.
Digitalis	ST depression T wave flattening or inversion Shortened QT interval, increased U wave amplitude

Quinidine
  Procainamide
  Disopyramide
  Phenothiazines
  Tricyclic antidepressants
	Prolonged QT interval, mainly due to prolonged T wave duration with flattening or inversion
	QRS prolongation
	Increased U wave amplitude

CNS insult (e.g., intracerebral hemorrhage)	Diffuse, wide, deeply inverted T waves with prolonged QT

Fig. 2-5   Metabolic and drug influences on the electrocardiogram. (From Andreoli TE [ed]: *Cecil essentials of medicine,* ed 5, Philadelphia, 2001, WB Saunders.)

EDEMA, IN CHILDREN

Edema, in children
ICD-9CM # 782.3 Edema NOS

BOX 2-81   Causes of Edema in Children

Cardiovascular

Congestive heart failure
Acute thrombi or emboli
Vasculitis of many types

Renal

Nephrotic syndrome
Glomerulonephritis of many types
End-stage renal failure

Endocrine or Metabolic

Thyroid disease
Starvation
Hereditary angioedema

Iatrogenic

Drugs (diuretics and steroids)
Water or salt overload

Hematologic

Hemolytic disease of the newborn

Gastrointestinal

Hepatic cirrhosis
Protein-losing enteritis
Lymphangiectasis
Cystic fibrosis
Celiac disease
Enteritis of many types

Lymphatic Abnormalities

Congenital (gonadal dysgenesis)
Acquired

From Hoekelman R (ed): *Primary pediatric care*, ed 3, St Louis, 1997, Mosby.

EDEMA, GENERALIZED

Edema, generalized
ICD-9CM # 782.3 Edema NOS

BOX 2-82   Causes of Generalized Edema

I. Common causes
  A. Congestive heart failure
  B. Cirrhosis of the liver
  C. Nephrotic syndrome
  D. Acute "nephritic" syndrome
  E. Pregnancy
    1. Normal pregnancy
    2. Toxemia of pregnancy
  F. Idiopathic edema
II. Unusual causes
  A. Arteriovenous fistulas
  B. Hypothyroidism

C. Diabetes mellitus
  1. Associated with microangiopathy (rare)
  2. Associated with insulin treatment of ketoacidosis
D. Drugs
  1. Nonsteroidal antiinflammatory drugs
  2. Estrogens
  3. Vasodilator antihypertensive drugs
  4. Hyperstimulation syndrome secondary to menotropins (Pergonal)

From Stein JH (ed): *Internal medicine*, ed 5, St Louis, 1998, Mosby.

EDEMA, LEG, UNILATERAL

Edema, leg, unilateral
ICD-9CM # 782.3

BOX 2-83   Causes of Unilateral Lower Extremity Edema

With Pain

Deep venous thrombosis
Postphlebitic syndrome
Popliteal cyst rupture
Gastrocenemius rupture
Cellulitis
Psoas or other abscess

Without Pain

Deep venous thrombosis
Postphlebitic syndrome

Other venous insufficiency
  After saphenous vein harvest
  Varicosities
Lymphatic obstruction/lymphedema
  Carcinoma, including cervical, colorectal, prostate
  Lymphoma
  Retroperitoneal fibrosis
  Sarcoidosis
  Filariasis

From Goldman L, Braunwald E (eds): *Primary cardiology*, Philadelphia, 1998, WB Saunders.

EDEMA OF LOWER EXTREMITIES

Edema of lower extremities
ICD-9CM # 782.3

BOX 2-84   Edema of Lower Extremities

Congestive heart failure (right-sided)
Hepatic cirrhosis
Nephrosis
Myxedema
Lymphedema

Pregnancy
Abdominal mass: neoplasm, cyst
Venous compression from abdominal
    aneurysm
Varicose veins

Bilateral cellulitis
Bilateral thrombophlebitis
Venous thrombosis
Retroperitoneal fibrosis

ELEVATED HEMIDIAPHRAGM

BOX 2-85   Elevated Hemidiaphragm

Neoplasm (bronchogenic carcinoma, mediastinal neo-
    plasm, intrahepatic lesion)
Substernal thyroid
Infectious process (pneumonia, empyema, tuberculosis,
    subphrenic abscess, hepatic abscess)
Atelectasis
Idiopathic
Eventration
Phrenic nerve dysfunction (myelitis, myotonia, herpes
    zoster)

Trauma to phrenic nerve or diaphragm (e.g., surgery)
Aortic aneurysm
Intraabdominal mass
Pulmonary infarction
Pleurisy
Radiation therapy
Rib fracture

Elevated hemidiaphragm
ICD-9CM # 519.4 Diaphragm disorder
            519.4 Diaphragm paralysis
            756.6 Diaphragm eventration, congenital

EMBOLI, ARTERIAL

Emboli, arterial
ICD-9CM # 444.22 Embolism, artery, lower extremity
             444.21 Embolism, artery, upper extremity

> **BOX 2-86   Sources of Arterial Emboli**
>
> Myocardial infarction with mural thrombi
> Atrial fibrillation
> Cardiomyopathies
> Prosthetic heart valves
> Chronic congestive heart failure
> Endocarditis
> Left ventricular aneurysm
> Left atrial myxoma
> Sick sinus syndrome
> Paradoxical embolus from venous thrombosis
> Aneurysms of large blood vessels
> Atheromatous ulcers of large blood vessels

From Noble J: *Primary care medicine*, ed 3, St Louis, 2001, Mosby.

EMESIS, PEDIATRIC AGE

Emesis, pediatric age
ICD-9CM # 787.03

> **BOX 2-87   Causes of Emesis (Arranged by Usual Age of Earliest Occurrence)**
>
> **Infancy**
> *Gastrointestinal Tract*
>
> Congenital
>   Regurgitation—chalasia, gastroesophageal reflux
>   Atresia—stenosis (tracheoesophageal fistula, prepyloric diaphragm, intestinal atresia)
>   Duplication
>   Volvulus (errors in rotation and fixation, Meckel's diverticulum)
>   Congenital bands
>   Hirschsprung's disease
>   Meconium ileus (cystic fibrosis), meconium plug
>
> **Acquired**
>
> Acute infectious gastroenteritis, food poisoning (staphylococcal, clostridial)
> Pyloric stenosis
> Gastritis, duodenitis
> Intussusception
> Incarcerated hernia—inguinal, internal secondary to old adhesions
> Cow's milk protein intolerance, food allergy, eosinophilic gastroenteritis
> Disaccharidase deficiency
> Celiac disease—presents after introduction of gluten in diet; inherited risk
> Adynamic ileus—the mediator for many nongastrointestinal causes
> Neonatal necrotizing enterocolitis
> Chronic granulomatous disease with gastric outlet obstruction
>
> *Non–Gastrointestinal Tract*
>
> Infectious—otitis, urinary tract infection, pneumonia, upper respiratory tract infection, sepsis, meningitis
> Metabolic—aminoaciduria and organic aciduria, galactosemia, fructosemia, adrenogenital syndrome, renal tubular acidosis, diabetic ketoacidosis, Reye's syndrome
> Central nervous system—trauma, tumor, infection, diencephalic syndrome, rumination, autonomic responses (pain, shock)
> Medications—anticholinergics, aspirin, alcohol, idiosyncratic reaction (e.g., codeine)
>
> **Childhood (Additional Causes)**
> *Gastrointestinal Tract*
>
> Peptic ulcer—vomiting is a common presentation in children younger than 6 years old
> Trauma—duodenal hematoma, traumatic pancreatitis, perforated bowel
> Pancreatitis—mumps, trauma, cystic fibrosis, hyperparathyroidism, hyperlipidemia, organic acidemias
> Crohn's disease
> Idiopathic intestinal pseudoobstruction
> Superior mesenteric artery syndrome
>
> *Non–Gastrointestinal Tract*
>
> Central nervous system—cyclic vomiting, migraine, anorexia nervosa, bulimia

From Hoekelman R (ed): *Primary pediatric care*, ed 3, St Louis, 1997, Mosby.

ENCEPHALOMYELITIS

Encephalomyelitis
ICD-9CM # 323.5 Encephalomyelitis postimmunization or postvaccinal
049.9 Encephalitis, viral

BOX 2-88   A. Viral Causes of Acute Encephalomyelitis

Direct Infection

Togaviridae
  Alphaviruses
    Eastern equine
    Western equine
    Venezuelan equine
Flaviviridae
  St. Louis
  Murray Valley
  West Nile
  Japanese
  Dengue
  Tick-borne complex
Bunyaviridae
  La Crosse
  Rift Valley
  Toscana
Paramyxoviridae
  Paramyxovirus
    Mumps
  Morbillivirus
    Measles
    Hendra
    Nipah (Hendra-like)
Arenaviridae
  Arenavirus
    Lymphocytic choriomeningitis
    Machupo
    Lassa
    Junin
Picornaviridae
  Enterovirus
    Poliovirus
    Coxsackievirus
    Echovirus
    Hepatitis A
Reoviridae
  Colorado tick fever
Rhabdoviridae
  Lyssavirus
  Rabies
Filoviridae
  Ebola
  Marburg
Retroviridae
  Lentivirus
    Human immunodeficiency virus
Herpesviridae
  Herpesvirus
    Herpes simplex virus types 1 and 2
    Varicella-zoster virus
    Herpes B virus
  Epstein-Barr virus
  Cytomegalovirus
  Human herpesvirus 6
Adenoviridae
  Adenovirus

Postinfection

Togaviridae
  Rubivirus
    Rubella
Orthomyxoviridae
  Influenza
Paramyxoviridae
  Rubulavirus
    Mumps
  Morbillivirus
    Measles
Poxviridae
  Orthopoxvirus
    Vaccinia
Herpesviridae
  Herpesvirus
    Varicella-zoster virus
    Epstein-Barr virus

B. Nonviral Causes of Encephalomyelitis

Rocky Mountain spotted fever
Typhus
Ehrlichia
Q fever
Chlamydia
Mycoplasma
Legionella
Brucellosis
Subacute bacterial endocarditis
Listeria
Whipple's disease
Cat-scratch disease
Syphilis (meningovascular)

Relapsing fever
Lyme disease
Leptospirosis
Nocardia
Actinomycosis
Tuberculosis
Cryptococcus
Histoplasma
Naegleria
Acanthamoeba
Ballamuthia mandrillaris
Toxoplasma
Plasmodium falciparum
Trypanosomiasis
Behçet's disease
Vasculitis

From Mandell GL: *Mandell, Douglas, and Bennett's principles and practice of infectious diseases*, ed 5, New York, 2000, Churchill Livingstone.

Encephalopathy, drug and toxin-induced
ICD-9CM # 349.82 Toxic encephalopathy

ENCEPHALOPATHY, DRUG AND TOXIN-INDUCED

BOX 2-89   Drugs and Toxins That Can Cause Encephalopathy

Alcohols

Ethyl, methyl, propyl, ethylene glycol

Analgesics, narcotics

All

Anticonvulsants

Diphenylhydantoin, bromides, all barbiturates, primidone, all benzodiazepines, sodium valproate

Antidepressants

Tricyclic drugs, lithium

Antineoplastic drugs

L-Asparaginase, methotrexate, mitotane, nitrogen mustards procarbazine, vidarabine, vinca alkaloids, interferon alpha-*n1*, recombinant IL-2 (aldesleukin)

Diuretics

All

Sedatives and Hypnotics

Miscellaneous

Acetaminophen	Bromocriptine	Gasoline	Prajamalium
Amantadine	Calcium salts	Gold	Propranolol
Aminophylline	Carbon disulfide	Heroin	Rifampin
Amphetamines	Carbon monoxide	Isoniazid	Steroids
Arsenic	Chloroquine	Insulin	Streptomycin
Aspirin	Chymopapain	Interferon	Strychnine
Atropine/belladonna alkaloids	Cimetidine	Lead	Sulfonamides
	Cycloserine	Methyl bromide	Sulfonylureas
Baclofen	Cyproheptadine	Methyl mercury	Thallium
Bismuth	Disulfiram	Metrizamide	Toluene
	L-Dopa	Organophosphorus	
	Digitalis	Penicillin	

From Noble J: *Primary care medicine*, ed 3, St Louis, 2001, Mosby.

II

Encephalopathy, metabolic
ICD-9CM # 291.2   Alcoholic encephalopathy
          572.2   Hepatic encephalopathy
          251.2   Hypoglycemic encephalopathy
          349.82 Toxic encephalopathy
          984.9   Lead encephalopathy
          293.9   Encephalopathy from dialysis

ENCEPHALOPATHY, METABOLIC

BOX 2-90   Causes of Acute Metabolic Encephalopathy

Substrate Deficiency

Hypoxia/ischemia
Carbon monoxide poisoning
Hypoglycemia

Cofactor Deficiency

Thiamine
Vitamin B_{12}
Pyridoxine (isoniazid administration)

Electrolyte Disorders

Hyponatremia
Hypercalcemia
Carbon dioxide narcosis
Dialysis disequilibrium syndrome

Endocrinopathies

Hyperglycemia
  Diabetic ketoacidosis
  Nonketotic hyperglycemic hyperosmolar coma
Hypothyroidism
Hyperadrenocorticism
Hyperparathyroidism

Endogenous Toxins

Liver disease
  Portal-systemic shunting
  Liver failure
Uremia
Porphyria

Exogenous Toxins

Drug overdose
  Sedative/hypnotics
  Ethanol
  Narcotics
  Salicylates
  Tricyclic antidepressants
Drug withdrawal
Toxicity of therapeutic medications
Industrial toxins (e.g., organophosphorus insecticides,
  heavy metals)
Sepsis

Heat Stroke

Epilepsy (Postictal)

From Stein J (ed): *Internal medicine,* ed 5, St Louis, 1998, Mosby.

ENTERIC FEVER

Enteric fever
ICD-9CM # Code varies with specific disorder

TABLE 2-57   Clinical, Epidemiologic, and Laboratory Clues to the Causes of Enteric Fever and Conditions That May Mimic Enteric Fever

ETIOLOGIC AGENT OR DISEASE	CLINICAL CLUES IN ADDITION TO FEVER	EPIDEMIOLOGIC CLUES	LABORATORY CLUES
Causes of Enteric Fever			
Salmonella typhi *Salmonella paratyphi A* *Salmonella schottmuelleri* *Salmonella choleraesuis*	Relative bradycardia, splenomegaly, rose spots, conjunctivitis	Young adults, travel, especially to India, Mexico, and other tropical areas,* exposure to known carrier	Cultures (B, BM, U, F), serology, leukopenia
Yersinia enterocolitica *Yersinia pseudotuberculosis*	Chronic liver or other underlying disease, arthritis, erythema nodosum	Older adults, ± pet exposure	Cultures (B, F, J), serology
Campylobacter fetus	Stigmata or chronic liver disease, phlebitis	Older adults, ± farm or small-animal contact	Cultures (B, F), serology
Brucellosis (*Brucella* spp.)	Paucity of physical findings	Occupation (abattoir employee, butcher), animal contact (goats, sheep, cattle), diet (unpasteurized cheese)	Cultures (B, BM), serology, leukopenia
Typhoidal tularemia (*Francisella tularensis*)	Severe prostration, splenomegaly	Animal contact (especially rabbits), vector exposure (ticks)	Serology
Conditions That May Mimic Enteric Fever			
Bacterial infections			
Septicemic plague (*Yersinia pestis*)	Severe prostration	Rodent contact, vector exposure (fleas), travel	Cultures (B), serology
Intestinal anthrax (*Bacillus anthracis*)	Severe prostration	Travel,* diet (undercooked meat)	Cultures (B, F)
Septicemia melioidosis (*Burkholderia pseudomallei*)	Severe prostration, pustular skin lesions	Travel,* especially Southeast Asia	Cultures (B), serology, chest radiograph
Acute bartonellosis (*Bartonella bacilliformis*)	Severe prostration, hemolysis, renal failure	Travel to Andean valleys in Peru, Ecuador, and Columbia,* vector exposure (sand fly)	Cultures (B), blood smear, acute hemolysis
Leptospirosis (*Leptospira* spp.)	Relative bradycardia, conjunctival suffusion	Occupation (farmers, abattoir and sewer workers, veterinarians), animal contact (especially cattle, dogs), swimming†	Cultures (B, CSF, U), serology, hepatorenal dysfunction
Relapsing fever (*Borrelia* spp.)	Fever pattern, conjunctival suffusion, splenomegaly, skin rash	Travel, especially to Southeast Asia, Far East, Ethiopia, and the western United States),* vector exposure (louse, tick)	Blood smear
Legionellosis (*Legionella* spp.)	Pneumonia, CNS symptoms	Normal or compromised host	Chest radiograph, purulent sputum, DFA of sputum, urine antigen
Intestinal tuberculosis (*Mycobacterium tuberculosis*, *Mycobacterium avium-intracellulare*)	Stigmata of tuberculosis or AIDs	Exposure to known case, ± travel* ± diet (unpasteurized milk and milk products), malnourished children, HIV infection	Cultures (S, G, BM, L), radiograph (UGI, SBFT)
Abdominal actinomycosis (*Actinomyces* spp.)	Abdominal mass, fistula	Men	Culture (FD, A), radiograph (UGI, SBFT), CT with oral contrast medium

From Mandell GL: *Mandell, Douglas, and Bennett's principles and practice of infectious diseases*, ed 5, New York, 2000, Churchill Livingstone.
A, Abscess; *AIDS*, acquired immunodeficiency syndrome; *ANA*, antinuclear antibody; *B*, blood; *BM*, bone marrow; *C´*, complement; *CNS*, central nervous system; *CSF*, cerebrospinal fluid; *CT*, computed tomography; *DFA*, direct fluorescent antibody test; *F*, feces; *FD*, fistula drainage; *G*, gastric aspirate; *HIV*, human immunodeficiency virus; *J*, joint fluid; *L*, liver; *LN*, lymph node; *MM*, mucous membrane; *N*, nasal; *O&P*, ova and parasite; *S*, sputum; *T*, throat; *U*, urine; *UGI, SBFT*, upper gastrointestinal tract with small bowel follow-through.
*Travel to endemic areas, either domestic or foreign.
†Swimming in contaminated surface water.

Continued

II

ENTERIC FEVER—cont'd

TABLE 2-57 **Clinical, Epidemiologic, and Laboratory Clues to the Causes of Enteric Fever and Conditions That May Mimic Enteric Fever**

ETIOLOGIC AGENT OR DISEASE	CLINICAL CLUES IN ADDITION TO FEVER	EPIDEMIOLOGIC CLUES	LABORATORY CLUES
Intraabdominal abscess	Spiking daily fever, reduced diaphragmatic excursion, intraabdominal or diaphragmatic pain	Previous surgery, bowel or biliary tract disease	Leukocytosis, CT, gallium scan, sonography, fluoroscopy
Rat bite fever			
Streptobacillus moniliformis	Headache, nausea, vomiting, rash, myalgia, polyarthritis	Rat bite or footborne outbreak	Culture (B, J), serology
Spirillum minus	Headache, nausea, adenopathy, roseolarurticarial rash	Rat bite	Serology
Mycoplasma pneumoniae	Cough, headache, bullous myringitis	Children and adolescents	Serology
Chlamydia psittaci	Headache, nausea, vomiting, arthralgias, cough	Exposure to parrots, parakeets, related birds	Serology
Bacterial pneumonia (*Streptococcus pneumoniae, Haemophilus influenzae* spp.)	Cough, sputum, rales, headache, delirium, pulmonary infiltrates	Older adults, smoking, underlying diseases	Sputum Gram stain, culture (S, B), chest radiograph
Viral infections			
Hepatitis	Jaundice, arthritis (with hepatitis B)	Exposure to known case, drug abuse, travel*	Liver dysfunction, antibody and/or antigen detection
Dengue	Relative bradycardia, myalgia, conjunctival suffusion, rash	Travel,* vector exposure (mosquito)	Culture (B), serology, leukopenia, thrombocytopenia
Infectious mononucleosis	Pharyngitis, lymphadenopathy, splenomegaly, rash	Young adults	Serology, lymphocyte morphology
Rickettsial infections			
Rocky Mountain spotted fever	Rash, headache, myalgias	Travel,* vector exposure (tick)	Serology, skin biopsy
Epidemic typhus	Conjunctival suffusion, rash, severe prostration	Travel,* vector exposure (louse)	Serology
Brill-Zinsser disease	Rash	Older adults, remote travel* history	Serology
Endemic typhus	Conjunctival suffusion, rash, splenomegaly	Rat contact, vector exposure (flea)	Serology
Scrub typhus	Conjunctival suffusion, rash, lymphadenopathy	Travel,* vector exposure (mites)	Serology
Q fever	Pneumonia, hepatitis	Animal contact (especially livestock), ± travel, ± diet (especially unpasteurized milk)	Serology, chest radiograph, liver dysfunction
Ehrlichiosis	Headache, myalgia, rash (occasional)	Travel,* vector exposure (tick)	Serology, leukopenia, thrombocytopenia
Mycotic infections			
Disseminated histoplasmosis	Mucocutaneous lesions, adrenal insufficiency	Travel,* animal contact (chicken, birds, bats), hobby (cave exploration)	Culture (B, BM, L, MM), biopsy (BM, L, MM), chest radiograph, urine antigen
Penicillium marneffei	Umbilicated skin lesions, lymphadenopathy, cough, hepatomegaly	Travel,* concurrent AIDS	Culture (B, BM, LN), chest radiograph

ENTERIC FEVER—cont'd

TABLE 2-57   Clinical, Epidemiologic, and Laboratory Clues to the Causes of Enteric Fever and Conditions That May Mimic Enteric Fever

ETIOLOGIC AGENT OR DISEASE	CLINICAL CLUES IN ADDITION TO FEVER	EPIDEMIOLOGIC CLUES	LABORATORY CLUES
Parasitic infections			
Malaria	Fever pattern, splenomegaly	Travel,* vector exposure (mosquito)	Blood smear
Amebiasis	Colitis, liver abscess	Travel*	Stool examination, serology, liver scan, sonography, CT, colon biopsy
Babesiosis	Paucity of physical findings	Travel,* splenectomy, vector exposure (tick)	Blood smear, serology
Toxoplasmosis	Lymphadenopathy	Animal contact (cat); diet (undercooked pork)	Serology, biopsy (lymph node)
Trichinosis	Periorbital edema, muscle tenderness	Diet (undercooked pork or bear meat)	Serology, eosinophilia, biopsy (muscle)
Katayama fever (acute schistosomiasis)	Urticaria, lymphadenopathy	Travel,* swimming or other freshwater exposure	Eosinophilia, serology, stool O&P
Visceral larva migrans	Hepatosplenomegaly, rash, bronchospasm, ocular lesions	Young children with history of pica, animal contact (dog, cat)	Serology, biopsy (L), eosinophilia
Noninfectious causes			
Malignancy	Adenopathy, anergy, weight loss	Family history or prior malignancy	Sonography, CT, gallium scan, biopsy
Collagen vascular or granulomatous disease (e.g., sarcoidosis, granulomatous hepatitis, ulcerative colitis, Crohn's disease, Still's disease, vasculitis, etc.)	Skin lesions, arthritis, serositis, multiple organ involvement	Family history	Biopsy of involved tissue, serology (ANA, C´), exclusion of other causes

ENTHESOPATHY

Enthesopathy
ICD-9CM # Code not available

BOX 2-91   Enthesopathy

Reactive arthritis
Ankylosing spondylitis
Psoriatic arthritis
Bacteremia
Viremia
Fluorosis
X-linked vitamin D–resistant rickets
Etetrinate treatment
Forestier's disease (DISH)
Fluoroquinolone treatment

From Canoso J: *Rheumatology in primary care,* Philadelphia, 1997, WB Saunders.

EOSINOPHILIA

Eosinophilia
ICD-9CM # 288.3

BOX 2-92 Causes of Significant Peripheral Blood Eosinophilia

Helminthic Parasites

Ascaris lumbricoides (invasive larval stage)
Hookworms (invasive larval stage)
Strongyloides stercoralis (initial infection and autoinfection)
Trichinosis
Filariasis
Echinococcus granulosus and *E. multilocularis*
Toxocara species
Animal hookworms
Angiostrongylus cantonensis and *A. costaricensis*
Schistosomiasis
Liver flukes
Fasciolopis buski
Anisakiasis
Capillaria philippinensis
Paragonimus westermani
"Tropical eosinophilia" (unidentified microfilariae)

Other Infections/Infestations

Pulmonary aspergillosis
Severe scabies

Allergies

Asthma
Hay fever
Drug reactions
Atopic dermatitis

Autoimmune and Related Disorders

Polyarteritis nodosa
Necrotizing vasculitis
Eosinophilic fasciitis
Pemphigus

Neoplastic Diseases

Hodgkin's disease
Mycosis fungoides
Chronic myelocytic leukemia
Eosinophilic leukemia

Polycythemia vera
Mucin-secreting adenocarcinomas

Immunodeficiency States

Hyperimmunoglobulin E with recurrent infection
Wiskott-Aldrich syndrome

Other

Addison's disease
Inflammatory bowel disease
Dermatitis herpetiformis
Toxic/chemical syndrome
Eosinophilic myalgia syndrome, tryptophan, toxic oil syndrome
Hypereosinophilic syndrome (unknown etiology)

From Noble J (ed): *Primary care medicine,* ed 3, St Louis, 2001, Mosby.

EPILEPSY

Epilepsy
ICD-9CM # 345.9 Epilepsy NOS

TABLE 2-58 Differential Diagnosis of Epilepsy

DISORDER	UNLIKE EPILEPSY	LIKE EPILEPSY
Syncope	Premonitory symptoms Precipitating factors Diffuse fading vision	Myoclonic jerks or tonic stiffening, on occasion
Transient ischemic attack	No "march" of symptoms No jerks, twitches No loss of consciousness, amnesia Brain stem symptoms	Focal electroencephalogram (EEG) slowing Normal examination between attacks
Migraine	Prominent headache Preserved consciousness	Focal symptoms Focal EEG slowing
Hypoglycemia	Temporal relationship to fasting Initial sympathetic discharge	Focal symptoms and EEG slowing Loss of consciousness Postictal headache, confusion
Paroxysmal vertigo	Preserved consciousness Monosymptomatic spells Auditory, vestibular abnormalities	Severe temporary disability
Narcolepsy	Cataplexy Appropriate sleep behavior with attacks	Hallucinations Inappropriate, unpredictable timing of attacks
Psychogenic spells	Event-related Stressful context Lack of autonomic features Lack of incontinence	Dramatic convulsive behavior

From Stein JH (ed): *Internal medicine,* ed 5, St Louis, 1998, Mosby.

ERECTILE DYSFUNCTION, ORGANIC

Erectile dysfunction, organic
ICD-9CM # 607.84

TABLE 2-59   Causes of Organic Erectile Dysfunction

VASCULOGENIC ABNORMALITIES	ARTERIAL INSUFFICIENCY, VENOUS INCOMPETENCE
Neurogenic abnormalities	Somatic nerve neuropathy, central nervous system abnormalities
Psychogenic causes	Depression, performance anxiety, marital conflict
Endocrinologic causes	Hyperprolactinemia, hypogonadotropic hypogonadism, testicular failure, estrogen excess
Trauma	Pelvic fracture, prostate surgery, penile fracture
Systemic disease	Diabetes mellitus, renal failure, hepatic cirrhosis
Medications	Diuretics, tricyclic antidepressants, H_2 blockers, exogenous hormones, alcohol, antihypertensives, nicotine abuse
Structural abnormalities	Peyronie's disease

From Rakel RE (ed): *Principles of family practice*, ed 6, Philadelphia, 2002, WB Saunders.

ERYTHROCYTE FRAGMENTATION SYNDROMES

Erythrocyte fragmentation syndromes
ICD-9CM # 283.19

BOX 2-93   Erythrocyte Fragmentation Syndromes

Disseminated intravascular coagulation
Hemolytic uremic syndrome
Thrombotic thrombocytopenic purpura
Malignant hypertension
Eclampsia
Vasculitis
Glomerulonephritis
Solid organ transplant rejection
Post–bone marrow transplantation thrombotic microangiopathy
Disseminated carcinoma, especially adenocarcinoma
Cavernous hemangioma
Hepatic hemangioendothelioma
Drugs
    Mitomycin C
    Cyclosporin A
    Quinidine
Aortic stenosis
Ruptured chordae tendineae
Aortic aneurysm
After surgical repair of heart and large vessel defects
Perivalvular leak
March hemoglobinuria

From Stein J (ed): *Internal medicine*, ed 5, St Louis, 1998, Mosby.

ESOPHAGEAL MOTOR DISORDERS

Esophageal motor disorders
ICD-9CM # 530.5 Esophageal spasm
530.0 Esophageal aperistalsis

TABLE 2-60   Esophageal Motor Disorders

	ACHALASIA	SCLERODERMA	DIFFUSE ESOPHAGEAL SPASM
Symptoms	Dysphagia Regurgitation of nonacidic material	Gastroesophageal reflux disease Dysphagia	Substernal chest pain (angina-like) Dysphagia with pain
X-ray appearance	Dilated, fluid-filled esophagus Distal "bird beak" stricture	Aperistaltic esophagus Free reflux Peptic stricture	Simultaneous noncoordinated contractions
Manometric findings			
Lower esophageal sphincter	High resting pressure Incomplete or abnormal relaxation with swallow	Low resting pressure	Normal pressure
Body	Low-amplitude, simultaneous contractions after swallow	Low-amplitude peristaltic contractions or no peristalsis	Some peristalsis Diffuse and simultaneous nonperistaltic contractions, occasionally high amplitude

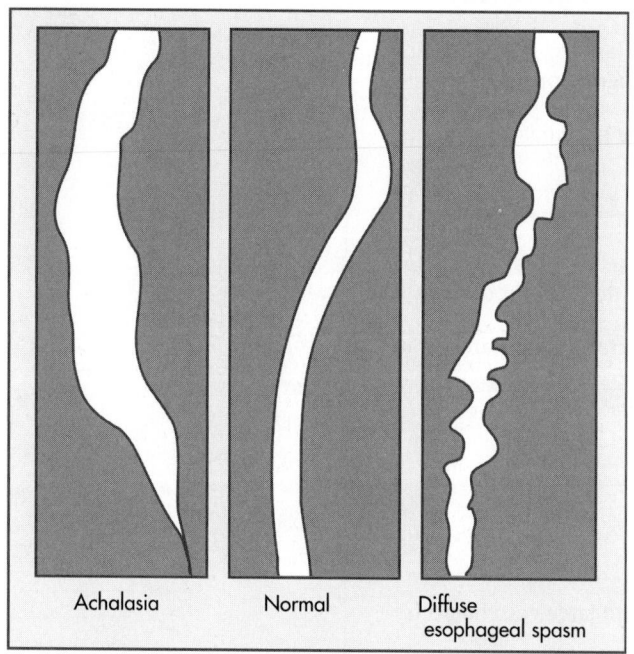

Achalasia   Normal   Diffuse esophageal spasm

Fig. 2-6   Radiologic appearance of achalasia *(left)* and diffuse esophageal spasm *(right)*. In achalasia the esophageal body is dilated and terminates in a narrowed segment or "bird beak." The appearance of numerous simultaneous contractions is typical of diffuse esophageal spasm. (Courtesy Dr. E.E. Templeton and Dr. C.A. Rohrmann. From Pope CE II: In Sleisenger MH, Fordtran JS [eds]: *Gastrointestinal disease,* ed 3, Philadelphia, 1983, WB Saunders.)

EXANTHEMS

TABLE 2-61   **Exanthems**

Exanthems
ICD-9CM # 782.1

DISEASE	AGE	PRODROME	SKIN MORPHOLOGY	DISTRIBUTION	OTHER FINDINGS	DIAGNOSIS
Measles	Infants Young adults	Fever, URI, conjunctivitis	Erythematous macules—papules become confluent	Face first Moves down over entire body	Koplik's spots, cough, photophobia, adenopathy	Clinical; acute/convalescent hemagglutinin serology
Rubella	Adolescents Young adults	Fever, malaise, cough	Rose-pink macules and papules Not confluent	Face first Moves downward	Forschheimer spots Postauricular adenopathy Headache	Rubella hemagglutinin inhibition or complement fixation titers acute/convalescent
Erythema infectiosum (fifth disease) (parvovirus B19)	5-15 yr	None or mild fever, malaise	Slapped red cheeks Reticulate erythema or maculopapular Not pruritic	Face—red cheeks Arm/legs reticulate	Rash waxes-wanes several weeks Arthritis; aplastic anemia	IgM antibody
Roseola exanthem HHV 6	6 mo–3 yr	High fever 3-5 days, then rash	Rose-pink, maculo-papular Appears after fever resolves	Neck, trunk with little involvement of face Lasts only hours to few days	Cervical and postauricular adenopathy HH6 may cause neonatal hepatitis	Clinical
Varicella chickenpox	1-14 yr	Fever, malaise	Vesicles (often umbilicated) or red base Very pruritic	Generalized involvement Lesions leave scars	Oral lesions Pneumonia in older patients	Tzanck viral culture
Enterovirus (coxsackie, ECHO)	Children	Fever, URI	Variable—maculopapular, petechial, vesicular	Generalized or acral (hand-foot-mouth)	Fever, myocarditis, meningitis, pleurodynia, mouth ulcers	Clinical, viral culture
Adenovirus	5 mo–5 yr	Fever, URI	Maculopapular, morbilliform, rubelliform, petechial roseola-like	Generalized	Fever, URI, conjunctivitis	Viral culture Acute/convalescent titer

Continued

II

TABLE 2-61 Exanthems—cont'd

DISEASE	AGE	PRODROME	SKIN MORPHOLOGY	DISTRIBUTION	OTHER FINDINGS	DIAGNOSIS
Epstein-Barr virus (infectious mononucleosis)	Children Adolescents	Fever, sore throat	Maculopapular, morbilliform, urticarial, erythema multiforme–like	Trunk Extremities	Cervical adenopathy Hepatosplenomegaly	Mono spot Acute/convalescent EBV nuclear Ag titers
Kawasaki disease	6 mo–6 yr	Fever, eye irritation	Papular, morbilliform, scarlatiniform Commonly desquamates as clears	Generalized with palm, sole, and perineal accentuation	Conjunctivitis, cheilitis, glossitis, adenopathy, peripheral edema, coronary artery abnormalities	Clinical
Staphylococcal scalded skin (*Staphylococcus* toxin)	Neonates, infants	Nikolsky's sign	Sudden onset, tender, red rash that exfoliates leaving raw surfaces	Generalized	Fever, conjunctivitis	Culture of coagulase + staphylococcus from systemic site Not skin
Scarlet fever (β-*Streptococcus* toxin)	School age	Fever, sore throat, malaise, headache	Diffuse, erythema with "sandpaper" texture Exfoliative as rash clears	Generalized, circumoral pallor Pastia's lines	Pharyngitis, palate perlèche, abdominal pain, strawberry tongue	Throat culture ↑ ASO titer
Staphylococcal scarlet fever (exfoliative toxin)	School age		Tender, red, erythroderma with sandpaper quality Does not desquamate		No pharyngitis	Negative throat culture No ASO ↑
Meningococcemia	<2 yr	Malaise, fever, URI	Papules, petechiae, large areas of purpura, purpura fulminans	Trunk, extremities, soles, palms	High fever, meningismus, shock	Blood culture, spinal tap
Rocky Mountain spotted fever (*Rickettsia rickettsii*)	Any age	Fever, malaise	Maculopapular, petechial rash	Acral areas first; trunk later	CNS, pulmonary, and cardiac involvement	Serology Weil-Felix test

From Noble J (ed): *Primary care medicine,* ed 3, St Louis, 2001, Mosby.
CNS, Central nervous system; *ECHO,* echocardiography; *HHV6,* Human herpesvirus 6; *URI,* upper respiratory infection.

EXTREMITY PAIN, VASCULAR CAUSES

TABLE 2-62 Important Vascular Causes of Extremity Pain

NAME OF CONDITION	HISTORY AND PHYSICAL	STUDIES	COMMENTS
Atherosclerosis	Older individuals, especially males, may present with lower extremity pain with exercise (claudication)	Noninvasive vascular studies; angiography if therapeutic procedure considered	Exclude pseudoclaudication
Thromboangiitis obliterans	Young male smokers		Buerger's disease
Leriche syndrome	Pain in legs, hips, buttocks; impotence	Angiography shows arteriosclerotic disease in iliac vessels	
Acute ischemia	From emboli or thrombosis; acute pain, often severe, throbbing; livedo or pallor in limb	Angiography if therapeutic procedure considered	Underlying reason for emboli or thrombosis (e.g., atrial fibrillation, vasculitis, hypercoagulable state) usually apparent
Raynaud's phenomenon	Cold- or stress-induced; three-color change; upper extremities more common		Idiopathic or associated with underlying reason (e.g., rheumatologic disease, drugs, or trauma)
Thrombophlebitis	Risk factors for deep vein thrombosis; pain at site, better with leg elevation	IPG or ultrasound examination shows clot	Pain is not usually severe and may be minimal
Postphlebitic syndrome	Aching pain after episode of deep vein thrombosis	Clinical diagnosis: IPG; ultrasound normal	Pain worse with dependency
Superficial thrombophlebitis	Local pain; tenderness at superficial vein site		May have symptoms or signs of underlying malignancy

From Conn R: *Current diagnosis*, ed 9, Philadelphia, 1997, WB Saunders.
IPG, Impedance plethysmography.

II

EYE PAIN

Eye pain
ICD-9CM # 379.91

BOX 2-94   Eye Pain

Foreign body
Herpes zoster
Trauma
Conjunctivitis
Iritis
Iridocyclitis
Uveitis
Blepharitis

Ingrown lashes
Orbital or periorbital cellulitis/abscess
Sinusitis
Headache
Glaucoma
Inflammation of lacrimal gland
Tic douloureux
Cerebral aneurysm

Cerebral neoplasm
Entropion
Retrobulbar neuritis
Ultraviolet light
Dry eyes
Irritation or inflammation from eye
   drops, dust, cosmetics, etc.

EYELID CYSTIC LESIONS

Eyelid cystic lesions
ICD-9CM # 374.84 Eyelid cyst

TABLE 2-63   Cystic Lesions of the Eyelids*

LESION	HISTORY	SIGNS	TREATMENT
Hidrocystomas (retention cysts either of the apocrine [Moll's gland] or eccrine sweat glands)	Common; chronic, painless lid margin cyst	Occasionally multiple, but usually solitary; lid margin translucent, cystic nodule; often bluish, transilluminates	Excise
Pilosebaceous cysts, milia	Asymptomatic, multiple white lid bumps	Rounded, white; sharply circumscribed, pinhead-sized, pearly nodules	Excision, diathermy, or electrolysis
Pilosebaceous cysts, sebaceous or pilar cysts	Subcutaneous lid bump; stable or grow slowly	Globular, subcutaneous masses, attached to skin, often of brow; plugged pore at the summit often	Excise
Epidermal inclusion cysts	After trauma or surgery; grow slowly	Firm, globular, painless, mobile, dermal or subcutaneous masses; skin intact	Excise

From Noble J: *Primary care medicine,* ed 3, St Louis, 2001, Mosby.
*Other cystic lesions include dermoid cysts, pilomatrixoma, cystic basal cell carcinoma, and dacryops (cysts from dilated ducts of accessory lacrimal glands from scarring or chronic inflammation).

EYELID INFECTIONS AND INFESTATIONS

TABLE 2-64 Eyelid Infections and Infestations

LID INFECTION	SYMPTOMS	SIGNS	TREATMENT
Viral			
Molluscum contagiosum	Mildly contagious; bumps on lids; more bumps coming; itchy eyes	One or many dome-shaped, skin-colored, umbilicated nodules, 1-3 mm diam; cheesy, sebum-like material expressed; may give follicular conjunctivitis	Incise Excise Curet Swab with alcohol
Verruca	Warty lid bumps; often from inoculation from warts on hands	Verruca vulgaris: round, warty Verruca plana: flat Verruca digitata: fingerlike, horny, capped filaments, grouped on narrow base Verruca filiformis: threadlike, normal skin covering	Excise
Herpex simplex	Spread by kissing, two infection peaks—6 mo-4 yr, 16-25 yr; blisters on lids; "cold sore" on lid	Primary: subclinical or unilateral crop of pinhead-sized vesicles on swollen, slightly red base, usually lower lid; may have fever; resolve in 7 days, leave no scars; may give keratitis or conjunctivitis; in atopic patients, may give severe systemic infection, Kaposi's varicelliform eruption Recurrent herpes (cold sore) may affect the eyelids; benign unless eye infected	Refer Acyclovir 400 mg PO five times daily Vidarabine 3% ointment five times daily
Herpes zoster	Headache, sudden fever, malaise; in 3-4 days swelling and blistering on lid and forehead; usually adults and aged, sometimes the young; at increased risk are immunosuppressed patients; postherpetic neuralgia may be helped with antidepressants	Vesicles in V1 or V2 distribution, respect midline, one third involve lids and eye; vesicles filled with clear, then turbid fluid, quickly burst, giving eschar in nerve distribution, inviting secondary infection, healing in a week or two; may be marked eye inflammation; pain often severe, may persist for years (*postherpetic*) in elderly; skin often left mildly numb, yet giving pain on the slightest provocation (anesthesia dolorosa)	Refer If early diagnosis: oral antiviral for 7 days (acyclovir, famciclovir, valacyclovir)
Bacterial			
Hordeolum (much less common than chalazia)	Stye: pain and lid margin swelling and redness	Rapidly forms abscess, may point and drain, often secondary to staphylococcal blepharitis External hordeolum, furuncle of lash follicles and adjacent glands Internal hordeola involve meibomian glands	Refer Hot compresses Oral penicillinase-resistant antibiotics Surgical drainage if necessary
Fungal			
Tinea corporis	Often spreads from face; red spot	Red spot with centrifugal extension and central healing; ring shape	Topical antifungal twice daily, continue for 10 days after lesions disappear
Infestation			
Crab lice (*Phthirus pubis*)	Often in children; chronic, itchy blepharitis	Blepharitis Dramatic: multiple nits (eggs) glued to lash bases, several lice gripping lash bases or crawling about the shafts Subtle; only one or two nits	Refer Wash all clothes and bed linen in hot, soapy water Use an anti-lice shampoo on all affected individuals Pick off the nits and lice at the slit lamp
Demodex mites	Red, itchy lids; infest the lid margin pilosebaceous units	Chronic blepharitis and meibomianitis	Lid scrubs Antibiotic ointment

From Noble J: *Primary care medicine*, ed 3, St Louis, 2001, Mosby.

EYELID INFLAMMATIONS

TABLE 2-65   Eyelid Inflammations

INFLAMMATION	HISTORY	SIGNS	TREATMENT
Staphylococcal marginal blepharitis	Often begins in childhood; may last a lifetime; women > men; irritated, red, crusting eyelids; recurrent styes, often associated with seborrhea and acne rosacea	Dilated skin vessels; brittle, yellow crusts at lash roots leaving a bleeding ulcer when removed; recurrent hordeolum	Dandruff shampoo if seborrheic Wash with warm, soapy water twice a day "Eyelid scrubs" with face cloth or cotton-tipped applicator twice a day; remove all crusts
		If chronic may give entropion or ectropion, lid thickening or notching; lash loss, misdirection or whitening; papillary conjunctivitis, keratitis	Flare-ups or resistant cases: scrubs, then massage antibiotic ointment into lid margin If severe: antibiotic/corticosteroid ointment; oral tetracycline
Seborrheic marginal blepharitis	Associated seborrheic dermatitis of the scalp, nasolabial folds, brow, retroauricular area, and presternum	Reddened lid margins, soft, greasy scales, not clustered at the lash roots, and not giving bleeding microulcers when removed, foamy tear meniscus, meibomian orifices swollen or plugged by oil globules, chalazia, secondary chronic papillary conjunctivitis, interpalpebral corneal epithelial punctate erosions	As above
Chalazion	Stye; one or many; variable growth rate; variable pain, less than hordeolum; sebaceous gland inflammation from duct obstruction, spontaneous or secondary lid margin disease; associated with seborrheic dermatitis or acne rosacea	Usually painless, rounded, slowly enlarging, subcutaneous lid mass that may wax and wane in size; may rupture posteriorly, giving a polypoid, conjunctival mass of granulation tissue on the conjunctiva, or anteriorly, giving a subcutaneous mass	For acne rosacea or seborrheic dermatitis For lids: hot, moist compresses for 15 min, four times a day For resistant or chronic chalazia: incision and curettage, with subconjunctival triamcinolone injection Marginal chalazia resist conservative treatment
Dermatitis	Common Acute: red, itches, burns, swollen, flakes; blisters if severe Chronic: itchy, thick, scaling skin	Red, irritated, thickened, scaling lid skin	Remove irritant Cool compresses Hydrocortisone 0.5% in Aquaphor four times a day Dermatologic referral if widespread
Atopic dermatitis	Personal or family history of asthma, hay fever, atopic dermatitis	As above	As above
Contact dermatitis	Cosmetics, aerosols, nail polish, soap, eye drops—especially neomycin	As above	As above
Foreign body granuloma	Lid lump, grows slowly; old injury	Quiet lid lump	Excise

From Noble J: *Primary care medicine*, ed 3, St Louis, 2001, Mosby.

EYELID MALPOSITIONS

TABLE 2-66   **Eyelid Malpositions**

MALPOSITION	SYMPTOMS	SIGNS	MANAGEMENT
Trichiasis: normal lid position, but lashes directed posteriorly	Irritation, tearing red eye	Eyelid: no entropion, scarring, inflammation Eyelash: against the eye Eye: red, corneal ulcer	Lid scrubs, hot compresses, antibiotics For lash: temporary epilation, permanent epilation Electroepilation: excision of root(s), cryodestruction
Entropion: can be congenital, acquired, cicatricial, mechanical, senile	Intermittent (?), irritation, tearing, red eye	Eyelid: lid flipped in lashes and skin against the eye Eye: red, corneal ulcer	For lid: temporary or permanent tape, restore anatomy For eye: lubricate
Ectropion: can be congenital, acquired, cicatricial, paralytic, senile	Irritation, tearing, red eye, red lid	Eyelid: eyelid flipped out, irritated, exposed conjunctiva Eye: dry, irritated	For lid: surgically restore anatomy

Blepharoptosis
  Neurogenic
  Neuromuscular junction: myogenic, aponeurotic, mechanical
	Upper lid droop	Frontalis contraction, brow elevation, excess skin, high lid crease, droopy lid	Surgically restore, suspend lid

Retraction: Graves' disease?	Stare, eye too big, irritation, tearing	Lid: upper > up, lower > down Eye: red, exposed	Surgically lower upper and/or raise lower
Blepharospasm	Eyes close involuntarily	Lid spasms, facial twitches	Botulinum toxin, surgery

From Noble J: *Primary care medicine,* ed 3, St Louis, 2001, Mosby.

EYELID VASCULAR LESIONS

TABLE 2-67   **Vascular Lesions of the Eyelids**

LESION	HISTORY	SIGNS	TREATMENT
Capillary hemangioma	Develops just after birth, grows rapidly for about 1 year, then stabilizes, then involutes until about age 5 years	Raised, dimpled, intensely red "strawberry mark"; bulges with Valsalva's maneuver; blanches with pressure	Observe and await involution if possible Treat if amblyopia threatens Local injections of steroid Excision
Nevus flammeus or port-wine stain (may be part of Sturge-Weber syndrome)	Always present at birth; does not enlarge; often becomes darker with time	Flat, port-wine colored mark of varying size; no bulging with Valsalva's maneuver; no blanching	Cosmetics Photoablation Check for ocular and intracranial involvement if Sturge-Weber syndrome
Cavernous hemangioma	Usually develops in the second to fourth decade; grows slowly; does not involute	Raised, red or purplish lesion	Excise
Pyogenic granuloma (most common acquired eyelid lesion)	Follows minor trauma or surgery; grows rapidly; bleeds easily	Scarlet, brown, or blue-black nodule; friable surface	Excise
Varices	Grow slowly; often with other facial venous anomalies	Dark blue, deeper, soft lesions	Debulk as necessary Often recur
Lymphangiomas	Grow slowly; no spontaneous regression, intralesional bleeding may cause enlargement	Yellowish-tan or reddish swelling; deep component	Observe Excise Often recur
Kaposi's sarcoma	In patients with AIDS	Reddish vascular nodule of conjunctiva or lid	Treat AIDS Biopsy and excise as necessary

From Noble J: *Primary care medicine,* ed 3, St Louis, 2001, Mosby.

FACIAL PAIN

Facial pain
ICD-9CM # 784.0

TABLE 2-68 **Facial Pain**

	LOCATION	NATURE	TIMING	ASSOCIATED PHYSICAL FINDINGS
Tic douloureux	V2, then V2-V3; rarely V1	Triggered	Brief jabs	None
Geniculate neuralgia	Ear	Not often triggered	Brief jabs, or long duration	Vesicles in ear, VII palsy, ± VIII findings
Glossopharyngeal neuralgia	Tonsillar fossa, ear	Triggered	Brief jabs	Episodes of syncope
Postherpetic neuralgia	One or more adjacent cranial or cervical nerves	Burning	Constant	Healed skin lesions, sensory loss, or hyperpathia
Posttraumatic neuralgia	Usually one cranial or cervical nerve	Burning, aching	Constant	Sensory disturbances
Cluster headache	Retroorbital, cheek, temple	Boring, deep, intense	Attacks of 30-120 min	Lacrimation, ptosis, rhinorrhea
"Lower-half headache"	Orbit, nose, cheek, mastoid; may spread to neck and arm	Boring, deep, intense	Attacks lasting 1 or more hr	Sometimes flushing, lacrimation, rhinorrhea
Carotidynia	One side of neck	Deep, aching	Several days	Tender carotid in neck
Atypical facial pain	Cheek, jaw, entire face	Aching, may be bizarre	Constant	Emotional disturbance

From Stein JH (ed): *Internal medicine,* ed 5, St Louis, 1998, Mosby.

FACIAL PARALYSIS

Facial paralysis
ICD-9CM # 351.0 Facial (7th nerve) palsy

BOX 2-95 **Etiology of Facial Paralysis**

Infection
  Bacterial
    Otitis media
    Mastoiditis
    Chronic suppurative otitis media
      (especially with cholesteatoma)
    Meningitis
    "Malignant otitis media"
    Lyme disease
  Viral
    Infectious mononucleosis
    Herpes zoster
    Varicella
    Rubella
    Mumps

Mycobacterial
  Tuberculous meningitis
  Leprosy
Miscellaneous
  Syphilis
  Malaria
Trauma
  Temporal bone fracture
  Facial lacerations
  Surgical
Neoplasm
  Malignant
    Squamous cell carcinoma
    Basal cell and adenocystic
      tumors

Leukemia
Parotid neoplasms
Metastatic tumors
Benign
  Vestibular schwannoma
  Congenital cholesteatoma
  Facial nerve neuroma
Immunologic
  Guillain-Barré syndrome
  Reaction to tetanus antiserum
  Periarteritis nodosa
Metabolic
  Pregnancy
  Hypothyroidism
  Diabetes mellitus

From Noble J (ed): *Primary care medicine,* ed 3, St Louis, 2001, Mosby.

FAILURE TO THRIVE

BOX 2-96   Causes of Failure to Thrive*

Improper Feeding—50%-90%

Economic—10%-40%
Education—10%-40%
Psychologic—30%-40%
Intolerance—<5%

Other Causes—10%-50%

Hypothyroidism
Cystic fibrosis
Subdural hematoma
Glycogen storage disease
Celiac disease
Methylmalonic acidemia
Maple syrup urine disease
Mental retardation, unspecified
Urinary tract disease
Diencephalic syndrome
Brain tumors
Chronic liver disease
Congenital heart disease
Ulcerative colitis

From Hoekelman R (ed): *Primary pediatric care*, ed 3, St Louis, 1997, Mosby.
*Compendium from various sources. Some obvious causes are missing because the complaint is not failure to thrive but rather is related to the diagnosis.

FAMILIAL CANCER SYNDROMES

TABLE 2-69   Familial Cancer Syndromes

CANCER SYNDROME	GENE	CHROMOSOMAL REGION	PRINCIPAL TUMORS	PROTEIN PRODUCT LOCALIZATION	MODE OF ACTION
Loss-of-Function Cases (DNA Repair Genes)					
Ataxia telangiectasia	*ATM*	11q22	Lymphoma	Nucleus	DNA repair; ?Induction of *p53*
Bloom's syndrome	*BLM*	15q26.1	Solid tumors	Nucleus	?DNA helicase
Xeroderma pigmentosum	*XPB, XPD, XPA*	Multiple	Skin cancer	Nucleus	DNA repair helicases, nucleotide excision repair
Fanconi's anemia	*FACC*	9q22.3	Acute myelogenous leukemia	Nucleus	?DNA repair
	FACA	16q24.3			?DNA repair
Hereditary nonpolyposis colorectal cancer					
1	*MSH2*	2p16 ⎤	Colorectal, endometrial, and gastric carcinoma	Nucleus	Mismatch repair
2	*MLH1*	3p21 ⎟			
3	*PMS1*	2q32 ⎟			
4	*PMS2*	7p22 ⎦			
Low-penetrance familial nonpolyposis colorectal cancer	*MSH6*			Nucleus	Mismatch repair
Nimegen's breakage syndrome	*NBS1*	8q21.3		Nucleus	Double-strand break repair

From Abeloff MD: *Clinical oncology*, ed 2, New York, 2000, Churchill Livingstone.

Continued

FAMILIAL CANCER SYNDROMES

Familial cancer syndromes
ICD-9CM # Code varies with specific disorder

TABLE 2-69   Familial Cancer Syndromes—cont'd

CANCER SYNDROME	GENE	CHROMOSOMAL REGION	PRINCIPAL TUMORS	PROTEIN PRODUCT LOCALIZATION	MODE OF ACTION
Loss-of-Function Cases ("Tumor Suppressor Genes")					
Adenomatous polyposis coli (Gardner's syndrome)	APC	5q21	Adenomatous polyps, desmoid fibromas, colon cancer	Cytoplasm	?Regulates β-catenin function
Cowden's disease	PTEN (MMAC1)	10q23	Breast cancer, thyroid cancer (follicular type)		Dual-specificity phosphatase with similarity to tensin
Familial melanoma and pancreatic cancer					
1	CDKN2A (p16)	9p21	Melanoma, pancreatic cancer, ?other	Nucleus	Inhibitor of cyclin-dependent kinase
2	CDK4	12q13	Melanoma	Nucleus	Cyclin-dependent kinase
Familial breast cancer	BRCA1	17q21	Breast and ovarian cancer	Nucleus	Unknown—repair?
	BRCA2	13q12	Breast and ?other	Unknown	Unknown—repair?
Hereditary papillary renal cancer	MET	7q31	Papillary renal cancer		Transmembrane receptor for HGF
Li-Fraumeni	p53	17p13	Sarcomas, breast and brain tumors	Nucleus	Transcription factor; cell death regulator
Multiple exostoses (Langer-Giedion syndrome)	EXT1	8q24.1	Colon cancer Chondrosarcomas	Unknown	Unknown
Nevoid basal cell carcinoma (Gorlin's syndrome)	PTC	9q22.3	Basal cell carcinoma, medulloblastomas, ovarian fibromas	Membrane	Receptor for signaling by Hedgehog
Neurofibromatosis type 1	NF-1	17q11	Neurofibromas, sarcomas, gliomas	Cytoplasm	GTPase activator (RAS signaling)
Neurofibromatosis type 2	NF-2	22q	Schwannomas, meningiomas	Cytoplasm (juxta-membrane)	Cytoskeleton membrane link
Retinoblastoma	RB1	13q14	Retinoblastoma, osteosarcoma	Nucleus	Cell cycle regulator
Tuberous sclerosis	TSC2		Renal and brain tumors	?Golgi	p21rap-GTPase activator
Von Hippel-Lindau	VHL	3p25	Renal cell (clear cell) pheochromocytomas, hemangiomas	Nucleus	Transcriptional elongation
Wiedeman-Beckwith syndrome	Unknown	11p15	Wilm's tumor, hepatoblastoma, adrenocortical cancer		
Wilms' tumor	WT-1	11p13	Nephroblastoma	Nucleus	Zinc-finger transcription factor
Gain-of-Function Case ("Activated Proto-oncogene")					
Multiple endocrine neoplasia	RET	10q11	Carcinoma of thyroid	Membrane	Growth factor receptor—tyrosine kinase
Uncharacterized Cases (as of 1998)					
Hereditary prostate cancer (HPC)	Unknown	1q25 ?Others	Prostate cancer		Unknown
Palmoplantar keratoderma	Unknown	17q25	Esophageal cancer		Unknown

FATIGUE

TABLE 2-70 Differential Diagnosis of Fatigue

Fatigue
ICD-9CM # 780.7 Fatigue NOS
300.5 Fatigue psychogenic
780.7 Chronic fatigue syndrome

TYPE	NATURE OF PATIENT	NATURE OF SYMPTOMS	ASSOCIATED SYMPTOMS	AMELIORATING FACTORS	PHYSICAL FINDINGS	DIAGNOSTIC STUDIES
Physiologic						
Prolonged physical activity	Usually recognizes cause of fatigue and does not complain to physician about it			Rest		Within normal limits
Overwork						
Inadequate sleep						
Dieting						
Pregnancy and post-partum period						
Sedentary lifestyle				Increased physical activity		
Functional						
	May appear depressed	Fatigue on arising; may diminish during day Onset with emotional stress (job insecurity, major life change, significant loss) Often chronic	Insomnia Vague GI symptoms Chronic pain			
Depression				Improvement in life situations	"Flat" affect	
Anxiety			Numerous somatic complaints Irritability Breathlessness	Removal of stress	No physical abnormalities	
Emotional stress		Of longer duration than that of organic origin Often present or worse in morning Improves during day Unrelated to exertion	Irritability Breathlessness	Removal of stress	No physical abnormalities	

From Seller RH (ed): *Differential diagnosis of common complaints*, ed 4, Philadelphia, 2000, WB Saunders.

Continued

TABLE 2-70　Differential Diagnosis of Fatigue—cont'd

TYPE	NATURE OF PATIENT	NATURE OF SYMPTOMS	ASSOCIATED SYMPTOMS	AMELIORATING FACTORS	PHYSICAL FINDINGS	DIAGNOSTIC STUDIES
Organic						
		Of shorter duration than that of functional origin; Related to exertion; Not present in morning but worsens during day; Often related to onset of physical ailment	Symptoms of disease causing fatigue: dyspnea on exertion (cardiorespiratory disease), fever (infections), muscle weakness (myasthenia), cold intolerance (hypothyroidism)		Signs of organic pathology causing fatigue: pallor (anemia), rales (pulmonary congestion), weight loss (cancer), tachycardia (hyperthyroidism)	If diagnosis not clinically apparent: CBC with differential, urinalysis, serum glucose, SMA panel, ESR, chest x-ray, PPD, monospot test, thyroid function tests, serum electrolytes
Acute						
Viral or bacterial infections	Most common cause of acute fatigue in all age groups	Fatigue usually subsides in 2 wk	Fever		Signs of particular infection	CBC with differential; Cultures
Depression	Common cause of fatigue in adults		Sleep disturbance		No physical abnormalities	
Anxiety	Tense, nervous		Somatic complaints		May be signs of mitral valve prolapse	
Serous organic illnesses (e.g., cancer, endocrine disorders)	Rare in children; Most common in elderly		Depends on organic illness			
Drugs and medications			Bizarre behavior; Drowsiness		Bradycardia from methyldopa and β-blockers	
Organic illnesses Anemia		May have acute onset but increases progressively over time	Breathlessness; Anorexia and weight loss; Pallor; Numbness of extremities (with pernicious anemia)		Conjunctival or skin pallor	Hemoglobin, hematocrit
Hypothyroidism			Weight gain		Coarse hair; Loss of outer third of eyebrow; Hoarse voice; "Doughy" skin; Myoclonic reflexes (especially "hungup" ankle jerk)	Thyroid function tests

Chronic

Condition	Nature of Patient	Nature of Symptoms	Associated Symptoms	Ameliorating Factors	Physical Findings	
Depression (not a diagnosis of exclusion)	Does not present with fatigue in children Often overlooked in elderly Adolescents may present with somatic complaints and "acting out" behavior (e.g., abuse, sexual misconduct) Most common cause of chronic fatigue in adults	In adults, worse in the morning, improves as day progresses Signs and symptoms may vary with age, gender, and socioeconomic status	*Children:* Somatic complaints "Acting out" Hyperactivity School, eating, and sleeping problems Withdrawal *Adults:* Feelings of guilt, helplessness, pessimism, sadness, loneliness, anxiety, dissatisfaction Decreased libido Insomnia Early-morning awakening Weight loss and decreased appetite Social withdrawal Crying spells Headache Vague GI symptoms Skin disorders Chronic pain syndromes		"Flat" affect	Should *not* perform multiple diagnostic studies to rule out all possible organic causes before diagnosing depression
Medications	Users of antihistamines, psychotropics, tranquilizers, antihypertensives (reserpine, methyldopa, clonidine, β-blockers)	Onset correlates with beginning of drug ingestion		Cessation of drugs		
Chronic anxiety or stress		Constant over weeks or months Shows no diurnal variation Is not aggravated by effort May be precipitated by psychosocial factors	Somatic complaints Restlessness Irritability Sweating Palpitations Paresthesias		With mitral valve prolapse, possible midsystolic click or late systolic murmur	

Continued

From Seller RH (ed): *Differential diagnosis of common complaints*, ed 4, Philadelphia, 2000, WB Saunders.

TABLE 2-70   Differential Diagnosis of Fatigue—cont'd

TYPE	NATURE OF PATIENT	NATURE OF SYMPTOMS	ASSOCIATED SYMPTOMS	FACTORS	AMELIORATING PHYSICAL FINDINGS	DIAGNOSTIC STUDIES
Organic illnesses Congestive heart failure Cancer Chronic infection	Adults		Vary with illness		Vary with illness	
Mononucleosis	Most common in adolescents and young adults				Posterior cervical adenopathy Hepatomegaly Splenomegaly	Monospot test
Hepatitis	Most common in alcoholics and IV drug users				Hepatomegaly with or without jaundice	Abnormal liver function tests and hepatitis antigens
Fibromyalgia	Adults, usually female	Fatigue may be severe; may occur after minimal exertion	Insomnia Nonrestorative sleep Nonarticular rheumatism	Often relieved by tricyclics of trazodone	Hyperalgesic tender sites: low cervical/lumbar spine, suboccipital muscles, lateral epicondyle, medial fat pad of knee	Abnormal sleep, electroencephalogram

From Seller RH (ed): *Differential diagnosis of common complaints*, ed 4, Philadelphia, 2000, WB Saunders.

FATTY LIVER AND STEATOHEPATITIS

Fatty liver and steatohepatitis
ICD-9CM # 571.8

BOX 2-97 Differential Diagnosis of Fatty Liver and Steatohepatitis

Macrovesicular Fat

Alcohol abuse
Obesity
Hepatitis C
Protein calorie malnutrition
Diabetes mellitus
Wilson's disease
Medications: amiodarone, glucocorticoids, estrogen,
  methotrexate

Microvesicular Fat

Alcoholic foamy degeneration
Acute fatty liver of pregnancy
Reye's syndrome
Medications: tetracycline, valproic acid

Steatohepatitis

Alcohol abuse
Nonalcoholic steatohepatitis
  Idiopathic
  Jejunoileal bypass and massive intestinal resection
  Wilson's disease
  Abetalipoproteinemia
  Diabetes mellitus
  Obesity
  Limb lipodystrophy
  Weber-Christian disease
  Parenteral nutrition
  Medications: methotrexate, amiodarone, cortico-
    steroids, high-dose estrogen, nifedipine
    Historical interest: perhexiline maleate, diethylami-
      noethoxyhexestrol

From Stein J (ed): *Internal medicine,* ed 5, St Louis, 1998, Mosby.

II

FEVER AND INFECTION

Fever and infection
ICD-9CM # 780.6

TABLE 2-71 Infections Presenting with Fever as Sole or Dominant Feature

INFECTIOUS AGENT	EPIDEMIOLOGY/EXPOSURE HISTORY	DISTINCTIVE CLINICAL AND LABORATORY FINDINGS	DIAGNOSIS
Viral			
Rhinovirus, adenovirus, parainfluenza virus, enterovirus, echovirus	None (adenovirus in epidemics) Summer, epidemic	Often URI symptoms Occasionally, aseptic meningitis, rash, pleurodynia, herpangina	Throat and rectal cultures, serologies
Influenza	Winter, epidemic	Headache, myalgias, arthralgias	Throat cultures, serologies
EBV, CMV	See Section I		
Colorado tick fever	Southwest, northwest, tick exposure	Biphasic illness, leukopenia	Blood, CSF cultures, erythrocyte-associated viral antigen (indirect immunofluorescence)
Bacterial			
Staphylococcus aureus	IV drug users, patients with IV plastic cannulas, hemodialysis, dermatitis	Must exclude endocarditis	Blood cultures
Listeria monocytogenes	Depressed cell-mediated immunity	One half have meningitis	Blood, CSF cultures
Salmonella typhi, S. paratyphi	Food or water contaminated by carrier or patient	Headache, myalgias, diarrhea or constipation, transient rose spots	Early blood, bone marrow cultures; late stool culture
Streptococci	Valvular heart disease	Low-grade fever, fatigue, anemia	Blood cultures
Post-Animal Exposure			
Coxiella burnetii (Q fever)	Infected livestock	Retrobulbar headache, occasionally pneumonitis, hepatitis, culture-negative endocarditis	Serologies
Leptospira interrogans	Water contaminated by urine from dogs, cats, rodents, small mammals	Headache, myalgias, conjunctival suffusion Biphasic illness Aseptic meningitis	Serologies
Brucella species	Exposure to cattle or contaminated dairy products	Occasionally epididymitis	Blood cultures, serologies
Ehrlichia chaffeensis	South and southeast; deer or dog tick exposure	Acute onset of headache, fever, myalgias; leukopenia and thrombocytopenia	PCR, serologies
Granulomatous Infection			
Mycobacterium tuberculosis	Exposure to patient with tuberculosis, known positive tuberculin skin test	Back pain suggests vertebral infection; sterile pyuria or hematuria suggests renal infection	Liver, bone marrow histology, cultures
Histoplasma capsulatum	Mississippi and Ohio River valleys	Pneumonitis, oropharyngeal lesions	Serologies; histology and cultures on liver, bone marrow, oral lesions

From Andreoli TE (ed): *Cecil essentials of medicine,* ed 5, Philadelphia, 2001, WB Saunders.
CMV, Cytomegalovirus; *CSF,* cerebrospinal fluid; *EBV,* Epstein-Barr virus; *IV,* intravenous; *PCR,* polymerase chain reaction; *URI,* upper respiratory infection.

FEVER AND RASH

TABLE 2-72   Identification of Life-Threatening Diseases Associated with Fever and Rash

Fever and rash
ICD-9CM # 782.1 Exanthem
057.9 Exanthem viral

DISEASE	HISTORY	CHARACTERISTICS OF RASH	DISTRIBUTION OF RASH	ASSOCIATED CLINICAL FINDINGS	DIAGNOSTIC AIDS
Rocky Mountain spotted fever (RMSF)	Tick exposure (75%) May-September occurrence in temperate-zone states Heaviest endemic area: middle Atlantic states and Southeast	Initial maculopapular petechiae appearing on second to sixth febrile day and usually painless.	Begins on wrists, ankles, forearms, spreading within 6-8 hr to palms, soles, trunk	Prodrome of fever, headache, myalgias Hyponatremia, normal to slightly increased WBC, thrombocytopenia, hypoalbuminemia	Biopsy of involved skin with immunofluorescence and other serologic tests. Serology: Complement-fixation more sensitive and more specific than Weil-Felix agglutination.
Meningococcemia*	Tends to occur in late winter, early spring Outbreaks in military recruits, crowded living conditions	*Acute:* May be maculopapular initially. Small petechiae with irregular borders ("smudging"), at times with vesicular or grayish ulcer. May coalesce. Painful. *Chronic:* Maculopapules, petechial vesicles, or pustules; tender nodules.	*Acute:* Extremities and trunk in random fashion *Chronic:* Extremities, particularly over joints	*Acute:* Meningitis, disseminated intravascular coagulation, shock, acidosis *Chronic:* Rash appears with recurrent cycles of fever over 2-3 mo	*Acute:* Aspiration of center of skin lesions for Gram stain, culture (up to 60% positive). Blood cultures. Cerebrospinal fluid culture and Gram stain. *Chronic:* Blood culture usually positive during febrile episode. Biopsy findings resemble leukocytoclastic angiitis.
Disseminated gonococcal infection	Incidence higher in women than in men Young, sexually active Onset often related to menstruation	Pustules on erythematous base most characteristic. Also, macules, papules, pustules, and bullae less commonly.	Over extremities, with relative sparing of face and trunk; usually few (5-40) lesions	Migratory polyarthralgia, tenosynovitis, septic arthritis	Gram stain of lesion. Blood, joint fluid culture (50%) prove diagnosis. Cervical, rectal, throat cultures support diagnosis.
Staphylococcal septicemia	Nosocomial: indwelling catheters, pacemakers, dialysis shunts, wound infections Drug abuse	Pustules, purulent purpura, subcutaneous nodules, infarcts	Widespread, with infarcts having predilection for distal extremities	Endocarditis, with valvular incompetence, meningitis, multiple-organ involvement	Aspiration of lesions for Gram stain culture. Blood, cerebrospinal fluid (where indicated) cultures. Teichoic acid antibody suggestive of deep-seated infection.

Continued

TABLE 2-72   Identification of Life-Threatening Diseases Associated with Fever and Rash—cont'd

DISEASE	HISTORY	CHARACTERISTICS OF RASH	DISTRIBUTION OF RASH	ASSOCIATED CLINICAL FINDINGS	DIAGNOSTIC AIDS
Pseudomonas septicemia	Hospitalized patients, especially with neutropenia or burns	*Vesicles:* Isolated or in small clusters rapidly becoming hemorrhagic. *Ecthyma gangrenosum:* Round, indurated, ulcerated painless lesion with central gray eschar. *Maculopapular lesion:* Small erythematous lesion resembling "rose spots." Gangrenous cellulitis.	Random Axillary or anogenital area, thigh Trunk Localized	Generally extremely toxic, with fever; septic picture	Aspiration of lesion for Gram stain, culture. Cultures of blood, urine, sputum, etc.
Candida septicemia	Broad-spectrum antibiotics, leukemia, immunosuppression, hyperalimentation, cardiac surgery	Multiple discrete pink maculopapular lesions 2-5 mm in diameter.	Trunk and extremities	Toxic state; associated ophthalmitis, esophagitis, cystitis	Punch biopsy of lesion with stains for fungus. Buffy coat of blood. Blood cultures (definitive diagnosis). Examination and culture of stool, urine, sputum (supportive of diagnosis with multiple-site involvement). Barium or endoscopic examination of esophagus.
Infective endocarditis	Indwelling catheters, pacemakers, dialysis shunts, valvular heart disease, prosthetic valves, intravenous drug abuse, preceding dental or surgical manipulations	*Petechiae:* Often in small groups. *Osler's nodes:* Pea-sized, tender, erythematous nodules. *Janeway's lesions:* Small erythematous or hemorrhagic macules.	Conjunctivae, palate, upper chest, distal extremities Pads of fingers and toes Palms and soles	Heart murmur, valvular incompetence, metastatic abscesses, Roth's spots, splenomegaly, hematuria, glomerulonephritis, etc.	Serology not yet reliable. Blood cultures (3-5 sets). Echocardiogram. Circulating immune complexes.

Toxic shock syndrome	Young female predominance 1-4 days prodrome of fever, myalgias, arthralgias, and diarrhea Onset during or soon after menses (has also been reported in men and unassociated with menses in women)	*Erythroderma:* Seen at presentation. Diffuse, blanching, macular (deep-red "sunburned" appearance). Resolves within 3 days, followed 5-12 days later by desquamation, most commonly of hands and feet. *Mucosal hyperemia:* Pharynx, conjunctivae, vagina.	Diffuse, hands and feet predominantly	Fever, severe hypotension, multisystem involvement (gastrointestinal, muscular, renal, hepatic, hematologic, CNS)	Clinical criteria. See Section I. Negative serology for RMSF, leptospirosis, measles. Identification of toxin producing strain of *S. aureus.*
Lyme disease	From endemic areas—Northeast, Midwest (Minnesota/Wisconsin), and West (California/Oregon) Usually begins in summer	*Erythema chronicum migrans:* Expanding annular erythema (median diameter 15 cm) from central macule or papule. Secondary annular lesions seen.	Commonly, thigh, groin, axilla. Any site can be involved.	Fever, chills, malaise, myalgias, lymphadenopathy Late (weeks to months) CNS, cardiac, and joint involvement	Primarily history and clinical criteria. Organism can be cultured (difficult, special media). Serology.

From Stein JH (ed): *Internal medicine,* ed 5, St Louis, 1998, Mosby.
CNS, Central nervous system.

II

FEVER IN RETURNING TRAVELERS AND IMMIGRANTS

BOX 2-98   Differential Diagnosis of Some Selected Systemic Febrile Illnesses to Consider in Returned Travelers and Immigrants*

Common

Acute respiratory tract infection (worldwide)
Gastroenteritis (worldwide) [foodborne, waterborne, fecal-oral]
Enteric fever, including typhoid (worldwide) [food, water]
Urinary tract infection (worldwide) [sexual contact]
Drug reactions [antibiotics, prophylactic agents, other] {rash frequent}
Malaria (tropics, limited areas of temperate zones) [mosquitoes]
Arboviruses (Africa; tropics) [mosquitoes, ticks, mites]
Dengue (Asia, Caribbean, Africa) [mosquitoes]
Viral hepatitis (worldwide)
Hepatitis A (worldwide) [food, fecal-oral]
Hepatitis B (worldwide, especially Asia, sub-Sahara Africa) [sexual contact] {long incubation period}
Hepatitis C (worldwide) [blood or sexual contact]
Hepatitis E (Asia, North Africa, Mexico, ?others) [food, water]
Tuberculosis (worldwide) [airborne, milk] {long period to symptomatic infection}
Sexually transmitted diseases (worldwide) [sexual contact]

Less Common

Filariasis (see Table 2-57) (Asia, Africa, South America) [biting insects] {long incubation period, eosinophilia}
Measles (developing world) [airborne] {in susceptible individual}
Amebic abscess (worldwide) [food]
Brucellosis (worldwide) [milk, cheese, food, animal contact]
Listeriosis (worldwide) [foodborne] {meningitis}
Leptospirosis (worldwide) [animal contact, open fresh water] {jaundice, meningitis}
Strongyloidiasis (warm and tropical areas) [soil contact] {eosinophilia}
Toxoplasmosis (worldwide) [undercooked meat]

Rare

Relapsing fever (western Americas, Asia, northern Africa) [ticks lice]
Hemorrhagic fevers (worldwide) [arthropod and nonarthropod transmitted]
Yellow fever (tropics) [mosquitoes] {hepatitis}
Hemorrhagic fever with renal syndrome (Europe, Asia, North America) [rodent urine] {renal impairment}
    Hantavirus pulmonary syndrome (western North America, ?other) [rodent urine] {respiratory distress syndrome}
Lassa fever (Africa) [rodent excreta, person to person] {high mortality rate}
Other-chikungunya, Rift Valley, Ebola-Marburg, etc. (various) [insect bites, rodent excreta, aerosols, person to person] {often severe}
Rickettsial infections {Rashes and eschars}
Leishmaniasis, visceral (Middle East, Mediterranean, Africa, Asia, South America) [biting flies] {long incubation period}
Acute schistosomiasis (Africa, Asia, South America, Caribbean) [fresh water]
Chagas' disease (South and Central America) [reduviid bug bites] {often asymptomatic}
African trypanosomiasis (Africa) [tsetse fly bite] {neurologic syndromes, sleeping sickness}
Bartonellosis (South America) [sandfly bite; cb {skin nodules}
HIV infection/AIDS (worldwide) [sexual and blood contact]
Trichinosis (worldwide) [undercooked meat] {eosinophilia}
Plague (temperate and tropical plains) [animal exposures and fleas]
Tularemia (worldwide) [animal contact, fleas, aerosols] {ulcers, lymph nodes}
Anthrax (worldwide) [animal, animal product contact] {ulcers}
Lyme disease (North America, Europe) [tick bites] {arthritis, meningitis, cardiac abnormalities}

From Noble J: *Primary care medicine,* ed 3, St Louis, 2001, Mosby.
*Diagnoses for which particular symptoms are indicative are in *italics.* Exposure to regions of the world that are most likely to be significant to the diagnosis are presented in (parentheses). Vectors, risk behaviors, and sources associated with acquisition are presented in [brackets]. Special clinical characteristics are listed within.

FILARIAL INFECTIONS IN HUMANS
TABLE 2-73   Filarial Infections in Humans

Filarial infections in humans
ICD-9CM # 125.9 Filariasis, unspecified

AGENT	DISTRIBUTION	VECTOR	RESIDENCE OF ADULT WORMS	MIGRATION OF MICROFILARIAE	DIAGNOSTIC PROCEDURE	TREATMENT
			CLINICAL MANIFESTATIONS RELATED TO:			
Wuchereria bancrofti	Asia, Latin America, Pacific islands	Mosquitoes	Lymphatic tissue, Lymphadenitis, Lymphadenopathy, Elephantiasis, Hydrocele, Chyluria	Blood, Eosinophilia, Allergic reactions, Usually nocturnal periodicity	Membrane filtration of blood	Diethylcarbamazine [DEC] PO, Day 1: 50 mg, once, Day 2: 50 mg, tid, Day 3: 100 mg, tid, Days 4-21: 2 mg/kg, tid
Brugia malayi, B. timori	Southeast Asia, India, China, Korea, Indonesia	Mosquitoes		Some subperiodicity		
Loa loa	West Africa, Central Africa	Tabanid horseflies (Chrysops sp.)	Migratory in subcutaneous tissue, Erythematous "Calabar" swellings, Visible subconjunctival migration	Blood (eosinophils), Diurnal periodicity	(At peak microfilaria parasitemia, when periodicity presents)	DEC, PO, Days 1-3: as above, Days 4-21: 3 mg/kg, tid
Mansonella perstans	Africa, South America	Midges	Body cavities, Asymptomatic to mild abdominal pain and swellings	Blood, Minimal to no symptoms, Nonperiodic		Mebendazole, PO 100 mg, bid for 30 days
M. ozzardi	South America, Central America	Midges	Body cavities, Mild systemic symptoms	Blood, Nonperiodic		Ivermectin, PO 150 µg/kg, once
M. streptocerca	Central Africa, West Africa	Midges	Skin	Skin, lymph nodes, Dermatitis	Skin biopsy	? DEC (see above)
Onchocerca volvulus	Africa, Central America, South America, Yemen	Black flies (Simulium sp.)	Soft tissue, Subcutaneous nodules	Skin and subcutaneous tissue, Rash, Keratitis, iritis, Blindness	Skin snips (larvae), Biopsy of nodule (adult)	Ivermectin, 150 µg/kg once, Repeat every 6 to 12 mo

From Noble J: *Primary care medicine*, ed 3, St Louis, 2001, Mosby.

FLUSHING

BOX 2-99   Differential Diagnosis of Flushing

Physiologic Flushing

Menopause
Ingestion of monosodium glutamate (Chinese restaurant syndrome)
Ingestion of hot drinks

Drugs

Alcohol (with or without disulfiram, metronidazole, or chlorpropamide)
Diltiazem
Nifedipine
Nicotinic acid
Levodopa

Bromocriptine
Thyrotropin-releasing hormone
Amyl nitrate

Neoplastic Disorders

Carcinoid syndrome
VIPoma syndrome
Medullary carcinoma of the thyroid
Systemic mastocytosis
Basophilic chronic myelocytic leukemia
Renal cell carcinoma

Agnogenic Flushing

From Moore WT, Eastman RC: *Diagnostic endocrinology*, ed 2, St Louis, 1996, Mosby.
VIPoma, Vasoactive intestinal peptide–secreting tumor.

FOODBORNE ILLNESSES

BOX 2-100   Differential Diagnosis

A variety of infectious and noninfectious agents must be considered in patients suspected of having a foodborne illness. Establishing a diagnosis can be difficult, however, particularly in patients with persistent or chronic diarrhea, those with severe abdominal pain, and when there is an underlying disease process. The extent of diagnostic evaluation depends on the clinical picture, the differential diagnosis considered, and clinical judgment.

If any of the following signs and symptoms occur, alone or in combination, laboratory testing may provide important diagnostic clues (particular attention should be given to very young and elderly patients and to immunocompromised patients, all of whom are more vulnerable):
• Bloody diarrhea
• Weight loss
• Diarrhea leading to dehydration
• Fever
• Prolonged diarrhea (3 or more unformed stools per day, persisting several days)
• Neurologic involvement such as paresthesias, motor weakness, cranial nerve palsies
• Sudden onset of nausea, vomiting, diarrhea
• Severe abdominal pain

In addition to foodborne causes, a differential diagnosis of gastrointestinal tract disease should include underlying medical conditions such as irritable bowel syndrome; inflammatory bowel diseases such as Crohn's disease or ulcerative colitis; malignancy; medication use (including antibiotic-related *Clostridium difficile* toxin colitis); gastrointestinal tract surgery or radiation; malabsorption syndromes; immune deficiencies; Brainerd diarrhea; and numerous other structural, functional, and metabolic etiologies. Consideration also should be given to exogenous factors such as the association of the illness with travel, occupation, emotional stress, sexual practices, exposure to other ill persons, recent hospitalization, child care center attendance, and nursing home residence.

The differential diagnosis of patients presenting with neurologic symptoms due to a foodborne illness is also complex. Possible food-related causes to consider include recent ingestion of contaminated seafood, mushroom poisoning, and chemical poisoning. Because the ingestion of certain toxins (e.g., botulinum toxin, tetrodotoxin) and chemicals (e.g., organophosphates) can be life-threatening, a differential diagnosis must be made quickly with concern for aggressive therapy and life support measures (e.g., respiratory support, administration of antitoxin or atropine), and possible hospital admission.

MMWR 50(RR-2):1, 2001.

BOX 2-101   Clinical Microbiology Testing

When submitting specimens for microbiologic testing, it is important to realize that clinical microbiology laboratories differ in protocols used for the detection of pathogens. To optimize recovery of a causative agent, physicians should understand routine specimen collection and testing procedures as well as circumstances and procedures for making special test requests. Some complex tests (e.g., toxin testing, serotyping, molecular techniques) may be available only from large commercial and public health laboratories. Contact your microbiology laboratory for more information.

Stool cultures are indicated if the patient is immunocompromised, febrile, has bloody diarrhea, has severe abdominal pain, or if the illness is clinically severe or persistent. Stool cultures are also indicated if many fecal leukocytes are present, which indicates diffuse colonic inflammation and is suggestive of invasive bacterial pathogens such as *Shigella, Salmonella,* and *Campylobacter* species, and invasive *E. coli.* In most laboratories, routine stool cultures are limited to screening for *Salmonella* and *Shigella* species, and *Campylobacter jejuni/coli.* Cultures for *Vibrio* and *Yersinia* species, *E. coli* O157:H7, and *Campylobacter* species other than *jejuni/coli* require additional media or incubation conditions and therefore require advance notification or communication with laboratory and infectious disease personnel.

Stool examination for parasites generally is indicated for patients with suggestive travel histories, who are immunocompromised, who suffer chronic or persistent diarrhea, or when the diarrheal illness is unresponsive to appropriate antimicrobial therapy. Stool examination for parasites is also indicated for gastrointestinal tract illnesses that appear to have a long incubation period. Requests for ova and parasite examination of a stool specimen will often enable identification of *Giardia lamblia* and *Entamoeba histolytica,* but a special request may be needed for detection of *Cryptosporidium parvum* and *Cyclospora cayetanensis.* Each laboratory may vary in its routine procedures for detecting parasites so it is important to contact your laboratory.

Blood cultures should be obtained when bacteremia or systemic infection are suspected.

Direct antigen detection tests and molecular biology techniques are available for rapid identification of certain bacterial, viral, and parasitic agents in clinical specimens. In some circumstances, microbiologic and chemical laboratory testing of vomitus or implicated food items also is warranted.

MMWR 50(RR-2):1, 2001.

BOX 2-102 Etiologic Agents to Consider for Various Manifestations of Foodborne Illnesses

CLINICAL PRESENTATION	POTENTIAL FOOD-RELATED AGENTS TO CONSIDER
Gastroenteritis (vomiting as primary symptom; diarrhea also may be present)	Viral gastroenteritis, most commonly rotavirus in an infant or Norwalk-like virus in an older child or adult; or food poisoning due to preformed toxins (e.g., vomitoxin, *Staphylococcus aureus* toxin, *Bacillus cereus* toxin) and heavy metals.
Noninflammatory diarrhea (acute watery diarrhea without fever/dysentery; some cases may present with fever)*	Can be caused by virtually all enteric pathogens (bacterial, viral, parasitic) but is a classic symptom of: Enterotoxigenic *E. coli* / *Vibrio cholerae* / Enteric viruses (astroviruses, caliciviruses, enteric adenovirus, rotavirus) / *Cryptosporidium parvum* / *Cyclospora cayetanensis*
Inflammatory diarrhea (invasive gastroenteritis; grossly bloody stool and fever may be present)†	*Shigella* species / *Campylobacter* species / *Salmonella* species / Enteroinvasive *E. coli* / Enterohemorrhagic *E. coli* / *Vibrio parahemolyticus* / *Entamoeba histolytica* / *Yersinia enterocolitica*
Persistent diarrhea (lasting ≥14 days)	Prolonged illness should prompt examination for parasites, particularly in travelers to mountainous or other areas where untreated water is consumed. Consider *Cyclospora cayetanensis*, *Cryptosporidium parvum*, *Entamoeba histolytica*, and *Giardia lamblia*.
Neurologic manifestations (e.g., paresthesias, respiratory depression, bronchospasm)	Botulism (*Clostridium botulinum* toxin) / Organophosphate pesticides / Thallium poisoning / Scombroid fish poisoning (histamine, saurine) / Ciguatera fish poisoning (ciguatoxin) / Tetrodon fish poisoning (tetrodotoxin) / Neurotoxic shellfish poisoning (brevitoxin) / Paralytic shellfish poisoning (saxitoxin) / Amnesic shellfish poisoning (domoic acid) / Mushroom poisoning / Guillain-Barré syndrome (associated with infectious diarrhea due to *C. jejuni*)
Systemic illness	*Listeria monocytogenes* / *Brucella* species / *Trichinella spiralis* / *Toxoplasma gondii* / *Vibrio vulnificus* / Hepatitis A virus

MMWR 50(RR-2):1, 2001.

* Noninflammatory diarrhea is characterized by mucosal hypersecretion or decreased absorption without mucosal destruction and generally involves the small intestine. Some affected patients may be dehydrated because of severe watery diarrhea and may appear seriously ill. This is more common in the young and the elderly. Most patients experience minimal dehydration and appear mildly ill with scant physical findings. Illness typically occurs with abrupt onset and brief duration. Fever and systemic symptoms usually are absent (except for symptoms related directly to intestinal fluid loss).

† Inflammatory diarrhea is characterized by mucosal invasion with resulting inflammation and is caused by invasive or cytotoxigenic microbial pathogens. The diarrheal illness usually involves the large intestine and may be associated with fever, abdominal pain and tenderness, headache, nausea, vomiting, malaise, and myalgia. Stools may be bloody and may contain many fecal leukocytes.

FOODBORNE ILLNESSES, BACTERIAL

TABLE 2-74   Foodborne Illnesses (Bacterial)

ETIOLOGY	INCUBATION PERIOD	SIGNS AND SYMPTOMS	DURATION OF ILLNESS	ASSOCIATED FOODS	LABORATORY TESTING	TREATMENT
Bacillus anthracis	2 days to weeks	Nausea, vomiting, malaise, bloody diarrhea, acute abdominal pain.	Weeks	Insufficiently cooked contaminated meat.	Blood.	Penicillin is first choice for naturally acquired gastrointestinal anthrax. Ciprofloxacin is second option.
Bacillus cereus (diarrheal toxin)	10-16 hr	Abdominal cramps, watery diarrhea, nausea.	24-48 hr	Meats, stews, gravies, vanilla sauce.	Testing not necessary, self-limiting (consider testing food and stool for toxin in outbreaks).	Supportive care, self-limiting.
Bacillus cereus (preformed enterotoxin)	1-6 hr	Sudden onset of severe nausea and vomiting. Diarrhea may be present.	24 hr	Improperly refrigerated cooked and fried rice, meats.	Normally a clinical diagnosis. Clinical laboratories do not routinely identify this organism. If indicated, send stool and food specimens to reference laboratory for culture and toxin identification.	Supportive care.
Brucella abortus, B. melitensis, and *B. suis*	7-21 days	Fever, chills, sweating, weakness, headache, muscle and joint pain, diarrhea, bloody stools during acute phase.	Weeks	Raw milk, goat cheese made from unpasteurized milk, contaminated meats.	Blood culture and positive serology.	*Acute:* Rifampin and doxycycline daily for ≥6 weeks. Infections with complications require combination therapy with rifampin, tetracycline and an aminoglycoside.
Campylobacter jejuni	2-5 days	Diarrhea, cramps, fever, and vomiting; diarrhea may be bloody.	2-10 days	Raw and undercooked poultry, unpasteurized milk, contaminated water.	Routine stool culture; *Campylobacter* requires special media and incubation at 42° C to grow.	Supportive care. For severe cases, antibiotics such as erythromycin and quinolones may be indicated early in the diarrheal disease. Guillain-Barré syndrome can be a sequala.
Clostridium botulinum children and adults (preformed toxin)	12-72 hr	Vomiting, diarrhea, blurred vision, diplopia, dysphagia, and descending muscle weakness.	Variable (from days to months). Can be complicated by respiratory failure and death.	Home-canned foods with a low acid content, improperly canned commercial foods, home-canned or fermented fish, herb-infused oils, baked potatoes in aluminum foil, cheese sauce, bottled garlic, foods held warm for extended periods of time (e.g., in a warm oven).	Stool, serum, and food can be tested for toxin. Stool and food can also be cultured for the organism. These tests can be performed at some State Health Department Laboratories and the CDC.	Supportive care. Botulinum antitoxin is helpful if given early in the course of the illness. Call 404-639-2206 or 404-639-3753 workdays, 404-639-2888 weekends and evenings.

MMRW 50(RR-2):1, 2001.
CDC, Centers for Disease Control and Prevention; *TMP-SMX,* trimethoprim-sulfamethoxazole.
Please call the state health department for more information on specific foodborne illnesses. These telephone numbers are available at: http://www2.cdc.gov/mmwr/international/relres.html.

Continued

TABLE 2-74   Foodborne Illnesses (Bacterial)—cont'd

ETIOLOGY	INCUBATION PERIOD	SIGNS AND SYMPTOMS	DURATION OF ILLNESS	ASSOCIATED FOODS	LABORATORY TESTING	TREATMENT
Clostridium botulinum infants	3-30 days	In infants <12 mo; lethargy, weakness, poor feeding, constipation, hypotonia, poor head control, poor gag and suck.	Variable	Honey, home-canned vegetables and fruits.	Stool, serum, and food can be tested for toxin. Stool and food can also be cultured for the organism. These tests can be performed at some State Health Department laboratories and the CDC.	Supportive care. Botulism immune globulin can be obtained from the Infant Botulism Prevention Program, Health and Human Services, California (510-540-2646). Botulinum antitoxin is generally not recommended for infants.
Clostridium perfringens toxin	8-16 hr	Watery diarrhea, nausea, abdominal cramps; fever is rare.	24-48 hr	Meats, poultry, gravy, dried or precooked foods.	Stools can be tested for enterotoxin and cultured for organism. Because *Clostridium perfringens* can normally be found in stool, quantitative cultures must be done.	Supportive care. Antibiotics not indicated.
Enterohemorrhagic *E. coli* (EHEC) including *E. coli* 0157:H7 and other Shigatoxin-producing *E. coli* (STEC)	1-8 days	Severe diarrhea that is often bloody, abdominal pain and vomiting. Usually, little or no fever is present. More common in children <4 yr.	5-10 days	Undercooked beef, unpasteurized milk and juice, raw fruits and vegetables (e.g., sprouts), salami, salad dressing, and contaminated water.	Stool culture; *E. coli* O157:H7 requires special media to grow. If *E. coli* O157:H7 is suspected, specific testing must be requested. Shiga toxin testing may be done using commercial kits; positive isolates should be forwarded to public health laboratories for confirmation and serotyping.	Supportive care, monitor renal function, hemoglobin, and platelets closely. Studies indicate that antibiotics may be harmful. *E. coli* O157:H7 infection is also associated with hemolytic uremic syndrome, which can cause lifelong complications.
Enterotoxigenic *E. coli* (ETEC)	1-3 days	Watery diarrhea, abdominal cramps, some vomiting.	3->7 days	Water or food contaminated with human feces.	Stool culture. ETEC requires special laboratory techniques for identification. If suspected, must request specific testing.	Supportive care. Antibiotics are rarely needed except in severe cases. Recommended antibiotics include TMP-SMX and quinolones.
Listeria monocytogenes	9-48 hr for gastrointestinal symptoms, 2-6 wk for invasive disease

At birth and infancy | Fever, muscle aches, and nausea or diarrhea. Pregnant women may have mild flulike illness, and infection can lead to premature delivery or stillbirth. Elderly or immunocompromised patients may have bacteremia or meningitis.

Infants infected from mother at risk for sepsis or meningitis. | Variable | Fresh soft cheeses, unpasteurized milk, inadequately pasteurized milk, ready-to-eat deli meats, hot dogs. | Blood or cerebrospinal fluid cultures. Asymptomatic fecal carriage occurs; therefore, stool culture usually not helpful. Antibody to listerolysin O may be helpful to identify outbreak retrospectively. | Supportive care and antibiotics; Intravenous ampicillin, penicillin, or TMP-SMX are recommended for invasive disease. |

TABLE 2-74   Foodborne Illnesses (Bacterial)—cont'd

ETIOLOGY	INCUBATION PERIOD	SIGNS AND SYMPTOMS	DURATION OF ILLNESS	ASSOCIATED FOODS	LABORATORY TESTING	TREATMENT
Salmonella spp.	1-3 days	Diarrhea, fever, abdominal cramps, vomiting. *S. typhi* and *S. paratyphi* produce typhoid with insidious onset characterized by fever, headache, constipation, malaise, chills, and myalgia; diarrhea is uncommon, and vomiting is usually not severe.	4-7 days	Contaminated eggs, poultry, unpasteurized milk or juice, cheese, contaminated raw fruits and vegetables (alfalfa sprouts, melons). *S. typhi* epidemics are often related to fecal contamination of water supplies or street-vended foods.	Routine stool cultures.	Supportive care. Other than for *S. typhi*, antibiotics are not indicated unless there is extraintestinal spread, or the risk of extraintestinal spread, of the infection. Consider ampicillin, gentamicin, TMP-SMX, or quinolones if indicated. A vaccine exists for *S. typhi*.
Shigella spp.	24-48 hr	Abdominal cramps, fever, and diarrhea. Stools may contain blood and mucus.	4-7 days	Food or water contaminated with fecal material. Usually person-to-person spread, fecal-oral transmission. Ready-to-eat foods touched by infected food workers, raw vegetables, egg salads.	Routine stool cultures.	Supportive care. TMP/SMX recommended in the U.S. if organism is susceptible; nalidixic acid or other quinolones may be indicated if organism is resistant, especially in developing countries.
Staphylococcus aureus (preformed enterotoxin)	1-6 hr	Sudden onset of severe nausea and vomiting. Abdominal cramps. Diarrhea and fever may be present.	24-48 hr	Unrefrigerated or improperly refrigerated meats, potato and egg salads, cream pastries.	Normally a clinical diagnosis. Stool, vomitus, and food can be tested for toxin and cultured if indicated.	Supportive care.
Vibrio cholerae (toxin)	24-72 hr	Profuse watery diarrhea and vomiting, which can lead to severe dehydration and death within hours.	3-7 days. Causes life-threatening dehydration.	Contaminated water, fish, shellfish, street-vended food.	Stool culture; *Vibrio cholerae* requires special media to grow. If *V. cholerae* is suspected, must request specific testing.	Supportive care with aggressive oral and intravenous rehydration. In cases of confirmed cholera, tetracycline or doxycycline is recommended for adults, and TMP-SMX for children (<8 yr).
Vibrio parahaemolyticus	2-48 hr	Watery diarrhea, abdominal cramps, nausea, vomiting.	2-5 days	Undercooked or raw seafood, such as fish, shellfish.	Stool cultures. *Vibrio parahaemolyticus* requires special media to grow. If *V. parahaemolyticus* is suspected, must request specific testing.	Supportive care. Antibiotics are recommended in severe cases: tetracycline, doxycycline, gentamicin, and cefotaxime.
Vibrio vulnificus	1-7 days	Vomiting, diarrhea, abdominal pain, bacteremia, and wound infections. More common in the immunocompromised, or in patients with chronic liver disease (presenting with bullous skin lesions).	2-8 days; can be fatal in patients with liver disease and the immunocompromised	Undercooked or raw shellfish, especially oysters; other contaminated seafood, and open wounds exposed to sea water.	Stool, wound, or blood cultures. *Vibrio vulnificus* requires special media to grow. If *V. vulnificus* is suspected, must request specific testing.	Supportive care and antibiotics; tetracycline, doxycycline, and ceftazidime are recommended.
Yersinia enterocolytica and *Y. pseudotuberculosis*	24-48 hr	Appendicitis-like symptoms (diarrhea and vomiting, fever, and abdominal pain) occur primarily in older children and young adults. May have a scarlitiniform rash with *Y. pseudotuberculosis*.	1-3 wk	Undercooked pork, unpasteurized milk, contaminated water. Infection has occurred in infants whose caregivers handled chitterlings, tofu.	Stool, vomitus or blood culture. *Yersinia* requires special media to grow. If suspected, must request specific testing. Serology is available in research and reference laboratories.	Supportive care, usually self-limiting. If septicemia or other invasive disease occurs, antibiotic therapy with gentamicin or cefotaxime (doxycycline and ciprofloxacin also effective).

II

FOODBORNE ILLNESSES, NONINFECTIOUS

Foodborne illnesses, noninfectious
ICD-9CM # 989.7

TABLE 2-75   Foodborne Illnesses (Noninfectious)

ETIOLOGY	INCUBATION PERIOD	SIGNS AND SYMPTOMS	DURATION OF ILLNESS	ASSOCIATED FOODS	LABORATORY TESTING	TREATMENT
Antimony	5 min-8 hr, usually <1 hr	Vomiting, metallic taste.	Usually self-limited	Metallic container.	Identification of metal in beverage or food.	Supportive care.
Arsenic	Few hr	Vomiting, colic, diarrhea.	Several days	Contaminated food.	Urine. May cause eosinophilia.	Gastric lavage, BAL (dimer-caprol).
Cadmium	5 min-8 hr, usually <1 hr	Nausea, vomiting, myalgia, increase in salivation, stomach pain.	Usually self-limited	Seafood, oysters, clams, lobster, grains, peanuts.	Identification of metal in food.	Supportive care.
Ciguatera fish poisoning (ciguatera toxin).	2-6 hr	GI: abdominal pain, nausea, vomiting, diarrhea.	Days to weeks to months	A variety of large reef fish; grouper, red snapper, amber-jack, and bar-racuda (most common).	Radioassay for toxin in fish or a consistent history.	Supportive care, IV mannitol. Children more vulnerable.
	3 hr	Neurologic: pares-thesias, reversal of hot or cold, pain, weakness.				
	2-5 days	Cardiovascular: bradycardia, hy-potension, in-crease in T wave abnormalities.				
Copper	5 min-8 hr, usually <1 hr	Nausea, vomiting, blue or green vomitus.	Usually self-limited	Metallic container.	Identification of metal in beverage or food.	Supportive care.
Mercury	1 wk or longer	Numbness, weak-ness of legs, spastic paralysis, impaired vision, blindness, coma. Pregnant women and the develop-ing fetus are espe-cially vulnerable.	May be pro-tracted	Fish exposed to organic mercury, grains treated with mercury fungicides.	Analysis of blood, hair.	Supportive care.
Mushroom toxins, short-acting (museinol, muscarine, psilocybin, coprius artemetaris, ibotenic acid)	<2 hr	Vomiting, diarrhea, confusion, visual disturbance, sali-vation, diaphore-sis, hallucinations, disulfiram-like re-action, confusion, visual distur-bance.	Self-limited	Wild mushrooms (cooking may not destroy these toxins).	Typical syndrome and mushroom identified or demonstration of the toxin.	Supportive care.
Mushroom toxin, long-acting (amanita)	4-8 hr diar-rhea; 24-48 hr liver failure	Diarrhea, abdomi-nal cramps, leading to hepatic and renal failure.	Often fatal	Mushrooms.	Typical syndrome and mushroom identified and/or demonstration of the toxin.	Supportive care; life-threatening, may need life support.

MMWR 50(RR-2):1, 2001.
BAL, Bronchoalveolar lavage; *GI,* gastrointestinal; *IV,* intravenous.
Please call the state health department for more information on specific foodborne illnesses. These telephone numbers are available at: http://www2.cdc.gov/mmwr/international/relres.html.

TABLE 2-75 Foodborne Illnesses (Noninfectious)—cont'd

ETIOLOGY	INCUBATION PERIOD	SIGNS AND SYMPTOMS	DURATION OF ILLNESS	ASSOCIATED FOODS	LABORATORY TESTING	TREATMENT
Nitrite poisoning	1-2 hr	Nausea, vomiting, cyanosis, headache, dizziness, weakness, loss of consciousness, chocolate-brown colored blood.	Usually self-limited	Cured meats, any contaminated foods, spinach exposed to excessive nitrification.	Analysis of the food, blood.	Supportive care, methylene blue.
Pesticides (organophosphates or carbamates)	Few min to few hr	Nausea, vomiting, abdominal cramps, diarrhea, headache, nervousness, blurred vision, twitching, convulsions.	Usually self-limited	Any contaminated food.	Analysis of the food, blood.	Atropine.
Puffer fish (tetrodotoxin)	<30 min	Paresthesias, vomiting, diarrhea, abdominal pain, ascending paralysis, respiratory failure.	Death usually in 4-6 hr	Puffer fish.	Detection of tetrodotoxin in fish.	Life-threatening, may need respiratory support.
Scombroid (histamine)	1 min-3 hr	Flushing, rash, burning sensation of skin, mouth and throat, dizziness, urticaria, paresthesias.	3-6 hr	Fish: bluefin, tuna, skipjack, mackerel, marlin, and mahi mahi.	Demonstration of histamine in food or clinical diagnosis.	Supportive care, antihistamines.
Shellfish toxins (diarrheic, neurotoxic, amnesic)	Diarrheic shellfish poisoning (DSP)—30 min to 2 hr	Nausea, vomiting, diarrhea, and abdominal pain accompanied by chills, headache, and fever.	Hours to 2-3 days	A variety of shellfish, primarily mussels, oysters, scallops, and shellfish from the Florida coast and the Gulf of Mexico.	Detection of the toxin in shellfish; high pressure liquid chromatography.	Supportive care, generally self-limiting. Elderly are especially sensitive to ASP.
	Neurotoxic shellfish poisoning (NSP)— few min to hours	Tingling and numbness of lips, tongue, and throat, muscular aches, dizziness, reversal of the sensations of hot and cold, diarrhea, and vomiting.				
	Amnesic shellfish poisoning (ASP)— 24-48 hr	Vomiting, diarrhea, abdominal pain and neurologic problems such as confusion, memory loss, disorientation, seizure, coma.				

Continued

TABLE 2-75   Foodborne Illnesses (Noninfectious)—cont'd

ETIOLOGY	INCUBATION PERIOD	SIGNS AND SYMPTOMS	DURATION OF ILLNESS	ASSOCIATED FOODS	LABORATORY TESTING	TREATMENT
Shellfish toxins (paralytic shellfish poisoning)	30 min-3 hr	Diarrhea, nausea, vomiting leading to paresthesias of mouth, lips, weakness, dysphasia, dysphonia, respiratory paralysis.	Days	Scallops, mussels, clams, cockles.	Detection of toxin in food or water where fish are located; high pressure liquid chromatography.	Life-threatening, may need respiratory support.
Sodium fluoride	Few min to 2 hr	Salty or soapy taste, numbness of mouth, vomiting, diarrhea, dilated pupils, spasms, pallor, shock, collapse.	Usually self-limited	Dry foods (such as dry milk, flour, baking powder, cake mixes) contaminated with sodium fluoride-containing insecticides and rodenticides.	Testing of vomitus or gastric washings. Analysis of the food.	Supportive care.
Thallium	Few hr	Nausea, vomiting, diarrhea, painful paresthesias, motor polyneuropathy, hair loss.	Several days	Contaminated food.	Urine, hair.	Supportive care.
Tin	5 min-8 hr, usually <1 hr	Nausea, vomiting, diarrhea.	Usually self-limited	Metallic container.	Analysis of the food.	Supportive care.
Vomitoxin	Few min to 3 hr	Nausea, headache, abdominal pain, vomiting.	Usually self-limited	Grains, such as wheat, corn, barley.	Analysis of the food.	Supportive care.
Zinc	Few hr	Stomach cramps, nausea, vomiting, diarrhea, myalgias.	Usually self-limited	Metallic container.	Analysis of the food, blood and feces, saliva or urine.	Supportive care.

FOODBORNE ILLNESSES, PARASITIC

TABLE 2-76 Foodborne Illnesses (Parasitic)

ETIOLOGY	INCUBATION PERIOD	SIGNS AND SYMPTOMS	DURATION OF ILLNESS	ASSOCIATED FOODS	LABORATORY TESTING	TREATMENT
Cryptosporidium parvum	7 days average (2-28 days)	Cramping, abdominal pain, watery diarrhea; fever and vomiting may be present and may be relapsing.	Days to weeks	Contaminated water supply, vegetables, fruits, unpasteurized milk.	Must be specifically requested. May need to examine water or food.	Supportive care, self-limited. If severe consider paromomycin for 7 days.
Cyclospora cayetanensis	1-11 days	Fatigue, protracted diarrhea, often relapsing.	May be protracted (several weeks to several months)	Imported berries, contaminated water, lettuce.	Request specific examination of the stool for *Cyclospora*. May need to examine water or food.	TMP/SMX for 7 days.
Entamoeba histolytica	2-3 days to 1-4 wk	Bloody diarrhea, frequent bowel movements (looks like *Shigella*), lower abdominal pain.	Months	Fecal-oral; may contaminate water and food.	Examination of stool for cysts and parasites—at least 3 samples. Serology for long-term infections.	Metronidazole and iodoquinol.
Giardia lamblia	1-4 wk	Acute or chronic diarrhea, flatulence, bloating.	Weeks	Drinking water, other food sources.	Examination of stool for ova and parasites—at least 3 samples.	Metronidazole.
Toxoplasma gondii	6-10 days	Generally asymptomatic, 20% may develop cervical lymphadenopathy and/or a flulike illness. *In immunocompromised patients:* central nervous system (CNS) disease, myocarditis, or pneumonitis is often seen.	Months	Accidental ingestion of contaminated substances (e.g., putting hands in mouth after gardening or cleaning cat litter box); raw or partly cooked pork, lamb, or venison.	Isolation of parasites from blood or other body fluids; observation of parasites in patient specimens, such as bronchoalveolar lavage material or lymph node biopsy. Detection of organisms is rare, but serology can be a useful adjunct in diagnosing toxoplasmosis. Toxoplasma-specific IgM antibodies should be confirmed by a reference laboratory. However, IgM antibodies may persist for 6-18 mo and may not indicate recent infection. For congenital infection: isolation of *T. gondii* from placenta, umbilical cord, or infant blood. PCR of WBCs, CSF, or amniotic fluid (reference laboratory). IgM and IgA serology (reference laboratory).	Asymptomatic healthy, but infected, persons do not require treatment. Spiramycin or pyrimethamine plus sulfadiazine may be used for immunocompromised persons or pregnant women, in specific cases.

MMWR 50(RR-2):1, 2001.
CSF, Cerebrospinal fluid; *IgA*, immunoglobulin A; *IgM*, immunoglobulin M; *PCR*, polymerase chain reaction; *TMP-SMX*, trimethoprim-sulfamethoxazole.
Please call the state health department for more information on specific foodborne illnesses. These telephone numbers are available at: http://www2.cdc.gov/mmwr/international/relres.html.

Continued

TABLE 2-76   Foodborne Illnesses (Parasitic)—cont'd

ETIOLOGY	INCUBATION PERIOD	SIGNS AND SYMPTOMS	DURATION OF ILLNESS	ASSOCIATED FOODS	LABORATORY TESTING	TREATMENT
Toxoplasma gondii (congenital infection)	In infants at birth	Treatment of the mother may reduce severity and/or incidence of congenital infection. Most infected infants have few symptoms at birth. Later, they will generally develop signs of congenital toxoplasmosis (mental retardation, severely impaired eyesight, cerebral palsy, seizures) unless the infection is treated.		Passed from mother (who acquired acute infection during pregnancy) to child.		
Trichinella spiralis	1-2 days to 2-8 wk	Nausea, vomiting, diarrhea, abdominal discomfort followed by fever, myalgias, periorbital edema.	Months	Raw or undercooked contaminated meat, usually pork or wild game meat (e.g., bear or moose).	Positive serology or demonstration of larvae via muscle biopsy. Increase in eosinophils.	Supportive care + mebendazole.

FOOT PAIN

Foot pain
ICD-9CM # Code varies with specific diagnosis

TABLE 2-77   Differential Diagnosis of Foot Pain

CAUSE	NATURE OF PATIENT	NATURE OF SYMPTOMS	PRECIPITATING AND AGGRAVATING FACTORS	PHYSICAL FINDINGS	DIAGNOSTIC STUDIES
Muscular and ligamentous strain	Physically active, especially those unaccustomed to exercise	Pain in region of strained muscles or ligaments	Trauma Unaccustomed or strenuous physical activity	Localized tenderness on palpation	
Foot strain	Older adults Overweight patients	Dull ache in foot, especially forefoot	New shoes Change in heel size Prolonged standing	Forefoot may splay with weight bearing	
Plantar warts and callosities		Pain in plantar surface in metatarsal region	Weight bearing	Plantar callosities	
Jogger's foot	Joggers	Burning in heel Aching in arch		Decreased sensation behind big toe	
Fractures	Patients with history of trauma Joggers		Trauma		May need radiographs or MRI scan to diagnose small fractures of ankle and march fractures of metatarsals
Calcaneal spur on plantar fasciitis		Pain on undersurface of heel Continuous 2.25 cm (1 inch) from back of heel	Worse with weight bearing	Worse with dorsiflexion of toes	Radiograph may show calcaneal spur
Achilles tendinitis or bursitis	Joggers	Heel pain over Achilles tendon	Trauma Running	Swelling and tenderness over Achilles tendon	
Calcaneal apophysitis	Adolescents	Pain in back of heel	Running and jumping	Pain on palpation of Achilles insertion	
Arterial insufficiency	Older adults Diabetics	Rest pain in heel or toes		Coolness Decreased pulses Cornification of heel skin	Arteriography
Gout	Males, especially over age 40 Postmenopausal females	Acute severe pain in big toe metatarsophalangeal joint, occasionally other toes or ankle	Trauma	Warm, violaceous, tender, swollen joints	Uric acid Radiographs

From Seller RH (ed): *Differential diagnosis of common complaints*, ed 4, Philadelphia, 2000, WB Saunders.
MRI, Magnetic resonance imaging.

FORGETFULNESS

Forgetfulness
ICD-9CM # 780.9 Memory disturbance (loss)
310.1 Memory disturbance mild organic

TABLE 2-78 Differential Diagnosis of Forgetfulness

CONDITION	NATURE OF PATIENT	NATURE OF SYMPTOMS	ASSOCIATED SYMPTOMS	PRECIPITATING AND AGGRAVATING FACTORS	AMELIORATING FACTORS	PHYSICAL FINDINGS	DIAGNOSTIC STUDIES
Age-associated memory impairment	Older than 50 yr	Gradual onset	Difficulty remembering names and tasks to be done Misplacing objects		Reassurance Making lists Other memory-assisting techniques	Healthy	Mental status examination in all patients
Depression	All ages	Usually a gradual onset	Loss of concentration Anhedonia Decreased libido Low self-esteem	Grieving process Severe loss	Antidepressant medications	Depressed affect Weight loss	Serial 7s Gresham Ward questionnaire Wechsler Memory Scale
Alcohol and substance abuse	All ages, especially adolescents and young adults	Usually a sudden onset					Toxicology screen
Medications	All ages	Usually a sudden onset		Ingestion of psychotropic agents (e.g., benzodiazepines, hypnotics)	Stopping all medications, including over-the-counter drugs		
Alzheimer's disease, multiinfarct dementia, other progressive dementing processes	Older patients	Gradual onset Progressive	Progressive decrease in cognitive skills			Disheveled appearance Abnormal behavior	CT scan MRI scan
Parkinson's disease	Older patients	Gradual onset Progressive	Resting tremor			Resting tremor Bradykinesia Festinating gait Masked facies	
Other intracranial pathology	All ages	Sudden onset	Severe headache Nausea Fever	Stroke (CVA) Infection AIDS Brain tumor Severe head trauma Repeated head trauma			CT scan Spinal tap

From Seller RH (ed): *Differential diagnosis of common complaints*, ed 4, Philadelphia, 2000, WB Saunders.
AIDS, Acquired immunodeficiency syndrome; *CI*, computed tomography; *CVA*, cardiovascular accident; *MRI*, magnetic resonance imaging.

Fungal infections in the central nervous system
ICD-9CM # 117.9 Fungal infection NEC
           112.83 Candidal meningitis
           117.5 Cryptococcal meningitis
           117.3 *Aspergillus* species meningitis
           115.1 *Histoplasma capsulatum* meningitis

FUNGAL INFECTIONS IN THE CENTRAL NERVOUS SYSTEM

TABLE 2-79   **Common Fungal Infections of the Central Nervous System**

ORGANISM	HOST FACTORS	COMMON NEUROLOGIC PRESENTATION	OTHER NEUROLOGIC PRESENTATION	COMMENT

Molds
  Aspergillus species
  Mucorales
  P. boydii
  Fusarium
  S. griseus
	Immunocompromised (defective neutrophil function, e.g., cytotoxic chemotherapy recipients)
	Injection drug use
	Acidosis
	Near drowning
		Rhinocerebral syndrome
		Strokelike syndrome
		Inflammatory mass
			Meningitis	Diabetics are predisposed to rhinocerebral syndrome caused by Mucorales
				Cytotoxic agents predispose to *Aspergillus*
				Desferoxamine predisposes to Mucorales

Cryptococcus species *C. neoformans*	Immunocompromised (defective T-cell function, HIV infection, corticosteroid use, inherited immune defects) Normal host	Meningitis	Cryptococcoma	Acute meningitis more common in immunosuppressed patients; more indolent course in immunocompetent persons *Cryptococcus* has high predilection for CNS involvement

Candida species
  C. albicans
  C. tropicalis
  C. parapsilosis
  T. glabrata
  C. krusei
	Immunocompromised (defective neutrophil function)
	Inherited immune defects
	Cytotoxic agents
	Injecting drug use
	Corticosteroid use
	Intravenous catheters
	Broad-spectrum antibiotics
	Prematurity
		Meningitis
		Abscess
			Infarct	Community-acquired pathogens

Dimorphic fungi
  B. dermatitidis
  P. brasiliensis
  H. capsulatum
  C. immitis
  S. schenckii
	Normal host
	Immunocompromised (defective T-cell function)
		Meningitis
		Abscess
				Community-acquired pathogens
				C. immitis has increased predilection for CNS

Dematiacious fungi
  X. bantiana
  Bipolaris species
  Exerohilum species
  Curvularia species
  F. pedrosi
  R. obovoideum
	Normal host
	Immunocompromised
		Abscess	Meningitis	Community-acquired pathogens

From Johnson RT, Griffin JW: *Current therapy in neurologic disease,* ed 5, St Louis, 1997, Mosby.
CNS, Central nervous system; *HIV,* human immunodeficiency virus.

GAIT ABNORMALITIES

Gait abnormalities
ICD-9CM # 781.2 Gait abnormality

TABLE 2-80   **Characteristics of Unexpected Gait Patterns**

GAIT PATTERN	CHARACTERISTICS
Spastic hemiparesis	The affected leg is stiff and extended with plantar flexion of the foot. Movement of the foot results from pelvic tilting upward on the involved side. The foot is dragged, often scraping the toe, or it is circled stiffly outward and forward (circumduction). The affected arm remains flexed and adducted and does not swing (see Fig. 2-3, *A*).
Spastic diplegia (scissoring)	The patient uses short steps, dragging the ball of the foot across the floor. The legs are extended, and the thighs tend to cross forward on each other at each step, due to injury to the pyramidal system (see Fig. 2-3, *B*).
Steppage	The hip and knee are elevated excessively high to lift the plantar flexed foot off the ground. The foot is brought down to the floor with a slap. The patient is unable to walk on the heels (see Fig. 2-3, *C*).
Dystrophic (waddling)	The legs are kept apart, and weight is shifted from side to side in a waddling motion due to weak hip abductor muscles. The abdomen often protrudes, and lordosis is common.
Tabetic	The legs are positioned far apart, lifted high and forcibly brought down with each step. The heel stamps on the ground.
Cerebellar gait (cerebellar ataxia)	The patient's feet are wide-based. Staggering and lurching from side to side are often accompanied by swaying of the trunk (see Fig. 2-3, *D*).
Sensory ataxia	The patient's gait is wide-based. The feet are thrown forward and outward, bringing them down first on heels, then on toes. The patient watches the ground to guide his or her steps. A positive Romberg sign is present (see Fig. 2-3, *E*).
Parkinsonian gait	The patient's posture is stooped and the body is held rigid. Steps are short and shuffling, with hesitation on starting and difficulty stopping (see Fig. 2-3, *C*).
Dystonia	Jerky dancing movements appear nondirectional.
Ataxia	Uncontrolled falling occurs.
Antalgic limp	The patient limits the time of weight bearing on the affected leg to limit pain.

From Seidel HM (ed): *Mosby's guide to physical examination,* ed 4, St Louis, 1999, Mosby.

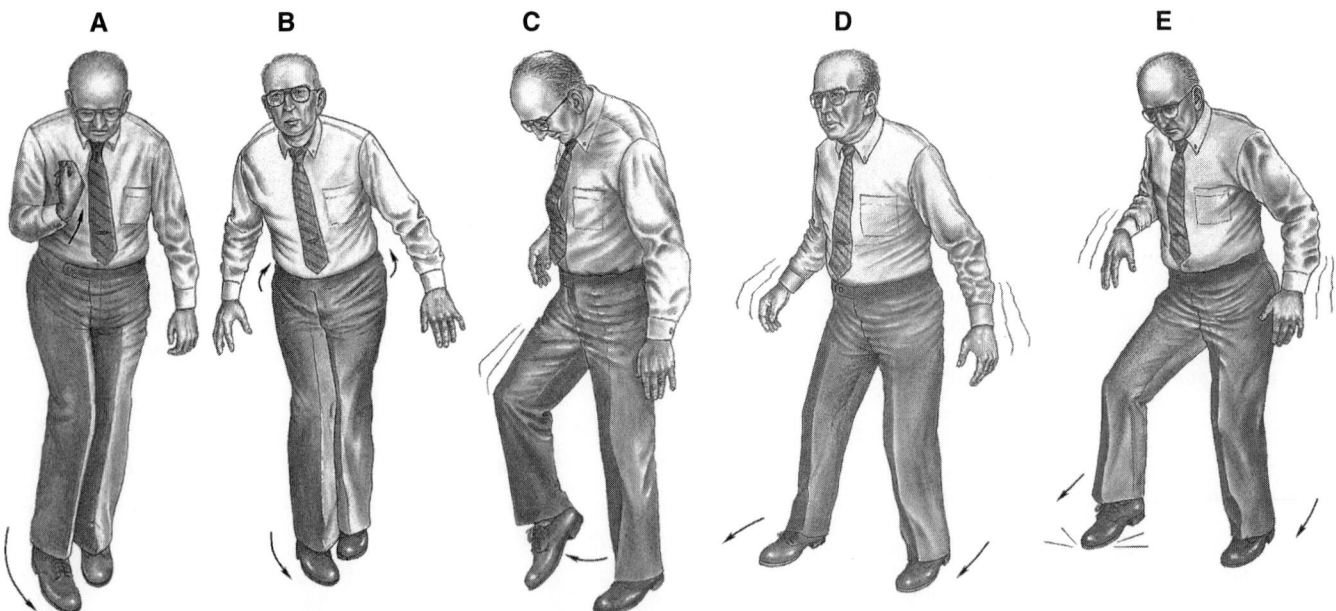

Fig. 2-7   Unexpected gait patterns. **A,** Spastic hemiparesis. **B,** Spastic diplegia (scissoring). **C,** Steppage gait. **D,** Cerebellar ataxia. **E,** Sensory ataxia. (From Seidel HM [ed]: *Mosby's guide to physical examination,* ed 4, St Louis, 1999, Mosby.)

GALACTORRHEA

Galactorrhea
ICD-9CM # 611.6

TABLE 2-81 **Causes of Galactorrhea**

CAUSES	MECHANISM
Prolonged suckling	Reduction in PIF from hypothalamus
Drugs (isoniazid, phenothiazines, reserpine derivatives, amphetamines, and tricyclic antidepressants)	Depletion of dopamine or blocked dopamine receptors
Major stressors (surgery, trauma)	Inhibition of hypothalamic PIF
Hypothyroidism	Thyrotropin-releasing hormone acts as prolactin-releasing factor
Pituitary tumors	Secretion of prolactin; tumor may compress pituitary and decrease products of other hormones

From Noble J (ed): *Primary care medicine,* ed 3, St Louis, 2001, Mosby.
PIF, Prolactin-inhibiting factor.

GASTRIC EMPTYING, DELAYED

Gastric emptying, delayed
ICD-9CM # 536.8 Gastric motility disorder

BOX 2-103 **Causes of Delayed Gastric Emptying**

Mechanical Causes

Peptic ulcer disease, scarred pylorus
Malignancy: gastric cancer, gastric lymphoma, pancreatic cancer
Gastric surgery: vagotomy, gastric resection, roux-en-Y anastomosis
Crohn's disease

Endocrine and Metabolic

Diabetes mellitus
Hypothyroidism
Hypoadrenal states
Electrolyte abnormalities
Chronic renal failure

Medications

Anticholinergics
Opiates
Dopamine agonists
Tricyclic antidepressants

Abnormalities of Gastric Smooth Muscle

Scleroderma
Polymyositis/dermatomyositis
Amyloidosis
Pseudo-obstruction
Myotonic dystrophy

Neuropathy

Scleroderma
Amyloidosis
Pseudo-obstruction
Autonomic neuropathy

Central Nervous System or Psychiatric Disorders

Brain stem tumors
Spinal cord injury
Anorexia nervosa
Stress

Miscellaneous

Idiopathic gastroparesis
Gastroesophageal reflux disease
Nonulcer (functional) dyspepsia
Cancer cachexia or anorexia

From Andreoli TE (ed): *Cecil essentials of medicine,* ed 5, Philadelphia, 2001, WB Saunders.

II

Gastrointestinal obstruction, pediatric age
ICD-9CM # 560.9 Intestinal obstruction NOS
777.1 Intestinal obstruction due to meconium
777.4 Intestinal obstruction, newborn transitory
560.2 Volvulus

GASTROINTESTINAL OBSTRUCTION, PEDIATRIC AGE

TABLE 2-82 Pediatric Gastrointestinal Obstruction: Clinical Findings

ETIOLOGY	VOMITING	PAIN	STOOL PATTERN	FINDINGS			
				DISTENTION	BOWEL SOUNDS	TENDERNESS	MASSES
Esophageal atresia	Nonbilious (saliva)	No	Normal meconium	No	Absent to normal	No	No
Gastric obstruction	Nonbilious (curdled formula)	Severe with gastric volvulus; none with antral web	Normal meconium	Epigastric	Absent to normal	Severe with volvulus	No
Hypertrophic pyloric stenosis	Nonbilious, projectile	No	Constipation (dehydration)	Epigastric	Hyperactive (epigastric)	No	Yes ("olive")
Duodenal obstruction	Bilious	Minimal	Small meconium stool	Epigastric	Absent to normal	No	No
Volvulus	Bilious	Severe	Hematochezia	Epigastric to generalized	Hyperactive	Yes (severe)	No
Jejunoileal atresia	Bilious	No	Small, hard, light-colored meconium stool	Generalized	Variable	No	No
Intussusception	Bilious	Yes (crampy)	Currant jelly stool	Generalized	Hyperactive	Yes	Yes ("sausage shaped")
Meconium ileus	Bilious	No	Obstipation	Generalized	Variable	No	Yes ("doughy beads")
Meconium plug	Bilious	No	Obstipation	Generalized	Variable	No	No
Congenital aganglionosis	Bilious	No	Obstipation, constipation, and intermittent diarrhea	Generalized	Hyperactive	No	Palpable stool
Obstipation of prematurity	Bilious	No	Obstipation	Generalized	Hyperactive	No	No
Incarcerated inguinal hernia	Bilious	Yes	Diarrhea or constipation	Generalized	Hyperactive	Yes	Inguinal or scrotal
Imperforate anus	Bilious	No	Obstipation	Generalized	Hyperactive	No	No

From Hoekelman R (ed): *Primary pediatric care*, ed 3, St Louis, 1997, Mosby.

GAY BOWEL SYNDROME

Gay bowel syndrome
ICD-9CM # 569.49 Anal infection

TABLE 2-83　Clinical Features of Gay Bowel Syndrome

DISEASE	SIGNS AND SYMPTOMS	DIAGNOSIS	TREATMENT
Anorectal gonorrhea	Creamy rectal discharge, constipation, pain	Culture of *Neisseria* on selective medium	Procaine penicillin, 4.8 million U IM, plus 1 g probenecid PO or Spectinomycin, 2 g IM
Herpes simplex infection	Extreme rectal pain and tenderness, bloody discharge; discrete on sigmoidoscopy	Viral isolation from stool, discharge, or acute and convalescent sera	Acyclovir, 5 mg/kg IV q8h
Anorectal syphilis	Mild or no symptoms	Darkfield examination of ulcer, serologic testing	Benzathine penicillin, 2.4 million U IM (single dose) or Tetracycline, 500 mg qid for 15 days
Amebiasis	Diarrhea with mucus or blood; diffuse proctitis with scattered ulcers at sigmoidoscopy	Motile trophozoites or cysts in stool, serologic studies	Metronidazole, 750 mg qid for 10 days
Lymphogranuloma venereum	Diarrhea, discharge; diffuse proctitis at sigmoidoscopy	Granulomas in rectal biopsy or stool	Tetracycline, 500 mg PO qid for 2-3 wk

From Noble J (ed): *Primary care medicine*, ed 3, St Louis, 2001, Mosby.
IM, Intramuscularly; *IV*, intravenously; *PO*, orally; *qid*, 4 times a day.

GENITAL DISCHARGE

BOX 2-104　Genital Discharge

Physiologic discharge	Menstrual cycle variation	IUD
Cervical mucus	Infection	Cervical ectropion
Vaginal transudation	Foreign body	Spermicide
Bacteria	Tampon	Nongenital causes
Squamous epithelial cells	Cervical cap	Urinary incontinence
Individual variation	Other	Urinary tract fistula
Pregnancy	Neoplasm	Crohn's disease
Sexual response	Fistula	Rectovaginal fistula

From Danakas G (ed): *Practical guide to the care of the gynecologic/obstetric patient*, St Louis, 1997, Mosby.

Genital discharge
ICD-9CM # 623.5 Vaginal discharge
　　　　　 788.7 Urethral discharge

GENITAL SORES

TABLE 2-84   Differentiation of Diseases Causing Genital Sores

Genital sores
ICD-9CM # 054.10 Genital herpes
          91.0 Genital syphilis
          078.11 Condyloma acuminatum
          099.0 Chancroid
          099.2 Granuloma inguinale
          099.1 Lymphogranuloma venereum
          629.8 Ulcer, genital site, female
          608.89 Ulcer, genital site, male

DISEASE	PRIMARY LESION	ADENOPATHY	SYSTEMIC FEATURES	DIAGNOSIS/RX
Herpes genitalis, primary 20% sexually active adults, caused by HSV-2	Incubation 2-7 days; multiple painful vesicles on erythematous base; persist 7-14 days	Tender, soft adenopathy, often bilateral	Fever	Tzanck smear positive; tissue culture isolation, HSV-2 antigen, fourfold rise in antibodies to HSV-2; Rx: acyclovir
Recurrent	Grouped vesicles on erythematous base, painful; last 3-10 days	None	None	Tzanck, HSV-2 antigen, tissue culture positive; titers not helpful; Rx: acyclovir
Syphilis, 90,000 cases in U.S. per year caused by *Treponema pallidum*	Incubation 10-90 days (m. 21); chancre: papule that ulcerates; painless, border raised, firm, ulcer indurated, base smooth; usually single; may be genital or almost anywhere; persists 3-6 wk, leaving thin, atrophic scar	1 wk after chancre appears; bilateral or unilateral; firm, discrete, movable, no overlying skin changes, painless, nonsuppurative; may persist for months	Later stages	Cannot be cultured; positive darkfield; VDRL positive, 77%; FTA-ABS positive, 86%
Chancroid, 2000 cases in U.S. per year caused by *Haemophilus ducreyi*	Incubation 3-5 days; vesicle or papule to pustule to ulcer; soft, not indurated; very painful	1 wk after primary in 50%; painful, unilateral (two thirds), suppurative	None	Organism in Gram stain of pus; can be cultured (75%) but direct yields highest from lymph node; Rx: ceftriazone, 250 mg once intramuscularly, or ciprofloxacin, 500 mg bid times 3 days

Granuloma inguinale, 50 cases in U.S. per year caused by *Calymmatobacterium granulomatis*	Incubation 9-50 days; at least one painless papule that gradually ulcerates; ulcers are large (1-4 cm), irregular, nontender, with thickened, rolled margins and beefy red tissue at base; older portions of ulcer show depigmented scarring, while advancing edge contains new papules	No true adenopathy; in one fifth, subcutaneous spread via lymphatics leads to indurated swelling or abscesses of groin—"pseudobuboes"	Metastatic infection of bones, joints, liver	Scraping or deep curetting at actively extending border—Wright's or Giemsa stain reveals short, plump, bipolar staining "Donovan's bodies" in macrophage vacuoles; Rx: tetracycline, 2 g/day times 21 days
Condyloma acuminatum (genital warts), frequent, due to human papillomavirus (HPV)	Characteristic large, soft, fleshy, cauliflower-like excrescences around vulva, glans, urethral orifice, anus, perineum	None	None per se; association with cervical dysplasia/neoplasia	Chief importance is distinction from syphilis and chancroid; Rx: topical podophyllin ± cryosurgery, laser resection
Lymphogranuloma venereum, 600-1000 cases per year in U.S. caused by *Chlamydia trachomatis*	Incubation 5-21 days; painless papule, vesicle, ulcer, evanescent (2-3 days), noted in only 10%-40%	5-21 days post primary, one third bilateral, tender, matted iliac/femoral "groove sign"; multiple abscesses; coalescent, caseating, suppurative, sinus tracts; thick yellow pus; fistulas; strictures; genital ulcerations	Fever, arthritis, pericarditis, proctitis, meningoencephalitis, keratoconjunctivitis, preauricular adenopathy, edema of eyelids, erythema nodosum	LGV CF positive 85%-90% (1-3 wk); must have high titer (>1:16), as cross-reacts with other *Chlamydia;* also positive STS, rheumatoid factor, cryoglobulins; Rx: doxycycline, 100 mg bid times 7 days

From Andreoli TE (ed): *Cecil essentials of medicine,* ed 4, Philadelphia, 1997, WB Saunders
CF, Complement fixation; *FTA-ABS,* fluorescent treponemal antibody absorption; *HSV,* herpes simplex virus; *LGV,* lymphogranuloma venereum; *Rx,* prescription; *STS,* serologic test for syphilis; *VDRL,* Venereal Disease Research Laboratory.

Goiter
ICD-9CM # 240.9 Goiter, unspecified
241.9 Goiter, adenomatous
246.1 Goiter, congenital
240.9 Goiter, nontoxic diffuse
241.1 Goiter, nontoxic multinodular
240.0 Simple goiter
242.1 Thyrotoxic goiter

GOITER

BOX 2-105   Goiter

Thyroiditis
Toxic multinodular goiter
Graves' disease
Medications (propylthiouracil, methimazole, sulfon-
    amides, sulfonylureas, ethionamide, amiodarone,
    lithium, etc.)

Iodine deficiency
Sarcoidosis, amyloidosis
Defective thyroid hormone synthesis
Resistance to thyroid hormone

GRANULOMATOUS DISORDERS

BOX 2-106   ## Classification of Granulomatous Disorders

Infections

Fungi

Histoplasma
Coccidioides
Blastomyces
Sporothrix
Aspergillus
Cryptococcus

Protozoa

Toxoplasma
Leishmania

Metazoa

Toxocara
Schistosoma

Spirochetes

Treponema pallidum
T. pertunue
T. carateum

Mycobacteria

M. tuberculosis
M. leprae
M. kanasasii
M. marinum
M. avian
Bacille Calmette-Guérin (BCG)
vaccine

Bacteria

Brucella
Yersinia

Other Infections

Cat scratch
Lymphogranuloma

Neoplasia

Carcinoma
Reticulosis
Pinealoma
Dysgerminoma
Seminoma
Reticulum cell sarcoma
Malignant nasal granuloma

Chemicals

Beryllium
Zirconium
Silica
Starch

Immunologic Aberrations

Sarcoidosis
Crohn's disease
Primary biliary cirrhosis
Wegener's granulomatosis
Giant-cell arteritis
Peyronie's disease
Hypogammaglobulinemia
Systemic lupus erythematosus
Lymphomatoid granulomatosis

Histiocytosis X
Hepatic granulomatous disease
Immune complex disease
Rosenthal-Melkersson syndrome
Churg-Strauss allergic granulomatosis

Leukocyte Oxidase Defect

Chronic granulomatous disease of childhood

Extrinsic Allergic Alveolitis

Farmer's lung
Bird fancier's
Mushroom worker's
Suberosis (cork dust)
Bagassosis
Maple bark stripper's
Paprika splitter's
Coffee bean
Spatlese lung

Other Disorders

Whipple's disease
Pyrexia of unknown origin
Radiotherapy
Cancer chemotherapy
Panniculitis
Chalazion
Sebaceous cyst
Dermoid
Sea urchin spine injury

From Schwarz MI, King TE: *Interstitial lung disease*, ed 2, St Louis, 1993, Mosby.

Granulomatous disorders
ICD-9CM # 446.4 Granulomatosis
              288.1 Granulomatous disease

GRANULOMATOUS LUNG DISEASE

TABLE 2-85   Differential Diagnosis of Granulomatous Lung Diseases

Granulomatous lung disease
ICD-9CM # 446.4 Granulomatosis, respiratory

FEATURE	WEGENER'S GRANULOMATOSIS		LYMPHOMATOID GRANULOMATOSIS	CHURG-STRAUSS SYNDROME	NECROTIZING SARCOID GRANULOMATOSIS	BRONCHOCENTRIC GRANULOMATOSIS		SARCOIDOSIS
	CLASSIC	LIMITED				ASTHMA	NO ASTHMA	
Sex	M/F	Equal	Affects men slightly more frequently	Same	Same	Same	Same	Same
Decade of incidence	50s	50s	30s-50s	50s	30s and 40s	30s	60s	30s and 40s
Presentation	Sinusitis Rhinorrhea Epistaxis	+	Cough Dyspnea Hemoptysis Arthralgia	Bronchitis Asthma Pneumonia	Fever Cough Pleurisy Malaise	Asthma	Cough Pleurisy Dyspnea	Insignificant symptoms
Ulcerated nose and nasal septum	+	+	–	–	–	Bronchiectasis Bronchial obstruction Eosinophilia	–	Only when associated with lupus pernio and SURT
Saddle nose								
Chest radiograph opacities	+	+	+	+	+	Particularly in upper lobes		+
Cavitation	++	+	+	Infiltration	+	Pulmonary fibrosis		Infiltration
Hilar adenopathy	–	–	–	–	–	–	–	+

Kidneys	Glomerulo-nephritis in 85%	–	Renal vasculitis	–	–	–	Nephrocalcinosis
Ocular	+	–	–	–	+	+	–
Allergy	±	±	–	–	–	–	+
Skin lesions	+	–	+	+	+	–	–
CNS	+	–	+	Rare	Rare	–	+
Cardiac	+	–	–	–	–	–	+
Characteristics	↑ESR ↑ANCA	–	–	Eosinophilia	Eosinophilia	Hypersensitivity to *Aspergillus* Eosinophilia	Increased SACE
Granulomas	±	±	Very rare	Always	Infrequent	+	Always
Vasculitis	++	++	Always	++	Always	±	Inconspicuous
Necrosis	Prominent and resemble infarcts	Prominent	Prominent	Prominent	Prominent	+	Inconspicuous
Treatment	Cyclophosphamide	Steroids, azathioprine	Cyclophosphamide Azathioprine	Steroids, azathioprine	Steroids, azathioprine	Corticosteroids	Steroids Azathioprine
Prognosis	Poor	Poor	Poor	Good	Good	Good	Good

From Schwarz MI, King TE: *Interstitial lung disease*, ed 2, St Louis, 1993, Mosby.
+, Present; ++, prominent; −, absent; ±, inconspicuous; *ANCA*, antineutrophil cycloplasmic antibody; *ESR*, erythrocyte sedimentation rate; *SACE*, serum angiotensin-converting enzyme; *SURT*, sarcoidosis of upper respiratory tract.

II

GROIN PAIN IN ACTIVE PEOPLE

Groin pain in active people
ICD-9CM # 959.1 Groin injury
848.8 Groin sprain

BOX 2-107   Differential Diagnosis of Groin Pain in Active People

Musculoskeletal

Avascular necrosis of the femoral head

Avulsion fracture (lesser trochanter, anterior superior iliac spine, anterior inferior iliac spine)

Bursitis (iliopectineal, trochanteric)

Entrapment of the ilioinguinal or iliofemoral nerve*

Gracilis syndrome

Muscle tear (adductors, iliopsoas, rectus abdominis, gracilis, sartorius, rectus femoris)

Myositis ossificans of the hip muscles

Osteitis pubis

Osteoarthritis of the femoral head

Slipped capital femoral epiphysis

Stress fracture of the femoral head or neck and pubis

Synovitis

Hernia-related

Avulsion of the internal oblique muscle in the conjoined tendon

Defect at the insertion of the rectus abdominis muscle

Direct inguinal hernia

Femoral ring hernia

Indirect inguinal hernia

Inguinal canal weakness

Urologic

Epididymitis

Fracture of the testis

Hydrocele

Kidney stone

Posterior urethritis

Prostatis

Testicular cancer

Torsion of the testis

Urinary tract infection

Varicocele

Gynecologic

Ectopic pregnancy

Ovarian cyst

Pelvic inflammatory disease

Torsion of the ovary

Vaginitis

Lymphatic Enlargement in Groin

From Swain R, Snodgrass: *Phys Sportsmed* 23:56, 1995.
*Usually postoperative.

GYNECOMASTIA

Gynecomastia
ICD-9CM # 611.1 Gynecomastia, nonpuerperal

BOX 2-108   Differential Diagnosis of Gynecomastia

Physiologic

Newborns

Puberty

Aging

Refeeding

Pathologic

Testosterone deficiency

Congenital anorchia

Klinefelter's syndrome

Defects in the structure or function of androgen receptors

Complete (testicular feminization syndrome)

Partial (Reifenstein, Lubs, Rosewater, and Dreyfus syndromes)

Defects in androgen synthesis

Primary Gonadal Failure

Viral orchitis, trauma, castration, granulomatous disease, varicocele

Secondary Hypogonadism

Increased Estrogen Production

Increased testicular estrogen secretion

hCG-producing tumor (especially lung, liver, and kidney cancer),

testicular tumor, bronchogenic carcinoma, gastrointestinal tumors, ectopic choriocarcinomas

True hermaphroditism

Estrogen-producing adrenal tumor

Increased Peripheral Conversion

Adrenal disease, liver disease (alcohol), starvation, thyrotoxicosis

Increase in Peripheral Aromatose Activity

Heredity, obesity

Increased Prolactin Level

Pituitary tumors (prolactinoma)

Drugs that deplete catecholamine or catecholamine antagonists—sulpiride, phenothiazine, methyldopa, reserpine, tricyclic antidepressant, metoclopramide

Drugs

Initiating or terminating exogenous androgens

Estrogen and estrogen-like substances (estradiol, diethylstilbestrol, digitalis)

Estrogen precursors—testosterone enanthate, testosterone propionate

GH therapy with elevated serum IGF-I level

Drugs that enhance endogenous estrogen formation—hCG, clomiphene

Drugs that inhibit testosterone synthesis and/or action, such as ketoconazole, alkylating agents, spironolactone, cimetidine, aminoglutethimide, flutamide, cyproterone

Others: amiodarone, busulfan, captopril, ethionamide, isoniazid, D-penicillamine, phenytoin, diazepam, marijuana, heroin, omeprazole, ranitidine, enalapril, nifedipine, verapamil

Idiopathic

From Moore WT, Eastman RC: *Diagnostic endocrinology*, ed 2, St Louis, 1996, Mosby.
GH, Growth hormone; *hCG,* human chorionic gonadotropin; *IGF,* insulin-like growth factor.

HALITOSIS

Halitosis
ICD-9CM # 784.9

BOX 2-109   Halitosis

Tobacco use
Alcohol use
Dry mouth (mouth breathing, insufficient fluid intake)
Foods (onion, garlic, meats, nuts)
Diseases of the mouth or nose (infections, cancer, inflammation)
Medications (antihistamines, antidepressants)

Systemic disorders (diabetes, uremia)
Gastrointestimal disorders (esophageal diverticula, hiatal hernia, gastroesophageal reflux disease)
Sinusitis
Pulmonary disorders (bronchiectasis, pneumonia, neoplasms, tuberculosis)

HAND, PAINFUL, SWOLLEN

Hand, painful, swollen
ICD-9CM # Code varies with specific diagnosis

BOX 2-110   Hand, painful, swollen

Gout
Pseudogout
Rheumatoid arthritis
Remitting seronegative symmetrical synovitis with pitting edema (RS3PE)
Polymyalgia rheumatica
Mixed connective tissue disease
Scleroderma
Rupture of the olecranon bursa

Medsger's syndrome (neoplasia)
The puffy hand of drug addiction
Reflex sympathetic dystrophy
Eosinophilic fasciitis
Sickle cell (hand-foot syndrome)
Leprosy
Factitial (the rubber band syndrome)

From Canoso J: *Rheumatology in primary care*, Philadelphia, 1997, WB Saunders.

II

HEADACHE

TABLE 2-86   **Clinical Characteristics of Common Headaches**

	TENSION	MIGRAINE	SINUSITIS	MASS LESION
Pain				
Location	Bilateral (frontal, occipital, bandlike)	Unilateral (but not always on same side)	Bifrontal (may be unilateral)	Unilateral (always on same side) or bilateral
Character	Pressure	Throbbing	Pressure	Pressure
Severity	Mild to moderate	Moderate to severe	Moderate	Progressively worse as mass expands
Time of occurrence	Late in day or anytime	Morning or anytime	Worse in morning	Constant (may be intermittent early in course)
Frequency	Several times per week	Less than weekly	Daily until resolved	Constant
Aura	No	Sometimes	No	No
Precipitants	Stress	Bright lights, menstruation, alcohol	None	None but pain aggravated by Valsalva-type provocation
Alleviating factors	Relaxation, sleep	Reclining in dark room, migraine-specific drug	Decongestants, antihistamines, antibiotics	None
Associated symptoms	None or stress related	Vomiting, photophobia	Nasal stuffiness or dripping, epistaxis	Projectile vomiting, neurologic symptoms
Age at onset	Any age	10-30 yr	Any age	Any age for primary brain tumor, older for metastatic brain tumor
Gender	Both	Majority female	Both	Both
Family history	Sometimes	Often	No	No
Chronicity	Several months to years	Several months to years	Acute except in allergic rhinitis (may be seasonal)	Progressive

From Wachtel T, Stein M: *Practical guide to the care of the ambulatory patient,* ed 2, St Louis, 2000, Mosby.

Headache
ICD-9CM # 784.0   Headache NOS
              307.81 Headache, tension
              346.2   Headache, cluster
              346.9   Headache, migraine
              784.0   Headache, vascular

HEADACHES AND FACIAL PAIN

Headache and facial pain
ICD-9CM # 784.0 Headache NOS
784.0 Facial pain

BOX 2-111   A Classification of Headaches and Facial Pain

I. Vascular headaches
  A. Migraine
    1. Migraine with headaches and inconspicuous neurologic features
      a. *Migraine without aura* ("common migraine")
    2. Migraine with headaches and conspicuous neurologic features
      a. With transient neurologic symptoms
        (1) *Migraine with typical aura* ("classic migraine")
        (2) *Sensory, basilar,* and *hemiplegic migraine*
      b. With prolonged or permanent neurologic features ("complicated migraine")
        (1) *Ophthalmoplegic migraine*
        (2) *Migrainous infarction*
    3. Migraine without headaches but with conspicuous neurologic features ("migraine equivalents")
      a. Abdominal migraine
      b. *Benign paroxysmal vertigo of childhood*
      c. *Migraine aura without headache* ("isolated auras," transient migrainous accompaniments)
  B. Cluster headaches
    1. *Episodic cluster headache* ("cyclic cluster headaches")
    2. *Chronic cluster headaches*
    3. *Chronic paroxysmal hemicrania*
  C. Other vascular headaches
    1. Headaches of reactive vasodilation (fever, drug-induced, postictal, hypoglycemia, hypoxia, hypercarbia, hyperthyroidism)
    2. *Headaches associated with arterial hypertension*
      a. Chronic severe hypertension (diastolic >120 mm Hg)
      b. Paroxysmal severe hypertension (pheochromocytoma, some coital headaches)
    3. Headaches caused by cranial arteritis
      a. *Giant cell arteritis* ("temporal arteritis")
      b. Other vasculitides
II. Headaches associated with demonstrable muscle spasm
  A. Headache caused by posturally induced or paralesional muscle spasm
    1. Headaches of sustained or impaired posture (e.g., prolonged close work, driving)
    2. Headaches associated with cervical spondylosis and other diseases of cervical spine
    3. Myofascial pain dysfunction syndrome *(headache or facial pain associated with disorders of teeth, jaws, and related structures, or "TMJ syndrome")*
  B. Headaches caused by psychophysiologic muscular contraction ("muscle contraction headaches," or *tension-type headache associated with disorder of pericranial muscles*)
III. Headaches and facial pain without demonstrable physical substrate
  A. Headaches of uncertain etiology
    1. "Tension headaches" *(tension-type headache unassociated with disorder of pericranial muscles)*
    2. Some forms of posttraumatic headache
  B. Psychogenic headaches (e.g., hypochondriacal, conversional, delusional, malingered)
  C. Facial pain of uncertain etiology ("atypical facial pain")
IV. Combined tension-migraine headaches
  A. Episodic migraine superimposed on chronic tension headaches
  B. Chronic daily headaches
    1. Associated with analgesic and/or ergotamine overuse ("rebound headaches")
    2. Not associated with drug overuse
V. Headaches and head pains caused by diseases of eyes, ears, nose, sinuses, teeth, or skull
VI. Headaches caused by meningeal inflammation
  A. Subarachnoid hemorrhage
  B. Meningitis and meningoencephalitis
  C. Others (e.g., meningeal carcinomatosis)
VII. Headaches associated with altered intracranial pressure ("traction headaches")
  A. Increased intracranial pressure
    1. Intracranial mass lesions (neoplasm, hematoma, abscess, etc.)
    2. Hydrocephalus
    3. Benign intracranial hypertension
    4. Venous sinus thrombosis
  B. Decreased intracranial pressure
    1. Post–lumbar puncture headaches
    2. Spontaneous hypoliquorrheic headaches
VIII. Headaches and head pains caused by cranial neuralgias
  A. Presumed irritation of superficial nerves
    1. Occipital neuralgia
    2. Supraorbital neuralgia
  B. Presumed irritation of intracranial nerves
    1. Trigeminal neuralgia ("tic douloureux")
    2. Glossopharyngeal neuralgia

From Stein JH (ed): *Internal medicine,* ed 5, St Louis, 1998, Mosby.

HEARING LOSS, ACUTE

Hearing loss, acute
ICD-9CM # 388.2

BOX 2-112   Common Causes of Sudden Hearing Loss

Infectious
Mumps
Measles
Influenza
Herpes simplex
Herpes zoster
Cytomegalovirus
Mononucleosis
Syphilis

Vascular
Macroglobulinemia
Sickle cell disease
Berger's disease
Leukemia

Polycythemia
Fat emboli
Hypercoagulable states

Metabolic
Diabetes
Pregnancy
Hyperlipoproteinemia

Conductive
Cerumen impaction
Foreign bodies
Otitis media
Otitis externa
Barotrauma
Trauma

Medications
Aminoglycosides (gentamicin,
  theomycin, vancomycin,
  kanamycin, streptomycin)
Loop diuretics (furosemide,
  ethacrynic acid)
Antineoplastics
Salicylates

Neoplasm
Acoustic neuroma

From Rosen P, Barkin R (eds): *Emergency medicine: concepts and clinical practice,* ed 5, St Louis, 2002, Mosby.

HEART SOUNDS, ABNORMAL INTENSITY

Heart sounds, abnormal intensity
ICD-9CM # 785.3

TABLE 2-87   Abnormal Intensity of Heart Sounds

	S_1	A_2	P_2
Loud	Short PR Interval Mitral stenosis with pliable valve	Systemic hypertension Aortic dilation Coarctation of the aorta	Pulmonary hypertension Thin chest wall
Soft	Long PR interval Mitral regurgitation Poor left ventricular function Mitral stenosis with rigid valve Thick chest wall	Calcific aortic stenosis Aortic regurgitation	Valvular or subvalvular pulmonic stenosis
Varying	Atrial fibrillation Heart block		

HEART SOUNDS, ABNORMAL SPLITTING OF S2

Heart sounds, abnormal splitting of S2
ICD-9CM # 785.3

TABLE 2-88   Abnormal Splitting of S_2

SINGLE S_2	WIDELY SPLIT S_2 WITH NORMAL RESPIRATORY VARIATION	FIXED SPLIT S_2	PARADOXICALLY SPLIT S_2
Aortic stenosis Pulmonic stenosis Systemic hypertension Coronary artery disease Any condition that can lead to paradoxical splitting of S_2	Right bundle branch block Left ventricular pacing Pulmonic stenosis Pulmonary embolism Idiopathic dilation of the pulmonary artery Mitral regurgitation Ventricular septal defect	Atrial septal defect Severe right ventricular dysfunction	Left bundle branch block Right ventricular pacing Angina, myocardial infarction Aortic stenosis Hypertrophic cardiomyopathy Aortic regurgitation

From Andreoli TE (ed): *Cecil essentials of medicine,* ed 5, Philadelphia, 2001, WB Saunders.

HEARTBURN AND INDIGESTION

TABLE 2-89   Differential Diagnosis of Heartburn and Indigestion

Heartburn and indigestion
ICD-9CM # 787.1 Heartburn
536.8 Indigestion

CAUSE	NATURE OF PATIENT	NATURE OF SYMPTOMS	ASSOCIATED SYMPTOMS	PRECIPITATING AND AGGRAVATING FACTORS	AMELIORATING FACTORS	PHYSICAL FINDINGS	DIAGNOSTIC STUDIES
Reflux esophagitis	Adults More common in pregnant women in later months	Severe heartburn Water brash with and without recumbency Recurrent pain radiates to back (40%), arms, or neck (5%)	Chest pain Dysphagia Belching (from aerophagia) Cough Asthma, especially nocturnal	Recumbency Straining or lifting Drinking alcoholic, caffeinated, or carbonated beverages Eating heavy meals or fatty, spicy, or acidic foods Smoking Pregnancy Exercise	Raising head of bed Antacids Small, frequent, low-fat meals Avoidance of tight garments		Pain often relieved by viscous lidocaine Esophagoscopy Upper GI radiograph Esophageal pH monitoring
Gastritis	Especially alcoholics	Abdominal pain Vague indigestion Heartburn	Decreased appetite Sense of fullness Nausea and vomiting	Alcohol Meals Drugs (aspirin, NSAIDs, corticosteroids, antibiotics, antiasthma agents)	Bile gastritis may be relived by vomiting	Tenderness to abdominal palpation or epigastric percussion	Endoscopy Upper GI radiograph Gastric biopsy
Active chronic gastritis	Especially older adults	Indigestion			Bismuth compounds (Pepto-Bismol) Antimicrobials		Gastric mucosal biopsy Urea breath test Serologic test of *H. pylori*
Nonulcer dyspepsia		Diffuse abdominal pain or discomfort	Nocturnal pain uncommon		Pain not usually relieved by antacids		Endoscopy

Continued

TABLE 2-89   Differential Diagnosis of Heartburn and Indigestion—cont'd

CAUSE	NATURE OF PATIENT	NATURE OF SYMPTOMS	ASSOCIATED SYMPTOMS	PRECIPITATING AND AGGRAVATING FACTORS	AMELIORATING FACTORS	PHYSICAL FINDINGS	DIAGNOSTIC STUDIES
Functional GI disorder	Children and adults	Distention Awareness of peristalsis and gurgling Intermittent symptoms Vague, nonspecific symptoms No weight loss Continuous pain	Significant emotional investment Other neurotic symptoms Belching (from aerophagia)	Social/environmental stresses		No signs of systemic disease	Studies normal
Excessive intestinal gas	Common in elderly	Vague feelings of indigestion	Abdominal bloating Belching Passing flatus	Increased ingestion of flatulogenic foods (e.g., bagels, legumes, high-fiber foods) GI Stasis Gut hypomotility Bacterial change Constipation Lack of exercise	Belching Passing flatus		
Gas entrapment (hepatic or splenic flexure syndrome)		Abdominal discomfort Pain often referred to chest	Chest pain	Bending over Wearing tight garments		Flexion of thigh on abdomen replicates symptoms	Abdominal radiograph shows trapped gas in hepatic or splenic flexure
Gallbladder disease		Vague abdominal discomfort Occasional distention Indigestion	Nausea Pain in right shoulder	Fatty foods			Cholecystograms Sonograms

HEEL PAIN, PLANTAR

BOX 2-113   Differential Diagnosis of Plantar Heel Pain

Skin

Keratoses
Verruca
Ulcer
Fissure

Connective Tissue

Fat

Atrophy
Panniculitis

Dense Connective Tissue

Inflammatory fasciitis
Fibromatosis
Enthesopathy
Bursitis

Bone (Calcaneus)

Stress fracture
Paget's disease
Benign bone cyst/tumor
Malignant bone tumor
Metabolic bone disease (osteopenia)

Nerve

Tarsal tunnel
Plantar nerve entrapment
S1 nerve root radiculopathy
Painful peripheral neuropathy

Infection

Dermatomycoses
Acute osteomyelitis
Plantar abscess

Miscellaneous

Foreign body
Nonunion calcaneus fracture
Psychogenic
Idiopathic

From Klippel J (ed): *Practical rheumatology,* London, 1995, Mosby.

HELMINTHIC INFECTIONS

TABLE 2-90   Helminthic Infections

HELMINTH	SETTING	VECTORS	DIAGNOSIS	TREATMENT
Endemic in United States				
Pinworm (enterobiasis)	Ubiquitous	Human	Direct exam for ova	Mebendazole, albendazole
Ascaris lumbricoides	Southeast	Human	Stool exam for ova	Mebendazole, albendazole
Trichuris trichiura	Southeast	Human	Stool exam for ova	Mebendazole, albendazole
Hookworm	Southeast	Human	Stool exam for ova	Mebendazole, albendazole
Common in Travelers and Immigrants				
Strongyloides stercoralis	Developing world	Human	Stool exam for larvae	Thiabendazole, ivermectin
Schistosoma sp.	Developing world	Snails	Stool exam for ova	Praziquantel
Wuchereria sp.	Asia	Mosquitos	Nocturnal blood exam	Ivermectin
Onchocerca volvulus	Africa, South and Central America	Blackfly	Biopsy	Ivermectin
Loa loa	Africa	Mosquitos	Blood exam, clinical setting	Ivermectin

From Andreoli TE (ed): *Cecil essentials of medicine,* ed 5, Philadelphia, 2001, WB Saunders.

HEMARTHROSIS

BOX 2-114   Differential Diagnosis of Hemarthrosis

Trauma with or without fractures
Pigmented villonodular synovitis
Synovioma, other tumors
Hemangioma
Charcot's joint or other severe joint
   destruction

von Willebrand's disease
Anticoagulant therapy
Myeloproliferative disease with
   thrombocytosis
Thrombocytopenia
Scurvy

Ruptured aneurysm
Arteriovenous fistula
Idiopathic

From Schumacher HR: Synovial fluid analysis and synovial biopsy. In Kelley WN, Harris ED Jr, Ruddy S, Sledge CB (eds): *Textbook of rheumatology,* ed 3, Philadelphia, 1989, WB Saunders.

HEMATURIA

Hematuria
ICD-9CM # 599.7 Hematuria, benign (essential)

BOX 2-115   Hematuria

Use the mnemonic TICS:

T (trauma): below to kidney, insertion of Foley catheter or foreign body in urethra, prolonged and severe exercise, very rapid emptying of overdistended bladder

(tumor): hypernephroma, Wilms' tumor, papillary carcinoma of the bladder, prostatic and urethral neoplasms

(toxins): turpentine, phenols, sulfonamides and other antibiotics, cyclophosphamide, NSAIDs

I (infections): glomerulonephritis, TB, cystitis, prostatitis, urethritis, *Schistosoma haematobium,* yellow fever, blackwater fever

(inflammatory processes): Goodpasture's syndrome, periarteritis, postirradiation

C (calculi): renal, ureteral, bladder, urethra

(cysts): simple cysts, polycystic disease

(congenital anomalies): hemangiomas, aneurysms, AVM

S (surgery): invasive procedures, prostatic resection, cystoscopy

(sickle cell disease and other hematologic disturbances): hemophilia, thrombocytopenia, anticoagulants

(somewhere else): bleeding genitals, factitious (drug addicts)

AVM, Arteriovenous malformation; *NSAIDs,* nonsteroidal anti-inflammatory drugs; *TB,* tuberculosis.

Helminthic infections
ICD-9CM # 127.9 Helminthic intestinal infections

TABLE 2-91   Key Laboratory Tests for Hematuria

FINDING	CLINICAL IMPLICATION
Dipstick	
Blood	Use only for screening—must confirm by presence of RBCs on microscopy
Leukocytes	Signifies infection or inflammation
Nitrites	Infection with urease-producing organisms
Heavy proteinuria	Suggests glomerulopathy
Microscopy	
RBCs	Hematuria is defined as presence of >3 RBC/hpf
Eumorphic RBCs	Implies epithelial origin of bleeding
Dysmorphic RBCs	Implies glomerular origin of bleeding
WBCs	Signifies infection or inflammation
Casts	Favor medical cause of bleeding
Crystals	Seen early in stone formation
Cytology	Aids in diagnosis of urothelial cancer
Culture	Needed to confirm suspected infection
Blood	
CBC	May see anemia, thrombocytopenia, or leukocytosis
Serum creatinine	Marker of renal function; required for IVP
Others (based on history)	Sickle cell panel
	Coagulation parameters
	Tumor markers

From Nseyo UO (ed): *Urology for primary care physicians,* Philadelphia, 1999, WB Saunders.
CBC, Complete blood count; *IVP,* intravenous pyelogram; *RBC,* red blood cell; *WBC,* white blood cell.

BOX 2-116 Most Frequent Causes of Hematuria by Age and Sex

0-20 yr

Acute glomerulonephritis
Acute urinary tract infections
Congenital urinary tract anomalies with obstruction

20-40 yr

Acute urinary tract infection
Bladder cancer
Urolithiasis

40-60 yr (women)

Acute urinary tract infection
Bladder cancer
Urolithiasis

40-60 yr (men)

Acute urinary tract infection
Bladder cancer
Urolithiasis

60 yr and older (women)

Acute urinary tract infection
Bladder cancer

60 yr and older (men)

Acute urinary tract infection
Benign prostatic hyperplasia
Bladder cancer

From Gillenwater JY et al (ed): *Adult and pediatric urology*, ed 3, St Louis, 1996, Mosby.

HEMIPARESIS/HEMIPLEGIA

Hemiparesis/Hemiplegia
ICD-9CM # 436.0 Acquired due to acute CVA, flaccid
436.1 Acquired due to CVA, acute, spastic

BOX 2-117 Hemiparesis/hemiplegia

Cerebrovascular accident
Transient ischemic attack
Cerebral neoplasm
Multiple sclerosis or other demyelinating disorder
CNS infection
Migraine
Subdural hematoma

Vasculitis
Todd's paralysis
Epidural hematoma
Metabolic (hyperosmolar state, electrolyte imbalance)
Psychiatric disorders
Congenital disorders
Leukodystrophies

HEMOPTYSIS

Hemoptysis
ICD-9CM # 786.3

BOX 2-118 Hemoptysis

Cardiovascular

Pulmonary embolism/infarction
Left ventricular failure
Mitral stenosis
AV fistula
Severe hypertension
Erosion of aortic aneurysm

Pulmonary

Neoplasm (primary or metastatic)
Infection
    Pneumonia: *Streptococcus pneumoniae, Klebsiella pneumoniae, Staphylococcus aureus, Legionella pneumophila*
    Bronchiectasis
    Abscess
    TB
    Bronchitis
    Fungal infections (aspergillosis, coccidioidomycosis)
Parasitic infections (amebiasis, ascariasis, paragonimiasis)

Vasculitis: Wegener's granulomatosis, Churg-Strauss syndrome, Henoch-Schönlein purpura
Goodpasture's syndrome
Trauma (needle biopsy, foreign body, right heart catheterization, prolonged and severe cough)
Cystic fibrosis, bullous emphysema
Pulmonary sequestration
Pulmonary AV fistula
SLE
Idiopathic pulmonary hemosiderosis
Drugs: aspirin, anticoagulants, penicillamine
Pulmonary hypertension
Mediastinal fibrosis

Other

Epistaxis, trauma
Laryngeal bleeding (laryngitis, laryngeal neoplasm)
Hematologic disorders (clotting abnormalities, DIC, thrombocytopenia)

HEPATIC CYSTS

Hepatic cysts
ICD-9CM # 751.62 Hepatic cyst, congenital
                122.8   Echinococcus infection, liver

BOX 2-119   Classification of Hepatic Cysts

I. Congenital hepatic cysts
   A. Parenchymal cysts
      1. Solitary cyst
      2. Polycystic disease
   B. Ductal cysts
      1. Localized dilation
      2. Multiple cystic dilations of intrahepatic ducts (Caroli's disease)
II. Acquired hepatic cysts
   A. Inflammatory cysts
      1. Retention cyst
      2. Echinococcal cyst
   B. Neoplastic cyst
   C. Peliosis hepatis

From Stein J (ed): *Internal medicine*, ed 5, St Louis, 1998, Mosby.

HEPATIC GRANULOMAS

Hepatic granulomas
ICD-9CM # 572.8

BOX 2-120   Diseases Associated with Hepatic Granulomas

Infections

Bacterial, spirochetal
   Tuberculosis and atypical *Mycobacterium* infections
   Tularemia
   Brucellosis
   Leprosy
   Syphilis
   Whipple's disease
   Listeriosis
Viral
   Infectious mononucleosis
   Cytomegalovirus infections
Rickettsial
   Q fever
Fungal
   Coccidioidomycosis
   Histoplasmosis
   Cryptococcal infections

   Actinomycosis
   Aspergillosis
   Nocardiosis
Parasitic
   Schistosomiasis
   Clonorchiasis
   Toxocariasis
   Ascariasis
   Toxoplasmosis
   Amebiasis

Hepatobiliary Disorders

Primary biliary cirrhosis
Granulomatous hepatitis
Jejunoileal bypass

Systemic Disorders

Sarcoidosis
Wegener's granulomatosis

Inflammatory bowel disease
Hodgkin's disease
Lymphoma

Drugs/Toxins

Beryllium
Parenteral foreign material (starch, talc, silicone, etc.)
Phenylbutazone
Alpha-methyldopa
Procainamide
Allopurinol
Phenytoin
Nitrofurantoin
Hydralazine

From Andreoli TE (ed): *Cecil essentials of medicine*, ed 5, Philadelphia, 2001, WB Saunders.

HEPATIC LESIONS, FOCAL

TABLE 2-92   Focal Hepatic Lesions

LESION	RISK FACTORS	RADIOGRAPHIC FINDINGS
Cystic		
Simple cyst	Genetic predisposition (polycystic disease)	Smooth cystic border with low-density contents
Pyogenic abscess	Biliary tract, intraabdominal infection; penetrating wounds or trauma	Low-density lesion containing echogenic material
Amebic abscess	Residence in or travel to endemic area; homosexual men	Elevated hemidiaphragm, pleural effusion, irregular cystic edge
Hydatid cyst	Travel to or residence in endemic regions	Elevated hemidiaphragm, cyst wall calcification, daughter cysts with detached membranes
Cystadenocarcinoma	Congenital cyst	Thick irregular cyst wall
Solid		
Benign tumors		
Adenoma	Oral contraceptives	Vascular hypodense lesions; no ^{99m}Tc uptake
Focal nodular hyperplasia	—	^{99m}Tc uptake; hypodense avascular lesions
Hemangioma	—	^{99m}Tc-tagged red blood cell study
Malignant		
Hepatocellular carcinoma	Hepatitis B or C, cirrhosis, mycotoxins	Hypodense lesion with nonhomogeneous contrast enhancement
Cholangiocarcinoma	*Clonorchis*, sclerosing cholangitis; polycystic disease; choledochal cyst; Thorotrast	Hypodense lesion; dilated intrahepatic ducts
Angiosarcoma	Vinyl chloride, anabolic steroids, Thorotrast	Hypodense vascular lesion
Metastasis	Primary tumor risk	Hypodense lesions; locality dependent or primary

From Gorbach SL: *Infectious diseases,* ed 2, Philadelphia, 1998, WB Saunders.

Hepatic lesions, focal
ICD-9CM # Code varies with specific diagnosis

Hepatitis, chronic
ICD-9CM # 571.40 Hepatitis, noninfectious, chronic
072.22 Hepatitis B, chronic
070.44 Hepatitis C, chronic

HEPATITIS, CHRONIC

BOX 2-121   Major Etiologies of Chronic Hepatitis

Chronic viral hepatitis
  Hepatitis B
  Hepatitis C
  Hepatitis D
Autoimmune hepatitis and variant syndromes
Hereditary hemochromatosis
Wilson's disease
α-Antitrypsin deficiency
Fatty liver and nonalcoholic steatohepatitis
Alcoholic liver disease
Drug-induced liver disease
Hepatic granulomas
  Infectious
  Drug induced
  Neoplastic
  Idiopathic

From Mandell GL: *Mandell, Douglas, and Bennett's principles and practice of infectious diseases,* ed 5, New York, 2000, Churchill Livingstone.

Gwendolyn R. Lee, M.D.
Internal Medicine

HEPATITIS, VIRAL

TABLE 2-93   **Features of the Six Hepatotropic Viruses**

	HAV	HBV	HCV	HDV	HEV	HGV
Nucleic acid	RNA	DNA	RNA	RNA	RNA	RNA
Incubation (mean)	30 days	100-120 days	7-9 wk	2-4 mo	40 days	Unknown
Transmission						
Percutaneous	Rare	Common	Common	Common	No	Common
Fecal-oral	Common	No	No	No	Common	No
Sexual	Rare	Common	Rare	Rare	Rare	Rare
Transplacental	No	Common	Rare	No	Probably no	Rare
Chronic infection	No	Yes	Yes	Yes	No	Yes
Fulminant disease	Rare	Yes	Rare	Yes	Rare	Probably no

From Behrman RE: *Nelson textbook of pediatrics,* ed 16, Philadelphia, 2000, WB Saunders.

Hepatitis, viral
ICD-9CM # 070.1   Hepatitis A
070.20 Hepatitis B, acute
070.4   Hepatitis C, acute

HEPATOMEGALY

Hepatomegaly
ICD-9CM # 789.1

BOX 2-122   **Hepatomegaly**

Frequent Jaundice

Infectious hepatitis
Toxic hepatitis
Carcinoma: liver, pancreas, bile ducts, metastatic neo-
    plasm to liver
Cirrhosis
Obstruction of common bile duct
Alcoholic hepatitis
Biliary cirrhosis
Cholangitis
Hemochromatosis with cirrhosis

Infrequent Jaundice

Congestive heart failure
Amyloidosis

Liver abscess
Sarcoidosis
Infectious mononucleosis
Alcoholic fatty infiltration
Lymphoma
Leukemia
Budd-Chiari syndrome
Myelofibrosis with myeloid metaplasia
Familial hyperlipoproteinemia type 1
Other: amebiasis, hydatid disease of liver, schistosomia-
    sis, kala-azar *(Leishmania donovani),* Hurler's syndrome,
    Gaucher's disease, kwashiorkor

HERMAPHRODITISM

Hermaphroditism
ICD-9CM # 752.7 Hermaphroditism, congenital

BOX 2-123 Etiologic Classification of Hermaphroditism

Female pseudohermaphroditism
  Androgen exposure
    Fetal source
      21-Hydroxylase (P450 c21) deficiency
      11β-Hydroxylase (P450 c11) deficiency
      3β-Hydroxysteroid dehydrogenase II (3β-HSD II)
        deficiency
      Aromatase ($P450_{arom}$) deficiency
    Maternal source
      Virilizing ovarian tumor
      Virilizing adrenal tumor
      Androgenic drugs
  Undetermined origin
    Associated with genitourinary and gastrointestinal
      tract defects
Male pseudohermaphroditism
  Defects in testicular differentiation
    Denys-Drash syndrome (mutation in WT1 gene)
    WAGR syndrome (*W*ilms tumor, *a*niridia, *g*enitouri-
      nary malformation, *r*etardation)
    Deletion of 11p13
    Camptomelic syndrome (autosomal gene at 17q24.3-
      q25.1) and SOX 9 mutation
    XY pure gonadal dysgenesis (Swyer syndrome)
      Mutation in SRY gene
      Unknown cause
    XY gonadal agenesis

Deficiency of testicular hormones
  Leydig cell aplasia
  Mutation in LH receptor
  Lipoid adrenal hyperplasia (P450 scc) deficiency; mu-
    tation in StAR (steroidogenic acute regulatory
    protein)
  3β-HSDII deficiency
  17-Hydroxylase/17, 20-lyase (P450 c17) deficiency
  Persistent müllerian duct syndrome
    Gene mutations, müllerian-inhibiting substance
      (MIS)
    Receptor defects for MIS
Defect in androgen action
  5α-Reductase II mutations
  Androgen receptor defects
    Complete androgen insensitivity syndrome
    Partial androgen insensitivity syndrome
    (Reinfenstein and other syndromes)
    Smith-Lemli-Opitz syndrome
      Defect in conversion of 7-dehydrocholesterol to
      cholesterol
True hermaphroditism
  XX
  XY
  XX/XY chimeras

From Behrman RE: *Nelson textbook of pediatrics*, ed 16, Philadelphia, 2000, WB Saunders.

HERNIAS

TABLE 2-94 Distinguishing Characteristics of Hernias

	INDIRECT INGUINAL	DIRECT INGUINAL	FEMORAL
Incidence	Most common type of hernia; both sexes are affected; often patients are children and young males	Less common than indirect inguinal; occurs more often in males than females; more common in those over age 40	Least common type of hernia; occurs more often in females than males; rare in children
Occurrence	Through internal inguinal ring; can remain in canal, exit the external ring, or pass into scrotum; may be bilateral	Through external inguinal ring; located in region of Hesselbach triangle; rarely enters scrotum	Through femoral ring, femoral canal, and fossa ovalis
Presentation	Soft swelling in area of internal ring; pain on straining; hernia comes down canal and touches fingertip on examination	Bulge in area of Hesselbach triangle; usually painless; easily reduced; hernia bulges anteriorly, pushes against side of finger on examination	Right side presentation more common than left; pain may be severe; inguinal canal empty on examination

Hernias
ICD-9CM # 553.9 Hernia NOS
       553.0 Hernia, femoral NOS
       550.9 Hernia, inguinal NOS

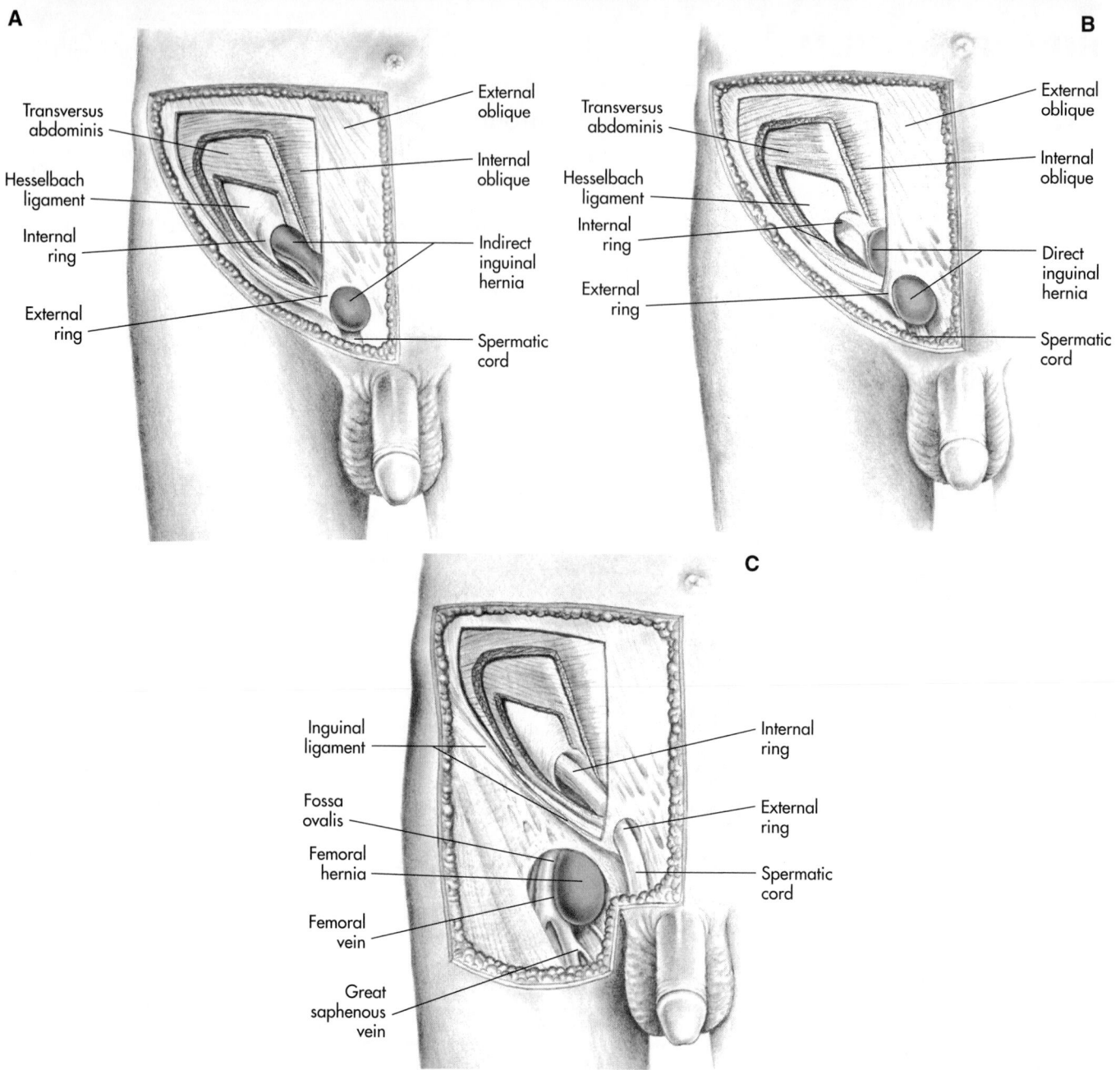

Fig. 2-8   Anatomy of region of common pelvic hernias. **A,** Indirect inguinal hernia. **B,** Direct inguinal hernia. **C,** Femoral hernia. (From Seidel HM [ed]: *Mosby's guide to physical examination,* ed 4, St Louis, 1999, Mosby.)

HICCUPS

BOX 2-124   Causes of Hiccups

Transient Hiccups

Sudden excitement, emotion
Gastric distention
Esophageal obstruction
Alcohol ingestion
Sudden change in temperature

Persistent or Chronic Hiccups

Toxic/metabolic: uremia, diabetes, hyperventilation, hypokalemia, hypocalcemia, hyponatremia, gout, fever

Drugs: benzodiazepines, steroids, α-methyldopa, barbiturates
Surgery/general anesthesia
Thoracic/diaphragmatic disorders: pneumonia, lung cancer, asthma, pleuritis, pericarditis, myocardial infarction, aortic aneurysm, esophagitis (peptic or infectious), esophageal obstruction, diaphragmatic hernia or irritation
Abdominal disorders: gastric ulcer or cancer, hepatobiliary or pancreatic

disease, inflammatory bowel disease, bowel obstruction, intra-abdominal or subphrenic abscess, prostatic infection or cancer
Central nervous system disorders: traumatic, infectious, vascular, structural
Ear, nose, and throat disorders: pharyngitis, laryngitis, tumor, irritation of auditory canal
Psychogenic disorders
Idiopathic disorders

From Kassirer J (ed): *Current therapy in adult medicine,* ed 4, St Louis, 1998, Mosby.

BOX 2-125   Treatment of Hiccups

Nonpharmacologic Methods

Irritation of uvula or nasopharynx
Counterirritation of vagal nerve
Interruption of respiratory rhythm
Counterirritation of diaphragm
Relief of gastric distention

Pharmacologic Agents

Baclofen

Chlorpromazine

Metoclopramide

Phenytoin

Quinidine sulfate

Examples

Tongue traction, lifting uvula, swabbing pharynx
Carotid sinus massage
Breath holding
Pulling knees up to chest
Nasogastric suction

Dosages

5 mg PO tid, increasing every 3 days to 80 mg/day maximum dose if needed
25-50 mg IV q6h
25-50 mg PO q6h
10 mg IV q4h
10 mg PO q6h
200 mg IV
100 mg PO qid
200 mg PO qid

From Kassirer J (ed): *Current therapy in adult medicine,* ed 4, St Louis, 1998, Mosby.
h, Hour; *IV,* intravenously; *PO,* orally; *q,* every; *qid,* four times a day; *tid,* three times a day.

HIRSUTISM AND HYPERTRICHOSIS

BOX 2-126   Differential Diagnosis of Excess Hair in Women

Hirsutism (Increased Sexual Hair)
Most Common

Polycystic ovary syndrome
Idiopathic hirsutism
Medications
   Danazol for endometriosis
   Androgenic oral contraceptives
      (norgestrel)
Hyperprolactinemia
Hyperthecosis

Less Common

Congenital adrenal hyperplasia
Ovarian tumors

Sertoli-Leydig cell tumors
Granulosa-theca cell tumors
Other tumors that stimulate
   ovarian stroma
Adrenal tumors
   Cushing's disease
   Other tumors of the adrenal cortex
Severe insulin resistance syndromes

**Hypertrichosis (Increased Total
Body Hair)—Rare**
Drugs

Dilantin
Streptomycin

Hexachlorobenzene
Penicillamine
Diazoxide
Minoxidil
Cyclosporine

Systemic Illness

Hypothyroidism
Anorexia nervosa
Malnutrition
Porphyria
Dermatomyositis

From Carlson KJ et al: *Primary care of women,* St Louis, 1995, Mosby.

HIV INFECTION, ANORECTAL LESIONS

BOX 2-127   Anorectal Lesions in the HIV Patient

Common Conditions

Anal fissure
Abscess and fistula
Hemorrhoids
Pruritus ani
Pilonidal disease

Common STDs

Gonorrhea
Chlamydia
Herpes
Chancroid
Syphilis
Condylomata acuminata

Atypical Conditions

Infectious: TB, CMV, actinomycosis,
   cryptococcus
Neoplastic: lymphoma, Kaposi's
   sarcoma, squamous cell carcinoma
Other: idiopathic and ulcer

From Rosen P (ed): *Emergency medicine,* ed 5, St Louis, 2002, Mosby.
CMV, Cytomegalovirus; *STDs,* sexually transmitted diseases; *TB,* tuberculosis.

HIV infection, anorectal lesions
ICD-9CM # 042 HIV infection, symptomatic
                V08 HIV infection, asymptomatic

HIV infection, chest radiographic abnormalities
ICD-9CM # 042 HIV infection, symptomatic
V08 HIV infection, asymptomatic

HIV INFECTION, CHEST RADIOGRAPHIC ABNORMALITIES

TABLE 2-95 **Chest Radiographic Abnormalities: Differential Diagnosis in the AIDS Patient**

FINDING	ETIOLOGIES
Diffuse interstitial infiltration	*Pneumocystis carinii* Cytomegalovirus *Mycobacterium tuberculosis* *Mycobacterium avium* complex Histoplasmosis Coccidioidomycosis Lymphoid interstitial pneumonitis
Focal consolidation	Bacterial pneumonia *Mycoplasma pneumoniae* *Pneumocystis carinii* *Mycobacterium tuberculosis* *Mycobacterium avium* complex
Nodular lesions	Kaposi's sarcoma *Mycobacterium tuberculosis* *Mycobacterium avium* complex Fungal lesions Toxoplasmosis
Cavitary lesions	*Pneumocystis carinii* *Mycobacterium tuberculosis* Bacterial infection
Pleural effusion	Kaposi's sarcoma (Small effusion may be associated with any infection)
Adenopathy	Kaposi's sarcoma Lymphoma *Mycobacterium tuberculosis* *Cryptococcus*
Pneumothorax	Kaposi's sarcoma

From Rosen P (ed): *Emergency medicine*, ed 5, St Louis, 2002, Mosby.

II

HIV INFECTION, COGNITIVE IMPAIRMENT

BOX 2-128   Differential Diagnosis of Cognitive Impairment

Early to Mid-Stage HIV Disease

Depression
Alcohol and substance abuse
Medication-induced cognitive impairment
Metabolic encephalopathies
HIV-related cognitive impairment

Advanced HIV Disease (CD4$^+$ <100/mm^3)

Opportunistic infection of CNS
Neurosyphilis
CNS lymphoma
Progressive multifocal leukoencephalopathy
Depression
Metabolic encephalopathies
Medication-induced cognitive impairment
Stroke
HIV dementia

From Mandell GL: *Mandell, Douglas, and Bennett's principles and practice of infectious diseases*, ed 5, New York, 2000, Churchill Livingstone.
CNS, Central nervous system; *HIV*, human immunodeficiency virus.

HIV infection, cutaneous manifestations
ICD-9CM # 042 HIV infection, symptomatic
V08 HIV infection, asymptomatic

HIV INFECTION, CUTANEOUS MANIFESTATIONS

TABLE 2-96   Common Cutaneous Manifestations in HIV Patients

CAUSE	CLINICAL FEATURES
Bacterial Infection	
Bacillary angiomatosis	Numerous angiomatous nodules associated with fever, chills, weight loss
Staphylococcus aureus	Folliculitis, ecthyma, impetigo, bullous impetigo, furuncles, carbuncles
Syphilis	May occur in different forms (primary, secondary, tertiary); chancre may become painful due to secondary infection
Fungal Infection	
Candidiasis	Mucous membranes (oral, vulvovaginal), less commonly candida intertrigo or paronychia
Cryptococcoses	Papules or nodules that strongly resemble molluscum contagiosum; other forms include pustules, purpuric papules, and vegetating plaques
Seborrheic dermatitis	Scaling and erythema in the hair-bearing areas (eyebrows, scalp, chest, and pubic area)
Arthropod Infestations	
Scabies	Pruritus with or without rash, usually generalized but can be limited to a single digit
Viral Infection	
Herpes simplex	Vesicular lesion in clusters; perianal, genital, orofacial, or digital; can be disseminated
Herpes zoster	Painful dermatomal vesicles that may ulcerate or disseminate
HIV	Discrete erythematous macules and papules on the upper trunk, palms, and soles are the most characteristic cutaneous finding of acute HIV infection
Human papillomavirus	Genital warts (may become unusually extensive)
Kaposi's sarcoma (herpesvirus)	Erythematous macules or papules; enlarge at varying rates; violaceous nodules or plaques; occasionally painful
Molluscum contagiosum	Discrete umbilicated papules commonly on the face, neck, and intertriginous sites (axilla, groin, or buttocks)
Noninfectious	
Drug reactions	More frequent and severe in HIV patients
Nutritional deficiencies	Mainly seen in children and patients with chronic diarrhea; diffuse skin manifestations, depending upon the deficiency
Psoriasis	Scaly lesions; diffuse or localized; can be associated with arthritis
Vasculitis	Palpable purpuric eruption (can resemble septic emboli)

From Kassirer J (ed): *Current therapy in adult medicine*, ed 4, St Louis, 1998, Mosby.

HIV INFECTION, ESOPHAGEAL DISEASE

HIV infection, esophageal disease
ICD-9CM # Code varies with specific diagnosis

TABLE 2-97   Esophageal Disease in Patients with Acquired Immunodeficiency Syndrome*

CHARACTERISTIC	*CANDIDA* Infection	CYTOMEGALOVIRUS INFECTION	APHTHOUS ULCER	HERPES SIMPLEX
Frequency (as cause of esophageal symptoms)	50%-70%	10%-20%	10%-20%	2.5%
Clinical features				
Dysphagia	++	+	+	+
Odynophagia	++	+++	+++	+++
Oral lesions	Thrush—70%	None	None	HSV >50%
Pain localization	Diffuse—esophageal	Focal—chest	Focal—chest	Focal—chest
Fever	None	Usually	None	Variable
Stage	CD4$^+$ cell count <100/mm^3	CD4$^+$ cell count <50/mm^3	CD4$^+$ cell count <50/mm^3	CD4$^+$ cell count <150/mm^3
Diagnosis				
Endoscopy	Usually treated empirically Pseudomembranous plaques	Ulcers—single or multiple discrete Biopsy—required to detect CMV	Ulcers—identical to those in CMV	Ulcers—shallow, small, confluent
Microbiology	Brush—yeast and pseudomycelia Culture for in vitro sensitivity test	Histopathology to show intranuclear inclusions; culture is inconclusive	Negative studies for alternative agents	Histopathology showing intracytoplasmic inclusions + multinucleated giant cells; HSV by fluorescent antibody stain or culture
Treatment				
Acute (2-3 wk)	Azoles; usually fluconazole Some require IV amphotericin	Ganciclovir Alternative is foscarnet	Systemic prednisone ± antifungal prophylaxis Thalidomide	Acyclovir by mouth or intravenously
Maintenance	Fluconazole or other azole only with repeated episodes	Arbitrary—some use only for recurrent disease	None	Arbitrary
Comment	Response to fluconazole: 85%	Should obtain ophthalmologic examination	May be severely debilitating	Relatively rare cause of esophageal ulcer Response to treatment is usually good

From Gorbach SL: *Infectious diseases*, ed 2, Philadelphia, 1998, WB Saunders.
*+, Modest; ++, moderate; +++, severe; *CMV*, cytomegalovirus; *HSV*, herpes simplex virus; *IV*, intravenous.

HIV INFECTION, HEPATIC DISEASE

BOX 2-129 Selected Causes of Hepatic Disease in Human Immunodeficiency Virus–Infected Persons

Viruses
  Hepatitis A
  Hepatitis B
  Hepatitis C
  Hepatitis D (with HBV)
  Epstein-Barr virus
  Cytomegalovirus
  Herpes simplex virus
  Adenovirus
  Varicella-zoster virus
Mycobacteria
  Mycobacterium avium complex
  Mycobcterium tuberculosis
Fungi
  Histoplasma capsulatum
  Cryptococcus neoformans
  Coccidioides immitis
  Candida albicans
  Pneumocystis carinii
  Penicillium marneffei

Protozoa
  Toxoplasma gondii
  Cryptosporidium parvum
  Microsporida spp.
  Schistosoma
Bacteria
  Bartonella henselae (peliosis hepatis)
Malignancy
  Kaposi's sarcoma (HHV-8)
  Non-Hodgkin's lymphoma
  Hepatocellular carcinoma
Medications
  Zidovudine
  Didanosine
  Ritonavir
  Other HIV-1 protease inhibitors
  Fluconazole
  Macrolide antibiotics
  Isoniazid
  Rifampin
  Trimethoprim-sulfamethoxazole

From Mandell GL: *Mandell, Douglas, and Bennett's principles and practice of infectious diseases,* ed 5, New York, 2000, Churchill Livingstone.
HBV, Hepatitis B virus; *HHV-8,* human herpesvirus type 8; *HIV-1,* human immunodeficiency virus type 1.

HIV INFECTION, INFECTIOUS DIARRHEA

HIV infection, infectious diarrhea
ICD-9CM # Code varies with specific diagnosis

TABLE 2-98   Acute Infectious Diarrhea in Patients with Acquired Immunodeficiency Virus

AGENT	FREQUENCY* (%)	CLINICAL FEATURES	DIAGNOSIS	TREATMENT
Salmonella	5-15	Watery diarrhea; fever; fecal white blood cells (WBCs) variable: CD4$^+$ cell count variable; increased frequency with low CD$^+$ cell count	Stool culture Blood culture	Ciprofloxacin (Cipro), 500-750 mg by mouth (PO) twice a day (bid) for 14 days Trimethoprim-sulfamethoxazole (TMP-SMX), 1-2 double-strength (DS) tablets PO bid for 14 days Ampicillin, 2 g/d PO or 6 g/d intravenously for 14 days (if sensitive) Third-generation cephalosporin or chloramphenicol Treatment may need to be extended in ≥4 wk
Shigella	1-3	Watery diarrhea or bloody flux; fever; fecal WBCs common; any CD4$^+$ cell count	Stool culture	Cipro, 500 mg PO bid for 3 days TMP-SMX, 1 DS tablet PO bid for 3 days
Campylobacter jejuni	4-8	Watery diarrhea or bloody flux; fever, fecal leukocytes variable; and CD4$^+$ cell count	Stool culture; most laboratories cannot detect C. *cinaedi*, C. *fennelli*, and others	Cipro, 500 mg PO bid for 3-5 days Erythromycin, 500 mg PO four times a day (qid) for 5 days
Clostridium difficile	10-15	Watery diarrhea; fecal WBCs variable; fever and leukocytosis common; antibacterial agent nearly always—especially clindamycin, ampicillin, and cephalosporins; any CD4$^+$ cell count	Endoscopy: pseudomembranous colitis, colitis, or normal Stool toxin assay: tissue culture of enzyme immunoassay preferred Computed tomographic scan: colitis with thickened mucosa	Metronidazole, 250-500 mg PO qid for 10-14 days Vancomycin, 125 mg PO qid for 10-14 days Antiperistaltic agents (diphenoxylate–atropine sulfate [Lomotil] or loperamide) contraindicated
Enteroadherent *Escherichia coli*	10-20	Watery diarrhea; acute, but may be chronic	Adherence to HEp-2 cells (research laboratories only)	Fluoroquinolone
Enteric viruses	15-30	Watery diarrhea; acute, but one third of cases become chronic; any CD4$^+$ cell count	Major agents: adenovirus, astrovirus, picobirnavirus, calcivirus, clinical laboratories cannot detect these viruses	Supportive treatment: Lomotil or loperamide
Idiopathic	25-40	Variable Noninfectious causes—rule out medications, diet, irritable bowel syndrome; any CD4$^+$ cell count	Negative studies including culture, ova and parasites examination, and C. *difficile* toxin assay	Severe acute diarrhea: Cipro, 500 mg PO bid or ofloxacin, 200-300 mg PO bid for 5 days ± metronidazole

From Gorbach SL: *Infectious diseases,* ed 2, Philadelphia, 1998, WB Saunders.
*Frequency among patients with acute diarrhea defined as three or more loose or watery stools for 3-10 days.

HIV INFECTION, LOWER GI TRACT DISEASE

HIV infection, lower GI tract disease
ICD-9CM # 042 HIV infection, symptomatic

BOX 2-130   Causes of Lower Gastrointestinal Tract Disease in Patients with Human Immunodeficiency Virus

Causes of Enterocolitis

Bacteria
  Campylobacter jejuni and other spp.
  Salmonella spp.
  Shigella flexneri
  Aeromonas hydrophila
  Plesiomonas shigelloides
  Yersinia enterocolitica
  Vibrio spp.
  Mycobacterium avium complex
  Mycobacterium tuberculosis
  Escherichia coli (enterotoxigenic, enteroadherent)
  Bacterial overgrowth
  Clostridium difficile (toxin)
Parasites
  Cryptosporidium parvum
  Microsporida *(Enterocytozoon bieneusi, Septata intestinalis)*
  Isospora belli
  Entamoeba histolytica
  Giardia lamblia
  Cyclospora cayetanensis
Viruses
  Cytomegalovirus
  Adenovirus
  Calicivirus
  Astrovirus
  Picobirnavirus
  Human immunodeficiency virus
Fungi
  Histoplasma capsulatum

Causes of Proctitis

Bacteria
  Chlamydia trachomatis
  Neisseria gonorrhoeae
  Treponema pallidum
Viruses
  Herpes simplex
  Cytomegalovirus

From Mandell GL: *Mandell, Douglas, and Bennett's principles and practice of infectious diseases,* ed 5, New York, 2000, Churchill Livingstone.

II

HIV infection, neurologic complications
ICD-9CM # 042 HIV infection, symptomatic
V08 HIV infection, asymptomatic

HIV INFECTION, NEUROLOGIC COMPLICATIONS

TABLE 2-99 Neurologic Complications Classified by Stage of HIV Disease

	EARLY HIV DISEASE (CD4 > 500)	LATE HIV DISEASE (CD4 < 200)
Encephalopathy	Aseptic meningitis Depressive pseudodementia Neurosyphilis*	HIV dementia CNS opportunistic processes†
Cranial neuropathy	Aseptic meningitis	CMV encephalitis Lymphomatous meningitis Cryptococcal meningitis
Chronic myelopathy	Coexisting HTLV-I infection*‡	Vacuolar myelopathy Toxoplasma myelitis
Acute paraparesis	AIDP Spinal cord compression* (e.g., epidural abscess)	Lumbosacral radiculomyelitis Toxoplasma myelitis
Peripheral neuropathy	CIDP Multiple entrapment neuropathies Mononeuritis multiplex	Toxic neuropathy (e.g., ddI, d4T) HIV-associated neuropathy Mononeuritis multiplex
Myopathy	Polymyositis	Toxic myopathy (AZT) Polymyositis

From Johnson R (ed): *Current therapy in neurologic disease*, ed 5, St Louis, 1997, Mosby.
AIDP, Acute inflammatory demyelinating polyneuropathy; *AZT*, zidovidine; *CIDP*, chronic inflammatory demyelinating polyneuropathy; *CMV*, cytomegalovirus; *CNS*, central nervous system; *ddI*, dideoxyinosine; *d4T*, stavudine; *HIV*, human immunodeficiency virus; *HTLV-I*, human T-cell lymphotrophic virus type 1.
*These conditions can occur at any stage of HIV infection but should be particularly suspected if the CD4 count is high and opportunistic processes are unlikely.
†Primary CNS lymphoma, progressive multifocal leukoencephalopathy, CNS toxoplasmosis, or CMV encephalitis.
‡Coexisting HTLV-I infection may falsely elevate CD4 count.

HIV INFECTION, OCULAR MANIFESTATIONS

BOX 2-131 Ocular Manifestations of Acquired Immunodeficiency Syndrome

Eyelids
Molluscum contagiosum
Kaposi's sarcoma

Cornea/Conjunctiva
Keratoconjunctivitis sicca
Bacterial/fungal ulcerative keratitis
Herpes simplex
Herpes zoster ophthalmicus
Conjunctival microvasculopathy
Kaposi's sarcoma

Retina, Choroid, and Vitreous
Microvasculopathy
Endophthalmitis

Cytomegalovirus retinitis
Acute retinal necrosis
Syphilis
Toxoplasmosis
Pneumocystis choroidopathy
Cryptococcosis
Mycobacterial infection
Intraocular lymphoma
Candidiasis
Histoplasmosis

Drugs Associated with Ocular Toxicity
Rifabutin
Didanosine

Neuroophthalmic
Disc edema
Primary or secondary optic neuropathy
Cranial nerve palsies

Orbital
Lymphoma
Infection
Pseudotumor

From Stein J (ed): *Internal medicine*, ed 5, St Louis, 1998, Mosby.

HIV infection, ocular manifestations
ICD-9CM # 042 HIV infection, symptomatic
V08 HIV infection, asymptomatic

HIV INFECTION, ORAL MANIFESTATIONS

HIV infection, oral manifestations
ICD-9CM # 042 HIV infection, symptomatic
V08 HIV infection, asymptomatic

TABLE 2-100   Oral Manifestations of HIV Infection

LESION	CHARACTERISTICS
Oral hairy leukoplakia	White, irregular lesions on lateral side of tongue or buccal mucosa; may have prominent folds or "hairy" projections
Angular cheilitis	Red, unilateral or bilateral fissures at corners of mouth
Candidiasis	Creamy white plaques on oral mucosa that bleed when scraped
Herpes simplex	Recurrent vesicular, crusting lesions on the vermilion border of the lip
Herpes zoster	Vesicular and ulcerative oral lesions in the distribution of the trigeminal nerve; may also be on gingiva
Human papillomavirus	Single or multiple, sessile or pedunculated nodules in the oral cavity
Aphthous ulcers	Recurrent circumscribed ulcers with an erythematous margin
Periodontal disease	In a mouth with little plaque or calculus, gingivitis with rapid bone and soft tissue degeneration accompanied by severe pain
Kaposi's sarcoma	In the mouth, incompletely formed blood vessels proliferate, forming lesions of various shades and size as blood extravasates in response to the malignant tumor of the epithelium

From Seidel HM (ed): *Mosby's guide to physical examination,* ed 4, St Louis, 1999, Mosby.

HIV INFECTION, PULMONARY DISEASE

TABLE 2-101   Causes of Pulmonary Disease
                Associated with Human
                Immunodeficiency Virus Infection

CATEGORY	PATHOGEN OR ENTITY
Mycobacterial	*M. tuberculosis*
	M. kansasii
	M. avium complex
	Other nontuberculous mycobacteria
Other bacterial	*Streptococcus pneumoniae*
	Staphylococcus aureus
	Haemophilus influenzae
	Enterobacteriaceae
	Pseudomonas aeruginosa
	Moraxella catarrhalis
	Group A *Streptococcus*
	Nocardia species
	Rhodococcus equi
	Chlamydia pneumoniae
Fungal	*Pneumocystis carinii*
	Cryptococcus neoformans
	Histoplasma capsulatum
	Coccidioides immitis
	Aspergillus species
	Blastomyces dermatitidis
	Penicillium marneffei
Viral	Cytomegalovirus
	Herpes simplex virus
	Adenovirus
	Respiratory syncytial virus
	Influenza viruses
	Parainfluenza virus
Other	*Toxoplasma gondii*
	Strongyloides stercoralis
	Kaposi's sarcoma
	Lymphoma
	Lung cancer
	Lymphocytic interstitial pneumonitis
	Nonspecific interstitial pneumonitis
	Bronchiolitis obliterans with organizing pneumonia
	Pulmonary hypertension
	Emphysema-like or bullous disease
	Pneumothorax
	Congestive heart failure
	Diffuse alveolar damage
	Pulmonary embolus

From Mandell GL: *Mandell, Douglas, and Bennett's principles and practice of infectious diseases,* ed 5, New York, 2000, Churchill Livingstone.

HIV INFECTION, RHEUMATIC SYNDROMES

HIV infection, rheumatic syndromes
ICD-9CM # 042 HIV infection, symptomatic

TABLE 2-102   Rheumatic Syndromes Associated with Human Immunodeficiency Virus (HIV) Infection

SYNDROME	INCIDENCE	PATTERNS OF INVOLVEMENT	SEVERITY	ASSOCIATED FEATURES
Arthralgias	33%	Intermittent; occurs at any stage; usually resolves in weeks to months	May be severe	Bone pain
Reiter's syndrome (RS)	1%-10%; unknown if HIV predisposes patient for RS	Usually develops around transformation to symptomatic AIDS; prominent peripheral arthritis, usually asymmetric, oligoarticular; predilection for lower extremity joint and entheses	Peripheral oligoarthritis and cutaneous manifestations often more severe than RS not associated with HIV	Severe axial involvement (sacroiliitis, spondylitis), conjunctivitis, and uveitis uncommon; hyperkeratotic skin lesions, particularly keratoderma blennorrhagicum, similar to pustular psoriasis
Psoriatic arthritis	Less common than RS	More often polyarticular than is RS; involvement of distal interphalangeal (DIP) joints		Pitting of nails, particularly adjacent to affected DIP joints; severe psoriasis
HIV-associated arthritis	Unknown	Oligoarthritis involving knees and ankles; short-lived, 1-6 wk	Severe, incapacitating symptoms; often more severe than objective findings	Synovial fluid and synovial histology mildly inflammatory
Septic arthritis/osteomyelitis	Not as common as might be expected	Includes opportunistic organisms		
Sicca complex	Unknown	Dry eyes and mouth at any stage of HIV infection; with parotid gland enlargement and lymphocyte infiltration of salivary glands, similar to Sjögren's syndrome; referred to as diffuse infiltrative lymphocytosis syndrome (DILS)		Many genetic, pathologic, and serologic differences between DILS and primary Sjögren's syndrome
Polymyositis	Unknown	Myopathy at any time during HIV infection; indistinguishable from idiopathic polymyositis		Must be distinguished from the myopathy associated with zidovudine
Vasculitis	Unknown	Inflammatory vascular disease similar to polyarteritis (necrotizing, medium-sized arteritis), leukocytoclastic vasculitis, and granulomatous vasculitis		

From Noble J: *Primary care medicine*, ed 3, St. Louis, 2001, Mosby.

HOARSENESS

BOX 2-132   Hoarseness

Allergic rhinitis
Infections (laryngitis, epiglottitis, tracheitis, croup)
Vocal cord polyps
Voice strain
Irritants (tobacco smoke)
Vocal cord trauma (intubation, surgery)
Neoplastic involvement of vocal cord (primary and
  metastatic)

Neurologic abnormalities (multiple sclerosis, amyotrophic lateral sclerosis, parkinsonism)
Endocrine abnormalities (puberty, menopause, hypothyroidism)
Other (laryngeal webs or cysts, psychogenic, muscle
  tension abnormalities)

HYPERCALCEMIA, LABORATORY DIFFERENTIAL DIAGNOSIS

TABLE 2-103   Laboratory Differential Diagnosis of Hypercalcemia

DIAGNOSIS	PLASMA TESTS					URINE TESTS			COMMENTS
	Ca	PO$_4$	PTH	25(OH)D	1,25(OH)$_2$D	cAMP	TmP/GFR	Ca	
Primary hyper-parathyroidism	↑	N/↓	↑	N	N/↑	↑	↓	↑	Parathyroid adenoma most common
MEN I									Parathyroid hyperplasia; also includes pituitary and pancreatic neoplasms
MEN IIa									Parathyroid hyperplasia; also includes medullary thyroid carcinoma and pheochromocytoma
MEN IIb									Parathyroid disease uncommon, primarily medullary thyroid carcinoma and pheochromocytoma
FHH	↑	N	N/↑	N	N	N/↑	N/↓	↓↓	Autosomal dominant inheritance; hypercalcemia present within first decade; benign
Malignancy									
Solid tumor— humoral	↑	N/↓	↓	N	N	↑	↓	↑↑	Primarily epidermoid tumors; PTH-related protein(s) is mediator
Solid tumor— osteolytic	↑	N/↑	↓	N	N	↓	↑	↑↑	
Lymphoma	↑	N/↑	↓	N/↓	↑	↓	↑	↑↑	
Granulomatous disease	↑	N/↑	↓	N/↓	↑↑	↓	↑	↑↑	Sarcoid most common etiology
Vitamin D intoxication	↑	N/↑	↓	↑↑	N	↓	↑	↑↑	
Hyperthyroidism	↑	N	↓	N	N	N	N	↑↑	Plasma concentrations of T$_4$ and/or T$_3$ are elevated

From Moore WT, Eastman RC: *Diagnostic endocrinology,* ed 2, St Louis, 1996, Mosby.
Ca, Calcium; *cAMP,* cyclic adenosine monophosphate; *FHH,* familial hypocalciuric hypercalcemia; *GFR,* glomerular filtration rate; *MEN,* multiple endocrine neoplasia; *25(OH)D,* 25 hydroxyvitamin D; *PO$_4$,* phosphate; *PTH,* parathormone; *T$_3$,* triiodothyronine; *T$_4$,* thyroxine; *TmP,* renal threshold for phosphorus.

HYPERCAPNIA

Hypercapnia
ICD-9CM # 786.09

BOX 2-133   Causes of Persistent Hypercapnia

1. With normal lungs:
   a. Central nervous system disturbances (e.g., cerebrovascular disease, Parkinson's disease, encephalitis)
   b. Metabolic alkalosis
   c. Myxedema
   d. Primary alveolar hypoventilation (Ondine's curse)
   e. Spinal cord lesions
2. Diseases of the chest wall (e.g., kyphoscoliosis, ankylosing spondylitis)
3. Neuromuscular disorders (e.g., myasthenia gravis, Guillain-Barré syndrome, amyotrophic lateral sclerosis, acid maltase disease, muscular dystrophy, poliomyelitis)
4. Chronic obstructive pulmonary disease

From Stein JH (ed): *Internal medicine,* ed 5, St Louis, 1998, Mosby.

HYPERCOAGULABLE STATES

Hypercoagulable states
ICD-9CM # 289.8 Hypercoagulation syndrome

II

BOX 2-134   Hypercoagulable States

Suspect when unusual, recurrent thromboses or thromboembolism in a young person with no predisposing factors (e.g., surgery)

Hereditary Disorders

Protein C Deficiency (Vitamin K–Dependent Clot Inhibitor)

Heterozygous autosomal dominant transmission
Prevalence of 1 in 300 individuals
Dx by functional and immunoassay of protein C
Causes disease in newborns, skin necrosis, purpura
Responsible for up to 10% of thromboses in patients <45 years of age

Protein S Deficiency (Vitamin K–Dependent Clot Inhibitor)

Codominant autosomal transmission
Prevalence of 1 in 15,000 individuals
Dx by functional and immunoassay of protein S
Responsible for 5% to 8% of thromboses in patients <45 years of age
Often starts in the early teen years

Antithrombin III (Inhibits Final Coagulation Cascade)

Autosomal dominant transmission
Measure antithrombin III levels, Dx if <60% of normal
Responsible for 2% to 4% of thromboses in patients <45 years of age
Often starts in early childhood

Dysfibrinogenemia

Can be inherited or spontaneous mutation
Prolonged thrombin time suggests this disorder

Other

Factor V Leiden mutation, hyperhomocystinemia, high levels of factor XI, G20210A prothrombin mutation, lupus anticoagulant, anticardiolipin antibody

Acquired Disorders

IgG Antiphospholipid Antibodies

Responsible for spontaneous abortion, arterial and venous thrombi
Lupus anticoagulant present
PTT that is prolonged and does not correct with a 1:1 mix suggests the diagnosis

Malignancy

Increased platelet adhesion
Procoagulant factors involved

Other Conditions

Surgery, trauma, estrogens, pregnancy, renal disease, sepsis, varicose veins, congestive heart failure, myeloproliferative disorder

Modified from Driscoll CE et al: *The family practice desk reference,* ed 3, St Louis, 1996, Mosby.

HYPERHIDROSIS

BOX 2-135 Causes of Hyperhidrosis

Cortical

Emotional
Familial dysautonomia
Congenital ichthyosilorm erythroderma
Epidermolysis bullosa
Nail-patella syndrome
Jadassohn-Lewandowsky syndrome
Pachyonychia congenita
Palmoplantar keratoderma

Hypothalamic

Drugs

Antipyretics
Emetics
Insulin
Meperidine

Exercise

Infection

Defervescence
Chronic illness

Metabolic

Debility
Diabetes mellitus
Hyperpituitarism
Hyperthyroidism
Hypoglycemia
Obesity
Porphyria
Pregnancy
Rickets
Infantile scurvy

Cardiovascular

Heart failure
Shock

Vasomotor

Cold injury
Raynaud phenomenon
Rheumatoid arthritis

Neurologic

Abscess
Familial dysautonomia
Postencephalitic
Tumor

Miscellaneous

Chédiak-Higashi syndrome
Compensatory
Phenylketonuria
Pheochromocytoma
Vitiligo

Medullary

Physiologic gustatory sweating
Encephalitis
Granulosis rubra nasi
Syringomyelia
Thoracic sympathetic trunk injury

Spinal

Cord transection
Syringomyelia

Changes in Blood Flow

Mallucci syndrome
Arteriovenous fistula
Klippel-Trenaunay syndrome
Glomus tumor
Blue rubber bleb nevus syndrome

From Behrman RE (ed): *Nelson textbook of pediatrics*, Philadelphia, 1996, WB Saunders.

HYPERINSULINISM

TABLE 2-104 Differential Diagnosis of Hyperinsulinism

	POSTABSORPTIVE VENOUS PLASMA GLUCOSE <45 MG/DL			
	INSULIN	C-PEPTIDE	INSULIN ANTIBODIES	OTHER
Exogenous hyperinsulinism	↑	↓†	+	
Endogenous hyperinsulinism				
Insulinoma	↑	↑	—	↑ Proinsulin
Sulfonylurea	↑	↑	—	Positive sulfonylurea assay
Autoimmune hypoglycemia				
Antibodies to insulin	↑↑↑*	↓†	+	
Antibodies to insulin receptor	↑	?	—	Insulin receptor antibodies present; associated autoimmune disorder

From Stein JH (ed): *Internal medicine*, ed 5, St Louis, 1998, Mosby.
*Insulin antibodies artifactually increase insulin levels measured by double-antibody radioimmunoassay.
†Free C-peptide levels are low, but total C-peptide levels may not be because of cross reactivity with antibody-bound proinsulin.

HYPERKALEMIA

Hyperkalemia
ICD-9CM # 276.7

BOX 2-136   Causes of Hyperkalemia

I. Pseudohyperkalemia
  A. Hemolysis of sample
  B. Thrombocytosis
  C. Leukocytosis
  D. Laboratory error
II. Increased potassium intake and absorption
  A. Potassium supplements (oral and parenteral)
  B. Dietary—salt substitutes
  C. Stored blood
  D. Potassium-containing medications
III. Impaired renal excretion
  A. Acute renal failure
  B. Chronic renal failure
  C. Tubular defect in potassium secretion
    1. Renal allograft
    2. Analgesic nephropathy
    3. Sickle cell disease
    4. Obstructive uropathy
    5. Interstitial nephritis
    6. Chronic pyelonephritis
    7. Potassium-sparing diuretics
    8. Miscellaneous (lead, systemic lupus erythematosus, pseudohypoaldosteronism)
  D. Hypoaldosteronism
    1. Primary (Addison's disease)
    2. Secondary
      a. Hyporeninemic hypoaldosteronism (type IV RTA)
      b. Congenital adrenal hyperplasia
      c. Drug-induced
        (1) Nonsteroidal antiinflammatory medications
        (2) ACE inhibitors
        (3) Heparin
        (4) Cyclosporine
IV. Transcellular shifts
  A. Acidosis
  B. Hypertonicity
  C. Insulin deficiency
  D. Drugs
    1. β-blockers
    2. Digitalis toxicity
    3. Succinylcholine
  E. Exercise
  F. Hyperkalemic periodic paralysis
V. Cellular injury
  A. Rhabdomyolysis
  B. Severe intravascular hemolysis
  C. Acute tumor lysis syndrome
  D. Burns and crush injuries

From Rosen P, Barkin R (eds): *Emergency medicine: concepts and clinical practice,* ed 5, St Louis, 2002, Mosby.

HYPERKINETIC MOVEMENT DISORDERS

TABLE 2-105   Hyperkinetic Movement Disorders

Hyperkinetic movement disorders
ICD-9CM # 314.8 Hyperkinetic syndrome
275.1 Choreoathetosis
335.5 Hemiballism
333.7 Dystonia due to drugs
333.6 Dystonia, idiopathic

DISORDER	CLINICAL MANIFESTATIONS	DIFFERENTIAL DIAGNOSIS	TESTS	TREATMENT
Chorea, choreoathetosis, tardive dyskinesia	Continuum of abnormal involuntary movements; jerky, nonrhythmic, semipurposive, predominantly in limbs; may affect head, neck, trunk; lips and tongue may participate (buccolingual dyskinesia); often mixed with writhing (choreoathetosis)	Drug-induced Phenothiazines L-Dopa Phenytoin Cocaine Amiphetamines Tricyclics Oral contraceptives	Urine toxic screen	Withdrawal of toxic drug Symptomatic treatment: clonazepam 0.5 mg bid up to 4-16 mg/day Haloperidol 0.5-1.0 mg tid up to 5-15 mg/day
		Liver failure	Liver function tests	Treatment of hepatic encephalopathy
		Wilson's disease: dyskinesia accompanied by dystonia, cerebellar ataxia, dysarthria, proximal limb tremor, emotional lability	Slit-lamp examination for Kayser-Fleischer rings; serum ceruloplasmin, serum copper	Penicillamine
		Thyrotoxicosis	Serum thyroxine, TSH	Antithyroid drugs
		Polycythemia	Hematocrit	Phlebotomy
		Systemic lupus erythematosus	Antinuclear antibody	Steroids
		Sydenham's chorea	—	Symptomatic
		Huntington's chorea	Brain CT/MRI, DNA analysis	Symptomatic
Hemiballismus	Large, flinging, ballistic limb movements; predominates in arm or leg	Lacunar CVA in vicinity of subthalamic nuclei in basal ganglia; other focal lesions: metastases and toxoplasmosis (in AIDS)	Brain CT/MRI	Therapy of underlying lesion Symptomatic treatment same as for chorea
Focal dystonia	Spasmodic torticollis	Idiopathic	Clinical	Anticholinergics (high dose): trihexyphenidyl (Artane), 2 mg bid up to 10-40 mg/day Benzodiazepines: clonazepam as above; diazepam, 5 mg bid up to 20-60 mg/day Botulin A toxin: focal injections Surgery: peripheral muscle denervation

Disorder	Clinical features	Etiology	Diagnostic tests	Treatment
	Spasmodic dysphonia (laryngeal)	Idiopathic	—	Botulin A toxin: injection into vocal muscles
	Essential blepharospasm: dystonia of orbicularis oculi muscle is principal feature; if accompanied by dystonia of facial, tongue, and neck muscles, called Meige's syndrome	Idiopathic	—	Clonazepam as above; Botulin A toxin: injection into appropriate muscles
Segmental and generalized dystonia	May affect different segments of body or be generalized or multifocal	Idiopathic; Hereditary; Drug induced: Phenothiazines, L-Dopa, Calcium channel blockers	—	Symptomatic treatment: anticholinergics, clonazepam; Baclofen: 10 mg bid up to 50-100 mg/day; Carbamazepine: 100 mg bid up to 600-1200 mg/day
		Wilson's disease; Diurnal dystonia: childhood-onset (Segawa disease type) may have parkinsonian features	Same as for chorea; Familial	Penicillamine plus symptomatic treatment; Dramatic response to L-dopa; Carbidopa/L-dopa: 25/100 mg bid or tid
Acute dystonic reaction	May be segmental or generalized with oculogyric crisis, torticollis, tongue protrusion, opisthotonus; children more susceptible	Drug-induced: Prochlorperazine, Metoclopramide	—	Benztropine (Cogentin): 1-2 mg IM; Diphenhydramine: 50 mg IM
Paroxysmal dystonia	Kinesigenic: brief attacks of dystonia triggered by sudden movements	Idiopathic or familial	—	Carbamazepine: 100-200 mg tid; Phenytoin: 100 mg tid
	Nonkinesigenic dystonia: prolonged paroxysm of dystonia unrelated to activity	Idiopathic or familial	—	Carbamazepine, clonazepam; Acetazolamide (Diamox): 250 mg tid

From Noble J (ed): *Primary care medicine*, ed 3, St Louis, 2001, Mosby.

AIDS, Acquired immunodeficiency syndrome; *CVA*, cerebrovascular accident; *DNA*, deoxyribonucleic acid; *MRI*, magnetic resonance imaging; *TSH*, thyroid-stimulating hormone.

HYPERMAGNESEMIA

Hypermagnesemia
ICD-9CM # 275.2

BOX 2-137   Causes of Hypermagnesemia

I. Decreased renal excretion
  A. Renal failure—glomerular filtration rate less than 30 ml/min
  B. Hyperparathyroidism
  C. Hypothyroidism
  D. Addison's disease
  E. Lithium intoxication
  F. Familial hypocalciuric hypercalcemia
II. Other causes: usually in association with decrease in glomerular filtration rate

A. Endogenous loads
  1. Diabetic ketoacidosis
  2. Severe tissue injury—burns
B. Exogenous loads
  1. Gastrointestinal
    a. Magnesium-containing laxatives and antacids
    b. High-dose vitamin D analogs
  2. Parenteral: management of toxemia of pregnancy

From Stein JH (ed): *Internal medicine*, ed 5, St Louis, 1998, Mosby.

HYPERPIGMENTATION

Hyperpigmentation
ICD-9CM # 709.00

BOX 2-138   Differential Diagnosis of Diffuse (Generalized) Hyperpigmentation

Addison's disease*
Arsenic ingestion
ACTH or MSH producing tumors (e.g., oat cell carcinoma of the lung)*
Drug induced (i.e., antimalarials, some cytotoxic agents)
Hemochromatosis ("bronze" diabetes)
Malabsorption syndrome (Whipple's disease and celiac sprue)
Melanoma
Melanotropic hormone injection*
Pheochromocytoma
Porphyrias (porphyria cutanea tarda and variegate porphyria)
Pregnancy
Progressive systemic sclerosis and related conditions
PUVA therapy (psoralen administration) for psoriasis and vitiligo*

From Callen JP (ed): *Color atlas of dermatology*, ed 2, Philadelphia, 2000, WB Saunders.
ACTH, Adrenocorticotropic hormone; *MSH*, melanocyte-stimulating hormone; *PUVA*, psoralen plus ultraviolet A.
*Accentuation on sun-exposed surfaces.

HYPERTENSION IN CHILDREN

BOX 2-139 Common Causes of Hypertension in Children

Renal Parenchymal Disease

Glomerulonephritis
Pyelonephritis
Henoch-Schönlein purpura (nephritis)
Hemolytic-uremic syndrome
Polycystic kidney disease
Dysplastic kidney
Obstructive uropathy
Autoimmune process: systemic lupus erythematosus, other vasculitides

Renal Vascular Disease

Arterial anomalies or thrombosis, especially in newborns
Venous anomalies or thrombosis

Vascular Disease

Coarctation of the aorta
Renal artery stenosis
Vasculitis
Aortic or mitral insufficiency

Neurologic Disease

Encephalitis
Brain tumor
Dysautonomia
Guillain-Barré syndrome
Stress, including major burns

Endocrine Disease

Pheochromocytoma

Steroid therapy—Cushing's disease, congenital adrenal hyperplasia, birth control pills
Hyperthyroidism
Neuroblastoma

Intoxication

Lead
Mercury
Amphetamine
Cocaine
LSD
Licorice
Steroids

Essential Hypertension

From Barkin RM, Rosen P: *Emergency pediatrics,* St Louis, 1999, Mosby.

Hypertension in children
ICD-9CM # 401.0 Hypertension, essential malignant
401.1 Hypertension, essential benign
405.91 Hypertension, renovascular secondary
405.1 Hypertension, secondary benign
405.0 Hypertension, secondary malignant

HYPERVENTILATION

Hyperventilation
ICD-9CM # 786.01

BOX 2-140 Causes of Persistent Hyperventilation

Fibrotic lung disease
Metabolic acidosis (e.g., diabetes, uremia)
CNS disorders (midbrain and pontine lesions)
Hepatic coma

Salicylate intoxication
Fever
Psychogenic (e.g., anxiety)

From Stein JH (ed): *Internal medicine,* ed 5, St Louis, 1998, Mosby.

HYPOCALCEMIA, LABORATORY DIFFERENTIAL DIAGNOSIS

Hypocalcemia, laboratory differential diagnosis
ICD-9CM # 275.41

TABLE 2-106 Laboratory Differential Diagnosis of Hypocalcemia

DIAGNOSIS	PLASMA TESTS					URINE TESTS					COMMENTS
	Ca	PO_4	PTH	25(OH)D	1,25$(OH)_2$D	cAMP	cAMP AFTER PTH	TmP/GFR	TmP/GFR AFTER PTH	Ca	
Hypoparathyroidism	↓	↑	N/↓	N	↓	↓	↑↑	↑	↓↓	N/↓	Deficiency of PTH
Pseudohypoparathyroidism											
Type I	↓	↑	↑↑	N	↓	↓	NC	↑	↑	N/↓	Resistance to PTH; patients may have Albright's hereditary osteodystrophy and resistance to multiple hormones
Type II	↓	N	↑↑	N	↓	↓	↑	↓	↑	N/↓	Renal resistance to cAMP
Vitamin D deficiency	↓	N/↓	↑↑	↓↓	N/↓	↑	↑	↓	↓	↓↓	Deficient supply (e.g., nutrition) or absorption (e.g., pancreatic insufficiency) of vitamin D
Vitamin D–dependent rickets											
Type I	↓	N/↓	↑↑	N	↓	↑		↓		↓↓	Deficient activity of renal 25(OH)D-1α-hydroxylase
Type II	↓	N/↓	↑↑	N	↑↑	↑		↓		↓↓	Resistance to 1,25$(OH)_2$D

From Moore WT, Eastman RC: *Diagnostic endocrinology*, ed 2, St Louis, 1996, Mosby.
Ca, Calcium; *cAMP*, cyclic adenosine monophosphate; *FHH*, familial hypocalciuric hypercalcemia; *GFR*, glomerular filtration rate; *MEN*, multiple endocrine neoplasia; *NC*, no change or small increase; *(OH)D*, hydroxycalciferol D; *PO₄*, phosphate; *PTH*, parathyroid hormone; *T₃*, triiodothyronine; *T₄*, thyroxine; *TmP*, renal threshold for phosphorus.

HYPOGLYCEMIA SYNDROMES, TEST RESULTS

TABLE 2-107 Hypoglycemia Syndromes, Test Results

Hypoglycemia syndromes, test results
ICD-9CM # 251.2 Hypoglycemia NOS
251.0 Hypoglycemia, iatrogenic
251.2 Hypoglycemia, reactive

CASE	GLUCOSE (MG/DL)	INSULIN (μU/ML, <6 μU/ML)	TOTAL CPR (NG/ML, <0.9 NG/ML)	FREE CPR (NG/ML, <0.9 NG/ML)	IA	SULFONYLUREA ASSAY	
						HPLC	GCMS
1 Insulinoma	35	10	2	2	Absent	Absent	—
2 Factitious insulin	39	5067	0.56	—	Present	Absent	—
3 Factitious insulin	25	4600	4.41	0.65	Present	Absent	—
4 Factitious sulfonylurea	35	25	9	9	Absent	Present	Present
5 Pseudofactitious sulfonylurea (insulinoma)	27	7	2.4	—	Absent	Present	Absent

From Moore WT, Eastman RC: *Diagnostic endocrinology*, ed 2, St Louis, 1996, Mosby.
CPR, C-peptide immunoreactivity; *GCMS,* gas chromatography mass spectroscopy; *HPLC,* high-performance liquid chromatography; *IA,* antiinsulin antibodies; —, not done.

Hypogonadism
ICD-9CM # 256.3 Female
          257.2 Male
          256.3 Ovarian
          253.4 Pituitary
          257.2 Testicular

HYPOGONADISM

BOX 2-141   Causes of Hypogonadism

Primary (Hypergonadotropic) Hypogonadism

Gonadal defects
  Genetic defect
    Klinefelter's syndrome
    Myotonic dystrophy
    Polyglandular autoimmune disease
    Other genetic syndromes
  Anatomic defect (including castration)
  Defect caused by toxins
    Drugs (cytotoxins and spironolactone)
    Radiation
    Alcohol
  Viral orchitis (mumps most common)
Hormone resistance
  Androgen insensitivity
  Luteinizing hormone insensitivity

Secondary (Hypogonadotropic) Hypogonadism

Organic causes
  Panhypopituitarism
    Idiopathic
    Pituitary or hypothalamic tumor

Miscellaneous
    Granulomatous disease
    Vasculitis
    Hemochromatosis
    Infarction
    Trauma
  Hyperprolactinemia
  Isolated gonadotropin deficiency
    Kallmann's syndrome variants
    Idiopathic hypothalamic hypogonadism
    Isolated deficiency of luteinizing hormone or
      follicle-stimulating hormone
  Genetic disorder
    Prader-Willi syndrome
    Laurence-Moon-Biedl syndrome
  Systemic disorder
    Chronic disease
    Nutritional deficiency or starvation
    Massive obesity
  Drugs
    Glucocorticoids
Constitutional cause (delayed puberty)

From Bagatell CJ, Bremner WJ: *N Engl J Med* 334:707, 1996.

HYPOKALEMIA

BOX 2-142   Causes of Hypokalemia

I. Decreased intake
   A. Decreased dietary potassium
   B. Impaired absorption of potassium
   C. Clay ingestion
   D. Kayexalate
II. Increased loss
   A. Renal
      1. Hyperaldosteronism
        a. Primary
          1. Conn's syndrome
          2. Adrenal hyperplasia
        b. Secondary
          1. Congestive heart failure
          2. Cirrhosis
          3. Nephrotic syndrome
          4. Dehydration
        c. Bartter's syndrome
      2. Glycyrrhizic acid (licorice, chewing tobacco)
      3. Excessive adrenal corticosteroids
        a. Cushing's syndrome
        b. Steroid therapy
        c. Adrenogenital syndrome
      4. Renal tubular defects
        a. Renal tubular acidosis
        b. Obstructive uropathy
        c. Salt-wasting nephropathy
      5. Drugs
        a. Diuretics
        b. Aminoglycosides
        c. Mannitol
        d. Amphotericin
        e. Cisplatin
        f. Carbenicillin

   B. Gastrointestinal
      1. Vomiting
      2. Nasogastric suction
      3. Diarrhea
      4. Malabsorption
      5. Ileostomy
      6. Villous adenoma
      7. Laxative abuse
   C. Increased losses from the skin
      1. Excessive sweating
      2. Burns
III. Transcellular shifts
   A. Alkalosis
      1. Vomiting
      2. Diuretics
      3. Hyperventilation
      4. Bicarbonate therapy
   B. Insulin
      1. Exogenous
      2. Endogenous response to glucose
   C. β_2-Agonists (albuterol, terbutaline, epinephrine)
   D. Hypokalemia periodic paralysis
      1. Familial
      2. Thyrotoxic
IV. Miscellaneous
   A. Anabolic state
   B. Intravenous hyperalimentation
   C. Treatment of megaloblastic anemia
   D. Acute mountain sickness

From Rosen P, Barkin R (eds): *Emergency medicine: concepts and clinical practice,* ed 5, St Louis, 2002, Mosby.

HYPOMAGNESEMIA

BOX 2-143   Causes of Hypomagnesemia

Alcoholic abuse
Diuretic use
Renal losses
   Acute and chronic renal failure
   Postobstructive diuresis
   Acute tubular necrosis
   Chronic glomerulonephritis
   Chronic pyelonephritis
   Interstitial nephropathy
   Renal transplantation
Gastrointestinal losses
   Chronic diarrhea
   Nasogastric suctioning
   Short bowel syndrome

Protein calorie malnutrition
Bowel fistula
Total parenteral nutrition
   Acute pancreatitis
Endocrine
   Diabetes mellitus
   Hyperaldosteronism
   Hyperthyroidism
   Hyperparathyroidism
   Acute intermittent porphyria
Pregnancy
Drugs
   Aminoglycosides
   Amphotericin

β-Agonists
Cisplatin
Cyclosporine
Diuretics
Foscarnet
Pentamidine
Theophylline
Congenital disorders
   Familial hypomagnesemia
   Maternal diabetes
   Maternal hypothyroidism
   Maternal hyperparathyroidism

From Rosen P et al (eds): *Emergency medicine: concepts and clinical practice,* ed 5, St Louis, 2002, Mosby.

HYPOTENSION, POSTURAL

Hypotension, postural
ICD-9CM # 458.0

BOX 2-144 Causes of Postural Hypotension

Antihypertensive medications
Diuretics
Antiarrhythmia drugs
Dehydration
Peripheral autonomic dysfunction
  Diabetes
  Guillain-Barré Syndrome
  Amyloidosis
  Familial dysautonomia
Central autonomic dysfunction
  Shy-Drager syndrome
  Hypothalamic disease
Peripheral venous disease
Central venous disease
Impaired cardiac output
  Aortic stenosis
  Constrictive pericarditis
  Congestive heart failure
  Atrial myxoma
Toxins
Idiopathic orthostatic hypotension

From Wiederholt WC: *Neurology for non-neurologists*, ed 4, Philadelphia, 2000, WB Saunders.

IMMUNODEFICIENCIES, CONGENITAL

Immunodeficiencies, congenital
ICD-9CM # Code varies with specific disorder

TABLE 2-108 Congenital Immunodeficiencies

CLINICAL DISEASE	AFFECTED GENE PRODUCT*	CHROMOSOMAL LOCATION	INHERITANCE	FUNCTIONAL DEFECT	IMPORTANT FINDINGS
T cells					
SCID					
X-linked SCID	Interleukin-2 receptor α-chain	Xq13k-21.1	X	T-cell proliferation, antibody production	Lymphopenia, hypogammaglobulinemia
Adenosine deaminase deficiency	Adenosine deaminase	20q13-ter	AR	T-cell functions, antibody production	Absent adenosine deaminase activity, lymphopenia, hypogammaglobulinemia
Purine nucleoside phosphorylase deficiency	Purine nucleoside phosphorylase	14q13.1	AR	T-cell functions	Absent purine nucleoside phosphorylase activity, low CD3$^+$ cells, increased natural killer cells, low uric acid
Defective MHC molecules	RF-X	19q13	AR	Cell-mediated immunity	B cells normal, Ig normal or low, absent MHC molecules
IL-2 deficiency	Nuclear factor-activated T cells	?	AR	Cell-mediated immunity, antibody production	Lymphopenia, hypogammaglobulinemia
Reticular dysgenesis	?	?	AR	Pancytopenia	Pancytopenia
DiGeorge syndrome	ufd1?	22q11.21-q11.23	AD	Anomalous development of the 3rd and 4th pharyngeal pouches	Thymic aplasia, parathyroid aplasia, cardiac anomalies, abnormal facies
Ataxia-telangiectasia	?	11q22.3	AR	DNA repair, T cells	Low IgA, low CD3$^+$ and CD4$^+$ cells
Wiskott-Aldrich syndrome	WASP	Xq11-11.3	X	T cells and platelets	Thrombocytopenia, low IgM, high IgA
B cells					
X-linked agammaglobulinemia	B-cell progenitor kinase	Xq22	X	B cells	Very low antibody levels
X-linked immunodeficiency with hyper-IgM syndrome	CD40 ligand (gp39)	Xq26	X	B cells	High IgM, low IgG, IgA
X-linked lymphoproliferative syndrome (Duncan's syndrome)	SLAM	Xq25	X	Epstein-Barr virus response	Low antibody to Epstein-Barr nuclear antigen
Common variable immunodeficiency	?	?	?	Antibody synthesis	Low IgG, poor antibody response, low IgA common
IgA deficiency	IgA	?6p21.3	AR	IgA	Associated with other immunodeficiencies
Phagocytes					
CGD					
X-linked CGD	gp91^{phox}	Xp21.1	X	Bacterial and fungal killing defective in all forms of CGD	Infections with catalase-positive microbes, granulomas, and absent NBT reduction and superoxide generation in 60% of CGD
Autosomal recessive CGD	p22^{phox}	16q24	AR		5% of CGD
	p47^{phox}	77q11.23	AR		30% of CGD
	p67^{phox}	1q25	AR		5% of CGD

From Mandell GL: *Mandell, Douglas, and Bennett's principles and practice of infectious diseases,* ed 5, New York, 2000, Churchill Livingstone.
AD, Autosomal dominant; *AR,* autosomal recessive; *CGD,* chronic granulomatous disease; *CH$_{50}$,* total hemolytic complement; *G-CSF,* granulocyte colony-stimulating factor; *MHC,* major histocompatibility complex; *NBT,* nitroblue tetrazolium; *SCID,* severe combined immunodeficiency; *WASP,* Wiskott-Aldrich syndrome protein; *X,* X-linked inheritance.
*The affected gene product is not always the gene in which the lesion has occurred. The genetic lesion may disable a regulatory gene required for expression or function of the affected gene product.

Continued

TABLE 2-108   Congenital Immunodeficiencies—cont'd

CLINICAL DISEASE	AFFECTED GENE PRODUCT*	CHROMOSOMAL LOCATION	INHERITANCE	FUNCTIONAL DEFECT	IMPORTANT FINDINGS
Cyclic neutropenia	?G-CSF	?5q	AR	Neutropenia	Cyclic hematopoiesis, cycle about 21 days
Chédiak-Higashi syndrome	Lyst, lysosomal transport protein	1q43	AR	Chemotactic defect, neutropenia	Giant granules in neutrophils, oculocutaneous albinism
Leukocyte adhesion deficiency type 1	CD18	21q22.3	AR	Absent integrins	Chronic leukocytosis, delayed umbilical cord separation, recurrent infections
Leukocyte adhesion deficiency type 2	Sialyl-Lewis X	?19q	AR	E-selectin ligand, ?fucose metabolism	Short stature, mental retardation
Neutrophil-specific granule deficiency	C/EBPϵ	14q11.2	AR	Neutrophil granule products	Absent neutrophil-specific granules, absent defensins
Myeloperoxidase deficiency	Myeloperoxidase	17q21-q23	AR	Conversion of superoxide to hydrogen peroxide	Absent myeloperoxidase, usually unassociated with infections
Interferon-γ receptor 1 deficiency	IFN γR1	6q23-q24	AR, AD	Absence of interferon-γ binding	Recurrent nontuberculous mycobacterial and salmonella infections
Interferon-γ receptor 2 deficiency	IFN γR2	21q22.1-q22.2	AR	Absence of interferon-γ signaling	Recurrent nontuberculous mycobacterial and salmonella infections
Interleukin-12 receptor β1 deficiency	IL-12RB1	19p13.1	AR	Absence of IL-12 signaling	Recurrent nontuberculous mycobacterial and salmonella infections
Hyper-IgE and recurrent infection syndrome (Job's syndrome)	?	4q	AD	Intermittently poor chemotaxis, ?CD8$^+$ T-cell dysfunction	Extremely high IgE, eczema; facial, dental, and bony abnormalities; pneumatocele formation
Interlukin-12 p40 deficiency	IL-12 p40	5q31-q33	AR	Absence of IL-12	Recurrent nontuberculous mycobacterial and salmonella infections
Complement					
Classic pathway		1p			
		12p13			
C1q deficiency	C1q	12p13	AR		
C1r deficiency	C1r	6p21.3	AR		
C1s deficiency	C1s	19p13.2-p	AR		
C2 deficiency	C2	13.11	AR		Low CH$_{50}$ is seen with all forms of classic complement component deficiency. Individual components are very low or absent. Autoimmune disease common in early component deficiencies (C1–C4). Bacteremia and meningitis are common in all types of complement deficiency
C3 deficiency	C3	6p21.3	AR		
C4A deficiency	C4A	6p21.3	AR		
C4B deficiency	C4B	9q22-q34	AR		
C5 deficiency	C5	5	AR		
C6 deficiency	C6	1p22	AR	Antibody-dependent complement lysis is depressed in all forms of classic complement component deficiencies	
C7 deficiency	C7	1p36.2-p2	AR		
C8 deficiency	C8	2.1	AR		
C9 deficiency	C9	5p14-p12	AR		
Alternative pathway					
Properdin deficiency	Properdin	Xp21-p11	X	Antibody-independent complement lysis is depressed in alternative complement component deficiencies	More severe susceptibility to infection than with classic component deficiencies
Factor H deficiency	Factor H	1q32	AR		
Factor I deficiency	Factor I	4q25	AR		

IMPOTENCE

BOX 2-145   **Causes of Impotence**

Psychogenic

Primary or secondary

Endocrine

Hypothalamic-pituitary-testicular axis
Thyroid: hyperthyroidism, hypothyroidism
Hyperprolactinemia
Diabetes mellitus
Cushing's syndrome

Vascular

Arterial insufficiency
Venous leakage
Arteriovenous malformation
Local trauma

Medications

Neurogenic

Peripheral neuropathy: autonomic or sensory neuropathy
Spinal cord: trauma, tumor
Central nervous system: stroke, multiple sclerosis, temporal lobe epilepsy
Neurotransmitters

Systemic illness

Renal failure
Chronic obstructive pulmonary disease
Cirrhosis of liver
Myotonic dystrophy

Peyronie's disease

Prostatectomy

Multiple causes

From Moore WT, Eastman RC: *Diagnostic endocrinology,* ed 2, St Louis, 1996, Mosby.

Impotence
ICD-9CM # 302.72 Psychosexual
          607.84 Organic
          997.99 Organic postprostatectomy

INCONTINENCE, DRUG-INDUCED

BOX 2-146   **Medications That Can Cause Incontinence**

Antihypertensives

Antiadrenergics

Clonidine, α-methyldopa, β-blockers: decreased sphincter tone, cognitive dysfunction, depression

Calcium Channel Blockers

Verapamil, nifedipine, diltiazem, others: decreased detrusor contractility, constipation, fecal impaction

Angiotensin-Converting Enzyme (ACE) Inhibitors

Captopril, others: drug-induced cough

Diuretics

Hydrochlorothiazide, furosemide, others: increased urine production, glucose intolerance

Sedative-Hypnotics

Benzodiazepines, chloral hydrate, antihistamines (e.g., diphenhydramine): cognitive dysfunction (delirium), anticholinergic effects

Antidepressants

Tricyclic agents (e.g., amitriptyline): anticholinergic side effects, cognitive dysfunction

Neuroleptics

Haloperidol, others: cognitive dysfunction, parkinsonism, anticholinergic effects, especially in low-potency neuroleptics (e.g., thioridazine)

Narcotic Analgesics

Various: cognitive dysfunction

Ethanol

Cognitive, motor dysfunction, increased urine production

Decongestants

Ephedrine, pseudoephedrine, phenylpropanolamine: sphincter dysfunction, decreased detrusor contractility

Antihistamines

Diphenhydramine, chlorpheniramine, others: anticholinergic effects

---

From Noble J: *Primary care medicine,* ed 3, St Louis, 2001, Mosby.

Incontinence, drug-induced
ICD-9CM # 788.30 Incontinence, unspecified

INFECTIOUS DISEASES IN COMPROMISED HOST

Infectious diseases in compromised host
ICD-9CM # 279.9 Immune mechanism disorder

TABLE 2-109   Patterns of Infection in Patients with Impaired Host Defense Mechanisms

HOST DEFENSE MECHANISM IMPAIRED	CAUSE OF IMPAIRMENT	SITE OF INFECTION	COMMON INFECTING AGENTS
I. Anatomic and physiologic barriers to infection		Recurrent at site of abnormality	
A. Skin	Dermatitis Burns IV catheters	Skin → blood	Staphylococci, streptococci, GNR
B. Skull	Skull fracture Cerebrospinal fluid leak	Meninges	Depends on site of leak: predominantly pneumococci but occasionally staphylococci or GNR if a dermal sinus is present
C. Mucociliary elevator	Alcohol Smoking Endotracheal tube Obstruction Immotile cilia (Kartagener's syndrome)	Bronchi, lungs	Colonizing flora
D. Gastric acid	Surgery, pernicious anemia, antacids	Intestine	*Salmonella* *Mycobacterium tuberculosis* Cholera
E. Intestinal motility or mucosal barrier	Blind loop syndrome, obstruction, tumor	Intestine → blood	Colonizing flora (*Streptococcus bovis*, clostridia, usually in the presence of a colonic neoplasm)
F. Urinary tract	Obstruction Catheterization Stones	Upper or lower urinary tract → blood	*Escherichia coli* "Urea splitters": *Proteus, Providencia*
G. Lymphatics	Obstruction	Lymphangitis	Group A streptococci
II. Immunologic barriers to infection			
A. Antibody IgG		Blood, meninges, bronchopulmonary tree, sinuses, ears, intestine	Encapsulated bacteria* Enteroviruses *Giardia lamblia* *Pneumocystis carinii*
IgM IgA	Acquired or inherited	Blood Bronchopulmonary tree, sinuses	Meningococci, GNR Colonizing flora
B. Complement	Acquired or inherited	Blood, meninges, bronchopulmonary tree, sinuses, ears	Encapsulated bacteria* Disseminated gonococcal infection

C. Cell-mediated immunity	Acquired or inherited	Lungs, meninges, gastrointestinal tract	Bacteria
			    Listeria
			    M. tuberculosis
			    Atypical mycobacteria
			Viruses
			    Herpes simplex
			    Cytomegalovirus
			    Varicella zoster (shingles)
			Fungi
			    Candida
			    Cryptococcus
			Protozoa
			    P. carinii
			    Toxoplasma gondii
			    Cryptosporidium

From Stein JH (ed): *Internal medicine*, ed 5, St Louis, 1998, Mosby.
GNR, Gram-negative rods; *IgA, IgG, and IgM*, immunoglobulins A, G, and M.
*Streptococcus pneumoniae, Haemophilus influenzae, Neisseria meningitidis.

TABLE 2-109 Patterns of Infection in Patients with Impaired Host Defense Mechanisms—cont'd

HOST DEFENSE MECHANISM IMPAIRED	CAUSE OF IMPAIRMENT	SITE OF INFECTION	COMMON INFECTING AGENTS
D. Phagocytic function			
1. Neutrophils			
Deficient numbers (<500/mm^3)	Neoplasia Cytotoxic chemotherapy Autoimmune neutropenia	Skin, soft tissue, lung, blood	Staphylococci, GNR, *Candida, Aspergillus*
Defective function	Chronic granulomatous disease	Skin, soft tissue, lung, blood, bone, liver	Staphylococci, GNR, *Nocardia, Candida, Aspergillus*
	Job's (hyperimmunoglob-ulinemia E) syndrome	Skin, soft tissue	Staphylococci
	Chediak-Higashi syndrome	Skin, soft tissue	Staphylococci
	Myeloperoxidase deficiency	Lung	*Candida*
2. Reticuloendothelial function	Asplenia Hemoglobinopathies	Blood	Encapsulated bacteria*
	Cirrhosis	Blood	GNR

From Stein JH (ed): *Internal medicine,* ed 5, St Louis, 1998, Mosby.

INFECTIOUS DISEASES IN TRAVELERS

Infectious diseases in travelers
ICD-9CM # 009.2 Traveler's diarrhea

TABLE 2-110 Infectious Disease in Travelers Categorized According to Approximate Time After Exposure When Patients Are Likely to Present with Evidence of Disease

3 DAYS OR LESS	3 TO 28 DAYS	1 TO 6 MO	6 TO 18 MO	SEVERAL YR
Cholera	Amebiasis	Amebiasis	Amebiasis	Amebiasis
Diarrhea from *Campylobacter, E. coli,* or *Vibrio* sp.	Bartonellosis	Ascariasis	Ascariasis	Chagas' disease, chronic phase
Plague	Brucellosis	Bartonellosis	Clonorchiasis	Clonorchiasis
Salmonellosis	Chagas' disease, acute phase	Brucellosis	Cutaneous leishmaniasis	Hookworm infection
Shigellosis	Dengue fever	Chagas' disease, acute phase	Fascioliasis	Mucocutaneous leishmaniasis
Viral gastroenteritis	Diarrhea from *Campylobacter*	Clonorchiasis	Fasciolopsiasis	Paragonimiasis
	Giardiasis	Cutaneous leishmaniasis	Loiasis	Schistosomiasis, chronic
	Hemorrhagic fevers	Fascioliasis	Malaria	Strongyloidiasis
	Hepatitis A	Fasciolopsiasis	Onchocerciasis	Tapeworm infection
	Leptospirosis	Hepatitis A	Paragonimiasis	Tropical sprue
	Malaria	Hepatitis B	Sleeping sickness	
	Meningococcal disease	Hookworm disease	Strongyloidiasis	
	Paragonimiasis	Kala-azar	Tropical sprue	
	Plague	Malaria		
	Polio	Paragonimiasis		
	Relapsing fever	Relapsing fever		
	Sleeping sickness	Schistosomiasis, acute		
	Tularemia	Sleeping sickness		
	Typhoid fever	Strongyloidiasis		
	Typhus	Tropical sprue		

From Stein JH (ed): *Internal medicine,* ed 5, St Louis, 1998, Mosby.

Insomnia
ICD-9CM # 780.52 Insomnia NOS
          307.42 Insomnia, chronic associated
                    with anxiety or depression
          780.51 Insomnia with sleep apnea

INSOMNIA

TABLE 2-111   Differential Diagnosis of Insomnia

CAUSE	NATURE OF PATIENT	NATURE OF SYMPTOMS	ASSOCIATED SYMPTOMS	PRECIPITATING AND AGGRAVATING FACTORS
Bedwetting (nocturnal enuresis) Nightmares and night terrors	Children (especially ages 3-15) More common in males More common in children	Arousal after deep sleep Arousal during REM sleep	Sleepwalking	Environmental or psychological stresses and fears
Painful or uncomfortable conditions Physical disorders	Any age	Delayed latency Poor sleep quality	Symptoms related to physical disorder or painful or uncomfortable condition	Toothache Pleurisy Arthritis Pregnancy Esophagitis Nocturnal asthma or seizures Congenital hip lesions Hyperthyroidism Nocturia
Change in sleep habits	Elderly people	Delayed sleep latency Poor sleep quality	Daytime naps or dozing	
Unipolar depression	Depressed	Delayed sleep latency Early-morning wakefulness	Anorexia Fatigue Lack of interest in activities Decreased libido Constipation Vague aches and pains	Conditions, medications, and situations that produce depression
Bipolar depression	Manic Manic-depressive	May not sleep at all during manic phases	Agitation Hyperactivity Flight of ideas	Worse just before and during manic phase
Anxiety	Any age	Delayed sleep latency	Somatic complaints Headaches Chest pain Palpitations Dizziness Gastrointestinal symptoms Nervousness Feelings of foreboding	Situations that produce anxiety
Sleep apnea	Adults Often obese males	Frequent awakening Poor sleep quality	Snoring Excess daytime sleepiness	Sleep apnea Obstruction Central apnea
Caffeine	Any age	Delayed sleep latency Poor sleep quality	May have previously tolerated caffeine well	Use of caffeine (especially after 6 PM)
Alcohol	Teenagers Adults Elderly	Delayed latency Frequent awakening	Nervousness Signs of alcoholism	Alcohol Alcoholic withdrawal Recovering alcoholics
Withdrawal of antidepressants or hypnotics	Any age	Similar to prior symptoms	May redevelop symptoms of anxiety, depression	
Medications and drugs	Any age	Poor sleep quality Prolonged sleep latency	Depends on drug responsible	Psychotropics β-blockers Bronchodilators Sympathomimetics Diuretics Hypnotics Appetite suppressants Amphetamines Cocaine

From Seller RH (ed): *Differential diagnosis of common complaints*, ed 4, Philadelphia, 2000, WB Saunders.

INTERVERTEBRAL DISC DISEASE

Intervertebral disc disease
ICD-9CM # 722.90

TABLE 2-112 **Common Root Syndromes of Intervertebral Disc Disease**

DISC SPACE	ROOT AFFECTED	MUSCLES AFFECTED	AREA OF PAIN/ PARESTHESIAS	REFLEX AFFECTED
C4-5	C5	Deltoid/biceps	Shoulder	Biceps
C5-6	C6	Wrist extensors	Radial forearm	Triceps
C6-7	C7	Triceps	Middle finger	Brachioradialis
C7-T1	C8	Hand intrinsics	Fourth and fifth fingers	Finger flexion
L3-4	L4	Quadriceps	Anterior thigh	Knee jerk
L4-5	L5	Peronei	Great toe/dorsum of foot	
L5-S1	S1	Gastrocnemius/glutei	Lateral foot/sole	Ankle jerk

From Andreoli TE (ed): *Cecil essentials of medicine,* ed 5, Philadelphia, 2001, WB Saunders.

II

INTESTINAL HELMINTHS

TABLE 2-113 Intestinal Helminths

FAMILY	SPECIES	TRANSMISSION	MAJOR CLINICAL PRESENTATION	EOSINOPHILIA	DIAGNOSIS (ADULTS)	TREATMENT
Strictly Intestinal Helminths						
Nematode	*Enterobius vermicularis* (pinworm)	Fecal-oral	Perianal pruritus	No	Cellophane tape applied to rectum	Mebendazole 100 mg once (repeat in 2 wk) or pyrantel pamoate 11 mg/kg (max, 1 g), or albendazole 400 mg/kg once
Nematode	*Trichuris trichiura* (whipworm)	Fecal-oral	Diarrhea, rectal prolapse	No	Stool O&P	Albendazole* 400-600 µg/kg once or 400 mg/kg daily for 3 days, or mebendazole 100 mg bid for 3 days
Cestode	*Taenia saginata* (beef tapeworm)	Ingestion of raw beef	Passage of proglottids	No	Proglottid in stool	Niclosamide 2 g once or praziquantel* 5-10 mg/kg once
Cestode	*Taenia solium* (pork tapeworm)	Ingestion of raw pork	Passage of proglottids	No (yes in cysticercosis)	Stool O&P for intestinal infection	Praziquantel 5-10 mg/kg once for intestinal infection
Cestode	*Diphyllobothrium latum* (fish tapeworm)	Ingestion of raw fish	Vitamin B_{12} deficiency	No	Stool O&P	Same as for *T. saginata*
Cestode	*Hymenolepsis nana* (dwarf tapeworm)	Fecal-oral	Diarrhea, dizziness in children	Yes	Stool O&P	Praziquantel 25 mg/kg once
Trematode	*Fasciolopis buski*	Ingestion of raw water chestnuts or bamboo	Diarrhea, intestinal or biliary obstruction	Yes	Stool O&P	Praziquantel 25 mg/kg tid for 1 day or niclosamide 2 g once
Trematode	*Heterophyes heterophyes*	Ingestion of raw fish	Diarrhea, abdominal pain	Yes	Stool O&P	Praziquantel 25 mg/kg tid for 1 day
Trematode	*Metagonimus yokogawai*	Ingestion of raw fish	Diarrhea	Yes	Stool O&P	Praziquantel 25 mg/kg tid for 1 day
Trematode	*Echinostoma ilocanum*	Ingestion of raw fish	Diarrhea	Yes	Stool O&P	Praziquantel* 25 mg/kg tid for 1 day
Nematode	*Ascaris lumbricoides* (giant roundworm)	Fecal-oral	PIE, intestinal or biliary	During migration, obstruction	Stool O&P	Mebendazole 100 mg PO bid for 3 days or albendazole* 400 µg/kg once or pyrentel pamoate 11 mg/kg once

From Stein JH (ed): *Internal medicine*, ed 5, St Louis, 1998, Mosby.
O&P, Ova and parasites; *PO*, orally; *bid*, twice a day; *tid*, three times a day.
*Considered an investigational drug by the U.S. Food and Drug Administration.

TABLE 2-113   Intestinal Helminths—cont'd

FAMILY	SPECIES	TRANSMISSION	MAJOR CLINICAL PRESENTATION	EOSINOPHILIA	DIAGNOSIS (ADULTS)	TREATMENT
Nematode	*Ancylostoma duodenale* (hookworm)	Skin penetration	PIE, iron deficiency anemia, dermatitis	During migration	Stool O&P	Mebendazole 100 mg PO bid for 3 days, albendazole 400 µg/kg once, or pyrantel pamoate* 11 mg/kg (max, 1 g) for 3 days
Nematode	*Necator duodenale* (hookworm)	Skin penetration	PIE, iron deficiency anemia, dermatitis	During migration	Stool O&P	Same as for *A. duodenale*
Nematode	*Strongyloides stercoralis*	Skin penetration	PIE, diarrhea, malabsorption Hyperinfection syndrome	Yes	Stool O&P	Thiabendazole 25 mg/kg bid for 2 days, 5 days for disseminated infection, or albendazole*† 400 mg daily for 3 days, or ivermectin* 200 µg/kg/day for 1-2 days

†Should be considered experimental treatment.

INTESTINAL PSEUDOOBSTRUCTION

BOX 2-147   Classification of Intestinal Pseudoobstruction

I. "Primary" (idiopathic intestinal pseudoobstruction)
   A. Hollow visceral myopathy
      1. Familial
      2. Sporadic
   B. Neuropathic
      1. Abnormal myenteric plexus
      2. Normal myenteric plexus
II. Secondary
   A. Scleroderma
   B. Myxedema
   C. Amyloidosis
   D. Muscular dystrophy
   E. Hypokalemia
   F. Chronic renal failure
   G. Diabetes mellitus
   H. Drug toxicity caused by
      1. Anticholinergics
      2. Opiate narcotics
   I. Ogilvie's syndrome

From Stein JH (ed): *Internal medicine*, ed 4, St Louis, 1994, Mosby.

Intestinal pseudoobstruction
ICD-9CM # 560.1 Adynamic intestinal obstruction
      564.9 Intestinal disorder, functional

ISCHEMIC COLITIS, NONOCCLUSIVE

Ischemic colitis, nonocclusive
ICD-9CM # 557.1

BOX 2-148 Causes of Nonocclusive Ischemic Colitis

Acute Diminution of Colonic Intramural Blood Flow

Small Vessel Obstruction

Collagen-vascular disease
Vasculitis, diabetes
Oral contraceptives

Nonocclusive Hypoperfusion

Hemorrhage
Congestive heart failure, myocardial infarction, arrhythmias
Sepsis
Vasoconstricting agents: digitalis, vasopressin, ergot, NSAIDs

Increased viscosity: polycythemia, sickle cell disease, thrombocytosis

Increased Demand on Marginal Blood Flow
Increased Motility

Mass lesion, stricture
Constipation

Increased Intraluminal Pressure

Bowel obstruction
Colonoscopy
Barium enema

From Kassirer J (ed): *Current therapy in adult medicine,* ed 4, St Louis, 1998, Mosby.

JAUNDICE

BOX 2-149 Jaundice

Predominance of Direct (Conjugated) Bilirubin

Extrahepatic obstruction:
    Common duct abnormalities: calculi, neoplasm, stricture, cyst, sclerosing cholangitis
    Metastatic carcinoma
    Pancreatic carcinoma, pseudocyst
    Ampullary carcinoma
Hepatocellular disease: hepatitis, cirrhosis
Drugs: estrogens, phenothiazines, captopril, methyl-testosterone, labetalol
Cholestatic jaundice of pregnancy

Hereditary disorders: Dubin-Johnson syndrome, Rotor's syndrome
Recurrent benign intrahepatic cholestasis

Predominance of Indirect (Unconjugated) Bilirubin

Hemolysis: hereditary and acquired hemolytic anemias
Inefficient marrow production
Impaired hepatic conjugation: chloramphenicol, pregnanediol
Neonatal jaundice
Hereditary disorders: Gilbert's syndrome, Crigler-Najjar syndrome

---

Jaundice
ICD-9CM # 782.4 Jaundice NOS
         576.8 Jaundice, obstructive
         277.4 Bilirubin excretion disorders

JAUNDICE IN NEONATE AND YOUNG INFANT

Jaundice in neonate and young infant
ICD-9CM # 774.6

BOX 2-150   Differential Diagnosis of Jaundice in the Neonate and Young Infant

Unconjugated Hyperbilirubinemia*
(Noncholestatic Jaundice)
Overproduction of Bilirubin

Sepsis
Rh/ABO incompatibility
Hematoma (birth trauma)
Drugs (e.g., vitamin K)
Polycythemia
    Maternal-fetal or twin-to-twin transfusion
    Delayed clamping of umbilical cord
Erythrocyte defects (e.g., congenital spherocytosis)
Hemoglobinopathies
Physiologic jaundice

Impaired Transport of Bilirubin

Hypoxia, acidosis
Drugs (e.g., sulfonamides, aminosalicylic acid)
Serum free fatty acids
    Breast milk
    Fat emulsions
Hypoalbuminemia of prematurity

Impaired Hepatic Uptake of Bilirubin

Decreased sinusoidal perfusion (e.g., diminished venous
    flow after birth)
Gilbert's syndrome
Physiologic jaundice

Impaired Conjugation of Bilirubin

Breast milk jaundice
Drugs (e.g., chloramphenicol)
Hypoglycemia
Hypothyroidism
High intestinal obstruction
Glucuronyl transferase deficiency (types I and II)
Physiologic jaundice

Enterohepatic Circulation of Bilirubin

Delayed passage of meconium
    Low intestinal obstruction
    Cystic fibrosis
Diminished intestinal motility

Physiologic jaundice
    Negligible intestinal bacterial flora
    Presence of intestinal beta-glucuronidase

**Conjugated Hyperbilirubinemia* (Cholestatic
Jaundice)**
Acquired Cholestatic Jaundice

Sepsis
Other infections
    Bacterial
    Congenital (TORCH)
    Viral (e.g., hepatitis A, B, or C; HIV)
    Parasitic (e.g., toxoplasmosis)
Chemical liver injury (e.g., drugs)
Total parenteral nutrition

Idiopathic Cholestatic Jaundice

Hepatocellular cholestatic jaundice
    Neonatal hepatitis
Ductal cholestatic jaundice
    Biliary atresia
    Biliary hypoplasia
    Paucity of intrahepatic bile ducts
    Choledochal cyst

Inherited Cholestatic Jaundice

Familial cholestatic syndromes (e.g., benign recurrent
    cholestasis)
Metabolic cholestasis
    Galactosemia
    Hereditary fructose intolerance
    Hereditary tyrosinemia
    Cystic fibrosis
    Alpha-1-antitrypsin deficiency
    Glycogen storage disease
    Inborn errors of bile acid metabolism
Other storage disease
    Niemann-Pick disease
    Gaucher's disease
"Noncholestatic" syndromes
    Dubin-Johnson syndrome
    Rotor syndrome

From Hoekelman R (ed): *Primary pediatric care*, ed 3, St Louis, 1997, Mosby.
*When this is the predominant form of bilirubin, the following diagnoses should be considered.

JAUNDICE DURING PREGNANCY

TABLE 2-114   Etiology of New-Onset Jaundice During Pregnancy

DIAGNOSIS	PREVALENCE	WHEN	SYMPTOMS	SIGNS	ASPARTATE AMINO-TRANSFERASE	ALKALINE PHOS-PHATASE	BILIRUBIN	OTHER LABORATORY STUDIES	MATERNAL OUTCOME	FETAL OUTCOME	THERAPY	RECURRENCE RATE
Viral hepatitis (leading cause of jaundice during pregnancy [50% of total])	Acute hepatitis A or C in 1 per 1000 pregnancies Acute hepatitis B in 2 per 1000 pregnancies	Any trimester	Usual symptoms of viral hepatitis	Usual signs of viral hepatitis	Typical of nonpregnant individuals with viral hepatitis	Typical of nonpregnant individuals with viral hepatitis	Typical of nonpregnant individuals with viral hepatitis	Serologic diagnosis is typical of nonpregnant individuals with viral hepatitis	Comparable to nonpregnant individuals	Potential for transmission at delivery is an indication for passive (hepatitis B immunoglobulin) and active (hepatitis B vaccine) immunization; utility passive immunization for hepatitis C not established	Supportive and similar to general guidelines for viral hepatitis	Natural history of viral hepatitides is unchanged by pregnancy
Intrahepatic cholestasis of pregnancy (IHCP) (second leading cause of jaundice during pregnancy)	Varies with ethnicity (0.1% in United States—20% in Chile)	Third trimester	Pruritus of entire body, usually beginning with palms and soles	30% become jaundiced ≈ 2 weeks after onset of pruritus	$2\text{-}10 \times \Uparrow$	$4 \times \Uparrow$	$\Uparrow$ but <6 mg/dl	$\Uparrow$ bile acids 30-100×	No increase in morbidity	$\Uparrow$ Prematurity, fetal distress, and peripartum fetal death	Vitamin K + cholestyramine; limited study of ursodeoxycholic acid, dexamethasone, and S-adenosyl-L-methione	Resolves 2 days-2 wk after delivery; recurs in most subsequent pregnancies
Preeclampsia's HELLP (hemolysis, elevated liver functions, and low platelets) syndrome	4%-12% of women with preeclampsia	Late second-third trimester (usually earlier in gestation than AFLP)	Nausea, vomiting, right upper quadrant pain; other findings of preeclampsia	Right upper quadrant tenderness, hypertension, diffuse edema, hyperreflexia	$2\text{-}10 \times \Uparrow$	$1\text{-}2 \times \Uparrow$	$\Uparrow$ but <5 mg/dl	Platelets <100,000, microangiopathic hemolytic anemia, disseminated intravascular coagulation	Maternal mortality 2%, $\Uparrow$ risk of hemorrhage and need for blood products	$\Uparrow$ Prematurity and perinatal mortality 5%-30%	Delivery and other therapeutic measures for preeclampsia	May transiently worsen, then improve over several days; recurrence rate 5%

Condition	Incidence	Timing	Symptoms	Signs					Maternal Mortality	Fetal Mortality	Treatment	Prognosis
Hepatic rupture (80% is associated with preeclampsia)	Five per 10,000 pregnancies	Third trimester and postpartum	Acute abdominal pain, nausea, vomiting	Right upper quadrant tenderness, shock; preexisting findings of preeclampsia	2-100 × ⇑	1-2 × ⇑	⇑ but <5 mg/dl	May see subcapsular hematoma on ultrasonography	Mortality 60%	Mortality 60%	Delivery, surgery where indicated	Data inadequate to predict outcome, one report of recurrence
Acute fatty liver of pregnancy (AFLP)	One per 13,000 pregnancies	Third trimester	Malaise, nausea, vomiting, epigastric pain	Right upper quadrant tenderness; may be findings of hepatic encephalopathy	1-5 × ⇑, usually <500 U/L	2-8 × ⇑	⇑ but <10 mg/dl	White blood cell count >15,000; platelets often <100,000; hypoglycemia; disseminated intravascular coagulation	Mortality 10%-18%	Mortality 18%-25%	Delivery and supportive care	Normal liver function restored postpartum; usually does not recur during next pregnancy

From Goldman L, Bennett JC (eds): *Cecil textbook of medicine,* ed 21, Philadelphia, 2000, WB Saunders.
Additional considerations are drug-induced hepatitis, cholelithiasis with common duct obstruction, Budd-Chiari syndrome, and chronic liver disease.

JOINT PAIN

BOX 2-151 Causes of Pain in Area of Joint

Anterior Hip, Medial Thigh, Knee

Acute

Acute rheumatic fever
Adductor muscle strain
Avascular necrosis
Crystal arthritis
Femoral artery (pseudo) aneurysm
Fracture (femoral neck or intertrochanteric)
Hemarthrosis
Hernia
Herpes zoster
Iliopectineal bursitis
Iliopsoas tendinitis
Inguinal lymphadenitis
Osteomalacia
Painful transient osteoporosis of hip
Septic arthritis

Subacute and chronic

Adductory muscle strain
Amyloidosis
Acute rheumatic fever
Femoral artery aneurysm
Hernia (inguinal or femoral)
Iliopectineal bursitis
Iliopsoas tendinitis
Inguinal lymphadenopathy
Osteochondromatosis
Osteomyelitis
Osteitis deformans (Paget's disease)
Osteomalacia (pseudofracture)
Postherpetic neuralgia
Sterile synovitis (e.g., rheumatoid arthritis, psoriatic, systemic lupus erythematosus)

Lateral Hip, Lateral Thigh

Acute

Herpes zoster
Iliotibial tendinitis

Impacted fracture of femoral neck
Lateral femoral cutaneous neuropathy (meralgia paresthetica)
Radiculopathy: L4-5
Trochanteric avulsion fracture (greater trochanter)
Trochanteric bursitis
Trochanteric fracture

Subacute and chronic

Lateral femoral cutaneous neuropathy (meralgia paresthetica)
Osteomyelitis
Postherpetic neuralgia
Radiculopathy: L4-5
Tumors

Posterior Hips, Thigh, Buttock

Acute

Gluteal muscle strain
Herpes zoster
Ischial bursitis
Ischial or sacral fracture
Osteomalacia (pseudofracture)
Sciatic neuropathy
Radiculopathy: L5-S1

Subacute and chronic

Gluteal muscle strain
Ischial bursitis
Lumbar spinal stenosis
Osteoarthritis of hip
Osteitis deformans (Paget's disease)
Osteomyelitis
Osteochondromatosis
Osteomalacia (pseudofracture)
Postherpetic neuralgia
Radiculopathy: L5-S1
Tumors

From Noble J: *Primary care medicine*, ed 3, St Louis, 2001, Mosby.

Joint pain
ICD-9CM # 719.4 Add 5th digit
  0. Site NOS
  1. Shoulder region
  2. Upper arm (elbow, humerus)
  3. Forearm (radius, wrist, ulna)
  4. Hand (carpal, metacarpal)
  5. Pelvic region and thigh
  6. Lower leg (fibula, patella, tibia)
  7. Ankle and/or foot

JUGULAR VENOUS DISTENTION

Jugular venous distention
ICD-9CM # 459.89 Increased venous pressure

BOX 2-152 Jugular Venous Distention

Right-sided heart failure
Cardiac tamponade
Constrictive pericarditis
Goiter

Tension pneumothorax
Pulmonary hypertension
Cardiomyopathy (restrictive)
Superior vena cava syndrome

Valsalva
Right atrial myxoma
Chronic obstructive pulmonary disease

Jugular venous pulse
abnormalities
ICD-9CM # not available

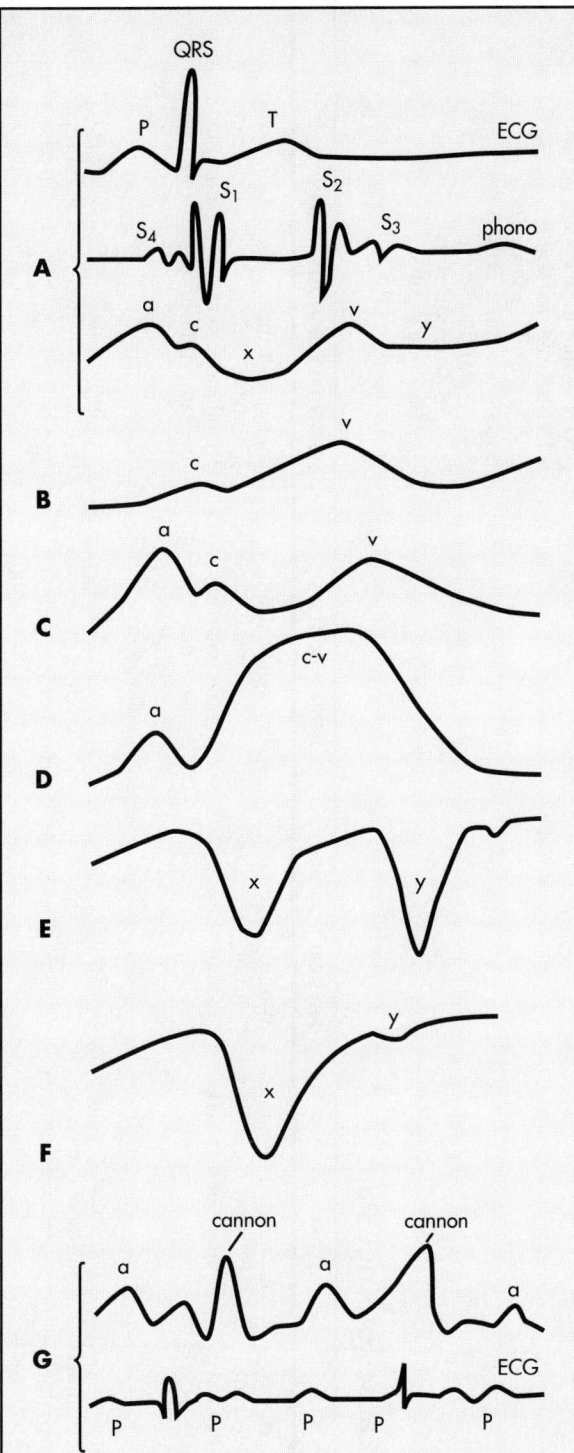

Fig. 2-9 Normal and abnormal jugular venous pulse tracings. **A,** Normal jugular pulse tracing with simultaneous electrocardiogram *(ECG)* and phonocardiogram. **B,** Loss of the a wave in atrial fibrillation. **C,** Large a wave in tricuspid stenosis. **D,** Large c-v wave in tricuspid regurgitation. **E,** Prominent x and y descents in constrictive pericarditis. **F,** Prominent x descent and diminutive y descent in pericardial tamponade. **G,** Jugular venous pulse tracing and simultaneous ECG during complete heart block demonstrating "cannon a waves" occurring when the atrium contracts against a closed tricuspid valve during ventricular systole. (From Andreoli TE [ed]: *Cecil essentials of medicine,* ed 5, Philadelphia, 2001, WB Saunders.)

KNEE PAIN

TABLE 2-115   Selected Causes of Knee Pain

Knee pain
ICD-9CM # 844.1   Collateral ligament sprain, medial
           844.2   Cruciate ligament sprain
           716.96 Knee inflammation
           959.7   Knee injury
           718.86 Knee instability
           836.1   Lateral meniscus tear
           836.0   Medial meniscus tear
           844.8   Patellar sprain
           719.56 Knee stiffness
           719.06 Knee swelling

DISORDER	EPIDEMIOLOGY	HISTORY	PHYSICAL EXAMINATION	DIAGNOSTIC TESTS	DIFFERENTIAL DIAGNOSIS	MANAGEMENT
Gout	Middle age, elderly, overproducers of urate, transplant patients	Acute onset of pain, often with previous attack in first MTP	Warmth, erythema, effusion, exquisite tenderness	High synovial WBC, urate crystals seen under polarizing microscope, "rat bite" erosions on radiograph	Rheumatoid arthritis, spondylitis, other crystal-induced arthropathy, infection	NSAIDs, colchicine, local corticosteroid injection acutely, allopurinol or uricosuric long-term
Pseudogout	Elderly, patients with metabolic disorders such as hypothyroidism, hypomagnesemia, ochronosis, hemochromatosis, Wilson's disease, hyperparathyroidism	Acute onset of pain; if metabolic disease, systemic complaints	Similar to gout	High synovial WBC, calcium pyrophosphate crystals seen under polarizing microscope, chondrocalcinosis on radiograph; if clinically indicated, serum iron studies, magnesium, phosphate, calcium, ceruloplasmin, thyroid studies	Gout, rheumatoid arthritis, spondylitis, infection	NSAIDs, colchicine, local corticosteroid injection acutely, daily colchicine as prophylaxis against further attacks
Rheumatoid arthritis	Age varies, usually female	Morning stiffness, involvement of joints of the hand, multiple joint involvement, fatigue, multiple attacks	Warmth, erythema with effusion, if long-standing "boggy" synovium, symmetric involvement of joints, decreased ROM	High synovial WBC, RF often positive, elevated ESR, anemia, consistent with chronic disease, bone erosions on radiographs	Crystal-induced arthropathy, spondylitis, infection	NSAIDs, local corticosteroid injection, second-line agents such as methotrexate and gold

Condition	Patient profile / History	Physical findings	Diagnostic findings	Differential diagnosis	Treatment
Spondyloarthropathy (reactive arthritis, Reiter's syndrome)	Young adults, male predominance; patients with associated disorders such as IBD, psoriasis, Chlamydia, Yersinia, or Shigella infection, ankylosing spondylitis; acute or subacute onset of pain, often associated with low back pain in other joints, may have a component of morning stiffness, may have systemic complaints related to underlying condition. Acute or subacute onset of pain, often associated with low back pain and pain in other joints, may have a component of morning stiffness, may have systemic complaints related to underlying condition	Warmth, erythema, with effusion; may have "boggy" synovium if disease is long-standing; may have evidence of underlying disease, such as oral ulcers, rash, nail changes, decreased ROM of spine	High synovial WBC, erosions on radiograph, sacroiliitis on radiograph, squaring of vertebral bodies, syndesmophytes	Rheumatoid arthritis, crystal-induced arthritis, infection	NSAIDs, local corticosteroid injection, sulfasalazine, methotrexate
Gonococcal infection	Young adults predominantly, but any age if sexually active. Acute onset of symptoms, may complain of GU symptoms, recent menses, general malaise	Warmth, erythema, with very large tense effusion, decreased ROM, maculopapular rash over trunk, fever, urethral or cervical discharge, arthritis of other joints, tenosynovitis	High synovial WBC, positive culture for Gc from GU tract, blood, or synovial fluid	Rheumatoid arthritis, spondylitis, crystal-induced arthropathy, nongonococcal infection, Lyme disease	Ceftriaxone or penicillin G for sensitive strains
Nongonococcal infection	IV drug abusers, severely debilitated, patients prone to fulminant sepsis or endocarditis. Acute onset of severe pain, swelling, redness, decreased ROM, may have associated systemic symptoms, may have arthritis in other joints	Warmth, erythema, effusion, decreased ROM, signs of source for bacteremia (e.g., pneumonia, UTI)	Very high synovial WBC, positive synovial or blood culture or Gram stain, high ESR, elevated peripheral blood WBC, periosteal elevation on radiograph suggests concomitant osteomyelitis	Rheumatoid arthritis, spondylitis, crystal-induced arthritis, gonococcal infection	IV antibiotic therapy guided by Gram stain, culture results, and sensitivities; drain with needle aspiration or arthroscopically, ROM exercises, and analgesics

From Noble J (ed): *Primary care medicine*, ed 3, St Louis, 2001, Mosby.
AVN, Avascular necrosis; *ECM*, erythema chronicum migrans; *ESR*, erythrocyte sedimentation rate; *Gc*, gonococci; *GU*, genitourinary; *IBD*, inflammatory bowel disease; *MRI*, magnetic resonance imaging; *MTP*, metatarsophalangeal joint; *NSAIDs*, nonsteroidal antiinflammatory drugs; *OA*, osteoarthritis; *PVNS*, pigmented villonodular synovitis; *RF*, rheumatoid factor; *ROM*, range of motion; *SLE*, systemic lupus erythematosus; *UTI*, urinary tract infection; *WBC*, white blood cell.

Continued

II

TABLE 2-115   Selected Causes of Knee Pain—cont'd

DISORDER	EPIDEMIOLOGY	HISTORY	PHYSICAL EXAMINATION	DIAGNOSTIC TESTS	DIFFERENTIAL DIAGNOSIS	MANAGEMENT
Lyme disease	Those who have traveled to or live in endemic areas	Subacute onset of symptoms, swelling, warmth, decreased ROM, pain, history of ECM skin lesion(s), Bell's palsy, other painful joints	Warmth, erythema, effusion, may have "boggy" synovium	Lyme titers, synovial fluid culture rarely positive, radiographs may eventually show erosions	Rheumatoid arthritis, spondylitis, gonococcal and other nongonococcal infection, crystal-induced arthropathy	IV penicillin G or ceftriaxone
Fracture	Any age, risk factors include steroid use, osteoporosis or other causes, metastatic malignancy	History of trauma, sudden-onset pain, swelling, warmth	Swelling, tenderness over affected area, pain on weight bearing, decreased ROM	Bloody synovial fluid, may show fat droplets under polarizing microscopy, fracture seen on radiograph, bone scan may detect stress fractures inapparent on radiograph	Meniscal tear, ligamentous tear, hemophilia, PVNS, anticoagulant therapy	Splinting to protect against additional neurovascular injury, reduction, and casting
Ligamentous injury	Young adults, athletes	Trauma with pivoting or hyperextension, feeling of "giving way," acute pain and swelling	Swelling, point tenderness medial or lateral joint line, positive anterior or posterior drawer sign, medial or lateral laxity depending on ligament disrupted	Bloody or serosanguineous noninflammatory synovial fluid, radiographs to rule out fracture, MRI reveals high T_2 signal in area of ligamentous tear	Meniscal tear, fracture, hemophilia, PVNS, anticoagulant therapy	Analgesics, knee immobilizer, orthopedic consultation for possible surgical repair for complete tears in patients who are active
Meniscal tear	Two groups: elderly with OA and young adults, athletes	Acute or subacute onset of pain, locking, painful popping	Swelling, tenderness over the lateral or medial joint line, positive McMurray's test	Bloody or serosanguineous synovial fluid, radiograph to rule out fracture, MRI, arthrography, or arthroscopy diagnostic	Fracture, ligamentous tear, hemophilia, PVNS, anticoagulant therapy, worsening osteoarthritis	Initial conservative (rest, NSAIDs); if unsuccessful, orthopedic referral for arthroscopic debridement, or total knee replacement if concomitant severe osteoarthritis
Osteonecrosis/avascular necrosis	Any age, patients with sickle cell anemia, chronic steroid use, alcoholism, decompression illness, trauma, SLE, dyslipoproteinemia	Acute onset of pain, swelling, rest pain, increased pain with weight bearing	Swelling, tenderness, decreased ROM	Area of subchondral collapse appears after weeks on plain radiograph, MRI most sensitive for AVN before subchondral collapse	Tumor, fracture, osteomyelitis, osteoarthritis, meniscal tear	Initial conservative (non-weight bearing, NSAIDs, analgesics); if unsuccessful, tibial osteotomy, hemiarthroplasty, or total knee replacement

Condition	Population	History/Symptoms	Physical findings	Diagnostic studies	Differential diagnosis	Treatment
Osgood-Schlatter syndrome	Young adolescents	Pain at the inferior aspect of the patella, subacute to chronic onset	Tenderness to palpation, occasionally swelling in region of tibial tubercle	None	Fracture, tendinitis of patellar tendon, tumor, osteomyelitis	Reassurance, analgesics
Chondromalacia	Young active persons, either gender	Subacute onset of patellar pain, worse walking stairs, little pain at rest	Reproduction of pain on pressing patella against femoral condyles	Synovial fluid noninflammatory, sunrise radiograph may reveal irregularity of articulating surface of patella	Tendinitis, bursitis, meniscal injury	Quadriceps isometric strengthening exercises, NSAIDs, or pure analgesics
Anserine bursitis	Middle age, elderly with OA, young active patients	Subacute onset of pain localized to the posteromedial aspect of the knee	Point tenderness over anserine bursa, rarely palpable swelling	None	Osteoarthritis, medial meniscus injury	NSAIDs, local heat, local corticosteroid injection
Prepatellar bursitis	Those who kneel on hard surfaces, especially carpenters, plumbers, roofers, carpet layers	Subacute onset of pain in prepatellar area, swelling, erythema, desquamation or purulent discharge suggests septic bursitis	Tenderness, erythema, fluctuant swelling of bursa anterior to patella, knee flexion may be limited but full extension possible without increased pain	Bursal aspirate, culture, Gram stain, crystal search	Cellulitis, gouty bursitis, hemobursa, septic bursitis, patellar fat necrosis, erythema nodosum	If septic: antibiotics, repeated needle aspiration for drainage; if nonseptic: NSAIDs, local heat, activity modification
Osteoarthritis	Middle-aged, elderly, athletes, obese, those with prior knee trauma	Progressive, slowly increasing pain, stiffness, decreased ROM over years, "cracking" of joint, no rest pain unless very advanced arthritis, short-lived morning stiffness (minutes)	Decreased ROM, swelling, crepitation, bony prominence	Synovial fluid noninflammatory, osteophyte formation, subchondral cysts, sclerosis, joint space narrowing seen on radiograph	Inflammatory arthritis, meniscal tear, anserine bursitis, secondary forms of osteoarthritis: hemochromatosis, Wilson's disease, ochronosis, gout, acromegaly, hypothyroidism, hyperparathyroidism	Analgesics or NSAIDs, quadriceps strengthening exercises, weight loss if appropriate, use of cane; Consider surgical intervention (tibial osteotomy or total knee replacement) for unremitting pain
Synovial chondromatosis	Wide age range, either gender	Slowly progressing pain, swelling, stiffness	Swelling with effusion, diffuse tenderness	Multiple calcific densities and effusion on plain radiograph, noncalcified chondral bodies may only be apparent on MRI, arthrography, or arthroscopy	Other synovial tumors, inflammatory arthritis, pigmented villonodular synovitis, avascular necrosis with loose osteochondral fragments	Surgical synovectomy, total knee replacement if advanced disease with articular cartilage destruction

Continued

From Noble J (ed): *Primary care medicine*, ed 3, St Louis, 2001, Mosby.
AVN, Avascular necrosis; *ECM*, erythema chronicum migrans; *ESR*, erythrocyte sedimentation rate; *Gc*, gonococci; *GU*, genitourinary; *IBD*, inflammatory bowel disease; *MRI*, magnetic resonance imaging; *MTP*, metarsophalangeal joint; *NSAIDs*, nonsteroidal antiinflammatory drugs; *OA*, osteoarthritis; *PVNS*, pigmented villonodular synovitis; *RF*, rheumatoid factor; *ROM*, range of motion; *SLE*, systemic lupus erythematosus; *UTI*, urinary tract infection; *WBC*, white blood cell.

II

TABLE 2-115   Selected Causes of Knee Pain—cont'd

DISORDER	EPIDEMIOLOGY	HISTORY	PHYSICAL EXAMINATION	DIAGNOSTIC TESTS	DIFFERENTIAL DIAGNOSIS	MANAGEMENT
Pigmented villonodular synovitis	Young adults	Recurrent knee pain and swelling	Erythema, swelling, limited ROM, and tenderness	Synovial fluid reddish brown, noninflammatory; effusion or soft tissue swelling, joint space narrowing, and erosions may be seen on plain radiograph; MRI suggestive, synovial biopsy definitive	Inflammatory arthritis, recurrent hemorrhage, synovial chondromatosis	Surgical synovectomy or radiation synovectomy
Malignancy	Metastatic cancer most common, primary bone and soft tissue sarcomas less likely, leukemia, lymphoma, and myeloma	Slowly worsening pain swelling, stiffness, prominent night pain is suggestive	Decreased ROM, diffuse tenderness, effusion	Synovial fluid with lymphocytic predominance, tumor cells sometimes seen, periosteal disruption or lytic bone lesions on plain radiograph; MRI defines bone and soft tissue involvement; biopsy if no known primary	Inflammatory arthritis, benign tumors, osteomyelitis	Primary tumors: surgical excision or amputation, adjuvant chemotherapy or radiation therapy Metastatic tumors: radiation therapy for pain control, other treatment based on type of malignancy

From Noble J (ed): *Primary care medicine*, ed 3, St Louis, 2001, Mosby.
AVN, Avascular necrosis; *ECM,* erythema chronicum migrans; *ESR,* erythrocyte sedimentation rate; *Gc,* gonococci; *GU,* genitourinary; *IBD,* inflammatory bowel disease; *MRI,* magnetic resonance imaging; *MTP,* metarsophalangeal joint; *NSAIDs,* nonsteroidal antiinflammatory drugs; *OA,* osteoarthritis; *PVNS,* pigmented villonodular synovitis; *RF,* rheumatoid factor; *ROM,* range of motion; *SLE,* systemic lupus erythematosus; *UTI,* urinary tract infection; *WBC,* white blood cell.

KNEE PAIN, BASED ON LOCATION

Knee pain, based on location
ICD-9CM # 844.1 Collateral ligament pain, medial
836.1 Lateral meniscus tear
836.0 Medial meniscus tear

BOX 2-153 Differential Diagnosis of Knee Pain Based on Location

Diffuse

Articular

Anterior

Prepatellar bursitis
Patellar tendon enthesopathy
Chondromalacia patellae
Patellofemoral osteoarthritis
Cruciate ligament injury
Medial plica syndrome

Medial

Anserine bursitis
Spontaneous osteonecrosis
Osteoarthritis
Medial meniscal tear

Medial collateral ligament bursitis
Referred pain from hip and L3
Fibromyalgia

Lateral

Iliotibial band syndrome
Meniscal cyst
Lateral meniscal tear
Collateral ligament
Peroneal tenosynovitis

Posterior

Popliteal cyst (Baker's cyst)
Tendinitis
Aneurysms, ganglions, sarcoma

From Noble J: *Primary care medicine*, ed 3, St Louis, 2001, Mosby.

LEG CRAMPS, NOCTURNAL

Leg cramps, nocturnal
ICD-9CM # 729.82 Muscle cramps

BOX 2-154 Nocturnal Leg Cramps

Diabetic neuropathy
Medications
Electrolyte abnormalities (hypokalemia, hyponatremia, hypoglycemia, hypocalcemia,
hyperkalemia, hypermagnesemia)

Respiratory alkalosis
Uremia
Hemodialysis
Peripheral nerve injury
Amyotrophic lateral sclerosis
Alcohol use

Heat cramps
Vitamin B_{12} deficiency
Hyperthyroidism
Contractures
Deep venous thrombosis
Peripheral vascular insufficiency

LEG LENGTH DISCREPANCIES

Leg length discrepancies
ICD-9CM # 736.81 Length discrepancy (acquired)
755.30 Length discrepancy (congenital)

BOX 2-155 Common Causes of Leg Length Discrepancies

Congenital

Proximal femoral local deficiency
Coxa vara
Hemiatrophy-hemihypertrophy (anisomelia)
Development dysplasia of the hip

Developmental

Legg-Calvé-Perthes disease

Neuromuscular

Polio
Cerebral palsy (hemiplegia)

Infectious

Pyogenic osteomyelitis with physeal damage

Trauma

Physeal injury with premature closure
Overgrowth
Malunion (shortening)

Tumor

Physeal destruction
Radiation-induced physeal injury
Overgrowth

Modified from Thompson GH: Gait disturbances. In Kliegman RM, Nieder ML, Super DM (eds): *Practical strategies of pediatric diagnosis and therapy*, Philadelphia, 1996, WB Saunders.

LEG PAIN WITH EXERCISE

Leg pain with exercise
ICD-9CM # 729.82 Muscle cramps

TABLE 2-116   Differential Diagnosis of Leg Pain with Exercise

	SEX	AGE	FREQUENCY	CAUSE	PULSES
Arteriosclerosis obliterans	M > F	Seventh decade	Very common	Occluded or stenosed large or medium size arteries; lower extremity involvement	Abnormal
Neurogenic	M = F	Sixth-seventh decade	Common	Spinal cord compression or ischemia	Normal
Thromboangiitis obliterans	M > F	Third-fourth decade	Rare	Vasculitis of medium to small arteries; upper and lower extremity involvement	Abnormal; loss of ulnar pulse
Adventitial cysts	M > F	Fourth decade	Rare	Unknown	Usually normal
Popliteal artery entrapment syndrome	M > F	Third-fourth decade	Rare	Abnormal origin of muscles	Usually normal
Venous claudication	M = F	Any age	Rare	Iliofemoral thrombophlebitis	Normal
McArdle's syndrome	M = F	Any age	Rare	Deficient muscle phosphorylases	Normal
Shin splints	M = F	Any age	Common	Swollen anterior tibial muscle	Normal

From Noble J (ed): *Primary care medicine*, ed 3, St Louis, 2001, Mosby.

Leg ulcers
ICD-9CM # 440.23 Lower limb arteriosclerotic
707.1   Lower limb chronic
707.1   Lower limb neurogenic
250.70 Lower limb, chronic, diabetes
mellitus type II
250.71 Lower limb, chronic, diabetes
mellitus type I

LEG ULCERS

BOX 2-156   Differential Diagnosis of Leg Ulcers

Vascular
Arterial
  Arteriosclerosis
  Thromboangiitis obliterans
  Cholesterol emboli
  Hypertension
  Arteriovenous malformation
Venous
  Superficial varicosities
  Deep venous thrombosis
  Incompetent perforators
  Lymphatics (elephantiasis nostra)

Vasculitis
Small vessel
  Hypersensitivity vasculitis (leukocytoclastic vasculitis)
  Lupus erythematosus
  Rheumatoid arthritis
  Scleroderma
  Livedo vasculitis (atrophie blanche)
  Pyoderma gangrenosa
  Antiphospholipid antibodies (anticardiolipin or lupus anticoagulant)
Medium and large vessel
  Polyarteritis nodosa
  Nodular vasculitis

Hematologic
Sickle cell anemia
Spherocytosis
Thalassemia
Polycythemia rubra vera
Leukemia
Dysproteinemias
  Cryoglobulinemia
  Cold agglutinin disease
  Macroglobulinemia
Deficiencies of coagulation inhibitors
  Protein C and S deficiency

Infectious
Fungus
  Blastomycosis
  Coccidioidomycosis
  Histoplasmosis
  Sporotrichosis
Bacterial
  Furuncle
  Ecthyma

Ecthyma gangrenosum
Septic emboli
Pseudomonas
Mycobacterial (typical and atypical)
Protozoal
  Leishmaniasis

Metabolic
Diabetes
  Necrobiosis lipoidica diabeticorum
Gout
Gaucher's disease
Prolidase deficiency
Calcinosis cutis
Localized bullous pemphigoid

Tumors
Basal cell carcinoma
Squamous cell carcinoma
Melanoma
Kaposi's sarcoma
Metastatic tumors
Lymphoproliferative
Cutaneous T-cell lymphoma (mycoses fungoides)

Trauma
Insect bites
Pressure
Cold injury (frostbite, lupus pernio)
Radiation dermatitis
Burns
Factitial

Neuropathic
Diabetic trophic ulcers
Tabes dorsalis
Syringomyelia

Drug
Halogens
Methotrexate
Coumarin necrosis
Ergotism
Hydroxyurea

Panniculitis
Weber-Christian disease
Pancreatic fat necrosis
α_1-Antitrypsinase deficiency

From Noble J (ed): *Primary care medicine,* ed 3, St Louis, 2001, Mosby.

LEISHMANIASIS

Leishmaniasis
ICD-9CM # 085.9

TABLE 2-117 Leishmaniasis: Summary of Epidemiologic and Clinical Features and Treatment

SPECIES	GEOGRAPHIC LOCATION	RESERVOIR	CLINICAL FEATURES	TREATMENT
Leishmania tropica L. tropica major	Desert areas of Central Asia, North Africa, Middle East	Desert rodents	Cutaneous: acute, wet, ulcerated lesions on extremities	Pentostam,* 20 mg/kg/day IV or IM for 20 days; repeated courses may be needed; alternative drugs; amphotericin B, ketoconazole, or pentamidine
L. tropica minor	Urban areas of Middle East, Mediterranean littoral areas, India, Pakistan, Africa	Dogs	Cutaneous: chronic, dry lesion that rarely ulcerates	Pentostam as for *L. tropica major*
L. mexicana	Yucatan peninsula, Belize, Guatemala, Venezuela, Dominican Republic, southern United States (rare)	Forest rodents	Cutaneous: chiclero ulcer; single or limited number of skin lesions; may cause diffuse cutaneous leishmaniasis or, rarely, mucocutaneous leishmaniasis	Pentostam as for *L. tropica major:* most cases resolve spontaneously; if needed. Pentostam or amphotericin B in various doses for various lengths of time
L. braziliensis	Panama, Costa Rica, South America, including Brazil, Venezuela, Bolivia, Peru, northern Argentina	Forest rodents and dogs	Cutaneous and mucocutaneous (especially Brazil)	Pentostam as for *L. tropica major.* Addition of allopurinol, 20 mg/kg/day in four divided doses for 15 days increased cure rates compared with Pentostam alone. Allopurinol alone at the same dose was also effective.
L. donovani	Mediterranean littoral areas, Middle East, India, Pakistan, China, South and Central America (*L. chagasi*), Asia, Africa	Dogs, foxes, rodents; no animal reservoir in India	Visceral leishmaniasis	Pentostam as for *L. tropica major*

From Stein J (ed): *Internal medicine,* ed 5, St Louis, 1998, Mosby.
IV, Intravenously; *IM,* intramuscularly.
*Dosage of Pentostam is calculated as milligrams of antimony per kilogram. In the United States, Pentostam is available from the Drug Service of the Centers for Disease Control and Prevention; telephone: (404) 639-3670 or (404) 639-2888.

LEUKOCYTOCLASTIC VASCULITIS

BOX 2-157   Leukocytoclastic Vasculitis (LCV): Differential Diagnosis and Associated Conditions

I. Entities that are manifest by palpable purpura and LCV histopathologically

Idiopathic

Henoch-Schönlein purpura (IgA-related LCV)

Non-IgA vasculitis

Acute hemorrhagic edema of infancy

Infections: Any infection can be associated; the following are perhaps more common:

Streptococcus

Hepatitis B

Influenza

Mononucleosis

Otitis media

Meningococcemia

Gonococcemia

Systemic Disease

Lupus erythematosus

Rheumatoid arthritis

Dermatomyositis

Chronic active hepatitis

Cryoglobulinemia or other paraproteinemia

Sjögren's syndrome

Scleroderma

Inflammatory bowel disease

Wegener's granulomatosis

Antiphospholipid antibody syndrome

Malignancy ("paraneoplastic vasculitis")

Leukemia and lymphoma

Multiple myeloma

Hodgkin's disease

Solid tumors

Drugs and chemicals: Any drug can be associated; the following are perhaps more common:

Penicillin

Quinidine

Propylthiouracil

Sulfonamides

Allopurinol

Food additives

II. Entities that demonstrate LCV histopathologically but may not exhibit palpable purpura

Hypocomplementemic (urticarial) vasculitis

Degos' disease

Erythema elevatum diutinum

III. Entities that may demonstrate palpable purpura but are not LCV histopathologically

Antiphospholipid antibody syndrome

Embolic phenomenon

Bacterial endocarditis

Atheroembolic

Cholesterol emboli

Left atrial myxoma

Purpura fulminans

Coumarin necrosis

Disseminated intravascular coagulopathy

From Callen JP (ed): *Color atlas of dermatology,* ed 2, Philadelphia, 2000, WB Saunders.
IgA, Immunoglobulin A.

II

Limp
ICD-9CM # 781.2 Gait abnormality
      719.75 Gait disorder due to joint
            abnormality in hip, buttock, or
            femur
      719.76 Gait disorder due to joint
            abnormality in lower leg
      719.77 Gait disorder due to joint
            abnormality in ankle and/or foot
      300.11 Hysterical gait disorder

LIMP

TABLE 2-118   Limp: Diagnostic Considerations

CONDITION	DIAGNOSTIC FINDINGS	ANCILLARY DATA	COMMENTS/MANAGEMENT
Trauma			
Sprain/contusion	History of trauma; local pain, tenderness, swelling, ecchymosis; variably unstable	X-ray study result negative	Support, restrict weight bearing
Fracture	Variable history of trauma; local pain, tenderness, swelling; may be occult	X-ray study result may be positive; if negative, do serial studies, looking for buckle fracture in the cortex of tibia, fibula, or femur; be certain x-ray study includes all potentially involved areas; technetium bone scan rarely needed	Orthopedic consultation; stress fracture may occur after repeated indirect trivial injuries; consider child abuse
Periostitis	Minor trauma to tibia, femur; local tenderness, fullness	X-ray study for subperiosteal hemorrhage (may be delayed)	Periosteum is loosely attached, with minor trauma; may have periosteal hemorrhage
Foreign body/splinter in foot	Acute onset pain, local tenderness, variable erythema	X-ray study rarely needed, but foreign body may localize if radiopaque	Remove; location will dictate need for consult
Poorly fitting shoe	Limp disappears when shoe is removed		
Vertebral disk injury	Motor defect—weakness, asymmetric reflexes; sensory defect	X-ray study may show injury	Orthopedic and neurosurgical consultation
Infection/Inflammation			
Toxic synovitis of hip	Preceding viral illness, nontoxic; hip rarely warm, tender, or limited range of motion	CBC, ESR: WNL; x-ray study: variable effusion; aspirate if question of septic arthritis	Self-limited; common in 1½- to 7-yr-old children
Osteomyelitis	Fever, variable systemic toxicity; local swelling, tenderness, warmth, monoarticular, long bones (femur, tibia)	↑ CBC, ↑ ESR; x-ray study; technetium bone scan; joint and bone aspirate	May have arthritis and osteomyelitis concurrently; antibiotics
Arthritis, septic	Febrile, monoarticular, large weight-bearing (knee, hip) joints; local swelling, warmth, tenderness	↑ WBC, ↑ ESR; x-ray study; bone scan; joint aspirate	Requires urgent drainage and antibiotics

Arthritis, viral
  Rubella
  Rubella vaccine
  Hepatitis
  Chickenpox
	Local swelling, warmth, tenderness; polyarticular, particularly large joints (knee); associated symptoms	CBC, viral titers, liver functions; x-ray study: effusion; joint aspirate	Usually self-limited

Arthritis, uncommon
  Mycobacterium
  Fungal
	Insidious, commonly hip with progression; leg is flexed, well abducted	Joint aspirate; CBC; variable syphilis serologic findings; tuberculin skin test	

Appendicitis	RLQ pain, psoas/obturator sign, limited hip movement	↑ WBC, variable pyuria	Important to consider in differential as well as other abdominal problems

Modified from Barkin RM, Rosen P: *Emergency pediatrics,* St Louis, 1999, Mosby.
CBC, Complete blood count; *CSF,* cerebrospinal fluid; *ESR,* erythrocyte sedimentation rate; *RLQ,* right lower quadrant; *WBC,* white blood cell count; *WNL,* within normal limits.
Continued

TABLE 2-118   Limp: Diagnostic Considerations—cont'd

CONDITION	DIAGNOSTIC FINDINGS	ANCILLARY DATA	COMMENTS/MANAGEMENT
Infection/Inflammation—cont'd			
Polio	Systemic disease with asymmetric flaccid paralysis, bulbar involvement	CSF pleocytosis; ↑ WBC; positive viral culture finding	Decreased incidence
Guillain-Barré syndrome	Ascending symmetric paralysis with pain, paresthesias and paralysis; may involve cranial nerves; preceding viral illness	CSF: high protein	Danger of respiratory insufficiency; associated with viral infection; supportive care with IV gamma globulin (? plasma exchange)
Vascular			
Legg-Calvé-Perthes disease	Insidious onset pain of hip with limp or limitation of motion	X-ray study: bulging capsule with widened joint space; technetium scan: ↓ uptake	Peak: 4:1 males; 4-10 yr; orthopedic consultation—treat hip in abduction and internal rotation
Discitis	Gait problem (<3 yr); local back, abdominal pain with limp (>3 yr); irritable, no systemic illness	X-ray study result normal for 4-8 wk; disk space may narrow by 3-4 wk; result of technetium scan abnormal after 7 days	Vascular disruption of epiphyseal end-plate of vertebrae; prognosis good; treatment: support, antibiotics controversial
Neurologic			
Cerebral vascular accident	Focal neurologic deficits	CT or MRI of brain diagnostic	See Section I
Multiple sclerosis	Spasticity, focal neurologic deficits	MRI of brain useful	See Section I
Neurodegenerative disorders	Focal neurologic deficits; ±spasticity	History of progressive impairment	See Section I
Degenerative			
Slipped capital femoral epiphysis	Unilateral or bilateral pain in knee (referred) or in medial aspect of thigh; hip or knee made worse by activity; limitation of abduction and internal rotation	X-ray study: widening epiphyseal growth plate	Peak: 12-15 yr; orthopedic consultation; surgical immobilization; child obese or tall and thin, with rapid growth spurt
Osgood-Schlatter disease	Pain in knee caused by patella tendonitis at insertion into tibial tubercle	X-ray study result: fragmentation of tibial tuberosity	Peak: 11-15 yr; symptomatic treatment, rest, avoid activities that cause pain
Osteochondroses Chrondomalacia patellae	Irregularity of patella, pain on compression of patella at intercondylar notch with contraction of quadriceps	X-ray study result: WNL	Teenagers, female > males; symptomatic; treatment: quadriceps strengthening
Osteochondritis dissecans	Pain, stiffness, swelling, clicking of knee	X-ray study result: tunnel view shows demineralization of medial femoral condyle	Teenagers; decreased activity, muscle strengthening
Neuromuscular disease	Associated motor and sensory findings		Often progressive
Degenerative joint disease	Pain and stiffness of involved joint; generally elderly patient; joint deformities may be evident	X-ray study: osteoarthritic changes of affected joints	NSAIDs are generally effective in relieving symptoms

Modified from Barkin RM, Rosen P: *Emergency pediatrics*, St Louis, 1999, Mosby.

Continued

TABLE 2-118   Limp: Diagnostic Considerations—cont'd

CONDITION	DIAGNOSTIC FINDINGS	ANCILLARY DATA	COMMENTS/MANAGEMENT
Congenital			
Hemophilia	Variable history of trauma; muscle bleeding; monoarticular joint swollen, tender with hemarthrosis	X-ray study result: variable bleeding screen	Factor replacement
Sickle cell disease	Systemic disease; bone pain; polyarticular joint involvement	X-ray study result; Hct; positive sickle preparation; variable technetium bone scan	May have concurrent infection; may be crisis or infarct
Dislocated hip	Normal newborn except for instability and range of motion of joint; positive hip click (abduction)	X-ray study	Orthopedic consult, splint hip in flexion and abduction
Unequal leg length	Unequal length from anterior iliac crest to medial malleolus		Orthopedic consultation
Testicular torsion	Acute onset of scrotal or groin pain; mass, tender swollen		Surgical emergency
Incarcerated hernia			
Autoimmune			
Neoplasm			
Osteochondroma	Local pain with exostosis		
Leukemia	Systemic disease with associated symptoms		
Neuroblastoma			
Ewing			
Spinal cord tumor			
Intrapsychic			
Attention getting	Inconsistent signs and symptoms		May be functional habit after resolution of physical problem, particularly in children under 5 yr
Hysteria			

Modified from Barkin RM, Rosen P: *Emergency pediatrics,* St Louis, 1999, Mosby.
CBC, Complete blood count; *CSF,* cerebrospinal fluid; *ESR,* erythrocyte sedimentation rate; *RLQ,* right lower quadrant; *WBC,* white blood cell count; *WNL,* within normal limits.

LIMPING, PEDIATRIC AGE

Limping, pediatric age
ICD-9CM # 781.2 Gait abnormality

TABLE 2-119   Common Causes of Limping According to Age

AGE	ANTALGIC	TRENDELENBURG	LEG LENGTH DISCREPANCY

Toddler (1-3 yr)	Infection
	  Septic arthritis
	    Hip
	    Knee
	  Osteomyelitis
	  Diskitis
	Occult trauma
	  Toddler's fracture
	Neoplasia
		Hip dislocation (DDH)
		Neuromuscular disease
		  Cerebral palsy
		  Poliomyetitis
			⊖

Childhood (4-10 yr)	Infection
	  Septic arthritis
	    Hip
	    Knee
	  Osteomyelitis
	  Diskitis
	  Transient synovitis, hip
	LCPD
	Tarsal coalition
	Rheumatologic disorder
	  JRA
	Trauma
	Neoplasia
		Hip dislocation (DDH)
		Neuromuscular disease
		  Cerebral palsy
		  Poliomyetitis
			⊕

Adolescence (11+ yr)	SCFE Rheumatologic disorder JRA Trauma Tarsal coalition Neoplasia		⊕

From Thompson GH: Gait disturbances. In Kliegman RM, Nieder ML, Super DM (eds): *Practical strategies of pediatric diagnosis and therapy,* Philadelphia, 1996, WB Saunders.
DDH, Developmental dysplasia of the hip; *JRA,* juvenile rheumatoid arthritis; *LCPD,* Legg-Calvé-Perthes disease; *SCFE,* slipped capital femoral epiphysis.
⊖, absent; ⊕, present.

LIPIDOSES

Lipidoses
ICD-9CM # 272.7

TABLE 2-120   Lipidoses

SYNDROME	DISTINGUISHING FEATURES	DEFECT
Farber lipogranulo-matosis	Joint swelling, stiffness, and pain in first year; widespread granu-loma in dermis and pulmonary tree	Ceramidase
Niemann-Pick	Acute: failure to thrive, cachexia, neurologic signs, and cherry-red spots in the macula Juvenile: gait changes and ataxia in first year Chronic: adult hepatosplenomegaly and respiratory disease with normal intellect	Sphingomyelinase
Gaucher's	Infantile: failure to thrive, hypertonia, and neurologic signs with death in first 2 years; Gaucher's cells Juvenile: as in infantile, with slower progression and survival into first decade; Gaucher's cells Chronic: adult hepatosplenomegaly, osteoporosis; Gaucher's cells	Glucocerebrosidase
Krabbe's	Increased startle reflex, progressing to hyperreflexia and opis-thotonos to vegetative state in first year; globoid cells	Galactocerebrosidase
Metachromatic leuko-dystrophy (MLD)	Infantile: gait changes progress to weakness and psychomotor disability and blindness in first years	Arylsulfatase A
Multiple sulfatase deficiency	MLD-like presentation in presence of MPS phenotype with uri-nary mucopolysaccharides	Arylsulfatase A, B, C
Fabry's	Angiectasis corporis diffusum, renal pain, renal and cardiac failure	Alpha-galactosidase
GM$_1$ gangliosidosis	Infantile: MPS-like phenotype with failure to thrive progressing to decerebrate rigidity and respiratory failure Juvenile: mild or no MPS features, psychomotor retardation in first decade Adult: ataxia and seizures	Beta-galactosidase
GM$_2$ gangliosidosis	Infantile (Tay-Sachs, Sandhoff): cherry-red retinal spots, exag-gerated startle reflex progressing to hyperactivity, psychomotor retardation, and a vegetative state with death in first years Juvenile (Tay-Sachs): delayed progression of infantile form through first and second decades Adult (Tay-Sachs): dystonia and spinocerebellar degeneration	Tay-Sachs: hexosaminidase A Sandhoff's hexosaminidase A and B

From Stein J (ed): *Internal medicine,* ed 5, St Louis, 1998, Mosby.
MPS, Mucopolysaccharidosis.

LIPODYSTROPHIC SYNDROMES

Lipodystrophic syndromes
ICD-9CM # 272.6

TABLE 2-121   Clinical Comparison of the Major Lipodystrophic Syndromes

CLINICAL FINDINGS	TOTAL LIPODYSTROPHIES			PARTIAL LIPODYSTROPHIES	
	LEPRECHAUNISM	CONGENITAL	ACQUIRED	ACQUIRED	FAMILIAL
Inheritance	Autosomal recessive	Autosomal recessive	Sporadic	Usually sporadic	Always familial More than one generation affected Autosomal dominant
Age at recognition	Infancy	Infancy	Childhood-adult	Childhood-adult	Puberty
Sex incidence	Female/male (2:1)	Female/male (2:1)	Female predominance	Female predominance	Female predominance
Sites of lipoatrophy	Generalized	Face, trunk, limbs	Face, trunk, limbs	Face, upper trunk, upper limbs	Trunk and limbs
Prominence of muscles	Absent	+	Absent	Absent	Absent
Genital enlargement	+++	+	+	Absent	Common
Hepatomegaly/cirrhosis	±	Common	Common	Usually absent	Absent
Acanthosis nigricans	+++	++	+	Rare	+
Hypertension	±	+→++	+	Absent	Common
Associated abnormalities	Absent	Hepatic, renal, neurologic, cardiac	None	Renal, neurologic	None

From Stein J (ed): *Internal medicine*, ed 5, St Louis, 1998, Mosby.
+, Mild; ++, moderate; +++, severe.

TABLE 2-122   Laboratory Comparison of the Major Lipodystrophic Syndromes

	TOTAL LIPODYSTROPHIES			PARTIAL LIPODYSTROPHIES	
	LEPRECHAUNISM	CONGENITAL	ACQUIRED	ACQUIRED	FAMILIAL
Hypertriglyceridemia	—	+++	++	±	++
Hypoglycemia	+++	—	—	—	—
Ketosis	—	—	—	—	—
Insulin resistance	+++	+++	++	+	+
Hyperinsulinemia	+++	+++	++	—	—
Insulin receptor abnormal	++	Affinity	—	—	—
Glucose intolerance	+++	++	++	++	++
Liver dysfunction	—	++	++	—	—
Hypothalamic-pituitary function	Normal	Normal	Normal	Normal	Normal
Bone age	Retarded	Accelerated	Normal	Normal	Normal

From Stein J (ed): *Internal medicine*, ed 5, St Louis, 1998, Mosby.
—, Absent; ±, mild; ++, moderate; +++, severe.

LIVEDO RETICULARIS, DIFFERENTIAL DIAGNOSIS

Livedo reticularis, secondary causes
ICD-9CM # Code varies with specific disorder

BOX 2-158   Differential Diagnosis of Livedo Reticularis

Congenital
   Cutis marmorata telangiectatica congenita
Physiologic
   Cutis marmorata
Blood vessel disease
   Arteriosclerosis
   Arteritis
   Leukocytoclastic vasculitis
   Cutaneous polyarteritis nodosa
   Lupus erythematosus
   Dermatomyositis
   Rheumatoid arthritis
   Pancreatitis
Intravascular obstruction
   Emboli—such as cholesterol emboli, left atrial
     myxoma, subacute bacterial endocarditis

Antiphospholipid antibody syndrome—primary or
   secondary
Cryoglobulinemia, cryofibrinogenemia
Oxalosis
Sneddon's syndrome
Thrombocythemia or polycythemia
Pharmacologic
   Amantadine
   Catecholamines
   Quinine
   Quinidine
Idiopathic
   Livedoid vasculitis

From Callen JP (ed): *Color atlas of dermatology,* ed 2, Philadelphia, 2000, WB Saunders.

LIVER DISEASE IN PREGNANCY

Liver disease in pregnancy
ICD-9CM # 646.73 Antepartum complication

TABLE 2-123   Characteristics of Liver Diseases in Pregnancy

DISEASE	SYMPTOMS	JAUNDICE	TRIMESTER	INCIDENCE IN PREGNANCY	LABORATORY VALUES*	ADVERSE EFFECTS
Hyperemesis gravidarum	Nausea, vomiting	Mild	1 or 2	0.3%-1.0%	Bilirubin <4 mg/dl, ALT <200 U/L	Low birth weight
Intrahepatic cholestasis of pregnancy	Pruritus	In 20%-60%, 1-4 wk after pruritus starts	2 or 3	0.1%-0.2% in U.S.	Bilirubin <6 mg/dl, ALT <300 U/L, increased bile acids	Stillbirth, prematurity, bleeding, fetal mortality 3.5%
Biliary tract disease	Right upper quadrant pain, nausea, vomiting, fever	With CBD obstruction	Any	Unknown	If CBD stone, increased bilirubin and GGT	Unknown
Drug-induced hepatitis	None or nausea, vomiting, pruritus	Early (in cholestatic hepatitis)	Any	Unknown	Variable	Unknown
Acute fatty liver of pregnancy	Upper abdominal pain, nausea, vomiting, confusion late in disease	Common	3	0.008%	ALT <500 U/L, low glucose, DIC in >75%, increased bilirubin and ammonia late in disease	Increased maternal mortality (≤20%) and fetal mortality (13%-18%)
Preeclampsia and eclampsia	Upper abdominal pain, edema, hypertension, mental status changes	Late, 5%-14%	2 or 3	5%-10%	ALT <500 U/L (unless infarction), proteinuria, DIC in 7%	Increased maternal mortality (~1%)
HELLP syndrome	Upper abdominal pain, nausea, vomiting, malaise	Late, 5%-14%	3	0.1% (4%-12% of women with preeclampsia)	ALT <500 U/L, platelets <100,000/mm³, hemolysis, increased LDH, DIC in 20%-40%	Increased maternal mortality (1%-3%) and fetal mortality (35%)
Viral hepatitis	Nausea, vomiting, fever	Common	Any	Same as general population	ALT greatly increased (>500 U/L), increased bilirubin, DIC rare	Maternal mortality increased with hepatitis E

From Knox TA, Olans LB: *N Engl J Med* 335:569-576, 1996.
ALT, Alanine aminotransferase; *CBD,* common bile duct; *DIC,* disseminated intravascular coagulation; *GGT,* γ-glutamyltranspeptidase; *LDH,* lactate dehydrogenase.
*To convert bilirubin values to micromoles per liter, multiply by 17.1.

LIVER FUNCTION TESTS IN LIVER DISEASE

TABLE 2-124　Liver Function Test Patterns in Hepatobiliary Disorders and Jaundice

Liver function tests in liver disease
ICD-9CM # 573.8 Liver disorder other specified

TYPE OF DISORDER	BILIRUBIN	AMINOTRANSFERASES	ALKALINE PHOSPHATASE	ALBUMIN	GLOBULIN	PROTHROMBIN TIME
Hemolysis Gilbert's syndrome	Normal to 5 mg/dl 85% caused by indirect fractions No bilirubinuria	Normal	Normal	Normal	Normal	Normal
Acute hepatocellular necrosis (viral and drug hepatitis, hepatotoxins, acute heart failure)	Both fractions may be elevated Peak usually follows aminotransferases Bilirubinuria	Elevated, often >500 IU ALT ≥ AST	Normal to <3 times normal elevation	Normal	Normal	Usually normal; if >5 sec above control and not corrected by parenteral vitamin K, suggests poor prognosis
Chronic hepatocellular disorders	Both fractions may be elevated Bilirubinuria	Elevated, but usually <300 IU	Normal to <3 times normal elevation	Often decreased	Increased gamma globulin	Often prolonged Fails to correct with parenteral vitamin K
Alcoholic hepatitis Cirrhosis	Both fractions may be elevated Bilirubinuria	AST/ALT >2 suggests alcoholic hepatitis or cirrhosis	Normal to <3 times normal elevation	Often decreased	Increased IGA and increased gamma globulin	
Intrahepatic cholestasis Obstructive jaundice	Both fractions may be elevated Bilirubinuria	Normal to moderate elevation Rarely >500 IU	Elevated, often >4 times normal elevation	Normal, unless chronic	Gamma globulin normal Beta globulin may be increased	Normal If prolonged, will correct with parenteral vitamin K
Infiltrative diseases (tumor, granulomata); partial bile duct obstruction	Usually normal	Normal to slight elevation	Elevated, often >4 times normal elevation Fractionate, or confirm liver origin with 5'-nucleotidase, γ-glutamyl transpeptidase	Normal	Usually normal Gamma globulin may be increased in granulomatous disease	Normal

From Stein JH (ed): *Internal medicine*, ed 5, St Louis, 1998, Mosby.

LUNG DISEASE, DRUG-INDUCED

Lung disease, drug-induced
ICD-9CM # 508.8

TABLE 2-125 Common Drug-Induced Lung Disease

DRUG	DOSE RELATION	MANIFESTATION
Chemotherapeutic		
Bleomycin	Acute/chronic, >450 U increased risk	Pneumonitis, fibrosis, BOOP
Busulfan	Chronic	Fibrosis, alveolar proteinosis
Cyclophosphamide	Chronic	Fibrosis, BOOP
Cytosine arabinoside	Acute	Pulmonary edema, ARDS
Methotrexate	Acute/chronic	Hypersensitivity pneumonitis, resolves with discontinuation, BOOP
Mitomycin C	Acute/delayed	Pneumonitis, ARDS, BOOP hemolytic uremic syndrome
Antimicrobial		
Nitrofurantoin	Acute/chronic	Acute pneumonitis, fibrosis
Sulfasalazine	Acute/chronic	Pulmonary infiltrate with eosinophilia/BOOP
Cardiovascular		
Amiodarone	Acute/chronic, >400 mg/day	Pneumonitis fibrosis
Flecainide	Acute	ARDS, LIP
Tocainide	Weeks/months	Pneumonitis
Procainamide	Subacute/chronic	Drug-induced systemic lupus erythematosus, pleural effusions, infiltrates
Antiinflammatory		
Aspirin	Acute	Pulmonary edema, bronchospasm
Illicit		
Opiates	Acute	Pulmonary edema
Cocaine	Acute	Pulmonary edema, diffuse alveolar damage, pulmonary hemorrhage, BOOP
Talc (in IV and inhaled illicit drugs)	Acute/chronic	Granulomatous interstitial fibrosis, granulomatous pulmonary artery occlusion, particulate embolization
Tocolytics		
Terbutaline, albuterol, ritodrine	Acute	Pulmonary edema

From Andreoli TE (ed): *Cecil essentials of medicine,* ed 5, Philadelphia, 2001, WB Saunders.
ARDS, Acute respiratory distress syndrome; *BOOP,* bronchiolitis obliterans with organizing pneumonia; *LIP,* lymphoid interstitial pneumonia.

LYMPH NODE ENLARGEMENT BY LOCATION

BOX 2-159   Causes of Lymph Node Enlargement by Location

Cervical nodes
  Infections of the head, neck, sinuses, ears, eyes, scalp,
    pharynx
  Mononucleosis syndromes (Epstein-Barr virus,
    cytomegalovirus, toxoplasmosis
  Rubella
  Tuberculosis (often suppurative nodes)
  Lymphoma (often unilateral)
  Head and neck malignancy (often unilateral)
Scalene/supraclavicular nodes
  Lung, retroperitoneal, or gastrointestinal malignancy
    (e.g., Virchow's node)
  Lymphoma
  Thoracic or retroperitoneal bacterial or fungal
    infections
Axillary nodes
  Infections, bites, trauma to the hands or arms
  Cat-scratch disease
  Lymphoma
  Breast carcinoma
  Brucellosis
  Melanoma
Epitrochlear nodes
  Infections of the hand (unilateral)
  Lymphoma (unilateral)
  Sarcoidosis (bilateral)
  Tularemia (often unilateral)
  Secondary syphilis (bilateral)
Inguinal nodes
  Infections of the leg or foot
  Lymphoma

Pelvic malignancy
  Venereal diseases (lymphogranuloma venereum,
    syphilis)
  Pasteurella pestis
Hilar nodes
  Sarcoidosis
  Tuberculosis
  Systemic fungal infections
  Lung carcinoma (unilateral)
Mediastinal nodes
  Mononucleosis syndromes
  Sarcoidosis
  Tuberculosis
  Histoplasmosis
  Lung carcinoma
  Lymphoma
Abdominal/retroperitoneal nodes
  Mesenteric lymphadenitis (tuberculosis)
  Lymphoma
  Germ cell tumors/seminoma
  Prostatic carcinoma and other malignancies
Generalized lymphadenopathy (more than two separate
    sites)
  Infections (Epstein-Barr virus, cytomegalovirus, toxo-
    plasmosis, tuberculosis, hepatitis, syphilis, HIV/AIDS,
    histoplasmosis)
  Malignancy (lymphoma, chronic myelogenous
    leukemia, chronic lymphocytic leukemia, acute
    leukemia)
  Drug reactions
  Systemic lymphadenopathy syndromes

From Faller DV: Diseases of lymph nodes and spleen. In Bennett JC, Plum F (eds): *Cecil textbook of medicine,* ed 20, Philadelphia, 1996, WB Saunders.
HIV/AIDS, Human immunodeficiency virus/acquired immunodeficiency syndrome.

LYMPHADENITIS, INFECTIOUS

Lymphadenitis, infectious
ICD-9CM # 683 Lymphadenitis, acute

TABLE 2-126   Clinical Patterns and Microbial Agents of Infectious Lymphadenitis

DISEASE	INFECTING ORGANISM	REGIONAL	REGIONAL WITH SUPPURATION (OR CASEATION)	INGUINAL BUBO FORMATION	ULCERO-GLAN-DULAR	OCULO-GLAN-DULAR	GENERALIZED
Bacterial							
Pyogenic	Group A or B streptococci; *Staphylococcus aureus*	+	+				
Scarlet fever	Group A streptococci	+	+				+
Diphtheria	*Corynebacterium diphtheriae*	+					
Fusospirochetal angina	*Prevotella melaninogenica;* peptostreptococci, etc.	+					
Scrofula	*Mycobacterium tuberculosis*	+	+				
	Mycobacterium scrofulaceum; Mycobacterium avium-intracellulare	+	+				
Miliary tuberculosis	*M. tuberculosis*						+
Brucellosis	*Brucella*						+
Leptospirosis	*Leptospira*						+
Syphilis	*Treponema pallidum*	+					+
Chancroid	*Haemophilus ducreyi*			+			
Plague	*Yersinia pestis*	+	+	+			
Tularemia	*Francisella tularensis*		+		+	+	
Rat-bite fever	*Streptobacillus moniliformis; Spirillum minus*	+			+		
Anthrax	*Bacillus anthracis*	+			+		
Listeriosis	*Listeria monocytogenes*					+	
Melioidosis	*Burkholderia pseudomallei*	+	+				+
Glanders	*Burkholderia mallei*	+	+				+
Cat-scratch fever	*Bartonella henselae*	+	+		±	+	
Typhoid fever	*Salmonella typhi* "						+
Mycotic							
Histoplasmosis	*Histoplasma capsulatum*						+
	H. capsulatum var. *duboisii*	+					
Coccidioidomycosis	*Coccidioides immitis*	+					
Paracoccidioidomycosis	*Paracoccidioides brasiliensis*	+					
Cryptococcosis	*Cryptococcus neoformans*	+					+
Rickettsial							
Boutonneuse fever, etc.	*Rickettsia conorii*					+	
Scrub typhus	*Rickettsia tsutsugamushi*	+					+
Rickettsialpox	*Rickettsia akari*	+					
Chlamydial							
Lymphogranuloma venereum	*Chlamydia trachomatis*			+		+	+

From Mandell GL: *Mandell, Douglas, and Bennett's principles and practice of infectious diseases,* ed 5, New York, 2000, Churchill Livingstone.
AIDS, Acquired immunodeficiency syndrome.

Continued

II

LYMPHADENITIS, INFECTIOUS

Lymphadenitis, infectious
ICD-9CM # 683 Lymphadenitis, acute

TABLE 2-126 **Clinical Patterns and Microbial Agents of Infectious Lymphadenitis—cont'd**

FORM OF LYMPHADENITIS

DISEASE	INFECTING ORGANISM	REGIONAL	REGIONAL WITH SUPPURATION (OR CASEATION)	INGUINAL BUBO FORMATION	ULCERO-GLAN-DULAR	OCULO-GLAN-DULAR	GENERALIZED
Viral							
Measles	Measles virus						+
Rubella	Rubella virus						+
Infectious mono-nucleosis	Epstein-Barr virus						+
Cytomegalovirus mononucleosis	Cytomegalovirus						+
Dengue fever	Dengue virus						+
West Nile fever	West Nile virus						+
Lassa fever	Lassa fever virus						+
Genital herpes infection	Herpes simplex virus type 2	+					
Pharyngocon-junctival fever	Adenovirus (types 3 and 7)	+				+	
Epidemic keratocon-junctivitis	Adenovirus (types 8 and 19)					+	
AIDS; AIDS-related complex	Human immunodefi-ciency virus						+
Protozoan							
Kala azar	*Leishmania donovani*						+
African trypanosomiasis	*Trypanosoma brucei*	+					+
Chagas disease	*Trypanosoma cruzi*						
Toxoplasmosis	*Toxoplasma gondii*					+	+
Helminthic							+
Filariasis	*Wucheria bancrofti*						+
	Brugia malayi						+
Loiasis	*Loa loa*			+			
Onchocerciasis	*Onchocerca volvulus*			+			

From Mandell GL: *Mandell, Douglas, and Bennett's principles and practice of infectious diseases,* ed 5, New York, 2000, Churchill Livingstone.
AIDS, Acquired immunodeficiency syndrome.

LYMPHADENOPATHY

Lymphadenopathy
ICD-9CM # 785.6

BOX 2-160 **Lymphadenopathy**

Generalized

AIDS
Lymphoma: Hodgkin's disease, non-Hodgkin's lymphoma
Leukemias, reticuloendotheliosis
Infectious mononucleosis, cytomegalovirus, and other viral infections
Diffuse skin infection: generalized furunculosis, multiple tick bites
Parasitic infections: toxoplasmosis, filariasis, leishmaniasis, Chagas disease
Serum sickness
Collagen vascular diseases (rheumatoid arthritis, systemic lupus erythematosus)
Dengue (arbovirus infection)

Sarcoidosis and other granulomatous diseases
Drugs: isoniazid, hydantoin derivatives, antithyroid and antileprosy drugs
Secondary syphilis
Hyperthyroidism, lipid storage diseases

Localized

Any of the causes of generalized lymphadenopathy
Draining lymphatics from local infection: infected furuncle, throat infection, dental abscess, lymphogranuloma venereum, brucellosis, parasitic infections, cat-scratch disease
Neoplasm
Tuberculosis (scrofula)

LYMPHOCYTE ABNORMALITIES IN PERIPHERAL BLOOD

TABLE 2-127 **Differential Diagnosis of Abnormal Lymphocytes in Peripheral Blood**

LYMPHOCYTE TYPE	USUAL DISEASE ASSOCIATION	CYTOLOGIC FEATURES	LABORATORY FEATURES	CLINICAL FEATURES
Small lymphocyte	Chronic lymphocytic leukemia	B-cell surface markers with low concentration of surface immunoglobulin, CD5 antigen	Hypogammaglobulinemia in 50%; positive direct Coombs' test in 15%; on node biopsy, diffuse, well-differentiated lymphocytic infiltrate	Elderly adults; presentation runs gamut from asymptomatic with lymphocytosis only to bulky disease with adenopathy, splenomegaly, and "packed" bone marrow
Atypical lymphocyte	Infectious mononucleosis, other viral illnesses	Suppressor T-cell markers	Heterophil agglutinin; positive serology for Epstein-Barr virus, cytomegalovirus, toxoplasma, HBsAg	Pharyngitis, fever, adenopathy, rash, splenomegaly, palatal petechiae, jaundice
Plasmacytoid lymphocyte	Waldenström's macroglobulinemia	Cytoplasmic IgM, periodic acid–Schiff (PAS) positivity	IgM paraprotein, rouleaux, cryoglobulins	Adenopathy, splenomegaly, absence of bone lesions, hyperviscosity syndrome, cryopathic phenomena
Lymphoblast	Acute lymphoblastic leukemia (ALL)	Terminal transferase positivity, common ALL antigen, B- or T-precursor markers	Anemia, granulocytopenia, thrombocytopenia, hyperuricemia, diffuse bone marrow infiltration	Peak incidence in childhood, acute onset, bone pain frequent
Lymphosarcoma cell	Lymphocytic lymphoma	B-cell surface markers with high concentration of monoclonal surface immunoglobulin	Nodular or diffuse, poorly differentiated lymphocytic lymphoma on node biopsy, patchy, peritrabecular bone marrow involvement	Middle-aged to older adults, generalized adenopathy, constitutional symptoms

From Stein JH (ed): *Internal medicine*, ed 5, St Louis, 1998, Mosby.

Continued

Lymphocyte abnormalities in peripheral blood
ICD-9CM # 288.8 Lymphocytopenia
         288.8 Lymphocytosis, symptomatic

TABLE 2-127   Differential Diagnosis of Abnormal Lymphocytes in Peripheral Blood—cont'd

LYMPHOCYTE TYPE	USUAL DISEASE ASSOCIATION	CYTOLOGIC FEATURES	LABORATORY FEATURES	CLINICAL FEATURES
Sézary cell	Cutaneous lymphomas	T-lymphocyte surface markers	Skin biopsy is diagnostic	Exfoliative erythroderma, cutaneous plaques or tumors
Hairy cell	Hairy cell leukemia	B-lymphocyte markers, cytoplasmic projections, tartrate-resistant acid phosphatase, interleukin-2 receptors, CD11 antigen	Pancytopenia	Middle-aged males, moderate to marked splenomegaly without adenopathy
Prolymphocyte	Prolymphocytic leukemia	B-cell surface markers with high concentration of surface immunoglobulin, CD5 negative	Marked lymphocytosis (frequently $>100 \times 10^9$/L)	Elderly adults, massive splenomegaly, minimum adenopathy, poor response to therapy

From Stein JH (ed): *Internal medicine,* ed 5, St Louis, 1998, Mosby.

Malabsorptive disorders
ICD-9CM # 579.9 Malabsorption syndrome
                579.8 Due to bacterial overgrowth
                579.8 Drug induced
                579.3 Postsurgical syndrome

MALABSORPTIVE DISORDERS

BOX 2-161   Classification of Malabsorptive Disorders (with Comments on Occurrence and Associated Abnormalities)

I. Inadequate mixing of food with bile salts and lipase—mild chemical steatorrhea common, but clinical steatorrhea uncommon. Actual diarrhea uncommon. Anemia in approximately 15%-35%; most often iron deficiency, rarely megaloblastic.
   A. Pyloroplasty
   B. Subtotal and total gastrectomy (occasional megaloblastic anemias reported)
   C. Gastrojejunostomy

II. Inadequate lipolysis—lack of lipase or normal stimulation of pancreatic secretion. Steatorrhea only in far-advanced pancreatic destruction, and diarrhea even less often.
   A. Cystic fibrosis of the pancreas
   B. Chronic pancreatitis
   C. Cancer of the pancreas or ampulla of Vater
   D. Pancreatic fistula
   E. Severe protein deficiency
   F. Vagus nerve section

III. Inadequate emulsification of fat—lack of bile salts. Clinical steatorrhea uncommon, sometimes occurs in very severe cases. Usually no diarrhea.
   A. Obstructive jaundice
   B. Severe liver disease

IV. Primary absorptive defect—small bowel
   A. Inadequate length of normal absorptive surface; unusual complication of surgery
      1. Surgical resection
      2. Internal fistula
      3. Gastroileostomy
   B. Obstruction of mesenteric lymphatics (rare)
      1. Lymphoma
      2. Hodgkin's disease
      3. Carcinoma
      4. Whipple's disease
      5. Intestinal tuberculosis
   C. Inadequate absorptive surface resulting from extensive mucosal disease; except for *Giardia* infection and regional enteritis, most of these diseases are uncommon; steatorrhea only if there is extensive bowel involvement

   1. Inflammatory
      a. Tuberculosis
      b. Regional enteritis or enterocolitis (diarrhea very common)
      c. *Giardia lamblia* infection (diarrhea common; malabsorption rare)
   2. Neoplastic
   3. Amyloid disease
   4. Scleroderma
   5. Pseudomembranous enterocolitis (diarrhea frequent)
   6. Radiation injury
   7. Pneumatosis cystoides intestinalis
   D. Biochemical dysfunction of mucosal cells
      1. "Gluten-induced" (steatorrhea and diarrhea very common)
         a. Celiac disease (childhood)
         b. Nontropical sprue (adult)
      2. Enzymatic defect
         a. Disaccharide malabsorption (diarrhea a frequent symptom)
         b. Pernicious anemia (deficiency of gastric "intrinsic factor")
      3. Cause unknown; uncommon except for tropical sprue (which is common only in the tropics)
         a. Tropical sprue (diarrhea and steatorrhea common)
         b. Severe starvation
         c. Diabetic visceral neuropathy
         d. Endocrine and metabolic disorder (e.g., hypothyroidism)
         e. Zollinger-Ellison syndrome (diarrhea common; steatorrhea may be present)
         f. Miscellaneous
V. Malabsorption associated with altered bacterial flora (diarrhea fairly common)
      1. Small intestinal blind loops, diverticula, anastomoses (rare)
      2. Drug (oral antibiotic) administration (infrequent but not rare)

From Ravel R: *Clinical laboratory medicine*, ed 6, St Louis, 1995, Mosby.

MALFORMATION SYNDROMES

TABLE 2-128   Common Abnormal Signs and Symptoms of Syndromes by System

Malformation syndromes
ICD-9CM # Code varies with specific syndrome

SYNDROME	PRINCIPAL FEATURES	OCULAR	IQ	NEURO	CARDIOVASCULAR		ENDO	GI	GU	MS	TUMOR	OTHER
					HYPERTENSION	ANOMALY						
Williams	Prominent lips, hoarse voice, cardiovascular defect	+	+	+	+	+	+	+	+	+	–	–
Noonan	Neck webbing, pectus excavatum, pulmonic stenosis	–	+	–	–	+	+	–	+	+	–	Hematologic
Beckwith-Wiedemann	Overgrowth, macrocrania, poor coordination	–	–	–	–	+	+	–	–	+	+	–
Sotos	Overgrowth, macrocrania, poor coordination	–	+	–	–	+	+	–	–	+	+	–
Prader-Willi	Obesity, hypogenitalism, behavioral abnormalities	+	+	–	+	–	+	–	+	+	–	–
Stickler	Flat facies, myopia, spondylo-epiphyseal dysplasia	+	–	–	–	+	–	–	–	+	–	Cleft palate Hearing loss
Fetal alcohol	Microcephaly, short palpebral fissures, long smooth philtrum	+	+	+	–	+	–	–	–	+	–	–
Velocardiofacial	Cleft palate, cardiac defect, characteristic facies	–	+	–	–	+	+	–	–	–	–	Psychosis Immune deficiency
Bardet-Biedl	Pigmentary retinopathy, obesity, renal abnormalities	+	+	–	+	+	+	–	+	+	–	–
Werner	Cataract, gray sparse hair, skin changes	+	–	+	+	+	+	+	+	+	+	Short stature Metastatic calcifications

From Goldman L, Bennett JC (eds): *Cecil textbook of medicine*, ed 21, Philadelphia, 2000, WB Saunders.

MEDIASTINAL MASSES

Mediastinal masses
ICD-9CM # 785.6 Adenopathy
519.3 Disease NEC
793.2 Shift (CXR)

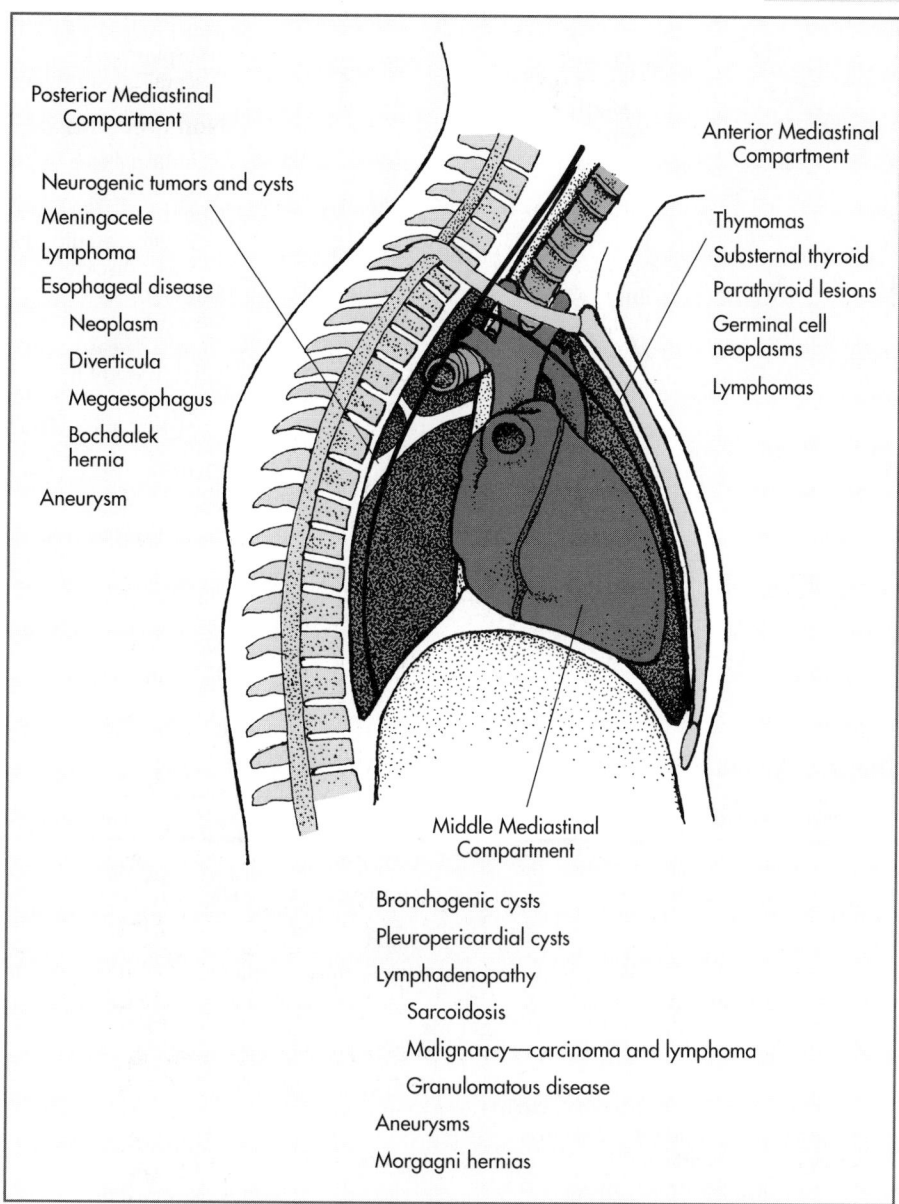

Posterior Mediastinal
Compartment

Neurogenic tumors and cysts
Meningocele
Lymphoma
Esophageal disease
    Neoplasm
    Diverticula
    Megaesophagus
    Bochdalek
    hernia
Aneurysm

Anterior Mediastinal
Compartment

Thymomas
Substernal thyroid
Parathyroid lesions
Germinal cell
neoplasms
Lymphomas

Middle Mediastinal
Compartment

Bronchogenic cysts
Pleuropericardial cysts
Lymphadenopathy
    Sarcoidosis
    Malignancy—carcinoma and lymphoma
    Granulomatous disease
Aneurysms
Morgagni hernias

Fig. 2-10 Masses of the mediastinum indicated by their anatomic location. (From Andreoli TE [ed]: *Cecil essentials of medicine,* ed 4, Philadelphia, 1997, WB Saunders.)

MENINGITIS, CHRONIC

BOX 2-162 Causes of Chronic Meningitis

Bacterial

Tuberculosis
Brucellosis
Nocardiosis
Syphilis
Lyme disease
Actinomycosis
Listeriosis
Subacute bacterial endocarditis
Tularemia
Leptospirosis
Meningococcal infection

Fungal

Cryptococcosis
Coccidioidomycosis
Histoplasmosis
Blastomycosis

Candida
Aspergillus
P. boydii
Zygomycetes
Sporothrix

Viral

Retroviruses
Herpesvirus
Enteroviruses
Lymphocytic choriomeningitis
Mumps

Parasitic

Cysticercosis
Schistosomiasis
Trichinosis
Paragonimiasis
Echinococcosis

Toxoplasmosis
Visceral larva migrans

Noninfectious

Neoplasm
Vasculitis
Chemical meningitis
Collagen vascular disease
Behcet's disease
Sarcoidosis
Systemic lupus erythematosus
Fabry's disease
Foreign body in the central nervous
   system
Vogt-Koyanagi-Harada syndrome

Other

Parameningeal focus
Chronic lymphocytic meningitis

From Rakel RE (ed): *Principles of family practice,* ed 6, Philadelphia, 2002, WB Saunders.

TABLE 2-129 Laboratory Evaluation for Chronic Meningitis

TYPE OF TEST	SPECIFIC EVALUATION
Blood	Complete blood count, differential
	Chemistries, erythrocyte sedimentation rate, antinuclear antibodies
	HIV serology
	RPR
	Consider angiotensin-converting enzyme (ACE), antineutrophilic cytoplasmic antibodies, specific serologies, blood smears
Cerebrospinal fluid	Cell count with differential, protein, glucose
	Cytology
	VDRL
	Cultures (TB, fungal, bacterial, viral)
	Stain (Gram's, acid fast, India ink)
	Cryptococcal antigen
	Oligoclonal bands, IgG index
	Consider ACE; PCR (viruses, mycobacteria, *T. whippelii*); histoplasma antigen, immunocytochemistry (*T. whippelii* and other selected agents); paired antibodies for *B. burgdorferi, Brucella,* histoplasma, *coccidioides,* other fungal agents; neoplastic markers
Neuroimaging	Brain MRI with contrast
	Consider CT, spinal MRI, angiography
Cultures	Blood (parasites, fungi, viruses, rare bacteria)
	Urine (mycobacteria, viruses, fungi)
	Sputum (mycobacteria, fungi)
	Consider gastric washings, stool, bone marrow, liver (mycobacteria, fungi)
Ancillary	Chest radiograph
	Electrocardiogram
	Selected testing (mammogram, CT chest/abdomen, etc.)
Biopsy	Extraneural sites (bone marrow, lymph node, peripheral nerve, liver, lung, skin, small bowel)
	Leptomeningeal/brain (± special stains)

From Coyle PK: Overview of acute and chronic meningitis. In Marra CM (ed): *Neurologic clinics,* Philadelphia, 1999, WB Saunders.
CT, Computed tomography; *HIV,* human immunodeficiency virus; *IgG,* immunoglobulin G; *MRI,* magnetic resonance imaging; *PCR,* polymerase chain reaction; *RPR,* rapid plasma regain; *TB,* tuberculosis; *VDRL,* Venereal Disease Research Laboratory.

MENINGITIS, RECURRENT

Meningitis, recurrent
ICD-9CM # 322.9

BOX 2-163 Causes of Recurrent Meningitis

Infectious

Recurrent infections (*Staphylococcus aureus, Neisseria meningitidis, Staphylococcus epidermidis, Haemophilus influenzae, Streptococcus pneumoniae, Brucella, Mycobacterium tuberculosis, Cryptococcus,* viruses)
Mollaret's meningitis (herpesvirus)
Familial Mediterranean fever
Parameningeal infection with seeding
Immune defects (recurrent bacterial infections)
  Complement deficiency
  Antibody deficiency
  Splenectomy

Noninfectious

Anatomic defects: traumatic, congenital, postoperative
Autoimmune disease
Drug-induced hypersensitivity
Behcet's disease
Migraine with pleocytosis
Vogt-Koyanagi-Harada syndrome
Chemical meningitis: endogenous (cyst or tumor) or exogenous (drug or dye)
Sarcoidosis
Whipple's disease
Systemic lupus erythematosus

From Rakel RE (ed): *Principles of family practice,* ed 6, Philadelphia, 2002, WB Saunders.

II

MENSTRUAL PAIN

Menstrual pain
ICD-9CM # 625.3 Dysmenorrhea
306.52 Dysmenorrhea psychogenic

TABLE 2-130 Differential Diagnosis of Menstrual Pain

CAUSE	NATURE OF PATIENT	NATURE OF SYMPTOMS	ASSOCIATED SYMPTOMS	PRECIPITATING AND AGGRAVATING FACTORS	AMELIORATING FACTORS	PHYSICAL FINDINGS	DIAGNOSTIC STUDIES
Premenstrual syndrome		Begins 2-12 days before menses and subsides at onset or during first days of period Diffuse, dull, pelvic ache May coexist with dysmenorrhea	Irritability Nervousness Headaches Swelling of breasts and extremities Bloating and weight gain Breast tenderness	Emotional stress Dysmenorrhea	Menses	Breasts tender to palpation	
Primary dysmenorrhea	30%-50% of young women 95% of adolescents	Most common menstrual disorder, especially in adolescents Begins within 3-12 mo of menarche with ovulatory cycles Becomes more severe with age *Pain:* Just precedes or begins with menstrual flow Lasts for 6 hr to 2 days Is crampy or a dull ache Is usually in midline of lower abdomen May radiate down thighs and to lower back	Nausea and vomiting Diarrhea Headache Fatigue Nervousness Dizziness	PMS IUD Emotional stress	Pain may lessen as menstrual cycles become regular Pregnancy Oral contraceptives Nonsteroidal antiinflammatory drugs	None	

Condition	Nature of Patient	Nature of Symptoms	Associated Symptoms	Precipitating Factors	Menses	Physical Findings	Diagnostic Studies
Secondary dysmenorrhea	Over age 20 Often a history of recurrent pelvic inflammatory disease	Secondary to organic disease Begins years after menarche; may occur with anovulatory cycles *Pain:* Begins several hours before menses Is a dull, continuous, diffuse, lower abdominal pain May be crampy Can radiate down thighs and into back		Cervical stenosis secondary to cervical conization or radiation IUD		Depends on cause of secondary dysmenorrhea	Papanicolaou test Gonorrhea and chlamydia culture Laparoscopy Ultrasound for myomas and ovarian cysts
Endometriosis	Usually over age 30 Uncommon in teenagers	Symptoms worsen with each cycle *Pain:* Begins 2-3 d before menses and persists for 2 d after May continued into intermenstrual period	Rectal pain with defecation Dyspareunia Tenesmus Backache Urgent micturition		Pregnancy Oral contraceptives	Pelvic examination best done in late luteal phase Nodularity felt in uterosacral ligaments or other sites of endometrial implants	Fern test Basal body temperature Laparoscopy Ultrasonography
Fibroids		Uncommon cause of dysmenorrhea	Menorrhagia			Uterine mass	Ultrasonography
Pelvic inflammatory disease		Pain is greatest premenstrually	Menorrhagia	Onset at menses		Cervical discharge Chandelier sign	Gonorrhea culture Leukocytosis Chlamydial culture

From Seller RH (ed): *Differential diagnosis of common complaints*, ed 4, Philadelphia, 2000, WB Saunders.
IUD, intrauterine device; *PMS*, premenstrual syndrome.

METASTASES, SKELETAL

Metastases, skeletal
ICD-9CM # 198.5

TABLE 2-131   Skeletal Metastasis: Radiographic Appearance and Incidence

PRIMARY FOCUS	USUAL TYPE OF SKELETAL METASTASIS	VERY COMMON	COMMON	INFREQUENT	RARE
Breast	Lytic, mixed, or blastic	X			
Lung					
Carcinoma	Predominantly lytic	X			
Carcinoid	Predominantly blastic		X		
Genitourinary system					
Kidney					
Carcinoma	Lytic, expansile	X			
Wilms' tumor	Lytic				X
Prostate	Predominantly blastic; lytic in older age group	X			
Urinary bladder	Predominantly lytic; blastic if prostate involved			X	
Adrenal gland					
Pheochromocytoma	Lytic, expansile				X
Carcinoma	Lytic				X
Male and female reproductive system					
Uterus					
Corpus	Lytic			X	
Cervix	Lytic or mixed			X	
Ovary	Predominantly lytic; occasionally blastic				X
Testis	Predominantly lytic; occasionally blastic			X	
Thyroid	Lytic, expansile		X		
Gastrointestinal tract					
Esophagus	Lytic				X
Stomach	Blastic or mixed			X	
Colon	Predominantly lytic; occasionally blastic		X		
Rectum	Predominantly lytic			X	
Biliary tree	Lytic				X
Pancreas	Lytic				X
Liver (hepatoma)	Lytic				X
Head, neck, and central nervous system					
Brain (medulloblastoma)	Lytic or blastic (usually after craniotomy)				X
Neuroblastoma	Lytic, mixed, or blastic	X			
Paranasal sinuses	Lytic				X
Nasopharynx	Lytic or blastic			X	
Salivary glands	Lytic				X
Chordoma	Lytic				X
Skin					
Squamous cell carcinoma	Lytic				X
Melanoma	Lytic, expansile			X	
Malignant neoplasms of bone or soft tissues					
Osteosarcoma	Lytic or blastic				X
Chondrosarcoma	Lytic or mixed				X
Ewing's tumor	Lytic, permeative	X			
Fibrosarcoma	Lytic				X
Vascular neoplasms (angiosarcoma, hemangiopericytoma)	Lytic				X

From Sartoris D: *Musculoskeletal imaging: the requisites,* St Louis, 1996, Mosby.

METASTATIC NEOPLASMS

Metastatic neoplasms
ICD-9CM # 198.5 Bone and bone marrow
            198.3 Brain and spinal cord
            197.7 Liver
            197.0 Lung

BOX 2-164   Metastatic Neoplasms

To Bone

Breast
Lung
Prostate
Thyroid
Kidney
Bladder
Endometrium
Cervix
Melanoma

To Brain

Lung
Breast
Melanoma
Genitourinary tract
Colon
Sinuses
Sarcoma
Skin
Thyroid

To Liver

Colon
Stomach
Pancreas
Breast
Lymphomas
Bronchus
Lung

To Lung

Breast
Colon
Kidney
Testis
Stomach
Thyroid
Melanoma
Sarcoma
Choriocarcinoma

II

MICROCEPHALY

Microcephaly
ICD-9CM # 742.1 Microcephalus

TABLE 2-132 Causes of Microcephaly

CAUSES	CHARACTERISTIC FINDINGS
Primary (Genetic)	
1. Familial (autosomal recessive)	• Incidence 1/40,000 births • Typical appearance with slanted forehead, prominent nose and ears; severely mentally retarded and prominent seizures; surface convolutional markings of the brain poorly differentiated and disorganized cytoarchitecture
2. Autosomal dominant	• Nondistinctive facies, up-slanting palpebral fissures, mild forehead slanting, and prominent ears • Normal linear growth, seizures readily controlled, and mild or borderline mental retardation
3. Syndromes	
Down (21-trisomy)	• Incidence 1/800 • Abnormal rounding of occipital and frontal lobes and a small cerebellum; narrow superior temporal gyrus, propensity for Alzheimer's neurofibrillary alterations, and ultrastructure abnormalities of cerebral cortex
Edward (18-trisomy)	• Incidence 1/6500 • Low birth weight, microstomia, micrognathia, low-set malformed ears, prominent occiput, rocker-bottom feet, flexion deformities of fingers, congenital heart disease, increased gyri, heterotopias of neurons
Cri-du-chat (5 p-)	• Incidence 1/50,000 • Round facies, prominent epicanthic folds, low-set ears, hypertelorism, and characteristic cry • No specific neuropathology
Cornelia de Lange	• Prenatal and postnatal growth delay; synophrys; thin, down-turning upper lip • Proximally placed thumb
Rubinstein-Taybi	• Beaked nose, downward slanting of palpebral fissures, epicanthic folds, short stature with broad thumbs and toes
Smith-Lemli-Opitz	• Ptosis, scaphocephaly, inner epicanthic folds, anteverted nostrils • Low birth weight, marked feeding problems
Secondary (Nongenetic)	
1. Radiation	• Microcephaly and mental retardation most severe if exposure before fifteenth wk of gestation
2. Congenital infections	
Cytomegalovirus	• Small for dates, petechial rash, hepatosplenomegaly, chorioretinitis, deafness, mental retardation, and seizures • Central nervous system calcification and microgyria
Rubella	• Growth retardation, purpura, thrombocytopenia, hepatosplenomegaly, congenital heart disease, chorioretinitis, cataracts, and deafness • Perivascular necrotic areas, polymicrogyria, heterotopias, subependymal cavitations
Toxoplasmosis	• Purpura, hepatosplenomegaly, jaundice, convulsions, hydrocephalus, chorioretinitis, and cerebral calcification
3. Drugs	
Fetal alcohol	• Growth retardation, ptosis, absent philtrum and hypoplastic upper lip, congenital heart disease, feeding problems, neuroglial heterotopia, and disorganization of neurons
Fetal hydantoin	• Growth delay, hypoplasia of distal phalanges, inner epicanthic folds, broad nasal ridge, and anteverted nostrils
4. Meningitis/encephalitis	• Cerebral infarcts, cystic cavitation, diffuse loss of neurons
5. Malnutrition	• Controversial cause of microcephaly
6. Metabolic	• Maternal diabetes mellitus and maternal hyperphenylalaninemia
7. Hyperthermia	• Significant fever during first 4-6 wk has been reported to cause microcephaly, seizures, and facial anomalies • Pathologic studies show neuronal heterotopias • Further studies showed no abnormalities with maternal fever
8. Hypoxic-ischemic encephalopathy	• Initially diffuse cerebral edema; late stages characterized by cerebral atrophy

From Behrman RE: *Nelson textbook of pediatrics*, ed 16, Philadelphia, 2000, WB Saunders.

MICROPENIS

BOX 2-165   Causes of Micropenis

Hypogonadotropic hypogonadism (hypothalamic or pituitary deficiencies)

Kallman's syndrome: autosomal dominant; associated with hyposmia

Prader-Willi syndrome: hypotonia, mental retardation, obesity, small hands and feet

Rud syndrome: hyposomia, ichthyosis, mental retardation

De Morsier's syndrome (septooptic dysplasia): hypopituitarism, hypoplastic optic discs, absent septum pellucidum

Hypergonadotropic hypogonadism

Primary testicular defect: disorders of testicular differentiation or inborn errors of testosterone synthesis

Klinefelter syndrome

Other X polysomies (i.e., XXXXY, XXXY)

Robinow's syndrome: brachymesomelic dwarfism, dysmorphic facies

Partial androgen insensitivity

Idiopathic

Defective morphogenesis of the penis

From Moore WT, Eastman RC: *Diagnostic endocrinology,* ed 2, St Louis, 1996, Mosby.

Micropenis
ICD-9CM # 752.69 Penile agenesis or atresia
607.89 Penile atrophy
752.64 Micropenis (congenital)

MIOSIS

Miosis
ICD-9CM # 379.42 Miosis persistent not due to miotics

BOX 2-166   Miosis

Medications (morphine, pilocarpine, etc.)

Neurosyphilis

Congenital

Iritis

CNS pontine lesion

CNS infections

Cavernous sinus thrombosis

Inflammation/irritation of cornea or conjunctiva

CNS, Central nervous system.

MONOCLONAL IMMUNOGLOBULIN SECRETION DISORDERS

Monoclonal immunoglobulin secretion disorders
ICD-9CM # code varies with specific disorder

TABLE 2-133   Classification of Disorders Associated with Monoclonal Immunoglobulin (M Protein) Secretion

DISORDER	M PROTEIN	ANTIBODY ACTIVITY OF M PROTEIN
Plasma Cell Neoplasms		
Multiple myeloma	IgG > IgA > IgD; ± free light chain or light chain alone (κ > λ)	
"Solitary" myeloma of bone	IgG > IgA > IgD; ± free light chain or light chain alone (κ > λ)	
Extramedullary plasmacytoma	IgG > IgA > IgD; ± free light chain or light chain alone (κ > λ)	
Waldenström's macroglobulinemia	IgM ± free light chain (κ > λ)	
Heavy-chain disease	γ, α, or μ heavy chain or fragment	
Primary amyloidosis	Free light chain (λ > κ)	
Monoclonal gammopathy of unknown significance	IgG > IgM > IgA, usually without urinary light chain secretion	
Other B-Cell Neoplasms		
Chronic lymphocytic leukemia	M protein occasionally secreted; IgM > IgG	
B-cell non-Hodgkin's lymphomas; Hodgkin's disease	M protein occasionally secreted; IgM > IgG	
Nonlymphoid Neoplasms		
Chronic myelogenous leukemia	No consistent patterns	
Carcinomas (e.g., colon, breast, prostate)	No consistent patterns	
Autoimmune or Aurtoreactive Disorders		
Cold agglutinin disease	IgMκ most common	Anti-I antigen
Mixed cryoglobulinemia	IgM or IgA	Anti-IgG
Sjögren's syndrome	IgM	
Miscellaneous Inflammatory, Storage, or Infectious Disorders		
Lichen myxedematosus	IgGλ	
Gaucher's disease	IgG	
Cirrhosis, sarcoid, parasitic diseases, renal acidosis	No consistent pattern	

Modified from Salmon SE: Plasma cell disorders. In Wyngaarden JB, Smith LH Jr (eds): *Cecil textbook of medicine,* ed 18, Philadelphia, 1988, WB Saunders.
IgA, Immunoglobulin A; *IgD,* immunoglobulin D; *IgG,* immunoglobulin G; *IgM,* immunoglobulin M.

MONONEUROPATHY AND MULTIPLE MONONEUROPATHY

Mononeuropathy and multiple mononeuropathy
ICD-9CM # 355.9

BOX 2-167   Common Causes of Mononeuropathy and Multiple Mononeuropathy

Mononeuropathy
    Compression
    Trauma
    Diabetes
    Vasculitis (systemic or nonsystemic)
    Other vascular
    Postinfectious or inflammatory
    Herpes zoster or herpes simplex
    Tumor
Multiple mononeuropathy
    Multiple compressions
    Demyelinating with conduction block
    Necrotizing vasculitis
    Diabetes
    Sarcoidosis
    Postinfectious or inflammatory
    Neurofibromatosis
    Leprosy
    Wegener's granulomatosis
    Lymphomatoid granulomatosis
    Malignant infiltration

From Wiederholt WC: *Neurology for non-neurologists*, ed 4, Philadelphia, 2000, WB Saunders.

MUSCLE DISEASE

Muscle disease
ICD-9CM # 359.9

BOX 2-168   Muscle Diseases

Muscular dystrophies
    Duchenne
    Becker
    Emery-Dreifuss
    Myotonic
    Facioscapulohumeral
    Scapuloperoneal
    Limb-girdle
    Ocular
    Oculocraniosomatic
    Distal
Congenital myopathies
    Central core
    Nemaline
    Mitochondrial
    Other
Inflammatory myopathies
    Polymyositis
    Dermatomyositis
    Inclusion body myositis
    Sarcoid myopathy
    Lupus
    Polyarteritis nodosa
    Rheumatoid arthritis
    Mixed connective tissue disease

Scleroderma
Sjögren's syndrome
Paraneoplastic syndrome
Infectious myopathies
    Toxoplasmosis
    Trichinosis
    Cysticercosis
    Viral myositis
    HIV
Toxic, metabolic, and endocrine myopathies
    Alcohol
    Emetine
    Chloroquine
    Vincristine
    McArdle disease (muscle phosphorlyase deficiency)
    Mitochondrial encephalomyopathy
    Several glycogen and lipid storage diseases
    Periodic paralyses
    Paroxysmal myoglobinuria
    Corticosteroid excess or deficiency
    Thyroid hormone excess or deficiency
    Acromegaly
Other
    Fibromyalgia

From Wiederholt WC: *Neurology for non-neurologists*, ed 4, Philadelphia, 2000, WB Saunders.
HIV, Human immunodeficiency virus.

MUSCLE WEAKNESS

Muscle weakness
ICD-9CM # 728.9

BOX 2-169   Causes of Muscle Weakness

I. Primary proximal weakness
   A. Muscle
      1. Endocrine: hyperthyroidism, hypothyroidism, subacute thyroiditis, hyperparathyroidism, acromegaly, Addison's disease (acute adrenal insufficiency), primary aldosteronism, steroid myopathy (Cushing's syndrome; iatrogenic), and male hypogonadism
      2. Metabolic: diabetes mellitus, insulin-induced hypoglycemia, glycogen storage diseases (acid maltase deficiency, muscle phosphorylase deficiency, muscle phosphofructokinase deficiency), lipid storage disease (carnitine deficiency), and alcoholic myopathy
      3. Muscular dystrophies: limb-girdle, Duchenne's, Becker's
      4. Inflammatory myopathies: polymyositis, dermatomyositis, other collagen-vascular diseases including rheumatoid arthritis, sarcoidosis, human immunodeficiency virus
      5. Hypercalcemia, hypophosphatemia, hypokalemia, and hyperkalemia of any cause
      6. Drug induced: colchine, chloroquine, cimetidine, amiodarone, β-blockers, D-penicillamine, cyclosporine
   B. Neuromuscular junction: myasthenia gravis, Eaton-Lambert syndrome, botulism, organophosphate poisoning
   C. Peripheral nerve: diabetic proximal neuropathy, Guillain-Barré syndrome, acute intermittent porphyria, tick paralysis, and arsenic poisoning
   D. Anterior horn cell: poliomyelitis, chronic spinal muscular atrophy
II. Primary distal weakness
   A. Muscle: myotonic dystrophy
   B. Peripheral nerve: beriberi, diphtheria, lead, porphyrins, carcinomatous neuropathy, chronic progressive demyelinating neuropathy, peroneal muscle atrophy (Charcot-Marie-Tooth disease), Guillain-Barré syndrome, Refsum's disease, compressive lesions (root, plexus, nerve)
   C. Anterior horn cell: poliomyelitis, motor neuron disease
III. Generalized weakness
   A. Decreased cardiac output (mitral stenosis, tricuspid stenosis, mitral regurgitation)
   B. Acute infectious diseases and chronic infectious diseases such as tuberculosis, brucellosis, and trichinosis
   C. Chronic glomerulonephritis and other causes of uremia, including generalized rhabdomyolysis
   D. Pernicious anemia (and other anemias)
   E. Hepatitis
   F. Neurosyphilis
   G. Psychiatric illnesses such as depression
   H. Multiple sclerosis
   I. Mitochondrial myopathy (genetic, zidovudine)
   J. L-Tryptophan (eosinophilia-myalgia)

From Stein JH (ed): *Internal medicine*, ed 5, St Louis, 1998, Mosby.

MUSCLE WEAKNESS, LOWER MOTOR NEURON VERSUS UPPER MOTOR NEURON

Muscle weakness, lower motor neuron versus upper motor neuron
ICD-9CM # 728.9

BOX 2-170   Lower Motor Neuron Versus Upper Motor Neuron Muscle Weakness

Lower Motor Neuron

Weakness, usually severe
Marked muscle atrophy
Fasciculations
Decreased muscle stretch reflexes
Clonus not present
Flaccidity
No Babinski sign
Asymmetric and may involve one limb only in the beginning to become generalized as the disease progresses

Upper Motor Neuron

Weakness, usually less severe
Minimal disuse muscle atrophy
No fasciculations
Increased muscle stretch reflexes
Clonus may be present
Spasticity
Babinski sign
Often initial impairment of only skilled movements.
   In the limbs the following muscles may be the only ones weak or weaker than the others: triceps; wrist and finger extensors; interossei; iliopsoas; hamstrings; and foot dorsiflexors, inverters and extroverters

From Wiederholt WC: *Neurology for non-neurologists*, ed 4, Philadelphia, 2000, WB Saunders.

MYDRIASIS

BOX 2-171   **Mydriasis**

Coma
Medications (cocaine, atropine, epinephrine, etc.)
Glaucoma

Cerebral aneurysm
Ocular trauma
Head trauma

Optic atrophy
Cerebral neoplasm

Mydriasis
ICD-9CM # 379.43 Mydriasis persistent not due to
mydriatics

Myelopathy and myelitis
ICD-9CM # 722.70 Myelopathy, discogenic
intervertebral NOS
336.9   Myelopathy, nondiscogenic
unspecified

MYELOPATHY AND MYELITIS

BOX 2-172   **Causes of Myelopathy and Myelitis**

Inflammatory
  Infectious
    Bacterial: spirochetal, tuberculous
    Viral: poliomyelitis; herpes, HTLV, HIV, zoster; rabies
    Other: rickettsial, fungal, parasitic
  Noninfectious
    Idiopathic transverse myelitis, multiple sclerosis
Toxic/metabolic
  Arsenic
  Pernicious anemia
  Pellagra
  Diabetes mellitus
  Chronic liver disease
Trauma
  Spinal fracture/dislocation
  Stab/bullet wound
  Herniated nucleus pulposus

Compression
  Spinal neoplasm
  Cervical spondylosis
  Extramedullary hematopoiesis
  Epidural abscess
  Epidural hematoma
Vascular
  Arteriovenous malformation
  Periarteritis nodosa
  Lupus erythematosus
  Dissecting aortic aneurysm
Physical agents
  Electrical injury
  Irradiation
Neoplastic
  Spinal cord tumors
  Paraneoplastic myelopathy

From Stein JH (ed): *Internal medicine,* ed 5, St Louis, 1998, Mosby.

MYELOPROLIFERATIVE DISORDERS

Myeloproliferative disorders
ICD-9CM # 238.7 Myeloproliferative disease or syndrome

TABLE 2-134 Clinical Features of Myeloproliferative Disorders

	ESSENTIAL THROMBOCYTOSIS	CHRONIC MYELOID LEUKEMIA	POLYCYTHEMIA VERA	MYELOFIBROSIS WITH MYELOID METAPLASIA
Symptoms and signs	Hemorrhage, thrombosis, increased platelets	Bone pain, fever/sweats, pruritus	Hemorrhage, thrombosis, portal HTN	Hemorrhage, thrombosis, massive spleen
Splenomegaly, megaly	30%-40%	95%	90%	100%
White blood cell count	10,000-20,000	20,000-600,000	10,000-20,000	10,000-25,000
Differential	Rare basophil	Immature myeloid cells, basophilia	Usually normal	Immature myeloid cells, basophilia
Red cell	Normal	Normal	Normal*	Teardrops, nucleated RBCs, polychro-matophilia
Hematocrit	Normal	Normal or decreased	Increased*	Decreased
LAP	→↑↓	↓	↑	↑
Cytogenetics, genetics	Normal	Ph^1 chromosome†	Normal	Normal*
Marrow	↑ Megakaryocytes	↑ All lines	↑ All lines	↑ All lines, fibrosis
Progression to leukemia	Rare	Most	1%-2% (13% if treated with radioactive phosphorus)	6%

From Noble J: *Primary care medicine*, ed 3, St Louis, 2001, Mosby.
HTN, Hypertension; *LAP*, leukocyte alkaline phosphatase; *RBCs*, red blood cells.
*Platelet defects may induce occult gastrointestinal blood loss, producing an artifactually normal or decreased hematocrit and morphologic changes consistent with iron deficiency.
†Gross chromosomal translocation may occasionally be absent, but genetic rearrangements involving the *bcr* locus on chromosome 22 and *c-abl* locus on chromosome 9 should be detectable on Southern Blot analysis.

MYOCARDIAL ISCHEMIA

Myocardial ischemia
ICD-9CM # 414.8 Ischemia (chronic)
              411.89 Ischemia, acute without MI

BOX 2-173 Causes of Myocardial Ischemia in Presence and Absence of Coronary Artery Disease

I. Atherosclerotic obstructive coronary artery disease
II. Nonatherosclerotic coronary artery disease
  A. Coronary artery spasm
  B. Congenital coronary artery anomalies
    1. Anomalous origin of coronary artery from pulmonary artery
    2. Aberrant origin of coronary artery from aorta or another coronary artery
    3. Coronary arteriovenous fistula
    4. Coronary artery aneurysm
III. Acquired disorders of coronary arteries
  A. Coronary artery embolism
  B. Dissection
    1. Surgical
    2. During percutaneous coronary angioplasty
    3. Aortic dissection
    4. Spontaneous, e.g., during pregnancy
  C. Extrinsic compression
    1. Tumors
    2. Granulomas
    3. Amyloidosis
  D. Collagen-vascular disease
    1. Polyarteritis nodosa
    2. Temporal arteritis
    3. Rheumatoid arthritis
    4. Systemic lupus erythematosus
    5. Scleroderma
  E. Miscellaneous disorders
    1. Irradiation
    2. Trauma
    3. Kawasaki disease
  F. Syphilis
IV. Hereditary disorders
  A. Pseudoxanthoma elasticum
  B. Gargoylism
  C. Progeria
  D. Homocystinuria
  E. Primary oxaluria
V. "Functional" causes of myocardial ischemia in absence of anatomic coronary artery disease
  A. Syndrome X
  B. Hypertrophic cardiomyopathy
  C. Dilated cardiomyopathy
  D. Muscle bridge
  E. Hypertensive heart disease
  F. Pulmonary hypertension
  G. Valvular heart disease; aortic stenosis, aortic regurgitation

From Stein J (ed): *Internal medicine*, ed 5, St Louis, 1998, Mosby.

MYOPATHIES, INFLAMMATORY

Myopathies, inflammatory
ICD-9CM # 359.9 Myopathy

BOX 2-174 Differential Diagnosis of Idiopathic Inflammatory Myopathies (IMs)

Collagen Vascular Disease

Fibromyalgia
Polyarteritis nodosa
Polymyalgia rheumatica
Rheumatoid arthritis
Scleroderma
Systemic lupus erythematosus
Temporal arteritis

Neurologic

Denervation
  Amyotrophic lateral sclerosis
Neuromuscular junction disorders
  Myasthenia gravis
  Eaton-Lambert syndrome
Muscular dystrophies
  Duchenne's
  Limb girdle
  Other
Neuropathies
  Guillain-Barré syndrome
  Diabetes mellitus
  Porphyria

Metabolic/Nutritional

Uremia
Hepatic failure
Malabsorption
Hypercalcemia or hypocalcemia
Hypernatremia or hyponatremia
Hyperkalemia or hypokalemia
Hypophosphatemia
Periodic paralysis
Vitamin E deficiency
Vitamin D deficiency

Endocrine

Hyperthyroidism or hypothyroidism
Hyperparathyroidism or hypoparathyroidism
Cushing's disease
Addison's disease
Hyperaldosteronism

Carcinomatous

Neuropathy
Neuromyopathy

Myositis
Microembolization

Drug Induced

Cimetidine
Clofibrate
Colchicine
Corticosteroids
ϵ-Aminocaproic acid
Emetine
Ethanol
Hydroxychloroquine
Ipecac
Lovastatin
Penicillamine
Vincristine
Zidovudine (AZT)

Infectious

Viral
  Influenza
  Epstein-Barr virus
  Coxsackieviruses A and B
  Human immunodeficiency virus
  Adenovirus
  Echovirus
  Rubella
Parasitic
  Toxoplasmosis
  Trichinosis
  Schistosomiasis
  Toxocariasis
  Cysticercosis
Bacterial
  Staphylococcal
  Streptococcal
  Clostridial
Rickettsial

Storage Diseases

Glycogen storage diseases
Lipid
  Carnitine deficiency
  Carnitine palmitoyltransferase deficiency
Purine
  Myoadenylate deaminase deficiency

Modified from Wortmann RL: Idiopathic inflammatory myopathies. In Bennett JC, Plum F (eds): *Cecil textbook of medicine,* ed 20, Philadelphia, 1996, WB Saunders.

MYOPATHIES, IDIOPATHIC INFLAMMATORY

Myopathies, idiopathic, inflammatory (addition to existing table)
ICD-9CM # 359.9

TABLE 2-135 Idiopathic Inflammatory Myopathies: Clinical and Laboratory Features

MYOPATHY	SEX	TYPICAL AGE AT ONSET	PATTERN OF WEAKNESS	CREATINE KINASE	MUSCLE BIOPSY	RESPONSE TO IMMUNOSUPPRESSIVE THERAPY
Dermatomyositis	F > M	Childhood and adult	Proximal > distal	Increased (up to 50× normal)	Perifascicular atrophy, MAC, immunoglobulin, complement deposition on vessels	Yes
Polymyositis	F > M	Adult	Proximal > distal	Increased (up to 50× normal)	Endomysial inflammation	Yes
Inclusion body myositis	M > F	Elderly (>50 yr)	Proximal and distal; predilection for finger/wrist flexors, knee extensors	Increased (<10× normal)	Endomysial inflammation, rimmed vacuoles; amyloid deposits; electron microscopy: 15-18 nm tubulofilaments	No

From Andreoli TE (ed): *Cecil essentials of medicine,* ed 5, Philadelphia, 2001, WB Saunders.
MAC, Membrane attack complex.

MYOPATHIES, METABOLIC AND MITOCHONDRIAL

Myopathies, metabolic and mitochondrial
ICD-9CM # 359.9

BOX 2-175   Metabolic and Mitochondrial Myopathies

Glycogen Metabolism Deficiencies

Type II	$\alpha_{1,4}$-Glucosidase (acid maltase)
Type III	Debranching enzyme
Type IV	Branching enzyme
Type V	Phosphorylase* (McArdle's)
Type VII	Phosphofructokinase* (Tarui's)
Type VIII	Phosphorylase B kinase*
Type IX	Phosphoglycerate kinase*
Type X	Phosphoglycerate mutase*
Type XI	Lactate dehydrogenase*

Lipid Metabolism Deficiencies

Carnitine palmitoyl transferase*
Primary systemic/muscle carnitine deficiency
Secondary carnitine deficiency

Mitochondrial Myopathies

Pyruvate dehydrogenase complex deficiencies
Progressive external ophthalmoplegia (PEO)
Kearns-Sayre syndrome
Myoclonic epilepsy and ragged-red fibers (MERRF)
Mitochondrial encephalopathy with lactic acidosis and stroke-like episodes (MELAS)
Mitochondrial neurogastrointestinal encephalomyopathy (MNGIE)
Mitochondrial depletion syndrome
Leigh's syndrome and neuropathy, ataxia, retinitis pigmentosa (NARP)
Succinate dehydrogenase deficiency*

From Andreoli TE (ed): *Cecil essentials of medicine,* ed 5, Philadelphia, 2001, WB Saunders.
*Deficiency can produce exercise intolerance and myoglobinuria.

MYOPATHIES, TOXIC

Myopathies, toxic
ICD-9CM # 359.9

BOX 2-176   Toxic Myopathies

Inflammatory: cimetidine, D-penicillamine
Noninflammatory necrotizing or vacuolar: cholesterol-lowering agents, chloroquine, colchicine
Acute muscle necrosis and myoglobinuria: cholesterol-lowering drugs, alcohol, cocaine
Malignant hyperthermia: halothane, ethylene, others; succinylcholine
Mitochondrial: zidovudine
Myosin loss: nondepolarizing neuromuscular blocking agents; glucocorticoids

---

From Andreoli TE (ed): *Cecil essentials of medicine,* ed 5, Philadelphia, 2001, WB Saunders.

MYOSITIS, IDIOPATHIC INFLAMMATORY

Myositis, idiopathic, inflammatory
ICD-9CM # 729.1

BOX 2-177   Differential Diagnosis of Idiopathic Inflammatory Myositis

Infectious

Viral myositis:
  Retroviruses (HIV, HTLV-I)
  Enteroviruses (echovirus, Coxsackievirus)
  Other viruses (influenza, hepatitis A and B, Epstein-Barr virus)
Bacterial: pyomyositis
Parasites: trichinosis, cysticercosis
Fungi: candidiasis

Idiopathic

Granulomatous myositis (sarcoid, giant cell)
Eosinophilic myositis
Eosinophilia-myalgia syndrome

Endocrine/Metabolic Disorders

Hypothyroidism
Hyperthyroidism
Hypercortisolism
Hyperparathyroidism
Hypoparathyroidism
Hypocalcemia
Hypokalemia

Metabolic Myopathies

Myophosphorylase deficiency (McArdle's disease)
Phosphofructokinase deficiency
Myoadenylate deaminase deficiency
Acid maltase deficiency
Lipid storage diseases
Acute rhabdomyolysis

Drug-Induced Myopathies

Alcohol
D-Penicillamine
Zidovudine
Colchicine
Chloroquine, hydroxychloroquine
Lipid-lowering agents
Cyclosporine
Cocaine, heroin, barbiturates
Corticosteroids

Neurologic Disorders

Muscular dystrophies
Congenital myopathies
Motor neuron disease
Guillain-Barré syndrome
Myasthenia gravis

From Andreoli TE (ed): *Cecil essentials of medicine,* ed 5, Philadelphia, 2001, WB Saunders.
HIV, Human immunodeficiency virus; *HTLV-I,* human T-cell lymphotropic virus–I.

NAIL DISORDERS

Nail disorders
ICD-9CM # 681.02 Infection (paronychia or onychia)
703.9   Disease unspecified
696.0   Psoriasis
697.0   Lichen planus

TABLE 2-136   **Differential Diagnosis of Nail Disorders**

CONDITION	PE/HISTORY	LABORATORY	MANAGEMENT
Onychomycosis	Hyperkeratosis of nail bed, yellow-brown discoloration, onycholysis. Usually chronic.	KOH positive Culture positive	Systemic or topical antifungal therapy
Paronychia, acute	Red, warm, tender nail. Often follows injury to nail fold.	Positive bacterial culture, usually *Staphylococcus*	Systemic antibiotic
Paronychia, chronic	Boggy, swollen, red, inflamed nail folds. Usually occurs in people who have wet-work jobs.	Pus is KOH positive and culture positive for *C. albicans*	Anticandida therapy, topical or systemic
Psoriasis	Usually associated with cutaneous psoriasis. Pitting, onycholysis, splinter hemorrhages, nail bed hyperkeratosis.	KOH negative	Topical or intralesional steroids
Lichen planus	Pitting and ridging early. Can eventuate in scarring and pterygium formation.	KOH negative	Systemic, topical, or intralesional steroids
Melanoma	Pigmented band in the nail that widens or darkens.	Biopsy nail bed or matrix depending on site of pigment	Wide excision
SCC	Hyperkeratosis, onycholysis.	Biopsy lesion	Excision, sometimes Mohs' surgery
Habit tic	Usually thumbs, horizontal parallel lines on nail plate. History of manipulating nail folds.	KOH negative	Explain cause to patient; occasionally wrapping nail
Mucous cyst	Occurs on proximal nail fold and over DIP joint.	Mucin expressed from punctured lesion	Excision, repeated liquid N_2, intralesional cortisone

From Noble J (ed): *Primary care medicine*, ed 3, St Louis, 2001, Mosby.
DIP, Distal interphalangeal; *KOH*, potassium hydroxide; *PE*, physical examination; *SCC*, squamous cell carcinoma.

NAUSEA AND VOMITING

Nausea and vomiting
ICD-9CM # 787.01

BOX 2-178   **Causes of Nausea and Vomiting**

Infections (viral, bacterial)
Intestinal obstruction
Metabolic (uremia, electrolyte abnormalities, DKA, acidosis, etc.)
Severe pain
Anxiety, fear
Psychiatric disorders (bulimia, anorexia nervosa)
Pregnancy

Medications (NSAIDs, erythromycin, morphine, codeine, aminophylline, chemotherapeutic agents, etc.)
Withdrawal from substance abuse (drugs, alcohol)
Head trauma
Vestibular or middle ear disease
Migraine headache

CNS neoplasms
Radiation sickness
Peptic ulcer disease
Carcinoma of GI tract
Reye's syndrome
Eye disorders
Abdominal trauma

CNS, Central nervous system; *DKA*, diabetic ketoacidosis; *GI*, gastrointestinal; *NSAIDs*, nonsteroidal antiinflammatory drugs.

NECK MASS

TABLE 2-137   Differential Diagnosis of Nonneoplastic Inflammatory Etiologies of a Neck Mass

ETIOLOGY	PATIENT CHARACTERISTICS, SIGNS, AND SYMPTOMS	TESTING STRATEGIES AND FINDINGS	TREATMENT
Adenopathy secondary to peritonsillar abscess	Sore throat Dysphagia Odynophagia Malaise Fever Drooling "Hot potato" voice Trismus Deviation of uvula Bulging of palate Fluctuance in peritonsillar region	Needle aspiration of peritonsillar space	Incision and drainage Antibiotics Hydration
Retropharyngeal abscess	Neck mass often not discrete Usually in pediatric age group Fever Malaise Dysphagia	Lateral neck x-ray Axial CT	Incision and drainage (after careful endotracheal intubation) in the OR Antibiotics
Parapharyngeal abscess	Spiking fever Rigors Malaise Trismus Dysphagia Odynophagia Aphasia Drooling Torticollis Neck rigidity and pain Paresthesias	Leukocytosis Anemia CT scan with contrast	IV antibiotics Hydration Incision and drainage
Salivary gland infections	Gland enlargement and tenderness ↑ Pain with eating Mucopurulent discharge from duct (if suppuration) Patients often elderly, dehydrated	X-ray for sialolith CT, if abscess suspected (Radionuclide scanning) (Sialogram)	Hydration Bland diet Analgesics Bed rest Antistaphylococcal antibiotics Warm compresses Gentle massage Surgical incision and drainage, if suppuration Gland excision for chronic/recurrent sialoadenitis or sialolithiasis
Jugular vein thrombus	Neck swollen, diffuse, usually tender Often H/O indwelling catheter (IJ or subclavian) If *suppurative* thrombophlebitis: Overlying erythema ↑ Tenderness Malaise Fever	CT with contrast or duplex Doppler ultrasound (Angiography)	Broad-spectrum antibiotics Hydration Supportive care Anticoagulants controversial Vein ligation if septic emboli
Mononucleosis	Mild and nonspecific URI 80% have triad: Sore throat Fever Lymphadenopathy Fatigue sometimes marked	CBC with differential Atypical lymphocytes Monospot Heterophile antibodies ↑ Serum liver enzymes	Supportive care: Hydration Bed rest (?) Antibiotics Steroids for prolonged or severe cases

AIDS, Acquired immunodeficiency syndrome; *CBC,* complete blood count; *ELISA,* enzyme-linked immunosorbent assay; *FTA-ABS,* fluorescent treponemal antibody absorption; *H/O,* history of; *IJ,* internal jugular; *PPD,* purified protein derivative; *sxs,* symptoms; *URI,* upper respiratory tract infection.

Continued

TABLE 2-137   Differential Diagnosis of Nonneoplastic Inflammatory Etiologies of a Neck Mass—cont'd

ETIOLOGY	PATIENT CHARACTERISTICS, SIGNS, AND SYMPTOMS	TESTING STRATEGIES AND FINDINGS	TREATMENT

	Exudative adenotonsillitis
	  Yellowish white
	  Confluent
	Adenopathy
	  Usually bilateral
	  Commonly posterior triangle
	  Tender
	  Can grow to impressive sizes
	Palatal petechiae
	Nonallergic rash to ampicillin
	Hepatosplenomegaly
			Endotracheal intubation or tonsillectomy if airway compromised

CMV	Mild URI sxs Similar to EBV, but less severe *No* exudative pharyngitis	Negative heterophile antibody Serologic test for CMV (+)	Supportive care

Tuberculosis	Nodes usually painless
	  Usually nonerythematous
	  Usually enlarging
	  Multiple (66%)
	  Posterior (70%)
	Overlying skin indurated and slightly brown
	Sinus tracts may open in skin
		Smear or pathologic examination of node or drainage
		Culture
			Systemic antituberculosis medication

Atypical mycobacterium	Unilateral cervical lymphadenitis, most commonly submandibular
	Skin erythematous
	  Usually nontender
	  Usually not warm
	  Changes in color from red to lilac pink
	Minimal systemic findings
	Not associated with pulmonary disease
		PPD negative or weakly positive	Surgical excision of infected nodes without antimicrobial chemotherapy

AIDS	Opportunistic infections Hairy leukoplakia Kaposi's sarcoma Candidiasis Verrucae Giant aphthous stomatitis	ELISA Western blot Helper/suppressor T-cell ratios	Treatment of underlying disease Biopsy of nodes if neoplasm suspected

Toxoplasmosis	Common cold sxs
	Asymptomatic or mildly tender posterior triangle adenopathy
	Nodes usually confined to one side
	  May fluctuate in size
	  Do not suppurate or develop fistulae
		Fluorescent antibody test
		Complement fixation test
		Hemagglutination
		Sabin-Feldman dye test
			Sulfonamides
			Pyrimethamine

Actinomyces	Neck mass: not true lymphadenitis
	  Blue
	  Rubbery
	  Nontender
	  Central loculation
	Discharge of water material
		Curettage and culture	High-dose penicillin G IV 4-6 wk followed by 12 mo of oral penicillin

Cat-scratch disease	Mild clinical symptoms Regional lymphadenopathy	Serologic test for *Rochalimaea henselae*	Supportive care

TABLE 2-138 **Differential Diagnosis of Congenital Anomalies Presenting as a Neck Mass**

ANOMALY	PATIENT CHARACTERISTICS, SIGNS, SYMPTOMS	TESTING STRATEGIES AND FINDINGS	TREATMENT
Syphilis	Cervical adenopathy	FTA-ABS	Penicillin
Tularemia	See Section I	See Section I	See Section I
Brucellosis	See Section I	See Section I	See Section I
Leptospirosis	See Section I	See Section I	See Section I

Thyroglossal duct cyst	Most patients <30 yr
	Midline mass
	  Usually inferior to hyoid
	  Soft
	Retraction of cyst on protrusion of tongue is pathognomonic
			Surgical excision
			Antibiotics if infection

Branchial apparatus anomalies	Usually present in childhood
	  Usually diagnosed by age 30 yr
	Mass
	  Along anterior border of SCM
	  Between ear canal and clavicle
	  Smooth
	  Fluctuant
	  Nontender
	  Ill-defined margins
	  Varies in size (associated with URIs)
		Needle aspiration results in decompression
		Thin or mucopurulent fluid
			Surgical excision

Cystic hygroma	Multiloculated cystic masses
	90% diagnosed before age 2 yr
	Often enlarge during URIs
	(Airway compromise)
	Transilluminate
		CT scan
		May have visible cysts
		(Aspiration → clear yellow fluid)
			Excision if:
			  Functional impairment
			  Recurrent infection
			  Severe cosmetic deformity

Hemangioma	Most diagnosed by age 6 mo
	Proliferate during first year
	(Airway obstruction)
	(High-output cardiac failure)
		CT scan	Surgical excision if:
			  No regression by age 5 yr
			  Impending complications

Dermoid cysts	Midline masses
	  Smooth
	  Not attached to larynx or hyoid
	  Doughy consistency
	  Commonly found in 20s
			Surgical excision

Teratomas	Mass
	  Irregular
	  Firm
	  Lateral
			Surgical excision

Laryngoceles	Very soft, compressible mass ↑ Size with Valsalva's maneuver Laryngeal component		Surgical excision (Antibiotics if infection)
Ranula	Soft, compressible mass Associated with sublingual gland	CT scan (Salivary amylase)	Surgical excision

From Noble J (ed): *Primary care medicine*, ed 3, St Louis, 2001, Mosby.
CT, Computed tomography; *FTA-ABS,* fluorescent treponemal antibody absorption; *SCM,* sternocleidomastoid muscle; *URI,* upper respiratory tract infection.

NECK PAIN

BOX 2-179 Differential Diagnosis of Cervical Neck Pain

Inflammatory Diseases

Rheumatoid arthritis (RA)
Spondyloarthropathies
Juvenile RA

Noninflammatory Disease

Cervical osteoarthritis
Diskogenic neck pain
Diffuse idiopathic skeletal hyperostosis
Fibromyalgia or myofascial pain

Infectious Causes

Meningitis
Osteomyelitis
Infectious diskitis

Neoplasms

Primary
Metastatic

Referred Pain

Temporomandibular joint pain
Cardiac pain
Diaphragmatic irritation
Gastrointestinal sources (gastric ulcer, gallbladder,
    pancreas)

From Noble J: *Primary care medicine*, ed 3, St Louis, 2001, Mosby.

NECROTIZING SOFT TISSUE INFECTIONS

TABLE 2-139   Necrotizing Soft Tissue Infections

> Necrotizing soft tissue infections
> ICD-9CM # Code varies with specific diagnosis

PARAMETER	GAS-FORMING CELLULITIS	SYNERGISTIC NECROTIZING CELLULITIS	GAS GANGRENE	"STREPTOCOCCAL" MYONECROSIS	NECROTIZING FASCIITIS	INFECTED VASCULAR GANGRENE	STREPTOCOCCAL INFECTION
Predisposing conditions	Traumatic	Diabetes, prior local lesions, perirectal lesions	Traumatic or surgical wound	Trauma, surgery	Diabetes, trauma, surgery, perineal infection	Arterial insufficiency	Traumatic or surgical wound
Incubation period	>3 days	3-14 days	1-4 days	3-4 days	1-4 days	>5 days	6 hr-2 days
Etiologic organisms	Clostridia, others	Mixed aerobic-anaerobic flora	Clostridia, especially *Clostridium perfringens*	Anaerobic streptococci	Mixed aerobic-anaerobic flora	Mixed aerobic-anaerobic flora	*Streptococcus pyogenes*
Systemic toxicity	Minimal	Moderate to severe	Severe	Minimal until late in course	Moderate to severe	Minimal	Severe
Course	Gradual	Acute	Acute	Subacute	Acute to subacute	Subacute	Acute
Wound findings Local pain	Minimal	Moderate to severe	Severe	Late only	Minimal to moderate	Variable	Severe
Skin appearance	Swollen, minimal discoloration	Erythematous or gangrene	Tense and blanched, yellow-bronze, necrosis with hemorrhagic bullae	Erythema or yellow-bronze	Blanched, erythema, necrosis with hemorrhagic bullae	Erythema or necrosis	Erythema, necrosis
Gas	Abundant	Variable	Usually present	Variable	Variable	Variable	No
Muscle involvement	No	Variable	Myonecrosis	Myonecrosis	No	Myonecrosis limited to area of vascular insufficiency	No
Discharge	Thin, dark, sweetish or foul odor	Dark pus or "dishwater," putrid	Serosanguineous, sweet or foul odor	Seropurulent	Seropurulent or dishwater, putrid	Minimal	None or sero-sanguineous
Gram stain	PMNs, gram-positive bacilli	PMNs, mixed flora	Sparse PMNs, gram-positive bacilli	PMNs, gram-positive cocci	PMNs, mixed flora	PMNs, mixed flora	PMNs, gram-positive cocci in chains
Surgical therapy	Débridement	Wide filleting incisions	Extensive excision, amputation	Excision of necrotic muscle	Wide filleting incisions	Amputation	Débridement of necrotic tissue

From Bartlett JG: Clostridial myonecrosis and other clostridial diseases. In Wyngaarden JB, Smith LH Jr, Bennett JC (eds): *Cecil textbook of medicine*, ed 19, Philadelphia, 1992, WB Saunders.
PMNs, Polymorphonuclear leukocytes.

II

NEMATODE TISSUE INFECTIONS

Nematode tissue infections
ICD-9CM # 128.9

TABLE 2-140 Nematode Tissue Infections

SPECIES OR DISEASE	EPIDEMIOLOGY	TRANSMISSION	MAJOR CLINICAL PRESENTATION	DIAGNOSIS	TREATMENT
Wuchereria bancrofti (lymphatic filariasis)	Tropics, subtropics	Mosquito	Lymphatic obstruction	Night blood	Diethylcarbamazine (DEC),* 50 mg first day, 50 mg tid second day, 100 mg tid third day, 2 mg/kg tid for 20 days; or ivermectin,†,‡,§ 400 μg/kg; or albendazole,†,‡,§ 400 mg for 21 days
Brugia malayi (lymphatic filariasis)	South and Southeast Asia	Mosquito	Lymphatic obstruction	Night blood	Same as for *W. bancrofti*
Onchocerca volvulus (river blindness)	Central and South America	Blackfly	Dermatitis, blindness	Skin snips	Ivermectin,§ 150 μg/kg once every 3 to 12 mo or every 4 mo
Loa loa (eyeworm)	West and Central Africa	Deerfly, horsefly	Calabar swellings	Day or night blood samples	DEC or ivermectin†‡§ as for *W. bancrofti*
Tropical pulmonary eosinophilia (TPE)	All the above areas	Unknown	Eosinophilia, pneumonitis	Serology and clinical picture	DEC, 2 mg/kg tid for 7-10 days; ivermectin or albendazole†,‡,§ as for *W. bancrofti*
Dracunculus medinensis (guinea worm)	Africa	Step-in wells	Painful boil in legs	Visualization of worm	Niridazole,† 25 mg/kg for 10 days, or metronidazole,† 250 mg tid for 10 days
Trichinella spiralis	Worldwide	Raw meat	Fever, myalgias, periorbital edema	Serology, muscle biopsy	Thiabendazole,‡ 25 mg/kg for 5 days (max, 3 g/day), or mebendazole,†‡ 200-400 mg tid for 3 days, 400-500 mg tid for 10 days, or albendazole,†‡ 400 mg bid for 10 days, and ?steroids
Angiostrongylus cantonensis	Southeast Asia, Pacific Islands	Raw mollusks or crustaceans	Eosinophilia, meningitis	Clinical picture	Surgical removal
Angiostrongylus costaricensis	Same as above	Same as above	Same as above	Same as above	Surgical removal; mebendazole, 100 mg bid for 5 days, or ?thiabendazole,†‡ 25 mg/kg tid for 3 days
Gnathostoma spinigerum	Thailand, Japan	Raw fish	Eosinophilia, meningitis, subcutaneous swellings	Serology	Surgical removal; mebendazole,‡ 200 mg every 3 hr for 6 days
Anisakis species	Japan, Scandinavia	Raw fish	Benign stomach "tumor"	Endoscopy with biopsy, serology	Surgical removal
Visceral larva migrans	Worldwide	Ingestion of soil (pica)	Fever, abdominal pain, optic involvement, diarrhea	Serology	Albendazole, 400 mg bid for 3-5 days, or thiabendazole, 25 mg/kg bid for 5 days (max, 3 g/day), or DEC,† 2 mg/kg bid for 10 days, or mebendazole,† 100-200 mg for 5 days, all with steroids‡
Cutaneous larva migrans	Worldwide	Skin penetration	Creeping eruption	Clinical picture	Thiabendazole, topically or 50 mg/kg/day (max, 3 g/day) for 2-5 days, or albendazole, 200 mg bid for 3 days or ivermectin,†§ 150-200 μg/kg once
Strongyloidosis	Worldwide, immunosuppressor	Fecal-oral	Gram-negative bacteremia, multiple organ involvement	Stool ova and parasites, tissue biopsy	Thiabendazole, 25 mg/kg bid for 2 days, 5 days for dissemination; or albendazole, 400 mg/day for 3 days,†,§ or ivermectin, 200 μg/kg/day for 1-2 days†,§

From Stein JH (ed): *Internal medicine,* ed 5, St Louis, 1998, Mosby.
bid, Twice a day; *tid,* three times a day.
*May precipitate severe reactions in infected individuals.
†Considered an investigational drug by the U.S. Food and Drug Administration.
‡Effectiveness not clearly established.
§Not available in the United States.

NEUROGENIC BLADDER

Neurogenic bladder
ICD-9CM # 396.54

BOX 2-180 Causes of Neurogenic Bladder

Supratentorial

CVA
Parkinson's disease
Alzheimer's disease
Cerebral palsy

Spinal Cord

Spinal cord injury
Spinal stenosis

Central cord syndrome
ALS
Multiple sclerosis
Myelodysplasia

Peripheral Neuropathy

Diabetes
Alcohol
Shingles
Syphilis

From Nseyo UO (ed): *Urology for primary care physicians*, Philadelphia, 1999, WB Saunders.
ALS, Amyotrophic lateral sclerosis; *CVA*, cerebrovascular accident.

NEUROLOGIC DEFICIT, FOCAL

Neurological deficit, focal
ICD-9CM # 436   CVA
435.9 TIA

BOX 2-181 Causes of Acute Focal Neurologic Deficit

Traumatic: intracranial, intraspinal
  Subdural hematoma
  Intraparenchymal hemorrhage
  Epidural hematoma
  Traumatic hemorrhagic necrosis
Infectious
  Brain abscess
  Epidural and subdural abscesses
  Meningitis
Neoplastic
  Primary central nervous system tumors
  Metastatic tumors
  Syringomyelia
  Vascular

Thrombosis
Embolism
Spontaneous hemorrhage: arteriovenous malforma-
  tion, aneurysm, hypertensive
Metabolic
  Hypoglycemia
  B_{12} deficiency
  Postseizure
  Hyperosmolar nonketotic
Other
  Migraine
  Bell's palsy
  Psychogenic

From Rosen P, Barkin R (eds): *Emergency medicine: concepts and clinical practice*, ed 5, St Louis, 2002, Mosby.

NEUROLOGIC DEFICIT, MULTIFOCAL

BOX 2-182 Causes of Multifocal Neurologic Deficit

Acute disseminated encephalomyelitis
  Postviral or postimmunization
Infectious encephalomyelitis
  Poliovirus, enteroviruses, arbovirus, herpes zoster,
    Epstein-Barr virus
Granulomatous encephalomyelitis
  Sarcoid

Autoimmune
  Systemic lupus erythematosus
Other
  Familial spinocerebellar degenerations

From Rosen P, Barkin R (eds): *Emergency medicine: concepts and clinical practice*, ed 5, St Louis, 2002, Mosby.

Neurological deficit, multifocal
ICD-9CM # 436   CVA
435.9 TIA

NEUROMUSCULAR JUNCTION DISORDERS

BOX 2-183   Disorders of the Neuromuscular Junction

Autoimmune

Myasthenia gravis
   Lambert-Eaton myasthenic syndrome

Congenital

Presynaptic defects in Ach resynthesis, packaging, or release
Synaptic defect: congenital end-plate AChE deficiency
Postsynaptic defects: slow-channel syndromes
Postsynaptic defects: decreased response to ACh
   Low-affinity fast channel syndromes
   Mode-switching kinetics of AChR
   AChR deficiency without kinetic abnormality
Familial limb girdle myasthenia

Toxic

Botulism
Drug-induced
Organophosphate intoxication

From Andreoli TE (ed): *Cecil essentials of medicine,* ed 5, Philadelphia, 2001, WB Saunders.
ACh, Acetylcholine; *AChE,* acetylcholinesterase; *AChR,* acetylcholine receptor.

NEUROMUSCULAR TRANSMISSION DISORDERS

BOX 2-184   Disorders of Neuromuscular Transmission

Myasthenia gravis
Myasthenic (Eaton-Lambert) syndrome
Congenital myasthenia
Botulism
Arthropod envenomation (tick, scorpion, black widow spider)
Snake envenomation (cobra, mamba, viper, sea snake, South American rattlesnake)
Induced by aminoglycoside antibiotics
Induced by anesthetic agents
Induced by organophosphate insecticides
Associated with polymyositis
Associated with amyotrophic lateral sclerosis

From Wiederholt WC: *Neurology for non-neurologists,* ed 4, Philadelphia, 2000, WB Saunders.

Neuropathies
ICD-9CM # 355.9   Neuropathy NOS
             357.5   Alcoholic
             357.8   Chronic progressive or relapsing
             356.2   Congenital sensory
             356.0   Dejerine-Sottas
             350.60 Diabetic polyneuropathy, type II
             350.61 Diabetic polyneuropathy, type I

NEUROPATHIES

TABLE 2-141   **Diseases Associated with Different Types of Neuropathy**

	AIDP	CIDP	AXONAL SMP	MN	MNMP	PLEX	SMALL
Metabolic							
Diabetes			+	+	+	+	+
Acromegaly*			+	+ (CTS)			
Hypothyroidism*		+	+	+ (CTS)			
Infectious							
AIDS*	+	+	+		+		
Leprosy			+		+		
Lyme disease	+		+	+	+		
Connective Tissue							
SLE*	+		+		+		
Rheumatoid arthritis			+	+	+		
Sjögren's syndrome			+		+		
Periarteritis nodosa*			+		+		
Wegener's granulomatosis*			+		+		
Cranial arteritis*			+		+		
Churg-Strauss syndrome			+		+		
Cryoglobulinemia			+		+		
Hypersensitivity angiitis			+		+		
Idiopathic							
Sarcoidosis*			+		+		

From Stein JH (ed): *Internal medicine*, ed 5, St Louis, 1998, Mosby.
AIDP, Acute inflammatory demyelinating polyneuropathy; *AIDS*, acquired immunodeficiency syndrome; *axonal SMP*, axonal sensorimotor polyneuropathy; *CIDP*, chronic idiopathic demyelinating polyradiculoneuropathy; *CTS*, carpal tunnel syndrome; *MN*, mononeuropathy; *MNMP*, mononeuropathy ultiplex; *plex*, plexopathy; *SLE*, systemic lupus erythematosus; *small*, small-fiber polyneuropathy.
*Central nervous system manifestations may be present.

NEUROPATHIES, CLASSIFICATION BASED ON TEMPORAL PRESENTATION

Neuropathies, classification based on temporal presentation
ICD-9CM # 355.9

TABLE 2-142   Neuropathies Classified by Temporal Presentation

ACUTE ONSET (WITHIN DAYS)	SUBACUTE ONSET (WEEKS TO MONTHS)	CHRONIC COURSE (MONTHS TO YEARS)	RELAPSING
GBS	Most toxins	CIDP	GBS
Vasculitis	Most drugs	Alcohol	HIV
Porphyria	Nutritional deficiencies	Diabetes	Porphyria
Diphtheria	Abnormal metabolic state	Hereditary neuropathies	Refsum's disease
Thallium toxicity	Diabetic plexopathy		CIDP
Ischemia	Neoplasms		
Penetrating trauma	Uremia		
Rheumatoid arthritis			
Diabetic plexopathy or cranial neuropathy			
Acute nerve compression			
Polyarteritis nodosa			
Burns			
Iatrogenic (e.g., improper injection techniques)			

From Rakel RE (ed): *Principles of family practice*, ed 6, Philadelphia, 2002, WB Saunders.
CIDP, Chronic inflammatory demyelinating polyradiculoneuropathy; *GBS*, Guillain-Barré syndrome; *HIV*, human immunodeficiency virus.

NEUROPATHIES, DRUG- AND TOXIN-INDUCED

Neuropathies, drug and toxin induced
ICD-9CM # 357.7

TABLE 2-143   Neuropathies Caused by Drugs and Toxins

DRUGS		TOXINS
Axonal	**Demyelinating**	**Industrial**
Alpha interferon	Amiodarone	Organophosphates
Amitriptyline	Colchicine	Lead, arsenic, mercury
Chloroquine	Gold	Thallium, methyl bromide
Cimetidine	Surmanin	Plastics, synthetic fabrics
Colchicine		Carbon monoxide
Dapsone	**Neuronopathy**	Ethylene oxide
Didanosine	Cisplatin	
Disulfram	Pyridoxine	**Euphorants**
Ethambutol	Thalidomide	Glue
Hydralazine		Solvents
Isoniazid		Nitrous oxide
Lithium		
Metronidazole		
Nitrous oxide		
Nitrofurantoin		
Paclitaxel		
Phenytoin		
Piridoxine		
Procainamide		
Vincristine		

From Rakel RE (ed): *Principles of family practice*, ed 6, Philadelphia, 2002, WB Saunders.

NEUROPATHIES, HEREDITARY

Neuropathies, hereditary
ICD-9CM # 356.9

TABLE 2-144   Major Hereditary Neuropathies

DISORDER	TYPE	CLINICAL FEATURES	PATHOPHYSIOLOGY	INHERITANCE	GENE DEFECT
Charcot-Marie-Tooth Disease					
CMT I		Slowly evolving motor-sensory neuropathies with high arches, hammertoes, hypertrophic nerves	Demyelination and re-myelination with onion bulbs		
	a			Dominant	Duplication of a segment of chromosome 17 encoding PMP-22
	b			Dominant	Point mutation in the myelin protein P_0
	x			X-linked	Mutation in connexin 32
Liability to pressure palsies			Tomaculous neuropathy	Dominant	Deletion of PMP-22 region of chromosome 17
CMT II		Similar, without hypertrophic nerves	Distally predominant axonal degeneration	Dominant	Unknown
CMT III (Dejerine-Scottas disease)		Early onset, severe motor-sensory neuropathy	Severe hypomyelination with onion bulbs	Recessive	Mutation in P_0

Familial Amyloidosis (Four Subtypes)

Porphyria
Others (Rare)
Fabry's disease
Leukodystrophies
Refsum's disease
Tangier disease
Abetalipoproteinemia
Mitochondrial
   neuropathies

From Andreoli TE (ed): *Cecil essentials of medicine,* ed 5, Philadelphia, 2001, WB Saunders.

Gwendolyn R. Lee, M.D.
Internal Medicine

NEUROPATHIES, PAINFUL

Neuropathies, painful
ICD-9CM # 355.9

BOX 2-185   Painful Neuropathies

Mononeuropathies
  Compressive neuropathy (carpal tunnel, meralgia
    paresthetica)
  Trigeminal neuralgia
  Ischemic neuropathy
  Polyarteritis nodosa
  Diabetic mononeuropathy
  Herpes zoster
  Idiopathic and familial brachial plexopathy
Polyneuropathies
  Diabetes mellitus
  Paraneoplastic sensory neuropathy
  Nutritional neuropathy
  Multiple myeloma
  Amyloid
  Dominantly inherited sensory neuropathy
  Toxic (arsenic, thallium, metronidazole)
  AIDS-associated neuropathy
  Tangier disease
  Fabry disease

From Wiederholt WC: *Neurology for non-neurologists*, ed 4, Philadelphia, 2000, WB Saunders.
AIDS, Acquired immunodeficiency syndrome.

NYSTAGMUS

Nystagmus
ICD-9CM # 379.50 Nystagmus NOS
          386.11 Benign positional
          386.2 Central positional
          379.51 Congenital

**TABLE 2-145   Types of Nystagmus with Localizing Value and the Common Location
and Cause of the Responsible Lesions**

TYPE	COMMON LOCATION	COMMON CAUSES
Up-beat nystagmus	Cerebellar vermis or brainstem, especially cervicomedullary junction	Alcoholic cerebellar degeneration, multiple sclerosis, neoplasm, anticonvulsants and sedatives
Down-beat nystagmus	Cervicomedullary junction, cerebellar vermis	Cranial malformation (Arnold-Chiari), multiple sclerosis, lithium toxicity, anticonvulsants and sedatives, infarction, alcoholic cerebellar degeneration
Periodic alternating nystagmus	Cervicomedullary junction	Cranial malformation, multiple sclerosis
Seesaw nystagmus	Anterior third ventricle	Neoplasm
Convergence-retraction nystagmus	Dorsal midbrain	Neoplasm, multiple sclerosis
Ocular myoclonus	Dentatorubroolivary triangle	Infarction, multiple sclerosis
Ocular flutter and opsoclonus	Cerebellum	Immunologically mediated cerebellar encephalitis, postinfectious, or as a remote effect of neoplasia
Ocular bobbing	Pons	Infarction, toxic or metabolic encephalopathy

From Stein J (ed): *Internal medicine*, ed 5, St Louis, 1998, Mosby.

OPHTHALMOPLEGIA

Ophthalmoplegia
ICD-9CM # 378.9   Ophthalmoplegia NOS
              378.52 Cerebellar ataxia syndrome
              376.22 Exophthalmic

TABLE 2-146   Major Causes of Acute (<48 Hr) Ophthalmoplegia

CONDITION	DIAGNOSTIC FEATURES
Bilateral	
Botulism	Contaminated food; high-altitude cooking; pupils involved
Myasthenia gravis	Fluctuating degree of paralysis; responds to edrophonium chloride (Tensilon) IV
Wernicke's encephalopathy	Nutritional deficiency; responds to thiamine IV
Acute cranial polyneuropathy	Antecedent respiratory infection; elevated CSF protein
Brainstem stroke	Other brainstem signs
Unilateral	
Carotid-posterior	Third cranial nerve, pupil involved communicating aneurysm
Diabetic-idiopathic	Third or sixth cranial nerve, pupil spared
Myasthenia gravis	As above
Brainstem stroke	As above

From Andreoli TE (ed): *Cecil essentials of medicine*, ed 4, Philadelphia, 1997, WB Saunders.
CSF, Cerebrospinal fluid; *IV,* intravenous.

ORAL MUCOSA, ERYTHEMATOUS LESIONS

Oral mucosa, erythematous lesions
ICD-9CM # 528.3 Oral abscess
              528.9 Oral disease (soft tissue)
              528.8 Hyperplasia tongue

TABLE 2-147   Erythematous Lesions

DISEASE	LOCATION	LESION CHARACTERISTICS	DIAGNOSIS	TREATMENT
Erythroplakia	Floor of mouth and retromolar trigone	Loss of surface keratin, painless, 50% invasive carcinoma	Biopsy	Wide local excision
Geographic tongue	Dorsum and lateral tongue	Loss of filiform papillae, appear as smooth erythematous patches with gray-white rims. Prominent fungiform papillae. Changing patterns	History—increased in patients with psoriasis and juvenile diabetes	Bland diet and anti-histamine mouthrinses if symptomatic, treatment does not eliminate condition
Stomatitis areata migrans	Buccal mucosa>labial and oral vestibules>floor of mouth>ventral tongue>soft palate>gingiva	Nonlingual form of geographic tongue; multiple flat, painless, irregularly shaped red patches; raised keratotic rims; heal and reappear	History—geographic tongue and fissured tongue associated with this condition	Antihistamine mouthrinses, antibiotics
Candidiasis	Dorsum of tongue and palate. Areas under dental prostheses	Erythematous or atrophic form—loss of epithelium and papillae	History Culture	Clotrimazole, nystatin
Allergy	Nonspecific oral cavity	Erythema multiforme. Lichenoid	Clinical	Remove offending agent
Plasma cell gingivitis (atypical allergic gingivostomatitis)	Gingiva>lips>buccal mucosa>tongue	Intense gingival erythema. Plasma cell infiltration	History—allergic reaction to ingredients in gum and toothpaste; biopsy	Remove offending agent
Pemphigus vulgaris	Nonspecific oral cavity or tongue. Skin	Intense erythema of oral cavity, geographic tongue, or small scattered white plaques	Clinical	Symptomatic

From Conn R: *Current diagnosis*, ed 9, Philadelphia, 1997, WB Saunders.
>, Greater than.

ORAL MUCOSA, PIGMENTED LESIONS

Oral mucosa, pigmented lesions
ICD-9CM # 528.3 Oral abscess
528.9 Oral disease (soft tissue)
528.8 Hyperplasia tongue

TABLE 2-148   Pigmented Lesions

DISEASE	LOCATION	LESION CHARACTERISTICS	DIAGNOSIS	TREATMENT
Racial pigmentation	Gingiva Buccal mucosa	Dark-skinned individuals; diffuse blue, black, brown color	Clinical	None, phenol peel for cosmesis
Oral melanotic macule	Lower lip>gingiva>buccal mucosa	Solitary dark lesion, <1 cm in diameter, light-skinned patients	Biopsy	None
Peutz-Jeghers syndrome	Lips, buccal mucosa, fingers, gingiva, palate, tongue	Autosomal dominant Oral melanosis, benign intestinal polyposis, macular deposits	Clinical	None
Neurofibromatosis	Lips and skin	Café au lait	Clinical	None
Albright's syndrome	Lips and skin—café au lait	Polyostotic fibrous dysplasia, precocious puberty, and cutaneous pigmentation	Clinical	None
Addison's disease	Diffuse/multifocal	Macular darkening of skin and mucosa	Clinical	None
Chloasma	Gingiva and skin	Macular darkening of skin and mucosa	Clinical	None
Drug reactions— quinacrine	Hard palate	Diffuse pigmentation	History	None
Drug reactions— Minocin, chlorpromazine, Myleran	Nonspecific oral pigmentation	Diffuse	History	None
Amalgam tattoo	Adjacent to dental silver restoration; buccal mucosa or gingiva	Solitary gray-black	Clinical	None
Lead line	Free gingival margin	Lead—precipitation of metal by sulfide-producing bacteria	Clinical	Remove offending agents/treat systemic disease
Argyria	Skin/mucous membrane	Silver—blue-gray		
Graphite	Submucosa	Graphite—black		
Smoker's melanosis	Anterior mandible and attached gingiva	Brown-black macules	Biopsy	None
Nevi	Hard palate>buccal mucosa>lip>gingiva>labial mucosa>soft palate>retromolar trigon>tongue	Flat or slightly raised gray, brown, or black macular lesions with irregular borders	Biopsy	Excision if lentigo maligna
Melanoma	Palate>maxillary gingiva>buccal mucosa>lip>mandibular gingival>tongue>floor of mouth	Pigmented macule or nodule, exophytic mass, 25% amelanotic, ulceration with irregular borders	Biopsy	Complete excision

From Conn R: *Current diagnosis*, ed 9, Philadelphia, 1997, WB Saunders.
>, Greater than; <, less than.

ORAL MUCOSA, PUNCTATE EROSIVE LESIONS

Oral mucosa, punctate erosive lesions
ICD-9CM # 528.3 Oral abscess
528.9 Oral disease, soft tissue
528.8 Hyperplasia tongue

TABLE 2-149   Punctate Erosive Lesions

DISEASE	LOCATION	LESION CHARACTERISTICS	DIAGNOSIS	TREATMENT
Herpes simplex virus	Lips and gingiva, may occur throughout the oral cavity	Vesicular phase, then ulcerative with erythematous halo; clustered on fixed mucosa	Tzanck preparation	Supportive and/or acyclovir for recurrent infection or immunosuppressed host
Coxsackievirus A and B	Predilection for posterior pharyngeal structures: tonsils, tonsillar pillars, soft palate	Multiple vesicles	Coxsackievirus B1-B5—throat swab with plating on PMK medium/serology; coxsackievirus A1-A10 and A27—exclusionary diagnosis	Supportive
Coxsackievirus A16	Lips, buccal mucosa, extremities (hands and feet)	Multiple vesicles	Clinical	Supportive
Herpes zoster	Extremities Palate	Exanthem, multiple vesicles	Tzanck preparation, serology, direct immunofluorescence	Supportive, acyclovir
Aphthous stomatitis	Affinity for lateral tongue, buccal mucosa, lips, floor of mouth	Solitary/multifocal shallow ulcers 2-5 mm, necrotic center with erythematous borders	Biopsy if lesions are large and persistent	Supportive, 1% triamcinolone I Orabase
Sutton's disease (giant aphthae)	As for aphthous stomatitis	Lesions may be 10-15 mm and can be associated with ulcerative colitis, Crohn's disease, gluten-sensitive enteropathy	As for aphthous stomatitis	As for aphthous stomatitis
Behçet's syndrome	Oral cavity, genitalia, eyes, and skin	Painful oral ulcerative lesions, yellow necrotic base, erythema	Clinical, HLA-B5	Supportive, prednisone, triamcinolone in Orabase, diphenhydramine syrup, colchicine
Reiter's syndrome	Soft palate, buccal mucosa, dorsum of tongue	Painless ulcers, arthritis, ocular and genital lesions	Culture to exclude gonorrhea, HLA-B27	NSAIDs, steroids
Neutropenia	Favors gingiva, but there may be diffuse oral cavity involvement	Ulcers with central necrosis	Medical and drug histories, CBC	Treat underlying condition
ANUG	Gingiva	Loss of interdental papillae, gray pseudomembrane with bleeding base	Clinical	Penicillin, oral rinses, gingival sealing, periodontal treatment
Drug reaction	Buccal mucosa, gingiva	Ulcerations of variable depth	Medical and drug histories	Remove offending agent
Crohn's disease and ulcerative colitis	Lips, gingiva, vestibular sulci	Small ulcers, fissures, angular cheilitis, hyperplastic lesions, glossitis	Medical history, biopsy, direct immunofluorescence	Steroids
Contact allergy	Adjacent to gold dental restoration	Erythematous, ulcerations	Clinical skin tests not reliable	Remove restoration

From Conn R: *Current diagnosis*, ed 9, Philadelphia, 1997, WB Saunders.
ANUG, Acute necrotizing ulcerative gingivostomatitis; *CBC,* complete blood count; *NSAIDs,* nonsteroidal antiinflammatory drugs.

ORAL MUCOSA, WHITE LESIONS

Oral mucosa, white lesions
ICD-9CM # 528.3 Oral abscess
528.9 Oral disease, soft tissue
528.8 Hyperplasia tongue

TABLE 2-150   White Lesions

DISEASE	LOCATION	LESION CHARACTERISTICS	DIAGNOSIS	TREATMENT
Leukoplakia	Buccal mucosa most common, but may occur anywhere in oral cavity	Histology—hyperkeratosis, parakeratosis, dyskeratosis, acanthosis. 2%-11% SCCA	Biopsy	Remove irritant, laser ablation, wide local excision
White, hairy leukoplakia	Lateral border of tongue more often than buccal or labial mucosa	Occurs exclusively in HIV-positive patients	HIV testing Biopsy	None
Squamous cell carcinoma	Tongue more often than floor of mouth	Hyperkeratotic, erythroplakic, granular, ulcerative with zone of central necrosis	Biopsy	Wide excision
Lichen planus	Skin and/or oral cavity, especially buccal mucosa	Reticular, ulcerative, erythematous, atrophic, bullous, plaque, and nummular forms	Biopsy Direct immuno-fluorescence	None
Stomatitis nicotina	Hard and soft palates	Microkeratotic papules with elevated red centers	Biopsy	None
Benign intra-epithelial dyskeratosis	Buccal mucosa, oral commissure, conjunctiva	Pathology—hyperkeratosis	Biopsy	None
White, spongy nevus of Cannon	Buccal mucosa, anogenital region	Onset—infancy Pathology—parakeratosis/acanthosis	Biopsy	None
Leukoedema	Bilateral buccal mucosa	Dark-skinned patients	Stretch mucosa with tongue blades	None
Darier-White disease	Predilection—buccal mucosa; also skin and genitalia	Broad areas of yellow-white papular keratotic lesions	Biopsy	Topical vitamin A
Pachyonychia congenita	Bilateral buccal lesions	Pathology—parakeratosis, acanthosis, dystrophic changes in nails, palmar/plantar hyperkeratosis	Biopsy	None
Candidiasis	Nonspecific oral cavity	Thick, white plaques that can be rubbed off to show bleeding base	Culture	Antifungals
Allergy	Mucosal area apposed to dental restoration	Lichenoid-type keratotic reaction	History	Remove offending agent
SLE	Buccal mucosa	Central atrophy or ulceration with peripheral radial hyperkeratotic striae	Biopsy ANA	Systemic steroids

From Conn R: *Curent diagnosis*, ed 9, Philadelphia, 1997, WB Saunders.
>, Greater than; *ANA*, antinuclear antibody test; *HIV*, human immunodeficiency virus; *SCCA*, squamous cell carcinoma; *SLE*, systemic lupus erythematosus.

ORAL VESICLES AND ULCERS

BOX 2-186   Oral Vesicles and Ulcers

Aphthous stomatitis
Primary herpes simplex infection
Vincent's stomatitis
Syphilis
Coxsackievirus A (herpangina)
Fungi (histoplasmosis)
Behçet's syndrome
Systemic lupus erythematosus
Reiter's syndrome
Crohn's disease
Erythema multiforme
Pemphigus
Pemphigoid

From Andreoli TE (ed): *Cecil essentials of medicine,* ed 5, Philadelphia, 2001, WB Saunders.

Oral vesicles and ulcers
ICD-9CM # 528.9

ORGASM DYSFUNCTION

BOX 2-187   Orgasm Dysfunction

Anorgasmia: inadequate stimulation or learning
Spinal cord lesion or injury
Multiple sclerosis
Alcoholic neuropathy
Amyotrophic lateral sclerosis
Spinal cord accident
Spinal cord trauma
Peripheral nerve damage
Radical pelvic surgery
Herniated lumbar disk
Hypothyroidism
Addison's disease
Cushing's disease
Acromegaly
Hypopituitarism
Pharmacologic agents (e.g., SSRIs, β-blockers)
Psychogenic

Modified from Danakas G (ed): *Practical guide to the care of the gynecologic/obstetric patient,* St Louis, 1997, Mosby.

Orgasm dysfunction
ICD-9CM # 302.73 Orgasm inhibited female
psychosexual
302.74 Orgasm inhibited male
psychosexual

OVULATORY DYSFUNCTION

Ovulatory dysfunction
ICD-9CM # 628.0 Anovulatory cycle
626.5 Ovulation pain

BOX 2-188   Ovulatory Dysfunction

Hyperandrogenic Anovulation

Polycystic ovarian syndrome
Late-onset congenital adrenal hyperplasias
Ovarian hyperthecosis
Androgen-producing ovarian tumors
Androgen-producing adrenal tumors
Cushing's syndrome

Hypoestrogenic Anovulation (Hypothalamic or Pituitary Etiology)

Hypogonadotropic Hypoestrogenic States

Reversible:
  Functional hypothalamic amenorrheas
    Eating disorders (anorexia nervosa, excessive weight loss)
    Excessive athletic training
  Neoplastic
    Craniopharyngioma
    Pituitary stalk compression
  Infiltrative diseases
    Histiocytosis-X
    Sarcoidosis
  Hypophysitis
  Pituitary adenomas
    Hyperprolactinemia
    Euprolactinemic galactorrhea

Endocrinopathies
  Hypothyroidism/hyperthyroidism
  Cushing's disease
Irreversible:
  Kallmann's syndrome
  Isolated gonadotropin deficiency (hypothalamic or pituitary origin)
  Panhypopituitarism/pituitary insufficiency
    Sheehan's syndrome, pituitary apoplexy
    Pituitary irradiation or ablation

Hypergonadotropic Hypoestrogenic States

Physiologic states
  Menopause
  Perimenopause
Premature ovarian failure
Immune-related
  Radiation/chemotherapy-induced
Ovarian dysgenesis
Turner's syndrome
46XX with mutations of X
Androgen insensitivity syndrome

Miscellaneous

Endometriosis
Luteal phase defect

From Kassirer J (ed): *Current therapy in adult medicine,* ed 4, St Louis, 1998, Mosby.

PALPITATIONS

Palpitations
ICD-9CM # 785.1 Palpitations

TABLE 2-151   Differential Diagnosis of Palpitations

CAUSE	NATURE OF PATIENT	NATURE OF SYMPTOMS	ASSOCIATED SYMPTOMS	PRECIPITATING AND AGGRAVATING FACTORS	PHYSICAL FINDINGS*	DIAGNOSTIC STUDIES†
Anxiety	Most common cause of palpitations in children and adolescents		Sweaty palms	Hyperventilation	Have patient hyperventilate for 3-4 min to see whether arrhythmias can be induced	
Ingestion of stimulants of drugs (caffeine, alcohol, amphetamines, cocaine)	Patients have decreased tolerance to these agents with increased age		Nervousness Tremor	Caffeine Alcohol Drugs (e.g., amphetamines, psychotropic agents, thyroid hormone)	Premature ventricular contractions Tachycardia	Toxicology screening tests
Digitalis glycosides			Nausea Anorexia	Increased digitalis dose Hypokalemia Hypomagnesemia Decreased renal function	Premature ventricular contractions Tachyarrhythmias Bradyarrhythmias Second- or third-degree heart block	Serum digitalis levels Electrocardiography Holter monitoring Serum potassium Serum magnesium Creatinine
β-blockers Antihypertensives Calcium channel blockers Hydralazine Minoxidil	Patients with angina or hypertension				Bradycardia	
					Sinus tachycardia	
Hypoglycemia	Insulin-dependent diabetics	Arrhythmias occur near time of peak insulin activity	Sweating Headache Tremor Weakness	Increased insulin Decreased carbohydrate	Premature ventricular contractions Tachycardia	Blood sugar
Hyperthyroidism	More common in older men	Atrial premature contractions May be silent	Nervousness Tremors Weight loss	Heart disease	Atrial fibrillation Premature contractions Tachycardias	Thyroid function tests
Exercise	Normal More frequent in patients with coronary heart disease, hypertension, mitral valve prolapse, and cardiomyopathy			Exercise		

From Seller RH (ed): *Differential diagnosis of common complaints*, ed 4, Philadelphia, 2000, WB Saunders.
*Arrhythmias are often absent.
†All arrhythmias should be documented by electrocardiography or Holter monitoring.

Continued

II

TABLE 2-151   Differential Diagnosis of Palpitations—cont'd

CAUSE	NATURE OF PATIENT	NATURE OF SYMPTOMS	ASSOCIATED SYMPTOMS	PRECIPITATING AND AGGRAVATING FACTORS	PHYSICAL FINDINGS*	DIAGNOSTIC STUDIES†
Reactive hypoglycemia		Recurrent arrhythmias in late afternoon and early evening; Arrhythmias occur several hours after ingestion of carbohydrates	Sweating Tremors Headache	Anxiety		5-hour glucose tolerance test
Cardiac disease						
Mitral valve prolapse	Most common in young women (average age, 38 yr)		Sticking chest pain	Exercise	Midsystolic click Late systolic murmur Premature ventricular contractions or premature atrial contractions Tachycardia	Echocardiography
Wolff-Parkinson-White syndrome	Often detected in children and adolescents	Recurrent palpitations Frequent paroxysmal tachycardia		Exercise Digitalis	Paroxysmal tachycardia	Electrocardiography Holter monitoring
Sick sinus syndrome	Older patients	Bradyarrhythmia Tachyarrhythmia	Chest pain Syncope Congestive heart failure Dizziness	Exercise Digoxin β-blockers Calcium channel blockers	Bradyarrhythmia Tachyarrhythmia	Electrocardiography Holter monitoring Electrophysiologic studies
Coronary artery disease	Older patients	Palpitations	Angina pectoris Congestive heart failure		Premature ventricular contractions Paroxysmal atrial fibrillation	Exercise electrocardiography Holter monitoring

From Seller RH (ed): *Differential diagnosis of common complaints,* ed 4, Philadelphia, 2000, WB Saunders.
*Arrhythmias are often absent.
†All arrhythmias should be documented by electrocardiography or Holter monitoring.

PANCYTOPENIA

Pancytopenia
ICD-9CM # 284.8

BOX 2-189   Causes of Pancytopenia

1. Pancytopenia with hypocellular bone marrow
   a. Acquired aplastic anemia
   b. Constitutional aplastic anemia
   c. Exposure to chemical or physical agents, including ionizing irradiation and chemotherapeutic agents
   d. Some hematologic malignancies, including myelodysplasia and aleukemic leukemia
2. Pancytopenia with normal or increased cellularity of hematopoietic origin
   a. Some hematologic malignancies, including myelodysplasia, and some leukemias, lymphomas, and myelomas
   b. Paroxysmal nocturnal hemoglobinuria
   c. Hypersplenism
   d. Vitamin B_{12}, folate deficiencies
   e. Overwhelming infection
3. Pancytopenia with bone marrow replacement
   a. Tumor metastatic to marrow
   b. Metabolic storage diseases
   c. Osteopetrosis
   d. Myelofibrosis

From Stein JH (ed): *Internal medicine,* ed 5, St Louis, 1998, Mosby.

PAPILLEDEMA

Papilledema
ICD-9CM # 377.00 Papilledema NOS
          377.02 With decreased ocular pressure
          377.01 With increased intracranial pressure
          377.03 With retinal disorder

BOX 2-190   Papilledema

CNS infections (viral, bacterial, fungal)
Medications (lithium, cisplatin, corticosteroids, tetracycline, etc.)
Head trauma
CNS neoplasm (primary or metastatic)
Pseudotumor cerebri
Cavernous sinus thrombosis
Systemic lupus erythematosus
Sarcoidosis

Subarachnoid hemorrhage
Carbon dioxide retention
Arnold-Chiari malformation and other developmental or congenital malformations
Orbital lesions
Central retinal vein occlusion
Hypertensive encephalopathy
Metabolic abnormalities

CNS, Central nervous system.

PARALYSIS

TABLE 2-152   Paralysis: Diagnostic Considerations

	GUILLAIN-BARRÉ SYNDROME	SECONDARY POLYNEUROPATHY	POLIOMYELITIS	TICK-BITE PARALYSIS	TRANSVERSE MYELITIS/ NEUROMYELITIS OPTICA
Etiology	Unknown; role of viral, mycoplasm infections unknown	Infectious or inflammatory: viral, bacterial (diphtheria, botulism), immunizations; autoimmune; intoxication	Poliovirus	Toxin release by tick	Unknown but may be inflammatory and related to multiple sclerosis
Prodrome	Nonspecific respiratory gastrointestinal symptoms 5-14 days before onset	Low-grade fever and other signs and symptoms reflecting the underlying disease	Fever, respiratory or gastrointestinal symptoms; may have meningism	1 wk after tick bites and remains attached; fatigue, irritability	
Neurologic findings	Symmetric flaccid ascending paralysis; greater involvement of lower extremities, greater proximally; facial diplegia, cranial nerve, bulbar involved; muscle tenderness; sensory-distal hyperesthesia with impaired position, vibration	Variable involvement; flaccid paralysis with loss of DTR and position and vibration senses; ataxia; cranial nerve involvement with dysphagia; generalized weakness	Flaccid, asymmetric paralysis with maximum deficit 3-5 days after onset; lower extremities more involved than upper; bulbar involvement may occur very early; sensory examination normal; marked muscle tenderness, pain, fasciculations, and twitching	Rapid progression of muscle pain with ascending flaccid symmetric paralysis; pain and paresthesias	Rapid progression; may have ataxia, weakness, multiple neurologic deficits; optic neuritis; paralysis develops with sensory loss below lesion and hyperesthesia above; bowel and bladder problems
Ancillary data	CSF: few WBC, high protein after 10 days	CSF: few monocytes with high protein; tests to determine underlying disease; nerve conduction velocity	CSF: pleocytosis (initially PMN, then monocytes), elevated protein level	CSF: normal	CSF: (not done routinely) pleocytosis, increased protein level; myelogram if indicated
Comments	Peaks in 5- to 9-yr-old children; usual recovery in 1-3 wk; supportive care and IV gamma globulin*	Major systemic illness reflects nature of underlying disease	May be asymptomatic or nonparalytic; summer epidemic; unimmunized individuals	Tick usually attached to head or neck; rapid improvement with removal of tick	Steroids (ACTH) may be useful in treatment

From Barkin RM, Rosen P: *Emergency pediatrics*, St Louis, 1999, Mosby.
ACTH, Adrenocorticotropic hormone; *CSF*, cerebrospinal fluid; *DTR*, deep tendon reflex; *WBC*, white blood cells.
*Gamma globulin, 400 mg/kg/24 hr q24hr IV.

Paralysis
ICD-9CM # 344.9 Paralysis unspecified
357.0 Guillain-Barré syndrome
045.1 Poliomyelitis, acute paralytic
357.5 Polyneuropathy, alcoholic
357.6 Polyneuropathy due to drugs
357.2 Diabetic polyneuropathy

PARANEOPLASTIC SYNDROMES, ENDOCRINE

TABLE 2-153   Endocrine Paraneoplastic Syndromes

SYNDROME	MEDIATOR	ASSOCIATED MALIGNANCY
Hypercalcemia	Parathyroid hormone (parathormone, PTH) or PTH-like substance Osteoclast-activating factors Prostaglandins Tumor growth factor, alpha Interleukin-1 Tumor necrosis factor Lymphotoxin	Breast cancer Squamous cell carcinoma of lung, head and neck, esophagus Multiple myeloma Renal cell carcinoma
Syndrome of inappropriate secretion of antidiuretic hormone	Antidiuretic hormone	Small cell carcinoma of lung Head and neck carcinomas Hodgkin's disease Non-Hodgkin's lymphoma
Hypoglycemia	Insulin Insulin-like peptides	Insulinoma Mesenchymal tumors, including mesothelioma, fibrosarcoma, neurofibrosarcoma, rhabdomyosarcoma
Zollinger-Ellison syndrome	Gastrin	Gastrinoma
Ectopic secretion of human chorionic gonadotropin	Human chorionic gonadotropin	Germ cell tumors containing trophoblastic elements
Cushing's syndrome	Adrenocorticotropic hormone	Lung carcinoma

From Stein J (ed): *Internal medicine*, ed 5, St Louis, 1998, Mosby.

Paraneoplastic syndromes, nonendocrine
ICD-9CM # Code varies with specific disorder

Paraneoplastic syndromes, endocrine
ICD-9CM # Code varies with specific disorder

PARANEOPLASTIC SYNDROMES, NONENDOCRINE

BOX 2-191   Nonendocrine Paraneoplastic Syndromes

Cutaneous

Dermatomyositis
Acanthosis nigricans
Sweet's syndrome
Erythema gyratum repens
Systemic nodular panniculitis (Weber-Christian disease)

Renal

Nephrotic syndrome
Nephrogenic diabetes insipidus

Neurologic

Subacute cerebellar degeneration
Progressive multifocal leukoencephalopathy
Subacute motor neuropathy
Sensory neuropathy
Ascending acute polyneuropathy (Guillain-Barré syndrome)
Myasthenic syndrome (Eaton-Lambert syndrome)

Hematologic

Microangiopathic hemolytic anemia
Migratory thrombophlebitis (Trousseau's syndrome)
Anemia of chronic disease

Rheumatologic

Polymyalgia rheumatica
Hypertrophic pulmonary osteoarthropathy

From Stein J (ed): *Internal medicine*, ed 5, St Louis, 1998, Mosby.

PARAPLEGIA

BOX 2-192 Paraplegia

Trauma: penetrating wounds to motor cortex, fracture-dislocation of vertebral column with compression of spinal cord or cauda equina, prolapsed disk, electrical injuries

Neoplasm: parasagittal region, vertebrae, meninges, spinal cord, cauda equina, Hodgkin's disease, non-Hodgkin's lymphoma, leukemic deposits, pelvic neoplasms

Multiple sclerosis and other demyelinating disorders

Mechanical compression of spinal cord, cauda equina, or lumbosacral plexus: Paget's disease, kyphoscoliosis, herniation of intervertebral disk, spondylosis, ankylosing spondylitis, rheumatoid arthritis, aortic aneurysm

Infections: spinal abscess, syphilis, tuberculosis, poliomyelitis, leprosy

Thrombosis of superior sagittal sinus

Polyneuritis: Guillain-Barré syndrome, diabetes, alcohol, beri-beri, heavy metals

Heredofamilial muscular dystrophies

Amyotrophic lateral sclerosis

Congenital and familial conditions: syringomyelia, myelomeningocele, myelodysplasia

Hysteria

Paraplegia
ICD-9CM # 344.1 Paraplegia, acquired
343.0 Paraplegia, congenital
438.50 Paraplegia, late effect of CVA

PARESTHESIAS

Paresthesias
ICD-9CM # 782.0

BOX 2-193 Paresthesias

Multiple sclerosis

Nutritional deficiencies (thiamin, vitamin B_{12}, folic acid)

Compression of spinal cord or peripheral nerves

Medications (isoniazid, lithium, nitrofurantoin, gold, cisplatin, hydralazine, amitriptyline, sulfonamides, amiodarone, metronidazole, dapsone, disulfiram, chloramphenicol, etc.)

Toxic chemicals (lead, arsenic, cyanide, mercury, organophosphates, etc.)

Diabetes mellitus

Myxedema

Alcohol

Sarcoidosis

Neoplasms

Infections (Human immunodeficiency virus, Lyme disease, herpes zoster, leprosy, diphtheria)

Charcot-Marie-Tooth disease and other hereditary neuropathies

Guillain-Barré neuropathy

PAROTID SWELLING

BOX 2-194 Differential Diagnosis of Parotid Swelling

Infectious

Mumps
Parainfluenza
Influenza
Cytomegalovirus infection
Coxsackievirus infection
Lymphocytic choriomeningitis
Echovirus infection
Suppuration (bacterial)
Actinomyces infection
Mycobacterial infection
Cat-scratch disease

Noninfectious

Drug hypersensitivity (thiouracil, phenothiazines, thiocyanate, iodides, copper, isoprenaline, lead, mercury, phenylbutazone)
Sarcoidosis
Tumors, mixed
Hemangioma, lymphangioma
Sialectasis

Sjögren syndrome
Mikulicz syndrome (scleroderma, mixed connective tissue disease, systemic lupus erythematosus)
Recurrent idiopathic parotitis
Pneumoparotitis
Trauma
Sialolithiasis
Foreign body
Cystic fibrosis
Malnutrition (marasmus, alcohol cirrhosis)
Dehydration
Diabetes mellitus
Waldenström macroglobulinemia
Reiter syndrome
Amyloidosis

Nonparotid Swelling

Hypertrophy of masseter muscle
Lymphadenopathy
Rheumatoid mandibular joint swelling
Tumors of jaw
Infantile cortical hyperostosis

Modified from Marks MI: Mumps. In Braude AI, Davis CE, Fierer J (eds): *Infectious diseases and medical microbiology*, ed 2, Philadelphia, 1986, WB Saunders.

Parotid swelling
ICD-9CM # 527.2 Allergic parotitis
72.9 Infectious parotitis
527.8 Salivary gland obstruction
527.5 Salivary gland obstruction with calculus
527.8 Salivary gland stricture
527.3 Salivary gland abscess
235.1 Salivary gland neoplasm

PELVIC MASS

Pelvic mass
ICD-9CM # 789.39

BOX 2-195 Differential Diagnosis of Pelvic Masses

Benign
Ovarian

Simple cyst (follicle or corpus luteum)
Hemorrhagic cyst
Cystadenoma
Endometrioma
Teratoma
Other benign tumors: papilloma, fibroma

Nonovarian

Leiomyoma
Paraovarian cyst
Hydrosalpinx
Tuboovarian abscess
Ectopic pregnancy
Intrauterine pregnancy

Diverticulitis
Appendiceal abscess
Peritoneal inclusion cyst

Malignant
Ovarian

Epithelial ovarian carcinoma
Germ cell tumors of the ovary
Borderline tumors

Nonovarian

Leiomyosarcoma
Endometrial cancer
Carcinoma of fallopian tube
Colorectal carcinoma

From Carlson KJ et al: *Primary care of women*, St Louis, 1995, Mosby.

PELVIC PAIN, CHRONIC

Pelvic pain, chronic
ICD-9CM # 625.9 Pelvic pain, female
789.09 Pelvic pain, male

BOX 2-196   Causes of Chronic Pelvic Pain

Gynecologic Disorders

Primary dysmenorrhea
Endometriosis
Adenomyosis
Adhesions
Fibroids
Retained ovary syndrome after hysterectomy
Previous tubal ligation
Chronic pelvic infection

Musculoskeletal Disorders

Myofascial pain syndrome

Gastrointestinal Disorders

Irritable bowel syndrome
Inflammatory bowel disease

Urinary Tract Disorders

Interstitial cystitis
Nonbacterial urethritis

From Carlson KJ et al: *Primary care of women*, St Louis, 1995, Mosby.

PELVIC PAIN, GENITAL ORIGIN

BOX 2-197   Causes of Acute Pelvic Pain of Genital Origin

Peritoneal Irritation

Ruptured ectopic pregnancy*
Ovarian cyst rupture*
Ruptured tuboovarian abscess*
Uterine perforation*

Torsion

Ovarian cyst or tumor*
Pedunculated fibroid*

Intratumor Hemorrhage or Infarction

Ovarian cyst*
Solid ovarian tumor*
Uterine leiomyoma*

Infection

Endometritis
Pelvic inflammatory disease
Trichomonas cervicitis or vaginitis
Tuboovarian abscess*

Pregnancy-Related
First Trimester

Ectopic pregnancy*
Abortion*
Corpus luteum hematoma*

Late Pregnancy

Placental problems*
Preeclampsia*
Premature labor*

Miscellaneous

Endometriosis
Foreign objects*
Pelvic adhesions
Pelvic neoplasm
Primary dysmenorrhea

From Rosen P (ed): *Emergency medicine*, ed 5, St Louis, 2002, Mosby.
*Potentially requires surgical management.

Pelvic pain, genital origin
ICD-9CM # 625.9 Pelvic pain, female
789.09 Pelvic pain, male

PERIPHERAL VASCULAR DISEASES

TABLE 2-154   Peripheral Vascular Diseases

Peripheral vascular diseases
ICD-9CM # 443.9 Peripheral vascular disease, NOS
250.7 Peripheral vascular disease, diabetic:
5th digit
  0. Type 2 diabetes mellitus, controlled
  1. Type 1 diabetes mellitus, controlled
  2. Type 2 diabetes mellitus, uncontrolled
  3. Type 1 diabetes mellitus, uncontrolled

DISEASE	PATHOLOGY	CLINICAL FEATURES	PHYSICAL FINDINGS	LABORATORY FINDINGS	TREATMENT
Atherosclerotic occlusive peripheral vascular disease	Atherosclerotic narrowing of large and medium-sized arteries of lower extremities; segmental with skip areas; occasionally involves upper extremities	Male > female Common in diabetics Exertional leg pain relieved with rest (claudication); rest pain with severe disease Buttock claudication and impotence with aortoiliac disease (Leriche's syndrome)	Decreased or absent lower extremity pulses Aortic, iliac, or femoral bruits Limb ischemia: cool, pale, cyanotic, shiny, hairless skin; ulcerations, gangrene	Decreased ankle:brachial index Arterial narrowing or obstruction on duplex examination or angiography	Intermittent claudication: Exercise as tolerated Stop smoking Avoid peripheral vaso-constricting drugs (e.g., β-blockers) Meticulous skin and nail care Pentoxifylline, cilostazol Severe claudication or rest ischemia: Percutaneous angioplasty or surgical bypass; amputation if gangrene
Thromboangiitis obliterans (Buerger's disease)	Intimal proliferation and thrombi in small to medium-sized vessels with inflammatory infiltrates Segmental involvement of arteries and veins Upper and lower extremity involvement	Male > female Usually <age 30 Symptoms related to smoking Cool extremities Raynaud's phenomenon Distal limb claudication (instep or hand) Sudden onset limb pain	Cool extremities Digital ulcers Migratory thrombophlebitis	Characteristic findings on angiogram	Smoking cessation Sympathectomy to prevent vasospasm Amputation of gangrenous digits
Arterial embolism	May originate from the aorta or heart	Sudden onset of painful extremity (occasionally more gradual)	Cool, pale, painful extremity with absent pulses distal to embolus	Pathologic examination of embolus may reveal etiology	Heparin Embolectomy for larger vessels Chronic anticoagulation if source cannot be removed

From Andreoli TE (ed): *Cecil essentials of medicine*, ed 5, Philadelphia, 2001, WB Saunders.

TABLE 2-154   Peripheral Vascular Diseases—cont'd

DISEASE	PATHOLOGY	CLINICAL FEATURES	PHYSICAL FINDINGS	LABORATORY FINDINGS	TREATMENT
Atheroembolism	Atheromatous debris ± thrombus, usually from aorta	Can be asymptomatic May follow intravascular procedures Digital (toe) ischemia common	Blue digits, livedo reticularis, renal insufficiency, guaiac + stool, abdominal petechiae	Eosinophilia, low complement levels Skin or renal biopsy may reveal cholesterol emboli	Resection of source of debris, if possible Heparin relatively contraindicated
Takayasu's arteritis	Probably immunologic Intimal proliferation and fibrosis of the aortic wall Involves the aortic arch and its branches May involve renal arteries	Women > men Systemic symptoms common (malaise, fever, weight loss)	Diminished or absent pulses Hypertension and aortic insufficiency common	Elevated erythocyte sedimentation rate Characteristic pattern on arteriogram	Glucocorticoids reduce symptoms Surgical or percutaneous revascularization for threatened vascular territories
Raynaud's phenomenon	Vasospasm of digital vessels precipitated by cold	Primary: Female > male; age <40; no underlying condition Secondary: Male > female; age >40; multiple underlying conditions (arterial occlusive disease, connective tissue disease, neurologic disease, vasoconstricting drugs, cryoglobulinemia, cold agglutinins, post frostbite)	Triphasic color changes: white on exposure to cold, followed by blue (cyanosis), followed by red on rewarming (hyperemia) Normal pulses unless underlying arterial occlusive disease Small areas of digital gangrene in severe cases, but amputation rare	Depends on underlying condition	Limitation of cold exposure Treat underlying condition Smoking cessation Vasodilators Regional sympathectomy in severe cases

PERSONALITY DISORDERS

TABLE 2-155 Schema for Personality Disorders

DSM-IV	COMMON PHYSICIAN REACTIONS	PATIENT CORE BELIEFS AND THOUGHTS	PATIENT FEARS	PATIENT BEHAVIOR
Paranoid	Fearful; sense of danger; mistrust; feeling accused, blamed, or threatened	Others are adversaries and are to blame; I am being examined; they are out to get me; I can't trust anyone	Exploitation, slights, betrayal, humiliation, physical intrusion from medical procedures	Wariness, suspicion, mistrust, jealousy, self-sufficiency, counterattacking, anger, violence
Schizoid	Detached or removed; wish to involve patient with others to break through the isolation	I need space; I need to be alone; people are replaceable or unimportant	Emotional contact, warmth, intimacy, caring, intrusion or violation of privacy	Withdrawal, seeking isolation and privacy
Schizotypal	Detached, removed, "weird and alone" feelings, wish to involve or to break through the isolation	Idiosyncratic, magical, or eccentric beliefs; I know what they're thinking/feeling; premonitions	Emotional contact; warmth, caring; violation of privacy	Withdrawal; odd, autistic and/or magical behavior and movements; seeks isolation and privacy
Antisocial	Used, exploited, or deceived; anger, wish to uncover lies, punish, or imprison	People are there to be used and exploited; I come before all others	Boredom; loss of prestige, power, or esteem	Lies, deceit, and manipulation; violence; seeks secondary gain
Histrionic	Flattered, captivated, seduced, aroused; wish to rescue, flooded by emotions, depleted	I need to impress, to be admired/loved; I need to be taken care of or helped	Loss of love, admiration, attention, or dependent care	Dramatics, exhibitionism, expressiveness, impressionistic
Borderline	Feeling manipulated, angry, impotent, depleted, self-doubting; wish to rescue or get rid of the patient; guilty	I am very bad or very good, who am I? I can't be alone	Separation, loss; emotional abandonment; not being loved and cared for; fluctuating self-esteem	Impulsive behavior; suicidal actions; cutting; anger/violence; panic; anxiety; poor reality; stormy relationships
Narcissistic	Devalued/overvalued; inferior/superior; fearful of patient's criticism or anger; wish to retaliate, get rid of, or devalue the patient	I am special. I am important. I come first. The world should revolve around me	Loss of prestige, image, power, or esteem	Self-aggrandizement, inflated/deflated self-view, entitled, devalue/idealize, viciousness, envy, competitive
Avoidant	Frustrated because the patient often can't articulate fears, annoyed at the patient's weakness	I must avoid harm and be cautious, or I may get rejected, exposed, or be humiliated	Rejection, embarrassment in social situations, humiliation, exposure of inadequacies	Avoidance, withdrawal, social timidity, caution, fear/anxiety
Dependent	Depleted, annoyed at the patient's dependence, may deny the patient's reasonable needs	I am helpless without others; I can't make a decision; I need constant reassurance and care	Separation, independence, making decisions, anger	Unusually submissive; clinging, indecisive, childlike, needing to be taken care of
Obsessive-compulsive	In a battle of control; negative reactions to patient stinginess, need for order, and stubbornness; distanced from feelings; bored with details	People should do better, try harder; I must be perfect, make no errors or mistakes; details rule, not feelings	Disorder, mistakes, imperfection; feelings, especially rage/anger; anxiety, self-doubt, dependency	Perfectionism, driven orderliness; logical, compulsions, controlling, critical; stubbornness, stinginess; workaholic; overly rational
DSM III-R self-defeating	Wish to rescue, sadistic fantasies that the patient will suffer or die, defeated; self-blame, self-doubt or hope, helplessness	I must suffer and sacrifice; I am a martyr; I should be punished	Loss of love, pleasure, recovery	Feels worse with good news, self-defeating and self-destructive

From Rakel RE (ed): *Principles of family practice*, ed 6, Philadelphia, 2002, WB Saunders. *DSM, Diagnostic and Statistical Manual of Mental Disorders.*

TABLE 2-156 Patient Defenses and Physician Interventions

DSM-IV	PATIENT DEFENSES	NEUROTIC BORDERLINE PSYCHOTIC	PHYSICIAN INTERVENTIONS
Paranoid	**Projection:** ascribe to others one's impulses. **Projective identification:** project one's impulse plus control of others as a way to control one's own impulses. **Denial:** refusal to admit painful realities. **Splitting:** self and others are seen as all good or all bad	PPO or BPO	(1) Empathize with patient's fear of being hurt. Acknowledge complaints w/o arguing or ignoring. (2) Openly and honestly explain medical illness. (3) Correct reality distortions and unreasonable patient expectations. (4) Gently question irrational thoughts and suggest more rational ones. (5) Don't confront delusions. (6) If the patient refuses care out of mistrust, rather than insist, ask if it's OK if you can disagree about the need for the test. (7) Interpret projection (blame) and other defenses
Schizoid	**Isolation of affect:** thoughts stored without emotion. **Intellectualization:** replace feelings with facts. **Denial** and **splitting:** see above. **Regression:** revert to childlike thoughts, feelings, and behavior	PPO or BPO	(1) Empathize with patient's need for both privacy and contact. (2) Accept the patient's unsociability. (3) Reduce the patient's isolation as tolerated. (4) Neutrally impart medical information. (5) Don't demand involvement or permit total withdrawal. (6) Correct reality distortions and unreasonable patient expectations. (7) Gently question irrational thoughts and suggest more rational ones. (8) Interpret isolation and other defenses
Schizotypal	**Schizoid fantasy:** retreat to idiosyncratic fantasy when faced with a painful experience. **Undoing:** symbolic magical action designed to reverse or cancel unacceptable thoughts or actions. **Regression, denial,** and **splitting:** see above	PPO or BPO	(1) Empathize with patient's idiosyncratic style, magical thinking, and perceptions without directly confronting patient. (2) Recognize the need for privacy and contact. (3) Accept the patient's unsociability and reduce the patient's isolation as tolerated. (4) Neutrally impart information. (5) Don't demand involvement or permit total withdrawal. (6) Correct reality distortions and unreasonable patient expectations. (7) Gently question irrational thoughts and suggest more rational ones. (8) Interpret regression and other defenses
Antisocial	**Acting out:** expression in action and behavior rather than words or emotions. **Splitting:** see above	BPO; with stress, PPO	(1) Empathize with patient's fear of exploitation and low self-esteem. (2) Determine if you are being used for secondary gain. Should you suspect dishonesty, verify symptoms and illness progression with others. (3) Don't moralize. Explain that deception results in your giving the patient poor care. (4) Correct reality distortions and unreasonable patient expectations. (5) Gently question irrational thoughts and suggest more rational ones. (6) Interpret defenses
Histrionic	**Sexualization:** functions or objects are changed into sexual symbols to avoid anxieties. **Regression, acting out,** and **splitting:** see above. **Dissociation:** disrupted perceptions or sensations, consciousness, memory, or personal identity. **Somatization:** physical symptoms caused by mental processes. **Repression:** involuntary forgetting of painful memories, feeling, or experience	BPO/NPO; with stress, PPO	(1) Empathize with patient's fear of losing love or care. (2) Interact in a friendly way, not too reserved or too warm. (3) Discuss the patient's fears; reassure when possible. (4) Use logic to counteract an emotional style of thinking. (5) Limit-set if patient regresses. (6) Correct reality distortions and unreasonable patient expectations. (7) Gently question irrational thoughts and suggest more rational ones. (8) Interpret sexualization, regression, and other specific defenses

From Rakel RE (ed): *Principles of family practice*, ed 6, Philadelphia, 2002, WB Saunders.
BPO, Borderline personality organization; *DSM, Diagnostic and Statistical Manual of Mental Disorders; NPO,* neurotic personality organization; *PPO,* psychotic personality organization.

TABLE 2-156 Patient Defenses and Physician Interventions—cont'd

DSM-IV	PATIENT DEFENSES	NEUROTIC BORDERLINE PSYCHOTIC	PHYSICIAN INTERVENTIONS
Borderline	**Splitting, projection, projective identification, dissociation/ regression, acting out:** see above. **Omnipotence:** seeing self or others as all-powerful. **Idealization/ devaluation:** vacillate between seeing self or others as ideal and then deprecating self or others. **Minipsychotic experiences**	BPO; with stress, PPO	(1) Empathize with patient's fear of abandonment/separation and plan for absences by arranging coverage. (2) Express a wish to help and satisfy reasonable needs. (3) Ask the patient to monitor impulsive behavior with a diary or log. (4) Set firm limits and do not punish. (5) Correct reality distortions and unreasonable patient expectations. (6) Gently question irrational thoughts and suggest more rational ones. (7) Interpret splitting and other defenses. (8) Negotiate emergency procedures in advance. If suicidal, the patient must go to the emergency room. If the patient refuses emergency help when offered, let the patient know in advance that this therapeutic breach may end the relationship
Narcissistic	**Splitting, projection, projective identification, acting out, denial,** and **regression:** see above	BPO/NPO; with stress, rarely PPO	(1) Empathize with patient's vulnerability and low self-esteem. (2) Don't mistake patient's superior attitude for real confidence and don't confront entitlement. (3) When you are devalued or attacked, acknowledge the patient's hurt and your mistakes and express your continued wish to help. (4) If devaluing continues, offer a referral as an option, not as punishment. (5) Correct reality distortions and unreasonable patient expectations. (6) Gently question irrational thoughts and suggest more rational ones. (7) Interpret splitting and other defenses
Avoidant	**Inhibition:** restriction of thoughts, feelings, and behavior to avoid shame, exposure or inadequacies, rejection, and humiliation. **Displacement:** transferring one's feelings from one person or object to another, which leads to phobias. **Phobias:** fears of objects, people, and/or situations that are avoided to prevent anxiety. **Avoidance/ withdrawal:** behavioral efforts to escape anxiety situations. **Regression** and **somatization:** see above	NPO/BPO; rarely PPO	(1) Empathize with patient's social fears, shame, shyness, and fears of revealing inadequacies, rejection, embarrassment, humiliation, and anger. (2) Help the patient describe in detail the feared situation(s). (3) Encourage and support the need for the patient to gradually face the fears and the tendency to avoid them. If this seems overwhelming, choose smaller fears to confront and/or refer. (4) If frustrated or unclear about the nature of the fears, ask for detailed descriptions of the problem. (5) Gently elicit irrational thoughts and suggest more rational ones. (6) Correct reality distortions. (7) Interpret avoidance/phobias and other defenses
Dependent	**Dependent:** yearning for care, clinging, and needing direction. **Passive-aggressive:** superficial compliance and passivity disguising stubbornness and anger. **Reaction formation:** unacceptable impulses expressed as the opposite. **Regression** and **splitting:** see above	NPO/BP; rarely PPO PPO or BPO	(1) Empathize with patient's need for care. (2) Frustrate total dependence. (3) Be careful to avoid telling the patient what to do. (4) Encourage independent thinking and action. (5) Realize that what the patient asks for (care taking) is not necessarily what is needed. (6) Ask the patient what it is about independence that is so frightening. (7) Don't abandon or threaten termination. Some very dependent patients need regular physician contact for life. (8) Correct reality distortions and unreasonable patient expectations. (9) Gently elicit irrational thoughts and suggest more rational ones. (10) Interpret regression and other specific defenses

Continued

TABLE 2-156 Patient Defenses and Physician Interventions—cont'd

DSM-IV	PATIENT DEFENSES	NEUROTIC BORDERLINE PSYCHOTIC	PHYSICIAN INTERVENTIONS
Obsessive-compulsive	**Isolation of affect, intellectualization, reaction formation,** and **undoing:** see above. **Controlling:** efforts to regulate objects or others to avoid anxiety. **Displacement:** transfer of feelings from one person to another. **Dependent:** see above. **Inhibition:** restricting thoughts, feelings, or behavior for fear that unacceptable impulses will erupt and create anxiety or damage. **Phobias** and **repression:** see above	BPO/NPO; rarely PPO	(1) Empathize with patient's logical, detailed, unemotional style of thinking. (2) If obsessive thoughts are interfering with medical care, ask about the patient's feelings. (3) Don't struggle with the patient over control and critical judgments. (4) Avoid abandoning the patient. (5) Correct reality distortions and unreasonable patient expectations. (6) Gently elicit irrational thoughts and suggest more rational ones. (7) Interpret specific defenses
DSM-III-R self-defeating	**Ambivalence:** coexistence of opposite feelings. **Displacement, denial, projective identification, reaction formation, passive-aggressive,** and **splitting:** see above	BPO/NPO; rarely PPO	(2) Empathize with patient's suffering. Acknowledge and appreciate the difficulty of the illness/treatments. (2) Emphasize that recovery may be a slow steady process. (3) The need for recovery can be presented as necessary to benefit others. (4) Inquire about obviously self-destructive or self-defeating behavior. (5) Don't abandon. (6) Correct reality distortions and unreasonable patient expectations. (7) Gently elicit irrational thoughts and suggest more rational ones. (8) Interpret specific defenses

PHOTOSENSITIVITY

Photosensitivity
ICD-9CM # 692.72

TABLE 2-157 Photosensitivity: Differential Considerations

	HISTORY	MORPHOLOGY AND PHYSICAL EXAMINATION	LABORATORY	MANAGEMENT
PML	26-yr-old woman: onset with extreme sun exposure; delayed onset 6-8 hr postexposure, lasts 7-10 days; pruritic	Papules, vesicles, or plaques; distribution includes face, neck, dorsal arms	Biopsy: superficial and deep mononuclear cell infiltrate	Topical corticosteroids, oral corticosteroids, β-carotene, PUVA, Trisoralen, antimalarial
Solar urticaria	Hives appear immediately with sun exposure, last 1-4 hr; pruritic	Urticaria appearing in sun-exposed areas	MED testing with UVA and UVB may reproduce lesions; biopsy: superficial perivascular mononuclear cell infiltrates	Antihistamines, UVB/UVA hardening, PUVA, oral corticosteroids
Phototoxic	Sunburn appears after minimal exposure; patient may have used new oral medications	Sunburn erythema with sharp cutoffs at non-exposed areas		Discontinue offending agent; oral corticosteroids; PUVA if becomes chronic
Photoallergic	Itchy dermatitis with sun exposure; patient may have used new topical product or oral medication	Eczematous dermatitis; may spread somewhat into non-sun-exposed areas	Reduced MED to UVA; biopsy: spongiosis in epidermis; superficial and deep mononuclear cell infiltrate	Same as above; topical corticosteroids
PCT	Estrogen or alcohol intake; history of skin fragility or blisters on hands	Vesicles and bullae on dorsal hands that heal with scarring and milia; mottled hypopigmentation of face; hyperpigmentation of the periorbital area	Biopsy: subepidermal bullae; increased uroporphyrin I and 7-carboxyl porphyrin III in urine; increased isocoproporphyrin in feces	Phlebotomy—500 ml/wk until clinical clearing occurs
SLE	Sunburn persists days or weeks with no further exposure; rash in butterfly distribution across nose; drugs associated with lupuslike syndrome	Long-lasting sunburn reaction; plaques in butterfly distribution of smaller area	Biopsy: positive ANA; positive Ro antigen; dif-band of fluorescent material at dermal epidermal junction	Chloroquine 125 to 250 mg twice weekly

From Noble J (ed): *Primary care medicine*, ed 3, St Louis, 2001, Mosby.
ANA, Antinuclear antibody; *MED*, minimum erythema dose; *PCT*, porphyria cutanea tarda; *PML*, polymorphous light eruption; *PUVA*, psoralen ultraviolet A; *SLE*, systemic lupus erythematosus; *UV*, ultraviolet.

II

PLATELET AGGREGATION DISORDERS

Platelet aggregation disorders
ICD-9CM # 287.1

TABLE 2-158   **Disorders Causing Abnormal Platelet Aggregation**

	RESPONSE TO AGONIST				
	EPINEPHRINE	ADP	COLLAGEN	ARACHADONIC ACID	RISTOCETIN
Aspirin/NSAIDs	#	#	NL, ↓*	↓	NL
Glanzmann's disease	Absent	Absent	Absent	Absent	#
Bernard-Soulier syndrome	NL	NL	NL	NL	Absent
Storage pool disease	↓	#	↓	NL, ↓	#
Hermansky-Pudlak syndrome	↓	#	↓	NL	#
Gray platelet syndrome	↓	↓	↓	NL	NL
vWD	NL	NL	NL	NL	↓, NL†

From Andreoli TE (ed): *Cecil essentials of medicine,* ed 5, Philadelphia, 2001, WB Saunders.

↓, Decreased; #, primary wave aggregation only; *NL,* normal; *NSAIDs,* nonsteroidal antiinflammatory drugs; *vWD,* von Willebrand's disease.

* Aspirin results in decreased aggregation with low-dose collagen, but aggregation is normal with high-dose collagen.

† In vWD type 2B, patients have increased aggregation with low-dose ristocetin, and decreased or normal aggregation with standard doses of ristocetin.

PLATELET FUNCTION INHIBITORS

Platelet function inhibitors
ICD-9CM # 287.1

BOX 2-198   **Drugs Affecting Platelet Function**

Strong Inhibitors

Abciximab (and other anti-gpIIb/IIIa or anti-RGD compounds)

Aspirin (often contained in over-the-counter medications)

Clopidogrel/ticlopidine (ADP receptor blockers)

Nonsteroidal antiinflammatory drugs

Moderate Inhibitors

Antibiotics (penicillins, cephalosporins, nitrofurantoin)

Dextran

Fibrinolytics

Heparin

Hetastarch

Weak Inhibitors

Alcohol

Nitroglycerin

Nitroprusside

From Andreoli TE (ed): *Cecil essentials of medicine,* ed 5, Philadelphia, 2001, WB Saunders.

PLEURAL EFFUSIONS

BOX 2-199   A. Causes of Pleural Effusions

Transudates

Common

Congestive heart failure
Cirrhosis

Less common

Nephrotic syndrome
Peritoneal dialysis
Urinothorax
Pulmonary embolism
Atelectasis
Superior venal caval obstruction

Exudates

Common

Parapneumonia
Malignancy
Pulmonary embolism

Less common

Tuberculosis
Nonbacterial infections: viral, fungal, parasitic
Pancreatitis, pseudocyst
Esophageal rupture
Endoscopic sclerotherapy
Subphrenic/liver abscess
Collagen vascular diseases
Dressler's syndrome
Drugs, including those causing drug-induced lupus
Benign asbestos effusion
Chylothorax
Uremia
Sarcoidosis
Meigs' syndrome
Yellow nail syndrome
Trauma
Amyloidosis
Vertebral osteomyelitis

B. Clues to the Cause of Pleural Effusion

History

Smoking
Asbestos exposure
Trauma
Drugs
Tuberculosis exposure
Cough with purulent sputum
Hemoptysis
Chills, fever
Joint pains, swelling, stiffness
Urinary obstruction
Present or recent subclavian venous line insertion
Recent abdominal surgery, orthopedic surgery, parturition, vomiting, abdominal pain, upper gastrointestinal endoscopy, sclerotherapy
History of congestive heart failure, nephrotic syndrome, cirrhosis, deep venous thrombosis, any malignant disease, cardiac surgery

Physical Examination

Clubbing of fingers
Yellow nails
Superior vena cava syndrome
Horner's syndrome
Cervical/supraclavicular/other lymphadenopathy
Rheumatoid subcutaneous nodules, joint swelling, deformity
Sclerodactyly, malar rash, Raynaud's phenomenon
Putrid breath, purulent sputum
Herpes labialis, fever
Jugular vein distention, S_3, rales, leg edema
Ascites
Abdominal tenderness, mass

From Noble J: *Primary care medicine*, ed 3, St Louis, 2001, Mosby.

PLEURAL EFFUSIONS, DRUG-INDUCED

BOX 2-200   Drugs That Can Cause a Pleural Effusion

Drugs that induce systemic lupus erythematosus, (diphenylhydantoin, hydralazine, isoniazid, procainamide)
Sclerosing agents for esophageal varices
Chemotherapeutic agents (e.g., procarbazine, methotrexate)
Tocolytics used for premature labor

Bromocriptine
Dantrolene
Methysergide
L-Tryptophan
Nitrofurantoin
Amiodarone

From Noble J (ed): *Primary care medicine*, ed 3, St Louis, 2001, Mosby.

Pleural effusions
ICD-9CM # 511.9 Pleural effusion, unspecified
        197.2 Pleural effusion, malignant
        997.3 Pleural effusion, post-op

PNEUMONIA, CHRONIC

BOX 2-201 Etiology of Chronic Pneumonia Syndrome

Infectious Agents That Typically Cause Chronic Pneumonia

Bacteria and actinomycetes
  Mixed aerobic-anaerobic bacteria
  Actinomyces spp.
  Propionibacterium propionicus
  Nocardia spp.
  Rhodococcus equi
  Burkholderia pseudomallei
Mycobacteria
  Mycobacterium tuberculosis
  Mycobacterium kansasii
  Mycobacterium avium complex
Fungi
  Aspergillus spp.
  Blastomyces dermatitidis
  Coccidioides immitis
  Cryptococcus neoformans
  Emmonsia
  Histoplasma capsulatum
  Sporothrix schenckii
  Paracoccidioides brasiliensis
Protozoa
  Entamoeba histolytica
Worms
  Echinococcus granulosus
  Schistosomes: *Schistosoma hematobium, Schistosoma japonicum, Schistosoma mansoni*
  Paragonimus westermani

Noninfectious Causes

Neoplasia
  Carcinoma (primary or metastatic)
  Lymphoma
Sarcoidosis
Amyloidosis
Vasculitis (autoimmune diseases)
  Systemic lupus erythematosus
  Polyarteritis nodosa

Allergic angiitis and granulomatosis (Churg-Strauss syndrome)
Progressive systemic sclerosis
Rheumatoid arthritis
Mixed connective tissue syndrome (overlap syndrome)
Wegener's granulomatosis
Lymphomatoid granulomatosis
Chemicals, drugs, or inhalation
Radiation
Recurrent pulmonary emboli
Bronchial obstruction with atelectasis (e.g., tumor, foreign body)
Pulmonary infiltration with eosinophilia syndrome
  Löffler syndrome—usually transient
  Tropical eosinophilia
  Pneumonia plus asthma (e.g., allergic bronchopulmonary aspergillosis)
  Bronchocentric granulomatosis
  Vasculitis
  Eosinophilic pneumonia—chronic
Pneumoconiosis
Chronic form of extrinsic allergic alveolitis (hypersensitivity pneumonitis)
Other lung disease—unknown cause
  Bronchiolitis obliterans organizing pneumonia
  Chronic interstitial pneumonia (fibrosing alveolitis, idiopathic pulmonary fibrosis)
    Usual interstitial pneumonia (UIP)
    Desquamative interstitial pneumonia (DIP)
    Lymphocytic interstitial pneumonia (LIP)
    Giant cell interstitial pneumonia (GIP)
  Eosinophilic granuloma (histiocytosis X)
  Lymphangioleiomyomatosis
  Goodpasture's syndrome
  Pulmonary alveolar proteinosis (phospholipoproteinosis)
  Pulmonary alveolar microlithiasis
  Idiopathic pulmonary hemosiderosis
  Angiocentric immunoproliferative lesions

From Mandell GL: *Mandell, Douglas, and Bennett's principles and practice of infectious diseases*, ed 5, New York, 2000, Churchill Livingstone.

PNEUMONIA, CHRONIC, RADIOLOGIC PATTERNS

Pneumonia, chronic, radiologic patterns
ICD-9CM # 486 Pneumonia, unspecified

TABLE 2-159 Radiologic Patterns of Diseases That Commonly Cause Chronic Pneumonia Syndrome

DISEASE	RADIOLOGIC CHARACTERISTICS
Diseases That Cause Patchy Infiltrates and/or Bronchopneumonia or Lobar Consolidation	
Infectious	
Aspiration pneumonia secondary to mixed aerobic and anaerobic infection	Usually dependent portions: superior or basilar segments of lower lobes or posterior segments of upper lobes; pleural involvement with empyema common
Necrotizing pneumonia secondary to infection by Enterobacteriaceae, *Psuedomonas aeruginosa,* or *Staphylococcus aureus*	Any lobe or segment Chronic *Klebsiella* pneumonia commonly involves upper lobes; may be multiple sites of pulmonary infection secondary to septic embolization
Actinomycosis	Commonly involves lower lobes; cavitation frequently present; pleural involvement with empyema common
Nocardiosis	No distinctive pattern; may involve single or multiple lobes; cavitation may be present; pleural involvement may occur
Tuberculosis exudative pneumonia	Not restricted to upper lobes; often bilateral with perihilar distribution
Blastomycosis	Often a dense area of lobar or segmental consolidation; cavitation infrequent
Cryptococcosis	Single or multiple patchy infiltrates; less commonly, lobar consolidation; occasionally, single or diffuse nodular lesions
Paracoccidioidomycosis	Asymptomatic bilateral fluffy infiltrates; may be extremely indolent
Noninfectious	
Chronic eosinophilic pneumonia	Rapidly progressive, dense infiltrates; usually peripheral (reverse pattern of pulmonary edema)
Bronchiolitis obliterans organizing pneumonia	Patchy nonsegmental areas of consolidation, often subpleural and bilateral; large irregular nodules
Diseases That Cause Pulmonary Cavitation	
Infectious	
Pyogenic lung abscess	
Complicating aspiration pneumonia	Usually single cavity; location same as aspiration pneumonia; air-fluid level common
Complicating necrotizing pneumonia	May involve any lobe; often multiple and bilateral, depending on route of acquisition of pneumonia
Tuberculosis-reactivation or adult type	Usually upper lobes; often bilateral; may be multiple; fibrosis and calcification common
Atypical mycobacterial disease	Radiologically indistinguishable from tuberculosis, except that cavitation may be more frequent
Melioidosis	Simulates tuberculosis, but may involve any lobe
Rhodococcal lung disease	Simulates tuberculosis or nocardiosis; cavitation common
Histoplasmosis, chronic cavitary	Mimics tuberculosis; upper lobes frequently involved but can involve any lobe; unilateral or bilateral
Coccidioidomycosis	Usually single, thin-walled cavity with minimum involvement of surrounding lung; occasionally thick-walled cavity surrounded by extensive parenchymal disease
Sporotrichosis	May mimic tuberculosis but can involve any lobe; cavitation is frequent; thin-walled cavity more likely than thick-walled cavity
Aspergillosis	Single or multiple areas of pneumonia with or without central cavitation; not to be confused with intracavitary fungus ball
Paragonimiasis	Cystlike lesions as well as cavities, usually associated with linear or patchy infiltrates, fibrosis, and/or calcification
Echinococcosis	Single or multiple discrete, sharply defined, round lesions (cysts) with little surrounding inflammatory response; cavitation and/or calcification may occur

From Mandell GL: *Mandell, Douglas, and Bennett's principles and practice of infectious diseases,* ed 5, New York, 2000, Churchill Livingstone.   *Continued*

II

TABLE 2-159   Radiologic Patterns of Diseases That Commonly Cause Chronic Pneumonia Syndrome—cont'd

DISEASE	RADIOLOGIC CHARACTERISTICS
Noninfectious	
Wegener's granulomatosis and lymphomatoid granulomatosis	Often multiple nodules with cavitation; may be unilateral or bilateral
Silicosis	Associated with conglomerate nodular densities, frequently in upper lobes; usually superimposed on background of diffuse nodulation; rarely, eggshell calcification of hilar nodes
Bronchogenic carcinoma	Eccentric cavitation more common in squamous cell type
Lymphoma, especially Hodgkin's disease	Cavitation may occur in peripheral parenchymal nodules
Kaposi's sarcoma	Small or large nodules associated with peribronchial cuffing and tram track opacities

Infectious and Noninfectious Diseases That Cause Chronic Diffuse Pulmonary Infiltration and Fibrosis

DISEASE	RADIOLOGIC CHARACTERISTICS
Bronchioloalveolar carcinoma Intrapulmonary bleeding (e.g., Goodpasture's syndrome) Pulmonary alveolar proteinosis	Alveolar pattern
Sarcoidosis Early asbestosis or berylliosis Bronchiolitis obliterans organizing pneumonia	Ground-glass interstitial pattern
Granulomatous infectious diseases (e.g., miliary tuberculosis, disseminated histoplasmosis) Sarcoidosis Lymphangitic carcinomatosis Wegener's granulomatosis Lymphomatoid granulomatosis Allergic angiitis and granulomatosis Rheumatoid lung disease Pneumoconiosis (including asbestosis, silicosis, and berylliosis)	Nodular interstitial pattern, including miliary spherical nodules
Chronic form of hypersensitivity pneumonitis Idiopathic pulmonary hemosiderosis Radiation injury—chronic Progressive systemic sclerosis Sarcoidosis	Linear interstitial pattern, including fine reticular markings and dense fibrosis
Advanced form of fibrosing alveolitis Bronchiectasis Eosinophilic granuloma (histiocytosis X) Sarcoidosis	Honeycombing (coarse reticular pattern with cystic airspaces)

From Mandell GL: *Mandell, Douglas, and Bennett's principles and practice of infectious diseases,* ed 5, New York, 2000, Churchill Livingstone.

Pneumonia, recurrent
ICD-9CM # 482.9 Bacterial pneumonia
          480.9 Viral pneumonia
          484.1 Fungal pneumonia
          485   Segmental pneumonia

PNEUMONIA, RECURRENT

BOX 2-202   Common Conditions Associated with Recurrent Pneumonia

Mechanical

Chronic obstructive pulmonary disease
Congestive heart failure
Asthma
Chronic sinusitis
Sarcoidosis*
Cerebral vascular accident
Pulmonary tuberculosis*
Kyphoscoliosis
Epilepsy
Bronchiectasis
Pulmonary resection
Systemic lupus erythematosus
Pulmonary fibrosis*
Silicosis

Immune

Alcoholism
Diabetes mellitus
Splenectomy
AIDS*
Malignancy
Systemic steroid use
Hemoglobinopathy

From Harrington J (ed): *Consultation in internal medicine*, ed 2, St Louis, 1997, Mosby.
*Designates diagnoses that can cause bronchiectasis.

PNEUMONITIDES, HYPERSENSITIVITY, OCCUPATIONAL

Pneumonitides, hypersensitivity, occupational
ICD-9CM # 495.9 Pneumonitis, hypersensitivity

TABLE 2-160 Occupational Hypersensitivity Pneumonitides

DISEASE	EXPOSURE	SPECIFIC INHALANT
Farmer's lung	Moldy hay	*Thermoactinomyces vulgaris*
		T. candidus
		T. viridis
		Micromonospora faeni
Bagassosis	Moldy sugar cane	*T. vulgaris*
		T. sacchare
Maple bark–stripper's lung	Contaminated maple logs	*Cryptostroma corticale*
Bird-breeder's lung	Avian droppings	Serum protein
Air conditioner, humidifier lung	Contaminated water	*T. vulgaris*
		T. candidus
		Amoeba species
		Endotoxin
Mushroom-worker's lung	Mushroom compost	*T. vulgaris*
		M. Faeni
Malt-worker's lung	Moldy barley	*Aspergillus clavatus*
		A. fumigatus
Bakers asthma	Flour dust	Wheat flour
Detergent-worker's lung	Detergent powder	*Bacillus subtilis*
Grain weevil (miller's) lung	Grain dust	*Sitophilus granarius*
	Flour	
Suberosis	Oak bark	*Penicillium frequentans*
	Cork dust	
Furrier's lung	Fox	Hair protein
Coffee-worker's lung	Coffee bean dust	Coffee bean protein
Vineyard-sprayer's lung	Spray solution	Copper sulfate
		T. viridis
Sequoiosis	Redwood sawdust	*Graphium* species
		Aureobasidium pullulans
Cheese-washer's lung	Cheese mold	*Penicillium caseii*
		P. roqueforti
Fish meal–handler's lung	Fish meal (pet food)	Fish proteins
Wood-dust disease	Mahogany and oak dust	Unknown
Wood pump–worker's lung	Moldy logs	*Alternaria tenuis*
Paprika-slicer's lung	Moldy paprika pods	*Mucor stolonifer*
Fog fever	Cattle	*T. candidus*
Feather-plucker's lung	Chicken products	Chicken proteins
Tobacco-grower's lung	Tobacco plants	Unknown
Tea-grower's lung	Tea plants	Unknown
Bible-printer's disease	Moldy typesetting water	Unknown
Plastics and resin makers	Plastics industry	Toluene diisocyanate
	Polyurethane	Methylene diphenyldiisocyanate
	Paints	Hexamethylene diisocyanate
Painters and paint makers	Sand binders	Trimellitic anhydride

From Noble J: *Primary care medicine,* ed 3, St Louis, 2001, Mosby.

Polycythemias
ICD-9CM # 790.0 Polycythemia NOS
          289.0 Acquired
          289.6 Erythrocytosis benign familial
          289.0 Due to high altitude
          238.4 Polycythemia vera

POLYCYTHEMIAS

TABLE 2-161   Differential Diagnosis of Relative Erythrocytosis, Secondary Erythrocytosis, and Polycythemia Vera

EXAMINATION	RELATIVE ERYTHROCYTOSIS	SECONDARY ERYTHROCYTOSIS	POLYCYTHEMIA VERA
Red blood cell mass	N	I	I
Plasma volume	D	N or I	N or I
Granulocytes	N	N	N or I
Platelets	N	N	N or I
Serum vitamin B_{12}	N	N	I
Transcobalamin 1	N	N	I
Serum iron	N	N	Usually D
Leukocyte alkaline phosphatase	N	N	N or I
Arterial oxygen saturation	N	N or D	N
Bone marrow	N	Erythroid hyperplasia	Panhyperplasia
Erythropoietin	N	I	N or D
Splenomegaly	Absent	Absent	Usually present

From Noble J (ed): *Primary care medicine,* ed 3, St Louis, 2001, Mosby.
D, Decreased; *I,* increased; *N,* normal.

POLYNEUROPATHY, COMMON CAUSES

Polyneuropathy, common causes
ICD-9CM # 357.9

BOX 2-203   Common Causes of Polyneuropathy

Predominantly motor
  Guillain-Barré syndrome
  Porphyria
  Diphtheria
  Lead
  Hereditary sensorimotor neuropathy, types I and II
  Paraneoplastic neuropathy
Predominantly sensory
  Diabetes
  Amyloidosis
  Leprosy
  Lyme disease
  Paraneoplastic neuropathy
  Vitamin B_{12} deficiency
  Hereditary sensory neuropathy, types I-IV
Predominantly autonomic
  Diabetes
  Amyloidosis
  Alcoholic neuropathy
  Familial dysautonomias

Mixed sensorimotor
  Systemic diseases
    Renal failure, hypothyroidism, acromegaly, rheumatoid arthritis, periarteritis nodosa, systemic lupus erythematosus, multiple myeloma, macroglobulinemia, remote effect of malignancy
  Medications
    Isoniazid, nitrofurantoin, ethambutal, chloramphenicol, chloroquine, vincristine, vinblastine, dapsone, disulfiram, diphenylhydantoin, cisplatin, 1-tryptophan
  Environmental toxins
    N-hexane, methyl *N*-butyl ketone, acrylamide, carbon disulfide, carbon monoxide, hexachlorophene, organophosphates
  Deficiency disorders
    Malabsorption, alcoholism, vitamin B_1 deficiency, Refsum's disease, metachromatic leukodystrophy

From Wiederholt WC: *Neurology for non-neurologists,* ed 4, Philadelphia, 2000, WB Saunders.

POLYNEUROPATHY, DRUG-INDUCED

Polyneuropathy, drug-induced
ICD-9CM # 357.6

BOX 2-204   Drugs That Cause Polyneuropathy

Drugs in oncology
  Vincristine
  Procarbazine
  Cisplatin
  Mesonidazole
  Metronidazole (Flagyl)
  Taxol
Drugs in infectious diseases
  Isoniazid
  Nitrofurantoin
  Dapsone
  ddC (dideoxycytidine)
  ddI (dideoxyinosine)

Drugs in cardiology
  Hydralazine
  Perhexiline maleate
  Procainamide
  Disopyramide
Drugs in rheumatology
  Gold salts
  Chloroquine
Drugs in neurology and psychiatry
  Diphenylhydantoin
  Glutethimide
  Methaqualone

Miscellaneous
  Disulfiram (Antabuse)
  Vitamin: pyridoxine (megadoses)

From Noble J (ed): *Primary care medicine*, ed 3, St Louis, 2001, Mosby.

POLYNEUROPATHY, SYMMETRIC

Polyneuropathy, symmetric
ICD-9CM # 357.9

BOX 2-205   A Classification of Chronic Symmetric Polyneuropathies

Acquired neuropathies
  Toxic
    Drugs
    Industrial toxins
    Heavy metals
    Abused substances
  Metabolic/endocrine
    Diabetes
    Chronic renal failure
    Hypothyroidism
    Polyneuropathy of critical illness
  Nutritional deficiency
    Vitamin B_{12} deficiency
    Alcoholism
    Vitamin E deficiency
  Paraneoplastic
    Carcinoma
    Lymphoma
  Plasma cell dyscrasia
    Myeloma, typical, atypical, and solitary forms
    Primary systemic amyloidosis

Idiopathic chronic inflammatory demyelinating
  polyneuropathies
Polyneuropathies associated with peripheral nerve
  autoantibodies
Acquired immunodeficiency sydrome
Inherited neuropathies
  Neuropathies with biochemical markers
    Refsum's disease
    Bassen-Kornzweig disease
    Tangier disease
    Metachromatic leukodystrophy
    Krabbe's disease
    Adrenomyeloneuropathy
    Fabry's disease
  Neuropathies without biochemical markers or systemic
    involvement
    Hereditary motor neuropathy
    Hereditary sensory neuropathy
    Hereditary sensorimotor neuropathy

From Noble J (ed): *Primary care medicine*, ed 2, St Louis, 1996, Mosby.

POLYURIA

BOX 2-206   Polyuria

Diabetes mellitus
Diabetes insipidus
Primary polydipsia (compulsive water drinking)
Hypercalcemia
Hypokalemia
Postobstructive uropathy

Diuretic phase of renal failure
Drugs: diuretics, caffeine, lithium
Sickle cell trait or disease, chronic pyelonephritis (failure
  to concentrate urine)
Anxiety, cold weather

POPLITEAL SWELLING

Popliteal swelling
ICD-9CM # 459.2 Venous obstruction
         747.4 Vein anomaly, lower limb vessel
         442.3 Artery aneurysm
         904.41 Artery injury
         447.8 Entrapment syndrome
         727.51 Baker's cyst
         451.2 Phlebitis, lower extremity
         727.67 Rupture of Achilles tendon

BOX 2-207   Popliteal Swelling

Phlebitis (superficial)
Lymphadenitis
Trauma: fractured tibia or fibula, contusion, traumatic
  neuroma
Deep vein thrombosis
Ruptured varicose vein
Baker's cyst

Popliteal abscess
Osteomyelitis
Ruptured tendon
Aneurysm of popliteal artery
Neoplasm: lipoma, osteogenic sarcoma, neurofibroma,
  fibrosarcoma

PORPHYRIAS

Porphyrias
ICD-9CM # 277.1

TABLE 2-162　Principal Clinical and Biochemical Manifestations in the Porphyrias

DISORDER	CUTANEOUS LESIONS	NEUROLOGIC DYSFUNCTION	HEPATIC DISEASE	MAJOR SITE OF PORPHYRIN OVERPRODUCTION	ERYTHROCYTES	URINE	FECES
Congenital erythropoietic porphyria	+	0	0	Bone marrow	↑ Uroporphyrin	↑ Uroporphyrin	↑ Uroporphyrin and coproporphyrin
Protoporphyria	+	0	+	Bone marrow and liver	↑ Protoporphyrin	—	↑ Protoporphyrin
Porphyria cutanea tarda	+	0	+	Liver	—	↑ Uroporphyrin	Isocoproporphyrin
Hepatoerythropoietic porphyria	+	0	+	Bone marrow and liver	↑ Zn-protoporphyrin	↑ Uroporphyrin	Isocoproporphyrin
Acute intermittent porphyria	0	+	0	Liver	—	↑ ALA and PBG	—
Variegate porphyria	+	+	0	Liver	—	↑ ALA, PBG, and coproporphyrin	↑ Protoporphyrin
Hereditary coproporphyria	+	+	0	Liver	—	↑ ALA, PBG, and coproporphyrin	↑ Coproporphyrin
ALA dehydrase deficiency	0	+	0	Liver	—	↑ ALA	—

From Stein J (ed): *Internal medicine,* ed 5, St Louis, 1998, Mosby.
ALA, γ-Aminolevulinic acid; *PBG,* porphobilinogen.
This table does not list all of the biochemical abnormalities and only serves as a guide to indicate which measurements are most critical in the evaluation of the porphyrias.

PORTAL HYPERTENSION

Portal hypertension
ICD-9CM # 572.3

BOX 2-208 **Causes of Portal Hypertension**

Increased resistance to flow
 Presinusoidal
  Portal or splenic vein occlusion (thrombosis, tumor)
  Schistosomiasis
  Congenital hepatic fibrosis
  Sarcoidosis
 Sinusoidal
  Cirrhosis (all causes)
  Alcoholic hepatitis
 Postsinusoidal
  Veno-occlusive disease
  Budd-Chiari syndrome
  Constrictive pericarditis
Increased portal blood flow
 Splenomegaly not due to liver disease
 Arterioportal fistula

From Andreoli TE (ed): *Cecil essentials of medicine*, ed 5, Philadelphia, 2001, WB Saunders.

PROPTOSIS

Proptosis
ICD-9CM # 376.30

TABLE 2-163 **Disorders Resulting in Proptosis**

ACUTE OR CHRONIC	UNILATERAL OR BILATERAL	CONJUNCTIVAL INJECTION (REDNESS)	PAIN	FEVER	OTHER FEATURES
Thyroid Eye Disease					
Subacute	Bilateral but possibly asymmetric	0-4+, variable depending on extent of disease	None	No	Possible association with systemic thyroid abnormalities
Orbital Pseudotumor					
Acute	Usually unilateral	3-4+	Severe pain, particularly with eye movement	No	Possible decreased vision and diplopia
Optic Nerve Tumor					
Chronic	Unilateral	0	None	No	Slow-onset visual field loss
Cavernous Sinus Arteriovenous Fistula					
Acute onset, chronic course	Unilateral	1-4+, variable depending on flow rate	Variable	No	Elevated intraocular pressure, double vision, possible visual loss, audible bruit, or pulsating exophthalmos
Cellulitis					
Acute	Unilateral	4+	Moderate to severe	Yes	Most common association with sinusitis, elevated white blood cell count

From Palay D (ed): *Ophthalmology for the primary care physician*, St Louis, 1997, Mosby.

PROSTATITIS SYNDROMES

Prostatitis syndromes
ICD-9CM # 601.0 Prostatitis, acute
601.1 Prostatitis, chronic

TABLE 2-164   Classification of Prostatitis Syndromes of the Basis of Lower Urinary Tract Localization Studies

CONDITION	BACTERIURIA*	INFECTION LOCALIZED TO PROSTATE	INFLAMMATORY RESPONSE†	ABNORMAL RECTAL EXAMINATION OF PROSTATE‡	SYSTEMIC ILLNESS§
Acute bacterial prostatitis	+	+	+	+	+
Chronic bacterial prostatitis	+	+	+	−	−
Chronic prostatitis/chronic pelvic pain syndrome					
Inflammatory subtype‖	−	−	+	−	−
Noninflammatory subtype¶	−	−	−	−	−
Asymptomatic inflammatory prostatitis	−	−	+	±	−

From Mandell GL: *Mandell, Douglas, and Bennett's principles and practice of infectious diseases*, ed 5, New York, 2000, Churchill Livingstone.
*Documented with an identical organism that is shown to localize to a prostatic focus when the midstream urine culture is negative.
†In expressed prostatic secretions, semen, post-massage urine, or prostate tissue.
‡Abnormal findings include exquisite tenderness and swelling that may be associated with signs of lower urinary tract obstruction.
§Systemic findings frequently include fever and rigors and may include signs of bacteremia.
‖Formerly termed "nonbacterial prostatitis."
¶Formerly termed "prostatodynia."

PROTEINURIA

Proteinuria
ICD-9CM # 791.0

BOX 2-209   Proteinuria

Nephrotic syndrome as a result of primary renal diseases
Malignant hypertension
Malignancies: multiple myeloma, leukemias, Hodgkin's disease
Congestive heart failure
Diabetes mellitus
Systemic lupus erythematosus, rheumatoid arthritis
Sickle cell disease
Goodpature's syndrome
Malaria
Amyloidosis, sarcoidosis

Tubular lesions: cystinosis
Functional (after heavy exercise)
Pyelonephritis
Pregnancy
Constrictive pericarditis
Renal vein thrombosis
Toxic nephropathies: heavy metals, drugs
Radiation nephritis
Orthostatic (postural) proteinuria
Benign proteinuria: fever, heat or cold exposure

PROTOZOAL INFECTIONS

Protozoal infections
ICD-9CM # 136.8 Protozoal disease
007.8 Protozoal intestinal disease

TABLE 2-165 Protozoal Infections

PROTOZOAN	SETTING	VECTORS	DIAGNOSIS	SPECIAL CONSIDERATIONS	TREATMENT
Endemic in United States					
Babesia microti	New England	Ixodid ticks, transfusions	Thick or thin blood smear	Severe disease in asplenic persons	Quinine and clindamycin
Giardia lamblia	Mountain states	Humans, ? small mammals	Microscopic examination of stool or duodenal fluid examination	Common in homosexual men, travelers, children in day care	Quinacrine or metronidazole
Toxoplasma gondii	Ubiquitous	Domestic cats, raw meat	Clinical; serologic confirmation	Pregnant women, immunosuppressed host (AIDS)	Pyrimethamine and sulfadiazine
Entamoeba histolytica	Southeast	Human	Microscopic examination of stool or "touch prep" from ulcer	Common in homosexual men, travelers, institutionalized persons	Metronidazole
Cryptosporidium sp.	Ubiquitous	Human	Acid-fast stain of stool	Severe in immunosuppressed hosts (AIDS)	None
Trichomonas vaginalis	Ubiquitous	Human	"Wet prep" of genital secretions	Common cause of vaginitis	Metronidazole
Primarily Seen in Travelers and Immigrants					
Plasmodium sp.	Africa, Asia, South America	*Anopheles* mosquito	Thick and thin blood smear	Consider in returning travelers with fever	Dependent upon regional resistance pattern
Leishmania donovani	Middle East	Sandfly	Tissue biopsy	Consider in immigrants with fever and splenomegaly	Pentostam
Trypanosoma sp.	Africa, South America	Reduviid bugs, transfusion	Direct examination of blood or cerebrospinal fluid	Very rare in travelers, transfusion associated	Supportive

From Andreoli TE (ed): *Cecil essentials of medicine,* ed 5, Philadelphia, 2001, WB Saunders.
AIDS, Acquired immunodeficiency syndrome.

II

PRURITUS

BOX 2-210   A. Generalized Pruritus Associated with Systemic Disease

Uremia
Obstructive biliary disease
  Primary biliary cirrhosis
    Chlorpropamide
    Contraceptive pills
  Extrahepatic biliary obstruction
  Intrahepatic cholestasis of pregnancy
Endocrine disorders
  Thyrotoxicosis
  Hypothyroidism
  Diabetes
  Carcinoid
Psychiatric disorders
Myeloproliferative disorders
  Hodgkin's disease
  Mycosis fungoides
  PCV
  Lymphoma
  Multiple myeloma
Visceral malignancies
  Breast carcinoma
  Gastric carcinoma
  Lung carcinoma
Iron deficiency anemia
Neurologic disorders
  Multiple sclerosis
  Brain abscess
  CNS infarct

B. Skin Diseases Associated with Pruritus

Xerosis
Scabies
Dermatitis herpetiformis
Atopic dermatitis
Pruritus vulvae
Pruritus ani
Miliaria
Insect bites
Pediculosis
Contact dermatitis
Drugs
Pruritic urticarial papular eruption of pregnancy
Psoriasis
Lichen planus
Urticaria
Folliculitis
Lichen simplex chronicus
Sunburn
Bullous pemphigoid
Fiberglass dermatitis
Trichinosis
Onchocerciasis
Echinococcosis

From Noble J: *Primary care medicine*, ed 3, St Louis, 2001, Mosby.

Pruritus
ICD-9CM # 698.9 Pruritus NOS
          697.0 Pruritus ani
          698.1 Pruritus, genital organs

PRURITUS ANI

BOX 2-211   Causes of Pruritus Ani

Dermatitis
Fecal Irritation

Poor hygiene
Anorectal conditions
    Fissure, fistula, hemorrhoids, skin tags, perianal
    clefts
Systemic
    Caffeine, tea, beer, spicy foods, citrus fruits, quini-
    dine, intravenous hydrocortisone, colchicine, tetra-
    cycline

Contact Dermatitis

Anesthetic agents, topical corticosteroids, perfumed
    soap

Systemic Diseases
Dermatologic

Psoriasis, seborrhea
Lichen simplex or sclerosus

Nondermatologic

Chronic renal failure, myxedema, diabetes mellitus,
    thyrotoxicosis, polycythemia vera
Vitamins A or D deficiency, iron deficiency
Cancers
    Bowen's, Paget's, Hodgkin's diseases

Infectious Agents
Sexually Transmitted Diseases

Syphilis
Herpes simplex virus
Human papillomavirus

Other Agents

Scabies
Pinworm
Bacterial infection
Fungal infection

From Rosen P (ed): *Emergency medicine,* ed 5, St Louis, 2002, Mosby.

Psychiatric disorders, postpartum
ICD-9CM # 648.44 Postpartum depression
296.24 Postpartum psychotic episode

PSYCHIATRIC DISORDERS, POSTPARTUM

TABLE 2-166   Postpartum Psychiatric Disorders

	SYMPTOMS	ONSET	RESOLUTION	MANAGEMENT
Postpartum Mood Disorders				
Maternity blues	Tearfulness Mood lability Anxiety Some difficulty with sleep	2-3 days post delivery	2-3 wk	Reassurance
Complicated blues	Same as above	Same as above	4-6 wk	Awareness for subsequent pregnancy
Major nonpsychotic depression	Agitation, anxiety Hopelessness Poor sleep Poor appetite Poor concentration Suicidal thoughts/plan	1-4 wk 8-12	After effective medications ? Hospitalization	Antidepressants Antianxiety drugs Counseling Contraception
Psychosis	Confusion/agitation Mania Hallucinations Delusions Paranoia	1-4 wk	Hospital	Mood stabilizers Antipsychotics Antianxiety drugs High recurrence rates—prophylaxis in future pregnancies
Postpartum Anxiety Disorders				
Panic disorder	Panic attacks Secondary mood disorder	1-6 wk	After effective medications	Antipanic medications Antidepressant
Obsessive-compulsive disorder	Thoughts of harming infant Avoidant behavior Nonpsychotic secondary mood disorder	1-6 wk ? Later	After effective medications	Selective serotonin reuptake inhibitors Clonazepam Counseling

From Carlson K (ed): *Primary care of women,* St Louis, 1995, Mosby.

PSYCHOSIS

Psychosis
CD-9CM # 298.9 Pychosis NOS
298.90 Psychosis, affective
291.0 Psychosis, alcoholic
290.41 Psychosis, acute, arteriosclerotic

BOX 2-212   Causes of Psychosis

Primary

Schizophrenia related*
Major depression
Dementia
Bipolar disorder

Secondary

Drug use†	Hypomagnesemia
Drug withdrawal‡	Epilepsy
Drug toxicity§	Meningitis
Charles Bonnet syndrome	Encephalitis
Infections (pneumonia)	Brain abscess
Electrolyte imbalance	Herpes encephalopathy
Syphilis	Hypoxia
Congestive heart failure	Hypercarbia
Parkinson's disease	Hypoglycemia
Trauma to temporal lobe	Thiamine deficiency
Postpartum psychosis	Postoperative states
Hypothyroidism/ hyperthyroidism	

From Noble J: *Primary care medicine,* ed 3, St Louis, 2001, Mosby.
*Includes schizophrenia, schizophreniaform disorder, brief reactive psychosis.
†Includes hypnotics, glucocorticoids, marijuana, phencyclidine, atropine, dopaminergic agents (e.g., amantadine, bromocriptine, L-dopa), immunosuppressants.
‡Includes alcohol, barbiturates, benzodiazepines.
§Includes digitalis, theophylline, cimetidine, anticholinergics, glucocorticoids, catecholaminergic agents.

PTOSIS

Ptosis
ICD-9CM # 374.30 Ptosis NOS
          743.61 Congenital
          374.33 Mechanical
          374.32 Myogenic
          374.31 Paralytic

TABLE 2-167   Disorders Causing Ptosis

HISTORY	DEGREE OF PTOSIS	MOTILITY	PUPIL
Third Nerve Palsy			
Double vision, possible severe pain	Moderate to severe	Decreased elevation, depression, and medial movement	Dilated and unreactive or normal
Horner's Syndrome			
Asymptomatic	Mild	Normal	Small
Myasthenia Gravis			
Fatigue, difficulty swallowing or breathing, double vision	Variable, possible worsening on sustained upgaze	Any abnormality or no abnormality	Normal
Senile Ptosis			
Possible history of recent eye surgery	Variable	Normal	Normal

From Palay D (ed): *Ophthalmology for the primary care physician,* St Louis, 1997, Mosby.

PUBERTY, DELAYED

Puberty, delayed
ICD-9CM # 259.0

BOX 2-213   Causes of Delayed Puberty

I. Normal or low serum gonadotropin levels
  A. Constitutional delay in growth and development
  B. Hypothalamic and/or pituitary disorders
    1. Isolated deficiency of growth hormone
    2. Isolated deficiency on Gn-RH
    3. Isolated deficiency of LH and/or FSH
    4. Multiple anterior pituitary hormone deficiencies
    5. Associated with congenital anomalies: Kallmann's syndrome; Prader-Willi syndrome; Laurence-Moon-Biedl syndrome; Friedreich's ataxia
    6. Trauma
    7. Postinfection
    8. Hyperprolactinemia
    9. Postirradiation
    10. Infiltrative disease (histiocytosis)
    11. Tumor
    12. Autoimmune hypophysitis
    13. Idiopathic
  C. Functional
    1. Chronic endocrinologic or systemic disorders
    2. Emotional disorders
    3. Drugs: cannabis
II. Increased serum gonadotropin levels
  A. Gonadal abnormalities
    1. Congenital
      a. Gonadal dysgenesis
      b. Klinefelter's syndrome
      c. Bilateral anorchism
      d. Resistant ovary syndrome
      e. Myotonic dystrophy in males
      f. 17-Hydroxylase deficiency in females
      g. Galactosemia
    2. Acquired
      a. Bilateral gonadal failure resulting from trauma or infection or after surgery, irradiation, or chemotherapy
      b. Oophoritis: isolated or with other autoimmune disorders
III. Uterine or vaginal disorders
  A. Absence of uterus and/or vagina
  B. Testicular feminization: complete or incomplete androgen insensitivity

From Moore WT, Eastman RC: *Diagnostic endocrinology,* ed 2, St Louis, 1996, Mosby.
FSH, Follicle-stimulating hormone; *Gn-RH,* gonadotropin-releasing hormone; *LH,* luteinizing hormone.

Puberty, precocious
CD-9CM # 259.1 Puberty, precocious NOS
255.2 Adrenocortical hyperfunction
256.1 Ovarian hyperfunction

PUBERTY, PRECOCIOUS

BOX 2-214   Conditions Causing Precocious Puberty

Gonadotropin-dependent puberty (true precocious puberty)
  Idiopathic (constitutional, functional)
  Organic brain lesions
    Hypothalamic hamartoma
    Brain tumors, hydrocephalus, severe head trauma
  Hypothyroidism, prolonged and untreated
Combined gonadotropin-dependent and gonadotropin-independent puberty
  Treated congenital adrenal hyperplasia
  McCune-Albright syndrome, late
  Familial male precocious puberty, late
Gonadotropin-independent puberty (precocious pseudopuberty)
  Females
    Isosexual (feminizing) conditions
      McCune-Albright syndrome
      Autonomous ovarian cysts
      Ovarian tumors
        Granulosa-theca cell tumor associated with Ollier disease
        Teratoma, chorionephithelioma
        Sex-cord tumor with annular tubules (SCTAT) associated with Peutz-Jeghers
          syndrome
        Feminizing adrenocortical tumor
        Exogenous estrogens
    Heterosexual (masculinizing) conditions
      Congenital adrenal hyperplasia
      Adrenal tumors
      Ovarian tumors
      Glucocorticoid receptor defect
      Exogenous androgens
  Males
    Isosexual (masculinizing) conditions
      Congenital adrenal hyperplasia
      Adrenocortical tumor
      Leydig cell tumor
      Familial male precocious puberty
      Isolated
      Associated with pseudohypoparathyroidism
      hCG-secreting tumors
        Central nervous system
        Hepatoblastoma
        Mediastinal tumor associated with Klinefelter syndrome
      Teratoma
      Glucocorticoid receptor defect
      Exogenous androgen
    Heterosexual (feminizing) conditions
      Feminizing adrenocortical tumor
      Sex-cord tumor with annular tubules (SCTAT) associated with Peutz-Jeghers
        syndrome
      Exogenous estrogens
  Incomplete (partial) precocious puberty
    Premature thelarche
    Premature adrenarche
    Premature menarche

From Behrman RE: *Nelson textbook of pediatrics,* ed 16, Philadelphia, 2000, WB Saunders.

PULMONARY CRACKLES

BOX 2-215   Causes of crackles

- Left ventricular failure
- Fibrosing alveolitis
- Extrinsic allergic alveolitis
- Pneumonia
- Bronchiectasis
- Chronic bronchitis
- Asbestosis

From Epstein O (ed): *Clinical examination,* ed 2, London, 1997, Mosby.

PULMONARY FUNCTION ABNORMALITIES

TABLE 2-168   **Basic Pattern of Pulmonary Function Abnormality**

TYPE OF IMPAIRMENT	PARAMETER					
	FEV$_1$	FVC	FEV$_1$/FVC	RV	TLC	DLCO
Obstruction	↓	→↓	↓	→↑*	→↑†	→↓‡
Restriction, extrinsic	→↓	↓	→↑	→↓	↓	→§
Restriction, intrinsic	→↓	↓	→↑	→↓	↓	↓
Combined obstruction and restriction	↓	↓	↓	→↓	↓	→↓
Consider: early interstitial lung disease, pulmonary embolism, anemia, and increased carboxyhemoglobin	→	→	→	→	→	↓
Consider: polycythemia, pulmonary hemorrhage, and left-to-right cardiac shunt	→	→	→	→	→	↑

From Ferri F: *Practical guide to the care of the medical patient,* ed 5, St Louis, 2001, Mosby.
↑, Greater than predicted; →, normal; ↓, less than predicted.
*An elevated residual volume is interpreted as "air trapping."
†An elevated total lung capacity is interpreted as "hyperaeration."
‡A low diffusion capacity in setting of severe airway obstruction would be consistent with pulmonary emphysema.
§When corrected for alveolar volume.
DLCO, Carbon monoxide diffusion in the lung; *FEV$_1$,* forced expiratory volume in 1 second; *FVC,* forced vital capacity; *RV,* respiratory volume; *TLC,* total lung capacity.

TABLE 2-169   **Pulmonary Function Test Patterns in Common Lung Disease**

DISORDER	PARAMETER						BRONCHODILATOR RESPONSE
	FVC	FEV$_1$	FEV$_1$/FVC	RV	TLC	DIFFUSION	
Asthma	↓	↓	↓	→↑	→↑	→	+
Chronic obstructive bronchitis	↓	↓	↓	→↑	→↑	→	−
Chronic obstructive bronchitis with bronchospasm	↓	↓	↓	→↑	→↑	→	+
Emphysema	↓	↓	↓	→↑	→↑	→↓	−
Interstitial fibrosis	↓	→↓	→↑	→↓	↓	↓	−
Obesity/kyphosis	↓	→↓	→↑	→↓	↓	→	−

From Ferri F: *Practical guide to the care of the medical patient,* ed 5, St Louis, 2001, Mosby.
↑, Greater than predicted; →, normal; ↓, less than predicted; *FEV$_1$,* forced expiratory volume in 1 second; *FVC,* forced vital capacity; *RV,* respiratory volume; *TLC,* total lung capacity.

Pulmonary lesions
ICD-9CM # 518.3   Pulmonary infiltrate
         518.89 Pulmonary nodule
         508.9   Pulmonary disorder due to
                 unspecified external agent
         861.20 Pulmonary injury NOS

PULMONARY LESIONS

BOX 2-216   Pulmonary Lesions

Tuberculosis
Legionella pneumonia
Mycoplasma pneumonia
Viral pneumonia
Pneumocystis carinii
Hypersensitivity pneumonitis

Aspiration pneumonia
Fungal disease (aspergillosis, histo-
   plasmosis)
Adult respiratory distress syndrome
   associated with pneumonia
Psittacosis

Sarcoidosis
Septic emboli
Metastatic cancer
Multiple pulmonary emboli
Rheumatoid nodules

PULMONARY NODULE, SOLITARY

Pulmonary nodule, solitary
ICD-9CM # 518.89

TABLE 2-170   Causes of Solitary Pulmonary Nodules

CAUSE	RANGE OF REPORTED INCIDENCE (%)	CAUSE	RANGE OF REPORTED INCIDENCE (%)
Malignant tumors		Granulomas–cont'd	
Bronchogenic carcinoma	16-52	Coccidioidomycosis	2-14
Bronchial adenoma (certain cell types	1-2	Cryptococcosis	0-1
seen are benign and have benign courses)		Miscellaneous	
Metastatic carcinoma	1-10	Bronchogenic cyst	1-3
Benign tumors	5-12	Arteriovenous malformation	0-1
Hamartoma	1-2	Bronchopulmonary sequestration	0-1
Fibroma	0-1	Sclerosing hemangioma	0-1
Granulomas		Intrapulmonary lymph node	0-1
Histoplasmosis	5-38		
Tuberculosis	10-15		

From Stein JH (ed): *Internal medicine*, ed 5, St Louis, 1998, Mosby.

PULSE ABNORMALITIES

PULSE

POSSIBLE CAUSE

Alternating pulse (pulsus alternans)

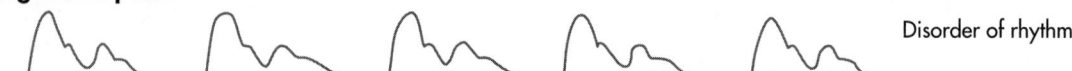

Left ventricular failure
(More significant if
pulse slow)

Pulsus alternans is characterized by alternation of a pulsation of small amplitude with the pulsation of large amplitude while the rhythm is normal.

Pulsus bisferiens

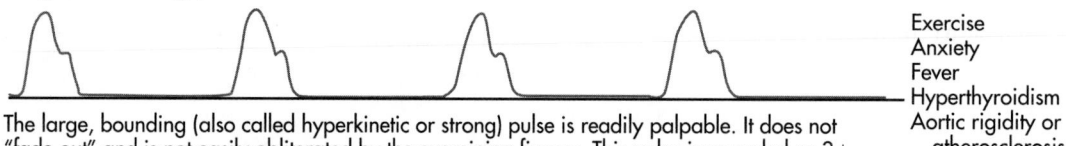

Aortic stenosis combined
with aortic insufficiency

Pulsus bisferiens is best detected by palpation of the carotid artery. This pulsation is characterized by two main peaks. The first is termed percussion wave and the second, tidal wave. Although the mechanism is not clear, the first peak is believed to be the pulse pressure and the second, reverberation from the periphery.

Bigeminal pulse

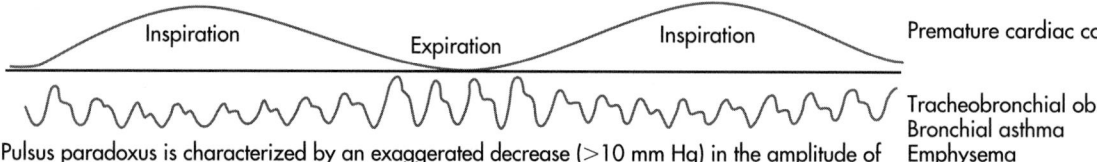

Disorder of rhythm

Bigeminal pulsations result from a normal pulsation followed by a premature contraction. The amplitude of the pulsation of the premature contraction is less than that of the normal pulsation.

Large, bounding pulse

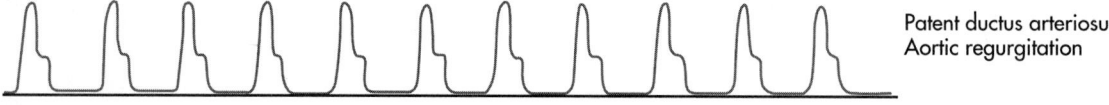

Exercise
Anxiety
Fever
Hyperthyroidism
Aortic rigidity or
  atherosclerosis

The large, bounding (also called hyperkinetic or strong) pulse is readily palpable. It does not "fade out" and is not easily obliterated by the examining fingers. This pulse is recorded as 3+.

Paradoxic pulse (pulsus paradoxus)

Inspiration   Expiration   Inspiration

Premature cardiac contraction

Tracheobronchial obstruction
Bronchial asthma
Emphysema
Pericardial effusion
Constrictive pericarditis

Pulsus paradoxus is characterized by an exaggerated decrease (>10 mm Hg) in the amplitude of pulsation during inspiration and increased amplitude during expiration. (See text for measurement with sphygmomanometer.)

Water-hammer pulse (Corrigan pulse)

Patent ductus arteriosus
Aortic regurgitation

The water-hammer pulse (also known as collapsing) has a greater amplitude than the normal pulse, a rapid rise to a narrow summit, and a sudden descent.

Small, weak pulse

Hypovolemia
Physical obstruction to
  left ventricular output,
  e.g., aortic stenosis

A weak pulse may be difficult to feel, and the vessel may be obliterated easily by the fingers. The pulse may "fade out" (be impalpable). This pulse is recorded as 1+. The pulsation is slower to rise, has a sustained summit, and falls more slowly than the normal. A pulse that is weak and variable in amplitude is called thready.

Fig. 2-11   Pulse abnormalities. (Modified from Barkauskas VH et al: *Health and physical assessment,* ed 2, St Louis, 1998, Mosby.)

PUPIL ABNORMALITIES

Pupil abnormalities
ICD-9CM # 379.40 Dysfunction
364.75 Deformity
379.43 Dilated
364.76 Fixed
379.46 Dysfunction tonic

TABLE 2-171   Descriptions of Various Pupil Abnormalities

ABNORMALITY	CONTRIBUTING FACTORS	APPEARANCE
Bilateral		
Miosis (pupillary constriction; usually less than 2 mm in diameter)	Iridocyclitis; miotic eye drops (such as pilocarpine given for glaucoma)	
Mydriasis (pupillary dilation; usually more than 6 mm in diameter)	Iridocyclitis; mydriatic or cycloplegic drops (such as atropine); midbrain (reflex arc) lesions or hypoxia; oculomotor (CN III) damage; acute-angle glaucoma (slight dilation)	
Failure to respond (constrict) with increased light stimulus	Iridocyclitis; corneal or lens opacity (light does not reach retina); retinal degeneration; optic nerve (CN II) destruction; midbrain synapses involving afferent pupillary fibers or oculomotor nerve (CN III) (consensual response is also lost); impairment of efferent fibers (parasympathetic) that innervate sphincter pupillae muscle	
Argyll Robertson pupil	Bilateral, miotic, irregularly shaped pupils that fail to constrict with light but retain constriction with convergence; pupils may or may not be equal in size; commonly caused by neurosyphilis or lesions in midbrain where afferent pupillary fibers synapse	
Unilateral		
Anisocoria (unequal size of pupils)	Congenital (approximately 20% of healthy people have minor or noticeable differences in pupil size, but reflexes are normal) or caused by local eye medications (constrictors or dilators), amblyopia, or unilateral sympathetic or parasympathetic pupillary pathway destruction (NOTE: Examiner should test whether pupils react equally to light; if response is unequal, examiner should note whether larger or smaller eye reacts more slowly [or not at all], since either pupil could represent the abnormal size)	Normal eye Affected eye
Iritis constrictive response	Acute uveitis is frequently unilateral; constriction of pupil accompanied by pain and circumcorneal flush (redness)	Normal eye Affected eye
Oculomotor nerve (CN III) damage	Pupil dilated and fixed; eye deviated laterally and downward; ptosis	Normal eye Affected eye
Adie pupil (tonic pupil)	Affected pupil dilated and reacts slowly or fails to react to light; responds to convergence; caused by impairment of postganglionic parasympathetic innervation to sphincter pupillae muscle or ciliary malfunction; often accompanied by diminished tendon reflexes (as with diabetic neuropathy or alcoholism)	

Modified from Thompson JM et al: *Mosby's clinical nursing*, ed 4, St Louis, 1997, Mosby.

PURPURA

Purpura
ICD-9CM # 287.2 Purpura NOS
287.0 Autoimmune
287.0 Henoch-Schönlein
287.3 Idiopathic thrombocytopenic
446.6 Thrombocytopenic thrombotic

BOX 2-217   Purpura

Trauma
Septic emboli, atheromatous emboli
Disseminated intravascular coagulation
Thrombocytopenia

Meningococcemia
Rocky Mountain spotted fever
Hemolytic-uremic syndrome
Viral infection: echo, coxsackie
Scurvy

Other: left atrial myxoma, cryoglobulinemia, vasculitis, hyperglobulinemic purpura

---

RADICULOPATHY, CERVICAL

Radiculopathy, cervical
ICD-9CM # 723.4

TABLE 2-172   Distribution of Symptoms and Signs of Cervical Root Damage

ROOT	PAIN	PARESTHESIAS	WEAKNESS	DEPRESSED REFLEXES
C5	Neck, shoulder, lateral arm (distal to elbow)	Shoulder	Deltoid, infraspinatus	Biceps, brachioradialis
C6	Neck, shoulder, scapula, thumb, radial forearm	Thumb	Biceps, brachioradialis, wrist extensors	Biceps, brachioradialis
C7	Neck, shoulder, dorsal or volar forearm	Middle finger	Triceps	Triceps
C8	Neck, shoulder, ulnar forearm	Little finger	Intrinsic hand muscles	Triceps or none

From Wiederholt WC: *Neurology for non-neurologists*, ed 4, Philadelphia, 2000, WB Saunders.

RADICULOPATHY, LUMBOSACRAL

Radiculopathy, lumbosacral
ICD-9CM # 724.4

TABLE 2-173   Distribution of Symptoms and Signs of Lumbosacral Root Damage

ROOT	PAIN	PARESTHESIAS	WEAKNESS	DEPRESSED REFLEXES
L4	Posterolateral hip, anterior thigh	Anterior thigh anterolateral leg	Quadriceps	Quadriceps
L5	Posterolateral thigh, leg, dorsum of foot	Lateral calf, dorsum of foot	Tibialis anterior, tibialis posterior, gastrocnemius	Hamstrings (internal)
S1	Posterior thigh, leg, heel	Posterior calf, lateral and plantar foot	Foot muscles, hamstrings, gastrocnemius	Hamstrings (external) Gastrocnemius

From Wiederholt WC: *Neurology for non-neurologists*, ed 4, Philadelphia, 2000, WB Saunders.

RECTAL PAIN

Rectal pain
ICD-9CM # 569.42

BOX 2-218   Rectal Pain

Anal fissure
Thrombosed hemorrhoid
Anorectal abscess
Foreign bodies
Fecal impaction

Endometriosis
Neoplasms (primary or metastatic)
Pelvic inflammatory disease
Inflammation of sacral nerves
Compression of sacral nerves

Prostatitis
Other: proctalgia fugax, uterine abnormalities, myopathies, coccygodynia

RED EYE

Red eye
ICD-9CM # 379.93

TABLE 2-174   **Red Eye: Differential Features**

	CONJUNCTIVITIS			KERATITIS		IRITIS	GLAUCOMA (ACUTE)
	BACTERIAL	VIRAL	ALLERGIC	BACTERIAL	VIRAL		
Blurred vision	0	0	0	+++	0 to ++	+ to ++	++ to +++
Pain	0	0	0	++	0 to +	++	++ to +++
Photophobia	0	0	0	++	++	+++	+ to ++
Discharge	Purulent + to +++	Watery + to ++	White, ropy +	Purulent +++	Watery +	0	0
Injection	+++	++	+	+++	+	0 to + (limbal)	+ to ++ (limbal)
Corneal haze	0	0	0	+++	+ to +++	0	+ to +++
Ciliary flush	0	0	0	+++	+	+++ to +++	+ to ++
Pupil	Normal	Normal	Normal	Normal or miotic (iritis)	Normal	Miotic	Mid-dilated Nonreactive
Pressure	Normal	Normal	Normal	Normal	Normal	Normal, low, or high	High
Preauricular nodes	Rare	Usual	0	0	0	0	0
Smear	Bacteria PMNs	Lymphs	Eosinophil	Bacteria PMNs	0	0	0
Therapy	Antibiotics	Nonspecific	Nonspecific	Antibiotics	Antivirals (if herpes)	Cycloplegia Topical steroids	Medical or surgical

From Kassirer J (ed): *Current therapy in adult medicine,* ed 4, St Louis, 1998, Mosby.
+, Mild; ++, moderate; +++, severe; *PMNs,* polymorphonuclear leukocytes.

Renal cystic diseases
ICD-9CM # 753.9 Multicystic renal disease, congenital
593.2 Renal cyst
753.13 Polycystic kidney disease, adult type
753.14 Polycystic kidney disease, childhood type

RENAL CYSTIC DISEASES

TABLE 2-175 **Features of Renal Cystic Diseases**

| | CORTEX AND MEDULLA | | | | MEDULLA | |
| | | | POLYCYSTIC | | | |
	SIMPLE	ACQUIRED	DOMINANT	RECESSIVE	SPONGE KIDNEY	MEDULLARY CYSTIC
Prevalence	Common	>50% of dialysis patients	1:1500-1:1000	Rare	1:5000-1:1000	Rare
Symptoms	Rare	Occasional	Common	Common	Occasional	Common
Inherited	No	No	Yes	Yes	Unknown	Dominant and recessive forms
Kidney size	Normal	Small to large	Large	Large	Normal	Small
Hypertension	Rare	Variable	Common	Common	Rare	Rare
Hematuria	Occasional	Occasional	Common	Occasional	Rare (except with stones)	Rare
Associated conditions						
Azotemia	No	Always	Common	Common	Rare	Common
Liver disease	No	No	40%-60%	100%	No	No
Arterial aneurysm	No	No	10%	No	No	No
Differential diagnosis	Tumor Diverticula of renal pelvis	ADPKD Simple cysts von Hippel-Lindau disease	ARPKD Tuberous sclerosis Multiple simple cysts	ADPKD Medullary sponge kidney	Medullary cystic kidney Renal tubular acidosis Idiopathic nephrocalcinosis	End-stage renal disease Medullary sponge kidney

From Stein JH (ed): *Internal medicine*, ed 5, St Louis, 1998, Mosby.
ADPKD, Autosomal dominant polycystic kidney disease; *ARPKD*, autosomal recessive polycystic kidney disease.

RENAL FAILURE, MEDICATION-INDUCED

Renal failure, medication-induced
ICD-9CM # 586

TABLE 2-176   Medications Associated with Acute Renal Failure

MEDICATION	POSSIBLE MECHANISM
Nonsteroidal antiinflammatory drugs, angiotensin-converting enzyme inhibitors, cyclosporin, tacrolimus, amphotericin, radiographic contrast media	Renal vasoconstriction
Aminoglycosides, radiographic contrast media, cisplatin, cyclosporin, tacrolimus, amphotericin, pentamidine	Direct tubular toxicity
Cocaine, ethanol, lovastatin	Rhabdomyolysis
Penicillin, cephalosporins, sulfonamides, nonsteroidal antiinflammatory drugs, rifampin	Acute interstitial nephritis
Acyclovir, sulfonamides, methotrexate	Intratubular obstruction

From Nseyo UO (ed): *Urology for primary care physicians,* Philadelphia, 1999, WB Saunders.

Renal insufficiency, reversible causes
ICD-9CM # 586

RENAL INSUFFICIENCY, REVERSIBLE CAUSES

BOX 2-219   Reversible Causes of Acute Deterioration in Renal Function

Decreased renal perfusion
   Intravascular volume depletion
   Heart failure
   Third spacing
Obstruction
Infection
   Urinary tract infection
   Sepsis
Nephrotoxins
   Endogenous: myoglobulin, hemoglobin, uric acid,
     calcium, phosphorus
   Exogenous: contrast media, drugs
Poorly controlled hypertension: malignant or acceler-
   ated hypertension

From Andreoli TE (ed): *Cecil essentials of medicine,* ed 5, Philadelphia, 2001, WB Saunders.

II

RESPIRATORY FAILURE, HYPOVENTILATORY

Respiratory failure, hypoventilatory
ICD-9CM # 518.81 Respiratory failure

BOX 2-220   Causes of Hypoventilatory Respiratory Failure

Abnormal Respiratory Capacity (Normal Respiratory Workloads)

Acute depression of central nervous system
  Various causes
Chronic central hypoventilation syndromes
  Obesity-hypoventilation syndrome
  Sleep apnea syndrome
  Hypothyroidism
  Shy-Drager syndrome (multisystem atrophy syndrome)
Acute toxic paralysis syndromes
  Botulism
  Tetanus
  Toxic ingestion or bites
  Organophosphate poisoning
Neuromuscular disorders (acute and chronic)
  Myasthenia gravis
  Guillain-Barré syndrome
  Drugs
  Amyotrophic lateral sclerosis
  Muscular dystrophies
  Polymyositis

Spinal cord injury
Traumatic phrenic nerve paralysis

Abnormal Pulmonary Workloads

Chronic obstructive pulmonary disease
  Chronic bronchitis
  Asthmatic bronchitis
  Emphysema
Asthma and acute bronchial hyperreactivity syndromes
Upper airway obstruction
Interstitial lung diseases

Abnormal Extrapulmonary Workloads

Chronic thoracic cage disorders
  Severe kyphoscoliosis
  After thoracoplasty
  After thoracic cage injury
Acute thoracic cage trauma and burns
Pneumothorax
Pleural fibrosis and effusions
Abdominal processes

From Noble J (ed): *Primary care medicine,* ed 3, St Louis, 2001, Mosby.

RESPIRATORY FAILURE, HYPOXEMIC

Respiratory failure, hypoxemic
ICD-9CM # 518.81 Respiratory failure, acute

BOX 2-221   Causes of Acute Hypoxemic Respiratory Failure

Diffuse Pulmonary Abnormalities

Cardiogenic pulmonary edema
Adult respiratory distress syndrome (ARDS)
Diffuse infectious pneumonitis
Alveolar hemorrhage
Pulmonary alveolar proteinosis

Focal Pulmonary Lesions

Lobar pneumonia
Atelectasis
Pulmonary contusion
Alveolar and pulmonary hemorrhage
Reperfusion pulmonary edema
Reexpansion pulmonary edema

From Noble J: *Primary care medicine,* ed 3, St Louis, 2001, Mosby.

RHINITIS, CHRONIC

TABLE 2-177   Classification and Therapy of Chronic Rhinitis

DIAGNOSTIC CLASSIFICATION	DIFFERENTIAL CLINICAL FINDINGS	NASAL CYTOLOGY	ALLERGY SKIN TESTS	PHARMACOLOGIC THERAPY	NONPHARMACOLOGIC THERAPY
I. Inflammatory rhinitis					
A. Eosinophilic allergic rhinitis	Onset typically in, but not limited to, childhood Sneezing, nasal itching, clear rhinorrhea, ocular symptoms Pale, swollen nasal mucosa Specific allergen precipitants (historically) Associated atopic disorders	↑ Eosinophils with or without ↑ basophils and/or mast cells	Positive and correlate with history	Antihistamines Antihistamine-decongestant combinations Intranasal corticosteroids Intranasal cromolyn	Antigen avoidance Immunotherapy
1. Seasonal	Hay fever Typically spring, summer, fall Extended asymptomatic intervals common				
2. Perennial	Typically daily Usually triggered by animals, dust mites, mold				
B. Eosinophilic nonallergic rhinitis	Onset in adulthood (usually) Perennial symptoms Prominent pale mucosal edema Aspirin may increase symptoms Anosmia common Frequent polyps and/or sinus disease	↑ Eosinophils with or without ↑ basophils and/or mast cells	Negative or coincidental (not correlated with history)	Antihistamine-decongestant combinations Intranasal corticosteroids Oral corticosteroids (for severe cases)	Saline lavage Exercise
C. Primary nasal mastocytosis	Onset adulthood (usually)	↑ Mast cells	Negative or coincidental	Intranasal corticosteroids	

From Stein JH (ed): *Internal medicine*, ed 5, St Louis, 1998, Mosby.

Continued

II

TABLE 2-177 Classification and Therapy of Chronic Rhinitis—cont'd

DIAGNOSTIC CLASSIFICATION	DIFFERENTIAL CLINICAL FINDINGS	NASAL CYTOLOGY	ALLERGY SKIN TESTS	PHARMACOLOGIC THERAPY	NONPHARMACOLOGIC THERAPY
	Perennial rhinorrhea and congestion May be associated with migraine headaches or asthma Nonspecific precipitants frequent			Intranasal cromolyn Systemic oral corticosteroids (for severe cases)	
D. Nasal polyps	Severe obstruction Anosmia Polyps on physical examination Sinus involvement common				Polypectomy with or without submucous resection Ethmoidectomy
1. Eosinophilic	Incidence, 85% Uncommon in children Seromucous secretion Associated with aspirin sensitivity, intrinsic asthma Role of allergy doubtful Steroid responsive	↑ Eosinophils with or without ↑ basophils and/or mast cells	Negative or coincidental	Intranasal corticosteroids Oral corticosteroids	
2. Neutrophilic	Incidence, 15% Purulent secretions Associated with cystic fibrosis, Kartagener's triad, ciliary disturbances, sinusitis, immune deficiency Steroid unresponsive	↑ Neutrophils with or without bacteria	Negative or coincidental	Antibiotics	
E. Neutrophilic nasopharyngitis or sinusitis	Prominent postnasal drip Frequent sinus pain or tenderness Purulent secretions in nose and throat Infection characteristic	↑ Neutrophils with prominent bacteria	Negative or when positive may be related to underlying allergic rhinitis	Control underlying rhinitis/polyps (if present) Topical decongestants (short courses) Antibiotic courses (2 to 3 wk)	Saline lavage Sinus irrigation Sinus surgery (especially ethmoidectomy with or without sphenoidectomy)

Diagnosis	Clinical features	Sinus films	Allergy/relation	Pharmacologic treatment	Other treatment
	Sinus films frequently abnormal (sinusitis) May complicate eosinophilic rhinitis or polyps or occur with immune deficiencies, foreign bodies, or trauma or without demonstrable cause			Possibly oral decongestants Sometimes longer-term antibiotics Possibly mucoevacuants Sometimes oral corticosteroids, plus antibiotics	
F. Atrophic rhinitis	Severe nasal obstruction Physiologically patent nasal passages Associated with aging, too extensive nasal tissue extirpation, Wegener's granulomatosis	Unremarkable unless infected	Unrelated	Antibiotics when appropriate	Saline lavage Lubricants (petrolatum) Surgical transplantation
II. Noninflammatory rhinitis A. Rhinitis medicamentosa 1. Topical	Obstruction (most prominent symptom) Associated with local sympathomimetic abuse	Unremarkable (usually)	Negative or related to underlying disorder	Discontinue topical decongestants Intranasal corticosteroid Oral corticosteroids (for severe cases)	Saline lavage Exercise
2. Systemic	Current antihypertensive therapy, oral decongestant (rare), β agonist, birth control pills			Consider reducing dosage or discontinuing (if possible) or switching to alternate effective medication or therapy Intranasal corticosteroids	

Continued

From Stein JH (ed): Internal medicine, ed 5, St Louis, 1998, Mosby.

II

TABLE 2-177 Classification and Therapy of Chronic Rhinitis—cont'd

DIAGNOSTIC CLASSIFICATION	DIFFERENTIAL CLINICAL FINDINGS	NASAL CYTOLOGY	ALLERGY SKIN TESTS	PHARMACOLOGIC THERAPY	NONPHARMACOLOGIC THERAPY
B. Vasomotor instability	Nonspecific hypersensitivity of nasal mucosal vasculature and glands apparently related to local autonomic nervous system imbalance	Unremarkable	Unrelated	Possibly oral decongestants Intranasal ipratropium for prominent rhinorrhea	Saline lavage Exercise Avoid precipitants
1. Associated with systemic conditions	Thyroid disorders Pregnancy			Correct disorder (if possible)	
2. Idiopathic vasomotor rhinitis (primary vasomotor instability)	Most common in young adult women				Exercise essential
III. Structurally related rhinitis	Frequent history of nasal trauma Unilateral obstruction Abnormality diagnosed on physical examination	Unremarkable	Unrelated		Surgery (including laser)

From Stein JH (ed): *Internal medicine*, ed 5, St Louis, 1998, Mosby.

RICKETTSIOSES

TABLE 2-178 Some Characteristics of the Major Human Rickettsioses

DISEASE	ORGANISMS (RICKETTSIA AND OTHERS)	VECTOR	VERTEBRATE HOST	MEANS OF TRANSMISSION TO HUMANS	GEOGRAPHIC DISTRIBUTION	MORTALITY RATE (%) UNTREATED	MORTALITY RATE (%) TREATED
Spotted Fever Group							
Rocky Mountain spotted fever	R. rickettsii	Ticks (e.g., Dermacentor variabilis, Dermacentor andersoni)	Rodents	Tick bite	North, Central, and South America	20-25	3
Boutonneuse fever	R. conorii	Ticks	Rodents	Tick bite	Africa, Asia, and Mediterranean basin	?	1-3†
North Asian tick typhus	R. sibirica	Ticks	Rodents	Tick bite	Asia	0	0
Queensland tick typhus	R. australis	Ticks	Rodents, marsupials	Tick bite	Eastern Australia	2	0
Rickettsial pox	R. akari	Mites	Mice	Mouse to mite to human	United States, Russia, possibly worldwide	0	0
Flinders Island spotted fever	R. honei	Unknown	Unknown	Presumed tick bite	Australia	0	0
Oriental spotted fever	R. japonica	Ticks	Unknown	Presumed tick bite	Japan	0	0
Typhus Group							
Epidemic typhus	R. prowazekii	Body louse	Humans	Human to louse to human	Worldwide	15-30*	5*
Murine typhus	R. typhi (R. mooseri)	Rat fleas	Rats	Rat to rat flea to human	Worldwide	1	0-1†
Cat flea typhus	R. felis	Cat fleas	Opossums	Cat flea to human	Texas and California	0	0
Scrub Typhus Group							
Scrub typhus	Orientia tsutsugamushi	Larvae of mites (chiggers)	Rats, other rodents, birds	Mite to human	Asia, Pacific islands, and Australia	5	1
Other Genera							
Q fever	Coxiella burnetii	Ticks (but usually by aerosol)	Cattle, goats, sheep, other mammals	Livestock to human, by aerosol	Worldwide	5	0‡
Human monocytic ehrlichiosis	Ehrlichia chaffeensis	Ticks (e.g., Amblyomma americanum)	Deer	Tick bite	North America and Europe, possibly worldwide	2-5	0-2
Human granulocytic ehrlichiosis	HGE agent	Ticks (e.g., Ixodes dammini)	Rodents, deer	Tick bite	North America, possibly worldwide	2-5	0-2

From Stein J (ed): *Internal medicine*, ed 5, St Louis, 1998, Mosby.
*Mortality can be high in debilitated, malnourished patients; otherwise, it is lower than mortality from Rocky Mountain spotted fever.
†In hospitalized patients.
‡Excluding Q fever endocarditis, which causes significant mortality.

II

SCLERODERMA-LIKE SYNDROMES

Scleroderma-like syndromes
ICD-9CM # varies with specific diagnosis

TABLE 2-179 Scleroderma-like Syndromes

	DISTINGUISHING FEATURES
Other Diseases	
Morphea	Patchy or linear distribution
Eosinophilic fasciitis	Sparing of hands, biopsy shows involvement extending to fascia and muscle
Scleredema (of Buschke)	Prominent involvement of neck, shoulders, and upper arms; hands spared; association with diabetes
Scleromyxedema	Association with gammopathy; skin lichenoid and thickened but not tethered; may have Raynaud's phenomenon
Graft-versus-host disease	Skin changes similar to scleroderma; vasculopathy
Environmental Agents and Drugs	
Bleomycin	Skin and lung fibrosis similar to scleroderma
L-Tryptophan	Eosinophilia-myalgia; from contaminant or metabolite
	Fever, eosinophilia, neurologic manifestations, pulmonary hypertension
Organic solvents	Trichloroethylene and others implicated
	Clinically indistinguishable from idiopathic systemic sclerosis
Pentazocine	Localized lesions at injection sites
Toxic oil syndrome	Contaminated rapeseed oil (Spanish epidemic 1981)
	Similar to eosinophilia myalgia syndrome
Vinyl chloride disease	Vascular lesions, acro-osteolysis, sclerodactyly
	No visceral disease

From Andreoli TE (ed): *Cecil essentials of medicine,* ed 5, Philadelphia, 2001, WB Saunders.

SCROTAL SWELLING

Scrotal swelling
ICD-9CM # 608.86

BOX 2-222   Causes of Scrotal Swelling

Acute, Painful Scrotal Swelling

Torsion of spermatic cord
Torsion of appendix, testis, epididymis
Acute epididymitis, orchitis
Mumps orchitis
Henoch-Schönlein purpura
Trauma
Insect bite
Thrombosis of spermatic vein
Fat necrosis
Hernia
Folliculitis
Dermatitis

Acute, Painless Scrotal Swelling

Tumor
Idiopathic scrotal edema
Hydrocele
Henoch-Schönlein purpura
Hernia

Chronic Scrotal Swelling

Hydrocele
Hernia
Varicocele
Spermatocele
Sebaceous cyst
Tumor

From Hoekelman R (ed): *Primary pediatric care,* ed 3, St Louis, 1997, Mosby.

SEIZURES, CLASSIFICATION

Seizures, classification
ICD-9CM # 780.39

BOX 2-223   Classification of Seizures

Generalized (bilaterally symmetrical and without focal onset)
  Tonic
  Clonic
  Tonic-clonic
  Absence
  Infantile spasms
  Myoclonus
  Akinetic
  Atonic
Partial seizures (seizures beginning focally)
  Partial with secondary generalization
  Partial elementary (without impairment of consciousness)

With motor symptoms
With somatosensory symptoms
With autonomic symptoms
Compound forms
Partial complex (with alteration of consciousness)
  With affective disturbances
  With cognitive disturbances
  With complex motor behavior
  With subjective visceral or sensory symptoms
Unilateral seizures
Miscellaneous
  Reflex seizures (stimulus-induced; e.g., pattern or photic-induced, musicogenic)

From Wiederholt WC: *Neurology for non-neurologists*, ed 4, Philadelphia, 2000, WB Saunders.

II

SEIZURES, DIFFERENTIAL DIAGNOSIS

Seizures, differential diagnosis
ICD-9CM # code varies with specific diagnosis

BOX 2-224   Differential Diagnosis of Seizures

Syncope
Breath-holding spells
Hyperventilation
TIAs
Complicated migraine
Hypoglycemia
Sleep myoclonus
Drug intoxication
Decerebrate-decorticate posturing
Clonus
Pseudoseizure

From Wiederholt WC: *Neurology for non-neurologists*, ed 4, Philadelphia, 2000, WB Saunders.
TIA, Transient ischemic attack.

SEIZURES, PEDIATRIC

Seizures, pediatric
ICD-9CM # 780.39 Infantile seizures
779.0   Seizures, newborn

BOX 2-225   Pediatric Seizures: Cause by Age of Onset

First Month of Life
First Day

Hypoxia
Drugs
Trauma
Infection
Hyperglycemia
Hypoglycemia
Pyridoxine deficiency

Day 2-3

Infection
Drug withdrawal
Hypoglycemia
Hypocalcemia
Developmental malformation
Intracranial hemorrhage
Inborn error of metabolism
Hyponatremia or hypernatremia

Day >4

Infection
Hypocalcemia

Hyperphosphatemia
Hyponatremia
Developmental malformation
Drug withdrawal
Inborn error of metabolism

1 to 6 Months

As above

6 Months to 3 Years

Febrile seizures
Birth injury
Infection
Toxin
Trauma
Metabolic disorder
Cerebral degenerative disease

>3 Years

Idiopathic
Infection
Trauma
Cerebral degenerative disease

Modified from Barkin RM, McClellan S, Knapp J, et al: *Pediatric emergency medicine: concepts and clinical practice,* St Louis, 1992, Mosby. In Rosen P (ed): *Emergency medicine,* ed 5, St Louis, 2002, Mosby.

SEXUAL PRECOCITY

Sexual precocity
ICD-9CM # 259.1

TABLE 2-180   Differential Diagnosis of Sexual Precocity

CONDITION	PLASMA GONADOTROPINS	LH RESPONSE TO LHRH	SERUM SEX STEROID CONCENTRATIONS	GONADAL SIZE	MISCELLANEOUS
True Precocious Puberty					
Premature reactivation of LHRH pulse generator	Prominent LH pulses, initially during sleep	Pubertal LH response	Pubertal values of testosterone or estradiol	Normal pubertal testicular enlargement or ovarian and uterine enlargement (by ultrasonography)	MRI of brain to rule out CNS tumor or other abnormality; skeletal survey for McCune-Albright syndrome
Incomplete Sexual Precocity					
(Pituitary Gonadotropin Independent)					
Males					
Chorionic gonadotropin-secreting tumor	High hCG, low LH	Prepubertal LH response	Pubertal value of testosterone	Slight to moderate uniform enlargement of testes	Hepatomegaly suggests hepatoblastoma; CT scan of brain if hCG-secreting CNS tumor suspected
Leydig cell tumor	Suppressed	No LH response	Very high testosterone	Irregular asymmetric enlargement of testes	

From Wilson JD et al (eds): *Williams textbook of endocrinology,* ed 9, Philadelphia, 1998, WB Saunders.
CNS, Central nervous system; *CT,* computed tomography; *CYP11B1,* 11-hydroxylase; *CYP21,* 21-hydroxylase; *DHEAS,* dehydroepiandrosterone; *FSH,* follicle-stimulating hormone; *hCG,* human chorionic gonadotropin; *LH,* luteinizing hormone; *LHRH,* LH-releasing hormone; *MRI,* magnetic resonance imaging; *17-OHP,* 17-hydroxyprogesterone; T_4, thyroxine; *TSH,* thyroid-stimulating hormone.

TABLE 2-180   Differential Diagnosis of Sexual Precocity—cont'd

CONDITION	PLASMA GONADOTROPINS	LH RESPONSE TO LHRH	SERUM SEX STEROID CONCENTRATIONS	GONADAL SIZE	MISCELLANEOUS
Males—cont'd					
Familial testotoxicosis	Suppressed	No LH response	Pubertal values of testosterone	Testes symmetric and larger than 2.5 cm but smaller than expected for pubertal development; spermatogenesis occurs	Familial; probably sex-limited, autosomal dominant trait
Virilizing congenital adrenal hyperplasia	Prepubertal	Prepubertal LH response	Elevated 17-OHP in CYP21 deficiency or elevated 11-deoxycortisol in CYP11B1 deficiency	Testes prepubertal	Autosomal recessive, may be congenital or late-onset form, may have salt loss in CYP21 deficiency or hypertension in CYP11B1 deficiency
Virilizing adrenal tumor	Prepubertal	Prepubertal LH response	High DHEAS and androstenedione values	Testes prepubertal	CT, MRI, or ultrasonography of abdomen
Premature adrenarche	Prepubertal	Prepubertal LH response	Prepubertal testosterone, DHEAS, or urinary 17-ketosteroid values appropriate for pubic hair stage II	Testes prepubertal	Onset usually after age 6 yr; more frequent in CNS-injured children
Females					
Granulosa cell tumor (follicular cysts may be manifested similarly)	Suppressed	Prepubertal LH response	Very high estradiol	Ovarian enlargement on physical examination, CT, or ultrasonography	Tumor often palpable on abdominal examination
Follicular cyst	Suppressed	Prepubertal LH response	Prepubertal to very high estradiol	Ovarian enlargement on physical examination, CT, or ultrasonography	Single or recurrent episodes of menses and/or breast development; exclude McCune-Albright syndrome
Feminizing adrenal tumor	Suppressed	Prepubertal LH response	High estradiol and DHEAS values	Ovaries prepubertal	Unilateral adrenal mass
Premature thelarche	Prepubertal	Prepubertal LH, pubertal estradiol response	Prepubertal or early	Ovaries prepubertal	Onset usually before age 3 yr
Premature adrenarche	Prepubertal	Prepubertal LH response	Prepubertal estradiol; DHEAS or urinary 17-ketosteroid values appropriate for pubic hair stage II	Ovaries prepubertal	Onset usually after age 6 yr; more frequent in brain-injured children
Late-onset virilizing congenital adrenal hyperplasia	Prepubertal	Prepubertal LH response	Elevated 17-OHP in basal or corticotropin-stimulated state	Ovaries prepubertal	Autosomal recessive
In Both Sexes					
McCune-Albright syndrome	Suppressed	Suppressed	Sex steroids pubertal or higher	Ovarian enlargement (on ultrasound); slight testicular enlargement	Skeletal survey for polyostotic fibrous dysplasia and skin examination for café au lait spots
Primary hypothyroidism	LH prepubertal; FSH may be slightly elevated	Prepubertal FSH may be increased	Estradiol may be pubertal	Testicular enlargement; ovaries cystic	TSH and prolactin elevated; T_4 low

SEXUALITY DISORDERS

BOX 2-226   Sexuality Disorders

Primary or secondary sexual trauma
Incest
Abuse
Depression
Pharmacologic agents
  Anticholinergics
  Antiandrogens
  α-blockers and β-blockers
  Narcotics
  Sedatives
  Antidepressants
  Antihistamines
Malignancy
Hepatic/renal disease

Chronic illness
Disfigurement
Mastectomy
Radical neck
Burns
Trauma
Multiple sclerosis
Cord injury
Diabetic neuropathy
Hypoadrenalism
Panhypopituitarism
Ovarian failure
Premenstrual syndrome

From Danakas G (ed): *Practical guide to the care of the gynecologic/obstetric patient,* St Louis, 1997, Mosby.

Sexuality disorders
ICD-9CM # 302.79 Sexual disorder (psychosexual)
V41.7   Sexual function problem

SEXUALLY TRANSMITTED DISEASES, ANORECTAL REGION

TABLE 2-181   **Sexually Transmitted Diseases of the Anorectum**

TYPE	FINDINGS	TREATMENT
Ulcerative		
Lymphogranuloma venereum	Unilateral inguinal adenopathy Fever, malaise Mucoid or bloody discharge	Doxycycline 100 mg PO bid × 21 days If pregnant or allergic to tetracyclines: erythromycin 500 mg PO qid × 21 days

Herpes simplex virus	Rectal pain, tenesmus, constipation
	Bloody, mucoid discharge
	Vesicles and ulcerations
	Fever, malaise, myalgias, paresthesias
		First episode:
		  Perianal: acyclovir 400 mg PO tid ×
		    7-10 days
		  Proctitis: acyclovir 800 mg PO tid ×
		    7-10 days
		  Recurrent: acyclovir 400 mg PO tid ×
		    5 days

Early (primary) syphilis	Chancre Tenesmus, pain, mucoid discharge Inguinal lymphadenopathy	Benzathine penicillin G 2.4 MU IM × 1 Alternatives: doxycycline or erythromycin
Chancroid (*Haemophilus ducreyi*)	Inflammatory lesion progresses to ulcer Inguinal adenitis-bubo	Erythromycin 500 mg PO qid × 7 days *or* Ceftriaxone 250 mg IM × 1 *or* Azithromycin 1 g PO once
Cytomegalovirus	Tenesmus, diarrhea, weight loss	Gancyclovir with appropriate disposition
Idiopathic (usually HIV+)	Eccentric, deep, poor healing, multiple	Symptomatic relief or surgical referral
Nonulcerative		

Condyloma acuminatum	Keratinized vegetative growths in anus
	  or skin
	Asymptomatic or pruritus ani and/or
	  bleeding
		Podophyllum topically for limited
		  involvement

Gonorrhea (*Neisseria gonorrhoeae*)	Pruritus ani
	Tenesmus
	Purulent yellow discharge
		Ceftriaxone 250 mg IM once
		Alternatives: cefixime, ofloxacin,
		  ciprofloxacin
		For pregnant patients: spectinomycin
		  2 g IM *plus*
		  erythromycin 500 mg PO qid × 7 days

Chlamydia (*Chlamydia trachomatis*)	Mucoid or bloody discharge Tenesmus	Doxycycline 100 mg PO × 7 days *or* Azithromycin 1 g PO once For pregnant patients: erythromycin 500 mg PO qid × 7 days
Syphilis (secondary)	Maculopapular rash Condyloma latum	Benzathine penicillin G 2.4 MU IM × 1 Alternatives: doxycycline or erythromycin

From Rosen P (ed): *Emergency medicine*, ed 5, St Louis, 2002, Mosby.
bid, Twice a day; *HIV*, human immunodeficiency virus; *IM*, intramuscularly; *PO*, orally; *qid*, four times a day; *tid*, three times a day.

Shock
ICD-9CM # 785.50 Shock NOS
              785.51 Cardiogenic
              785.59 Septic
              308.9 Neurogenic
              785.59 Hypovolemic

SHOCK

BOX 2-227 Causes of Shock

Hypovolemic Shock

I. Inadequate circulating blood volume
  A. Acute hemorrhage (e.g., trauma, gastrointestinal bleeding, retroperitoneal bleeding, hemoptysis, hemothorax, ruptured aortic aneurysm)
  B. Plasma volume loss
    1. Intestinal obstruction
    2. Peritonitis, pancreatitis, rapid accumulation of ascites
    3. Splanchnic ischemia
    4. Extensive burns or exudative skin disease
    5. Increased capillary permeability (prolonged hypoxia and ischemia, extensive tissue injury, anaphylaxis)
  C. Excessive water and electrolyte losses
    1. Inadequate fluid and salt intake
    2. Excessive sweating
    3. Severe vomiting or diarrhea
    4. Excessive urinary losses (e.g., diabetes mellitus, diabetes insipidus, nephrotic syndrome, salt-losing nephropathy, postobstructive uropathy, diuretic phase of acute renal failure, excessive diuretic use)
    5. Acute adrenocortical insufficiency

Septic Shock

Gram-negative septicemia

Cardiogenic Shock

I. Impaired contractility/excessive preload
  A. Acute myocardial infarction
  B. Dilated cardiomyopathy
  C. Mitral insufficiency (subacute, chronic)
  D. Aortic insufficiency (subacute, chronic)
  E. Ventricular septal rupture
  F. Tachyarrhythmias/bradyarrhythmias
II. Decreased preload
  A. Right ventricular infarction
  B. Pericardial tamponade
  C. Pulmonary embolism
  D. Hypovolemia resulting from blood loss (e.g., ruptured aneurysm)
  E. Cardiac myxoma
  F. Tension pneumothorax
  G. Mitral stenosis
III. Excessive afterload
  A. Malignant hypertension
  B. Coarctation of the aorta
  C. Aortic stenosis
  D. Hypertrophic cardiomyopathy (preload may also be reduced)

Neurogenic Shock (Loss of Vasomotor Tone)

I. Spinal anesthesia
II. Spinal cord or brain damage
III. Drugs (ganglionic or adrenergic blocking agents)
IV. Anaphylaxis
V. Addisonian crisis

From Stein J (ed): *Internal medicine,* ed 5, St Louis, 1998, Mosby.

SHORT STATURE

TABLE 2-182 Differential Diagnosis of Short Stature

TYPE OF GROWTH PATTERN	CHRONOLOGIC AGE, HEIGHT AGE, AND BONE AGE	GROWTH RATE	DIFFERENTIAL DIAGNOSIS
Intrinsic short stature	CA = BA > HA	Normal range*	Familial short stature Intrauterine growth retardation Chromosomal anomalies, especially Turner's syndrome or one of its variants Bone dysplasias Dysmorphic syndromes Secondary to spinal irradiation
	CA > BA > HA		Constitutional delay in growth and puberty with familial short stature Intrauterine growth retardation Chromosomal anomalies
Delayed growth	CA > BA = HA	Normal range†	Constitutional delayed growth and puberty Chronic disorders Malnutrition

Acquired growth failure	CA > HA ≥ BA	Subnormal	Endocrinopathies
			  GH deficiency
			  Non–GH deficient, GH-responsive growth failure (biologic inactive GH or GH and/or somatomedin-C resistance)
			Hypothyroidism
			Cushing's syndrome
			Sex hormone deficiency after 10 yr of age
			Severe chronic organic diseases
			Severe malnutrition
			Psychosocial short stature

	CA > HA ≥ BA	Subnormal	Hypopituitarism Hypothyroidism

From Moore WT, Eastman RC: *Diagnostic endocrinology,* ed 2, St Louis, 1996, Mosby.
BA, Bone age; *CA,* chronologic age; *GH,* growth hormone; *HA,* height age.
*Slightly subnormal growth rate may occur occasionally.
†Slightly subnormal growth rate may occur occasionally.

Shoulder pain
ICD-9CM # 952.2 Shoulder injury
               718.81 Shoulder instability
               726.19 Shoulder ligament or muscle instability
               840.9 Shoulder strain, site unspecified

SHOULDER PAIN

BOX 2-228   Differential Diagnosis of Shoulder Pain

Intraarticular Processes

Synovitis secondary to rheumatoid arthritis or spondy-
  loarthropathies
Infection
Adhesive capsulitis
Osteoarthritis
Internal derangement (labral tears)
Avascular necrosis
Benign or malignant tumors (bone or synovial)

Periarticular Processes

Impingement syndrome: rotator cuff or bicipital
Calcific tendinitis
Tears of rotator cuff or biceps tendons
Myofascial pain
Acromioclavicular arthritis

Referred Pain

Sternoclavicular joint processes
Cervical radiculopathy
Pancoast's tumor
Subdiaphragmatic processes (abscess or gallbladder
  disease)
Myocardial infarction
Mediastinal tumors (pain localized to axilla)

Others

Reflex sympathetic dystrophy
Brachial neuritis
Thoracic outlet syndrome
Suprascapular nerve entrapment

Modified from Thornhill TS. In Kelley WN et al (eds): *Textbook of rheumatology*, ed 5, Philadelphia, 1993, WB Saunders.

Shoulder pain by location
ICD-9CM # 952.2 Shoulder injury
               726.19 Shoulder ligament or muscle instability
               840.8 Shoulder separation

SHOULDER PAIN BY LOCATION

BOX 2-229   Differential Diagnosis of Shoulder Pain by Location

Top of Shoulder (C4)

Cervical source
Acromioclavicular
Sternoclavicular
Diaphragmatic

Superolateral (C5)

Rotator cuff tendinitis
Impingement
Adhesive capsulitis
Glenohumeral arthritis

Anterior

Bicipital tendinitis and rupture
Glenoid labral tear
Adhesive capsulitis
Glenohumeral arthritis
Osteonecrosis

Axillary

Neoplasm (Pancoast's, mediastinal)
Herpes zoster

From Noble J: *Primary care medicine*, ed 3, St Louis, 2001, Mosby.

Sickle cell variants
ICD-9CM # 282.60 Anemia unspecified
          282.63 HbC disease, HbS/HbC disease
          282.69 HbD, HbE, HbS/HbD, HbS/HbE
                  disease

SICKLE CELL VARIANTS

TABLE 2-183   **Some Clinical Effects and Laboratory Values in Sickle Cell Disease**

GENOTYPE	MAJOR CLINICAL EFFECTS	AVERAGE HEMATOLOGIC PROFILE		HEMOGLOBIN ELECTROPHORESIS RESULTS (%)
S/S	Severe hemolytic anemia	Hb 6-9 g/dl*	A	0
	Stroke in childhood	PCV 18%-30%*	S	80-95
	Splenic sequestration crises	MCV 85-110 fl	A_2	2-3.5*
	Aplastic crises		F	1-20
	Vasoocclusive crises			
	Avascular necrosis of the femoral and humeral heads			
	Gallstones			
	Ankle ulcers			
S/β°thal	Moderate to severe anemia	Hb 7-10 g/dl	A	0
	Vasoocclusive crises	PCV 20%-35%	S	80-90
	Highest incidence of femoral head necrosis	MCV 65-80 fl	A_2	3-6
			F	10-20
S/C	Proliferative retinopathy	Hb 10-14 g/dl	A	0
	Occasional vasoocclusive crises	PCV 30%-35%	S	50
	Aseptic necrosis of femoral head in about 5% of cases	MCV 75-90 fl	C	50
	Mild splenomegaly			
S/β⁺thal	Mild anemia	Hb 10-14 g/dl	A	10-25
	Rare vasoocclusive crises	PCV 35%-45%	S	70-85
	Avascular necrosis in about 5% of cases	MCV 65-80 fl	A_2	3.5-6
	Risk of proliferative retinopathy		F	1-15
S/dβ-thal	Mild anemia	Hb 10-12 g/dl	A	0
	Rare vasoocclusive crises	PCV 36%-40%	S	70-80
	Rare complications	MCV 75-85 fl	A_2	1-3
			F	15-30

From Kassirer J (ed): *Current therapy in adult medicine,* ed 4, St Louis, 1998, Mosby.
*S/S patients with concomitant alpha-thalassemia have Hb A_2 levels of 4% to 5%, a decreased mean corpuscular volume (MCV) of 75 to 65 fl, and a slightly higher hemoglobin and packed cell volume (PCV).

II

SKIN LESIONS, PRIMARY

Skin lesions, primary
ICD-9CM # 709.9 Skin disorder
707.9 Skin ulcer unspecified

TABLE 2-184 Primary Skin Lesions

DESCRIPTION	DIFFERENTIAL DIAGNOSIS	
Macule		

A circumscribed flat discoloration, that may be brown, blue, red, or hypopigmented 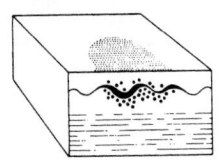	Brown
	  Becker's nevus
	  Café-au-lait spot
	  Erythrasma
	  Fixed drug eruption
	  Freckle
	  Junction nevus
	  Lentigo
	  Lentigo maligna
	  Melasma
	  Photoallergic drug eruption
	  Phototoxic drug eruption
	  Stasis dermatitis
	  Tinea nigra palmaris
	Blue
	  Ink (tattoo)
	  Maculae caeruleae (lice)
	  Mongolian spot
	  Ochronosis
		Red
		  Drug eruptions
		  Juvenile rheumatoid arthritis
		    (Still's disease)
		  Rheumatic fever
		  Secondary syphilis
		  Viral exanthems
		Hypopigmented
		  Idiopathic guttate hypomelanosis
		  Piebaldism
		  Postinflammatory (psoriasis)
		  Radiation dermatitis
		  Nevus anemicus
		  Tinea versicolor
		  Tuberous sclerosis
		  Vitiligo

Pustule		
A circumscribed collection of leukocytes and free fluid that varies in size 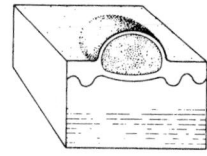	Acne Candidiasis Dermatophyte infection Dyshidrosis Folliculitis Gonococcemia Hidradenitis suppurativa	Herpes simplex Herpes zoster Impetigo Psoriasis Pyoderma gangrenosum Rosacea Varicella
Vesicle		
A circumscribed collection of free fluid up to 0.5 cm in diameter 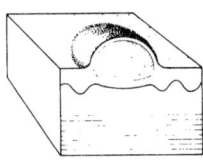	Benign familial chronic pemphigus Cat-scratch disease Chicken pox Dermatitis herpetiformis Eczema (acute) Erythema multiforme Herpes simplex	Herpes zoster Impetigo Lichen planus Pemphigus foliaceus Porphyria cutanea tarda Scabies
Bulla		
A circumscribed collection of free fluid more than 0.5 cm in diameter	Fixed drug eruption Herpes gestationis Lupus erythematosus Pemphigus	Bullae in diabetics Bullous pemphigoid Cicatricial pemphigoid Epidermolysis bullosa acquisita
Wheal		
A firm, edematous plaque resulting from infiltration of the dermis with fluid; it is transient and may last only a few hours 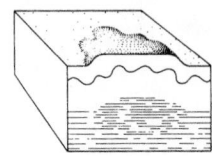	Angioedema Dermographism Hives Insect bites Urticaria pigmentosa (mastocytosis)	

From Habif TP: *Clinical dermatology: a color guide to diagnosis and therapy,* ed 2, St Louis, 1990, Mosby.

TABLE 2-184   Primary Skin Lesions—cont'd

DESCRIPTION	DIFFERENTIAL DIAGNOSIS

Papule

An elevated solid lesion up to 0.5 cm in diameter; color varies; papules may become confluent and form plaques

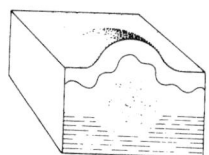

Flesh colored, yellow, or white
  Adenoma sebaceum
  Basal cell epithelioma
  Closed comedone (acne)
  Flat warts
  Granuloma annulare
  Lichen nitidus
  Lichen sclerosus et atrophicus
  Molluscum contagiosum
  Milium
  Nevi (dermal)
  Neurofibroma
  Pearly penile papules
  Pseudoxanthoma elasticum
  Sebaceous hyperplasia
  Skin tags
  Syringoma
Brown
  Dermatofibroma
  Keratosis follicularis
  Melanoma
  Nevi
  Seborrheic keratosis
  Urticaria pigmentosa
  Warts

Red
  Acne
  Atopic dermatitis
  Cholinergic urticaria
  Chondrodermatitis nodularis chronica helicis
  Eczema
  Folliculitis
  Insect bites
  Keratosis pilaris
  Leukocytoclastic vasculitis
  Miliaria
  Polymorphic light eruption
  Psoriasis
  Pyogenic granuloma
  Scabies
  Urticaria
Blue or violaceous
  Angiokeratoma
  Blue nevus
  Lichen planus
  Lymphoma
  Kaposi's sarcoma
  Melanoma
  Mycosis fungoides
  Venous lake

Plaque

A circumscribed, elevated, superficial, solid lesion more than 0.5 cm in diameter, often formed by the confluence of papules

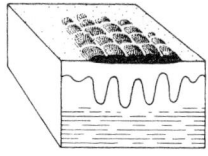

Eczema
Mycosis fungoides
Papulosquamous (papular and scaling)
  Discoid lupus erythematosus
  Lichen planus
  Pityriasis rosea
  Psoriasis
  Seborrheic dermatitis
  Syphilis (secondary)
  Tinea corporis
  Tinea versicolor

Nodule

A circumscribed, elevated, solid lesion more than 0.5 cm in diameter; a large nodule is referred to as a tumor

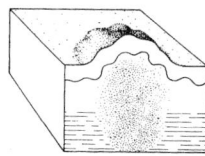

Basal cell epithelioma
Erythema nodosum
Furuncle
Hemangioma
Kaposi's sarcoma
Keratoacanthoma
Lipoma
Lymphoma
Melanoma

Metastatic carcinoma
Mycosis fungoides
Neurofibromatosis
Prurigo nodularis
Sporotrichosis
Squamous cell carcinoma
Warts
Xanthoma

Continued

Skin lesions, secondary
ICD-9CM # 709.9 Skin disorder
707.9 Skin ulcer unspecified

SKIN LESIONS, SECONDARY

TABLE 2-185   Secondary Skin Lesions

DESCRIPTION	DIFFERENTIAL DIAGNOSIS

Scale

Excess dead epidermal cells that are produced by abnormal keratinization and shedding

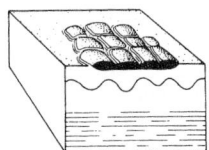

Fine to stratified
  Eczema craquele
  Ichthyosis (quadrangular)
  Lupus erythematosus (carpet tack)
  Pityriasis rosea (collarette)
  Psoriasis (silvery)
  Scarlet fever (fine on trunk)
  Seborrheic dermatitis (greasy)
  Syphilis (secondary)
  Tinea (dermatophytes)
  Tinea versicolor
  Xerosis (dry skin)
Scaling in sheets
  Scarlet fever (hands and feet)
  Staphylococcal scalded skin syndrome

Crust

A collection of dried serum and cellular debris; a scab

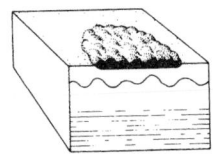

Acute eczematous inflammation
Atopic (face)
Impetigo (honey colored)
Pemphigus foliaceus
Tinea capitis

Erosion

A focal loss of epidermis; it does not penetrate below dermal-epidermal junction and therefore heals without scarring

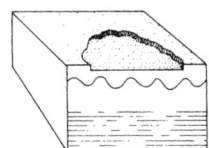

Candidiasis
Dermatophyte infection
Eczematous diseases
Intertrigo
Perlèche
Senile skin
Toxic epidermal necrolysis
Vesiculobullous diseases

Ulcer

A focal loss of epidermis and dermis; it heals with scarring

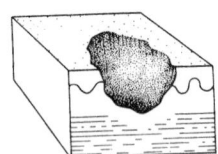

Aphthae
Chancroid
Decubitus
Factitial
Ischemic
Necrobiosis lipoidica diabeticorum
Neoplasms
Pyoderma gangrenosum
Radiodermatitis
Stasis ulcers
Syphilis (chancre)

From Habif TP: *Clinical dermatology: a color guide to diagnosis and therapy,* ed 2, St Louis, 1990, Mosby.

TABLE 2-185 Secondary Skin Lesions—cont'd

DESCRIPTION	DIFFERENTIAL DIAGNOSIS
Fissure	
A linear loss of epidermis and dermis with sharply defined nearly vertical walls 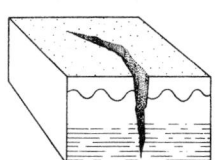	Chapping (hands, feet) Eczema (fingertip) Intertrigo Perlèche
Atrophy	
A depression in skin resulting from thinning of epidermis or dermis 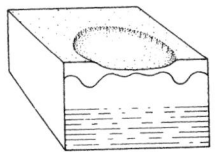	Aging Dermatomyositis Discoid lupus erythematosus Lichen sclerosus et atrophicus Morphea Necrobiosis lipoidica diabeticorum Radiodermatitis Striae Topical and intralesional steroids
Scar	
An abnormal formation of connective tissue implying dermal damage; when following injury or surgery, it is initially thick and pink but with time becomes white and atrophic 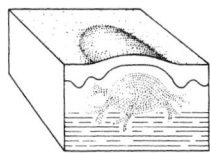	Acne Burns Herpes zoster Hidradenitis suppurativa Porphyria Varicella

SKIN LESIONS, SPECIAL

Skin lesions, special
ICD-9CM # 709.9 Skin disorder
        707.9 Skin ulcer unspecified

TABLE 2-186 Special Skin Lesions

DESCRIPTION	DIFFERENTIAL DIAGNOSIS
Excoriation	—
An erosion caused by scratching; often linear	
Comedone	—
A plug of sebaceous and keratinous material lodged in the opening of a hair follicle; the follicular orifice may be dilated (blackhead) or narrowed (whitehead) or closed (comedone)	
Milia	—
Small superficial keratin cysts with no visible openings	
Cyst	—
A circumscribed lesion having a wall and a lumen; the lumen may contain fluid or solid matter	
Burrow	—
A narrow, elevated, tortuous channel produced by a parasite	
Lichenification	—
An area of thickened epidermis induced by scratching; the skin lines are accentuated so the surface looks like a washboard	
Telangiectasia	
Dilated superficial blood vessels	Actinically damaged skin
	Adenoma sebaceum
	Ataxia-telangiectasia
	Basal cell carcinoma
	Bloom's syndrome
	CRST syndrome
	Hereditary hemorrhagic telangiectasia
	Keloid
	Lupus erythematosus
	Necrobiosis lipoidica diabeticorum
	Of the proximal nail fold
	Dermatomyositis
	Lupus erythematosus
	Scleroderma
	Poikiloderma
	Radiodermatitis
	Rosacea
	Scleroderma
	Vascular spiders
	Pregnancy
	Cirrhosis
	Xeroderma pigmentosum
Petechia	Gonococcemia
A circumscribed deposit of blood less than 0.5 cm in diameter	Leukocytoclastic vasculitis
	Meningococcemia
Purpura	Platelet abnormalities
A circumscribed deposit of blood greater than 0.5 cm in diameter	Progressive pigmentary purpura
	Rocky Mountain spotted fever
	Scurvy
	Senile (traumatic)

From Habif PF: *Clinical dermatology: a color guide to diagnosis and therapy,* ed 2, St Louis, 1990, Mosby.
CRST, Calcinosis, Raynaud's phenomenon, sclerodactyly, telangiectasia.

SOMATOFORM DISORDERS

Somatoform disorders
ICD-9CM # 300.81

TABLE 2-187   **Somatoform Disorders**

DIAGNOSIS	CLINICAL FEATURES	EPIDEMIOLOGY	DIAGNOSTIC CONSIDERATIONS
Somatization disorder	Multiple physical symptoms in multiple organ systems	Lifetime prevalence of 0.2% Women outnumber men 5- to 20-fold Onset before age 30 yr Commonly coexists with other mental disorders	Onset before age 30 yr Functional impairment Somatic symptoms in multiple organ systems Medical illness is excluded
Conversion disorder	One or more symptoms or deficits suggesting neurologic or general medical condition	Conversion symptoms in up to one third of population Women outnumber men 2- to 5-fold Onset at any age Common in poorly educated, rural, lower socioeconomic populations	Symptom or deficit is symbolic of intrapsychic conflict Symptom or deficit is not intentionally produced Medical illness is excluded
Hypochondriasis	Preoccupation with fear of disease or illness	Prevalence of 5% in clinic populations Men and women equally affected Onset in 20s	Preoccupation with disease exists despite evaluation and reassurance Preoccupation is not delusional in nature Duration of at least 6 mo
Body dysmorphic disorder	Preoccupation with imagined defect in appearance	Poorly studied but likely rare Onset in late teens Commonly coexists with other mental disorders (major depression, anxiety disorder)	Concern with physical defect is excessive and associated with significant distress
Pain disorder	Pain in one or more anatomic sites severe enough to warrant clinical attention	Pain syndromes are common in clinical practice Women outnumber men 2-fold Onset in 50s to 60s Commonly coexists with other psychiatric disorders	Pain causes significant distress and impairment in functioning Closely associated with psychologic factors Symptom is not intentionally produced

From Conn R: *Current diagnosis,* ed 9, Philadelphia, 1977, WB Saunders.

II

SORE THROAT

TABLE 2-188　Differential Diagnosis of Sore Throat

Sore Throat
ICD-9CM # 462　Pharyngitis
075　Mononucleosis
472.1　Chronic pharyngitis
487.1　Pharyngitis, influenzal
074.0　Coxsackie virus pharyngitis

TYPE OF PHARYNGITIS	NATURE OF PATIENT	NATURE OF SYMPTOMS	PREDISPOSING FACTORS	PHYSICAL FINDINGS	DIAGNOSTIC STUDIES
Without pharyngeal ulcers					
Viral	All ages	Pain in throat Rapid onset Systemic symptoms		Exudate less likely than with streptococcal infections	
Infectious mononucleosis	Adolescents and young adults Uncommon in elderly	Gradual onset		Low-grade temperature Occasional exudate Enanthem Posterior cervical adenopathy Hepatosplenomegaly	Monospot test
Streptococcal pharyngitis	Patients younger than age 25, especially ages 6-12	Pain in throat Rapid onset Few systemic symptoms	Fall and winter Streptococcal infection in family Diabetes	Marked erythema and throat swelling Temperature >101° F Tender anterior cervical nodes Scarlatiniform rash Tonsillar exudate more likely than with viral infection	Culture Rapid streptococcal antigen screening Increased ASO titer
Gonococcal pharyngitis	Most common in male homosexuals and those with anogenital gonorrhea	Often no symptoms	Orogenital sex		Culture
Sinusitis with postnasal drip	Adults	Mild throat soreness Symptoms often worse with recumbency		Evidence of sinusitis Postnasal drip	Sinus radiographs
Allergic pharyngitis			Seasonal allergies	No fever Intermittent postnasal drip Swollen pharynx with minimal injection	Eosinophils in nasal secretions

With pharyngeal ulcers

Herpangina	More common in children	Painful ulcers on tonsils, pillars, or uvula	Immunosuppression Summer and autumn	Vesicles 1-2 mm ulcers	Serologic tests
Fusospirochetal infection (Vincent's angina)	Children and those with poor oral hygiene	Painful ulcers Bleeding gums Foul breath		No vesicles Ulcerative gingivitis Gray necrotic ulcers 2-30 mm ulcers Pseudomembrane	Gram stain; spirochetes
Candidiasis	Children Immunosuppressed patients Those taking antibiotics		Immunosuppression Antibiotics	3-11 mm ulcers No vesicles	KOH smear; *Candida* Culture
Herpes simplex	Most common in children	Not usually a cause of sore throat	Immunosuppression	1-2 mm painful ulcers Vesicles present on lips, gingivae, buccal mucosa, or tongue	Tzanck smear show multinucleated giant cells

From Seller RH (ed): *Differential diagnosis of common complaints*, ed 4, Philadelphia, 2000, WB Saunders.

SPHEROCYTOSIS

BOX 2-230   **Causes of Spherocytosis**

ABO hemolytic disease of newborn
Acute transfusion reactions (especially ABO type)
Hereditary spherocytosis
Transfused stored bank blood
Autoimmune hemolytic anemia
Thermal injury, especially in first 24 hr

Physical red blood cell injury (as a component of microangiopathic hemolytic anemia)
Toxins (*Clostridium welchii* sepsis and certain snake venoms)
Hereditary elliptocytosis (10%-20% of cases)
Occasionally in severe Heinz body hemolytic anemias

From Ravel R: *Clinical laboratory medicine,* ed 6, St Louis, 1995, Mosby.

SPLENOMEGALY

Splenomegaly
ICD-9CM # 789.2 Splenomegaly unspecified
             289.51 Chronic congestive
             759.0 Congenital
             789.2 Unknown origin

BOX 2-231   Causes of Splenomegaly

Infectious Causes

Infectious mononucleosis
Endocarditis
Human immunodeficiency virus infection
Abscess
Salmonella infection
Brucellosis
Mycobacterial infection
Spirochetal infection
Rickettsial infection
Psittacosis
Histoplasmosis
Tularemia
Listeriosis
Toxocariasis
Malaria and other tropical diseases

Hematologic Causes

Lymphoproliferative disorders
Chronic lymphocytic leukemia
Hodgkin's disease
Non-Hodgkin's lymphoma
Waldenström's macroglobulinemia
Heavy-chain disease
Angioimmunoblastic lymphadenopathy
Acute lymphocytic leukemia
Myeloproliferative disorders
Chronic myelogenous leukemia
Polycythemia vera
Myeloid metaplasia
Essential thrombocythemia
Chronic myelomonocytic leukemia
Acute myelogenous leukemia
Red blood cell disorders
Hereditary spherocytosis
Thalassemia
Hemoglobin SC
Other hemoglobinopathy or hemolytic syndrome
Histiocytosis
Systemic mastocytosis
Malignant hypereosinophilic syndrome

Immune Causes

Collagen-vascular diseases
Rheumatoid arthritis
Systemic lupus erythematosus
Behçet's syndrome
Granulomatous diseases
Sarcoidosis
Crohn's disease
Berylliosis
Hypersensitivity reaction
Phenytoin

Endocrine Causes

Hyperthyroidism

Infiltrative Causes

Lipoidosis
Gaucher's disease
Niemann-Pick disease
Hyperlipidemias
Amyloidosis

Congestive Causes

Hepatic cirrhosis (Banti's syndrome)
Splenic or portal venous thrombosis
Congestive heart failure (rarely)

Tumors or Cysts, or Both

Tumors
Metastatic (melanoma, carcinoma of the lung, breast,
    pancreas)
Locally invasive (carcinoma of the pancreas, left kidney,
    stomach)
Primary
Cysts
Epithelial
Lymphangiomatous
Posttraumatic

Unknown Etiology

Idiopathic nontropical (Dacie's syndrome)
Chronic renal failure in patients on hemodialysis
Idiopathic portal hypertension

From Harrington J (ed): *Consultation in internal medicine,* ed 2, St Louis, 1997, Mosby.

SPONDYLOARTHROPATHIES

Spondyloarthropathies
ICD-9CM # 720.7

BOX 2-232   Differential Diagnosis for Spondyloarthropathies

Axial arthritis
  Discogenic back pain
  Osteoarthritis
    Facet disease
    Diffuse idiopathic hypertrophic osteoarthropathy
    Osteoarthritis of sacroiliac joints
  Osteitis condensans ilii
  Infection (sacroiliitis)
    Tuberculosis, brucellosis*
    Bacteremia from intravenous drug abuse
  Others
    Whipple's disease*
    Behçet's syndrome*
    Relapsing polychondritis
    Secondary hyperparathyroidism
Peripheral arthritis
  Other inflammatory arthritides
    Rheumatoid arthritis
    Crystals
  Infections
    Borrelia burgdorferi (Lyme disease)
    Gonococcal

Poststreptococcal, acute rheumatic fever*
HIV
Chronic fungal or tuberculous
Noninflammatory arthritides
  Osteoarthritis, particularly inflammatory osteo-
    arthritis
  Mechanical derangement
Synovial neoplasia
  Pigmented villonodular synovitis*
  Osteogenic sarcoma*
  Synovial osteochondromatosis*
Others
  Sarcoidosis
Axial and peripheral arthritis
  Osteoarthritis
  Rheumatoid arthritis
  Whipple's disease*
  Behçet's syndrome*
  Relapsing polychondritis*
  Familial Mediterranean fever*

From Noble J (ed): *Primary care medicine*, ed 3, St Louis, 2001 Mosby.
*Rare occurrences.

SPONDYLOARTHROPATHIES, SERONEGATIVE

Spondyloarthropathies, seronegative
ICD-9CM # 720.7

TABLE 2-189   Comparison of Seronegative Spondyloarthropathies

SPONDYLOARTHROPATHY	ANKYLOSING SPONDYLITIS	REITER'S SYNDROME	PSORIATIC ARTHRITIS	ARTHRITIS ASSOCIATED WITH GI DISEASE
Characteristics and presentation	Insidious onset of constant back pain lasting longer than 3 mo in patient less than 40 yr of age Pain and stiffness are improved by exercise; patients often walk around at night to gain relief from nocturnal back pain Associated with anterior uveitis (25%), aortitis (5%)	Arthritis usually follows episode of urethritis Eye involvement: bilateral conjunctivitis, uveitis, keratitis, retinitis Dermatitis: usually painless mucocutaneous lesions on glans penis and mouth, hyperkeratotic lesions on palms and soles (keratoderma blenorrhagicum)	Arthritis usually involves DIP joints, often resulting in "sausage" digits Skin lesions usually precede arthritis Nail changes (pitting) often accompany psoriatic arthritis	Occurs with: Whipple's disease (up to 90% of patients), Crohn's disease (20%) After intestinal bypass Ulcerative colitis (10%) Remission of underlying disorder usually results in complete remission of the arthritis May be associated with erythema nodosum, pyoderma gangrenosum, anterior uveitis

DIP, Distal interphalangeal; *GI*, gastrointestinal; *NSAIDs*, nonsteroidal antiinflammatory drugs.

TABLE 2-189 Comparison of Seronegative Spondyloarthropathies—cont'd

SPONDYLOARTHROPATHY	ANKYLOSING SPONDYLITIS	REITER'S SYNDROME	PSORIATIC ARTHRITIS	ARTHRITIS ASSOCIATED WITH GI DISEASE
Association with HLA-B27	Strong association	Strong association	No significant association	No significant association except in patients with inflammatory bowel disease and sacroiliitis
Characteristic radiographic patterns of spine	Radiographs of spine initially show straightening of lumbar part of spine; in advanced disease, diffuse syndesmophyte formation may result in fusion of entire spine (bamboo spine)	Unlike ankylosing spondylitis, distribution of syndesmophytes is asymmetric and non-marginal	Similar to Reiter's syndrome	Radiographic evaluation may be normal or may reveal sacroiliitis
Peripheral arthritis	Oligoarticular Hips, shoulder	Oligoarticular Asymmetric Lower extremities	DIP joints Usually asymmetric and oligoarticular but can be variable	Large joints (knees, ankles) Symmetric
Therapy	NSAIDs, physical therapy	Joint immobilization, NSAIDs Topical corticosteroids for conjunctivitis, corticosteroid therapy, physical therapy	Treat skin disease NSAIDs Methotrexate Gold therapy	Treat underlying disorder Sulfasalazine (Azulfidine) for sacroiliitis associated with inflammatory bowel disease

DIP, Distal interphalangeal; *GI,* gastrointestinal; *NSAIDs,* nonsteroidal antiinflammatory drugs.

ST SEGMENT ELEVATION

**ST segment elevation
ICD-9CM # 794.31 Abnormal electrocardiogram**

TABLE 2-190 Differential Diagnosis of ST Segment Elevation (by Degree, Morphology, and Associated Findings)*

	MYOCARDIAL ISCHEMIA	EARLY REPOLARIZATION	ACUTE (SIMPLE) PERICARDITIS
ST elevation (over 5 mm)	+	0	0
Reciprocal ST depression	+	±	±
Convex ST	+	0	±
Concave ST	+	+	+
Prominent T (over 5 mm)	+	+	0
Same lead ST elevation and T depression	+	±	±
Pathologic Q waves	+	0	0
Special findings	Atrioventricular block	0	Electrical alternans

From Rosen P et al (eds): *Emergency medicine: concepts and clinical practice,* St Louis, 1992, Mosby.
*Only positive findings are classified; negative findings do not exclude ischemia or pericarditis; +, often found; ±, not often found or restricted to certain leads; 0, reliably absent.

ST-T WAVE CHANGES

ST-T wave changes
ICD-9CM # 794.31 Abnormal electrocardiogram

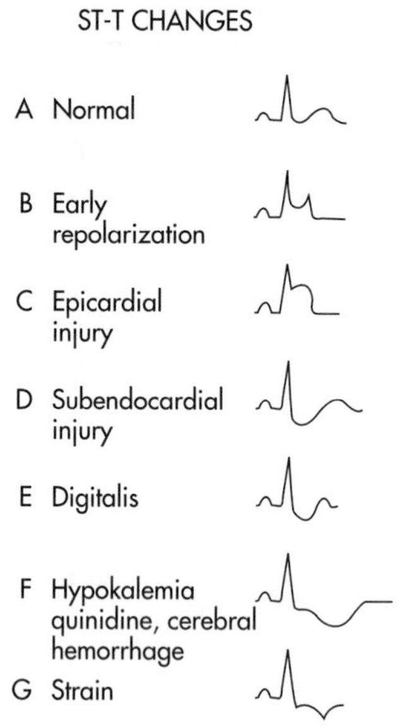

ST-T CHANGES

A Normal

B Early repolarization

C Epicardial injury

D Subendocardial injury

E Digitalis

F Hypokalemia quinidine, cerebral hemorrhage

G Strain

Fig. 2-12   ST-T wave changes in normal and abnormal conditions. (From Gazes PC: *Clinical cardiology: a bedside approach,* ed 2, Chicago, 1983, Mosby.)

STRIDOR, PEDIATRIC AGE

Stridor, pediatric age
ICD-9CM # 786.1 Stridor
              748.3 Stridor laryngeal congenital

BOX 2-233   Causes of Recurrent or Persistent Stridor in Children

Recurrent

Allergic (spasmodic) croup
Respiratory infections in a child with otherwise asymptomatic anatomic narrowing of the large airways
Laryngomalacia

Persistent

Laryngeal obstruction
  Laryngomalacia
  Papillomas, other tumors
  Cysts and laryngoceles
  Laryngeal webs
  Bilateral abductor paralysis of the cords
  Foreign body
Tracheobronchial disease
  Tracheomalacia
  Subglottic tracheal webs
  Endotracheal, endobronchial tumors
  Subglottic tracheal stenosis
    Congenital
    Acquired

Extrinsic masses
  Mediastinal masses
  Vascular ring
  Lobar emphysema
  Bronchogenic cysts
  Thyroid enlargement
  Esophageal foreign body
Tracheoesophageal fistulas
Other
  Gastroesophageal reflux
  Macroglossia, Pierre Robin syndrome
  Cri du chat syndrome
  Hysterical stridor
  Hypocalcemia

From Behrman RE: *Nelson textbook of pediatrics,* ed 16, Philadelphia, 2000, WB Saunders.

STROKE

Stroke
ICD-9CM # 436 Acute stroke

BOX 2-234   Differential Diagnosis of Stroke

Migraine
Syncope
Hyperventilation
Metabolic encephalopathy
Drug overdose or intoxication
Transient global amnesia
Vestibular vertigo
Seizures
Hypoglycemia
Hysterical conversion reaction

From Stein J (ed): *Internal medicine,* ed 5, St Louis, 1998, Mosby.

STROKE, YOUNG ADULT

Stroke, young adult
ICD-9CM # 436

BOX 2-235   Causes of Stroke in Young Adults

Migraine
Arterial dissection
Drugs (cocaine, heroin, oral contraceptive pill)
Premature atherosclerosis (homocystinuria, hyperlipidemia)
Postpartum angiopathy
Cardiac factors
  Atrial septal defect
  Patent foramen ovale
  Mitral valve prolapse
  Endocarditis
Hematologic factors
  Deficiency states (antithrombin III, protein S, protein C)
  Disseminated intravascular coagulation
  Thrombotic thrombocytopenic purpura
Inflammatory factors
  Systemic lupus erythematosus
  Polyarteritis nodosa
  Neurosyphilis
  Cryoglobulinemia
Other factors
  Fibromuscular dysplasia
  Moyamoya syndrome

From Andreoli TE (ed): *Cecil essentials of medicine,* ed 5, Philadelphia, 2001, WB Saunders.

STROKE, PEDIATRIC AGE

BOX 2-236   Causes of Stroke in Children

I. Cardiac Disease
  A. Congenital
    1. Aortic stenosis
    2. Mitral stenosis; mitral prolapse
    3. Ventricular septal defects
    4. Patent ductus arteriosus
    5. Cyanotic congenital heart disease involving right-to-left shunt
  B. Acquired
    1. Endocarditis (bacterial, SLE)
    2. Kawasaki disease
    3. Cardiomyopathy
    4. Atrial myxoma
    5. Arrhythmia
    6. Paradoxical emboli through patent foramen ovale
    7. Rheumatic fever
    8. Prosthetic heart valve
II. Hematologic Abnormalities
  A. Hemoglobinopathies
    1. Sickle cell (SS) disease
    2. Sickle (SC) disease
  B. Polycythemia
  C. Leukemia/lymphoma
  D. Thrombocytopenia
  E. Thrombocytosis
  F. Disorders of coagulation
    1. Protein C deficiency
    2. protein S deficiency
    3. Factor V Leiden
    4. Antithrombin III deficiency
    5. Lupus anticoagulant
    6. Oral contraceptive pill use
    7. Pregnancy and the postpartum state
    8. Disseminated intravascular coagulation
    9. Paroxysmal nocturnal hemoglobinuria
    10. Inflammatory bowel disease (thrombosis)
III. Inflammatory Disorders
  A. Meningitis
    1. Viral
    2. Bacterial
    3. Tuberculosis
  B. Systemic infection
    1. Viremia
    2. Bacteremia
    3. Local head and neck infections

C. Drug-induced inflammation
    1. Amphetamine
    2. cocaine
  D. Autoimmune disease
    1. Systemic lupus erythematosus
    2. Juvenile rheumatoid arthritis
    3. Takayasu arteritis
    4. Mixed connective tissue disease
    5. Polyarteritis nodosum
    6. Primary CNS vasculitis
    7. Sarcoidosis
    8. Behçet's syndrome
    9. Wegener granulomatosis
IV. Metabolic Disease Associated with Stroke
  A. Homocystinuria
  B. Pseudoxanthoma elasticum
  C. Fabry disease
  D. Sulfite oxidase deficiency
  E. Mitochondrial disorders
    1. MELAS
    2. Leigh syndrome
  F. Ornithine transcarbamylase deficiency
V. Intracerebral Vascular Processes
  A. Ruptured aneurysm
  B. Arteriovenous malformation
  C. Fibromuscular dysplasia
  D. Moyamoya disease
  E. Migraine headache
  F. Postsubarachnoid hemorrhage vasospasm
  G. Hereditary hemorrhagic telangiectasia
  H. Sturge-Weber syndrome
  I. Carotid artery dissection
  J. Post varicella
VI. Trauma and Other External Causes
  A. Child abuse
  B. Head trauma/neck trauma
  C. Oral trauma
  D. Placental embolism
  E. ECMO therapy

From Riukin M: In Kliegman R (ed): *Practical strategies in pediatric diagnosis and therapy*, Philadelphia, 1996, WB Saunders.
CNS, Central nervous system; *ECMO*, extracorporeal membrane oxygenation; *MELAS*, mitochondrial encephalomyopathy, lactic acidosis, and stroke.

SUDDEN DEATH, PEDIATRIC AGE

Sudden death, pediatric age
ICD-9CM # Code varies with specific disorder

BOX 2-237   Potential Causes of Sudden Death in Infants, Children, and Adolescents

SIDS and SIDS "Mimics"

SIDS
Long Q-T syndromes
Inborn errors of metabolism
Child abuse
Myocarditis
Duct-dependent congenital heart disease

Corrected or Unoperated Congenital Heart Disease

Aortic stenosis
Tetralogy of Fallot
Transposition of great vessels (postoperative atrial switch)
Mitral valve prolapse
Hypoplastic left heart syndrome
Eisenmenger's syndrome

Coronary Arterial Disease

Anomalous origin
Anomalous tract
Kawasaki disease
Periarteritis
Arterial dissection
Marfan syndrome
Myocardial infarction

Myocardial Disease

Myocarditis
Hypertrophic cardiomyopathy
Dilated cardiomyopathy
Arrhythmogenic right ventricular dysplasia

Conduction System Abnormality/Arrhythmia

Long Q-T syndromes
Proarrhythmic drugs
Preexcitation syndromes
Heart block
Commotio cordis
Idiopathic ventricular fibrillation
Heart tumor

Miscellaneous

Pulmonary hypertension
Pulmonary embolism
Heat stroke
Cocaine
Anorexia nervosa
Electrolyte disturbances

From Behrman RE: *Nelson textbook of pediatrics,* ed 16, Philadelphia, 2000, WB Saunders.
SIDS, Sudden infant death syndrome.

SWOLLEN LIMB

Swollen limb
ICD-9CM # 729.81 Swollen arm or hand
729.81 Swollen leg or foot

TABLE 2-191   **Differential Diagnosis of the Swollen Limb**

	PAIN	INFLAMMATORY SIGNS	VARICOSE VEINS	NONINVASIVE VENOUS STUDIES	CLUES TO DIAGNOSIS
Thrombophlebitis	+	+	±	+	Acute onset of swelling
Lymphedema	Usually absent	0	0	Negative	Gradual onset of swelling
Postphlebitic syndrome	+	±	+	Negative	Stasis pigmentation, subcutaneous tissue induration
Ruptured popliteal synovial membrane	+	+	0	Negative	Fluid in the knee joint, history of arthritis
Ruptured calf	+	+	0	Negative	Ecchymoses around ankle, tender knot in muscle, sudden onset during exercise—may feel a pop
Myositis ossificans	+	+	0	Negative	Indurated area in thigh with localized swelling; positive bone scan

From Noble J (ed): *Primary care medicine,* ed 3, St Louis, 2001, Mosby.

SYNOVIAL FLUID ABNORMALITIES

Synovial fluid abnormalities
ICD-9CM # 792.9 Abnormal synovial fluid

TABLE 2-192 Classification and Interpretation of Synovial Fluid Analysis

GROUP	DISEASES	APPEARANCE	VISCOSITY	MUCIN CLOT	WBC/MM³	%PMN	GLUCOSE (MG/DL) (BLOOD–SYNOVIAL FLUID)	PROTEIN (G/DL)
Normal	—	Clear	↑	Firm	<200	<25	<10	<2.5
I (noninflammatory)	Osteoarthritis, aseptic necrosis, traumatic arthritis, erythema nodosum, osteochondritis dissecans	Clear, yellow (may be xanthochromic if traumatic arthritis)	↑	Firm	↑ Up to 10,000	<25	<10	<2.5
II (inflammatory)	Crystal-induced arthritis, rheumatoid arthritis, Reiter's syndrome, collagen-vascular disease, psoriatic arthritis, serum sickness, rheumatic fever	Clear, yellow, turbid	↓	Friable	↑↑ Up to 100,000	40-90	<40	>2.5
III (septic)	Bacterial (staphylococcal, gonococcal, tuberculosis)	Turbid	↓/↑	Friable	↑↑↑ Up to 5 million	40-100	20-100	>2.5

↑, Elevated; ↑↑, markedly high; ↓, decreased; *PMN*, polymorphonuclear leukocytes. Note that there is considerable overlap in the numbers listed above.

T WAVE CHANGES

T wave changes
ICD-9CM # 794.31 Abnormal electrocardiogram

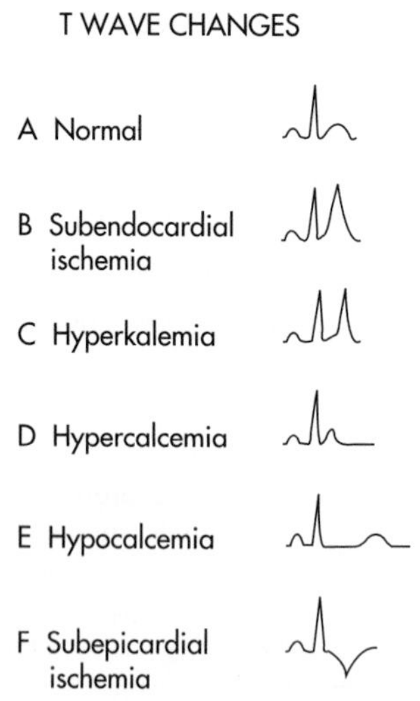

T WAVE CHANGES

A Normal

B Subendocardial ischemia

C Hyperkalemia

D Hypercalcemia

E Hypocalcemia

F Subepicardial ischemia

Fig. 2-13 T wave changes in normal and abnormal conditions. (From Gazes PC: *Clinical cardiology: a bedside approach,* ed 2, Chicago, 1983, Mosby.)

TALL STATURE

BOX 2-238   Causes of Tall Stature

Constitutional (familial or genetic)—most common
  cause
Endocrine causes
  Growth hormone excess—gigantism
  Sexual precocity (tall as children, short as adults)
    True sexual precocity
    Pseudosexual precocity
  Androgen deficiency
    Klinefelter's syndrome
    Bilateral anorchism
Genetic causes
  Klinefelter's syndrome
  Syndromes of XYY, XXYY
Miscellaneous syndromes and disorders
  Cerebral gigantism or Sotos' syndrome: prominent
    forehead, hypertelorism, high arched palate,
    dolichocephaly, mental retardation, large hands and
    feet, and premature eruption of teeth. Large at birth,
    with most rapid growth in first 4 years of life.

Marfan's syndrome: disorder of mesodermal tissues,
  subluxation of the lenses, arachnodactyly, and aortic
  aneurysm
Homocystinuria: same phenotype as Marfan's syndrome
Obesity: tall as infants, children, and adolescents
Total lipodystrophy: large hands and feet, generalized
  loss of subcutaneous fat, insulin-resistant diabetes
  mellitus, and hepatomegaly
Beckwith-Wiedemann syndrome: neonatal tallness,
  omphalocele, macroglossia, and neonatal hypoglycemia
Weaver-Smith syndrome: excessive intrauterine
  growth, mental retardation, megalocephaly, widened
  bifrontal diameter, hypertelorism, large ears, micrognathia, camptodactyly, broad thumbs, and limited
  extension of elbows and knees
Marshall-Smith syndrome: excessive intrauterine
  growth, mental retardation, blue sclerae, failure to
  thrive, and early death

From Moore WT, Eastman RC: *Diagnostic endocrinology,* ed 2, St Louis, 1996, Mosby.

Tall stature
**ICD-9CM # 253.0 Growth hormone overproduction,
           gigantism**

Tardive dyskinesia
ICD-9CM # 781.3 Dyskinesia
**   300.11 Hysterical dyskinesia**
**   333.82 Orofacial dyskinesia**
**   307.9 Psychogenic dyskinesia**

TARDIVE DYSKINESIA

BOX 2-239   Differential Diagnosis of Tardive Dyskinesia

Neurologic Disorders

Brain neoplasms
Fahr's syndrome
Huntington's disease
Idiopathic dystonias (tics, blepharospasm, aging)
Ill-fitting dentures
Meige's syndrome (spontaneous oral dyskinesia)
Postanoxic extrapyramidal syndrome
Postenecephalitic extrapyramidal syndrome
Torsion dystonia
Wilson's disease

Drugs

Amphetamines
Anticholinergics
Antidepressants
Heavy metals
L-Dopa
Lithium
Magnesium
Phenytoin

From Goldberg RJ (ed): *The care of the psychiatric patient,* ed 2, St Louis, 1998, Mosby.

TASTE AND SMELL LOSS

Taste and smell loss
ICD-9CM # 781.1 Smell and taste disturbance
of sensation

TABLE 2-193   Common Causes of Sustained Loss of Taste and Smell

	TASTE	SMELL
Local	Radiation therapy	Allergic rhinitis, sinusitis, nasal polyposis, bronchial asthma
Systemic	Cancer, renal failure, hepatic failure, nutritional deficiency (vitamin B_{12}, zinc), Cushing's syndrome, hypothyroidism, diabetes mellitus, infection (influenza), drugs (antirheumatic and antiproliferative)	Renal failure, hepatic failure, nutritional deficiency (vitamin B_{12}), Cushing's syndrome, hypothyroidism, diabetes mellitus, infection (viral hepatitis, influenza), drugs (nasal sprays, antibiotics)
Neurologic	Bell's palsy, familial dysautonomia, multiple sclerosis	Head trauma, multiple sclerosis, Parkinson's disease, frontal brain tumor

From Baloh RW: Smell and taste. In Andreoli TE (ed): *Cecil essentials of medicine,* ed 4, Philadelphia, 1997, WB Saunders.

TELANGIECTASIA

Telangiectasia
ICD-9CM # 448.9

BOX 2-240   Differential Diagnosis of Telangiectasia

Primary telangiectasia
Angioma serpiginosum
Ataxia telangiectasia
Generalized essential telangiectasia
Hereditary hemorrhagic telangiectasia
Spider telangiectases
Unilateral nevoid telangiectasia syndrome
Secondary telangiectasia
Poikiloderma
Chronic graft-versus-host disease
Corticosteroid induced (systemic or topical)
Dermatomyositis

Drug induced
Hepatic cirrhosis
Lupus erythematosus
Mastocytosis (telangiectasia macularis eruptiva perstans)
Bloom syndrome
Oral contraceptive agents
Pregnancy
Radiation induced x-ray, ultraviolet or natural sunlight
Rosacea, varicose veins
Systemic sclerosis
Trauma
Xeroderma pigmentosa

From Callen JP (ed): *Color atlas of dermatology,* ed 2, Philadelphia, 2000, WB Saunders.

TENDINITIS SYNDROMES

Tendinitis syndromes
ICD-9CM # 726.90

TABLE 2-194   Tendinitis Syndromes

LOCATION	SYMPTOM	FINDING
Extensor pollicis brevis and abductor pollicis longus (DeQuervain's tenosynovitis)	Wrist pain	Pain on ulnar deviation of the wrist, with the thumb grasped by the remaining four fingers (Finkelstein's test)
Flexor tendons of fingers	Triggering or locking of fingers in flexion	Tender nodule on flexor tendon On palm over metacarpal joint
Medial epicondyle	Elbow pain	Tenderness of medial epicondyle
Lateral epicondyle	Elbow pain	Tenderness of lateral epicondyle
Bicipital tendon	Shoulder pain	Tenderness along bicipital groove
Patellar	Knee pain	Tenderness at insertion of patellar tendon
Achilles	Heel pain	Tender Achilles tendon
Tibialis posterior	Medial ankle pain	Tenderness under medial malleolus with resisted inversion of the ankle
Peroneal	Lateral mid-foot or ankle pain	Tenderness under lateral malleolus with passive inversion

From Andreoli TE (ed): *Cecil essentials of medicine,* ed 5, Philadelphia, 2001, WB Saunders.

TERATOGENS

Teratogens
ICD-9CM # not available

BOX 2-241   **Human Teratogens**

Maternal infections
  Rubella
  Cytomegalovirus
  Toxoplasmosis
  Varicella
  Herpes simplex
  Venezuela equine encephalitis
  Syphilis
  Parvovirus
  Lymphocytic choriomeningitis virus
Maternal conditions
  Diabetes mellitus
  Phenylketonuria
  Maternal hyperthermia
  Graves' disease
  Systemic lupus erythematosus
Drugs and chemicals
  Ethanol
  Thalidomide
  Diethylstilbestrol

Warfarin
Hydantoin
Trimethadione
Valproic acid
Aminopterin/methotrexate
Tetracycline
Retinoic acid/isotretinoin
Angiotensin-converting enzyme inhibitors
Penicillamine
Antithyroid agents
Androgens
Masculinizing progestins
Methyl mercury
Polychlorobiphenyls
Tobacco
Chloroquine
Cocaine/crack
Streptomycin
Ionizing radiation

From Rakel RE (ed): *Principles of family practice,* ed 6, Philadelphia, 2002, WB Saunders.

TESTICULAR FAILURE

Testicular failure
ICD-9CM # 257.1 Testicular failure

BOX 2-242 Primary and Secondary Testicular Failure

Primary

Klinefelter's syndrome (XXY)
XYY
Vanishing testes syndrome (in utero or early postnatal torsion)
Noonan's syndrome
Varicocele
Myotonic dystrophy
Orchitis (mumps, gonorrhea)
Cryptorchidism
Chemical exposure
Irradiation to testes
Spinal cord injury
Polyglandular failure
Idiopathic oligospermia or azoospermia
Germinal cell aplasia (Sertoli cell–only syndrome)
Idiopathic testicular failure
Testicular torsion
Testicular trauma
Diethylstilbestrol (maternal use during pregnancy resulting in in utero estrogen exposure)
Testicular tumor with subsequent irradiation therapy, chemotherapy, or surgery (retroperitoneal lymph node dissection or orchiectomy)

Secondary

Delayed puberty
Kallmann's syndrome
Isolated gonadotropin deficiency
Prader-Labhart-Willi syndrome
Lawrence-Moon-Biedl syndrome
Central nervous system irradiation
Prepubertal panhypopituitarism
Postpubertal panhypopituitarism
Hypogonadism secondary to hyperprolactinemia
Adrenogenital syndrome
Chronic liver disease
Chronic renal failure/uremia
Hemochromatosis
Cushing's syndrome
Malnutrition
Massive obesity
Sickle cell anemia
Hyper/hypothyroidism
Anabolic steroid use

From Copeland LJ: *Textbook of gynecology,* ed 2, Philadelphia, 2000, WB Saunders.

TESTICULAR PAIN

Testicular pain
ICD-9CM # 608.9

TABLE 2-195 Testicular Pain: Diagnostic Considerations

CONDITION	DIAGNOSTIC FINDINGS	ANCILLARY DATA
Testicular torsion	Sudden onset; may follow trauma or occur during sleep or vehicle ride; nausea, vomiting Physical examination: tender testicle with horizontal lie; abdominal or flank pain; palpable cord twist Peak incidence 13 yr of age; uncommon in those over 30 yr of age	Urine: normal Technetium scan: decreased activity Doppler examination: decreased flow
Trauma	Sudden onset with history of trauma Physical examination: pain and swelling of testicle; hematoma may be present; findings reflect injury	Urine: normal Technetium scan: variable Doppler examination: variable
Epididymitis	Usually gradual onset; uncommon in boys before puberty; groin pain; may be associated with trauma, lifting, exercise; recent instrumentation Physical examination: tender epididymis present early with a soft normal testicle whereas later, diffuse tenderness of epididymis and testicle is noted; febrile; prostatic tenderness	Urine: pyuria, bacteriuria Technetium scan: increased activity Doppler examination: normal or increased flow
Tumor	Gradual onset unless hemorrhage Physical examination: hard, irregular, and usually painless testicle	Urine: normal Technetium scan: normal Doppler examination: normal

From Barkin RM, Rosen P: *Emergency pediatrics: a guide to ambulatory care,* ed 5, St Louis, 1999, Mosby.

TESTICULAR SIZE VARIATIONS

BOX 2-243   Causes of Variations in Testicular Size

Small Testes

Hypothalamic-pituitary dysfunction
    Gonadotropin deficiency
    Growth hormone deficiency
Normal variant
Primary hypogonadism
    Autoimmune destruction, chemotherapy, cryptorchid-
    ism, irradiation, Klinefelter's syndrome, orchiditis,
    testicular regression syndrome, torsion, trauma

Large Testes

Adrenal rest tissue
Compensatory
Fragile X syndrome
Idiopathic
Tumor

From Moore WT, Eastman RC: *Diagnostic endocrinology,* ed 2, St Louis, 1996, Mosby.

Testicular size variations
ICD-9CM # 608.3   Testicular atrophy
**   608.89 Testicular mass**
**   257.2   Hypogonadism**

THALASSEMIC SYNDROMES

Thalassemic syndromes
ICD-9CM # 348.8

TABLE 2-196   Thalassemic Syndromes

DISORDER	GENOTYPIC ABNORMALITY	CLINICAL PHENOTYPE
β-Thalassemia		
Thalassemia major (Cooley's anemia)	Homozygous β^0 thalassemia	Severe hemolysis, ineffective erythropoiesis, transfusion dependency, iron overload
Thalassemia intermedia	Compound heterozygous β^0 and β^+ thalassemia	Moderate hemolysis, severe anemia, but not transfusion dependent; main life-threatening complication is iron overload
Thalassemia minor	Heterozygous β^0 or β^+ thalassemia	Microcytosis, mild anemia
α-Thalassemia		
Silent carrier	$\alpha-/\alpha\alpha$	Normal complete blood count
α-Thalassemia trait	$\alpha\alpha/-$ (α-thalassemia 1) OR $\alpha-/\alpha-$ (α-thalassemia 2)	Mild microcytic anemia
Hemoglobin H	$\alpha-/-$	Microcytic anemia and mild hemolysis; not transfusion dependent
Hydrops fetalis	$-/-$	Severe anemia, intrauterine anasarca from congestive heart failure; death in utero or at birth

From Andreoli TE (ed): *Cecil essentials of medicine,* ed 5, Philadelphia, 2001, WB Saunders.

THROMBOCYTOPENIA

Thrombocytopenia
ICD-9CM # 287.3 Congenital or primary
287.4 Secondary
287.5 Thrombocytopenia NOS

BOX 2-244   Major Causes of Thrombocytopenia

I. Decreased platelet production
  A. Megakaryocyte hypoplasia
    1. Aplastic anemia
    2. Myelofibrosis
    3. Leukemia
    4. Marrow invasion by metastatic tumor, granulomas
    5. Viral infection
    6. Radiation myelosuppression
    7. Toxic agents, drugs, antineoplastic chemotherapy
  B. Ineffective thrombopoiesis
    1. Vitamin B_{12} deficiency
    2. Folate deficiency
II. Splenic sequestration, hypersplenism

III. Increased platelet destruction
  A. Non–immune-mediated platelet destruction
    1. Disseminated intravascular coagulation
    2. Prosthetic intravascular devices
    3. Extracorporeal circulation
    4. Thrombotic thrombocytopenic purpura
  B. Immune-mediated platelet destruction
    1. Drug-induced immune thrombocytopenia
    2. Alloimmune thrombocytopenia
      a. Neonatal
      b. Posttransfusion purpura
    3. Autoimmune thrombocytopenia
      a. Idiopathic thrombocytopenic purpura
      b. Secondary to rheumatic diseases, infections, lymphoproliferative disorders

---

From Stein JH (ed): *Internal medicine,* ed 4, St Louis, 1994, Mosby.

THROMBOPHILIA, INHERITED CAUSES

Thrombophilia, inherited causes
ICD-9CM # code varies with specific diagnosis

BOX 2-245   Inherited Causes of Thrombophilia

Activated protein C resistance/factor V Leiden (20-60%)*
Homocyst(e)inemia (10-15%)
Prothrombin 20210A (5-15%)
Antithrombin III deficiency (1-4%)
Protein C deficiency (2-6%)
Protein S deficiency (2-5%)
Tissue plasminogen activator deficiency (rare)
Plasminogen activator inhibitor excess (rare)
Dysfibrinogenemia (rare)
Decreased plasminogen (very rare)

From Andreoli TE (ed): *Cecil essentials of medicine,* ed 5, Philadelphia, 2001, WB Saunders.
* Prevalence in patients presenting with deep venous thrombosis or pulmonary embolism.

THROMBOSIS, ACQUIRED

Thrombosis, acquired
ICD-9CM # 453.9

BOX 2-246 Acquired Causes of Thrombosis

Medical and Surgical Illnesses

Antiphospholipid antibody/lupus anticoagulant
Artificial heart valves
Atrial fibrillation
Hemolytic anemia (sickle cell, thrombotic thrombo-
  cytopenic purpura)
Hyperlipidemia
Immobilization
Malignancy
Myeloproliferative disorders/thrombocytosis
Nephrotic syndrome
Orthopedic procedures
Pregnancy
Trauma/fat embolism

Medications

Heparin-induced thrombocytopenia
Oral contraceptives
Prothrombin complex concentrates

From Andreoli TE (ed): *Cecil essentials of medicine,* ed 5, Philadelphia, 2001, WB Saunders.

THYROID NODULE, COLD

BOX 2-247 Differential Diagnosis of the Cold Thyroid Nodule

Common Causes

Follicular adenoma—with or without cystic/hemorrhagic
  degeneration
Hyperplastic nodule
Thyroiditis—subacute, "silent," or chronic (rarely acute)
Thyroid carcinoma—papillary, follicular, or anaplastic
Colloid cyst
Previous surgery

Rare Causes

Hemiagenesis
Primary thyroid lymphoma

Medullary thyroid carcinoma
Branchiogenic cyst
Parathyroid adenoma, carcinoma, or cyst
Malignancy metastatic to thyroid
Tuberculoma
Amyloidosis
Postradiation fibrosis
Marine-Lenhart syndrome

From Moore WT, Eastman RC: *Diagnostic endocrinology,* ed 2, St Louis, 1996, Mosby.

Thyroid nodule, cold
ICD-9CM # 226   Thyroid adenoma
              241.0 Nontoxic uninodular goiter

TICK-BORNE VIRAL DISEASES

TABLE 2-197   Tick-Borne Viral Diseases

Tick-borne viral diseases
ICD-9CM # code varies with specific diagnosis

VIRUS	TAXONOMIC GROUP	MAJOR VECTOR	ANIMAL HOSTS	GEOGRAPHIC DISTRIBUTION	HUMAN ILLNESS	FREQUENCY OF RECOGNIZED DISEASE	RISK FACTORS
Colorado tick fever	Reoviridae, genus *Orbivirus*	*Dermacentor andersoni*	Rodents, other small mammals	Mountain highland areas of western United States and Canada	Biphasic FI, ME especially in children, in prolonged viremia	Sporadic, common in endemic areas	Occupational and recreational pursuits in mountain areas
Kemerovo	Reoviridae, genus *Orbivirus*	*Ixodes ricinus*, *I. persulcatus*	Domestic and wild mammals, birds	Siberia, Czech and Slovak Republics	Mild FI, occasional ME, not fatal	Sporadic, rare	Occupational and recreational pursuits in forested areas
Tick-Borne Encephalitis Complex							
Powassan encephalitis	Togaviridae, genus *Flavivirus*	*I. marxi*, *I. cookei*	Small mammals	Northern United States, Canada	FI, ME: possible sequelae and death especially in young	Sporadic, rare	Rural areas, pets?
Louping ill		*I. ricinus*	Goats, sheep, cattle, small mammals	Central and eastern Europe	Biphasic ME	Sporadic, common in endemic areas	Agricultural and forestry workers, drinking goat's milk
Russian spring-summer encephalitis		*I. ricinus*, *I. persulcatus*	Goats, sheep, cattle, small mammals	Siberia	Biphasic ME, possibly severe, with 20% mortality	Sporadic, common in endemic areas	Agricultural and forestry workers
Kyasanur Forest disease		*Haemaaphysalis spinigera*	Monkeys, small mammals	Southern India	FI, ME, possible hemorrhagic complications	Sporadic, epidemics occur	Residence in or travel to endemic areas
Omsk hemorrhagic fever		*Dermacentor pictus?*	Muskrats	Western Siberia	FI, hemorrhagic complications	Rare	Direct contact with muskrats
Crimean-Congo hemorrhagic fever	Bunyaviridae, genus *Nairovirus*	*Hyalomma marginatum*, *H. anatolicum*, others	Domestic and wild mammals	Southern Russia, Middle East, India, Pakistan, central Africa	FI, petechialecchymotic rash, hemorrhage, 3%-30% mortality	Sporadic, epidemics occur	Agricultural workers
Dugbe	Bunyaviridae, genus *Nairovirus*	Ixodid species	Cattle	Nigeria, Central African Republic	Acute FI	Rare, primarily children	Herding or caring for livestock
Bhanja	Probably Bunyaviridae	Ixodid species	Domestic and wild mammals	Yugoslavia, Italy, Kenya, Nigeria, India	FI, ME	Rare	Agricultural workers
Thogoto	Possibly Orthomyxoviridae	Ixodid species	Ruminants	Egypt, Kenya, Nigeria	FI, ME, optic neuritis	Rare	Herding or caring for livestock
Quaranfil	Unclassified	*Argas arboreus*	Pigeons, wild birds	Africa, Iran, Afghanistan	FI	Rare	Residence in endemic areas

From Auerbach PS: *Wilderness medicine*, ed 4, St Louis, 2001, Mosby.
FI, Febrile illness; *ME*, meningoencephalitis.

TICK-RELATED INFECTIONS

Tick-related infections
ICD-9CM # 082.0 Rocky Mountain spotted fever
         066.1 Colorado tick fever
        088.82 Babesiosis
        082.8 Ehrlichiosis
        088.81 Lyme disease

TABLE 2-198   **Tick-Related Infections in the United States**

DISEASE	ORGANISM	VECTOR	RESERVOIR	GEOGRAPHIC DISTRIBUTION	TYPE OF ILLNESS
Babesiosis	*Babesia microti*	*Ixodes scapularis*	*Peromyscus lueco-pus* (white-footed mouse)	Islands of Massachusetts, Rhode Island, New York	Malaria-like; fever, anemia, renal failure
Lyme disease	*Borrelia burgdorferi*	*I. scapularis, I. pacificus*	Rodents, deer	Northeastern, midwestern, and western U.S.	Fever, erythema migrans, headache, myalgias; multiple stages
Tularemia	*Francisella tularensis*	*Ambylomma americanum, Dermacentor andersoni, D. variabilis*	Rabbits, dogs, rodents	Southern, southeastern, midwestern U.S.	Fever, lymphadenopathy, pneumonia
Rocky Mountain spotted fever	*Rickettsia rickettsii*	*D. variabilis, D. andersoni*	Dogs, cats, rodents	Southeastern U.S., western hemisphere	Fever, headache, rash, toxic appearance
Ehrlichiosis	*Ehrlichia chaffeensis*	*D. variabilis, A. americanum*	Dogs	South-central and south Atlantic U.S.	Fever, chills, hematologic abnormalities
	Human granulocytic ehrlichiosis	*D. variabilis, A. americanum, I. scapularis*	Unknown	Northeastern, midwestern U.S.	Fever, chills, hematologic abnormalities
Relapsing fever	*Borrelia hermsii, B. turicatae, B. parkeri*	*Ornithodoros hermsii, O. turicata, O. parkeri*	Rodents	Grand Canyon, western mountains in U.S.	Fever, chills, relapsing course
Q fever	*Coxiella burnetii*	Inhalation of infected aerosols	Cattle, sheep, cats, ticks	Nova Scotia, Europe, Australia	Fever, headache, pneumonia
Colorado tick fever	Coltivirus	*D. andersoni*	Squirrels, rabbits, deer	Rocky Mountain states	Fever, headache, leukopenia
Tick paralysis	Neurotoxin	*D. andersoni, D. variabilis, A. americanum, A. maculatum, I. scapularis*		Pacific Northwest, Rocky Mountain states	Ascending flaccid paralysis, ataxia

From Kassirer J (ed): *Current therapy in adult medicine*, ed 4, St Louis, 1998, Mosby.

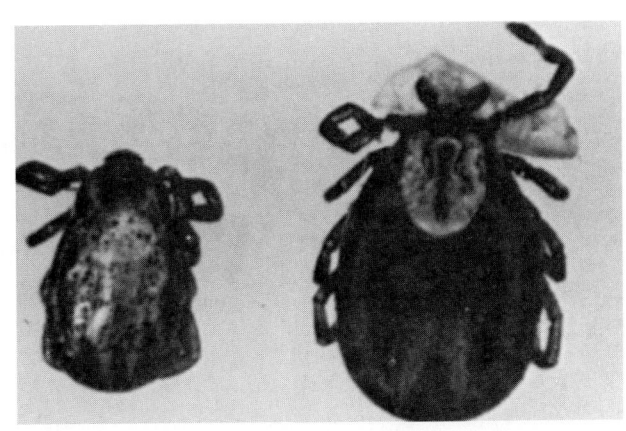

Fig. 2-14   Nymph and adult dog ticks *(Dermacentor variabilis)*. The adult female dog tick is approximately twice as large as the adult female deer tick.
(From Mandell GL: *Mandell, Douglas, and Bennett's principles and practice of infectious diseases,* ed 5, New York, 2000, Churchill Livingstone.)

Tick-related infections
ICD-9CM # 082.0 Rocky Mountain spotted fever
 088.81 Lyme disease
 088.82 Babesiosis
 082.8 Ehrlichiosis

TABLE 2-199 Some Ticks of Medical Importance in the United States

SPECIES NAME, COMMON NAME	DESCRIPTION	DISTRIBUTION	DISEASES	COMMENTS
Ixodidae, hard ticks				
Ixodes scapularis, black-legged tick	Dark brown with long mouth parts	Northern form from southern Ontario south through eastern and central United States to Virginia; southern form to northern Mexico	Northern form transmits Lyme disease, babesiosis, and human granulocytic ehrlichiosis; Lyme transmission requires >24 hr for nymphs, 36 hr for adults	Adults active in fall, winter, and spring; immature forms active in spring and summer; favors edges of paths, roads; nymphs important vectors
Ixodes pacificus, western black-legged tick	Similar to *I. scapularis*	Canadian Pacific coast south through California to Mexico	Lyme disease; Lyme transmission requires 96 hr for nymphs	May cause type I sensitivity reactions
Dermacentor variabilis, American dog tick	Dark brown with rounded mouth parts	Throughout United States except Rocky Mountains; southern Canada; northern Mexico	RMSF, tularemia; RMSF transmission requires ≥24 hr	Handling ticks picked off dogs may be risky; favor trails or roadsides near clearings
Dermacenter andersoni, Rocky Mountain wood tick	Dark brown with white markings on scutum	Rocky Mountains and adjacent areas of United States and Canada	RMSF, Colorado tick fever, tularemia, tick paralysis	Favors brushy vegetation
Ambylomma americanum, Lone Star tick	Red-brown with long mouth parts; females have white spot on back	Central Texas north and east to Iowa and New York; northern Mexico	Tularemia, human monocytic ehrlichiosis, Lyme or Lyme-like disease in southeastern United States	Bites aggressively in southern areas; nymphs are common seed ticks
Ambylomma maculatum, Gulf Coast tick	Brown females have metallic markings on scutum; long mouth parts	Southeastern Atlantic and Gulf coasts, south to South America	None	Bites aggressively
Argasidae, soft ticks				
Ornithodoros hermsi	Characteristic soft tick morphology, gray, mammalated, up to 1 cm	Western United States and Canada	Relapsing fever	Painless bite; often found in cabins
Ornithodoros turicata, relapsing fever tick	Similar to *O. hermsi*	Southwestern and south-central United States to northern Florida, eastern Mexico	Relapsing fever	Painless bite but intense local reaction may occur

From Mandell GL: *Mandell, Douglas, and Bennett's principles and practice of infectious diseases,* ed 5, New York, 2000, Churchill LIvingstone.
RMSF, Rocky Mountain spotted fever.

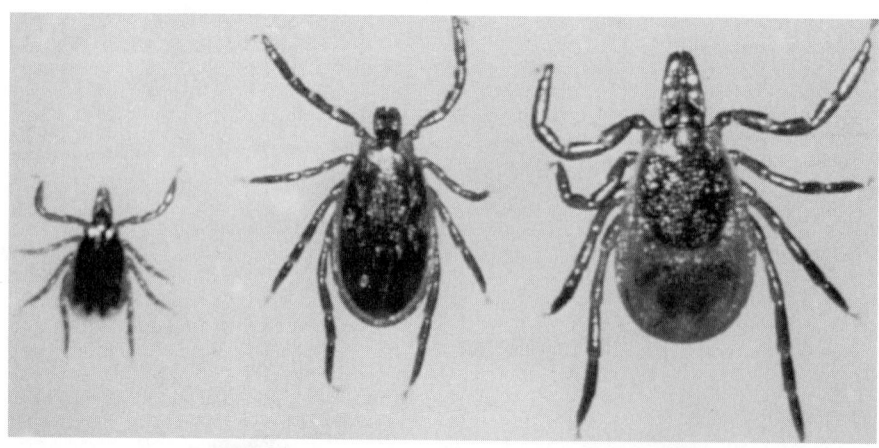

Fig. 2-15 Nymph, adult male, and adult female ticks *(Ixodes scapularis [dammini]).* (From Mandell GL: *Mandell, Douglas, and Bennett's principles and practice of infectious diseases,* ed 5, New York, 2000, Churchill Livingstone.)

TOXIC SYNDROMES, FISH- AND ALGAE-RELATED

Toxic syndromes, fish- and algae-related
ICD-9CM # code varies with specific diagnosis

TABLE 2-200   Summary of Fish- and Algae-Related Toxic Syndromes

TOXIDROME	SEAFOOD INVOLVED	AREAS COMMONLY SEEN	CAUSATIVE ORGANISMS	TOXIN PRODUCED
Fish-Related Toxic Syndromes				
Scombroid	Albacore, tuna, wahoo, mackerel, shipjack, bonito, mahimahi	Worldwide	Bacteria within the fish transform histidine to histamine	Histamine, saurine
Tetrodotoxin	Puffer fish, "fugu," porcupine fish, sunfish	Tropical and subtropical	? *Pseudomonas* species	Tetrodotoxin
Algae Bloom-Related Toxic Syndromes				
Ciguatera	Tropical and semi-tropical reef fish such as barracuda, grouper, snapper, jack	Worldwide, most common in Indian Ocean, South Pacific, Caribbean	*Gambierdiscus toxicus* and other species	Ciguatoxin, maito-toxin, GT1-4, palytoxin
Clupeotoxin	Herring, sardines, anchovies, tarpons, bonefish	Caribbean, Indo-Pacific, Africa	*Ostreopis siamensis*	Palytoxin
PSP	Shellfish	NE and NW coast of US, Philippines, Alaska, North Sea	*Protogonyaulax, Alexandrium catarella, Pyrodinium, Saxidomus, Gonyaulax*	Saxitoxin, neosaxitoxins, gonyautoxins
NSP	Shellfish	Gulf of Mexico, Florida, Texas, North Carolina, New Zealand	*Ptychodiscus breve*	Brevetoxins
DSP	Shellfish	Japan, Spain, Netherlands, Chile	*Dinophysis, Prorocentrum*	Okadaic acid and others
Domoic acid	Shellfish	Canada, Japan, NE and NW USA	*Nitzschia pungens, Pseudonitzschia australis*	Domoic acid
Pfiesteria syndrome	Estuarine fish	Coastal waterways in eastern USA and Gulf coast	*Pfiesteria piscicida*	Unidentified
Haff disease	Buffalo fish	USA, Russia, Sweden	? Blue-green algae	Unknown

From Auerbach PS: *Wilderness medicine*, ed 4, St Louis, 2001, Mosby.
ATPase, Adenosine triphosphatase; *AV*, atrioventricular; *DSP*, diarrhetic shellfish poisoning; *IVF*, intravenous fluid; *NSP*, neurotoxic shellfish poisoning; *PSP*, paralytic shellfish poisoning.

TREMATODE TISSUE INFECTIONS

TABLE 2-201   Trematode Tissue Infections

SPECIES	EPIDEMIOLOGY	TRANSMISSION	LOCATION OF ADULT WORMS	MAJOR CLINICAL PRESENTATION	DIAGNOSIS	TREATMENT
Schistosoma spp.						
S. mansoni	Africa, South America, Middle East, Caribbean	Contact with fresh water	Mesenteric vasculature	Portal hypertension, hepatosplenomegaly	Stool O&P, rectal snips	Praziquantel, 20 mg/kg bid for 1 day, or praziquantel, 40 mg/kg once, or oxamniquine, 10 mg/kg bid for 1 day
S. japonicum	China, Philippines, Indonesia	Contact with fresh water	Mesenteric vasculature	Same as for *S. mansoni* plus seizures	Same as for *S. mansoni*	Praziquantel, 20 mg/kg tid for 1 day
S. mekongi	Thailand, Laos, Cambodia	Contact with fresh water	Mesenteric vasculature	Same as for *S. japonicum*	Same as for *S. mansoni*	Praziquantel, 20 mg/kg tid for 1 day
S. haematobium	Africa, Middle East	Contact with fresh water	Vesical venules	Hematuria, hydronephrosis, carcinoma of bladder	Urine O&P	Praziquantel, 20 mg/kg bid for 1 day, or praziquantel 40 mg/kg once
Clonorchis sinensis	Japan, China, Korea	Raw fish	Biliary tree	Cholangitis, portal hypertension, cholangiocarcinoma	Stool O&P	Praziquantel,* 25 mg/kg tid for 2 days
Fasciola hepatica	Worldwide where sheep are raised	Raw watercress	Bile ducts, liver tissue	Right upper quadrant pain and fever, biliary obstruction, hepatic fibrosis	Stool O&P serology	Albendazole* 10 mg/kg for 7 days or bithionol,† 30-50 mg/kg every other day for 15 days
Paragonimus westermani	Orient, India, Central Africa	Raw crab	Lungs	Cough, sputum production, resembling tuberculosis	Sputum, stool O&P	Praziquantel,* 25 mg/kg tid for 2 days, or bithionol† as for *F. hepatica*
Opisthorchis viverrini	Europe, Asia, Southeast Asia	Raw freshwater fish	Biliary tree	Same as for *C. sinensis*	Stool O&P	Praziquantel,* 25 mg/kg tid for 1 wk

From Stein JH (ed): *Internal medicine*, ed 5, St Louis, 1998, Mosby.
bid, Twice a day; *O&P,* ova and parasites; *tid,* three times a day.
*Considered an investigational drug by the U.S. Food and Drug Administration.
†Available only from the Centers for Disease Control and Prevention in the United States.

TREMORS

Tremors
ICD-9CM # 781.0 Tremor NOS
            333.1 Benign essential tremor
            333.1 Familial tremor

TABLE 2-202   **Characteristics of Common Tremors**

	ASSOCIATED DISORDER	POSITION	FREQUENCY, CHARACTER
Essential	Normal or anxiety-accentuated	Sustained posture	8-12 Hz Oscillating, distal extremities
Familial	Autosomal pattern of inheritance; linked to essential tremor	Sustained posture Intention	8-12 Hz Oscillating head-neck, distal extremities
Parkinson's	Basal ganglia disease Wilson's disease	Resting or postural Not intention	4-7 Hz Reciprocally alternating Tongue, facial muscles, distal extremities

Cerebellar	Vermis, anterior cerebellar	Action-intention tremor;
		   rhythmic regular
		   titubation of trunk,
		   lower extremities
			Coarse, 3-6 Hz
			Oscillating

	Spinobulbar cerebellar input Neocerebellar dentate outflow	Distal lower extremity Distal upper extremity	Coarse, somewhat irregular ataxia Often irregular. Increases as target is approached

Asterixis	Metabolic encephalopathy,
	   particularly hepatic
		Outstretched tongue or,
		   more often, hands;
		   flaplike appearance
			Coarse, 1-3 Hz
			Rapid twitches with variable intervals
			   between

From Andreoli TE (ed): *Cecil essentials of medicine,* ed 4, Philadelphia, 1997, WB Saunders.

UPPER EXTREMITY PAIN

TABLE 2-203　Differential Diagnosis of Upper Extremity Pain

Upper extremity pain
ICD-9CM # 739.7 Upper extremity segmental or somatic dysfunction
840.8 Upper extremity strain
912.8 Upper extremity injury other and unspecified

CAUSE	NATURE OF PATIENT	NATURE OF SYMPTOMS	ASSOCIATED SYMPTOMS	PRECIPITATING AND AGGRAVATING FACTORS	AMELIORATING FACTORS	PHYSICAL FINDINGS
Shoulder						
Supraspinatus tendinitis	Over age 40	Pain in lower part of deltoid region, which is referral area for pain from supraspinatus tendon		Reaching overhead and lying on affected shoulder		Pain worse with resisted abduction and with abduction to 60 degrees and internal rotation
Subacromial bursitis	Under age 40	Severe pain with marked limitation of motion Pain may radiate to distal arm and even forearm		Lifting objects or combing hair		Point tenderness over subacromial bursa, which may be warm and swollen
Bicipital tendinitis		Generalized tenderness anteriorly in region of long head of biceps (anterior subacromial bursa)				Resisted forearm supination causes anterior shoulder pain Free abduction and forward flexion
Calcific tendinitis	Younger adults	Usually a sequela to acute bursitis				
Rotator cuff tear	Adults	Sudden onset Pain in deltoid area that intensifies 6-12 hr after initial trauma	Recurrent pain		Arm hanging limp	Restricted motion in one plane at glenohumeral joint Weakness and atrophy of supraspinatus and infraspinatus Pain over greater tuberosity
Teres minor or infraspinatus tendinitis		Diffuse shoulder pain	No pain radiation into arm or neck		Arm dependent	Pain on moving humerus posteriorly
Subscapularis tendinitis		Diffuse shoulder pain	No pain radiation into arm or neck	Prolonged immobilization	Arm dependent	Pain with resisted medial rotation
Frozen shoulder		Gradual onset of pain with limitation of motion at glenohumeral and scapulothoracic joints Limitation of abduction, extension, rotation, and forward flexion Pain may radiate into neck and down arm to elbow	Some atrophy of shoulder muscles			Marked restriction of motion of shoulder in all directions

Impingement syndrome	Athletes (e.g., baseball, swimming, tennis)	Tendinitis of biceps and/or supraspinatus tendon progressing to subacromial bursitis and inflammation of acromioclavicular joint			Pain on forward flexion of arm with elbow extended
Fibrositis syndrome	Ages 20-60	Pain at midpoint of upper border of trapezius, origin of supraspinatus near medial border of scapula, 2-3 cm distal to lateral epicondyle of humerus	Sleep disturbance; Diffuse musculoskeletal pain	Tricyclic antidepressants	Multiple tender points
Lesion of cervical spine and cord	Referred pain to upper extremity: back of neck, back of shoulder, down arm, forearm				Pain and hypesthesia along dermatome distribution
Elbow					
Lateral epicondylitis	Often in tennis players, especially those over age 40	Pain over lateral epicondyle that may radiate down back of forearm	Resisted extension of wrist and supination of forearm		Tender to palpation over lateral epicondyle
Bursitis		Pain in back of elbow			Swelling, warmth, and tenderness over back of elbow
Radial head dislocation	Child		Swing child around by arms		Radial head palpable in displaced position

Continued

TABLE 2-203 Differential Diagnosis of Upper Extremity Pain—cont'd

CAUSE	NATURE OF PATIENT	NATURE OF SYMPTOMS	ASSOCIATED SYMPTOMS	PRECIPITATING AND AGGRAVATING FACTORS	AMELIORATING FACTORS	PHYSICAL FINDINGS
SHand and Wrist						
Tenosynovitis of abductors and extensors of wrist (de Quervain's disease)		Pain at base of thumb		Flexing thumb	ts	
Tenosynovitis of flexors of fingers (Dupuytren's contracture)		Pain in palm at base of third and fourth digits				Catching or fixation of third or fourth digits in flexion; Painless thickening of palmar fascia or tendon sheath
Thoracic outlet syndrome	More common in middle-aged women	Hand pain, weakness, or numbness (usually left) after arms are hyperabducted or on awakening	Numbness of ulnar distribution or whole hand	Prolonged hyperabduction		Decreased radial pulse with Adson's and other maneuvers
Gout and pseudogout	Adults	Wrist often involved in pseudogout				
Carpal tunnel syndrome	More common in women	Pain in wrist radiating to hand and forearm				Tinel and Phalen tests may be positive; Thenar wasting

From Seller RH (ed): *Differential diagnosis of common complaints*, ed 4, Philadelphia, 2000, WB Saunders.

URETERAL CALCULUS COLIC

Ureteral calculus colic
ICD-9CM # 594.2

BOX 2-248   **Differential Diagnosis for Ureteral Calculus Colic**

Renal colic secondary to noncalculus etiology
    Passage of blood or clot
    Passage of necrotic material (sloughed papilla)
    Stricture or compression of ureter (extrinsic) or excessive angulation of ureter
Other causes of abdominal/flank pain
    Gastrointestinal: appendicitis (retrocecal), terminal ileitis, diverticulitis, cholecystitis, cholelithiasis, duodenal or ventricular ulceration, pancreatitis
    Vascular: infarction of kidney, spleen, or bowel, renal vein thrombosis, abdominal aortic aneurysm
    Gynecologic: ovarian cysts, adnexitis, ectopic pregnancy, endometriosis
Rare causes: psoas abscess, retroperitoneal masses, cardiac infarction, porphyria, heavy metal intoxication, diabetes mellitus, pheochromocytoma, Addison's disease, metastatic breast cancer

From Nseyo UO (ed): *Urology for primary care physicians,* Philadelphia, 1999, WB Saunders.

Gwendolyn R. Lee, M.D.
Internal Medicine

URETHRAL DISCHARGE AND DYSURIA

TABLE 2-204   Differential Diagnosis of Urethral Discharge and Dysuria

Urethral discharge and dysuria
ICD-9CM # 788.7 Urethral discharge
599.9 Urethral discharge bloody
788.1 Dysuria

CAUSE	NATURE OF PATIENT	NATURE OF SYMPTOMS	ASSOCIATED SYMPTOMS	PRECIPITATING AND AGGRAVATING FACTORS	AMELIORATING FACTORS	PHYSICAL FINDINGS	DIAGNOSTIC STUDIES
Cystitis	Most common in women ages 15-34	Dysuria (worse at end of flow) Urgency Frequency "Internal" discomfort Acute onset of symptoms with bacterial infection	Hematuria Nocturia Fever	Meatal stenosis may cause recurrent UTI in children Drugs (e.g., NSAIDs, cyclophosphamide)	Avoidance of urinating Warm baths	Suprapubic tenderness to palpation or percussion Fever	Urine culture positive Cystoscopy Special test for *Chlamydia* Pyuria by urinalysis or leukocyte esterase test
Interstitial cystitis	Women ages 20-50	Dysuria Marked frequency of small volume of urine	Nocturia Bladder pain Urgency	Some relief of pain with voiding		Tenderness of bladder base	Urine culture: sterile Cystoscopy: Hunner's ulcers
Female urethral syndrome		Dysuria Urgency Frequency Gradual onset of symptoms over 2-7 days	Suprapubic pain			Suprapubic pain No fever	Minimal pyuria Urine culture usually negative
Vaginitis	Candidiasis more common in diabetic patients	Dysuria "External burning"	Vaginal itching			Vaginal discharge on pelvic examination	KOH and saline wet mounts for *Candida* and *Trichomonas* Gram stain and culture for gonococci
Chemical vaginitis	Common cause of dysuria and urethral discharge in young girls	Dysuria "External burning" Urethral discharge (minimal)		Bubble baths Vaginal sprays and douches		Vaginitis	
Prostatitis	Men over age 50	Dysuria Frequency	Backache Fever Decreased or intermittent stream	Abrupt change in frequency of ejaculation (e.g., after a vacation)		May be costovertebral tenderness Prostate tender to palpation on rectal examination	Examination and culture of prostatic secretions

Condition		Symptoms	Predisposing factors	Discharge	Laboratory
Meatal stenosis	Children	Dysuria Recurrent UTI symptoms			
Urethritis					
Gonorrheal	Most common in men	Sexually transmitted Urethral discharge is moderate to large, purulent, mucoid, or mucopurulent and develops 1-3 wk after coitus with infected partner Dysuria (worse at beginning of urine flow)	Sexual contact	Urethral discharge is spontaneous or elicited by penile stripping	Gram stain and culture of urethral smear
Nongonorrheal (chlamydial or trichomonal)	Most common in men	Sexually transmitted Symptoms usually minimal or absent Discharge (if present) is observed on awakening, thin and clear or whitish Dysuria (ranges in severity) Urgency Frequency	Multiple sexual partners Meatal or urethral irritant	Thin, scanty, and whitish Urethral discharge appears on penile stripping	Gram stain and culture of urethral smear Special test for *Chlamydia* Saline wet mount for *Trichomonas*
Mechanical	Most common in young boys and girls	Dysuria Minimal urethral discharge	Horseback or bike riding Masturbation Foreign body		

From Seller RH (ed): *Differential diagnosis of common complaints*, ed 4, Philadelphia, 2000, WB Saunders. *KOH*, Potassium hydroxide; *NSAIDs*, nonsteroidal antiinflammatory drugs; *UTI*, urinary tract infection.

II

URINARY RETENTION, ACUTE

**TABLE 2-205 Acute Urinary Retention:
Etiologic Classifications**

CLASSIFICATION	ETIOLOGIC FACTORS
Anatomic	Urethral stricture
	Benign prostatic enlargement
	Acute prostatic hematoma
	Prostate cancer
	Bladder neck contracture
	Urethral stone
	Foreign body (iatrogenic)
Functional	Neurogenic
	Neurogenic bladder
	Neurologic diseases
	Multiple sclerosis, Parkinson's disease
	DESD, tabes dorsalis, Alzheimer's disease
	Spinal cord injury, stroke, brain tumor
	Spinal bifida occulta
	Abdominal pelvic resection
	Posterior pelvic exenteration
	Spinal anesthesia
	Postoperative pain
	Viral infection
	Echovirus (primarily in female children)
	Encephalitis
	Lower urinary tract instrumentation
	Pregnancy
	Drug toxicity
	Alcohol toxicity
	Traumatic pain
Psychogenic	Hinman's syndrome
	Emotional derangement

From Nseyo UO (ed): *Urology for primary care physicians*, Philadelphia,
1999, WB Saunders.
DESD, Detrusor external sphincter dyssynergia.

URINE, RED

BOX 2-249 Causes of Red Urine

With a Positive Dipstick
1. Hematuria
2. Hemoglobinuria: negative urinalysis
3. Myoglobinuria: negative urinalysis
With a Negative Dipstick
Drugs
  Aminosalicylic acid
  Deferoxamine mesylate
  Ibuprofen
  Phenacetin
  Phenolphthalein
  Phensuximide
  Rifampin
  Anthraquinone laxatives
  Doxorubicin

  Methyldopa
  Phenazopyridine
  Phenothiazine
  Phenytoin
Dyes
  Azo dyes
  Eosin
Foods
  Beets, berries, maize
  Rhodamine B
Metabolic
  Porphyrins
  Serratia marcescens (red diaper syndrome)
  Urate crystalluria

From Nseyo UO (ed): *Urology for primary care physicians*, Philadelphia, 1999, WB Saunders.

UROPATHY, OBSTRUCTIVE

Uropathy, obstructive
ICD-9CM # 599.6

BOX 2-250   Causes of Obstructive Uropathy

I. Intrinsic Causes

A. Intraluminal
1. Intratubular deposition of crystals (uric acid, sulfas)
2. Stones
3. Papillary tissue
4. Blood clots

B. Intramural
1. Functional
   a. Ureter (ureteropelvic or ureterovesical dysfunction)
   b. Bladder (neurogenic): spinal cord defect or trauma, diabetes, multiple sclerosis, Parkinson's disease, cerebrovascular accidents
   c. Bladder neck dysfunction
2. Anatomic
   a. Tumors
   b. Infection, granuloma
   c. Strictures

II. Extrinsic Causes

A. Originating in the reproductive system
1. Prostate: benign hypertrophy or cancer
2. Uterus: pregnancy, tumors, prolapse, endometriosis
3. Ovary: abscess, tumor, cysts

B. Originating in the vascular system
1. Aneurysms (aorta, iliac vessels)
2. Aberrant arteries (ureteropelvic junction)
3. Venous (ovarian veins, retrocaval ureter)

C. Originating in the gastrointestinal tract: Crohn's disease, pancreatitis, appendicitis, tumors

D. Originating in the retroperitoneal space
1. Inflammations
2. Fibrosis
3. Tumor, hematomas

From Stein JH (ed): *Internal medicine*, ed 5, St Louis, 1998, Mosby.

UTERINE BLEEDING, ABNORMAL

Uterine bleeding, abnormal
ICD-9CM # 626.9

BOX 2-251   Abnormal Uterine Bleeding

Pregnancy

Threatened abortion
Incomplete abortion
Complete abortion
Molar pregnancy
Ectopic pregnancy
Retained products of conception

Ovulatory

Vulva: infection, laceration, tumor
Vagina: infection, laceration, tumor, foreign body
Cervix: polyps, cervical erosion, cervicitis, carcinoma
Uterus: fibroids (submucous fibroids most likely to cause abnormal bleeding), polyps, adenomyosis, endometritis, intrauterine device, atrophic endometrium
Pregnancy complications: ectopic pregnancy; threatened, incomplete, complete abortion; retained products of conception
Abnormality of clotting system
Midcycle bleeding

Halban's disease (persistent corpus luteum)
Menorraghia
Pelvic inflammatory disease

Anovulatory

Physiologic causes
   Puberty
   Perimenopausal
Pathologic causes
   Ovarian failure (FSH over 40 IU/ml)
   Hyperandrogenism
   Hyperprolactinemia
   Obesity
   Hypothalamic dysfunction (polycystic ovaries); LH/FSH ratio greater than 2:1
   Hyperplasia
   Endometrial carcinoma
   Estrogen-producing tumors
   Hypothyroidism

From Danakas G (ed): *Practical guide to the care of the gynecologic/obstetric patient*, St Louis, 1997, Mosby.
FSH, Follicle-stimulating hormone; *LH*, luteinizing hormone.

VAGINAL BLEEDING ABNORMALITIES

Vaginal bleeding abnormalities
ICD-9CM # 626.6 Irregular vaginal bleeding

TABLE 2-206 Differential Diagnosis:
Abnormal Vaginal Bleeding

FACTORS	DIAGNOSIS
General	Trauma
	Neoplasia
Specific to Reproductive Cycle	
Pregnancy	
First trimester	Miscarriage
	Ectopic implantation
Third trimester	Placenta previa
	Placental abruption
	Premature labor
Ovulatory Cycles Present	Shortened follicular luteal phase
	Anatomic lesion
	Endometrial polyps
	Cervical polyps
	Adenomyosis
	Fibroids
	Systemic disease
	Coagulopathies
	Intrauterine device
	Cervical cancer
	Sarcomas
	Pelvic inflammatory disease
Anovulatory Cycles	Immature hypothalamic regulation
	Polycystic ovary syndrome
	Perimenopausal changes
	Endometrial hyperplasia
	Endometrial carcinoma
	Postmenopausal hormone replacement
	Dysfunctional uterine bleeding (no pelvic organ disease or systemic disorder)
	Endometriosis

From Carlson KJ et al: *Primary care of women*, St Louis, 1995, Mosby.

Vaginal bleeding, pregnancy
ICD-9CM # 640.93 Antepartum (<22 weeks)
641.23 Abruptio placentae
641.13 Placenta previa

VAGINAL BLEEDING, PREGNANCY

BOX 2-252   Differential Diagnosis of Abnormal Vaginal Bleeding in Pregnant Women

First Trimester

Implantation bleeding
Abortion
   Threatened
   Complete
   Incomplete
   Missed
Ectopic pregnancy
Neoplasia
   Hydatidiform mole
   Cervix

Third Trimester

Placenta previa
Placental abruption
Premature labor
Choriocarcinoma

From Carlson KJ et al: *Primary care of women,* St Louis, 1995, Mosby.

VAGINAL DISCHARGE, PREPUBERTAL GIRLS

Vaginal discharge, prepubertal girls
ICD-9CM # 623.5 Vaginal discharge

BOX 2-253   Causes of Vaginal Discharge in Prepubertal Girls

Irritative (bubble baths, sand)
Poor perineal hygiene
Foreign body
Associated systemic illness (group A streptococci, chickenpox)
Infections
   Escherichia coli with foreign body
   Shigella organisms
   Yersinia organisms
Infections (consider sexual abuse)
   Chlamydia trachomatis
   Neisseria gonorrhoeae
   Trichomonas vaginalis
Tumor (rare)

From Hoekelman R (ed): *Primary pediatric care,* ed 3, St Louis, 1997, Mosby.

VAGINAL DISCHARGES AND INFECTIONS

Vaginal discharges and infections
ICD-9CM # 623.5 Vaginal discharge
616.10 Vaginitis NOS

TABLE 2-207 **Vaginal Discharges and Infections**

CONDITION	HISTORY	PHYSICAL FINDINGS	DIAGNOSTIC TESTS
Physiologic vaginitis	Increase in discharge No foul odor, itching, or edema	Clear or mucoid discharge; pH <4.5	Wet mount: up to 3-5 WBCs; epithelial cells
Bacterial vaginosis (*Gardnerella vaginalis*)	Foul-smelling discharge; complains of "fishy odor"	Homogenous thin, white or gray discharge; pH >4.5	+ KOH "whiff" test; wet mount: + clue cells
Candida vulvovaginitis (*Candida albicans*)	Pruritic discharge; itching of labia; itching may extend to thighs	White, curdy discharge; pH 4.0-5.0; cervix may be red; may have erythema of perineum and thighs	KOH prep: mycelia, budding, branching yeast, pseudohyphae
Trichomoniasis (*Trichomonas vaginalis*)	Watery discharge foul odor; dysuria and dyspareunia with severe infection	Profuse, frothy, greenish discharge; pH 5.0-6.6; red friable cervix with petechiae ("strawberry" cervix)	Wet mount: Round or pear-shaped protozoa; motile "gyrating" flagella
Gonorrhea (*Neisseria gonorrhoeae*)	Partner with sexually transmitted disease; often asymptomatic or may have symptoms of pelvic inflammatory disease	Purulent discharge from cervix; Skene/Bartholin inflammation; cervix and vulva may be inflamed	Gram stain Culture DNA probe
Chlamydia (*Chlamydia trachomatis*)	Partner with nongonococcal urethritis; often asymptomatic; may complain of spotting after intercourse or urethritis	+/− purulent discharge; cervix may or may not be red or friable	DNA probe
Atrophic vaginitis	Dyspareunia; vaginal dryness; perimenopausal or postmenopausal	Pale thin vaginal mucosa; pH >4.5	Wet mount: folded clumped epithelial cells
Allergic vaginitis	New bubble bath, soap, douche, or other hygiene products	Foul smell, erythema, pH <4.5	Wet mount: WBCs
Foreign body	Red and swollen vulva; vaginal discharge; history of use of tampon, condom, or diaphragm	Bloody or foul-smelling discharge	Wet mount: WBCs

From Seidel HM (ed): *Mosby's guide to physical examination,* ed 4, St Louis, 1999, Mosby.
DNA, Deoxyribonucleic acid; *KOH,* potassium hydroxide; *WBCs,* white blood cells.

VALVULAR HEART DISEASE, ACQUIRED

Valvular heart disease, acquired
ICD-9CM # code varies with specific diagnosis

TABLE 2-208 Characteristic Physical, ECG, and Chest Radiographic Findings in Chronic Acquired Valvular Heart Disease

	PHYSICAL FINDINGS*	ECG	RADIOGRAPH
Aortic stenosis	Pulsus parvus et tardus (may be absent in older patients or with associated aortic regurgitation); carotid "shudder" (coarse thrill) Ejection murmur radiates to base of neck; peak late in systole if stenosis severe Sustained but not markedly displaced LV impulse A_2 decreased, S_2 single or paradoxically split S_4 gallop, often palpable	LV hypertrophy; left bundle branch block also common Rare heart block from calcific involvement of conduction system	LV prominence without dilation Poststenotic aortic root dilation Aortic valve calcification
Aortic regurgitation	Increased pulse pressure Bifid carotid pulses Rapid pulse upstroke and collapse LV impulse hyperdynamic and displaced laterally Diastolic decrescendo murmur; duration related to severity Systolic flow murmur S_3G common	LV hypertrophy, often with narrow deep Q waves	LV and aortic dilation
Mitral stenosis	Loud S_1 Opening snap (OS) (S_2-OS interval inversely related to stenosis severity) S_1 not loud, and OS absent if valve heavily calcified Signs of pulmonary arterial hypertension	Left atrial abnormality Atrial fibrillation common RV hypertrophy pattern may develop if associated pulmonary arterial hypertension	Large LA: double-density, posterior displacement of esophagus, elevation of left mainstem bronchus Straightening of left heart border due to enlarged left appendage Small or normal size LV Large pulmonary artery Pulmonary venous congestion
Mitral regurgitation	Hyperdynamic LV impulse S_3 Widely split S_2 may occur Holosystolic apical murmur radiating to axilla (murmur may be atypical with acute mitral regurgitation, papillary muscle dysfunction, or mitral valve prolapse—see text)	Left atrial abnormality LV hypertrophy Atrial fibrillation	Enlarged LA and LV Pulmonary venous congestion
Mitral valve prolapse	One or more systolic clicks—often midsystolic—followed by late systolic murmur Auscultatory findings dynamic—see text Patients may exhibit tall thin habitus, pectus excavatum, straight back syndrome	Often normal Occasionally ST segment depression and/or T wave changes in inferior leads	Depends on degree of valve regurgitation and presence or absence of those abnormalities
Tricuspid stenosis	Jugular venous distention with prominent a wave if sinus rhythm Tricuspid OS and diastolic rumble at left sternal border—may be overshadowed by concomitant mitral stenosis Tricuspid OS and rumble increased during inspiration	Right atrial abnormality Atrial fibrillation common	Large RA
Tricuspid regurgitation	Jugular venous distention with large regurgitant (systolic) wave Systolic murmur at left sternal border, increased with inspiration Diastolic flow rumble RV S_3 increased with inspiration Hepatomegaly with systolic pulsation	RA abnormality Findings often related to cause of the tricuspid regurgitation	RA and RV enlarged Findings often related to cause of the tricuspid regurgitation

From Andreoli TE (ed): *Cecil essentials of medicine*, ed 5, Philadelphia, 2001, WB Saunders.
ECG, Electrocardiogram; *LA*, left atrium; *LV*, left ventricle; *RA*, right atrium; *RV*, right ventricle.
* Findings are influenced by the severity and chronicity of the valve disorder.

II

VASCULITIS, DIFFERENTIAL DIAGNOSIS

Vasculitis, differential diagnosis
ICD-9CM # 447.6 Vasculitis, NOS
            287.0 Vasculitis, allergic
            273.2 Vasculitis cryoglobulinemic
            446.29 Leukoclastic vasculitis

BOX 2-254   Diseases That Mimic Vasculitis

Embolic Disease

Infectious or marantic endocarditis
Cardiac mural thrombus
Atrial myxoma
Cholesterol embolization syndrome

Noninflammatory Vessel Wall Disruption

Atherosclerosis
Arterial fibromuscular dysplasia
Drug effects (vasoconstrictors, anticoagulants)
Radiation
Genetic disease (neurofibromatosis, Ehler-Danlos
    syndrome)
Amyloidosis
Intravascular malignant lymphoma

Diffuse Coagulation

Disseminated intravascular coagulation
Thrombotic thrombocytopenic purpura
Hemolytic-uremic syndrome
Protein C and S deficiencies, factor V/Leiden
    mutation
Antiphospholipid syndrome

From Noble J: *Primary care medicine,* ed 3, St Louis, 2001, Mosby.

VENTRICULAR FAILURE

Ventricular failure
ICD-9CM # 429.9 Ventricular dysfunction

BOX 2-255   Ventricular Failure

Left Ventricular Failure

Systemic hypertension
Valvular heart disease (AS, AR, MR)
Cardiomyopathy, myocarditis
Bacterial endocarditis
Myocardial infarction
Idiopathic hypertrophic subaortic stenosis

Right Ventricular Failure

Valvular heart disease (mitral stenosis)
Pulmonary hypertension
Bacterial endocarditis (right-sided)
Right ventricular infarction

Biventricular Failure

Left ventricular failure
Cardiomyopathy
Myocarditis
Arrhythmias
Anemia
Thyrotoxicosis
Arteriovenous fistula
Paget's disease
Beri-beri

VERTIGO

BOX 2-256   Vertigo

Peripheral

Otitis media
Acute labyrinthitis
Vestibular neuronitis
Benign positional vertigo
Meniere's disease
Ototoxic drugs: streptomycin, gentamycin
Lesions of the eighth nerve: acoustic neuroma, meningioma, mononeuropathy, metastatic carcinoma
Mastoiditis

CNS or Systemic

Vertebrobasilar artery insufficiency
Posterior fossa tumor or other brain tumors
Infarction/hemorrhage of cerebral cortex, cerebellum, or brainstem
Basilar migraine
Metabolic: drugs, hypoxia, anemia, fever
Hypotension/severe hypertension
Multiple sclerosis
CNS infections: viral, bacterial
Temporal lobe epilepsy
Arnold-Chiari malformation, syringobulbia
Psychogenic: ventilation, hysteria

CNS, Central nervous system.

Vertigo
ICD-9CM # 780.4 Vertigo NOS
        386.11 Benign paroxysmal positional
        386.2 Central origin
        386.10 Peripheral
        386.12 Vestibular (neuronitis)

VESICLES AND PUSTULES, INTRAEPIDERMAL

Vesicles and pustules, intraepidermal
ICD-9CM # 709.8

TABLE 2-209   Differential Diagnosis of Intraepidermal Vesicles and Pustules

LOCATION OF THE BLISTER	DISORDER
Intracorneal or subcorneal	Staphylococcal scalded skin syndrome
	Toxic shock syndrome
	Impetigo
	Candidiasis
	Subcorneal pustular dermatosis
	Transient pustular melanosis of infancy
	Pemphigus foliaceus or pemphigus erythematosus
Suprabasilar	Eczematous dermatoses
	Epidermolysis bullosa simplex group
	Friction blisters
	Herpes virus infections
	Incontinentia pigmenti
	Pemphigus vulgaris and pemphigus vegetans
	Hailey-Hailey disease (chronic benign familial pemphigus)
	Darier's disease (keratosis follicularis)
	Transient acantholytic dermatosis (Grover's disease)
	Epidermolytic hyperkeratosis
	Acropustulosis of infancy

From Callen JP (ed): *Color atlas of dermatology,* ed 2, Philadelphia, 2000, WB Saunders.

VESTIBULAR DYSFUNCTION

Vestibular dysfunction
ICD-9CM # 386.12

TABLE 2-210   Symptoms and Signs That May Distinguish Peripheral from Central Vestibular Dysfunction

SYMPTOM OR SIGN	PERIPHERAL	CENTRAL
Direction of nystagmus	Mainly unidirectional	Bi- or unidirectional
Hallucination of movement	Definite	Less definite
Severity of vertigo	Marked	Mild
Autonomic nervous system symptoms	Definite	Less definite
Direction of falling	Toward slow phase	Variable
Influenced by head position	Frequent	Seldom
Effect of head turning	Present	No effect
Vertical nystagmus	Never present	May be present
Disturbance of consciousness	Rare	May be present
Duration of symptoms	Finite	Often chronic
Tinnitus or deafness	Often	Usually absent
Other neurologic signs	Usually absent	Frequently present
Common causes	Labyrinthitis, positional vertigo, trauma	Vascular, MS, tumor

From Wiederholt WC: *Neurology for non-neurologists,* ed 4, Philadelphia, 2000, WB Saunders.
MS, Multiple sclerosis.

VISION LOSS, ACUTE, PAINFUL

Vision loss, acute, painful
ICD-9CM # 368.11 Vision loss, sudden

TABLE 2-211   Acute, Painful Loss of Vision

The following group of disorders cause acute visual loss and are associated with severe pain. In addition, marked injection of the conjunctiva often occurs as a result of ocular inflammation:

ADDITIONAL HISTORY

KEY EXAM FEATURES

Corneal Ulcer

A history of recent trauma or contact lens wear is usually reported. Sleeping in contact lenses greatly increases the risk of developing an infectious corneal ulcer.

The penlight examination may show a corneal abrasion, but an early corneal infiltrate can be difficult to identify. As the infection progresses, a white infiltrate is seen in the cornea. With extensive infections, a layering of white cells may be seen in the anterior chamber (hypopyon).

Uveitis

The origin of uveitis is often idiopathic. Common systemic associations include sarcoidosis, syphilis, tuberculosis, and HLA-B27–associated disorders (e.g., Reiter's syndrome, ankylosing spondylitis, inflammatory bowel disease, psoriasis). A history of sensitivity to light is also noted.

The pupil may be small, sluggish, or nonreactive to light. A circular injection of the eye surrounding the cornea (circumlimbal flush) is seen. The red reflex may be diminished, particularly with corneal edema and vitreous inflammation. Uveitis is usually unilateral but may affect both eyes.

Acute Angle-Closure Glaucoma

Acute angle-closure glaucoma usually occurs in older individuals and more commonly in those who are farsighted. It may be precipitated by an advancing cataract. A full-blown attack may be preceded by a history of blurred vision, halos around lights, and pain precipitated by dark conditions (e.g., after being in a movie theater). Markedly elevated intraocular pressure can cause a headache and nausea and vomiting. Systemic symptoms may be out of proportion to visual symptoms, so patients can be misdiagnosed.

In its acute form, it is always unilateral. The eye is red, and the pupil is middilated and nonreactive. Vision is usually diminished initially because of corneal edema, but it may be subsequently diminished by optic nerve damage from prolonged elevated intraocular pressure. Intraocular pressure is usually elevated to levels above 50 mm Hg.

Endophthalmitis

Most cases of endophthalmitis are associated with recent eye surgery. Rarely, patients may develop endophthalmitis (e.g., fungal endophthalmitis) from another source of infection in the body.

In addition to markedly decreased vision and injection of the eye, a mucopurulent discharge may be present. A layering of white cells in the anterior chamber (hypopyon) is common. The red reflex is diminished because of vitreous inflammation. In fungal endophthalmitis, the anterior segment exam may be entirely normal.

From Palay D (ed): *Ophthalmology for the primary care physician,* St Louis, 1997, Mosby.

VISION LOSS, ACUTE, PAINLESS

Vision loss, acute, painless
ICD-9CM # 368.11 Vision loss, sudden

TABLE 2-212 Acute, Painless Loss of Vision

In cases of acute, painless loss of vision, no injection of the conjunctiva occurs. The following provides information on these types of disorders:

ADDITIONAL HISTORY	KEY EXAM FEATURES
Vitreous Hemorrhage	
Patients report the sensation of spider webs clouding their vision or have recent-onset floaters. Associated systemic diseases include diabetes, sickle cell anemia, and blood dyscrasias.	If the vitreous hemorrhage is extensive, decreased red reflex and poor visualization of the retina are found. Mild vitreous hemorrhages may be difficult to see with the direct opthalmoscope.
Retinal Detachment	
Retinal detachment commonly occurs in highly nearsighted individuals or may occur after eye surgery or trauma. The onset may be preceded by acute symptoms of flashes or floaters. Patients report a loss of visual field or a loss of a certain part of their vision.	Detachment may be difficult to recognize with the direct ophthalmoscope. Indirect ophthalmoscopic evaluation is indicated.
Retinal Artery Occlusion	
Occlusion is caused by emboli and may be associated with carotid artery disease and valvular heart disease. It may be associated with previous episodes of a cloud interfering with the vision that eventually clears (amaurosis fugax). The visual loss is abrupt and almost complete.	With central retinal artery occlusion, vision is often limited to hand motions or light perception. Emboli may be visualized in the retinal arterioles. With central retinal artery occlusion, diffuse retinal whitening occurs and a cherry-red spot is present in the macula.
Retinal Vein Occlusion	
Occlusion is most commonly associated with hypertension and rarely with blood dyscrasias.	Occlusion results from a thrombosis of the retinal veins. Ophthalmoscopic findings include numerous retinal hemorrhages and occasional cotton-wool spots. The veins are tortuous and dilated.
Exudative Macular Degeneration	
Macular degeneration usually occurs in older individuals (over the age of 60 years) and may progressively worsen over several days. It is associated with an abnormal distortion of straight lines (metamorphopsia).	Retinal hemorrhage is noted in the macular region.
Ischemic Optic Neuropathy	
Visual loss is usually sudden. The disorder is often associated with giant cell arteries, and patients may have symptoms of jaw claudication, scalp tenderness, neck pain, and weight loss (age usually 60 years or older). It may also be associated with hypertension and diabetes (age usually 40 years or older).	An afferent pupillary defect is present. The optic nerve head is swollen on ophthalmoscopic examination.
Optic Neuritis	
Visual loss usually occurs over several days. Pain with eye movement may be present. The disorder is usually associated with multiple sclerosis (in patients 15 to 45 years of age).	An afferent pupillary defect is present. Two thirds of patients have a normal optic disc; one third have optic disc edema.
Cerebral Infarct	
A history of previous vascular disease or strokes may be reported.	A bilateral loss of visual field usually occurs. If the infarct involves the occipital lobe, visual acuity may be reduced. Ocular examination findings are normal.
Functional Visual Loss	
A history of recent stress or earlier psychologic problems is usually reported.	Examination findings are normal.

From Palay D (ed): *Ophthalmology for the primary care physician*, St Louis, 1997, Mosby.

VISION LOSS, CHRONIC, PROGRESSIVE

Vision loss, chronic, progressive
ICD-9CM # 369.9 Vision loss NOS

TABLE 2-213 Chronic, Progressive Loss of Vision

The following disorders cause chronic, progressive loss of vision:

ADDITIONAL HISTORY	KEY EXAM FEATURES
Refractive Error	
The patient may already wear contacts or glasses.	The visual acuity is near normal when the patient looks through a pinhole.
Cataract	
Cataract is one of the most common causes of chronic, progressive visual loss and may be associated with a family history of cataracts, diabetes, or chronic corticosteroid use. Patients may complain of multiple images when looking with only one eye. As the cataract progresses, objects become blurred and distinguishing objects up close and at a distance is difficult.	The visual acuity may be slightly improved with the pinhole. Pupil responses are normal. The normal red reflex is diminished, and visualizing the fundus with a direct ophthalmoscope can be difficult.
Open-Angle Glaucoma	
Open-angle glaucoma is more common in patients with a family history of glaucoma, nearsighted patients, patients with diabetes, and African-American patients. Visual acuity may remain normal until very late in the disease process, so patients with severe glaucoma may be relatively asymptomatic.	Elevated intraocular pressure greater than or equal to 22 mm Hg and increased optic nerve cupping of 0.6 or greater are significant.
Atrophic Macular Degeneration	
Atrophic macular degeneration is usually seen in patients older than age 60 years. It may be associated with a family history of macular degeneration.	With early disease, multiple hyaline nodules (drusen) are seen in the fundus. With advancing disease, retinal atrophy occurs, leaving a large scar or an atrophic area in the central macula.
Brain Tumor	
Headache, nausea upon awakening, and variable neurologic symptoms and signs can be seen.	The pattern of visual field loss varies with the location of the tumor. Tumors posterior to the optic nerve chiasm do not produce optic nerve atrophy or afferent pupillary defects. Tumors involving the chiasm or intrinsic to the optic nerve produce afferent pupillary defects and optic nerve atrophy.

From Palay D (ed): *Ophthalmology for the primary care physician,* St Louis, 1997, Mosby.

VISION LOSS, MONOCULAR, TRANSIENT

Vision loss, monocular, transient
ICD-9CM # 368.9

TABLE 2-214 Common Causes of Transient Monocular Vision Loss

CATEGORY/(TYPICAL DURATION)	CAUSES	DIFFERENTIAL FEATURES
Thromboembolism (1-5 min)	Atherosclerosis	Other atherosclerotic vascular disease, associated crossed hemiparesis, angiography (carotid atheromata)
	Cardiac	Valvular disease, mural thrombi, atrial fibrillation, recent MI
	Blood dyscrasia	Blood tests + for sickle cell anemia, macroglobulinemia, multiple myeloma, polycythemia, etc.
Vasospasm (5-30 min)	Migraine	Ipsilateral headache, other classic aura, and family history
Vascular compression (few sec)	Increased intracranial pressure	Precipitated by position change, Valsalva maneuver, or pressure waves
	Tumor	Associated slowly progressive monocular visual loss
Vasculitis (1-5 min)	Temporal arteritis	Associated headache, polymyalgia rheumatica, palpable temporal artery, elevated sedimentation rate

From Goldman L, Bennett JC (eds): *Cecil textbook of medicine,* ed 21, Philadelphia, 2000, WB Saunders.
MI, myocardial infarction.

VISUAL FIELD DEFECTS

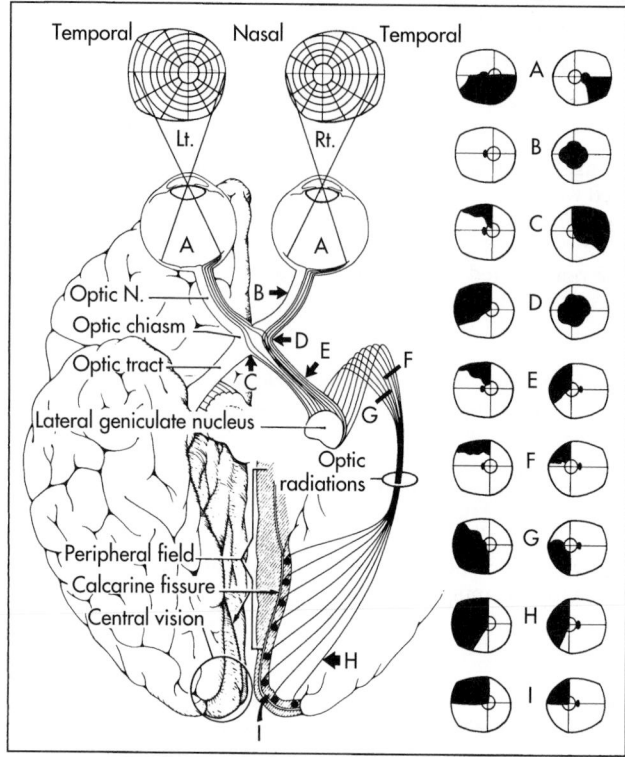

Fig. 2-16   A, Two examples of *altitudinal visual field defects* that could be caused either by occlusion of a superior branch of the central retinal artery or by an episode of ischemic optic neuropathy involving the superior optic disc. On the left is a large field defect involving both lower quadrants. On the right the injury is more limited, and the defect involves only the temporal quadrant, but it connects with the blind spot and does not go to fixation or have a border at the vertical meridian. **B,** A *central scotoma* in the visual field of the right eye caused by a lesion of the right optic nerve. **C,** *Bitemporal hemianopia* caused by a lesion of the optic chiasm. The asymmetry is typical of chiasmal field defects until a late stage, when the hemianopia may be complete in both eyes. **D,** *Junctional scotoma,* that is, a central scotoma on the side of a lateral chiasmal lesion with a temporal hemianopia in the visual field of the opposite eye. **E,** Markedly incongruous *homonymous hemianopia* seen with a lesion of the optic tract. **F,** *Homonymous superior quadrantanopia* seen with lesions of the optic radiations in the temporal lobe. **G,** *Homonymous inferior quadrantanopia* seen with lesions of the superior optic radiations in the low parietal or parietotemporal lobe junction. **H,** *Congruous homonymous hemianopia* seen with lesions, either of the optic radiations close to their termination or of the calcarine cortex itself. **I,** *Precise inferior quadrantanopia* seen if an occipital lobe lesion involves just the superior bank of the calcarine cortex. (From Stein JH [ed]: *Internal medicine,* ed 5, St Louis, 1998, Mosby.)

Vocal cord paralysis
ICD-9CM # 478.30 Unspecified
            478.31 Unilateral partial
            478.32 Unilateral complete
            478.33 Bilateral partial
            478.34 Bilateral complete

VOCAL CORD PARALYSIS

BOX 2-257   **Etiology of Vocal Cord Paralysis**

Neoplasm (35.8%)

Pulmonary
Laryngeal
Thyroid, parathyroid
Jugular foramen tumors
Central nervous system tumors
Carotid sheath and parapharyngeal space tumors
Mediastinal

Postsurgical (24.6%)

Thyroidectomy
Parathyroidectomy
Cervical spine surgery
Carotid endarterectomy
Neck dissection
Cervical esophageal surgery
Cardiac surgery

Idiopathic (14.3%)

Medical/Inflammatory (13.3%)

Rheumatoid arthritis
Toxic neuropathy
Viral and bacterial infection
Congestive heart failure (Ortner's syndrome)

Trauma (6.0%)

Intubation injury
Blunt or penetrating neck or chest injury
Birth trauma

Central Nervous System (6.0%)

Arnold-Chiari malformation
Hydrocephalus
Meningomyelocele
Stroke, vascular insufficiency
Multiple sclerosis
Parkinson's disease

From Noble J: *Primary care medicine*, ed 3, St Louis, 2001, Mosby.

II

VOICE DISORDERS, MEDICAL CAUSES

Voice disorders, medical causes
ICD-9CM # 784.40

TABLE 2-215　Voice Disorders, Medical Causes

DISORDER	SYMPTOMS	DIFFERENTIAL DIAGNOSIS	TESTING	MANAGEMENT
Endocrine				
Hypothyroidism	Mild hoarseness (early), decreased pitch, loss of range, loss of fine control	Overuse/Misuse	Thyroid function tests	Thyroid hormone
Sex hormone				
Premenstrual syndrome	Loss of range Mild raspiness		Characteristic history is diagnostic	Supportive conservation
Pregnancy	Decreased pitch, voice fatigue third trimester			Speech evaluation Voice instruction
Diabetes	Voice changes late in disease	Rule out other causes of dysphonia		Voice instruction
Neurologic Disorders				
Vocal fold paralysis	Breathiness Loss of volume	Vocal fold masses Viral upper respiratory infection	Otolaryngology assessment after 2 wk of hoarseness	Treat underlying cause Surgery
Multiple sclerosis	Hoarseness Difficulty swallowing	Other neurologic disorders	MRI, Lumbar puncture	Voice therapy, supportive
Amyotrophic lateral sclerosis	Progressive loss of voice Difficulty swallowing	Vocal fold paralysis		Supportive voice, swallowing instruction
Myasthenia gravis	Increased breathiness with use		Tensilon test	Voice improves with treatment

From Noble J (ed): *Primary care medicine,* ed 3, St Louis, 2001, Mosby.
MRI, Magnetic resonance imaging.

VOLUME DEPLETION

Volume depletion
ICD-9CM # 276.5

BOX 2-258 Causes of Volume Depletion

Gastrointestinal losses
  Upper: bleeding, nasogastric suction, vomiting
  Lower: bleeding, diarrhea, enteric or pancreatic fistula, tube drainage
Renal losses
  Salt and water: diuretics, osmotic diuresis, post-obstructive diuresis, acute tubular necrosis (recovery phase), salt-losing nephropathy, adrenal insufficiency, renal tubular acidosis
  Water loss: diabetes insipidus
Skin and respiratory losses
  Sweat, burns, insensible losses
Sequestration without external fluid loss
  Intestinal obstruction, peritonitis, pancreatitis, rhabdomyolysis, internal bleeding

---

From Andreoli TE (ed): *Cecil essentials of medicine,* ed 5, Philadelphia, 2001, WB Saunders.

VOLUME EXCESS

Volume excess
ICD-9CM # code varies with specific diagnosis

BOX 2-259 Causes of Volume Excess

Primary Renal Sodium Retention (Increased Effective Circulating Volume)

Acute renal failure
Acute glomerulonephritis
Severe chronic renal failure
Nephrotic syndrome
Primary hyperaldosteronism
Cushing's syndrome
Liver disease

Secondary Renal Sodium Retention (Decreased Effective Circulating Volume)

Heart failure
Liver disease
Nephrotic syndrome (minimal change disease)
Pregnancy

From Andreoli TE (ed): *Cecil essentials of medicine,* ed 5, Philadelphia, 2001, WB Saunders.

VOMITING

Vomiting
ICD-9CM # 787.03

BOX 2-260   Vomiting

Gastrointestinal disturbances
    Obstruction: esophageal, pyloric, intestinal
    Infections: viral or bacterial enteritis, viral hepatitis, food poisoning
    Pancreatitis
    Appendicitis
    Biliary colic
    Peritonitis
    Perforated bowel
    Diabetic gastroparesis
    Other: gastritis, peptic ulcer disease, inflammatory bowel disease, gastrointestimal tract neoplasms
Drugs: morphine, digitalis, cytotoxic agents, bromocriptine
Severe pain: myocardial infarction, renal colic
Metabolic disorders: uremia, acidosis/alkalosis, hyperglycemia, diabetic ketoacidosis, thyrotoxicosis

Trauma: blows to the testicles, epigastrium
Vertigo
Reye's syndrome
Increased intracranial pressure
Central nervous system disturbances: trauma, hemorrhage, infarction, neoplasm, infection, hypertensive encephalopathy, migraine
Radiation sickness
Vomiting associated with pregnancy
Motion sickness
Bulimia, anorexia nervosa
Psychogenic: emotional disturbances, offensive sights or smells
Severe coughing
Pyelonephritis

VULVAR LESIONS

BOX 2-261   Vulvar Lesions

Red Lesion

Infection

1. Fungal infection
    a. Candida
    b. Tinea cruris
    c. Intertrigo
    d. Pityriasis versicolor
2. *Sarcoptes scabiei*
3. Erythrasma: *Corynebacterium minutissimum*
4. Granuloma inguinale: *Calymmatobacterium granulomatis*
5. Folliculitis: *Staphylococcus aureus*
6. Hidradenitis suppurativa
7. Behçet's syndrome

Inflammation

1. Reactive vulvitis
2. Chemical irritation
    a. Detergent
    b. Dyes

    c. Perfume
    d. Spermicide
    e. Lubricants
    f. Hygiene sprays
    g. Podophyllum
    h. Topical 5-FU
    i. Saliva
    j. Gentian violet
    k. Semen
3. Mechanical trauma: scratching
4. Vestibular adenitis
5. Essential vulvodynia
6. Psoriasis
7. Seborrheic dermatitis

Neoplasm

1. Vulvar intraepithelial neoplasia (VIN)
    a. Mild dysplasia
    b. Moderate dysplasia
    c. Severe dysplasia
    d. Carcinoma-in-situ

From Danakas G (ed): *Practical guide to the care of the gynecologic/obstetric patient,* St Louis, 1997, Mosby.

Vulvar lesions
ICD-9CM # 625.8   Vulvar mass
        098.0   Vulvar ulcer, gonococcal
        091.0   Vulvar ulcer, syphilitic
        616.51 Behcet's
        624.0   Leukoplakia
        624.8   Dysplasia
        233.3   Carcinoma in situ
        616.9   Inflammatory lesion
        624.4   Vulvar scar (old)
        624.1   Vulvar atrophy

BOX 2-261   Vulvar Lesions—cont'd

Neoplasm—cont'd

2. Vulvar dystrophy
3. Bowen's disease
4. Invasive cancer
   a. Squamous cell carcinoma
   b. Malignant melanoma
   c. Sarcoma
   d. Basal cell carcinoma
   e. Adenocarcinoma
   f. Paget's disease
   g. Undifferentiated

White Lesion

1. Vulvar dystrophy
   a. Lichen sclerosus
   b. Vulvar dystrophy
   c. Vulvar hyperplasia
   d. Mixed dystrophy
2. VIN
3. Vitiligo
4. Partial albinism
5. Intertrigo
6. Radiation treatment

Dark Lesion

1. Lentigo
2. Nevi (mole)
3. Neoplasm (see Neoplasm, Vulvar, below)
4. Reactive hyperpigmentation
5. Seborrheic keratosis
6. Pubic lice

Ulcerative Lesion

1. Infection
   a. Herpes simplex
   b. Vaccinia
   c. *Treponema pallidum*
   d. Granuloma inguinale
   e. Pyoderma
   f. Tuberculosis

2. Noninfection
   a. Behçet's disease
   b. Crohn's disease
   c. Pemphigus
   d. Pemphigoid
   e. Hidradenitis suppurativa (see Neoplasm, Vulvar, below)

Neoplasm

1. Basal cell carcinoma
2. Squamous cell carcinoma
3. Vulvar tumor <1 cm
   a. Condyloma acuminatum
   b. Molluscum contagiosum
   c. Epidermal inclusion
   d. Vestibular cyst
   e. Mesenephric duct
   f. VIN
   g. Hemangioma
   h. Hidradenoma
   i. Neurofibroma
   j. Syringoma
   k. Accessory breast tissue
   l. Acrochordon
   m. Endometriosis
   n. Fox-Fordyce disease
   o. Pilonidal sinus
4. Vulvar tumor >1 cm
   a. Bartholin cyst or abscess
   b. Lymphogranuloma venereum
   c. Fibroma
   d. Lipoma
   e. Verrucous carcinoma
   f. Squamous cell carcinoma
   g. Hernia
   h. Edema
   i. Hematoma
   j. Acrochordon
   k. Epidermal cysts
   l. Neurofibromatosis
   m. Accessory breast tissue

II

WEAKNESS

Weakness
ICD-9CM # 780.7

TABLE 2-216 **Partial Differential Diagnosis of Weakness**

ILLNESS	AUTONOMIC INVOLVEMENT	SENSORY CHANGES	FEVER	FASCICULATIONS/ MUSCLE CRAMPS	CRANIAL NERVE INVOLVEMENT
Myasthenia gravis	No	No	No	No	Yes
Guillain-Barré	Possible	Yes	No	No	Rare, pupil reactivity maintained
Botulism	Dry mouth	No	No	No	Yes, early
Tick paralysis	No	Paresthesias	No	No	No
Diphtheria	No	Occasional	Yes	No	Pharyngeal followed by other cranial nerves; may resolve before generalized weakness
Eaton-Lambert	No	No	No	No	Yes
Organophosphate poisoning (or pyridostigmine overdose)	Prominent sweating, bradycardia, other cholinergic signs	No	No	Yes	Yes
Subacute multifocal motor neuropathy	No	Occasionally	No	No	No
ALS	No	No	No	Prominent but disappear in advanced disease	Early
Polymyositis/ dermatomyositis	No	No	No	No	Pharyngeal only; ocular usually intact

From Graber MA: *The family practice handbook,* ed 4, St Louis, 2001, Mosby.
ALS, Amyotrophic lateral sclerosis.

WEIGHT GAIN

BOX 2-262 Weight Gain

Sedentary lifestyle
Fluid overload
After discontinuation of tobacco abuse
Endocrine disorders: hypothyroidism, hyperinsulinism associated with maturity-onset diabetes mellitus, Cushing's syndrome, hypogonadism, insulinoma, hyperprolactinemia, acromegaly

Medications: nutritional supplements, oral contraceptives, glucocorticoids, etc.
Anxiety disorders with compulsive eating
Laurence-Moon-Biedl syndrome, Prader-Willi syndrome, other congenital diseases
Hypothalamic injury (rare; <100 cases reported in medical literature)

Weight gain
ICD-9CM # 783.1   Abnormal weight gain
**   278.00 Obesity**

WEIGHT LOSS

Weight loss
ICD-9CM # 783.2 Abnormal weight loss

BOX 2-263 Causes of Weight Loss

I. Weight loss with normal to increased food intake associated with unimpaired appetite
 A. Insulin-dependent diabetes mellitus
 B. Thyrotoxicosis
 C. Pheochromocytoma
 D. Carcinoid
 E. Malabsorption and maldigestion
 F. Intestinal parasite infestation
 G. Diencephalic syndrome
 H. Malignancy (uncommon)
 I. Luft's syndrome
II. Weight loss with normal or decreased food intake
 A. Impaired appetite that in some cases may be coupled with an increased caloric requirement
  1. Malignancy
  2. Psychiatric disorders (including anorexia nervosa)
  3. Acquired immunodeficiency syndrome

 4. Liver disease
 5. Addison's disease
 6. Uremia
 7. Chronic infection
 8. Chronic lung disease
 9. Chronic inflammatory disease
 10. Cardiac cachexia
 11. Diabetic neuropathic cachexia
 12. Hypothalamic tumor (very rare)
 B. Unimpaired appetite but decrease of food intake secondary to other factors
  1. Gastric ulcer
  2. Duodenal ulcer with outlet obstruction
  3. Postgastrectomy syndrome
  4. Regional enteritis
  5. Ulcerative colitis
  6. Food faddism
  7. Social isolation

From Stein JH (ed): *Internal medicine,* ed 5, St Louis, 1998, Mosby.

WHEEZING

Wheezing
ICD-9CM # 786.09

BOX 2-264   Wheezing

Asthma
Chronic obstructive pulmonary
  disease
Interstitial lung disease
Infections: pneumonia, bronchitis,
  bronchiolitis, epiglottitis

Cardiac asthma
Gastroesophageal reflux disease with
  aspiration
Foreign body aspiration
Pulmonary embolism
Anaphylaxis

Obstruction in airway: neoplasm,
  goiter, edema or hemorrhage from
  trauma, aneurysm, congenital abnormalities, strictures, spasm
Carcinoid syndrome

WHEEZING, PEDIATRIC AGE

Wheezing, pediatric age
ICD-9CM # 786.09 Wheezing

BOX 2-265   Causes of Recurrent or Persistent Wheezing in Children

Reactive airways disease
  Atopic asthma
  Infection-associated airway reactivity
  Exercise-induced asthma
  Salicylate-induced asthma and nasal polyposis
  Asthmatic bronchitis
  Other hypersensitivity reactions
    Hypersensitivity pneumonitis
    Tropical eosinophilia
    Visceral larva migrans
    Allergic bronchopulmonary aspergillosis
Aspiration
  Foreign body
  Food, saliva, gastric contents
  Laryngotracheoesophageal cleft
  Tracheoesophageal fistula, H-type
  Pharyngeal incoordination or neuromuscular
    weakness
Cystic fibrosis
Primary ciliary dyskinesia
Cardiac failure
Bronchiolitis obliterans
Extrinsic compression of airways
  Vascular ring
  Enlarged lymph node
  Mediastinal tumor
  Lung cysts
Tracheobronchomalacia
Endobronchial masses
Gastroesophageal reflux
Pulmonary hemosiderosis
Sequelae of bronchopulmonary dysplasia
"Hysterical" glottic closure
Cigarette smoke, other environmental insults

From Behrman RE: *Nelson textbook of pediatrics,* ed 16, Philadelphia, 2000, WB Saunders.

Xanthomas
ICD-9CM # 272.7 Bone
        277.8 Craniohypophyseal
        272.7 Cutaneotendinous dissemination
        374.51 Eyelid
        272.0 Hypercholesterinemic
        272.4 Hyperlipemic
        272.2 Tuberosum

XANTHOMAS

TABLE 2-217   **Xanthomas**

TYPE	CLINICAL FEATURES	LIPID ABNORMALITY
Xanthelasma	Periocular, flat-topped, or papular	Apo E, hyperapo β-lipoproteinemia; occasionally, no abnormality found
Plane xanthoma	Palms, face, neck	Biliary cirrhosis: type III
Eruptive xanthoma	Eruptive crops of papular lesions on buttocks, extremities	Hypertriglyceridemia: primary types I, III, IV, V, or secondary (diabetes mellitus)
Tuberous	Large nodular lesions on elbows and knees	Hypertriglyceridemia: familial types II, III
Tendinous	Deep nodules over tendons: knees, elbows, hands, Achilles	Hypercholesterolemia: familial types II, III

Modified form Habif TP: *Clinical dermatology,* ed 3, St Louis, 1996, Mosby.

XEROSTOMIA AND XEROPHTHALMIA

Xerostomia and xerophthalmia
ICD-9CM # 527.7 Xerostomia
         372.53 Xerophthalmia

BOX 2-266   **Causes of Xerostomia and Xerophthalmia**

Xerostomia

Medications
  Tricyclic antidepressants: amitriptyline (Elavil), doxepin (Sinequan)
  Antihistamines: diphenhydramine (Benadryl), chlorpheniramine (Chlor-Trimeton), promethazine (Phenergan), and many cold and decongestant preparations
  Anticholinergic agents: antiemetics such as scopolamine, antispasmodic agents such as oxybutynin chloride (Ditropan)
Dehydration
  Debility
  Fever
Polyuria
  Alcohol intake
  Arrhythmia
  Diabetes
Previous head and neck irradiation
Systemic diseases
  Sjögren's syndrome
  Sarcoidosis
  Amyloidosis
  Human immunodeficiency virus (HIV) infection
  Graft-vs.-host disease

Xerophthalmia

See medications and systemic diseases listed above
Abnormalities of eyelid function
  Neuromuscular disorders
  Aging
  Thyrotoxicosis
Abnormalities of tear production
  Hypovitaminosis A
  Stevens-Johnson syndrome
  Familial diseases affecting sebaceous secretions
Abnormalities of corneal surfaces: scarring from past injuries and herpes simplex infection

From Noble J: *Primary care medicine,* ed 3, St Louis, 2001, Mosby.

Clinical Algorithms

PLEASE NOTE: These algorithms are designed to assist clinicians in the evaluation and treatment of patients. They may not apply to all patients with a particular condition and are not intended to replace a clinician's individual judgment.

ABDOMINAL PAIN

Abdominal path
ICD-9CM # 789.0 Unspecified site
789.1 Upper right quadrant
789.2 Upper left quadrant
789.3 Lower right quadrant
789.4 Lower left quadrant
789.5 Periumbilic
789.6 Epigastric
789.7 Generalized
789.8 Other specified site (multiple)

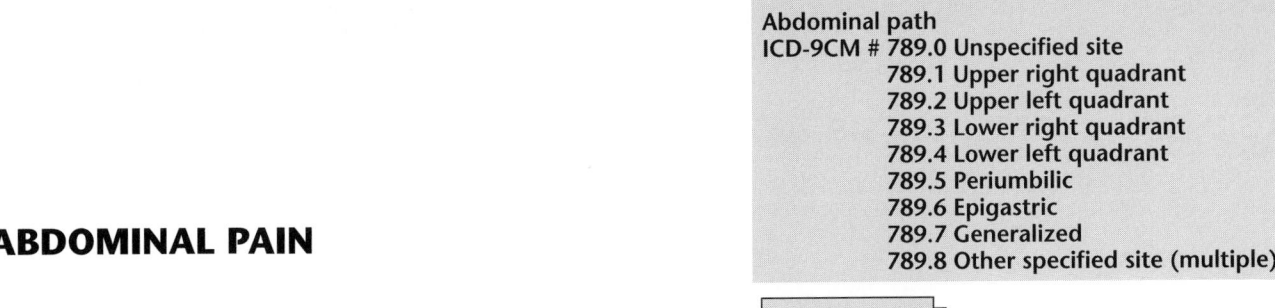

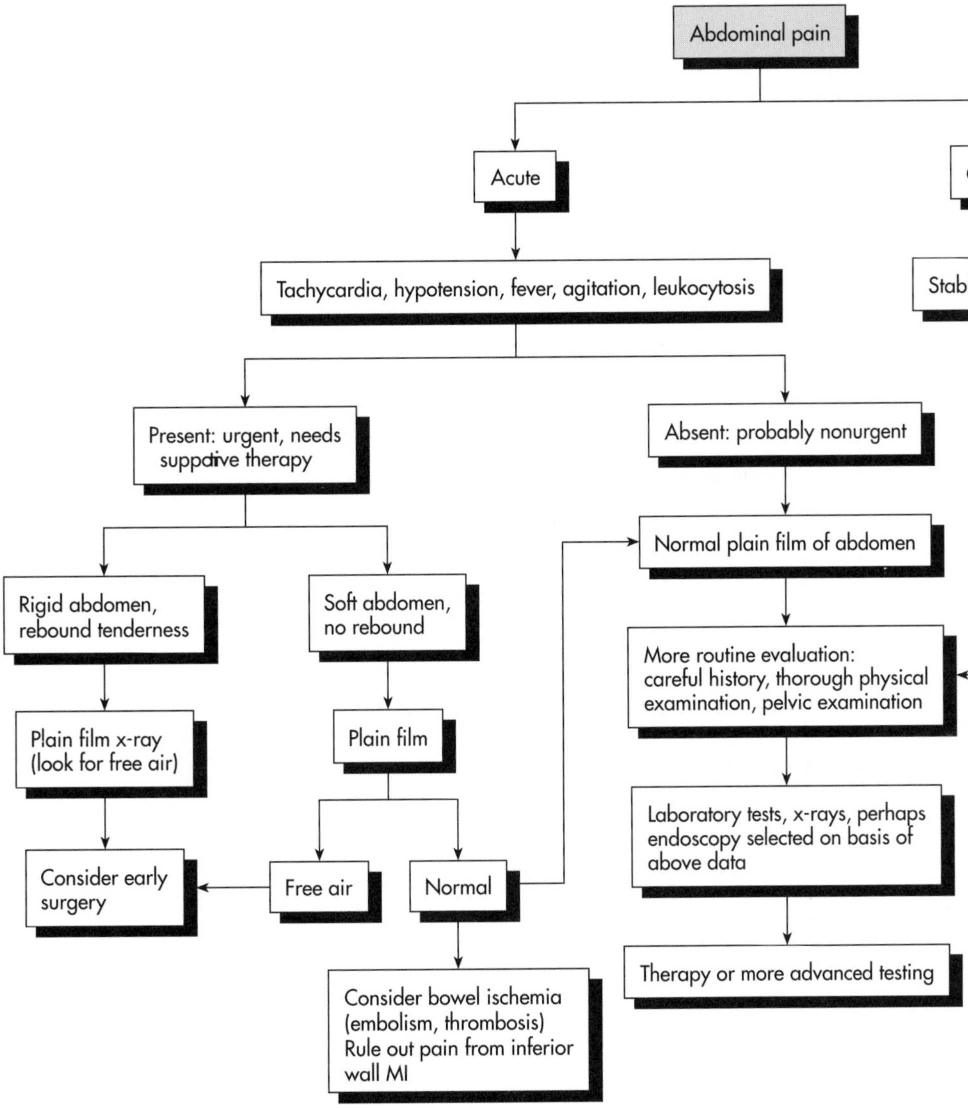

Fig. 3-1 **Evaluation of patients with abdominal pain.** (From Stein JH [ed]: *Internal medicine,* ed 5, St Louis, 1998, Mosby.)

ACID-BASE HOMEOSTASIS

Acid-base homeostasis
ICD-9CM # 276.2 Lactic acidosis
               276.2 Metabolic acidosis
               276.2 Respiratory acidosis
               276.3 Respiratory alkalosis
               276.3 Metabolic alkalosis

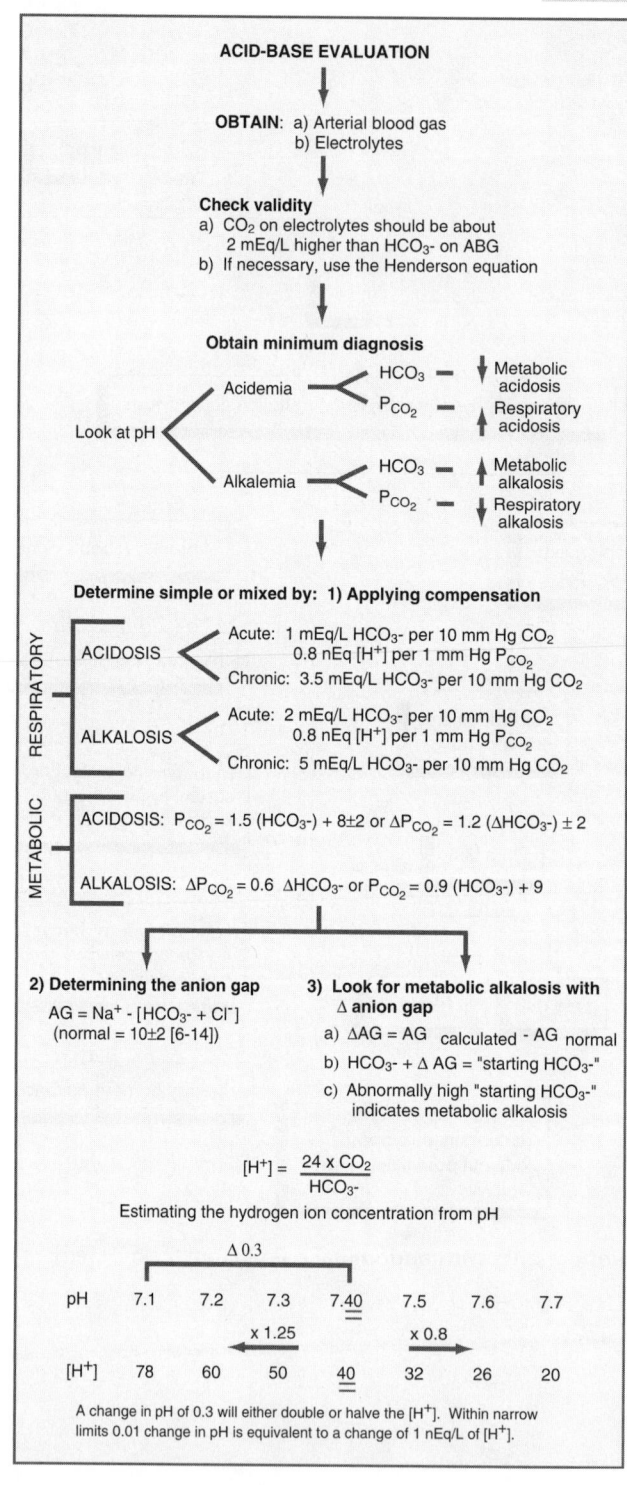

Fig. 3-2   Scheme for assessing acid-base homeostasis. (From Andreoli TE [ed]: *Cecil essentials of medicine,* ed 4, Philadelphia, 1997, WB Saunders.)

ACIDOSIS, METABOLIC

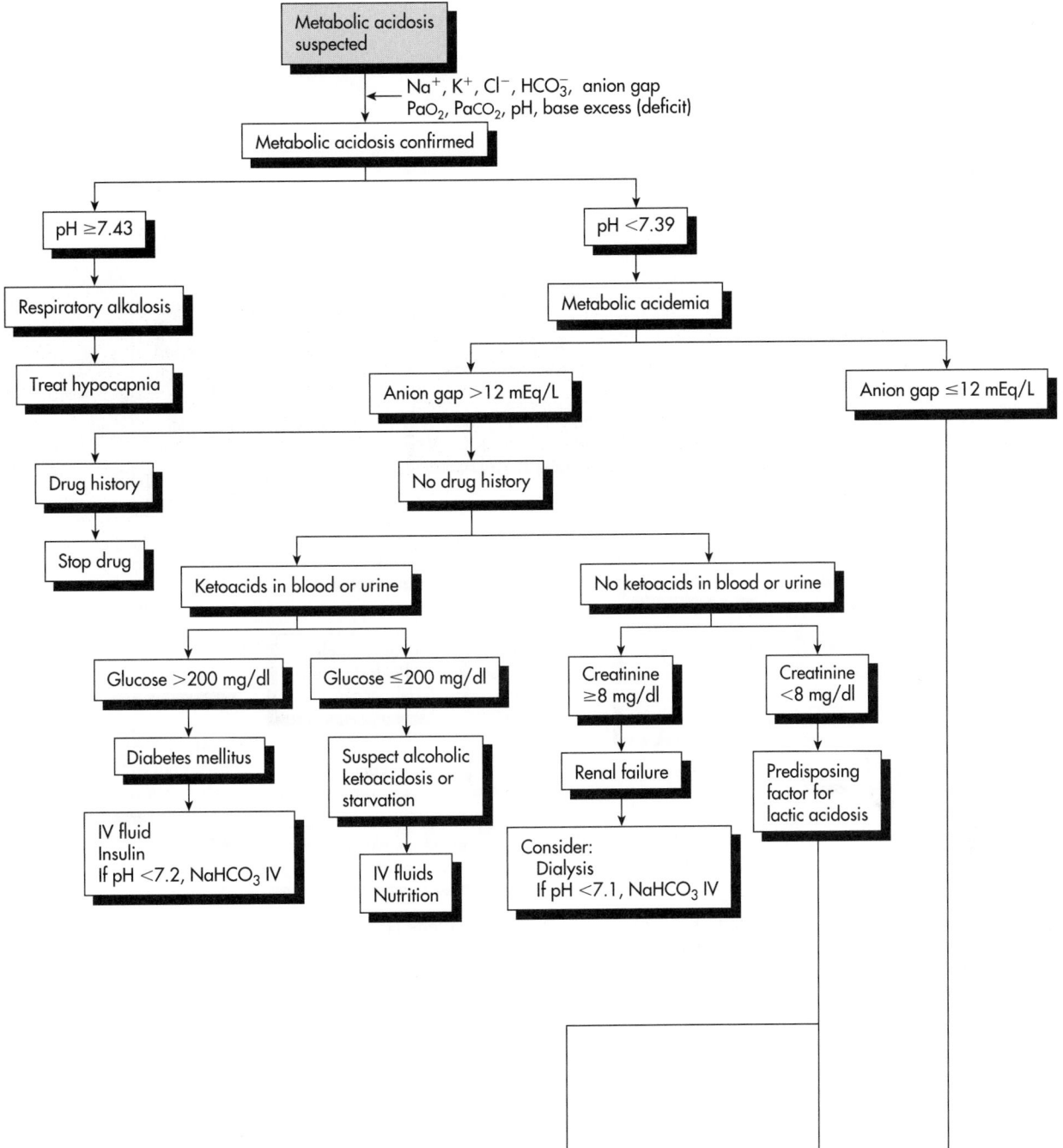

Fig. 3-3   Suspected metabolic acidosis. (From Greene HL, Johnson WP, Lemke D [eds]: *Decision making in medicine,* ed 2, St Louis, 1998, Mosby.)

ACIDOSIS, METABOLIC—cont'd

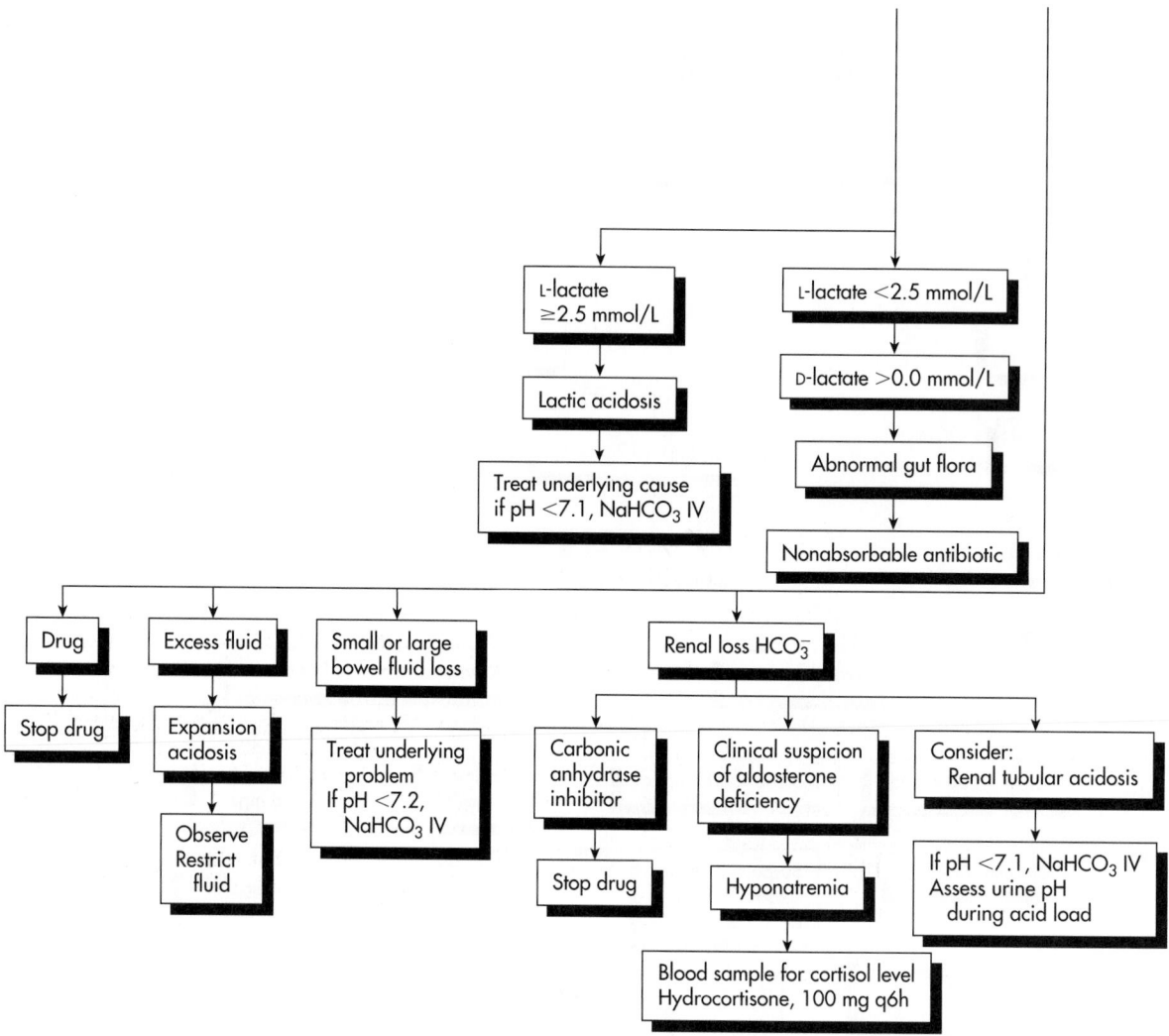

Fig. 3-3, cont'd   Suspected metabolic acidosis. (From Greene HL, Johnson WP, Lemke D [eds]: *Decision making in medicine*, ed 2, St Louis, 1998, Mosby.)

ADRENAL INCIDENTALOMA

Adrenal incidentaloma
ICD-9CM # 255.9

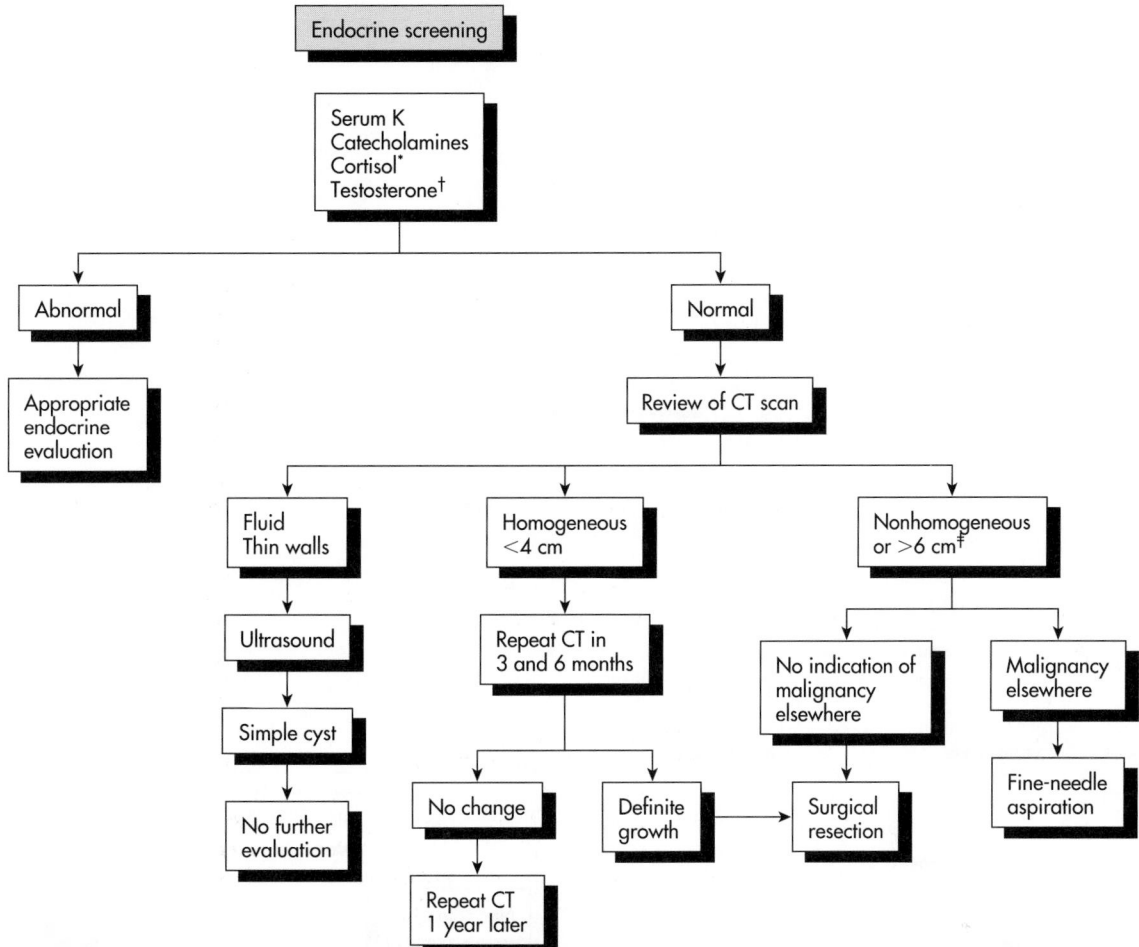

Fig. 3-4   Algorithm for evaluation of an adrenal incidentaloma. *Only if there are clinical indications of excess cortisol. †Only in women with hirsutism. ‡Measure dehydroepiandrosterone sulfate, a marker of primary adrenal carcinoma. (From Nseyo UO [ed]: *Urology for primary care physicians,* Philadelphia, 1999, WB Saunders.)

ADRENAL MASS

Adrenal mass
ICD-9CM # 194.0 Adrenal cortical carcinoma site NOS
M8370/3
255.8 Adrenal hyperplasia

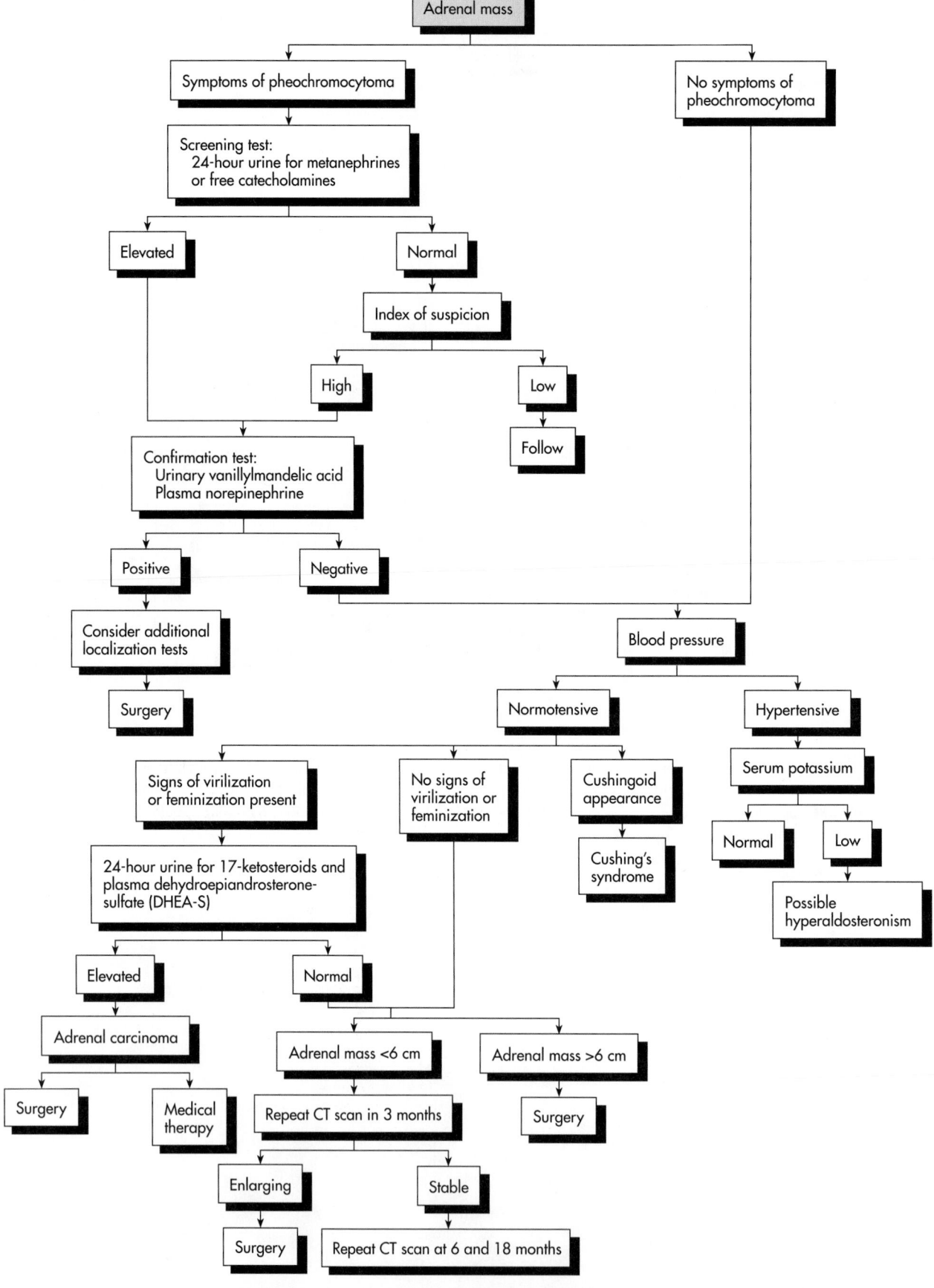

Fig. 3-5 **Evaluation of adrenal mass.** *CT,* Computed tomography. (From Greene HL, Johnson WP, Lemcke D [eds]: *Decision making in medicine,* ed 2, St Louis, 1998, Mosby.)

ALKALOSIS, METABOLIC

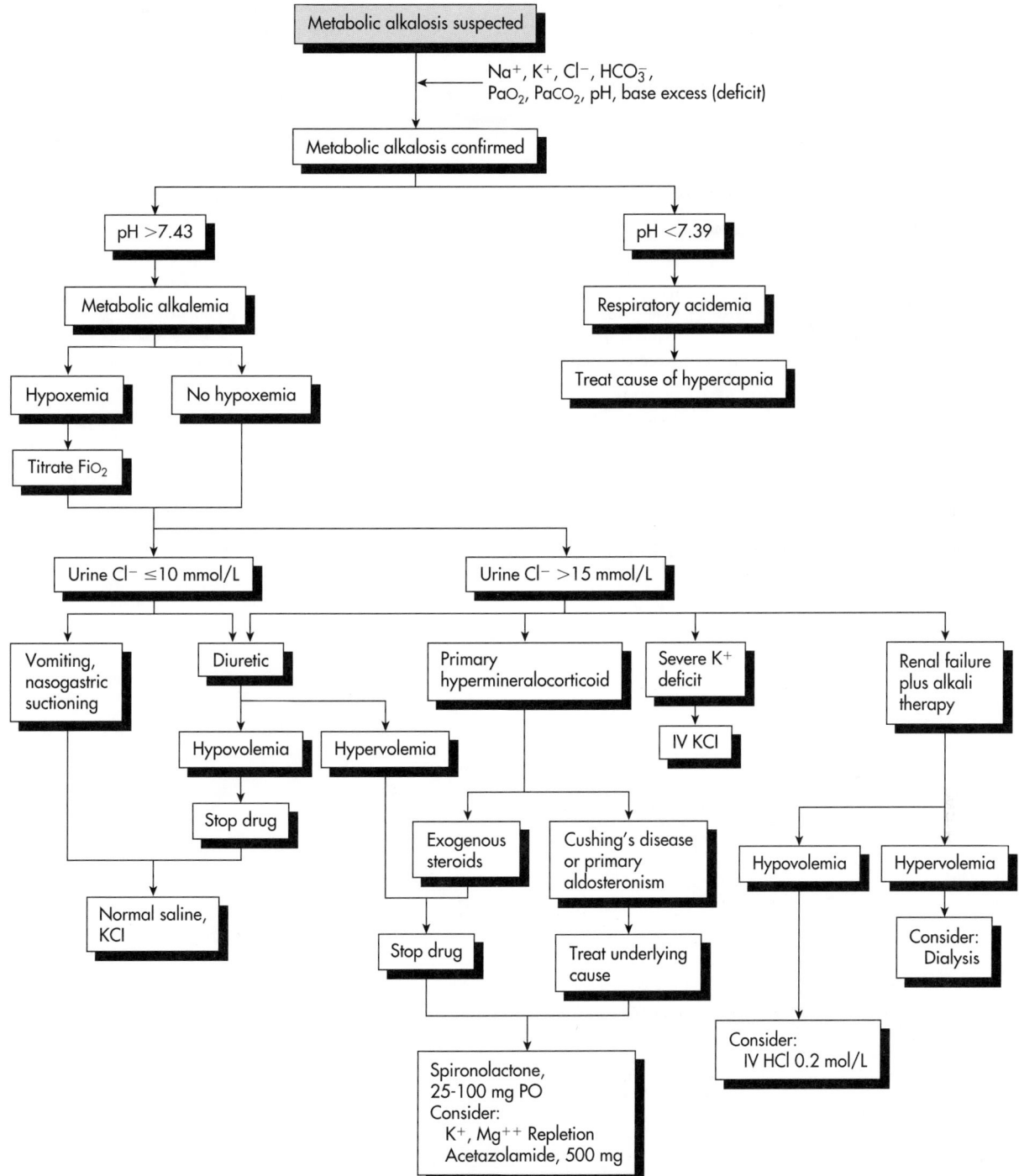

Fig. 3-6   Suspected metabolic alkalosis. (From Greene HL, Johnson WP, Lemke D [eds]: *Decision making in medicine,* ed 2, St Louis, 1998, Mosby.)

ALOPECIA

ICD-9CM # 704.01 Androgenic alopecia or alopecia
areata
757.4 Congenital alopecia
316 Psychogenic alopecia
091.82 Syphilitic alopecia

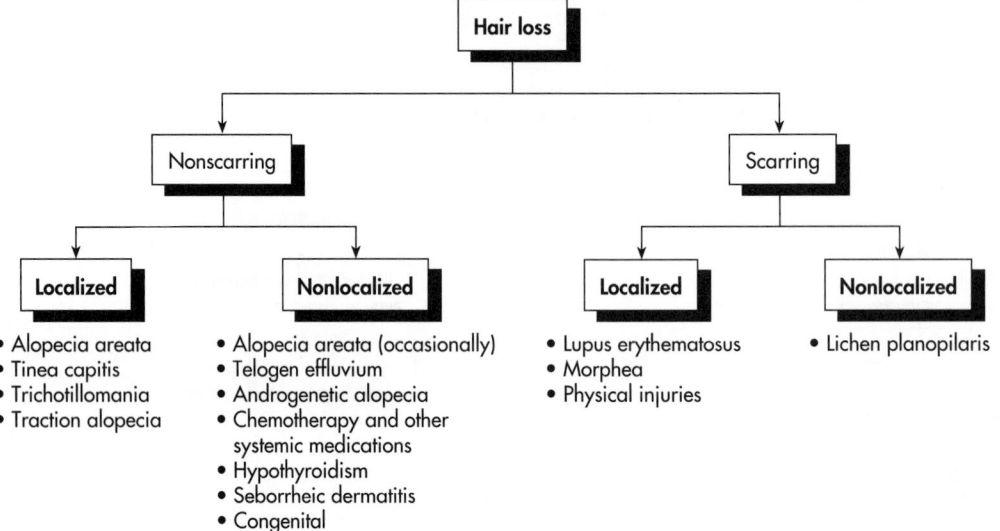

Fig. 3-7 An approach to the diagnosis of the cause of alopecia. (From Goldman L, Bennett JC [eds]: *Cecil textbook of medicine,* ed 21, Philadelphia, 2000, WB Saunders.)

AMENORRHEA, PRIMARY

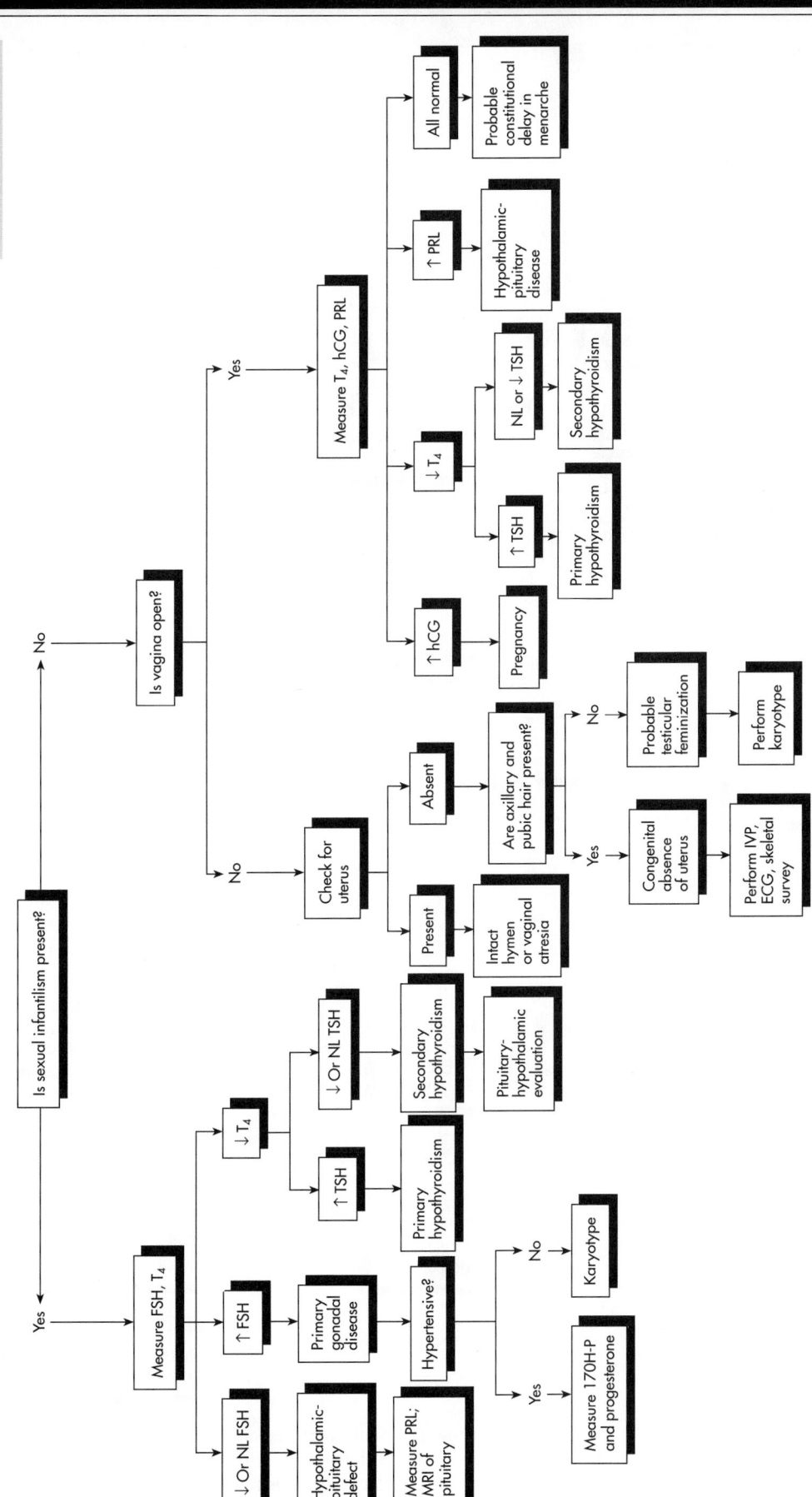

Fig. 3-8   Diagnostic evaluation of primary amenorrhea. *ECG*, Electrocardiogram; *FSH*, follicle-stimulating hormone; *hCG*, human chorionic gonadotropin; *IVP*, intravenous pyelogram; *MRI*, magnetic resonance imaging; *NL*, normal; *17OH-P*, 17 α-hydroxyprogesterone; *PRL*, prolactin; *T₄*, thyroxine; *TSH*, thyroid-stimulating hormone; ↓, decreased; ↑, increased. (From Andreoli TE [ed]: *Cecil essentials of medicine*, ed 5, Philadelphia, 2001, WB Saunders.)

AMENORRHEA, SECONDARY

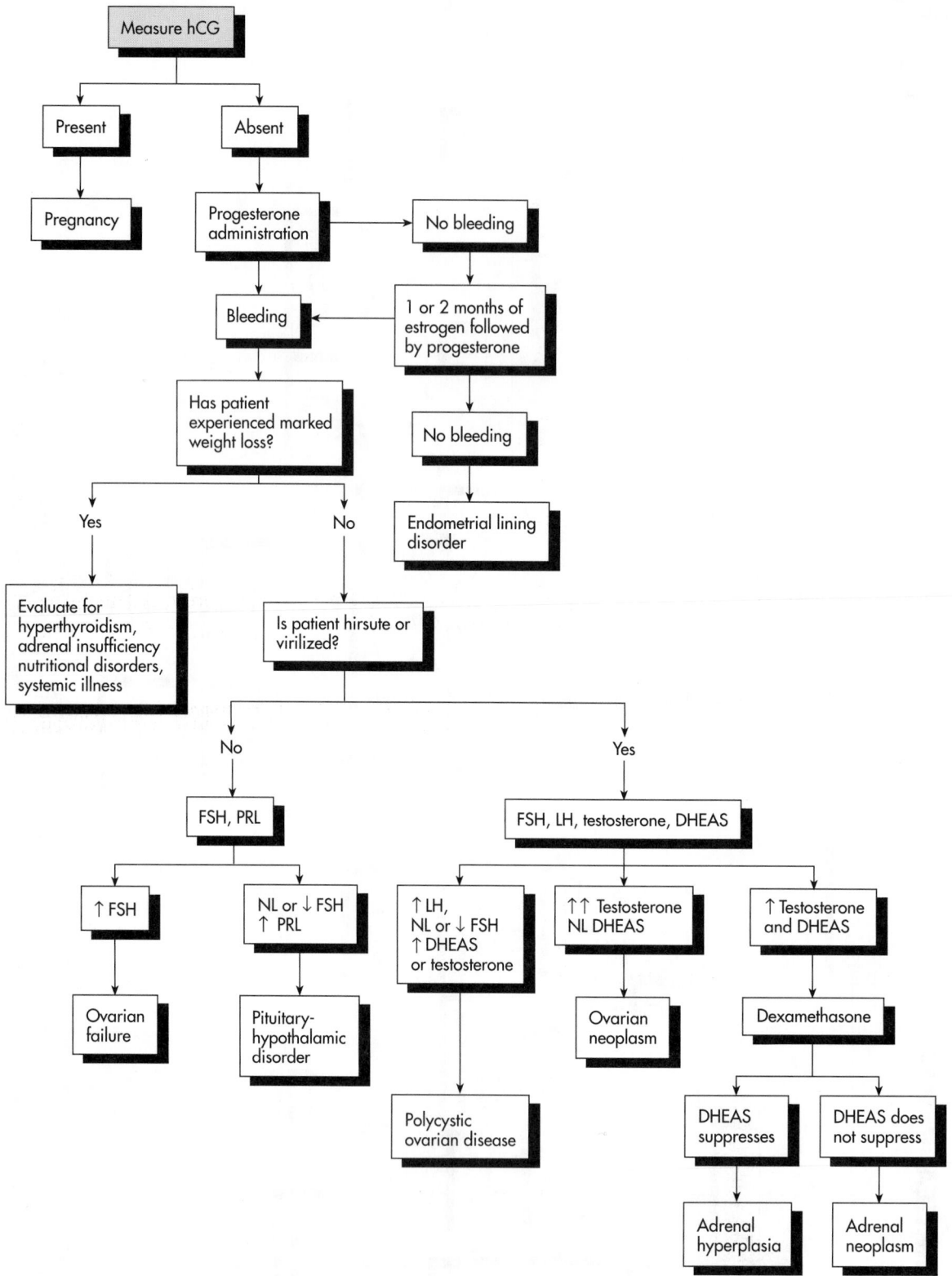

Fig. 3-9   Evaluation of secondary amenorrhea. *DHEAS,* Dehydroepiandrosterone-sulfate; *FSH,*
follicle-stimulating hormone; *hCG,* human chorionic gonadotropin; *LH,* luteinizing hormone;
NL, normal; *PRL,* prolactin; ↑, increased; ↑↑, markedly increased; ↓, decreased. (From Andreoli TE
[ed]: *Cecil essentials of medicine,* ed 5, Philadelphia, 2001, WB Saunders.)

ANEMIA

Anemia
ICD-9CM # 285.9 Anemia NOS

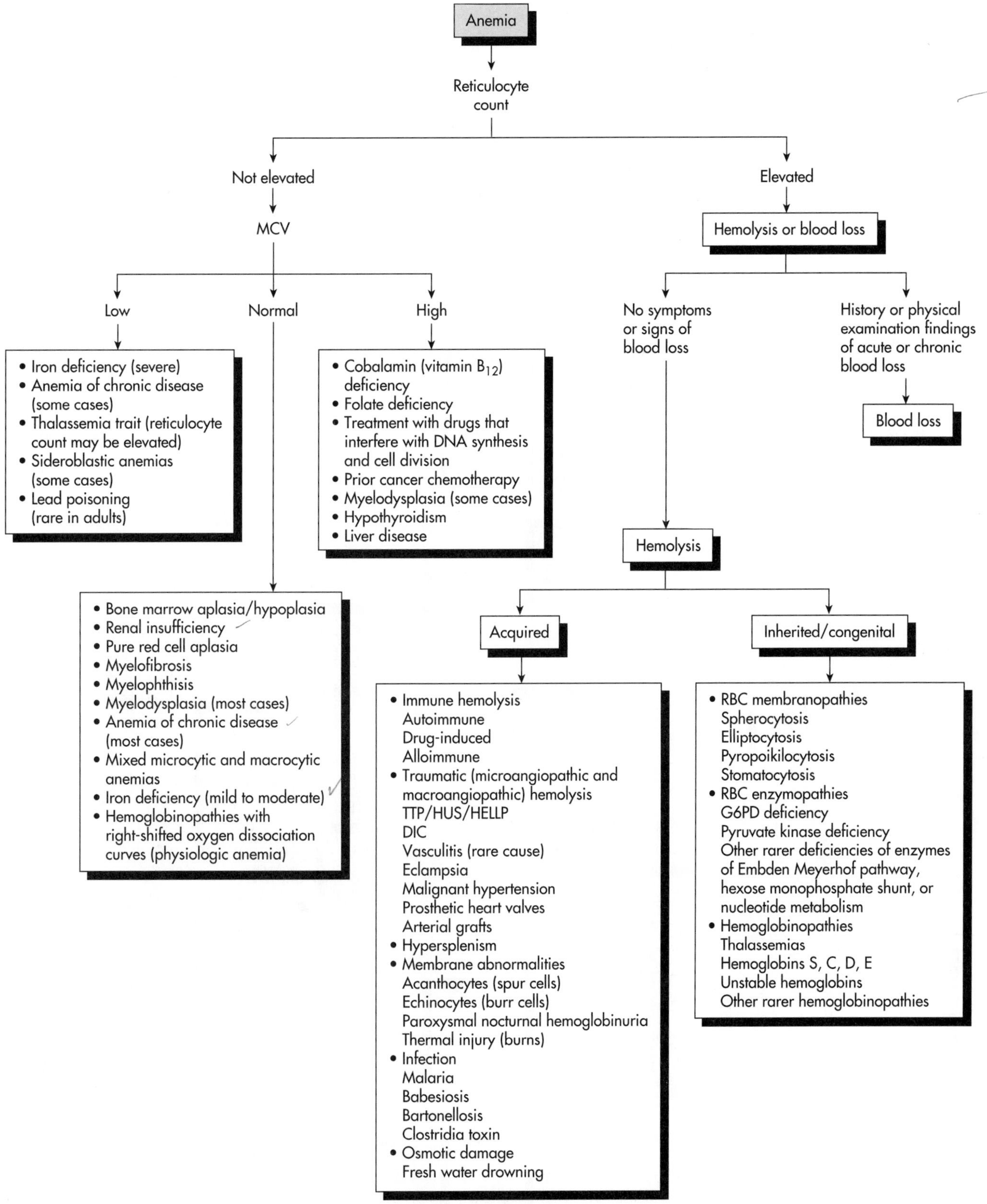

Fig. 3-10   Algorithm for diagnosis of anemias. *DIC,* Disseminated intravascular coagulation; *HELLP, h*epatomegaly-*e*levated *l*iver (function tests)-*l*ow *p*latelets; *HUS,* hemolytic-uremic syndrome; *MCV,* mean corpuscular volume; *RBC,* red blood cell; *TTP,* thrombotic thrombocytopenic purpura. (From Goldman L, Bennett JC [eds]: *Cecil textbook of medicine,* ed 21, Philadelphia, 2000, WB Saunders.)

ANEMIA, MACROCYTIC

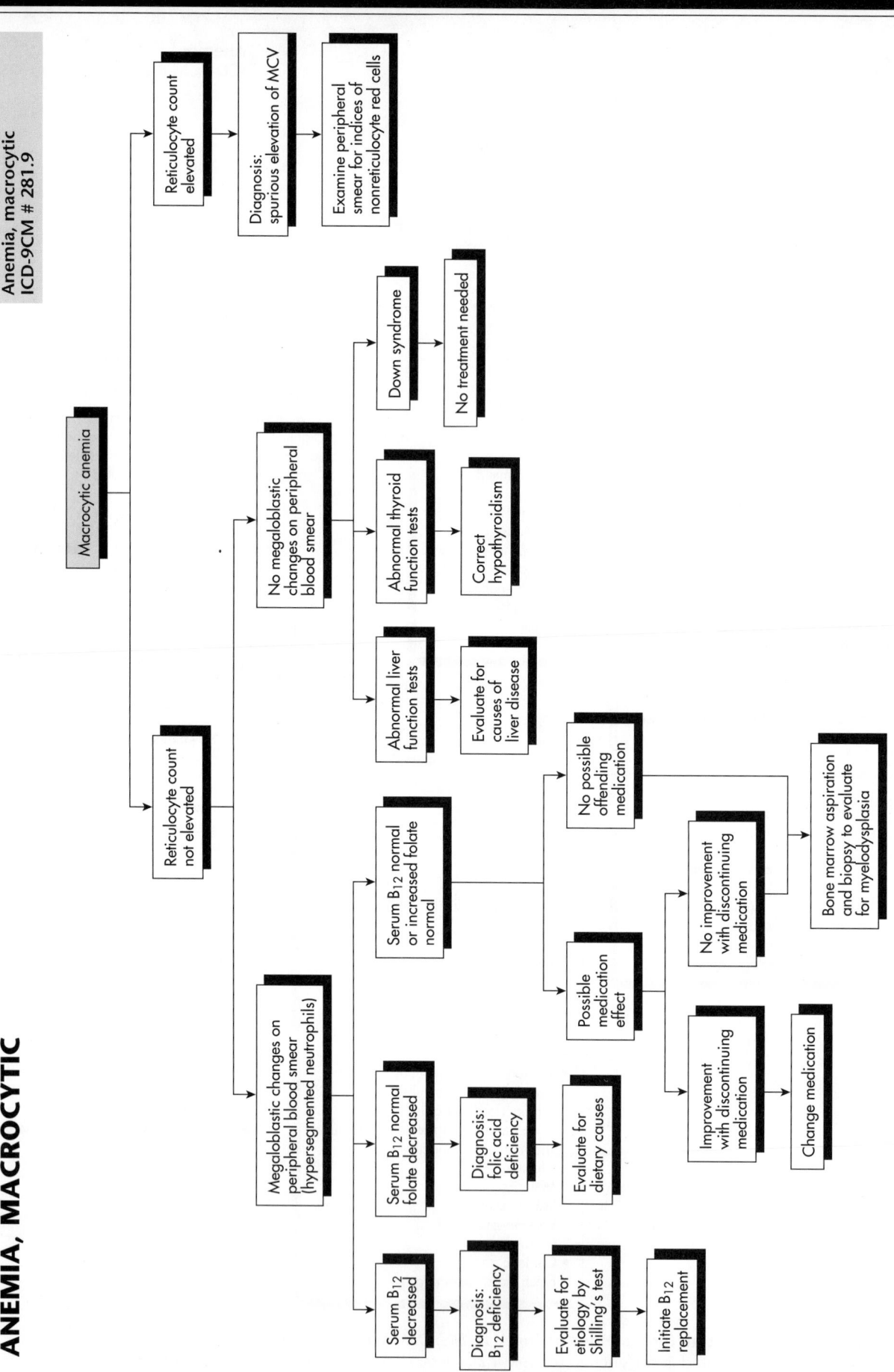

Fig. 3-11   Differential diagnosis of macrocytic anemia. (From Rakel RE [ed]: *Principles of family practice*, ed 6, Philadelphia, 2002, WB Saunders.)

ANEMIA, MICROCYTIC

Anemia, microcytic
ICD-9CM # 282.4

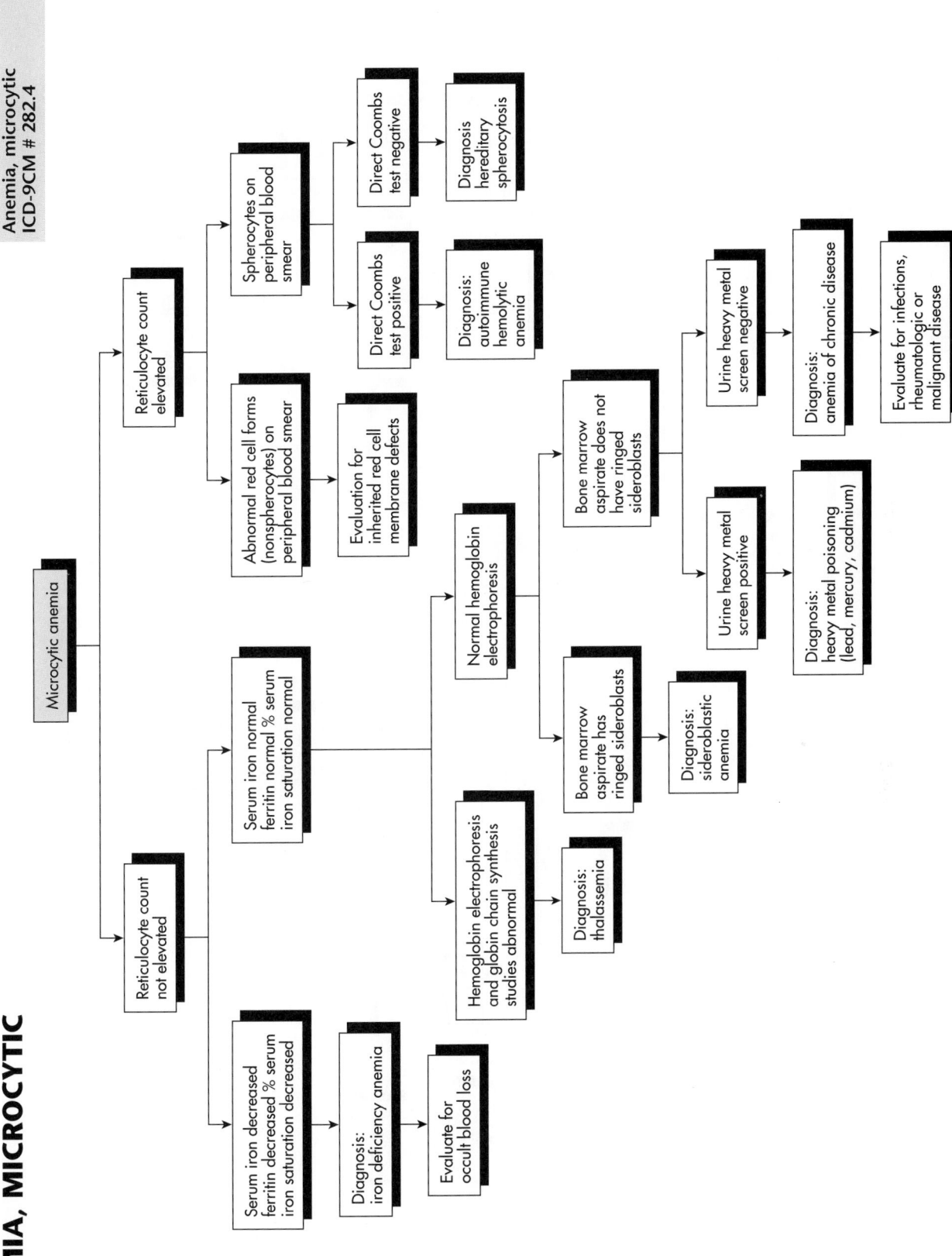

Fig. 3-12 Differential diagnosis of microcytic anemia. (From Rakel RE [ed]: *Principles of family practice*, ed 6, Philadelphia, 2002, WB Saunders.)

ANEMIA, WITH RETICULOCYTOSIS

Anemia with reticulocytosis
ICD-9CM # 790.99

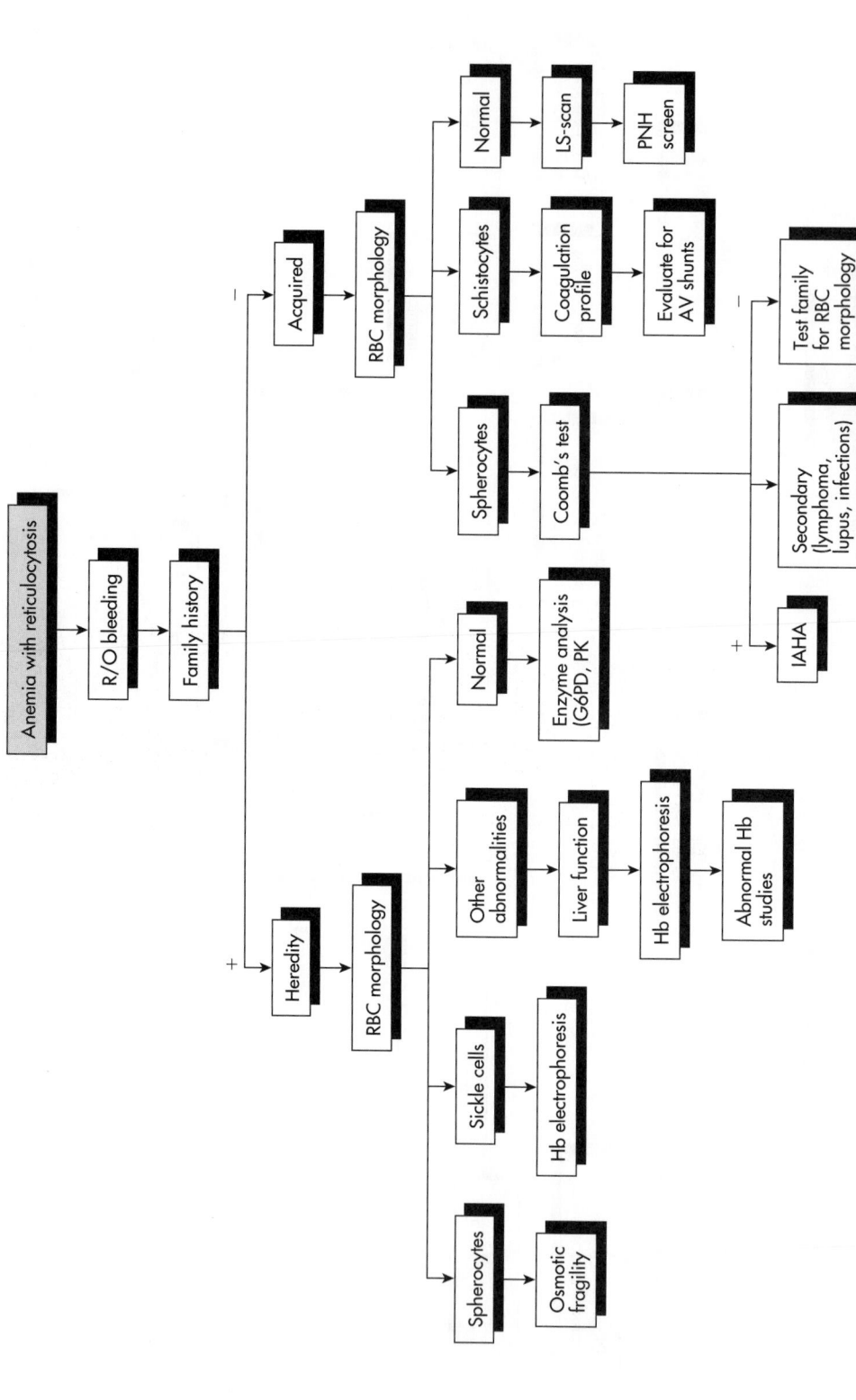

Fig. 3-13   Evaluations of patients with hemolytic anemia. *AV,* Arteriovenous; *Hb,* hemoglobin; *IAHA,* idiopathic autoimmune hemolytic anemia; *LS,* liver spleen; *PK,* pyruvate kinase; *PNH,* paroxysmal nocturnal hemoglobinuria; *RBC,* red blood cell. (From Stein JH: *Internal medicine,* ed 5, St Louis, 1997, Mosby.)

ANISOCORIA

Anisocoria
ICD-9CM # 379.41

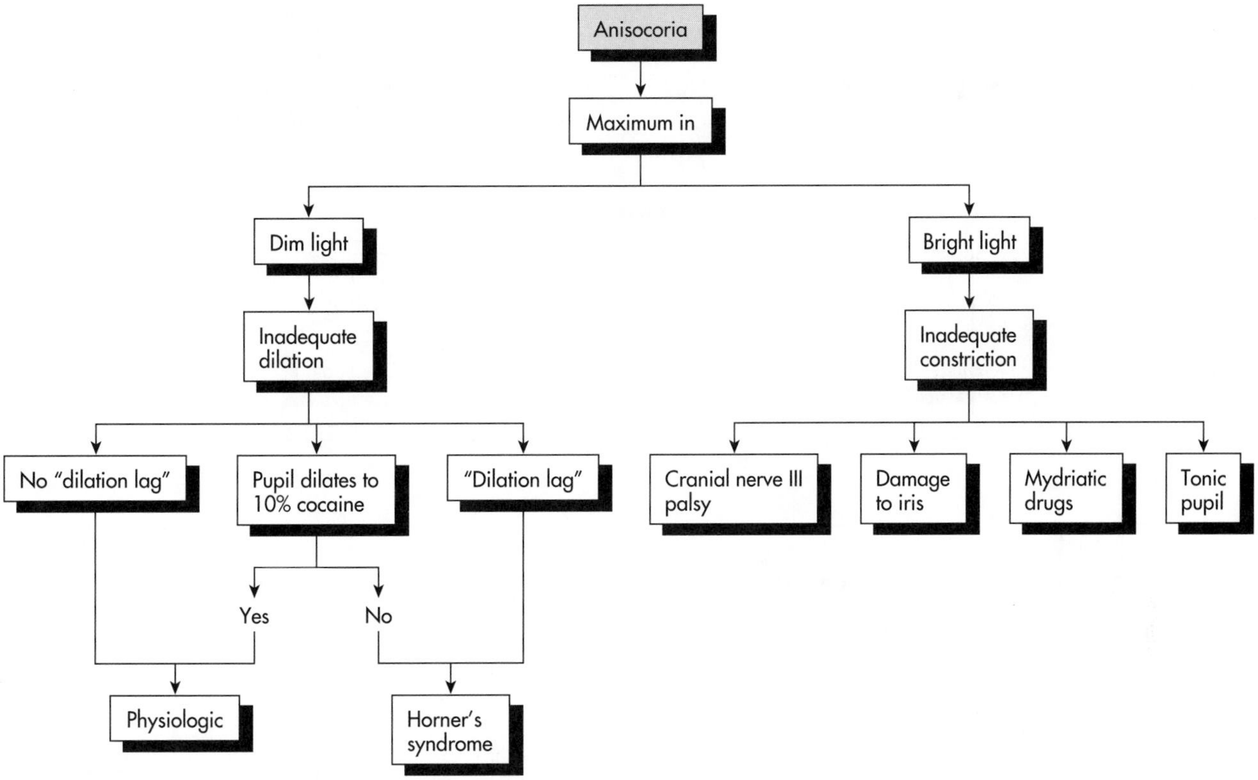

Fig. 3-14   Algorithm for the approach to unequal pupils (anisocoria). (From Andreoli TE [ed]: *Cecil essentials of medicine,* ed 5, Philadelphia, 2001, WB Saunders.)

III

Anorectal complaints
ICD-9CM # 569.49 Anal inflammation or infection
           569.42 Anal pain
           959.1   Anal injury
           564.6   Anal spasm
           569.2   Anal stenosis
           787.99 Anal swelling
           569.41 Anal ulcer

ANORECTAL COMPLAINTS

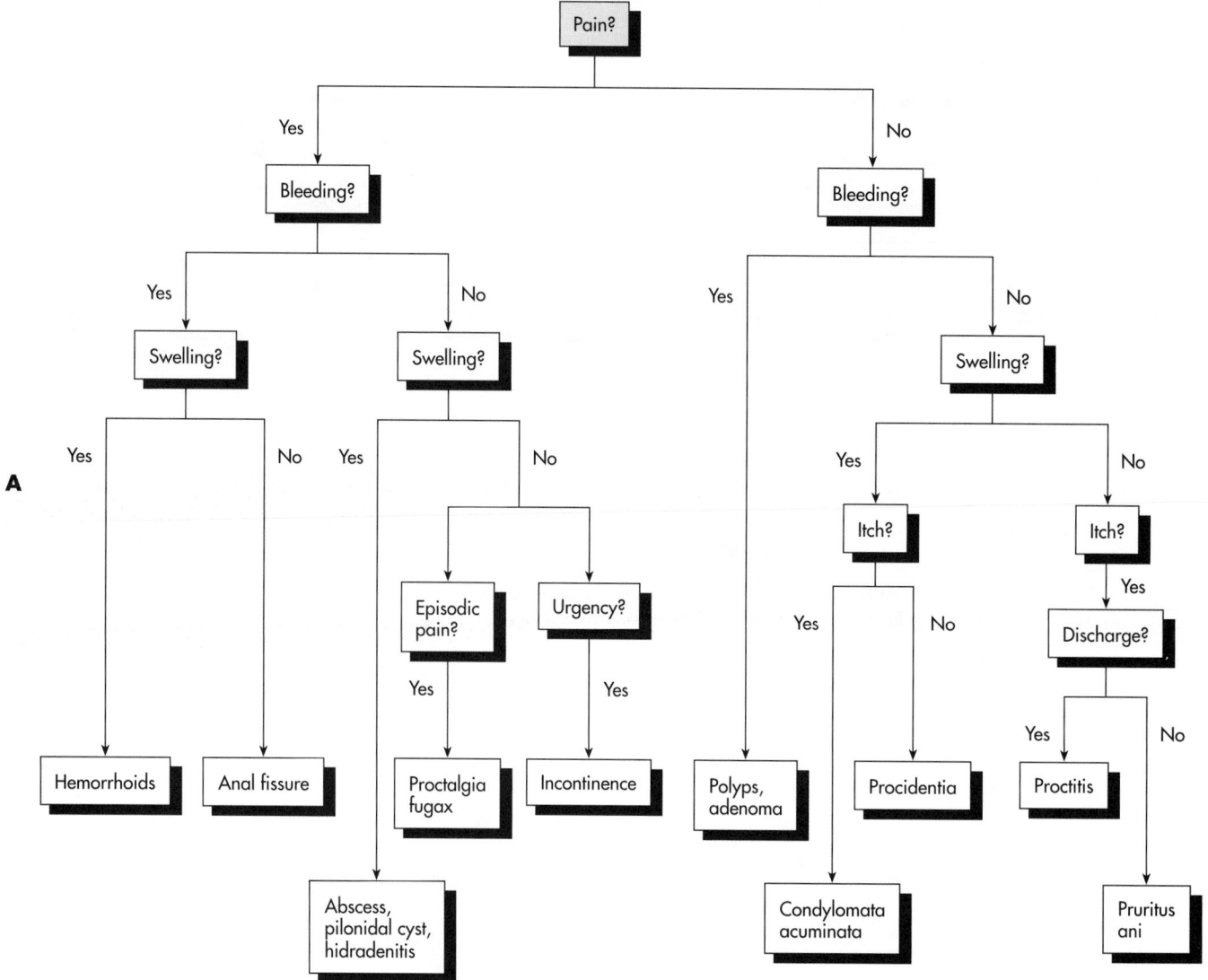

Fig. 3-15   A, Anorectal complaints. (From Rosen P [ed]: *Emergency medicine,* ed 5, St Louis, 2002, Mosby.)

ANORECTAL COMPLAINTS—cont'd

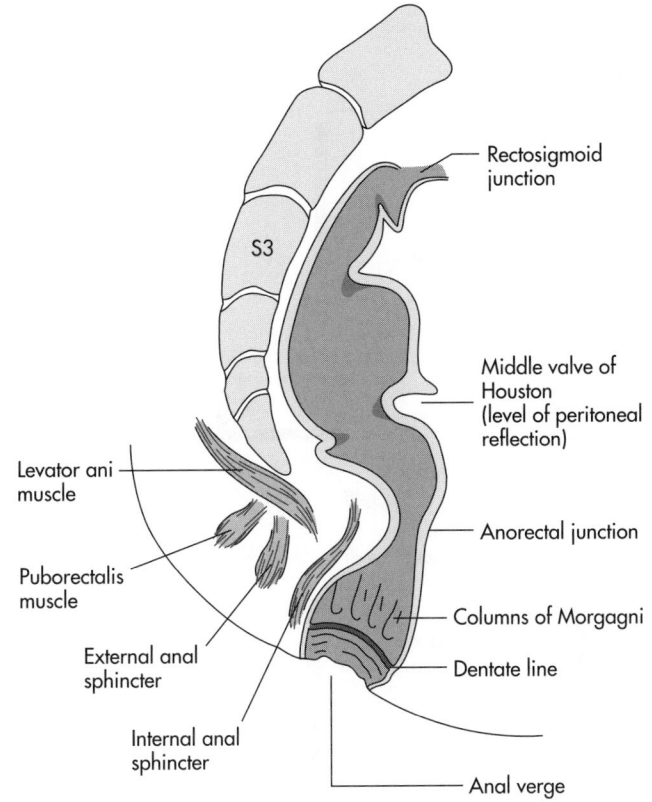

B

- Rectosigmoid junction
- S3
- Middle valve of Houston (level of peritoneal reflection)
- Levator ani muscle
- Anorectal junction
- Puborectalis muscle
- Columns of Morgagni
- External anal sphincter
- Dentate line
- Internal anal sphincter
- Anal verge

Fig. 3-15, cont'd **B, Anorectal anatomy.** (From Rosen P [ed]: *Emergency medicine,* ed 5, St Louis, 2002, Mosby.)

BOX 3-1 **Medical History**

Anorectal History

Pain
Bleeding
Swelling
Itching
Discharge

Gastrointestinal History

Change in bowel habits (straining, flatus, color, consistency, frequency)
Nausea or vomiting
Incontinence of stool
Underlying gastrointestinal disease (Crohn's disease, cancer, polyps)

Systemic Disease History

Diabetes mellitus
Coagulopathy
Cancer
Human immunodeficiency virus

Sexual History of the Anus

Penetration
Known sexually transmitted diseases

From Rosen P (ed): *Emergency medicine,* ed 5, St Louis, 2002, Mosby.

III

ANOREXIA

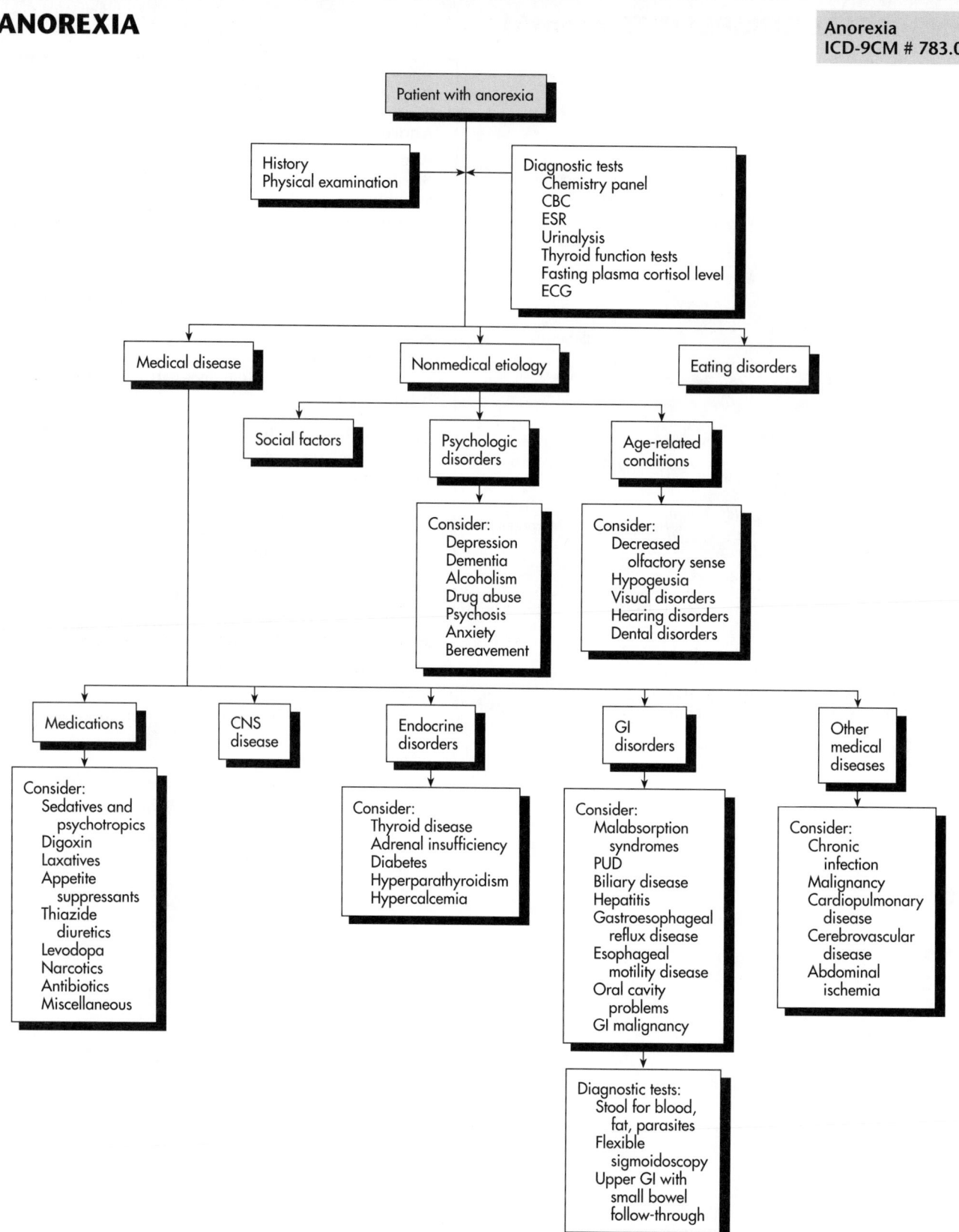

Fig. 3-16 **Evaluation of anorexia.** *CBC,* Complete blood count; *CNS,* central nervous system; *ECG,* electrocardiogram; *ESR,* erythrocyte sedimentation rate; *GI,* gastrointestinal; *PUD,* peptic ulcer disease. (From Greene HL, Johnson WP, Lemcke D [eds]: *Decision making in medicine,* ed 2, St Louis, 1998, Mosby.)

ANTINUCLEAR ANTIBODY ABNORMALITY

Antinuclear antibody abnormality
ICD-9CM # 795.79

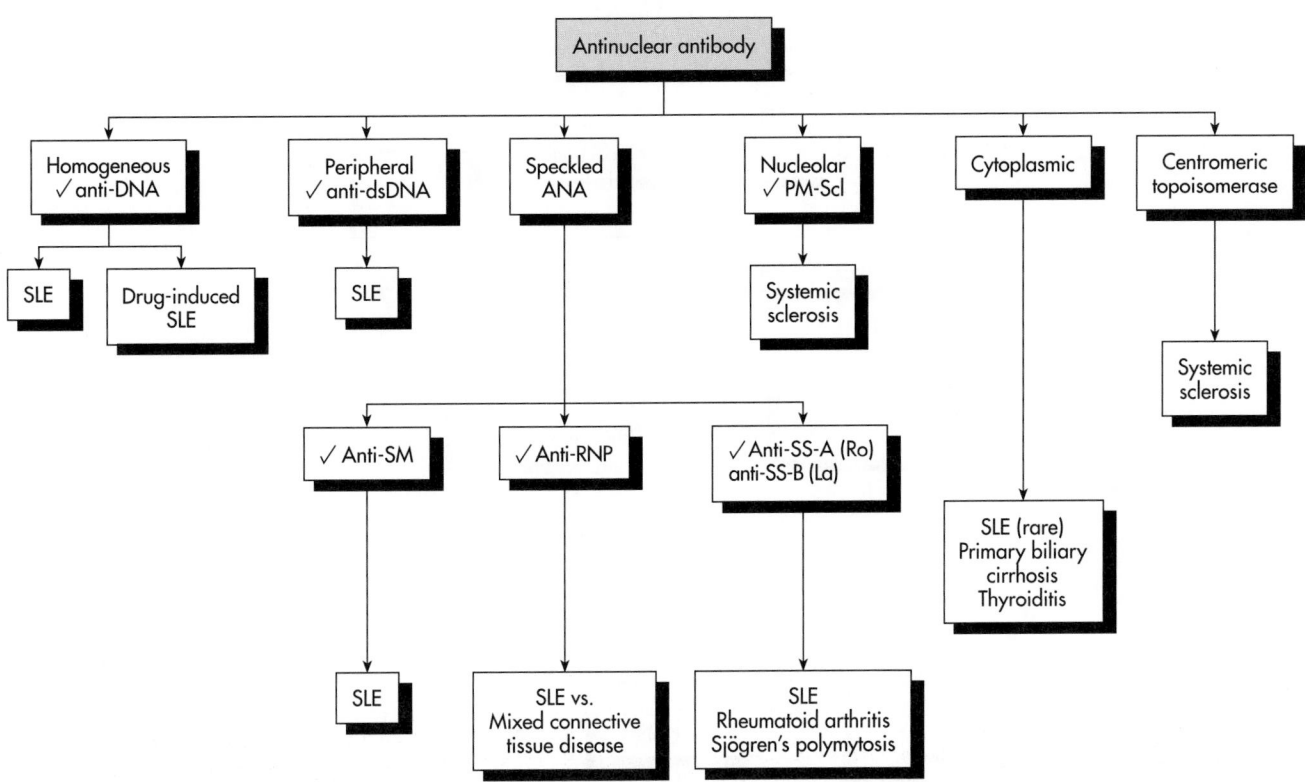

Fig. 3-17   **Diagnostic tests and diagnoses to consider from antinuclear antibody pattern.**
ANA, Antinuclear antibody; *SLE,* systemic lupus erythematosus. (From Carlson KJ et al: *Primary care of women,* St Louis, 1995, Mosby.)

ARTHRALGIA LIMITED TO ONE OR FEW JOINTS

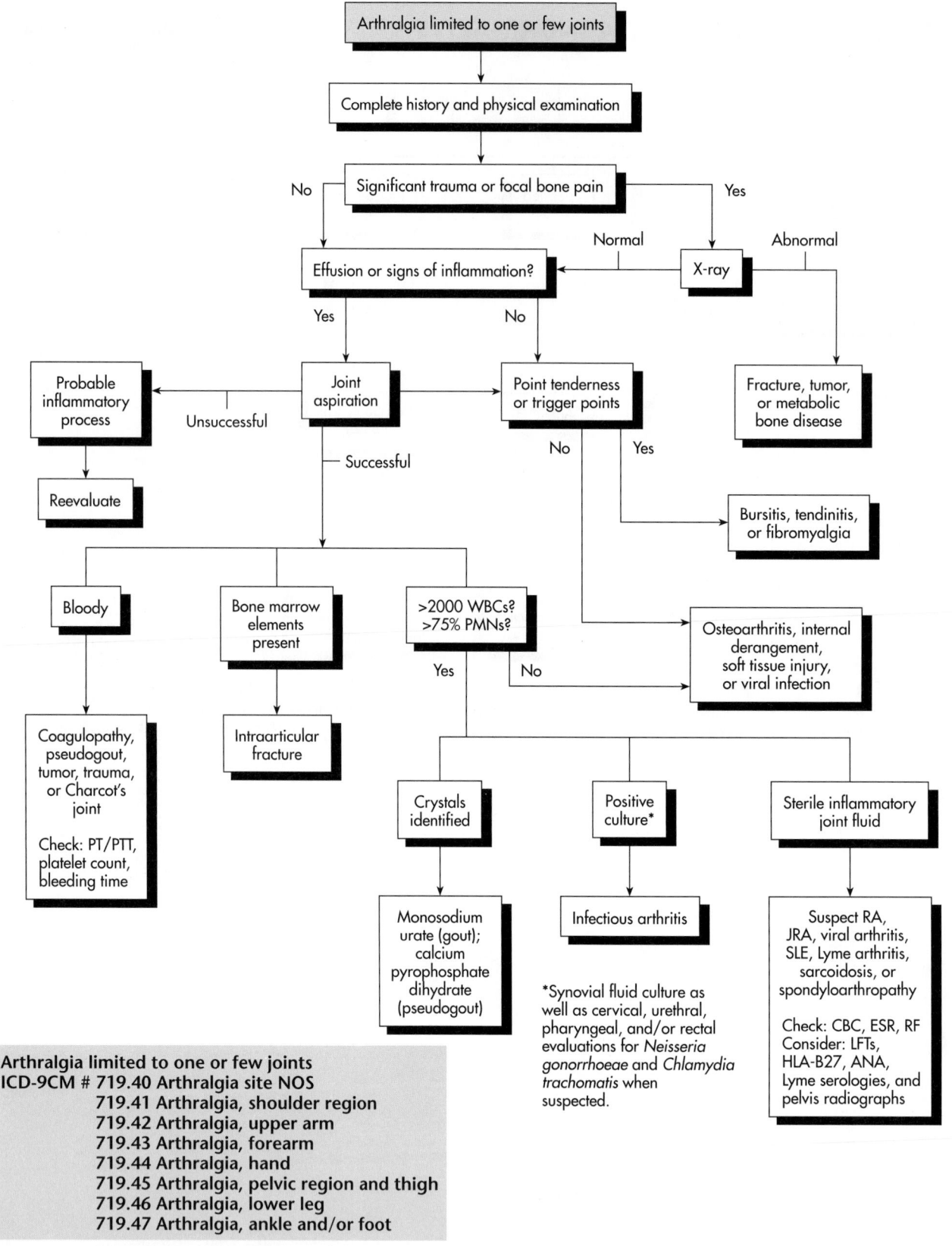

Fig. 3-18   A diagnostic approach to arthralgia in a few joints. *ANA,* Antinuclear antibodies; *CBC,* complete blood count; *ESR,* erythrocyte sedimentation rate; *JRA,* juvenile rheumatoid arthritis; *LFTs,* liver function tests; *PMNs,* polymorphonuclear neutrophils; *PT,* prothrombin time; *PTT,* partial thromboplastin time; *RA,* rheumatoid arthritis; *RF,* rheumatoid factor; *SLE,* systemic lupus erythematosus; *WBCs,* white blood cells. (Modified from American College of Rheumatology Ad Hoc Committee on Clinical Guidelines: *Arthritis Rheum* 39:1, 1996.)

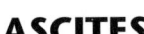

Ascites
ICD-9CM # 789.5 Ascites NOS
            197.6 Ascites, cancerous (malignant)
                  M8000/6
            457.8 Chylous
            014.0 Tuberculous

ASCITES

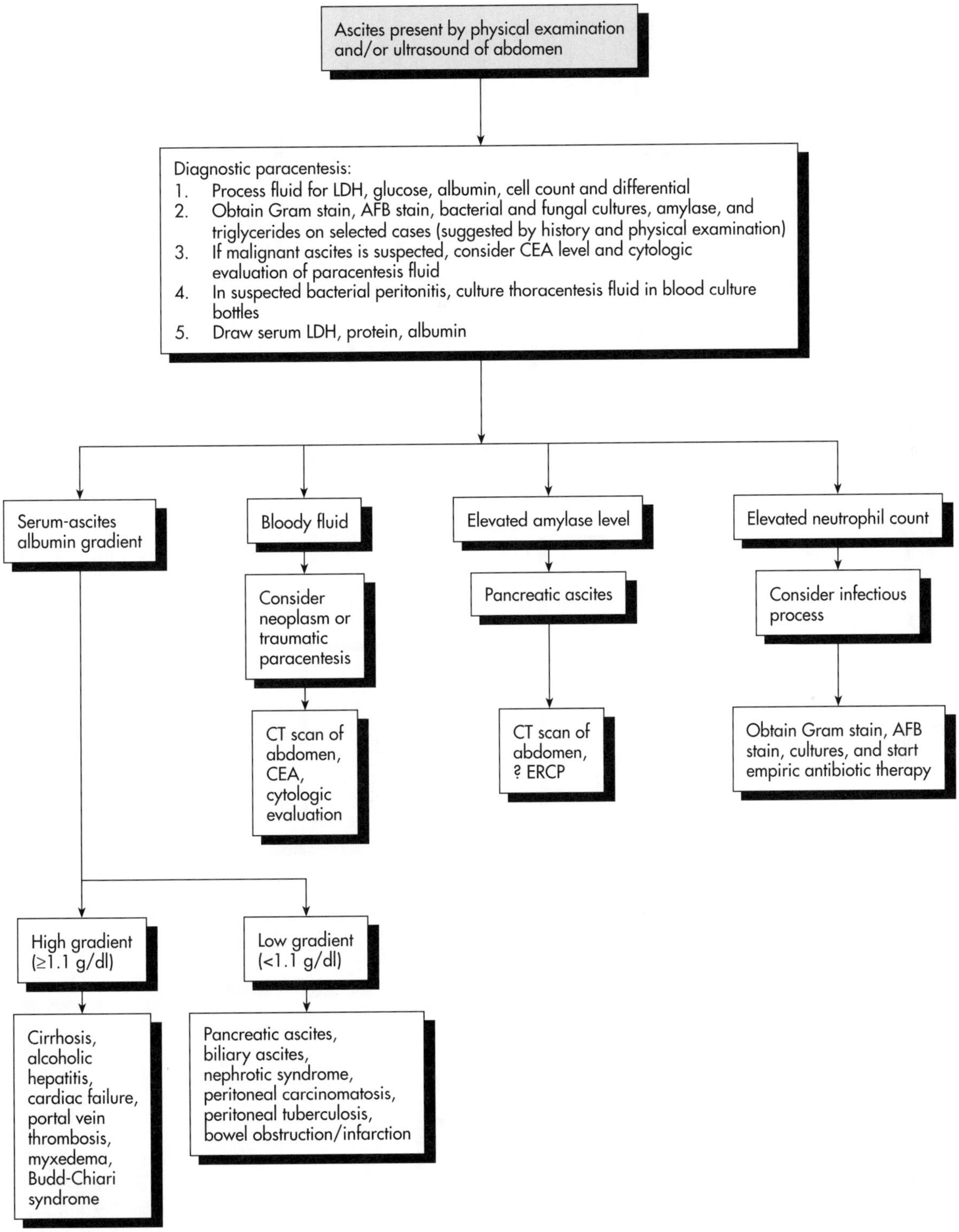

Ascites present by physical examination and/or ultrasound of abdomen

Diagnostic paracentesis:
1. Process fluid for LDH, glucose, albumin, cell count and differential
2. Obtain Gram stain, AFB stain, bacterial and fungal cultures, amylase, and triglycerides on selected cases (suggested by history and physical examination)
3. If malignant ascites is suspected, consider CEA level and cytologic evaluation of paracentesis fluid
4. In suspected bacterial peritonitis, culture thoracentesis fluid in blood culture bottles
5. Draw serum LDH, protein, albumin

Serum-ascites albumin gradient

Bloody fluid

Consider neoplasm or traumatic paracentesis

CT scan of abdomen, CEA, cytologic evaluation

Elevated amylase level

Pancreatic ascites

CT scan of abdomen, ? ERCP

Elevated neutrophil count

Consider infectious process

Obtain Gram stain, AFB stain, cultures, and start empiric antibiotic therapy

High gradient (≥1.1 g/dl)

Low gradient (<1.1 g/dl)

Cirrhosis, alcoholic hepatitis, cardiac failure, portal vein thrombosis, myxedema, Budd-Chiari syndrome

Pancreatic ascites, biliary ascites, nephrotic syndrome, peritoneal carcinomatosis, peritoneal tuberculosis, bowel obstruction/infarction

III

Fig. 3-19   Evaluation of ascites. *AFB,* Acid-fast bacillus; *CEA,* carcinoembryonic antigen; *CT,* computed tomography; *ERCP,* endoscopic retrograde cholangiopancreatography; *LDH,* lactate dehydrogenase.

ASPIRATION, GASTRIC CONTENTS

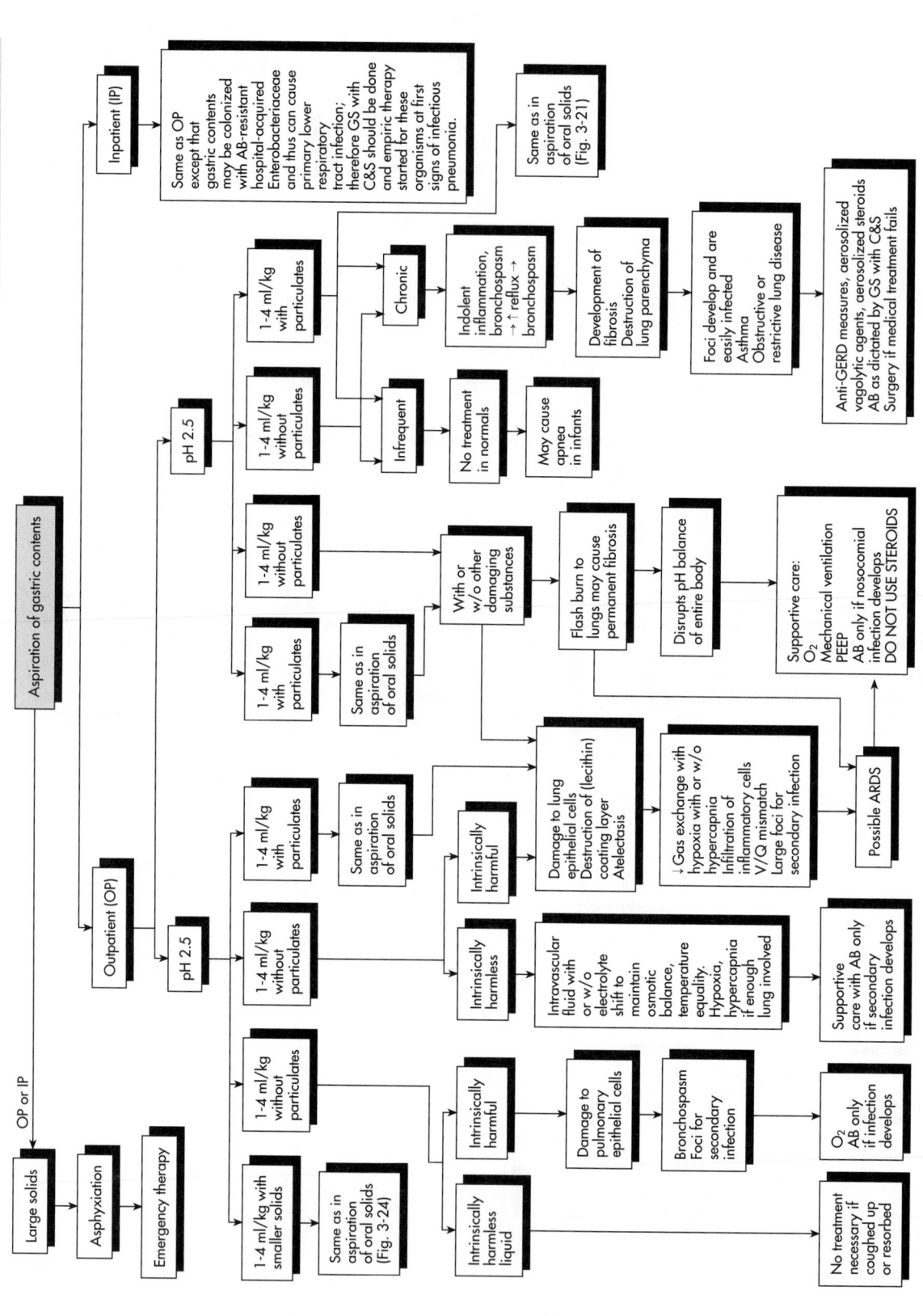

Fig. 3-20   Management of aspiration of gastric contents. *AB,* Antibiotics; *C&S,* culture and sensitivity; *GERD,* gastroesophageal reflux disease; *GS,* Gram's stain; *PEEP,* positive end-expiratory pressure; *V/Q,* ventilation-perfusion. (From Kassirer J [ed]: *Current therapy in adult medicine,* ed 4, St Louis, 1998, Mosby.)

ASPIRATION, ORAL CONTENTS

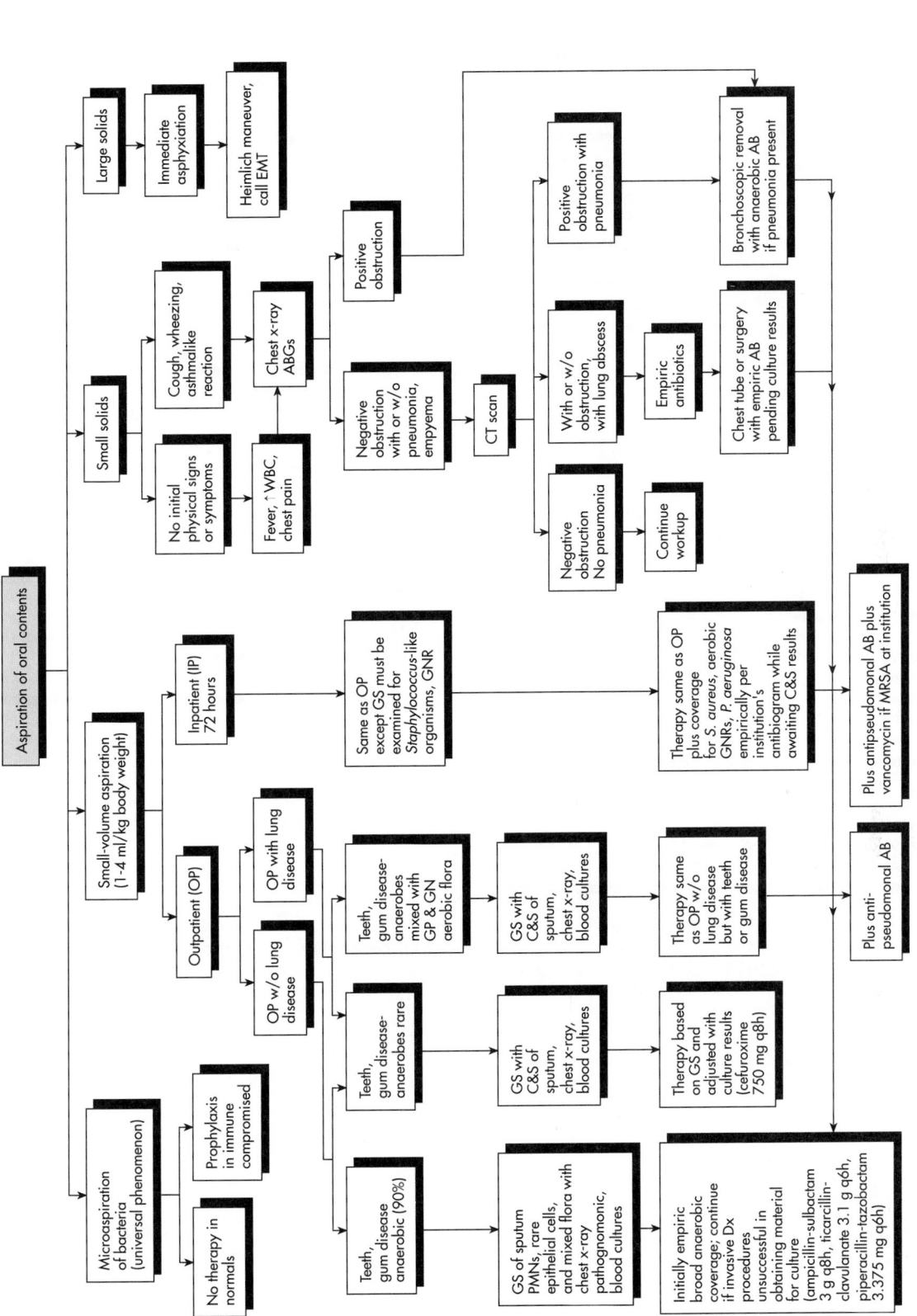

Fig. 3-21 Management of aspiration of oral contents. *AB,* Antibiotics; *ABG,* arterial blood gases; *C&S,* culture and sensitivity; *CT,* computed tomography; *Dx,* diagnostic; *EMT,* emergency medical technician; *GN,* gram-negative; *GNRs,* gram-negative rods; *GP,* gram-positive; *GS,* Gram stain; *MRSA,* methicillin-resistant *Staphylococcus aureus; PMNs,* polymorphonuclear leukocytes; *WBC,* white blood cells. (From Kassirer J [ed]: *Current therapy in adult medicine,* ed 4, St Louis, 1998, Mosby.)

ASYSTOLE

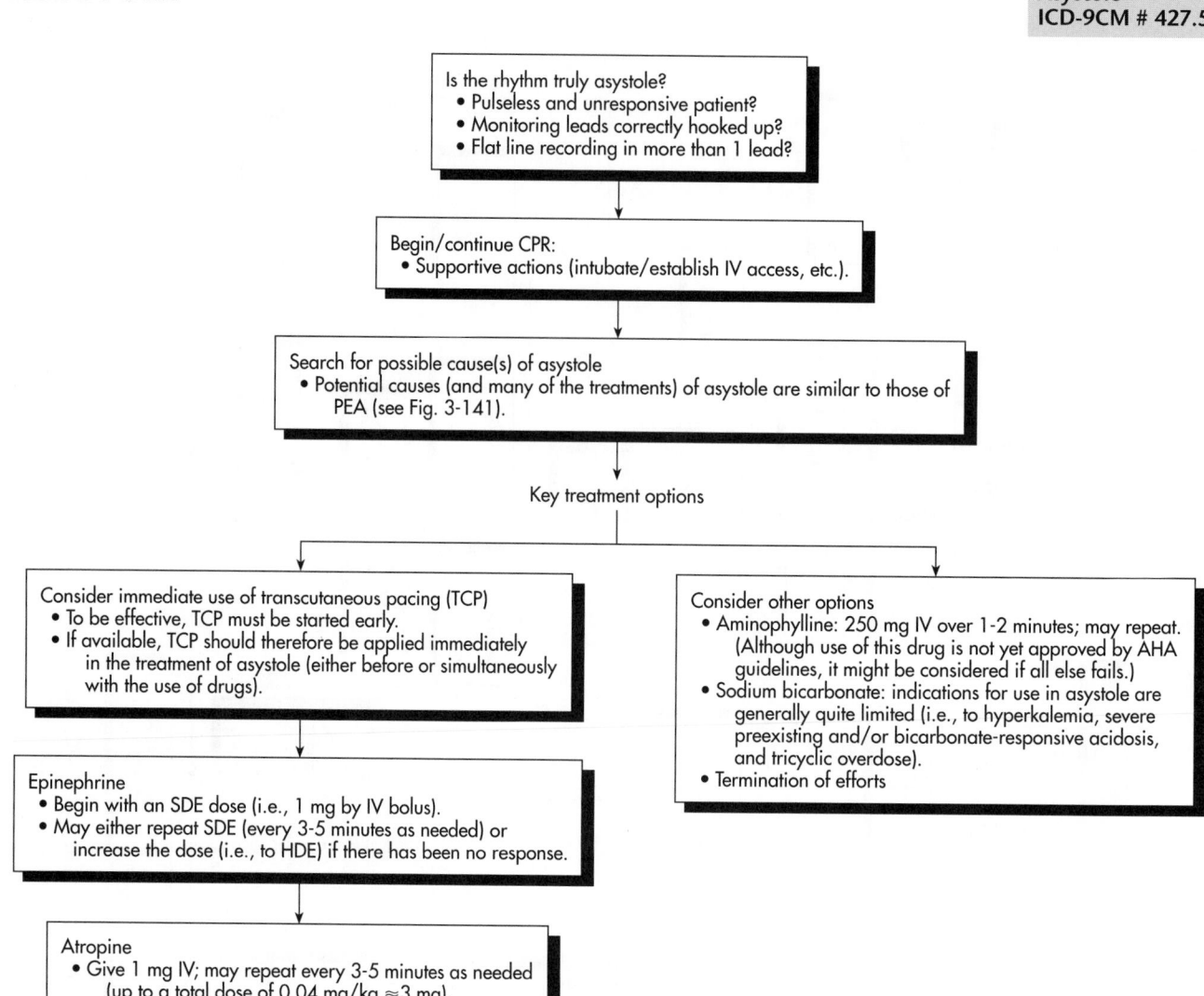

Is the rhythm truly asystole?
- Pulseless and unresponsive patient?
- Monitoring leads correctly hooked up?
- Flat line recording in more than 1 lead?

Begin/continue CPR:
- Supportive actions (intubate/establish IV access, etc.).

Search for possible cause(s) of asystole
- Potential causes (and many of the treatments) of asystole are similar to those of PEA (see Fig. 3-141).

Key treatment options

Consider immediate use of transcutaneous pacing (TCP)
- To be effective, TCP must be started early.
- If available, TCP should therefore be applied immediately in the treatment of asystole (either before or simultaneously with the use of drugs).

Epinephrine
- Begin with an SDE dose (i.e., 1 mg by IV bolus).
- May either repeat SDE (every 3-5 minutes as needed) or increase the dose (i.e., to HDE) if there has been no response.

Atropine
- Give 1 mg IV; may repeat every 3-5 minutes as needed (up to a total dose of 0.04 mg/kg ≈3 mg).

Consider other options
- Aminophylline: 250 mg IV over 1-2 minutes; may repeat. (Although use of this drug is not yet approved by AHA guidelines, it might be considered if all else fails.)
- Sodium bicarbonate: indications for use in asystole are generally quite limited (i.e., to hyperkalemia, severe preexisting and/or bicarbonate-responsive acidosis, and tricyclic overdose).
- Termination of efforts

Fig. 3-22   Asystole. *AHA,* American Heart Association; *CPR,* cardiopulmonary resuscitation; *HDE,* high-dose epinephrine; *IV,* intravenous; *PEA,* pulseless electrical activity; *SDE,* standard-dose epinephrine. (Modified from Grauer K, Cavallaro D: *ACLS: Rapid review and case scenarios,* ed 4, St Louis, 1996, Mosby.)

BACK PAIN

Back pain
ICD-9CM # 724.5 Back pain, postural
            307.89 Back pain, psychogenic
            847.9 Back strain
            959.1 Back injury

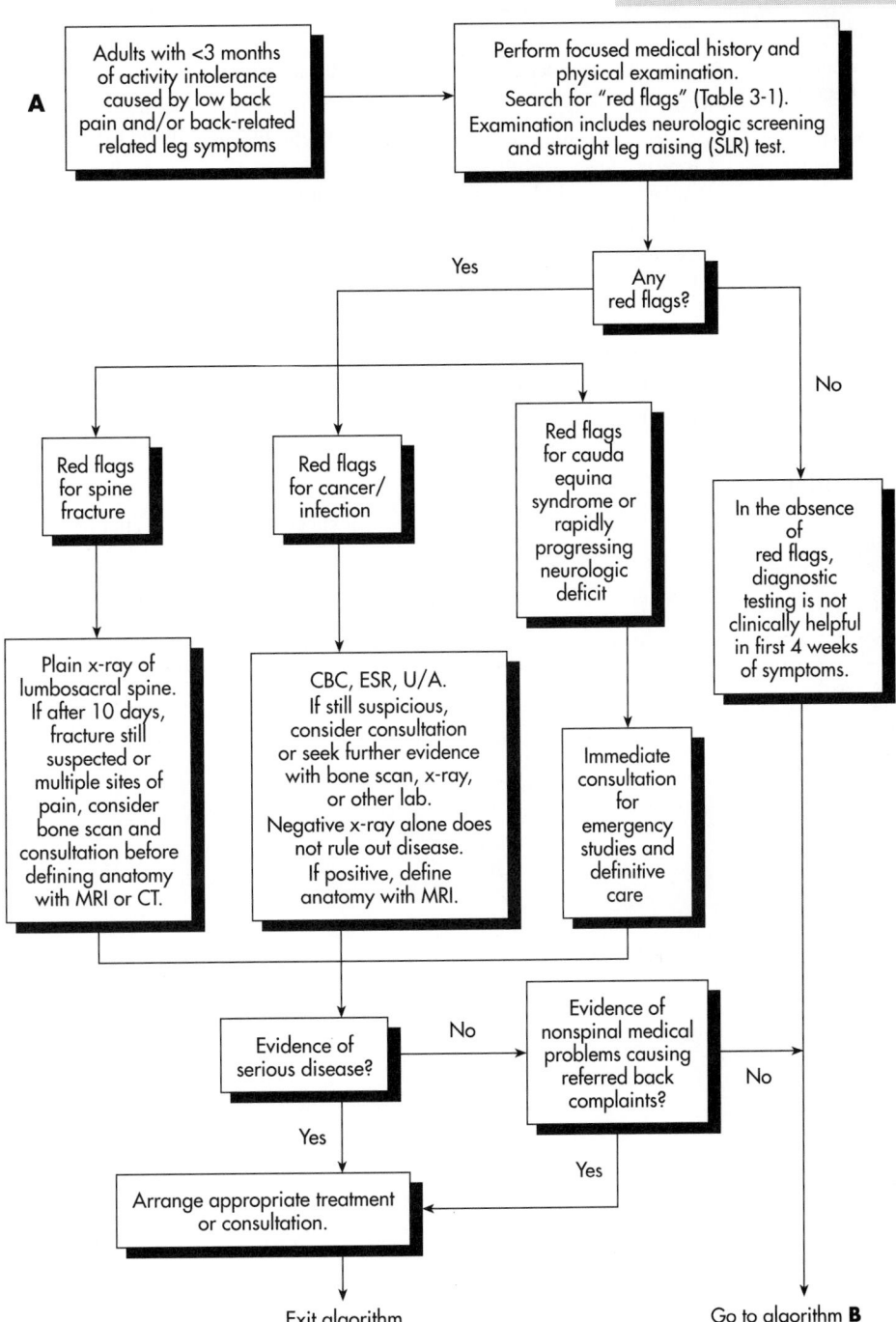

Fig. 3-23 Low back pain. A, Initial evaluation of acute low back problem. *CBC,* Complete blood count; *CT,* computed tomography; *ESR,* erythrocyte sedimentation rate; *MRI,* magnetic resonance imaging; *U/A,* urinalysis. (From Bigos S et al: *Acute low back problems in adults,* Clinical Practice Guideline, Quick Reference Guide Number 14, Rockville, Md, US Department of Health and Human Services, Public Health Service, Agency for Health Care Policy and Research, AHCPR Pub No 95-0643, Dec 1994.)

BACK PAIN—cont'd

TABLE 3-1 Red Flags for Potentially Serious Conditions

POSSIBLE FRACTURE	POSSIBLE TUMOR OR INFECTION	POSSIBLE CAUDA EQUINA SYNDROME
From Medical History		
Major trauma, such as vehicle accident or fall from height	Age over 50 or under 20 yr	Saddle anesthesia
	History of cancer	Recent onset of bladder dysfunction, such as urinary retention, increased frequency, or overflow incontinence
Minor trauma or even strenuous lifting (in older or potentially osteoporotic patient)	Constitutional symptoms, such as recent fever or chills or unexplained weight loss	Severe or progressive neurologic deficit in the lower extremity
	Risk factors for spinal infection: recent bacterial infection (e.g., urinary tract infection); intravenous drug abuse; or immune suppression (from steroids, transplant, or human immunodeficiency virus)	
	Pain that worsens when supine; severe nighttime pain	
From Physical Examination		
		Unexpected laxity of the anal sphincter
		Perianal/perineal sensory loss
		Major motor weakness: quadriceps (knee extension weakness); ankle plantar flexors, evertors, and dorsiflexors (foot drop)

BACK PAIN—cont'd

B Initial visit

Adults with low back problem and no underlying serious condition (see algorithm **A**) → Provide assurance; education about back problems.

↓

Does patient require help relieving symptoms? — Yes → Recommend/prescribe comfort options based on risk/benefits and patient preference (Table 3-2).

No ↓

Recommend activity alterations to avoid back irritation.
Review activity limitations (if any) caused by back problem; encourage to continue or return to normal activities (including work, with or without restrictions) as soon as possible.
Encourage low-stress aerobic exercise.

↓

Symptoms improving? — Yes → Return to normal activities

No ↓

Follow-up visits

Change in symptoms? — Yes → Review history and physical findings.

No ↓

Provide assurance that recovery is expected.
Recommend activities to avoid debilitation and reduce risk of recurrence.
Support return to work or required daily activities.
Can begin muscle conditioning exercises after a few weeks.

No ← Any red flags?

↓

Has reasonable activity tolerance returned within 4 weeks?

Yes → Symptom recurrence? — Yes →

No ↓   No ↓   Yes ↓

Go to algorithm **C**   Return to normal activities   Return to algorithm **A**

Fig. 3-23, cont'd   B, Treatment of acute low back problem on initial and follow-up visits.

III

BACK PAIN—cont'd

TABLE 3-2 Symptom Control Methods

RECOMMENDED		

Nonprescription Analgesics

Acetaminophen (safest)

NSAIDs (aspirin,* ibuprofen*), COX-2 inhibitors

Prescribed Pharmaceutical Methods	Prescribed Physical Methods	
Nonspecific Low Back Symptoms and/or Sciatica	*Nonspecific Low Back Symptoms*	*Sciatica*
Other NSAIDs*	Manipulation (in place of medication or a shorter trial if combined with NSAIDs)	

	Options	
Nonspecific Low Back Symptoms and/or Sciatica	*Nonspecific Low Back Symptoms*	*Sciatica*
Muscle relaxants†,‡,§	Physical agents and modalities† (heat or cold modalities for home programs only)	Manipulation (in place of medication or a shorter trial if combined with NSAIDs)
Opioids	Shoe insoles†	Physical agents and modalities† (heat or cold modalities for home programs only)
		Few days' rest§
		Shoe insoles†

NSAID, Nonsteroidal antiinflammatory drug.
*Aspirin and other NSAIDs are not recommended for use in combination with one another because of the risk of gastrointestinal complications.
†Equivocal efficacy.
‡Significant potential for producing drowsiness and debilitation; potential for dependency.
§Short course (few days only) for severe symptoms.

BACK PAIN—cont'd

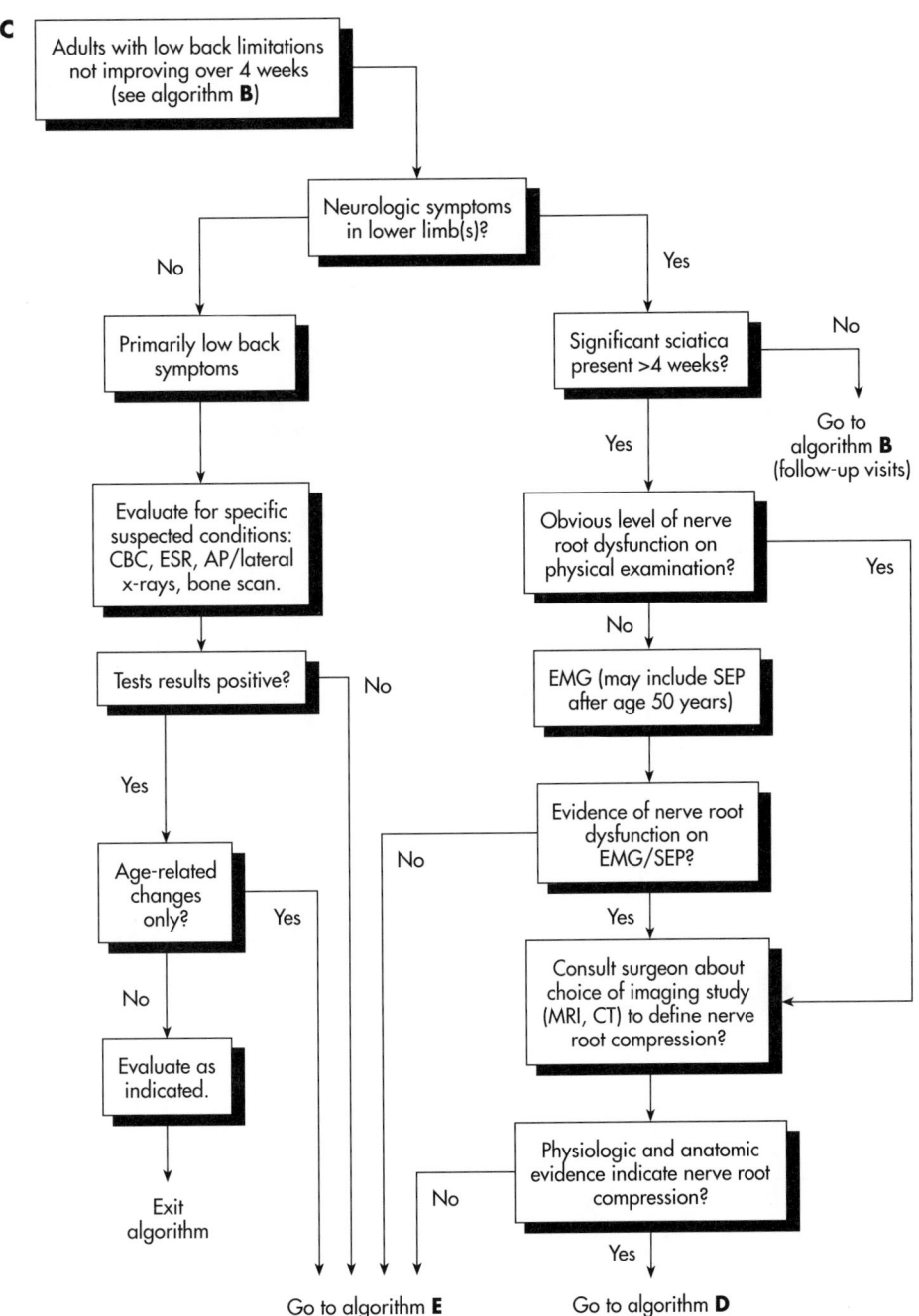

Fig. 3-23, cont'd **C, Evaluation of the slow-to-recover patient (symptoms >4 weeks).**
AP, Anteroposterior; *CBC,* complete blood count; *CT,* computed tomography; *EMG,* electromyography; *ESR,* erythrocyte sedimentation rate; *MRI,* magnetic resonance imaging; *SEP,* somatosensory evoked potential.

BACK PAIN—cont'd

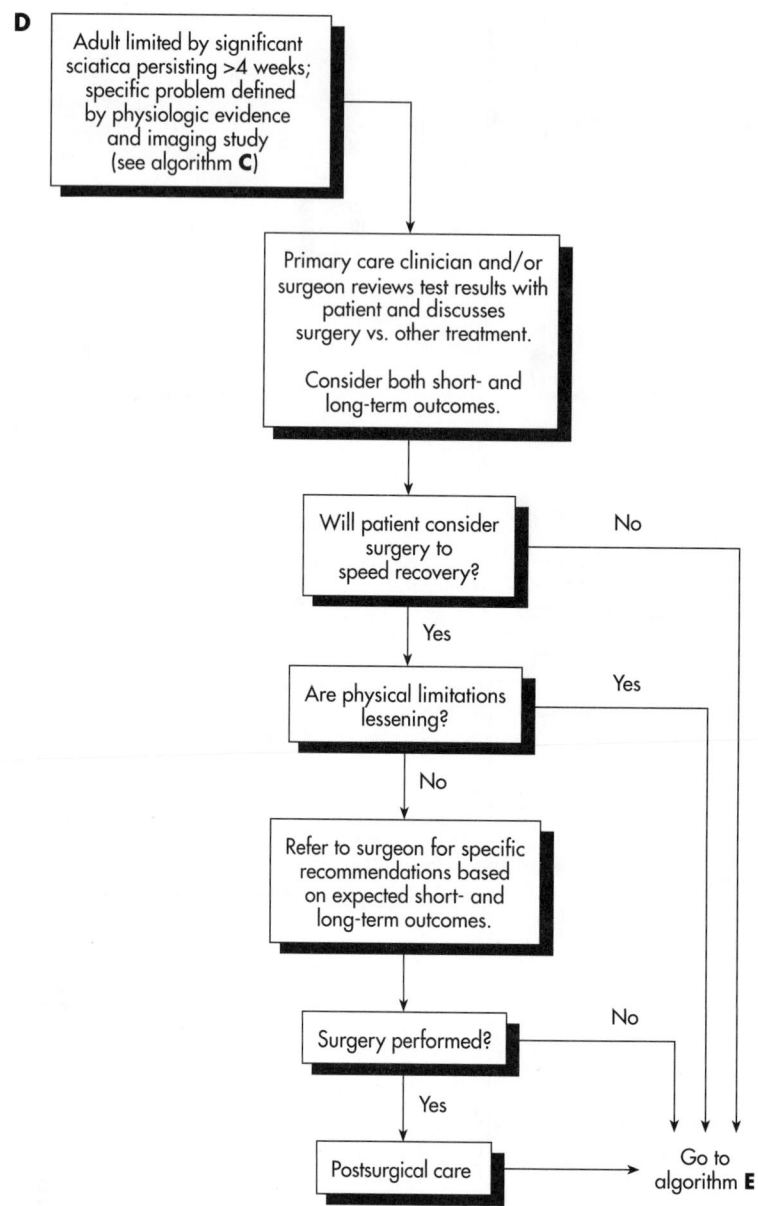

D

Adult limited by significant sciatica persisting >4 weeks; specific problem defined by physiologic evidence and imaging study (see algorithm **C**)

Primary care clinician and/or surgeon reviews test results with patient and discusses surgery vs. other treatment.

Consider both short- and long-term outcomes.

Will patient consider surgery to speed recovery?   No

Yes

Are physical limitations lessening?   Yes

No

Refer to surgeon for specific recommendations based on expected short- and long-term outcomes.

Surgery performed?   No

Yes

Postsurgical care → Go to algorithm **E**

Fig. 3-23, cont'd   D, Surgical considerations for patients with persistent sciatica.

BACK PAIN—cont'd

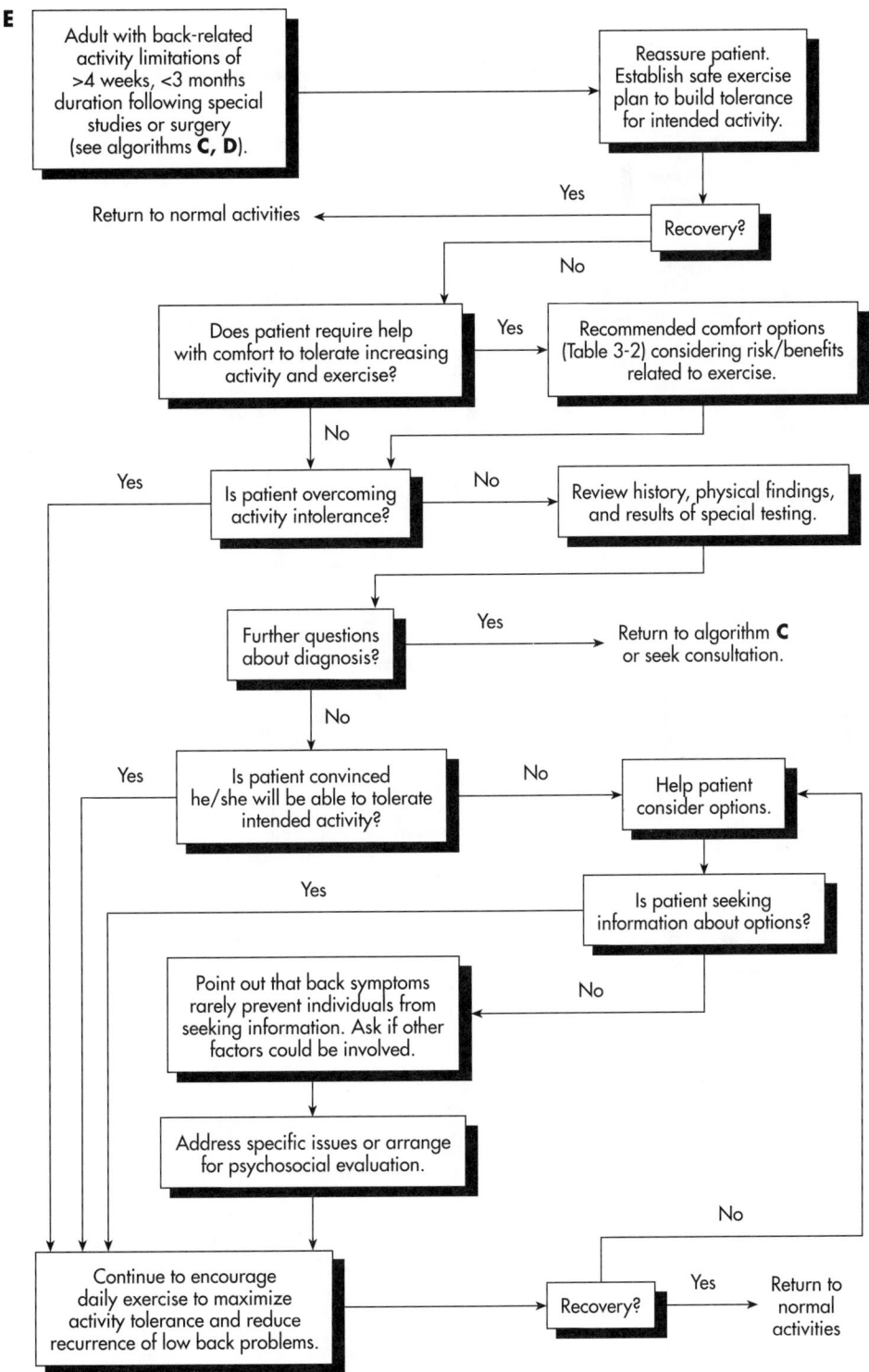

E

Adult with back-related activity limitations of >4 weeks, <3 months duration following special studies or surgery (see algorithms **C, D**).

Reassure patient. Establish safe exercise plan to build tolerance for intended activity.

Recovery?

Yes → Return to normal activities

No

Does patient require help with comfort to tolerate increasing activity and exercise?

Yes → Recommended comfort options (Table 3-2) considering risk/benefits related to exercise.

No

Is patient overcoming activity intolerance?

Yes

No → Review history, physical findings, and results of special testing.

Further questions about diagnosis?

Yes → Return to algorithm **C** or seek consultation.

No

Is patient convinced he/she will be able to tolerate intended activity?

Yes

No → Help patient consider options.

Is patient seeking information about options?

Yes

No → Point out that back symptoms rarely prevent individuals from seeking information. Ask if other factors could be involved.

Address specific issues or arrange for psychosocial evaluation.

Continue to encourage daily exercise to maximize activity tolerance and reduce recurrence of low back problems.

Recovery?

Yes → Return to normal activities

No

Fig. 3-23, cont'd   E, Further management of acute low back problem.

III

BLEEDING, EARLY PREGNANCY

Bleeding, early pregnancy
ICD-9CM # 641.9 Vaginal bleeding NOS in pregnancy

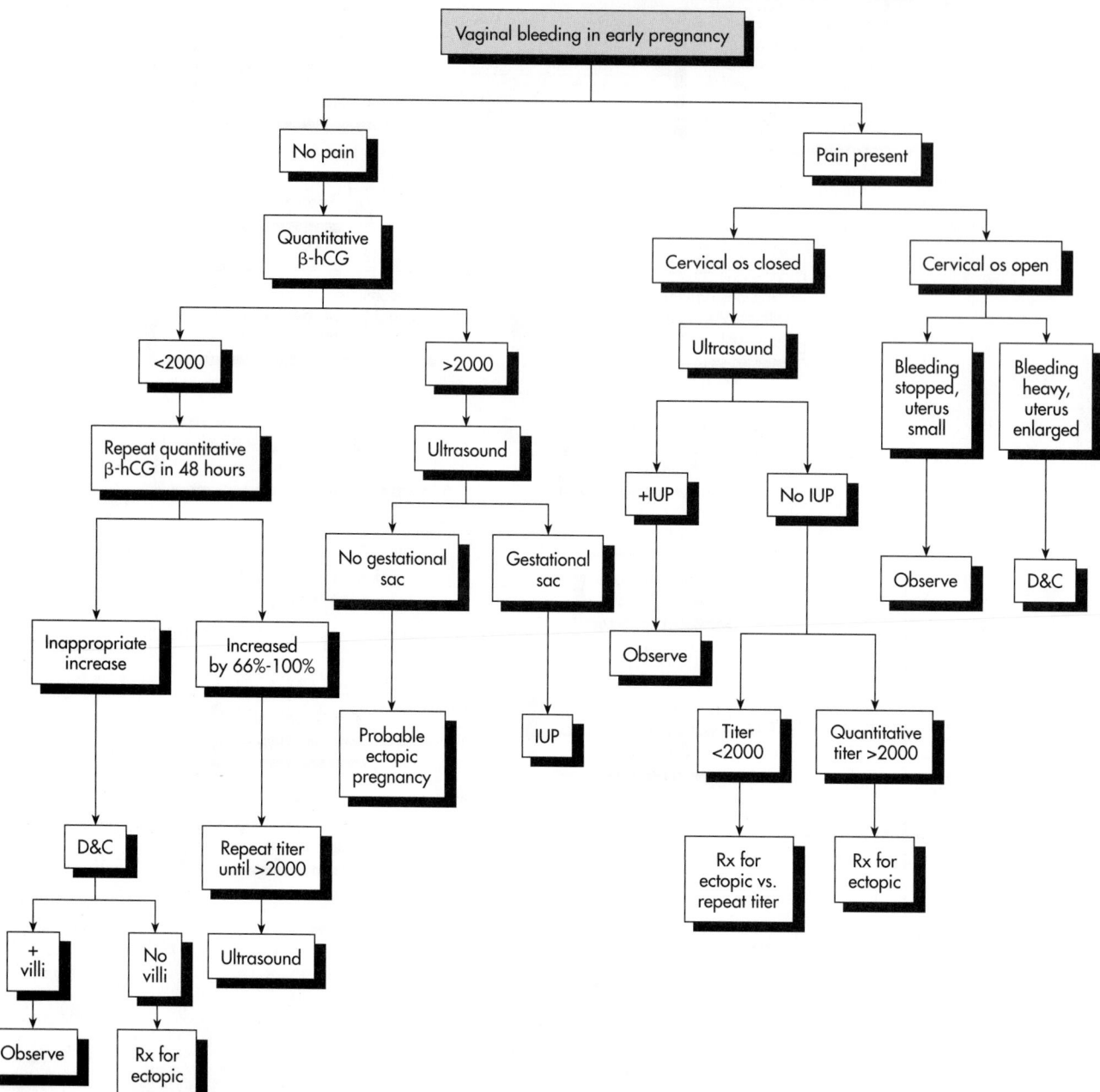

Fig. 3-24   Diagnosis of vaginal bleeding in early pregnancy. *D&C,* Dilation and curettage; *β-hCG,* β-human chorionic gonadotropin; *IUP,* intrauterine pregnancy. (From Carlson KJ et al: *Primary care of women,* St Louis, 1995, Mosby.)

BLEEDING, GASTROINTESTINAL

Bleeding, gastrointestinal
ICD-9CM # 578.9 GI bleeding, cause unspecified

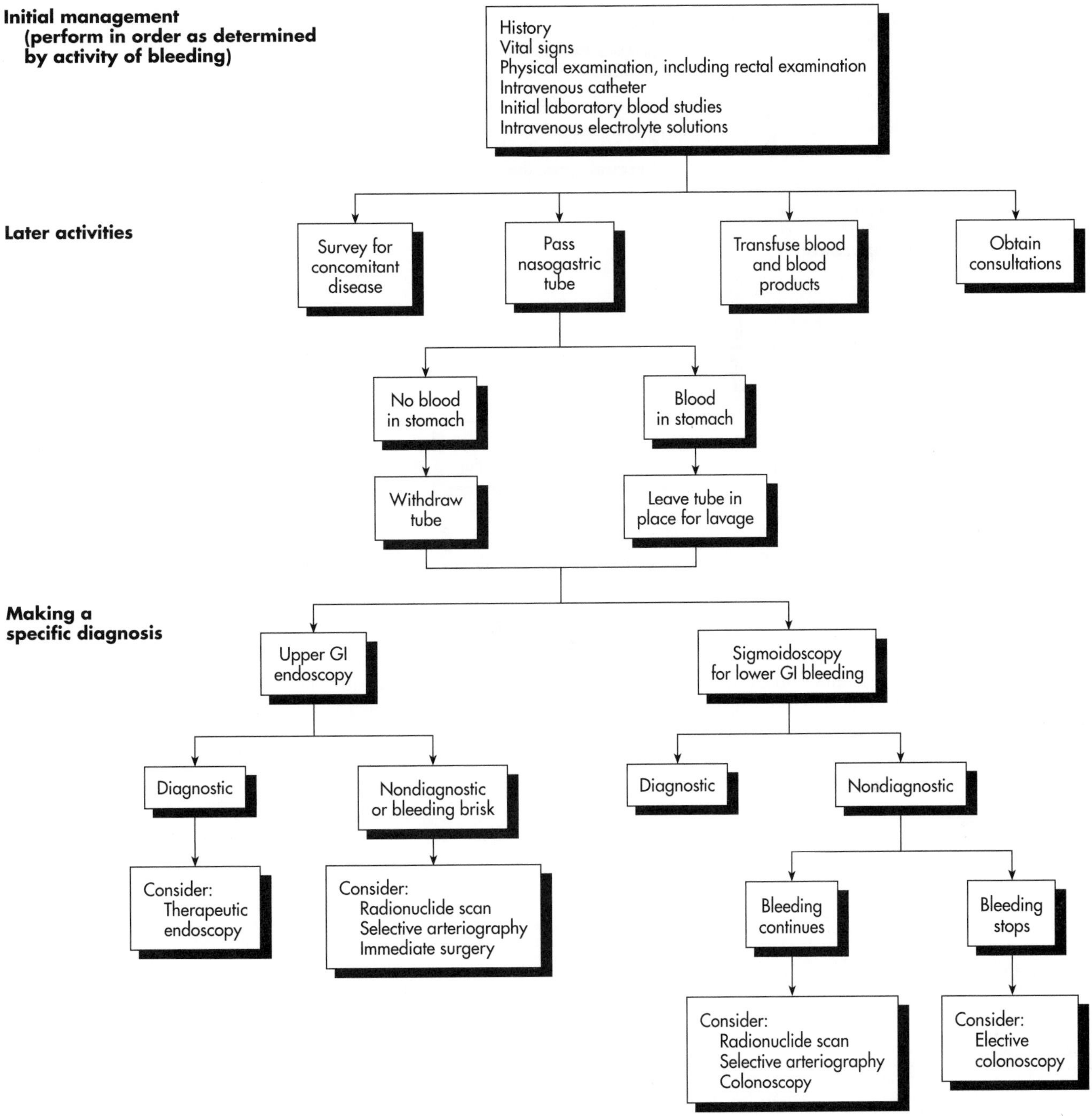

Initial management
(perform in order as determined
by activity of bleeding)

History
Vital signs
Physical examination, including rectal examination
Intravenous catheter
Initial laboratory blood studies
Intravenous electrolyte solutions

Later activities

Survey for concomitant disease

Pass nasogastric tube

Transfuse blood and blood products

Obtain consultations

No blood in stomach

Blood in stomach

Withdraw tube

Leave tube in place for lavage

Making a
specific diagnosis

Upper GI endoscopy

Sigmoidoscopy for lower GI bleeding

Diagnostic

Nondiagnostic or bleeding brisk

Diagnostic

Nondiagnostic

Consider:
Therapeutic endoscopy

Consider:
Radionuclide scan
Selective arteriography
Immediate surgery

Bleeding continues

Bleeding stops

Consider:
Radionuclide scan
Selective arteriography
Colonoscopy

Consider:
Elective colonoscopy

III

Fig. 3-25 **Management of acute gastrointestinal bleeding.** *GI,* Gastrointestinal. (From Stein JH [ed]: *Internal medicine,* ed 5, St Louis, 1998, Mosby.)

BLEEDING, VAGINAL

Bleeding, vaginal
ICD-9CM # 623.8 Vaginal bleeding NOS

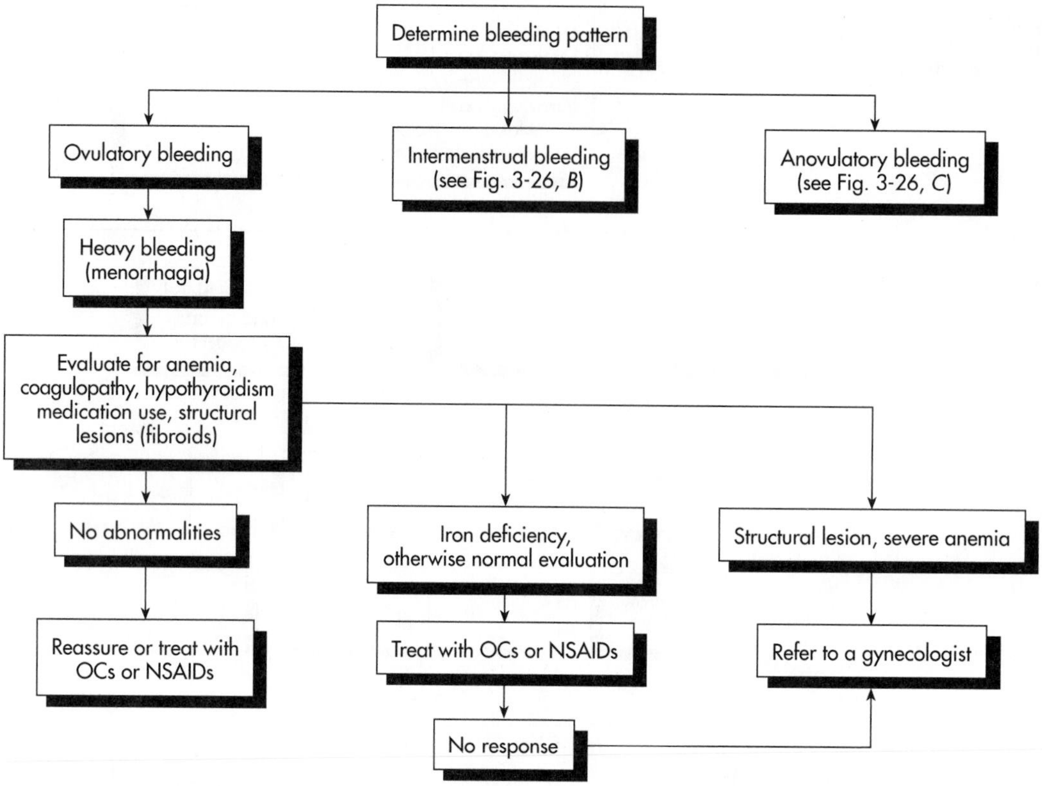

Fig. 3-26 A, Evaluation of ovulatory bleeding. *NSAIDs,* Nonsteroidal antiinflammatory drugs; *OCs,* oral contraceptives. (From Appleby J, Henderson M, Wathen PI: *Intern Med* Sept:17, 1996.)

BLEEDING, VAGINAL—cont'd

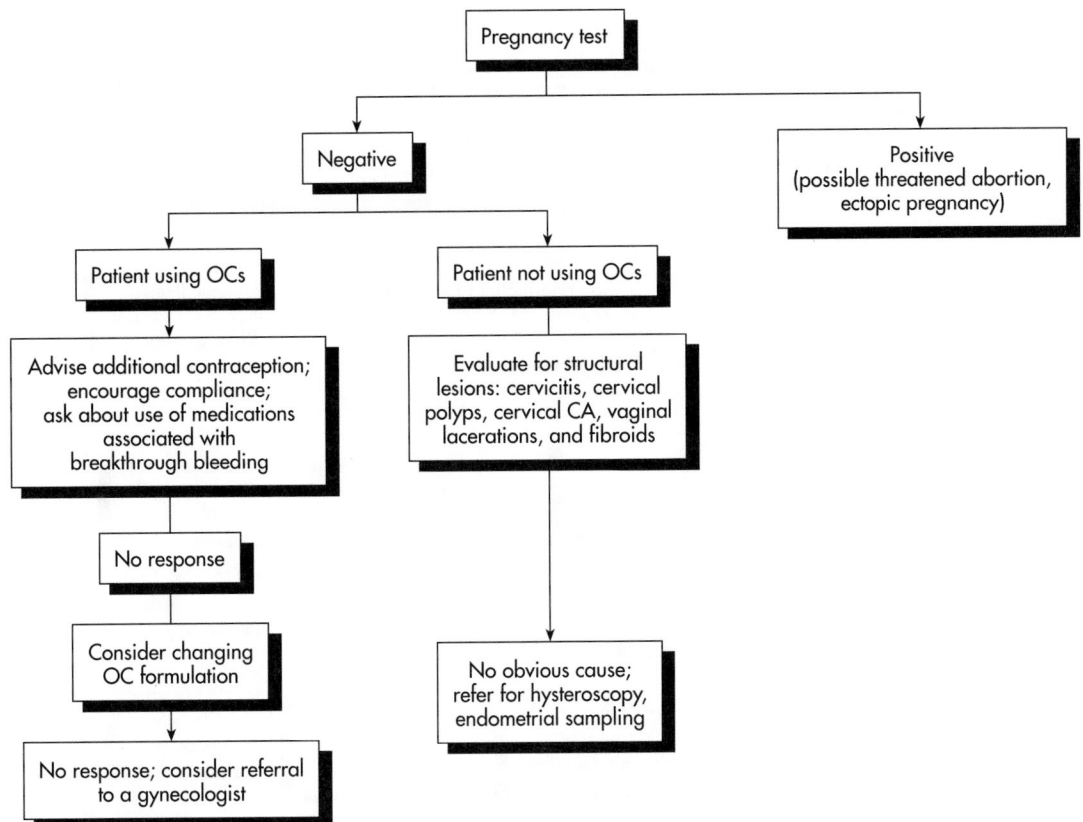

Fig. 3-26, cont'd   B, Evaluation of intermenstrual bleeding. *CA,* Cancer; *OCs,* oral contraceptives.
(From Appleby J, Henderson M, Wathen PI: *Intern Med* Sept:17, 1996.)

III

BLEEDING, VAGINAL—cont'd

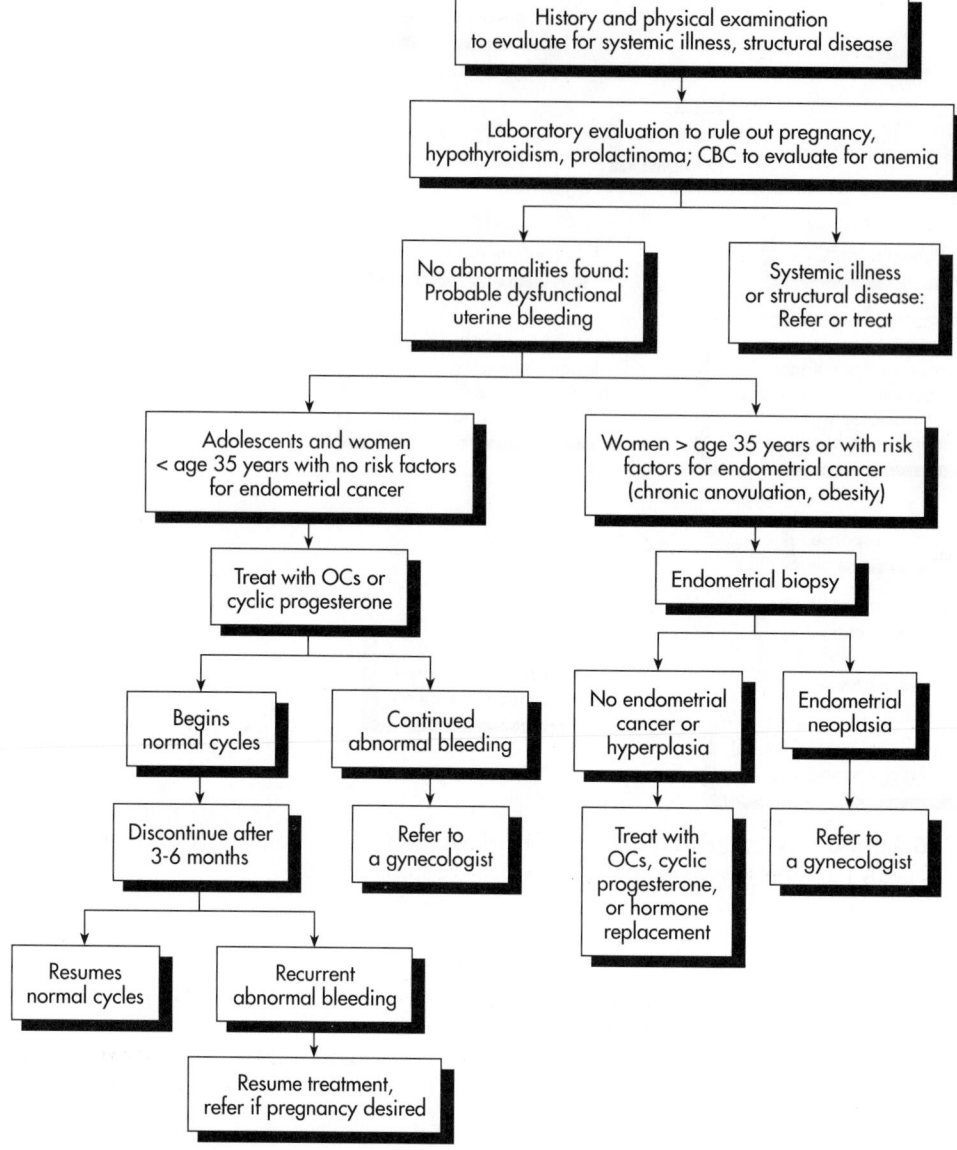

Fig. 3-26, cont'd   C, Evaluation of anovulatory bleeding. *CBC,* Complete blood count; *OCs,* oral contraceptives. (From Appleby J, Henderson M, Wathen Pl: *Intern Med* Sept:17, 1996.)

BLEEDING, VARICEAL

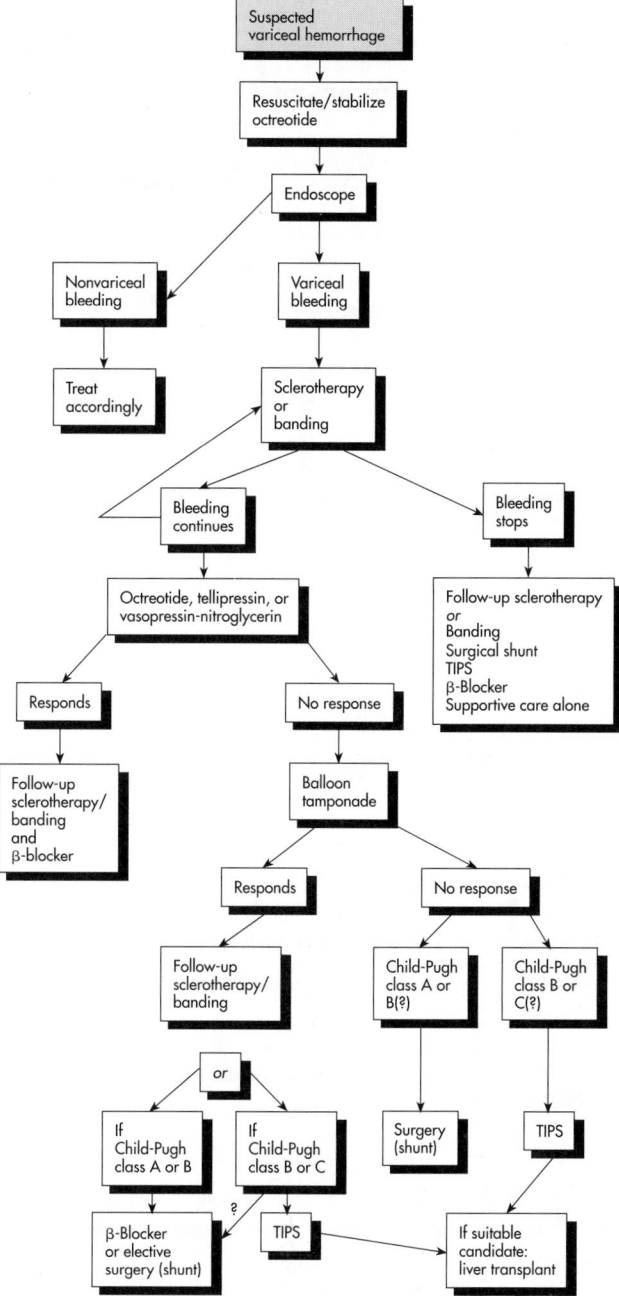

Fig. 3-27   Management of bleeding varices. Practice may vary according to local resources, personnel, expertise, and preference. Where hepatic transplant is available, candidates may undergo placement of transjugular intrahepatic portosystemic shunt (TIPS) sooner, especially if sclerotherapy or banding for esophageal varices fails (gastric varices are generally not readily amenable to these procedures). Those who are not transplant candidates may benefit from portacaval shunt (side-to-side if ascites is present) to stop active bleeding or from distal splenorenal shunt if the patient is not actively bleeding and without ascites. (From Stein J [ed]: *Internal medicine,* ed 5, St Louis, 1998, Mosby.)

TABLE 3-3   Child-Pugh classes

PROGNOSTIC VARIABLES	CHILD-PUGH SCORE* POINTS		
	1	2	3
Bilirubin (mg/dl)	>1.1-2.0	>2.0-3.0	>3.0
Albumin (g/dl)		2.8-3.5	<2.8
Prothrombin time (seconds above control)	1-3	4-6	>6
Encephalopathy		Grade 1-2	Grade 3-4
Ascites		Mild	Moderate
Age (years)			
Edema (± diuretics)			
Splenomegaly			
Histologic stage			

From Stein J (ed): *Internal medicine,* ed 5, St Louis, 1998, Mosby.
*Child-Pugh classes: A, score 1-6; B, score 7-9; C, score 10-15.

III

BLEEDING DISORDER, CONGENITAL

Bleeding disorder, congenital
ICD-9CM # 286.9

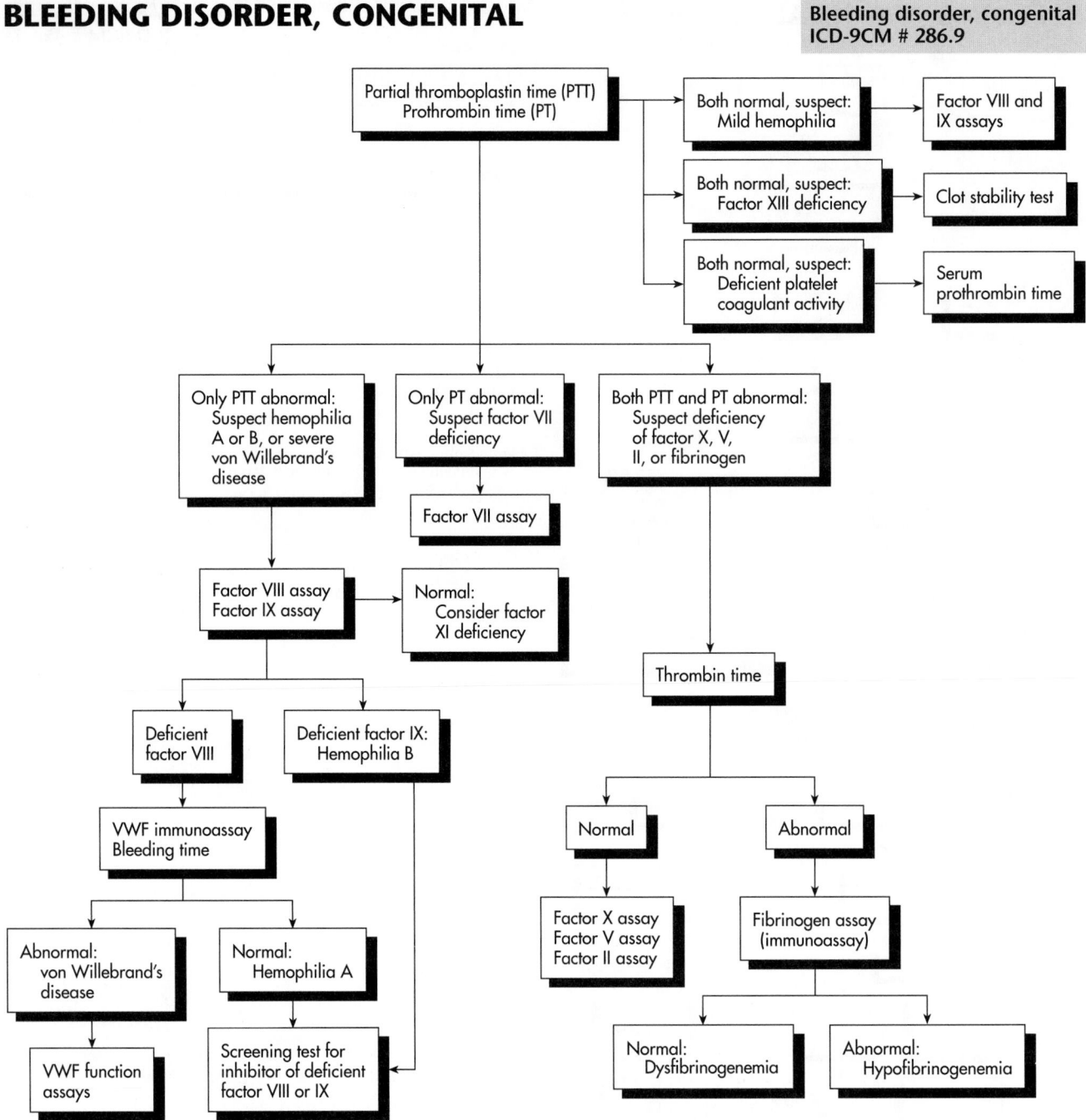

Fig. 3-28   Laboratory evaluation of a patient with a bleeding disorder in whom the history and physical examination suggest a congenital coagulation disorder. *VWF,* von Willebrand factor. (From Stein JH [ed]: *Internal medicine,* ed 5, St Louis, 1998, Mosby.)

BLEEDING TIME, PROLONGED

ICD-9CM 790.92 Bleeding time, abnormal finding
        286.9   Bleeding time prolonged
                coagulation defect

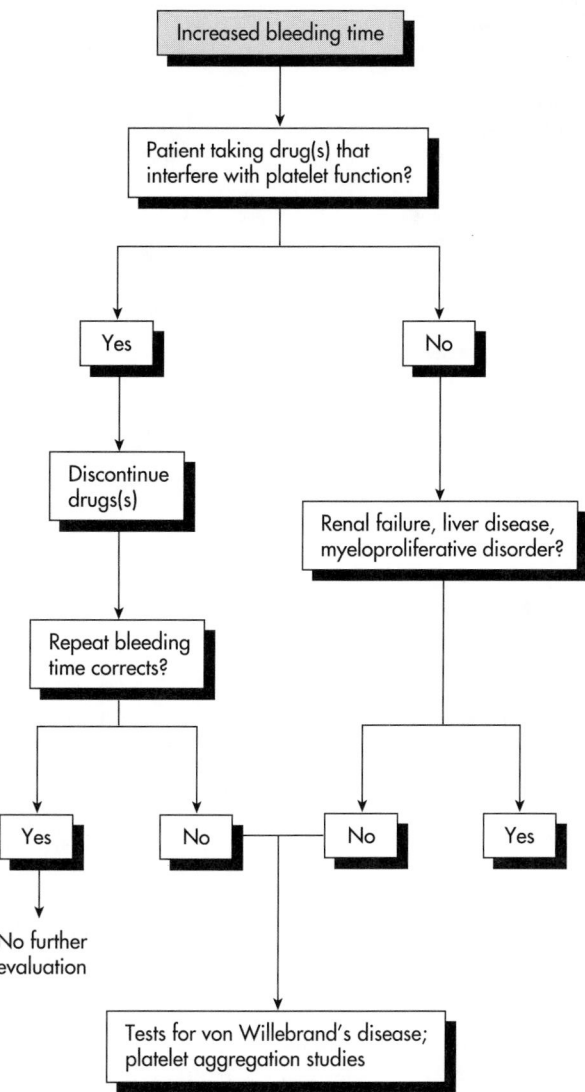

Fig. 3-29   An algorithm for diagnostic decisions in evaluating patients with a prolonged bleed-ing time. The scheme assumes that the platelet count is normal, because thrombocytopenia itself can prolong the bleeding time. (From Goldman L, Bennett JC [eds]: *Cecil textbook of medicine,* ed 21, Philadelphia, 2000, WB Saunders.)

BONE METASTASES

Bone metastases
ICD-9CM # 198.5

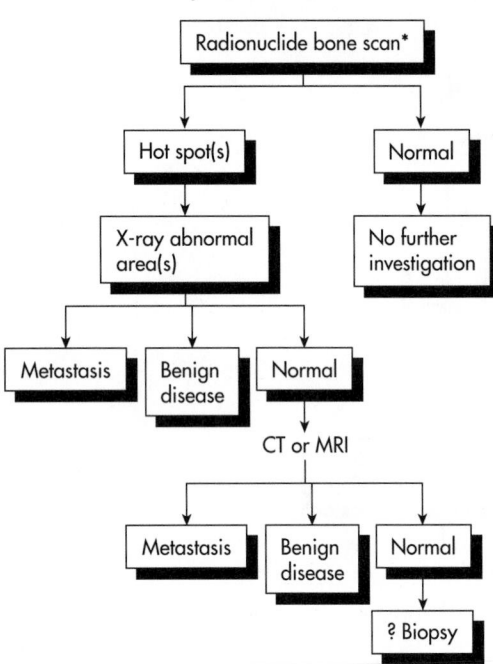

Schema for the
investigation of a patient with
possible bone metastases

*Patients with multiple myeloma are best
investigated by performing a skeletal survey.

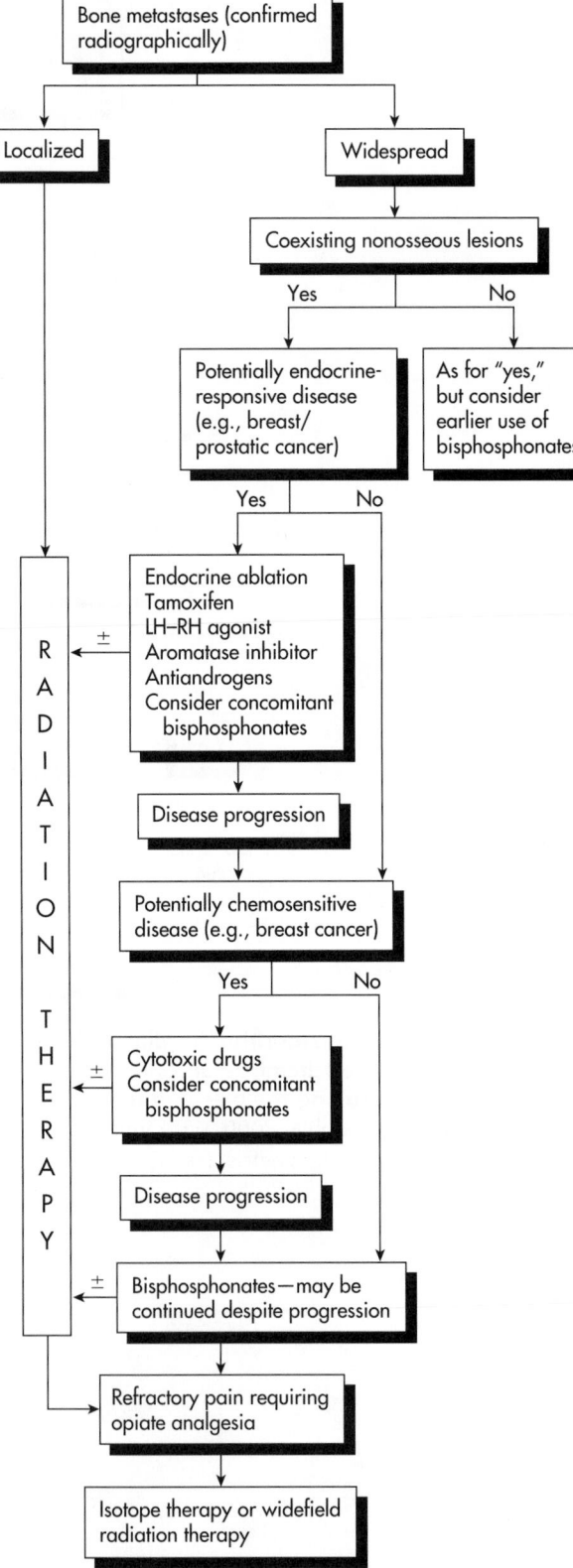

Treatment of bone metastases

Fig. 3-30   Bone metastases. (From Abeloff MD: *Clinical oncology*, ed 2, New York, 2000, Churchill Livingstone.)

ICD-9CM # 427.89 Unspecified bradycardia
427.81 Chronic bradycardia
770.8 Newborn bradycardia
427.89 Postoperative bradycardia
337   Reflex bradycardia
427.89 Sinus bradycardia

BRADYCARDIA

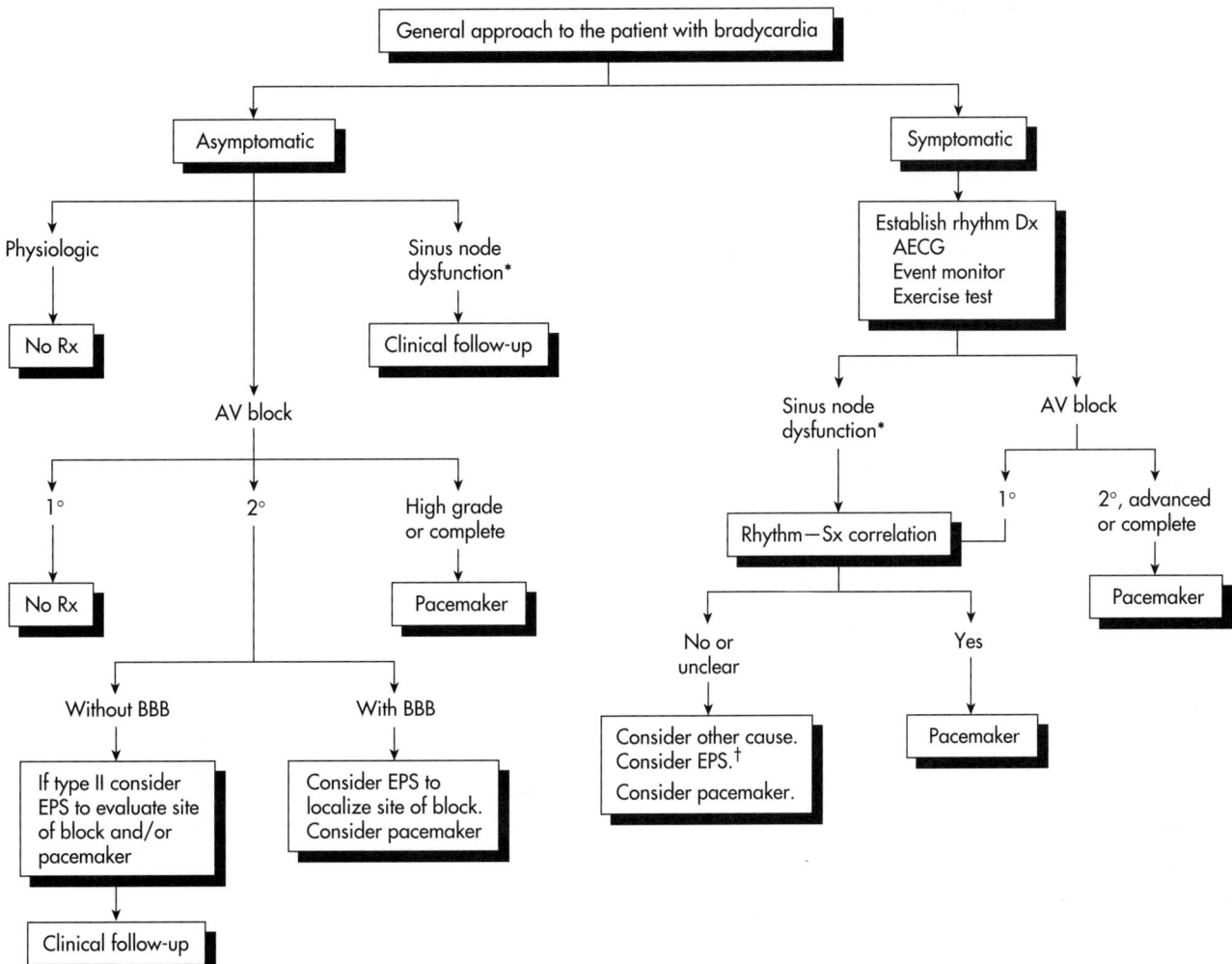

*Includes bradycardia-tachycardia syndrome.
†EPS includes sinus node function and ventricular arrhythmia induction studies.

Fig. 3-31   General approach to the patient with bradycardia. *AECG,* Ambulatory electrocardi-ography; *AV,* atrioventricular: *BBB,* bundle branch block; *Dx,* diagnostic; *EPS,* electrophysiologic study; *Rx,* treatment; *Sx,* symptoms; 1°, first-degree; 2°, second-degree. (From Goldman L, Braunwald E [eds]: *Primary cardiology,* Philadelphia, 1998, WB Saunders.)

III

BREAST, NIPPLE DISCHARGE EVALUATION*

Breast, nipple discharge evaluation
ICD-9CM # 611.79

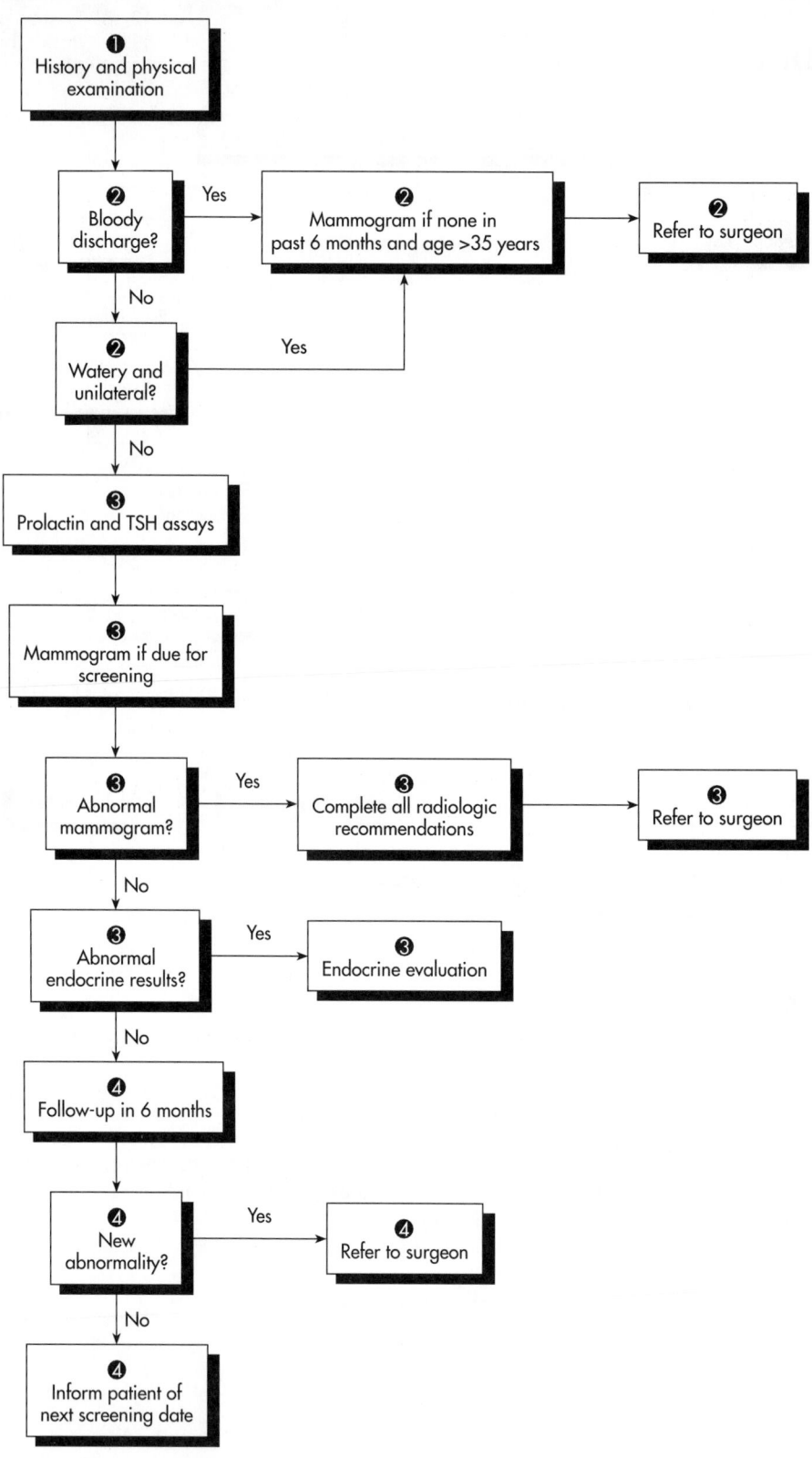

*Without palpable mass.

Fig. 3-32   Breast cancer screening and evaluation. (From Institute for Clinical Systems Integration, Minneapolis: *Postgrad Med* 100:182, 1996.)

1. **History and physical examination.*** Patients who present with a complaint of nipple discharge should be evaluated with breast-related history taking and a physical examination. History taking is aimed at uncovering and characterizing any other breast-related symptom. A risk assessment should also be undertaken for identified risk factors, including patient age over 50 years, any past personal history of breast cancer, history of hyperplasia on previous breast biopsies, and family history of breast cancer in first-degree relatives (mother, sister, daughter). Physical examination should include inspection of the breast for any evidence of ulceration or contour changes and inspection of the nipple for Paget's disease. Palpation should be performed with the patient in both the upright and the supine positions to determine the presence of any palpable mass.

2. **Bloody discharge?** If the discharge appears frankly bloody, the patient should be referred to a surgeon for evaluation. At the time of referral, a mammogram of the involved breast should be obtained if the patient is over 35 years of age and has not had a mammogram within the preceding 6 months. Similarly, patients with a watery, unilateral discharge should be referred to a surgeon for evaluation and possible biopsy.

3. **Endocrine tests. Mammogram.** If the discharge appears frankly milky or is bilateral, serum prolactin and serum thyroid-stimulating hormone (TSH) assays should be performed to rule out the presence of an endocrinologic basis for the symptoms. At the time of that visit, a mammogram should also be performed if the patient is due for routine mammographic screening according to the recommended intervals. A patient with an abnormal mammogram should be further evaluated radiologically to better characterize the lesion and then be referred to a surgeon if appropriate. Make certain that all recommended additional views, ultrasound examinations, and follow-up studies have been obtained before referral to a surgeon. Should the mammogram appear normal, results of the assays for TSH and prolactin should be reviewed. If the results are abnormal the patient should undergo appropriate evaluation for etiology, either by a primary care physician or by an endocrinologist.

4. **Six-month follow-up results.** If results of the mammogram and the endocrinologic screening studies are normal, the patient should return for a follow-up visit in 6 months to ensure that there has been no specific change in the character of the discharge, such as development of frank bleeding or Paget's disease, that would warrant surgical evaluation. If the evaluation at that follow-up visit fails to reveal any palpable or visible abnormalities, the patient should be returned to the routine screening process with studies performed at the recommended intervals.

III

---

*ICSI healthcare guidelines are designed to assist clinicians by providing an analytic framework for the evaluation and treatment of patients. They are not intended either to replace a clinician's judgment or to establish a protocol for all patients with a particular condition. A guideline will rarely establish the only approach to a problem. In addition, guidelines are "living documents" that are expected to be imperfect and are subject to annual review and revision.

ICSI is a nonprofit organization that provides healthcare quality improvement services to 20 medical groups affiliated with HealthPartners in central and southern Minnesota and western Wisconsin. The guidelines are developed through a process that involves physicians, nurses, and other healthcare professionals from beginning to end, and healthcare purchasers are included in decision making. To order any of the more than 40 guidelines ICSI has developed, contact the ICSI Publications Fulfillment Center, in care of the ARDEL Group, 6518 Walker St., Suite 150, Minneapolis, MN 55426; 612-927-6707.

BREAST, RADIOLOGIC EVALUATION

Breast, radiologic evaluation
ICD-9CM # V76.10

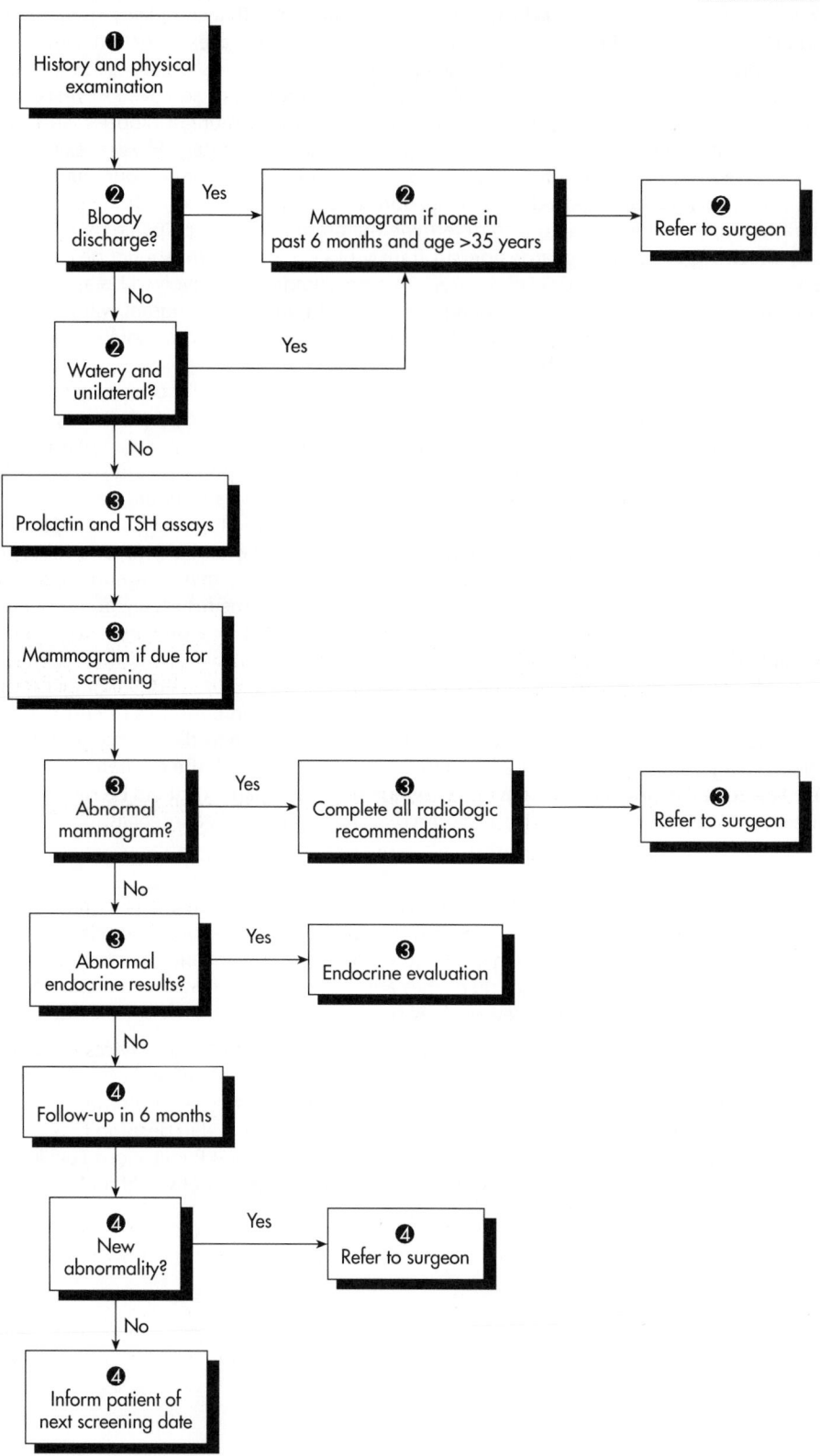

Fig. 3-33   Breast cancer screening and evaluation. (From Institute for Clinical Systems Integration, Minneapolis: *Postgrad Med* 100:182-187, 1996.)

Fig. 3-33, cont'd

1. **Screening mammogram.*** Patients are most commonly referred to a radiologist for screening mammography. Occasionally, however, patients are referred for diagnostic mammography based on symptoms or findings on breast exam. In the event of an abnormal finding on the mammogram, complete evaluation under the direction of a radiologist is recommended. It is the responsibility of the radiologist to complete the radiologic assessment so that the best possible characterization of the abnormality can be provided in an expeditious fashion to the primary care physician who ordered the original study. Any recommendations for referral to a surgeon for possible biopsy should be made directly to the primary care physician. The ultimate responsibility to make the referral will rest with the primary care physician.

2. **Abnormal mammogram. Sorting abnormalities. Suspicious for cancer?** On obtaining an abnormal finding on a mammogram, the radiologist determines whether further mammographic images are required for completion of the evaluation process. This may include a repeated image of the involved breast at 6 months to document stability of a low-risk, probably benign lesion. Alternatively, spot compression, magnification, or both may be necessary to obtain further characterization of indeterminate breast lesions. These additional studies should be done with the radiologist present to reduce the risk of patient recall for further studies necessary to evaluate the same lesion.

   On completion of these views, each and every abnormality uncovered for each independent lesion of the breast studied should be sorted according to the nature of the abnormality. The radiologist should classify the lesion as representing either suspicious microcalcifications, architectural distortion, or a soft-tissue mass. For any lesions identified as demonstrating microcalcifications that suggest cancer, biopsy will be recommended. It is up to the primary care physician to make the referral to a surgeon for biopsy. If a soft-tissue mass is identified on the mammogram, it should be studied further to determine its relative risk for malignancy. Any suspect lesions identified as having associated microcalcifications, architectural distortion, or interval growth when compared with the previous mammogram should likewise be referred to a surgeon for possible biopsy.

3. **Ultrasound results.** When the mass is not immediately suggestive of cancer, an ultrasound should be performed to determine whether the lesion is solid. A solid mass should be further characterized for its level of benignity according to three criteria:
   - Size less than 15 mm
   - Three or fewer lobulations
   - More than 50% of the margin of the lesion appearing well circumscribed in any view

   Patients who have lesions that fit all three criteria may be observed and then evaluated with a 6-month follow-up study. Any lesion that does not fit all three criteria for benignity should be characterized as indeterminate, and biopsy should be considered. Likewise, any solid mass that is palpable should be referred to a surgeon for possible open biopsy. Finally, any lesion that appears to be new since the last screening mammogram should be considered for biopsy.

4. **Aspiration and results.** If the ultrasound of the soft-tissue mass demonstrates that it is a cystic lesion, the cyst should be further categorized by the criteria listed in the algorithm: irregular wall, as seen on ultrasonography; internal echoes; complex, septated appearance; and palpability within the region of the ultrasound-proven cyst. A positive finding for any of these criteria would be an indication for ultrasound-directed aspiration of the cyst. Aspiration should also be offered if the patient requests it.

   After cyst aspiration, a single-view mammogram should be obtained to demonstrate complete resolution of the lesion. If the lesion is sufficiently complex, a cyst pneumogram may be performed. Should any residual mass be present or if the cyst pneumogram findings are abnormal, biopsy should be recommended. If, on the other hand, the mass is a simple cyst that does not fit any of the previously listed criteria, the patient should be returned to the screening process, and completion of this evaluation should be reported to the ordering health care provider.

---

*ICSI healthcare guidelines are designed to assist clinicians by providing an analytic framework for the evaluation and treatment of patients. They are not intended either to replace a clinician's judgment or to establish a protocol for all patients with a particular condition. A guideline will rarely establish the only approach to a problem. In addition, guidelines are "living documents" that are expected to be imperfect and are subject to annual review and revision.

ICSI is a nonprofit organization that provides healthcare quality improvement services to 20 medical groups affiliated with HealthPartners in central and southern Minnesota and western Wisconsin. The guidelines are developed through a process that involves physicians, nurses, and other healthcare professionals from beginning to end, and healthcare purchasers are included in decision making. To order any of the more than 40 guidelines ICSI has developed, contact the ICSI Publications Fulfillment Center, in care of the ARDEL Group, 6518 Walker St., Suite 150, Minneapolis, MN 55426; 612-927-6707.

BREAST, ROUTINE SCREEN OR PALPABLE MASS EVALUATION

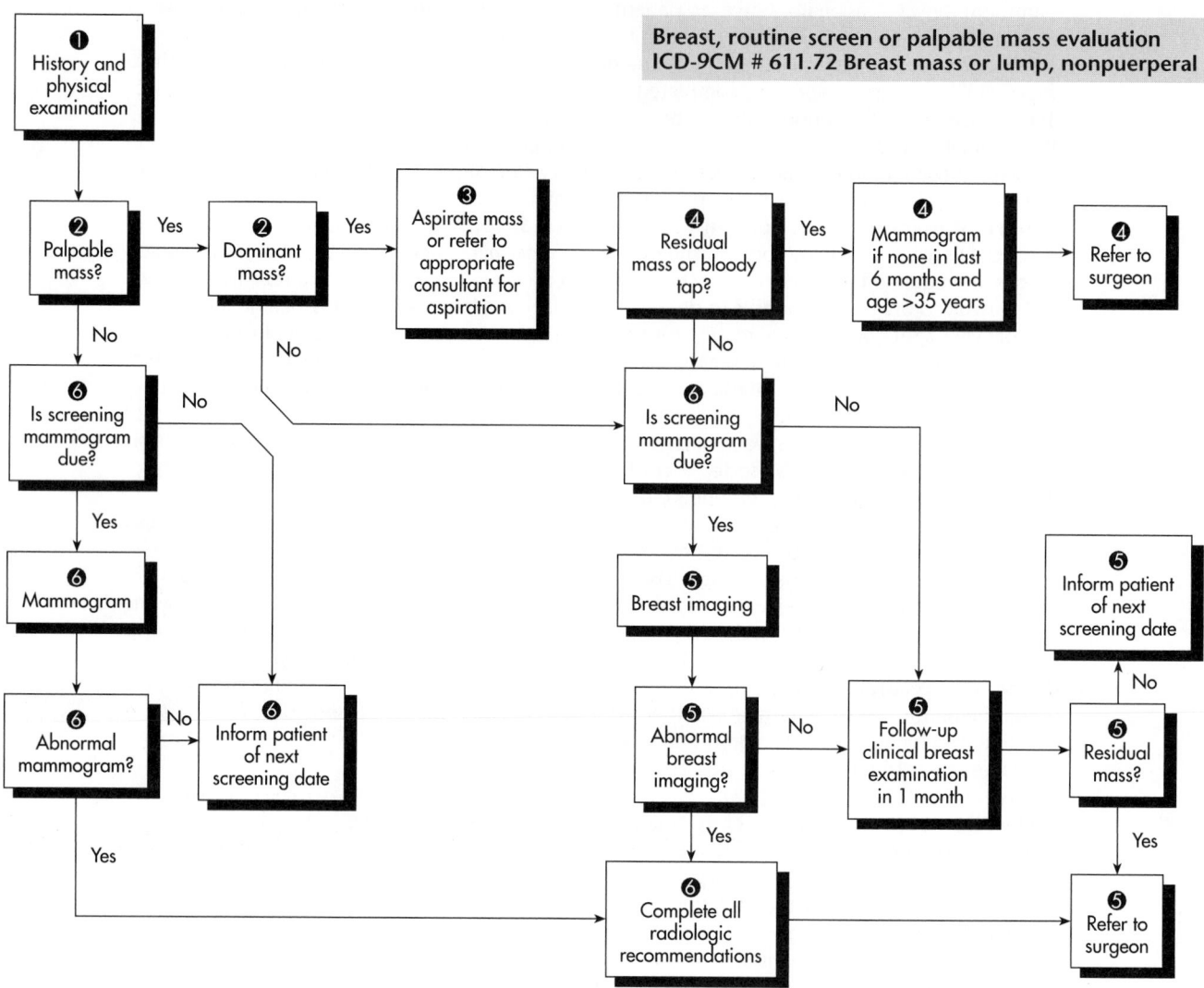

Breast, routine screen or palpable mass evaluation
ICD-9CM # 611.72 Breast mass or lump, nonpuerperal

Fig. 3-34 **Breast cancer screening and evaluation.** (From Institute for Clinical Systems Integration, Minneapolis: *Postgrad Med* 100:182, 1996.)

1. **History and physical examination.*** Primary care evaluation is initiated with history taking aimed at uncovering and characterizing any breast-related symptom. A risk assessment should also be undertaken for identified risk factors, including patient age over 50 years, any past personal history of breast cancer, history of hyperplasia on previous breast biopsies, and family history of breast cancer in first-degree relatives (mother, sister, daughter). Physical examination should include inspection of the breast for any evidence of ulceration or contour changes and inspection of the nipple for Paget's disease. Palpation should be performed with the patient in both the upright and supine positions to determine the presence of any palpable mass.

2. **Palpable mass? Dominant mass?** A dominant mass is a palpable finding that is discrete and clearly different from the surrounding parenchyma. If a palpable mass is identified, it should be determined whether it represents a dominant (i.e., discrete) mass, which requires immediate evaluation. The primary care physician or appropriate consultant should attempt to aspirate any dominant mass because a simple cyst may be uncovered, in which case aspiration completes the evaluation process.

3. **Aspirate mass or refer for aspiration.** Aspiration of a dominant palpable mass should be performed by the primary care physician or by the appropriate consultant. The breast skin is prepped with alcohol. Then, with the lesion immobilized by the nonoperating hand, an 18- to 25-gauge needle mounted on a 10-ml syringe is directed to the central portion of the mass for a single attempt at aspiration. Successful aspiration of a simple cyst would yield a nonbloody fluid with complete resolution of the dominant mass. Typical watery fluid may be discarded. However, cyst fluid that is bloody or unusually tenacious should be examined cytologically.

Fig. 3-34, cont'd

4. **Residual mass or bloody tap? Mammogram if none in past 6 months. Refer to surgeon.** Should the mass remain after the attempt at aspiration or should frank blood be aspirated during the process, the presence of a malignant process cannot be ruled out. Patients with a residual mass or bloody tap should be referred to a surgeon for possible biopsy. Before the referral, a mammogram should be obtained for any patient over age 35 years who has not had a mammogram within the preceding 6 months. In patients 35 years and under, obtaining any other breast-imaging studies should be left to the discretion of the surgeon or radiologist.

5. **Is screening mammogram due? Breast imaging. Follow-up clinical breast examination. Refer to surgeon.** Should physical examination demonstrate a palpable mass that is not clearly a discrete and dominant mass, its size, location, and character should be documented in anticipation of a follow-up examination. A screening mammogram should be obtained if one has not been done within the recommended interval. If no mammogram is required or if a required mammogram demonstrates no abnormality, a follow-up examination in 1 month is indicated. Should any residual mass be identified, the patient should be referred to a surgeon for possible biopsy. Patients with a persisting nondominant palpable mass that does not resolve within 1 month and those with any recurring cystic mass should be referred for surgical evaluation. If no mass is apparent at the time of the follow-up examination, the patient should then be informed of the appropriate date for her next screening examination, according to the recommended intervals.

6. **Screening mammogram and results.** After completion of the physical examination, the appropriateness of a routine screening mammogram should be determined. If a mammogram is done, the radiologist should provide the results to the primary care physician for reporting to the patient. Should any abnormalities be uncovered, it will be the responsibility of the radiologist to complete any additional imaging studies required for the complete radiographic characterization of the lesion. The radiologist should make certain that all recommended additional views, follow-up studies, and ultrasound examinations have been completed before referral to a surgeon. However, it is important that the primary care physician who ordered the mammogram review the results of these studies to understand fully the opinion of the radiologist and to ensure that all recommendations of the radiologist have been completed. Should the radiologist recommend that surgical consultation is warranted, it will be the responsibility of the primary care physician to establish this referral.

   NOTE: *The importance of communication between the surgical consultant and the primary care physician cannot be overstated. Biopsy results should be reported both to the surgeon and to the primary care physician. More important, patients who do not require biopsy after surgical consultation should be returned to the routine screening process. This process is under the supervision of the primary care physician. Therefore it is absolutely necessary for the primary care physician to know when the patient reenters the routine screening population. In the event that new symptoms arise during the screening interval, the patient should be evaluated by the primary care physician using the primary care evaluation process of this guideline.*

III

---

*ICSI healthcare guidelines are designed to assist clinicians by providing an analytic framework for the evaluation and treatment of patients. They are not intended either to replace a clinician's judgment or to establish a protocol for all patients with a particular condition. A guideline will rarely establish the only approach to a problem. In addition, guidelines are "living documents" that are expected to be imperfect and are subject to annual review and revision.

ICSI is a nonprofit organization that provides healthcare quality improvement services to 20 medical groups affiliated with HealthPartners in central and southern Minnesota and western Wisconsin. The guidelines are developed through a process that involves physicians, nurses, and other healthcare professionals from beginning to end, and healthcare purchasers are included in decision making. To order any of the more than 40 guidelines ICSI has developed, contact the ICSI Publications Fulfillment Center, in care of the ARDEL Group, 6518 Walker St., Suite 150, Minneapolis, MN 55426; 612-927-6707.

BREASTFEEDING DIFFICULTIES

Breastfeeding difficulties
ICD-9CM # 676.8

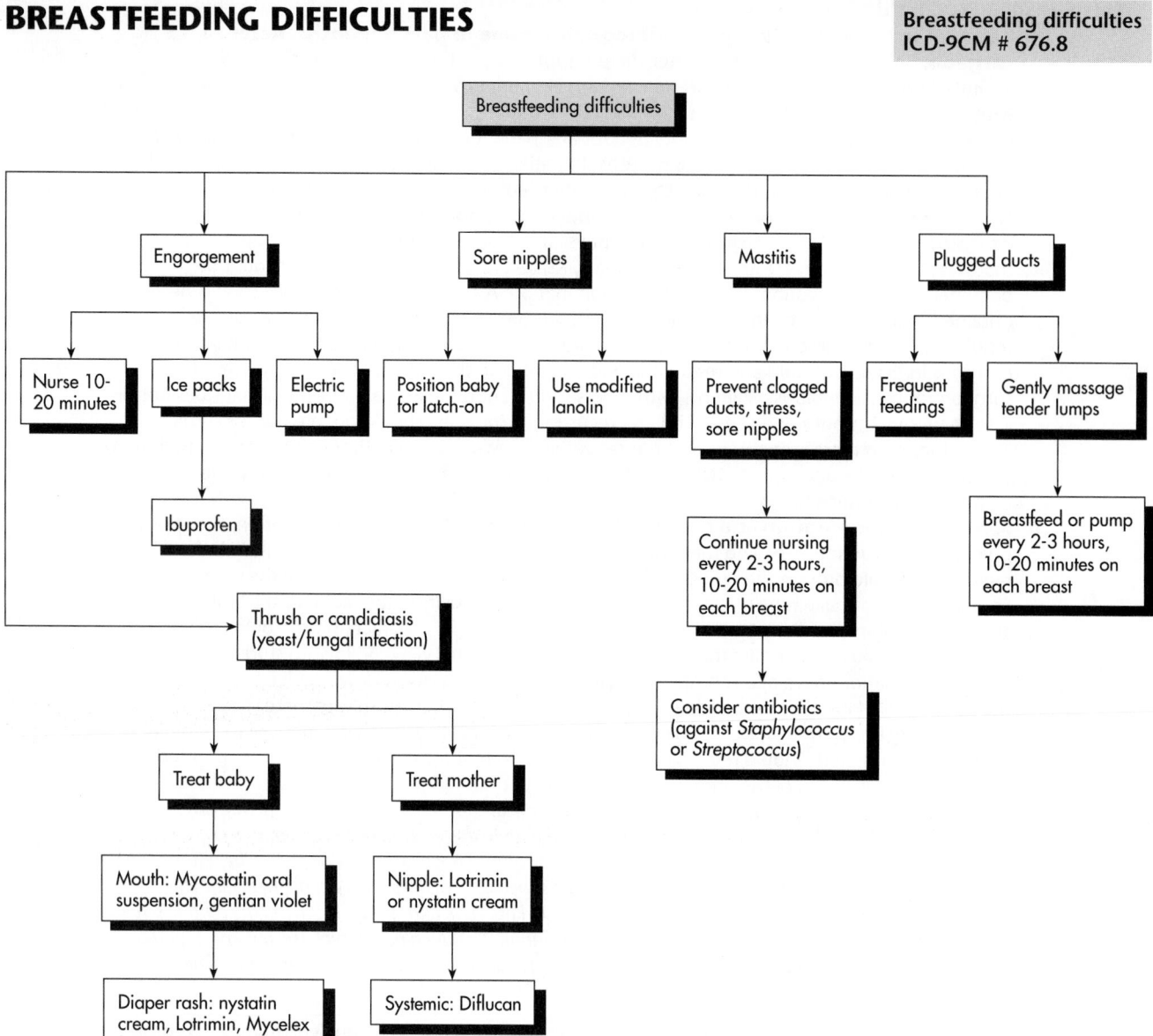

Fig. 3-35   Management of breastfeeding difficulties. (From Zuspan FP [ed]: *Handbook of obstetrics, gynecology, and primary care,* St Louis, 1998, Mosby.)

CACHEXIA, CANCER PATIENT

Cachexia, cancer patient
ICD-9CM # 799.4

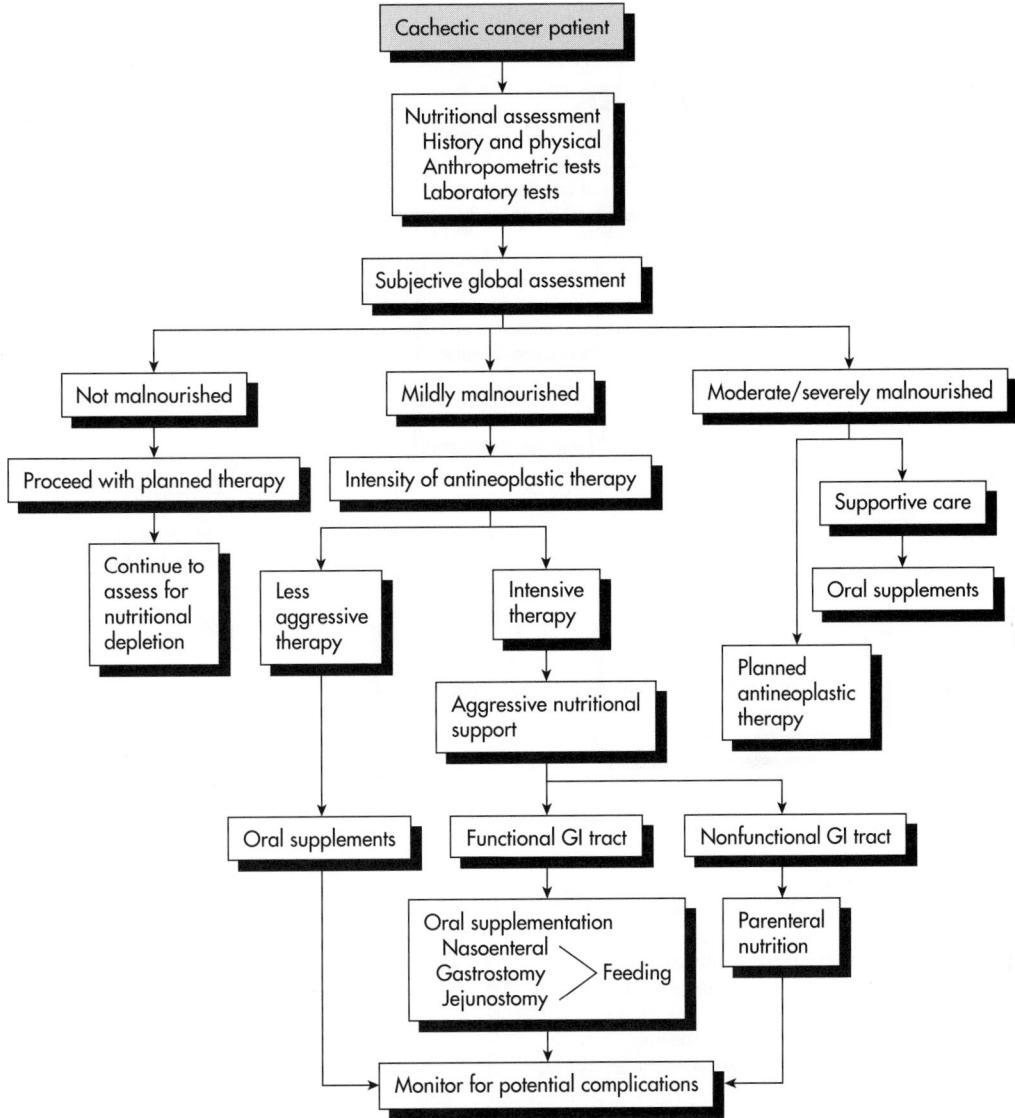

Fig. 3-36   An approach to the cachectic cancer patient. *GI,* Gastrointestinal. (From Abeloff MD: *Clinical oncology,* ed 2, New York, 2000, Churchill Livingstone.)

III

CARDIOMEGALY ON CHEST X-RAY

Cardiomegaly
ICD-9CM # 429.3 Idiopathic cardiomegaly
746.89 Congenital cardiomegaly
402.0 Hypertensive cardiomegaly, malignant
402.1 Hypertensive cardiomegaly, benign
402.11 Hypertensive cardiomegaly with congestive heart failure

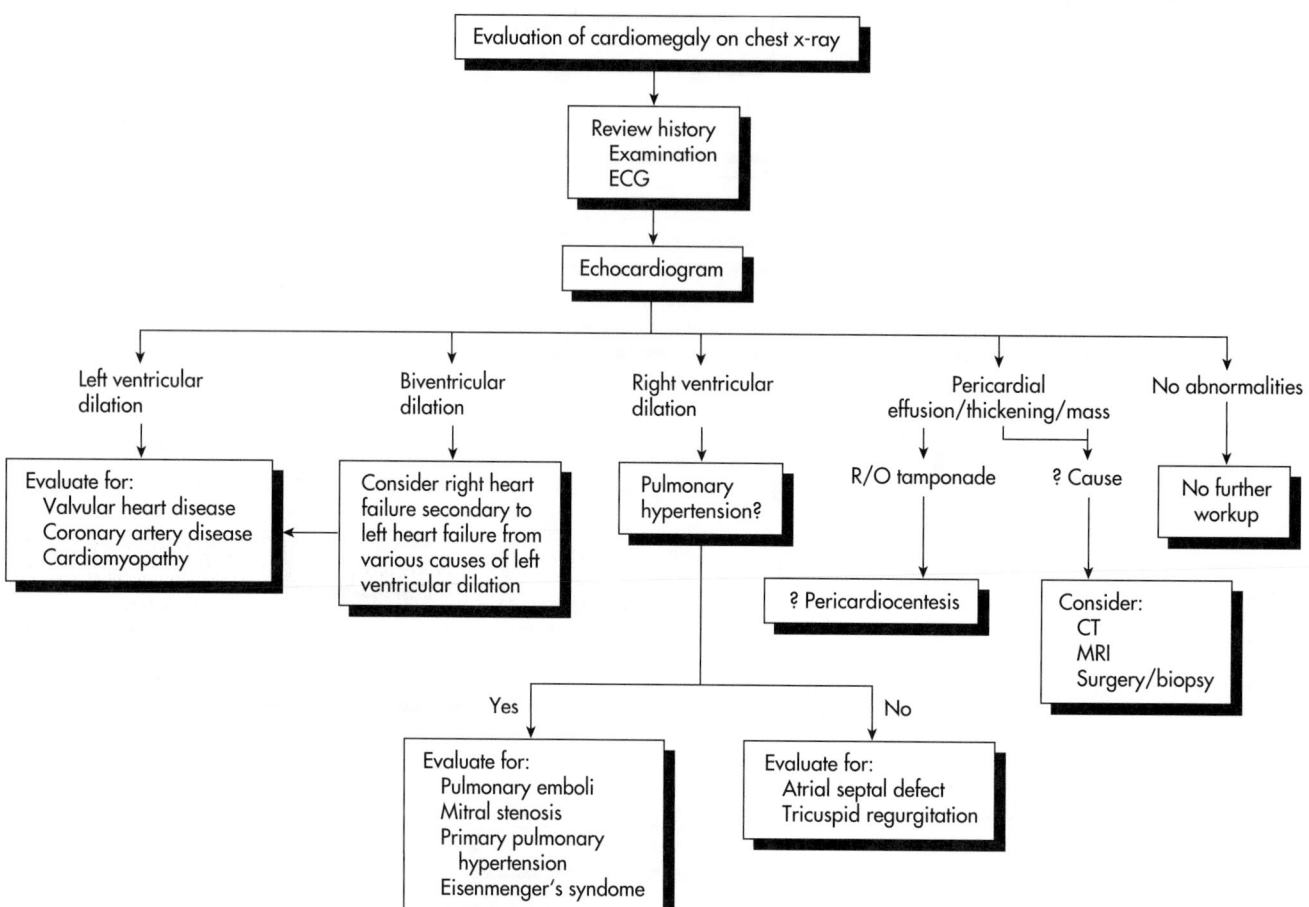

Fig. 3-37   Approach to the patient with cardiomegaly. When cardiomegaly is found on the chest radiograph, the history and physical examination should be reviewed and an electrocardiogram (ECG) performed before obtaining a two-dimensional Doppler echocardiographic study. Cardiomegaly may be explained by left ventricular dilation, biventricular dilation, right ventricular dilation, or pericardial abnormalities, or it may be found to be spurious on the echocardiogram. Rarely, isolated abnormalities of the atrium, particularly the left atrium, may cause abnormalities on the chest radiograph but will not cause true cardiomegaly. Depending on the echocardiographic findings, further tests can help elucidate the cause of echocardiographically confirmed cardiomegaly. *CT,* Computer tomography; *MRI,* magnetic resonance imaging; *R/O,* rule out. (From Goldman L, Branwald E [eds]: *Primary cardiology,* Philadelphia, 1998, WB Saunders.)

CEREBRAL ISCHEMIA

Cerebral ischemia
ICD-9CM # 437.1 Cerebral ischemia (chronic)
435.9 Cerebral ischemia intermittent
(transient)

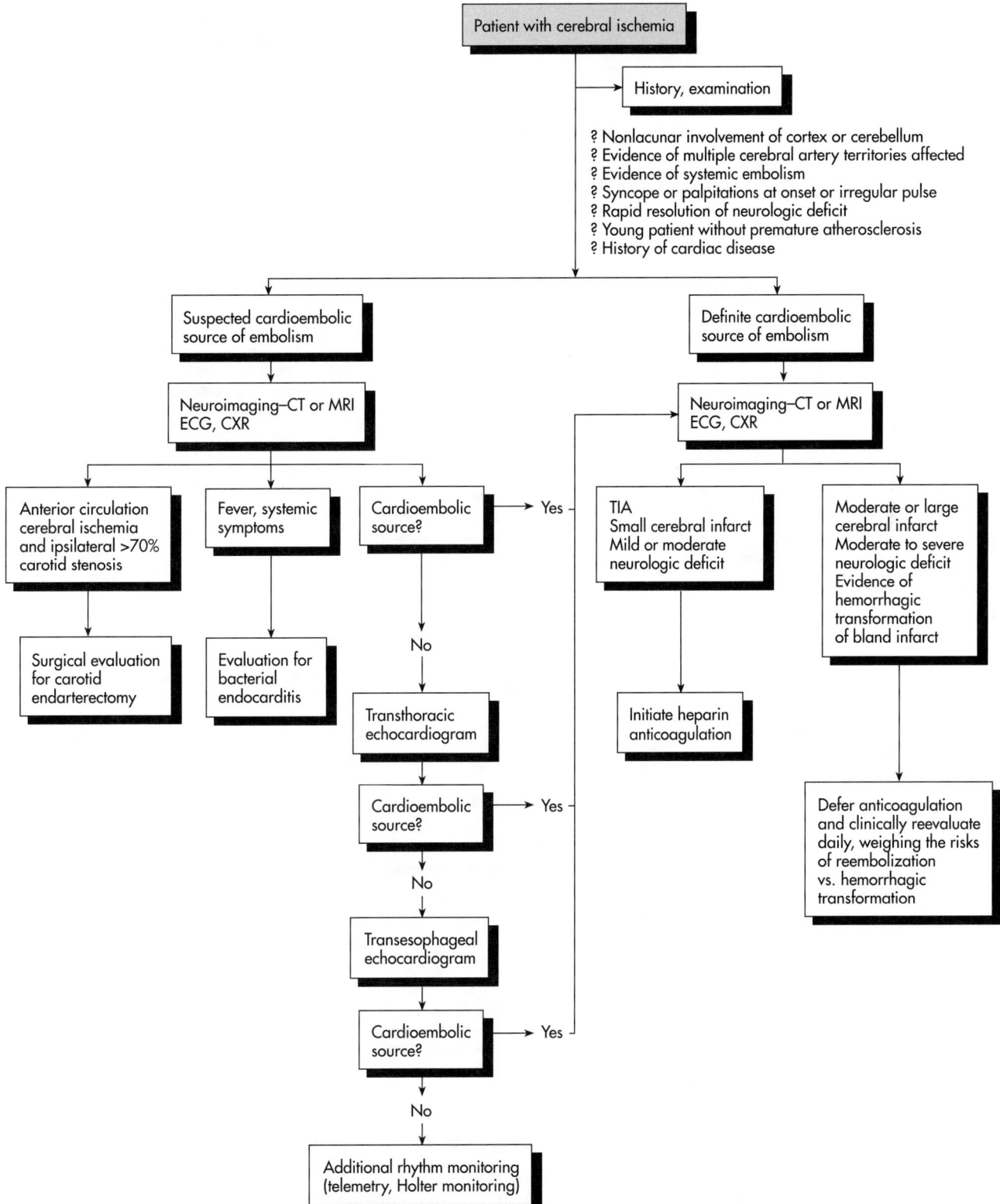

Fig. 3-38   Evaluation of patients with cerebral ischemia for a cardioembolic source. *CT,* computed tomography; *CXR,* chest radiograph; *ECG,* electrocardiogram; *MRI,* magnetic resonance imaging; *TIA,* transient ischemic attack. (From Johnson R [ed]: *Current therapy in neurologic disease,* ed 5, St Louis, 1997, Mosby.)

CODE STATUS DETERMINATION BEFORE CARDIAC ARREST

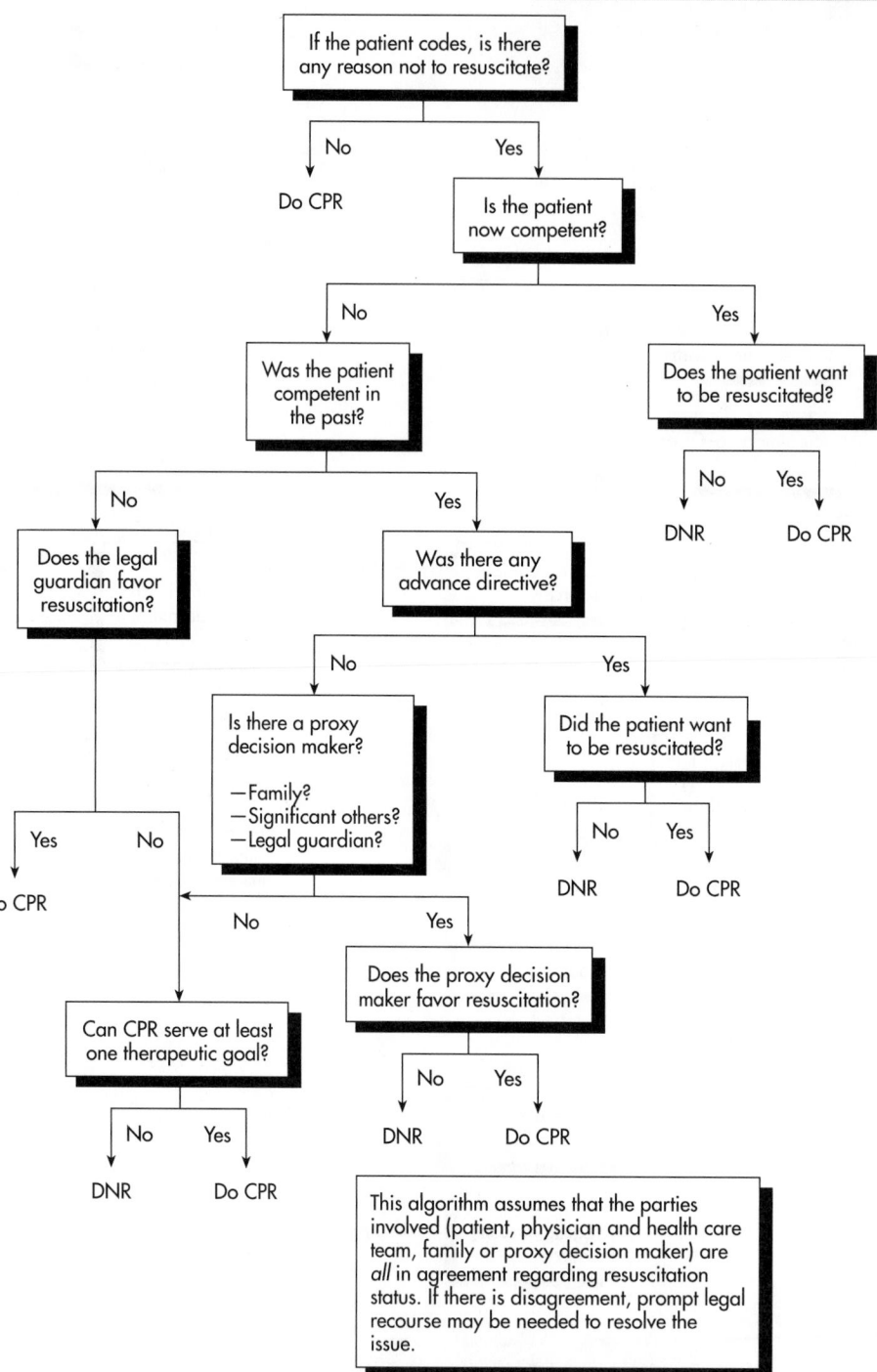

Fig. 3-39　Determination of code status before cardiac arrest. *CSR,* Cardiopulmonary resuscitation; *DNR,* do not resuscitate. (From Grauer K, Cavallaro D [eds]: *ACLS certification preparation,* St Louis, 1993, Mosby.)

CONSTIPATION

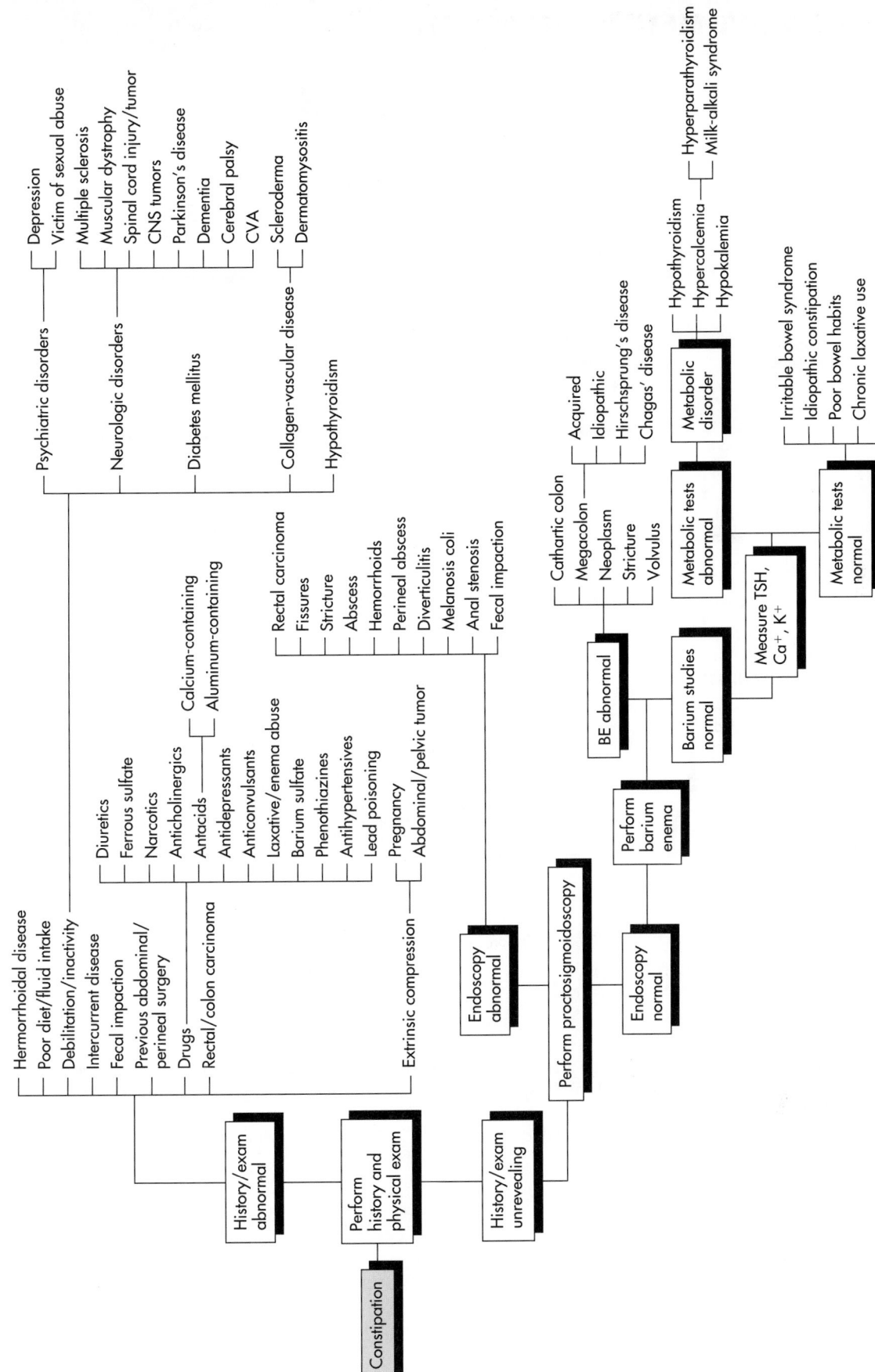

Fig. 3-40 **Constipation.** *BE,* Barium enema; *CNS,* central nervous system; *CVA,* cerebral vascular accident; *TSH,* thyroid-stimulating hormone. (From Healey PM: *Common medical diagnosis: an algorithmic approach,* ed 3, Philadelphia, 2000, WB Saunders.)

III

CONTRACEPTIVE METHOD SELECTION

Contraceptive method selection
ICD-9CM # V25.09

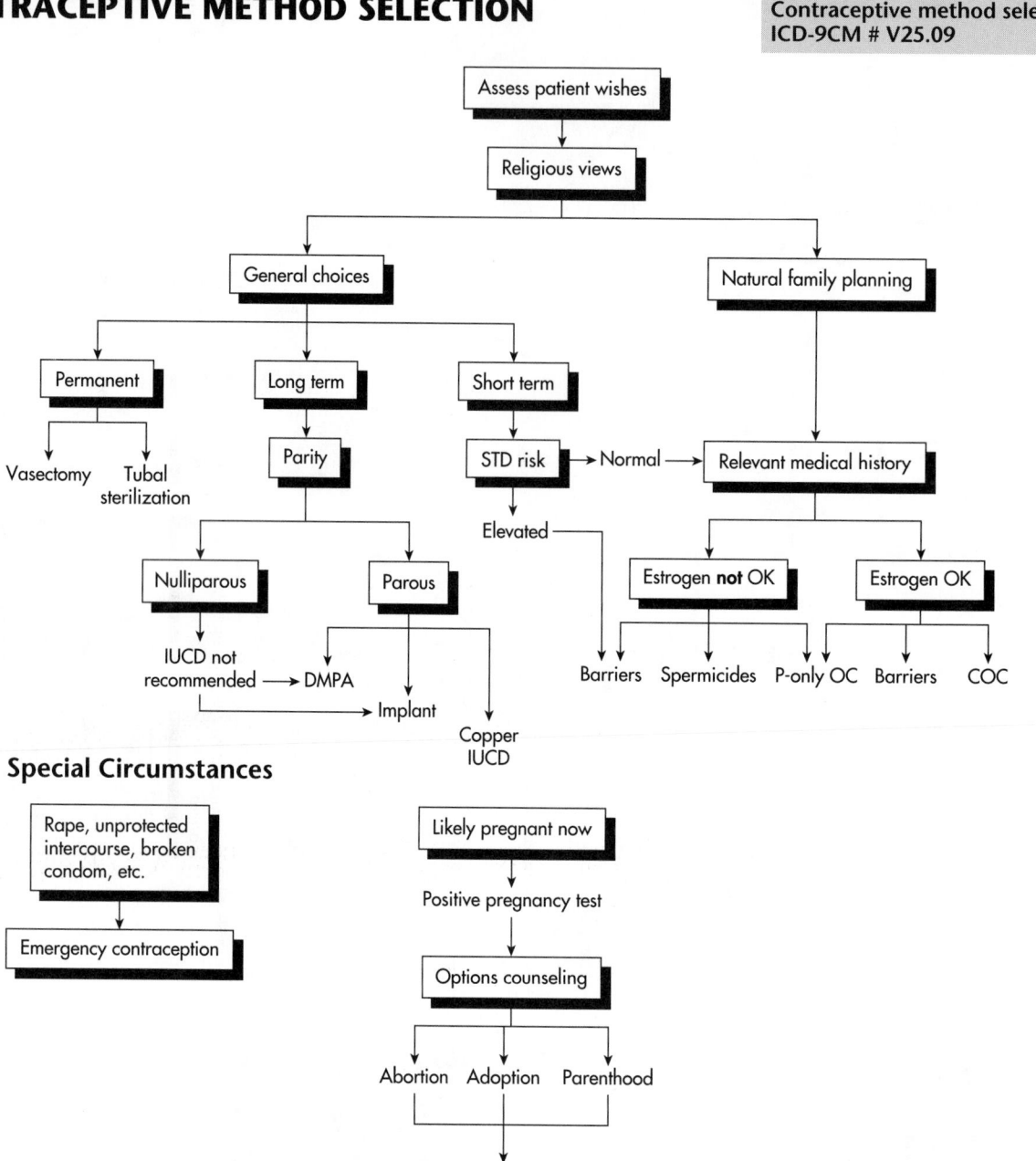

Special Circumstances

Fig. 3-41　**Helping couples select a contraceptive method.** *COC,* Combination estrogen-progestin oral contraceptive; *DMPA,* depot medroxyprogesterone acetate; *IUCD,* intrauterine contraceptive device; *P-only OC,* progestin-only oral contraceptive; *STD,* sexually transmitted disease. (From Copeland LJ: *Textbook of gynecology,* ed 2, Philadelphia, 2000, WB Saunders.)

CONTRACEPTIVE USE, ORAL

Contraceptive use, oral
ICD-9CM # V25.01 Prescription or use, oral
contraceptive

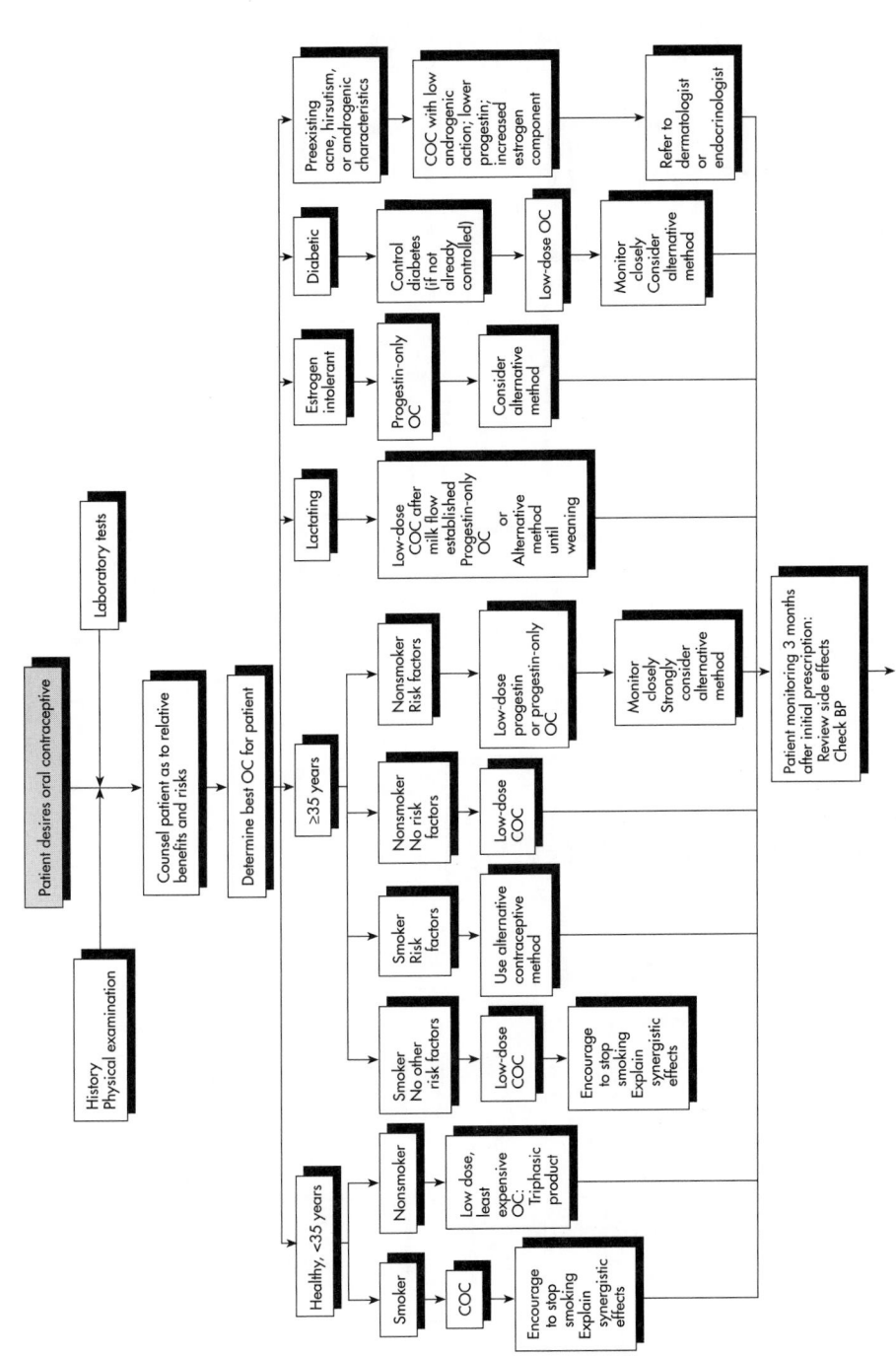

Fig. 3-42 **Contraceptive use.** *BP,* Blood pressure; *BTB,* breakthrough bleeding; *COC,* combination oral contraceptives; *CVA,* cerebrovascular accident; *OC,* oral contraceptive. (From Robles TA: Use of oral contraceptives. In Greene HL, Johnson WP, Lemcke D [eds]: *Decision making in medicine,* ed 2, St Louis, 1998, Mosby.) *Continued*

CONTRACEPTIVE USE, ORAL—cont'd

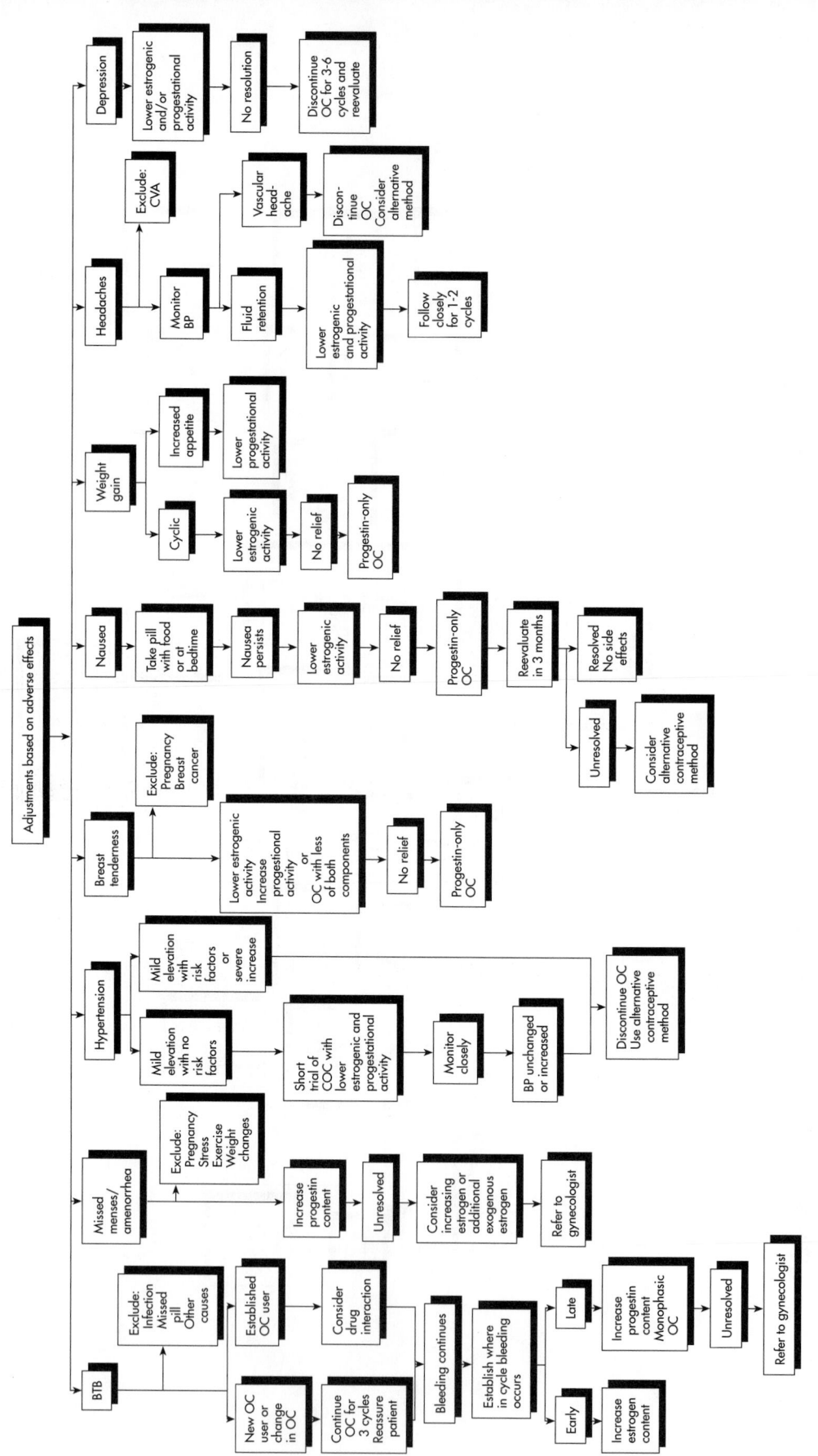

Fig. 3-42, cont'd

CONVULSIVE DISORDER, PEDIATRIC AGE

Convulsive disorder
ICD-9CM # 780.39

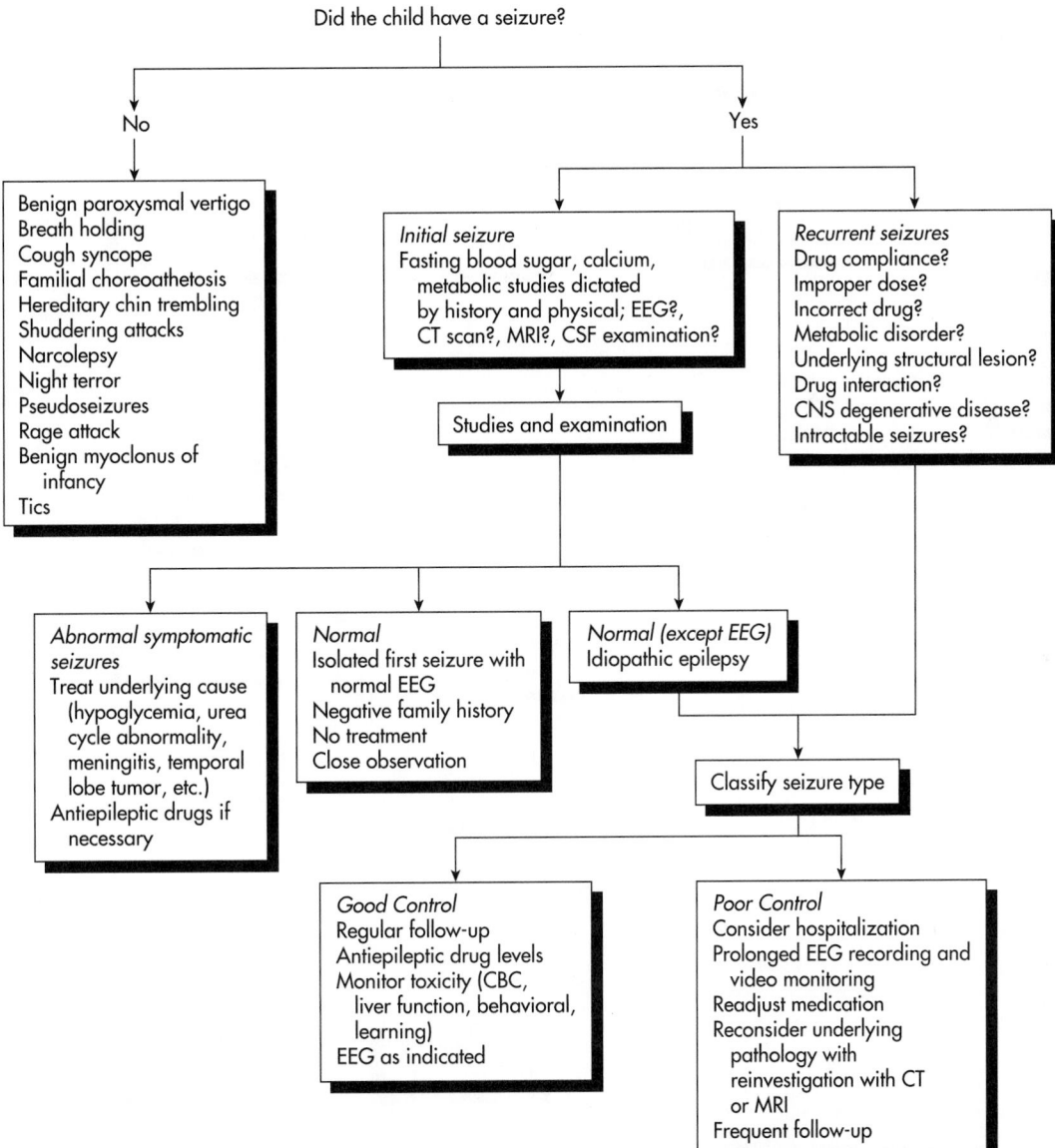

Fig. 3-43   An approach to the child with a suspected convulsive disorder. *CBC,* Complete blood count; *CNS,* central nervous system; *CSF,* cerebrospinal fluid; *CT,* computed tomography; *EEG,* electroencephalogram; *MRI,* magnetic resonance imaging. (From Behrman RE: *Nelson textbook of pediatrics,* ed 16, Philadelphia, 2000, WB Saunders.)

CORNEAL DISORDERS

Corneal disorders
ICD-9CM # 918.1 Corneal abrasion
743.9 Corneal anomalies NOS

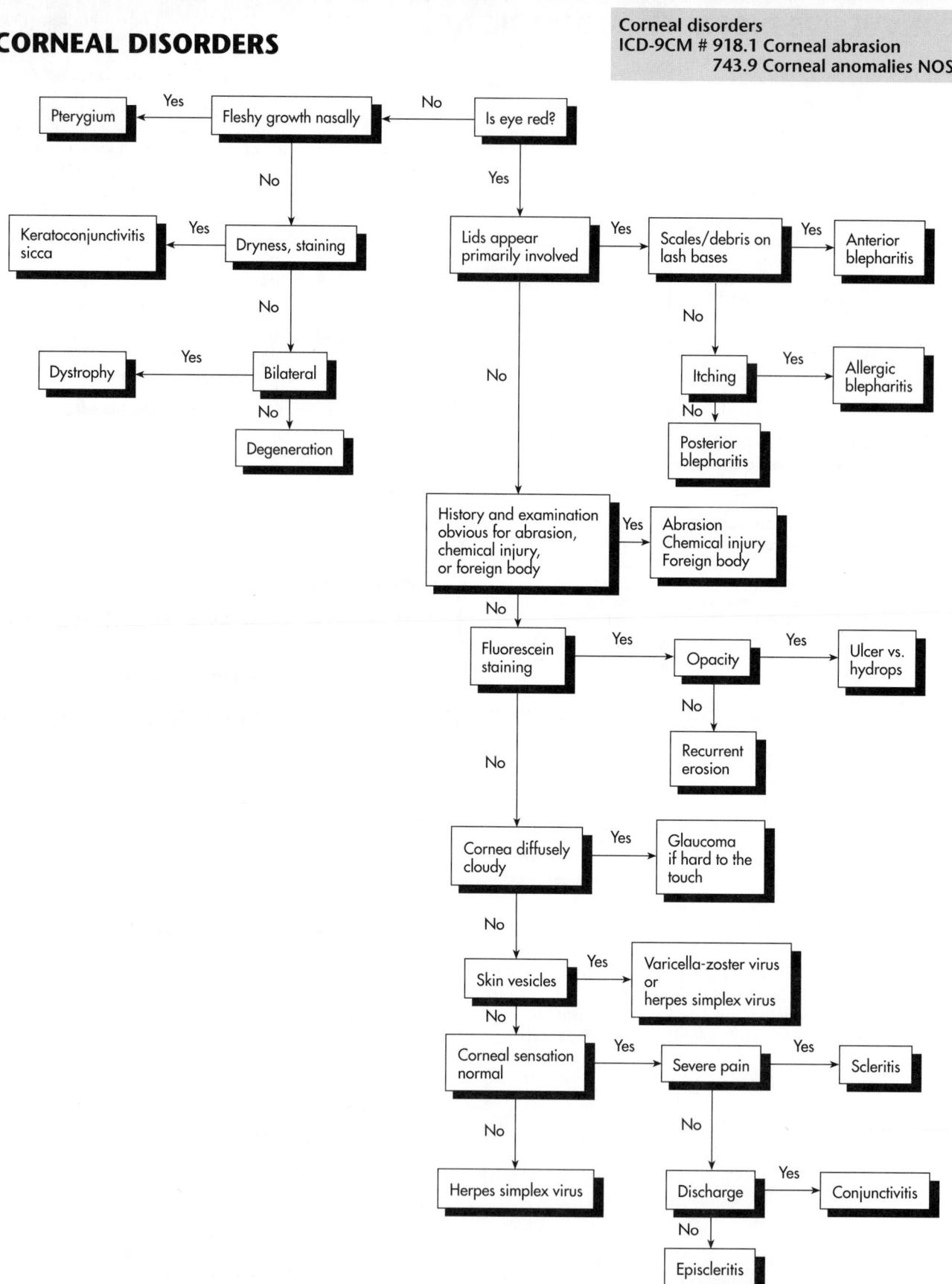

Fig. 3-44 Approach to the patient with corneal disorders. (From Noble J [ed]: *Primary care medicine,* ed 3, St Louis, 2001, Mosby.)

COUGH

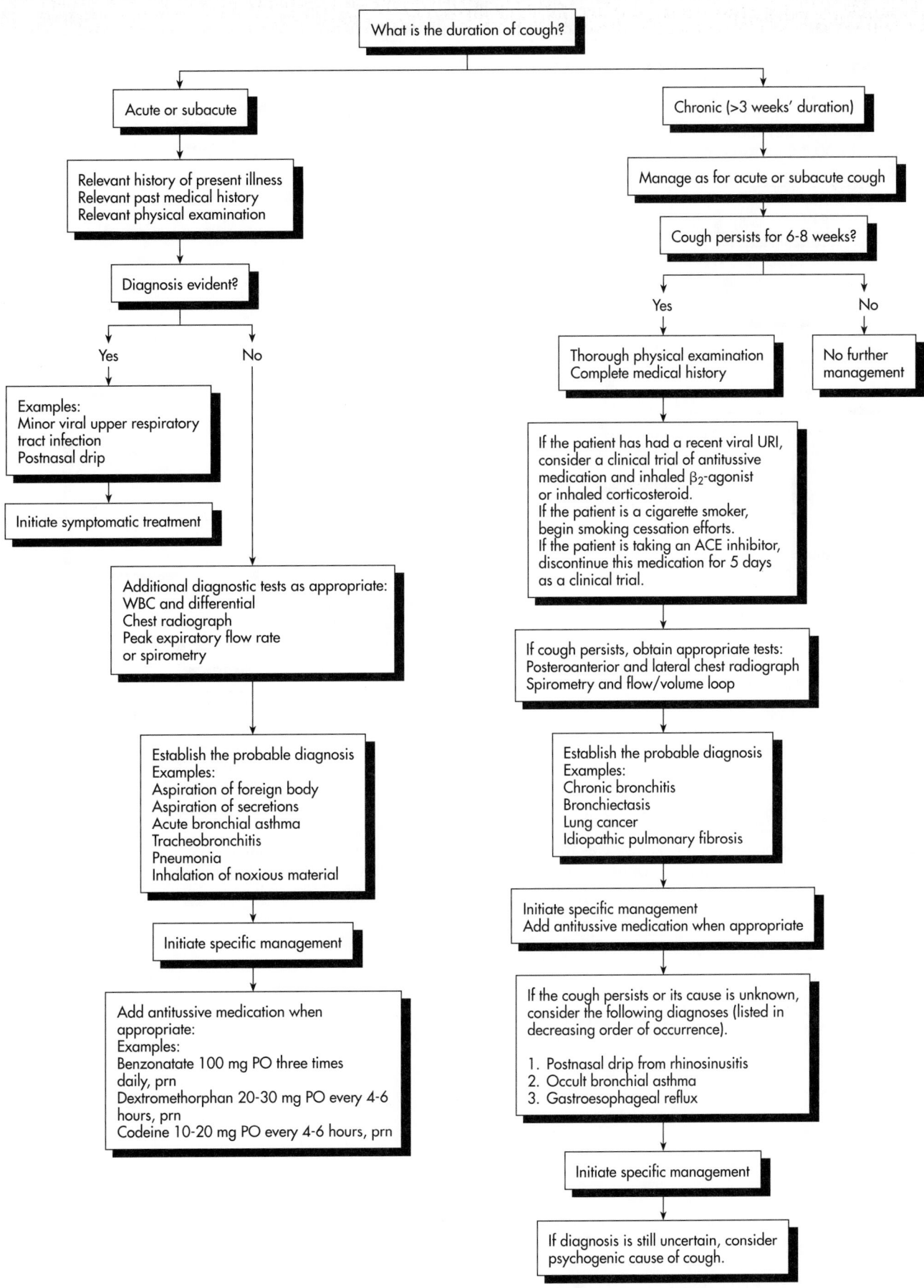

Fig. 3-45   Evaluation and treatment of the patient with cough. *ACE,* Angiotensin-converting enzyme; *URI,* upper respiratory infection; *WBC,* white blood count. (From Stein J [ed]: *Internal medicine,* ed 5, St Louis, 1998, Mosby.)

CREATINE KINASE ELEVATION

Creatine kinase elevation
ICD-9CM # V72.6 Laboratory exam

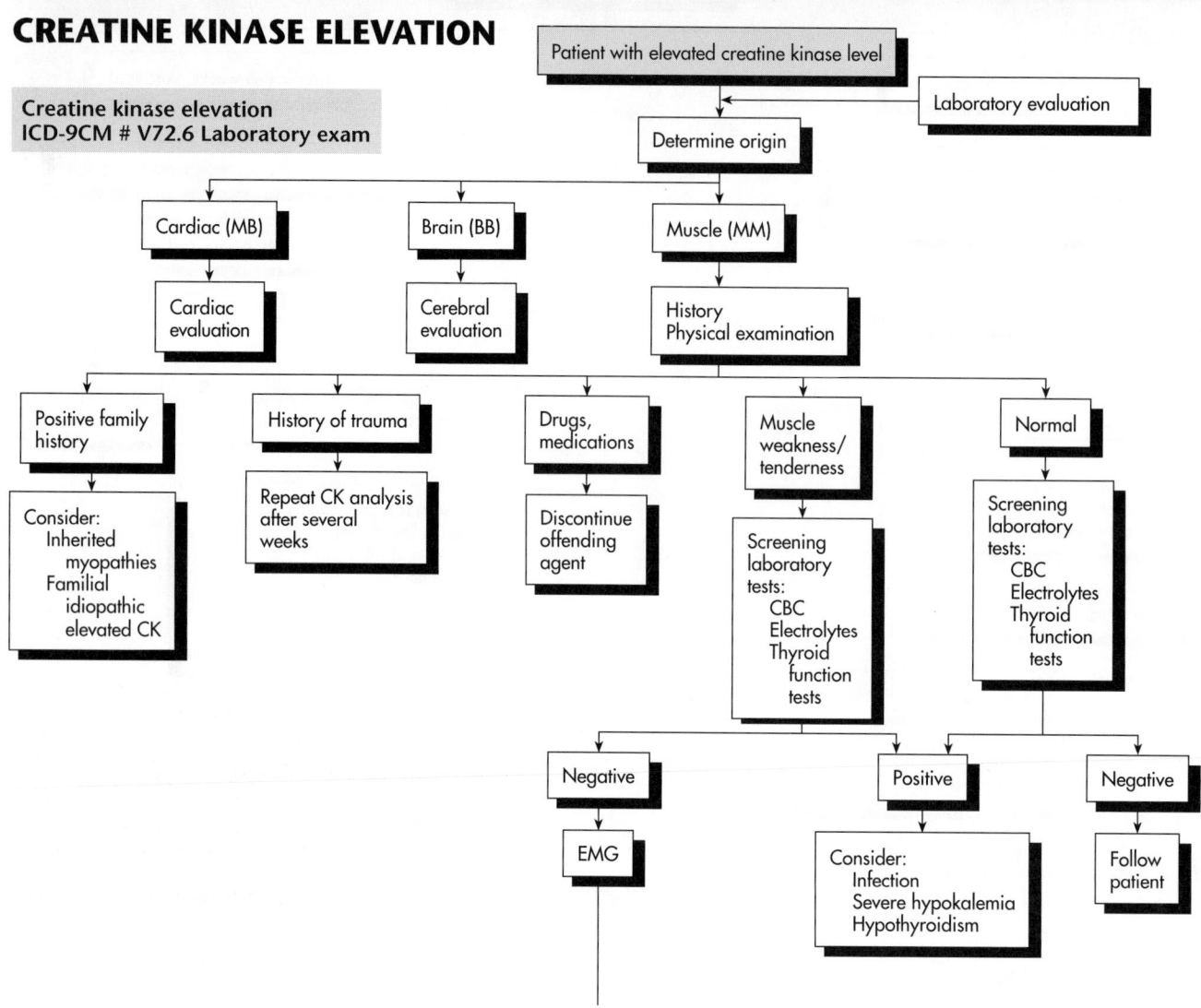

Fig. 3-46   Evaluation of creatine kinase elevation. *CBC,* Complete blood count; *CK,* creatine kinase; *EMG,* electromyography. (From Greene HL, Johnson WP, Lemcke D [eds] : *Decision making in medicine,* ed 2, St Louis, 1998, Mosby.)

CREATINE KINASE ELEVATION—cont'd

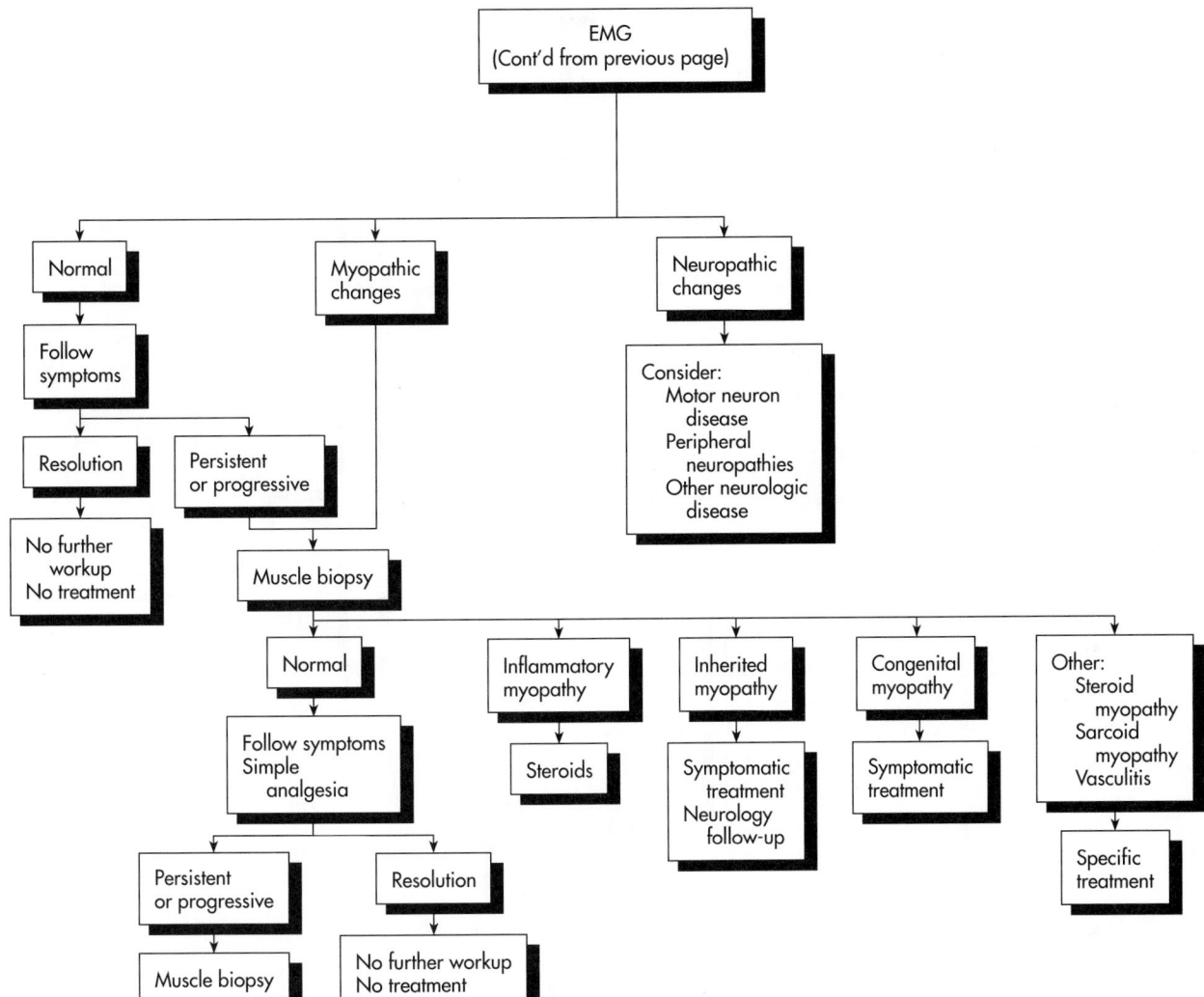

Fig. 3-46, cont'd

CYANOSIS

Cyanosis
ICD-9CM # 782.5 Cyanosis NOS

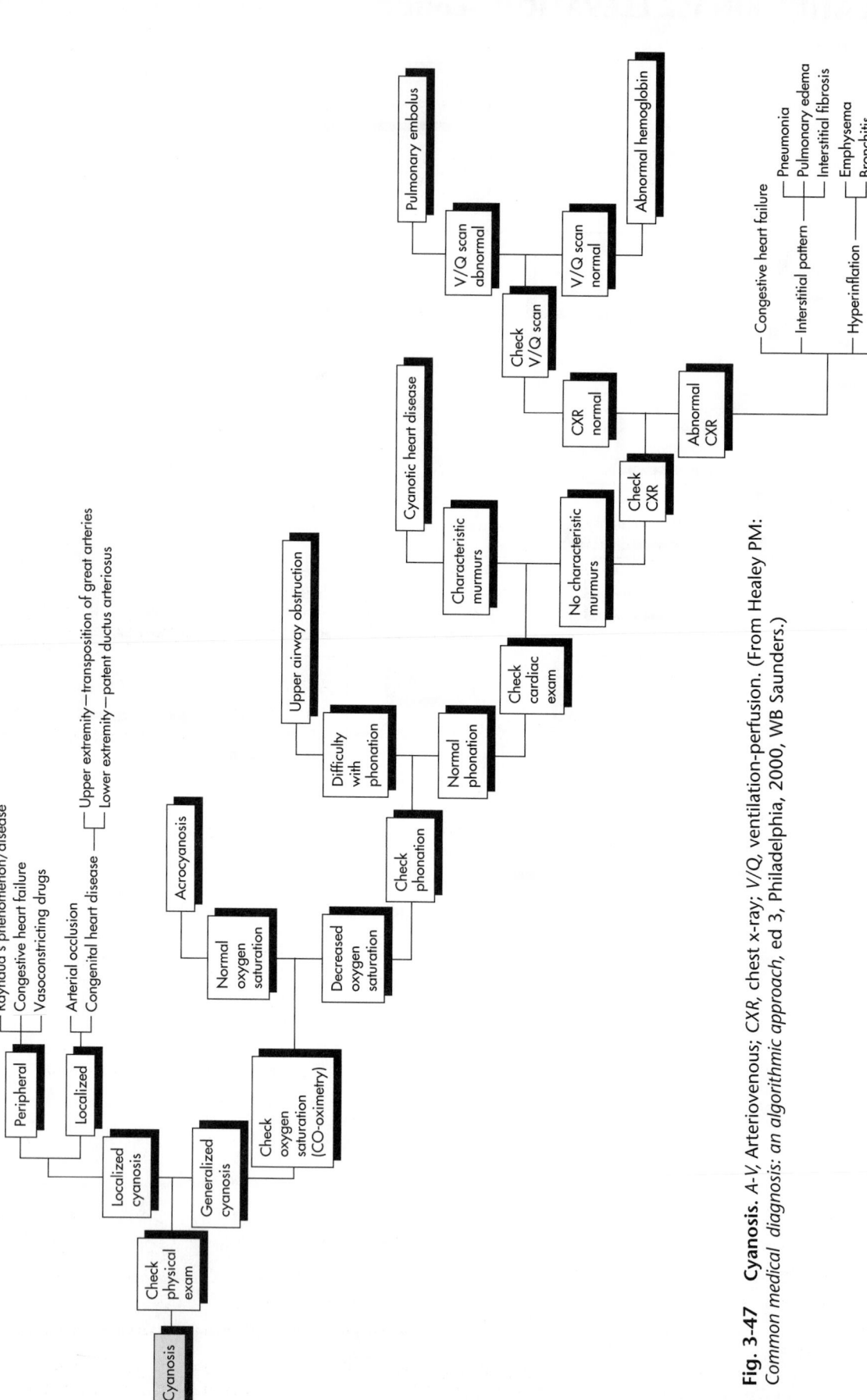

Fig. 3-47 **Cyanosis.** *A-V,* Arteriovenous; *CXR,* chest x-ray; *V/Q,* ventilation-perfusion. (From Healey PM: *Common medical diagnosis: an algorithmic approach,* ed 3, Philadelphia, 2000, WB Saunders.)

DELIRIUM, GERIATRIC PATIENT

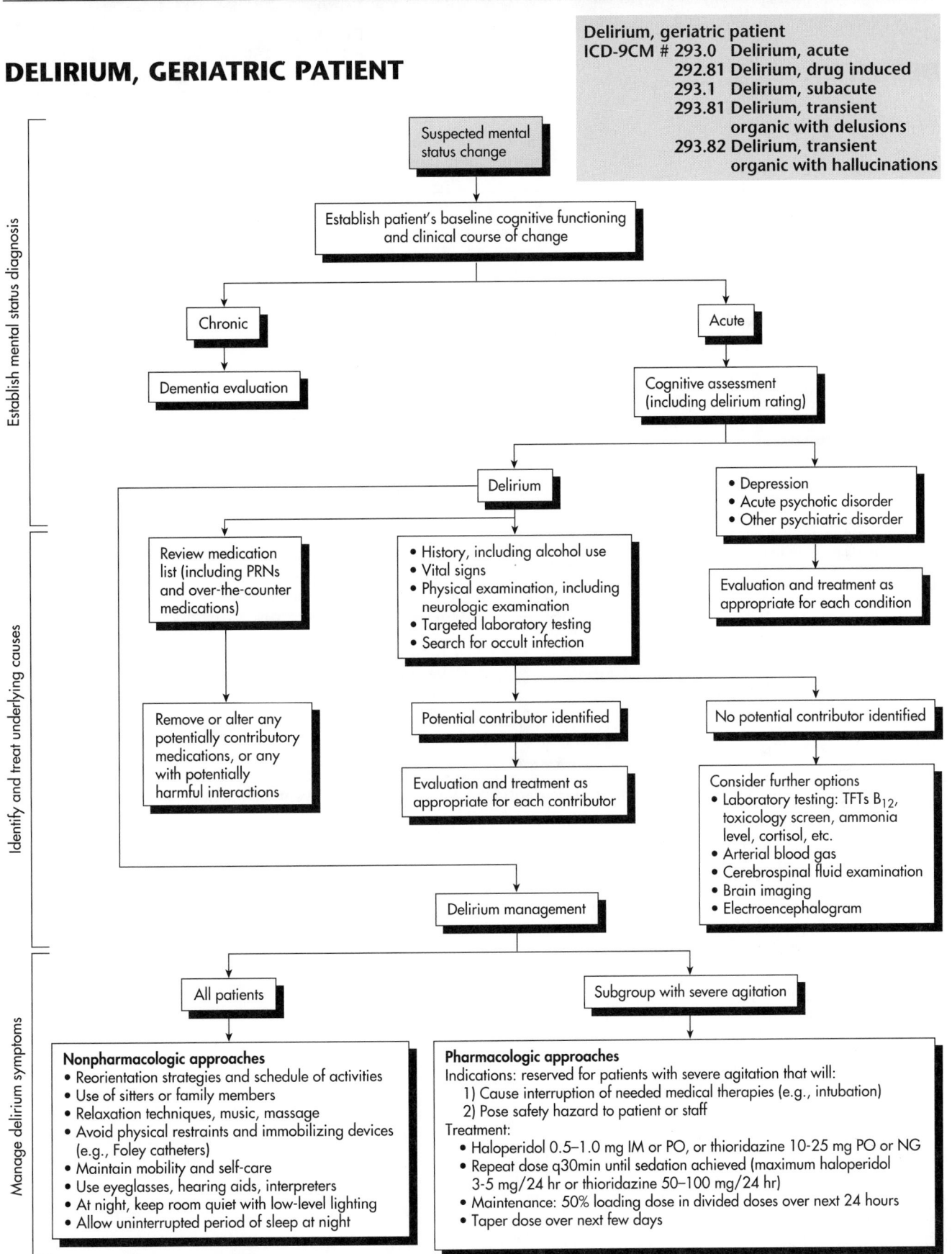

Delirium, geriatric patient
ICD-9CM # 293.0 Delirium, acute
          292.81 Delirium, drug induced
          293.1 Delirium, subacute
          293.81 Delirium, transient
                 organic with delusions
          293.82 Delirium, transient
                 organic with hallucinations

Establish mental status diagnosis

Suspected mental status change

Establish patient's baseline cognitive functioning and clinical course of change

Chronic → Dementia evaluation

Acute → Cognitive assessment (including delirium rating)

Delirium

- Depression
- Acute psychotic disorder
- Other psychiatric disorder

Evaluation and treatment as appropriate for each condition

Identify and treat underlying causes

Review medication list (including PRNs and over-the-counter medications)

- History, including alcohol use
- Vital signs
- Physical examination, including neurologic examination
- Targeted laboratory testing
- Search for occult infection

Remove or alter any potentially contributory medications, or any with potentially harmful interactions

Potential contributor identified → Evaluation and treatment as appropriate for each contributor

No potential contributor identified → Consider further options
- Laboratory testing: TFTs B$_{12}$, toxicology screen, ammonia level, cortisol, etc.
- Arterial blood gas
- Cerebrospinal fluid examination
- Brain imaging
- Electroencephalogram

Delirium management

Manage delirium symptoms

All patients

Subgroup with severe agitation

Nonpharmacologic approaches
- Reorientation strategies and schedule of activities
- Use of sitters or family members
- Relaxation techniques, music, massage
- Avoid physical restraints and immobilizing devices (e.g., Foley catheters)
- Maintain mobility and self-care
- Use eyeglasses, hearing aids, interpreters
- At night, keep room quiet with low-level lighting
- Allow uninterrupted period of sleep at night

Pharmacologic approaches
Indications: reserved for patients with severe agitation that will:
  1) Cause interruption of needed medical therapies (e.g., intubation)
  2) Pose safety hazard to patient or staff
Treatment:
- Haloperidol 0.5–1.0 mg IM or PO, or thioridazine 10-25 mg PO or NG
- Repeat dose q30min until sedation achieved (maximum haloperidol 3-5 mg/24 hr or thioridazine 50–100 mg/24 hr)
- Maintenance: 50% loading dose in divided doses over next 24 hours
- Taper dose over next few days

III

Fig. 3-48 Algorithm for evaluation of suspected mental status change in an older patient. *IM,* Intramuscular; *NG,* nasogastric; *PO,* by mouth; *PRNs,* as needed; *TFTs,* thyroid function tests. (From Goldman L, Bennett JC [eds]: *Cecil textbook of medicine,* ed 21, Philadelphia, 2000, WB Saunders.)

DEMENTIA

Dementia
ICD-9CM # 290.10 Dementia, presenile
                   290.0   Dementia, senile
                   437.0   Dementia, arteriosclerotic

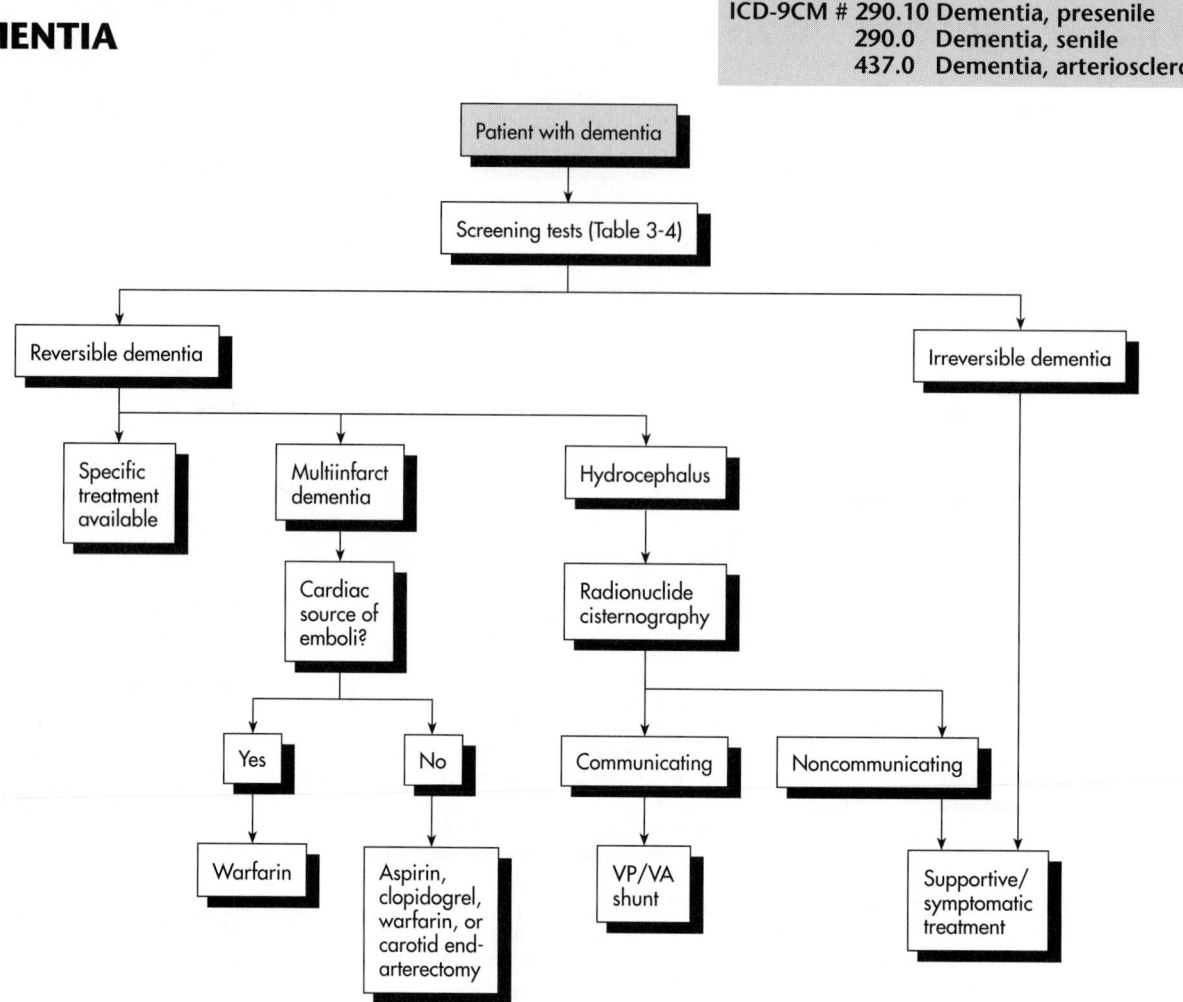

Fig. 3-49   Management of dementia. *VA,* Ventriculoatrial; *VP,* ventriculoperitoneal.

DEMENTIA—cont'd

TABLE 3-4 Screening Tests for Diagnosis of Dementia

TEST	RATIONALE	REMARKS
Blood Test		
Complete blood count	Assess general nutritional status	
Serum B_{12} level	Exclude vitamin B_{12} deficiency	Schilling's test if B_{12} level is low
TSH + free T_4 *or* TSH + FTI	Exclude primary and secondary hypothyroidism	
HIV serology	Exclude HIV infection	Perform only if indicated; consent from patient required
Cerebrospinal Fluid		
Cell count/protein level	Exclude chronic meningitis	Perform only if indicated
Cytology	Exclude carcinomatous meningitis	Perform only if indicated
VDRL	Exclude neurosyphilis	Perform only if indicated; check serum TPHA and HIV serology if CSF VDRL is positive
CT Scan/MRI of the Brain		
	Identify infarcts and white matter changes; exclude presence of neoplasm, demyelinating disease, and hydrocephalus; location of atrophy may suggest the diagnosis (e.g., parahippocampal atrophy in Alzheimer's disease, frontotemporal atrophy in Pick's disease)	
Electroencephalogram		
	Exclude metabolic encephalopathies; useful if Creutzfeldt-Jakob disease or status epilepticus is suspected	Perform only if indicated
Neuropsychologic Evaluation		
	Help to characterize pattern of cognitive impairment, which may aid in the classification of dementia; rule out pseudodementia from depression	

From Johnson RT, Griffin JW: *Current therapy in neurologic disease,* ed 5, St Louis, 1997, Mosby.
CSF, Cerebrospinal fluid; *CT,* computed tomography; *FTI,* free thyroxine index; *HIV,* human immunodeficiency virus; *MRI,* magnetic resonance imaging; *T_4,* thyroxine; *TPHA, Treponema pallidum* hemagglutination assay; *TSH,* thyroid-stimulating hormone; *VDRL,* Venereal Disease Research Laboratory test.

III

Developmental delay
ICD-9CM # 783.4 Developmental delay, physiological

DEVELOPMENTAL DELAY

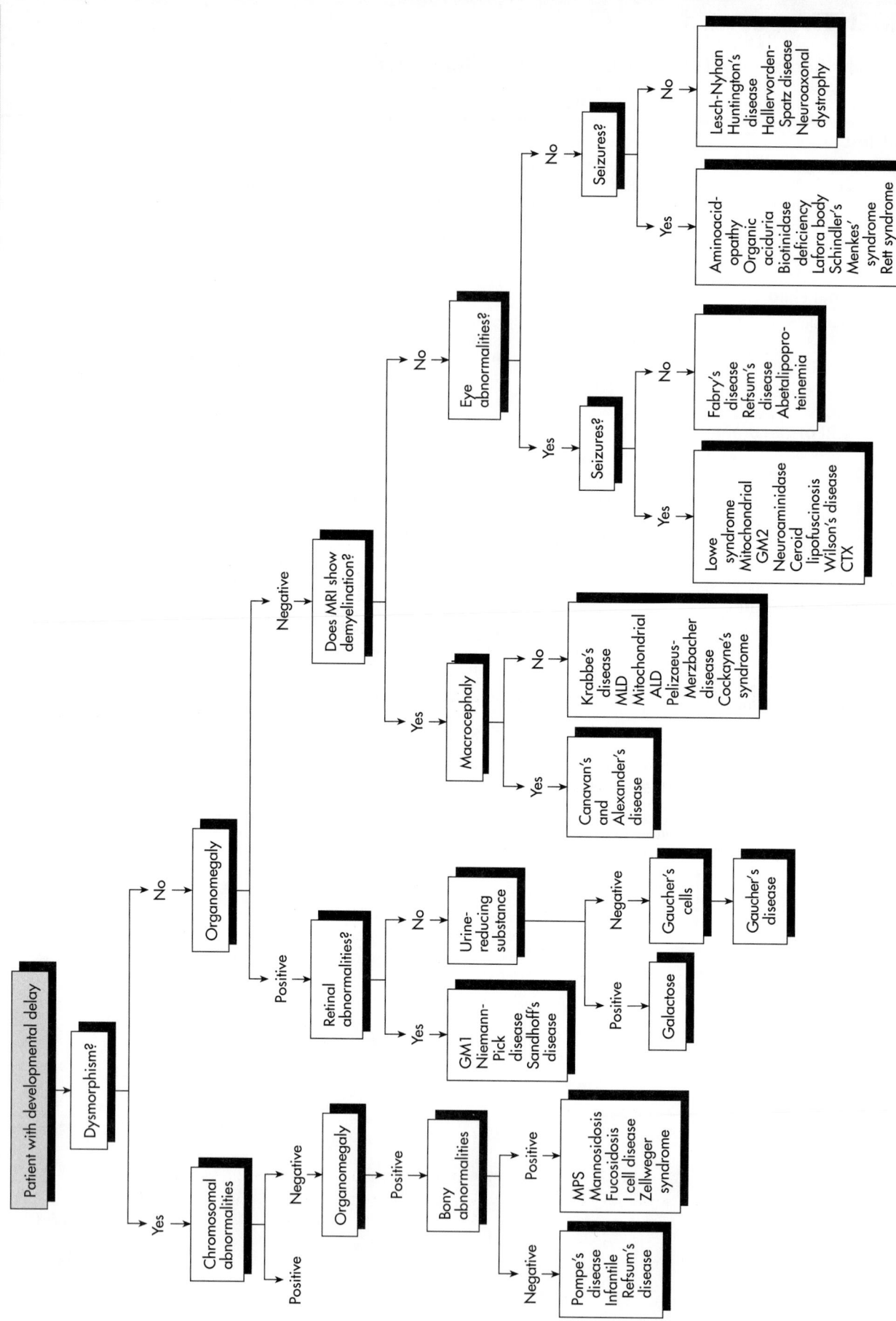

Fig. 3-50   Workup for developmental delay. *ALD,* Adrenoleukodystrophy; *CTX,* cerebrotendinous xanthomatosis; *MLD,* metachromatic leukodystrophy; *MPS,* mucopolysaccharidosis; *MRI,* magnetic resonance imaging. (From Johnson RT, Griffin JW: *Current therapy in neurologic disease,* ed 5, St Louis, 1997, Mosby.)

DIARRHEA, ACUTE

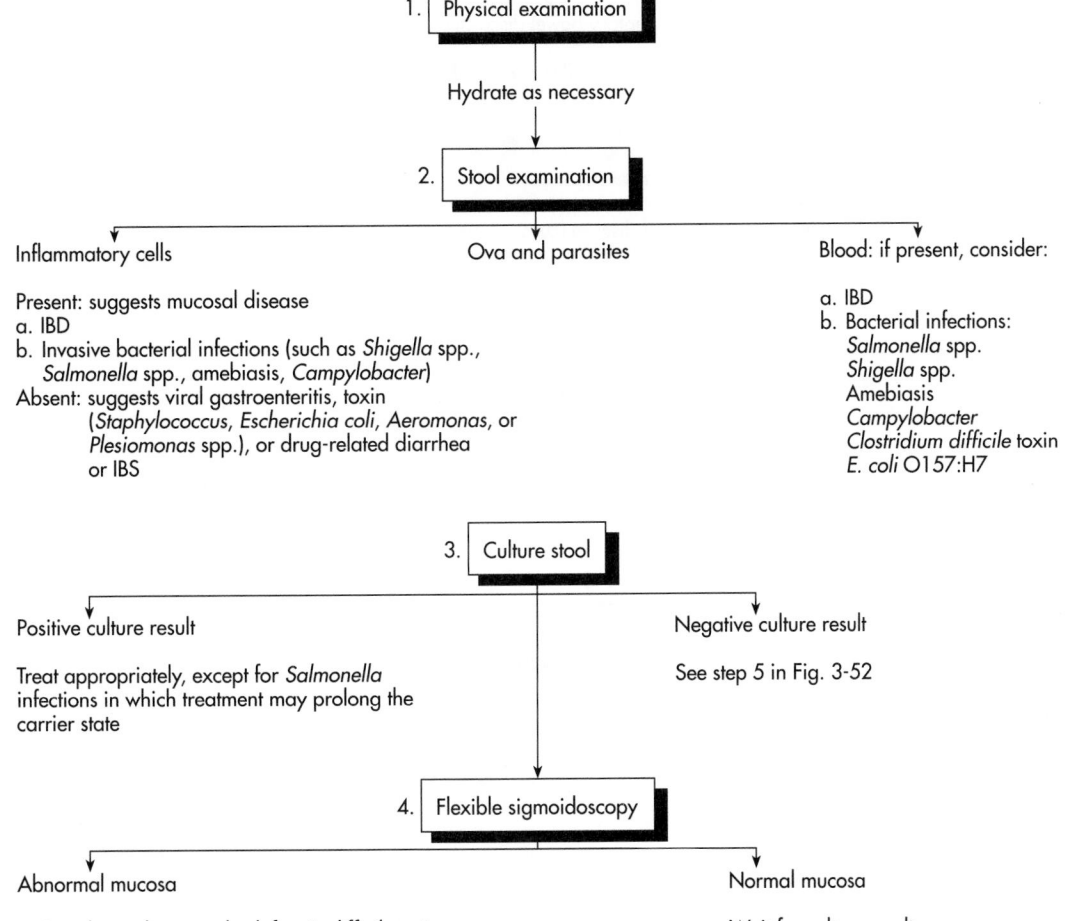

1. Physical examination

Hydrate as necessary

2. Stool examination

Inflammatory cells

Present: suggests mucosal disease
a. IBD
b. Invasive bacterial infections (such as *Shigella* spp.,
 Salmonella spp., amebiasis, *Campylobacter*)
Absent: suggests viral gastroenteritis, toxin
 (*Staphylococcus, Escherichia coli, Aeromonas,* or
 Plesiomonas spp.), or drug-related diarrhea
 or IBS

Ova and parasites

Blood: if present, consider:

a. IBD
b. Bacterial infections:
 Salmonella spp.
 Shigella spp.
 Amebiasis
 Campylobacter
 Clostridium difficile toxin
 E. coli O157:H7

3. Culture stool

Positive culture result

Treat appropriately, except for *Salmonella*
infections in which treatment may prolong the
carrier state

Negative culture result

See step 5 in Fig. 3-52

4. Flexible sigmoidoscopy

Abnormal mucosa

a. Pseudomembranes: check for *C. difficile* toxin:
 treat with metronidazole, vancomycin, or bacitracin
b. Ulcerations/granularity
 (1) Proctitis only: culture for *Chlamydia trachomatis, Neisseria gonorrhoeae*; Gram stain and culture urethra and
 pharynx; biopsy as in (2)
 (2) More extensive: culture; biopsy to look for amebae, granulomas, or nonspecific finding of IBD

Normal mucosa

Wait for culture results

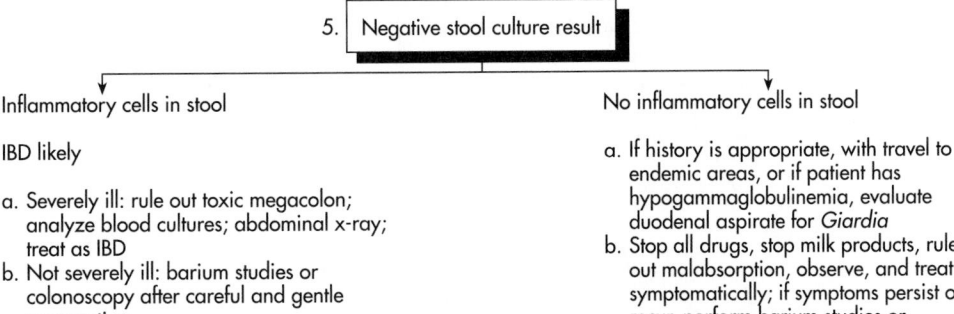

5. Negative stool culture result

Inflammatory cells in stool

IBD likely

a. Severely ill: rule out toxic megacolon;
 analyze blood cultures; abdominal x-ray;
 treat as IBD
b. Not severely ill: barium studies or
 colonoscopy after careful and gentle
 preparation

No inflammatory cells in stool

a. If history is appropriate, with travel to
 endemic areas, or if patient has
 hypogammaglobulinemia, evaluate
 duodenal aspirate for *Giardia*
b. Stop all drugs, stop milk products, rule
 out malabsorption, observe, and treat
 symptomatically; if symptoms persist or
 recur, perform barium studies or
 colonoscopy

Fig. 3-51   Diagnostic steps in the assessment of acute diarrhea. *IBD,* Inflammatory bowel
disease; *IBS,* irritable bowel syndrome. (From Stein JH [ed]: *Internal medicine,* ed 5, St Louis, 1998,
Mosby.)

III

DIARRHEA, CHRONIC

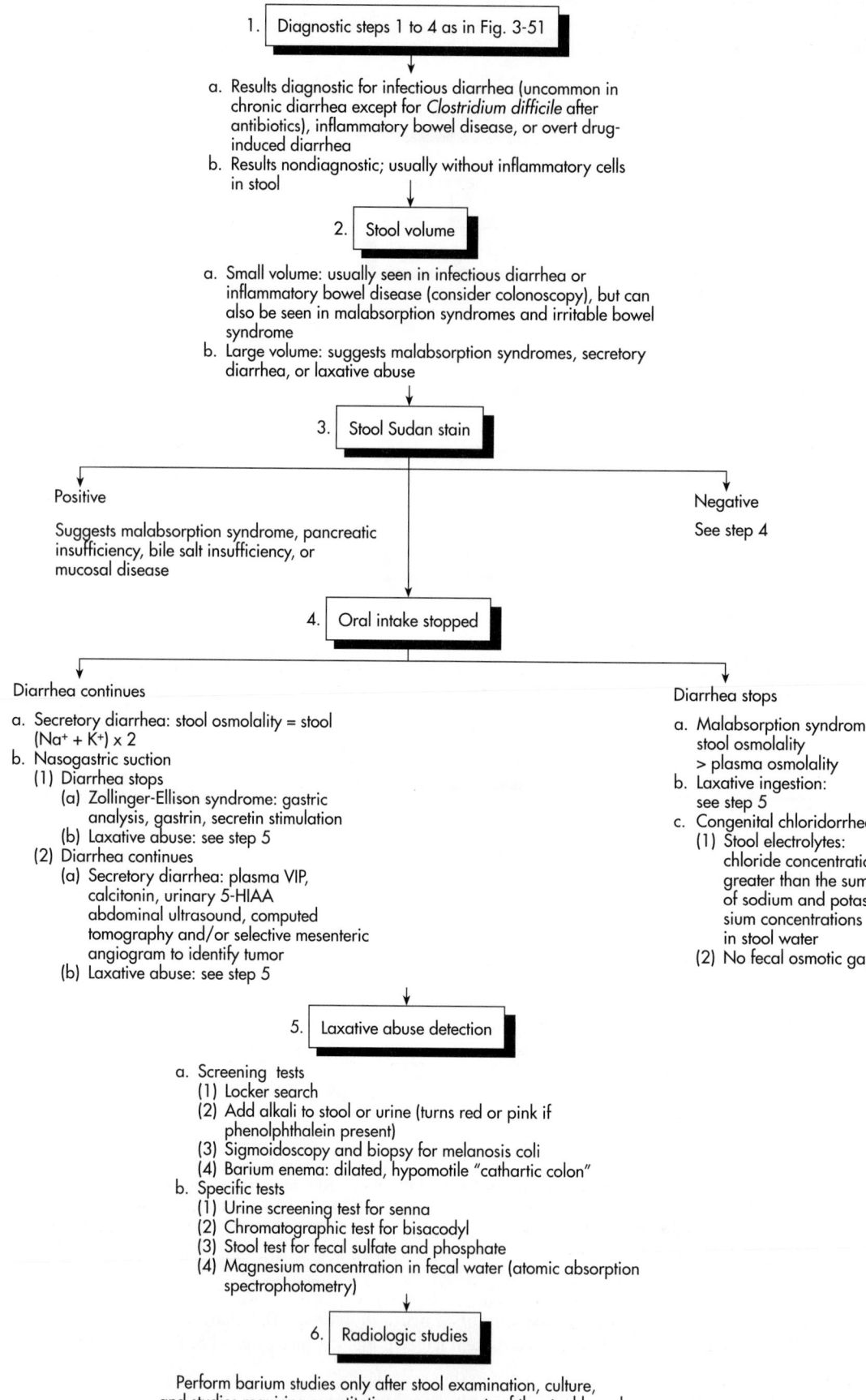

Fig. 3-52 **Diagnostic approach to the patient with chronic diarrhea.** *5-HIAA,* 5-Hydroxyin-doleacetic acid; *VIP,* vasoactive intestinal polypeptide. (From Stein JH [ed]: *Internal medicine,* ed 5, St Louis, 1998, Mosby.)

DIARRHEA, CHRONIC, IN PATIENTS WITH HIV INFECTION

Diarrhea, chronic, in patients with HIV infection
ICD-9CM # 787.1 Diarrhea, chronic

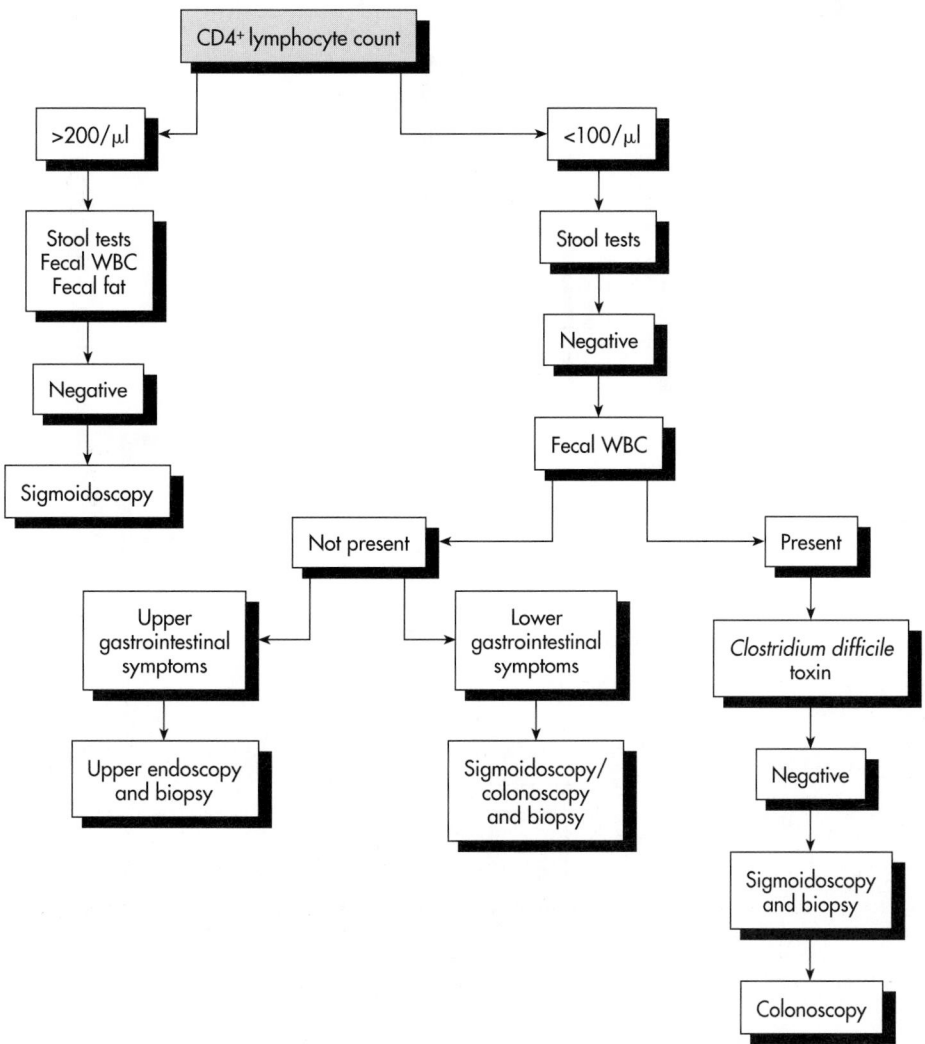

Fig. 3-53   Approach to evaluating chronic diarrhea in patients with HIV infection. *WBC,* White blood cell count. (From Wilcox CM: *Gastrointest Dis Today* 5:9, 1996.)

TABLE 3-5   Common Gastrointestinal Pathogens Associated With HIV Infection

PATHOGEN	CD4+ CELLS/μl	STOOL VOLUME AND FREQUENCY	ABDOMINAL PAIN	WEIGHT LOSS	FEVER	FECAL LEUKOCYTES
Cytomegalovirus*	<100	Mild to moderate	++	++	++	+
Cryptosporidiosis	<100	Moderate to severe	−	++	−	−
Microsporidiosis	<100	Mild to moderate	−	+	−	−
Mycobacterium avium complex†	<100	Mild to moderate	+	+++	+++	−

From Wilcox CM: *Gastrointest Dis Today* 5:9, 1996.
*Can have proctitis symptoms when involving the distal colon.
†Typical presentation is fever and wasting; diarrhea is usually secondary.
+++, Very common; ++, frequent; +, can occur; −, absent.

DILATED PUPIL

Dilated pupil
ICD9-CM # 379.43 Pupil dilation

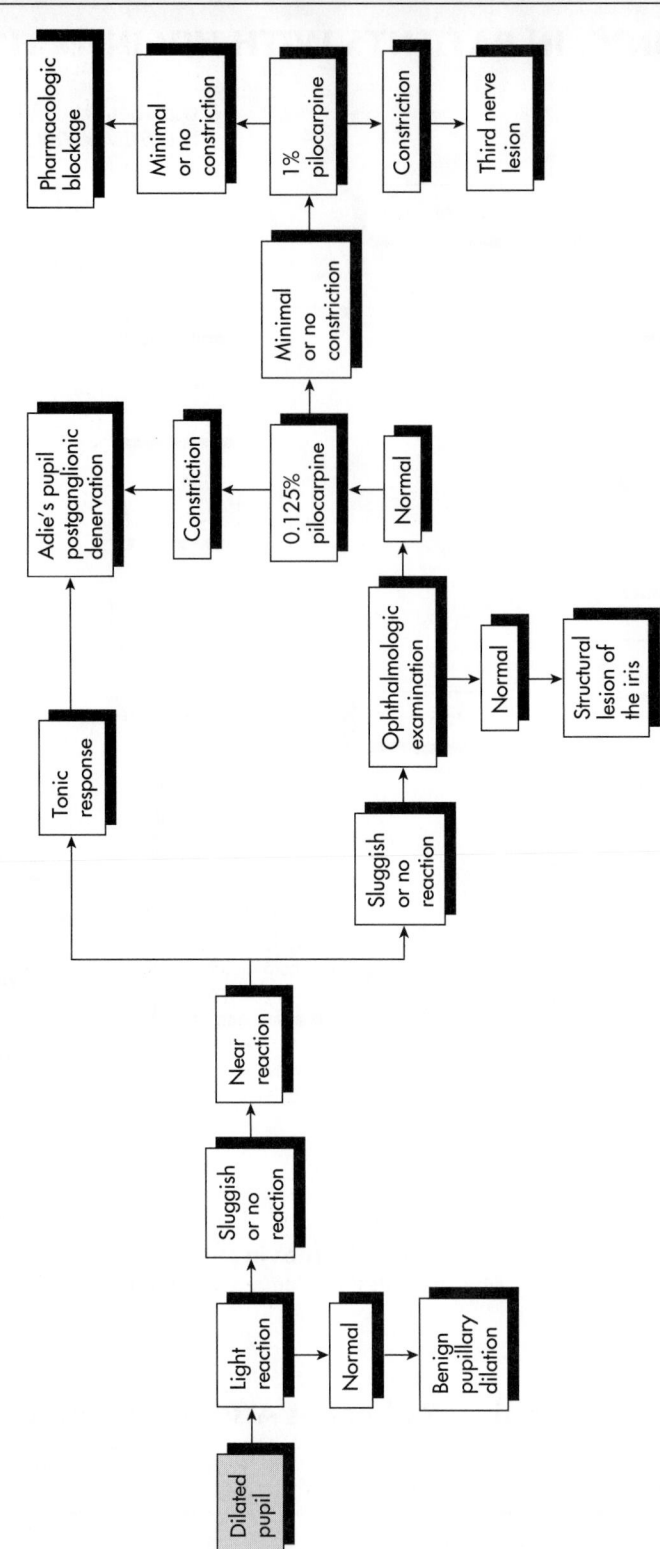

Fig. 3-54 Use of pilocarpine to help differentiate between different causes of a dilated pupil. (From Goldman L, Bennett JC [eds]: *Cecil textbook of medicine*, ed 21, Philadephia, 2000, WB Saunders.)

Domestic violence
ICD-9CM # 995.80 Adult maltreatment unspecified
       995.81 Adult physical abuse, battery
       995.82 Adult emotional/psychological
         abuse
       995.83 Adult sexual abuse
       995.84 Adult neglect (nutritional),
         desertion
       995.50 Child abuse, unspecified
       995.51 Child abuse, emotional/
         psychological
       995.52 Child neglect (nutritional),
         desertion
       995.53 Child abuse, sexual
       995.54 Child abuse, physical
       995.55 Shaken infant syndrome

DOMESTIC VIOLENCE

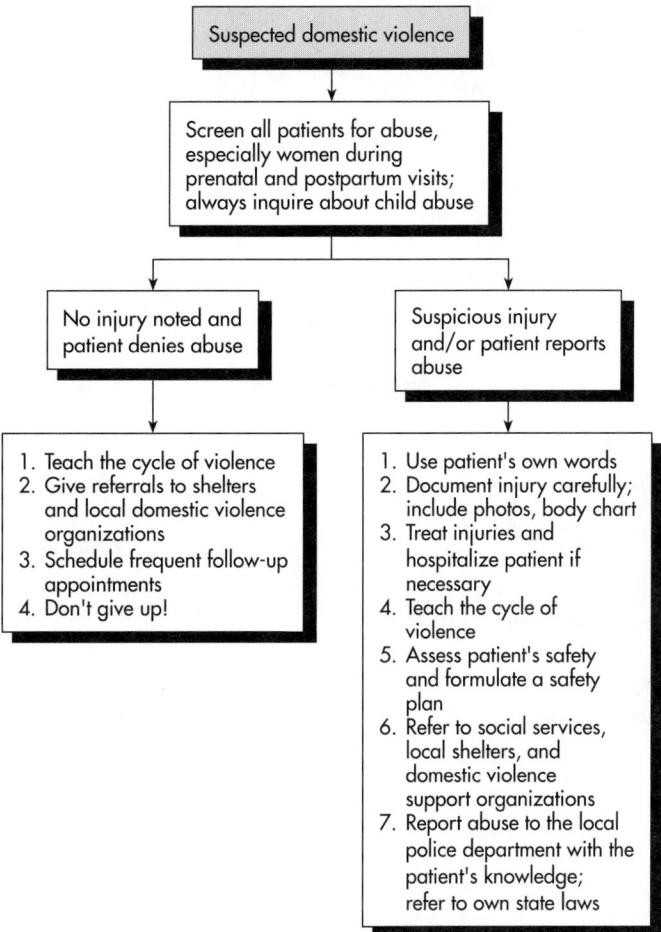

Fig. 3-55   Management of suspected domestic violence. (From Zuspan FP [ed]: *Handbook of obstetrics, gynecology, and primary care,* St Louis, 1998, Mosby.)

DYSPEPSIA

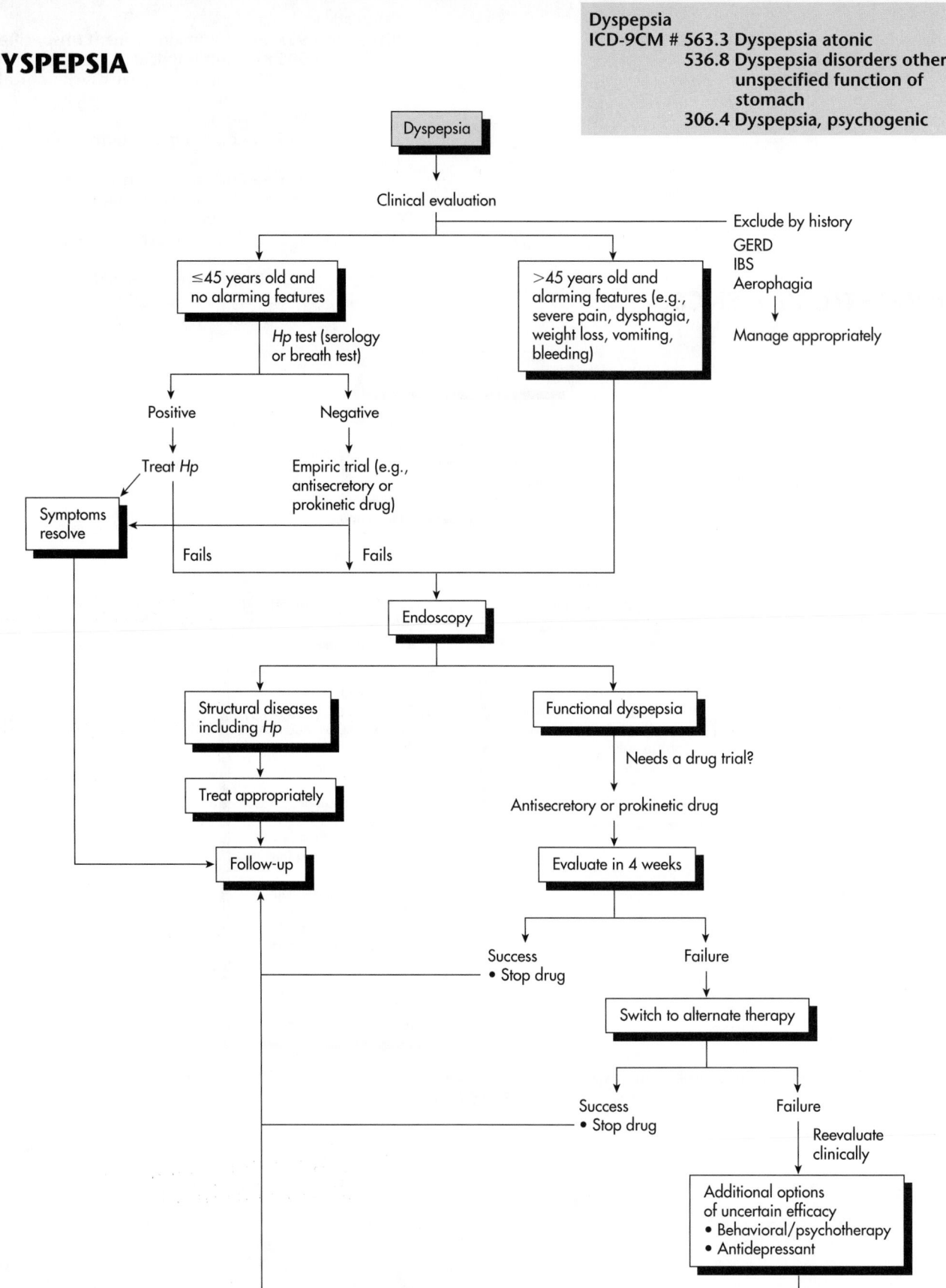

Dyspepsia
ICD-9CM # 563.3 Dyspepsia atonic
536.8 Dyspepsia disorders other
unspecified function of
stomach
306.4 Dyspepsia, psychogenic

Fig. 3-56   **Algorithm for the evaluation of dyspepsia.** *GERD,* Symptomatic gastroesophageal reflux disease; *Hp,* Helicobacter pylori; *IBS,* irritable bowel syndrome. (From Goldman L, Bennet JC [eds]: *Cecil textbook of medicine,* ed 21, Philadelphia, 2000, WB Saunders.)

DYSPHAGIA

Dysphagia
ICD-9CM # 787.2

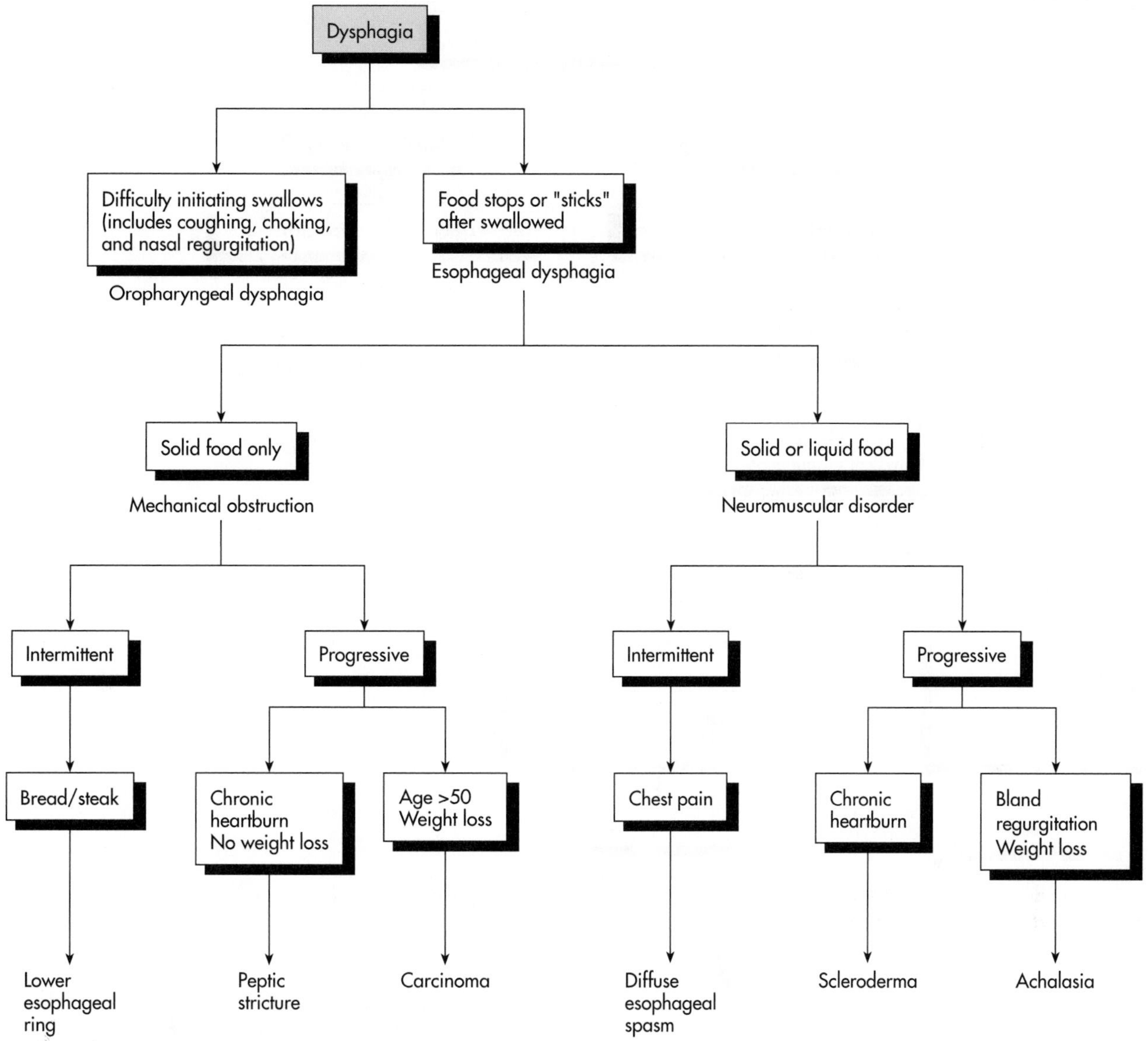

Fig. 3-57 **Differential diagnosis of dysphagia.** (From Andreoli TE [ed]: *Cecil essentials of medicine,* ed 5, Philadelphia, 2001, WB Saunders.)

Gwendolyn R. Lee, M.D.
Internal Medicine

DYSPNEA, ACUTE

Dyspnea, acute
ICD-9CM # 786.00

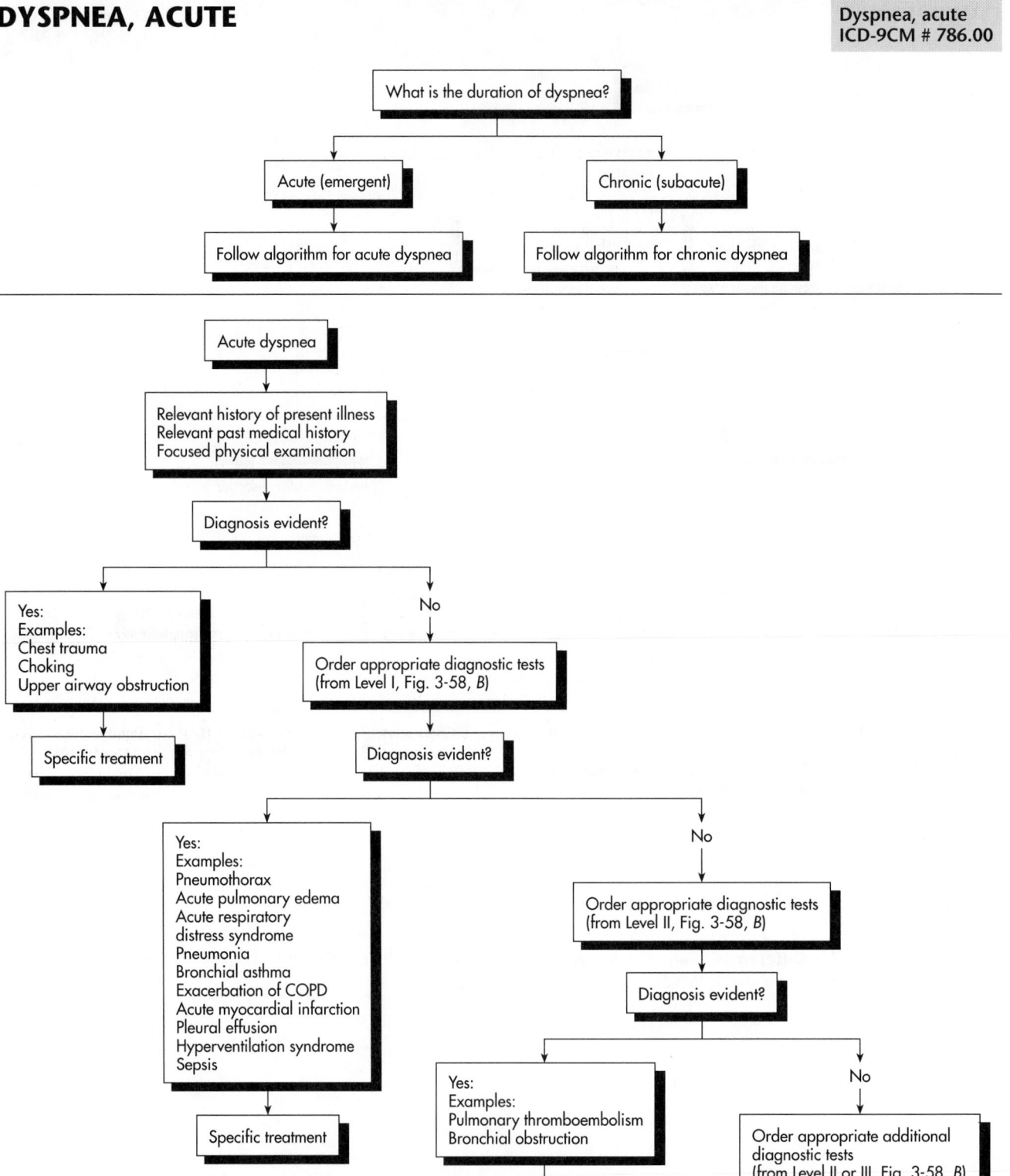

Fig. 3-58   A, Evaluation of the patient with dyspnea. *COPD,* Chronic obstructive pulmonary disease. (From Stein J [ed]: *Internal medicine,* ed 5, St Louis, 1998, Mosby.)

DYSPNEA, ACUTE—cont'd

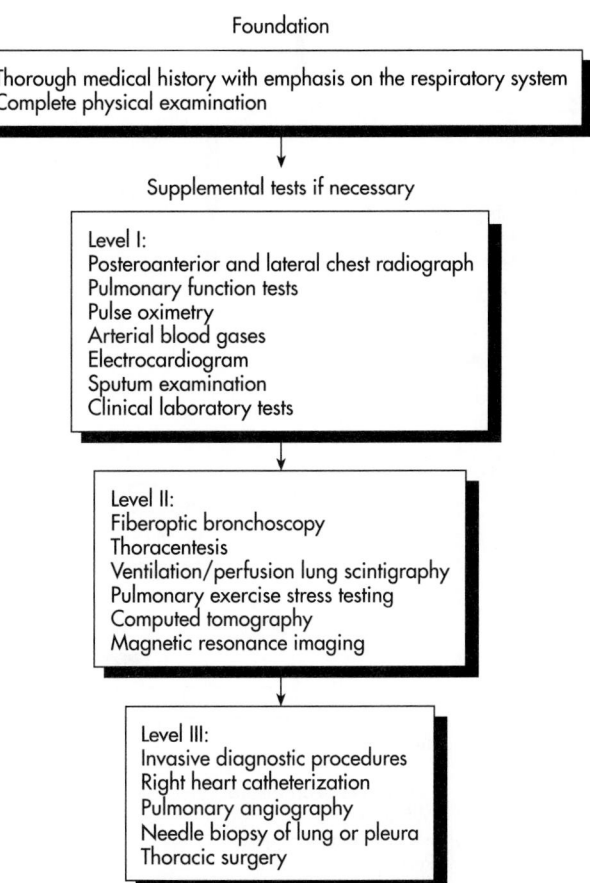

Foundation

Thorough medical history with emphasis on the respiratory system
Complete physical examination

Supplemental tests if necessary

Level I:
Posteroanterior and lateral chest radiograph
Pulmonary function tests
Pulse oximetry
Arterial blood gases
Electrocardiogram
Sputum examination
Clinical laboratory tests

Level II:
Fiberoptic bronchoscopy
Thoracentesis
Ventilation/perfusion lung scintigraphy
Pulmonary exercise stress testing
Computed tomography
Magnetic resonance imaging

Level III:
Invasive diagnostic procedures
Right heart catheterization
Pulmonary angiography
Needle biopsy of lung or pleura
Thoracic surgery

Fig. 3-58, cont'd   B, Medical history and physical examination are the foundation for the diagnosis of respiratory system disease. Diagnostic tests of increasing levels of complexity and invasiveness are performed if necessary to supplement the initial history and physical examination. (From Stein J [ed]: *Internal medicine,* ed 5, St Louis, 1998, Mosby.)

III

DYSPNEA, CHRONIC

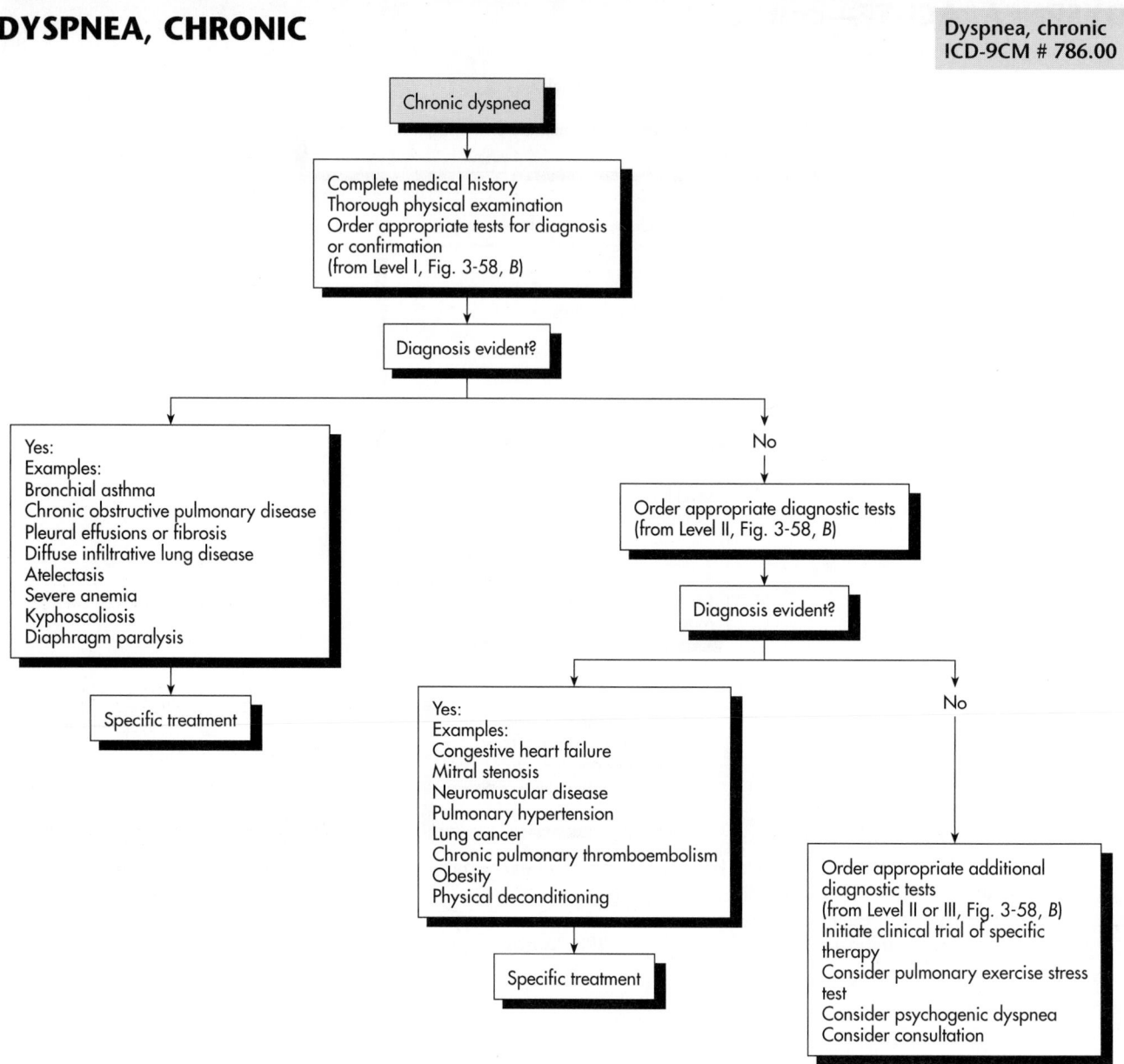

Fig. 3-59   **Chronic dyspnea.** (From Stein J [ed]: *Internal medicine,* ed 5, St Louis, 1998, Mosby.)

DYSURIA AND/OR URETHRAL/VAGINAL DISCHARGE

Dysuria and/or urethral/vaginal discharge
ICD-9CM # 788.1 Dysuria
788.7 Urethral discharge
623.5 Vaginal discharge

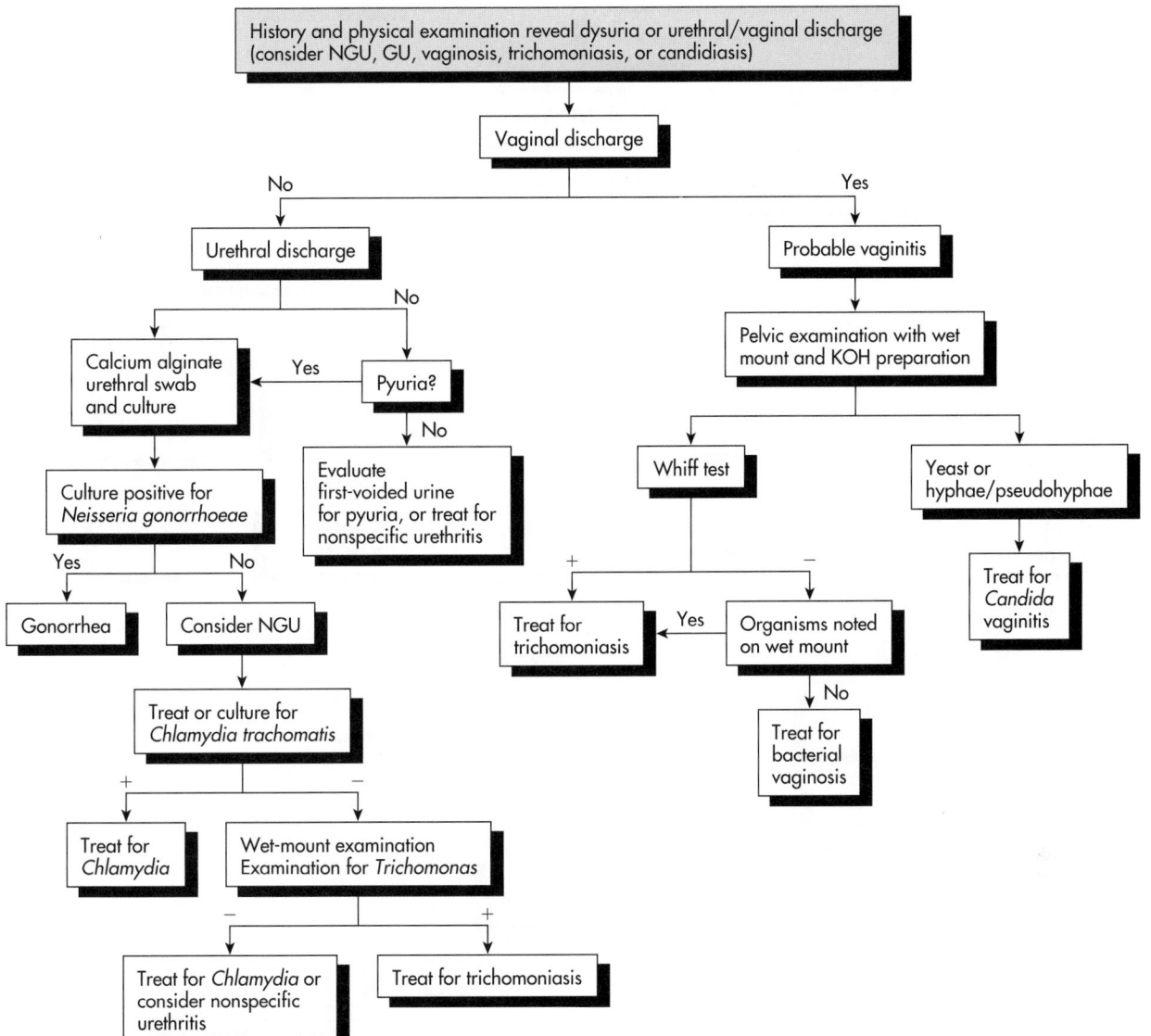

Fig. 3-60　Evaluation of patients with dysuria and/or urethral/vaginal discharge. *GU,* Gonococcal urethritis; *KOH,* potassium hydroxide; *NGU,* nongonococcal urethritis. (From Nseyo UO [ed]: *Urology for primary care physicians,* Philadelphia, 1999, WB Saunders.)

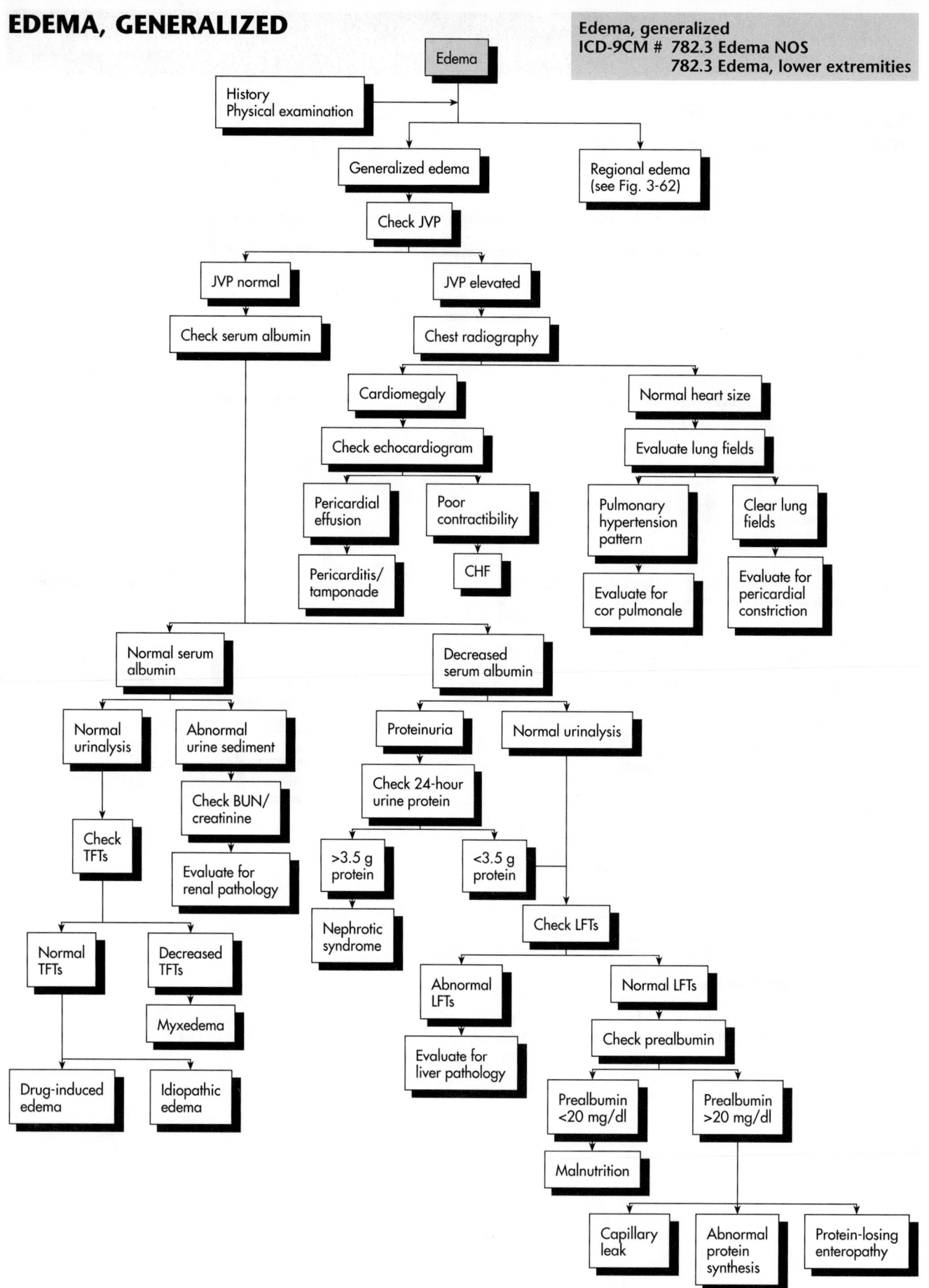

Fig. 3-61   Evaluation of generalized edema. *BUN,* Blood urea nitrogen; *CHF,* congestive heart failure; *JVP,* jugular venous pressure; *LFT,* liver function tests; *TFT,* thyroid function tests. (From Greene HL, Johnson WP, Lemcke D [eds]: *Decision making in medicine,* ed 2, St Louis, 1998, Mosby.)

EDEMA, REGIONAL

Edema, regional
ICD-9CM # 782.3   Edema, lower extremities
629.8   Edema, genitalia, female
608.86 Edema, genitalia, male
376.33 Edema, orbital
518.4   Edema, pulmonary, acute
514   Edema, pulmonary, chronic
782.3   Edema, unknown etiology

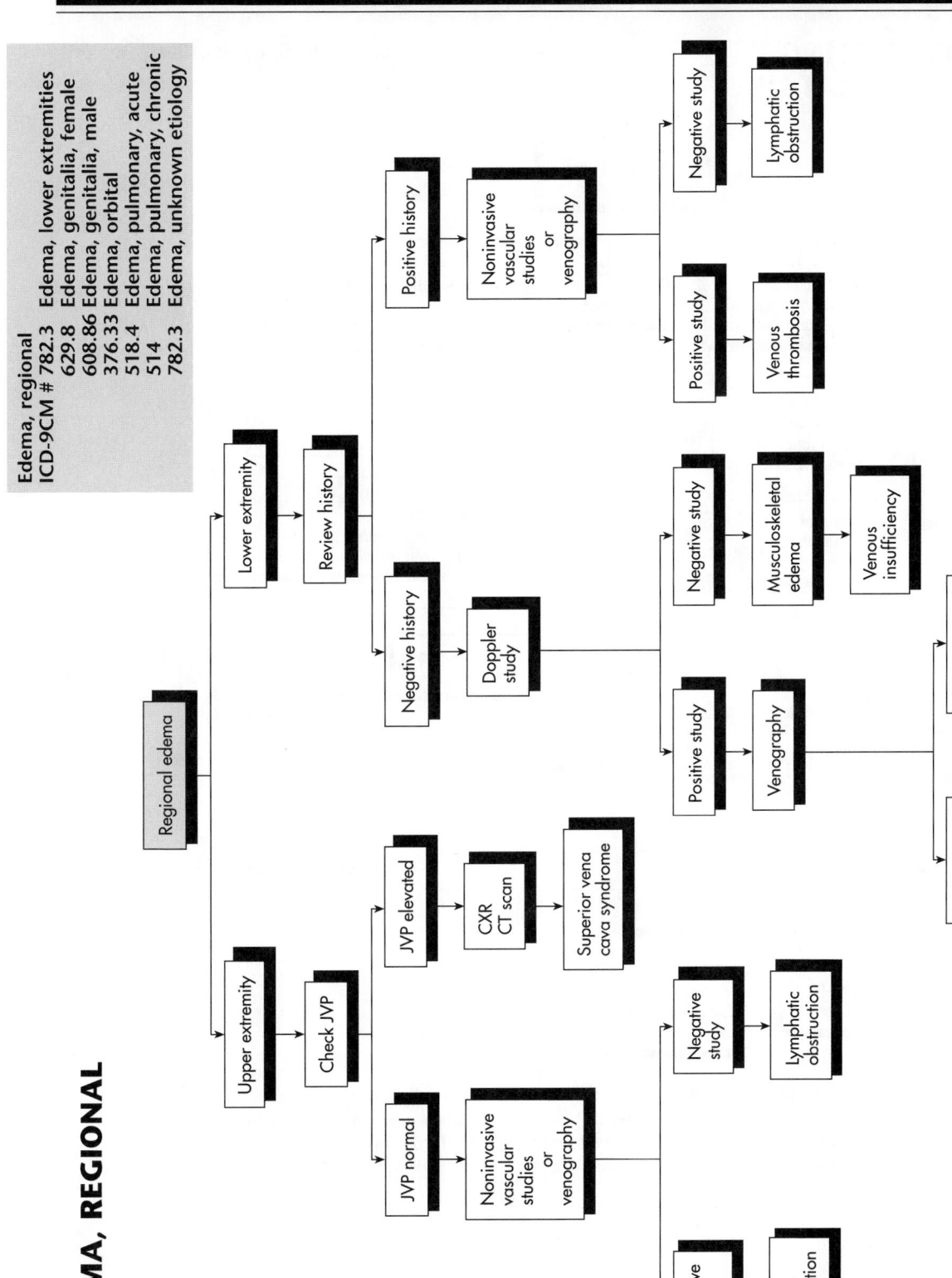

Fig. 3-62   Evaluation of regional edema. *CT,* Computed tomography; *CXR,* chest x-ray examination; *JVP,* jugular venous pressure. (From Greene HL, Johnson WP, Lemcke D [eds]: *Decision making in medicine,* ed 2, St Louis, 1998, Mosby.)

III

ENURESIS AND VOIDING DYSFUNCTION, PEDIATRIC

Enuresis and voiding dysfunction, pediatric
ICD-9CM # 788.30

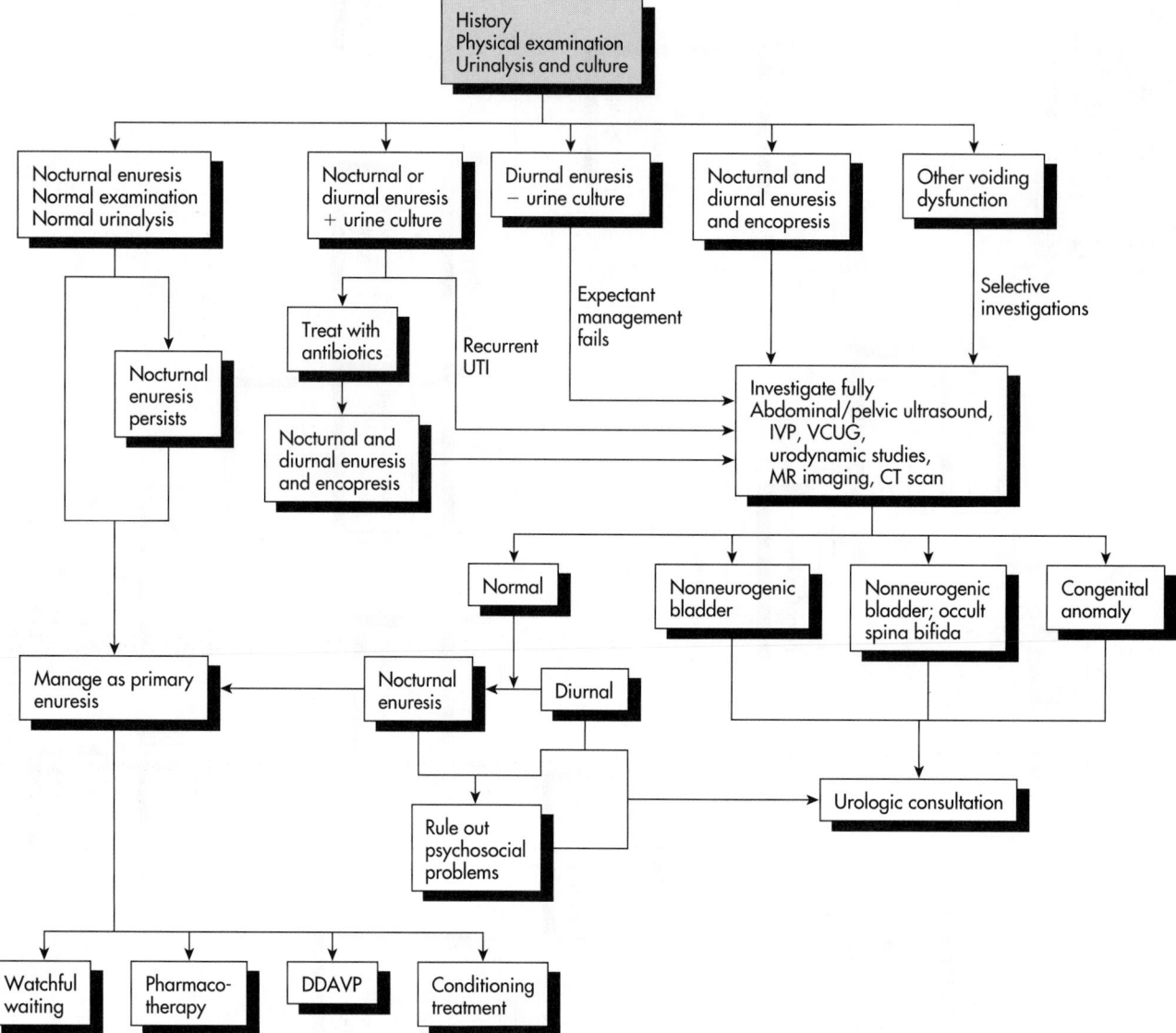

Fig. 3-63   Algorithm of management of pediatric enuresis and voiding dysfunction. *CT,* Computed tomography; *DDAVP,* desmopressin acetate; *IVP,* intravenous pyelogram; *MR,* magnetic resonance; *UTI,* urinary tract infection; *VCUG,* voiding cystourethrogram. (From Nseyo UO [ed]: *Urology for pirmary care physicians,* Philadelphia, 1999, WB Saunders.)

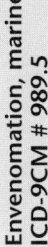

ENVENOMATION, MARINE

Envenomation, marine
ICD-9CM # 989.5

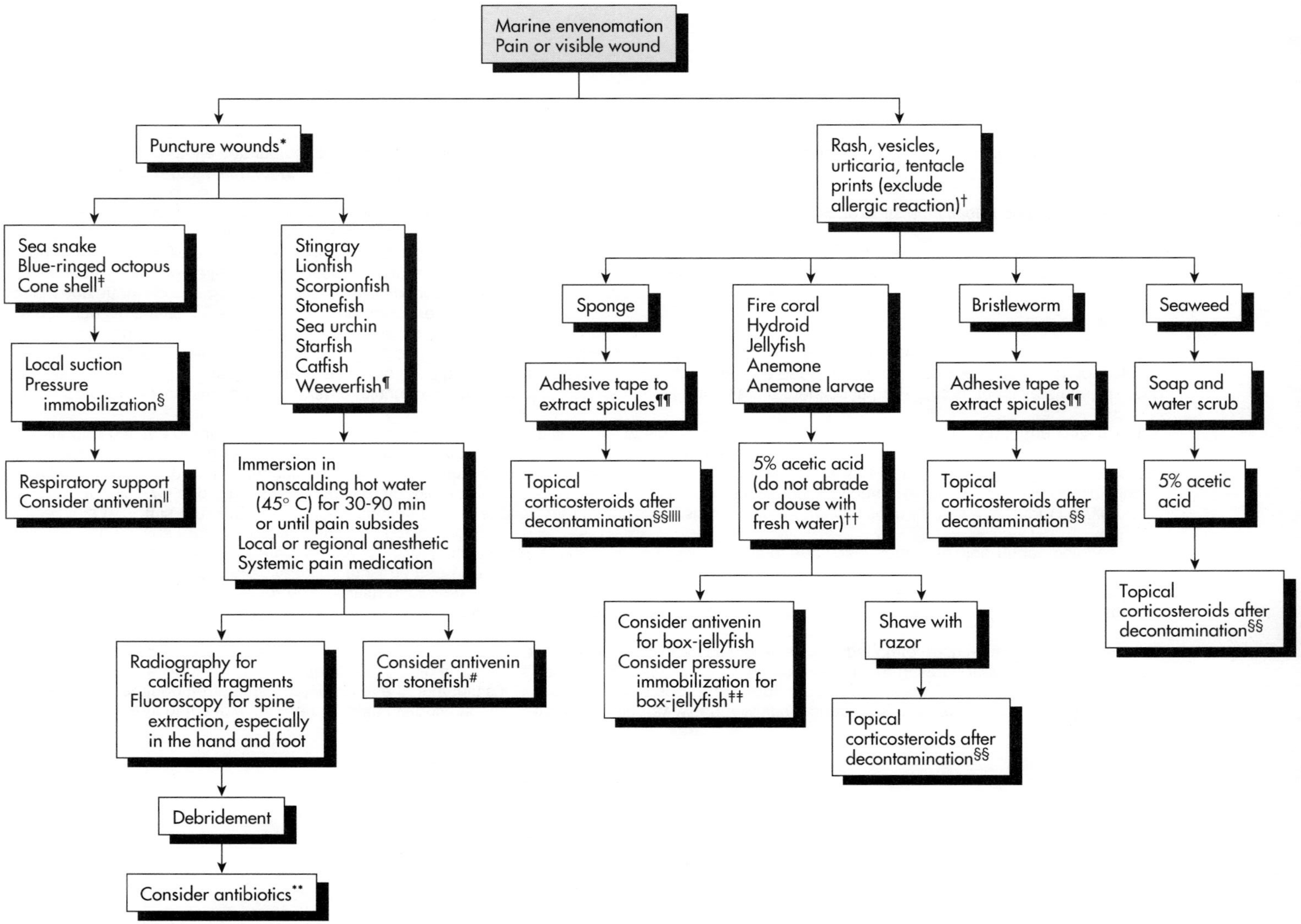

Marine envenomation
Pain or visible wound

Puncture wounds*

Sea snake
Blue-ringed octopus
Cone shell‡

→ Local suction
Pressure immobilization§

→ Respiratory support
Consider antivenin‖

Stingray
Lionfish
Scorpionfish
Stonefish
Sea urchin
Starfish
Catfish
Weeverfish¶

→ Immersion in nonscalding hot water (45° C) for 30-90 min or until pain subsides
Local or regional anesthetic
Systemic pain medication

→ Consider antivenin for stonefish#

→ Radiography for calcified fragments
Fluoroscopy for spine extraction, especially in the hand and foot

→ Debridement

→ Consider antibiotics**

Rash, vesicles, urticaria, tentacle prints (exclude allergic reaction)†

Sponge

→ Adhesive tape to extract spicules¶¶

→ Topical corticosteroids after decontamination§§‖‖

Fire coral
Hydroid
Jellyfish
Anemone
Anemone larvae

→ 5% acetic acid (do not abrade or douse with fresh water)††

→ Shave with razor

→ Topical corticosteroids after decontamination§§

→ Consider antivenin for box-jellyfish
Consider pressure immobilization for box-jellyfish##

Bristleworm

→ Adhesive tape to extract spicules¶¶

→ Topical corticosteroids after decontamination§§

Seaweed

→ Soap and water scrub

→ 5% acetic acid

→ Topical corticosteroids after decontamination§§

Fig. 3-64 Algorithmic approach to marine envenomation. (From Auerbach PS: *Wilderness medicine,* ed 4, St Louis, 2001, Mosby.)

Continued

III

*A gaping laceration, particularly of the lower extremity, with cyanotic edges suggests a stingray wound. Multiple punctures in an erratic pattern with or without purple discoloration or retained fragments are typical of a sea urchin sting. One to eight (usually two) fang marks are usually present after a sea snake bite. A single ischemic puncture wound with an erythematous halo and rapid swelling suggests scorpionfish envenomation. Blisters often accompany a lionfish sting. Painless punctures with paralysis suggest the bite of a blue-ringed octopus; the site of a cone shell sting is punctate, painful, and ischemic in appearance.

†Wheal and flare reactions are nonspecific. Rapid (within 24 hours) onset of skin necrosis suggests an anemone sting. "Tentacle prints" with cross-hatching or a frosted appearance are pathognomonic for box-jellyfish (*Chironex fleckeri*) envenomation. Ocular or intraoral lesions may be caused by fragmented hydroids or coelenterate tentacles. An allergic reaction must be treated promptly.

‡Sea snake venom causes weakness, respiratory paralysis, myoglobinuria, myalgias, blurred vision, vomiting, and dysphagia. The blue-ringed octopus injects tetrodotoxin, which causes rapid neuromuscular paralysis.

§If *immediately* available (which is rarely the case), local suction can be applied without incision using a plunger device, such as The Extractor (Sawyer Products, Safety Harbor, Fla.). As soon as possible, venom should be sequestered locally with a proximal venous-lymphatic occlusive band of constriction or (preferably) the pressure immobilization technique, in which a cloth pad is compressed directly over the wound by an elastic wrap that should encompass the entire extremity at a pressure of 9.33 kPa (70 mm Hg) or less. Incision and suction are not recommended.

‖Early ventilatory support has the greatest influence on outcome. The minimal initial dose of sea snake antivenin is one to three vials; up to ten vials may be required.

¶The wounds range from large lacerations (stingrays) to minute punctures (stonefish). Persistent pain after immersion in hot water suggests a stonefish sting or a retained fragment of spine. The puncture site can be identified by forcefully injecting 1% to 2% lidocaine or another local anesthetic agent without epinephrine near the wound and observing the egress of fluid. Do not attempt to crush the spines of sea urchins if they are present in the wound. Spine dye from already-extracted sea urchin spines will disappear (be absorbed) in 24 to 36 hours.

#The initial dose of stonefish antivenin is one vial per two puncture wounds.

**The antibiotics chosen should cover *Staphylococcus*, *Streptococcus*, and microbes of marine origin, such as *Vibrio*.

††Acetic acid 5% (vinegar) is a good all-purpose decontaminant and is mandated for the sting from a box-jellyfish. Alternatives, depending on the geographic region and indigenous jellyfish species, include isopropyl alcohol, bicarbonate (baking soda), ammonia, papain, and preparations containing these agents.

‡‡The initial dose of box-jellyfish antivenin is one ampule intravenously or three ampules intramuscularly.

§§If inflammation is severe, steroids should be given systematically (beginning with at least 60 to 100 mg of prednisone or its equivalent) and the dose tapered over a period of 10 to 14 days.

‖‖An alternative is to apply and remove commercial facial peel materials.

¶¶An alternative is to apply and remove commercial facial peel materials followed by topical soaks of 30 ml of 5% acetic acid (vinegar) diluted in 1 L of water for 15 to 30 minutes several times a day until the lesions begin to resolve. Anticipate surface desquamation in 3 to 6 weeks.

ERYTHROCYTOSIS, ACQUIRED

Erythrocytosis, acquired
ICD-9CM # 289.0 Polycythemia, acquired

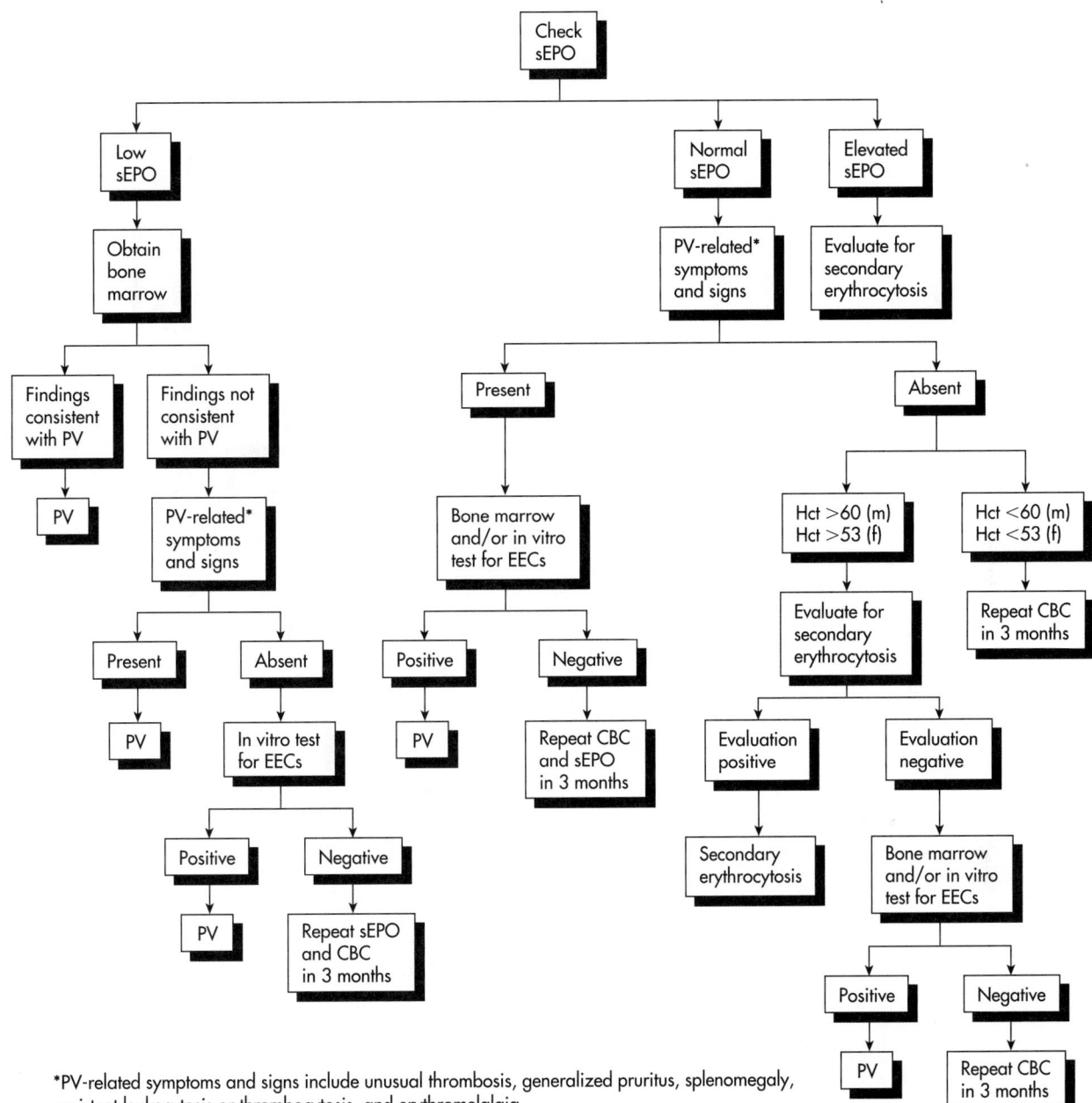

*PV-related symptoms and signs include unusual thrombosis, generalized pruritus, splenomegaly, peristent leukocytosis or thrombocytosis, and erythromelalgia.

Fig. 3-65   A diagnostic approach to acquired erythrocytosis. *CBC,* Complete blood cell count; *EEC,* endogenous (spontaneous) erythroid colonies; *f,* female; *Hct,* hematocrit; *m,* male; *PV,* poly-cythemia vera; *sEPO,* serum erythropoietin level. (From Goldman L, Bennett JC [eds]: *Cecil textbook of medicine,* ed 21, Philadelphia, 2000, WB Saunders.)

FATIGUE

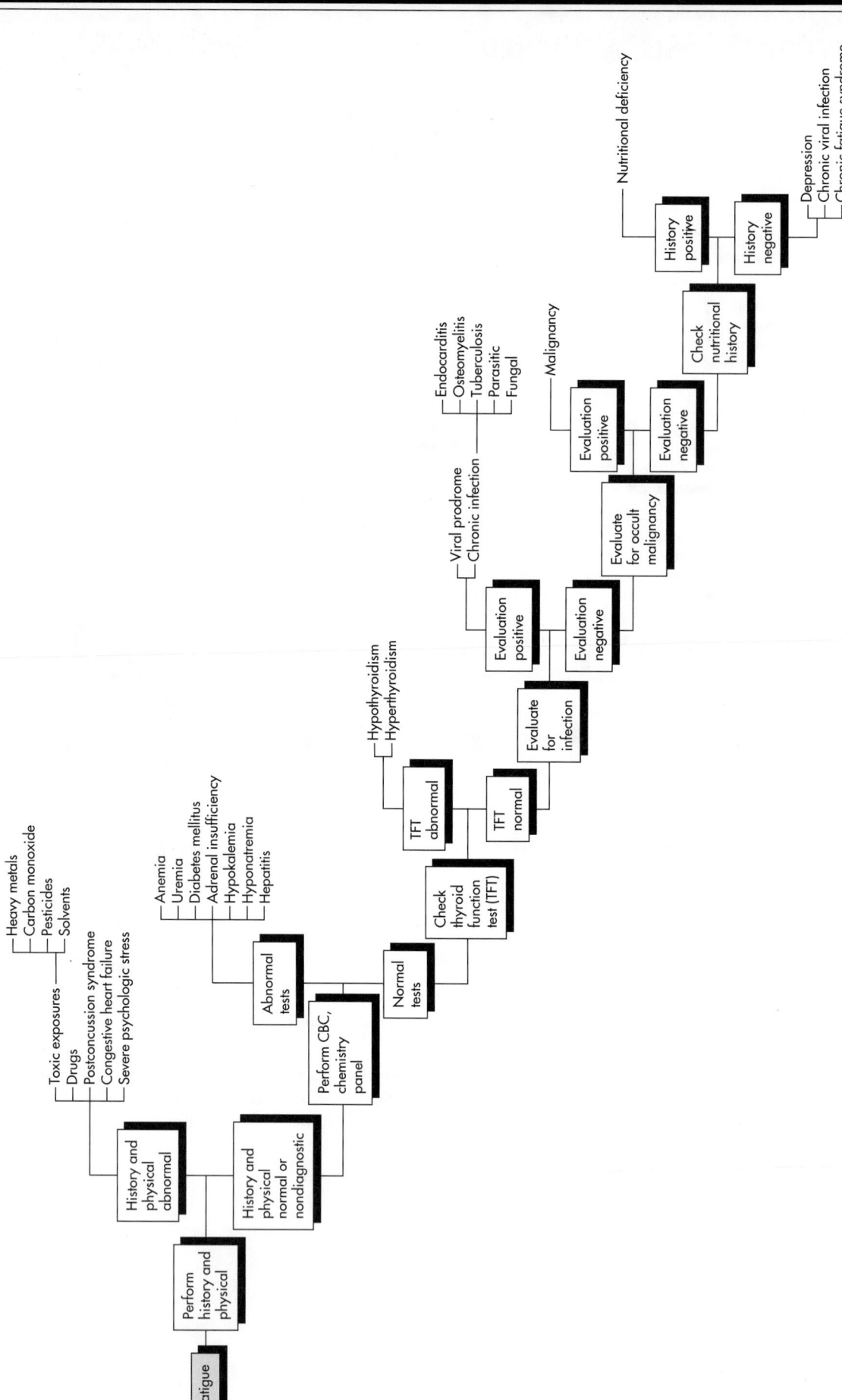

Fig. 3-66 Evaluation of fatigue. *CBC*, Complete blood count. (From Healey PM: *Common medical diagnosis: an algorithmic approach*, ed 3, Philadelphia, 2000, WB Saunders.)

FECAL OCCULT BLOOD EVALUATION

**Fecal occult blood evaluation
ICD-9CM # 792.1 Occult blood in stool**

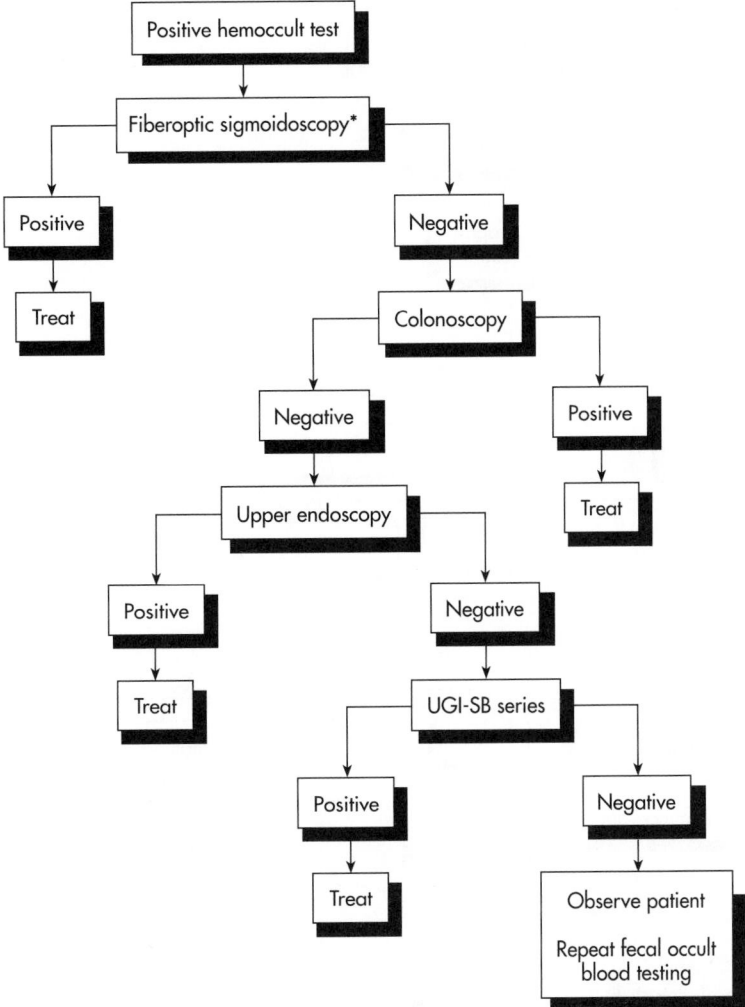

*Flexible sigmoidoscopy may be preferred as the initial study in patients under age 40 without risk factors for colon cancer. In older patients and in those with risk factors for colon cancer, colonoscopy should be the initial diagnostic study.

Fig. 3-67   Evaluation of asymptomatic patients with positive fecal occult blood. *UGI-SB,* Upper gastrointestinal–small bowel. (From Ferri FF: *Practical guide to the care of the medical patient,* ed 5, St Louis, 2001, Mosby.)

FRACTURE, BONE

Fracture, bone
ICD-9CM # 829.0 Fracture bone(s) NOS closed
829.1 Fracture bone(s) NOS open

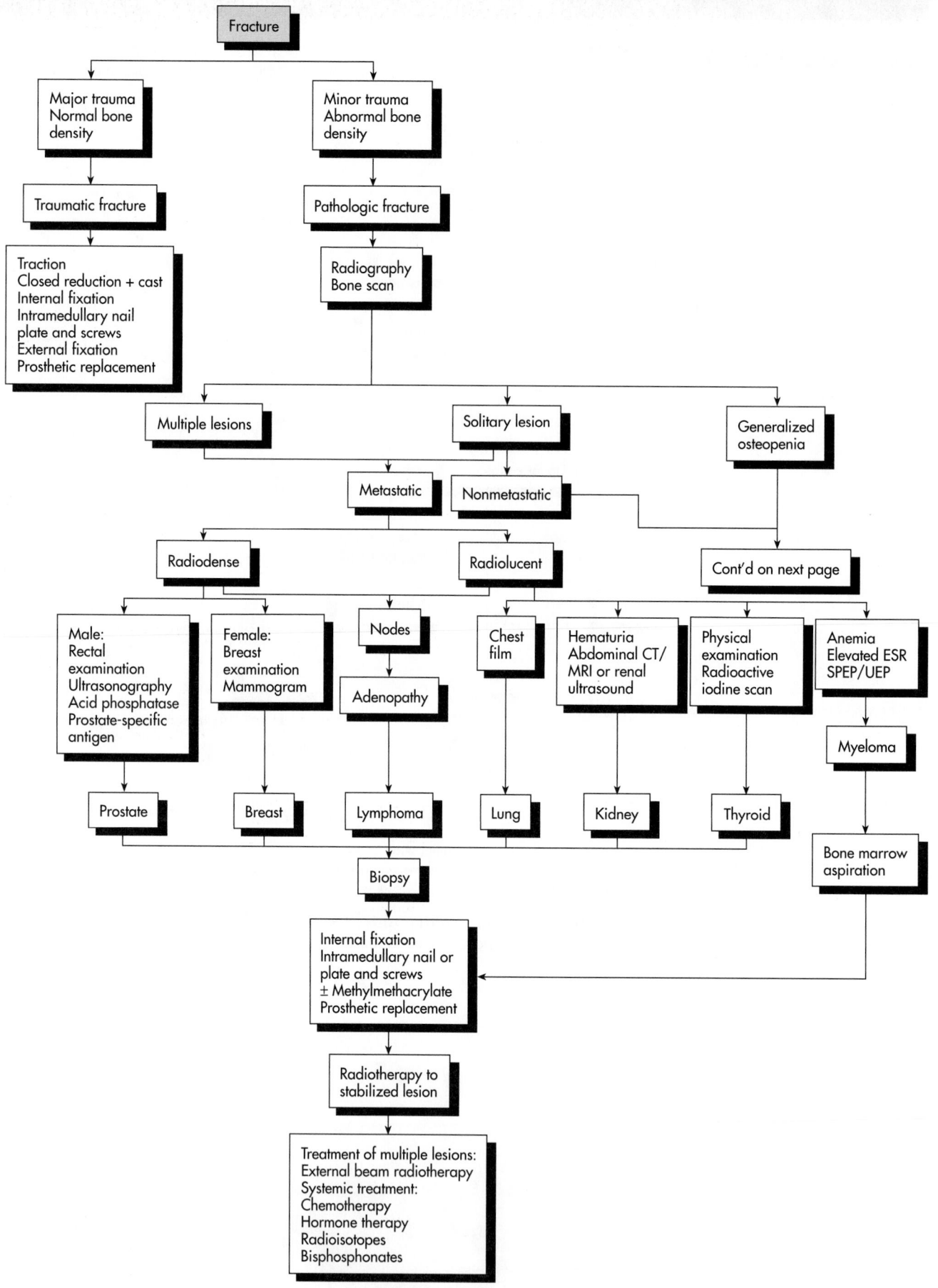

Fig. 3-68 **Bone fracture.** *CT,* Computed tomography; *ESR,* erythrocyte sedimentation rate; *MRI,* magnetic resonance imaging; *SPEP,* serum protein electrophoresis; *UEP,* urine electrophoresis. (From Greene HL, Johnson WP, Lemcke D [eds]: *Decision making in medicine,* ed 2, St Louis, 1998, Mosby.)

FRACTURE, BONE—cont'd

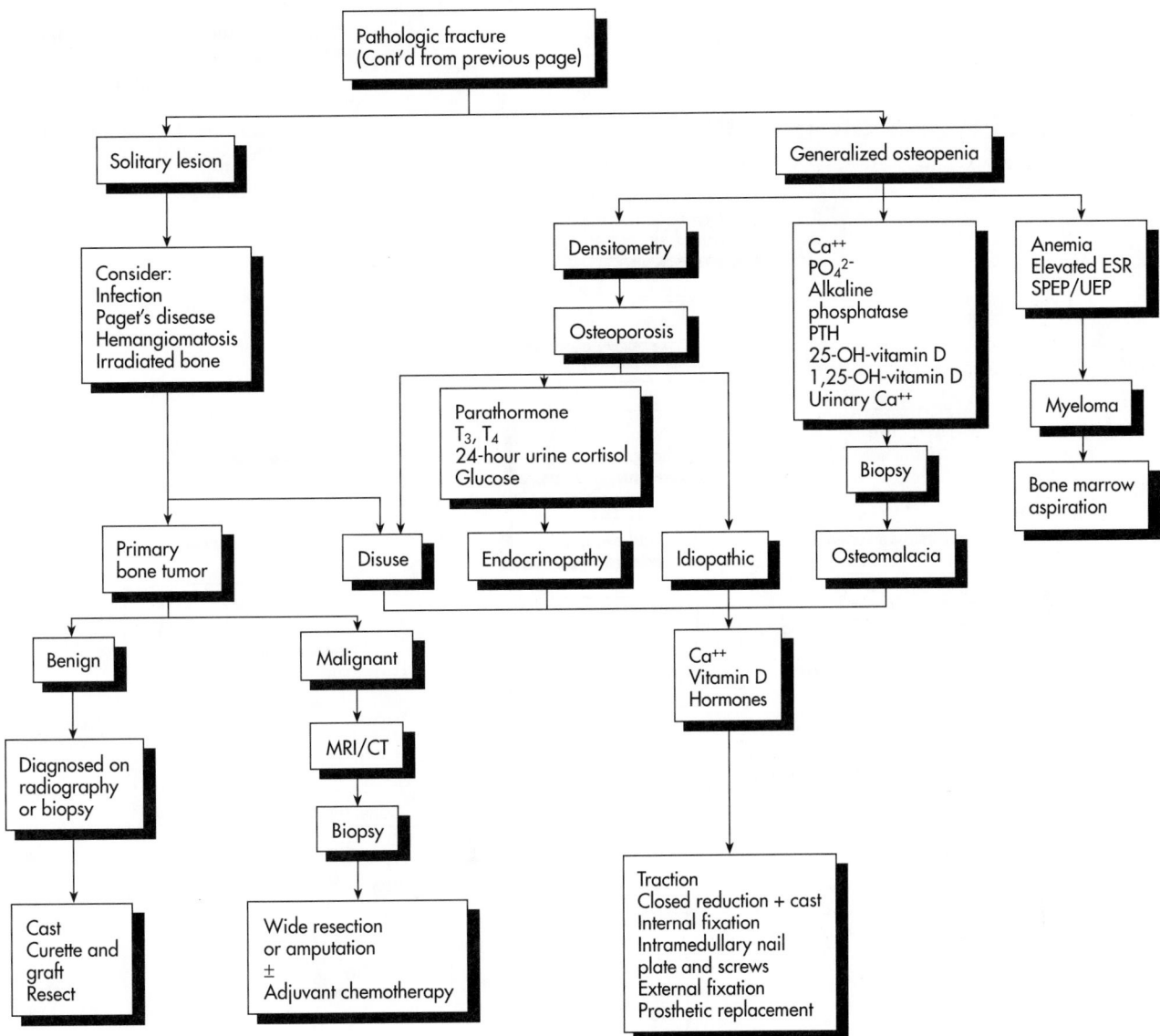

Fig. 3-68, cont'd

Genital sores
ICD-9CM # 054.10 Genital herpes
             91.0 Genital syphilis
             078.11 Condyloma acuminatum
             099.0 Chancroid
             099.2 Granuloma inguinale
             099.1 Lymphogranuloma venereum
             629.8 Ulcer, genital site, female
             608.89 Ulcer, genital site, male

GENITAL LESIONS OR ULCERS

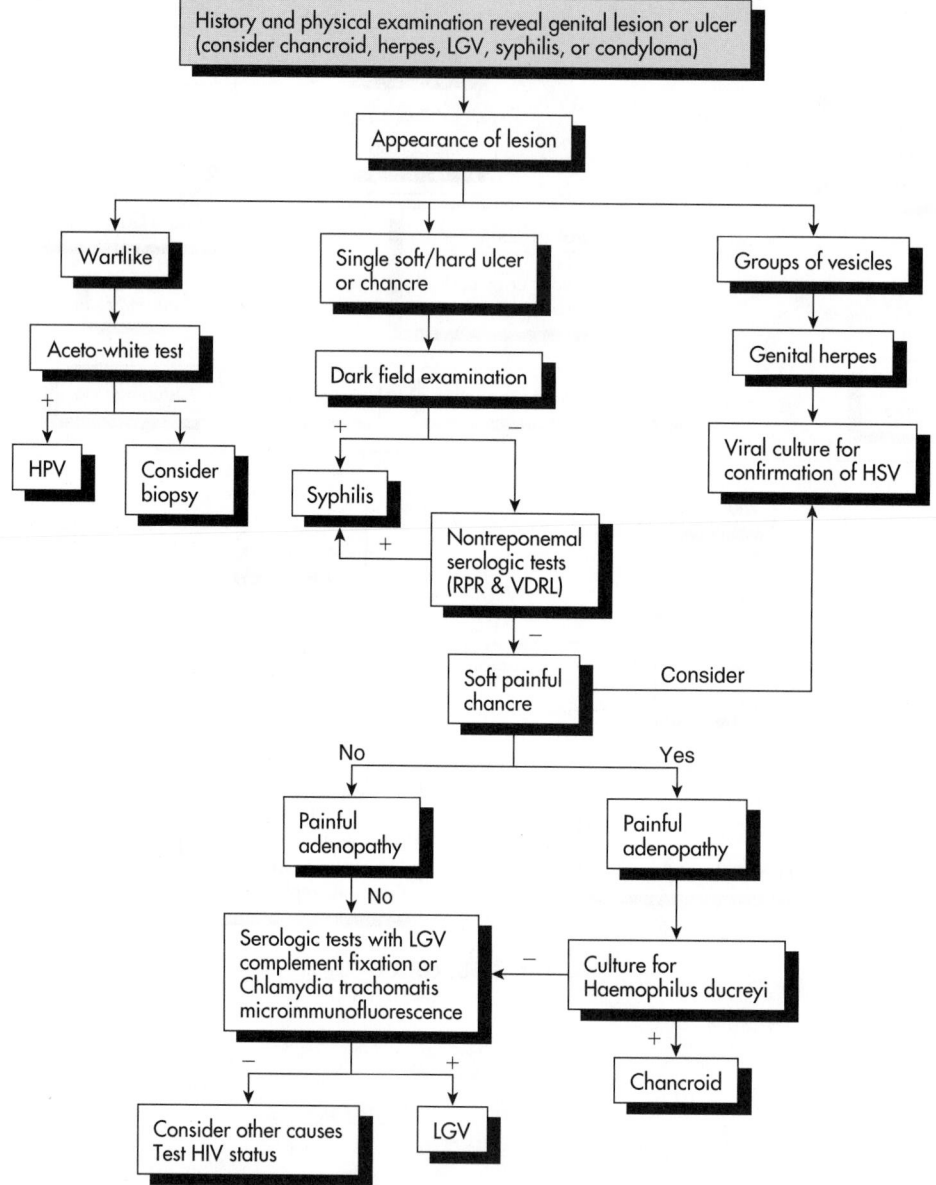

Fig. 3-69   Evaluation of patients with genital lesions or ulcers. *HIV,* Human immunodeficiency virus; *HPV,* human papillomavirus; *HSV,* herpes simplex virus; *LGV,* lymphogranuloma venereum; *RPR,* rapid plasma reagin; *VDRL,* Venereal Disease Research Laboratory. (From Nseyo UO [ed]: *Urology for primary care physicians,* Philadelphia, 1999, WB Saunders.)

GOITER EVALUATION AND MANAGEMENT

Goiter evaluation and management
ICD-9CM # 240.9 Goiter, unspecified
240.0 Goiter, simple
241.9 Goiter, adenomatous
246.1 Goiter, congenital
242.1 Goiter, uninodular with thyrotoxicosos
242.2 Goiter, multinodular with thyrotoxicosos

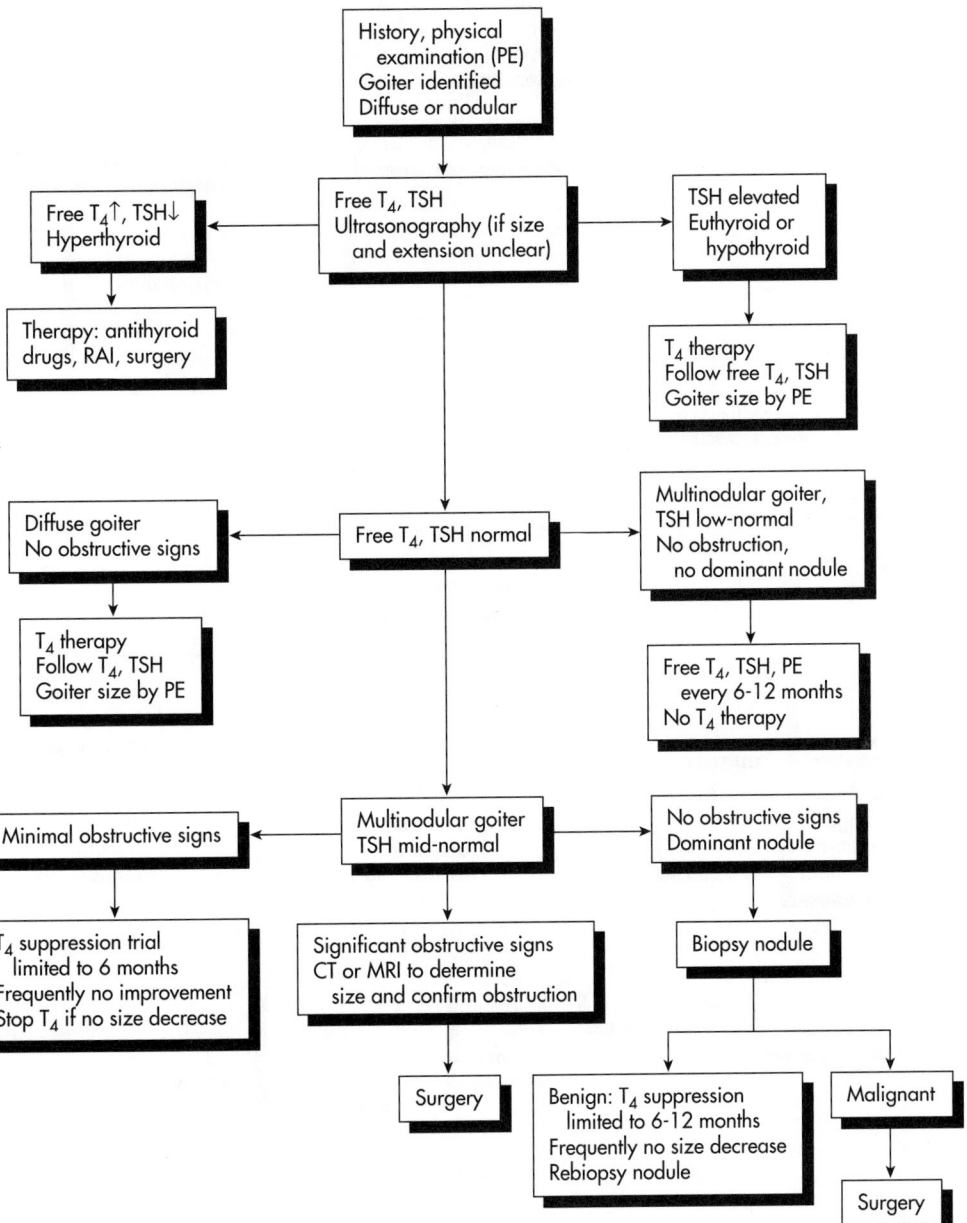

Fig. 3-70 *Evaluation and management of patients with nontoxic diffuse and nodular goiter and undetermined thyroid status.* *CT,* Computed tomography; *MRI,* magnetic resonance imaging; *RAI,* radioactive iodine; *TSH,* thyroid-stimulating hormone. (From Goldman L, Bennett JC [eds]: *Cecil textbook of medicine,* ed 21, Philadelphia, 2000, WB Saunders.)

GYNECOMASTIA

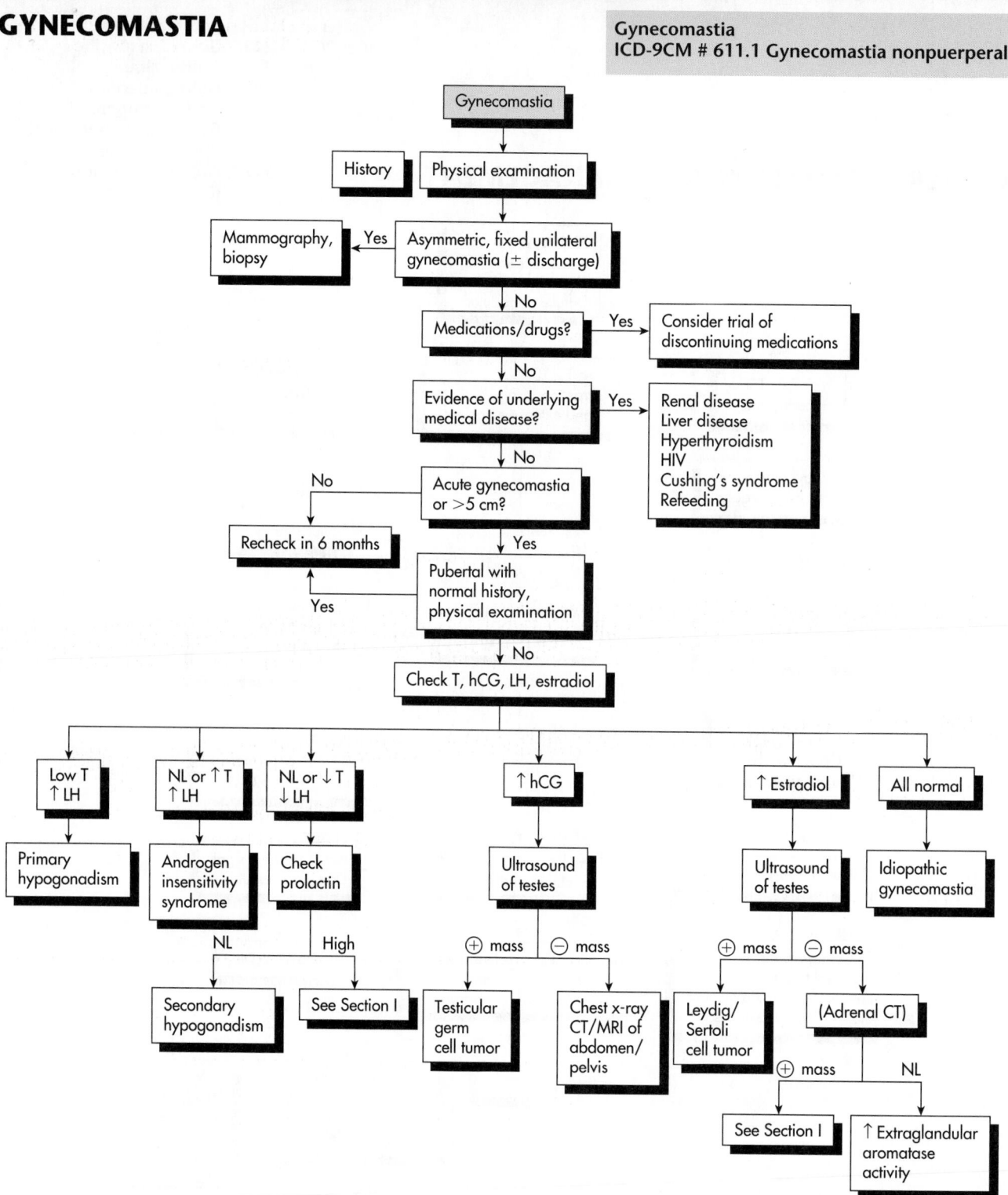

Fig. 3-71 Evaluation of gynecomastia. *CT,* Computed tomography; *hCG,* human chorionic gonadotropin; *HIV,* human immunodeficiency syndrome; *LH,* luteinizing hormone; *MRI,* magnetic resonance imaging; *NL,* normal limits; *T,* testosterone. (From Noble J: *Primary care medicine,* ed 3, St Louis, 2001, Mosby.)

HEAD INJURY

Head injury
ICD-9CM # 959.01 Head injury, NOS

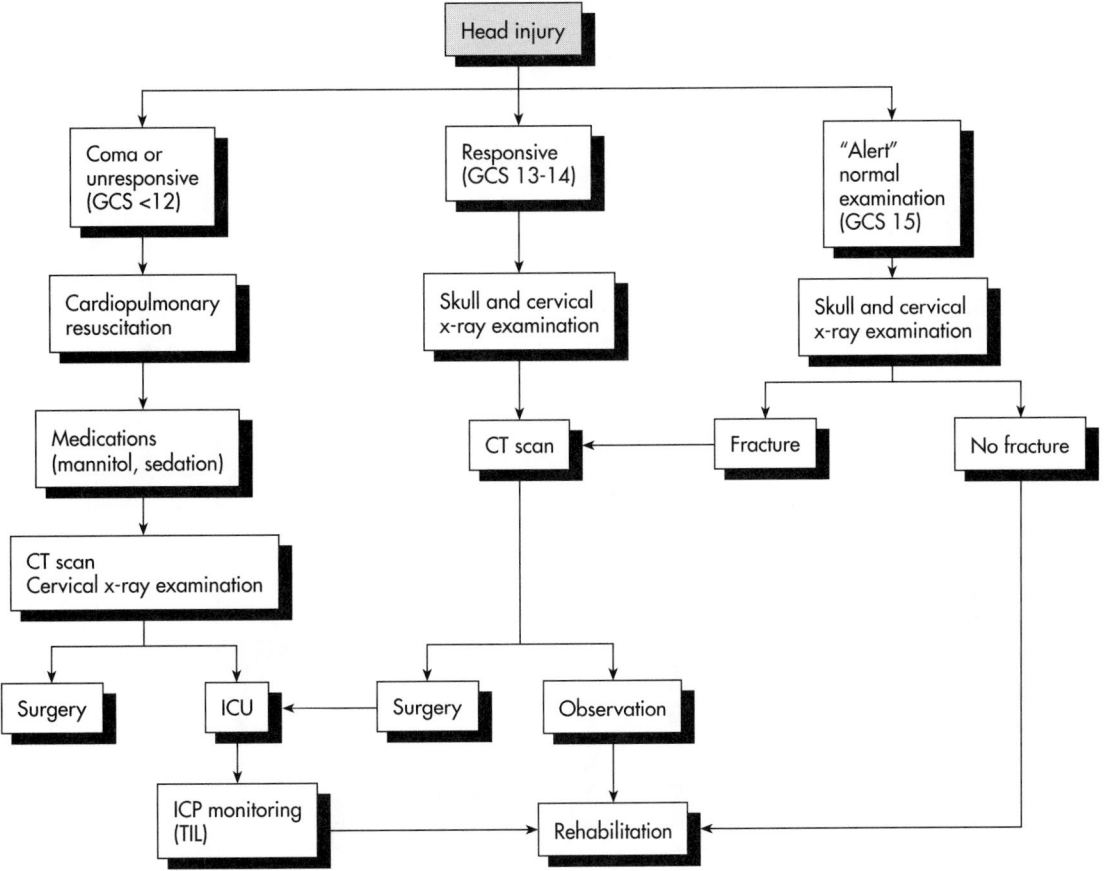

Fig. 3-72   Management of head injury. *CT,* Computed tomography; *GCS,* Glasgow Coma Scale score; *ICP,* intracranial pressure; *ICU,* intensive care unit; *TIL,* therapeutic intensity level. (From Johnson RT, Griffin JW: *Current therapy in neurologic disease,* ed 5, St Louis, 1997, Mosby.)

TABLE 3-6   Glasgow Coma Scale*

EYE OPENING	BEST MOTOR RESPONSE	BEST VERBAL RESPONSE	SCORE
No response	None	None	1
Opens with painful stimulus	Extension (decerebrate rigidity) with painful stimulus	Unintelligible sounds	2
Opens with verbal command	Flexion (decorticate rigidity) with painful stimulus	Use of inappropriate words	3
Opens spontaneously	Withdrawal from noxious stimulus	Confused, disoriented conversation	4
	Localization of pain, pushes away noxious stimulus	Oriented, able to converse	5
	Obeys simple verbal commands	Alert and oriented	6

*Total score is determined by adding the best score from each category (eye opening, best motor response, best verbal response). For example, a patient may:

Open eyes with verbal command	3
Obey simple verbal commands	6
Use inappropriate words	3
TOTAL SCORE	12

III

HEARING LOSS

Hearing loss
ICD-9CM # 389.00 Conductive NOS
389.10 Sensorineural NOS

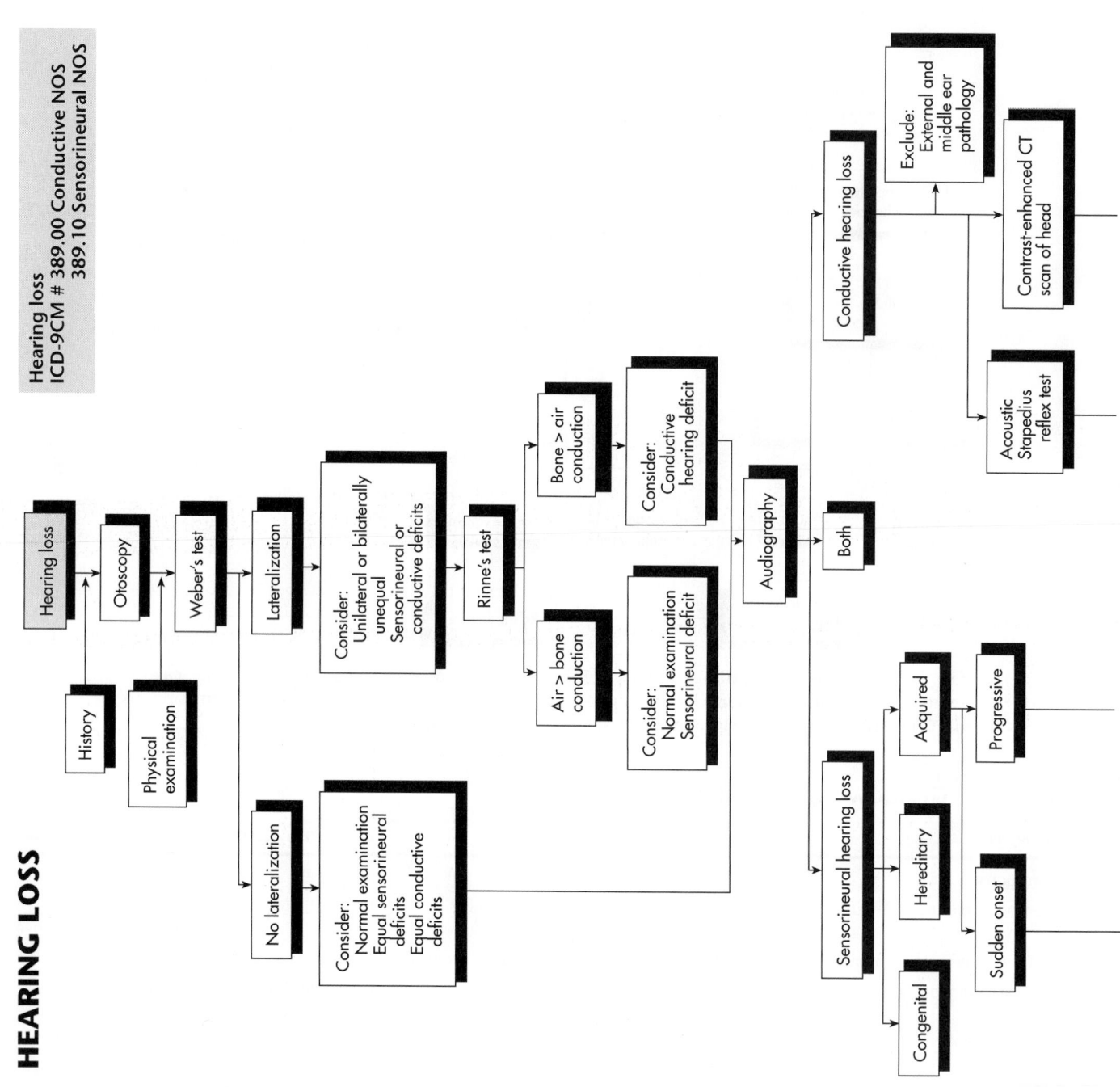

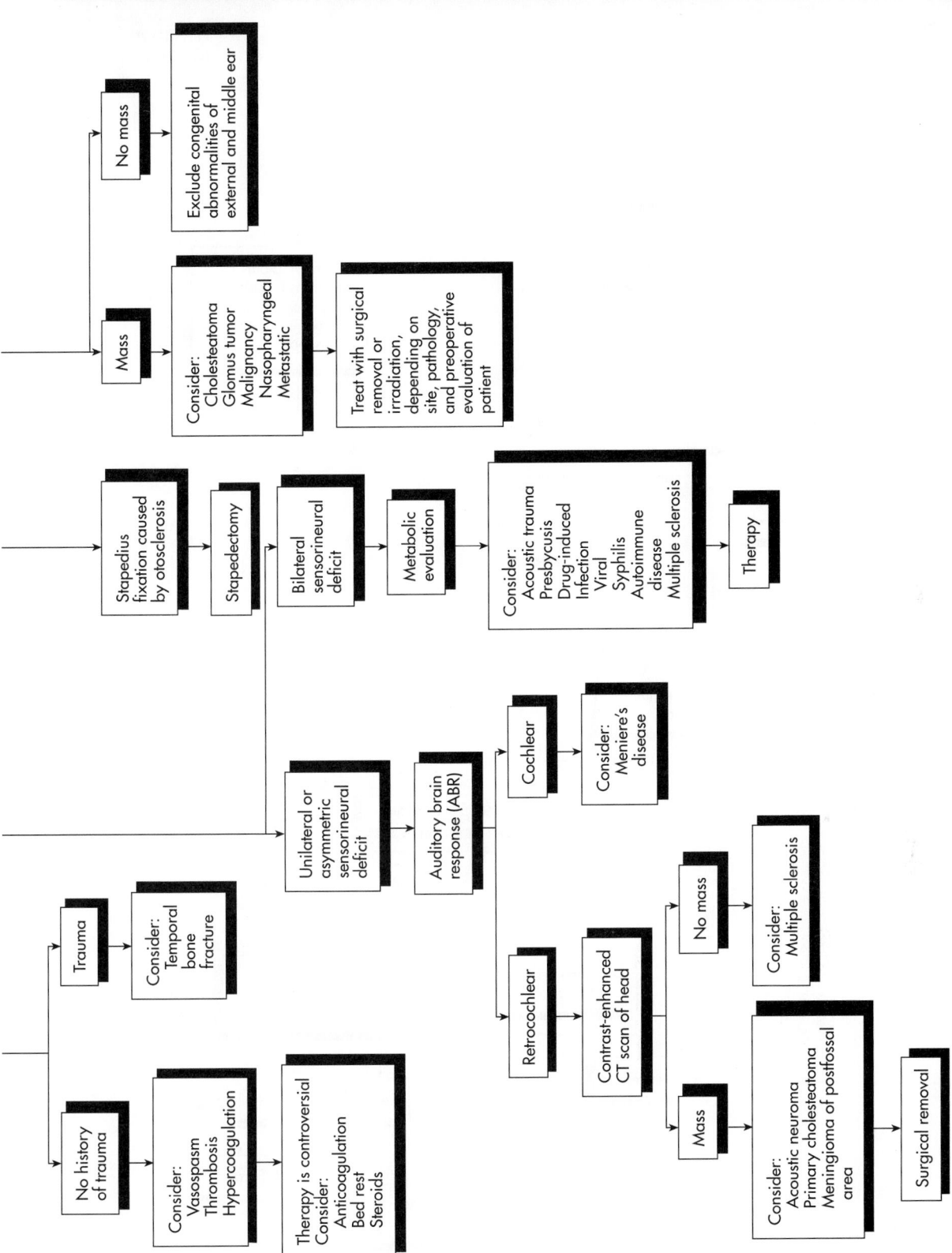

Fig. 3-73 **Evaluation of hearing loss.** *CT,* Computed tomography. (From Greene HL, Johnson WP, Lemcke D [eds]: *Decision making in medicine,* ed 2, St Louis, 1998, Mosby.)

HEARTBURN

Heartburn
ICD-9CM # 787.1

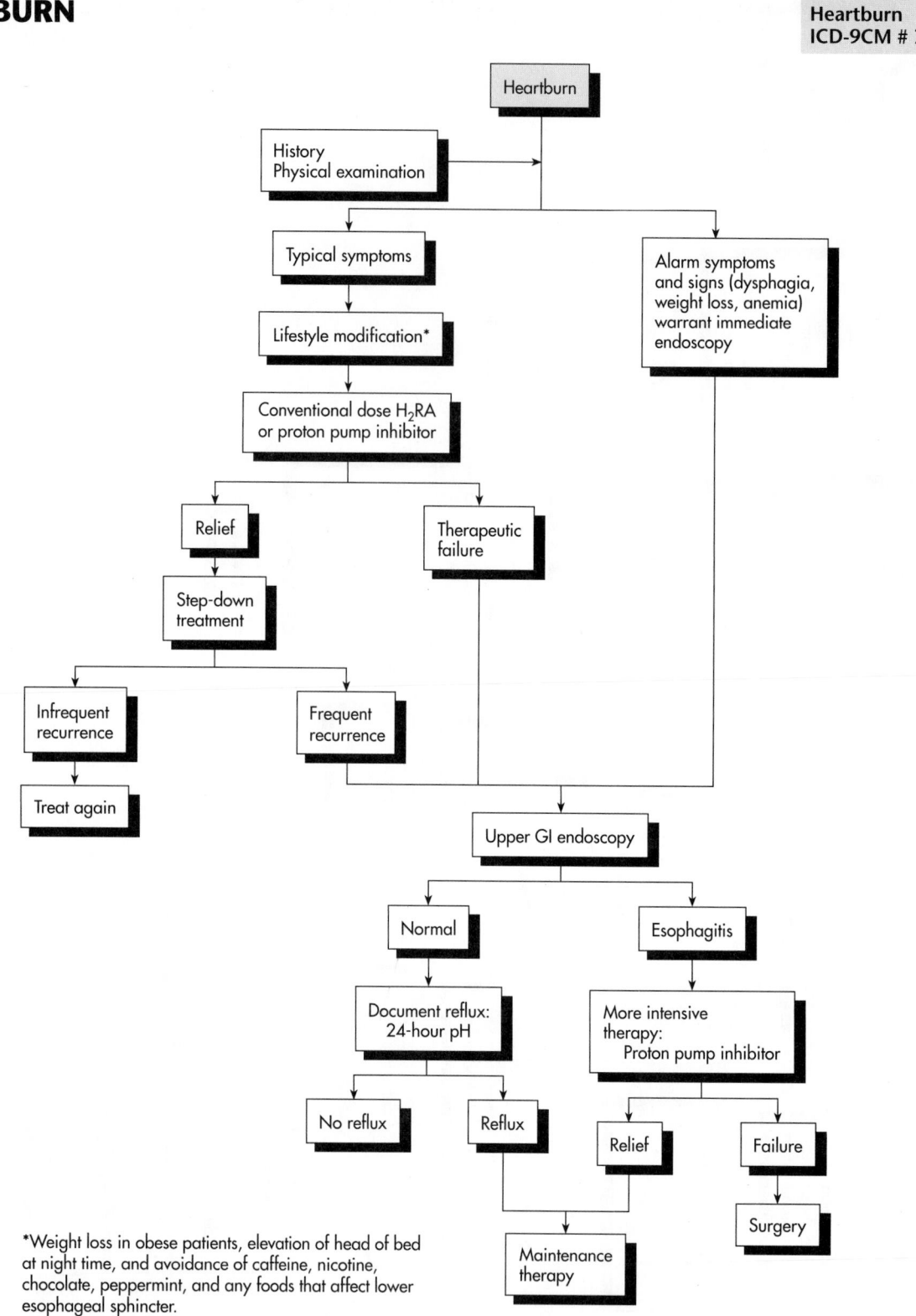

Fig. 3-74   Treatment of a patient with heartburn. *GI,* Gastrointestinal; *H₂RA,* H₂ receptor antagonist.
(Modified from Sampliner RE: Heartburn. In Greene HL, Johnson WP, Lemcke D [eds]: *Decision making in medicine,* ed 2, St Louis, 1998, Mosby.)

HEMATURIA, MICROSCOPIC, ASYMPTOMATIC

Hematuria, microscopic, asymptomatic
ICD-9CM # 599.7

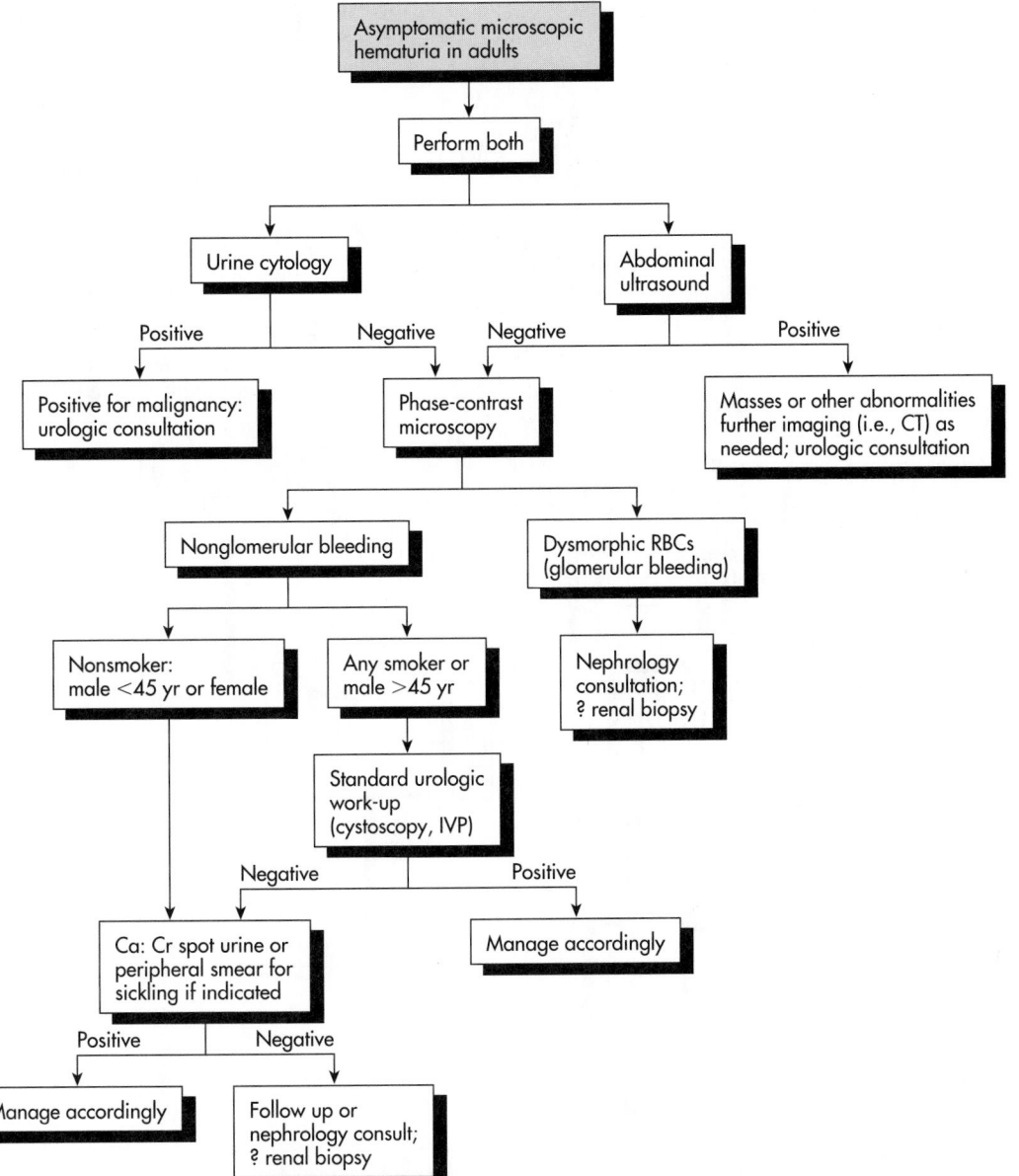

Fig. 3-75   Suggested algorithm for the evaluation of adult asymptomatic microscopic hematuria. These patients must have no symptoms referable to the hematuria and a negative urinalysis except for red blood cells (RBCs). Adults with gross hematuria require a full urologic evaluation. *Ca:Cr*, Calcium:creatinine ratio; *IVP*, intravenous pyelogram. (From Nseyo UO [ed]: *Urology for primary care physicians*, Philadelphia, 1999, WB Saunders.)

III

HEMOPTYSIS

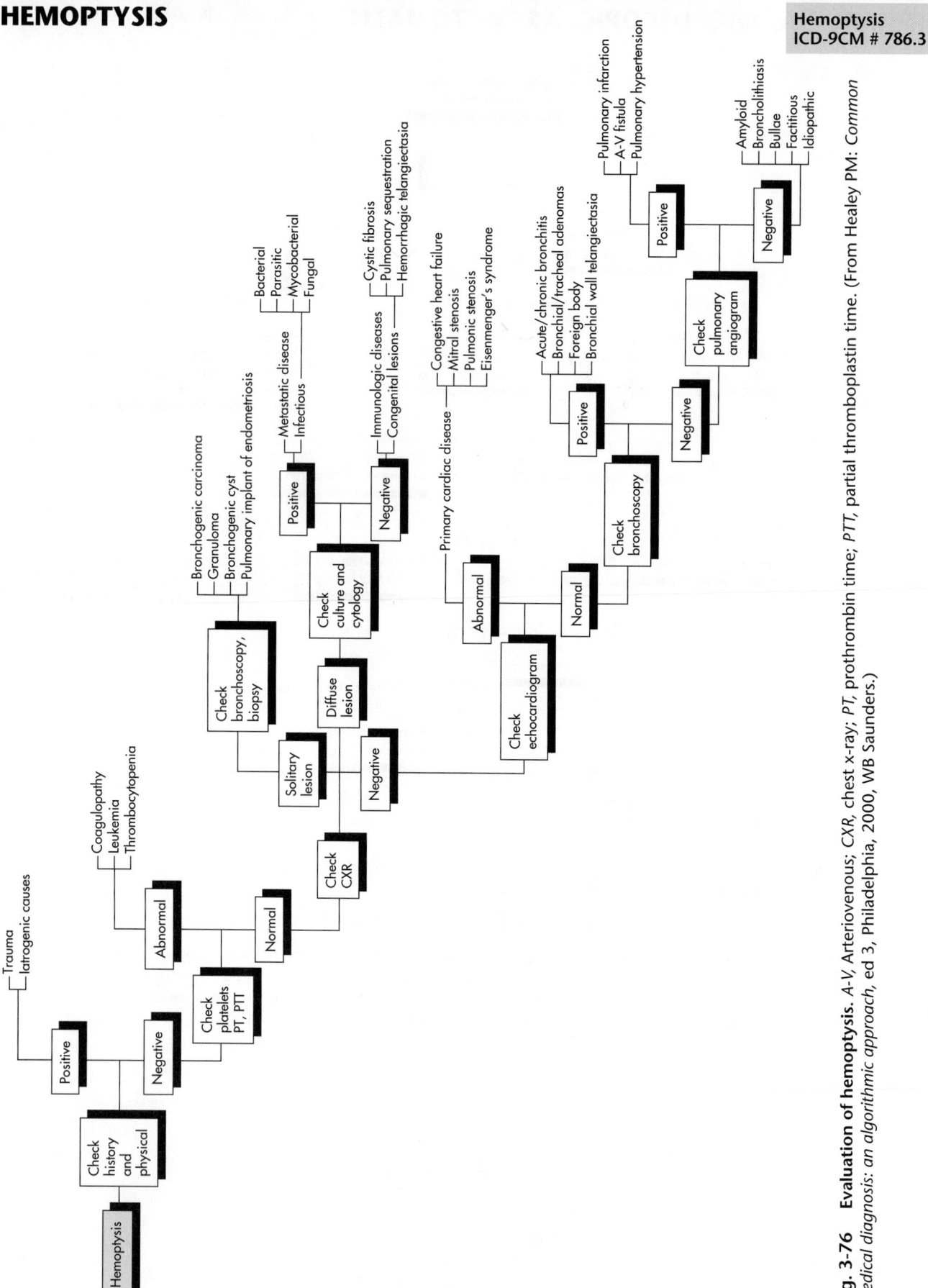

Fig. 3-76 Evaluation of hemoptysis. *A-V,* Arteriovenous; *CXR,* chest x-ray; *PT,* prothrombin time; *PTT,* partial thromboplastin time. (From Healey PM: *Common medical diagnosis: an algorithmic approach,* ed 3, Philadelphia, 2000, WB Saunders.)

HEPATITIS, VIRAL

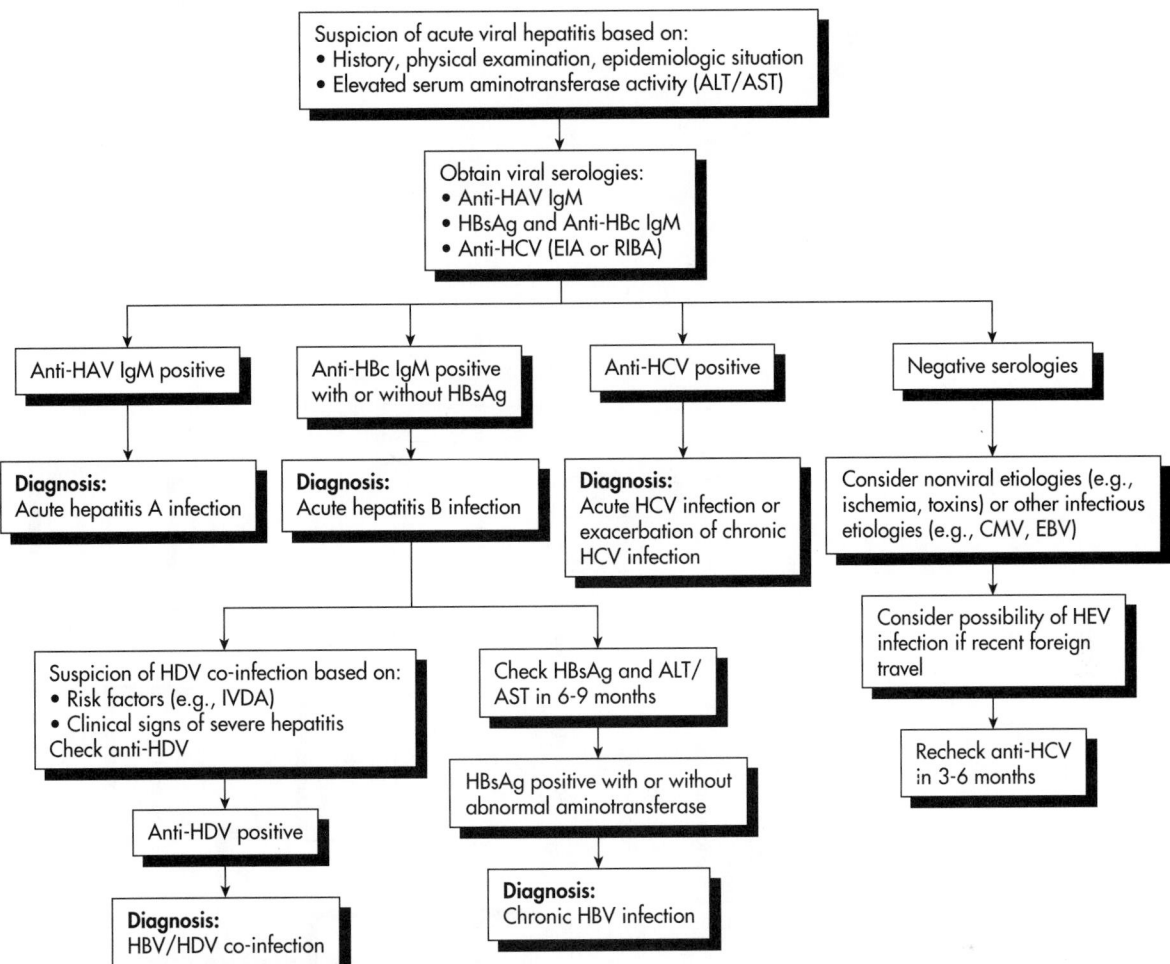

Fig. 3-77   A flow diagram showing the use of specific serologic tests for the diagnosis of acute viral hepatitis in relation to the clinical and epidemiologic setting. Co-infections and superinfections of chronic hepatitis B or C patients should always be considered in cases that do not fit well with the clinical or serologic picture. *CMV,* Cytomegalovirus; *EBV,* Epstein-Barr virus; *EIA,* enzyme immunoassay; *HBV,* hepatitis B virus; *HCV,* hepatitis C virus; *HDV,* hepatitis D virus; *HEV,* hepato-encephalomyelitis virus; *IVDA,* intravenous drug abuse; *RIBA,* recombinant immunoblot assay. (From Mandell GL: *Mandell, Douglas, and Bennett's principles and practice of infectious diseases,* ed 5, New York, 2000, Churchill Livingstone.)

III

HEPATOMEGALY

Hepatomegaly
ICD-9CM # 789.1

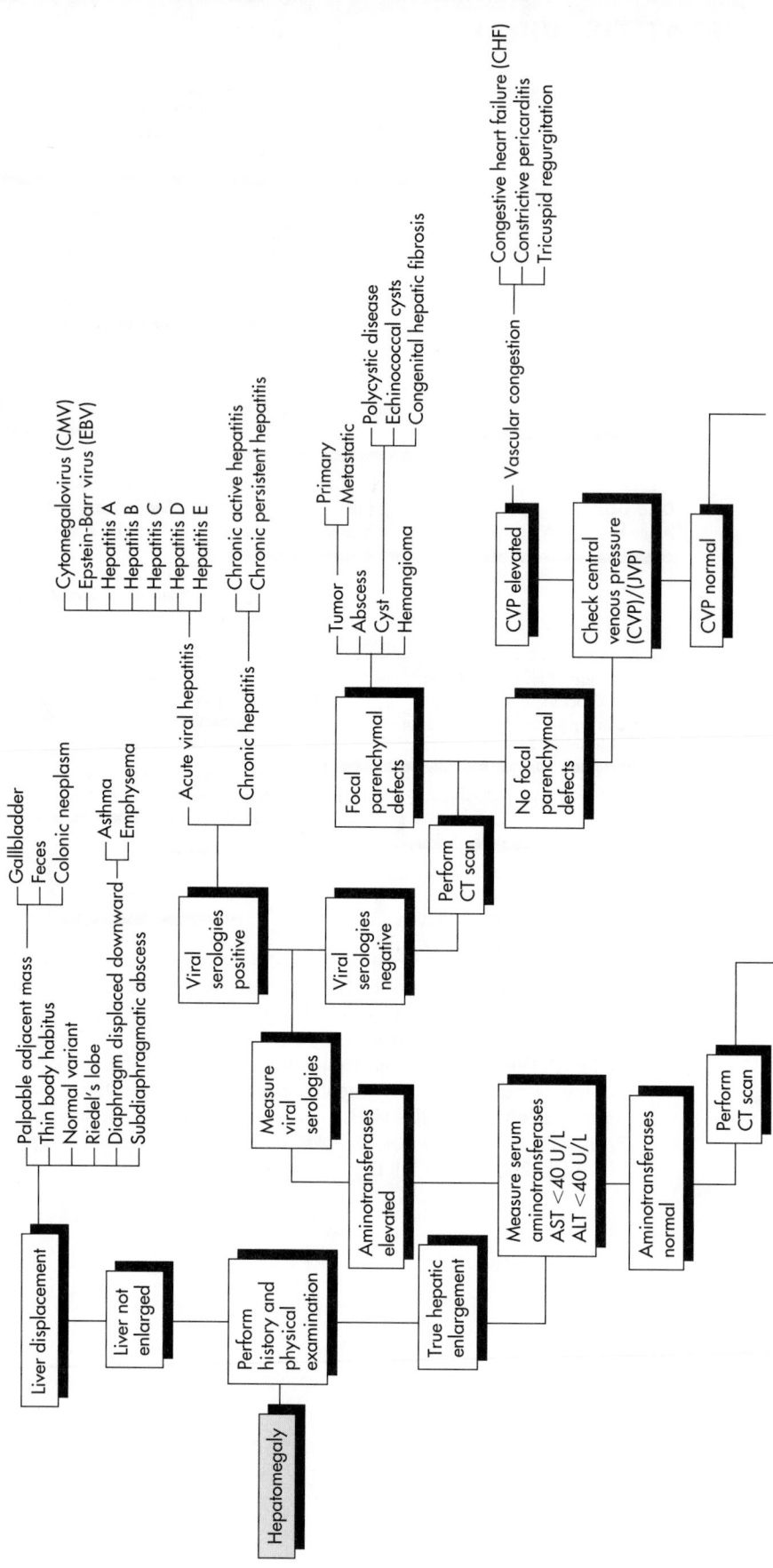

Hepatomegaly

Perform history and physical examination

Liver displacement
— Palpable adjacent mass — Gallbladder
— Feces
— Colonic neoplasm
— Thin body habitus
— Normal variant
— Riedel's lobe
— Diaphragm displaced downward — Asthma
— Emphysema
— Subdiaphragmatic abscess

Liver not enlarged

True hepatic enlargement

Aminotransferases elevated

Measure viral serologies

Viral serologies positive
— Acute viral hepatitis — Cytomegalovirus (CMV)
— Epstein-Barr virus (EBV)
— Hepatitis A
— Hepatitis B
— Hepatitis C
— Hepatitis D
— Hepatitis E
— Chronic hepatitis — Chronic active hepatitis
— Chronic persistent hepatitis

Viral serologies negative

Perform CT scan

Focal parenchymal defects
— Tumor — Primary
— Metastatic
— Abscess
— Cyst — Polycystic disease
— Echinococcal cysts
— Congenital hepatic fibrosis
— Hemangioma

No focal parenchymal defects

Measure serum aminotransferases
AST <40 U/L
ALT <40 U/L

Aminotransferases normal

Perform CT scan

Check central venous pressure (CVP)/(JVP)

CVP elevated
— Vascular congestion — Congestive heart failure (CHF)
— Constrictive pericarditis
— Tricuspid regurgitation

CVP normal

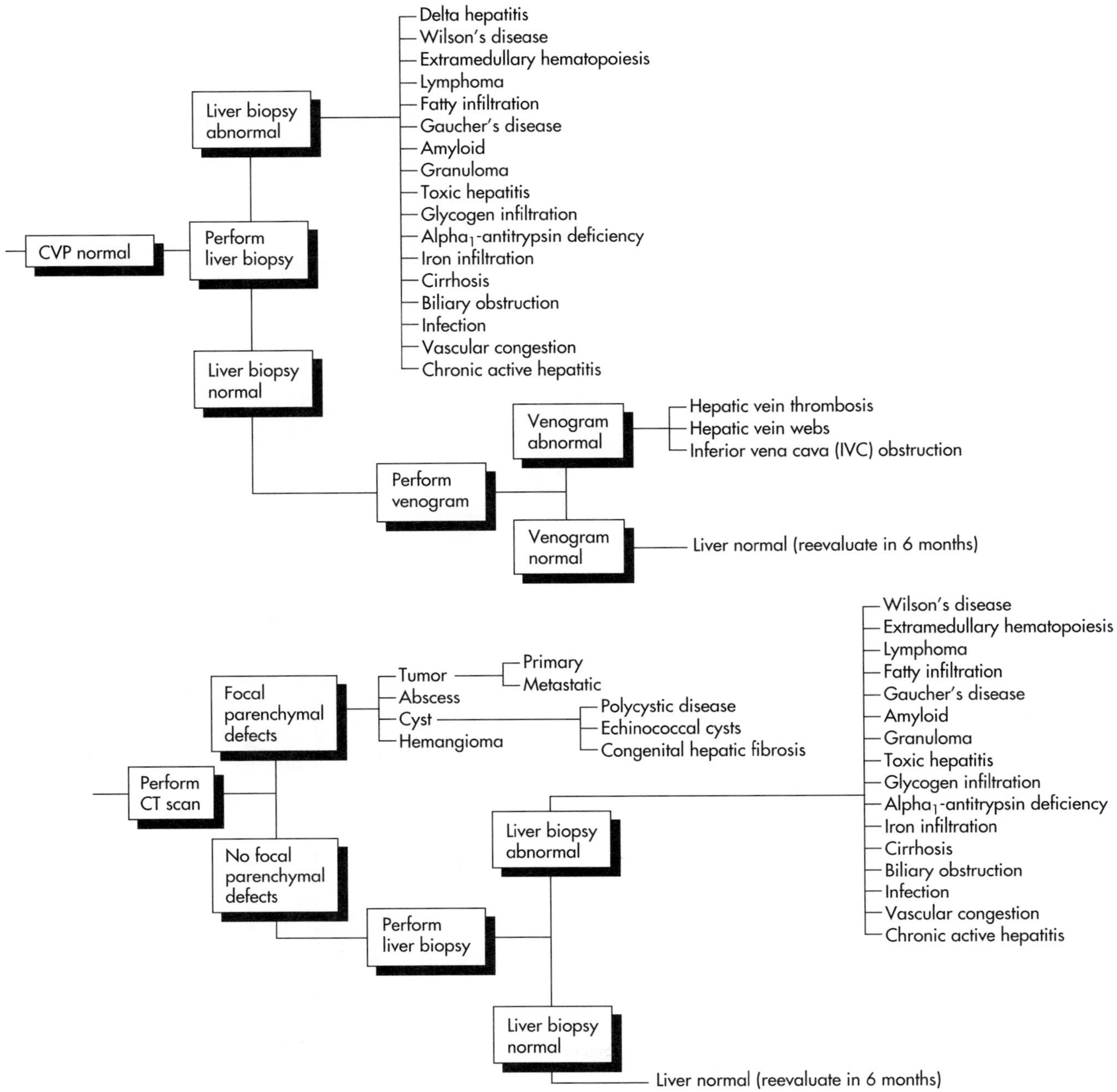

Hepatomegaly.

Delta hepatitis
Wilson's disease
Extramedullary hematopoiesis
Lymphoma
Fatty infiltration
Gaucher's disease
Amyloid
Granuloma
Toxic hepatitis
Glycogen infiltration
Alpha₁-antitrypsin deficiency
Iron infiltration
Cirrhosis
Biliary obstruction
Infection
Vascular congestion
Chronic active hepatitis

Liver biopsy abnormal
Perform liver biopsy
Liver biopsy normal
CVP normal

Hepatic vein thrombosis
Hepatic vein webs
Inferior vena cava (IVC) obstruction

Venogram abnormal
Venogram normal
Liver normal (reevaluate in 6 months)
Perform venogram

Wilson's disease
Extramedullary hematopoiesis
Lymphoma
Fatty infiltration
Gaucher's disease
Amyloid
Granuloma
Toxic hepatitis
Glycogen infiltration
Alpha₁-antitrypsin deficiency
Iron infiltration
Cirrhosis
Biliary obstruction
Infection
Vascular congestion
Chronic active hepatitis

Tumor — Primary / Metastatic
Abscess
Cyst — Polycystic disease / Echinococcal cysts / Congenital hepatic fibrosis
Hemangioma

Focal parenchymal defects
No focal parenchymal defects
Perform CT scan

Liver biopsy abnormal
Perform liver biopsy
Liver biopsy normal
Liver normal (reevaluate in 6 months)

Fig. 3-78 **Hepatomegaly.** *ALT,* Alanine aminotransferase; *AST,* aspartate aminotransferase; *CT,* computed tomography; *JVP,* jugular venous pressure. (From Healey PM: *Common medical diagnosis: an algorithmic approach,* ed 3, Philadelphia, 2000, WB Saunders.)

III

HIRSUTISM

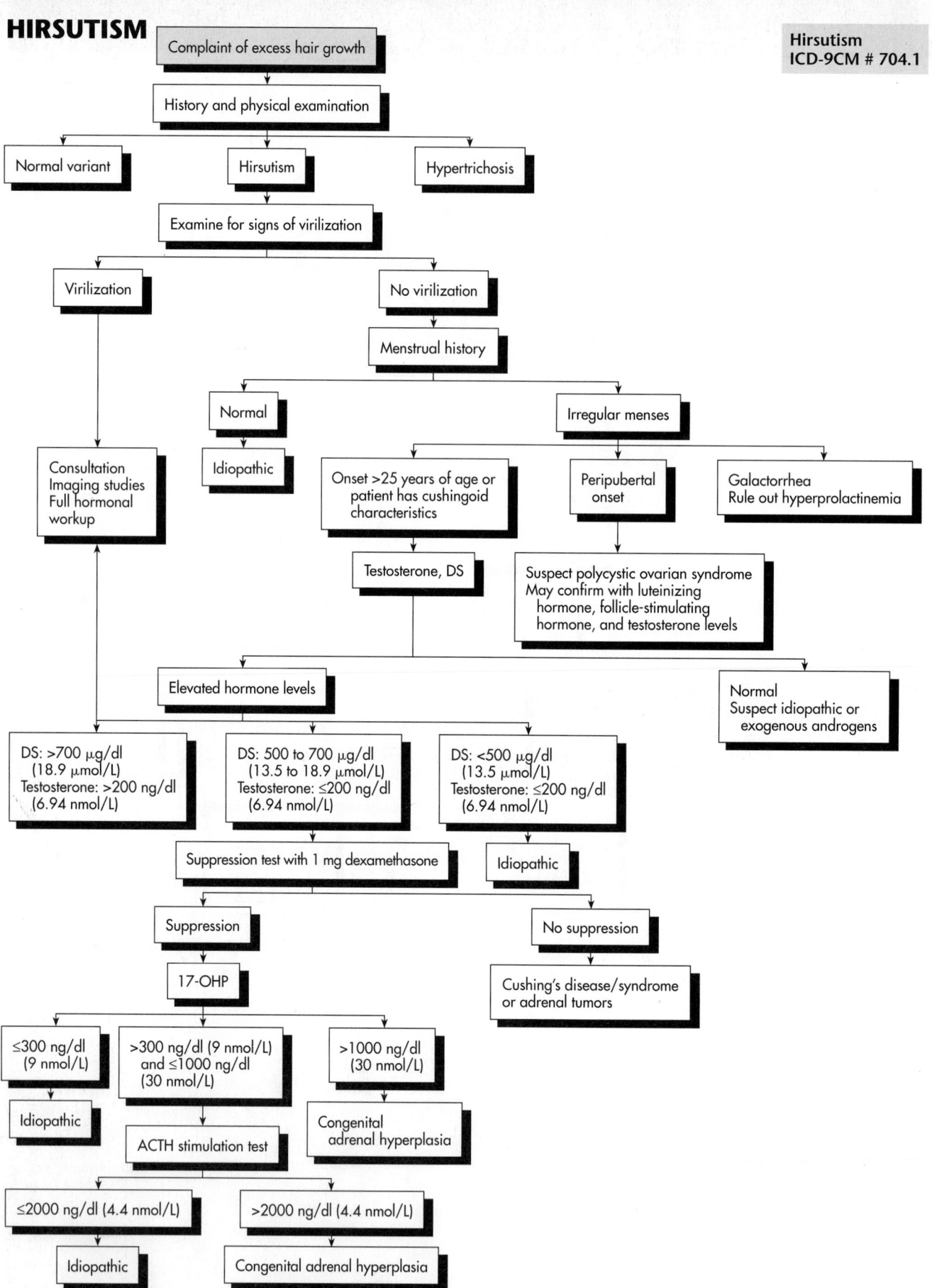

Fig. 3-79 **Algorithm showing the evaluation and treatment of hirsutism.** *ACTH,* Adrenocorti-cotropic hormone; *DS,* dehydroepiandrosterone; *17-OHP,* 17-hydroxyprogesterone. (From Gilchrist VJ, Hecht BR: *Am Fam Physician* 52:1837, 1995.)

HIV-INFECTED PATIENT, ACUTELY ILL

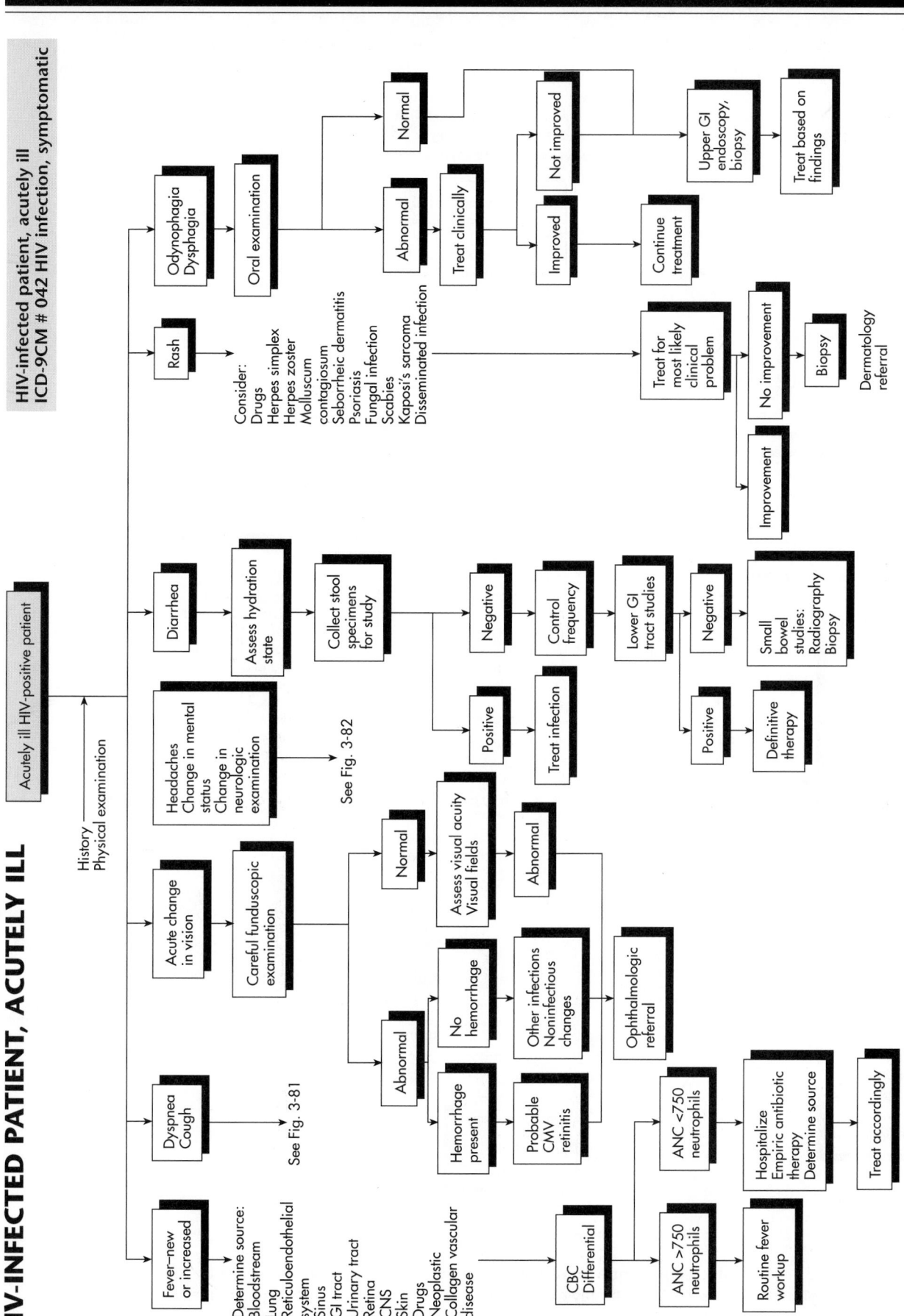

Fig. 3-80 Acutely ill HIV-positive patient. *ANC,* Absolute neutrophil count; *CBC,* complete blood count; *CMV,* cytomegalovirus; *CNS,* central nervous system; *GI,* gastrointestinal. (From Greene HL, Johnson WP, Lemcke D [eds]: *Decision making in medicine,* ed 2, St Louis, 1998, Mosby.)

III

HIV-INFECTED PATIENT WITH RESPIRATORY COMPLAINTS

HIV-infected patient with respiratory complaints
ICD-9CM # 042 HIV infection, symptomatic

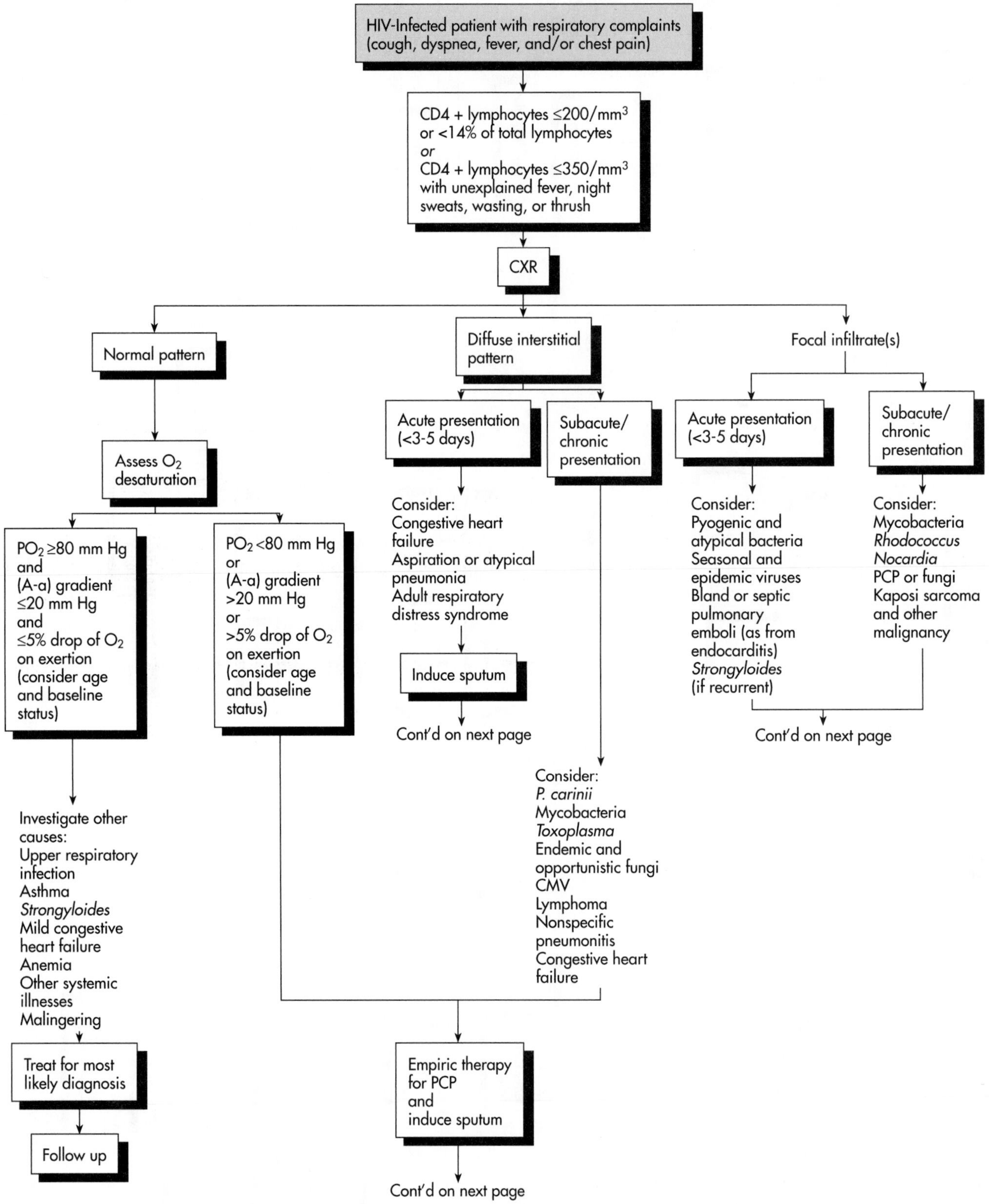

HIV-Infected patient with respiratory complaints (cough, dyspnea, fever, and/or chest pain)
CD4 + lymphocytes ≤200/mm³ or <14% of total lymphocytes *or* CD4 + lymphocytes ≤350/mm³ with unexplained fever, night sweats, wasting, or thrush
CXR
Normal pattern
Diffuse interstitial pattern
Focal infiltrate(s)
Assess O_2 desaturation
PO_2 ≥80 mm Hg and (A-a) gradient ≤20 mm Hg and ≤5% drop of O_2 on exertion (consider age and baseline status)
PO_2 <80 mm Hg or (A-a) gradient >20 mm Hg or >5% drop of O_2 on exertion (consider age and baseline status)
Investigate other causes: Upper respiratory infection Asthma *Strongyloides* Mild congestive heart failure Anemia Other systemic illnesses Malingering
Treat for most likely diagnosis
Follow up
Acute presentation (<3-5 days)
Subacute/ chronic presentation
Consider: Congestive heart failure Aspiration or atypical pneumonia Adult respiratory distress syndrome
Induce sputum
Cont'd on next page
Consider: *P. carinii* Mycobacteria *Toxoplasma* Endemic and opportunistic fungi CMV Lymphoma Nonspecific pneumonitis Congestive heart failure
Empiric therapy for PCP and induce sputum
Cont'd on next page
Acute presentation (<3-5 days)
Subacute/ chronic presentation
Consider: Pyogenic and atypical bacteria Seasonal and epidemic viruses Bland or septic pulmonary emboli (as from endocarditis) *Strongyloides* (if recurrent)
Consider: Mycobacteria *Rhodococcus* *Nocardia* PCP or fungi Kaposi sarcoma and other malignancy
Cont'd on next page

Fig. 3-81 HIV-infected patient with respiratory complaints. *BAL,* Bronchoalveolar lavage; *CMV,* cytomegalovirus; *CXR,* chest x-ray examination; *PCP, Pneumocystis carinii* pneumonia; *TBB,* transbronchial biopsy. (From Greene HL, Johnson WP, Lemcke D [eds]: *Decision making in medicine,* 2, St Louis, 1998, Mosby.)

HIV-INFECTED PATIENT WITH RESPIRATORY COMPLAINTS—cont'd

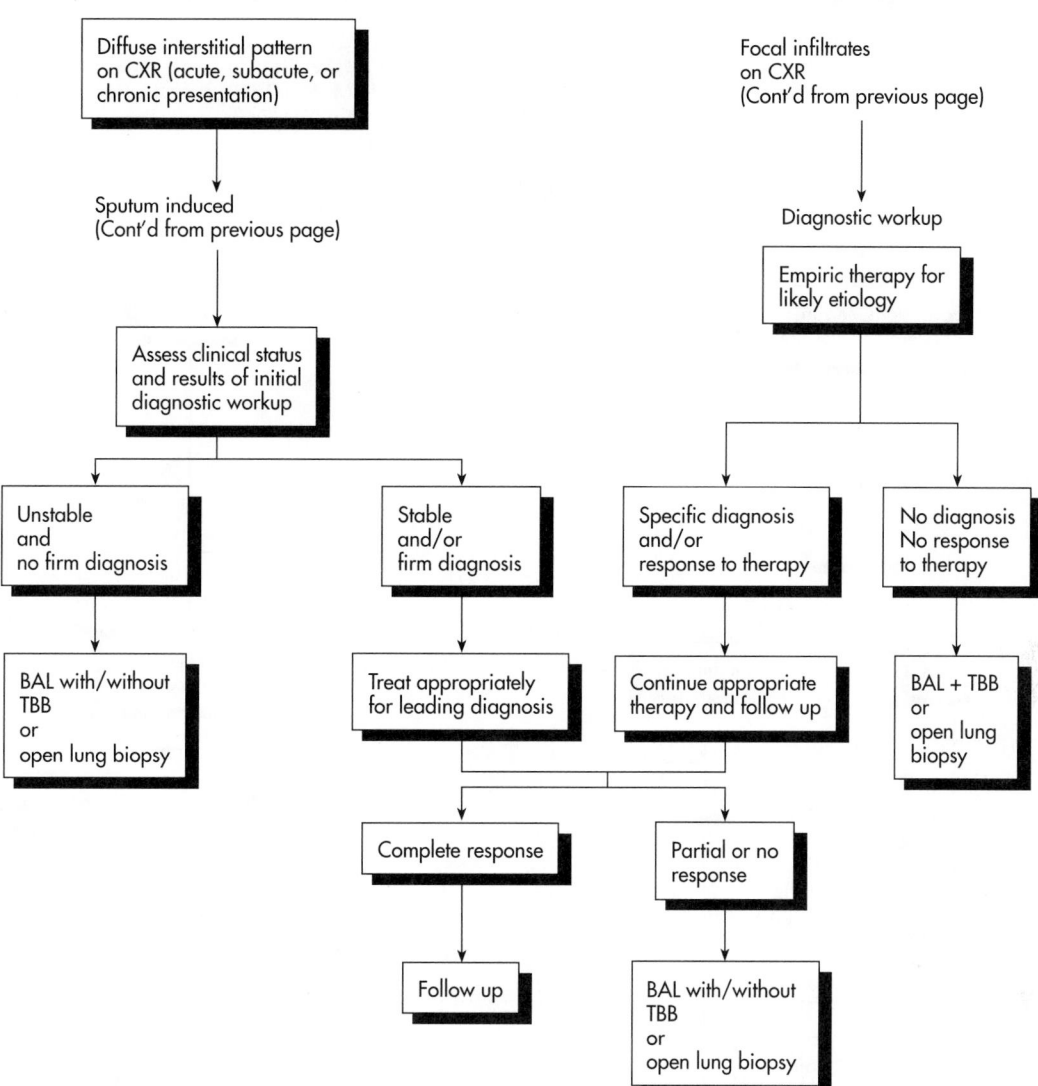

Fig. 3-81, cont'd

HIV-INFECTED PATIENT WITH SUSPECTED CENTRAL NERVOUS SYSTEM INFECTION

**HIV-infected patient with suspected CNS infection
ICD-9CM # 042 HIV infection, symptomatic**

History
Physical examination
with detailed
neurologic examination

Focal signs, seizures,
or altered mental status

Nonfocal

CT scan

Masses

No masses

Lumbar puncture
Laboratory tests

Single
lesion

Other

Normal

Abnormal

MRI

Watchful
waiting

Multiple ring-enhancing
lesions

Single
lesion

Positive
VDRL test

Positive
cryptococcal
antigen test

Bacterial
infection

Aseptic
meningitis

Empiric therapy
for toxoplasmosis

Treat for
neurosyphilis

Treat with
appropriate
antibiotics

No response to
therapy after
14 days

Biopsy

Treat for
cryptococcal
meningitis

Consider:
Viral, fungal, AFB,
syphilis

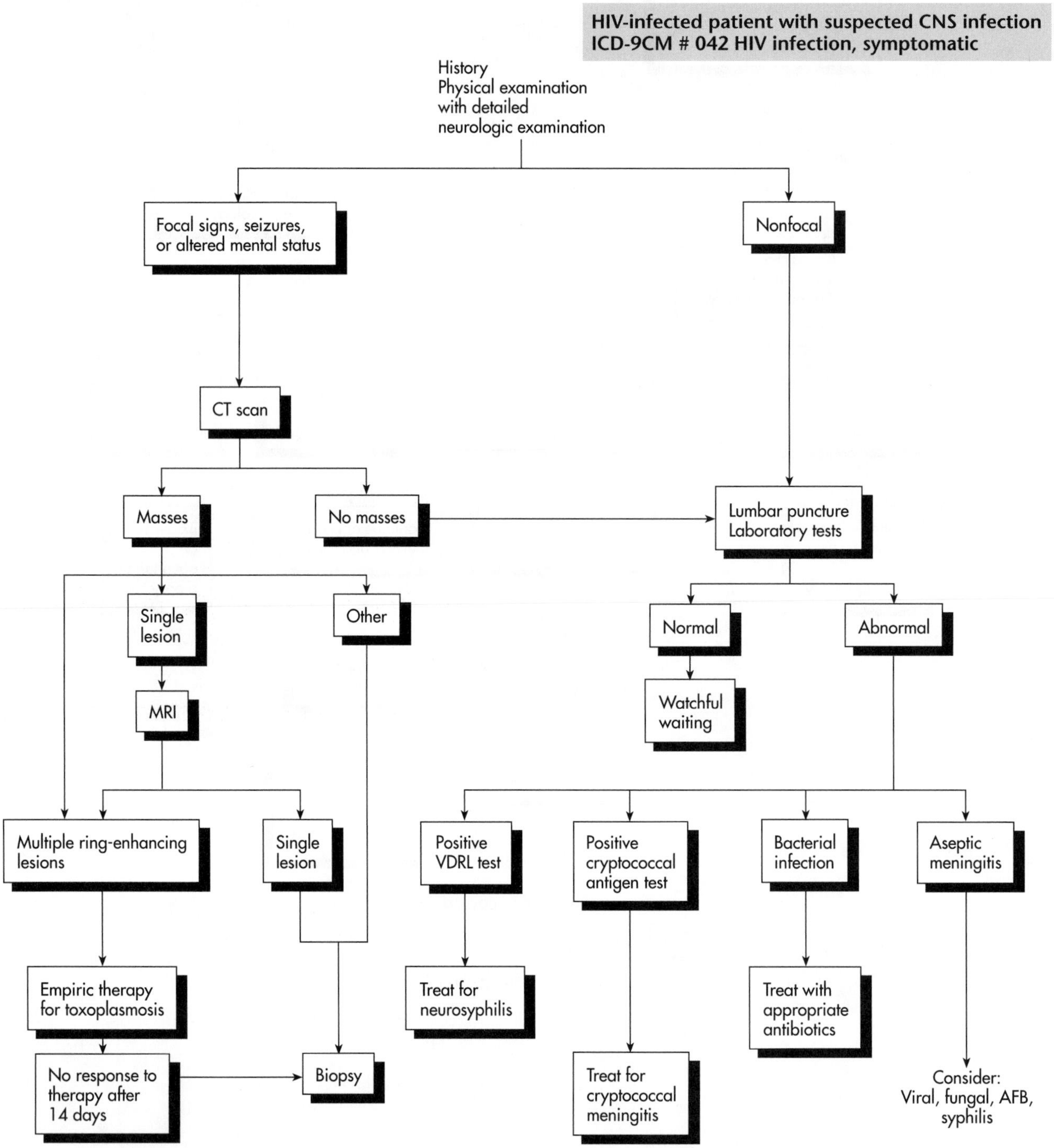

Fig. 3-82   HIV-positive patient with suspected central nervous system infection. *AFB,* Acid-fast bacilli; *CNS,* central nervous system; *CT,* computed tomography; *MRI,* magnetic resonance imaging; *VDRL,* Venereal Disease Research Laboratory. (From Greene HL, Johnson WP, Lemcke D [eds]: *Decision making in medicine,* ed 2, St Louis, 1998, Mosby.)

HYPERCALCEMIA

A

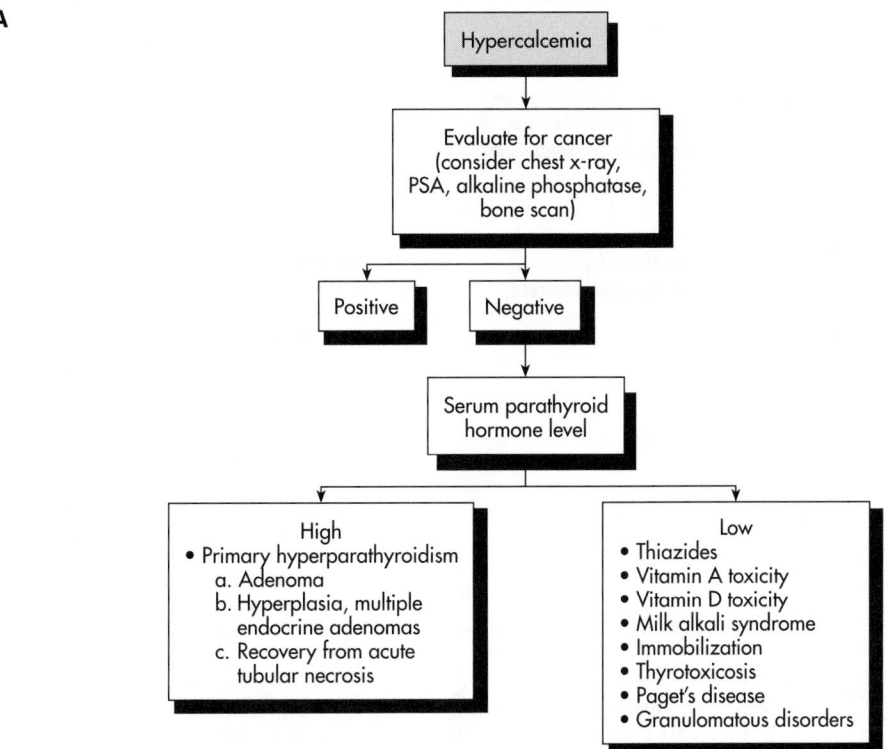

Fig. 3-83 **A, Evaluation of hypercalcemia.** *PSA,* Prostate-specific antigen. (From Wachtel TJ, Stein MD: *Practical guide to the care of the ambulatory patient,* St Louis, 1995, Mosby.)

B

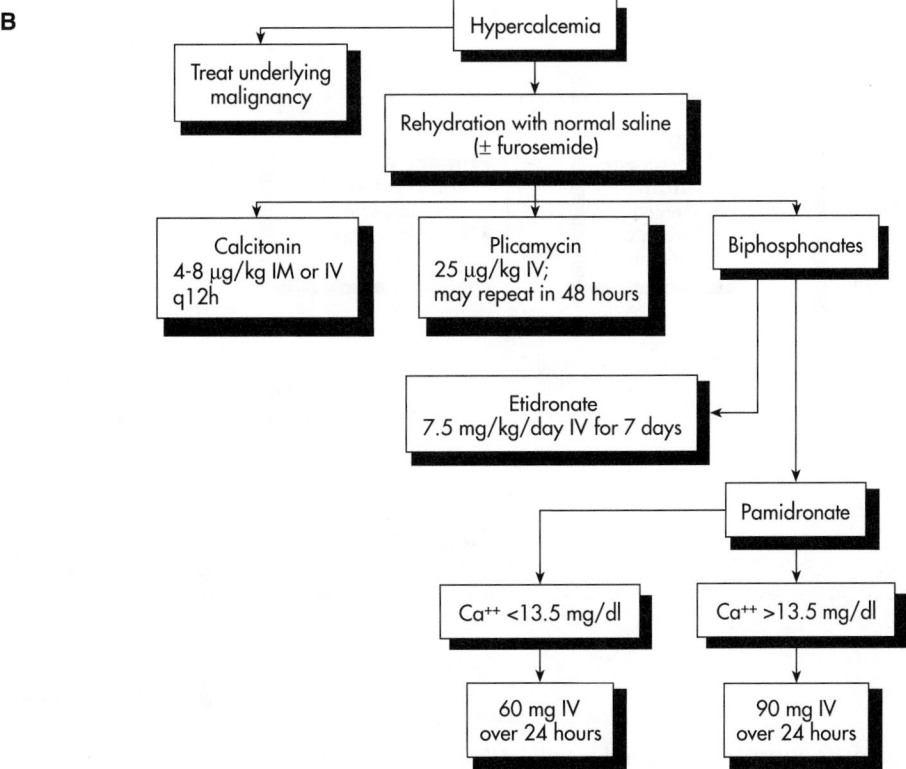

Fig. 3-83, cont'd **B, Therapy for hypercalcemia.** *IM,* Intramuscularly; *IV,* intravenously. (From Noble J [ed]: *Primary care medicine,* ed 3, St Louis, 2001, Mosby.)

HYPERKALEMIA, EVALUATION

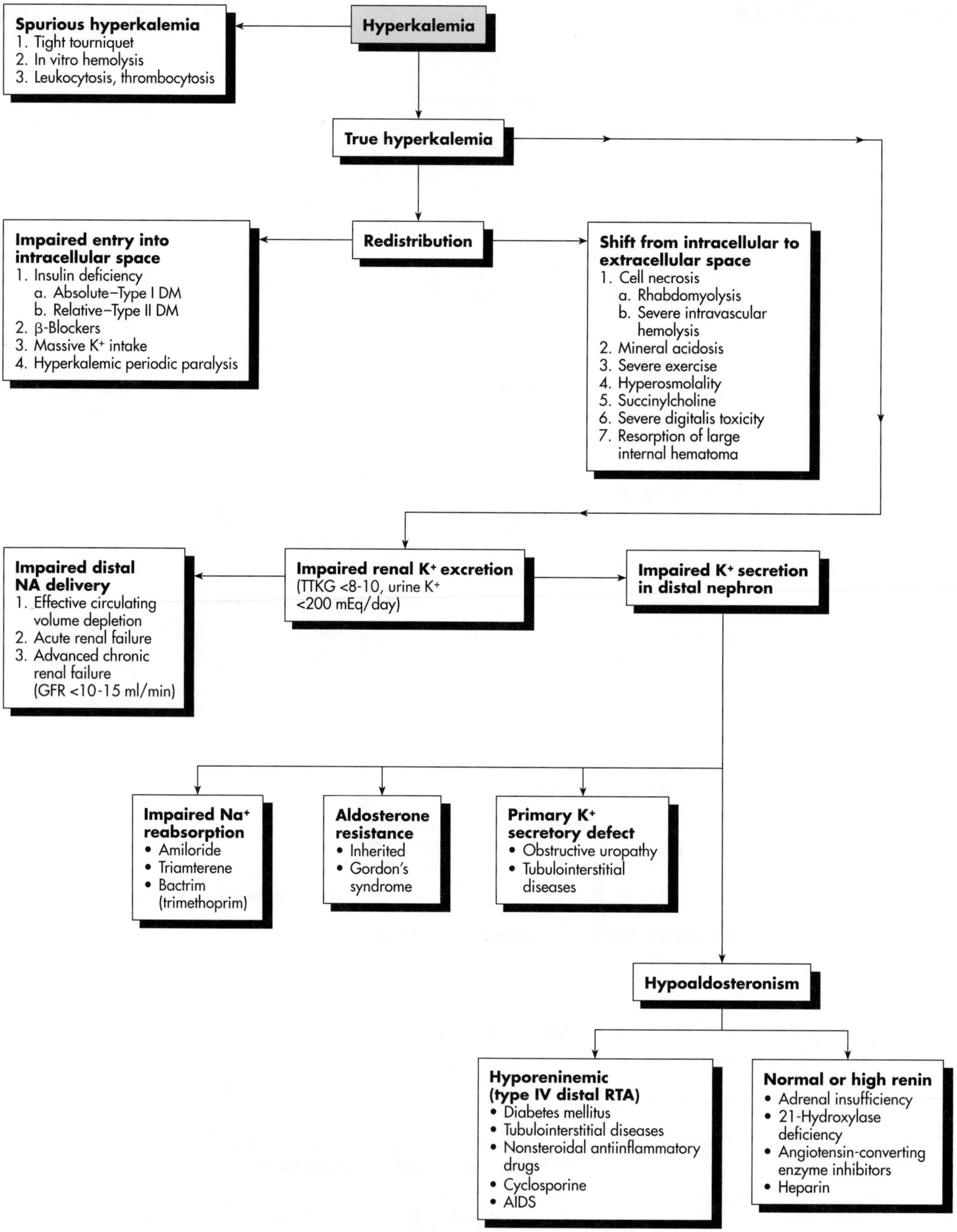

Hyperkalemia

Spurious hyperkalemia
1. Tight tourniquet
2. In vitro hemolysis
3. Leukocytosis, thrombocytosis

True hyperkalemia

Redistribution

Impaired entry into intracellular space
1. Insulin deficiency
   a. Absolute—Type I DM
   b. Relative—Type II DM
2. β-Blockers
3. Massive K+ intake
4. Hyperkalemic periodic paralysis

Shift from intracellular to extracellular space
1. Cell necrosis
   a. Rhabdomyolysis
   b. Severe intravascular hemolysis
2. Mineral acidosis
3. Severe exercise
4. Hyperosmolality
5. Succinylcholine
6. Severe digitalis toxicity
7. Resorption of large internal hematoma

Impaired distal NA delivery
1. Effective circulating volume depletion
2. Acute renal failure
3. Advanced chronic renal failure (GFR <10-15 ml/min)

Impaired renal K+ excretion
(TTKG <8-10, urine K+ <200 mEq/day)

Impaired K+ secretion in distal nephron

Impaired Na+ reabsorption
- Amiloride
- Triamterene
- Bactrim (trimethoprim)

Aldosterone resistance
- Inherited
- Gordon's syndrome

Primary K+ secretory defect
- Obstructive uropathy
- Tubulointerstitial diseases

Hypoaldosteronism

Hyporeninemic (type IV distal RTA)
- Diabetes mellitus
- Tubulointerstitial diseases
- Nonsteroidal antiinflammatory drugs
- Cyclosporine
- AIDS

Normal or high renin
- Adrenal insufficiency
- 21-Hydroxylase deficiency
- Angiotensin-converting enzyme inhibitors
- Heparin

Fig. 3-84   Diagnostic approach to hyperkalemia. *AIDS,* Acquired immunodeficiency syndrome; *DM,* diabetes mellitus; *GFR,* glomerular filtration rate; *RTA,* renal tubular acidosis; *TTKG,* transtubular potassium gradient. (From Andreoli TE [ed]: *Cecil essentials of medicine,* ed 4, Philadelphia, 1997, WB Saunders.)

HYPERKALEMIA, TREATMENT

A

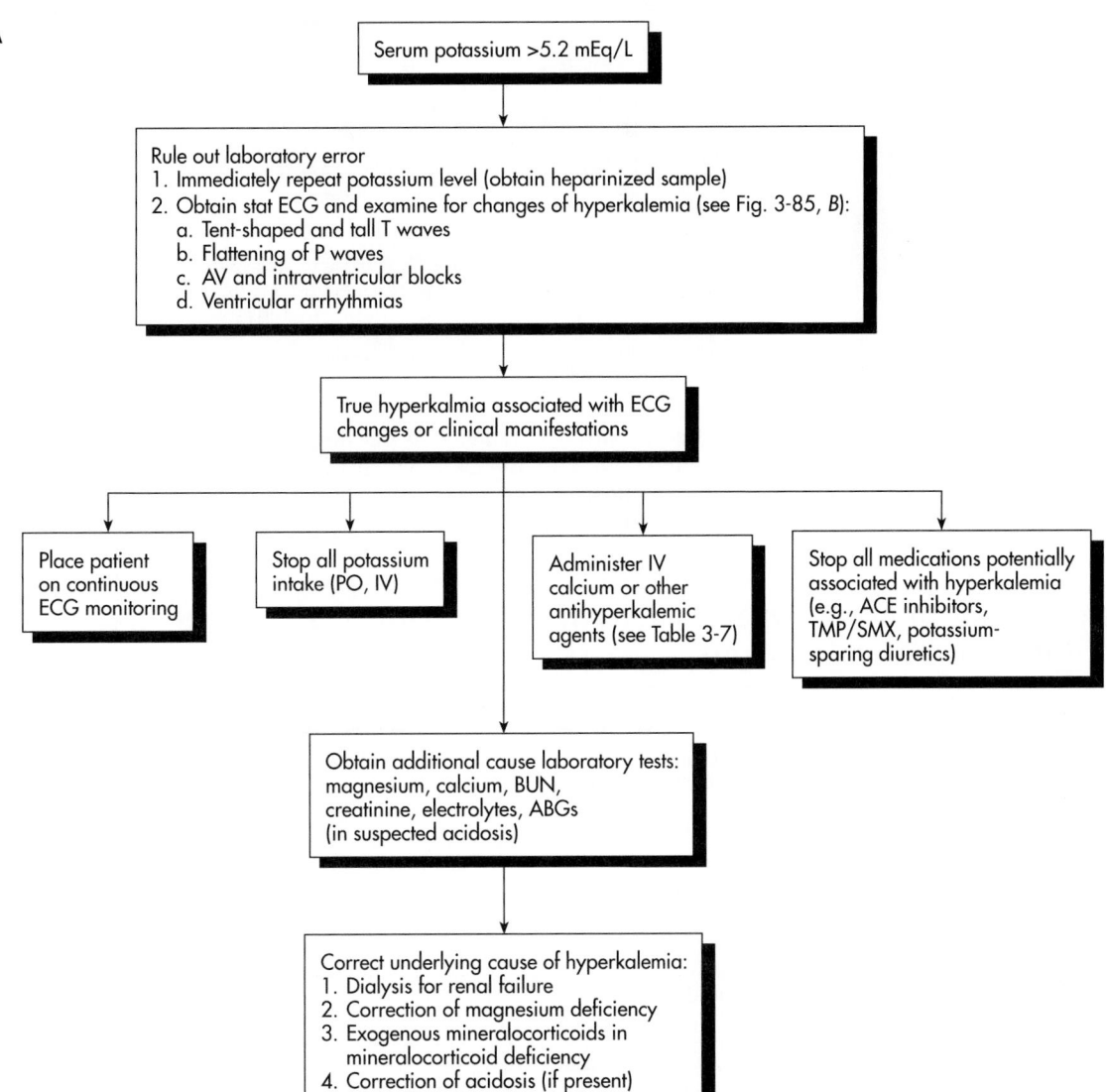

Fig. 3-85   A, Evaluation and treatment of hyperkalemia. *ABGs,* Arterial blood gases; *ACE,* angiotensin-converting enzyme; *AV,* atrioventricular; *BUN,* blood urea nitrogen; *ECG,* electrocardiogram; *IV,* intravenous; *PO,* oral; *TMP/SMX,* trimethoprim-sulfamethoxazole. (From Ferri F: *Practical guide to the care of the medical patient,* ed 5, St Louis, 2001, Mosby.)

Continued

HYPERKALEMIA, TREATMENT—cont'd

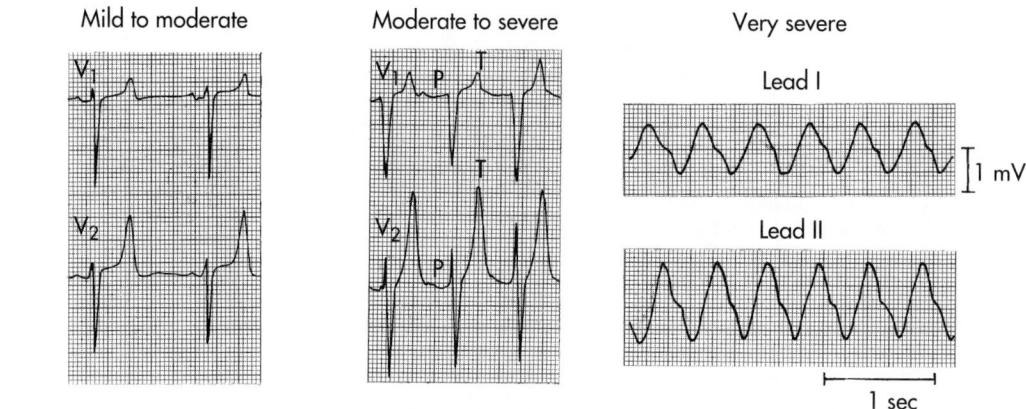

B   Mild to moderate   Moderate to severe   Very severe

Fig. 3-85, cont'd   B, The earliest change with hyperkalemia is peaking ("tenting") of the T waves. With progressive increases in serum potassium, the QRS complexes widen, the P waves decrease in amplitude and may disappear and, finally, a sine-wave pattern leads to asystole. (From Goldberger AL [ed]: *Clinical electrocardiography,* ed 6, St Louis, 1999, Mosby.)

TABLE 3-7   Therapy of Acute Hyperkalemia Associated with ECG Changes or Clinical Manifestations*

TREATMENT OPTIONS	ONSET OF ACTION	DURATION OF ACTION
Glucose, 50 g IV bolus or IV infusion of 500 ml of 10% dextrose solution, *plus* insulin, 10 U regular insulin IV	Approximately 30 min	3 hr
Calcium gluconate† (10% solution), 5-10 ml IV over 3 min	5 min	<1 hr
Dialysis (hemodialysis or peritoneal)	5 min after start of dialysis	3 hr after end of dialysis
Sodium bicarbonate (NaHCO$_3$), 1 amp (44 mEq) over 5 min	Approximately 30 min	3 hr
Sodium polystyrene sulfonate (Kayexalate), PO or via NG tube: 20-50 g Kayexalate plus 100-200 ml of 20% sorbitol Retention enema: 50 g Kayexalate in 200 ml of 20% sorbitol	1-2 hr	3 hr
Diuretics Furosemide 40-160 mg IV over 30 min or bumetanide 1-8 mg IV over 30 min	At onset of diuresis	

From Ferri F: *Practical guide to the care of the medical patient,* ed 5, St Louis, 2001, Mosby.
*Cardiac monitoring is recommended.
†Use with caution in patients receiving digitalis.

HYPERMAGNESEMIA

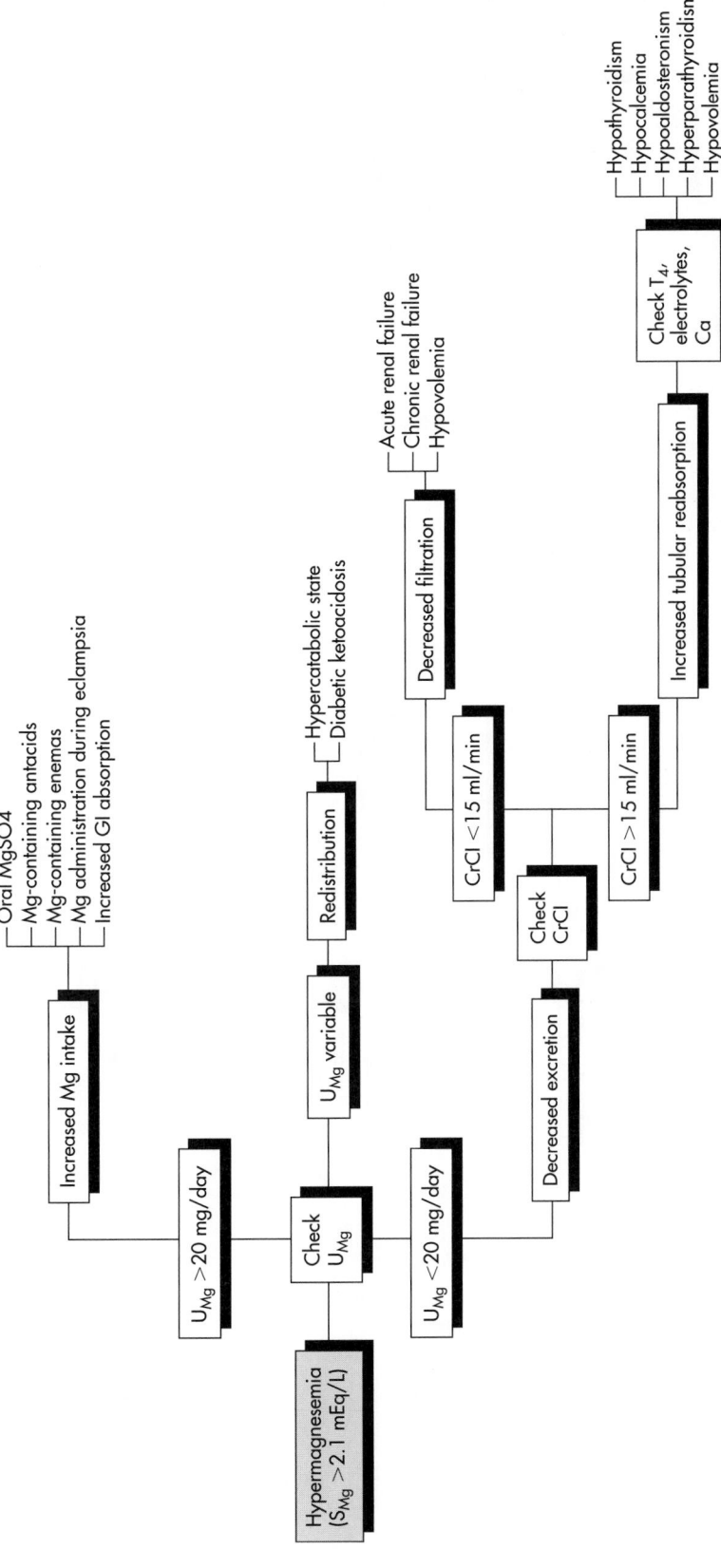

Fig. 3-86 **Hypermagnesemia.** *CrCl,* Creatinine clearance; *GI,* gastrointestinal; *MgSO₄,* magnesium sulfate. (From Healey PM: *Common medical diagnosis: an algorithmic approach,* ed 3, Philadelphia, 2000, WB Saunders.)

HYPERNATREMIA

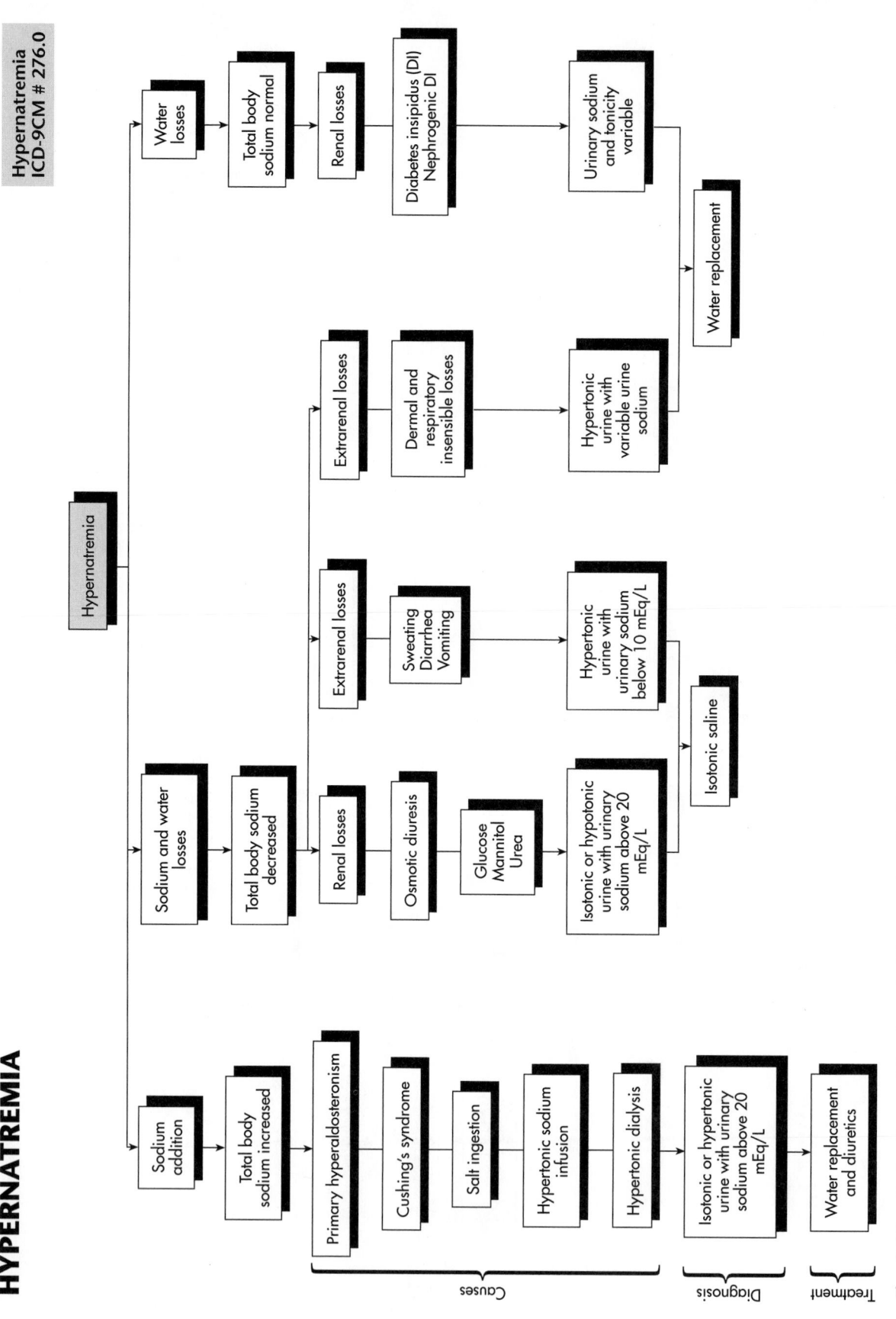

Fig. 3-87   **Evaluation and treatment of hypernatremia.** (From Rosen P et al [eds]: *Emergency medicine: concepts and clinical practice*, ed 5, St Louis, 2002, Mosby.)

HYPERPHOSPHATEMIA

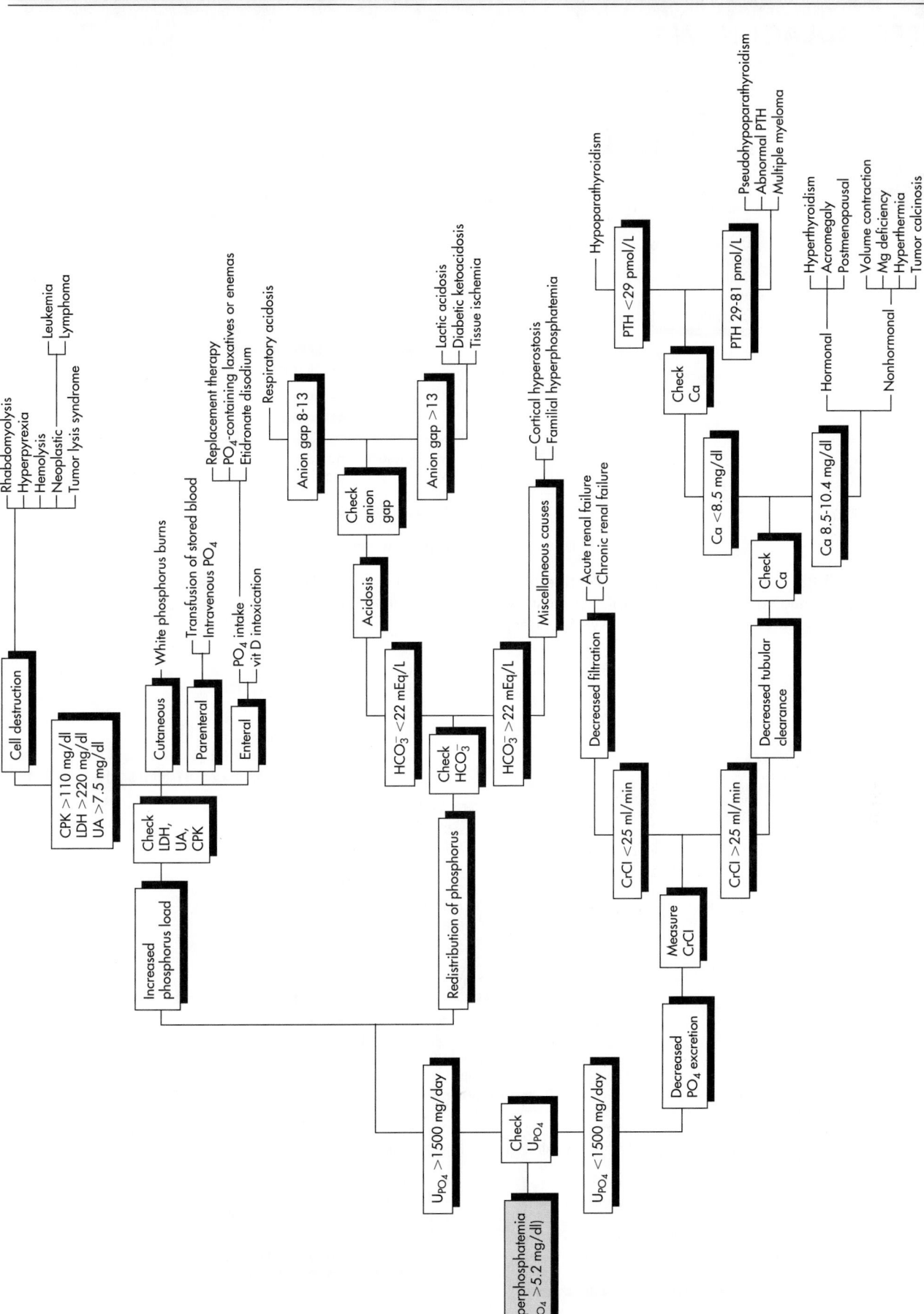

Fig. 3-88   Approach to hyperphosphatemia. *CT,* Computerized tomography; *MRI,* magnetic resonance imaging; *T₄,* thyroxine; *TSH,* thyroid-stimulating hormone. (From Copeland LJ: *Textbook of gynecology,* ed 2, Philadelphia, 2000, WB Saunders.)

HYPERPROLACTINEMIA

Hyperprolactinemia
ICD-9CM # 253.1

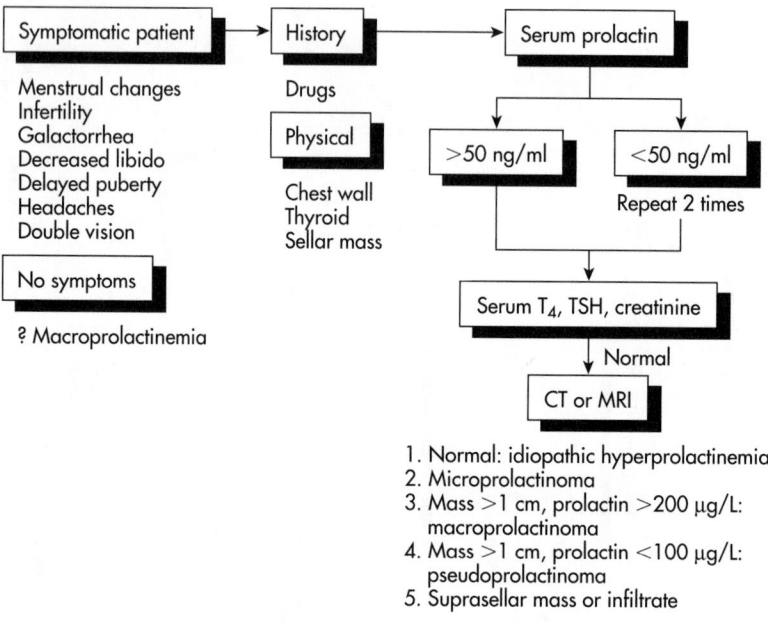

Fig. 3-89   Approach to hyperprolactinemia. *CT,* Computed tomography; *MRI,* magnetic resonance imaging; *T₄,* thyroxine; *TSH,* thyroid-stimulating hormone. (From Copeland LJ: *Textbook of gynecology,* ed 2, Philadelphia, 2000, WB Saunders.)

HYPOCALCEMIA

Hypocalcemia
ICD-9CM # 275.41 Hypocalcemia NOS

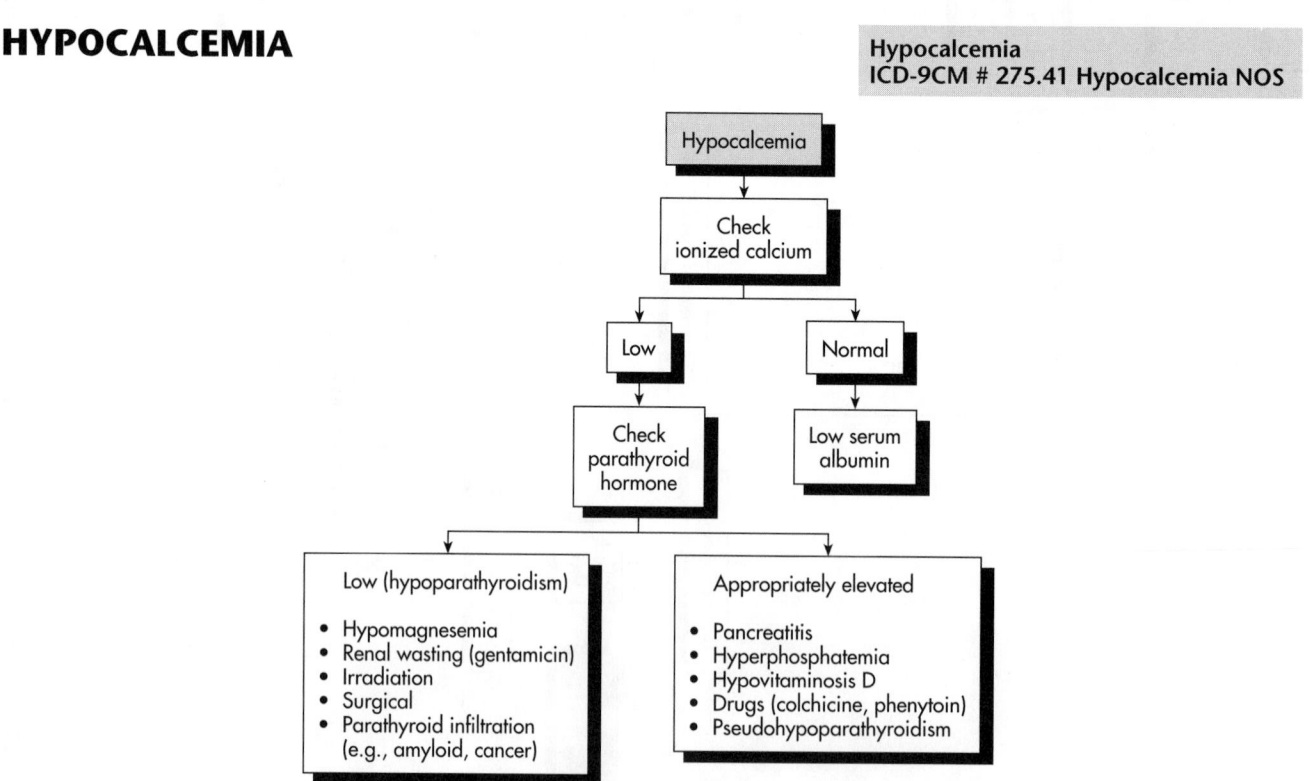

Fig. 3-90   Evaluation of hypocalcemia. (From Wachtel TJ, Stein MD: *Practical guide to the care of the ambulatory patient,* ed 2, St Louis, 2000, Mosby.)

HYPOGLYCEMIA, FASTING

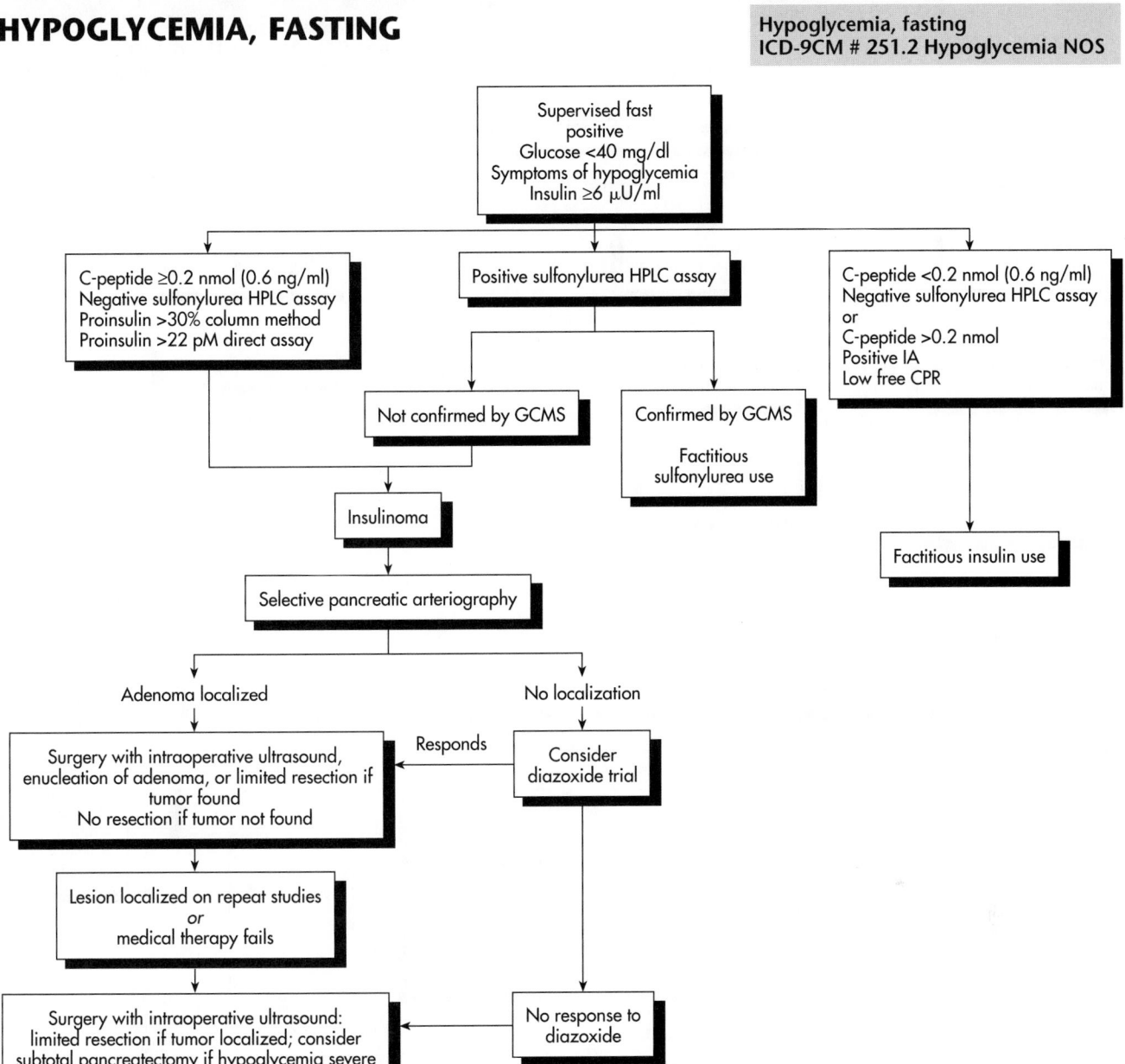

Fig. 3-91 **Diagnostic evaluation of patients with documented hypoglycemia and elevated insulin.** *CPR,* C-peptide immunoreactivity; *GCMS,* gas chromatography mass spectrometry; *HPLC,* high-pressure liquid chromatography; *IA,* insulin antibodies. (From Moore WT, Eastman RC: *Diagnostic endocrinology,* ed 2, St Louis, 1996, Mosby.)

III

HYPOGONADISM

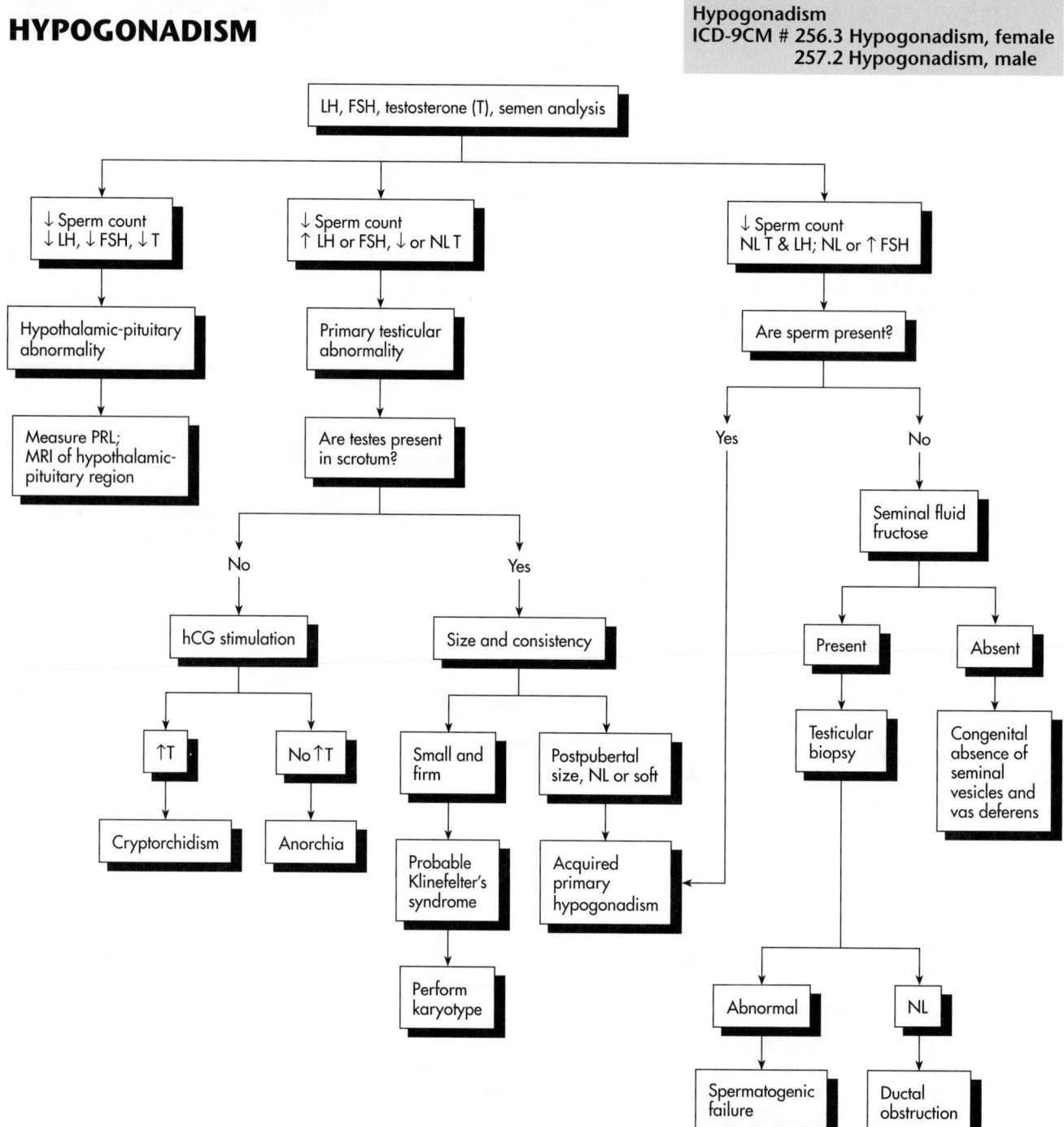

Fig. 3-92   Laboratory evaluation of hypogonadism. *FSH,* Follicle-stimulating hormone; *hCG,* human chorionic gonadotropin; *LH,* luteinizing hormone; *MRI,* magnetic resonance imaging; *NL,* normal; *PRL,* prolactin; ↑, elevated; ↓, decreased or low. (From Andreoli TE [ed]: *Cecil essentials of medicine,* ed 5, Philadelphia, 2001, WB Saunders.)

HYPOGONADISM—cont'd

BOX 3-2 Classification of Male Hypogonadism

Hypothalamic-Pituitary Disorders (Secondary Hypogonadism)

Panhypopituitarism
Isolated gonadotropin deficiency
Complex congenital syndromes

Gonadal Disorders (Primary Hypogonadism)

Klinefelter's syndrome and associated chromosomal defects
Myotonic dystrophy
Cryptorchidism
Bilateral anorchia
Seminiferous tubular failure
Adult Leydig cell failure
Androgen biosynthesis enzyme deficiency

Defects in Androgen Action

Testicular feminization (complete androgen insensitivity)
Incomplete androgen insensitivity
5α-Reductase deficiency

From Andreoli TE (ed): *Cecil essentials of medicine,* ed 4, Philadelphia, 1997, WB Saunders.

HYPOKALEMIA

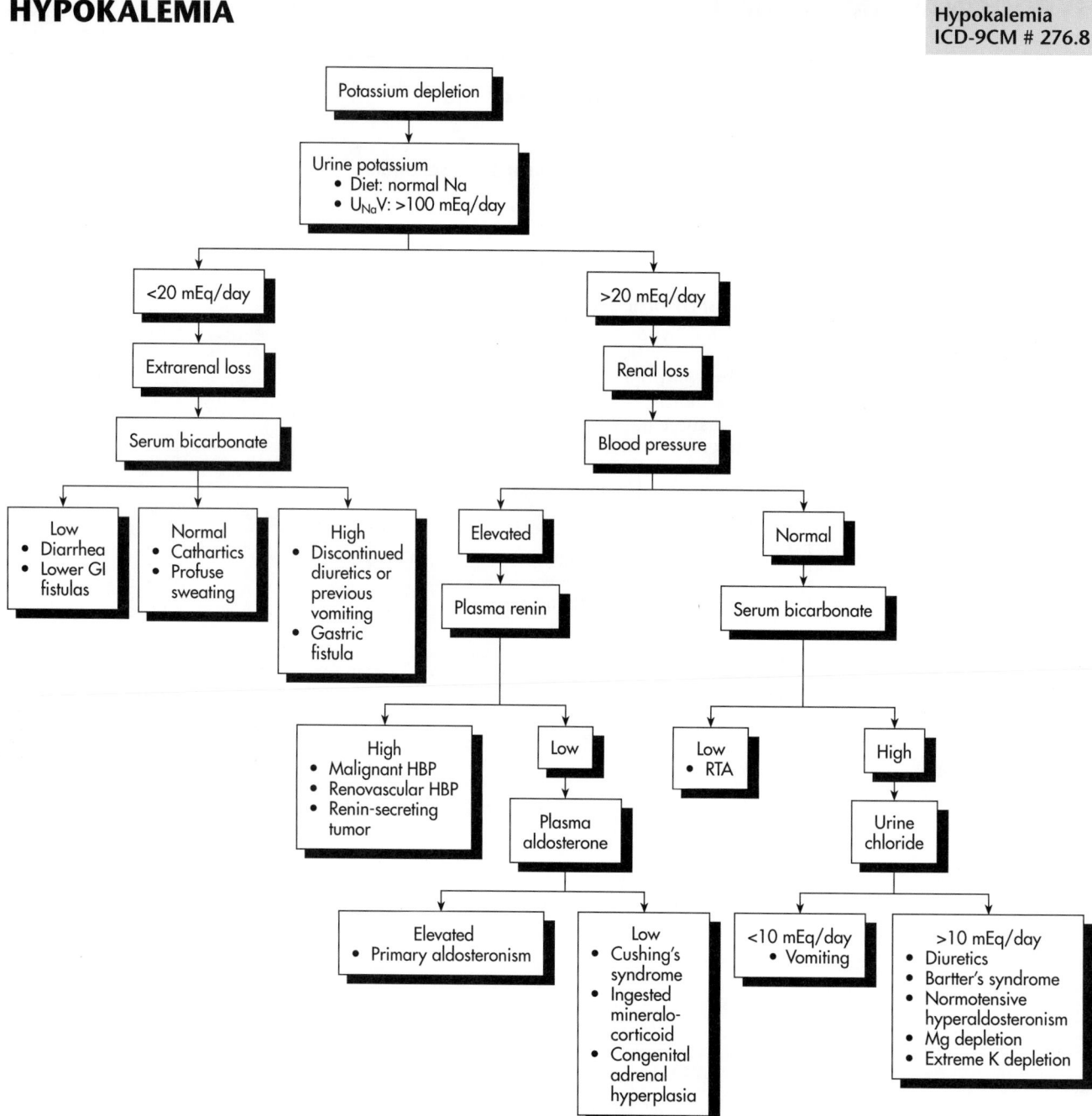

Fig. 3-93   Diagnostic approach to hypokalemia. Because renal potassium wasting may improve during sodium restriction, diminished potassium excretion is indicative of extrarenal loss only when the diet (and therefore the urine) is rich in sodium. *GI,* Gastrointestinal; *HBP,* high blood pressure; *RTA,* renal tubular acidosis; $U_{Na}V$, urinary sodium volume. (From Stein JH [ed]: *Internal medicine,* ed 5, St Louis, 1998, Mosby.)

HYPOMAGNESEMIA

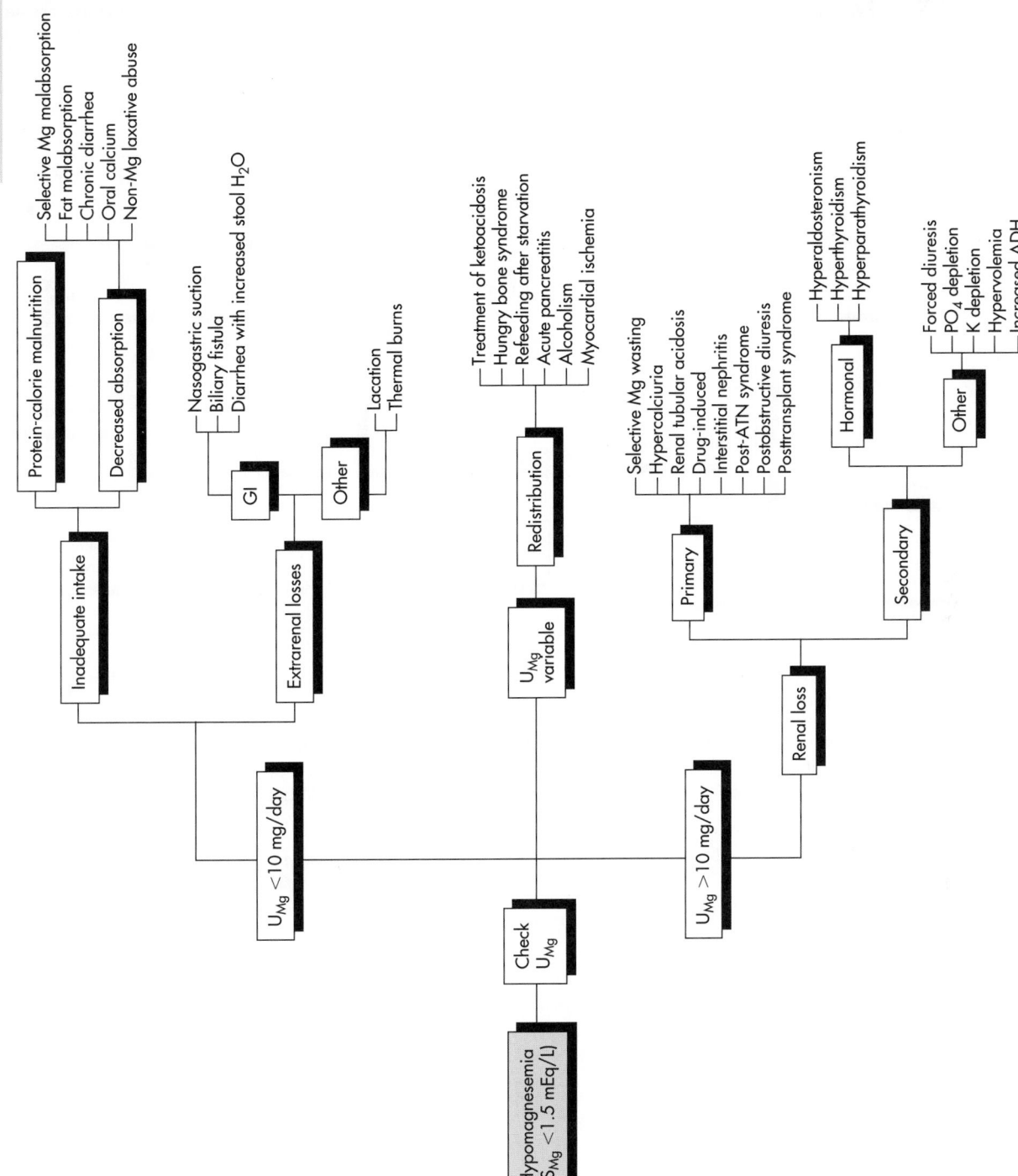

Fig. 3-94 Hypomagnesemia. *ADH,* Antidiuretic hormone; *GI,* gastrointestinal; *post-ATN,* post acute tubular necrosis. (From Healy PM: *Common medical diagnosis: an algorithmic approach,* ed 3, Philadelphia, 2000, WB Saunders.)

HYPONATREMIA

Hyponatremia
ICD-9CM # 276.1

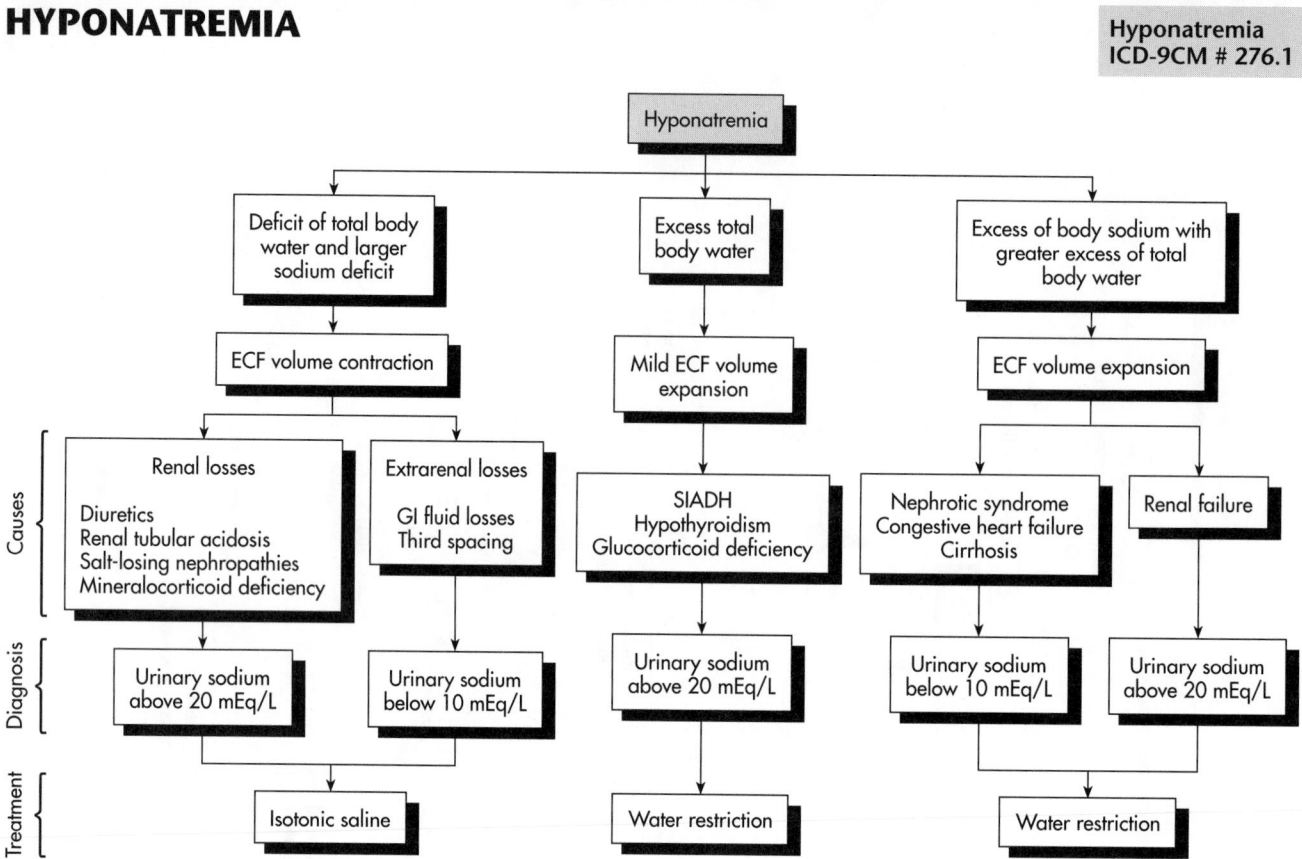

Fig. 3-95   Evaluation and treatment of asymptomatic, mild hyponatremia. *ECF,* Extracellular fluid; *GI,* gastrointestinal; *SIADH,* syndrome of inappropriate secretion of antidiuretic hormone. (From Rosen P et al [eds]: *Emergency medicine: concepts and clinical practice,* ed 5, St Louis, 2002, Mosby.)

HYPOPHOSPHATEMIA

Hypophosphatemia
ICD-9CM # 275.3

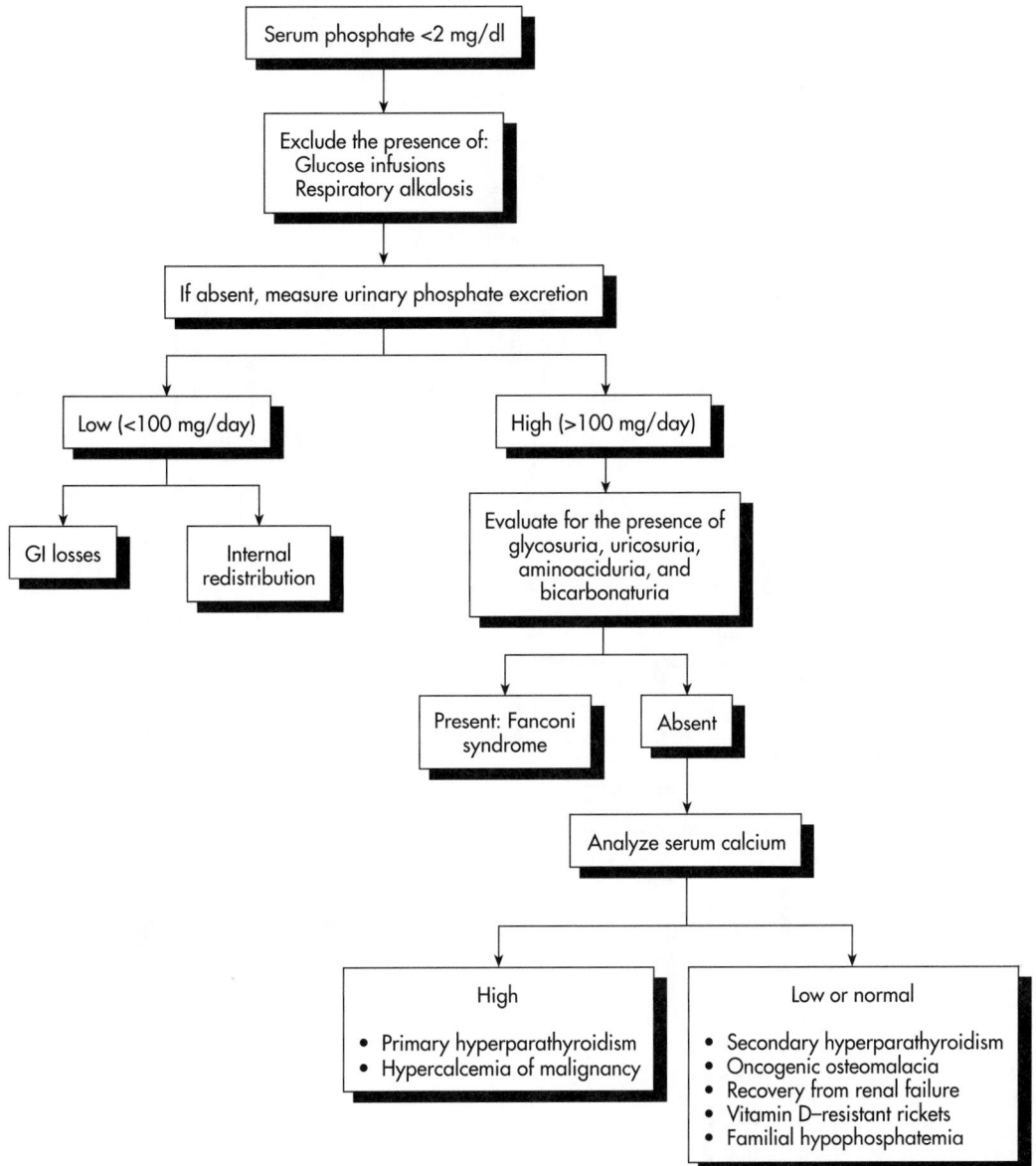

Fig. 3-96   Diagnostic workup of hypophosphatemia. *GI,* Gastrointestinal. (From Stein JH [ed]: *Internal medicine,* ed 5, St Louis, 1998, Mosby.)

HYPOTENSION

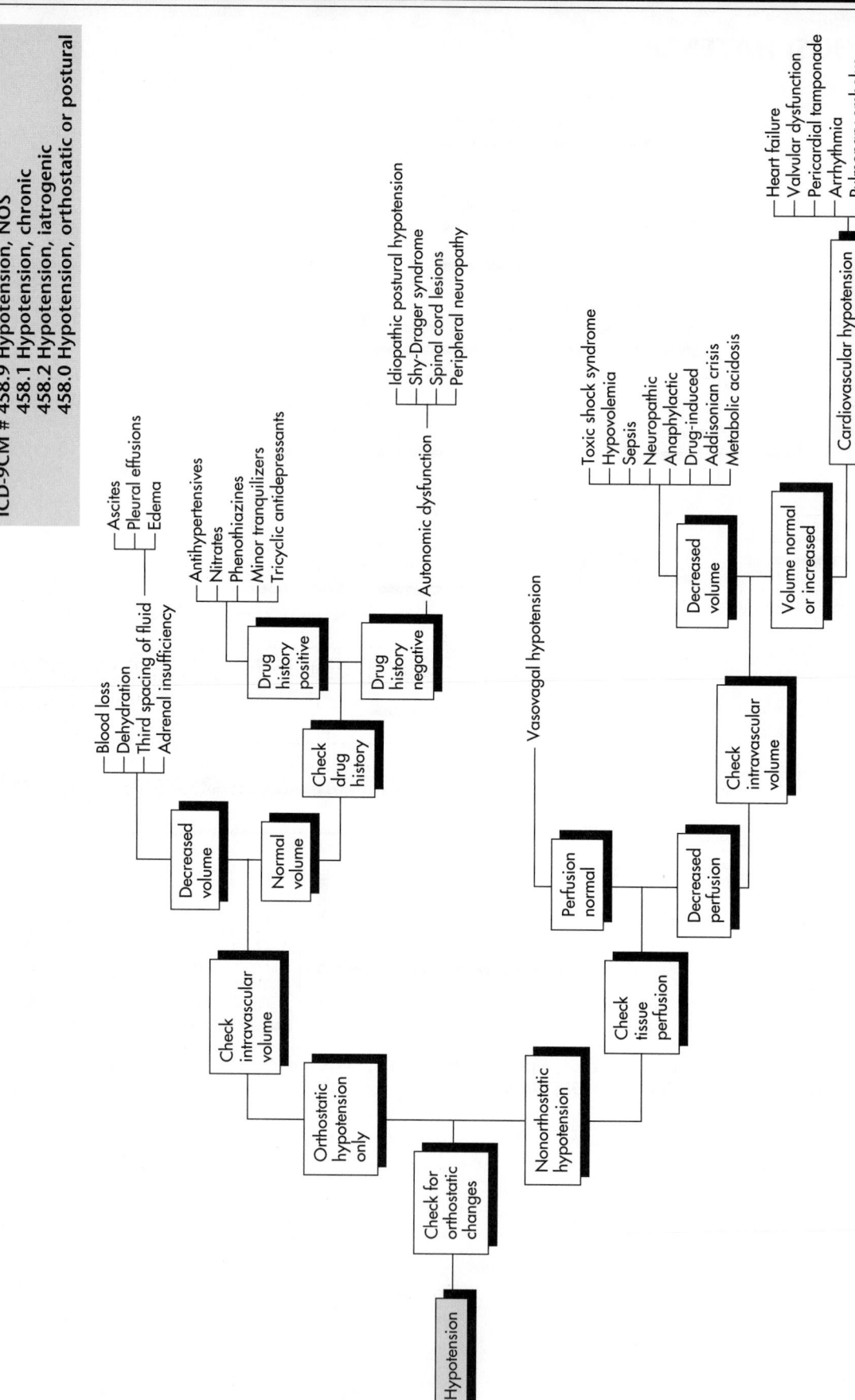

Hypotension
ICD-9CM # 458.9 Hypotension, NOS
458.1 Hypotension, chronic
458.2 Hypotension, iatrogenic
458.0 Hypotension, orthostatic or postural

Fig. 3-97   **Hypotension.** (From Healey PM: *Common medical diagnosis: an algorithmic approach,* ed 3, Philadelphia, 2000, WB Saunders.)

INFERTILITY

Infertility
ICD-9CM # 628.9 Infertility, female, unspecified
606.9 Infertility, male, unspecified

A

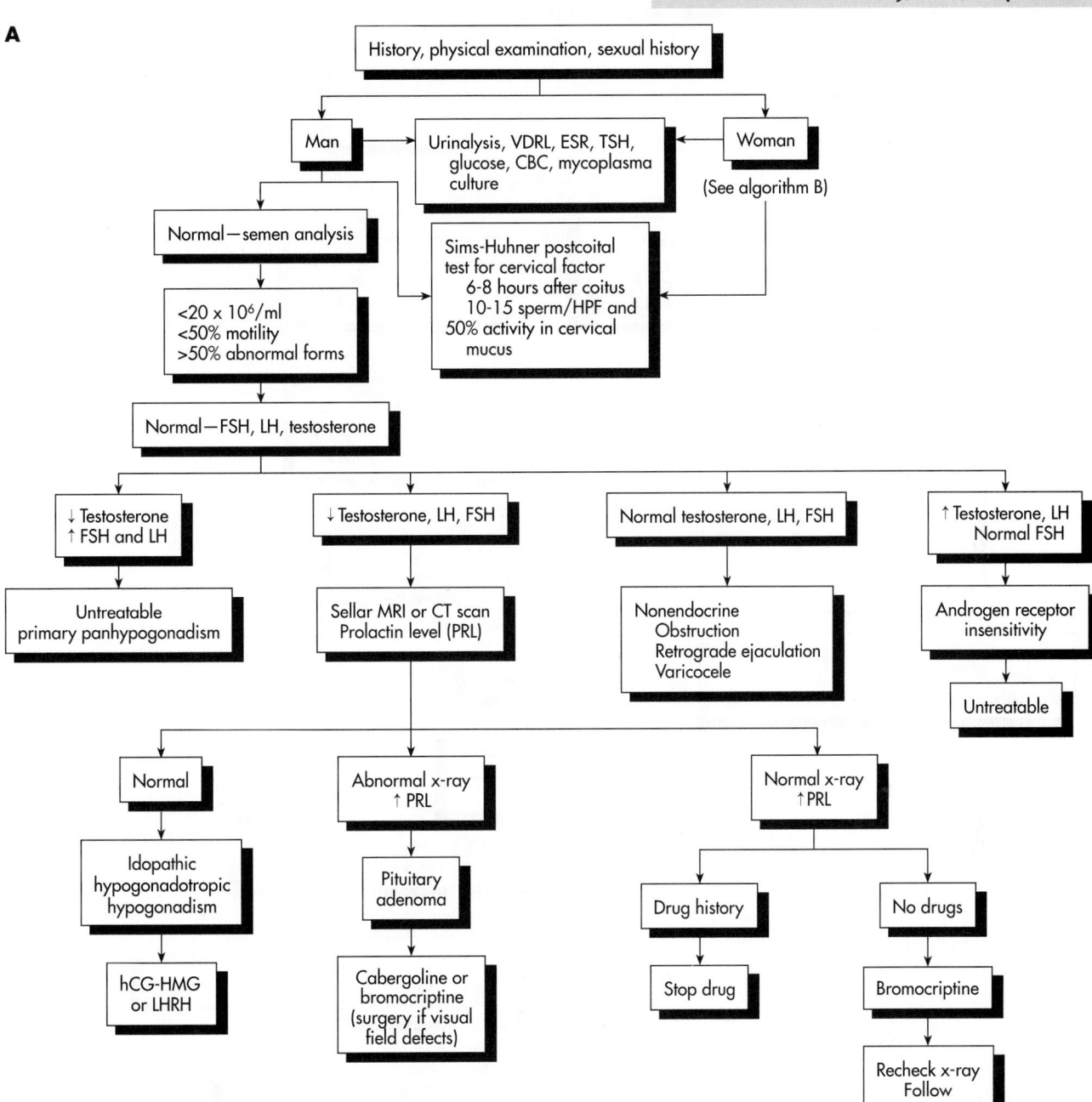

Fig. 3-98   A, Evaluating infertility in the man. *CBC,* Complete blood count; *CT,* computed tomography; *ESR,* erythrocyte sedimentation rate; *FSH,* follicle-stimulating hormone; *hCG-HMG,* human chorionic gonadotropin/human menopausal gonadotropin; *HPF,* high-power field; *LH,* luteinizing hormone; *LHRH,* luteinizing hormone–reducing hormone; *PRL,* prolactin level; *TSH,* thyroid-stimulating hormone; *VDRL,* Venereal Disease Research Laboratory. (Modified from Driscoll CE et al: *The family practice desk reference,* ed 3, St Louis, 1996, Mosby.)

Continued

B

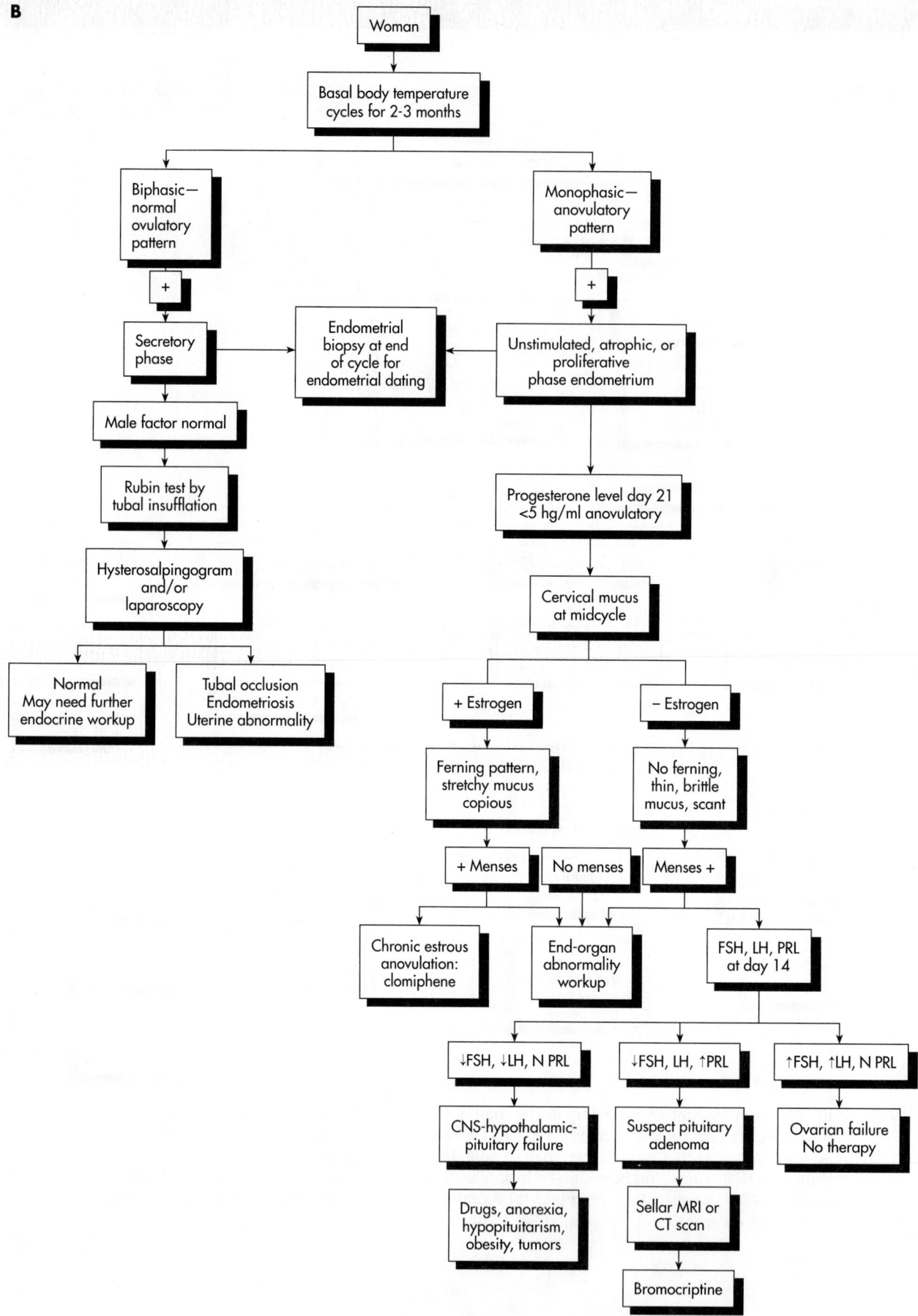

Fig. 3-98, cont'd **B, Evaluating infertility in the woman.** *CNS,* Central nervous system; *CT,* computed tomography; *FSH,* follicle-stimulating hormone; *LH,* luteinizing hormone; *N,* normal; *PRL,* prolactin level. (Modified from Driscoll CE et al: *The family practice desk reference,* ed 3, St Louis, 1996, Mosby.)

JAUNDICE AND HEPATOBILIARY DISEASE

Jaundice and hepatobiliary disease
ICD-9CM # 782.4 Jaundice NOS
277.4 Bilirubin excretion disorders
576.8 Jaundice, obstructive

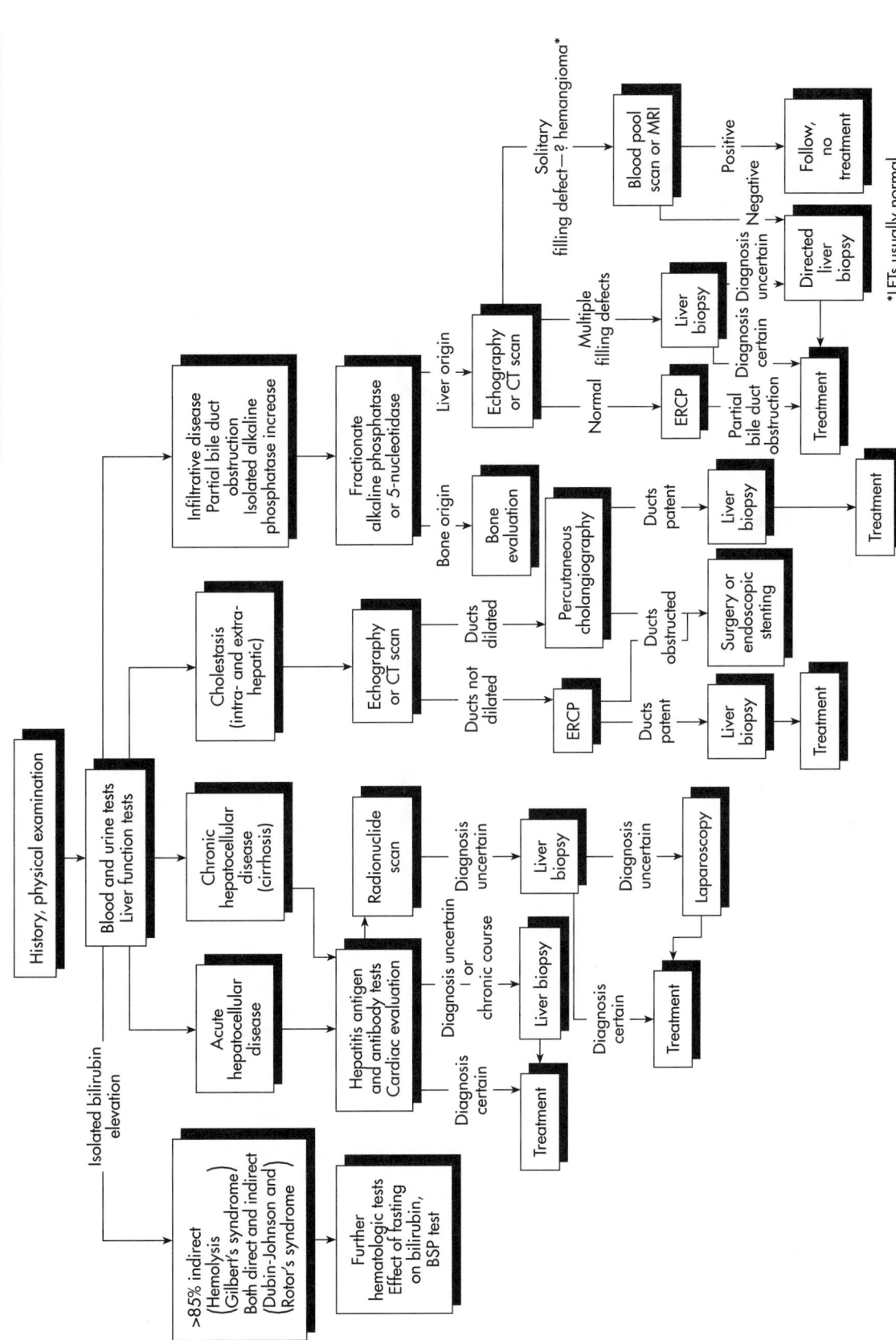

Fig. 3-99 **Evaluation of jaundice and hepatobiliary disease.** *BSP,* Bromsulphalein; *CT,* computed tomography; *ERCP,* endoscopic retrograde cholangiopancreatography; *LFTs,* liver function tests; *MRI,* magnetic resonance imaging. (From Stein JH [ed]: *Internal medicine,* ed 5, St Louis, 1998, Mosby.)

JAUNDICE, NEONATAL

Jaundice, neonatal
ICD-9CM # 774.6 Jaundice neonatal, NOS
            773.1 ABO reaction perinatal
            774.1 Hemolytic perinatal
            773.0 RH reaction perinatal
            751.61 Bile duct obstruction, congenital

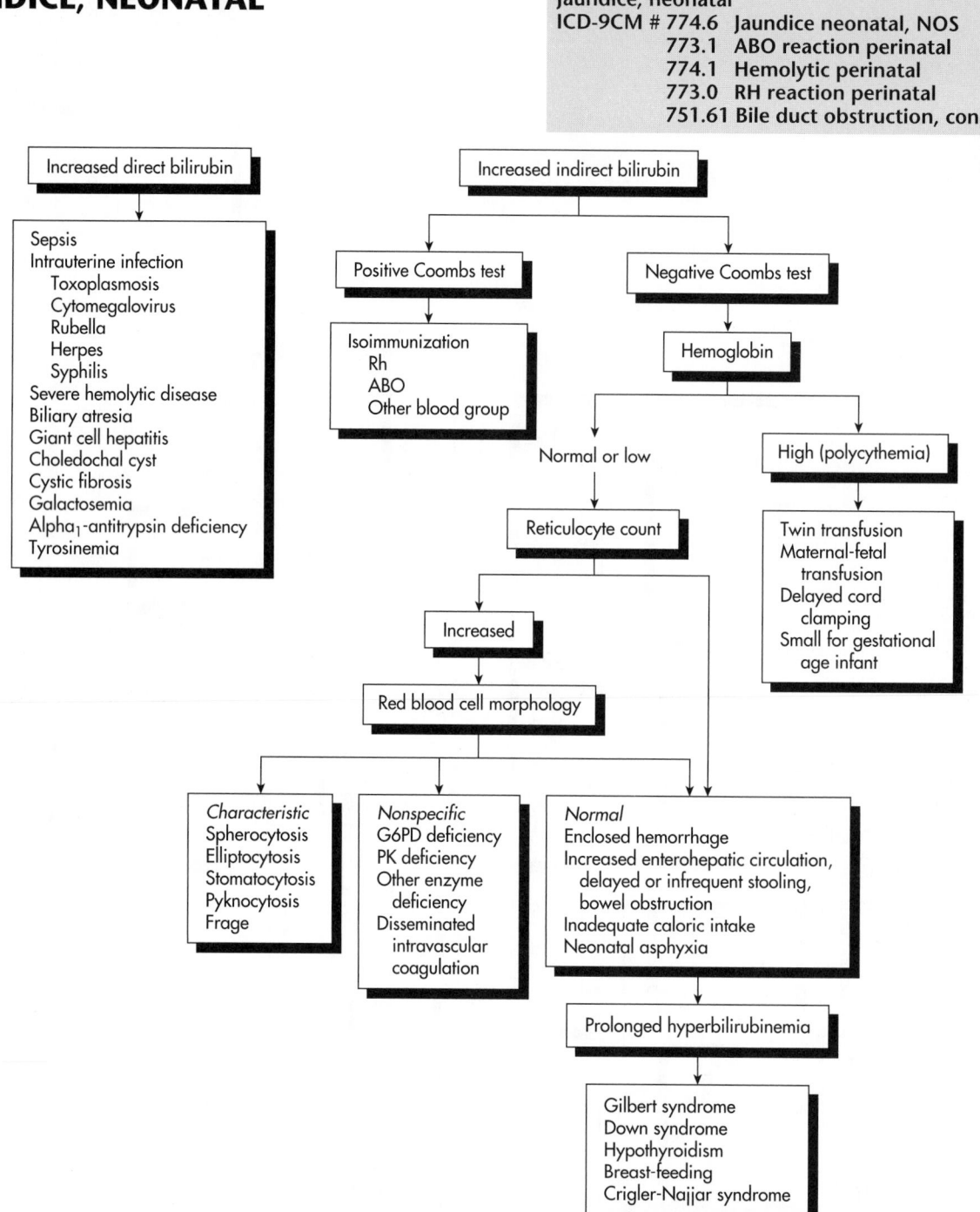

Fig. 3-100 Schematic approach to the diagnosis of neonatal jaundice. *G6PD*, Glucose-6-phosphate dehydrogenase; *PK*, pyruvate kinase. (From Oski FA: Differential diagnosis of jaundice. In Taeusch HW, Ballard RA, Avery MA [eds]: *Schaffer and Avery's diseases of the newborn*, ed 6, Philadelphia, 1991, WB Saunders.)

Knee pain, anterior
ICD-9CM # 716.96 Knee inflammation
959.7   Knee injury
719.56 Knee stiffness
719.06 Knee swelling

KNEE PAIN, ANTERIOR

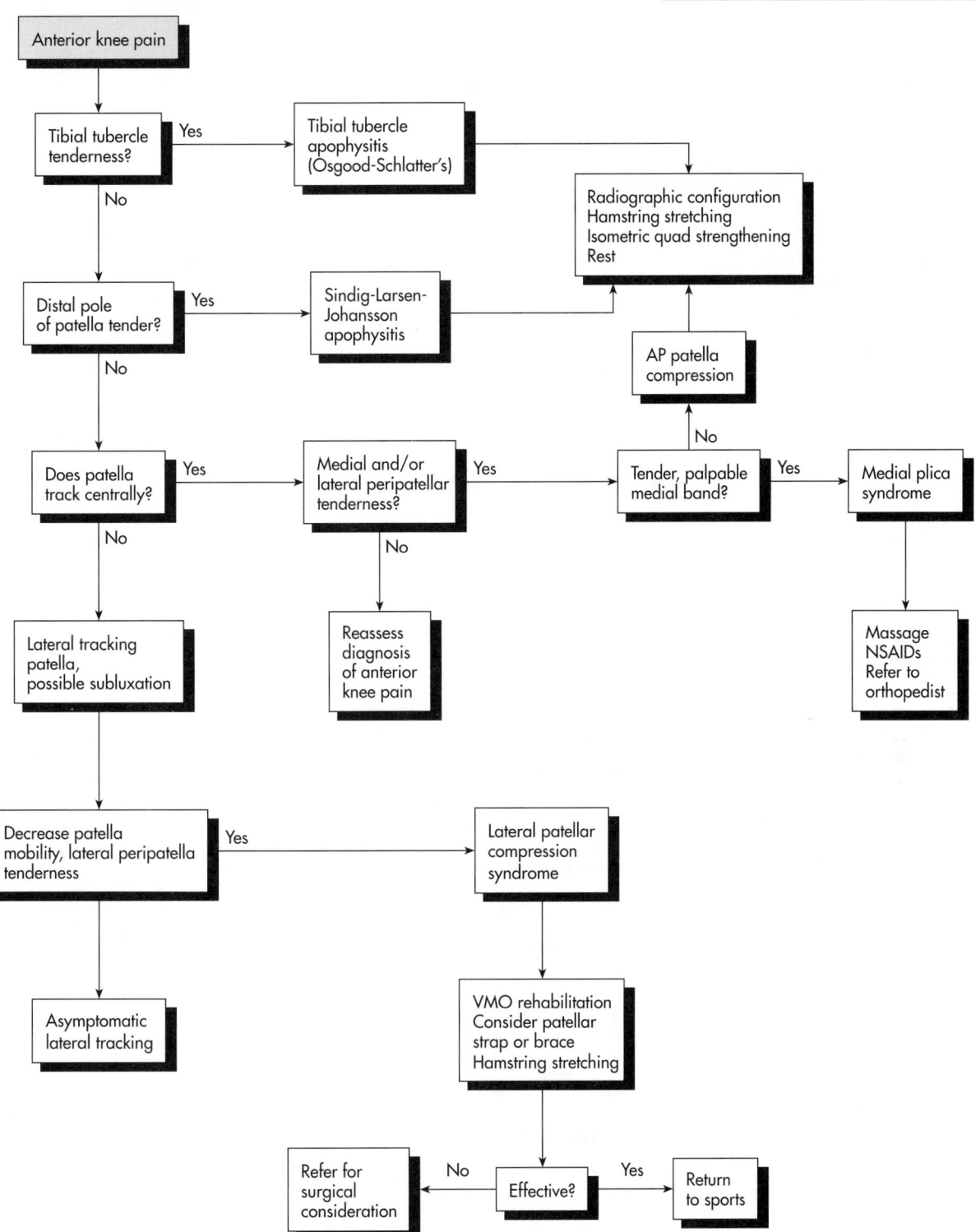

Fig. 3-101   Evaluation and management of knee extensor mechanism pain. Focused treatment based on specific etiology will prevent recurrence. *AP,* Anteroposterior; *NSAIDs,* nonsteroidal antiin-flammatory drugs; *VMO,* vastus medialis obliquus muscle. (From Scudieri G [ed]: *Sports medicine, principles of primary care,* St Louis, 1997, Mosby.)

Leg ulcer
ICD-9CM # 440.23 Ulcer, lower limb, arteriosclerotic
          707.1 Ulcer, lower limb, chronic
          707.1 Ulcer, lower limb, neurogenic
          707.9 Ulcer, non-healing
          707.0 Pressure ulcer

LEG ULCER

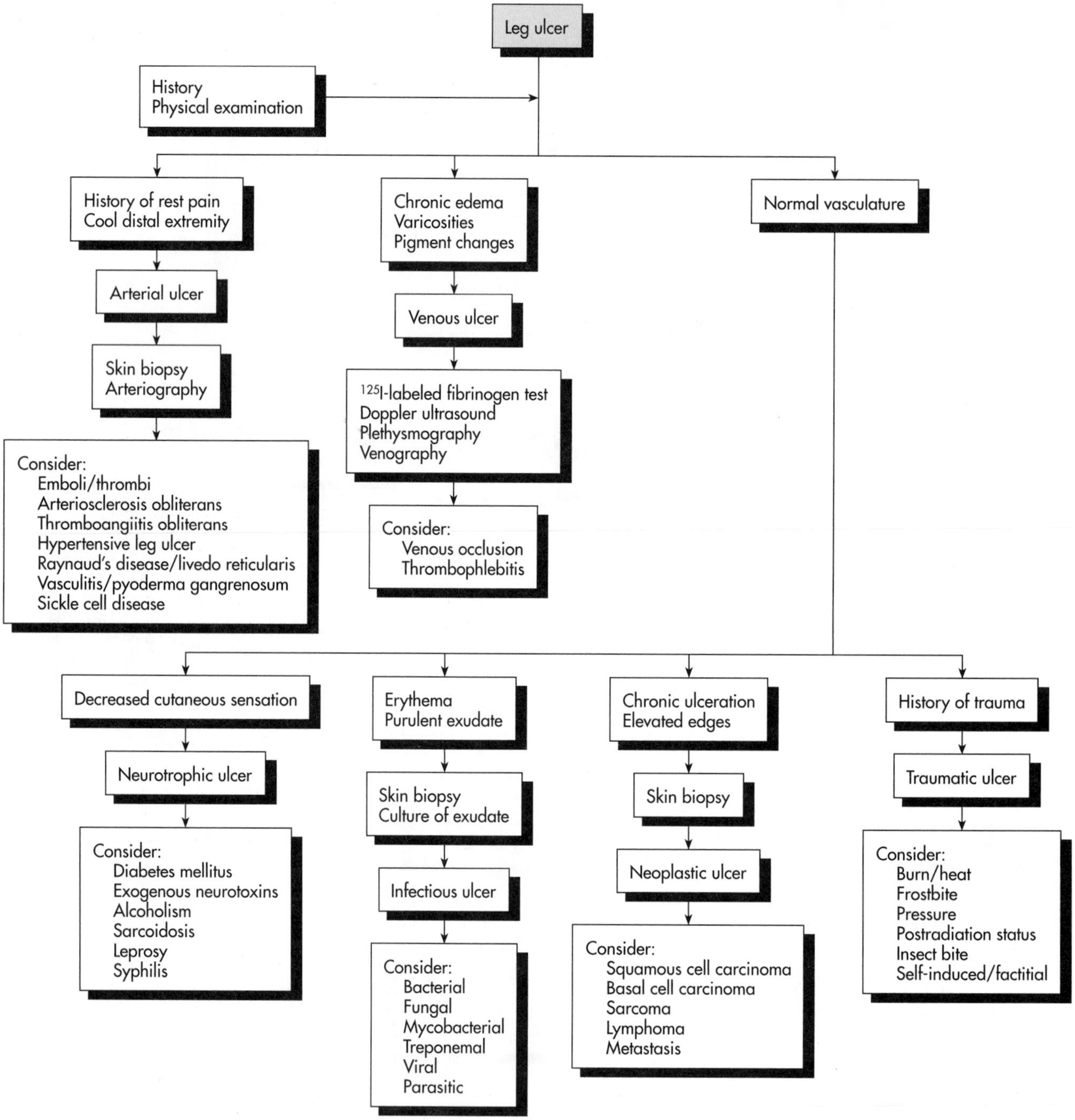

Leg ulcer

History
Physical examination

History of rest pain
Cool distal extremity

Chronic edema
Varicosities
Pigment changes

Normal vasculature

Arterial ulcer

Venous ulcer

Skin biopsy
Arteriography

^{125}I-labeled fibrinogen test
Doppler ultrasound
Plethysmography
Venography

Consider:
  Emboli/thrombi
  Arteriosclerosis obliterans
  Thromboangiitis obliterans
  Hypertensive leg ulcer
  Raynaud's disease/livedo reticularis
  Vasculitis/pyoderma gangrenosum
  Sickle cell disease

Consider:
  Venous occlusion
  Thrombophlebitis

Decreased cutaneous sensation

Erythema
Purulent exudate

Chronic ulceration
Elevated edges

History of trauma

Neurotrophic ulcer

Skin biopsy
Culture of exudate

Skin biopsy

Traumatic ulcer

Consider:
  Diabetes mellitus
  Exogenous neurotoxins
  Alcoholism
  Sarcoidosis
  Leprosy
  Syphilis

Infectious ulcer

Neoplastic ulcer

Consider:
  Burn/heat
  Frostbite
  Pressure
  Postradiation status
  Insect bite
  Self-induced/factitial

Consider:
  Bacterial
  Fungal
  Mycobacterial
  Treponemal
  Viral
  Parasitic

Consider:
  Squamous cell carcinoma
  Basal cell carcinoma
  Sarcoma
  Lymphoma
  Metastasis

Fig. 3-102   **Leg ulcer.** (From Greene HL, Johnson WP, Lemcke D [eds]: *Decision making in medicine,* ed 2, St Louis, 1998, Mosby.)

LEUKOCYTOSIS, NEUTROPHILIC

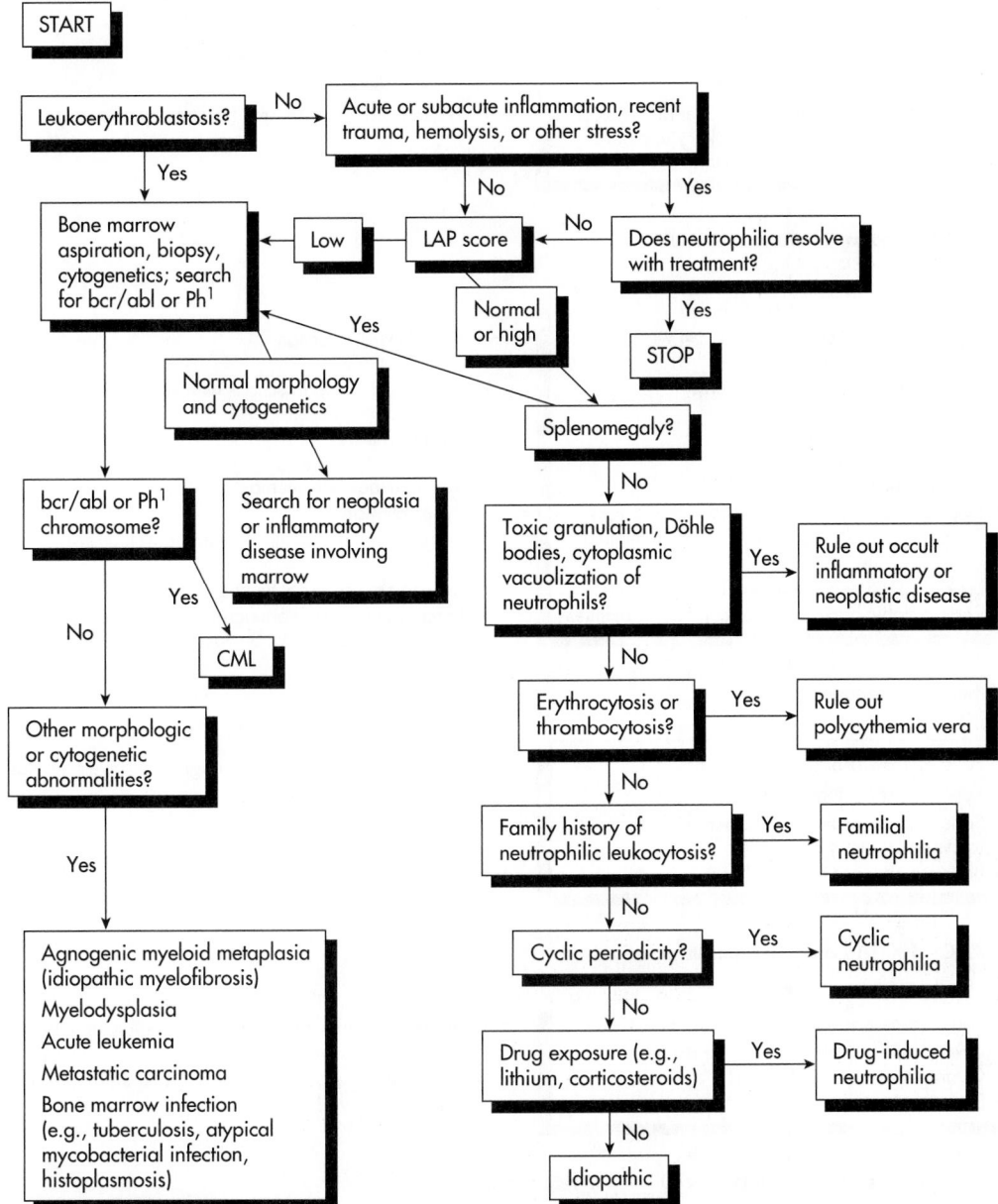

Fig. 3-103   Evaluation of patients with neutrophilic leukocytosis. *bcr/abl,* The translocation of the *c-abl* gene from chromosome 9 to the *bcr* gene on chromosome 22q; *CML,* chronic myelogenous leukemia; *LAP,* leukocyte alkaline phosphatase; *Ph[1],* Philadelphia chromosome. (From Goldman L, Bennett JC [eds] *Cecil textbook of medicine,* ed 21, Philadelphia, 2000, WB Saunders.)

III

LEUKOPENIA OR RECURRENT UNUSUAL BACTERIAL INFECTIONS

Leukopenia or recurrent unusual bacterial infection ICD-9CM # 288.0

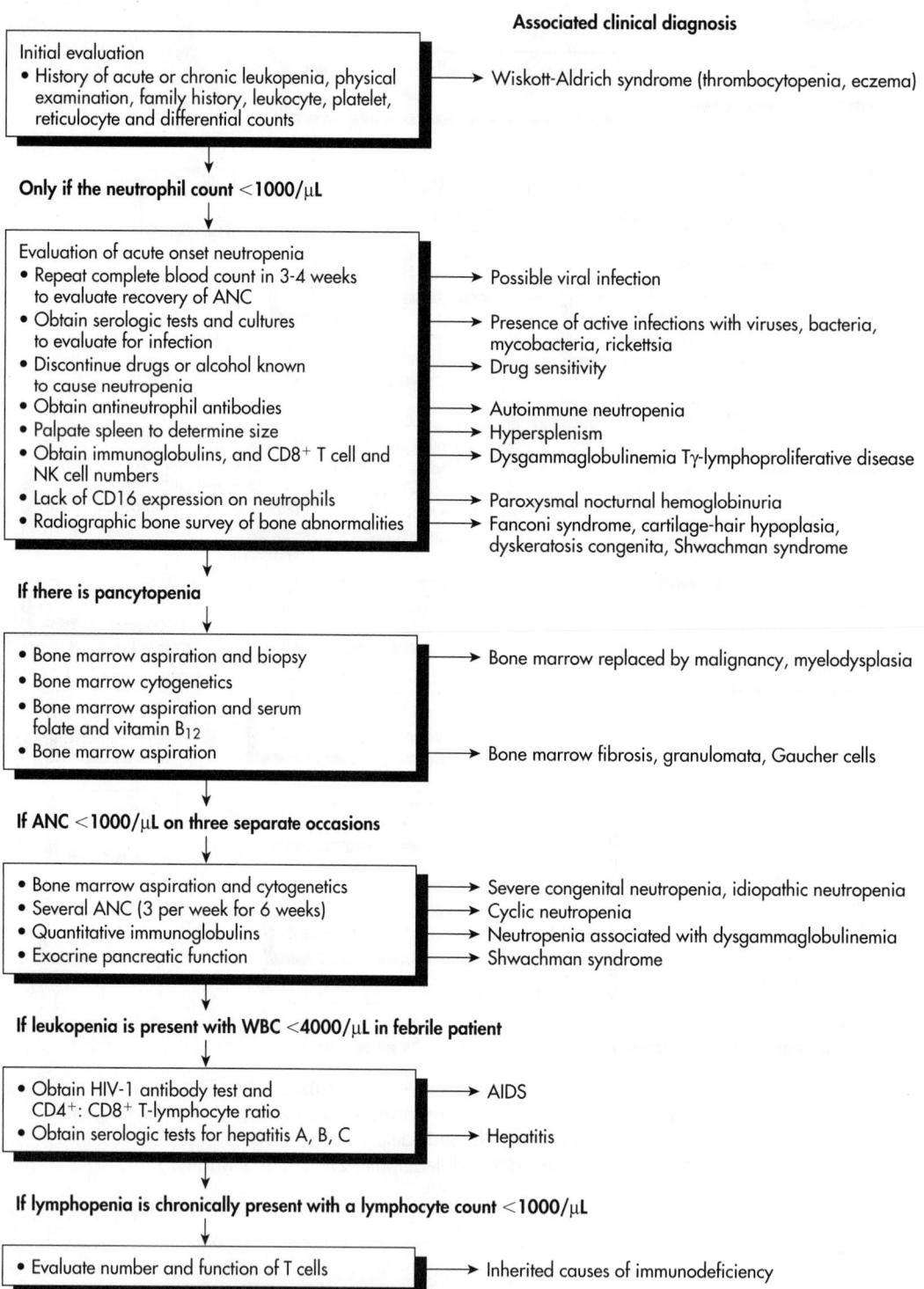

Associated clinical diagnosis

Initial evaluation
• History of acute or chronic leukopenia, physical examination, family history, leukocyte, platelet, reticulocyte and differential counts
→ Wiskott-Aldrich syndrome (thrombocytopenia, eczema)

Only if the neutrophil count <1000/μL

Evaluation of acute onset neutropenia
• Repeat complete blood count in 3-4 weeks to evaluate recovery of ANC
→ Possible viral infection
• Obtain serologic tests and cultures to evaluate for infection
→ Presence of active infections with viruses, bacteria, mycobacteria, rickettsia
• Discontinue drugs or alcohol known to cause neutropenia
→ Drug sensitivity
• Obtain antineutrophil antibodies
→ Autoimmune neutropenia
• Palpate spleen to determine size
→ Hypersplenism
• Obtain immunoglobulins, and CD8+ T cell and NK cell numbers
→ Dysgammaglobulinemia Tγ-lymphoproliferative disease
• Lack of CD16 expression on neutrophils
→ Paroxysmal nocturnal hemoglobinuria
• Radiographic bone survey of bone abnormalities
→ Fanconi syndrome, cartilage-hair hypoplasia, dyskeratosis congenita, Shwachman syndrome

If there is pancytopenia

• Bone marrow aspiration and biopsy
• Bone marrow cytogenetics
→ Bone marrow replaced by malignancy, myelodysplasia
• Bone marrow aspiration and serum folate and vitamin B12
• Bone marrow aspiration
→ Bone marrow fibrosis, granulomata, Gaucher cells

If ANC <1000/μL on three separate occasions

• Bone marrow aspiration and cytogenetics
→ Severe congenital neutropenia, idiopathic neutropenia
• Several ANC (3 per week for 6 weeks)
→ Cyclic neutropenia
• Quantitative immunoglobulins
→ Neutropenia associated with dysgammaglobulinemia
• Exocrine pancreatic function
→ Shwachman syndrome

If leukopenia is present with WBC <4000/μL in febrile patient

• Obtain HIV-1 antibody test and CD4+: CD8+ T-lymphocyte ratio
→ AIDS
• Obtain serologic tests for hepatitis A, B, C
→ Hepatitis

If lymphopenia is chronically present with a lymphocyte count <1000/μL

• Evaluate number and function of T cells
→ Inherited causes of immunodeficiency

Fig. 3-104   Algorithm for the evaluation of the patient with leukopenia or recurrent or unusual bacterial infections. *AIDS,* Acquired immunodeficiency syndrome; *ANC,* absolute neutrophil count; *HIV,* human immunodeficiency virus; *NK,* natural killer; *WBC,* white blood cell count. (From Copeland LJ: *Textbook of gynecology,* ed 2, Philadelphia, 2000, WB Saunders.)

Liver function test abnormalities
ICD-9CM # 571.0 Fatty liver, alcoholic
                571.8 Fatty liver, non-alcoholic
                751.60 Liver anomaly NOS
                571.9 Liver disease, chronic
                573.3 Liver disease, drug induced
                571.3 Liver disease, alcoholic
                573.9 Liver disorder

LIVER FUNCTION TEST ABNORMALITIES

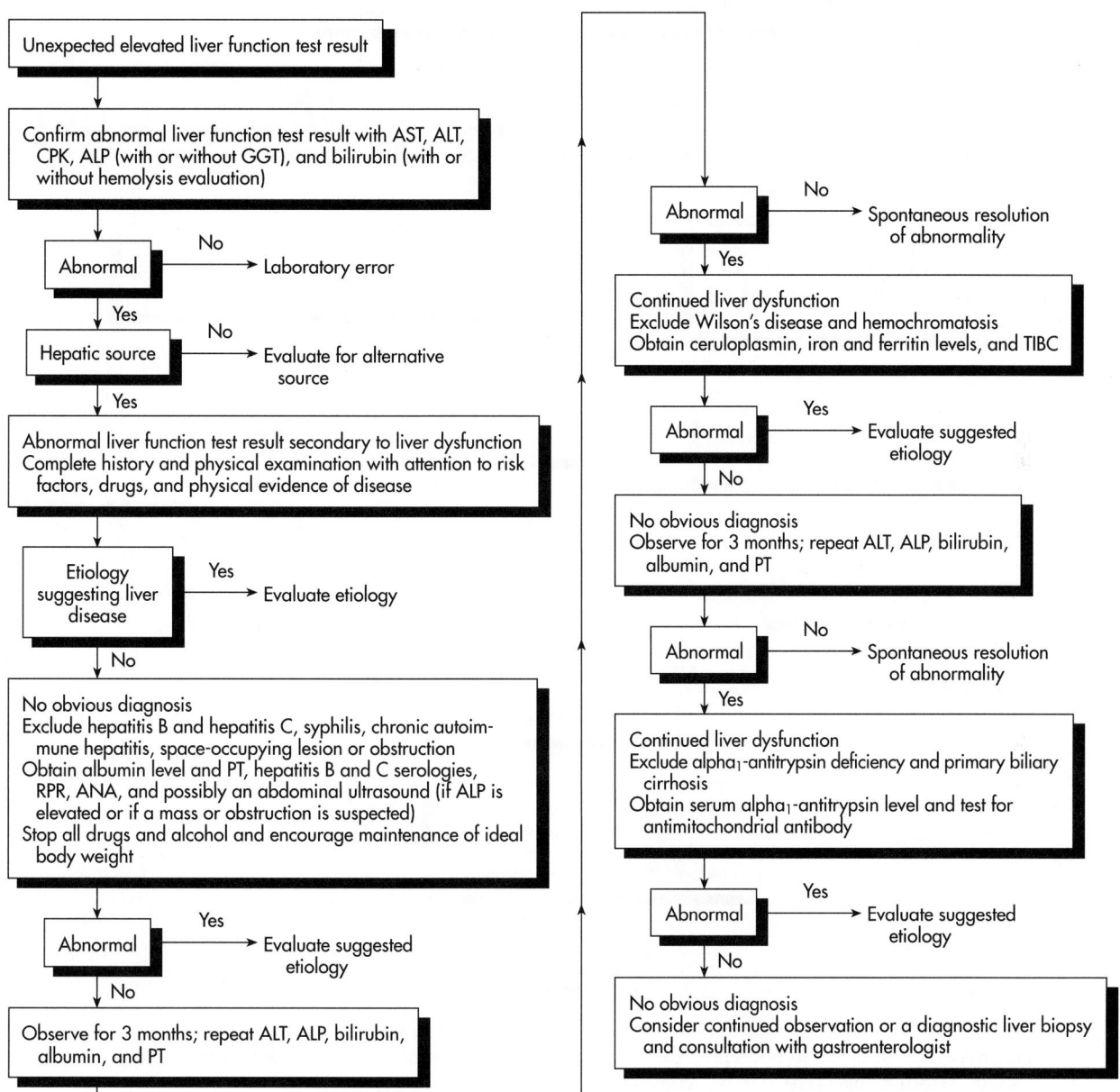

Fig. 3-105   Evaluation of a patient with abnormal results on liver function tests. *ALP,* Alkaline phosphatase; *ALT,* alanine transaminase; *ANA,* antinuclear antibody; *AST,* aspartate transaminase; *CPK,* creatine phosphokinase; *GGT,* gamma glutamyltransferase; *PT,* prothrombin time; *RPR,* rapid plasma reagent; *TIBC,* total iron-binding capacity. (From Theal RM, Scott K: *Am Fam Physician* 53:2111, 1996.)

LYMPHADENOPATHY, GENERALIZED

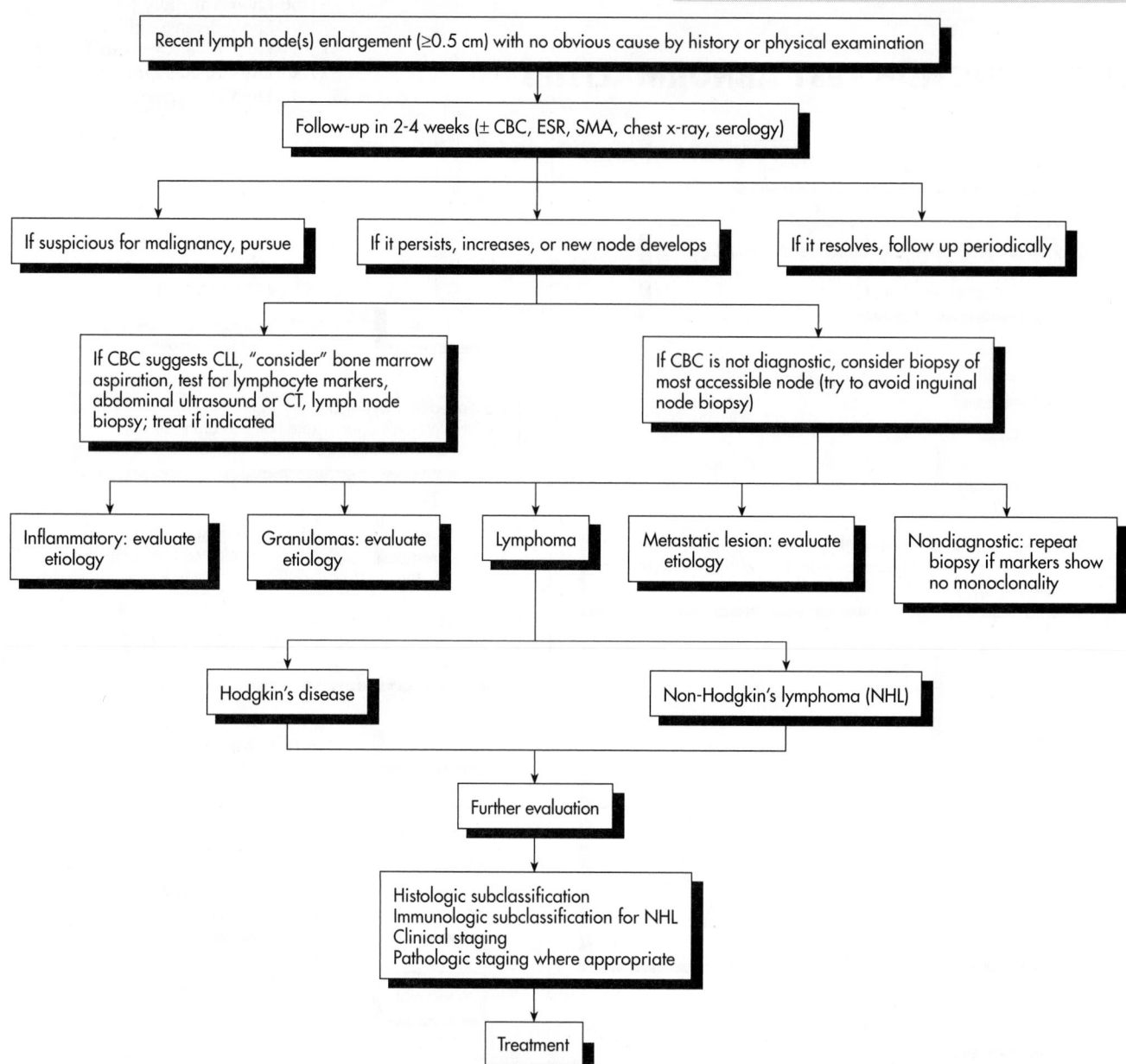

Fig. 3-106 **Workup of lymphadenopathy.** *CBC*, Complete blood count; *CLL*, chronic lymphocytic leukemia; *CT*, computed tomography; *ESR*, erythrocyte sedimentation rate; *SMA*, sequential multiple analysis. (From Noble J [ed]: *Primary care medicine*, ed 3, St Louis, 2001, Mosby.)

LYMPHADENOPATHY, LOCALIZED

Lymphadenopathy, localized
ICD-9CM # 785.6 Lymphadenopathy, unknown
etiology

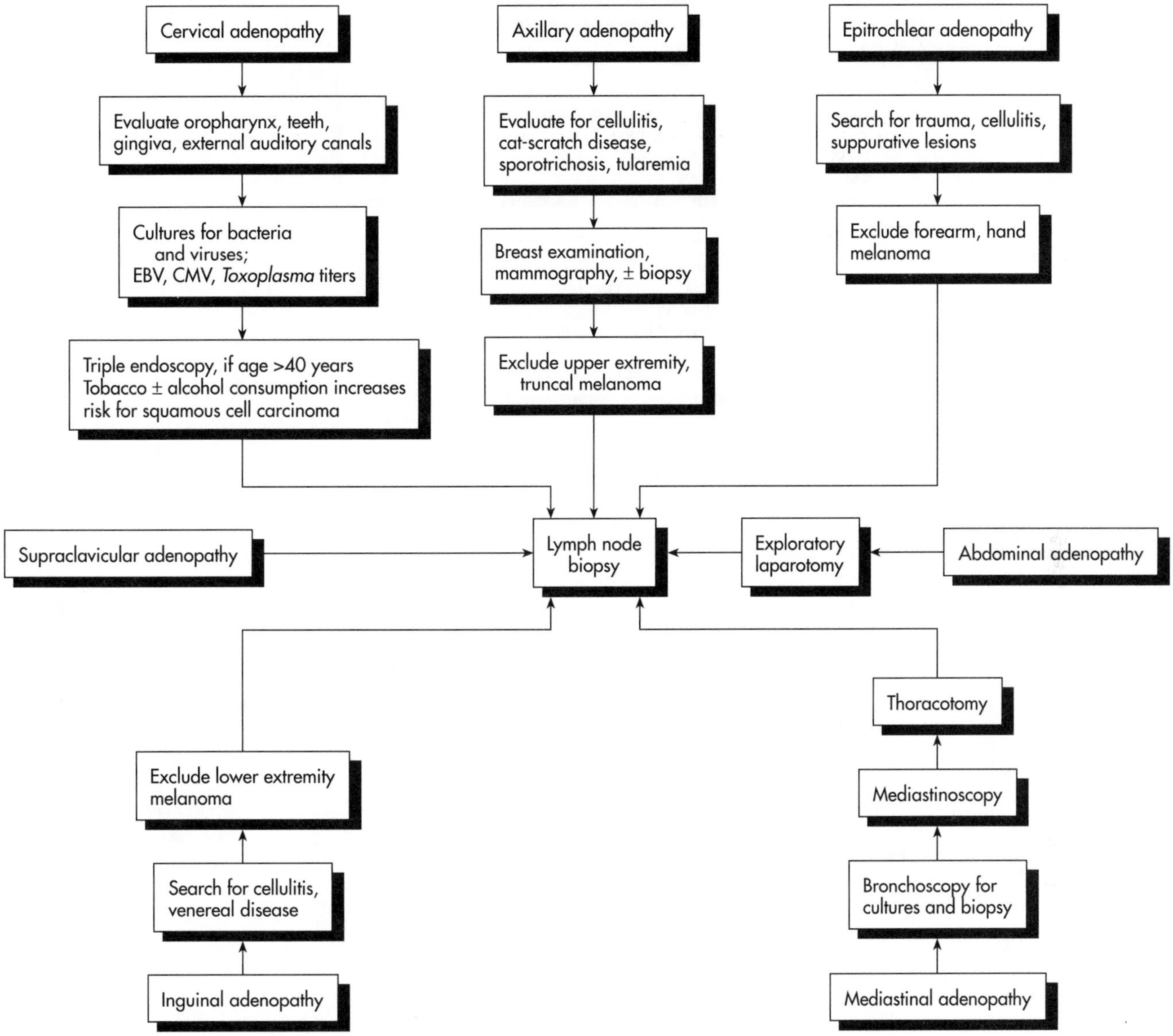

Cervical adenopathy

Evaluate oropharynx, teeth, gingiva, external auditory canals

Cultures for bacteria and viruses; EBV, CMV, *Toxoplasma* titers

Triple endoscopy, if age >40 years Tobacco ± alcohol consumption increases risk for squamous cell carcinoma

Axillary adenopathy

Evaluate for cellulitis, cat-scratch disease, sporotrichosis, tularemia

Breast examination, mammography, ± biopsy

Exclude upper extremity, truncal melanoma

Epitrochlear adenopathy

Search for trauma, cellulitis, suppurative lesions

Exclude forearm, hand melanoma

Supraclavicular adenopathy

Lymph node biopsy

Exploratory laparotomy

Abdominal adenopathy

Exclude lower extremity melanoma

Search for cellulitis, venereal disease

Inguinal adenopathy

Thoracotomy

Mediastinoscopy

Bronchoscopy for cultures and biopsy

Mediastinal adenopathy

Fig. 3-107   Clinical approach to the patient with localized lymphadenopathy. *CMV,* Cytomegalovirus; *EBV,* Epstein-Barr virus. (From Stein JH [ed]: *Internal medicine,* ed 5, St Louis, 1998, Mosby.)

III

MACROCYTOSIS

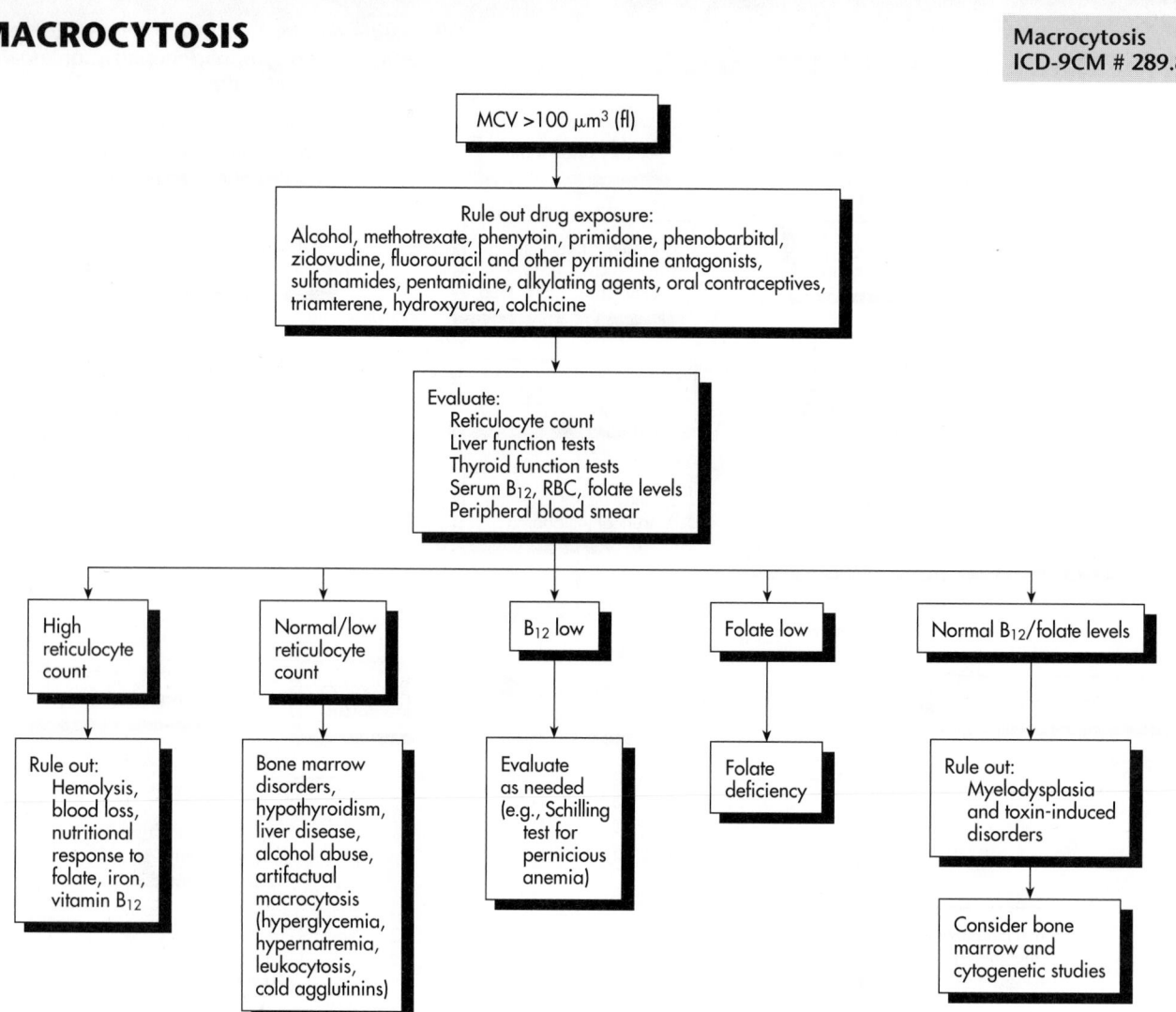

Fig. 3-108   Evaluation of macrocytosis. *MCV,* Mean corpuscular volume.

MALABSORPTION, SUSPECTED

Malabsorption, suspected
ICD-9CM # 579.9

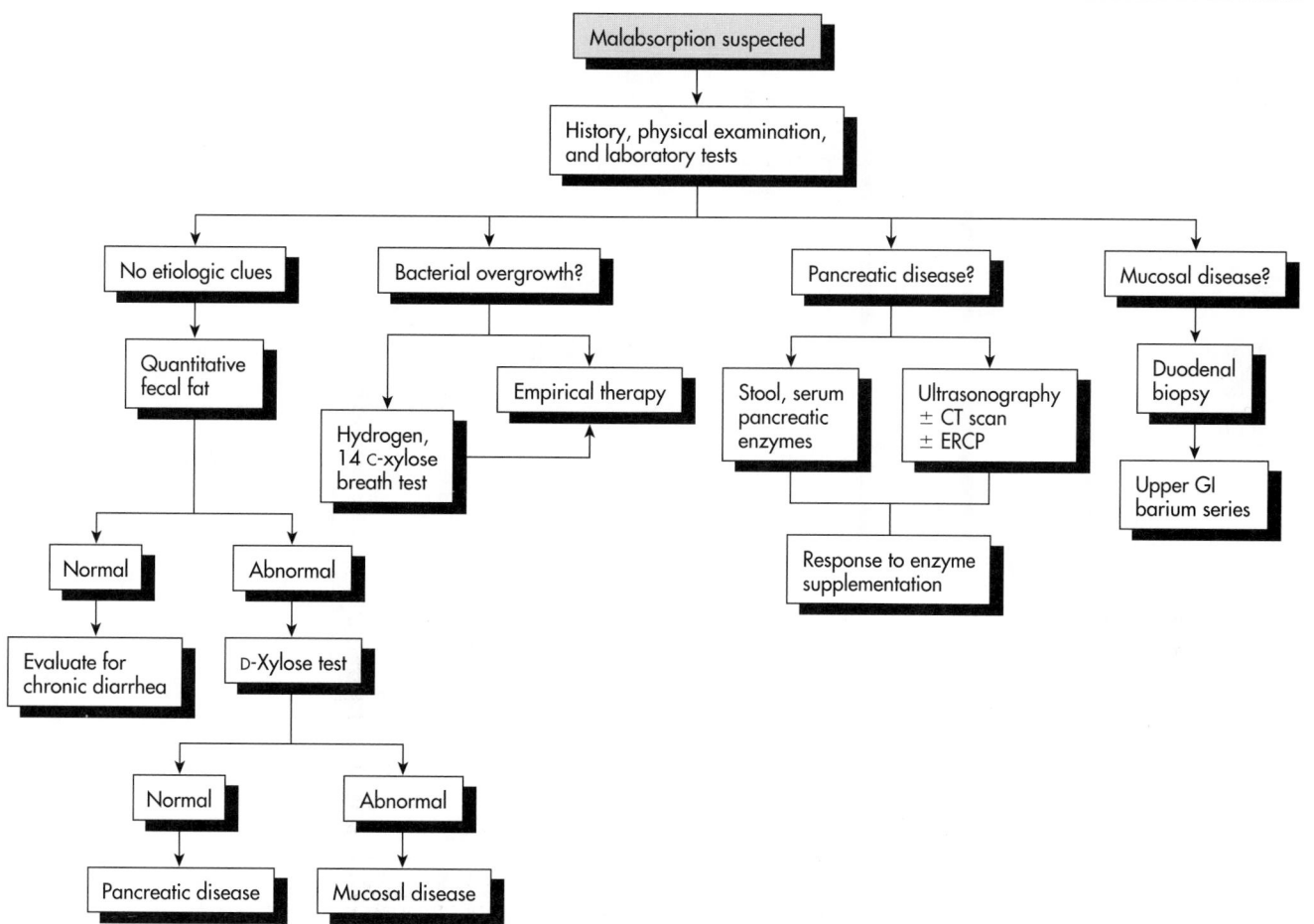

Fig. 3-109   Approach to the patient with suspected malabsorption. *CT,* Computed tomography; *ERCP,* endoscopic retrograde cholangiopancreatography; *GI,* gastrointestinal. (Adapted from Riley SA, Marsh MN: Maldigestion and malabsorption. In Feldman M, Scharschmidt BF, Sleisenger MH [eds]: *Sleisenger and Fordtran's gastrointestinal and liver diseases: pathophysiology/diagnosis/management,* ed 6, Philadelphia, 1998, WB Saunders.)

III

MESENTERIC ISCHEMIA, ACUTE

Mesenteric ischemia, acute
ICD-9CM # 557.0 Mesentery artery embolism
557.0 Mesenteric artery infarction

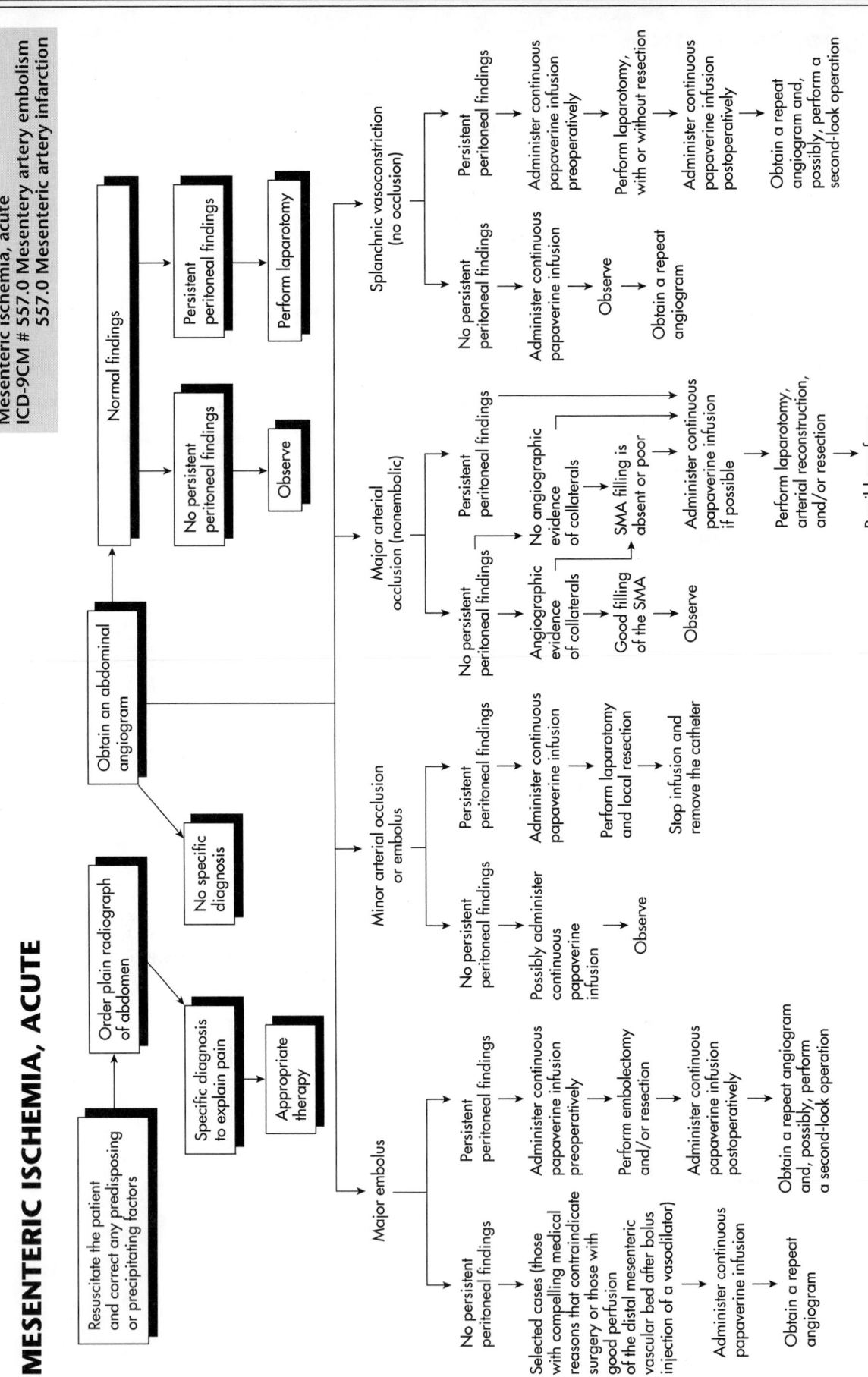

Fig. 3-110   Algorithm for managing patients with suspected acute mesenteric ischemia. *SMA*, Superior mesenteric artery. (From Goldman L, Bennett JC [eds]: *Cecil textbook of medicine*, ed 21, Philadelphia, 2000, WB Saunders.)

MESOTHELIOMA

Mesothelioma
ICD-9CM # 229.9 Epithelioid benign site NOS
199.1 Epithelioid malignant site NOS

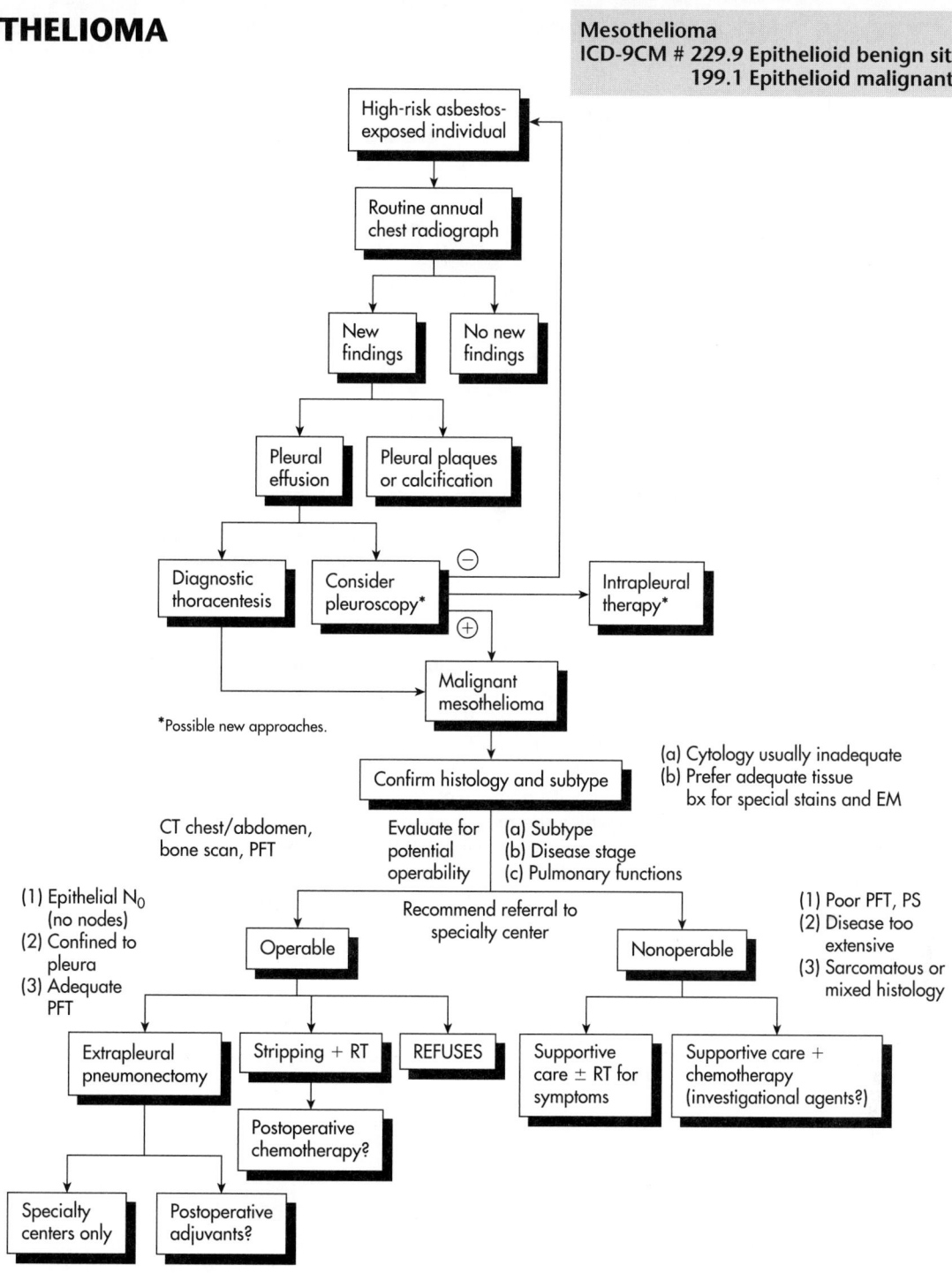

Fig. 3-111   Evaluation and treatment of mesothelioma. *bx,* Biopsy; *CT,* computed tomography; *EM,* electron microscopy; *PFT,* pulmonary function test; *PS,* pleural sclerosis; *RT,* respiratory therapy. (From Abeloff MD: *Clinical oncology,* ed 2, New York, 2000, Churchill Livingstone.)

MICROCYTOSIS AND HYPOCHROMIA

Microcytosis and hypochromia → Fe, TIBC, or ferritin

Normal

$\downarrow$ Fe
$\uparrow$ TIBC — Fe deficiency anemia
$\downarrow$ Ferritin

Hemoglobin electrophoresis

Normal
possible α-thalassemia
(confirmation, if desirable, requires family study or gene mapping)

$\uparrow$ HbA$_2$
Heterozygous β-thalassemia

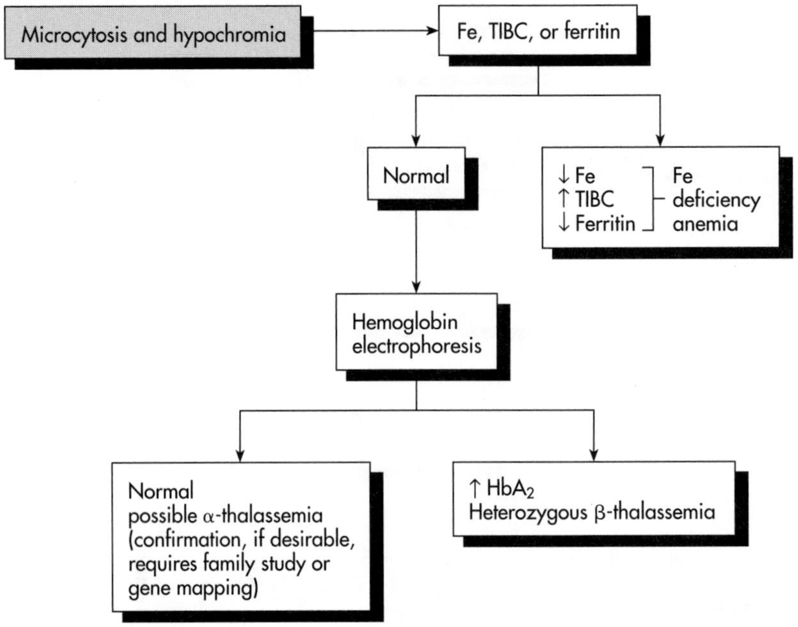

Fig. 3-112   Evaluation of microcytosis and mild thalassemias. Microcytosis, best detected by electronic cell counters, may result from many causes. Iron deficiency is excluded by measuring serum iron level and iron-binding capacity or ferritin level. If these values are normal, hemoglobin electrophoresis should be performed, with measurement of the level of adult hemoglobin A$_2$ (HbA$_2$) and fetal hemoglobin (HbF). An elevated HbA$_2$ level is consistent with heterozygous β-thalassemia. If HbA$_2$ and HbF levels are normal, microcytosis with minimal or no anemia suggests α-thalassemia. This diagnosis is more likely in populations in which the prevalence of this disorder is high. *TIBC,* Total iron-binding capacity. (From Stein J [ed]: *Internal medicine,* ed 5, St Louis, 1998, Mosby.)

MURMUR, DIASTOLIC

Murmur, diastolic
ICD-9CM # 785.2 Murmur heart

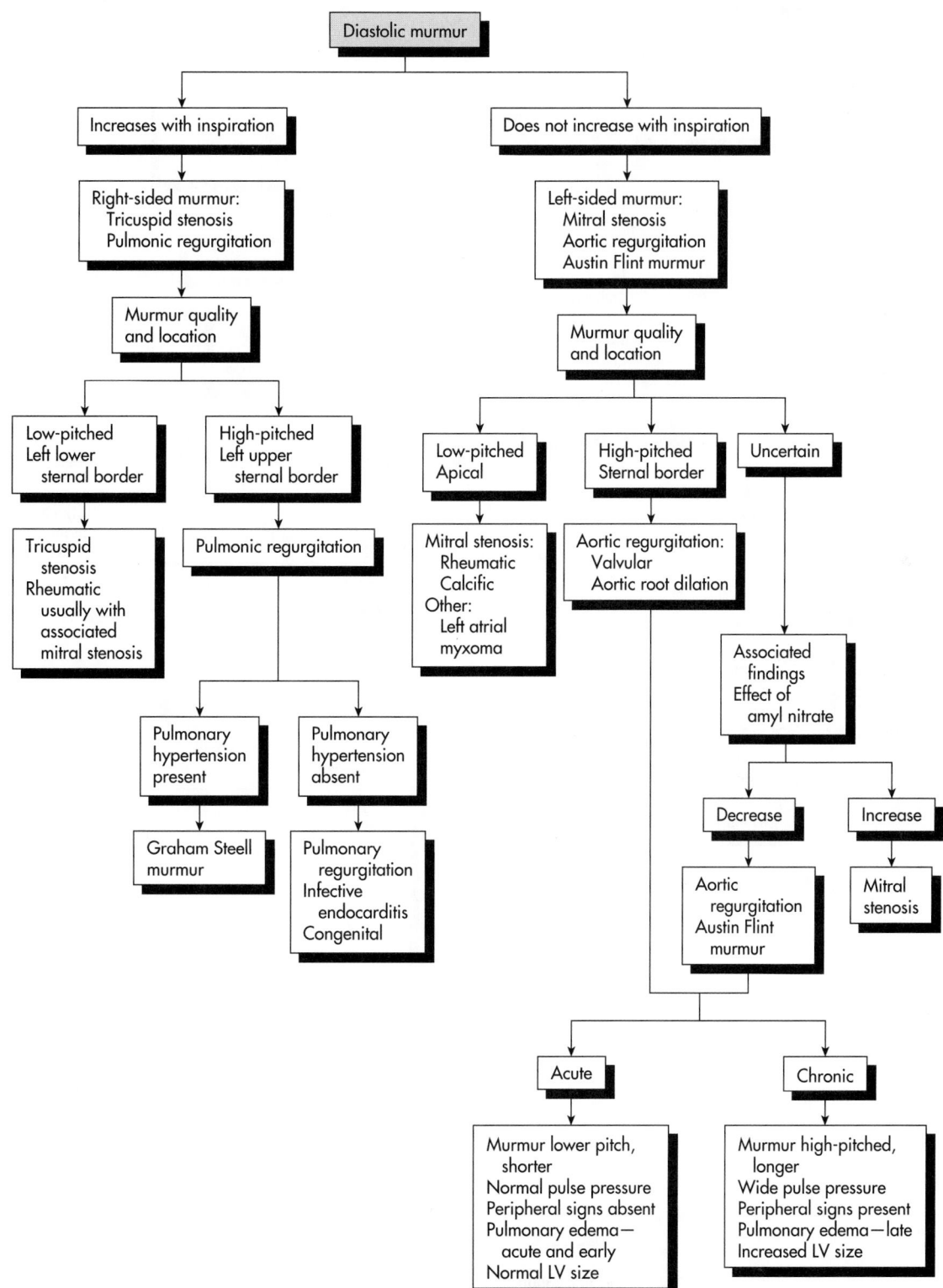

Fig. 3-113 **Diastolic murmur.** *LV,* Left ventricle. (From Greene HL, Johnson WP, Lemke D [eds]: *Decision making in medicine,* ed 2, St Louis, 1998, Mosby.)

MURMUR, SYSTOLIC

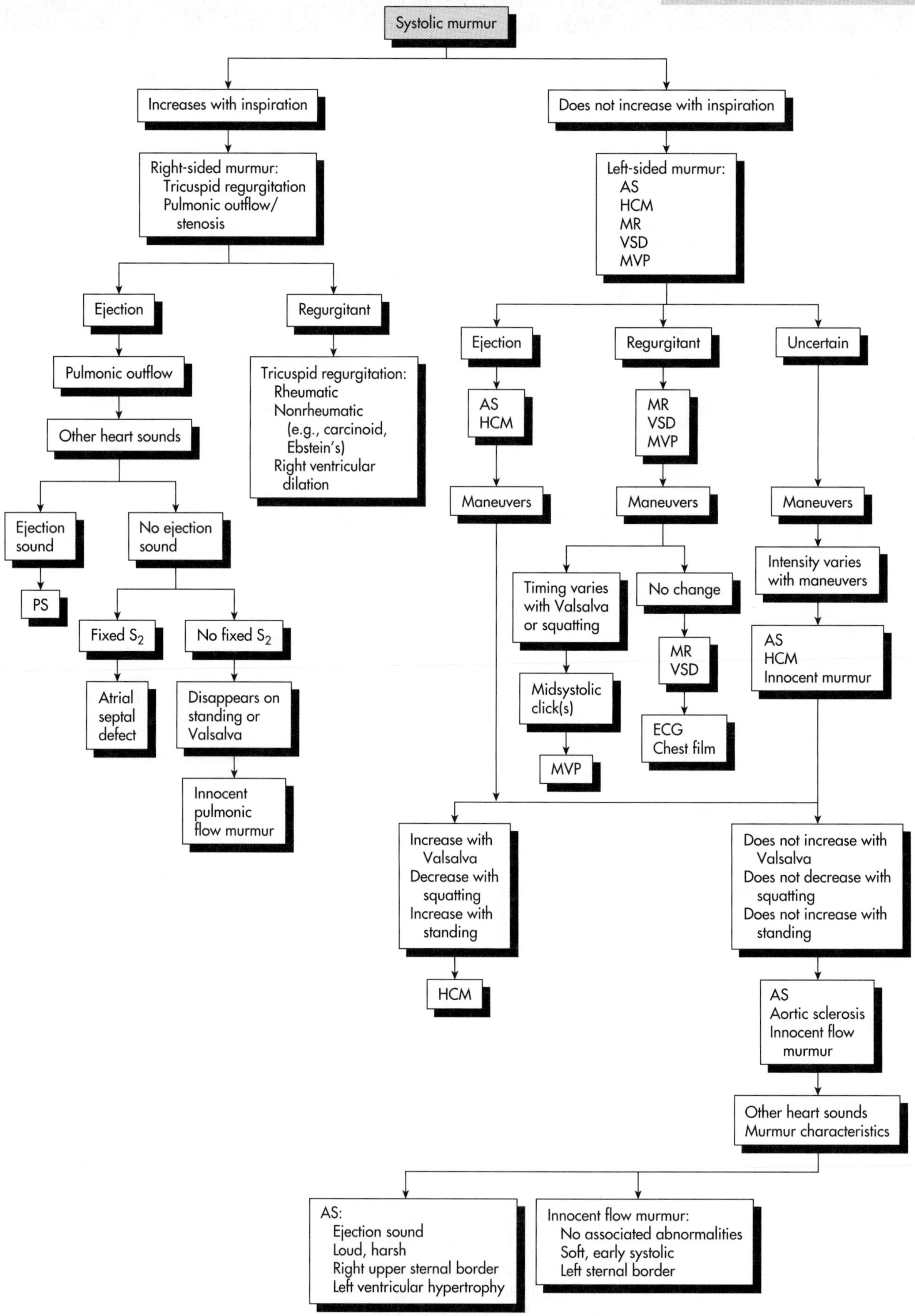

Fig. 3-114 **Systolic murmur.** *AS,* Aortic stenosis; *ECG,* electrocardiogram; *HCM,* hypertrophic cardiomyopathy; *MR,* mitral regurgitation; *MVP,* mitral valve prolapse; *PS,* pulmonary stenosis; *VSD,* ventricular septal defect. (From Greene HL, Johnson WP, Lemke D [eds]: *Decision making in medicine,* ed 2, St Louis, 1998, Mosby.)

MUSCLE CRAMPS AND ACHES

Muscle cramps and aches
ICD-9CM # 729.82

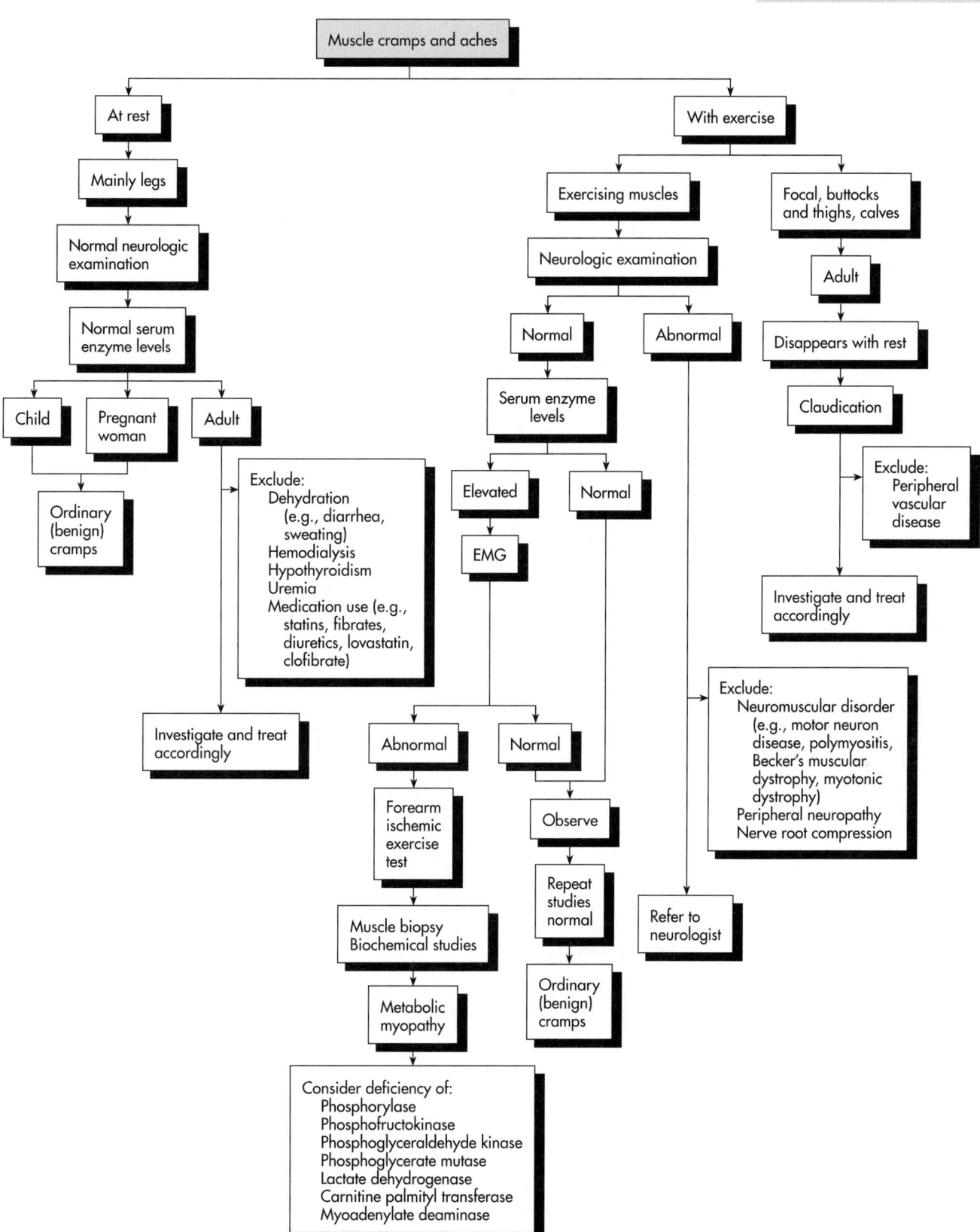

Fig. 3-115 **Evaluation of muscle cramps and aches.** *EMG,* Electromyography. (From Greene HL, Johnson WP, Lemcke D [eds]: *Decision making in medicine,* ed 2, St Louis, 1998, Mosby.)

MUSCLE WEAKNESS

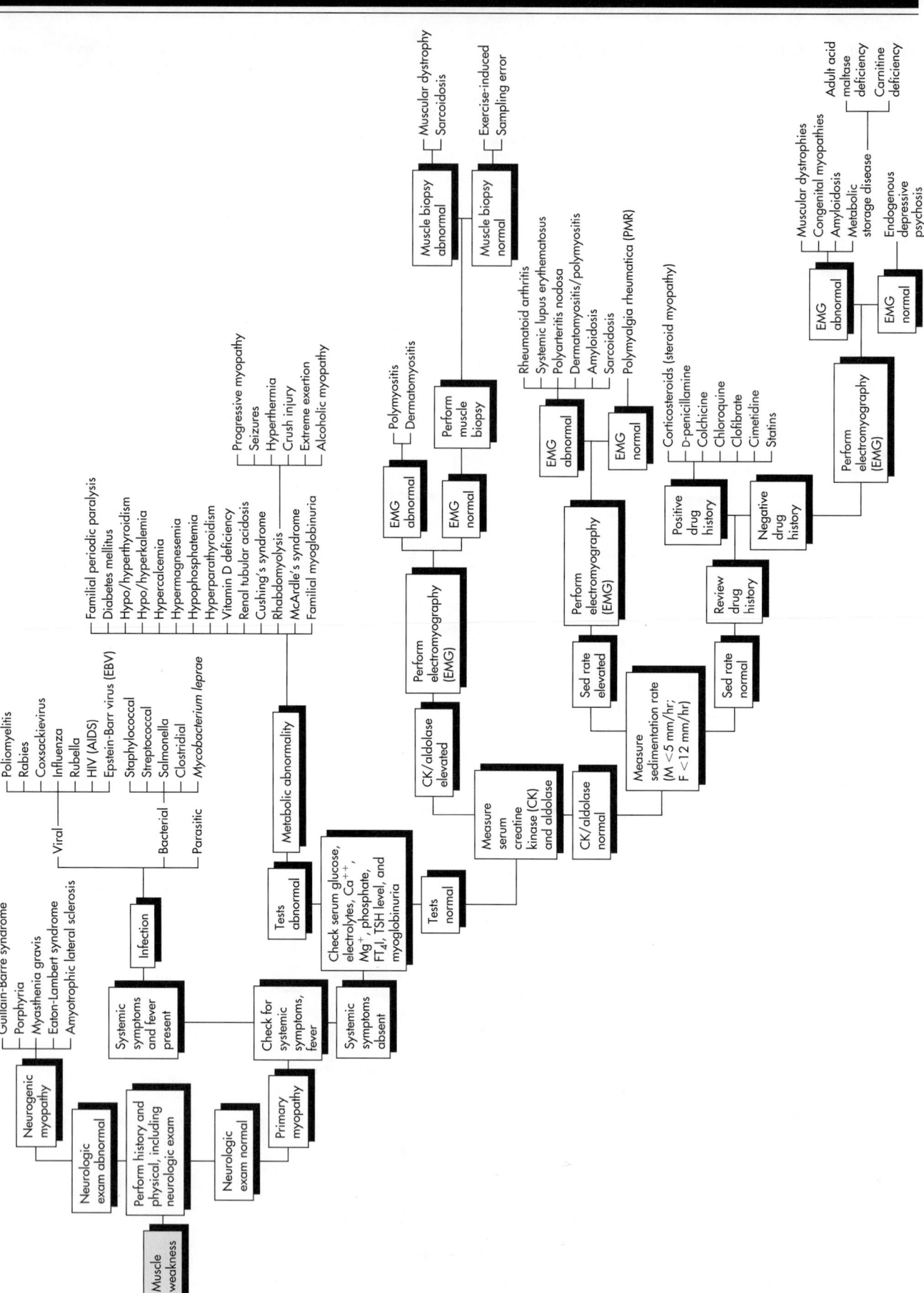

Fig. 3-116   **Muscle weakness.** *AIDS,* Acquired immunodeficiency syndrome; *EBV,* Epstein-Barr virus; *F,* female; *HIV,* human immunodeficiency virus; *M,* male. (From Healey PM: *Common medical diagnosis: an algorithmic approach,* ed 3, Philadelphia, 2000, WB Saunders.)

MUSCULOSKELETAL TUMOR

Musculoskeletal tumor
ICD-9CM # 239.2

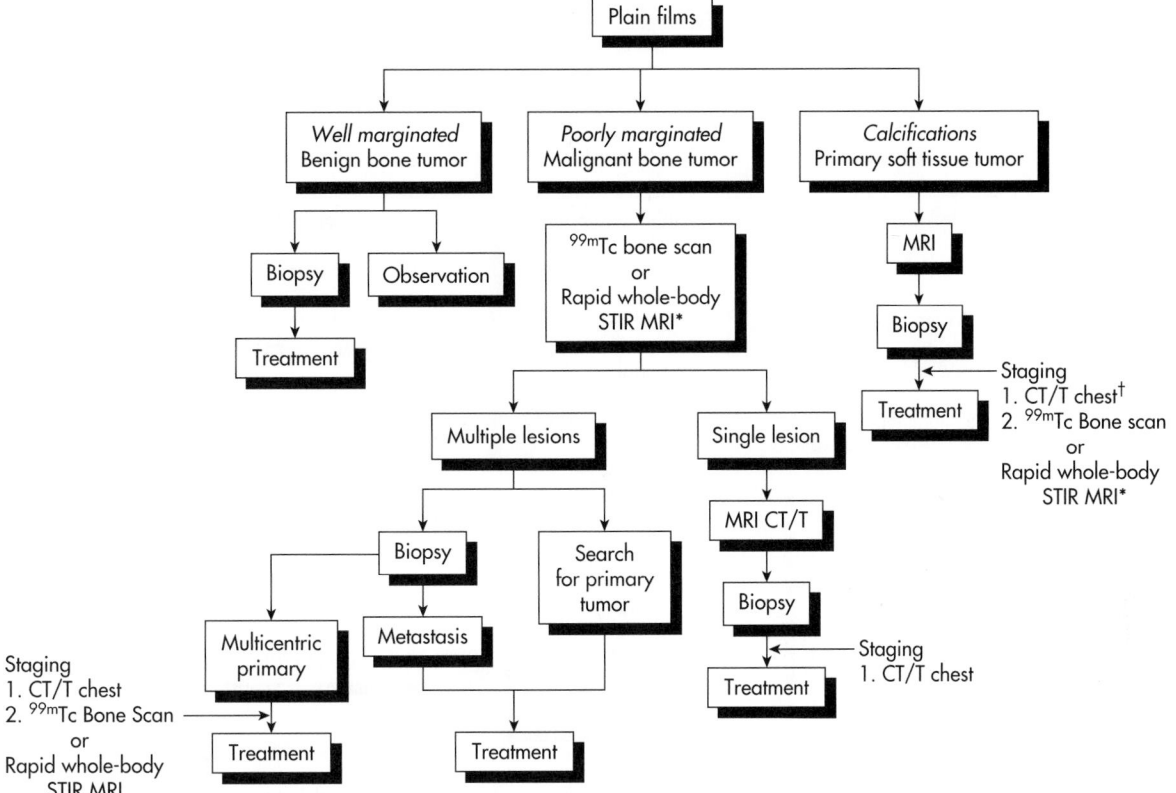

*The majority of bone and soft-tissue lesions are best evaluated by a single well-planned MRI using specific predetermined planes and images with specialized sequences. This requires excellent communication and consultation among the radiologist, orthopedic surgeon, and pathologist before initiating and designing the study. The T_1-weighted images produce superior anatomic detail, whereas T_2-weighted images best characterize the structure and composition of the lesion (solid, homogeneous, heterogeneous, cystic, or combinations of these characteristics). There should be very few if any "routine" MRI studies that do not involve considerable interaction with the supervising radiologist.

†Metastases to bone become detectable only after 50% of the bone mineral content has been lost with conventional plain film technology. Cortical destruction can often be detected with CT/T by imaging of contiguous tomographic planes. Bone scintigraphy, however, is more sensitive than either plain x-ray or CT/T when using ^{99m}Tc-methylene diphosphonate. Bone scintigraphy allows for a total body imaging assessment, thereby providing valuable noninvasive staging data. Although scintigraphy is very sensitive, it lacks diagnostic specificity. Numerous studies comparing scintigraphy with regional MRI have demonstrated both superior sensitivity and specificity of MRI.

Fig. 3-117   Approach to musculoskeletal tumor evaluation. (From Abeloff MD: *Clinical oncology,* ed 2, New York, 2000, Churchill Livingstone.)

NECK MASSES

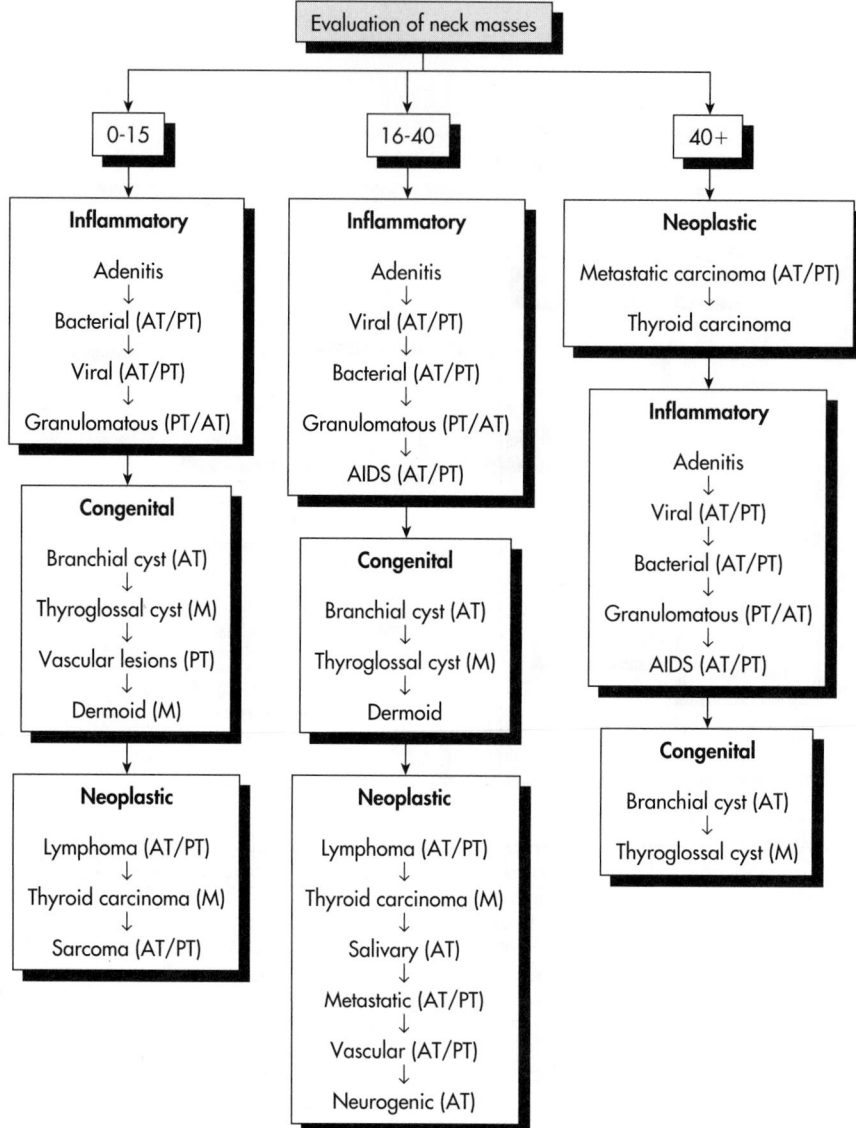

Fig. 3-118   Relative frequency of specific neck masses within causative groups by age. *AIDS,* Acquired immunodeficiency syndrome; *AT,* anterior; *M,* midline; *PT,* posterior. (From McGuirt FW: In Cummings CW et al [eds]: *Otolaryngology: head and neck surgery,* ed 3, St Louis, 1998, Mosby.)

Neck pain
ICD-9CM # 723.5 Stiff neck
847.0 Neck strain
723.5 Neck spasm
959.9 Neck injury

NECK PAIN

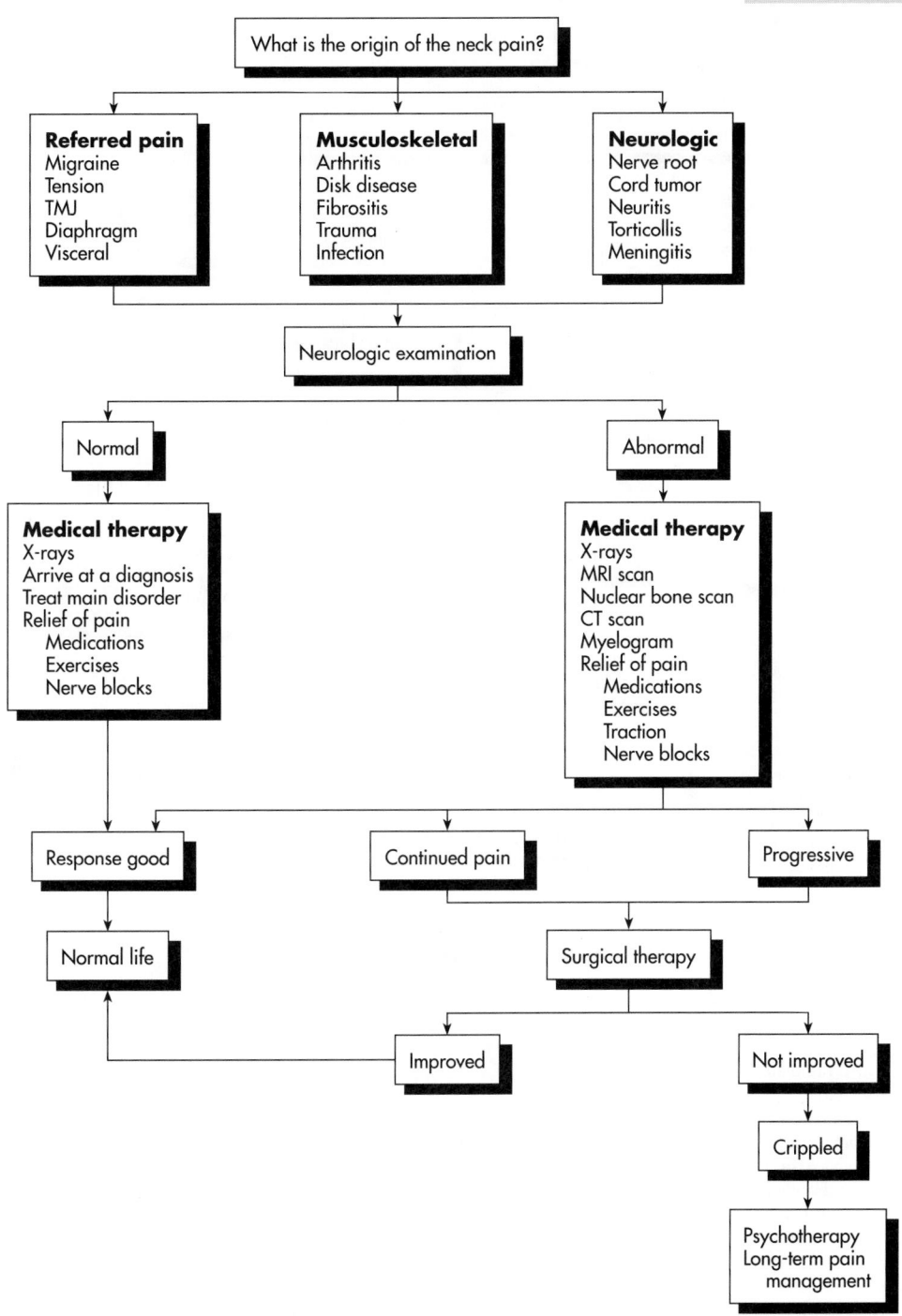

Fig. 3-119   Diagnosis and therapy for neck pain. *CT,* Computed tomography; *MRI,* magnetic resonance imaging; *TMJ,* temporomandibular joint. (From Stein JH [ed]: *Internal medicine,* ed 5, St Louis, 1998, Mosby.)

NEUTROPENIA

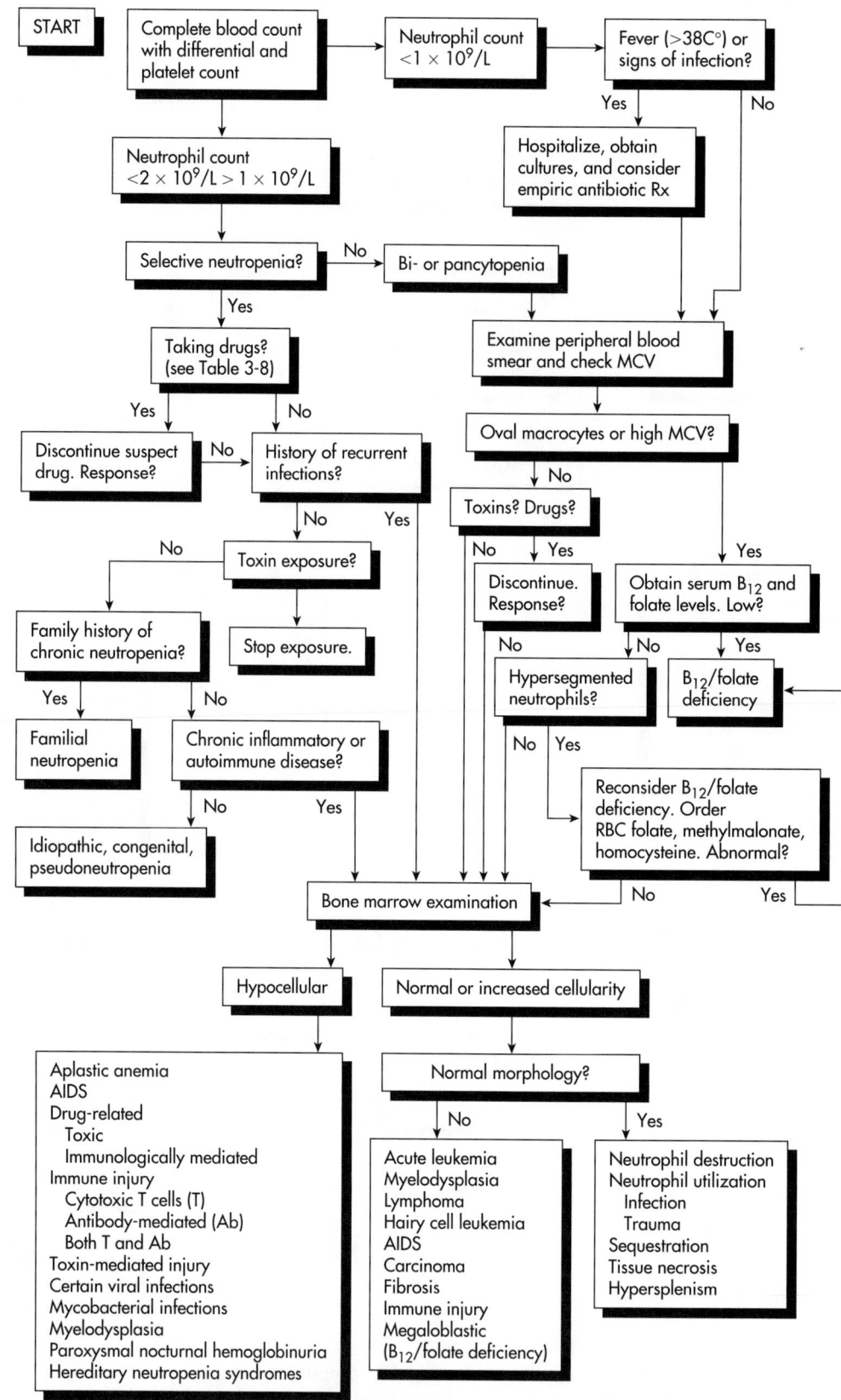

Fig. 3-120   A practical algorithm for the evaluation of patients with neutropenia. The fundamental diagnostic principle is that for patients with severe neutropenia or for those with bicytopenia or pancytopenia, bone marrow examination will likely be necessary unless the following diagnoses are made: (1) a nutritional (folate or vitamin B_{12}) deficiency or (2) drug or toxin-induced neutropenia in a patient whose neutropenia resolves after discontinuation of the offending agent. *AIDS,* Acquired immunodeficiency syndrome; *MCV,* mean corpuscular volume; *RBC,* red blood cell. (From Goldman L, Bennett JC [eds]: *Cecil textbook of medicine,* ed 21, Philadelphia, 2000, WB Saunders.)

NEUTROPENIA—cont'd

TABLE 3-8   Drugs That Cause Neutropenia

Antiarrhythmics
  Tocainide, procainamide, propranolol, quinidine

Antibiotics
  Chloramphenicol, penicillins, sulfonamides, p-aminosalicylic acid (PAS), rifampin, vancomycin, isoniazid, nitrofurantoin

Antimalarials
  Dapsone, quinine, pyrimethamine

Anticonvulsants
  Phenytoin, mephenytoin, trimethadione, ethosuximide, carbamazepine

Hypoglycemic agents
  Tolbutamide, chlorpropamide

Antihistamines
  Cimetidine, brompheniramine, tripelennamine

Antihypertensives
  Methyldopa, captopril

Antiinflammatory agents
  Aminopyrine, phenylbutazone, gold salts, ibuprofen, indomethacin

Antithyroid agents
  Propylthiouracil, methimazole, thiouracil

Diuretics
  Acetazolamide, hydrochlorothiazide, chlorthalidone

Phenothiazines
  Chlorpromazine, promazine, prochlorperazine

Immunosuppressive agents
  Antimetabolites

Cytotoxic agents
  Alkylating agents, antimetabolites, anthracyclines, *Vinca* alkaloids, cisplatin, hydroxyurea, dactinomycin

Other agents
  Recombinant interferons, allopurinol, ethanol, levamisole, penicillamine, zidovudine, streptokinase, carbamazepine, clopidogrel, ticlopidine

Modified from Goldman L, Bennett JC (eds): *Cecil textbook of medicine,* ed 21, Philadelphia, 2000, WB Saunders.

III

NEUTROPHILIA

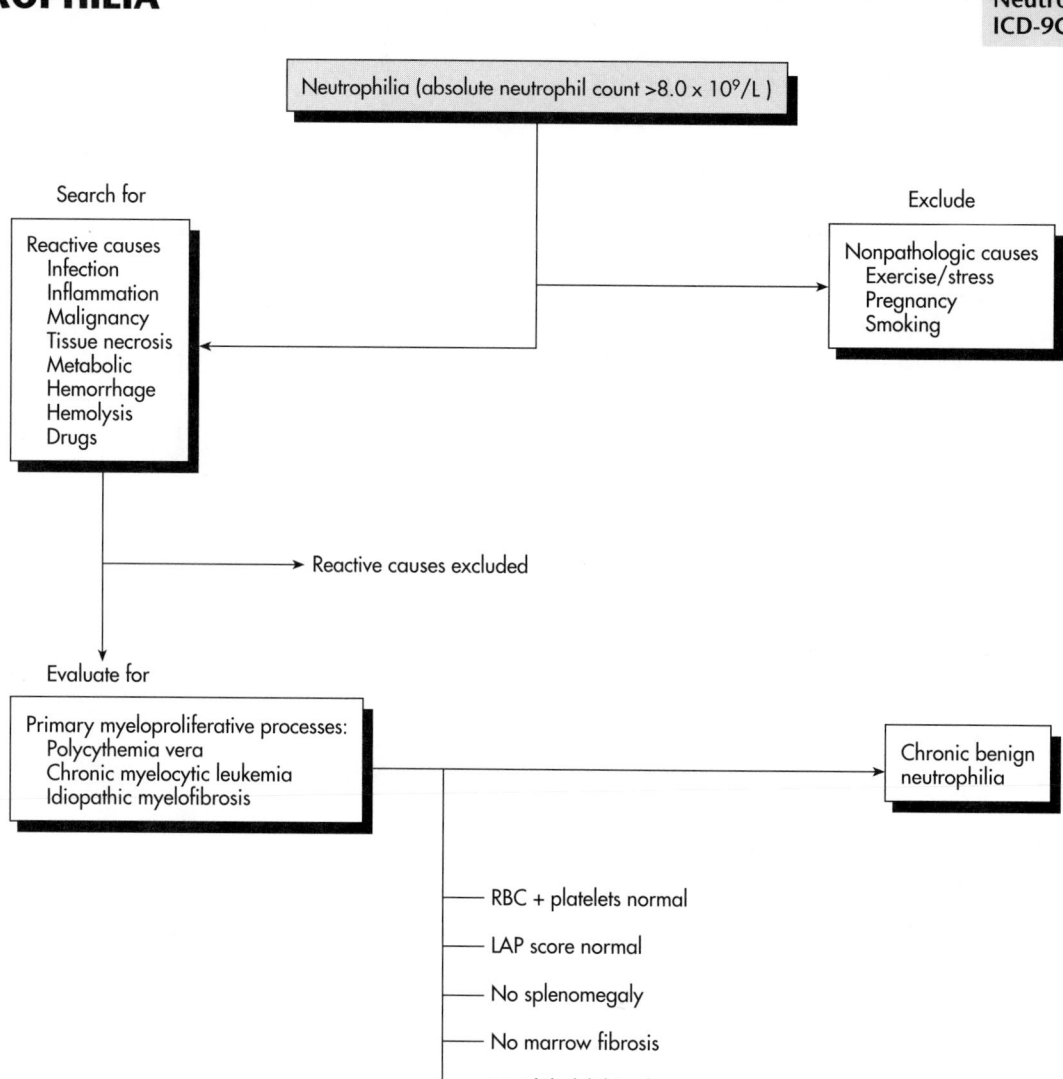

Fig. 3-121   General approach to neutrophilia. *LAP,* Leukocyte alkaline phosphatase. (From Stein JH [ed]: *Internal medicine,* ed 5, St Louis, 1998, Mosby.)

OLIGURIA

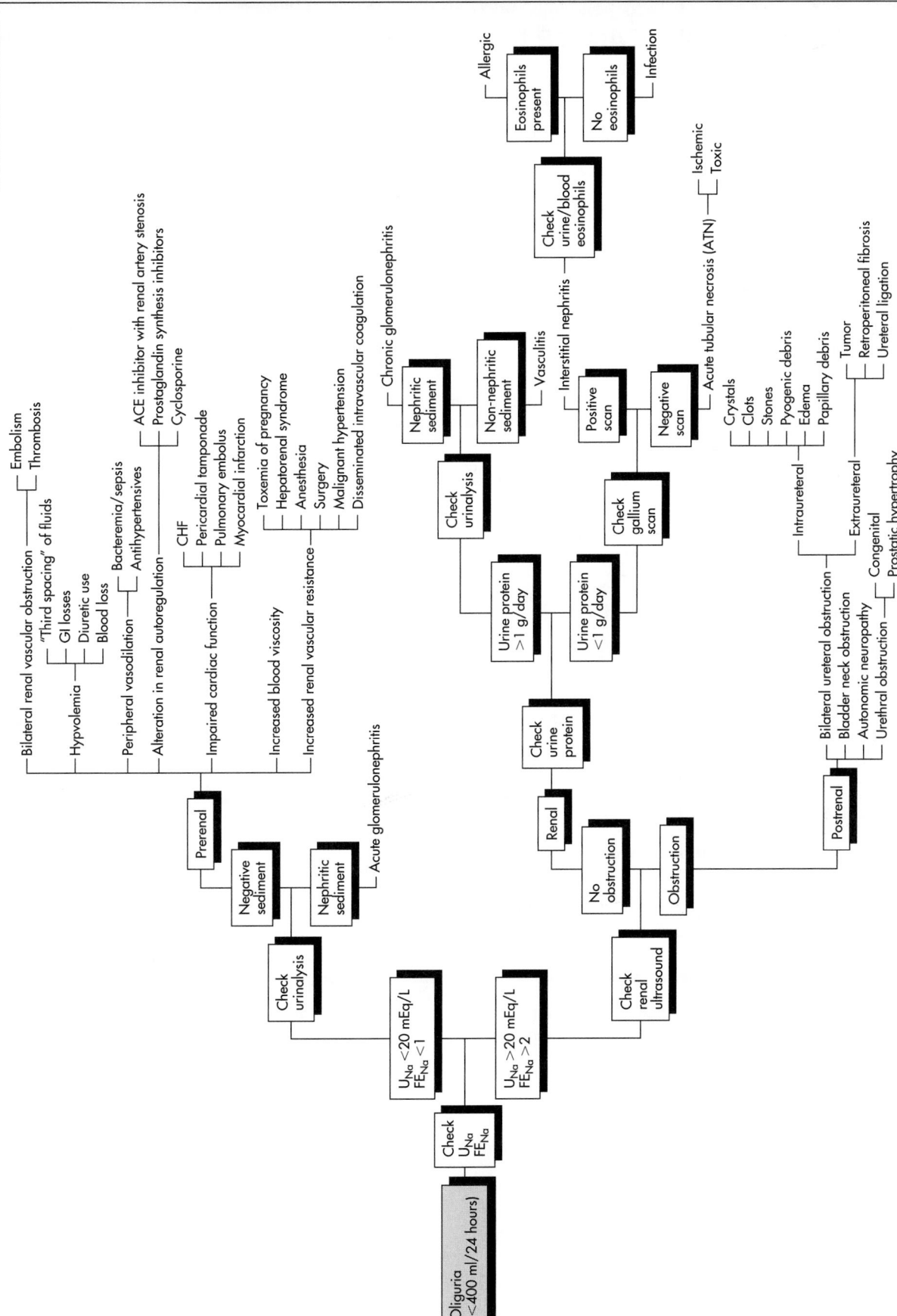

Fig. 3-122   Evaluation of oliguria. *ACE,* Angiotensin-converting enzyme; *CHF,* congestive heart failure; *GI,* gastrointestinal. (From Healey PM: *Common medical diagnosis: an algorithmic approach,* ed 3, Philadelphia, 2000, WB Saunders.)

PAIN MANAGEMENT, CANCER PATIENT

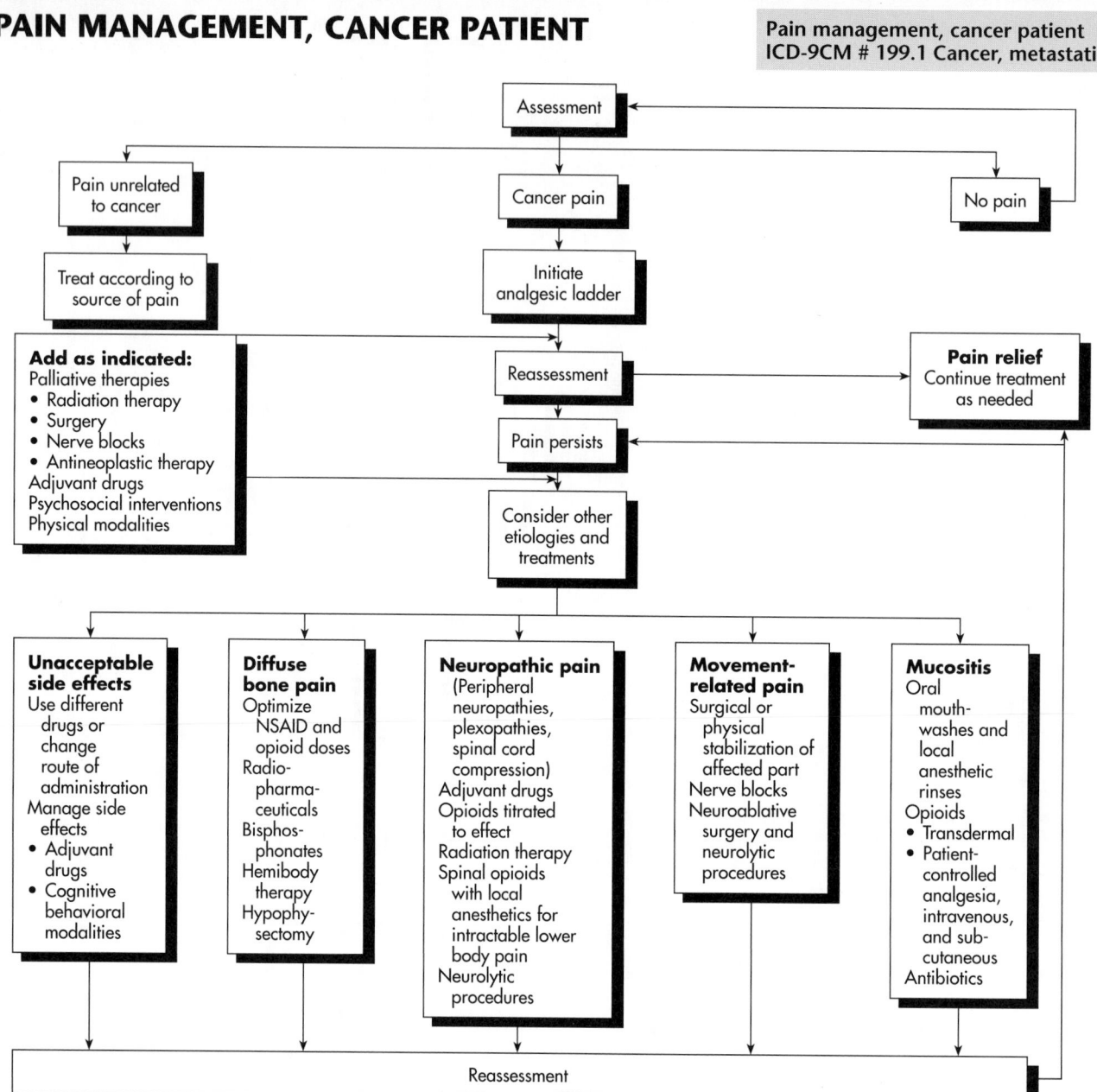

Fig. 3-123   Pain management in patients with cancer. *NSAID,* Nonsteroidal antiinflammatory drug. (From Noble J [ed]: *Primary care medicine,* ed 3, St Louis, 2001, Mosby.)

PALPITATIONS

Palpitations
ICD-9CM # 785.1 Palpitations

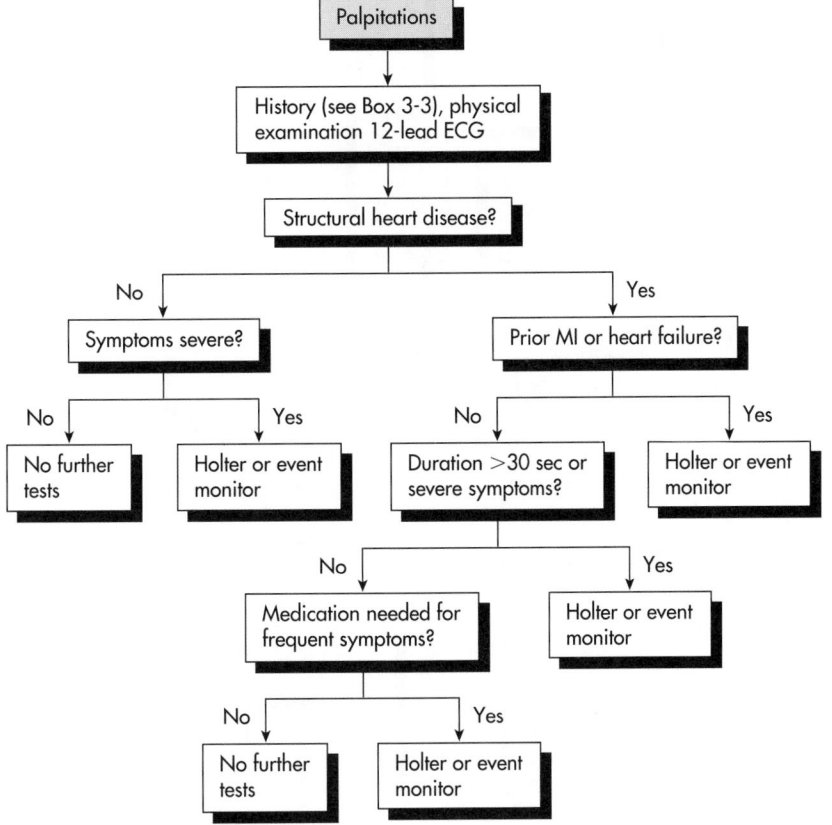

Fig. 3-124   Diagnostic approach to the patient with palpitations. *ECG,* Electrocardiogram; *MI,* myocardial infarction. (From Goldman L, Braunwald E [eds]: *Primary cardiology,* Philadelphia, 1998, WB Saunders.)

BOX 3-3   Clinical History in Evaluation of Palpitations

Symptoms of Palpitations

Duration of episode
Frequency of episodes
Associated chest pain, dyspnea, lightheadedness?
How does episode start? How does episode stop?

Underlying Heart Disease

Angina, prior myocardial infarction
Valvular heart disease
Congenital heart disease
Cardiomyopathy
Coronary risk factors
Congestive heart failure
Prior antiarrhythmic therapy

Precipitating Factors

Psychologic stress
Exercise
Caffeine, alcohol, cocaine, amphetamines
Thyroid disease
Anemia, hypoxemia

From Goldman L, Braunwald E (eds): *Primary cardiology,* Philadelphia, 1998, WB Saunders.

PANCREATIC ISLET CELL TUMORS

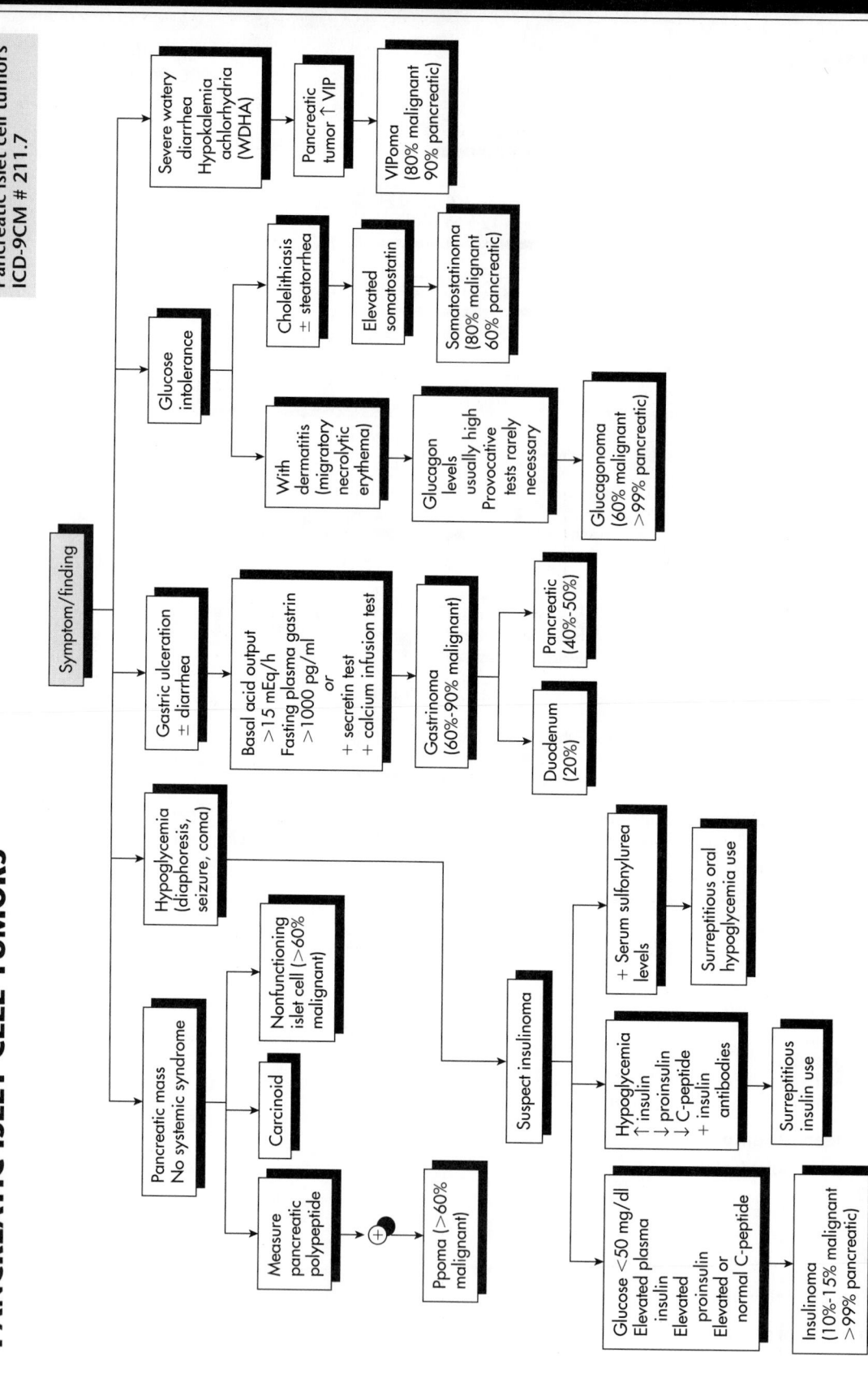

Fig. 3-125   Diagnosis of pancreatic islet cell tumors. *Ppoma,* Islet cell tumor secreting pancreatic polypeptide; *VIP,* vasoactive intestinal peptide; *VIPoma,* islet cell tumor secreting vasoactive intestinal peptide. (From Abeloff MD: *Clinical oncology,* ed 2, New York, 2000, Churchill Livingstone.)

PAP SMEAR ABNORMALITY

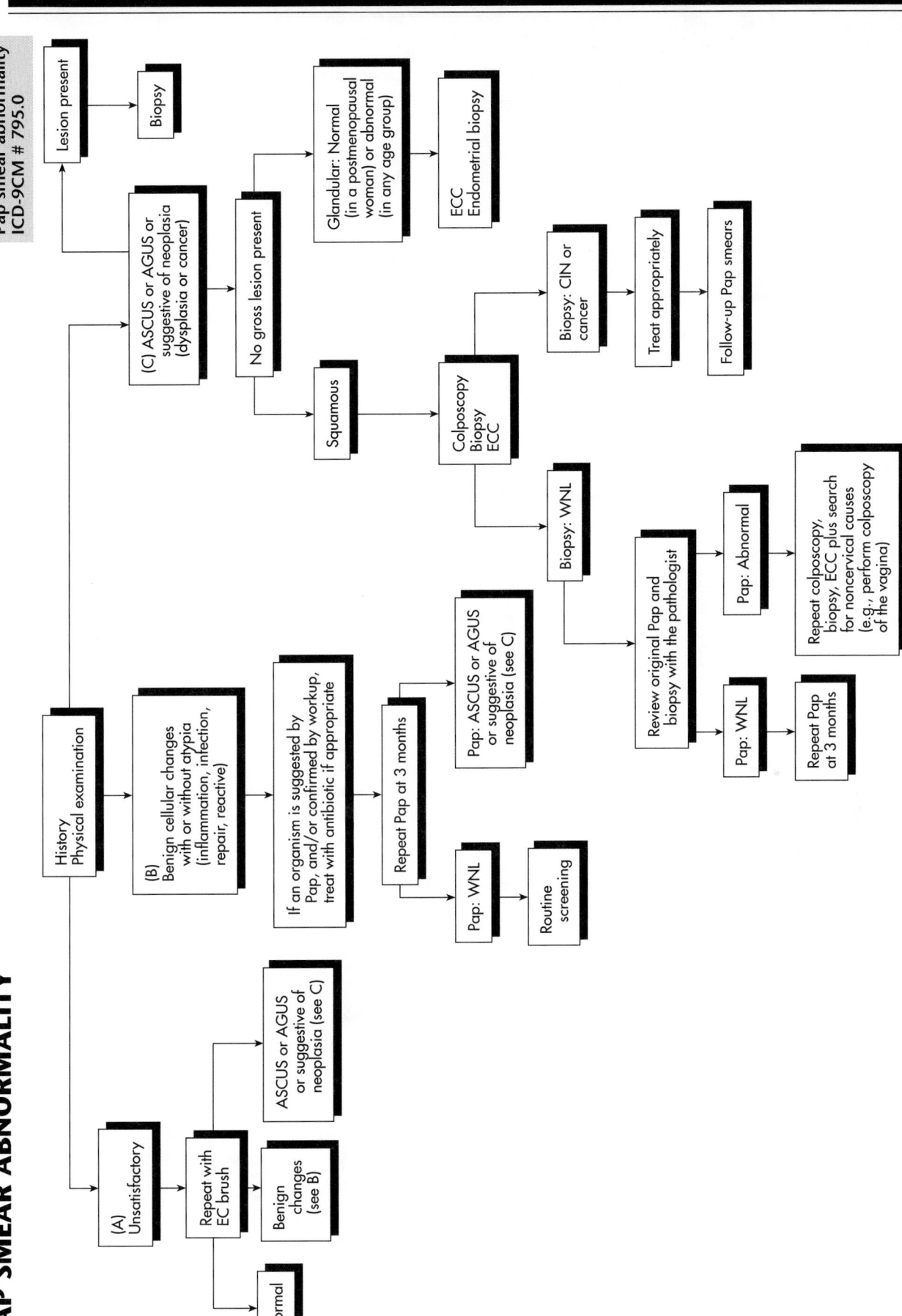

Fig. 3-126   Workup of an abnormal Pap smear. *ASCUS* or *AGUS,* Atypical squamous cells or atypical glandular cells of undetermined significance; *CIN,* cervical intraepithelial neoplasia; *EC,* endocervical; *ECC,* endocervical curettage; *WNL,* within normal limits. (From Noble J [ed]: *Primary care medicine,* ed 3, St Louis, 2001, Mosby.)

PATIENT WITH ILL-DEFINED PHYSICAL COMPLAINTS

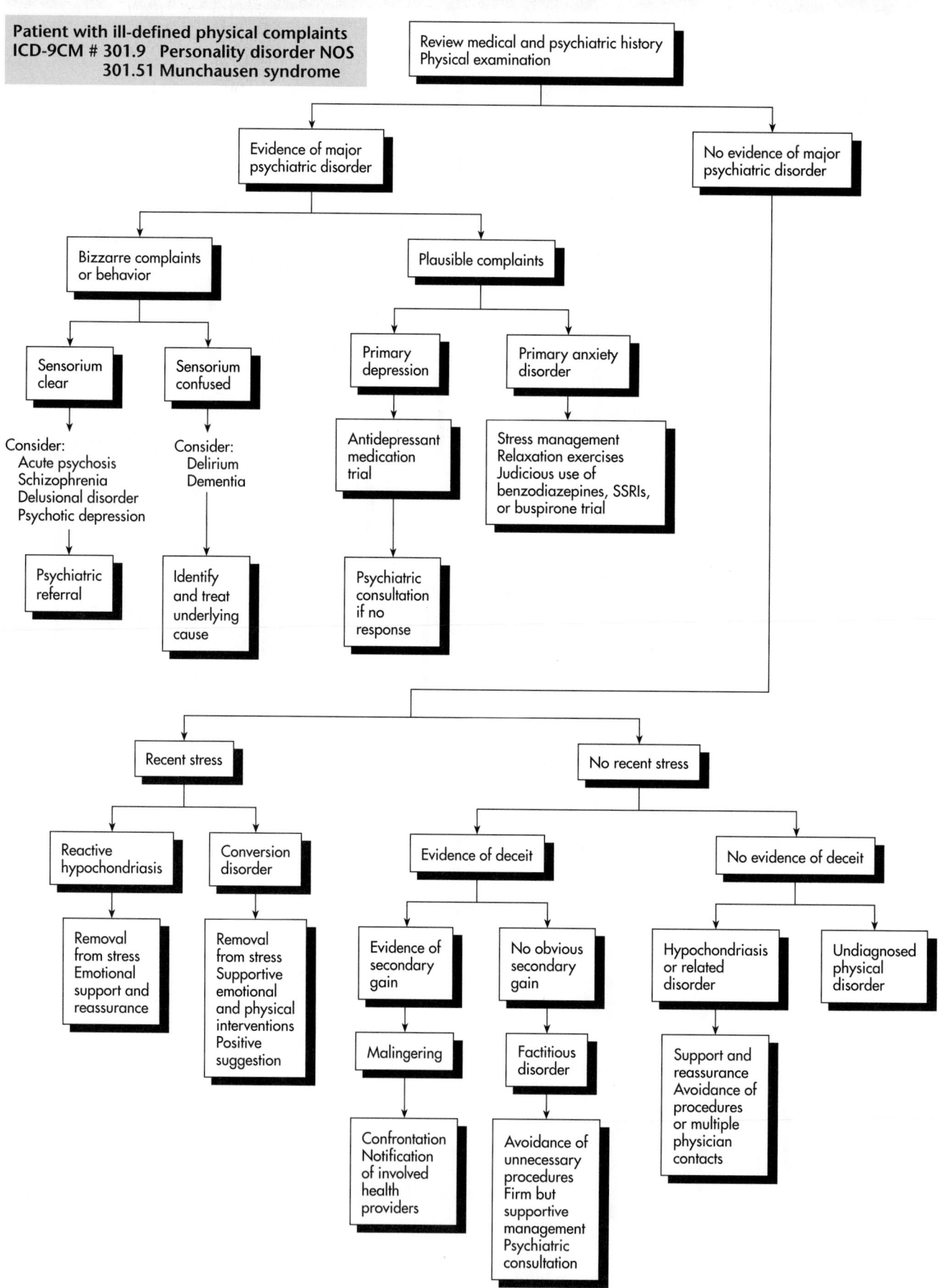

Patient with ill-defined physical complaints
ICD-9CM # 301.9   Personality disorder NOS
301.51 Munchausen syndrome

Review medical and psychiatric history
Physical examination

Evidence of major psychiatric disorder

No evidence of major psychiatric disorder

Bizzarre complaints or behavior

Plausible complaints

Sensorium clear

Sensorium confused

Primary depression

Primary anxiety disorder

Consider:
Acute psychosis
Schizophrenia
Delusional disorder
Psychotic depression

Consider:
Delirium
Dementia

Antidepressant medication trial

Stress management
Relaxation exercises
Judicious use of benzodiazepines, SSRIs, or buspirone trial

Psychiatric referral

Identify and treat underlying cause

Psychiatric consultation if no response

Recent stress

No recent stress

Reactive hypochondriasis

Conversion disorder

Evidence of deceit

No evidence of deceit

Removal from stress
Emotional support and reassurance

Removal from stress
Supportive emotional and physical interventions
Positive suggestion

Evidence of secondary gain

No obvious secondary gain

Hypochondriasis or related disorder

Undiagnosed physical disorder

Malingering

Factitious disorder

Support and reassurance
Avoidance of procedures or multiple physician contacts

Confrontation
Notification of involved health providers

Avoidance of unnecessary procedures
Firm but supportive management
Psychiatric consultation

Fig. 3-127   Patient with ill-defined physical complaints. Previous or recent evaluations are noncontributory. *SSRIs,* Selective serotonin reuptake inhibitors. (From Greene H, Johnson WP, Lemcke D [eds]: *Decision making in medicine,* ed 2, St Louis, 1998, Mosby.)

PELVIC MASS

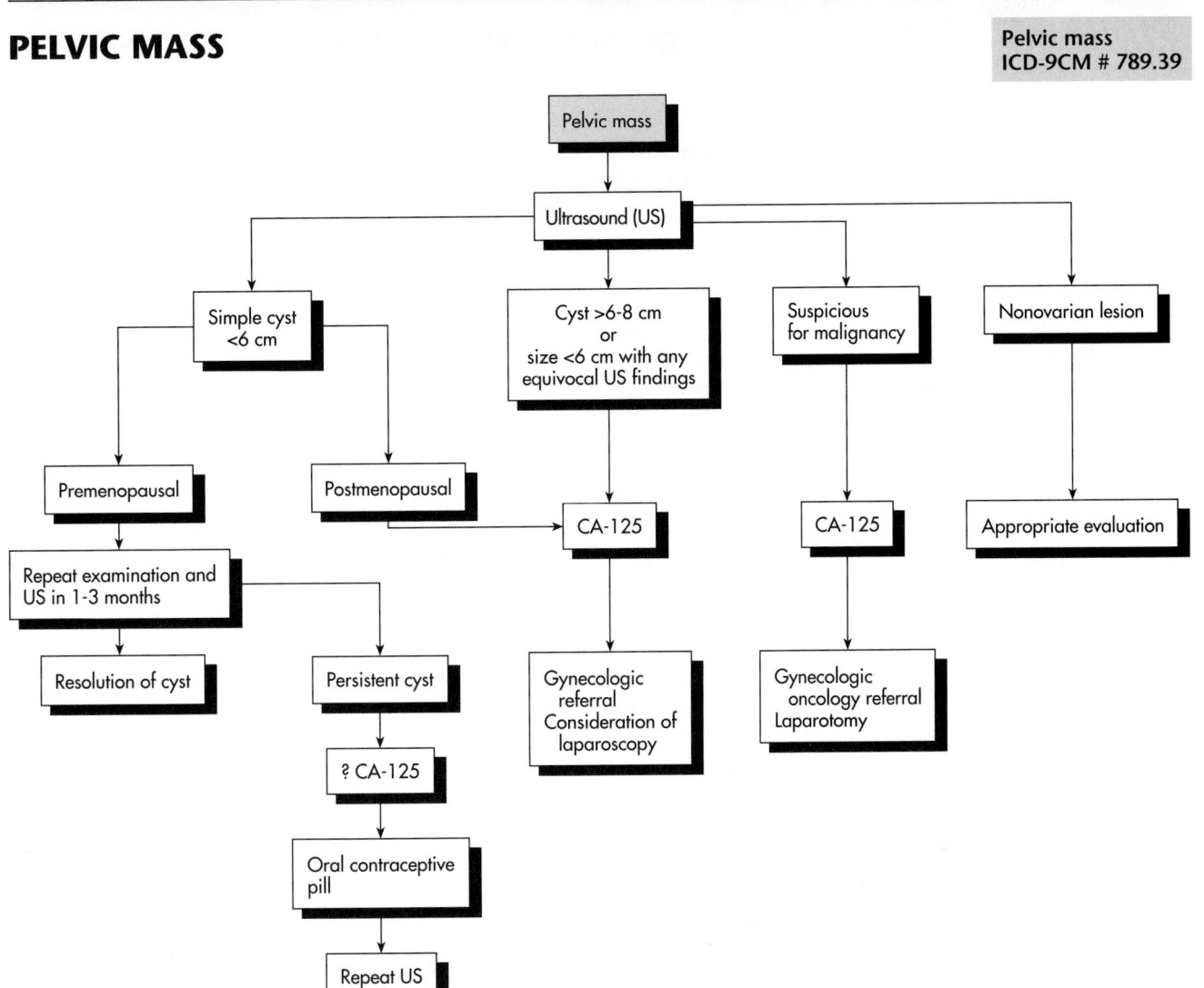

Fig. 3-128 **Approach to the patient with a pelvic mass.** *US,* Ultrasound. (From Carlson KJ et al: *Primary care of women,* St Louis, 1995, Mosby.)

PELVIC PAIN, REPRODUCTIVE-AGE WOMAN

1. Rapid history and external abdominal examination

- **If surgical abdomen**: consider early ob/gyn/surgery consultation
    - Rupture (ectopic, cyst, abscess)
    - Torsion (adnexal, fibroid)
    - Perforation (uterine)
    - Appendicitis

2. Vital signs

- **If unstable**: Establish venous access and administer fluid bolus
    Spin Hct, type and crossmatch blood as needed
    Consider early ob/gyn/surgery consult without ultrasound
    - Rupture (ectopic, cyst)
    - Septic (abortion, abscess)
    - Placental (previa, abruptio)

3. Complete history and physical examination, and perform pelvic examination

- **If obvious abortion**: consult obstetrician and consider ultrasound
    - Abortion (incomplete, septic)

- **If late pregnancy**: forego pelvic exam
            Check for fetal heart tones
            Consider ultrasound followed by ob/gyn consultation
    - Placenta previa or abruptio
    - Premature labor contractions

4. Laboratory diagnostic workup (pregnancy test, CBC, UA/micro)

- **If pregnant**: consider ultrasound followed by ob/gyn consultation
    - R/I viable intrauterine gestation
    - R/O ectopic pregnancy, abortion, placental problems
    - R/O free intraperitoneal fluid, abscess formation

- **If not pregnant**: consider ultrasound and ob/gyn/surgery consultation
    - R/O gynecologic surgical problems
    - Ovarian cyst rupture, hemorrhage
    - Tubo-ovarian abscess rupture
    - Adnexal or fibroid torsion
    - Uterine perforation

    - Consider nonsurgical gynecologic problems
    - PID, pelvic adhesions, endometriosis, neoplasm, menstrual

    - R/O general surgery problems
    - Appendicitis and complications
    - Other, GI, GU, vascular, orthopedic surgery problems

    - Consider nonsurgical nongynecologic problems
    - Systemic illnesses

Fig. 3-129   Evaluation and management of reproductive-age women with acute pelvic pain.
CBC, Complete blood count; *GI,* gastrointestinal; *GU,* genitourinary; *Hct,* hematocrit; *PID,* pelvic inflammatory disease; *UA/micro,* urinalysis with microscopy. (From Rosen P et al [eds]: *Emergency medicine: concepts and clinical practice,* ed 5, St Louis, 2002, Mosby.)

PERICARDIAL EFFUSION

Pericardial effusion
ICD-9CM # 423.9   Pericardial effusion
            420.90 Pericardial effusion, acute

A

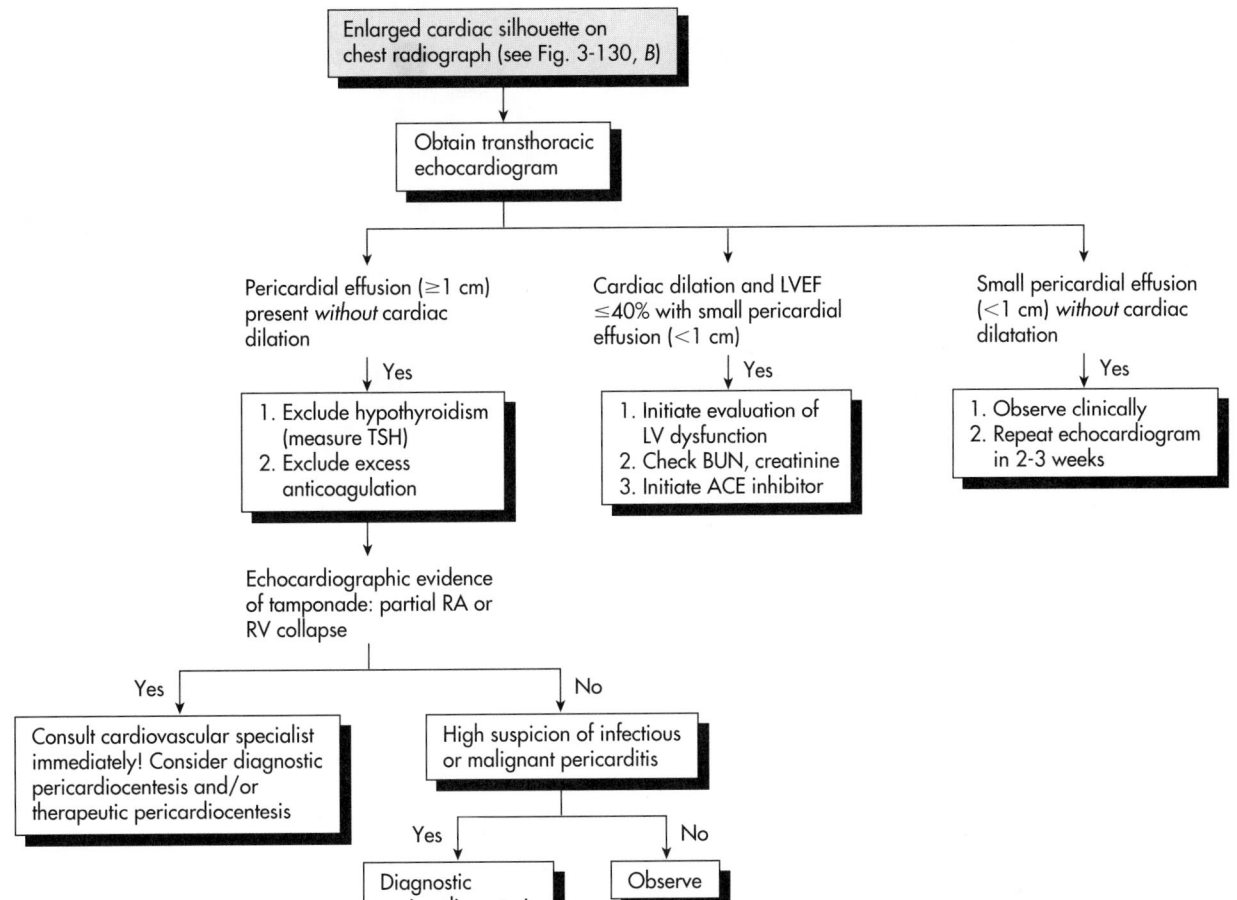

Fig. 3-130   A, Management of asymptomatic pericardial effusion in patients with a normal physical examination. *ACE,* Angiotensin-converting enzyme; *BUN,* blood urea nitrogen; *EF,* ejection fraction; *LV,* left ventricular; *RA,* right atrial; *RV,* right ventricular; *TSH,* thyroid-stimulating hormone. (From Goldman L, Braunwald E [eds]: *Primary cardiology,* Philadelphia, 1998, WB Saunders.)

Continued

III

PERICARDIAL EFFUSION—cont'd

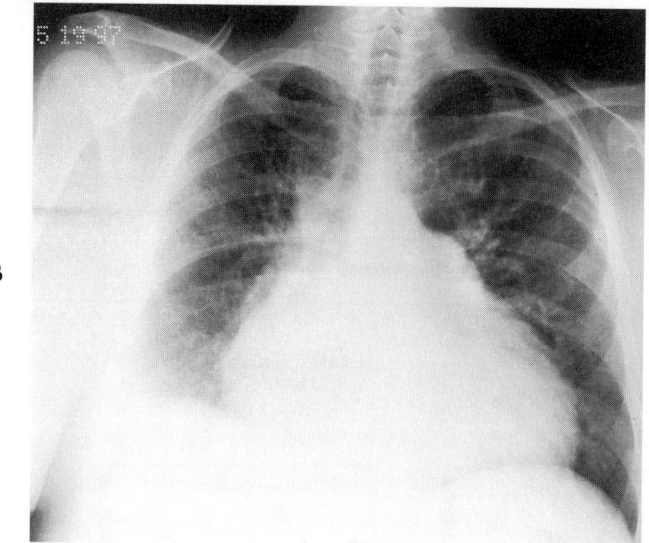

B

Fig. 3-130, cont'd   B, Posteroanterior chest radiograph from a patient with a large circumferential pericardial effusion. Note the flask-shaped contour of the cardiac silhouette. (From Andreoli TE [ed]: *Cecil essentials of medicine,* ed 5, Philadelphia, 2001, WB Saunders.)

Peripheral arterial disease
ICD-9CM # 440.20 Peripheral arteriosclerosis,
                unspecified
        440.21 Peripheral arteriosclerosis with
                intermittent claudication
        440.22 Peripheral arteriosclerosis with rest
                pain
        440.23 Peripheral arteriosclerosis with
                ulceration
        440.24 Peripheral arteriosclerosis with
                ischemic gangrene
        440.29 Other arteriosclerosis of extremities

PERIPHERAL ARTERIAL DISEASE

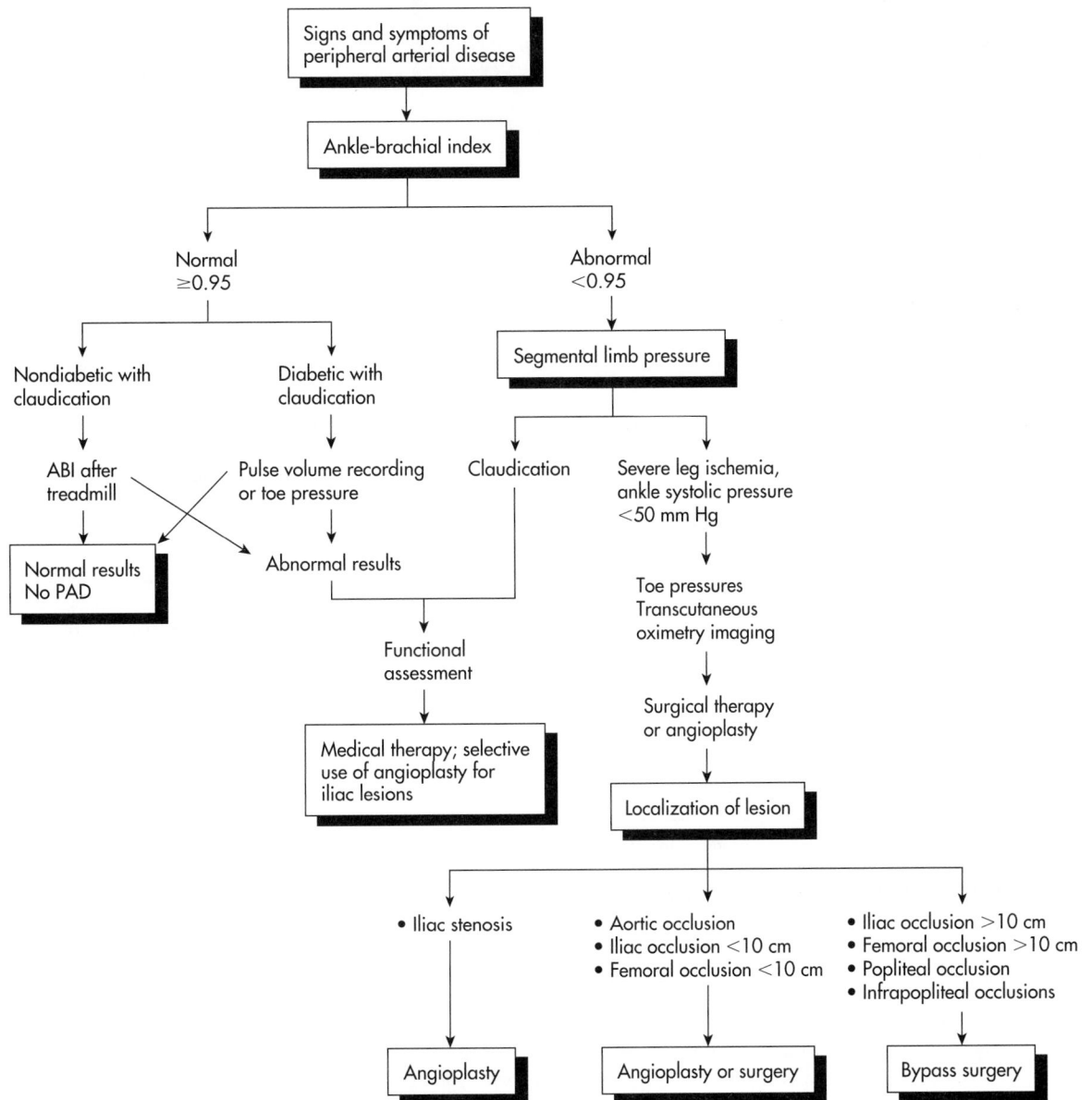

Fig. 3-131   Peripheral vascular diagnosis. *ABI,* Ankle/brachial index; *PAD,* peripheral arterial
disease. (From Goldman L, Bennett JC [eds] *Cecil textbook of medicine,* ed 21, Philadelphia, 2000,
WB Saunders.)

PLEURAL SPACE FLUID

Pleural space fluid
ICD-9CM # 511.9 Pleural effusion, unspecified

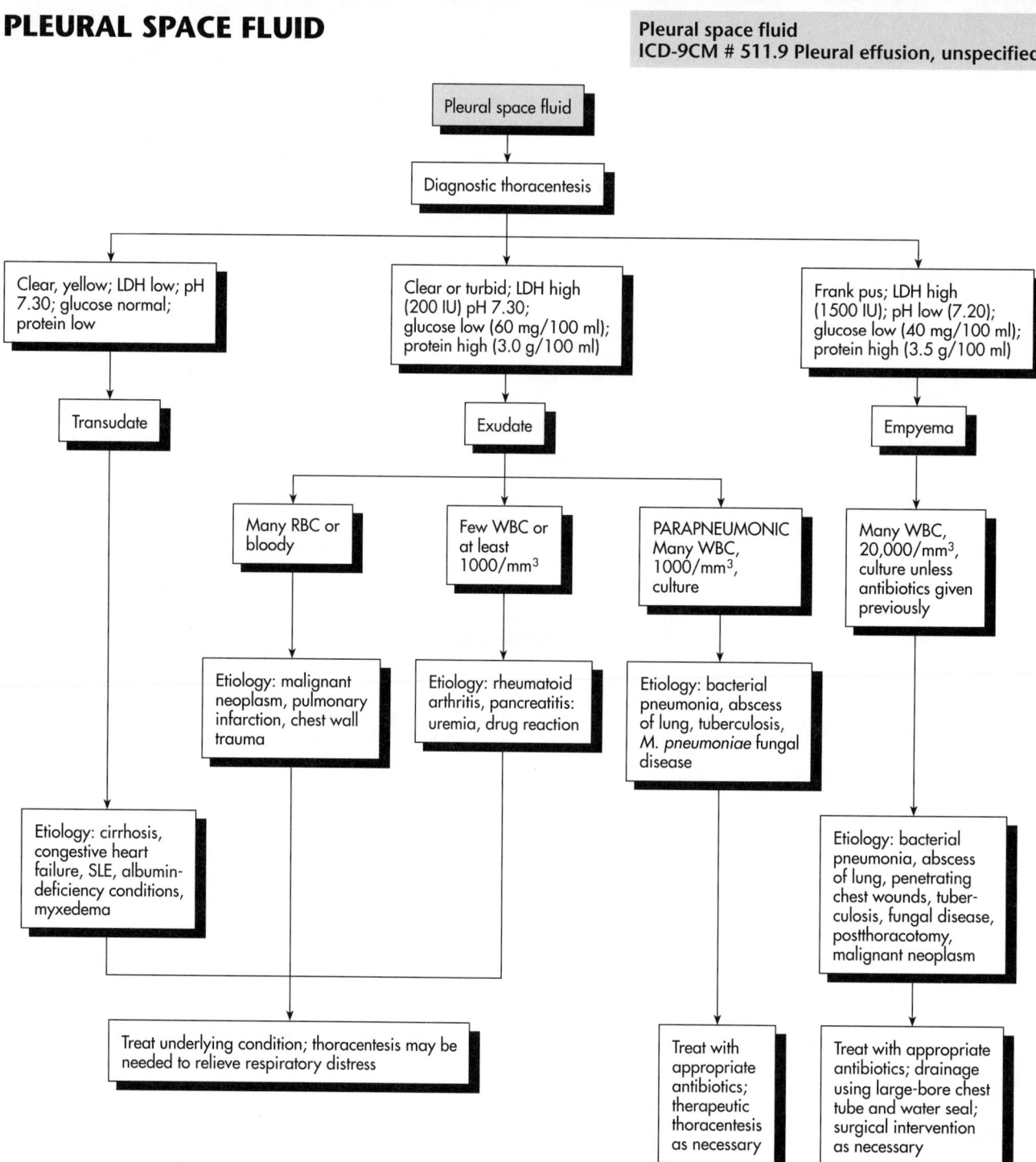

Fig. 3-132　Evaluation, common etiologies, and management of pleural effusion and empyema. *LDH,* Lactate dehydrogenase; *RBC,* red blood cells; *SLE,* systemic lupus erythematosus; *WBC,* white blood cells. (From Kassirer J [ed]: *Current therapy in adult medicine,* ed 4, St Louis, 1998, Mosby.)

PREOPERATIVE EVALUATION, PATIENT WITH CORONARY HEART DISEASE

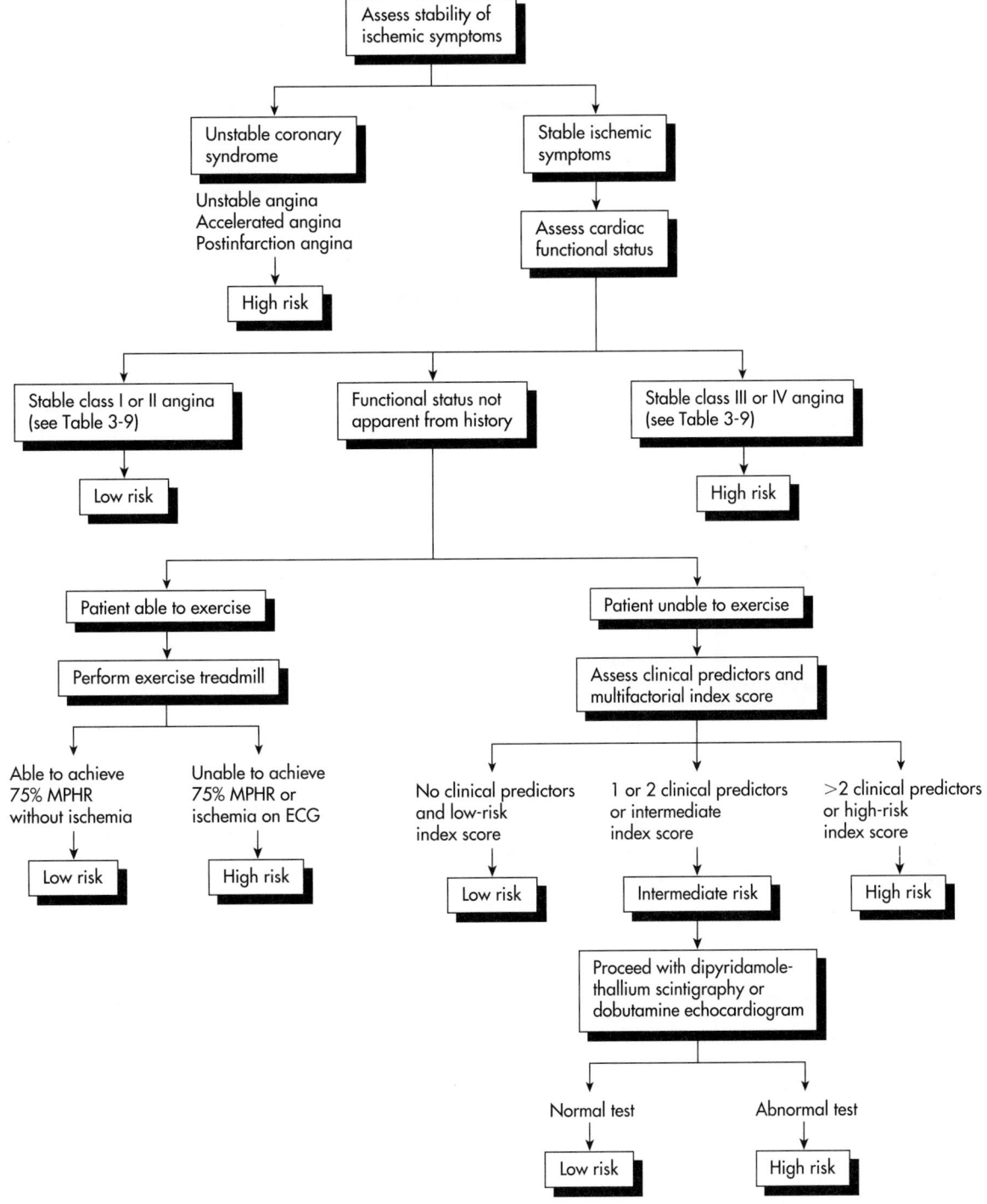

Fig. 3-133 **Preoperative evaluation of patients with known or suspected coronary artery disease.** (From Goldman L, Braunwald E [eds]: *Primary cardiology*, Philadelphia, 1998, WB Saunders.)

TABLE 3-9 **New York Heart Association Functional Classification**

Class I	No limitation	Ordinary physical activity does not cause symptoms
Class II	Slight limitation	Comfortable at rest Ordinary physical activity causes symptoms
Class III	Marked limitation	Comfortable at rest Less than ordinary activity causes symptoms
Class IV	Inability to carry on any physical activity	Symptoms present at rest

PROTEINURIA

Proteinuria
ICD-9CM # 791.0 Proteinuria, NOS

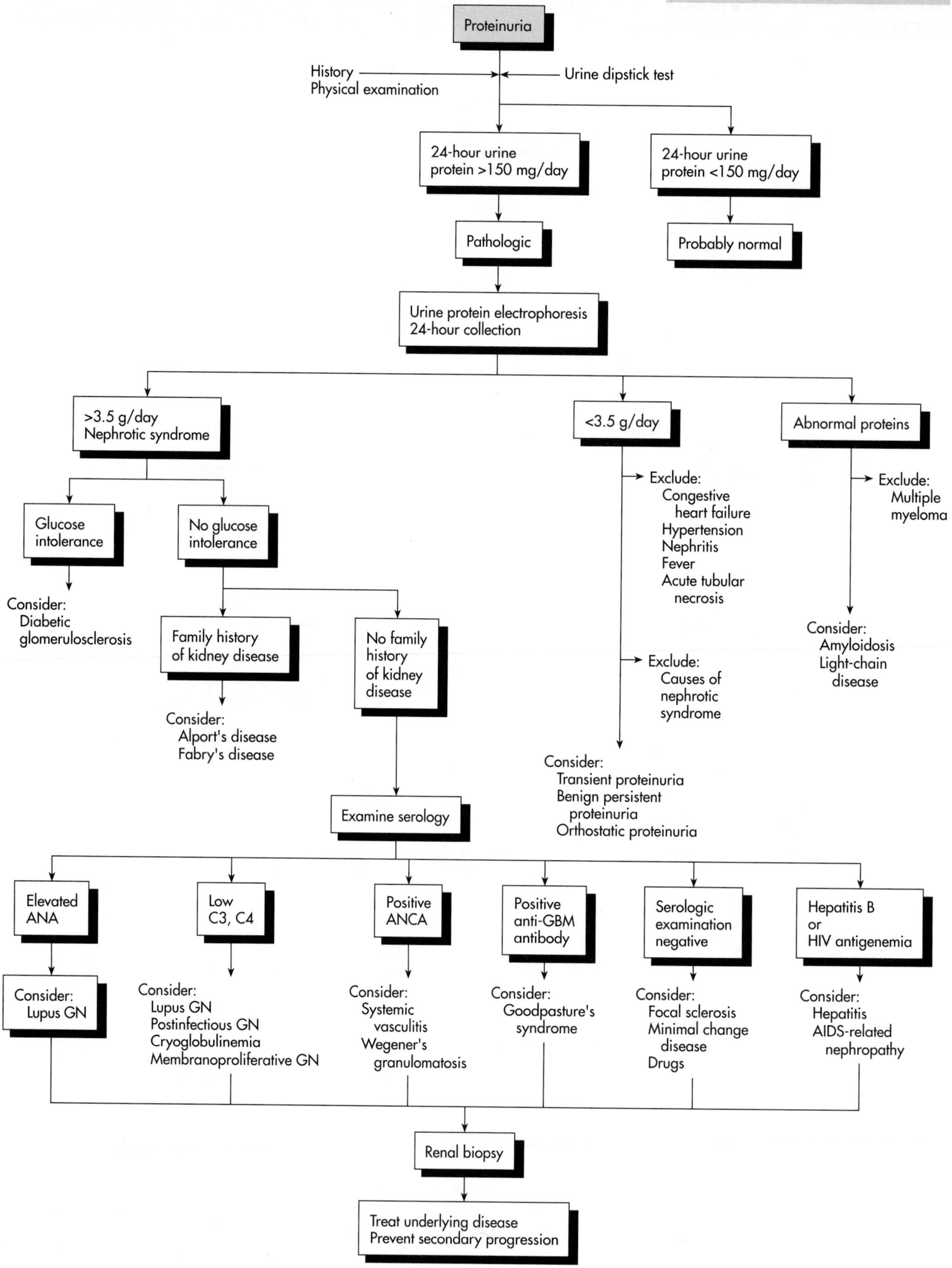

Fig. 3-134 Proteinuria. *AIDS,* *Acquired immunodeficiency syndrome; ANA, antinuclear antibody; ANCA,* antineutrophil cytoplasmic autoantibody; *anti-GBM,* anti–glomerular basement membrane; *GN,* glomerulonephritis. (From Greene HL, Johnson WP, Lemcke D [eds]: *Decision making in medicine,* ed 2, St Louis, 1998, Mosby.)

PRURITUS, GENERALIZED

Pruritus, generalized
ICD-9CM # 698.9 Pruritus NOS

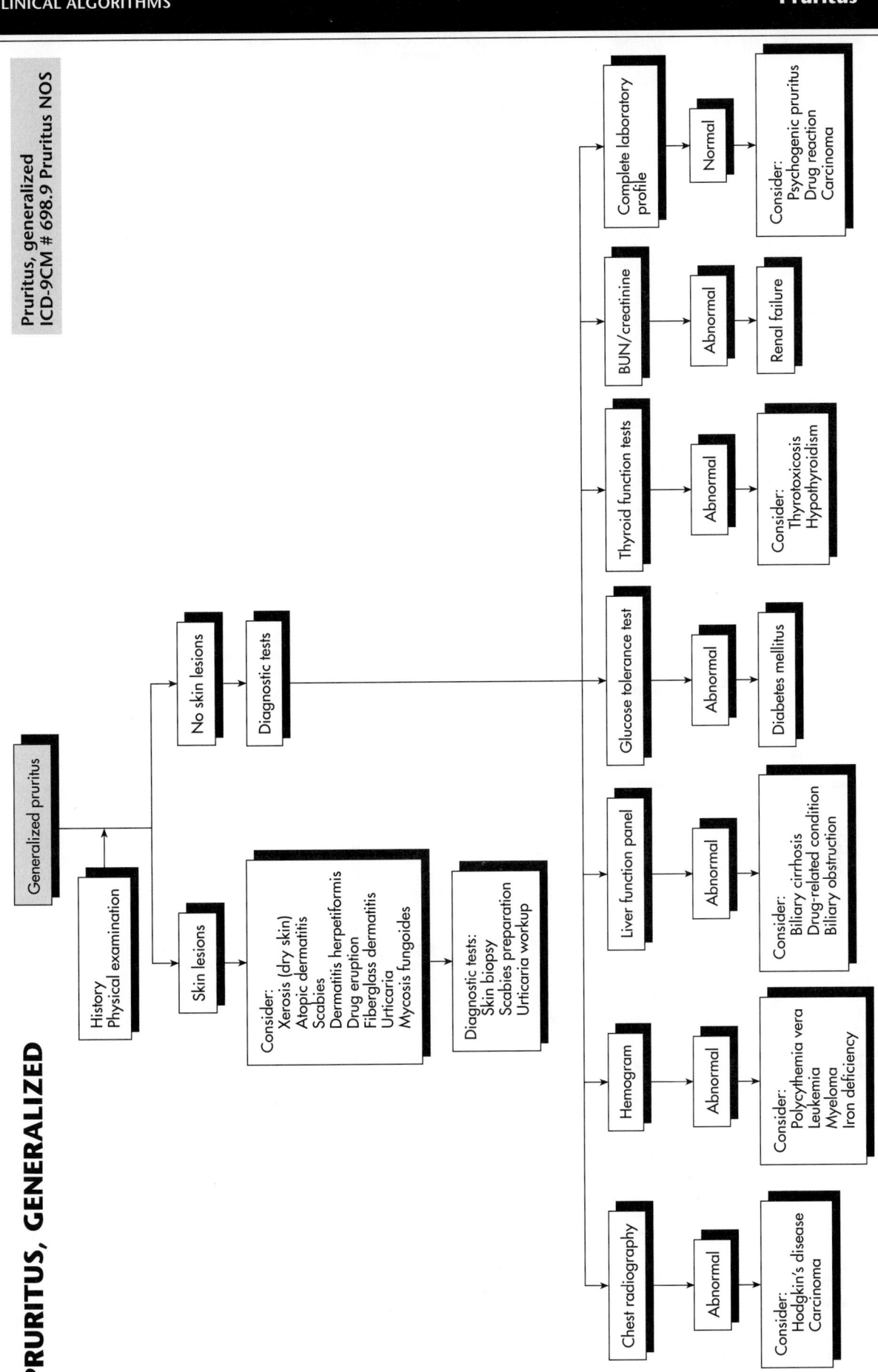

Fig. 3-135 **Evaluation of generalized pruritus.** *BUN,* Blood urea nitrogen. (From Greene HL, Johnson WP, Lemcke D [eds]: *Decision making in medicine,* ed 2, St Louis, 1998, Mosby.)

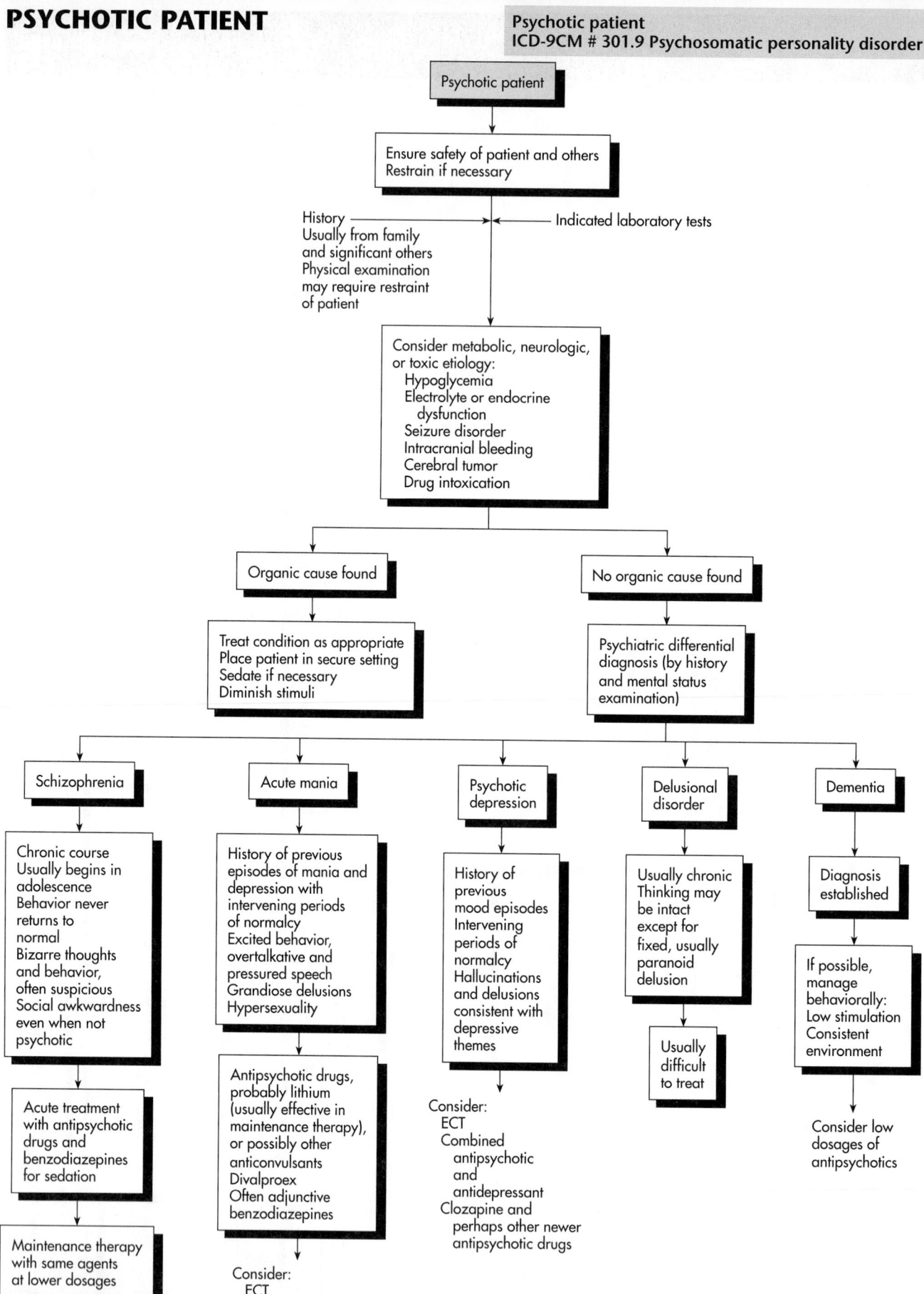

Fig. 3-136   Evaluation of psychotic patient. *ECT,* Electroconvulsive therapy. (From Greene HL, Johnson WP, Lemcke D [eds]: *Decision making in medicine,* ed 2, St Louis, 1998, Mosby.)

PUBERTY, DELAYED

Puberty, delayed
ICD-9CM # 259.0

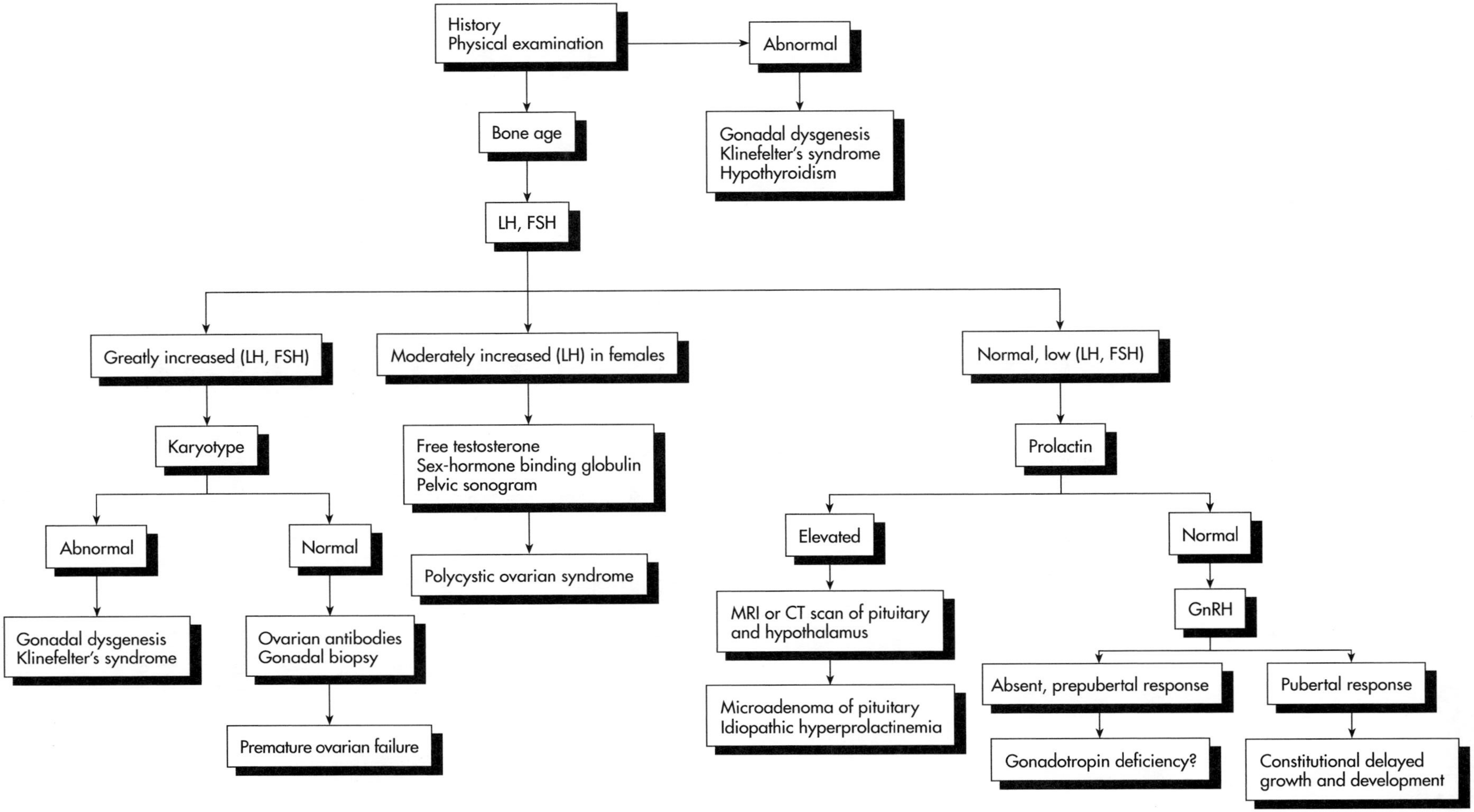
History
Physical examination
Abnormal
Gonadal dysgenesis
Klinefelter's syndrome
Hypothyroidism
Bone age
LH, FSH
Greatly increased (LH, FSH)
Moderately increased (LH) in females
Normal, low (LH, FSH)
Karyotype
Abnormal
Normal
Gonadal dysgenesis
Klinefelter's syndrome
Ovarian antibodies
Gonadal biopsy
Premature ovarian failure
Free testosterone
Sex-hormone binding globulin
Pelvic sonogram
Polycystic ovarian syndrome
Prolactin
Elevated
Normal
MRI or CT scan of pituitary
and hypothalamus
Microadenoma of pituitary
Idiopathic hyperprolactinemia
GnRH
Absent, prepubertal response
Pubertal response
Gonadotropin deficiency?
Constitutional delayed
growth and development

Fig. 3-137 Evaluation of patient with delayed puberty. *CT,* Computed tomography; *FSH,* follicle-stimulating hormone; *GnRH,* gonadotropin-releasing hormone; *LH,* luteinizing hormone; *MRI,* magnetic resonance imaging. (From Moore WT, Eastman RC: *Diagnostic endocrinology,* ed 2, St Louis, 1996, Mosby.)

III

PUBERTY, PRECOCIOUS

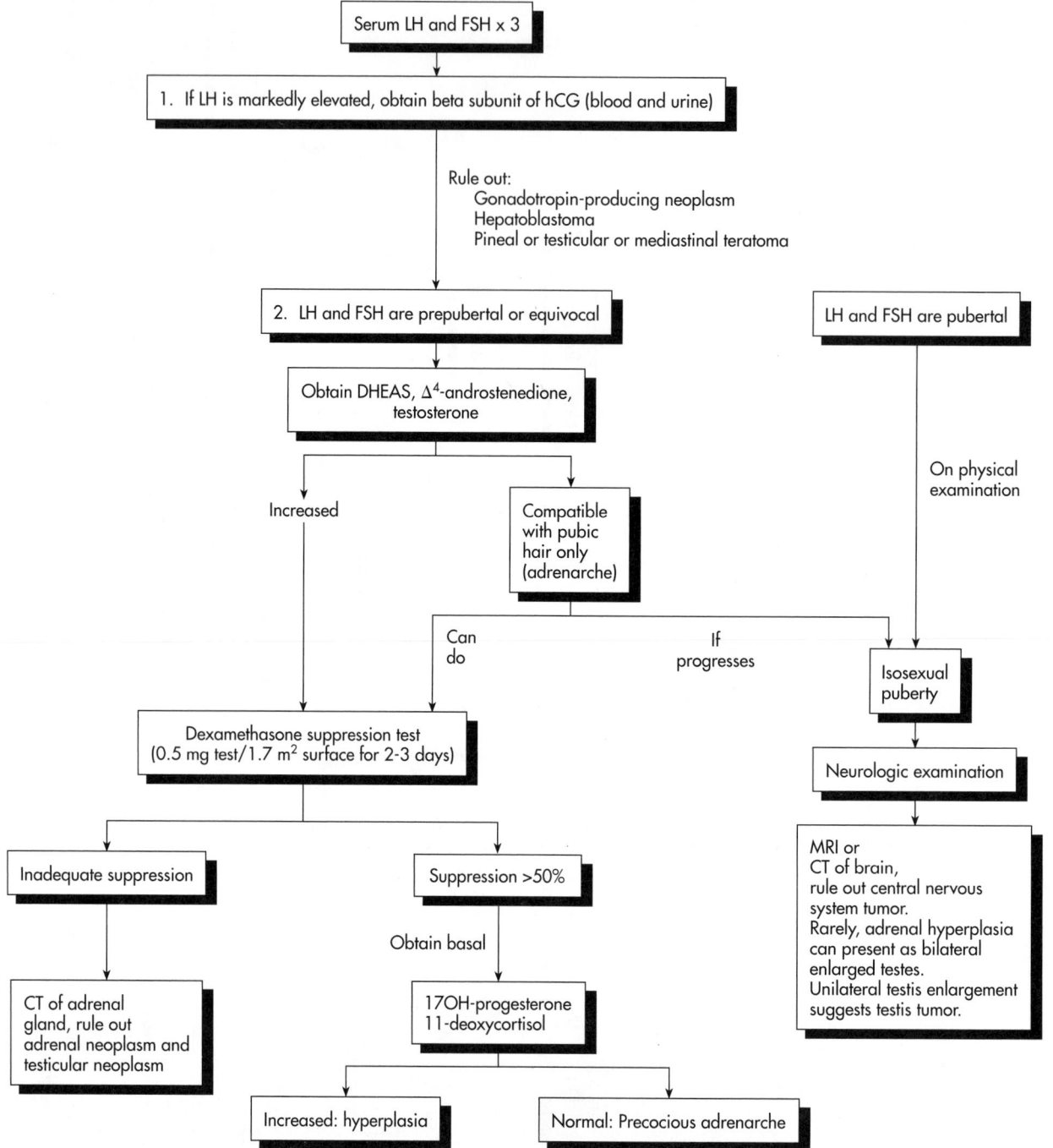

Fig. 3-138   Evaluation of precocious puberty, excluding factitious and iatrogenic causes. *CT,* Computed tomography; *DHEAS,* dehydroepiandrosterone sulfate; *FSH,* follicle-stimulating hormone; *hCG,* human chorionic gonadotropin; *LH,* luteinizing hormone; *MRI,* magnetic resonance imaging. (Modified from Odell WD: The physiology of puberty: disorders of the pubertal process. In DeGroot LJ et al [eds]: *Endocrinology,* vol 3, New York, 1979, Grune & Stratton.)

PULMONARY INFECTIONS, RECURRENT

Pulmonary infections, recurrent
ICD-9CM # 518.3 Pulmonary infiltrate

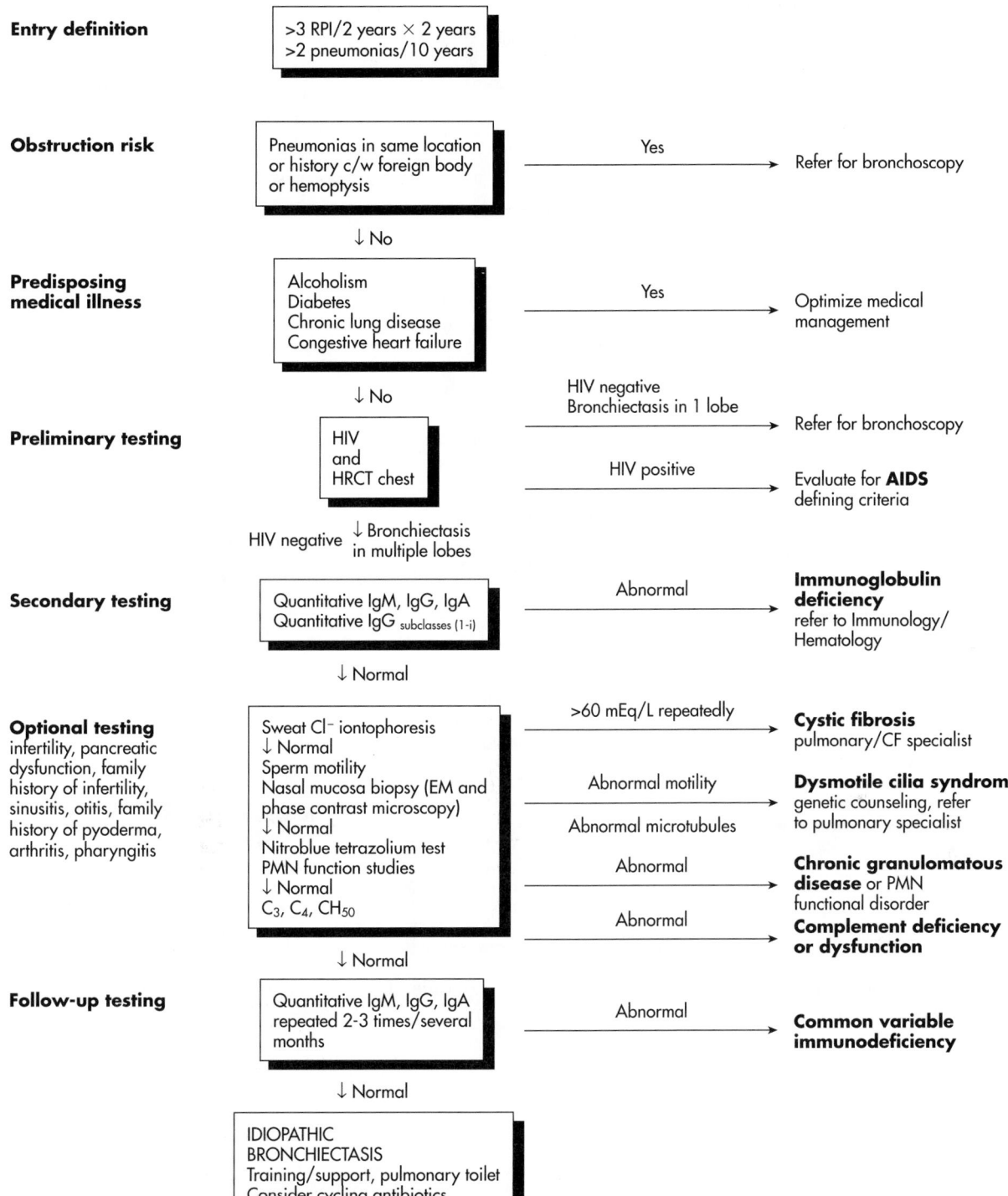

Entry definition

>3 RPI/2 years × 2 years
>2 pneumonias/10 years

Obstruction risk

Pneumonias in same location
or history c/w foreign body
or hemoptysis

→ Yes → Refer for bronchoscopy

↓ No

**Predisposing
medical illness**

Alcoholism
Diabetes
Chronic lung disease
Congestive heart failure

→ Yes → Optimize medical management

↓ No

Preliminary testing

HIV
and
HRCT chest

HIV negative
Bronchiectasis in 1 lobe → Refer for bronchoscopy

HIV positive → Evaluate for **AIDS** defining criteria

HIV negative ↓ Bronchiectasis in multiple lobes

Secondary testing

Quantitative IgM, IgG, IgA
Quantitative IgG subclasses (1-i)

→ Abnormal → **Immunoglobulin deficiency** refer to Immunology/Hematology

↓ Normal

Optional testing
infertility, pancreatic
dysfunction, family
history of infertility,
sinusitis, otitis, family
history of pyoderma,
arthritis, pharyngitis

Sweat Cl⁻ iontophoresis
↓ Normal
Sperm motility
Nasal mucosa biopsy (EM and
phase contrast microscopy)
↓ Normal
Nitroblue tetrazolium test
PMN function studies
↓ Normal
C_3, C_4, CH_{50}

>60 mEq/L repeatedly → **Cystic fibrosis** pulmonary/CF specialist

Abnormal motility → **Dysmotile cilia syndrome** genetic counseling, refer to pulmonary specialist
Abnormal microtubules

Abnormal → **Chronic granulomatous disease** or PMN functional disorder

Abnormal → **Complement deficiency or dysfunction**

↓ Normal

Follow-up testing

Quantitative IgM, IgG, IgA
repeated 2-3 times/several
months

→ Abnormal → **Common variable immunodeficiency**

↓ Normal

IDIOPATHIC
BRONCHIECTASIS
Training/support, pulmonary toilet
Consider cycling antibiotics

Fig. 3-139   Evaluating patients presenting with recurrent pulmonary infections. *AIDS,* Acquired immunodeficiency syndrome; *EM,* electron microscopy; *HIV,* human immunodeficiency virus; *HRCT,* high-resolution, thin-section computerized tomography; *Ig,* immunoglobulin; *PMN,* polymorphonuclear; *RPI,* recurrent pulmonary infections. (From Harrington J [ed]: *Consultation in internal medicine,* ed 2, St Louis, 1997, Mosby.)

III

PULMONARY NODULE

Pulmonary nodule
ICD-9CM # 518.89

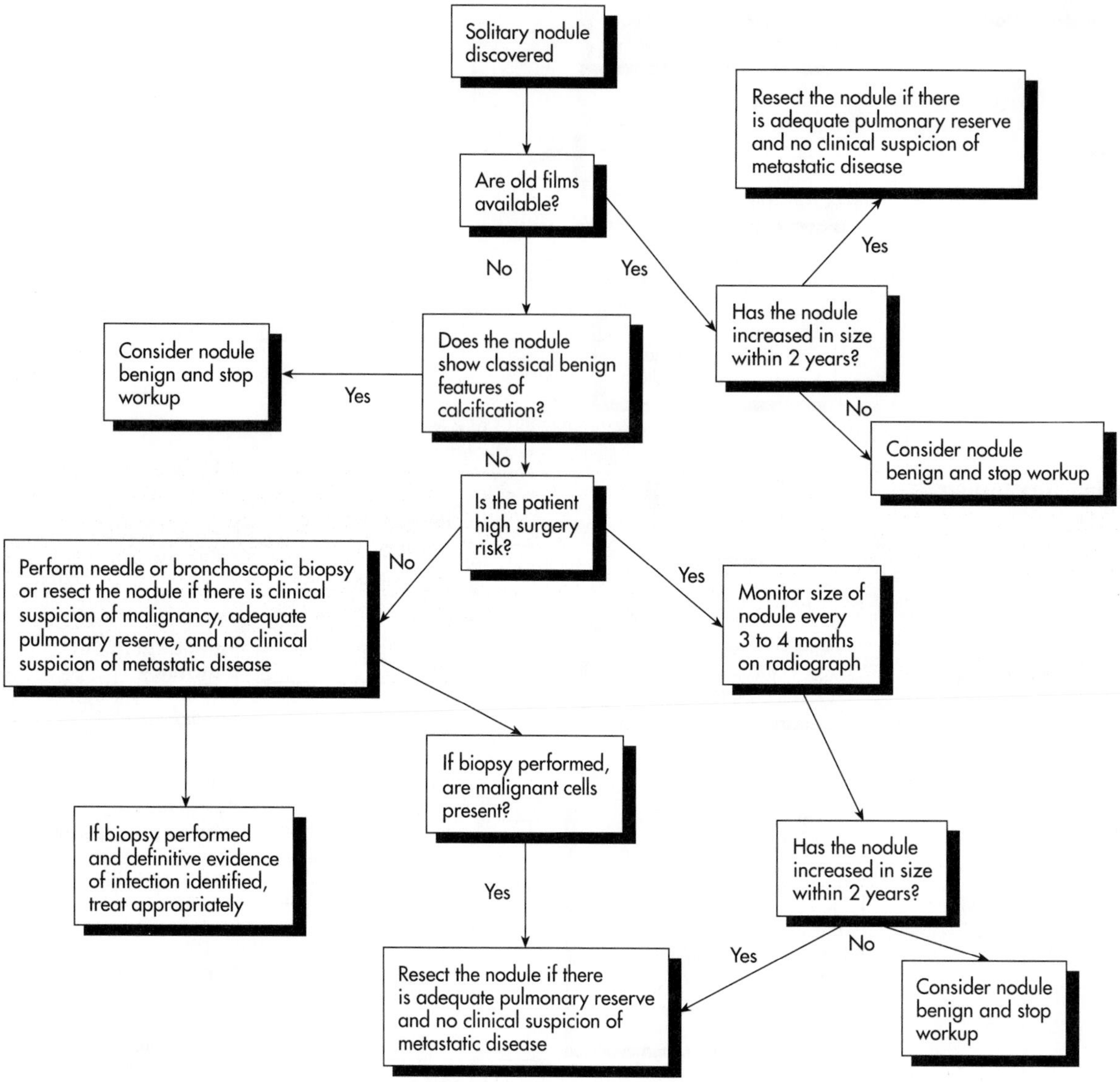

Fig. 3-140 Approach to the patient with a solitary nodule. (From Stein J [ed]: *Internal medicine,* ed 5, St Louis, 1998, Mosby.)

PULSELESS ELECTRICAL ACTIVITY

Pulseless electrical activity (PEA)
ICD-9CM # 427.5 Cardiac arrest, NOS

The term PEA (pulseless electrical activity) has been added to AHA guidelines in an attempt to *unify* an otherwise complex group of cardiac rhythms. Similarities among the entities included in this group are that they all share a common list of potential etiologies and that they generally respond to the same treatment protocol. It should be noted that this newer term encompasses many rhythms that had previously been designated as EMD (ElectroMechanical Dissociation).

Clinically, the meaning of the term *PEA* is suggested by its name. Thus the term is used to describe a group of diverse electrocardiographic rhythms that by definition manifest evidence of electrical activity (since they all produce an ECG rhythm) but which are unified by the clinical finding of pulselessness. According to this definition, PEA rhythms must therefore be *nonperfusing* — or at most no more than *minimally* perfusing — (because they are by definition associated with the pulseless state).

Many types of ECG rhythms have been associated with the clinical entity known as PEA. Most of these rhythms can be classified into one of the following groups:

- **EMD Rhythms** — in which there is an *organized* ECG rhythm (usually with a *narrow* QRS complex) — but no pulse.

- **Pseudo-EMD Rhythms** — in which the ECG rhythm is associated with at least some *meaningful* mechanical contraction (as might be evidenced by obtaining a pulse with doppler that is too faint to palpate clinically).

- **Idioventricular** or **Ventricular Escape Rhythms** — in which the QRS complex of the escape rhythm is widened. Atrial activity is absent. There is no pulse. Included in this group are *postdefibrillation* idioventricular rhythms.

- **Bradyasystolic Rhythms** — in which there is profound bradycardia, often with prolonged periods of asystole. There is no pulse.

Key treatment options

Begin/continue CPR
- Early performance of CPR is essential (since by definition PEA is a *nonperfusing or poorly perfusing rhythm*).
- Supportive actions (intubate/establish IV access, etc.).
- Assess blood flow and other clinical parameters (i.e., use of doppler, end-tidal CO2, arterial line as possible).

Epinephrine
- Begin with an SDE dose (i.e., 1.0 mg by IV bolus).
- May either repeat SDE (every 3-5 minutes as needed) or increase the dose (i.e., to HDE) if there has been no response.

Search for the cause of PEA
- Consider the most common causes
   - a) Inadequate ventilation?
   - b) Inadequate circulation?
   - c) Metabolic disorder?
- Once detected, try to correct the underlying/precipitating cause.
- Consider empiric volume infusion (since hypovolemia is probably the most common potentially correctable cause of PEA).

Consider other options
- Atropine is likely to be helpful only if the PEA rhythm is associated with absolute or relative bradycardia. Give 1 mg IV; may repeat every 3-5 minutes (as needed); up to a total dose of 0.04 mg/kg (= 3 mg).
- Pacing is likely to be helpful only if PEA is due to temporarily disturbed conduction (as may occur in some cases of drug overdose).

Conditions most likely to cause a PEA rhythm

Inadequate ventilation
- Intubation of right mainstem bronchus or other cause of hypoxemia
- Tension pneumothorax (trauma, asthma, patient on ventilator)
- Bilateral pneumothorax (trauma)

Inadequate circulation
- Pericardial effusion with tamponade (trauma, pericarditis, uremia, too vigorous CPR)
- Myocardial rupture or rupture of aortic aneurysm
- Massive pulmonary embolism
- Hypovolemia caused by
   - Acute blood loss (trauma, GI bleeding)
   - Dehydration
   - Septic shock
   - Cardiogenic shock (acute MI, myocardial contusion)
   - Anaphylactic shock
   - Neurogenic shock (cervical spine fracture)

Metabolic disorders
- Electrolyte disturbance (severe hyperkalemia, hypokalemia, hypomagnesemia)
- Persistent severe acidosis (diabetic ketoacidosis, lactic acidosis)
- Overdose of cardiac depressant drugs (tricyclic antidepressants)
- Hypothermia

NOTE: The ECG appearance of a PEA rhythm may provide insight as to the relative likelihood that the condition can be reversed. In general, prognosis tends to be better if the ECG rhythm manifests organized atrial activity (in the form of P waves that conduct), a rate that is not excessively slow, and narrow QRS complexes, provided (of course) that the underlying cause of the PEA rhythm can be identified and corrected.

In contrast, PEA is much more likely to be a preterminal rhythm when organized atrial activity is absent, the QRS complex is wide, and/or bradycardia persists despite medical treatment.

Fig. 3-141 Pulseless electrical activity (PEA). *CO2,* Carbon dioxide; *CPR,* cardiopulmonary resuscitation; *ECG,* electrocardiogram; *GI,* gastrointestinal; *HDE,* high-dose epinephrine; *IV,* intravenous; *MI,* myocardial infarction; *SDE,* standard-dose epinephrine. (Modified from Grauer K, Cavallaro D: *ACLS: Rapid review and case scenarios,* ed 4, St Louis, 1996, Mosby.)

III

PURPURA, PALPABLE

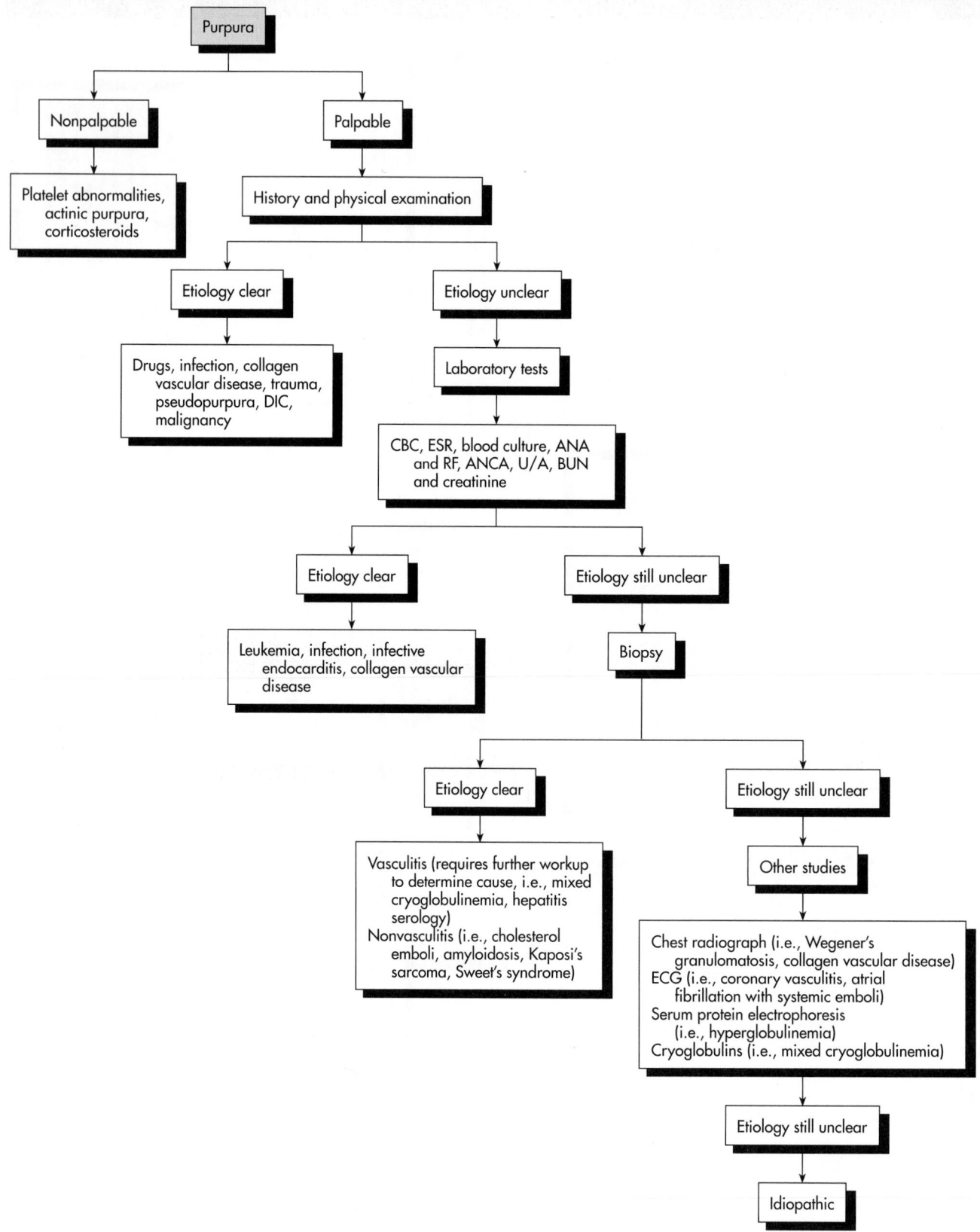

Fig. 3-142 **Diagnostic algorithm for palpable purpura.** *AIDS, Acquired immunodeficiency syndrome; ANA, antinuclear antibody; ANCA, antineutrophil cytoplasmic antibody test; BUN, blood urea nitrogen; CBC, complete blood cell count; DIC, disseminated intravascular coagulation; ECG, electrocardiogram; ESR, erythrocyte sedimentation rate; MCV, mean corpuscular volume; RF, rheumatoid factor; U/A, urinalysis.* (From Stevens GL, Adelman HM, Wallach PM: *Am Fam Physician* 52:1355, 1995.)

RED EYE, ACUTE

Red eye, acute
ICD-9CM # 379.93

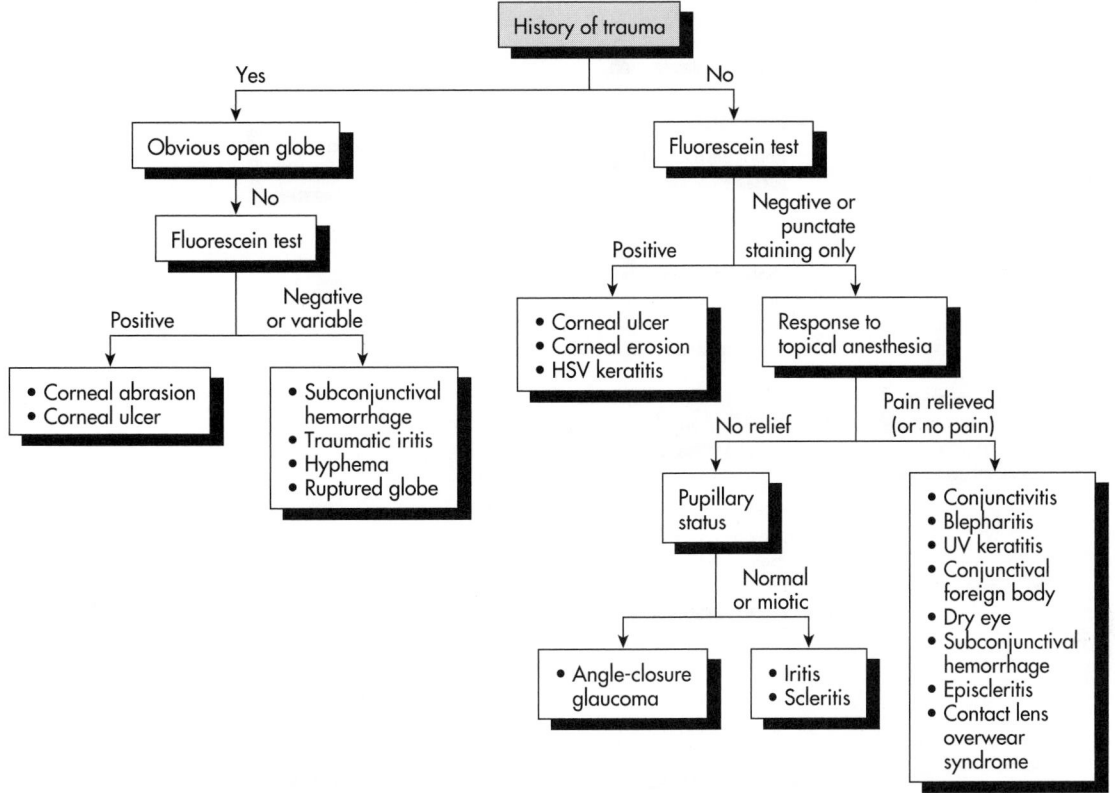

Fig. 3-143 Algorithm showing wilderness diagnostic procedure for the acute red eye. *HSV*, Herpes simplex virus; *UV*, ultraviolet. (From Auerbach PS: *Wilderness medicine,* ed 4, St Louis, 2001, Mosby.)

III

RENAL MASS

```
                    ┌──────────────────┐        ┌──────────────────┐
                    │ Renal mass on    │ ◄───── │ Symptoms or      │
                    │ IVP/tomography   │        │ hematuria        │
                    └──────────────────┘        └──────────────────┘
                             │
┌──────────────┐   ┌──────────────────┐        ┌──────────────────────┐
│ Cystic       │   │                  │        │ Mass not identified  │
│ Smooth wall  │◄──│ Renal ultrasound │───────►│ (confirmed with CT   │
│ No internal  │   │                  │        │ scan)                │
│ echoes       │   └──────────────────┘        └──────────────────────┘
└──────────────┘            │
       │           ┌──────────────────┐
       ▼           │ Solid/complex    │
┌──────────┐       │ Internal echoes  │
│ Observe  │       │ Irregular wall   │
└──────────┘       └──────────────────┘
                            │
┌──────────────────┐   ┌──────────┐
│ Negative CT      │◄──│ CT scan  │
│ number           │   └──────────┘
│ Fat density      │      │      \
│ Angiomyolipoma   │      │       \
└──────────────────┘      │        \
       │                  │         \
       ▼          ┌──────────────────┐   ┌──────────────────┐   ┌──────────────┐
┌──────────┐      │ Complex mass     │   │ Solid            │   │ Suspected    │
│ Observe  │      │ No contrast      │   │ Contrast         │──►│ caval        │
└──────────┘      │ enhancement      │   │ enhancement      │   │ thrombus     │
                  │ Indeterminate    │   │ Vascular tumor   │   └──────────────┘
                  └──────────────────┘   └──────────────────┘          │
                            │                  │                        ▼
                            │             ┌──────────┐            ┌──────────┐
                            │             │ Surgery  │◄───────────│   MRI    │
                            │             └──────────┘            └──────────┘
                            │
┌──────────────┐   ┌──────────────────┐   ┌──────────────────┐
│ Avascular    │◄──│ Renal arteriogram│──►│ Neovascularity   │
│ Inconclusive │   └──────────────────┘   └──────────────────┘
└──────────────┘                                  │
       │                                          ▼
       ▼                                   ┌──────────┐
┌──────────────────┐                       │ Surgery  │
│ Needle aspiration│                       └──────────┘
└──────────────────┘
       │
       ▼
┌──────────────────┐
│ Malignant cells  │
└──────────────────┘
       │
       ▼
┌──────────┐
│ Surgery  │
└──────────┘
```

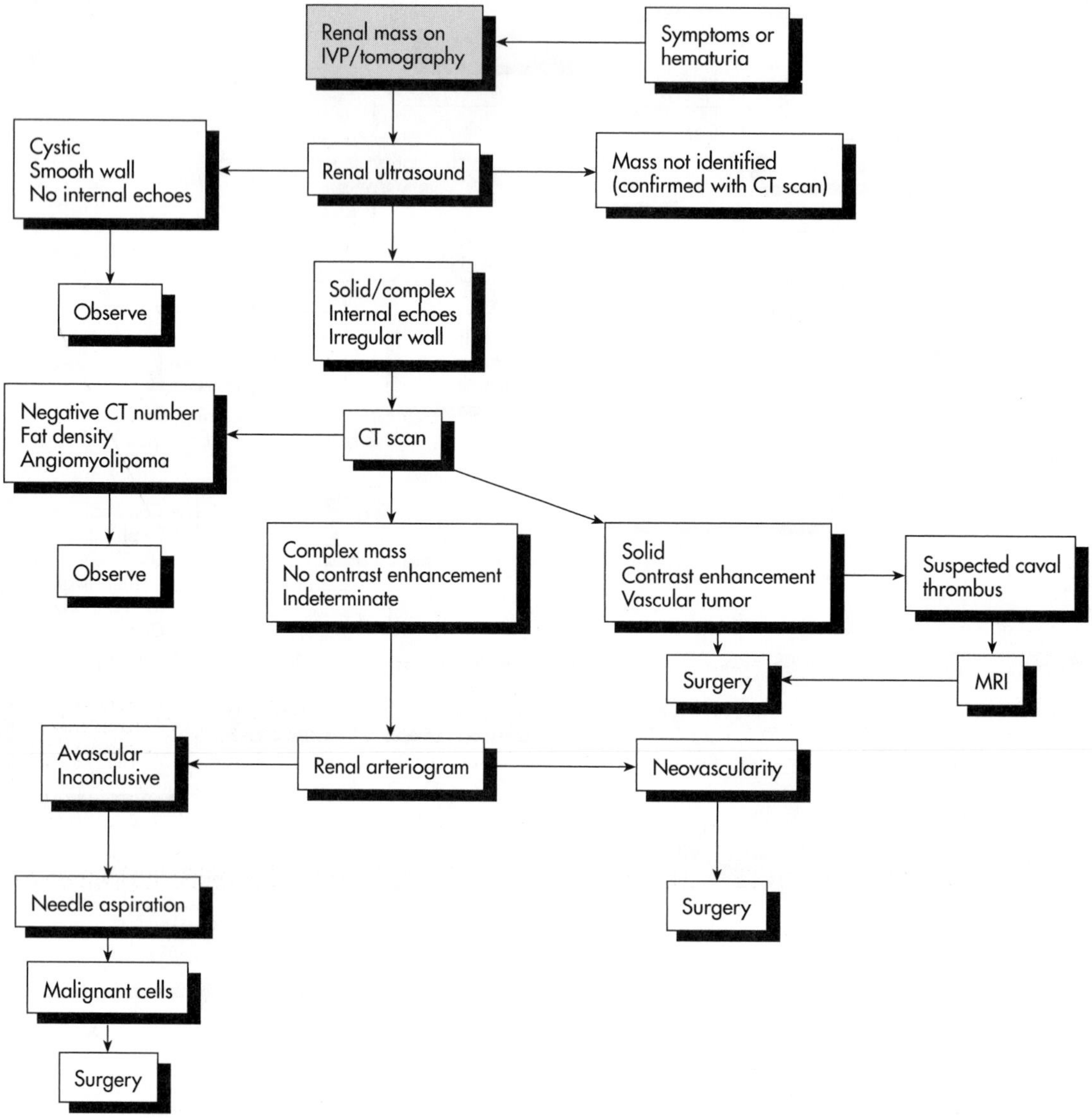

Fig. 3-144   Evaluation of a patient with a renal mass. *CT,* Computed tomography; *IVP,* intravenous pyelogram; *MRI,* magnetic resonance imaging. (Modified from Williams RD: Tumors of the kidney, ureter, and bladder. In Wyngaarden JB, Smith JL, Jr, Bennett JC [eds]: *Cecil textbook of medicine,* ed 19, Philadelphia, 1992, WB Saunders.)

RESPIRATORY DISTRESS

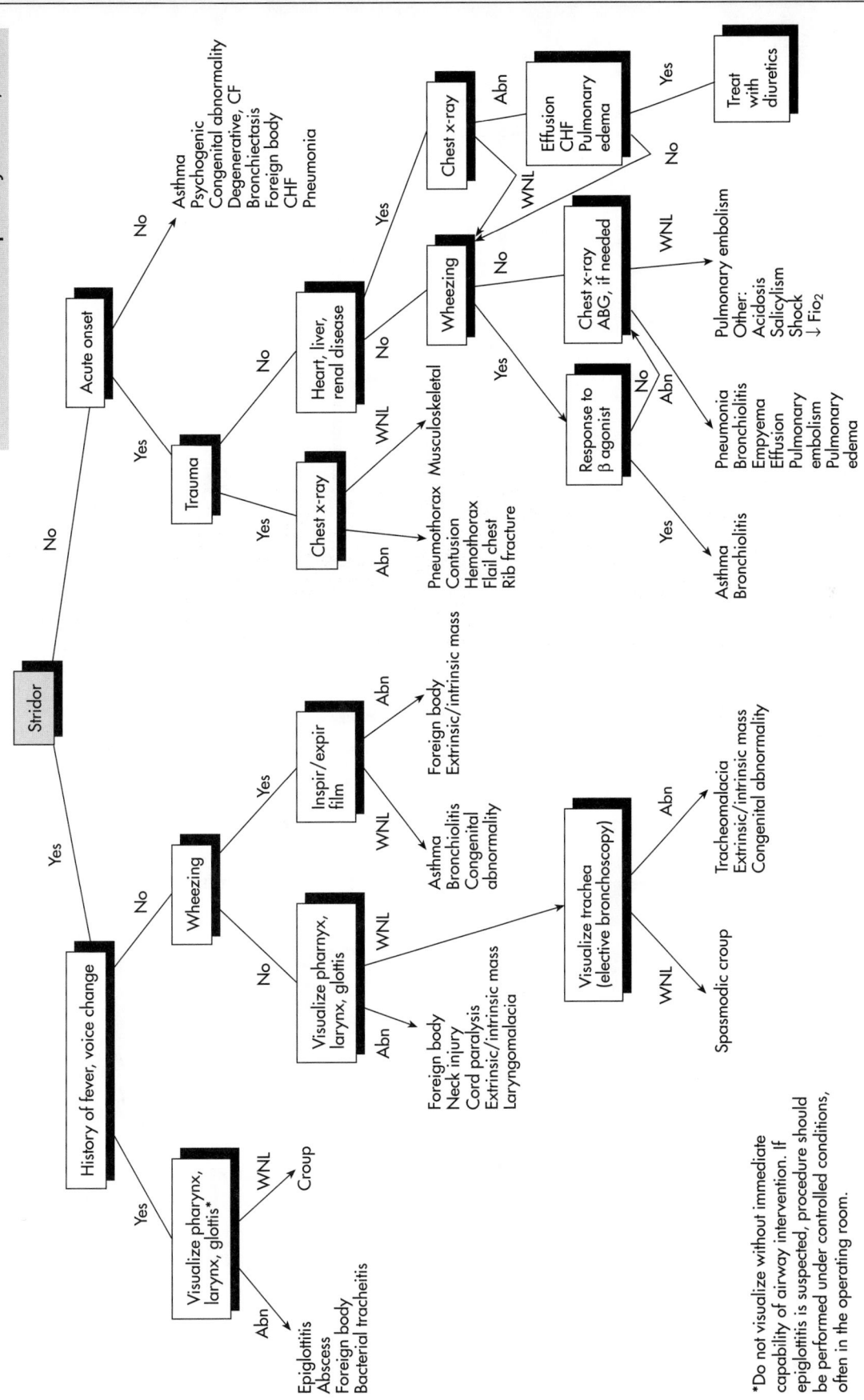

Respiratory distress
ICD-9CM # 786.09 Respiratory distress NOS
518.82 Respiratory distress, acute

*Do not visualize without immediate capability of airway intervention. If epiglottitis is suspected, procedure should be performed under controlled conditions, often in the operating room.

Fig. 3-145 Respiratory distress. *ABG,* Arterial blood gas; *Abn,* abnormal; *CF,* cystic fibrosis; *CHF,* congestive heart failure; *WNL,* within normal limits. (From Barkin RM, Rosen P: *Emergency pediatrics,* St Louis, 1999, Mosby.)

RETICULOCYTE COUNT ELEVATION

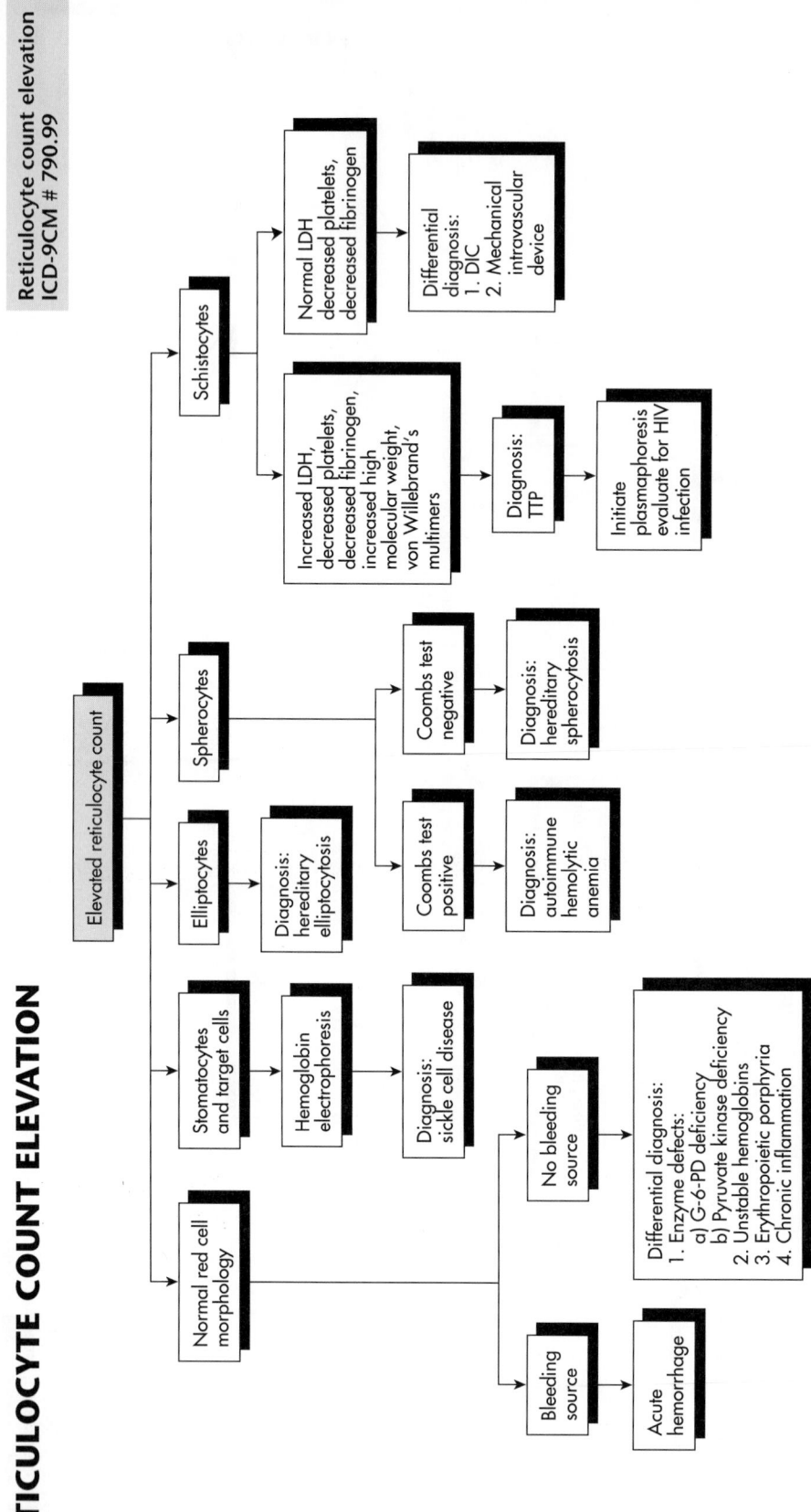

Fig. 3-146   Differential diagnosis of elevated reticulocyte count. *DIC,* Disseminated intravascular coagulation; *G6PD,* glucose-6-phosphate dehydrogenase; *HIV,* human immunodeficiency virus; *LDH,* lactic dehydrogenase; *TTP,* thrombotic thrombocytopenic purpura. (From Rakel RE [ed]: *Principles of family practice,* ed 6, Philadelphia, 2002, WB Saunders.)

RHINORRHEA

Rhinorrhea
ICD-9CM # 478.1

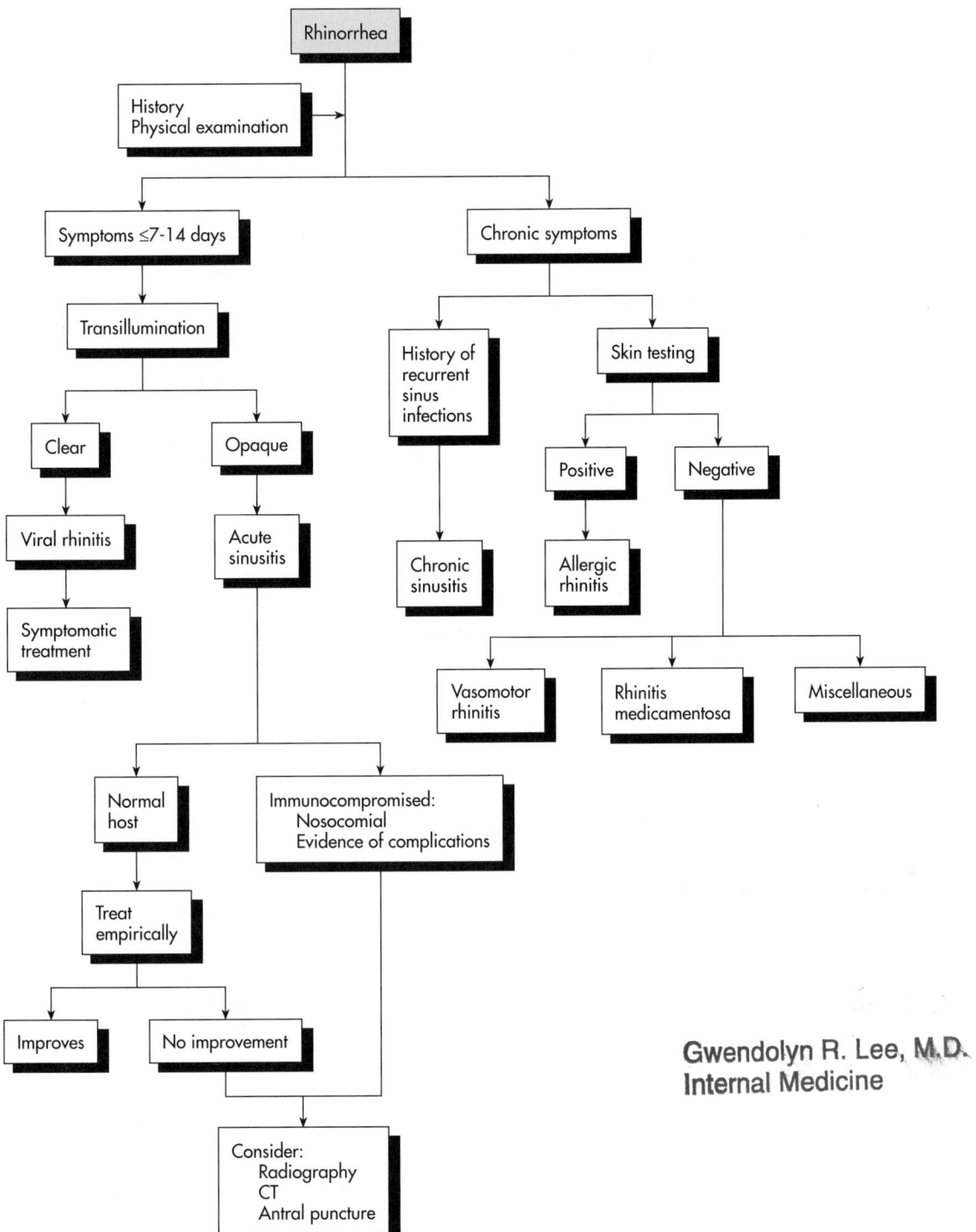

Fig. 3-147 **Approach to a patient with rhinorrhea.** *CT,* Computed tomography. (From Noble J [ed]: *Primary care medicine,* ed 3, St Louis, 2001, Mosby.)

SCHILLING TEST

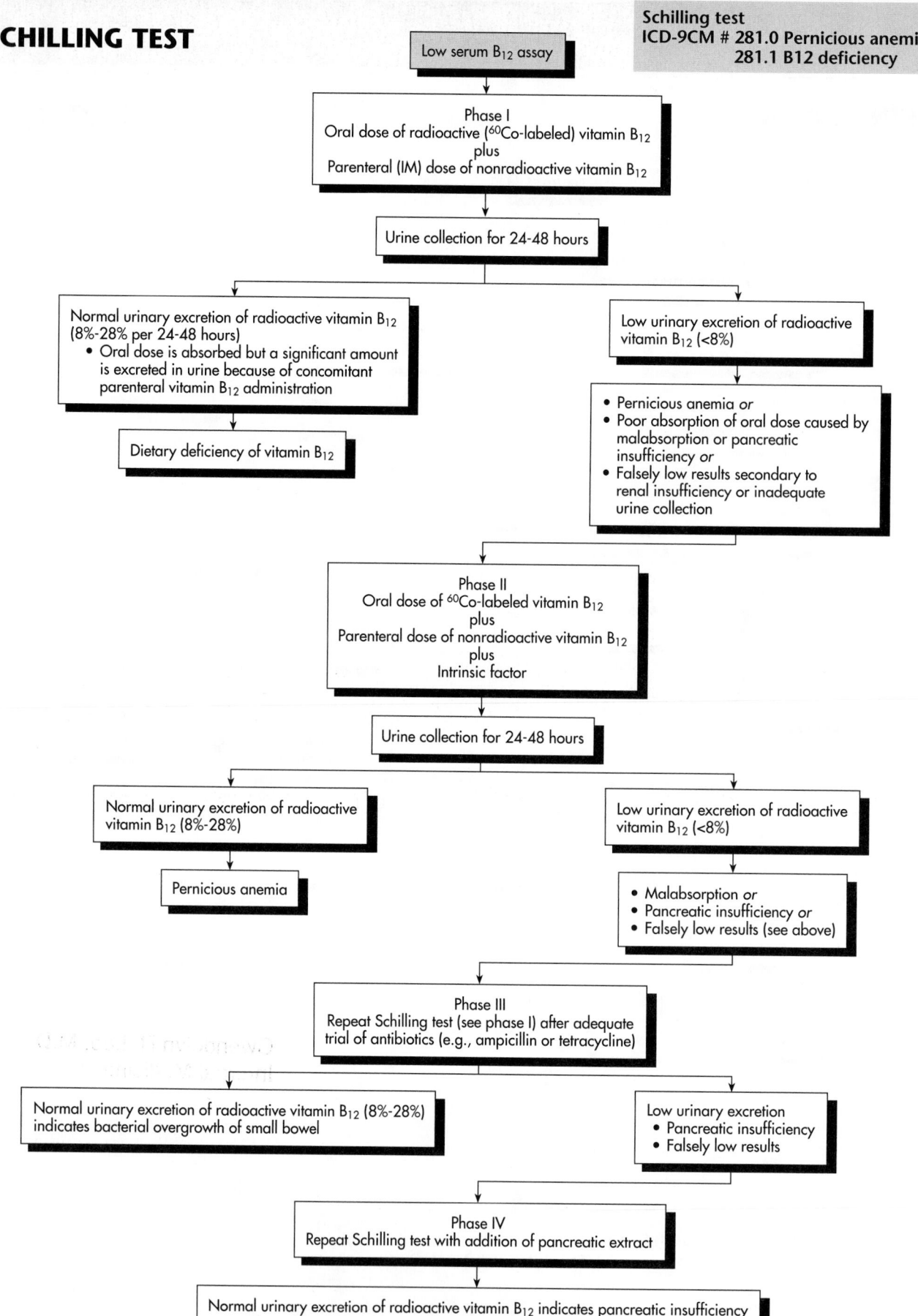

Fig. 3-148 **Schilling test.** *IM,* Intramuscular. (From Ferri FF: *Practical guide to the care of the medical patient,* ed 5, St Louis, 2001, Mosby.)

SCROTAL MASS

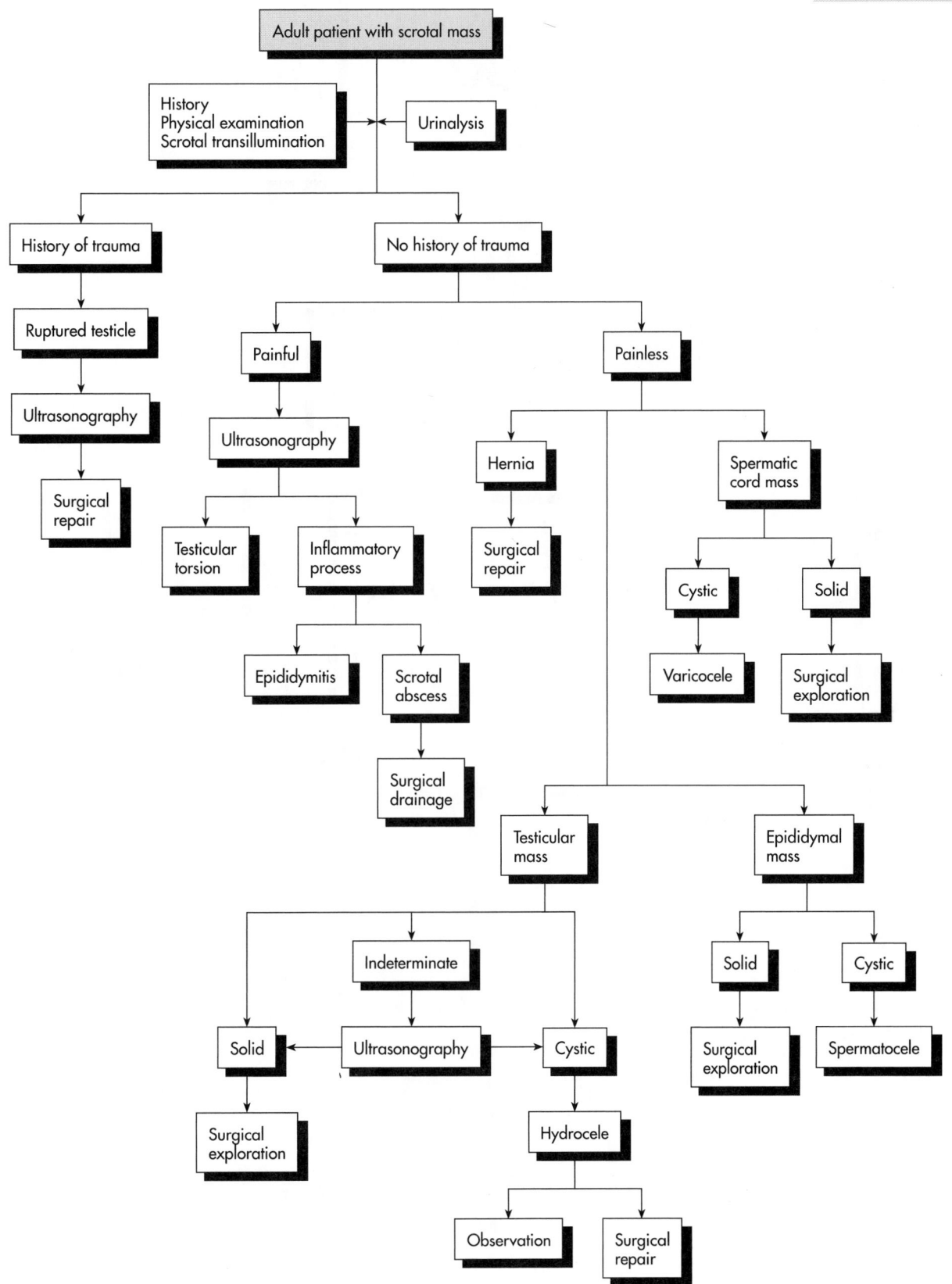

Fig. 3-149 **Evaluation of scrotal mass.** (From Greene HL, Johnson WP, Lemcke D [eds]: *Decision making in medicine,* ed 2, St Louis, 1998, Mosby.)

SEXUAL DYSFUNCTION

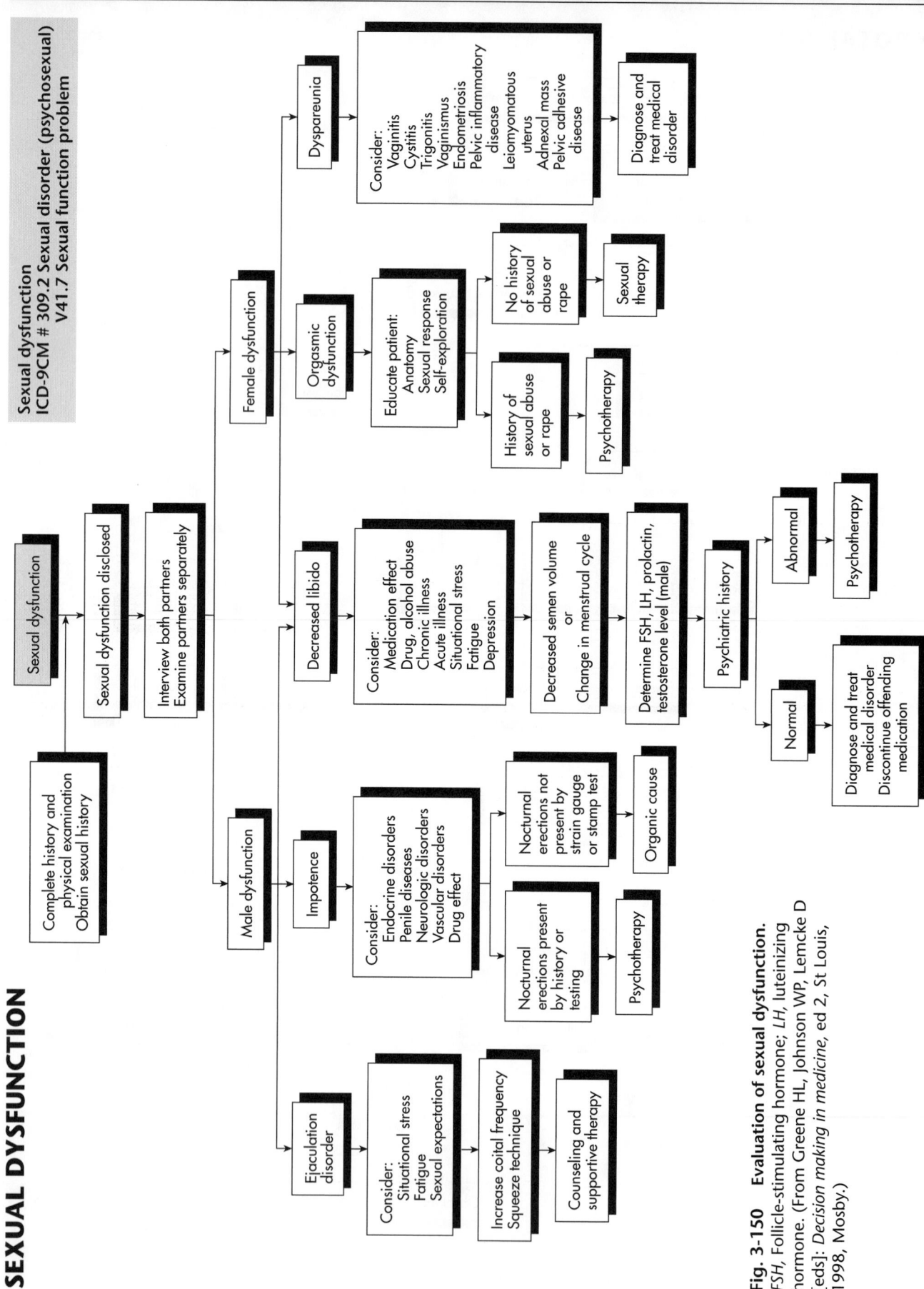

Fig. 3-150   Evaluation of sexual dysfunction.
FSH, Follicle-stimulating hormone; *LH,* luteinizing hormone. (From Greene HL, Johnson WP, Lemcke D [eds]: *Decision making in medicine,* ed 2, St Louis, 1998, Mosby.)

SHIN SPLINTS

Shin splints
ICD-9CM # 844.9

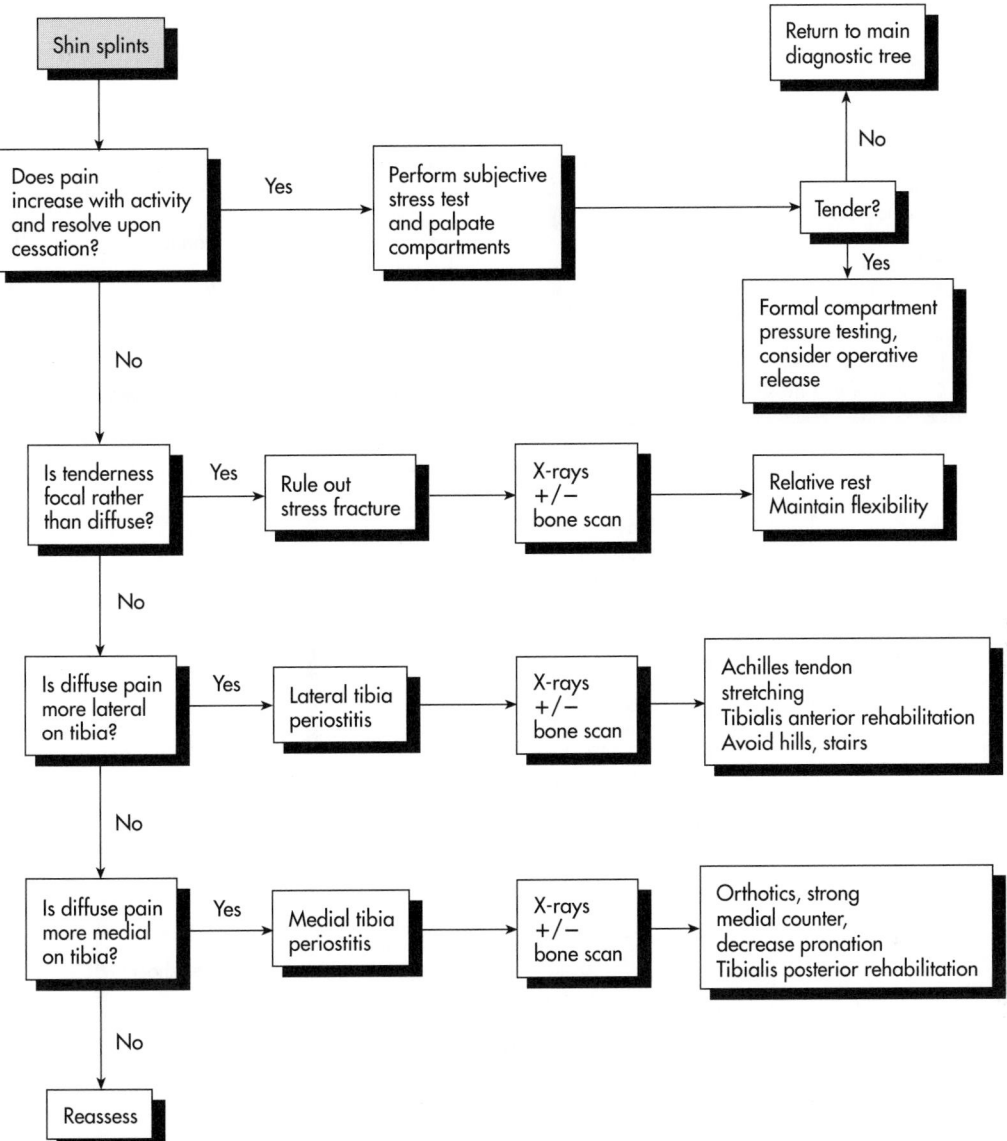

Fig. 3-151   Evaluation and management of shin splints. (From Scudieri G [ed]: *Sports medicine, principles of primary care,* St Louis, 1997, Mosby.)

SHORT

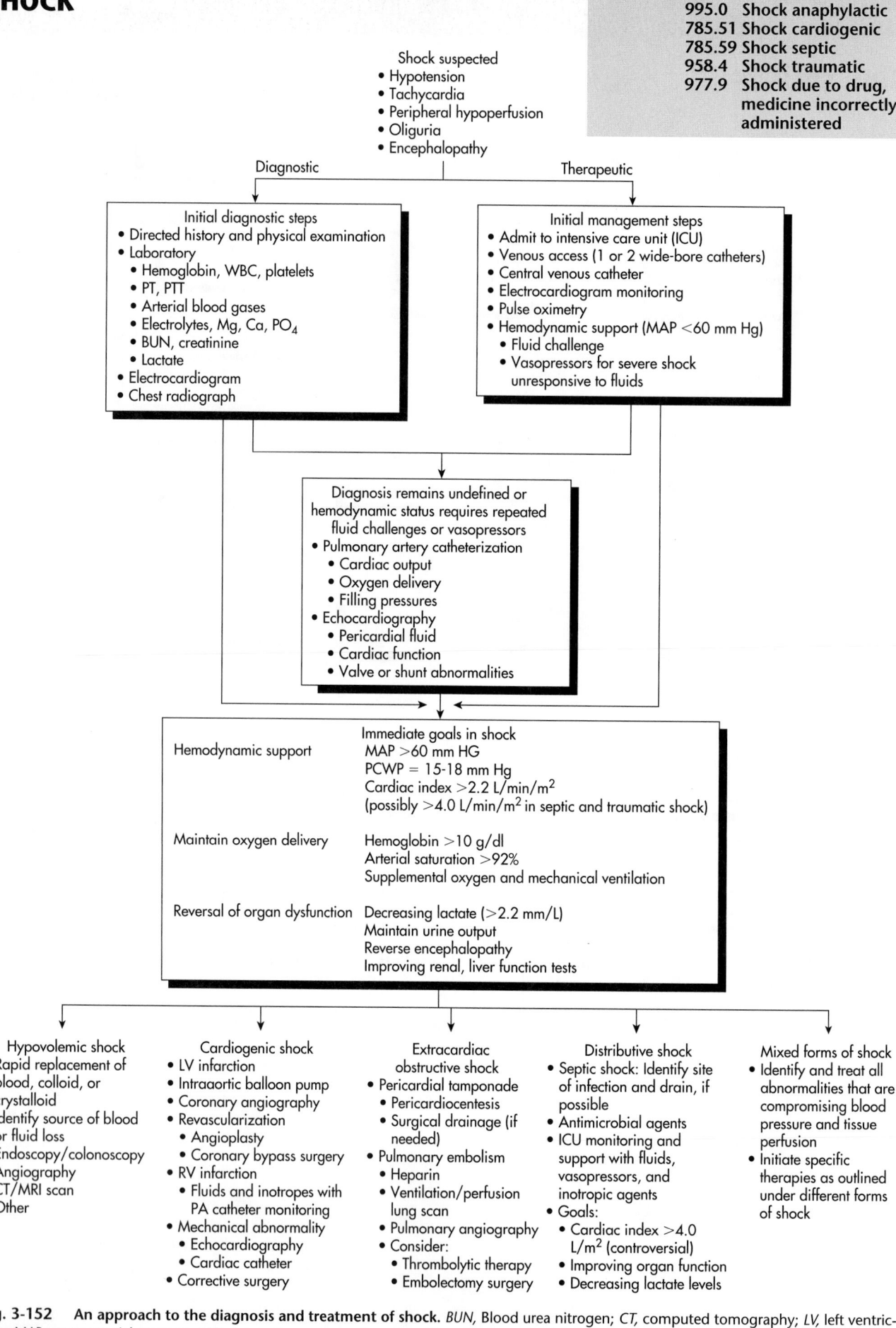

Fig. 3-152 **An approach to the diagnosis and treatment of shock.** *BUN,* Blood urea nitrogen; *CT,* computed tomography; *LV,* left ventricular; *MAP,* mean arterial pressure; *MRI,* magnetic resonance imaging; *PA,* pulmonary arterial; *PCWP,* pulmonary capillary wedge pressure, *PT,* prothrombin time; *PTT,* partial thromboplastin time; *RV,* right ventricular; *WBC,* white blood cell count. (From Goldman L, Bennett JC [eds]: *Cecil textbook of medicine,* ed 21, Philadelphia, 2000, WB Saunders.)

SLEEP DISORDERS

Sleep disorders
ICD-9CM # 780.50 Sleep disorder, unspecified cause

A

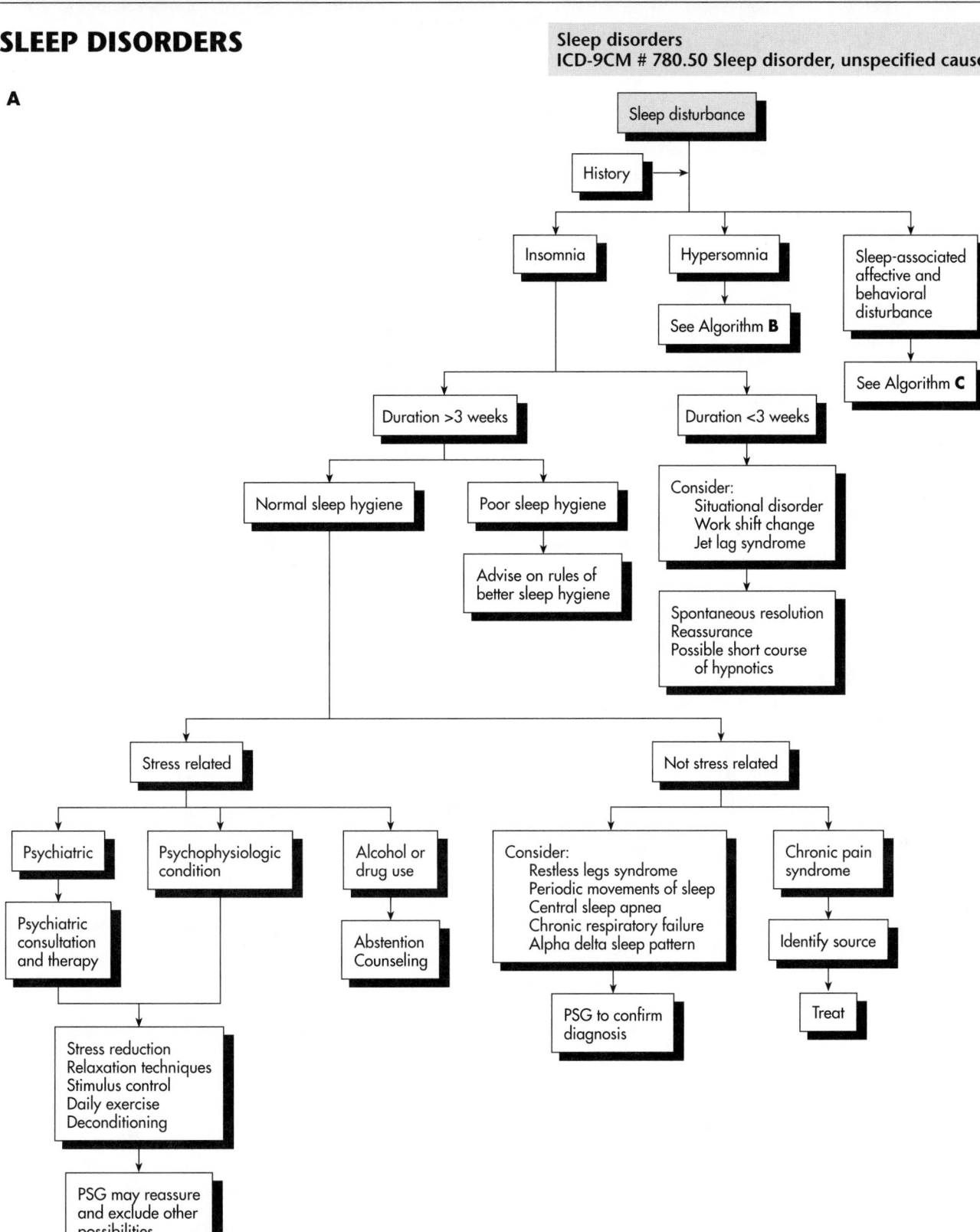

Fig. 3-153   **A, Patient with sleep disturbance.** *MSLT,* Multiple sleep latency tests; *PSG,* polysomnography. (From Greene HL, Johnson WP, Lemcke D [eds]: *Decision making in medicine,* ed 2, St Louis, 1998, Mosby.)

Continued

SLEEP DISORDERS—cont'd

B

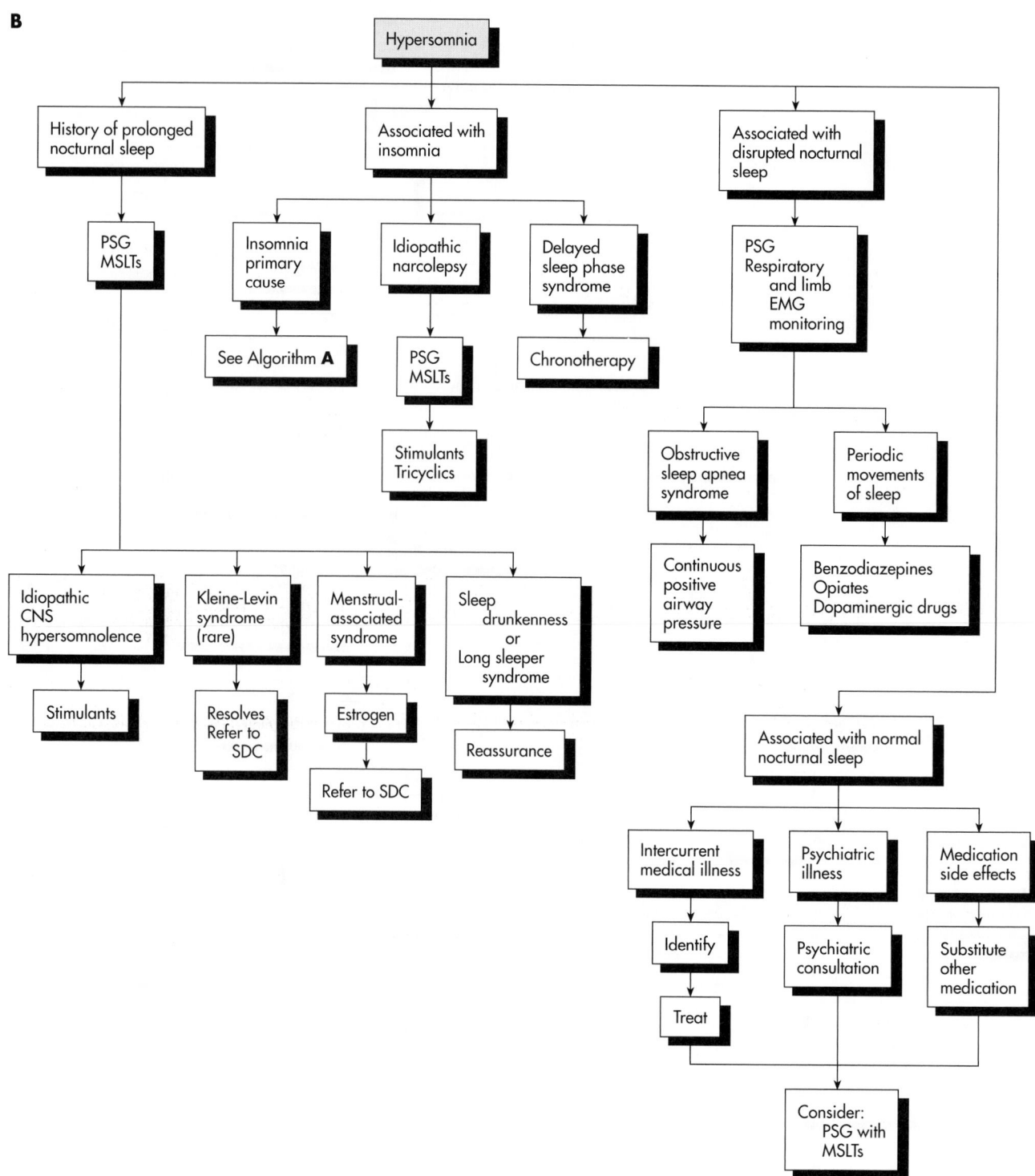

Fig. 3-153, cont'd   B, Hypersomnia. *CNS,* Central nervous system; *EMG,* electromyelogram; *MSLTs,* multiple sleep latency tests; *PSG,* polysomnography; *SDC,* sleep disorders clinic.

SLEEP DISORDERS—cont'd

C

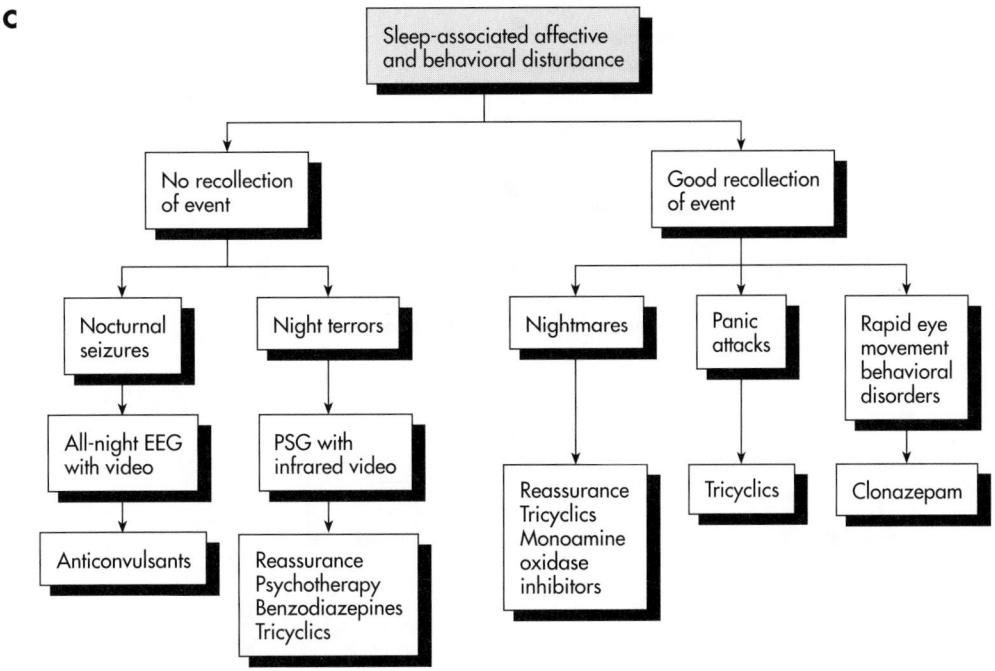

Fig. 3-153, cont'd   C, Sleep-associated affective and behavioral disturbance. *EEG,* Electroencephalogram; *PSG,* polysomnography.

SPINAL INJURY, CERVICAL

Spinal injury, cervical
ICD-9CM # 952.9 Spinal cord injury, site unspecified

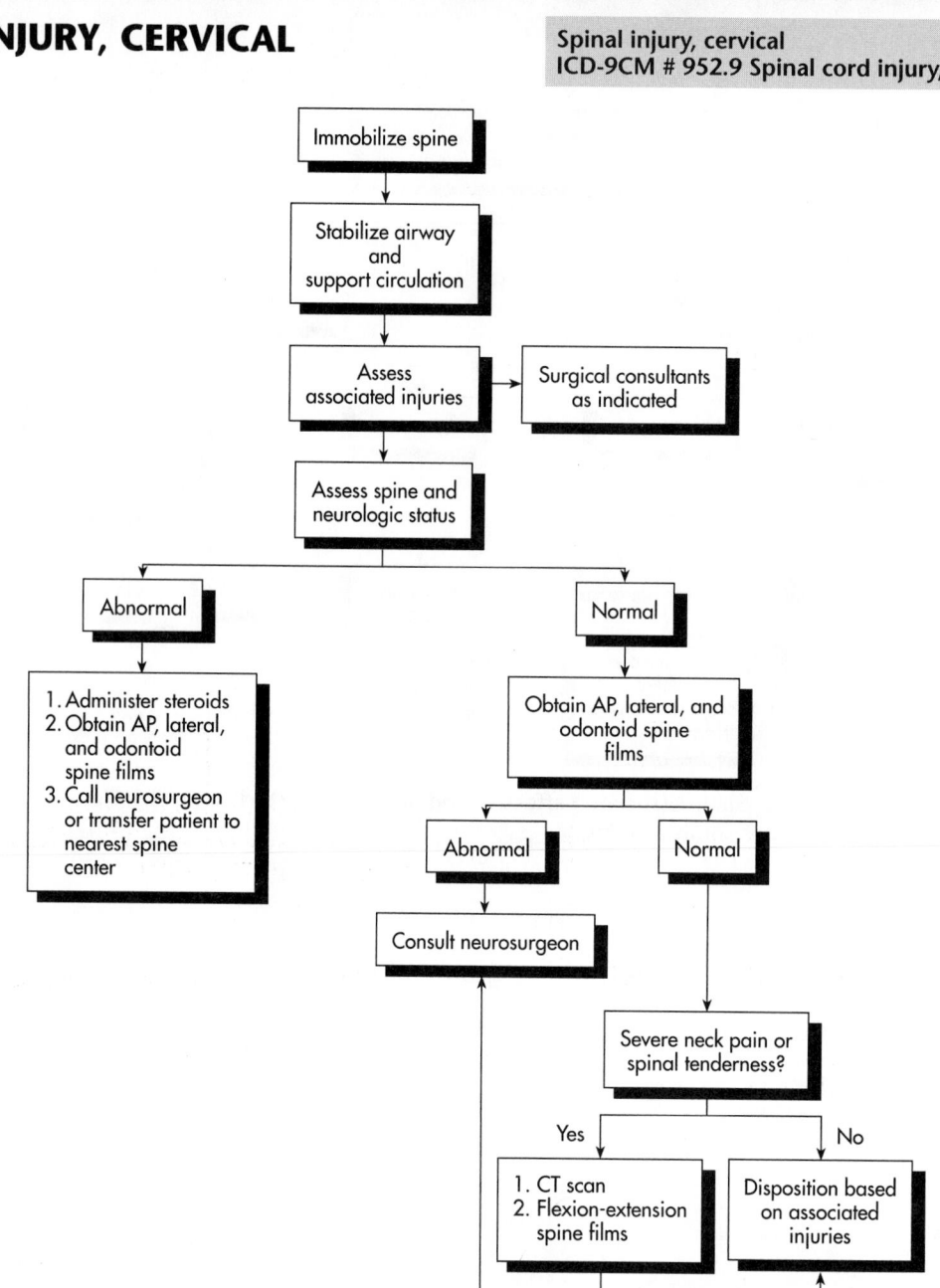

Fig. 3-154   Approach to patient with suspected cervical spinal injury. *AP,* Anteroposterior; *CT,* computed tomography. (From Rosen P et al [eds]: *Emergency medicine: concepts and clinical practice,* ed 5, St Louis, 2002, Mosby.)

SPINE TUMORS

Spine tumors
ICD-9CM # 225.3 spine tumor, benign
237.5 spinal cord tumor, uncertain behavior

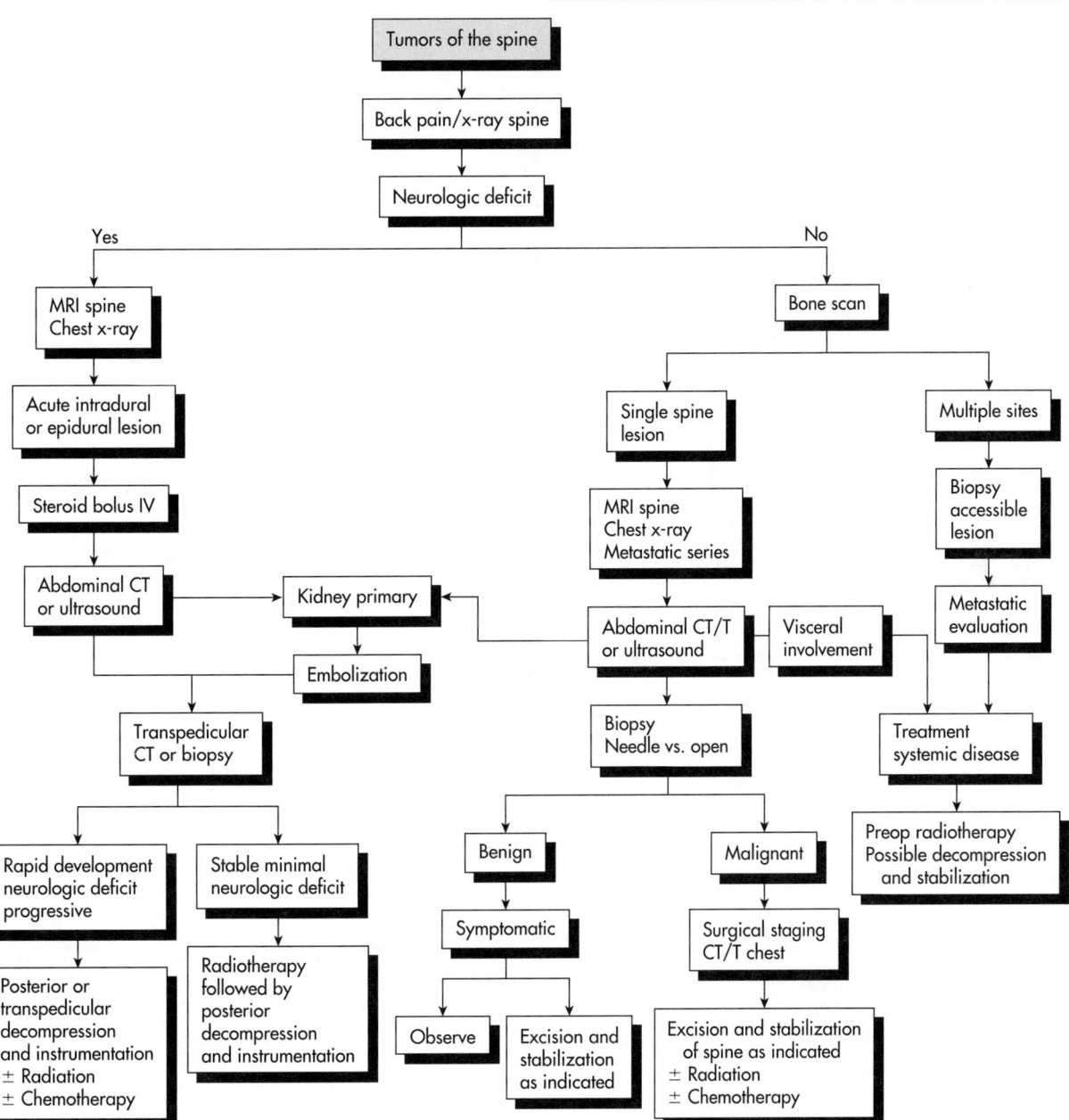

Fig. 3-155 *CT,* Computed tomography; *IV,* intravenous; *MRI,* magnetic resonance imaging. (From Abeloff MD: *Clinical oncology,* ed 2, New York, 2000, Churchill Livingstone.)

SPLENOMEGALY

Splenomegaly
ICD-9CM # 789.2 Splenomegaly, unspecified
289.51 Splenomegaly, chronic congestive
759.0 Splenomegaly, congenital
789.2 Splenomegaly, unknown etiology

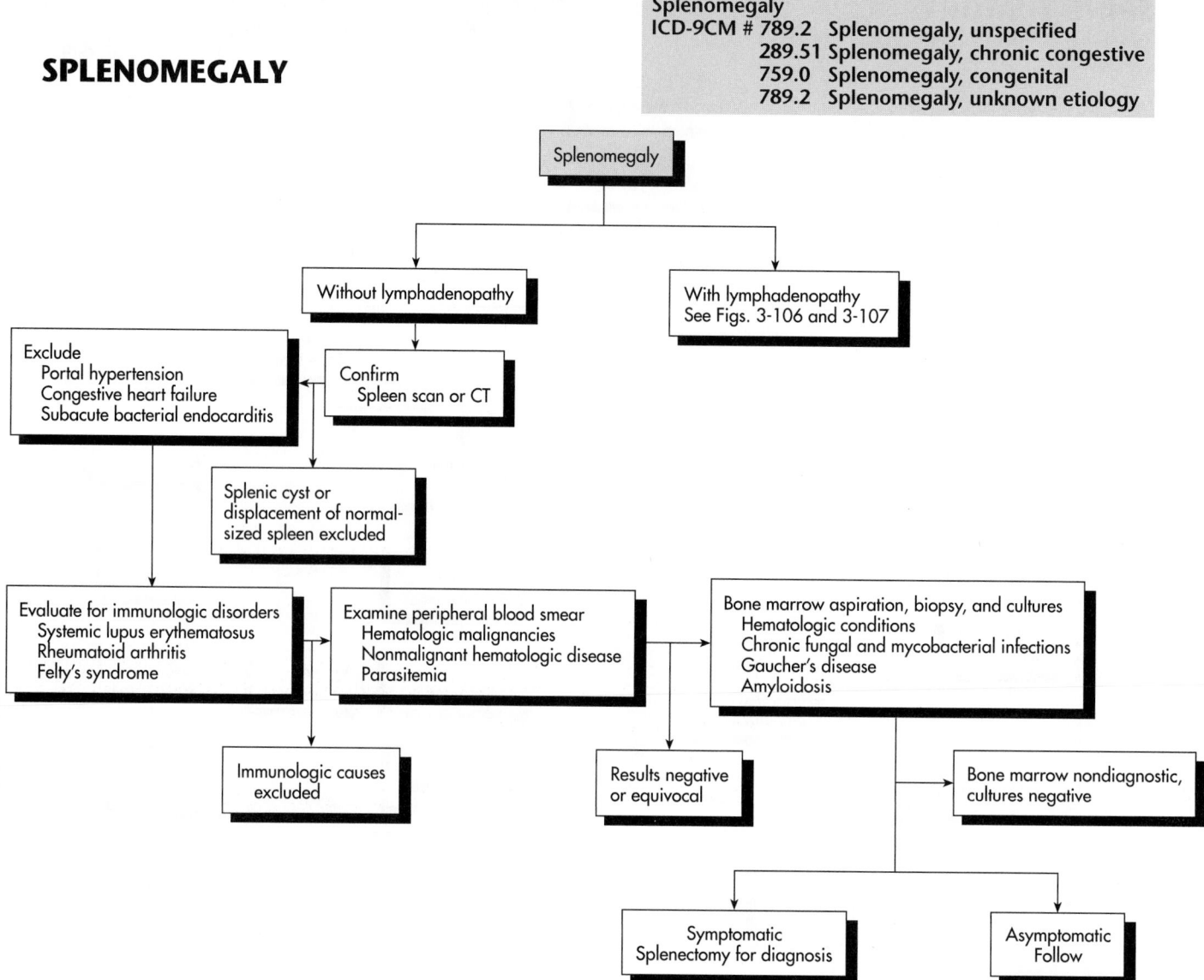

Fig. 3-156 **Clinical approach to patient with splenomegaly.** *CT,* Computed tomography. (From Stein JH [ed]: *Internal medicine,* ed 5, St Louis, 1998, Mosby.)

SPONDYLOARTHROPATHY, DIAGNOSIS

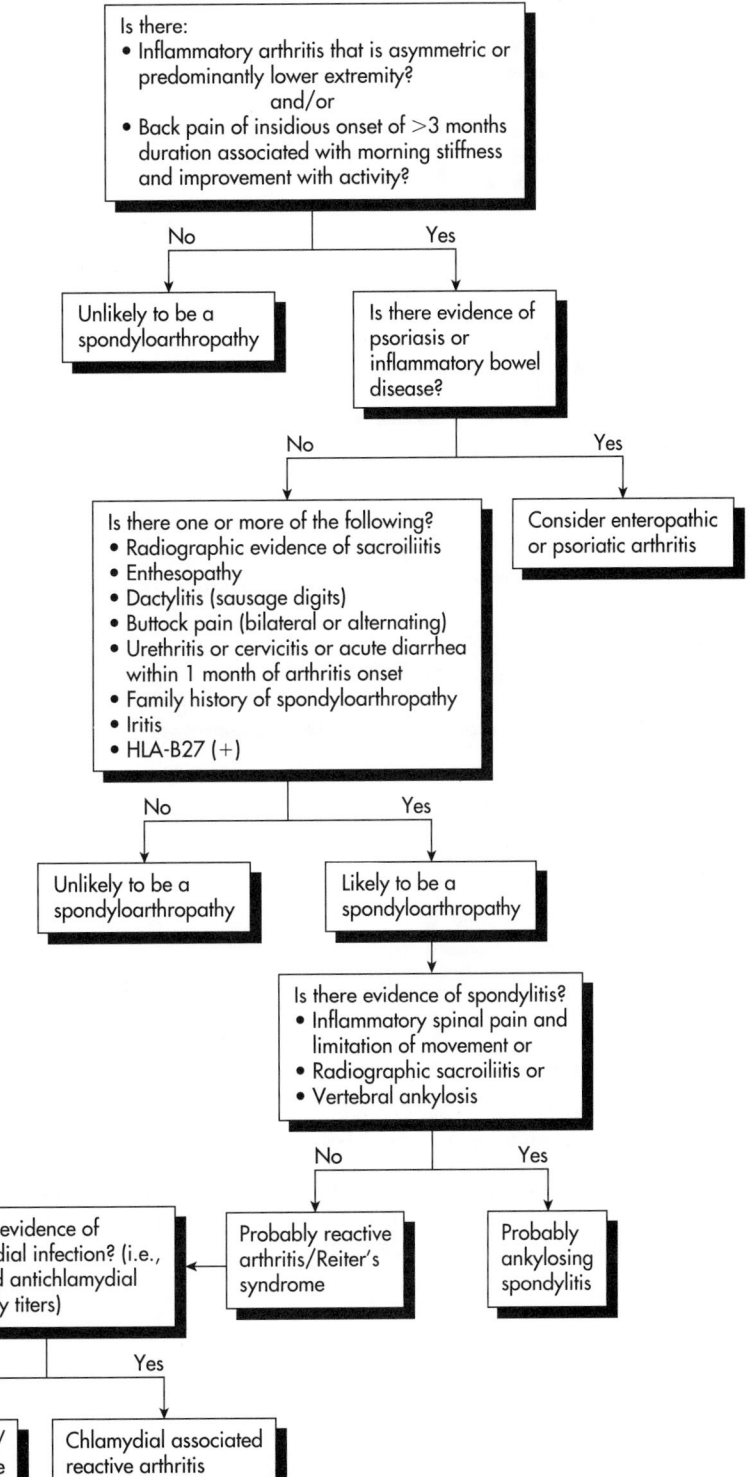

Fig. 3-157   Algorithm for diagnosis of the spondyloarthropathies. (From Goldman L: *Cecil textbook of medicine,* ed 21, Philadelphia, 2000, WB Saunders.)

SPONDYLOARTHROPATHY, TREATMENT

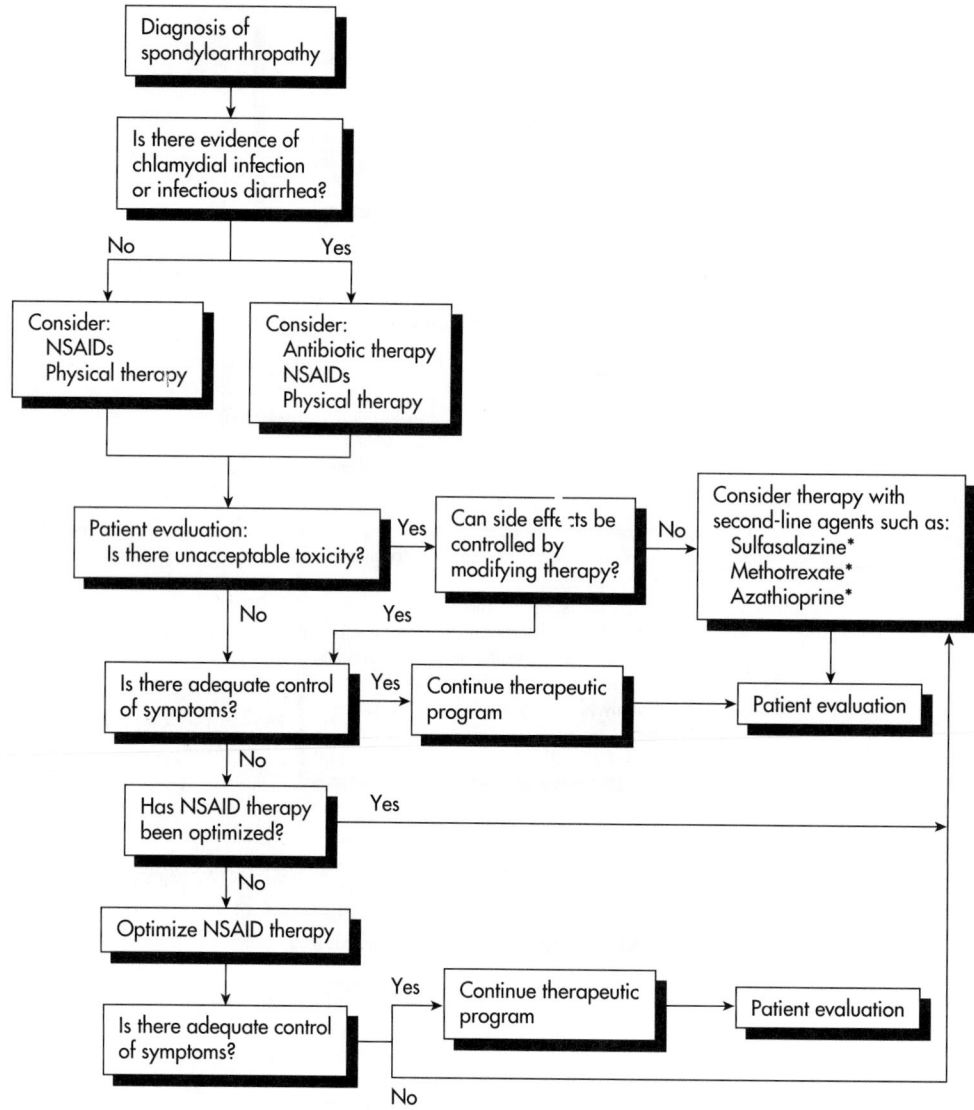

*Not approved by the FDA for treatment of spondyloarthropathies.

Fig. 3-158   Treatment algorithm for patients with a spondyloarthropathy. *FDA,* Food and Drug Administration; *NSAID,* nonsteroidal antiinflammatory drug. (From Goldman L: *Cecil textbook of medicine,* ed 21, Philadelphia, 2000, WB Saunders.)

SPONDYLOSIS, CERVICAL

Spondylosis, cervical
ICD-9CM # 721.0

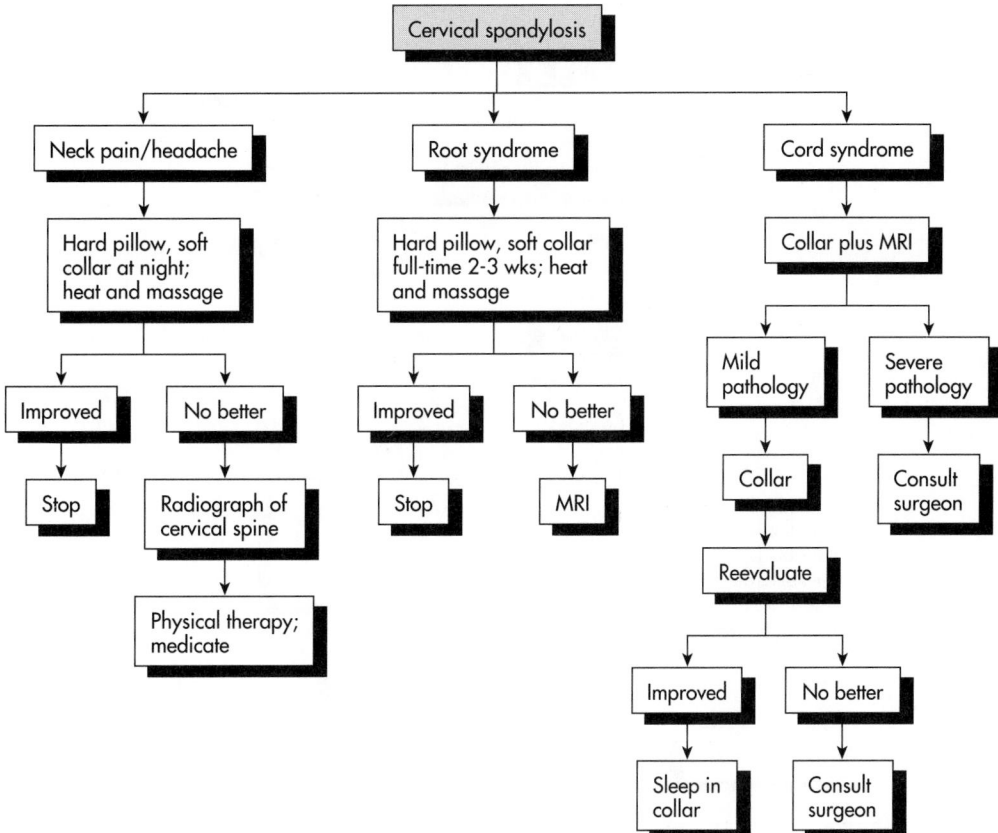

Fig. 3-159   Algorithm for the treatment of cervical spondylosis. *MRI,* Magnetic resonance imaging. (From Ronthal M, Rachlin JR: Cervical spondylosis. In Johnson RT, Griffin JW [eds]: *Current therapy in neurologic disease,* ed 5, St Louis, 1997, Mosby.)

III

TACHYCARDIA, NARROW COMPLEX

Tachycardia, narrow complex
ICD-9CM # 427.2 Paroxysmal tachycardia
427.0 Supraventricular paroxysmal
tachycardia
427.42 Ventricular flutter
427.1 Ventricular paroxysmal tachycardia
427.89 Atrial tachycardia

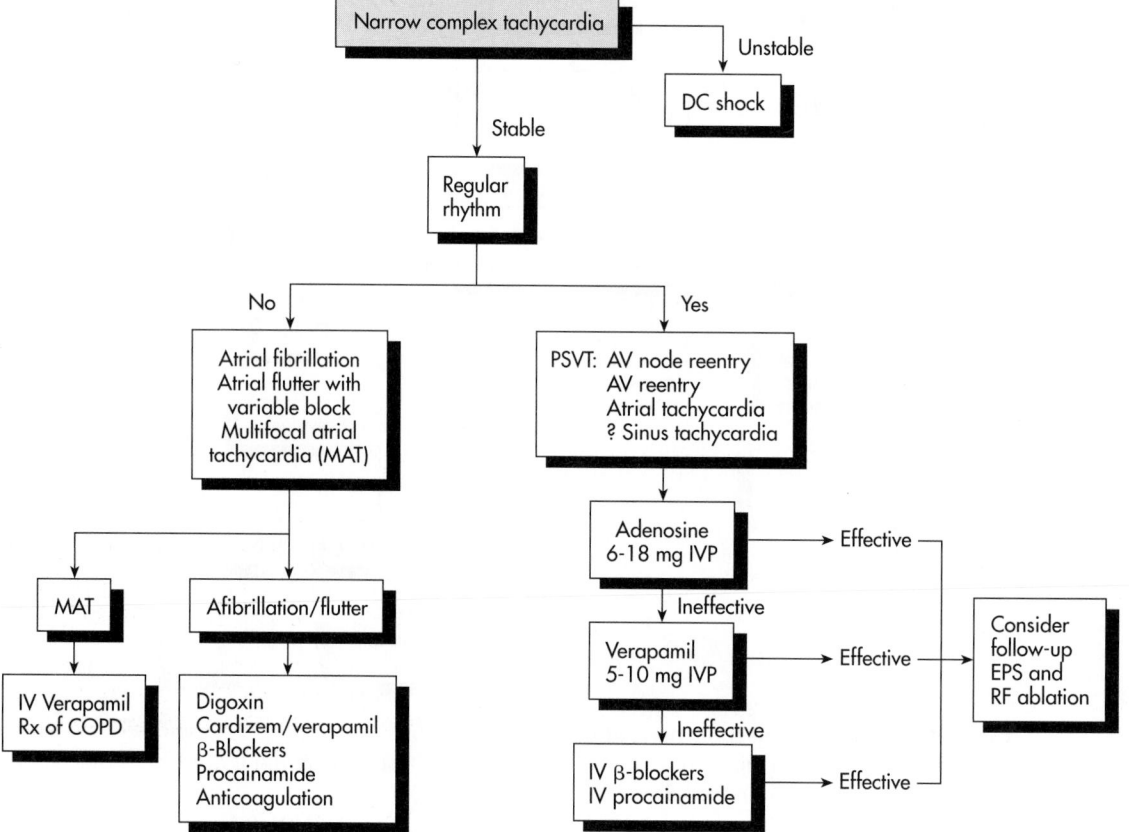

Fig. 3-160 **Evaluation and management of narrow complex tachycardia.** *AV,* Atrioventricular; *COPD,* chronic obstructive pulmonary disease; *EPS,* electrophysiologic studies; *IV,* intravenous; *IVP,* intravenous push; *PSVT,* paroxysmal supraventricular tachycardia; *RF,* radiofrequency. (From Driscoll CE et al: *The family practice desk reference,* ed 3, St Louis, 1996, Mosby.)

TACHYCARDIA, WIDE COMPLEX

Tachycardia, wide complex
ICD-9CM # 427.2 Paroxysmal tachycardia
      427.0 Supraventricular paroxysmal
             tachycardia
      427.42 Ventricular flutter
      427.1 Ventricular paroxysmal tachycardia
      427.89 Atrial tachycardia

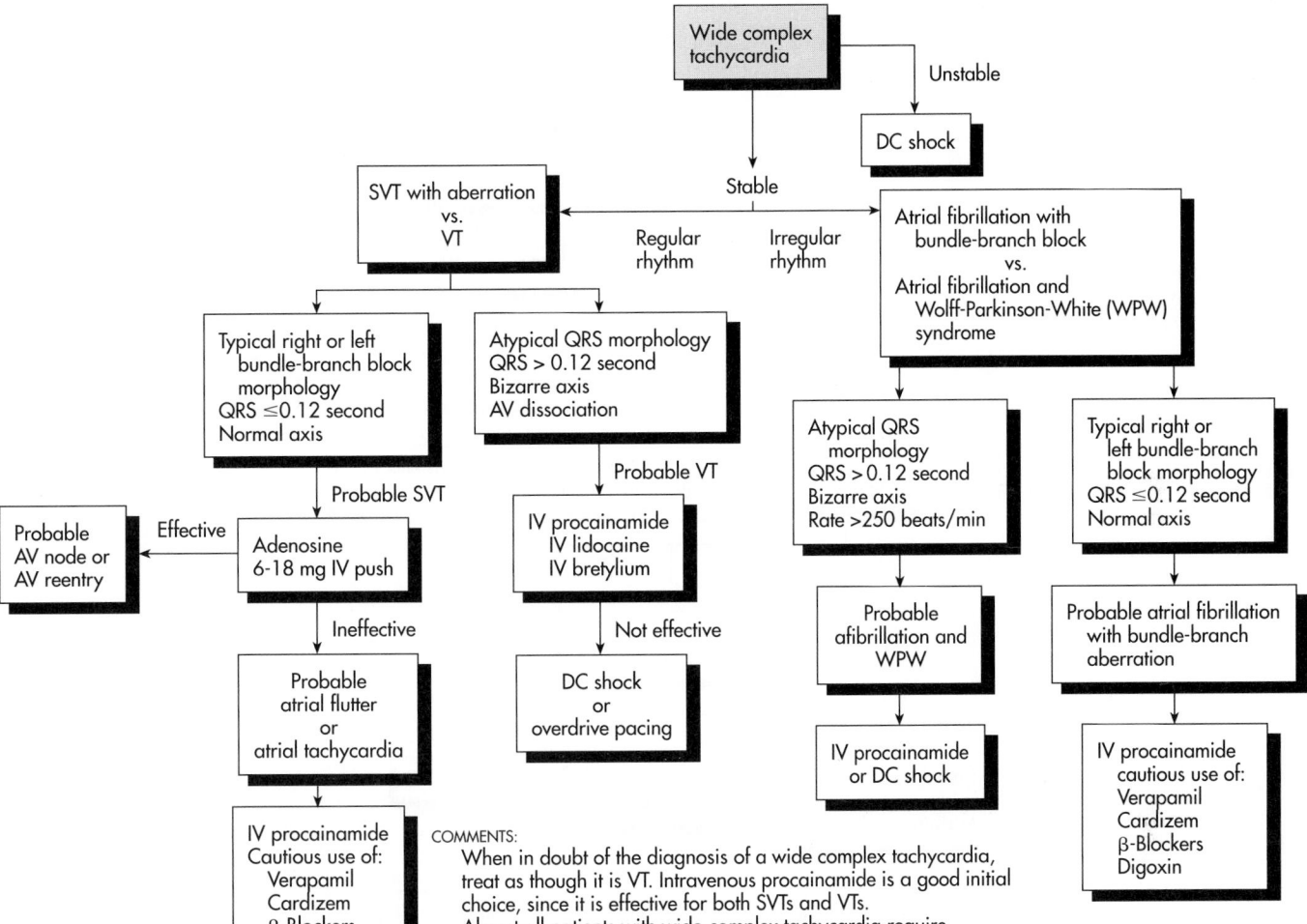

COMMENTS:
When in doubt of the diagnosis of a wide complex tachycardia, treat as though it is VT. Intravenous procainamide is a good initial choice, since it is effective for both SVTs and VTs.
Almost all patients with wide complex tachycardia require follow-up EP testing for long-term management.

Fig. 3-161 **Evaluation and management of wide complex tachycardia.** *AV,* Atrioventricular; *EP,* electrophysiologic; *IV,* intravenous; *SVT,* supraventricular tachycardia; *VT,* ventricular tachycardia. (From Driscoll CE et al: *The family practice desk reference,* ed 3, St Louis, 1996, Mosby.)

TESTICULAR GERM CELL TUMOR

Testicular germ cell tumor
ICD-9CM # 186.9 Testicular neoplasm

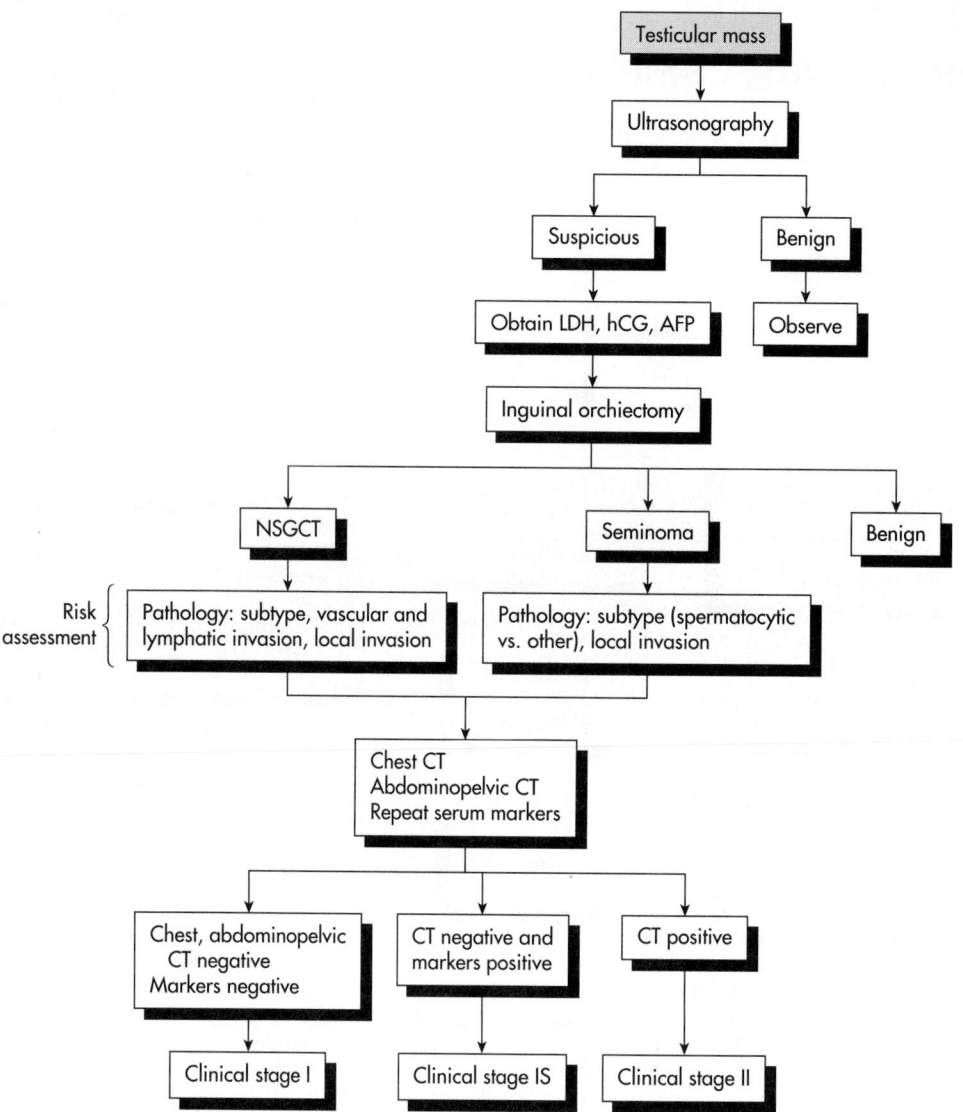

Fig. 3-162 **Diagnosis, staging, and risk assessment of patients with testicular germ cell tumor.** *AFP,* Alpha-fetoprotein; *CT,* computed tomography; *hCG,* human chorionic gonadotropin; *LDH,* lactic dehydrogenase; *NSGCT,* nonseminoma germ cell tumor. (From Abeloff MD: *Clinical oncology,* ed 2, New York, 2000, Churchill Livingstone.)

THROMBOCYTOPENIA

Thrombocytopenia
ICD-9CM # 287.5 Thrombocytopenia NOS
287.3 Thrombocytopenia, primary
287.4 Thrombocytopenia, secondary

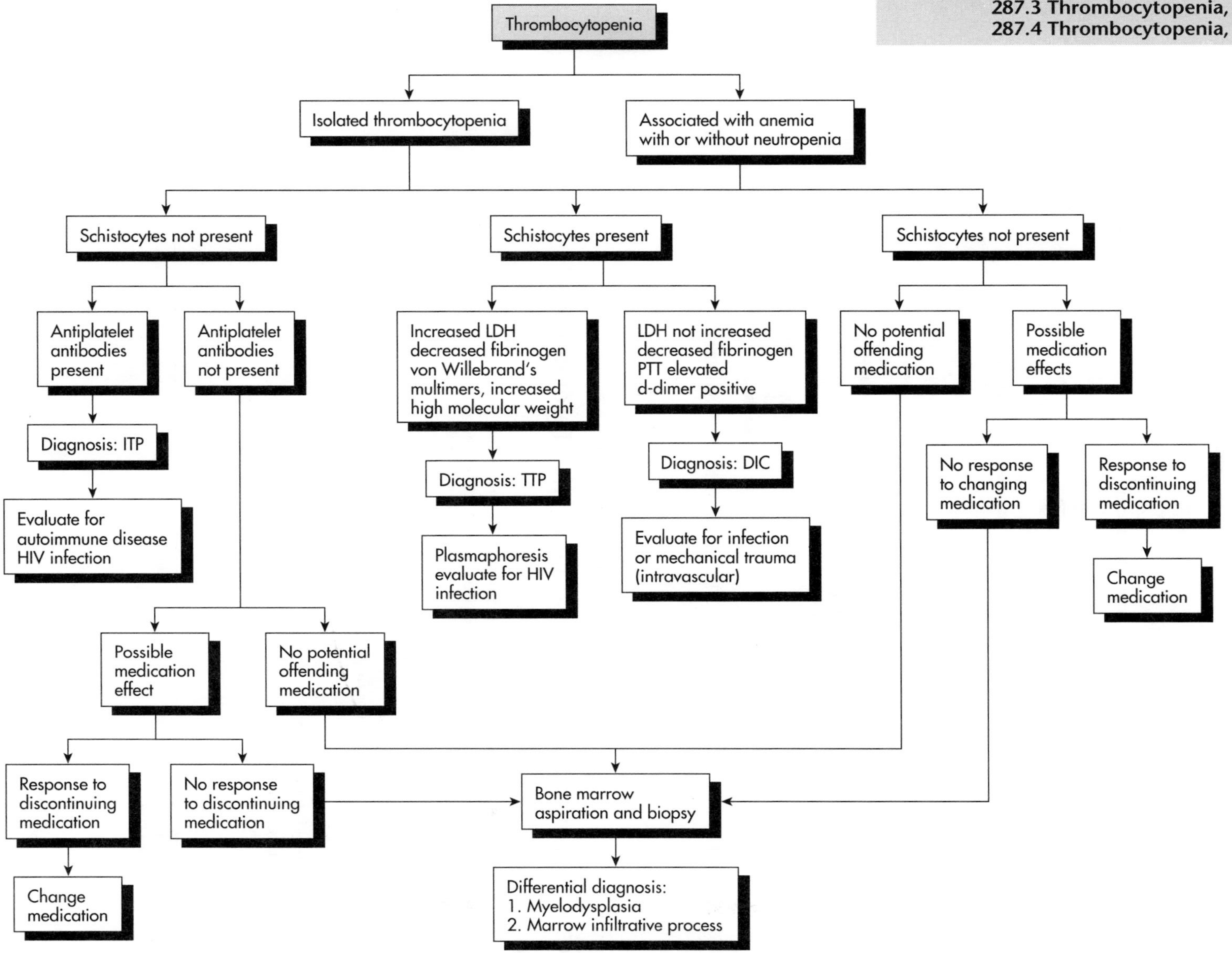

Fig. 3-163   Differential diagnosis of thrombocytopenia. *DIC,* Disseminated intravascular coagulation; *HIV,* human immunodeficiency virus; *ITP,* idiopathic thrombocytopenic purpura; *LDH,* lactic dehydrogenase; *PTT,* partial thromboplastin time; *TTP,* thrombotic thrombocytopenic purpura. (From Rakel RE [ed]: *Principles of family practice,* ed 6, Philadelphia, 2002, WB Saunders.)

THROMBOCYTOSIS

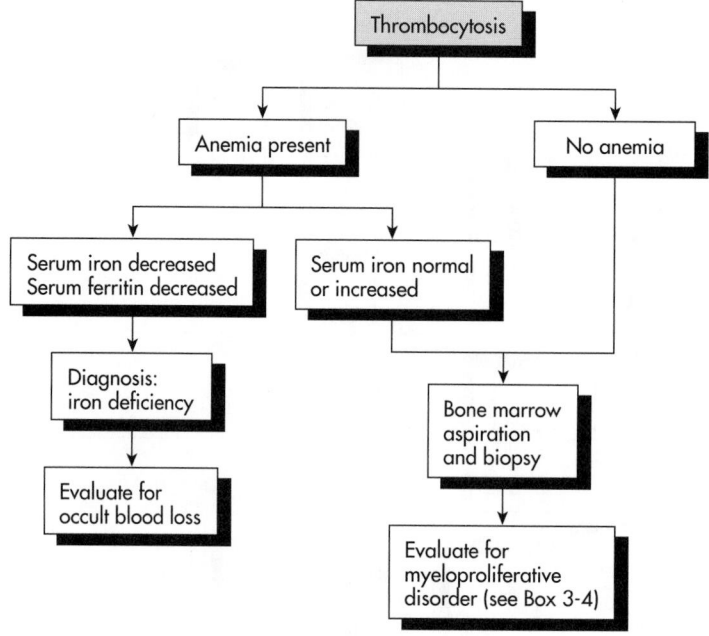

Fig. 3-164 Differential diagnosis of thrombocytosis. (From Rakel RE [ed]: *Principles of family practice,* ed 6, Philadelphia, 2002, WB Saunders.)

BOX 3-4 Etiologic Conditions Associated with Thrombocytosis

Reactive Thrombocytosis

Infections or inflammatory states—vasculitis, allergic reactions, etc.
Surgery and tissue damage—myocardial infarction, pancreatitis, etc.
Postsplenectomy state
Malignancy—solid tumors, lymphoma
Iron deficiency anemia, hemolytic anemia, acute blood loss
Uncertain etiology
Rebound effect after chemotherapy or immune thrombocytopenia
Renal disorders—renal failure, nephrotic syndrome

Myeloproliferative Disorders

Chronic myeloid leukemia
Primary thrombocythemia
Polycythemia vera
Idiopathic myelofibrosis

Modified from Hoffman R: Primary thrombocythemia. In Hoffman R et al (eds): *Hematology: basic principles and practice,* ed 3, New York, 2000, Churchill Livingstone.

THYROID, PAINFUL

Thyroid, painful
ICD-9CM # 245.0 Acute thyroiditis

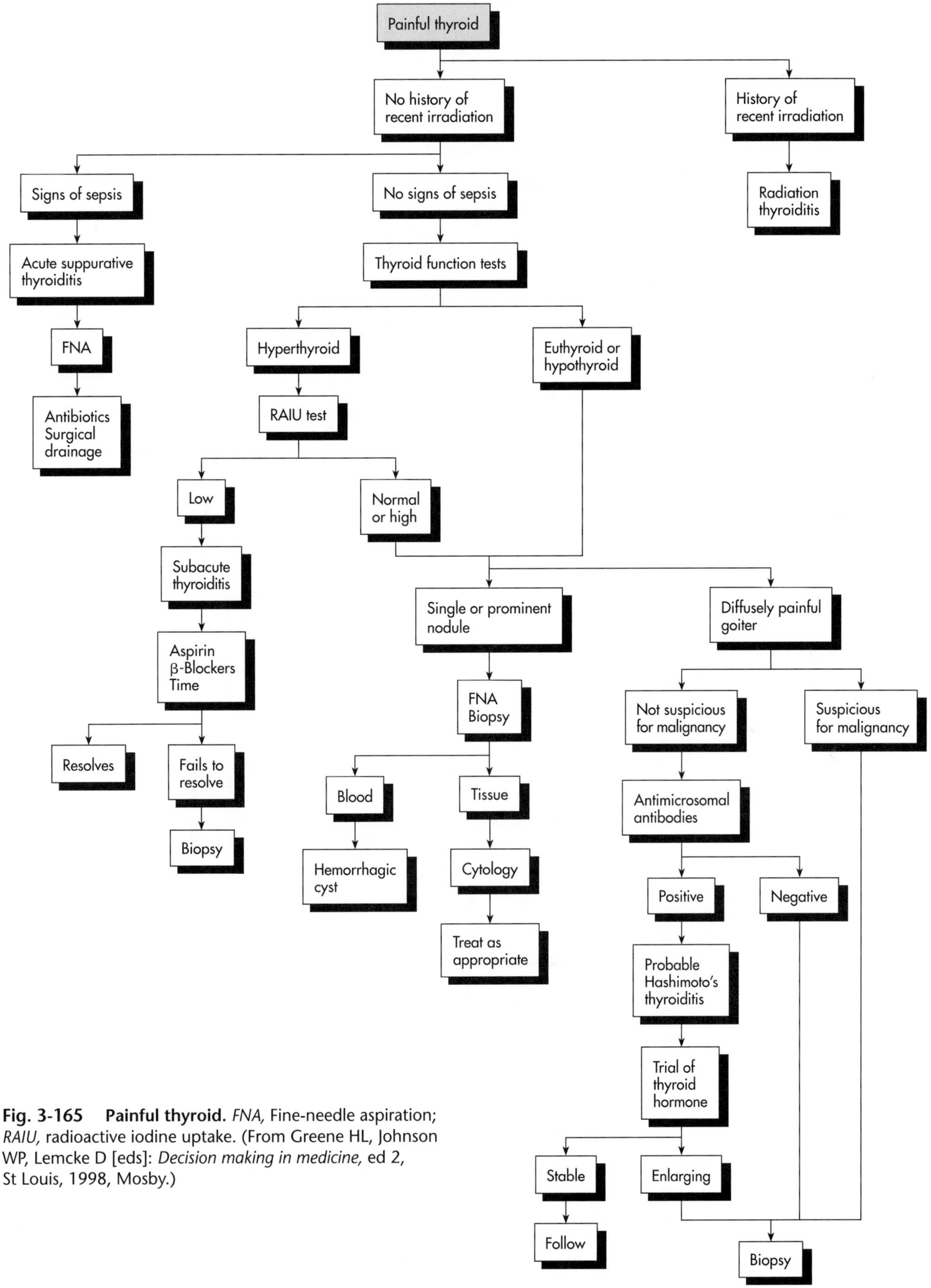
Painful thyroid
No history of recent irradiation
History of recent irradiation
Radiation thyroiditis
Signs of sepsis
No signs of sepsis
Acute suppurative thyroiditis
FNA
Antibiotics Surgical drainage
Thyroid function tests
Hyperthyroid
Euthyroid or hypothyroid
RAIU test
Low
Normal or high
Subacute thyroiditis
Aspirin β-Blockers Time
Resolves
Fails to resolve
Biopsy
Single or prominent nodule
Diffusely painful goiter
FNA Biopsy
Blood
Tissue
Hemorrhagic cyst
Cytology
Treat as appropriate
Not suspicious for malignancy
Suspicious for malignancy
Antimicrosomal antibodies
Positive
Negative
Probable Hashimoto's thyroiditis
Trial of thyroid hormone
Stable
Enlarging
Follow
Biopsy

Fig. 3-165 Painful thyroid. *FNA,* Fine-needle aspiration; *RAIU,* radioactive iodine uptake. (From Greene HL, Johnson WP, Lemcke D [eds]: *Decision making in medicine,* ed 2, St Louis, 1998, Mosby.)

THYROID TESTS, DIAGNOSTIC APPROACH

Thyroid tests, diagnostic approach
ICD-9CM # V77.0 Thyroid disorder screening

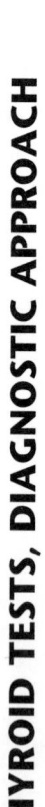

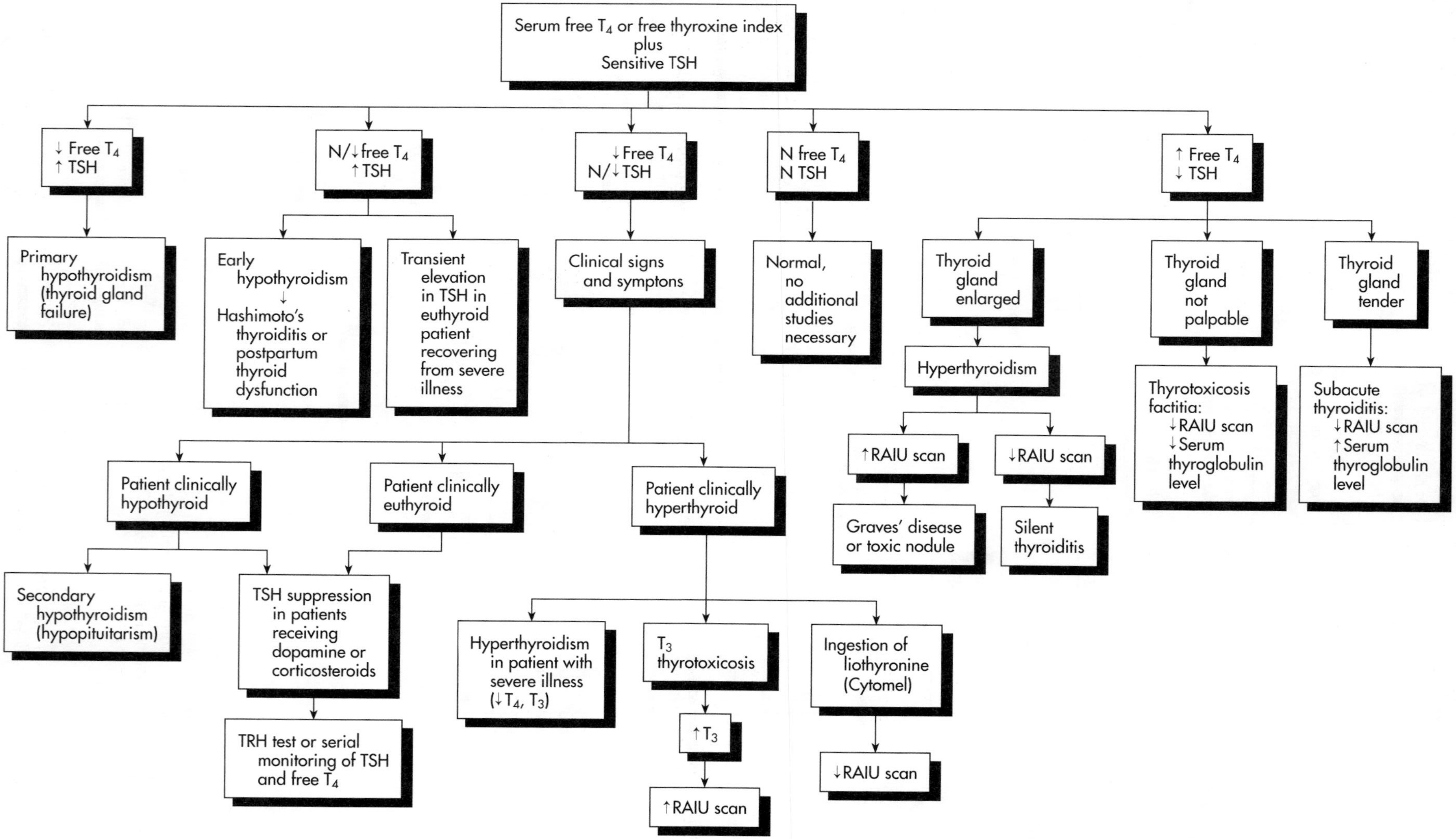

Fig. 3-166 Diagnostic approach to thyroid testing. *N,* Normal; *RAIU,* radioactive iodine uptake; *TRH,* thyrotropin-releasing hormone; *TSH,* thyroid-stimulating hormone. (From Ferri FF: *Practical guide to the care of the medical patient,* ed 5, St Louis, 2001, Mosby.)

Serum free T₄ or free thyroxine index plus Sensitive TSH

↑ Free T₄
↓ TSH

Thyroid gland tender → Subacute thyroiditis: ↓RAIU scan ↑Serum thyroglobulin level

Thyroid gland not palpable → Thyrotoxicosis factitia: ↓RAIU scan ↓Serum thyroglobulin level

Thyroid gland enlarged → Hyperthyroidism → ↓RAIU scan → Silent thyroiditis

↑RAIU scan → Graves' disease or toxic nodule

N free T₄
N TSH → Normal, no additional studies necessary

↓ Free T₄
N/↓ TSH → Clinical signs and symptoms

Patient clinically hyperthyroid → T₃ thyrotoxicosis → ↑ T₃ → ↑RAIU scan

Hyperthyroidism in patient with severe illness (↓T₄, T₃)

Ingestion of liothyronine (Cytomel) → ↓RAIU scan

N/↓ free T₄
↑ TSH

Transient elevation in TSH in euthyroid patient recovering from severe illness

Early hypothyroidism → Hashimoto's thyroiditis or postpartum thyroid dysfunction

Patient clinically euthyroid

Patient clinically hypothyroid → TSH suppression in patients receiving dopamine or corticosteroids → TRH test or serial monitoring of TSH and free T₄

Secondary hypothyroidism (hypopituitarism)

↓ Free T₄
↑ TSH → Primary hypothyroidism (thyroid gland failure)

TINNITUS

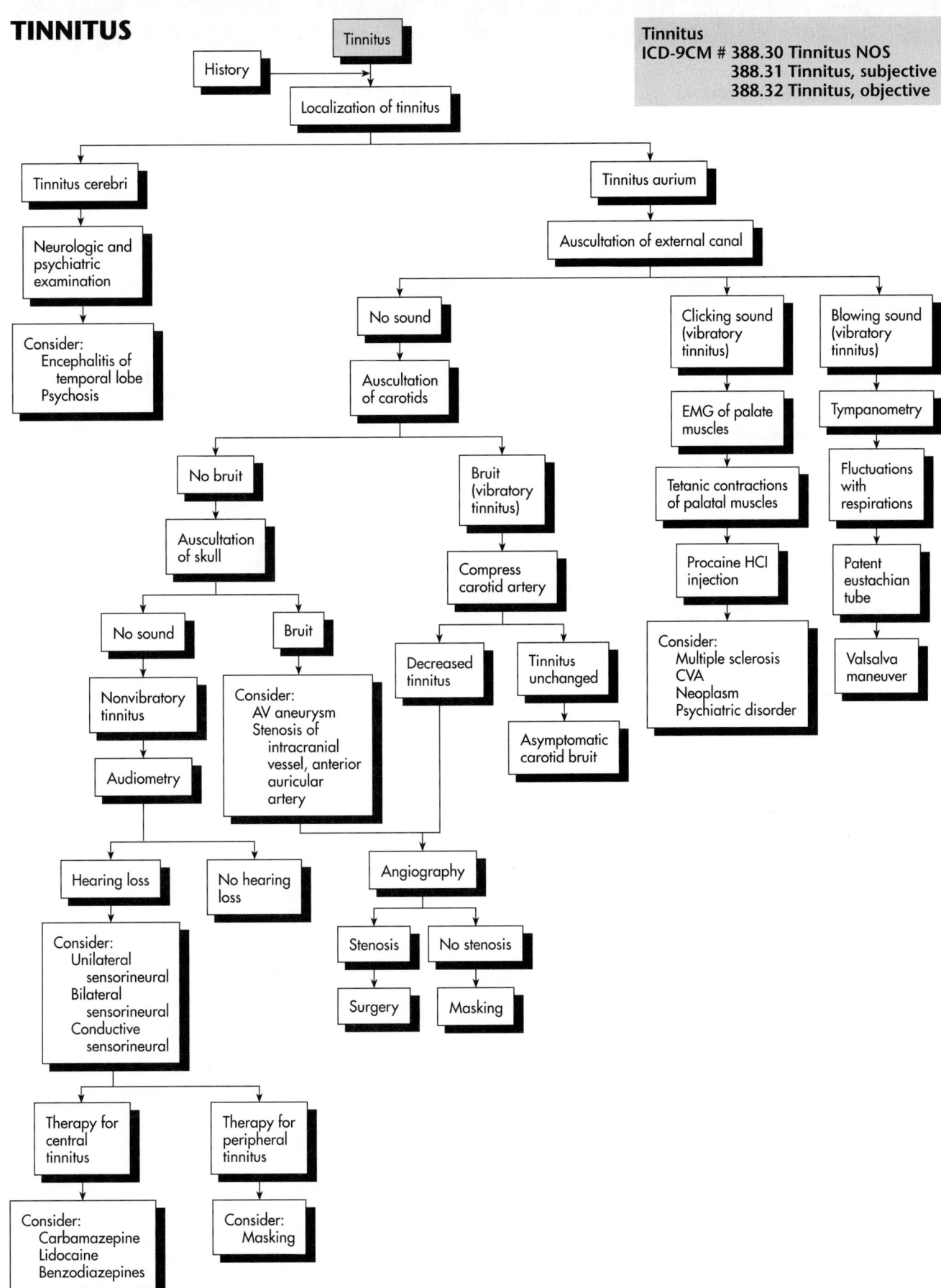

Fig. 3-167 Evaluation of tinnitus. *AV,* Atrioventricular; *CVA,* cerebrovascular accident; *EMG,* electromyography. (From Greene HL, Johnson WP, Lemcke D [eds]: *Decision making in medicine,* ed 2, St Louis, 1998, Mosby.)

TRAUMA, ABDOMEN

Trauma, abdomen
ICD-9CM # 868.00 Abdomen injury, unspecified site

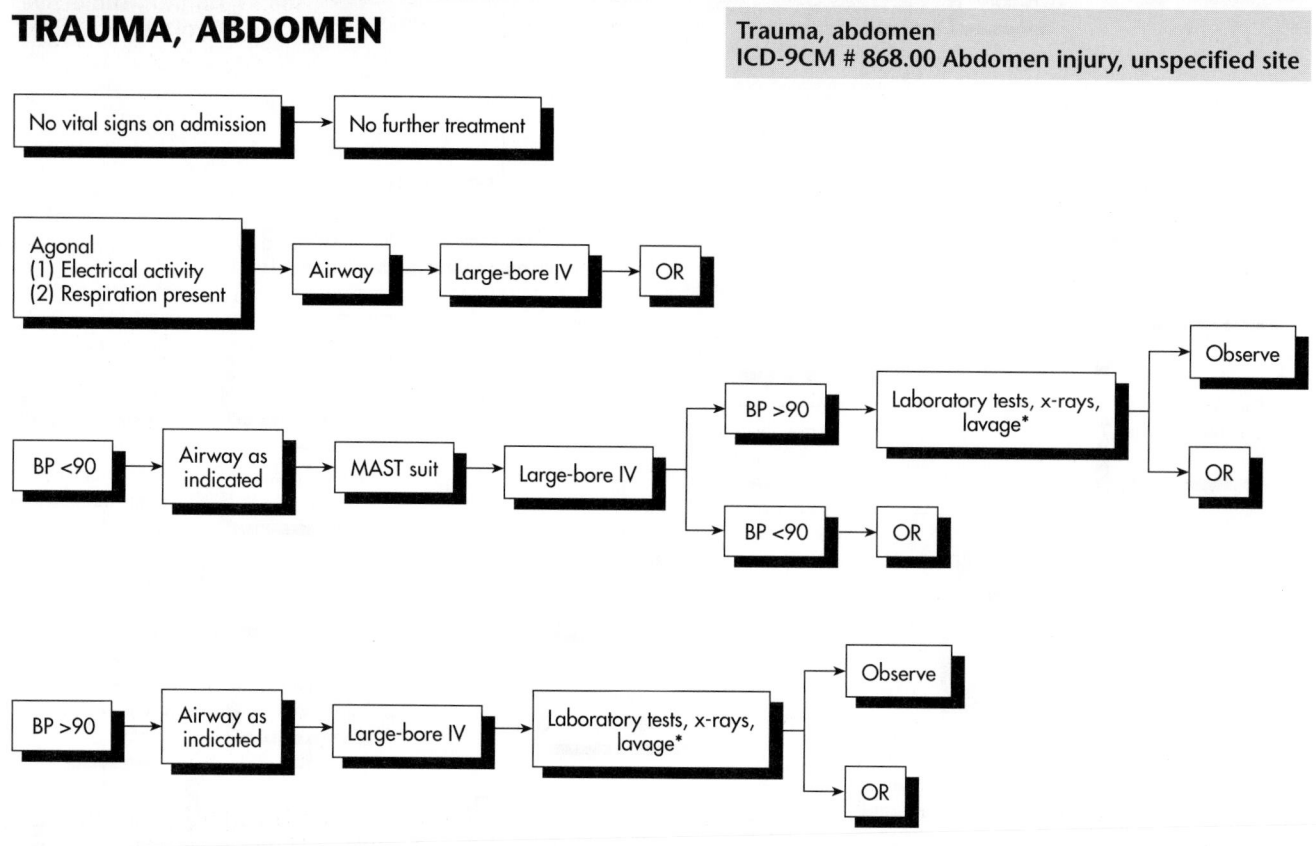

*Indications:
(1) ETOH intoxication
(2) Drug intoxication
(3) Head injury
(4) Cord injury
(5) Equivocal examination
(6) Significant trauma on both sides of diaphragm

Fig. 3-168　**Blunt abdominal trauma.** *BP,* Blood pressure; *ETOH,* ethyl alcohol; *IV,* intravenous; *MAST,* military antishock trousers; *OR,* operating room. (From Berry SM [ed]: *The Mont Reid surgical handbook,* ed 4, St Louis, 1997, Mosby.)

Trauma, chest
ICD-9CM # 862.8 Trauma (with injury to intrathoracic
organs)
862.9 Trauma with open wound (with
injury to intrathoracic organs)
862.8 Crushed chest

TRAUMA, CHEST

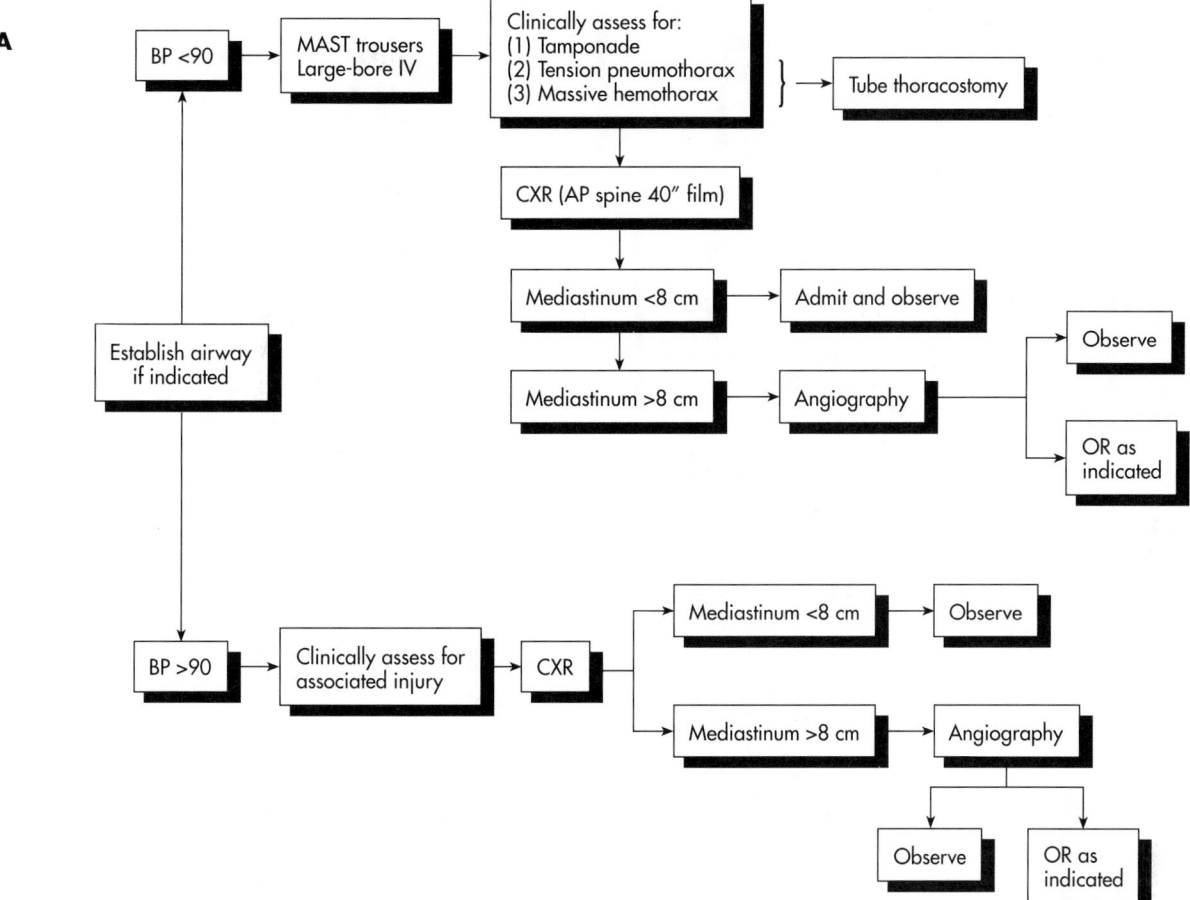

Fig. 3-169   A, Blunt chest trauma. *AP,* Anteroposterior; *BP,* blood pressure; *CT,* computed tomography; *CVP,* cardioventricular pacing; *CXR,* chest x-ray; *ED,* emergency department; *IV,* intravenous; *MAST,* military antishock trousers; *OR,* operating room. (From Berry SM [ed]: *The Mont Reid surgical handbook,* ed 4, St Louis, 1997, Mosby.)

Continued

TRAURA, CHEST—cont'd

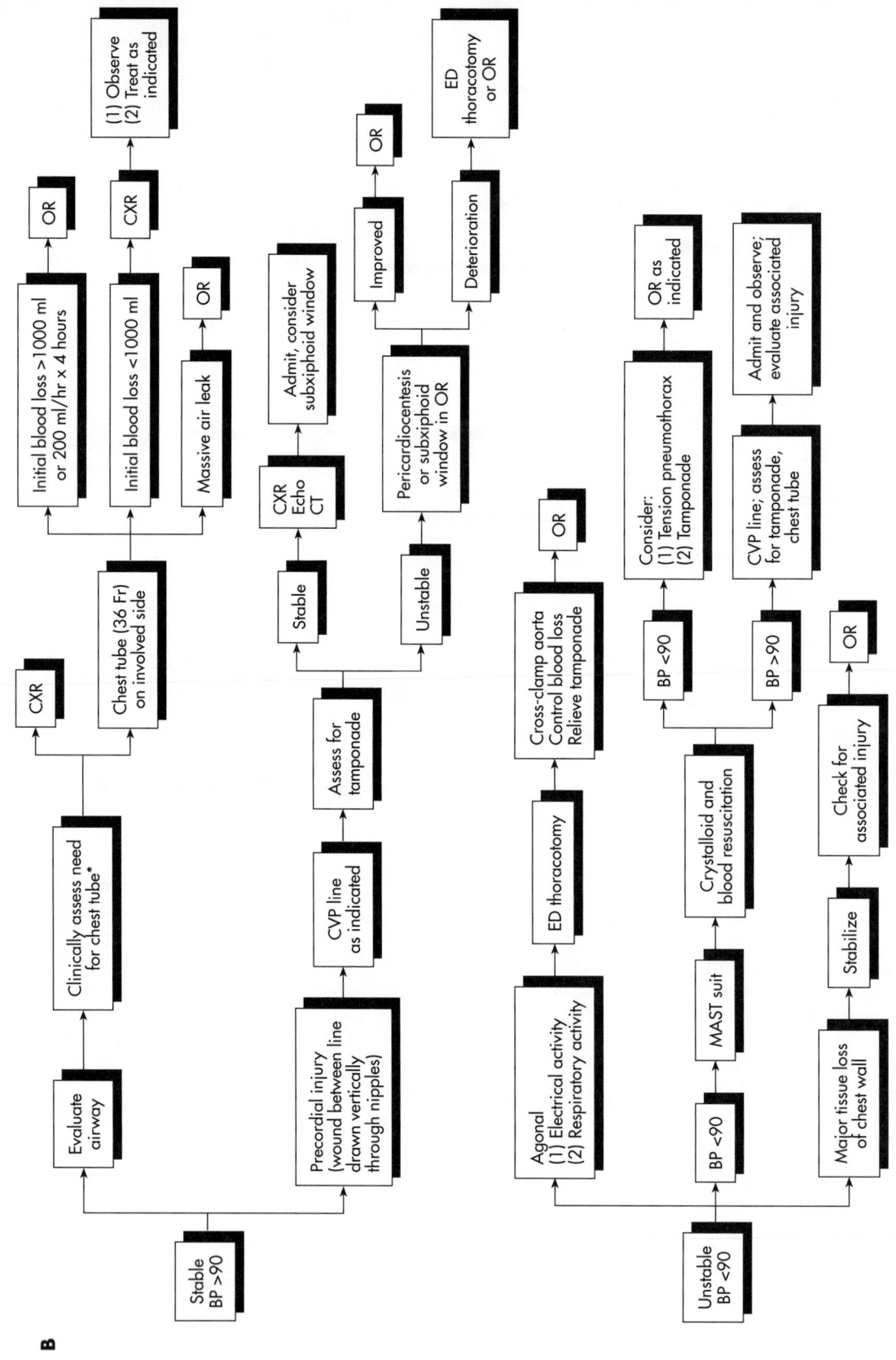

B

*(1) Tension pneumothorax; (2) sucking chest wound; (3) hemothorax.

Fig. 3-169, cont'd   B, Penetrating chest trauma. (From Berry SM [ed]: *The Mont Reid surgical handbook,* ed 4, St Louis, 1997, Mosby.)

TRAUMA, GENITOURINARY

Trauma, genitourinary
ICD-9CM # 867.6

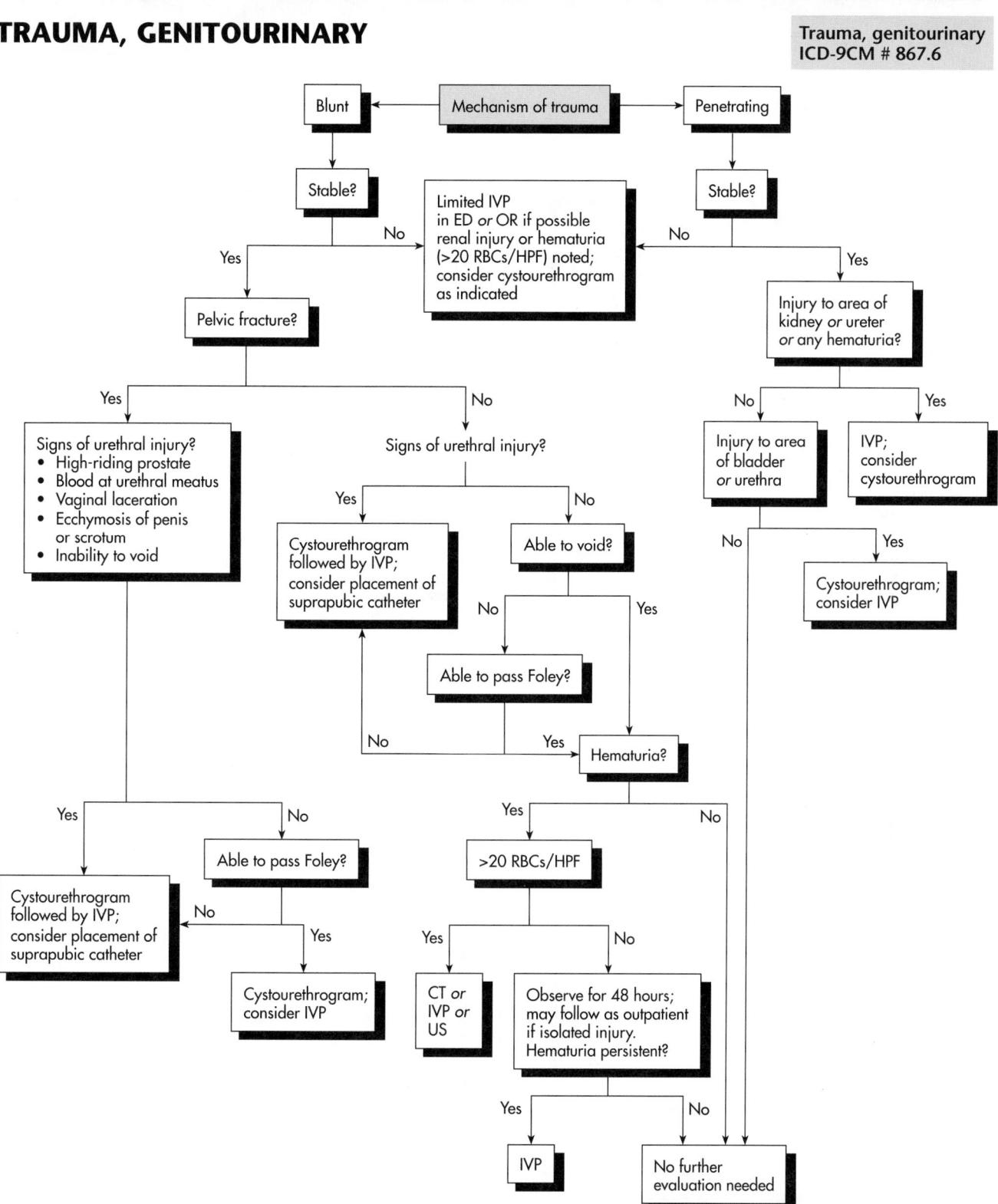

Fig. 3-170   Evaluating the trauma patient for genitourinary injury. *CT,* Computed tomography; *ED,* emergency department; *HPF,* high-power field; *IVP,* intravenous pyelogram; *OR,* operating room; *RBCs,* red blood cells; *US,* ultrasound. (From Barkin RM: *Pediatric emergency medicine: concepts and clinical practice,* ed 2, St Louis, 1997, Mosby.)

TRAUMA, KIDNEYS

Trauma, kidneys
ICD-9CM #866.0 Kidney injury, closed
   866.1 Kidney injury with open wound into cavity

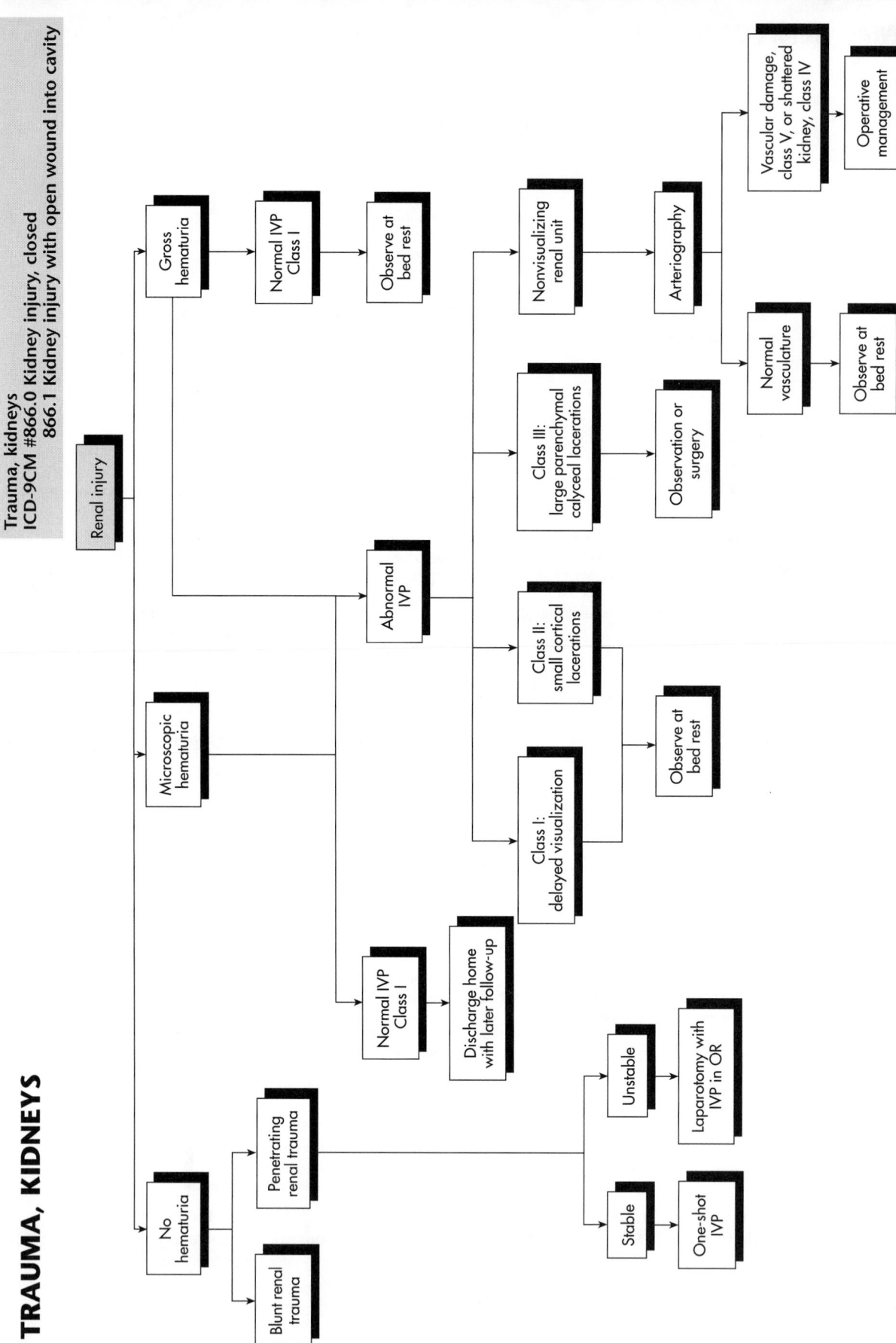

Fig. 3-171   Treatment of renal trauma. *IVP,* Intravenous pyelogram; *OR,* operating room. (From Rosen P et al [eds]: *Emergency medicine: concepts and clinical practice,* ed 5, St Louis, 2002, Mosby.)

UNCONSCIOUS PATIENT

Unconscious patient
ICD-9CM # 780.09

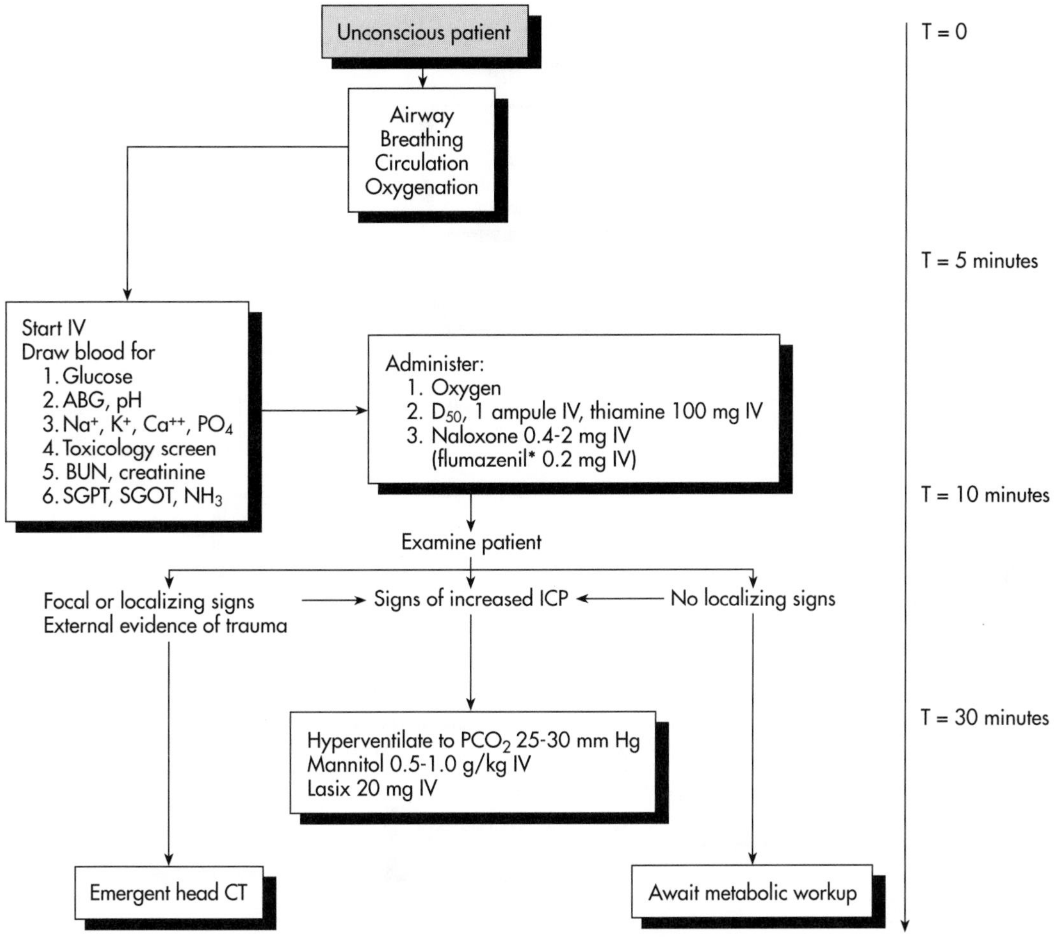

* Use of flumazenil should not be considered routine because it can precipitate seizures in certain subsets of patients.

Fig. 3-172 Approach to the unconscious patient. *ABG,* Arterial blood gas; *BUN,* blood urea nitrogen; *CT,* computed tomography; *ICP,* intracranial pressure; *SGOT,* serum glutamic oxaloacetic transaminase; *SGPT,* serum glutamic pyruvic transaminase. (From Johnson RT, Griffin JW: *Current therapy in neurologic disease,* ed 5, St Louis, 1997, Mosby.)

VAGINAL DISCHARGE

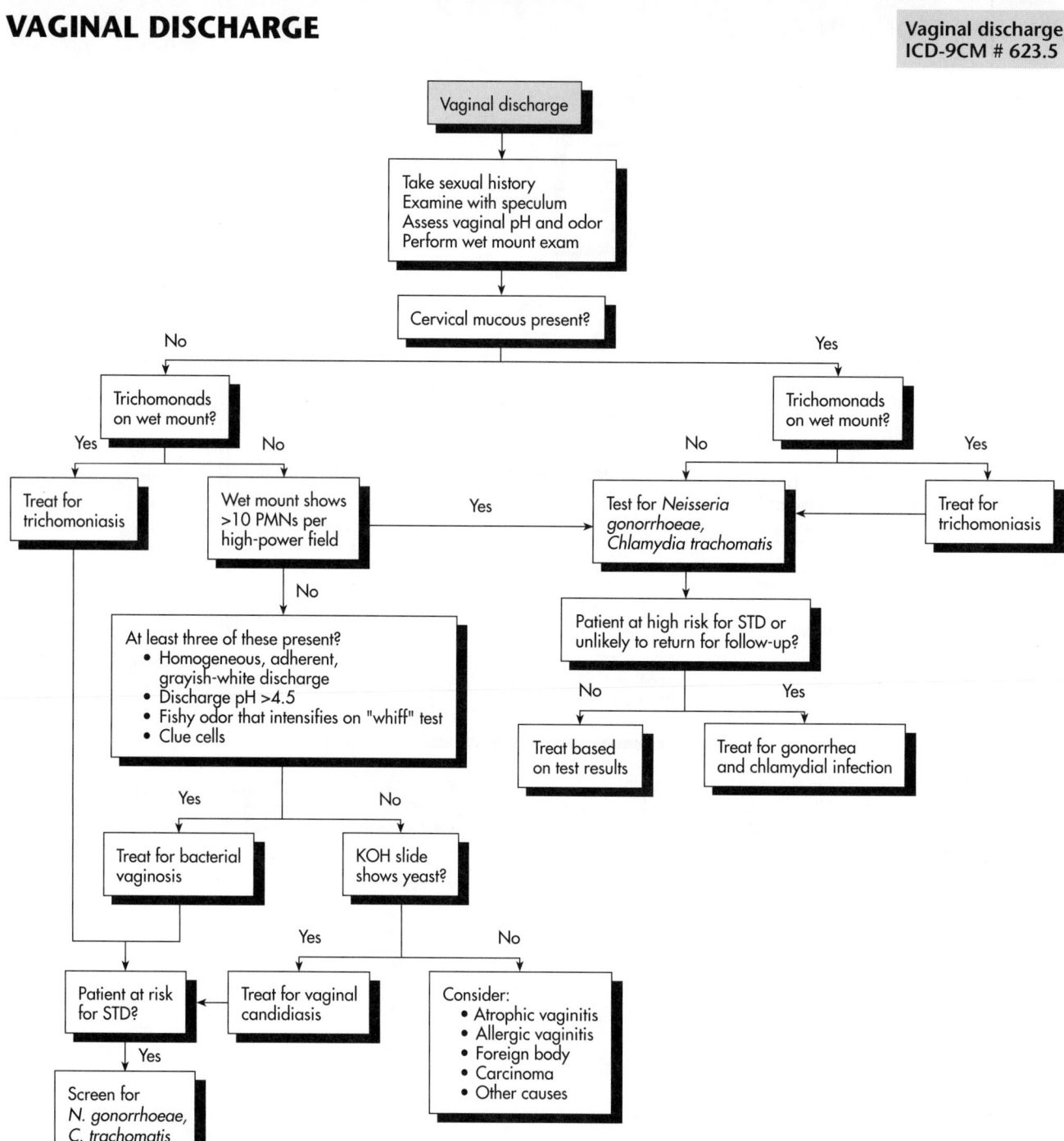

Fig. 3-173   Evaluation of vaginal discharge. *KOH,* Potassium hydroxide; *PMN,* polymorphonuclear leukocyte; *STD,* sexually transmitted disease. (From Fox KK, Behets FMT: *Postgrad Med* 98:87, 1995.)

VAGINAL PROLAPSE

Vaginal prolapse
ICD-9CM # 618.0

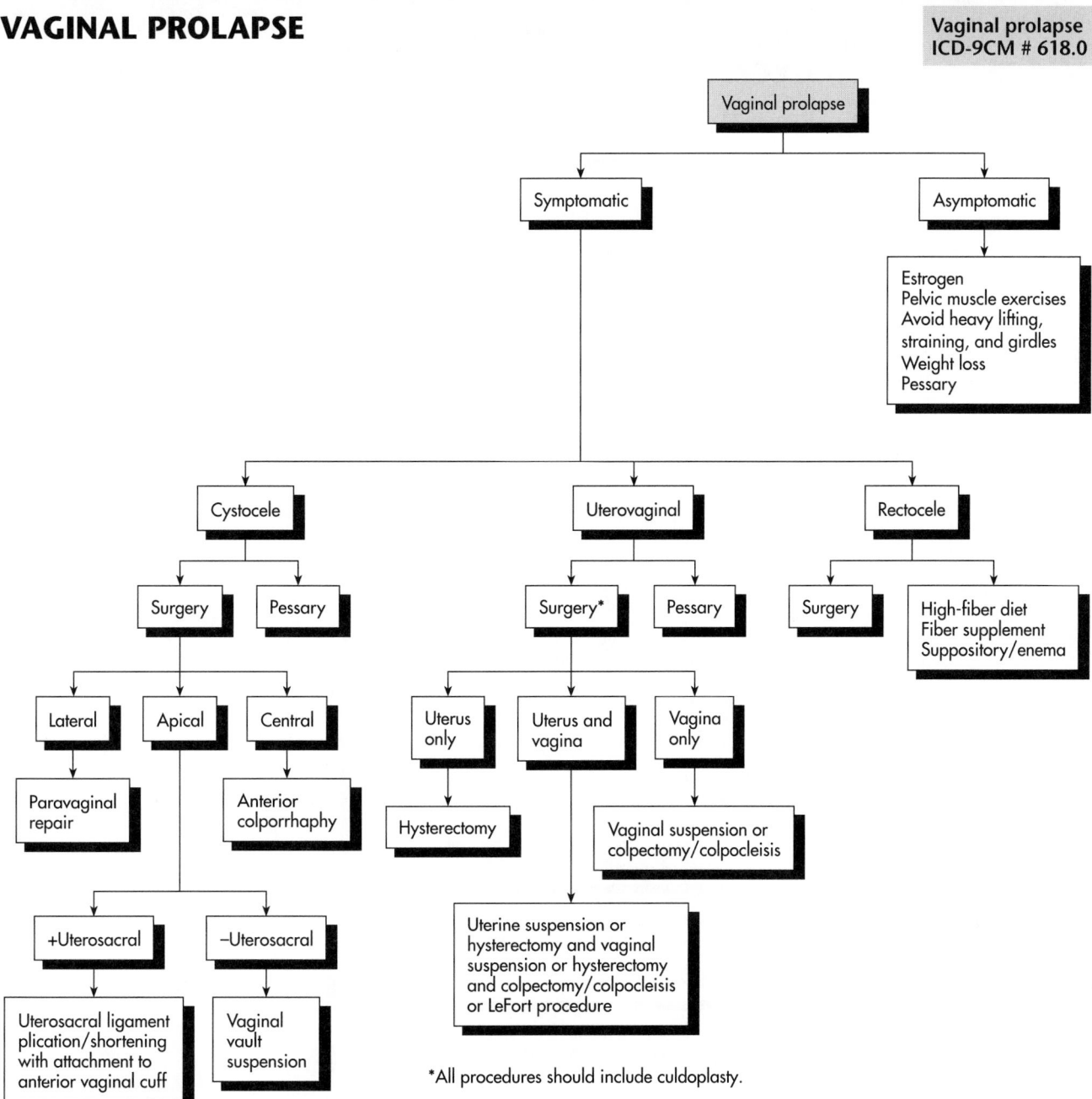

Fig. 3-174 **Management of vaginal prolapse.** (From Zuspan FP [ed]: *Handbook of obstetrics, gynecology, and primary care,* St Louis, 1998, Mosby.)

VENTRICULAR FIBRILLATION OR PULSELESS VENTRICULAR TACHYCARDIA

Ventricular fibrillation or pulseless ventricular tachycardia
ICD-9CM # 427.41 Ventricular fibrillation
427.1 Ventricular tachycardia

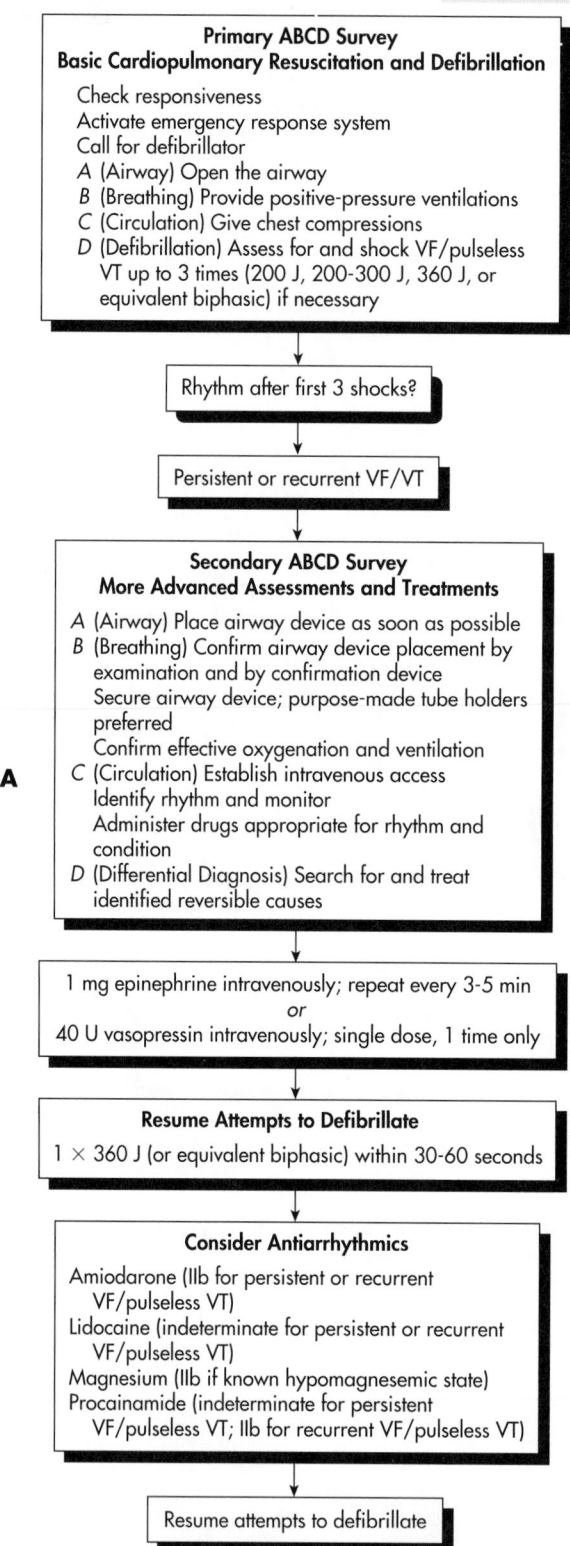

Primary ABCD Survey
Basic Cardiopulmonary Resuscitation and Defibrillation

Check responsiveness
Activate emergency response system
Call for defibrillator
A (Airway) Open the airway
B (Breathing) Provide positive-pressure ventilations
C (Circulation) Give chest compressions
D (Defibrillation) Assess for and shock VF/pulseless VT up to 3 times (200 J, 200-300 J, 360 J, or equivalent biphasic) if necessary

Rhythm after first 3 shocks?

Persistent or recurrent VF/VT

Secondary ABCD Survey
More Advanced Assessments and Treatments

A (Airway) Place airway device as soon as possible
B (Breathing) Confirm airway device placement by examination and by confirmation device
Secure airway device; purpose-made tube holders preferred
Confirm effective oxygenation and ventilation
C (Circulation) Establish intravenous access
Identify rhythm and monitor
Administer drugs appropriate for rhythm and condition
D (Differential Diagnosis) Search for and treat identified reversible causes

A

1 mg epinephrine intravenously; repeat every 3-5 min
or
40 U vasopressin intravenously; single dose, 1 time only

Resume Attempts to Defibrillate
1 × 360 J (or equivalent biphasic) within 30-60 seconds

Consider Antiarrhythmics

Amiodarone (IIb for persistent or recurrent VF/pulseless VT)
Lidocaine (indeterminate for persistent or recurrent VF/pulseless VT)
Magnesium (IIb if known hypomagnesemic state)
Procainamide (indeterminate for persistent VF/pulseless VT; IIb for recurrent VF/pulseless VT)

Resume attempts to defibrillate

Fig. 3-175 **Ventricular fibrillation (VF)/pulseless ventricular tachycardia (VT) algorithm.** (A from American Heart Association: Guidelines 2000 for cardiopulmonary resuscitation and emergency cardiovascular care, *Circulation* 102(suppl):I 1, 2000.)

VENTRICULAR FIBRILLATION OR PULSELESS VENTRICULAR TACHYCARDIA—cont'd

Search for a potentially correctable cause of V Fib

Persistence of V Fib at this point in the code should prompt consideration of other factors that could account for the patient's refractory condition. This might include a problem with the ABCs (i.e., a nonpatent airway, asymmetric or absent breath sounds, lack of a pulse with CPR), and/or some other predisposing cause.

- Potentially correctable predisposing causes of refractory V Fib to consider include underlying metabolic disturbance (such as diabetic ketoacidosis or hyperkalemia), hypothermia, hypovolemia, drug overdose (especially of cocaine, tricyclic antidepressants, or narcotics) and/or development of a complication of CPR (such as tension pneumothorax or pericardial tamponade).
- V Fib may also be the end result of (i.e., caused by) many other kinds of processes such as cardiogenic shock (from extensive myocardial infarction), massive pulmonary embolism, ruptured aortic aneurysm, or severe trauma with exsanguinating hemorrhage. Practically speaking, specific diagnosis of these types of conditions is much less important clinically because of the improbability that V Fib resulting from any of these conditions will be amenable to any form of treatment at this point in the code.

B

Refractory V Fib: other measures to consider

Clinically, it may be helpful to realize that if V Fib persists despite implementation of the actions listed that remaining therapeutic options are relatively limited. There simply is not that much more that can be done. At this point in the process, we suggest consideration of the following measures:

- Continuing epinephrine: Recovery from prolonged cardiopulmonary arrest is unlikely unless coronary perfusion pressure (CPP) is adequate (i.e., ≥ 15 mm Hg). In the arrested heart, it appears that epinephrine is needed in sufficient amount to achieve such pressures. As a result, the drug should be repeated at least every 3-5 minutes for as long as the patient remains in cardiac arrest. Consideration might also be given to the use of higher doses of drug (i.e., HDE) if the patient fails to respond to SDE doses.
- Considering sodium bicarbonate: Although sodium bicarbonate has been freely used in the past for the treatment of cardiac arrest, recent data strongly question this practice. In fact, a strong case could be made for never administering any sodium bicarbonate at all during cardiopulmonary resuscitation, regardless of what the pH value happens to be. Instead, efforts at correcting acidosis are probably better directed at optimizing ventilation, especially during the early minutes of a code when the major component of acidosis is likely to be respiratory in nature (from hypoventilation). Practically speaking, acceptable indications for use of sodium bicarbonate in the setting of cardiac arrest are limited. They include:
  - Severe metabolic acidosis (usually to a pH value of less than 7.20) that persists beyond the initial phase (i.e., beyond the first 5-15 minutes) of the arrest.
  - Cardiac arrest in a patient known to have a severe preexisting metabolic acidosis before the arrest.

NOTE: A number of special resuscitation situations exist in which use of bicarbonate is both appropriate and likely to be helpful. These include hyperkalemia and drug overdose with tricyclic antidepressants or phenobarbital.

Fig. 3-175, cont'd   (**B** Modified from Grauer K, Cavallaro D: *ACLS: Rapid review and case scenarios,* ed 4, St Louis, 1996, Mosby.)

III

VENTRICULAR TACHYCARDIA

Ventricular tachycardia
ICD-9CM # 427.1 Ventricular tachycardia

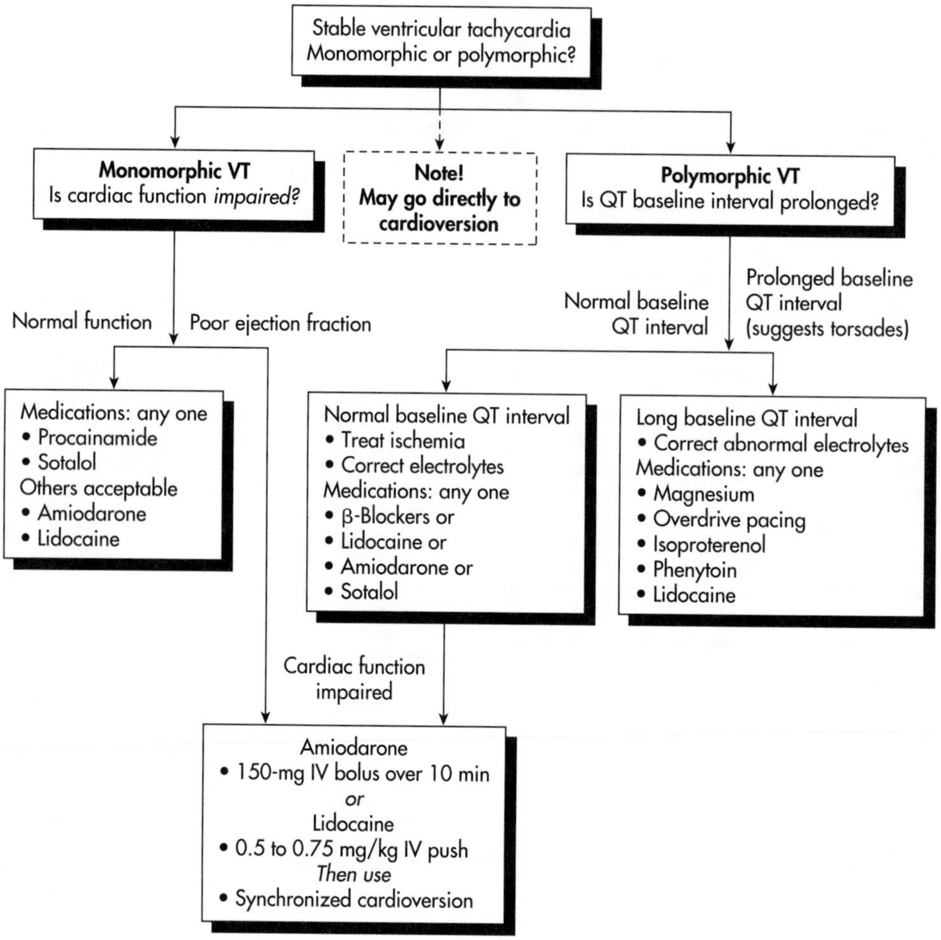
Stable ventricular tachycardia
Monomorphic or polymorphic?
Monomorphic VT
Is cardiac function impaired?
Note!
May go directly to cardioversion
Polymorphic VT
Is QT baseline interval prolonged?
Normal function
Poor ejection fraction
Normal baseline QT interval
Prolonged baseline QT interval (suggests torsades)
Medications: any one
• Procainamide
• Sotalol
Others acceptable
• Amiodarone
• Lidocaine
Normal baseline QT interval
• Treat ischemia
• Correct electrolytes
Medications: any one
• β-Blockers or
• Lidocaine or
• Amiodarone or
• Sotalol
Long baseline QT interval
• Correct abnormal electrolytes
Medications: any one
• Magnesium
• Overdrive pacing
• Isoproterenol
• Phenytoin
• Lidocaine
Cardiac function impaired
Amiodarone
• 150-mg IV bolus over 10 min
or
Lidocaine
• 0.5 to 0.75 mg/kg IV push
Then use
• Synchronized cardioversion

Fig. 3-176 Stable ventricular tachycardia (monomorphic or polymorphic) algorithm. (From American Heart Association: Guidelines 2000 for cardiopulmonary resuscitation and emergency cardiovascular care, *Circulation* 102(suppl): I 1, 2000.)

VERTIGO

Vertigo
ICD-9CM # 780.4   Vertigo NOS
          386.11 Benign paroxysmal positional
          386.2   Vertigo, central origin
          386.10 Vertigo, peripheral

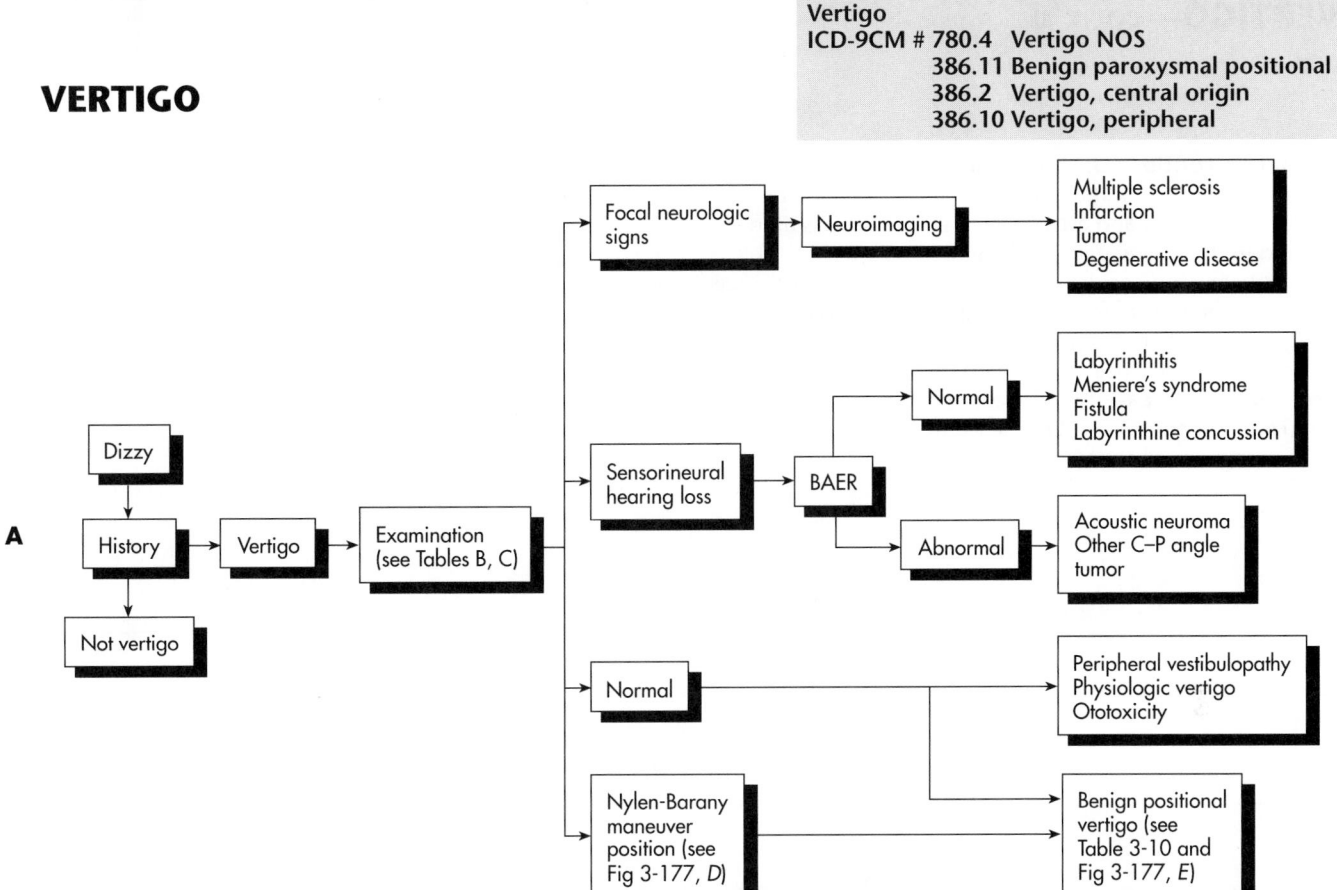

A

Fig. 3-177   **A, Evaluation of vertigo.** *BAER,* Brain stem auditory evoked response. (Modified from Baloh RW: Hearing and equilibrium. In Andreoli TE [ed]: *Cecil essentials of medicine,* ed 4, Philadelphia, 1997, WB Saunders.)

B

SYMPTOM OR SIGN	PERIPHERAL	CENTRAL
Severity	4+	1-4+
Onset	Sudden	Nonparoxysmal
Nausea and vomiting	Common	Uncommon
Nystagmus	*Always* present	Present or absent
Tinnitus and hearing loss	Often present	Very rare
Visual fixation	Inhibits	No effect

B, Symptoms suggestive of central versus peripheral vertigo. (From Andreoli TE [ed]: *Cecil essentials of medicine,* ed 5, Philadelphia, 2001, WB Saunders.)

C

CHARACTERISTIC	PERIPHERAL	CENTRAL
Direction	Usually horizontal, may have rotary component	Any direction (pure vertical is always central)
Symmetry between eyes	Always symmetric	Dissociation between eyes possible
Lesion side	Fast component away from injured labyrinth	No relation between direction and lesion location
Duration of problem	Minutes to weeks	Days to years
Visual fixation	Decreases	No effect

C, Characteristics of central versus peripheral nystagmus. (From Andreoli TE [ed]: *Cecil essentials of medicine,* ed 5, Philadelphia, 2001, WB Saunders.)

VERTIGO—cont'd

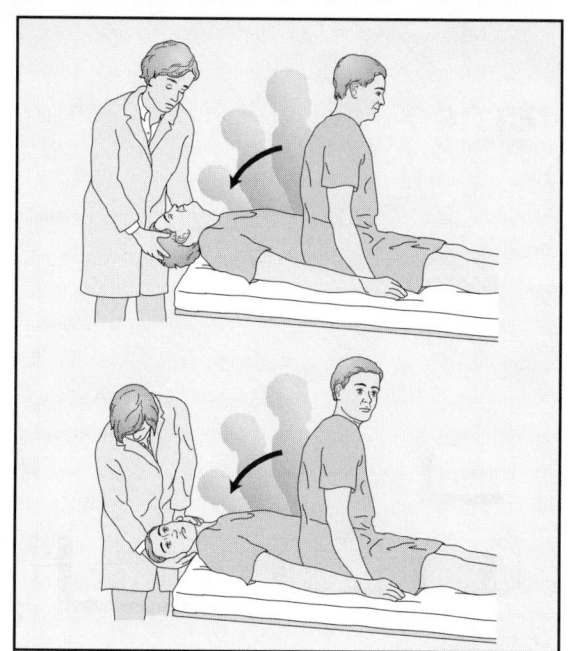

Fig. 3-177, cont'd **D,** Nylen Bárány or Dix-Hallpike maneuver to test for position nystagmus. *Top,* The patient is seated on an examining table with head and eyes directed forward and is then quickly lowered to the supine position with the head over the table edge, 45 degrees below the horizontal. The patient is instructed to keep eyes open; nystagmus is observed for, and the patient is asked to report vertigo. When the test is positive, the affected ear is down; the fast phase of nystagmus beats toward the affected ear. *Bottom,* The test is repeated with the patient's head turned to the right and again to the left. (From Simon RP et al: *Clinical neurology,* ed 4, Stamford, Conn, 1999, Appleton & Lange.)

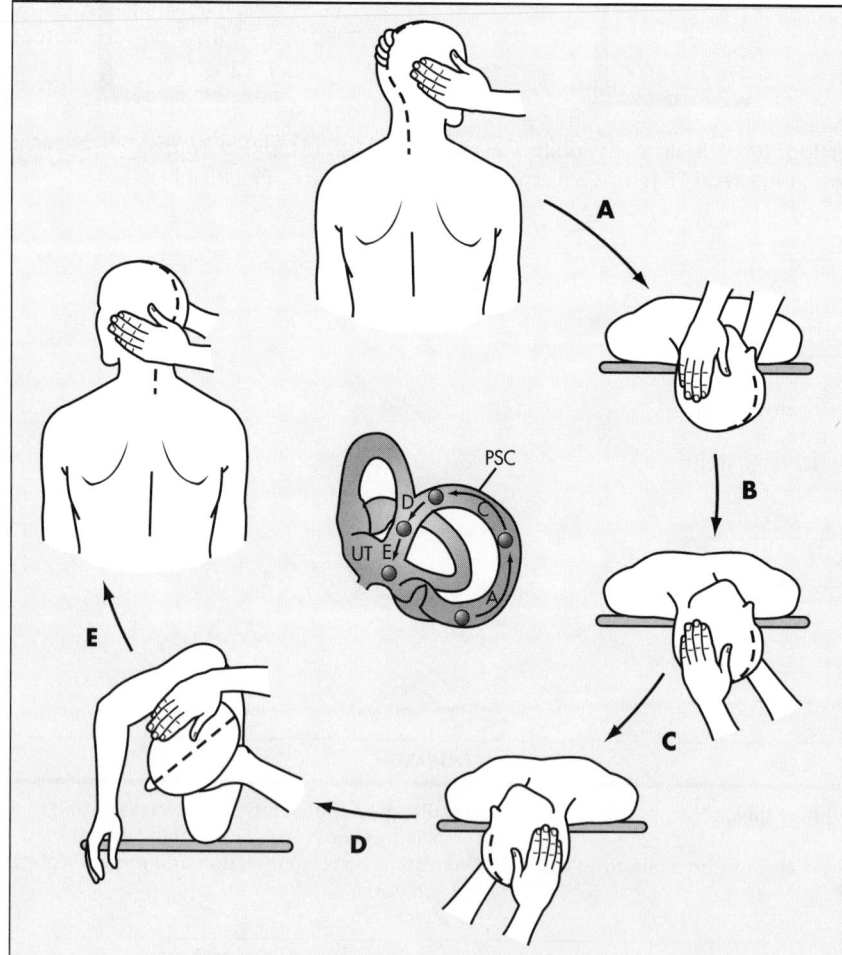

Fig. 3-177, cont'd **E,** Repositioning treatment for benign positional vertigo designed to move endolymphatic debris out of the posterior semicircular canal (PSC) of the right ear and into the utricle (UT). Th epatient is seated, and the head is turned 45 degrees to the right **(A).** The head is lowered rapidly to below the horizontal **(B).** The examiner shifts hand positions **(C),** and the patient's head is rotated rapidly 90 degrees in the opposite direction, so it now points 45 degrees to the left, where it remains for 30 seconds **(D).** The patient then rolls onto the left side without turning the head in relation to the body and maintains this position for another 30 seconds **(E)** before sitting up. The treatment is repeated until nystagmus is abolished. The procedure is reversed for treating the left ear. The patient must avoid the supine position for 2 days. (Modified from Foster CA, Baloh RW: Episodic vertigo. In Rakel RE [ed]: *Conn's current therapy,* Philadelphia, 1995, WB Saunders.)

VERTIGO—cont'd

TABLE 3-10   Exercises for Benign Positional Vertigo

Eyes

Look up and down, slowly at first, then quickly, 20 times.
Look from side to side, slowly at first, then quickly, 20 times.
Focus on one's finger at arm's length. Move the finger to the side about 1 foot and then back 20 times.

Head

With eyes open, bend head forward and backward. Move slowly at first and more quickly later. Do this 20 times.
Turn head side to side 20 times
When the dizziness improves, try the head exercises with eyes closed.

Sitting

Shrug shoulders 20 times.
Turn shoulders right and left 20 times.
Bend forward to pick up an object and then sit up 20 times.

Standing

Sit and stand 20 times with eyes open.
Sit and stand 20 times with eyes closed.
Toss a ball from hand to hand above eye level 20 times.
Toss a ball from hand to hand under one knee 20 times.

Moving

Walk across the room with eyes open 10 times.
Walk across the room with eyes closed 10 times.
Walk up and down the steps with eyes open 10 times.
Walk up and down the steps with eyes closed 10 times.

From Rakel RE (ed): *Principles of family practice,* ed 6, Philadelphia, 2002, WB Saunders.
These exercises should be performed twice daily. Initially, the exercises should be performed for 15 minutes. Each exercise session should gradually increase to 30 minutes.
These exercises may need to be modified for elderly patients, especially if they have existing motor, sensory, or cognitive impairments.

III

WEAKNESS, BILATERAL, AND SYMMETRIC, INFECTIOUS CAUSES

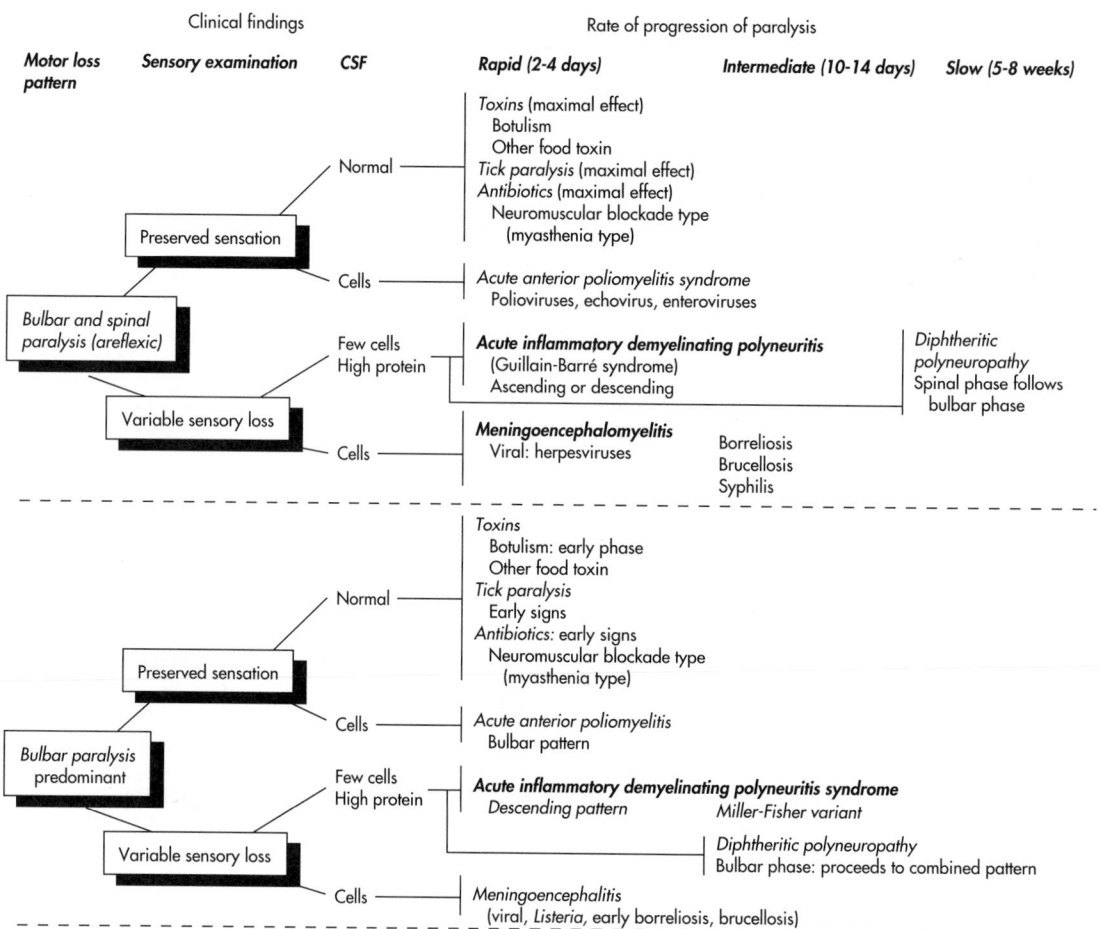

Fig. 3-178   Evaluation of patient with bilateral symmetric weakness or paralysis for possible infection-related cause. *AJ,* Ankle jerk; *CMV,* cytomegalovirus; *CSF,* cerebrospinal fluid; *CT,* computed tomography; *HIV,* human immunodeficiency virus; *HSV,* herpes simplex virus; *HTLV-I,* human T-cell lymphotropic virus type I; *KJ,* knee jerk; *MRI,* magnetic resonance imaging; *PMN,* polymorphonuclear leukocytes; *VZV,* varicella-zoster virus. (From Gorbach SL: *Infectious diseases,* ed 2, Philadelpia, 1998, WB Saunders.)

WEAKNESS, BILATERAL, AND
SYMMETRIC, INFECTIOUS CAUSES—cont'd

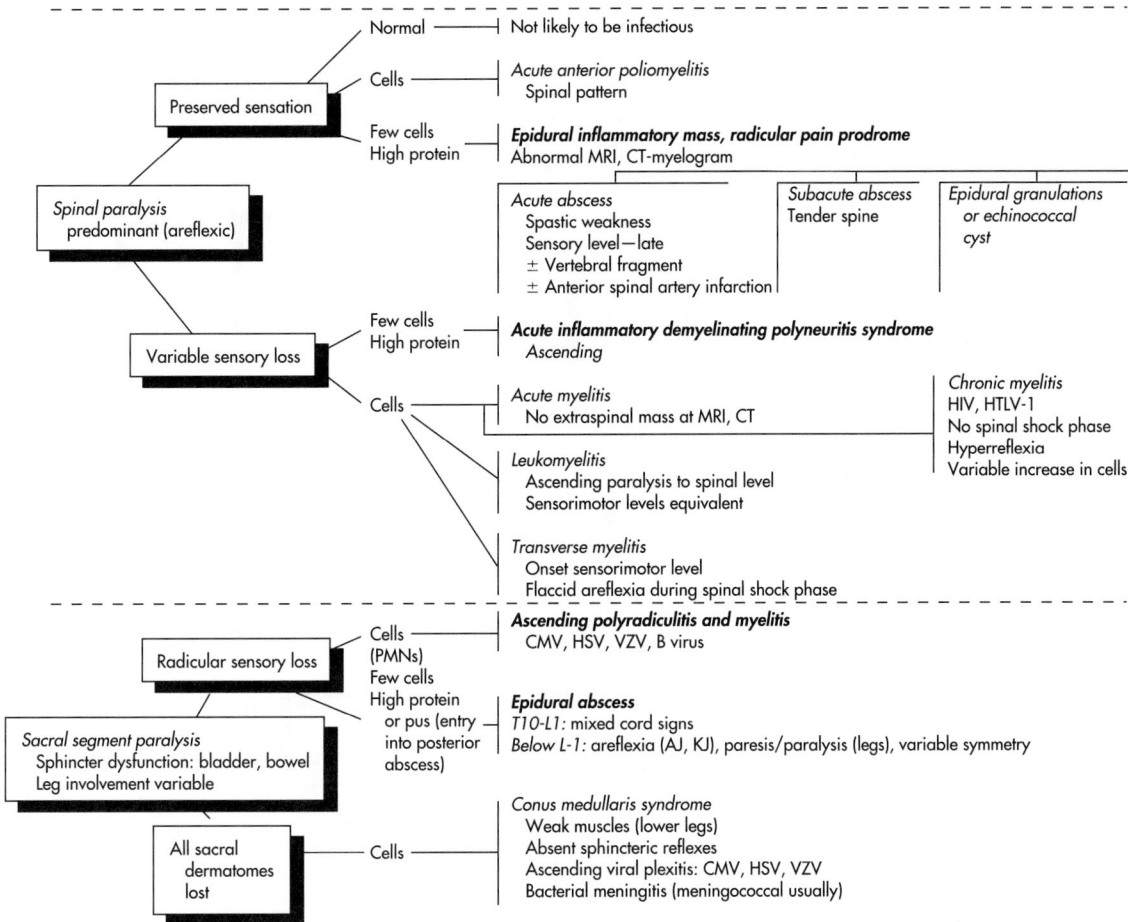

Fig. 3-178, cont'd

WEIGHT GAIN

Weight gain
ICD-9CM # 783.1 Abnormal weight gain
278.00 Obesity

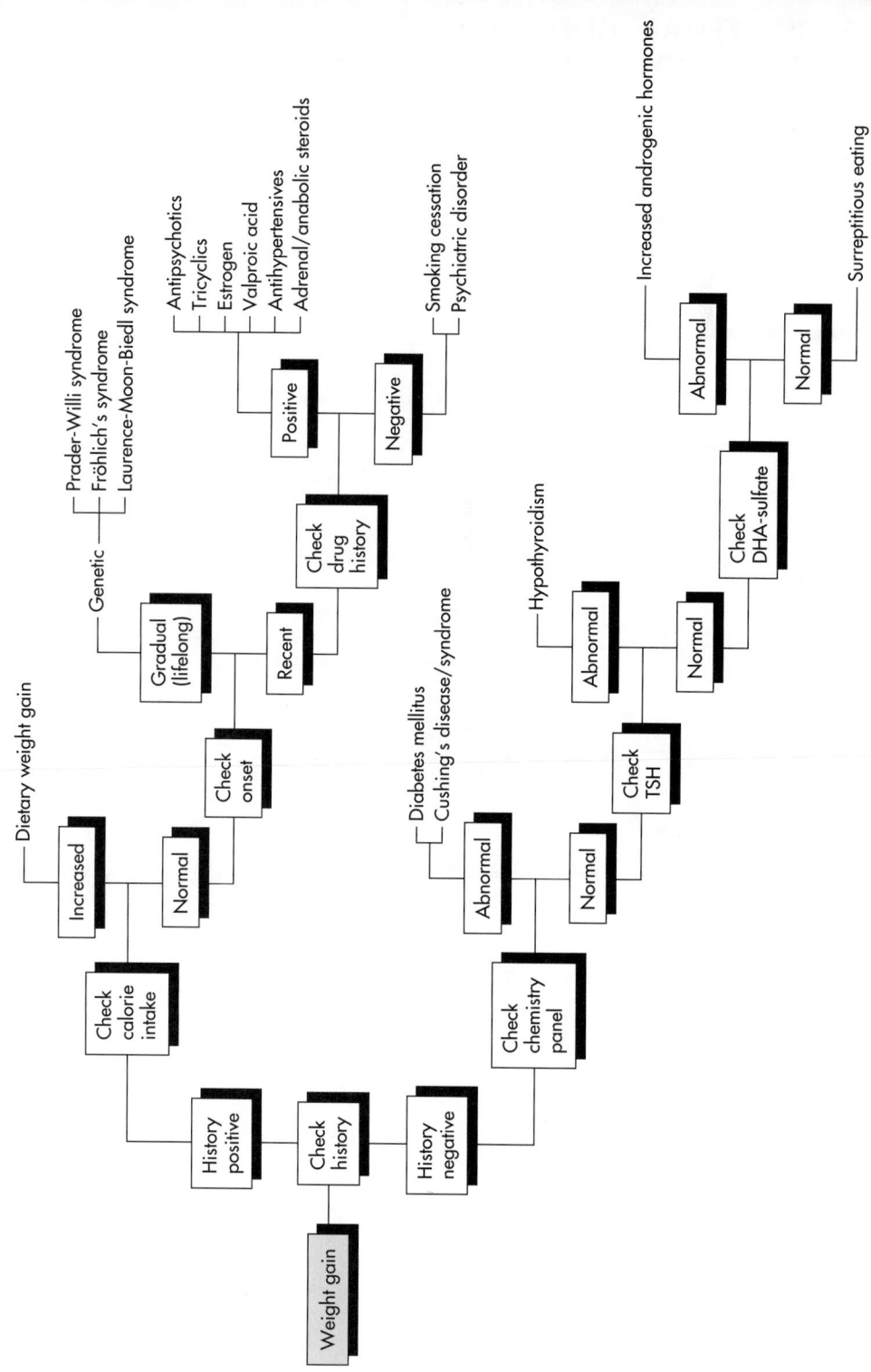

Fig. 3-179   Weight gain. *DHA,* Dehydroepiandrosterone; *TSH,* thyroid-stimulating hormone. (From Healey PM: *Common medical diagnosis: an algorithmic approach,* ed 3, Philadelphia, 2000, WB Saunders.)

WEIGHT LOSS, INVOLUNTARY

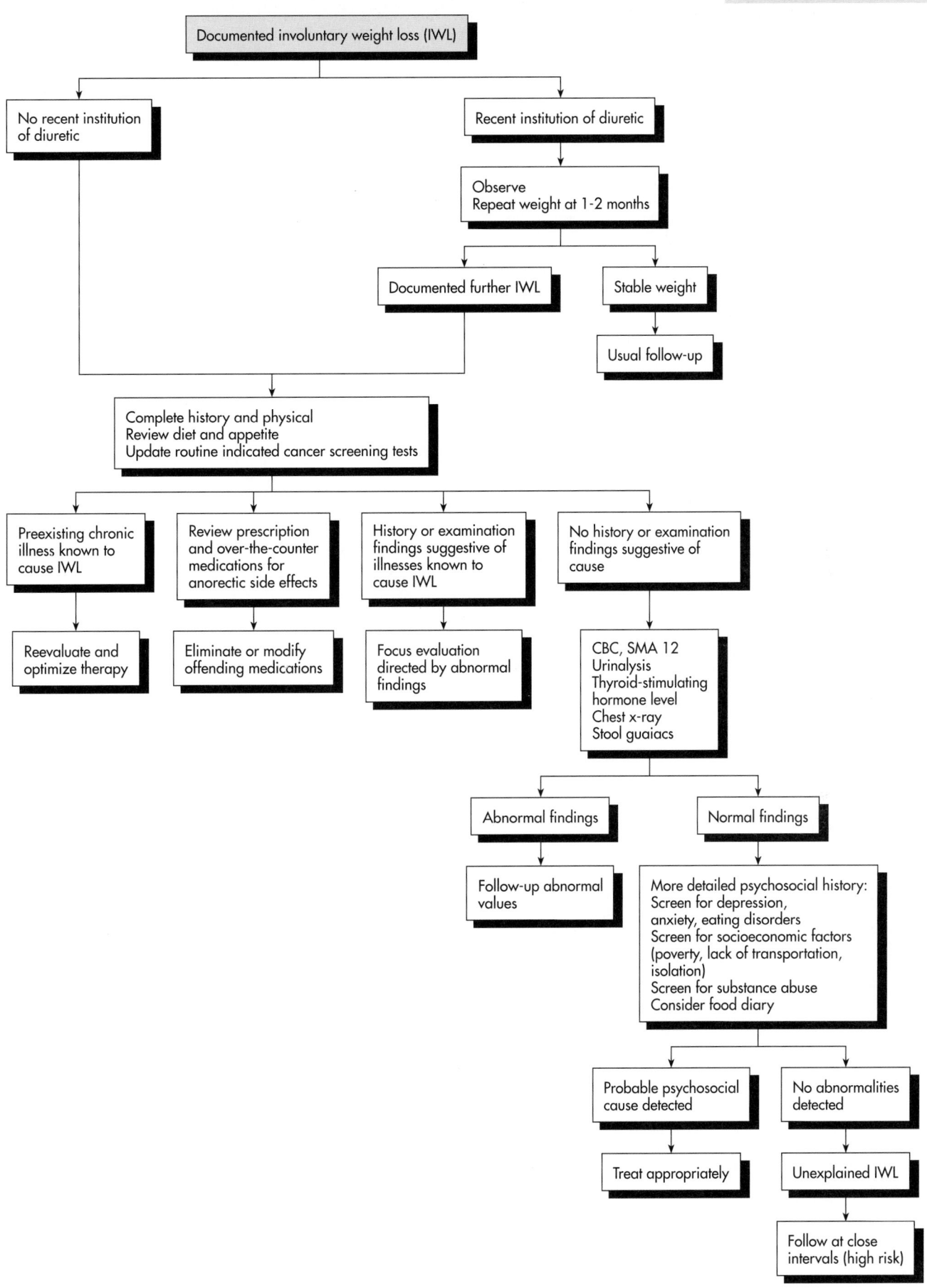

Fig. 3-180   Involuntary weight loss. *CBC,* Complete blood count. (From Greene HL, Johnson WP, Lemcke D [eds]: *Decision making in medicine,* ed 2, St Louis, 1998, Mosby.)

Laboratory Tests and Interpretation of Results

This section contains more than 200 commonly performed laboratory tests. In general, the tests are approached with the following format:

1. Laboratory test
2. Normal range in adult patients
3. Cost
4. Common abnormalities, such as positive test, increased or decreased value
5. Causes of abnormal result

The normal ranges may differ slightly, depending on the laboratory. The reader should be aware of the "normal range" of the particular laboratory performing the test. Every attempt has been made to present current laboratory test data, with emphasis on practical considerations. Normal values are given using the present (traditional) reference interval, followed by the Système Internationale (SI) reference interval, the conversion factor (CF), and the suggested minimum increment (SMI). For example,

TEST	PRESENT REFERENCE INTERVAL	SI REFERENCE INTERVAL	CF	SMI
Fasting glucose	70-110 mg/dl	3.6-6.1 mmol/L	0.05551	0.1 mmol/L

LABORATORY TEST COSTS

Please note that the cost of each laboratory test noted in the following list is a national average based on the charge submitted by most laboratories. Reimbursement for each laboratory test will vary regionally and with the type of medical insurance of the patient. The current cost assumes that the laboratory test is ordered individually. When tests are ordered as part of a test panel the charge will vary.

Acetone (serum or plasma) ($40)
Acid-base reference values
Acid phosphatase (serum) ($24)
Alanine aminotransferase (ALT, SGPT) ($23)
Albumin (serum) ($23)
Aldolase (serum) ($37)
Aldosterone ($123)
Alkaline phosphatase (serum) ($23)
Ammonia (serum) ($57)
Amylase (serum) ($26)
Angiotensin-converting enzyme (ACE level) ($58)
Anion gap
Anti-DNA ($51)
Antimitochondrial antibody ($41)
Antineutrophil cytoplasmic antibody (ANCA) ($89)
Antinuclear antibody (ANA) ($49)
Anti-streptolysin O titer (Streptozyme, ASLO titer) ($32)
Antithrombin III ($38)
Aspartate aminotransferase (AST, SGOT) ($23)
Basophil count
Bilirubin, direct (conjugated bilirubin) ($23)
Bilirubin, indirect (unconjugated bilirubin) ($24)
Bilirubin, total ($24)
Bleeding time (modified Ivy method) ($31)
Calcitonin (serum) ($123)
Calcium (serum) ($23)
Cancer antigen 125 ($76)
Carboxyhemoglobin ($47)
Carcinoembryonic antigen (CEA) ($79)
Carotene (serum) ($50)
CD4+ T-lymphocyte count (CD4+ T-cells) ($111)
Cerebrospinal fluid (CSF)
Ceruloplasmin (serum) ($40)
Chloride (serum) ($23)
Cholesterol, total ($23)
Chromosome abnormalities in malignancy
Circulating anticoagulant (lupus anticoagulant) ($98)
Coagulation factors
Cold agglutinins titer ($28)
Complement
Complete blood count (CBC) ($22)
Coombs, direct ($23)
Coombs, indirect ($23)
Copper (serum) ($89)
Cortisol, plasma ($55)
C-peptide ($89)
C-reactive protein ($26)
C-reactive protein, high sensitivity (hs-CRP, Cardio-CRP)
Creatine kinase (CK, CPK) ($27)

Creatine kinase isoenzymes ($60)
Creatinine (serum) ($23)
Creatinine clearance ($31)
Cryoglobulins (serum) ($29)
Drug monitoring
Eosinophil count
Epstein-Barr viral infection ($53)
Erythrocyte sedimentation rate (ESR; Westergren method) ($24)
Estrogen ($79)
Extractable nuclear antigen (ENA complex, anti-RNP antibody, anti-Sm, anti-Smith) ($158)
Fecal fat, quantitative (72-hr collection) ($42)
Ferritin (serum) ($45)
α-1Fetoprotein ($66)
Fibrin degradation product (FDP) ($40)
Fibrinogen ($38)
Folate (folic acid) ($52)
Follicle-stimulating hormone (FSH) ($58)
Free thyroxine index
Gastrin (serum) ($62)
Glomerular basement membrane (GBM) antibody ($89)
Glucose, fasting ($23)
Glucose, postprandial ($23)
Glucose tolerance test ($43)
Glucose-6-phosphate dehydrogenase screen (blood) ($79)
γ-Glutamyl transferase (GGT) ($23)
Glycated (glycosylated) hemoglobin (HbA_{1c}) ($39)
Ham test (acid serum test) ($79)
Haptoglobin (serum) ($44)
Hematocrit ($20)
Hemoglobin ($20)
Hemoglobin electrophoresis ($45)
Hepatitis A antibody ($54)
Hepatitis A viral infection
Hepatitis B surface antigen (HBsAg) ($37)
Hepatitis B viral infection
Hepatitis C viral infection
Hepatitis D viral infection
Heterophil antibody ($30)
High-density lipoprotein (HDL) cholesterol ($24)
HLA antigens ($80)
Human chorionic gonadotropin (hCG) ($34)
Human immunodeficiency virus antibody, type 1 (HIV-1) ($59)

Human immunodeficiency virus type 1 (HIV-1) antigen (p24), qualitative (p24 antigen) ($105)
Human immunodeficiency virus type 1 (HIV-1) viral load ($105)
Immune complex assay ($86)
Immunoglobulins ($81)
International normalized ratio (INR) ($23)
Iron-binding capacity, total (TIBC) ($45)
Lactate dehydrogenase (LDH) ($23)
Lactate dehydrogenase isoenzymes ($69)
Legionella titer ($69)
Leukocyte alkaline phosphatase ($47)
Lipase ($23)
Low-density lipoprotein (LDL) cholesterol ($58)
Luteinizing hormone ($58)
Lyme disease antibody titer ($67)
Lymphocytes
Magnesium (serum) ($23)
Mean corpuscular volume (MCV)
Monocyte count
Neutrophil count
5' nucleotidase ($42)
Oncogenes
Osmolality (serum) ($31)
Partial thromboplastin time (PTT), activated partial thromboplastin time (APTT) ($32)
Phosphate (serum) ($23)
Platelet count ($22)
Potassium (serum) ($23)
Prolactin ($80)
Prostatic specific antigen (PSA) ($49)
Protein (serum) ($23)
Protein electrophoresis (serum) ($52)
Prothrombin time (PT) ($23)
Protoporphyrin (free erythrocyte) ($49)
Red blood cell (RBC) count ($20)
Red blood cell distribution width (RDW)
Red blood cell mass (volume) ($129)
Red blood cell morphology
Renin (serum) ($125)
Reticulocyte count ($22)
Rheumatoid factor (RF) ($18)
Semen analysis ($50)
Smooth muscle antibody ($40)
Sodium (serum) ($23)
Sucrose hemolysis test (sugar water test) ($42)

T_3 (triiodothyronine) ($49)
T_4, free (free thyroxine) ($53)
Testosterone (total testosterone) ($79)
Thrombin time (TT) ($32)
Thyroid-stimulating hormone (TSH) ($65)
Thyroxine (T_4) ($25)
Transferrin ($36)
Triglycerides ($23)
Tuberculin test (PPD) ($18)
Tumor markers
Urea nitrogen, blood (BUN) ($23)
Uric acid (serum) ($23)
Urinalysis ($22)
Urine amylase ($26)
Urine bile
Urine calcium ($23)
Urine cAMP ($89)
Urine catecholamines ($50)
Urine chloride ($24)
Urine copper ($58)
Urine cortisol, free ($125)
Urine creatinine (24 hr) ($23)
Urine eosinophils
Urine glucose (qualitative)
Urine hemoglobin, free
Urine hemosiderin
Urine 5-hydroxyindole-acetic acid (urine 5-HIAA) ($79)
Urine indican
Urine ketones (semiquantitative)
Urine metanephrines ($79)
Urine myoglobin
Urine nitrite
Urine occult blood
Urine osmolality ($31)
Urine pH
Urine phosphate ($23)
Urine potassium ($23)
Urine protein (quantitative) ($23)
Urine sediment
Urine sodium (quantitative) ($23)
Urine specific gravity
Urine vanillylmandelic acid (VMA) ($50)
VDRL ($49)
Viscosity (serum) ($34)
Vitamin B_{12} ($52)
Wet-mount microscopic procedures
D-Xylose absorption ($52)

MEDICAL NECESSITY – ICD CODES

Carriers have developed local medical review policies that limit coverage for some tests to specified medical conditions. Medicare will pay only for those services that it determines to be "reasonable and necessary" under section 1862 (a) (1) of the Medicare law. "Limited Coverage Tests" (LCTs) have been established for which Medicare will pay only if the patient has one of a limited number of diagnoses that are defined by the carrier as justifying payment of the test. When carriers develop local medical review policies for certain laboratory tests, they issue carrier bulletins to inform physicians and laboratories about their limited coverage policies.

To facilitate the payment process, laboratories submit with the claim all of the diagnosis codes (ICD codes) provided by the physician. The Balanced Budget Act of 1997 amended the Social Security Act to require physicians to provide these ICD codes to laboratories as a way to ensure that laboratory claims will be accurate.

The CPT Codes provided are based on American Medical Association (AMA) guidelines and are for informational purposes only. Current procedural terminology (CPT) coding is the sole responsibility of the billing party. Please direct any questions regarding coding to the payor being billed.

PANELS

In a continuing effort to control federal healthcare spending, the U.S. government mandated that all laboratory tests ordered for a Medicare/Medicaid assisted patient be medically necessary for the diagnosis or treatment of that patient. Medicare/Medicaid will pay only for those laboratory tests they determine to be "reasonable and necessary."

As a result of these changes in reimbursement and their impact on the way physicians practice medicine, the American Medical Association has revised their organ/disease related panels.

Com, Comments; *CPT,* CPT code; *NA,* not available; *NLA,* reflects 2001 Medicare national limitation amount.

Test Information

Electrolyte Panel
Carbon dioxide
Chloride
Potassium
Sodium
CPT: 80051
NLA: $9.69

Hepatic Function Panel
A/G ratio
Albumin
Alkaline phosphatase
ALT
AST
Bilirubin, direct
Bilirubin, total
Globulin, calculated
Protein, total
CPT: 80076
NLA: $11.29

Test Information

Basic Metabolic Panel
BUN
BUN/creatinine ratio
Calcium
Carbon dioxide
Chloride
Creatinine
Glucose
Potassium
Sodium
CPT: 80048
NLA: $11.70

Hepatitis Panel, Acute, with Reflex#
Hepatitis A antibody, IgM
Hepatitis B core antibody, IgM
Hepatitis B surface antigen with reflex confirmation
Hepatitis C antibody
Spec: 1 spun barrier tube
CPT: 80074
NLA: NA
If Hepatitis B surface antigen is borderline or positive, confirmation by neutralization will be performed
(CPT 87341 NLA: $14.27).

IV

Test Information

Lipid Panel
Cholesterol
Cholesterol/HDL ratio
HDL Cholesterol
LDL Cholesterol, calculated
Triglycerides
Spec: 2 ml serum (12 hr fasting sample required)
CPT: 80061
NLA: NA

Test Information

Comprehensive Metabolic Panel
A/G ratio
Albumin
Alkaline phosphatase
ALT
AST
Bilirubin, total
BUN
BUN/creatinine ratio
Calcium
Carbon dioxide
Chloride
Creatinine
Globulin, calculated
Glucose
Potassium
Protein, total
Sodium
CPT: 80053
NLA: $14.61

Obstetric Panel with Reflex#
Antibody screen, RBC with reflex identification
and titer blood group and Rh type
CBC; includes differential and platelet count
Hepatitis B surface antigen (HB s Ag) with reflex
confirmation
RPR with reflex titer and confirmation
Rubella screen
Spec: 1 lavender top tube (EDTA), 2 peripheral
        blood smears, 1 yellow top tube (ACD Solu-
        tion B), 1 spun barrier tube
CPT: 80055
NLA: NA
If hepatitis B surface antigen is borderline or posi-
tive, confirmation by neutralization will be per-
formed (CPT 87341 NLA: $14.27).
If RPR is reactive, a titer will be performed (CPT
86593 NLA: $6.09) and confirmation will be per-
formed (CPT 86781 NLA: $18.30).
If the antibody screen is positive, antibody identifi-
cation and titer will be performed (CPT 86870/
86886 NLA: NA/$7.15). If abnormal cells are noted

on a manual review of the peripheral blood smear
or if the automated differential information indicates a possible discrepancy, a full manual differential will be performed. The manual differential will
replace the automated differential if, (1) there is an
elevation above the normal range for bands, or (2)
there are ≥1% immature or abnormal cells, or (3)
the results of a manual differential indicate a discrepancy which exceeds the limits or (4) the difference between the basophil counts is ≥2% in the
absence of basophilia on smear review.

CPT Codes for Individual Tests and Medicare National Limitation Amounts

Test Information

Acetylcholine Receptor Binding Antibody, Serum
CPT: 84238
NLA: $50.53

Acid Phosphatase, Prostatic (PAP), Serum
CPT: 84066
NLA: $13.35

Activated Partial Thromboplastin Time (aPTT), Plasma
CPT: 85730
NLA: $8.30

Adenovirus Culture
Virus identification may require additional studies
(CPT: 87253 NLA: $27.91)
CPT: 87252
NLA: $36.02

Adrenocorticotropic Hormone (ACTH), Plasma
CPT: 82024
NLA: $53.38

Alanine Aminotransferase (ALT), Serum
CPT: 84460
NLA: $7.32

Albumin, Serum
CPT: 82040
NLA: $6.85

Albumin (Microalbumin), Random Urine
CPT: 82043
NLA: $8.00

Albumin (Microalbumin), Timed Urine
CPT: 82043
NLA: $8.00

Alcohol, Ethyl, without Confirmation, Blood
CPT: 82055
NLA: $14.93

Alcohol, Ethyl, without Confirmation, Gastric
CPT: 82055
NLA: $14.93

Aldolase, Serum
CPT: 82085
NLA: $13.42

Test Information

Aldosterone, Serum
CPT: 82088
NLA: $56.32

Aldosterone, Urine
CPT: 82088
NLA: $56.32

Alkaline Phosphatase, Serum
CPT: 84075
NLA: $7.15

Alkaline Phosphatase, Bone Specific
CPT: 84075
NLA: $7.15

Alpha-1-Antitrypsin, Serum
CPT: 82103
NLA: $18.56

Alpha Fetoprotein (AFP), Amniotic Fluid
Acetylcholinesterase (CPT: 84999 NLA: NA) and
fetal hemoglobin (CPT: 83033 NLA: $8.24) will be
performed when MoM is >2.0.
CPT: 82106
NLA: $23.18

Alpha Fetoprotein (AFP), Maternal Serum
Not recommended for Down syndrome screening.
ACOG has recommended multiple marker screen-
ing for this purpose.
Com: *No laboratory assay has been approved by the*
FDA for screening of Down syndrome. Any es-
timate of risk for Down syndrome based on
AFP results is for investigational use only.
CPT: 82105
NLA: $23.18

Alpha Fetoprotein (AFP), Tumor Marker, Serum
CPT: 82105
NLA: $23.18

Amikacin, Peak, Serum
CPT: 80150
NLA: $20.83

Amikacin, Trough, Serum
CPT: 80150
NLA: $20.83

Amiodarone and Desethylamiodarone, Serum
CPT: 80299
NLA: $18.92

Amitriptyline and Nortriptyline, Serum
CPT: 80152
NLA: $24.74

Ammonia, Plasma
CPT: 82140
NLA: $20.14

Amylase, Fluid
CPT: 82150
NLA: $8.96

Test Information

Amylase, Serum
CPT: 82150
NLA: $8.96

Amylase, Urine
CPT: 82150
NLA: $8.96

Angiotensin Converting Enzyme (ACE), Serum
CPT: 82164
NLA: $20.17

Angiotensin II
CPT: 82163
NLA: $28.37

Anti-Nuclear Antibody (ANA), Serum
If positive, a titer and pattern will be performed
(CPT: 86039 NLA: $15.43).
CPT: 86038
NLA: $16.70

Anti-Streptolysin O (ASO), Serum
CPT: 86060
NLA: $10.09

Anti-Thrombin III, Antigenic, Plasma
CPT: 85301
NLA: $14.95

Anti-Thrombin III, Functional, Plasma
CPT: 85300
NLA: $16.38

Antibiotic Sensitivity & Identification
Antibiotic Sensitivity
Each pathogen: (CPT: 87186 or 87184 or 87181 or
  87185 NLA: $11.94 or $9.53 or $6.56 or $6.56)
Identification
Salmonella serogrouping: (CPT: 87147 NLA: $7.15)
Shigella serotyping: (CPT: 87147 NLA: $7.15)
Streptococci serogrouping: (CPT: 87147 NLA: $7.15)
Neisseria gonorrhoeae (direct probe): (CPT: 87149
  NLA: $27.71)
Non-urine pathogens: (CPT: 87077 or 87076 or
  87140 or 87143 NLA: $11.16 or $11.16 or $7.71
  or $17.32)
Urine pathogens: (CPT: 87077 or 87147 or 87143
  NLA: $11.16/$7.15/$17.32)

Antibody Identification and Titer
CPT: 86870/86886
NLA: NA/$7.15

**Antibody Screen, RBC with Reflex to Antibody
Identification and Titer, Blood**
If screen is positive, antibody identification and
titer will be performed (CPT: 86870/86886 NLA:
NA/$7.15).
CPT: 86850
NLA: NA

Test Information

Apolipoprotein A-1, Serum
CPT: 82172
NLA: $21.41

Apolipoprotein B, Serum
CPT: 82172
NLA: $21.41

Aspartate Aminotransferase (AST), Serum
CPT: 84450
NLA: $7.14

Basic Metabolic Panel
(Includes calcium, carbon dioxide [CO_2] chloride, creatinine, glucose, potassium, sodium, urea nitrogen [BUN] and BUN/creatinine ratio)
CPT: 80048
NLA: $11.70

Beta-2-Microglobulin, Serum
CPT: 82232
NLA: $22.36

Beta-2-Microglobulin, Urine
CPT: 82232
NLA: $22.36

Bilirubin, Direct
CPT: 82248
NLA: $6.94

Bilirubin, Total, Serum
CPT: 82247
NLA: $6.94

Blood Group
CPT: 86900
NLA: $4.12

Blood Group and Rh Type
CPT: 86900/86901
NLA: $4.12/NA

Bordetella pertussis Antigen, DFA
CPT: 87265
NLA: $16.58

Bordetella pertussis Culture
Fluorescent antibody smear is highly recommended and should be ordered with culture.
Identification on positive cultures will be performed (CPT: 87077 NLA: $11.16).
CPT: 87081
NLA: $9.16

Borrelia burgdorferi Antibody, Early or Stage Unknown, with Confirmation by Western Blot, Serum
Borrelia burgdorferi Antibody IgG and IgM by Western blot will be performed on all samples with positive or equivocal results (CPT: 86617 (×2) NLA: $21.40 (×2)).
CPT: 86618
NLA: $23.54

Test Information

Borrelia burgdorferi Antibody IgG & IgM by Western Blot
CPT: 86617 (×2)
NLA: $21.40 (×2)

Borrelia burgdorferi Antibody, Late Stage with Reflex to Late Disease (IgG) by Western Blot, Serum
Borrelia burgderferi antibody IgG by Western blot will be performed on all samples with positive or equivocal results (CPT: 86617 NLA: $21.40).
CPT: 86618
NLA: $23.54

BUN
See Urea Nitrogen (BUN), Serum

CA 19-9, Serum
CPT: 86301
NLA: NA

CA 27.29, Serum
CPT: 86300
NLA: $28.76

CA 125, Serum
CPT: 86304
NLA: $28.76

Calcium, Ionized, Serum
CPT: 82330
NLA: $18.88

Calcium, Serum
CPT: 82310
NLA: $7.12

Calcium, 24 Hour Urine
CPT: 82340
NLA: $8.34

Carbamazepine, Serum
CPT: 80156
NLA: $20.12

Carbon Dioxide (CO_2), Serum
CPT: 82374
NLA: $6.76

Carcinoembryonic Antigen (CEA), Serum
CPT: 82378
NLA: $26.22

Cardio CRP
CPT: 86140
NLA: $7.15

Carotene, Serum
CPT: 82380
NLA: $12.75

Catecholamines, Fractionated, Plasma
(Includes dopamine, epinephrine, and norepinephrine)
CPT: 82384
NLA: $34.90

Test Information

Catecholamines, Fractionated, Urine
(Includes dopamine, epinephrine, and norepinephrine)
CPT: 82384
NLA: $34.90

CBC includes Differential and Platelet Count
(Includes WBC, RBC, HGB, HCT, MCV, MCH, MCHC, RDW (red cell distribution width), MPV (mean platelet volume), platelet count, plus automated differential cell count with manual differential reflex. See Page 3 for parameters.)
CPT: 85025
NLA: $10.74

Cell Count and Differential, CSF
CPT: 89051
NLA: $7.61

Cell Count and Differential, Fluids
(Pleural or peritoneal)
CPT: 89051
NLA: $7.61

Ceruloplasmin, Serum
CPT: 82390
NLA: $14.84

Chlamydia trachomatis, DNA Probe (Female Endocervical or Male Urethral)
CPT: 87490
NLA: $27.71

Chlamydia trachomatis/Neisseria gonorrhoeae DNA Probe (Female Endocervical or Male Urethral)
If positive, individual probe confirmation will be performed (CPT: 87490/87590 NLA: $27.71/$27.71).
CPT: 87800
NLA: $27.71

Chlamydia trachomatis Direct Antigen, Direct Immunofluorescence Staining
CPT: 87270
NLA: $16.58

Chlamydia trachomatis Culture
CPT: 87110/87140
NLA: $27.08/$7.71

Chlamydia trachomatis, PCR, Endocervical
CPT: 87491
NLA: $48.50

Chlamydia trachomatis, PCR, Male Urethral
CPT: 87491
NLA: $48.50

Chlamydia trachomatis, PCR, Male Urine
CPT: 87491
NLA: $48.50

Chloride, Serum
CPT: 82435
NLA: $6.35

Test Information

Chloride, Urine
CPT: 82436
NLA: $6.95

Chlorpromazine, Serum
CPT: 84022
NLA: $21.53

Cholesterol, Serum
CPT: 82465
NLA: $6.02

Cholinesterase, Plasma
(For monitoring of insecticide poisoning)
CPT: 82480
NLA: $10.89

Chromosome Study, Amniotic Fluid
CPT: 88235/88269/88280/88291
NLA: $203.50/$229.85/$34.68/$5.54

Citrate, Urine
CPT: 82507
NLA: $38.43

Clomipramine and Metabolite, Serum
CPT: 80299
NLA: $18.92

Clostridium difficile Toxins A and B, Stool
CPT: 87324
NLA: $16.58

Clostridium difficile Toxin B, Screen
CPT: 87230
NLA: $27.28

Clozapine, Plasma
CPT: 80154
NLA: $25.56

Coccidioides Antibody, Immunodiffusion, Serum
CPT: 86635
NLA: $15.85

Collagen Cross-Linked N-Telopeptide, (The NTx Assay), Urine
CPT: 82523
NLA: $25.83

Complement C3, Fluid
CPT: 86160
NLA: $16.59

Complement C3, Serum
CPT: 86160
NLA: $16.59

Complement C4, Fluid
CPT: 86160
NLA: $16.59

Complement C4, Serum
CPT: 86160
NLA: $16.59

IV

Test Information

Complement, Total (CH50), Serum
CPT: 86162
NLA: $28.08

Comprehensive Metabolic Panel
(Includes albumin, alanine aminotransferase (ALT), alkaline phosphatase, aspartate aminotransferase (AST), calcium, carbon dioxide (CO_2), chloride, creatinine, glucose, potassium, sodium, total bilirubin, total protein, urea nitrogen (BUN), albumin/globulin ratio, BUN/creatinine ratio, and globulin)
CPT: 80053
NLA: $14.61

Coombs' Direct, Polyspecific with Reflex
If positive with polyspecific antisera, the sensitization component will be identified as IgG or C3d (CPT: 86880 ($\times$2) NLA: $7.42 ($\times$2)).
CPT: 86880
NLA: $7.42

Cortisol, Free, Urine
CPT: 82530
NLA: $23.10

Cortisol, Serum (Single Specimen)
CPT: 82533
NLA: $22.53

Cortisol, Serum (Two Specimens, A.M. and P.M.)
CPT: 82533 ($\times$2)
NLA: $22.53 ($\times$2)

Cortisol Stimulation by Adrenocorticotropic Hormone (ACTH), Serum
CPT: 82533 ($\times$ # of specimens received)
NLA: $22.53 ($\times$ # of specimens received)

C-Peptide, Plasma
CPT: 84681
NLA: $28.75

C-Reactive Protein (CRP), Serum
CPT: 86140
NLA: $7.15

Creatine Kinase (CK), Serum
CPT: 82550
NLA: $9.01

Creatinine, Serum
CPT: 82565
NLA: $7.07

Creatinine, Urine
CPT: 82570
NLA: $7.15

Creatinine Clearance
CPT: 82575
NLA: $13.06

Cryptococcus Antigen, CSF
CPT: 87327
NLA: $16.58

Test Information

Cryptococcus Antigen Titer, Serum
CPT: 86406
NLA: $14.70

Cryptosporidium Ag, Stool
CPT: 87015/87272
NLA: $9.23/$16.58

Crystal Identification, Synovial Fluid
(Includes identification of uric acid and calcium pyrophosphate)
CPT: 89060
NLA: $9.88

Culture, Aerobic, Miscellaneous
Source must be indicated on requisition form. Antibiotic sensitivities and identification will be performed on each pathogen isolated. See Antibiotic Sensitivity and Identification.
CPT: 87070
NLA: $11.90

Culture, Anaerobic
(Includes Gram stain smear) Identification will be performed on each pathogen isolated. See Antibiotic Sensitivity and Identification.
CPT: 87075/87205
NLA: $13.08/$5.90

Culture, Blood
Antibiotic sensitivities and identification will be performed on each pathogen isolated. See Antibiotic Sensitivity and Identification.
CPT: 87040
NLA: $14.27

Culture, CSF
(Includes Gram Stain Smear) Antibiotic sensitivities and identification will be performed on each pathogen isolated. See Antibiotic Sensitivity and Identification.
CPT: 87070/87205
NLA: $11.90/$5.90

Culture, Ear
Antibiotic sensitivities and identification will be performed on each pathogen isolated. See Antibiotic Sensitivity and Identification.
CPT: 87070
NLA: $11.90

Culture, Eye
Antibiotic sensitivities and identification will be performed on each pathogen isolated. See Antibiotic Sensitivity and Identification.
CPT: 87070
NLA: $11.90

Test Information

Culture, Fluid

(Includes aerobic bacterial culture and Gram stain smear. For anaerobic culture see Culture, Anaerobic.)

> Antibiotic sensitivities and identification will be performed on each pathogen isolated. See Antibiotic Sensitivity and Identification.

CPT: 87070/87205
NLA: $11.90/$5.90

Culture, Fungus, Blood

Identification will be performed for each pathogen isolated. See Culture, Fungus, Identification and Susceptibility.

CPT: 87103
NLA: $12.46

Culture, Fungus, Miscellaneous, Source other than Blood or Skin

(Includes calcofluor/KOH exam)
Identification will be performed for each pathogen isolated. See Culture, Fungus, Identification and Susceptibility.

CPT: 87206/87102
NLA: $7.42/$11.61

Culture, Fungus, Skin, Nail or Hair

(Includes calcofluor/KOH exam)
Identification will be performed for each pathogen isolated. See Culture, Fungus, Identification and Susceptibility.

CPT: 87220/87101
NLA: $5.90/$10.66

Culture, Fungus, Identification and Susceptibility

Identification
Yeast: (CPT: 87106 NLA: $14.27)
Mold: (CPT: 87107 NLA: $14.27)
Probe: (CPT: 87149 NLA: $27.71)
Exoantigen testing: (CPT: 87158 NLA: $7.23)
Yeast Susceptibility
Broth microdilution: (CPT: 87186 NLA: $11.94)

Culture, Genital

> Antibiotic sensitivities and identification will be performed on each pathogen isolated. See Antibiotic Sensitivity and Identification.

CPT: 87070
NLA: $11.90

Culture, Herpes simplex Virus, Rapid Method

CPT: 87254
NLA: $6.76

Culture, Herpes simplex Virus, Rapid with Type

Typing of positive culture isolates will automatically be performed (CPT: 87140 NLA: $7.71).
CPT: 87254
NLA: $6.76

Test Information

Culture, Nasopharyngeal

> Antibiotic sensitivities and identification will be performed on each pathogen isolated. See Antibiotic Sensitivity and Identification.

CPT: 87070
NLA: $11.90

Culture, Sputum

(Includes Gram stain smear)

> Antibiotic sensitivities and identification will be performed on each pathogen isolated. See Antibiotic Sensitivity and Identification.

CPT: 87070/87205
NLA: $11.90/$5.90

Culture, Stool

See Culture, Stool, Slamonella and Shigella Only and Culture, Stool, Campylobacter Only.

Culture, Stool, Salmonella and Shigella Only

CPT: 87045
NLA: $13.04

Culture, Stool, Campylobacter Only

CPT: 87046
NLA: $3.26

Culture, Throat

> Antibiotic sensitivities and identification will be performed on each pathogen isolated. See Antibiotic Sensitivity and Identification.

CPT: 87070
NLA: $11.90

Culture, Tissue

(Includes aerobic and anaerobic culture and Gram stain smear)

> Antibiotic sensitivities and identification will be performed on each pathogen isolated. See Antibiotic Sensitivity and Identification.

CPT: 87070/87075/87205
NLA: $11.90/$13.08/$5.90

Culture, Urine, Routine

Use for clean catch urine and urine from indwelling catheters.

> Antibiotic sensitivities and identification will be performed on each pathogen isolated. See Antibiotic Sensitivity and Identification.

CPT: 87088
NLA: $11.18

IV

Test Information

Culture, Urine, Special
Use for in-and-out or straight catheter collected specimens, suprapubic aspirates, and urine specimens following prostatic massages or by cystoscope.

Antibiotic sensitivities and identification will be performed on each pathogen isolated. See Antibiotic Sensitivity and Identification.

CPT: 87088
NLA: $11.18

Culture, Wound, Superficial
Antibiotic sensitivities and identification will be performed on each pathogen isolated. See Antibiotic Sensitivity and Identification.

CPT: 87070
NLA: $11.90

Culture, Wound, Deep
(Includes aerobic and anaerobic culture and Gram stain smear)

Antibiotic sensitivities and identification will be performed on each pathogen isolated. See Antibiotic Sensitivity and Identification. Anaerobic sensitivities will be performed, upon request (CPT: 87186 NLA $11.94).

CPT: 87070/87075/87205
NLA: $11.90/$13.08/$5.90

Cyclospora and Isospora Examination
CPT: 87015/87207
NLA: $9.23/$8.28

Cystine, Plasma
CPT: 82131
NLA: $23.31

Cytology, Breast Ductal Lavage
If cell block preparation is required (CPT: 88305 NLA: NA).

CPT: 88108
NLA: NA

Cytology, Breast Fine Needle Aspiration (FNA)
If cell block preparation is required (CPT: 88305 NLA: NA).

CPT: 88173
NLA: NA

Cytology, Breast Nipple Discharge
CPT: 88160
NLA: NA

Cytology, Fluid, Washings or Brushings (miscellaneous site)
If cell block preparation is required (CPT: 88305 NLA: NA).

CPT: 88104
NLA: NA

Test Information

Cytology, Direct Smears, (miscellaneous site)
Use for cytology discharges and scrapings. If cell block preparation is required (CPT: 88305 NLA: NA).

CPT: 88160
NLA: NA

Cytology, Fine Needle Aspiration (FNA) (miscellaneous site)
If cell block preparation is required (CPT: 88305 NLA: NA).

CPT: 88173
NLA: NA

Cytology, Pap Smear
The CPT and NLA listed is for one slide. Pap results requiring physician interpretation will be performed at an additional charge (CPT: 88141 Diagnostic/P3001 Screening NLA: NA/NA).

CPT: Diagnostic 88164, Screening P3000
NLA: $14.60

Cytology, Sutum
CPT: 88161
NLA: NA

Cytology, ThinPrep Pap Test
Pap results requiring physician interpretation will be performed for an additional charge (*CPT:* 88141 Diagnostic/G0124 Screening NLA: NA/NA).

CPT: Diagnostic 88142, Screening G0123
NLA: NA/NA

Cytology, ThinPrep Pap Test with reflex to High-Risk HPV DNA
Pap results requiring physician interpretation will be performed for an additional charge (CPT: 88141 Diagnostic/G0124 Screening NLA: NA/NA). ThinPrep Pap Test results of ASCUS, atypical metaplasia, or atypical cells not otherwise specified, will be automatically reflexed to testing for high-risk HPV DNA for an additional charge (CPT: 87621 NLA: $48.50).

CPT: Diagnostic 88142, Screening G0123
NLA: NA/NA

Cytology, Thyroid Fine Needle Aspiration (FNA)
If cell block preparation is required (CPT: 88305 NLA: NA).

CPT: 88173
NLA: NA

Cytology, Urine
CPT: 88104
NLA: NA

Cytomegalovirus (CMV) Antibody IgM, Serum
Recommended for diagnosis of acute infection only.

CPT: 86645
NLA: $23.28

Test Information

Cytomegalovirus (CMV) Antibody IgG, Serum
CPT: 86644
NLA: $19.89

Cytomegalovirus (CMV) Culture, Rapid
CPT: 87254
NLA: $6.76

Dehydroepiandrosterone (DHEA) Unconjugated, Serum
CPT: 82626
NLA: $34.93

Dehydroepiandrosterone Sulfate (DHEA Sulfate), Serum
CPT: 82627
NLA: $30.72

11-Deoxycortisol (Compound S), Serum
CPT: 82634
NLA: $40.46

Desipramine, Serum
CPT: 80160
NLA: $23.79

Differential, Manual
(Includes RBC morphology & platelet estimation)
CPT: 85007
NLA: $4.76

Digoxin, Serum
CPT: 80162
NLA: $18.35

Dilantin (Phenytoin), Serum
CPT: 80185
NLA: $18.32

Dilantin (Phenytoin), Free, Serum
CPT: 80186
NLA: $19.03

Disopyramide, Serum
CPT: 80299
NLA: $18.92

DNA Antibody, Double-Stranded, Serum
CPT: 86225
NLA: $18.99

DNase-B, Serum
CPT: 86215
NLA: $18.32

Doxepin and Metabolite, Serum
CPT: 80166
NLA: $21.42

Drug Screen 10 Drug, without Confirmation
(Includes amphetamines, barbiturates, benzodiazepines, cocaine, methadone, methaqualone, opiates, phencyclidine, propoxyphene, THC)
CPT: 80101 ($\times$10)
NLA: $19.03 ($\times$10)

Test Information

Electrolyte Panel
(Includes carbon dioxide (CO_2), chloride, potassium, and sodium)
CPT: 80051
NLA: $9.69

Entamoeba histolytica Antibody, Serum
CPT: 86753
NLA: $17.12

Eosinophils, Nasal Smear
CPT: 89190
NLA: $6.56

Epstein-Barr Virus (EBV) Capsid Antigen, Antibody IgG, Serum
CPT: 86665
NLA: $25.07

Epstein-Barr Virus (EBV) Capsid Antigen, Antibody IgM, Serum
CPT: 86665
NLA: $25.07

Epstein-Barr Virus (EBV) Nuclear Antigen, Antibody IgG, Serum
CPT: 86664
NLA: $21.14

Erythrocyte Sedimentation Rate (ESR), Westergren
CPT: 85652
NLA: $3.73

Erythropoietin (EPO)
CPT: 82668
NLA: $25.97

Escherichia coli Shiga Toxins, EIA, Stool
CPT: 87427
NLA: $16.58

Estradiol (E2), Non-Pregnancy, Serum
CPT: 82670
NLA: $38.62

Estrogen Receptor Assay (ER-ICA), Paraffin Block
CPT: 84233
NLA: $89.01

Estrone (E1), Serum
CPT: 82679
NLA: $34.50

Ethosuximide, Serum
CPT: 80168
NLA: $22.58

Extractable Nuclear Antigen (ENA), Antibody, Serum
(Includes anti-Sm and anti-RNP antibodies)
CPT: 86235 ($\times$2)
NLA: $24.78 ($\times$2)

Factor VIII, Functional, Plasma
CPT: 85240
NLA: $24.75

IV

Test Information

Factor XI, Functional, Plasma
CPT: 85270
NLA: $24.75

Fatty Acids, Free, Plasma
CPT: 82725
NLA: $18.40

Fecal Fat, Qualitative
CPT: 82705
NLA: $7.04

Fecal Leukocyte Stain
CPT: 87205
NLA: $5.90

Ferritin, Serum
CPT: 82728
NLA: $18.83

Fibrin Degradation Products (FDP), Blood
CPT: 85362
NLA: $9.52

Fibrinogen, Clottable, Plasma
CPT: 85384
NLA: $11.74

Fibrinogen Antigen
CPT: 85384
NLA: $11.74

FK506 (Tacrolimus), Blood
CPT: 80197
NLA: $18.97

Fluoride, Serum
CPT: 82735
NLA: $25.63

Folate, Serum
CPT: 82746
NLA: $20.32

Folate, RBC
(Includes hematocrit)
CPT: 82747/85014
NLA: $23.93/$3.27

Follicle Stimulating Hormone (FSH), Serum
CPT: 83001
NLA: $25.69

Fructosamine, Serum
CPT: 82985
NLA: $20.83

Fungal Direct Examination (KOH Preparation)
CPT: 87200 (hair, skin, nails)/87206 (other sources)
NLA: $5.90/$7.42

Gabapentin, Plasma
CPT: 80299
NLA: $18.92

Test Information

Gamma Glutamyltransferase (GGT), Serum
CPT: 82977
NLA: $9.95

Gastrin, Serum
CPT: 82941
NLA: $24.38

Gentamicin, Peak, Serum
CPT: 80170
NLA: $22.65

Gentamicin, Trough, Serum
CPT: 80170
NLA: $22.65

Giardia Antigen, EIA, Stool
CPT: 87328
NLA: $16.58

Glucose, CSF
CPT: 82945
NLA: $5.42

Glucose, Fluid
CPT: 82945
NLA: $5.42

Glucose, Quantitative, Urine
CPT: 82945
NLA: $5.42

Glucose, Serum or Plasma
CPT: 82947
NLA: $5.42

Glucose, 2 Hour Postprandial, Plasma
CPT: 82947
NLA: $5.42

Glucose for Gestational Diabetes, One Hour Challenge, Plasma (Single Specimen)
CPT: 82950
NLA: $6.56

Glucose Tolerance Test (GTT) for Gestational Diabetes, Plasma
(4 tests)
CPT: 82951/82952
NLA: $17.80/$5.42

Glucose Tolerance Test (GTT), Plasma
(3 tests)
CPT: 82951
NLA: $17.80

Glucose-6-Phosphate Dehydrogenase (G-6-PD), RBC
CPT: 82955
NLA: $13.40

Gram Stain Smear
(Not to be used for diagnosis of gonorrhea in females)
CPT: 87205
NLA: $5.90

Test Information

Growth Hormone (hGH), Serum
CPT: 83003
NLA: $23.04

Haloperidol, Serum
CPT: 80173
NLA: $20.12

Haptoglobin, Serum
CPT: 83010
NLA: $17.38

hCG (Human Chorionic Gonadotropin), Qualitative, Serum
CPT: 84703
NLA: $10.38

hCG (Human Chorionic Gonadotropin), Qualitative, Urine
CPT: 84703
NLA: $10.38

hCG, (Human Chorionic Gonadotropin), Total, Quantitative, Serum
CPT: 84702
NLA: $20.80

HDL Cholesterol, Serum
CPT: 83718
NLA: $11.31

Helicobacter pylori Antibody IgG, Serum
CPT: 86677
NLA: $20.05

Helicobacter pylori Antibody IgM, Serum
CPT: 86677
NLA: $20.05

Helicobacter pylori Antigen, Stool
CPT: 87338
NLA: NA

Hematocrit, Blood
CPT: 85014
NLA: $3.27

Hemoglobin A$_{1c}$, Blood
CPT: 83036
NLA: $13.42

Hemoglobin and Hematocrit, Blood
CPT: 85014/85018
NLA: $3.27/$3.27

Hemoglobin, Blood
CPT: 85018
NLA: $3.27

Hemoglobin F (Fetal), Blood
CPT: 83021
NLA: $24.96

Hemogram without Platelet Count
CPT: 85021
NLA: $7.72

Test Information

Hemogram includes Platelet Count
(Includes WBC, RBC, HGB, HCT, MCV, MCH, MCHC, RDW [red cell distribution width], MPV [mean platelet volume], and platelet count)
CPT: 85027
NLA: $8.95

Hemosiderin, Urine
CPT: 83070
NLA: $6.56

Hepatic Function Panel
(Includes A/G ratio, alanine aminotransferase [ALT], albumin, alkaline phosphatase, aspartate aminotransferase [AST], direct bilirubin, total bilirubin, globulin, and total protein)
CPT: 80076
NLA: $11.29

Hepatitis A Antibody, Total, Serum
CPT: 86708
NLA: $17.12

Hepatitis A Antibody IgM, Serum
CPT: 86709
NLA: $15.55

Hepatitis B Core Antibody, Serum
CPT: 86704
NLA: $16.66

Hepatitis B Core Antibody IgM, Serum
CPT: 86705
NLA: $16.27

Hepatitis B Surface Antibody, Serum
CPT: 86706
NLA: $14.84

Hepatitis B Surface Antibody, Qualitative, Serum
CPT: 86706
NLA: $14.84

Hepatitis B Surface Antigen, Serum
If borderline or positive, confirmation by neutralization will be performed (CPT: 87341 NLA: $14.27).
CPT: 87340
NLA: $14.27

Hepatitis B Viral DNA (Viral Load), Quantitative, Serum
CPT: 87517
NLA: NA

Hepatitis Be Antibody, Serum
CPT: 86707
NLA: $15.98

Hepatitis Be Antigen, Serum
CPT: 87350
NLA: $15.92

Hepatitis C Antibody, RIBA
CPT: 86804
NLA: $21.40

IV

Test Information

Hepatitis C Antibody, Serum
CPT: 86803
NLA: $19.73

Hepatitis C Viral RNA, Qualitative PCR
CPT: 87521
NLA: NA

Hepatitis C Viral RNA (Viral Load), Quantitative, bDNA, Serum
CPT: 87522
NLA: NA

Hepatitis C Viral RNA (Viral Load), Quantitative, PCR, Serum
CPT: 87522
NLA: NA

Hepatitis Panel, Acute, with Reflex
(Includes hepatitis A antibody, IgM, hepatitis B surface antigen, hepatitis B core antibody, IgM, and hepatitis C antibody)
> If hepatitis B surface antigen is borderline or positive, confirmation by neutralization will be performed (CPT: 87341 NLA: $14.27).

CPT: 80074
NLA: NA

Histamine, Urine
CPT: 83088
NLA: NA

HIV-1 Antibody Confirmation by Western Blot
CPT: 86689
NLA: $26.75

HIV-1 Antibody with Reflex to Confirmation of Positive Results by Western Blot
If positive, Western blot confirmation will be performed (CPT: 86689 NLA: $26.75).

HIV-1 Culture
(Includes antigen capture EIA test)
CPT: 87390/87252
NLA: $24.38/$36.02

HIV-1 DNA, Qualitative PCR
CPT: 87535
NLA: NA

HIV-1 RNA, PCR, 1st Generation
CPT: 87536
NLA: $117.59

HIV-1 RNA, Quantitative PCR, 2nd Generation
CPT: 87536
NLA: $117.59

HLA-B8, Blood
CPT: 86812
NLA: $35.66

HLA-B27, Blood
CPT: 86812
NLA: $35.66

Test Information

HLA A and B Typing, Blood
CPT: 86813
NLA: $80.13

Homocysteine (Cardio), Serum
CPT: 83090
NLA: $23.31

HPV (Human Papillomavirus), DNA
(Includes low and intermediate/high risk probes)
CPT: 87621 (×2)
NLA: $48.50 (×2)

HTLV-I/II Antibody, Serum
Com: There is no FDA-approved confirmatory test for HTLV-I or HTLV-II antibody.
CPT: 86790
NLA: $17.81

5-Hydroxyindoleacetic Acid (5-HIAA), Urine
CPT: 83497
NLA: $17.82

17-Hydroxyprogesterone, Serum
CPT: 83498
NLA: $37.54

Ibuprofen, Serum
CPT: 80299
NLA: $18.92

IgA, Serum
CPT: 82784
NLA: $12.85

IgD, Serum
CPT: 82784
NLA: $12.85

IgE, Serum or Plasma
CPT: 82785
NLA: $22.76

IGF-I (Somatomedin-C), Serum
CPT: 84305
NLA: $29.38

IgG, CSF
CPT: 82784
NLA: $12.85

IgG/Albumin Ratio, CSF
(Includes IgG and albumin)
CPT: 82042/82784
NLA: $7.15/$12.85

IgG, Serum
CPT: 82784
NLA: $12.85

IgM, Serum
CPT: 82784
NLA: $12.85

Imipramine and Desipramine, Serum
CPT: 80174/80160
NLA: $23.79/$23.79

Test Information

Immunofixation, Serum
CPT: 86334
NLA: $30.87

Immunofixation, Urine
CPT: 86334
NLA: $30.87

Immunoglobulins IgG, IgA and IgM, CSF
CPT: 82784 (×3)
NLA: $12.85 (×3)

Immunoglobulins IgG, IgA and IgM, Serum
CPT: 82784 (×3)
NLA: $12.85 (×3)

Influenza Antibodies
(Includes types A and B)
CPT: 86710 (×2)
NLA: $18.74 (×2)

Inhibin, Serum
CPT: 83520
NLA: NA

Insulin, Serum
CPT: 83525
NLA: $15.81

Interleukin 2 (IL-2), Serum
CPT: 83520
NLA: NA

Interleukin 2 Receptor (IL-2R), Serum
CPT: 84238
NLA: NA

Iron, Serum
CPT: 83540
NLA: $8.95

Iron and Total Iron Binding Capacity, Serum
(Includes transferring percent saturation)
CPT: 83540/83550
NLA: $8.95/$12.08

Jo-1 Antibody, Serum
CPT: 86235
NLA: $24.78

Lactate Dehydrogenase (LD), Serum
CPT: 83615
NLA: $8.35

Lactate Dehydrogenase (LD), Fluid
CPT: 83615
NLA: $8.35

Lactate Dehydrogenase Isoenzymes (LDI), Serum
(Includes total lactate dehydrogenase (LD))
CPT: 83625/83615
NLA: $17.69/$8.35

Lamotrigine, Serum
CPT: 80299
NLA: $18.92

Test Information

Lead, Blood
CPT: 83655
NLA: $16.72

Lecithin/Sphingomyelin (L/S) Ratio, Amniotic Fluid
CPT: 83661
NLA: $30.38

Legionella Antigen, Urine
CPT: 87449
NLA: $16.58

Legionella pneumophila Antibody, Serum
CPT: 86713
NLA: $21.15

Leukocyte Alkaline Phosphatase (LAP)
CPT: 85540
NLA: $11.88

Lidocaine, Serum
CPT: 80176
NLA: $20.30

Lipase, Serum
CPT: 83690
NLA: $9.52

Lipid Panel
(Includes cholesterol, HDL cholesterol, calculated LDL cholesterol, triglycerides, and cholesterol/HDL ratio)
CPT: 80061
NLA: NA

Lithium, Serum
CPT: 80178
NLA: $9.13

Lorazepam, Serum
CPT: 80154
NLA: $25.56

Low-Density Lipoprotein (LDL) Cholesterol, Direct, Serum
CPT: 83721
NLA: $13.18

Luteinizing Hormone (LH), Serum
CPT: 83002
NLA: $25.60

Lyme
see Borrelia burgdorferi

Magnesium, Serum
CPT: 83735
NLA: $9.26

Malaria, Blood Smear
CPT: 87207
NLA: $8.28

IV

Test Information

Maternal Serum Biochemical Double Marker
(Includes alpha fetoprotein (AFP) and chorionic gonadotropin (hCG))
Com: No laboratory assay has been approved by the FDA for screening of Down syndrome. Any estimate of risk for Down syndrome based on AFP results is for investigational use only.
CPT: 82105/84702
NLA: $23.18/$20.80

Maternal Serum Biochemical Triple Marker
(Includes alpha fetoprotein (AFP), chorionic gonadotropin (hCG), and free estriol)
Com: No laboratory assay has been approved by the FDA for screening of Down syndrome. Any estimate of risk for Down syndrome based on AFP results is for investigational use only.
CPT: 82105/84702/82677
NLA: $23.18/$20.80/$33.43

Meprobamate, Serum
CPT: 83805
NLA: $24.36

Metanephrines, Fractionated, Urine
CPT: 83835
NLA: $23.41

Methotrexate, Serum
CPT: 80299
NLA: $18.92

Microsporidia, Body Fluid or Stool
CPT: 87207
NLA: $8.28

Mitochondrial Antibody, Serum
If screen is positive, a titer will automatically be performed (CPT: 86256 NLA: $16.66).
CPT: 86255
NLA: $16.66

Mononucleosis Screen, Serum
CPT: 86308
NLA: $7.15

Mumps Virus Antibody IgG, Serum
CPT: 86735
NLA: $18.03

Mycobacteria Culture, Blood
(Includes acid fast bacilli smear) positive isolates are identified by nucleic acid hybridization or conventional methods when appropriate (CPT: 87118 or 87149 NLA: $15.13 or $27.71). Antibiotic sensitivities for *M. tuberculosis* isolates will be performed (CPT: 87190 ($\times$5) NLA: $7.81 ($\times$5)).
CPT: 87116/87206
NLA: $14.93/$7.42

Test Information

Mycobacteria Culture, Sputum
(Includes acid fast bacilli smear) Positive isolates are identified by nucleic acid hybridization or conventional methods when appropriate (CPT: 87118 or 87149 NLA: $15.13 or $27.71). Antibiotic sensitivities for *M. tuberculosis* isolates will be performed (CPT: 87190 ($\times$5) NLA: $7.81 ($\times$5).
CPT: 87015/87116/87206
NLA: $9.23/$14.93/$7.42

Mycobacteria Culture, Urine
(Includes acid fast bacilli smear) Positive isolates are identified by nucleic acid hybridization or conventional methods when appropriate (CPT: 87118 or 87149 NLA: $15.13 or $27.71). Antibiotic sensitivities for *M. tuberculosis* isolates will be performed (CPT: 87190 ($\times$5) NLA: $7.81 ($\times$5).
CPT: 87015/87116/87206
NLA: $9.23/$14.93/$7.42

Mycobacterium Stain
Additional charge if concentration is required (CPT: 87015 NLA: $9.23)
CPT: 87206
NLA: $7.42

Mycoplasma pneumoniae Antibody (IgG), EIA, Serum
CPT: 86738
NLA: $18.31

Mycoplasma pneumoniae Antibody (IgM), Serum
CPT: 86738
NLA: $18.31

Mycoplasma pneumoniae Culture, Respiratory
CPT: 87109
NLA: $21.26

Myoglobin, Urine
CPT: 83874
NLA: $17.84

Neisseria gonorrhoeae, Anal Culture
Antibiotic sensitivities and identification will be performed on *Neisseria gonorrhoeae* isolated. See Antibiotic Sensitivity and Identification.
CPT: 87081
NLA: $9.16

Neisseria gonorrhoeae, Genital Culture
Antibiotic sensitivities and identification will be performed on *Neisseria gonorrhoeae* isolated. See Antibiotic Sensitivity and Identification.
CPT: 87081
NLA: $9.16

Neisseria gonorrhoeae, DNA Probe, (Female Endocervical or Male Urethral)
CPT: 87590
NLA: $27.71

Test Information

Neopterin, Serum
CPT: 83519
NLA: NA

Neuron Specific Enolase (NSE), Serum
CPT: 83520
NLA: $17.89

Nortriptyline, Serum
CPT: 80182
NLA: $18.72

5'Nucleotidase, Serum
CPT: 83915
NLA: $15.41

Obstetric Panel with Reflex
(Includes antibody screen with reflex, blood group and Rh type; CBC includes differential and platelet count with reflex to manual differential, hepatitis B surface antigen with reflex, RPR with reflex, and Rubella antibody, IgG [immune status])

     If antibody screen is positive, antibody identification and titer will be performed (CPT: 86870/86886 NLA: NA/$7.15).
     If hepatitis B surface antigen is borderline or positive, confirmation by neutralization will be performed (CPT: 87341 NLA: $14.27).
     If RPR screen is reactive, a titer will be performed (CPT: 86593 NLA: $6.09) and confirmation by FTA-ABS will be performed (CPT: 86781 NLA: $18.30).

CPT: 80055
NLA: NA

Occult Blood, Stool, Diagnostic (1 Paper Slide)
CPT: 82270
NLA: $4.49

Occult Blood, Stool, Screening (1 Paper Slide)
CPT: G0107
NLA: $3.50

Occult Blood, Stool, Diagnostic (3 Paper Slides)
CPT: 82270
NLA: $4.49

Occult Blood, Stool, Screening (3 Paper Slides)
CPT: G0107
NLA: $3.50

Oligoclonal Bands, CSF
CPT: 83916
NLA: $27.79

Osmolality, Serum
CPT: 83930
NLA: $9.13

Osmolality, Urine
CPT: 83935
NLA: $9.42

Test Information

Osteocalcin, Serum
CPT: 83937
NLA: NA

Ova and Parasites, Single Set, Stool
(Includes concentration and stain)
CPT: 87177/88312
NLA: $12.30/NA

Ova and Parasites, Three Sets, Stool
(Includes concentration and stain. Testing performed on 3 sets of paired samples.)
CPT: 87177 (×3)/88312 (×3)
NLA: $12.30 (×3)/NA

Oxalate, Urine
CPT: 83945
NLA: $17.80

Oxazepam, Serum
CPT: 80154
NLA: $25.56

Parathyroid Hormone (PTH), Intact, Serum
(Includes calcium)
CPT: 83970/82310
NLA: $57.04/$7.12

Parietal Cell Antibody, Serum
If screen is positive, a titer will automatically be performed (CPT: 86256 NLA: $16.66).
CPT: 86255
NLA: $16.66

Parvovirus B-19 Antibody IgG and IgM, Serum
CPT: 86747 (×2)
NLA: $20.77 (×2)

Pentobarbital, Serum
CPT: 82205
NLA: $15.83

Phenobarbital, Serum
CPT: 80184
NLA: $15.83

Phenothiazines, Qualitative, Urine
CPT: 80101
NLA: $19.03

Phenotype, Red Blood Cell Antigens, Blood
The CPT and NLA listed is for one antigen.
CPT: 86905
NLA: $5.28

Phenotype, Red Blood Cell Rh Antigens, Blood
(Includes red blood cell antigens D, C, c, E, e)
CPT: 86906
NLA: $10.71

Phenylalanine, Plasma
CPT: 84030
NLA: $7.61

IV

Test Information

Phenytoin (Dilantin), Serum
CPT: 80185
NLA: $18.32

Phosphate (as Phosphorus), Serum
CPT: 84100
NLA: $6.56

Phosphate (as Phosphorus), Urine
CPT: 84105
NLA: $7.15

Platelet Antibody, Indirect, IgG
CPT: 86022
NLA: $25.38

Platelet Count, Blood
CPT: 85595
NLA: $6.18

Porphobilinogen, Quantitative, Urine
CPT: 84110
NLA: $11.68

Porphyrins, Fractionated, Urine
(Includes coproporphyrin, heptacarboxyporphyrin, hexacarboxyporphyrin, pentacarboxyporphyrin, porphobilinogen, total porphyrins, and uroporphyrin)
CPT: 84120/84110
NLA: $20.33/$11.68

Porphyrins, Stool
(Includes coproporphyrin (tetracarboxyl), uroporphyrin (octacarboxyl), heptacarboxyporphyrin, and protoporphyrin (dicarboxyporphyrin))
CPT: 84126
NLA: $35.20

Potassium, Fluid
CPT: 84999
NLA: NA

Potassium, Serum
CPT: 84132
NLA: $6.35

Potassium, Urine
CPT: 84133
NLA: $5.94

Prealbumin, Serum
CPT: 84134
NLA: $20.16

Procainamide and N-Acetylprocainamide, Serum
CPT: 80192
NLA: $23.15

Progesterone, Serum
CPT: 84144
NLA: $28.83

Prolactin, Serum
CPT: 84146
NLA: $26.78

Test Information

Propoxyphene and Norpropoxyphene, Serum or Plasma
CPT: 80299
NLA: $18.92

Propranolol, Serum
CPT: 80299
NLA: $18.92

Prostate Specific Antigen (PSA), Serum, Diagnostic
CPT: 84153
NLA: $25.42

Prostate Specific Antigen (PSA), Serum, Screening
CPT: G0103
NLA: $25.42

Prostate Specific Antigen (PSA), Free, Serum
(Includes total prostate specific antigen)
CPT: 84153/84154
NLA: $25.42/$25.42

Protein C, Antigenic, Plasma
CPT: 85302
NLA: $16.61

Protein C, Functional, Plasma
CPT: 85303
NLA: $19.11

Protein S, Antigenic, Plasma
CPT: 85305
NLA: $16.02

Protein S, Functional, Plasma
CPT: 85306
NLA: $21.18

Protein, Total, Serum
CPT: 84155
NLA: $5.06

Protein, Total, Urine
CPT: 84155
NLA: $5.06

Protein Electrophoresis, Serum
(Includes quantitative total protein)
CPT: 84165/84155
NLA: $14.84/$5.06

Protein Electrophoresis, Random Urine
(Includes quantitative total protein)
CPT: 84165/84155
NLA: $14.84/$5.06

Prothrombin Time (PT) (INR), Blood
CPT: 85610
NLA: $5.43

Quinidine, Serum
CPT: 80194
NLA: $20.17

Renin Activity (PRA), Plasma
CPT: 84244
NLA: $30.40

Test Information

Respiratory Syncytial Virus (RSV), Direct Antigen
CPT: 87420
NLA: $16.58

Respiratory Syncytial Virus (RSV) Culture
If culture is positive, a fluorescent antibody stain will be performed (CPT: 87253 NLA: $27.91).
CPT: 87252
NLA: $36.02

Reticulocyte Count, Blood
CPT: 85045
NLA: $5.54

Rh Type, Blood
CPT: 86901
NLA: NA

Rheumatoid Factor, Serum
CPT: 86431
NLA: $7.85

Rotavirus Antigen, Stool
CPT: 87425
NLA: $16.58

RPR, (Rapid Plasma Reagin), Serum, Diagnostic
If RPR screen is reactive, a titer will be performed (CPT: 86593 NLA: $6.09) and confirmation will be performed (CPT: 86781 NLA: $18.30).
CPT: 86592
NLA: $5.90

RPR, (Rapid Plasma Reagin), Serum, Monitoring
If RPR screen is reactive, a titer will be performed (CPT: 86593 NLA: $6.09).
CPT: 86592
NLA: $5.90

Rubella Antibody IgG, Immune Status, Serum
CPT: 86762
NLA: $19.89

Rubella Antibody IgG, Serum
(Use this test in conjunction with rubella AB IgM to help in the diagnosis of acute infection)
CPT: 86762
NLA: $19.89

Rubella Antibody IgM, Serum
CPT: 86762
NLA: $19.89

Rubeola (Measles) Antibody IgG, Serum
Recommended test for immune status
CPT: 86765
NLA: $17.81

Salicylates, Serum
CPT: 80196
NLA: $9.81

Scl-70 Antibody, EIA, Serum
CPT: 86235
NLA: $24.78

Test Information

Secobarbital, Serum
CPT: 82205
NLA: $15.83

Sedimentation Rate
see Erythrocyte Sedimentation Rate (ESR), Westergren

Serotonin, Blood
CPT: 84260
NLA: $42.81

Sickle Cell Screen, Blood
Com: Test not recommended for patients less than 6 months of age.
CPT: 85660
NLA: $7.63

Sjögren's Antibody, Serum
(Includes SS-A and SS-B)
CPT: 86235 (×2)
NLA: $24.78 (×2)

Smooth Muscle Antibody, Serum
If screen is positive, a titer will automatically be performed (CPT: 86256 NLA: $16.66).
CPT: 86255
NLA: $16.66

Sodium, Serum
CPT: 84295
NLA: $6.65

Sodium, Urine
CPT: 84300
NLA: $6.72

Stool Examination, Qualitative
CPT: 82705
NLA: $7.04

Streptococci Group A Culture, Throat
Serological grouping of streptococci isolated will be performed (CPT: 87147 NLA: $7.15).
CPT: 87081
NLA: $9.16

Streptococci Group A, DNA Probe
CPT: 87650
NLA: $27.71

Streptococci Group A Antigen
A negative result is only presumptive, and a culture should be performed to reasonably exclude the diagnosis of group A streptococcal infection.
CPT: 87430
NLA: $16.58

Streptococci Group B Culture
Serological grouping of streptococci isolated will be performed (CPT: 87147 NLA: $7.15).
CPT: 87081
NLA: $9.16

IV

Test Information

Streptozyme (Streptococcal Exoenzymes), Serum
CPT: 86403
NLA: $14.08

Streptozyme Titer, Serum
CPT: 86406
NLA: $14.70

Striated Muscle Antibody, Serum
If screen is positive, a titer will automatically be performed (CPT: 86256 NLA: $16.66).
CPT: 86255
NLA: $16.66

Syphilis Confirmation, Serum
CPT: 86781
NLA: $18.30

T3 (Triiodothyronine), Free, Serum
CPT: 84481
NLA: $23.41

T3 (Triiodothyronine), Total, Serum
CPT: 84480
NLA: $19.60

T3 Uptake, Serum
CPT: 84479
NLA: $8.95

T4, Free, Serum
CPT: 84439
NLA: $12.46

T4 (Thyroxine), Total, Serum
CPT: 84436
NLA: $9.50

Testosterone, Total, Serum
CPT: 84403
NLA: $35.68

Testosterone, Total and Free, Serum or Plasma
(Includes total testosterone, free testosterone, and percent free testosterone)
CPT: 84402/84403
NLA: $35.19/$35.68

Theophylline, Serum
CPT: 80198
NLA: $19.56

Thrombin Time (TT), Blood
CPT: 85670
NLA: $7.98

Thyroglobulin Antibody, Serum
CPT: 86800
NLA: $21.98

Thyroglobulin and Anti-Thyroglobulin Antibodies, Serum
CPT: 86800/84432
NLA: $21.98/22.20

Test Information

Thyroid Peroxidase Antibody (Anti-TPO), Serum
CPT: 86376
NLA: $20.11

Thyroid-Stimulating Hormone (TSH), Serum
CPT: 84443
NLA: $23.21

Thyroid-Stimulating Hormone (TSH) with Free T4 Reflex, Serum
If TSH is ≤ 0.10 **or** ≥ 10.00 mU/L, Free T4 will be performed (CPT: 84439 NLA: $12.46).
CPT: 84443
NLA: $23.21

Thyroid-Stimulating Immunoglobulin (TSI), Serum
CPT: 84445
NLA: $70.28

Thyroxine-Binding Globulin (TBG), Serum
CPT: 84442
NLA: $20.44

Tissue Pathology
Complexity Level
CPT: 88302, 88304, 88305, 88307, 88309
NLA: NA
When bony tissue is received, there is an additional charge (CPT: 88311 NLA: NA) which will be applied for the decalcification process.
If, in the opinion of the pathologist, special stains or studies (including immunocytochemistry) are essential, those tests will be performed at an additional charge.

Tissue Pathology, Immunocytochemistry
Com: CPT and NLA listed is for one antigen; an additional charge will be applied for added antigens.
CPT: 88342
NLA: NA

Tobramycin, Peak, Serum
CPT: 80200
NLA: $22.27

Tobramycin, Trough, Serum
CPT: 80200
NLA: $22.27

Toxoplasma gondii Antibody IgG, Serum
CPT: 86777
NLA: $19.89

Toxoplasma gondii Antibody IgG & IgM, Serum
CPT: 86777/86778
NLA: $19.89/$19.90

Transferrin, Serum
CPT: 84466
NLA: $17.65

Trichomonas vaginalis Culture
(Includes smear)
CPT: 87081/87210
NLA: $9.16/$5.90

Test Information

Trichomonas vaginalis, Direct Identification
CPT: 87299
NLA: $16.58

Triglycerides, Serum
CPT: 84478
NLA: $7.95

Trimethadione and Dimethadione, Serum or Plasma
CPT: 82654
NLA: $19.14

Trimipramine, Serum
CPT: 80299
NLA: $18.92

Troponin I (cTnI), Serum
CPT: 84484
NLA: $13.60

Urea Nitrogen (BUN), Serum
CPT: 84520
NLA: $5.45

Urea Nitrogen, 24 Hour Urine
CPT: 84540
NLA: $6.56

Ureaplasma urealyticum and Mycoplasma hominis Culture, Genital
CPT: 87109
NLA: $21.26

Uric Acid, Joint Fluid
CPT: 84560
NLA: $6.56

Uric Acid, Serum
CPT: 84550
NLA: $6.25

Uric Acid, Urine
CPT: 84560
NLA: $6.56

Urinalysis, Screen
(Includes macro and dipstick)
(Includes bilirubin, blood, glucose, ketone, leukocyte esterase, nitrite, pH, protein, and specific gravity)
CPT: 81003
NLA: $3.10

Urinalysis, Screen with Reflex Microscopic
(Includes macro and dipstick)
If nitrite, leukocyte esterase, blood, or protein are not negative, microscopic exam will be performed and the CPT code will change to 81001 (NLA: $4.37).
CPT: 81003
NLA: $3.10

Urinalysis, Complete
(Includes macro, dipstick, and microscopic)
CPT: 81001
NLA: $4.37

Test Information

Urogram
see Urinalysis screen (includes macro and dipstick)

Valproic Acid, Serum
CPT: 80164
NLA: $18.72

Vancomycin, Peak, Serum
CPT: 80202
NLA: $18.72

Vancomycin, Trough, Serum
CPT: 80202
NLA: $18.72

Vanillylmandelic Acid (VMA), Urine
CPT: 84585
NLA: $21.42

Varicella-Zoster Virus (VZV) Antibody IgG, Serum
Recommended test for immune status due to a previous infection but is unsuitable for the detection of post-vaccination immune status.
CPT: 86787
NLA: $17.81

Varicella-Zoster Virus (VZV) Antibody IgM, Serum
CPT: 86787
NLA: $17.81

VDRL, CSF
CPT: 86592
NLA: $5.90

Viral Culture
Detection of virus may require additional tests (CPT: 87253 NLA: $27.91) and/or typing of positive culture (CPT: 87140 NLA: $7.71).
CPT: 87252
NLA: $36.02

Vitamin A (Retinol), Serum or Plasma
CPT: 84590
NLA: $16.02

Vitamin B6 (Pyridoxine), Serum or Plasma
CPT: 84207
NLA: $38.82

Vitamin B12 (Cyanocobalamin), Serum
CPT: 82607
NLA: $20.83

Vitamin C (Ascorbic Acid), Serum
CPT: 82180
NLA: $13.66

Vitamin D, 25-Hydroxy, Serum or Plasma
CPT: 82306
NLA: $40.91

Vitamin D, 1,25-Dihydroxy, Serum
CPT: 82652
NLA: $53.19

IV

Test Information

WBC Count

CPT: 85048
NLA: $3.52

Xylose Absorption, 2 Hour Blood

CPT: 84620
NLA: $16.37

Xylose Absorption, 5 Hour Urine

CPT: 84620
NLA: $16.37

Yeast Culture

Identification on each pathogen isolated will be performed (CPT: 87106/87107 NLA: $14.27/$14.27).

CPT: 87102
NLA: $11.61

Test Information

Yersinia Culture

Antibiotic sensitivities and identification will be performed on each pathogen isolated. See Antibiotic Sensitivity and Identification.

CPT: 87046
NLA: $3.26

Zinc Protoporphyrin (FEP, Free Erythrocyte Protoporphyrin)

CPT: 84202
NLA: $19.83

- **ACE LEVEL;** see ANGIOTENSIN-CONVERTING ENZYME
- **ACETONE** (serum or plasma)
  Normal:
  Negative
  Cost: $40
  Elevated in:
  DKA, starvation, isopropanol ingestion
- **ACID-BASE REFERENCE VALUES;** *see* Tables 4-1 and 4-2.
- **ACID PHOSPHATASE** (serum)
  Normal range:
  0-5.5 U/L (0-90 nkat/L) [CF: 16.67; SMI: 2 nkat/L]
  Cost: $24

Elevated in:
Carcinoma of prostate, other neoplasms (breast, bone), Paget's disease, osteogenesis imperfecta, malignant invasion of bone, Gaucher's disease, multiple myeloma, myeloproliferative disorders, benign prostatic hypertrophy, prostatic palpation or surgery, hyperparathyroidism, liver disease, chronic renal failure, idiopathic thrombocytopenic purpura, bronchitis
- **ACID SERUM TEST;** *see* HAM TEST
- **ACTIVATED PARTIAL THROMBOPLASTIN TIME** (APTT, aPTT); *see* PARTIAL THROMBOPLASTIN TIME

TABLE 4-1 Commonly Used Acid-Base Reference Values for Arterial and Venous Plasma or Serum (Averaged from Various Sources)

	ARTERIAL		VENOUS	
	CONVENTIONAL UNITS	SI UNITS*	CONVENTIONAL UNITS	SI UNITS*
pH	7.40 (7.35-7.45)	7.40 (7.35-7.45)	7.37 (7.32-7.42)	7.37 (7.32-7.42)
P_{CO_2}	40 mm Hg (35-45)	5.33 kPa (4.67-6.10)	45 mm Hg (45-50)	6.10 kPa (5.33-6.67)
P_{O_2}	80-100 mm Hg	10.66-13.33 kPa	40 mm Hg (37-43)	5.33 kPa (4.93-5.73)
HCO_3 (CO_2 combining power)	24 mEq/L (20-28)	24 mmol/L (20-28)	26 mEq/L (22-30)	26 mmol/L (22-30)
CO_2 content	25 mEq/L (22-28)	25 mmol/L (22-28)	27 mEq/L (24-30)	27 mmol/L (24-30)

From Ravel R: *Clinical laboratory medicine,* ed 6, St Louis, 1995, Mosby.
*International system.

TABLE 4-2 Summary of Laboratory Findings in Primary Uncomplicated Respiratory and Metabolic Acid-Base Disorders*

DISORDER	P_{CO_2}	pH	BASE EXCESS
Acute primary respiratory hypoactivity (respiratory acidosis)	Increase	Decrease	Normal/positive
Acute primary respiratory hyperactivity (respiratory alkalosis)	Decrease	Increase	Normal/negative
Uncompensated metabolic acidosis	Normal	Decrease	Negative
Uncompensated metabolic alkalosis	Normal	Increase	Positive
Partially compensated metabolic acidosis	Decrease	Decrease	Negative
Partially compensated metabolic alkalosis	Increase	Increase	Positive
Chronic primary respiratory hypoactivity (compensated respiratory acidosis)	Increase	Normal	Positive
Fully compensated metabolic alkalosis	Increase	Normal	Positive
Chronic primary respiratory hyperactivity (compensated respiratory alkalosis)	Decrease	Normal	Negative
Fully compensated metabolic acidosis	Decrease	Normal	Negative

From Ravel R: *Clinical laboratory medicine,* ed 6, St Louis, 1995, Mosby.
*Base excess results refer to negative (−) values more than −2 and positive (+) values more than +2.

IV

- **ALANINE AMINOTRANSFERASE** (ALT, SGPT)
Normal range:
0-35 U/L (0.058 μkat/L) [CF: 0.02 μkat/L]
Cost: $23
Elevated in:
Liver disease (hepatitis, cirrhosis, Reye's syndrome), hepatic congestion, infectious mononucleosis, myocardial infarction, myocarditis, severe muscle trauma, dermatomyositis/polymyositis, muscular dystrophy, drugs (antibiotics, narcotics, antihypertensive agents, heparin, labetalol, statins, NSAIDs, amiodarone, chlorpromazine, phenytoin), malignancy, renal and pulmonary infarction, convulsions, eclampsia, shock liver

- **ALBUMIN** (serum)
Normal range:
4-6 g/dl (40-60 g/L) [CF: 10; SMI: 1 g/L]
Cost: $23
Elevated in:
Dehydration (relative increase)
Decreased in:
Liver disease, nephrotic syndrome, poor nutritional status, rapid IV hydration, protein-losing enteropathies (inflammatory bowel disease), severe burns, neoplasia, chronic inflammatory diseases, pregnancy, oral contraceptives, prolonged immobilization, lymphomas, hypervitaminosis A, chronic glomerulonephritis

- **ALDOLASE** (serum)
Normal range:
0-6 U/L (0-100 nkat/L) [CF: 16.67; SMI: 20 nkat/L]
Cost: $37
Elevated in:
Muscular dystrophy, rhabdomyolysis, dermatomyositis/polymyositis, trichinosis, acute hepatitis and other liver diseases, myocardial infarction, prostatic carcinoma, hemorrhagic pancreatitis, gangrene, delirium tremens, burns
Decreased in:
Loss of muscle mass, late stages of muscular dystrophy

- **ALDOSTERONE**
Normal range:
Recumbent: 50-150 ng/L
Upright: 150-300 ng/L

(Highest levels in neonates, decreasing over time to adult levels)
Cost: $123
Elevated in:
Primary aldosteronism, secondary aldosteronism, pseudoprimary aldosteronism
Decreased in:
Patient with hypertension: diabetes mellitus, Turner's syndrome, acute alcohol intoxication, excess secretion of deoxycorticosterone, corticosterone, and 18-hydroxycorticosterone
Patient without hypertension: Addison's disease, hypoaldosteronism resulting from renin deficiency, isolated aldosterone deficiency

- **ALKALINE PHOSPHATASE** (serum)
Normal range:
30-120 U/L (0.5-2 μkat/L) [CF: 0.01667; SMI: 0.1 μkat/L]
Cost: $23
Elevated in:
Biliary obstruction, cirrhosis (particularly primary biliary cirrhosis), liver disease (hepatitis, infiltrative liver diseases, fatty metamorphosis), Paget's disease of bone, osteitis deformans, rickets, osteomalacia, hypervitaminosis D, hyperparathyroidism, hyperthyroidism, ulcerative colitis, bowel perforation, bone metastases, healing fractures, bone neoplasms, acromegaly, infectious mononucleosis, cytomegalovirus infections, sepsis, pulmonary infarction, congestive heart failure, hypernephroma, leukemia, myelofibrosis, multiple myeloma, drugs (estrogens, albumin, erythromycin and other antibiotics, cholestasis-producing drugs [phenothiazines]), pregnancy, puberty, others (Boxes 4-1 and 4-2)
Decreased in:
Hypothyroidism, pernicious anemia, hypophosphatemia, hypervitaminosis D, malnutrition

- **ALPHA-1-FETOPROTEIN** (serum); *see* α-1 FETOPROTEIN
- **ALT;** *see* ALANINE AMINOTRANSFERASE
- **AMMONIA** (serum)
Normal range:
10-80 μg/dl (5-50 μmol/L) [CF: 0.5872; SMI: 5 μmol/L]

BOX 4-1 **Isolated Elevation of Alkaline Phosphatase**

ALP Level Increased
AST Level Normal
Total Bilirubin Level Normal

Liver space-occupying lesions
Bone osteoblastic activity increased

Drug-induced (Dilantin most common)
Intrahepatic cholestatic process in advanced stage of resolution
Pregnancy (third trimester)
Hyperthyroidism
Hyperparathyroidism

From Ravel R: *Clinical laboratory medicine,* ed 6, St Louis, 1995, Mosby.

BOX 4-2   Most Common Causes for Alkaline Phosphatase Elevation

Liver and Biliary Tract Origin

Extrahepatic bile duct obstruction
Intrahepatic biliary obstruction
   Liver cell acute injury
   Liver passive congestion
   Drug-induced liver cell dysfunction
Space-occupying lesions
Primary biliary cirrhosis
Sepsis

Bone Origin (Osteoblast Hyperactivity)

Physiologic (rapid) bone growth (childhood and adolescent)
Metastatic tumor with osteoblastic reaction

Fracture healing
Paget's disease of bone

Capillary Endothelial Origin

Granulation tissue formation (active)

Placental Origin

Pregnancy
Some parenteral albumin preparations

Other

Thyrotoxicosis
Benign transient hyperphosphatasemia
Primary hyperparathyroidism

From Ravel R: *Clinical laboratory medicine,* ed 6, St Louis, 1995, Mosby.

Cost: $57
Elevated in:
Hepatic failure, hepatic encephalopathy, Reye's syndrome, portacaval shunt, drugs (diuretics, polymyxin B, methicillin)
Decreased in:
Drugs (neomycin, lactulose, tetracycline), renal failure

- **AMYLASE** (serum)
Normal range:
0-130 U/L (0-2.17 μkat/L) [CF: 0.01667; SMI: 0.01 μkat/L]
Cost: $26
Elevated in:
Acute pancreatitis, pancreatic neoplasm, abscess, pseudocyst, ascites, macroamylasemia, perforated peptic ulcer, intestinal obstruction, intestinal infarction, acute cholecystitis, appendicitis, ruptured ectopic pregnancy, salivary gland inflammation, peritonitis, burns, diabetic ketoacidosis, renal insufficiency, drugs (morphine), carcinomatosis (of lung, esophagus, ovary), acute ethanol ingestion, mumps, prostate tumors, post–endoscopic retrograde cholangiopancreatography, bulimia, anorexia nervosa
Decreased in:
Advanced chronic pancreatitis, hepatic necrosis, cystic fibrosis

- **AMYLASE, URINE;** *see* URINE AMYLASE
- **ANA;** *see* ANTINUCLEAR ANTIBODY
- **ANCA;** *see* ANTINEUTROPHIL CYTOPLASMIC ANTIBODY
- **ANGIOTENSIN-CONVERTING ENZYME** (ACE level)
Normal range:
<40 nmol/ml/min (<670 nkat/L) [CF: 16.67; SMI: 10 nkat/L]
Cost: $58

Elevated in:
Sarcoidosis, primary biliary cirrhosis, alcoholic liver disease, hyperthyroidism, hyperparathyroidism, diabetes mellitus, amyloidosis, multiple myeloma, lung disease (asbestosis, silicosis, berylliosis, allergic alveolitis, coccidioidomycosis), Gaucher's disease, leprosy

- **ANION GAP**
Normal range:
9-14 mEq/L
Elevated in:
Lactic acidosis, ketoacidosis (diabetes, alcoholic starvation), uremia (chronic renal failure), ingestion of toxins (paraldehyde, methanol, salicylates, ethylene glycol), hyperosmolar nonketotic coma, antibiotics (carbenicillin)
Decreased in:
Hypoalbuminemia, severe hypermagnesemia, IgG myeloma, lithium toxicity, laboratory error (falsely decreased sodium or overestimation of bicarbonate or chloride), hypercalcemia of parathyroid origin, antibiotics (e.g., polymyxin)

- **ANTICOAGULANT;** *see* CIRCULATING ANTICOAGULANT
- **ANTI-DNA**
Normal range:
Absent
Cost: $51
Present in:
Systemic lupus erythematosus, chronic active hepatitis, infectious mononucleosis, biliary cirrhosis

- **ANTIGLOMERULAR BASEMENT ANTIBODY;** *see* GLOMERULAR BASEMENT MEMBRANE ANTIBODY
- **ANTIMITOCHONDRIAL ANTIBODY**
Normal range:
<1:20 titer
Cost: $41

IV

Elevated in:

Primary biliary cirrhosis (85% to 95%), chronic active hepatitis (25% to 30%), cryptogenic cirrhosis (25% to 30%)

■ **ANTINEUTROPHIL CYTOPLASMIC ANTIBODY** (ANCA)

Positive test:

Cytoplasmic pattern (cANCA): positive in Wegener's granulomatosis

Perinuclear pattern (pANCA): positive in inflammatory bowel disease, primary biliary cirrhosis, primary sclerosing cholangitis, autoimmune chronic active hepatitis, crescenteric glomerulonephritis

Cost: $89

■ **ANTINUCLEAR ANTIBODY** (ANA)

Normal range:

<1:20 titer

Cost: $49

Positive test:

Systemic lupus erythematosus (more significant if titer >1:160), drugs (phenytoin, ethosuximide, primidone, methyldopa, hydralazine, carbamazepine, penicillin, procainamide, chlorpromazine, griseofulvin, thiazides), chronic active hepatitis, age over 60 years (particularly age over 80 years), rheumatoid arthritis, scleroderma, mixed connective tissue disease, necrotizing vasculitis, Sjögren's syndrome, tuberculosis, pulmonary interstitial fibrosis. Table 4-3 describes diseases associated with ANA subtypes. Fig. 4-1 illustrates various fluorescent ANA test patterns.

■ **ANTI-RNP ANTIBODY;** *see* EXTRACTABLE NUCLEAR ANTIGEN

■ **ANTI-SM (ANTI-SMITH) ANTIBODY;** *see* EXTRACTABLE NUCLEAR ANTIGEN

■ **ANTI-SMOOTH MUSCLE ANTIBODY;** *see* SMOOTH MUSCLE ANTIBODY

■ **ANTISTREPTOLYSIN O TITER** (Streptozyme, ASLO titer)

Normal range for adults:

<160 Todd units

Cost: $32

Elevated in:

Streptococcal upper airway infection, acute rheumatic fever, acute glomerulonephritis, increased levels of β-lipoprotein

NOTE: A fourfold increase in titer between acute and convalescent specimens is diagnostic of streptococcal upper airway infection regardless of the initial titer.

■ **ANTITHROMBIN III**

Normal range:

81% to 120% of normal activity; 17-30 mg/dl

Cost: $38

Decreased in:

Hereditary deficiency of antithrombin III, disseminated intravascular coagulation, pulmonary embolism, cirrhosis, thrombolytic therapy, chronic liver failure, postsurgery, third trimester of pregnancy, oral contraceptives, nephrotic syndrome, IV heparin >3 days, sepsis, acute leukemia, carcinoma, thrombophlebitis

Elevated in:

Warfarin drugs, post–myocardial infarction

■ **ASLO TITER:** *see* ANTISTREPTOLYSIN O TITER

■ **ASPARTATE AMINOTRANSFERASE** (AST, SGOT)

Normal range:

0-35 U/L (0-0.58 μkat/L) [CF: 0.01667, SMI: 0.01 μkat/L]

Cost: $23

Elevated in:

Liver disease (hepatitis, cirrhosis, Reye's syndrome), hepatic congestion, infectious mononucleosis, myocardial infarction, myocarditis, severe muscle trauma, dermatomyositis/polymyositis,

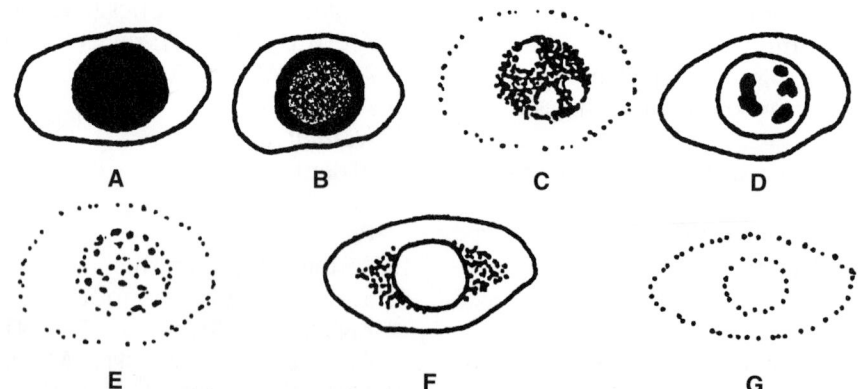

Fig. 4-1   Fluorescent antinuclear antibody test patterns (HEP-2 cells). **A,** Solid (homogeneous). **B,** Peripheral (rim). **C,** Speckled. **D,** Nucleolar. **E,** Anticentromere. **E,** Antimitochondrial. **G,** Normal (nonreactive). (From Ravel R [ed]: *Clinical laboratory medicine,* ed 6, St Louis, 1995, Mosby.)

TABLE 4-3 Disease-Associated ANA Subtypes

NUCLEAR LOCATION	DISEASE(S)
"Native" DNA (dsDNA, or dsDNA/ssDNA complex)	SLE (60%-70%; range, 35%-75%) —also PSS (5%-55%), MCTD (11%-25%), RA (5%-40%), DM (5%-25%), SS (5%)
sNP	SLE (50%) —also other collagen diseases
DNP (DNA-histone complex)	SLE (52%) —also MCTD (8%), RA (3%)
Histones	Drug-induced SLE (95%) —also SLE (30%), RA (15%-24%)
ENA	
Sm	SLE (30%-40%; range, 28%-40%) —also MCTD (0%-8%)
RNP (U1-RNP)	MCTD (in high titer without any other ANA subtype present: 95%-100%) —also SLE (26%-50%), PSS (11%-22%), RA (10%), SS (3%)
SS-A (Ro)*	SS without RA (60%-70%) —also SLE (26%-50%), neonatal SLE (over 95%), PSS (30%), MCTD (50%), SS with RA (9%), PBC (15%-19%)
SS-B (La)	SS without RA (40%-60%) —also SLE (5%-15%), SS with RA (5%)
Scl-70*	PSS (15%-43%)
Centromere*	CREST syndrome (70%-90%; range 57%-96%) —also PSS (4%-20%), PBC (12%)
Nucleolar	PSS (scleroderma) (54%-90%) —also SLE (25%-26%), RA (9%)
RAP (RANA)	SS with RA (60%-76%) —also SS without RA (5%)
Jo-1	Polymyositis (30%)
PM-1	Polymyositis or PMS/PSS overlap syndrome (60%-90%) —also DM (17%)
ssDNA	SLE (60%-70%) —also CAH, infectious mononucleosis, RA, chronic GN, chronic infections, PBC

CYTOPLASMIC LOCATION	DISEASE(S)
Mitochondrial	Primary biliary cirrhosis (90%-100%) —also CAH (7%-30%), cryptogenic cirrhosis (30%), acute hepatitis, viral hepatitis (3%), other liver diseases (0%-20%), SLE (5%), SS and PSS (8%)
Microsomal†	Chronic active hepatitis (60%-80%), Hashimoto's thyroiditis (97%)
Ribosomal	SLE (5%-12%)
Smooth muscle‡	Chronic active hepatitis (60%-91%) —also cryptogenic cirrhosis (28%), acute hepatitis, viral hepatitis (5%-87%), infectious mononucleosis (81%), MS (40%-50%), malignancy (67%), PBC (10%-50%)

From Ravel R: *Clinical laboratory medicine*, ed 6, St Louis, 1995, Mosby.
CAH, Chronic active hepatitis; *DM,* dermatomyositis; *GN,* glomerulonephritis; *MS,* multiple sclerosis; *PBC,* primary biliary cirrhosis; *SS,* Sjögren's syndrome.
*Not detected using rat or mouse liver or kidney tissue method.
†Not detected by cultured cell method.
‡Detected by cultured cells but better with rat or mouse tissue.

muscular dystrophy, drugs (antibiotics, narcotics, antihypertensive agents, heparin, labetalol, statins, NSAIDs, phenytoin, amiodarone, chlorpromazine), malignancy, renal and pulmonary infarction, convulsions, eclampsia, other (Boxes 4-3 and 4-4).

■ BASOPHIL COUNT
Normal range:
0.4% to 1% of total WBC; 40-100/mm³
Elevated in:
Leukemia, inflammatory processes, polycythemia vera, Hodgkin's lymphoma, hemolytic anemia, after splenectomy, myeloid metaplasia, myxedema

IV

BOX 4-3   Some Etiologies for Aspartate Aminotransferase Values Over 1000 IU/ml

Liver Origin

Acute hepatitis, viral hepatitis
Chronic active hepatitis (occasional patients; 16% in one study)
Reye's syndrome
Severe liver passive congestion or hypoxia (with or without acute MI, shock, or sepsis)

Drug-induced (e.g., acetaminophen)
HELLP syndrome of pregnancy (some patients)

Other

First 2-3 days of acute common bile duct obstruction

Acute myocardial infarct (occasional patients)
Severe rhabdomyolysis

From Ravel R: *Clinical laboratory medicine,* ed 6, St Louis, 1995, Mosby.

BOX 4-4   Some Etiologies for Aspartate Aminotransferase Elevation

Heart

Acute myocardial infarction
Pericarditis (active: some cases)

Liver

Hepatitis virus, Epstein-Barr, or cytomegalovirus infection
Active cirrhosis
Liver passive congestion or hypoxia
Alcohol or drug-induced liver dysfunction
Space-occupying lesions (active)
Fatty liver (severe)

Extrahepatic biliary obstruction (early)
Drug-induced

Skeletal Muscle

Acute skeletal muscle injury
Muscle inflammation (infectious or noninfectious)
Muscular dystrophy (active)
Recent surgery
Delirium tremens

Kidney

Acute injury or damage
Renal infarct

Other

Intestinal infarction
Shock
Cholecystitis
Acute pancreatitis
Hypothyroidism
Heparin therapy (60%-80% of cases)

From Ravel R: *Clinical laboratory medicine,* ed 6, St Louis, 1995, Mosby.

Decreased in:
Stress, hypersensitivity reaction, steroids, pregnancy, hyperthyroidism, postirradiation

■ **BILE, URINE;** *see* URINE BILE

■ **BILIRUBIN, DIRECT** (conjugated bilirubin)
Normal range:
0-0.2 mg/dl (0-4 μmol/L) [CF: 17.10; SMI: 2 μmol/L]
Cost: $23
Elevated in:
Hepatocellular disease, biliary obstruction, drug-induced cholestasis, hereditary disorders (Dubin-Johnson syndrome, Rotor's syndrome)

■ **BILIRUBIN, INDIRECT** (unconjugated bilirubin)
Normal range:
0-1.0 mg/dl (2-18 μmol/L) [CF: 17.10; SMI: 2 μmol/L]
Cost: $24
Elevated in:
Hemolysis, liver disease (hepatitis, cirrhosis, neoplasm), hepatic congestion secondary to congestive heart failure, hereditary disorders (Gilbert's disease, Crigler-Najjar syndrome), other (Box 4-5)

■ **BILIRUBIN, TOTAL**
Normal range:
0-1.0 mg/dl (2-18 μmol/L) [CF: 17.10, SMI: 2 μmol/L]
Cost: $24
Elevated in:
Liver disease (hepatitis, cirrhosis, cholangitis, neoplasm, biliary obstruction, infectious mononucleosis), hereditary disorders (Gilbert's disease, Dubin-Johnson syndrome), drugs (steroids, diphenylhydantoin, phenothiazines, penicillin, erythromycin, clindamycin, captopril, amphotericin B, sulfonamides, azathioprine, isoniazid, 5-aminosalicylic acid, allopurinol, methyldopa, indomethacin, halothane, oral contraceptives, procainamide, tolbutamide, labetalol), hemolysis, pulmonary embolism or infarct, hepatic congestion secondary to congestive heart failure

■ **BILIRUBIN, URINE:** *see* URINE BILE

■ **BLEEDING TIME** (modified Ivy method)
Normal range:
2 to 9½ min

BOX 4-5 Unconjugated Hyperbilirubinemia

A. **Result of increased bilirubin production** (if normal liver, serum unconjugated bilirubin is usually less than 4 mg/100 ml)
1. Hemolytic anemia
   a. Acquired
   b. Congenital
2. Resorption from extravascular sources
   a. Hematomas
   b. Pulmonary infarcts
3. Excessive ineffective erythropoiesis
   a. Congenital (congenital dyserythropoietic anemias)

b. Acquired (pernicious anemia, severe lead poisoning; if present, bilirubinemia is usually mild)

B. **Defective hepatic unconjugated bilirubin clearance** (defective uptake or conjugation)
1. Severe liver disease
2. Gilbert's syndrome
3. Crigler-Najjar type I or II
4. Drug-induced inhibition
5. Portacaval shunt
6. Congestive heart failure
7. Hyperthyroidism (uncommon)

From Ravel R: *Clinical laboratory medicine,* ed 6, St Louis, 1995, Mosby.

BOX 4-6 Selected Etiologies of Hypercalcemia

Relatively Common

Neoplasia (noncutaneous)
  Bone primary
    Myeloma
    Acute leukemia
  Nonbone solid tumors
    Breast
    Lung
    Squamous nonpulmonary
    Kidney
  Neoplasm secretion of parathyroid hormone-related protein (PTHrP, "ectopic PTH")

Primary hyperparathyroidism
Thiazide diuretics
Tertiary (renal) hyperparathyroidism
Idiopathic
Spurious (artifactual) hypercalcemia
  Dehydration
  Serum protein elevation
  Laboratory technical problem

Relatively Uncommon

Neoplasia (less common tumors)
Sarcoidosis
Hyperthyroidism

Immobilization (mostly seen in children and adolescents)
Diuretic phase of acute renal tubular necrosis
Vitamin D intoxication
Milk-alkali syndrome
Addison's disease
Lithium therapy
Idiopathic hypercalcemia of infancy
Acromegaly
Theophylline toxicity

From Ravel R: *Clinical laboratory medicine,* ed 6, St Louis, 1995, Mosby.

Cost: $31

Elevated in:

Thrombocytopenia, capillary wall abnormalities, platelet abnormalities (Bernard-Soulier disease, Glanzmann's disease), drugs (aspirin, warfarin, antiinflammatory medications, streptokinase, urokinase, dextran, β-lactam antibiotics, moxalactam), disseminated intravascular coagulation, cirrhosis, uremia, myeloproliferative disorders, von Willebrand's disease

■ BRCA ANALYSIS

Description of Analysis

Comprehensive BRACAnalysis:

BRCA1: Full sequence determination in both forward and reverse directions of approximately 5500 base pairs comprising 22 coding exons and one noncoding exon (exon 4) and approximately 800 adjacent base pairs in the noncoding intervening sequence (intron). Exon 1, which is noncoding, is not analyzed. The wild-type *BRCA1* gene encodes a protein comprising 1863 amino acids.

BRCA2: Full sequence determination in both forward and reverse directions of approximately 10,200 base pairs comprising 26 coding exons and approximately 900 adjacent base pairs in the noncoding intervening sequence (intron). Exon 1, which is noncoding, is not analyzed. The wild-type *BRCA2* gene encodes a protein comprising 3418 amino acids.

The noncoding intronic regions of *BRCA1* and *BRCA2* that are analyzed do not extend more than 20 base pairs proximal to the 5′ end and 10 base pairs distal to the 3′ end of each exon.

Single-site **BRACAnalysis:** DNA sequence analysis for a specified mutation in *BRCA1* and/or *BRCA2*.

Multisite 3 BRACAnalysis: DNA sequence analysis of specific portions of *BRCA1* exon 2, *BRCA1* exon 20 and *BRCA2* exon 11 designed to detect only mutations 187delAG and 5385insC in *BRCA1* and 6174delT in *BRCA2*.

IV

Interpretive Criteria

"Positive for a deleterious mutation": Includes all mutations (nonsense, insertions, deletions) that prematurely terminate ("truncate") the protein product of *BRCA1* at least 10 amino acids form the C-terminus, or the protein product of *BRCA2* at least 110 amino acids from the C-terminus (based on documentation of deleterious mutations in *BRCA1* and *BRCA2*).

In addition, specific missense mutations and noncoding intervening sequence (IVS) mutations are recognized as deleterious on the basis of data derived from linkage analysis of high-risk families, functional assays, biochemical evidence and/or demonstration of abnormal mRNA transcript processing.

"Genetic variant, suspected deleterious": Includes genetic variants for which the available evidence indicates a likelihood, but not proof, that the mutation is deleterious. The specific evidence supporting such an interpretation will be summarized for individual variants on each such report.

"Genetic variant, favor polymorphism": Includes genetic variants for which available evidence indicates that the variant is highly unlikely to contribute substantially to cancer risk. The specific evidence supporting such an interpretation will be summarized for individual variants on each such report.

"Genetic variant of uncertain significance": Includes missense mutations and mutations that occur in analyzed intronic regions whose clinical significance has not yet been determined, as well as chain-terminating mutations that truncate *BRCA1* and *BRCA2* distal to amino acid positions 1853 and 3308, respectively.

"No deleterious mutation detected": Includes nontruncating genetic variants observed at an allele frequency of approximately 1% of a suitable control population (providing that no data suggest clinical significance), as well as all genetic variants for which published data demonstrate absence of substantial clinical significance. Also includes mutations in the protein-coding region that neither alter the amino acid sequence nor are predicted to significantly affect exon splicing, and base pair alterations in noncoding portions of the gene that have been demonstrated to have no deleterious effect on the length or stability of the mRNA transcript.

There may be uncommon genetic abnormalities in *BRCA1* and *BRCA2* that will not be detected by BRACAnalysis. This analysis, however, is believed to rule out the majority of abnormalities in these genes, which are believed responsible for most hereditary susceptibility to breast and ovarian cancer.

"Specific variant/mutation not identified": Specific and designated deleterious mutations or variants of uncertain clinical significance are not present in the individual being tested. If one (or rarely two) specific deleterious mutations have been identified in a family member, a negative analysis for the specific mutation(s) indicates that the tested individual is at the general population risk of developing breast or ovarian cancer.
(From Myriad Genetic Laboratories, 320 Wakara Way, Salt Lake City, UT 84108-9930.)

- **BUN**; *see* UREA NITROGEN
- **C282Y and H63D MUTATION ANALYSIS**
  Procedure: Detection of the C282Y and H63D mutations is accomplished by amplification of exons 2 and 4 of the HFE gene on chromosome 6 by polymerase chain reaction (PCR) followed by allele-specific hybridization and chemiluminiscent detection of hybridized probes. H63D is viewed by some as a polymorphism rather than a mutation due to its prevalence in the population because 15% of the individuals affected with hereditary hemochromatosis (HH) are compound heterozygotes for C282Y and H63D and about 1% of patients are H63D homozygotes, which suggests that H63D may be causative in the development of the disorder at reduced penetrance. The test is performed by Quest diagnostics pursuant to a license agreement with Roche Molecular systems, Inc.
  Interpretation: Homozygosity for the C282Y mutation has been associated with an increased risk of being affected with hereditary hemochromatosis (HH) compared with the general population. The genotype is observed in 60% to 90% of individuals affected with HH and occurs in less than 1% of the general population. However, approximately 25% of asymptomatic individuals with this genotype do not develop the disorder.
- **C3**; *see* COMPLEMENT C3
- **C4**; *see* COMPLEMENT C4
- **CALCITONIN** (serum)
  Normal range:
  <100 pg/ml (<100 ng/L) [CF: 1; SMI: 10 ng/L]
  Cost: $123
  Elevated in:
  Medullary carcinoma of the thyroid (particularly if level >1500 pg/ml), carcinoma of the breast, APUDomas, carcinoids, renal failure, thyroiditis
- **CALCIUM** (serum)
  Normal range:
  8.8-10.3 mg/dl (2.2-2.58 mmol/L) [CF: 0.2495; SMI: 0.02 mmol/L]
  Cost: $23

See Boxes 4-6 and 4-7 for causes of elevated or decreased serum calcium levels. Laboratory findings in conditions affecting serum calcium and phosphorus levels are described in Table 4-4.

- **CALCIUM, URINE;** *see* URINE CALCIUM
- **CANCER ANTIGEN 125**
  Normal range:
  Less than 1.4%
  Cost: $176
  The cancer antigen 125 (CA 125) test uses an antibody against antigen from tissue culture of an ovarian tumor cell line. Various published evaluations report sensitivity of about 75%-80% in patients with ovarian carcinoma. There is also an appreciable incidence of elevated values in nonovarian malignancies and in certain benign conditions (Box 4-8). Test values may transiently increase during chemotherapy.

BOX 4-7 Selected Etiologies of Hypocalcemia

Artifactual	Renal failure	Drug-induced hypocalcemia
Hypoalbuminemia	Magnesium deficiency	Large doses of magnesium sulfate
Hemodilution	Sepsis	Anticonvulsants
Primary hypoparathyroidism	Chronic alcoholism	Mithramycin
Pseudohypoparathyroidism	Tumor lysis syndrome	Gentamicin
Vitamin D–related	Rhabdomyolysis	Cimetidine
Vitamin D deficiency	Alkalosis (respiratory or metabolic)	
Malabsorption	Acute pancreatitis	

From Ravel R: *Clinical laboratory medicine,* ed 6, St Louis, 1995, Mosby.

TABLE 4-4 Classic Laboratory Findings in Selected Conditions Affecting Serum Calcium and Phosphorus Levels*

	SERUM CALCIUM	SERUM PHOSPHORUS	ALKALINE PHOSPHATASE	ACIDOSIS	URINE CALCIUM
PHPT	H	N/L†	N/H†		H
Ectopic PTH syndrome	H	L	H		H
Vitamin D excess	H	N/L	N/H		H
Sarcoidosis	N/H	N	H		N/H
Secondary hyperparathyroidism	L/N	H	H	+	H
Tertiary hyperparathyroidism	H	H	H		
Renal acidosis	L/N	N/L	H	+	H
Sprue	L/N	N/L	H		L
Osteomalacia	L/N	L/N	H		L
Paget's disease	N‡	N	H‡		N/H
Metastatic neoplasm to bone§	N/H	N	N/H		N/H
Hypoparathyroidism	L	H	N		L
Osteoporosis	N	N	N		N/H
Hyperthyroidism	N/H	N/H	N/H		N/H

From Ravel R: *Clinical laboratory medicine,* ed 6, St Louis, 1995, Mosby.
PHPT, Pseudohypoparathyroidism; *PTH,* parathyroid hormone.
*Incidence of these findings varies in individual patients. *H, N,* and *L,* High, normal, and low; second letter, if present, indicates less common finding.
†Alkaline phosphatase level is high and serum phosphate level is low in "textbook cases" of PHPT.
‡PTH normal; alkaline phosphatase normal in 15% of early monostotic stage; calcium occasionally small increase from immobilization.
§Depends on primary tumor and type of bone lesion produced. Metastatic carcinoma to calcium is a common etiology of hypercalcemia, perhaps the most common.

IV

BOX 4-8   Elevated CA 125 Levels in Various Conditions

Malignant

Epithelial ovarian carcinoma, 75%-80% (range 25%-92%, better in serous than mucinous cystadenocarcinoma)
Endometrial carcinoma, 25%-48% (2%-90%)
Pancreatic carcinoma, 59%
Colorectal carcinoma, 20% (15%-56%)
Endocervical adenocarcinoma, 83%
Squamous cervical or vaginal carcinoma, 7%-14%
Lung carcinoma, 32%
Breast carcinoma, 12%-40%
Lymphoma, 35%

Benign

Cirrhosis, 40%-80%
Acute pancreatitis, 38%
Acute peritonitis, 75%
Endometriosis, 88%
Acute pelvic inflammation disease, 33%
Pregnancy first trimester, 2%-24%
During menstruation (occasionally)
Renal failure (?frequency)
Normal persons, 0.6%-1.4%

From Ravel R: *Clinical laboratory medicine*, ed 6, St Louis, 1995, Mosby.

■ **CARBON MONOXIDE;** *see* CARBOXYHEMOGLOBIN
■ **CARBOXYHEMOGLOBIN**
Normal range:
Saturation of hemoglobin <2%; smokers <9% (coma: 50%; death: 80%)
Cost: $47
Elevated in:
Smoking, exposure to smoking, exposure to automobile exhaust fumes, malfunctioning gas-burning appliances

■ **CARCINOEMBRYONIC ANTIGEN** (CEA)
Normal range:
Nonsmokers: 0-2.5 ng/ml (0-2.5 μg/L) [CF: 1; SMI: 0.1 μg/L]
Smokers: 0-5 ng/ml (0-5 μg/L) [CF: 1; SMI: 0.1 μg/L]
Fig. 4-2 describes the clinical role of CEA testing.
Cost: $79
Elevated in:
Colorectal carcinomas, pancreatic carcinomas, and metastatic disease (usually produce higher elevations: >20 ng/ml)
Carcinomas of the esophagus, stomach, small intestine, liver, breast, ovary, lung, and thyroid (usually produce lesser elevations)
Benign conditions (smoking, inflammatory bowel disease, hypothyroidism, cirrhosis, pancreatitis, infections) (usually produce levels <10 ng/ml)

■ **CAROTENE** (serum)
Normal range:
50-250 μg/dl (0.9-4.6 μmol/L) [CF: 0.01863; SMI: 0.1 μmol/L]
Cost: $50
Elevated in:
Carotenemia, chronic nephritis, diabetes mellitus, hypothyroidism, nephrotic syndrome, hyperlipidemia
Decreased in:
Fat malabsorption, steatorrhea, pancreatic insufficiency, lack of carotenoids in diet, high fever, liver disease

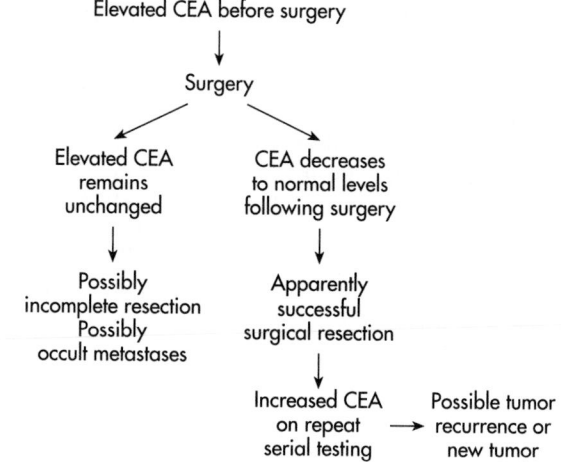

Fig. 4-2   Role of carcinoembryonic antigen. (From Ferri F [ed]: *Practical guide to the care of the medical patient,* ed 5, St Louis, 2001, Mosby.)

■ **CATECHOLAMINES, URINE;** *see* URINE CATECHOLAMINES
■ **CBC;** *see* COMPLETE BLOOD COUNT
■ **CD4+ T-LYMPHOCYTE COUNT** (CD4+ T-cells)
Cost: $111
Calculated as total WBC × % lymphocytes × % lymphocytes stained with CD4.
This test is used primarily to evaluate immune dysfunction in HIV infection and should be done every 3-6 months in all HIV-infected persons. It is useful as a prognostic indicator and as a criterion for initiating prophylaxis for several opportunistic infections that are sequelae of HIV infection. Progressive depletion of CD4+ T-lymphocytes is associated with an increased likelihood of clinical complications (Table 4-5). Adolescents and adults with HIV are classified as having AIDS if their CD4+ lymphocyte count is under 200/μL and/or if their CD4+ T-lymphocyte percentage is less than 14%. HIV-infected patients whose CD4+

count is less than 200/μL and who acquire certain infectious diseases or malignancies are also classified as having AIDS. Corticosteroids decrease CD4+ T-cell percentage and absolute number.

- **CEA**; *see* CARCINOEMBRYONIC ANTIGEN
- **CEREBROSPINAL FLUID** (CSF)
  Normal range:
  Appearance: clear
  Glucose: 40-70 mg/dl (2.2-3.9 mmol/L) [CF: 0.055; SMI: 0.1 mmol]
  Protein: 20-45 mg/dl (0.20-0.45 g/L) [CF: 0.01; SMI: 0.1 g/L]
  Chloride: 116-122 mEq/L (116-122 mmol/L) [CF: 1; SMI: 1 mmol/L]
  Pressure: 100-200 mm H_2O
  Cell count (cells/mm^3) and cell type: <6 lymphocytes, no polymorphonucleocytes
  Table 4-6 describes CSF abnormalities in various conditions.

- **CERULOPLASMIN** (serum)
  Normal range:
  20-35 mg/dl (200-350 mg/L) [CF: 10; SMI: 10 mg/L]
  Cost: $40
  Elevated in:
  Pregnancy, estrogens, oral contraceptives, neoplastic diseases (leukemias, Hodgkin's lymphoma, carcinomas), inflammatory states, systemic lupus erythematosus, primary biliary cirrhosis, rheumatoid arthritis
  Decreased in:
  Wilson's disease (values often <10 mg/dl), nephrotic syndrome, advanced liver disease, malabsorption, total parenteral nutrition, Menkes' syndrome

TABLE 4-5   Relation of CD4 Lymphocyte Counts to the Onset of Certain, HIV-Associated Infections and Neoplasms in North America

CD4 COUNT (CELLS/MM³)*	OPPORTUNISTIC INFECTION OR NEOPLASM	FREQUENCY (%)†
>500	Herpes zoster, polydermatomal	5-10
200-500	*Mycobacterium tuberculosis* infection, pulmonary and extrapulmonary	2-20
	Oral hairy leukoplakia	40-70
	Candida pharyngitis (thrush)	40-70
	Recurrent *Candida* vaginitis	15-30 (F)
	Kaposi's sarcoma, mucocutaneous	15-30 (M)
	Bacterial pneumonia, recurrent	15-20
	Cervical neoplasia	1-2 (F)
100-200	*Pneumocystis carinii* pneumonia	15-60
	Herpes simplex, chronic, ulcerative	5-10
	Histoplasma capsulatum infection, disseminated	0-20
	Kaposi's sarcoma, visceral	3-8 (M)
	Progressive multifocal leukoencephalopathy	2-3
	Lymphoma, non-Hodgkin's	2-5
<100	*Candida* esophagitis	15-20
	Mycobacterium avium-intracellulare, disseminated	25-40
	Toxoplasma gondii encephalitis	5-25
	Cryptosporidium enteritis	2-10
	Cytomegalovirus (CMV) retinitis	20-35
	Cryptococcus neoformans encephalitis	2-5
	CMV esophagitis or colitis	6-12
	Lymphoma, central nervous system	4-8

From Andreoli TE (ed): *Cecil essentials of medicine,* ed 4, Philadelphia, 1997, WB Saunders.
F, Exclusively in women; *HIV,* human immunodeficiency virus; *M,* almost exclusively in men.
*Table indicates CD4 count at which specific infections or neoplasms generally begin to appear. Each infection may recur or progress during the subsequent course of HIV disease.
†Even within the United States, great regional differences in the incidence of specific opportunistic infections are apparent. For example, disseminated histoplasmosis is common in the Mississippi River drainage area, but very rare in individuals who have lived exclusively on the East or West Coast.

IV

TABLE 4-6 Cerobrospinal Fluid Abnormalities in Various Central Nervous System Conditions

	APPEARANCE	GLUCOSE (MG/DL)	PROTEIN (MG/DL)	CELL COUNT (CELLS/MM³) AND CELL TYPE	PRESSURE (MM HG)
Normal	Clear	50-80	20-45	<6 lymphocytes	100-200
Acute bacterial meningitis	Cloudy	↓↓	↑↑	↑↑ PMN	↑↑
Aseptic (viral) meningitis	Clear/cloudy	N	↑	↑, usually mononuclear cells May be PMN in early stages	N/↑
Hemorrhage	Bloody/xanthochromic	N/↓	↑	↑↑ RBC	↑
Neoplasm	Clear/xanthochromic	N/↓	N/↑	N/↑ lymphocytes	↑↑
Tuberculous meningitis	Cloudy	↓	↑	↑ PMN (early) ↑ lymphocytes (later)	↑
Fungal meningitis	Clear/cloudy	↓	↑	↑ monocytes	↑
Neurosyphilis	Clear/cloudy	N	↑	↑ monocytes	N/↑
Guillain-Barré syndrome	Clear/cloudy	N	↑↑	N/↑ lymphocytes	N

↑, Increased; ↑↑, markedly increased; ↓, decreased; ↓↓, markedly decreased; *N*, normal; *PMN*, polymorphonucleocytes; *RBC*, red blood cells.

■ **CHLORIDE** (serum)
Normal range:
95-105 mEq/L (95-105 mmol/L) [CF: 1; SMI: 1 mmol/L]
Cost: $23
Elevated in:
Dehydration, excessive infusion of normal saline solution, cystic fibrosis (sweat test), hyperparathyroidism, renal tubular disease, metabolic acidosis, prolonged diarrhea, drugs (ammonium chloride administration, acetazolamide, boric acid, triamterene)
Decreased in:
Congestive heart failure, syndrome of inappropriate antidiuretic hormone secretion, Addison's disease, vomiting, gastric suction, salt-losing nephritis, continuous infusion of D_5W, thiazide diuretic administration, diaphoresis, diarrhea, burns, diabetic ketoacidosis
■ **CHLORIDE, URINE;** *see* URINE CHLORIDE
■ **CHOLESTEROL, TOTAL**
Normal range:
Varies with age
Generally <200 mg/dl (<5.20 mmol/L) [CF: 0.02586; SMI: 0.05 mmol/L]
Cost: $23
Elevated in:
Primary hypercholesterolemia, biliary obstruction, diabetes mellitus, nephrotic syndrome, hypothyroidism, primary biliary cirrhosis, high-cholesterol diet, pregnancy third trimester, myocardial infarction, drugs (steroids, phenothiazines, oral contraceptives)
Decreased in:
Starvation, malabsorption, sideroblastic anemia, thalassemia, abetalipoproteinemia, hyperthyroidism, Cushing's syndrome, hepatic failure, multiple myeloma, polycythemia vera, chronic myelocytic leukemia, myeloid metaplasia, Waldenström's macroglobulinemia, myelofibrosis
■ **CHOLESTEROL, HIGH-DENSITY LIPOPROTEIN;** *see* HIGH-DENSITY LIPOPROTEIN CHOLESTEROL
■ **CHOLESTEROL, LOW-DENSITY LIPOPROTEIN;** *see* LOW-DENSITY LIPOPROTEIN CHOLESTEROL
■ **CHROMOSOME ABNORMALITIES IN MALIGNANCY;** *see* Table 4-7
■ **CIRCULATING ANTICOAGULANT** (lupus anticoagulant)
Normal:
Negative
Cost: $98
Detected in:
Systemic lupus erythematosus, drug-induced lupus, long-term phenothiazine therapy, multiple myeloma, ulcerative colitis, rheumatoid arthritis, postpartum, hemophilia, neoplasms, chronic inflammatory states, AIDS, nephrotic syndrome
NOTE: The name is a misnomer because these patients are prone to hypercoagulability and thrombosis.
■ **CK;** *see* CREATINE KINASE

TABLE 4-7 Some Important Chromosome Abnormalities in Hematopoietic Malignancies

MALIGNANCY	CHROMOSOME ABNORMALITIES	OTHER
CML	t(9;22) (q34;q11)	98% of CML; 25%-33% of adult ALL
CML blast crisis	t(9;22) (q34;q11) with trisomy 8	70% of cases
ANLL (general)	Trisomy 8	Most common ANLL abnormality
ANLL-M2	t(8;21) (q22.1;q27)	10%-18% of patients, often with loss of one sex chromosome
ANLL-M3	t(15;17) (q22;q11)	50%-70% (range 40%-100%) of cases
ANLL-M4	inv(16) (p13;q22)	30% of cases
ANLL-M5	t(9;11) (p22;q23)	35% of cases
ALL-L1	t(1;19) (q23;q13)	Pre-B-cell origin Pre–pre-B-cell origin
ALL-L2	t(4;11) (q21;q23) del (6) (q21;q25)	"Common" B-cell origin
ALL-L3	t(8;14) (q24;q32)	B-cell origin
Myelodysplasia	del (5q)	Most common chromosome abnormality
Burkitt's lymphoma	t(8;14) (q;24;32)	80% of cases, also some cases of small noncleaved non-Burkitt's
Follicular (nodular) lymphoma	t(14;18) (q32;q21)	80%-90% of cases by chromosome analysis, nearly 100% by DNA probe; involves Bcl-2 oncogene on chromosome 18
CLL	Trisomy 12	Most common abnormality
Therapy-related ANLL	del (5q) or del (7q)	90% of cases

From Ravel R: *Clinical laboratory medicine*, ed 6, St Louis, 1995, Mosby.
ANLL, Acute nonlymphocytic leukemia; *ALL,* acute lymphocytic leukemia; *CLL,* chronic lymphocytic leukemia; *CML,* chronic myelogenous leukemia. *M* and *L* followed by a number refer to FAB categories of acute leukemia.

■ **CO;** *see* CARBOXYHEMOGLOBIN
■ **COAGULATION FACTORS;** *see* Table 4-9 for characteristics of coagulation factors
Factor reference ranges:
V: >10%
VII: >10%
VIII: 50% to 170%
IX: 60% to 136%
X: >10%
XI: 50% to 150%
XII: >30%
• Fig. 4-3 describes the blood coagulation pathways.
• Table 4-8 describes screening laboratory results in coagulation factor deficiencies.
■ **COLD AGGLUTININS TITER**
Normal range:
<1:32
Cost: $28
Elevated in:
Primary atypical pneumonia (mycoplasma pneumonia), infectious mononucleosis, CMV infection
Others: hepatic cirrhosis, acquired hemolytic anemia, frostbite, multiple myeloma, lymphoma, malaria
■ **COMPLEMENT**
Normal range:
C3: 70-160 mg/dl (0.7-1.6 g/L) [CF: 0.01; SMI: 0.1 g/L]

C4: 20-40 mg/dl (0.2-0.4 g/L) [CF: 0.01; SMI: 0.1 g/L]
Abnormal values:
See Table 4-13.
• Fig. 4-3 describes the complement system.
• Table 4-10 describes complement receptors.
• The biologic function of complement proteins is described in Table 4-11.
• Measurement of complement is described in Table 4-12.
• Hereditary deficiencies of complement proteins are described in Table 4-13.
■ **COMPLETE BLOOD COUNT** (CBC)
Cost: $22
White blood cells 3200-9800 mm^3 (3.2-9.8 × 10^9/L) [CF: 0.001; SMI: 0.1 × 10^9/L]
Red blood cells
  Male: 4.3-5.9 × 10^6/mm^3 (4.3-5.9 × 10^{12}/L) [CF: 1; SMI: 0.1 × 10^{12}/L]
  Female: 3.5-5 × 10^6/mm^3 (3.5-5 × 10^{12}/L) [CF: 1; SMI: 0.1 × 10^{12}/L]
Hemoglobin
  Male: 13.6-17.7 g/dl (136-172 g/L) [CF: 10; SMI: 1 g/L]
  Female: 12-15 g/dl (120-150 g/L) [CF: 10; SMI: 1 g/L]
Hematocrit
  Male: 39% to 49% (0.39-0.49) [CF: 0.01; SMI: 0.01]

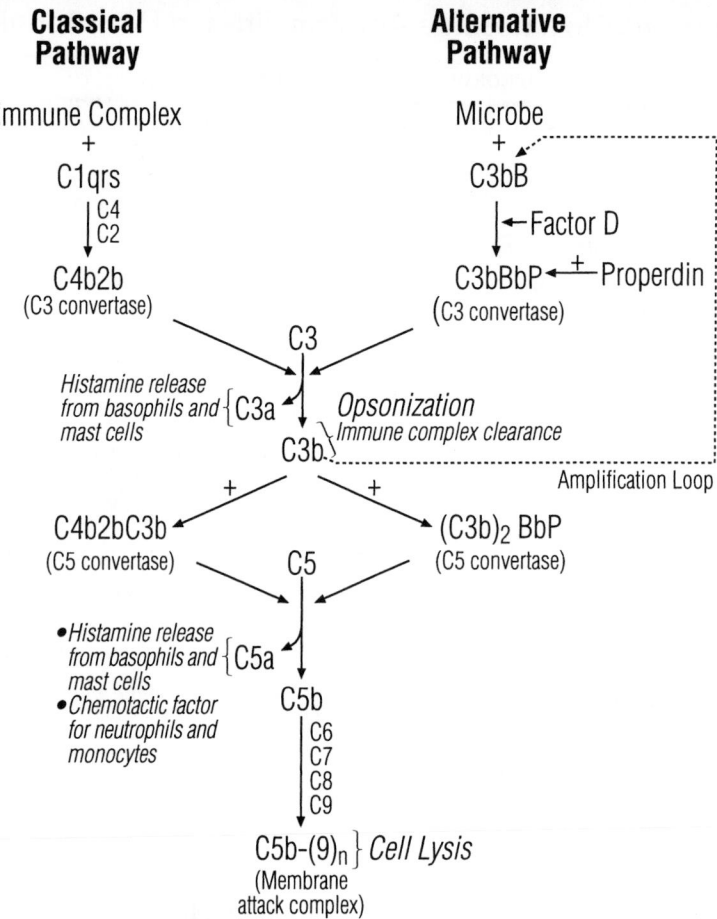

Classical Pathway   **Alternative Pathway**

Fig. 4-3   The complement system. The two major pathways of complement activation are the classical and alternative pathways. Each pathway forms separate but functionally identical C3 and C5 convertases that cleave C3 and C5 respectively, leading to the formation of C3b and C5b and the release into the plasma of biologically active fragments C3a and C5a. The formation of C5b initiates the assembly and insertion of the terminal components into the cell membrane, resulting in cell lysis. (From Altman LV [ed]: *Allergy in primary care,* Philadelphia, 2000, WB Saunders.)

TABLE 4-8   **Screening Laboratory Results in Coagulation Factor Deficiencies**

DEFICIENT FACTOR	FREQUENCY	PT	PTT	TT
I (fibrinogen)	Rare	↑	↑	↑
II (prothrombin)	Very rare	↑	↑	↑
V	1:1,000,000	↑	↑	NL
VII	1:500,000	↑	NL	NL
VIII	1:5000 (male)	NL	↑	NL
IX	1:30,000 (male)	NL	↑	NL
X	1:500,000	↑	↑	NL
XI	Rare*	NL	↑	NL
XII† or HMWK† or PK†	Rare	NL	↑	NL
XIII	Rare	NL	NL	NL

From Andreoli TE (ed): *Cecil essentials of medicine,* ed 5, Philadelphia, 2001, WB Saunders.
↑, Increased over normal range; *HMWK,* high-molecular-weight kininogen; *NL,* normal; *PK,* prekallikrein; *PT,* prothrombin time; *PTT,* partial thromboplastin time; *TT,* thrombin time.
*Except in those of Ashkenazi Jewish descent (approximately 4% are heterozygous for factor XI deficiency).
†Not associated with clinical bleeding.

TABLE 4-9 **Characteristics of Coagulation Factors**

FACTOR	DESCRIPTIVE NAME	SOURCE	APPROXIMATE HALF-LIFE (HR)	FUNCTION
I	Fibrinogen	Liver	120	Substrate for fibrin clot (CP)
II	Prothrombin	Liver (VKD)	60	Serine protease (CP)
V	Proaccelerin, labile factor	Liver	12-36	Cofactor (CP)
VII	Serum prothrombin conversion accelerator, proconvertin	Liver (VKD)	6	(?) Serine protease (EP)
VIII	Antihemophilic factor or globulin	Endothelial cells and (?) elsewhere	12	Cofactor (IP)
IX	Plasma thromboplastin component, Christmas factor	Liver (VKD)	24	Serine protease (IP)
X	Stuart-Prower factor	Liver (VKD)	36	Serine protease (CP)
XI	Plasma thromboplastin antecedent	(?) Liver	40-84	Serine protease (IP)
XII	Hageman factor	(?) Liver	50	Serine protease contact activation (IP)
XIII	Fibrin-stabilizing factor	(?) Liver	96-180	Transglutaminase (CP)
Prekallikrein	Fletcher factor	(?) Liver	?	Serine protease contact activation (IP)
High–molecular weight kininogen	Fitzgerald factor, Flaujeac or Williams factor	(?) Liver	?	Cofactor, contact activation (IP)

From Noble J (ed): *Primary care medicine,* ed 3, St Louis, 2001, Mosby.
CP, Common pathway; *EP,* extrinsic pathway; *IP,* intrinsic pathway; *VKD,* vitamin K dependent.

TABLE 4-10 **Complement Receptors**

RECEPTOR PROTEIN	SPECIFICITY	EXPRESSED ON THESE CELLS	FUNCTION
C1qR	C1q	Neutrophils, monocytes, B lymphocytes	Enhances phagocytosis
CR1	C3b/C4b	Erythrocytes, neutrophils, monocytes/macrophages, follicular dendritic cells, B lymphocytes	Clearance of immune complexes, enhances phagocytosis
CR2	C3d, C3dg	B lymphocytes, follicular dendritic cells	Lowers threshold of B lymphocyte activation
CR3	iC3b	Neutrophils, monocytes/macrophages, natural killer cells	Mediates adhesion of leukocytes to endothelium, enhances phagocytosis
CR4	iC3b	Neutrophils, monocytes/macrophages, dendritic cells and natural killer cells	Mediates adhesion of leukocytes to endothelium

From Altman LV (ed): *Allergy in primary care,* Philadelphia, 2000, WB Saunders.

IV

TABLE 4-11 Biologic Functions of Complement

COMPLEMENT PROTEIN	FUNCTION
C2 fragment	Kinin-like activity: venular permeability and vasodilation; contributes to the swelling in hereditary angioedema
C3a, C5a	Anaphylatoxins: release of histamine from mast cells and basophils; C3a inhibits antibody production; C5a stimulates antibody production
C5a	Chemotactic factor for neutrophils and monocytes; increases adhesiveness and is a potent activator of inflammatory mediators from these cells; stimulates oxidative burst in neutrophils
C3b	Enhances phagocytosis and clearance of immune complexes
C5b-9	Membrane attack complex: produces cell injury and lysis

From Altman LV (ed): *Allergy in primary care,* Philadelphia, 2000, WB Saunders.

TABLE 4-12 Measurement of Complement

CONDITION	C1 INH	C1	C4	C3	CH$_{50}$
Classical pathway activation (e.g., SLE, SBE, mixed cryoglobulinemia)	NA	NA	↓	↓	↓
Alternative pathway activation (e.g., membranoproliferative glomerulonephritis type II and partial lipodystrophy associated with the C3 nephritic factor)	NA	NA	N*	↓	N
Deficiency of a complement component (e.g., C2). May be associated with lupus-like disorder or recurrent bacterial infections depending on the absent complement component	NA	N	N	N	Absent
Hereditary angioedema	↓†	N	↓	N	N or sl ↓
Acquired angioedema	↓	↓	↓	N	N or sl ↓

From Altman LV (ed): *Allergy in primary care,* Philadelphia, 2000, WB Saunders.
NA, Not applicable (measurement is not of clinical value in these disorders); *SBE,* subacute bacterial endocarditis; *SLE,* systemic lupus erythematosus.
*Normal
†Protein measurement of C1 INH may be normal but protein is nonfunctional. Functional assay of C1 INH is required.

TABLE 4-13 Hereditary Deficiencies of Complement Proteins

PROTEIN	PATTERN OF INHERITANCE	CLINICAL FEATURES
C1q, C1r, or C1s	Autosomal recessive	Lupus-like illness, susceptibility to bacterial infections
C4 or C2	Autosomal recessive	SLE and lupus-like illness, dermatomyositis, glomerulonephritis, vasculitis
C3	Autosomal recessive	Recurrent, pyogenic infections, lupus-like illness
C5, C6, C7, or C8	Autosomal recessive	Lupus-like illness, recurrent *Neisseria* infections
Properdin	X-linked	Recurrent *Neisseria* infections, recurrent pyogenic infections
Factor D	Autosomal recessive	*Neisseria* infections
Factor H or I	Autosomal recessive	Recurrent pyogenic infections
C1 inhibitor	Autosomal dominant	Hereditary angioedema

From Altman LV (ed): *Allergy in primary care,* Philadelphia, 2000, WB Saunders.
SLE, Systemic lupus erythematosus.

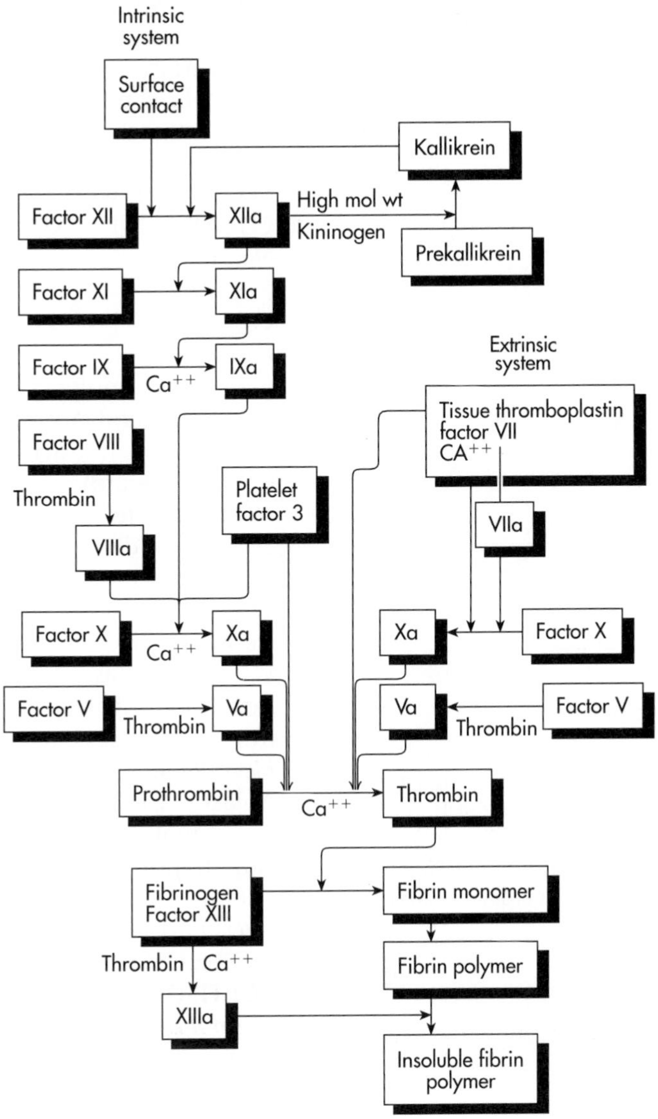

Fig. 4-4   Blood coagulation pathways. *a,* Activated. (From Ravel R: *Clinical laboratory medicine,* ed 6, St Louis, 1995, Mosby.)

IV

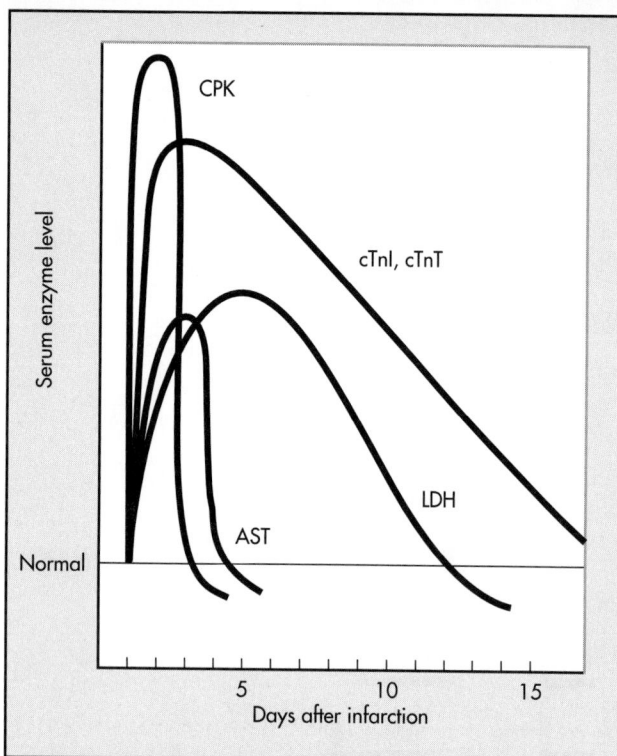

Fig. 4-5 Typical time course for the detection of enzymes released after myocardial infarction. (From Andreoli TE [ed]: *Cecil essentials of medicine,* ed 5, Philadelphia, 2001, WB Saunders.) *AST,* Serum aspartate aminotransferase; *CPK,* creatine kinase; *cTnI,* cardiac troponin I; *cTnT,* cardiac troponin T; *LDH,* lactate dehydrogenase.

Female: 33% to 43% (0.33-0.43) [CF: 0.01; SMI: 0.01]

Mean corpuscular volume (MCV): 76-100 μm^3 (76-100 fL) [CF: 1; SMI: 1 fL]

Mean corpuscular hemoglobin (MCH): 27-33 pg (27-33 pg) [CF: 1; SMI: 1 pg]

Mean corpuscular hemoglobin concentration (MCHC): 33-37 g/dl (330-370 g/L) [CF: 10; SMI: 10 g/L]

Red blood cell distribution width index (RDW): 11.5% to 14.5%

Platelet count: 130-400 × 10^3/mm^3 (130-400 × 10^9/L) [CF: 1; SMI: 5 × 10^9/L]

Differential:

2-6 stabs (bands, early mature neutrophils)
60-70 segs (mature neutrophils)
1-4 eosinophils
0-1 basophils
2-8 monocytes
25-40 lymphocytes

Table 4-14 describes normal hematologic blood values at various ages.

■ **CONJUGATED BILIRUBIN;** *see* BILIRUBIN, DIRECT

■ **COOMBS, DIRECT**

Normal:

Negative

Cost: $23

Positive:

Autoimmune hemolytic anemia, erythroblastosis fetalis, transfusion reactions, drugs (α-methyldopa, penicillins, tetracycline, sulfonamides, levodopa, cephalosporins, quinidine, insulin)

False positive:

May be seen with cold agglutinins

■ **COOMBS, INDIRECT**

Normal:

Negative

Cost: $23

Positive:

Acquired hemolytic anemia, incompatible cross-matched blood, anti-Rh antibodies, drugs (methyldopa, mefenamic acid, levodopa)

■ **COPPER** (serum)

Normal range:

70-140 μg/dl (11-22 μmol/L) [CF: 0.1574, SMI: 0.2 μmol/L]

Cost: $89

Decreased in:

Wilson's disease, Menkes' syndrome, malabsorption, malnutrition, nephrosis, total parenteral nutrition, acute leukemia in remission

Elevated in:

Aplastic anemia, biliary cirrhosis, systemic lupus erythematosus, hemochromatosis, hyperthyroidism, hypothyroidism, infection, iron deficiency anemia, leukemia, lymphoma, oral contraceptives, pernicious anemia, rheumatoid arthritis

■ **COPPER, URINE;** *see* URINE COPPER

■ **CORTISOL, PLASMA**

Normal range:

Varies with time of collection (circadian variation):

8 AM: 4-19 μg/dl (110-520 nmol/L) [CF: 27.59; SMI: 10 nmol/L]

4 PM: 2-15 μg/dl (50-410 nmol/L) [CF: 27.59; SMI: 10 nmol/L]

Cost: $55

Elevated in:

Ectopic adrenocorticotropic hormone production (i.e., oat cell carcinoma of lung), loss of normal diurnal variation, pregnancy, chronic renal failure iatrogenic, stress, adrenal, or pituitary hyperplasia or adenomas

Decreased in:

Primary adrenocortical insufficiency, anterior pituitary hypofunction, secondary adrenocortical insufficiency, adrenogenital syndromes

■ **C-PEPTIDE**

Cost: $89

Elevated in:

Insulinoma, sulfonylurea administration

Decreased in:

Insulin-dependent diabetes mellitus, factitious insulin administration

■ **CPK;** *see* CREATINE KINASE

TABLE 4-14 **Normal Hematologic Blood Values at Various Ages***

| | CORD | DAY | | | | | |
		1	2	3	7	14	30
Hb (g/100 ml, venous blood)	17.0 (13.5-22)	19.0† (14.5-23)	18.5 (15-23)	18 (14-23)	17.5 (13.5-22)	16.5 (13-21.5)	13.5 (10-17.5)
MCV (Fl)	110 (99-120)	109 (98-119)	115 (101-129)	116 (106-126)	114 (88-140)	106 (86-126)	102 (84-121)
Retics (%)	3-7	1.5-6.5	1.5-6.5	1-5	0-1	0-1	0-1
Nucleated RBCs (% of 100 WBCs)	2-5	1-3	0-1	0	0	0	
Platelets (1000s)	100-290	140-300	150-400		200-470		150-450
WBCs (1000s)	18.1 (9.0-30.0)	18.9 (9.4-34.0)			12.2 (5.0-21.0)	11.4 (5.0-20.0)	10.8 (5.0-19.5)
Neutrophils (% 100 WBCs)	55	60‡			50	40	35
Lymphocytes (% 100 WBCs)	30	30			35	50	55

| | MONTH | | | | YEAR | | |
	2	3	6	12	5	10	ADULT
Hb (g/100 ml, venous blood)	12.0 (10-13.5)	11.3 (9.7-13)	12.0 (10.1-14)	12.0 (10.5-13.5)	12.5 (10.7-14.7)	13.0 (10.8-15.5)	M: 14-18 F: 12-16
MCV (FL)	96 (80-118)		88 (73-100)	79 (71-86)	80 (73-86)	81 (75-87)	90 (80-100)
Retics (%)	0-1						0-1.5
Nucleated RBCs (% of 100 WBCs)	0						0
Platelets (1000s)							150-400
WBCs (1000s)			11.9 (6.0-17.5)	11.4 (6.0-17.5)	8.5 (5.0-14.5)	8.1 (4.5-13.5)	7.5 (4.5-10.5)
Neutrophils (% 100 WBCs)			30	30	50	55	60
Lymphocytes (% 100 WBCs)			60	60	40	40	40

From Ravel R: *Clinical laboratory medicine*, ed 6, St Louis, 1995, Mosby.
Hb, Hemoglobin; *MCV*, mean corpuscular volume; *RBC*, red blood cell; *Retic*, reticulocyte; *WBC*, white blood cell.
*Compiled from various sources. Numbers represent average values; numbers in parentheses indicate reference range.
†Capillary hemoglobin is about 2 g higher than venous; the gap then narrows and disappears by day 7. Neonatal Hb is influenced by amount of blood received from the umbilical cord at delivery.
‡Normal neutrophil count is about 25% higher in capillary than in venous blood on day 1 and about 10% higher on day 2.

IV

■ **C-REACTIVE PROTEIN**
Normal range:
6.8-820 μg/dl (68-8200 μg/L) [CF: 10; SMI: 10 μg/L]
Cost: $26
Elevated in:
Rheumatoid arthritis, rheumatic fever, inflammatory bowel disease, bacterial infections, myocardial infarction, oral contraceptives, pregnancy third trimester (acute phase reactant), inflammatory and neoplastic diseases

■ **C-REACTIVE PROTEIN, HIGH SENSITIVITY**
(hs-CRP, Cardio-CRP)
is a new test used as a cardiac risk marker. It is increased in patients with silent atherosclerosis years before a cardiovascular event and is independent of cholesterol level and other lipoproteins. It can be used to help stratify cardiac risk.

Interpretation of results:

CARDIO-CRP RESULT (mg/L)	RISK
≤0.6	Lowest risk
0.7-1.1	Low risk
1.2-1.9	Moderate risk
2.0-3.8	High risk
3.9-4.9	Highest risk
≥5.0	Results may be confounded by acute inflammatory disease. If clinically indicated, a repeat test should be performed in 2 or more weeks.

■ CREATINE KINASE (CK, CPK)

Normal range:

0-130 U/L (0-2.16 μkat/L) [CF: 0.01667; SMI: 0.01 μkat/L]

Cost: $27

Elevated in:

Myocardial infarction, myocarditis, rhabdomyolysis, myositis, crush injury/trauma, polymyositis, dermatomyositis, vigorous exercise, muscular dystrophy, myxedema, seizures, malignant hyperthermia syndrome, IM injections, cerebrovascular accident, pulmonary embolism and infarction, acute dissection of aorta

Decreased in:

Steroids, decreased muscle mass, connective tissue disorders, alcoholic liver disease, metastatic neoplasms

■ CREATINE KINASE ISOENZYMES

Cost: $60

CK-BB:

Elevated in: cerebrovascular accident, subarachnoid hemorrhage, neoplasms (prostate, gastrointestinal tract, brain, ovary, breast, lung), severe shock, bowel infarction, hypothermia, meningitis

CK-MB:

Elevated in: myocardial infarction (MI), myocarditis, pericarditis, muscular dystrophy, cardiac defibrillation, cardiac surgery, extensive rhabdomyolysis, strenuous exercise (marathon runners), mixed connective tissue disease, cardiomyopathy, hypothermia

NOTE: CK-MB exists in the blood in two subforms. MB_2 is released from cardiac cells and converted in the blood to MB_1. Rapid assay of CK-MB subforms can detect MI (CK-MB_2 ≥1.0 U/L, with a ratio of CK-MB_2/CK-MB_1 ≥1.5) within 6 hours of onset of symptoms.

Fig. 4-5 illustrates the time course of CK and LDH activity after acute MI. Table 4-15 describes serum enzyme changes after acute MI.

CK-MM:

Elevated in: crush injury, seizures, malignant hyperthermia syndrome, rhabdomyolysis, myositis, polymyositis, dermatomyositis, vigorous exercise, muscular dystrophy, IM injections, acute dissection of aorta

■ CREATININE (serum)

Normal range:

0.6-1.2 mg/dl (50-110 μmol/L) [CF: 88.4; SMI: 10 μmol/L]

Cost: $23

Elevated in:

Renal insufficiency (acute and chronic), decreased renal perfusion (hypotension, dehydration, congestive heart failure), urinary tract infection, rhabdomyolysis, ketonemia

Drugs (antibiotics [aminoglycosides, cephalosporins], hydantoin, diuretics, methyldopa)

Falsely elevated in:

Diabetic ketoacidosis, administration of some cephalosporins (e.g., cefoxitin, cephalothin)

TABLE 4-15 **Serum Enzyme Concentration Changes After Acute Myocardial Infarction**

ENZYME	RISE	PEAK	RETURN TO NORMAL
CK	2-8 hr	12-36 hr	3-4 days
LDH	12-48 hr	3-6 days	8-14 days

From Ferri F (ed): *Practical guide to the care of the medical patient,* ed 4, St Louis, 1998, Mosby.
CK, Creatine kinase; *LDH,* lactate dehydrogenase.

Decreased in:
Decreased muscle mass (including amputees and older persons), pregnancy, prolonged debilitation
- **CREATININE CLEARANCE**
Normal range:
75-124 ml/min (1.24-2.08 ml/sec) [CF: 0.01667; SMI: 0.02 ml/sec]
Box 4-9 describes a formula for calculation of creatinine clearance.
The Cockcroft-Gault formula to calculate creatinine clearance is described in Box 4-10.
Cost: $31
Elevated in:
Pregnancy, exercise
Decreased in:
Renal insufficiency, drugs (cimetidine, procainamide, antibiotics, quinidine)
- **CREATININE, URINE;** *see* URINE CREATININE
- **CRYOGLOBULINS** (serum)
Normal range:
Not detectable
Cost: $29
Present in:
Collagen-vascular diseases, chronic lymphocytic leukemia, hemolytic anemias, multiple myeloma, Waldenström's macroglobulinemia, chronic active hepatitis, Hodgkin's disease
- **CSF;** *see* CEREBROSPINAL FLUID
- **CYTOKINES**
Cytokines and their activities are described in Table 4-16.
Cytokines with a potential role in systemic inflammatory response syndrome are described in Table 4-17.
- **DRUG MONITORING;** *see* Table 4-18
- **ELECTROLYTES, URINE;** *see* URINE ELECTROLYTES
- **ELECTROPHORESIS, HEMOGLOBIN;** *see* HEMOGLOBIN ELECTROPHORESIS
- **ELECTROPHORESIS, PROTEIN;** *see* PROTEIN ELECTROPHORESIS
- **ENA-COMPLEX;** *see* EXTRACTABLE NUCLEAR ANTIGEN
- **EOSINOPHIL COUNT**
Normal range:
1%-4% eosinophils (0-440/mm^3)
Elevated in:
Allergy, parasitic infestations (trichinosis, aspergillosis, hydatidosis), angioneurotic edema, drug reactions, warfarin sensitivity, collagen-vascular diseases, acute hypereosinophilic syndrome, eosinophilic nonallergic rhinitis, myeloproliferative disorders, Hodgkin's lymphoma, radiation therapy, non-Hodgkin's lymphoma, L-tryptophan ingestion, urticaria, pernicious anemia, pemphigus, inflammatory bowel disease, bronchial asthma

- **EPSTEIN-BARR VIRAL INFECTION;** *see* Table 4-9, Fig. 4-6, and Box 4-11 for test interpretation
Cost: $53
- **ERYTHROCYTE SEDIMENTATION RATE** (ESR; Westergren)
Normal range:
Male: 0-15 mm/hr
Female: 0-20 mm/hr
Cost: $24
Elevated in:
Collagen-vascular diseases, infections, myocardial infarction, neoplasms, inflammatory states (acute phase reactant), hyperthyroidism, hypothyroidism, rouleaux formation
Decreased in:
Sickle cell disease, polycythemia, corticosteroids, spherocytosis, anisocytosis, hypofibrinogenemia, increased serum viscosity
- **ESTROGEN**
Normal range:
Serum: Males: 20-80 pg/ml
         Females: Follicular: 60-200 pg/ml
                 Luteal: 160-400 pg/ml
                 Postmenopausal: <130 pg/ml
Urine: Males: 4-23 µg/g creatinine
        Females: Follicular: 7-65 µg/g creatinine
                Midcycle: 32-104 µg/g creatinine
                Luteal: 8-135 µg/g creatinine
Cost: $79
Elevated in:
Hyperplasia of adrenal cortex, ovarian tumors producing estrogen, granulosa and thecal cell tumors, testicular tumors
Decreased in:
Menopause, hypopituitarism, primary ovarian malfunction, anorexia nervosa, hypofunction of adrenal cortex, ovarian agenesis, psychogenic stress, gonadotropin-releasing hormone deficiency
- **EXTRACTABLE NUCLEAR ANTIGEN** (ENA complex, anti-RNP antibody, anti-Sm, anti-Smith)
Normal:
Negative
Cost: $158
Present in:
Systemic lupus erythematosus, rheumatoid arthritis, Sjögren's syndrome, mixed connective tissue disease
- **FDP;** *see* FIBRIN DEGRADATION PRODUCT
- **FECAL FAT, QUANTITATIVE** (72-hr collection)
Normal range:
2-6 g/24 hr (7-21 mmol/dl) [CF: 3.515; SMI: 1 mmol/dl]
Cost: $42
Elevated in:
Malabsorption syndrome

IV

BOX 4-9   Calculation of the Creatinine Clearance

$C_{cr} = U_{cr} \times V/P_{cr}$
where C_{cr} = clearance of creatinine (ml/min)
         U_{cr} = urine creatinine (mg/dl)
         V = volume of urine (ml/min) (for 24-hr
             volume: divide by 1440)
         P_{cr} = plasma creatinine (mg/dl)

Normal range: 95 to 105 ml/min/1.75m^2

BOX 4-10   Cockroft-Gault Formula to Calculate Creatinine Clearance (C_{cr})

$$C_{cr} = \frac{(140 - \text{age in years}) \times (\text{lean body weight in kg})}{S_{cr} \text{ in mg/dl} \times 72}$$

For women multiply final value by 0.85

Scr, Serum creatinine.

TABLE 4-16   Cytokines and Their Activities

ABBREVIATION	NAME	EFFECTS ON HEMATOPOIESIS
EPO	Erythropoietin	Stimulation of proliferation and maturation of erythroid progenitors; produced by the kidney in response to anemia/hypoxia; important clinically for treatment of anemia associated with low EPO levels (renal failure, some anemia of chronic disease)
G-CSF	Granulocyte colony-stimulating factor	Stimulation of proliferation and maturation of granulocytes; more broad-based effect, because also increases release of "stem cells" in peripheral blood; clinically important for treatment of neutropenia and mobilization of stem cells for transplant
GM-CSF	Granulocyte-monocyte colony-stimulating factor	Proliferation of granulocyte and monocyte precursors; role unclear in steady-state hematopoiesis, because knockout has no hematopoietic phenotype
TPO	Thrombopoietin	Proliferation of megakaryocytes; results in disappointing clinical studies
M-CSF	Monocyte colony-stimulating factor	Proliferation of monocytes
IL-2	Interleukin-2	Proliferation of T cells
IL-3	Interleukin-3 (multi-CSF)	Proliferation of granulocytes, monocytes; broad-based effects, appearing to increase the proliferation of "stem cells"; not in use clinically
IL-4	Interleukin-4	Proliferation of B cells
IL-5	Interleukin-5	Proliferation of T cells, B cells; proliferation and differentiation of eosinophils
IL-11	Interleukin-11	Proliferation of megakaryocytes; undergoing clinical testing
LIF	Leukemia inhibitory factor	Proliferation of stem cells and megakaryocytes
SCF	Stem cell factor (kit ligand)	Proliferation of progenitor cells; broad-based effects on multiple lineages

From Andreoli TE (ed): *Cecil essentials of medicine,* ed 5, Philadelphia, 2001, WB Saunders.

TABLE 4-17 Cytokines with a Potential Role in Systemic Inflammatory Response Syndrome

CYTOKINE	SOURCE	TARGET CELL	FUNCTION
Granulocyte-macrophage colony-stimulating factor (GM-CSF)	T cells, macrophages, endothelial cells, fibroblasts	Myeloid precursor cells, neutrophils, eosinophils, macrophages	Proliferation of progenitor cells Differentiation and maturation of neutrophils and macrophages
Granulocyte colony-stimulating factor (G-CSF)	Monocytes, endothelial cells, fibroblasts, neutrophils	Neutrophils, promyelocytes	Proliferation of myeloid progenitor cells Enhanced neutrophil survival and function
Interleukin-1 (IL-1) (α and β)	Macrophages, fibroblasts, T cells, endothelial cells, hepatocytes	Fibroblasts, T cells, monocytes, neutrophils	Induces cytokines (IL-2, IL-3, IL-6, TNF). Induces B- and T-cell activation, growth, and differentiation Synthesis of acute phase reaction, induces fever, catabolism
Interleukin-2 (IL-2)	Activated T cells	Activated lymphoid cells	Enhances T- and B-cell immune responses Promotes cytotoxic T cells Induces INF-γ and TNF
Interleukin-4 (IL-4)	TH2 T cells	B and T cells, macrophages, mast cells	Induces B-cell activation, proliferation and differentiation and IgGI and IgE production Enhances MHC CI and II receptors
Interleukin-6 (IL-6)	Macrophages, fibroblasts, TH2 T cells	Lymphocytes, monocytes	Stimulates B-cell growth, differentiation, and activation Induces synthesis of acute phase reactivants
Interleukin-8 (IL-8)	Monocytes, fibroblasts, endothelial cells	Neutrophils, monocytes	Enhanced neutrophil activity and histamine release
Interleukin-12 (IL-12)	Macrophages, B cells	T cells	Induces differentiation of TH1 cells Initiates production of IFN-α
Interferon gamma (INF-γ)	T cells	Macrophages, monocytes, T and B cells	Pronounced monocyte/macrophage activation Increased MHC class II expression
Tumor necrosis factor: TNF-α (cachectin) TNF-β (lymphotoxin)	Monocytes, macrophages, lymphocytes, mast cells	Monocytes, macrophages, lymphocytes, neutrophils, fibroblasts	Induces cascade of inflammatory reactions (fever, catabolism, acute phase reactants) Induces multiple cytokines (IL-1, GM-CSF) Increases MHC class I expression Enhances B-cell proliferation and immunoglobulin production

From Andreoli TE (ed): *Cecil essentials of medicine,* ed 5, Philadelphia, 2001, WB Saunders.
MHC, Major histocompatibility complex.

IV

TABLE 4-18   Therapeutic Drug Monitoring Data*

	% PROTEIN BOUND	HALF-LIFE ADULTS	HALF-LIFE CHILDREN	TIME TO PEAK PLASMA LEVEL†	LIVER METABOLISM	TIME TO STEADY STATE ADULTS	TIME TO STEADY STATE CHILDREN	THERAPEUTIC RANGE ADULTS	THERAPEUTIC RANGE CHILDREN	TOXIC LEVELS
Lithium carbonate	0	8-35 hr	—	1-3 hr	No	2-7 days	—	0.8-1.4 mEq/L	—	2.0 mEq/L
Amitriptyline	82-96	17-40 hr	—	4-8 hr	Yes	4-8 days	—	120-250 ng/ml	—	500 ng/ml
Desipramine	73-92	12-54 hr	—	2-8 hr	Yes	2.5-11 days	—	150-250 ng/ml	—	500 ng/ml
Imipramine	80-95	9-24 hr	—	1-2 hr	Yes	2-5 days	—	150-250 ng/ml	—	500 ng/ml
Nortriptyline	93-95	18-93 hr	—	4-8 hr	Yes	4-19 days	—	50-150 ng/ml	—	500 ng/ml
Acetylsalicylic acid	50-90	2-4.5 hr	2-3 hr	1-2 hr	Yes	10-22.5 hr	10-15 hr	Depends on use	Same	300 µg/ml
Acetaminophen	20-30	2-4 hr	2-4 hr	0.5-1.0 hr	Yes	10-20 hr	10-20 hr	Depends on use	Same	250 µg/ml
Theophylline	55-65	3-8 hr	1-8 hr	1-3 hr	Yes	15-20 hr	5-40 hr	10-20 µg/ml	Same	20 µg/ml
Methotrexate	50-70	1.5-15 hr	1.5-15 hr	1-2 hr	No	Varies	Varies	>0.01 µmol	—	10 µmol/24 hr
Carbamazepine	65-85	10-30 hr	8-19 hr	6-18 hr	Yes	2-6 days	2-4 days	8-12 µg/ml	Same	15 µg/ml
Ethosuximide	0	40-60 hr	30-50 hr	1-2 hr	Yes	8-12 days	6-10 days	40-100 µg/ml	Same	150 µg/ml
Phenobarbital	45-50	50-120 hr	40-70 hr	6-18 hr	Yes	11-25 days	8-15 days	15-40 µg/ml	Same	50 µg/ml
Phenytoin	87-93	18-30 hr	12-22 hr	4-8 hr	Yes	4-6 days	2-5 days	10-20 µg/ml	Same	20 µg/ml
Primidone	0-20	4-12 hr	4-6 hr	2-4 hr	Yes	16-60 hr	20-30 hr	5-12 µg/ml	Same	15 µg/ml
Valproic acid	90-95	8-15 hr	6-15 hr	0.5-1.5 hr	Yes	40-75 hr	30-75 hr	50-100 µg/ml	Same	200 µg/ml
Digoxin	10-40	32-51 hr	11-50 hr	1.5-5 hr	20%	7-11 days	2-10 days	0.1-2.0 ng/ml	Same	2.4 ng/ml
Disopyramide	10-80	5-6 hr	—	1-3 hr	Yes	25-30 hr	—	2-5 µg/ml	—	7 µg/ml
Lidocaine	60-70	1-2 hr	—	15-30 min (IM)	Yes	5-10 hr	—	1.5-5.0 µg/ml	—	7 µg/ml
Procainamide (PA)	15	2.2-4 hr	—	1-2 hr	Yes	11-20 hr	—	4-10 µg/ml	—	16 µg/ml
N-Acetyl procainamide (NAPA)	10	4-8 hr	—	—	No	22-40 hr	—	9-20 µg/ml	—	—
PA + NAPA	—	—	—	—	—	—	—	10-30 µg/ml	—	30 µg/ml
Propranolol	90-96	2-6 hr	—	1-2 hr	Yes	10-30 hr	—	50-100 ng/ml	—	Variable
Quinidine sulfate	80-90	4-7 hr	—	1.5-2 hr	Yes	20-35 hr	—	2-5 µg/ml‡	—	10 µg/ml
Amikacin	0-11	2-3 hr	—	1 hr (IM)	No	10-15 hr	—	15-25 µg/ml	—	35 µg/ml peak 5 µg/ml residual
Gentamicin	0-10	2-3 hr	2-3 hr	1 hr (IM) 0.5 hr (IV)	No	10-15 hr	10-15 hr	5-10 µg/ml	—	12 µg/ml peak 2 µg/ml residual
Tobramycin	0-10	2-3 hr	—	1 hr (IM)	No	10-15 hr	—	5-10 µg/ml	—	Same as gentamicin
Vancomycin	50	4-8 hr	2-3 hr	15 min (IV)	Minor component	—	—	5-10 µg/ml trough 30-40 µg/ml peak	—	80-100 mg/L

From Ravel R: *Clinical laboratory medicine*, ed 6, St Louis, 1995, Mosby.
IM, Intramuscular; *IV*, intravenous.
*Compiled from various sources.
†Oral dose unless otherwise specified.
‡More specific methods (high-power liquid chromatography, enzyme multiplied immunoassay

TABLE 4-19   Antibody Tests in Epstein-Barr Viral Infection

	APPEARANCE	PEAK	DISAPPEARS
Heterophil Ab	3-5 days after onset of Sx (range, 0-21 days)	During second wk after onset of Sx (1-4 wk)	2-3 mo after onset of Sx (still found at 1 yr in 20% of cases)
VCA-IgM	Beginning of Sx (1 wk before to 1 wk after Sx begin)	During first wk after onset of Sx (0-21 days)	2-3 mo after onset of Sx (1-6 mo)
VCA-IgG	3 days after onset of Sx (0-2 wk)	During second wk after onset of Sx (1-3 wk)	Decline to lower level, then persists for life
EBNA-IgG	3 wk after onset of Sx (1-4 wk)	8 mo after appearance (3-12 mo)	Lifelong
EA-D	5 days after onset of Sx (during first 1-2 wk after onset of Sx)	14-21 days after onset of Sx (1-4 wk)	9 wk after appearance (2-6 mo)
(EBNA-IgM)	(Same as VCA-IgM)	(Same as VCA-IgM)	(Same as VCA-IgM)

From Ravel R: *Clinical laboratory medicine,* ed 6, St Louis, 1995, Mosby.
Ab, Antibody; *EA,* early antigen; *EBNA,* Epstein-Barr virus nuclear antigen; *Sx,* symptoms; *VCA,* viral capsid antigen.

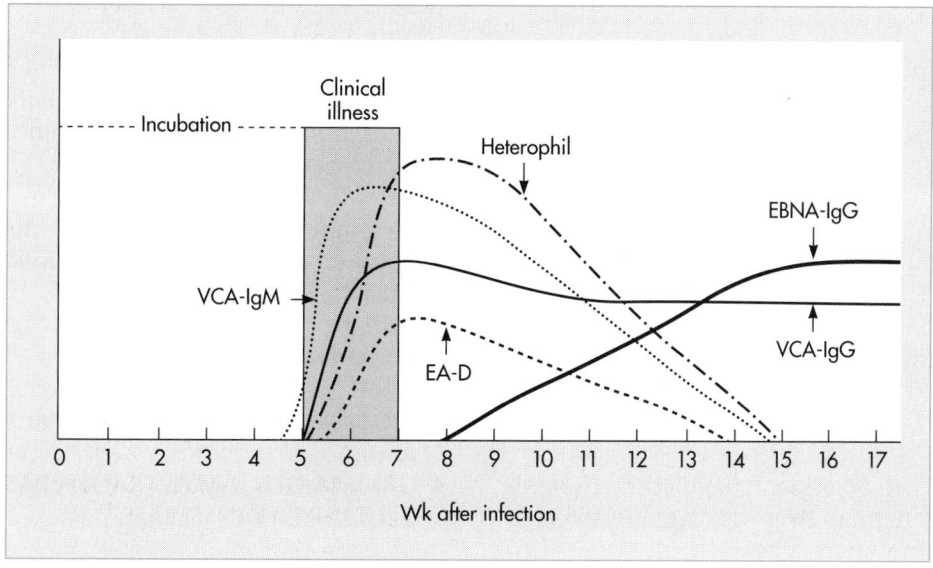

Fig. 4-6   Tests in Epstein-Barr viral infection. See Table 4-19 for abbreviations. (From Ravel R: *Clinical laboratory medicine,* ed 6, St Louis, 1995, Mosby.)

IV

BOX 4-11   Summary of Epstein-Barr Antibody Test Interpretation

Never infected (susceptible): VCA-IgM and IgG both negative

Presumptive primary infection: clinical symptoms, heterophil positive

Primary infection: VCA-IgM positive (EBNA-IgG negative; heterophil positive or negative)

Reactivated infection: VCA-IgG positive; EBNA-IgG positive; EA-D positive (heterophil negative, VCA-IgM negative)

Old previous infection: VCA-IgG positive; EBNA-IgG positive; EA-D negative (VCA-IgM negative, heterophil negative)

From Ravel R: *Clinical laboratory medicine,* ed 6, St Louis, 1995, Mosby.
See Table 4-19 for abbreviations.

■ **FERRITIN** (serum)
Normal range:
18-300 ng/ml (18-300 μg/L) [CF: 1; SMI: 10 μg/L]
Cost: $45

Elevated in:
Hyperthyroidism, inflammatory states, liver disease (ferritin elevated from necrotic hepatocytes), neoplasms (neuroblastomas, lymphomas, leukemia, breast carcinoma), iron replacement therapy, hemochromatosis, hemosiderosis

Decreased in:
Iron deficiency anemia

- **α-1 FETOPROTEIN**

Normal range:
0-20 ng/ml (0-20 µg/L) [CF: 1; SMI: 1 µg/L]

Cost: $66

Elevated in:
Hepatocellular carcinoma (usually values >1000 ng/ml), germinal neoplasms (testis, ovary, mediastinum, retroperitoneum), liver disease (alcoholic cirrhosis, acute hepatitis, chronic active hepatitis), fetal anencephaly, spina bifida, basal cell carcinoma, breast carcinoma, pancreatic carcinoma, gastric carcinoma, retinoblastoma, esophageal atresia

- **FIBRIN DEGRADATION PRODUCT** (FDP)

Normal range:
<10 µg/ml

Cost: $40

Elevated in:
Disseminated intravascular coagulation, primary fibrinolysis, pulmonary embolism, severe liver disease
NOTE: The presence of rheumatoid factor may cause falsely elevated FDP.

- **FIBRINOGEN**

Normal range:
200-400 mg/dl (2-4 g/L) [CF: 0.01; SMI: 0.1 g/L]

Cost: $38

Elevated in:
Tissue inflammation or damage (acute phase protein reactant), oral contraceptives, pregnancy, acute infection, myocardial infarction

Decreased in:
Disseminated intravascular coagulation, hereditary afibrinogenemia, liver disease, primary or secondary fibrinolysis, cachexia

- **FOLATE** (folic acid)

Normal range:
Plasma: 2-10 ng/ml (4-22 nmol/L) [CF: 2.266; SMI: 2 nmol/L]
Red blood cells: 140-960 ng/ml (550-2200 nmol/L) [CF: 2.266; SMI: 10 nmol/L]

Cost: $52

Decreased in:
Folic acid deficiency (inadequate intake, malabsorption), alcoholism, drugs (methotrexate, trimethoprim, phenytoin, oral contraceptives, azulfidine), vitamin B_{12} deficiency (defective red cell folate absorption), hemolytic anemia

Elevated in:
Folic acid therapy

- **FOLLICLE-STIMULATING HORMONE** (FSH)

Normal range:
5-20 mIU/mL

Cost: $58

Elevated in:
Menopause, primary gonadal failure, alcoholism, castration, Klinefelter's syndrome, gonadotropin-secreting pituitary hormones

Decreased in:
Pregnancy, polycystic ovary disease, anorexia nervosa, anterior pituitary hypofunction

- **FREE T_4;** *see* T_4, FREE
- **FREE THYROXINE INDEX**

Normal range:
1.1-4.3
See Boxes 4-12 and 4-13 for causes of abnormal results.

- **GAMMA-GLUTAMYL TRANSFERASE** (GGT); *see* γ-GLUTAMYL TRANSFERASE

BOX 4-12   Causes for Increased Thyroxine or Free Thyroxine Values

Laboratory error
Primary hyperthyroidism (T_4/T_3 type)
Severe thyroxine-binding globulin elevation; some patients with some FT_4 kits
Excess therapy of hypothyroidism
Excessive dose of levothyroxine
Active thyroiditis (subacute, painless, early active Hashimoto's disease); some patients
Familial dysalbuminemic hyperthyroxinemia (some FT_4 kits, especially analog types)
Peripheral resistance to T_4 syndrome
Amiodarone or propranolol; some patients
Postpartum transient toxicosis
Factitious hyperthyroidism
Jod-Basedow (iodine-induced) hyperthyroidism
Severe nonthyroid illness, occasional patients
Acute psychosis (especially paranoid schizophrenia); some patients

T_4 sample drawn 2-4 hr after Synthroid dose
Struma ovarii
Pituitary thyroid-stimulating hormone–secreting tumor; some patients
Certain x-ray contrast media (Telepaque and Oragrafin)
Acute porphyria; some patients
Heparin effect (some T_4 and FT_4 kits)
Amphetamine, heroin, methadone, and phencyclidine abuse; some patients
Perphenazine or 5-fluorouracil; some patients
Antithyroid or anti-IgG heterophil (HAMA) autoantibodies (some sandwich-method monoclonal antibody kits); occasional patients
"T_4" hyperthyroidism
Hyperemesis gravidarum; about 50% of patients
High altitudes, some patients

From Ravel R: *Clinical laboratory medicine*, ed 6, St Louis, 1995, Mosby.
FT_4, Free thyroxine; *HAMA,* human antimouse antibodies; *T_3,* triiodothyronine; *T_4,* thyroxine.

BOX 4-13   Causes for Decreased Thyroxine or Free Thyroxine Values

Laboratory error
Primary hypothyroidism
Severe nonthyroid illness*; many patients
Lithium therapy; some patients
Severe thyroxine-binding globulin decrease (congenital, disease, or drug-induced) or severe albumin decrease*
Dilantin, Depakene, or high-dose salicylate drugs*
Pituitary insufficiency
Large doses of inorganic iodide (e.g., saturated solution of potassium iodide)

Moderate or severe iodine deficiency
Cushing's syndrome
High-dose glucocorticoid drugs; some patients
Pregnancy, third trimester (low normal or small decrease)
Addison's disease; some patients (30%)
Heparin effect (a few FT_4 kits)
Desipramine or amiodarone drugs; some patients
Acute psychiatric illness; a few patients

From Ravel R: *Clinical laboratory medicine,* ed 6, St Louis, 1995, Mosby.
*FT_4 less affected than T_4; two-step FT_4 method affected less than analog FT_4 method.

BOX 4-14   Clinical Situations in Which Measurement of Serum Gastrin Levels Is Indicated

Family history of peptic ulcer
Ulcer associated with hypercalcemia or other manifestations of multiple endocrine neoplasia type I
Multiple ulcers
Peptic ulceration of postbulbar duodenum or jejunum

Peptic ulceration associated with diarrhea*
Chronic unexplained diarrhea*
Enlarged gastric folds on upper gastrointestinal x-ray
Before surgery for "intractable" ulcer
Recurrent ulcer after ulcer surgery

Modified from Schiller LR: Peptic ulcer: epidemiology, clinical manifestations, and diagnosis. In Andreoli TE (ed): *Cecil essentials of medicine,* ed 4, Philadelphia, 1997, WB Saunders.
*Not due to antacid ingestion.

- **GASTRIN** (serum)
  Normal range:
  0-180 pg/ml (0-180 ng/L) [CF: 1; SMI: 10 ng/L]
  Cost: $62
  Elevated in:
  Zollinger-Ellison syndrome (gastrinoma), pernicious anemia, hyperparathyroidism, retained gastric antrum, chronic renal failure, gastric ulcer, chronic atrophic gastritis, pyloric obstruction, malignant neoplasms of the stomach, H_2-blockers, omeprazole, calcium therapy, ulcerative colitis, rheumatoid arthritis
  Box 4-14 describes clinical situations in which measurement of serum gastrin levels is indicated.

- **GLOMERULAR BASEMENT MEMBRANE** (GBM) **ANTIBODY**
  Normal:
  Negative
  Cost: $89
  Present in:
  Goodpasture's syndrome

- **GLUCOSE, FASTING**
  Normal range:
  70-110 mg/dl (3.9-6.1 mmol/L) [CF: 0.05551; SMI: 0.1 mmol/L]
  Cost: $23

  Elevated in:
  Diabetes mellitus, stress, infections, myocardial infarction, cerebrovascular accident, Cushing's syndrome, acromegaly, acute pancreatitis, glucagonoma, hemochromatosis, drugs (glucocorticoids, diuretics [thiazides, loop diuretics]), glucose intolerance

- **GLUCOSE, POSTPRANDIAL**
  Normal range:
  <140 mg/dl (<7.8 mmol/L) [CF: 0.05551; SMI: 0.1 mmol/L]
  Cost: $23
  Elevated in:
  Diabetes mellitus, glucose intolerance
  Decreased in:
  Postgastrointestinal resection, reactive hypoglycemia, hereditary fructose intolerance, galactosemia, leucine sensitivity

- **GLUCOSE TOLERANCE TEST**
  Normal values above fasting:
  30 min: 30-60 mg/dl (1.65-3.3 mmol/L) [CF: 0.05551; SMI: 0.1 mmol/L]
  60 min: 20-50 mg/dl (1.1-2.75 mmol/L) [CF: 0.05551; SMI: 0.1 mmol/L]
  120 min: 5-15 mg/dl (0.28-0.83 mmol/L) [CF: 0.05551; SMI: 0.1 mmol/L]
  180 min: fasting level or below

IV

Abnormal in:
Glucose intolerance, diabetes mellitus, Cushing's syndrome, acromegaly, pheochromocytoma, gestational diabetes
Cost: $43

■ **GLUCOSE-6-PHOSPHATE DEHYDROGENASE SCREEN** (blood)
Normal:
G_6PD enzyme activity detected
Cost: $79
Abnormal:
If a deficiency is detected, quantitation of G_6PD is necessary; a G_6PD screen may be falsely interpreted as "normal" after an episode of hemolysis because most G_6PD deficient cells have been destroyed.

■ **γ-GLUTAMYL TRANSFERASE (GGT)**
Normal range:
0-30 U/L (0.050 μkat/L) [CF: 0.01667; SMI: 0.01 μkat/L]
Cost: $23
Elevated in:
Chronic alcoholic liver disease, neoplasms (hepatoma, metastatic disease to the liver, carcinoma of the pancreas), systemic lupus erythematosus, congestive heart failure, trauma, nephrotic syndrome, sepsis, cholestasis, drugs (phenytoin, barbiturates), other (Box 4-15 lists additional causes of GGT elevation.)

■ **GLYCATED (GLYCOSYLATED) HEMOGLOBIN** (HbA_{1c})
Normal range:
4.0% to 6.7%
Cost: $39
Elevated in:
Uncontrolled diabetes mellitus (glycated hemoglobin levels reflect the level of glucose control over the preceding 120 days), lead toxicity, alcoholism, iron deficiency anemia, hypertriglyceridemia

Decreased in:
Hemolytic anemias, decreased red blood cell survival, pregnancy, acute or chronic blood loss, chronic renal failure, insulinoma, congenital spherocytosis, hemoglobin S, C, and D diseases

■ **HAM TEST** (acid serum test)
Normal:
Negative
Cost: $79
Positive in:
Paroxysmal nocturnal hemoglobinuria
False positive in:
Hereditary or acquired spherocytosis, recent transfusion with aged red blood cells, aplastic anemia, myeloproliferative syndromes, leukemia, hereditary dyserythropoietic anemia type II

■ **HAPTOGLOBIN** (serum)
Normal range:
50-220 mg/dl (0.50-2.2 g/L) [CF: 0.01; SMI: 0.01 g/L]
Cost: $44
Elevated in:
Inflammation (acute phase reactant), collagen-vascular diseases, infections (acute phase reactant), drugs (androgens), obstructive liver disease
Decreased in:
Hemolysis (intravascular more than extravascular), megaloblastic anemia, severe liver disease, large tissue hematomas, infectious mononucleosis, drugs (oral contraceptives)

■ **HDL;** *see* HIGH-DENSITY LIPOPROTEIN CHOLESTEROL

■ **HEMATOCRIT**
Normal range:
Male: 39% to 49% (0.39-0.49) [CF: 0.01; SMI: 0.01]
Female: 33% to 43% (0.33-0.43) [CF: 0.01; SMI: 0.01]
Cost: $20

BOX 4-15 Some Etiologies for γ-Glutamyl Transferase (GGT) Elevation

Liver space-occupying lesions (M-H)* (88%, 45%-100%)†
Alcoholic active liver disease (M, occasionally H) (85%, 63%-100%)
Common bile duct obstruction (M-H) (90%, 62%-100%)
Intrahepatic cholestasis (M-H) (90%, 83%-94%)
Biliary tract acute inflammation (M-H) (95%, 90%-100%)
Acute hepatitis virus hepatitis (M, occasionally H) (95%, 89%-100%)
Infectious mononucleosis (M/S, occasionally H) (90%)
Cytomegalovirus acute infection (S/M) (75%)
Acute pancreatitis (M, occasionally H) (85%, 71%-100%)
Active granulation tissue formation (S-M)
Acetaminophen overdose (S/M)

Dilantin therapy (S, occasionally M) (70%, 58%-90%)
Phenobarbitol (similar to Dilantin)
Severe liver passive congestion (S) (60%)
Reye's syndrome (S) (63%)
Other; all usually S elevations
  Acute myocardial infarction (5%-30%)
  Tegretol (30%)
  Hyperthyroidism (0%-62%)
  Epilepsy (50%-85%)
  Brain tumor (57%)
  Diabetes mellitus (24%-57%)
  Nonalcohol fatty liver

From Ravel R: *Clinical laboratory medicine,* ed 6, St Louis, 1995, Mosby.
**H,* High (over 5×); *M,* moderate (3-5×); *S,* small (1-3× upper limit).
†Percentage of patients, with literature range.

Elevated in:

Polycythemia vera, smoking, chronic obstructive pulmonary disease, high altitudes, dehydration, hypovolemia

Decreased in:

Blood loss (gastrointestinal, genitourinary) anemia

■ **HEMOGLOBIN**

Normal range:

Male: 13.6-17.7 g/dl (136-172 g/L) [CF: 10; SMI: 1 g/L]

Female: 12.0-15.0 g/dl (120-150 g/L) [CF: 10; SMI: 1 g/L]

Cost: $20

Elevated in:

Hemoconcentration, dehydration, polycythemia vera, chronic obstructive pulmonary disease, high altitudes, false elevations (hyperlipemic plasma, white blood cells >50,000/mm^3), stress

Decreased in:

Hemorrhage (gastrointestinal, genitourinary) anemia Fig. 4-7 describes a diagnostic approach to low hemoglobin/hematocrit levels.

■ **HEMOGLOBIN A$_{1C}$,** *see* GLYCATED HEMOGLOBIN

■ **HEMOGLOBIN ELECTROPHORESIS**

Normal range:

HbA$_1$: 95%-98%

HbA$_2$: 1.5%-3.5%

HbF: <2%

HbC: absent

HbS: absent

Cost: $45

■ **HEMOGLOBIN, GLYCATED;** *see* GLYCATED HEMOGLOBIN

■ **HEMOGLOBIN, GLYCOSYLATED;** *see* GLYCATED HEMOGLOBIN

■ **HEMOGLOBIN, URINE;** *see* URINE HEMOGLOBIN

■ **HEMOSIDERIN, URINE;** *see* URINE HEMOSIDERIN

■ **HEPATITIS A ANTIBODY**

Normal:

Negative

Cost: $54

Present in:

Viral hepatitis A; can be IgM or IgG (if IgM, acute hepatitis A; if IgG, previous infection with hepatitis A); *see* Boxes 4-16 through 4-18 and Fig. 4-8

■ **HEPATITIS A VIRAL INFECTION;** *see above*

■ **HEPATITIS B SURFACE ANTIGEN** (HBsAg)

Normal:

Not detected

Cost: $37

Detected in:

Acute viral hepatitis type B, chronic hepatitis B (Boxes 4-19 through 4-27 and Figs. 4-9 through 4-12)

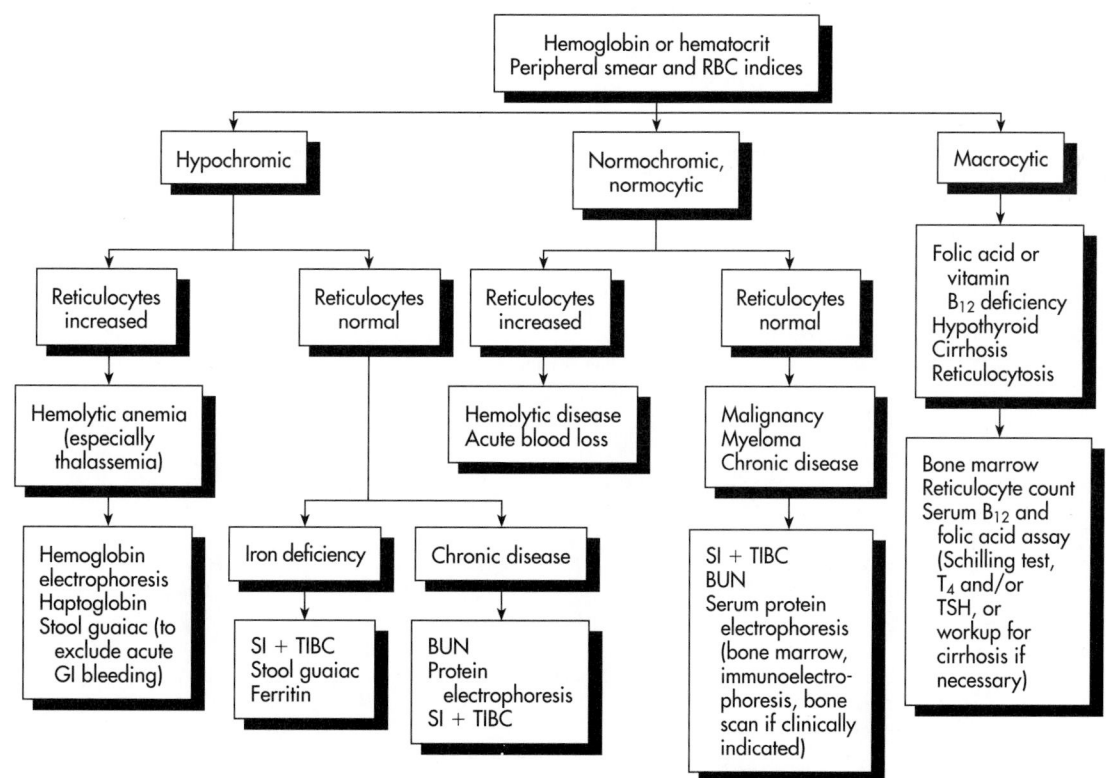

Fig. 4-7   Simplified guide to anemia diagnosis using a minimum of tests aimed at most important disease categories. *BUN,* Blood urea nitrogen; *GI,* gastrointestinal; *RBC,* red blood cell; *SI,* serum iron; *TIBC,* total iron-binding capacity. (From Ravel R: *Clinical laboratory medicine,* ed 6, St Louis, 1995, Mosby.)

IV

BOX 4-16   HAV Antibodies

HAV-IgM Antibody

Appearance

About the same time as clinical symptoms (3-4 wk after exposure, range 14-60 days), or just before beginning of AST/ALT elevation (range 10 days before–7 days after)

Peak

About 3-4 wk after onset of symptoms (1-6 wk)

Becomes Nondetectable

3-4 mo after onset of symptoms (1-6 mo). In a few cases HAV-IgM antibody can persist as long as 12-14 mo.

HAV-Total Antibody

Appearance

About 3 wk after IgM becomes detectable (therefore about the middle of clinical symptom period to early convalescence)

Peak

About 1-2 mo after onset

Becomes Nondetectable

Remains elevated for life, but can slowly fall somewhat

From Ravel R: *Clinical laboratory medicine,* ed 6, St Louis, 1995, Mosby.

BOX 4-17   Hepatitis A Antigen and Antibodies

HAV-Ag by EM (in stool)
  Shows presence of virus in stool early in infection

HAV-Ab (IgM)
  Current or recent HAV infection
HAV-Ab (total)
  Convalescent or old HAV infection

From Ravel R: *Clinical laboratory medicine,* ed 6, St Louis, 1995, Mosby.

BOX 4-18   Summary: Diagnosis of HAV Infection

Best all-purpose test(s) to diagnose acute HAV infection = HAV-Ab (IgM)

Best all-purpose test(s) to demonstrate past HAV infection/immunity = HAV-Ab (total)

From Ravel R: *Clinical laboratory medicine,* ed 6, St Louis, 1995, Mosby.

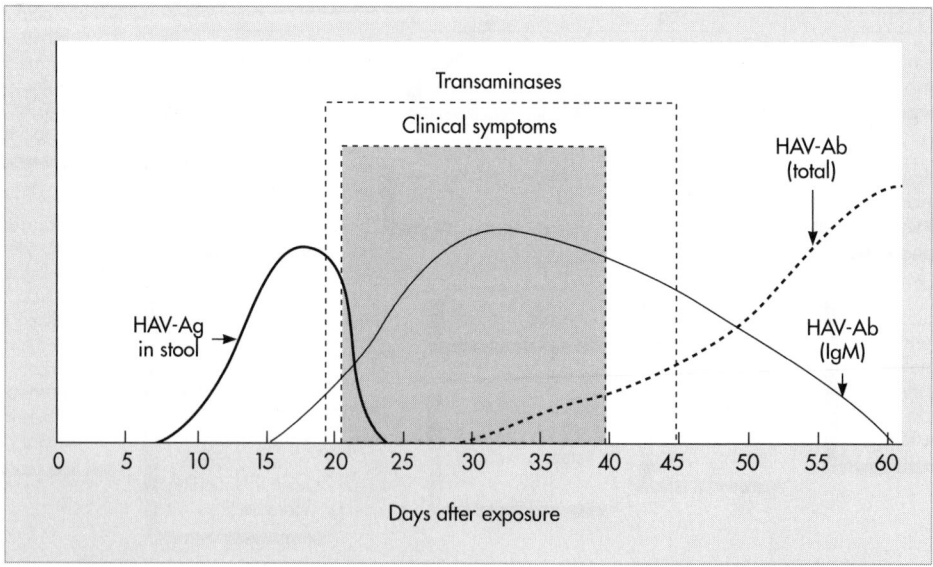

Fig. 4-8   Serologic tests in HAV infection. (From Ravel R: *Clinical laboratory medicine,* ed 6, St Louis, 1995, Mosby.)

BOX 4-19   Interpretation of Hepatitis B Serologic Tests

I. HB$_S$Ag positive, HB$_C$Ab negative*
   About 5% (range 0%-17%) of patients with early stage HBV acute infection (HB$_C$Ab rises later)

II. HB$_S$Ag positive, HB$_C$Ab positive, HB$_S$Ab negative
   a. Most of the clinical symptom stage
   b. Chronic HBV carriers without evidence of liver disease ("asymptomatic carriers")
   c. Chronic HBV hepatitis (chronic persistent type or chronic active type)

III. HB$_S$Ag negative, HB$_C$Ab positive,* HB$_S$Ab negative
   a. Late clinical symptom stage or early convalescence stage (core window)
   b. Chronic HBV infection with HB$_S$Ag below detection levels with current tests
   c. Old previous HBV infection

IV. HB$_S$Ag negative, HB$_C$Ab positive, HB$_S$Ab positive
   a. Late convalescence to complete recovery
   b. Old infection

From Ravel R: *Clinical laboratory medicine,* ed 6, St Louis, 1995, Mosby.
*HB$_C$Ab, Combined IgM + IgG. In some cases (e.g., category III), selective Hb$_C$Ab-IgM assay is useful to differentiate recent and old infection.

BOX 4-20   HB$_S$Ag by Immunoassay

Appearance

2-6 wk after exposure (range 6 days–6 mo). 5%-15% of patients are negative at onset of jaundice

Peak

1-2 wk before to 1-2 wk after onset of symptoms

Becomes Nondetectable

1-3 mo after peak (range 1 wk-5 mo)

From Ravel R: *Clinical laboratory medicine,* ed 6, St Louis, 1995, Mosby.

BOX 4-21   Summary: HBV Surface Antigen and Antibody

HB$_S$Ag by immunoassay
1. Means current active HBV infection.
2. Persistence over 6 mo indicates carrier/chronic HBV infection.

HB$_S$Ag by nucleic acid probe
1. Same significance as detection by immunoassay.
2. Present before and longer than HB$_S$Ag by immunoassay.

3. More reliable marker for increased infectivity than HB$_S$Ag by immunoassay and/or HB$_e$Ag.

From Ravel R: *Clinical laboratory medicine,* ed 6, St Louis, 1995, Mosby.

■ **HEPATITIS B VIRAL INFECTION;** *see above*

■ **HEPATITIS C VIRAL INFECTION;** *see* Boxes 4-28 through 4-30 and Fig. 4-13

■ **HEPATITIS D VIRAL INFECTION;** *see* Boxes 4-31 through 4-33 and Fig. 4-14

■ **HETEROPHIL ANTIBODY**
Normal:
Negative
Cost: $30
Positive in:
Infectious mononucleosis

■ **HIGH-DENSITY LIPOPROTEIN** (HDL) **CHOLESTEROL**
Normal range:
Male: 45-70 mg/dl (0.8-1.8 mmol/L) [CF: 0.02586; SMI: 0.05 mmol/L]
Female: 45-90 mg/dl (0.8-2.35 mmol/L) [CF: 0.02586; SMI: 0.05 mmol/L]
Cost: $24

Increased in:
Use of gemfibrozil, statins, fenofibrate, nicotinic acid, estrogens, regular aerobic exercise, small (1 oz) daily alcohol intake
Decreased in:
Deficiency of apoproteins, liver disease, probucol ingestion, Tangier disease
NOTE: A cholesterol/HDL ratio ±4.5 is associated with increased risk of coronary artery disease.

■ **HLA ANTIGENS**
Cost: $80
Associated disorders:
see Table 4-20.

■ **HUMAN CHORIONIC GONADOTROPIN** (hCG)
Normal range:
Varies with gestational stage
1st week: 5-50 mU/ml
1-2 wk: 50-550 mU/ml
2-3 wk: up to 5000 mU/ml

IV

BOX 4-22   Summary of Hepatitis Test Applications

HB$_S$

-Ag

HB$_S$Ag: shows current active HBV infection.
Persistence over 6 mo indicates carrier/chronic HBV infection.
HBV nucleic acid probe: present before and longer than HB$_S$Ag.
More reliable marker for increased infectivity than HB$_S$Ag and/or HB$_e$Ag.

-Ab

HB$_S$Ab-total: shows previous healed HBV infection and evidence of immunity.

HB$_C$

-Ab

HB$_C$Ab-IgM: shows either acute or very recent infection by HBV.
In convalescent phase of acute HBV, may be elevated when HB$_S$Ag has disappeared (core window).
Negative HB$_C$Ab-IgM with positive HB$_S$Ag suggests either very early acute HBV or carrier/chronic HBV.
HB$_C$Ab-total: only useful to show past HBV infection if HB$_S$Ag and HB$_C$Ab-IgM are both negative.

HB$_e$

-Ag

HB$_e$-AbAg: when present, especially without HB$_e$Ab, suggests increased patient infectivity.
HB$_e$Ab-total: when present, suggests less patient infectivity.

HDV

-Ag

HDV-Ag: shows current infection (acute or chronic) by HDV.

HDV nucleic acid probe: detects antigen before and longer than HDV-Ag by EIA.

-Ab

HDV-Ab (IgM): high elevation in acute HDV; does not persist.
Low or moderate elevation in convalescent HDV; does not persist.
Low to high persistent elevation in chronic HDV (depends on degree of cell injury and sensitivity of the assay).
HDV-Ab (total): high elevation in acute HDV; does not persist.
High persistent elevation in chronic HDV.

HCV

-Ag

HCV nucleic acid probe: shows current infection by HCV (especially using PCR amplification).

-Ab

HCV-Ab (IgG): current, convalescent, or old HCV infection.

HAV

-Ag

HAV-Ag by EM: Shows presence of virus in stool early in infection.

-Ab

HAV-Ab (IgM): current or recent HAV infection.
HAV-Ab (total): convalescent or old HAV infection.

From Ravel R: *Clinical laboratory medicine,* ed 6, St Louis, 1995, Mosby.

BOX 4-23   HB$_C$Ab-IgM

Appearance	Peak	Becomes Nondetectable
About 2 wk (range, 0-6 wk) after HB$_S$Ag appears	About 1 wk after onset of symptoms	3-6 mo after appearance (range 2 wk–2 yr)

From Ravel R: *Clinical laboratory medicine,* ed 6, St Louis, 1995, Mosby.

BOX 4-24   HB$_C$Ab-Total

Appearance	Peak	Becomes Nondetectable
3-4 wk (range 2-10 wk) after HB$_S$Ag appears	3-4 wk after first detection	Elevated throughout life; may have slow decline to lower titers over many years

From Ravel R: *Clinical laboratory medicine,* ed 6, St Louis, 1995, Mosby.

BOX 4-25 HB_eAg

Appearance

About 3-5 days after appearance of HB_SAg

Peak

About the same time as HB_SAg peak

Becomes Nondetectable

About 2-4 wk before HB_SAg disappears in about 70% of cases

About 1-7 days after HB_SAg disappears in about 20% of cases

Accompanies persistent HB_SAg in 30%-50% or more patients who become chronic HBV carriers or have chronic HBV infection; however, may eventually convert to antibody in up to 40% of these patients

From Ravel R: *Clinical laboratory medicine,* ed 6, St Louis, 1995, Mosby.

BOX 4-26 HB_eAb-Total

Appearance

At the same time as or within 1-2 wk (range, 0-4 wk) after e antigen disappears (2-4 wk before HB_SAg loss to 2 wk after HB_SAg loss)

Peak

During HBV core window

Becomes Nondetectable

Persists for several years (4-6 yr)

From Ravel R: *Clinical laboratory medicine,* ed 6, St Louis, 1995, Mosby.

BOX 4-27 Summary: HBV e Antigen and Antibody

HB_eAg
When present, especially without HB_eAb, suggests increased patient infectivity

HB_eAb-total
When present, suggests less patient infectivity

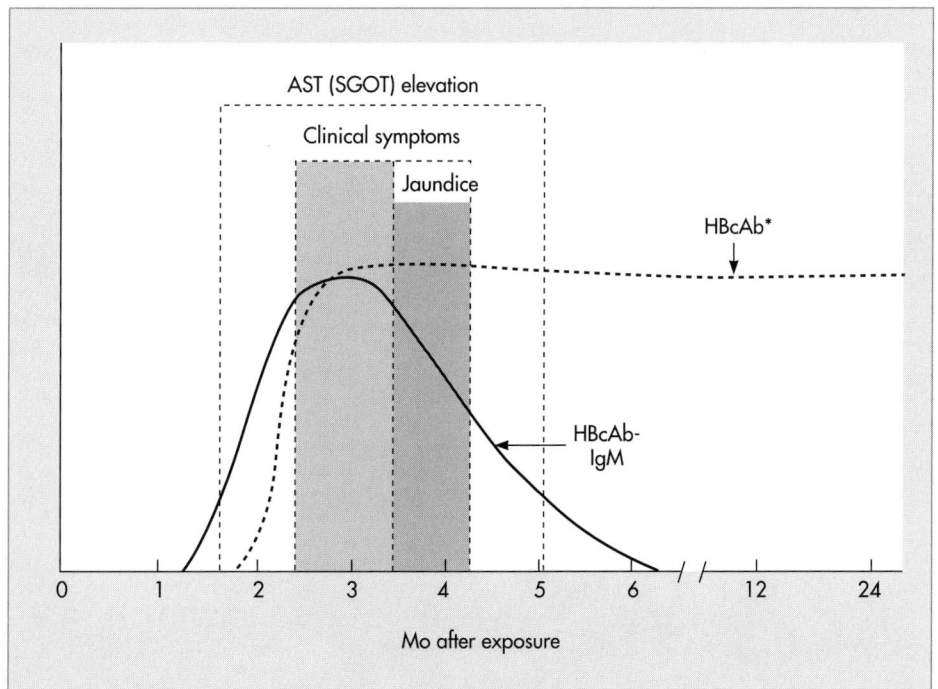

Fig. 4-9 HBV core antibodies. *HB_CAb = HB_CAb-IgM + HB_CAb-IgG (combined). (From Ravel R: *Clinical laboratory medicine,* ed 6, St Louis, 1995, Mosby.)

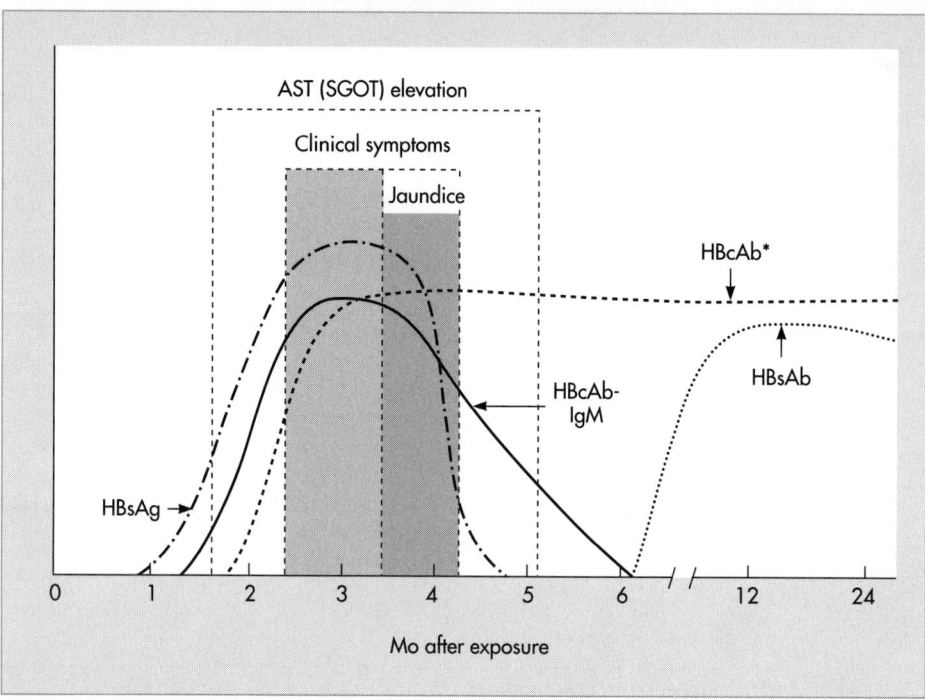

Fig. 4-10 **HBV surface antigen-antibody and core antibodies** (note "core window"). *HB$_C$Ab = HB$_C$Ab-IgM + HB$_C$Ab-IgG (combined). (From Ravel R: *Clinical laboratory medicine,* ed 6, St Louis, 1995, Mosby.)

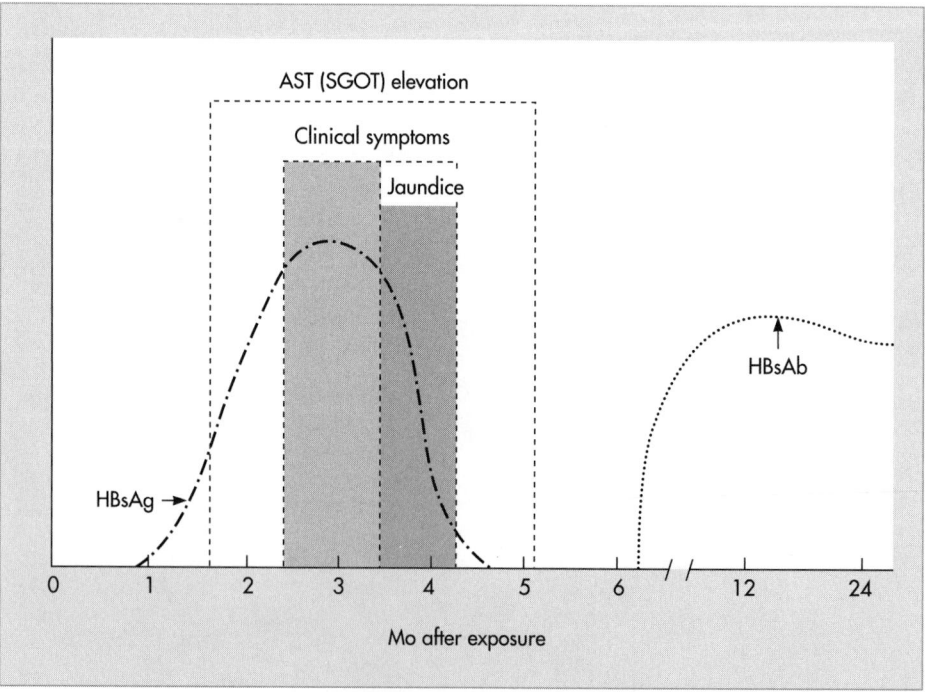

Fig. 4-11 **HBV surface antigen and antibody** (HB$_S$Ag and HB$_S$Ab-total). (From Ravel R: *Clinical laboratory medicine,* ed 6, St Louis, 1995, Mosby.)

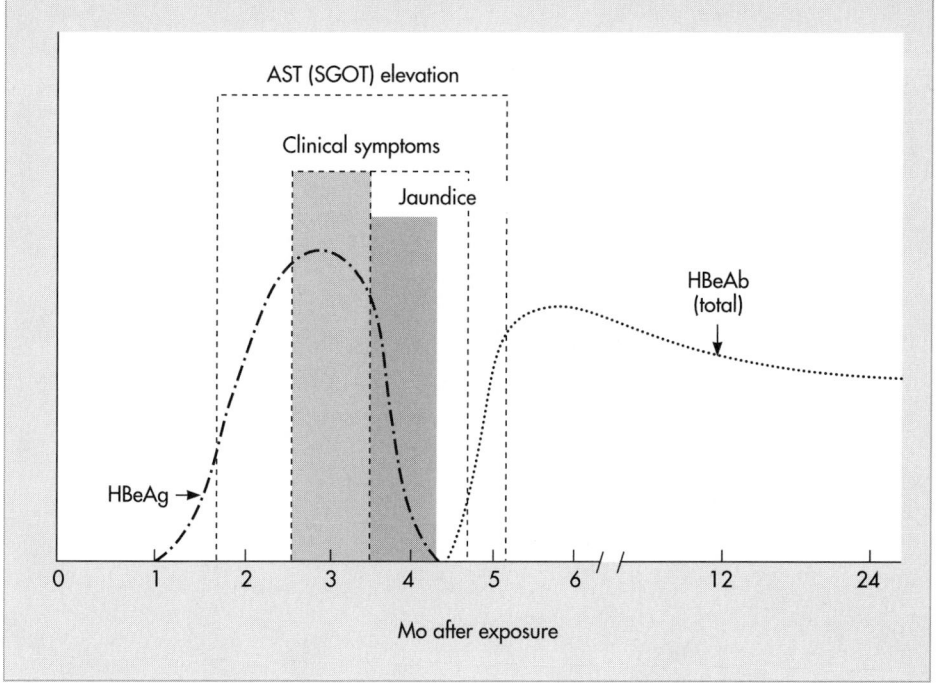

Fig. 4-12   HBV e antigen and antibody. (From Ravel R: *Clinical laboratory medicine,* ed 6, St Louis, 1995, Mosby.)

BOX 4-28   HCV-Ag

Nucleic Acid Probe (Without PCR)

Appearance: about 3-4 wk after infection (about 1-2 wk later than PCR-enhanced probe)
Becomes nondetectable: near the end of active infection, beginning of convalescence

Nucleic Acid Probe (with PCR)

Appearance: as early as the second week after infection
Becomes nondetectable: end of active infection, beginning of convalescence

From Ravel R: *Clinical laboratory medicine,* ed 6, St Louis, 1995, Mosby.
PCR, Polymerase chain reaction.

BOX 4-29   HCV-Ab (IgG)

Second-Generation ELISA

Appearance: about 3-4 mo after infection (about 2-4 wk before first-generation tests); 80% by 5-6 wk after symptoms
Becomes nondetectable: 7% lose detectable antibody by 1.5 yr; 7%-66% negative by 4 yr (by first-generation tests; more remain elevated and for longer time by second-generation tests)

From Ravel R: *Clinical laboratory medicine,* ed 6, St Louis, 1995, Mosby.

IV

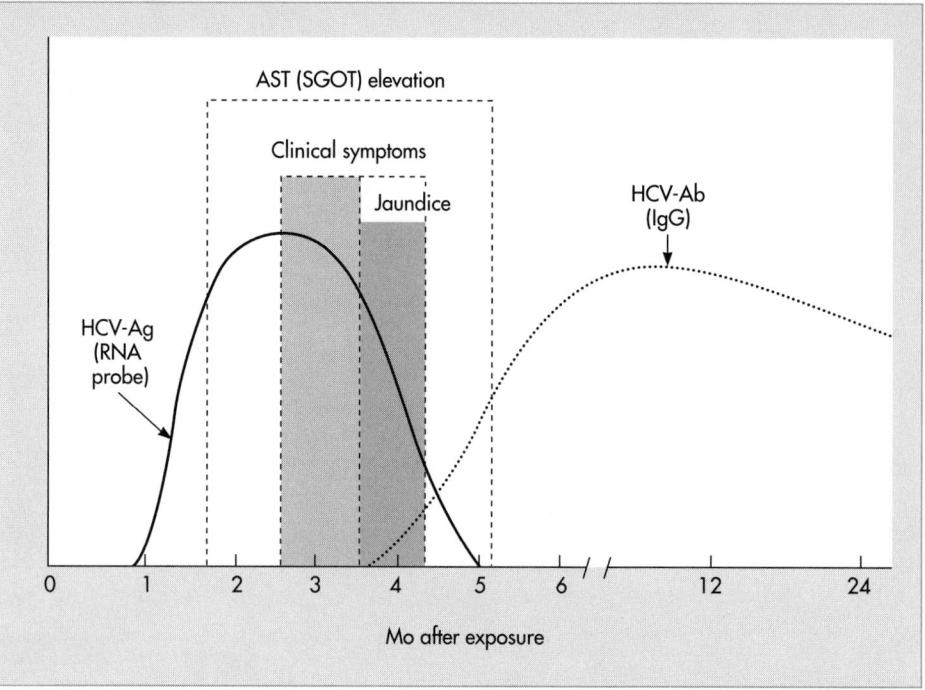

Fig. 4-13   HCV antigen and antibody. (From Ravel R: *Clinical laboratory medicine,* ed 6, St Louis, 1995, Mosby.)

BOX 4-30   Summary: Hepatitis C Antigen and Antibody

HCV-Ag by nucleic acid probe
  Shows current infection by HCV (especially using polymerase chain reaction amplification)

HCV-Ab (IgG)
  Current, convalescent, or old HCV infection (behaves
  more like IgM or "total" Ab than usual IgG Ab)

From Ravel R: *Clinical laboratory medicine,* ed 6, St Louis, 1995, Mosby.

BOX 4-31   Delta Hepatitis Coinfection (Acute HDV + Acute HBV) or Superinfection (Acute HDV + Chronic HBV)

HDV-AG

Detected by DNA probe, less often by immunoassay
Appearance: Prodromal stage (before symptoms); just at
  or after initial rise in ALT (about a week after appearance of HB_SAg and about the time HB_CAb-IgM level
  begins to rise)
Peak: 2-3 days after onset
Becomes nondetectable: 1-4 days (may persist until
  shortly after symptoms appear)

HDV-AB (IgM)

Appearance: about 10 days after symptoms begin (range
  1-28 days)

Peak: about 2 wk after first detection
Becomes nondetectable: about 35 days (range 10-80
  days) after first detection (most other IgM antibodies
  take 3-6 mo to become nondetectable)

HDV-AB (Total)

Appearance: about 50 days after symptoms begin (range
  14-80 days); about 5 wk after HDV-Ag (range 3-11 wk)
Peak: About 2 wk after first detection
Becomes nondetectable: about 7 mo after first detection
  (range 4-14 mo)

From Ravel R: *Clinical laboratory medicine,* ed 6, St Louis, 1995, Mosby.

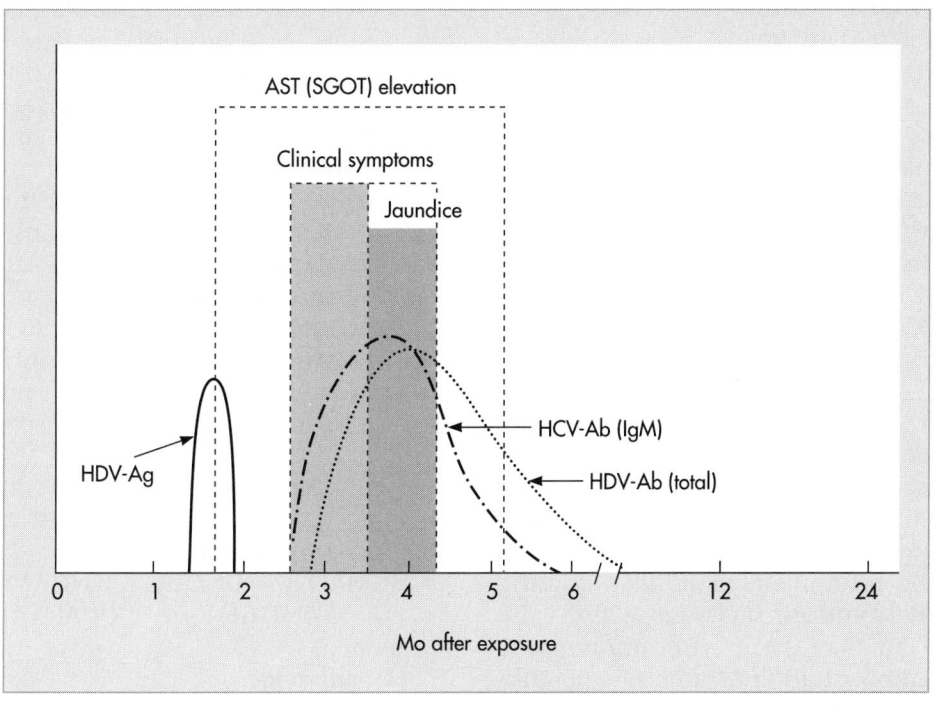

Fig. 4-14   HDV antigen and antibodies. (From Ravel R: *Clinical laboratory medicine,* ed 6, St Louis, 1995, Mosby.)

Gwendolyn R. Lee, M.D.
Internal Medicine

BOX 4-32   Delta Hepatitis Chronic Infection (Chronic HDV + Chronic HBV)

HDV-Ag

Detectable in serum by nucleic acid probe

HDV-Ab (IgM)

Detectable (may need sensitive method; titer depends on degree of virus activity)

HDV-Ab (Total)

Detectable, usually in high titer

From Ravel R: *Clinical laboratory medicine,* ed 6, St Louis, 1995, Mosby.

BOX 4-33   Summary: Diagnosis of HDV Infection

Best current all-purpose screening test = ADV-Ab (total)

Best test to differentiate acute from chronic infection = HDV-Ab (IgM)

From Ravel R: *Clinical laboratory medicine,* ed 6, St Louis, 1995, Mosby.

TABLE 4-20   HLA Antigens Associated with Specific Diseases

ANTIGEN	CONDITION	ANTIGEN	CONDITION
HLA-B27	Ankylosing spondylitis	HLA-B8, Dw3	Celiac disease
	Reiter's syndrome	HLA-B8, Dw3	Dermatitis herpetiformis
	Psoriatic arthritis	HLA-B8	Myasthenia gravis
HLA-A10, B18, Dw2	C2 deficiency	HLA-B8	Chronic active hepatitis in children
HLA-A2, B40, Cw3	C4 deficiency	HLA-Drw4	Active chronic hepatitis in adults
HLA-B7, Dw2	Multiple sclerosis	HLA-B13, Bw17	Psoriasis
HLA-A3	Hemochromatosis		

From Cerra FB: *Manual of critical care,* St Louis, 1987, Mosby.

3-4 wk: up to 10,000 mU/ml
4-5 wk: up to 50,000 mU/ml
2-3 mo: 10,000-100,000 mU/ml
Cost: $34
Elevated in:
Normal pregnancy, hydatidiform mole, chorio-carcinoma, germ cell tumors of testicle, some nontrophoblastic neoplasms (e.g., neoplasms of cervix, gastrointestinal tract, ovary, lung, breast)

■ **HUMAN IMMUNODEFICIENCY VIRUS ANTIBODY, TYPE 1 (HIV-1)**
Normal range:
Not detected
Cost: $59
Abnormal result:
HIV antibodies usually appear in the blood 1-4 mo after infection.
Testing sequence:
1. ELISA is the recommended initial screening test. Sensitivity and specificity are >99%. False positive ELISA may occur with autoimmune disorders, administration of immune globulin manufactured before 1985 within 6 wk of testing, presence of rheumatoid factor, presence of DLA-DR antibodies in multigravida female, administration of influenza vaccine within 3 mo of testing, hemodialysis, positive plasma reagin test, certain medical disorders (hemophilia, hypergammaglobulinemia, alcoholic hepatitis)

2. A positive ELISA is confirmed with Western blot. False positive Western blot may result from connective tissue disorders, human leukocyte antigen antibodies, polyclonal gammopathies, hyperbilirubinemia, presence of antibody to another human retrovirus, or cross reaction with other non-virus-derived proteins in healthy persons. Undetermined Western blot may occur in AIDS patients with advanced immunodeficiency (caused by loss of antibodies), and in recent HIV infections.
3. Polymerase chain reaction is used to confirm indeterminate Western blot results or negative results in persons with suspected HIV infection.
Fig. 4-15 describes tests in HIV infection.
Indications for plasma HIV RNA testing are described in Table 4-21.

■ **HUMAN IMMUNODEFICIENCY VIRUS TYPE 1 (HIV-1) ANTIGEN (p24), QUALITATIVE (p24 antigen)**
Normal range:
Negative
Cost: $105
This test detects uncomplexed HIV-1 p24 antigen. The core protein p24 is the first detectable protein encoded by the group-specific antigen *(gag)* gene. This protein is a marker for viremia. This test should not be used in place of HIV-1 antibody testing as a screen for HIV-1 infection. HIV-1 p24

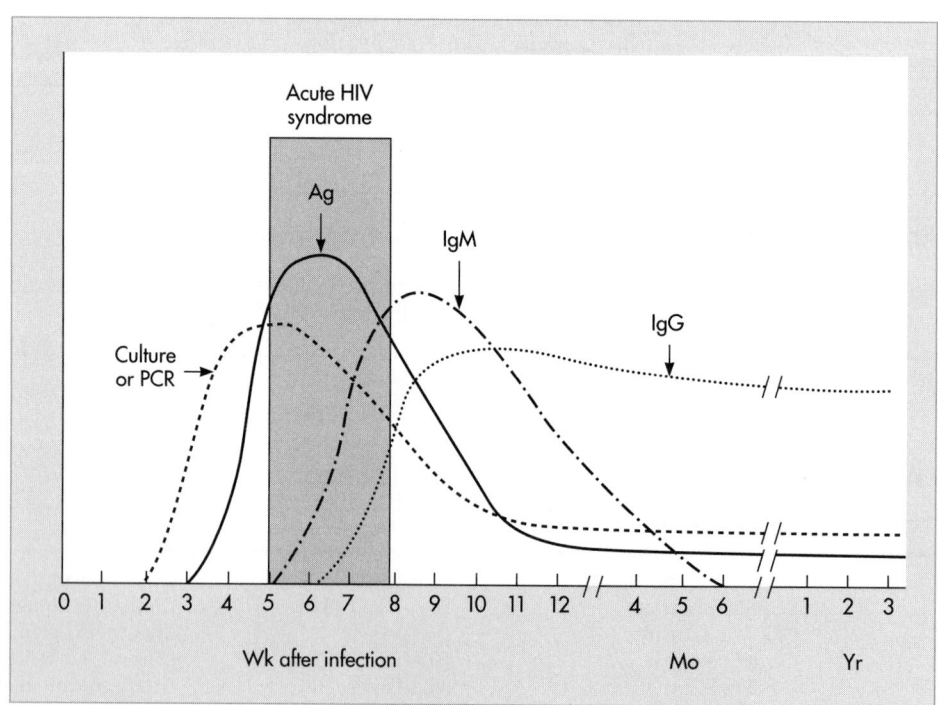

Fig. 4-15   Tests in HIV-1 infection. (From Ravel R: *Clinical laboratory medicine*, ed 6, St Louis, 1995, Mosby.)

TABLE 4-21   Indications for Plasma HIV RNA Testing*

CLINICAL INDICATION	INFORMATION	USE
Syndrome consistent with acute HIV infection	Establishes diagnosis when HIV antibody test is negative or indeterminate	Diagnosis†
Initial evaluation of newly diagnosed HIV infection	Baseline viral load "set point"	Decision to start or defer therapy
Every 3-4 mo in patients not on therapy	Changes in viral load	Decision to start therapy
4-8 wk after initiation of anti-retroviral therapy	Initial assessment of drug efficacy	Decision to continue or change therapy
3-4 mo after start of therapy	Maximal effect of therapy	Decision to continue or change therapy
Every 3-4 mo in patients on therapy	Durability of antiretroviral effect	Decision to continue or change therapy
Clinical event or significant decline in CD4+ T cells	Association with changing or stable viral load	Decision to continue, initiate, or change therapy

From *MMWR*, vol 47, no RR-5, Apr 24, 1998.
*Acute illness (e.g., bacterial pneumonia, tuberculosis, HSV, PCP) and immunizations can cause increase in plasma HIV RNA for 2-4 wk; viral load testing should not be performed during this time. Plasma HIV RNA results should usually be verified with a repeat determination before starting or making changes in therapy. HIV RNA should be measured using the same laboratory and the same assay.
†Diagnosis of HIV infection determined by HIV RNA testing should be confirmed by standard methods (e.g., Western blot serology) performed 2-4 mo after the initial indeterminate or negative test.

may be detectable in the first month of acute HIV-1 infection and generally falls to undetectable levels during the asymptomatic stage of HIV-1 infection. A negative result does not exclude the possibility of infection or exposure to HIV-1. It is recommended that a negative result be followed with repeat testing at least 8 weeks after the original test. This test is used primarily for screening of donated blood and plasma and as an aid for the prognosis of HIV-1 infection.

- **HUMAN IMMUNODEFICIENCY VIRUS TYPE 1 (HIV-1) VIRAL LOAD**
Normal range:
HIV-1 RNA, quant. bDNA 3: less than 50 copies/ml or less than 1.7 log copies/ml
Cost: $105
This test should be used only in individuals with documented HIV-1 infection for monitoring the progression of infection, response to antiretroviral therapy, and disease prognosis. It is not indicated for diagnosis of HIV infection.

- **5-HYDROXYINDOLE-ACETIC ACID, URINE;** *see* URINE 5-HYDROXYINDOLE-ACETIC ACID

- **IMMUNE COMPLEX ASSAY**
Normal:
Negative
Cost: $86
Detected in:
Collagen-vascular disorders, glomerulonephritis, neoplastic diseases, malaria, primary biliary cirrhosis, chronic acute hepatitis, bacterial endocarditis, vasculitis

- **IMMUNOGLOBULINS**
Normal range:
IgA: 50-350 mg/dl (0.5-3.5 g/L) [CF: 0.01; SMI: 0.01 g/L]
IgD: <6 mg/dl (<60 mg/L) [CF: 0.01; SMI: 0.01 g/L]
IgE: <25 μg/dl (<0.00025 g/L) [CF: 0.01; SMI: 0.01 g/L]
IgG: 800-1500 mg/dl (8-15 g/L) [CF: 0.01; SMI: 0.01 g/L]
IgM: 45-150 mg/dl (0.45-1.5 g/L) [CF: 0.01; SMI: 0.01 g/L]
Table 4-22 describes properties of human immunoglobulins.
Cost: $81
Elevated in:
IgA: lymphoproliferative disorders, Berger's nephropathy, chronic infections, autoimmune disorders, liver disease
IgE: allergic disorders, parasitic infections, immunologic disorders, IgE myeloma
IgG: chronic granulomatous infections, infectious diseases, inflammation, myeloma, liver disease
IgM: primary biliary cirrhosis, infectious diseases (brucellosis, malaria), Waldenström's macroglobulinemia, liver disease
Decreased in:
IgA: nephrotic syndrome, protein-losing enteropathy, congenital deficiency, lymphocytic leukemia, ataxia-telangiectasia, chronic sinopulmonary disease
IgE: hypogammaglobulinemia, neoplasma (breast, bronchial, cervical), ataxia-telangiectasia

IV

TABLE 4-22   Properties of Human Immunoglobulins

	IgG	IgA	IgM	IgD	IgE
H chain class	γ	α	μ	δ	ε
Molecular weight (approximate)	150,000	170,000	900,000	180,000	190,000
Complement fixation (classic)	++	0	++++	0	0
Opsonic activity (for binding)	++++	++	0	0	0
Reaginic activity	0	0	0	0	++++
Serum concentration (approximate mg/dL)	1500	150-350	100-150	2	2
Serum half-life (days)	23	6	5	3	2.5
Major functions	Recall response; opsonization; transplacental immunity	Secretory immunity	Primary response; complement fixation	?	Allergy; anthelmintic immunity

From Andreoli TE (ed): *Cecil essentials of medicine*, ed 5, Philadelphia, 2001, WB Saunders.
Ig, Immunoglobulin.

IgG: congenital or acquired deficiency, lymphocytic leukemia, phenytoin, methylprednisolone, nephrotic syndrome, protein-losing enteropathy
IgM: congenital deficiency, lymphocytic leukemia, nephrotic syndrome

■ **INTERNATIONAL NORMALIZED RATIO** (INR)
The INR is a comparative rating of prothrombin time (PT) ratios. The INR represents the observed PT ratio adjusted by the International Reference Thromboplastin. It provides a universal result indicative of what the patient's PT result would have been if measured using the primary World Health Organization International Reference reagent. For proper interpretation of INR values, the patient should be on stable anticoagulant therapy.
Cost: $23
Recommended INR ranges:
Proximal deep vein thrombosis: 2-3
Pulmonary embolism: 2-3
Transient ischemic attacks: 2-3
Atrial fibrillation: 2-3
Mechanical prosthetic valves: 3-4.5
Recurrent venous thromboembolic disease: 3-4.5

■ **IRON-BINDING CAPACITY, TOTAL** (TIBC)
Normal range:
250-460 μg/dl (45-82 μmol/L) [CF: 0.1791; SMI: 1 μmol/L]
Cost: $45
Elevated in:
Iron deficiency anemia, pregnancy, polycythemia, hepatitis, weight loss
Decreased in:
Anemia of chronic disease, hemochromatosis, chronic liver disease, hemolytic anemias, malnutrition (protein depletion)

Table 4-23 describes TIBC and serum iron abnormalities.
■ **LACTATE DEHYDROGENASE** (LDH)
Normal range:
50-150 U/L (0.82-2.66 μkat/L) [CF: 0.01667; SMI: 0.02 μkat/L]
Cost: $23
Elevated in:
Infarction of myocardium, lung, kidney
Diseases of cardiopulmonary system, liver, collagen, central nervous system
Hemolytic anemias, megaloblastic anemias, transfusions, seizures, muscle trauma, muscular dystrophy, acute pancreatitis, hypotension, shock, infectious mononucleosis, inflammation, neoplasia, intestinal obstruction, hypothyroidism

■ **LACTATE DEHYDROGENASE ISOENZYMES**
Normal range:
LDH_1: 22% to 36% (cardiac, red blood cell) (0.22-0.36) [CF: 0.01, SMI: 0.01]
LDH_2: 35% to 46% (cardiac, red blood cell) (0.35-0.46)
LDH_3: 13% to 26% (pulmonary) (0.15-0.26)
LDH_4: 3% to 10% (striated muscle, liver) (0.03-0.1)
LDH_5: 2% to 9% (striated muscle, liver) (0.02-0.09)
Normal ratios:
$LDH_1 < LDH_2$
$LDH_5 < LDH_4$
Abnormal values:
$LDH_1 > LDH_2$: myocardial infarction (can also be seen with hemolytic anemias, pernicious anemia, folate deficiency, renal infarct)
$LDH_5 > LDH_4$: liver disease (cirrhosis, hepatitis, hepatic congestion)
Cost: $69

TABLE 4-23   Serum Iron and Total Iron-Binding Capacity Patterns

SI↓	TIBC↓	Chronic diseases Uremia
SI↓	TIBC↑	Chronic iron deficiency anemia Pregnancy in third trimester
SI↑	TIBC↓	Hemachromatosis Iron therapy overload (TIBC may be normal) Hemolytic anemia; thalassemia; lead poisoning; megaloblastic anemia; aplastic, pyridoxine deficiency, or other sideroblastic anemias
SI↑	TIBC↑	Oral contraceptives Acute hepatitis (some report TIBC is low normal) Chronic hepatitis (some patients)
SI↑	TIBC NL	B_{12} or folate deficiency
SI↓	TIBC NL	Chronic iron deficiency (some patients) Acute infection, surgery, tissue damage
SI NL	TIBC↑	B_{12}/folate deficiency plus iron deficiency

From Ravel R: *Clinical laboratory medicine,* ed 6, St Louis, 1995, Mosby.
NL, Normal; *SI,* serum iron; *TIBC,* total iron-binding capacity.

- **LAP SCORE;** *see* LEUKOCYTE ALKALINE PHOSPHATASE
- **LDH;** *see* LACTATE DEHYDROGENASE
- **LDL;** *see* LOW-DENSITY LIPOPROTEIN CHOLESTEROL
- *LEGIONELLA* **TITER**
  Normal:
  Negative
  Cost: $69
  Positive in:
  Legionnaire's disease (presumptive: ≥1:256 titer; definitive: fourfold titer increase to ≥1:128)
- **LEUKOCYTE ALKALINE PHOSPHATASE**
  Normal range:
  13-100 (33-188 U)
  Cost: $47
  Elevated in:
  Leukemoid reactions, neutrophilia secondary to infections (except in sickle cell crisis—no significant increase in LAP score), Hodgkin's disease, polycythemia vera, hairy cell leukemia, aplastic anemia, Down's syndrome, myelofibrosis
  Decreased in:
  Acute and chronic granulocytic leukemia, thrombocytopenic purpura, paroxysmal nocturnal hemoglobinuria, hypophosphatemia, collagen disorders
- **LEUKOCYTE COUNT;** *see* COMPLETE BLOOD COUNT
- **LIPASE**
  Normal range:
  0-160 U/L (0-2.66 μkat/L) [CF: 0.01667; SMI: 0.02 μkat/L]
  Cost: $23

Elevated in:
Acute pancreatitis, perforated peptic ulcer, carcinoma of pancreas (early stage), pancreatic duct obstruction, bowel infarction, intestinal obstruction
- **LIPOPROTEIN CHOLESTEROL, HIGH-DENSITY;** *see* HIGH-DENSITY LIPOPROTEIN CHOLESTEROL
- **LIPOPROTEIN CHOLESTEROL, LOW-DENSITY;** *see* LOW-DENSITY LIPOPROTEIN CHOLESTEROL
- **LOW-DENSITY LIPOPROTEIN (LDL) CHOLESTEROL**
  Normal range:
  50-130 mg/dl (1.30-1.68 mmol/L) [CF: 0.02586; SMI: 0.05 mmol/L]
  LDL cholesterol

<100	Optimal
100-129	Near or above optimal
130-159	Borderline high
160-189	High
≥190	Very high

  Cost: $58
- **LUPUS ANTICOAGULANT;** *see* CIRCULATING ANTICOAGULANT
- **LUTEINIZING HORMONE**
  Normal range:
  5-25 mIU/ml
  Cost: $58
  Elevated in:
  Postmenopause, pituitary adenoma, primary gonadal dysfunction, polycystic ovary syndrome
  Decreased in:
  Severe illness, anorexia nervosa, malnutrition, pituitary or hypothalamic impairment, severe stress

IV

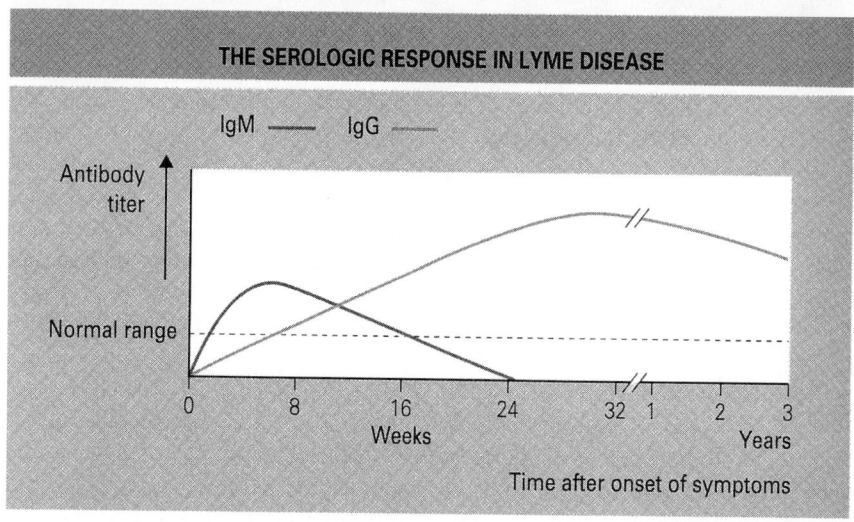

Fig. 4-16 **Usual serologic response in Lyme disease.** Specific IgM becomes detectable 1 to 2 weeks after symptom onset and the appearance of erythema chronicum migrans. The later appearance of IgG is frequently concurrent with systemic manifestations. IgG is nearly always elevated in late disease. Typically, and even in untreated patients, IgM falls over 4 to 6 months; persistence for longer than this predicts later manifestations. (From Klippel J, Dieppe P, Ferri R [eds]: *Primary care rheumatology,* London, 1999, Mosby.)

■ **LYME DISEASE ANTIBODY TITER**
Normal range:
Negative
Cost: $67
Positive result:
Fig. 4-16 illustrates the usual serologic response in Lyme disease.
A serologic test is not necessary or helpful for several days after a tick bite, because it is only 40%-50% sensitive in this stage and a negative test does not rule out the diagnosis.

■ **LYMPHOCYTES**
Normal range:
15% to 40%: Total lymphocyte count = 800-2600/mm^3
Total T lymphocyte = 800-2200/mm^3
CD4 lymphocytes = ≥400/mm^3
CD8 lymphocytes = 200-800/mm^3
Normal CD4/CD8 ratio is 2.0
Elevated in:
Chronic infections, infectious mononucleosis and other viral infections, chronic lymphocytic leukemia, Hodgkin's disease, ulcerative colitis, hypoadrenalism, idiopathic thrombocytopenia
Decreased in:
AIDS, bone marrow suppression from chemotherapeutic agents or chemotherapy, aplastic anemia, neoplasms, steroids, adrenocortical hyperfunction, neurologic disorders (multiple sclerosis, myasthenia gravis, Guillain-Barré syndrome)
CD4 lymphocytes are calculated as total white blood cells × % lymphocytes × % lymphocytes

stained with CD4. They are decreased in AIDS and other immune dysfunction.

■ **MAGNESIUM** (serum)
Normal range:
1.8-3.0 mg/dl (0.80-1.20 mmol/L) [CF: 0.4114; SMI: 0.02 mmol/L]. See Box 4-34 for description of magnesium abnormalities.
Cost: $23

■ **MEAN CORPUSCULAR VOLUME** (MCV)
Normal range:
76-100 μm^3 (76-100 fL) [CF: 1; SMI: 1 fL]
See Tables 4-24 and 4-25 for description of MCV abnormalities.

■ **METANEPHRINES, URINE;** *see* URINE METANEPHRINES

■ **MONOCYTE COUNT**
Normal range:
2% to 8%
Elevated in:
Viral diseases, parasites, infections, neoplasms, inflammatory bowel disease, monocytic leukemia, lymphomas, myeloma, sarcoidosis
Decreased in:
Aplastic anemia, lymphocytic leukemia, glucocorticoid administration

■ **MYOGLOBIN, URINE;** *see* URINE MYOGLOBIN

■ **NEUTROPHIL COUNT**
Normal range:
50% to 70%
Subsets
Stabs (bands, early mature neutrophils): 2% to 6%
Segs (mature neutrophils): 60% to 70%

BOX 4-34 **Magnesium Disorders**

Magnesium Deficiency

Alcoholism
Malabsorption
Malnutrition
IV fluids without magnesium
Severe diarrhea
Diabetic ketoacidosis
Hemodialysis
Hypercalcemia
Congestive heart failure
Artifact (hypoalbuminemia)

Certain medications
  Loop and thiazide diuretics
  Cyclosporine
  Cisplatin
  Gentamicin

Magnesium Excess

Oliguric renal failure
Overuse of magnesium-containing compounds
Artifactual (specimen hemolysis)

From Ravel R: *Clinical laboratory medicine*, ed 6, St Louis, 1995, Mosby.

TABLE 4-24   Some Causes of Increased Mean Corpuscular Volume (Macrocytosis)

CAUSES	% OF ALL MACROCYTOSIS PATIENTS*	% OF MACROCYTOSIS IN EACH DISEASE†
Common		
Folate or B$_{12}$ deficiency	20-30 (5-50)‡	80-90 (4-100)
Chronic liver disease	15-20 (6-28)	25-30 (8-65)
Chronic alcoholism	10-12 (3-15)	60 (26-90)
Cytotoxic chemotherapy	10-15 (2-20)	30-40 (13-82)
Cardiorespiratory abnormality	8 (7-9.5)	?
Reticulocytosis	6-7 (0-15)	Depends on severity
Myelodysplastic syndromes	Frequent over age 40 yr	>60 in RAEB and RARS
Unexplained	25 (22.5-27)	—
Normal newborn		
Less Common	<4%	
Noncytotoxic drugs		
Zidovudine		
Phenytoin		30 (14-50)
Azathioprine		
Hypothyroidism		20-30 (8-55)
Chronic leukemia/myelofibrosis		
Radiotherapy for malignancy		
Chronic renal disease (occasional patients)		
Distance-runner macrocytosis (some persons)		
Down syndrome		
Artifactual (e.g., cold agglutinins)		

From Ravel R: *Clinical laboratory medicine*, ed 6, St Louis, 1995, Mosby.
RAEB, Refractory anemia with excessive blasts; *RARS,* refractory anemia with ring sideroblasts (formerly called IASA, or idiopathic acquired sideroblastic anemia).
*Percentage of all patients with macrocytosis.
†Percentage of patients with each condition listed who have macrocytosis.
‡Numbers in parentheses are literature range.

TABLE 4-25   Some Causes of Decreased Mean Corpuscular Volume (Microcytosis)

COMMON	LESS COMMON
Chronic iron deficiency	Some cases of polycythemia
α- or β-thalassemia (minor)	Some cases of lead poisoning
Anemia of chronic disease	Some cases of congenital spherocytosis
	Some cases of sideroblastic anemia
	Certain abnormal Hbs (Hb E, Hb Lepore)

From Ravel R: *Clinical laboratory medicine*, ed 6, St Louis, 1995, Mosby.

IV

Elevated in:
Acute bacterial infections, acute myocardial infarction, stress, neoplasms, myelocytic leukemia
Decreased in:
Viral infections, aplastic anemias, immunosuppressive drugs, radiation therapy to bone marrow, agranulocytosis, drugs (antibiotics, antithyroidals, clopidogrel), lymphocytic and monocytic leukemias

- **5'-NUCLEOTIDASE**
  Normal range:
  2-16 IU/L ($3-27 \times 10^{-8}$ kat/L) [CF: 1.67×10^{-8}; SMI: 1×10^{-8} kat/L]
  Cost: $42
  Elevated in:
  Biliary obstruction, metastatic neoplasms to liver, primary biliary cirrhosis, renal failure, pancreatic carcinoma, chronic active hepatitis
- **ONCOGENES**
  See Table 4-26 for description of common oncogene abnormalities.

TABLE 4-26 Some Currently Important Oncogenes

ONCOGENE	CHROMOSOME LOCATION	OTHER
Neu (HER-2; c-erbB2) (rat neuroblastoma)	17q21	Amplification in 10%-40% of primary cancers; especially breast, ovary, prostate, thyroid, neuroblastoma
bcl-2 (acute B-cell leukemia)	18q21	Involved in translocation t(14;18) (q32q21) in 80%-90% of acute follicular (nodular) non-Hodgkin's lymphoma by chromosome analysis (nearly 100% by DNA probe)
Rb (retinoblastoma)	13q14	Tumor suppressor gene; deletion or mutation results in increased incidence of retinoblastoma, osteosarcoma, breast, endometrial, lung small cell CA*
ras oncogene group (rat sarcoma virus)		
Harvey (c-Ha-ras, H-ras)	11p15	
Kirsten (c-Ki-ras, K-ras)	12p12	
Neuroblastoma (N-ras)	1p22	Mutational activation of ras group member is estimated to occur in 10%-20% of human malignancies; especially lung non–small-cell, kidney, breast, colorectal, prostate; in neuroblastoma, H-ras amplification is paradoxically associated with better prognosis
myc oncogene group (avian myelocytomatosis virus)		
L-myc	1p32	
N-myc	2p	
C-myc	8q24	Amplification in breast CA (37%), neuroblastoma (25%-30%), Burkitt's lymphoma, acute lymphoblastic leukemia of L-3 type
p53	17p13	Tumor suppressor gene; deletion or mutation produces defective gene; increase in colorectal CA (70%-80%), endometrial CA, early-onset breast CA, various others
FAP (familial adenomatous polyposis; also called APC)	5q21	Suppressor gene for familial polyposis and Gardner's syndrome
DCC (deleted in colon cancer)	18q21	Suppressor gene; when deleted, increase in colorectal CA (75%), especially if FAP gene is present
mcc (mutated in colon cancer)	5q21	40% of colon cancer
wt-1 (Wilms' tumor)	11p13	Suppressor gene deletion found in Wilms' tumor; also some cases of breast CA, rhabdomyosarcoma, hepatoblastoma, urinary bladder CA
nf = 1 (neurofibroma)	17q11	Suppressor or gene in von Recklinghausen's disease
RCC (renal cell carcinoma)	3p14	Gene area break in most RCC patients
Meningioma	22q	Partial or full monosomy 22 (specific defect)
Neuroblastoma (83% cases)	del(1p)	Deletion causes loss of suppressor gene
abl (Abelson)	9q	Part of 9, 22 translocation of Philadelphia chromosome

From Ravel R: *Clinical laboratory medicine*, ed 6, St Louis, 1995, Mosby.
*CA, Carcinoma.

- **OSMOLALITY** (serum)

Normal range:

280-300 mOsm/kg (280-300 mmol/kg) [CF: 1; SMI: 1 mmol/kg]

It can also be estimated by the following formula:

$$2([Na] + [K]) + \frac{Glucose}{18} + \frac{BUN}{2.8}$$

Cost: $31

Elevated in:

Dehydration, hypernatremia, diabetes insipidus, uremia, hyperglycemia, mannitol therapy, ingestion of toxins (ethylene glycol, methanol, ethanol), hypercalcemia, diuretics

Decreased in:

Syndrome of inappropriate diuretic hormone secretion, hyponatremia, overhydration, Addison's disease, hypothyroidism

- **OSMOLALITY, URINE;** *see* URINE OSMOLALITY

- **PARTIAL THROMBOPLASTIN TIME** (PTT), **ACTIVATED PARTIAL THROMBOPLASTIN TIME** (APTT)

Normal range:

25-41 sec

Cost: $32

Elevated in:

Heparin therapy, coagulation factor deficiency (I, II, V, VIII, IX, X, XI, XII), liver disease, vitamin K deficiency, disseminated intravascular coagulation, circulating anticoagulant, warfarin therapy, specific factor inhibition (PCN reaction, rheumatoid arthritis), thrombolytic therapy, nephrotic syndrome

NOTE: Useful to evaluate the intrinsic coagulation system.

- **pH, URINE;** *see* URINE pH

- **PHOSPHATASE, ACID;** *see* ACID PHOSPHATASE

- **PHOSPHATASE, ALKALINE;** *see* ALKALINE PHOSPHATASE

- **PHOSPHATE** (serum)

Normal range:

2.5-5 mg/dl (0.8-1.6 mmol/L) [CF: 0.3229; SMI: 0.05 mmol/L]

Cost: $23

See Box 4-35 for description of phosphate abnormalities.

- **PLATELET COUNT**

Normal range:

$130\text{-}400 \times 10^3/\text{mm}^3$ ($130\text{-}400 \times 10^9/\text{L}$) [CF: 1; SMI: $5 \times 10^9/\text{L}$]

Cost: $22

Elevated in:

Neoplasms (gastrointestinal tract), chronic myelocytic leukemia, polycythemia vera, myelofibrosis with myeloid metaplasia, infections, after splenectomy, postpartum, after hemorrhage, hemophilia, iron deficiency, pancreatitis, cirrhosis

Decreased:

A. Increased destruction

  1. Immunologic

    a. Drugs: quinine, quinidine, digitalis, procainamide, thiazide diuretics, sulfonamides, phenytoin, aspirin, penicillin, heparin, gold, meprobamate, sulfa drugs, phenylbutazone, NSAIDs, methyldopa, cimetidine, furosemide, INH, cephalosporins, chlorpropamide, organic arsenicals, chloroquine

    b. Idiopathic thrombocytopenic purpura

    c. Transfusion reaction: transfusion of platelets with platelet antigen HPA-1a (PL^{A1}) in recipients without PL^{A1}

    d. Fetal/maternal incompatibility

    e. Vasculitis (e.g., systemic lupus erythematosus)

IV

BOX 4-35   Selected Disorders Associated with Serum Phosphate Abnormality

Phosphate Decrease*

Parenteral hyperalimentation
Diabetic acidosis
Alcohol withdrawal
Severe metabolic or respiratory alkalosis
Antacids that bind phosphorus
Malnutrition with refeeding using low-phosphorus nutrients
Renal tubule failure to reabsorb phosphate (Fanconi's syndrome; congenital disorder; vitamin D deficiency)
Glucose administration
Nasogastric suction
Malabsorption

Gram-negative sepsis
Primary hyperthyroidism
Chlorothiazide diuretics
Therapy of acute severe asthma
Acute respiratory failure with mechanical ventilation

Phosphate Excess

Renal failure
Severe muscle injury
Phosphate-containing antacids
Hypoparathyroidism
Tumor lysis syndrome

From Ravel R: *Clinical laboratory medicine*, ed 6, St Louis, 1995, Mosby.
*Low-phosphate diet can magnify effect of phosphorus-lowering disorders.

f. Autoimmune hemolytic anemia
g. Lymphoreticular disorders (e.g., chronic lymphocytic leukemia)
2. Nonimmunologic
a. Prosthetic heart valves
b. Thrombotic thrombocytopenic purpura
c. Sepsis
d. Disseminated intravascular coagulation
e. Hemolytic-uremic syndrome
f. Giant cavernous hemangioma
B. Decreased production
1. Abnormal marrow
a. Marrow infiltration (e.g., leukemia, lymphoma, fibrosis)
b. Marrow suppression (e.g., chemotherapy, alcohol, radiation)
2. Hereditary disorders
a. Wiskott-Aldrich syndrome: X-linked disorder characterized by thrombocytopenia, eczema, and repeated infections
b. May-Hegglin anomaly: increased megakaryocytes but ineffective thrombopoiesis
3. Vitamin deficiencies (e.g., vitamin B$_{12}$, folic acid)
C. Splenic sequestration, hypersplenism
D. Dilutional, secondary to massive transfusion

■ **POTASSIUM** (serum)
Normal range:
3.5-5 mEq/L (3.5-5 mmol/L) [CF: 1; SMI: 0.1 mmol/L]
Cost: $23
See Box 4-36 for causes of potassium abnormalities.

■ **POTASSIUM, URINE;** *see* URINE POTASSIUM
■ **PROLACTIN**
Normal range:
<20 ng/ml (<20 µg/L) [CF: 1; SMI: 1 µg/L]

Cost: $80
Elevated in:
Prolactinomas (level >200 highly suggestive), drugs (phenothiazines, cimetidine, tricyclic antidepressants, metoclopramide, estrogens, antihypertensives [methyldopa], verapamil, haloperidol), postpartum, stress, hypoglycemia, hypothyroidism

■ **PROSTATE SPECIFIC ANTIGEN** (PSA)
Normal range:
0-4 ng/ml
Table 4-28 describes age-specific reference ranges for PSA.
Cost: $49
Elevated in:
Benign prostatic hypertrophy, carcinoma of prostate, postrectal examination, prostate trauma Factors affecting serum PSA are described in Table 4-27.

■ **PROTEIN** (serum)
Normal range:
6-8 g/dl (60-80 g/L) [CF: 10; SMI: 1 g/L]
Cost: $23
Elevated in:
Dehydration, multiple myeloma, Waldenström's macroglobulinemia, sarcoidosis, collagen-vascular diseases
Decreased in:
Malnutrition, low-protein diet, overhydration, malabsorption, pregnancy, severe burns, neoplasms, chronic diseases, cirrhosis, nephrosis

■ **PROTEIN ELECTROPHORESIS** (serum)
Normal range:
Albumin: 60% to 75% (0.6-0.75) [CF: 0.01; SMI: 0.01]
α-1: 1.7% to 5% (0.02-0.05)
α-2: 6.7% to 12.5% (0.07-0.13)
β: 8.3% to 16.3% (0.08-0.16)
γ: 10.7% to 20% (0.11-0.2)

BOX 4-36   Clinical Conditions Commonly Associated with Serum Potassium Abnormalities

Hypokalemia
Inadequate intake (cachexia or severe illness of any type)
Intravenous infusion of potassium-free fluids
Renal loss (diuretics; primary aldosteronism)
Gastrointestinal loss (protracted vomiting; severe prolonged diarrhea; gastrointestinal drainage)
Severe trauma
Treatment of diabetic acidosis without potassium supplements
Treatment with large doses of adrenocorticotropic hormone; Cushing's syndrome
Cirrhosis; some cases of secondary aldosteronism

Hyperkalemia
Renal failure
Dehydration
Excessive parenteral administration of potassium
Artifactual hemolysis of blood specimen
Tumor lysis syndrome
Hyporeninemic hypoaldosteronism
Spironolactone therapy
Addison's disease and salt-losing congenital adrenal hyperplasia
Thrombocythemia

From Ravel R: *Clinical laboratory medicine*, ed 6, St Louis, 1995, Mosby.

TABLE 4-27 Factors Affecting Serum Prostate-Specific Antigen (PSA)

FACTORS AFFECTING SERUM PSA	DURATION OF EFFECT
Prostate cell number	Not applicable
Prostate size	Not applicable
Recent ejaculation	6-48 hours
Prostate manipulation	
Vigorous massage	1 week
Cystoscopy	1 week
Prostate biopsy	4-6 weeks
Prostatitis	
Acute	3-6 months
Chronic	Unknown
Prostate cancer	Not applicable
Drugs: finasteride (Proscar)*	3-6 months

From Nseyo UO (ed): *Urology for primary care physicians,* Philadelphia, 1999, WB Saunders.
*Lowers PSA for as long as patient is on the medication.

TABLE 4-28 Age-Specific Reference Ranges for PSA

AGE (YR)	SERUM PSA (NG/ML)		
	WHITES	JAPANESE	AFRICAN AMERICAN
40-49	0-2.5	0-2.0	0-2.0
50-59	0-3.5	0-3.0	0-4.0
60-69	0-4.5	0-4.0	0-4.5
70-79	0-6.5	0-5.0	0-5.5

From Nseyo UO (ed): *Urology for primary care physicians,* Philadelphia, 1999, WB Saunders.
PSA, Prostate-specific antigen.

Albumin: 3.6-5.2 g/dl (36-52 g/L) [CF: 0.01; SMI: 1 g/L]
α-1: 0.1-0.4 g/dl (1-4 g/L)
α-2: 0.4-1 g/dl (4-10 g/L)
β: 0.5-1.2 g/dl (5-12 g/L)
γ: 0.6-1.6 g/dl (6-16 g/L)
Cost: $52
Elevated in:
Albumin: dehydration
α-1: neoplastic diseases, inflammation
α-2: neoplasms, inflammation, infection, nephrotic syndrome
β: hypothyroidism, biliary cirrhosis, diabetes mellitus
γ: *see* IMMUNOGLOBULINS
Decreased in:
Albumin: malnutrition, chronic liver disease, malabsorption, nephrotic syndrome, burns, systemic lupus erythematosus
α-1: emphysema (α-1 antitrypsin deficiency), nephrosis
α-2: hemolytic anemias (decreased haptoglobin), severe hepatocellular damage
β: hypocholesterolemia, nephrosis
γ: *see* IMMUNOGLOBULINS
Fig. 4-17 describes serum protein electrophoretic patterns.

■ **PROTHROMBIN TIME** (PT)
Normal range:
10-12 sec
Cost: $23
Elevated in:
Liver disease, oral anticoagulants (warfarin), heparin, factor deficiency (I, II, V, VII, X), disseminated intravascular coagulation, vitamin K deficiency, afibrinogenemia, dysfibrinogenemia, drugs

(salicylate, chloral hydrate, diphenylhydantoin, estrogens, antacids, phenylbutazone, quinidine, antibiotics, allopurinol, anabolic steroids)
Decreased in:
Vitamin K supplementation, thrombophlebitis, drugs (glutethimide, estrogens, griseofulvin, diphenhydramine)

■ **PROTOPORPHYRIN** (free erythrocyte)
Normal range:
16-36 μg/dl of red blood cells (0.28-0.64 μmol/L) [CF: 0.0177; SMI: 0.02 μmol/L]
Cost: $49
Elevated in:
Iron deficiency, lead poisoning, sideroblastic anemias, anemia of chronic disease, hemolytic anemias, erythropoietic protoporphyria

■ **PSA;** *see* PROSTATE SPECIFIC ANTIGEN
■ **PT;** *see* PROTHROMBIN TIME
■ **PTT;** *see* PARTIAL THROMBOPLASTIN TIME
■ **RDW;** *see* RED BLOOD CELL DISTRIBUTION WIDTH
■ **RED BLOOD CELL** (RBC) **COUNT**
Normal range:
Male: 4.3-5.9 $\times$ 10^6/mm^3 (4.3-5.9 $\times$ 10^{12}/L) [CF: 1; SMI: 0.1 $\times$ 10^{12}/L]
Female: 3.5-5 $\times$ 10^6/mm^3 (3.5-5 $\times$ 10^{12}/L) [CF: 1; SMI: 0.1 $\times$ 10^{12}/L]
Cost: $20
Elevated in:
Polycythemia vera, smokers, high altitude, cardiovascular disease, renal cell carcinoma and other erythropoietin-producing neoplasms, stress, hemoconcentration/dehydration
Decreased in:
Anemias, hemolysis, chronic renal failure, hemorrhage, failure of marrow production

IV

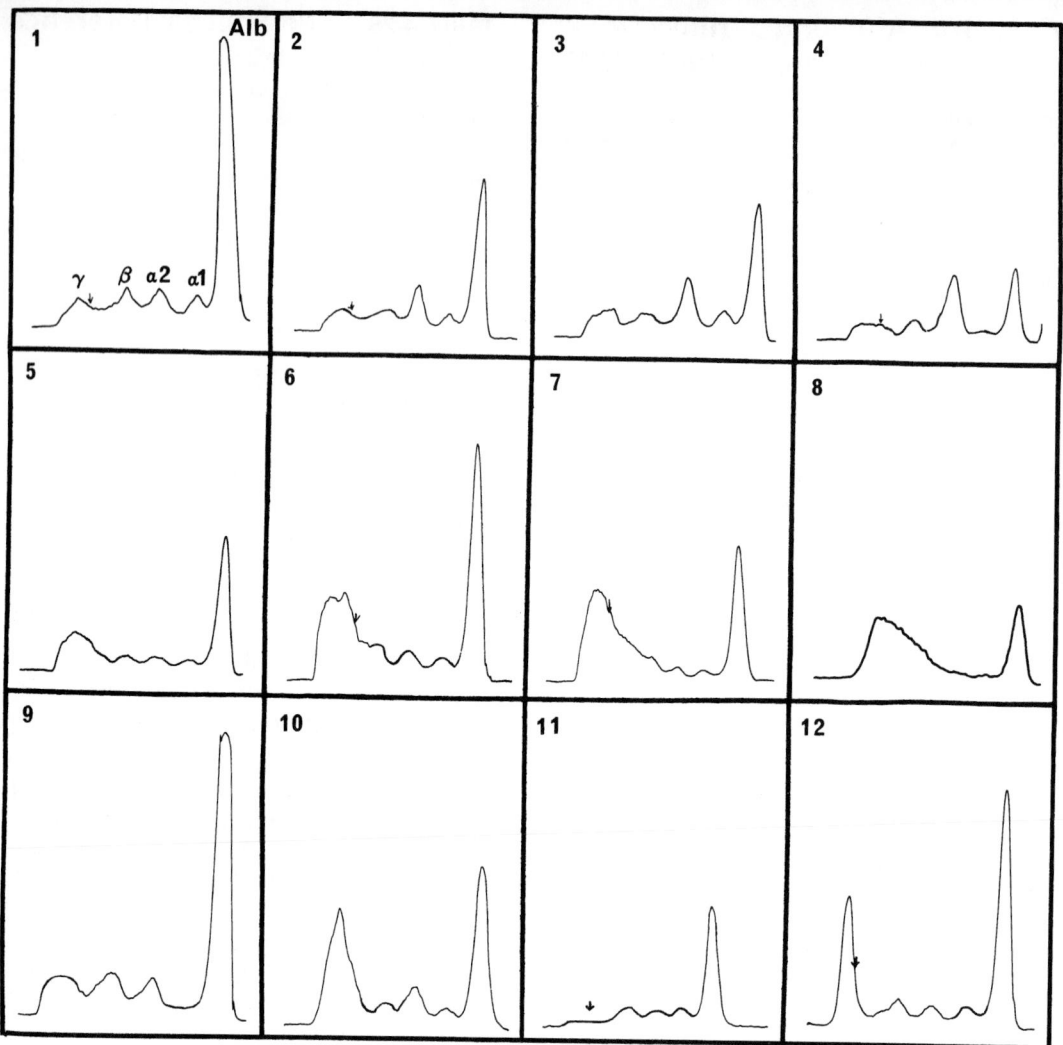

Fig. 4-17 **Typical serum protein electrophoretic patterns.** *1,* Normal (*arrow* near γ region indicates serum application point). *2,* Acute reaction pattern. *3,* Acute reaction or nephrotic syndrome. *4,* Nephrotic syndrome. *5,* Chronic inflammation, cirrhosis, granulomatous diseases, rheumatoid-collagen group. *6,* Same as *5,* but γ elevation is more pronounced. There is also partial (but not complete) β-γ fusion. *7,* Suggestive of cirrhosis but could be found in the granulomatous diseases or the rheumatoid-collagen group. *8,* Characteristic pattern of cirrhosis. *9,* α-1 Antitrypsin deficiency with mild γ elevation suggesting concurrent chronic disease. *10,* Same as *5,* but the γ elevation is marked. The configuration of the γ peak superficially mimics that of myeloma, but is more broad-based. There are superimposed acute reaction changes. *11,* Hypogammaglobulinemia or light-chain myeloma. *12,* Myeloma, Waldenström's macroglobulinemia, idiopathic or secondary monoclonal gammopathy. (From Ravel R: *Clinical laboratory medicine,* ed 6, St Louis, 1995, Mosby.)

■ RED BLOOD CELL DISTRIBUTION WIDTH (RDW)

Measures variability of red cell size (anisocytosis)

Normal range:

11.5-14.5

Normal RDW and:

Elevated mean corpuscular volume (MCV): aplastic anemia, preleukemia

Normal MCV: normal, anemia of chronic disease, acute blood loss or hemolysis, chronic lymphocytic leukemia (CLL), chronic myelocytic leukemia, nonanemic enzymopathy or hemoglobinopathy

Decreased MCV: anemia of chronic disease, heterozygous thalassemia

Elevated RDW and:

Elevated MCV: vitamin B_{12} deficiency, folate deficiency, immune hemolytic anemia, cold agglutinins, CLL with high count, liver disease

Normal MCV: early iron deficiency, early vitamin B_{12} deficiency, early folate deficiency, anemic globinopathy

Decreased MCV: iron deficiency, red blood cell fragmentation, HbH disease, thalassemia intermedia

- **RED BLOOD CELL FOLATE;** *see* FOLATE, RED BLOOD CELL

- **RED BLOOD CELL MASS** (volume)

Normal range:

Male: 20-36 ml/kg of body weight (1.15-1.21 L/m^2 body surface area)

Female: 19-31 ml/kg of body weight (0.95-1.00 L/m^2 body surface area)

Cost: $129

Elevated in:

Polycythemia vera, hypoxia (smokers, high altitude, cardiovascular disease), hemoglobinopathies with high oxygen affinity, erythropoietin-producing tumors (renal cell carcinoma)

Decreased in:

Hemorrhage, chronic disease, failure of marrow production, anemias, hemolysis

- **RED BLOOD CELL MORPHOLOGY;** *see* Fig. 4-18

- **RENIN** (serum)

Cost: $125

Elevated in:

Drugs (thiazides, estrogen, minoxidil), chronic renal failure, Bartter's syndrome, pregnancy (normal), pheochromocytoma, renal hypertension, reduced plasma volume, secondary aldosteronism

Decreased in:

Adrenocortical hypertension, increased plasma volume, primary aldosteronism, drugs (propranolol, reserpine, clonidine)

Table 4-24 describes typical renin-aldosterone patterns in various conditions.

- **RETICULOCYTE COUNT**

Normal range:

0.5% to 1.5%

Cost: $22

Elevated in:

Hemolytic anemia (sickle cell crisis, thalassemia major, autoimmune hemolysis), hemorrhage, postanemia therapy (folic acid, ferrous sulfate, vitamin B_{12}), chronic renal failure

Decreased in:

Aplastic anemia, marrow suppression (sepsis, chemotherapeutic agents, radiation), hepatic cirrhosis, blood transfusion, anemias of disordered maturation (iron deficiency anemia, megaloblastic anemia, sideroblastic anemia, anemia of chronic disease)

- **RHEUMATOID FACTOR**

Normal:

Negative

Cost: $18

Present in titer > 1:20

Rheumatoid arthritis, systemic lupus erythematosus, chronic inflammatory processes, old age, infections, liver disease, multiple myeloma, sarcoidosis, pulmonary fibrosis, Sjögren's syndrome, other (Box 4-37)

- **RNP;** *see* EXTRACTABLE NUCLEAR ANTIGEN

- **SEDIMENTATION RATE;** *see* ERYTHROCYTE SEDIMENTATION RATE

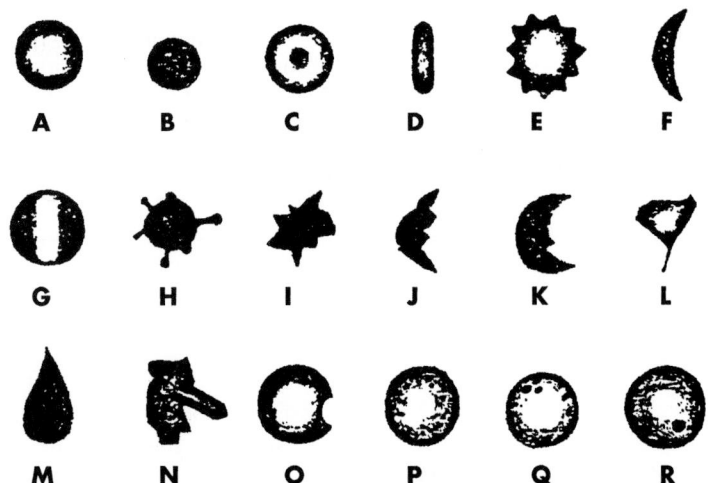

Fig. 4-18   Abnormal red blood cells (RBCs). A, Normal RBC. **B,** Spherocyte. **C,** Target cell. **D,** Elliptocyte. **E,** Echinocyte. **F,** Sickle cell. **G,** Stomatocyte. **H,** Acanthocyte. **I** to **L,** Schistocytes. **M,** Teardrop RBC. **N,** Distorted RBC with Hb C crystal protruding. **O,** Degmacyte. **P,** Basophilic stippling. **Q,** Pappenheimer bodies. **R,** Howell-Jolly body. (From Ravel R: *Clinical laboratory medicine,* ed 6, St Louis, 1995, Mosby.)

TABLE 4-24   **Typical Renin-Aldosterone Patterns in Various Conditions**

	PLASMA RENIN	ALDOSTERONE
Primary aldosteronism	Low	High
"Low-renin" essential hypertension	Low	Normal
Cushing's syndrome	Low	Low-normal
Licorice ingestion syndrome	Low	Low
High-salt diet	Low	Low
Oral contraceptives	High	Normal
Cirrhosis	High	High
Malignant hypertension	High	High
Unilateral renal disease	High	High
"High-renin" essential hypertension	High	High
Pregnancy	High	High
Diuretic overuse	High	High
Juxtaglomerular tumor (Bartter's syndrome)	High	High
Low-salt diet	High	High
Addison's disease	High	Low
Hypokalemia	High	Low

From Ravel R: *Clinical laboratory medicine,* ed 6, St Louis, 1995, Mosby.

BOX 4-37   **Diseases in Which Rheumatoid Factor Is Commonly Present**

Rheumatic Diseases

Rheumatoid arthritis
Sjögren's syndrome
Systemic lupus erythematosus
Polymyositis/dermatomyositis
Mixed connective tissue disease
Scleroderma

Infectious Diseases

Subacute bacterial endocarditis
Tuberculosis
Infectious mononucleosis
Hepatitis
Syphilis
Leprosy
Influenza

Malignancies

Lymphoma
Multiple myeloma
Waldenström's macroglobulinemia
Postradiation or postchemotherapy

Miscellaneous

Normal adults, especially the elderly
Sarcoidosis
Chronic pulmonary disease (interstitial fibrosis)
Chronic liver disease (chronic active hepatitis, cirrhosis)
Mixed essential cryoglobulinemia
Hypergammaglobulinemic purpura

From Noble J (ed): *Primary care medicine,* ed 3, St Louis, 2001, Mosby.

■ **SEMEN ANALYSIS**
Cost: $50
- Table 4-30 describes semen analysis reference ranges.
- The frequency of various categories of semen analysis results among men being evaluated for infertility is described in Table 4-31.

■ **SGOT;** *see* ASPARTATE AMINOTRANSFERASE
■ **SGPT;** *see* ALANINE AMINOTRANSFERASE
■ **SMOOTH MUSCLE ANTIBODY**
Normal:
Negative
Cost: $40

Present in:
Chronic acute hepatitis ($\geq$1:80), primary biliary cirrhosis ($\leq$1:80), infectious mononucleosis

■ **SODIUM** (serum)
Normal range:
135-147 mEq/L (135-147 mmol/L) [CF: 1; SMI: 1 mmol/L]
Cost: $23
Abnormal:
see Box 4-38

■ **STREPTOZYME;** *see* ANTI-STREPTOLYSIN O TITER

TABLE 4-30   **Semen Analysis Reference Ranges**

Color	Grayish white
pH	7.3-7.8 (literature range, 7.0-7.8)
Volume	2.0-5.0 ml (literature range, 1.5-6.0 ml)
Sperm count	20-250 million/ml (literature range for upper limit varies from 100-250 million/ml)
Motility	>60% motile <3 hours after specimen is obtained (literature range, >40% to >70%)
% Normal sperm	>60% (literature range, >60% to >70%)
Viscosity	Can be poured from a pipet in droplets rather than a thick strand

From Ravel R (ed): *Clinical laboratory medicine,* ed 6, St Louis, 1995, Mosby.

BOX 4-38   **Clinical Situations Frequently Associated with Serum Sodium Abnormalities**

I. Hyponatremia

  A. Sodium and water depletion (deficit hyponatremia)
    1. Loss of gastrointestinal secretions with replacement of fluid but not electrolytes
      a. Vomiting
      b. Diarrhea
      c. Tube drainage
    2. Loss from skin with replacement of fluids but not electrolytes
      a. Excessive sweating
      b. Extensive burns
    3. Loss from kidney
      a. Diuretics
      b. Chronic renal insufficiency (uremia) with acidosis
    4. Metabolic loss
      a. Starvation with acidosis
      b. Diabetic acidosis
    5. Endocrine loss
      a. Addison's disease
      b. Sudden withdrawal of long-term steroid therapy
    6. Iatrogenic loss from serous cavities
      a. Paracentesis or thoracentesis
  B. Excessive water (dilution hyponatremia)
    1. Excessive water administration
    2. Congestive heart failure
    3. Cirrhosis
    4. Nephrotic syndrome
    5. Hypoalbuminemia (severe)
    6. Acute renal failure with oliguria
  C. Inappropriate antidiuretic hormone (IADH) syndrome
  D. Intracellular loss (reset osmostat syndrome)
  E. False hyponatremia (actually a dilutional effect)
    1. Marked hypertriglyceridemia*
    2. Marked hyperproteinemia*
    3. Severe hyperglycemia

II. Hypernatremia

Dehydration is the most frequent overall clinical finding in hypernatremia.
    1. Deficient water intake (either orally or intravenously)
    2. Excess kidney water output (diabetes insipidus, osmotic diuresis)
    3. Excess skin water output (excess sweating, loss from burns)
    4. Excess gastrointestinal tract output (severe protracted vomiting or diarrhea without fluid therapy)
    5. Accidental sodium overdose
    6. High-protein tube feedings

From Ravel R: *Clinical laboratory medicine,* ed 6, St Louis, 1995, Mosby.
*Artifact in flame photometry, not in ISE.

IV

■ **SUCROSE HEMOLYSIS TEST** (sugar water test)
Normal:
Absence of hemolysis
Cost: $42
Positive in:
Paroxysmal nocturnal hemoglobinuria
False positive: autoimmune hemolytic anemia, megaloblastic anemias
False negative: may occur with use of heparin or EDTA

■ **T₃** (triiodothyronine)
Normal range:
75-220 ng/dl (1.2-3.4 nmol/L) [CF: 0.01536; SMI: 0.1 nmol/L]
Cost: $49
Abnormal values:
see Table 4-32

■ **T₄, FREE** (free thyroxine)
Normal range:
0.8-2.8 ng/dl (10-36 pmol/L) [CF: 12.87; SMI: 1 pmol/L]
Cost: $53

Abnormal values:
see Table 4-32

■ **TESTOSTERONE** (total testosterone)
Normal range:
(Variable with age and sex)
Serum/plasma: Males: 280-1100 ng/dl
Females: 15-70 ng/dl
Urine: Males: 50-135 μg/day
Females: 2-12 μg/day
Cost: $79
Elevated in:
Testicular tumors, ovarian masculinizing tumors
Decreased in:
Hypogonadism
The use of testosterone levels in the endocrine evaluation of infertile men is described in Table 4-33.

■ **THROMBIN TIME** (TT)
Normal range:
11.3-18.5 sec
Cost: $32

TABLE 4-31 Frequency of Various Categories of Semen Analysis Results Among Men Being Evaluated for Infertility

CATEGORY	FREQUENCY (%)
Normal	14
Azoospermia	14
Multiple parameters abnormal	49
Single abnormal parameter	23
Volume	7
Sperm count	4
Motility	6
Morphology	4
Pyospermia	2

From Nseyo UO (ed): *Urology for primary care physicians,* Philadelphia, 1999, WB Saunders.

TABLE 4-32 Findings in Thyroid Function Tests in Various Clinical Conditions

CONDITION	T₄	FT₄I	T₃	FT₃I	TSH	TSI	TRH STIMULATION
Hyperthyroidism							
Graves' disease	↑	↑	↑	↑	↓	+	↓
Toxic nodular goiter	↑	↑	↑	↑	↓	−	↓
Pituitary TSH-secreting tumors	↑	↑	↑	↑	↑	−	↓
T₃ thyrotoxicosis	N	N	↑	↑	↓	+, −	↓
T₄ thyrotoxicosis	↑	↑	N	N	↓	+, −	↓
Hypothyroidism							
Primary	↓	↓	↓	↓	↑	+, −	↑
Secondary	↓	↓	↓	↓	↓, N	−	↓
Tertiary	↓	↓	↓	↓	↓, N	−	N
Peripheral unresponsiveness	↑, N	↑, N	↑, N	↑	↑, N	−	N, ↑

From Tilton RC, Barrows A: *Clinical laboratory medicine,* St Louis, 1992, Mosby.
N, Normal; ↑, increased; ↓, decreased; +, − variable.

TABLE 4-33 Endocrine Evaluation of Infertile Men

DIAGNOSIS	T	LH	FSH
Secondary hypogonadism	↓	↓	↓
Primary hypogonadism	↓	↑	↑
Germ cell abnormalities	NL	NL	↑
Obstruction	NL	NL	NL

From Nseyo UO (ed): *Urology for primary care physicians*, Philadelphia, 1999, WB Saunders.
FSH, Follicle-stimulating hormone; *LH,* luteinizing hormone; *NL,* normal; *T,* testosterone.

BOX 4-39 Conditions That Increase Serum Thyroid-Stimulating Hormone Values

Laboratory error
Primary hypothyroidism
Synthroid therapy with insufficient dose; some patients
Lithium or amiodarone; some patients
Hashimoto's thyroiditis in later stage; some patients
Large doses of inorganic iodide (e.g., SSKI)
Severe nonthyroid illness in recovery phase; some patients
Iodine deficiency (moderate or severe)
Addison's disease
TSH specimen drawn in evening (peak of diurnal variation)

Pituitary TSH-secreting tumor
Therapy of hypothyroidism (3-6 wk after beginning therapy [range, 1-8 wk]; sometimes longer when pretherapy TSH is over 100 μU/ml); some patients
Acute psychiatric illness; few patients
Peripheral resistance to T_4 syndrome; some patients
Antibodies (e.g., HAMA) interfering with monoclonal sandwich method of TSH assay
Telepaque (iopanic acid) and Oragrafin (ipodate) x-ray contrast media; some patients
Amphetamines; some patients
High altitudes; some patients

From Ravel R: *Clinical laboratory medicine*, ed 6, St Louis, 1995, Mosby.
HAMA, Human antimouse antibodies; *SSKI,* saturated solution of potassium iodide; *TSH,* thyroid-stimulating hormone.

Elevated in:
Thrombolytic and heparin therapy, disseminated intravascular coagulation, hypofibrinogenemia, dysfibrinogenemia

■ **THYROID-STIMULATING HORMONE** (TSH)
Normal range:
2-11 μU/ml (2-11 mU/L) [CF: 1; SMI: 1 mU/L]
Cost: $65
Abnormal:
see Boxes 4-39 and 4-40 and Table 4-32

■ **THYROXINE** (T_4)
Normal range:
4-11 μg/dl (51-142 nmol/L) [CF: 12.87; SMI: 1 nmol/L]
Cost: $25
Abnormal values:
see Table 4-32

■ **TIBC;** *see* IRON-BINDING CAPACITY
■ **TRANSFERRIN**
Normal range:
170-370 mg/dl (1.7-3.7 g/L) [CF: 0.01; SMI: 0.01 g/L]
Cost: $36
Elevated in:
Iron deficiency anemia, oral contraceptive administration, viral hepatitis, late pregnancy
Decreased in:
Nephrotic syndrome, liver disease, hereditary deficiency, protein malnutrition, neoplasms, chronic inflammatory states, chronic illness, thalassemia, hemochromatosis, hemolytic anemia

■ **TRIGLYCERIDES**
Normal range:
<160 mg/dl (<1.80 mmol/L) [CF: 0.01129; SMI: 0.02 mmol/L]
Cost: $23

Elevated in:

Hyperlipoproteinemias (types I, IIb, III, IV, V), hypothyroidism, pregnancy, estrogens, acute myocardial infarction, pancreatitis, alcohol intake, nephrotic syndrome, diabetes mellitus, glycogen storage disease

Decreased in:

Malnutrition, congenital abetalipoproteinemias, drugs (e.g., gemfibrozil, nicotinic acid, clofibrate)

- **TRIIODOTHYRONINE;** *see* T_3
- **TSH;** *see* THYROID-STIMULATING HORMONE
- **TT;** *see* THROMBIN TIME
- **TUBERCULIN TEST** (PPD)
  Abnormal results:
  see Boxes 4-41 and 4-42 for interpretation
- **TUMOR MARKERS;** *see* Table 4-34 for description of common tumor markers
- **UNCONJUGATED BILIRUBIN;** *see* BILIRUBIN, INDIRECT

BOX 4-40   Conditions That Decrease Serum Thyroid-Stimulating Hormone Values*

Laboratory error
T_4/T_3 toxicosis (diffuse or nodular etiology)
Excessive therapy for hypothyroidism
Active thyroiditis (subacute, painless, or early active Hashimoto's disease); some patients
Multinodular goiter containing areas of autonomy; some patients
Severe nonthyroid illness (especially acute trauma, dopamine, or glucocorticoid); some patients
T_3 toxicosis
Pituitary insufficiency
Cushing's syndrome (and some patients on high-dose glucocorticoid)

Jod-Basedow (iodine-induced) hyperthyroidism
Thyroid-stimulating hormone drawn 2-4 hr after levothyroxine dose; few patients
Postpartum transient toxicosis
Factitious hyperthyroidism
Struma ovarii
Radioimmunoassay, surgery, or antithyroid drug therapy for hyperthyroidism; some patients, 4-6 wk (range 2 wk–2 yr) after the treatment
Interleukin-2 drugs (3%-6% of cases) or α-interferon therapy (1% of cases)
Hyperemesis gravidarum
Amiodarone therapy; some patients

From Ravel R: *Clinical laboratory medicine,* ed 6, St Louis, 1995, Mosby.
*High-sensitivity TSH method is assumed.

BOX 4-41   PPD Reaction Size Considered "Positive" (Intracutaneous 5 TU Mantoux Test at 48 hr)

5 mm or More

HIV infection or risk factors for HIV
Close recent contact with active TB case
Persons with chest x-ray consistent with healed TB

10 mm or More

Foreign-born persons from countries with high TB prevalence in Asia, Africa, and Latin America
IV drug users
Medically underserved low-income population groups (including Native Americans, Hispanics, and blacks)

Residents of long-term care facilities (nursing homes, mental institutions)
Medical conditions that increase risk for TB (silicosis, gastrectomy, undernourished, diabetes mellitus, high-dose corticosteroids or immunosuppression Rx, leukemia or lymphoma, other malignancies)
Employees of long-term care facilities, schools, child-care facilities, health care facilities

15 mm or More

All others not already listed

TB, Tuberculosis; *TU,* tuberculin units.

BOX 4-42   Factors Associated with False-Negative Tuberculin Tests

Technical Errors

Improper administration
Inaccurate reading
Loss of potency of antigen

Patient-Related Factors (Anergy)

Age (elderly)
Nutritional status

Medications—corticosteroids, immunosuppressive agents
Severe tuberculosis
Coexisting diseases
  HIV infection
  Viral illness or vaccination
  Lymphoreticular malignancies
  Sarcoidosis
  Solid tumors

Lepromatous leprosy
Sjögren's syndrome
Ataxia telangiectasia
Uremia
Primary biliary cirrhosis
Systemic lupus erythematosus
Severe systemic disease of any etiology

From Stein JH (ed): *Internal medicine,* ed 4, St Louis, 1994, Mosby.

TABLE 4-34   Tumor Markers

General Uses:

1. Monitor serial titers before and after therapy. For example, a high preoperative CEA titer that falls to the normal range postoperatively is associated with a better prognosis in breast or colon cancer than is one that remains elevated after local therapy.

2. Serial values are also of use in monitoring (a) the clinical course of disease after local therapy and (b) the response to systemic chemotherapy. A decline in elevated values is usually consistent with tumor regression. Tumor markers are most valuable in monitoring disease not readily assessable by physical examination or simple radiographs.

	CHARACTERISTICS	PRESENCE IN NORMAL SERUM/PLASMA	CONDITIONS IN WHICH ELEVATED SERUM/PLASMA CONCENTRATIONS OCCUR	
			NEOPLASTIC	NONNEOPLASTIC
I. Oncofetal proteins				
1. Carcinoembryonic antigen (CEA)	Glycoprotein (MW 200,000)	<2.5 ng/ml	GI, breast, lung cancers	Inflammatory bowel disease, pancreatitis, gastritis, smoker's chronic bronchitis, alcoholic liver disease, hepatitis
2. Alpha fetoprotein (AFP)	α-Globulin (MW 70,000)	<40 ng/ml	Hepatoma, nonseminomatous testicular cancers	Pregnancy, regenerating liver tissue after viral hepatitis, chemically induced liver necrosis, partial hepatectomy
II. Hormones				
1. Human chorionic gonadotropin, β subunit (β-hCG)	Glycoprotein (MW 45,000); β subunit provides specificity versus LH, FSH, TSH	0	Choriocarcinoma, nonseminomatous testicular cancer, giant cell carcinoma of lung	Pregnancy
2. Ectopic hormones	ACTH, ADH, PTH		Lung, breast, head and neck, cervical cancers	
III. Serum enzymes				
1. Prostatic acid phosphatase (PAP)	Radioimmunoassay detects prostatic isozyme and distinguishes it from acid phosphatases of other organs (e.g., liver, spleen, kidney, small intestine), red and white blood cells, and platelets	0	Prostatic carcinoma	
2. Placental alkaline phosphatase	Biochemically and immunologically similar to that produced by the placenta	0	Seminoma, ovarian cancer	Pregnancy
3. Lactic dehydrogenase (LDH)	Tetramer, two distinct polypeptide chains: H (heart) and M (muscle)		Lymphoma	Hepatitis, MI, muscle injury
IV. Immunoglobulins	Monoclonal elevation (M spike) of complete protein, light or heavy chain, or portions		Multiple myeloma, B cell lymphoma	Monoclonal gammopathy of unknown significance (M-GUS)
V. Tumor-associated antigens				
1. CA-125			Ovarian, lung cancers	Benign gynecologic disease, cirrhosis
2. CA-15.3			Breast, ovarian, lung cancers	
3. Prostate-specific antigen	Glycoprotein (MW 30,000-40,000)		Prostatic carcinoma	Benign prostatic hypertrophy

From Stein JH (ed): *Internal medicine*, ed 4, St Louis, 1994, Mosby.
ACTH, Adrenocorticotropic hormone; *ADH*, antidiuretic hormone; *FSH*, follicle-stimulating hormone; *GI*, gastrointestinal; *LH*, luteinizing hormone; *MI*, myocardial infarction; *MW*, molecular weight; *PTH*, parathormone (parathyroid hormone); *TSH*, thyroid-stimulating hormone.

IV

■ **UREA NITROGEN, BLOOD** (BUN)
Normal range:
8-18 mg/dl (3-6.5 mmol/L) [CF: 0.357; SMI: 0.5 mmol/L]
Box 4-43 describes factors affecting BUN level independent of renal function.
Cost: $23
Elevated in:
Drugs (aminoglycosides and other antibiotics, diuretics, lithium, corticosteroids), dehydration, gastrointestinal bleeding, decreased renal blood flow (shock, congestive heart failure, myocardial infarction), renal disease (glomerulonephritis, pyelonephritis, diabetic nephropathy), urinary tract obstruction (prostatic hypertrophy)
Decreased in:
Liver disease, malnutrition, pregnancy third trimester, overhydration, acromegaly, celiac disease

■ **URIC ACID** (serum)
Normal range:
2-7 mg/dl (120-420 μmol/L) [CF: 59.48; SMI: 10 μmol/L]
Cost: $23
Elevated in:
Renal failure, gout, excessive cell lysis (chemotherapeutic agents, radiation therapy, leukemia, lymphoma, hemolytic anemia), hereditary enzyme deficiency (hypoxanthine-guanine-phosphoribosyl transferase), acidosis, myeloproliferative disorders, diet high in purines or protein, drugs (diuretics, low doses of ASA, ethambutol, nicotinic acid), lead poisoning, hypothyroidism, Addison's disease, nephrogenic diabetes insipidus, active psoriasis, polycystic kidneys

Decreased in:
Drugs (allopurinol, high doses of ASA, probenecid, warfarin, corticosteroid), deficiency of xanthine oxidase, syndrome of inappropriate antidiuretic hormone secretion, renal tubular deficits (Fanconi's syndrome), alcoholism, liver disease, diet deficient in protein or purines, Wilson's disease, hemochromatosis

■ **URINALYSIS**
Normal range:

Color: light straw	Protein: absent
Appearance: clear	Ketones: absent
pH: 4.5-8 (average, 6)	Glucose: absent
Specific gravity: 1.005-1.030	Occult blood: absent

Microscopic examination:
Red blood cells: 0-5 (high-power field)
White blood cells: 0-5 (high-power field)
Bacteria (spun specimen): absent
Casts: 0-4 hyaline (low-power field)
Cost: $22
Abnormalities in the microscopic examination of urine are described in Table 4-35.

TABLE 4-35 Microscopic Examination of the Urine

FINDING	ASSOCIATIONS
Casts	
Red blood cell	Glomerulonephritis, vasculitis
White blood cell	Interstitial nephritis, pyelonephritis
Epithelial cell	Acute tubular necrosis, interstitial nephritis, glomerulonephritis
Granular	Renal parenchymal disease (nonspecific)
Waxy, broad	Advanced renal failure
Hyaline	Normal finding in concentrated urine
Fatty	Heavy proteinuria
Cells	
Red blood cell	Urinary tract infection, urinary tract inflammation
White blood cell	Urinary tract infection, urinary tract inflammation
Eosinophil	Acute interstitial nephritis
(Squamous) epithelial cell	Contaminants
Crystals	
Uric acid	Acid urine, acute uric acid nephropathy, hyperuricosuria
Calcium phosphate	Alkaline urine
Calcium oxalate	Acid urine, hyperoxaluria, ethylene glycol poisoning
Cystine	Cystinuria
Sulfur	Sulfa-containing antibiotics

From Andreoli TE (ed): *Cecil essentials of medicine*, ed 5, Philadelphia, 2001, WB Saunders.

BOX 4-43 Factors Affecting Blood Urea Nitrogen Level Independent of Renal Function

Disproportionate Increase in Blood Urea Nitrogen

Volume depletion "prerenal azotemia"
Gastrointestinal hemorrhage
Corticosteroid or cytotoxic agents
High-protein diet
Obstructive uropathy
Sepsis
Catabolic states tissue breakdown

Disproportionate Decrease in Blood Urea Nitrogen

Low-protein diet
Liver disease

From Andreoli TE (ed): *Cecil essentials of medicine*, ed 5, Philadelphia, 2001, WB Saunders.

■ **URINE AMYLASE**
Normal range:
35-260 U Somogyi/hr (6.5-48.1 U/hr) [CF: 0.185; SMI: 1 U/hr]
Cost: $26
Elevated in:
Pancreatitis, carcinoma of the pancreas

■ **URINE BILE**
Normal:
Absent
Abnormal:
Urine bilirubin: hepatitis (viral, toxic, drug-induced), biliary obstruction
Urine urobilinogen: hepatitis (viral, toxic, drug-induced), hemolytic jaundice, liver cell dysfunction (cirrhosis, infection, metastases)

■ **URINE CALCIUM**
Normal range:
<250 mg/24 hr (<6.2 mmol/dl) [CF: 0.02495; SMI: 0.1 mmol/dl]
Cost: $23
Elevated in:
Primary hyperparathyroidism, hypervitaminosis D, bone metastases, multiple myeloma, increased calcium intake, steroids, prolonged immobilization, sarcoidosis, Paget's disease, idiopathic hypercalciuria, renal tubular acidosis
Decreased in:
Hypoparathyroidism, pseudohypoparathyroidism, vitamin D deficiency, vitamin D–resistant rickets, diet low in calcium, drugs (thiazide diuretics, oral contraceptives), familial hypocalciuric hypercalcemia, renal osteodystrophy, potassium citrate therapy

■ **URINE cAMP**
Cost: $89
Elevated in:
Hypercalciuria, familial hypocalciuric hypercalcemia, primary hyperparathyroidism, pseudohypoparathyroidism, rickets
Decreased in:
Vitamin D intoxication, sarcoidosis

■ **URINE CATECHOLAMINES**
Normal range:
Norepinephrine: <100 μg/24 hr (<590 nmol/day) [CF: 5.911; SMI: 10 nmol/day]
Epinephrine: <10 μg/24 hr (55 nmol/day) [CF: 5.458; SMI: 5 nmol/day]
Cost: $50
Elevated in:
Pheochromocytoma, neuroblastoma, severe stress

■ **URINE CHLORIDE**
Normal range:
110-250 mEq/day (110-250 mmol/day) [CF: 1; SMI: 1 mmol/day]
Cost: $24

Elevated in:
Corticosteroids, Bartter's syndrome, diuretics, metabolic acidosis, severe hypokalemia
Decreased in:
Chloride depletion (vomiting), colonic villous adenoma, chronic renal failure, renal tubular acidosis

■ **URINE COPPER**
Normal range:
<40 μg/24 hr (<0.6 μmol/day) [CF: 0.01574; SMI: 0.2 μmol/day]
Cost: $58

■ **URINE CORTISOL, FREE**
Normal range:
10-110 μg/24 hr (30-300 nmol/day) [CF: 2.759; SMI: 10 nmol/day]
Cost: $125
Elevated:
See CORTISOL, PLASMA

■ **URINE CREATININE** (24 hr)
Normal range:
Male: 0.8-1.8 g/day (7-16 mmol/day) [CF: 8.840; SMI: 0.1 mmol/day]
Female: 0.6-1.6 g/day (5.3-14 mmol/day)
Cost: $23
NOTE: Useful test as an indicator of completeness of 24 hr urine collection.

■ **URINE EOSINOPHILS**
Normal:
Absent
Present:
Interstitial nephritis, acute tubular necrosis, urinary tract infection, kidney transplant rejection, hepatorenal syndrome

■ **URINE GLUCOSE** (qualitative)
Normal:
Absent
Present in:
Diabetes mellitus, renal glycosuria (decreased renal threshold for glucose), glucose intolerance

■ **URINE HEMOGLOBIN, FREE**
Normal:
Absent
Present in:
Hemolysis (with saturation of serum haptoglobin binding capacity and renal threshold for tubular absorption of hemoglobin)

■ **URINE HEMOSIDERIN**
Normal:
Absent
Present in:
Paroxysmal nocturnal hemoglobinuria, chronic hemolytic anemia, hemochromatosis, blood transfusion, thalassemias

IV

- **URINE 5-HYDROXYINDOLE-ACETIC ACID** (urine 5-HIAA)
  Normal range:
  2-8 mg/24 hr (10-40 μmol/day) [CF: 5.23; SMI: 5 μmol/day]
  Cost: $79
  Elevated in:
  Carcinoid tumors, after ingestion of certain foods (bananas, plums, tomatoes, avocados, pineapples, eggplant, walnuts), drugs (monoamine oxidase inhibitors, phenacetin, methyldopa, glycerol guaiacolate, acetaminophen, salicylates, phenothiazines, imipramine, methocarbamol, reserpine, methamphetamine)

- **URINE INDICAN**
  Normal:
  Absent
  Present in:
  Malabsorption secondary to intestinal bacterial overgrowth

- **URINE KETONES** (semiquantitative)
  Normal:
  Absent
  Present in:
  Diabetic ketoacidosis, alcoholic ketoacidosis, starvation, isopropanol ingestion

- **URINE METANEPHRINES**
  Normal range:
  0-2.0 mg/24 hr (0-11.0 μmol/day) [CF: 5.458; SMI: 0.5 μmol/day]
  Cost: $79
  Elevated in:
  Pheochromocytoma, neuroblastoma, drugs (caffeine, phenothiazines, monoamine oxidase inhibitors), stress

- **URINE MYOGLOBIN**
  Normal:
  Absent
  Present in:
  Severe trauma, hyperthermia, polymyositis/dermatomyositis, carbon monoxide poisoning, drugs (narcotic and amphetamine toxicity), hypothyroidism, muscle ischemia

- **URINE NITRITE**
  Normal:
  Absent
  Present in:
  Urinary tract infections

- **URINE OCCULT BLOOD**
  Normal:
  Negative
  Positive in:
  Trauma to urinary tract, renal disease (glomerulonephritis, pyelonephritis), renal or ureteral calculi, bladder lesions (carcinoma, cystitis), prostatitis, prostatic carcinoma, menstrual contamination, hematopoietic disorders (hemophilia, thrombocytopenia), anticoagulants, ASA

- **URINE OSMOLALITY**
  Normal range:
  50-1200 mOsm/kg (50-1200 mmol/kg) [CF: 1; SMI: 1 mmol/kg]
  Cost: $31
  Elevated in:
  Syndrome of inappropriate antidiuretic hormone secretion, dehydration, glycosuria, adrenal insufficiency, high-protein diet
  Decreased in:
  Diabetes insipidus, excessive water intake, IV hydration with D_5W, acute renal insufficiency, glomerulonephritis

- **URINE pH**
  Normal range:
  4.6-8 (average 6)
  Elevated in:
  Bacteriuria, vegetarian diet, renal failure with inability to form ammonia, drugs (antibiotics, sodium bicarbonate, acetazolamide)
  Decreased in:
  Acidosis (metabolic, respiratory), drugs (ammonium chloride, methenamine mandelate), diabetes mellitus, starvation, diarrhea

- **URINE PHOSPHATE**
  Normal range:
  0.8-2.0 g/24 hr
  Cost: $23
  Elevated in:
  Acute tubular necrosis (diuretic phase), chronic renal disease, uncontrolled diabetes mellitus, hyperparathyroidism, hypomagnesemia, metabolic acidosis, metabolic alkalosis, neurofibromatosis, adult-onset vitamin D–resistant hypophosphatemic osteomalacia
  Decreased in:
  Acromegaly, acute renal failure, decreased dietary intake, hypoparathyroidism, respiratory acidosis

- **URINE POTASSIUM**
  Normal range:
  25-100 mEq/24 hr (25-100 mmol/day) [CF: 1; SMI: 1 mmol/day]
  Cost: $23
  Elevated in:
  Aldosteronism (primary, secondary), glucocorticoids, alkalosis, renal tubular acidosis, excessive dietary potassium intake
  Decreased in:
  Acute renal failure, potassium-sparing diuretics, diarrhea, hypokalemia

■ **URINE PROTEIN** (quantitative)
Normal range:
<150 mg/24 hr (<0.15 g/day) [CF: 0.001; SMI: 0.01 g/day]
Cost: $23
Elevated in:
Renal disease (glomerular, tubular, interstitial), congestive heart failure, hypertension, neoplasms of renal pelvis and bladder, multiple myeloma, Waldenström's macroglobulinemia

■ **URINE SEDIMENT;** *see* Fig. 4-19 for evaluation of common abnormalities

■ **URINE SODIUM** (quantitative)
Normal range:
40-220 mEq/day (40-220 mmol/day) [CF: 1; SMI: 1 mmol/day]
Cost: $23
Elevated in:
Diuretic administration, high sodium intake, salt-losing nephritis, acute tubular necrosis, vomiting, Addison's disease, syndrome of inappropriate antidiuretic hormone secretion, hypothyroidism, congestive heart failure, hepatic failure, chronic renal failure, Bartter's syndrome, glucocorticoid deficiency, interstitial nephritis caused by analgesic abuse, mannitol, dextran, or glycerol therapy, milk-alkali syndrome, decreased renin secretion, postobstructive diuresis
Decreased in:
Increased aldosterone, glucocorticoid excess, hyponatremia, prerenal azotemia, decreased salt intake

■ **URINE SPECIFIC GRAVITY**
Normal range:
1.005-1.03
Elevated in:
Dehydration, excessive fluid losses (vomiting, diarrhea, fever), x-ray contrast media, diabetes mellitus, congestive heart failure, syndrome of inappropriate antidiuretic hormone secretion, adrenal insufficiency, decreased fluid intake
Decreased in:
Diabetes insipidus, renal disease (glomerulonephritis, pyelonephritis), excessive fluid intake or IV hydration

■ **URINE VANILLYLMANDELIC ACID** (VMA)
Normal range:
<6.8 mg/24 hr (<35 μmol/day) [CF: 5.046; SMI: 1 μmol/day]
Cost: $50
Elevated in:
Pheochromocytoma, neuroblastoma, ganglioblastoma, drugs (isoproterenol, methocarbamol, levodopa, sulfonamides, chlorpromazine), severe stress, after ingestion of bananas, chocolate, vanilla, tea, coffee

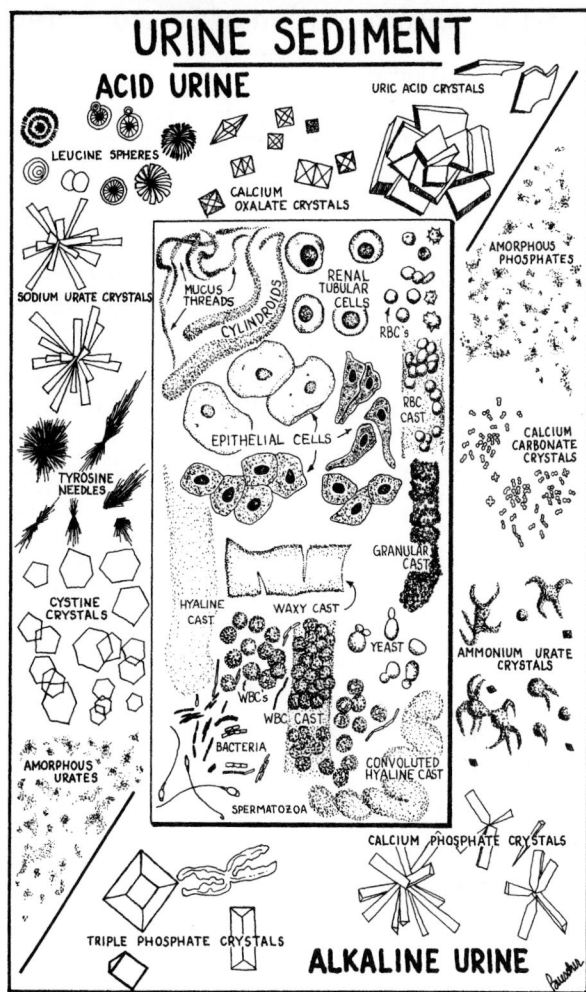

Fig. 4-19   Microscopic examination of urinary sediment. (From Grigorian Greene M: *The Harriet Lane handbook: a manual for pediatric house officers,* ed 12, St Louis, 1991, Mosby.)

Decreased in:
Drugs (monoamine oxidase inhibitors, reserpine, guanethidine, methyldopa)

■ **VDRL**
Normal range:
Negative
Cost: $49
Positive test:
Syphilis, other treponemal diseases (yaws, pinta, bejel)
NOTE: A false-positive test may be seen in patients with systemic lupus erythematosus and other autoimmune diseases, infectious mononucleosis, HIV, atypical pneumonia, malaria, leprosy, typhus fever, rat-bite fever, relapsing fever.
NOTE: see Table 4-36 for interpretation of serologic tests for syphilis.

IV

TABLE 4-36   Interpretation of Serologic Tests for Syphilis*

FINDING		
NONTREPONEMAL TESTS	TREPONEMAL TESTS	INTERPRETATION OF FINDING: IS SYPHILIS PRESENT?*
Nonreactive	Nonreactive	*Early primary syphilis is not ruled out by negative serologic tests.* *Early syphilis* is present in 13%-30% of patients who have a negative microhemagglutination–*Treponema pallidum* test; in about 30% of patients who present with chancre but have a nonreactive reagin test; and in about 10% of patients who have a negative FTA-ABS test. *Late syphilis* is present in a very small fraction of patients. *Adequately treated syphilis in remote past* may produce these results, but treponemal tests usually remain reactive.
	Reactive	Observed in about 10% of patients with chancre. The treponemal tests may turn positive shortly before the reagin tests. Reagin tests repeated after several days are generally positive. *In adequately treated early syphilis,* the reagin test may return to nonreactive within 1-2 yr, whereas the treponemal tests generally do not. *Late syphilis* is not ruled out by a negative reagin test. The sensitivity of the reagin tests is lower than that of treponemal tests in untreated late syphilis. In *secondary syphilis,* rarely, a highly reactive serum appears negative when tested undiluted with a reagin test because flocculation is inhibited by relative antibody excess. Not reported to occur with treponemal tests. Quantitative reagin tests are positive. False-positive treponemal tests occur in 40% of patients with Lyme disease.
Reactive	Nonreactive borderline (FTA-ABS)	Finding is not diagnostic of syphilis but constitutes a classic biologic false-positive reaction. Not diagnostic of syphilis: most patients (90%) with this pattern do not develop clinical or serologic evidence of syphilis. Repeat test is indicated. Chronic borderline results are associated with a variety of conditions other than syphilis.
	Beaded (FTA-ABS)	Not diagnostic of syphilis. Seen with collagen-vascular disease.
	Reactive	Findings diagnostic of syphilis or other treponemal disease. *In adequately treated syphilis,* one would expect (1) a sustained fourfold drop in titer of reagin test, although reagin test may remain positive after adequate therapy; (2) treponemal tests remain positive after adequate therapy. Concurrent false-positive results on both nontreponemal and treponemal tests could occur in rare instances. It may be impossible to rule out syphilis in an individual with this test profile.

From Stein JH (ed): *Internal medicine*, ed 4, St Louis, 1994, Mosby.
FTA-ABS, Fluorescent treponemal antibody, absorbed.
*Serologic data must always be interpreted in the light of a total clinical evaluation. Diagnosis based on serologic criteria alone is fraught with error. Serologic tests apparently in conflict with clinical diagnosis should be confirmed by repetition or possibly referral to a reference laboratory.

BOX 4-44   Wet-Mount Microscopic Procedures

India Ink Preparation

1. Place a drop of specimen on a clean glass slide.
2. Cover with coverslip, preferably a larger size.
3. Place a small drop of India ink on the slide, touching the coverslip; it will be drawn under the coverslip and provide a gradient suspension of the ink particles.
4. Examine using bright-field microscopy; scan the slide to find the point at which suspension is optimal for observing capsules or organisms.

Potassium Hydroxide Preparation

1. Place a small portion of specimen on a clean glass slide.
2. Add a drop of 10% potassium hydroxide solution; if necessary, mix with specimen using an applicator stick.

3. Cover with a coverslip, then heat gently by passing through a flame (do not heat excessively; several minutes or more of setting may be necessary to dissolve material composed of keratin).
4. Examine using bright-field microscopy; adjust substage condenser to optimize contrast.

Methylene Blue Stain for Fecal Leukocytes

1. Place a small portion of liquid stool on a clean glass slide.
2. Add a drop of methylene blue stain and mix with the specimen; place coverslip.
3. Let stand several minutes, then examine with bright-field microscopy.

From Stein JH (ed): *Internal medicine*, ed 5, St Louis, 1998, Mosby.

■ **VISCOSITY** (serum)

Normal range:

1.4-1.8 relative to water (1.10-1.22 centipoise)

Cost: $34

Elevated in:

Monoclonal gammopathies (Waldenström's macro-globulinemia, multiple myeloma), hyperfibrino-genemia, systemic lupus erythematosus, rheuma-toid arthritis, polycythemia, leukemia

■ **VITAMIN B₁₂**

Normal:

190-900 ng/ml

Cost: $52

Vitamin B₁₂ deficiency

Etiology

1. Pernicious anemia (antibodies against intrinsic factor and gastric parietal cells)
2. Dietary (strict lacto-ovovegetarians, food fad-dists)
3. Malabsorption (achlorhydria, gastrectomy, ileal resection, pancreatic insufficiency, drugs [omeprazole, cholestyramine])

Falsely low levels occur in patients with severe folate deficiency, in patients using high doses of ascorbic acid, and when cobalamin levels are mea-sured after nuclear medicine studies (radioactivity interferes with cobalamin radioimmunoassay).

Falsely high or normal levels in patients with cobalamin deficiency can occur in severe liver disease and chronic granulocytic leukemia.

The absence of anemia or macrocytosis does not exclude the diagnosis of cobalamin deficiency.

■ **WBC;** *see* COMPLETE BLOOD COUNT

■ **WESTERGREN;** *see* ERYTHROCYTE SEDIMENTATION RATE

■ **WET-MOUNT MICROSCOPIC PROCEDURES;** *see* Box 4-44

■ **WHITE BLOOD COUNT;** *see* COMPLETE BLOOD COUNT

■ **ᴅ-XYLOSE ABSORPTION**

Normal range:

21% to 31% excreted in 5 hr (0.21-0.31) [CF: 0.01; SMI: 0.01]

Cost: $52

Decreased in:

Malabsorption syndrome

IV

Clinical Preventive Services

*Data modified from US Preventive Services Task Force: *Guide to clinical preventive services: report of the US Preventive Services Task Force,*
ed 2, Washington, DC, 1996 (revised 2001), US Department of Health and Human Services. Text downloaded from Internet site:
http://text.nlm.nih.gov

V

THE PERIODIC HEALTH EXAMINATION
Age-Specific Charts

TABLE 5-1 Birth to 10 Years

Interventions considered
  and recommended for the
  Periodic Health Examination

Leading causes of death
  Conditions originating in perinatal period
  Congenital anomalies
  Sudden infant death syndrome (SIDS)
  Unintentional injuries (non–motor vehicle)
  Motor vehicle injuries

Interventions for the General Population

Screening

Height and weight

Blood pressure

Vision screen (age 3-4 yr)

Hemoglobinopathy screen (birth)[1]

Phenylalanine level (birth)[2]

T_4 and/or TSH (birth)[3]

Counseling

Injury prevention
Child safety car seats (age <5 yr)

Lap/shoulder belts (age ≥5 yr)

Bicycle helmet; avoid bicycling near traffic

Smoke detector, flame retardant sleepwear

Hot water heater temperature <120°-130°F

Window/stair guards, pool fence

Safe storage of drugs, toxic substances, firearms, and matches

Syrup of ipecac, poison control phone number

CPR training for
  parents/caretakers
Diet and exercise
Breast-feeding, iron-enriched formula and foods (infants and
  toddlers)

Limit fat and cholesterol; maintain caloric balance; emphasize
  grains, fruits, vegetables (age ≥2 yr)

Regular physical activity*
Substance use
Effects of passive smoking*

Antitobacco message*
Dental health
Regular visits to dental care provider*

Floss, brush with fluoride toothpaste daily*

Advice about baby bottle tooth decay*

Immunizations

Diphtheria-tetanus-pertussis (DTP)[4]

Inactivated poliovirus vaccine (IPV)[5]

Measles-mumps-rubella (MMR)[6]

H. influenzae type b (Hib) conjugate[7]

Hepatitis B[8]

Varicella[9]

Pneumococcal vaccine[10]

Chemoprophylaxis

Ocular prophylaxis (birth)

Interventions for High-Risk Populations

Population	Potential Interventions (See detailed high-risk definitions)
Preterm or low birth weight	Hemoglobin/hematocrit (HR1)
Infants of mothers at risk for HIV	HIV testing (HR2)
Low income; immigrants	Hemoglobin/hematocrit (HR1); PPD (HR3)
TB contacts	PPD (HR3)
Native American/Alaska Native	Hemoglobin/hematocrit (HR1); PPD (HR3); hepatitis A vaccine (HR4); pneumococcal vaccine (HR5)
Travelers to developing countries	Hepatitis A vaccine (HR4)
Residents of long-term care facilities	PPD (HR3); hepatitis A vaccine (HR4); influenza vaccine (HR6)
Certain chronic medical conditions	PPD (HR3); pneumococcal vaccine (HR5); influenza vaccine (HR6)
Increased individual or community lead exposure	Blood lead level (HR7)
Inadequate water fluoridation	Daily fluoride supplement (HR8)
Family hx of skin cancer; nevi; fair skin, eyes, hair	Avoid excess/midday sun, use protective clothing* (HR9)

[1]Whether screening should be universal or targeted to high-risk groups will depend on the proportion of high-risk individuals in the screening area, and other considerations. [2]If done during first 24 hr of life, repeat by age 2 wk. [3]Optimally between day 2 and 6, but in all cases before newborn nursery discharge. [4]2, 4, 6, and 12-18 mo; once between ages 4-6 yr (DTaP may be used at 15 mo and older). [5]2, 4, 6-18 mo; once between ages 4-6 yr. [6]12-15 mo and 4-6 yr. [7]2, 4, 6 and 12-15 mo; no dose needed at 6 mo if PRP-OMP vaccine is used for first 2 doses. [8]Birth, 1 mo, 6 mo; or, 0-2 mo, 1-2 mo later, and 6-18 mo. If not done in infancy: current visit, and 1 and 6 mo later. [9]12-18 mo; or any child without hx of chickenpox or previous immunization. Include information on risk in adulthood, duration of immunity, and potential need for booster doses. [10]The 7-Valent conjugate vaccine (PCV) can be administered at the same time as the other childhood vaccines at a separate site.
*The ability of clinician counseling to influence this behavior is unproven.

V

HR1 = Infants age 6-12 mo who are living in poverty, black, Native American or Alaska Native, immigrants from developing countries, preterm and low birth weight infants, infants whose principal dietary intake is unfortified cow's milk.

HR2 = Infants born to high-risk mothers whose HIV status is unknown. Women at high risk include past or present injection drug use; persons who exchange sex for money or drugs, and their sex partners; injection drug–using, bisexual, or HIV-positive sex partners currently or in past; persons seeking treatment for STDs; blood transfusion during 1978-1985.

HR3 = Persons infected with HIV, close contacts of persons with known or suspected TB, persons with medical risk factors associated with TB, immigrants from countries with high TB prevalence, medically underserved low-income populations (including homeless), residents of long-term care facilities.

HR4 = Persons ≥2 yr living in or traveling to areas where the disease is endemic and where periodic outbreaks occur (e.g., countries with high or intermediate endemicity; certain Alaska Native, Pacific Island, Native American, and religious communities). Consider for institutionalized children aged ≥2 yr. Clinicians should also consider local epidemiology.

HR5 = Immunocompetent persons ≥2 yr with certain medical conditions, including chronic cardiac or pulmonary disease, dia-
betes mellitus, and anatomic asplenia. Immunocompetent persons ≥2 yr living in high-risk environments or social settings (e.g., certain Native American and Alaska Native populations).

HR6 = Annual vaccination of children ≥6 mo who are residents of chronic care facilities or who have chronic cardiopulmonary disorders, metabolic diseases (including diabetes mellitus), hemoglobinopathies, immunosuppression, or renal dysfunction.

HR7 = Children about age 12 mo who: (1) live in communities in which the prevalence of lead levels requiring individual intervention, including residental lead hazard control or chelation, is high or undefined; (2) live in or frequently visit a home built before 1950 with dilapidated paint or with recent or ongoing renovation or remodeling; (3) have close contact with a person who has an elevated lead level; (4) live near lead industry or heavy traffic; (5) live with someone whose job or hobby involves lead exposure; (6) use lead-based pottery; or (7) take traditional ethnic remedies that contain lead.

HR8 = Children living in areas with inadequate water fluoridation (<0.6 ppm).

HR9 = Persons with a family history of skin cancer, a large number of moles, atypical moles, poor tanning ability, or light skin, hair, and eye color.

TABLE 5-2 Ages 11-24 Years

Interventions considered
  and recommended for the
   Periodic Health Examination

Leading causes of death
  Motor vehicle/other unintentional injuries
  Homicide
  Suicide
  Malignant neoplasms
  Heart diseases

Interventions for the General Population

Screening

Height and weight

Blood pressure[1]

Papanicolaou (Pap) test[2] (females)

Chlamydia screen[3] (females <25 yr)

Lipid panel (in high-risk young adults only)

Rubella serology or vaccination hx[4] (females >12 yr)

Assess for problem drinking

Counseling

Injury prevention
Lap/shoulder belts

Bicycle/motorcycle/ATV helmets*

Smoke detector*

Safe storage/removal of firearms*
Substance use
Avoid tobacco use

Avoid underage drinking and illicit drug use*

Avoid alcohol/drug use while driving, swimming, boating, etc.*

Sexual behavior
STD prevention: abstinence*; avoid high-risk behavior*;
  condoms/female barrier with spermicide*
Unintended pregnancy: contraception

Diet and exercise
Limit fat and cholesterol; maintain caloric balance; emphasize
  grains, fruits, vegetables

Adequate calcium intake (females)

Regular physical activity*
Dental health
Regular visits to dental care provider*

Floss, brush with fluoride toothpaste daily

Immunizations

Tetanus-diphtheria (Td) boosters (11-16 yr)

Hepatitis B[5]

MMR (11-12 yr)[6]

Varicella (11-12 yr)[7]

Rubella[4] (females >12 yr)

Chemoprophylaxis

Multivitamin with folic acid (females)

Interventions for High-Risk Populations

Population	Potential Interventions (See detailed high-risk definitions)
High-risk sexual behavior	RPR/VDRL (HR1); screen for gonorrhea (female) (HR2), HIV (HR3), chlamydia (female) (HR4); hepatitis A vaccine (HR5)
Injection or street drug use	RPR/VDRL (HR1); HIV screen (HR3); hepatitis A vaccine (HR5); PPD (HR6); advice to reduce infection risk (HR7)
TB contacts; immigrants; low income	PPD (HR6)
Native Americans/Alaska Natives	Hepatitis A vaccine (HR5); PPD (HR6); pneumococcal vaccine (HR8)
Travelers to developing countries	Hepatitis A vaccine (HR5)
Certain chronic medical conditions	PPD (HR6); pneumococcal vaccine (HR8); influenza vaccine (HR9)
Settings where adolescents and young adults congregate	Second MMR (HR10)
Susceptible to varicella, measles, mumps	Varicella vaccine (HR11); MMR (HR12)
Blood transfusion between 1975-1985	HIV screen (HR3)
Institutionalized persons; health care/lab workers	Hepatitis A vaccine (HR5); PPD (HR6); influenza vaccine (HR9)
Family hx of skin cancer; nevi; fair skin, eyes, hair	Avoid excess/midday sun, use protective clothing* (HR13)
Prior pregnancy with neural tube defect	Folic acid 4.0 mg (HR14)
Inadequate water fluoridation	Daily fluoride supplement (HR15)

V

[1]Periodic BP for persons aged ≥21 yr. [2]If sexually active at present or in the past: q ≤3 yr. If sexual history is unreliable, begin Pap tests at age 18 yr. [3]If sexually active. [4]Serologic testing, documented vaccination history, and routine vaccination against rubella (preferably with MMR) are equally acceptable alternatives. [5]If not previously immunized: current visit, 1 and 6 mo later. [6]If no previous second dose of MMR. [7]If susceptible to chickenpox.
*The ability of clinician counseling to influence this behavior is unproven.

HR1 = Persons who exchange sex for money or drugs, and their sex partners; persons with other STDs (including HIV); and sexual contacts of persons with active syphilis. Clinicians should also consider local epidemiology.

HR2 = Females who have two or more sex partners in the last year; a sex partner with multiple sexual contacts; exchanged sex for money or drugs; or a history of repeated episodes of gonorrhea. Clinicians should also consider local epidemiology.

HR3 = Males who had sex with males after 1975; past or present injection drug use; persons who exchange sex for money or drugs, and their sex partners; injection drug–using, bisexual, or HIV-positive sex partner currently or in the past; blood transfusion during 1978-1985; persons seeking treatment for STDs. Clinicians should also consider local epidemiology.

HR4 = Sexually active females with multiple risk factors including history of prior STD; new or multiple sex partners; age under 25; nonuse or inconsistent use of barrier contraceptives; cervical ectopy. Clinicians should consider local epidemiology of the disease in identifying other high-risk groups.

HR5 = Persons living in, traveling to, or working in areas where the disease is endemic and where periodic outbreaks occur (e.g., countries with high or intermediate endemicity; certain Alaska Native, Pacific Island, Native American, and religious communities); men who have sex with men; injection or street drug users. Vaccine may be considered for institutionalized persons and workers in these institutions, military personnel, and day-care, hospital, and laboratory workers. Clinicians should also consider local epidemiology.

HR6 = HIV positive, close contacts of persons with known or suspected TB, health care workers, persons with medical risk factors associated with TB, immigrants from countries with high TB prevalence, medically underserved low-income populations (including homeless), alcoholics, injection drug users, and residents of long-term facilities.

HR7 = Persons who continue to inject drugs.

HR8 = Immunocompetent persons with certain medical conditions, including chronic cardiac or pulmonary disease, diabetes mellitus, and anatomic asplenia. Immunocompetent persons who live in high-risk environments or social settings (e.g., certain Native American and Alaska Native populations).

HR9 = Annual vaccination of residents of chronic care facilities; persons with chronic cardiopulmonary disorders, metabolic diseases (including diabetes mellitus), hemoglobinopathies, immunosuppression, or renal dysfunction; and health care providers for high-risk patients.

HR10 = Adolescents and young adults in settings where such individuals congregate (e.g., high schools and colleges), if they have not previously received a second dose.

HR11 = Healthy persons aged ≥13 yr without a history of chickenpox or previous immunization. Consider serologic testing for presumed susceptible persons aged ≥13 yr.

HR12 = Persons born after 1956 who lack evidence of immunity to measles or mumps (e.g., documented receipt of live vaccine on or after the first birthday, laboratory evidence of immunity, or a history of physician-diagnosed measles or mumps).

HR13 = Persons with a family or personal history of skin cancer, a large number of moles, atypical moles, poor tanning ability, or light skin, hair, and eye color.

HR14 = Women with prior pregnancy affected by neural tube defect who are planning pregnancy.

HR15 = Persons aged <17 yr living in areas with inadequate water fluoridation (<0.6 ppm).

TABLE 5-3   Ages 25-64 Years

Interventions considered
  and recommended for the
  Periodic Health Examination

Leading causes of death
  Malignant neoplasms
  Heart diseases
  Motor vehicle and other unintentional injuries
  Human immunodeficiency virus (HIV) infection
  Suicide and homicide

Interventions for the General Population

Screening

Blood pressure

Height and weight

Lipid panel (men age 35-64, women age 45-64)

Papanicolaou (Pap) test (women)[1]

Fecal occult blood test[2] and/or colonoscopy (≥50 yr)

Mammogram ± clinical breast exam[3] (women 50-69 yr)

Assess for problem drinking

Rubella serology or vaccination hx[4] (women of childbearing age)

Counseling

Substance use
Tobacco cessation

Avoid alcohol/drug use while driving, swimming, boating, etc.*
Diet and exercise
Limit fat and cholesterol; maintain caloric balance; emphasize grains, fruits, vegetables

Adequate calcium intake (women)

Regular physical activity*
Injury prevention
Lap/shoulder belts

Motorcycle/bicycle/ATV helmets*

Smoke detector*

Safe storage/removal of firearms*
Sexual behavior
STD prevention: avoid high-risk behavior*; condoms/female barrier with spermicide*

Unintended pregnancy: contraception
Dental health
Regular visits to dental care provider*

Floss, brush with fluoride toothpaste daily*

Immunizations

Tetanus-diphtheria (Td) boosters

Rubella[4] (women of childbearing age)

Influenza vaccine for people over age 50

Chemoprophylaxis

Multivitamin with folic acid (women planning or capable of pregnancy)

Discuss hormone prophylaxis (peri- and postmenopausal women)

Interventions for High-Risk Populations

Population	*Potential Interventions (See detailed high-risk definitions)*
High-risk sexual behavior	RPR/VDRL (HR1); screen for gonorrhea (female) (HR2), HIV (HR3), chlamydia (female) (HR4); hepatitis B vaccine (HR5); hepatitis A vaccine (HR6)
Injection or street drug use	RPR/VDRL (HR1); HIV screen (HR3); hepatitis B vaccine (HR5); hepatitis A vaccine (HR6); PPD (HR7); advice to reduce infection risk (HR8)
Low income; TB contacts; immigrants; alcoholics	PPD (HR7)
Native Americans/Alaska Natives	Hepatitis A vaccine (HR6); PPD (HR7); pneumococcal vaccine (HR9)
Travelers to developing countries	Hepatitis B vaccine (HR5); hepatitis A vaccine (HR6)
Certain chronic medical conditions	PPD (HR7); pneumococcal vaccine (HR9); influenza vaccine (HR10)
Blood product recipients	HIV screen (HR3); hepatitis B vaccine (HR5)
Susceptible to measles, mumps, or varicella	MMR (HR11); varicella vaccine (HR12)
Institutionalized persons	Hepatitis A vaccine (HR6); PPD (HR7); pneumococcal vaccine (HR9); influenza vaccine (HR10)
Health care/lab workers	Hepatitis B vaccine (HR5); hepatitis A vaccine (HR6); PPD (HR7); influenza vaccine (HR10)
Family hx of skin cancer; fair skin, eyes, hair	Avoid excess/midday sun, use protective clothing* (HR13)
Previous pregnancy with neural tube defect	Folic acid 4.0 mg (HR14)

V

[1]Women who are or have been sexually active and who have a cervix: q ≤3 yr. [2]Annually. [3]Mammogram q1-2 yr, or mammogram q1-2 yr with annual clinical breast examination. [4]Serologic testing, documented vaccination history, and routine vaccination (preferably with MMR) are equally acceptable.
*The ability of clinician counseling to influence this behavior is unproven.

HR1 = Persons who exchange sex for money or drugs, and their sex partners; persons with other STDs (including HIV); and sexual contacts of persons with active syphilis. Clinicians should also consider local epidemiology.

HR2 = Women who exchange sex for money or drugs, or who have had repeated episodes of gonorrhea. Clinicians should also consider local epidemiology.

HR3 = Men who had sex with men after 1975; past or present injection drug use; persons who exchange sex for money or drugs, and their sex partners; injection drug–using, bisexual, or HIV-positive sex partner currently or in the past; blood transfusion during 1978-1985; persons seeking treatment for STDs. Clinicians should also consider local epidemiology.

HR4 = Sexually active women with multiple risk factors including history of STD; new or multiple sex partners; nonuse or inconsistent use of barrier contraceptives; cervical ectopy. Clinicians should also consider local epidemiology.

HR5 = Blood product recipients (including hemodialysis patients), persons with frequent occupational exposure to blood or blood products, men who have sex with men, injection drug users and their sex partners, persons with multiple recent sex partners, persons with other STDs (including HIV), travelers to countries with endemic hepatitis B.

HR6 = Persons living in, traveling to, or working in areas where the disease is endemic and where periodic outbreaks occur (e.g., countries with high or intermediate endemicity; certain Alaska Native, Pacific Island, Native American, and religious communities); men who have sex with men; injection or street drug users. Consider for institutionalized persons and workers in these institutions, military personnel, and day-care, hospital, and laboratory workers. Clinicians should also consider local epidemiology.

HR7 = HIV positive, close contacts of persons with known or suspected TB, health care workers, persons with medical risk factors associated with TB, immigrants from countries with high TB prevalence, medically underserved low-income populations (including homeless), alcoholics, injection drug users, and residents of long-term care facilities.

HR8 = Persons who continue to inject drugs.

HR9 = Immunocompetent institutionalized persons aged ≥50 yr and immunocompetent persons with certain medical conditions, including chronic cardiac or pulmonary disease, diabetes mellitus, and anatomic asplenia. Immunocompetent persons who live in high-risk environments or social settings (e.g., certain Native American and Alaska Native populations).

HR10 = Annual vaccination of residents of chronic care facilities; persons with chronic cardiopulmonary disorders, metabolic diseases (including diabetes mellitus), hemoglobinopathies, immunosuppression or renal dysfunction; and health care providers for high-risk patients.

HR11 = Persons born after 1956 who lack evidence of immunity to measles or mumps (e.g., documented receipt of live vaccine on or after the first birthday, laboratory evidence of immunity, or a history of physician-diagnosed measles or mumps).

HR12 = Healthy adults without a history of chickenpox or previous immunization. Consider serologic testing for presumed susceptible adults.

HR13 = Persons with a family or personal history of skin cancer, a large number of moles, atypical moles, poor tanning ability, or light skin, hair, and eye color.

HR14 = Women with previous pregnancy affected by neural tube who are planning pregnancy.

TABLE 5-4   Age 65 and Older

Interventions considered
 and recommended for the
 Periodic Health Examination

Leading causes of death
 Heart diseases
 Malignant neoplasms (lung, colorectal, breast)
 Cerebrovascular disease
 Chronic obstructive pulmonary disease
 Pneumonia and influenza

Interventions for the General Population

Screening

Blood pressure

Height and weight

Fecal occult blood test[1] and/or colonoscopy

Mammogram ± clinical breast exam[2] (women ≤69 yr)

Papanicolaou (Pap) test (women)[3]

Vision screening

Assess for hearing impairment

Assess for problem drinking

Counseling

Substance use
Tobacco cessation

Avoid alcohol/drug use while driving, swimming, boating, etc.*

Diet and exercise
Limit fat and cholesterol; maintain caloric balance; emphasize
 grains, fruits, vegetables

Adequate calcium intake (women)

Regular physical activity*
Injury prevention
Lap/shoulder belts

Motorcycle and bicycle helmets*

Fall prevention*

Safe storage/removal of firearms*

Smoke detector*

Set hot water heater to <120°-130°F

CPR training for household members
Dental health
Regular visits to dental care provider*

Floss, brush with fluoride toothpaste daily*
Sexual behavior
STD prevention: avoid high-risk sexual behavior*; use
condoms

Immunizations

Pneumococcal vaccine

Influenza[1]

Tetanus-diphtheria (Td) boosters

Chemoprophylaxis

Discuss hormone prophylaxis (peri- and postmenopausal
 women)

Interventions for High-Risk Populations

Population	*Potential Interventions (See detailed high-risk definitions)*
Institutionalized persons	PPD (HR1); hepatitis A vaccine (HR2); amantadine/rimantadine (HR4)
Chronic medical conditions; TB contacts; low income; immigrants; alcoholics	PPD (HR1)
Persons ≥75 yr, or ≥70 yr with risk factors for falls	Fall prevention intervention (HR5)
Cardiovascular disease risk factors	Consider cholesterol screening (HR6)
Family hx of skin cancer; nevi; fair skin, eyes, hair	Avoid excess/midday sun, use protective clothing* (HR7)
Native Americans/Alaska Natives	PPD (HR1); hepatitis A vaccine (HR2)
Travelers to developing countries	Hepatitis A vaccine (HR2); hepatitis B vaccine (HR8)
Blood product recipients	HIV screen (HR3); hepatitis B vaccine (HR8)
High-risk sexual behavior	Hepatitis A vaccine (HR2); HIV screen (HR3); hepatitis B vaccine (HR8); RPR/VDRL (HR9)
Injection or street drug use	PPD (HR1); hepatitis A vaccine (HR2); HIV screen (HR3); hepatitis B vaccine (HR8); RPR/VDRL (HR9); advice to reduce infection risk (HR10)
Health care/lab workers	PPD (HR1); hepatitis A vaccine (HR2); amantadine/rimantadine (HR4); hepatitis B vaccine (HR8)
Persons susceptible to varicella	Varicella vaccine (HR11)

[1]Annually. [2]Mammogram q1-2 yr, or mammogram q1-2 yr with annual clinical breast exam. [3]All women who are or have been sexually active and who have a cervix. Consider discontinuation of testing after age 65 yr if previous regular screening with consistently normal results.
*The ability of clinician counseling to influence this behavior is unproven.

V

HR1 = HIV positive, close contacts of persons with known or suspected TB, health care workers, persons with medical risk factors associated with TB, immigrants from countries with high TB prevalence, medically underserved low-income populations (including homeless), alcoholics, injection drug users, and residents of long-term care facilities.

HR2 = Persons living in, traveling to, or working in areas where the disease is endemic and where periodic outbreaks occur (e.g., countries with high or intermediate endemicity; certain Alaska Native, Pacific Island, Native American, and religious communities); men who have sex with men; injection or street drug users. Consider for institutionalized persons and workers in these institutions, and day-care, hospital, and laboratory workers. Clinicians should also consider local epidemiology.

HR3 = Men who had sex with men after 1975; past or present injection drug use; persons who exchange sex for money or drugs, and their sex partners; injection drug–using, bisexual, or HIV-positive sex partner currently or in the past; blood transfusion during 1978-1985; persons seeking treatment for STDs. Clinicians should also consider local epidemiology.

HR4 = Consider for persons who have not received influenza vaccine or are vaccinated late; when the vaccine may be ineffective due to major antigenic changes in the virus; for unvaccinated persons who provide home care for high-risk persons; to supplement protection provided by vaccine in persons who are expected to have a poor antibody response; and for high-risk persons in whom the vaccine is contraindicated.

HR5 = Persons aged 75 years and older; or aged 70-74 with one or more additional risk factors including use of certain psychoactive and cardiac medications (e.g., benzodiazepines, antihypertensives); use of ≥4 prescription medications; impaired cognition, strength, balance, or gait. Intensive individualized home-based multifactorial fall prevention intervention is recommended in settings where adequate resources are available to deliver such services.

HR6 = Although evidence is insufficient to recommend routine screening in elderly persons, clinicians should consider cholesterol screening on a case-by-case basis for persons aged 65-75 with additional risk factors (e.g., smoking, diabetes, or hypertension).

HR7 = Persons with a family or personal history of skin cancer, a large number of moles, atypical moles, poor tanning ability, or light skin, hair, and eye color .

HR8 = Blood product recipients (including hemodialysis patients), persons with frequent occupational exposure to blood or blood products, men who have sex with men, injection drug users and their sex partners, persons with multiple recent sex partners, persons with other STDs (including HIV), travelers to countries with endemic hepatitis B.

HR9 = Persons who exchange sex for money or drugs and their sex partners; persons with other STDs (including HIV); and sexual contacts of persons with active syphilis. Clinicians should also consider local epidemiology.

HR10 = Persons who continue to inject drugs.

HR11 = Healthy adults without a history of chickenpox or previous immunization. Consider serologic testing for presumed susceptible adults.

TABLE 5-5   Pregnant Women*

Interventions considered and recommended for the Periodic Health Examination

Interventions for the General Population

Screening

First visit

Blood pressure

Hemoglobin/hematocrit

Hepatitis B surface antigen (HBsAg)

RPR/VDRL

Chlamydia screen (<25 yr)

Rubella serology or vaccination history

D(Rh) typing, antibody screen

Offer CVS (<13 wk)[1] or amniocentesis (15-18 wk)[1] (age ≥35 yr)

Offer hemoglobinopathy screening

Assess for problem or risk drinking

Offer HIV screening[2]

Follow-up visits

Blood pressure

Urine culture (12-16 wk)

Offer amniocentesis (15-18 wk)[1] (age ≥35 yr)

Offer multiple marker testing[1] (15-18 wk)

Offer serum α-fetoprotein[1] (16-18 wk)

Counseling

Tobacco cessation; effects of passive smoking

Alcohol/other drug use

Nutrition, including adequate calcium intake

Encourage breast-feeding

Lap/shoulder belts

Infant safety car seats

STD prevention: avoid high-risk sexual behavior†; use condoms†

Chemoprophylaxis

Multivitamin with folic acid[3]

Interventions for High-Risk Populations

Population	*Potential Interventions (See detailed high-risk definitions)*
High-risk sexual behavior	Screen for chlamydia (1st visit) (HR1), gonorrhea (1st visit) (HR2), HIV (1st visit) (HR3); HBsAg (3rd trimester) (HR4); RPR/VDRL (3rd trimester) (HR5)
Blood transfusion 1978-1985	HIV screen (1st visit) (HR3)
Injection drug use	HIV screen (HR3); HBsAg (3rd trimester) (HR4); advice to reduce infection risk (HR6)
Unsensitized D-negative women	D(Rh) antibody testing (24-28 wk) (HR7)
Risk factors for Down syndrome	Offer CVS[1] (1st trimester), amniocentesis[1] (15-18 wk) (HR8)
Prior pregnancy with neural tube defect	Offer amniocentesis[1] (15-18 wk), folic acid 4.0 mg[3] (HR9)

[1]Women with access to counseling and follow-up services, reliable standardized laboratories, skilled high-resolution ultrasound, and, for those receiving serum marker testing, amniocentesis capabilities. [2]Universal screening is recommended for areas (states, counties, or cities) with an increased prevalence of HIV infection among pregnant women. In low-prevalence areas, the choice between universal and tangled screening may depend on other considerations. [3]Beginning at least 1 mo before conception and continuing through the first trimester.
*See Tables 5-2 and 5-3 for other preventive services recommended for women of this age group.
†The ability of clinician counseling to influence this behavior is unproven.

HR1 = Women with history of STD or new or multiple sex partners. Clinicians should also consider local epidemiology. Chlamydia screen should be repeated in 3rd trimester if at continued risk.

HR2 = Women under age 25 with two or more sex partners in the last year, or whose sex partner has multiple sexual contacts; women who exchange sex for money or drugs; and women with a history of repeated episodes of gonorrhea. Clinicians should also consider local epidemiology. Gonorrhea screen should be repeated in the third trimester if at continued risk.

HR3 = In areas where universal screening is not performed due to low prevalence of HIV infection, pregnant women with the following individual risk factors should be screened: past or present injection drug use; women who exchange sex for money or drugs; injection drug–using, bisexual, or HIV-positive sex partner currently or in the past; blood transfusion during 1978-1985; persons seeking treatment for STDs.

HR4 = Women who are initially HBsAg negative who are at high risk due to injection drug use, suspected exposure to hepatitis B during pregnancy, multiple sex partners.

HR5 = Women who exchange sex for money or drugs, women with other STDs (including HIV), and sexual contacts of persons with active syphilis. Clinicians should also consider local epidemiology.

HR6 = Women who continue to inject drugs .

HR7 = Unsensitized D-negative women.

HR8 = Prior pregnancy affected by Down syndrome, advanced maternal age (≥35 yr), known carriage of chromosome rearrangement.

HR9 = Women with previous pregnancy affected by neural tube defect.

V

PART B
IMMUNIZATIONS AND CHEMOPROPHYLAXIS
Childhood Immunizations

TABLE 5-6 Recommended Childhood Immunization Schedule, United States, 2002

Vaccine ▼ \ Age ▶	Birth	1 mo	2 mos	4 mos	6 mos	12 mos	15 mos	18 mos	24 mos	4-6 yrs	11-12 yrs	13-18 yrs
				range of recommended ages			catch-up vaccination			preadolescent assessment		
Hepatitis B[1]	Hep B #1	only if mother HBsAg (-)								Hep B series		
			Hep B #2			Hep B #3						
Diphtheria, Tetanus, Pertussis[2]			DTaP	DTaP	DTaP		DTaP			DTaP	Td	
Haemophilus influenzae Type b[3]			Hib	Hib	Hib	Hib						
Inactivated Polio[4]			IPV	IPV		IPV				IPV		
Measles, Mumps, Rubella[5]						MMR #1				MMR #2	MMR #2	
Varicella[6]						Varicella				Varicella		
Pneumococcal[7]			PCV	PCV	PCV	PCV				PCV	PPV	
Vaccines below this line are for selected populations												
Hepatitis A[8]										Hepatitis A series		
Influenza[9]					Influenza (yearly)							

This schedule indicates the recommended ages for routine administration of currently licensed childhood vaccines, as of December 1, 2001, for children through age 18 years. Any dose not given at the recommended age should be given at any subsequent visit when indicated and feasible. Indicates age groups that warrant special effort to administer those vaccines not previously given. Additional vaccines may be licensed and recommended during the year. Licensed combination vaccines may be used whenever any components of the combination are indicated and the vaccine's other components are not contraindicated. Providers should consult the manufacturers' package inserts for detailed recommendations.

1. Hepatitis B vaccine (Hep B). All infants should receive the first dose of hepatitis B vaccine soon after birth and before hospital discharge; the first dose may also be given by age 2 months if the infant's mother is HBsAg-negative. Only monovalent hepatitis B vaccine can be used for the birth dose. Monovalent or combination vaccine containing Hep B may be used to complete the series; four doses of vaccine may be administered if combination vaccine is used. The second dose should be given at least 4 weeks after the first dose, except for Hib-containing vaccine which cannot be administered before age 6 weeks. The third dose should be given at least 16 weeks after the first dose and at least 8 weeks after the second dose. The last dose in the vaccination series (third or fourth dose) should not be administered before age 6 months.

Infants born to HBsAg-positive mothers should receive hepatitis B vaccine and 0.5 ml hepatitis B immune globulin (HBIG) within 12 hours of birth at separate sites. The second dose is recommended at age 1-2 months and the vaccination series should be completed (third or fourth dose) at age 6 months.

Infants born to mothers whose HBsAg status is unknown should receive the first dose of the hepatitis B vaccine series within 12 hours of birth. Maternal blood should be drawn at the time of delivery to determine the mother's HBsAg status; if the HBsAg test is positive, the infant should receive HBIG as soon as possible (no later than age 1 week).

2. Diphtheria and tetanus toxoids and acellular pertussis vaccine (DTaP). The fourth dose of DTaP may be administered as early as age 12 months, provided 6 months have elapsed since the third dose and the child is unlikely to return at age 15-18 months. **Tetanus and diphtheria toxoids (Td)** is recommended at age 11-12 years if at least 5 years have elapsed since the last dose of tetanus and diphtheria toxoid-containing vaccine. Subsequent routine Td boosters are recommended every 10 years.

3. *Haemophilus influenzae* type b (Hib) conjugate vaccine. Three Hib conjugate vaccines are licensed for infant use. If PRP-OMP (PedvaxHIB or ComVax [Merck] is administered at ages 2 and 4 months, a dose at age 6 months is not required. DTaP/Hib combination products should not be used for primary immunization in infants at ages 2, 4, or 6 months, but can be used as boosters following any Hib vaccine.

4. Inactivated polio vaccine (IPV). An All-IPV schedule is recommended for routine childhood polio vaccination in the United States. All children should receive four doses of IPV at ages 2 months, 4 months, 6-18 months, and 4-6 years.

5. Measles, mumps, and rubella vaccine (MMR). The second dose of MMR is recommended routinely at age 4-6 years but may be administered during any visit, provided at least 4 weeks have elapsed since the first dose and that both doses are administered beginning at or after age 12 months. Those who have not previously received the second dose should complete the schedule by the 11-12-year-old visit.

6. Varicella vaccine. Varicella vaccine is recommended at any visit at or after age 12 months for susceptible children, i.e., those who lack a reliable history of chickenpox. Susceptible persons aged ≥ 13 years should receive two doses, given at least 4 weeks apart.

7. Pneumococcal vaccine. The heptavalent **pneumococcal conjugate vaccine (PCV)** is recommended for all children age 2-23 months. It is also recommended for certain children age 24-59 months. **Pneumococcal polysaccharide vaccine (PPV)** is recommended in addition to PCV for certain high-risk groups. See MMWR 2000;49(RR-9):1-35.

8. Hepatitis A vaccine. Hepatitis A vaccine is recommended for use in selected states and regions, and for certain high-risk groups; consult your local public health authority. See MMWR 1999;48(RR-12):1-37.

9. Influenza vaccine. Influenza vaccine is recommended annually for children age ≥ 6 months with certain risk factors (including, but not limited to, asthma, cardiac disease, sickle cell disease, HIV, diabetes; see MMWR 2001;50(RR-4):1-44, and can be administered to all others wishing to obtain immunity. Children aged ≤ 12 years should receive vaccine in a dosage appropriate for their age (0.25 ml if age 6-35 months or 0.5 ml if aged ≥ 3 years). Children aged ≤ 8 years who are receiving influenza vaccine for the first time should receive two doses separated by at least 4 weeks.

For additional information about vaccines, vaccine supply, and contraindications for immunization, please visit the National Immunization Program Web site at www.cdc.gov/nip or call the National Immunization Hotline at 800-232-2522 (English) or 800-232-0233 (Spanish). Approved by the Advisory Committee on Immunization Practices (www.cdc.gov/nip/acip), the American Academy of Pediatrics (www.aap.org), and the American Academy of Family Physicians (www.aafp.org).

Minimal Age for Initial Childhood Vaccinations and Minimal Interval Between Vaccine Doses by Type of Vaccine*

VACCINE TYPE	MINIMAL AGE FOR DOSE 1	MINIMAL INTERVAL BETWEEN DOSES 1 AND 2	MINIMAL INTERVAL BETWEEN DOSES 2 AND 3	MINIMAL INTERVAL BETWEEN DOSES 3 AND 4
Hepatitis B	Birth	1 mo	2 mo	†
DTaP (DT)‡	6 wk	4 wk	4 wk	6 mo
Combined DTwP–Hib§	6 wk	1 mo	1 mo	6 mo
Hib (primary series)				
HbOC	6 wk	1 mo	1 mo	§
PRP-T	6 wk	1 mo	1 mo	§
PRP-OMP	6 wk	1 mo	§	
Inactivated poliovirus	6 wk	4 wk	4 wk‖	¶
Pneumococcal conjugate	6 wk	1 mo	1 mo	§
MMR	12 mo**	1 mo		
Varicella	12 mo	4 wk		

Modified from *Epidemiology and prevention of vaccine-preventable diseases,* ed 6, Atlanta, 2000, Centers for Disease Control and Prevention.

DTaP (DT), Diphtheria and tetanus toxoids and acellular pertussis vaccine (diphtheria and tetanus toxoids vaccine); *DTwP–Hib,* diphtheria and tetanus toxoids and whole-cell pertussis vaccine–*Haemophilus influenzae* type b conjugate vaccine; *HbOC,* oligosaccharides conjugated to diphtheria CRM_{197} toxin protein; *PRP-T,* polyribosylribitol phosphate polysaccharide conjugated to tetanus toxoid; *PRP-OMP,* polyribosylribitol phosphate polysaccharide conjugated to a meningococcal outer membrane protein; *MMR,* measles-mumps-rubella.

*The minimal acceptable ages and intervals may not correspond with the optimal recommended ages and intervals for vaccination. For current recommended routine schedules, see the annual Recommended Childhood Immunization Schedule on the facing page.

†This final dose of hepatitis B vaccine is recommended at least 4 months after the first dose and no earlier than 6 months of age.

‡The total number of doses of diphtheria and tetanus toxoids should not exceed six each before the seventh birthday.

§The booster doses of Hib and pneumococcal vaccines that are recommended following the primary vaccination series should be administered no earlier than 12 months of age and at least 2 months after the previous dose.

‖For unvaccinated adults at increased risk of exposure to poliovirus with less than 3 months but more than 2 months available before protection is needed, 3 doses of IPV should be administered at least 1 month apart.

¶If the third dose is given after the third birthday, the fourth (booster) dose is not needed.

**Although the age for measles vaccination may be as young as 6 months in outbreak areas where cases are occurring in children younger than 1 year, children initially vaccinated before the first birthday should be revaccinated at 12 to 15 months of age and an additional dose of vaccine should be administered at the time of school entry or according to local policy. Doses of MMR or other measles-containing vaccines should be separated by at least 1 month.

TABLE 5-7   Accelerated Schedule of Routine Childhood Immunizations if Necessary for Travel

VACCINE	ROUTINE SCHEDULE	ACCELERATED SCHEDULE
Diphtheria, tetanus, pertussis	DTaP: 2, 4, 6, 15-18 mo of age	DTaP: 6 wk of age, with 4 wk between 1st, 2nd, and 3rd doses, and 6 mo between 3rd and 4th doses
	DTaP: 4-6 yr of age (booster) dT every 10 yr	DTaP: 4 yr of age dT every 5 yr if at high risk
Poliomyelitis	IPV: at 2 and 4 mo, 6-18 mo and 4-6 yr	IPV: 6 wk of age, with 1 mo between 1st and 2nd doses and 6 mo between 2nd and 3rd doses
	No additional boosters unless traveling to an endemic area	A single IPV lifetime booster for adolescents and adults who have completed primary immunization
Measles, mumps. rubella	MMR: 12-15 mo of age, with second dose at age 4-6 yr	Two doses at ≥12 mo of age, 4 wk apart
	Not routinely recommended for children <12 mo of age	May give first measles as early as age 6 mo, with additional two doses ≥12 mo of age
Haemophilus influenzae type b	2, 4, 6 (if HbOC or PRP-T), and 12-15 mo	HbOC and PRP-T: 6 wk of age, with 1 mo between the 1st and 2nd and the 2nd and 3rd doses; booster at ≥12 mo of age (≥2 mo from the 3rd dose)
		PRO-OMP: 6 wk of age, with 1 mo between the 1st and 2nd doses; booster at ≥12 mo of age (≥2 mo from the 3rd dose)
Hepatitis B	Birth, 1-2 mo, 6 mo	0, 1, and 4 mo of age
Varicella	12-18 mo of age	12 mo of age (two doses 1 mo apart for persons age ≥13 yr)
Rotavirus	2, 4, 6 mo of age	6 wk of age, with 2nd and 3rd doses each separated by 3 wk

From Behrman RE: *Nelson textbook of pediatrics,* ed 16, Philadelphia, 2000, WB Saunders.

TABLE 5-8   Immunizations for Immunocompromised Infants and Children

VACCINE	ROUTINE	HIV/AIDS	SEVERE IMMUNO-SUPPRESSION*	ASPLENIA	RENAL FAILURE	DIABETES
Routine Infant Immunizations						
DTaP/DTP (DT/T/Td)	Recommended	Recommended	Recommended	Recommended	Recommended	Recommended
IPV	Recommended	Recommended	Recommended	Use as indicated	Use as indicated	Use as indicated
MMR/MR/M/R	Recommended	Recommended/considered	Contraindicated	Recommended	Recommended	Recommended
Hib	Recommended	Recommended	Recommended	Recommended	Recommended	Recommended
Hepatitis B	Recommended	Recommended	Recommended	Recommended	Recommended	Recommended
Varicella	Recommended	Contraindicated/considered§	Contraindicated	Contraindicated	Use if indicated	Use if indicated
Rotavirus	Recommended	Contraindicated	Contraindicated	Contraindicated	Use if indicated	Use if indicated
Other Childhood Immunizations						
Pneumococcus†	Use if indicated	Recommended	Recommended	Recommended	Recommended	Recommended
Influenza‡	Use if indicated	Recommended	Recommended	Recommended	Recommended	Recommended

Modified from Centers for Disease Control and Prevention: Recommendations of the Advisory Committee on Immunization Practices (ACIP): Use of vaccines and immune globulins in persons with altered immunity, *MMWR* 42 (RR-4):15, 1993.
*Severe immunosuppression can result from congenital immunodeficiency, HIV infection, leukemia, lymphoma, aplastic anemia, generalized malignancy, alkylating agents, antimetabolites, radiation, or large amounts of corticosteroids.
†Recommended for persons ≥2 yr of age.
‡Not recommended for infants <6 mo of age.
§Varicella vaccine should be considered for asymptomatic or mildly symptomatic HIV-infected children in CDC class N1 or A1 with age-specific CD4+ T-lymphocyte percentages of ≥25%. Eligible children should receive two doses of varicella vaccine with a 3-month interval between doses.

TABLE 5-9 Recommended Immunization Schedule for HIV-Infected Children*

AGE ▶ VACCINE ▼	BIRTH	1 MO	2 MOS	4 MOS	6 MOS	12 MOS	15 MOS	18 MOS	24 MOS	4-6 YRS	11-12 YRS	14-16 YRS
☛ Recommendations for these vaccines are the same as those for immunocompetent children ☛												
Hepatitis B†	Hep B-1										Hep B‡	
		Hep B-2		Hep B-3								
Diphtheria, Tetanus, Pertussis¶		DTaP or DTP	DTaP or DTP	DTaP or DTP		DTaP or DTP			DTaP or DTP		
											Td	
*Haemophilus** influenzae* type b			Hib	Hib	Hib	Hib						
☛ Recommendations for these vaccines differ from those for immunocompetent children ☛												
Polio††			IPV	IPV		IPV				IPV		
Measles, Mumps, Rubella§§						MMR	MMR					
Influenza¶¶					Influenza (a dose is required every year)							
*Streptococcus pneumoniae***									Pneumo-coccal			
Varicella					CONTRAINDICATED in all HIV-infected persons							

Modified from *MMWR* 46(RR-12), 1997.

Note: Modified from the immunization schedule for immunocompetent children. This schedule also applies to children born to HIV-infected mothers whose HIV infection status has not been determined. Once a child is known not to be HIV-infected, the schedule for immunocompetent children applies. This schedule indicates the recommended age for routine administration of currently licensed childhood vaccines. Some combination vaccines are available and may be used whenever administration of all components of the vaccine is indicated. Providers should consult the manufacturers' package inserts for detailed recommendations.

*Vaccines are listed under the routinely recommended ages. Bars indicate range of acceptable ages for vaccination. Shaded bars indicate catch-up vaccination: at 11-12 yrs of age, hepatitis B vaccine should be administered to children not previously vaccinated.

†*Infants born to HBsAg-negative mothers* should receive 2.5 µg of Merck vaccine (Recombivax HB) or 10 µg of SmithKline Beecham (SB) vaccine (Engerix-B). The 2nd dose should be administered >1 mo after the 1st dose.

Infants born to HBsAg-positive mothers should receive 0.5 ml of hepatitis B immune globulin (HBIG) within 12 hr of birth and either 5 µg of Merck vaccine (Recombivax HB) or 10 µg of SB vaccine (Engerix-B) at a separate site. The 2nd dose is recommended at 1-2 mo of age and the 3rd dose at 6 mo of age.

Infants born to mothers whose HBsAg status is unknown should receive either 5 µg of Merck vaccine (Recombivax HB) or 10 µg of SB vaccine (Engerix-B) within 12 hr of birth. The 2nd dose of vaccine is recommended at 1 mo of age and the 3rd dose at 6 mo of age. Blood should be drawn at the time of delivery to determine the mother's HBsAg status; if it is positive, the infant should receive HBIG as soon as possible (no later than 1 wk of age). The dosage and timing of subsequent vaccine doses should be based upon the mother's HBsAg status.

§Children and adolescents who have not been vaccinated against hepatitis B in infancy may begin the series during any childhood visit. Those who have not previously received three doses of hepatitis B vaccine should initiate or complete the series during the 11- to 12-year-old visit. The 2nd dose should be administered at least 1 mo after the 1st dose, and the 3rd dose should be administered at least 4 mo after the 1st dose and at least 2 mo after the 2nd dose.

¶DTaP (diphtheria and tetanus toxoids and acellular pertussis vaccine) is the preferred vaccine for all doses in the vaccination series, including completion of the series in children who have received > one dose of whole-cell DTP vaccine. Whole-cell DTP is an acceptable alternative to DTaP. The 4th dose of DTaP may be administered as early as 12 mo of age, provided 6 mo have elapsed since the 3rd dose, and if the child is considered unlikely to return at 15-18 mo of age. Td (tetanus and diphtheria toxoids, adsorbed, for adult use) is recommended at 11-12 yr of age if at least 5 yr have elapsed since the last dose of DTP, DTaP, or DT. Subsequent routine Td boosters are recommended every 10 yr.

**Three *H. influenzae* type b (Hib) conjugate vaccines are licensed for infant use. If PRP-OMP (PedvaxHIB [Merck]) is administered at 2 and 4 mo of age, a dose at 6 mo is not required. After the primary series has been completed, any Hib conjugate vaccine may be used as a booster.

††Inactivated poliovirus vaccine (IPV) is the only polio vaccine recommended for HIV-infected persons and their household contacts. Although the 3rd dose of IPV is generally administered at 12-18 mo, the 3rd dose of IPV has been approved to be administered as early as 6 mo of age. Oral poliovirus vaccine (OPV) should NOT be administered to HIV-infected persons or their household contacts.

§§MMR should not be administered to severely immunocompromised children. HIV-infected children without severe immunosuppression should routinely receive their first dose of MMR as soon as possible upon reaching the 1st birthday. Consideration should be given to administering the second dose of MMR vaccine as soon as 1 mo (i.e., minimum 28 days) after the 1st dose, rather than waiting until school entry.

¶¶Influenza virus vaccine should be administered to all HIV-infected children >6 mo of age each year. Children aged 6 mo-8 yr who are receiving influenza vaccine for the first time should receive two doses of split virus vaccine separated by at least 1 mo. In subsequent years, a single dose of vaccine (split virus for persons ≤12 yr of age, whole or split virus for persons >12 yr of age) should be administered each year. The dose of vaccine for children aged 6-35 mo is 0.25 ml; the dose for children aged ≥3 yr is 0.5 ml.

***Pneumococcal vaccine should be administered to HIV-infected children at 24 mo of age. Revaccination should generally be offered to HIV-infected children vaccinated 3-5 yr (children aged ≤10 yr) or >5 yr (children aged >10 yr) earlier.

V

TABLE 5-10 Contraindications to and Precautions in Routine Childhood Vaccinations

TRUE CONTRAINDICATIONS AND PRECAUTIONS	NOT CONTRAINDICATIONS (VACCINES MAY BE ADMINISTERED)
GENERAL FOR ALL ROUTINE VACCINES (DTAP/DTP, OPV, IPV, MMR, HIB, HEPATITIS B, VARICELLA, ROTAVIRUS)	

Contraindications

Anaphylactic reaction to a vaccine contraindicates further doses of that vaccine

Anaphylactic reaction to a vaccine constituent contraindicates the use of vaccines containing that substance

Moderate or severe illnesses with or without a fever

Not Contraindications

Mild to moderate local reaction (soreness, redness, swelling), after a dose of an injectable antigen

Low-grade or moderate fever after a prior vaccine dose

Mild acute illness with or without low-grade fever

Current antimicrobial therapy

Convalescent phase of illness

Prematurity (same dose and indications as for normal full-term infants)

Recent exposure to an infectious disease

History of penicillin or other nonspecific allergies or fact that relatives have such allergies

Pregnancy of mother or household contact

Unvaccinated household contact

DTaP/DTP

Contraindications

Encephalopathy within 7 days of administration of previous dose of DTaP/DTP

Precautions*

Temperature of ≥40.5° C (105° F) within 48 hr after vaccination with a prior dose of DTaP/DTP and not attributable to another identifiable cause

Collapse or shocklike state (hypotonic-hyporesponsive episode) within 48 hr of receiving a prior dose of DTaP/DTP

Convulsions within 3 days of receiving a prior dose of DTaP/DTP†

Persistent, inconsolable crying lasting ≥3 hr, within 48 hr of receiving a prior dose of DTaP/DTP

Guillain-Barré syndrome within 6 wk after a dose‡

Not Contraindications

Temperature of <40.5° C (105° F) after a previous dose of DTaP/DTP

Family history of convulsions†

Family history of sudden infant death syndrome

Family history of an adverse event after DTaP/DTP administration

---

OPV

Contraindications

Infection with HIV or a household contact with HIV infection

Known immunodeficiency (hematologic and solid tumors; congenital immunodeficiency; long-term immunosuppressive therapy)

Immunodeficient household contact

Precaution*

Pregnancy

Not Contraindications

Breast-feeding

Current antimicrobial therapy

Mild diarrhea

IPV

Contraindications

Anaphylactic reaction to neomycin, streptomycin, or polymyxin B

Precaution*

Pregnancy

MMR

Contraindications

Anaphylactic reaction to neomycin or gelatin

Pregnancy

Known immunodeficiency (hematologic and solid tumors; congenital immunodeficiency; long-term immunosuppressive therapy; HIV infection with evidence of severe immunosuppression)

Not Contraindications

Tuberculosis or positive PPD test result

Simultaneous tuberculin skin testing§

Breast-feeding

Pregnancy of mother or household contact of vaccine recipient

Immunodeficient family member or household contact

HIV infection without evidence of severe immunosuppression

Allergic reaction to eggs‖

Nonanaphylactic reactions to neomycin

Recent (within 3-11 mo, depending on product and dose)
  administration of a blood product or immune globulin
  preparation
Thrombocytopenia*
History of thrombocytopenic purpura¶

HIB

Contraindications

None

Precautions

None

HEPATITIS B

Contraindications

Anaphylactic reaction to common baker's yeast

Not contraindications

Pregnancy

Precautions

None

VARICELLA

Contraindications

Anaphylactic reaction to neomycin or gelatin
Pregnancy
HIV infection with evidence of severe immunosuppression
Known immunodeficiency (hematologic and solid tumors;
  congenital immunodeficiency; long-term immuno-
  suppressive therapy)

Not Contraindications

Breast-feeding
Immunodeficiency in a household contact
HIV infection in a household contact
Pregnancy of mother or household contact of vaccine recipient

Precautions*

Recent (within 3-11 mo, depending on product and dose)
  administration of a blood product or immune globulin
  preparation
Family history of immunodeficiency**

ROTAVIRUS

Contraindications

Hypersensitivity to aminoglycosides, amphotericin B, or
  monosodium glutamate
Moderate or severe febrile illness
Known immunodeficiency (hematologic and solid tumors;
  congenital immunodeficiency; long-term immunosuppressive therapy)
Children of HIV-infected mothers, until tests for HIV infection
  in the infant are negative at ≥2 mo of age by PCR or culture

Not Contraindications

Breast-feeding
Immunodeficiency in a household contact
HIV infection in a household contact

Precautions*

Acute vomiting or diarrhea

This information is based on the recommendations of the Advisory Committee on Immunization Practices (ACIP) and of the Committee on Infectious Diseases of the American Academy of Pediatrics (AAP). Some recommendations may vary from those in the manufacturer's product label. For more detailed information, health care providers should consult the published recommendations of the ACIP, AAP, the American Academy of Family Physicians (AAFP), and the manufacturer's product label. These guidelines have been adapted and updated from Centers for Disease Control and Prevention: Update: vaccine side effects, adverse reactions, contraindications, and precautions. Recommendations of the Advisory Committee on Immunization Practices (ACIP), MMWR 45(RR-12):1, 1996.

DTaP, Diphtheria and tetanus toxoids plus acellular pertussis vaccine; DTP, diphtheria, tetanus, and pertussis vaccine; PPd, purified protein derivative; PCR, polymerase chain reaction; MMR, measles, mumps, and rubella vaccine; OPV, oral poliovirus vaccine; IPV, inactivated poliovirus vaccine; VZIG, varicella-zoster immune globulin.

*The events or conditions listed as precautions, although not contraindications, should be carefully reviewed. The benefits and risks of administering a specific vaccine to an individual under the circumstances should be considered. If the risks are believed to outweigh the benefits, the vaccine should be withheld; if the benefits are believed to outweigh the risks (e.g., during an outbreak or foreign travel), the vaccine should be administered. Whether and when to administer DTaP/DTP to children with proven or suspected underlying neurologic disorders should be decided individually. Avoiding administration of certain vaccines to pregnant women is prudent on theoretic grounds. If immediate protection against poliomyelitis is needed, either OPV or IPV is recommended.

†Acetaminophen administered before DTaP or DTP vaccination and thereafter every 4 hr for 24 hr should be considered for children with a personal or family history of convulsions in siblings or parents.

‡The decision to give additional doses of DTaP or DTP should be based on consideration of the benefit of further vaccination vs the risk of recurrence of Guillain-Barré syndrome. For example, completion of the primary vaccination series in children is justified.

§Measles vaccination may temporarily suppress tuberculin skin test reactivity. MMR vaccine may be administered after or on the same day as Mantoux tuberculin skin testing. If MMR has been given recently, the tuberculin test should be postponed until 4-6 wk after administration of MMR.

‖Recent data suggest that most anaphylactic reactions to measles- and mumps-containing vaccines are not associated with hypersensitivity to egg antigens but to other components of the vaccines, such as gelatin. Because the risk of anaphylactic reactions after administration of measles- or mumps-containing vaccines by persons who are allergic to eggs is extremely low, and skin testing with vaccine is not predictive of allergic reactions to these vaccines, skin testing and desensitization are no longer required before administration of MMR vaccine to persons who are allergic to eggs.

¶The decision to vaccinate should be based on consideration of the benefits of immunity to measles, mumps, and rubella vs the risk of recurrence or exacerbation of thrombocytopenia after vaccination, or from natural infections of measles or rubella. In most instances, the benefits of immunity are much greater than the potential risks and justify giving MMR, particularly in view of the even greater risk of thrombocytopenia after measles or rubella disease. However, if a prior episode of thrombocytopenia occurred in close temporal proximity to vaccination, avoiding a subsequent dose may be prudent.

**Varicella vaccine should not be administered to a member of a household with a family history of immunodeficiency until the immune status of the recipient and other children in the family is documented.

TABLE 5-11 Vaccines for Children Who Travel

VACCINE	DESCRIPTION	DOSING	COMMENTS/ CONTRAINDICATIONS	LENGTH OF TRAVEL		
				BRIEF (<2 WK)	INTERMEDIATE (2 WK TO 3 MO)	LONG TERM RESIDENTIAL (>3 MO)
Routine						
Polio*	OPV: live attenu- ated, oral IPV: inactivated, in- jection	IPV at 2, 4 mo; OPV at 12-18 mo, 4-6 yr; may accelerate to q 4-8 wk × 3 doses	IPV at 2 and 4 mo de- creases risk of polio in undiagnosed immuno- compromised infants; AAP recommendation may change to IPV only	+	+	+
Diphtheria-tetanus- pertussis*	DPT: D, T toxoid + whole cell P DtaP: DT toxoid + acellular P Td: booster	DtaP recommended at 2, 4, 6, 15-18 mo and 4-6 yr; Td booster at age 12, then q10yr	May accelerate to dose every 4 wk × 3 doses if necessary; decreased in- cidence of vaccine- related reactions with DTaP	+	+	+
Haemophilus B*	Hib polysaccha- ride: protein conjugate	0.5 ml IM at 2, 4, 6, 12-15 mo	Typically given as combi- nation with DTaP	+	+	+
Hepatitis B	Recombivax HB: inactivated viral antigen Engerix-B: same	3 doses: 0, 1, 6 mo <11 yr: 0.25 ml IM >11 yr: 0.5 ml IM 3 doses 0, 1, 6 mo <11 yr: 0.5 ml IM >11 yr: 1.0 ml IM	Some protection after just 1 or 2 doses; may accel- erate Engerix-B to 0, 1, 2, 12 mo	+	+	+
Measles-mumps- rubella†	Live attenuated viruses	0.25 ml IM at 12-15 mo, then booster at 4-6 or 11-12 yr	May accelerate to 6-12 mo, repeat 1 mo later, then per usual schedule; give at least 2-3 wk before IgG	+	+	+
Varicella	Live attenuated virus	12 mo-12 yr: 0.5 ml SC as single dose >12 yr: 2 doses 4-8 wk apart	Give at lest 2-3 wk before IgG; may be given with MMR using different sites; avoid if immuno- compromised	+	+	+
Routine for Travel						
Hepatitis A	Havrix: inactive virus (720ELU) Vaqta (24U)	>2 yr: 2 × 0.5 ml doses 6-12 mo apart	Preferred for hepatitis A protection if over age 2 yr Protects in 4 wk after dose 1	+	+	+
Immune globulin (IgG)	Antibodies	<2 yr: 0.02 ml/kg for <3 mo of travel; 0.06 ml/kg q5mo and 3 days before travel	Hepatitis A protection for those under age 2 yr; beware of timing with live virus vaccines			

Consult Centers for Disease Control and Prevention (CDC) for current and specific vaccine recommendations for destination country. From Auerbach PS: *Wilderness medicine*, ed 4, St Louis, 2001, Mosby.
+, Recommended; ±, consider; *AAP*, American Academy of Pediatrics; *DTaP*, diphtheria and tetanus toxoids plus acellular pertussis vaccine; *IM*, intramus- cularly; *q*, every; *SC*, subcutaneously.

TABLE 5-11   Vaccines for Children Who Travel—cont'd

VACCINE	DESCRIPTION	DOSING	COMMENTS/ CONTRAINDICATIONS	BRIEF (<2 WK)	INTERMEDIATE (2 WK TO 3 MO)	LONG TERM RESIDENTIAL (>3 MO)
Required or Geographically Indicated						
Yellow fever	Live virus	>9 mo: 0.5 ml SC at least 10 days before departure; booster q10yr	Required for parts of sub-Saharan Africa, of tropical South America; may give at 4-9 mo if traveling to epidemic area; under 9 mo: risk of vaccine-related encephalitis	+	+	+
Typhoid	Heat inactivated	6 mo-2 yr: 2 × 0.25 ml SC 4 wk apart, booster q3yr	Fever, pain with heat killed: significantly fewer side effects with ViCPS and Ty21a; important for Latin America, Asia, Africa; vaccine not a substitute for eating and drinking cleanly	±	+	+
	ViCPS: polysaccharide Ty21a: oral live attenuated	2-6 yr: 0.5 ml IM × 1 booster q2yr >6 yr: 1 capsule q 2 days × 4; booster q 5 yr				
Meningococcal	Serogroups A, C, Y, W-135: polysaccharide	>2 years: 0.5 ml SC; booster in 1 yr if 1st dose after age 4 yr, otherwise in 5 yr	Use for central Africa, Saudi Arabia for the Hajj, Nepal, and epidemic areas; minimal efficacy under age 2 yr	±	±	±
Japanese encephalitis	Inactivated virus	1-3 yr: 0.5 ml SC at 0, 7, 14-30 days >3 years: 1.0 ml SC at 0, 7, 14-30 days Last dose >10 days before travel	Indicated for parts of India and rural Asia if stay > 1 mo; no safety data for under age 1 yr; high rate of hypersensitivity	±	±	+
Cholera	Inactivated bacteria	>6 mo: 0.2 ml SC	Vaccine of questionable efficacy; not recommended by CDC or WHO; do not use under 6 mo			
Lyme disease	LYMErix: antigenic protein*	>15 yr: 0.5 ml IM at 0, 1, 12 mo	Indicated for frequent, prolonged exposure to Lyme-endemic area, not brief exposures			
Extended Stay						
Rabies	HDCV: human diploid cell	1 ml IM in deltoid muscle at 0, 7, 21-28 days if >1 mo stay	If exposed and immunized: give vaccine, 1 ml IM at 0, 3 days. If exposed and unimmunized: give rabies Ig (RIG), 20 IU/kg half at site and half IM; give vaccine, 1 ml IM at 0, 3, 7, 14, 28 days	±	+	+

*Not readily available.

V

TABLE 5-12   Schedule for Catch-Up Administration of PCV (Prevnar) in Unvaccinated Infants and Children

AGE AT FIRST DOSE	PRIMARY SERIES	BOOSTER DOSE
2-6 mo	Three doses, 2 mo apart*	One dose at 12-15 mo†
7-11 mo	Two doses, 2 mo apart*	One dose at 12-15 mo†
12-23 mo	Two doses, 2 mo apart	—
24-59 mo		
Healthy children	One dose	—
Children with sickle cell disease, asplenia, HIV infection, chronic illness, or immunocompromising condition‡	Two doses, 2 mo apart	—

Modified from *MMWR Morb Mortal Wkly Rep* 49(RR-9):24, 2000.
HIV, Human immunodeficiency virus; *PCV,* pneumococcal conjugate vaccine.
*For the primary series in children vaccinated before 12 mo of age, the minimum interval between doses is 4 wk.
†The booster dose should be administered at least 8 wk after the primary series is completed.
‡Recommendations do not include children who have undergone bone marrow transplant.

TABLE 5-13   Administration Schedule for PCV (Prevnar) When a Lapse in Immunization Has Occurred

AGE AT PRESENTATION (MONTHS)	PREVIOUS PCV IMMUNIZATION HISTORY	RECOMMENDED REGIMEN
7 to 11	One dose	One dose at 7 to 11 mo followed by a booster at 12 to 15 mo with a minimal interval of 2 mo
	Two doses	One dose at 7 to 11 mo followed by a booster at 12 to 15 mo with a minimal interval of 2 mo
12 to 23	One dose before 12 mo	Two doses at least 2 mo apart
	Two doses before 12 mo	One dose at least 2 mo following the most recent dose
24 to 59	Any incomplete schedule	One dose*

Modified from *MMWR Morb Mortal Wkly Rep* 49(RR-9):24, 2000.
PCV, Pneumococcal conjugate vaccine.
*Children with certain chronic illnesses or immunosuppressing conditions should receive two doses at least 2 mo apart.

TABLE 5-14   Using PPV in High-Risk Children 2 Years and Older Who Have Been Immunized with PCV (Prevnar)

HEALTH STATUS	PPV SCHEDULE	REVACCINATE WITH PPV
Healthy	None	No
Sickle cell disease, anatomic or functional asplenia, HIV-infection, immunocompromising conditions	1 dose PPV given at least 2 mo after PCV	Yes*
Chronic illness	1 dose PPV given at least 2 mo after PCV	No

Modified from *MMWR Morb Mortal Wkly Rep* 49(RR-9):24, 2000.
HIV, Human immunodeficiency virus; *PCV,* pneumococcal conjugate vaccine; *PPV,* pneumococcal polysaccharide vaccine.
* If patient is older than 10 yr, a single revaccination should be given at least 5 yr after previous dose; if patient is 10 yr or younger, revaccinate 3 to 5 yr after previous dose. Regardless of when administered, a second dose of PPV should not be given less than 3 yr following the previous PPV dose.

Immunizations for Adolescents and Adults

TABLE 5-15 Summary of Adolescent/Adult Immunization Recommendations

AGENT	INDICATIONS	PRIMARY SCHEDULE	CONTRAINDICATIONS	COMMENTS
Tetanus and diphtheria toxoids combined (Td)	All adults All adolescents should be assessed at 11-12 or 14-16 yr of age and immunized if no dose was received during the previous 5 yr.	Two doses 4-8 wk apart, third dose 6-12 mo after the second. No need to repeat doses if the schedule is interrupted. Dose: 0.5 ml intramuscular (IM) Booster: At 10-yr intervals throughout life	Neurologic or severe hypersensitivity reaction to prior dose	WOUND MANAGEMENT: Patients with three or more previous tetanus toxoid doses: (a) give Td for clean minor wounds only if more than 10 yr since last dose; (b) for other wounds, give Td if over 5 yr since last dose. Patients with less than three or unknown number of prior tetanus toxoid doses, give Td for clean, minor wounds and Td and TIG (tetanus immune globulin) for other wounds.
Influenza vaccine	a. Adults 50 yr of age and older b. Residents of nursing homes or other facilities for patients with chronic medical conditions c. Persons ≥6 mo of age with chronic cardiovascular or pulmonary disorders, including asthma d. Persons ≥6 mo of age with chronic metabolic diseases (including diabetes), renal dysfunction, hemoglobinopathies, immunosuppressive or immunodeficiency disorders e. Women in their second or third trimester of pregnancy during influenza season f. Persons 6 mo-18 yr of age receiving long-term aspirin therapy g. Groups, including household members and care givers, who can infect high-risk persons	Dose: 0.5 ml, intramuscular (IM) Given annually, each fall	Anaphylactic allergy to eggs Acute febrile illness	Depending on season and destination, persons traveling to foreign countries should consider vaccination. Any person ≥6 mo of age who wishes to reduce the likelihood of becoming ill with influenza should be vaccinated. Avoiding subsequent vaccination of persons known to have developed GBS within 6 wk of a previous vaccination seems prudent; however, for most persons with a GBS history who are at high risk for severe complications, many experts believe the established benefits of vaccination justify yearly vaccination.

Modified from the recommendations of the Advisory Committee on Immunization Practices (ACIP). Foreign travel and less commonly used vaccines such as typhoid, rabies, and meningococcal are not included.

V

TABLE 5-15 Summary of Adolescent/Adult Immunization Recommendations—cont'd

AGENT	INDICATIONS	PRIMARY SCHEDULE	CONTRAINDICATIONS	COMMENTS
Hepatitis B vaccine	a. Persons with occupational risk of exposure to blood or blood-contaminated body fluids b. Clients and staff of institutions for the developmentally disabled c. Hemodialysis patients d. Recipients of clotting-factor concentrates e. Household contacts and sex partners of those chronically infected with HBV f. Adoptees from countries where HBV infection is endemic g. Certain international travelers h. Injecting drug users i. Men who have sex with men j. Heterosexual men and women with multiple sex partners or recent episode of a sexually transmitted disease k. Inmates of long-term correctional facilities l. All unvaccinated adolescents	Three doses: second dose 1-2 mo after the first, third dose 4-6 mo after the first. No need to start series over if schedule interrupted. Can start series with one manufacturer's vaccine and finish with another. Dose (*Adult*): intramuscular (IM) Recombivax HB: 10 µg/1.0 ml (green cap) Engerix-B: 20 µg/1.0 ml (orange cap) Dose (*Adolescents 11-19 yr*): intramuscular (IM) Recombivax HB: 5 µg/0.5 ml (yellow cap) Engerix-B: 10 µg/0.5 ml (light blue cap) Booster: None presently recommended	Anaphylactic allergy to yeast	a. Persons with serologic markers of prior or continuing hepatitis B virus infection do not need immunization. b. For hemodialysis patients and other immunodeficient or immunosuppressed patients, vaccine dosage is doubled or special preparation is used. c. *Pregnant women should be sero-screened for HBsAg and, if positive, their infants should be given postexposure. prophylaxis beginning at birth.* d. Postexposure prophylaxis: consult ACIP recommendations, or state or local immunization program.
Poliovirus vaccine	Routine vaccination of those ≥18 yr of age residing in the U.S. is not necessary. Vaccination is recommended for the following high-risk adults: a. Travelers to areas or countries where poliomyelitis is epidemic or endemic b. Members of communities or specific population groups with disease caused by wild polioviruses c. Laboratory workers who handle specimens that may contain polioviruses d. Health care workers who have close contact with patients who may be excreting wild polioviruses e. Unvaccinated adults whose children will be receiving OPV	Unimmunized adolescents/adults: IPV is recommended—two doses at 4 to 8-wk intervals, third dose 6-12 mo after second (can be as soon as 2 mo) Dose: 0.5 ml subcutaneous (SC) or intramuscular (IM) Partially immunized adolescents/adults: Complete primary series with IPV or OPV only in selected circumstances (see *MMWR Morb Mortal Wkly Rep* 49[RR-5]:1, 2000.) (IPV schedule shown above). OPV scheduleis three doses given 6-8 wk apart; if accelerated protection is needed, minimal interval between doses is 4 wk.	*IPV:* Anaphylactic reaction following previous dose or to streptomycin, polymyxin B or neomycin *OPV:* a. Anaphylactic reaction following previous dose b. Immunodeficiency disorders or altered immune states resulting from malignant disease, or compromised immune systems, such as radiation or HIV infection	In instances of potential exposure to wild poliovirus, adults who have had a primary series of OPV or IPV may be given one more dose of either vaccine. Although no adverse effects have been documented, vaccination of pregnant women should be avoided. However, if immediate protection is required, pregnant women may be given OPV or IPV in accordance with the recommended schedule for adults. If inadvertent administration of OPV to a household contact of an immunocompromised person occurs, avoid close contact for 4-6 wk.

IPV, Inactivated vaccine; *OPV,* oral (live) vaccine.

Continued

AGENT	INDICATIONS	PRIMARY SCHEDULE	CONTRAINDICATIONS	COMMENTS
Pneumococcal polysaccharide vaccine (PPV)	a. Adults 65 yr of age and older b. Persons ≥2 yr with chronic cardiovascular or pulmonary disorders including congestive heart failure, diabetes mellitus, chronic liver disease, alcoholism, CSF leaks, cardiomyopathy, COPD, or emphysema c. Persons ≥2 yr with splenic dysfunction or asplenia, hematologic malignancy, multiple myeloma, renal failure, organ transplantation, or immunosuppressive conditions, including HIV infection d. Alaskan Natives and certain American Indian populations	One dose for most people Dose: 0.5 ml intramuscular (IM) or subcutaneous (SC) Persons vaccinated before age 65 should be vaccinated at age 65 if 5 or more yr have passed since the first dose. For all persons with functional or anatomic asplenia, transplant patients, patients with chronic kidney disease, immunosuppressed or immunodeficient persons, and others at highest risk of fatal infection, a second dose should be given at least 5 yr after first dose.	The safety of PPV during the first trimester of pregnancy has not been evaluated. The manufacturer's package insert should be reviewed for additional information.	If elective splenectomy or immunosuppressive therapy is planned, give vaccine 2 wk ahead, if possible. When indicated, vaccine should be administered to patients with unknown vaccination status. All residents of nursing homes and other long-term care facilities should have their vaccination status assessed and documented.
Measles and mumps vaccines*	a. Adults born after 1956 without written documentation of immunization on or after the first birthday b. Health care personnel born after 1956 who are at risk of exposure to patients with measles should have documentation of two doses of vaccine on or after the first birthday or of measles seropositivity c. HIV-infected persons without severe immunosuppression d. Travelers to foreign countries e. Persons entering post-secondary educational institutions (e.g., college)	At least one dose. (Two doses if in college, in health care profession, or traveling to a foreign country with second dose at least 1 mo after the first.) Dose: 0.5 ml subcutaneous (SC)	a. Immunosuppressive therapy or immunodeficiency, including HIV-infected persons with severe immunosuppression b. Anaphylactic allergy to neomycin c. Pregnancy d. Immune globulin preparation or blood/blood product received in preceding 3-11 mo	Women should be asked if they are pregnant before receiving vaccine, and advised to avoid pregnancy for three months after immunization.
Rubella vaccine*	a. Persons (especially women) without written documentation of immunization on or after the first birthday or of seropositivity b. Health care personnel who are at risk of exposure to patients with rubella and who may have contact with pregnant patients should have at least one dose	One dose Dose: 0.5 ml subcutaneous (SC)	Same as for measles and mumps vaccines	Same as for measles and mumps vaccines

Modified from the recommendations of the Advisory Committee on Immunization Practices (ACIP). Foreign travel and less commonly used vaccines such as typhoid, rabies, and meningococcal are not included.
*These vaccines can be given in the combined form measles-mumps-rubella (MMR). Persons already immune to one or more components can still receive MMR.

V

TABLE 5-15 **Summary of Adolescent/Adult Immunization Recommendations—cont'd**

AGENT	INDICATIONS	PRIMARY SCHEDULE	CONTRAINDICATIONS	COMMENTS
Varicella vaccine	a. Persons of any age without a reliable history of varicella disease or vaccination, or who are seronegative for varicella b. All susceptible health care workers c. Susceptible family contacts of immuno-compromised persons d. Susceptible persons in the following groups who are at high risk for exposure: persons – who live or work in environments in which transmission of varicella is likely (e.g., teachers of young children, day care employees, residents and staff in institutional settings) or can occur (e.g., college students, inmates and staff of correctional institutions, military personnel) – nonpregnant women of childbearing age – international travelers	For persons <13 yr of age, one dose For persons 13 yr of age and older, two doses separated by 4-8 wk. If >8 wk elapse following the first dose, the second dose can be administered without restarting the schedule. Dose: 0.5 ml subcutaneous (SC)	a. Anaphylactic allergy to gelatin or neomycin b. Untreated, active TB c. Immunosuppressive therapy or immunodeficiency (including HIV infection) d. Family history of congenital or hereditary immunodeficiency in first-degree relatives, unless the immune competence of the recipient has been clinically substantiated or verified by a laboratory e. Immune globulin preparation or blood/blood product received in preceding 5 mo f. Pregnancy	Women should be asked if they are pregnant before receiving varicella vaccine, and advised to avoid pregnancy for 1 mo following each dose of vaccine.
Hepatitis A vaccine	a. Persons traveling to or working in countries with high or intermediate endemicity of infection b. Men who have sex with men c. Injecting and non-injecting illegal drug users d. Persons who work with HAV-infected primates or with HAV in a research laboratory setting e. Persons with chronic liver disease f. Persons with clotting factor disorders g. Consider food handlers, where determined to be cost-effective by health authorities or employers	HAVRIX: Two doses, separated by 6-12 mo. Adults (19 of age and older)—Dose: 1.0 ml intramuscular (IM); Persons 2-18 yr of age: Dose: 0.5 ml (IM) VAQTA: Adults (18 yrs of age and older): Two doses, separated by 6 mo. Dose: 1.0 ml intramuscular (IM); Persons 2-17 yr of age: Two doses, separated by 6-18 mo; Dose: 0.5 ml (IM)	A history of hypersensitivity to alum or the preservative 2-phenoxyethanol	The safety of hepatitis A vaccine during pregnancy has not been determined, though the theoretical risk to the developing fetus is expected to be low. The risk of vaccination should be weighed against the risk of hepatitis A in women who may be at high risk of of exposure to HAV.

Modified from the recommendations of the Advisory Committee on Immunization Practices (ACIP). Foreign travel and less commonly used vaccines such as typhoid, rabies, and meningococcal are not included.
HAV, Hepatitis A virus; *HIV,* human immunodeficiency virus; *TB,* tuberculosis.

VACCINATION OF PREGNANT WOMEN

"Risk from vaccination during pregnancy is largely theoretical. The benefit of vaccination among pregnant women usually outweighs the potential risk when (a) the risk for disease exposure is high, (b) infection would pose a special risk to the mother or fetus, and (c) the vaccine is unlikely to cause harm." ACIP General Recommendations on Immunization, p. 20.

Generally, live-virus vaccines are contraindicated for pregnant women because of the theoretical risk of transmission of the vaccine virus to the fetus. If a live-virus vaccine is inadvertently given to a pregnant woman or if a woman becomes pregnant within 3 months after vaccination, she should be counseled about the potential effects on the fetus. However, it is not ordinarily an indication to terminate the pregnancy.

Whether live or inactivated vaccines are used, vaccination of pregnant women should be considered on the basis of risks vs. benefits (i.e., the risk of the vaccination vs. the benefits of protection in a particular circumstance). Table 5-16, A, may be used as a general guide.

TABLE 5-16, A   Guidelines for Vaccinating Pregnant Women

VACCINE	SHOULD BE CONSIDERED IF OTHERWISE INDICATED	CONTRAINDICATED DURING PREGNANCY	SPECIAL OR ABSENT RECOMMENDATION[b]
Routine			
Hepatitis A			"The safety of hepatitis A vaccination during pregnancy has not been determined; however, because hepatitis A vaccine is produced from inactivated [hepatitis A virus], the theoretical risk to the developing fetus is expected to be low. **The risk associated with vaccination should be weighed against the risk for hepatitis A in women who may be at high risk for exposure to [hepatitis A virus].**"[c]
Hepatitis B	✓		"On the basis of limited experience, there is no apparent risk of adverse effects to developing fetuses when hepatitis B vaccine is administered to pregnant women (CDC, unpublished data). The vaccine contains noninfectious HBsAg particles and should cause no risk to the fetus. [Hepatitis B virus] infection affecting a pregnant woman may result in severe disease for the mother and chronic infection for the newborn. **Therefore, neither pregnancy nor lactation should be considered a contraindication to vaccination of women.**"[d] "Hepatitis B vaccine is recommended for women at risk for hepatitis B infection . . ."[e]
Influenza	✓		"On the basis of . . . data that suggest that influenza infection may cause increased morbidity in women during the second and third trimesters of pregnancy, the [ACIP] recommends that **women who will be beyond the first trimester of pregnancy (≥ 14 weeks' gestation) during the influenza season be vaccinated.**"[f] "**Pregnant women who have medical conditions that increase their risk for complications from influenza should be vaccinated before the influenza season—regardless of the state of pregnancy.**"[f] "Studies of influenza immunization of more than 2,000 pregnant women have demonstrated no adverse fetal effects associated with influenza vaccine; however, more data are needed."[f]
Measles[a]		✓	"**MMR and its component vaccines should not be administered to women known to be pregnant.** Because a risk to the fetus from administration of these live virus vaccines cannot be excluded for theoretical reasons, women should be counseled to avoid becoming pregnant for 30 days after vaccination with measles or mumps containing vaccines and for 3 months after administration of MMR or other rubella-containing vaccines."[g] "If a pregnant woman is vaccinated or if she becomes pregnant within 3 months after vaccination, she should be counseled about the theoretical basis of concern for the fetus, but MMR vaccination during pregnancy should not ordinarily be a reason to consider termination of pregnancy."[g]

[a]Live, attenuated vaccine.
[b]Relevant passages from ACIP recommendations are reprinted for each vaccine. Material in quotation marks is taken verbatim from ACIP (emphasis in **bold type** added); material not in quotation marks is paraphrased.
[c]Centers for Disease Control and Prevention: Prevention of hepatitis A through active or passive immunization: recommendations of the Advisory Committee on Immunization Practices (ACIP), *MMWR* 45 (No. RR-15):20, 1996.
[d]Centers for Disease Control and Prevention: Hepatitis B virus: a comprehensive strategy for eliminating transmission in the United States through universal childhood vaccination: recommendations of the Immunization Practices Advisory Committee (ACIP), *MMWR* 40 (No. RR-13):4, 1991.
[e]Centers for Disease Control and Prevention: General recommendations on immunization: recommendations of the Advisory Committee on Immunization Practices (ACIP), *MMWR* 43 (No. RR-1):21, 1994.
[f]Centers for Disease Control and Prevention: Prevention and control of influenza: recommendations of the Advisory Committee on Immunization Practices (ACIP), *MMWR* 47 (No. RR-6):6, 1998.
[g]Centers for Disease Control and Prevention: Measles, mumps, and rubella—vaccine use and strategies for elimination of measles, rubella, and congenital rubella syndrome and control of mumps: recommendations of the Immunization Practices Advisory Committee (ACIP), *MMWR* 47 (No. RR-8):32-33, 1998.

Continued

V

TABLE 5-16, A   Guidelines for Vaccinating Pregnant Women—cont'd

VACCINE	SHOULD BE CONSIDERED IF OTHERWISE INDICATED	CONTRAINDICATED DURING PREGNANCY	SPECIAL OR ABSENT RECOMMENDATION[b]
Routine—cont'd			
Mumps[a]		✓	"**MMR and its component vaccines should not be administered to women known to be pregnant.** Because a risk to the fetus from administration of these live virus vaccines cannot be excluded for theoretical reasons, women should be counseled to avoid becoming pregnant for 30 days after vaccination with measles or mumps containing vaccines and for 3 months after administration of MMR or other rubella-containing vaccines."[g] "If a pregnant woman is vaccinated or if she becomes pregnant within 3 months after vaccination, she should be counseled about the theoretical basis of concern for the fetus, but MMR vaccination during pregnancy should not ordinarily be a reason to consider termination of pregnancy."[g]
Pneumococcal			"The safety of pneumococcal polysaccharide vaccine during the first trimester of pregnancy has not been evaluated, although no adverse consequences have been reported among newborns whose mothers were inadvertently vaccinated during pregnancy."[h]
Polio (OPV[a] and IPV)			"Although no adverse effects of OPV or IPV have been documented among pregnant women or their fetuses, **vaccination of pregnant women should be avoided.** However, if a pregnant woman requires immediate protection against poliomyelitis, she may be administered OPV or IPV in accordance with the recommended schedules for adults."[i]
Rubella[a]		✓	"**MMR and its component vaccines should not be administered to women known to be pregnant.** Because a risk to the fetus from administration of these live virus vaccines cannot be excluded for theoretical reasons, women should be counseled to avoid becoming pregnant for 30 days after vaccination with measles or mumps containing vaccines and for 3 months after administration of MMR or other rubella-containing vaccines."[g] "If a pregnant woman is vaccinated or if she becomes pregnant within 3 months after vaccination, she should be counseled about the theoretical basis of concern for the fetus, but MMR vaccination during pregnancy should not ordinarily be a reason to consider termination of pregnancy."[g] "Rubella-susceptible women who are not vaccinated because they state they are or may be pregnant should be counseled about the potential risk for CRS and the importance of being vaccinated as soon as they are no longer pregnant."[g] A registry of susceptible women vaccinated with rubella vaccine between 3 months before and 3 months after conception—the "Vaccine in Pregnancy (VIP) Registry"—was kept between 1971 and 1989. No evidence of CRS occurred in the offspring of the 226 women who received the current RA 27/3 rubella vaccine and continued their pregnancy to term.[g]
Tetanus/Diphtheria	✓		"**Combined tetanus and diphtheria toxoids are . . . routinely indicated for susceptible pregnant women.** Previously vaccinated pregnant women who have not received a Td vaccination within the last 10 years should receive a booster dose."[j] "Pregnant women who are unimmunized or only partially immunized against tetanus should complete the primary series."[j] "Although no evidence exists that tetanus and diphtheria toxoids are teratogenic, waiting until the second trimester of pregnancy to administer Td is a reasonable precaution for minimizing any concern about the theoretical possibility of such reactions."[k]

[h]Centers for Disease Control and Prevention: Prevention of pneumococcal disease: recommendations of the Advisory Committee on Immunization Practices (ACIP), *MMWR* 46 (No. RR-8):6, 1997.

[i]Centers for Disease Control and Prevention: Poliomyelitis prevention in the United States: introduction of a sequential vaccination schedule of inactivated poliovirus vaccine followed by oral poliovirus vaccine: recommendations of the Advisory Committee on Immunization Practices (ACIP), *MMWR* 46 (No. RR-3):18, 1997.

[j]Centers for Disease Control and Prevention: General recommendations on immunization: recommendations of the advisory committee on immunization practices (ACIP), *MMWR* 43 (No. RR-1):20-21, 1994.

[k]Centers for Disease Control and Prevention: Diphtheria, tetanus, and pertussis: recommendations for vaccine use and other preventive measures: recommendations of the Immunization Practices Advisory Committee (ACIP), *MMWR* 40 (No. RR-10):14, 1991.

TABLE 5-16, A   Guidelines for Vaccinating Pregnant Women—cont'd

VACCINE	SHOULD BE CONSIDERED IF OTHERWISE INDICATED	CONTRAINDICATED DURING PREGNANCY	SPECIAL OR ABSENT RECOMMENDATION[b]
Routine—cont'd			
Varicella[a]		✓	"The effects of the varicella virus vaccine on the fetus are unknown; therefore, **pregnant women should not be vaccinated.** Non-pregnant women who are vaccinated should avoid becoming pregnant for 1 month following each injection. For susceptible persons, having a pregnant household member is not a contraindication to vaccination."[l] "If a pregnant woman is vaccinated or becomes pregnant within 1 month of vaccination, she should be counseled about potential effects on the fetus."[l] "Because the virulence of the attenuated virus used in the vaccine is less than that of the wild-type virus, the risk to the fetus, if any, should be even lower."[l] "In most circumstances, the decision to terminate a pregnancy should not be based on whether vaccine was administered during pregnancy."[l] "VZIG [Varicella Zoster Immune Globulin] should be strongly considered for susceptible, pregnant women who have been exposed."[l] The manufacturer and CDC have established a VARIVAX Pregnancy Registry to monitor outcomes of women who got the vaccine 3 months before or any time during pregnancy. Call **1-800-986-8999.**
Travel & Other			
BCG[a]		✓	"Although no harmful effects to the fetus have been associated with BCG vaccine, **its use is not recommended during pregnancy.**"[m]
Cholera			"No specific information exists on the safety of cholera vaccine during pregnancy. Its use should be individualized to reflect actual need."[n]
Japanese Encephalitis			"No specific information is available on the safety of JE vaccine in pregnancy. Vaccination poses an unknown but theoretical risk to the developing fetus, and **the vaccine should not be routinely administered during pregnancy.**"[o] "Pregnant women who must travel to an area where risk of JE is high should be vaccinated when the theoretical risks of immunization are outweighed by the risk of infection to the mother and developing fetus."[o]
Meningococcal	✓		Studies have shown the vaccine to be both safe and efficacious when given to pregnant women. While high antibody levels were found in umbilical cord blood following vaccination during pregnancy, antibody levels in the infants decreased during the first few months after birth. Subsequent response to meningococcal vaccination was not affected. "Based on data from studies involving use of meningococcal vaccines administered during pregnancy, **altering meningococcal vaccination recommendations during pregnancy is unnecessary.**"[p]

[l]Centers for Disease Control and Prevention: Prevention of varicella: recommendations of the Advisory Committee on Immunization Practices (ACIP), *MMWR* 45 (No. RR-11):19, 1996.

[m]Centers for Disease Control and Prevention: The role of BCG vaccine in the prevention and control of tuberculosis in the United States: a joint statement by the Advisory Council for the Elimination of Tuberculosis and the Advisory Committee on Immunization Practices, *MMWR* 45 (No. RR-4):13, 1996.

[n]Centers for Disease Control and Prevention: Cholera vaccine: recommendations of the Immunization Practices Advisory Committee (ACIP), *MMWR* 37 (No. 40):2, 1988.

[o]Centers for Disease Control and Prevention: Inactivated Japanese encephalitis vaccine: recommendations of the Advisory Committee on Immunization Practices (ACIP), *MMWR* 42 (No. RR-1):12-13, 1993.

[p]Centers for Disease Control and Prevention: Control and prevention of meningococcal disease and control and prevention of serogroup C meningococcal disease: evaluation and management of suspected outbreaks: recommendations of the Advisory Committee on Immunization Practices (ACIP), *MMWR* 46 (No. RR-5):5, 1997.

Continued

V

TABLE 5-16, A   Guidelines for Vaccinating Pregnant Women—cont'd

VACCINE	SHOULD BE CONSIDERED IF OTHERWISE INDICATED	CONTRAINDICATED DURING PREGNANCY	SPECIAL OR ABSENT RECOMMENDATION[B]
Travel & Other—cont'd			
Plague			"The effects of plague vaccine on the developing fetus . . . are unknown. Pregnant women who cannot avoid high-risk situations should be advised of risk-reduction practices and **should be vaccinated only if the potential benefits of vaccination outweigh potential risks to the fetus.**"[q]
Rabies	✓		"Because of the potential consequences of inadequately treated rabies exposure, and because there is no indication that fetal abnormalities have been associated with rabies vaccination, **pregnancy is not considered a contraindication to postexposure prophylaxis.**"[r] "**If there is substantial risk of exposure to rabies, preexposure prophylaxis may also be indicated during pregnancy.**"[r]
Typhoid (Parenteral and Ty21a[a])			"No data have been reported on the use of any of the three typhoid vaccines among pregnant women."[s]
Vaccinia[a]		✓	"**Vaccinia should not be administered to pregnant women.**"[t] "On rare occasions, almost always after primary vaccination, vaccinia virus has been reported to cause fetal infection. . . . Vaccinia vaccine is not known to cause congenital malformations."[t]
Yellow Fever[a]			"If international travel requirements constitute the only reason to vaccinate a pregnant woman, rather than an increased risk of infection, efforts should be made to obtain a waiver letter from the traveler's physician."[u] "**Pregnant women who must travel to areas where the risk of yellow fever is high should be vaccinated.** Under these circumstances, for both mother and fetus, the small theoretical risk from vaccination is far outweighed by the risk of yellow fever infection."[u]

[q]Centers for Disease Control and Prevention: Prevention of plague: recommendations of the Advisory Committee on Immunization Practices (ACIP), *MMWR* 45 (No. RR-14):10, 1996.

[r]Centers for Disease Control and Prevention: Rabies prevention—United States, 1991: Recommendations of the Immunization Practices Advisory Committee (ACIP), *MMWR* 40 (No. RR-3):11-12, 1991.

[s]Centers for Disease Control and Prevention: Typhoid immunization: recommendations of the Advisory Committee on Immunization Practices (ACIP), *MMWR* 43 (No. RR-14):7, 1994.

[t]Centers for Disease Control and Prevention: Vaccinia (Smallpox) vaccine: recommendations of the Immunization Practices Advisory Committee (ACIP), *MMWR* 40 (No. RR-14):6, 1991.

[u]Centers for Disease Control and Prevention: Yellow fever vaccine: recommendations of the Immunization Practices Advisory Committee (ACIP), *MMWR* 39 (No. RR-6):3, 1990.

PASSIVE IMMUNIZATION DURING PREGNANCY
"There is no known risk to the fetus from passive immunization of pregnant women with immune globulin preparations." ACIP *General Recommendations on Immunization,* p. 21.

PRENATAL SCREENING FOR VACCINE-PREVENTABLE DISEASES
The ACIP currently recommends prenatal screening for rubella and hepatitis B:
    "Prenatal serologic screening . . . is indicated for all pregnant women who lack acceptable evidence of rubella immunity. Upon completion or termination of their pregnancies, women who do not have serologic evidence of rubella immunity or documentation of rubella vaccination should be vaccinated with MMR before discharge from the hospital, birthing center, or abortion clinic." ACIP, *Measles, Mumps, and Rubella—Vaccine Use and Strategies for Elimination of Measles, Rubella, and Congenital Rubella Syndrome and Control of Mumps,* p. 18.
    "All pregnant women should be routinely tested for HBsAg during an early prenatal visit in each pregnancy. . . . HBsAg-positive mothers identified during screening may have HBV-related acute or chronic liver disease and should be evaluated by their physicians." ACIP, *Protection Against Viral Hepatitis,* p. 14.

VACCINATING WOMEN WHO ARE BREASTFEEDING
"Neither killed nor live vaccines affect the safety of breast-feeding for mothers or infants. Breastfeeding does not adversely affect immunization and is not a contraindication for any vaccine." ACIP, *General Recommendations on Immunization,* p. 20.
    The following applies to varicella vaccine, which was licensed after the ACIP General Recommendations were published: "Whether attenuated vaccine VZV is excreted in human milk and, if so, whether the infant could be infected are not known. Most live vaccines have not been demonstrated to be secreted in breast milk. Attenuated rubella vaccine virus has been detected in beast milk but has produced only asymptomatic infection in the nursing infant. Therefore, varicella vaccine may be considered for a nursing mother." ACIP, *Prevention of Varicella,* pp. 19-20.

For More Information

More detailed information about vaccination of pregnant women can be found in:

ACIP statements for specific diseases.

The ACIP's *Update on Adult Immunization* (*MMWR* Vol. 40, No. RR-12, November 15, 1991). See especially p. 9 and Appendix 5, pp. 82-88.

Current ACIP recommendations can be found on the National Immunization Program's website at <http://www.cdc.gov/nip.> Or call the National Immunization Program's Information Center at (404) 639-8226.

The American College of Obstetricians and Gynecologists (ACOG) Technical Bulletin Number 160, October 1991. This publication is available from the American College of Obstetricians and Gynecologists, Attn: Resource Center, 409 12th Street SW, Washington, DC 20024-2188.

The American College of Physicians' *Guide for Adult Immunization,* ed 3, pp. 25-29. Customer Service for the American College of Physicians can be contacted at (215) 351-2600 or (800) 523-1546.

Information on "Vaccination of Pregnant Women" and Table 5-16, *A,* from http://www.cdc.gov/nip/publications/preg_guide.pdf downloaded May 15, 2002.

TABLE 5-16, B Immunization in Pregnancy

INFECTION	VACCINE TYPE*	USE IN PREGNANCY
Diphtheria	Bacterial toxoid	No contraindications to use.
Hepatitis A	Inactivated virus	There is no evidence of a risk to the fetus, but the vaccine should not be given in the absence of a specific indication.
Hepatitis B	Inactivated virus	No contraindications to use.
Influenza	Inactivated virus	There is no evidence of a risk to the fetus, but the vaccine should not be given in the absence of a specific indication.
Measles	Live-attenuated virus	Contraindicated.
Meningococcal infection	Bacterial antigen	There is no evidence of a risk to the fetus, but the vaccine should not be given in the absence of a specific indication (i.e., a genuine risk of infection, such as during an outbreak).
Mumps	Live-attenuated virus	Contraindicated.
Pneumococcal infection	Bacterial antigen	Not recommended (although there is probably little or no risk to the fetus).
Poliomyelitis	(1) Live-attenuated virus (2) Inactivated virus	(1) Not recommended *unless* the woman is traveling to an endemic area when the risk of immunization is outweighed by the risk of infection. (2) No contraindications to use.
Rabies	Live-attenuated virus	Preexposure immunization is not recommended *unless* the woman is at high risk of exposure to rabies. Postexposure immunization should not be withheld, as the risk of infection outweighs the risk of immunization.
Rubella	Live-attenuated virus	Contraindicated.
Tetanus	Bacterial toxoid	No contraindication to use.
Tuberculosis	Live-attenuated bacteria	Do not use until after delivery (although the risk to the fetus is probably very small).
Typhoid	(1) Whole cell killed bacteria (2) Bacterial antigen (3) Live attenuated bacteria	(1) and (2) There is no evidence of a risk to fetus, but the vaccine should not be given in the absence of a specific indication. (3) Probably should be avoided until after delivery.
Yellow fever	Live-attenuated virus	Not recommended *unless* the woman is traveling to a high-risk area when the risk of immunization is outweighed by the risk of infection.

From Department of Health: Immunisation against infectious disease, London, 1996, HMSO. In Barron WM, Lindheimer MD: *Medical disorders during pregnancy,* ed 3, St Louis, 2000, Mosby.
*All the vaccines listed here are placed in FDA pregnancy category C.

V

TABLE 5-17 Immunizing Agents and Immunization Schedules for Health-Care Workers (HCWs)*

GENERIC NAME	PRIMARY SCHEDULE AND BOOSTER(S)	INDICATIONS	MAJOR PRECAUTIONS AND CONTRAINDICATIONS	SPECIAL CONSIDERATIONS
Immunizing Agents Strongly Recommended for Health-Care Workers				
Hepatitis B (HB) recombinant vaccine	Two doses IM 4 wk apart; third dose 5 mo after second; booster doses not necessary.	**Preexposure:** HCWs at risk for exposure to blood or body fluids.	Based on limited data no risk of adverse effects to developing fetuses is apparent. Pregnancy should *not* be considered a contra-indication to vaccina-tion of women. Previous anaphylactic reaction to common baker's yeast is a contraindication to vaccination.	The vaccine produces neither therapeutic nor adverse effects on HBV-infected persons. Prevaccination serologic screening is not indicated for persons being vaccinated because of occupational risk. HCWs who have contact with pa-tients or blood should be tested 1-2 mo after vacci-nation to determine serologic response.
Hepatitis B immune globulin (HBIG)	0.06 ml/kg IM as soon as possible after exposure. A second dose of HBIG should be administered 1 mo later if the HB vaccine series has not been started.	**Postexposure** prophylaxis: For per-sons exposed to blood or body fluids containing HBsAg and who are not im-mune to HBV infection—0.06 ml/kg IM as soon as pos-sible (but no later than 7 days after exposure).		
Influenza vaccine (inactivated whole-virus and split-virus vaccines)	Annual vaccination with current vaccine. Administered IM.	HCWs who have con-tact with patients at high risk for influenza or its complications; HCWs who work in chronic care facilities; HCWs with high-risk medical conditions or who are aged ≥65 yr	History of anaphylactic hypersensitivity to egg ingestion.	No evidence exists of risk to mother or fetus when the vaccine is administered to a pregnant woman with an underlying high-risk condi-tion. Influenza vaccination is recommended during second and third trimesters of preg-nancy because of increased risk for hospitalization.
Measles live-virus vaccine	One dose SC; second dose at least 1 mo later.	HCWs† born during or after 1957 who do not have document-ation of having re-ceived two doses of live vaccine on or after the first birthday **or** a history of physician-diagnosed measles or serologic evidence of immunity. Vaccina-tion should be con-sidered for all HCWs who lack proof of im-munity, including those born before 1957.	Pregnancy; immuno-compromised persons‡, including HIV-infected persons who have evidence of severe immunosup-pression; anaphylaxis after gelatin ingestion or administration of neomycin; recent administration of immune globulin.	MMR is the vaccine of choice if recipients are likely to be susceptible to rubella and/or mumps as well as to measles. Persons vaccinated during 1963-1967 with a killed mea-sles vaccine alone, killed vaccine followed by live vac-cine, or with a vaccine of un-known type should be revac-cinated with two doses of live measles virus vaccine.

Modified from *MMWR* 46(RR-18), 1998.

HBsAg, Hepatitis B surface antigen; *HBV,* hepatitis B virus; *HIV,* human immunodeficiency virus; *IM,* intramuscular; *MMR,* measles, mumps, rubella vaccine; *SC,* subcutaneous.

*Persons who provide health care to patients or work in institutions that provide patient care (e.g., physicians, nurses, emergency medical personnel, dental professionals and students, medical and nursing students, laboratory technicians, hospital volunteers, and administrative and support staff in health-care institutions).

†All HCWs (i.e., medical or nonmedical, paid or volunteer, full time or part time, student or nonstudent, with or without patient-care responsibilities) who work in health-care institutions (e.g., inpatient and outpatient, public and private) should be immune to measles, rubella, and varicella.

‡Persons immunocompromised because of immune deficiency diseases, HIV infection, leukemia, lymphoma or generalized malignancy or immunosup-pressed as a result of therapy with corticosteroids, alkylating drugs, antimetabolites, or radiation.

TABLE 5-17 **Immunizing Agents and Immunization Schedules for Health-Care Workers (HCWs)*—cont'd**

GENERIC NAME	PRIMARY SCHEDULE AND BOOSTER(S)	INDICATIONS	MAJOR PRECAUTIONS AND CONTRAINDICATIONS	SPECIAL CONSIDERATIONS
Mumps live-virus vaccine	One dose SC; no booster	HCWs† believed to be susceptible can be vaccinated. Adults born before 1957 can be considered immune.	Pregnancy; immunocompromised persons‡; history of anaphylactic reaction after gelatin ingestion or administration of neomycin	MMR is the vaccine of choice if recipients are likely to be susceptible to measles and rubella as well as to mumps.
Hepatitis A vaccine	Two doses of vaccine either 6-12 mo apart (HAVRIX), or 6 mo apart (VAQTA)	Not routinely indicated for HCWs in the United States. Persons who work with HAV-infected primates or with HAV in a research laboratory setting should be vaccinated.	History of anaphylactic hypersensitivity to alum or, for HAVRIX, the preservative 2-phenoxyethanol. The safety of the vaccine in pregnant women has not been determined; the risk associated with vaccination should be weighed against the risk for hepatitis A in women who may be at high risk for exposure to HAV.	
Meningococcal polysaccharide vaccine (tetravalent A, C, W135, and Y)	One dose in volume and by route specified by manufacturer; need for boosters unknown	Not routinely indicated for HCWs in the United States	The safety of the vaccine in pregnant women has not been evaluated; it should not be administered during pregnancy unless the risk for infection is high.	
Typhoid vaccine, IM, SC, and oral	*IM vaccine:* One 0.5-ml dose, booster 0.5 ml every 2 yr. SC vaccine: two 0.5 ml doses, ≥4 wk apart, booster 0.5 ml SC or 0.1 ID every 3 yr if exposure continues *Oral vaccine:* Four doses on alternate days. The manufacturer recommends revaccination with the entire four-dose series every 5 yr	Workers in microbiology laboratories who frequently work with *Salmonella typhi*	Severe local or systemic reaction to a previous dose. Ty21a (oral) vaccine should not be administered to immunocompromised persons† or to persons receiving antimicrobial agents.	Vaccination should not be considered an alternative to the use of proper procedures when handling specimens and cultures in the laboratory.
Vaccinia vaccine (smallpox)	One dose administered with a bifurcated needle; boosters administered every 10 yr	Laboratory workers who directly handle cultures with vaccinia, recombinant vaccinia viruses, or orthopox viruses that infect humans	The vaccine is contraindicated in pregnancy, in persons with eczema or a history of eczema, and in immunocompromised persons† and their household contacts.	Vaccination may be considered for HCWs who have direct contact with contaminated dressings or other infectious material from volunteers in clinical studies involving recombinant vaccinia virus.

*Persons who provide health care to patients or work in institutions that provide patient care (e.g., physicians, nurses, emergency medical personnel, dental professionals and students, medical and nursing students, laboratory technicians, hospital volunteers, and administrative and support staff in health-care institutions).

†All HCWs (i.e., medical or nonmedical, paid or volunteer, full time or part time, student or nonstudent, with or without patient-care responsibilities) who work in health-care institutions (e.g., inpatient and outpatient, public and private) should be immune to measles, rubella, and varicella.

‡Persons immunocompromised because of immune deficiency diseases, HIV infection, leukemia, lymphoma or generalized malignancy or immunosuppressed as a result of therapy with corticosteroids, alkylating drugs, antimetabolites, or radiation.

V

Continued

TABLE 5-17   Immunizing Agents and Immunization Schedules for Health-Care Workers (HCWs)*—cont'd

GENERIC NAME	PRIMARY SCHEDULE AND BOOSTER(S)	INDICATIONS	MAJOR PRECAUTIONS AND CONTRAINDICATIONS	SPECIAL CONSIDERATIONS
Other Vaccine-Preventable Diseases				
Tetanus and diphtheria (toxoids [Td])	Two IM doses 4 wk apart; third dose 6-12 mo after second dose; booster every 10 yr	All adults	Except in the first trimester, pregnancy is not a precaution. History of a neurologic reaction or immediate hypersensitivity reaction after a previous dose. History of severe local (Arthus-type) reaction after a previous dose. Such persons should not receive further routine or emergency doses of Td for 10 yr.	Tetanus prophylaxis in wound management‡
Pneumococcal polysaccharide vaccine (23 valent)	One dose, 0.5 ml, IM or SC; revaccination recommended for those at highest risk ≥5 yr after the first dose	Adults who are at increased risk of pneumococcal disease and its complications because of underlying health conditions; older adults, especially those age ≥65 who are healthy	The safety of vaccine in pregnant women has not been evaluated; it should not be administered during pregnancy unless the risk for infection is high. Previous recipients of any type of pneumococcal polysaccharide vaccine who are at highest risk for fatal infection or antibody loss may be revaccinated ≥5 yr after the first dose.	
Rubella live-virus vaccine	One dose SC; no booster	Indicated for HCWs,† both men and women, who do not have documentation of having received live vaccine on or after their first birthday **or** laboratory evidence of immunity. Adults born before 1957, **except women who can become pregnant,** can be considered immune.	Pregnancy; immunocompromised persons†; history of anaphylactic reaction after administration of neomycin	The risk for rubella vaccine–associated malformations in the offspring of women pregnant when vaccinated or who become pregnant within 3 mo after vaccination is negligible. Such women should be counseled regarding the theoretic basis of concern for the fetus. MMR is the vaccine of choice if recipients are likely to be susceptible to measles or mumps, as well as to rubella.
Varicella zoster live-virus vaccine	Two 0.5-ml doses SC 4-8 wk apart if ≥13 yr of age	Indicated for HCWs† who do not have either a reliable history of varicella or serologic evidence of immunity	Pregnancy, immunocompromised persons,‡ history of anaphylactic reaction following receipt of neomycin or gelatin. Avoid salicylate use for 6 wk after vaccination.	Vaccine is available from the manufacturer for certain patients with acute lymphocytic leukemia (ALL) in remission. Because 71%-93% of persons without a history of varicella are immune, serologic testing before vaccination is likely to be cost-effective.

Modified from *MMWR* 46(RR-18), 1998.

TABLE 5-17   **Immunizing Agents and Immunization Schedules for Health-Care Workers (HCWs)*—cont'd**

GENERIC NAME	PRIMARY SCHEDULE AND BOOSTER(S)	INDICATIONS	MAJOR PRECAUTIONS AND CONTRAINDICATIONS	SPECIAL CONSIDERATIONS
Varicella-zoster immune globulin (VZIG)	Persons <50 kg: 125 μ/10 kg IM; persons ≥50 kg: 625 μ§	Persons known or likely to be susceptible (particularly those at high risk for complications, e.g., pregnant women) who have close and prolonged exposure to a contact case or to an infectious hospital staff worker or patient		Serologic testing may help in assessing whether to administer VZIG. If use of VZIG prevents varicella disease, patient should be vaccinated subsequently.

BCG Vaccination

Bacille Calmette Guérin (BCG) vaccine (tuberculosis)	One percutaneous dose of 0.3 ml; no booster dose recommended	Should be considered only for HCWs in areas where multidrug tuberculosis is prevalent, a strong likelihood of infection exists, and where comprehensive infection control precautions have failed to prevent TB transmission to HCWs	Should not be administered to immunocompromised persons,‡ pregnant women	In the United States tuberculosis-control efforts are directed toward early identification, treatment of cases, and preventive therapy with isoniazid.

Other Immunobiologics That Are or May Be Indicated for Health-Care Workers

Immune globulin (hepatitis A)	**Postexposure**—One IM dose of 0.02 ml/kg administered ≤2 wk after exposure	Indicated for HCWs exposed to feces of infectious patients	Contraindicated in persons with IgA deficiency; do not administer within 2 wk after MMR vaccine, or 3 wk after varicella vaccine. Delay administration of MMR vaccine for ≥3 mo and varicella vaccine ≥5 mo after administration of IG	Administer in large muscle mass (deltoid, gluteal).

§Some experts recommend 125 μ/10 kg regardless of total body weight.

V

TABLE 5-18 Recommendations for Persons with Medical Conditions Requiring Special Vaccination Considerations

CONDITION	TD	MMR	VARICELLA	HBV	HAV	PNEUMOVAX§	INFLUENZA‖	HbCV	MENINGOCOCCAL	IPV	OTHER LIVE VACCINES#	OTHER KILLED VACCINES**
HIV infection	Rou	Rou/Contr*	Contr†	Rou‡	Rou	Rec	Rec	Cons	Rou	Rou	Contr	Rou
Severe immunocompromise††	Rou	Contr	Contr†	Rou‡	Rou	Rec	Rec	Rou‡‡	Rou	Rou	Contr	Rou
Renal failure	Rou	Rou	Rou	Rec‡	Rou	Rec	Rec	Rou	Rou	Rou	Rou	Rou
Diabetes	Rou	Rou	Rou	Rou	Rou	Rec	Rec	Rou	Rou	Rou	Rou	Rou
Chronic liver disease	Rou	Rou	Rou	Rou	Rec	Rec	Rec	Rou	Rou	Rou	Rou	Rou
Cardiac disease	Rou	Rou	Rou	Rou	Rou	Rec	Rec	Rou	Rou	Rou	Rou	Rou
Pulmonary disease	Rou	Rou	Rou	Rou	Rou	Rec	Rec	Rou	Rou	Rou	Rou	Rou
Alcoholism	Rou	Rou	Rou	Rou	Rou	Rec	Rec	Rou	Rou	Rou	Rou	Rou
Functional/anatomic asplenia	Rou	Rou	Rou	Rou	Rou	Rec§§	Rec	Rec§§	Rec§§	Rou	Rou	Rou
Terminal complement deficiency	Rou	Rou	Rou	Rou	Rou	Rou	Rou	Rou	Rec	Rou	Rou	
Clotting factor disorders	Rou	Rou	Rou	Rec	Rec	Rou	Rou	Rou	Rou	Rou	Rou	Rou

Modified and updated from CDC: *MMWR* 42(RR-4):16 and 17, 1993.

Cons, Consider vaccination; *Contr,* contraindicated; *Rec,* recommended; *Rou,* routine as outlined for all adults.

*For asymptomatic, nonseverely immunocompromised persons with human immunodeficiency virus (HIV), MMR can be used; it is contraindicated in severely immunocompromised persons. MMR can be considered in symptomatic HIV patients without severe immunocompromise.

†Varicella can be given to household members and caregivers, but if varicella-like rash develops after vaccination, contact should be avoided.

‡Recommended for persons with severe chronic renal failure approaching or already receiving dialysis, and higher doses should be given. Antibody titers should be measured after vaccination in these patients and in those with HIV or severe immunocompromise (who may require higher doses) to ensure adequate response. Yearly titers should be measured in dialysis patients.

§Pneumovax should be repeated in 5 years for patients in whom vaccine is recommended. Asthma without chronic obstructive pulmonary disease is not an indication for the vaccine.

‖Influenza vaccine should also be given to caregivers and household members.

#Includes bacille Calmette-Guérin, vaccinia, oral typhoid, yellow fever (if exposure cannot be avoided, persons with HIV can be given yellow fever vaccine; see text).

**Includes rabies (check postvaccination titers in HIV or severely immunocompromised persons), Lyme, inactivated typhoid, cholera, plague, and anthrax.

††Severe immunocompromise can result from congenital immunodeficiency, leukemia, lymphoma, malignancy, organ transplant, chemotherapy, radiation therapy, or high-dose corticosteroids.

‡‡Only for persons with Hodgkin's disease.

§§Give at least 2 weeks in advance of elective splenectomy.

Administration of Vaccines and Immune Globulins

TABLE 5-19   Administration of Multiple Vaccines and Immune Globulins

VACCINE COMBINATION	RECOMMENDED MINIMAL INTERVAL BETWEEN DOSES
≥2 killed vaccines	None. May be administered simultaneously or at any interval between doses. (If possible, cholera, parenteral typhoid, and plague vaccines should be given on separate occasions to avoid accentuating their side effects.)
Killed and live vaccines	None. May be administered simultaneously or at any interval between doses. (Cholera vaccine with yellow fever vaccine is the exception. These vaccines should be given separately at least 3 wk apart; otherwise the antibody response to each may be suboptimal.)
≥2 live vaccines	May be administered simultaneously. If given separately, there must be an interval of at least 4 wk between them. However, OPV can be administered at any time before, with, or after an MMR or oral typhoid, if indicated.
Live vaccine and PPD	May be administered simultaneously. If given separately, the PPD should be given 4 to 6 wk after the live vaccine.
Immune globulin and killed vaccine	None. May be administered simultaneously or at any interval between doses.
Immune globulin and live vaccine	Should not be given together. The live vaccine should be given a minimum of 2 wk before the immune globulin. If the live vaccine is to be given after the immune globulin, the minimum time that should elapse between administration is dose dependent and is outlined in Table 5-17. Of note, OPV, oral typhoid, and yellow fever are exceptions to these recommendations and can be given any time before, during, or after an immune globulin–containing product.

Modified from *MMWR* 43(RR-1):15-16, 1994.

TABLE 5-20   Minimal Interval Between Vaccine Doses for Use When Immunization Is Behind Schedule*

VACCINE TYPE	MINIMAL INTERVAL BETWEEN DOSE 1 AND 2	MINIMAL INTERVAL BETWEEN DOSE 2 AND 3	MINIMAL INTERVAL BETWEEN DOSE 3 AND 4
Hepatitis B	1 mo	2 mo†	
DTP/DTaP (DT)‡	4 wk	4 wk	6 mo
Hib (primary series)			
HbOC	1 mo	1 mo	2 mo and ≥ 12 mo old§
PRP-T	1 mo	1 mo	2 mo and ≥ 12 mo old§
PRP-OMP	1 mo	2 mo and ≥ 12 mo old§	
Poliovirus	4 wk	4 wk	No earlier than 4 yr
MMR‖	1 mo‖		

Modified from Centers for Disease Control and Prevention: *Epidemiology and prevention of vaccine-preventable diseases*, ed 5, Atlanta, 1999, CDC.
DTP/DTaP (DT), Diphtheria and tetanus toxoids and whole-cell pertussis vaccine/diphtheria and tetanus toxoids and acellular pertussis vaccine (diphtheria and tetanus toxoids vaccine); *HbOC*, oligosaccharides conjugated to diphtheria CRM_{197} toxin protein; Hib, *Haemophilus influenzae* type b conjugate vaccine; *MMR*, measles-mumps-rubella vaccine; *PRP-OMP*, polyribosylribitol phosphate polysaccharide conjugated to a meningococcal outer membrane protein; *PRP-T*, polyribosylribitol phosphate polysaccharide conjugated to tetanus toxoid.
*The minimal acceptable intervals may not correspond with the optimal recommended ages and intervals for vaccination.
†This final dose of hepatitis B vaccine is recommended at least 4 mo after the first dose and no earlier than 6 mo of age.
‡The total number of doses of diphtheria and tetanus toxoids should not exceed six each before the seventh birthday.
§The booster dose of Hib vaccine that is recommended following the primary vaccination series should be administered no earlier than 12 mo of age and at least 2 mo after the previous dose of Hib vaccine.
‖Although the age for measles vaccination may be as young as 6 mo in outbreak areas where cases are occurring in children less than 1 yr of age, children initially vaccinated before the first birthday should be revaccinated at 12 to 15 mo of age and an additional dose of vaccine should be administered at the time of school entry or according to local policy.

V

TABLE 5-21 Suggested Intervals Between Administration of Immune Globulin Preparations for Various Indications and Vaccines*

INDICATIONS	DOSE	INTERVAL (MO) BEFORE MEASLES VACCINATION
Tetanus prophylaxis (TIG)	250 units (10 mg IgG per kg) IM	3
Hepatitis A prophylaxis (IG)		
Contact prophylaxis	0.02 ml/kg (3.3 mg IgG per kg) IM	3
International travel	0.06 ml/kg (10 mg IgG per kg) IM	3
Hepatitis B prophylaxis (HBIG)	0.06 ml/kg (10 mg IgG per kg) IM	3
Rabies prophylaxis (HRIG)	20 IU/kg (22 mg IgG per kg) IM	4
Varicella prophylaxis (VZIG)	125 units per 10 kg (20 to 40 mg IgG per kg) IM (maximum: 625 units)	5
Measles prophylaxis (IG)		
Standard (i.e., nonimmunocompromised) contact	0.25 ml/kg (40 mg IgG per kg) IM	5
Immunocompromised contact	0.50 ml/kg (80 mg IgG per kg) IM	6
Blood transfusion		
RBCs, washed	10 ml/kg (negligible IgG per kg) IV	0
RBCs, adenine-saline added	10 ml/kg (10 mg IgG per kg) IV	3
Packed RBCs (hematocrit: 65%)†	10 ml/kg (60 mg IgG per kg) IV	6
Whole blood (hematocrit: 35% to 50%)†	10 ml/kg (80 to 100 mg IgG per kg) IV	6
Plasma/platelet products	10 ml/kg (160 mg IgG per kg) IV	7
Replacement therapy for immune deficiencies‡	300 to 400 mg/kg IV (as IVIG)	8
Respiratory syncytial virus prophylaxis	750 mg/kg IV (as RSV-IGIV)	9
Immune thrombocytopenic purpura	400 mg/kg IV (as IGIV)	8
	1000 mg/kg IV (as IGIV)	10
Kawasaki disease	2 g/kg IV (as IGIV)	11

Modified from *MMWR* 47(RR-8):24, 1998.

HBIG, Hepatitis B immune globulin; *HRIG,* human rabies immune globulin; *IG,* serum immune globulin; *IGIV,* immune globulin, intravenous; *IM,* intramuscularly; *IV,* intravenously; *RBCs,* red blood cells; *RSV-IGIV,* respiratory syncytial virus immune globulin, intravenous; *TIG,* tetanus immune globulin; *VZIG,* varicella zoster immune globulin.

*This table is not intended for determining the correct indications and dosage for the use of immune globulin preparations. Unvaccinated persons may not be fully protected against measles during the entire suggested time interval, and additional doses of immune globulin or measles vaccine, or both, may be indicated after measles exposure. The concentration of measles antibody in a particular immune globulin preparation can vary by lot. The rate of antibody clearance after receipt of an immune globulin preparation can vary. The recommended intervals are extrapolated from an estimated half-life of 30 days for passively acquired antibody and an observed interference with the immune response to measles vaccine for 5 mo after a dose of 80 mg IgG per kg.

†Assumes a serum IgG concentration of 16 mg per ml.

‡Measles vaccination is recommended for children infected with human immunodeficiency virus who do not have evidence of severe immunosuppression, but is contraindicated for patients who have congenital disorders of the immune system.

TABLE 5-22   Vaccinations for International Travel

DISEASE*	AREAS AFFECTED†	PROPHYLAXIS RECOMMENDED	IDEAL TIME BETWEEN LAST VACCINE DOSE AND TRAVEL
Tetanus	All	All travelers; vaccine series/booster.	Probably 30 days for series Anamnestic response to booster
Measles	All	Born after 1956; ensure immunity by antibody titer, diagnosed measles, or two doses of vaccine.	As MMR, 7-14 days
Rubella	All	Born after 1956 and any female of childbearing age; rubella titer or one dose of vaccine.	As MMR, 7-14 days
Mumps	All	Born after 1956; ensure immunity by antibody titer, diagnosed mumps, or one dose of vaccine.	As MMR, 7-14 days
Varicella	All	All travelers; antibody titer, reported illness, or vaccine series.	7-14 days
Hepatitis B	5%-20% of population are carriers in Africa, Middle East except Israel, all Southeast Asia, Amazon basin, Haiti, and Dominican Republic; 1%-5% of population are carriers in south-central and southwest Asia, Israel, Japan, Americas, Russia, and eastern and southern Europe.	Travelers for more than 6 mo in close contact with population or for less time but with high-risk activities (close household contact, seeking dental or medical care, sex); vaccine series.	Probably 30 days
Hepatitis A	Developing countries.	Travelers to rural areas; eating and drinking in settings of poor sanitation; vaccine or pooled immune globulin (IG).	Vaccine, 30 days Pooled IG, 2 days
Influenza	Tropics throughout the year; southern hemisphere from April to September.	Travelers for whom vaccine is otherwise indicated; give current vaccine and revaccinate in fall as usual.	7-14 days
Meningococcus*	Sub-Saharan Africa "belt" (Senegal to Ethiopia) from December to June; required for pilgrims to Saudi Arabia during Hajj; epidemics reported in other African nations, India, Nepal, and Mongolia.	All travelers; vaccine.	7-10 days
Rabies	Endemic dog rabies exists in Mexico, El Salvador, Guatemala, Peru, Colombia, Ecuador, India, Nepal, Philippines, Sri Lanka, Thailand, and Vietnam.	Travelers staying for more than 30 days or at high risk of exposure to domestic or wild animals; vaccine series/booster.	7-14 days
Poliomyelitis	Developing countries not in western hemisphere; at risk all year in tropics; in temperate zones, incidence increases in summer and fall.	All travelers; vaccine series/booster.	Parenteral vaccine series, 28 day (see text) Anamnestic response to booster

Continued

V

TABLE 5-22 **Vaccinations for International Travel—cont'd**

DISEASE*	AREAS AFFECTED†	PROPHYLAXIS RECOMMENDED	IDEAL TIME BETWEEN LAST VACCINE DOSE AND TRAVEL
Typhoid fever	Many countries in Asia, Africa, Central America, and South America.	Travelers with prolonged stay in rural areas with poor sanitation; vaccine series/booster.	Oral vaccine, 7 days Parenteral vaccine, probably 14 days
Yellow fever*	North and central South America, forest-savannah zones of Africa; some countries in Africa, Asia, and Middle East require travelers from endemic areas to be vaccinated.	All travelers; vaccine/booster at approved yellow fever vaccination center.	10 days
Japanese encephalitis	Seasonally in most areas of Asia, Indian subcontinent, and western Pacific islands; in temperate zones, incidence increases in summer and early fall; in tropics, year-round incidence.	Travelers staying for more than 30 days in high-risk rural areas; staying outdoors during transmission season; vaccine series.	10 days
Cholera*	Certain undeveloped countries.	If required by local authorities, one dose usually suffices; primary series only for those living in high-risk areas under poor sanitary conditions or those with compromised gastric defense mechanisms (achlorhydria, antacid therapy, pervious ulcer surgery); booster every 6 mo.	Probably 30 days
Plague	Africa, Asia, and Americas in rural mountainous or upland areas.	Travelers whose research or field activities bring them in contact with rodents; vaccine series/booster; consider taking tetracycline (500 mg four times a day) for chemoprophylaxis (inferred from clinical experience in treating plague).	Probably 30 days

From Noble J: *Primary care medicine,* ed 3, St Louis, 2001, Mosby.
*Only yellow fever vaccine is required for entry by any country; cholera vaccine may be required by some local authorities; and meningococcus vaccine is required for pilgrims to Mecca, Saudia Arabia, during Haj. However, it is important to follow CDC recommendations for all vaccines to prevent disease. If a required vaccine is contraindicated or withheld for any reason, attempts should be made to obtain a waiver from the country's consulate or embassy.
†Because areas affected can change, and for more specific details, consult CDC's traveler's hotline.

TABLE 5-23   Recommended Schedule of Hepatitis B Immunoprophylaxis to Prevent Perinatal Transmission

POPULATION GROUP	VACCINE DOSE*	AGE OF INFANT
Infants born to HBsAg-positive mothers	First dose	Birth (within 12 hr)
	HBIG†	Birth (within 12 hr)
	Second dose	1 mo
	Third dose	6 mo‡
Infants born to mothers not screened for HBsAg§	First dose	Birth (within 12 hr)
	HBIG‡	If mother is HBsAg positive, administer HBIG to infant as soon as possible, not later than 1 wk after birth
	Second dose	1-2 mo‖
	Third dose	6 mo‡

Modified from *MMWR* 40(RR-13):12, 1991.
HbsAg, Hepatitis B surface antigen; *HBIG*, hepatitis B immune globulin.
*See Table 5-20 for appropriate vaccine dose.
†HBIG is given in a dose of 0.5 ml, administered intramuscularly at a site different from that used for vaccine.
‡If four-dose schedule (Engerix-B) is used, the third dose is administered at 2 mo of age and the fourth dose at 12-18 mo.
§First vaccine dose is the same as the dose for an HBsAg-positive mother (see Table 5-20). If mother is HBsAg positive, continue that dose; if mother is HBsAg negative, use appropriate dose from Table 5-20.
‖Infants of women who are HBsAg negative can be vaccinated at 2 mo of age.

TABLE 5-24   Recommended Doses of Currently Licensed Hepatitis B Vaccines

POPULATION GROUP	RECOMBIVAX HB* DOSE IN μG (DOSE IN ml)	ENGERIX-B* DOSE IN μG (DOSE IN ml)
Infants of HbsAg-negative mothers and children <11 yr	2.5 (0.25)	10 (0.5)
Infants of HbsAg-positive mothers; prevention of perinatal infection	5 (0.5)	10 (0.5)
Children and adolescents 11-19 yr	5 (0.5)	20 (1.0)
Adults ≥20 yr	10 (1.0)	20 (1.0)
Dialysis patients and other immunocompromised persons	40†	40‡

Modified from *MMWR* 40(RR-13):7, 1991.
*Both vaccines are routinely administered in a three-dose series at 0, 1, and 6 mo. Engerix-B is also licensed for a four-dose series administered at 0, 1, 2, and 12 mo.
†Special formulation.
‡Two 1.0-ml doses administered at one site in a four-dose schedule at 0, 1, 2, and 6 mo.

Endocarditis Prophylaxis

BOX 5-1   Cardiac Conditions Associated with Endocarditis

Endocarditis Prophylaxis Recommended
High-Risk Category

Prosthetic cardiac valves, including bioprosthetic and homograft valves
Previous bacterial endocarditis
Complex cyanotic congenital heart disease (e.g., single ventricle states, transposition of the great arteries, tetralogy of Fallot)
Surgically constructed systemic pulmonary shunts or conduits

Moderate-Risk Category

Most other congenital cardiac malformations (other than above and below)
Acquired valvar dysfunction (e.g., rheumatic heart disease)
Hypertrophic cardiomyopathy
Mitral valve prolapse with valvar regurgitation and/or thickened leaflets

Endocarditis Prophylaxis Not Recommended
Negligible-Risk Category (No Greater Risk Than the General Population)

Isolated secundum atrial septal defect
Surgical repair of atrial septal defect, ventricular defect, or patent ductus arteriosus (without residua beyond 6 mos)
Previous coronary artery bypass graft surgery
Mitral valve prolapse without valvar regurgitation
Physiologic, functional, or innocent heart murmurs
Previous Kawasaki disease without valvar dysfunction
Previous rheumatic fever without valvar dysfunction
Cardiac pacemakers (intravascular and epicardial) and implanted defibrillators

---

From Dajani AS et al: *JAMA* 277:1794-1801, 1997.

V

BOX 5-2 Dental Procedures and Endocarditis Prophylaxis

Endocarditis Prophylaxis Recommended*

Dental extractions

Periodontal procedures including surgery, scaling and root planing, probing, and recall maintenance

Dental implant placement and reimplantation of avulsed teeth

Endodontic (root canal) instrumentation of surgery only beyond the apex

Subgingival placement of antibiotic fibers or strips

Initial placement of orthodontic bands—but not brackets

Intraligamentary local anesthetic injections

Prophylactic cleaning of teeth or implants where bleeding is anticipated

Endocarditis Prophylaxis Not Recommended

Restorative dentistry† (operative and prosthodontic) with or without retraction cord‡

Local anesthetic injections (nonintraligamentary)

Intracanal endodontic treatment; postplacement and buildup

Placement of rubber dams

Postoperative suture removal

Placement of removable prosthodontic or orthodontic appliances

Taking of oral impressions

Fluoride treatments

Taking of oral radiographs

Orthodontic appliance adjustment

Shedding of primary teeth

From Dajani AS et al: *JAMA* 277:1794-1801, 1997.
*Prophylaxis is recommended for patients with high- and moderate-risk cardiac conditions.
†This includes restoration of decayed teeth (filling cavities) and replacement of missing teeth.
‡Clinical judgment may indicate antibiotic use in selected circumstances that may create significant bleeding.

BOX 5-3 Other Procedures and Endocarditis Prophylaxis

Endocarditis Prophylaxis Recommended
Respiratory tract

Tonsillectomy and/or adenoidectomy

Surgical operations that involve respiratory mucosa

Bronchoscopy with a rigid bronchoscope

*Gastrointestinal Tract***

Sclerotherapy for esophageal varices

Esophageal stricture dilation

Endoscopic retrograde cholangiography* with biliary obstruction

Biliary tract surgery

Surgical operations that involve intestinal mucosa

Genitourinary Tract

Prostatic surgery

Cystoscopy

Urethral dilation

Endocarditis Prophylaxis Not Recommended
Respiratory Tract

Endotracheal intubation

Bronchoscopy with a flexible bronchoscope, with or without biopsy†

Tympanostomy tube insertion

Gastrointestinal Tract

Transesophageal echocardiography†

Endoscopy with or without gastrointestinal biopsy†

Genitourinary Tract

Vaginal hysterectomy†

Vaginal delivery†

Cesarean section

In uninfected tissue:
    Urethral catheterization
    Uterine dilation and curettage
    Therapeutic abortion
    Sterilization procedures
    Insertion or removal of intrauterine devices

Other

Cardiac catheterization, including balloon angioplasty

Implanted cardiac pacemakers, implanted defibrillators, and coronary stents

Incision or biopsy of surgically scrubbed skin

Circumcision

From Dajani AS et al: *JAMA* 277:1794-1801, 1997.
*Prophylaxis is recommended for high-risk patients; optional for medium-risk patients.
†Prophylaxis is optional for high-risk patients.

TABLE 5-25 **Prophylactic Regimens for Dental, Oral, Respiratory Tract, or Esophageal Procedures**

SITUATION	AGENT	REGIMEN*
Standard general prophylaxis	Amoxicillin	Adults: 2.0 g; children: 50 mg/kg orally (PO) 1 hr before procedure
Unable to take oral medications	Ampicillin	Adults: 2.0 g intramuscularly (IM) or intravenously (IV); children: 50 mg/kg IM or IV within 30 min before procedure
Allergic to penicillin	Clindamycin *or*	Adults: 600 mg; children: 20 mg/kg PO 1 hr before procedure
	Cephalexin† or cefadroxil† *or*	Adults: 2.0 g; children: 50 mg/kg PO 1 hr before procedure
	Azithromycin or clarithromycin	Adults: 500 mg; children: 15 mg/kg PO 1 hr before procedure
Allergic to penicillin and unable to take oral medications	Clindamycin *or*	Adults: 600 mg; children: 20 mg/kg IV within 30 min of procedure
	Cefazolin†	Adults 1.0 g; children: 25 mg/kg IM or IV within 30 min of procedure

From Dajani AS et al: *JAMA* 277:1794-1801, 1997.
*Total children's dose should not exceed adult dose.
†Cephalosporins should not be used in individuals with immediate-type hypersensitivity reaction (urticaria, angioedema, or anaphylaxis) to penicillins.

TABLE 5-26 **Prophylactic Regimens or Genitourinary Gastrointestinal (Excluding Esophageal) Procedures**

SITUATION	AGENTS*	REGIMEN†
High-risk patients	Ampicillin plus gentamicin	Adults: ampicillin 2.0 g intramuscularly (IM) or intravenously (IV) plus gentamicin 1.5 mg/kg (not to exceed 120 mg) within 30 min of starting the procedure; 6 hr later, ampicillin 1 g IM/IV or amoxicillin 1 g orally (PO)
		Children: ampicillin 50 mg/kg IM or IV (not to exceed 2.0 g) plus gentamicin 1.5 mg/kg within 30 min of starting the procedure; 6 hr later, ampicillin 25 g/kg IM/IV or amoxicillin 25 mg/kg PO
High-risk patients allergic to ampicillin	Vancomycin plus gentamicin	Adults: vancomycin 1.0 g IV over 1-2 hr plus gentamicin 1.5 mg/kg IV/IM (not to exceed 120 mg); complete injection/infusion within 30 min of starting the procedure
		Children: vancomycin 20 mg/kg IV over 1-2 hr plus gentamicin 1.5 mg/kg IV/IM; complete injection/infusion within 30 min of starting the procedure
Moderate-risk patients	Amoxicillin or ampicillin	Adults: amoxicillin 2.0 g PO 1 hr before procedure, or ampicillin 2.0 g IV/IV within 30 min of starting the procedure
		Children: amoxicillin 50 mg/kg PO 1 hr before procedure, or ampicillin 50 mg/kg IM/IV within 30 min of starting the procedure
Moderate-risk patients allergic to ampicillin/amoxicillin	Vancomycin	Adults: vancomycin 1.0 g IV over 1-2 hr; complete infusion within 30 min of starting the procedure
		Children: vancomycin 20 mg/kg IV over 1-2 hr; complete infusion within 30 min of starting the procedure

From Dajani AS et al: *JAMA* 277:1794-1801, 1997.
*Total children's dose should not exceed adult dose.
†No second dose of vancomycin or gentamicin is recommended.

V

TABLE 5-27　**Recommended Daily Dosage of Influenza Antiviral Medications for Treatment and Prophylaxis**

ANTIVIRAL AGENT	AGE GROUPS				
	ONE TO SIX YEARS	SEVEN TO NINE YEARS	10 TO 12 YEARS	13 TO 64 YEARS	65 YEARS AND OLDER
Amantadine[a]					
Treatment	5 mg per kg per day up to 150 mg in two divided doses[b]	5 mg per kg per day up to 150 mg in two divided doses[b]	100 mg bid[c]	100 mg bid[c]	100 mg or less per day
Prophylaxis	5 mg per kg per day up to 150 mg in two divided doses[b]	5 mg per kg per day up to 150 mg in two divided doses[b]	100 mg bid[c]	100 mg bid[c]	100 mg or less per day
Rimantadine[d]					
Treatment[e]	NA	NA	NA	100 mg bid[c]	100 or 200[f] mg per day
Prophylaxis	5 mg per kg per day up to 150 mg in two divided doses[b]	5 mg per kg per day up to 150 mg in two divided doses[b]	100 mg bid[c]	100 mg bid[c]	100 or 200[f] mg per day
Zanamivir[g,h]					
Treatment	NA	10 mg bid	10 mg bid	10 mg bid	10 mg bid
Oseltamivir					
Treatment[i]	Dose varies by child's weight[j]	Dose varies by child's weight[j]	Dose varies by child's weight[j]	75 mg bid	75 mg bid
Prophylaxis	NA	NA	NA	75 mg per day	75 mg per day

From *MMWR Morb Mortal Wkly Rep* 50(RR-4):1, 2001.
NA, Not applicable.
[a]The drug package insert should be consulted for dosage recommendations for administering amantadine to persons with creatinine clearance of 50 mL or less per min per 1.73m^2.
[b]5 mg per kg of amantadine or rimantadine syrup = 1 tsp/22 lb.
[c]Children 10 yr of age or older who weigh less than 40 kg (88 lb) should be administered amantadine or rimantadine at a dosage of 5 mg per kg per day.
[d]A reduction in dosage to 100 mg per day of rimantadine is recommended for persons who have severe hepatic dysfunction or those with creatinine clearance of 10 ml or less per min. Other persons with less severe hepatic or renal dysfunction taking 100 mg per day of rimantadine should be observed closely, and the dosage should be reduced or the drug discontinued, if necessary.
[e]Only approved for treatment in adults.
[f]Elderly residents of nursing homes should be administered only 100 mg per day of rimantadine. A reduction in dosage of 100 mg per day should be considered for all persons 65 yr of age or older if they experience side effects when taking 200 mg per day.
[g]Zanamivir is administered via inhalation by using a plastic device included in the package with the medication. Patients will benefit from instruction and demonstration of correct use of the device.
[h]Zanamivir is not approved for prophylaxis.
[i]A reduction in the dose of oseltamivir is recommended for persons with creatinine clearance of less than 30 ml per min.
[j]The dose recommendation for children who weigh less than 15 kg (33 lb) is 30 mg bid; for children weighing 15 to 23 kg (33 to 50.6 lb), the dose is 45 mg bid; for children weighing 23 to 40 kg (50.6 to 88 lb), the dose is 60 mg bid; and for children weighing more than 40 kg (88 lb), the dose is 75 mg bid.

BOX 5-4 Recommendations for the Contents of the Occupational Exposure Report

- Date and time of exposure
- Details of the procedure being performed, including where and how the exposure occurred; if related to a sharp device, the type and brand of device and how and when in the course of handling the device the exposure occurred
- Details of the exposure, including the type and amount of fluid or material and the severity of the exposure (e.g., for a percutaneous exposure, depth of injury and whether fluid was injected; for a skin or mucous membrane exposure, the estimated volume of material and the condition of the skin [e.g., chapped, abraded, intact])
- Details about the exposure source (e.g., whether the source material contained HBV, HCV, or HIV; if the source is HIV-infected, the stage of disease, history of antiretroviral therapy, viral load, and antiretroviral resistance information, if known)
- Details about the exposed person (e.g., hepatitis B vaccination and vaccine-response status)
- Details about counseling, postexposure management, and follow-up

---

From *MMRW* 50(RR-11), 2001.
HBV, Hepatitis B virus; *HCV,* hepatitis C virus; *HIV,* human immunodeficiency virus.

BOX 5-5 Factors to Consider in Assessing the Need for Follow-up of Occupational Exposures

- Type of exposure
  — Percutaneous injury
  — Mucous membrane exposure
  — Nonintact skin exposure
  — Bites resulting in blood exposure to either person involved
- Type and amount of fluid/tissue
  — Blood
  — Fluids containing blood
  — Potentially infectious fluid or tissue (semen; vaginal secretions; and cerebrospinal, synovial, pleural, peritoneal, pericardial, and amniotic fluids)
  — Direct contact with concentrated virus
- Infectious status of source
  — Presence of HbsAg
  — Presence of HCV antibody
  — Presence of HIV antibody
- Susceptibility of exposed person
  — Hepatitis B vaccine and vaccine response status
  — HBV, HCV, and HIV immune status

From *MMRW* 50(RR-11), 2001.
HBsAg, Hepatitis B surface antigen; HBV, hepatitis B virus; *HCV,* hepatitis C virus; *HIV,* human immunodeficiency virus.

BOX 5-6 Evaluation of Occupational Exposure Sources

Known sources

- Test known sources for HBsAg, anti-HCV, and HIV antibody
  — Direct virus assays for routine screening of source patients are **not** recommended
  — Consider using a rapid HIV-antibody test
  — If the source person is **not** infected with a bloodborne pathogen, baseline testing or further follow-up of the exposed person is **not** necessary
- For sources whose infection status remains unknown (e.g., the source person refuses testing), consider medical diagnoses, clinical symptoms, and history of risk behaviors
- Do not test discarded needles for bloodborne pathogens

Unknown sources

- For unknown sources, evaluate the likelihood of exposure to a source at high risk for infection
  — Consider likelihood of bloodborne pathogen infection among patient sin the exposure setting

---

HbsAg, Hepatitis B surface antigen; *HCV,* hepatitis C virus; *HIV,* human immunodeficiency virus.

TABLE 5-28   Recommended Postexposure Prophylaxis for Exposure to Hepatitis B Virus

VACCINATION AND ANTIBODY RESPONSE STATUS OF EXPOSED WORKERS*	TREATMENT		
	SOURCE HBsAg POSITIVE	SOURCE HBsAg NEGATIVE	SOURCE UNKNOWN OR NOT AVAILABLE FOR TESTING
Unvaccinated	HBIG† × 1 and initiate HB vaccine series‡	Initiate HB vaccine series	Initiate HB vaccine series
Previously vaccinated			
Known responder§	No treatment	No treatment	No treatment
Known nonresponder‖	HBIG × 1 and initiate revaccination or HBIG × 2¶	No treatment	If known high-risk source, treat as if source were HBsAg positive
Antibody response unknown	Test exposed person for anti-HBs¶ 1. If adequate,§ no treatment is necessary 2. If inadequate,‖ administer HBIG × 1 and vaccine booster	No treatment	Test exposed person for anti-HBs 1. If adequate,‡ no treatment is necessary 2. If inadequate,‡ administer vaccine booster and recheck titer in 1-2 mo

Anti-HBs, Antibody to HBsAg; *HB,* hepatitis B; *HBIG,* hepatitis B immune globulin; *HBsAg,* hepatitis B surface antigen.
*Persons who have previously been infected with HBV are immune to reinfection and do not require postexposure prophylaxis.
†Hepatitis B immune globulin; dose is 0.06 ml/kg intramuscularly.
‡Hepatitis B vaccine.
§A responder is a person with adequate levels of serum antibody to HBsAg (i.e., anti-HBs ≥10 mIU/ml).
‖A nonresponder is a person with inadequate response to vaccination (i.e., serum anti-HBs <10 mIU/ml).
¶The option of giving one dose of HBIG and reinitiating the vaccine series is preferred for nonresponders who have not completed a second 3-dose vaccine series. For persons who previously completed a second vaccine series but failed to respond, two doses of HBIG are preferred.

TABLE 5-29   Recommended HIV Postexposure Prophylaxis for Percutaneous Injuries

EXPOSURE TYPE	INFECTION STATUS OF SOURCE				
	HIV-POSITIVE CLASS 1*	HIV-POSITIVE CLASS 2*	SOURCE OF UNKNOWN HIV STATUS†	UNKNOWN SOURCE‡	HIV-NEGATIVE
Less severe§	Recommend basic 2-drug PEP	Recommend expanded 3-drug PEP	Generally, no PEP warranted; however, consider basic 2-drug PEP‖ for source with HIV risk factors††	Generally, no PEP warranted; however, consider basic 2-drug PEP‖ in settings where exposure to HIV-infected persons is likely	No PEP warranted
More severe#	Recommend expanded 3-drug PEP	Recommend expanded 3-drug PEP	Generally, no PEP warranted; however, consider basic 2-drug PEP‖ for source with HIV risk factors¶	Generally, no PEP warranted; however, consider basic 2-drug PEP‖ in settings where exposure to HIV-infected persons is likely	No PEP warranted

HIV, Human immunodeficiency virus; *PEP,* postexposure prophylaxis (see Box 5-10).
*HIV-Positive, Class 1—asymptomatic HIV infection or known low viral load (e.g., <1500 RNA copies/ml). HIV—Positive, Class 2-symptomatic HIV infection, acquired immunodeficiency syndrome, acute seroconversion, or known high viral load. If drug resistance is a concern, obtain expert consultation. Initiation of PEP should not be delayed pending expert consultation, and, because expert consultation alone cannot substitute for face-to-face counseling, resources should be available to provide immediate evaluation and follow-up care for all exposures.
†Source of unknown HIV status (e.g., deceased source person with no samples available for HIV testing).
‡Unknown source (e.g., a needle from a sharps disposal container).
§Less severe (e.g., solid needle and superficial injury).
‖The designation "consider PEP" indicates that PEP is optional and should be based on an individualized decision between the exposed person and the treating clinician.
¶If PEP is offered and taken and the source is later determined to be HIV-negative, PEP should be discontinued.
#More severe (e.g., large-bore hollow needle, deep puncture, visible blood on device, or needle used in patient's artery or vein).

TABLE 5-30 **Recommended HIV Postexposure Prophylaxis for Mucous Membrane Exposures and Nonintact Skin[a] Exposures**

	INFECTION STATUS OF SOURCE				
EXPOSURE TYPE	HIV-POSITIVE CLASS 1[b]	HIV-POSITIVE CLASS 2[b]	SOURCE OF UNKNOWN HIV STATUS[c]	UNKNOWN SOURCE[d]	HIV-NEGATIVE
Small volume[e]	Consider basic 2-drug PEP[f]	Recommend basic 2-drug PEP	Generally, no PEP warranted; however, consider basic 2-drug PEP[f] for source with HIV risk factors[g]	Generally, no PEP warranted; however, consider basic 2-drug PEP[f] in settings where exposure to HIV-infected persons is likely	No PEP warranted
Large volume[h]	Recommend basic 2-drug PEP	Recommend expanded 3-drug PEP	Generally, no PEP warranted; however, consider basic 2-drug PEP[f] for source with HIV risk factors[g]	Generally, no PEP warranted; however, consider basic 2-drug PEP[f] in settings where exposure to HIV-infected persons is likely	No PEP warranted

HIV, Human immunodeficiency virus; *PEP,* postexposure prophylaxis (see Box 5-10).
[a]For skin exposures, follow-up is indicated only if there is evidence of compromised skin integrity (e.g., dermatitis, abrasion, or open wound).
[b]HIV-Positive, Class 1—asymptomatic HIV infection or known low viral load (e.g., <1,500 RNA copies/mL). HIV-Positive, Class 2—symptomatic HIV infection, acquired immunodeficiency syndrome, acute seroconversion, or known high viral load. If drug resistance is a concern, obtain expert consultation. Initiation of PEP should not be delayed pending expert consultation, and, because expert consultation alone cannot substitute for face-to-face counseling, resources should be available to provide immediate evaluation and follow-up care for all exposures.
[c] Source of unknown HIV status (e.g., deceased source person with no samples available for HIV testing).
[d]Unknown source (e.g., splash from inappropriately disposed blood).
[e]Small volume (i.e., a few drops).
[f]The designation, "consider PEP," indicates that PEP is optional and should be based on an individualized decision between the exposed person and the treating clinician.
[g]If PEP is offered and taken and the source is later determined to be HIV-negative, PEP should be discontinued.
[h]Large volume (i.e., major blood splash).

BOX 5-7 **Situations for Which Expert* Consultation for HIV Postexposure Prophylaxis Is Advised**

- Delayed (i.e., later than 24-36 hr) exposure report
  — the interval after which there is no benefit from postexposure prophylaxis (PEP) is undefined
- Unknown source (e.g., needle in sharps disposal container or laundry)
  — decide use of PEP on a case-by-case basis
  — consider the severity of the exposure and the epidemiologic likelihood of HIV exposure
  — do not test needles or other sharp instruments for HIV
- Known or suspected pregnancy in the exposed person
  — does not preclude the use of optimal PEP regimens
  — do not deny PEP solely on the basis of pregnancy
- Resistance of the source virus to antiretroviral agents
  — influence of drug resistance on transmission risk is unknown
  — selection of drugs to which the source person's virus is unlikely to be resistant is recommended, if the source person's virus is known or suspected to be resistant to ≥1 of the drugs considered for the PEP regimen
  — resistance testing of the source person's virus at the time of the exposure is not recommended
- Toxicity of the initial PEP regimen
  — adverse symptoms, such as nausea and diarrhea are common with PEP
  — symptoms often can be managed without changing the PEP regimen by prescribing antimotility and/or antiemetic agents
  — modification of dose intervals (i.e., administering a lower dose of drug more frequently throughout the day, as recommended by the manufacturer), in other situations, might help alleviate symptoms

HIV, Human immunodeficiency virus.
*Local experts and/or the National Clinicians' Postexposure Prophylaxis Hotline (PEPline [1-888-448-4911]).

V

BOX 5-8   Occupational Exposure Management Resources

National Clinicians' Postexposure Prophylaxis Hotline (PEPline)

Run by University of California–San Francisco/San Francisco General Hospital staff; supported by the Health Resources and Services Administration Ryan White CARE Act, HIV/AIDS Bureau, AIDS Education and Training Centers, and CDC.

Phone: (888) 448-4911
Internet: http://www.ucsf.edu/hivcntr

Needlestick!

A website to help clinicians manage and document occupational blood and body fluid exposures. Developed and maintained by the University of California, Los Angeles (UCLA), Emergency Medicine Center, UCLA School of Medicine, and funded in party by CDC and the Agency for Healthcare Research and Quality.

Internet: http://www.needlestick.mednet.ucla.edu

Hepatitis Hotline

Phone: (888) 443-7232
Internet: http://www.cdc.gov/ncidod/diseases/hepatitis/index.htm
Phone: (800) 893-0485

Reporting to CDC: Occupationally acquired HIV infections and failures of PEP.

HIV Antiretroviral Pregnancy Registry

Phone: (800) 258-4263
Fax: (800) 800-1052
Address:
    1410 Commonwealth Drive
    Suite 215
    Wilmington, NC 28405
Internet:
    http://www.glaxowellcome.com/preg_reg/antiretroviral

Food and Drug Administration

Report unusual or severe toxicity to antiretroviral agents.

Phone: (800) 332-1088
Address:
    MedWatch
    HF-2, FDA
    5600 Fishers Lane
    Rockville, MD 20857
    Internet: http://www.fda.gov/medwatch

HIV/AIDS Treatment Information Service

Internet: http://www.hivatis.org

BOX 5-9   Management of Occupational Blood Exposures

Provide immediate care to the exposure site:

- Wash wounds and skin with soap and water
- Flush mucous membranes with water

Determine risk associated with exposure:

- Type of fluid (e.g., blood, visibly bloody fluid, other potentially infectious fluid or tissue, and concentrated virus)
- Type of exposure (i.e., percutaneous injury, mucous membrane or nonintact skin exposure, and bites resulting in blood exposure)

Evaluate exposure source:

- Assess the risk of infection using available information
- Test known sources for HBsAg, anti-HCV, and HIV antibodies (consider using rapid testing)
- For unknown sources, assess risk of exposure to HBV, HCV, or HIV infection
- Do not test discarded needles or syringes for virus contamination

Evaluate the exposed person:

- Assess immune status for HBV infection (i.e., by history of hepatitis B vaccination and vaccine response)

Give PEP for exposures posing risk of infection transmission:

- HBV: See Table 5-28
- HCV: PEP not recommended
- HIV: See Tables 5-29 and 5-30
  - — Initiate PEP as soon as possible, preferably within hours of exposure
  - — Offer pregnancy testing to all women of childbearing age not known to be pregnant
  - — Seek expert consultation if viral resistance is suspected
  - — Administer PEP for 4 wk if tolerated

Perform follow-up testing and provide counseling:

- Advise exposed persons to seek medical evaluation for any acute illness occurring during follow-up

HBV exposures

- Perform follow-up anti-HBs testing in persons who receive hepatitis B vaccine
  - — Test for anti-HBs 1-2 mo after last dose of vaccine
  - — Anti-HBs response to vaccine cannot be ascertained if HBIG was received in the previous 3-4 mo

HCV exposures

- Perform baseline and follow-up testing for anti-HCV and alanine amino-transferase (ALT) 4-6 mo after exposures
- Perform HCV RNA at 4-6 wk if earlier diagnosis of HCV infection desired
- Confirm repeatedly reactive anti-HCV enzyme immunoassays (EIAs) with supplemental tests

HIV exposures

- Perform HIV-antibody testing for at least 6 mo postexposure (e.g., at baseline, 6 wk, 3 mo, and 6 mo)
- Perform HIV antibody testing if illness compatible with an acute retroviral syndrome occurs
- Advise exposed persons to use precautions to prevent secondary transmission during the follow-up period
- Evaluate exposed persons taking PEP within 72 hr after exposure and monitor for drug toxicity for at least 2 wk

HBIG, Hepatitis B immune globulin; *HBsAg,* hepatitis B surface antigen; *HBV,* hepatitis B virus; *HCV,* hepatitis C virus; *HIV,* human immunodeficiency virus; *PEP,* postexposure prophylaxis; *RNA,* ribonucleic acid.

V

BOX 5-10   Basic and Expanded HIV Postexposure Prophylaxis Regimens

Basic Regimen
- **Zidovudine (Retrovir; ZDV; AZT) and Lamivudine (Epivir; 3TC); available as Combivir**
  — ZDV: 600 mg per day, in two or three divided doses
  — 3TC: 150 mg bid

Advantages
  — ZDV is associated with decreased risk of HIV transmission in the CDC case-control study of occupational HIV infection
  — ZDV has been used more than the other drugs for PEP in HCP
  — Serious toxicity is rare when used for PEP
  — Side effects are predictable and manageable with antimotility and antiemetic agents
  — Probably a safe regimen for pregnant HCP
  — Can be given as a single tablet (Combivir) bid

Disadvantages
  — Side effects are common and might result in low adherence
  — Source patient virus might have resistance to this regimen
  — Potential for delayed toxicity (oncogenic/teratogenic) is unknown

Alternative Basic Regimens
- **Lamivudine (3TC) and Stavudine (Zerit; d4T)**
  — 3TC: 150 mg bid
  — d4T: 40 mg (if body weight is <60 kg, 30 mg) bid

Advantages
  — Well tolerated in patients with HIV infection, resulting in good adherence
  — Serious toxicity appears to be rare
  — Twice daily dosing might improve adherence

Disadvantages
  — Source patient virus might be resistant to this regimen
  — Potential for delayed toxicity (oncogenic/teratogenic) is unknown

- **Didanosine (Videx, chewable/dispersable buffered tablet; Videx EC, delayed-release capsule; ddI) and Stavudine (d4T)**
  — ddI: 400 mg (if body weight is <60 kg, 125 mg bid) daily, on an empty stomach
  — d4T: 40 mg (if body weight is <60 kg, 30 mg bid) bid

Advantages
  — Likely effective against HIV strains from source patients who are taking ZDV and 3TC

Disadvantages
  — ddI is difficult to administer and unpalatable.
  — Chewable/dispersable buffered tablet formulation of ddI interferes with absorption of some drugs (e.g., quinolone antibiotics, and indinavir).
  — Serious toxicity (e.g., neuropathy, pancreatitis, or hepatitis) can occur. Fatal and nonfatal pancreatitis has occurred in HIV-positive, treatment-naive patients. Patients taking ddI and d4T should be carefully assessed and closely monitored for pancreatitis, lactic acidosis, and hepatitis.
  — Side effects are common; anticipate diarrhea and low adherence.
  — Potential for delayed toxicity (oncogenic/teratogenic) is unknown.

Expanded Regimen
Basic regimen plus one of the following:

- **Indinavir (Crixivan; IDV)**
  — 800 mg every 8 hr, on an empty stomach

Advantages
  — Potent HIV inhibitor

Disadvantages
  — Serious toxicity (e.g., nephrolithiasis) can occur; must take 8 glasses of fluid per day
  — Hyperbilirubinemia common; must avoid this drug during late pregnancy
  — Requires acid for absorption and cannot be taken simultaneously with ddI in chewable/dispersable buffered tablet formulation (doses must be separated by at least 1 hr)
  — Concomitant use of astemizole, terfenadine, dihydroergotamine, ergotamine, ergonovine, methylergonovine, rifampin, cisapride, St. John's Wort, lovastatin, simvastatin, pimozide, midazolam, or triazolam is not recommended
  — Potential for delayed toxicity (oncogenic/teratogenic) is unknown

BOX 5-10   Basic and Expanded HIV Postexposure Prophylaxis Regimens—cont'd

- **Nelfinavir (Viracept; NFV)**
  - 750 mg tid, with meals or snack, or
  - 1250 mg bid, with meals or snack

Advantages

  - Potent HIV inhibitor
  - Twice dosing per day might improve adherence

Disadvantages

  - Concomitant use of astemizole, terfenadine, dihydroergotamine, ergotamine, ergonovine, methylergonovine, rifampin, cisapride, St. John's Wort, lovastatin, simvastatin, pimozide, midazolam, or triazolam is not recommended
  - Might accelerate the clearance of certain drugs, including oral contraceptives (requiring alternative or additional contraceptive measures for women taking these drugs)
  - Potential for delayed toxicity (oncogenic/teratogenic) is unknown

- **Efavirenz (Sustiva; EFV)**
  - 600 mg daily, at bedtime

Advantages

  - Does not require phosphorylation before activation and might be active earlier than other antiretroviral agents (Note: this might be only a theoretical advantage of no clinical benefit)
  - One dose daily might improve adherence

Disadvantages

  - Drug is associated with rash (early onset) that can be severe and might rarely progress to Stevens-Johnson syndrome.
  - Differentiating between early drug-associated rash and acute seroconversion can be difficult and cause extraordinary concern for the exposed person.
  - Nervous system side effects (e.g., dizziness, somnolence, insomnia, and/or abnormal dreaming) are common. Severe psychiatric symptoms are possible (dosing before bedtime might minimize these side effects).
  - Should not be used during pregnancy because of concerns about teratogenicity.
  - Concomitant use of astemizole, cisapride, midazolam, triazolam, ergot derivatives, or St. John's Wort is not recommended because inhibition of the metabolism of these drugs could create the potential for serious and/or life-threatening adverse events (e.g., cardiac arrhythmias, prolonged sedation, or respiratory depression).
  - Potential for oncogenic toxicity is unknown.

- **Abacavir (Ziagen; ABC); available as Trizivir, a combination of ZDV, 3TC, and ABC**
  - 300 mg bid

Advantages

  - Potent HIV inhibitor
  - Well tolerated in patients with HIV infection

Disadvantages

  - Severe hypersensitivity reactions can occur, usually within the first 6 wk of treatment
  - Potential for delayed toxicity (oncogenic/teratogenic) is unknown

Antiretroviral Agents for Use as PEP Only With Expert Consultation

- **Retonavir (Norvir; RTV)**

Disadvantages

  - Difficult to take (requires dose escalation)
  - Poor tolerability
  - Many drug interactions

- **Saquinavir (Fortovase, soft-gel formulation; SQV)**

Disadvantages

  - Bioavailability is relatively poor, even with new formulation

Continued

V

BOX 5-10   Basic and Expanded HIV Postexposure Prophylaxis Regimens—cont'd

- **Amprenavir (Agenerase; AMP)**
Disadvantages

— Dosage consists of eight large pills taken bid
— Many drug interactions

- **Delavirdine (Rescriptor; DLV)**
Disadvantages

— Drug is associated with rash (early onset) that can be severe and progress to Stevens-Johnson syndrome
— Many drug interactions

- **Lopinavir/Ritonavir (Kaletra)**

— 400/100 mg bid

Advantages

— Potent HIV inhibitor
— Well tolerated in patients with HIV infection

Disadvantages

— Concomitant use of flecainide, propafenone, astemizole, terfenadine, dihydroergotamine, ergotamine, ergonovine, methylergonovine, rifampin, cisapride, St. John's Wort, lovastatin, simvastatin, pimozide, midazolam, or triazolam is not recommended because inhibition of the metabolism of these drugs could create the potential for serious and/or life-threatening adverse events (e.g., cardiac arrhythmias, prolonged sedation, or respiratory depression)
— May accelerate the clearance of certain drugs, including oral contraceptives (requiring alternative or additional contraceptive measures for women taking these drugs)
— Potential for delayed toxicity (oncogenic/teratogenic) is unknown

Antiretroviral Agents Generally Not Recommended for Use as PEP

- **Nevirapine (Viramune; NVP)**

— 200 mg daily for 2 wk, then 200 mg bid

Disadvantages

— Associated with severe hepatotoxicity (including at least one case of liver failure requiring liver transplantation in an exposed person taking PEP)
— Associated with rash (early onset) that can be severe and progress to Stevens-Johnson syndrome
— Differentiating between early drug-associated rash and acute seroconversion can be difficult and cause extraordinary concern for the exposed person
— Concomitant use of St. John's Wort is not recommended because this might result in suboptimal antiretroviral drug concentrations

Definitions of Complementary/ Alternative Therapies

Acupuncture Thin needles are inserted superficially on the skin at locations throughout the body. These points are located along "channels" of energy. Heat can be applied by burning (moxibustion), electric current (electroacupuncture), or pressure (acupressure). Healing is proposed by the restoration of a balance of energy flow called *Qi*. Another explanation suggests that, possibly, the stimulation activates endorphin receptors.

Alexander Technique A body work technique in which rebalancing of "postural sets" (i.e., physical alignment) is taught by mentally focusing on the way correct alignments should look and feel and through verbal and tactile guidance by the practitioner.

Antineoplastons Naturally occurring peptides, amino acid derivatives, and carboxylic acids are proposed to control neoplastic cell growth using the patient's own "biochemical defense system," which works jointly with the immune system.

Applied Kinesiology A form of treatment that uses nutrition, physical manipulation, vitamins, diets, and exercise to restore and energize the body. Weak muscles are proposed to be a source of dysfunctional health.

Aromatherapy A form of herbal medicine that uses various oils from plants. Route of administration can be through absorption in the skin or inhalation. The action of antiviral and antibacterial agents is proposed to aid in healing. The aromatic biochemical structures of certain herbs are thought to act in areas of the brain related to past experiences and emotions (e.g., limbic system).

Ayurveda A major health system that emphasizes a preventive approach to health by focusing on an inner state of harmony and spiritual realization for self-healing. Includes special types of diets, herbs, and mineral parts and changes based on a system of constitutional categories in lifestyle. The use of enemas and purgation is to cleanse the body of excess toxins.

Biofeedback A mind-body therapy procedure in which sensors are placed on the body to measure muscle, heart rate, and sweat responses or neural activity. Information is provided by visual, auditory, or body-muscle cell activation so as to teach either to increase or decrease physiologic activity which, when reconstituted, is proposed to improve health problems (i.e., pain, anxiety, or high blood pressure). In some cases, relaxation exercises complement this procedure.

Brachytherapy Ionizing radiation therapy with the source applied to the surface of the body or located a short distance from the treated area.

Bristol Cancer Help Center (BCHC) Diet A stringent diet of raw and partly cooked vegetables with proteins from soy; claimed to enhance the quality of life and attitude toward illness in cancer patients.

Cell Therapy Healthy cellular material from fetuses, embryos, or organs of animals is directly injected into human patients to stimulate healing in dysfunctional organs. May also include blood transfusions or bone marrow transplantations.

Chelation Therapy Involves the removal—through intravenous infusion of a chelating agent (synthetic amino acid ethylenediamine tetraacetic acid [EDTA])—of metal, toxins, lead, mercury, nickel, copper, cadmium, and plaque as a way to treat certain diseases (e.g., cardiovascular). Ancillary treatments include the use of vitamins, changes in diet, and exercise.

Cognitive Therapy Psychologic therapy in which the major focus is on altering and changing irrational beliefs through a type of "socratic" dialogue and self-evaluation of certain illogical thoughts. Conditioning and learning are important components of this therapy.

Craniosacral Therapy A form of gentle manual manipulation used for diagnosis and for making corrections in a system made up of cerebrospinal fluid, cranial and dural membranes, cranial bones, and sacrum. This system is proposed to be dynamic with its own physiologic frequency. Through touch and pressure, tension is proposed to be reduced and cranial rhythms normalized, leading to improvement in health and disease.

Dance Therapy A movement-based therapy that aids in promoting feeling and awareness. The goal is to integrate body, mind, and self-esteem. It uses different parts of the body such as fingers, wrists, and arms to respond to music.

Diathermy The use of high-frequency electrical currents as a form of physical therapy and in surgical procedures. The term *diathermy*, derived from the Greek words *dia* and *therma*, literally means "heating through." The three forms of diathermy used by physical therapists are shortwave, ultrasound, and microwave.

Dimethylaminoethanol (DMAE) Pharmacologic therapy that uses a natural substance found in certain foods and the human brain. It is a precursor to the transmitter

From Spencer JW: *Complementary/alternative medicine: an evidence-based approach*, St Louis, 1999, Mosby.

acetylcholine. It is proposed to have a stimulant effect on the central nervous system if used as a supplement.

Electrochemical Treatment (ECT) A method using direct current to treat cancer. It involves inserting platinum electrodes into tumors and applying a constant voltage of less than 10 V to produce a 40- to 80-mA current between the anodes and cathodes for 30 minutes to several hours.

Electroencephalographic Normalization Gross neural activity is recorded from the scalp as an electroencephalogram (EEG) to assist in "restoring a balance in health" by training patients to produce more uniform and consistent EEG frequencies throughout certain or all areas of the brain (occipital, frontal, temporal, and parietal).

Environmental Medicine A practice of medicine in which the major focus is on cause-and-effect relationships in health. Evaluations are made of factors such as eating and living habits and types of air breathed. Testing in the patient's own environment is performed to determine what precipitators are present that may be related to disease or other health problems. A treatment protocol is developed from this information.

Eye Movement Desensitization and Reprocessing (EMDR) A technique that proposes to remove painful memories by behavioral techniques. Rhythmic, multisaccadic eye movements are produced by allowing the patient to track and follow a moving object while imaging a stressful memory or event. By using deconditioning, including verbal interaction with the therapist, the painful memory is extinguished and health improved.

Feldenkrais Method A bodywork technique in which its founder used the integration of physics, judo, and yoga. The practitioner directs sequences of movement using verbal or hands-on techniques or teaches a system of self-directed exercise to treat physical impairments through the learning of new movement patterns.

Hallucinogens The use of lysergic acid diethylamide (LSD) to produce at certain doses anticraving for certain illicit drugs such as cocaine, or ibogaine, a stimulant, to assist in developing tolerance and decreasing symptoms of dependence.

Hatha Yoga The branch of yoga practice that involves physical exercise, breathing practices, and movement. These exercises are designed to have a salutary effect on posture, flexibility, and strength, and are intended ultimately to prepare the body to remain still for long periods of meditation.

Hellerwork A bodywork technique that treats and improves proper body alignment through the development of a more complete awareness of the physical body. The goal is to realign fascia for improvement in standing, sitting, and breathing using "body energy," verbal feedback, and changing emotions and attitudes.

Herbal Medicine Herbs are used to treat various health conditions. Herbal medicine is a major form of treatment for more than 70% of the world's population.

Homeopathy A form of treatment in which substances (minerals, plant extracts, chemicals, or disease-producing germs), which in sufficient doses would produce a set of illness symptoms in healthy individuals, are given in microdoses to produce a "cure" of those same symptoms. The *symptom* is not thought to be part of the illness but part of a curative process.

Hydergine A phytotherapeutic method that combines extracts from the ergot fungus. Originally proposed to be used as an antihypertensive agent.

Hydrazine Sulfate A pharmacologic treatment proposed to treat certain cancers.

Hyperbaric Oxygen A therapy in which 100% oxygen is given at or above atmospheric pressure. An increase in oxygen in the tissue is proposed to increase blood circulation and improve healing and health and influence the course of disease.

Hyperthermia The use of various heating methods (such as electromagnetic therapy) to produce temperature elevations of a few degrees in cells and tissues, leading to a proposed antitumor effect. This is often used in conjunction with radiotherapy or chemotherapy for cancer treatment.

Immunoaugmentative Therapy A cancer treatment that proposes that cancer cells can be arrested by the use of four different blood proteins; this approach is also proposed to restore the immune system. Can be used as an adjunctive therapy.

Jin Shin Jyutsu A bodywork technique that uses specific "healing points" at the body surface, which are proposed to overlie energy flowing (Qi). The therapist's fingers are used to "redirect, balance, and provide a more efficient energy flow" to and throughout the body.

Laetrile A pharmacologic treatment using apricot pits that has been proposed to treat certain cancers.

Light Therapy Natural light or light of specified wavelengths is used to treat disease. This may include ultraviolet light, colored light, or low-intensity laser light. The eye generally is the initial entry point for the light because of its direct connection to the brain.

Magnetic Therapy Magnets are placed directly on the skin, stimulating living cells and increasing blood flow by ionic currents that are created from polarities on the magnets. Both acute and chronic health conditions are suggested to be treatable by this procedure.

Manual Manipulation A group of therapies with different assumptions and, in part, different areas of treatment. The major focus includes both stimulation and body manipulation, which are proposed to improve health or arrest disease, or both. Includes soft-tissue manipulation through stroking, kneading, friction, and vibration. Types include *massage,* adjustment of the spinal column *(chiropractic),* and tissue and musculoskeletal *(osteopathic)* manipulation.

Mediterranean Diet A diet that is thought to provide optimal distribution of daily caloric intake of different nutrients and includes 50% to 60% carbohydrates, 30% fats, and 10% proteins. The diet is derived from the eating habits of people in the Mediterranean area, who were shown to have reduced rates of cardiovascular disease.

Mind-Body Therapies A group of therapies that emphasize using the mind or brain in conjunction with the body to assist healing. Mind-body therapies can involve varying degrees of levels of consciousness, including *hypnosis,* in which selective attention is used to induce a specific altered state (trance) for memory retrieval, relaxation, or suggestion; *visual imagery,* in which the focus is on a target visual stimulus; *yoga,* which involves integration of posture and controlled breathing, relaxation, and/or meditation; *relaxation,* which includes lighter levels of altered states of consciousness through indirect or direct focus; and *meditation,* in which there is an intentional use of posture, concentration, contemplation, and visualization.

Muscle Energy Technique A manual therapy with components of both passive mobilization and muscle reeducation. Diagnosis of somatic dysfunction is performed by the practitioner after which the patient is guided to provide corrective muscle contraction. This is followed by further testing and correction.

Music Therapy The use of music either in an active or passive mode. Proposed to help allow for the expression of feelings, which helps to reduce stress. Other types of "vibratory" sounds can be used mainly to reduce stress, anxiety, and pain.

Native American Therapies Therapies used by many Native American Indian tribes, including their own healing herbs and ceremonies that use components with a spiritual emphasis.

Naturopathy A major health system that includes practices that emphasize diet, nutrition, homeopathy, acupuncture, herbal medicine, manipulation, and various mind-body therapies. Focal points include self-healing and treatment through changes in lifestyle and emphasis on health prevention.

Neuroelectric Therapy Transcranial or cranial neuroelectric stimulation (TENS), once called "electrosleep"; originally used in the 1950s to treat insomnia. In a typical TENS session, surface electrodes are placed in the mastoid region (behind the ear) and, similar to electroacupuncture, stimulated using a low-amperage, low-frequency alternating current. It has been suggested that TENS stimulates endogenous neurotransmitters such as endorphins that produce symptomatic relief.

Ornish Diet A life-choice program based on eating a vegetarian diet containing less than 10% fat. The diet is high in complex carbohydrates and fiber. Animal products and oils are avoided.

Orthomolecular Therapy A therapeutic approach that uses naturally occurring substances within the body, such as proteins, fat, and water, that promote restoration or balance (or both) by using vitamins, minerals, or other forms of nutrition to subsequently treat disease or promote healing, or both.

Oslo Diet An eating plan that emphasizes increased intake of fish and reduced total fat intake. Diet is combined with regular endurance exercise.

Pilates An educational and exercise approach using the proper body mechanics, movements, truncal and pelvic stabilization, coordinated breathing, and muscle contractions to promote strengthening. Attention is paid to the entire musculoskeletal system.

Piracetam A pharmacologic treatment proposed to be useful in the treatment of dementia. Uses a cyclic relative of the transmitter gamma-aminobutyric acid (GABA).

Prayer The use of prayer(s) that are offered to "some higher being" or authority to heal and/or arrest disease. May be practiced by the individual patient, by groups, or by other(s) with or without the patient's knowledge (e.g., intercessory).

Pritkin Diet A weight management plan that is based on a vegetarian framework. Meals are low in fat, high in fiber, and high in complex carbohydrates.

Qi Gong A form of Chinese exercise-stimulation therapy that proposes to improve health by redirecting mental focus, breathing, coordination, and relaxation. The goal is to "rebalance" the body's own healing capacities by activating proposed electrical or energetic currents that flow along meridians located throughout the body. These meridians, however, do not follow conventional nerve or muscle pathways. In Chinese medical training and practice this therapy includes "external Qi," which is energy transmitted from one person to another so as to heal.

Raja Yoga Yoga practice that includes all of the other forms of yoga practice. The practitioner is instructed to follow moral directives, physical exercises, breathing exercises, meditation, devotion, and service to others to facilitate religious awakening.

Reconstructive Therapy A nonsurgical therapy for arthritis that involves the injection of nutritional substances into the supporting tissues around an injured joint. The intent is to cause the dilation of blood vessels, which will allow fibroblasts to form around the injury and begin the healing process.

Reflexology A bodywork technique that uses reflex points on the hands and feet. Pressure is applied at points that correspond to various body parts, to eliminate blockages thought to produce pain or disease. The goal is to bring the body into balance.

Reiki Comes from the Japanese word meaning "universal life force energy." The practitioner serves as a conduit for healing energy directed into the body or energy field of the recipient without physical contact with the body.

Restricted Environmental Stimulation Therapy (REST) A procedure that uses a completely sensory-deprived environment to increase physical or mental healing through a nonreactive state.

Rolfing A bodywork technique that involves the myofascia. The body is realigned by using the hands to apply a deep pressure and friction that allows more sufficient posture, movement, and the "release" of emotions from the body.

Shark Cartilage A cancer therapy that proposes that shark cartilage can interrupt blood supply to a tumor(s) and subsequently "starve" it of any nutrients by using the antiangiogenic properties and other substances contained in the cartilage.

Shiatsu A bodywork technique involving finger pressure at specific points on the body mainly to balance "energy" in the body. The major focus is on prevention by keeping the body healthy. The therapy uses more than 600 points on the skin that are proposed to be connected to pathways through which energy flows. A Japanese form of acupressure.

T'ai Chi A technique that uses slow, purposeful motor-physical movements of the body to control and achieve a more balanced physiologic and psychologic state.

Therapeutic Riding A form of animal-assisted therapy in which either passive or active movements are produced to aid in approximating the human gait. In certain cases, physiotherapeutic exercises are performed.

Therapeutic Touch A body energy field technique in which hands are passed over the body without actually touching the body to recreate and change proposed "energy imbalances" for restoring innate healing forces. Verbal interaction between patient and therapist helps to maximize effects.

Traditional Chinese Medicine An ancient form of medicine that focuses on prevention and secondarily treats disease with an emphasis on maintaining balance through the body by stimulating a constant, smooth-flowing Qi energy. Herbs, acupuncture, massage, diet, and exercise are also used.

Trager Psychophysical Integration A bodywork technique in which the practitioner enters a meditative state and guides the client through gentle, light, rhythmic, nonintrusive movements. "Mentastics" exercises using self-healing movements are taught to the clients.

Transcranial Electrostimulation Pulsed electrical stimulation of 50 microamperes or less is applied between two electrodes attached to the ear. The stimulation is proposed to activate endogenous opioid activity, which may assist in the treatment of certain health problems such as substance abuse and physical pain.

Twelve-Step Program A program such as Alcoholics Anonymous that is based on a series of 12 steps, or tasks, that participants are asked to complete. As members progress through the 12 steps, they are expected to gain courage to attempt personal change and develop a greater acceptance of themselves. Programs emphasize the group process through the sharing of stories and experiences and through social interactions with other group members. Most 12-step programs incorporate a spiritual component and ask members to turn their lives over to a higher power.

The definitions listed above are not complete; for additional information, the interested reader should consult books such as Micozzi's *Fundamentals of complementary and alternative medicine* and Spencer JW: *Complementary/alternative medicine: an evidence-based approach.*

Commonly Used Herbals with Documented or Suspected Risks

Commonly Used Herbals with Documented or Suspected Risks

HERBAL	PLANT SOURCE	COMMON USE	COMMENTS
Aconite (Monkshood)	*Aconitum napellus*	Analgesic, antipyretic, wound healing	Side effects include cardiac arrhythmia and respiratory paralysis.
Aloe (internally)	*Aloe barbadenis, Aloe vera,* various Aloe species	Constipation, general tonic, wound healing	Side effects include gastrointestinal (GI) cramping, diarrhea, nephritis, hypokalemia, albuminuria, and hematuria with chronic use.
Borage	*Borago officinalis*	Antidiarrheal, diuretic	Contains low levels of pyrrolizidine alkaloids (lycopsamine, amabiline, thesinine) that are potentially hepatotoxic and carcinogenic.
Calamus	*Acorus calamus*	Antipyretic, digestive aid	Some calamus species contain beta asarone, which may be carcinogenic.
Chaparral	*Larrea tridentata*	Anticancer	Case reports of liver toxicity have been associated with use.
Coltsfoot	*Tussilago farfara*	Antitussive, demulcent	Contains pyrrolizidine alkaloids that are potentially hepatotoxic and carcinogenic.
Comfrey	*Symphytum officinale,* various Smphytum species	Bruises, sprains, wound healing	Contains pyrrolizidine alkaloids that are potentially hepatotoxic and carcinogenic.
Ephedra (Ma-huang)	*Ephedra sinica,* various *Ephedra* species	Appetite suppressant, bronchodilator, athletic performance enhancement (often combined with caffeine-containing herbals)	Side effects include insomnia, irritability, GI disturbances, urinary retention, and tachycardia. Misuse can lead to hypertension and arrhythmias.
Germander	*Teucrium chamaedrys*	Appetite suppressant	Contains diterpneoid derivatives that are potentially hepatotoxic.
Licorice	*Glycyrrhiza glabra*	Antiulcer, expectorant	Should only be used in small doses for short duration (<4 wk). With high doses, hypertension, hypokalemia, and sodium and water retention may occur.
Life root	*Senecio aureus*	Emmenagogue	Contains pyrrolizidine alkaloids that are potentially hepatotoxic and carcinogenic.
Pokeroot	*Phytolacca americana*	Anticancer, antirheumatic	Contains a saponin mixture, phytolaccatoxin, and PWM (a proteinaceous mitogen), which can cause gastroenteritis, hypotension, and diminished respiration.
Sassafras	*Sassafras albidum*	Antirheumatic, antispasmodic, stimulant	Contains the volatile oil safrole, which is potentially carcinogenic.
Yohimbe	*Pausinystalia yohimbe*	Impotence	Side effects include anxiety, nervousness, nausea, vomiting, and tachycardia.

From Novey DW: *A clinician's guide to complementary & alternative medicine,* St Louis, 2000, Mosby.

Commonly Used Herbal Medicines

HERBAL MEDICINE	SCIENTIFIC NAME	COMMON USE	POTENTIAL INTERACTIONS	POTENTIAL ADVERSE EFFECTS	CONTRAINDICATIONS
Aloe vera (external only)	Aloe barbendenis, Aloe vera, various Aloe species	External: first-degree burns, cuts, abrasions	None known	Contact dermatitis	May delay healing of deep vertical (surgical) wounds
Arnica (external only)	Arnica montana	External: wound healing, inflammation	None known	Contact dermatitis; can damage skin with prolonged use	None unknown
Astragalus (or Tragacanth)	Astragalus membranaceus	Colds, flu, minor infections; hyperlipidemia, hyperglycemia (unproven)	None known	None known	None known
Bearberry	Arctostaphylos uva-ursi	Urinary tract inflammation	Any substance that acidifies the urine	Nausea and vomiting	Pregnancy, lactation, children under age 12 yr
Bilberry	Vaccinium myrtillus	Atherosclerosis, bruising, diarrhea, local inflammation of mucous membranes	Anticoagulants and antiplatelet drugs (possible)	Excessive consumption of berries; constipation	None known
Black cohosh	Cimicifuga racemosa	Dysmenorrhea, menopausal symptoms, premenstrual syndrome	None known	Gastric discomfort, dizziness, nervous system and visual disturbances, hypotension, bradycardia, increased perspiration	Pregnancy, lactation
Blessed thistle	Centaurea enedictus	Appetite stimulant, dyspepsia	None known	Allergies	Allergies to blessed thistle
Blue cohosh	Caulophyllum thalictroides	Menstrual difficulties; uterine stimulant	None known	Hypertension, respiratory stimulation, stimulation of intestinal motility	Should not be used without medical supervision; pregnancy, lactation, in children
Calendula	Calendula officinalis	External: wound healing	None known	None known	None known
Cascara sagrada	Rhamnus purshiana	Constipation	With chronic use due to potassium loss: cardiac glycoside, thiazide diuretics, corticosteroids, licorice root	Abdominal cramps	Intestinal obstruction, acute intestinal inflammation
Cat's claw	Unicaria tomentosa, U. guianesis	Cancer (anecdotal)	None known	None known	None known
Cayenne (Capsicum)	Capsicum frutescens	External: muscle spasms, chronic pain associated with herpes zoster, trigeminal neuralgia, surgical trauma	None known	Local burning sensation, hypersensitivity reaction	Injured skin, allergy
Chamomile	Matricaria recutita (formerly M. chamomile, Chamomile recutita)	External: skin and mucous membrane inflammation; internal: GI spasm and GI inflammatory disease	May delay concomitant drug absorption from the gut	Allergies (rare)	Allergies to chamomile (and other herbs of the daisy family); avoid in pregnancy

Common name	Scientific name	Uses	Drug interactions	Potential adverse effects	Contraindications/cautions
Cranberry	Vaccinium macrocarpon	Prevention of urinary tract infection	None known	Overuse: diarrhea	None known
Dandelion	Tanaxacum officinale	Appetite stimulant, dyspepsia	None known	Contact dermatitis, gastric discomfort	None known
Devil's claw	Arpagophytum procumbens	Appetite stimulant, supportive therapy for degenerative disorder of the locomotor system	None known	None known	Gastric and duodenal ulcers; gallstone (use only after consultation with health care provider)
Dong-quai	Angelica sinensis	CNS stimulant, suppression of immune system, analgesia, uterus stimulant (effectiveness is controversial)	Contains courmarin derivatives, monitor with warfarin; possible synergism with calcium channel blockers	Photosensitivity; lowers blood pressure, possible CNS stimulation; possible carcinogenic (contains safrole)	Pregnancy
Echinacea	Echinacea angustifolia, E. pallida, E. purpurea	Supportive therapy for colds and flu	None known	Local tingling and numbing sensation with fresh juice	Long-term use not recommended; progressive systemic illness such as tuberculosis, leucosis, collagenosis, multiple sclerosis, AIDS and HIV infection, and other autoimmune diseases; allergy to plants in the daisy family
Eleuthero	Eleutherococcus senticosus	Improvement in well-being	Digitalis glycosides	High doses: irritability, insomnia, anxiety; skin eruptions, headache, diarrhea, hypertension, pericardial pain in rheumatic heart disease	Similar to ginseng
Evening primrose	Oenothera biennis	Hyperlipidemia, atopic eczema	None known	Nausea, GI disturbances, headache	None known
Eyebright	Euphrasia officinalis	Topical: conjunctivitis, eye irritations	None known	None known; cannot be recommended because of risk of potential contamination with homemade, nonsterile preparations	See "Potential Adverse Effects"
Fenugreek	Trigonella foenumgraecum	External: inflammation; internal: appetite stimulant	None known	Skin reactions with repeated external application	None known
Feverfew	Tanacetum parthenium	Migraine prophylaxis	Anticoagulants, antiplatelet drugs, thrombolytics	Mouth ulceration with chewing leaves, oral irritation, GI disturbances, increase in heart rate	Allergy to feverfew and other plants in the daisy family; pregnancy
Fo-ti	Polygonum multiforum	Rejuvenation, decreased liver and kidney function, insomnia, hyperlipidemia, immunosuppression, antimicrobial	None known	None known	Pregnancy

Commonly Used Herbal Medicines—cont'd

HERBAL MEDICINE	SCIENTIFIC NAME	COMMON USE	POTENTIAL INTERACTIONS	POTENTIAL ADVERSE EFFECTS	CONTRAINDICATIONS
Garlic	*Allium sativum*	Hyperlipidemia; other uses: antibacterial, anticancer, antifungal, antihypertensive, antiinflammatory agent, hypoglycemic	Anticoagulants, antiplatelet drugs	GI disturbances, garlic odor; may increase insulin level, producing decrease in blood glucose; high dose: anemia	Pregnancy and lactation
Ginger	*Zingiber officinale*	Dyspepsia, prevention of motion sickness	Anticoagulants, antiplatelet drugs; calcium channel blocker (possible)	None; GI irritation and discomfort with high dose	Gallstones (use only after consultation with health care provider); pregnancy (controversial)
Ginkgo	*Ginkgo biloba*	Symptomatic treatment of age-related organic brain syndrome, peripheral arterial occlusive disease (stage II of Fontaine), SSRI-induced sexual dysfunction, tinnitus, vertigo	Anticoagulants, antiplatelet drugs, thrombolytics	GI upset, headache, allergic skin reaction; cases of spontaneous bleeding have been reported	None known
Ginseng	*Panax ginseng, P. quinquefolia*	Improvement in well-being	Anticoagulants, antiplatelet drugs, thrombolytics; may potentiate MAOIs; stimulants (including caffeine), antipsychotic drugs, hormone therapy	High dose: breast tenderness, nervousness, excitation; estrogenic effects in women, hypotension, hypertension	Chronic use (should use 2 wk on and 2 wk off); acute illnesses, any form of hemorrhage; pregnancy and lactation
Goldenseal	*Hydrastis canadensi*	Inflammation of mucous membranes (unproven); does not mask illegal drugs in urine drug screens	May interfere with the ability of colon to manufacture B vitamins and may decrease their absorption; heparin (possible)	Hypoglycemia	Pregnancy and lactation
Gotu kola	*Centella asiatica (formerly Hydrocotyle asiatica)*	External: wound healing	None known	Hypersensitivity	None known
Grape seed	*Vitis vinifera*	Antioxidant	None known	None known	None known
Hawthorn	*Crataegus* spp.	Congestive heart failure; stage II of NYHA	Cardiotonic drugs, antihypertensive drugs	High dose: hypotension and sedation; nausea, fatigue, sweating, rash; none	Pregnancy, lactation
Horse chestnut	*Aeculus hippocastanum*	Chronic venous insufficiency	None known	GI disturbances, nausea, pruritus	None known
Hyssop	*Hyssopus officinalis*	Pharyngitis, expectorant	None known	None known	None known
Kava-Kava	*Piper methysticum*	Anxiety, restlessness, sleep induction	Potentiation of CNS depressants and alcohol	Chronic use: kavaism with dry, flaking, discolored skin and reddened eyes; numbness of mouth with chewing, CNS depression	Pregnancy, nursing, endogenous depression

Common Name	Scientific Name	Reported Uses	Drug Interactions	Side Effects	Contraindications
Licorice	*Glycyrrhiza glabra*	Gastric/duodenal ulcers	Due to potassium loss; digitalis glycosides, thiazide diuretics, corticosteroids, licorice	With prolonged use and with high doses: mineralocorticoid effects including sodium and water retention, hypokalemia, myoglobinuria	Gall bladder disease, kidney disease, pheochromocytoma and other adrenal tumors, diseases that cause low serum potassium livers, fasting, anorexia, bulimia, untreated hypothyroidism
Marshmallow	*Althaea officinalis*	Ingestion, irritation of oral and pharyngeal mucosa	May delay absorption of other drugs taken simultaneously	None known	None known
Milkthistle	*Silbum marianum*	Dyspepsia, supportive therapy for toxic liver damage	None known	Mild diarrhea	None known
Passion flower	*Passiflora incarnata*	Anxiety, insomnia (unproven)	None known	None known; may have MAOI activity	None known
Pau d'arco	*Tabebuia impetiginosa*	Cancer	Vitamin K	Chronic use: anemia	Bleeding disorders
Peppermint	*Mentha X piperita*	External: myalgia and neuralgia; internal: GI spasms, nausea, inflammation of oral mucosa	External: irritation of mucous membranes; overuse: heartburn, relaxation of esophageal sphincter	External: contact dermatitis; internal: mouth irritation, muscle tremor, hypersensitivity reaction, heartburn, bradycardia	Obstruction of bile ducts, gallbladder inflammation, severe liver damage, pregnancy
Plantain	*Plantago major*	External: inflammation of skin; internal: cough, oral and pharyngeal mucosa inflammation	None known	None known	None known
Pygeum	*Pygeum africanum*	Benign prostatic hyperplasia	None known	GI disturbance	None known
Saw palmetto	*Serenoa repens*	Benign prostatic hyperplasia, stages I and II	Hormone therapy	GI disturbance	Pregnancy, lactation, children, breast cancer
Slippery elm	*Scutellaria lateriflora*	Pharyngitis, GI inflammatory disorders	None known	Contact dermatitis	None known
St. John's wort	*Hypericum perforatum*	External: oil preparation for mild wounds and burns; internal: mild to moderate depression	MAOIs; SSRIs and other antidepressants, sympathomimetics	Possible photosensitization, GI disturbance	Pregnancy and lactation
Stinging nettle	*Urtica dionica*	Benign prostatic hyperplasia	None known	Allergy	Pregnancy; cardiac and renal dysfunction
Tea tree	*Melaleuca alternifolia*	External: bacteriostatic	None known	Allergic contact dermatitis	None known
Tumeric	*Curuma longa*	Dyspepsia	None known	None known	Obstruction of bile passages
Valerian	*Valeriana officinalis*	Restlessness, sleeping disorders	Possible with CNS depressants and alcohol	Strong, disagreeable odor; headache, excitability, cardiac disturbances, rare morning drowsiness	None known
Vitex (or Chaste Tree Berry)	*Vitex agnus-castus*	Menstrual disorders	May interfere with dopamine-receptor antagonists	GI disturbances, itching, urticaria	None known

AIDS, Acquired immunodeficiency syndrome; *CNS,* central nervous system; *GI,* gastrointestinal; *HIV,* human immunodeficiency virus; *MAOI,* monoamine oxidase inhibitor; *NYHA,* New York Heart Association; *SSRI,* selective serotonin reuptake inhibitors.

APPENDIX 3

Relaxation Techniques

Relaxation Techniques

RELAXATION TECHNIQUE	SUMMARY	FURTHER RESOURCES
Breathing exercise	This is the foundation of most relaxation techniques. Have patients place one hand on the chest and the other on the abdomen. Instruct them to take a slow, deep breath, as if they were sucking in all the air in the room. While doing this, the hand on the abdomen should rise higher than the hand on the chest. This promotes diaphragmatic breathing that increases alveolar expansion in the bases of the lungs. Have them hold the breath for a count of 7 and then exhale. Exhalation should take twice as long as inhalation. Repeat this for a total of five breaths, and encourage patients to do this three times a day.	*Conscious Breathing* by Gay Hendricks is one of many good resources on using breathing for relaxation and health.
Meditation		
Transcendental/The relaxation response	To prevent distracting thoughts, the subject repeats a mantra (a word or sound) over and over again while sitting in a comfortable position. If a distracting thought comes to mind, it is accepted and let go, with the mind focusing again on the mantra.	www.mindbody.harvard.edu or *The Relaxation Response* by Herbert Benson; www.tm.org for information on transcendental meditation
Mindful meditation	This represents the philosophy of living in the present or in the moment. The *body scan* is one technique where the subject uses breathing to obtain a relaxed state while lying or sitting. The mind progressively focuses on different parts of the body, where it feels any and all sensations intentionally but nonjudgmentally before moving on to another part of the body. A patient with back pain may focus on the quality and characteristics of the pain as if to better understand it and bring it under control.	*Full Catastrophe Living* by Jon Kabat-Zinn describes this technique in full and the program for stress reduction at the University of Massachusetts Medical Center.
Centering prayer	This is a form similar to transcendental meditation that has a more religious foundation. The subject repeats a "sacred word" similar to a mantra. As thoughts come to mind, they are accepted and let go, clearing the mind to become more centered on the spirit within, as if the mind's preoccupied thoughts are the layers of an onion that are peeled away, allowing better understanding of the spirit at the core.	www.Centeringprayer.com; look under "method of centering prayer" for a nondenominational discussion.

From Rakel RE (ed): *Principles of family practice*, ed 6, Philadelphia, 2002, WB Saunders.

Continued

Relaxation Techniques—cont'd

RELAXATION TECHNIQUE	SUMMARY	FURTHER RESOURCES
Progressive muscle relaxation (PMR)	A form of relaxation in which the subject is attuned to the difference in feeling when the muscles are tensed and then relaxed. In a comfortable position, start by tensing the whole body from head to toe. While doing this, notice the feelings of tightness. Take a deep breath in and as you let it out, let the tension release and the muscles relax. This is then followed by progressive tension and relaxation throughout the body. One may start by clenching the fists and then tensing the arms, shoulders, chest, abdomen, hips, legs, and so on, with each step followed by relaxation.	www.uaex.edu/publications/pub/ fshei28.htm is a good review of PMR as well as other relaxation exercises. It is sponsored by the University of Arkansas. *You Must Relax* is a book by the founder of this technique, Edmund Jacobson.
Visualization/ Self-hypnosis	The subject uses visualization to recruit images that create a relaxed state. For example, if a person is anxious, visualizing images of a place and a time that were peaceful and comforting would help induce relaxation. This is best used in conjunction with a breathing exercise.	There are many audiocassettes that can guide people through a visualization "script" that can result in relaxation. Emmett Miller is one well-known author.
Autogenic training	This induces a physiologic response by using simple phrases. For example, "My legs are heavy and warm" is meant to increase the blood flow to this area, resulting in relaxation. This is done progressively from head to toe with the use of deep breathing and repetition of the phrase. After completing this, focus attention on any body part that may still be tense, and then focus the breath and phrase to that area until the whole body is relaxed.	The British Autogenic Society at www.autogenictherapy.org.uk is a good resource for more information.
Exercise/Movement Aerobic	While performing an aerobic exercise, focus attention on a phrase, sound, word, or prayer and passively disregard other thoughts that may enter the mind. Some may focus on their breathing, saying to themselves, "In" with inhalation and "Out" with exhalation, or repeating "one-two, one-two" with each step they take with jogging. Doing this will help the mind focus, preventing other thoughts that may cause tension.	*Beyond the Relaxation Response* by Herbert Benson includes discussion of his research on inducing the relaxation response while exercising.
Yoga	This has been practiced for thousands of years in India. In America, it has been divided into three aspects: breathing (pranayama yoga), bodily postures or asanas (hatha yoga), and meditation to maintain balance and health. Regular practice induces relaxation.	For the following therapies, it is best to encourage your patients to take a class at a local community center or gym and to pick up an introductory book at a library or bookstore.
Tai chi	An ancient Chinese martial art that uses slow, graceful movements combined with inner mindfulness and breathing techniques to help bring balance between the mind and body.	See above.
Qigong	A traditional Chinese practice that uses movement, meditation, and controlled breathing to balance the body's vital energy force, chi.	See above.

APPENDIX 4

Selected Resources for Complementary/Alternative Medicine

ORGANIZATIONS

American Academy of Medical Acupuncturists
5820 Wilshire Blvd., Suite 500
Los Angeles, CA 90032
Phone: (213) 937-5514

American Association of Naturopathic Physicians
601 Valley St., Suite 105
Seattle, WA 98109
Phone: (206) 328-8510

American Chiropractic Association
1701 Clarendon Blvd.
Arlington, VA 22209
Phone: (703) 276-8800

American Massage Therapy Association
820 Davis St., Suite 100
Evanston, IL 60201
Phone: (847) 864-0123

PUBLICATIONS

Advances: The Journal of Mind-Body Health
John E. Fetzer Institute
9292 West KL Avenue
Kalamazoo, MI 49009
Phone: (616) 375-2000

Alternative Therapies in Health and Medicine
InnoVision Communications
101 Columbia Street
Aliso Viejo, CA 92656
Phone: (800) 899-1712

HerbalGram
American Botanical Council
P.O. Box 2016600
Austin, TX 78720

Journal of Alternative and Complementary Medicine: Research on Paradigm, Practice and Policy
Mary Ann Liebert, Inc.
2 Madison Ave.
Larchmont, NY 10538
Phone: (914) 834-3100; (800) MLIEBERT

OTHER RESOURCES

American Botanical Council
P.O. Box 201660
Austin, TX 78720-1660
(512) 331-8861; (800) 373-7105
Commission E monographs (monographs published by the German government's Commission E, an expert committee of physicians, pharmacologists, toxicologists, and other authorities, charged with writing monographs on a number of commonly used herbal medicines) have been translated by and are available from the Council.
Web site: **http://www.herbalgram.org/ commission_e/index.html**

Centers for the Study of Complementary and Alternative Medicine

Addictions
Center for Addiction and Alternative Medicine Research (CAMMR)
University of Minnesota Medical School
914 S. 8th St., Suite D917
Minneapolis, MN 55404
Thomas J. Kiresuk, PhD, Principal Investigator
Web site: **http://www.winternet.com/~caamr/**

Aging
Complementary and Alternative Medicine Program at Stanford University (CAMPS)
730 Welch Road, Suite B
Palo Alto, CA 94304-1583
William L. Haskell, PhD, Principal Investigator
Web site: **http://scrdp.stanford.edu/camps.html**

From Spencer JW: *Complementary/alternative medicine: an evidence-based approach*, St Louis, 1999, Mosby.

Asthma, Allergy, and Immunology
Center for Alternative Medicine Research in
Asthma and Immunology
University of California at Davis
TB 192, Division of Rheumatology-Clinical
Immunology
Davis, CA 95616
Merrill Gershwin, MD, principal Investigator
Web site: **http://www-camra.ucdavis.edu**

Cancer
University of Texas Center for Alternative and
Complementary Medicine Research in Cancer
P.O. Box 20186, No. W430
Houston, TX 77225
Guy Parcel, PhD, Principal Investigator
Web site: **http://www.sph.uth.tmc.edu/utcam**

Chiropractic
Consortorial Center for Chiropractic Research
741 Brady St.
Davenport, IA 52803-5260
William Meeker, DC, MPH, Principal Investigator
Web site: **http://www.c3r.org**

General Medical Conditions
Center for Alternative Medicine Research at Beth
Israel Hospital/Deaconess Medical Center
330 Brookline Ave.
Boston, MA 02215
David Eisenberg, MD, Principal Investigator
Web site: **http://www.bidmc.harvard.edu/
medicine/camr**

Human Immunodeficiency Virus/Acquired Immunodeficiency Syndrome
Bastyr University AIDS Research Center
14500 Juanita Dr., NE
Bothell, WA 98011
Leanna Standish, ND, PhD, Principal Investigator
Web site: **http://www.bastyr.edu/resarch/
research.html**

Pain
Center for Alternative Medicine Pain Research
and Evaluation
Kernan Hospital Mansion
2200 Kernan Dr.
Baltimore, MD 21207
Brian Berman, MD, Principal Investigator
Web site: **http://www.compmed.ummc.ab.umd.edu**

University of Virginia Center for the Study of
Complementary and Alternative Therapies
University of Virginia School of Nursing
McLeod Hall
15th and Lane St.
Charlottesville, VA 22903-3395
Ann Gill Taylor, EdD, Principal Investigator
Web site: **http://www.med.virginia.edu/nursing/
centers/alt-ther.html**

Stroke and Neurologic Conditions
Center for Research in Complementary and Alternative
Medicine for Stroke and Neurologic Disorders
Kessler Medical Rehabilitation Research and Education
Corporation (KMRREC)
1199 Pleasant Valley Way
West Orange, NJ 07052
Samual Schiflett, PhD, Principal Investigator
Web site: **http://www.umdnj.edu/altmdweb**

Women's Health
Center for Complementary/Alternative Medicine Research
in Women's Health
Columbia University College of Physicians and Surgeons
630 West 168th St., Box 75
New York, NY 10032
Fredi Kronenberg, PhD, Principal Investigator
Web site: **http://cpmcnet.columbia.edu/
dept/rosenthal/**

Index

Page references followed by f indicate figures; t, tables; b, boxes. Page references in **boldface** indicate main disease and disorder discussions.

Gwendolyn R. Lee, M.D.
Internal Medicine

Immunosuppression
agents that cause neutropenia, 1441t
-associated Kaposi's sarcoma, 472
CMV in, 248
immunizations for infants and children with, 1608t
Immunotherapy
for condyloma acuminatum, 225
for renal cell adenocarcinoma, 698
Imodium, 748
Impedance plethysmography, 801t
Imperforate anus, 1050t
Impetigo, **457**
differential diagnosis of, 956t
of ear, 591
Impetigo vulgaris. *See* Impetigo.
Impingement syndrome. *See* Rotator cuff syndrome.
Impotence. *See* Erectile dysfunction.
Imuran. *See* Azathioprine (Imuran).
Inappropriate secretion of antidiuretic hormone, **458**
differential diagnosis of, 1181t
Incarcerated hernia, 1126t
Inclusion body myositis, **459**
Incontinence
clinical, psychologic, and social impact of, 460
conditions that predispose to surgical failure, 461
drug-induced, 1101b
extraurethral, 461
functional, 460, 461
medications that cause, 1101b
mixed stress and urge, 460, 461
overflow, 460, 461
sensory, 460, 461
sphincteric, 460
of stool, functional, **297**
stress, 460, 461
transient, 460, 461
urge, 460, 461
urinary, **304, 460-461**
India ink preparation, 1592b
Indican, urine, 1590
Indigestion, 1063t-1064t
Indinavir (Crixivan), 27t
Indomethacin
for ankylosing spondylitis, 74
for Behçet's disease, 127
for hypertrophic osteoarthropathy, 446
for pericarditis, 619
for Reiter's syndrome flares, 695
Infant botulism, 150
Infantile autism, early, **117**
Infantile paralysis. *See* Poliomyelitis.
Infantile spasms, 741, 741t
Infants. *See also* Pediatric age.
abdominal pain in, 899b
appetite loss in, 920b
bacterial meningitis in, 524
benign ovarian tumors in, 597
decreased hepatic glucose output in, 468
emesis in, causes of, 1003b

Infants—cont'd
immunocompromised, 1608t
jaundice in, 1109b
sudden death in, 1251b
Turner's syndrome in, 841
urinary tract infection in, 848
Infected vascular gangrene, 1163t
Infections. *See also specific agents, infections.*
abnormal female genital tract bleeding with, 944b
anaerobic, **51-52**
associated with hepatic granulomas, 1068b
bacterial. *See* Bacterial infections.
bone, **363,** 363f
bone pain, 950b
causes of noisy breathing, 955b
of central nervous system, 1400f
childhood amaurosis (blindness), 946b
chronic pneumonia, 1194b
in compromised host, 1102t-1103t
Coxsackievirus. *See* Hand-foot-mouth disease.
cranial nerve syndromes, 982t-983t
ear, 997t
eyelid, 1017t
fever as sole or dominant feature, 1028t
filarial, 1033t
fungal. *See* Fungal infections.
fusospirochetal, 1243t
genital, *Chlamydia,* **203**
granulomatous, 1055b
helminthic parasites, 1010b, 1065t
intestinal, 1106t-1107t
HIV-associated, 1543t, 1544t
bacterial, 1081b
of central nervous system, 1400f
mycobacterial, 1084t
opportunistic, 28t-29t
parasitic, 1081b
viral, 1081b
with impaired host defense mechanism, 1102t-1103t
of intervertebral disk space, 925t
in knee, 1115t
limp considerations, 1124t-1125t
mycobacterial, 1084t
mycosis fungoides, **552-553**
mycotic, 1008t
deep-seated, 767
neonatal. *See* Neonatal infections.
neuropathies associated with, 621
nosocomial. *See* Nosocomial infections.
opportunistic, HIV-related prophylaxis of, 29t
therapy for, 28t-29t
parasitic. *See* Parasitic infections.

Infections—cont'd
peripheral blood eosinophilia, 1010b
postinfectious glomerulonephritis, **352-354,** 354t
protozoal, 1205t
chronic pneumonia, 1194b
pruritus ani, 674, 1207b
pulmonary
recurrent, 1461f
viral, 1084t
recurrent
hyper-IgE and (Job's syndrome), 1100t
pulmonary, 1461f
red flags for, 1322t
with rheumatoid factor present, 1582b
salivary gland, 1159t
of soft tissue
necrotizing, 1163t
nematode, 1164t
tick-related, 1260t-1261t
in travelers, 1103t
urinary tract. *See* Urinary tract infection.
vaginal discharges and, 1276t
viral. *See* Viral infections.
Infectious (bacterial) arthritis
associated with HIV infection, 1085t
diagnostic considerations, 1124t
Infectious diarrhea, acute, 1080t
Infectious hepatitis. *See* Hepatitis A.
Infectious keratitis. *See* Corneal ulcers.
Infectious lymphadenitis, 1135t-1136t
Infectious mononucleosis. *See also* Epstein-Barr virus infection; Mononucleosis.
differential diagnosis of, 1014t, 1242t
lymphadenitis, 1136t
Infective endocarditis, **298-299**
rash associated with, 1030t
Infertile male syndrome, 915t
Infertility
differential diagnosis of, 465
endocrine evaluation of infertile men, 1585t
endometriosis-associated, 302
etiology of, 465
female
etiology of, 465
evaluation of, 1418f
imaging studies of, 465
laboratory tests, 465
male
etiology of, 465
evaluation of, 1417f
workup for, 465
Infestations. *See also specific organisms.*
eyelid, 1017t
helminthic parasites, 1010b, 1065t
mites, 721
differential diagnosis of, 1017t
that cause peripheral blood eosinophilia, 1010b

Inflammation
cerebrovascular disease, ischemic, 965b
eyelid, 1018t
limp considerations, 1124t-1125t
systemic inflammatory response syndrome. *See* Septicemia.
Inflammatory bowel disease. *See* Crohn's disease; Ulcerative colitis.
Inflammatory carcinoma, of breast, 153
Inflammatory demyelinating polyneuritis syndrome, acute, 1506f
Inflammatory enterocolitis, 995b
Inflammatory joint diseases, 929t
Inflammatory lesions
of breast, 953b
of choroid. *See* Retinal detachment.
Inflammatory myopathy, idiopathic. *See also* Dermatomyositis.
differential diagnosis of, 1155b
inclusion body myositis, **459**
Inflammatory prostatitis, asymptomatic, 1204t
Infliximab, for Crohn's disease, 240
Influenza, **462-463**
acute general treatment of, 644
"classic" flu, 462
CPT code, 1525
differential diagnosis of, 974t
HIV-related, 29t
incidence of, 643
nonpharmacologic therapy for, 644
physical findings and clinical presentation of, 643
predominant age of, 643
treatment of, 156, 156t
vaccinations for. *See* Influenza vaccine.
yuppie flu, **208**
Influenza vaccine, 462
for adolescents and adults, 1615t
for health-care workers, 1624t
for HIV-infected children, 1609t
for HIV-related opportunistic infections, 29t
for immunocompromised infants and children, 1608t
for international travel, 1631t
during pregnancy, 1620t
recommendations for persons with medical conditions requiring special considerations, 1628t
for Reye's syndrome, 714
Infrainguinal bypass, 217
Infraspinatus tendinitis, 1266t
Inguinal hernia
direct, 1071t, 1072f
incarcerated, 1050t
indirect, 1071t, 1072f